NURSING CARE PLANS

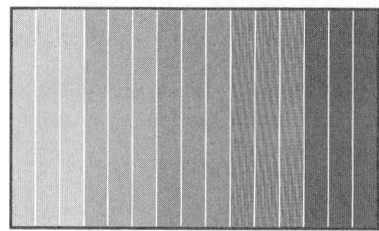

Contributors

CHARLOTTE R. ABBINK, RN, PhD

Assistant Professor, College of Nursing
University of New Mexico
Albuquerque, New Mexico

JOANN FETT ALLISON, RN, MSN

Director of Quality Assurance
Visiting Nurse Association of Manchester
and Southern New Hampshire, Inc
Manchester, New Hampshire;
Former Perioperative Isntructor
Rockford Memorial School of Nursing
Rockford, Illinois

JUDITH J. BARROWS, RN, MSN, CCRN

Instructor, Cape Cod Community College
Hyannis, Massachusetts

CATHERINE M. BENDER, RN, MN

Assistant Professor, Graduate Program
Medical-Surgical Nursing, University of Pittsburgh
Responsible for the Oncology Component
Pittsburgh, Pennsylvania

BARBARA J. BOSS, RN, PhD

Professor of Nursing, School of Nursing
University of Mississippi Medical Center
Jackson, Mississippi

LINDA C. CARNAGO, RN, MSN

Instructor of Nursing, Henry Ford Community College
Dearborn, Michigan

GAYLE ZIEGLER CASTERLINE, RN, MS

Instructor, Samuel Merritt College
Oakland, California

M. CAROLYN CECERE, RN, MSN, CPNP, JD

Associate Professor, Indiana University School of Nursing
Parent-Child Nursing, Indianapolis, Indiana

IDOLIA COX COLLIER, DNSc, RNCS

Associate Professor, College of Nursing
University of New Mexico
Albuquerque, New Mexico

CECELIA C. DAIL, BS, MT (ASCP), CLS

Instructor, Medical Laboratory Sciences
Department of Pathology, School of Medicine
University of New Mexico
Albuquerque, New Mexico

KERRY A. DALEN, RN, MSN, CCRN

Trauma Nurse Specialist
Staff Nurse, Regional Burn Unit
University of New Mexico Hospital
Albuquerque, New Mexico

GLADYS ELIZABETH DETERS, RN, MS

Assistant Professor, University of Virginia School of Nursing
Charlottesville, Virginia

JEANNE E. DOYLE, RN, BS

Nurse Consultant, Peripheral Vascular Surgery
The University Hospital, Boston, Massachusetts;
Executive Director, Society for Peripheral Vascular Nursing
Norwood, Massachusetts

ELLEN STOETZNER DUKE, RN, MSN, CCRN

Instructor of Nursing
Stephen F. Austin State University
Nacogdoches, Texas

PATSY L. ORTH DUPHORNE, RN, MN

Assistant Professor, College of Nursing
University of New Mexico
Albuquerque, New Mexico

RACHEL ELROD, RN, MS

Professor, Front Range Community College
Westminster (Denver)
Faculty Member, University of Phoenix, Colorado Campus
Denver, Colorado

SUE E. ELSTER, RN, PhD

Clinical Assistant Professor
Department of Administrative Studies in Nursing
University of Illinois College of Nursing
Chicago, Illinois

LINDA GRIEGO, RN, MSN, CCRN

Clinical Nurse Specialist, Medical-Cardiac Intensive Care
University of New Mexico Hospital
Albuquerque, New Mexico

LINDA B. HAAS, RN, PhD, CDE

Clinical Nurse Specialist, Endocrinology
Seattle Department of Veteran Affairs Medical Center
Seattle, Washington

BARBARA HENZEL, RN, BSN, CGC

Clinical Supervisor, GI Endoscopy Suite
Gastrointestinal Department
Hospital of the University of Pennsylvania
Philadelphia, Pennsylvania

PATRICIA ROBERTSON HERCULES, RN, MS

Manager, Nursing Education, The Methodist Hospital
Houston, Texas

LESLIE A. HOFFMAN, RN, PhD

Professor, Pulmonary Nursing
University of Pittsburgh School of Nursing
Pittsburgh, Pennsylvania

MARY ANN CAMMARANO HOUSE, RN, MSN, CCRN, CS

Assistant Professor, Graduate School
College of Nursing, University of Florida
Gainesville, Florida

BONNIE MOWINSKI JENNINGS, RN, DNSc, LTC(P), AN

Lieutenant Colonel, US Army Nurse Corps
Nursing Education Branch
US Army Surgeon General's Office
Falls Church, Virginia

CAROLYN I. JOHNS, RN, MS, CANP

Cardiology Nurse Practitioner, Lovelace Medical Center
Albuquerque, New Mexico

NANCY STOETZNER KUPPER, RN, MSN

Associate Professor of Nursing, Tarrant County Junior College
Fort Worth, Texas

SHARON MANTIK LEWIS, RN, PhD

Associate Professor, College of Nursing
Research Assistant Professor, Department of Pathology
School of Medicine, University of New Mexico
Albuquerque, New Mexico

CAROL WIKOFF LOVE, RN, MS

Regional Supervisor, Illinois Department of Public Aid
Bureau of Long-Term Quality Care
Rockford, Illinois

JAN D. MANZETTI, RN, MN, CRNP

Lung Transplant Coordinator
University of Pittsburgh Medical Center
Pittsburgh, Pennsylvania

KATHERYN ELLEN McCASH, RN, MS

Lecturer, College of Nursing
University of New Mexico, College of Nursing
Albuquerque, New Mexico

MARY E. MEANS, RN, BSN

Clinical Nurse Specialist I, Department of Nursing
The University of Iowa Hospitals and Clinics
Iowa City, Iowa

CINDY MEREDITH, RN, MSN

Urology Nurse Consultant, Private Practice;
Instructor, University of Michigan, School of Nursing
Flint, Michigan

JOYCE TREMPER MITCHELL, RN, MS, NS, CS

Pulmonary Clinical Nurse Specialist
Quality Management Specialist
Tucson Veterans Administration Medical Center
Tucson, Arizona

CHRISTINA M. MUMMA, RN, PhD, CRRN

Assistant Professor, Chairperson
Department of Physiological Nursing
University of Alaska — Anchorage
College of Nursing and Health Sciences
Anchorage, Alaska

ELLEN FRANCES OLSHANSKY, RNC, DNSc

Associate Professor, Department of Parent and Child Nursing
University of Washington
Seattle, Washington

SUSAN ERIN O'NEILL, RN, MS

Assistant Professor of Nursing
California State University — Sacramento
Sacramento, California

JUDITH M. OZUNA, RN, MN, CNRN

Clinical Nurse Specialist, Neurology
Veterans Administration Center
Seattle, Washington

M. KENT POWELL, RN, BSN, CRNA

Department Head, Department of Anesthesia
Coon Memorial Hospital
Dalhart, Texas

JACQUELINE RHOADS, RN, PhD

Tennessee State University, Nashville, Tennessee;
Lieutenant Colonel, US Army Nurse Corps,
1st Armor Division
Saudi Arabia

BARBARA D. RICKERT, RN, PhD

Assistant Professor, College of Nursing
University of New Mexico
Albuquerque, New Mexico

SUSAN C. RUDA, MS, RN, ONC

Nurse Clinician, Parkview Orthopaedic Group
Palos Heights, Illinois

BETH RUNNELS, BS, MT(ASCP)

Graduate Student, Anatomy-Pathology
Instructor, Medical Laboratory Sciences, School of
  Medicine
University of New Mexico
Albuquerque, New Mexico

PAMELA S. SCHREMP, RN, MSN, CRNO

Clinical Nurse Specialist, University Hospital of Cleveland;
Clinical Instructor, Frances Payne Bolton School of Nursing
Case Western Reserve University
Cleveland, Ohio

JOANN SEPPELT, RN

Transplant Coordinator, University of New Mexico Hospital
Albuquerque, New Mexico

CAROL COX SMITH, BS, MA

Career and Education Writer;
Former Instructor, Technical-Vocational Institute
Albuquerque, New Mexico

CAROL E. SMITH, RN, PhD

Associate Professor, School of Nursing and Health
Sciences Center, University of Kansas
Kansas City, Kansas

SALLY D. SPERRY, BS, MT (ASCP)

Instructor, Medical Laboratory Sciences, School of Medicine
University of New Mexico
Albuquerque, New Mexico

PATRICIA PALMER STEPHENS, RN, MS, MA

Director of Nursing Programs
Albuquerque Technical-Vocational Institute
Albuquerque, New Mexico

JUDITH HEFFRON SWEENEY, RN, MSN

Assistant Professor of Nursing
Vanderbilt University School of Nursing
Nashville, Tennessee

VIRGINIA VALENTINE, RN, MS, CDE

Private Practice Diabetes Educator
Diabetes Center of New Mexico
Albuquerque, New Mexico

TRISCH VAN SCIVER, RN, MS, NS, CCRN

Pulmonary Clinical Nurse Specialist
Lovelace Medical Center
Albuquerque, New Mexico

SHARON WALKER, RN, MSN, CCRN, CNRN

Critical Care Nurse Specialist
Lovelace Medical Center
Albuquerque, New Mexico

CONNIE A. WALLECK, RN, MS, CNRN, FCCN

Interim Director of Nursing
University Hospital, SUNY Health Science Center
Syracuse, New York

TERRI E. WEAVER, RN, PhD, CS

Assistant Professor
School of Nursing
University of Pennsylvania
Philadelphia, Pennsylvania

JOAN STEHLE WERNER, RN, DNSc

Associate Professor, Department of Adult Health Nursing
School of Nursing, University of Wisconsin—Eau Claire
Eau Claire, Wisconsin

DINA D'ADDIO WILSON, RN, MN

Instructor of Nursing
Johnson County Community College
Overland Park, Kansas

BARBARA WOOD, RN

Home Training Coordinator
New Mexico Artificial Kidney Center
Albuquerque, New Mexico

JOYCE M. YASKO, RN, PhD, FAAN

Professor and Program Director, Medical-Surgical Nursing;
Associate Director, Nursing and Patient Care Services Division
Pittsburgh Cancer Institute, University of Pittsburgh
Pittsburgh, Pennsylvania

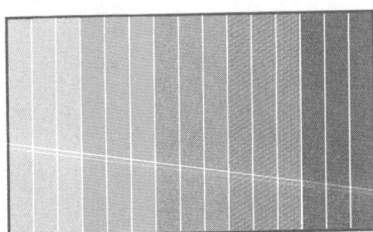

Acknowledgments for Previous Contributions

Larry L. Burden, RN, MSN, CCRN

Michael A. Carter, RN, DNSc, FAAN

Katherine L. Chipman, RN, MSN

Dorothy Hendel Clough, RN, PhD

Marie E. Folk-Lighty, RN, MSN, CCRN

Anita A.W. Garman, RN, MSN

Diane Germain, RN, BS

Charlene Harrington, RN, PhD

Virginia M. Hunter, RD

Susan Searle Jackson, RN, MSN

Phyllis Gappa Jensen, RNC, MSN (deceased)

Carol Fair Keith, RN, MS

Melva Kravitz, RN, PhD

Barbara J. Lockwood, RN, MS

Karen H. May McArdle, RN, MA

Martha J. Price, RNC, MSN

Donna J. Rodriguez, RD

Susan Walker, RN, EdD

Earnestine Huffman White, RN, EdD (deceased)

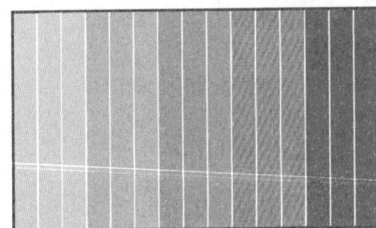

Reviewers

Lucy Bradley-Springer, RN, PhD
Albuquerque, New Mexico

Debra Broadwell-Jackson, RN, PhD, CETN
Atlanta, Georgia

Sally Brozenec, RN, PhD
Chicago, Illinois

Evelyn Butera, RN, MSN, CNN
Seattle, Washington

Cynthia Chernecky, RN, MN
Cleveland, Ohio

Kathy Clark, RN, MS
Lincoln, Nebraska

Joan Colgin, RN, BSN, CDE
Dallas, Texas

Amanda Conley, RN, MSN
Albuquerque, New Mexico

Carol Dolan, RN, MSN, OCN
Albuquerque, New Mexico

Tana Durnbaugh, RN, EdD
Elgin, Illinois

Joan Enggaard, RN, MSN
Grayslake, Illinois

Victora Fahey, RN, MSN
Chicago, Illinois

Sharon Fought, RN, PhD
Bellevue, Washington

Florencetta Gibson, RN, MSN, CNS
Monroe, Louisiana

Michele Goodman, RN, MS
Oak Park, Illinois

Linda Griego, RN, MSN, CCRN
Albuquerque, New Mexico

Marsha Halfman-Franey, RN, MSN
Scottsdale, Arizona

Lynn Hanson, RN, NP, MS
Larkspur, California

Marilyn Hopkins, RN, DNSc
Sacramento, California

Beverly Hydo, RN, MSN
Troy, Michigan

Frances Jackson, RN, PhD
Detroit, Michigan

Patricia Long, RN, EdD, CS, CARN
Freeport, New York

Donna Bernocchi Losey, RN, MA
Redwood City, California

Sr. Regina Maibusch, RN, MS
Milwaukee, Wisconsin

Sandi Martin, RN, BSN, CCRN
Houston, Texas

Peggy Mayfield, RNC, MSN
Fort Worth, Texas

Nancy Molter, RN, MN, CCRN
San Antonio, Texas

Mary Lou Muwaswes, RN, MS
San Francisco, California

Judith Paice, RN, MS
Chicago, Illinois

Kathy Patterson, RN, CNM, PhD
Honolulu, Hawaii

Jan Pigg, RN, BSN, MS
Milwaukee, Wisconsin

Virginia Printz-Feddersen, RNC, MSN, CNRN
Albuquerque, New Mexico

Beth Pulliam, RN, MSN
Nashville, Tennessee

Kathleen Puntillo, RN, MS
San Anselmo, California

Julia Robinson, RN, MS, FNP-C
Bakersfield, California

Brenda Robison, RN, CRNA, MAE
Albuquerque, NM

Carolyn Sabo, RN, EdD
Las Vegas, Nevada

Nancy Munn Short, RN, BSN, CCRN
Durham, North Carolina

Hilary Sigmon, RN, PhD
Washington, DC

Jan Smith, RN, MS
Aurora, Colorado

Sandra Somma, RN, BSN
New Haven, Connecticut

Steve Toussiant, RN, MSN
Portland, Oregon

Sharon Walker, RN, MSN, CCRN, CNRN
Albuquerque, New Mexico

Janice Zeller, RN, PhD
Chicago Illiois

To the profession of nursing
and
to the important people in our lives

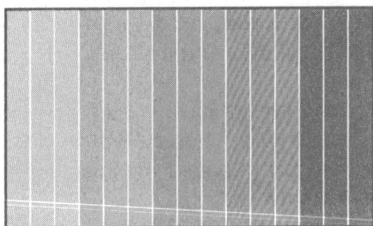

Preface

The knowledge base on which nurses make decisions changes rapidly. To accommodate these changes, we have prepared a revised edition of *Medical-Surgical Nursing: Assessment and Management of Clinical Problems*. The strengths of the first two editions have been retained, including the use of the nursing process as an organizational thread for nursing management, and a commitment to support the role of nurses on the health care team.

Contributors have again been selected for their acknowledged excellence in a specific content area. The two editors have undertaken final rewriting and editing to achieve internal consistency. In addition, one or more specialists in the subject area thoroughly reviewed each chapter.

ORGANIZATION

Content is organized into two major divisions. The first division (Section I: Chapters 1 through 6) discusses general nursing concepts related to adult clients. We have intentionally omitted material usually covered in nursing fundamentals textbooks to avoid overlap in content. The second division (Sections II through IX: Chapters 7 through 60) presents nursing assessment and the nursing role in management of medical-surgical problems.

To promote the reader's understanding of the body as an integrated whole, we have grouped the various body systems to reflect their interrelated functions. Each section is organized around two main themes: assessment and management. Chapters dealing with the first theme, *assessment of a body system,* include a discussion of the following:

1. Anatomy and physiology in brief review focusing on information that will promote understanding of nursing care
2. Health history and noninvasive physical assessment skills to expand the data base on which decisions are made
3. Common diagnostic studies, expected results, and related nursing responsibilities

The second theme is the *nursing role in management* of the various disorders of body systems. Chapters embracing this theme focus on the significance of the problem, pathogenesis and/or pathophysiological bases, and expected abnormalities of diagnostic studies. In addition, each chapter presents a concise discussion of the usual therapeutic and nursing management for major diseases and problems.

Levels of care continue to be the organizational theme for nursing management, enabling the nurse to provide care related to the following:

1. Health maintenance and promotion
2. Acute intervention
3. Rehabilitative or chronic management

This approach is used in discussing nursing management of all major health problems.

SPECIAL FEATURES

The third edition offers expanded content devoted to the older adult in both the assessment and management chapters. This focus reflects the changing population demographics related to increasing numbers of older adults.

Content has been expanded in all areas related to nursing management of health problems. Phases of the nursing process have been delineated more specifically in this edition and include greatly expanded content on problem-specific nursing diagnoses. Additional tables facilitate nursing assessment (both subjective and objective data) for all major health problems. The theoretical background for the nursing process and its specific components are presented in Chapters 2 and 3. Defining characteristics for nursing diagnoses have been added to all nursing care plans.

To assist the nurse in delivering optimal care, this edition offers several other features. Client education, a major aspect of all areas of nursing care, receives expanded attention. Each of the more than 80 nursing care plans found in this edition include nursing diagnoses, defining characteristics, nursing interventions, and evaluation criteria. Coverage of each major medical-surgical problem contains specific discussion of pharmacological and nutritional intervention. Critical care content is included where appropriate.

LEARNING AIDS

Learning objectives precede each chapter to focus on essential content, and review questions follow each chapter to enable the reader to assess mastery of the content. Each management chapter includes a case study with discussion questions. Sample charting for normal assessment findings for each body system is included in tabular format.

The authors recognize that learning occurs in a variety of ways. This book intentionally addresses both the verbally oriented and the visually oriented learner. Accordingly, the authors use both approaches and have selected many tables and figures to supplement the textual content. Readability has been analyzed, and when necessary, text has been rewritten to ensure an appropriate and consistent reading level throughout the book.

ANCILLARIES

Accompanying the third edition is an enhanced ancillary package. There are 48 illustrations reproduced as transparency acetates that make the book's most informative figures available for use in the classroom.

The new Instructor's Resource Manual provides key terms, chapter outlines with suggested teaching strategies, case studies with discussion questions, and review sheets formatted for reproduction and distribution to students. There are 50 transparency masters included in the Instructor's Resource Manual for conversion to transparencies.

An NCLEX-formatted Test Bank, which includes approximately 50 case studies with 400 related questions, is bound in the manual. The Test Bank is also available in IBM-computerized form.

ACKNOWLEDGMENTS

The editors are especially grateful to many people at Mosby–Year Book, Inc. who assisted with this major revision effort. In particular, we wish to thank the editorial team of Jeanne Rowland, Terry Van Schaik, and Don Ladig.

Our persevering typists have earned our special thanks and include Eleanor Orth, Loretta Milberger, and Christa Cooper. Kay McCash provided invaluable assistance as a consultant on nursing diagnosis and revision of nursing care plans. Sharon Walker provided excellent new material for the nursing assessment tables and the Instructor's Manual.

We are particularly grateful to the nurses and student nurses who have put their faith in our book to assist them on their path to excellence. The increasing use of this book throughout the United States and Canada has been gratifying. We are grateful to the many users who shared their comments and suggestions on the first two editions.

We also wish to thank our contributors and the reviewers for their conscientious attention to detail throughout the revision process. Their commitment to nursing kept them at their tasks until the job was done. We sincerely hope that this book will assist both students and clinicians in practicing truly professional nursing.

Sharon Mantik Lewis
Idolia Cox Collier

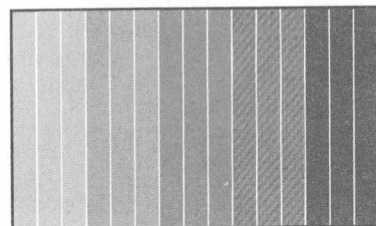

Contents

38 Nursing Role in Management: Problems of the Liver, Biliary Tract, and Pancreas, 1121

Rachel Elrod

SECTION VII

PROBLEMS WITH URINARY FUNCTION

39 Nursing Assessment: Urinary System, 1168

Sharon Mantik Lewis

40 Nursing Role in Management: Renal and Urological Problems, 1185

Sharon Mantik Lewis

41 Nursing Role in Management: Acute and Chronic Renal Failure, 1221

Sharon Mantik Lewis
Barbara Wood
JoAnn Seppeit

SECTION VIII

PROBLEMS RELATED TO REGULATORY MECHANISMS

42 Nursing Assessment: Endocrine System, 1258

Linda B. Haas

43 Nursing Role in Management: The Client with Diabetes, 1282

Virginia Valentine

44 Nursing Role in Management: Endocrine Problems, 1319

Linda B. Haas

52 Nursing Role in Management: Intracranial Problems, 1521

Connie A. Walleck

53 Nursing Role in Management: Stroke Client, 1557

Christina M. Mumma

54 Nursing Role in Management: Chronic Neurological Problems, 1579

Judith M. Ozuna

55 Nursing Role in Management: Peripheral Nerve and Spinal Cord Problems, 1615

Connie A. Walleck

56 Nursing Assessment: Musculoskeletal System, 1645

Susan C. Ruda

MEDICAL-SURGICAL NURSING
Assessment and Management of Clinical Problems

GENERAL CONCEPTS OF NURSING PRACTICE

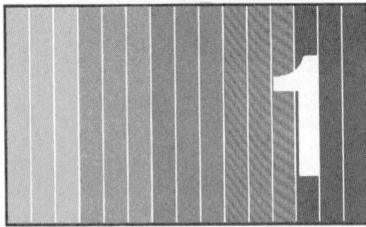

CHAPTER

1

General Concepts

Experience of Health and Illness

Patricia Palmer Stephens

Learning Objectives

1. Define health, wellness, and illness.
2. Describe modern theories of disease causation.
3. Differentiate among behaviors that promote health or result in illness.
4. Describe behaviors characteristic of illness and the sick role.
5. Differentiate between acute and chronic illness.
6. Explain the stages of acute illness.
7. Explain special concerns and tasks of the chronically ill person.

Illness is the nightside of life, a more onerous citizenship. Everyone who is born holds dual citizenship, in the kingdom of the well and in the kingdom of the sick. Although we all prefer to use only the good passport, sooner or late each of us is obliged, at least for a spell, to identify ourselves as citizens of that other place.[1]

Sonntag

The focus of this chapter is the experience of health and illness. The meaning of health and illness and common role changes that may occur with illness are discussed. To manage clients well, nurses must begin with an understanding of how health and illness are defined and experienced. General knowledge comes from health theories and research studies, and specific information gained from a client's nursing history is added. General knowledge and specific information provide the data base for implementing the nursing process with a client. (The nursing process is discussed in Chapter 2.)

Reviewed by Carolyn E. Sabo, R.N., Ed.D., Associate Professor, Department of Nursing, University of Nevada, Las Vegas, Nevada.

HEALTH AND ILLNESS
Conceptual Definitions of Health

An easily understood and usable definition of health is not easy to achieve. Sometimes the terms *health* and *wellness* are used interchangeably. However, there is an important difference. *Health* is often defined as the absence of illness. The phrase "state of health" may be used to refer to excellent or poor health. However, *wellness* is often given a more positive connotation, suggesting that it involves more than absence of illness.

Definition of health. The most commonly quoted definition of health may be that of the World Health Organization (WHO). This definition states that health is "a state of complete physical, mental, and social well-being and not merely the absence of disease or infirmity."[2] To be healthy, an individual must be in a state of well-being physically, mentally, and socially. Thus according to the WHO definition, people considered physically and mentally healthy are not truly healthy if they are deprived access to basic education because this statement assumes that basic education is necessary for social health. Many health professionals also have difficulty in agreeing with definitions of health in the physical, mental, and social dimensions, and there is a scarcity of resources available to meet the goals of WHO's definition.

High-level wellness. In the late 1950s, Halbert Dunn described the concept of high-level wellness.[3] This concept is based on a grid with two axes (Fig. 1-1). The health axis includes death and peak wellness, and the environmental axis includes a very unfavorable environment and a very favorable environment. The health axis includes physical and mental health. The environmental axis includes socioeconomic and biophysical factors in the environment that may affect health. Thus high-level wellness refers to peak physical and mental health in a very favorable biophysical and socioeconomic environment.

Dunn further stated that "high-level wellness for the individual is an integrated method of functioning which is oriented toward maximizing the potential of which the individual is capable, within the environment where he is functioning."[4] He described wellness as a dynamic process

Table 1-1 Comparison of Health and Wellness: Process and Product

Wellness	Health
A process of moving toward greater awareness of oneself and the environment, leading toward ever-increasing planned interactions with the dimensions of nutrition, fitness, stress, environment, interpersonal relationships, and self-care responsibility.	A state; either it exists or it does not. Occurs throughout life between periods of illness and disease.
A positive striving; no guilt involved because the important factor is striving, not attainment.	Guilt or negative associations may be attached to not being able to measure up to states attained by others or prescribed by others.
Unique to the individual.	An average; primarily associated with the absence of disease.
Purposeful in direction, working to become the best one can be.	Thought to be severely restricted by factors such as age, race, genetics.
The individual self-assesses the need for a wellness goal; the wellness practitioner acts as a facilitator for learning and change; individuals striving toward wellness may be medically uninteresting.	An expert is consulted and asked to provide an evaluation and prescription for what is needed to attain health.
Can be ill and still have wellness if there is a life purpose and a deep appreciation for and joy of living.	Illness and health are oppositional states.

From Clark CC: Wellness nursing: concepts, theory, research, and practice, New York, 1986, Springer Publishing Co, p 3.

moving toward a higher level of functioning and health as a passive state in which the individual is free from disease in a peaceful environment. In Dunn's view, an individual is considered to be body, mind, and spirit, which are interdependent and balanced. Ideally, individuals work to achieve interdependence and balance as they progress toward self-fulfillment and maturity.

An example of high-level wellness is a 38-year-old college professor who is free of disease and who jogs regularly. She experiences personal satisfaction from her career and involvement in her church. She lives in a quiet town, relatively free from pollution and crime. This individual experiences high-level wellness even though she has a chronic illness, hypertension, which she keeps under control through appropriate diet, exercise, medication, and lifestyle management.

Developing wellness. In the mid-1970s, Bruhn and others[5] stressed the wellness process. They stated that good health is a static position that is the consequence of avoiding behaviors or circumstances producing illness. However, wellness is a constantly evolving process in which individuals actively arrange their lifestyles and behavior. Fig. 1-2 depicts the health continuum from illness to wellness. Good health, as frequently defined by health professionals, is in the middle of the continuum. Thus the health continuum in Fig. 1-2 demonstrates that clients are only halfway toward experiencing wellness when they have been rehabilitated from specific illnesses. Table 1-1 compares the differences between wellness and health. Wellness is a dynamic process, whereas health is a state of being.

Sociological definition of health. Sociology is a source for another definition of health. Sociologists see health as bodily and emotional conditions that sup-

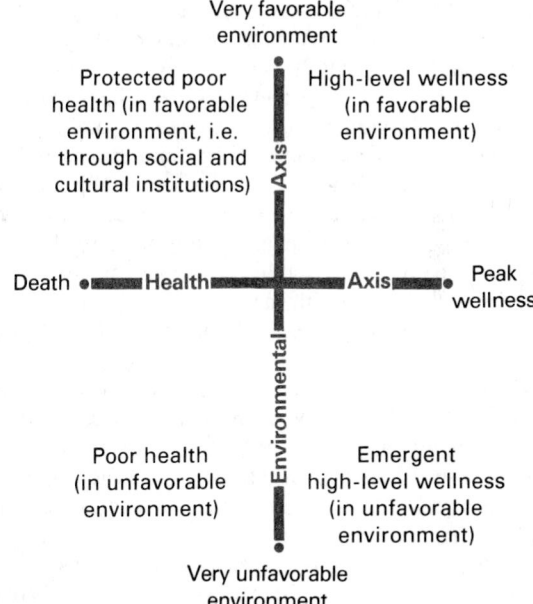

Fig. 1-1 The health grid, its axes, and quadrants. (From US Department of HEW, Public Health Service, National Office of Statistics.)

port or complement the pursuit and enjoyment of prized cultural values; examples might include being employed or rearing a family.[6] Thus illness is any condition that interferes with the pursuit and enjoyment of desired cultural values.

Holistic health care. Increased recognition that high-level wellness considers the needs of the whole person has

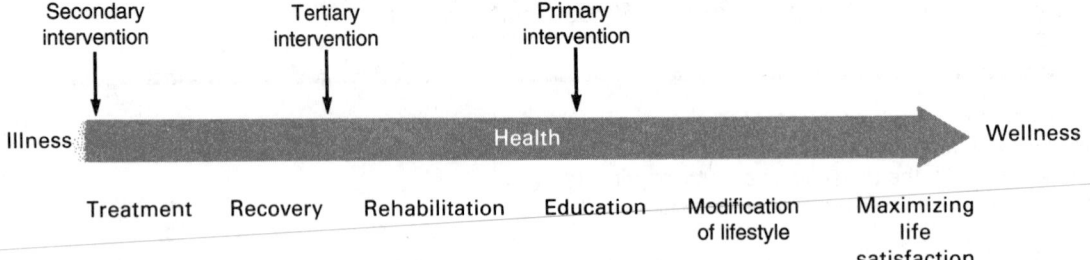

Fig. 1-2 A linear health continuum demonstrating the three areas of intervention for prevention. (Modified from Bruhn JG and others: The wellness process, J Community Health 2:210, 1977.)

led to the growth of holistic health (sometimes called *holistic medicine*). Holistic health practitioners, including nurses, focus on the promotion of health, the prevention of illness, and the healing process.[5] They emphasize the personal responsibility of clients in achieving high-level wellness. In addition, care is focused on bringing the whole person (mind, body, and spirit) into harmony with the environment. Holistic health practitioners also see illness (a lack of harmony between the whole person and the environment) as an opportunity for personal growth. Health-promoting measures recommended by holistic care providers include meditation, prayer, massage, rolfing, music and art therapy, good nutrition, exercise, imagery, biofeedback, and therapeutic touch.[7]

These health-promoting measures are called *alternative health care measures* because they are an alternative to traditional Western medicine. With more emphasis being placed on health, a variety of alternative health care centers where individuals may receive assistance in carrying out these practices have opened. Chiropractors, long disparaged by the medical establishment, have increased their emphasis on holistic health measures. In addition, homeopathic physicians are increasingly being regulated by state government.

When illness is present, holistic health measures may be used with traditional Western medical treatments. This may be done by one person or by a team made up of practitioners with different skills. Recognizing the importance of the spiritual care of clients, many hospitals now have hospital chaplains on their staffs. In addition, there is greater acceptance of religious advisors or lay leaders from outside the hospital to minister to the spiritual needs of clients.

Sociocultural Considerations in Defining Health and Illness

Definitions of health and illness vary according to the social and cultural orientation of individuals. The nurse must recognize that these differences exist and that nursing intervention must be planned accordingly.

Little evidence has been found to support differences in the definitions of health and illness among American socioeconomic groups of the majority culture. However, there is a difference in help-seeking behavior. Generally, persons from higher socioeconomic levels tend to seek help earlier when they suspect the presence of illness. Other variables, such as personal values and accessibility of health care (financial state or geographical location), affect this behavior.

There are more obvious variations in the definitions of health and illness by ethnic groups in the United States. Ethnic minority groups include Black Americans, Hispanic Americans, Native Americans (e.g., Eskimo, Iroquois, Seminole, Sioux, Navajo, Pueblo groups), and Asian-Americans. Accessibility and traditional values and ethics significantly affect health-seeking behaviors. People who identify more closely with their ethnic group are called *traditional*. Those who identify more closely with the majority culture are called *acculturated*. The beliefs of many ethnic people are somewhere on a continuum between traditional beliefs and acculturated beliefs. Table 1-2 presents examples of the way three ethnic minority groups traditionally define health and describe causation of disease. It also describes traditional healers and methods of treatment.

Theories of Illness Causation

Part of the science of medicine has been directed toward identifying the cause of disease. Great advances have been made in this area. Today health care professionals recognize that diseases may be caused by the following:

1. Inherited genetic defects
2. Developmental defects because of factors such as exposure to viral substances or certain chemicals or drugs during pregnancy
3. Biological agents or toxins
4. Physical agents such as temperature extremes, chemicals, or radiation
5. Generalized response of tissues to injury or irritation
6. Physiological and psychological reactions to various stressors
7. Biochemical imbalances within the body

Many of these factors are interrelated. However, the causes of many diseases are still unknown. For many diseases, there is not a direct cause-and-effect relationship between a specific disease-producing agent and the onset of disease.

Historical theories of disease causation. Claude Bernard (a nineteenth-century physiologist) and Walter Cannon (an early-twentieth-century physician) described theo-

Table 1-2 Variations in Defining and Treating Health and Disease by Ethnic Groups*

Definition of Health	Causation of Disease	Traditional Treatment Method	Traditional Healer
BLACK AMERICANS			
Harmony with nature exists because things influence each other. No separation between mind, body, and spirit occurs.	Illness is disharmony due primarily to demons and evil spirits.	Voodoo: a belief system using white magic and black magic; good *grisgris* (pleasantly scented oils and powders) to prevent illness, causing success; bad *grisgris* (vile-smelling oils and powders) to cause illness, leading to failure; use of candles and Catholic relics Many folk remedies Faith healers: emphasis on healing power of religion	Women voodoo leaders who do *rooting* (determining source and treatment of a disease) Faith healers (pray over the individual for healing; stress faith of the sick person)
HISPANIC AMERICANS			
Chicano (Mexican-American descent)			
Balance or harmony in body is from "luck," good behavior, or gift from God.	Imbalances of hot or cold, wet or dry, in body are due to punishment for wrongdoing. Dislocation of body parts occurs. Magic causes outside of the body such as witchcraft or *malojo* (bad eye). Strong emotions (e.g., *susto* from fright) occur.	Use of certain religious rituals and artifacts such as confession, laying on of hands, lighting candles Massage *Cleanings,* or passing an unbroken egg or herbal bunch over the body Classification of treatments as hot or cold and application for the opposite type of illness Magic and religious practices such as pilgrimages, offering medals, lighting candles, making promises Variety of herbs	*Curandero:* a holistic healer who has ties to the "world of the sacred" and shares responsibility for recovery with the ill person and family Herbalist: skilled in using herbs for treatment
Puerto Rican Same as Chicano.	Similar to above. See illnesses as hot or cold. Consider people who see visions as special people, not mentally ill.	Similar to Chicanos. Use of special herbs, foods, lotion Use of charms for prevention Classification of treatments as *frio* (cold), *fresco* (cool), or *caliente* (hot)	*Esperitista* or *curendera:* a sophisticated folk practitioner *Santero:* treater of mental illness
ASIAN-AMERICANS			
Spiritual and physical harmony occur with nature. Balance is maintained between *yin* (female, negative, cold, dark, inside of the body) and *yang* (male, positive, warm, light, outside of the body) by following *Tao,* the order or way of nature. *Yen* stores the vital strength of life. *Yang* protects the body from outside sources.	Upset in *yin* and *yang* balance is present.	Acupuncture (cold treatment): puncturing of certain areas of the skin to cure disease or pain Moxibustion (hot treatment): application of heated pulverized wormwood to specific areas of the skin to restore balance of *yin* and *yang* Wide variety of herbal remedies (ginseng most common)	First-class physician: preventer of occurrence of disease, plus treater of disease Second-class physician: treater only to those with disease

Modified from Spector RE: Cultural diversity in health and illness, New York, 1985, Appleton-Century-Crofts, pp 127-179.
*The reader is cautioned to use this background information only as a guideline in implementing the nursing process. The beliefs of each client need to be assessed and incorporated into the nursing process.

Table 1-3 Possible Psychosomatic Disorders

Bronchial asthma	Paroxysmal tachycardia
Essential hypertension	Peptic ulcers
Hyperthyroidism	Raynaud's disease
Migraine headaches	Rheumatoid arthritis
Neurodermatitis	Ulcerative colitis

ries of disease causation that underlie modern theories. Bernard was the first to describe the internal environment of the body and the necessity for it to be maintained in a relatively constant state for health. He hypothesized that disease is the result of an upset in the internal environment, an interruption of the normal link between the internal and external environment of the body, and an overreaction of the body's attempt to adapt to the changes in the

Table 1-4 Social Readjustment Rating Scale

No. Life Event	Mean Value
1 Death of spouse	100
2 Divorce	73
3 Marital separation from mate	65
4 Detention in jail or other institution	63
5 Death of a close family member	63
6 Major personal injury or illness	53
7 Marriage	50
8 Being fired at work	47
9 Marital reconciliation with mate	45
10 Retirement from work	45
11 Major change in health of a family member	44
12 Pregnancy	40
13 Sexual difficulties	39
14 Gaining a new family member (e.g., through birth, adoption, moving in)	39
15 Major business readjustment (e.g., merger, reorganization, bankruptcy)	39
16 Major change in financial state (e.g., a lot worse off or a lot better off than usual)	38
17 Death of a close friend	37
18 Changing to different line of work	36
19 Major change in number of arguments with spouse (e.g., either a lot more or a lot less than usual regarding child-rearing, personal habits)	35
20 Taking out a mortgage or loan for a major purchase (e.g., for a home, business)	31
21 Foreclosure on a mortgage or loan	30
22 Major change in responsibilities at work (e.g., promotion, demotion, lateral transfer)	29
23 Son or daughter leaving home (e.g., marriage, attending college)	29
24 Trouble with in-laws	29
25 Outstanding personal achievement	28
26 Spouse beginning or ceasing work outside the home	26
27 Beginning or ceasing normal schooling	26
28 Major change in living conditions (e.g., building a new home, remodeling, deterioration of home or neighborhood)	25
29 Revision of personal habits (e.g., dress, manners, associations)	24
30 Trouble with boss	23
31 Major change in working hours or conditions	20
32 Change in residence	20
33 Changing to a new school	20
34 Major change in usual type and/or amount of recreation	19
35 Major change in church activities (e.g., a lot more or a lot less than usual)	19
36 Major change in social activities (e.g., clubs, dancing, movies, visiting)	18
37 Taking out a mortgage or loan for a lesser purchase (e.g., for a car, TV, freezer)	17
38 Major change in sleeping habits (a lot more or a lot less sleep, or change in part of day when asleep)	16
39 Major change in number of family get-togethers (e.g., a lot more or a lot less than usual)	15
40 Major change in eating habits (a lot more or a lot less food intake, or very different meal hours or surroundings)	15
41 Vacation	13
42 Christmas	12
43 Minor violation of law (e.g., traffic tickets, jaywalking, disturbing the peace)	11

Modified from Holmes TH and Rahe RH: Social readjustment rating scale, J Psychosom Res 11:216, 1967.

internal environment. Cannon was the first to use the term *homeostasis* when referring to physiological processes within the body. He defined homeostasis as dynamic equilibrium in which a constant change occurs in bodily processes; these changes are so balanced that the result is a constant environment. The support for his theory came from his study of self-regulating mechanisms in the body such as blood levels of oxygen and carbon dioxide, blood pressure, and body temperature.

General adaptation syndrome or stress syndrome.
Hans Selye, a physician, drawing from the work of Bernard on adaptive responses, hypothesized that the stress syndrome was present in all diseases. As a young medical student he observed the "syndrome of being sick." He was struck more by the similarities of appearance and nonspecific symptoms of ill individuals than he was by their differences.

Selye defines *stress* as "the state manifested by a specific syndrome which consists of all the non-specifically induced changes within a biologic system."[8] Stress is caused by a stressor, any agent such as physical exertion, emotional tension, or temperature extremes that stresses the body. Selye calls the response the *general adaptation syndrome (GAS)* because it involves nonspecific changes, mediated by the sympathetic nervous system and adrenal cortices, that are directed toward adaptation of the body to the stressor. In his early work, Selye emphasizes acute stressors and physiological responses. In his recent work, Selye has put more emphasis on psychological stressors. (A more detailed discussion of the stress syndrome is discussed in Chapter 5.)

Disease as maladaptation. In the 1950s and 1960s, Harold Wolff, a psychiatrist, built on the work of Bernard and Selye. He emphasized psychological and physiological responses to chronic stressors. Thus he proposed that the entire life of an individual may be involved in disease causation. He noted that, because of a highly developed central nervous system, humans react not only to actual stressors but to symbols and threats of danger as if they were actual stressors. Therefore reactions to symbolic danger may be inappropriate. In addition, he noted that certain organs may react inappropriately to stressors. Often, different organs react inappropriately in different individuals.[9] For example, one person is more apt to have physiological changes in the stomach when stressed, whereas another individual might have changes in the respiratory tract. Wolff proposed that these individual, specific organ reactions are the cause of psychosomatic diseases. Psychosomatic diseases or disorders have physiological or structural changes thought to result at least partially from psychological or mental influences. Experts in psychosomatic medicine continue to look at the role emotions play in disease causation. A list of disorders thought to be caused partly by psychological factors is provided in Table 1-3.

Life changes and illness. A large number of life changes may cause disease. Much of the research in this area has been done by Rahe and others.[10,11] In one study, Rahe and Holmes defined a life change as any positive or negative event in a person's life that requires the person to expend energy to adapt to the change. In this study, various socioeconomic and cultural groups ranked a number of

Table 1-5 LCUs and Incidence of Major Illness*

Number	Amount of Change	Incidence of Major Illness
0-149	Insignificant	Minimal
150-199	Mild	33%
200-299	Moderate	50%
300+	Major	80%

Modified from Holmes T and Rahe E: The social readjustment rating scale, J Psychosom Res 11:213, 1967.
*This table describes the amount of stress as measured by LCUs, followed by the statistical incidence of disease according to the number of LCUs. The chance of illness is based on the number of LCUs over 1 to 2 years.

life changes according to the amount of energy needed to adapt to the changes. The social readjustment rating scale (SRRS), Table 1-4, shows the results of this ranking and the number of life change units (LCUs) assigned to each event. (Marriage was given an arbitrary score of 50.) This rating system is still being researched to determine whether the number of life changes is the important factor when determining the amount of stress a person experiences or whether a combination of factors, such as social support, perception, and coping styles, are the factors that allow the person to cope.[12-14]

Additional research studies using the SRRS have found a significant relationship between life changes and the development of physical and mental illnesses. The reason that illness develops because of many life changes is that changes require adaptive behavior. Adaptive behaviors cause major alterations in an individual's psychophysiological systems, thus lowering the resistance of the body to illness.[15] Table 1-5 describes the incidence of illness according to the number of life changes over 1 to 2 years. Other studies have shown that the higher the average number of LCUs over 2 years, the more serious the illness. For example, the LCUs before developing bronchitis were around 320, whereas the LCUs before developing cancer were 780.[16]

Other factors such as health habits, social assets (family and financial security and academic achievement), and psychological well-being may have as much influence on health status as life changes. However, Pesznecker and McNeil found that the number of LCUs was the strongest variable predicting health status. However, all variables were weakly associated with maintaining health status.[6] Research regarding factors affecting health status is still being done.[17-19]

There are many factors involved in the causation of disease in an individual. These factors are found in the external and internal environment. In addition, both physical and psychological factors can cause illness. Recent research findings regarding the stress of life changes are especially significant for health promotion and maintenance in our rapidly changing society. This is especially true when the physiological impact of stress is considered (see Chapter 5).

Table 1-6 Decision-Making Phase of Preventive Health Behavior

Motivating Perceptions	Basis
PERSONAL	
Importance of health to the person	Activities it allows a person to do
Perceived level of internal and external control	Individuals with internal locus of control having a history of more preventive health behaviors than those having external loci of control
Perceived vulnerability to a specific disease	Family history of certain diseases, present health status of the individual, and incidence of disease in the general population
Perceived seriousness of the disease	Degree of discomfort the disease threatens, degree of visibility, degree of disruption in the family or occupation, and degree of communicability of the disease to others
Perceived efficacy of specific actions	Choice of actions perceived to lower threat of illness with the least amount of risk and inconvenience
Perceived value of early detection	Belief of the benefit of a technique for early detection for a specific illness (e.g., Pap smear for cervical cancer or blood pressure screening for hypertension)
PSYCHOSOCIAL	
Concern of significant others	Individuals with strong social support being more likely to initiate and continue a preventive health behavior (e.g., an exercise program)
Family patterns of health behavior	High maternal influence with a positive correlation between the level of education of the dominant female in the home and the level of preventive health behavior
Societal group norms and pressures	Compliance with societal norms giving satisfaction
Cultural acceptance of health behaviors	Preventive health behavior occurring when a culture sanctions it as a responsible action (Some cultures sanction seeking medical attention for serious illness only.)
Expectations of health professionals	The greater the credibility of the person giving the information, the greater the motivating factor
Information from media	Use of media increasing the perceived vulnerability of the individual

Adapted from Kozier B and Erb G: Fundamentals of nursing, ed 3, Menlo Park, Calif, 1987, Addison-Wesley, pp 59-60; and from Zindler-Wernet P and Weiss SJ: Health locus of control and preventive health behavior, West J Nurs Res 9:160-179, 1987.

BEHAVIORS THAT PROMOTE HEALTH
Health Practices

Some behaviors seem to promote and maintain health. Certain health practices are positively correlated with health. These include the following[20]:

1. Sleeping regularly 7 to 8 hours per night
2. Eating breakfast
3. Eating regular meals with minimal or no snacking
4. Eating moderately to maintain an ideal weight
5. Exercising moderately
6. Drinking no more than a moderate amount of alcohol
7. Not smoking (best if have never smoked)

These behaviors help people maintain good health regardless of their sex, age, and economic status. These behaviors are also cumulative; that is, the greater the number of these factors habitually practiced by individuals, the better their health.[21]

Good mental health practices are important for good health as well. These practices primarily result in a realistic, positive self-concept and the ability to problem solve.

Preventive Health Behavior

Preventive health behavior is a voluntary* action taken by individuals or a group to decrease the threat of illness. This action is not curative or remedial because it is taken while the person has no symptoms for any disease.[22]

Preventive health behavior has decision-making and action phases. The phases relate to primary prevention and early detection. *Primary prevention* refers to measures such as proper diet, proper exercise, and immunizations that may prevent the occurrence of a specific disease. *Early detection* refers to measures such as blood pressure screening and breast self-examination that may detect the early onset of disease so that early treatment may be instituted.

Sometimes, health care providers make the false assumption that people do what is best for their health. Unfortunately, health care providers themselves disprove this assumption, as evidenced by the number who smoke and

*Required school immunizations are the major exception to this definition.

Table 1-7 Nursing Measures for Health Promotion

Nursing Measure	Example
Inform clients of daily activities that help to maintain optimum health.	Inform client that a proper diet to maintain an ideal weight and adequate sleep and exercise are important in health maintenance.
Inform clients of the characteristics of a disease for which they are at risk.	Tell client that a history of deaths of parents at 40 years of age due to coronary artery disease is usually familial.
Explain the consequences of the disease for which clients are at risk.	Explain that client may also have coronary artery disease at a young age because of the family history.
Give clients specific information about how they can reduce their vulnerability to the disease.	Counsel client about early detection measures by having lipid screening. Also counsel about moderate eating, regular exercise, and cessation of smoking.
Use societal group norms and peer pressure.	For example, say, "I talked to your younger brother yesterday. He has cut down on desserts and started jogging every other day."

Modified from Pender NJ: Health promotion in nursing practice, ed 2, Norwalk, Conn, 1987, Appleton & Lange, pp 75–90, 213–281.

who are overweight, underexercised, and overstressed. Most human beings make the easiest and not necessarily the most healthy choices about health practices. However, in recent years, the changes in the lifestyle of many Americans indicate the positive value of education aimed at prevention. Table 1-6 outlines the factors affecting the decision-making process in preventive health behavior. After people have decided to perform preventive health behaviors, they need cues to initiate action. These cues may be a perception of aging, advertisements stressing healthy behavior, or a recent illness.

■ Nursing Management of Health-Promoting Behaviors

The role of nursing in encouraging preventive behavior for better health should be directed to helping the client make informed decisions. Nurses should first take steps to ensure that the client has the knowledge to select options. Nurses may also need to help clients find the resources needed to change behavior. Table 1-7 lists nursing measures that can be used to promote healthy behaviors. When carrying out such nursing measures, nurses should consider the whole person, including the biophysical, psychological, sociocultural, and environmental dimensions. Many disorders can be prevented if the seven health practices listed previously are followed. Thus nursing care should begin by emphasizing these basic health habits.

TYPES OF ILLNESS

The two major categories of illness are acute and chronic. Acute illness is an illness or disease (deviation from normal) of relatively rapid onset and short duration. It is usually self-limiting or responds readily to a specific treatment. Most acute illnesses allow individuals who develop no complications to return to their previous level of functioning after recovery.

Chronic illnesses are illnesses that lead to at least some of the following characteristics: (1) permanent impairments or deviations from normal, (2) irreversible pathological changes, (3) a residual disability, (4) special rehabilitation, and (5) long-term medical and/or nursing management.[22] Chronic illnesses may have acute exacerbations during which clients move from a level of optimum functioning, with the illness in good control, to physiological instability in which others may need to provide assistance.

Although both types of illnesses require nursing management, nursing skills needed vary for each. In this book, nursing is divided into health promotion and maintenance, acute intervention, and chronic or rehabilitative management. Nurses need skills and knowledge to meet the needs of clients in each of these categories. The specific skills for acute and chronic nursing interventions will be described with the problem to which they are most applicable.

EXPERIENCE OF ILLNESS
Illness Behavior

The experience of illness as described by the terms *illness behavior* and *sick role* focuses attention on the individual rather than on the disease. An understanding of the processes involved in illness enables the nurse to provide care that considers the total person in the biophysical, psychological, sociocultural, and environmental dimensions.

Illness behavior is the way people deal with organic malfunctioning such as pain, discomfort, or fever. It includes the perception of symptoms, the evaluation of the significance (seriousness) of these symptoms, and the way individuals respond to the symptoms and their evaluations of them. Each component of illness behavior is influenced by the severity of the symptoms and the individual's sociocultural environment.

People's responses to illness fall into the following categories: (1) taking action, (2) taking no action, or (3) taking counteraction.[23]

Taking action. Taking action to relieve symptoms may involve self-diagnosis and self-treatment or seeking help from a health care provider. Billions of dollars are spent annually by Americans on over-the-counter drugs (drugs not requiring a prescription) to alleviate symptoms that ill persons have self-diagnosed and decided to treat. This behavior is influenced by media advertising, as well as social grouping. Other ill persons may choose to treat themselves by using home or folk remedies. Other forms of self-treatment include activities such as rest, change in diet, and exercise.

If self-treatment does not work, individuals probably seek out a health care provider. The health care provider selected will depend primarily on the clients' sociocultural backgrounds. One person may choose to go to a physician, whereas another may choose to go to an herbalist, a chiropractor, or a spiritual healer. Sometimes the choice of health care provider depends on the symptoms experienced. For instance, an individual may go to a chiropractor for back problems or headache but will go to a physician for a fever or abdominal pain.

Taking no action. Taking no action is another behavioral response to illness. It may be the result of a "wait-and-see" attitude or denial of the significance of the symptoms. Persons may wait to see whether the symptoms subside or worsen before deciding to take action. For example, a person may say, "I will wait 2 or 3 days to see if my stomach pain will go away." On the other hand, the symptom may be so frightening that the individual denies it; for example, a man may completely ignore rectal bleeding although his father died of cancer of the colon. Some individuals delay action because they are unwilling to admit that they are sick or fear the consequences of their illness. Others may delay because they do not know which physician to see.

The individual's lack of action is rewarded if the symptoms disappear. However, if the symptoms persist or worsen, the person is forced to take action, possibly because of pressure from family or friends, because the symptoms interfere with usual activities, or because the person is responding constructively to a health-threatening symptom.

Taking counteraction. Taking counteraction refers to those behaviors that attempt to disprove the existence of symptoms. An example might be the man who decides to lift weights to work the "soreness" out of his left arm when the symptom suggests myocardial ischemia. Another example is an individual who has been diagnosed with leukemia but who then shops around to find a health practitioner who will tell him that he does not have leukemia. Taking counteraction is an example of deviant illness behavior because individuals want to be defined as healthy when they are ill. They are not open to seeking help, and thus their conditions may worsen and possibly cause death.

Sick Role Behavior

After individuals admit that they are ill, they enter the sick role. They take on the expected behaviors of a sick person as defined by their sociocultural group. Twaddle[24] defines *sickness* as the judgment of the health of one person by others. (He also sees illness as the symptoms the person experiences and disease as physical changes that shorten life or reduce the individual's capacity to function.) Thus for individuals to function in a sick role, the people around them must perceive that they are ill.

The classic components of the sick role were defined by Parsons in the early 1950s. They follow[25]:
1. The right of the individual to not be held responsible for the illness
2. The right of the individual to be released from usual responsibilities
3. The duty of the individual to try to get well and to see illness as undesirable
4. The duty of the individual to seek medically competent help and to cooperate with the treatment plan

These expectations have been debated and analyzed over the last 40 years but have been found to be an accurate description of the major components of sick role expectations,[25] especially when they are applied to acute illness.

The relationship between illness behavior and the sick role is diagrammed in Fig. 1-3, which demonstrates an overlap between seeking help (illness behavior) and assumption of the sick role. It also points out that sick people need to receive validation of the sick role from those around them and legitimization of it from a health care provider. Some individuals may find the sick role very stressful because they may have to temporarily give up other family or group roles. This change often produces a lot of stress for family members or significant others as well.

Stages of Acute Illness

Individuals with acute illnesses usually experience a specific sequence of events from onset to recovery, assuming that they are restored to health. They may even experience a higher level of wellness because of health teaching received during the illness. The stages of acute illness combine illness behavior and the sick role behavior.

Every person experiences forms of acute illness. Fig. 1-3 demonstrates the ways the stages of acute illness fit throughout life into a health-illness continuum. This illustration is based on Suchman's analysis of behavior patterns in illness.[26]

Symptom experience. Clients experience symptoms of the acute illness during the first stage. They recognize that they have sensations incompatible with their concept of health. If the symptoms subside while they take no action, they skip the steps in the circle and return to the optimum level of wellness. The symptoms may also subside after the use of folk remedies or over-the-counter medications. However, if symptoms persist or worsen, they move on to the next stage.

The most significant symptom suggesting illness is pain. Examples of other symptoms are fever, chills, and shortness of breath. If the symptoms are severe, the person seeks professional health care more rapidly than if they are mild or moderate. People's emotional responses to symptoms are other factors in their response to the symptoms.

Assumption of the sick role. When individuals perceive their symptoms as illness, they relinquish their normal duties and activities. They seek validation of their illness from family, friends, or co-workers. If the others agree that they are ill, the ill individuals are allowed to enter the sick role. For many, this validation is acceptable only for 1 or 2 days because American society requires professional validation of illness (Fig. 1-4).

As individuals assume the sick role, they usually be-

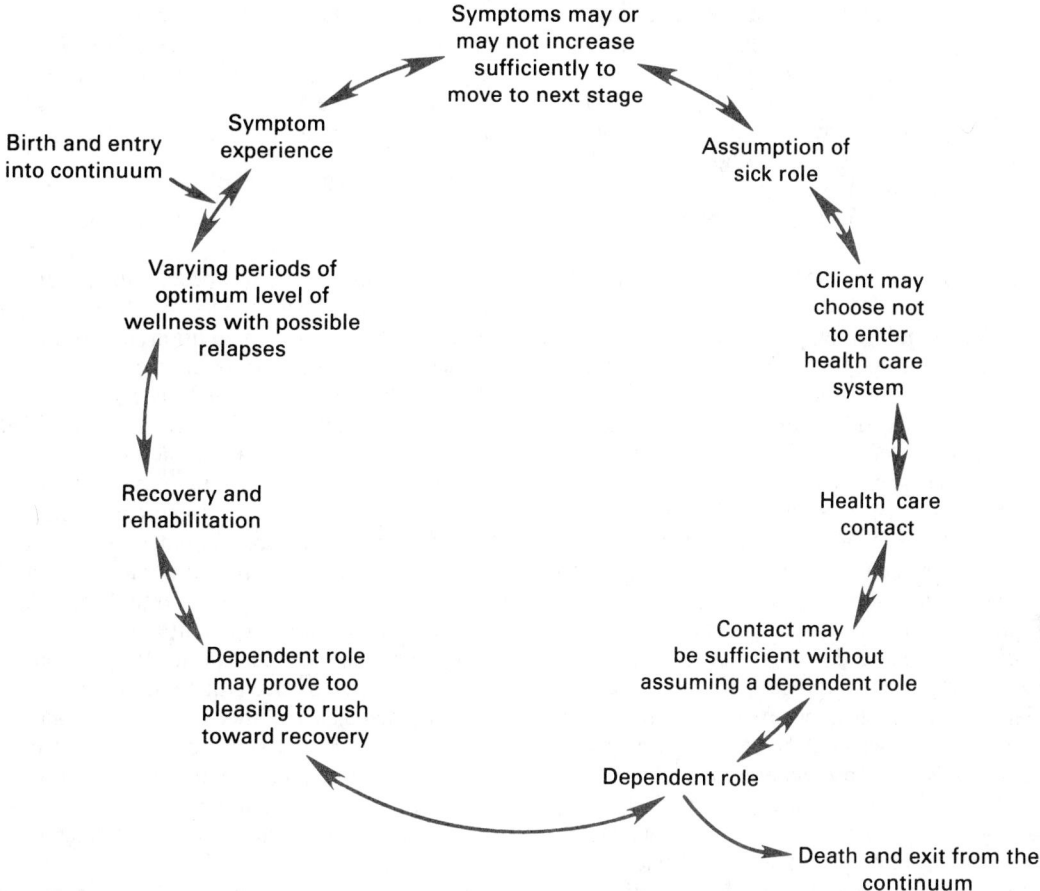

Fig. 1-3 This circular health-illness continuum demonstrates the relationship between illness behavior and the sick role. Individuals may move around the circle many times during their lives. They may stop at the different places for varying times and may reverse their direction. (Modified from Fromer MJ: Community health care and the nursing process, ed 2, St Louis, 1983, The CV Mosby Co, p 203.)

come preoccupied with their symptoms and other bodily functions. This behavior is shown by the ill persons' thoughts and conversations, which focus on minor variations in pulse, elimination patterns, and temperature. Attention is directed inward. Thus if ill persons go to work, their performance tends to suffer because of this preoccupation.

Health care contact. Some people may choose not to seek professional health care. However, most people seek professional health care to legitimize the sick role and to ease the intensity and personal significance of the symptoms. They make the medical contact (usually with a physician) for diagnosis, treatment, and prognosis of the illness (Fig. 1-4). If the illness is validated, they continue in the sick role. If it is not validated, they may decide to return to their normal role or seek out another medical person who will validate the illness; this is called *shopping around*. Either response may be valid, depending on the circumstances.

Dependent role. Individuals enter the dependent role stage after deciding to accept the diagnosis and treatment plan of the physician. Less energy is available to many

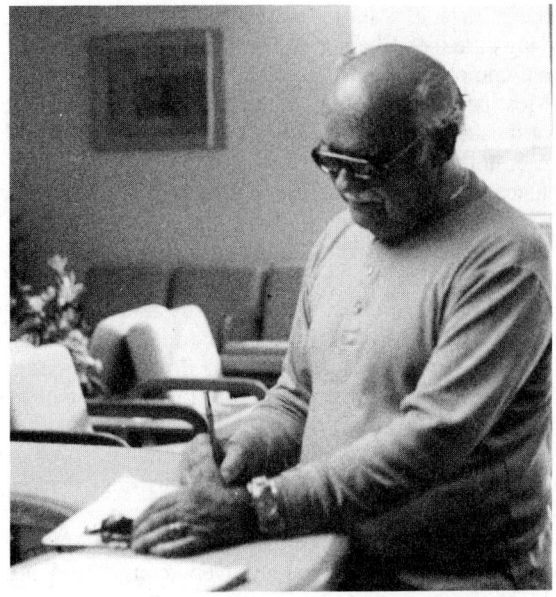

Fig. 1-4 Ill person seeking validation.

persons with acute illnesses because of the physiological effects of illness (for example, fever, blurred vision, pain, and cloudy thinking), so these people are less able to function independently; thus they become dependent. The more severe the illness, the greater the dependency of individuals. At this stage clients may be hospitalized. Dependency falls into the following categories[23]:

1. Compliance with or conformity to opinions and demands of others
2. The need for physical assistance in activities of daily living
3. The need for emotional support in the form of approval, reassurance, physical closeness, and protection

People may at first be reluctant to enter this dependent role because it is usually viewed as undesirable. On the other hand, it may also be seen as the only way to restore health. Nurses often play an important part in helping sick individuals adapt to this role. (Acute nursing interventions, described in the management chapters in this book, focus on assisting clients in this stage.)

An important component of the dependent role is compliance. *Compliance* refers to the cooperation of the client with the treatment regimen prescribed. Treatment may include a special diet, a modification in activity (change in type such as special exercises or an increase or decrease in level), or medications. Clinical experience and research have shown that total compliance rarely occurs.

Clients comply with treatment regimens for many reasons. Clients' relationships with medical providers are very important. Clients must perceive the caregiver as friendly and understanding, must agree with the caregiver about the nature of the illness, and must perceive the treatment as appropriate to the illness. In addition, clients must perceive their personal susceptibility to recurrence of the illness, the seriousness of the illness, and the effectiveness of the treatment in alleviating symptoms.[27] Thus compliance involves good rapport between caregivers and clients, effective treatment plans, and knowledge of the illness by clients. There is a strong emphasis on client education in nursing care (see Chapter 6) because of this correlation between compliance and education.

Most people recover from their illnesses. When moving toward recovery, clients may experience some secondary gain or enjoyment of the dependency role because they experience a release from the normal responsibilities and pressures of daily living and enjoy the attention they are receiving. Thus recovery is often experienced physically before it is experienced emotionally. However, because individuals perceive the sick role as undesirable, health care providers and family members and friends encourage recovered clients to recover. If clients do not, they are considered *malingerers*—a deviant role in which persons pretend to be sick to avoid responsibilities.

Recovery and rehabilitation. The final stage of acute illness is recovery and rehabilitation. This stage may begin in the hospital but concludes in the home. Individuals choose to give up the sick role and resume normal tasks and responsibilities. They may even return to an higher level of wellness than experienced before the illness be-

cause of the health education that resulted in better health practices. Thus persons should receive assistance with health promotion and maintenance practices, as well as treatment, to prevent recurrence of disease. Nurses are in an ideal position to accomplish this task.

Special Tasks and Problems of the Chronically Ill

Since there have been many advances in the treatment of acute illnesses that have resulted in their decreased incidence, chronic illness has become increasingly significant. Today the incidence of chronic illness is a major health problem (Table 1-8). In addition, each chronically ill individual usually suffers from an average of two chronic conditions. Some diseases, such as hypertension, congestive heart failure, and renal failure, are related. Others such as arthritis and emphysema may be unrelated.

The incidence of chronic illness increases with age. Therefore people with the highest incidence of chronic illness are 65 years of age and older. Because this population group has been increasing in number, the health care and Medicare systems are having trouble in adapting to meet the needs of the chronically ill elderly client.

People who have chronic illnesses do not fit neatly into the five stages of acute illness. When a chronic illness such as diabetes mellitus is in good control, the person may experience no signs or symptoms of the disease. However, to remain symptom-free, the chronically ill individual needs to maintain contact with a medical caregiver and to comply with the treatment regimen (a degree of dependency found in the sick role). Depending on the disease and the stage it is in, there is a varying impact on lifestyle. However, a chronic illness requires adaptation by the individual. Anselm L. Strauss, a medical sociologist, has identified the following tasks of the chronically ill individual[22]:

1. Preventing and managing crisis
2. Carrying out prescribed regimens
3. Controlling symptoms
4. Reordering time
5. Adjusting to changes in the course of disease
6. Preventing social isolation
7. Attempting to normalize interactions with others

These tasks were identified as common themes in the lives of chronically ill persons who participated in several research studies conducted by Strauss and others.[22] The following is a summary of their work.

Table 1-8 Incidence of Chronic Illness

Age	Incidence of Chronic Illness*	Illness Limiting Major Activity*
Under 17 years	23	1
17–44 years	54	5
45–64 years	71	14
65 years and above	84	40

Modified from Strauss AL and others: Chronic illness and the quality of life, ed 2, St Louis, 1984, The CV Mosby Co.
*Percentage.

Preventing and managing a medical crisis. Most chronic illnesses have the potential of an acute exacerbation of symptoms, which may result in increased disability or death. Examples include the client with cardiac disease who may have another myocardial infarction or the client with asthma who may have a severe attack. Thus chronically ill persons and their families must learn to prevent or manage crises. This involves learning the potential of a crisis and ways to prevent it or modify its threat, which usually involves compliance with a prescribed medical regimen. They also need to know the clues or signs and symptoms of the onset of a crisis. These may occur rapidly, as with a seizure, or slowly, as with hyperglycemia in a person with diabetes.

Clients should also make a plan of how to deal with the crisis. This may involve a diabetic person carrying some candy in case of a sudden onset of hypoglycemia or a plan to never leave alone an individual prone to sudden choking seizures. Factors affecting the organization of a plan to manage a crisis are the possible occurrence of the crisis, association of a medical crisis with the original onset of disease, distance in time from an actual crisis, and the possibility of a breakdown in organization due to disruption in the lives of those who will manage the crisis.

Managing regimens. Chronically ill individuals must learn to live with medical treatment regimens. Regimens vary in degree of difficulty and the impact they have on lifestyle. Clients should evaluate their regimens and adapt it to meet their needs. Characteristics of regimens include the following:

1. Degree of difficulty involved in learning the regimen: This may range in difficulty from remembering to take a tablet once a day to learning to run a hemodialysis unit at home.
2. Amount of time required to implement the regimen: Does it involve an activity lasting 1 minute three times a day or 2 hours three times a day?
3. Amount of discomfort and energy associated with the implementation of the regimen in its prescribed form: If a regimen is uncomfortable and takes a considerable amount of energy, there is less chance that it will be carried out as prescribed. Thus an insulin-dependent diabetic may decide to forgo an injection because it hurts. Another consideration affecting compliance is uncomfortable or undesirable side effects, such as impotence from some antihypertensive drugs.
4. Visibility of the regimen to other people and the social acceptability of the disease the regimen suggests: For example, a seeing-eye dog with a blind person in a restaurant is generally considered more socially acceptable than the frequent expectoration that occurs with chronic obstructive lung disease.
5. Effectiveness and speed of the regimen in treating or preventing symptoms of the disease: Some clients erroneously assume that they may stop taking their medication if the signs or symptoms disappear. A common example is the client with hypertension who stops medicines "because my blood pressure is normal now."

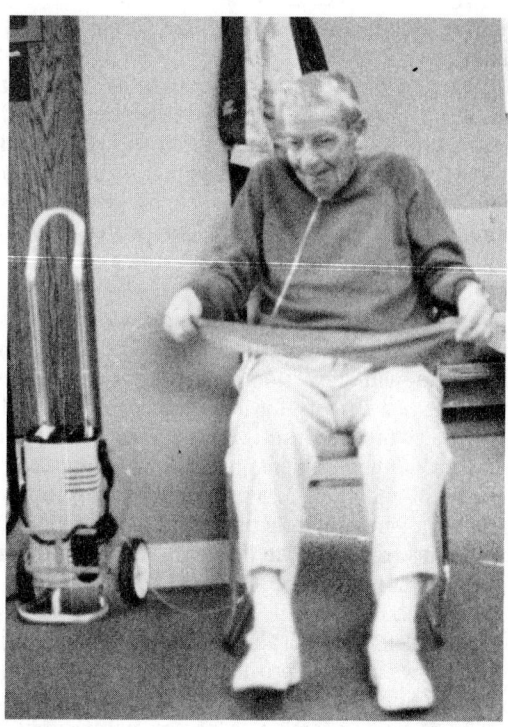

Fig. 1-5 People with chronic illnesses may need specialized equipment to assist them in daily activities.

Controlling symptoms. Clients must also learn to control symptoms so that they can continue desired activities. Methods of managing the visibility of symptoms may also be included. Some individuals redesign their lifestyle by learning to plan ahead; for example, a person with ulcerative colitis may choose to go only to events where there are restrooms near the seating area. Others may make changes in their environment or use special tools to assist them in daily activities; for example, a person with severe emphysema may need to adjust to the use of portable oxygen (Fig. 1-5). A person with arthritis may select clothing having zippers with large pull tabs rather than small buttons. Some people rearrange work schedules for times when their symptoms, such as coughing up a large amount of sputum, are less severe.

Individuals should learn about the pattern of symptoms (typical onset, duration, and severity) and whether they can affect their duration and intensity. Chronically ill persons must also learn the limits of their abilities in controlling symptoms. Finally, they must learn to use the good times when symptoms are less severe to do things they cannot do when symptoms are present; for example, a client with decreased levels of energy due to cardiac disease may elect to have sexual relations in the morning after a good night's sleep.

Reordering of time. The use of time is another problem for chronically ill persons. They may have too much or too little available time. For example, individuals forced to retire because of a chronic illness may find too much time on their hands and have to find activities that they enjoy to fill the empty hours. On the other hand, many regimens take tremendous amounts of time for the chronically ill and their helpers.

Adjusting to changes in the course of the disease. Chronically ill individuals must also learn to live with the course of a chronic illness. Some diseases such as multiple sclerosis have unpredictable courses that make adjustments difficult. Other diseases such as controlled diabetes are more predictable. Part of the task also involves developing a personal identity that includes the chronic illness and the lifestyle changes it necessitates.

Preventing social isolation. As indicated earlier, social isolation may occur with chronic illness because individuals choose to withdraw from activities. For example, a man who has had surgery for lung cancer might avoid coffee breaks at work because everyone else smokes and he has stopped. Other persons might also withdraw from chronically ill individuals. For example, the co-workers might avoid a person with partially controlled epilepsy.

Attempting to normalize interactions with others. Finally, an ill individual must normalize interactions with others. Most chronically ill individuals attempt to manage symptoms and to hide disabilities or disfigurement. This may involve wearing a prosthesis or demonstrating that they can function like a "normal" person (i.e., one without the disability). For example, a person with chronic lung problems might stop walking to catch his breath but looks as if he is inspecting a plant or looking in a store window. Closely related to this is the desire of many dying individuals to be treated as being among the living, with normal interests and desires.

■ Nursing Management of the Chronically Ill

These seven tasks of the chronically ill focus on managing disease and managing life. Nurses may use these tasks to plan the management of chronically ill clients.

Family members are important to chronically ill clients. They may help or hinder the management of the chronic illness. Ideally, family members, frequently spouses, work together in managing the disease or diseases. This collaboration should be initiated under the direction of the health care team at diagnosis to prevent difficulties later.[28] When the family member is an elderly spouse, the caregiver may also have a chronic illness, which complicates the situation.

Tasks of the family member may include assuming an increased physical burden of work because of the need to add tasks previously assumed by the chronically ill person, dealing with the changes in the progress of the disease, coping with feelings of being psychologically and physically overwhelmed, and dealing with changes in social roles and the identity of themselves and the family member because of the illness.[22] (Chapter 4 further explores the developmental tasks of the chronically ill adult.)

As clients and family members are assisted in achieving these tasks, clients will move toward their potential for high-level wellness. (Specific points of how to deal with a chronic illness will be covered in the management chapters.) However, nurses may gain additional insights by asking their chronically ill clients how they deal with specific problems. Information gained in this manner may then be shared with other clients with similar problems.

Gaining information from clients with a specific chronic illness has been formalized into a number of self-help groups. These groups, such as Alcoholics Anonymous, ostomy clubs, and Mended Heart clubs, are organized specifically to assist people with the same disorders. Such groups have the support of many health professionals and voluntary health agencies. Nurses may recommend one of these groups or assist in the organization of one.

SUMMARY

Although health is defined in a variety of ways, there seems to be a consensus that it involves the whole person—mind, body, and spirit—functioning at full energy levels. Conversely, illness may be caused by physical, emotional, and spiritual factors. As factors associated with the onset of illness have been identified, more measures that promote health have been communicated to the public. (The important role of nursing related to health education is detailed in the various management chapters.)

People go through specific stages when deciding whether they are ill and have typical behaviors (roles). These stages provide a framework that the nurse can use in understanding the experience of an individual with a specific illness. However, the nurse must not force an individual into a specific role pattern but recognize that illness changes the person's ability to function in various roles.

The special tasks of the chronically ill person are especially significant because of the correlation between the increased incidence of chronic illness and the increasing average age of the population. Nurses assist clients in learning to manage these tasks so that these clients have time and energy for quality living.

⊞ eview Questions

The number of the question corresponds to the same-numbered objective at the beginning of the chapter.

1. Wellness is
   a. a dynamic condition in which a person functions in mind, body, and spirit to achieve full potential
   b. a static condition that is the result of a person avoiding factors that cause illness
   c. a state of complete physical, mental, and social well-being
   d. the absence of any symptoms of illness
2. Which one of the following individuals was one of the first to articulate the theory that disease is partially due to an upset in the internal environment of the body?
   a. Cannon
   b. Selye
   c. Bernard
   d. Rahe
3. Factors positively correlated with preventive health behaviors include all the following *except*
   a. a mother with a college education as compared to a mother with a grade-school education
   b. the belief that one is invulnerable to lung cancer despite a 60 pack-year history

c. the use of media to highlight the risk of cancer and pulmonary and heart disease from smoking

d. a perception that it is important to one's health to participate in activities such as skiing

4. Which of the following is an example of taking action when symptoms of an illness exist?
   a. deciding to wait 2 or 3 days to see whether a pain in the eye will disappear
   b. taking an over-the-counter medication for stomach pains
   c. changing dietary intake because "sodium is bad for you"
   d. increasing jogging "to work soreness out of my left leg and help decrease the swelling"

5. A characteristic of a chronic disease is that it
   a. results in permanent deviation from normal
   b. has a rapid onset
   c. is self-limiting
   d. has a short duration

6. An example of the dependent role in an acutely ill person is
   a. taking an antibiotic for pharyngitis
   b. returning to work after appendicitis
   c. omitting a morning dose of a diuretic
   d. seeing the physician because "I sprained my ankle"

7. All the following statements about living with chronic illness are true *except*
   a. chronically ill persons need to have a plan to deal with exacerbations of the acute stages of their illness
   b. chronically ill persons learn to control symptoms of their disease to minimize their social implications
   c. the major problem of chronically ill persons is extra time on their hands due to social isolation
   d. chronically ill persons attempt to normalize their interactions with others by disguising evidence of their illness

REFERENCES

1. Sonntag S: Illness as metaphor, as quoted by Mathiessen in Unsurance, Hippocrates 6:36, 1989.
2. World Health Organization: Constitution of the World Health Organization, Chronicle of the World Health Organization p 1, 1947.
3. Dunn HL: High-level wellness for man and society, Am J Public Health 49:786, 1959.
4. What high-level wellness means: Health, Values 1:9, 1977.
5. Bruhn JG and others: The wellness process, J Community Health 2:209, 1977.
6. Pesznecker BL and McNeil J: Relationship among health habits, social assets, psychological well-being, life change and alterations in health status, Nurs Res 24:297, 1975.
7. Flynn PAR: Holistic health, Bowie, Md, 1980, Brady.
8. Selye H: The stress of life, New York, 1976, McGraw-Hill, Inc.
9. Wolff HG: Stress and disease, ed 2, Springfield, Ill, 1968, Charles C Thomas.
10. Holmes TH and Rahe RH: Social readjustment rating scale, J Psychosom Res 11:216, 1967.
11. Gunderson EK and Rahe RH, eds: Life stress and illness, Springfield, Ill, 1974, Charles C Thomas.
12. Lynn BL and Werner JS: Stress, Annu Rev Nurs Res 5:3, 1987.
13. Pender NJ: Health promotion and illness prevention, Annu Rev Nurs Res 2:83, 1984.
14. Doswell WM: Physiologic response to stress, Annu Rev Nurs Res 8:51, 1989.
15. Ruch LO: A multidimensional analysis of the concept of life change, J Health Soc Behav 18:71, 1977.
16. Dudley DL and Welke E: How to survive being alive, New York, 1977, Doubleday & Co.
17. Richard EJ and Gerwin JM: Life change stress factors in hospitalized otolaryngolic patients, South Med J 9:79, 1986.
18. Zimmerman M, O'Hara MW, and Corenthal CP: Symptom contamination of life events scales, Health Psychol 3:77, 1984.
19. Kiecolt-Glasser JK and others: Psychosocial modifiers of immunocompetence in medical students, Psychosom Med 46:7, 1984.
20. Belloc NB and Breslow L: Relationship of physical health status and health practices, Prev Med 1:409, 1972.
21. Strauss AL and others: Chronic illness and the quality of life, ed 2, St Louis, 1984, The CV Mosby Co.
22. Zindler-Wernet P and Weiss SJ: Health locus of control and preventive health behavior, West J Nurs Res 9:160, 1987.
23. Wu R: Behavior and illness, Englewood Cliffs, NJ, 1973, Prentice Hall.
24. Twaddle AC: Sickness: a sociological view. In Folta JR and Deck ES, eds: A sociological framework for patient care, ed 2, New York, 1979, John Wiley & Sons, Inc.
25. Arluke A, Kennedy L, and Kersler RC: Re-examining the sick role concept: an empirical assessment, J Health Soc Behav 20:30, 1979.
26. Suchman EA: Stages of illness and medical care, J Health Human Behav 6:128, 1965.
27. Hover J and Juelsgaard N: The sick role reconceptualized, Nurs Forum 17:412, 1978.
28. Corbin JM and Strauss AL: Collaboration: couples working together to manage chronic illness, Image 16:115, 1984.

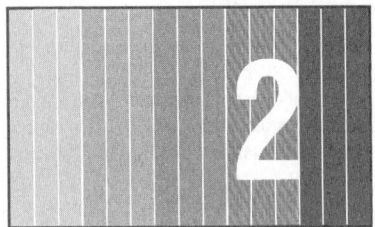

CHAPTER

2

General Concepts
Nursing Process

Katheryn Ellen McCash

The nursing process is a tool used by the nurse to identify the health care needs of the client and to organize and deliver nursing care. Once learned, the nursing process becomes an inherent part of nursing care and is actualized in the unique style of each nurse.

NURSING YESTERDAY AND TODAY

In primitive times, there was no distinction between nursing and medicine. The sick and injured were merely cared for by those with nurturant instincts.[1] In more recent times, society has tried to differentiate between nursing and medical practice. However, even today there is not a clear delineation between nursing and medical practice.

We now recognize that caregivers in medicine are primarily concerned with the diagnosis and treatment of ill-

ness or injury, whereas nurses deal with "the diagnosis and treatment of human responses to actual or potential health problems."[2] The emphasis for nursing is the response of an individual or group to an actual or potential health problem rather than the disease process itself. For example, a nurse focuses on the self-care limitations of a person with a spinal cord injury rather than on the injury itself.

Nursing's Territory

Many modern theorists such as Johnson, Newman, Orem, Rogers, and Roy are attempting to precisely define nursing's territory.[3] Although such work is needed, many of the current issues in nursing were previously concerns of Florence Nightingale. In 1893, she addressed holistic health when she emphasized that one must nurse the whole person rather than the disease.[4] Health maintenance and promotion, health teaching, family and community nursing, establishment of trust, use of good communication skills, and stress reduction techniques were all an integral part of nursing as defined by Florence Nightingale.[5]

In the 1960s the team concept of nursing care delivery became popular. Fragmentation of client care occurred as nurses and health care workers descended on the client to complete their designated tasks. Nursing professionals were not satisfied with this system of fragmented care. Nursing roles are changing in response to client and nurse dissatisfaction, as well as to technological advances, increased hospital costs, decreased length of hospital stays, changing societal attitudes toward the physician, changing needs of clients, a longer life span, and more leisure time. Primary nursing care is once again seen as a means to deliver quality health care. Primary nursing care is a continuous and coordinated nursing process in which a primary nurse ensures that all the basic needs of clients are met on a 24-hour basis.[6]

Expanded Roles

Today, those in the health care system also talk of "expanded roles" for nurses. These roles emphasize health assessment, diagnosis, and treatment of conditions usually considered only within the physician's domain. Some

Reviewed by Donna Bernocchi Losey, R.N., M.A., former Instructor of Nursing, University of Nevada, Las Vegas, Nevada.

nursing leaders dislike the term "expanded role." Mauksch states,[5]

I do not believe there are expanded roles for nurses. I believe my role as a nurse clinician or practitioner is a new role because it encompasses new behaviors. These behaviors are risk taking, decision making, being accountable, and being assertive.

But are these expanded roles really new behaviors for nurses? Nursing leaders of the past such as Florence Nightingale, Esther Lucile Brown, and Margaret Sanger would not have made such strides for the profession lacking these assertive kinds of behaviors. A closer look at nursing history indicates that rather than expanding into totally new areas, nurses are merely reclaiming old territory once held.

Nurses have always assessed their clients' health status. However, today, due to scientific and technological advances, there are new methods available requiring new equipment and skills. Nurses today are asserting that they have the right to learn and apply skills that enhance their abilities to determine health status. By increasing their assessment skills, nurses increase their data base on which they make sound judgments. The thermometer was at one time the private domain of the chief physician. Today, no one questions whether the nurse should use this instrument to assess temperature.[5]

Scientific and technological advances have made an impact on health care and care of the sick. Nursing is in a state of evolution in response to these advances. In its attempt to keep pace, nursing would do well to remember what the Queen in *Through the Looking Glass* said to Alice[7]:

Now *here,* you see, it takes all the running *you* can do to keep in the same place. If you want to get somewhere else, you must run at least twice as fast as that.

Increasing emphasis on assertiveness, persistence, risk taking, and decision making are essential if nursing is to "get somewhere else."

Definitions of Nursing

A basic question revolves around how the profession of nursing views itself. Several well-known definitions of nursing indicate that a basic theme of health, illness, and caring has existed since Florence Nightingale. Note the commonalities in the following definitions:

The unique function of the nurse is to assist the individual, sick or well, in the performance of those activities contributing to health or its recovery (or to peaceful death) that he would perform unaided if he had the necessary strength, will or knowledge. And to do this in such a way as to help him gain independence as rapidly as possible[8] (1969 International Council of Nurses, Geneva.)
Nursing is putting the patient in the best condition for nature to act.[4]
Nursing is a direct service, goal oriented, and adaptable to the needs of the individual, the family and community during health and illness.[9]

In this textbook, nursing is defined broadly as assisting the client in any setting, through the application of the

nursing process, to maintain or attain a state of dynamic equilibrium at the highest possible level of wellness with the least possible expenditure of energy.[10]

In this definition the terms used are further defined as follows:

1. Client: Any individual, family, or group requiring nursing intervention
2. Nursing process: The systematic use of the steps of assessment, diagnosis, planning, implementation, and evaluation when providing nursing care
3. Dynamic equilibrium: A relative state of balance, or homeostasis, in which basic needs are met by minimal output of energy
4. Level of wellness: The degree of physiological and psychological adaptation
5. Assist: Implies doing with, not doing for, to facilitate independence to the greatest degree possible

Nursing's View of Humanity

Nursing's view of humanity must be considered when describing nursing. Although different terms have been used, there is widespread agreement among nursing theorists that an individual has physiological (or biophysical), psychological (or emotional), sociocultural (or interpersonal), spiritual, and environmental components or dimensions.[10] In this text the human individual is considered "a biopsychosocial being in constant interaction with a changing environment."[11] The dimensions composing the individual in actuality are not separate entities but are interrelated. Thus, a problem in one dimension generally affects one or more of the other dimensions. Psychological anxiety, for instance, affects the autonomic nervous system, a part of the biophysical dimension.

Growth and development are influenced by interactions with others. No two individuals are ever exactly alike. No one individual remains the same from moment to moment. Each individual therefore has value as an irreplaceable member of humanity. Inherent in this individuality is the right to develop unique potentials according to a personal value system to the extent that the exercise of this right does not deny it to others.[10]

The individual's behavior is meaningful and oriented toward fulfilling needs and coping with environmental stresses. At times, however, the individual needs assistance to meet these needs and to cope successfully.

THE NURSING PROCESS

Nursing can best accomplish its goal of assisting others to resolve actual or potential problems[12] by use of the nursing process. The nursing process is a problem-solving approach based on the scientific method. The use of this process enables the nurse to provide care in an organized and scientific manner in each of the following areas:

1. Health maintenance and promotion
2. Acute intervention
3. Rehabilitative or chronic management

Phases of the Nursing Process

The nursing process consists of five phases: assessment, diagnosis, planning, implementation, and evaluation (Fig.

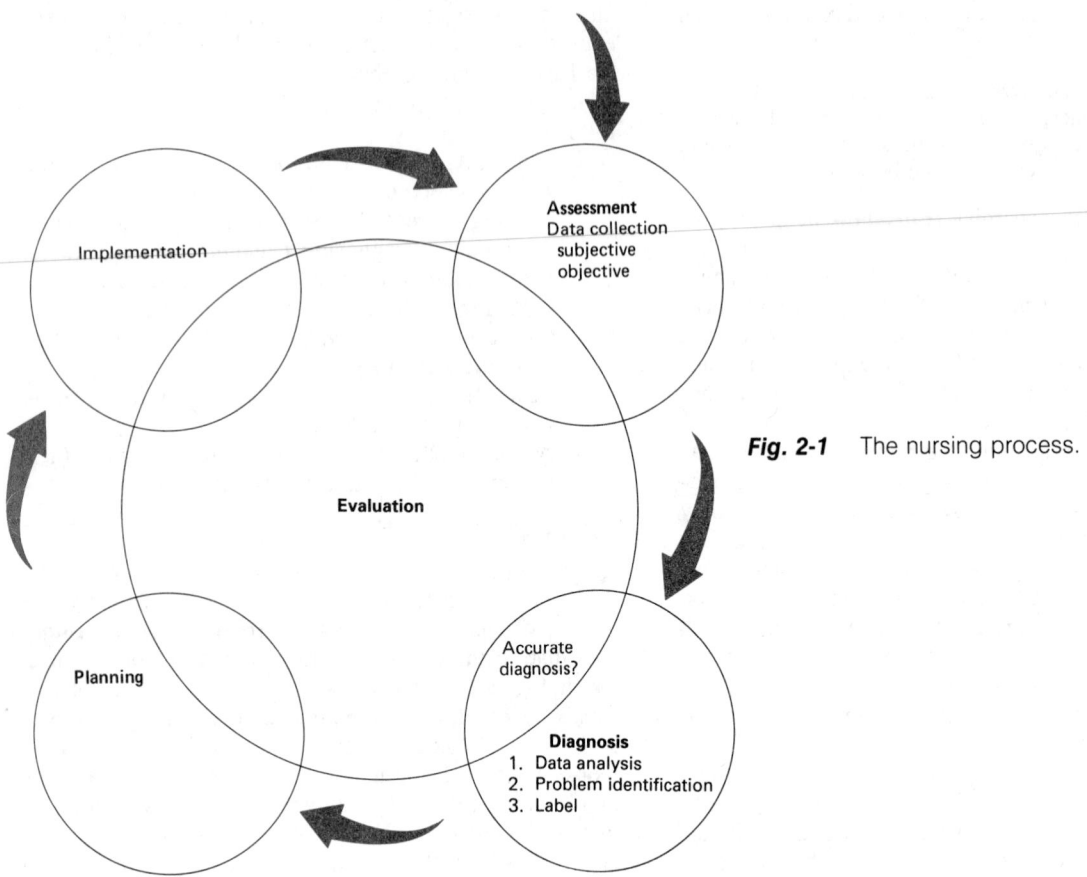

Fig. 2-1 The nursing process.

2-1). However, numerous other terms or phrases are being used in nursing to describe the steps of the nursing process. Table 2-1 lists these other terms. Assessment involves collecting subjective and objective information. The diagnosis phase involves analyzing the information, drawing conclusions from the information, and labeling the human response. Planning consists of setting goals and determining strategies for accomplishing the goals. Implementation is the plan set in action. Evaluation is the analysis of the effectiveness of the assessment, diagnosis, planning, and implementation phases.

Interrelatedness of Phases

The five phases of the nursing process do not occur in isolation from one another. For example, nurses may gather data about the wound condition (assessment) as they change the soiled dressing (intervention). There is, however, a basic order to the nursing process, beginning with assessment. This provides the data on which to base the plan. Implementation follows a careful plan based on the nursing diagnosis. Once begun, the nursing process is not only continuous but cyclical in nature. There is no limit to the number of times the cycle can be reinitiated. Evaluation continues throughout the cycle. This continuous evaluation provides feedback on the effectiveness of the plan or the need for revision. Revision may be needed in the data collection method, the diagnosis, the goals, the plan, or the intervention method.

Application of the nursing process requires sound knowledge of the physical and behavioral sciences and a repertoire of intellectual, interpersonal, and technical skills. Note the similarity of the nursing process and scientific method as compared in Table 2-2.

The nursing profession and the medical profession use a problem-solving process. The uniqueness of nursing's problem-solving approach stems from the goals of nursing and the means of accomplishing these goals. A comparison of the goals of medicine and nursing is made in Table 2-3.

Independent and Dependent Functions

Nursing practice has dependent, interdependent, and independent functions. As the profession has become more autonomous, the nurse independently initiates nursing interventions such as health teaching, counseling, and other measures that assist clients in meeting their basic needs. However, dependent and interdependent functions are also encompassed in the practice of nursing.

When nurses carry out medical orders, they function dependently. Dependent functions may include administering medications, performing or assisting with certain medical treatments, and assisting with diagnostic tests and procedures. The exact lines are often determined by individual state and agency policies. The theoretical division of nursing into dependent and independent roles may no longer be functional.[13] The nurse's role in most cases is

Table 2-1 Commonly Used Terms for Components of the Nursing Process

ASSESSMENT PHASE

	Data collection
	Data gathering
	Assessment
	Collection of information
	History and physical examination

DIAGNOSIS PHASE

Step I:	Data analysis
	Assessment
	Judgment
	Decision making
	Clustering information
	Determination of strengths and weaknesses
	Determination of unmet needs
	Determination of assets and limitations
Step II:	Nursing diagnosis
	Assessment
	Problem identification
	Etiology determination
	Determining cause of problem
	Labeling the problem
	Naming the problem
	Classification of problem

PLANNING PHASE

Step I:	Priority setting
Step II:	Expected outcome determined
	Goal setting
	Objective setting, subgoals
	Desired behaviors
Step III:	Planning interventions
	Planning nursing actions
	Nursing orders
	Planning strategies of care

IMPLEMENTATION

	Application
	Intervention
	Nursing care
	Implementation
	Reassessment
	Audit

Table 2-2 Similarities of the Nursing Process and the Scientific Method

Scientific Method	Nursing Process	
Defining a problem	Client identified	General problem areas are identified through health screening.
Collecting data	Assessment	Subjective and objective data are obtained in depth.
Forming the hypothesis	Diagnosis	Data are analyzed. The problem is identified and labeled.
	Planning	The expected outcome is stated. Strategies are considered. Interventions are selected.
Testing the hypothesis	Implementation	Interventions are tried.
Forming conclusions	Evaluation	Results of the entire process are analyzed.

Table 2-3 Comparison of Primary Goals: Nursing and Medicine

Nursing	Medicine
Determines responses to health problems, level of wellness, and need for assistance	Determines illness or injury
Provides physical care, emotional care, teaching, guidance, and counseling	Provides medical treatments and surgery
Interventions aimed at assisting the client to meet own needs	Interventions aimed at preventing and curing injury or illness

one of "interdependence and coparticipation" with the client and other health team members.[14] In general, the nurse is expected to have the following intellectual, interpersonal, and technical skills:

Health assessment skills
History taking
Physical examination
Psychosocial assessment
Analytical skills
Diagnostic skills
Decision-making skills
Creativity and the ability to improvise
Teaching skills
Therapeutic skills
Counseling and referral skills
Technical skills
Administrative skills
Leadership and management skills

Recording and reporting skills
Research skills

Some or all of these skills are used during the various phases of the nursing process.

ASSESSMENT PHASE
Data Collection

A sound data base is the foundation for the entire nursing process. Collection of data is a prerequisite to making a diagnosis, to planning, and to intervening. A human being as a biopsychosocial being has needs and problems in all dimensions. A nursing diagnosis made without supporting data in all dimensions can lead to incorrect conclusions and depersonalized care. For example, a client who does not sleep all night may be mistakenly diagnosed as having a sleep pattern disturbance. In fact he may have worked nights his entire adult life, and it is normal for him to be awake at night. This information about his sleeping habits would be necessary to individualize his care so that he did not receive a sleep medication at 10 PM. The importance of assessment to the process of clinical decision making cannot be overemphasized.[15] The use of a nursing data base, rather than a medical history, is recommended to facilitate the collection of data most useful to the nurse.

Subjective and objective data. A sound data base includes subjective and objective data. Subjective data are what the client or family members state spontaneously or by direct questioning. Objective data are what the nurse and other members of the health team gather directly by such methods as inspection, palpation, percussion, and auscultation. The client's chart, diagnostic tests, and other health team members also provide additional useful subjective and objective data. An easy way to remember the common abbreviations, "S" and "O," is the following:

S = Subjective statements
O = Objective observations

In the initial assessment phase, most of the subjective data are obtained through the nursing history. However, while interviewing, the nurse also observes the client's general appearance and nonverbal behavior. These observations provide some objective data. The majority of the objective data are obtained through physical examination of the client. The nurse continues to obtain subjective data as the client makes statements during the examination procedures, especially in regard to pain during palpation. (The nursing history and physical examination are described in detail in Chapter 3.)

Because nursing interventions are only as sound as the data base on which they are formulated, it is critical that the data base be accurate. Therefore information gained from sources such as the chart, other health care workers, the client's family, and the nurse's observations should be validated with the client when possible. Likewise, questionable statements by the client should be validated by a knowledgeable person when possible.

Interviewing skills. Several factors affect success in obtaining information:

1. Rapport with the client
2. The timing of the interview
3. The surrounding environment
4. The amount of time available
5. The condition of the client

Each factor will be considered as basic generalizations related to interviewing techniques are presented. Because an in-depth discussion of communication is beyond the scope of this text, the student is encouraged to refer to a specialty book on this topic.

First, nurses should identify themselves and their roles and inform the client about what information is needed and why. Clients cannot be expected to discuss personal health concerns without a sound reason. Seemingly nonpersonal questions may be perceived by the client as very private information.

The time of the interview should be carefully selected. Pain, fear, fatigue, anxiety, and other common stressors associated with illness are examples of situations that should alert nurses to defer an interview until a more appropriate time. A calm, comfortable client is more likely to share information.

Careful attention should be directed to the environment. If necessary, the environment should be altered to make it more conducive to sharing information. For example, nurses should provide for privacy, close the door to eliminate distractions, and change the lighting or temperature in the room as necessary for the client's age and condition. The client's and nurses' attention are required for an interaction to be successful. The client should be informed of the approximate amount of time the interview will take. The amount of time should be realistic, considering nurses' responsibilities and the client's condition. If additional time is required, the client should be consulted for a suitable time.

The client's condition must be a primary concern when planning a data-gathering session. If acutely ill, the client will be unable to expend energy on nonemergency questions. Other sources of information such as old charts, family members, or friends may need to be used in such a situation. The nurse must be attuned to the needs of the client when directing an interview. For instance, the nurse may want to determine the learning needs of a preoperative client, whereas the client may only care to discuss what medication will be used postoperatively to control pain.

Nurses should begin an interview with easily answered, impersonal questions. As rapport is established, they should advance to the more personal questions. Nurses' comfort level with the topic, as well as a genuine concern for the client, promotes rapport. Nurses need to know the reason certain information is necessary and must have insight into personal attitudes and feelings about asking personal questions.

Nurses should listen to rather than anticipate the client's comments. If nurses are mentally planning how to respond to the client, they cannot listen to what is being said. While listening, nurses should closely observe the client, noting any incongruency between verbal and nonverbal behaviors. Before beginning a purposeful interview, nurses should take time to hear the client's concerns. This not only helps to establish rapport, but can also provide important additional information. It is neither necessary nor wise to strictly adhere to a rigid interviewing format because much psychosocial data are obtained as the individual is allowed time to share concerns. Open-ended rather than closed questions (closed questions can be answered by a yes or no or short statement) provide the most information. Nurses should always give the client time to answer.

The number of questions asked during the history can give the client a sense of urgency that discourages communication. Nurses should select words carefully, based on the client's apparent ability to understand. Underestimating or overestimating a client's ability to comprehend can negatively affect communication. The purpose is an interview, not an interrogation. It is important to use simple language. The author vividly remembers an English-speaking client who asked what a low hematocrit was. When the author explained that it meant the number of red blood cells were decreased, the client asked, "What's a cell?" Nurses should never assume they are being understood; they should look for nonverbal and verbal clues and ask the client to request clarification of unfamiliar terms.

DIAGNOSIS PHASE
Data Analysis and Problem Identification

The diagnostic process begins with the collection of information and ends with an evaluative judgment about a client's health status.[16] That evaluative judgment is reached after analysis of the assessment data. Gordon has described a set of health patterns (functional health patterns) specifying areas of basic information that are collected regardless of the conceptual framework being used. Analysis of each functional health pattern facilitates the nursing diagnosis process (Table 2-4).[15]

The diagnoses phase of the diagnostic process begins when the nurse mentally sorts through and organizes or clusters the information, determining unmet needs,

strengths, and discrepancies between the two. The findings are then compared to documented norms to determine whether anything is interfering or could interfere with the client's needs or ability to maintain a state of dynamic equilibrium.

After a thorough analysis of all available information, one of two possible conclusions results: (1) there are no problems that require intervention, or (2) the client needs assistance to solve a potential or actual problem. The final conclusions about the problems are the diagnoses.

Nursing Diagnosis

In 1980 the Congress for Nursing Practice of the American Nurses' Association (ANA) defined *nursing* as "the diagnosis and treatment of human responses to actual or potential health problems."[2] Although the routine use of the term *nursing diagnosis* is relatively recent, the act of diagnosing was routinely performed by Florence Nightingale and her colleagues.[15]

Definition. The term *nursing diagnosis* has many different meanings. To some, it merely connotes the identification of a health problem. More commonly today, a nursing diagnosis is viewed as the conclusion about an identified cluster of signs and symptoms. The diagnosis is generally expressed as concisely as possible.

Gordon restricts her definition of a nursing diagnosis to only clinical diagnoses that nurses are "capable and licensed to treat."[16] Guzzetta suggests that this definition may be too restrictive because it does not include all health problems encountered by nurses.[14]

Throughout this book, the term *nursing diagnosis* will mean (1) the process of identifying actual and potential health problems and (2) the label or concise statement that describes "a clinical judgment about an individual, family, or community response to actual or potential health problems/life processes. Nursing diagnoses provide the basis

Table 2-4 Typology of Health Patterns

Pattern	Characteristics
Health perception–health management	Describes client's perceived pattern of health and well-being and how health is managed
Nutritional-metabolic	Describes pattern of food and fluid consumption relative to metabolic need and pattern indicators of local nutrient supply
Elimination	Describes patterns of excretory function (bowel, bladder, and skin)
Activity-exercise	Describes pattern of exercise, activity, leisure, and recreation
Cognitive-perceptual	Describes sensory-perceptual and cognitive pattern
Sleep-rest	Describes patterns of sleep, rest, and relaxation
Self-perception–self-concept	Describes self-concept pattern and perceptions of self (e.g., body comfort, body image, feeling state)
Role-relationship	Describes pattern of role-engagements and relationships
Sexuality-reproductive	Describes client's patterns of satisfaction and dissatisfaction with sexuality pattern; describes reproductive patterns
Coping–stress tolerance	Describes general coping pattern and effectiveness of the pattern in terms of stress tolerance
Value-belief	Describes patterns of values, beliefs (including spiritual), or goals that guide choices or decisions

Modified from Gordon M: Nursing diagnosis: process and application, ed 2, St Louis, 1987, The CV Mosby Co.

for selection of nursing interventions to achieve outcomes for which the nurse is accountable."[17] Collaborative problems, on the other hand, are health problems that nurses treat with other health care providers, most frequently, physicians.

There is some healthy controversy about what constitutes a nursing diagnosis as opposed to a medical diagnosis, especially with the more physiological diagnoses. Most nurses agree that a nursing diagnosis is not the diagnosis of disease. A look at the primary goals of nursing (Table 2-3) helps in differentiating between nursing and medical diagnoses. Diagnosis is an act of identifying and labeling human responses to actual or potential health problems or stressors. The human responses identified, however, frequently result from the disease process. For example, a client may have the medical diagnosis of chronic obstructive pulmonary disease (COPD). The nursing diagnosis, however, would relate to how the COPD affects daily functioning (e.g., activity intolerance related to imbalance between oxygen supply and demand).

A number of other terms or situations are not nursing diagnoses but are often mislabeled as such. These include the following[18]:

Medical pathology (hypertension)
Diagnostic tests or studies (upper gastrointestinal series)
Equipment (has nasogastric tube)
Signs (restlessness)
Symptoms (feels tired)
Surgical procedures (hysterectomy)
Treatments (decubiti care)
Therapeutic goals (should perform own oral care)
Nursing problems (difficult to turn)
Therapeutic needs (needs more rest)
Staff problems (Mr. Jones is too demanding)

The North American Nursing Diagnosis Association. Nursing is moving toward standardized nomenclature for classifying clients' responses or problems. The identification and development of a classification system of nursing diagnoses began formally in 1973 when Kristine Gebbie and Mary Ann Lavin of St. Louis University called the First National Conference on Classification of Nursing Diagnosis. At this time, a National Task Force, a voluntary group of nurses from the United States and Canada, was appointed to continue development of diagnoses. The task force also developed a Clearinghouse for Nursing Diagnoses, which still serves as a depository of materials on nursing diagnosis and disseminates information about the National Conference Group's activities. National Conferences have been held about every 2 years since 1973.[19]

The National Group for the Classification of Nursing Diagnosis has evolved since the Fifth National Conference into a formal organization and has been renamed the North American Nursing Diagnosis Association (NANDA). The development of the diagnostic classification system continues under NANDA. A list of diagnoses accepted by NANDA for clinical testing is found in Appendix A.

The accepted diagnoses are evolving as research results are interpreted. In addition, the list is not all-inclusive, and the nurse will encounter "nursing problems" not cited on the list. Nurses are encouraged to submit refinements of accepted diagnoses to NANDA.* The terminology from the NANDA list of accepted nursing diagnoses will be used in this text when possible.

The Diagnostic Process

There are three components in a nursing diagnosis, known as the PES format:

Problem (P): A brief statement of the client's potential or actual health problem

Etiology (E): A brief description of the probable cause of the problem

Signs/symptoms (S): A list of the cluster of the objective and subjective data that lead the nurse to pinpoint a problem

It is important to remember that gathering the (S) comes first in the diagnostic process even though the format has been described as PES. Although the (S) is not usually listed with the diagnostic statement on a problem list or care plan, it is helpful to do so for learning purposes.

Identifying the problem. The NANDA list of accepted nursing diagnoses has been categorized into 11 functional patterns listed in Appendix A. This framework is extremely useful when analyzing the data for actual, high-risk, and possible nursing diagnoses. Clustered data are analyzed to generate diagnostic hypotheses. These hypotheses may include nursing diagnoses, as well as collaborative problems.

However, the nurse should not force a problem to fit accepted terminology. At times the nurse may need to use a new word or phrase that should then be used consistently with the same problem.

It is also important not to state an untreatable condition, instead of the client's underlying problem, as the (P). "Inability to turn related to traction" is not treatable as such, whereas "high risk for altered skin integrity related to effects of traction or immobility" is treatable. Table 2-5 suggests ways to evaluate the components of a nursing care plan.

Etiology. The etiology of a nursing diagnosis should be included in the diagnostic statement and separated from the defining characteristics.[20] Defining characteristics are signs and/or symptoms commonly associated with a nursing diagnosis. Taking the time to refine the problem with its proper etiology directs the nurse to the correct interventions. The etiology can be a pathophysiological, maturational, situational, or treatment-related factor. The etiology of the problem most often determines the intervention. The etiology is written after the diagnostic label. These two components are separated by the statement, "related to." A correctly written nursing diagnosis might be "feeding self-care deficit related to lethargy." The etiology directs the nurse to select the appropriate intervention. When the etiology is not included in the diagnosis, the nurse may not plan the correct intervention to treat the specific cause of the problem. The etiology should be validated with the client when possible. When the etiology is unknown, the statement reads, "related to unknown etiology."

*NANDA, % Clearinghouse for Nursing Diagnoses, St. Louis University School of Nursing, 3525 Caroline Street, St. Louis, MO 63104.

Table 2-5 Guidelines for Evaluating Nursing Care Plans

Met Expectations*	Unmet Expectations†
NURSING DIAGNOSIS	
Is the cause or possible etiology of the problem identified? Example: Ineffective individual coping related to depression in response to identifiable stressors as manifested by helplessness, frequent crying, and poor personal hygiene	Does the nurse get an answer other than that which was written down when asked how the nurse knew this was a problem? If so, the nurse has stated an inference or is too general. Example: Demanding client
Are potential high-risk problems, as well as present problems, included? Example: High risk for impaired mobility of right shoulder related to pain during movement and loss of muscle mass	Does the nurse create new problems when asked what other problems the present problem causes? If so, the problem may be too general. Example: Radical mastectomy
Is the diagnosis specific? Do the problem and etiology refer to different findings (not redundant)? Is the problem treatable? Example: Sleep pattern disturbance related to high caffeine intake	Is this the nurse's problem? Example: Time consuming due to frequent requests
	Is this an intervention? Example: IV in left arm
	Is this a client's need? Example: Need for fluids
	Is this an untreatable condition? Example: Amputated leg due to gangrene
	Is the etiology redundant? Example: Rape trauma syndrome related to rape
	Is there a legally inadvisable statement? Example: Potential for injury related to lack of supervision
	Is it difficult to tell whether the expected outcome is accomplished?
PLAN OF ACTION	
Are very specific steps given? Would a nurse new to the unit understand exactly how to do the activity? Did the nurse note how, when, how long, how often, where, by whom, with what, and when appropriate? Was the nurse specific to the clients? Tailored to meet their particular problems? Example: Uninterrupted 15 minutes a day with client discussing concerns; stating nursing concerns before beginning	Was the nurse too general so that different people might interpret the plan differently? Example: Reassure the client bid
	Did the nurse use good-intention words such as *support, encourage, help, reassure, explain, explore* with client? If so, the nurse is too general; these words may only be used when answered in the plan by *how, when, where,* and so on.

*Expectations are met if the nurse answers "yes" to the questions.
†Expectations are unmet if the nurse answers "yes" to the questions.

Continued.

—

Multiple etiologies become more common as expertise in the use of nursing diagnoses increases. There is often no single cause of a problem. Most nursing diagnoses presented in the general care plans of this book contain multiple etiologies. They can be used to provide a checklist of possible causative factors to be considered when determining the nursing diagnosis specific to the client.

PLANNING PHASE
Priority Setting

After the nursing diagnoses and collaborative problems are identified, the nurse must decide on the urgency of intervention needed. Diagnoses of the highest priority require immediate intervention. Those of lower priority can be dealt with at a later time.

Table 2-5 Guidelines for Evaluating Nursing Care Plans—cont'd

Met Expectations*	Unmet Expectations†
EVALUATION CRITERIA	
Did the nurse gather subjective data to indicate the achievement of the expected outcome? (S) Example: Clients stating they understand why they do not want to be alone	Did the nurse forget to mention that the expected outcome was accomplished or not accomplished? Is the plan outdated?
Did the nurse gather objective data to indicate the effectiveness of each intervention and movement toward the expected outcome? (O) Example: Client asking nurse three times to bring items within reach	
Did the nurse state whether the expected outcome was accomplished? (A) Example: Expected outcome accomplished—clients discussing horror at having only one breast, feeling no one could like them that way	
Did the nurse note whether to revise, continue, or discontinue the expected outcome or interventions? (P) Example: Clients needing longer periods of uninterrupted time before expressing feelings; nurse spending 20 minutes per day instead of 15 with client	

*Expectations are met if the nurse answers "yes" to the questions.
†Expectations are unmet if the nurse answers "yes" to the questions.

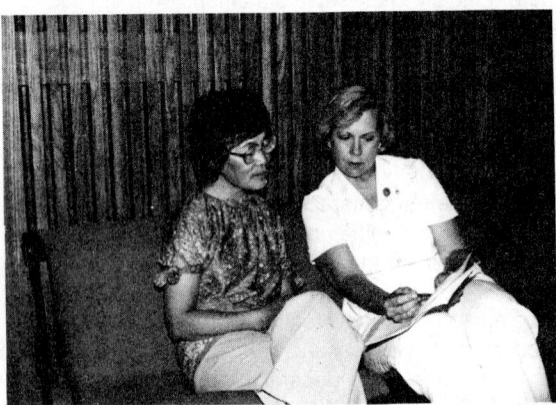

Fig. 2-2 Cooperation between the client and the nurse is necessary in setting goals.

When setting priorities, nurses should first intervene for life-threatening problems. Then they may use several guidelines to assist in priority setting. One is the client's own perception of what is important. Nurses may need to give explanations or do some teaching to help the client understand the need to do one thing before another.

Another suggestion is to identify nursing diagnoses that may be managed simultaneously. For example, nurses may assess the condition of a pressure sore (impaired skin integrity) while giving morning care (bathing self-care deficit).[21]

Maslow's hierarchy of needs also acts as a useful guide to determining priorities. These needs include physical needs, safety, love and belonging, esteem, and self-actualization.[22] As in climbing a mountain, the lower level must be reached before a higher level can be attained.

Identified priorities change as clients' levels of wellness fluctuate. For example, the clients' highest priorities in the morning may be a need for information about diabetes because they are going home and must care for themselves. During the teaching session a client does not feel well and the nurse suspects that there is a high risk of insulin shock because the client has not eaten breakfast. The session is interrupted so that the nurse can get the client a glass of orange juice. High-risk problems may have a higher priority than existing (actual) problems.

Setting Goals

After priorities are established, the client and nurse mutually decide on expected outcomes or goals (Fig. 2-2). Long-term and short-term goals need to be set.

Although the ultimate goal for the client is to maintain or attain a state of dynamic equilibrium at the highest possible level of wellness, the setting of more specific goals, both short- and long-term, is necessary for systematic evaluation of the client's progress. Short-term goals can be met relatively quickly (i.e., in less than a week). Long-term goals may take weeks or months to achieve.[21] In today's acute-care setting where the length of stay is often very short, there is a predominance of short-term goals.

Long-term goals may then be addressed by a home health care nurse. Short-term goals may also be small steps toward achieving a long-term goal. For example, a short-term goal might be, "Mr. Smith will ambulate with crutches 1 day postoperatively," whereas a long-term goal might be "Mr. Smith will ambulate unassisted by discharge."

Thus, goals must be worded as expected outcomes and worded specifically enough that everyone caring for the client will be able to agree whether the goals have been achieved. Wording the goals in terms of desired, observable behaviors and specifying a date by when the expected outcome should be accomplished facilitates this process. To be worthwhile, written short-term goals should fit the following criteria:

1. Be realistic and achievable
2. Be measurable, observable, behavioral
3. Be client-centered (the client's expected outcome)
4. Have a time designation (*Example:* The client will state he has no pain by 10-1-91)
5. Be mutually set

Short-term goals can serve as motivators for the client and nurse, especially when a goal takes a great deal of time and effort to reach. For example, for the nursing diagnosis, "altered health maintenance related to lack of knowledge regarding oral hygiene," the long-term goal for the client is to attain healthy gums and teeth. Short-term goals could be that after teaching sessions the client does the following:

1. Demonstrates proper brushing technique after each meal
2. Demonstrates proper flossing of teeth before going to bed at night
3. Permanently refrains from chewing gum containing sugar
4. Visits the dentist by 11-9-91

Planning Interventions

After expected outcomes are determined, nursing actions to accomplish these desired behaviors should be planned. The nurse should use available resources when determining possible nursing interventions. The client often has a wealth of information about measures that were successful or that failed in the past. A lot of time and effort are saved by asking the client what has already been tried and discarded as ineffective. The client's family can also be consulted regarding the feasibility of the plan.

Other nurses and health care providers can be valuable sources for intervention ideas. Because members of the health team share common goals for the client, sharing ideas to reach these goals should be encouraged. A client-centered conference is a good way to foster such sharing.

Literature and research provide valuable suggestions and information that can facilitate the process of determining a means to accomplish the goals. Nurses need to foster the use of a research-based approach to interventions. Intuition should no longer be the mainstay of intervention.

Sound knowledge, good judgment, and decision-making ability are required to effectively choose the methods the nurse will use to intervene. Interventions should be based on sound rationales from the behavioral and physical sciences. In addition, the nurse must use ingenuity, creativity, and past experience when tailoring a plan to meet a client's needs. The benefits of the intervention must outweigh the disadvantages. Factors such as availability of help, equipment, time, money, and other resources must also be considered. As in the case of goal determination, the final selection of strategies remains the prerogative of the client.

When recording the plan on the chart or Kardex, the nurse needs to be very specific. This enables everyone concerned with the client to understand precisely what is to be accomplished. The plan should be tailored to meet each client's needs and should note particulars such as how, when, how long, how often, where, by whom, and with what. For example, "Wound care qid" is not an adequate plan. The following plan communicates much more: "The nurse *(who)* is to irrigate the leg wound *(where)* with 200 ml ½ H_2O_2 and ½ NS *(with what)* @ 9-1-5-9 *(how often)*." These specific, individualized interventions are sometimes called *nursing orders*.

IMPLEMENTATION PHASE

Carrying out a specific, individualized plan constitutes the implementation phase. The planned activities that the nurse performs to accomplish the implementation phase are called *nursing interventions*. The nurse may carry out the interventions or designate others who are qualified to intervene (Fig. 2-3).

A nursing intervention is any direct action that a nurse performs (or designates to others to perform) on behalf of a client. These actions include nurse-initiated treatments resulting from nursing diagnoses, physician-initiated treatments resulting from medical diagnoses, and daily, essential activities that the client cannot perform independently.[23] When choosing an intervention, the nurse considers the following[23]:

1. Characteristic of the nursing diagnosis. Will the intervention facilitate the client's progress toward a desired outcome?
2. Research base associated with the intervention

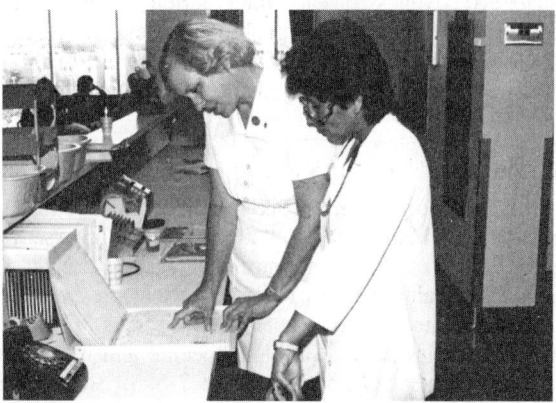

Fig. 2-3 Even though the nurse may designate another to implement a nursing activity, the nurse maintains responsibility for the client's welfare.

3. Feasibility of successfully implementing the intervention
4. Acceptability of the intervention to the client
5. Capability of the nurse

There are a variety of nursing interventions from which one may choose. Examples follow[21]:

1. Directly performing an activity for a client
2. Assisting the client
3. Supervising the client and family
4. Teaching
5. Counseling
6. Monitoring

Throughout this phase the nurse must evaluate the effectiveness of the method chosen to implement the plan. For example, the nurse may determine that the nursing assistant caring for a client with a mastectomy should not continue to be the person who implements the client's exercise plan. Perhaps the client is more depressed than anticipated and would benefit from contact with a nurse who is knowledgeable about changes in body image. The exercise plan might essentially remain the same, but the implementor of the plan would be different and would use different skills to carry out the plan. Referrals to other professionals may also be made when the nurse anticipates that expertise in specialized areas would help the client.

EVALUATION PHASE

A look at the diagram of the nursing process (Fig. 2-1) indicates that all phases must be evaluated. Evaluation not only occurs after implementation of the plan but is ongoing throughout the process.

The nurse evaluates whether sufficient assessment data have been obtained to allow a nursing diagnosis to be made. The diagnosis is in turn evaluated for accuracy. For example, was the pain actually related to the wound itself or related to pressure from a constricting dressing?

Next the nurse evaluates whether the expected outcomes and interventions are realistic and achievable. If not, a new plan should be formulated. This may involve revision of goals and interventions. Consideration must be given to whether the plan should be maintained, modified, or totally revised in light of the client's status.

The effectiveness of each intervention and its contribution to progress toward the goal are also evaluated. In addition, the nurse considers whether a different method of implementation of the same plan would provide better results.

Progress Notes

It is critical that client progress be documented in a systematic way. Many documentation methods are used, depending on personal preference and agency policy. One method of evaluating and recording client progress is the problem-oriented progress note, referred to as SOAP. This type of progress note is problem-specific and incorporates the components described in Table 2-6. In some institutions, SOAP notes constitute the "Nurses' Notes" portion of the nurses' charting.

The SOAP term "assessment" has a slightly different meaning than when the term is used to describe the first

Table 2-6 Components of a Problem-Oriented Progress Note

	Explanation
Subjective (S)	Information supplied by client or knowledgeable other
Objective (O)	Information obtained by nurse directly, from client records, or through diagnostic studies
Assessment (A)	Tentative conclusion or diagnosis based on subjective and objective data
Plan (P)	Specific interventions related to a problem or diagnosis considering diagnostic, therapeutic, and client education needs

phase of the nursing process. With SOAP, *assessment* connotes data analysis and diagnosis. The process of SOAP evaluation is as follows:

1. Additional subjective and objective data are gathered about the area of concern.
2. Based on old and new data, an assessment of the client's progress toward the goal and the effectiveness of each intervention is made.
3. Based on the reassessment of the situation, the initial plan is maintained, revised, or discontinued.

For example, a diagnosis is high risk for infection related to traumatized tissue secondary to surgery. States wound is more painful today is *S*. Elevated temperature, facial grimacing, and dressing saturated with purulent drainage is *O*. Possible postsurgical wound infection is *A*. Notify surgeon, take temperature q 2 hr, and reinforce dressing is *P*.

Use of this SOAP format helps avoid conflict or duplication in services and allows all members of the health team to quickly evaluate the client's progress. This written evaluation should occur regardless of whether the client appears to be progressing satisfactorily, appears unchanged, or appears to be regressing.

WRITTEN CARE PLANS

An individualized nursing care plan is recorded to facilitate continuity of care and to help avoid duplication of services. When it is kept as a permanent part of the client's chart, it can aid in the evaluation of nursing care. It also documents the client's nursing care requirements and directs nursing care. All nursing diagnoses identified and dealt with by nurses are included in the nursing care plan.

Generally, only the more unusual or unexpected problems are addressed in the care plan. Predictable routine problems experienced by many clients with the same diagnosis should be planned for but are not necessarily recorded on the care plan. Actual (or existing) and high-risk problems should be considered appropriate for the written care plan.

Sometimes the care plan is written in pencil so that the outdated interventions can be erased. Then only the cur-

Table 2-7

SAMPLE NURSING CARE PLAN		
Defining Characteristics	Nursing Interventions	Evaluation Criteria
NURSING DIAGNOSIS: Impaired verbal communication related to decreased ability to articulate words		
Inability to speak words, ability to understand others and write words	Provide client with paper and pencil or magic slate. Allow client to ask questions. Do not anticipate answers. Keep writing arm free of IV lines. Refer client to speech therapist.	Absence of frustration when communicating; by time of discharge, use of alternative communication techniques

rent plan remains, avoiding confusion. However, this method should not be used without some kind of permanent record of the plan because the nurse also needs a source of information about which interventions were unsuccessful so that they are not repeated. The permanent care plan is considered to be a part of the legal medical record. Some nurses use a "highlighter pen" over completed or changed items. Table 2-5 presents a useful guideline for evaluating nursing care plans.

Institutions continually experiment with various methods of recording the care plan, and there are many formats available. An example of the nursing care plan format used in this text is shown in Table 2-7.

Some institutions write the care plan in ink and retain the entire plan as a part of the client's record. This kind of care plan often has a fourth column for evaluation, where comments about the progress toward the expected outcome and the effectiveness of the interventions are recorded. The evaluation portion of the care plan is not generally necessary if the SOAP method of charting is used because evaluation is ongoing with this system. A column to note discontinued nursing orders helps avoid confusion.

Standardized care plans are often used as guides for routine nursing care and for developing individualized care plans. The care plans throughout this book are general or standardized care plans. This type of plan lists nursing actions, or broad interventions, that are applicable to any number of clients having the particular problem. When planning individualized care, a standardized care plan should be personalized and made very specific based on assessment data.

SUMMARY

Nursing roles continually evolve as our society changes and we learn to apply new technology. Although nursing is defined in different ways by today's nursing theorists, the various definitions of nursing have commonalities of health, illness, and caring.

Nursing care is provided through the application of the nursing process: assessment, diagnosis, planning, implementation, and evaluation. Assessment involves collecting data by chart review, performing an interview, and doing a nursing history and physical. Good interviewing skills are essential for obtaining these data. The nurse's skill at collecting subjective and objective data affects the quality of the data base.

There are two major steps to the diagnosis phase: data analysis and nursing diagnosis (or problem identification). The planning phase also has three major steps: priority setting, goal formulation, and planning interventions. The plan of action must be founded on a sound data base. Implementation, the actual carrying out of the plan, may be performed by the nurse or by someone the nurse designates. It continues throughout the nursing process.

Several methods of record keeping are used to promote continuity of client care and facilitate the nursing process. Two such methods are the SOAP progress notes and the written care plan.

The nursing process is a form of scientific method application. It differs from medicine's problem-solving approach in its goals and means of accomplishing its goals. Knowledge of the physical and behavioral sciences and specific skills such as teaching, counseling, and technical skills are required to be able to apply the nursing process. Through the systematic use of the nursing process, nursing can best accomplish its goal of assisting others to maintain or attain optimal functioning.

R eview Questions

The number of the question corresponds to the same-numbered objective at the beginning of the chapter.

1. A commonality in definitions of nursing is that nursing is
   a. client-centered
   b. an independent function
   c. a dependent function
   d. restorative in nature
2. The phases of the nursing process are
   a. assessment, problem solving, diagnosis, evaluation
   b. subjective, objective, assessment, plan
   c. assessment, diagnosis, planning, implementation, evaluation
   d. problem identification, goal setting, intervention, evaluation

3. Subjective data are
   a. what the nurse observes
   b. what the nurse states
   c. what the client exhibits
   d. what the client states
4. Which of the following would be considered a nursing diagnosis?
   a. needs suctioning
   b. sleep pattern disturbance
   c. diabetes
   d. restlessness
5. A part of nursing's primary goal is to
   a. diagnose the illness or injury
   b. provide medical treatment
   c. assist the physician with the medical plan
   d. assist the client to meet his needs
6. Which of the following most affects success in obtaining an accurate, detailed nursing history?
   a. a cool, calm manner
   b. the ability to establish rapport
   c. self-confidence
   d. the client's age
7. A progress note should include
   a. a conclusion about the data
   b. a goal
   c. a summary of past treatment
   d. a medical diagnosis
8. To be useful, the nursing care plan should
   a. be general
   b. be specific
   c. be idealistic
   d. be a legal part of the chart

REFERENCES

1. Goodnow M: Outlines of nursing history, ed 6, Philadelphia, 1938, WB Saunders Co.
2. American Nurses' Association, Congress for Nursing Practice: Nursing: a social policy statement, Kansas City, Mo, 1980, The Association.
3. The Nursing Theories Conference Group: Nursing theories: the base for professional nursing practice, ed 2, Englewood Cliffs, NJ, 1985, Prentice Hall.
4. Nightingale F: Notes on nursing: what it is and what it is not, facsimile edition, Philadelphia, 1946, JB Lippincott Co.
5. Bower FL and Bevis EO: Fundamentals of nursing practice, St. Louis, 1979, The CV Mosby Co.
6. Manthey M: Can primary nursing survive? Am J Nurs 88:644, 1988.
7. Carroll L: Alice's adventures in wonderland and through the looking glass, New York, 1973, Collier Books.
8. Henderson V: The nature of nursing, New York, 1966, Macmillan Publishing Co.
9. American Nurses' Association: Standards of practice, Kansas City, Mo, 1973, The Association.
10. UNM Curriculum Overview, Albuquerque, 1985, University of New Mexico.
11. Roy SC: Introduction to nursing: an adaptation model, Englewood Cliffs, NJ, 1976, Prentice Hall.
12. Yura H and Walsh M: The nursing process: assessing, planning, implementing, evaluation, ed 5, East Norwalk, Conn, 1988, Appleton & Lange.
13. Kim MJ and others: Clinical use of nursing diagnosis in cardiovascular nursing. In Kim JMJ and Moritz DA, eds: Classification of nursing diagnosis: proceedings of the third and fourth national conferences, New York, 1982, McGraw-Hill, Inc.
14. Guzzetta C and others: Clinical assessment tools for use with nursing diagnoses, St Louis, 1989, The CV Mosby Co.
15. Wilson CM, Holkola PM, and Jones DA: Validation of a screening assessment tool and generation of diagnostic hypotheses. In Carroll-Johnson RM, ed: Classification of nursing diagnoses: proceedings of the eighth conference, Philadelphia, 1989, JB Lippincott Co.
16. Gordon M: Nursing diagnosis: process and application, New York, 1987, McGraw-Hill, Inc.
17. Editorial, Nurs Diagn 1:50, 1990.
18. Carpenito L: Nursing diagnosis: application to clinical practice, Philadelphia, 1989, JB Lippincott Co.
19. Gordon M: Historical perspective: the national conference group for classification of nursing diagnoses (1978, 1980). In Kim MJ and others: Classification of nursing diagnosis: proceedings of the third and fourth national conferences, New York, 1982, McGraw-Hill, Inc.
20. Kim MJ: Future direction and concluding remarks. In Carroll-Johnson RM, ed: Classification of nursing diagnoses: proceedings of the eighth conference, Philadelphia, 1989, JB Lippincott Co.
21. Alfaro R: Application of nursing process, Philadelphia, 1986, JB Lippincott Co.
22. Maslow A: Motivation and personality, New York, 1954, Harper & Row, Publishers, Inc.
23. Bulechek G and McCloskey J: Nursing interventions: treatments for potential nursing diagnoses. In Carroll-Johnson RM, ed: Classification of nursing diagnoses: proceedings of the eighth conference, Philadelphia, 1989, JB Lippincott Co.

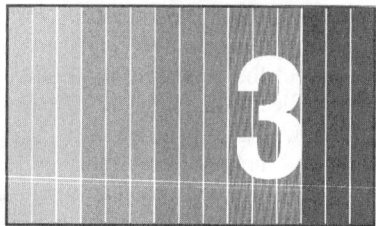

CHAPTER

3

Nursing Assessment
Health History and Physical Examination

M. Carolyn Cecere
Katheryn Ellen McCash

L *earning Objectives*

1. *Explain the purpose, components, and techniques related to the health history and physical examination.*
2. *Differentiate between a nursing history and a health history.*
3. *Describe the appropriate use and techniques of inspection, palpation, percussion, and auscultation.*
4. *Identify the equipment needed to perform a physical examination.*
5. *Describe the indications, purposes, and components of the branching or regional examination.*
6. *Describe a routine format for recording the health history and physical examination.*

The client history, general survey, and physical examination are part of the assessment phase of the nursing process. This information provides a data base of a client's health, including potential and actual health problems, on which the other phases of the nursing process are based.[1] Numerous formats exist for taking histories in the health care setting. The nurse and physician may use different formats and analyze the data differently because of each discipline's different focus. Basically, these histories are described as *health history* and *nursing history*.

Both subjective and objective information is gathered. A health history provides subjective data about the state of the client's health. Subjective data are supplied by the client either as spontaneously offered information or as a response to direct questioning by the nurse. Knowledgeable others can also contribute subjective data about the client. The *general survey* statement provides a comprehensive descriptive statement about the client. The *physical exam-*

Reviewed by Peggy Mayfield, R.N.C., M.S.N., Adult Nurse Practitioner, Associate Professor, Harris College of Nursing, Texas Christian University, Fort Worth, Texas.

ination provides objective data related to the health status of the client. Objective data are gathered by the nurse through inspection, palpation, percussion, and auscultation. Additional sources of objective data include the findings of other health care providers and the results of diagnostic studies.

INTERVIEWING CONSIDERATIONS

Effective communication is a key factor in the interview process. Establishing a relationship and obtaining information are the goals of the communication process. Nurses should remember that individuals communicate not only in their verbal responses but in their manner of dress, gestures, and body language.

Collection of data assists the examiner and the client in identifying health problems, as well as client assets and resources. The nurse can use the data to identify areas where the client may be unable to meet personal needs and may require nursing assistance. Clients perceive this encounter as an indication of how the health care system will assist them. *Contracting* is one method that can be used to promote a nurse-client relationship. Contracting involves a mutual agreement of the behaviors that the client and nurse will expect of each other. The emphasis is placed on the client's needs, which gives the nurse direction for the interaction.[2]

The timing of a complete health history may vary with the format used and the experience of the nurse. It may be completed in one or several sessions, depending on the setting and the client. In the case of an older adult client with a low energy level, several short sessions may need to be scheduled. Allowing time for the client to volunteer information about particular areas of concern enables the nurse to work *with* the client to identify existing and potential health problems. When a client is unable to provide the necessary data (e.g., is unconscious or aphasic), the nurse asks the person who has assumed responsibility for the client's welfare to provide as much information as possible.

Before beginning the health history, the nurse should

explain to the client that the purpose of a detailed history is to collect information that will provide a health profile for comprehensive health care, including health maintenance and promotion. This information is collected at the initial visit, and only updates are needed subsequently. The nurse should also explain that personal and social data are needed to individualize the plan of care. This explanation is necessary because clients may not be accustomed to sharing personal information about themselves and need to know the purpose of such questioning. The nurse should assure the client that all information will be kept confidential.

A health history form indicates *what to ask,* not *how to ask it.* In addition to understanding the principles of effective communication, each nurse must develop a personal style of relating to clients. Although no single style fits all people, wording specific questions in certain ways will increase the probability of eliciting the needed information. Ease at asking questions, particularly those related to sensitive areas such as sexual functioning and income, comes with experience. Videotaping the health history is effective in self-critiquing communication techniques.

To obtain accurate social and personal information, the nurse must communicate acceptance of the client as an individual. When asking sensitive questions, the nurse can communicate the acceptance or normalcy of behaviors by prefacing questions with "most people" or "frequently." For example, stating, "Most people have sexual concerns; are there any you would like to discuss?" shows the client that a personal situation may not be unique. Another method of putting the client at ease is to word the question so that an affirmative answer appears expected. An example of this technique is to ask "What do you like to drink at a party?" instead of "Do you drink?" "How often do you drink alcohol?" is another way of obtaining information related to alcohol intake. These questions are open ended, encouraging the client to speak freely and showing concern for what worries the client most.[3]

For example, factors such as a prolonged response time or visual and hearing impairment may give a false impression of an older adult client's mental status. The complaints may seem multifaceted due to long-lasting and complex health problems. Assisting the client in identifying priority concerns is often helpful.[4] The nurse cannot assume the relative importance of a problem without validating this with the client.

The amount of information that should be collected on initial contact with the client is a nursing judgment based on the client, the problem, and the setting. Interviews with older adult clients, clients with long-term chronic disease, and emergency room admissions are examples of situations in which the nurse must use this judgment. The nurse may choose to ask only those questions that are pertinent to a specific problem, deferring the complete history until a more appropriate time.

HEALTH HISTORY AND NURSING HISTORY

A health history is designed to collect data to be used primarily by the physician to diagnose a health problem. However, much of this history is used by nurses and other health care providers. In an inpatient setting, members of the medical team (physician, resident, and medical student) usually collect the health history. Often, the admitting nurse also collects this same information during the admission interview. There is increasing disapproval of the nurse repeating this process; credibility is lost when the nurse repeats the same questions that others have already asked. In other settings, such as clinics and physicians' offices, the nurse may be primarily responsible for collecting the health history.

A nursing history has a different focus—the client's response to the health problems. A nursing history provides information that assists the nurse in more accurately identifying nursing diagnoses.

Health History

The format for collecting a health history is fairly standardized (Table 3-1). The components include the following:

1. Demographic or identifying data
2. Chief complaint or motivation for seeking health care
3. History of present illness or present health status
4. Past health history
5. Family health history
6. Review of systems

Demographic data. The first part of the health history, the *demographic data,* consists of identifying data such as name, date, and age. When recording the data, the nurse should note who supplied the information (informant) and how accurate the information is considered to be (reliability). The nurse should also note any discrepancies or inconsistencies.

Chief complaint. The *chief complaint* (CC) is the term used to describe what has motivated the client to seek health care. It should be recorded in the client's own words whenever possible. Quotation marks indicate that the client's words have been used. When a health problem is involved, the chief complaint should describe the problem and its duration. For example, "nausea for 36 hours" is a properly recorded chief complaint. If the client does not have a health problem or chief complaint, the reason for entering the health care system at this time should be noted. For example, "I need an insurance physical" gives direction to the interview that follows.

Dealing with the client's perceived problems initially is important. Although the provider may view other problems as more important, the client's concerns must be addressed before progress can be made in other areas.

History of present illness or present health status. The *history of present illness* (HPI) provides detailed data about the chief complaint or reason for entering the health care system. Reasons for entry into a health care system vary, and the provider should determine if the client is seeking health maintenance and promotion information or acute care management.

The provider should be quite directive in this phase. If the client has entered the health care system with a particular problem, very specific information about the client's symptoms should be gathered. This is done systematically

Table 3-1 Health History Form

DEMOGRAPHIC DATA

Dates of assessment
Client's name
Parent's, guardian's, or caretaker's name (if client is a minor)
Address
Age, birth date

Birthplace
Primary language
Marital status
Occupation and place of employment
Health insurance coverage
Informant/reliability

CHIEF COMPLAINT

Client's subjective statement about problem, duration, reason for seeking health care

HISTORY OF PRESENT ILLNESS

Investigation of a symptom:
　Bodily location
　Quality
　Chronology
　Setting
　Aggravating and alleviating factors
List significant positive and negative findings related to the chief complaint

Associated manifestations
Effect on eating, sleeping, elimination, and activity
　patterns
Meaning to individual

PAST HEALTH HISTORY

General health statement
Childhood illnesses: Rubella, mumps, pertussis, scarlet fever, rheumatic fever, chickenpox, polio, measles, strep throat, asthma
Adult illnesses: Rheumatic fever, hepatitis, cystitis, strep throat, pneumonia, anemia, tuberculosis
Immunization: Type and dates

Injuries, hospitalization, and operations: Type and dates
Therapeutic regimens: Medications, diet, psychotherapy (past and present)
Allergies: Environmental, ingestion, drugs, other
Travel in last 5 years: Dates, locations, related illness
Habits: Smoking, alcohol, caffeine, recreational drugs
Supportive devices: Cane, walker, eyeglasses, dentures

FAMILY HEALTH HISTORY

Specific information about the following:
　Tuberculosis
　Diabetes
　Glaucoma
　Hypertension
　Heart disease
　Strokes
　Renal disease
　Alcoholism
　Sexually transmitted diseases

Arthritis
Gout
Ulcers
Cancer
Epilepsy
Depression
Mental illness
Other

Genetic chart*: Record all significant positives and negatives, including mental retardation, congenital abnormalities, hereditary diseases, and family allergies

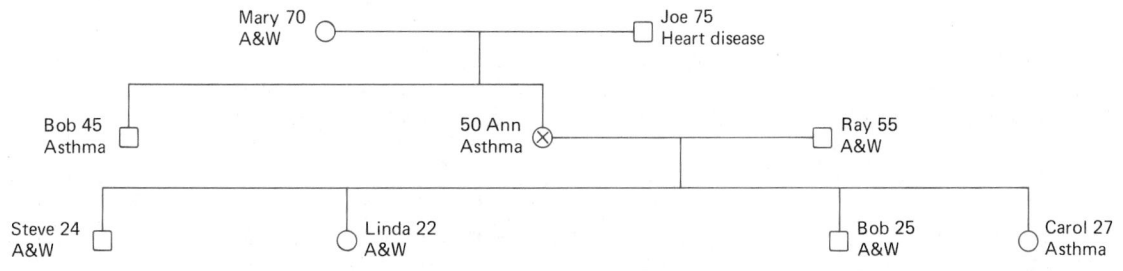

*Code: ○, female; □, male; ●, ■, deceased; x, client; *A & W*, alive and well.　　　　　　　　　　　　　*Continued.*

Table 3-1   Health History Form—cont'd

REVIEW OF SYSTEMS
General

Present weight (loss or gain of 10 lb)
Weakness
Fatigue
Malaise
Sleep patterns
Fever

Chills
Sweats or night sweats
Dizziness
Fainting
Headache

Vision and hearing

Eyes
Pain
Vision
Glasses or contacts
Spots or floaters
Recent change in acuity
Diplopia
Infection
Glaucoma
Cataract
Date of last examination

Ears
Earaches
Hearing
Tinnitus
Discharge
Infection
Mastoiditis
Ears pierced
Vertigo
Sensitivity to noise
Date of audiometric testing (if ever)

Integumentary

Pruritus
Pigmentary and other color changes
Lesions/rashes
Tendency to bruising

Excessive dryness
Texture or moisture
Character of hair and nails
Use of hair dyes or other possibly toxic agents

Respiratory

Nose
Sinus pain
Nasal obstruction
Rhinorrhea/discharge
Postnasal drip
Frequent colds
Sneezing
Mouth/throat
Pain
Difficulty chewing
Hoarseness
Expectoration
Frequent sore throats
Condition of teeth
Voice changes

Lungs
Chest pain
Pleurisy
Cough
Sputum
Hemoptysis
Dyspnea
Wheezing
Bronchitis
Pneumonia
Tuberculosis or contact with individual with TB
Exercise pattern
Date of last chest x-ray examination
TB skin test (date and results)

Hematological

Bleeding tendencies of skin or mucous membranes
Anemia and treatment
Blood transfusion and reaction
Blood type

Blood dyscrasia
Exposure to toxic agents or radiation
Lymph node enlargement

Cardiovascular

Chest pain or distress
Palpitations
Dyspnea on exertion
Orthopnea
Paroxysmal nocturnal dyspnea

History of heart murmur
Rheumatic fever
Hypertension
Coronary artery disease
Anemia

Table 3-1 Health History Form—cont'd

REVIEW OF SYSTEMS—cont'd
Cardiovascular—cont'd

Nocturia (awakens client or client awakens and then voids)
Cyanosis

Heart attack
Date of last ECG
Other cardiac work-up

Peripheral vascular

Intermittent claudication
Thrombophlebitis
Varicose veins or complications
Peripheral edema

Raynaud's disease
Cyanosis
Hair loss
Chronic coldness of extremities

Gastrointestinal

Appetite
Food intolerances
Dysphagia (solids, liquids)
Heartburn
Indigestion
Postprandial pain or distress
Use of antacids
Other abdominal pain or distress
Belching
Nausea and vomiting
Hematemesis
Distention
Flatulence
Abdominal masses

Use of laxatives
Character of stool
Melena
Change in bowel habits
Rectal conditions (pruritus, hemorrhoids, fissures, fistulas)
Gallbladder disease
Hepatitis
Jaundice
Appendicitis
Abdominal surgery
Colitis
Parasites
Hernia
Date of previous x-rays

Genitourinary

Renal colic/stones
Frequency of urination
Nocturia
Polyuria
Oliguria
Dysuria
Hematuria
Albuminuria
Pyuria

Urination (hesitancy, urgency, narrow or weak stream, dribbling, incontinence)
Kidney disease
Facial edema
Cystoscopy
Infections
Gonorrhea or syphilis (common name and signs, date, treatment, complications)
Herpes simplex type 1 or type 2

Reproductive/sexual

Sexual
  Drive
  Activity
  Pleasure
  Discomfort
  Impotence
  Frigidity
  Sterility
  Contraceptive methods (type, how long, methods, effectiveness)
Pregnancies
  Gravida
  Parity
  Abortions
  Spontaneous or therapeutic
  Stillbirths
  Premature births
  Number of living children

Women
  Menstrual history (last normal menstrual period [LNMP], menarche, cycle and duration, amount of flow, premenstrual tension/pain, dysmenorrhea, intermenstrual bleeding)
  Vaginal discharge
  Menopause and associated symptoms
  Vaginal or uterine surgery
  Date of last Pap smear/results
  Breast masses
  Breast self-exam: Knows how? How often?
  Nipple discharge
Men
  Impotence
  Premature ejaculation
  Prostate problems
  Rashes/lesions on penis or scrotum

Continued.

Table 3-1   Health History Form—cont'd

REVIEW OF SYSTEMS—cont'd

Endocrine

Nutritional and growth history

Thyroid function (tolerance to heat and cold, changes in skin, relationship between appetite and weight, nervousness, tremors, drowsiness, results of previous tests)

Hair distribution/hirsutism

Sexual vigor

Goiter

Diabetes or its symptoms (polyuria, polydipsia, polyphagia)

Sugar in blood or urine

Excessive sweating

Hormone therapy

Neurological

Headache

Nervousness

Sleep disturbance

Vertigo

Syncope

Loss of consciousness

Convulsions/fits

Stroke

Sensory or motor disturbance (speech disturbance, tremor, weakness, paralysis, clumsiness of movement)

Paresthesia

Memory loss

Disorientation

Musculoskeletal

Muscles

  Muscle weakness

  Pain

  Cramps

  Trauma

  Aches

  Atrophy

  Spasms

Bones

  Dislocation

  Fractures

  Osteomyelitis

  Flat feet

Joints

  Pain

  Stiffness

  Swelling

  Rheumatoid arthritis

  Osteoarthritis

  Gout

  Bursitis

  Back (pain, stiffness, limitation of motion, sciatica, disk disease)

---

and is referred to as the *investigation of a symptom*. The information obtained helps determine the cause of the problem. Table 3-2 lists the eight areas that must be investigated if a symptom is present.

For example, if a client stated that he had "pain in his leg at times," the provider may obtain and record the following information:

Has right midcalf pain *(location)*, described as "like being stabbed with a knife" *(quality)*. Pain is so severe that it is not possible for the client to continue walking *(quantity)*. Onset is abrupt, lasting for 1 to 2 minutes, it occurs once or twice daily, and it last occurred on 5-5-92 *(onset, duration, frequency)*. Generally occurs at work when climbing stairs after lunch, but last occurred when cutting lawn *(setting)*. Pain is alleviated by rest for 2 to 3 minutes. The client has been salting his food "more heavily" than he used to, but "it doesn't help" *(alleviating factor)*. Leg pain is sometimes accompanied by chest pain that causes some nausea *(associated manifestations)*. The client has not altered his lifestyle because of the intermittent pain. He thinks it is caused by "muscle cramps from lack of salt" *(personal meaning)*.

Throughout the health history, any *positive findings* are explored using the same criteria as the investigation of a symptom. A positive finding indicates that the client has had or does have a particular problem or symptom posed by the provider. For example, if the client answers "yes" to the question of chest pain, this indicates a positive finding. Relevant information about this problem should then be gathered.

Negative findings may also be significant. A negative finding is the absence of a symptom usually associated with a problem. For example, peripheral edema is common with congestive heart failure. If edema is not present in a client with congestive heart failure, this should be noted. Another type of negative finding includes the absence of usual health promotion practices. Lack of tetanus immunization is a negative finding and should be recorded.

Past health history. The *past health history* (PHH) provides information about the client's prior state of health. The client is specifically questioned about major childhood and adult illnesses, immunizations, injuries, hospitalizations, operations, therapeutic regimens, allergies, travel, habits, and the use of supportive devices. This procedure

Table 3-2 Investigation of a Symptom

LOCATION

Ask:	"Where do you feel it? Where is it located?"
Record:	Region of the body
	If local or radiating
	If superficial or deep

QUALITY

Ask:	"What does it (feel, look) like?"
Record:	The client's analogy (e.g., "Like being burned")

QUANTITY

Ask:	"How often do you have this feeling? How bad is it? How much is it? How big is it?"
Record:	Frequency (mild, moderate, severe), volume, size, extent, or number

CHRONOLOGY

Ask:	"When was the first time it occurred? Any particular time of day, week, month, or year?"
Record:	Time of onset
	Duration
	Periodicity and frequency
	Course of symptoms

SETTING

Ask:	"Where are you when this occurs? What were you doing?"
Record:	Where the client is when the symptom occurs
	What the client is doing
	If the symptom is related to anything

AGGRAVATING OR ALLEVIATING FACTORS

Ask:	"What makes it better? Worse? Is there any activity that seems to cause it? What have you done for it? Did it help? Was there some reason you didn't do anything about it?"
Record:	The influence of physical and emotional activities
	The client's attempts to alleviate (or treat) the symptom

ASSOCIATED MANIFESTATIONS

Ask:	"What other things do you see or feel when it occurs? Has it affected your appetite? Elimination? Sleeping?"
Record:	Other symptoms

MEANING OF THE SYMPTOM TO THE CLIENT

Ask:	"How has it affected you? Your life? Why have you sought care now? What do you think may be the cause?"
Record:	Client's statements about the effect of the symptom and the cause of the symptom

is more effective than simply asking if the client has had any illness. Many illnesses are long forgotten or considered irrelevant. If there is a positive finding, the nurse needs to determine when the client had the problem, how it was treated, and whether the client still experiences any health problems related to the illness. In some instances the client may not know about childhood illnesses. This should be indicated on the history.

The nurse also determines if the client's immunizations are current. A current immunization schedule from the local health department can serve as a checklist. Specific immunizations to ask about include polio, measles, mumps, tetanus, pertussis, rubella, and diphtheria. With an older adult client, recent immunizations against influenza and pneumonia should be noted.[5]

All injuries, hospitalizations, and surgeries are recorded, along with a note of the date of the event, the treatment, and the outcome (whether the problem was completely resolved). Blood transfusions received by the client are also noted.

Specific details related to past or present therapeutic regimens are obtained. This includes use of prescription or over-the-counter medications. Examples of specific medications to ask about include steroids, birth control pills, antibiotics, diuretics, aspirin, antacids, and laxatives. Older adult clients, in particular, need to be questioned about medication routines. Changes in absorption, metabolism, reaction to, and elimination of drugs as well as surgery and concurrent disease make drug-related problems a serious potential problem in older adults.[6]

Data related to special diets, either prescribed or self-selected, should be obtained. Examples of common special diets to specifically ask about include restricted-calorie, low-salt, and low-cholesterol diets.

The client is questioned regarding allergies, including known allergens, specific reactions, and treatments. Information related to desensitization regimens should also be obtained. History of travel in the past 5 years is included in the questioning, since different geographic locations may expose the client to new and different health hazards.

Habits related to smoking, alcohol intake, caffeine, and recreational drugs should be noted. The type, quantity, and duration of use should be specifically elicited and recorded. For example, cigarette smoking history is documented by recording the age when regular smoking started, the number of cigars or cigarettes smoked per day, and the age when smoking was given up. The number of packs of cigarettes times the years smoked is then recorded as "pack years."

Finally, the client needs to be questioned about the use of supportive devices such as a cane, walker, eyeglasses, contact lenses, or hearing aid. The reason and duration of use should be included.

Family health history. A *family health history* (FHH) notes illnesses that have an environmental, genetic, or familial tendency or that are communicable. The presence or absence of such conditions or problems should be noted. Again, stating the most common diseases can help the client to remember which illnesses various family members have had.

Generally, obtaining a detailed family history on an older adult is not necessary. A genetic disease would not likely require intensive consideration in advanced age. Asking questions about grandchildren, however, can yield important information. If grandchildren are experiencing medical or social problems, it can cause grave concern in the older client.[7]

A genetic chart or family tree of three generations can be developed to illustrate the family's health history.[8] The provider notes the ages of family members and whether the family members are alive and well (A & W) or have a health problem.

The genetic history can provide significant information. It reveals (1) a picture of the family or relational composition, (2) the way the client's health affects and is affected by health conditions and illnesses of other family members, and (3) health trends and predispositions of hereditary and constitutional factors.[8] In some situations, including information on roommates, sexual partners, and significant others may be appropriate.

Review of systems. The *review of systems* (ROS) is the final portion of the health history. It is the systematic collection of specific information about the client's past and present health status related to common problems of body systems. It is considered subjective data because the information is supplied by the client. Leading, directed questions are posed to the client in an orderly manner using a systems approach.

In addition to questioning the client about current or past health problems, health promotion and maintenance practices—such as breast self-examination (BSE), eye ex-aminations, ECG testing, testicular examination, dental examinations, tuberculin screening, and chest x-ray study—are recorded with the appropriate system.

Before beginning the lengthy list of review-of-systems questions, the client should be told the importance of this information in planning health care. Generally, "yes" or "no" answers are satisfactory. If the client answers affirmatively to a symptom or problem, it should be investigated using the criteria presented under history of present illness.

Responses that have already been elicited in previous portions of the health history need not be repeated. Avoiding repetitive questions is important. This can lead the client to believe that the nurse is not listening to what is being said. It is also important to use common, easily understood words to describe medical problems. If not, the client may give inaccurate information because of lack of understanding.

Recording of responses should be standardized if a printed review-of-systems form is used. This ensures that all care providers have asked the same questions to elicit the recorded responses. For example, all positive responses are circled, all negative responses are crossed out, and information-not-available responses are underlined. The directions should clearly indicate the system to be followed.

General Survey

Following the health history a general survey statement is made. The *general survey* is a statement of the provider's general impression of a client, including behavioral observations. This initial survey is considered a scanning procedure and begins with the provider's first encounter with the client and continues during the health history.

Although the provider may include other data that seem pertinent, the major areas usually included in the general survey statement are (1) body features, (2) state of consciousness and arousal, (3) speech, (4) body movements, (5) physical signs, (6) nutritional status, and (7) behavior. Vital signs, height, and weight are often included in the general survey statement. Observations of these areas provide the data for the general survey statement. The following is a sample of a general survey statement:

Mrs. H. is a 34-year-old Mexican-American female, BP 130/84/80, P 88, R 18. No distinguishing body features. Alert but anxious. Speech rapid with trailing thoughts. Wringing hands and shuffling feet during interview. Skin flushed, hands clammy. Overweight in proportion to height. Sits with eyes downcast and shoulders slumped and avoids eye contact.

Many nurses believe that the information in the general survey has been added to the health history to elicit data nurses need to provide care. Use of a nursing history obtains this as well as other data that are important in planning the client's care.

Nursing History

A conceptual model of nursing should be used to guide the development of a nursing data base.[9] However, because of the many conceptual models available to nursing, as well as the difficulty in translating theory into practice, nurses have not standardized a nursing data base. Numerous nursing history/data base formats are available in the literature.[9-11]

What are the goals and concerns of nursing? Nursing is concerned with "the diagnosis and treatment of human responses to actual or potential health problems."[12] Nurses need to ask questions that elicit information related to the individual's responses to actual or potential problems. Information obtained in these questions will provide the necessary data to support the identification of nursing diagnoses.

The format used in this text for gathering a nursing history is organized around a client's functional health patterns (see Tables 2-4 and 3-3). It is designed to gather information systematically to determine the presence of actual, high-risk, or possible nursing diagnoses. Both subjective and objective data are collected related to each functional health pattern.

Health perception–health management pattern. Assessment of the health perception–health management functional health pattern focuses on the client's perceived level of health and well-being and on personal practices for maintaining health. This includes preventive screening activities such as breast and testicular examinations; colorectal cancer, hypertension, and cardiac risk factor screening; and Papanicolaou testing.[1]

The questions for this pattern also seek to identify risk factors by obtaining a family history, history of health habits (for example, smoking, alcohol, and drug use), and exposure to environmental hazards.

Subjective data. There are several ways to identify the client's perceived level of health and well-being. When questioning the client, the nurse determines the client's feelings of effectiveness at staying healthy—what helps and what hinders.

The client is asked to describe personal health and any concerns about it. This information should be recorded in the client's own words.

The client is asked about a family history of major problems such as cardiovascular disease, hypertension, cancer, diabetes mellitus, psychiatric illness, and genetic disorders. Information about sexual abuse, violence, and drug and alcohol abuse should also be obtained.

Determining what the client does when not well is also important. This question elicits information about a client's knowledge of the health problem, awareness of what should be done, and ability to use certain resources to manage the problem.

The nurse also assesses the client's developmental stage in this pattern. This ensures that care appropriate for the developmental capabilities of the client is planned.

Objective data. Objective data collected in this pattern include the results of breast, testicular, pelvic, and rectal exams. Observations of general appearance, hygiene, dress, and attitude in regard to health management should also be noted.

Nutritional-metabolic pattern. The processes of ingestion, digestion, absorption, transport, and metabolism are assessed in this pattern.

Subjective data. A 24-hour dietary recall should be obtained from the client. From this information the nurse can evaluate the quantity and quality of foods and fluids eaten and drunk. Questions regarding weight gain, weight loss, and energy level should be asked to evaluate metabolism.

The impact of psychological factors such as depression, anxiety, and self-concept is assessed. For example, "How is your appetite affected by anxiety?" is an appropriate question. Sociocultural factors such as food budget, the preparer of the meals, and food preferences are also assessed.

Determining how the client's present condition has interfered with eating and appetite is important. If the client's present condition has produced symptoms such as nausea, gas, or pain, the effect of these symptoms on appetite should be determined. Food allergies and the need for a special or restricted diet should also be noted. The person's knowledge of nutrition can be determined by asking specific questions such as, "Tell me which of the four food groups you had today."

Objective data. The client's overall nutritional status, including weight, body mass, and skin appearance, should be assessed. Specifically, the presence of edema, fat depletion, and muscle wasting should be observed. Anthropometric measurements (weight, midarm muscle circumference, and skinfold thickness) are taken to evaluate nutritional status.

The skin, hair, and nails are assessed within this pattern by inspection and palpation. The oral cavity should be inspected and palpated for any abnormalities.

Physical examination findings of the abdomen may provide objective data for this pattern. The abdomen is inspected for any pulsations, visible masses, or vascular changes. (See Chapter 33 for physical assessment of the abdomen, and Chapter 16 for physical assessment of the skin, hair, and nails.)

Elimination pattern. Within this pattern the nurse assesses bowel and bladder function.

Subjective data. The nurse asks about the frequency of each function, the description of each, whether any discomfort is related to the function, whether there are problems with control, and usual practices such as taking laxatives or enemas. If any devices are used, such as catheter or colostomy equipment, the nurse asks about their care.

Objective data. The bowel and bladder patterns of the client should be assessed for frequency, amount, and the relationship of output to fluid intake. Physical examination may reveal gastrointestinal, neurological, or musculoskeletal abnormalities that may contribute to problems with elimination. The assessment chapters for these specific systems should be consulted.

The results of laboratory work and diagnostic tests that relate to the gastrointestinal or renal systems should be evaluated. Examples include stool guaiac, proctoscopy, sigmoidoscopy, intravenous pyelogram, urinalysis, and serum electrolytes.

Activity-exercise pattern. Within this pattern the nurse assesses the client's usual pattern of exercise, activity, leisure, and recreation.

Subjective data. The client should be questioned about ability to perform activities of daily living. Table 3-3 outlines the grading scale for self-care abilities. If the client is unable to perform activities of daily living, such as toilet-

Table 3-3 Nursing Data Base: Functional Health Pattern Approach

DEMOGRAPHIC DATA

Name, address, age, occupation

CURRENT MEDICATIONS

Name and dosage

PAST HEALTH-SURGICAL HISTORY

Subjective data	**Objective data**
Health perception–health management pattern	
1. How has general health been?	1. General appearance, hygiene, dress, attitude about health
2. Any colds in past year?	2. Results of breast, testicular, pelvic, rectal exams
3. Most important things to keep healthy? Think these things make a difference to health (include family folk remedies, if appropriate)? Use of cigarettes, alcohol, drugs? Breast self-exam?	
4. In past, been easy to find ways to follow things doctors or nurses suggest?	
5. What do you think caused this illness? Actions taken when symptoms perceived? Results of action?*	
6. Things important to you while you're here? How can we be most helpful?*	
7. Family health history	
8. Illness and injury risk factors	
Nutritional-metabolic pattern	
1. Typical daily food intake (describe)? Supplements?	1. Height, weight
2. Typical daily fluid intake (describe)?	2. Desirable weight
3. Weight loss/gain (amount, time span)?	3. Triceps skin fold
4. Appetite?	4. Skin (edema, muscle wasting)
5. Food or eating: Discomfort? Diet restrictions?	5. Oral cavity
6. Heal well or poorly?	6. IV, drains (specify)
7. Skin problems: Lesions? Dryness?	7. Temperature
8. Dental problems?	8. Lymph nodes
9. How is appetite affected by anxiety?	9. Abdominal exam
10. Food preferences?	10. Hair, nails
11. Food allergies?	
Elimination pattern	
1. Bowel elimination pattern (describe): Frequency? Character? Discomfort?	1. Stool check for occult blood
2. Urinary elimination pattern (describe): Frequency? Problem in control?	2. Urinary output
3. Excess perspiration? Odor problems?	3. Body odor and skin moisture
4. Care of any external devices	4. Diagnostic tests
Activity-exercise pattern	
1. Sufficient energy for desired/required activities?	1. Musculoskeletal system
2. Exercise pattern? Type? Regularity?	a. ROM
3. Spare time (leisure) activities?	b. Strength of grip
4. Perceived ability for (code for level):	c. Gait
Feeding _____	d. Posture, stability
Grooming _____	2. Cardiovascular system
Bathing _____	a. Pulse rate, rhythm
General mobility _____	b. Edema
Toileting _____	c. PMI
Cooking _____	d. Blood pressure

Modified from Fuller J and Schaller-Ayers J: Health assessment, a nursing approach, New York, 1989, JB Lippincott Co.
*If appropriate.
†For women.

Table 3-3 Nursing Data Base: Functional Health Pattern Approach—cont'd

PAST HEALTH-SURGICAL HISTORY—cont'd

Subjective data—cont'd

    Bed mobility _____
    Home maintenance _____
    Dressing _____
    Shopping _____

Functional levels code

Level 0: Full self-care
Level I: Requires use of equipment or device
Level II: Requires assistance or supervision from another person
Level III: Requires assistance or supervision from another person and equipment or device
Level IV: Is dependent and does not participate

Sleep-rest pattern

1. Generally rested and ready for daily activities after sleep? If not, why?
2. Sleep onset problems? Aids? Dreams (nightmares)? Early awakening?
3. Usual sleep rituals?
4. Usual sleep pattern?

Cognitive-perceptual pattern

1. Hearing difficulty? Aid?
2. Vision? Wear glasses? Last checked?
3. Any recent change in memory?
4. Easiest way to learn things?
5. Any discomfort? Pain? How managed?

Self-perception–self-concept pattern

1. How would you describe yourself most of the time? Do you feel good (not so good) about yourself?
2. Changes in your body or the things you can do? Problems to you?
3. Changes in way you feel about yourself or your body (since illness started)?
4. Find things frequently make you angry? Annoyed? Fearful? Anxious? Depressed? What helps relieve these feelings?

Role-relationship pattern

1. Live alone? Family? Family structure diagram?
2. Any family problems you have difficulty handling (nuclear/extended)?
3. How does family usually handle problems?
4. Family depend on you for things? How managing?
5. How family/others feel about your illness/hospitalization?*
6. Problems with children? Difficulty handling?*
7. Belong to social groups? Close friends? Feel lonely (frequency)?

Objective data—cont'd

3. Respiratory system
    a. Breath sounds
    b. Depth, rhythm, rate
4. Vital signs
    a. Before activity
    b. After activity
5. Diagnostic tests
    a. CBC
    b. ECG
    c. Other

1. Mental alertness
2. Sleep environment
3. Behavior while sleeping
4. Napping during day

1. Eye exam (Snellen)
2. Reads newsprint, glasses needed
3. PERRLA
4. Conjunctiva
5. Cornea, lens
6. Whisper heard
7. Attention span
8. Recent and remote memory
9. Communication pattern
10. Pain assessment
11. Level of consciousness
12. Taste, touch, smell

1. Appearance during interview
2. Eye contact
3. Affect
4. Data from other assessment tools

1. Interaction with family, others
2. Assertive or passive (rate from 1 to 5)
3. Communication with family or significant others

Continued.

Table 3-3 Nursing Data Base: Functional Health Pattern Approach—cont'd

PAST HEALTH-SURGICAL HISTORY—cont'd
Subjective data—cont'd

8. Things generally go well for you at work? (school)? Income sufficient for needs?*
9. Feel part of or isolated in neighborhood where living?

Sexuality-reproductive pattern
1. Any changes or problems in sexual relations?*
2. Use of contraceptives? Problems?*
3. When menstruation started? Last menstrual period. Menstrual problems? Para? Gravida?†
4. What is the effect of client's present condition or treatment on sexuality?

Coping–stress-tolerance pattern
1. Tense a lot of the time? What helps? Use any medicines, drugs, alcohol?
2. Who's most helpful in talking things over? Available to you now?
3. Any big changes in your life in the last year or two?
4. When (if) you have big problems (any problems) in your life, how do you handle them?
5. Most of the time, is this (are these) way(s) successful?

Value-belief pattern
1. Generally get things you want out of life?
2. Religion important in your life? Does this help when difficulties arise?*
3. Will being here interfere with any religious practices?*

Other
1. Any other things that we have not talked about that you would like to mention?
2. Questions?

Objective data—cont'd

1. Women
   a. Breast exam
   b. External genitalia
   c. Pelvic exam
2. Men
   a. Testicular exam
   b. Male genital exam

1. Nervous or relaxed (rate from 1 to 5)
2. Vital signs
3. Active defense mechanisms, other coping strategies
4. Cues of suicide

1. Ethnic background
2. Religious articles

*If appropriate.
†For women.

ing, eating, and moving independently, the specific problems that limit an activity should be noted. For example, chest pain, dyspnea, dizziness, claudication, musculoskeletal pain, fatigue, and weakness are problems that commonly result in some degree of self-care deficit.

Objective data. If possible, the nurse should observe the client's ability to perform activities of daily living. Vital signs should be monitored before and after activity. Mobility should be assessed related to range of motion and possible problems of other body systems, such as the musculoskeletal and neurological systems.

Laboratory tests to be analyzed in this pattern are the complete blood count, electrocardiogram and other cardiac studies, pulmonary function studies, and arterial blood gases. (See Chapters 19, 24, 26, and 56 for a complete description of the respiratory, hematological, cardiovascular, and musculoskeletal assessments.)

Sleep-rest pattern. This pattern describes the client's pattern of sleep, rest, and relaxation in a 24-hour period. The individual's perception of the effectiveness of sleep and relaxation is pertinent. Most people take sleep for granted unless they have a problem with sleeping.[1]

Subjective data. The client's usual activities related to bedtime and the usual sleep pattern should be determined. Particular routines, position, and environmental factors used to foster sleep should also be elicited. The client should be questioned about feelings after sleeping well or sleeping poorly.

Objective data. The client's sleep environment should be evaluated for noise level, temperature, and other comfort measures. The client should be observed while sleeping for restlessness, wakefulness, rapid eye movement, dreaming, and the timing of sleep-wake cycles. Napping patterns during daytime hours should also be noted.

Cognitive-perceptual pattern. Assessment of this pattern involves a description of all senses (vision, hearing, taste, touch, smell, and pain) and the cognitive functions (such as communication, memory, and decision making).

Subjective data. The client should be asked about any sensory deficits that affect the ability to perform activities of daily living. Routine eye care, including the date of the last examination, should be elicited. Ways in which the client compensates for any sensory-perceptual problems should be discussed and noted.

Objective data. During the interview, the nurse should note the status of the client's senses and the ability to communicate and follow directions. The client's communication skills, attention span, level of consciousness, and general response to the interview should also be assessed. (See Chapter 51 for a complete assessment of pain and Chapters 15 and 52 for assessment of sensory organs and level of consciousness.)

Self-perception–self-concept pattern. This pattern describes the client's self-concept, which is critical in determining the way the person interacts with others. Included are attitudes about self, perception of personal abilities, body image, and general sense of worth.[13]

Subjective data. The nurse should ask the client for a self-description and how the health condition affects self-attitude. Nurses should avoid making value judgments about how people perceive themselves. What concerns the client about a personal situation may differ from what concerns the nurse.

Objective data. The client's general appearance, body language, and interactions with others should be observed. The effect of personal possessions such as pictures and religious articles should be noted. The congruence of behavior with statements about self and the client's response to any threats from the environment should also be noted. Assessment tools are available to measure certain aspects of self-concept if the nurse feels a more definitive assessment is indicated.

Role-relationship pattern. This pattern describes the roles and relationships, including major responsibilities, of the individual. It examines the person's self-evaluation of the performance of the expected behaviors related to these roles.

Subjective data. The client should describe family, social, and work relationships. The nurse should determine if events in these relationships are satisfactory or if strain is evident in these relationships. The client's feelings about the role in these relationships and the effect the present condition has on the role/relationship should be noted.

Objective data. The nurse should observe the client's interactions with significant others. The presence or absence of support from significant others and communication patterns should be noted.

Sexuality-reproductive pattern. This pattern describes satisfaction or dissatisfaction with personal sexuality and describes the reproductive pattern. Assessing this pattern is important because many illnesses, surgical procedures, and medications affect sexual function. Clients' sexual and reproductive concerns may be expressed, teaching needs and treatable problems may be identified, and normal growth and development may be monitored through information obtained via this pattern.[13]

Subjective data. The interview should be appropriate to the developmental stage of the client. This area is often difficult for the inexperienced nurse. A beginning nurse, untrained in the area of sexuality, may take a health history and screen for sexual function and dysfunction. Based on this history, this nurse may be able to provide limited sex education or refer the client for specific suggestions and intensive therapy to a more experienced professional.

Specifically, the nurse should determine if there is lack of knowledge in relation to sexuality and reproduction. Whether the client perceives a problem in the area of sexuality should also be determined. The effect of the client's present condition or treatment on personal sexuality should also be noted.

Objective data. For women, physical examination involves a genital and pelvic examination and a breast examination. For men a genital examination is required. (See Chapter 45 for a detailed description of these examinations.)

Coping–stress tolerance pattern. This pattern describes the general coping pattern and the effectiveness of the coping mechanisms. Assessment of this pattern involves analyzing the specific stressors or problems that confront the client, the client's perception of the stressor, and the person's response to the stressor.[13]

Subjective data. The major losses or changes experienced by the client in the previous year are important to document. Current major stressors confronting the client are also important. The strategies used by the client to deal with stressors and relieve tension should be noted. The presence of a person on whom the client can rely when problems arise should be recorded.

Objective data. The nurse should observe for potential stressors in the client's environment. Documentation of active defense mechanisms or other coping strategies should be done.

Physiological manifestations of stress, such as diaphoresis, increased heart rate, and increased blood pressure, should be assessed. The nurse should be vigilant for cues that may be signs of a crisis or suicide attempt.

Value-belief pattern. This pattern describes the values, goals, and beliefs (including spiritual) that guide health-related choices.[1]

Subjective data. The client's ethnic background as well as the effects of culture and beliefs on health practices should be noted. The client's belief about health and illness should be documented. The client's wishes about continuation of religious practices and use of religious articles should be noted and honored.

Objective data. The nurse can note cultural cues by the client's appearance and communication pattern. The presence of religious articles should be noted.

PHYSICAL EXAMINATION

The *physical examination* is the systematic assessment of the physical and mental status of a client and is considered objective data. It is observable data that are not distorted by the client's perception.[14] During the physical examination, additional subjective data may be obtained from the client. This may occur from direct questioning by the nurse regarding a finding or be coincidental to the client remembering a forgotten piece of information. Combining the review of systems with the physical examination is not advisable. The review of systems gives valuable direction to the physical examination. Also, the two activities of questioning and examining can be confusing to both the client and the nurse. An exception to this might be an emergency situation in which time is a factor.

Types

There are two types of physical examinations: the screening physical examination and the branching or regional examination. The *screening physical examination* is performed for screening situations, health surveillance, and health maintenance purposes. It is an organized, purposeful check of major body systems to detect any possible problems. If a problem is detected in the course of the screening physical, a more detailed branching examination of the involved system should be done.

A *branching* or *regional examination* is a more detailed assessment of a particular system. The client's clinical manifestations should alert the nurse to the appropriate branching exam. For example, abdominal pain indicates the need to do a branching exam of the abdomen. Some problems necessitate more than one branching exam. A complaint of headache indicates the need to do musculoskeletal, neurological, head and neck, and psychiatric exams.

Techniques

Four major techniques are used in performing the physical examination: inspection, palpation, percussion, and auscultation.

Inspection. Inspection is the visual examination of a part or region of the body to assess normal conditions or deviations from normal. Inspection is more than just looking. This technique is deliberate, systematic, and focused. The nurse needs to compare what is seen with the known, generally visible characteristics of the part being inspected. For example, most 30-year-old men have hair on their legs. Absence of hair may indicate a vascular problem and signals the need for further investigation. This same absence of hair in a 70-year-old man may represent a normal skin change of aging.

Palpation. Palpation is the examination of the body through the use of touch. The use of light and deep palpation can yield information related to masses, pulsatility, organ enlargement, tenderness or pain, swelling, muscular spasm or rigidity, elasticity, vibration of voice sounds, crepitus, moisture, and differences in texture.[15] The nurse

will learn that different parts of the hand are more sensitive for specific assessments. For example, the tips of the fingers are used to palpate lymph nodes, the dorsa of hands and fingers are used to assess temperatures, and the palmar surface is best suited for feeling vibrations (Fig. 3-1).

Percussion. Percussion is an assessment technique involving the production of sound to obtain information about the underlying area. The percussion sound may be produced directly or indirectly. Direct percussion is performed by directly tapping the body with one or two fingers to elicit a sound. Indirect or mediated percussion is the more common percussion technique. The middle finger *(pleximeter)* of the nondominant hand is placed firmly against the body surface. The tip of the middle finger of the dominant hand *(plexor)* strikes the distal phalanx of the pleximeter finger (Fig. 3-2). A relaxed wrist and rapid strike produce the best sounds. The sounds and the vibrations produced are evaluated relative to the underlying structures. Deviation from an expected sound may indicate a problem. For example, the usual percussion sound in the right lower quadrant of the abdomen is tympany. Dullness in this area may indicate a problem and needs to be investigated. (Specific percussion sounds of various body parts and regions are discussed in the appropriate assessment chapters.)

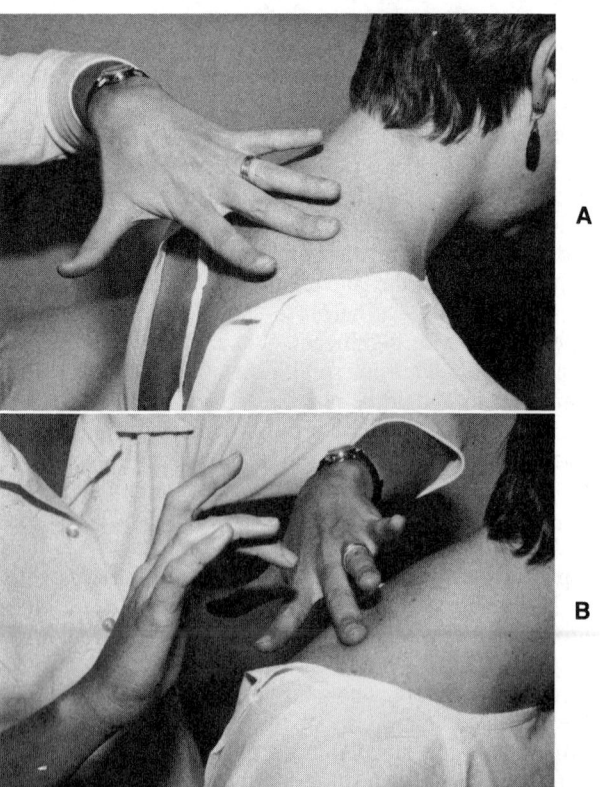

Fig. 3-2 Percussion. **A,** Placement of the pleximeter finger. **B,** Plexor finger striking the pleximeter finger to produce sound.

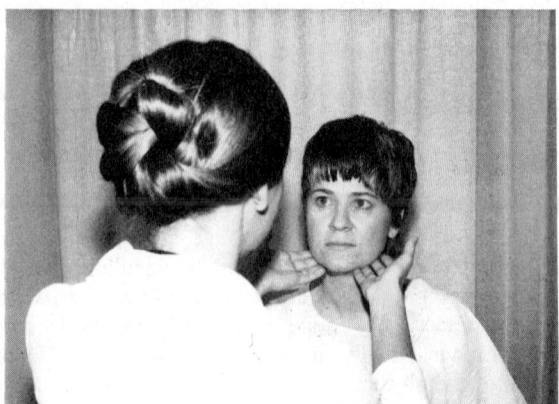

Fig. 3-1 Palpation is the examination of the body through the use of touch.

Auscultation. Auscultation is the listening to sounds produced by the body to assess normal conditions and deviations from normal. Auscultation is usually indirect, using a stethoscope to amplify sounds (Fig. 3-3). The bell of the stethoscope is more sensitive to low-pitched sounds. The diaphragm of the stethoscope is more sensitive to high-pitched sounds. Auscultation is particularly useful in evaluating sounds from the heart, lungs, abdomen, and vascular system. (Specific auscultatory sounds are discussed in the appropriate assessment chapters.)

Not all assessment techniques are appropriate for all body parts and systems. The nurse will learn which technique to use to elicit the most information. The physical assessment techniques are usually performed in the sequence of inspection, palpation, percussion, and auscultation. The only exception to this sequence is for the abdominal exam. In this situation, the sequence is inspection, auscultation, percussion, and palpation. Palpation and percussion of the abdomen before auscultation can alter bowel sounds and produce false findings.

Table 3-4   Equipment for Screening Physical Examination

Stethoscope (with bell and diaphragm, tubing 15-18 inches)
Wrist watch (with second hand)
Blood pressure cuff
Ophthalmoscope/otoscope set
Eye chart (wall chart or Snellen pocket eye card)
Pocket flashlight
Tongue blades
Cotton balls
Percussion hammer
Tuning fork
Alcohol swabs
Client gown
Paper cup with water
Examining table or bed

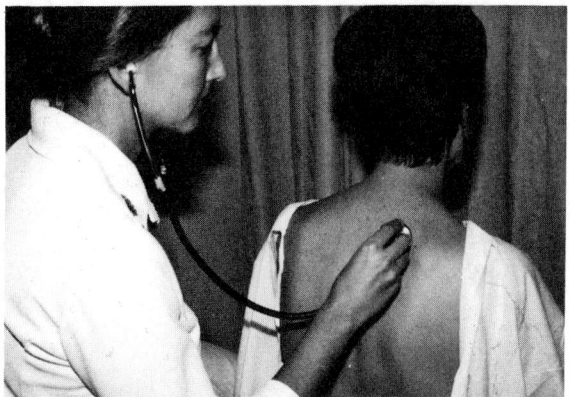

Fig. 3-3   Auscultation is listening to sounds produced by the body to assess normal and deviations from normal.

Equipment

The equipment needed for the screening physical should be easily accessible during the examination (Table 3-4). Organizing equipment before the exam saves the time and energy of the client and the nurse. Lack of organization can discourage the client from the trust and confidence the nurse needs to collect the data base. (The use of specific pieces of equipment is discussed in the appropriate assessment chapters.)

Developing a System

The screening physical should be performed systematically and efficiently. Explanations should be given to the client as the examination proceeds. The factors to be considered are efficiency, client comfort, safety, and privacy. In developing a routine method, the examiner is less likely to forget a procedure, a step in the sequence, or a portion of the body if the same sequence is followed every time. Table 3-5 suggests an outline for the screening physical examination that is organized, logical, and complete. Adaptations of the process of performing the physical examinations are often useful for the older adult who has decreased mobility and energy level and perceptual changes.[16] A limited outline listing some of the adaptations is found in Table 3-6.

Recording the Screening Physical Examination

Only abnormal findings should be recorded during the actual examination. This prevents needless interruptions in the examination to write lengthy normal findings. At the conclusion of the examination, the nurse should combine the normal and abnormal findings in a carefully recorded physical examination. Table 3-7 is an example of how to record a screening physical on a healthy adult. (Table 4-8, Anatomical and Physiological Changes with Aging, and reference to the age-related assessment findings in each chapter dealing with assessment will be helpful in recording findings occurring with age.)

PROBLEM IDENTIFICATION AND THE NURSING DIAGNOSIS

After completing the history and physical examination, the nurse is ready to develop a list of *nursing diagnoses* and collaborative problems. Fig. 3-4 illustrates the problem identification phase of the nursing process.

Nursing diagnoses are health-related problems that respond primarily to nursing care. (Chapter 2 explains the process of establishing nursing diagnoses.)

In this text, nursing diagnoses are presented in two formats. For major health problems, a full nursing care plan has been developed. The nursing diagnosis statement is presented first and includes the problem and etiological statement. Next, the defining characteristics that cue the nurse to this specific diagnosis are listed. Specific nursing interventions that address the nursing diagnosis are then specified. Finally, one or more evaluation criteria are described that aid the nurse in determining if the goals of treatment have been met.

A listing of nursing diagnosis is used in this text for less common health problems. Nursing diagnoses are presented

Text continued on p. 49.

Table 3-5 Outline for Screening Physical Examination

GENERAL SURVEY

Observe general state of health (client is seated):

Body features

State of consciousness and arousal

Speech

Body movements

Physical signs

Nutritional status

Stature

VITAL SIGNS

Record vital signs:

Blood pressure

Radial pulse

Respiration

Record height and weight

INTEGUMENTARY SYSTEM

Inspect and palpate skin for the following:

Color

Lesions

Scars

Bruises

Edema

Moisture

Texture

Temperature

Turgor

Vascularity

Inspect and palpate nails for the following:

Color

Lesions

Size

Flexibility

Shape

Angle

HEAD AND NECK

Inspect and palpate head for the following:

Shape and symmetry of skull

Masses

Tenderness

Hair

Scalp

Skin

Temporal arteries

Temporomandibular joint

Sensory (CN V, light touch and pain)

Motor (CN VII, shows teeth, purses lips, raises eyebrows)

Inspect and palpate eyes for the following:

Visual acuity

Eyebrows

Position and movement of eyelids

Visual fields

Extraocular movements (CN III, IV, VI)

Cornea, sclera, conjunctiva

PERRLA

Red reflex

Eyeball tension

Inspect and palpate ears for the following:

Placement

Pinna

Auditory acuity (Weber or Rinne, whispered voice, ticking watch)

Mastoid process

Auditory canal

Tympanic membrane

Inspect and palpate nose and sinuses for the following:

External nose

  Shape

  Blockage

Internal nose

  Patency of nasal passages

  Shape

  Turbinates/polyps

Discharge

Discharge

Frontal and maxillary sinuses

Inspect and palpate mouth for the following:

Lips (symmetry, lesions, color)

Buccal mucosa (Stensen's and Wharton's ducts)

Teeth (absent, state of repair, color)

Gums

Tongue for strength (asymmetry, ability to stick out tongue, side to side, fasciculations)

Palates

Tonsils and pillars

Uvular elevation (CN IX)

Posterior pharynx

Gag reflex (CN X)

Jaw strength (CN XI)

Table 3-5   Outline for Screening Physical Examination—cont'd

HEAD AND NECK—cont'd

Moisture
Color
Floor of mouth

Looking up and wrinkling forehead (CN VII)
Raise shoulders against resistance (CN XI)

Inspect and palpate (occasionally ausculate) neck for the following:

Skin (vascularity and visible pulsations)
Symmetry
Postural alignment
Range of motion
Pulses (carotid)

Midline structure (trachea, thyroid gland and cartilage)
Lymph nodes (preauricular, postauricular, occipital, mandibular, tonsillar, submental, anterior and posterior cervical, infraclavicular, supraclavicular)

Inspect neurological status:

Motor status observations:
　Gait
　Toe walk
　Heel walk
　Drift

Coordination
　Finger to nose
　Romberg's sign
Spine (scoliosis)

EXTREMITIES

Observe size and shape, symmetry and deformity, involuntary movements

Inspect and palpate arms, fingers, wrists, elbows, and shoulders for the following:

Strength
Range of motion
Crepitus

Joint pain
Swelling
Fluid

Test reflexes:
　Biceps
　Triceps
　Brachioradialis

Patellar
Achilles
Plantar

Inspect and palpate legs for the following:

Strength of hips
Edema

Hair distribution
Pulses (dorsalis pedis, posterior tibialis)

POSTERIOR THORAX

Inspect for muscular development, respiratory movement, approximation of A–P diameter
Palpate for symmetry of respiratory movement, tenderness of CVA, spinous processes, tumors or swelling, tactile fremitus

Percuss for pulmonary resonance
Ausculate for breath sounds

ANTERIOR THORAX

Assess breasts for configuration, symmetry, dimpling of skin
Assess nipples for rash, direction, inversion, retraction
Initiate teaching or review of breast self-exam
Perform upright examination

Palpate axillae
Inspect, palpate, check breasts for discharge (client is supine)
Complete teaching of breast self-exam

Chest
　Inspect for PMI, other precordial pulsations
　Palpate for thrills, lifts, heaves, tenderness over precordium

Ausculate for rate and rhythm, character of S_1 and S_2; S_1 and S_2 in the aortic, pulmonic, Erb's point, tricuspid, mitral areas; bruits at carotid, epigastrium; breath sounds at RML

Neck
　Inspect for venous distention, pulsations, waves

ABDOMEN

Inspect for scars, shape, symmetry, bulging, muscular development, position and condition of umbilicus, movements (respiratory, pulsations, presence of peristaltic waves)
Ausculate for peristalsis, femoral bruits

Percuss border of liver, all quadrants
Palpate to confirm positive findings; check liver (size, surface contour, tenderness); spleen, kidney (size, contour, consistency, tenderness, mobility); urinary bladder (distention); femoral pulses; inguinofemoral nodes

Continued.

Table 3-5 Outline for Screening Physical Examination—cont'd

COMPLETION OF EXAMINATION OF EXTREMITIES

Observe the following:

Range of motion of hips, ankles, feet	Muscle development
Crepitus	Coordination (heel to shin)
Joint pain	Homans' sign
Swelling	Proprioception (position sense of great toe)
Fluid	

GENITALIA*

Male external genitalia

Inspect penis, noting hair distribution, prepuce, glans, urethral meatus, scars, ulcers, eruptions, structural alterations	Inspect skin of scrotum; palpate for descended testes, masses, pain
Inspect epidermis of perineum, rectum	

Female external genitalia

Inspect hair distribution; mons pubis, labia (minora and majora); urethral meatus; Bartholin, urethral, Skene's glands (may also be palpated, if indicated); introitus	Assess for presence of cystocele, rectocele, prolapse (client bears down)
	Inspect perineum, rectum

*If the nurse has the appropriate training, the speculum and bimanual examination of women and the prostate gland examination of men should be performed after this inspection.

Table 3-6 Adaptations in Physical Assessment Techniques for Older Adult Clients

GENERAL APPROACH

Keep client warm and comfortable because loss of subcutaneous fat decreases ability to stay warm. Adapt positioning to physical limitations. Avoid unnecessary changes in position. Perform as many activities as possible in the position of comfort for the client.

SKIN

Handle with care because of fragility and loss of subcutaneous fat.

HEAD AND NECK

Provide a quiet and distraction-free environment because of sensory deficits such as decreased vision, touch, and hearing.

EXTREMITIES

Use nonvigorous movements and reinforcement techniques. Avoid having client hop on one foot or perform deep knee bends because older adults have limited range of motion of the extremities, decreased reflexes, and diminished sense of balance.

THORAX

Adapt examination for changes resulting from decrease in force of expiration, weakened cough reflex, and shortness of breath.

ABDOMEN

Be cautious in palpating client's liver because it is easily palpated with increased size. Older adult client may have diminished pain perception in abdominal wall.

GENITALIA

Use a well-lubricated or smaller speculum for vaginal exam because dryness and atrophy of the female genitalia may cause discomfort.

Table 3-7 Recording a Screening Physical Examination

Client's Name _____   Date _____
        Age _____   Vital Signs: BP _____ P _____ R _____

GENERAL STATUS

Well-nourished, well-hydrated, well-developed white ♀ (female) or ♂ (male) in NAD, appears stated age, looks pleasant, smiles readily, speech clear and evenly paced; is alert and oriented ×3; cooperative, calm

HAIR

Thick, brown; normal distribution

EYES

Visual fields intact on gross confront
VA: OD 20/20
    OS 20/20
    OU 20/20
    s̄ glasses
  EOM: Intact on all gazes ō ptosis, nystagmus
Fundi: Red reflex present bilat no opacities; fundi WNLs
Pupils: PERRLA; cover/uncover test neg; Hirschberg test neg

SINUSES

Nontender

MOUTH

Moist, pink; soft and hard palates intact; uvula rises midline on "ahh"

THROAT

Tonsils surgically removed; no redness

TONGUE

Moist, pink; size appropriate for mouth

LYMPH NODES

Supraclavicular: Nonpalpable
Inguinal: Nonpalpable
Cervical: Nonpalpable
Axillary: Nonpalpable

LUNGS

No increase in A-P diameter; resp rate 18; reg rhythm; no ↑ in tactile fremitus; no tenderness; lungs resonant throughout; diaphragmatic excursion 4 cm; lung fields clear throughout

AXILLA

Hair present, shaved; no lesions; nontender

SKIN

Clear ō lesions; warm and dry; trunk warmer than extremities; turgor returns quickly; no ↑ vascularity; no varicose veins

NAILS

Well-groomed; round, 160-degree angle ō lesions; nail beds pink; nails flexible

EARS

Pinna intact, in proper alignment; external canal patent; TMs intact; pearly gray LM, LR visible, not bulging

NOSE

Patent bilaterally; turbinates pink, no swelling; smell intact bilaterally

HEARING

Rinne: AC > BC; Weber: does not lateralize, whisper heard about 4 feet

HEAD

Normocephalic

NECK

Supple, ō masses, ō bruits; nontender
Thyroid: Palpable, smooth; not enlarged
ROM: Full, intact, strong
Trachea: Midline, nontender

TEETH

24 present, in good repair; gums pink

BREASTS

Soft, nonpendulous, ō venous pattern; ō dimpling, puckering
Nipples: ō inversion, point in same direction, areola dark and sizes sym, no discharge, no masses, nontender

HEART

Rate 82, reg rate and rhythm; no lifts, heaves
PMI: within MCL 5th ICS; L nonpalpable; nonpalpable thrills S_1, S_2 louder, softer in appropriate locations; no S_3, S_4; no murmurs, rubs, clicks
Cartoid, femoral, pedal, radial: All present; equal, strong bilaterally

---

NAD, No acute distress; *ō,* without; *VA,* visual acuity; *EOM,* extraocular movements; *PERRLA,* pupils equal, round, reactive to light and accommodation; *FN,* finger to nose; *BUS,* Bartholin's gland, urethral meatus, Skene's duct; *TM,* tympanic membrane; *LM,* landmarks; *LR,* light reflex; *AC>BC,* air conduction greater than bone conduction.   *Continued.*

ABDOMEN

No pulsations visible, rounded; bowel sounds present, active; no bruits ō CVA tenderness

LIVER

Edge palpable, smooth, nontender; approx 9 cm in size

MASSES

None palpable

SPLEEN

Nonpalpable, nontender; no inguinal hernia palpable

NEUROLOGICAL SYSTEM

Cranial nerves I-XII intact
Motor (drift, toe stand) intact
Coord (FN, Romberg) intact
Reflexes: See diagram
Sensation (touch, vibration, prop) intact

MUSCULOSKELETAL SYSTEM

Well developed, no muscle wasting; ō crepitus, nodules, swelling
ROM: Full, intact head to toe; no scoliosis
Strength: Equal, strong bilaterally
Gait: Walks erect 2-foot steps; arms swinging at side ō staggering

FEMALE GENITALIA

External genitalia: No swelling, redness, tenderness in BUS; normal hair distribution; no cysts, rectocele
Vagina: No lesions, discharge; pink
Cervix: Os closed; no lesions, erosions; nontender
Uterus: Small, firm, nontender; pink
Adnexa: No enlargement; nontender
Rectovaginal: Sphincter intact; confirms above findings

MALE GENITALIA

Normal male hair distribution
Penis: Urethral opening patent; no redness, swelling, discharge; no lesions, structural alterations
Scrotum: Testes descended; no redness, masses, tenderness
Rectal: No lesions, redness; sphincter intact; prostate small, nontender

PSYCHOLOGICAL STATUS

Affect appropriate; eye contact
Orientation: Oriented ×3—time, place, person
Mood: Pleasant, appropriate
Thought content: Intelligent, coherent
Memory: Remote and recent intact
Serial sevens: Not done or intact

Signature _____

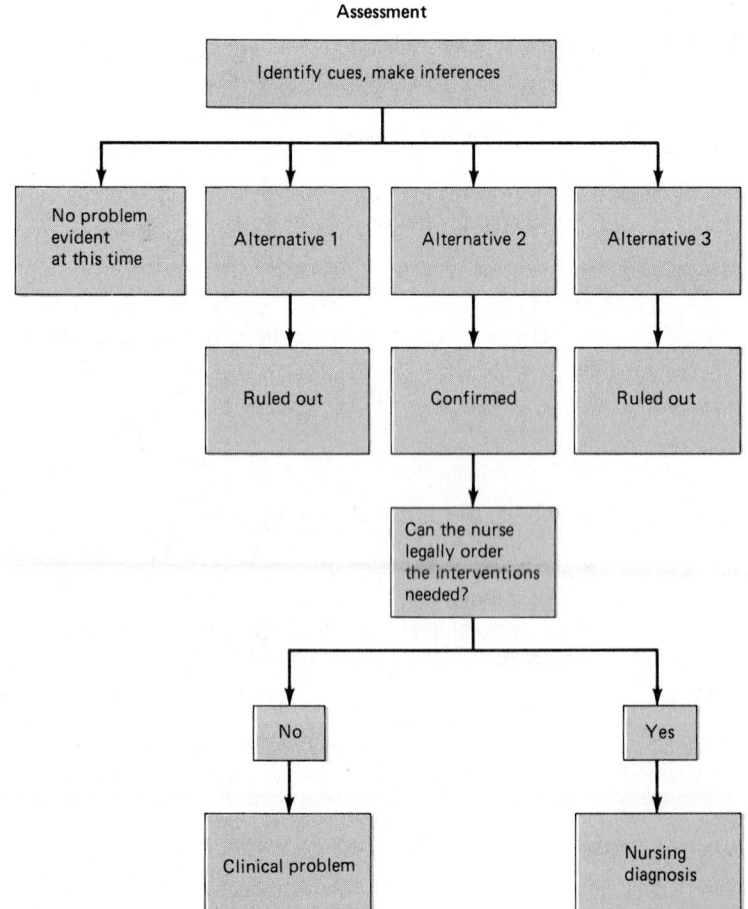

Fig. 3-4   Problem identification phase of the nursing process. (From Carpenito LJ: Nursing diagnosis: application to clinical practice, Philadelphia, 1989, JB Lippincott Co, p 54.)

before the nursing interventions are addressed in the written text.

Following the identification of the nursing diagnoses, the nurse is ready to proceed to the planning phase of establishing therapeutic goals and interventions in the nursing process.

R eview Questions

The number of the question corresponds to the same-numbered objective at the beginning of the chapter.

1. The health history is considered to be a part of the
   a. objective data
   b. subjective data
   c. general survey
2. Data in a nursing history focus on
   a. past health history
   b. client's response to present condition or treatment
   c. physical examination
   d. pathophysiology of client's condition
3. Examination of the body through the use of touch is called
   a. inspection
   b. palpation
   c. auscultation
4. The proper length for a stethoscope is
   a. 10 inches
   b. 15 inches
   c. 22 inches
   d. 25 inches
5. A branching examination is an examination of
   a. a region of the body
   b. the four extremities
   c. mental status
   d. a system of the body
6. In a screening history and physical, the first information to record is the
   a. health history
   b. problem list
   c. general survey
   d. physical examination
7. A general survey statement is recorded
   a. after the physical examination
   b. after the mental status examination
   c. after collection of demographic data
   d. before the physical examination

REFERENCES

1. Gordon M: Nursing diagnosis: process and application, ed 2, New York, 1987, McGraw-Hill, p 8.
2. Sundeen S and others: Nurse-client interaction, ed 4, St Louis, 1989, The CV Mosby Co, p 114.
3. Morton P: Health assessment in nursing, Springhouse, Penn, 1989, Springhouse Corp, p 39.
4. Gress L and Bahr R Sr: The aging person, a holistic perspective, St Louis, 1984, The CV Mosby Co, p 3.
5. Burggraf V and Stanley M: Nursing the elderly: a care plan approach, Philadelphia, 1989, JB Lippincott Co, p 6.
6. Esberger K and Hughes S Jr: Nursing care of the aged, Norwalk, Conn, 1989, Appleton & Lange, p 36.
7. Steel K: History taking from elderly patients, Hosp Pract 20:71, 1985.
8. Malasanos L and others: Health assessment, ed 3, St Louis, 1986, The CV Mosby Co, p 41.
9. Guzzetta C and others: Clinical assessment tools for use with nursing diagnosis, St Louis, 1989, The CV Mosby Co, p 4.
10. Carpenito L: Nursing diagnosis, application to clinical practice, ed 3, Philadelphia, 1989, JB Lippincott Co, p 831.
11. Christensen P and Kenney J: Nursing process: application of conceptual models, ed 3, St Louis, 1990, Mosby–Year Book, Inc, p 75.
12. American Nurses' Association, Congress for Nursing Practice: Nursing: a social policy statement, Kansas City, Mo, 1980, The Association.
13. Fuller J and Schaller-Ayers J: Health assessment: a nursing approach, Philadelphia, 1990, JB Lippincott Co, p 371.
14. Hickey P: Nursing process handbook, St Louis, 1990, Mosby–Year Book, Inc, p 7.
15. Grimes J and Burns E: Health assessment in nursing practice, ed 2, Boston, 1987, Jones & Bartlett Publishers, Inc, p 135.
16. Jones D, Lepley M, and Baker B: Health assessment across the life span, New York, 1984, McGraw-Hill, Inc, p 793.

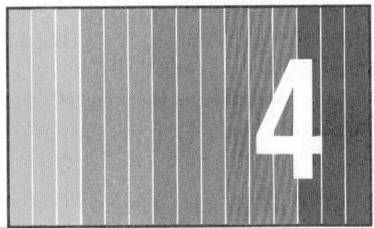

CHAPTER

4

General Concepts
Adult Development and the Impact of Disruption

Charlotte R. Abbink

L *earning Objectives*

1. *Explain the major concepts in the adult developmental theories proposed by Erikson, Peck, Havighurst, and Levinson.*
2. *Contrast the disengagement, activity, and identity continuity psychosocial aging theories.*
3. *Describe the major psychodynamic concerns of young, middle, and older adults in terms of self-concept, intellectual processes, and sexuality.*
4. *List the major family developmental tasks for young, middle, and older adults.*
5. *Compare the community activities of young, middle, and older adults in terms of work, leisure, and civic participation.*
6. *Describe important health maintenance concerns for young, middle, and older adults related to changes from the process of aging.*
7. *Describe the impact of illness on young, middle, and older adults related to their developmental status.*

WHY CONSIDER DEVELOPMENTAL STAGES?

For many nurses and nursing students, the first and sometimes only mental picture when reading the words "developmental stages" is of children. However, the entire human life span is a dynamic sequence of biological, psychological, and social changes that occur in predictable patterns. Like childhood, adulthood can be divided into developmental stages, although adult stages have not been as comprehensively described as childhood stages.

The following discussion of adulthood describes predictable patterns in adult growth and development. Understanding these patterns gives the nurse insight into what may be happening in a client's life at given points in the life cycle. Assessing growth and developmental status is just as crucial in planning appropriate nursing care for an adult as it is for a child. Nursing care is superficial and incomplete if it separates the experiences of illness from what the client is experiencing in all other areas of life.

Reviewed by Joan B. Enggaard, R.N., M.S.N., Associate Professor, Associate Degree Nursing Program, College of Lake County, Grayslake, Illinois.

Although predictable developmental patterns exist, caution must be used in imposing these patterns on a specific client before first validating the unique developmental processes the client is experiencing. For example, the nurse cannot determine that an unmarried young adult is not mastering the intimacy tasks until a complete developmental assessment is made and validated.

CONCEPTUAL APPROACHES TO ADULT DEVELOPMENT

Theorists have proposed models for understanding adult development based on the following premises:
1. Adult development continues to occur in definable, predictable, and sequential patterns.
2. Critical periods occur throughout the life span when physical and psychosocial growth undergoes reorganization.
3. Within each stage of development, there are certain normative activities or tasks to be accomplished.
4. Mastering the tasks of preceding stages is fundamental to transition and mastery of tasks in future stages.

The adult development models of Erikson, Peck, Levin-

Table 4-1   Adult Developmental Stage Theories

Theorist	Young Adulthood	Middle Adulthood	Older Adulthood
Erikson	Intimacy versus isolation	Generativity versus self-absorption	Ego integrity versus despair
Peck		Valuing wisdom versus physical power Socializing versus sexualizing relationships Emotional flexibility versus emotional impoverishment Mental flexibility versus mental rigidity	Ego differentiation versus work role preoccupation Body transcendence versus body preoccupation Ego transcendence versus ego preoccupation
Havighurst	Mate selection and marriage adjustments Establishing family and child rearing Home management Occupation launching Beginning civic responsibility	Launching teenage children Maturing relationship with spouse Adjusting to aging parents Career and occupational maturity Adult social and civic responsibility Developing leisure activities Adjusting to physiological changes	Adjusting to health decline Adjusting to retirement Adjusting to social role changes Establishing satisfactory living arrangements Adjusting to death of spouse
Levinson	Early adult transition Entering the adult world Thirties transition Settling down	Midlife transition Payoff years	

son, and Havighurst use this stage approach. Table 4-1 summarizes the adult developmental stages according to these theorists.

Erikson's Theory: Psychosocial Developmental Conflicts

Erikson views personality development as resulting from the confrontations between ego and social milieu.[1] He identifies points in the life cycle where specific developmental conflicts become paramount because a person's capacities or experiences dictate that a major self-adjustment and adjustment to the environment must be made. In the process of making this adjustment, the individual moves toward one of two opposing positions, such as toward intimacy or toward isolation. When a person successfully masters a core conflict (such as intimacy), the negative sense (isolation) remains as a dynamic counterpart and may be demonstrated in new situations in which this conflict needs to be mastered again at a higher level. Although critical times for mastery of each core conflict exist, all conflicts are present throughout the life span. For example, autonomy is especially important to a toddler; however, adolescents striving for identity need some independent space, and older adults frequently suffer loss of autonomy when limitations are placed on their decision-making prerogatives.

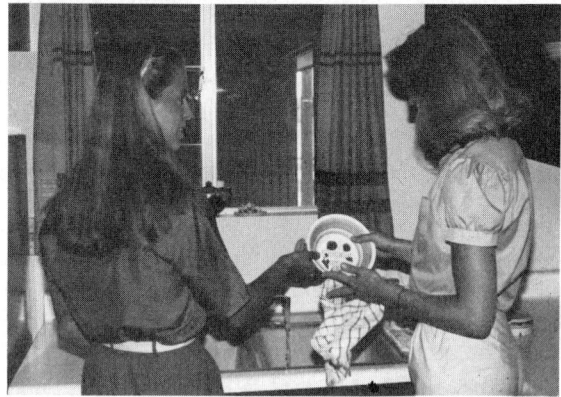

Fig. 4-1   The sharing of everyday tasks by roommates can be an expression of intimacy for young adults.

Intimacy versus isolation.   In Erikson's model, the young adult task is *intimacy* (Fig. 4-1). This involves fusing self-identity with the identities of others in friendships, for causes or creative efforts, or in close personal relationships, including sexual union. Intimacy requires a degree of commitment that necessitates sacrifice, compromise, and self-abandonment for the benefit of others. The young adult who avoids making this commitment to others, fearing the loss of self-identity, will experience a sense of isolation and, consequently, self-absorption.

Generativity versus stagnation. During middle adulthood, the primary task is *generativity*. Generative adults are concerned with establishing the next generation by nurturing and guiding either their children or other young people. A sense of productivity in work and creativity in living are also important components of this task. This core conflict probably arises out of an altruistic need to leave some mark that will make the world a better place in which to live. If generativity does not occur, adults experience a sense of *stagnation* and turn inward, becoming self-preoccupied and overly concerned with physical and psychological health needs. Self-absorbed people's focus on physical changes of middle age may result in either invalidism or inappropriate youthfulness in an attempt to stay young. Regression to an obsessive need for pseudointimacy may occur, which may be expressed through affairs with younger members of the opposite sex.

Ego integrity versus despair. Old age is a time for reviewing the past and rearranging the "photo album of life." This bringing together of all the previous life stages should result in a sense of wholeness, purpose, and a life well lived, or a sense of *ego integrity*, according to Erikson. When a person accepts and approves of a unique life, death can also be accepted as a meaningful part of life. However, if the life review is laden with opportunities missed or wrong directions taken, a sense of *despair* arises. At this point the person knows life is too short to correct the failures. Death is faced with anxiety because it steals away the chance to make changes. In this last stage of ego integrity versus despair, each person must face adjustments and come to a final conflict resolution that is the product of all previous developmental conflict resolutions.

Peck's Theory: Developmental Tasks

Building on Erikson's work, Robert Peck has further defined psychosocial tasks of middle and old age.[2]

Middle adult tasks. Peck has identified four tasks relevant to middle adulthood. The first two tasks, *valuing wisdom versus physical power* and *socializing versus sexualizing relationships*, reflect the biological changes of middle age. With a general decline in physical and sexual functioning, the middle-aged adult's self-esteem can suffer if it is heavily based on these attributes. However, judgmental abilities tend to increase with experience, so valuing the use of one's "head" becomes a positive alternative for maintaining esteem. The progression to a socializing relationship is appropriate as sexual motivations decline. This allows a love relationship to focus on total personalities and companionship rather than sexual performance.

Tasks three and four, *emotional flexibility versus emotional impoverishment* and *mental flexibility versus mental rigidity*, arise from the need for adjusting to life changes and new events that occur in the middle years. When children leave home, parents die, jobs change, and friends die or move away, adults must be flexible enough to shift attachments and reinvest emotions in other people and pursuits. People also need the mental flexibility to allow for new solutions to life problems, rather than being dogmatic and governed by past experiences or judgments.

Older adult tasks. Peck delineated three tasks for old age. The first, *ego differentiation versus work preoccupation*, is important for maintaining a sense of self-esteem after retirement. This is achieved by reassigning the value of the work role to other roles and dimensions of life. The task of *body transcendence versus body preoccupation* involves recognizing physical decline but rising above aches and pains so that happiness is not defined by physical well-being. This task is exemplified by the person who experiences suffering but retains a zest and pleasure in life. The final task of old age, *ego transcendence versus ego preoccupation*, is very similar to Erikson's ego-integrity task. It denotes an ability to accept personal death without fear. It is neither a denial nor a passive resignation to death but an acceptance that moves the individual to be actively and emotionally involved in a legacy that continues. In contrast, the ego-preoccupied individual mires in the thought of personal death, unable to let go of life and immediate gratification.

Havighurst's Theory: Developmental Tasks

Havighurst has also proposed specific developmental tasks for each life stage.[3] (See Table 4-1 for the list of tasks. The listed order does not imply hierarchical arrangement.) Like Erikson, he contends that there are optimal points in life to master these tasks and that current mastery is contingent on having successfully mastered the tasks of previous life stages. Unlike Erikson and Peck, who focused on individual developmental tasks, Havighurst also included family-oriented tasks that are significant to individual development.

Levinson's Theory: Evolution of Life Structures

Levinson's basic concept, *individual life structure,* is the pattern of a given life at any point in time.[4] Life structure is formed by the interactions of self-system (for example, judgments, motives, and values), the social and cultural context of life (such as family, ethnicity, religion, occupation, and social events such as war and inflation), and the particular set of roles a person assumes (for example, husband/wife, worker, and friend). When any component changes, the life structure must reorganize (Fig. 4-2). Levinson considers some aspects of life structure, such as family and occupation, as central because they hold great significance to the individual; other aspects are peripheral because they are less critical and more fluid.

Life structure is dynamic, with predictable changes occurring as the individual moves through life. There are four major periods in adult life: early adulthood (age 20 to 40), middle adulthood (age 40 to 60), late adulthood (age 60 to 80), and late-late adulthood (beyond 80). Within each period the individual experiences alternating times of transition and stability in life structure. *Transitions* are a time of evaluating and making changes that permit growth and redirection of life toward identified goals and values. *Stable times* are those times for building on changes while maintaining an intact life structure to focus on the goals and values of that life period.

Early adult transition. The first transition is the *early adult transition,* which occurs between the ages of 18 and 22. The major concerns of this time are to terminate or

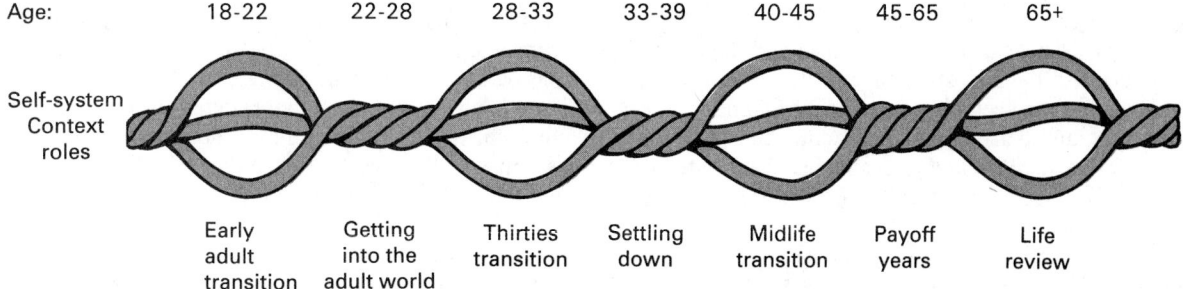

Age: 18-22   22-28   28-33   33-39   40-45   45-65   65+

Self-system
Context
roles

Early   Getting   Thirties   Settling   Midlife   Payoff   Life
adult   into the   transition down   transition years   review
transition   adult world

Fig. 4-2   An individual's life structure. According to Levinson's theory, life structure may be seen as a "life rope" in which the interacting strands are taken apart and individually reviewed during transition periods and are then rewoven in stable periods.

modify existing life structures and to make preliminary adult choices that move an individual toward new life structures, consolidating an initial adult identity. This transition includes breaking away from the family of origin; making an initial career choice; establishing new intimate relationships; and selecting personal goals, values, and a lifestyle (Fig. 4-3).

Entering the adult world. From ages 22 to 28, the young adult is *entering the adult world*. This is a time to grasp onto the adult world by doing what "should be done" as defined by external models such as family, peers, culture, and media. Concurrently, the young adult is working out a balance between building on previous choices and exploring alternative opportunities to avoid cementing the future prematurely. Because of this exploring, the occupational choices and relationships that are being established at this time may have a transient quality.

The thirties transition. The transition experienced between ages 28 and 33 may bring enrichment or dramatic changes to the life structure of the twenties. Previous commitments made to a mate, career, friends, and goals are evaluated with greater realism and a focus on self-directed rather than externally directed decisions. Single persons may consider marriage, unhappy marriages may terminate, childless couples may conceive or adopt, and careers may be left or reconfirmed with new vigor.

Settling down. During the thirties, there is a calm period referred to as *settling down*. This is a time of investing into those areas of life that are of primary importance, for example, family, work, friends, and community. During this time, establishing a place in society as a full-fledged adult is important so that an individual can advance and attain the goals that have been set. There is a striving toward exerting authority and gaining status and recognition with respect and reward from others.

Midlife transition. The *midlife transition,* occurring between ages 40 and 45, is the gateway into middle adulthood. This usually involves a profound reappraisal of life goals and values, with a concurrent emotional upheaval. Self-identity and authenticity are questioned and stripped of the illusions of young adulthood. All life structures are renegotiated, including marriage, friendships, occupation, and social roles. Time is realigned relative to the amount of time left to live. For some individuals, this transition results in a continuance of the previous lifestyle, but with

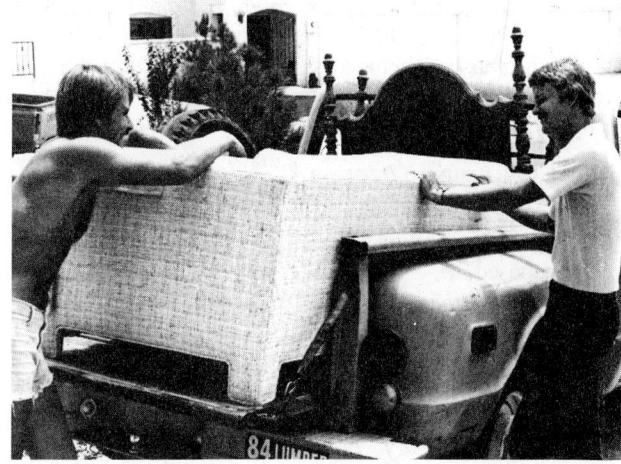

Fig. 4-3   The move from home to an apartment is an external sign of the early adult transition.

new confirmation and enthusiasm for the current life structure. For others, there are varying degrees of change and, in some cases, dramatic reorganization of life structures. For example, a person may return to school to complete previously aborted educational plans.

The payoff years. As middle adults emerge from the transitional stage, having reorganized or reaffirmed the direction of life, they enter into a time that may be very satisfying and creative. Ages 45 to 65 become the *payoff years* when people experience a time of maximum influence, heightened self-perception, self-approval, and self-direction. Middle adults can demonstrate wisdom and sound judgment as well as vision and innovation. Levinson projects that beyond middle age there is a continued growth process involving transition and stability based on previous life structures.

Psychosocial Aging Theories

Because developmental theories are least explicit about the later years of life, other theoretical approaches have been taken to explain the processes of aging. The *disengagement theory* proposes that successful psychosocial aging is characterized by a reciprocal decline in the involvement of the individual with society and society with the individual.[5] The criticism of this theory has focused on the proposition that disengagement is intrinsic and therefore a norm for successful aging. Disengagement will vary in old people depending on factors such as health, abilities, previous lifestyle, and personality type. Contrasting with disengagement, the *activity theory* maintains that continued productivity and social interaction are necessary for successful aging.[6] Although forms of activity may need to change because of reductions in physical health and strength, the level of activity with society should be commensurate with lifelong patterns. To remain engaged, the aging person will compensate for lost roles and activities by replacing them with new ones. The *identity continuity theory* proposes that adaptation to aging is correlated with the ability to maintain the same behavior patterns and lifestyle that existed before old age.[7] This continuity is maintained by selectively attending to those things that fit previously established behavioral patterns. However, in the present change-oriented society, maintaining consistencies in lifestyle is increasingly difficult.

Biological Aging Theories

No single set of theories can describe the multidimensional process of aging. Various biological theories have been proposed.

The *somatic mutation* and *intrinsic mutagenesis* theories postulate that aging is a result of life-long genetic damage.[8] This damage may include the progressive accumulation of faulty copying in dividing cells or the accumulation of errors in information-containing molecules. According to somatic mutation theory, body cells develop spontaneous mutations in the same way germ cells do. These mutations are presumably a result of life-long background radiation of various types. Subsequent cell divisions perpetuate the mutations until organs become inefficient and ultimately fail. The intrinsic mutagenesis theory suggests that the increase in mutational cells occurs because of a breakdown of genetic regulatory mechanisms. The basic premise is that the regulatory capacity of the human genetic constitution diminishes throughout life, and thus more mutations occur with aging that will ultimately result in functional failure. Although both theories are attractive, little evidence exists to support or deny them.

The *neuroaging theory* proposes that aging occurs because of functional decrements in neurons and associated hormones.[9] It suggests that neural and endocrine changes may be pacemakers for many cellular and physiological aspects of aging. This approach relates aging to the organism's loss of responsiveness of neuroendocrine tissue to various signals. In some cases, this is due to a loss of receptors, but in others, it is due to changes in neurotransmission beyond the receptors. An important focus of this theory is on the functional changes of the hypothalamic-pituitary system, which are accompanied by a decline in functional capacity in all systems.

The *immunological theory* proposes declining functional capacity of the immune system as the basis for the aging process.[10] It suggests that aging is not a passive wearing out of systems but an active self-destruction mediated by the immune system. This theory is based on ob-

serving an age-associated decline in T-cell functioning, accompanied by decreased resistance, and an increase in autoimmune diseases with aging. Whether the immunological changes are genetically determined, regulated by environment, or influenced by endocrine factors remains to be defined. However, some studies of cell division suggest that the cells of the immune system become more diversified with age and demonstrate a progressive loss of self-regulatory patterns between the body and the cell. The result is an auto-aggressive phenomenon in which cells normal to the body are mistaken as foreign and are attacked by the immune system or in which impaired surveillance by lymphocytes occurs.

PSYCHODYNAMIC ISSUES OF ADULTHOOD

Psychodynamic issues arise from confrontation between inner development and the demands of the social world. People continually try to find a comfortable fit between themselves and their world, attempting to integrate their sense of who they are and who they are becoming.

Self-Concept

Self-concept and self-esteem are interdependent constructs. *Self-concept* may be defined as the totality of ideas people hold about themselves, and *self-esteem* is self-evaluation, that is, satisfaction or dissatisfaction with these ideas.

Young adulthood. During the young adult years, a strong theme in self-concept is "I can handle it." A sense of mastery and self-control over life events and the environment prevails. The actions of young adults convey the attitude that self-will and boldness are the components of success. This confidence is a reflection of the high energy levels and the increasing power and control young adults experience over life when moving out of adolescence.

Middle adulthood. During the middle adult years, self-concept may vary greatly, depending on the perceived balance between positive and negative aspects of middle age. This perception is partially determined by culture, social class, personality, and health status. In some cultures, people are preprogrammed to consider themselves "old" at the age of 40; in others, people have just "made it" at this age. It has been found that working-class men may consider themselves old at 40, whereas professionals perceive old as after 70. Some middle-age people have the time of their life, with an increased sense of self-approval because of peak family and career investments in terms of power, prestige, and income and continued good health. In contrast, if people experience a decline in career or health, self-esteem may also decline.

The sense of self-control continues into middle age; however, during middle adulthood, people recognize the finiteness of life and shift to a more realistic appraisal of the limits of self-will. Recognizing that willpower alone does not overcome life circumstances, people become aware that help and advice from others can be valuable rather than allowing it to threaten self-esteem. With this new insight regarding self-will, middle-aged adults may also reevaluate a personal spiritual position, determining that placing trust in God is not a crutch for the weak per-

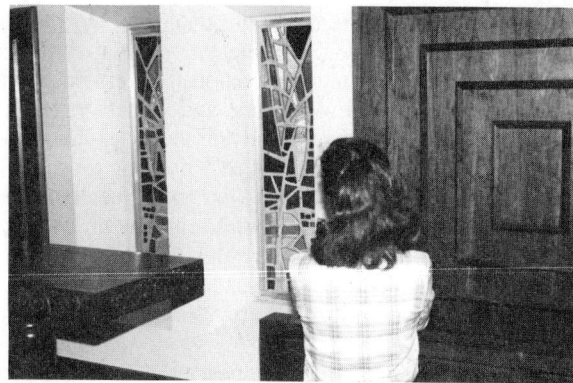

Fig. 4-4 An increasing awareness of spiritual needs often occurs in the middle years.

Table 4-2 Effects of Aging on Adult Mental Functioning

Function	Effect of Aging
Fluid intelligence	Declines during middle age
Crystallized intelligence	Improves
Vocabulary/verbal reasoning	Improves
Spatial perception	Constant or improves
Synthesis of new information	Declines during middle age
Mental performance speed	Declines during middle age
Short-term recall memory	Declines during old age
Long-term recall memory	Constant

sonality but a desire for living beyond human finiteness (Fig. 4-4).

Older adulthood. Although self-concept is usually stable from middle age to old age, it is not static. Life events experienced with aging (poor health, loss of income, loss of roles, isolation, relocation, and institutionalization) all serve to decrease the older adult's sense of control and may threaten self-esteem. However, it has been found that older people have compensatory mechanisms to offset some threats brought on by aging changes. A paradox exists in that age perception decreases with age. Older adults may think of other cohorts as being old according to social stereotypes attributed to old people. They may not perceive themselves, however, as old and will refuse to respond to others' suggestions that they are aging or need help or care. Another compensatory mechanism is that many older adults retain their middle-age self-concepts by thinking of themselves in their former roles. A retired farmer still thinks of himself as a farmer, or a school teacher as a teacher. Maintaining a consistent sense of self, making decisions, and managing life are clearly important to well-being at this stage of life. Autonomy and dignity are essential elements to an older adult's positive self-esteem.

Mental Functioning

Intelligence. Traditionally it has been held that intelligence declines after age 30. However, longitudinal research indicates that intellectual abilities can be improved or at least sustained until late adulthood.[11] In the months before death an older adult's intellectual abilities may decrease sharply. This change is part of a complex phenomenon called *terminal decline.*

The patterns of change in adult intelligence vary with the specific mental abilities measured (Table 4-2). *Fluid intelligence* consists of those abilities that are related to neurological development and includes associative power, memory, figural relationships, and visual-motor flexibility. Because of degenerative neurological changes, fluid intelligence may decline during middle age. *Crystallized intelligence* consists of those abilities that arise out of experience and the accumulation of learning and includes verbal comprehension, formal reasoning, and general information. Crystallized intelligence improves with age.

Several environmental and individual variables such as education, social class, illness, personality, and motivation affect adult intelligence. Generally, individuals who have had above-average IQs as young adults, who have obtained more years of formal education, and who have continued to use intellectual processes demonstrate greater increases in intelligence throughout adulthood.[12]

Nurses must recognize that speed in mental functioning may be a major problem for older adults. Because of central nervous system decline and sensory deficits such as poor eyesight, some older persons have trouble with quick thinking and performance. Old people perform equally as well as young people when time is not a factor. Because of this, any teaching or skills practice should be carefully planned to allow the older client adequate time for comprehension and performance without the pressure of hurrying.

Memory. Although many middle adults fear becoming forgetful, no real decline in memory has been demonstrated until old age. *Short-term memory* deteriorates first. This refers to immediate recall that requires information retention for a few seconds to a few minutes. An example is remembering how to dial an unfamiliar phone number after having read it in the phone book. The decline in short-term memory may be related to neurotransmission interference or temporary storage integration problems. Because neurotransmission is slower, older adults become vulnerable to interference from other stimuli, which impede acquisition and storage of information. Thus information cannot be retrieved later because it was inadequately registered. This short-term memory problem can have significant effects on the learning process, since learning new material often requires speed in acquisition, comprehension, and registration.

Long-term memory seems quite resistant to aging. It is often noted that older adults can describe in minute detail past life events yet forget recent ones. This recall ability for past events may be attributed to the fact that once information is registered, people retain a sound memory for it. It is also likely that the memory for past events is firmly consolidated because the details have been previously re-called and rehearsed by the person.

Another memory difficulty in older adults is the inability to recall specifics after recognizing a person or a place. For example, a grandmother may recognize her grandchild but call him by another family member's name. In this case, she has placed the child in the family, recognizing the person, but cannot recall the name. This problem seems to be in the retrieval process rather than in registration of information.

In addition to aging changes, the memory of an older adult is affected by health status, drugs, education, amount of stimulation, motivation, and the meaningfulness of the material.

Sexuality

Sexuality is a broad concept that incorporates physiological characteristics, attitudes, values, and behaviors related to gender perceptions. The task of developing a compatibility between gender identity and self-expression of sex-related roles is vital to self-concept integration during adulthood. This is an ongoing task that pervades practically all aspects of adult life, including mate selection, career choices, friendships, and all forms of self-expression.

Young adulthood. For the young adult, gender identity and sexual relationships are primary concerns in achieving a sexual self-concept and sense of intimacy. Although intimacy transcends a sexual relationship to include affiliative sharing, for the sexually active young adult intimacy is usually established by commitment to a relationship that includes an expression of affection and physical sexuality. Sexual performance in a marriage relationship represents more than physical pleasure. It becomes an expression of caring and closeness, which helps the couple find satisfaction in sharing their work, play, childbearing, and child-rearing activities. It has been found that young couples who are satisfied with their sexual relationship are most often satisfied with their overall marriage and vice versa.

For some, a homosexual relationship provides a feeling of intimacy and comfort. Just as in heterosexual individuals, homosexual men and women vary greatly in their emotional and social adjustments. The increased incidence and identification of the life-threatening disease AIDS appears to have caused a drastic change in the lifestyles of those homosexuals who were accustomed to multiple partners.

Young adults are in the prime of physical and reproductive performance. Many of their biosocial concerns center around sexual activity, including cyclic changes in sexual arousal and orgasm, use and selection of contraceptives, sexual changes with pregnancy and postpartum, abortion, infertility, and sexually transmitted diseases. It has been found that in men the peak sexual drive and responsiveness occurs during the late teens and early twenties, whereas this peak occurs between the ages of 30 to 45 in women. However, most healthy adults maintain a strong sex drive beyond the age of 70.

Middle adulthood. During the middle years, both men and women experience hormonal declines that produce physiological changes affecting sexual desire and respon-

siveness. However, more important than the physiological changes are the psychological expectations related to these changes. It has been found that menopausal and postmenopausal women have fewer fears and negative feelings about the effects of menopause on their sexuality than young adult women. Rather than experiencing a decline in sexual capacity, postmenopausal women frequently experience an increased libido and greater enjoyment. With the male climacteric, the decline in testosterone may result in a decreased libido and a slower sexual arousal and climax, but these changes do not necessarily lessen the pleasure of sexual intercourse.

Factors probably more important than hormonal changes that negatively affect sexual activity in the middle years include monotony in a repetitious sexual pattern, boredom with a relationship, career and economic preoccupation, mental and physical fatigue, excessive eating or drinking, and fear of sexual failure. Becoming a victim to the myth that a youthful body is equated with sexual desirability and potency also negatively affects sexual activity. Middle-aged adults are at risk for the potential onset of chronic illnesses that may affect libido. Also, they may be taking a variety of prescribed drugs that can reduce sexual responsiveness.

Sexual activity continues to be a very important part of middle adult life. Satisfaction with sexual life in the middle years is not as related to frequency of intercourse as to vitality in the relationship and enjoyment derived from all sexual experiences in younger years.

Older adulthood. Although our society attributes sexlessness to the older adult, people are sexual beings throughout their lives. Most studies attest to continued sexual activity well into the last decades of life for men and women who have been sexually active as young and middle adults. Physical changes in the sexual organs should not be considered as biological limiters of sexual activity, nor should they reduce the satisfaction experienced by sexual partners. The most important criteria for remaining sexually active in old age are a receptive partner, reasonable physical health, and a positive attitude about regular sexual activity.

Because society has been slow to recognize the sexual needs of older adults and most older adults have been socialized to not talk about sex, identifying and intervening in sex-related problems is difficult for caregivers. It has been suggested that sex education programs be developed for older adults to inform them of normal changes and to help them cope with unmet sexual needs and with social and familial attitudes about continued sexual activity.

Intimacy. In a broad context, *intimacy* incorporates the concept of attachment or seeking a relationship in which an individual can maintain contact or proximity to the object of attachment. From this perspective, intimacy is a need that is manifest from conception to death and does not decrease in intensity or significance throughout adulthood. Intimacy is maintained *physically* by touching, stroking, patting, hugging, kissing, and usually through sexual intercourse. It is maintained *emotionally* by sharing joys, sorrows, affection, ideas, and values.

Throughout life, touch plays an important role in receiving and expressing intimacy. However, as hearing and sight decline with age, reaching out to touch becomes an even more important way to make intimate physical contact. Old people often attempt to touch and be touched by others to experience some sense of physical closeness. The response to their touch communicates a message of acceptance or nonacceptance that may never have been expressed verbally.

The need for expressing physical intimacy in behaviors having sexual connotations is often disregarded for older adults. Although these expressions are accepted as normal in younger adults, they may be viewed with disdain and disapproval or as an amusing and childish behavior when expressed by old people. This disregard is seen in some institutional structures and policies. Many nursing homes provide little opportunity for expression of sexual needs. Private rooms and locked doors often are neither provided nor respected. Older adult couples may be segregated and placed on separate men's and women's units or, if in the same room, may have single beds. Is it any wonder that an older person, who has for years shared a bed with a spouse, becomes disoriented at night and wanders around or gets into bed with someone else? The youth-oriented society has developed skewed ideas about appropriate sexual behavior in older adults and as a result has placed severe restrictions on intimate relationships during old age.

SOCIAL PROCESSES IN ADULTHOOD

Adulthood is lived out in a social context with major developmental tasks being determined by the interaction of individuals with their social systems. Adult social concerns primarily involve the family, work and leisure, and community responsibilities.

Family and Adult Development

Throughout life the family is the major socializing institution for its members. A global survey of people representing 70 nations found that family life is overwhelmingly the greatest source of satisfaction and happiness for most people.[13] The family is a focal source for adults in meeting their needs for emotional security, belonging, love, companionship, esteem, and approval from others. The process of family development reflects the developmental changes occurring in the adult members. (See Table 4-3 for a summary of family tasks during adulthood.)

Young adulthood. Emancipation from the family of origin is the first family task of young adulthood. This usually occurs as a gradual process that includes physical, economic, and emotional independence from parents. However, emancipation is not the end of a relationship with the family but rather the first step to establishing an interdependent adult relationship between young adults and their parents.

Often concurrent with emancipation from the family of origin, the young adult establishes a new family system in which roles, relationships, and expectations are being determined. This usually includes adjusting to an intimate relationship requiring a high level of communication and compromise and adapting to the predictable crises of childbearing. Stress is frequently high in the emerging young adult family because of the multiplicity of changing relationships and structures. Also, the work trajectories for both husband and wife are often launched and new outside demands are placed on adult family members. Because of these changes, the emerging family may easily become dysfunctional. This is reflected in the fact that the highest divorce rate occurs during the first 3 to 5 years of marriage for young adults under the age of 30.

Following the initial family transition, young adults move into a more stable, comfortable family life period. Commitment to the success of the family is high, and there is less turmoil with children, who are usually now in middle childhood. Couples without children also find this to be a time for strengthening relationships with each other and their social group.

Middle adulthood. Middle adults find themselves caught in the "family sandwich" between the needs of their children and their aging parents. Family life can be stressful because it is a complex chore to concurrently work through a midlife identity transition, the identity confusion of teenagers, and the redefinition of family roles and relationships in both the families of origin and marriage and parenthood.

Disenchantment with the marital relationship is frequently experienced by middle-aged adults. Research has demonstrated that married couples are least satisfied with each other when they are between the ages of 40 and 50. There are multiple contributing factors to this dissatisfaction. A husband or wife may be preoccupied or confused about occupational goals and blame the spouse for per-

Table 4-3 Family Tasks in Adult Development

Young Adulthood	Middle Adulthood	Older Adulthood
Emancipating from family of origin	Assisting teenage children to become responsible adults	Establishing satisfactory living arrangements with limited income
Establishing interdependent adult relationship with parents	Restructuring relationship with spouse as children leave home	Restructuring family roles and responsibilities after retirement
Selecting mate and adjusting to intimate relationship	Restructuring relationship with aging parents	Adapting living arrangements to meet problems caused by physical decline
Adapting family system to demands of childbearing	Adjusting to death of parents	Adjusting to death of spouse
Finding balance to family, work, and social demands	Defining roles and responsibilities of grandparent	

sonal dissatisfaction. Some middle-aged adults may feel that self-development needs were sacrificed for a spouse's job and the family. Also, the financial and emotional strain of having adolescent children may come between a husband and wife. Although the divorce rate is not quite as high during middle adulthood as during early young adulthood, it does increase again during the years shortly after children leave home.

Middle-aged couples who recommit themselves to their spouses and a continuing marriage find marital satisfaction frequently hits a new high. Although much discussion has been heard about the crisis of the "empty nest," many middle-aged men and women experience a new sense of self and unity as a couple after the children leave home. They again define their relationship as lovers and companions, rather than as parents. In many ways the postparental years become the payoff for investing in a mutual relationship with shared problems and joys, if the couple survives the trials of the midlife marriage.

During middle age, adults often come to appreciate their parents and understand the problems of old people in a new way. When the aging parent is in good health and basically self-reliant, the parent-child relationship is usually characterized by a friendship that is quite satisfactory to both. If aging parents are confronted with problems such as inadequate finances, ill health, or death of a spouse that make it impossible for them to remain independent, the parent-child relationship and roles may be restructured. A very difficult and sometimes necessary role reversal occurs when a middle-aged child must become the parent to a parent. This requires giving up feelings of dependency on the parent and often assuming an uncomfortable authority role, which the older adult parent may find difficult to relinquish. The manner in which the middle-aged adult responds to the parent's dependency needs will be determined by the previous relationship, available resources, and the other responsibilities of the middle-aged adult. Eventually, many middle-aged adults must deal with their feelings about the death of parents. Although little has been done to study the family changes at this time, becoming a member of the family's oldest generation because of the death of parents is an important phase in family life.

Grandparenting. An increasing number of adults today become grandparents during middle adulthood (Fig. 4-5). This new social role may have a positive or negative impact on the grandparent's self-esteem. To some it is met with excitement and anticipation; for others it represents "growing old," which conflicts with how the grandparent wants to feel.

Older adulthood. The onset of this final period in family life is generally considered to be marked by retirement and poses new and unique developmental tasks for the aging family. The first task is to establish satisfactory living arrangements within a limited income, considering the role changes brought on by retirement and the physical incapacities of aging. In terms of living arrangements, most older adults live in their own households[14] (see Table 4-4). Presently, the majority of the older generation prefer independent living rather than living with children. However,

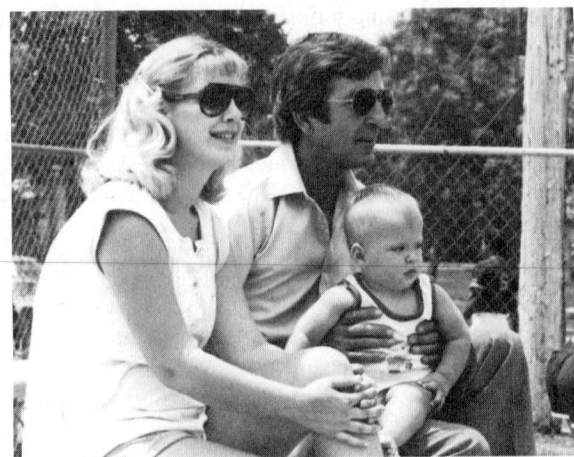

Fig. 4-5 The active grandparent plays a positive role in the lives of the child and the grandchild.

Table 4-4 Living Arrangements for Persons over 65 Years of Age

	Percentage of Men	Percentage of Women
Living in household	99.7	99.5
Living alone	15.4	40.9
Spouse present	76.7	38.7
Living with someone else	7.6	19.9
Not in household (e.g., institutions)	0.3	0.5

From US Department of Commerce, US Bureau of Commerce: Statistical abstract of the United States 1985, Washington, DC, 1985.

contact with children is frequent; 73% of older adults have at least one child living less than 30 minutes away, and 77% have contact with a child each week.[15] For older adults who are in relatively good health and have an adequate income, living in their own homes rather than with family members allows them to maintain a sense of privacy, competency, and independence (Fig. 4-6).

Being able to adjust family responsibilities and routines becomes an important part of the adaptation a couple must make following retirement. Schedules and activities are readjusted, and a retiree will frequently turn to family members to meet self-esteem needs that were previously met by the referent work group.

Loss of a spouse. The loss of a spouse is a major crisis at any stage in life. The reaction to a spouse's death may vary, depending on how compatible the relationship was; the circumstances of the death; the available support systems, including family and religious beliefs; the physiological independence of the survivor; and the adequacy of financial resources. Although the degree of marital happiness varies for older adults, couples who have had a long marriage have generally established an interdependent symbiotic relationship that gives them a great deal of pleasure during their later years.

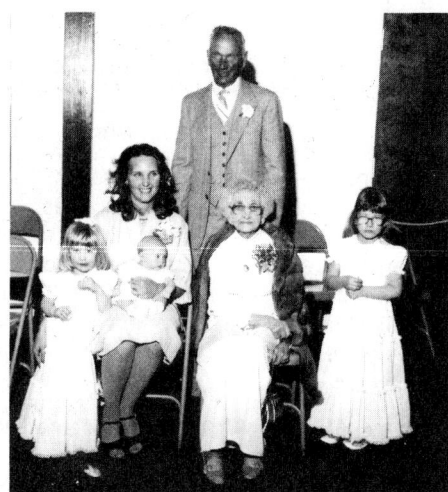

Fig. 4-6 This four-generation family demonstrates that the children of an older grandparent may themselves be old.

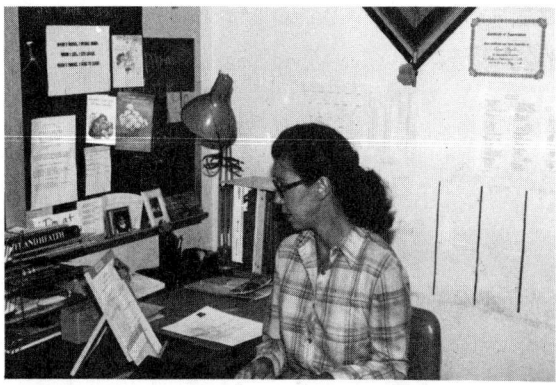

Fig. 4-7 The middle-aged woman may experience the same career clock as a man because of economic concerns and greater life choices.

Developing a new social identity and adjusting living arrangements are major tasks of adjusting to loss of a spouse. For many, this is a time when they are socially marooned unless they actively seek out activities they can participate in without a spouse. Some older adults choose to move in with family members; others move to smaller apartments, trailers, or a community for older adults. In any case, relocation may be an additional trauma.

Remarriage becomes an alternative to living alone or to living with children or friends. Most older adults remarry for companionship, and although there is the danger of idealizing the deceased mate and making unrealistic comparisons with the new spouse, most of these remarriages are happy.

Singlehood and single parenting. Single adults include the never-married, separated, and divorced and those who have lost a spouse. Some people choose not to marry or remarry because of personal freedom and development; career goals; family responsibilities to parents, siblings, or children; ill health; or the inability to find a compatible mate. Those who prefer to remain single value their roles and contributions to society. They do not see the unmarried state as a period of waiting.

A change in the traditional American family is the single-parent family. Most often, single parenting results from divorce or death of the spouse. However, some single persons choose to have children by adoption, artificial insemination, surrogate parenting, or pregnancy. A major stress for single parents is playing all the roles of mother and father that are necessary for discipline and socialization of the child. Some of this role overload may be relieved by joint child custody in the case of divorce and by other members of the extended family. Downward economic mobility is a frequent problem faced by the single-parent mother.

Divorce. Multiple social and individual factors contribute to family dissolution. Divorce is a source of personal crisis for all family members and as such affects their physical and mental health status. Developmentally, it re-quires that a reorientation process be started. Each family member must make adjustments in self-identity and establish new social roles. This process is harder for middle-aged and older adults, since life patterns and the incorporation of a spouse into personal identity have been well established.

Community Life in Adulthood

Participating in community life is a major developmental task of adulthood. Personal and family well-being strongly depends on successful interactions with the community via work, leisure, and civic participation.

Work and young adulthood. Work provides more than just the financial means to support a standard of living. It becomes a salient feature of personal identity and self-concept. Launching a career is the first point in the work cycle and occurs in young adulthood for most men and women. This entry point confronts the young adult with many potentially stressful role adjustments on the job and within the family. The interactions of family and work life cycles become more complex in a two-career family in which husband and wife are seeking career advancements.

Work and the middle-age career clock. The second major occupational crisis occurs during middle age when people assess if they are "on time" or "behind time" according to their personal career clock (Fig. 4-7). With the perspective of time until retirement, occupational goals often need to be revised toward more realistic expectations.

Since the middle-aged adult is frequently at the peak of job performance, work may become the pivot around which all relationships and activities are ordered. Because the job is so central, job stresses and dissatisfaction can have profound effects on physical and mental health. Also, the person who develops health problems that impede the ability to work or threaten career timing will experience less job satisfaction, thus producing a vicious, stressful circle. Frequently, nurses must help middle-aged clients adjust to job restrictions created by hospitalization and medical regimens.

Table 4-5 Work Cycle

Work	Young Adulthood	Middle Adulthood	Older Adulthood
Focus	Career launch	Midlife career crisis	Retirement
Expectations	Reorganization of time Job role adjustments Family role adjustments	Measurement of accomplishments against goals Revision of unrealistic career goals with the perspective of time until retirement If desired, change of jobs and/or careers before it is "too late"	Reorganization of time and daily activities Family role adjustments Establishment of referent group other than co-workers
Major problems	Expectations for job not congruent with reality "Now is the time to make it" attitude with an imbalance between work, family, and personal development needs	Sense of occupational failure and frustration if unable to give up idealistic young adult goals and set realistic current goals Ego deflation with being at the "entry level" of a new career when changing careers at midlife	Lowered income and standard of living Loss of self-esteem if unable to transfer status from the work role to other roles Psychological mark of old age

Retirement. Retirement is the third major event in the occupation cycle. The significant issues adults must face with retirement include a lowered income, which can have profound effects on lifestyle; loss of work role and associated relationships, which are part of the individual's personal identity and social status; a readjustment of time and restructuring of daily activities; a change in family roles and arrangements; and the psychological mark of old age, which increases awareness of the aging process. However, with improved retirement benefits and better pension plans, more individuals are choosing to retire early. They view retirement as a reward for past productivity and an opportunity to pursue new goals and satisfy previously unmet needs.

The transition from employed to retired is less stressful when the person has comprehensively planned for retirement. Gerontological nurses should take significant roles in preparing clients for the predictable stresses that occur with retirement and thus lessen some of the potential crises of this major life change. Table 4-5 further describes the work cycle.

Leisure During Adulthood

The concept of leisure is becoming more important in society. It is of interest not only to the retiree but also to young and middle-aged adults who are experiencing more nonwork time and need to determine how to spend this time in a satisfying manner. In general, the amount of available leisure time increases as an individual moves from young adulthood to retirement (Table 4-6). During any life stage, the occupational choice and leisure are interdependent. The job heavily influences the amount of leisure time available, as do financial resources and the physical and mental energy left for leisure activities.

Young adulthood. Young adults often have very busy schedules with little time for leisure. Attempts to balance work, school, family responsibilities, and leisure often result in frustration. The forms of leisure they engage in are affected by personal interests and social factors, including marriage and parenting roles, new friendships, occupational choices, and financial resources.

Middle adulthood. The leisure patterns in middle adulthood change slightly from young adulthood because of physical and social changes in this stage of life. The use of leisure time is an important concern for middle-aged adults because they are beginning to prepare for retirement. During this time, they can develop interests that can be continued into the retirement years and bridge the gap from the working life to full-time leisure.

Older adulthood. Older adults tend to continue to fill their time with the leisure activities they enjoyed in middle age, as long as their health and finances remain adequate. However, as more older adults have opportunities to participate in a variety of programs such as those provided by senior centers, they can increase their scope of activities and do the things they have never tried before. Government programs at federal, state, and local levels as well as private enterprise have joined to help provide and make leisure activities more accessible to older people. The Older American Act has established funds and programs such as multipurpose senior citizens' centers, which provide a variety of activities including classes, recreational activities, arrangements for discount tickets for entertainment programs and travel, and special education programs.

Older adults use their leisure time in self-oriented activities and they also contribute much to society through their volunteer services. Volunteering provides older adults with an opportunity to share their talents and to participate in meaningful activities that fill a need in society.

With continued aging and decline in health, older people may engage in more homebound solitary activities, such as relaxing in a rocking chair, thinking, daydream-

Table 4-6 Adult Leisure Time

	Young Adulthood	Middle Adulthood	Older Adulthood
Time factor	Minimal pure leisure time because of holding second job or going to school and working full time	Increasing amounts of available time because of usually greater occupational stability and less time spent on child-rearing activities	Possibly too much available time
Cost factor	Financial resources limiting time spent and type of leisure activities pursued	More money available for leisure because of higher earning power	Reduced and fixed incomes limiting activities Reduction of cost of leisure activities for retired citizens because of government programs
General types of leisure	Activities that sustain marital and family closeness such as family outings and home entertainment Activities with other young families Activities with same-sex friends such as sports and arts and crafts	Less home-centered activities because of greater freedom; traveling, going out with friends Activities that are less physically demanding and do not require quick reflexes Activities oriented toward health maintenance; swimming, jogging, exercising	Activities enjoyed during middle adulthood if health and finances permit Creative arts and crafts and recreational activities such as cards and dancing Activities with family members and friends Volunteer services such as Foster Grandparents

ing, people watching, and patting a pet. In general, the leisure activities of older adults are determined by their health, previous activities, money, and current expectations about what they can do (Fig. 4-8).

Civic Participation

Participation in community through civic and governmental organizations, church groups, professional groups, and special interest groups begins in young adulthood, peaks in middle adulthood, and generally declines during old age. Because young adults are very involved with the commitments of establishing an overall lifestyle, including a family, career, and friendships, their time and energy are limited for consistent participation in community activities.

Although society is youth oriented, the control is held by middle-aged and older adults. This becomes apparent when examining the ages of individuals who are in high decision-making positions at all levels of government and private enterprise. Middle-aged adults not only participate in more community and professional activities, they also have developed the expertise and leadership qualities to participate at higher organizational levels. The increase in political activism among middle-aged women has become especially prominent because of their successful election attempts. In general, middle-aged men and women are at the peak of their influence and responsibility for the affairs of society in local, national, and international arenas. Older people who have been active in their communities will usually remain active as long as their health and income permit.

With the growing population of older adults, various forms of retirement communities have arisen. These in-

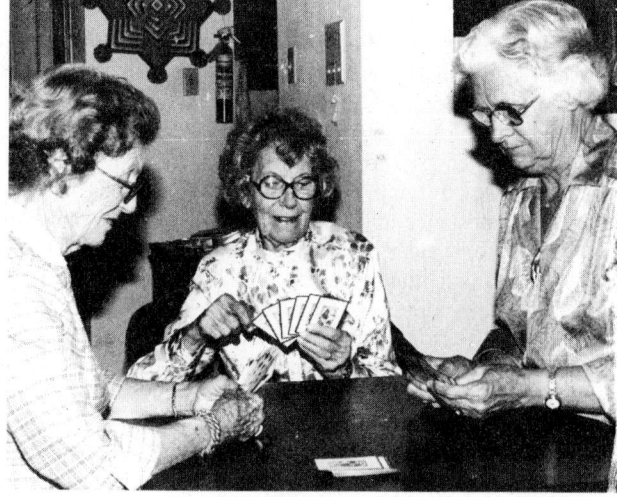

Fig. 4-8 Good friends and pleasant activities help fill the lives of active older adults.

clude communities with private homes, condominiums, apartment complexes, and recreational vehicles in organized private campgrounds for retired people. Older adults who live in these communities become very involved with all aspects of their community's life. Older adults also remain politically active and organize for their own causes, in groups such as the American Association of Retired Persons, National Council of Senior Citizens, and the Gray Panthers. Most politicians recognize the political strength of older adults as a group because of their organizations and the fact that they vote. In a recent presidential election the population over the age of 65 represented

Table 4-7 Civic Participation in Adulthood

	Young Adulthood	Middle Adulthood	Older Adulthood
Factors encouraging/ discouraging involvement	Time and energy for civic involvement limited because of family and career commitments	Concern for future of society fostering civic participation as a priority	Available time, resources, and special interest causes encouraging civic participation Declining health reducing ability to participate
Type of participation	Activities perceived as having direct bearing on day-to-day lives, such as labor unions, PTA, church activities Participation usually at the local level	Increased political and professional activity Leadership and decision-making positions at all levels of government and private enterprise	Civic involvements begun during the middle-adult years continuing Retirement community activities Political involvement, including political action groups that promote legislation for causes of special interest to older adults

15.4% of the total potential voters but cast 16.8% of the total votes.[15] Table 4-7 further describes civic activities.

PHYSIOLOGICAL PROCESSES IN ADULTHOOD

Having a healthy body is truly an asset and can be a major factor in having positive or negative feelings.

Physiological Changes during Adulthood

The young adult body is generally at its peak of health and performance. Although the physical changes associated with aging are beginning at this time, the effects are not yet great enough to require attention. Extrinsic factors such as accidents and physical stressors such as lack of sleep and substance abuse are the most common source of disabling biophysical problems in young adults.

Structural and functional body changes that were unnoticed in young adulthood may begin to be apparent during middle age. The rate and expression of physiological aging changes are highly individual. Frequently, changes in physical appearance such as dry skin, wrinkles, thinning and graying hair, and inches on the waist and hips are the first noticeable clues of aging. Sometime during the middle years, most adults notice that muscle strength and agility are declining, but on a day-to-day basis, most people make small compensations that minimize the effects of these changes. While the middle-aged individual is aware of these signs of aging, changes in the vital organs are often going on unnoticed. Table 4-8 describes physiological changes resulting from the aging process.[16,17] Because these changes involve aging rather than a pathological process, they begin insidiously in young adulthood, becoming more apparent in middle adulthood, and culminating in death, when the body can no longer compensate for or adapt to the changes.

Although many older people remain vigorous beyond the age of 80, the general decline in all systems and reduction of normally functioning cells caused by aging decrease the older person's overall ability to withstand and adapt to physical or emotional stress. When one system is placed under stress, there is a domino effect; without the ability to compensate, all systems may collapse. For example, the older person who breaks a hip and is immobilized is more vulnerable to urinary problems due to reduced renal function; respiratory problems due to weakened muscles and rigid respiratory tissue; circulatory problems due to decreased cardiac output; skin problems due to thin skin and decreased peripheral circulation; gastrointestinal problems due to decreased esophageal, stomach, and bowel motility; and confusion due to decreased sensory input. Thus, maintaining physical and emotional integrity in the older person can be very precarious.

Considerations for Health Maintenance

Young adulthood. Although the young adult years are a time of generally good physical and emotional health, the young adult lifestyle may hold potential health hazards. Accidents, sleep deprivation, substance abuse, inactivity, obesity, exposure to environmental and occupational hazards, and stress-related illnesses such as ulcers, depression, and suicide are important health problems during this time of life. Chronic illnesses such as hypertension, coronary artery disease, and diabetes may have their onset in young adulthood without being known to the young adult but become serious health threats later.

Middle adulthood. The middle-aged lifestyle should be assessed for areas that are detrimental to health. With a decline in strength and stamina, daily exercise is essential; however, sporadic weekend exercise or competitive physical overexertion can lead to injury (Fig. 4-9). Reducing caloric intake is often necessary to prevent weight gain. This may be particularly difficult for middle-aged adults whose social and business lifestyles encourage overindulgence at dinners and parties. Life pressures frequently mount during middle age, and a variety of substances may be used and overconsumed to cope, including cigarettes, alcohol, and tranquilizers. Rather than relying on these, the individual may need assistance to deal with the sources of pressure.

Table 4-8   Anatomical and Physiological Changes with Aging

System	Normal Aging Changes	Outcomes
CARDIOVASCULAR		
Cardiac function	Decreased force of contraction Decreased stroke volume Decreased cardiac volume	Decreased cardiac output by 1% per year after the age of 30 Decreased peripheral circulation Decreased blood flow to liver, GI tract, kidneys; maximum supply to brain and heart Decreased physical endurance (increased fatigue)
Cardiac rate	Unchanged resting state rate with age Increase in output with exercise but to reduced maximal rate Slowed response to stress with only slightly increased rate Slowed return to basal levels	Maximum attained rate (20-year-old, 200/min; 80-year-old, 120/min) Decreased ability to compensate for stress Absence of increased pulse rate masking shock or infection
Blood vessels	Straightening, fragmentation of elastic fibers Accumulation of collagen and calcium	Decreased resilience and distensibility Normal increase in BP (20-year-old, 120/80; 65-year-old, 160/90)
RESPIRATORY	Thickening of alveolar walls; decreased recoil Loss of interalveolar septi; decreased number of alveoli/larger size Decreased maximal breathing capacity Increased residual air and dead space Decreased ciliary movement Decreased strength of expiratory muscles Increased thoracic wall rigidity	Decreased endurance; easily fatigued Decreased capacity for deep breathing and coughing Increased potential for lower respiratory tract infection
EXCRETORY		
Kidney	Decline in kidney function 50% from age 20 to age 90 Decreased nephrons, 40% fewer by age 85 Decreased renal plasma flow Decreased glomerular filtration rate (age 40, normal GFR 120 mL/min; age 85, normal GFR 60–70 mL/min)	Increased protein in urine Increased BUN Increased drug toxicity Increased potential for electrolyte imbalance Increased potential for dehydration
Bladder	Decreased muscle tone Decreased sphincter control Decreased capacity	Urinary retention, dribbling Increased potential for infection
GASTROINTESTINAL	Loss of teeth/dentures Decreased taste buds Decreased saliva volume and salivary amylase Decreased tone and motility of esophagus, stomach, intestines Decreased gastric acid production Decreased external intestinal sphincter reflex Increased biliary stones	Soft diet necessary Increased potential for hiatal hernia Difficulty swallowing, especially in supine position Increased potential for aspiration Increased potential for food intolerances, malnutrition Increased potential for constipation Increased potential for fecal incontinence
ENDOCRINE		
Pancreas	Delayed insulin release Reduced peripheral sensitivity to insulin	Decreased glucose tolerance Slower return to fasting level
Gonads Male	Decreased testosterone production	Decreased libido; reproductive capacity remaining
Female	Decreased estrogen/progesterone levels after menopause	No reproductive capacity Atrophy of reproductive structures

Continued.

Table 4-8 Anatomical and Physiological Changes with Aging—cont'd

System	Normal Aging Changes	Outcomes
IMMUNOLOGICAL	Thymic atrophy Decreased response to antigens Decreased natural antibodies Decreased immune surveillance Increased autoantibodies	Decreased T lymphocytes Increased susceptibility to infections Increased incidence of malignancies Increased autoimmune disease
MUSCULOSKELETAL		
Muscles	Decreased mass; replacement of muscle cells with adipose tissue More rigid collagen fibers	Decreased strength, endurance, agility 10% decline age 30–60 Flabby appearance
Bones	Decreased mass, demineralization, protein matrix loss (greatest in postmenopausal women)	Increased brittleness and fractures Potential osteoporosis
Joints	Cartilage erosion Increased calcium deposits Decreased water in cartilage	Painful articulation, crepitation Decreased range of motion Narrowing of joint spaces Shortened vertebral column, decreased height Kyphosis
INTEGUMENTARY		
Skin	Decreased subcutaneous fat Decreased sweat glands Decreased extracellular water Decreased melanin Decreased receptors Decreased circulation to extremities	Wrinkles; bags under eyes Decreased homeostatic balance Thin, dry skin; easily bruised Liver spots Decreased pain sensitivity Nonhealing skin lesions
Hair	Thinning/loss Decreased pigment and oil	Alopecia Gray, dry hair
Nails	Decreased peripheral blood supply Increased keratin	Thickened, brittle nails Ridging, callus formation
NERVOUS		
Brain	Decreased number of cells Decreased pyramidal tract function Decreased blood flow and oxygen utilization Increased plaque/pigment accumulation	Reduced speed of mental processing Impaired proprioception Loss of balance/coordination Decreased CNS integration; more prolonged response to stress
Nerves	Decreased conduction velocity	Slower response/reaction time
Receptors	Decreased number/function	Decreased sensory input Potential depression
SENSORY		
Vision	Decreased acuity/accommodation/visual fields Decreased pupil size/dark adaptation Decreased cones in retina Decreased lens clarity (lens yellows with age) Decreased lacrimal secretion	Decreased visual input Decreased binocular depth perception Decreased color discrimination at blue spectrum Increased sensitivity to glare
Hearing	Decreased acuity/pitch discrimination Decreased sensitivity to higher frequency Increased keratin/cerumen Tympanic membrane sclerosis Vestibular cone degeneration	Potential hearing loss; depression Impaired speech reception Diminished sound conduction Tinnitus Body sway/dizziness
Taste	Decreased number/function of taste buds	Increased taste-threshold level
Smell	Fiber loss in olfactory bulb Cellular degeneration in parietal lobe	Diminished sense of smell; food less pleasing
Touch	Decreased receptors	Less sensitive to tactile environment

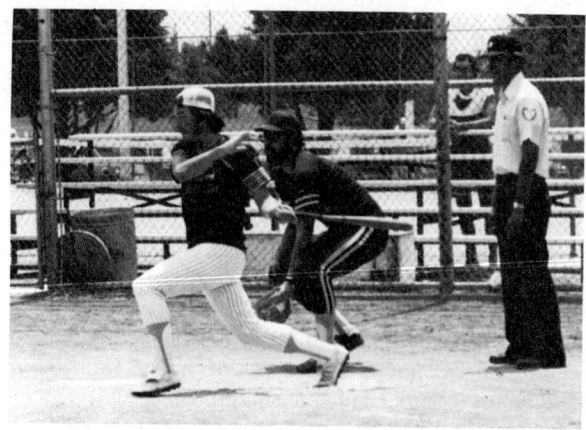

Fig. 4-9 Both young and middle-aged adults are subject to injuries associated with sporadic activity.

Middle-aged adults need to be encouraged to seek routine medical and dental examinations directed toward disease prevention and early treatment of problems. The Surgeon General's Report recommends annual dental and biannual physical examinations for healthy middle-aged adults. It also recommends Pap smears every 3 years, unless estrogen therapy or oral contraceptives are being used, and yearly mammography after the age of 40 for women with a family history of breast cancer. After the age of 50, mammography is recommended yearly when the personal and family history are negative for breast cancer.[18] Nurses have a fundamental role in health maintenance care by educating and promoting self-care responsibility among middle-aged adults.

Although many middle-aged adults feel they are in the prime of life, a rising incidence of chronic illnesses is associated with middle age. In addition to those that continue into middle age from young adulthood, some major health concerns are heart and vascular disease, cancer, liver cirrhosis, diabetes, and sexual dysfunctions.

Older adulthood. An estimated 86% of the population over 65 has one or more chronic conditions with varying degrees of disability.[19] The health problems of older people reflect past health and lifestyle influences. The major problems include chronic or recurrent conditions from earlier adult stages, chronic brain syndrome, degenerative bone and joint diseases, malnutrition, acute and chronic respiratory diseases, renal diseases, drug-induced problems, and mental disorders.

The health of older adults is influenced not only by pathophysiological disease processes but also by the process of aging. Although the aging process cannot be stopped, the effects can be reduced by good health habits, including proper nutrition, activity and rest, safety, and correct drug usage.

Nutrition. Maintaining adequate nutrition can be a problem for older adults for multiple physical and social reasons. Physiologically, food may be less appealing with the decline in taste and smell, and chewing is more difficult with dentures or loss of teeth. Swallowing and digestive problems may also accompany eating because of decreases in saliva, gastric motility, and enzyme production. So-

cially, if a person eats alone, snacking on quick foods is easier than preparing meals. The lack of transportation or access to a grocery store, inability to see the merchandise, and financial poverty may be additional factors in poor nutrition. However, obesity is a problem for some older adults. Usually this problem has arisen earlier in adulthood and continues because of difficulty in changing lifelong eating patterns.

Sleep. Sleep is often a concern to older adults because of changed sleep patterns. Older people no longer experience the stage IV deep sleep and are easily aroused. As a result, they cannot maintain a prolonged night sleep. Even though the demand for sleep decreases with age, older adults may be disturbed by insomnia and complain that they spend more time in bed but still feel tired. Frequently, older persons prefer to spread their sleep throughout the 24 hours with short naps providing adequate rest.

Safety. Environmental safety is crucial in health maintenance for older people. With normal sensory changes, slowed reaction time, decreased thermal and pain sensitivity, changes in gait and balance, and medication effects, older adults are prone to accidents. Most accidents occur in or around the home. Falls, motor vehicle accidents, and fires are the common causes for accidental death in older adults.[16] Another environmental problem arises from an impaired thermoregulating system that cannot adapt to extremes in environmental temperatures. An older adult's body can neither conserve nor dissipate heat efficiently; therefore, both hypothermia and heat prostration occur more readily. This age group accounts for the majority of mortality statistics during severe cold spells and heat waves.

Medications. Medication use poses a number of potential health problems for older adults. Because of altered drug metabolism and excretion, individual sensitivities and side effects occur more readily. Drug interactions can occur because many older adults take multiple prescription and nonprescription drugs. Self-medication is often a hazard in that leftover drugs may be saved and used again after they are outdated or may be shared with a friend or family member who reports similar symptoms. Dosages may be increased because if "a little does some good, more will do better," or dosages may be reduced so that an expensive medication will last longer. With memory changes, drugs may be taken sporadically, some doses being missed and others taken twice. Polypharmacy, overdose, and addiction to prescription drugs have become recognized as major causes of illness in older adults. To accurately assess drug use and knowledge, many nurses ask their older adult clients to bring to the health care appointment all medications (both over-the-counter and prescription) that they take regularly or occasionally. This allows the nurse to accurately assess all medications the client is taking and prevents omissions of drugs that the client may have thought were unimportant.

Stress of Illness during Adulthood

Illness is a situational crisis that can disrupt adult life at any time. The extent of the disruption may vary from a minor annoyance to a complete lifestyle change. The significance that "being ill" holds for an individual is determined by multiple variables: the type of illness and its perceived threat, the personality type, socioeconomic resources, family or significant other support, and possible restrictions on current lifestyle or structure. With Levinson's model, the impact of illness will differ depending on whether the individual is in a transitional or stable period of development. During stable periods when life is generally going smoothly, people have more energy to cope with illness. In contrast, with the changes being made in overall life structure during transitional periods, there is less energy to cope with illness, and illness and its potential effects add new variables to consider in the restructuring process. Because transitional stages represent a time of uncertainty, role changes, and anxiety, the individual is also more vulnerable to becoming ill. Conversely, the stable periods, which are typically times of commitment, confidence, and success, foster health. The presence of illness, either personal illness or illness in a significant other, can also trigger movement from a stable period into a transitional stage. This may be characteristically seen in the midlife transition during which an illness can initiate the "time left" thinking that is fundamental to the profound reassessment of life at this time.

Illness of an individual member may also pose a developmental threat to the family's integrity. The nurse must consider the family as a unit of care, identifying family needs and supporting family strengths and positive coping mechanisms.

Young adulthood. The most frequent acute conditions in young adults are minor accidents, drug abuse, respiratory infections, influenza, gastroenteritis, urinary tract infections, and minor surgery. These conditions may be developmentally significant to young adults for several reasons. First, with the hectic schedules of young adults, an acute minor illness is annoying because of disruption in life activities. With an acute disability, young adults may know that the effects are short term; however, they may be impatient with the healing process and concerned that long-term problems will result. Family rearrangements can be stressful, especially when hospitalization is required. Hospitalization is also frustrating because of forced dependency and limitations posed by treatment regimens. Maintaining control is very important for young adults, so they need to be informed and involved with decisions about care. Young adults are generally strongly motivated toward recuperation to resume life activities.

Although chronic conditions are not common in young adulthood, they can occur. Disabilities caused by accidents, multiple sclerosis, rheumatoid arthritis, and cancer are the common long-term conditions faced by young adults. Chronic illness and disability in young adulthood strike at the very core of developmental tasks and can result in delayed development. With the onset of chronic illness or disability, the threat to the young adult's independence may precipitate multiple crises when personal, family, and career goals need to change. The nurse must identify and direct nursing intervention toward potential developmental problems in the areas of identity reorganization; establishment of independence; and reorganization of intimate relationships, family structure, and launching of a chosen career.

Middle adulthood. The characteristics of acute illness are much the same in middle adulthood as in young adulthood. However, recuperative power in middle adulthood slows. Injuries and acute conditions that were rapidly resolved in young adulthood may have a longer recovery period and are more likely to become chronic problems.

Chronic conditions during middle age interfere with the individual's sense of generativity. This task requires outward-directed concerns and activities. Long-term recurrent illness often forces an interiority that can lead to physical and psychological self-absorption. When middle-aged adults develop a chronic illness or disability, they may feel unable to influence their destiny, let alone influence and provide for others. The impact on generativity includes changes in family, job, and community involvement.

With the onset of chronic illness in middle age, established family roles are often forced to change. The psychological trauma of these role changes is caused by the strong emotional component to roles, which is based on the value placed on a role as a part of self-identity and the vested power the role holds. The nurse should be perceptive to the potential for family dysfunction and should serve as a resource to the entire family, helping them to seek counseling and therapy as necessary.

Career or occupational orientation may need to change as a result of chronic illness. This is particularly stressful during the middle years because it confounds the career timing and readjustment of goals that occur with the midlife occupational crisis. When the illness is severely disruptive, the person may need to change occupations or jobs or may need to face an early forced retirement. Both these options may be a source of great stress and a threat to generativity because of occupational regression or being denied the gratification that comes from closing a career with the feeling of a job well done.

Older adulthood. The distinction between acute and chronic illness in older adults is less precise, since acute conditions may become chronic or may be an exacerbation of chronic problems. However, acute problems such as gastroenteritis, primary pneumonia, removable tumors, and noncomplicated accidental injuries can have a short course with complete recovery. The difficulties such illnesses pose for older adults are that they add stress to a body system with a decreased physiological and psychological ability to compensate for stress. The ability to perform self-care is an important problem for older adults when an acute illness occurs. If the person lives alone or with a frail spouse or housemate and does not have adequate support systems, an acute illness can precipitate a life disorganization that results in a move from the home and toward dependency.

When an older adult is hospitalized, many situations occur that threaten ego integrity and cause the hospitalization to be a very disorganizing experience. New situations and environments often normally produce anxiety, and when combined with the stress of being sick, the unfamiliar becomes confusing. When giving care, the nurse needs to carefully orient and reorient the older adult to the hospital environment. Allowing the older adult client to keep personal belongings within reach and visible will also help maintain a sense of orientation, as well as reduce the depersonalized feeling that accompanies hospitalization. Nursing care should be paced to allow older adult clients an opportunity to participate without hurrying so that they can maintain control and have time to understand and cooperate with what is being done.

Family situations are an important concern in caring for the hospitalized older adult. The nurse must recognize when role reversals are occurring between an older parent and the adult children. Children who have problems with this reversal may respond by withdrawing or by becoming overprotective and smothering. In either case, the parent's self-worth is threatened. The nurse should also be perceptive to other family concerns of the hospitalized older adult, such as worry over a spouse being home alone or concern for pets and plants or household maintenance if the client lives alone.

Chronic conditions are very common problems in health that older adults learn to manage. Part of this process includes incorporating the accoutrements of aging such as canes, wheelchairs, dentures, and hearing aids into a healthy self-esteem. Chronic conditions also have social implications if the illness imposes an involuntary disengagement process. When this occurs, transcending the physical problems is increasingly difficult. The social isolation that is experienced may reduce self-esteem and the physical and emotional strength needed to cope with the stresses of disease and aging.

R eview Questions

The number of the question corresponds to the same-numbered objective at the beginning of the chapter.

1. Erikson's developmental conflicts are based on
   a. biological changes during adulthood
   b. adjustments of self and social environment
   c. changes in the individual life structure
   d. instinctual energies and drives
2. Disengagement
   a. is a developmental stage theory
   b. occurs in all people over 65 years of age
   c. assumes that older adults cannot adapt to aging
   d. varies according to health, abilities, and previous lifestyle
3. Significant changes in mental functioning during middle and older adulthood include
   a. improved fluid intelligence
   b. declining verbal comprehension and reasoning skill
   c. declining speed in mental performance
   d. improved synthesis of new information
4. Young adult family tasks involve
   a. establishing a new family system that focuses on internal structure and relationships
   b. adapting a family system to outside demands
   c. modifying the relationship with the families of origin
   d. all of the above
5. Select the one correct statement about work and adulthood.
   a. The only significance work has to an adult is as a means of financial support.
   b. The important role changes when launching a career are those related to the job.
   c. Resolution of the middle-aged occupational crisis requires self-evaluation of goals.
   d. Retirement is not stressful if the preretirement standard of living can be maintained.
6. Physical changes associated with aging in adulthood
   a. arise from extrinsic factors
   b. are pathological in origin
   c. can be halted by proper health maintenance
   d. have an insidious beginning in young adults
7. Hospitalization can be a disorganizing experience for the older adult client because
   a. new environments produce anxiety and are difficult to manage
   b. disorientation may occur when personal belongings are out of sight and out of reach
   c. a hurried place reduces the older adult's ability to participate and maintain control
   d. all the above

REFERENCES

1. Erikson E: Childhood and society, ed 2, New York, 1963, WW Norton & Co, Inc.
2. Peck RC: Psychological developments in the second half of life. In Neugarten BL, ed: Middle-age and aging: a reader in social psychology, Chicago, 1986, University of Chicago Press.
3. Havighurst RJ: Developmental tasks and education, ed 3, New York, 1973, David McKay Co, Inc.
4. Levinson DJ: The seasons of a man's life, New York, 1978, Alfred A Knopf, Inc.
5. Cummings E and Henry WE: Growing old: the process of disengagement, New York, 1961, Basic Books, Inc, Publishers.
6. Carnevali DL and Patrick M: Nursing management for the elderly, ed 2, Philadelphia, 1986, JB Lippincott Co.
7. Atchley RC: A continuity theory of normal aging, Gerontologist 29:183, 1989.
8. Birren JE and Bengston V: Emergent theories of aging, New York, 1988, Springer Publishing Co, Inc.
9. Kane RL, Ouslander JG, and Abrass IB: Essentials of clinical geriatrics, ed 2, New York, 1989, McGraw-Hill, Inc.
10. Ebersole P and Hess P: Toward healthy aging: human needs and nursing response, ed 2, St Louis, 1985, The CV Mosby Co.
11. Cristofalo VJ: An overview of theories of biological aging. In Birren J and Bengston V, eds: Emergent theories of aging, New York, 1988, Springer Publishing Co, Inc.
12. Schaie KW: Middle life influences upon intellectual functioning in old age, Int J Behav Dev 7:463, 1984.
13. Gallup GH: Human needs and satisfaction: a global survey, Public Opinion Q 40:459, 1976.
14. US Department of Commerce, US Bureau of Commerce: Statistical abstract of the United States, 1985, Washington, DC, 1985, US Government Printing Office.
15. Schick FL, ed: Statistical handbook on aging Americans, Phoenix, 1986, The Oryx Press.
16. Goodman R: Aging changes in structure and function. In Carnevali DL and Patrick M: Nursing management for the elderly, ed 2, Philadelphia, 1986, JB Lippincott Co.
17. Yurick AG and others: The aged person and the nursing process, ed 2, East Norwalk, Conn, 1984, Appleton-Century-Crofts.
18. US Surgeon General's Report: Healthy people, Washington, DC, 1979, US Government Printing Office.
19. Gilford DM, ed: The aging population in the 21st century: statistics for health policy, Washington, DC, 1988, National Academy Press.

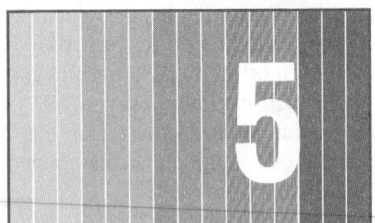

CHAPTER 5

Nursing Assessment and Role in Management

Stress

Joan Stehle Werner
Susan Erin O'Neill

Joan Stehle Werner
Susan Erin O'Neill

Learning Objectives

1. *Define stressor, stress, demands, primary appraisal, secondary appraisal, coping, and adaptation.*
2. *Describe the three stages of Selye's general adaptation syndrome.*
3. *Describe the role of cognitive appraisal in the stress process.*
4. *Describe the role of the nervous system in the stress process.*
5. *Describe the role of the endocrine system in the stress process.*
6. *Describe coping behaviors evidenced by a client experiencing stress.*
7. *List variables that may influence the experience of stress.*
8. *Describe the nursing assessment and management of a client experiencing stress.*

Interest in the study of stress has intensified as investigators have begun to identify its role in relation to physical and emotional health. Most contemporary approaches to the study of stress have been influenced by three different but complementary types of stress theories. The first type of theory conceptualizes stress as a response to some kind of environmental stressor. The major theory of this type was first proposed by Selye, who identified *stress* as "the nonspecific response of the body to any demand made upon it."[1] Selye called these stress-inducing demands

Reviewed by Marilyn Brolin Hopkins, R.N., D.N.Sc., Professor, Division of Nursing, California State University, Sacramento, California. A portion of this chapter was reviewed by Norma J. Briggs, R.N., Ph.D., Associate Professor, University of Wisconsin-Eau Claire School of Nursing, Eau Claire, Wisconsin.

Table 5-1 Examples of Stressors

Physical	Emotional
Noise	Diagnosis of cancer
Amphetamines	Promotion at work
Burns	Watching a loved one die
Running a marathon	Failing an exam
Infectious diseases	Financial loss
Pain	Winning a beauty contest

stressors. They could be physical or emotional, pleasant or unpleasant, as long as they required the individual to adapt (Table 5-1). Whether the stressor was physical in nature, such as a burn, or psychological in nature, such as the death of a loved one, a series of physiological responses resulted. Selye called this pattern of responses the *general adaptation syndrome.*

The second type of stress theory views stress as a stimulus that causes a disrupted response. This work originated with Holmes and Masuda and Holmes and Rahe, who developed methods to assess effects of life changes on health.[2,3] *Life changes* are defined as infrequent conditions ranging from minor violations of the law to death of a loved one (see Table 1-4). The major assumption of this type of theory is that frequent life changes make people vulnerable to illness.

The third type of stress theory is called *transactional* or *interactional.* This type of theory is concerned with person-environment transactions.[4,5] The most notable theory of this type was proposed by Lazarus, who emphasized the role of cognitive appraisal in assessing stressful situations and selecting coping options. Lazarus and Folkman defined *psychological stress* as "a particular relationship between the person and the environment that is appraised by the person as taxing or exceeding his or her resources and

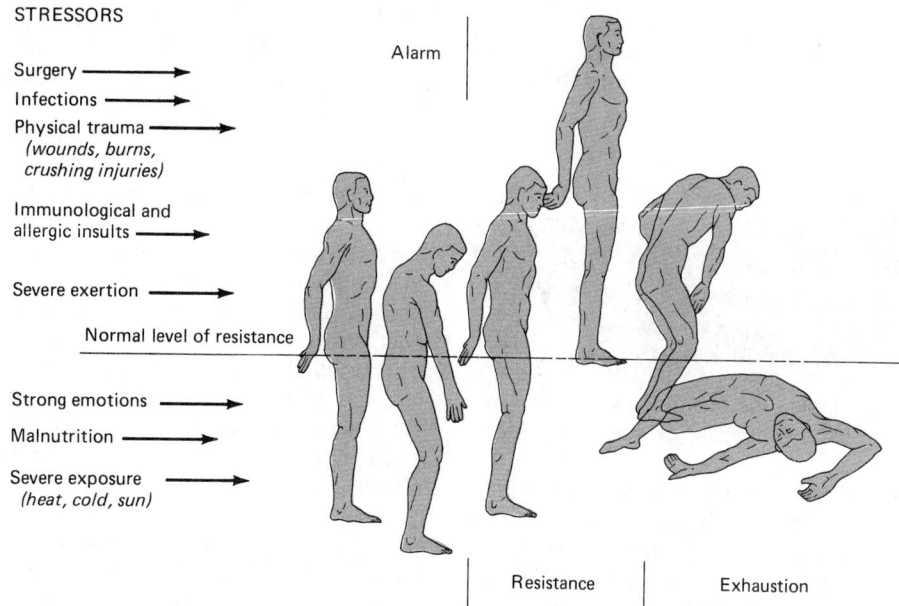

STRESSORS

Surgery ⟶
Infections ⟶
Physical trauma ⟶
(*wounds, burns,*
crushing injuries)

Immunological and ⟶
allergic insults

Severe exertion ⟶

Normal level of resistance

Strong emotions ⟶
Malnutrition ⟶
Severe exposure ⟶
(*heat, cold, sun*)

Alarm

Resistance   Exhaustion

Fig. 5-1   Phases of the stress intensification process. (From Byrne ML and Thompson LF: Concepts for the study and practice of nursing, St Louis, 1978, The CV Mosby Co, p 75.)

endangering his or her well-being."[6] These three types of theories are discussed in more detail in the remainder of this chapter.

STRESS AS A RESPONSE

Historically, Selye's early research using animals supported his theory that different stressors resulted in a similar response pattern. He called the bodily responses the *general adaptation syndrome* (GAS), which was made up of three stages: *alarm reaction, stage of resistance,* and *stage of exhaustion* (Fig. 5-1). Stressors of lesser magnitude were likely to result in a local response (*local adaptation syndrome* [LAS]), which is considered equivalent to the inflammatory reaction. Once the stressor or stimulus is integrated into the central nervous system, multiple responses occur in the pituitary-hypothalamic-adrenal axis. The nature of these responses, in which the stimulus and its effects successively cause changes in specific tissues in the nervous and endocrine systems, is fundamental to understanding the physiological and behavioral changes occurring in the individual experiencing stress.

Alarm Reaction

In the alarm reaction of the GAS, the individual perceives a stressor physically or mentally, and the "fight-or-flight" mechanism is initiated. When the stressor is of sufficient intensity to threaten the steady state of the individual, it requires a reallocation of energy so that adaptation can occur. This temporarily decreases the individual's resistance to stress and may even result in death if prolonged and severe.

Physical symptoms of the alarm reaction are generally those of sympathetic nervous system stimulation. These symptoms include an increased rate and force of heartbeat, increased blood pressure and respiratory rate, anorexia or nausea, pupil dilatation, and increased perspiration.

Stage of Resistance

Ideally, the individual quickly moves from the alarm reaction to the stage of resistance in which physiological forces are mobilized to increase resistance to stress. This is when adaptation occurs. It may involve modification of the external and internal environment. Resistance is high at this time as compared to the normal state. The amount of resistance varies among individuals depending on the level of physical functioning, coping abilities, and the total number and intensity of stressors they are experiencing. For example, a person who has been jogging regularly will have more ability to adapt to the stress of emergency surgery than a person who has been very sedentary.

Although few overt physical symptoms usually occur in this stage as compared to the alarm stage, the person is expending energy to adapt. This adaptive energy is limited by the resources of the individual. For example, a client may successfully recover from surgery and return to a normal coping state or may move to the next phase of the GAS, which is the stage of exhaustion.

Stage of Exhaustion

The stage of exhaustion is the final stage of the GAS; it occurs when all the energy for adaptation has been expended. Physical symptoms of the alarm reaction may briefly reappear in a final effort by the body to survive. This is exemplified by a terminally ill person who becomes alert and has stronger vital signs shortly before death. The individual in the stage of exhaustion usually becomes ill and may die if assistance from outside sources is not available. This stage can often be reversed by external sources of adaptive energy, such as medication, blood transfusions, and psychotherapy.

Refinements in Selye's Stress Theory

Selye's work addressed the importance of conditioning factors that may affect the stress response. These include proposed internal conditioning factors such as age, genetics, and previous experience with the stressors, as well as external conditioning factors such as diet and climate.[7] Selye created the term *eustress* to refer to stress associated with positive events such as winning a tennis match. However, he never fully explained the health consequences of eustress versus stress. This relationship is currently under investigation.

Selye's description of stress focused on the nonspecific physiological changes of the nervous and endocrine systems that occurred as an organism responded to a specific stressor. This nonspecificity implied a predictable uniform pattern in the physiological responses to various stressors. Present research supports different patterns of the physiological changes that occur during stress.[8] Illustrating this view is an early classic study conducted by Lacey and Lacey in 1958.[9] These investigators subjected 42 subjects to four mild stressors. Stressors included: (1) the cold pressor test, in which one arm is placed in ice water, (2) anticipating the cold pressor test, (3) a mental math problem, and (4) a test of word fluency. A number of physiological stress responses were assessed. Findings indicated substantial variability in blood pressure, heart rate, pulse pressure, and other measures among subjects in response to the same stressor. The investigators labeled these individual physiological responses *individual response stereotypy*. Based on similar findings, different stressors will probably produce different complex profiles of hormonal and tissue changes in different individuals. This may help to explain why a variety of the so-called diseases of adaptation exist (Table 5-2). Some diseases have been comprehensively studied to explore the way adaptive failure results in illness.[10]

Table 5-2 Diseases of Adaptation

High blood pressure
Diseases of the heart and blood vessels
Diseases of the kidney
Eclampsia
Rheumatoid arthritis
Inflammatory diseases of the skin and eyes
Infections
Allergic and hypersensitivity diseases
Nervous and mental diseases
Sexual dysfuntions
Digestive diseases
Metabolic diseases
Cancer

STRESS AS A STIMULUS

Another approach to the study of stress is to view stress as the stimulus or the event that results in a disrupted response. Stress defined in this way is similar to Selye's term of stressor. Historically, this approach stems from attempts to develop questionnaires to measure stress in terms of life changes or life events.[2,3] Two questionnaires are the Social Readjustment Rating Scale (SRRS) (see Table 1-4) and the Schedule of Recent Experiences (SRE). Life events questionnaires such as the SRRS and the SRE have been developed that attempt to numerically weight the impact (stress) of various life changes, including the death of a spouse and financial changes. A life event is regarded as stressful if it is "associated with some adaptive or coping behavior on the part of the involved individual."[3] Each event, whether desirable or not, is "indicative or requires a significant change in the ongoing life pattern of the individual." It was originally proposed that the more events managed over a specific period of time, the greater the vulnerability to illness. Of particular interest was the research that reported an association between the number and intensity of life events and the resulting probability of physical and emotional illness in the near future.[11] Although several studies have resulted in statistically significant relationships between life events and illness onset, these relationships are often weak. Findings contrary to this relationship have also been reported.[12] Life events scaling has raised methodological issues, such as what other factors must be taken into account when considering life events.

Leventhal and Tomarken summarize the factors that have been shown to affect an individual's response to life events such as cultural bias, personality, clustering of events, biological variables, socioeconomic status, and interpersonal support systems.[12] Another important factor is timing, since some undetected diseases developing over lengthy periods of time may actually produce psychological changes or precipitate stressful life events. A third important factor is the issue of the outcome. Often, disease outcomes (biological processes and disease diagnoses) are confused with illness outcomes (total effect of disease on an individual), leading to inconclusive results.[12] This mounting evidence supports the importance of using a holistic approach when assessing the client.

Of interest is the research that identifies some individuals who experience high scores in terms of life events changes but do not succumb to the expected illness outcome. Kobasa and others have described *hardiness* as a mediating factor in the stress-illness relationship.[13,14] The hardy person has (1) a clear sense of personal values and goals, (2) a strong tendency toward interaction with the

Table 5-3 Examples of Daily Hassles

Misplacing or losing things	Not seeing enough people
Inconsiderate smokers	Having to wait
Planning meals	Unchallenging work
Concerns about job security	

environment, (3) a sense of meaningfulness, and (4) an internal rather than external locus of control.

Recent developments have continued to improve the predictability of health and illness outcomes related to stressor impact. Daily hassle scores have been found to be an important supplement to the life events approach. *Daily hassles* are "experiences and conditions of daily living that have been appraised as salient and harmful or threatening to the endorser's well-being."[15] The frequency and intensity of daily hassles has a stronger relationship with somatic illness than the life events scale.[16,17] Items addressed on the daily hassles scale (Table 5-3) reflect the content areas of work, family, social activities, the environment, practical considerations, finances, and health.[18]

As an adjunct to hassles, *uplifts* are defined as positive experiences that are likely to occur in everyday life.[16] This concept seems comparable to the eustress described earlier by Selye. Further investigation is needed in this area, since most research has looked at stressors or demands and negative outcomes.

STRESS AS A TRANSACTION

In contrast to Selye's theory and the life change approach, Lazarus' theory focuses on the person-environment transaction and the cognitive appraisal of demands and coping options.[6] A multitude of internal and external data is received on a neurocognitive level. Lazarus proposed that these data are interpreted during the process of cognitive appraisal. *Appraisal* is a judgment process that includes recognizing the degree of *demands* (another term for stressors) placed on the individual (Fig. 5-2). The appraisal process also involves the recognition of available resources or options that help to deal with the potential or actual demands.

During *primary appraisal*, demands are assessed according to the possible impact on the individual's well-being. Demands can be judged as *irrelevant*, *benign-positive*, or *stressful*. If demands are appraised as stressful,

they can be classified as representing *threat, harm-loss,* and *challenge*. Challenge demands differ from threat and harm-loss demands in that they are viewed as a potential for personal gain or growth. For example, hiking in the wilderness may place demands on the individual that will give the person the opportunity to test and exhibit strength and endurance. Harm or loss demands involve actual damage, and threat demands involve anticipated harm or loss.

Therefore, stress is a situation in which demands exceed the individual's adaptive resources. Demands can be either *external* (environmental) or *internal*. A demand is labeled *external* if the event requires an adaptive response. If the adaptive response does not occur, negative consequences will result. *Internal* demands are composed of "goals, values, commitments, programs, or tasks acquired by an individual (or social system or tissue system) whose thwarting or postponement would have negative consequences or implications."[19]

Secondary appraisal refers to the process of recognizing the coping resources and options that are available. Primary and secondary appraisal often occur simultaneously and interact with each other in determining stress. *Cognitive reappraisal* is the process of continuously relabeling cognitive appraisals.

Certain factors influence the labeling of appraisals.[20] Situational factors include (1) the intensity of the external demands, (2) the immediacy of the expected impact, and (3) ambiguity. Person-related factors include (1) motivational characteristics, (2) belief systems, and (3) intellectual resources and skills.

Theoretical Summary

The role of perception is the key to understanding the difference between the three major types of stress theories presented. In Lazarus' theory, the cognitive appraisal process, which is the individual's perception of demands and recognition of coping resources, determines whether the demands will be assessed as stressful. In the life change type of theory, perceived stressfulness is not considered, since each individual receives the same score for a certain stressor. In Selye's theory, all demands are stressors with the capacity to elicit the GAS. Conditioning factors in individuals influence the stress response.

Through cognitive appraisal, individuals experience different outcomes in dealing with demands, not only because of conditioning factors, but also as a result of how the demand is perceived and labeled during the person-stressor impact. What is stressful to one individual may be benign to another. The same holds true as the individual recognizes available resources.

PHYSIOLOGICAL MECHANISM OF STRESS

To simplify a description of the physiological events involved regarding the body's stress response, the following discussion is divided into the role of the nervous system and the role of the endocrine system. These systems affect and are affected by the other body systems. Understanding the physiological changes associated with stress will help provide the foundation for the assessment of the client experiencing stress and the implications for health outcomes.

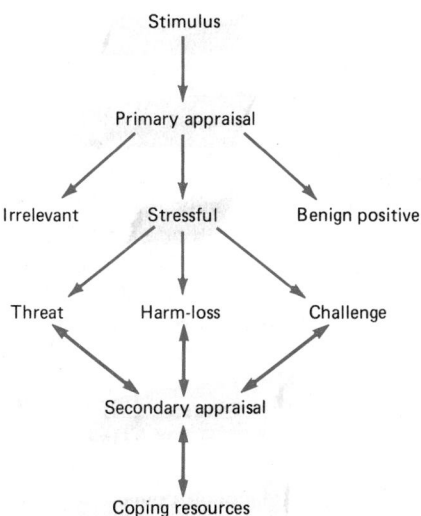

Fig. 5-2 Cognitive appraisal process.

Nervous System

Stressors (demands) may be physical, psychological, or social. (see also Chapter 1). They may be actually or symbolically present for the body to respond physiologically. The complex process by which an event is perceived as a stressor and by which the body responds is not fully understood. However, neural control of emotions by the hypothalamus is known to coordinate the many mechanisms of the stress response. This control is significant because most stressors precipitate an emotional reaction. The major parts of the brain involved in the neural control of emotion are the reticular formation, the hypothalamus, the limbic system, and the cerebral cortex. Their functions are very closely interrelated.

Cerebral cortex. Afferent input that an external event has occurred is sent to the cerebral cortex via sensory pathways from the peripheral nervous system, the eyes, and the ears. For example, the pressure of a restraint that is applied too tightly may be a stressor. While the afferent impulse is traveling upward, sensory impulses are sent to the reticular formation in the area of the brainstem. The reticular formation also sends input to the thalamus and cerebral cortex. Activities associated with these afferent impulses are called the *reticular activating system* (RAS). The RAS functions to maintain wakefulness and alertness.

The somatic, auditory, and visual associative areas of the cerebral cortex receive data from these senses and make some interpretation. The prefrontal area serves to reduce the speed of the associative functions so that the person has time to evaluate the information in light of past experiences and future consequences (primary and secondary appraisal) and to plan a course of action. All these functions are involved in the perception of a stressor.

The temporal lobes contain the auditory association areas, which produce fear when stimulated. Stimulation of the temporal lobes has resulted in sounds seeming louder or softer, visual displays seeming nearer or farther, and experiences seeming familiar or strange. These effects modify perception.

Limbic system. The limbic system, which lies in the inner midportion of the brain near the base, includes the septum, the cingulate gyrus, the amygdala, the hippocampus, and the anterior nuclei of the thalamus. (The hypothalamus is located in the center of these structures but is not considered a part of the limbic system.) The function of the limbic system is thought to be primarily involved with behavior. When stimulated, these structures lead to emotions, feelings, and behaviors that ensure survival and self-preservation, such as feeding, sociability, and sexuality. The cerebral cortex and limbic systems interact to serve the experiential and executive functions of emotion. Endorphins are also found in structures of the limbic system. (See Chapter 51.) They are known to reduce the perception of painful stimuli.

Reticular formation. The reticular formation is located between the lower end of the brainstem and the thalamus. It contains the RAS. The RAS sends impulses contributing to alertness to the limbic system as well as the cerebral cortex and thalamus. Impulses from the hypothalamus stimulate the RAS to increase its output of impulses lead-

Table 5-4 Hypothalamic Functions

COORDINATES IMPULSES

Autonomic nervous system
Body temperature regulation
Food intake
Water intake
Urine formation
Cardiovascular function

SECRETES RELEASING FACTORS

Various hormones of the adenohypophysis
Regulation of adenohypophyseal secretions

AFFECTS BEHAVIOR

Rage
Alertness
Psychosomatic disorders

ing to wakefulness. Perceived stress usually increases the degree of wakefulness.

Hypothalamus. The hypothalamus lies just above the pituitary gland. It serves many functions in the body (Table 5-4). The hypothalamus is a major pathway by which the limbic system sends messages. Since the hypothalamus secretes substances that regulate the release of hormones by the anterior pituitary, it is central to the connection between the nervous and endocrine systems in responding to stress (Fig. 5-3).

In addition, the hypothalamus regulates the function of both the sympathetic and parasympathetic systems of the autonomic nervous system. Thus, when an individual perceives the existence of a stressor, the hypothalamus mediates the response. It does this by activating the sympathetic nervous system and by releasing corticotropin-releasing factor (CRF) to stimulate the pituitary to release adrenocorticotropic hormone (ACTH) (see Chapters 42 and 50).

Endocrine System

Once the hypothalamus begins the response to stress, the endocrine system becomes involved. The sympathetic nervous system stimulates the adrenal medullae to release the hormones epinephrine and norepinephrine (catecholamines). These prepare the body for the fight-or-flight response (Fig. 5-4). The level of catecholamines can be measured in the blood or urine. Because of this, numerous research studies have used blood and urine tests to determine the impact of various stressors. It has been found that the greater the stressor, the higher the level of catecholamines.

The hypothalamus also secretes CRF, which stimulates the pituitary to release ACTH. ACTH, in turn, stimulates the adrenal cortex to release glucocorticoids, aldosterone, and androgens. The glucocorticoids are released in the greatest amounts. Aldosterone acts to increase extracellular fluid (ECF). Neural stimulation of the posterior pitu-

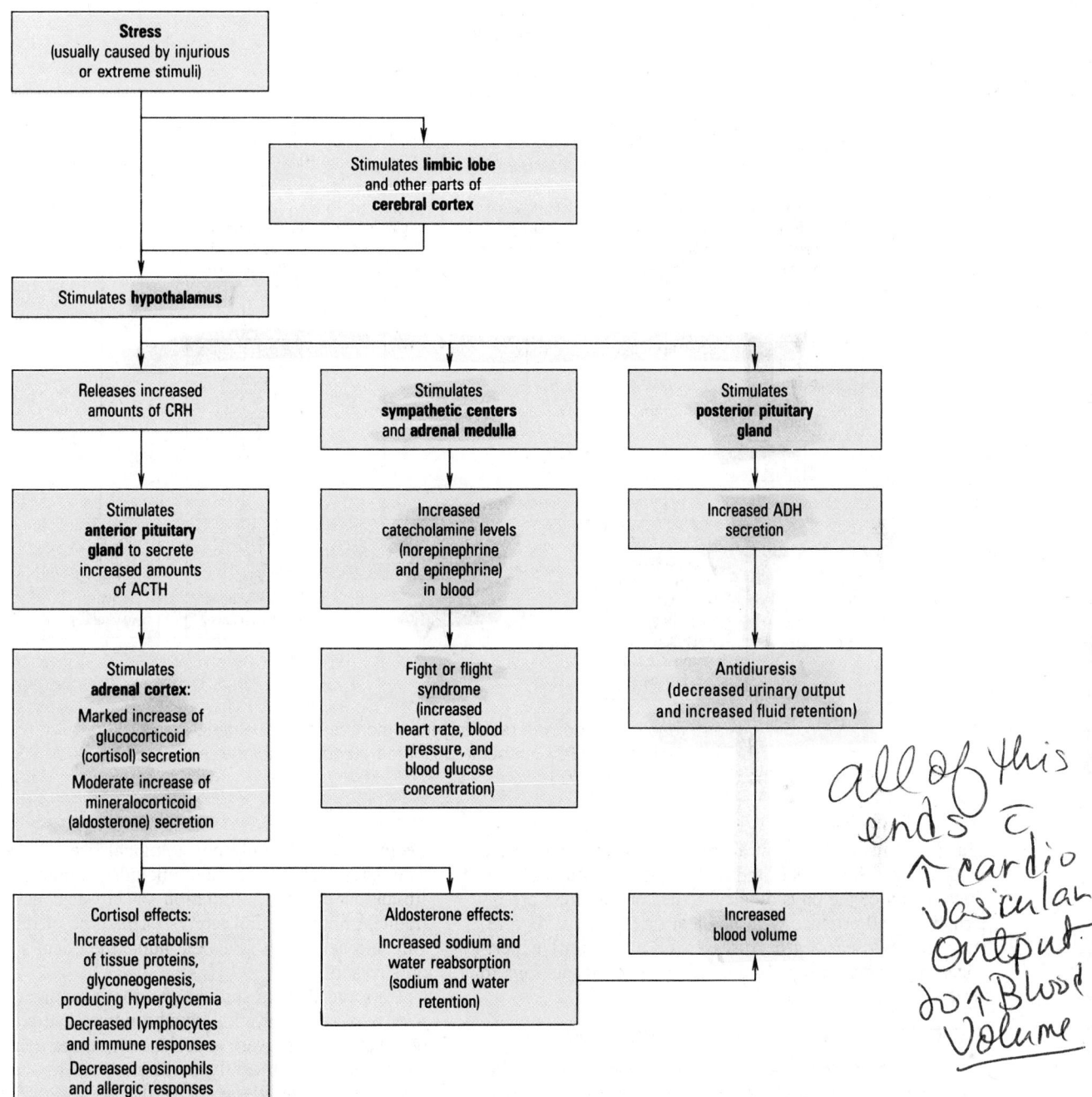

Fig. 5-3 Current concepts of the stress syndrome. (From Anthony CP and Thibodeau GA: Textbook of anatomy and physiology, St Louis, 1987, The CV Mosby Co, p 789.)

itary results in the secretion of antidiuretic hormone (ADH), which also promotes water retention.

Stimulating both the adrenal medullae and cortex results in an increased blood glucose level. This provides the additional fuel for the increased metabolism needed for fighting or fleeing.

The increased cardiac output (resulting from the increased heart rate, increased ECF, and increased blood pressure), increased blood glucose levels, and increased metabolic rate make the physical response possible. In ad-

dition, dilatation of blood vessels and resulting increased blood supply to the large muscles and the brain provide for quick movement and increased alertness. The increased blood volume (from increased ECF and the shunting of blood from the gastrointestinal system) and increased clotting time function to help maintain adequate blood volume in case of traumatic blood loss. These are some mechanisms of the physiological response to stress that illustrate the complex and interrelated processes involved.

The physiological response to stressors seems better

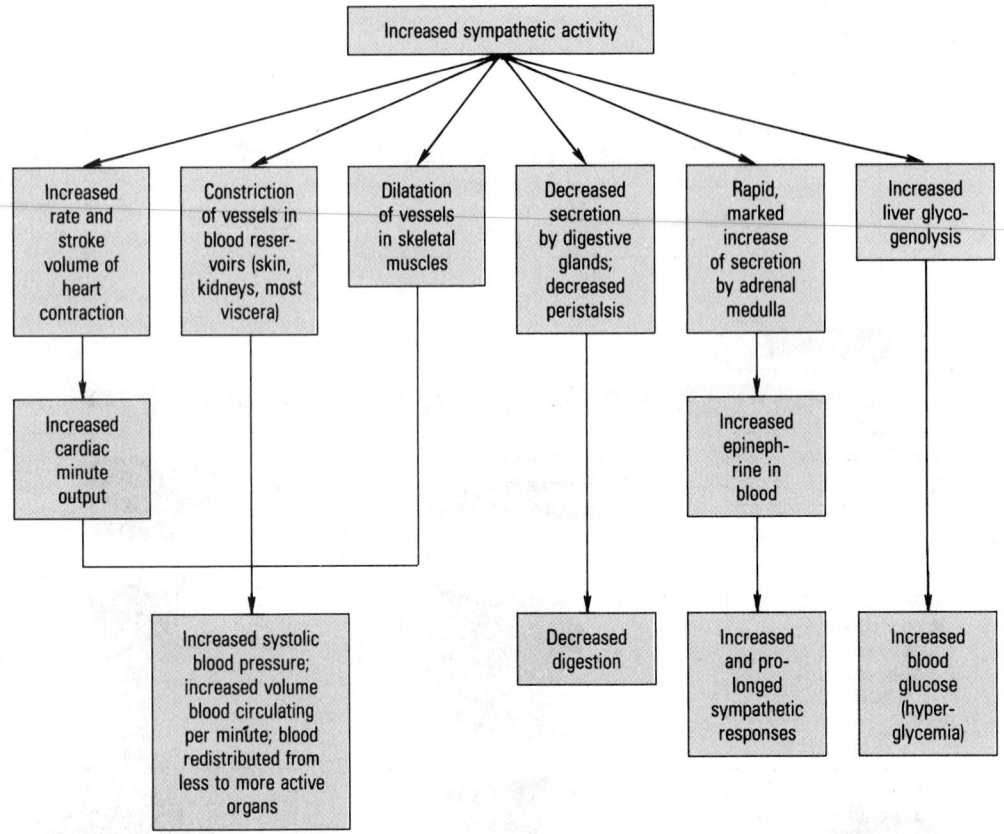

Fig. 5-4 Alarm reaction responses resulting from increased sympathetic activity. (From Anthony CP and Thibodeau GA: Textbook of anatomy and physiology, ed 12, St Louis, 1987, The CV Mosby Co, p 789.)

suited to persons living in a primitive society than in the industrialized societies of today. Because of social conventions, many of the physiological indicators of stress are internalized and produce wear and tear on the body. As a result, many diseases (the diseases of adaptation) experienced by modern people are considered maladaptations to stress.

IDENTIFYING STRESSORS OR DEMANDS

Nurses should become familiar with the types of stressors experienced by various populations and individuals in particular circumstances. For example, work-related stressors are often discussed in the literature.[21,22] Some demands are intrinsic to the job, such as poor working conditions, work overload, and time pressures. Other demands stem from the individual's role in the organization (role conflict), career development (overpromotion or underpromotion), relationships at work (difficulties in delegating responsibilities), and the organizational climate (restrictions on behavior). The extensive research on these factors and their effects validates including occupation as an essential factor in assessment.[23,24]

Another major source of stress relates to illness experienced by a client, which often also causes stress in family members.[25,26] For example, in clients receiving hemodialysis, the five most frequently ranked stressors included one physiological stressor and four psychosocial stressors.

Feeling tired, the only physiological stressor, ranked first. The psychosocial stressors included limitation of fluid, limitation of food, limitation of physical activities, and frequent hospital admissions.[27] This type of information is valuable because it gives the nurse the client's perspective on stressors.

Carr and Powers studied stressors associated with coronary bypass surgery.[28] Although nurses and clients agreed on what stressors were experienced, nurses generally rated all items as significantly more stressful for coronary bypass clients than did the clients themselves.[28] The stressors were categorized into illness-related stressors (I) and hospital-related stressors (H). The most severe of the stressors included having cardiac surgery (I), resuming lifestyle (I), experiencing pain/discomfort (I), having a fear of dying because of illness/surgery (I), and being absent from home/business (H).[28] This emphasizes the need for understanding the client's perception of the situation.

A hospital stress rating scale has been developed based on stressors identified by medical-surgical clients.[29] In developing the scale, clients rank-ordered 49 events related to the experience of hospitalization from the most to the least stressful. Events ranked as mildly stressful included having to wear a hospital gown and being awakened in the night by the nurse. Not knowing when to expect that certain tests would be done and having the staff in too much of a hurry were ranked as moderately stressful events. The five most stressful events in descending order of stressfulness included the possibility of losing sight, anticipated diagnosis of cancer, possibility of losing a kidney or other organ, knowing the illness is serious, and the possibility of losing the sense of hearing.[30] Knowledge of these and other stressors cited on the scale can further assist the nurse in identifying potential and actual sources of stress for this group of clients. Awareness of these stressors may further assist the nurse in identifying potential and actual sources of stress for similar groups of clients.

Nurses and student nurses have also been studied as groups experiencing stress and burnout. Stressors such as heavy workload, lack of adequate rewards, and lack of participation in decision making have been identified in various practice settings. Knowledge of these stressors is important if nurses do not want to become victims of stress in the work environment. The problem of burnout has been widely addressed in the literature.[31-33]

COPING

The concept of *coping* has been described by numerous authors. One definition is "constantly changing cognitive and behavioral efforts to manage specific external and/or internal demands that are appraised as taxing or exceeding the resources of the person."[34] Defense processes (for example, denial) may also be included as a coping process, since both defensive and coping processes mesh and are intrinsic to the psychological integrity of the individual.[54] *Coping resources,* defined as characteristics or actions drawn on to manage stress (Table 5-5), include factors within the person or environment that encompass categories such as (1) health/energy/morale, (2) positive beliefs, (3) problem-solving skills, (4) social skills, (5) social networks, and (6) material resources.

Coping efforts function broadly in two ways, as problem-solving (problem-focused) and emotion-regulating (emotion-focused) efforts (Table 5-6). As an individual attempts to deal with demands (internal or environmental) or obstacles that create the demands, the person is said to be using the *problem-focused coping* efforts. When the individual's effort is concentrated on methods of regulating the emotional response to the problem, the coping is said to be an *emotion-focused* effort. For example, a person with diabetes mellitus who learns to give injections is engaged in problem-focused coping. This person is using emotion-focused coping when the distress of being diagnosed with diabetes is lessened by the thought that it would be worse if the diagnosis had been cancer. Combinations of emotion-focused and problem-focused coping can be used.

Modes of coping have been described.[35,36] As an individual begins to deal with a stressor, the coping process may involve the following:

1. Information seeking (gathering data about the problem and possible solutions to the problem)
2. Direct actions (performing concrete acts to alter self or environment)
3. Inhibition of action (refraining from any action)
4. Intrapsychic processes (reappraising the situation; cognitive activity aimed at improving feelings)
5. Turning to others (obtaining social support)

The choice of coping strategies depends on various factors. Variables have been identified that affect an individual's choice of coping strategies, including degrees of uncertainty, threat or helplessness, and the presence of conflict.[37] The impact of each variable on choosing coping strategies can be clarified. If uncertainty is high, direct action is less likely to be selected as a coping strategy. If the degree of appraised threat is severe, more primitive coping modes (such as panic) are more likely to occur. In the presence of conflict, direct actions will likely be frozen. Helplessness promotes total immobilization. The strategy chosen may also be influenced by the outcome of the cognitive appraisal that categorizes the stressor as harm/loss, threat, or challenge.

Table 5-5 Examples of Coping Resources

PERSON-PROPERTIES

Health/energy/morale	Problem-solving skills
Robust health	Collection of information
High energy level	Identification of problem
High morale	Generation of alternatives

Positive beliefs	Social skills
Self-efficacy	Communication skills
Faith in God	Compatibility

ENVIRONMENT-PROPERTIES

Social networks	Utilitarian resources
Family members	Finances
Co-workers	Instructional manuals
Social contacts	Social agencies

Table 5-6 Examples of Demands and Coping

Demands	Coping
Being diagnosed with diabetes	Attending diabetic education classes (P-S)
	Taking a short vacation (E-R)
Failing an exam	Obtaining a tutor (P-S)
	Having dinner with friends (E-R)
Being told that more work will be required as part of the job	Learning to use a word processor (P-S)
	Venting negative feelings about paperwork to spouse (E-R)
Being notified of an appointment for an IRS audit	Reviewing tax records with accountant (P-S)
	Practicing deep breathing exercises (E-R)
Giving a public speech for the first time	Practicing in front of family members (P-S)
	Jogging the morning of the speech (E-R)

P-S, Problem-solving; *E-R*, emotion-regulation.

Specific strategies labeled as coping activities have been identified by studying groups of individuals assumed to be dealing with specific stressors.[38] For example, in looking at the coping methods used by hemodialysis clients, the most frequently cited coping methods were praying and trusting in God, trying to maintain control over the situation, accepting the situation as it is, and hoping that things would get better.[27] Cardiac transplant clients and other population groups are being tested to assess the use and effectiveness of eight coping styles. The proposed styles include the following:

1. Confrontive: Facing the problem
2. Evasive: Avoiding activities
3. Optimistic: Thinking positively
4. Fatalistic: Feeling hopeless
5. Emotive: Expressing emotions
6. Palliative: Making self feel better
7. Supportant: Using support systems
8. Self-reliant: Depending on self[39]

In the next decade, precise patterns in coping activities may become evident and thus more predictable. The results compiled to date have generated lists of coping strategies. Findings about which coping strategies are the most beneficial or adaptive are inconclusive.

■ Nursing Management of Stress

Nursing assessment

Clients face an array of potential stressors (demands) that can have health consequences. The nurse needs to be aware of situations that are likely to result in stress and must also assess the client's appraisal of the situation. In addition to the stress itself, specific coping mechanisms have health consequences and therefore must be included in the assessment.

Although the manifestations of stress may vary from person to person, the nurse should assess the client for the signs and symptoms of the stress reaction that occur as a result of changes in the nervous and endocrine systems. (See Chapters 42 and 50.)

Three major areas are important in assessment of stress with a client. These areas provide the nurse with a useful guide in the assessment process. The areas include demands, effects or human responses, and coping:

1. Demands
   a. Stressors or demands on the client may include major life changes, events, or situations, such as changes in family constellation or daily hassles the client is experiencing. Demands may be categorized as external (environmental) or internal, such as perceived tasks, goals, and commitments. Internal demands may also include physical demands resulting from disease or injury.

      In addition, the number of simultaneous demands, the duration of these demands, and previous experience with similar demands should be assessed. Specific assessment guides for particular types of clients are also available.[40]
   b. Primary appraisal or perception of the demands should be assessed. Demands may be categorized as representing harm or loss, threat, or challenge.

2. Effects or human responses
   a. Physiological effects of a demand that is appraised as stressful include the effects of sympathetic nervous system activity. Responses such as increased heart rate, increased blood pressure, loss of appetite, sweating, and dilated pupils are included. In addition, clients may exhibit some of the diseases of adaptation, for example, asthma, headaches, and allergies (Table 5-2).
   b. Behavioral human responses include observable actions and cognitions of the client. Behavioral effects may include responses such as accident proneness, impaired speech, anxiety, crying, and shouting. Behavior in other aspects of life such as occupation may include absenteeism or tardiness at work, lowered productivity, and job dissatisfaction. Observable cognitive responses include self-reports of excessive demand, inability to make decisions, and forgetfulness.

3. Coping
   a. Secondary appraisal of the client, or the client's evaluation of coping resources and options, should be assessed. Resources such as socially supportive family members, adequate finances, and the ability to solve problems are examples (see Table 5-5).
   b. Coping strategies include cognitive and behavioral efforts to meet demands. Coping use and effectiveness of problem-focused and emotion-focused efforts should be addressed (Table 5-6). These efforts may be categorized as direct action, avoidance of action, seeking information, defense mechanisms, and seeking assistance of others.[36] The probability that a certain coping strategy will bring about the desired result is another important aspect to be assessed.[41]

Nursing interventions

Adaptation refers to "a complex process involving numerous internal and external factors that influence response and the subsequent level of adaptation established."[42] The role of the nurse is to facilitate and enhance the processes of coping and adaptation.

Nursing interventions depend on the severity of the stress experience or demand. In the multiple trauma client, the human organism expends all energy in the attempt to physically survive. The nurse's efforts are directed to life-supporting interventions and to the inclusion of approaches aimed at the reduction of additional stressors to the client. For example, the multiple trauma client is much less likely to adapt (recover) if faced with additional stressors such as sleep deprivation or an infection.

The importance of cognitive appraisal in the stress experience should prompt the nurse to assess if changes in the way the client perceives and labels particular events or situations (cognitive reappraisal) are possible. Some experts also propose that the positive effects resulting from successfully meeting stressful demands be considered more and that more emphasis be placed on the part of cultural values and beliefs enhancing or constraining various coping options.[43]

Table 5-7 Conditioning Factors Altering the Stress Response

Age	Personality
Nutrition	Circadian rhythms
Heredity	Previous experiences

Since dealing with physical, social, and psychological demands is an integral part of daily experiences, the coping behaviors that are used should be adaptive and should not be a source of additional stress to the individual. Researchers have concluded that generalizing about which coping strategies are the most adaptive is not yet possible. However, in evaluating coping behaviors, the nurse should look at the short-term outcomes—the impact of the strategy on the reduction or mastery of the demands and the regulation of the emotional response—and the long-term outcomes that relate to health, morale, and social and psychological functioning.

Conditioning factors affect the response to various stressors (Table 5-7). Resistance to stress can be increased with a healthy lifestyle (see Chapter 1).

Stress-reducing activities have been studied for use in nursing practice. The activities suggested can also be viewed as conditioning factors, since the person is developing a sense of control with resulting increased self-esteem as the practices are incorporated into daily activities. A sense of control is an important mediator in the stress process.[44,45]

The nurse should recognize when the client or family situation needs to be referred to a professional with advanced training in counseling. A psychiatric nursing text should be consulted for additional information.

However, nurses can assume a primary role in planning stress-reducing interventions. Specific stress-reducing activities within the scope of nursing practice (some of which may require additional training) include relaxation training, cognitive reappraisal, music therapy exercise, decisional control, massage, and humor.

Identifying diagnoses

The importance of stress and coping to nurses is shown by the amount of attention these concepts receive related to nursing diagnoses. A coping-stress-tolerance pattern has been identified as one of 11 functional health patterns.[46] This pattern includes 9 diagnoses (Table 5-8). Assessment of the health pattern results in a description of the coping-stress-tolerance patterns of a client. Stressors can be identified at the individual, family, and community level.

Two specific nursing diagnoses have been identified related to stress: ineffective individual coping and ineffective family coping. *Ineffective individual coping* is defined as a state of "impairment of adaptive behaviors and problem-solving abilities for meeting life's demands and roles. (Methods of handling stressful life situations are insufficient to control anxiety, fear, or anger.)"[47] Potential etiologies include situational or maturational crises, personal vulnerability, knowledge deficit, and problem-solving deficit.

Table 5-8 Nursing Diagnoses in Coping-Stress-Tolerance Pattern

Ineffective coping (individual)
Avoidance coping
Defensive coping
Ineffective denial or denial
Impaired adjustment
Post-trauma response
Family coping: potential for growth
Ineffective family coping: disabled
Ineffective family coping: compromised

From Gordon M: *Manual of nursing diagnoses, 1991-1992,* St Louis, 1991, The CV Mosby Co.

Ineffective family coping: compromised refers to "usually supportive primary person (family member or close friend) providing insufficient, ineffective, or compromised support, comfort, assistance, or encouragement which may be needed by client to manage or master adaptive tasks related to health challenge."[48] In addition, two nursing diagnoses have been identified that support strengths aimed at wellness in the coping-stress-tolerance functional pattern. They are *crisis resolution, effective* and *effective individual coping.*[49]

In summary, a knowledge of stress and coping theories provides the nurse with useful concepts that are applicable to all phases of the nursing process. Keeping abreast of the current research in this sphere is a challenge. The models and concepts proposed are useful to nurses who choose to establish a research- and theory-based practice that recognizes the relationships among stress, coping, and health.

 ase Study

STRESS DURING HOSPITALIZATION

Mr. R. Ranson, a 20-year-old college student and starting basketball guard, was admitted for an emergency appendectomy the night before his basketball team entered the final playoffs. His past health history is negative except for exertional asthma that has been controlled by medications. His brother visited him during his first postoperative night and mentioned to the nurse that Ranson's diet has consisted of Coke and pizza since he made the first-string team last year.

Discussion Questions

1. Explain the physiological changes that would be expected in Mr. Ranson during the first 24 hours postoperatively as a result of the demand of surgery.
2. Explain how Ranson's previous diet may have affected his current adaptability.
3. What physiological and psychological stressors can be identified or predicted in Ranson's situation? Describe the possible effects on his asthma.
4. What factors will Mr. Ranson's secondary appraisal process focus on?
5. What specific nursing interventions can be included in Ranson's management that will enhance his adaptability?

a. anxiety
b. forgetfulness
c. decreased blood pressure
d. impaired speech

R eview Questions

The number of the question corresponds to the same-numbered objective at the beginning of the chapter.

1. Choose the false statement regarding stress.
   a. It occurs when demands exceed the adaptive resources of an individual.
   b. It occurs only as a result of physiological stressors.
   c. What is stressful to one individual may be benign to another.
   d. It may result from a perceived threat.
2. All the following statements are true about the GAS *except*
   a. It was first defined by Hans Selye and is different from the local response to a stressor.
   b. It involves the central and autonomic nervous systems and the pituitary, thyroid, and adrenal glands.
   c. Symptoms of the state of resistance are caused by stimulation of the sympathetic nervous system.
   d. Symptoms of the stage of exhaustion may initially mimic those of the stage of alarm.
3. All the following statements regarding cognitive appraisal are true *except* it is a judgment process that
   a. occurs on a cognitive level
   b. recognizes the degree of demands placed on the individual
   c. occurs only during perceived threats
   d. recognizes available resources
4. When an individual perceives the existence of a stressor, the response is mediated by the part of the central nervous system called the
   a. hypothalamus
   b. reticular formation
   c. limbic system
   d. temporal lobes
5. The part of the nervous system that connects it to the endocrine system is the
   a. hypothalamus
   b. cerebral cortex
   c. reticular formation
   d. limbic system
6. Choose the false statement regarding coping behaviors.
   a. They may include efforts to regulate emotion.
   b. Some coping behaviors are problem focused.
   c. Denial is a form of coping.
   d. If uncertainty is high, direct action is usually the selected coping strategy.
7. All the following statements regarding hardiness are true *except*
   a. It involves having a clear sense of goals.
   b. It involves having an external rather than internal locus of control.
   c. There is a strong tendency toward interaction with the environment.
   d. The person has a sense of meaningfulness.
8. Examples of the signs and symptoms exhibited by the client experiencing stress include all *except*
   a. anxiety
   b. forgetfulness
   c. decreased blood pressure
   d. impaired speech

REFERENCES

1. Selye H: The stress concept: past, present, and future. In Cooper CL: Stress research: issues for the eighties, New York, 1983, John Wiley & Sons, Inc, p 2.
2. Holmes T and Masuda M: Magnitude estimations of social readjustments, J Psychosom Res 11:219, 1966.
3. Holmes T and Rahe R: The social readjustment rating scale, J Psychosom Res 12:213, 1967.
4. Cox T: Stress, Baltimore, 1978, University Park Press, pp 18–24.
5. Lyon BL and Werner JS: Stress. In Fitzpatrick J and Taunton R, eds: Annual review of nursing research, vol 5, New York, 1987, Springer Publishing Co, Inc, pp 8–10.
6. Lazarus R and Folkman S: Stress, appraisal, and coping, New York, 1984, Springer Publishing Co, Inc, p 19.
7. Selye H: The stress of life, New York, 1956, McGraw-Hill, Inc, p 97.
8. Suter S: Health psychophysiology, Hillsdale, NJ, 1986, Lawrence Erlbaum Associates, Inc, p 67.
9. Lacey JI and Lacey BC: Verification and extension of the principle of autonomic response stereotype, Am J Psychol 71:50, 1958.
10. Suter S: Health psychophysiology, Hillsdale, NJ, 1986, Lawrence Erlbaum Associates, Inc, pp 193-240.
11. Holmes TH and Masuda M: Life change and illness susceptibility. In Dohrenwend BA and Dohrenwend BP, eds: Stressful life events: their nature and effects, New York, 1974, John Wiley & Sons, Inc, p 45.
12. Leventhal H and Tomarken A: Stress and illness: perspectives from health psychology. In Kasl SV and Cooper CL, eds: Stress and health: issues in research methodology, New York, 1978, John Wiley & Sons, Inc, pp 27–55.
13. Kobasa SC: Stressful life events, personality, and health: an inquiry into hardiness, J Pers Soc Psychol 37:2, 1979.
14. Madi S and Kobasa S: The hardy executive-health under stress, Chicago, 1984, The Dorsey Press.
15. Lazarus RS: Puzzles in the study of daily hassles, J Behav Med 7:376, 1984.
16. Lazarus R and Folkman S: Stress, appraisal, and coping, New York, 1984, Springer Publishing Co, Inc, pp 311-313.
17. Rowlison RT and Felner RD: Major life events, hassles, and adaptation in adolescence: confounding in the conceptualization and measurement of life stress and adjustment revisited, J Pers Soc Psychol 55:432, 1988.
18. Kanner AD and others: Comparison of two modes of stress measurement: daily hassles and uplifts versus major life events, J Behav Med 4:1, 1981.
19. Lazarus RS and Launier R: Stress-related transactions between person and environment. In Pervin LA and Lewis M, eds: Perspectives in international psychology, New York, 1978, Plenum Publishing Corp, p 296.
20. Lazarus R and Folkman S: Stress, appraisal, and coping, New York, 1984, Springer Publishing Co, Inc, pp 82-116.
21. Crabbs MA, Black KU, and Morton SP: Stress at work: a comparison of men and women, J Employment Counseling 3:2, 1986.
22. Hendrix WH: Behavioral and physiological consequences of stress and its antecedent factors, J Appl Psychol 2:188, 1985.
23. Motowidlo SJ, Packard JS, and Manning MR: Occupational stress: its causes and consequences, J Appl Psychol 11:618, 1986.
24. Osipow SH, Doty RE, and Spokane AR: Occupational stress, strain and coping across the life span, J Vocational Behav 17:98, 1985.
25. Walker CL: Stress and coping in siblings of childhood cancer patients, Nurs Res 37:208, 1988.

26. Northouse LL: Social support in patients' and husbands' adjustment to breast cancer, Nurs Res 37:91, 1988.

27. Gurklis JA and Menke EM: Identification of stressors and use of coping methods in chronic hemodialysis patients, Nurs Res 37:236, 1988.

28. Carr JA and Powers MJ: Stressors associated with coronary bypass surgery, Nurs Res 35:243, 1986.

29. Volicer BJ: Perceived stress levels of events associated with the experience of hospitalization: development and testing of a measurement tool, Nurs Res 22:491, 1973.

30. Volicer BJ and Bohannon MW: A hospital stress rating scale, Nurs Res 24:352, 1975.

31. Keane A, Ducette J, and Adler D: Stress in ICU and non-ICU nurses, Nurs Res 34:231, 1985.

32. Scalzi C: Role stress and coping strategies of nurse executives, J Nurs Adm 18:34, 1988.

33. Van Amerigen MR, Arsenault A, and Dolan SL: Intrinsic job stress and diastolic blood pressure among female hospital workers, J Occup Med 30:93, 1988.

34. Lazarus R and Folkman S: Stress, appraisal, and coping, New York, 1984, Springer Publishing Co, Inc, p 141.

35. Cohen F and Lazarus RS: Coping and adaptation in health and illness. In Mechanic D, ed: Handbook of health, health care, and the health professions, New York, 1983, Free Press, p 613.

36. Cohen F: Measurement of coping. In Kasl SV and Cooper CL, eds: Stress and health: issues in research methodology, New York, 1987, John Wiley & Sons, Inc, pp 283–305.

37. Lazarus RS and Launier R: Stress-related transactions between person and environment. In Pervin LA and Lewis M, eds: Perspectives in interactional psychology, New York, 1978, Plenum Publishing Corp, pp 319-320.

38. Anderson LP and Rehm LP: The relationship between strategies of coping and perception of pain in three chronic pain groups, J Clin Psychol 40:1170, 1984.

39. Jalowiec A: Revision and testing of the Jalowiec Coping Scale. Proceedings of the thirteenth annual conference of the Midwest Nursing Research Society 13:150, 1989.

40. Miller VSL: Identification of stressors related to patients' psychologic responses to the surgical intensive care unit, Heart Lung 16:267, 1978.

41. Musil CM and Abraham IL: Coping, thinking, and mental health nursing: cognitions and their application to psychosocial intervention, Issues Ment Health Nurs 8:191, 1986.

42. Pollock SE: The hardiness characteristic: a motivating factor in adaptation, Adv Nurs Sci 11:53, 1989.

43. Lazarus R and Folkman S: Stress, appraisal, and coping, New York, 1984, Springer Publishing Co, Inc, p 165.

44. Hull J, Treuren R, and Virnelli S: Hardiness and health: a critique and alternative approach, J Pers Soc Psychol 54:518, 1987.

45. Dennis K: Dimensions of client control, Nurs Res 36:151, 1987.

46. Gordon M: Manual of nursing diagnosis, 1990-1991, St Louis, 1991, The CV Mosby Co, p vii.

47. Gordon M: Manual of nursing diagnosis, 1990-1991, St Louis, 1991, The CV Mosby Co, p 329.

48. Gordon M: Manual of nursing diagnosis, 1990-1991, St Louis, 1991, The CV Mosby Co, p 345.

49. Houldin Ad, Saltstein SW, and Ganley KM: Nursing diagnoses for wellness: supporting strengths, New York, 1987, JB Lippincott Co, pp 135-139.

CHAPTER

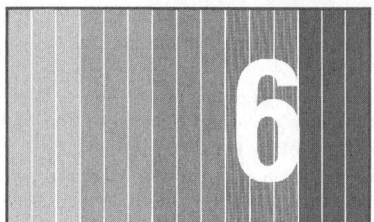

General Concepts
Client Teaching

Carol Cox Smith

L *earning Objectives*

1. *Identify nine attainable goals of client teaching.*
2. *Discuss effective ways of reducing stressors faced by the nurse-teacher.*
3. *Identify four common characteristics of the adult learner.*
4. *Identify factors contributing to successful teaching.*
5. *Differentiate among the three domains of learning.*
6. *List and describe the four steps in the teaching-learning process.*

7. *Identify four dimensions of assessment related to the teaching-learning process.*
8. *Discuss and give examples of barriers to learning.*
9. *Identify correctly written learning objectives.*
10. *Describe seven common teaching strategies.*
11. *Describe methods of short-term and long-term evaluation.*
12. *Select appropriate teaching strategies based on assessment of client needs and learning styles.*

The nurse has many teaching opportunities in hospitals and clinics, health care institutions, the community, schools, industry and offices, and the home. A client may experience specific and immediate needs, such as those associated with acute illness or hospitalization. At this time, the nurse-teacher can be particularly effective because the client is very receptive.

Learning helps the client cope with the stress of illness and the traumatic events surrounding hospitalization or surgery. It assists the client with handling outside factors (for example, family and job) and self-management. It can also make the client's treatment more effective and less costly.

Learning helps a client comply with treatment. A compliant client follows health plan instructions and cooperates with the health team. Compliance provides the client with the full benefit of prescribed medications and procedures, nutritional advice, and recommended lifestyle and activity adjustments.[1] Learning about specific information can increase the client's adaptation to change, and when the family is involved in the teaching process, it can reduce family stress.[2] By teaching correct procedures and

self-care, the nurse can help the client reduce the number of costly doctor's office visits and the length of a hospital stay.[2]

However, simply giving information is not teaching. The nurse-teacher must understand teaching-learning theory and be able to apply appropriate strategies for achieving learning objectives. No two clients are alike. The nurse-teacher must learn to individualize teaching to provide the right information at the right time and pace, under the right circumstances, and in the right manner.

ATTAINABLE GOALS OF CLIENT TEACHING

The short length of hospital stays often limits what the nurse-teacher can accomplish. However, even in a few days, the client and family can benefit when the nurse accomplishes one or more teaching goals:

1. Forewarn: Probably the most helpful teaching is forewarning. This teaching informs the client about normal sensations and situations associated with procedures and recovery. The nurse should provide information concerning any procedures or equipment the client will encounter, as well as any position the client may be asked to assume. The nurse should also explain what sensations the client may experience and offer suggestions for coping with anxiety-provoking circumstances.

Reviewed by Kathleen A. Clark, R.N., M.S., Curriculum Manager, Medical-Surgical Nursing, Bryan Memorial Hospital School of Nursing, Lincoln, Nebraska.

Sensory information should be given in specific terms, such as *cold, sharp,* or *dry.* Vague descriptions, such as *easy* or *painless,* should be avoided because they can be misinterpreted. Relaxation techniques and exercises can be explained and practiced to enhance the client's cooperation and confidence.[2] Preparation helps to relieve tension and reduce restlessness during and after procedures.

2. Teach skills: The nurse-teacher may teach motor skills ranging from simple (such as drinking from a straw) to complex (such as suctioning a tracheostomy). Teaching the skill and providing for practice and evaluation should be an ongoing process.

3. Assist in decision making: The nurse-teacher can provide information to help the client and family more fully understand the illness and judge its effects. This information allows the client and family to make informed decisions when several alternatives or choices are available.

4. Involve the family: The care and support of family members can help the recovery process. By involving the family in client teaching sessions, the nurse-teacher can soothe their concerns while building the client's confidence and positive attitude toward recovery.

5. Reinforce: An important factor in recovery is the client's confidence in the treatment and the practitioner. Often, clients do not feel well during treatment, such as with early ambulation following surgery. Calm encouragement from the nurse-teacher can minimize doubts and fears and help the client to remain calm and have a positive outlook.

6. Explain: Medical terminology and procedures are often mystifying to clients. A common medical term such as *catheter* may frighten an anxious client. The nurse-teacher must constantly guard against using terms that are unfamiliar or that can be misunderstood. A brief definition or explanation can greatly aid the client's coping mechanisms and conserve energy.

7. Discuss: After certain operations and procedures, the client may wish to discuss both present and future situations. For example, after a hysterectomy, women are often concerned about sexuality and resuming sexual relations. The nurse-teacher will find many opportunities to reassure the client that these questions are valid and answerable.

8. Advise: The nurse-teacher can advise the client and family concerning nursing or home care, community services, volunteer organizations, and support groups that can assist recovery. Advice on ways the family can monitor changes in the client's condition and suggestions for the client regarding self-care are important, particularly when a chronic illness is involved.

9. Change: By explaining behavioral goals and selecting the best teaching strategies and circumstances, the nurse-teacher can change client attitudes, help solve problems, and increase self-sufficiency. Although many teaching opportunities occur spontane-

ously, the best results will be achieved when goals are systematically planned and evaluated.

NURSE-TEACHER STRESSORS

Most nurses agree that client teaching is essential and that they would like to function more effectively in this role. However, nurses may become discouraged and decide to reduce their teaching efforts because of continuing problems and stress (Table 6-1). Two stressors experienced by the nurse-teacher are lack of time and insecurity

Table 6-1 Approaches to Overcoming Nurse-Teacher Stressors

Stressor	Approach
Lack of time	Preplan; set realistic goals; use time with client efficiently; break teaching and practice into small time periods
Lack of knowledge	Broaden knowledge base; read, study, ask questions; screen teaching materials; participate in other teaching sessions, observe more experienced nurse-teachers, attend classes
Disagreement with client	Establish agreed-on, written goals; develop a plan and discuss with client before teaching begins; introduce a role model to help illustrate therapeutic expectations; enlist the aid of significant others; revise expectations; learn to be satisfied with small achievements
Powerlessness, frustration	Recognize personal reactions to stress; develop a support system; rely on friends and family for positive encouragement; join a nurse-oriented support group; express feelings to others, but avoid griping and other negative interactions; improve communications with other professionals
Personal health problems	Take relaxation training; learn progressive muscular relaxation, biofeedback, self-hypnosis; practice self-suggestion, meditation; focus on the present; experiment with relaxers, such as music, exercise, positive imagery, assertiveness training

about self-knowledge and competence.[3] Another stressor is disagreement between nurse-teacher and client. Their values, needs, and expectations of teaching results may differ, causing tension in the teaching relationship.

The nurse-teacher should remember that the client is responsible for learning. The nurse-teacher cannot *force* a client to change a behavior or attitude. For many reasons, the client may not want to change. The nurse-teacher's job is to provide the information the client needs in ways that promote successful learning. The client must assume responsibility for the rest of the learning process.

Perhaps the nurse-teacher's most serious problem is accepting powerlessness. The client may not be willing to face problems or talk about the illness. The client's values may be vague, conflicting, or so outdated that the nurse-teacher cannot communicate. Family members or significant others may hold preset ideas that override the nurse-teacher's efforts. Sometimes, the nurse-teacher may face hostility, resentment, and verbal abuse. The nurse-teacher's frustration can cause personal health problems such as headache and backache.

Complicating these problems may be the health-care system itself. The nurse-teacher may face role ambiguity and conflict; that is, it may not be clear who should be responsible for client teaching and who should make teaching decisions. Lack of teaching facilities and materials can hinder teaching plans, and lack of communication with other professionals can cause duplication and omission of information, confusion, or oversights. However, the nurse-teacher can manage or overcome these stressors using several techniques.

CHARACTERISTICS OF THE ADULT LEARNER

The same general principles of learning apply, whether the client is a child or an adult. One principle is that learning cannot take place without perception—the mental grasp of information through the senses. For example, if a client cannot hear, verbal instructions cannot be followed. Other principles of learning include the following:
1. Learning is more effective when the client recognizes a need for it.
2. Learning must be reinforced (rewarded).
3. Learning is retained longer when it is put into immediate use.

However, four specific characteristics of adult learners affect the way in which the nurse-teacher uses these general principles.[2] These principles are (1) self-directed, (2) life experienced, (3) socially motivated, and (4) application oriented.

Self-Directed

The first characteristic of adult learners is that an adult's self-concept demands self-direction. That is, adults usually want to choose what and how they will learn. They prefer to control the method and rate of their learning. The nurse-teacher can take advantage of this characteristic by getting the client actively involved in the learning process.

For example, the nurse-teacher and client should discuss and agree on desired outcomes ("We agree that you need to be able to administer your own insulin injections" or "We want you to be able to successfully change your own colostomy bag"). The nurse-teacher may establish a written contractual agreement with the client based on agreed-on goals.

The client should also participate in the selection of reading or audiovisual materials. ("Which pamphlet is most interesting to you?") New teaching aids, such as programmed self-instruction and interactive computerized instruction, may give adult learners the control they need.

Although children often learn out of respect for authority, adults do not.[2] Adults will freely challenge the teacher's knowledge, methods, experience, and conclusions. They will always want to discuss what is taught from their own perspective and take control of the teaching session. The nurse-teacher should not feel threatened or defensive but should encourage the client to ask questions and provide input—making sure to stay on the topic and cover planned learning material.

Life Experienced

Adults have a vast fund of life experience on which the nurse-teacher can build. If clients feel they already "know" something about the subject from past experience, such as when a friend or relative has had a similar condition, they may be more willing to discuss it. However, if previous experience has been negative, the nurse may encounter resistance. In these cases, the nurse-teacher should discuss past experiences and try to correct misinformation. Clients may be more receptive to learning from other adults with a similar condition; seeing another person's progress will help relieve anxiety. Adults like to share life experiences, and the nurse-teacher is wise to take advantage of this characteristic.

If adults think they do not need the material or that it does not relate to their situation, they may resist or refuse instruction. The nurse-teacher can assist learning by finding out what the client needs to know and already knows. Unnecessary, irrelevant material should be omitted. Only those printed or audiovisual materials that target the specific problem should be used, and discussions and demonstrations should be limited to necessary content. Agreed-on goals that relate directly to what the client needs to know should be set.

Socially Motivated

Adults tend to learn more readily when they can apply what they learn to their social roles. That is, if learning a new skill will help a man become a better husband or employee, he is more likely to be receptive. However, if the learner believes that a skill is unnecessary because it does not apply to personal circumstances, attention to the lesson and motivation to learn will decrease.

The nurse-teacher can use this characteristic by determining the client's social roles and related concerns about fulfilling these roles. For example, the client may be concerned about caring for an elderly parent. This client may learn more readily if the nurse-teacher shows the way the new knowledge, attitude, or skill will help the parent. The client's support systems may be helpful in this process. The nurse-teacher can enlist the client's family, friends, and co-workers to encourage the client to learn, while praising the client's successes.

Application Oriented

Another characteristic of the adult learner is the need to apply learning immediately. Long-term goals have little appeal. The nurse-teacher should provide short-term, reachable goals and frequent opportunity for practice and review. Whenever possible, the nurse should allow the client to perform a task or procedure with the nurse's supervision and feedback.

A good idea is to briefly quiz the client verbally during each visit. ("Can you name the four basic food groups?" or "Review for me how to correctly draw up an insulin injection" or "Are you having any problems with your injections?") Once the nurse is satisfied that previously given instruction is retained, new content can begin. Rewards, such as praise, a treat, or a privilege, help reinforce new learning.

FACTORS CONTRIBUTING TO SUCCESSFUL TEACHING

Many factors combine to achieve or hinder the desired teaching outcomes. First, the nurse-teacher should be aware of the learner's unique characteristics. The nurse-teacher should also consider other factors that influence learning. These factors include the following:
1. The three domains of learning
2. Time and timing
3. The learning environment
4. Barriers to learning
5. Motivation

Domains of Learning

Learning takes place in three domains: cognitive, affective, and psychomotor. Depending on the client's needs, the nurse-teacher may plan learning experiences in all three.

The *cognitive domain* involves the learner's knowledge and understanding. It responds to facts and concepts conveyed in written materials, audiovisual aids, lectures, and discussions.[4] Cognitive learning also occurs by observing others, such as in peer support groups, film or video dramas, and case studies. This type of observation tends to decrease the client's inhibitions and self-consciousness and increase confidence, since the client sees that others are successfully dealing with similar situations.[4]

Knowledge and understanding can cause change. For example, after learning that an elevated cholesterol contributes to hypertension, a client is motivated to change cooking and eating patterns to reduce fat intake.

The *affective domain* involves the learner's attitudes, emotions, and ways of adjusting to illness. Bringing about change in the affective domain may be the nurse-teacher's most difficult challenge because the client must believe that the change is important. If a client refuses a vital blood transfusion because of fears of becoming infected with HIV, the nurse-teacher must try to change resistance to compliance and fear to confidence.

The affective domain can be influenced by the cognitive domain; knowledge and understanding can help change attitudes and emotions. For example, informing the client about protections against HIV infection and the positive implications of transfusion can reduce fear.

Other ways to bring about change in the affective domain include the following:
1. Allow the client to talk about feelings.
2. Help the client gain new insights into feelings.
3. Provide positive role models.
4. Encourage the client to take action.
5. Reinforce action with encouragement and support.

For example, talking to someone who has adjusted well to a colostomy can help a client face and overcome feelings of disfigurement. The nurse-teacher should look for positive experiences to help the client develop new attitudes.

The *psychomotor domain* involves learning motor skills such as walking with a prosthesis or changing a dressing. The ability to learn motor skills varies with the individual client's strength, reaction time, speed, balance, precision, and flexibility.[4] It is also influenced by factors such as the client's self-image and motivation. For example, a client may not want to learn to walk with the aid of a walker or cane; being dependent on a wheelchair may bring more sympathy from others. Such benefits are known as *secondary gains*.

The psychomotor domain is influenced by the cognitive and affective domains. In the cognitive domain, the nurse-teacher should demonstrate the skill and give cues for correct performance. A cue is a visual or audio clue, such as the snap of a correctly affixed hypodermic needle. The nurse-teacher should also give feedback in response to the client's skill performance. Routine repetition and consistent teaching are important.

The affective component of learning a motor skill requires that the nurse-teacher consider the client's attitude toward self-efficacy (the ability for self-care). For example, to a man who has undergone a leg amputation, walking may seem an impossible task. If he cannot walk, he cannot take care of himself, or so he believes. His preference for being dependent on others can cause him to resist learning even simple motor skills, such as getting in and out of bed without aid.

To overcome negative attitudes, the nurse-teacher should divide motor skills into short, achievable actions; this technique allows the client to succeed in small ways before proceeding to more difficult actions.[1] The nurse-teacher should use verbal persuasion to help the client believe in personal ability. The nurse-teacher should also be aware that vicarious experiences, those that occur when a client sees others achieving similar learning goals, raise the client's expectations of self-efficacy: "If others can do it, I can too!"

Time and Timing

Another factor contributing to successful learning is *time*. As people get older, their rate of learning changes. Since it takes an older person longer to learn a new skill than a younger person, more time must be allowed. Time limits and pressures imposed on the adult client may produce negative results. Best results usually occur when the adult client can set the rate of learning. However, proceeding at the client's rate may not always be possible due to many factors such as early discharge. In this case, the nurse should plan to refer the client to a home care program, visiting nurse, or another follow-up agency.

Incorporated in the concept of time is *timing:* knowing when to teach and when not to teach. The nurse needs to be attuned to each client's needs because these needs change from hour to hour and day to day. Planning ahead and knowing the client's schedule are helpful. For example, if a client is being discharged but needs to know how to change a dressing, the nurse should plan to teach this skill as far ahead of discharge as possible. In this way, the client will have time to practice and review the skill and feel confident after discharge.

Learning Environment

Another factor is the *learning environment.* From the moment the client enters the hospital until discharge— even before initial assessment is complete—the nurse must work to develop a feeling of trust, respect, and support. The client will learn best in an atmosphere of warmth, comfort, and caring. When the nurse and client establish rapport, the teaching-learning transaction will be more successful. (See Chapter 3 for interviewing principles and developing rapport.)

The learning environment is also a physical climate. Since distractions can reduce the efficiency of teaching and learning, the nurse should eliminate, rearrange, or control noise, lighting, ventilation, and odors. The window should be closed if too much traffic noise is coming from the street. The classroom door should be shut to eliminate visual distractions from passersby. The television set or radio should be turned off, and the privacy curtain should be pulled. Remembering that adult clients may have reduced visual or auditory ability, the nurse should provide clear visual cues (adequate illumination, larger print, reduced glare) and adequate auditory cues (speaking clearly, facing the client, and slightly increasing speech volume).

Barriers to Learning

Regardless of the many positive experiences the nurse-teacher provides, learning may be blocked by several barriers.[2] The nurse-teacher should be aware of these barriers and try to remove them so that learning can take place freely. However, not all barriers can be removed; those that remain need to be overcome with creative solutions.

Time can be a barrier if it is limited. The client may not have enough time to learn and practice a new skill or become comfortable with a new attitude. The nurse-teacher will need to set objectives based on short-term goals and make take-home materials available. In addition, the nurse-teacher should be prepared for "teachable moments" during which the client is available and receptive.[2]

The client may have other priorities, such as work or child care. For example, a woman may be unwilling to attend a class to learn a new skill at a clinic until she can get a babysitter. The learning level or reading level of the material may be too difficult, creating another barrier. Psychological deterrents, such as a learning disability, may interfere with learning.

Finally, the nurse-teacher may unknowingly create teaching barriers. Teaching may be unclear or confusing. The nurse-teacher may fail to show respect for the client's personhood and may not recognize the client's fears or mistaken health beliefs. Important visual cues, such as body positioning and facial expressions that indicate learning difficulty, may be overlooked.

The nurse-teacher can discuss priorities with clients and suggest ways to make necessary arrangements such as time off from work. The nurse-teacher should seek appropriate materials to fit each client's individual learning ability. Finally, the nurse-teacher should undertake the most difficult task of all—improving teaching performance.

One helpful technique for self-improvement is videotaping a teaching session and getting evaluation from a knowledgeable co-worker or supervisor. Another technique is observing effective teachers; copying their methods; and practicing on family, friends, and fellow nurses. Teaching is a skill and an art; it takes practice to improve.

Motivation

Learning will not take place without motivation. Motivation is the client's willingness to participate in the learning process by extending effort. Clients are motivated when they are convinced that they need to know something because it will reduce the threat of illness or increase their ability to take care of themselves.

Readiness to learn is the extent that a person is motivated to learn at a particular time. The nurse-teacher evaluates readiness to learn during the assessment step of the teaching-learning process. The client may not be ready to learn if the client is extremely anxious or is having difficulty adapting to the illness. Financial or family pressures that affect the client's attitude negatively and personal or family values that conflict with health care values will also decrease the client's readiness to learn. In these cases the nurse-teacher may recommend counseling, social services referral, or other intermediate steps before attempting to begin the teaching process.

Many people are motivated to learn, not so much from external forces (for example, peer pressure) as from *internal standards*. They set incentives for themselves based on their self-concept. For example, a self-made individual may be highly motivated to learn self-care to maintain independence. Other people are motivated by *external influences*, such as a positive learning environment, learning activities, rewards or other reinforcements, and the expectation of success.

For many clients, the most motivating factor is the nurse-teacher's support. The nurse-teacher is the client's "cheerleader," the one person who always maintains a positive attitude and believes totally in the client's ability to learn and accomplish. The nurse-teacher will not abandon the client when problems arise. A client's spouse or friends may be too critical or too complimentary, and the nurse-teacher may be the only person who will communicate realistically and nonjudgmentally. The nurse-teacher may be the only real support a person has (Fig. 6-1).

Other suggestions for enhancing motivation are (1) organize the material and present it in logical order from the *simple to the complex;* (2) always present a warm, caring, nonthreatening image to the client, using positive, *supportive communication;* and (3) provide frequent *measures of success*. A client who knows that learning is occurring

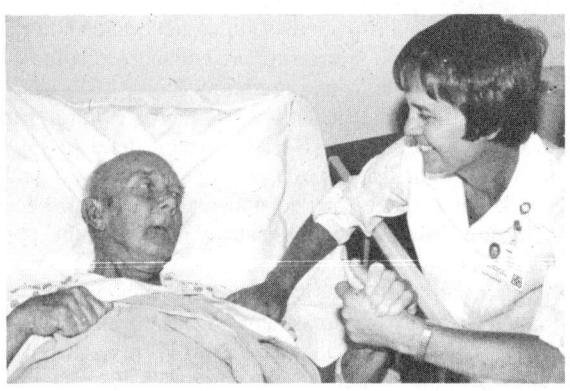

Fig. 6-1 A touch and a smile give warm support.

and experiences success is strongly motivated to learn more. Immediate experiences of success in the learning process help overcome the fear of failure, which is a learning block for many adults.

TEACHING-LEARNING PROCESS

The nurse-teacher should be able to follow these four basic steps in the teaching-learning process: (1) assessment, (2) planning, (3) implementation, and (4) evaluation.

Assessment

Assessment as a process may be defined as a systematic method of gathering relevant information about a particular client. Assessment for the purpose of developing a teaching plan includes collecting a complete data base identifying the client's strengths and weaknesses and determining personal characteristics, learning characteristics, and experiential characteristics of the client. Even during a brief hospital stay or short office visit, a quick interview can reveal what the client needs to know, already knows, and is ready to learn.

Biophysical dimension. Assessment begins when the nurse considers the client's *biophysical dimension.* How old is the client? Age will provide cues to the nurse concerning the rate of learning; past experiences; memory ability; mastery of developmental tasks; and possible impairments of vision, hearing, and reaction time.

The physiological condition and physical health of an adult client can determine readiness to learn. Sensory impairment such as poor vision or hearing loss can decrease ability to learn because of restricted sensory input. Learning requires an adequately functioning nervous system. Therefore, a client with problems such as a cerebral vascular accident, poor cardiac perfusion, or severe muscular or nervous system trauma may easily forget; the nurse may need to repeat information frequently to facilitate learning. In some cases the nurse may need to postpone teaching until the client is physiologically ready to learn, that is, until a certain amount of healing has taken place.

Pain and fatigue will also influence a client's readiness to learn. No one can learn efficiently when in severe pain. To clients experiencing intense pain, the nurse should give only a brief explanation and then follow with more detailed instruction when pain has been managed.

The nurse must also be aware of the client's energy level. A tired or weak client cannot learn effectively because the level of concentration is low. The nurse should wait until the client is rested and has more energy before beginning instruction.

Medications may also influence a client's readiness to learn. Barbiturates, tranquilizers, and narcotic analgesics can cause drowsiness, clouding of consciousness, and a general decrease in mental alertness. The nurse must continuously evaluate the client's physical condition, including response to medications, and reassess readiness to learn.

Psychological dimension. A second aspect of assessment is the *psychological dimension.* This involves the nurse assessing the client's personal adjustment to the illness and the learning situation. Is the client anxious? Although mild anxiety increases the learner's perceptual and recall abilities, excessive anxiety may block learning.[5] The nurse-teacher can help the client overcome anxiety by encouraging the open expression of fears.[6] The nurse-teacher's nonjudgmental understanding is better than superficial "pep talks."

Is the client depressed? The client may be grieving the loss of a valued ability or self-concept. The nurse-teacher should allow the client time to grieve and set only short, reachable teaching goals until the psychological state improves.

Is the client more internally or externally oriented? People who have an internal locus of control (they believe they control their lives) tend to want more knowledge about their health.[5] In contrast, persons who have an external locus of control (they believe that luck, chance, or powerful others control their life) may want less information.

Is the client a risk-taker? Some people do not want to try anything new and find change extremely threatening. Security and sameness may have more appeal than the unknown outcome of new knowledge, attitudes, and skills. When assessing this aspect, the nurse-teacher may note that the client's support system must participate in the learning process to lessen the client's feelings of risk.

Is the client denying or minimizing the illness or condition? Is the client showing self-blame for not following preventive health practices? Is the client regressing to a childlike state? Is the client overly cheerful, hiding depression or despair? These coping styles affect the individual's ability to process information. The nurse-teacher should not attempt to change the client's coping style drastically; rather, an understanding manner and a sensitive teaching plan that considers coping style will help reduce anxiety and motivate the client to learn.[6] (See Chapter 5 for a discussion of coping styles.)

Other psychological factors that can influence learning are the client's personality, the ways of adapting to illness, and outlook on life. The client's vulnerability, hopelessness, or defensiveness may decrease the desire to learn. Illness itself or the threat of illness can force the individual to reassess goals and reevaluate life.

In addition, if the client does not adapt well to illness, learning will not be effective. How well the individual adapts depends on self-concept before the illness, the severity of illness, life changes due to illness, and the meaning the illness has to the client and family, friends, and coworkers. Pertinent information can help the client adapt well if the nurse intervenes at the appropriate time.

Sociocultural dimension. The *sociocultural dimension* must also be assessed. Basically, this means that the nurse must examine the client's lifestyle (life situation). Lifestyle influences how the client perceives the hospital setting and the entire learning experience. Lifestyle includes many elements: occupation, education, income, housing arrangement, living location (rural or urban), dietary pattern, sleep pattern, exercise, sexuality, and stressors. The client's values and beliefs can also influence views of health and illness and therefore the response to the teaching-learning process.

For example, a person who values a youthful figure can be taught to diet and exercise to retain that figure while at the same time bringing an ulcer under control. However, being fat is valued as a sign of financial success and sexuality in many cultures. A client from such a culture would probably reject the concept of diet and exercise for weight control or any other reason.

The client's stage of life should be assessed. A person in midlife, newly aware of self-mortality, may be motivated or threatened by illness. The nurse-teacher should assess what help this client needs in coping with life changes such as menopause, decreasing sexual activity, and stress. An older adult may face the nurse-teacher's own prejudices—the attitude that teaching older adults is a "waste of time." The nurse-teacher must make a special effort to avoid stereotyping; the teaching plan should include topics related to lifestyle changes, prevention, nutrition, and quality of life, as well as information directly related to the client's present condition.

Learning is closely related to the wider culture and the subculture to which the client belongs. Health beliefs and actions vary by religious belief, ethnic group, and family group. The nurse must assess and understand the client's cultural background and must develop a teaching plan that considers this element.

For example, a middle-aged, upper-income woman may belong to a subculture in which "popping pills" is widely accepted. She may therefore be willing to take prescribed pills but unwilling to learn to self-administer an injection. When assessing the client's needs, the nurse must take a holistic approach and see the client as a total person within her subculture. The nurse's teaching plan must include ways to change the client's attitudes or show the client how her new skill will fit into her existing lifestyle.

Persons from various subcultures make up the client's support network. Family members, co-workers, supervisors, neighbors, classmates, religious advisors, interest groups, and team members can help the client cope with the stress of illness and the need for change. The nurse-teacher should assess the quality of the client's support network. The nurse-teacher should assess support persons' concerns and involve them in the learning process. When-

ever possible, support persons should encourage and praise the client's progress. Such support enhances readiness to learn, information gain, and retention.[5]

An interesting element within the client's cultural group is the *leadership pattern*. Because people tend to follow the advice of their leaders, the nurse should try to identify and work with leaders or decision makers within the client's culture group. Their assistance may help the client accept new ideas and techniques.

Environmental dimension. The *environmental dimension* is another part of assessment. A basic teaching motto is "Begin with what the learner knows." Previous life experiences will determine where the nurse-teacher should begin instruction. Since learning is a process by which individuals add to or modify their previously existing knowledge, skills, and attitudes, past experiences and types of informal and formal instruction should be determined. The nurse should ask questions related to previous hospital experiences, previous experiences with diet, medications, and other family illnesses. Has the client known anyone in the past with this illness? Has the client read any material about the illness? Have previous hospital experiences been positive or negative? Have any previous treatments familiarized the client with similar equipment or processes? For example, previous experience with allergy desensitization would have familiarized the client with syringes.

The nurse should also determine what educational experiences the client has had. If past educational situations have been negative (overly critical teachers, "waste of time" attitude, poor or failing grades, nonsupportive family or friends), the nurse-teacher will need to provide continuous encouragement and the earliest possible experiences of success.

Learning styles. A related concept that the nurse should assess is the client's *learning style*. Everyone has a distinct style of learning, as individual as personality. The three learning styles are (1) visual (reading), (2) aural (listening), and (3) physical (doing things). People often use more than one learning style. To determine the client's learning style, the nurse might ask the following questions:

1. In what kind of environment do you learn best? Formal classroom? Informal setting, such as home or office? Among a group of peers?
2. Do you learn best when you are alone or in a group?
3. Do you prefer to read information, hear it from a tape, listen to a lecture, or watch a film or slide presentation? Would you rather physically do something?
4. How do you feel that most of your learning has taken place? Have you learned primarily from classes, personal experience, discussion groups, personal reading, or television?

Answers to questions such as these help both the nurse and the client focus on the most appropriate teaching strategies to fit the learning style. Based on the assessment information, the nurse may recognize that lack of knowledge is an etiological factor for a specific nursing diagnosis such as anxiety, fear, or altered health maintenance.[7] The nurse should specify the exact nature of the knowledge deficiency so that a specific teaching plan can be developed.

For example, the nursing diagnosis of altered health maintenance related to lack of knowledge of insulin administration provides the nurse with a clear direction for the teaching-learning process.

Planning

The second step in the teaching-learning process follows detailed assessment. In this step the nurse involves the client in *determining objectives* and *planning the learning experience.* Together, they determine the gap between what the client knows and needs to know. Then the nurse organizes simple to complex objectives. Clients will feel motivated and ready to learn if objectives seem within their intellectual, educational, or physical ability.

Planning should be divided into short-term and long-term objectives. The nurse-teacher should plan short-term objectives that the client needs to use for self-care or discharge. These should include the client's understanding of normal changes in the course of illness, potential problems and risks, and self-monitoring skills. Because of time constraints, these may be the only objectives the nurse-teacher can accomplish. Long-term objectives may need to be referred to other health care professionals.

The use of standardized teaching plans for common major illnesses and surgeries has become an accepted method for developing a teaching plan. Standardized teaching plans contain widely accepted information and skills that a client needs to know concerning a specific medical illness or surgical procedure. The nurse should individualize these plans to meet the specific client's needs.

Because individuals tend to feel more committed to a decision or activity when they participate in making or planning it, the client and the nurse should mutually agree on learning objectives. If the physical or psychological condition of the client prevents active participation, the nurse must assume the major role of designing the learning experience. The client's family or significant others can assist the nurse in this process, and the client can be involved as soon as possible.

Learning objectives describe intended results of instruction, guide the selection of teaching strategies and materials, and help evaluate client and teacher progress. These objectives should be written down and made readily available to all members of the health care team. To communicate clearly to those who need to know, the nurse should acquire skill in writing clear, specific, measurable teaching objectives.

Writing specific learning objectives. Learning objectives are written statements defining exactly what learners must do to show that they have mastered the content. The objectives contain the following four elements:

1. The individual who will perform the activity or acquire the desired behavior:
   The client will . . .
   The spouse will . . .
   The client's family will . . .
2. The actual behavior that the learner will exhibit to demonstrate mastery of the objective:
   List the symptoms . . .
   Self-administer an insulin injection . . .
   Identify from a hospital menu . . .
3. The conditions under which the behavior is to be demonstrated (how and where the learner will perform):
   In front of the nurse . . .
   At home . . .
   Select from a random list . . .
   Choose from a restaurant menu . . .
4. The specific criteria that will be used to measure the client's success such as time and degree of accuracy:
   With 100% accuracy . . .
   Using correct technique . . .
   Within 3 minutes . . .

Well-written learning objectives contain very precise descriptions, using terms with few interpretations. When writing objectives, nurses should use verbs such as *identify, list, describe, demonstrate, name, recognize,* or *compare and contrast.* They should avoid terms with vague, ambiguous meanings, such as *appreciate, learn, understand, enjoy, feel,* or *value.*

Poorly written and well-written objectives. The following is an example of a poorly written learning objective:

The client will appreciate the importance of proper foot care.

How will the client demonstrate "appreciation"? When and to whom will this behavior be demonstrated? What criteria will be used? In the above objective, these questions are not answered.

The following are examples of well-written learning objectives:

The client will be able to demonstrate to the nurse the correct technique for changing a colostomy bag.

The client will self-administer in front of the nurse a subcutaneous injection of insulin using correct technique.

The client will select a 1000-mg Na diet from the hospital menu for breakfast, lunch, and dinner for 3 consecutive days with 90% accuracy.

Given a list of symptoms of hyperglycemia and hypoglycemia, the client will be able to identify the early symptoms of hypoglycemia with 80% accuracy.

When learning objectives are clear and specific and when they are written down and available in the client's record, all members of the health care team can work together to accomplish the same objectives. This type of communication will ensure good results.

Implementation

Implementation has two aspects: determination of teaching strategies and presentation of learning material to the client.

Teaching strategies. After the objectives are clearly stated, the nurse and client (with input from other members of the health care team as available and appropriate) can develop the teaching plan. Together, they can select content and materials and decide on strategies and learning tasks. Selecting a particular teaching strategy is determined by at least three factors: (1) the character of the learner (learning style, educational background, and culture and subculture), (2) the subject matter, and (3) available facilities. The nurse and client must choose the strategy or strategies that can be used most effectively and that are most beneficial.

There are seven common teaching strategies that the nurse-teacher can use to achieve learning objectives. Each has advantages and disadvantages that make it more suitable to a particular learning situation.

Lecture. For rapid learning when time is short, the *lecture* is an efficient, versatile, and economical teaching strategy. The nurse presents a series of related ideas or facts to one person or a group. Usually, the lecture is short (from 15 to 20 minutes), and some visual reinforcement such as a diagram on a blackboard emphasizes key points. Some disadvantages of the lecture are that it often has a negative "school learning" connotation, and individual learning is difficult to evaluate. In addition, the nurse-teacher is active but the clients are passive unless they are allowed to participate or ask questions.

Lecture-discussion. A second teaching strategy is the *lecture-discussion*, which can overcome some disadvantages of the straight lecture. With this strategy, the nurse presents specific information by using the lecture technique, followed by a period during which clients ask questions and exchange views with the nurse. This strategy assists the client in becoming an active participant in the learning process and creates a more informal give-and-take learning environment.

Discussion. A third strategy is *discussion*, and its purpose is to exchange views concerning a topic or question or to arrive at a decision or conclusion. The nurse can discuss content with an individual or a group, keeping the specific learning objectives in mind and clarifying information as needed. This strategy is a good choice when the client or clients have previous experience with a subject and have information to share, such as in smoking cessation, postcoronary, or preoperative teaching classes. The discussion allows the client to actively participate and to apply experiences and observations to the learning process. However, one disadvantage is that the discussion will take longer to cover a given amount of material than other methods. The informal sharing and nonthreatening environment of discussion are positive factors, but the time and difficulty of reaching desired objectives may be disadvantages.

Group teaching. Two kinds of *group teaching* exist. In the first, the nurse acts as a *facilitator* for group sharing about a common problem. The nurse does not teach or participate but keeps information moving among all group members. The nurse may introduce the client to an existing group or may form a group of persons with similar problems such as clients whose older parents live at home with them.

A second kind of *group teaching* involves peer teaching as found in *support groups*. A support group is a self-help organization that can provide continuing information, shared experiences, acceptance, understanding, and useful suggestions about a problem or concern. Clients with problems such as impotence, sexual self-destructiveness, suicide, cancer, alcoholism, Parkinson's disease, compul-

sive overeating, diabetes, hypoglycemia, heart surgery, child abuse, and drug addiction can find help from the support group approach. In many cases, support groups have proven to be the most effective form of teaching. Therefore, the nurse should actively look for opportunities to refer a client and concerned family and friends to a support group. This action should be taken in addition to but not instead of the nurse's planned teaching sessions.

Demonstration/return demonstration. *Demonstration/return demonstration* is probably the most common strategy a nurse-teacher uses. One purpose is to show the way something works and the procedure to follow when doing it. Another purpose is to illustrate to the client how a skill is performed or to demonstrate ideas, problem solving, or motor skills. The focus is on correct procedure and application. To handle this strategy correctly, the nurse should tell the client the purpose of the demonstration and ensure that the client can see and hear clearly. The nurse presents the demonstration informally, defines unfamiliar terms, and watches for signs of confusion from the client. The nurse clarifies and repeats as needed, and the client returns the demonstration with the nurse as observer. The entire process should last no more than 15 to 20 minutes and should be briefly repeated during the nurse's next teaching session with the client.

Role playing. Another strategy that the nurse may use, depending on teaching objectives, is *role playing*. This strategy may be effective when clients need to examine their attitudes and behaviors; understand viewpoints and attitudes of others; or practice carrying out thoughts, ideas, or decisions. The nurse is in a difficult and delicate position when using this strategy. The nurse must define the problem, determine goals, set the climate, and determine the situation and roles to be played. Information and instructions must be given to role players and observers, and time must be provided for feedback and evaluation. At the same time the nurse must keep the role playing from deteriorating into an emotional scene. Few clients are mature enough, confident enough, and flexible enough to role play successfully. More often, clients feel uncomfortable and inhibited with this method. Again, time can be a negative factor, and results are difficult to evaluate. However, this strategy is ideal for some situations. For example, a wife may need to rehearse how to talk to her husband about his need to quit smoking. In this case, "play acting" the discussion ahead of time is a helpful strategy.

Audiovisual material. A final strategy for the nurse to consider is the use of *audiovisual materials,* including movies, film strips, slides, posters, charts, videotapes, audiotapes, and simple transparencies. Innovative computer-assisted programs allow the client to interact with the subject matter. This strategy can be used to effectively present most information, and the presentation is more interesting because more than one sense is being used. To use this strategy, the nurse must know what materials are available within the care facility, from support agencies, and from professional groups. These materials must be previewed and evaluated for accuracy, completeness, and appropriateness to the learning objectives before being shown to

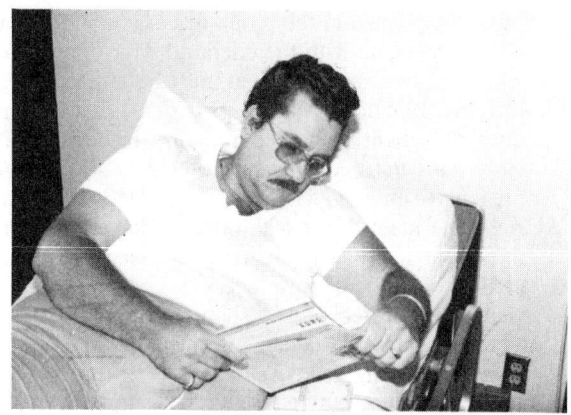

Fig. 6-2 Any teaching strategy can be reinforced with written material selected for the client's reading level.

the client. Unfortunately, many audiovisual items are expensive, and viewing or listening space may be difficult to obtain. Additionally, audiovisual equipment such as projectors and viewers must be in good repair and available for the nurse's use. The nurse must also be able to operate the equipment alone. However, in spite of these disadvantages, this strategy can be extremely beneficial, particularly when teaching content is largely visual, such as the steps, processes, and results of a surgical procedure.

Use of printed material with strategies. Many *printed materials* are available for the nurse-teacher, and these should be considered for use with each of the seven teaching strategies (Fig. 6-2). For example, after a lecture on the physiological effects of smoking, the nurse can distribute a pamphlet from the American Cancer Society that reviews and reinforces the topic. The nurse-teacher may select a book or magazine article written by a woman who has had a mastectomy and instruct the client to read this material before viewing a film on the same topic.

Nurses should always consider the learning style of the client. Many people prefer to read material in private at their own pace, before or after a learning experience. The care facility's library, the pharmacy, members of the health care team, the public library, federal and state agencies, universities, and research centers are some of the major resources for the nurse seeking relevant printed materials.

The nurse should evaluate the materials using nine criteria: (1) accuracy; (2) completeness; (3) the effectiveness of the materials in meeting specific learning goals; (4) vocabulary and sentence length suitable to the client's educational level; (5) use of pictures or diagrams to stimulate interest; (6) use of one main idea or concept per pamphlet; (7) use of terminology that the client understands rather than undefined medical terminology; (8) the amount of information contained that the client would like to know; and (9) the relevance of the material to the client's values (for example, same material may reflect values specific to the middle class).[4]

Presentation. Presentation is the second aspect of implementation. To present effectively, the nurse must have an attitude of interest, enthusiasm, respect, and belief in the client's ability to learn. The client should not be placed in the position of passive recipient. Based on the assessment of the client's physical and psychological condition, the nurse should determine the amount of active participation the client can assume. The time spent in the teaching-learning transaction should be based on the client's energy level. In most cases, short learning sessions are much more conducive to learning than long learning sessions. The nurse can incorporate teaching into routine nursing care or schedule separate sessions. Either way, the nurse should continuously reassess the client's condition so that the teaching situation remains flexible and adaptable as the client's needs change.

When implementing the teaching plan, the nurse should remember the basic concepts for successful teaching:

1. Keep the physical environment relaxed and nonthreatening to reduce client's anxiety.
2. Maintain a warm, enthusiastic, and respectful attitude. Maintain eye contact and a caring demeanor.
3. Involve the client in the teaching-learning process as fully as possible. Emphasize active participation.
4. Use and build on the client's previous experiences. Encourage questions.
5. Emphasize the practical application of the learned material to the client's lifestyle and immediate solution to problems.
6. When necessary, assist the client with unlearning poor habits or negative attitudes.
7. Allow the adult client to select the time for learning. Consider factors such as medications, fatigue, and family participation when scheduling a teaching session.
8. Individualize the teaching-learning transaction, even if standardized teaching plans are used.
9. Identify what the client wants to learn first to provide direction for learning activities.
10. Give positive feedback. Be aware of verbal and visual cues that reveal the client's concerns.
11. Allow the client to pace learning when possible.
12. Keep information relevant to the client's needs and goals.
13. Consider counseling intervention if the client is not ready to learn.
14. Preview and summarize each session.

Evaluation

Evaluation is the final step in the teaching-learning process and is a measure of the degree to which the client has mastered the learning objectives. The nurse must be aware of the performance level of the client so that changes can be made as needed. The nurse may find that the client has achieved the goals; however, if certain goals were not reached, the nurse may need to develop a new teaching plan. If the client has developed new needs, the nurse should plan new goals, content, and strategies.

For example, an older man with diabetes entered the hospital with a blood sugar of 320 mg/dL. When the student nurse began to prepare his insulin injection, the head nurse asked, "Are you going to have him give his own insulin and observe his technique?" "Oh, no," replied the student nurse, "He has been a diabetic for 20 years!" The assumption was that a client with diabetes would know how to perform this task correctly. The two nurses returned to the client's room and asked him to draw up his injection. They were astonished to see the client fill the syringe with 20 units of insulin and 20 units of air instead of 40 units of insulin. After correcting the dose and questioning the client more fully, the nurses concluded that the client could not accurately see the markings on the syringe; they believed that the client may have been self-administering insufficient insulin for a long time. The client's vision was not as good as it had been 20 years ago (his needs had changed), and special equipment was now necessary for him to safely and accurately administer the insulin.

Short-term evaluation techniques. Evaluation techniques may be short or long term. Short-term evaluation techniques may involve the client and nurse, the client's family, significant others, and/or members of the health care team. Nurses can quickly evaluate the client's mastery of a skill or behavior change in the following ways:

1. Observing the client directly: "Show me how you will change your dressing." "Let me see how you administer your injection." By observation, the nurse determines if a task has been mastered, if further instruction is needed, or if the client is ready for new or additional content.
2. Observing verbal and nonverbal clues: If the client asks questions, asks for repeat instructions, shakes the head, loses eye contact, slumps or droops in the chair or bed, becomes restless and fidgety, or otherwise expresses doubt about understanding, the client is indicating that further instruction is needed or a different approach should be taken. Nurses should be alert and watch and listen to the client carefully for correct evaluation.
3. Asking the client direct questions: "What are the four major food groups?" "How often must you change your dressing?" "What are the warning signs of a heart attack?" Nurses should ask questions that require more than a "yes" or "no" answer.
4. Using a written measurement tool (a test, essay, or list) that can be graded for accuracy: Written tests tend to bring about or increase anxiety in adult clients and therefore may not produce accurate evaluation. Often, adult clients will "freeze" when given a test, or they "go blank" when asked to write something that they know will be graded. Nurses need to assess the client's learning style before using this evaluation method.
5. Talking to the client's family, culture group members, group leaders, or other health professionals involved with care: "Is the client eating regularly?" "How is the client handling the walker?" "Did the

client participate in the group discussion?" Since the nurse cannot be with the client all day, other people who visit or assist the client must be utilized.

6. Helping the client evaluate progress: What evidence does the client have that progress is being made? How does the client feel: confident or unsure? Apprehensive or ready to go forward with new material? The main thrust with this technique is to determine whether the client believes that there is self-control of the learning process.

These short-term techniques should be used frequently and interchangeably to keep informed of the client's progress and changing needs.

Long-term evaluation techniques. Long-term evaluation requires follow-up by the nurse, the care facility, or an outside agency or program. A home visit may be possible in some care settings. In other situations, regular phone calls may ensure that movement toward long-term goals is being made. The client can also be evaluated on future visits to the health care facility when practical. The nurse's role is to emphasize to the client the need for regular evaluation and monitoring by an individual or group familiar with the client's needs and to act as a bridge between the client's needs and the program's focus.[8]

In some settings a referral may be necessary to accomplish long-term evaluation. Before making a referral, the nurse should assess the client's needs for further teaching and follow-up, locate a referral resource, and determine how the referral source matches the client's needs. The nurse should also consider factors such as eligibility requirements, teacher qualifications, subjects offered, focus, location, and cost. In addition, a client may self-refer to meet a particular need.

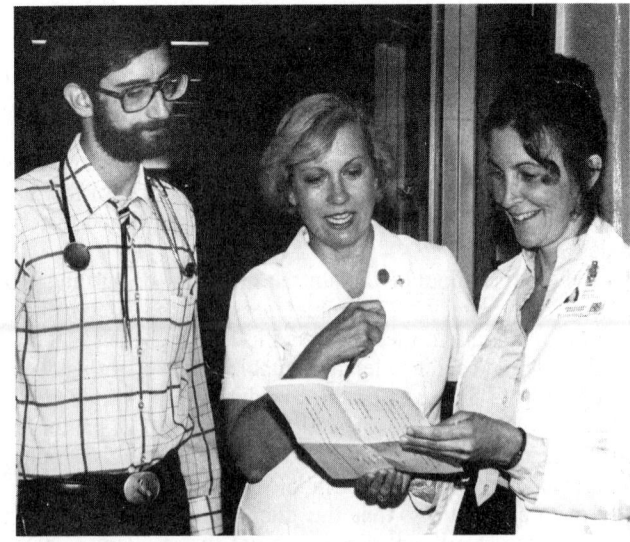

Fig. 6-3 Health team members should cooperate in setting objectives and evaluating client progress.

When a referral has been made, the nurse should telephone, visit, or write the referral source and request updated information on the client's progress. Once obtained, these data should be added to the client's records for future use.

Documentation is an essential component of the entire teaching-learning transaction. Documentation reminds the nurse and other health professionals what has been taught and what needs to be covered. It helps coordinate health care for a consistent approach to client teaching.[6] The nurse must record everything from the assessment through evaluation and each follow-up contact in detail. However, documentation should be kept simple. A checklist on the client's chart or a note on the client's records is usually sufficient. The documentation should be forwarded to the agency that will provide long-term follow-up for the client. Since many different members of the health care team will need to examine these records in many different places, and for many different reasons, the teaching objectives, content, strategies, and evaluation results should be written as clearly and completely as possible. Health team members should be encouraged to add comments and observations to these records, and conferences should be held whenever possible to review the teaching-learning plan (Fig. 6-3).

Teaching the adult client in an acute-care setting is a challenging and rewarding experience for the nurse. It is a dynamic process that begins when the client is first seen, continues with each contact, and remains an integral part of the client's care over a long period. The following case study illustrates many of the principles related to client education.

 ## ase Study

EXAMPLE OF THE TEACHING-LEARNING PROCESS

Mrs. A. has been admitted to the hospital for preliminary testing and preparation for a hysterectomy. The nurse is aware that a client scheduled for a hysterectomy is often deeply concerned about her self-concept as a woman. The nurse also knows that clients need to express their feelings in an atmosphere of support and understanding. Therefore the nurse has listened and asked questions carefully to assess the client's feelings about and knowledge of her forthcoming hysterectomy. The nurse has asked open-ended questions such as "How do you feel about having this hysterectomy?" and "What concerns do you have about your hysterectomy?" By establishing a climate of trust and a counseling relationship, the nurse has completed the following assessment:

Biophysical Dimension

Age: 44
Occupation: High school English teacher. Also sponsors girls' varsity cheerleaders.
Physiological condition and physical health: No sensory impairment. Good general health. Height/weight proportion average for age. Client states that she jogs 3 to 4 times a week and works out with the school cheerleading squad. Vision, hearing, and reaction time are normal. Since the client's energy level seems low, the nurse decides to begin teaching after the client has had a period of rest.

Psychological Dimension

Client appears mildly anxious about the surgery and worried about her husband's acceptance of her sexually. She is also worried about missing work and leaving her classes to a substitute teacher. She states that she does not "let physical problems get me down" and that she dislikes "pills and hospitals."

Client is accustomed to teaching, not to being taught, and tries to dominate any conversation or input from the nurse-teacher.

Sociocultural Dimension

Marital status: Married. One child, a 23-year-old son named Christopher.
Family: Mother had a mastectomy at age 51; no further medical problems. Father, healthy. Two younger sisters; both experienced difficult pregnancies and are using birth control pills. Client feels that family communication is good.
Client states that her lifestyle is work oriented and that her friends are primarily teaching associates. Her Italian heritage and Roman Catholic religion stress the importance of family and children. Among her friends, her hysterectomy is accepted as a health consideration, not as a moral or religious issue.

Environmental Dimension

The client has been in a hospital only once for the birth of her son. She has had no previous serious illnesses. She knows no other woman who has had a hysterectomy well enough to discuss details. She is almost totally unfamiliar with basic hospital procedures.
Learning style: Responds well to formal lectures and related personal reading. Also enjoys group discussion "if we stick to the subject and don't turn it into a gossip session."

Determining Objectives

After a brief period of rest and adjustment to the unfamiliar hospital environment, Mrs. A. states that she would like to learn more about the hysterectomy. Although many short-term and long-term objectives can be identified for any surgical experience, Mrs. A. and the nurse identified the following objectives in cognitive (C), affective (A), and psychomotor (P) domains.

Short-term objectives
1. Describe to the nurse what a hysterectomy is (C).
2. Express to the nurse concerns about sexuality (A).
3. Describe to the nurse steps the hospital takes for this procedure (C).
4. Complete arrangements with family and employer for convalescence and return to normal activities (P).

Long-term objectives
1. Differentiate expected from unexpected postoperative experiences to know when to seek medical advice (C).
2. Identify ways to avoid constipation, weight gain, and periods of depression (C).
3. Identify ways to comfortably return to normal sexual activities (C) (A).
4. Schedule follow-up appointment with doctor (P).

Table 6-2 is a sample teaching plan that includes objectives, content, strategy, and evaluation.

Table 6-2

SAMPLE TEACHING PLAN

Client Objectives	Content	Nurse Strategy	Client Evaluation
SHORT TERM			
Describe to the nurse what a hysterectomy is	Provide brief review of female reproductive system; explain procedure, forewarning normal sensory experiences	Provide simple pencil diagram, pamphlets related to procedure	Repeat pencil diagram and explanation; pass self-quizzes accompanying pamphlets
Express to the nurse concerns regarding sexuality	Validate client's feelings; review basic information about effects of hysterectomy, emphasizing that procedure should not affect sex life	Act as facilitator at peer group discussion; provide film on topic of procedure and discuss content; observe client's response during discussion	Review discussion content with nurse
Describe to the nurse steps the hospital takes for this procedure	Describe basic hospital procedures	Perform hospital tour, orientation	Describe step-by-step events before and after hysterectomy
Complete arrangements with family and employer for convalescence and return to normal activities	Describe methods to promote early recovery; address lifting, overexertion, proper rest	Assist client with preparation of checklist of necessary arrangements	Prepare written schedule of activities for 30 days after release
LONG TERM			
Differentiate expected from unexpected postoperative experiences to know when to seek medical advice	Explain normal symptoms, such as tiredness, emotional lows; discuss unusual or abnormal symptoms for which medical advice should be sought	Provide information sheet prepared by hospital or other resource	Accurately list five normal and five abnormal symptoms of recovery
Identify ways to avoid constipation, weight gain, and periods of depression	Provide suggestions for avoiding common problems	Promote discussion with nurse and peers	Correctly identify good practices from list of good and poor recovery practices
Identify ways to comfortably return to normal sexual activities	Provide suggestions for relieving common problems, such as vaginal dryness, back discomfort	Promote discussion with nurse; encourage discussion with husband on one-to-one basis	Ask questions and show improved communication with husband
Schedule follow-up appointment with doctor	Suggest follow-up times	Ask client to provide appointment date; note appointment date	Confirm follow-up appointment made

R eview Questions

The number of the question corresponds to the same-numbered objectives at the beginning of the chapter.

1. Which of the following statements is *not* a realistic goal of client teaching?
   a. Prepare the client for sensory experiences.
   b. Teach and practice skills needed for successful self-care.
   c. Change client's basic morals and values to agree with modern standards.
   d. Explain medical terminology that may be confusing to client.

2. Which of these statements concerning nurse-teacher stressors is most accurate?
   a. Most nurses feel that client teaching should be done by the doctor or others on the health team.
   b. The nurse-teacher may have difficulty accepting powerlessness in the face of client resistance to change.
   c. Agreed-on, written goals are too time consuming and lack practical value in teaching.
   d. The nurse-teacher should not express self-doubts and insecurities; seeking the support of others is unprofessional.

3. A characteristic of the adult learner is that
   a. adults do not need to practice a skill until they return to their normal surroundings
   b. most adults prefer to be a passive recipient in the learning process
   c. adults can often learn best from other adults with similar experiences
   d. adults enjoy learning new information and attitudes, even if they cannot see the relevance to their lives

4. Considering the factors contributing to successful teaching, which of the following statements is true?
   a. The nurse should plan teaching sessions when the work schedule permits.
   b. If the client is not ready to learn because of financial or family pressures, the nurse should consider referring the client for counseling or other intermediate intervention.
   c. Since learning takes place in only one domain at a time, the nurse should limit a teaching session to one subject, idea, or skill.
   d. The nurse should maintain a cool, impersonal demeanor toward the client to retain a teacher-student relationship.

5. Referring to the three domains of learning, which statement is true?
   a. Information (knowledge gain) is not necessary to teach a psychomotor skill.
   b. Attitudes can change when the client is allowed to express feelings and concerns.
   c. Awareness of the client's attitudes is not necessary when teaching a motor skill.
   d. Feedback is effective only in the psychomotor domain.

6. By identifying certain personality characteristics of the client, the nurse is incorporating principles from which dimension?
   a. biophysical
   b. psychological
   c. sociocultural
   d. environmental

7. Which of the following is *not* a dimension of assessment?
   a. biophysical
   b. implementation
   c. environmental
   d. sociocultural

8. Which of the following nursing interventions would *not* reduce a barrier to learning?
   a. using standardized materials for all clients
   b. helping the client rearrange priorities so that health needs can be met
   c. assessing the client's reading/educational level and selecting appropriate materials
   d. improving the nurse-teacher's communication skills

9. Which of the following learning objectives is properly written?
   a. The client should understand the implications of the condition.
   b. The client will read two pamphlets on the subject of breast self-examination.
   c. The client's spouse will demonstrate to the nurse how to correctly change a gastrostomy bag before discharge.
   d. The client will lose 25 pounds in 6 weeks.

10. Which of the following statements is *not* true concerning teaching strategies?
    a. The most effective strategy is lecture.
    b. Lecture-discussion is often preferred by adults because it allows greater participation than lecture alone.
    c. Adults can learn from each other in groups, but the nurse must be present to supervise.
    d. Audiovisual materials provide multisensory learning experiences, increasing the client's confusion.

11. Which of the following statements regarding evaluation is not usually the nurse's responsibility?
    a. observing whether the client can perform a psychomotor skill
    b. quizzing the client about previously learned material
    c. undertaking a long-term counseling program when barriers to learning occur
    d. suggesting appropriate agencies and programs to meet the client's long-term needs

12. Considerations in selecting appropriate teaching strategies include three of the following. Which answer is *not* a consideration?
    a. determining the client's learning style
    b. determining the client's ability to pay
    c. assessing available resources at the present health care facility
    d. assessing the client's visual, auditory, and verbal skills

REFERENCES

1. Luder E and Gilbride JA: Teaching self-management skills to cystic fibrosis patients and its effect on their caloric intake, J Am Diet Assoc 89:359, 1989.
2. Smith C: Patient education: nurses in partnership with other health professionals, Orlando, Fla, 1987, Grune & Stratton, Inc.
3. Jacobson SF: Nurses' stress in intensive and nonintensive care units. In Jacobson SF and McGrath HM: Nurses under stress, New York, 1983, John Wiley & Sons, Inc.
4. Redman B: The process of patient education, ed 6, St Louis, 1988, The CV Mosby Co.
5. Murphy MC, Fishman J, and Shaw RE: Education of patients undergoing coronary angioplasty: factors affecting learning during a structured educational program, Heart Lung 18:37, 1989.
6. Falvo D: Effective patient education: a guide to increased compliance, Rockville, Md, 1985, Aspen Publishers, Inc.
7. Carpenito LJ: Nursing diagnosis: application to clinical practice, ed 3, Philadelphia, 1989, JB Lippincott Co.
8. Harrison LL: Focus on patient teaching: the patient education bridge, Am J Maternal/Child Nurs, p 51, Jan/Feb 1989.

SECTION I BIBLIOGRAPHY
BOOKS

Bower AC and Thompson JM: Clinical manual of health assessment, ed 3, St Louis, 1988, The CV Mosby Co.

Buchanan JH: Patient encounters: the experience of disease, Charlottesville, NC, 1989, The University Press of Virginia.

Christensen P and Henney JW: The nursing process: application of theories, frameworks, and models, ed 3, St Louis, 1990, Mosby–Year Book, Inc.

Committee on Diet and Health, Food and Nutrition Board, Commission on Life Sciences, National Research Council: Diet and health: implications for reducing chronic disease risk, Washington, DC, 1989, National Academy Press.

Cooper CL and Payne R: Causes, coping and consequences of stress at work, New York, 1988, John Wiley & Sons, Inc.

Cox HC and others: Clinical applications of nursing diagnosis: adult health, child health, women's health, mental health, home health, Baltimore, 1989, Williams & Wilkins.

Dolan JT: Critical care nursing: clinical management through nursing process, Philadelphia, 1991, FA Davis Co.

Doswell WM: Physiological responses to stress. In Fitzpatrick J, Taunton RL, and Benoliel JQ: Annual review of nursing research, vol 7, New York, 1989, Springer Publishing Co, Inc, p 511.

Edelman CL and Mandle CL: Health promotion throughout the life span, ed 2, St Louis, 1990, Mosby–Year Book, Inc.

Eliopoulos C: Health assessment of the older adult, Redwood City, Calif, 1990, Addison-Wesley Publishing Co, Inc.

Fitzpatrick JJ and Whall AL, eds: Conceptual models of nursing: analysis and application, Norwalk, Conn, 1989, Appleton & Lange.

Gordon M: Nursing diagnosis: process and application, ed 2, New York, 1987, McGraw-Hill, Inc.

Gordon M: Manual for nursing diagnosis, St Louis, 1989, The CV Mosby Co.

Griffith HW: Instructions for patients, ed 4, Philadelphia, 1989, WB Saunders Co.

Guzzetta CE and others: Clinical assessment tools for use with nursing diagnoses, St Louis, 1989, The CV Mosby Co.

Hickey PW: Nursing process handbook, St Louis, 1990, Mosby–Year Book, Inc.

Kasl SV and Cooper CL: Stress and health: issues in research methodology, New York, 1987, John Wiley & Sons, Inc.

Kim MJ and MacFarland G: Pocket guide to nursing diagnosis, ed 3, St Louis, 1989, The CV Mosby Co.

Leuner JC and others: Mastering the nursing process: a case method approach, Philadelphia, 1990, FA Davis Co.

Lowenberg JS: Caring and responsibility: the crossroads between holistic practice and traditional medicine, Philadelphia, 1989, University of Pennsylvania Press.

Lyon BL and Werner JS: Stress. In Fitzpatrick J and Taunton RL: Annual review of nursing research, vol 5, New York, 1987, Springer Publishing Co, Inc, p 3.

Malasanos L, Barkauskas V, and Stoltenberg-Allen K: Health assessment, ed 4, St Louis, 1990, Mosby–Year Book, Inc.

McFarland G and McFarlane E: Nursing diagnosis and intervention, St Louis, 1989, The CV Mosby Co.

Neufeld RW: Advances in the investigation of psychological stress, New York, 1989, John Wiley & Sons, Inc.

Potter PA: Fundamentals of nursing: concepts, process, and practice, St Louis, 1989, The CV Mosby Co.

Potter PA: Pocket guide to physical assessment, ed 2, St Louis, 1990, Mosby–Year Book, Inc.

Redman B: The process of patient education, ed 6, St Louis, 1989, The CV Mosby Co.

Snyder M: Independent nursing interventions, New York, 1985, John Wiley & Sons, Inc.

Sundeen SJ, Stuart GW, and Rankin E: Nurse-client interaction: implementing the nursing process, ed 4, St Louis, 1989, The CV Mosby Co.

Suter S: Health psychophysiology: mind-body interactions in wellness and illness, Hillsdale, NJ, 1986, Lawrence Erlbaum Associates, Inc.

Talbot L and Meyer-Marquardt M: Pocket guide to critical care assessment, St Louis, 1989, The CV Mosby Co.

Thompson JM and Bowers AC: Health assessment: an illustrated pocket guide, ed 2, St Louis, 1988, The CV Mosby Co.

JOURNALS

Baille V: Stress, social support, and psychological distress of family caregivers of the elderly, Nurs Res 37:217, 1988.

Becker KL: Performing in-depth abdominal assessment, Nursing 18:59, 1988.

Biley FC: Stress in high dependency units, Intensive Care Nurs 5:134, 1989.

Bolles JR: The videodisc in health sciences education: a perspective on a powerful medium, J Biocommun 15:5, 1988.

Boynton P: Health maintenance alteration: a nursing diagnosis of the elderly, Clin Nurse Spec 3:5, 1989.

Buchan T and Smith R: Nursing process in community psychiatric nursing, Aust J Adv Nurs 6:5, 1989.

Buchanan M and Gerrity PL: Community wellness outreach: family health through empowerment, NLN Publ 21-2311:111, 1989.

Christman NJ and others: Uncertainty, coping, and distress following myocardial infarction: transition from hospital to home, Res Nurs Health 11:71, 1988.

Cunningham H: An exercise in formulating a nursing health history assessment tool, Nurse Educ 13:39, 1988.

Dixon JP, Dixon JK, and Spinner J: Perceptions of life-pattern disintegrity as a link in the relationship between stress and illness, Adv Nurs Sci 11:1, 1989.

Eisenhauer LA and Gendrop S: Review of research on creative problem solving in nursing, NLN Publ 15:2339:79, 1990.

Fowler MD: Ethical decision making in clinical practice, Nurs Clin North Am 24:955, 1989.

Grizmer JT and others: Self-directed learning: the wizard-of-oz syndrome, J Biocommun 15:10, 1988.

Guyon L: Prevention and health promotion. Has the die already been cast for the nursing profession? Nurs Que 8:35, 1988.

Harris RB: Reviewing nursing stress according to a proposed coping-adaptation framework, Adv Nurs Sci 11:12, 1989.

Harrison LL: A health promotion model for wellness education, MCN 15:191, 1990.

Hert M: The ophthalmic nurse and physical exam, Insight 14:19, 1989.

Holden-Lund C: Effects of relaxation with guided imagery on surgical stress and wound healing, Res Nurs Health 11:235, 1988.

Hull J, Treuren R, and Virnelli S: Hardiness and health: a critique and alternative approach, J Pers Soc Psychol 45:518, 1987.

Hyman RB: Measures of stress and related constructs: a guide for research and clinical practice, Scholar Inq Nurs Pract 2:4, 1988.

Johnson JE and Lauver DR: Alternative explanations of coping with stressful experiences associated with physical illness, Adv Nurs Sci 11:39, 1989.

Jones LH: How to assess stress: a significant step for the nursing student, J Nurs Educ 27:227, 1988.

Koldjeski D: Toward a theory of professional nursing caring: a unifying perspective, NLN Pub 41-2308:45, 1990.

Kruger S: A review of patient education in nursing, J Nurs Staff Dev 6:71, 1990.

Leidy NK: A physiological analysis of stress and chronic illness, J Adv Nurs 14:868, 1989.

Littlewood J: A model for nursing using anthropological literature, Int J Nurs Stud 26:221, 1989.

Lowery BJ: Stress research: some theoretical and methodological illues, Image J Nurs Sch 19:42, 1987.

Maglacas AM: Health for all: nursing's role, Nurs Outlook 36:66, 1988.

McCain NL and Lynn MR: Meta-analysis of a narrative review: studies evaluating patient teaching, West J Nurs Res 12:347, 1990.

McConnell EA: Getting the feel of lymph node assessment, Nursing 18:55, 1988.

Merry JA: Take your assessment all the way down to the toes, RN 51:60, 1988.

Miller T: Advances in understanding the impact of stressful life events on health, Hosp Community Psychiatry, 1988, p 615.

Packard JS and Motowidlo SJ: Subjective stress, job satisfaction, and job performance of hospital nurses, Res Nurs Health 10:253, 1987.

Padberg RM and Padberg LF: Strengthening the effectiveness of patient education: applying principles of adult education, Oncol Nurs Forum 17:65, 1990.

Perry K and Kirmer D: Wellness education for clients receiving psychiatric care in a partial hospital program, Holistic Nurs Pract 4:72, 1990.

Pollock SE: The hardiness characteristic: a motivating factor in adaptation, Adv Nurs Sci 11:53, 1989.

Porter Y: Evaluation of nursing documentation of patient teaching, J Contin Educ Nurs 21:134, 1990.

Rankin WW: Gratitude and wellness, J Pediatr Nurs 5:138, 1990.

Rew L and Barrow EM: Nurses' intuition. Can it coexist with the nursing process? AORN J 50:353, 1989.

Rice EM: Geriatric assessment (continuing education credit), AD Nurse 4:8, 1989.

Riegel B: Social support and psychological adjustment to chronic coronary heart disease: operationalization of Johnson's behavioral system model, Adv Nurs Sci 11:74, 1989.

Ritter M: Assisting staff nurses in patient teaching, Ostomy/Wound Management 25:24, 1989.

Santo-Novak DA: Seven keys to assessing the elderly, Nursing 18:60, 1988.

Selleck CS, Sirles AT, and Newman KD: Health promotion at the workplace, AAOHN J 37:412, 1989.

Sherman JB, Clark L, and McEwen MM: Evaluation of a worksite wellness program: impact on exercise, weight, smoking, and stress, Pub Health Nurs 6:114, 1989.

Stevens SA and Becker KL: How to perform picture-perfect respiratory assessment, Nursing 18:57, 1988.

Stokes SA and Gordon SE: Development of an instrument to measure stress in the older adult, Nurs Res 37:16, 1988.

Thatcher RM: Community support: promoting health and self-care, Nurs Clin North Am 24:725, 1989.

The journal of infection control nursing: universal precautions—how they can work in practice, Nurs Times 86:65, 12-18, 1990.

Tipton JF: A hospital-based approach to physical assessment, J Nurs Staff Dev 5:70, 1989.

Van Amerigen MR, Arsenault A, and Dolan SL: Intrinsic job stress and diastolic blood pressure among female hospital workers, J Occup Med 30:93, 1988.

ORGANIZATIONS

Administration on Aging
Office of Human Development Services
US Department of Health and Human Services
Washington, DC 20201

American Academy of Ambulatory Nursing Administration
North Woodbury Road, Box 56
Pitman, NJ 08071

American Association of Critical-Care Nurses
One Civic Plaza
Newport Beach, CA 92669

American Association of Occupational Health Nurses
50 Lenox Pointe
Atlanta, GA 30324

American Association of Nurse Anesthetists
216 West Higgins Road
Park Ridge, IL 60068

American Association of Retired Persons
1901 K Street, NW
Washington, DC 20049

American Holistic Nurses' Association
1100 Raleigh Building
5 West Hargett Street
Raleigh, NC 27601

American Hospital Association
840 North Lake Shore Drive
Chicago, IL 60611

American Medical Association
535 North Dearborn Street
Chicago, Il 60610

American Nurses Association
2420 Pershing Road
Kansas City, MO 64108

American Organization of Nurse Executives
840 North Lake Shore Drive
Chicago, IL 60611

Association of Operating Room Nurses
10170 East Mississippi Avenue
Denver, CO 80231

Center for Disease Control
Bureau of Health Education
1600 Clifton Road, NE
Atlanta, GA 30333

Concern for Dying
250 West 57th Street
New York, NY 10107

International Council of Nurses
3, Place Jean-Marteau
CH-1201 Geneva, Switzerland

National Association for Healthcare Recruitment
PO Box 5769
Akron, OH 44372

National Association of Hispanic Nurses
2300 West Commerce, Suite 304
San Antonio, TX 78207

National Black Nurses Association
PO Box 1823
Washington, DC 20013

National Council on Aging
West Wing, Suite 100
600 Maryland Ave, S.W.
Washington, DC 20024

National League for Nursing
350 Hudson Street
New York, NY 10014

National Student Nurses' Association
555 West 57th Street
New York, NY 10019

Nurses' Christian Fellowship
PO Box 7895
Madison, WI 53707

Nurses' Coalition for Political Action
c/o American Nurses' Association
2420 Pershing Road
Kansas City, MO 64108

Sigma Theta Tau
International Honor Society of Nursing
550 West North Street
Indianapolis, IN 46202

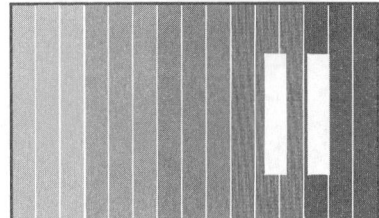

SECTION II

PATHOPHYSIOLOGICAL MECHANISMS OF DISEASE

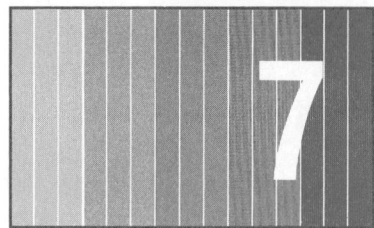

CHAPTER

7

Nursing Role in Management
Cell Injury and Inflammation

Sharon Mantik Lewis

Learning Objectives

1. Describe the structures and functions of the normal cell.
2. Explain the cellular adaptive mechanisms to sublethal injury.
3. Describe the causes and mechanisms of lethal cell injury.
4. Differentiate among types of cell necrosis.
5. Describe the components and functions of the mononuclear phagocyte system.
6. Describe the inflammatory response, including vascular and cellular responses and exudate formation.
7. Explain local and systemic manifestations of inflammation and their physiological bases.
8. Differentiate among healing by primary, secondary, and tertiary intention.
9. Describe factors that delay wound healing and common complications of wound healing.
10. Describe the pharmacological, dietary, and nursing management of inflammation.

The major work of the body occurs at the cellular level in the form of chemical reactions. Each cell has a specific function and, together with other cells, makes up body tissues, organs, and systems. Cellular reactions synthesize new products for growth and energy and break down used products. Understanding the structure and function of an individual cell is necessary to comprehend the functioning of tissues, organs, and systems.

The cell's response to adverse conditions depends on its ability to adapt to changing conditions. Adaptations include responses such as atrophy, hypertrophy, degeneration, inflammation, regeneration, and repair. When the cell fails to adapt, it undergoes a series of changes that can result in cell death (necrosis) and eventually tissue death.

THE HUMAN CELL
Cell Structure

The cell is the basic unit of structure in any living organism (Fig. 7-1). Each cell is surrounded by a semiper-

Reviewed by Janice M. Zeller, R.N., Ph.D., Professor, Department of Medical Nursing; Associate Professor, Department of Immunology/Microbiology, Rush-Presbyterian-St. Luke's Medical Center, Chicago, Illinois.

meable plasma membrane. The two basic parts of a cell are the cytoplasm and the nucleus.

Cytoplasm. Cytoplasm is composed of viscous protoplasm, which consists of water, protein, lipid, carbohydrate, and inorganic solutes. *Organelles* located within the cytoplasm perform cellular functions, which are shown in Table 7-1 (see p. 100).

Nucleus. The nucleus is present in all cells that can divide and consists mainly of *chromosomes*. (The tangled threads of chromosomes found when the cell is not actively dividing are called *chromatin*.) There are 23 pairs of chromosomes in human somatic cells. The basic unit of the chromosome is the *gene*. Deoxyribonucleic acid (DNA) is the building block of the gene. The sequence of nucleotides of the large, complex DNA molecule is the genetic information, the heredity unit of the cell. DNA also directs synthesis of specific proteins by the cell (Fig. 7-2), thus determining its special characteristics.

Ribonucleic acid (RNA) is also found in the nucleus. It transmits the information from DNA to ribosomes in the cytoplasm. Ribosomes are the site of protein synthesis of the cell. The protein products may be used for cellular metabolism (e.g., enzymes) or secreted for use in other parts of the body (e.g., insulin).

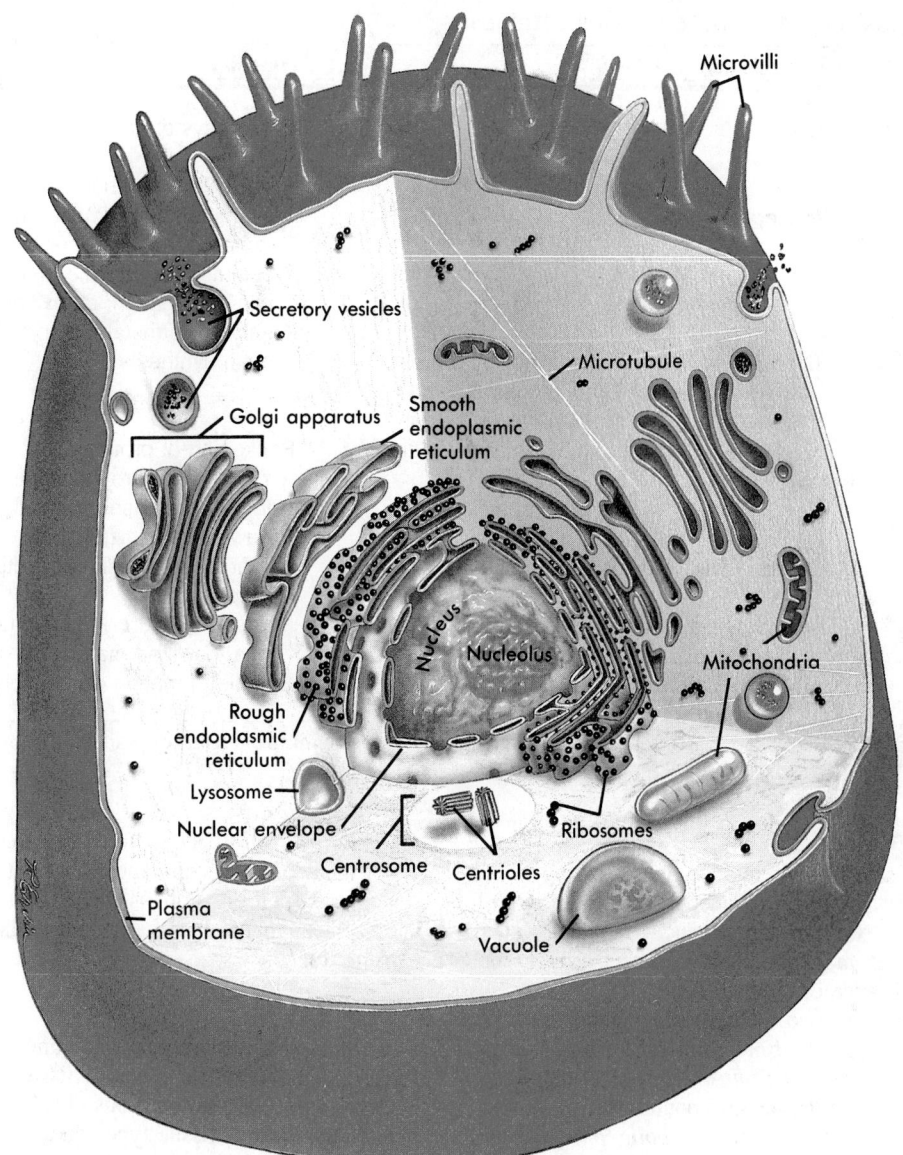

Fig. 7-1 Human cell and organelles. (From Seeley R, Stephens T, and Tate P: Anatomy and physiology, St Louis, 1989, Times Mirror/Mosby College Publishing, p 58.)

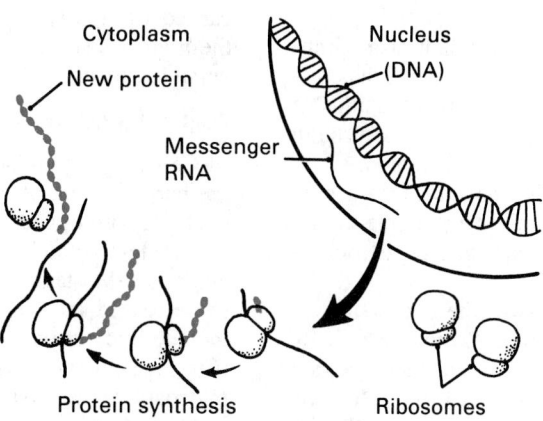

Fig. 7-2 Protein synthesis directed by DNA.

Table 7-1 Composition and Function of Cell Organelles

Organelle	Composition	Function
Nucleus	DNA	Control system of cell, site of cellular reproduction
	RNA	Site for RNA synthesis
	Nucleolus	Transmittal of information to ribosomes
Endoplasmic reticulum*	Network of tubular structures	Communication between nucleus cytoplasm, cell membrane; lipid and steroid synthesis; bile conjugation; detoxification of unnecessary cell substances; protein synthesis
Ribosomes	Granules of RNA held together by protein, which may merge into clumps (polyribosomes)	Protein synthesis
Golgi complex	Flattened collection of tubules and vesicles	Packaging of proteins (hormones and enzymes) that are stored as secretion granules for later release from cell, packaging of newly synthesized lipids
Mitochondria	Layered cristae (folds) formed into small, oval bodies	Powerhouse of cell, production of ATP, cellular respiration
Lysosome	Membrane-surrounded sac containing enzymes	Release of hydrolytic enzymes on contact with phagocytized material to degrade it
Centrosome	Pair of centrioles	Spindle formation during cell division

*Includes smooth endoplasmic reticulum (SER or agranular) and rough endoplasmic reticulum (RER or granular).

Cellular Processes

The basic processes of cells include the following:

1. *Transport of metabolites:* Transport of metabolites is the movement of substances such as electrolytes across the cell membrane actively or passively or with the assistance of a carrier.
2. *Metabolism:* The two phases of metabolism are *anabolism* and *catabolism.* Both take place within the cells. In the *anabolic phase,* simpler compounds are converted into larger compounds (e.g., amino acids into proteins). In the *catabolic phase* these larger compounds are broken down into simpler compounds and the energy necessary for cell function is released.
3. *Movement:* Many body cells (especially muscle cells) work together in a coordinated manner to permit body movement.
4. *Conduction:* Conduction is transmission of a stimulus from one part of the body to another. Transmission of a nerve impulse through nerve and muscle cells and passage of heat and sound waves through parts of the body are examples of conduction.
5. *Absorption:* Absorption is the movement of a substance through a cell membrane. An example is glucose absorption by the lining cells of the gastrointestinal (GI) tract.
6. *Body protection:* Certain cells of the body (such as the epithelial cells of the epidermis) protect the body against injury from penetration or abrasion. Other cells, such as white blood cells (WBCs), protect the body against invading agents by means of the inflammatory and immune responses.
7. *Reproduction:* New cells are necessary for replacement of aged cells and for growth of the body. *Mitosis* (cell division) is the process by which cells replace themselves. Not all cells are capable of mitosis.

TISSUE TYPES

Cells similar in structure and function are organized to form tissues. The four types of tissue are epithelial, connective, muscular, and nervous. Table 7-2 discusses examples of the various tissue types and their regenerative ability.

CELL INJURY

Cell injury can be sublethal or lethal. *Sublethal* injury alters function without causing cell death. The changes caused by this type of injury are potentially reversible if the injurious stimulus is removed. *Lethal* injury is an irreversible process that causes cell death.

Cell Adaptation to Sublethal Injury

Cell adaptations to sublethal injuries are common and are part of many physiological and disease processes. For example, prolonged exposure to sunlight stimulates melanin production and thus provides protection of deeper skin layers by skin tanning. Lack of muscular activity can lead to decreased muscle tone. Adaptive processes of the cell include hypertrophy, hyperplasia, atrophy, and metaplasia (Fig. 7-3). Other adaptive responses that are considered maladaptive are dysplasia and anaplasia.

Hypertrophy. *Hypertrophy* refers to an increase in the size of cells without cell division. For example, a pregnant

***Table* 7-2** Major Tissue Types

Tissue Type	Regenerative Ability
EPITHELIAL	
Skin, linings of blood vessels, mucous membranes	Cells readily divide and regenerate
CONNECTIVE TISSUE	
Bone	Active tissue heals rapidly
Cartilage	Regeneration is possible but slow
Tendons and ligaments	Regeneration is possible but slow
Blood	Cells actively regenerate
MUSCLE	
Smooth	Regeneration is usually possible (particularly in GI tract)
Cardiac	Damaged muscle is replaced by connective tissue
Skeletal	Connective tissue replaces severely damaged muscle; some regeneration in moderately damaged muscle occurs
NERVE	
Neuron	Cells do not divide; cells regenerate only if cell body is not injured
Glial	Cells regenerate; scar tissue is often formed when neurons are damaged

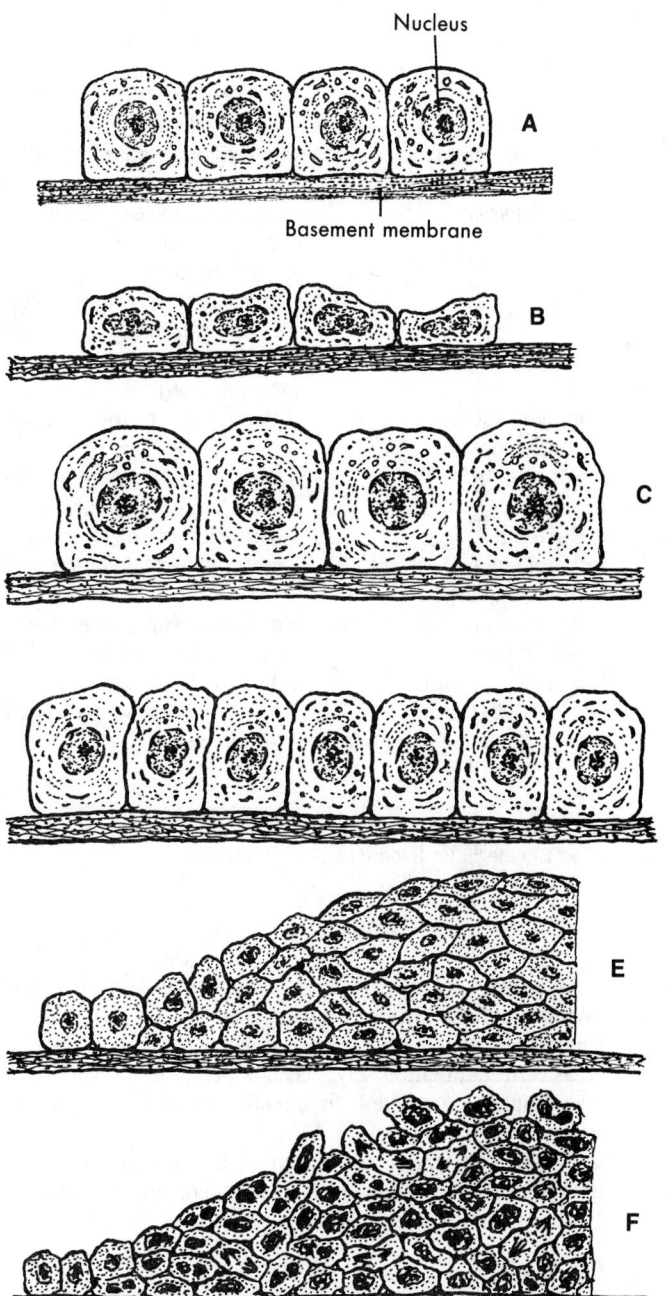

***Fig.* 7-3** Adaptive alterations in simple cuboidal epithelial cells. **A,** Normal. **B,** Atrophy. **C,** Hypertrophy. **D,** Hyperplasia. **E,** Metaplasia. **F,** Dysplasia. (From McCance KL and Huether SE: Pathophysiology: the biological basis for disease in adults and children, St Louis, 1990, Mosby–Year Book, Inc, p 49.)

uterus enlarges from hormonal stimulation. The heart of a person with severe hypertension enlarges to compensate for the increased resistance to its pumping action. Muscle hypertrophy results from an increase in the size of muscle fibers.

Hyperplasia. *Hyperplasia* refers to the actual increase in the number of cells. This process is reversible when the stimulus is removed. The female breast experiences hyperplasia during lactation. Hyperplasia of the liver may restore damaged liver tissue.

Atrophy. *Atrophy* refers to a decrease in the size of a tissue or organ caused by a decreased number of cells or reduction in the size of the individual cells. It frequently occurs as a result of disease (decreased muscle activity), lack of blood supply (thrombus formation), natural aging process (decreased breast size after menopause), and nutritional deficiency.

Metaplasia. *Metaplasia* is the transformation of one cell type into another. An example of physiological metaplasia is when circulating monocytes change to macrophages as they migrate into inflamed tissues. An example of pathophysiological metaplasia is when the normal pseudostratified columnar epithelium of the bronchi changes to stratified squamous epithelium in response to chronic cigarette smoking.

Table 7-3 Causes of Lethal Cell Injury

Cause	Effect on Cell
Physical agents	
Heat	Denaturation of protein, acceleration of metabolic reactions
Cold	Decreased blood flow from vasoconstriction, slowed metabolic reactions, thrombosis of blood vessels, freezing of cell content that forms crystals and can burst cell
Radiation	Alteration of cell structure and activity, alteration of enzyme systems, mutations
Electrothermal injury	Interruption of neural conduction, fibrillation of cardiac muscle, coagulative necrosis of skin and skeletal muscle
Mechanical trauma	Transfer of excess kinetic energy to cells causing rupture of cells, blood vessels, tissue; examples include:
	Abrasion: Scraping of skin or mucous membrane
	Laceration: Severing of vessels and tissue
	Contusion (bruise): Crushing of tissue cells causing hemorrhage into skin
	Puncture: Piercing of body structure or organ
	Incision: Surgical cutting
Chemical injury	Alteration of cell metabolism, interference with normal enzymatic action within cells
Microbial injury	
Viruses	Taking over of cell metabolism and synthesis of new particles that may cause cell rupture, cumulative effect possibly producing clinical disease
Bacteria*	Destruction of cell membrane or cell nucleus, production of lethal toxins
Ischemic injury	Compromised cell metabolism, acute or gradual cell death
Immunological†	
Antigen-antibody response	Release of substances (histamine, complement) that can injure and damage cells
Autoimmune	Activation of complement, which destroys normal cells and produces inflammation
Neoplastic growth	Cell destruction from abnormal and uncontrolled cell growth
Normal substances (e.g. digestive enzymes, uric acid)	Release into abdomen causing peritonitis, crystallization of excess accumulation in joints and renal tissue

*Bacteria are commonly classified as gram-negative or gram-positive.
†See Chapter 8 for a more detailed discussion.

Dysplasia. *Dysplasia* is an abnormal differentiation of dividing cells resulting in changes in the size, shape, and appearance of the cells. Minor dysplasia is found in some areas of inflammation. Dysplasia is potentially reversible if the stimulus is removed. Frequently, dysplasia is a precursor of malignancy.

Anaplasia. *Anaplasia* is cell differentiation to a more immature or embryonic form. Malignant tumors are often characterized by anaplastic cell growth.

Causes of Lethal Cell Injury

Many different agents and factors can cause lethal cell injury (Table 7-3). The mechanism of actual cell death varies. Examples include pyknosis (nuclear condensation and shrinking), karyolysis (dissolution of nucleus and contents), rupture of cell membrane, and alteration in cell metabolism.

Microbial invasion frequently, but not always, results in cell injury and death. Infection occurs when *pathogens* (microorganisms capable of producing disease) invade and multiply in body tissues. (Common viruses and bacteria that cause diseases in humans are listed in Tables 7-4 and

7-5.) *Opportunistic* organisms are microorganisms that are not usually considered pathogens. However, they may cause injury if the resistance of the host is decreased from events such as trauma or illness.

Cell Necrosis

Necrosis is the death of cells within a living organism. Different types of necrosis tend to occur in different organs or tissues.

Coagulative necrosis. Necrotic cells maintain their outline (lytic enzymes are somewhat inhibited). Proteins are denatured, and enzymes lose their function. *Coagulative necrosis* is commonly due to lack of blood supply.

Liquefactive necrosis. Necrotic cells rapidly disappear as lytic enzymes digest tissues. *Liquefactive necrosis* commonly occurs in the brain where the supply of lytic enzymes is abundant.

Caseous necrosis. Necrotic cells disintegrate, but cell fragments remain for long periods of time. This type of necrosis is called *caseous* (cheeselike) because of its crumbly appearance. It is frequently found in tuberculosis of the lung.

Table 7-4 Common Viruses Causing Disease

Type	Disease Caused
DNA VIRUSES	
Herpesviruses	
Varicella-zoster	Chickenpox; shingles
Herpes simplex	
Type 1	Herpes labialis ("fever blisters"), genital herpes infection
Type 2	Genital herpes infection
Epstein-Barr	Mononucleosis, Burkitt's lymphoma (possibly)
Cytomegalovirus (CMV)	Pneumonia in immunosuppressed individuals, infectious mononucleosislike syndrome
Pox viruses	Smallpox
Adenoviruses	Upper respiratory tract infection, pneumonia
Parvovirus	Gastroenteritis
Papovavirus	Warts
RNA VIRUSES	
Picornaviruses	
Coxsackie viruses A and B	Upper respiratory tract infection, gastroenteritis, acute myocarditis, aseptic meningitis
Echoviruses	Upper respiratory tract infection, gastroenteritis, aseptic meningitis
Rhinovirus	Upper respiratory tract infection, pneumonia
Poliovirus	Poliomyelitis
Myxoviruses	
Influenza A, B, C	Upper respiratory tract infection
Parainfluenza 1-4	Upper respiratory tract infection
Respiratory syncytial virus	Upper respiratory tract infection
Mumps	Parotitis, orchitis in postpubertal males
Measles (rubeola)	Measles
Arbovirus	Syndrome of fever, malaise, headache, myalgia; aseptic meningitis; encephalitis
Rhabdovirus	Rabies
Togaviruses	German measles
Reoviruses	
Reoviruses 1, 2, 3	Gastroenteritis, respiratory tract infection
Rotaviruses	Gastroenteritis
Coronavirus	Upper respiratory tract infection

Table 7-5 Common Bacteria Causing Disease

Type	Diseases Caused
GRAM-POSITIVE	
Staphylococcus aureus	Skin infections, pneumonia, urinary tract infections, acute osteomyelitis, toxic shock syndrome
Streptococci	
S. pyogenes (group A β-hemolytic streptococci)	Pharyngitis, scarlet fever, rheumatic fever, acute glomerulonephritis, erysipelas, pneumonia
S. pyogenes (group B β-hemolytic streptococci)	Urinary tract infections
S. pneumoniae	Pneumococcal pneumonia
S. viridans	Bacterial endocarditis
S. faecalis	Genitourinary infection, infection of surgical wounds
Neisseriae	
N. meningitidis	Meningococcemia, meningitis
N. gonorrhoeae	Gonorrhea, pelvic inflammatory disease
Corynebacterium diphtheriae	Diphtheria
Clostridia	
C. tetani	Tetanus (lockjaw)
C. botulinum	Food poisoning with progressive muscle paralysis
Mycobacteria	
M. tuberculosis	Tuberculosis
M. leprae	Leprosy (Hansen's disease)
Treponema pallidum	Syphilis
GRAM-NEGATIVE	
Pseudomonas aeruginosa	Urinary tract infections, meningitis
Klebsiella-Enterobacter organisms	Urinary tract infections, peritonitis; pneumonia
Proteus species	Urinary tract infections, peritonitis
Escherichia coli	Urinary tract infections, peritonitis
Salmonella species	
S. typhi	Typhoid fever
Other *Salmonella* organisms	Food poisoning, gastroenteritis
Haemophilus organisms	
H. influenzae	Nasopharyngitis, meningitis, pneumonia
H. pertussis	Whooping cough
Shigella species	Shigellosis, diarrhea with abdominal pain and fever (dysentery)
Legionella pneumophila	Pneumonia (Legionnaire's disease)

Gangrenous necrosis. *Gangrenous necrosis* results from severe hypoxia and subsequent ischemic injury, which is common after impaired circulation in the lower legs. *Dry* gangrene refers to the dry, shriveled, darkened area (Fig. 7-4), and *wet* gangrene refers to the liquefied underlying necrotic tissue.

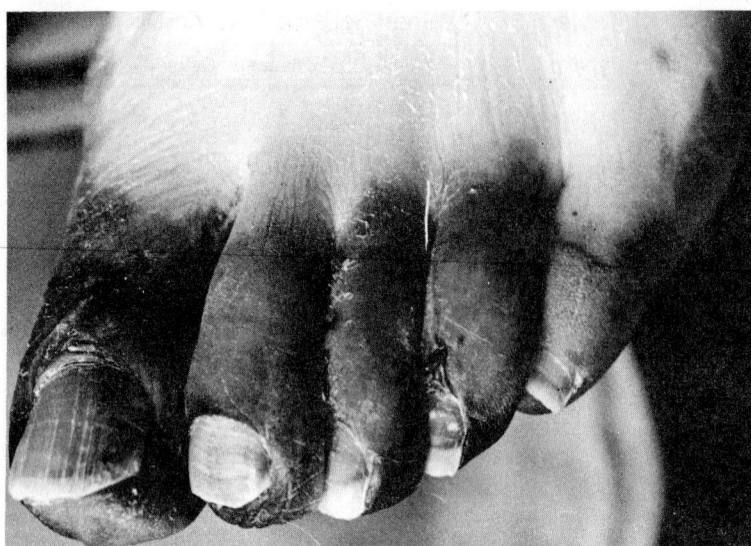

Fig. 7-4 Gangrene of the toes. (From Price S and Wilson L: Pathophysiology: clinical concepts of disease processes, ed 3, St Louis, 1991, Mosby–Year Book, Inc.)

DEFENSE AGAINST INJURY

To protect against injury, the body has various defense mechanisms. These defense mechanisms are (1) the skin and mucous membranes, which is the first line of defense (see Chapter 16); (2) the mononuclear phagocyte system; (3) the inflammatory response; and (4) the immune system (see Chapter 8).

Mononuclear Phagocyte System

The mononuclear phagocyte system (MPS) consists of monocytes and macrophages and their precursor cells. In the past the MPS system was called the *reticuloendothelial system* (RES). It is not a body system with distinctly defined tissues and organs. It consists of phagocytic cells located in various tissues and organs (Table 7-6). The phagocytic cells are either *fixed* or *free* (mobile). The macrophages of the liver, spleen, bone marrow, lungs, and lymph nodes are fixed phagocytes. The monocytes (in blood) and macrophages found in connective tissue, known as *histiocytes,* are mobile or wandering phagocytes.

Monocytes and macrophages originate in the bone marrow. Monocytes spend a few days in the blood and then enter tissues and change into macrophages. Tissue macrophages are larger and more phagocytic than monocytes.

The functions of the macrophage system include (1) recognition and phagocytosis of foreign material such as microorganisms, (2) removal of old or damaged cells from circulation, and (3) participation in the immune response (see Chapter 8).

Inflammatory Response

The inflammatory response is a sequential reaction to cell injury. It neutralizes the inflammatory agent, removes necrotic materials, and establishes an environment suitable for healing and repair. The term *inflammation* is often but incorrectly used as a synonym for the term *infection.* Inflammation is always present in infection, but infection is not always present with inflammation. An infection involves invasion of tissues or cells by microorganisms such

Table 7-6   Location and Name of Macrophages*

Location	Name
Connective tissue	Histiocytes
Liver	Kupffer cells
Lung	Alveolar macrophages
Spleen	Free and fixed macrophages
Bone marrow	Fixed macrophages
Lymph nodes	Free and fixed macrophages
Bone tissue	Osteoclasts
Central nervous system	Microglial cells
Peritoneal cavity	Peritoneal macrophages
Pleural cavity	Pleural macrophages
Skin	Histiocyte, Langerhans' cells
Synovium	Type A cells

*In addition, monocytes become macrophages once they leave the blood and enter the tissues.

as bacteria, fungi, and viruses. In contrast, inflammation can also be caused by nonliving agents such as heat, radiation, and trauma (see Table 7-3). If infection is also present, it is from an additional invasion of microorganisms.

The mechanism of inflammation is basically the same regardless of the injuring agent. The intensity of the response depends on the extent and severity of injury and on the reactive capacity of the victim. The inflammatory response can be divided into a vascular response, cellular response, formation of exudate, and healing.

Vascular response. After the cell injury the capillaries in the area briefly undergo vasoconstriction. After release of histamine and other chemicals by the injured cells, the vessels dilate. This vasodilatation results in *hyperemia* (increased blood supply), which raises filtration pressure. Vasodilatation and the effect of chemical mediators also make the capillaries more permeable. Movement of fluid from capillaries into tissue spaces is thus facilitated. Ini-

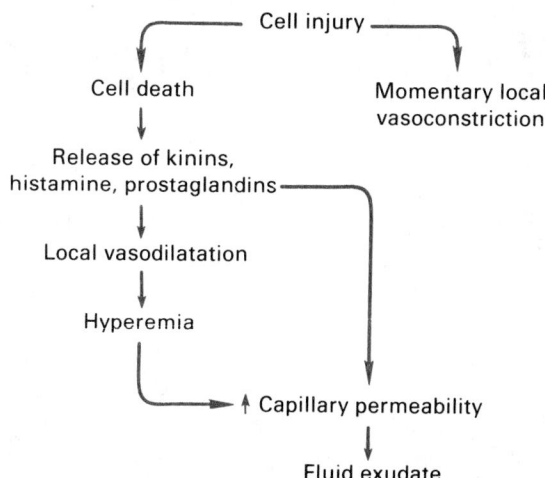

Fig. 7-5 Vascular response in inflammation.

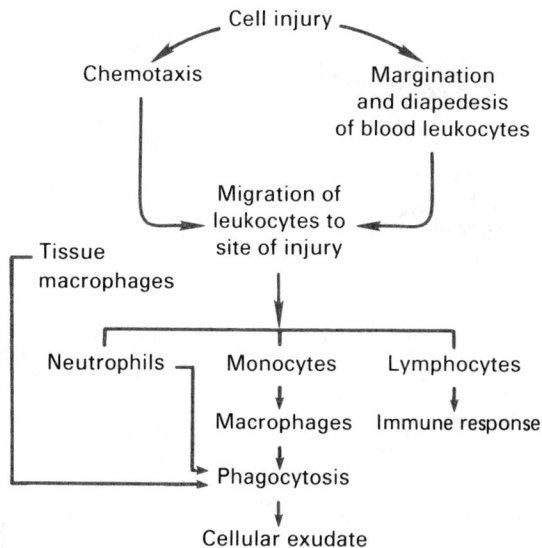

Fig. 7-6 Cellular response in inflammation.

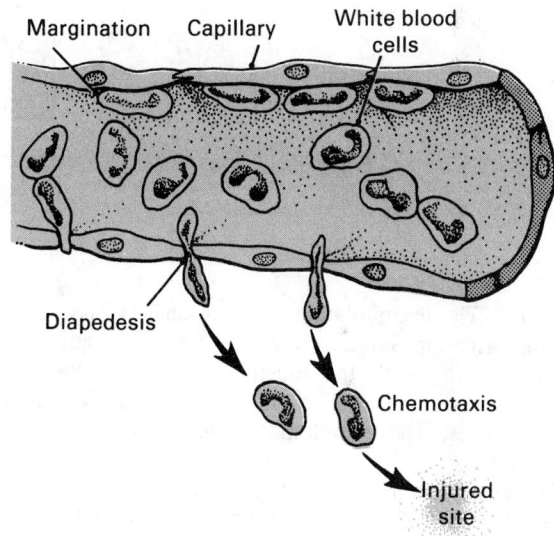

Fig. 7-7 Margination, diapedesis, and chemotaxis of white blood cells.

tially composed of serous fluid, this *inflammatory exudate* is later joined by plasma proteins, primarily albumin. The proteins exert oncotic pressure that further draws fluid from blood vessels. The tissue becomes edematous. This response is illustrated in Fig. 7-5.

As the plasma protein fibrinogen leaves the blood, it is activated to *fibrin* by the products of the injured cells. Fibrin strengthens a blood clot formed by platelets. The clot functions to trap bacteria, preventing their spread, and serves as a framework for the healing process.

Cellular response. The cellular response to injury is illustrated in Fig. 7-6. The blood flow through capillaries in the area slows as fluid is lost and viscosity rises. Neutrophils and monocytes move to the inner surface of the capillaries *(margination)* and then, in ameboid fashion, through the capillary wall *(diapedesis)* and to the site of injury (Fig. 7-7).

Chemotaxis is the directional migration of WBCs along a concentration gradient of chemoattractant. Chemotaxis is the mechanism for ensuring accumulation of neutrophils and monocytes at the focus of injury. Chemotactic factors include bacterial-derived chemotactic factors, complement-derived chemotactic factor (C5a), lipid-derived chemotactic factors (leukotriene B_4, 5-HETE, platelet-activating factor), platelet-derived chemotactic factors, and coagulation-related chemotactic factors.

Neutrophils. Neutrophils are the first leukocytes to arrive (usually by 12 to 24 hours).[1] They phagocytize bacteria, other foreign material, and damaged cells. With their short life span (24 to 48 hours), dead neutrophils soon accumulate. In time the mixture of dead neutrophils, digested bacteria, and other cell debris accumulate as a creamy substance known as *pus.*

To keep up with the demand for neutrophils, the bone marrow releases more into circulation. This results in an elevated WBC count (especially the neutrophil count). Sometimes the demand for neutrophils increases so much that the bone marrow releases immature forms of neutrophils *(bands)* into circulation. (Mature neutrophils are called *segmented neutrophils*). The finding of increased numbers of band neutrophils in circulation is called a *shift to the left.*

Monocytes. Monocytes are the second type of phagocytic cells that migrate from circulating blood. On entering the tissue spaces, monocytes transform into macrophages. Together with the tissue macrophages, these macrophages assist in phagocytosis of the inflammatory debris. The macrophage role is very important in cleaning the area before healing can occur. Macrophages have a long life span; they can multiply and may stay in the damaged tissues for weeks. These long-lived cells are very important in orchestrating the healing process.

In some cases, macrophages perform tasks other than phagocytosis. They may accumulate and fuse to form a multinucleated *giant cell.* The giant cell serves to wall off

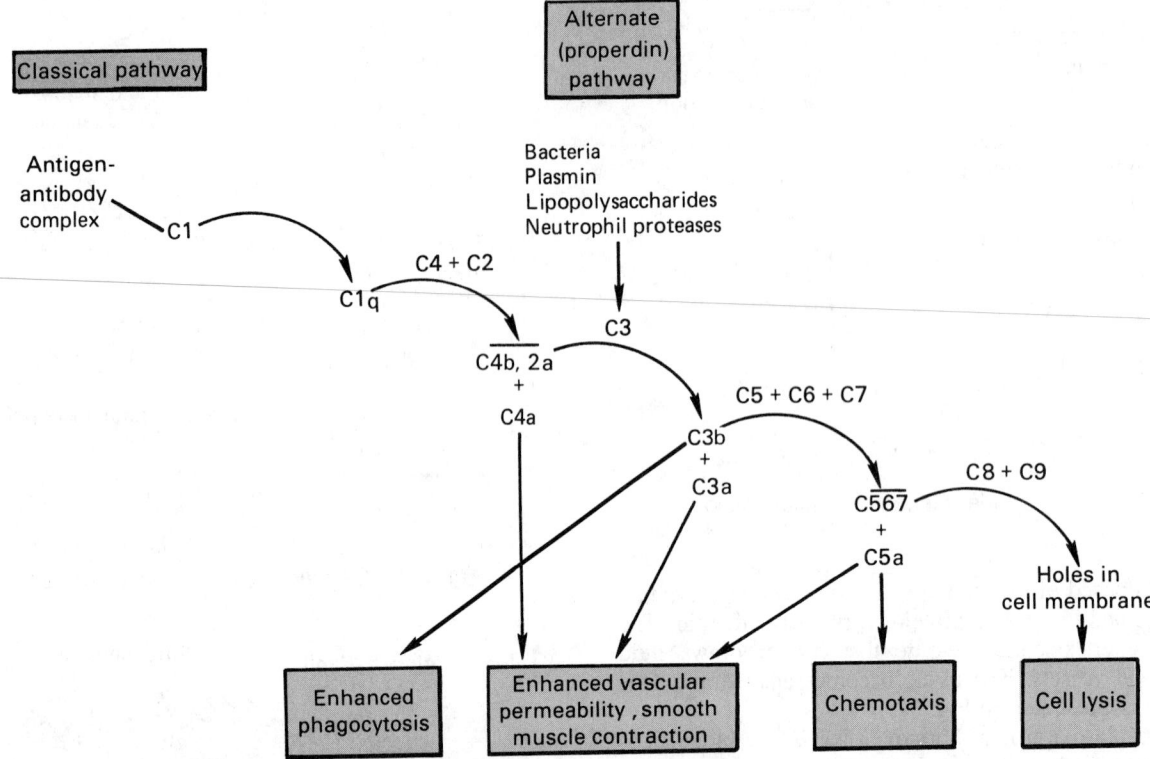

Fig. 7-8 Sequential activation and biological effects of the complement system.

infection. The accumulation of macrophages may lead to nodule formation *(granulomata)*. A classic example of this process occurs with the tubercle bacillus in the lung. While the bacillus is walled off, a chronic state of inflammation exists. The granuloma formed is a cavity of necrotic tissue.

Lymphocytes. Lymphocytes arrive later at the site of injury. Their primary role is related to cell-mediated immunity (see Chapter 8).

Eosinophils and basophils. Eosinophils and basophils are also phagocytic leukocytes but appear to have a more selective role in inflammation. Eosinophils are released in large quantities during an allergic reaction. They are involved in phagocytosis of the allergen-antibody complex. The histamine and heparin that basophils carry in their granules are released during inflammation. Histamine is a potent vasodilator.

Chemical mediators

Complement system. The complement system is a major mediator of the inflammatory response. When activated, the components occur in the sequential order of C1, C4, C2, C3, C5, C6, C7, C8, and C9 (Fig. 7-8). (The numbering reflects the order of their discovery.) Some components have subparts designated by lowercase letters (e.g., C3a, C3b, and C5a). The primary pathway for activation of the complement system is through fixation of component C1 to an antigen-antibody complex. The immunoglobulins IgG and IgM are responsible for fixing

complement. Each activated complex can act on the next component, creating a cascade effect.

An alternate pathway, the *properdin pathway,* exists in which C3 is activated without prior antigen-antibody fixation. Bacterial products, lipopolysaccharides, plasmin, and neutrophil proteases can stimulate the complement sequence at the C3 level with activation of C5 to C9.

Major functions of the complement system are enhanced phagocytosis, increased vascular permeability, chemotaxis, and cellular lysis. All of these activities are important to the inflammatory response.

Complement increases phagocytosis through opsonization and chemotaxis. Immune adherence and opsonization occur when the antigen, in combination with complement factor C3 and specific antibodies, sticks to the surface of phagocytic cells. This adherence leads to more rapid phagocytosis. In addition, complement component C5a promotes chemotaxis.

C3a, C5a, and C4a are called *anaphylatoxins,* which bind to receptors on mast cells and basophils, triggering histamine release. Histamine causes smooth muscle contraction and an increase in vascular permeability.

The entire complement sequence of C1 to C9 must be activated for cell lysis to occur. The final component (C8,9) acts on the cell surface causing rupture of the cell membrane and lysis. Bacteria, red blood cells (RBCs), and nucleated cells are susceptible to the lysis.

Prostaglandins and leukotrienes. Prostaglandins (PGs)

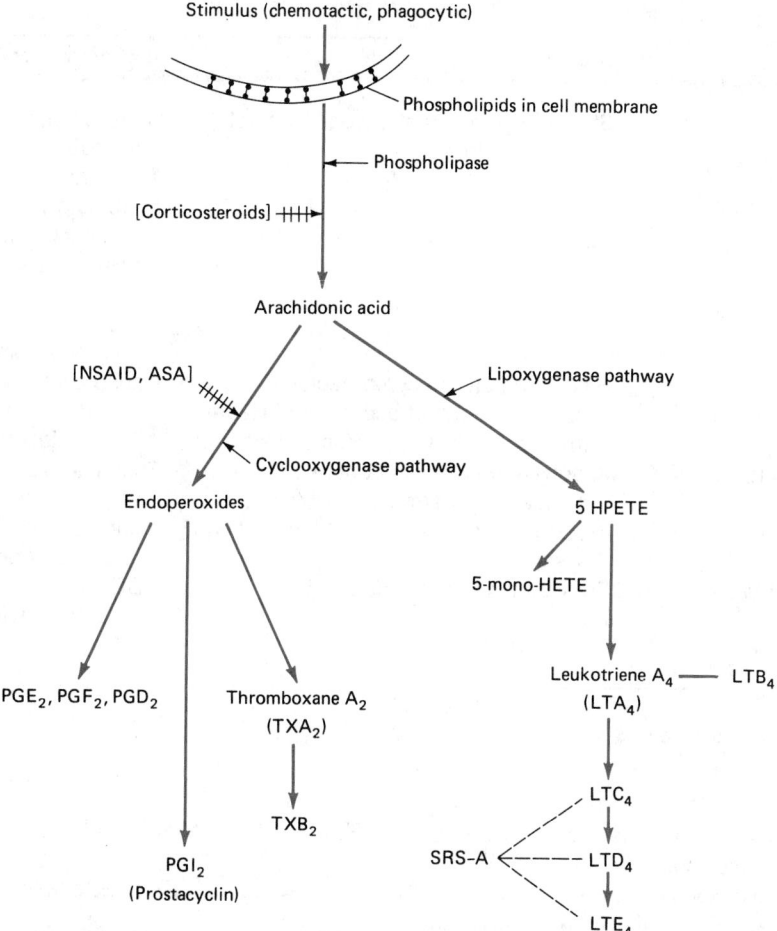

Fig. 7-9   Pathway of arachidonic acid oxygenation and generation of prostaglandins and leukotrienes. Corticosteroids, nonsteroidal antiinflammatory drugs, and acetylsalicylic acid act to inhibit various steps in this pathway. LTC$_4$, LTD$_4$, and LTE$_4$ form the slow-reacting substance of anaphylaxis, an important mediator of allergic responses, by causing bronchoconstriction and increased vascular permeability.

are substances that can be synthesized from the phospholipids of cell membranes of most body tissues, including blood cells. On stimulation by chemotactic factors or phagocytosis or after cell injury, phospholipids can be converted to arachidonic acid (a 20-carbon polyunsaturated fatty acid), which is then oxidized by two different pathways (Fig. 7-9.)

The *cyclooxygenase* metabolic pathway leads to the production of prostaglandins of the E, I, and F series and thromboxanes (formed on activation of platelets). Prostaglandins of the E and I series are potent vasodilators and inhibit platelet and neutrophil aggregation. PGF$_2$ can also sensitize pain receptors to arousal by stimuli that would normally be painless. PGF$_2$ is also a potent pyrogen, acting on the temperature-regulating area of the hypothalamus. Thromboxane A$_2$ is a potent vasoconstrictor and platelet-aggregating agent. PG are generally considered proinflammatory, contributing to increased blood flow, edema, and pain. Metabolism of arachidonic acid by the

lipoxygenase pathway leads to the production of leukotrienes (LT). LTB$_4$ is a potent chemotactic factor. LTC$_4$, LTD$_4$, and LTE$_4$ form the slow-reacting substance of anaphylaxis (SRS-A), which constricts smooth muscles of bronchi and increases blood vessel permeability.

Drugs that inhibit PG synthesis are useful clinically. Nonsteroidal antiinflammatory drugs (NSAID) are a prototype drug treatment of rheumatoid arthritis and other inflammatory conditions. Acetylsalicylic acid (ASA) blocks platelet aggregation; it also has antiinflammatory action. Prostacyclin (PGI$_2$) has been used experimentally to prevent platelet deposition in extracorporeal systems, such as hemodialysis and heart-lung bypass oxygenators. Corticosteroid drugs are valuable in the treatment of asthma because they inhibit leukotriene production and thus prevent bronchoconstriction. (Other mediators of the inflammatory response are described in Table 7-7.)

Exudate formation. Exudate is formed from the fluid and the cells that move to the site of injury. The nature

Table 7-7 Mediators of Inflammation*

Mediator	Source	Mechanisms of Action
Histamine	Stored in granules of basophils, mast cells, platelets	Causes vasodilatation and increased vascular permeability by stimulating contraction of endothelial cells and creating widened gaps between cells
Serotonin	Stored in platelets	Causes vasodilatation and increased vascular permeability by stimulating contraction of endothelial cells and creating widened gaps between cells; stimulates smooth muscle contraction
Kinins (e.g., bradykinin)	Produced from precursor factor kininogen as a result of activation of Hageman factor (XII) of clotting system	Cause contraction of smooth muscle and dilatation of blood vessels; result in stimulation of pain
Complement components (C3a, C4a, C5a)	Anaphylatoxic agents generated from complement pathway activation	Stimulate histamine release; stimulate chemotaxis
Fibrinopeptides	Produced from activation of the clotting system	Increase vascular permeability; stimulate chemotaxis for neutrophils
Prostaglandins and leukotrienes	Produced from arachidonic acid*	PGE_1 and PGE_2 cause vasodilation; LTB_4 stimulates chemotaxis
Lymphokines†		

*See Fig. 7-9.
†For information on lymphokines, see Table 8-4.

and quantity of exudate depend on the type and severity of the injury and the tissues involved.

Serous exudate. Serous exudate results from the outpouring of fluid that contains few cells and has a low protein content. It is seen in the early stages of inflammation or when the injury is mild. Examples include skin blisters and pleural effusion.

Fibrinous exudate. This type of exudate occurs with increasing vascular permeability and fibrinogen leakage into the interstitial spaces. If fibrin is formed in excessive amounts, it may coat tissue surfaces and cause them to adhere. Adhesions may develop in the healing process and bind surfaces together (e.g., the pleura adhering secondary to pneumonia).

Purulent exudate. Purulent exudate (pus) consists of leukocytes, microorganisms (dead and alive), liquefied dead cells, and other debris. A *furuncle* (boil) and *abscess* are localized forms of purulent exudates. *Cellulitis* is a diffuse inflammation involving the connective tissue.

Catarrhal exudate. Catarrhal exudate is found in tissues in which cells have the ability to produce mucus. The inflammatory response accelerates mucus production. Catarrhal exudate occurs in the nasopharynx (e.g., the runny nose common with upper respiratory infection), lungs, and GI tract.

Hemorrhagic exudate. This type of exudate results from rupture and/or necrosis of the blood vessel walls. It consists of erythrocytes that escape into the tissues.

Healing. Normally, inflammation is followed by healing (see p. 110). If the cause of the inflammation is not effectively removed, the inflammation becomes chronic.

Table 7-8 Local Manifestations of Inflammation

Manifestations	Cause
Redness (rubor)	Hyperemia from vasodilatation
Heat (calor)	Increased metabolism at inflammatory site
Pain (dolor)	Change in pH; change in local ionic concentration; nerve stimulation by chemicals (e.g., histamine, prostaglandins); pressure from fluid exudate
Swelling (tumor)	Fluid shift to interstitial spaces; fluid exudate accumulation
Loss of function (functio laesa)	Swelling and pain

Clinical manifestations. The *local response* to inflammation includes the manifestations of (1) redness, (2) heat, (3) pain, (4) swelling, and (5) loss of function (Table 7-8).

Systemic manifestations of inflammation include (1) fever, (2) leukocytosis with a shift to the left, (3) malaise, (4) nausea and anorexia, (5) weight loss, and (6) increased pulse and respiratory rate.

Fever is caused by endogenous pyrogens—interleukin 1 (IL-1) and tumor necrosis factor (TNF)—which are released from monocytes and act on the temperature-regulating center in the hypothalamus to raise the core body temperature (Fig. 7-10). Prostaglandins (e.g., PGE_2) act directly to increase the thermostatic set point. The febrile re-

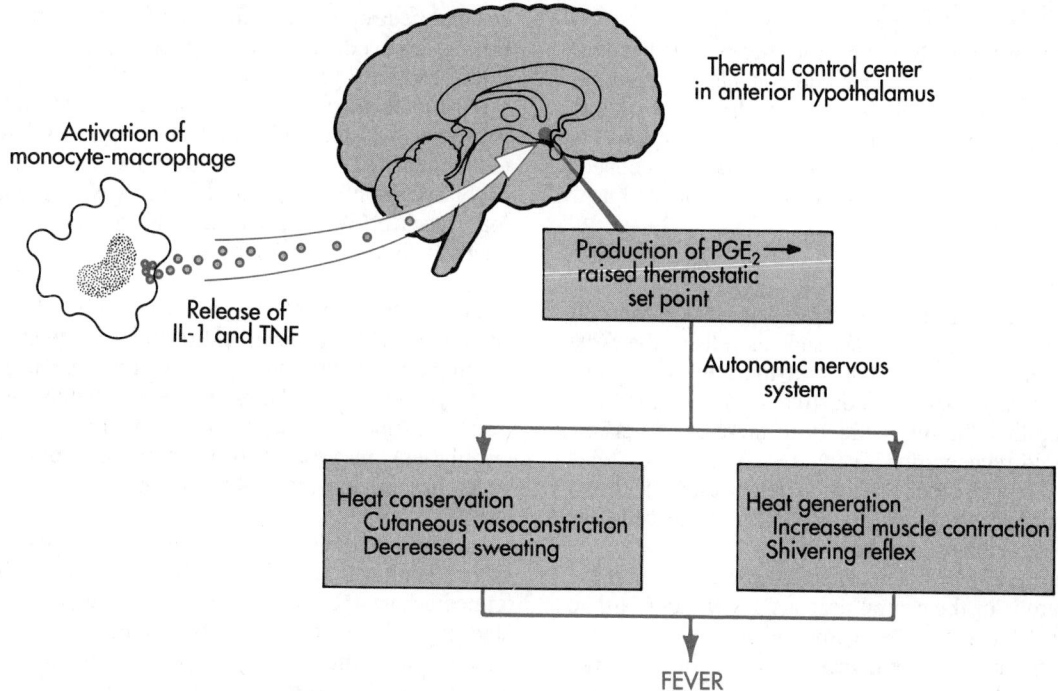

Fig. 7-10   When monocytes/macrophages are activated, they secrete interleukin-1 and tumor necrosis factor, which reach the hypothalamic thermoregulatory center by the arterial blood supply. They induce synthesis and secretions of prostaglandins in the anterior hypothalamus. Prostaglandins increase the thermostatic set point, and the autonomic nervous system is stimulated, resulting in shivering, muscle contraction, and peripheral vasoconstriction.

sponse is classified into four stages (Table 7-9). IL-1 and TNF and the fever they trigger activate the body's defense mechanisms. IL-1 and TNF enhance immunity by increasing the proliferation of T lymphocytes. Higher body temperatures may also enhance the activity of interferon, the body's natural virus-fighting substance (see Chapter 8).

Leukocytosis results from the increased release of leukocytes from the bone marrow. An increase in the circulating numbers of one or more types of leukocytes may be found. Inflammatory reactions are accompanied by the vaguely defined constitutional symptoms of malaise, nausea, anorexia, and fatigue. The causes of these systemic changes are poorly understood. An increase in pulse and respiration follows the rise in metabolism as a result of an increase in body temperature.

Types of inflammation. The basic types of inflammation are acute, subacute, and chronic. In *acute inflammation* the healing occurs within 2 to 3 weeks and usually leaves no residual damage. Neutrophils are the predominant cell type. A *subacute inflammation* has the features of the acute process but lasts longer. For example, subacute bacterial endocarditis is a smoldering infection with acute inflammation but persists over weeks or months.

Chronic inflammation lasts for weeks, months, or even years. The injurious agent persists or repeatedly injures tissue. The predominant cell types are lymphocytes, plasma

Table 7-9   Stages of the Febrile Response

Stage	Characteristics
Prodromal	Nonspecific complaints such as mild headache, fatigue, general malaise, muscle aches
Chill	Cutaneous vasoconstriction, "goose pimples," pale skin; feeling of being cold; generalized, shaking chill; shivering causing body to reach new temperature set by control center in hypothalamus
Flush	Sensation of warmth throughout body; cutaneous vasodilatation; warming and flushing of skin
Defervescence	Sweating; decrease in body temperature

cells, and macrophages. Examples of chronic inflammation include rheumatoid arthritis and tuberculosis. Tuberculosis is a type of chronic granulomatous inflammation.

A chronic inflammatory process is debilitating and can be devastating over the long term. The prolongation and chronicity of any inflammation may be due to an alteration in the immune response.

THE HEALING PROCESS

The final phase of the inflammatory response is healing. Healing includes the two major components of regeneration and repair. *Regeneration* is the replacement of lost cells and tissues with cells of the same type. *Repair* is healing as a result of lost cells being replaced by connective tissue. It is the more common type of healing and usually results in scar formation.

Regeneration

The ability of cells to regenerate depends on the cell type (see Table 7-2). *Labile cells,* such as cells of the skin, lymphoid organs, bone marrow, and mucous membranes of the GI, urinary, and reproductive tracts, divide constantly during their lifetimes. Injury to these organs is followed by rapid regeneration.

Stable cells retain their ability to regenerate but do so only if the organ is injured. Examples of stable cells are liver, pancreas, kidney, and bone cells.

Permanent cells do not regenerate. Examples of these cells are neurons of the central nervous system and cardiac muscle cells. Damage to heart muscle or central nervous system neurons leads to permanent loss. Healing will occur by repair with scar tissue.

Repair

Repair is a more complex process than regeneration. Most injuries heal by connective tissue repair. Repair healing occurs by primary, secondary, or tertiary intention (Fig. 7-11).

Primary intention. Primary intention healing takes place when wound margins are neatly approximated, such as in a surgical incision. A continuum of processes is associated with primary healing (Table 7-10). These processes include three phases.

Initial phase. The initial phase lasts for 3 to 5 days. The edges of the incision are first aligned and sutured in place. The incision area fills with blood from the cut blood vessels, and blood clots form. An acute inflammatory reaction occurs because of the exudate and necrotic cells. The area of injury is composed of fibrin clots, erythrocytes, neutrophils (both dead and dying), and other debris. Macrophages ingest and digest cellular debris, fibrin fragments, and RBCs. Extracellular enzymes derived from macropha-

ges and neutrophils help to digest fibrin. As the wound debris is removed, the fibrin clot serves as a meshwork for future capillary growth and migration of epithelial cells.

Granulation phase. The granulation (fibroplasia) phase is the second step and lasts from 5 days to 4 weeks. The components of granulation tissue include proliferating fibroblasts; proliferating capillary sprouts (angioblasts); various types of WBCs; exudate; and loose, semifluid, connective–tissue ground substance.

Fibroblasts are immature connective tissue cells that migrate into the healing site and secrete collagen. Over time the collagen is organized and restructured to strengthen the healing site. At this stage it is called *fibrous* or *scar tissue*.

During the granulation phase the wound is pink and very vascular. Numerous red granules (young budding capillaries) are present. At this point the wound is very friable, has an anesthetic quality, and is resistant to infection.[3]

Surface epithelium at the wound edges begins to regenerate. Within a few days a thin layer of epithelium migrates across the wound surface. The epithelium thickens and begins to mature, and the wound now closely resembles the adjacent skin. In a superficial wound, reepithelialization may take 3 to 5 days.

Scar contraction and maturation phase. The scar contraction and maturation phase overlaps with the granulation phase. It may begin 7 days after the injury and continue for several months. Collagen fibers are further organized, and the remodeling process occurs. Fibroblasts disappear as the wound becomes stronger. The active movement of the myofibroblasts causes contraction of the healing area, helping to close the defect and bring the skin edges closer together. A mature scar is then formed. In contrast to granulation tissue, a mature scar is virtually avascular and pale, and it may be more painful at this phase than in the granulation phase.

Secondary intention. Wounds that occur from trauma, ulceration, and infection and have large amounts of exudate and wide, irregular wound margins may not have edges that can be approximated. The inflammatory reaction may be greater than in primary healing. This results in more debris, cells, and exudate. The debris may have to be cleaned away *(debrided)* before healing can take place.

In some instances a primary incision may become infected, creating additional inflammation. The wound may reopen, and healing by secondary intention takes place.

The process of healing by secondary intention is essentially the same as by primary healing. The major differences are the greater defect and the gaping wound edges. Healing and granulation take place from the edges inward and from the bottom of the wound upward until the defect is filled. There is more granulation tissue, and the result is a much larger scar.

Wound classification. The red-yellow-black concept is sometimes used to describe open wounds.[4,5] This concept is based on the color of the open wound—red, yellow, or black—rather than on the depth of tissue destruction (Table 7-11). It can be applied to any wound allowed to heal by secondary intention, including surgically induced wounds left to heal without skin closure because of a high

Table 7-10 Phases in Primary Intention Healing

Phase	Activity
Initial (3–5 days)	Approximation of incision edges; migration of epithelial cells; clot serving as meshwork for starting capillary growth
Granulation (5 days–4 weeks)	Migration of fibroblasts; secretion of collagen; abundance of capillary buds; fragility of wound
Scar contracture (7 days–several months)	Remodeling of collagen; strengthening of scar

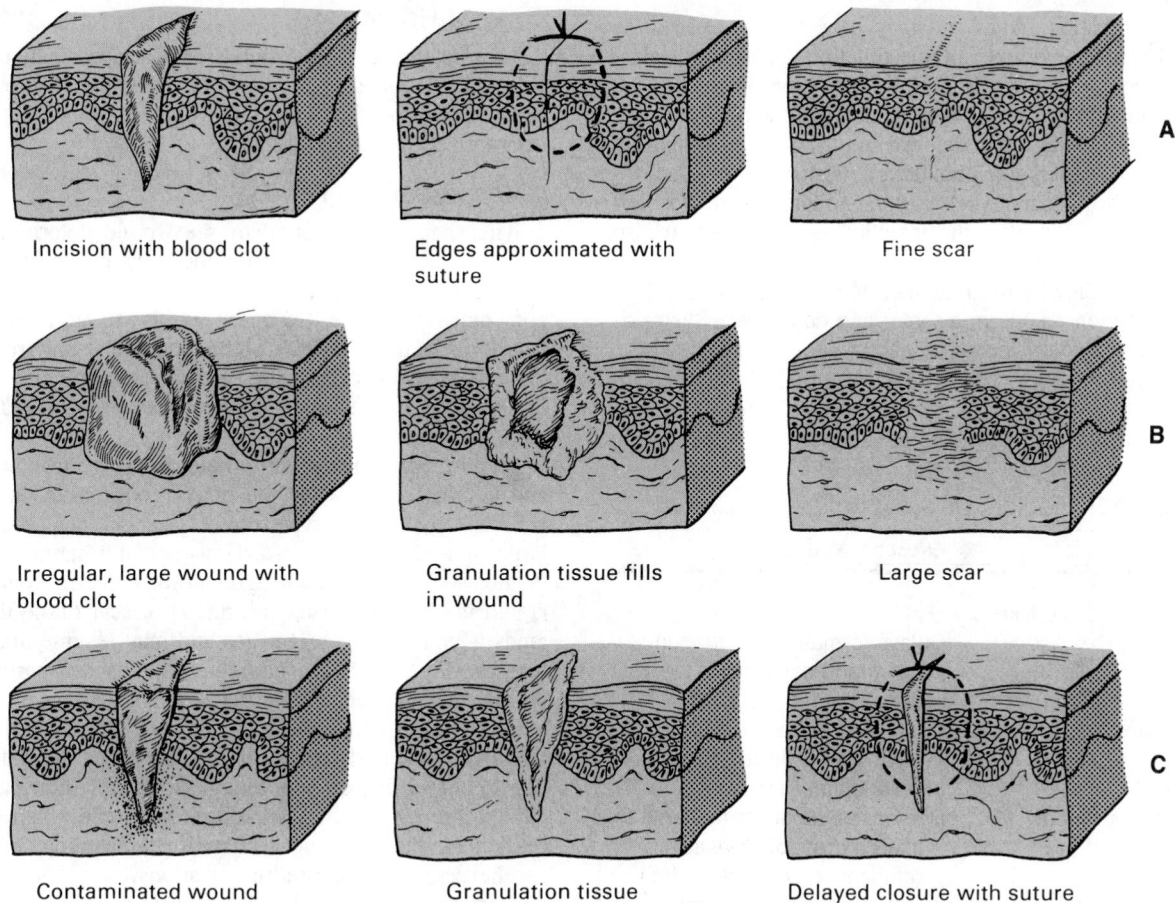

Incision with blood clot

Edges approximated with suture

Fine scar

A

Irregular, large wound with blood clot

Granulation tissue fills in wound

Large scar

B

Contaminated wound

Granulation tissue

Delayed closure with suture

C

Fig. 7-11 Types of wound healing. **A,** Primary intention. **B,** Secondary intention. **C,** Tertiary intention.

Table 7-11 Red-Yellow-Black Concept of Wound Care

Red Wound	Yellow Wound	Black Wound
CHARACTERISTICS		
Traumatic or surgical wound, possible presence of serosanguineous drainage, pink to bright or dark red healing or chronic wounds with granulating tissue	Presence of slough or soft necrotic tissue, liquid to semiliquid slough with exudate ranging from creamy ivory to yellow-green	Black, gray, or brown adherent necrotic tissue; possible presence of pus
PURPOSE OF TREATMENT		
Protection and gentle atraumatic cleansing	Wound cleansing to remove nonviable tissue and absorb excess drainage	Debridement of eschar and nonviable tissue
DRESSINGS/THERAPY		
Transparent film dressing (e.g., Tegaderm, Opsite), hydrocolloid dressing (e.g., Duoderm), hydrogels (e.g., Vigilon), gauze dressing with antimicrobial ointment/solution, Telfa dressing with antibiotic ointment	Wound irrigations, hydrotherapy in conjunction with wet-to-dry dressings, moist gauze dressing with or without antibiotic/antimicrobial agent, hydrocolloidal dressing, hydrogel covered with gauze, hydrophilic products (e.g., Debrisan beads and paste)	Topical enzyme debridement, surgical debridement, hydrotherapy, chemical debridement (e.g., Dakin's solution), moist gauze dressing, hydrogel covered with gauze, hydrophilic bead, powder, or paste covered with gauze

risk of infection. A wound may have two or even three colors at the same time. In this situation the wound is classified according to the least-desirable color present.

Tertiary intention. Tertiary intention (delayed primary intention) occurs with delayed suturing of a wound in which two layers of granulation tissue are sutured together. This occurs when a contaminated wound is left open and sutured after the infection is controlled. It also occurs when a primary wound becomes infected, is opened, is allowed to granulate, and is then sutured. Tertiary intention results in a larger and deeper scar than primary or secondary intention.

Table 7-12 Factors Delaying Wound Healing

Factor	Effect on Wound Healing
Nutritional deficiencies	
Vitamin C	Delays formation of collagen fibers and capillary development
Protein	Decreases supply of amino acids for tissue repair
Zinc	Impairs epithelialization
Inadequate blood supply	Decreases supply of nutrients to injured area, decreases removal of exudative debris, inhibits inflammatory response
Corticosteroid drugs	Impair phagocytosis by WBCs, inhibit fibroblast proliferation and function, depress formation of granulation tissue, inhibit wound contraction
Infection	Increases inflammatory response and tissue destruction
Mechanical friction on wound	Destroys granulation tissue, prevents apposition of wound edges
Advanced age	Slows collagen synthesis by fibroblasts, impairs circulation, requires longer time for epithelialization of skin, alters phagocytic and immune responses
Obesity	Decreases blood supply in fatty tissue
Diabetes mellitus	Decreases collagen synthesis, retards early capillary growth, impairs phagocytosis (result of hyperglycemia)
Poor general health	Causes generalized absence of factors necessary to promote wound healing
Anemia	Supplies less oxygen at tissue level

Delay of Healing

In a healthy person, wounds heal at a normal, predictable rate. Little can be done to accelerate this process. However, some factors delay wound healing. These are summarized in Table 7-12.

Complications of Healing

The shape and location of the wound determine how well the wound will heal. Complications result from interference with wound healing.[6] These factors may include poor nutrition, decreased blood supply, tissue trauma, denervation, and infection. Complications that may result include hypertrophic scars and keloids, contracture, dehiscence, excess granulation tissue, adhesions, and major organ dysfunction.

Hypertrophic scars and keloids. Hypertrophic scars and keloids occur when the body produces an excess of collagen tissue. A hypertrophic scar is inappropriately large, red, raised, and hard. However, it remains confined to the wound edges and regresses in time. In contrast, a keloid is an even greater protrusion of scar tissue that extends beyond the wound edges and may assume tumorlike masses (Fig. 7-12). In addition, keloids are permanent, without any tendency to subside. Clients with keloids often complain of tenderness, pain, and hyperesthesia, particularly in the early stages of development.[7] A predisposition to keloid formation is thought to be hereditary and occurs more often in dark-skinned people, particularly blacks. Neither complication is life threatening, but both can have serious cosmetic implications.

Contracture. Wound contraction is necessary for healing. This process may become abnormal when there is excessive contraction resulting in deformity or contracture. A shortening of muscle or scar tissue results from excessive fibrous formation, especially if the wound is near a joint. Contracture frequently occurs in burns in which a great loss of skin and subcutaneous tissue occurs (see Chapter 18).

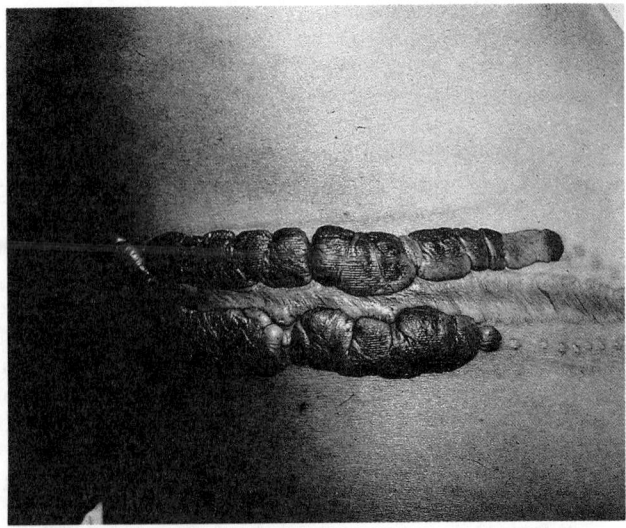

Fig. 7-12 Keloid formation resulting from suture marks.

Dehiscence. Dehiscence is separation and disruption of previously joined wound edges. It usually occurs when a primary healing site bursts open. There are two possible causes of dehiscence. First, an infection may cause an inflammatory process. Second, the granulation tissue may not be strong enough to withstand the forces imposed on the wound. *Evisceration* occurs when wound edges separate to the extent that intestinal contents protrude through the wound.

Excess granulation tissue. Excess granulation tissue ("proud flesh") protrudes above the surface of the healing wound. If the granulation tissue is cauterized or cut off, healing continues in a normal manner.

Adhesions. Adhesions are bands of scar tissue between or around organs. Adhesions may occur in the abdominal cavity or between the lungs and pleura. Adhesions in the abdomen may cause an intestinal obstruction. Adhesions between the lungs and pleura require *decortication* (stripping of pleura) to permit normal ventilation.

Major organ dysfunction. Major organ dysfunction results when an acute inflammation of any organ (such as the heart, kidney, or brain) occurs. The resulting scar tissue causes an alteration in the physiological function of the organ. The scar tissue "patch" will never function like the original tissue.

THERAPEUTIC MANAGEMENT

The actual therapeutic management of injury and inflammation is highly variable. It depends on the causative agent, the degree of injury, and the client's condition. Superficial skin injuries may need only cleansing. Deeper skin wounds can be closed by suturing the edges together. Adhesive strips may be used instead of sutures. If the wound is contaminated, it needs to be converted into a clean wound before healing can occur normally. Surgical debridement of a wound that has multiple fragments or devitalized tissue may be necessary. If the source of injury or inflammation is an internal organ (e.g., the appendix, a ruptured spleen), surgical removal of the organ is the treatment of choice.

PHARMACOLOGICAL MANAGEMENT

Pharmacological agents are used in all types of inflammation. Drugs are used for the specific purposes of reducing fever (antipyretic agents), reducing the inflammatory response (antiinflammatory agents), and destroying the infectious agent (antibiotics) (Table 7-13). Antihistamine drugs may also be used to antagonize the action of histamine and prevent vasodilator effects. (Antihistamines are discussed in Chapter 8.)

NUTRITIONAL CONSIDERATIONS

There are special nutritional measures to consider to facilitate wound healing. A high fluid intake is needed to replace fluid loss from perspiration and exudate formation. An increased metabolic rate intensifies water loss. There is a 7% increase in metabolism for every 0.3° C increase in temperature.

A diet high in protein, carbohydrate, and vitamins with moderate fat intake is necessary to promote healing. *Protein* is needed to correct the negative nitrogen balance re-

Table 7-13 Pharmacological Agents Used to Treat Inflammation

Drug	Mechanisms of Action
ANTIPYRETIC DRUGS	
Salicylates (aspirin)	Lower temperature by action on heat-regulating center in hypothalamus, resulting in peripheral dilatation and heat loss; interfere with formation and release of PGs; selectively depress central nervous system
Acetaminophen (Tylenol)	Lowers temperature by action in heat-regulating center in hypothalamus
Nonsteroidal antiinflammatory agents (e.g., ibuprofen [Motrin, Advil])	Inhibit synthesis of prostaglandins
ANTIINFLAMMATORY DRUGS	
Salicylates	Inhibit synthesis of PGs, reduce capillary permeability
Corticosteroids	Interfere with tissue granulation, induce immunosuppressive effects (decreased synthesis of lymphocytes), prevent liberation of lysosomes
Nonsteroidal antiinflammatory agents (e.g., ibuprofen [Motrin], piroxicam [Feldene])	Inhibit synthesis of PGs
ANTIBIOTIC AND ANTIMICROBIAL DRUGS	
Penicillin	Interferes with formation of bacteria cell wall, is bacteriostatic and bactericidal
Cephalosporins	Interfere with formation of bacteria cell wall, are bactericidal
Erythromycin	Inhibits synthesis of bacterial protein, is bacteriostatic
Tetracycline	Inhibits synthesis of bacterial protein, is bacteriostatic
Aminoglycosides	Inhibit synthesis of bacterial protein, are bactericidal
Sulfonamides	Interfere with incorporation of para-aminobenzoic acid (PABA) into folic acid, are bacteriostatic
VITAMINS	
Vitamin A	Accelerates epithelialization
Vitamin B complex	Acts as coenzymes
Vitamin C	Assists in synthesis of collagen and angiogenesis
Vitamin D	Facilitates calcium absorption

sulting from the increased metabolic rate. Protein is also necessary for synthesis of immune factors, leukocytes, fibroblasts, and collagen. *Carbohydrate* is needed for the increased metabolic energy required in inflammation and healing. If there is a carbohydrate deficit, the body will break down protein for the needed energy. *Fats* are also a necessary component in the diet to help in the synthesis of fatty acids and triglycerides, which are part of the cellular membrane. *Vitamin C* is necessary for capillary synthesis, capillary formation, and resistance to infection. The *B-complex vitamins* are necessary as coenzymes for many metabolic reactions. If a vitamin B deficiency develops, a disruption of protein, fat, and carbohydrate metabolism will occur. *Vitamin A* is also needed in healing because it aids in the process of epithelialization. It increases collagen synthesis and tensile strength of the healing wound.

■ Nursing Management of Inflammation

Health promotion and maintenance

The best management of inflammation is the prevention of infection, trauma, surgery, and contact with potentially harmful agents. This is not always possible. A simple mosquito bite causes an inflammatory response. Since occasional injury is inevitable, concerted efforts to combat inflammation are needed.

Adequate nutrition is essential so that the body has the necessary factors to promote healing when injury occurs. Individuals at risk for wound-healing problems are those with malabsorption problems (e.g., Crohn's disease, GI surgery, liver disease), deficient intake or high energy demands (e.g., malignancy, major trauma or surgery, sepsis, fever), and diabetes. Individuals should always be considered at risk for wound healing problems if they have experienced a loss of 20% or more of their total body weight in the preceding 6 months or 10% loss in the preceding 2 months.[8]

Early recognition of manifestations of inflammation is necessary so that appropriate treatment can begin. This treatment may be rest, pharmacological treatment, or specific treatment of the injured site. Immediate treatment may prevent the extension and complications of inflammation.

Acute intervention

Observation and vital signs. The ability to recognize the clinical manifestations of inflammation is important. Observation and recording of wound healing are also essential. The consistency, color, and odor of any drainage should be recorded and reported if abnormal for the situation. *Staphylococcus* and *Pseudomonas* species are common organisms that produce purulent, draining wounds.

Vital signs are important to note with any inflammation and especially when an infectious process is present. When infection is present, temperature may rise and pulse and respiration rates may increase. If a wound infection develops in a postoperative client, vital signs will show a change 4 to 5 days after surgery.

Fever. Although fever is usually regarded as "bad," an increase in body temperature is an important defense mechanism. In addition to the beneficial effects of fever, the elevated temperature can also inhibit the growth or even kill a variety of microorganisms. In the seventeenth century, Thomas Sydenham noted that "fever is a mighty engine which nature brings into the world for the conquest of her enemies."[9]

Steps are frequently taken to lower temperatures to relieve the anxiety of medical personnel and the client. However, fever (especially if greater than 40° C [104° F]) can be damaging to body cells, and delirium and convulsions can occur.[10] At temperatures greater than 41° C (105.8° F), regulation by the hypothalamic temperature control center becomes impaired and damage can occur to the internal structures of many cells, including those in the brain.

Several drugs are commonly used to lower the body temperature set point in the hypothalamus. ASA specifically blocks prostaglandin synthesis in the hypothalamus, as well as elsewhere in the body. Acetaminophen acts on the heat-regulating center in the hypothalamus. Some nonsteroidal antiinflammatory agents (e.g., ibuprofen [Motrin, Advil]) have antipyretic effects (Fig. 7-9). The action of these drugs results in dilatation of superficial blood vessels, increased skin temperatures, and sweating. Sponge baths decrease fever by increasing evaporative losses, and cooling blankets (mattresses) increase conductive losses. (The nursing care of the client with a fever is presented in Table 52-19.)

Rest and immobilization. Rest and immobilization of the inflamed area promote healing by decreasing the inflammatory process, assisting in the repair process, and decreasing metabolic needs. Immobilization with a cast, splint, or bandage lessens wound debris and the possibility of hemorrhage. The repair process is facilitated by allowing fibrin and collagen to form across the wound edges with little disruption. Rest helps the body better use its nutrients and oxygen for the healing process.

Elevation. Elevating the injured extremity will reduce the edema at the inflammatory site and increase venous return. This helps reduce pain and improve the circulation of blood, which provides the oxygen and nutrients needed for healing.

Oxygenation. Adequate oxygenation of the inflamed area is essential because oxygen promotes the differentiation of fibroblasts and collagen synthesis. Oxygen is also essential for cell growth and division. People with arterial disease, hypovolemia, and hypotension are at greatest risk for infection and may benefit from oxygen administration.

Heat and cold. Application of heat and cold are controversial interventions. Cold application is usually appropriate at the time of the initial trauma to cause vasoconstriction. This decreases swelling, pain, and the congestion from increased metabolism in the area of inflammation. Heat may be used later to promote healing by increasing the circulation to the inflamed site and subsequent removal of debris. Heat is also used to localize the inflammatory agents. Warm, moist heat may help debride the wound site if necrotic material is present.

Wound management. The type of wound management and dressings required depend on the type, extent, and characteristics of the wound. The purposes of wound management include (1) cleaning a dirty, infected wound to

Table 7-14

Prehospital Emergency Care of the Client with a Skin Wound*

Possible etiologies: Penetrating objects, avulsions, contusions, incised wounds, abrasions

CLINICAL MANIFESTATIONS

Redness, swelling
Bleeding
Pain
Surrounding nerve and vascular impairment
Discoloration of skin
Fear and anxiety

MANAGEMENT

Assess for bleeding areas; rule out any other injuries.
Check wound for impaled objects, pieces of glass, debris.
Do not attempt to remove any penetrating object; stabilize for removal under controlled environment.
Cleanse wound with isotonic solution if available.
For an avulsed part, fold the skin flap back into normal position and then control bleeding.
Apply bulky, sterile dressing to area and immobilize injured part.

*See Chapter 59 for a general discussion on measures related to prehospital emergency care.

prepare it for healing and (2) protecting a clean wound until it can heal normally. Prehospital care of the client with a skin wound is shown in Table 7-14.

For wounds that heal by primary intention, it is common to cover the incision with a dry, sterile dressing that is removed as soon as the drainage stops or within 2 to 3 days. Medicated sprays that form a transparent film on the skin may be used for dressings on a clean incision or injury. Sometimes a surgeon will leave a surgical wound uncovered.

Management of wounds healing by secondary intention is described as the red-yellow-black concept of wound care (see Table 7-11).

RED WOUND. A red wound can be a superficial wound if it is clean and pink in appearance. Examples include skin tears, pressure necrosis sores (stage 2), partial-thickness or second-degree burns, and wounds created surgically that are allowed to heal by secondary intention. The purpose of treatment is protection of the wound and gentle cleansing (if indicated). Clean wounds that are granulating and reepithelializing should be kept slightly moist and protected from further trauma until they heal naturally. A dressing material that keeps the wound surface clean and slightly moist is optimal to promote epithelialization. Adhesive semipermeable dressings (e.g., Op-Site, Tegaderm, Vigilon) are occlusive dressings that are permeable to oxygen. Antimicrobials such as bacitracin, neomycin, and povidone-iodine ointment can be used for application on clean wounds, which are then usually covered with a sterile

dressing. Unnecessary manipulation during dressing changes may destroy new granulation tissue and break down fibrin formation.

YELLOW WOUND. After the black eschar is removed, a yellow wound results. This type of wound can also result from surgical or traumatic injuries. The moist environment resulting from wound drainage creates an ideal situation for bacterial growth. The purpose of treatment is continual cleansing to remove nonviable tissue and to absorb excessive drainage. A type of dressing used in yellow wounds is hydrophilic beads, gels, or pastes (e.g., Debrisan), which absorb exudate and cleanse the wound surface. They work by drawing excess drainage from the wound surface. After these preparations are saturated with exudate, they should be washed off with sterile saline or water. The amount of wound secretions determines the number of dressing changes (usually two to three daily).

Occlusive dressings such as Duoderm are also used to treat yellow wounds. The inner part of these dressings interacts with the exudate, forming a hydrated gel over the wound. When the dressing is removed, the gel separates and stays over the wound, thus preventing damage to newly formed tissue. These types of dressings are designed to be left in place for up to 7 days or until leakage occurs around the dressing.

BLACK WOUND. A black wound is covered with thick necrotic tissue (eschar). Examples of black wounds include full-thickness or third-degree burns, pressure necrosis sores (stages 3 or 4), and gangrenous ulcers. The risk of wound infection increases in proportion to the amount of necrotic tissue present. The immediate treatment is debridement of the eschar and nonviable tissue. The debridement method used depends on the amount of debris and the condition of the wound tissue. There are three approaches to debridement:

1. *Surgical debridement:* This method is indicated when large amounts of nonviable tissue are present.
2. *Mechanical debridement:* This method is used when minimal debris is present. A common form of mechanical debridement is wet-to-dry dressings in which open-mesh gauze is moistened with normal saline or an antimicrobial solution, packed on or into the wound surface, and allowed to dry. Wound debris adheres to the dressing. When the dressing is removed, the coarse debris is entrapped in the gauze. Topical antimicrobials/antibactericidals used on wet-to-dry dressings include povidone-iodine (Betadine), Dakin's solution (sodium hypochlorite), hydrogen peroxide (H_2O_2), and chlorhexidine (Hibiclens). Topical antimicrobials should be used with caution in wound care, since they can damage healing tissue (e.g., H_2O_2 damages new epithelium). Semiocclusive or occlusive dressings may be used to promote eschar softening by autolysis. These types of dressings are used in open wounds with minimal necrotic debris and no contamination. Another method of mechanical debridement is wound irrigation. This method may be appropriate when wounds are contaminated. However, irrigation should be used with caution because high pressure can interfere with fi-

Table 7-15 Category-Specific Isolation Precautions

Type	Private Room	Gown	Mask	Handwashing
Strict isolation	Yes (with door closed)	Yes	Yes	After touching client or contaminated articles and before taking care of another client
Contact isolation	Yes	Yes (if soiling is likely)	Yes (for those in close contact with client)	Same as for strict isolation
Respiratory isolation	Yes	No	Yes (for those in close contact with client)	Same as for strict isolation
Tuberculosis isolation	Yes (with special ventilation; door closed)	Yes (to prevent gross contamination of clothing)	Yes (if client is coughing and does not cover mouth)	Same as for strict isolation
Enteric precautions	Yes (if client hygiene is poor)	Yes (if soiling is likely)	No	Same as for strict isolation
Drainage and secretion precautions	No	Yes (if soiling likely)	No	Same as for strict isolation
Blood and body fluid precautions*	Yes (if client hygiene is poor); puncture-resistant container available for needles	Yes (if soiling of clothing with blood or body fluids is likely)	Yes (if performing procedures where contamination with blood or body fluids is likely)	Yes (if potentially contaminated with blood or body fluids [done immediately] and before taking care of another client)

*See also Table 8-28.

broblast formation and macrophage function.

3. *Enzymatic debridement:* This method uses agents such as sutilains (Travase) in conjunction with normal, saline-moistened dressings. These enzyme products may be indicated for fragile and extremely sensitive wounds with minimal debris.

Infection control. The nurse and the client must scrupulously follow aseptic procedures for keeping the wound free from infection. The client should not be allowed to touch a recently injured area. The client's environment should be as free as possible from contamination from items introduced by roommates and visitors. Antibiotics may be administered prophylactically to some clients. If an infection develops, a culture and sensitivity test should be done to determine the most effective antibiotic for the specific organism.

If the client develops an infection that is considered a risk to others, *isolation* may be needed. The purpose of isolation is to prevent the spread of the infection. Isolation precautions in hospitals are recommended by the Centers for Disease Control (CDC) in Atlanta, Georgia. Individual hospitals then modify the guidelines to meet their own needs. In the past, *category-specific* precautions were rec-

ommended to prevent transmission of the most infectious diseases in each category (e.g., respiratory isolation, enteric isolation). This frequently meant more isolation precautions than necessary to prevent transmission of a certain organism. A new system, *disease-specific* isolation precautions, handles each infectious disease or condition separately. With this system, it is possible to list only those precautions necessary to interrupt transmission of the specific organism. Hospitals decide which system to use. A complete listing of category- and disease-specific isolation precautions is available.[11,12] A summary of category-specific isolation precautions is found in Table 7-15.

The CDC has recently published a document recommending that blood and body fluid precautions be consistently used for all clients, regardless of their blood-borne infection status.[13] This extension of blood and body fluids precautions is referred to as "Universal Blood and Body Fluid Precautions" or "Universal Precautions" (see Table 8-28). Universal precautions are intended to prevent parenteral, mucous membrane, and nonintact skin exposure of health care workers to blood-borne pathogens. In addition, immunization with hepatitis B vaccine is recommended as an important adjunct to universal precautions for health

Gloves	Handling of Contaminated Articles	Diseases
Yes	Discard or bag and label, then disinfect or sterilize	Diphtheria (pharyngeal), pneumonic plague, chickenpox
Yes (if touching infective material)	Same as for strict isolation	Disseminated herpes simplex, rabies, major skin, wound, or burn infection, pneumonia (*S. aureus* or group A *Streptococcus* species), endometritis (group A *Streptococcus* species), cutaneous diphtheria
No	Same as for strict isolation	Measles, meningitis, meningococcal pneumonia, mumps, whooping cough
No	Clean, disinfect, or discard	Pulmonary tuberculosis (with positive sputum smear or chest x-ray)
Yes (if touching infective material)	Same as for strict isolation	Amebic dysentery, viral hepatitis A, viral meningitis, acute diarrhea (with suspected infectious etiology), gastroenteritis (caused by *Giardia, Salmonella, Shigella* species or by viruses such as Norwalk agent, rotaviruses)
Yes (if touching infective material)	Same as for strict isolation	Minor or limited skin wound or burn infections
Yes (if touching blood or body fluids and performing venipuncture; avoid needle-stick injuries)	Discard or bag and label, then disinfect or sterilize; clean blood spills promptly with disinfectant	AIDS, viral hepatitis B, viral hepatitis (non-A and non-B), syphilis (primary and secondary), malaria

care workers who are exposed to blood and blood products.

A low WBC count and depressed immune responses (for example, in clients undergoing cancer chemotherapy, clients with neutropenia, or clients with leukemias and lymphomas) may indicate a need for another type of isolation called *reverse (protective)* isolation. The purpose of reverse isolation is to protect the vulnerable client from environmental sources of infection. Institutional policies related to reverse isolation should be followed when the client's condition warrants this intervention. (Reverse isolation is discussed in Chapter 25.)

Psychological implications. The client may be distressed at the thought or sight of an incision or wound because of fear of scarring or disfigurement. Drainage from a wound often causes increased alarm. The client needs to understand the healing process and the normal changes that occur as the wound heals. When a nurse is changing a dressing, inappropriate facial expressions can alert the client to problems with the wound or the nurse's ability to care for it. Wrinkling of the nose may convey disgust. A nurse should also be careful not to focus on the wound to the extent that the client is not treated as a total person.

Chronic management

Wound healing may not be complete for 4 to 6 weeks or longer. Adequate rest and good nutrition should be continued throughout this time. Physical and emotional stress should be minimal. Observing for wound complications such as contractures, adhesions, and secondary infection is important during the rehabilitative stage.

Medications will often be taken for a period of time after recovery from the acute infection. Awareness of the necessity to continue the drugs for the specified time is an important point to teach the client. For example, a client who is to take an antibiotic for 10 days may stop taking the medication after 5 days because of decreased symptoms. However, the organism may not be entirely eliminated, and it may increase in number and virulence if the medication is not continued. The organism may also become resistant to the antibiotic in this situation.

The client may also need teaching in some areas of personal care, including changing dressings and caring for the wound. The client may need to take medication and observe for any adverse side effects. Manifestations of abnormal wound healing should be taught so that the client can report any findings to the health care provider.

C ase Study

INJURY AND INFLAMMATION

Roger, a 20-year-old man, was admitted to the hospital emergency room with burns estimated to be second degree that involved his face, neck, and upper trunk. He also had a lacerated right leg. He was alert and his voice was slightly hoarse. An IV was started immediately, and an indwelling catheter was inserted into the bladder. His right leg was splinted and the lacerated wound was cleaned and debrided.

By the third day postburn, Roger had marked edema throughout his body and developed a temperature of 39° C. On the sixth day postburn the leg wound became infected and pus developed. His white blood cell count was 26,400/μl and a differential showed the following:

Neutrophils 75%   Basophils   0.5%   Monocytes 3%
Eosinophils 2%   Lymphocytes 20%

By the third week, the burn sites and leg wound were healing well. When Roger complained of stiffness of his neck, the nurse noticed contractures developing in the neck area.

Discussion Questions

1. What clinical manifestations of inflammation did Roger exhibit and what are their pathophysiological mechanisms?
2. What type of exudate formation did he develop?
3. What is the basis for the development of the temperature?
4. What is the significance of his WBC count and differential?
5. Because his wound was deep, primary tissue healing was not possible. How would you expect healing to take place?
6. What is the cause of the contracture development?
7. What problems might Roger have with self-concept or body image? What concerns or problems might a nurse have in caring for Roger?

R eview Questions

The number of the question corresponds to the same-numbered objective at the beginning of the chapter.

1. What is the function of DNA?
   a. to transmit all genetic information
   b. to determine the occurrence of cell division
   c. to build RNA
   d. to regulate the sequence of genes on chromosomes
2. Physiological hyperplasia is commonly found in
   a. the bronchi of a chronic cigarette smoker
   b. a distended urinary bladder
   c. the female breast during lactation
   d. an enlarged myocardium in congestive heart failure
3. Which of the following describes a mechanism of cell death?
   a. cytoplasm becoming more granular
   b. rupture of cell membrane
   c. increase in size of cell
   d. embryonic differentiation
4. Which of the following is a common cause of coagulation necrosis?
   a. autophagocytosis
   b. granulomatous inflammation
   c. lack of blood supply
   d. malignant brain tumor
5. A major function of the mononuclear phagocyte system is to
   a. stimulate fibrin formation
   b. synthesize neutrophils
   c. release histamine
   d. phagocytize foreign material
6. Which of these best describes inflammation?
   a. an antigen-antibody reaction
   b. a sequential reaction to cell injury
   c. a secondary defense mechanism
   d. a detrimental defense mechanism of body
7. Which of the following are local manifestations of inflammation?
   a. contractures and adhesions
   b. pain and ulceration
   c. boil and cyanosis
   d. swelling and loss of function
8. Wound healing by primary intention involves all the following *except*
   a. abundant collagen formation
   b. an inflammatory reaction
   c. regenerating epithelium
   d. blood clot formation
9. Contractures frequently occur after burn healing because of
   a. weakness of connective tissue
   b. lack of adequate blood supply
   c. excess fibrous tissue formation
   d. secondary infection
10. Rest and immobilization are important measures of acute care for wound healing because
    a. the production of leukocytes will be decreased
    b. the inflammatory response will be decreased
    c. they are known mechanisms to increase the rate of healing
    d. they increase the body's production of corticosteroids

REFERENCES

1. Orgill D and Demling RH: Current concepts and approaches to wound healing, Crit Care Med 16:899–908, 1988.
2. Dinarello C: The endogenous pyrogens in host-defense interactions, Hosp Pract 24:111-128, 1989.
3. Hunt TK: The physiology of wound healing, Ann Emerg Med 17:1265-1273, 1988.
4. Cuzzell JZ: The new RYB color code, Am J Nurs 88:1342-1346, 1988.
5. Stotts NA: Seeing red and yellow and black: the three-color concept of wound care, Nurs 20:59-61, 1990.
6. Robson MC: Disturbances of wound healing, Ann Emerg Med 17:1274-1278, 1988.
7. Habif TP: Clinical dermatology, ed 2, St Louis, 1990, Mosby–Year Book, Inc, p 509.
8. Meser MS: Wound care, Crit Care Nurs Q 11:17-27, 1989.
9. Atkins E: Fever: its history, cause and function, Yale J Biol Med 55:283-289, 1982.
10. Enright T and Hill EMG: Treatment of fever, Focus Crit Care 16:96-102, 1989.
11. Guidelines for isolation precautions in hospitals, Infect Control 4:249-349, 1983.
12. CDC guidelines for isolation precautions in hospitals, Superintendent of Documents, Washington, DC.
13. Centers for Disease Control: Update: universal precautions for prevention of transmission of human immunodeficiency virus, hepatitis B virus, and other bloodborne pathogens in health-care settings, MMWR 37:377, 1988.

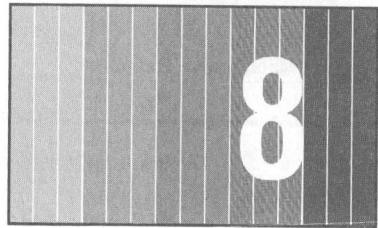
Nursing Role in Management
Altered Immune Responses

Sharon Mantik Lewis
Barbara D. Rickert

---

1. Describe the functions and components of the immune system.
2. Differentiate between natural and acquired immunity.
3. Compare and contrast humoral and cell-mediated immunity regarding lymphocytes involved, types of reactions, and effects on antigens.
4. Identify the five types of immunoglobulins and their characteristics.
5. Differentiate among the four types of hypersensitivity reactions in terms of immunological mechanism, time sequence, and disease manifestations.
6. Identify the clinical manifestations and emergency treatment for a systemic anaphylactic reaction.
7. Describe the assessment and management of a client with chronic allergies.

8. Describe the pharmacological intervention for the client with allergies.
9. Describe the etiological factors, clinical manifestations, and treatment modalities of autoimmune diseases.
10. Explain the relationship between the HLA system and certain diseases.
11. Describe the etiological factors, categories, and treatment for immunodeficiency disorders.
12. Describe the etiology, populations at risk, and treatment of acquired immunodeficiency syndrome.
13. Identify the clinical course of an individual with an HIV infection.
14. Describe the nursing management of a client with an HIV infection.

The human body has always had to protect itself from invasion by microorganisms. A complex defense system has evolved to withstand these constant attacks. The defense system in humans consists of a nonspecific inflammatory response (including phagocytosis) and a specific immune response (humoral immunity and cell-mediated immunity). (The inflammatory response is discussed in Chapter 7.)

Immunocompetence exists when the body's immune system can identify and inactivate or destroy foreign sub-stances. When the immune system is incompetent or underresponsive, immunodeficiency diseases and malignancies occur. When the immune system overreacts, hypersensitivity disorders such as allergies and autoimmune diseases occur.

NORMAL IMMUNE RESPONSE
Immunity

Immunity is a state of responsiveness to invading organisms and foreign or tumor protein. Immune responses serve three functions[1] (Table 8-1):

1. *Defense:* The body resists invasions by microorganisms and prevents infection from developing by attacking foreign pathogens.
2. *Homeostasis:* Damaged cellular substances that are constantly being catabolized in the body are removed. Through this mechanism the specific cell type remains uniform and unchanged.

Reviewed by Janice M. Zeller, R.N., Ph.D., Professor, Department of Medical Nursing; Associate Professor, Department of Immunology/Microbiology, Rush-Presbyterian-St Luke's Medical Center, Chicago, Illinois and Lucy Bradley-Springer, R.N., Ph.D., Education Coordinator, New Mexico AIDS Education and Training Center, University of New Mexico, Albuquerque, New Mexico.

Table 8-1 Functions of the Immune System

Function	Adaptive Response	Maladaptive Response	
		Hyper	Hypo
Defense	Destruction of viruses, bacteria, fungi	Allergic disorders	Immunodeficiency disorders
Homeostasis	Removal of damaged cells	Autoimmune diseases	—
Surveillance	Removal of cell mutants	—	Malignant diseases

Modified from Bellanti JA: Immunology III, Philadelphia, 1985, WB Saunders Co, p 7.

3. *Surveillance:* Mutations continually arise in the body but are normally recognized as foreign cells and destroyed.

Properties of the Immune Response

The immune system has three important properties that make its protection diverse and long lasting. They are the following:

1. *Specificity:* When an antigen (foreign substance) enters the body, a series of cellular changes occurs. These changes result in the formation of a specific antibody or sensitized lymphocyte that attaches to the surface of the antigen.
2. *Memory:* The immune system has the unique ability to remember the antigen. Therefore, a secondary immune response is faster and stronger.
3. *Self-recognition:* Since there frequently is little difference between the body's own proteins and foreign proteins, the body must distinguish between the two. When the body fails to recognize self-proteins, autoantibodies develop, leading to tissue destruction.

Types of immunity. Immunity is classified as *natural* or *acquired.* Natural immunity exists in a person without prior contact with an antigen. It may be related to a species, race, or genetic tendency. Acquired immunity implies the development of immunity in a human being, either actively or passively (Table 8-2).

Active acquired immunity. Active acquired immunity results from invasion of the body by microorganisms and subsequent development of antibodies and sensitized lymphocytes. With each reinvasion of the microorganisms, the body responds more rapidly and vigorously to fight off the invader. Active acquired immunity may result naturally from a disease or artificially through inoculation of a less virulent antigen. Because antibodies are synthesized, immunity takes time to develop but is long lasting.

Passive acquired immunity. Passive acquired immunity implies that the host receives antibodies to an antigen rather than synthesizes them. This may take place naturally through the transfer of immunoglobulins across the placental membrane from mother to fetus. Artificial passive acquired immunity occurs through injection with γ-globulin (serum antibodies). The benefit of this immunity is its immediate effect. Unfortunately, the immunity is short lived, since the host did not synthesize the antibodies and consequently does not retain memory cells for the antigen.

Antigens

An *antigen* is a foreign substance that elicits an immune response by the body. Most antigens are composed of protein. However, other substances such as large-size polysaccharides, lipoproteins, and nucleic acids can act as antigens. *Haptens* (low molecular weight substances) are harmless alone but form complexes that are antigenic when combined with high molecular weight carriers. Common haptens include dust, animal danders, drugs, and industrial chemicals. Once antibodies are produced, future exposure to the hapten alone can elicit an immune response. Haptens are important in hypersensitivity reactions.

Most antigens are not chemically pure substances but rather have multiple antigenic determinants on their surface with which antibodies can combine. Physical or chemical irritation of normal body cells may stimulate the expression of new antigenic determinants. This process results in hypersensitivity, autoimmunity, and neoplasia.

Components of the Immune System

Lymphoid organs function in production of lymphocytes, one of the essential cells of the immune response. The mononuclear phagocyte system is also involved in the production of a normal immune response.

Lymphoid organs. The lymphoid system is composed of central and peripheral lymphoid organs. The *central lymphoid organs* are the thymus gland and bone marrow. The *peripheral lymphoid organs* are the tonsils; gut-, genital-, bronchial-, and skin-associated lymphoid tissues; lymph nodes; and spleen (Fig. 8-1).

Lymphocytes are produced in bone marrow and eventually migrate to the peripheral organs. The thymus is important for the differentiation and maturation of T lymphocytes and is therefore essential for a cell-mediated immune response. During childhood the gland is large. The gland shrinks with age and is a collection of reticular fibers, lymphocytes, and connective tissue in older persons.

Lymphoid tissue is found in the submucosa of the respiratory (bronchial-associated), genitourinary (genital-associated), and gastrointestinal (gut-associated) tracts. This tissue protects the body surface from external microorganisms. The tonsils are a typical example of lymphoid tissue.

The skin-associated lymph tissue primarily consists of lymphocytes and Langerhans cells (bone marrow–derived macrophages) found in the epidermis of skin. When Langerhans cells are depleted, the skin can neither initiate

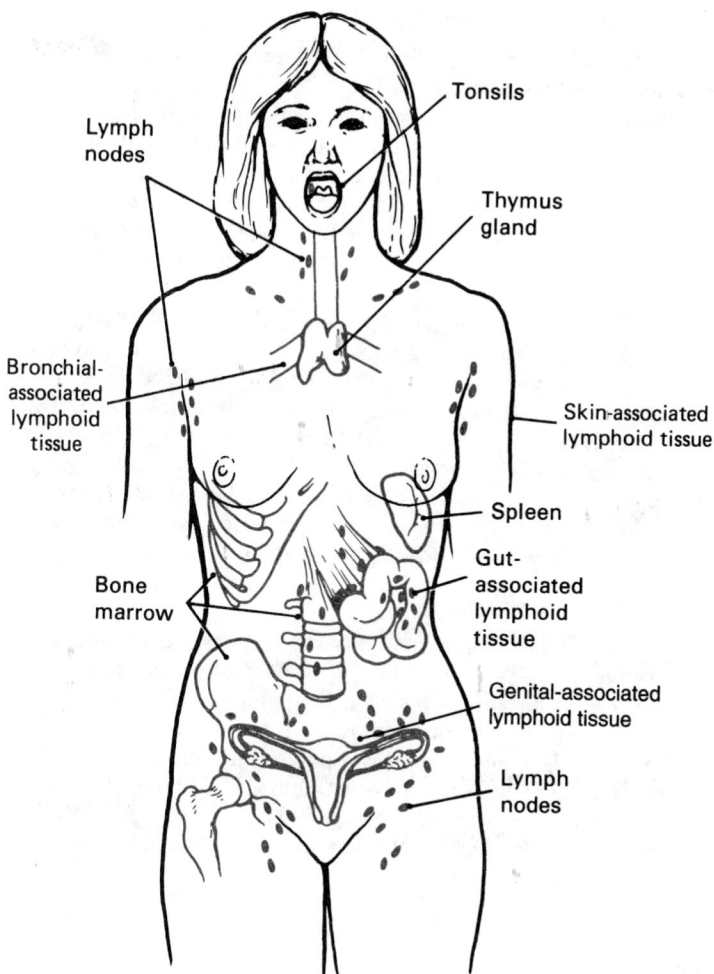

Fig. 8-1 Organs of the immune system.

an immune response nor support a skin-localized delayed hypersensitivity response.

When antigens are introduced into the body, they may be carried by the bloodstream or lymph channels to regional *lymph nodes*. The antigens interact with B and T lymphocytes and macrophages in the lymph node. The two important functions of lymph nodes are (1) filtration of foreign material brought to the site and (2) circulation of lymphocytes.

The spleen is important as the primary site for filtering foreign substances from the blood. It consists of two kinds of tissue: *white pulp* containing B and T lymphocytes and *red pulp* containing erythrocytes. Macrophages line the pulp and sinuses of the spleen. If the spleen is removed in children, it can predispose them to life-threatening septicemia.

Mononuclear phagocyte system. The mononuclear phagocyte system includes macrophages found throughout the body. (See Chapter 7 for a more complete description.) Macrophages have a critical role in the immune system. They are responsible for capturing, processing, and presenting the antigen to the lymphocytes. This stimulates a

Table 8-2 Types of Acquired Specific Immunity

Acquisition of Immunity	Protection
ACTIVE	
Natural	
Natural contact with antigen through clinical or sub-clinical case; for example, recovery from childhood diseases (e.g., chicken-pox, measles, mumps)	**Development** Develops slowly; protective levels reached in few weeks **Duration** Long term, often lifetime **Spectrum** Specific to antigen con-tacted
Artificial	
Immunization with antigen; for example, immuniza-tion with live or killed vac-cines, toxoid immunization	**Development** Develops slowly; protective levels reached in few weeks **Duration** Several years; extended protection with "booster" doses **Spectrum** Specific to antigen targeted by immunization
PASSIVE	
Natural	
Transplacental and colos-trum transfer from mother to child; for example, ma-ternal immunoglobulins in neonate	**Development** Immediate **Duration** Temporary; several months **Spectrum** All antigens to which mother has immunity
Artificial	
Injection of serum from im-mune human or animal; for example, injection of pooled human gamma globulin, injection of ani-mal hyperimmune sera	**Development** Immediate **Duration** Temporary; several weeks **Spectrum** All antigens to which source has immunity

From Phipps WJ, Long BC, and Woods NF: Medical-surgical nurs-ing: concepts and clinical practice, ed 3, St Louis, 1987, The CV Mosby Co, p 1886.

humoral or cell-mediated immune response. Capturing is accomplished through phagocytosis. The macrophage-bound antigen, which is highly immunogenic, is presented to circulating T or B lymphocytes and thus triggers an immune response (Fig. 8-2).

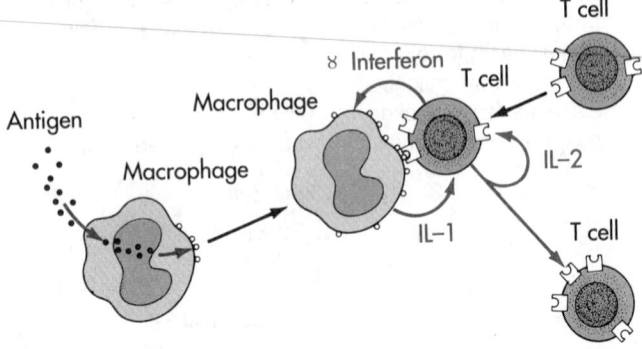

Fig. 8-2 Schematic representation of the cellular events involved in T-cell activation. In the early phase of the immune response, foreign antigen is taken up by mononuclear phagocytes, processed, and reexpressed on the macrophage cell membrane where it is recognized by specific T cells. In the presence of monocyte-derived mediators such as interleukin-1, this series of events leads to proliferation and activation of T cells. The activated T cells secrete various lymphokines (e.g., interleukin-2, γ-interferon) that mediate responses involving lymphocytes and mononuclear phagocytes.

Lymphocyte Production

Lymphocytes arise from undifferentiated stem cells in the fetal liver and later from the bone marrow (Fig. 8-3). Lymphocytes differentiate into B and T lymphocytes.

In birds, B lymphocytes (bursa-equivalent or thymus-independent cells) mature under the influence of the bursa of Fabricius. However, this lymphoid organ does not exist in humans. The equivalent of the bursa has not yet been identified. Several sites have been suggested, including the bone marrow and the fetal liver and spleen.

Cells that migrate from the bone marrow to the thymus differentiate into T lymphocytes (thymus-dependent cells). The thymus secretes thymic hormones, including thymosin. It stimulates the maturation and differentiation of T lymphocytes. T cells compose 70% to 80% of the circulating lymphocytes and are primarily responsible for immunity to intracellular viruses, tumor cells, and fungi. These T cells live from a few months to the life span of an individual and account for long-term immunity.

Humoral Immunity

A successful humoral immune response leads to humoral immunity. Production of antibodies (immunoglobulins) is an essential step in a humoral immune response. Immunoglobulins are composed of amino acids arranged on two light and two heavy polypeptide chains. Differences in the heavy chain configuration differentiate the five classes of immunoglobulins, which are IgG, IgA, IgM, IgD, and IgE. Each class of immunoglobulins has specific characteristics (Table 8-3).

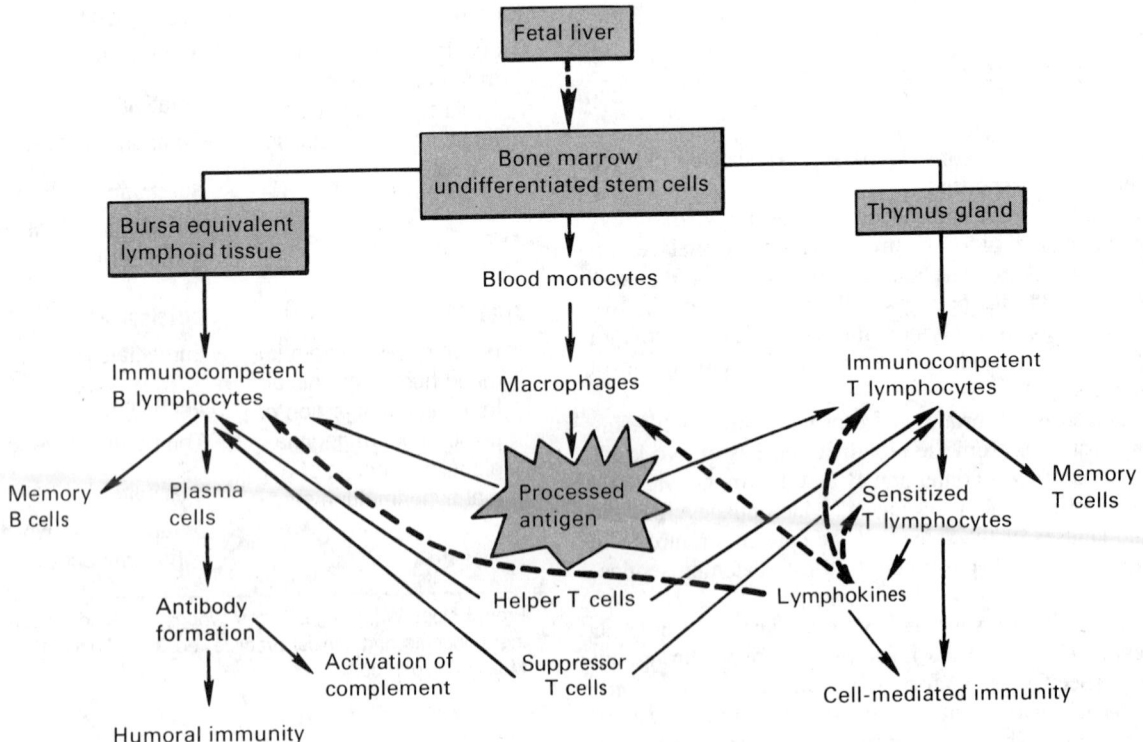

Fig. 8-3 Relationships and functions of macrophages, B lymphocytes, and T lymphocytes in an immune response.

Table 8-3 Characteristics of Immunoglobulins

Class	Relative Serum Concentration (%)	Location	Characteristics
IgG	76	Plasma, interstitial fluid	Exists as only immunoglobulin that crosses placenta
			Fixes complement
			Is responsible for secondary immune response
IgA	15	Body secretions, including tears, saliva, breast milk, colostrum	Lines mucous membranes and protects body surfaces
IgM	8	Plasma	Fixes complement
			Is responsible for primary immune response
			Provides specific antitoxin action when with IgG
			Forms antibodies to ABO blood antigens
IgD	1	Plasma	Is present on lymphocyte surface
			Assists in the differentiation of B lymphocytes
IgE	0.002	Plasma, interstitial fluids, exocrine secretions	Causes symptoms of allergic reactions
			Fixes to mast cells and basophils
			Assists in defense against parasitic infections

Humoral immune response. When an antigen (especially bacteria) enters the body, it may encounter a B lymphocyte specific for that antigen. The B lymphocyte recognizes the antigen because it has cell surface receptors specific for the antigen. After contact with the antigen, most B lymphocytes differentiate into plasma cells (Fig. 8-3). The mature plasma cell secretes immunoglobulins. Each plasma cell produces only one type of immunoglobulin. Some stimulated B lymphocytes remain as memory cells.

The *primary immune response* is evident 4 to 8 days after initial exposure to the antigen. IgM is the first type of antibody formed. Because of the large size of the IgM molecule, this immunoglobulin is confined to the intravascular space. As the immune response progresses, IgG is produced and can move from intravascular to extravascular spaces.

When the individual is exposed to the antigen the second time, a *secondary antibody response* occurs. This response occurs faster (1 to 2 days), is stronger, and lasts for a longer time than a primary response. Memory cells account for the memory of the first exposure to the antigen and the more rapid production of antibodies. IgG is the primary antibody found in a secondary immune response.

During gestation, the fetus has some immunity to protect against in utero infections. However, the lymph nodes and spleen are underdeveloped at birth. Fortunately, IgG crosses the placental membrane and provides the newborn with passive acquired immunity for at least 3 months. Infants may also get some immunity from IgA concentrated in breast milk and colostrum. By 9 months of age, a baby's IgM level is at normal concentration and the lymph nodes and spleen are well developed.

Antigen-antibody interactions. Antigen-antibody interactions result in elimination or destruction of the antigen. The five kinds of interactions are the following:

1. *Precipitation:* Soluble antigens combine with antibodies to form a lattice formation of insoluble complexes that precipitate.
2. *Agglutination:* Particulate antigens (e.g., red blood cells [RBCs]) may combine with antibodies to form clumps.
3. *Opsonization:* Bacteria are coated with molecules that allow them to be recognized and ingested by neutrophils and monocytes. The opsonization mechanism involves IgG and complement-derived C3b. Opsonized particles attach to receptors on the surface of neutrophils and monocytes.
4. *Lysis:* Lysis occurs after complement acts on the antigen cell membrane to cause rupture and spillage of cell contents. (The complement system is discussed in Chapter 7.)
5. *Neutralization:* Antibodies neutralize some toxins released from bacteria. The mononuclear phagocyte system phagocytizes the antigen-antibody complex and removes it from the body.

Monoclonal antibodies. Monoclonal antibody technology is a form of genetic engineering resulting in the production of specific antibodies by specialized tissue culture lines. Monoclonal antibodies are homogeneous populations of identical antibody molecules. The procedure uses simple cell fusion techniques and standard in vitro tissue culture systems. The two essential biological components are immunized mice or rats and tumor cell lines of lymphoid origin called *myelomas*. Single antibody-forming cells (lymphocytes) from rodents previously immunized with antigen are fused with myeloma cells to create hybrid cells with properties of both parent cell types. The hybrids have an unlimited capacity to grow similar to that of the myeloma parent, and they produce the single type of antibody molecule that they inherited from the normal, antibody-forming cell parent. Hybrid cells derived in this way can produce unlimited quantities of specific antibody. With appropriate selection techniques, producing monoclonal antibodies to virtually any antigen is possible. Because the monoclonal antibodies are a completely homogeneous population, their use incurs fewer problems than conventional polyclonal antisera. Because most antigens (immunogens) have multiple antigenic determinants that stimulate B lymphocytes to proliferate, most humoral immune responses are polyclonal with multiple antibodies produced.

Monoclonal antibodies are finding wide application in many areas of medicine and biological science. Thousands of monoclonal antibodies have been made against many different types of antigens. They have begun to replace conventional antibodies in blood banking and are used in the identification of organisms in the bacteriology laboratory. Monoclonals have also been extensively used in radioimmunoassays to measure serum levels of various substances (e.g., parathyroid hormone). They have been very useful in quantitating types of white blood cells (WBCs) and subgroups of lymphocytes. They are also used in the diagnosis of leukemias. More recently, they have been used to identify tumors in vivo and, in certain instances, to treat leukemias and lymphomas. They have been used to treat transplant rejection episodes (see Chapter 41), purge bone marrow of tumor cells in bone marrow transplants, and remove mature T cells that cause graft-versus-host disease in bone marrow transplants (see p. 142). Recently, human hybridomas have been produced using human myelomas. These hybrids synthesize human monoclonals and are therefore advantageous for in vivo use in diagnosis and therapy.

Cell-Mediated Immunity

The immune response may involve interactions of the cells of the immune system with the antigen; these interactions are called *cell-mediated immunity*. Although these reactions were initially considered to be mediated by T cells, several cell types and factors are involved in cell-mediated immunity. The cell types involved include T lymphocytes, macrophages, and natural killer cells. Cell-mediated immunity is of primary importance in (1) immunity against viral infections, fungal infections, and some bacterial intracellular obligate infections including those caused by *Mycobacterium* species; (2) rejection of transplanted tissues; (3) contact hypersensitivity reactions; and (4) tumor immunity.

T lymphocytes. T lymphocytes can be categorized into T-cytotoxic, T-helper or inducer, and T-suppressor cells.

T-cytotoxic cells. T-cytotoxic cells are involved in attacking the cell membrane of foreign antigens and releasing cytolytic substances that destroy the antigen. These cells have antigen specificity and are sensitized by exposure to the antigen. Similar to B lymphocytes, some sensitized T cells do not attack the antigen but remain as memory T cells. As in the humoral immune response, a second exposure to the antigen will result in a more intense and rapid cell-mediated immune response.

T-helper and T-suppressor cells. T-helper or inducer cells and T-suppressor cells are involved in the regulation of the humoral antibody response and cell-mediated immunity, providing a positive and negative signal, respectively. These two cell types are often referred to as *immu-*

Table 8-4   Mediators of Cellular Immunity

Cytokine	Effect
Interleukin-1, tumor necrosis factor, lymphotoxin	Activate T and B lymphocytes; enhance interleukin-2 production, local and systemic inflammation, hematopoiesis, acute phase responses, thrombosis
Interleukin-2	Promotes antibody production by B cells; stimulates T-cell proliferation and activation; activates T-cytotoxic cells*
Interleukin-3	Supports growth of several types of bone marrow stem cells giving rise to different kinds of blood cells
Interleukin-4	Stimulates B-cell growth; stimulates resting T cells
Interleukin-5	Stimulates B-cell growth
Interleukin-6	Promotes B-cell differentiation; stimulates hepatocytes
Interferons†	Interfere with viral growth; stimulate phagocytic action of macrophages; stimulate killing activity of sensitized lymphocytes and natural killer cells
Colony-stimulating factor, granulocyte-macrophage colony–stimulating factor, granulocyte colony-stimulating factor	Regulate proliferation and differentiation of hematopoietic cells, recruit and activate leukocytes
Lymphocyte-derived chemotactic factor	Attracts macrophages and neutrophils to area of antigen
Macrophage-activating factor, macrophage-inhibiting factor	Increase macrophage tumoricidal and microbicidal function; inhibit migration of macrophages

*See Fig. 8-2.
†See Table 8-5.

noregulatory cells. With many autoimmune diseases the number of T-suppressor cells decreases in proportion to the number of T-helper cells, thus resulting in an overaggressive immune response.

Natural killer cells. Natural killer cells are also involved in cell-mediated immunity. These cells are not T or B cells, and unlike these types of lymphocytes, they have granules in the cytoplasm. Thus, they are often referred to as *large granular lymphocytes*. Natural killer cells occur naturally and do not require prior sensitization for their generation. These cells are probably involved in nonspecific killing of virally transformed cells, transplanted grafts, resistance to some infections, and tumor rejection. They may have a significant role in immune surveillance of malignant diseases in humans.

Cytokines. The immune response involves complex interactions of T cells, B cells, and monocytes. These interactions depend on *cytokines* (soluble factors secreted by these cells) acting as messengers between the cell types. These cytokines can be classified as *lymphokines* (secreted by lymphocytes) and *monokines* (secreted by monocytes or macrophages). Various kinds of cytokines that act as mediators of the immune response are summarized in Table 8-4.

Interferon. Interferon, one type of lymphokine, was identified in 1957 as a substance that helps the body's natural defenses attack tumors and viruses. Three types of interferon have now been identified and are classified according to the cell of origin and functional characteristics (Table 8-5). In addition to their direct antiviral properties, interferons have immunoregulatory functions (e.g., enhancement of natural killer cell production and activation as well as inhibition of tumor cell growth).

Interferon is not directly antiviral but produces an antiviral effect in cells by reacting with them and inducing the formation of a second protein called *antiviral protein* (Fig. 8-4). This protein mediates the antiviral action of interferon by altering the cell's protein synthesis and preventing new viruses from becoming assembled. Interferons are currently being tested in clinical trials to evaluate their effectiveness in treating malignancies (see Chapter 9).

Macrophages. Lymphokines attract and activate macrophages in the area of the immune reaction. These macrophages release lysosomal enzymes that damage surrounding tissues.

Summary of Immune Responses

Humans need humoral and cell-mediated immunity to remain healthy. Each type of immunity has unique properties and different methods of action; each reacts against particular antigens. Table 8-6 compares humoral and cell-mediated immunity.

Effects of Aging on the Immune System

With advancing age there is a decline in the immune system. The primary clinical evidence for this immunosenescence is the high incidence of tumors in older adults. A greater susceptibility to infections (such as influenza and pneumonia) from pathogens that an older person has been relatively immunocompetent against earlier in life also occurs.[2]

Aging does not affect all aspects of the immune system. The bone marrow is relatively unaffected by increasing age. However, aging has a pronounced effect on the thymus, which involutes proportional to aging. This involution is probably a primary cause of immunosenescence. Both T and B cells show deficiencies in activation, transit

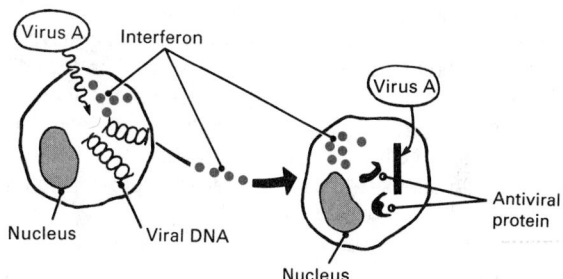

Fig. 8-4 Mechanism of action of interferon. Virus A attacks a cell. The cell begins to synthesize viral DNA and interferon. Interferon serves as an intercellular messenger. Interferon induces the production of antiviral proteins. Virus A is not able to replicate in the cell.

Table 8-5 Types of Interferon

Type	Cell of Origin	Activity
α-Interferon	T lymphocytes	Acts as antiviral agent; activates natural killer cells; stimulates interleukin-1 production
β-Interferon	Fibroblasts, epithelial cells, macrophages	Acts as antiviral agent
γ (immune)-Interferon	T lymphocytes, natural killer cells	Stimulates natural killer cell activity; activates macrophages; enhances B-cell differentiation; prevents proliferation of neoplastic cells

Table 8-6 Comparison of Humoral Immunity and Cell-Mediated Immunity

Cells	Products	Memory Cells	Reaction	Protection	Examples
HUMORAL IMMUNITY					
B lymphocytes	Antibodies	Present	Immediate	Bacteria, viruses (extra-cellular), respiratory and gastrointestinal pathogens	Anaphylactic shock, atopic diseases, transfusion reaction, neutralization of exo-toxins, bacterial in-fections
CELL-MEDIATED IMMUNITY					
T lymphocytes, macro-phages	Sensitized T cells, lym-phokines	Present	Delayed	Fungus, viruses, (intra-cellular), chronic in-fectious agents, tumor cells	Tuberculosis, fungal infections, contact dermatitis, graft re-jection, destruction of cancer cells

Table 8-7 Effects of Aging on the Immune System

Thymic involution	Deficient expression of interleukin-2 receptors
Normal peripheral T- and B-cell counts	
Decreased percentage of T cells	Decreased activation poten-tial of T and B cells
Decreased percentage of T-helper cells	Decreased proliferative re-sponse of T and B cells
Decreased percentage of T-suppressor cells	Decreased primary and secondary antibody re-sponses
Decreased interleukin-1 synthesis	Increased autoantibodies
Decreased interleukin-2 synthesis	

time through the cell cycle, and subsequent differentia-tion.[3] The most significant alterations seem to involve T cells. As thymic output of T cells diminishes, the differen-tiation of T cells in peripheral lymphoid structures in-creases. Consequently, there is an accumulation of mem-ory cells rather than new precursor cells responsive to pre-viously unencountered antigens. The effects of aging on the immune system are summarized in Table 8-7.

ALTERED IMMUNE RESPONSE

The immune system normally reacts protectively against the invasion of antigens. However, sometimes the response is overreactive and results in tissue damage. This is called a *hypersensitivity reaction*. A type of hypersensi-tivity response occurs when the body fails to recognize self-proteins and reacts against its own protein. Tissue damage resulting from this mechanism is called *autoimmu-nity*. Finally, tissue damage may occur if the immune sys-tem is deficient. The immunodeficiency state may be pri-mary or secondary to other diseases.

Hypersensitivity Reactions

Classification of hypersensitivity reactions may be done according to the source of the antigen (exogenous, homol-ogous, or autologous), time sequence (immediate or de-layed), or the basic immunological mechanisms causing the injury (Gell and Coombs classification). The Gell and Coombs classification is the most comprehensive.

Basically, four types of hypersensitivity reactions exist. Types I, II, and III are immediate and are examples of hu-moral immunity. Type IV is a delayed hypersensitivity re-action and is related to cell-mediated immunity. See Table 8-8 for a summary of the four types of hypersensitivity re-actions.

The manifestations of hypersensitivity reactions depend on many etiological factors. Among the most important are the following:

1. Degree of exposure to the allergen—The effect is more serious if the client ingested, inhaled, or touched a large amount of the allergen.
2. The type of antibody involved in the reaction.
3. Target organs and tissues affected—Especially vul-nerable are the skin and gastrointestinal (GI) and respiratory tracts.
4. Release of chemical mediators on target organs.

Type I-anaphylactoid reactions. Anaphylactoid reac-tions are type I reactions that occur *only* in susceptible per-sons who are highly sensitized from previous exposure to allergens. On subsequent exposure to a challenge allergen, IgE immediately reacts with the allergen and triggers the release of chemical mediators from mast cells and baso-phils. The mediators act on target cells of the body, caus-ing tissue damage. Common allergic reactions include ana-phylactic shock (anaphylaxis), allergic asthma, allergic rhinitis, atopic dermatitis, urticaria, and angioedema.

The IgE immunoglobulins have a characteristic property of attaching to mast cells and basophils (Fig. 8-5). Within these cells are granules containing potent chemical media-

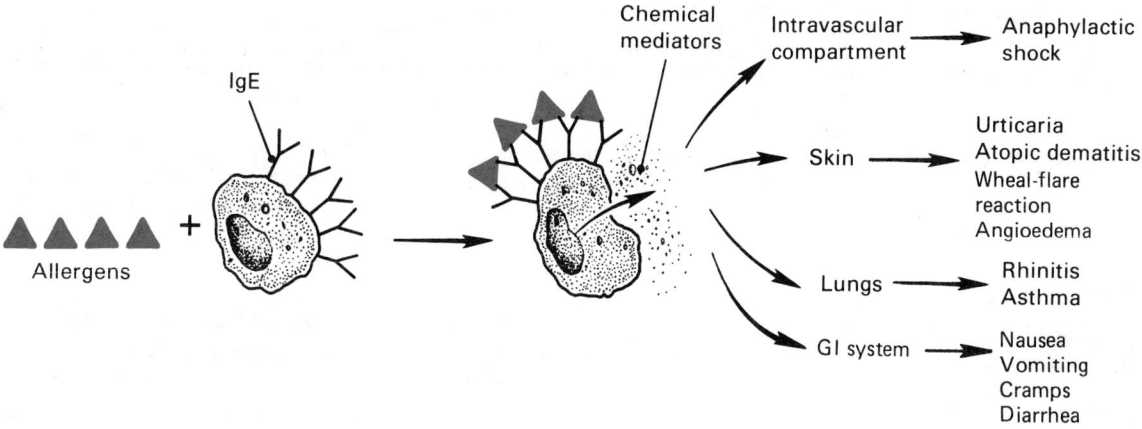

Fig. 8-5   Steps in an allergic type I reaction.

Table 8-8   Hypersensitivity Reactions

Type	Antigen	Antibody	Complement Involved	Mediators of Injury	Examples	Skin Test
I. Anaphylactic	Exogenous pollen, food, drugs, dust	IgE	No	Histamine, SRS-A	Allergic rhinitis, asthma	Wheal and flare
II. Cytotoxic	Cell surface of RBC, basement membrane	IgG, IgM, or IgA	Yes	Complement lysis, neutrophils	Transfusion reaction, Goodpasture's syndrome	None
III. Immune-complex-mediated	Extracellular fungal, viral, bacterial	IgG, IgM, or IgA	Yes	Neutrophils, complement lysis	Serum sickness, systemic lupus erythematosus, rheumatoid arthritis	Erythema and edema in 3 to 8 hours
IV. Delayed-hypersensitivity (cell-mediated)	Intracellular or extracellular	None	No	Lymphokines, T-cytotoxic cells, monocytes/ macrophages, lysosomal enzymes	Contact dermatitis, allograft or tumor rejection	Erythema and edema in 24 to 48 hours (e.g., TB test)

SRS-A, Slow-reacting substance of anaphylaxis.

tors (histamine, serotonin, slow-reacting substance of anaphylaxis [SRS-A], ECF-A, kinins, and bradykinin). (Leukotriene components [LTC$_4$, LTD$_4$, and LTE$_4$] of slow-reacting substance of SRS-A are discussed in Chapter 7 and Fig. 7-9.) When IgE-bound mast cells or basophils react with an allergen, the cell is degranulated. In this process, mediators are released, which then attack target organs, causing clinical allergy symptoms. These effects include smooth muscle contraction, increased vascular permeability, vasodilatation, hypotension, increased secretion of mucus, and itching. Fortunately, the mediators are short

acting and their effects are reversible. (The mediators and their effects are summarized in Table 8-9.)

A genetic predisposition for the development of allergic diseases exists. The capacity to become sensitized to an allergen appears to be the inherited trait rather than the specific allergic disorder. For example, a father with asthma may have a son who has allergic rhinitis.

The clinical manifestations of an anaphylactoid reaction depend on whether the mediators remain local or become systemic or whether they affect particular organs. When the mediators remain localized, a cutaneous response

Table 8-9 Chemical Mediators of Allergic Response

Source and Storage	Biological Activity	Pathological Outcomes
HISTAMINE		
Mast cell and basophil granules	Increases vascular permeability; constricts smooth muscle; stimulates irritant receptors	Edema of airways and larynx; bronchial constriction; urticaria, angioedema, pruritus; nausea, vomiting, diarrhea; shock
LEUKOTRIENES		
Metabolites of arachidonic acid by lipoxygenase pathway*	Constrict bronchial smooth muscle; increase vascular permeability	Bronchial constriction; enhanced effect of histamine on smooth muscle
PROSTAGLANDINS		
Metabolites of arachidonic acid by cyclooxygenase pathway	Stimulate vasodilation; constrict smooth muscle	Wheal-and-flare reaction on skin; hypotension; bronchospasm
PLATELET-ACTIVATING FACTOR		
Mast cell	Aggregates platelets; stimulates vasodilation	Increase in pulmonary artery pressure; systemic hypotension
KININS		
Kininogen	Stimulate slow, sustained smooth muscle contraction; increase vascular permeability; stimulate secretion of mucus; stimulate pain	Angioedema with painful swelling; bronchial constriction
SEROTONIN		
Platelets	Increases vascular permeability; stimulates smooth muscle contraction	Mucosal edema; bronchial constriction
EOSINOPHIL CHEMOTACTIC FACTOR		
Mast cells	Promotes chemotaxis of eosinophils	Influx of eosinophils
ANAPHYLATOXINS		
C3a, C4a, C5a from complement activation	Stimulate histamine release	Same as for histamine

*See Fig. 7-9.

called the *wheal-and-flare reaction* occurs. This reaction is characterized by a pale wheal containing edematous fluid surrounded by a red flare from the hyperemia. The reaction occurs in minutes or hours and is usually not dangerous. A classic example of a wheal-and-flare reaction is the mosquito bite. The reaction serves a positive purpose as a means of demonstrating allergic reactions to specific allergens during skin tests.

Anaphylactic shock. Anaphylactic shock (anaphylaxis) occurs when mediators are released systemically (e.g., after injection of a drug or after an insect sting). The reaction occurs within minutes and is life threatening because of respiratory obstruction and vascular collapse. The target organs affected are seen in Fig. 8-6. Initial symptoms include edema and itching at the site of the allergen. Within minutes, shock manifested by rapid, weak pulse; hypotension; dilated pupils; dyspnea; and cyanosis may occur. This is compounded by bronchial edema and angioedema.

Death will occur if emergency treatment is not initiated. Some of the important allergens leading to anaphylactic shock in hypersensitive persons are listed in Table 8-10.

Atopic reactions. An estimated 20% of the population is *atopic,* an inherited tendency to become sensitive to environmental allergens.[4] The atopic diseases that can result are allergic rhinitis, allergic asthma, atopic dermatitis, urticaria, and angioedema.

Allergic rhinitis or hay fever is the most common type I hypersensitivity reaction. It may occur year round (perennial allergic rhinitis), or it may be seasonal (seasonal allergic rhinitis). Persons afflicted with allergic rhinitis often have sensitive nasal mucosa and are susceptible to respiratory infections. Airborne substances (aeroallergens) are the primary cause of allergic rhinitis. The target areas affected are the conjunctiva of the eyes and the upper respiratory tract mucosa. Symptoms include nasal discharge; sneezing; lacrimation; mucosal swelling with airway obstruc-

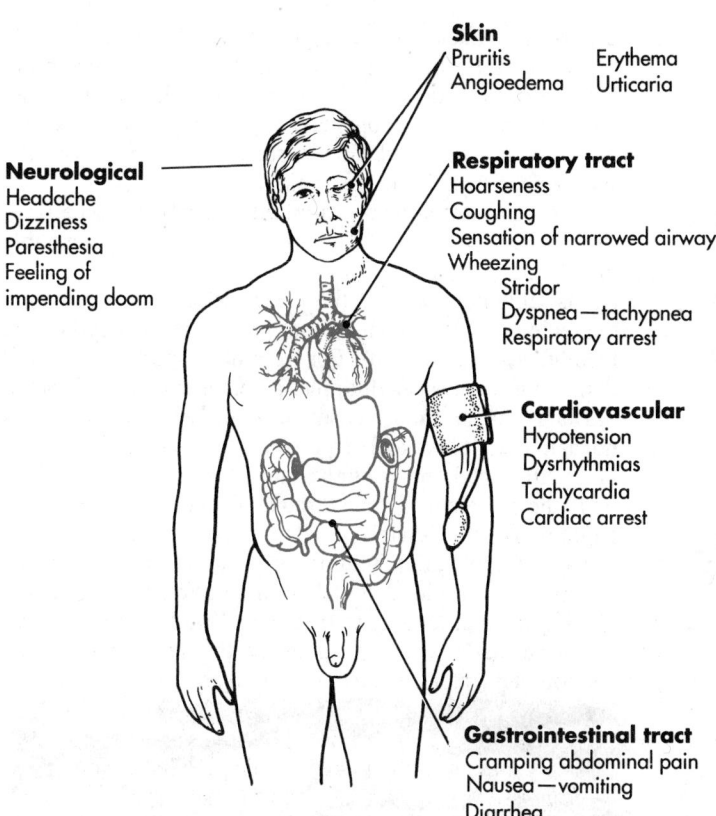

Skin
Pruritis   Erythema
Angioedema   Urticaria

Neurological
Headache
Dizziness
Paresthesia
Feeling of
impending doom

Respiratory tract
Hoarseness
Coughing
Sensation of narrowed airway
Wheezing
Stridor
Dyspnea—tachypnea
Respiratory arrest

Cardiovascular
Hypotension
Dysrhythmias
Tachycardia
Cardiac arrest

Gastrointestinal tract
Cramping abdominal pain
Nausea—vomiting
Diarrhea

Fig. 8-6 Clinical manifestations of a systemic anaphylactic reaction.

tion; and pruritus around the eyes, nose, throat, and mouth. (Treatment of allergic rhinitis is discussed in Chapter 20.)

Approximately 50% of asthmatics have asthma caused by hypersensitivity to allergens.[4] The asthma may be *extrinsic* if caused by environmental allergens (foods, seasonal pollens, dust, and danders) or *intrinsic* if due to bacterial or viral infections of the respiratory tract. Most clients with extrinsic asthma present a past history of atopic disorders (e.g., infantile eczema, allergic rhinitis, or food intolerances). Clients with intrinsic asthma have no atopic history. Extrinsic asthma usually starts in people aged 5 to 30; intrinsic asthma starts as an adult disorder.[5]

In allergic asthma, SRS-A and histamine are primarily responsible for action on the bronchioles. These mediators produce bronchial smooth muscle constriction, excessive secretion of viscoid mucus, edema of the mucous membranes of the bronchi, and decreased lung compliance. Because of these physiological alterations, clients manifest dyspnea, severe expiratory wheezing, coughing, tightness in the chest, thick sputum, and a fear of suffocation. (Treatment of asthma is discussed in Chapter 22.)

Atopic dermatitis is a chronic, inherited skin disorder characterized by exacerbations and remissions.[6] It is caused by several environmental allergens that are difficult to identify. Children with infantile eczema frequently have allergic respiratory disorders, although the relationship between the two is not fully understood. Although clients with atopic dermatitis have elevated IgE levels and positive skin tests, the histopathological features do not repre-

Table 8-10   Allergens Causing Anaphylactic Shock

DRUGS

Penicillins	Sulfonamides
Insulins	Aspirin
Tetracycline	Local anesthetics
Chemotherapeutic agents	Cephalosporins
Nonsteroidal antiinflammatory agents	

INSECT VENOMS

Hymenoptera*

FOODS

Eggs	Milk
Nuts	Peanuts
Shellfish	Fish
Chocolate	Strawberries

ANIMAL SERUMS

Tetanus antitoxin	Rabies antitoxin
Diphtheria antitoxin	Snake venom antitoxin

TREATMENT MEASURES

Blood products (whole blood and components)	Iodine-contrast media dye for IVP or angiogram test
Allergenic extracts in hyposensitization therapy	

*Wasps, hornets, yellow jackets, bumblebees, and ants.

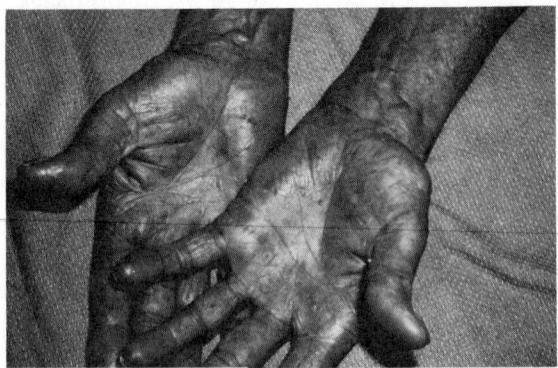

Fig. 8-7 Chronic lesions of atopic dermatitis on the hands of a woman; erythema, crusts, and cracks are evident.

sent the typical, localized wheal-and-flare type I reactions. The skin lesions are more generalized and involve vasodilation of blood vessels, resulting in intracellular edema with vesicle formation (Fig. 8-7). (Dermatitis is discussed in Chapter 17.)

Urticaria (hives) is a cutaneous lesion occurring in atopic persons. It is characterized by transient wheals (pink, raised, edematous pruritic areas) that vary in size and shape and may occur throughout the body. Urticaria develops rapidly after exposure to an allergen and may last minutes or hours. Histamine causes (1) localized vasodilation (erythema), (2) transudation of fluid (wheal), and (3) stimulation of local axon reflexes (flaring). Internal urticaria is characterized by edema in internal organs. Histamine is also responsible for the numbness and pruritus associated with the lesions. (Urticaria is discussed in Chapter 17.)

Angioedema is a localized cutaneous lesion similar to urticaria but involving deeper layers of the skin and the submucosa. The principal areas of involvement include the eyelids, lips, tongue, larynx, hands, feet, GI tract, and genitalia. Swelling usually occurs in only one area at a time. Dilation and engorgement of the capillaries secondary to release of histamine cause the diffuse swelling. Welts are not apparent as in urticaria; the outer skin appears normal or has a reddish hue. The lesions may burn, sting, or itch and will cause no discomfort or cause acute pain if in the GI tract. The swelling may occur suddenly or over 2 hours and it usually lasts for 24 hours.

Type II—cytotoxic and cytolytic reactions. Cytotoxic and cytolytic reactions are type II hypersensitivity reactions involving the direct binding of IgG, IgM, or IgA antibodies to an antigen on the cell surface. IgG or IgM activates the complement system and helps mediate the reaction. Cellular tissue is destroyed in one of three ways: (1) activation of the complement cascade resulting in cytolysis, (2) enhanced phagocytosis from complement fixation, and (3) a cytotoxic reaction independent of complement involvement.

Target cells frequently destroyed in type II reactions are erythrocytes, platelets, and leukocytes. Some of the antigens involved are the ABO blood group, Rh factor, and drug haptens such as chloramphenicol. Pathophysiological

disorders characteristic of type II reactions include ABO incompatibility transfusion reaction, Rh incompatibility transfusion reaction, autoimmune and drug-related hemolytic anemias, leukopenias, thrombocytopenias, erythroblastosis fetalis, and Goodpasture's syndrome. The tissue damage usually occurs rapidly.

Hemolytic transfusion reactions. A classical type II reaction occurs when a recipient receives ABO-incompatible blood from a donor. Natural antibodies (agglutinins) to antigens (agglutinogens) of the ABO blood group are within the recipient's serum but are not present on the erythrocyte membranes (Table 24-6). For example, a person with type A blood has anti-B agglutinins, a person with type B blood has anti-A agglutinins, a person with type AB blood has no antiagglutinins, and a person with type O blood has both anti-A and anti-B agglutinins.

If the recipient is transfused with incompatible blood, agglutinins immediately coat the foreign erythrocytes, causing agglutination (clumping). The clumping of cells blocks all small blood vessels in the body and depletes the clotting factors, leading to bleeding. Within hours, neutrophils and macrophages phagocytize the agglutinated cells. As complement is fixed to the antigen, cytolysis occurs. Cellular lysis causes the release of hemoglobin into the urine and plasma. In addition, a cytotoxic reaction causes vascular spasms in the kidney, which further block the renal tubules. Acute renal failure can result from the hemoglobinuria. (Blood transfusions are discussed in Chapter 25.)

Goodpasture's syndrome. Goodpasture's syndrome is a rare disorder involving the lungs and kidneys. An antibody-mediated autoimmune reaction occurs with the glomerular and alveolar basement membranes. The circulating antibodies combine with tissue antigen to activate complement, which causes deposits of IgG to form along the basement membranes of the lungs or kidney. This reaction may result in pulmonary hemorrhage and glomerulonephritis.

The disease is usually rapidly progressive and fatal. Corticosteroids may induce temporary remission but will not prevent death. Plasmapheresis offers the most hope. (Goodpasture's syndrome is discussed in more detail in Chapter 40.)

Type III—immune-complex reactions. Tissue damage in immune-complex reactions, which are type III reactions, occur secondary to antigen-antibody complexes. Soluble antigens combine with immunoglobulins of the IgG and IgM classes to form complexes that are too small to be effectively removed by the mononuclear phagocyte system. Therefore, the complexes deposit in tissue or small blood vessels. They cause the fixation of complement and the release of chemotactic factors that lead to inflammation and phagocytosis of the involved tissue.

Type III reactions may be local or systemic and immediate or delayed. The clinical manifestations depend on the number of complexes and the location in the body. Common sites for deposit are the kidneys, skin, joints, and blood vessels. Severe type III reactions are associated with some autoimmune disorders such as systemic lupus erythematosus, acute glomerulonephritis, and rheumatoid arthritis. Two classic disorders that illustrate type III reactions are the Arthus reaction and serum sickness.

Arthus reaction. The Arthus reaction is a localized inflammatory response resulting from antigen-antibody complexes deposited in the small vessels of the skin. It may occur from inhalation of dust or spores, resulting in pneumonitis or farmer's lung.

The underlying defect that triggers an Arthus reaction appears to be the production of *excess IgG* to specific antigens. On subsequent exposure to soluble antigens, antigen-antibody complexes form, leading to a type III reaction. Because of the chemotactic substances released by complement, neutrophils infiltrate to the site of the complex. The neutrophils that phagocytize the cells are the primary factor responsible for tissue damage.

Arthus reactions are manifested by edematous, hemorrhagic, and necrotic lesions that develop over 6 to 12 hours. Most classic Arthus reactions are not clinically significant because strong antigenic substances are not ordinarily given repeatedly to a hypersensitive individual. However, allergic vasculitis to drugs (e.g., penicillin, sulfonamides) resembles the Arthus reaction.

Serum sickness. Serum sickness is another type III reaction that involves deposits of antigen-antibody complexes in blood vessel walls of the skin, joints, and especially the renal glomeruli. In contrast to an Arthus reaction, this disorder is systemic. It develops slowly, 10 to 14 days after exposure to an antigen, and is self-limiting. Although the reaction is delayed, serum sickness is considered a humoral hypersensitivity reaction because of the presence of antibodies causing tissue damage.

The critical factor in serum sickness is the presence of *excess soluble antigen.* Common antigens triggering the reaction are horse antitoxin serums and certain drugs (e.g., penicillins, sulfonamides). Unlike clients with a type I reaction, the person does not need to be previously sensitized to react to the antigen. Rather, a single dose of the antigen that remains at high levels in the body for several days reacts with antibodies formed about 2 weeks after initial exposure to the antigen. The antigen-antibody complex then triggers complement to deposit in vessels, resulting in an intravascular inflammation. The predominant signs and symptoms of serum sickness are urticaria, angioedema, fever, muscle soreness, malaise, lymphadenopathy, joint pain, polyarthritis, and nephritis.

Fortunately, serum sickness reactions can be avoided by using human serums. However, watching for drug sensitivities is still critical. The actual treatment of serum sickness depends on the severity of the reaction. For mild reactions, aspirin is prescribed for the fever and arthritis, and antihistamines are given for urticaria and angioedema. Corticosteroids are prescribed for more severe reactions, especially when renal or neurological changes are present.

Type IV-delayed hypersensitivity reactions. A delayed hypersensitivity reaction—a type IV reaction—is also called a *cell-mediated immune response.* However, a cell-mediated response is a protective mechanism; tissue damage occurs in delayed hypersensitivity reactions.

The tissue damage in a type IV reaction does not occur in the presence of antibodies or complement. Rather, sen-

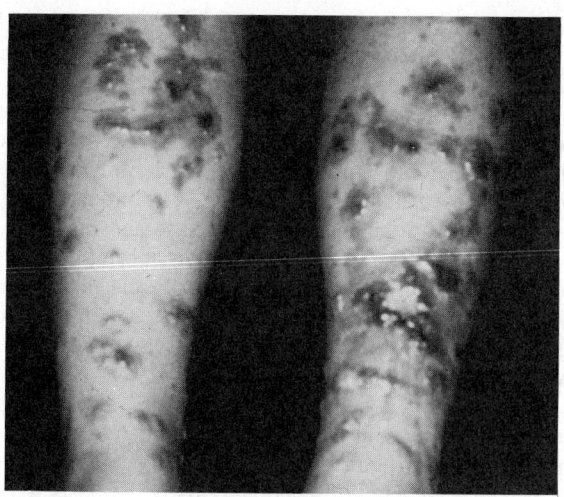

Fig. 8-8 Acute contact dermatitis on lower extremities. Note the edema, erythema, papules, bullae, and weeping vesicles.

sitized T lymphocytes directly attack antigens or indirectly release lymphokines to interact with specific antigens. The lymphokines attract macrophages into the area. The macrophages and enzymes released by them are responsible for most of the tissue destruction. The delayed hypersensitivity response takes 24 to 48 hours for a reaction to occur.

Clinical examples of a delayed hypersensitivity reaction include (1) contact dermatitis; (2) hypersensitivity reactions to bacterial, fungal, and viral infections; and (3) transplant rejections. Some drug sensitivity reactions also fit this category.

Contact dermatitis. Allergic eczematous contact dermatitis is an example of a delayed hypersensitivity reaction involving the skin. The reaction occurs when the skin is exposed to haptens. The haptens easily penetrate the skin to combine with epidermal proteins. The hapten-carrier substance then becomes antigenic. Over a period of 7 to 14 days, memory cells form to the antigen. On subsequent exposure to the hapten, a sensitized person develops eczematous skin lesions within 48 hours. The most common haptens encountered are metal compounds (e.g., nickel, mercury); rubber compounds; catechols present in poison ivy, poison oak, and sumac; cosmetics; and some dyes.

In acute contact dermatitis the skin lesions appear erythematous and edematous and are covered with papules, vesicles, and bullae. The involved area is very pruritic but may also burn or sting. When contact dermatitis becomes chronic, the lesions resemble atopic dermatitis because they are thickened, scaly, and lichenified. The main difference between contact dermatitis and atopic dermatitis is that contact dermatitis is localized and restricted to the area exposed to the allergens, and atopic dermatitis is widespread (Fig. 8-8).

Microbial hypersensitivity reactions. Although cell-mediated immunity plays an important defensive role in destroying viruses, bacteria, and fungi, delayed hypersensitivity reactions do occur as the surrounding tissue is damaged. Examples of infectious delayed hypersensitivity reactions include skin rashes of measles and smallpox, lesions of leprosy and herpes simplex virus, and the generalized toxemia and caseous necrosis with tuberculosis.

The classic example of a bacterial cell-mediated immune reaction is the body's defense against the tubercle bacillus. Tuberculosis results from invasion of lung tissue by highly resistant tubercle bacillus. The organism itself does not directly damage the lung tissue and may live in the host for some time before symptoms appear. However, antigenic material released from the tubercle bacilli react with T lymphocytes over time, initiating a cell-mediated response. The resulting lymphocytotoxicity causes extensive caseous necrosis of the lung.

After the initial cell-mediated reaction, memory cells persist, so subsequent contact with the tubercle bacillus or an extract of purified protein from the organism causes a delayed hypersensitivity reaction. This is the basis for the PPD tuberculosis skin test read 48 to 72 hours after the injection. (Tuberculosis is discussed in Chapter 21.)

Transplant rejection. Rejection of organs occurs by cell-mediated immunity if the donor organ does not perfectly match the recipient's human leukocytic antigens, also called *histocompatibility antigens*. The rejection can be prevented by closely matching ABO, Rh, and HLA antigens between donor and recipient. Unfortunately, many different HLA antigens exist, and a perfect match is nearly impossible unless the tissue is *autograftic* (self) or *isograftic* (identical twin).

Graft rejection is a complicated process that involves sensitized T lymphocytes (see Fig. 41-6). If the tissue is mismatched, sensitized T lymphocytes arrive at regional lymph nodes within 6 to 10 days. The clinical signs of rejection appear in about 14 days when sensitized T lymphocytes attack the site. At this time the vascularization stops and the tissue becomes necrosed. Common manifestations of transplant rejection include fever, malaise, localized graft tenderness, hypertension, leukocytosis, elevated sedimentation rate, and elevated enzyme studies.

Drugs that interfere with cell-mediated immune responses are given to recipients of transplanted organs. (Some of the agents used are summarized in Table 41-11.) Unfortunately, the use of immunosuppressant drugs can result in major complications including (1) increased susceptibility to infection, (2) increased risk of developing cancer, and (3) graft-versus-host disease.

ALLERGIC DISORDERS

Although an alteration of the immune system may be manifested in many ways, allergies or type I hypersensitivity reactions are seen most frequently.

Assessment

For a thorough assessment of a client with allergies, a complete data base must be obtained. This consists of a comprehensive client history, physical examination, diagnostic workup, and skin testing for allergens.

Health history. A comprehensive history that covers family allergies, past and present allergies, and social and environmental factors is essential. The information may be obtained from the client or the client's caregiver.

Family history, including information about atopic reactions in relatives, is especially important in identifying high-risk clients. The specific disorder, clinical manifestations, and treatments prescribed should be assessed.

Past and present allergies must be noted. Identifying the allergens that may have triggered a reaction is essential to control allergic reactions. Table 8-11 lists four major categories of allergens that should be evaluated. Determination of the time of year that an allergic reaction occurs can be a clue to a seasonal allergen.

In addition to identification of the allergen, information about the clinical manifestations and course of allergic reaction should be obtained. If the client is a woman, assessment of symptoms during pregnancy, menstruation, or menopause may be important.

Social and environmental factors, especially the physical environment, are very important. Questions about pets, trees, and plants on property; pollutants in the air; and cooling and heating systems in the home can provide valuable information about allergens. In addition, a daily or weekly food diary with a description of any untoward reaction is important. Of particular interest is a screening for any reaction to medication. Finally, questions about the client's lifestyle and stress level should be reviewed in connection with the appearance of allergic symptoms.

Physical examination. A comprehensive head-to-toe physical exam should be given to each allergy client, with particular attention focused on the site of the allergic manifestations. A comprehensive assessment that includes objective and subjective data should be obtained from the client (Table 8-12).

Table 8-11 Categories of Allergens

Inhalants	Contactants	Ingestants	Injectables
Pollens	Plants	Foods	Drugs
Molds	Drugs	Food additives	Vaccines
Spores	Metals	Drugs	Insect stings
Animal dander	Cosmetics		
House dust	Dyes		
Mites	Fibers		
	Various chemicals		

Diagnostic Studies

Many specialized immunological techniques can be done to detect abnormalities of lymphocytes, eosinophils, and immunoglobulins. A complete blood count (CBC) and blood serology tests are commonly done.

The CBC is required with an absolute lymphocyte count and eosinophil count. Cellular immunodeficiency is diagnosed if the lymphocyte count is below 1200/μL. T- and B-cell quantification is used to diagnose immunodeficiency syndromes. The eosinophil count is elevated with type I hypersensitivity reactions involving IgE immunoglobulins. Serum IgE level is also generally elevated in type I hyper-

Table 8-12

Nursing Assessment of the Client with Allergies

SUBJECTIVE DATA

History
Positive family history; recurrent respiratory problems; seasonal exacerbations; unusual reactions to insect bites/stings; past and present allergies; environmental factors including pets
Medications
Unusual reactions to any drugs or medications; use of over-the-counter medication
General
Malaise; fatigue
Integumentary
Itching
Respiratory
Hoarseness; dyspnea; cough
Gastrointestinal
Colic; cramping; vomiting; diarrhea; food intolerances

OBJECTIVE DATA

Integumentary
Rashes (note symmetry and location); dryness; scaliness; irritations; scratches; urticaria
Respiratory
Wheezing; stridor
EENT
Eyes: Allergic shiners; conjunctivitis; lacrimation; rubbing or excessive blinking; styes
Ears: Diminished hearing; immobile or scarred tympanic membranes
Nose: Allergic salute; nasal polyps; nasal voice; nose twitching; rhinitis; pale, boggy mucous membranes; sniffling; sneezing; swollen nasal passages; recurrent nosebleeds
Throat: Continual throat clearing; swollen lips or tongue; red throat; orofacial and dental deformities; mouth wrinkling with facial grimaces; palpable neck lymph nodes
Possible findings
Eosinophilia; elevated serum IgE levels; positive skin tests; abnormal chest and sinus x-rays

sensitivity reactions and serves as a diagnostic indicator of atopic diseases. Radioallergosorbent test (RAST) is an in vitro diagnostic test for IgE antibodies to an allergen. The RAST involves the measurement of IgE with a specific antigen. Although expensive, it is safe but less sensitive than skin tests for detecting allergens.

Sputum, nasal, and bronchial secretions also may be tested for the presence of eosinophils. If asthma is suspected, pulmonary function tests for vital capacity, forced expiratory volume, and maximum midexpiratory flow rates are helpful.

Skin tests. Skin testing is generally used to confirm specific sensitivity in clients with atopic disease after the history has suggested possible allergens for testing.

Procedure. Skin testing may be done by one of two methods: (1) a cutaneous scratch or prick or (2) an intracutaneous injection. The areas of the body usually used in testing are the arms and back. Allergen extracts are applied to the skin in rows with a corresponding control site opposite the test site. Saline or another diluent is applied to the control site.

In the *scratch test* the epidermis skin layer is scratched with a lancet and the allergen extract is applied at the site. The *prick test* involves placing a drop of allergen extract on the skin and then piercing the underlying epidermis with a needle.

In the *intracutaneous method* the allergen extract is injected intradermally in rows, usually on the arm. Since the allergic reaction is more severe, the test is used only for persons who did not react to cutaneous methods.

Results. If the person is hypersensitive to the allergen, a positive reaction will occur within minutes after insertion in the skin and may last for 8 to 12 hours. A positive reaction is manifest by a local wheal-and-flare response. The size of the positive reaction does not always correlate with the severity of allergy symptoms. False-positive and false-negative results may occur. Negative results from skin testing do not necessarily mean the person does not have an allergic disorder, and positive results do not necessarily mean that the allergen was causing the clinical manifestations. Positive results imply that the person is sensitized to that allergen. Therefore, correlating skin test results with the client's history is very important.

Precautions. A highly sensitive person is always at risk for developing an anaphylactic reaction to skin tests. Therefore, a client should never be left alone during the testing period. Sometimes skin testing is completely contraindicated and the RAST test is used. If a severe reaction does occur with a cutaneous test, the extract is immediately removed and antiinflammatory topical cream is applied to the site. For intracutaneous testing, the arm is used so that a tourniquet can be applied during a severe reaction. A subcutaneous injection of epinephrine may also be necessary.

Therapeutic Management

After an allergic disorder is diagnosed, the therapeutic treatment is aimed at (1) reducing exposure to the offending allergen, (2) treating the symptoms, and (3) desensitizing the person through immunotherapy. All health care workers must be prepared for the rare but life-threatening anaphylactic reaction, which requires immediate medical and nursing interventions.

Anaphylaxis. Anaphylactic reactions occur suddenly in hypersensitive clients after exposure to the allergen. They may occur following parenteral injection of drugs (especially antibiotics) and insect stings. The cardinal principle in therapeutic management is *speed* in (1) recognition of signs and symptoms of an anaphylactic reaction, (2) maintenance of a patent airway, (3) prevention of spread of the allergen by using a tourniquet, (4) administration of drugs, and (5) treatment for shock.[7] Table 8-13 summarizes treatment of anaphylactic shock.

The drug of choice is epinephrine, 1:1000 strength, administered subcutaneously every 5 to 10 minutes according to the physician's orders or a hospital emergency drug protocol. The drug may be discontinued when anaphylactic signs and symptoms disappear. If the reaction is severe, antihistamine drugs (e.g., diphenhydramine, ranitidine, cimetidine) are administered parenterally to counteract the effects of histamine on the body tissues. Theophylline ethylenediamine (aminophylline) may be used to relax the bronchial smooth muscle spasms. Although not effective immediately, ACTH and corticosteroids may be used to suppress the immune and inflammatory responses.

Hypovolemic shock may occur because of the loss of intravascular fluid into interstitial spaces. Peripheral vasoconstriction and stimulation of the sympathetic nervous system occur to compensate for the fluid shift. However, unless shock is treated early, the body will no longer be able to compensate, and irreversible tissue damage will occur, leading to death. Therefore, the following emergency measures should be undertaken immediately:[8]

1. Intravenous administration of volume expanders (e.g., plasma, dextran, and normal saline) should be done to correct the hypotension. Nurses must carefully monitor for signs of circulatory overload.
2. Vasopressor drugs are necessary to raise the blood pressure. However, these drugs can be very dangerous when administered intravenously. Levarterenol bitartrate (Levophed) may cause severe hypertension if the infusion rate is too rapid. Severe sloughing of tissue may occur if the IV infiltrates. Therefore, the nurse must continually monitor the client at the bedside during intravenous administration of a vasopressor. Vital signs should be monitored every 15 minutes, and the IV flow rate should be adjusted to maintain a stable blood pressure as prescribed by the physician.

Chronic allergies. Most allergic reactions are chronic and are characterized by remissions and exacerbations of symptoms. Treatment focuses on identification and control of allergens, relief of symptoms through pharmacological interventions, and hyposensitization of a client to an offending allergen.

Allergen recognition and control. The nurse plays an important role in helping a client adjust lifestyle so that there is minimal exposure to offending allergens. The nurse must reinforce that even with drug therapy and immunotherapy, the client will never be desensitized or completely symptom-free. The nurse can initiate various preventive measures that will help control the allergic symptoms.

Of primary importance is the need to identify the offending allergen. Sometimes this is done through skin testing. In the case of food allergies, an elimination diet is valuable. If an allergic reaction occurs, all food eaten should be eliminated and gradually reintroduced one at a time until the offending food is detected. In the case of infants with a strong family history of atopic disorders, new solid foods should be introduced one at a time. The elimination system may also be used to detect fabric and cosmetic allergens.

Many allergic reactions, especially asthma and urticaria, may be aggravated by fatigue and emotional stress. The nurse can be instrumental in initiating a stress management program with clients. Relaxation techniques can be practiced when clients come for frequent immunotherapy treatments.

Sometimes control of allergic symptoms requires environmental control, including changing an occupation, moving to a different climate, or giving up a favorite pet. In the case of aeroallergens, sleeping in an air-conditioned room, damp dusting daily, and wearing a mask outdoors may be helpful.

If the allergen is a drug, the client should be instructed to avoid the drug. The client also has the responsibility to make the drug intolerance well known to all health care providers. The client should wear a medical-alert bracelet listing the particular drug allergy and have the offending drug listed on all medical and dental records.

Table 8-13

Therapeutic Management: Anaphylactic Shock

Establish and maintain airway; administer epinephrine by inhaler or nebulizer if laryngeal edema is present.

When possible, apply tourniquet to decrease blood flow from source of antigen; remove stinger if an insect sting; remove tourniquet every 15 minutes.

Place client in a recumbent position; elevate legs; keep client warm; provide oxygen.

Administer epinephrine 1:1000, 0.3–0.5 ml subcutaneously.

Administer diphenhydramine (Benadryl) IM or IV.

Administer ranitidine (Zantac) or cimetidine (Tagamet) IV.

Maintain blood pressure with fluids, volume expanders, vasopressors (e.g., dopamine [Intropin], levarterenol [Isuprel]).

If wheezing is present, administer aminophylline IV.

For prolonged reactions, repeat epinephrine and give hydrocortisone IV.

Modified from McBride PT and Kaliner MA: Current idiopathic and cryptogenic anaphylaxis. In Lichtenstein LM and Fauci AS: Current therapy in allergy, immunology, and rheumatology, vol 3, St Louis, 1988, The CV Mosby Co, p 100.

For clients allergic to insect stings, commercial bee-sting kits containing preinjectable epinephrine and a tourniquet are available. The nurse has the responsibility to instruct the client about the technique of applying the tourniquet and self-injecting the subcutaneous epinephrine. These clients also should wear medical-alert bracelets and carry bee-sting kits with them whenever they go outdoors.

Pharmacological management. The major categories of drugs used in symptomatic relief of chronic allergic disorders include (1) sympathomimetic drugs, (2) antipruritic drugs, (3) bronchodilators, and (4) antihistamines. Many of these drugs may be obtained over the counter and are often misused by clients. The drugs are summarized in Table 8-14.

Sympathomimetic drugs. The major sympathomimetic drug is epinephrine (Adrenalin), which is the drug of choice to treat an anaphylactic reaction. Epinephrine is a hormone produced by the adrenal medulla that stimulates α- and β-adrenergic receptors. Stimulation of the α receptors causes vasoconstriction of peripheral blood vessels. β-Receptor stimulation relaxes bronchial smooth muscle spasms. These drugs also act directly on mast cells to stabilize them against further degranulation. The action of epinephrine lasts only a few minutes. The drug must be given parenterally (usually subcutaneously).

Several specific, minor sympathomimetic drugs differ from epinephrine because they can be taken orally or na-

sally and last for several hours. Included in this category are isoproterenol (Isuprel), phenylephrine (Neo-Synephrine), and pseudoephedrine (Sudafed, Isoephedrine). The minor sympathomimetic drugs are used primarily to treat chronic asthma and allergic rhinitis. The action of these drugs includes bronchodilation, nasal decongestion, reduction in nasal edema, elevation of blood pressure, and cardiac stimulation.

Of the drugs used in the management of chronic allergy clients, ephedrine is abused most frequently. Since these drugs may be bought over the counter, clients tend to overmedicate themselves. *Rhinitis medicamentosa,* a rebound effect in which nasal mucosa becomes more edematous and congested after medicating, may develop from the local overuse of nasal sprays containing ephedrine.

Antipruritic drugs. Antipruritic drugs are most effective when the skin is not broken. These drugs protect the skin and provide relief from itching. Common over-the-counter drugs include calamine lotion, coal tar solutions, and camphor. Menthol and phenol may be added to other lotions to produce an antipruritic effect. Some more potent drugs that require a prescription include methdilazine (Tacaryl) and trimeprazine (Temaril). These drugs should be used with great caution because of the associated risk of agranulocytosis.

Bronchodilators. The most common bronchodilator is theophylline (aminophylline), which acts directly on bronchial smooth muscle to promote bronchodilatation. This drug may be given by mouth, intramuscularly, or intravenously. However, for an acute asthma attack the intravenous method is recommended. One of the side effects from theophylline preparations is myocardial stimulation. Therefore, vital signs should be frequently monitored by the nurse during intravenous administration, and the IV drip rate should be slowed as necessary.

Antihistamines. Antihistamines are the best drugs for treatment of allergic rhinitis and urticaria. They are less effective for severe allergic reactions. The drugs may be given intravenously or orally; applied topically; inhaled; or used as a nasal spray. They act by combining with histamine receptors on cell surfaces. Since the drugs inhibit further release of histamine from mast cells, best results are achieved if they are taken immediately after allergy signs and symptoms appear. Antihistamines have no effect on histamine after it is released from mast cells or basophils. Antihistamines are effective antagonists of edema and pruritus but relatively ineffective in preventing bronchoconstriction. With seasonal rhinitis, antihistamines should be taken during peak pollen seasons.

A number of side effects are associated with antihistamines, especially drowsiness, sedation, and disturbed coordination. Therefore, clients should be cautioned about driving and operating machinery. Other side effects include dryness of mouth, GI upset, blurred vision, and dizziness.

Because of the difficulties with side effects, a new generation of antihistamines has been developed. Terfenadine (Seldane) and astemizole (Hismanal) do not readily cross the blood-brain barrier. Therefore, the central nervous system depression and anticholinergic side effects seen with

Table 8-14 Common Drugs Used for Treatment of Allergic Symptoms

Generic Name	Trade Name
ANTIHISTAMINES	
Diphenhydramine	Benadryl
Azatadine maleate	Optimine
Carbinoxamine maleate	Clistin
	Histadyl
Triprolidine	Actidil
Brompheniramine maleate	Dimetane, Dimetapp
Chlorpheniramine maleate	Coricidin, Chlor-Trimeton, Teldrin
Terfenadine	Seldane
Astemizole	Hismanal
ANTIPRURITICS	
Diphenhydramine	Benadryl
ZnCO$_3$	Calamine lotion
Methdilazine	Tacaryl
SYMPATHOMIMETICS	
Epinephrine	Adrenalin
Isoproterenol	Isuprel
Pseudoephedrine	Sudafed, Isoephedrine
Phenylephrine	Dristan, Demazin, Neo-Synephrine
Propylhexedrine	Benzedrex
Oxymetazoline	Afrin

other types of antihistamines are not frequently observed with these newer antihistamines. In addition, these drugs require administration only 1 to 2 times per day.

Cromolyn. Cromolyn (Intal, Fivent, Opticrom) is a mast cell–stabilizing agent that inhibits the release of histamine, leukotrienes, and other agents from the mast cell. It is available as an inhalant, a nasal spray, and eye drops. It is used in the prophylactic management of asthma (see Chapter 22) and treatment of allergic rhinitis and allergic eye disorders. For effective results, this drug needs to be used 4 to 6 times daily. An important feature of cromolyn is a very low incidence of side effects.

Immunotherapy. Immunotherapy is the recommended treatment for control of allergic symptoms when the allergen cannot be avoided and drug therapy is not effective. Immunotherapy is absolutely indicated only in individuals with anaphylactic reactions to hymenopteran venom. It involves administration of small titers of an allergen extract in increasing strengths until hyposensitivity to the specific allergen is achieved. For best results the client should continue only limited exposure to the offending allergen because complete *desensitization* is impossible.

Mechanism of action. The IgE immunoglobulin level is elevated in atopic individuals. When IgE combines with an allergen in a hypersensitive person, a chemical reaction occurs, releasing histamine in various body tissues. Allergens more readily combine with IgG immunogobulin than with other immunoglobulins. Therefore, immunotherapy involves injecting allergen extracts that will stimulate increased IgG levels. The binding of IgG to allergen-reactive sites interferes with allergen binding to mast cell–bound IgE, preventing most cell degranulation, and thus reduces the number of chemical reactions that cause tissue damage. The goal of long-term immunotherapy is to keep "blocking" IgG levels high. In addition, allergen-specific T-suppressor cells develop in individuals receiving immunotherapy.[9]

Method of administration. Immunotherapy involves the subcutaneous injection of titered amounts of allergen extracts biweekly or weekly. The dose is small at first and is increased slowly until a maintenance dosage is reached. The maintenance dosage is given every 2 to 8 weeks for several years. For clients with severe allergies and/or sensitivity to insect stings, maintenance therapy is continued indefinitely. Best results are achieved when immunotherapy is administered throughout the year.

■ Nursing Management of Immunotherapy

Nurses are often primarily responsible for giving immunotherapy. Adverse reactions should always be anticipated, especially when opening a new-strength vial, after a previous reaction, or after a missed dose. Early signs and symptoms indicative of a systemic reaction include pruritus, urticaria, sneezing, laryngeal edema, and hypotension. Emergency measures for anaphylactic shock should be initiated immediately. A local reaction should be described according to the degree of redness and swelling at the injection site. If the area is greater than the size of a nickel in a child or a fifty-cent piece in an adult, the reaction should be reported to the physician so that the allergen dosage may be decreased.

Immunotherapy always carries the risk of a severe anaphylactic reaction. Therefore, a physician, emergency equipment, and essential drugs should be available whenever injections are given. Important emergency equipment includes an oral pharyngeal airway, laryngeal scope and endotracheal tubes, oxygen, tourniquet, intravenous therapy equipment and fluids, and a cardiac monitor with a defibrillator. The essential drugs are epinephrine 1:1000 in an injectable syringe, antihistamines, corticosteroids, and vasopressor drugs.

Record keeping must be accurate and can be invaluable in preventing an adverse reaction to the allergen extract. Before giving an injection, the nurse should check the client's name with the name on the vial. Next the vial strength, amount of last dose, date of last dose, and any reaction information should be screened.

The physician should be consulted about the amount of allergen to administer whenever a previous severe reaction has occurred or the client has missed the previous appointment. The dosage will have to be adjusted before administering the next dose.

The nurse should always administer the allergen extract in an extremity away from a joint so that a tourniquet can be applied for a severe reaction. The site should be rotated for each injection. The nurse must aspirate for blood before giving an injection to ensure that the allergen extract is not injected into a blood vessel. An injection directly into the bloodstream can potentiate an anaphylactic reaction. After the injection is given, the client should be carefully observed for 20 minutes because systemic reactions are most likely to occur immediately. However, clients should be warned that a delayed reaction can occur as long as 24 hours later.

AUTOIMMUNE PHENOMENA

Autoimmunity is a state of responsiveness to certain self-proteins; the body no longer differentiates self from nonself with respect to these substances. For some unknown reason, cells that are normally unresponsive (tolerant to self-antigens) are activated. Both T and B cells have the ability for tolerance to self-antigens. Therefore, an alteration in T cells alone or in both B cells and T cells can produce autoantibodies and autosensitized T cells to cause pathophysiological tissue damage. The particular autoimmune diseases manifested depend on which self-antigen is damaged.

Theories of Causation

The cause of autoimmune diseases is still unknown. Age plays some role, since the number of circulating autoantibodies increases in persons over age 50. It appears that no one theory is conclusive. A combination of etiological factors must be considered.[10]

Forbidden clone theory. Through somatic mutation, a clone of mutant T or B cells may survive. These new clone cells may become reactive against the body's own tissue, resulting in an autoimmune process.

Sequestered antigen theory. During embryonic development (when immune tolerance develops), certain tissues are normally separated or sequestered from the circulatory and lymph systems. These tissues include the lens of the eye, the thyroid, the testes, and the central nervous system. If later trauma, infection, or chemical exposure results in the cells' release into circulation, these cells will not be recognized as "self" and an autoimmune response will occur. Examples of this reaction include Hashimoto's thyroiditis and autoantibody formation against sperm after vasectomy and cardiac muscle after myocardial infarction.

Immunological deficiency theory. Persons with a hypoactive immune system have a higher incidence of developing an autoimmune disease. In animal experiments the tissue injury occurs because of autoreactive mutant lymphocytes or because of persistent antigens.

Viral mutation of cells theory. Viral infections can cause alteration of tissue substances not normally antigenic. There is evidence that hepatitis B virus is found in clients with polyarteritis nodosa, an autoimmune disease.

Tissue injury theory. After severe trauma, necrosis, radiation, drugs, and infections, the body tissue is sometimes altered so that the body no longer recognizes it as "self." An example is hemolytic anemia secondary to methyldopa (Aldomet) administration.

Cross-reacting antigen theory. Autoimmunity sometimes develops because of the close structural resemblance between the body's own antigens and foreign antigens. The antibodies synthesized in response to the foreign invasion cross-react with healthy tissue. This appears to be the cause of rheumatic heart disease. Antibodies developed against group A β-hemolytic streptococcus cross-react with heart muscle, heart valves, and synovial membrane, causing tissue damage.

Genetic instruction theory. For an unknown reason the genetic instruction for antibody production is altered. There appears to be a genetic predisposition to develop autoimmune diseases within some families. Most of the research work in this area correlates certain HLA types with an autoimmune condition.[11]

Diminished T-suppressor cell function theory. Decreased T-suppressor cells have been found in individuals with autoimmune disease. Suppressor cells are short lived and may become less numerous with aging. The incidence of autoantibodies increases with age, presumably because atrophy of the thymus results in a decreased ability to produce new T-suppressor cells. If decreased T-suppressor cells are present, immunoregulation is altered and antibody levels or T-cell responses are increased.

Autoimmune Diseases

Generally, autoimmune diseases are grouped according to *organ-specific* and *systemic* diseases. (See Table 8-15 on p. 138 for a summary of autoimmune diseases.)

Autoimmune hemolytic anemia. Autoimmune hemolytic anemia (AHA) is an organ-specific disease involving the erythrocytes. The autoimmune disease may be primary or secondary to other diseases such as systemic lupus erythematosus and lymphocytic leukemia. Regardless of the cause, the immune response is similar. The cause is unknown, but drugs and viruses may alter the antigenic structure of the erythrocyte membrane, making it more susceptible to hemolysis. In addition, some people appear to have a genetically determined susceptibility to form autoantibodies.

Clients with AHA present with signs and symptoms of pallor, fatigue, fever, jaundice, splenomegaly, and hepatomegaly. Diagnosis is based on a positive Coombs' test and the presence of spherically shaped erythrocytes on a smear.

Systemic lupus erythematosus. Systemic lupus erythematosus is a classic example of a systemic autoimmune disease characterized by vasculitic damage to multiple organs. It occurs most frequently in women aged 20 to 40 years. The etiology is unknown, but there appears to be a loss of self-tolerance for the body's own DNA antigens. Viruses, drugs, and genetic factors are believed to affect the self-tolerance.

Systemic lupus erythematosus meets the criteria of an autoimmune disease. Laboratory analysis reveals (1) elevated serum immunoglobulins because of hyperactive humoral immunity, (2) defective T-cell function, (3) deposition of immune antigen-antibody complexes in small blood vessels of diseased organs, and (4) low serum-complement levels.

In systemic lupus erythematosus, tissue injury appears to be the result of the formation of antinuclear antibodies. For some reason (possibly a viral infection), the cell membrane is damaged and DNA is released into the systemic circulation where it is viewed as "non-self." This DNA is normally sequestered inside the nucleus of cells. On release into circulation the DNA antigen reacts with an antibody. Some antibodies are involved in immune complex formation, and others may cause damage directly. Once the complexes are deposited, complement is activated and further damages the tissue, especially the renal glomerulus. (Systemic lupus erythematosus is discussed in more detail in Chapter 58.)

Apheresis

Apheresis indicates the use of a procedure to separate components of the blood followed by the removal of one or more of these components. Compound words are used to describe any particular apheresis procedure, depending on the blood components being collected. *Cytapheresis* is a general term for cell separation and removal. *Leukocytapheresis* is a general term indicating the removal of WBCs and is used in chronic myelogenous leukemia to remove high numbers of leukemic cells. *Lymphocytapheresis* is used to decrease high lymphocyte counts in individuals with chronic lymphocytic leukemia. *Plasmapheresis* is the removal of plasma. When plasma is removed, it is replaced by substitution fluids such as saline or albumin. Therefore, the term *plasma exchange* more accurately describes this procedure, although both terms are used simultaneously.

Plasmapheresis has been used to treat antibody- or immune complex–mediated diseases such as systemic lupus erythematosus, Goodpasture's syndrome, myasthenia gravis, thrombocytopenic purpura, rheumatoid arthritis, and Guillain-Barré syndrome.[12] Apheresis procedures are also done on healthy donors to obtain plasma and selected blood components to administer as replacement therapy for clients.

The rationale for performing therapeutic plasmapheresis in autoimmune disorders is to remove pathophysiological

Table 8-15   Autoimmune Diseases

Disease	Autoantigen	Comments
SYSTEMIC DISEASES		
Systemic lupus erythematosus	DNA, DNA proteins	Circulating antinuclear antibodies attack DNA
Rheumatoid arthritis	IgG	Rheumatoid factor is an IgM that reacts with IgG
Progressive systemic sclerosis or scleroderma	DNA proteins	—
Mixed connective tissue disease	DNA proteins	—
ORGAN-SPECIFIC DISEASES		
Blood		
Autoimmune hemolytic anemia	RBC surface	Drugs and trauma may alter the RBC surface antigens
Idiopathic thrombocytopenic purpura	Platelet surface	—
Central nervous system		
Multiple sclerosis	Myelin sheath around nervous tissue	Possibly triggered by a viral infection; T-helper cells appear uncontrolled because of very reduced levels of T-suppressor cells*
Guillain-Barré syndrome	Myelin sheath	Peripheral nerve damage
Muscle		
Myasthenia gravis*	Muscle cells and thymus cells	—
Heart		
Rheumatic fever	Cross-reactive streptoccocal antigens	Occurs secondary to strep throat infection
Endocrine system†		
Addison's disease	Adrenal cell	
Thyroiditis	Thyroid cell surface	—
Hypothyroidism	Thyroid globulin	
Type I diabetes mellitus	Islet cell antigens	
Gastrointestinal tract‡		
Pernicious anemia	Intrinsic factor of parietal cells	—
Ulcerative colitis	Colon mucosal cells	
Kidney§		
Goodpasture's syndrome	Glomerular basement membrane	—
Glomerulonephritis	Cross-reactive streptococcal antigens	
Liver		
Primary biliary cirrhosis	Mitochondria	—
Chronic active hepatitis	Virally infected liver cells	
Eye		
Uveitis‖	Uvea	—

RBC, Red blood cell.
*See Chapter 54.
†See Chapter 44.
‡See Chapter 37.
§See Chapter 40.
‖See Chapter 15.

substances present in plasma. Many disorders for which plasmapheresis is being used are characterized by circulating autoantibodies (usually of the IgG class) and antigen-antibody complexes. Immunosuppressive therapy has been used to prevent recovery of IgG production, and plasmapheresis has been used to prevent antibody rebound.

In addition to removing antibodies and antigen-antibody complexes, plasmapheresis may also remove inflammatory mediators (such as complement) that are responsible for tissue damage. In the treatment of systemic lupus erythematosus, plasmapheresis is reserved for clients in an acute attack who are unresponsive to conventional therapy. Plasmapheresis seems to lower the level of DNA antibodies and immune complexes, allowing the mononuclear phagocyte system to take control of removing immune complexes.

The procedure involves removal of whole blood through a needle inserted in one arm and circulation of the blood through a cell separator. Inside the separator the blood is divided into plasma and its cellular components by centrifugation or membrane filtration. A needle is inserted into the opposite arm for return of the blood to the client. Plasma, platelets, WBCs, or red blood cells (RBCs) can be separated selectively. The undesirable component is removed, and the remainder is returned to the client. The plasma is generally replaced with physiological saline, fresh-frozen plasma, plasma protein fractions, reconstituted dried plasma, or albumin. When blood is manually removed, only 500 ml may be taken at one time. However, with the use of apheresis procedures, over 4 L of plasma can be pheresed in 2 to 3 hours.

As with administration of other blood products, nurses need to be aware of side effects associated with plasmapheresis. The most common complications are hypotension and citrate toxicity. Hypotension is usually the result of vagovagal reaction or transient volume changes. Citrate is used as an anticoagulant and may cause hypocalcemia, which may present as headache, paresthesias, and dizziness. Other complications that may arise are hepatitis (especially when fresh frozen plasma is used as replacement fluid), infections, depletion of coagulation factors, and electrolyte imbalances.

Human Leukocyte Antigen System

The human leukocyte antigen (HLA) system consists of a series of linked genes that occur together on the sixth chromosome in humans. The products of these genes include the cell membrane antigens of the HLA series. Because of its importance in the study of tissue matching in transplant rejection, the chromosomal region incorporating the HLA genes is referred to as the *major histocompatibility complex*. The genes determining the products recognized as the HLA-A, HLA-B, HLA-C, HLA-D, and HLA-DR antigens are clustered together (Fig. 8-9). HLA antigens are present on all nucleated cells and platelets.

A very important characteristic of HLA genes is that they are highly polymorphic. Each HLA locus has many alleles (antigens) with at least 20 at A (e.g., A1, A21), 40 at B (e.g., B17, B49), 8 at C (e.g., C1, C8), 18 at D (e.g., D1, D18), and 15 at DR (e.g., DR1, DR7). With so

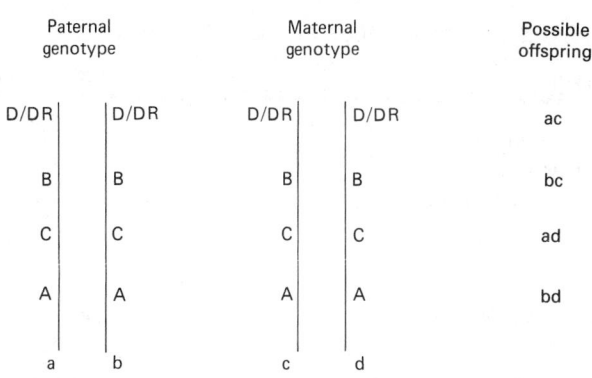

Paternal genotype		Maternal genotype		Possible offspring
D/DR	D/DR	D/DR	D/DR	ac
B	B	B	B	bc
C	C	C	C	ad
A	A	A	A	bd
a	b	c	d	

Fig. 8-9 Patterns of HLA inheritance. The two haplotypes of the father are labeled *a* and *b* and the haplotypes of the mother are labeled *c* and *d*. Each child inherits two haplotypes, one from each parent. Therefore, only four combinations—*ac, bc, ad,* and *bd*—are possible, and 25% of the offspring will have identical HLA haplotypes.

Table 8-16 Characteristics of Diseases Showing HLA Associations

1. Hereditary or familial tendencies
2. Immune or autoimmune features
3. Poorly understood etiology and pathophysiology
4. Subacute or chronic course
5. Little or no effect on reproductive capacity
6. Association with HLA-B or HLA-DR loci

many alleles possible at each HLA locus, many combinations exist. Each person has two antigens for each locus. Both antigens of a locus are expressed independently (i.e., they are codominant). The entire set of A, B, C, D, and DR antigens located on one chromosome is called a *haplotype*. A complete set of antigens located on a chromosome is usually inherited as a unit (haplotype). Fig. 8-9 illustrates the inheritance of HLA haplotypes in a family.

Because of the polymorphic nature of the HLA system, it is an ideal marker for genetic studies. This characteristic also makes it a useful tool in settling paternity disputes. The frequencies of HLA antigens vary considerably among different races. For example, HLA-B8 is relatively high (17.1%) in American Caucasians, drops to 6% in Mexicans, 2.9% in American Indians, and 0.2% in Japanese.[13]

HLA and disease associations. The early interest in HLA was stimulated by its potential role in matching donors and recipients of organ transplants. (Its role in transplantation is discussed in Chapter 41.) During the last few years, interest in the association between HLA and disease has grown (Table 8-16). Some very strong associations between HLA type and susceptibility to certain diseases have been demonstrated (Table 8-17). The discovery of HLA associations with certain diseases is a major breakthrough in understanding the genetic basis of these diseases. It is now known that at least part of the genetic basis of HLA-associated diseases lies in the HLA region, but the actual

Table 8-17   HLA Types and Disease Associations

Disease	HLA Type
Ankylosing spondylitis	B27
Reiter's syndrome	B27
Rheumatoid arthritis	DR4
	B27
Diabetes mellitus, type I	DR4
	DR3
Multiple sclerosis	DR2
	B7
Goodpasture's syndrome	DR2
Graves' disease	B35
	DR3
Celiac disease	DR3
	DR7
	B8
Narcolepsy	DR2
Myasthenia gravis	B8
Systemic lupus erythematosus	B8
	DW3
Sjögren's syndrome	B8
	DW3
Acute anterior uveitis	B27
Dermatitis herpetiformis	DR3
Idiopathic hemochromatosis	A3

Modified from Tiwari JL and Terasaki PI: HLA and disease associations, New York, 1985, Springer-Verlag New York, Inc, p 33.

Table 8-18   Explanations for HLA and Disease Association

Mechanism	Description
Receptor theory	HLA antigens act as cell-surface receptor for pathophysiological organisms (e.g., viruses) that cause disease
Molecular mimicry	Molecular structure of infectious agent of disease resembles particular HLA antigen of host so closely that no immune response is mounted
Interaction of HLA molecules with nonimmunological factors	HLA molecules have structures similar to those on receptors for certain hormones (e.g., insulin, glucagon) that cause competition between HLA and receptor molecules for hormone
Involvement of genes closely linked with HLA complex	Specific disease gene linked to HLA complex results in disease susceptibility (especially with B locus)
	Immune response gene or genes linked to HLA complex results in abnormal immune response to specific antigens (especially associated with D or DR loci); may explain relationship with autoimmune diseases

mechanism or mechanisms involved in these associations are still unknown. Various hypotheses have been proposed, and these are briefly described in Table 8-18.

Diseases showing strong associations with A, B, and C antigens involve T-cytotoxic cells, whereas diseases strongly associated with DR antigens involve T-helper or T-suppressor lymphocytes. A possible hypothesis about the way DR-associated factors convey susceptibility to insulin-dependent diabetes mellitus is the following: A β-cell tropic virus infects the pancreatic islet cells of a DR3-positive person. The DR3 molecules on macrophages or other cells present the virus to T-helper cells. Strong activation of T-cytotoxic cells and subsequent destruction of virus-infected B cells occur. The individual experiences loss of insulin-producing cells.

The association between HLA and certain diseases is presently of little practical clinical importance. Nevertheless, there is promise for the development of clinical applications in the future. For example, in certain autoimmune diseases, indicating members of a family at greatest risk for developing the same or a related autoimmune disease may be possible. These individuals would need close medical supervision, preventive measures implemented (if possible), and early diagnosis and treatment instituted to prevent chronic complications.

IMMUNODEFICIENCY DISORDERS

When the immune system does not adequately protect the body, an *immunodeficient* state exists. The immunodeficiency disorders involve an impairment of one or more immune mechanisms, which include (1) phagocytosis, (2) humoral response, (3) cell-mediated response, (4) complement, and (5) a combined humoral and cell-mediated deficiency. Immunodeficiency disorders are *primary* if the immune cells are improperly developed and *secondary* if an interference with the immune system develops. Primary immunodeficiency disorders are rare and often serious, whereas secondary disorders are more common and less severe.

Table 8-19 Immunodeficiency Disorders

Disorder	Affected Cells	Genetic Basis
Chronic granulomatous disease	PMN, monocytes	Sex-linked
Job's syndrome	PMN, monocytes	
Bruton's X-linked hypogammaglobulinemia	B	Sex-linked
Common variable hypogammaglobulinemia	B	
Selective IgA, IgM, or IgG deficiency	B	Some sex-linked
DiGeorge syndrome (thymic hypoplasia)	T	
Severe combined immunodeficiency disease	Stem, B,T	Sex-linked
Ataxia telangiectasia	B,T	Autosomal recessive
Wiskott-Aldrich syndrome	B,T	Sex-linked
Graft-versus-host disease	B,T	
Acquired immunodeficiency syndrome	T	

Primary Immunodeficiency Disorders

The basic categories of primary immunodeficiency disorders include (1) phagocytic defects, (2) B-cell deficiency, (3) T-cell deficiency, and (4) a combined B- and T-cell deficiency (Table 8-19).

Hypogammaglobulinemia. The defect in B cells can range from the complete absence of all immunoglobulin classes (*agammaglobulinemia*) to a defect in only one immunoglobulin class. *Hypogammaglobulinemia* refers to a decreased level of the circulating immunoglobulins. The disorder may be congenital or acquired. Congenital hypogammaglobulinemia (Bruton's disease) is a rare sex-linked recessive disorder that occurs only in males. It is characterized by a deficiency of B cells and immunoglobulins and an intact thymus gland and normal T-cell immune response. The disorder usually is first manifest in the infant at approximately 3 months of age when the IgG antibody from the mother is depleted and the infant develops recurrent respiratory tract and pyrogenic bacterial infections.

Acquired hypogammaglobulinemia (common variable hypogammaglobulinemia) is a more common disorder that is characterized by the presence of T and B cells but no plasma cells. There appears to be a defect in differentiation of B cells to plasma cells. A possible cause of acquired hypogammaglobulinemia is an abundance of T-suppressor cells that suppress B-cell maturation into plasma cells. The disorder resembles Bruton's disease except that the recurrent bacterial infections (primarily of the respiratory tract) do not occur until clients are 15 to 35 years of age. The treatment includes γ-globulin injections or transfusions of plasma.

DiGeorge syndrome. DiGeorge syndrome (also known as congenital thymic hypoplasia) is a condition in which neither the thymus nor parathyroid gland develops. B-cell function is normal, but T-cell function is absent. The disorder is manifest by recurrent viral, fungal, and protozoan infections; inability to reject allografts; and inability to have a delayed skin test reaction. Symptoms of oral candidiasis and chronic diarrhea develop in the first year of life. Microscopically, no thymus-dependent areas in the spleen or lymph nodes are seen. Because T-helper cells are missing, the circulation levels of some antibodies may also be reduced. Hypocalcemic tetany is also present due to the absence of the parathyroid gland. Treatment consists of administration of calcium and a fetal thymus transplant. A fetal thymus gland (from a fetus less than 14 weeks' gestational age) can be locally implanted intramuscularly or minced and injected intraperitoneally. Once it is in place, mature T cells are produced.

Severe combined immunodeficiency disease. This condition includes a group of inherited disorders in which B- and T-cell functions are abnormal. The most common form of severe combined immunodeficiency disease is sex-linked Swiss type agammaglobulinemia. The etiology of the disorder is unknown but seems to represent a bone marrow stem defect or a failure in normal development of thymus and bursa equivalent tissue. Microscopically, the thymus gland is hypoplastic and lymph nodes contain no B and T cells. The disorder is manifest by severe viral, bacterial, fungal, or protozoan infections that occur within the first 2 years of life. Treatment consists of controlling the infection with antibiotics and placing the client in protective isolation. Histocompatible bone marrow transplants have been somewhat successful. Other treatments include thymus transplant, γ-globulin injections, fetal liver transplant, and administration of thymic epithelium. Even with treatment, the prognosis is guarded.

Secondary Immunodeficiency Disorders

Some of the important factors that may cause secondary immunodeficiency disorders are listed in Table 8-20. Drug-induced immunosuppression is the most common. It is prescribed for clients to treat autoimmune disorders and to prevent transplant rejection. In addition, immunosuppression is a serious side effect of cytotoxic drugs used in cancer chemotherapy. Generalized leukopenia often results, leading to a decreased humoral and cell-mediated response. Therefore, secondary infections are common in immunosuppressed clients. (Refer to Table 41-11 for a summary of the specific action of the various drugs on the immune system.)

Stress appears to alter the immune response by neural

Table 8-20 Causes of Secondary Immunodeficiency

Drug-induced	Surgery and trauma
Antineoplastic agents	Infections
Corticosteroids	Burns
Stress	Chronic renal failure
Age	Diabetes
Infants	Alcoholic cirrhosis
Older adults	Systemic lupus erythema-
Malnutrition	tosus
Dietary deficiency	Anesthesia
Cirrhosis	Malignancies
Cancer cachexia	Acquired immunodeficiency
Radiation	syndrome

interruption from the hypothalamus, which ultimately alters function of the thymus gland. Stress also increases the release of glucocorticoids, which suppress the inflammatory response (see Chapter 5).

A hypofunctional state of the immune system exists in young children and older adults. Laboratory studies have demonstrated that immunoglobulin levels decrease with age and therefore lead to a suppressed humoral immune response in older adults. Thymic involution occurs in senescence along with decreased numbers of T and B cells. The incidence of malignancies and autoimmune diseases increases with aging and may be related to immunological deterioration.

Malnutrition impairs cell-mediated immune responses. When protein is deficient over a prolonged period, atrophy of the thymus gland occurs and lymphoid tissue decreases. In addition, an increased susceptibility to infections always exists.

Irradiation destroys lymphocytes either directly or through depletion of stem cells. As the radiation dose is increased, more bone marrow atrophies, leading to severe pancytopenia and severe suppression of immune function.

Surgical removal of lymph nodes, thymus, or spleen can suppress the immune response. Splenectomy in children is especially dangerous and may lead to septicemia from simple respiratory infections.

Hodgkin's disease greatly impairs the cell-mediated immune response, and clients may die from severe viral or fungal infections. Viruses, especially rubella, may cause immunodeficiency by direct cytotoxic damage to lymphoid cells. Systemic infections can place such a load on the defense system that further antigenic stimulation can result in a decreased resistance.

Graft-Versus-Host Disease

Graft-versus-host (GVH) disease occurs when an immunoincompetent (immunodeficient) client is transfused or transplanted with immunocompetent cells. A GVH response may result from the infusion of any blood product containing viable lymphocytes, such as in therapeutic blood transfusions; plasma replacement; and transplantation of fetal thymus, fetal liver, or bone marrow. Unlike most other transplantation situations, the host's rejection of the graft is not as serious as the graft's rejection of the host.

The GVH response may have its onset 7 to 30 days following infusion of viable lymphocytes. Once the reaction is started, little can be done to modify its course. The exact mechanism involved in this reaction is not completely understood; however, it involves donor T cells attacking and destroying vulnerable host cells.

The target organs for the GVH phenomenon are the skin, gut, and liver. The skin disease may be a maculopapular rash, which can progress to a generalized erythema with bullous formation and desquamation. The liver disease may range from mild jaundice to hepatic coma. The intestinal disease may be represented by mild-to-severe diarrhea, severe abdominal pain, and malabsorption. The biggest problem with GVH disease is infection, with different types of infections seen in different periods. Bacterial and fungal infections predominate immediately after transplantation when granulocytopenia exists. The development of interstitial pneumonitis is the predominant problem later. There is no adequate treatment of GVH disease once it is established. Although corticosteroids are often used, they enhance the susceptibility to infection. The use of methotrexate and cyclosporine have been most effective as preventive rather than treatment measures. Radiation of blood products before they are administered is another measure to prevent T-cell replication.

Human Immunodeficiency Virus Infection

The clinical spectrum of infection related to human immunodeficiency virus (HIV) ranges from an asymptomatic state to the severe immunosuppression and related opportunistic diseases associated with acquired immunodeficiency syndrome (AIDS). This virus was presumably introduced into the United States in the 1970s. In 1981 the disease syndrome associated with AIDS first came to the attention of the Centers for Disease Control (CDC) when there were simultaneous outbreaks of *Pneumocystis carinii* pneumonia associated with immune dysfunction in homosexual men in New York City and Los Angeles. A nationwide survey revealed that similar cases had occurred since 1979.

Since 1981, more than 180,000 cases of AIDS in adults and children have been reported in the United States.[14] An estimated 1 to 1.5 million people in the United States are infected with the virus, and many more people are at risk for the infection.

The virus is transmitted through specific sexual practices and exposure to infected blood. Persons at high risk for developing AIDS include homosexual and bisexual men, intravenous drug users, hemophiliacs, heterosexuals who have sexual contact with infected persons, infants of mothers who are infected, and recipients of blood or blood-product transfusions. Fig. 8-10 illustrates the percentage of AIDS cases in each risk group.

Epidemiology. AIDS has reached epidemic proportions in the United States, and the epidemic has only begun. The long latency period from infection to immune dysfunction, which averages 10 to 12 years, makes it very difficult to predict the number of persons who will develop the disease. In addition, only estimates of the number of

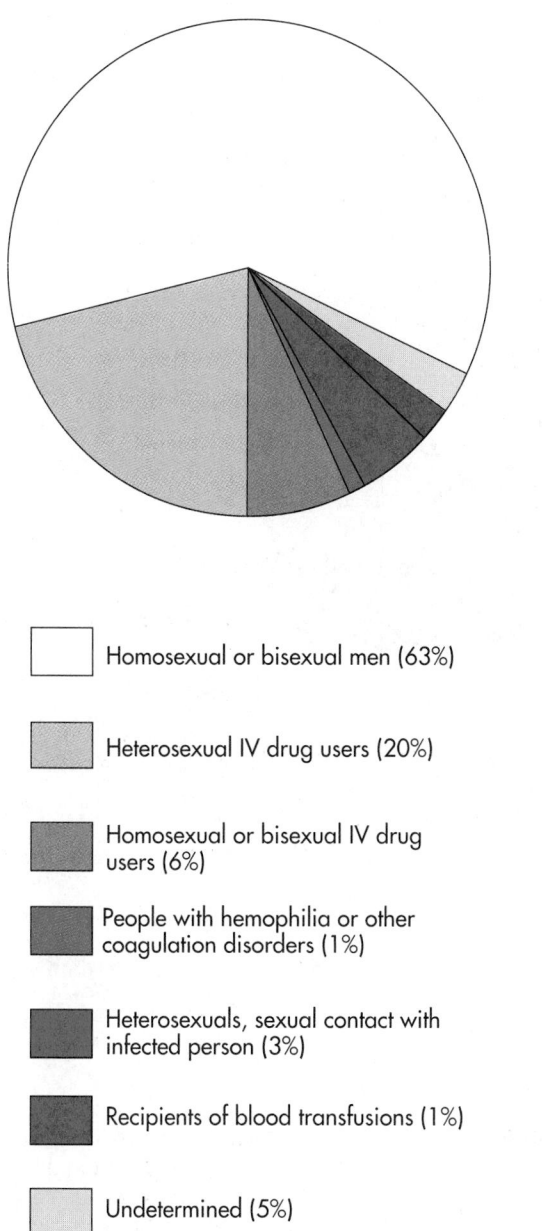

Homosexual or bisexual men (63%)

Heterosexual IV drug users (20%)

Homosexual or bisexual IV drug users (6%)

People with hemophilia or other coagulation disorders (1%)

Heterosexuals, sexual contact with infected person (3%)

Recipients of blood transfusions (1%)

Undetermined (5%)

Fig. 8-10 Population groups accounting for adult cases of AIDS. (From Centers for Disease Control, Atlanta, 1991.)

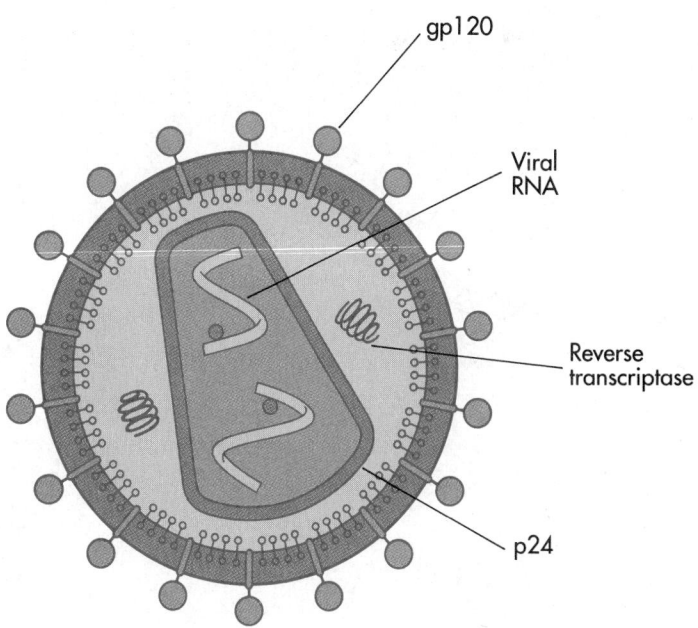

gp120

Viral RNA

Reverse transcriptase

p24

Fig. 8-11 HIV is surrounded by an envelope made up of proteins (including gp120 proteins) and contains a core of viral RNA and proteins (including p24 antigens).

persons who have been infected exist. Testing for the presence of HIV antibody among persons in high-risk groups has confirmed that the AIDS cases reported constitute a small proportion of the total number of people infected with the virus.[15] Although homosexual and bisexual men currently represent the largest number of infected individuals in the United States, the proportion of this group who are infected is decreasing, but HIV infection among IV drug users is rising sharply. In addition, the incidence of infection in women and children is increasing.

Blacks and Hispanics represent a disproportionate number of AIDS cases. The cumulative incidence of AIDS per 100,000 persons in 1989 was 83.8 in blacks and 73 in Hispanics, and the incidence was 26.3 in whites.[16] The higher number of cases in these ethnic groups is related to intravenous drug use and heterosexual transmission.[15,17,18]

Pathophysiology. The primary defect in clients with AIDS is depletion of T-helper (T4) cells. The etiological agent of AIDS, the human immunodeficiency virus (Fig. 8-11), is an RNA virus and a member of the family of retroviruses. HIV invades the T-helper lymphocytes by binding to the CD4 antigen on the cell surface[19] (Fig. 8-12). Once bound, the virus is internalized and its genetic material is uncoated. The viral genetic material (RNA) is subsequently transcribed into DNA by the action of the viral enzyme reverse transcriptase. Viral DNA can enter the nucleus of the T4 cell and become integrated into its genome. The virus may remain latent for long periods until it is activated to reproduce.[20]

The major pathophysiological mechanisms of HIV are replication of the virus in the T4 cells. Thus, the infected cells become "viral factories" and are ultimately destroyed. The destruction of T4 cells results in a severely compromised immune system (Fig. 8-13).

When HIV enters lymphocytes, it remains present for life. The virus ultimately destroys the T4 cells. There are several mechanisms by which T4 cells are destroyed. First, as the virus buds from the cell surface of the infected cell, the cell ruptures and dies because of a massive increase in the permeability of the cell membrane. Second, a single infected cell can fuse with other infected or uninfected cells. This fusion process continues until a large number of cells have combined into a large multinucleated cell called a *syncytium*. This syncytial formation kills all affected cells. A third process of destruction is initiated by the infected person's immune system. Antibodies are produced against the HIV virus. An infected T4 cell displays the viral protein on its cell surface. The circulating antibodies bind to the cell-surface viral proteins and activate

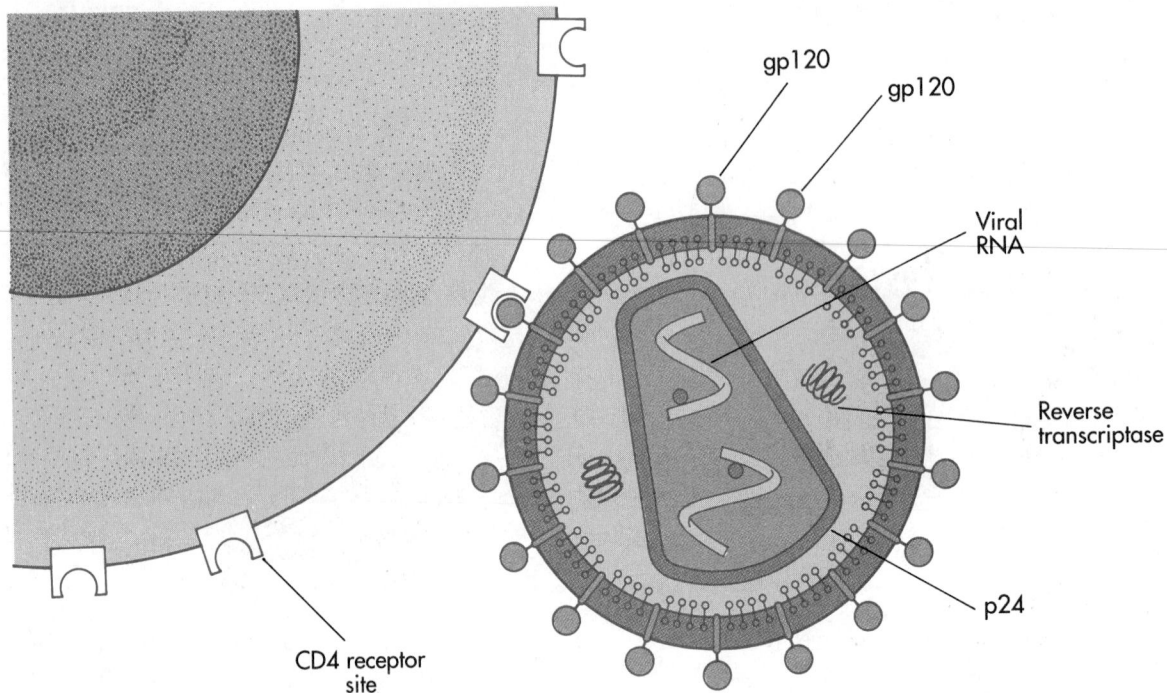

Fig. 8-12   HIV has gp120 proteins that attach to the CD4 receptors on the surface of T-helper cells.

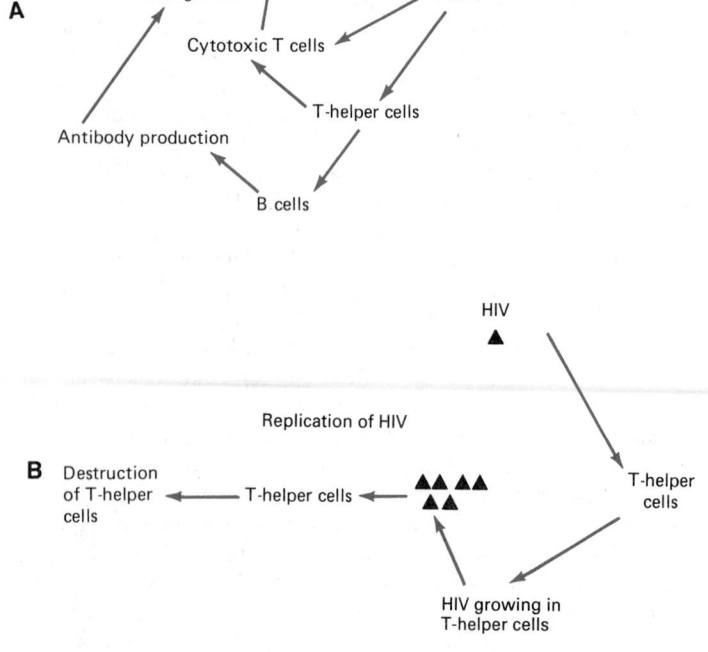

Fig. 8-13   **A,** Normal response to a virus. Normally when viruses enter a healthy body, they are detected and identified by macrophages that present the virus to the T cells. The T cells are activated and multiply into several kinds of T cells. The T-helper cells stimulate B cells to make antibodies and T-cytotoxic cells, which results in the killing and destruction of the invading virus. **B,** Response to attack by HIV. T-helper cells are infected with HIV, and the damaged T cells produce more HIV, which invades other T-helper cells. The damaged T-helper cells are unable to perform their normal functions and die.

the complement system, which ultimately promotes lysis of the infected T4 cells.

The mechanisms by which dormant HIV-infected T4 cells are stimulated to produce HIV remains unclear. However, cofactors may influence the progression of the infection. Individuals whose immune systems were compromised before infection with the virus may have a more rapid progression of the disease.[20] In addition, when the immune response is stimulated by later infections, the disease process is hastened.[20] Other diseases or pathogens, such as the herpes virus and hepatitis B, may interact with the virus and cause its activation. Repeated exposure to HIV may also increase the risk of progression of the disease.[21]

Other cofactors hypothesized in the progression of the disease include age (i.e., infants and older homosexual men have more rapid progression) and time (i.e., those persons infected the longest time have the highest risk of progression to AIDS). Communicability of the virus appears to be facilitated in the presence of other sexually transmitted diseases.[22] Moreover, host susceptibility may influence whether the virus is acquired, as well as the rate of disease progression.[23] Positive cofactors such as a healthy lifestyle, good nutritional status, and the management of stress may impede the progression of the disease process, although this relationship has not been confirmed.[24]

HIV can also infect monocytes by attaching to the CD4 receptor that is present on certain subsets of the cells or by phagocytic ingestion. Monocytes that are infected with HIV do not undergo significant cytopathic changes, suggesting they may be important viral reservoirs.

The monocyte/macrophage may play an important role in the development of neurological disease in HIV-infected individuals. Neuropsychiatric abnormalities are a significant complication of HIV infection, occurring in at least 60% of infected clients.[25] HIV-infected monocytes may cross the blood-brain barrier and thus cause the spread of the virus to the central nervous system.

Transmission. HIV is transmitted to others by individuals infected with the virus. An infected individual who is asymptomatic may transmit the virus. There is evidence that as HIV infection progresses, infectivity also increases.[15,22] Individuals who have AIDS or who have become symptomatic with HIV infection are more prone to transmitting the virus than persons who are asymptomatic. In addition, some individuals may transmit the virus more readily than others and their degree of infectivity varies over time.[15]

HIV is not spread casually. The virus cannot be transmitted from hugging, kissing, shaking hands, or sharing drinking glasses.[26] In addition, there is no evidence that the virus can be transmitted by insects.[27] Repeated studies have failed to demonstrate transmission of the virus by respiratory droplets, enteric routes, or any casual encounter in any setting. Health workers have a very low risk of acquiring the virus, even with needle stick injury.[23]

HIV is a very fragile virus that requires blood, semen, or vaginal secretions for transmission. Three modes of transmission have been recognized: (1) sexual intercourse, (2) contact with blood and blood products, and (3) perinatal transmission.[24,27]

Sexual intercourse. Transmission of HIV is primarily through sexual contact. The virus is communicated through specific sexual practices. Anal intercourse, a common practice among homosexual men and many heterosexual couples, may result in trauma to the rectal mucosa. This increases the likelihood of infection with HIV because tearing of the mucous membrane provides a portal of entry for the virus into the systemic circulation. While it appears that the risk of infection is considerably less for the insertive partner, infection may still occur. "Fisting," a practice among some homosexual men in which the fist is inserted into the anus of the partner, may result in infection if an infected partner then ejaculates into the rectum. In addition, a large number of different sexual partners increases the risk of exposure to the virus.[17,21,22]

Although homosexual and bisexual men constitute the majority of AIDS cases, infection also results from heterosexual intercourse.[17] Sexual contact with an HIV-infected partner creates a risk of infection whether the partner was infected through blood products, needle sharing, or sexual practices. IV drug use is creating a new epidemic of HIV infection among sexual partners of drug users and their children. The crack/cocaine epidemic has created a new group of high-risk heterosexual women who trade sex for the drug.

Contact with blood and blood products. HIV is transmitted by exposure to contaminated blood through the sharing of needles and syringes. Infection with the virus by IV drug users is a particularly important mode of transmission because it is the primary method of transmission to the heterosexual population and ultimately to children from perinatal infection.

Transfusion of infected blood and blood products has caused AIDS in 2% of adult cases and 12% of pediatric cases.[27] Approximately 1% of the infections were acquired by hemophiliacs who were treated with blood products. In 1985, screening of blood donors to identify individuals in high-risk groups and testing the blood for the presence of HIV antibodies were implemented, improving the safety of the blood supply. Routine screening of blood donors is crucial to ensure that the blood supply is uninfected. Although transmission of HIV from blood transfusions is very unlikely today, it is still possible because some individuals may not develop detectable antibodies for a period of time.

Perinatal transmission. Transmission of the virus to children may occur from an infected woman during pregnancy, delivery, or breast feeding.[21,27] The mother's infection is most commonly associated with IV drug use.[15,21,27] The incidence of the infection in children is increasing at an alarming rate, particularly in areas with large numbers of IV drug users. If the current trend of AIDS in children continues, it will soon be among the top five leading causes of death in children.[28]

Clinical course. Infection with HIV produces clinical manifestations that vary from asymptomatic infection to life-threatening cancers and opportunistic infections. The majority of individuals infected with HIV follow a progressive course that culminates in AIDS. (The timeline from exposure to the virus to the development of AIDS is shown in Fig. 8-14.) Detectable levels of antibodies de-

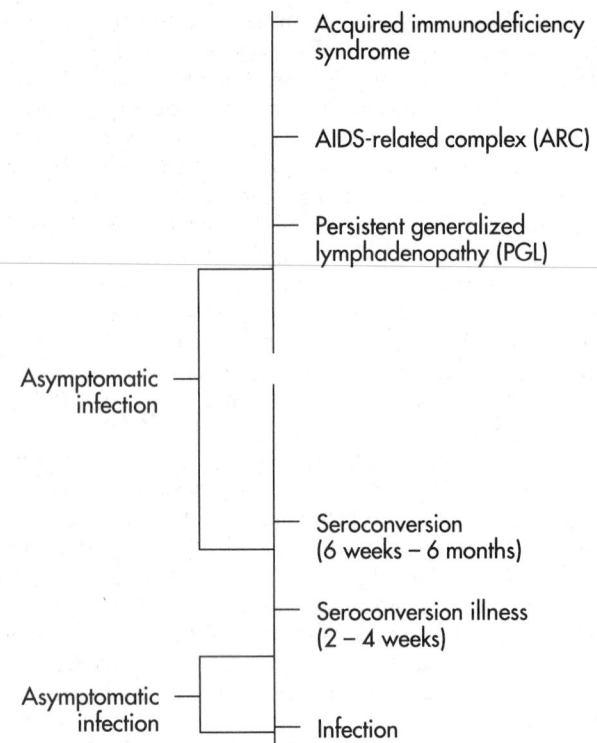

Fig. 8-14 Timeline for HIV infection. The timeline represents the course of the illness from the time of infection to clinical manifestations of disease. The broken line in the middle of the vertical line represents the long latency period. (Modified from Mountain-Plains Regional AIDS Education and Training Center: Curriculum manual, ed 2, 1989. Produced under HRSA Grant Number 000041.)

velop in an average of 6 weeks to 6 months after exposure to the virus. However, antibodies may not develop for 6 or more months in some cases.[29] One research study demonstrated that antibodies to HIV may not develop for as long as 3 years in some people, but the implications of this study are unclear.[30]

Most individuals are asymptomatic following infection with HIV. However, approximately 20% of persons develop a seroconversion illness 2 to 4 weeks after exposure to the virus. The illness resembles the clinical manifestations of the flu or mononucleosis, including fever, arthralgia, myalgia, lethargy, rash, enlarged lymph nodes, sore throat, nausea, and vomiting. These signs and symptoms last approximately 1 to 2 weeks, although fatigue may persist for months.

During the asymptomatic period, transmission of the virus can occur. The average time before symptoms appear is 10 to 12 years. However, the time is extremely variable. Some individuals become symptomatic in 5 years; others may not become ill for as long as 10 years. Since the disease has been followed for a relatively short time, some individuals who have been exposed to the virus may never become ill, although this appears to be unlikely. As the disease progresses, some infected individuals develop *persistent generalized lymphadenopathy* (PGL). This stage is

defined as two or more enlarged lymph nodes of 1 cm or larger size located in areas other than the inguinal area and persistence of the enlarged nodes for at least 3 months. PGL can persist for several years before further progression of the disease occurs.

AIDS-related complex (ARC) is the last stage on the timeline before the appearance of AIDS. ARC is defined as the presence of clinical symptoms that are suggestive of immunodeficiency in the absence of any known underlying cause except exposure to HIV but that do not fit the CDC criteria for AIDS.[31]

The clinical manifestations in ARC are referred to as *constitutional symptoms*. These include cyclical fevers; recurrent drenching night sweats; diarrhea, fatigue, anorexia, and weight loss; oral hairy leukoplakia; and AIDS-dementia complex.

Oral hairy leukoplakia (HL), an infection by the Epstein-Barr virus, has been found to be highly predictive of progression to AIDS. About one third of HIV-infected individuals will progress to AIDS within a year of development of HL. It produces painless, white, raised lesions over the lateral aspect of the tongue. The lesions subside and return spontaneously. Candidiasis is also an important predictor of disease progression. It is more common than HL and is diagnostic for ARC.

Neurological manifestations. HIV infection of the central or peripheral nervous system produces dementia, myelopathy, and peripheral neuropathy. Approximately 10% of individuals develop neurological problems as the first manifestation of the disease. As many as 80% of individuals infected with HIV develop neurological manifestations.[32]

AIDS-dementia complex (ADC) is the most common neurological disorder. It may result from direct invasion of the brain by HIV, although lymphomas, toxoplasmosis, cytomegalovirus, herpes virus (type I and II), papovavirus, and *Cryptococcus* also invade the brain and produce symptoms that resemble ADC. The clinical manifestations of ADC include cognitive, behavioral, and motor abnormalities.[32,33] Manifestations of ADC may occur early in the course of the disease before any other clinical signs of HIV infection develop.

A variety of neurological symptoms have been associated with HIV infection. *Distal sensory polyneuropathy* is the most common neuropathy in individuals with AIDS, although it can occur early in the disease process. It is manifested by burning pain and hypersensitivity in the feet. The feet become weak and sensitive to touch, and walking becomes difficult. The reflex in the Achilles tendon disappears. *Acute inflammatory demyelinating sensorimotor polyradiculopathy (Guillain-Barré syndrome)* produces an ascending paralysis that may progress to quadriplegia and necessitate respiratory support. It can develop at any point during HIV infection.

A chronic inflammatory *demyelinating polyneuropathy* may also occur before the onset of other symptoms of HIV infection or after other symptoms appear. Manifestations include muscle weakness or paralysis, some sensory deficits, and disappearance of deep tendon reflexes. A *progressive polyradiculopathy* is frequently seen in individuals with AIDS. However, it may occur earlier in the disease process. This neuropathy produces an asymmetrical muscle weakness and affects the anal and urinary sphincters. Deep tendon reflexes are obliterated. The syndrome is unresponsive to treatment and ultimately results in death. *Mononeuritis multiplex* causes random inflammation of spinal, cranial, and peripheral nerves, which leads to sensory or motor deficits, lower leg pain, and weakness. The symptoms may be manifest during the early period of ARC and AIDS.[32]

Polymyositis is a common muscle disease in HIV-infected individuals. Its appearance during the course of HIV infection is highly variable. It may occur as the first symptom of HIV infection or in the last stages of AIDS. In this disease a sudden onset of weakness and occasionally pain in the muscles of the thighs and upper arms occur. *Amyotrophic lateral sclerosis* may occur at the time of seroconversion. Vacuolar myelopathy with associated ataxia and weakness in the legs may also develop with the AIDS-dementia complex.[32]

Classification. The CDC and Walter Reed Army Medical Center have developed classification systems for HIV infection[34] (Tables 8-21 and 8-22). Classification systems provide a useful reference in providing treatment to individuals with the infection by grouping persons who are infected according to the stage of infection. The CDC classification system corresponds to the timeline in Fig. 8-14. Acute infection (stage I) represents the seroconversion illness that occurs in some individuals. Asymptomatic infection (stage II) is present during the latent period, and persistent generalized lymphadenopathy (stage III) occurs before the onset of ARC and AIDS. Stage IV, which includes constitutional, neurological, and secondary or other conditions, represents ARC and AIDS.

In the Walter Reed Army Medical Center classification system, stage 0 is exposure to the virus. When the presence of HIV is detected, the individual is in stage 1. As the disease progresses, the first sign of infection is often chronically swollen lymph nodes. This stage may last 3 to 5 years. The appearance of chronic lymphadenopathy places the person in stage 2. The beginning of stage 3 is marked by a drop in the number of T4 cells. This stage lasts until evidence of impaired cell-mediated immunity arises. The individual enters stage 4 when failure to respond to three out of four skin tests occurs. The tests mea-

sure the ability of an individual's immune system to respond to specific proteins injected under the skin. Progression to stage 5 occurs when a detectable immune response to the skin tests is completely absent. At this stage the first sign of impaired immunity usually occurs, which is thrush on the tongue or mucous membrane in the oral cavity and

Table 8-21   CDC Classification System

I. Acute infection
II. Asymptomatic infection
III. Persistent generalized lymphadenopathy
IV. Constitutional, neurological, and secondary or other conditions
    Constitutional disease (fever, weight loss, diarrhea)
    Neurologic disease (dementia, myelopathy, neuropathy)
    Secondary or other conditions
    1. CDC case definition
       a. Protozoal: *Pneumocystis* pneumonia, toxoplasmosis, cryptosporidiosis, isosporiasis
       b. Viral: Cytomegalovirus infection, mucocutaneous herpes simplex; progressive multifocal leukoencephalopathy
       c. Bacterial: Nontuberculous mycobacteriosis, extrapulmonary tuberculosis, *Salmonella* bacteremia, recurrent pyogenic infections
       d. Neoplastic: Kaposi's sarcoma, primary lymphoma of brain, non-Hodgkin's lymphoma
       e. Fungal: Candidiasis, cryptococcosis, histoplasmosis, coccidioidomycosis
       f. HIV-related: Wasting syndrome, AIDS-dementia complex, lymphoid interstitial pneumonia
    2. Other
       a. Hairy leukoplakia, multidermatomal herpes zoster, *Salmonella* bacteremia, nocardiosis, tuberculosis, thrush
       b. Secondary cancers (Kaposi's sarcoma, non-Hodgkin's lymphoma, primary lymphoma of the brain, lymphoid interstitial pneumonitis)

Modified from Centers for Disease Control: CDC surveillance case definition for acquired immunodeficiency syndrome, MMWR 36:3S-15S, 1987.

Table 8-22   Walter Reed Army Medical Center Classification System

Stage	HIV Antibody	Chronic Lymphadenopathy	T4 Cells/μl	Delayed Hypersensitivity	Thrush	Opportunistic Infections
WR 0	−	−	>400	Normal	−	−
WR 1	+	−	>400	Normal	−	−
WR 2	+	+	>400	Normal	−	−
WR 3	+	+/−	<400	Normal	−	−
WR 4	+	+/−	<400	Partial defect	−	−
WR 5	+	+/−	<400	Fails to respond	+/−	−
WR 6	+	+/−	<400	Fails to respond	+/−	+

Table 8-23 Opportunistic Infections: Clinical Manifestations, Diagnostic Tests, and Treatment

Organism/Disease	Clinical Manifestations	Diagnostic Tests	Treatment
RESPIRATORY SYSTEM			
Pneumocystis carinii	Pneumonia, fever, night sweats, nonproductive cough	Chest x-ray, sputum culture, pulmonary function tests	Pentamidine, dapsone-trimethoprim, sulfamethoxazole
Cytomegalovirus	Shortness of breath, cough, dyspnea	Bronchoscopy	Ganciclovir
Cryptococcus species	Pneumonia, fever, malaise	Chest x-ray, sputum culture	Amphotericin B
Histoplasmosis	Pneumonia, fever, symptoms of sepsis	Sputum culture, bronchoscopy, lung biopsy	Amphotericin B
Aspergillus organisms	Pneumonia, fever, cough with or without sputum	Chest x-ray, sputum culture, biopsy	Amphotericin B, steroids
Mycobacterium tuberculosis	Productive, purulent cough; fever	Chest x-ray, AFB smears	INH, ethambutol, rifampin
Herpes simplex (type 1)	Vesicular eruptions of tracheobronchial mucosa	Viral cultures	Acyclovir
Kaposi's sarcoma	Dyspnea	Chest x-ray, biopsy of lesion	Radiation, chemotherapy
Non-Hodgkin's lymphoma	Dyspnea	Chest x-ray, lymph node biopsy	Chemotherapy, steroids, radiation
INTEGUMENTARY SYSTEM			
Herpes simplex (type 1)	Vesicular eruptions on lips	Viral cultures	Acyclovir, vidarabine
Herpes simplex (type 2)	Vesicular eruptions around perianal area	Viral cultures	Acyclovir
Herpes zoster	Erythematous macules, pain, pruritus, paresthesia	Viral cultures	Acyclovir, vidarabine
Candida albicans	Erythematous skin rash, yellowish-brown lesions of skin and mucous membrane, fissured nails	Microscopic exam of material from lesion	Nystatin, ketoconazole
Kaposi's sarcoma	Purplish-blue multicentric lesions	Biopsy of lesions	Radiation, chemotherapy
EYE			
Cytomegalovirus	Lesions on retina, blurry vision, loss of vision	Opthalmoscopic exam	Ganciclovir
Herpes simplex (type 1)	Blurring of vision, corneal lesions	Opthalmoscopic exam	Acyclovir, vidarabine
Herpes zoster	Ocular lesion	Opthalmoscopic exam	Acyclovir, vidarabine

oral hairy leukoplakia. Most individuals in stage 5 have T4 cell counts of less than 200/μl. Stage 5 may last 1 to 2 years. A severe decline in immune function usually ensues, and the individual enters stage 6. In the last stage of the disease, AIDS occurs with its many manifestations of opportunistic diseases. The T4 cell count is often less than 100/μl. Most people infected with HIV infection follow the same course and move from stage to stage.[34]

Opportunistic diseases. As HIV infection progresses, the immune system becomes increasingly more compromised and less functional. Numerous infections, a variety of cancers, and wasting result from this impairment. Organisms that are nonvirulent or cause limited or localized diseases in immunocompetent individuals can cause se-

vere, debilitating, disseminated, and life-threatening opportunistic infections in AIDS. Table 8-23 summarizes the clinical manifestations, diagnosis, and treatment of common opportunistic diseases and cancers associated with AIDS.

Pneumocystis carinii pneumonia (PCP) occurs in as many as 85% of clients with AIDS. The infection is usually fatal without treatment. Individuals with T4 cell counts less than 200/μl are particularly vulnerable to this infection. Several prophylactic therapies are now available to prevent or delay the onset of PCP. (PCP is discussed in Chapter 21.)

Kaposi's sarcoma was a rare form of skin cancer before the AIDS epidemic. It is recognized as one of the cancers

Table 8-23 Opportunistic Infections: Clinical Manifestations, Diagnostic Tests, and Treatment—cont'd

Organism/Disease	Clinical Manifestations	Diagnostic Tests	Treatment
GASTROINTESTINAL SYSTEM			
Cryptosporidium muris	Watery diarrhea, abdominal pain, fever	Stool culture, biopsy of bowel	Spiramycin, antispasmodic drugs .
Cytomegalovirus	Diarrhea	Stool culture	Ganciclovir
Herpes simplex (type 1)	Vesicular eruptions on tongue, buccal mucosa, pharyngeal, esophageal mucosa	Viral cultures	Acyclovir, vidarabine
Candida albicans	Whitish-yellow patches in mouth; present in esophagus, GI tract	Microscopic exam of tissue from lesion	Nystatin, ketoconazole, Mycelex
Mycobacterium avium-intracellulare	Watery diarrhea	Stool culture	INH, ethambutol, streptomycin, cycloserine
Kaposi's sarcoma	Diarrhea	GI series	Radiation, chemotherapy
Non-Hodgkin's lymphoma	Abdominal pain, fever, night sweats, weight loss	Lymph node biopsy	Chemotherapy, steroids
NEUROLOGICAL SYSTEM			
Toxoplasma gondii	Cognitive dysfunction, motor impairment, headaches, seizures	CT scan, MRI	Pyrimethamine, sulfadiazine, clindamycin
Cytomegalovirus	Personality changes, motor impairment	Biopsy, CSF analysis	Ganciclovir
JC papovavirus	Progressive decline in mental acuity resulting in dementia, motor impairment	CT scan, MRI, EEG, CSF analysis	Cytarabine
Herpes simplex (type 1 and 2)	Personality changes, cognitive dysfunction, motor and sensory deficits, seizures	Viral cultures, CSF analysis, CT scan	Acyclovir, vidarabine
Cryptococcal meningitis	Cognitive impairment, motor dysfunction	CT scan, MRI	Amphotericin B
Aspergillus organisms	Sudden onset speech difficulty, motor impairment, seizures	CT scan	Amphotericin B, steroids
Non-Hodgkin's lymphoma	Cognitive dysfunction, motor impairment	CSF analysis, CT scan	Chemotherapy, radiation
CNS lymphoma	Personality changes, motor impairment, headaches, seizures	CT scan, MRI	Radiation

occurring in AIDS. Previously, Kaposi's sarcoma had appeared primarily in individuals whose immune systems were suppressed by chemotherapy for treatment of cancer or in those who received immunosuppressive therapy to prevent rejection of organ transplants. Kaposi's sarcoma occurs predominantly in male homosexuals and bisexuals, leading scientists to suggest that it is sexually transmitted.

The lesions in Kaposi's sarcoma may have the appearance of bruises, moles, or birthmarks. They are often described as purplish-red, but they may be violet, dark purple, pink, red, or red-brown. Lesions often occur in different areas at the same time. They may occur on any skin surface, and they frequently invade organ systems such as the GI system, liver, lungs, lymph nodes, heart, spleen,

testes, pancreas, and adrenal glands. The tip of the nose, buccal mucosa, hard and soft palate, the gums, and tonsils may be affected. Clients with Kaposi's sarcoma usually die from an opportunistic infection rather than from the cancer.

Treatment of Kaposi's sarcoma in clients with AIDS is usually based on the overall clinical status of the individual, since treatment does not improve survival.[35] The goals of therapy are to relieve pain, decrease cosmetic problems, reduce large obstructive lesions, decrease edema, and improve pulmonary status. When lesions are limited and the client is relatively asymptomatic, no treatment may be initiated. Radiation therapy can control local disease and provide an improvement in appearance. Chemotherapeutic agents and immune modulators (e.g., α-interferon) are used to achieve systemic effects when the disease becomes problematic. However, side effects of chemotherapy may further suppress the immune system.

Diagnostic studies. An enzyme-linked immunosorbent assay (ELISA) is used as a screening test to detect the presence of antibodies to HIV. Although the ELISA is highly sensitive and specific (i.e., it detects the presence of antibodies to HIV), it is not 100% accurate. A small percentage of uninfected individuals will have a positive test and, conversely, some infected people will test negative. Therefore, the Western blot test is used to confirm all positive ELISA tests because it is more specific. Because viral cultures are expensive and time consuming and require specialized facilities, they are not suitable for screening purposes but are useful in research and clinical diagnosis in some situations (Table 8-24).

The progression of the disease process in HIV can be predicted by laboratory tests. As the disease progresses, the T4 lymphocyte count decreases and the ratio of T4 to T8 cells (helper to suppressor cell) gradually reverses. Normally, there are about twice as many helper cells as there are suppressor cells. In HIV infection, T4 cells are destroyed, and the ratio is reversed, with more T-suppressor cells than T-helper cells. There may also be an associated anemia, elevated erythrocyte sedimentation rate, thrombocytopenia, and high levels of β-2 microglobulin.[29]

Therapeutic management. Asymptomatic HIV-positive individuals need close medical supervision. The T4 cells are usually monitored every 3 to 6 months. Although there is no cure for HIV infection, zidovudine—also known as azidothymidine (AZT) and Retrovir—is effective in slowing the progression of the disease.[36] The FDA has approved the use of AZT in asymptomatic clients whose T4-cell count is reduced to 500/μl or lower. Fewer side effects result from the drug when the individual is still healthy. The drug's effectiveness results from its ability to inhibit reverse transcriptase and thus the production of viral DNA. A major toxic effect of AZT is bone marrow suppression resulting in severe anemia. Clients may require repeated blood transfusions.[37] WBCs and platelets may also be reduced. As many as 30% to 35% of persons with AIDS are unable to take AZT because of bone marrow suppression.[38] Other side effects of the drug include nausea, abdominal pain, and headaches.

Several drugs that have shown promise in slowing the progression of HIV infection and/or possibly preventing AIDS are currently being tested. The drugs include soluble CD4, which prevents the virus from entering cells by binding directly to the virus; d4T, ddI, and ddA, which suppress viral DNA synthesis; and ddC, which inhibits reverse transcriptase. Another category of drugs that inhibits the maturation of viral particles are being investigated. These drugs include castanospermine (SC-48334) and hypericin. In addition, several products that occur naturally in the body and act to bolster antiviral defenses in the immune system are undergoing research. These drugs are interleukin-1, interleukin-2, and the interferons.[38] Numerous drugs are available to treat the various opportunistic diseases associated with AIDS. However, there is no effective therapy for restoring the T-helper cells and correcting the severe immunodeficiency.[38]

Considerable research is in progress to develop a vaccine for AIDS. Vaccine development is difficult due to the heterogeneity of HIV and the fact that it is an intracellular pathogen. Two types of whole-virus vaccines are being investigated for possible use. These vaccines contain either a killed whole virus or a virus genetically engineered so that disease cannot be produced. Other vaccine attempts have used several proteins from HIV that serve as antigenic stimuli and generate a protective immune response. Other researchers are using parts of proteins or peptides from HIV to develop a vaccine. In addition, researchers are investigating vaccines that would be used as a treatment for individuals already infected with the virus. Vaccines are currently being tested in animals.[39]

Table 8-24

Diagnostic Studies for HIV Infection	
Test	**Method**
ANTIBODY	
ELISA	Detects serum antibodies that bind to HIV antigens in test plates
Western blot	Uses electrophoresis to separate viral antigens and measures serum antibody reaction to specific viral core and envelope proteins
VIRUS	
Cell culture	Grows virus in vitro by putting lymphocytes into cell culture system
ANTIGEN (CORE P24)	
ELISA	Detects viral antigen p24 in serum by binding to antibody in test plates
HIV-DNA SEQUENCES	
Polymerase chain reaction	Analyzes DNA extracted from lymphocytes using in vitro amplification procedure
LYMPHOCYTE NUMBER	
T4 and T8 lymphocyte counts	Determines percentage of T4 and T8 cells in peripheral blood by using monoclonal antibodies specific for these lymphocytes

Table 8-25

Nursing Assessment of Client with HIV Infection

SUBJECTIVE DATA

History
Male homosexual or bisexual activity; prostitution; sex with prostitute; intravenous drug user, male homosexual, bisexual; history of intravenous drug use and sharing of needles; history of blood transfusion or infusion of anti-hemophilia factors in last 10 years

General
Chronic fatigue; malaise; low-grade fever; drenching night sweats; unexplained weight loss

Head and Neck
Headache; stiff neck

Oral
Whitish-yellow patches in mouth; white, painless coating on lateral surface of tongue; painful lesions in mouth and on lips; difficulty swallowing; pain in throat

Eyes
Blurring of vision

Respiratory
Persistent symptoms of upper respiratory infection; cough (productive or nonproductive); progressive shortness of breath

Integumentary
Painful eruptions; rash; lesions; discolorations

Gastrointestinal
Anorexia; nausea; vomiting; persistent diarrhea; appetite loss; hydration status; rectal pain, lesions, or ulcerations

Neurological
Confusion; changes in mental status; short-term memory loss; paresthesia, hypersensitivity in feet

Musculoskeletal
Difficulty with walking; muscle weakness

OBJECTIVE DATA

General
Weight, vital signs

Eyes
Presence of exudate; retinal hemorrhage; lesions; papilledema

Oral
Presence of lesions; white coating on lateral surfaces of tongue; purplish lesions; vesicular eruptions; gingivitis

Neck
Enlarged lymph nodes

Integumentary
Integrity; appearance; presence of lesions, eruptions, or discoloration; enlarged lymph nodes

Respiratory
Presence of rales; dry or productive cough; dyspnea

Gastrointestinal
Tenderness; masses; enlarged spleen and/or liver; lymphadenopathy

Neuromuscular
Hemiparesis; aphasia; ataxia; motor incoordination; sensory loss; tremors in extremities; slurred speech; unilateral or bilateral weakness; loss of deep tendon reflexes

Neurological
Confusion; forgetfulness; slurred speech; short-term memory loss; apathy; agitation; social withdrawal; inappropriate behavior

■ Nursing Management of HIV Infection

The majority of individuals with HIV infection are persons who have been stigmatized by society, that is, gay and bisexual men and intravenous drug users. When the individual becomes ill with AIDS, tremendous discrimination often occurs. Unfortunately, the societal attitude may be one of "they are getting what they deserve." Persons with AIDS often lose their jobs and their homes. They may be denied insurance and are often estranged from their friends and families. Effective nursing care must consider the psychosocial problems that affect the individual who is infected.

Reactions to a positive HIV-antibody test or a diagnosis of AIDS are similar to those in persons with cancer or other life-threatening illnesses. They include anxiety, fear, denial, anger, and guilt. As the disease progresses, the individual must confront issues associated with life-threatening illness, such as feelings of powerlessness, social isolation, depression, grief, disturbances in self-concept, al-

tered sexual practices, the possibility of impending death, and thoughts of suicide. When involvement of the central nervous system occurs, nursing management is more complex. Determining whether behavioral manifestations are from HIV infection or from the psychological response to the illness is often difficult.

Nursing assessment
Subjective and objective data that should be obtained from an individual who has HIV infection are shown in Table 8-25.

Nursing diagnoses
Nursing diagnoses specific to the client with HIV infection include but are not limited to those presented in Table 8-26.

Nursing interventions
Health maintenance and promotion. In the absence of a vaccine to prevent AIDS and the lack of a cure, changes in behavior to prevent the disease are crucial. Clients in all settings need to be assessed for risk and provided with in-

Text continued on p. 156.

Table 8-26

NURSING CARE PLAN FOR THE CLIENT WITH HIV INFECTION

Defining Characteristics	Nursing Interventions	Evaluation Criteria
NURSING DIAGNOSIS: Chronic and acute pain related to peripheral neuropathies; effects of pressure on nerve endings; muscle aches; pneumonia; headaches; or oral, vaginal, or perianal excoriation		
Complaint of pain, assumption of protective posture	Assess need for medications; administer analgesics promptly as needed; encourage use of nonsteroidal anti-inflammatory agents to potentiate effects of analgesics. Teach and encourage use of alternate methods of pain relief—massage, visualization, warm bath, talking, touching. Assist in titrating medication for pain relief.	Verbalization of satisfaction with level of pain relief; notification when relief from medications not obtained; use of alternate methods of pain relief
NURSING DIAGNOSIS: Anxiety related to lack of knowledge of client/family of disease process transmission and prevention, medications and their side effects, alternative treatment modalities, infection control measures in the hospital and home, safe sex and/or needle use, and available community resources		
Frequent and multiple questions asked about course and treatment of disease, appearance of agitation	Instruct client/caregivers on infection control measures related to transmission of HIV infection. Instruct/supervise caregivers' ability to comply with recommendations on infection control. Provide written, specific instructions for caregivers in home. Educate client and family about signs of opportunistic infections and malignancies. Teach about action and common side effects of medications; provide written list of medications with times, dose, and possible side effects.	Verbalization of understanding of HIV infection and AIDS; display of knowledge of action and side effects of drugs; use of appropriate infection control measures and community resources; verbalization of feeling less anxious
NURSING DIAGNOSIS: Sensory/perceptual alterations: confusion related to neurological changes, opportunistic central nervous system infections, central nervous system malignancy, side effects of medications, and stress		
Inappropriate responses, disorientation	Assess onset and progression of confusion. If client is confused, speak in simple, short sentences; provide written instructions. Instruct caregiver in memory cues: calendar, clock, log to reorient client. Provide nonstimulating environment. Discuss need for 24-hour care as mental status deteriorates. Teach stress reduction techniques.	Correct orientation to person, place, time; participation in daily care as able; maintenance of maximal level of sensory/perceptual function

ADL, Activities of daily living.
*For nursing care plan related to nausea and vomiting, see Table 36-3.
†See Table 8-29 for nutritional intervention.
‡See Table 8-29 for nutritional management.

Table 8-26

NURSING CARE PLAN FOR THE CLIENT WITH HIV INFECTION—cont'd

Defining Characteristics	Nursing Interventions	Evaluation Criteria

NURSING DIAGNOSIS: **Altered nutrition: less than body requirements related to opportunistic infections, anorexia, nausea/vomiting/diarrhea, impaired swallowing, esophagitis, or lack of knowledge regarding appropriate anabolic diet**

Weight loss; presence of anorexia, nausea, vomiting, diarrhea*; difficulty in swallowing	Monitor weight, intake and output, caloric intake; increase intake of calories and protein. Teach client to prepare and store food properly to decrease possibility of opportunistic infections from food. Encourage intake of 40 to 45 kcal/kg, 1 to 1.5 g/kg of protein.†	Increase of nutritional intake; improved skin turgor and condition of skin, hair, nails, and mucous membranes; verbalization of satisfaction with diet

NURSING DIAGNOSIS: **Total self-care deficit related to motor and/or cognitive deficits; fatigue, weakness, and debilitation; or emotional reactions to illness**

Inability to perform ADL independently	Assess functional ability and determine need for assistance. Instruct and supervise caregivers in physical care. Provide emotional support to client and significant others. Refer to physical or occupational therapy as indicated. Provide information about community resources. Initiate referrals as appropriate.	Completion of self-care as able; acceptance of care unable to provide for self; expression of satisfaction with care

NURSING DIAGNOSIS: **Hyperthermia related to HIV or opportunistic infectious processes and drug reaction**

Fever, diaphoresis, chills, tachycardia	Administer antipyretics and evaluate efficacy. Note that acetaminophen should not be used in client taking AZT. Evaluate need for cooling measures—ice packs, tepid baths, cooling blanket. encourage fluid intake to maintain hydration. Bathe and change linens as needed to promote comfort and evaluate skin integrity. Monitor temperature.	Afebrile, verbalization of feeling comfortable

NURSING DIAGNOSIS: **Diarrhea related to opportunistic bowel infection(s), adverse medication reaction, and tube feeding intolerance**

Frequent diarrheal stools	Encourage fluids (juices, broths, water) to prevent dehydration. Cleanse and dry rectal area after each bowel movement; apply vaseline, A & D, or other ointment to prevent skin breakdown. Provide sitz baths for perianal excoriation.‡	Maintenance of stable bowel function, decrease in number of stools/day, balanced intake and output, expression of feeling of comfort, no skin breakdown

Continued.

Table 8-26

 NURSING CARE PLAN FOR THE CLIENT WITH HIV INFECTION—cont'd

Defining Characteristics	Nursing Interventions	Evaluation Criteria

NURSING DIAGNOSIS: Potential impaired gas exchange related to hypoxemia, decreased air exchange, decreased tidal volume, viscous secretions, ineffective or severe cough, and dyspnea

Dyspnea, tachypnea, cyanosis, wheezing, cough; inability to raise secretions; use of accessory muscles	Suction as indicated. Administer antibiotics as ordered, evaluate for side effects. Monitor use and effectiveness of therapies such as oxygen, mechanical ventilation, humidification, chest tubes, and medications. Assist client with clearance of secretions by effective coughing. Prevent stasis of secretions by deep breathing, ambulation, postural drainage. Encourage fluid intake to prevent dehydration and to assist in liquification of secretions. Teach positioning to facilitate breathing; teach relaxation techniques to decrease anxiety.	Decreased symptoms of dyspnea and air hunger, expectoration of secretions, relief of symptoms causing discomfort, blood gases within normal limits, improved respiratory function

NURSING DIAGNOSIS: Impaired skin integrity related to immobility, poor nutritional status, prolonged skin contact with body excretions, opportunistic infections such as *Candida*, herpes simplex§

Presence of broken, draining skin areas	Leave dry lesions open to air. Clean draining lesions with soap and water, pat dry, apply normal saline dressing. Apply topical antiobiotic such as polymyxin B, bacitracin, or neomycin and nonadhering dressing.	No areas of skin breakdown, client verbalization of comfort

NURSING DIAGNOSIS: Altered oral mucous membrane related to mucocutaneous lesions and mucositis

Painful, raw oral lesions	Give oral hygiene before topical antifungals used. Scrub gums gently with soft toothbrush or toothette 3 to 4 times a day, then rinse mouth with dilute mouthwash, saline gargle, or lemon water rinse. Obtain dental consultation. Encourage client to get dental prophylaxis every 3 months.	No or decreased areas of oral mucous membrane breakdown

§See also skin care—diarrhea.

Table 8-26

 NURSING CARE PLAN FOR THE CLIENT WITH HIV INFECTION—cont'd

Defining Characteristics	Nursing Interventions	Evaluation Criteria
NURSING DIAGNOSIS: High risk for secondary infection related to immunosuppression; neutropenia related to medication, treatment, or infection; lack of knowledge regarding infection control; and impaired skin integrity		
Fever, fatigue; swollen lymph nodes	Monitor skin integrity for signs of infection; monitor vital signs and laboratory tests for signs of infection. Inform client not to clean cat litter boxes, eat foods that could be spoiled, or drink unpasteurized milk. Assess medication regimen to determine if causing low WBC. Wash hands before caring for client. Do not place two AIDS clients in same room (may acquire infections from each other). Teach infection control measures to client, visitors, and family; teach client to monitor for signs of infection.	Free of nosocomial infections; no unnecessary isolation due to inappropriate infection control; identification of ways to reduce risk of opportunistic infections
NURSING DIAGNOSIS: Dysfunctional grieving related to diagnosis of terminal illness and anticipated death		
Possible responses—total avoidance to total preoccupation	Establish a caring relationship with client and family. Promote grief work with open sharing; refer if reactions are excessive. Inquire if client desires clergy visit.	Sharing of feelings among client and family about impending death, expression of meaning of death by client
NURSING DIAGNOSIS: High risk for infection transmission related to lack of knowledge of appropriate precautions		
Questioning of ways to reduce risk of transmission, verbalization of practice of activities known to transmit HIV	Teach facts about at-risk population, modes of transmission, disinfecting equipment, and safe sex.	Verbalization of correct knowledge of facts related to risk factors, transmission, and prevention techniques; correct disinfection of equipment; demonstration of condom use on model
NURSING DIAGNOSIS: Impaired social interaction related to fear of AIDS by general population, isolation required to prevent spread of disease to others or infection of client from others, presence of terminal illness		
Absence of sufficient support system, hopelessness, social isolation	Assure client of self-worth. Teach significant others regarding mode of transmission. Plan meaningful interactions and diversional activities.	Verbalization of satisfaction with social interactions and support system

Table 8-27   Safer Sex Practices to Reduce Risks for HIV Infection

SAFE	POSSIBLY SAFE	UNSAFE
Mutual masturbation	French kissing (wet)	Anal intercourse without condom
Kissing (dry, social)	Anal intercourse with condom*	Fisting (inserting the hand into vagina
Body massage	Vaginal intercourse with condom*	or rectum) followed by ejaculation
Body-to-body rubbing (frottage)	Oral sex with condom*	Oral sex without condom
Using own sex toys		Contact with blood
Fantasy, voyeurism		Vaginal intercourse without condom
		Rimming (oral/anal contact)
		Ingestion of urine or semen

CORRECT USE OF CONDOMS

1. Only latex condoms should be used. The "natural skin" condoms have pores that are large enough for HIV to pass through. The condom should contain 5% nonoxynol-9, which has been shown to kill HIV and prevent other sexually transmitted diseases. The expiration date on the condom package should be inspected to ensure that the nonoxynol-9 is still effective and that the latex is intact. Condoms should not be exposed to heat or carried in a back pocket because they can be damaged.
2. If condoms that are not already impregnated with nonoxynol-9 are being used, a small amount of 5% nonoxynol-9 should be placed inside the tip of the condom and on the outside of the condom.
3. The condom should be placed on the erect penis. As the condom is rolled onto the penis, the tip of the condom should be held to squeeze out the air, leaving space for the ejaculate.
4. The tip of the condom is grasped while it is unrolled over the entire penis down to the hair.
5. The condom must be placed on the penis before entering the partner.
6. Only water-soluble lubricants such as K-Y jelly or 5% nonoxynol-9 should be used. Oil-based lubricants such as Vaseline cause disintegration of the condom and allow it to leak.
7. After ejaculation, the condom must be removed while the penis is still erect to prevent leakage of semen. A new condom must be used with each sexual encounter.
8. Unlubricated condoms should be used during oral sex. Nonoxynol-9 may be placed inside the condom before oral sex but should *not* be placed on the outside of the condom.

*Condoms must be used correctly.

formation to prevent the acquisition of HIV infection. To reduce the likelihood of acquiring and transmitting the virus, clients in high-risk groups should be advised to do the following:

1. Be tested for the presence of HIV infection
2. Reduce the number of sexual partners
3. Participate only in safer sexual practices (Table 8-27)
4. Use condoms correctly during all sexual encounters
5. Not give blood, donate organs, or donate semen for artificial insemination
6. Not share razors, toothbrushes, or other household items that may contain blood or other body fluids
7. Inform dentists and other health care workers that they are a member of a high-risk group so that proper precautions can be taken
8. Use birth control measures to avoid spreading the virus to offspring
9. Avoid having sexual intercourse with prostitutes
10. Avoid sexual contact with persons who are known to have or are suspected of having AIDS or who use intravenous drugs
11. Avoid sexual contact with persons who have had multiple sex partners
12. Clean equipment with 1:10 bleach and not share drug paraphernalia (if intravenous drug user)

Although HIV is a fragile virus and is not readily transmittable, nurses must protect themselves by adhering to CDC's "Universal Precaution Guidelines" when coming into contact with any body fluids (Table 8-28). In addition, needles should not be recapped or bent but should be promptly disposed of in a puncture-resistant container. Any spills of body excrements or secretions should be wiped up with disposable material, and the contaminated area should be disinfected with a 1:10 solution of bleach.

Acute intervention. The nurse should assist the client with an HIV infection to obtain as high a level of health and well-being as possible. Asymptomatic HIV-infected persons may not progress to AIDS if they begin taking drugs that inhibit the reproduction of the virus early in the infection process and engage in a healthy lifestyle. Nursing care plans should include dietary recommendations (see Chapter 35), stress reduction strategies (see Chapter 5), abstinence from alcohol and recreational drugs, and cessation of smoking. Moreover, in stressing optimum health, the nurse should assist the person with gaining some control over the events in life. Facilitating empowerment is particularly important because the individual with HIV infection often experiences many losses.

Avoiding repeated exposure to HIV and other infectious diseases is crucial. Repeated T-cell stimulation from viral infections increases the likelihood of progression of the

Table 8-28 Universal Precautions*

GLOVES

Gloves should be worn for contact with blood or body fluids and when the skin is not intact.
Double gloves should be worn if tearing is likely during a procedure.
Gloves should be worn to perform venipuncture but will not protect against needle stick injuries.

GOWNS

Gowns should be worn when soiling of clothing with blood or body fluids is anticipated and during procedures that are likely to generate splashes of blood or other body fluids.

MASKS

A mask should be worn during procedures that are likely to generate droplets of blood or other body fluids to prevent exposure of mucous membranes of the mouth, nose, and eyes or tuberculosis.
A mask should be worn when the client has a productive cough.

PROTECTIVE EYEWEAR

Goggles should be worn when splattering of blood, bloody secretions, or body fluids is possible.

NEEDLES AND SYRINGES

Needles and syringes should be discarded in rigid-wall, puncture-resistant containers.
Disposable equipment should be used whenever possible.
Needles should not be recapped, bent, or broken by hand (a common cause of needle stick injury).
Parenteral injections, blood drawing, and starting of IV should be done by experienced personnel.

LINEN

Linen should be double bagged and labeled *Infectious Waste.*

NONDISPOSABLE ARTICLES

Nondisposable articles contaminated with blood or body fluids should be bagged, labeled, and sent for decontamination.

ROOM

A private room is desirable to protect the client from infection.

GENERAL MEASURES

HIV-infection precautions are similar to those for hepatitis B.
All specimens should be labeled.
Handwashing is mandatory before and after contact.
Hands should be washed immediately and thoroughly if they become contaminated with blood.
If the environment is contaminated, a 5.25% sodium hypochlorite (household bleach) in a 1:10 dilution should be used for disinfection.
Clients being transported require no special precautions other than blood and body fluid precautions.

*Since clients infected with HIV or other blood-borne pathogens may not be identified, blood and body fluid precautions should be consistently used for *all* clients.

---

disease.[40] The client should be counseled about clinical manifestations that may indicate progression of the disease and urged to seek prompt medical care. Early manifestations may include unexplained weight loss, night sweats, diarrhea, fever, swollen lymph nodes, oral hairy leukoplakia, and oral candidiasis. Referral to support groups may be useful to assist the HIV-infected person to deal with the disease and to derive support from others in similar circumstances.

The individual who has ARC or AIDS should also be encouraged to practice healthy habits. The client should be advised to continue usual activities as long as health permits. Specific information should be provided on preventing infection, such as wearing gloves when cleaning the litter box of cats, fish tanks, and bird cages; drinking only pasteurized milk; and eating well-cooked meat.

When the individual develops an opportunistic infection, symptomatic nursing care, education, and emotional support are necessary. For example, when *Pneumocystis carinii* pneumonia occurs, intensive nursing intervention is required (see Chapter 21). Nursing care includes careful monitoring of the respiratory status, administering medications and oxygen, positioning to facilitate breathing, performing relaxation exercises to decrease anxiety, and performing techniques to conserve energy to decrease oxygen demand. Since a high mortality rate is associated with the

Table 8-29 Clinical Problems and Nutritional Interventions

Dietary Recommendation	Intervention
DIARRHEA	
Lactose-free, low-fat, low-fiber, and high-potassium foods	Avoid dairy products, red meat, margarine, butter, eggs, dried beans, peas, raw fruits and vegetables. Cooked or canned fruits and vegetables will provide needed vitamins. Encourage potassium-rich foods such as bananas and apricot nectar. Discontinue foods, nutritional supplements, and medications that may make diarrhea worse (e.g., Ensure, antacids, stool softeners). Avoid gas-producing foods. Serve warm, not hot foods. Plan small, frequent meals. Drink plenty of fluids between meals.
CONSTIPATION	
High-fiber foods	Eat beans, peas, fruits, and vegetables, cereal, and whole wheat bread. Gradually increase fiber. Drink plenty of fluids. Exercise.
NAUSEA AND VOMITING	
Low-fat foods	Avoid dairy products and red meat. Plan small, frequent meals. Prepare nonodorous foods. Eat dry, salty foods. Serve food cold or at room temperature. Drink liquids between meals. Avoid gas-producing, greasy, spicy foods. Eat slowly in a relaxed atmosphere. Rest after meals with head elevated.
CANDIDIASIS	
Soft or pureed foods	Serve moist foods. Drink plenty of fluids. Avoid acidic and spicy foods. Use straw and tilt head back and forth when drinking. Eat soft diet, such as puddings and yogurt, to decrease discomfort.
FEVER	
High-caloric, high-protein foods	Use nutritional supplements. Increase fluid intake.
ALTERED TASTE	
Diet as tolerated	Try herbs and spices. Marinate meat, poultry, and fish. Serve food cold or at room temperature. Drink plenty of fluids. Add salt or sugar. Introduce alternative protein sources.
ANEMIA	
High-iron foods	Eat red meat, organ meats, and raisins. Drink orange juice when taking iron supplements to facilitate absorption.
FATIGUE	
High-caloric foods	Cook in large quantities and freeze in meal-size packets. Use microwave and convenience foods. Use easy-to-fix snack foods. Encourage social support system to assist with meal planning and preparation. Provide in-home homemaker services. Access community Meals-on-Wheels programs.

disease, emotional support for the client and caregiver is particularly important.

Chronic management. Many chronic problems occur in HIV infection. Diarrhea is often a long-term problem. Nursing management includes recommending dietary interventions (Table 8-29), encouraging a high fluid intake to prevent dehydration, instructing the client about skin care, and managing excoriation around the perianal area. The nurse can recommend the use of incontinent materials to prevent soiling of the clothes. In addition, the nurse should assess for factors that may trigger the diarrhea, such as anxiety and medications. Relaxation techniques and alterations in the diet may provide some relief.

Severe weight loss, referred to as the *HIV-wasting syn-*drome, occurs in some individuals. The etiology is unclear, but it is probably related to an organism producing chronic diarrhea, malabsorption in the intestines, and the hypermetabolic state caused by the infectious processes associated with HIV. HIV-infected clients begin to take on the typical physical appearance of older adults. Severe emaciation occurs, the hair turns gray and becomes thinner, posture slumps, and gait becomes unsteady. Caring for the person with HIV-wasting syndrome is a tremendous nursing challenge. Extreme disturbance occurs in self-concept and self-image. Useful interventions include creating an atmosphere of acceptance and reassurance, encouraging a focus on past accomplishments and personal strengths, and facilitating the use of positive affirmations.

Review Questions

The number of the question corresponds to the same-numbered objective at the beginning of the chapter.

1. Which of the following is not a component of the immune system?
   a. spleen
   b. thymus
   c. bone marrow
   d. connective tissue
2. Administration of the MMR (mumps, measles, rubella) vaccine is done to promote which type of immunity?
   a. active natural immunity
   b. passive natural immunity
   c. passive acquired immunity
   d. active acquired immunity
3. All the following statements are characteristic of cell-mediated immunity except
   a. effective in fighting fungal infections
   b. response occurs immediately within minutes
   c. surveys the body for invasion by tumor cells
   d. sensitized lymphocytes directly attack antigens
4. The reason newborns are protected for the first 6 months of life from bacterial infections is because of the maternal transmission of
   a. IgG
   b. IgA
   c. IgM
   d. IgE
5. In a type I hypersensitivity reaction, the primary immunological disorder appears to be
   a. binding of IgG to an antigen on a cell surface
   b. deposit of antigen-antibody complexes in small vessels
   c. release of lymphokines to interact with specific antigens
   d. release of chemical mediators from IgE-bound mast cells
6. The treatment of choice for an acute anaphylactic reaction is
   a. theophylline (aminophylline)
   b. diphenhydramine (Benadryl)
   c. epinephrine (Adrenalin)
   d. corticosteroids (Solu-Cortef)
7. All the following are true about skin testing except
   a. a positive reaction is manifested by a wheal-and-flare reaction
   b. a highly sensitive person may develop an anaphylactic reaction
   c. the preferred site for intracutaneous testing is the back
   d. it may be done to determine initial titer of allergen extracts
8. Antihistamines are most effectively used in treating
   a. systemic lupus erythematosus
   b. intrinsic asthma
   c. allergic rhinitis
   d. anaphylactic shock
9. Autoimmunity is defined as a phenomenon involving

   a. production of endotoxins that destroy B lymphocytes
   b. inability to differentiate self from nonself
   c. overproduction of reagin antibody
   d. depression of the immune response
10. Association between HLA antigens and diseases is most commonly found in what disease conditions?
    a. Infectious diseases
    b. Autoimmune disorders
    c. Neurological diseases
    d. Malignancies
11. Congenital hypogammaglobulinemia is characterized by all the following except
    a. deficiency of T lymphocytes
    b. recurrent otitis media infections
    c. symptoms manifest after age 3 months
    d. sex-linked recessive disorder
12. Which of the following is not characteristic of AIDS?
    a. Decreased number of T-helper cells
    b. Associated with opportunistic infections
    c. Easily transmissible by casual contact
    d. Very difficult to treat
13. An early indication of the progression to AIDS is the development of
    a. hairy leukoplakia
    b. amyotrophic lateral sclerosis
    c. AIDS-wasting syndrome
    d. recurrent diarrhea
14. Nursing care of the client with AIDS includes all of the following except
    a. administering analgesics as needed
    b. providing care for anal excoriations
    c. monitoring of T-lymphocyte counts
    d. encouraging the use of dairy products

REFERENCES

1. Bellanti JA: Immunology III, Philadelphia, 1985, WB Saunders Co, p 7.
2. Weigle WO: Effects of aging on the immune system, Hosp Pract 24:112-119, 1989.
3. Thoman ML and Weigle WO: The cellular and subcellular bases of immunosenescence, Adv Immunol 46:221-261, 1989.
4. Kaliner M, Eggleston PA, and Mathews KP: Rhinitis and asthma, JAMA 258:2851-2873, 1987.
5. McFadden ER: Asthma. In Braunwald E and others, eds: Harrison's principles of internal medicine, ed 11, New York, 1987, McGraw-Hill, Inc, pp 1060-1065.
6. Slavin RG and Ducomb DF: Allergic contact dermatitis, Hosp Pract 24:39-51, 1989.
7. Wasserman SI and Marquardt DL: Anaphylaxis. In Middleton E and others: Allergy: principles and practices, ed 3, St Louis, 1988, The CV Mosby Co, pp 1365-1376.
8. Randall BJ: Reacting to anaphylaxis, Nurs 16:34-40, 1986.
9. Norman PS: Immunotherapy of IgE-mediated disease, Hosp Pract 25:81-92, 1990.
10. Kantor FS: Autoimmunities: diseases of dysregulation, Hosp Pract 23:75-84, 1988.
11. Arnett FC: HLA genes and predisposition to rheumatic diseases, Hosp Pract 25:89-100, 1990.
12. Kresevic DM and Kralik K: Understanding therapeutic plasma exchange, Nurs 20:68-71, 1990.
13. Tiwari JL and Terasaki PL: HLA and disease associations, New York, 1985, Springer-Verlag New York, Inc, p 9.

14. Centers for Disease Control: AIDS and human immunodeficiency virus infection in the United States: 1991, personal communication.

15. Heyward WL and Curran JW: The epidemiology of AIDS in the U.S., Sci Am 259:72-81, 1988.

16. Centers for Disease Control: HIV/AIDS surveillance: AIDS cases reported through April, 1989, U.S. Department of Health and Human Services, 1989.

17. Curran JW and others: Epidemiology of HIV infection and AIDS in the United States, Science 239:610-616, 1988.

18. Selik RM, Castro KG, and Pappaioanou M: Racial/ethnic differences in the risk of AIDS in the United States, Am J Public Health 75:1539-1545, 1988.

19. Weber JN and Weiss RA: HIV infection: the cellular picture, Sci Am 259:101-109, 1988.

20. Gallo RC and Montagnier L: AIDS in 1988, Sci Am 259:41-48, 1988.

21. Francis DP and Chin J: The prevention of acquired immunodeficiency syndrome in the United States, JAMA 257:1357-1366, 1987.

22. Mann JM and others: The international epidemiology of AIDS, Sci Am 259:82-89, 1988.

23. Kay K: The global struggle against AIDS: WHO's strategy, Int Nurs Rev 35:35-41, 1988.

24. Allen JR and Curran JW: Prevention of AIDS and HIV infection: needs and priorities for epidemiologic research, Am J Public Health 78:381-386, 1988.

25. Rosenberg AS and Fauci A: Immunopathogenic mechanisms of HIV infection, Clin Immunol Immunopathol 50:S149-S156, 1989.

26. Meisenhelder JB and LaCharite CL: Comfort in caring: nursing the person with HIV infection, Glenview, Ill, 1989, Scott, Foresman & Co.

27. Friedland GH and Klein RS: Transmission of the human immunodeficiency virus: an updated review, Int Nurs Rev 35:44-54, 1988.

28. American Public Health Association: AIDS may soon be among top 5 killers of US children, The Nation's Health, Jan 1989.

29. Lifson AR, Rutherford GW, and Jaffe HW: The natural history of human immunodeficiency virus infection, J Infect Dis 159:1360-1367, 1988.

30. Imagawa DT and others: Human immunodeficiency virus type 1 infection in homosexual men who remain seronegative for prolonged periods, N Engl J Med 320:1458-1462, 1989.

31. Abrams DI: AIDS-related conditions, Clin Immunol Allergy 6:581-599, 1986.

32. Scherer P: How HIV attacks the peripheral nervous system, Am J Nurs May 1990, pp 67-70.

33. Grabbe L and Brown L: Identifying neurological complications of AIDS, Nurs 89:66-70, 1989.

34. Redfield RR and Burke DS: HIV infection: the clinical picture, Sci Am 259:90-98, 1988.

35. Gee G and Moran T: AIDS: concepts in nursing practice, Baltimore, 1988, Williams & Wilkins.

36. Volberding PA and others: Zidovudine in asymptomatic human immunodeficiency virus infection: a controlled trial in persons with fewer than 500 CD4-positive cells per cubic millimeter, N Engl J Med 322:941-949, 1990.

37. Yarchoan R, Mitsuya H, and Broder S: AIDS therapies, Sci Am 259:110-119, 1988.

38. Marx JL: AIDS drugs coming but not here, Res News 21:287, 1989.

39. Barnes D: AIDS vaccines: exploring the options for protection and therapy, J NIH Res 1:81-88, 1989.

40. Cummings D: Caring for the HIV-infected adult, Nurse Pract 13:28-47, 1988.

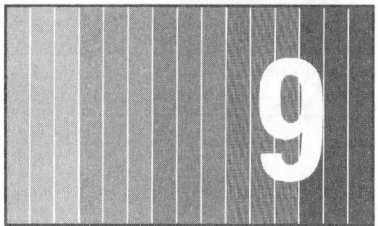

CHAPTER 9

Nursing Role in Management
Problems with Abnormal Cell Growth

Catherine M. Bender
Joyce M. Yasko

L earning Objectives

1. *Describe the prevalence and incidence of cancer in the United States.*
2. *Describe the processes involved in the biology of cancer.*
3. *Explain the three phases of the development of cancer.*
4. *Describe the role of the immune system related to cancer.*
5. *Describe the use of the classification systems for cancer.*
6. *Explain the role of the nurse in the prevention and detection of cancer.*
7. *Explain the use of surgery, radiation therapy, chemotherapy, and biological response modifier therapy in the treatment of cancer.*
8. *Differentiate between external and internal radiation.*
9. *Identify the classifications of chemotherapeutic agents and methods of administration.*
10. *Describe the effects of radiation therapy and chemotherapy on normal tissues.*
11. *Describe the nursing management for the client receiving radiation therapy and chemotherapy.*
12. *Describe the types of nursing management related to biological response modifier therapy.*
13. *Describe the nutritional problems of the client with cancer and appropriate management.*
14. *Explain the role of the nurse related to unproven methods of cancer treatment.*
15. *Describe complications that can occur in advanced cancer.*
16. *Describe appropriate psychological support of the client with cancer and the family.*

SIGNIFICANCE

It is believed that all multicellular organisms have the potential to develop cancer at some point in their lifetime. Hippocrates coined the word *carcinoma,* meaning a tumor that spread and destroyed the host. However, Galen was the first to describe cancer as being crablike in nature.

Cancer is a group of more than 200 diseases characterized by unregulated growth of cells. It can occur in persons of all ages and all races and is a major health problem in the United States. An estimated 30% of Americans now living will experience cancer at some point in their lives. The overall incidence of cancer has been steadily increasing since 1970. It is estimated that cancer (excluding non-

melanoma skin cancer and carcinoma in situ) will be diagnosed in 1,010,000 persons in 1991.[1] Some cancers, such as cancer of the stomach, uterus, and rectum, have decreased in incidence in recent times whereas others, such as cancer of the lung, colon, prostate, breast, and bladder, have increased in incidence.[2] A most notable increase in incidence of melanoma is occurring at a rate of 3.4% per year.[1] Differences are noted in the incidence of certain cancers in males and females (Table 9-1).

Considerable progress has been made in controlling cancer for long periods of time. More than 5 million Americans alive today have a history of cancer; in 3 million of these the cancer was initially diagnosed 5 or more years ago. Many of these 3 million persons now show *no evidence of disease* (NED). NED usually means that the person has remained free of disease and has the same life expectancy as a person who has never had cancer.[1] This

Reviewed by Cynthia Chernecky, R.N., M.N., Doctoral Candidate, Case Western Reserve University; Clinical Nurse Specialist in Oncology, Marymount Hospital, Garfield Heights, Ohio.

Table 9-1 Cancer Incidence by Site and Sex in 1989*

Male	Percentage	Female	Percentage
Prostate	21	Breast	28
Lung	20	Colon/rectum	15
Colon/rectum	14	Lung	11
Urinary tract	10	Uterus	9
Leukemia/ lymphoma	8	Leukemia/ lymphoma	7

From Cancer Facts and Figures 1989, American Cancer Society, 1989.
*Excluding nonmelanoma skin cancer and cancer in situ.

Table 9-2 Estimates of Cancer Deaths by Site and Sex in 1989*

Male	Percentage	Female	Percentage
Lung	35	Lung	21
Colon/rectum	11	Breast	18
Prostate	11	Colon/rectum	13
Leukemia/ lymphoma	9	Leukemia/ lymphoma	9

From Cancer Facts and Figures 1989, American Cancer Society, 1989.
*Excluding nonmelanoma skin cancer and cancer in situ.

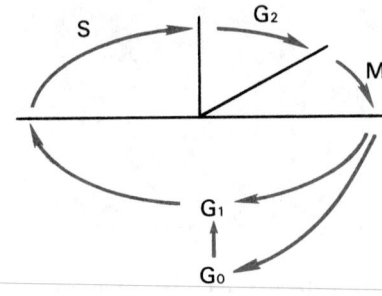

G_1 = relatively dormant with some RNA and protein synthesized
S = DNA is synthesized; RNA and protein synthesis continue
G_2 = some RNA synthesized
M = mitosis (cellular division)
G_0 = resting phase, cells are not in the process of cellular division

Fig. 9-1 Cell life cycle and metabolic activity. Generation time is the period from M phase to M phase. Cells not in the cycle, but capable of division, are in the resting phase *(G_0)*.

BIOLOGY OF CANCER*

Cancer is a group of many diseases of multiple causes that can arise in any cell of the body capable of evading regulatory controls over proliferation and/or differentiation. Two major dysfunctions present in the process of cancer are: (1) defective cellular proliferation (growth) and (2) defective cellular differentiation.

Defect in Cellular Proliferation

Normally, most tissues of the human adult contain a population of predetermined undifferentiated cells known as *stem cells. Predetermined* means that the stem cells of a particular tissue will ultimately differentiate and become mature, functioning cells of that tissue and only that tissue.

Cell proliferation originates in the stem cell and begins when the stem cell enters the cell cycle (Fig. 9-1). The time from the birth of a new cell to the time the cell divides into two identical cells is called the *generation time* of the cell. A mature cell continues to function until it degenerates and dies. At any time, there are cells at various stages of the cell cycle in all body tissues.

All cells of a tissue are controlled by an intracellular mechanism that determines when cellular proliferation is necessary. Under normal conditions, a state of dynamic equilibrium is constantly maintained (i.e., cellular proliferation equals cellular degeneration or death). The process

term is frequently substituted for the term *cured,* which is used cautiously because of the slow-developing nature of some forms of cancer.

Cancer is the second most common cause of death in the United States (heart disease is first). One of every five deaths is due to cancer, with one half of these deaths occurring before the age of 65. The death rate is leveling off or decreasing except for an increasing rate of deaths from lung cancer in women (Table 9-2). In 1989, approximately 502,000 Americans died of cancer. The cancer incidence and death rate are higher in blacks than in whites. This is especially apparent among black males. Most of the differences in cancer rates between blacks and whites are attributed to environmental and social rather than biological factors.[1]

Statistics cannot reveal the physiological, psychological, and sociological impact of cancer. Cancer is known to be the most feared disease, feared far more than heart disease. The word *cancer* is viewed as being synonymous with death, pain, disfigurement, and dependency. However, attitudes toward cancer do not fit the present status of the treatment and control of cancer. Education of health professionals and the public is essential if current attitudes surrounding cancer and cancer care are to become more positive and realistic.

*This section was reviewed by Ronald Goldfarb, Ph.D., Associate Director, Pittsburgh Cancer Institute, Division of Basic Research; Associate Professor of Pathology, University of Pittsburgh; Senior Lecturer in Biomedical Engineering, Carnegie-Mellon University, Pittsburgh, Pennsylvania.

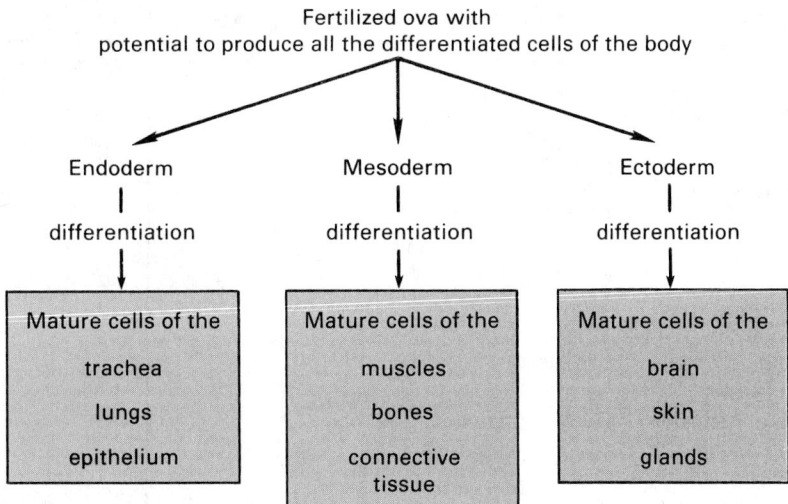

Fig. 9-2 Normal cellular differentiation.

of cellular division and proliferation is activated only in the presence of cellular degeneration or death. Cellular proliferation will also occur if the body has a physiological need for more cells. For example, a normal increase in white blood cells occurs in the presence of infection.

Another explanation for the phenomenon of proliferation control of normal cells is *contact inhibition*. Normal cells respect the boundaries and territory of the cells surrounding them. They will not invade a territory that is not their own. The neighboring cells are thought to inhibit cellular growth through the physical contact of the surrounding cell membranes.

The rate of normal cellular proliferation (from the time of cellular birth to the time of cellular death) differs in each body tissue. In some tissues, such as bone marrow, hair follicle, and epithelial lining of the gastrointestinal tract, the rate of cellular proliferation is rapid. In other tissues, such as liver, myocardium, brain, and cartilage, the rate of cellular proliferation is much slower. In fact, in adulthood the proliferation rate of these cells is so slow that it is barely perceptible.

Cancer cells usually proliferate in the manner and at the rate of the normal cells of the tissue from which they arise. However, cancer cells respond differently than normal cells to the intracellular signals that regulate the state of dynamic equilibrium. Cancer cells divide indiscriminately and haphazardly. Sometimes they produce more than two cells at the time of mitosis. Several authorities have postulated that the loss of intracellular control of proliferation is due to a mutation of the stem cells.[2] The stem cells are viewed as the target or the origin of cancer development. The DNA of the stem cell is substituted for or permanently rearranged. When this happens, the stem cell is mutated and has the potential to become malignant. It will usually proliferate at the rate of the tissue of origin, and some subpopulations can promote tumor progression to generate malignant cells (i.e., cells with invasive and metastatic potential). The stem cell theory of cancer development is not complete, since it has been noted that malignant stem cells can differentiate to form normal tissue cells.[3]

A common misconception regarding the characteristics of cancer cells is that their rate of proliferation is more rapid than that of any normal body cell. In most situations, cancer cells proliferate at the same rate as the normal cells of the tissue from which they originate. The difference is that proliferation of the cancer cells is indiscriminate and continuous. In this way, with each cell division creating two or more offspring cells, there is continuous growth of a tumor mass: $1 \rightarrow 2 \rightarrow 4 \rightarrow 8 \rightarrow 16$ and so on. This is referred to as the *pyramid effect*. The time required for a tumor mass to double in size is known as its *doubling time*.

Cancer cells grown in tissue culture are also characterized by loss of contact inhibition. They have no regard for cellular boundaries and will grow on top of one another and also on top of or between normal cells.

Defect in Cellular Differentiation

Cellular differentiation is an orderly process that progresses from a state of immaturity to a state of maturity. Since all body cells are derived from the fertilized ova, all cells have the potential to perform all body functions. As cells differentiate, this potential is repressed and the mature cell is capable of performing only specific functions (Fig. 9-2).

With cellular differentiation there is a stable and orderly phasing out of cellular potential. Under normal conditions the differentiated cell is stable and will not differentiate (that is, revert to a previous undifferentiated state).

The exact mechanism that controls cellular differentiation and proliferation is not completely understood. Genes that are important regulators of these normal cellular processes are the *protooncogenes*. Mutations that alter the expression of genes or their products can activate protooncogenes to function as *oncogenes* (tumor-inducing genes) by inducing mitosis but inhibiting differentiation of the cell.

The protooncogene has been described as the genetic

Table 9-3 Comparison of Benign and Malignant Growths

	Malignant Tumor	Benign Tumor
Encapsulated	Rarely	Usually
Differentiated	Poorly	Partially
Metastasis	Frequently present	Absent
Recurrence	Frequent	Rare
Vascularity	Moderate to marked	Slight
Mode of growth	Infiltrative and expansive	Expansive
Cell characteristics	Cells abnormal and become more unlike parent cells	Fairly normal and similar to parent cells

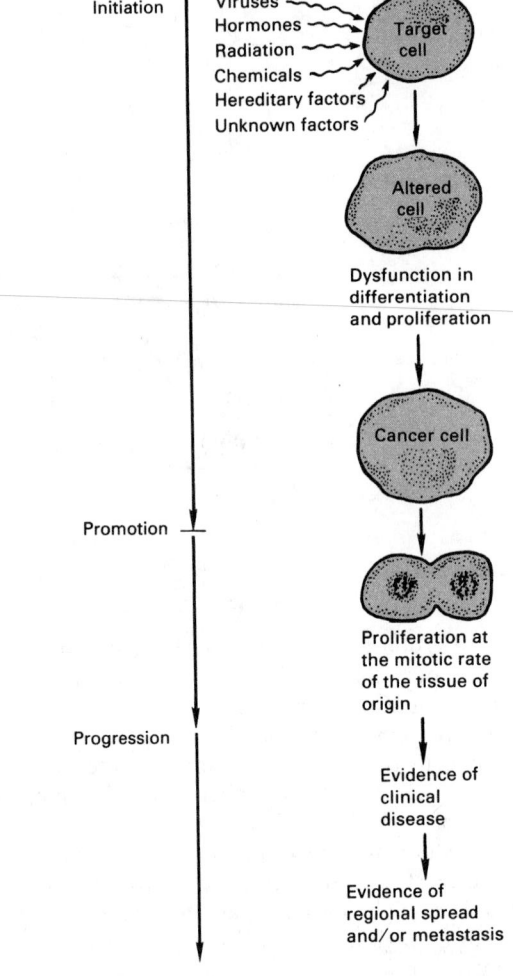

Fig. 9-3 Process of cancer development.

lock that keeps cells in their mature functioning state. When this lock is "unlocked," as may occur through exposure to carcinogens (agents that cause cancer) or oncogenic viruses, genetic alterations and mutations occur. The abilities and properties that the cell had in fetal development are again expressed. This process is referred to as *derepression* and leads to *dedifferentiation* of the cell. Although oncogenes and oncogenic products contribute to normal cell function, oncogenes interfere with normal cell expression under some conditions, causing the cell to become malignant. This derepressed cell regains a fetal appearance and function. For example, some cancer cells produce new proteins, such as those characteristic of the embryonic and fetal periods of life. These proteins located on the cell membrane include carcinoembryonic antigen and alpha-fetoprotein. They can be detected in human blood by laboratory studies (see section on Role of the Immune System). Other cancer cells, such as oat-cell carcinoma of the lung, produce hormones (see section on Complications Resulting from Cancer) that are ordinarily produced by cells arising from the same germ cell layer as the tumor cells.[2]

Tumors can be classified as *benign* or *malignant*. In general, benign neoplasms are well differentiated and malignant neoplasms range from well differentiated to undifferentiated. The ability of malignant tumor cells to invade and metastasize is the major difference between benign and malignant cells. Other differences between benign and malignant cells are presented in Table 9-3.

Development of Cancer

The following is a theoretical model of the development of cancer. The cause and development of each type of cancer are likely to be multifactorial; it is not known how many tumors have a chemical, environmental, genetic, immunological, or viral origin. Cancers may arise spontaneously from causes that are thus far unexplained.

It is a common belief that the development of cancer is a rapid, haphazard event. The natural history of cancer is an orderly process comprising several stages and occurring over a period of time. These stages include (1) initiation, (2) promotion, and (3) progression (Fig. 9-3).

Initiation. The first stage, *initiation,* is an irreversible alteration in the cell's genetic structure resulting from the action of a chemical, physical, or biological agent. This altered cell thus has the potential for developing into a clone of neoplastic cells.[2] Most carcinogens (agents capable of producing these cellular alterations) are detoxified by protective enzymes and are harmlessly excreted. If this protective mechanism fails, however, carcinogens enter the cell's nucleus and may irreversibly bind to DNA. DNA repair is possible. However, if it does not occur before cell division, the cell will replicate into daughter cells, each with the same genetic alteration.[4]

Carcinogens may be chemical, physical, or genetic in nature. Common characteristics of carcinogens are that their effects in the stage of initiation are irreversible and additive. In addition, there exists no known threshold below which their effects are not exhibited.[5]

Chemical carcinogens. Chemicals were identified as

Table 9-4 Occupational and Environmental Carcinogens

Carcinogen	Associated Neoplasm
Cigarette smoke	Lung, upper respiratory tract, bladder, cervix, and other cancers
Asbestos	Mesothelioma, lung
Arsenic	Skin, lung, liver
Cadmium	Prostate, kidney
Chromium compounds	Lung
Nickel	Lung, nasal sinuses
Uranium	Lung
Aflatoxin	Liver
Nitrites	Stomach
Chloromethyl ethers	Lung
Isopropyl oil	Nasal sinuses
Benzidine	Bladder
Vinyl chloride	Angiosarcoma of liver
Benzene	Acute myelogenous leukemia
Radiation	Numerous locations
Polycyclic hydrocarbons	Lung, skin
Mustard gas	Lung

Table 9-5 Cancers Related to Drug Exposures in Humans

Drug	Cancer
RADIOISOTOPES	
Phosphorus (^{32}P)	Acute leukemia
Radium, mesothorium	Osteosarcoma and sinus carcinoma
Thorotrast	Hemangioendothelioma of liver
IMMUNOSUPPRESSIVE AGENTS	
Antilymphocyte serum	Reticulum-cell sarcoma, epithelial cancer of skin and viscera, acute myelocytic leukemia
Antimetabolites	
Alkylating agents	
Corticosteroids	
CYTOTOXIC DRUGS	
Phenylalanine mustard	Bladder cancer
Cyclophosphamide	Acute myelogenous leukemia
HORMONES	
Synthetic estrogens	
Prenatal	Vaginal and cervical adenocarcinoma (clear-cell type)
Postnatal	Endometrial carcinoma (adenosquamous type)
Androgenic-anabolic steroids	Hepatocellular carcinoma
OTHERS	
Arsenic	Skin cancer
Phenacetin-containing drugs	Renal pelvis carcinoma
Coal for ointments	Skin cancer
Diphenylhydantoin (?)	Lymphoma
Chloramphenicol (?)	Leukemia
Amphetamines (?)	Hodgkin's disease

cancer-causing agents in the latter part of the eighteenth century when Percival Pott noted that chimney sweeps, especially those with poor personal hygiene, had a higher incidence of cancer of the scrotum associated with exposure to soot residues in chimneys. As the years went on, more chemical agents were identified as actual and potential carcinogens as statistical evidence showed that persons exposed to certain chemicals over a period of time had a greater incidence of certain cancers than others. The long latency period from the time of exposure to the development of cancer makes it difficult to identify cancer-causing chemicals. Also, those chemicals that cause cancer in animals may or may not cause the same specific cancer in human beings. Some chemicals are cancer causative in their environmental form, but others must first undergo certain metabolic changes.[2] Chemical carcinogens thought to cause cancer in human beings are included in Table 9-4.

Certain drugs have also been identified as carcinogens (Table 9-5). Drugs that are capable of interacting with DNA (e.g., alkylating agents) as well as immunosuppressive agents have the potential to cause neoplasms in human beings. The use of alkylating agents (e.g., cyclophosphamide and nitrogen mustard), either alone or in combination with radiation therapy, has been associated with an increased incidence of acute myelogenous leukemia in persons treated for Hodgkin's disease, non-Hodgkin's lymphomas, and multiple myeloma. These secondary leukemias are relatively refractory to induction of remission with combination chemotherapy. Secondary leukemia has also been observed in persons who have undergone transplant surgery and have taken immunosuppressive drugs.

Chemical carcinogens associated with lifestyle have also been identified. For example, dietary factors have been demonstrated to play a role in the development of cancer. A major factor is caloric intake. Persons who are overweight have a higher incidence of certain malignant conditions, such as breast and colon cancer. Although evidence does not support dietary factors as capable of genetic alteration, their role is believed to be one of tumor promotion.[2]

Physical carcinogens. Three classifications of physical carcinogens exist: (1) ionizing radiation, (2) ultraviolet radiation, and (3) foreign bodies. Since the turn of the century, it has been known that ionizing radiation can cause cancer in almost any human body tissue. At the present time, the dose of radiation that causes cancer is not known, and there is considerable debate surrounding the effect of exposure to low-dose radiation over a period of time.[2] When cells are exposed to a source of radiation, damage occurs to one or both strands of DNA (see p.179). Certain disorders have been correlated with radiation as a carcinogenic agent:

1. Leukemia, lymphoma, thyroid cancer, and other cancers increased in incidence in the general population of Hiroshima and Nagasaki after the atomic bomb explosions.
2. A higher incidence of bone cancer occurs in persons exposed to radiation in certain occupations, such as radiologists, radiation chemists, and uranium miners.
3. Thyroid cancer has a higher incidence in those persons who have received radiation to the head and neck area for treatment of a variety of disorders, such as acne, tonsillitis, sore throat, or enlarged thyroid gland.
4. A higher incidence of childhood cancer occurs in children exposed to radiation during fetal life.

Ultraviolet radiation has long been associated with squamous or basal cell carcinoma of the skin. Skin cancer is the most common type of cancer among white persons in the United States. Of great concern is the relatively recent increase in the incidence of melanoma, a skin cancer that is much less responsive to treatment. It is the second most rapidly increasing type of cancer in the United States.[1] Though definite evidence of a causal relationship between exposure to sunlight (ultraviolet radiation) and melanoma does not exist, the mounting evidence regarding sunlight exposure is strongly suggestive.[6]

Foreign bodies that are not biodegradable, such as Bakelite disc and cellophane implants, can induce the development of cancer by stimulating reactions to constant tissue damage such as scar formation, thus increasing the probability of neoplastic formations. The exact mechanism of this neoplastic transformation is as yet unknown. However, in general, the greater the surface area of the foreign body, the greater the probability of neoplastic transformation.[2]

Certain DNA and RNA viruses, termed *oncogenic,* can transform the cells they infect and induce malignant transformation. Viruses have been identified as causative agents of cancer in animals. In human beings this causative link has not been proved, since ethical considerations preclude the inoculation of human subjects with viruses that are thought to be cancer-causing agents. A cancer found in human beings, Burkitt's lymphoma, has consistently shown evidence of the presence of the Epstein-Barr virus (EBV) in vitro. This virus is also present in infectious mononucleosis, but the explanation of why an infectious disease develops in some persons and a lymphoma in others is not known.[2] Persons with acquired immunodeficiency syndrome (AIDS), which is caused by a virus, have a very high incidence of Kaposi's sarcoma (see Chapter 8). Other viruses that have been linked to the development of cancer include hepatitis B virus, associated with hepatocellular carcinoma, and human papillomavirus, which is capable of inducing lesions that may progress to squamous cell carcinomas, such as cervical cancers.[7]

Genetic susceptibility. In actuality, none of the specific types of cancer are truly considered hereditary in the Mendelian sense. However, what is inherited in relatively few cases is a strong predisposition to cancer. An example of such an inherited predisposing condition is familial polyposis coli. The incidence of carcinoma of the colon in persons with such a syndrome is 1000 times the average incidence. Several preneoplastic syndromes can be inherited and can increase the probability of certain cancers. Xeroderma pigmentosum is a preneoplastic syndrome that can be a precursor of certain skin cancers, especially with exposure to sunlight.[4]

"Cancer families" have also been identified in which several family members develop one or several specific cancers at a very early age. The specific cancers usually involve the colon and the uterus. Multiple-site cancers or cancers that occur at an early age are thought to have a genetic link. Most authorities believe that the occurrence of cancer in these instances is due to inherited chromosomal abnormalities.

For many years, scientists have searched for genetic patterns in the most common cancer sites. A few patterns have emerged:

1. The incidence of postmenopausal breast cancer is three times higher and the incidence of premenopausal breast cancer is five times higher in women with a family history of this disease. Breast cancer is rare in Asian women and common in American women.
2. The incidence of lung cancer is greater in smokers with a family history of this disease than in smokers without a family history of the disease.
3. The incidence of leukemia is greater in an identical twin of a person with the disease.
4. Neuroblastoma occurs with increased frequency among siblings.

Promotion. A single alteration of the genetic structure of the cell is not sufficient to result in cancer. At least one more mutation must occur in cells in which a mutation has already occurred. The chances of this occurring, given the billions of cells in the human body, seem highly unlikely. However, the odds of cancer development are increased with the presence of promoting agents.[2] *Promotion,* the second stage in the development of cancer, is characterized by the reversible proliferation of the altered, initiated cells and thus, with increasing numbers in the initiated cell population, the likelihood of a second cell mutation occurring is increased.

An important distinction between initiation and promotion is that the activity of promoters is reversible. This is a key concept in cancer prevention. Promoting factors include such agents as dietary fat, high caloric intake, cigarette smoking, and alcohol consumption (Table 9-6). Prolonged stress may also be a promoter. (For a complete discussion of stress, see Chapter 5.) The withdrawal of these factors can reduce the risk of neoplastic formation. This characteristic is giving new insight into the existence of threshold doses for promoters below which these agents cannot exert their effects.

Several promoting agents exert their activity against specific types of body tissues or organs. Therefore, they tend to promote specific kinds of cancer. For example,

Table 9-6 Factors Promoting Cancer Development

Factor	Effect
Age	↑ Incidence of cancer in the very young and in persons over the age of 55 years
Hormones	↑ Progression of endometrial cancer in the presence of estrogen
	↓ Progression of certain cancers with removal of the thyroid, adrenal, ovaries, and/or pituitary gland
Coping potential	↑ Progression of cancer in person with inadequate coping, who exhibits feelings of hopelessness, helplessness, and being out of control (not scientifically proved at the present time)
Dietary fat, high-caloric intake	↑ Incidence and progression of cancer in persons who are 25% or more over their recommended weight
	↑ Incidence and progression of breast and gallbladder cancers in the presence of a high-fat diet
	↑ Incidence and progression of colon cancer in the presence of a low-fiber diet
	↑ Progression of cancer in persons with protein deficiency
Cigarette smoke	↑ Incidence of bronchogenic, esophageal, and bladder cancers
Alcoholic beverages	↑ Incidence of oral, liver, and esophageal cancer
Combination of alcohol consumption and cigarette smoke	↑ Incidence of head, neck, esophageal, and bladder cancer

cigarette smoke is a promoting agent in bronchogenic carcinoma and, in conjunction with alcohol intake, promotes esophageal and bladder cancer. Some carcinogens (complete carcinogens) are capable of both initiating and promoting the development of cancer. Cigarette smoke is an example of a complete carcinogen capable of initiating as well as promoting cancer.

A period of time, ranging from 1½ to 40 years, elapses between the initial genetic alteration and the actual clinical evidence of cancer. This period, termed the *latent period,* is now theorized to comprise both the initiation and the promotion stages in the natural history of cancer.[8] The variation in the length of time that elapses before the cancer becomes clinically evident is associated with the mitotic rate of the tissue of origin and environmental factors.

For the disease process to become clinically evident, the cells must reach a critical mass. A 1 cm tumor (the size usually detectable by palpation) contains 10^9 (1 billion) cancer cells. A 0.5 cm tumor is the smallest that can be detected by current diagnostic measures, such as magnetic resonance imaging (MRI).

Progression. *Progression* is the final stage in the natural history of a cancer. This stage is characterized by increased growth rate of the tumor as well as by increased invasiveness and metastasis. Certain biochemical and morphological alterations also take place during this stage, enabling the tumor to survive and thrive in this primary environment and throughout the process of metastasis.

One possible result of genetic change in tumor cells is that tumor cells begin to produce their own growth factor. The growth of the primary tumor may cause damage within the organ, thus causing the release of growth factor. As the tumor increases in size, it develops its own blood supply. The process of the formation of blood vessels within the tumor itself is called *tumor angiogenesis.* As the tumor grows, it can begin to mechanically invade sur-

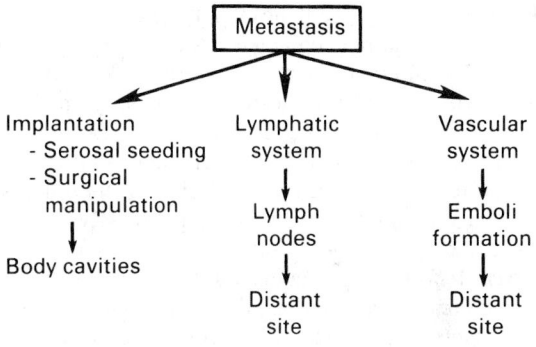

Fig. 9-4 Routes of metastasis.

rounding tissues, growing into those areas of least resistance.[9]

A unique and tragic characteristic of malignant tumor cells is their ability to metastasize or spread to distant parts of the body. *Metastasis* is the major cause of death in persons with cancer. Some cancers metastasize early in the process of development (e.g., premenopausal breast cancer), whereas others spread regionally and rarely metastasize (e.g., glioblastoma multiforme and basal cell carcinoma of the skin). Certain cancers seem to have an affinity for a particular tissue or organ as a site of metastasis; other cancers are unpredictable in their pattern of metastasis. Certain cancers ("seed") require a particular site for proliferation ("soil"). The most frequent sites of metastasis are the lungs, brain, bone, and liver. Most metastatic lesions are multiple and widely disseminated, but a few cancers such as adenocarcinoma of the kidney usually produce a single metastatic lesion.

Metastasis can occur via the (1) vascular system, (2) lymphatic system, and (3) process of implantation (Fig. 9-4).

Vascular spread. Metastasis via the vascular system occurs in a variety of ways:

1. Proliferating cancer cells in draining lymph nodes may enter a large collecting lymphatic vessel, such as the thoracic duct, that empties into the larger veins leading to the heart.
2. Surrounding tissue may be invaded from the primary site of the cancer cells. The cancer cells penetrate the blood vessels and are released into the bloodstream.
3. Cancer cell aggregates are trapped in the small capillaries of the tissues and/or organs.
4. Through the secretion of lytic substances (usually proteases), cancer cells penetrate the walls of the capillary and enter the adjacent tissue where they begin to proliferate.
5. A capillary bed is developed, and the cancer cells in the metastatic site continue to proliferate.

Lymphatic spread. Lymphatic spread occurs in a manner similar to vascular spread. Lymphatic vessels drain all intracellular fluid spaces in the body, conducting particles and fluid into lymph nodes. Cancer cells that break free from tissue or invade a lymph vessel almost always become trapped in the meshwork in the draining lymph node. If these cancer cells proliferate, the result is lymphadenopathy (abnormal enlargement of the lymph node). Continued proliferation may result in the release of cancer cells into the lymph vessel leading from the lymph node to the next lymph node up the chain.

Clinically, prognosis is best when there is no detectable spread to the lymph nodes in the region of the primary tumor. The prognosis becomes poorer when lymph nodes are involved.

Implantation. Implantation may occur when cancer cells become embedded along the serosal surfaces of body organs, such as the peritoneal cavity or the pleural cavity. During surgical procedures, implantation may also occur in the primary organ or the regional area if the environment is suitable.

Mechanisms. It was formerly believed that metastasis was a passive process, with tumor cells breaking off the expanding tumor and being swept through the blood vessels or the lymphatic system to a final resting place in a distant organ. However, it is an active process, involving only a small number of cells within the original tumor. Metastatic tumor cells must be able to penetrate the extracellular matrix surrounding the tumor, burrow through the wall of a nearby blood vessel or lymph canal, and travel to some distant site, where they must again penetrate a vessel or canal wall, settle, and begin to grow into a new tumor.

For the metastatic cells to penetrate vessel walls, they must secrete certain enzymes that dissolve holes in the basement membrane (a tough barrier surrounding tissues and blood vessels). The tumor cells can now migrate through the openings in the membrane. These cells produce their own migration factors, which ultimately attract the cells through the holes in the basement membrane. Once they enter the bloodstream, many metastatic cells are destroyed either by the host's immune system or by mechanical trauma caused by the turbulent flow of blood.

It is clear that an individual metastasis develops from a single cell or a group of identical cells (clone). However, as the metastatic site develops, the cells quickly become more heterogeneous. This change occurs as a result of spontaneous genetic mutations that take place in the tumor cells. The heterogeneous nature of the cells in the metastatic tumor makes it difficult to treat. Surgical removal of metastatic tumors is of value only if there is a small number of tumors. Some cells of heterogeneous, metastatic tumors have the ability to become resistant to chemotherapy and radiation therapy. Biological response modifiers are a promising form of therapy because research indicates that tumor cells do not develop resistance to this type of therapy (see p. 203).

Role of the Immune System

This section is limited to a discussion of the role of the immune system in the recognition and destruction of tumor cells. (For a detailed discussion of immune system function, see Chapter 8.)

Both normal and abnormal cells have a complex array of antigenic determinants (markers) on the surface of their cell membranes as well as within the cells. These antigenic determinants differ from one cell type to another. When foreign cells are transplanted from one individual to another individual, these antigenic determinants elicit an immunological response. This is the basis for rejection of a transplanted organ.

Some cancer cells have changes on their cell surface antigens as a result of malignant transformation. These antigens are called *tumor-associated antigens* (TAA) (Fig. 9-5). A TAA is an antigen that is found on a tumor cell and is undetected on the cells of a normal adult but may be found on normal cells under special circumstances (e.g., fetal antigens that are normally expressed during embryonic development). In addition to the retrogenetic expression of oncofetal antigens, TAA may result from mutations in the cell's DNA (e.g., by chemical carcinogens) or the expression of new genetic material introduced by a virus (e.g., oncogenic DNA or RNA viruses).

It is believed that one of the functions of the immune system is to respond to these tumor-associated antigens. The response of the immune system to antigens of the ma-

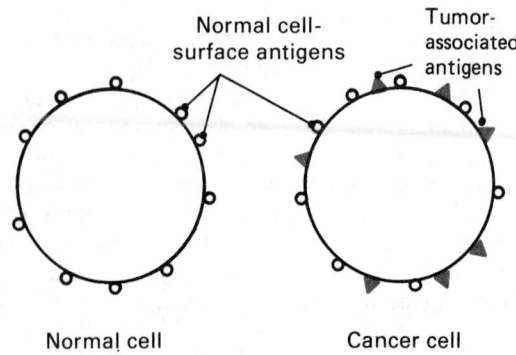

Fig. 9-5 Tumor-associated antigens appear on the cell surface of malignant cells.

lignant cells is called *immunological surveillance*. Lymphocytes are continually checking cell surface antigens and are capable of detecting and destroying cells with abnormal or altered antigenic determinants. It has been proposed that malignant transformation occurs continuously and that the malignant cells are destroyed by the immune response. (The immune system is discussed in Chapter 8.) Under most circumstances, immune surveillance will prevent these transformed cells from developing into clinically detectable tumors.

Virtually every cell type involved in normal immune responses and every effector function used to inactivate or remove antigens has been demonstrated in immune responses to tumors. These immune responses involve (1) T-cytotoxic cells, (2) natural killer cells, (3) macrophages, and (4) B lymphocytes.

T-cytotoxic cells are thought by many to play the dominant role in in vivo resistance to tumor growth. These cells are capable of killing tumor cells that express antigens for which they are specific. In addition to their cytotoxic function, T cells are also very important in the production of lymphokines (e.g., interleukin-2 and γ-interferon), which stimulate T cells, natural killer cells, B cells, and macrophages.

Natural killer (NK) cells are able to directly lyse tumor cells spontaneously without any prior sensitization. These cells are stimulated by γ-interferon and interleukin-2 (released from T cells), resulting in increased cytotoxic activity and cell growth.

Monocytes and *macrophages* have several important roles in tumor immunity (Fig. 9-6). Macrophages can be activated by γ-interferon (produced by T cells) to become nonspecifically lytic for tumor cells. Macrophages also secrete cytokines including (1) interleukin-1,[10] (2) α-interferon, (3) tumor necrosis factor (TNF), and (4) colony-stimulating factors. The release of interleukin-1, coupled with the presentation of the processed antigen, stimulates T-lymphocyte activation and production. α-Interferon augments the killing ability of NK cells.[11] Tumor necrosis factor causes hemorrhagic necrosis of tumors and exerts

cytocidal or cytostatic actions against tumor cells. Finally, colony-stimulating factors regulate the production of various blood cells in the bone marrow.[12]

B lymphocytes may produce specific antibodies that bind to tumor cells and may kill these cells by complement fixation and lysis (see Chapter 7). These antibodies are often detectable in the serum and saliva of the client. In some persons, antibodies that are apparently specific for both the person's own tumor and a similar tumor in other persons have been found.

Certain groups of people have a higher incidence of cancer than the general population.[13] Cancer occurs in nearly 10% of children with congenital immunodeficiencies. These cancers are derived primarily from cells of the lymphoid system. Persons receiving high doses of immunosuppressive drugs have an 80- to 100-fold increased risk of developing cancer. The types of cancer found in immunosuppressed persons are primarily epithelial or lymphoid in origin. These findings are mostly reported in persons treated with immunosuppressive agents for transplanted kidneys (see Chapter 41).

Other groups at an increased risk of cancer are the very young and older adults. In the very young person the immune system is immature. The incidence of cancer increases dramatically in persons 40 to 60 years of age. The reasons for this are not known. It is possible that their immunological surveillance system is working less effectively. It is also known that the thymus undergoes involution and atrophy with aging. In addition, the functional efficiency of T cells decreases with aging.

Escape mechanisms from immunological surveillance. Tumor development has often been referred to as *immunological escape*. In many persons with cancer, there is evidence of an active immunological response, and yet the tumor survives. Some theoretical explanations for immunological escape that have been proposed follow.

Sneaking through. The process of sneaking through is thought to occur when the cell-surface antigens are weak. Cancer cells in the early phase of growth may not excite an immunological response because the transformed cell-

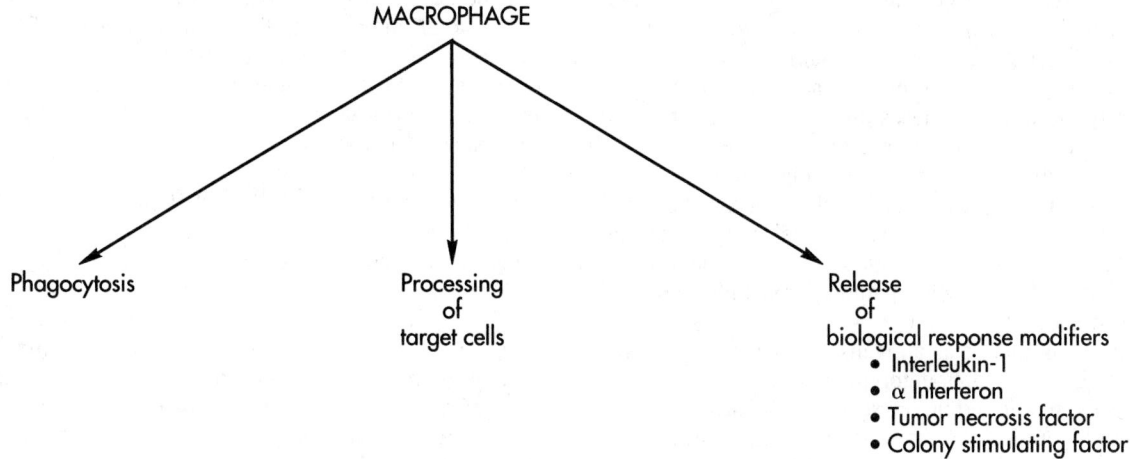

Fig. 9-6   Macrophage functioning in response to malignant target cells.

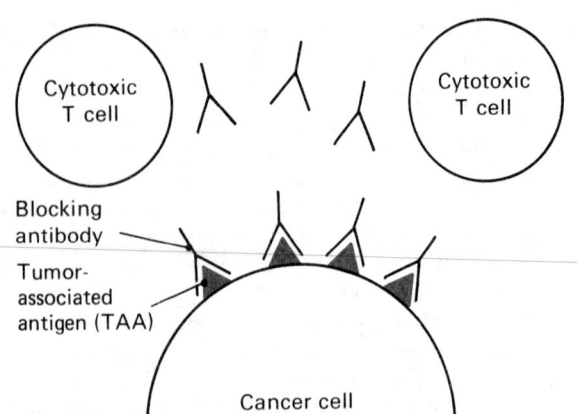

Fig. 9-7 Blocking antibodies prevent the T cells from interacting with tumor-associated antigens and destroying the malignant cell.

surface markers are of low antigenicity. By the time the immune system is alerted, the cancer is well established and too large for the immune system to destroy.

Antigenic modulation. The malignant cell has the ability to change or lose antigenic determinants during or after a response by the immune system. The cell may then express a new set of antigens. This process is known as *antigenic modulation*. The new set of antigens on the malignant cell fails to adequately stimulate the immune system.

Overwhelming antigen exposure. Cancers may escape attack by flooding the body with tumor antigen. The antigens bind to specific antibodies or to receptors on lymphocytes and prevent them from recognizing and destroying the cancer cells. The excess of antigens paralyzes the host immune system. Therefore, tumor growth is enhanced.

Blocking factors. Blocking factors may prevent attack of the tumor-associated antigens by T lymphocytes. For example, blocking antibodies may bind with TAA and prevent their recognition by T cells (Fig. 9-7). Another possibility is that free antigen produced and released by the malignant cell may bind with the T cell and prevent it from recognizing the malignant cell. These blocking factors related to the immune system may actually enhance tumor growth. This is known as *immunological enhancement*.

Oncofetal antigens. Oncofetal antigens, also called *carcinofetal antigens*, represent a type of tumor antigen. They are found on the surfaces and inside cancer cells as well as fetal cells. These antigens are an expression of the shift of cancerous cells to a more immature metabolic pathway, one usually associated with embryonic or fetal periods of life. The reappearance of fetal antigens in malignant disease is not well understood, but it is believed to occur as a result of the cell regaining the cellular potential that it once had.

Examples of oncofetal antigens are carcinoembryonic antigen (CEA) and alpha-fetoprotein (AFP). Carcinoembryonic antigen is found on the surfaces of cancer cells derived from the gastrointestinal tract as well as normal cells from the fetal gut, liver, and pancreas. Normally, it disappears during the last 3 months of fetal life. CEA was orig-

inally isolated from colon cancer. However, elevated CEA levels have also been found in nonmalignant conditions (e.g., cirrhosis of the liver, ulcerative colitis, and heavy smoking). Presently, the major value of CEA is its use as an indicator of the success of cancer treatment. For example, the persistence of elevated preoperative CEA titers after surgery indicates that the tumor was not completely removed. A rise in CEA levels after chemotherapy or radiation therapy may indicate recurrence or spread of the cancer.

AFP is produced by malignant liver cells as well as fetal liver cells. AFP levels have also been found to be elevated in testicular carcinoma, viral hepatitis, and nonmalignant liver disorders. AFP is of diagnostic value in primary cancer of the liver (hepatoma), but it is also produced when metastatic liver growth occurs. The detection of AFP is of value in tumor detection and determination of tumor progression.

Other examples of oncofetal antigens currently being studied are fetal sulfated glycopeptide found in gastric carcinoma, pregnancy-specific β_1-glycoprotein (SP$_1$) found in testicular cancer, human chorionic gonadotropin (HCG), CA-125 found in ovarian carcinoma, CA-19-9 found in pancreatic cancer, and pancreatic oncofetal antigen (POA) found in pancreatic and lung cancers.

Virus-induced antigens. Tumor-associated antigens may be induced by certain viruses. In experimental animals, DNA and RNA viruses induce unique nuclear and cell-surface antigens in cells. Establishing these findings in human beings is difficult. The DNA viruses include various herpesviruses and adenovirus. The three major candidates for human DNA virus–induced tumors are Burkitt's lymphoma, nasopharyngeal carcinoma, and cancer of the cervix. RNA viruses have been correlated with leukemia in mice and other animals as well as with mouse mammary tumors. Presently, conclusive evidence that human leukemia is a virus-induced disease does not exist.

CLASSIFICATION OF CANCER

Tumors can be classified according to: *anatomical site, histological analysis* (grading), and *extent of disease* (staging). Tumor classification systems are intended to provide a standardized way (1) to communicate the status of the cancer to all members of the health care team, (2) to assist in determining the most effective treatment plan, (3) to evaluate the treatment plan, (4) to serve as a factor in determining the prognosis, and (5) to compare like groups for statistical purposes.

Anatomical Site Classification

In the anatomical classification of tumors the tumor is identified by the tissue of origin, the anatomical site, and the behavior of the tumor (i.e., benign or malignant) (Table 9-7). *Carcinomas* originate from embryonal ectoderm (skin and glands) and endoderm (mucous membrane linings of the respiratory tract, gastrointestinal tract, and genitourinary tract). *Sarcomas* originate from embryonal mesoderm (connective tissue, muscle, bone, and fat). Lymphomas and leukemias originate from the hematopoietic system.

Table 9-7 Anatomical Classification of Tumors

Site	Benign	Malignant
EPITHELIAL TISSUE TUMORS*	**-OMA**	**-CARCINOMA**
Surface epithelium	Papilloma	Carcinoma
Glandular epithelium	Adenoma	Adenocarcinoma
CONNECTIVE TISSUE TUMORS†	**-OMA**	**-SARCOMA**
Fibrous tissue	Fibroma	Fibrosarcoma
Cartilage	Chondroma	Chondrosarcoma
Striated muscle	Rhabdomyoma	Rhabdomyosarcoma
Bone	Osteoma	Osteosarcoma
NERVOUS TISSUE TUMORS‡	**-OMA**	**-OMA**
Meninges	Meningioma	Meningeal sarcoma
Nerve cells	Ganglioneuroma	Neuroblastoma
HEMATOPOIETIC TISSUE TUMORS		
Lymphoid tissue	—	Hodgkin's disease, malignant lymphoma
Plasma cells		Multiple myeloma
Bone marrow		Lymphocytic and myelogenous leukemia

*Body surfaces, lining of body cavities, and glandular structures.
†Supporting tissue, fibrotic tissues, and blood vessels.
‡Brain nerves and retina.

Histological Analysis Classification

In histological grading of tumors the appearance of cells and their degree of differentiation are evaluated. For many tumor cells, four grades are used:

Grade I: Cells differ slightly from normal cells (mild dysplasia) and are well differentiated.

Grade II: Cells are more abnormal (moderate dysplasia) and moderately differentiated.

Grade III: Cells are very abnormal (severe dysplasia) and poorly differentiated.

Grade IV: Cells are immature and primitive (anaplasia) and undifferentiated; cell of origin is difficult to determine.

Extent of Disease Classification

The extent of disease classification is often called *staging.* This classification system is based on a description of the extent of the disease rather than on cell appearance. Although there are similarities in the staging of cancers, there are many differences based on a thorough knowledge of the natural history of each specific type of cancer.

Clinical staging. The clinical staging classification system determines the extent of the disease process of cancer by stages:

Stage 0: Cancer in situ

Stage I: Tumor limited to the tissue of origin: localized tumor growth

Stage II: Limited local spread

Stage III: Extensive local and regional spread

Stage IV: Metastasis

This classification system has been used as a basis for staging in cancer of the cervix (see Chapter 48) and non-Hodgkin's lymphoma (Table 25-33).

Table 9-8 TNM Classification System

PRIMARY TUMOR (T)

T_0	No evidence of primary tumor
T_{is}	Carcinoma in situ
T_{1-4}	Ascending degrees of increase in tumor size and involvement

REGIONAL LYMPH NODES (N)

N_0	No evidence of disease in lymph nodes
N_{1-4}	Ascending degrees of nodal involvement
N_x	Regional lymph nodes unable to be assessed clinically

DISTANT METASTASES (M)

M_0	No evidence of distant metastases
M_{1-4}	Ascending degrees of metastatic involvement of the host, including distant nodes

TNM classification system. The TNM classification system represents the standardization of the clinical staging of cancer by the International Union against Cancer (IUCC). This classification system (Table 9-8) is used to determine the extent of the disease process of cancer according to three parameters: tumor size (T), degree of regional spread to the lymph nodes (N), and absence of metastasis (M). (This system has been applied to cancer of the breast in Chapter 46.)

Staging of the disease can be done initially and at several intervals. Clinical diagnostic staging is done at the time of diagnosis to determine the most effective treatment

Table 9-9 Karnofsky Performance Scale

100	Normal, no complaints, no evidence of disease
90	Ability to carry on normal activity, minor signs or symptoms of disease
80	Normal activity with effort, some signs or symptoms of disease
70	Ability to care for self, inability to carry on normal activity or do active work
60	Occasional assistance necessary but ability to care for most needs
50	Considerable assistance and frequent medical care necessary
40	Disabled, special care and assistance necessary
30	Severely disabled, indication for hospitalization although death not imminent
20	Very sick, hospitalization necessary, active supportive treatment necessary
10	Moribund, fatal processes progressing rapidly
0	Dead

plan. Examples of diagnostic studies that may be performed to assess for spread of disease include bone and liver scans, ultrasonography, computerized tomography (CT) scans, and MRI.

Surgical evaluative staging is used to describe the extent of the disease process after biopsy or surgical exploration. For example, a laparotomy and a splenectomy may be performed in staging of Hodgkin's disease. During a staging laparotomy, areas of lymph node biopsy and margins of any masses may be marked with metal clips. These clips are used as markers when radiotherapy is used as a treatment modality.

Postsurgical treatment pathological staging is used after pathological examination of the surgical specimen. The presence of residual tumor should be recorded at this time. The stages are R_0, no residual tumor; R_1, microscopic residual tumor; and R_2, macroscopic residual tumor.

After the extent of the disease is determined, the stage classification is not changed. The original description of the extent of the tumor remains part of the original record. If additional treatment is needed, or if treatment fails, re-treatment staging is done to determine the extent of the disease process at the time of re-treatment.

Carcinoma in situ is a commonly used term in classification of cancer. It is defined as a lesion with all the histological features of cancer except invasion. If left untreated, carcinoma in situ will eventually become invasive.

In addition to tumor classification systems, there are also classification systems used to describe the status of the client with cancer. The status of the client is recorded at the time of diagnosis, treatment, and re-treatment and at each follow-up examination. The Karnofsky performance scale is an example of a method used to evaluate the performance status of the client (Table 9-9).

PREVENTION AND DETECTION OF CANCER

The nurse plays a prominent role in the prevention and detection of cancer. Early detection and prompt treatment are directly responsible for increased survival rates in clients with cancer. One important aspect is to educate the public to do the following:

1. Reduce or avoid exposure to known or suspected carcinogens and cancer-promoting agents.
2. Eat a balanced diet that includes vegetables (green, yellow, and orange), fresh fruits, whole grains, adequate amounts of fiber, and low levels of fats and preservatives.
3. Participate in a regular exercise regimen.
4. Obtain adequate, consistent periods of rest (at least 6 to 8 hours per night).
5. Have a health examination on a consistent basis; this should include a health history, a physical examination, and specific diagnostic tests for common cancers in accordance with the guidelines published by the American Cancer Society (Table 9-10).
6. Eliminate, reduce, or change the perceptions of stressors and increase the ability to cope with stressors.
7. Enjoy consistent periods of relaxation and leisure.
8. Know the seven warning signs of cancer as identified by the American Cancer Society (Table 9-11).
9. Learn and practice self-examination (e.g., breast self-examination and testicular examination).
10. Seek immediate medical care if cancer is suspected. Early detection of cancer has a positive impact on prognosis.

When the public is educated regarding the disease process of cancer, care should be taken to minimize the fear that surrounds cancer. Tactics that increase fear should never be used. The facts should be taught in an accurate, low-key manner at the level of the learner. The goal of public education is to *motivate* the learner to change the pattern of behavior as necessary to achieve and maintain an optimal state of health. The nurse can play a significant role in meeting this goal. Although the general public must be taught, those who are at an increased risk of cancer are the target population for effective cancer control (Table 9-10). The nurse can have a definite impact in convincing people that a change in lifestyle patterns will have a positive influence on health. If the nurse is to have a significant impact, the challenge needs to be recognized and strategies must be developed to teach effectively (see Chapter 6).

Diagnosis

When a client is admitted to a health care agency with the possible diagnosis of cancer, it is a very stressful time for the client and the family. The client typically undergoes several days of diagnostic studies. During this time the fear of the unknown is often more stressful than ultimately being told of a positive diagnosis of cancer.

During the time the client is waiting for the results of the diagnostic studies, the nurse needs to be available to

Table 9-10 Screening for Specific Cancer Sites

High-Risk Profile	Screening	Medium- and Low-Risk Profile	Screening
LUNG CANCER			
History of 20 pack-years of smoking (1 pack a day for 20 years); exposure to airborne carcinogens, especially asbestos, uranium, hydrocarbons; age range 40 to 80 years; chronic lung disease	Early detection method not available; annual chest x-rays (advised by some physicians); observation by client for change in respiratory status: increased frequency of infections and change in cough, sputum, breathing, voice	History of less than 20 pack-years of smoking, nonsmokers, former smokers after 10 years	Early detection method not available
COLON AND RECTAL CANCER			
History of familial polyposis, ulcerative colitis, Crohn's disease; personal or family history of colon or rectal cancer; diet high in fat and low in fiber; age range 40 to 75 years	Guaiac test on stools and digital rectal examination annually after age 40; sigmoidoscopic examination every 3 to 5 years beginning at age 40 based on advice of physician; observation by client for changes in bowel pattern: diarrhea, constipation, pain, flatus, black tarry stools, bleeding	Persons with no known risk factors	Guaiac test on stools and digital rectal examination annually after age 40; sigmoidoscopy as a baseline at age 50; after two normal examinations, repeated proctosigmoidoscopic examination every 3 to 5 years
PROSTATIC CANCER			
Presence of prostatic hypertrophy, presence of prostatic infection, black, increased risk with age	Rectal examination every year; observation by client for dysuria, blood in urine, difficulty in producing stream of urine	Presence of one risk factor, excluding age	Rectal examination annually after age 40
CERVICAL CANCER			
Early intercourse (before age 20) with multiple partners, poor personal hygiene, history of herpesvirus type II infection, cervical dysplasia	Pap test and pelvic examination every year for those who are or have been sexually active or who have reached age 18; colposcopy if suspicious area is noted; observation by client for abnormal vaginal bleeding or discharge, pain or bleeding with sexual intercourse	No known risk factors	Pap test and pelvic examination every year after age 18; after 3 or more normal examinations in a row, at least every 3 years
ENDOMETRIAL CANCER			
Infertility, ovarian dysfunction, obesity, uterine bleeding, estrogen therapy over long period of time, diabetes, age range 30 to 80 years	Pap test every year; pelvic examination every year; endometrial biopsy every year for women at menopause and at high risk; observation by client for abnormal uterine bleeding, pain, change in menstrual pattern	Presence of one risk factor, excluding estrogen therapy, over long period of time	Pap test and pelvic examination, endometrial tissue sample at menopause

Based on the American Cancer Society 1988 Recommendations.[14]

Continued.

Table 9-10 Screening for Specific Cancer Sites—cont'd

High-Risk Profile	Screening	Medium- and Low-Risk Profile	Screening
SKIN CANCER			
Prolonged exposure to sun; previous radiation exposure; fair, thin skin; positive family history of dysplastic nevus syndrome (DNS)	Self-examination monthly; physical examination every year; observation by client for sore that does not heal, change in wart or mole	Presence of one risk factor, excluding prolonged exposure to sun	Self-examination, physical examination each year
BREAST CANCER			
White, early menarche, late menopause, fibrocystic breast disease, infertility, over age 30 for first pregnancy, personal history of breast cancer, mother or sister with history of breast cancer, obesity, age range 35 to 65 years	Monthly breast self-examination; breast examination by health professional every 3 years for women age 20 to 40 and every year after age 40; baseline mammogram between ages 35 and 40, every 1 to 2 years between ages 40 and 49, and every year after age 50; observation by client for lump or thickening discharge from nipple, pain in breast	Excluding family history of breast cancer, fewer than two risk factors	Monthly breast self-examination; breast examination by health professional every year; baseline mammogram between ages 35 and 40, every 1 to 2 years for women aged 40 to 49 years, and every year after age 50

Table 9-11 Seven Warning Signs of Cancer

C hange in bowel or bladder habits
A sore that does not heal
U nusual bleeding or discharge from any body orifice
T hickening or a lump in the breast or elsewhere
I ndigestion or difficulty in swallowing
O bvious change in a wart or mole
N agging cough or hoarseness

actively listen to the client's concerns. False reassurance that everything will be all right is inappropriate and is an effective way to shut off further communication with the client. During this time of high anxiety the client may need repeated explanations regarding the diagnostic workup. Explanations should include as much information as is needed by the client and the family, should be given in clear, understandable terms, and should be reinforced as necessary.

A diagnostic plan for the person in whom cancer is suspected includes a health history, identification of risk factors, physical examination, and specific diagnostic studies. (The specifics of the health history and the screening physical examination are presented in Chapter 3.)

The health history includes particular emphasis on risk factors, such as family history of cancer, exposure to or use of known carcinogens (e.g., cigarette smoking and exposure to occupational pollutants or chemicals), diseases characterized by chronic irritation (e.g., ulcerative colitis), and drug ingestion (e.g., hormone therapy). Other important information relates to dietary habits, ingestion of alcohol, lifestyle, and patterns and degree of coping with perceived stressors.

The physical examination should be thorough, and attention should be given to the respiratory system, the gastrointestinal system (including colon, rectum, and liver), the lymphatic system (including the spleen), breasts, skin, the reproductive system of the male (testicles, prostate gland) and of the female (cervix, uterus, ovary), and the musculoskeletal and neurological systems.

Diagnostic studies to be performed will depend on the suspected primary or metastatic site(s) of the cancer. (Specific procedures as they relate to each body system are discussed in the respective assessment chapters.) Examples of diagnostic studies related to cancer detection include the following:

1. Cytology studies (e.g., Pap smear)
2. Chest x-ray study
3. Complete blood count
4. Proctoscopic examination
5. Liver function studies
6. Radiographic studies (e.g., mammogram)
7. Radioisotope scans (liver, brain, bone, lung)
8. CT scan
9. Presence of oncofetal antigens such as CEA, AFP, and POA
10. Bone marrow examination (if a hematolymphoid malignancy is suspected)
11. Lymphangiography (if a lymphoid cancer is suspected)
12. Biopsy

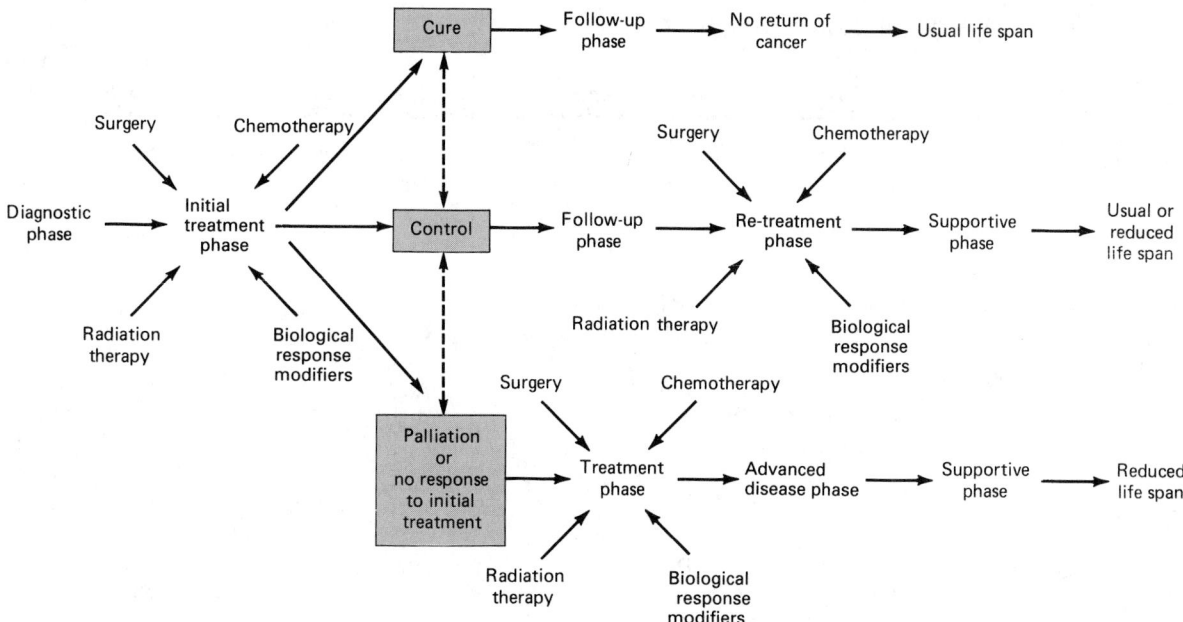

Fig. 9-8 Goals of cancer treatment.

Biopsy. The biopsy procedure is the definitive means of diagnosing cancer. It involves the histological examination by a pathologist of a piece of tissue from the suspicious area. A biopsy is essential to planning of a treatment regimen for the client. A biopsy will determine (1) whether the tissue is benign or malignant, (2) the anatomical tissue from which the tumor arises, and (3) the degree of cellular differentiation of the cancer cells present in the tumor.

The procedure may be a *needle biopsy,* an *incisional biopsy,* or an *excisional biopsy.* A needle biopsy specimen can be obtained by aspiration (e.g., bone marrow aspiration) or by the use of a large-bore needle. These needles are used in obtaining samples of prostate gland, breast, liver, and kidney tissues.

Incisional biopsy performed with a scalpel or dermal punch is a common technique used for making a diagnosis of cancer. The premise that incisional biopsy may contribute to the spread of cancer has not been proved.

Excisional biopsy involves removal of the entire tumor. It is usually used for small tumors (less than 2 cm in size), skin lesions, intestinal polyps, and breast tumors. This procedure can be considered therapeutic as well as diagnostic. Often when a tumor is not easily accessible, a major surgical procedure (laparotomy, thoracotomy, craniotomy) is necessary to obtain a piece of the tumor tissue. Biopsy specimens of the gastrointestinal, respiratory, and genitourinary systems can usually be obtained by endoscopic procedures.

TREATMENT
Goals and Modalities

The goal of cancer treatment is *cure, control,* or *palliation* (Fig. 9-8). Factors that determine the treatment modality are the cell type of the cancer, the location and size of the tumor, and the extent of the disease. The physiolog-

ical and psychological status and the expressed needs of the client also have an important part in determining the treatment plan. These factors influence the modalities chosen for treatment and the length of time the treatment is administered.

When caring for the client with cancer, the nurse should know the goals of the treatment plan to appropriately communicate with and support the client. When cure is the goal, it is expected that after treatment the client will be free of disease and will have a normal life span. Many kinds of cancer have the potential to go into permanent remission with an initial course of treatment or with treatment that extends for several weeks, months, or years. Basal cell carcinoma of the skin is usually cured by surgical removal of the lesion or by several weeks of radiation therapy. Acute lymphocytic leukemia (ALL) in children has the potential for cure. The treatment plan for ALL includes the administration of several chemotherapy drugs on a scheduled basis over a time span of 6 months to several years. Some forms of testicular cancer are also treated for cure.

Until a few years ago, a 5-year disease-free period was thought to be indicative of a cancer cure. This is not true for all cancers. Clients with tumors that have a rapid mitotic rate (e.g., testicular cancer) are considered in remission if cancer is not detected in a 2-year time span. Clients with tumors that have a slower mitotic rate (e.g., postmenopausal breast cancer) need 20 or more disease-free years before they can be considered cured of cancer.

Control is the goal of the treatment plan for many cancers that are considered to be chronic. The client undergoes the initial course of therapy and either is continued on maintenance therapy for a period of time or is followed closely so that early signs and symptoms of recurrence can be detected. These cancers are usually not cured, but they

Table 9-12 Treatment Modalities Used in Cancer

Original Cancer	Surgery	Radiotherapy	Chemotherapy	Biological Response Modifiers
Breast (Stage I)	P	Adj, I	Adj, I	ND
Ovary (Stage I)	P	Adj, I	Adj, I	I
Uterine cervix				
Stage II	P	P	I	ND
Lung				
Small (oat) cell	NU	Adj, I	P	I
Adenocarcinoma	P	Adj	I	I
Gastrointestinal				
Colon	P	Adj	Adj, I	I
Stomach	P	Adj	Adj	ND
Melanoma				
Stage I	P	I	I	I
Head and neck	P	P	I	I
Testes				
Seminoma (Stage I)	P	P	Adj	ND
Prostate	P	Alt	I	ND
Kidney	P	Adj, I	I	I
Brain	P	Alt, I	I	I
Lymphomas				
Hodgkin's disease				
Stage I	NU	P	Adj	ND
Stage III	NU	Alt	P	ND

P, Considered an integral part of standard primary treatment programs. *Alt,* An alternate, although less commonly used, method of primary treatment for which data are already available indicating results equivalent to more common approaches. *Adj,* Adjuvant therapy used after localized tumor is treated by a primary method; routine use is not considered essential. *I,* Investigational. The role in treatment is under examination in controlled clinical trials. Either a new approach to treatment or an older approach, which in the absence of sufficient data to support its frequent use, is being evaluated in controlled clinical trials. *NU,* No use in primary treatment program. Control rate of tumor in question may be sufficiently high with other forms of treatment to preclude testing of this modality. *ND,* No data available to evaluate this form of treatment.

are controlled by therapy for long periods of time. They are controlled in a manner similar to other chronic illnesses, such as diabetes mellitus, chronic lung disease, and congestive heart failure. An example of this type of cancer is chronic lymphocytic leukemia (see Chapter 25).

Palliation can also be a goal of the treatment plan. With this treatment goal, relief of symptoms and the maintenance of a high quality of life are the primary goals rather than cure or control of the disease process. Radiation therapy given to relieve the pain of bone metastasis is an example of treatment with a goal of palliation.

The goals of cure, control, and palliation are achieved through the use of four treatment modalities for cancer: surgery, radiation therapy, chemotherapy, and biological response modifiers. Surgery, radiation therapy, and chemotherapy can be used alone or in any combination in the initial treatment phase as well as in the re-treatment phase(s) of cancer. Biological response modifiers are currently being investigated for use alone or in combination with other treatment modalities.

In many cancer sites, two or more of the treatment modalities are used to achieve the goal of cure or control for a long period of time. Table 9-12 gives examples of the use of the treatment modalities to achieve cure or control of the disease process of cancer.

Clinical Trials

A clinical trial is a research study conducted with clients and is usually designed with the intent of evaluating new treatments. The evaluation of treatments in cancer research begins in the laboratory and with animal studies. From these studies, those treatments determined to be most effective, with reasonable levels of toxicity, are further evaluated in a series of studies on clients with cancer. New drugs or treatments, evaluated for the first time in human beings, usually go through three phases:

Phase I clinical trials: Determine dosage and route of administration of an agent and assess potential toxicities.

Phase II clinical trials: Evaluate the effect of a particular treatment on various types of cancer.

Phase III clinical trials: Compare the new treatment with standard therapy to determine which is more effective and which is associated with less morbidity.

Phase I clinical trials of biological response modifiers may be further delineated into phase I-A and phase I-B. Phase I-A clinical trials investigate the toxicity and maximum-tolerated dose of the biological response modifier agent. The intent of phase I-B clinical trials is to determine the optimum biological response modifying dose.

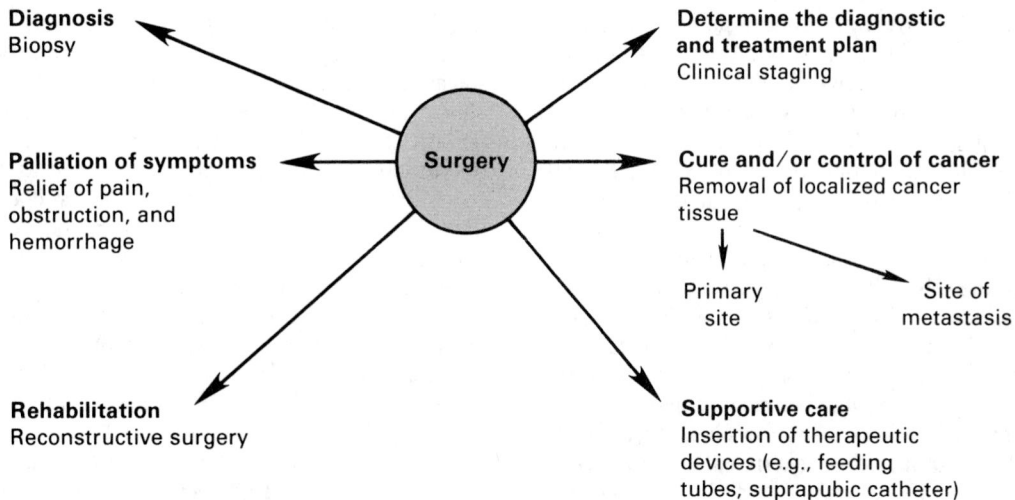

Fig. 9-9   Role of surgery in the treatment of cancer.

The rights of clients who participate in clinical trials are closely guarded by institutional review boards (IRBs) in each agency conducting such research. IRBs not only review clinical trials at their inception but continue to review and monitor the study until its completion. Informed consent is a process in which information is fully disclosed to the client by a physician and a nurse regarding the nature of the treatment being evaluated and the potential risks and benefits of entering the clinical trial. Clients must understand that they may elect to leave a clinical trial at any time.

Surgical Interventions

Surgery is the oldest form of cancer treatment and for many years it was the only effective method of cancer diagnosis and treatment. The treatment of choice for many years was to remove the cancer and as much of the surrounding tissue as possible. Therefore, most of the surgical procedures used were considered to be radical in nature. In the mid-1950s, it was statistically observed that even though the radical procedures were technically sophisticated, the mortality rates associated with certain cancer sites were not improving (e.g., breast cancer). Many cancers that were thought to be local disease processes were found to be systemic diseases with metastatic lesions located in anatomical sites other than the site of the primary disease. On analysis of these statistics, it became obvious that surgery alone, regardless of the extent of the procedure, was not an effective treatment for every type of cancer. Presently, surgery plays several roles in the diagnosis and treatment of cancer (Fig. 9-9).

Cure and control. Several principles are applicable when surgery is used to cure or control the disease process of cancer:

1. Cancer that arises from a tissue with a slow rate of cellular proliferation or replication is most amenable to surgical treatment.
2. A margin of normal tissue must surround the tumor at the time of resection.

3. Only as much tissue as necessary is removed and adjuvant therapy is used. The present trend among health care personnel is toward less radical surgery.
4. Preventive measures are used to reduce the surgical seeding of cancer cells.
5. The usual sites of regional spread may be surgically removed.

Examples of surgical procedures used for cure or control of cancer include radical neck dissection, lumpectomy, mastectomy, pneumonectomy, thyroidectomy, and bowel resection.

A *debulking procedure* may be used if the tumor cannot be completely removed (e.g., is attached to a vital organ). When this occurs, as much as possible of the tumor is removed and the client is given chemotherapy and/or radiation therapy. This type of surgical procedure makes the adjuvant therapy more effective.

Supportive care. Surgical procedures can also be used to provide supportive care throughout the disease process of cancer. Examples of supportive surgical procedures include the following:

1. Insertion of feeding tubes in the esophagus or stomach
2. Creation of a colostomy to allow a rectal abscess to heal
3. Suprapubic cystostomy for clients with advanced prostatic cancer

Palliation of symptoms. When cure or control of cancer is no longer possible, the quality of life must be maintained at the highest possible level for the longest possible period of time. Examples of surgical procedures done for palliative care include the following:

1. Relief of pain by a cordotomy or rhizotomy (see Chapter 51)
2. Colostomy for the relief of a bowel obstruction (see Chapter 38)
3. Laminectomy for the relief of a spinal cord compression (see Chapter 54)

Rehabilitative management. Cancer surgery often mutilates and produces a change in the body image. It is often difficult for the client to cope with this while attempting to maintain usual lifestyle patterns. As the treatment for certain cancers becomes more effective, the length of time the client must live with an alteration created by surgery will be increased. If quality of life is to be maintained, the body image must be one that the client is able to accept and cope with on a daily basis. A greater emphasis has been placed on the rehabilitative role of surgery in cancer care to increase the quality of life. Mammoplasty after a mastectomy is an example of a rehabilitative surgical procedure. The new appliances and the care of ostomies are other major focuses of rehabilitative management.

A nursing challenge is to assist the client to think of cancer as a chronic rather than a terminal illness. Many people with chronic illnesses, such as arthritis and diabetes mellitus, learn to cope with their disease and live a high quality of life. This is also the goal for the person with cancer.

Radiation Therapy*

Radiation therapy is a local treatment modality for cancer that can be administered externally (brachytherapy). The route of administration depends on the cell type; the location, size, and age of the cancer; the client being treated; and the current thinking regarding the most effective treatment plan for the specific cancer. Radiation therapy is a frequently used treatment modality. It is estimated that more than 50% of clients with cancer will be treated with radiation therapy.

Radiation is the emission of tiny particles or waves of energy from radioactive sources. Radiation from these sources has the ability to release electrons from the outer shell of an atom. This process changes the atom to an ionized state. When living cells become ionized, physical and chemical changes occur within the cells.

Types. Radiation therapy is the clinical use of various forms of ionizing radiation. Two types of radiation used in the treatment of cancer are (1) electromagnetic radiation (gamma rays and x rays) and (2) particulate radiation (alpha particles, beta particles, protons, neutrons, and pi mesons). Gamma rays and x rays, which have similar properties, are produced when electrons are liberated from their orbits in an x-ray vacuum tube or during nuclear disintegration (e.g., cobalt 60 and radium). Radium is an example of naturally occurring radiation. Artificial radioactive isotopes such as cobalt 60 are produced in a nuclear reactor. The range and penetration of gamma rays and x-rays are great, and dense material such as lead or concrete is necessary to shield tissue from this type of radiation. Electromagnetic radiation is used extensively in radiation therapy.

Particulate radiation has characteristics that are different from those of electromagnetic radiation. The depth to which these particles can penetrate depends on the energy with which they are propelled and the density of the substance to be penetrated. A thin sheet of paper or a piece of cloth will stop all alpha rays, and a piece of wood or plastic will stop beta rays. The other particulates are stopped by substances of a higher density, such as lead or concrete. Protons and negative pi mesons produce denser ionizing beams, transfer energy to a smaller area, and produce a greater effect on tumor and normal tissue.

Measurement. Several different units are used to measure radiation (Table 9-13). Grays and centigrays are the units currently used in clinical practice.

Detection. Special methods are available to detect the presence of radiation. The film badge is the most familiar device for detecting radiation, and it is widely used to monitor the exposure of health care personnel to radiation in the work setting. Radiation causes a change in the density of the film, which is detected when the film is processed. The film is then compared to film of known radiation exposure to determine the amount of radiation exposure experienced by the person wearing the badge.

The film badge is a monitoring device and offers no protection from radiation for the person wearing it. Nurses who are exposed to sources of radiation in the work setting must do the following:

1. Wear the film badge at all times during the time of potential or actual exposure to a source of radiation.
2. Keep the badge away from sources of heat or moisture, since these substances will alter the validity of the film reading.
3. Wear only the film badge that has been assigned to them. Personnel must not interchange film badges, since the film badge provides the only record of exposure to radiation over time.

Pocket dosimeters are also used to record exposure. These instruments register visually with each successive period of contact; therefore, they can be passed among caregivers. They are less expensive and must be read and documented after each contact.

An instrument used to measure the amount of ionizing radiation present in the environment is the Geiger-Müller

*This section was reviewed by Linda A. Dudjak, R.N., M.S.N., Instructor, Medical-Surgical Nursing, University of Pittsburgh, and Clinical Director, Inpatient Services, Pittsburgh Cancer Institute, Pittsburgh, Pennsylvania.

Table 9-13 Measurement of Radiation

Unit	Definition
Curie (Ci)	A measure of the number of atoms of a particular radioisotope that disintegrate in 1 second
Roentgen (R)	A measure of the radiation required to produce a standard number of ions in air; a unit of exposure to radiation
Rad	Measurement of radiation dosage absorbed by the tissues
Rem	Measurement of the biological effectiveness of various forms of radiation on the human cell (1 rem = 1 rad)
Gray (Gy)	100 rads = 1 Gy

detector. This instrument is used to determine the presence of a source of radiation and to measure the levels of radiation. When an internal source of radiation is used in the treatment of a client, a Geiger detector is always used to determine whether the radiation source has been dislodged or whether the entire source of radiation has been removed on completion of treatment.

Effect on cells. The interaction of radiation with human cells results in a variety of biological effects. Radiation interacts with the molecules of the tissues and produces activated molecules through the processes of excitation and ionization. The unstable activated molecules undergo secondary reactions to produce chemically active free radicals. These free radicals, such as OH^-, H^+, and H_3O^+, form from the water molecule and are powerful reducing or oxidizing agents that cause further chemical reactions within the cell. The cellular changes that occur involve primarily the interaction of these free radicals with the DNA, RNA, and enzymes of the cell.

The DNA of the cell is seen as the target of the radiation effect. It is now known that the chemically active hydroxyl radical (OH^-) causes most of the DNA alterations. The principal lesion produced by radiation is a single chromosomal strand break (Fig. 9-10). This lesion becomes lethal when it combines with another single-strand break of a cell that has also been exposed to radiation. In normal cells a single chromosomal strand break is usually repairable. However, repair of this alteration in cancer cells is at

best difficult. Radiation often produces a double chromosomal strand break, which is lethal to both normal cells and cancer cells.

The amount and degree of DNA damage are greatly influenced by the amount of oxygen available in the cellular environment. The greater the amount of oxygen, the greater the amount of damage to DNA. Studies are being conducted to determine the effectiveness of radiosensitizers (e.g., drugs such as nitroimidazole [misonidazole]) that are thought to biochemically mimic the action of oxygen. Other studies are being conducted to determine whether hyperbaric oxygenation and/or hyperthermia before or during the time of the radiation treatment will increase the cellular effect of radiation.

The effect of radiation on the tissues represents a summation of the effect of radiation on the cells forming the tissue. The cells of any tissue depend on the cellular arrangement of that tissue for their life, replication, and functioning. Therefore, cellular damage or death in a critical area may result in death of the entire tissue. In addition to the effect on the cells of a given tissue, the capillaries supplying the tissues with blood are also sensitive to the effects of radiation. The cellular destruction of a tissue that occurs from a decreased blood supply may be greater than the cellular destruction that occurs from exposure to radiation.

External radiation. Radiation therapy is the delivery of a high dose of radiation to a small amount of tissue in a short period of time. The radiation treatment plan is determined by the radiosensitivity of the tumor cells, the therapeutic ratio, and the volume of tissue that must be irradiated.

Radiosensitivity. By clinical definition, a radiosensitive tumor is one that is eradicated by radiation in a dose that is well tolerated by the surrounding normal tissues. Cells with a rapid generation time, such as those of the bone marrow, ovaries, testes, epithelial cells of the lining of the gastrointestinal and genitourinary tracts, the hair follicles, and the lymphatic tissue, are said to be radiosensitive (Table 9-14). The effect of radiation on these tissues is dramatic. Cells are destroyed and an inflammatory response occurs. As more cells are destroyed, cells may slough, causing the tissue to become thin, denuded, or ulcerated. This process causes side effects, such as mucositis, nausea, vomiting, diarrhea, and cystitis. Alopecia, leukopenia, thrombocytopenia, and sterility may also occur when

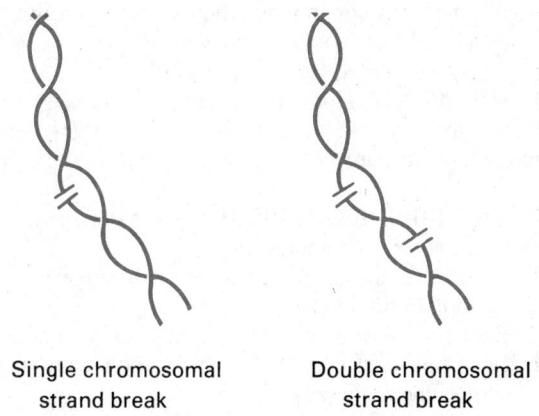

Single chromosomal strand break Double chromosomal strand break

Fig. 9-10   Lesions produced in cells by radiation.

Table 9-14   Tumor Radiosensitivity

High Radiosensitivity	Moderate Radiosensitivity	Mild Radiosensitivity	Poor Radiosensitivity
Ovarian dysgerminoma	Skin carcinoma	Soft tissue sarcomas (e.g., chondrosarcoma)	Osteosarcoma
Testicular seminoma	Oropharyngeal carcinoma	Gastric adenocarcinoma	Malignant melanoma
Hodgkin's disease	Esophageal carcinoma	Renal adenocarcinoma	Malignant gliomas
Non-Hodgkin's lymphoma	Breast adenocarcinoma	Colon adenocarcinoma	
Wilms' tumor	Uterine and cervical carcinoma		
Neuroblastoma	Prostate carcinoma		
	Bladder carcinoma		

a sufficient number of normal cells of these tissues begin to repair the cellular damage. However, the tissues may never return to their original state. This is due to the formation of fibrosis, which is a normal consequence of cellular repair. These changes in the tissue structure continue to occur for several months or even years after the exposure to radiation.

In tissues that have a slow generation time, such as those of the muscles, tendons, and nerves, the response to radiation is less dramatic. Little if any cellular destruction occurs in these tissues, since few cells are in the process of cellular division at any one point in time. These cells are said to be *radioresistant*. However, even though little cellular destruction occurs when radioresistant tissues are exposed to radiation, the capillaries of these tissues will be destroyed, with resulting edema and inflammation of the surrounding tissue. The degree of atrophy, fibrosis, and necrosis depends on the adequacy of the blood supply to these tissues.

Therapeutic ratio. The second determining factor of radiation dose, the *therapeutic ratio*, is defined as the relationship between the radiation dose that normal tissues in the area of the tumor can tolerate and the radiation dose necessary to destroy the tumor cells:

$$\text{Therapeutic ratio} = \frac{\text{Normal tissue tolerance dose}}{\text{Tumor-lethal dose}}$$

If the therapeutic ratio is greater than 1, it is likely that the tumor can be successfully eradicated. If the therapeutic ratio is less than 1, radiation therapy will not be effective. Radiation will affect the normal cells as well as the cancer cells in the treatment field.

If the entire tumor-lethal dose of radiation were given in one treatment, the exposure would be classified as an acute radiation exposure, similar to that of an atomic bomb blast or a nuclear power plant accident. By dividing the total tumor-lethal radiation dose into smaller doses (called *fractionation*) given on a daily basis until the total tumor-lethal dose is reached, radiation exposure that would be detrimental to the health of a client is prevented.

The usual course of external radiation therapy involves a series of treatments given over a period of 2 to 8 weeks on a 5-days-a-week schedule. Since most tumors require a radiation dose of between 4500 and 7500 rads, most clients receive a daily fractionated radiation dose of 200 ± 50 rads and a weekly radiation dose of 1000 ± 250 rads.

The immediate effect of radiation therapy occurs within the first 2 hours after exposure to a source of radiation. After this time, the normal cells as well as the tumor cells in the treatment field will attempt to repair themselves. The repair process will continue during the 24-hour period from one radiation treatment to the next. The normal cells in the treatment field have a greater capacity for cellular repair, in terms of both the rate and the quality of repair. Cancer cells can repair themselves, but the rate and quality of repair are slower and less accurate than in normal cells.

Radiation therapy is sometimes given as a *split course* of therapy to further enhance the repair of normal tissues. In this plan the treatments are given for 2 to 4 weeks, discontinued for several weeks so that the normal cells can repair themselves, and resumed for another 2 to 4 weeks. The client should receive each of the scheduled radiation treatments. If a treatment is omitted, the radiation therapist may add another treatment to the end of the treatment plan or increase the daily dose of each remaining radiation treatment. The client is usually reevaluated during and near the end of the course of treatment. Depending on the tumor response to radiation or the side effects of radiation therapy experienced by the client, the number of treatments may be increased or decreased and/or the daily dose of radiation may be altered.

Volume of tissue. The third factor to be considered in radiation therapy is the *volume* of tissue exposed to the source of radiation. The volume of tissues irradiated is known as the *treatment field*, and it includes the tumor and the smallest possible amount of surrounding normal tissue. The tumor-lethal dose delivered to the treatment field must be one that is high enough to destroy the cancer cells but that will not have a highly detrimental effect on the normal cells present in the field. If the volume of tissue irradiated is small, the tumor-lethal dose of radiation can be increased, the rate of tumor cell destruction will be greater, and the side effects experienced by the client will be fewer and less severe.

Goals of treatment. The goals of radiation therapy are cure, control, or palliation. To accomplish these treatment goals, radiation therapy can be used alone or as an adjuvant treatment modality in combination with surgery, chemotherapy, and/or biological response modifiers.

Cure is the goal when radiation therapy is used alone as a curative modality for treating clients with the following:
1. Basal cell carcinoma of the skin
2. Tumors confined to the vocal cords
3. Stage I or IIA Hodgkin's disease

Radiation therapy can be combined with surgery and/or chemotherapy to cure certain cancers such as the following:
1. Stage IIB, IIIA, and IIIB Hodgkin's disease in combination with chemotherapy
2. Wilms' tumor in combination with surgery and/or chemotherapy
3. Ewing's sarcoma in combination with chemotherapy
4. Head and neck cancer in combination with surgery and/or chemotherapy
5. Stage I and II breast cancer

Control of the disease process of cancer for a period of time is considered to be a reasonable goal in some situations. Initial treatment is offered at the time of diagnosis, and additional treatment is instituted each time symptoms of disease recur. Most clients enjoy a high quality of life during the symptom-free period. Radiation therapy can be combined with surgery to further enhance the local control of cancer. It can be given preoperatively to reduce the size of the tumor so that it can be more easily resected or postoperatively to destroy any remaining tumor cells. Intraoperative radiation therapy is now being given at some research centers. In this procedure, radiation is administered directly to the site of the tumor during surgery.

Inoperable tumors can be treated with radiation therapy. These tumors are large and have extended regionally. An example of an inoperable cancer treated for control with radiation therapy is oat-cell cancer of the lung.

Palliation is often the goal of radiation therapy. The client can be treated to control the distressing symptoms that are occurring as a result of the disease process. Tumors can be reduced in size to relieve symptoms such as pain and obstruction. Examples of the use of radiation therapy for palliation include the relief of the following:

1. Pain associated with bone metastasis
2. Pain and neurological symptoms associated with brain metastasis
3. Spinal cord compression
4. Intestinal obstruction
5. Superior vena cava obstruction
6. Bronchial or tracheal obstruction
7. Bleeding (e.g., bladder and intrabronchial)

Types of radiation therapy machines. The kilovoltage machine, the first available radiation therapy machine, delivers x-rays at a low energy level and is similar to machines used for diagnostic x-rays. The depth of the maximum-delivered dose of radiation is on the skin surface. A problem experienced when this machine is used is that the radiation scatters when it strikes the skin surface, causing the skin surrounding the treatment field to experience radiation exposure. The kilovoltage machine is rarely used today.

The cobalt 60 machine is a megavoltage machine that emits high-energy gamma rays as the source of radiation (Fig. 9-11). Because radioactive cobalt is a high-energy source of radiation, the penetration of the radiation is greater and the maximum radiation dose occurs below the surface of the skin. Therefore, this machine is used to treat tumors located below the skin surface with minimal radiation exposure of the skin surface and less radiation scatter. Although this machine is gradually being replaced by higher-voltage machines, its widespread use continues.

The large, high-energy supervoltage machine is the linear accelerator. It uses x-rays and/or electrons as a source of radiation to the treatment fields (Fig. 9-12). Since the penetration of the radiation from this machine is great and the radiation scatter is minimal, tumors located several centimeters below the skin surface can be effectively treated. These machines are currently popular and are supplementing or replacing the cobalt 60 machine.

Cyclotrons and betatrons are other examples of supervoltage machines. The betatron machine uses electrons, and the cyclotron uses protons, neutrons, or electrons as a source of radiation. These machines are being used in several cancer centers.

Effects on normal tissues. Side effects of radiation therapy are common. They are caused by destruction of irradiated normal tissues in the area of the tumor. Not all clients who receive radiation in a particular anatomical site will experience the same side effects, and the side effects will not be experienced to the same degree. In some clients the side effects are so slight that they are hardly noticed; in others the side effects seriously alter the usual lifestyle patterns.

Many side effects depend on the site being irradiated. For example, radiation therapy to the scalp will usually cause alopecia. Some side effects are more general in nature and are common to clients receiving radiation, regardless of the area being irradiated. These include skin reactions, fatigue, and anorexia.

Skin reactions. During each treatment, radiation passes through the skin. Since megavoltage or supravoltage machines are now used to deliver the source of radiation to the treatment field, the maximum effect of radiation therapy occurs below the skin surface and the skin is said to be spared. However, the epithelial cells of the skin have a rapid rate of cellular division, so some epithelial cells of the skin will be destroyed as the radiation enters the treat-

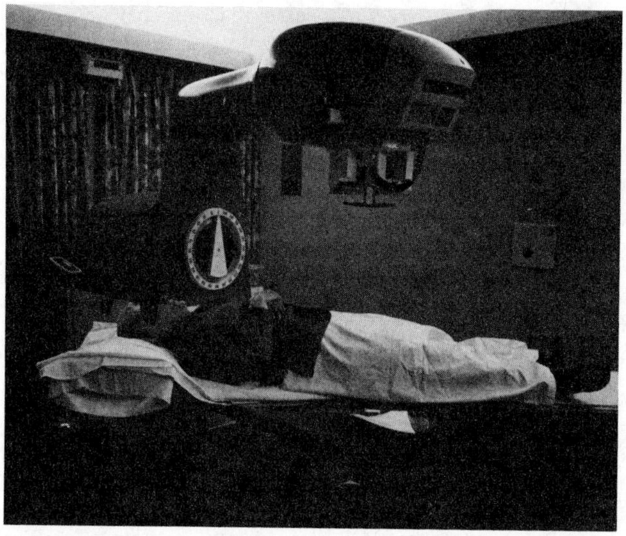

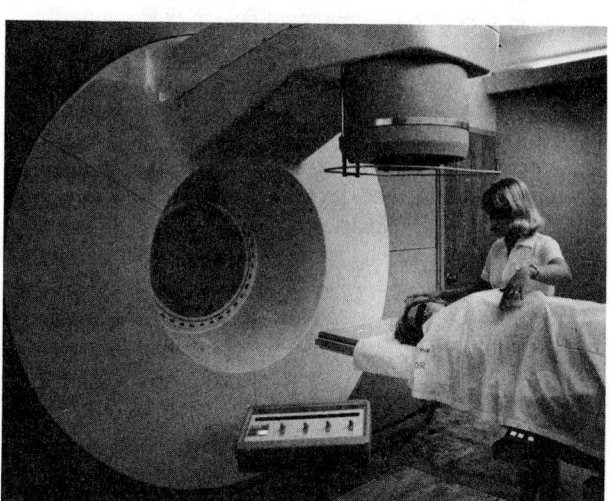

Fig. 9-11 Cobalt 60 radiation therapy machine. (From Yasko J: Care of the client receiving external radiation therapy, Reston, Va, 1982, Reston Publishing.)

Fig. 9-12 Linear accelerator. (From Yasko J: Care of the client receiving external radiation therapy, Reston, Va, 1982, Reston Publishing.)

Table 9-15

Nursing Management of Radiation Skin Reactions

1. Gently cleanse the skin in the treatment field using a mild soap (Ivory, Dove), tepid water, a soft cloth, and a gentle patting motion. Rinse thoroughly and pat dry.
2. Apply nonmedicated, nonperfumed, moisturizing lotion or creams, such as baby lotion/oil or aloe gel/cream to alleviate the dry skin of a level II skin reaction. This substance must be gently cleansed from the treatment field before each treatment and reapplied. (Note: Care differs from institution to institution.) Dusting with cornstarch may reduce itching.
3. Cleanse the area involved with half-strength hydrogen peroxide and normal saline solution if a level III reaction is present. The solution is best applied with an irrigating syringe to avoid friction. Rinse the area with saline solution. Expose the area to air as often as possible. If copious drainage is present, nonadhesive absorbent dressings are warranted, and they must be changed as soon as they become wet. Observe the area daily for signs of infection.
4. Instruct the client to avoid wearing tight-fitting clothing such as brassieres, girdles, and belts over the treatment field.
5. Instruct the client to avoid wearing harsh fabrics, such as wool and corduroy. A light-weight cotton garment is best. If possible, expose the treatment field to air.
6. Instruct the client to use gentle detergents such as Dreft and Ivory Snow to wash clothing that will come in contact with the treatment field.
7. Instruct the client to avoid direct exposure to the sun. If the treatment field is in an area that is exposed to the sun, protective clothing such as a wide-brimmed hat should be worn during exposure to the sun.
8. Avoid all sources of heat (hot water bottles, heating pads, and sun lamps) on the treatment field.
9. Avoid exposing the treatment field to cold temperatures (ice bags or cold weather).
10. Instruct the client to avoid swimming in salt water or in chlorinated pools during the time of treatment.
11. Instruct the client to avoid the use of all medications, deodorants, perfumes, powders, or cosmetics on the skin in the treatment field. Tape, dressings, and adhesive bandages should also be avoided unless permitted by the radiation therapist. Avoid shaving the hair in the treatment field.
12. Sensitive skin must continue to be protected after the treatment is completed. Teach the client to do the following:
    a. Avoid direct exposure to the sun. A sunscreen agent and/or protective clothing must be worn if the potential of exposure to the sun is present.
    b. Use an electric razor if shaving is necessary in the treatment field.

From Yasko J: Care of the client receiving external radiation therapy—a self-learning module for the nurse caring for the client with cancer, Reston, Va, 1982, Reston Publishing.

ment field. The greater the dose of radiation used in therapy, the more likely the skin reaction. Fair-skinned persons are usually more sensitive than those with darker skin.

There are four degrees or levels of skin reaction. Most clients will remain at level I or II throughout the course of treatment:

Level I: Erythema of the skin in the treatment field occurs. The skin in this area will be pink to red in color and will resemble a first-degree reaction of the skin to the sun.

Level II: Dry desquamation of the skin in the treatment field occurs. The skin becomes dry and scaly, and the client may complain of itching.

Level III: Wet desquamation of the skin in the treatment field occurs. The skin may become blistered, and the superficial layers may be lost through peeling. This reaction resembles a second-degree reaction of the skin to the sun. The damage to the skin is reversible, but it may be necessary to discontinue the radiation treatment until healing occurs.

Level IV: Loss of hair on the skin in the treatment field occurs. Permanent loss of hair in the treatment field as well as suppression of sweat glands occurs with high doses of radiation therapy. Late side effects may occur 6 months to 5 years after completion of treatment. These include (1) fibrosis of the skin and telangiectasis due to dilatation of capillaries in the treatment field, (2) impairment of the lymphatic drainage in the treatment field and the development of lymphedema due to fibrosis of the lymph glands, (3) pulmonary fibrosis, and (4) colonic necrosis.

The skin reaction must not be referred to as a radiation burn. A skin reaction is usually expected. When the word *burn* is used, it suggests that a mistake has been made, resulting in a burn.

With increased sophistication in technology and treatment planning, these side effects are much less common today. *Radiation recall* is a skin reaction that can occur when chemotherapy is given several weeks or even months after radiation therapy has ended. It involves the skin in the area that was previously treated with radiation therapy and may include any of the four levels of skin reaction. Nursing management of skin reactions to radiation is presented in Table 9-15.

■ Nursing Management of the Client Receiving External Radiation

To effectively care for the client who is undergoing external radiation therapy, the nurse must be aware of what the client will experience while being treated with radiation. Problems caused by radiation therapy are presented in Table 9-16.

Once the preliminary examinations (e.g., history and physical examination and review of medical records) are completed, the client is prepared for radiation therapy. This preparation is known as *treatment simulation*. The client is placed in the anticipated treatment position on a treatment table under a machine called the *simulator*, which is a diagnostic x-ray machine that can mimic the treatment capabilities of the radiation therapy machine.

Table 9-16 Problems Caused by Radiation Therapy and Chemotherapy

Problem	Etiology and Comments
GASTROINTESTINAL	
Dryness of the mucous membranes of the mouth	When salivary glands are located in the radiation treatment field, they are frequently damaged. This may be a permanent side effect of radiation therapy and it can be quite disturbing to the client because it is difficult to eat, swallow, and/or talk when the mucous membranes are dry. Artificial saliva is available.
Stomatitis and mucositis	Occurs when epithelial cells of the oral mucosa and intraoral soft tissue structures are destroyed by chemotherapy or radiation therapy. These cells are extremely sensitive because of their normal high cell turnover rate. Mucositis can precipitate complications of infection and hemorrhage.
Esophagitis	Inflammation and ulceration of mucous membranes of esophagus due to rapid cell destruction occur as a side effect of chemotherapy and radiation therapy to the area of the neck, chest, and/or back.
Nausea and vomiting	The vomiting center in the brain is stimulated by products of cellular breakdown that occur in response to chemotherapy and radiation therapy. The drugs used in chemotherapy also stimulate the vomiting center. Destruction of the epithelial lining of the gastrointestinal tract occurs in response to chemotherapy and radiation therapy to chest, abdomen, and back. A strong psychological impact is associated with nausea and vomiting and the high stress level associated with cancer and cancer treatment.
Anorexia	Site-specific side effects of radiation therapy—dry mouth, mucositis, esophagitis, nausea, vomiting, and diarrhea—occur. Side effects of chemotherapy include nausea, vomiting, stomatitis, esophagitis, diarrhea. Fatigue, pain, and infection are present. Alteration in the sensation of taste occurs when tumors release waste products into the bloodstream. Psychological and social impact of cancer and cancer therapy result in an increased level of stress and changes in the usual lifestyle pattern.
Altered taste sensation	Destruction of the taste buds in the treatment field occurs with radiation therapy. The amount of taste alteration or loss depends on the radiation dosage and the extent of the treatment field. Complete loss of taste often occurs. Taste changes may be a permanent outcome of therapy. Waste products occur in response to cellular destruction from radiation therapy and chemotherapy. These waste products are thought to be responsible for alterations in the sensation. Reduction in the amount of saliva occurs because of the location of the salivary glands in the treatment field. Food must be in solution to be tasted.
Diarrhea	Denuding of the epithelial lining of the small intestines occurs as a side effect of chemotherapy and as a side effect of radiation therapy to the abdomen and/or the lower back.
Constipation	Dysfunction of the autonomic nervous system from neurotoxic effects of plant alkaloids (vincristine, vinblastine) occurs.
Hepatotoxicity	Toxic effects of certain chemotherapy drugs such as methotrexate, mitomycin, 6-MP, and cytosine arabinoside are present.
HEMATOPOIETIC SYSTEM	
Anemia	Depressant effect on bone marrow function occurs because of chemotherapy and radiation therapy. Malignant infiltration of bone marrow by cancer is present. Ulceration, necrosis, and bleeding of neoplastic growth occur.
Leukopenia	Depressant effect on bone marrow activity is present due to chemotherapy and radiation therapy. Effect is especially significant because of the short life span of white blood cells. Infection is the most frequent cause of morbidity and death in the client with cancer. Usual sites of infection are the respiratory and genitourinary systems.
Thrombocytopenia	Depressant effect on bone marrow function is present due to chemotherapy and radiation therapy. Malignant infiltration of the bone marrow occurs. Abnormal destruction of circulating platelets is present. When the platelet count is less than 20,000/μl, spontaneous bleeding can occur.
INTEGUMENTARY	
Alopecia	Alopecia occurs as a side effect of some chemotherapy agents and radiation therapy to the skull. Hair loss that occurs in response to chemotherapy is usually temporary, and hair loss that occurs in response to radiation therapy is usually permanent. The hair begins to fall out during the first week of therapy, and this may progress to complete hair loss.
Skin reactions	Extravasation of vesicant chemotherapeutic drugs (e.g., doxorubicin) given intravenously causes severe necrosis of tissues exposed to the drug (see text).

Continued.

Table 9-16   Problems Caused by Radiation Therapy and Chemotherapy—cont'd

Problem	Etiology and Comments
GENITOURINARY	
Cystitis	Problem occurs when the epithelial cells of the lining of the bladder are destroyed as a side effect of chemotherapy (e.g., cyclophosphamide) and as a side effect of radiation therapy when the bladder is located in the treatment field. Clinical manifestations of urgency, frequency, and hematuria are present.
Sexual dysfunction	Chemotherapy on the cells of the testes or ova or radiation therapy when the cells of the testes or ova are located in the treatment field causes the problem. Symptoms of cancer and cancer therapy include fatigue, diarrhea, nausea, vomiting, anxiety, fear, and pain.
Nephrotoxicity	Necrosis of proximal renal tubules is present due to an accumulation of drugs (e.g., cisplatin) in the kidney.
NERVOUS SYSTEM	
Increased intracranial pressure	Problem may result from radiation edema in the central system. This phenomenon is not well understood but is easily controlled with steroids and pain medication.
Peripheral neuropathy	Paresthesias, areflexia, skeletal muscle weakness, and smooth muscle dysfunction (e.g., paralytic ileus, constipation) can occur as a side effect of the plant alkaloids (e.g., vinblastine, vincristine) and cisplatin.
RESPIRATORY SYSTEM	
Pneumonitis	When the lungs are located in the treatment field, radiation pneumonitis may develop 2 to 3 months after the start of treatment. It is characterized by a dry, hacking cough, fever, and exertional dyspnea. After 6 to 12 months, fibrosis will occur and will be persistently evident on x-ray. The client with fibrosis is more susceptible to respiratory infection. Problem can also occur as a result of chemotherapy (e.g., bleomycin and busulfan).
CARDIOVASCULAR	
Pericarditis and myocarditis	Problem is an infrequent complication when chest wall is irradiated. It may occur up to 1 year after treatment.
Cardiotoxicity	Chemotherapeutic agents such as doxorubicin and daunorubicin can cause nonspecific electrical changes (i.e., low voltage) and rapidly progressive heart failure. The drug therapy needs to be modified if these effects occur.
BIOCHEMICAL	
Hyperuricemia	Increase in uric acid levels occurs because of cell destruction by chemotherapy. Problem can cause a secondary form of gout.
Hypomagnesemia	Problem occurs with cisplatin therapy.
PSYCHOEMOTIONAL	
Fatigue	Increase in the metabolic rate occurs when cancer is present, with resultant increase in the amount of energy used. Destruction of cancer cells and normal cells by chemotherapy and radiation therapy occurs, with the release of waste products into the bloodstream. Increase in anabolic processes of cellular proliferation and differentiation are necessary to repair the normal cells and tissues destroyed by chemotherapy and radiation therapy.
Pain	Compression or infiltration of the blood vessels, the lymphatic vessels, and the nerves occurs. Obstruction of the gastrointestinal and/or genitourinary system occurs. Inflammation, ulceration, or necrosis of the tissues and/or organs is present. Fear, anxiety, and depression are experienced in response to the diagnosis and treatment of cancer.

The client will be asked to lie very still while a series of measurements and x rays is performed. To duplicate the exact position the client must assume during treatment, various immobilization devices may be used. Immobilization devices can be in the form of clamps or plaster of Paris molds or casts. The measurements and x-rays are necessary to determine the dose of radiation; the volume of tissue to be irradiated; and the length, number, and frequency of the radiation treatments. All computations are done with the aid of a computer.

When the treatment field is determined, the area is marked with indelible dye or ink as felt-tipped markers, gentian violet, and India ink. Dye or ink that is visible only under black light is also used and is particularly beneficial for clients who have tumors in exposed areas of the body, such as in the region of the head or neck.

Another treatment aid used to delineate the treatment field is the placement of lead blocks over the radiation source within the machine. The lead blocks shield the vital organs and normal tissue from exposure to radiation. The client is placed in exactly the same position for each treatment, and the lead blocks permit radiation exposure only to the treatment field. The skin markings are necessary to ensure that during each radiation treatment the source of radiation is directed to exactly the same area of the body.

In some cases the stress and inconvenience of skin markings can be minimized by placement of tiny permanent dots on the skin at the corners of the treatment field. These are known as *tattoos* and are made with indelible ink and a small-gauge needle. These markings are nearly invisible and resemble a tiny freckle or mole on the skin. The skin markings must not be washed off or removed in any way. If they are accidentally removed, the client must be cautioned not to attempt to redraw them. The radiation technician should be notified that the skin markings have been removed so that they can be redrawn according to the treatment plan. Many times the skin markings are a source of stress for the client. If they are visible, they become a constant reminder that the client has cancer and is being treated for it.

Before the start of treatment, it is helpful to have the client meet the radiation therapy personnel and see the actual machine that will be used so that many of the fears of the unknown will be minimized. If a pretreatment visit is not possible, a picture of the machine should be shown to the client and the family. The strange-looking machines often trigger many fears, concerns, and misconceptions.

Undergoing a radiation treatment is very similar to having an x-ray taken. Although the client is alone in the room during the treatment, visual and auditory communication is provided by a television monitor and an intercom system. The client should be assured that radiation is invisible, silent, and painless. However, some machines make unusual whirring or clicking sounds, and the client should be informed that it is the machine and not the source of radiation that causes these sounds.

The client should also be informed that lying immobile on the hard, flat treatment table may be uncomfortable. If the client experiences pain, pain medications should be administered 1 hour before the time of treatment to ensure comfort.

Clients will often ask if they are radioactive and a danger to others or if their clothing is radioactive. They must be assured that once the radiation therapy machine is turned off, radiation is no longer being emitted. Clients must also be reassured that the number of radiation treatments is not reflective of the severity of disease or the likelihood of cure.

Periodically throughout the course of the treatment the client will be evaluated by the radiation therapist and nurse. The effect as well as the side effects of radiation therapy will be assessed. Interventions to prevent or mini-mize the side effects of radiation therapy will be planned and implemented (Table 9-17). Adjustments of the original treatment plan will occur if warranted. The client should be aware that it is expected that changes in the original treatment plan may be necessary.

Clients who undergo radiation therapy should have regularly scheduled follow-up care for the rest of their lives. They should understand that follow-up care is an essential part of the treatment plan. After completion of treatment, the radiation therapist initially examines the client every 4 to 6 weeks. If the cancer appears to be cured or controlled, the time period for follow-up care is extended to every 6 months to 1 year. Consistent long-term follow-up care is also necessary to evaluate the late side effects of radiation therapy, some of which will not be evident for 5 to 10 years after completion of the course of treatment.

Internal radiation.* Internal radiation therapy (brachytherapy) involves the placement of a source of radiation in a specific area within or on the body. The source of radiation used in internal radiation therapy is either a mechanically positioned (sealed) radiation source or an unsealed radiation source. The selection of the type of internal radiation therapy used in the treatment plan is determined by the size, cell type, and location of the cancer. Table 9-18 lists the characteristics of the various sources of radiation used in internal radiation therapy.

Mechanically placed therapy. Mechanically placed internal radiation therapy or sealed internal therapy involves (1) the placement of a source of radiation in an externally placed mold, (2) interstitial placement (directly into the tissues of the tumor), or (3) intracavitary placement (within a body cavity). When a mold containing a source of radiation is externally placed, it is made to fit a particular anatomical site and the source of radiation is embedded within the mold. The mold is then applied directly over the skin or mucous membranes covering the tumor. The sources of radiation used in this form of internal radiation therapy include cobalt 60, tantalum 182, and strontium 90. The usual anatomical sites of treatment are the nostrils, lips, ears, scalp, mouth, larynx, skin, and penis.

In the interstitial placement of a radiation source, the source of radiation is in the form of a seed, needle, wire, or tube that is implanted within the tissues of the tumor. When possible, the catheter or device in which in the radioactive source will be placed is surgically positioned in the operating room. The radioactive source is then placed in the catheter or device in the client's room to decrease exposure to personnel. If placement of the radioactive source requires an open, operative procedure, the sources are placed directly into the tissue in the operating room. Cobalt 60, cesium 137, iridium 192, gold 198, iodine 125, radon 222, and tantalum 182 are the sources of radiation used in this placement technique (Table 9-18). All these radiation sources emit gamma rays. The *half-life* of the particular isotope used in the treatment plan determines whether the interstitial placement will be temporary (re-

---

*This section was modified from Yasko J: Internal radiation in cancer care. In Donovan DL, ed: A guide to patient education, New York, 1981, Appleton-Century-Crofts.

Table 9-17

NURSING CARE PLAN FOR THE CLIENT WITH CANCER*

Defining Characteristics	Nursing Interventions	Evaluation Criteria
NURSING DIAGNOSIS: Altered nutrition: less than body requirements related to anorexia, nausea, and vomiting		
Reported or observed inadequate food intake relative to minimum daily requirements with or without weight loss, fatigue	Avoid punitive or judgmental statements about food intake or weight loss. Administer antiemetic protocols as prescribed (e.g., begin 12 hr before chemotherapy or radiation therapy and continue every 4 to 6 hr for at least 24 hr) and evaluate efficacy of drug, dose, and time administered. Maintain a quiet, restful environment. Modify diet to include bland, lukewarm, high-calorie, high-protein foods. Try small, frequent feedings rather than fewer large meals. Teach client to eat and drink slowly. Offer client chewing gum, warm lemon-lime soda pop, cola syrup, sour candy, soda crackers, tepid tea, or anything the client associates with a positive outcome. Remove all sights, sounds, or smells that have the potential for initiating nausea, such as an emesis basin and unpleasant odors. Use techniques such as relaxation response and distraction. Provide a well-balanced diet that includes the basic four with increased protein-calorie intake. Provide a small amount of food every few hours. The client should be gently encouraged to eat, but nagging at mealtime must be avoided. Teach the client what to eat rather than stressing the fact that more food should be eaten. (Home-prepared items are often more appealing.) Set realistic goals for consumption. Avoid foods that are filling or gas forming, such as salads, gas-forming vegetables (cabbage, broccoli), fruits, and beer. Serve all foods attractively and in a pleasant environment. Augment dietary intake with nutritional supplements. Serve these cold in a container other than a can. Teach the client to sip the nutritional supplement slowly between meals.	Adequate nutritional intake, maintenance of body weight, adequate energy for ADL
NURSING DIAGNOSIS: Altered health maintenance related to lack of knowledge of long-term management of cancer		
Frequent questions by client and/or caregiver regarding self-care, treatment, side effects; observed inability of client and/or caregiver to manage technical aspects of long-term care	Determine knowledge and technical skills needed by client/caregiver. Assess current level of knowledge and skill. Teach required knowledge and skill. Provide opportunity for follow-up evaluation and teaching.	Verbalization by client/caregiver of confidence in ability and demonstration of ability to manage long-term care; demonstration of adequate knowledge base to provide safe self-care

*Only nursing diagnoses that apply to all types of cancer are included in this care plan.

†Level I: Walk, regular pace, on level indefinitely; one flight or more but more short of breath than normally. Level II: Walk one city block 500 feet on level; climb one flight slowly without stopping. Level III: Walk no more than 50 feet on level without stopping; unable to climb one flight of stairs without stopping. Level IV: Dyspnea and fatigue at rest.

Table 9-17

NURSING CARE PLAN FOR THE CLIENT WITH CANCER*—cont'd

Defining Characteristics	Nursing Interventions	Evaluation Criteria

NURSING DIAGNOSIS: Altered oral mucous membrane related to chemotherapy and oral cavity radiation

Verbalization or signs of pain or discomfort in oral mucous membranes, decrease or lack of saliva, coated tongue, xerostomia (dry mouth), halitosis, edema of membranes; hyperemia, oral lesions; ulcers, desquamation, vesicles, hemorrhagic gingivitis, leukoplakia, stomatitis	Assess oral mucosa daily. Teach client to inspect oral cavity. Remove dentures at night. Observe for dryness, redness, and white or yellow membrane and the presence of any breaks in integrity of tissues. If client wears dentures, assess to determine whether the dentures fit properly. Distinguish stomatitis from candidiasis and other oral problems, such as xerostomia and herpes. Maintain good oral hygiene. Use mouthwashes of baking soda, H_2O_2 (1:2), or normal saline solution every 2 hr. Use soft-bristle toothbrushes, sponge-tipped applicators, or an irrigation syringe as cleansing agents. Avoid the use of lemon and glycerin swabs for mouth care. Apply topical anesthetics, such as viscous Xylocaine or oxethazaine, as ordered. Modify diet to avoid hot, spicy, acidic foods. Discourage use of irritants such as tobacco and alcohol. Encourage drinking of water or other liquids at frequent intervals throughout the day or use of an artificial saliva to keep mucous membranes moist. Moisten lips regularly with a small amount of petroleum jelly, baby oil, or cocoa butter.	Absence of oral pain, absence of infections in the oral mucosa, maintenance of body weight and adequate nutritional intake, no break in integrity of oral mucosa

NURSING DIAGNOSIS: Activity intolerance: Level I, II, III, or IV related to the effects of cancer or treatment†

Verbal report of fatigue or weakness, exertional discomfort or dyspnea; abnormal responses to activity—heart rate, blood pressure, or electrocardiographic changes reflecting ischemia or dysrhythmias	Inform the client that fatigue is an expected side effect of therapy and that it usually begins during the first week of therapy, reaches its peak in 2 weeks, continues, and then gradually disappears 2 to 4 weeks after treatment has ended. Encourage client to rest when fatigued, to maintain usual lifestyle patterns as closely as possible, and to pace activities in accordance with energy level.	Maintenance of satisfactory activity level relative to phase of treatment

NURSING DIAGNOSIS: Ineffective individual coping related to depression in response to diagnosis and treatment, uncertain outcome, disruption in lifestyle, and/or financial burden of illness

Verbalized or observed inability to manage affective component of diagnosis and resulting symptoms; presence of threats or attempts to commit suicide; concerns over financial implications of disease stated	Have client direct own care when possible. Provide information to allow client to make informed choices regarding treatment regimen and plan of care. Facilitate communication between client and family. Assess and mobilize client's support system. Refer client to social services for financial assistance if appropriate. Assess need for further counseling.	Demonstration of appropriate response to problems; seeking and/or accepting of outside support and assistance

Continued.

Table 9-17

NURSING CARE PLAN FOR THE CLIENT WITH CANCER*—cont'd

Defining Characteristics	Nursing Interventions	Evaluation Criteria
NURSING DIAGNOSIS: Body-image disturbance related to hair loss, disfiguring surgery, and weight loss		
Expressions of concern with changes in body; refusal to interact with visitors; isolation of self, frequent crying; refusal to care for self or to look in mirror	Provide psychological support and prepare client for expected hair loss. Encourage client to select a wig and begin to wear it before hair loss begins and to wear a scarf or turban to conceal hair loss. Use a mild, protein-based shampoo, cream rinse, and hair conditioner every 4 to 7 days. Excessive shampooing should be avoided. Avoid excessive brushing and combing of hair. Avoid use of electric hair dryers, curlers, curling rods, and hair spray. When administering drugs that induce alopecia, reduce or occlude blood flow to hair follicles by using ice-packs, scalp tourniquets, or scalp sphygmomanometers (see text). Help client select clothing and colors that minimize weight loss and/or effects of disfiguring surgery. Assure client that value as a person is not associated with external appearance. Discuss expected physical changes with family members and advise them of ways to assist client with acceptance.	Verbalization of acceptance of changes in body appearance and function
NURSING DIAGNOSIS: Altered family processes related to cancer diagnosis of family member		
Observed communication problems among family members; lack of family support related to physical, emotional, and/or spiritual needs of client	Assess family structure and support system. Teach needed skills to family members. Provide opportunity for discussion of caregiving and emotional implications of role changes. Assist family members to set realistic expectations for client and selves. Provide guidance on course of disease and anticipated outcome.	Open communication among family members; cooperation of family members in care of client; seeking of outside help when needed
NURSING DIAGNOSIS: Potential complication: hyperuricemia related to chemotherapy		
High level of uric acid excretion in urine (normal 6.5 mg/kg/day), high serum uric acid (>7 mg/dl), obstructive uropathy, decreased urine output, nausea, vomiting, lethargy	Monitor uric acid levels. Record intake and output every shift. Force fluids to prevent uric acid crystals from causing obstruction. Evaluate urine pH, BUN, creatinine levels. Monitor for nausea, vomiting, hematuria, oliguria, elevated blood pressure, muscle twitching. Administer allopurinol (Zyloprim) as ordered. Observe for development of rash as an indication of significant drug reaction.	Maintenance of uric acid levels within normal limits

NURSING DIAGNOSIS: High risk for infection related to leukopenia, inadequate immune system function, and multiple exposure to infection‡

NURSING DIAGNOSIS: Potential complication: bleeding related to thrombocytopenia§

‡See Table 25-24.
§See Table 25-16.

Table 9-18   Sources of Radiation Used in Internal Radiation Therapy

Isotope	Emission	Half-Life	External Hazard	Use	Administration
^{131}I (iodine)	Gamma rays	8.05 days	Yes	Thyroid cancer	By mouth
^{32}P (phosphorus)	Beta particles	14.3 days	No	Malignant pleural or peritoneal effusion	Intracavitary in colloidal form
^{226}Ra (radium)	Alpha particles Beta particles Gamma rays	1602 years	Yes	Cancer of the uterus, cervix, nasopharynx, bladder	Intracavitary in an applicator
^{192}Ir (iridium)	Beta particles Gamma rays	74.4 days	Yes	Cancers of head and neck Breast cancer	Interstitial Intracavitary in an applicator
^{125}I (iodine)	Gamma rays	60.2 days	Yes	Cancer of neck, tongue, bladder, muscle	Interstitial
^{222}Rn (radon)	Alpha particles Beta particles Gamma rays	3.82 days	Yes	Gynecological cancer	Intracavitary in an applicator
^{137}Cs (cesium)	Beta particles Gamma rays	30.0 years	Yes	Gynecological cancer	Intracavitary in an applicator

maining in place for 24 to 72 hours) or permanent. Half-life is used to indicate the rate of decay. It is defined as the amount of time needed for a radioisotope to decay to one half its original radioactivity. The permanent interstitial radiation sources have a short half-life, which results in an inert substance in a short period of time. Radon, gold, and iodine seeds are the radiation sources generally used in permanent implants.

Intracavitary placement of a radiation source is the placement of a source of radiation within a particular body cavity by either preloading or afterloading. In *preloading* placement, the radiation source is placed within a capsule or applicator, and the capsule or applicator is then placed within a particular body cavity. This is done in the operating room. In *afterloading* placement, the empty capsule or applicator is placed in the particular body cavity in the operating room and then the radiation source is placed within the capsule or applicator in the client's room. The advantage of the afterloading placement is that it minimizes the number of persons exposed to the radiation source during the time of placement. In both forms of intracavitary placement an x-ray is taken to determine whether the applicator is in the correct position for the treatment. The usual sources of radiation for this placement technique are cesium, cobalt, and radon, all of which emit gamma rays. This form of internal radiation therapy is used in the treatment of cancer of the uterus, cervix, or vagina (Fig. 9-13). The intracavitary placement of a source of radiation is always temporary, and the source of radiation usually remains in place for 24 to 72 hours.

Safety precautions. Specific safety precautions *must* be observed to ensure minimum exposure of persons coming in contact with the client who is being treated with an internal source of radiation emitting gamma rays. These safety precautions include the following:

1. Admitting the client to a private room (preferably lead lined) that is fully equipped with everything (in-

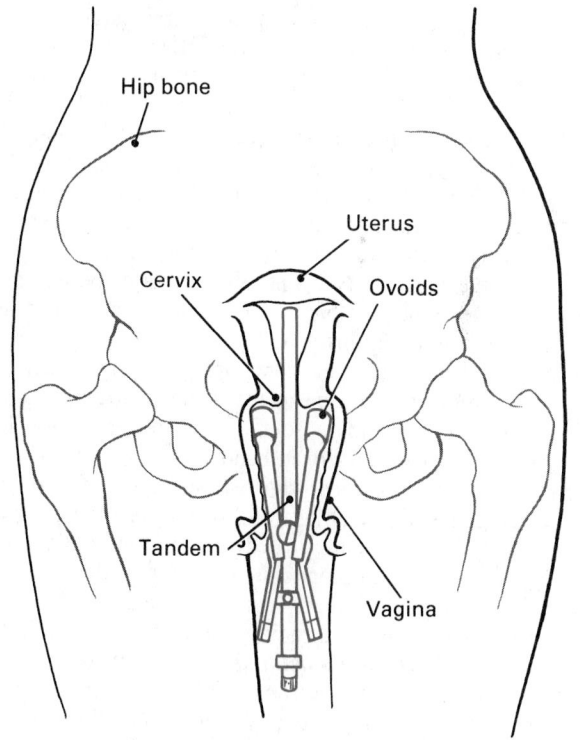

Fig. 9-13   Placement of tandem and ovoids into vagina for internal radiation therapy.

cluding bathroom facilities) the client will need during the time the source of radiation remains in place. The client will remain confined to the room until the source of radiation is removed.

2. Informing all persons coming in contact with the client that an internal source of radiation is being used in the treatment plan and that certain specific safety precautions will be necessary.

Fig. 9-14 Radiation area warning sign.

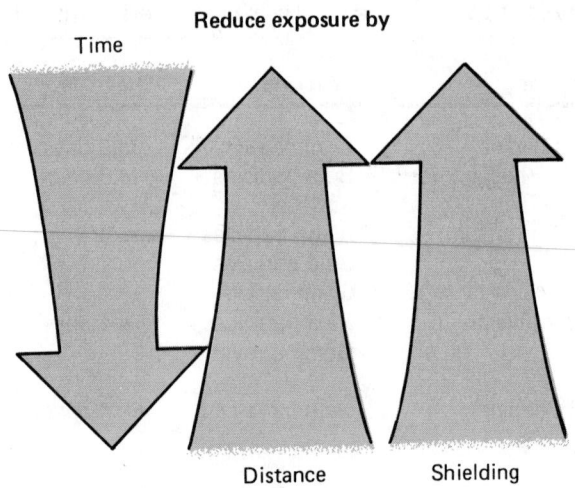

Fig. 9-15 Exposure to ionizing radiation can be reduced by decreasing the time spent near the source, increasing the distance from the source, and/or increasing the amount of shielding between the source and the object irradiated.

3. Placing a "Caution—Radiation Area" sign with the radiation symbol on the door of the client's room and on the client's chart (Fig. 9-14). These yellow and magenta signs and tags are standard and are used by all health care agencies that administer internal radiation therapy.
4. Placing a written list of instructions and precautionary measures in the chart (by the radiation safety officer). The list includes type of radiation, time inserted, and removal time, as well as name and telephone number of the radiation safety officer and any special precautions.
5. Having a lead-lined container and long forceps in the room to be used in the event dislodgement occurs. The radiation source must never be touched with the bare or gloved hand.
6. Restricting persons who are under the age of 18, pregnant, or lactating from visiting or caring for the client who is being treated with internal radiation.
7. Using radiation monitors or film badges for caretakers who will regularly come in contact with clients undergoing internal radiation therapy.

Time, distance, and shielding. All persons coming in contact with the client must observe the principles of time, distance, and shielding (Fig. 9-15). *Time* refers to the amount of time that a person can safely spend in the same room with the client. All client contacts should be arranged so that the greatest amount of care can be accomplished in the shortest period of time. The greatest amount of radiation exposure occurs over the anatomical area of the body that contains the source of radiation. All persons should limit contact with this anatomical site.

Distance, or the amount of space between the client and another person, has the greatest influence on the maximum time each person can remain in contact with the client. A source of radiation is known to lose its intensity according to the inverse square law. This means that if a person remains twice as far from the source of radiation, the person will receive one fourth of the amount of radiation exposure. For example, if the maximum exposure time is 6 hours, 40 minutes at a distance of 3 feet from a particular source of radiation, the maximum exposure time will increase to 26 hours, 40 minutes when the distance from the source is increased to 6 feet. The only time any person should be 3 feet or less from the source of radiation is when direct care is being given. At all other times the person in the room must remain 6 feet or more from the source of radiation.

Some health care agencies use the principle of *shielding*. Shielding refers to the placement of a thick lead shield between the caregivers and the source of radiation. The shield can be portable or permanent. Some caregivers believe that shielding equipment is very heavy and difficult to manage and that it actively reduces efficiency and increases the time needed to provide care. Therefore, the issue of shielding remains controversial. No practical amount of shielding will completely protect a person from the penetrating gamma rays. The principles of time and distance must be followed exactly and consistently.

The body excreta (urine, feces, vomitus, and perspiration) and soiled linen and dressings are not radioactive. In some health agencies, they are collected in the client's room until monitoring determines they do not contain a source of radiation that has become dislodged from the site of placement. A sealed lead-lined container should be present in the client's room at all times for immediate use if a dislodgement should occur. When a dislodgement is noted, the source of radiation must be picked up with a pair of long-handled forceps or tongs and placed in the lead container. The radiation source must *never* be picked up with the bare hands, and the radiation source must *never* be placed in the sewage system via the sink or toilet.

The radiation safety officer and/or the radiation therapist must be notified *immediately* if dislodgement occurs.

The removal of a radiation source must occur at the exact time designated in the treatment plan. The radiation source is gently removed and placed in the sealed lead container present in the client's room. The radiation source is then taken to the radiation therapy department, and the client and the room are surveyed to ensure that all the radiation source has been removed. After the radiation source is removed, all safety precautions are discontinued, since the client is no longer radioactive.

Unsealed therapy. Unsealed internal radiation therapy involves the use of a liquid source of radiation that is administered orally, intravenously, or by instillation into a specific body cavity. This form of internal radiation is metabolized and absorbed by the body and then concentrated in a specific body organ, often referred to as the *target organ*. Because the source of radiation is absorbed systemically in the body and metabolized, all body fluids and excreta are considered contaminated by the source of radiation used.

Iodine 131 is the most commonly encountered and most widely used absorbed radiation source. It is used to treat thyroid cancer as well as the benign diseases of hyperthyroidism and Graves' disease. This isotope is administered orally, and the client is asked to sip the liquid containing iodine 131 through a straw. Gamma rays with a half-life of 8 days are emitted. The same precautions used to avoid radiation exposure for mechanically placed internal radiation sources are used. The body fluids and excreta containing the greatest amount of contamination from the radiation source are saliva, perspiration, blood, vomitus, and urine. Considering the half-life of the isotope, the excretion rate of 50% in the first 24 hours, and the fact that it takes 3 to 5 days for the isotope to become concentrated in the thyroid gland (target organ), the time of greatest danger from radiation contamination of the body fluids is the first 24 to 96 hours after administration of the isotope. During this time, special precautions must be taken when other persons, equipment, and supplies come in contact with the radioactive body fluids and excreta of the treated client. After 96 hours, it can be assumed that the greatest portion of the radioactivity will be concentrated in the thyroid gland, so special precautions will not be necessary for the remainder of the time the isotope remains radioactive. Since the major portion of the isotope will be excreted by the kidneys, kidney function must be monitored before, during, and after administration of the isotope. If the kidneys are not functioning within normal limits, it may take a longer time to rid the body of the isotope than was predicted by the half-life. Care of the client with unsealed radioactive iodine is outlined in Table 9-19.

Radioactive phosphorus (phosphorus 32) is an isotope that emits beta particles and has a half-life of 14 days. Beta particles present no external hazard to persons coming in contact with the client as long as the isotope is contained within the client. Even though beta particles can penetrate several layers of skin, the particles are shielded by the body fluids and tissues. Phosphorus is administered orally or intravenously in multiple doses over several

Table 9-19 Care of the Client Treated with Radioactive Iodine

DAYS 1 THROUGH 4

1. Use the safety measures discussed for sealed mechanically placed radiation (see text).
2. If vomiting occurs, the vomitus will be highly contaminated with gamma radiation. All persons coming in contact with the vomitus are considered contaminated.
3. Take precautionary measures with the client's urine in accordance with the standards of the health care agency.
4. If the urine is to be deposited directly into the sewage system, the client must flush the toilet three times after each use, making sure that no urine is deposited on the toilet seat.
5. If the urine is to be decontaminated before disposal in the sewage system, the client uses a bedpan and the urine is collected in lead containers and stored for 10 to 40 days before placement in the sewage system.
6. Thoroughly wash the hands or anything contaminated with the urine with soap, water, and friction for 5 minutes or longer. Use rubber gloves and effective hand-washing techniques when coming in contact with the client's urine.
7. Instruct the client to use paper plates and plastic eating utensils and discard them after meals.
8. Wear hospital gown and store all soiled linen in tightly closed plastic bags. The linen is stored for 10 to 40 days before washing.
9. Monitor all articles coming in contact with the client. If contamination is present, all articles must be stored for 10 to 40 days and then checked again for contamination before being used or discarded.

DAYS 5 THROUGH 14

1. Continue to flush the toilet three times after voiding, and use effective hand-washing techniques.
2. Instruct the client to sleep alone.

Modified from Yasko J: Radiotherapy: a patient/significant other teaching plan. In Donovan DL, ed: A guide to patient education, New York, 1981, Appleton-Century-Crofts, pp 101-102.

weeks and is usually used in the treatment of the metastatic lesions of primary breast and prostate cancer. Soluble phosphorus 32 is given in multiple doses over several weeks. A frequently occurring side effect of soluble phosphorus is leukopenia. Phosphorus 32 in the soluble form is present in all body fluids and is excreted by the kidneys in the urine. All precautions associated with body fluids and urine that were used for iodine 131 are to be used when soluble phosphorus 32 is administered.

Chemotherapy

Chemotherapy is the systemic treatment of cancer with chemicals (drugs). In the 1940s, chemotherapy was in its infancy. Nitrogen mustard, a chemical warfare agent in

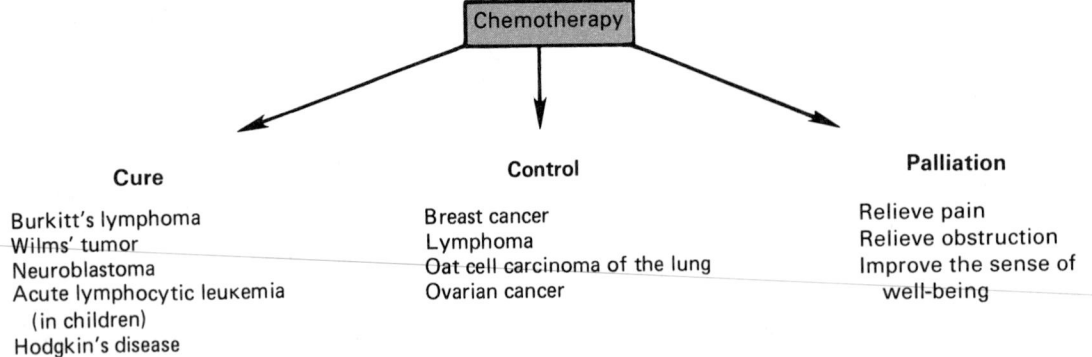

Fig. 9-16 Goals of chemotherapy.

World War II, was used in the treatment of acute leukemia, and a folic acid antimetabolite (5-FU) was found to have antitumor activity. In the 1950s, considerable experimentation with single-drug therapy began, and in the 1960s the emphasis was on the development and use of combination chemotherapy. In the 1970s, chemotherapy was established as an effective treatment modality for cancer. By the 1980s, clinical studies looked at the effect of high doses of chemotherapy used in the treatment of cancers previously resistant to therapy. Chemotherapy is now used in the treatment of many solid tumors, and it is the primary therapy for leukemias and some lymphomas. Chemotherapy has gone from a palliative, "last-ditch effort" treatment modality to one that can cure certain cancers, control other cancers for long periods of time, and offer palliative relief of symptoms when cure or control no longer is possible (Fig. 9-16).

Effect on cells. The effect of chemotherapy is at the cellular level. All cells (cancer cells and normal cells) enter the cell cycle for replication and proliferation (see Fig. 9-1). The effects of the chemotherapeutic agents are described in relationship to the cell cycle. The two major categories of chemotherapeutic drugs are *cell cycle–nonspecific* and *cell cycle–specific*.

Cell cycle–nonspecific chemotherapeutic drugs have their effect on the cells that are in the process of cellular replication and proliferation as well as on the cells that are in the resting phase (G_0).

Cell cycle–specific chemotherapeutic drugs have their effect on cells that are in the process of cellular replication/proliferation (G_1, S_1, G_2, or M). The cell cycle–specific chemotherapeutic drugs can be categorized more specifically into *phase-specific* chemotherapeutic agents. These drugs are effective at only one specific phase of the cell cycle.

Cell cycle–specific and cell cycle–nonspecific agents are often administered in combination with one another. The aim of this approach is to effect a better response using agents that function by differing mechanisms.

The goal of chemotherapy is to reduce the number of cancer cells present in the primary tumor site(s) and in metastatic tumor sites. Several factors will determine the response of cancer cells to chemotherapy:

1. Mitotic rate of the tissue from which the tumor arises: The more rapid the mitotic rate, the greater the response to chemotherapy. Chemotherapy is the treatment of choice for acute leukemia, choriocarcinoma of the placenta, Wilms' tumor (used in conjunction with surgery), and neuroblastoma. These cancer cells have a rapid rate of cellular proliferation.
2. Size of the tumor: The smaller the number of cancer cells, the greater the response to chemotherapy.
3. Age of the tumor: The younger the tumor, the greater the response to chemotherapy. Young tumors have a greater percentage of proliferating cells.
4. Location of the tumor: Certain anatomical sites provide a protected environment from the effects of chemotherapy. For example, only a few drugs (nitrosoureas and bleomycin) cross the blood-brain barrier.
5. Presence of resistant tumor cells: Mutation of cancer cells within the tumor mass can result in variant cells that are resistant to chemotherapy. Resistance can also occur because of the biochemical inability of some cancer cells to convert the drug to its active form.
6. Physiological and psychological status of the host: A state of optimum health and a positive attitude will allow the client to better withstand aggressive chemotherapy.

When the cancer first begins to grow, most of the cells are actively dividing. As the tumor increases in size, more and more cells become inactive and convert to a resting state (G_0). Since most chemotherapeutic agents are most effective against dividing cells, cells can escape death by staying in the G_0 phase. The main problem in cancer chemotherapy is the presence of drug-resistant resting and noncycling cells.

One way to prevent the existence of drug-resistant tumor cells is with the use of high-dose chemotherapy. The aim of this approach is to maximize the effects of the drug at the cellular level before the problem of resistance occurs. An example of high-dose chemotherapy is the use of cytarabine (ara-C) for the treatment of leukemia. The standard dose of this agent is 100 mg/m^2. However, the intensified regimen of this agent includes a dose of 3 g/m^2.

Classification. Chemotherapy drugs are categorized or classified according to their structure and mechanisms of action (Table 9-20 and Fig. 9-17). Each drug in a particu-

Table 9-20 Classification of Chemotherapy Drugs

Mechanisms of Action	Examples	Mechanisms of Action	Examples
ALKYLATING AGENTS **Cycle nonspecific** Damage DNA by causing breaks in the double-strand helix (similar to the effect of radiation therapy); if repair does not occur, cells will die immediately (cytocidal) or when they attempt to divide (cytostatic)	Mechlorethamine (nitrogen mustard), cyclophosphamide (Cytoxan), chlorambucil (Leukeran), melphalan (Alkeran), triethylene thiophosphoramide (Thiotepa), busulfan (Myleran), dacarbazine (DTIC)	**CORTICOSTEROIDS** **Cycle nonspecific** Disrupt the cell membrane and inhibit synthesis of RNA to protein; lyse circulating lymphocytes; inhibit mitosis; depress immune system; increase feeling of well-being	Prednisone (Merticorten), dexamethasone (Decadron)
ANTIMETABOLITES **Cycle specific** Interfere with synthesis of DNA by mimicking certain essential cellular metabolites that cell incorporates into synthesis of DNA; cells will die immediately (cytocidal)	Methotrexate (Amethopterin), cytosine arabinoside (ara-C, Cytosar), 5-fluorouracil (5-FU), 6-mercaptopurine (6-MP), thioguanine (6-TG), floxuridine (FUDR), vidarabine (Vira-A), 5-azacitidine, hexamethylmelamine	**HORMONES** **Cycle nonspecific** Stimulate the process of cellular differentiation; metastatic lesions are less able to survive in unfavorable environment; decrease the process of cellular proliferation	Androgens (testosterone, fluoxymesterone [Halotestine]), estrogens (diethylstibestrol [DES]), progestins (Provera, Delalutin, Megace)
ANTITUMOR ANTIBIOTICS **Cycle nonspecific** Modify function of DNA and interfere with transcription of RNA; cells will die immediately (cytocidal) or when they attempt to divide (cytostatic)	Doxorubicin (Adriamycin), bleomycin (Blenoxane), mitomycin (Mutamycin), daunorubicin (Daunomycin), actinomycin D	**MISCELLANEOUS** Heavy metal effect on DNA similar to alkylating agents Destroys exogenous supply of L-asparagine, which is needed for cellular proliferation; normal cells can synthesize but cannot be synthesized by cancer cells	Cisplatin (Platinol), carboplatin (JM-8, CBDCA) L-Asparaginase (Elspar)
PLANT ALKALOIDS **Cycle specific** Interrupt cellular replication in mitosis at metaphase; cells will die immediately (cytocidal)	Vinblastine (Velban), vincristine (Oncovin)	Has effect on DNA similar to alkylating agents; also blocks incorporation of thymidine into DNA Suppresses mitosis at interphase; also has effect similar to alkylating agents Antiestrogens used in breast cancer Antiadrenal drug blocks adrenal steroid production	Hydroxyurea (Hydrea) Procarbazine (Matulane, Natulan) Tamoxifen (Nolvadex) Aminoglutethimide (Cytadren)
NITROSUREAS **Cycle nonspecific** Has similar effect to alkylating agents and also blocks specific enzymes needed for the synthesis of purine; cells will die immediately (cytocidal) or when they attempt to divide (cytostatic)	Carmustine (BCNU), lomustine (CCNU), semustine (Methyl CCNU), streptozotocin (STZ), chlorozotozin (DCNU)		

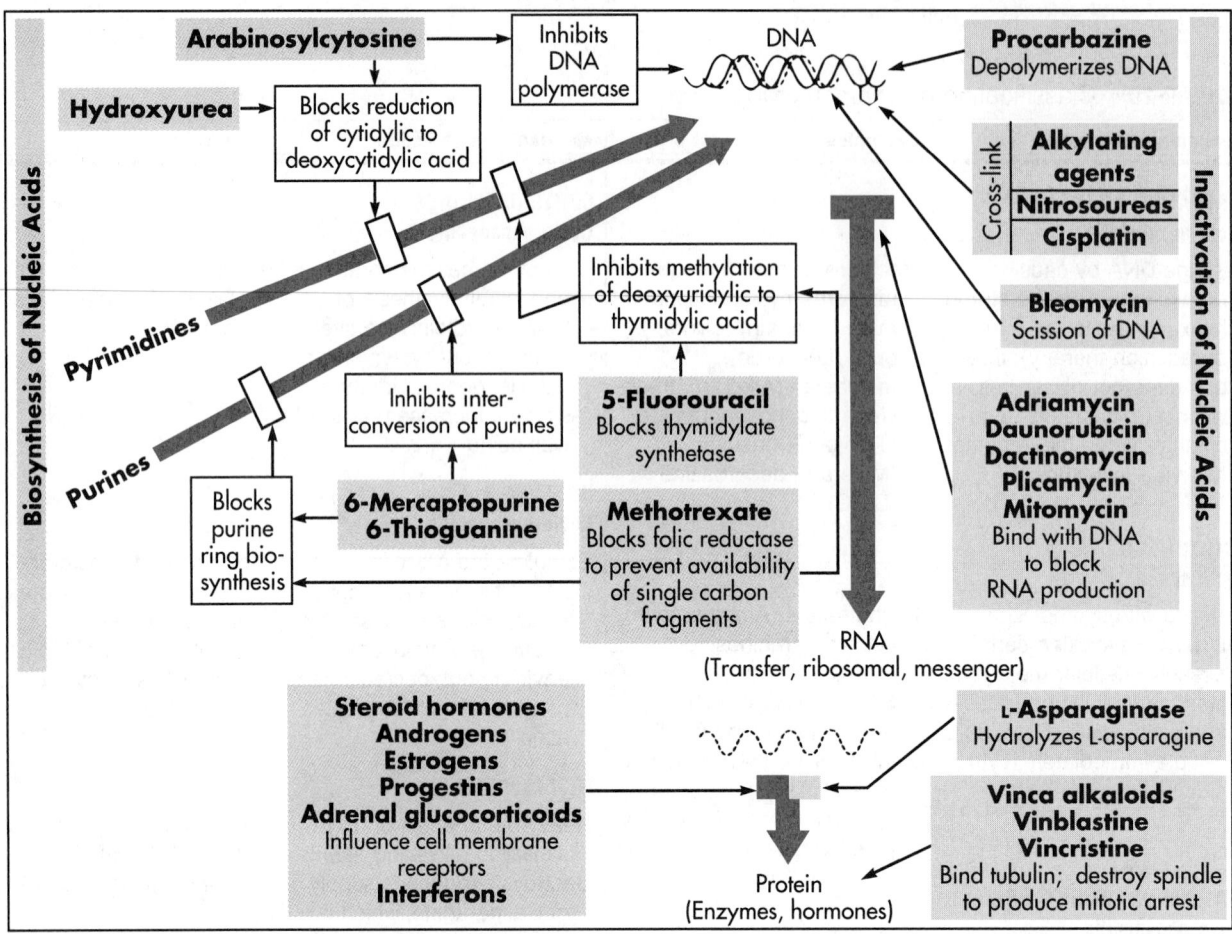

Fig. 9-17 Actions of chemotherapeutic drugs. (From Krakoff I: Cancer chemotherapeutic agents, CA 37:97, 1987.)

lar classification has many similarities, but major differences in the drugs are also evident.

Methods of administration. Chemotherapy can be administered by several routes (Table 9-21). The oral and intravenous routes are the most common. One of the major concerns with the intravenous administration of antineoplastic drugs is possible irritation of the vessel wall by the drug or, even worse, extravasation (infiltration of drugs into tissues surrounding the infusion site) causing local tissue damage. Many chemotherapeutic drugs are vesicants—agents that when accidentally infiltrated into the skin cause severe local tissue breakdown and necrosis. Some guidelines to promote safe use of the chemotherapeutic drugs by intravenous administration follow:

1. Obtain a knowledge base for the safe administration of chemotherapy.
2. Start an intravenous infusion of normal saline solution or 5% dextrose in water or saline solution with a small-lumen short needle or catheter. Ensure that recent venipunctures have not been performed proximal to the intravenous site. Avoid using an arm that has poor lymphatic drainage or that has previously received radiation therapy.

3. Select a vein that is large enough to promote infusion without irritating the intima of the vein. When a vesicant is administered, avoid the veins in the hand, wrist, and antecubital area.
4. Instruct the client to report immediately any changes in sensation, especially burning or stinging pain.
5. Check for a blood return before infusing the chemotherapy drug. However, a blood return does not always indicate an intact vein.
6. Administer vesicant agents first, when the vein is at its optimum integrity. (Note: This is controversial. Some believe that vesicants should be administered last or sandwiched between two nonvesicants to reveal the presence of vein fragility or spasm.)
7. Slowly push those drugs that are to be given by the push or bolus method. Pause 30 to 60 seconds and allow the intravenous infusion to flush the vein, check blood return, and again gently push 0.5 to 1 ml of the medication. Repeat until the medication has been given and allow the intravenous infusion to flush the vein for several minutes.
8. Stop the intravenous infusion immediately if the client complains of a burning or stinging pain or if you

Table 9-21 Methods of Chemotherapy
Administration

Method	Examples
Oral	Cyclophosphamide
Intramuscular	Bleomycin
Intravenous	Doxorubicin, vincristine
Intracavitary (pleural, peritoneal)	Radioisotopes, alkylating agents
Intrathecal	Methotrexate, cytosine arabinoside
Intraarterial	DTIC, 5-FU, methotrexate, floxuridine
Perfusion	Alkylating agents
Continuous infusion	5-FU, methotrexate, cytosine arabinoside
Subcutaneous	Cytosine arabinoside
Topical	5-FU cream
Intraperitoneal	Methotrexate, 5-FU

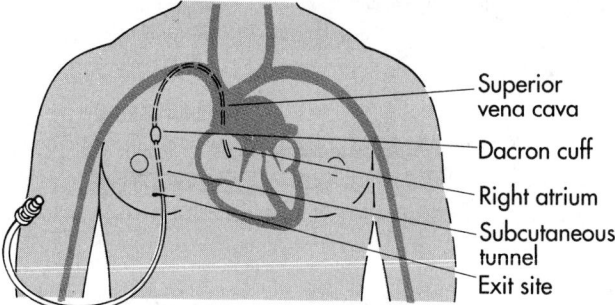

Fig. 9-18 Silastic right atrial catheter placement. Note tip of the catheter in the right atrium. (From Yasko JM and Bender CM: Trends in chemotherapy administration, Cancer Nurs Suppl 1:34-39, 1987.)

suspect there has been an infiltration. If the drug is an irritant, check for blood return and, if present, continue to administer the drug. If it is a vesicant, stop the infusion and begin appropriate extravasation procedures.

9. If extravasation occurs
   a. Stop the intravenous infusion immediately; notify the physician or use the standing written orders.
   b. Remove the intravenous infusion tubing and aspirate any remaining drug with a new syringe.
   c. Inject the prescribed antidote if one exists in the infusion needle and/or in a "pincushion" fashion in the skin surrounding the needle site.
   d. Apply a topical corticosteroid cream.
   e. Elevate the site.
   f. Apply cold compresses for the first 24 to 48 hours unless a *Vinca* alkaloid has been infiltrated. Heat is applied following extravasation of *Vinca* alkaloids.
   g. Document the extravasation.
   h. Observe site at designated intervals.
   i. A plastic surgeon may be consulted, depending on the extent of anticipated damage.

Pain is the cardinal symptom of extravasation, although extravasation has been known to occur without causing pain. Swelling, redness, and the presence of vesicles on the skin are other early signs of extravasation. After a few days, the tissue may begin to ulcerate and necrose. The process has the potential to progress to a deep, wide crater that often warrants closure with skin grafts. This is a very serious problem that may be life threatening if infection occurs.

Chemotherapy can also be administered by means of a vascular access device. Vascular access devices are placed in large vessels (venous or arterial) and permit frequent, continuous, or intermittent administration of chemotherapy and other products, thus avoiding multiple punctures for vascular access. These devices are indicated in instances of limited vascular access, intensive chemotherapy, and projected long-term need for vascular access. In addition to their usefulness in administration of chemotherapy, vascular access devices can be used to administer additional fluids, such as blood products, parenteral nutrition, and other medications, and for venous blood sampling. The advantages of vascular access devices are that they provide for rapid dilution of chemotherapy, decreased incidence of extravasation, and reduced need for venipuncture. Three major types of vascular access devices include Silastic right atrial catheters, implanted infusion ports, and infusion (external and implanted) pumps.

Silastic right atrial catheters. Silastic right atrial catheters (Hickman, Broviac, Raaf, and Corcath) are single-, double-, or triple-lumen catheters approximately 90 cm in length with internal diameters ranging from 1 to 2 mm (Fig. 9-18). These catheters are placed with the aid of local or general anesthesia through a central vein with the tip resting in the right atrium of the heart. The other end of the catheter is tunneled through subcutaneous tissue and exits through a separate incision on the chest or abdominal wall. A Dacron cuff on the catheter serves to stabilize the catheter and may also decrease the incidence of infection. Care requirements include cap change, cleansing, heparin flush, and dressing change. The exact frequency and procedures for these requirements vary from institution to institution. Reported complications with these catheters include clotting, sepsis, bleeding, thrombosis, technical problems, and local infection at the exit site.

The Groshong catheter is a distinct type of Silastic right atrial catheter. The unique features of this catheter are the existence of a pressure-sensitive valve near the distal end, which precludes the need for heparin flushing and clamping, and its placement 2 to 3 cm above the right atrium in the superior vena cava.

Implanted infusion ports. Implanted infusion ports (Infus-A-Port, Port-A-Cath, Vascular Access Port, and Medi-Port) consist of a central venous catheter connected to an implanted subcutaneous injection port (Fig. 9-19). The catheter is placed into the desired vein and the other end is connected to a port that is surgically implanted in a subcu-

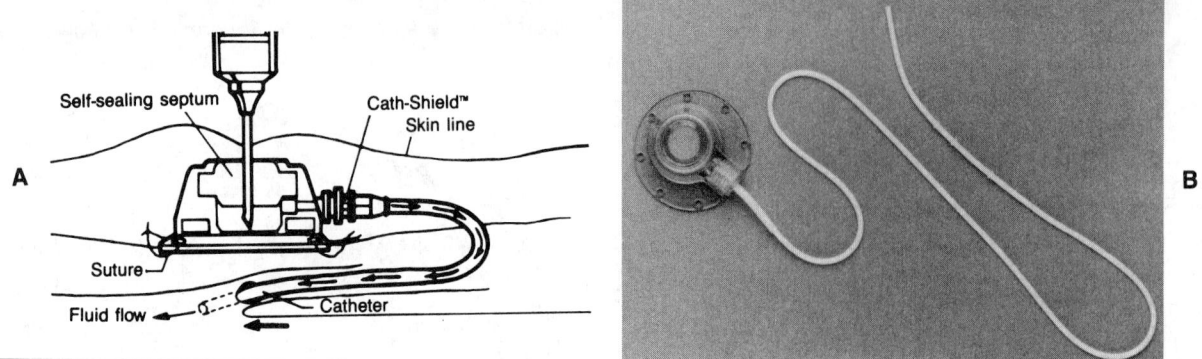

Fig. 9-19 **A,** Cross-section of implantable port displaying access of the port with the Huber needle. Note the deflected point of the Huber needle, which prevents coring of the port's septum. (Courtesy Pharmacia Deltec, Inc, St. Paul, Minn.) **B,** Infusaport. (Courtesy Shiley Infusaid Inc., Norwood, Mass.)

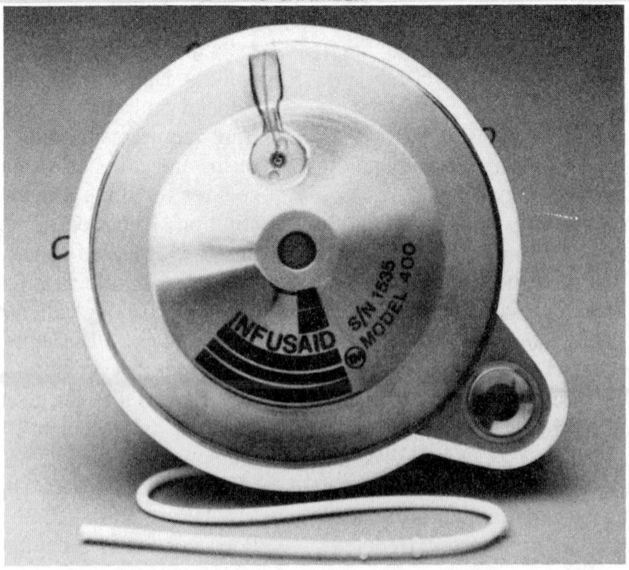

Fig. 9-20 **A,** Cross-section of the implantable pump displaying its two chambers: the drug chamber (inner) and the charging fluid chamber (outer). As the drug chamber is filled, the bellows expand, compressing the charging fluid in the outer chamber. The resulting increased pressure in the outer chamber forces the drug through a membrane filter and preset flow restrictor, thus ensuring a nearly constant flow. (Courtesy Shiley Infusaid, Norwood, Mass.) **B,** Infusaid Pump. (Courtesy Shiley Infusaid Inc., Norwood, Mass.)

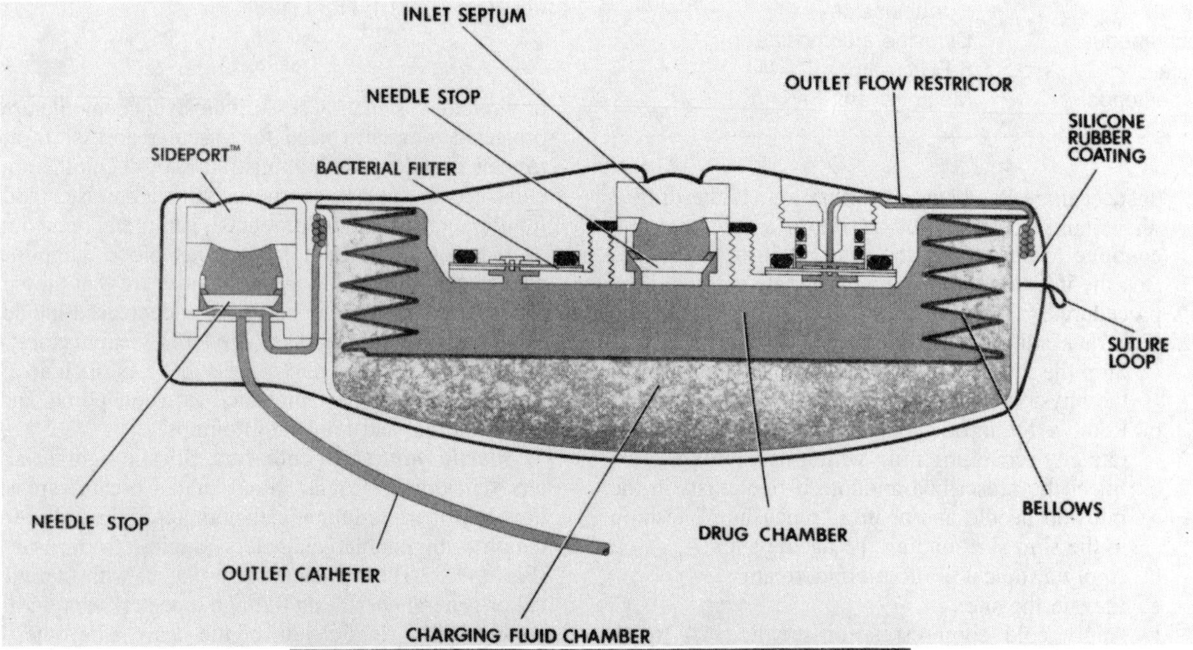

taneous pocket on the chest wall. The port consists of a metal sheath with a self-sealing silicone septum. It is accessed via the septum by means of a special Huber-point needle that has a deflected tip to prevent coring of the septum. Care requirements include dressing change, cleansing, and flushing. Complications attributed to implanted infusion ports include clotting, catheter migration, infection, bleeding, thrombosis, air embolism, and infection at the exit site or in the pocket.

Infusion pumps. Infusion pumps are used in cancer treatment primarily for the continuous infusion of chemotherapy by intravenous, subcutaneous, intraarterial, and epidural routes. Infusion pumps can be worn externally or implanted surgically. The various types of external infusion pumps (Autosyringe, Cormed, Infumed 200, Deltec-Pharmacia, Pancreatec, Travenol Infusor) differ in terms of their mechanisms of action, components, and capabilities.

Implanted infusion pumps (Infusaid) are used primarily for intraarterial administration of chemotherapy (Fig. 9-20). This approach permits continuous infusion of the chemotherapeutic agent directly to the area of the tumor while sparing the client the systemic effects of the drug. The most common use of this method of chemotherapy administration has been hepatic artery infusion in the treatment of liver metastasis, usually from primary colon cancer.

Implanted pumps also consist of a catheter that is threaded into the designated artery. The catheter is attached to a pump apparatus that consists of two chambers: an inner chamber that serves as the drug reservoir and an outer chamber that contains vapor pressure providing a source of power for the pump. The pump is implanted surgically in a subcutaneous pocket. Access to the pump is via a silicone septum with a Huber-point needle. Complications that have been associated with implanted infusion pumps include infection, thrombosis, clotting of the catheter, and pump malfunction.[15]

Other access devices used in the treatment of persons with cancer include the Tenckhoff catheter used in the administration of intraperitoneal chemotherapy and the Ommaya reservoir, which delivers agents directly to the central nervous system.

Effects on normal tissues. Chemotherapeutic agents cannot selectively distinguish between normal cells and cancer cells. When normal cells are destroyed, the client experiences certain signs and symptoms that are the expected side effects or toxic effects of chemotherapy. Effects of chemotherapy are due to (1) destruction of cells with a rapid rate of cellular proliferation (Table 9-22), (2) response of the body to the products of cellular destruction (cellular waste products in circulation may cause fatigue, anorexia, and taste alterations), and (3) specific drug toxicities (Table 9-23).

The adverse effects of these drugs can be classified as acute, delayed, or chronic. Acute toxicity includes vomiting, allergic reactions, and dysrhythmias. Delayed effects include mucositis, alopecia, and bone marrow depression. Mucositis can result in mouth sores, gastritis, and diar-

Table 9-22 Cells with Rapid Rate of Proliferation

Cells and Generation Time	Effect of Cell Destruction
Bone marrow stem cell, 6-24 hr	Myelosuppression; infection/ bleeding/anemia
Neutrophils, 12 hr	Leukopenia, infection
Epithelial cells lining the gastrointestinal tract, 12-24 hr	Anorexia, stomatitis, esophagitis, nausea/vomiting, diarrhea
Cells of the hair follicle, 24 hr	Alopecia
Ova/testes, 24-36 hr	Sexual dysfunction

rhea. Chronic toxicities involve damage to organ systems such as the heart, liver, kidneys, and lungs.

Treatment plan. When chemotherapy is used in the treatment of cancer, several drugs are usually given in combination. Single-drug chemotherapy is rarely chosen for a treatment plan today. The drugs given are carefully selected to most effectively kill the cancer cells while allowing the normal cells to repair themselves and proliferate. The dose of each drug is carefully calculated according to the body weight or the body surface area of the client being treated. The choice of the drugs selected to be given together to treat a particular cancer is based on the following principles of combination chemotherapy:

1. The drugs used in the treatment plan are effective against the cancer being treated.
2. When drugs are given in combination, a synergistic effect occurs.
3. The drug combination includes drugs that are cycle specific and cycle nonspecific and that have different mechanisms of action.
4. The drugs combined include drugs that have different toxic side effects.
5. The drug combination includes drugs whose nadir occurs at different time intervals. The nadir is the lowest level of the peripheral blood cell counts (particularly white blood cells) that occurs secondary to bone marrow depression. The nadir of most drugs ranges from 7 to 28 days, with recovery by 21 to 28 days after administration of chemotherapy.

The MOPP protocol, the first combination protocol for the treatment of Hodgkin's disease, is an example of a combination chemotherapy treatment regimen:

Nitrogen mustard (M)
Cycle nonspecific
Alkylating agent
Toxic side effects: myelosuppression, nausea, vomiting, alopecia
Nadir: 7 to 14 days

Oncovin (O)
Phase specific
Plant alkaloid
Toxic side effects: neurotoxicity, alopecia
Nadir: unknown

Table 9-23 Toxic Side Effects of Chemotherapy

Chemotherapeutic Agent	Myelosuppression	Mucositis	Nausea and vomiting	Alopecia	Vesicant	Allergic Reaction	Other Specific Toxicities
Actinomycin D (Cosmegen)	+	+	+	+	+	0	Diarrhea
5-Azacytidine	+	+	+	0	0	0	Hepatotoxicity
Bleomycin (Blenoxane)	±	+	±	+	0	+	Pulmonary toxicity, skin rash
Busulfan (Myleran)	+	0	±	0	0	0	Pulmonary fibrosis
Carmustine (BCNU)	+	+	+	0	+	0	Hepatotoxicity
Chlorambucil (Leukeran)	+	0	±	0	0	0	
Cisplatin (Platinol)	+	0	+	0	0	+	Nephrotoxicity / Peripheral neuropathy / Ototoxicity
Cyclophosphamide (Cytoxan)	+	0	+	+	0	0	Sterile hemorrhagic cystitis / Heart failure
Cytosine arabinoside (Cytosar, ara-C)	+	+	+	+	0	0	Hepatotoxicity
Dacarbazine (DTIC)	+	0	+	0	+	+	Hypotension
Daunorubicin (Daunomycin)	+	+	+	+	+	0	Cardiotoxicity / Hepatotoxicity
Diethylstilbestrol (DES)	0	0	+	0	0	0	CHF
Doxorubicin (Adriamycin)	+	+	+	+	+	0	Cardiotoxicity / Diarrhea
Floxuridine (FUDR)	+	+	+	+	0	0	Diarrhea, rash
5-Fluorouracil	+	+	±	±	0	0	Diarrhea, photosensitivity
Fluoxymesterone (Halotestin)	0	0	+	0	0	0	Masculinization
Hexamethylmelamine (HXM, HMM)	+	0	+	±	0	0	Peripheral neuropathy
Hydroxyurea (Hydrea)	+	+	+	+	0	0	
L-Asparaginase (Elspar)	0	0	+	0	0	+	Major organ failure
Lomustine (CCNU)	+	+	+	±	0	0	Hepatotoxicity
Megestrol acetate (Megace)	0	0	0	+	0	0	Fluid retention
Melphalan (Alkeran)	+	±	±	0	0	0	
Mechlorethamine (nitrogen mustard)	+	0	+	+	+	0	
6-Mercaptopurine (6-MP)	+	+	+	0	0	0	Hepatotoxicity
Methotrexate (MTX, Amethopterin)	+	+	±	±	0	0	Nephrotoxicity
Mithramycin (Mithracin)	+	+	+	0	+	0	Hemorrhagic tendency
Mitomycin (Mutamycin)	+	+	+	+	+	0	Nephrotoxicity, pulmonary toxicity

+, Common; ±, infrequent; 0, uncommon.

Modified from Lane C and others: Cancer chemotherapy guidelines, ed 5, Oncology Research Center, Bowman Gray School of Medicine, Wake Forest University, Winston-Salem, NC, 1985.

Table 9-23 Toxic Side Effects of Chemotherapy—cont'd

Chemotherapeutic Agent	Myelosuppression	Mucositis	Nausea and vomiting	Alopecia	Vesicant	Allergic Reaction	Other Specific Toxicities
							Hepatotoxicity
Oxymethalone (Androl-50)	0	0	+	0	0	0	Hepatotoxicity
Piperazinedione	+	0	+	0	+	0	
Prednisolone	0	0	0	0	0	0	Steroid side effects
Prednisone	0	0	0	0	0	0	Steroid side effects
Procarbazine hydro-chloride (Matulane)	+	±	+	0	0	0	Monoamine oxidase inhibitor
Semustine (Methyl CCNU)	+	+	+	0	0	0	
Streptozotocin (SRZ, Zanosar)	+	0	+	±	+	0	Nephrotoxicity
Tamoxifen (Nolvadex)	±	0	+	0	0	0	
6-Thioguanine (6-TG)	+	+	+	0	0	0	Hepatotoxicity
Uracil mustard	+	0	+	±	0	0	
Vinblastine (Velban)	+	+	+	±	+	0	Neurotoxicity
Vincristine (Oncovin)	0	0	0	+	+	0	Neurotoxicity
VP-16	+	0	+	+	0	+	Hypotension

Table 9-24 MOPP Chemotherapeutic Drug Schedule

	DAYS														
DRUG	1	2	3	4	5	6	7	8	9	10	11	12	13	14	15-28
Nitrogen mustard (intravenous adminis-tration)	↔							↔							
Oncovin (intravenous administration)	↔							↔							No drugs given
Procarbazine (oral administration)	←————————————————————————→														
Prednisone (oral administration)	←————————————————————————→														

Procarbazine (P)
Cycle specific
MAO inhibitor
Toxic side effects: myelosuppression, nausea, vomiting
Nadir: 2 to 8 weeks

Prednisone (P)
Corticosteroid
Toxic side effects: steroid effects
Nadir: unknown

The agents in this drug protocol differ in mechanisms of action, toxic side effects, and nadir, but the combination is synergistic in nature and effectively destroys the cancer cells present in the early stages of Hodgkin's disease.

The drugs are given according to a specific schedule that includes a time of drug administration and a time of rest from drug administration. The rest period is necessary to allow the normal body cells that have been destroyed to proliferate and repair the damaged tissue. The example in Table 9-24 describes a typical MOPP schedule. This drug schedule is repeated a specific number of times. Most chemotherapy treatment plans extend for 6 months or longer. The client is evaluated before the administration of each course of chemotherapy to determine whether the normal cells have proliferated to a sufficient degree.

Often the most difficult decision to make is when to stop the administration of chemotherapy. The client is evaluated according to the following criteria:

1. Complete remission: Complete absence of all evidence of cancer and a return to the usual performance status occur. The duration of a complete remission must exceed 1 month.
2. Partial remission: Regression of 50% or more of the disease process without evidence of progression and with subjective improvement noted. The duration of a partial remission is usually several months.
3. Improvement: Regression of 25% to 50% of the disease process with subjective improvement noted.
4. No response: Regression of 25% or less of the disease with no subjective improvement noted.
5. Progression: Progression of the disease process noted.

With a complete remission that has extended for a time, the chemotherapy is usually discontinued and the client is evaluated at frequent intervals. When partial remission or improvement occurs, the same treatment plan or a revised treatment plan is followed over a long period (several years) and the client is evaluated frequently. No response or progression of disease warrants a change in the treatment plan or a decision to use treatment for palliation.

Safe preparation, administration, and disposal of chemotherapeutic agents. An important issue in cancer care is that working with antineoplastic agents may be hazardous for health professionals. It is suspected that the person preparing or giving chemotherapy may absorb the drug through inhalation of particles when reconstituting a powder in an open ampule and through skin contact. There may also be some risk in handling the vomitus and excreta of persons receiving chemotherapy. At present, data regarding health risks for the professional working with chemotherapy are not conclusive.

Table 9-25   Guidelines for Safe Handling of Chemotherapeutic Agents

PREPARATION

Prepare all chemotherapeutic agents in a central area and under a Class II vertical laminar-flow biological safety cabinet, vented to the outside.

Agents should be prepared by a pharmacist, who should do the following:

Wear a disposable, protective gown with long sleeves and elastic cuffs and disposable, surgical, latex gloves.
Place a disposable, plastic-backed liner on work surface.
Post hazardous warning signs in the mixing area.
Avoid puncturing gloves or inoculating self.
Use Luer-Lok fittings where possible.
Vent all vials.
Wrap gauze around neck of ampule when opening.
Prime tubing under safety cabinet.
Place all exposed waste in an approved disposal container.

ADMINISTRATION AND DURING EXPOSURE TO EXCRETA/VOMITUS

Wear disposable latex surgical gloves.
Wear gown/mask if desired (remains controversial).
Place a disposable, plastic-backed liner under client's extremity.

DISPOSAL

Place all disposable items (needles, syringes, vials, and ampules) coming in contact with antineoplastic agents in an approved leak-proof container.
Discard waste containers in an approved incinerator.
Place contaminated linen in an approved container; linen must be washed separately.

SPILLS

Wear disposable, surgical, latex gloves.
Wear disposable gown with elastic cuffs.
Use "Spill Kits" containing all materials necessary for proper handling.

PERSONNEL RECOMMENDATIONS

Teach all persons likely to be exposed to antineoplastic agents or excreta the necessary precautions.
Prevent contact of pregnant or lactating women with chemotherapeutic agents.
Distribute workload to minimize employee exposure to chemotherapeutic agents.
Provide periodic health screening for exposed persons.
Document patterns of exposure.

The only well-known hazard associated with chemotherapy is that of cutaneous reactions following skin contact with certain drugs including BCNU (Carmustine), mechlorethamine (nitrogen mustard), doxorubicin (Adriamycin), and other vesicants. The literature accompanying these drugs specifically cautions against skin and eye contact to prevent possible skin reactions and corneal damage.

Guidelines for the safe handling of chemotherapeutic agents have been developed by the United States Occupational Safety and Health Administration and the Oncology Nursing Society. These guidelines are summarized in Table 9-25.

■ Nursing Management of the Client Receiving Chemotherapy

The role of the nurse in cancer chemotherapy has greatly expanded during the past decade. Regardless of the health care agency setting, the nurse will meet individuals who are receiving or who have received chemotherapy. One of the most important responsibilities of the nurse is that of differentiating between toxic effects of the drug and progression of the malignant process. The nurse also needs to differentiate between tolerable side effects and acute toxic effects of chemotherapeutic agents. For example, nausea and vomiting are expected and controllable side effects of many drugs. However, if paresthesia occurs with the use of vincristine or signs of heart failure appear with the use of doxorubicin, these serious reactions need to be reported to the physician so that drug dosages can be modified or discontinued. Some toxicities associated with chemotherapy may not be reversible. For example, ototoxicity may be an irreversible effect of cisplatin therapy, especially at higher doses. Periodic testing of hearing may be necessary to monitor for this toxicity. Specific nursing measures related to problems associated with chemotherapy are presented in the nursing care plan for the client with cancer (Table 9-17).

Nausea and vomiting are the most commonly observed gastrointestinal side effects. Vomiting may occur within 1 hour of administration and may last for 24 hours or more. Several antiemetic drugs are available. (See Chapter 36 and Table 36-2.) Metoclopramide (Reglan) and dexamethasone (Decadron) have also been used to decrease the nausea and vomiting caused by chemotherapy. Nursing management related to nausea and vomiting is presented in Table 9-17.

Results of laboratory studies of the client who is receiving chemotherapy should be monitored. Particular attention should be given to the white blood cell, platelet, and red blood cell counts. If the white blood cell count falls to less than 2000/μl, the drug regimen may need to be modified or discontinued. Every measure possible needs to be taken to prevent infections in a client with leukopenia (see Table 25-24). If the platelet count falls to less than 50,000/μl, the client must be assessed for any signs of bleeding, and measures should be taken to prevent bleeding (see Table 25-16). Platelet transfusions may be necessary. Red blood cell transfusions may also be indicated for treatment of symptomatic anemia. However, anemia is an uncommon problem in clients receiving chemotherapy.

Uric acid and creatinine levels are usually monitored weekly. Optimum hydration is important to prevent uric acid crystals from causing obstructive uropathy. Allopurinol is often administered as a prophylactic measure if a great degree of cell breakdown is expected. Other diagnostic monitoring depends on the type of drug. For example, an electrocardiogram is performed and cardiac ejection fractions are measured to monitor the potential cardiotoxic effects of doxorubicin and daunorubicin.

Client education

Education of the client is an extremely important part of the nurse role as related to the use of chemotherapy. To decrease the fear and anxiety often associated with chemotherapy, clients must be taught what to expect during a course of treatment. Clients' attitudes toward treatment should be explored so that any misconceptions or fears can be discussed. They need to be told of the possible side effects of chemotherapy that may be experienced during treatment. This may be a discouraging revelation. Therefore, good nursing judgment is essential to determine the amount of information clients can assimilate. Clients must be reassured that this is a temporary situation and that they should be feeling better within a few weeks after chemotherapy is discontinued. The client should also be informed that supportive care (e.g., antiemetics and antidiarrheals) will be provided as needed.

Management of hair loss

Many emotions are experienced and expressed when hair loss occurs; these include anger, grief, embarrassment, and fear. For some persons the loss of hair is one of the most stressful events experienced during the course of the illness. Alopecia due to the administration of chemotherapeutic agents is usually reversible. The degree and duration of hair loss depend on the dose of the chemotherapeutic agent, the duration of the treatment, and the nutritional status of the client. Sometimes the hair begins to grow back while the client is still receiving chemotherapeutic agents, but generally the hair cells do not grow back until the agents are discontinued. Often the new hair has a different color and texture than the hair that was lost.

Hair loss caused by certain chemotherapeutic drugs (e.g., cyclophosphamide and doxorubicin) administered by the bolus intravenous route can be minimized or prevented by the use of a scalp sphygmomanometer, a tourniquet, and/or hypothermia. The scalp tourniquet or sphygmomanometer is applied around the hairline to decrease the blood flow through the superficial scalp arteries before, during, and for 20 minutes after infusion of the drug. (This technique protects hair follicles from high concentrations of cytotoxic drugs.) When the sphygmomanometer is used, the cuff should never be more than 70 mm Hg above the normal systolic blood pressure to prevent tissue damage. When hypothermia is used, the hypothermic agent is applied at least 10 minutes before, during, and for 20 to 30 minutes after infusion of the chemotherapeutic agent. Several more sophisticated devices (Cryogel bags, Thermocirculator, Chemocap, Kold Kap) have been developed and provide vasocontriction by pressure and/or hypothermia. The degree of protection against hair loss varies with the individual client and with the drug administered.

Scalp tourniquets and hypothermia should not be used for clients undergoing chemotherapy for hematopoietic cancer. When these devices are used, chemotherapeutic agents may be prevented from reaching the cancer cells circulating in the vascular system of the scalp and these cancer cells are thus protected from the effects of the chemotherapeutic agents. Other nursing interventions for dealing with alopecia are presented in Table 9-17.

Counseling regarding sexual and reproductive function

Sexual dysfunction may be manifested as temporary or permanent sterility, disruption in the menstrual cycle (in women), temporary or permanent impotence (in men), or chromosomal damage leading to possible genetic mutation.

All clients should be instructed to use an effective means of birth control during the time of chemotherapy and/or radiation therapy and for up to 2 years after treatment. This is necessary to avoid birth defects due to chromosomal damage, to allow the sperm count to return to normal, and to determine the expected prognosis of the client. Sexual or genetic counseling is necessary before the conception of a child to determine the risk of chromosomal damage.

Sexual relations can be continued in the usual patterns during and after treatment if an effective method of birth control is used. It may be necessary to alter the time of day chosen for sexual relations if fatigue is a problem. Early morning may be the time the client feels most rested.

Denuding of the epithelial lining of the vagina may result in inflammation, edema, and ulceration. Sexual intercourse should be avoided if mucositis or ulceration is present. Sitz baths or sitting in a tub of warm water will provide some degree of comfort. A steroid-based cream available by prescription may also provide comfort. A water-based lubricant may be used at the time of intercourse to increase vaginal lubrication, which is necessary to prevent trauma to the vaginal lining and to prevent discomfort or pain.

The client should be encouraged to use other forms of physical contact to obtain sexual pleasure during the period of disruption in sexual functioning. Hugging, caressing, touching, and quiet talking can provide sexual pleasure when sexual intercourse is not possible. The client's partner must be included in all teaching and counseling sessions to be fully informed of the temporary or permanent changes in the client's sexual functioning. Both client and partner must understand that adjustments in sexual functioning patterns will take time, patience, and understanding.

Late Effects of Radiation and Chemotherapy

Cancer survivors are achieving long-term remission and survival rates because of advancements in treatment modalities. However, these forms of therapy (especially radiation and chemotherapy) may produce long-term sequelae known as *physiological late effects* that occur months to years after cessation of therapy. Every body system can be affected to some extent by chemotherapy and/or radiation

therapy. The effects of radiation on the body's tissues are due to cellular hypoplasia of stem cells and to alterations in the fine vasculature and fibroconnective tissues. In addition to the acute toxicities, chemotherapy can have long-term effects related to the loss of cells' proliferative reserve capacity. The additive effects of multiagent chemotherapy before, during, or after a course of radiotherapy can significantly increase the resulting physiological late effects. Some physiological late effects of radiation and chemotherapy are summarized in Table 9-26.

Cancer survivors may also be at risk for leukemias and other secondary malignancies resulting from therapy for their primary cancer. However, the potential risk for developing a second malignancy does not contraindicate the use of cancer treatment because the overall risk of developing neoplastic complications is low and the latency period may be long.

The cancer treatments most frequently implicated in causing secondary malignancy are the alkylating chemotherapeutic agents and high-dose radiation, which can induce cancers at the exposure site. The exact mechanism of oncogenesis of radiation and chemotherapy remains unclear. It could be related to interactions between immunosuppressive factors, direct cellular damage, and oncocarcinogenic effects with other environmental carcinogens.

Acute leukemias occurring as secondary malignancies have been most widely reported after treatment for Hodgkin's disease, but they also occur in survivors of ovarian, lung, and breast cancers. Secondary malignancies other than leukemias include multiple myeloma after radi-

Table 9-26 Possible Late Effects of Radiation and Chemotherapy

Body System	Effect
Cardiac	Chronic cardiomyopathy
	Myocardial fibrosis
Pulmonary	Diffuse alveolar damage
	Pneumonitis
	Fibrosis
Gastrointestinal	Hepatotoxicity
	Enteritis
	Esophagitis
	Fistula formation
Renal/urological	Nephrotoxicity
	Nephritis
	Hemorrhagic cystitis
	Acute tubular necrosis
Neurological	Neuropathy
	Autonomic nervous system disorders
	Hearing loss
	Myelopathy
	Necrotizing leukoencephalopathy
Endocrine	Gonadal impairment
	Ovarian destruction
	Infertility
	Disturbances in sexual functioning

ation therapy for breast cancer; non-Hodgkin's lymphoma after treatment for Hodgkin's disease; and cancers of the bladder, kidney, and ureters after the use of cyclophosphamide. Radiation therapy for breast, lung, ovarian, uterine, and thyroid cancers; non-Hodgkin's lymphoma; and Hodgkin's disease has been linked to secondary osteosarcoma of the rib, scapula, clavicle, humerus, sternum, ilium, and pelvis. Fibrosarcomas have been reported several years after radiation therapy for astrocytoma, glioblastoma, and pituitary adenoma. Unfortunately, secondary malignancies are very resistant to therapy.[16]

Biological Response Modifiers

Biological response modifiers (BRMs) are agents that modify the relationship between the host and the tumor by altering the biological response of the host to the tumor cells. Three categories of BRMs exist: (1) agents that have direct antitumor effects; (2) agents that restore, augment, or modulate host immune system mechanisms; and (3) agents that have other biological effects, such as interfering with the cancer cells' ability to metastasize or differentiate.[17]

Although the use of most BRMs in the treatment of cancer is in an early investigational stage, knowledge and experience with these agents are rapidly being gained with increased understanding of the immune system, advancements in molecular biology, development of hybridoma technology, and modern technological equipment. Current clinical studies with BRMs are being conducted to investigate their effectiveness as single agents; in combination with other BRMs; and with other treatment modalities such as chemotherapy, radiotherapy, and surgery.

Interferons. Interferons are naturally occurring complex proteins of which there are three types: (1) alpha (α) interferon, produced by lymphocytes; (2) beta (β) interferon, produced by fibroblasts and macrophages; and (3) gamma (γ) interferon produced by T lymphocytes. Interferons are cytokines that have antiviral, antiproliferative, and immunomodulatory properties (see Table 8-5). The antiviral activity of interferons was first identified in 1957. Interferons protect cells infected by viruses from attack by other viruses, and they inhibit replication of viral DNA (Fig. 8-4). The antiproliferative effects of interferons are unclear. However, they have been shown to inhibit DNA and protein synthesis in tumor cells and to stimulate the expression of tumor-associated antigens on tumor cell surfaces, thus increasing the potential for an immune response. Interferons modulate the immune response by their direct interaction with T lymphocytes. Interferons have also been shown (in vitro) to increase the cytotoxic activity and killing potential of NK cells.[18]

Because of the protein nature of interferons, they cannot be administered orally. Therefore, they are administered intravenously, intramuscularly, and subcutaneously. To date, the best dose, route, and frequency of administration have not been determined.

Clinical studies have demonstrated some effectiveness in the use of interferon to treat hematological malignancies. In 1986, α-interferon was approved by the FDA for use in the treatment of hairy cell leukemia. Interferons have also demonstrated effectiveness in the treatment of renal cell carcinoma, chronic myelogenous leukemia, T-cell lymphomas, malignant melanoma, multiple myeloma, Kaposi's sarcoma, ovarian carcinoma, and carcinoid tumors. Clinical trials continue to investigate the use of interferons to treat other malignancies.

Interleukin-2. Interleukin-2 (IL-2) is a cytokine or lymphokine produced by T lymphocytes that was first identified as an agent capable of stimulating division of T lymphocytes. It was later found to activate NK cells and T-cytotoxic lymphocytes. IL-2 also stimulates lymphocyte release of other lymphokines, including γ-interferon. Activated NK cells make up part of a group of cytotoxic lymphocytes that mediate lymphokine-activated killing (LAK).

IL-2 has been administered in clinical trials by various means, including intravenous bolus, continuous infusion, subcutaneous injection, and peritoneal infusion. As with other BRM agents, the optimum dose, route, and frequency of administration are yet to be determined.

Clinical trials are currently under way to investigate new approaches to the administration of IL-2. One approach involves the adoptive transfer of LAK cells to the client. It is based on the ability of IL-2 to activate LAK cells. This process involves the following:

1. Infusion of IL-2 to increase the number of lymphocytes
2. Lymphopheresis—a mechanical process designed to remove the lymphocytes from circulation
3. Incubation of the host lymphocytes with IL-2 in vitro
4. Reinfusion of the cultured lymphocytes to the host as LAK cells, which are capable of lysing tumor cells
5. Simultaneous administration of IL-2

Clinical responses with IL-2 and LAK cells have been reported in clients with metastatic renal cell cancer, colorectal cancer, melanoma, and non-Hodgkin's lymphoma.

A recent approach to the use of IL-2 involves the isolation of lymphocytes from the tumor itself. These cells are called *tumor-infiltrating lymphocytes* (TIL) and can be cultured with IL-2 and then reinfused into the client. These cells have been found to be more tumoricidal than LAK cells.

In addition to its use with LAK and TIL cells, IL-2 has been administered alone or in conjunction with other lymphokines such as α-interferon and tumor necrosis factor. Research on uses of IL-2 in cancer therapy is continuing.

Monoclonal antibodies. Monoclonal antibodies are antibodies or immunoglobulins produced by B lymphocytes that are capable of binding to specific target cells, including tumor cells. Various monoclonal antibodies (MoAbs) are currently being investigated for diagnostic as well as treatment capabilities. (Hybridoma technology for the production of MoAbs is described in Chapter 8.) The diagnostic use of MoAbs is primarily for the imaging of tumors to locate areas of metastatic disease and for radioimmunoassay in laboratory studies. This involves attachment of a radioactive substance to an antibody targeted to a specific antigen. The outcome of this process is a radiolabeled antibody that is useful in radiological scanning and laboratory analysis.[19]

MoAbs have also demonstrated limited effectiveness in treating cancers such as lymphomas, acute and chronic lymphocytic leukemias, T-cell leukemia, gastric and colon cancer, and melanoma. Clinical studies are investigating the use of MoAbs as "immunoconjugates" by binding the MoAb to radioisotopes, toxins, chemotherapeutic agents, and other BRMs. The goal of this approach is for the antibody to deliver the immunoconjugate directly to the targeted cancer cells for their ultimate destruction. MoAbs have also been used as single agents in the treatment of cancers, including melanoma and gastrointestinal malignancies. MoAbs are administered by the infusion method.

Tumor necrosis factor. Tumor necrosis factor (TNF) is a cytokine released by macrophages, and it ultimately binds to specific receptors located on cell membranes. The exact functions of TNF are unclear. However, it is known that, in vitro, TNF is toxic to animal and human tumor cells by exerting a necrotizing effect. Studies also suggest that TNF may activate cells of the immune system, as in increased neutrophil and T- and B-cell lymphocyte activity.

In clinical trials, TNF has been administered by intravenous, intramuscular, subcutaneous, and intratumor methods. Studies are currently being conducted to test the efficacy of this BRM in the treatment of ovarian and renal cancers and melanoma. These studies are investigating the potential use of this agent alone or in combination with other therapies such as chemotherapy.[20]

Colony-stimulating factors. Colony-stimulating factors (CSFs) are a group of glycoproteins, produced by various cells, which stimulate production, maturation, and function of cells of the hematological system. After release of CSFs, they attach to receptors on the cell surface of hematopoietic precursors (precursors of mature blood cells). CSFs then stimulate cellular production, maturation, release from the bone marrow, and bactericidal and other activities. Various CSFs have been isolated. These include granulocyte-CSF (G-CSF), granulocyte-macrophage colony CSF (GM-CSF), and macrophage CSF (M-CSF or CSF-1). Interleukin-3 (IL-3), also called *multi-CSF,* has been used as a multipotential stimulator of hematopoietic stem cells.

There are a number of potential clinical uses of CSFs. They may hasten recovery from bone marrow depression after standard and high-dose chemotherapy and bone marrow transplantation. These agents may also be used to strengthen host defenses against infection and malignancy. Finally, CSFs may act as differentiating and recruiting agents in preleukemia and leukemia.[21]

Toxic and side effects of BRM therapy. The administration of one cytokine usually induces the release of other cytokines. The release and action of these cytokines result in systemic immune and inflammatory responses. The toxicities and side effects of BRMs are related to dose and schedule. Common side effects include constitutional flulike symptoms, including headache, fever, chills, myalgias, fatigue, malaise, weakness, anorexia, and nausea. With interferons the flulike symptoms almost invariably

appear. CSFs do not produce these symptoms except for GM-CSF, which causes fever. Tachycardia and orthostatic hypotension are also commonly reported. TNF and IL-2 can cause capillary leak syndrome, which can result in pulmonary edema. Other toxic and side effects may involve the central nervous system, the renal and hepatic systems, and the cardiovascular system. These effects are found particularly with interferons and IL-2.

■ Nursing Management of the Client Receiving Biological Response Modifiers

Some problems experienced by clients who are receiving BRMs are quite different from those observed with more traditional forms of cancer therapy. For example, capillary leak syndrome and pulmonary edema, observed with high doses of IL-2, are problems that require critical care nursing. These critical care requirements are new to many oncology nurses. Other problems, such as bone marrow depression and fatigue, are more familiar but exist at different levels of severity than those customarily associated with other forms of cancer therapy. Bone marrow depression occurring with BRM administration is generally more transient and less severe than that observed with chemotherapy. Fatigue associated with BRM therapy can be so severe that it can constitute a dose-limiting toxicity.

Nursing interventions for flulike syndrome include the administration of acetaminophen before treatment and every 4 hours after treatment. Intravenous meperidine has been used to control the severe chills (rigors) associated with some BRMs. Other nursing measures include monitoring of vital signs and temperature, planning for periods of rest for the client, and assisting with activities of daily living.

A wide range of neurological deficits have been observed with interferon and IL-2 therapy. The nature and extent of these problems have not been completely elucidated. However, these problems are understandably frightening to clients and their families, who must be taught to observe for neurological problems (e.g., headache, lethargy, confusion, insomnia), report their occurrence, and institute appropriate safety and support measures.

Bone Marrow Transplantation

Bone marrow transplantation is a treatment option for some clients with cancer. Two types of bone marrow transplantation are performed. Both require the use of high-dose chemotherapy and/or total body irradiation aimed at complete eradication of the client's bone marrow. Subsequently, bone marrow is infused into the client.

In *allogeneic marrow transplantation* the infused bone marrow is acquired from a donor who has been determined to be closely matched to the recipient in terms of tissue antigen typing. This type of transplantation is used in the treatment of leukemias, lymphomas, and aplastic anemia. The goal of allogeneic transplantation is the engraftment and subsequent normal proliferation and differentiation of the donated marrow in the host. In *autologous marrow transplantation,* clients receive their own bone marrow. The aim of this approach is to enable clients to receive intensive chemotherapy and/or radiation while supporting

Table 9-27 Protein Foods with High Biological Value

MILK

1 cup of whole milk = 9 g protein
  Double-strength milk—1 quart of whole milk plus 1 cup of dried skim milk blended and chilled: 1 cup = 14 g protein
Milk shake—1 cup of ice cream plus 1 cup of milk = 15 g protein, 416 calories
Use evaporated milk, double-strength milk, or half-and-half to make casseroles, hot cereals, sauces, gravies, puddings, milk shakes, and soups.
Yogurt (regular and frozen)—check labels and purchase the brand with the highest protein content: 1 cup = 10 g protein

EGGS

Egg = 6 g protein
Eggnog (1 cup) = 15.5 g protein
  Add eggs to salads, casseroles, and sauces. Deviled eggs are especially well tolerated.
Desserts that contain eggs include angel food cake, sponge cake, custard, and cheesecake.

CHEESE

Cottage	½ cup	15 g protein
American	1 slice	3 g protein
Cheddar	1 slice	6 g protein
Cream	1 tbsp	1 g protein

Use cheese in a sandwich or as a snack.
Add cheese to salads, casseroles, sauces, and baked potatoes.
Cheesecake is usually a welcome treat.
Cheese spread with crackers is a wholesome snack that can be made and stored in the refrigerator for easy accessibility.

MEAT/POULTRY/FISH

Beef	3 oz	approx. 21 g protein
Pork	3 oz	approx. 19 g protein
Chicken	½ breast	approx. 26 g protein
Fish	3 oz	approx. 30 g protein
Tuna fish	6½ oz	approx. 44.5 g protein

Add meat, poultry, and fish to salads, casseroles, and sandwiches.
Add strained and junior baby meats to soups and casseroles.
Cocktail wieners or deviled ham on crackers are wholesome snacks. These snacks can be made and stored in the refrigerator for easy accessibility.

Modified from Yasko J: Care of the client receiving external radiation therapy—a self-learning module for the nurse caring for the client with cancer, Reston, VA, 1982, Reston Publishing and Donoghue M, Nunnally C and Yasko J: Nutritional aspects of cancer—a self-learning module for the nurse caring for the client with cancer, Reston, VA, 1982, Reston Publishing.

them with their own bone marrow. Chapter 25 contains a complete discussion of bone marrow transplantation.

Nutritional Considerations

Nutritional problems that most frequently occur in clients with cancer are malnutrition, anorexia, altered taste sensation, nausea, vomiting, diarrhea, stomatitis, and mucositis. These problems can be caused by a combination of many factors: drug toxicity, effects of radiation therapy, tumor involvement, recent surgery, emotional distress, or difficulty with ingestion or digestion of food. If the client is inadequately nourished, the normal cells will not be able to recover from the effects of therapy and the immune system will be depressed because of depletion of protein stores.

Malnutrition. The client with cancer usually experiences calorie and protein malnutrition characterized by fat and muscle depletion. (Assessment of the degree of malnutrition is discussed in Chapter 35.) Foods suggested for increasing the protein intake to facilitate repair and regeneration of cells are presented in Table 9-27. High-calorie foods for energy and to minimize weight loss are presented in Table 9-28. A sample high-calorie, high-protein diet is presented in Table 35-11.

Table 9-28 High-Calorie Foods

Mayonnaise	1 tbs = 101 cal
Butter/margarine	1 tsp = 35 cal
Sour cream	1 tbs = 72 cal
Peanut butter	1 tbs = 94 cal
Whipped cream	1 tbs = 53 cal
Corn oil	1 tbs = 119 cal
Jelly	1 tbs = 49 cal
Ice cream	1 cup = 256 cal
Honey	1 tbs = 64 cal

The nurse should suggest the need for a nutritional supplement to the physician as soon as a 5% weight loss is noted or if the client has the potential for protein and calorie malnutrition. Once a 10-pound weight loss occurs, it is very difficult to maintain the nutritional status. The client can be taught to use nutritional supplements in place of milk when cooking or baking. Foods to which nutritional supplements can be easily added include scrambled eggs, pudding, custard, mashed potatoes, cereal, and cream sauces. "Instant Breakfast" can be used as indicated on the package or sprinkled on cereals, desserts, and casseroles.

If the malnutrition cannot be treated with dietary intake, it may be necessary to use enteral or parenteral nutrition as an adjunct nutritional measure. (Enteral and parenteral nutrition is discussed in Chapter 35.)

Anorexia. It is important to realize that the anorexia experienced by the client with cancer is a challenging problem. An intervention may be effective one day and ineffective the next. Continual assessment and intervention are necessary to successfully manage this problem. The nurse must develop the philosophy that something can be done to prevent or minimize anorexia, evaluate each intervention, and continue to use those that have been successful in the past. Some suggestions are presented in the nursing care plan for the client with cancer (Table 9-17).

Altered taste sensation. It is theorized that cancer cells release substances that resemble amino acids and stimulate the bitter-taste buds. Clients have also experienced an alteration in the sweet taste sensation as well as in the sour and salty taste sensations. Meat may also taste bitter to some clients. At this time the physiological basis of these varied taste alterations is unknown. Other causes of altered taste sensation are presented in Table 9-16.

Clients with this problem should be instructed to avoid foods for which they have a strong dislike. Frequently, clients may feel compelled to eat certain foods because they believe they are good for them. They can be taught to experiment with spices and other seasoning agents in an attempt to mask the taste alterations that are occurring. Lemon juice, onion, mint, basil, and fruit juice marinades may improve the taste of certain meats and fish. Bacon bits, onion, and pieces of ham may enhance the taste of vegetables. An additional amount of a spice or seasoning agent is usually not an effective way to enhance the taste.

Unproven Methods of Cancer Treatment

Unproven methods of cancer treatment, sometimes referred to as *cancer quackery,* are as old as the disease itself. Cancer quackery is defined as the intentional misrepresentation and/or misapplication of measures that delay or impede the entry of the client into the health care system for treatment. Today, cancer quackery is a multimillion-dollar business in the United States. Fear appears to be the major factor that motivates clients to seek "miracle cures." Other factors include (1) impatience with the progress of their present cancer treatment, (2) the need to exercise control over their daily lives, (3) the impersonal approach of health care workers, (4) a need for hope when terminal illness is a reality, (5) lack of information on methods that are proven versus those that are not, and (6) suspicion that the health care system is not providing the most effective treatment plan available.[22]

The major hazard of cancer quackery is that it delays or prevents the client from receiving proven methods of cancer diagnosis and treatment. This delay may make the difference between cure or control and terminal illness. The nurse can play a significant role in preventing or minimizing the use of cancer quackery by doing the following:

1. Providing the client with accurate information concerning the benefits of the proven methods of cancer treatment
2. Informing the American Cancer Society, the local medical association, the health department, and the local consumer protection office when it is learned that clients are being approached by persons promoting unproven methods of cancer treatment
3. Discussing the fallacies of the unproven methods of cancer treatment with the client and the family

The current methods of cancer quackery include chemicals and drugs, dietary alterations, occult techniques, and mechanical devices.

Chemicals and drugs. Two drugs that have been associated with cancer quackery are krebiozin (the wonder drug of the 1950s and 1960s) and laetrile (the wonder drug of the 1970s and 1980s). A National Cancer Institute study on a large number of clients who used krebiozin failed to demonstrate any anticancer effects of this drug. Chemical analysis revealed that the major ingredient of krebiozin is mineral oil, with minute amounts of creatine and amyl alcohol.

Laetrile, also known as vitamin B-17 and Cyto H-3, has been actively used as a treatment for cancer for the past 25 to 30 years. The active ingredient of laetrile is hydrogen cyanide, and it is derived from apricot or peach pits. It is available in parenteral and tablet form, and the parenteral form contains 30 to 40 times as much cyanide as the oral form. Several studies have been conducted by some of the major cancer centers, and all have failed to show evidence of an anticancer effect of this drug.

Since laetrile is frequently used by clients with cancer and until recently has been thought a harmless drug, the nurse must be aware of the possible toxic effects that may be experienced. The cyanide content of laetrile is released in the presence of hydrolyzine β-glucosidase enzymes. These enzymes are present in raw fruits and vegetables, such as lettuce, mushrooms, green peppers, celery, and sweet almonds. When these foods are eaten after the ingestion of laetrile, cyanide intoxication may occur. The bacteria of the intestinal tract are also thought to contain this enzyme. When the cyanide is released, it inhibits cellular respiration and the resulting hypoxia produces symptoms such as dizziness, nausea or vomiting, hypotension, and shock. Because the drug is not controlled by the FDA, many impurities may exist that have the potential for causing systemic bacterial, viral, and fungal infections.

Dietary alterations. Books that propose cures for cancer enumerate the foods to eat and to avoid, offer special recipes, and usually recommend the use of an expensive blender to ensure the proper potency of the food mixture. Examples of nutritional alterations that have been used are eating raw foods; fasting for long periods of time; following the grape diet, the carrot juice diet, or the coffee and Coke diet; and using coffee, buttermilk, and/or yogurt enemas while on a special diet. None of these diets has been found effective in treating cancer. Nutritional alterations can have a profound effect on the client with cancer, since a great amount of protein and many calories are needed to maintain weight and prevent a negative nitrogen balance.

Occult techniques. The most commonly used occult form of cancer quackery is "psychic surgery." This surgery is performed by a healer without an incision. The client presents the problem, has the healing surgery, and leaves believing that the tumor has been removed. During the surgery the area where the problem exists is massaged and rubbed with animal blood. At some point, the client is shown a piece of animal tissue and told that it is the diseased tissue or organ. This tissue is thrown away, the massage with blood continues, and the client is told that the tumor is gone and the cancer is cured.

Mechanical devices. Mechanical devices are an old form of cancer quackery that have lost their popularity recently. These devices are usually nothing more than light bulbs, vibrators, a low-voltage generator, dials, and knobs. The client is told to place the device on or in front of the area of cancer for a certain period of time each day and the device will destroy the cancer.

Supportive care. One of the cancer quack's greatest assets is the emotional support given to the client and the client's family. This should demonstrate to the nurse the need to provide psychological support, caring, and active listening to the cancer client and the family. The nurse needs to be available, listen, and counsel the client during times when side effects are being experienced, when treatment is not effective, and when the client is experiencing fear, anger, and depression.

If the client chooses an unproven method of cancer treatment, the nurse needs to support the client and assume a nonjudgmental attitude. The nurse should attempt to persuade the client to continue the proven treatment plan and to maintain the nutritional status while using an unproven method of cancer treatment. Belief in the treatment may provide a placebo effect that may offer some benefits. It is important that all doors remain open to clients so that they can return to the health care system without feelings of fear or guilt.

COMPLICATIONS RESULTING FROM CANCER

The client may develop complications related to the continual growth of the malignancy or the side effects of treatment.

Infection

Infection is the most frequent cause of death in the client with cancer. The usual sites of infection include the lungs, genitourinary system, mouth, rectum, peritoneal cavity, and blood (septicemia). Infection occurs as a result of the ulceration and necrosis of the tumor, compression by the tumor of vital organs, and the state of neutropenia caused by the disease process or the treatment of cancer. Fungi and gram-negative bacteria are the usual causative organisms.

Many clients are neutropenic when an infection develops. In these individuals, infection may cause significant morbidity and may be rapidly fatal if not treated promptly. The classic manifestations of infection are often not present in a client with neutropenia.

Paraneoplastic Syndrome

Paraneoplastic syndrome includes all the physiological effects that occur as the result of the release of certain hormones by cancer cells in the primary and/or metastatic sites. Hormone secretion from cancer cells arising from tissues that do not normally release this hormone is caused by the process of depression. This process allows the stored potential of all cells to become evident. Paraneoplastic syndrome can occur during all phases of the cancer process, but it is commonly associated with the advanced illness phase. The most common paraneoplastic syndromes include the following:

1. Syndrome of inappropriate antidiuretic hormone (SIADH), caused by cancer cells located in the lung, pancreas, or prostate gland that produce ADH
2. Secretion of ACTH by a tumor of the lung, thymus, pancreas, thyroid, stomach, or ovary
3. Secretion of insulin by a tumor of the pancreas, liver, adrenal glands, stomach, or ovary
4. Hypercalcemia, which occurs when a parathormone-like substance and/or calcitonin is secreted by the cancer cells and is most frequent in clients with lung, breast, kidney, colon, or thyroid cancer

Hypercalcemia

Hypercalcemia is a serious electrolyte disorder that occurs in cancer. In addition to paraneoplastic syndrome, hypercalcemia may also occur in tumors characterized by extensive bone involvement, such as multiple myeloma and bony metastasis. Hypercalcemia may also result from immobilization with or without metastasis. Serum levels of calcium in excess of 12 mg/dl can be life threatening. Chronic hypercalcemia can result in nephrocalcinosis and irreversible renal failure. The long-term treatment of hypercalcemia is aimed at the primary disease. Acute hypercalcemia is treated by hydration (3 L/day), diuretic administration, and mithramycin if the client has severe symptoms.

Superior Vena Cava Syndrome

Superior vena cava syndrome results from obstruction of the superior vena cava by a tumor. The clinical manifestations include facial edema, periorbital edema, distention of veins of the neck and chest, headache, and convulsions. The presence of a mediastinal mass is often visible on a chest x-ray. The most common causes are Hodgkin's disease, non-Hodgkin's lymphoma, and lung cancer. Superior vena cava syndrome is considered a serious medical problem, and management usually involves radiation therapy to the site of obstruction and treatment of the primary tumor.

Hemorrhage

Hemorrhage can be due to the presence of thrombocytopenia, tumor invasion of a blood vessel causing the vessel to rupture, or the development of an ulcer. Petechiae, epistaxis, hematuria, and melena may signal the possibility of an impending major hemorrhage. The usual sites of massive hemorrhage are the brain, the gastrointestinal tract, the major vessels of the neck, the lungs, and the peritoneal cavity. Disseminated intravascular coagulation (DIC) can also occur in persons with cancer. It is due to the release of thromboplastic substances from cancer cells. (DIC is discussed in Chapter 25.)

Infarction and Organ Failure

Infarction occurs as a result of the formation of thrombi composed of tumor cells. When the thrombi occlude vessels in major body organs, they cause necrosis of vital organ tissue. The major sites of infarction are the lungs, heart, and brain. Organ failure is the result of primary or metastatic disease involvement of a vital organ, such as the brain, liver, kidney, or lung. The involvement is sufficient to cause physiological dysfunction, failure, or death.

Spinal Cord Compression

Spinal cord compression is a result of the presence of a malignant tumor in the epidural space of the spinal cord. The most common primary tumors that produce this problem are in the breast, lung, prostate, and kidney. It is also a recognized problem with lymphomas. The manifestations are back pain that is intense, localized, and persistent, accompanied by vertebral tenderness and aggravated by the Valsalva maneuver; motor weakness and dysfunction; sensory paresthesia and loss; and automatic dysfunction. Radiation therapy is used for clients with slowly progressive neurological deficits and radiosensitive tumors. Surgery is usually recommended for clients with rapidly progressive neurological signs, especially if their tumors are relatively radioresistant.

PSYCHOLOGICAL SUPPORT

Psychological support of the client is an important aspect of cancer care. Because of the effectiveness of cancer treatment, many clients with cancer are cured or their disease is controlled for long periods of time. In light of this trend in cancer treatment, emphasis must be placed on maintaining an optimal quality of life after the diagnosis of cancer. A positive attitude of client, family, and caregivers toward cancer has a significant positive impact on the quality of life the client experiences. Some authorities have stated that a positive attitude may also influence the prognosis of the client with cancer.

The diagnosis of cancer is viewed by most persons as a crisis. The most common fears experienced by clients with cancer include disfigurement, dependency, pain, emaciation, financial depletion, death, and abandonment.

To cope with these fears, the client with cancer will use and experience different behavioral patterns: shock, anger, denial, bargaining, depression, helplessness, hopelessness, rationalization, acceptance, and intellectualization. These behavioral patterns may occur at any time during the process of cancer. However, some patterns appear to occur more frequently or at a greater intensity at certain specific stages of the disease process. Several factors may determine how the client will cope with the diagnosis of cancer:

1. Ability to cope with stressful events in the past (e.g., loss of job, major disappointment): By simply asking how the client has coped with stressful events, the nurse can gain an understanding of the client's coping patterns, the effectiveness of the usual coping patterns, and the usual coping time framework.
2. Availability of significant others: Clients who have effective support systems tend to cope more effectively than clients who do not have a meaningful, available support system.
3. Ability to express feelings and concerns: Clients who are able to express their feelings and needs and who seek and ask for help appear to cope more effectively than those who internalize their feelings and needs.
4. Age at the time of diagnosis: Age determines the coping strategies to a great degree. A young mother with cancer will have concerns that differ from those of a 70-year-old woman with cancer.
5. Extent of disease: Cure or control of the disease process is usually easier to cope with than the reality of terminal illness.
6. Disruption of body image: Disruption of the body image (e.g., radical neck dissection, alopecia, mastectomy) may intensify the psychological impact of cancer.
7. Presence of symptoms: Symptoms such as fatigue, nausea, diarrhea, and pain may intensify the psychological impact of cancer.
8. Past experience with cancer: If past experiences with cancer have been negative, the client will probably view the personal status as negative.
9. Attitude associated with the cancer: A client who feels in control and has a positive attitude about cancer and cancer treatment is better able to cope with the diagnosis and treatment of cancer than the client who feels hopeless, helpless, and out of control.

To facilitate the development of a hopeful attitude about cancer and to support the client and the family during the various stages of the process of cancer, the nurse should do the following:

1. Be available and continue to be available, especially during difficult times.
2. Exhibit a caring attitude.
3. Listen actively to fears and concerns.
4. Provide relief of distressing symptoms.
5. Provide essential information regarding cancer and cancer care.
6. Maintain a relationship based on trust and confidence, being open, honest, and caring in the approach.
7. Use touch to exhibit caring. A squeeze of the hand or a hug may at times be more effective than words.
8. Assist the client in setting realistic, reachable short-term and long-term goals.
9. Assist the client in maintaining usual lifestyle patterns.
10. Maintain hope, the key to effective cancer care. Hope varies, depending on the status of the client—hope that the symptoms are not serious, hope that the treatment is curative, hope for indepen-

dence, hope for relief of pain, hope for a longer life, or hope for a peaceful death. Hope provides control over what is occurring and is the basis of a positive attitude toward cancer and cancer care.

Most clients with advanced cancer know that they are dying. Attempts at circumventing the truth are usually recognized by them and cause feelings of distrust and hostility toward the person who makes such attempts. Honesty and openness are the best approaches. Most clients will surprise their caregivers by expressing relief at a willingness to discuss what is foremost in their minds, their imminent death.

It is unnecessary for clients with cancer to experience severe, uncontrollable pain. Pain is most common in those with bone disease. Narcotics, tranquilizers, alcohol, and sedatives should be used liberally and often. The proper dose is whatever is enough to control the client's discomfort. Fear of addiction is not warranted and not worth considering. (Other measures to relieve pain are discussed in Chapter 51.)

Organizations and journals available as resources for nurses are listed in the bibliography at the end of this section. In many cities, there are local units of the American Cancer Society that provide a wide variety of services.

Hospice Care

A hospice is not a place but a concept of care that provides compassion, concern, support, and skilled professional care for the dying. Hospice care seeks to enhance the remaining time for those persons who are living with a dying body. The term *hospice* is derived from a medieval word that means a place of shelter for people on a difficult journey. The hospice concept of care has existed in England for many years. During the 1970s the idea took hold in the United States, and by the end of the decade, every state had existing hospice programs.

The National Hospice Organization has defined hospice as a centrally administered program of palliative and supportive services that provides physical, psychological, social, and spiritual care for dying persons and their families. Services are provided by a medically supervised interdisciplinary team of professionals and volunteers.

Hospice programs are organized under a variety of models. Some are based in hospitals or in home health agencies, while others are freestanding or community-based, volunteer-intensive programs. The National Hospice Organization publishes an annual directory that lists hospice programs in the United States. The directory not only provides the name, address, and phone number of the hospice but also its organizational type, the scope of its services, and the geographical service area.

Admission to a hospice program is on the basis of client and family need. Home care is provided on a part-time, intermittent, regularly scheduled, or round-the-clock on-call basis. Hospice services are available on a 24-hour basis 7 days a week to provide help to clients and families in their homes. Some hospice programs also have an inpatient unit in a hospital. Usually the in-hospital units have been deinstitutionalized to make the atmosphere as free and homelike as possible. Staff and volunteers are available to the client and family. A multidisciplinary team approach provides holistic personal care.

Bereavement care is a natural extension of the hospice structure. Because the client and family are the focus of hospice care, providing grief support to family members or to significant others after the death of the client is incorporated into the organizational structure and into treatment plans. The objective of a bereavement program is to provide support and to assist survivors in the transition to a life without the deceased person.

Regulation and reimbursement. A great deal of controversy surrounds the increasing bureaucratization of the American hospice movement. New sources of financial reimbursement for the benefit of clients now exist that were unheard of only 5 years ago.

Section 122 of the Tax Equity and Fiscal Responsibility Act of 1982 created the hospice Medicare benefit. In addition to the usual services covered by Medicare, the hospice benefit also covers drugs and BRMs for home use; home care service (including continuous care), whether or not the client is homebound; counseling; bereavement; and homemaker services. The Medicare benefit is available to clients through certified hospice programs.

There has been an increase in third-party payers in providing hospice-care benefits. These payers have added to the regulations and requirements to which hospice programs are obligated. In addition, at least half of all states currently have hospice-licensing regulations and laws in existence or in the planning stages.

Philosophy of hospice care. There is often a point in terminal disease when curative treatment is no longer possible. It is at this time that the hospice philosophy of promoting the quality of life and providing palliative care is appropriate. Palliative care controls symptoms and provides comfort but does not cure. Palliative care does not prolong life but provides comfort.

Hospice care represents a return to previous times when the dying were helped to remain at home and to die at home, if possible, surrounded by familiar sights, sounds, and smells and by the love of those who care. Hospice exists to provide support and care for persons in the last phases of incurable diseases so that they might live as fully and as comfortably as possible.

Although hospice programs initially were primarily volunteer programs of love and goodwill, hospice today is a health care program faced with a myriad of ethical and legal issues. Some of the issues include nonresuscitation orders, artificial feeding and hydration, the debate over "killing" or "letting die," and the right to truth and self-determination. Only time will tell whether hospice is greater than the ethical and legal issues it faces. The hospice movement is facing a challenging future.

Differences between traditional and hospice care. Hospice care differs from traditional care in a number of ways. The goals of traditional hospital and medical care are to (1) treat and cure disease, (2) prolong life, (3) use all appropriate technology, and (4) treat pain with limited, well-defined amounts of medication. Traditional medical care views death as a treatment failure.

In hospice care, the client and the family are the focus

of care. Preparation for dying is a task with which the family as well as the client must deal. Hospice provides a milieu in which this is more easily accomplished. Hospice recognizes dying as a normal process. It neither hastens nor postpones death. Hospice exists in the hope and belief that, through appropriate care and the promotion of a caring community sensitive to their needs, clients and families may be free to attain a degree of mental and spiritual preparation for death satisfactory to them.

Hospice care is not technology oriented. Rather, it is intensive personal care that provides skilled bedside nursing and focuses attention on the emotional, social, spiritual, and familial aspects of the client. Hospice offers little opportunity to do things *to* clients but offers great opportunity to do things *with* clients and families.

Pain is a common concern among terminally ill clients. In hospice, pain is considered a total experience rather than a physiological event. Adequate medication (usually narcotics) is used to provide relief. The prn order for pain is not found in hospice. Analgesia is routinely given in an attempt to eliminate the pain and, more important, to prevent its recurrence and to erase the memory of pain. Attention is also given to all the other factors that contribute to pain or to its increasing intensity: fear, loneliness, anxiety, insomnia, spiritual doubts or concerns, financial concerns, and depression.

When the client dies, the hospice team continues to follow the family and significant others through the bereavement period. The hospice team makes itself available to aid survivors through the grief period.

Support groups are available to hospice staff and volunteers. Crises and grief result in varying forms of stress for caregivers. To give to clients and families, the staff and volunteers must also have a means to be nourished and refreshed. Various means of stress relief are used by different hospices. Professionally assisted groups, informal rap sessions, flexible time schedules, and additional time off are a few ways to decrease stress. The needs of the caregiver must be considered important, or the care receiver will receive less of what is needed.

R eview Questions

The number of the question corresponds to the same-numbered objective at the beginning of the chapter.

1. Which type of cancer is increasing in incidence?
   a. uterine cancer
   b. esophageal cancer
   c. stomach cancer
   d. lung cancer
2. Cancer is a name for a large group of diseases, all of which are characterized by
   a. cell growth that escapes normal control
   b. rapid, explosive proliferation of cells
   c. production of toxins that alter cells
   d. a long and painful course
3. A characteristic of the stage of progression in the development of cancer is
   a. mutation of stem cell

b. continual steady growth facilitated by promoting factors
   c. proliferation of cancer cells in spite of host control mechanisms
   d. oncogenic viral transformation of target cells
4. The primary protective role of the immune system related to malignant cells is
   a. immunological surveillance
   b. immunological enhancement
   c. antigenic blindfolding
   d. antigenic modulation
5. The primary difference between benign and malignant neoplasms is
   a. rate of cell proliferation
   b. requirements for cellular nutrients
   c. characteristic of tissue invasiveness
   d. site of malignant tumor
6. Important nursing roles related to prevention and detection of cancer include all the following *except*
   a. teaching people self-examination of breast and testicles
   b. instructing people to eat low-fiber, refined-carbohydrate diets
   c. instructing persons on ways to increase capacity to cope with stress
   d. teaching people to obtain regular health care
7. The only definitive means of diagnosing cancer is by
   a. radiological study
   b. culture
   c. chemical testing
   d. biopsy
8. Which of the following is a radiation hazard when a client has radium needles implanted in a tongue lesion?
   a. saliva
   b. bed linen
   c. urine
   d. displaced needle
9. Which of the following sets of drug classifications and examples are incorrect?
   a. alkylating agent—nitrogen mustard
   b. antibiotic—actinomycin D
   c. antimetabolite—5-fluorouracil
   d. plant alkaloid—L-asparaginase
10. Stomatitis, a common side effect of chemotherapeutic agents, occurs because the
    a. general health of the client with cancer is poor
    b. rapidly dividing cells of the mucous membranes of the mouth are being destroyed
    c. chemotherapeutic drugs have an external, local, and irritating effect
    d. site of the malignancy is near the oral cavity
11. Radiation precautions on the clinical unit must be observed by the nurse caring for a client
    a. receiving supervoltage radiation therapy for lung cancer
    b. who has ingested radioactive iodine for diagnostic brain scan

c. having cobalt teletherapy for esophageal cancer

d. who has implanted radium needles in the breast

12. Which of the following is not characteristic of biological response modifiers?

   a. have no side or toxic effects

   b. augment the body's natural defenses

   c. most therapies are still under investigation

   d. monoclonal antibodies can be made to be antigen specific

13. The most common nutritional problems found in cancer clients include all the following *except*

   a. malnutrition

   b. anorexia

   c. altered taste sensation

   d. hypernatremia

14. If a client decides to take Laetrile, the nurse should inform the client that

   a. foods with hydrolyzine β-glucosidase enzymes should be avoided

   b. chemotherapy and Laetrile should not be taken simultaneously

   c. a pulmonary fungal infection will probably develop

   d. buttermilk should be drunk simultaneously to avoid toxic effects

15. Paraneoplastic syndrome that occurs in certain types of cancer is primarily due to

   a. invasiveness of cancer cells

   b. gram-negative septicemia

   c. ectopic hormonal production

   d. autoimmune reaction

REFERENCES

1. Cancer facts and figures, Atlanta, 1989, American Cancer Society.

2. DeVita VT, Helman S, and Rosenberg SA, eds: Cancer: principles and practice of oncology, Philadelphia, 1989, JB Lippincott Co, p 200.

3. Klein G and Klein E: Evolution of tumors and the impact of molecular oncology, Nature 315:190-195, 1985.

4. Rensberger B: Cancer: the new synthesis, cause, Science 84:28-33, 1984.

5. Pitot H: The natural history of neoplastic development: the relation of experimental models to human cancer, Cancer 49:1206-1211, 1982.

6. Fitzpatrick TB and Sober AJ: Sunlight and skin cancer, N Engl J Med 373:818-819, 1985.

7. Knudson AG: Hereditary cancer, oncogenes, and antioncogenes, Cancer Res 45:1437-1443, 1985.

8. Marx JL: How cancer cells spread in the body, Science 244:147-148, 1989.

9. Rawls RL: In search to control cancer: understanding metastasis is crucial, Clin Exp Neurol 22:10-17, 1985.

10. Grady C: Host defense mechanisms: an overview, Semin Oncol Nurs 4:86-94, 1988.

11. Huffer T, Kanapa D, and Stevenson G: Introduction to human immunology, Boston, 1986, Jones & Bartlett Publishers, Inc, p 114.

12. Dupere SL, O'Connor TE, and Oldham RK: Lymphokines/cytokines: biotherapeutic applications, J Immunopharmacol 8:201-209, 1988.

13. Gallucci B: The immune system and cancer, Oncol Nurs Forum Suppl 14:3-12, 1987.

14. The health professional and cancer prevention and detection, Atlanta, 1988, American Cancer Society Publication.

15. Fischer DS and Knobf MT: The cancer chemotherapy handbook, ed 3, Chicago, 1989, Year Book Medical Publishers, Inc.

16. Fraser M and Tucker M: Late effects of cancer therapy: chemotherapy-related malignancies, Oncol Nurs Forum 15:67-77, 1988.

17. Clark J and Longo D: Biological response modifiers, Mediguide to Oncology 6:1-10, 1986.

18. Hahn MB and Jassak P: Nursing management of patients receiving interferon, Semin Oncol Nurs 4:95-101, 1988.

19. Dullman JB: Toxicity of monoclonal antibodies in the treatment of cancer, Semin Oncol Nurs 4:107-111, 1988.

20. Moldawer NP and Figlin RA: Tumor necrosis factors: current clinical status and implications for nursing management, Semin Oncol Nurs 4:120-125, 1988.

21. Vadhan-Raj S: Clinical applications of colony-stimulating factors, Oncol Nurs Forum 16:21-26, 1989.

22. Howard RJ and Miller N: Unproven methods of cancer management, Parts I and II, Oncol Nurs Forum 10:46-54, 1983.

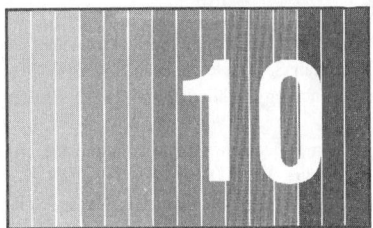

CHAPTER

10

Nursing Role in Management
Fluid, Electrolyte, and Acid-Base Imbalances

Judith Heffron Sweeney

Learning Objectives

1. Identify the major fluid compartments and the electrolytes in each compartment.
2. Describe the mechanisms controlling fluid and electrolyte movement.
3. Describe the mechanisms and causes of extracellular fluid shifts.
4. Explain the physiological mechanisms that regulate fluid and electrolyte balance.
5. Describe the common causes, clinical manifestations, and therapeutic and nursing management of fluid and electrolyte imbalances.
6. Describe pH and the mechanisms that regulate acid-base balance.
7. Describe the common causes, pathophysiology, compensatory mechanisms, and clinical manifestations of respiratory and metabolic acidosis and alkalosis.
8. Identify the significant assessment data and common abnormal assessment findings related to fluid and electrolyte imbalances.
9. Compare and contrast the types of solutions available for fluid and electrolyte therapy, including osmolarity and indications for use.

HOMEOSTASIS

The cells that make up body tissue exist in a chemically constant but physiologically dynamic internal environment. Physiological processes function to regulate this environment so that responses to stimuli minimally affect the body. The chemical consistency achieved through fluid, electrolyte, and acid-base balance is essential to the maintenance of homeostasis.[1] *Homeostasis* is the term used to describe the stable state produced by physiological processes that interact "to keep a physical or chemical parameter in the body relatively constant."

As long as life exists, the body is affected by stressors. Stressors such as disease and injury alter the normal balance. A stress state is produced by failure to satisfy a psychological or physiological need. Homeostatic compensatory mechanisms participate in the adjustment to stressors so that the body efficiently and effectively reestablishes a steady state.

The homeostatic mechanisms that regulate fluid and electrolyte balance represent an interaction between chemical and physiological processes. The challenge to the health professional is to understand how these processes control fluid and electrolyte movement and concentrations within the body. This knowledge is necessary to understand not only the pathophysiological effects of diseases but also the way treatments affect this delicate balance.

WATER CONTENT OF THE BODY

Water is the primary body fluid. It is the solvent used to transport nutrients to cells and to remove waste products produced by cellular metabolism. Temperature regulation is assisted by evaporation of water on the body's surface.

Variations

The adult human body is about 60% water. The water content varies with sex, lean body mass, and age. Males generally have a larger water content because they have more lean body mass than females. Adipose tissue contains less water than an equivalent amount of muscle tissue. Age also influences the body's water content (Fig. 10-1). In the older adult, body water content averages 45% to 55% of body weight. For an infant, water content is 70% to 80% of the body weight. Therefore, the young are at risk for fluid problems because of the large percentage of their body weight that is water. Older adults are at risk because they have less fluid reserve.

Reviewed by Julia Guenzi Marostice Robinson, R.N., M.S., F.N.P.-C., Doctoral Candidate, Associate Professor, Department of Nursing, California State University, Bakersfield, California.

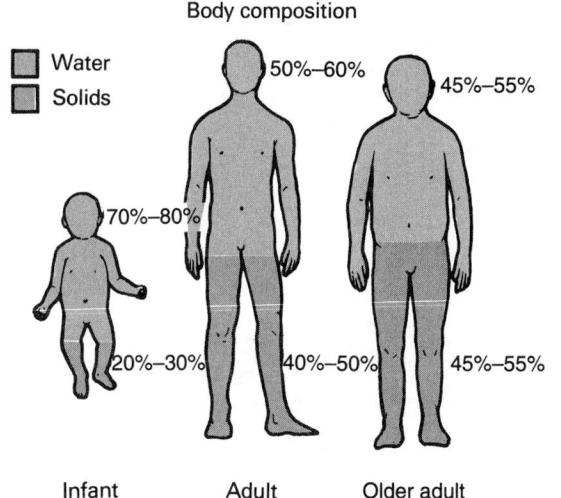

Fig. 10-1   Changes in body water content correlated with age.

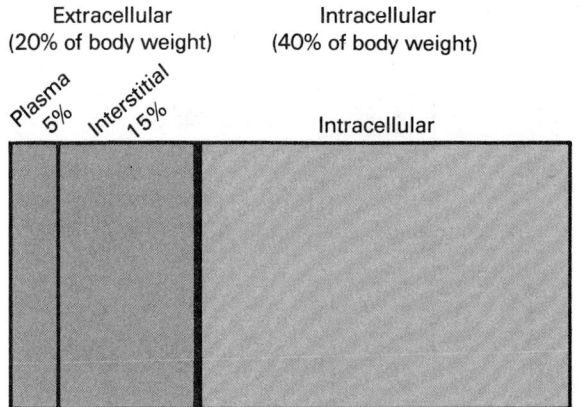

Fig. 10-2   Fluid compartments within the body.

Body Fluid Compartments

The two main fluid compartments in the body are *intracellular* and *extracellular* (Fig. 10-2). The intracellular fluid (ICF), located within cells, constitutes about 40% of body weight or 70% of the total body water. The extracellular fluid (ECF) constitutes about 20% of body weight or 30% of total body water.

The extracellular fluid consists of interstitial (between cells), intravascular (plasma), cerebrospinal, and intraocular fluid and secretions of the gastrointestinal tract. Sometimes the term *transcellular* (a product of secretion and diffusion from cells) is used to refer to cerebrospinal fluid, intraocular fluid, and gastrointestinal secretions together.

Fluid spacing is a term used to classify the distribution of body water. *First spacing* means that there is a normal distribution of fluid in both the extracellular and intracellular compartments. *Second spacing* refers to an excess accumulation of interstitial fluid (edema). *Third spacing* is

Table 10-1   Terminology Related to Body Fluid Chemistry

Anion	Ion that carries a negative charge
Cation	Ion that carries a positive charge
Electrolyte	Substance that dissociates in solution into ions (charged particles); a molecule of sodium chloride (NaCl) in solution becomes Na$^+$ and Cl$^-$
Nonelectrolyte	Substance that does not dissociate into ions in solution; examples include glucose and urea
Osmolality	A measure of the total solute concentration per kilogram of solvent
Osmolarity	A measure of the total solute concentration per liter of solution
Solute	Substance that is dissolved in a solvent
Solution	Homogeneous mixture of solutes dissolved in a solvent
Solvent	Substance that is capable of dissolving a solute (liquid or gas)

fluid accumulation in areas that normally have no fluid or a minimum amount of fluid. Some examples of third spacing are ascites, sequestration of fluid in the bowel with peritonitis, and edema associated with burns. Third spacing is a concern because it takes fluid away from the normal fluid compartments and may produce hypovolemia.

Calculation of Fluid Gain or Loss

One liter of water weighs 1 kg (2.2 pounds). If a client drank 240 ml of fluid, weight gain would be 0.24 kg (0.5 pound). A client under diuretic therapy and no dietary changes who loses 2 kg in 24 hours has experienced a fluid loss of about 2 liters. A sudden weight change is the best indicator of fluid volume deficit or excess.

ELECTROLYTES

Electrolytes are substances whose molecules dissociate or split into ions when placed in water. *Ions* are electrically charged particles. *Cations* are positively charged ions. Examples include sodium (Na$^+$), potassium (K$^+$), calcium (Ca^{2+}), and magnesium (Mg^{2+}). *Anions* are negatively charged ions. Examples include bicarbonate (HCO$_3^-$), chloride (Cl$^-$), and phosphate (PO$_4^{3-}$). (Terminology related to body fluid chemistry is presented in Table 10-1.)

Measurement

Electrolytes can be measured by weight or combining power. The unit of weight is milligrams per deciliter (mg/dl), and combining power is milliequivalents per liter (mEq/L). Milliequivalents equal weight (in milligrams) divided by the atomic weight and multiplied by the valence:

$$mEq = \frac{Weight\ (mg)}{Atomic\ weight} \times Valence$$

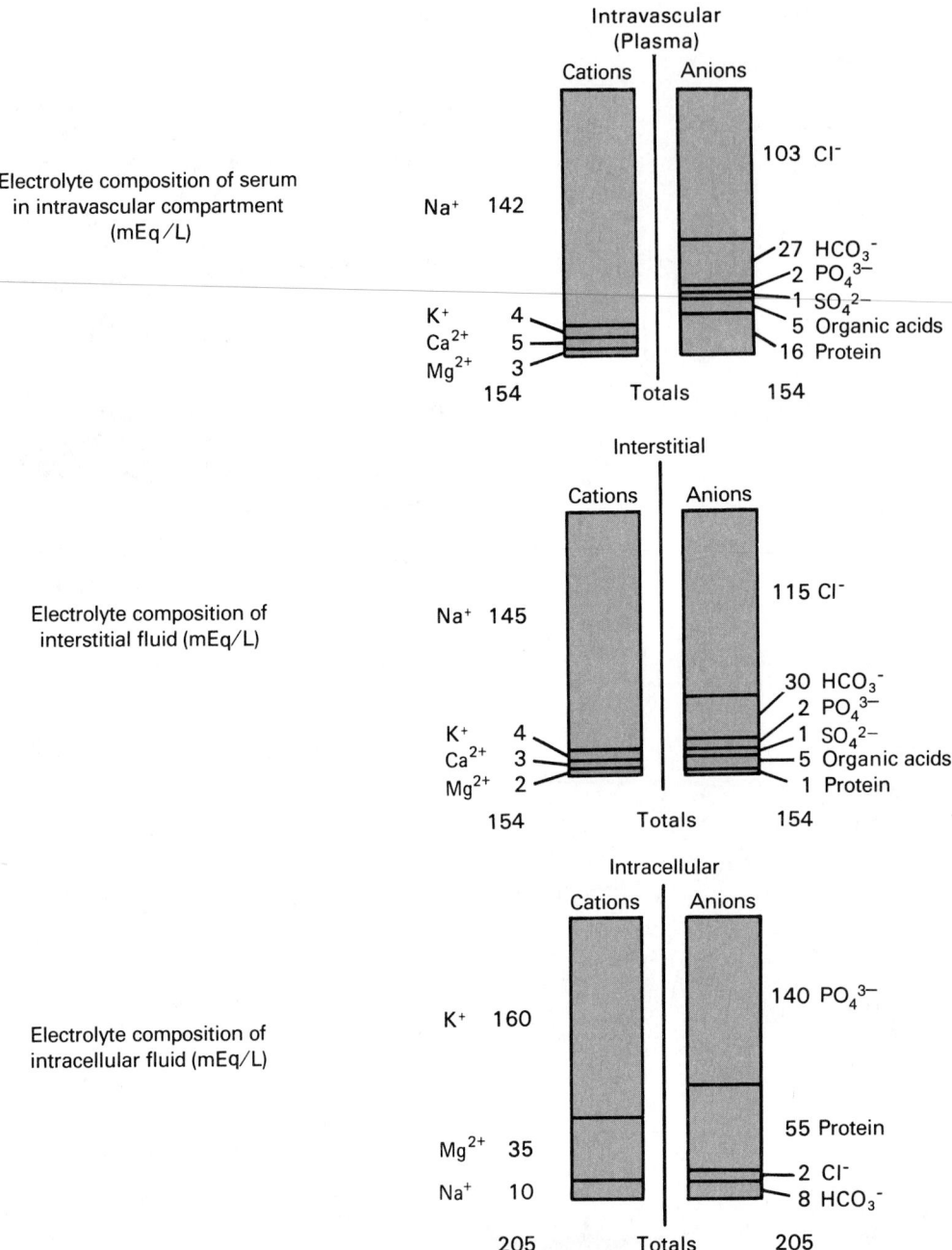

Fig. 10-3   Electrolyte content of fluid compartments.

The weight of an electrolyte gives no direct information regarding the number of ions or the number of charges carried by an electrolyte. Milliequivalents express the chemical activity of an electrolyte. For example, 1 mEq of sodium combines with 1 mEq of chloride, whereas 1 mEq of calcium combines with 2 mEq of chloride.

Electrolyte Composition of Fluid Compartments

The electrolytes found in the ECF and ICF are essentially the same. However, their concentrations vary somewhat between the compartments (Fig. 10-3). The primary intracellular cation is potassium, and the primary extracellular cation is sodium. The primary intracellular anion

is phosphate, and the primary extracellular anion is chloride. The main difference between plasma fluid and interstitial fluid is a higher concentration of protein in the plasma.

Functions

The roles of electrolytes in cellular function include the following:

1. Regulation of water distribution
2. Transmission of nerve impulses
3. Clotting of blood
4. Generation of adenosine triphosphate
5. Regulation of acid-base balance

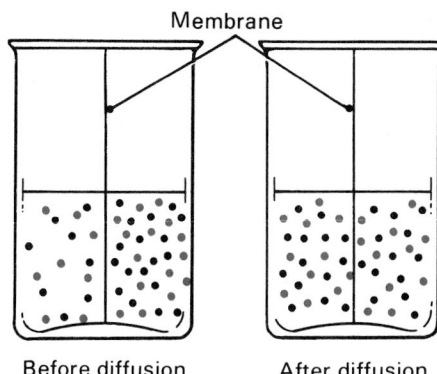

Fig. 10-4 Diffusion is the movement of molecules from an area of higher concentration to an area of lower concentration.

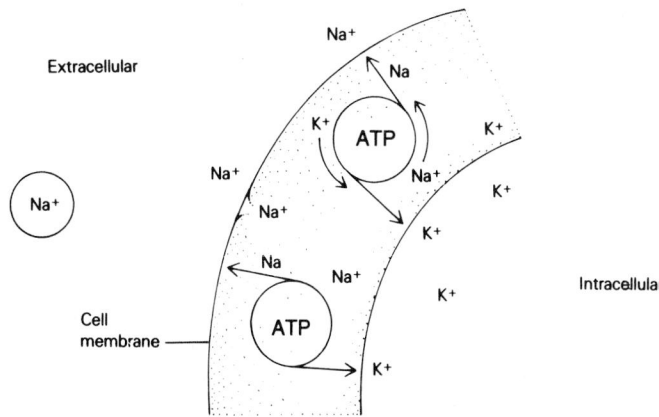

Fig. 10-5 Sodium-potassium pump. As sodium diffuses into the cell and potassium out of the cell, an active transport system supplied with energy delivers sodium back to the extracellular compartment and potassium to the intracellular compartment.

MECHANISMS CONTROLLING FLUID AND ELECTROLYTE MOVEMENT

Many different processes control the movement of fluid and electrolytes between the intracellular and extracellular spaces. These include simple diffusion, facilitated diffusion, active transport, osmosis, hydrostatic pressure, and oncotic pressure.

Diffusion

Diffusion is a movement of molecules from an area of higher concentration to one of lower concentration (Fig. 10-4). It occurs in liquids, gases, and solids. Net movement of molecules stops when the concentrations are equal in both areas. The membrane separating the two areas must be permeable to the diffusing substance for the process to occur. External energy is not required to move these molecules. Diffusion is an efficient mechanism for the movement of molecules in and out of cells.

Facilitated Diffusion

Because of the composition of cellular membranes, some molecules diffuse very slowly into the cell. However, when they are combined with a specific carrier molecule, the rate of diffusion is accelerated. Like simple diffusion, facilitated diffusion moves molecules from an area of high concentration to one of low concentration. Glucose transport into the cell is an example of facilitated diffusion in which insulin is the carrier molecule.

Active Transport

Active transport is a process in which molecules are moved from areas of low concentration to areas of high concentration. External energy is required for this process, since molecules are being moved against a concentration gradient. The concentrations of sodium and potassium differ markedly intracellularly and extracellularly (Fig. 10-3). By active transport, sodium is moved out of the cell and potassium is moved in to maintain this concentration difference (Fig. 10-5). The energy source for the pump is adenosine triphosphate (ATP), which is produced in the mitochondria.

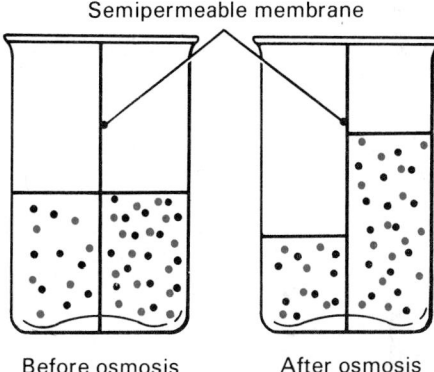

Fig. 10-6 Osmosis is the process of water movement through a semipermeable membrane from an area of low solute concentration to an area of high solute concentration.

Osmosis

Osmosis is a special type of diffusion. It is the flow of water between two compartments separated by a membrane permeable to water but not to a solute. Water moves through the membrane from an area of low solute concentration to an area of high solute concentration (Fig. 10-6). That is, water moves from the compartment that is more dilute (has more water) to the side that is more concentrated (has less water). The semipermeable membrane prevents movement of solute particles. Osmosis requires no outside energy sources and stops when concentration differences disappear. In addition to diffusion, osmosis is very important for maintaining the chemical stability of body cells.

Osmotic pressure or *force* is a term used to describe the movement of water by the process of osmosis. It can be described as a "pulling" of water. Osmolarity and osmolality are both measurements of osmotic pressure. *Osmolality* measures the osmotic force of solute per unit of weight of solvent (mOsm/kg). Osmotic force is measured in units of milliosmoles. *Osmolarity* measures the total milliosmoles of solute per unit of total volume of solution (mOsm/L).

For body fluids, the acceptable term is *osmolality* because it allows for the comparison of fluids such as plasma and urine, which do not have the same weight for an equal volume.[3] Osmolarity is used to compare solutions of equal weight and volume, such as plasma, with an intravenous solution.

Measurement of osmolality. Osmolality is measured in milliosmoles per kilogram of water (mOsm/kg). Normal osmolality of body fluids is somewhere between 275 and 295 mOsm/kg. The major determinants of plasma osmolality are sodium, glucose, and urea. Increases in the concentration of these substances in the plasma cause fluid movement into plasma because of its increased osmotic pressure.

The kidneys are mainly responsible for maintaining the concentration of body fluids within this narrow range of osmolality. When the plasma osmolality becomes abnormal, changes in the level of antidiuretic hormone (ADH) cause the kidneys to conserve or increase the excretion of water to return the osmolality to normal. The osmolality of urine may vary from 300 to 1300 mOsm/kg.

Osmotic movement of fluids. Cells are affected by the osmolality of the fluid that surrounds them. When fluids are added to the body, those that have the same osmolality as the cell interior are called *isotonic*. Solutions that contain more water than the cell are *hypotonic* (hypoosmolar), and those with less water than the cell are *hypertonic* (hyperosmolar) (Table 10-2).

Normally, the ECF and ICF are isotonic to one another; hence no net movement of water occurs. In the metabolically active cell there is a constant exchange of substances between the compartments, but no net gain or loss of water occurs.

If a cell is surrounded by hypotonic fluid, water moves into the cell, causing it to swell and possibly to burst. If a cell is surrounded by hypertonic fluid, water leaves the cell to dilute the ECF. The cell shrinks and may eventually die.

Hydrostatic Pressure

Hydrostatic pressure is the force exerted by a fluid against the walls of its container. The heart is a main component in generating pressure within blood vessels. Hydrostatic pressure in the vascular system gradually decreases as the blood moves through the arteries until it is about 32 mm Hg at the arterial end of a capillary. Because of the size of the capillary bed and fluid movement into the interstitium, the pressure decreases to about 15 mm Hg at the

Table 10-2 Definitions of Tonicity

Tonicity	Osmolality	Effects on Cell Size
Hypotonic	Less than 270 mOsm/kg	Swelling
Isotonic	275-295 mOsm/kg	None
Hypertonic	More than 300 mOsm/kg	Shrinking

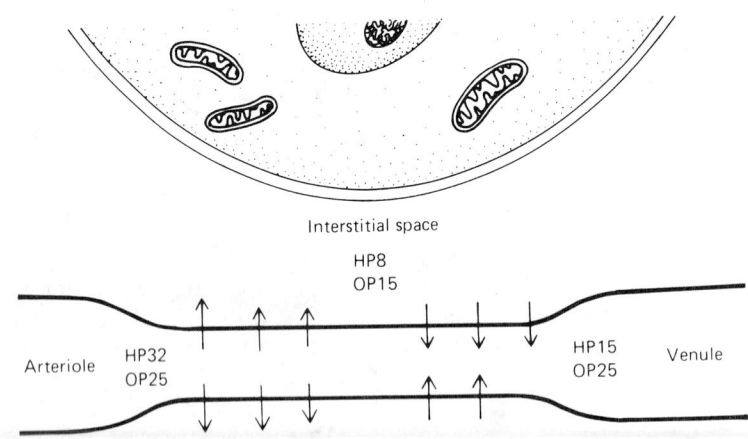

Fig. 10-7 Dynamics of fluid exchange between the vascular volume and the interstitial space. The arrow indicates direction of filtration flow. *HP,* hydrostatic pressure; *OP,* oncotic pressure. At the arteriolar end an HP of 32 mm Hg forces outward filtration, whereas an OP of 25 mm Hg resists this flow. The result is a 7 mm Hg filtration gradient. The tissue resists this capillary flow with an HP of 8 mm Hg but enhances the filtration with 15 mm Hg OP, resulting in a 7 mm Hg drawing force. The net arteriolar filtration gradient is 14 mm Hg. At the venule end, HP decreases to 15 mm Hg but the OP remains the same, so there is an inward capillary pull of 10 mm Hg. The tissue pressures remain the same with 7 mm Hg resistance. Therefore, fluid is reabsorbed into the capillary pressure gradient of 3 mm Hg. (From Barry J: Emergency nursing, New York, 1978, McGraw-Hill, Inc, p 12.)

venous end of the vessel. Hydrostatic pressure is the major force that moves water out of the vascular system at the capillary level.

Oncotic Pressure

Oncotic pressure (colloidal osmotic pressure) is osmotic pressure exerted by colloids in solution. In plasma, protein molecules attract water and contribute to the total osmotic pressure within the vascular system. Unlike electrolytes, the large molecular size of proteins prevents them from leaving the vascular space through pores in capillary walls. Plasma oncotic pressure is approximately 25 mm Hg. Some proteins are found in the interstitial space, and they exert an oncotic pressure of about 5 mm Hg.

FLUID MOVEMENT IN CAPILLARIES

There is normal movement of fluid between the capillary and the interstitium. The amount and direction of movement are determined by the interaction of the following pressures: (1) capillary hydrostatic pressure, (2) plasma oncotic pressure, (3) interstitial hydrostatic pressure, and (4) interstitial oncotic pressure.

Capillary hydrostatic pressure and interstitial oncotic pressure influence the movement of water *out of* the capillary. Plasma oncotic pressure and interstitial hydrostatic pressure attract and bring fluid *into* the capillary. At the arterial end of the capillary (Fig. 10-7), capillary hydrostatic pressure exceeds plasma oncotic pressure and fluid is moved to the interstitium. Capillary hydrostatic pressure is lower than plasma oncotic pressure at the venous end of the capillary, and fluid is drawn back into the capillary by plasma proteins.

Fluid Shifts

If capillary and/or interstitial pressures are altered, fluid may shift abnormally from one compartment to another. *Clinically,* the two shifts of fluid seen most often are (1) plasma to interstitial, as is seen in persons with edema, and (2) interstitial to plasma, as is seen in persons with dehydration.

Shifts of plasma to interstitial fluid. Accumulation of fluid in the interstitium (edema) occurs if venous hydrostatic pressure rises, plasma oncotic pressure decreases, or interstitial oncotic pressure rises.

Elevation of venous hydrostatic pressure. Increasing the pressure at the venous end of the capillary inhibits fluid movement back into the capillary. Causes of increased venous pressure include fluid overload, congestive heart failure, obstruction of venous return to the heart (e.g., tourniquets, restrictive clothing, venous thrombosis), and venous insufficiency (e.g., varicose veins).

Decrease in plasma oncotic pressure. Fluid remains in the interstitium if the plasma oncotic pressure is too low to draw it back into the capillary. Decreased oncotic pressure can result from excess protein loss (nephrotic syndrome), deficient protein synthesis (liver disease), and deficient protein intake (malnutrition).

Elevation of interstitial oncotic pressure. Trauma, burns, and inflammation can damage capillary walls and allow plasma proteins to accumulate in the interstitium.

The resultant increased interstitial oncotic pressure draws fluid into the interstitium and retains it there.

Shifts of interstitial fluid to plasma. Fluid moves from the interstitium in abnormally large quantities whenever there is an increase in the plasma osmotic-oncotic pressure. This is often therapeutically induced by the administration of colloids, dextran, mannitol, or hypertonic solutions. The hyperglycemia of uncontrolled diabetes mellitus also causes this shift.

Increasing the tissue hydrostatic pressure is another way of causing a shift of fluid into plasma. The wearing of elastic wraps or hose to decrease peripheral edema is a therapeutic use of this concept.

Hypovolemic shock acutely decreases the hydrostatic pressure at the arterial and the venous ends of the capillary, causing a rapid movement of interstitial fluid into plasma. The resultant increase in vascular volume is a way to temporarily compensate for the problem.

REGULATION OF FLUID AND ELECTROLYTES
Hypothalamic Regulation

Water ingestion in the conscious client is regulated by the hypothalamus. The thirst mechanism is stimulated by hypotension and increased serum osmolality. A dry mouth will cause the client to drink, even when there is no measurable body water deficit. Water ingestion will equal water excretion in a client who has free access to water, a normal antidiuretic hormone (ADH) mechanism, and normally functioning kidneys.

Pituitary Regulation

The posterior pituitary secretes ADH, which regulates water retention by the kidneys. The distal tubules and collecting ducts in the kidney respond to ADH by becoming more permeable to water so that water is reabsorbed into the blood and not excreted.

Normally, an increase in plasma osmolality or a decrease in circulating volume will stimulate ADH secretion. When there is a normal plasma osmolality and normal circulating plasma volume, ADH secretion is called *syndrome of inappropriate antidiuretic hormone* (SIADH) (see Chapter 44). Causes of SIADH include stress, trauma, tumors, surgery, ventilation with a positive-pressure respirator, and certain drugs. The inappropriate ADH causes water retention, which produces a decrease in plasma osmolality below the normal value and an increase in urine osmolality with a decrease in volume.

Absence of ADH produces diabetes insipidus (see Chapter 44). A copious amount of dilute urine is excreted because the renal tubules and collecting ducts do not reabsorb water. These clients exhibit extreme polyuria and polydipsia. They have symptoms of dehydration and hypernatremia if the water losses are not replaced.

Adrenal Cortical Regulation

ECF volume is maintained by a combination of hormonal influences. ADH affects only water reabsorption. The adrenal cortex secretes two groups of hormones: glucocorticoids and mineralocorticoids. The glucocorticoids have an antiinflammatory effect, whereas the mineralocor-

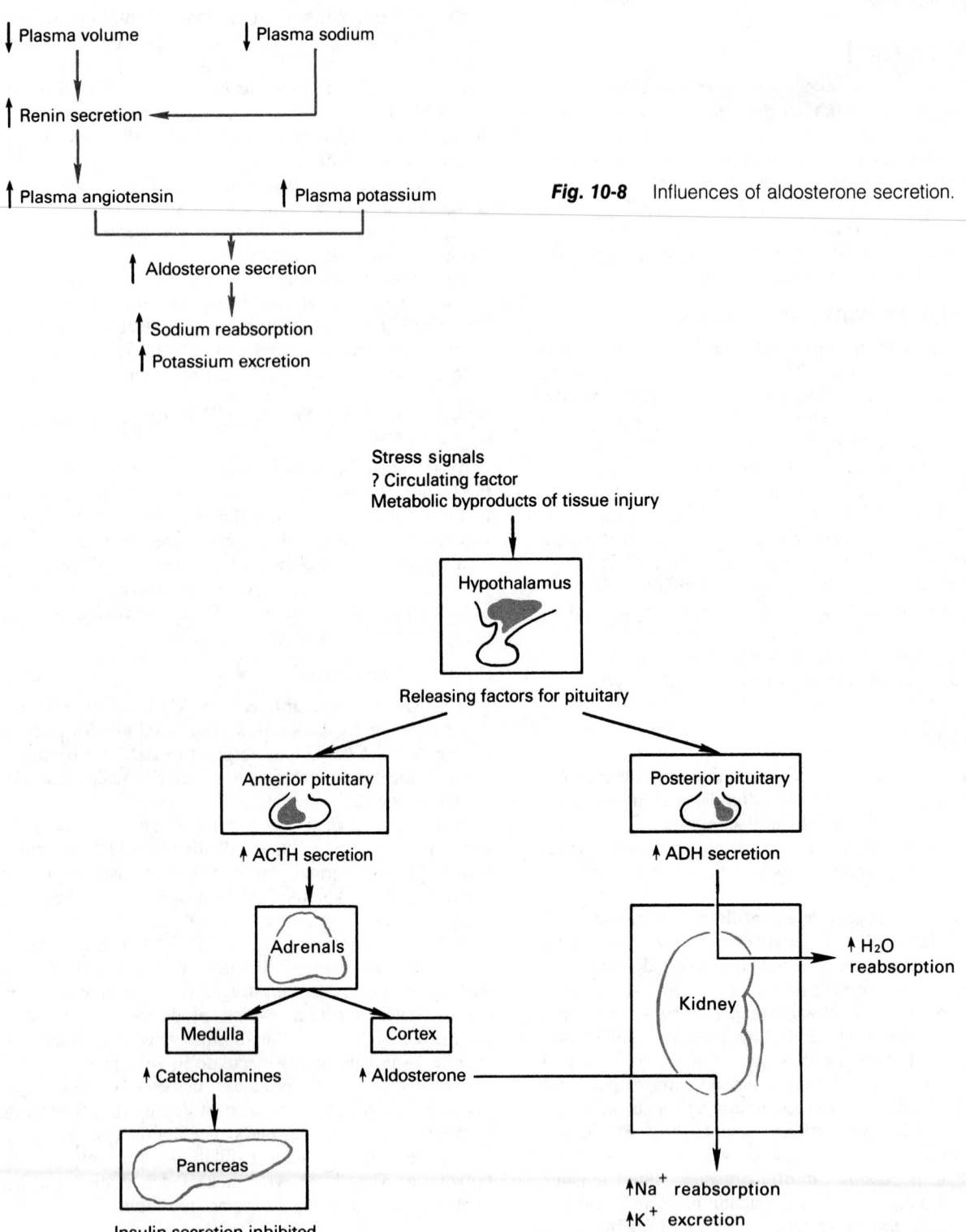

↓ Plasma volume   ↓ Plasma sodium

↑ Renin secretion ←

↑ Plasma angiotensin   ↑ Plasma potassium

↑ Aldosterone secretion

↑ Sodium reabsorption

↑ Potassium excretion

Fig. 10-8   Influences of aldosterone secretion.

Stress signals
? Circulating factor
Metabolic byproducts of tissue injury

Hypothalamus

Releasing factors for pituitary

Anterior pituitary

Posterior pituitary

↑ ACTH secretion

↑ ADH secretion

Adrenals

Kidney

↑ H_2O reabsorption

Medulla   Cortex

↑ Catecholamines   ↑ Aldosterone

Pancreas

↑ Na^+ reabsorption
↑ K^+ excretion

Insulin secretion inhibited
↑ Glycogen breakdown to glucose

Fig. 10-9   Effects of stress on fluid and electrolyte balance.

ticoids are known for their enhancement of sodium retention and potassium excretion (Fig. 10-8). When sodium is reabsorbed, some water is also reabsorbed because of the osmotic effect of sodium.

Cortisol is the most common example of a naturally occurring adrenocortical steroid. In large doses, cortisol has both glucocorticoid (antiinflammatory) and mineralocorticoid (sodium-retention) properties. The adrenocortical hormone cortisol is secreted whenever the body experiences stress. Many body systems, including fluid and electrolyte balance, are affected by stress (Fig. 10-9).

Aldosterone is the naturally occurring mineralocorticoid with the most potent sodium-retention and potassium-excreting capability. The secretion of aldosterone is stimulated by a decrease in plasma volume and a decrease in serum sodium. The kidney responds by secreting renin into the plasma. Angiotensinogen produced in the liver is acted on by the renin to form angiotensin, which stimulates the adrenal cortex to secrete aldosterone (Fig. 10-8). An increase in plasma potassium stimulates the adrenal cortex directly to secrete aldosterone.

Renal Regulation

The primary organ for regulation of fluid and electrolyte balance is the kidney (see Chapter 39). Normally, the kidney reabsorbs 99% of the glomerular filtrate.

Selective reabsorption and secretion of fluid and electrolytes function to maintain normal plasma osmolality and blood volume and acid-base balance. The renal tubules are the site for the hormonal action of ADH and aldosterone.

With impaired renal function, the kidneys cannot maintain fluid and electrolyte balance. This results in edema, potassium retention, impaired bicarbonate reabsorption, and many other problems (see Chapter 41).

Gastrointestinal Regulation

Daily water intake and output are between 2000 and 3000 ml (Table 10-3). The gastrointestinal tract accounts for most of the water intake. Water intake includes fluids, water from food metabolism, and the water present in solid foods. Fruits and vegetables are 50% to 60% water, whereas the water content of lean meats approaches 70%.

Most of the body water is excreted by the kidneys. A small amount of water is eliminated by the gastrointestinal tract in feces.

Insensible Water Loss

Insensible water loss is unavoidable vaporization from the lungs and skin, which assists in regulating body temperature. Normally, about 900 ml/day is lost. The amount of water loss is increased by accelerated body metabolism, which occurs with increased body temperature and exercise.

Insensible perspiration should not be confused with the vaporization of water excreted by sweat glands. Only water is lost by insensible perspiration. Excessive sweating (perspiration) caused by fever or high environmental temperatures may lead to large losses of water and sodium chloride.

FLUID AND ELECTROLYTE IMBALANCES

Fluid and electrolyte imbalances occur to some degree in most clients with a major illness or injury because illness disrupts the normal homeostatic mechanism. Some fluid and electrolyte imbalances are directly caused by the illness or disease (e.g., burns, congestive heart failure). At other times, therapeutic measures (e.g., intravenous fluid replacement, diuretics) cause or contribute to fluid and electrolyte imbalances.

The imbalances are commonly classified as *deficits* or *excesses*. Each imbalance is discussed separately. (For normal values, see Table 10-4.) In actual clinical situations, finding more than one imbalance in the same client is common. For example, a client with prolonged nasogastric suction may lose Na^+, K^+, and HCl. This may result in a deficiency of both sodium and potassium as well as metabolic alkalosis.

WATER AND SODIUM IMBALANCES

Sodium is the major cation in ECF. It participates in the generation and transmission of nerve impulses, is an essential electrolyte in the sodium-potassium pump, regulates osmotic pressure, and controls distribution of water throughout the body.

Table 10-3 Normal Fluid Balance in the Adult

Intake	
Fluids	1200 ml
Solid food	1000 ml
Water from oxidation	300 ml
	2500 ml
Output	
Insensible loss (skin and lungs)	900 ml
In feces	100 ml
Urine	1500 ml
	2500 ml

Table 10-4 Normal Serum Electrolyte Values

Anions	Normal Value	Cations	Normal Value
Bicarbonate (HCO_3^-)	20-30 mEq/L	Potassium (K^+)	3.5-5.5 mEq/L
Chloride (Cl^-)	96-106 mEq/L	Magnesium (Mg^{2+})	1.5-2.5 mEq/L
Phosphate (PO_4^{3-})	2.8-4.5 mg/dl	Sodium (Na^+)	135-145 mEq/L
Protein	6-8 g/dl	Calcium (Ca^{2+})	9-11 mg/dl 4.5-5.5 mEq/L

Table 10-5 Primary Water Imbalances: Causes and Clinical Manifestations

Primary Water Deficiency	Primary Water Excess
CAUSES	
Impaired thirst mechanism (injury)	Psychiatric disorder of large ingestion of H_2O
Swallowing problems	Renal failure
Diabetes insipidus	Excess administration of hypotonic fluids
Decreased water intake	
Coma	Excess tap water enemas
Debility	Inappropriate secretion of ADH
Decreased availability	
Watery diarrhea	
APPEARANCE	
Decreased skin turgor	Weight gain
Dehydrated	Edema
Dry, sticky mucous membranes	Good skin turgor
Rough, dry tongue	
Weight loss	
Fever	
BEHAVIOR	
Agitation	Confusion
Restlessness	Lethargy
Weakness	Weakness
	Seizures
CARDIOVASCULAR	
Orthostatic hypotension	Full, bounding pulse
↓ CVP	↑ CVP
Rapid, weak pulse	Jugular venous distention
GASTROINTESTINAL	
Hard stools	Nausea
	Vomiting
	Liquid stools
URINARY FINDINGS	
Urine volume ↓	Urinary volume ↑
Specific gravity >1.030	Specific gravity <1.010
Urine osmolality ↑	Urine osmolality ↓
SERUM VALUES	
Na^+ ↑	Na^+ ↓
Protein ↑	Protein ↓
Hematocrit ↑	Hematocrit ↓
Serum osmolality ↑	Serum osmolality ↓

The gastrointestinal tract absorbs sodium from foods that are consumed. The kidney regulates the ECF concentration of sodium by excreting or retaining sodium under the influence of aldosterone. A frequent saying is "where sodium goes, water goes." For this reason, sodium and water problems are often not differentiated. This can be very confusing because primary water problems require significantly different treatment than primary sodium problems. For example, a pure water gain produces a decreased serum sodium because the added water dilutes the sodium. Treatment with a normal saline solution would overload the client with both sodium and water. The appropriate treatment for a low serum sodium level (hyponatremia) caused by an excess of water is restriction of fluid.

Sodium and water alterations can be classified into primary water imbalances, primary sodium imbalances, and extracellular imbalances.

Primary Water Imbalances

Common causes of primary water imbalances are listed in Table 10-5.

Water deficit. Water deficit (dehydration or hypertonicity) is not a problem in an alert person who has access to water and is able to swallow. Primary water deficiency is often the result of an impaired level of consciousness and/or an inability to ingest oral fluids. Clients who receive only high-protein tube feedings will become water deficient. Often older adults, especially if they are ill, do not drink enough fluids.

Several clinical states can produce hypertonicity and dehydration. A deficiency in the synthesis or release of ADH from the posterior pituitary gland (diabetes insipidus) or a decrease in kidney responsiveness to ADH can result in profound diuresis resulting in dehydration. More common causes are thick tube feedings used in unconscious clients and osmotic diuresis, which occurs with uncontrolled diabetes mellitus (hyperglycemia) or after the administration of osmotic diuretics (mannitol, urea). Other causes are excessive pulmonary water loss in high fever states and diarrhea in infants, leading to excessive gastrointestinal fluid loss. Excessive sweating without water replacement also leads to dehydration.

The clinical manifestations of primary water deficiency are listed in Table 10-5. With persistent water deficiency, the vascular volume falls and ADH is released to increase water reabsorption by the kidneys as a compensatory mechanism.

Water excess. Water excess can lead to overhydration and hypotonicity. Overhydration involves an excess of fluids in the body in which more solvent than solute has been gained, so the expanded compartments become diluted and thus hypotonic. In the normal adult, water excess does not occur until fluid intake exceeds 20 L/day.

Common causes of water excess with hypotonicity are regular intravenous fluid administration or unchecked oral intake in unrecognized renal failure and excess of free water (glucose and water) administration during the first few days after major surgery or after another major traumatic event. Clinical manifestations of water excess include rapid weight gain, decreased serum sodium and hematocrit values, and increased central venous pressure (CVP).

Therapeutic management. The goal of treatment in both types of water imbalance is to treat the underlying cause. In primary water deficit, the continued water loss must be prevented and water replacement must be provided. If oral fluids cannot be ingested, intravenous solutions of 5% dextrose in water are given initially. If adequate renal function is present, electrolytes can be added to the intravenous solution.

In primary water excess, fluid restriction is often all that is needed to treat the problem. If severe symptoms (e.g., convulsions) develop, small amounts of hypertonic saline solution may be given to restore the serum sodium level while the body is returning to a normal water balance.

Primary Sodium Imbalances

Sodium in the ECF is measured in milliequivalents per liter (mEq/L) of water as it is concentrated or diluted in water. The common causes of sodium imbalances are included in Table 10-6. Sodium imbalances are usually directly related to water imbalances. Hyponatremia (low serum sodium level) may result from sodium loss or from water excess. Hypoosmolar and hypotonic states and hyponatremia all reflect low sodium levels. Sodium loss greater than water loss or water gain greater than sodium gain leads to a low concentration of sodium. The excessive use of hypotonic intravenous solutions causes hyponatremia because of water gain greater than sodium gain in the ECF compartment.

Hypernatremia (increased serum sodium levels) may result from excess sodium, water loss, or insufficient water intake.[2] If the sodium intake is greater than the water intake, a hypernatremia and a hyperosmolar or hypertonic state will result. The clinical manifestations of sodium imbalances are similar to those of water imbalances (Table 10-6).

Therapeutic management. Treatment of sodium imbalances needs to be directed at the underlying cause. Figs. 10-10 and 10-11 illustrate the underlying causes and fluid shifts that occur with water and sodium imbalances.

The goal of treatment for sodium deficit is to restore the sodium level without causing fluid volume excess. If the client also has a fluid excess (dilutional hyponatremia), therapy is aimed at restricting fluids. If there is a fluid deficit or normal fluid balance associated with the hyponatremia, intravenous isotonic saline solution (0.9% NaCl) is usually given. Occasionally, intravenous hypertonic saline solution (3% NaCl) is given.

The goal of treatment for sodium excess is to dilute the sodium concentration and promote excretion of the excess sodium. Intravenous solutions of 5% dextrose in water are usually given. Diuretics may be used to remove excess sodium and water.

Extracellular Fluid Volume Imbalances

The terms *extracellular fluid volume deficit* (hypovolemia) and *extracellular fluid volume excess* (hypervolemia) are commonly used in describing isotonic fluid imbalances

Table 10-6 Sodium Imbalances: Causes and Clinical Manifestations

Hyponatremia (Na⁺ <135 mEq/L)	Hypernatremia (Na⁺ >145 mEq/L)
CAUSES	
Excess sweating and increased water intake	Decreased water intake
Diuretic excess	Excess intake of saline or salt tablets
Adrenal insufficiency	Adrenal hyperfunction
Gastrointestinal suction with H_2O irrigations	Heatstroke
Edema (water retention exceeds sodium retention)	High fever
Cirrhosis	Saltwater drowning
Congestive heart failure	Rapid breathing with H_2O vapor loss
Excess IV administration of 5% dextrose in water	Excess IV administration of 0.9% NaCl
Freshwater drowning	Watery, profuse diarrhea
APPEARANCE	
Clammy skin	Flushed skin
Dehydration	Weight gain
Shocky	
Weakness	
BEHAVIOR	
Anxiety	Weakness
Lethargy	Lethargy
Stupor→coma	Restlessness
CARDIOVASCULAR	
Rapid, thready pulse	Hypertension (can deteriorate into congestive heart failure)
Postural hypotension	
↓ CVP	↑ CVP
Decreased jugular venous filling	Distended veins
GASTROINTESTINAL	
Anorexia, nausea	Thirst
Vomiting	Dry, swollen tongue
Abdominal pain	
NEUROMUSCULAR	
Muscle weakness	Depressed reflexes
Lower extremity muscle cramps	Possible seizures
SERUM VALUES	
Serum Na⁺ ↓	Serum Na⁺ ↑
Hematocrit ↑	Hematocrit ↓
Serum protein ↑	Serum protein ↓

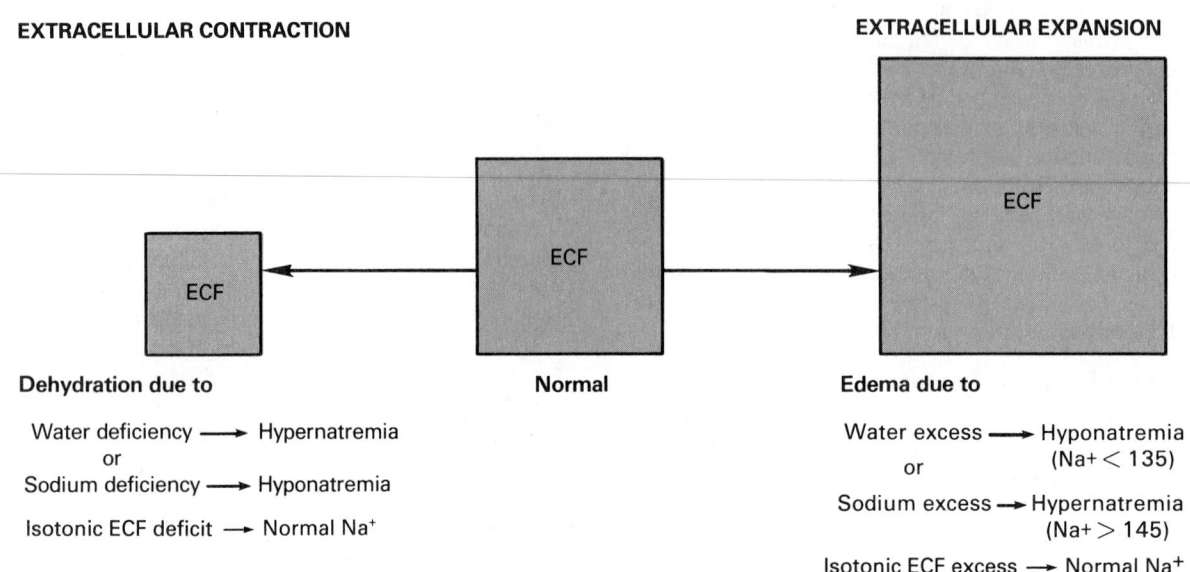

Fig. 10-10   Differential assessment of ECF volume.

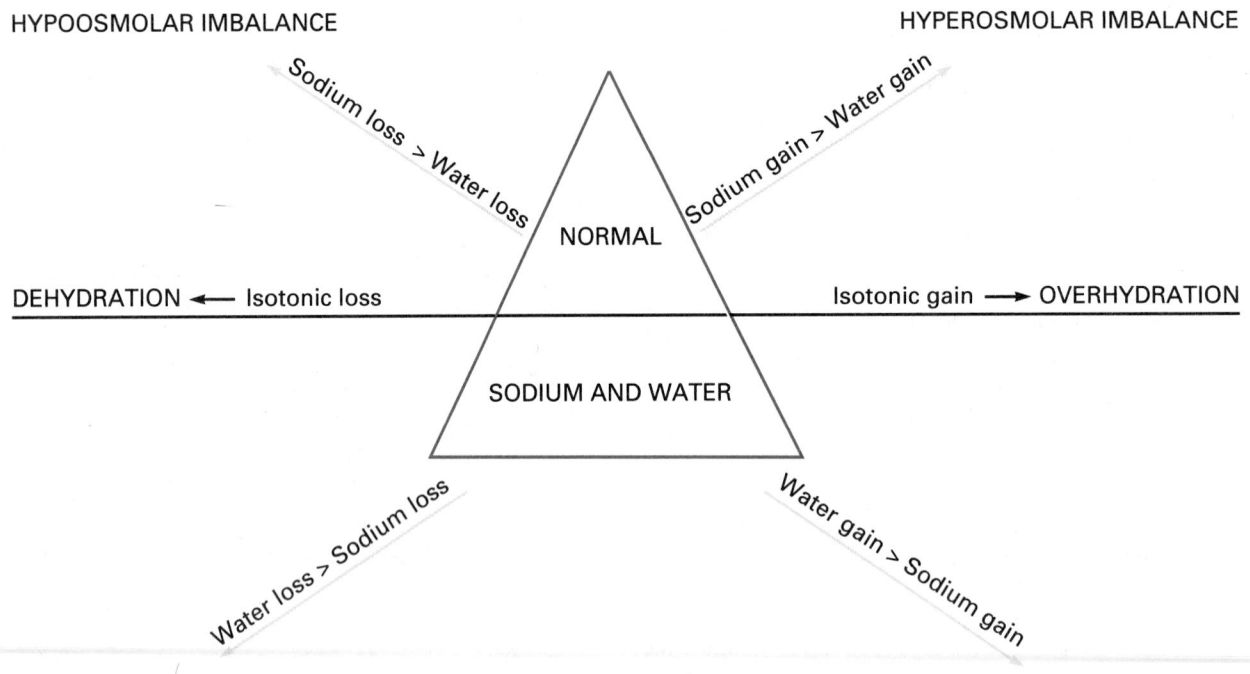

Fig. 10-11   Isotonic gains and losses affect mainly the ECF compartment with little or no water movement into the cells. Hypertonic imbalances cause water to move from inside the cell into the ECF to dilute the concentrated sodium, causing cell shrinkage. Hypotonic imbalances cause water to move into the cell, causing cell swelling.

Table 10-7 Causes of ECF Volume Imbalances

ECF Volume Deficit	ECF Volume Excess
INCREASED LOSS	**DECREASED LOSS**
Vomiting	Congestive heart failure
Diarrhea	Cushing's syndrome
Fistula drainage	Chronic liver disease with portal hypertension
GI suction	
Excessive sweating	Long-term use of corticosteroids
Fever	
Third-space fluid shifts (e.g., burns, intestinal obstruction)	Renal failure
	Excessive IV administration of isotonic fluids
Overuse of diuretics	
DECREASED INTAKE	**INCREASED INTAKE**
Nausea	Rare with adequate renal function
Anorexia	
Inability to drink	
Inability to obtain water	

(Table 10-7). These terms refer to a deficit or excess not just of water but of both water and electrolytes (primarily sodium) in approximately the same proportion. ECF deficit may result from severe diarrhea or fistula drainage in which both water and electrolytes are lost. ECF excess may result from excessive infusion of isotonic fluids. The clinical manifestations of ECF imbalances are similar to those of both water and sodium imbalances.

Therapeutic management. The goal of treatment for fluid volume deficit is to correct the underlying cause (e.g., vomiting, diarrhea) and to replace both water and electrolytes, especially if the problem has existed for several days. Balanced intravenous solutions such as lactated Ringer's solution are usually given.

The goal of treatment for fluid volume excess is removal of sodium and water without producing abnormal changes in electrolyte osmolality or composition of ECF. The primary cause needs to be identified and treated. Intravenous therapy is usually not indicated for this type of fluid imbalance. Usually diuretic therapy is indicated. Reduction of oral sodium intake may also be indicated. If the fluid excess leads to problems of ascites or pleural effusion, an abdominal paracentesis or thoracentesis may be indicated.

■ **Nursing Management of Sodium and Water Imbalances**

Nursing diagnoses

Nursing diagnoses specific to the client with the various fluid and sodium imbalances include, but are not limited to, the following:

Extracellular fluid volume excess
1. ECF volume excess related to increased sodium and water retention
2. Potential complication: edema (peripheral and pulmonary) related to an excess circulating fluid secondary to an expanded ECF volume

3. Impaired gas exchange related to decreased diffusion of oxygen secondary to pulmonary vascular congestion occurring with an increase in ECF
4. High risk for impairment of skin and tissue integrity related to edema secondary to fluid volume excess

Extracellular fluid volume deficit
1. Fluid volume deficit related to decreased circulatory volume secondary to excessive ECF losses or decreased fluid intake
2. Altered tissue perfusion (cerebral and peripheral) related to decreased circulation secondary to fluid volume deficit

Hypernatremia
High risk for injury related to altered sensorium and seizures secondary to cerebral edema

Hyponatremia
High risk for injury related to altered sensorium and LOC secondary to severe hyponatremia

Nursing interventions

Intake and output. The use of 24-hour intake and output records gives valuable information regarding fluid and electrolyte problems. Sources of excessive intake or fluid losses can be identified on a properly recorded intake-and-output flowsheet. Intake should include oral, intravenous, and tube feedings. Output includes urine, excess perspiration, wound or tube drainage, vomitus, and diarrhea. Fluid loss from wounds and perspiration should be estimated. Specific gravity measurements can be done. Readings of greater than 1.025 indicate a concentrated urine, whereas those of less than 1.010 indicate a dilute urine.

Vital signs. Signs and symptoms of ECF volume excess (expansion) and deficit (contraction) are reflected in changes in blood pressure, heart rate, respiratory rate, central venous pressure (CVP) readings, and lung sounds. In ECF volume excess, tachycardia secondary to sympathetic nervous system stimulation occurs. The pulse is rapid and bounding. Because of the expanded intravascular volume, it is not easily obliterated. The respiratory rate is increased. Blood pressure is usually elevated secondary to the increased volume, as is central venous pressure. With pulmonary congestion and edema, the client will experience shortness of breath and moist rales will be heard.

In ECF volume deficit, vital signs are similar to those seen in shock. With a decrease in the volume of ECF, initially there is sympathetic nervous system stimulation of the heart and vasoconstriction. Stimulation of the heart increases heart rate, and initially, the vasoconstriction maintains blood pressure within normal limits. As compensatory vasoconstriction fails, hypotension secondary to the reduced volume occurs. Because of the hypovolemia, the pulse is weak and thready and easily obliterated. The decreased volume is also reflected in a lowered CVP. Respiratory rate increases as a result of decreased tissue perfusion and hypoxia.

Neurological changes. Changes in neurological function may occur with sodium and water imbalances. With increased water volume and hyponatremia, water is osmotically "pulled" from the extracellular space into the cerebral cells because the tonicity of the cerebral cells is comparatively higher than that of the ECF. With swelling of the cerebral cells, dysfunction occurs. Alternatively, decreased water volume and hypernatremia (hypertonicity of the ECF) cause water to shift out of the cerebral cells with a resultant shrinkage.

Assessment of neurological function includes evaluation of (1) the level of consciousness, which includes responses to verbal and/or painful stimuli and determination of a person's orientation to time, place, and person; (2) pupillary response to light and equality of pupil size; and (3) voluntary movement of the extremities and degree of muscle strength.

Daily weights. Accurate daily weights are known to provide the best bedside measurement of hydration status. An increase of 1 kg is equal to 1000 ml fluid retention (provided the person has maintained usual dietary intake or has not been on NPO status). However, weight changes can be relied on only if obtained under standardized conditions. An accurate weight requires the client to be weighed at the same time every day and on the same carefully calibrated scale. Excess clothing and bedding should be removed and all drainage bags emptied before the weighing. If bulky dressings or tubes that may not necessarily be used every day are present, a notation regarding these variables should be recorded on the flowsheet or nursing notes.

Skin assessment and care. Dehydration and overhydration can be detected by inspection of the skin. Skin

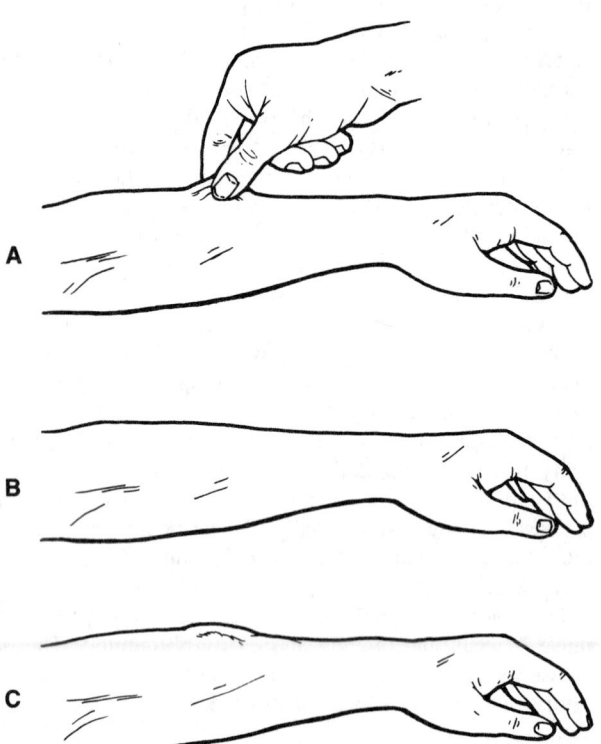

Fig. 10-12 Assessment of skin turgor. **A** and **B,** When normal skin is pinched, it resumes shape within seconds. **C,** If the skin remains wrinkled for 20 to 30 seconds, the client has poor skin turgor.

should be examined for turgor and mobility. Normally, a fold of skin when pinched will readily move and, on release, will rapidly return to its former position. Skin areas over the sternum, abdomen, and anterior forearm are the usual sites for evaluation of tissue turgor (Fig. 10-12).

In dehydration, skin turgor is diminished so that there is a lag in the pinched skin fold's return to its original state. The skin may be cool and moist if there is sympathetic vasoconstriction to compensate for the decreased fluid volume. Mild dehydration usually does not stimulate this compensatory response, so the skin will be warm and dry. Dehydration may also cause the skin to appear dry and wrinkled. This sign may be difficult to evaluate in older adults because their skin may be normally dry, wrinkled, and nonelastic.

Skin that is edematous may feel cool due to fluid accumulation and a decrease in blood flow secondary to the pressure of the fluid. The fluid can also stretch the skin so that it feels taut and hard. *Pitting edema* is the term used to describe edema when the examiner's thumb leaves an indentation over the edematous area. The areas to be evaluated for pitting edema are those where soft tissues overlie a bone. Skin areas over the tibia, fibula, and sacrum are the preferred sites.

Good skin care for the overhydrated and the dehydrated person is very important. Edematous tissues need to be protected from extremes of heat and cold, prolonged pressure, and trauma. Frequent skin care and changes in position will protect the client from skin breakdown. Elevation of edematous extremities helps to promote venous return. Dehydrated skin needs frequent care without the use of soap. The application of moisturizing creams or oils will increase moisture retention and stimulate circulation.

Other nursing measures. The rates of infusion of intravenous fluid solutions should be carefully monitored. Attempts to "catch up" should be approached with extreme caution, particularly when large volumes of fluid are involved. This is especially true in clients with heart, renal, or neurological problems. The nurse needs to encourage and often assist the older adult or debilitated client to maintain an adequate oral intake. Clients receiving tube feedings may need to have supplementary water added to their regular tube feedings.

Clients with nasogastric suction should not be allowed to drink water because it will be suctioned out along with electrolytes. Occasionally, the client may be given limited ice chips to suck. A nasogastric tube should always be irrigated with isotonic saline solution and not with water. Water causes diffusion of sodium into the stomach; this is suctioned out and can lead to hyponatremia.

POTASSIUM IMBALANCES

Potassium is the major cation in ICF. Its functions include maintenance of the regular cardiac rhythm, transmission and conduction of nerve impulses, and use of glucose by cells. Moreover, K^+ is part of the enzyme system necessary for cell energy production.[3]

Potassium enters the body via foods consumed and is readily absorbed from the gastrointestinal tract. The kid-

Table 10-8 Potassium Imbalances: Causes and Clinical Manifestations

Hypokalemia ($K^+ < 3.5$ mEq/L)	Hyperkalemia ($K^+ > 5.5$ mEq/L)	Hypokalemia ($K^+ < 3.5$ mEq/L)	Hyperkalemia ($K^+ > 5.5$ mEq/L)
CAUSES		**CARDIOVASCULAR—cont'd**	
Vomiting	Renal failure	Bradycardia, first- and second-degree heart block, atrial dysrhythmias	Complete heart block
Diarrhea	Early stage of burns		Ectopic beats
Potent diuretics	Adrenal insufficiency	PVCs, especially for clients on digitalis	Ventricular fibrillation → ventricular standstill
Aldosterone-producing tumor	Massive crushing injury	Postural hypotension	
Potassium-free IV solutions	Excess IV administration of K^+		
Recovery phase of diabetic acidosis	Metabolic acidosis	**GASTROINTESTINAL**	
Fistulas		Anorexia, nausea	Nausea
Metabolic alkalosis		Paralytic ileus	Vomiting
Anorexia			Intestinal colic
Starvation			Diarrhea
Malnutrition			
		NEUROMUSCULAR	
APPEARANCE		Hyporeflexia	Twitching
Drowsiness	No specific findings	Muscle weakness→paralysis	Seizures
		Muscle cramps and paresthesias	Paresthesias
BEHAVIOR			
Confusion	No alteration in mentation	**URINARY FINDINGS**	
Irritability	Irritability	Urinary output ↑	Urine potassium ↑
Lethargy		Specific gravity ↓	
Depression		May have decreased output because of urinary retention	
CARDIOVASCULAR			
ECG changes	ECG changes	**SERUM VALUES**	
ST depression	Peaked T waves	Serum potassium ↓	Serum potassium ↑
T wave inversion or flattening	PR interval prolongation	pH ↑	pH ↓
U waves	Disappearance of P wave		
	Widening of QRS		

neys play the primary role in K^+ excretion. The gastrointestinal tract and skin account for only a small amount of potassium loss. If kidney function is impaired, toxic levels of K^+ may result. The kidney is able to conserve sodium much more effectively than it does potassium. Aldosterone acts to retain sodium and excrete potassium. During periods of diuresis, large quantities of potassium may be excreted.

The laboratory measurement of potassium measures the amount in ECF. Since serum potassium is only a small fraction of total body potassium, it is only an indirect indicator of the level of intracellular K^+. Causes of potassium imbalance are presented in Table 10-8.

Hyperkalemia

Hyperkalemia occurs after massive cell destruction (e.g., burns or a crush injury), rapid transfusion of aged blood, and massive catabolic states (e.g., severe infec-

tions) and is due to the release of intracellular K^+ into the plasma. Increased intake or decreased excretion (renal failure) of potassium also elevates serum potassium levels. Metabolic acidosis causes a shift of K^+ from the ICF to the ECF as hydrogen ions move into the cell and K^+ exits. The resultant hyperkalemia is corrected either by increased renal excretion of K^+ or by correction of the acidosis. Adrenal insufficiency leads to retention of K^+ in the serum because of aldosterone deficiency.

Clinical manifestations. Hyperkalemia (high serum potassium) increases cell excitability but produces a weaker cardiac contraction. Cardiac cells demonstrate the most clinically significant changes with potassium imbalances. Fig. 10-13 illustrates the electrocardiographic (ECG) effects of hypokalemia and hyperkalemia. Clinical manifestations of hyperkalemia include cardiac dysrhythmias, muscle twitching, seizures, intestinal colic, and diarrhea. Other clinical manifestations are listed in Table 10-8.

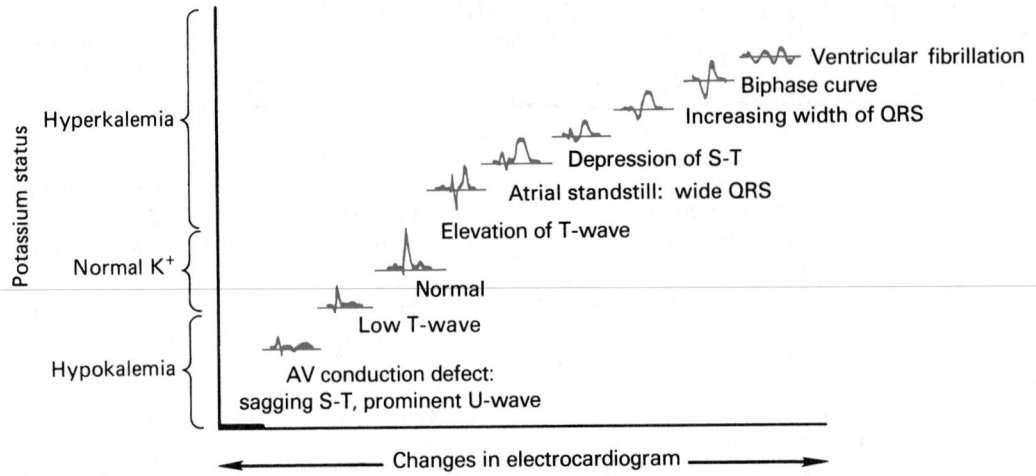

Fig. 10-13 ECG changes associated with alterations in potassium status.

■ Therapeutic and Nursing Management of Hyperkalemia

Nursing diagnoses

Nursing diagnoses specific to the client with hyperkalemia include, but are not limited to, the following:

1. High risk for decreased cardiac output related to decreased myocardial contractility and risk of ventricular dysrhythmias
2. Sensory/perceptual alteration related to excitable neuromuscular activity secondary to severe hyperkalemia

Nursing interventions

Treatment of hyperkalemia consists of the following:

1. Decrease in dietary sources of potassium (see Table 41-8)
2. Administration of sodium bicarbonate intravenously
3. Administration of calcium gluconate
4. Infusion of glucose and insulin intravenously
5. Use of cation exchange resins (Kayexalate)
6. Dialysis

Sodium bicarbonate corrects acidosis and facilitates potassium movement into the ICF. Calcium stabilizes cell membranes and antagonizes the effect of potassium on the heart. Glucose and insulin infusion may be used in the acute management of symptomatic hyperkalemia because insulin enhances the movement of potassium into the cell. Kayexalate binds potassium in exchange for sodium, and the resin is excreted in feces (see Chapter 41).

Hypokalemia

Hypokalemia (low serum potassium) can result from loss of potassium in intestinal tract fluids, excretion in urine, or a shift of potassium from the ECF to the ICF. Metabolic alkalosis causes potassium to move intracellularly in exchange for hydrogen ions. This type of hypokalemia will usually correct itself with treatment of the alkalosis.

Hypokalemia may be associated with the treatment of diabetic ketoacidosis. When glucose and insulin move intracellularly, they take potassium with them and decrease the ECF potassium. Causes of hypokalemia (reflecting a decrease in total body potassium) include diuretic therapy, increased aldosterone secretion, stress, and gastrointestinal losses in diarrhea, vomiting, and ileostomy drainage.

Extreme malnutrition and starvation can also cause hypokalemia by decreasing potassium intake. Anabolic states of cell repair lower extracellular potassium as it moves into the cell.

Clinical manifestations. Hypokalemia slows depolarization of cardiac cells and thus slows conduction velocity of the heart. Hypokalemia has been implicated in some cases of sudden cardiac death in persons with compromised cardiac function. Clinical manifestations of hypokalemia are presented in Table 10-8.

■ Therapeutic and Nursing Management of Hypokalemia

Nursing diagnoses

Nursing diagnoses specific to the client with hypokalemia include, but are not limited to, the following:

1. High risk for decreased cardiac output related to risk of ventricular dysrhythmias secondary to hypokalemia
2. High risk for ineffective breathing pattern related to weakness or paralysis of respiratory muscles secondary to severe hypokalemia
3. Sensory/perceptual alterations related to depressed mentation
4. Impaired physical mobility related to muscle weakness and paralysis

Nursing interventions

Hypokalemia is treated by giving potassium chloride supplements and increasing dietary intake of potassium. Potassium chloride (KCl) supplements can be given orally or intravenously. KCl should never be given unless there is urine output of at least 30 ml/hour. KCl supplements added to intravenous solutions should never exceed 60 mEq/L. The preferred level is 40 mEq/L. The rate of intravenous administration of KCl should not exceed 20-40 mEq/hr to prevent hyperkalemia and cardiac arrest. When

Table 10-9 Calcium Imbalances: Causes and Clinical Manifestations

Hypocalcemia (<9 mg/dl)	Hypercalcemia (>11 mg/dl)	Hypocalcemia (<9 mg/dl)	Hypercalcemia (>11 mg/dl)
CAUSES		**CARDIOVASCULAR**	
Acute pancreatitis	Excess milk-product ingestion	ECG changes	ECG changes
Primary hypoparathyroidism		Prolonged QT	Depressed T waves
Steatorrhea	Hyperparathyroidism	Dysrhythmias	Shortened QT interval
Generalized peritonitis	Prolonged immobilization		Hypertension
Chronic renal failure	Multiple myeloma		Cardiac arrest
Vitamin D deficiency	Thyrotoxicosis		
Surgical removal of parathyroids	Vitamin D excess	**GASTROINTESTINAL**	
		Colicky discomfort	Anorexia
Excess administration of citrated blood		Diarrhea	Nausea
			Constipation
Diuretic therapy			Paralytic ileus
Alcoholism			
Malabsorption		**NEUROMUSCULAR**	
Total parenteral nutrition		Hyperreflexia	Decreased muscle strength
		Muscle cramps	Depressed reflexes
APPEARANCE		Numbness and tingling in extremities	
Tonic and clonic convulsions	Lethargic	Carpopedal spasms	
	Weight loss	Chvostek's sign	
	Dehydrated	Trousseau's sign	
		Seizures	
BEHAVIOR		**RESPIRATORY**	
Personality changes	Decreased intellectual function	Laryngeal spasm	Hypoventilation
Depression		Respiratory arrest	
Irritability	Malaise	**URINARY FINDINGS**	
Easy fatigability	Confusion	No specific findings	Increased urinary output
Anxiety	Coma		
Confusion	Increased thirst	**SERUM VALUES**	
	Impaired memory	Overcorrection of acid pH (may precipitate symptomatic hypocalcemia)	↑ Serum albumin (client may not have symptoms despite increased Ca^{2+})
	Fatigue		

potassium is given intravenously, it may cause pain in the area of the vein where it is entering. Central intravenous lines should be used when rapid correction of hypokalemia is necessary.

Clients who are taking diuretics (especially thiazide and loop diuretics) need to be aware of the need to increase dietary potassium intake (Table 41-8). It may be necessary for them to take oral KCl supplements or salt substitutes that contain potassium. People should be taught which foods are high in potassium. They should also be instructed to recognize the clinical manifestations of hypokalemia and report them to their health care provider. If a client is also taking digitalis preparations, the serum potassium level must be closely monitored because hypokalemia enhances the action of digitalis.

CALCIUM IMBALANCES

Calcium is obtained from ingested foods. However, only about 30% is absorbed in the gastrointestinal tract.

The functions of calcium include transmission of nerve impulses, blood clotting, formation of teeth and bone, and muscle contraction. Normally, the amount of calcium and phosphorus found in the body is in an inverse relationship. Calcium is usually present in the body either in an ionized form or bound to protein. The ionized form is the biologically active form.

Serum calcium levels as usually reported reflect only the ionized form. Serum pH levels affect calcium binding to albumin. Acidosis decreases calcium binding, leading to more ionized calcium, and alkalosis increases calcium binding. More than 99% of the body's calcium is concentrated in the skeletal system. The bone serves as a readily available store of calcium. Thus, large vacillations in serum calcium levels are avoided.

Calcium balance depends on the proper functioning of three hormones: vitamin D, parathyroid hormone, and calcitonin (Table 10-9). Vitamin D is formed through the action of ultraviolet rays on a precursor found in the skin or is ingested in the diet. Vitamin D is essential for absorption of calcium from the gastrointestinal tract.

Parathyroid hormone is produced by the parathyroid gland. Its production and release are stimulated by low serum calcium levels. Parathyroid hormone increases bone resorption (movement of calcium out of bones), increases gastrointestinal absorption of calcium, and increases renal tubule reabsorption of calcium.

Calcitonin is produced by the thyroid gland and is stimulated by high serum calcium levels. It opposes the action of parathyroid hormone and thus lowers the serum calcium level by decreasing gastrointestinal absorption, increasing bone mineralization, and promoting renal excretion. Causes of calcium imbalance are listed in Table 10-9.

Hypercalcemia

Hypercalcemia is most commonly associated with malignancy, with or without skeletal metastasis, multiple myeloma, hyperparathyroidism, vitamin D overdose, and prolonged immobilization.[4] Hypercalcemia rarely occurs from increased ingestion of calcium-rich foods or antacids containing calcium.

Clinical manifestations. Excess serum calcium causes decreased memory span, confusion, disorientation, fatigue, muscle weakness, constipation, and cardiac dysrhythmias.

■ Therapeutic and Nursing Management of Hypercalcemia

Nursing diagnoses

Nursing diagnoses specific to the client with hypercalcemia include, but are not limited to, the following:

1. High risk for injury related to neuromuscular and sensorium changes secondary to hypercalcemia
2. Altered patterns of urinary elimination: dysuria, urgency, frequency, and polyuria secondary to administration of diuretics and changes in renal function occurring with hypercalcemia
3. Sensory/perceptual alteration related to hypercalcemia as evidenced by depressed levels of consciousness or psychotic behavior

Nursing interventions

The basic treatment of hypercalcemia is promotion of excretion of calcium in urine by administration of a loop diuretic (furosemide or ethacrynic acid) and hydration of the client with normal saline infusions. In hypercalcemia the client needs to drink 3000 to 4000 ml of fluid daily to promote the renal excretion of calcium and to decrease the possibility of renal calculi formation.

Synthetic calcitonin can also be administered to lower serum calcium levels. Mithramycin, a cytotoxic antibiotic, inhibits bone resorption and thus lowers the serum calcium level. Corticosteroids can also be given to decrease bone turnover and tubular reabsorption. A diet low in calcium is prescribed. Mobilization with weight-bearing activity is encouraged to enhance bone mineralization.

Hypocalcemia

Hypocalcemia is commonly associated with hypoparathyroidism caused by surgical removal of the parathyroids. Surgical removal of the parathyroids may be done primarily for treatment of tumors, or it may occur inadvertently

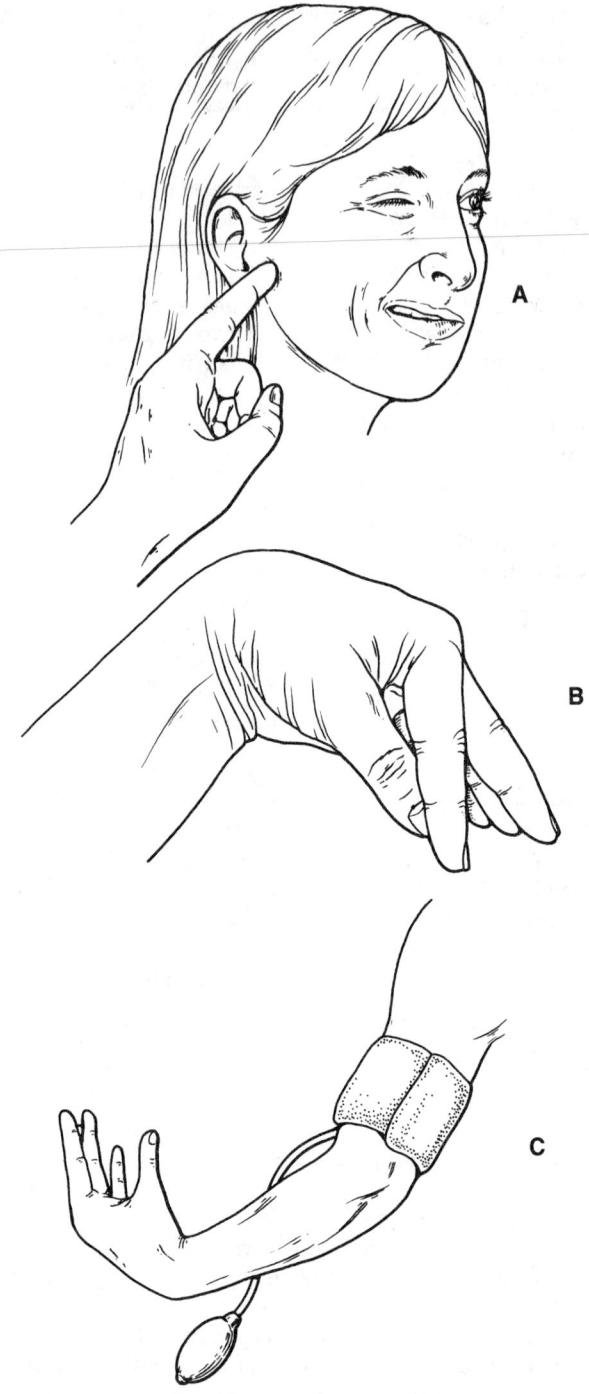

Fig. 10-14 **A,** Chvostek's sign is a contraction of facial muscles in response to a light tap over the facial nerve in front of the ear. **B,** Trousseau's sign is a carpal spasm. **C,** It is induced by inflating a blood pressure cuff above the systolic pressure for a few minutes.

during thyroid surgery. Acute pancreatitis is another common cause of hypocalcemia. Clients who receive multiple blood transfusions can become hypocalcemic because the citrate used to anticoagulate the blood binds with the calcium.[5] Hypocalcemia can also occur if the diet is low in calcium or if there is increased loss of calcium with laxative abuse and malabsorption syndromes. (See Table 10-9 for the clinical manifestations and etiologies of hypocalcemia.)

Clinical manifestations. Since calcium is essential for conduction of nerve impulses and muscle contraction, procedures that evaluate neuromuscular irritability are useful for assessing a low serum calcium level. *Trousseau's sign* refers to carpal spasms induced by inflating a blood pressure cuff on the arm (Fig. 10-14). The blood pressure cuff is inflated above the systolic pressure. Carpal spasms are evident within 3 minutes if hypocalcemia is present. *Chvostek's sign* is contraction of facial muscles in response to a tap over the facial nerve in front of the ear (Fig. 10-14).

Tetany refers to the increased neuroexcitability and sustained muscle contraction associated with hypocalcemia. Manifestations of tetany include wrist and carpopedal spasms (Fig. 10-14), laryngeal stridor, dysphagia, dysarthria, cardiac dysrhythmias, and convulsions.

■ Therapeutic and Nursing Management of Hypocalcemia

Nursing diagnoses

Nursing diagnoses specific to the client with hypocalcemia include, but are not limited to, the following:
1. High risk for injury related to tetany and seizures secondary to severe hypocalcemia
2. High risk for impaired gas exchange related to decreased availability of oxygen secondary to laryngeal spasm occurring with severe hypocalcemia
3. Decreased cardiac output related to cardiac contractility secondary to hypocalcemia or digitalis toxicity caused by calcium replacement

Nursing interventions

Hypocalcemia is managed as an emergency, particularly if laryngeal spasms and respiratory arrest are imminent. Any client who has had thyroid surgery must be observed closely for manifestations of hypocalcemia. The primary goal in treatment of hypocalcemia is aimed at treating the cause. Hypocalcemia can be treated with oral or intravenous calcium supplements. Calcium carbonate (oral) and calcium gluconate (intravenous) are commonly used as supplements. Care must be taken because infiltration of intravenous calcium can cause sloughing of the tissue. Calcium is not given intramuscularly because it will precipitate in the muscle. A diet high in calcium-rich foods is ordered, along with vitamin D supplements, for the client with hypocalcemia. Synthetic parathyroid hormone (parathormone) can also be given.

Phosphate Imbalances

Phosphorus is a primary anion in the ICF and is essential to the function of muscle, red blood cells, and the nervous system. It is deposited with calcium for bone and tooth structure. It is also involved in the acid-base buffering system, in the mitochondrial energy production of ATP, in cellular uptake and utilization of glucose, and as an intermediary in the metabolism of carbohydrates, proteins, and fats.

Maintenance of normal phosphate balance requires adequate renal functioning because the kidneys are the major

Table 10-10 Causes of Phosphate Imbalances

Hypophosphatemia	Hyperphosphatemia
Malabsorption syndrome	Renal failure
Nutritional recovery syndrome	Chemotherapeutic agents
Glucose administration	Enemas containing phosphorus (e.g., Fleet's)
Hyperalimentation	Excessive ingestion (e.g., milk, phosphate-containing laxatives)
Alcohol withdrawal	
Phosphate-binding antacids	
Diabetic ketoacidosis	Large vitamin D intake
Respiratory alkalosis	Hypoparathyroidism

route of phosphate excretion. A small amount is lost in the feces. There is a reciprocal relationship between phosphorus and calcium in that a high serum phosphate level tends to cause a low calcium concentration in the serum.

Hyperphosphatemia. The major condition that can lead to hyperphosphatemia is acute or chronic renal failure due to an altered ability of the kidney to excrete phosphate. Other causes include chemotherapy for certain malignancies (e.g., lymphomas), excessive ingestion of milk or phosphate-containing laxatives, and large intakes of vitamin D (which increase gastrointestinal absorption of phosphorus) (Table 10-10).

Clinical manifestations of hyperphosphatemia are primarily related to metastatic calcium-phosphate precipitates. Ordinarily, calcium and phosphate are deposited only in bone. However, an increased serum phosphate concentration along with calcium precipitates readily, and calcified deposits can occur in soft tissue such as joints, arteries, skin, kidney, and cornea (see in Chapter 41). Other manifestations of hyperphosphatemia are neuromuscular irritability and tetany, which are related to the low serum calcium levels often associated with high serum phosphate levels.

Management of hyperphosphatemia is aimed at identifying and treating the underlying cause. Ingestion of foods and fluids high in phosphorus (e.g., milk and dairy products) should be restricted. Adequate hydration and correction of hypocalcemic conditions can enhance the renal excretion of phosphate. For clients with renal failure, measures to reduce serum phosphate levels include phosphate-binding agents or gels and dietary phosphate restrictions (see Chapter 41).

Hypophosphatemia. Hypophosphatemia (low serum phosphate) is seen in clients who are malnourished or have malabsorption syndromes. Other causes include alcohol withdrawal, hyperalimentation without adequate phosphorus replacement, phosphate-binding antacids, and nutritional recovery syndrome (refeeding after starvation) (Table 10-10). During the anabolic phase of metabolism an influx of phosphorus into the cells occurs.

Most clinical manifestations of hypophosphatemia are related to a deficiency of ATP or 2,3-diphosphoglycerate (2,3-DPG), an enzyme in red blood cells. These conditions result in impaired cellular energy resources and oxygen delivery to tissues. Hemolytic anemia may occur because of the fragility of the red blood cells. Acute manifestations include CNS depression, confusion, and other mental changes. Other manifestations include muscle weakness and pain, dysrhythmias, and cardiomyopathy.

Management of a mild phosphorus deficiency may involve oral supplementation (e.g., Neutra-Phos) and ingestion of foods high in phosphorus (e.g., milk). Severe hypophosphatemia can be serious and requires intravenous administration of sodium phosphate or potassium phosphate. Frequent monitoring of serum phosphate levels is necessary to guide intravenous therapy.

Magnesium Imbalances

About 50% to 60% of the body's magnesium is contained in bone. Magnesium is the second most abundant intracellular cation. It functions as a coenzyme in the metabolism of carbohydrates and protein. It is also involved in metabolism of cellular nucleic acid and proteins. Regulation of magnesium is not well understood, but many of the factors that regulate calcium balance (e.g., parathyroid hormone, vitamin D) influence magnesium balance. The kidneys are the primary route of magnesium excretion. Causes of magnesium imbalance are listed in Table 10-11.

Neuromuscular excitability is profoundly affected by alterations in serum magnesium. Hypomagnesemia (a low serum magnesium level) produces neuromuscular and central nervous system hyperirritability. A high serum magnesium level (hypermagnesemia) depresses neuromuscular and central nervous system functions.

Hypermagnesemia. Hypermagnesemia usually occurs only with an increase in magnesium intake accompanied by renal insufficiency. Clients with chronic renal failure who ingest products containing magnesium (e.g., Maalox, milk of magnesia) will have a problem with excess magnesium. Magnesium excess could develop in the pregnant woman who receives magnesium sulfate for the management of eclampsia.

Initial clinical manifestations of a mildly elevated serum magnesium concentration include lethargy, drowsiness, and nausea and vomiting. As the levels of serum magnesium increase, deep tendon reflexes are lost, followed by somnolence; then respiratory and, ultimately, cardiac arrest can occur.

Management of hypermagnesemia should focus on prevention. Clients with renal failure should not take magnesium-containing medication. The emergency treatment of hypermagnesemia is intravenous administration of calcium chloride or calcium gluconate to physiologically oppose the effects of the magnesium on cardiac muscle. Promoting urinary excretion with fluid will decrease serum magnesium. Clients with impaired renal function will require dialysis, since the kidney is the major route of excretion for magnesium.

Hypomagnesemia. Hypomagnesemia develops gradually. Prolonged intravenous feeding without magnesium supplementation and excessive losses of fluids from the gastrointestinal tract are common causes.[6] The significant clinical manifestations are hyperactive deep tendon reflexes, tremors, and convulsions. Magnesium deficiency also predisposes to cardiac dysrhythmias. Clinically, hypomagnesemia resembles hypocalcemia. Mild magnesium deficiencies can be treated with oral supplements and increased dietary intake of foods high in magnesium (e.g., green vegetables, nuts, bananas, oranges, peanut butter, chocolate). If the condition is severe, parenteral (intravenous or intramuscular) magnesium (e.g., magnesium sulfate) should be administered. Too rapid administration of magnesium can lead to cardiac or respiratory arrest.

Protein Imbalances

Plasma proteins are a significant determinant of ECF content. Because of their large molecular size, they attract water and contribute to the colloidal oncotic pressure within the vascular system. Causes of protein imbalance are listed in Table 10-12.

Hypoproteinemia can occur over time. Causes related to intake are anorexia, malnutrition, poor economic environments, starvation, fad dieting, and true vegetarian diets. Poor absorption of protein can occur in certain gastrointestinal malabsorptive diseases. Protein can shift out of the ECF with cell membrane changes with inflammation. Ascites is an example of third-space shifting. Increased breakdown of proteins occurs with elevated basal metabolic rates and catabolic states, such as fever, infection, and certain malignancies. Increased use of protein occurs with cell growth and repair after surgical wounds or burns. Hemorrhage with loss of red blood cells can be a cause of protein deficit. The kidneys can lose large amounts of protein, especially albumin, in nephrotic syndrome.[7]

Clinical manifestations of protein deficit include edema

Table 10-11 Causes of Magnesium Imbalances

Hypomagnesemia	Hypermagnesemia
Diarrhea	Renal failure (especially if client is given magnesium products)
Vomiting	
Chronic alcoholism	
Impaired gastrointestinal absorption	Excessive administration of magnesium for treatment of eclampsia
Malabsorption syndrome	
Prolonged malnutrition	Adrenal insufficiency
Large urine outputs	
Nasogastric suction	
Diabetic ketoacidosis	
Hyperaldosteronism	

Table 10-12 Causes of Protein Imbalances

Hypoproteinemia	Hyperproteinemia
Decreased food intake	Dehydration
Starvation	Hemoconcentration
Diseased liver	
Massive burns	
Loss of albumin in renal disease	
Major infection	

(from decreased oncotic pressure), slow healing, anorexia, fatigue, anemia, and muscle loss resulting from the breakdown of body tissue to meet the body's need for protein.

Management of protein deficit includes providing a high-carbohydrate, high-protein diet and dietary protein supplements. If the client cannot meet the needs for protein orally, hyperalimentation may be used. (Protein-calorie malnutrition is discussed in Chapter 35.)

Hyperproteinemia is usually very rare, but it can occur with dehydration and hemoconcentration.

ACID-BASE IMBALANCES
Hydrogen Ion Concentration

The acidity or alkalinity of a solution depends on its hydrogen ion (H^+) concentration. An increase in H^+ concentration leads to acidity; a decrease leads to alkalinity. (Definitions related to acid-base balance are presented in Table 10-13.)

The weight of ionized hydrogen in water is about 0.0000001 g/L. This quantity may be expressed as 10^{-7}. Hydrogen ion concentration (symbolized as pH) is usually written as a negative logarithm. The pH may range from 1 to 14. The use of the negative logarithm means that the lower the pH, the higher the hydrogen ion concentration. In contrast to a pH of 7, a pH of 8 represents a tenfold decrease in hydrogen ion concentration.

A solution with a pH of 7 is considered neutral. An acid solution has a pH less than 7, and an alkaline solution has a pH greater than 7. Blood is slightly alkaline (pH 7.35 to 7.45); yet if it drops below 7.35, the person has *acidosis*, even though the blood may never become truly acidic. If the blood pH is greater than 7.45, the person has *alkalosis* (Fig. 10-15). The pH of blood is computed through the use of the Henderson-Hasselbalch equation (Table 10-14).

Table 10-13   Terms in Acid-Base Physiology

Acid	Donor of hydrogen ions (H^+); separation of an acid into hydrogen ion and its accompanying anion in solution
Acidemia	Signifying an arterial blood pH of less than 7.35
Acidosis	Process that adds acid or eliminates base from body fluids
Alkalemia	Signifying an arterial blood pH of more than 7.45
Alkalosis	Process that adds base or eliminates acid from body fluids
Base	Acceptor of hydrogen ions; chemical combining of acid and base when hydrogen ions are added to a solution containing a base; bicarbonate (HCO_3^-) most abundant base in body fluids
Buffer	Substance that reacts with an acid or base to prevent a large change in pH
pH	Negative logarithm of the hydrogen ion concentration; a pH of 7 signifying 10^{-7} or 0.0000001 g/L of hydrogen ion

Acid-Base Regulation

The body's metabolic processes constantly produce acids. These acids must be neutralized and excreted to maintain acid-base balance.

Normally, the body has three mechanisms by which it regulates acid-base balance to maintain the pH between 7.35 and 7.45. These mechanisms are (1) the buffer systems, (2) the respiratory system, and (3) the renal system.

The regulatory mechanisms react at different speeds; buffers react immediately. The respiratory system responds within minutes and reaches maximum effectiveness within hours. The renal response takes 2 to 3 days to respond maximally, but the kidneys can maintain balance for a long period of time.

Buffer system. The buffer system is the fastest-acting system and the primary regulator of acid-base balance. Buffers act chemically to alter strong acids into weaker acids or to bind acids to neutralize their effect. The buffers in the body are (1) carbonic acid-bicarbonate, (2) monohydrogen-dihydrogen phosphate, (3) intracellular and plasma proteins, and (4) hemoglobin.

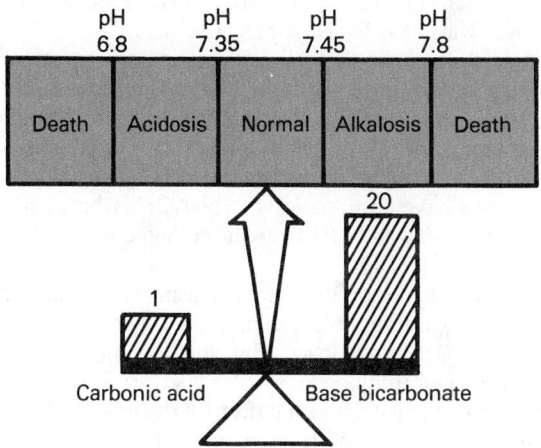

Fig. 10-15   The normal range of plasma pH is from 7.35 to 7.45. A normal pH is maintained by a ratio of 1 part carbonic acid to 20 parts base bicarbonate.

Table 10-14   Henderson-Hasselbalch Equation

$$pH = pK \text{ (constant)} + \log \frac{base}{acid}$$

$$= 6.1 + \log \frac{HCO_3^- \text{ (renal)}}{H_2CO_3 \text{ (lung)}}$$

$$= 6.1 + \log \frac{25.4 \text{ mEq}}{1.27}$$

$$= 6.1 + \log \frac{20}{1}$$

$$= 6.1 + 1.3$$

$$= 7.4$$

A buffer consists of a weakly ionized acid or a base and its salt. The mechanisms of buffering function to minimize the effect of acids on blood pH until they can be excreted from the body. The carbonic acid (H_2CO_3)-bicarbonate (HCO_3^-) buffer system neutralizes hydrochloric acid (HCl) in the following manner:

$$H^+Cl^- + Na^+HCO_3^- \rightarrow NaCl + H_2CO_3$$
$$\text{strong} \qquad \text{strong} \qquad \text{salt} \qquad \text{weak}$$
$$\text{acid} \qquad \text{base} \qquad \qquad \text{acid}$$

In this way, hydrochloric acid is prevented from making a large change in the solution's pH, and more H_2CO_3 is formed. The carbonic acid, in turn, is broken down to H_2O and CO_2. The CO_2 is excreted by the lungs. In this process the buffer system maintains the 20:1 ratio between bicarbonate and carbonic acid and the normal pH.

The phosphate buffer system is composed of sodium and other cations in combination with $H_2PO_4^-$ and HPO_4^{2-}. This buffer system acts in the same manner as the bicarbonate system. Strong acids are neutralized to form a weak acid of sodium biphosphate (which can be excreted in the urine) and sodium chloride: $Na_2HPO_4 + HCl \rightarrow NaCl + NaH_2PO_4$. When a strong base is added to the system, it is neutralized to form a weak base and H_2O: $NaOH + NaH_2PO_4 \rightarrow Na_2HPO_4 + H_2O$.

Intracellular and extracellular proteins are an effective buffering system throughout the body. The protein buffering system acts much like the bicarbonate system. Some of the amino acids of proteins contain free acid radicals, $-COOH$, which can dissociate into CO_2 and H. Other amino acids have basic radicals, $-NH_3OH$, which can dissociate into NH_3 and OH that can combine with a hydrogen ion to form H_2O.

Using the "chloride shift" mechanism, hemoglobin regulates pH by shifting chloride in and out of red blood cells in exchange for bicarbonate. This shift is regulated by the level of oxygen in blood.

The cell can also act as a buffer by shifting hydrogen in and out of the cell. With an accumulation of H^+ in the ECF, the intracellular compartment can accept hydrogen in exchange for another cation (e.g., sodium or potassium).

The body buffers an acid load better than it neutralizes base excess. Buffers cannot maintain pH without the adequate functioning of the respiratory and renal systems.

Respiratory system. The lungs excrete carbon dioxide and water, which are byproducts of cell metabolism. When released into circulation, CO_2 enters red blood cells and combines with H_2O to form H_2CO_3. The carbonic acid dissociates into hydrogen ions and bicarbonate. The free hydrogen is buffered by hemoglobin molecules, and the bicarbonate diffuses into the plasma. In the pulmonary capillaries, this process is reversed and CO_2 is formed and excreted by the lungs. The overall reversible reaction is expressed as the following:

$$CO_2 + H_2O \rightleftharpoons H_2CO_3 \rightleftharpoons H^+ + HCO_3^-$$

The amount of CO_2 in the blood is directly related to carbonic acid concentration and subsequently to hydrogen ion concentration. With increased respirations, less CO_2 remains in the blood. This leads to less carbonic acid and fewer H^+ ions. With decreased respirations, more CO_2 remains in the blood. This leads to increased carbonic acid and more hydrogen ions.

The rate of excretion of CO_2 is controlled by the respiratory center in the medulla of the brain. If increased amounts of CO_2 or hydrogen ions are present, the respiratory center stimulates an increased rate and depth of breathing. Respirations are inhibited if the center senses low H^+ or CO_2 levels.

As a compensatory mechanism the respiratory system acts on the $CO_2 + H_2O$ side of the reaction by altering the rate and depth of breathing to "blow off" or to "retain" carbon dioxide. If it is an etiological factor of an acid-base imbalance (e.g., respiratory failure), the respiratory system loses its ability to correct a pH alteration.

Renal system. The kidneys reabsorb and conserve most of the bicarbonate. In addition, the kidneys can eliminate excess hydrogen ions. The three mechanisms of acid elimination include (1) secretion of small amounts of free hydrogen into the renal tubule, (2) combination of hydrogen ions with ammonia (NH_3) to form ammonium (NH_4^+), and (3) excretion of weak acids.

The kidneys normally excrete an acidic urine (average pH equals 6). The kidneys are able to act on the $H^+ + HCO_3^-$ side of the reaction. As a compensatory mechanism, the pH of the urine can decrease to 4 and increase to 8. If the renal system is the cause of an acid-base imbalance (e.g., in renal failure), it loses its ability to correct a pH alteration. In clients with renal failure, metabolic acidosis is the usual finding.

Alterations in Acid-Base Balance

An acid-base imbalance is produced when the ratio of 1:20 between acid and base content is altered (Table 10-15). A primary disease or process may alter one side of the ratio (e.g., CO_2 retention in pulmonary disease). The compensatory process attempts to maintain the other side of the ratio (e.g., increased renal bicarbonate reabsorption). When the compensatory mechanism fails, an acid-base imbalance results. The compensatory process may be inadequate because either the pathophysiological process is overwhelming or there is insufficient time for the compensatory process to function.

Acid-base imbalances are classified as *respiratory* and *metabolic*. Respiratory imbalances affect carbonic acid concentrations; metabolic imbalances affect the base bicarbonate. Therefore, acidosis can be caused by an increase in carbonic acid (respiratory acidosis) or a decrease in bicarbonate (metabolic acidosis), and alkalosis can be caused by a decrease in carbonic acid (respiratory alkalosis) or an increase in bicarbonate (metabolic alkalosis).

Respiratory acidosis. Respiratory acidosis (carbonic acid excess) occurs whenever there is hypoventilation (Table 10-15). Carbon dioxide and subsequently carbonic acid accumulate in the blood. Carbonic acid dissociates, liberating H^+, and there is a decrease in pH. If carbon dioxide is not eliminated from the blood, acidosis results from the accumulation of carbonic acid (Fig. 10-16, *A*).

The kidneys conserve bicarbonate and secrete into the urine increased concentrations of hydrogen ion. In acute

Table 10-15 Acid-Base Imbalances

Common Causes	Pathophysiology	Laboratory Findings
RESPIRATORY ACIDOSIS		
Chronic obstructive pulmonary disease Barbiturate or sedative overdose Chest wall abnormality (e.g., obesity) Pneumonia Atelectasis Respiratory muscle weakness (e.g., Guillain-Barré syndrome) Mechanical underventilation	CO_2 retention from hypoventilation Impaired respiratory efforts due to airway obstruction, weakened respiratory muscles, or depressed respiratory center Compensatory response of HCO_3^- retention by kidney	Plasma pH ↓ P_{CO_2} ↑ HCO_3^- normal (uncompensated) HCO_3^- ↑ (compensated) Urine pH <6 (compensated)
RESPIRATORY ALKALOSIS		
Hyperventilation due to hypoxia, high altitudes, anxiety, fear, pain, exercise, fever Stimulated respiratory center due to septicemia, encephalitis, brain injury, salicylate poisoning Mechanical overventilation	Increased CO_2 excretion from hyperventilation Compensatory response of HCO_3^- excretion by kidney	Plasma pH ↑ P_{CO_2} ↓ HCO_3^- normal (uncompensated) HCO_3^- ↓ (compensated) Urine pH >6 (compensated)
METABOLIC ACIDOSIS		
Diabetic ketoacidosis Lactic acidosis Starvation Severe diarrhea Renal tubular acidosis Renal failure Gastrointestinal fistulas Shock	Gain of fixed acid, inability to excrete acid, loss of base Compensatory response of CO_2 excretion by lungs	Plasma pH ↓ P_{CO_2} ↓ (compensated) HCO_3^- ↓ Urine pH <6 (compensated)
METABOLIC ALKALOSIS		
Severe vomiting Excess gastric suctioning Diuretic therapy Potassium deficit Excess $NaHCO_3$ intake Excessive mineralocorticoids	Loss of strong acid or gain of base Compensatory response of CO_2 retention by lungs	Plasma pH ↑ P_{CO_2} ↑ (compensated) HCO_3^- ↑ Urine pH >6 (compensated)

respiratory acidosis the renal compensatory mechanisms begin to operate within 24 hours. Therefore, a low or normal serum bicarbonate level is usually found until the kidneys have compensated for the imbalance.

Respiratory alkalosis. Respiratory alkalosis (carbonic acid deficit) occurs with hyperventilation (Table 10-15). Anxiety, central nervous system disease, and mechanical overventilation all increase ventilation and decrease the P_{CO_2} level. This leads to decreased carbonic acid and alkalosis (Fig. 10-16, *A*).

Compensated respiratory alkalosis is not usually seen unless the client has been maintained on a ventilator or has a central nervous system problem. A decreased bicarbonate level differentiates compensated respiratory alkalosis from acute or uncompensated respiratory alkalosis.

Metabolic acidosis. Metabolic acidosis (base bicarbonate deficit) occurs when an acid other than carbonic acid accumulates in the body or when bicarbonate is lost from body fluids (Table 10-15 and Fig. 10-16, *B*). In both cases a bicarbonate deficit results. Acetoacetic acid accumulation in diabetic ketoacidosis and lactic acid accumulation with shock are examples of accumulation of acids. Severe diarrhea results in loss of bicarbonate. In renal disease the kidneys lose their ability to reabsorb bicarbonate and secrete hydrogen ions.

The compensatory response is to increase CO_2 excretion by the lungs. The client often develops Kussmaul breathing (deep, rapid breathing). In addition, the kidneys attempt to excrete additional acid.

Metabolic alkalosis. Metabolic alkalosis (base bicarbonate excess) occurs when a loss of acid (from prolonged vomiting or gastric suction) or a gain in bicarbonate (e.g., self-ingestion of baking soda) occurs (Table 10-15 and Fig. 10-16, *B*). The compensatory mechanism is a de-

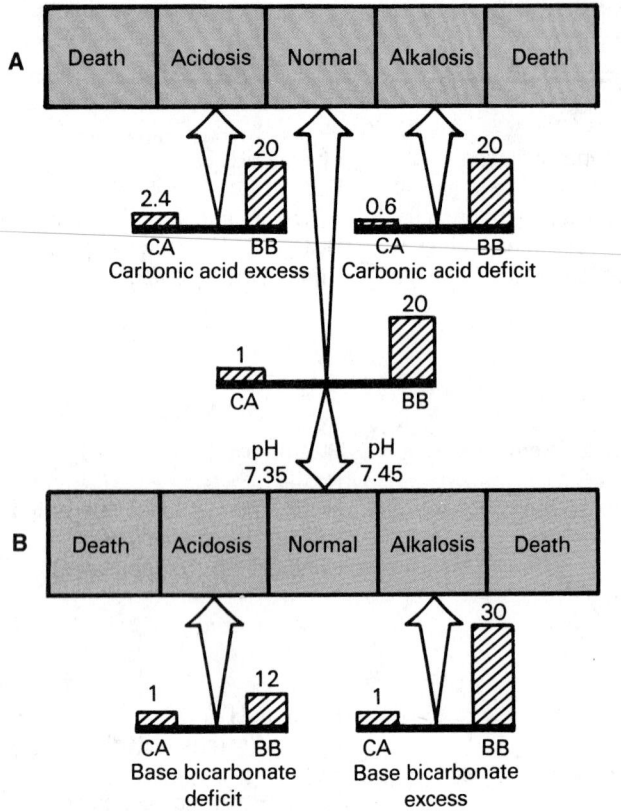

Fig. 10-16 Kinds of acid-base imbalances. **A,** Respiratory imbalances due to carbonic acid excess and carbonic acid deficit. **B,** Metabolic imbalances due to base bicarbonate deficit and base bicarbonate excess.

Table 10-16 Clinical Manifestations of Acidosis

Respiratory ($\uparrow$ P_{CO_2})	Metabolic ($\downarrow$ HCO_3^-)
APPEARANCE	
Drowsiness	Drowsiness
Unconscious	Coma
	Dehydration
BEHAVIOR	
Disorientation	Disorientation
Dizziness	
CARDIOVASCULAR	
Decreased blood pressure	Bradycardia
Ventricular fibrillation	Peripheral vasodilatation
Peripheral vasodilatation	
GASTROINTESTINAL	
No significant findings	Nausea, vomiting, diarrhea, abdominal pain
NEUROMUSCULAR	
Headache	Headache
Muscular twitching	Muscular twitching
Convulsions	
RESPIRATORY	
Rapid, shallow breaths or hypoventilation with hypoxia	Deep, rapid respirations

creased respiratory rate to increase CO_2. Renal excretion of bicarbonate also occurs.

Clinical Manifestations

Clinical manifestations of acidosis and alkalosis are summarized in Tables 10-16 and 10-17. Because a normal pH is vital to all cellular reactions, the clinical manifestations of acid-base imbalances are generalized and nonspecific. The actual compensatory mechanisms also produce some clinical manifestations. For example, the deep, rapid respirations of a client with metabolic acidosis are an example of respiratory compensation. In alkalosis, hypocalcemia may concurrently be found and accounts for many of the clinical manifestations.

Blood gas values. Blood gas values provide essential information for evaluation of acid-base problems.[8] These include pH, P_{CO_2}, and HCO_3^-. Diagnosis of acid-base disturbances and identification of compensatory processes are done by correlating the pH with the P_{CO_2} and HCO_3^-. First, it is necessary to determine whether the pH is alkalotic (>7.45) or acidotic (<7.35) and then whether the P_{CO_2} level or HCO_3^- is the primary cause of the pH change. For example, acidosis is caused by high carbon dioxide levels or low bicarbonate levels. Next, determining whether the body is attempting to compensate for the

pH change should be done. For example, if the primary problem is respiratory acidosis (low pH with an elevated P_{CO_2}), are the kidneys compensating by reabsorbing more bicarbonate? If compensatory mechanisms are functioning, the pH will return toward 7.40. The body will not overcompensate for pH changes.

Mixed acid-base problems are also possible. An example of a mixed acidosis appears in a client in cardiopulmonary arrest. Hypoventilation elevates the carbon dioxide level, and anaerobic metabolism produces lactic acid. Circulating bicarbonate levels fall as the HCO_3^- buffers the lactic acid. The blood gases of this client reflect an acidotic pH, an increased P_{CO_2}, and a decreased HCO_3^-. An example of a mixed alkalosis is the case of a client who is hyperventilating because of postoperative pain and is also losing acid secondary to nasogastric suctioning. (Refer to the laboratory findings section of Table 10-15 for the blood gas findings of the four major acid-base disturbances.)

Blood gas analysis will also show the P_{O_2} and oxygen saturation. Either arterial or venous blood can be used for sampling as long as one is consistently used for comparison. The arterial method is usually preferred. The values of blood gases differ slightly between arterial and venous samples (Table 10-18).

Table 10-17 Clinical Manifestations of Alkalosis

Respiratory ($\downarrow P_{CO_2}$)	Metabolic ($\uparrow HCO_3^-$)
APPEARANCE	
Lethargy	Confusion
	Dizziness
BEHAVIOR	
Lightheadedness	Irritability
Confusion	Nervousness
	Confusion
CARDIOVASCULAR	
Tachycardia	Tachycardia
Dysrhythmias	Dysrhythmias
GASTROINTESTINAL	
Nausea	Anorexia
Vomiting	Nausea
Epigastric pain	Vomiting
NEUROMUSCULAR	
Tetany	Tremors
Numbness	Hypertonic muscles
Tingling of extremities	Muscle cramps
Hyperreflexia	Tetany
	Tingling of fingers and toes
	Seizures
RESPIRATORY	
Hyperventilation	Hypoventilation

Table 10-18 Normal Arterial and Venous Blood Gas Values

Parameter	Arterial	Venous
pH	7.35-7.45	7.35-7.45
P_{CO_2}	35-45 mm Hg	40-45 mm Hg
Bicarbonate	20-30 mEq/L	20-30 mEq/L
P_{O_2}*	80-100 mm Hg	40-50 mm Hg†
Oxygen saturation	96%-100%	60%-85%
Base excess	±2.0	±2.0

*Decreases above sea level and with increasing age.
†Oxygen tension is defined as the significant difference between the P_{O_2} concentrations of arterial and venous blood.

ASSESSMENT OF FLUID, ELECTROLYTE, AND ACID-BASE IMBALANCES
Subjective Data

Health history. An assessment of the client's current and past use of medications is very important. The ingredients in many drugs (especially over-the-counter drugs) are often overlooked as sources of sodium, potassium, calcium, magnesium, and other electrolytes. Many prescription drugs can cause fluid and electrolyte problems. Examples include diuretics, corticosteroids, and electrolyte supplements. The client should be questioned about any primary disease or condition that can cause fluid and electrolyte imbalances, such as renal disease, diabetes mellitus, ulcerative colitis, and respiratory disease.

Social and personal history. Extremes of climate and activity markedly alter the body's fluid requirement. Some clients who live alone (e.g., older adults) may not satisfy their need for balanced fluid and electrolytes because they may not adequately prepare their meals. Clients should be questioned regarding their diet, especially whether they have been on a special diet (e.g., reducing, low-sodium, or fad diet).

Objective Data

Physical examination. There is no unique physical examination to assess fluid and electrolyte balance. Common abnormal assessment findings of major body systems give clues to possible fluid and electrolyte imbalances (Table 10-19).

Laboratory values. Normal serum electrolyte values are a good starting point for identifying fluid and electrolyte imbalance (Table 10-4). However, they often provide only cursory information. For example, the majority of the potassium in the body is found intracellularly. Serum potassium values only indirectly reflect the total body potassium.

A serum sodium value of 120 mEq/L reflects a low serum sodium level. The value may indicate a total body sodium depletion, as occurs when sodium losses exceed water loss, or a low serum sodium level, since normal sodium content is diluted with an excess of water. A reduced hematocrit value could indicate anemia, or it could be caused by fluid volume excess.

Therapeutic Management

In all cases of fluid, electrolyte, and acid-base imbalances the treatment is directed toward correction of the underlying cause. (The specific diseases or disorders that cause these imbalances are discussed in various chapters throughout this text.) Intravenous fluid and electrolyte therapy are commonly used to treat many different fluid and electrolyte imbalances.

INTRAVENOUS FLUID AND ELECTROLYTE REPLACEMENT

Many clients need *maintenance* intravenous fluid therapy only while they cannot take oral fluids (e.g., during and after surgery). Other clients need *corrective* or *replacement* therapy for losses that have already occurred.[9] The amount and type of solution are determined by the normal daily maintenance requirements and by imbalances identified by laboratory results. The normal daily requirement for fluids and electrolytes is as follows:

Electrolytes: Na^+—100 to 150 mEq; K^+—40 to 60 mEq

Glucose: 150 to 200 g (1 g equals 4 kcal)

Fluid: 1500 ml/m² body surface (2650 ml for a 70 kg adult with 1.76 m² body surface)

Table 10-19 Common Assessment Abnormalities of Fluid and Electrolyte Imbalances

Finding	Possible Cause
SKIN	
Poor skin turgor	Fluid volume deficit
Cold, clammy skin	Sodium deficit, shift of plasma to interstitial fluid
Pitting edema	Fluid volume excess
Flushed, dry skin	Sodium excess
PULSE	
Bounding pulse	Fluid volume excess, shift of interstitial fluid to plasma
Rapid, weak, thready pulse	Shift of plasma to interstitial fluid, sodium deficit, fluid volume deficit
Weak, irregular, rapid pulse	Severe potassium deficit
Weak, irregular, slow pulse	Severe potassium excess
BLOOD PRESSURE	
Hypotension	Fluid volume deficit, shift of plasma to interstitial fluid, sodium deficit
Hypertension	Fluid volume excess, shift of interstitial fluid to plasma
RESPIRATIONS	
Deep, rapid breathing	Metabolic acidosis
Shallow, slow, irregular breathing	Metabolic alkalosis
Shortness of breath	Fluid volume excess
Moist rales	Fluid volume excess, shift of interstitial fluid to plasma
SKELETAL MUSCLE	
Cramping of exercised muscle	Calcium deficit
Carpal spasm (Trousseau's sign)	Calcium deficit
Flabby muscles	Potassium deficit
Positive Chvostek's sign	Calcium deficit
BEHAVIOR OR MENTAL	
Picking at bedclothes	Potassium deficit, magnesium deficit
Indifference	Fluid volume deficit, sodium deficit
Apprehension	Shift of plasma to interstitial fluid
Extreme restlessness	Potassium excess, fluid volume deficit
Confusion and irritability	Potassium deficit, fluid volume excess

An example of normal daily maintenance intravenous therapy is presented in Table 10-20.

Solutions

Hypotonic. A hypotonic solution dilutes the ECF. Osmosis then produces a movement of water from the ECF to the ICF. After osmotic equilibrium has been achieved, the ICF and the ECF have the same osmolality. Total body water is increased by the amount of fluid infused or ingested. Examples of hypotonic fluids are given in Table 10-21. One liter of a 5% dextrose solution provides 50 grams of dextrose or 200 calories (1 g equals 4 cal). Although this amount of glucose is not enough to provide for caloric requirements, it should be adequate to prevent ketosis associated with starvation.

Isotonic. Administration of an isotonic solution produces no net movement between the ICF and the ECF. An isotonic fluid is ideal fluid replacement for a client with an extracellular fluid volume deficit. Examples of isotonic solutions are lactated Ringer's and 0.9% NaCl. Lactated Ringer's solution contains sodium, potassium, chloride, calcium, and lactate (the precursor of bicarbonate) in about the same concentrations as those of the ECF.

Hypertonic. A hypertonic solution initially raises the osmolality of ECF. Total body water is increased. In addition, the higher osmotic pressure draws water out of the cell into the ECF. (Examples are listed in Table 10-21.) Hypertonic solutions should be used with great caution and require frequent monitoring of blood pressure, lung sounds, and serum sodium levels.

Intravenous additives. In addition to the basic solutions that provide water and a minimum amount of calories and electrolytes, there are additives to replace specific losses. These additives have been mentioned previously during the discussion of the particular electrolyte deficiencies. Potassium chloride, calcium chloride, magnesium sulfate, and bicarbonate are the common additives that are added to the basic intravenous solutions.

Recommendations for giving potassium vary, but in general no more than 10 mEq/hour is considered safe for routine administration. Potassium can be safely diluted as 40 mEq/L of solution with a maximum of 60 mEq/L.

Plasma expanders. Plasma expanders stay within the vascular space and increase the oncotic pressure. Plasma expanders include colloids and dextran. Colloids are protein solutions such as plasma, albumin, and commercial plasmas (e.g., Plasmanate). Dextran is a complex synthetic sugar. Since dextran is metabolized slowly, it remains in the vascular system for a prolonged period but not as long as the colloids.

If the client has lost blood, whole blood or packed red blood cells are necessary to restore the hemoglobin. Packed red blood cells have the advantage of giving the client primarily red blood cells; the blood bank can use the plasma for blood components. Also, packed cells have a decreased plasma volume, which may be a significant consideration in a client who has received plasma expanders in emergency treatment of blood loss. Whole blood with its additional fluid volume may cause circulatory overload.

Table 10-20 Normal Daily Maintenance Requirements for Fluids and Electrolytes

Maintenance IVs	Volume	NaCl	K+	Glucose
5% dextrose and 0.45% normal saline with 20 mEq KCl	2000 ml	77 mEq/L	20 mEq/L	50 g/L
10% dextrose in water (D₁₀W)	1000 ml			100 g/L
	3000 ml	154 mEq	40 mEq	200 g

Table 10-21 Indications and Complications of Intravenous Therapy Solutions

Type	Indications for Use	Complications
HYPOTONIC 0.2% NaCl (¼% saline) 0.45% NaCl (½% saline) D₂₁/₂W (2½% dextrose in water)	Maintenance of water balance Dilution of ECF (e.g., in hypernatremia) Insensible water loss Dehydration	Osmotic movement of water into interstitial space and ICF can cause edema and cell swelling and lysis, particularly with red blood cells Primary water gain in ECF can cause dilutional hyponatremia and hypokalemia
ISOTONIC 0.9% NaCl (normal saline) Lactated Ringer's solution Ringer's solution D₅/0.2% NaCl (dextrose and saline) D₅W (5% dextrose in water)	Replacement of water and electrolyte lost from ECF (e.g., dehydration, shock, gastrointestinal loss, surgical loss, burns) Maintenance IV fluid	Fluid gain in ECF can cause fluid overload, hypertension, congestive heart failure
HYPERTONIC 10% dextrose in water or normal saline 20% dextrose in water 50% dextrose in water 3% or 5% saline	Sodium replacement (e.g., in hyponatremia) Water intoxication Provision of increased caloric intake	Osmotic pull of water out of intracellular space can cause cell dehydration and contraction Hypernatremia and ECF overload can occur Vein irritation can occur

C ase Study

FLUID AND ELECTROLYTE IMBALANCE

Susan R., a 65-year-old woman, was brought to the hospital by her sister. The sister stated that Susan had the flu for about a week and that she had been complaining of severe nausea, vomiting, and heart palpitations. Susan's sister became very concerned when she noticed that Susan was lethargic and confused.

Physical Assessment Findings

Neurological: Client slow to respond to questioning, oriented only to person.
Cardiovascular: Blood pressure 90/58, heart rate 110 and irregular, peripheral pulses weak. ECG: Sinus tachycardia with frequent premature ventricular contractions and the presence of a U wave.
Pulmonary: Respirations 20 per minute and shallow. Fine rales heard throughout all lung fields.
Additional findings: Decreased skin turgor, oral temperature 38.3° C (101° F).

Significant Laboratory Results

Serum electrolytes		Arterial blood gases	
Na+	155 mEq/L	pH	7.58
K+	2.6 mEq/L	Po₂	80 mm Hg
Cl⁻	115 mEq/L	Pco₂	34 mm Hg
BUN	40	HCO₃⁻	32 mEq/L
Hematocrit	52%		

Discussion Questions

1. Discuss the probable causes of Susan's fluid imbalance.
2. Is the hypernatremia due to a primary fluid or sodium imbalance? What symptoms can be related to the elevated sodium level?
3. Explain the reasons for Susan's ECG changes.
4. Identify the acid-base disturbance in this case and discuss its etiology. Is the body compensating for this disturbance?
5. Discuss the means by which the body conserves water.
6. Discuss the appropriate type of fluid replacement therapy for Susan, including the fluid's tonicity and electrolyte composition.

Review Questions

The number of the question corresponds to the same-numbered objective at the beginning of the chapter.

1. The major intracellular cation is
   a. sodium
   b. magnesium
   c. potassium
   d. calcium

2. Diffusion can best be defined as
   a. movement of molecules from an area of lesser concentration to an area of greater concentration
   b. movement of molecules from an area of greater concentration to an area of lesser concentration
   c. movement of water from an area of lesser concentration to an area of greater concentration
   d. movement of water from an area of greater concentration to an area of lesser concentration

3. A client is admitted to the hospital in congestive heart failure. The finding of severe generalized edema can be explained by
   a. a shift of interstitial fluid to plasma
   b. a shift of plasma to interstitial fluid
   c. a shift of extracellular to intracellular fluid
   d. a shift of interstitial to intracellular fluid

4. Body water loss from the skin and lungs is known as
   a. obligatory loss
   b. insensible water loss
   c. partial water loss
   d. essential water loss

5. Three days post burn, a client started to have diuresis and urinary output was 6000 ml in 2 days. The next day the nurse found him picking his bedclothes. His grasp was weak, and reflexes were absent. What electrolyte imbalance might these symptoms suggest?
   a. potassium deficit
   b. potassium excess
   c. sodium excess
   d. sodium deficit

6. To maintain a normal pH, the body must keep a ratio of
   a. 10 parts bicarbonate to 1 part carbonic acid
   b. 15 parts bicarbonate to 1 part carbonic acid
   c. 20 parts bicarbonate to 1 part carbonic acid
   d. 20 parts carbonic acid to 1 part bicarbonate

7. Hyperventilation causes an acid-base imbalance. The body compensates for this respiratory alkalosis primarily by
   a. lungs retaining CO_2
   b. kidneys retaining bicarbonate
   c. lungs eliminating CO_2
   d. kidneys eliminating bicarbonate

8. What is the possible cause of a bounding pulse that is not easily obliterated?
   a. sodium deficit
   b. potassium deficit
   c. fluid volume deficit
   d. fluid volume excess

9. If hypertonic saline is injected intravenously, in which of the following ways will body water shift?
   a. intracellular to intravascular
   b. interstitial to intracellular
   c. intravascular to interstitial
   d. intravascular to intracellular

REFERENCES

1. Metheny NM: Nurse's handbook of fluid balance, Philadelphia, 1987, JB Lippincott Co, pp 8-10.
2. Buckalew VM: Hyponatremia: pathogenesis and management, Hosp Pract 21:49-58, 1986.
3. Linshaw MA: Potassium homeostasis and hypokalemia, Pediatr Clin North Am 34:649-676, 1987.
4. Levine MM and Kleeman CR: Hypercalcemia: pathophysiology and treatment, Hosp Pract 22:93-110, 1987.
5. Zaloga GP and Chernow B: Hypocalcemia in critical illness, JAMA 256:1924-1929, 1986.
6. Flink EB: Magnesium deficiency: causes and effects, Hosp Pract 22:116A-116P, 1987.
7. Maxwell MH, Kleeman CR, and Narins RG: Clinical disorders of fluid and electrolyte metabolism, New York, 1987, McGraw-Hill Book Co.
8. Anderson S: Six easy steps to interpreting blood gases, Am J Nurs 90:42-45, 1990.
9. Metheny NM: Why worry about IV fluids? Am J Nurs 90:50-57, 1990.

SECTION II REFERENCES

BOOKS

Aloisi RM: Principles of immunology and immunodiagnostics, Philadelphia, 1988, Lea & Febiger.

Chabner BA and Collins JM, eds: Cancer chemotherapy: principles and practice, Philadelphia, 1990, JB Lippincott Co.

Cohen PT, Sande MA, and Volberding PA, eds: The AIDS knowledge base: a text book on HIV disease from the University of California, San Francisco, and the San Francisco General Hospital, Waltham, Mass, 1990, Medical Publishing Group.

Cossman J, ed: Molecular genetics in cancer diagnosis, New York, 1990, Elsevier Science Publishing Co, Inc.

Gallo RC and Wong-Staal F, eds: Retrovirus biology and human disease, New York, 1990, Marcel Dekker, Inc.

Gautherie M, ed: Biological basis of oncologic thermotherapy, New York, 1990, Springer-Verlag.

Grimes DE: Infectious diseases, St Louis, 1990, Mosby–Year Book, Inc.

Haskell CM, ed: Cancer treatment, ed 3, Philadelphia, 1990, WB Saunders Co.

Horne MM and Heitz UE: Fluid, electrolyte and acid-base balance, St Louis, 1990, Mosby–Year Book, Inc.

Johnson RJ, Eddleston B, and Hunter RD, editors: Radiology in the management of cancer, Edinburgh, New York, 1990, Churchill Livingstone.

Leukefeld RJ and Batljes ZA, eds: AIDS and intravenous drug use: future directions for community-based prevention research, National Institute on Drug Abuse Research, Monograph series 93, DHHS Pub No (ADM) 89-1627, Rockville, Mo, 1990, US Department of Health and Human Services, Public Health Services, Alcohol, Drug Abuse and Mental Health Administration, National Institute on Drug Abuse.

Misztal BA and Moss D, eds: Action on AIDS: national policies in comparative perspective, New York, 1990, Greenwood Press, Inc.

Oppenheim JJ and Shevach EM: Immunophysiology: the role of cells and cytokines in immunity and inflammation, New York, 1990, Oxford University Press.

Rottenberg RA, ed: Neurological complications of cancer treatment, Boston, 1991, Butterworth Publishers.

Smith SL: AACV organ and tissue transplantation: implications for professional nursing practices, St Louis, 1990, Mosby–Year Book, Inc.

Talmage DW and Samter M, eds: Immunological diseases, Boston, 1988, Little, Brown & Co, Inc.

US Congress, Office of Technology Assessment: Unconventional cancer treatment, Washington DC, 1990.

Weldy NJ: Body fluid, and electrolytes: a programmed presentation, ed 5, St Louis, 1988, The CV Mosby Co.

JOURNALS

Baer C, Penilton DD, and Lerch T: Nursing care of adults, NLN Publ 15-2232:211, 1989.

Bowell B: Assessing infection risks, Nursing 4:19, 1990.

Brown P and Chekryn J: The dying patient and dehydration, Can Nurs 85:14, 1989.

Burkinshaw L and others: Models of the distribution of protein, water and electrolytes in the human body, Infusionstherapie 17:21, 1990.

Campbell-Forsyth L: Patients' perceived knowledge and learning needs concerning radiation therapy, Cancer Nursing 13:81, 1990.

Dicks B: Palliative care: a vital cornerstone, Nurs Times 85:45, 1989.

Dobratz MC: Hospice nursing: present perspectives and future directives, Cancer Nursing 13:116, 1990.

Fontaine DK: Physical, personal, and cognitive responses to trauma, Crit Care Nurs Clin North Am 1:11, 1989.

Gauthier DK and Turner JG: Anti-HIV antibody testing: procedures and precautions, Am J Infect Control 17:213, 1989.

Goodinson SM: Keeping the flora out. Reducing risk of infection in IV therapy, Prof Nurse 5:572, 1990.

Grant M: The effect of nursing consultation on anxiety, side effects, and self-care of patients receiving radiation therapy, Oncol Nurs Forum 17(suppl 3)31, 1990.

Gurka AM: The immune system: implications for critical care nursing, Crit Care Nurse 9:24, 1989.

Hogan CM: Advances in the management of nausea and vomiting, Nurs Clin North Am 25:475, 1990.

Kinrade LC: Typhlitis: a complication of neutropenia, Pediatr Nurs 14:291, 1988.

Metheny NM: Why worry about IV fluids?, Am J Nurs 90:50, 1990.

Metzger JT and Hoffman LA: Cardiac transplantation: the changing faces of immunosuppression, Heart Lung 17:414, 1988.

Mueller KD and Boisen AM: Keeping your patient's water level up, RN 52:65, 1989.

Myles S: Monitoring patient outcomes in an oncology unit, J Nurs Qual Assur 4:35, 1989.

Nail LM and others: Nursing care by telephone: describing practice in an ambulatory oncology center, Oncol Nurs Forum 16:387, 1989.

Patterson LM and Noroian EL: Diabetes insipidus versus syndrome of inappropriate antidiuretic hormone, Dimens Crit Care Nurs 8:226, 1989.

Prim RG: Water intoxication and psychosis syndrome: clinical cautions, J Psychosoc Nurs Ment Health Serv 26:16, 1988.

Rutherford C: Fluid and electrolyte therapy: considerations for patient care, J Intraven Nurs 12:173, 1989.

Rutledge DN and Holtzclaw BJ: Amphotericin B-induced shivering in patients with cancer: a nursing approach, Heart Lung 17:432, 1988.

Selekman J: The multiple faces of immune deficiency in children, Pediatr Nurs 16:351, 1990.

Tribett D: Immune system function: implications for critical care nursing practice, Crit Care Nurs Clin North Am Dec 1989, p 25.

Ufema J: Death and dying, Nursing 20:22, 1990.

Warren B and Pohl JM: Cancer screening practices of nurse practitioners, Cancer Nurs 13:143, 1990.

Witt ME, McDonald-Lynch A, and Lydon J: Enhancing skin comfort during radiation therapy, Oncol Nurs Forum 17:276, 1990.

Woodson CD and Sachs GA: Prevention, diagnosis, and management of infection in the nursing home, Clin Geriatr Med 4:507, 1988.

Workman ML: Immunologic late effects in children and adults, Semin Oncol Nurs 5:36, 1989.

ORGANIZATIONS

American Cancer Society
1599 Clifton Road, NE
Atlanta, GA 30329

Association for Practitioners in Infection Control
505 East Hawley Street
Mundelein, IL 60060

Asthma and Allergy Foundation of America
1717 Massachusetts Avenue, Suite 305
Washington, DC 20036

Cancer Information Service
NIH Bldg. 31, Rm. 10A 24
Bethesda, MD 20892
Telephone: 1-800-4-CANCER

Centers for Disease Control
1600 Clifton Road, NE
Atlanta, GA 30333

Concern for Dying
250 West 57th Street
New York, NY 10843

Institute of Allergy and Infectious Disease
9000 Rockville Pike
Bethesda, MD 20892

National Hospice Organization
1901 North Moore Street, Suite 901
Arlington, VA 22209

Oncology Nursing Society
1016 Greentree Road, Third floor
Pittsburgh, PA 15220

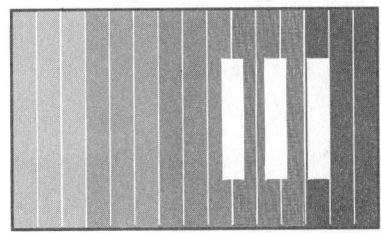

THE SURGICAL EXPERIENCE

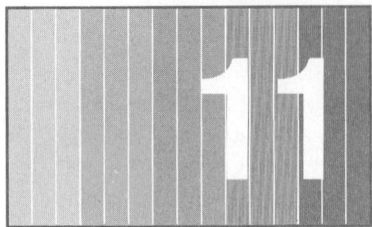

Nursing Role in Management
Preoperative Client

JoAnn Fett Allison
Carol Wikoff Love

L earning Objectives

1. Identify the usual purposes of surgery.
2. Describe the psychosocial and physiological nursing assessment of the preoperative client.
3. Interpret the significance of data related to the preoperative client's health status and operative risk.
4. Identify the baseline nursing data to be recorded preoperatively as a basis for postoperative management.
5. Explain the components of informed consent for surgery.
6. Describe the nursing role in the psychological and educational preparation of the surgical client.
7. Describe the nursing role in the physical preparation of the surgical client.
8. Explain the rationale for preoperative nursing management of the surgical client.
9. Identify the special considerations of preoperative preparation for the older adult surgical client.

Surgery can be defined as the art and science of treating diseases, injuries, and deformities by operation and instrumentation. The surgical procedure involves the interaction of the client, the surgeon, and the nurse.[1,2] Surgery may be performed for any of the following purposes:

1. *Diagnosis:* For example, lymph node biopsy or exploratory incision (laparotomy)
2. *Cure:* For example, removal of diseased part or total hip replacement to restore function of lower limb
3. *Palliation:* For example, cutting a nerve root (rhizotomy) to remove symptoms of pain or creating an artificial anus (colostomy) to alleviate bowel obstruction
4. *Cosmetic improvement:* For example, repairing a burn scar or changing breast shape (mammoplasty)
5. *Prevention:* For example, removal of moles before they become malignant or removal of the colon in familial polyposis to prevent cancer

Specific suffixes are commonly used in combination with identifying a body part or organ in naming surgical procedures (Table 11-1).

Surgery may be a carefully planned and anticipated event in a person's life. The need for surgery may sometimes arise with sudden and unanticipated urgency (Table 11-2). Both emergency and elective surgery may be performed in a variety of settings. The setting in which a surgical procedure may be safely and effectively performed is influenced by the extent of the surgery, the possible complications, and the general condition of the client.

In the past, surgery was usually performed in a hospital operating room and involved a hospital stay of several days. Today, because of increased interest in cost containment stimulated by the implementation of diagnosis related groups (DRGs), as well as by advances in technology and skill, many surgical clients are admitted to the hospital on the day of surgery instead of the evening or day before the scheduled procedure.[3]

An increasing number and type of today's surgical procedures are being performed as ambulatory procedures in emergency rooms, doctor's offices, freestanding surgical clinics, and outpatient (day care or same day) surgery units in hospitals. Ambulatory surgical procedures can be performed with the use of general or local anesthesia, usually

Table 11-1 Suffixes Describing Surgical Procedures

Suffix	Meaning	Example
-ectomy	Excision or removal of	Appendectomy
-lysis	Destruction of	Electrolysis
-orrhaphy	Repair or suture of	Herniorrhaphy
-oscopy	Looking into	Endoscopy
-ostomy	Creation of permanent opening into	Colostomy
-otomy	Cutting into or incision of	Tracheotomy
-plasty	Repair or reconstruction of	Mammoplasty

Table 11-2 Types of Surgery According to Need

Type	Example
EMERGENCY	
Immediate (without delay)	Ruptured aortic aneurysm, gunshot wound, acute appendicitis, epidural hematoma
Urgent (within 24-48 hours)	Ureteral calculi, bleeding uterine fibroids, obstructed duodenal ulcer
ELECTIVE	
Required (within weeks or months)	Cataract extraction, benign prostatic hypertrophy, chronic cholecystitis
Recommended	Simple hemorrhoids, rectocele or cystocele, simple hernias
Optional or cosmetic	Face-lift, rhinoplasty, breast plastic operations

Modified from Rothenberg RE: The complete surgical guide, New York, 1974, Simon & Schuster, Inc, pp 6-7.

take less than an hour, require less than a 2-hour stay in the postanesthesia recovery room, and do not require an overnight hospital stay.

The popularity of ambulatory surgery has steadily increased over the last decade. In some cases this concept has been mandated by third-party payers: private insurance companies, government insurers (Medicare/Medicaid), and health management organizations.[4] It is generally preferred by clients, physicians, and third-party payers for several reasons. Clients like the convenience, physicians prefer the flexibility in scheduling, and the cost is usually less for both the client and the insurer. Ambulatory surgery generally involves fewer laboratory tests and pharmacy items, fewer preoperative and postoperative medications, less psychological stress (especially in young children and older adults), and less susceptibility to hospital-acquired infections.

Regardless of where the surgery is performed, the nurse plays a significant role in preparing the client for surgery, maintaining surveillance of the client during surgery, preventing complications, and facilitating recovery following surgery. To perform this role effectively, the nurse must have certain basic information. First, the nature of the disorder requiring surgery and of any coexisting disease processes must be established. Second, the nurse must know the individual client's response to a stressful situation. Third, results of appropriate diagnostic tests done preoperatively must be assessed. Finally, the bodily alterations and possible risks and complications associated with the surgical procedure must be considered.

The preoperative nursing measures included in this chapter are those that are applicable to the preparation of any surgical client. Specific measures in preparation for particular surgical procedures (such as intestinal, thoracic, or orthopedic surgery) are covered in other chapters of this text.

When a client is to undergo emergency surgery, the nurse must establish priorities, respond to those elements that are life threatening, and include the essential preparation possible in the situation. Although nursing assessment and intervention are discussed separately, they are done simultaneously in practice.

ASSESSMENT OF THE PREOPERATIVE CLIENT
Psychosocial Aspects

Even when planned well in advance, surgery is a psychological and a physiological experience that elicits the stress response. The stress response is a desirable mechanism that enables the body to adapt and heal in the postoperative period. However, anxiety and fear are also stressors, as are client and family perceptions and life experiences.[4-9] If stressors are excessive, the stress response can be magnified, defensive stores can be depleted, and recovery can be affected. The nurse who is aware of a client's perceived or actual stressors can provide support and the needed information during the preoperative period so that stress will not become distress. (See Chapter 5 for a discussion of stress.)

Emotional reactions to impending surgery and hospitalization are often intensified in older persons. Hospitalization emphasizes the client's physical decline and loss of health, mobility, and independence. Older adults may view hospitals as places to die or as stepping-stones to nursing home placement. The nurse can be instrumental in allaying anxieties and fears and maintaining and restoring their self-esteem during the surgical experience.

Common fears. *Fear of pain and discomfort* is nearly universal. It includes concern about feeling pain during and after surgery. The nurse can reassure the client that surgery will not begin before the anesthetic has taken effect and that adequate anesthesia is maintained throughout the procedure. The nurse can encourage the client to talk with the anesthetist or anesthesiologist for clarification. The nurse can help the client who fears postoperative pain by emphasizing the availability of drugs for pain relief.

Fear of the unknown is also extremely common. It is based on lack of information about what to expect during the surgical experience as well as on uncertainty about the outcome of surgery. The dread of cancer, so prevalent in society, often contributes to this fear, both when the surgery is for diagnostic purposes and when the diagnosis is known. The client may have totally unrealistic expectations of what surgery will be like. This may be a result of past experiences or the vicarious experiences provided by friends' stories and the mass media, especially television. The nurse can relieve the client's fear of the unknown by providing accurate, specific information about what to expect. The surgeon should be informed if the client requires any additional information or if the fear seems excessive.

Fear of mutilation or alteration of body image may be a factor, not only when radical surgery or amputation is to be performed but also when much less extensive surgery is required. The prospect of their blood being shed provokes anxiety in some persons. The presence of even a small scar on the body is abhorrent to others. A person's body image and perception of a threat to it are unique. The nurse must listen to and assess the client's concern about this aspect of surgery with an open, nonjudgmental attitude.

Fear of death may be greater when clients know that they have a malignancy or are a poor surgical risk. However, it may be experienced by others who are contemplating even minor procedures. Surgery may be postponed if the client is convinced that it will lead to death. Attitude and emotional state are known to influence the surgical outcome. The nurse should inform the surgeon if a client expresses fear related to survival.

Fear of anesthesia may include concern about an unpleasant induction or aftereffects, hazards or complications (such as brain damage or paralysis), or loss of control while under its influence. The nurse can reassure the client that anesthesia does not have the effect of "truth serum." The client also needs to know that it is not usual for persons to reveal their deepest secrets while under anesthesia. The anesthesiologist can provide detailed information about what the client can expect to experience with the particular agents to be used.

Fear of disruption of life pattern may be present in varying degrees. It may range from fear of permanent disability to concern about not being able to play golf for a few weeks. Concerns about separation from family and about how spouse or children are managing are common. Financial concerns may be related either to an anticipated loss of income or to the costs of surgery.

Assessment procedure. A psychosocial assessment of the preoperative client should be carried out to gather information about how the client perceives the surgical experience (Table 11-3). This information can be gathered by the nurse during the admission nursing interview as well as throughout the ongoing nurse-client relationship.

For the older adult client, the factors listed in Table 11-3 are often intensified. Adding to situational change and loss, the perceived threat or loss of health associated with surgery may be overwhelming to the older adult. This overwhelming loss, which can affect independence, lifestyle, and self-esteem, may result in ineffective coping.

The nurse must remember that the thought processes and cognitive abilities may be slowed or impaired in some older adults. In addition, vision and hearing may be diminished. Consequently, the nurse must allow additional time

Table 11-3 Psychosocial Assessment of the Preoperative Client

SITUATIONAL CHANGES

Determine support systems, including family, significant others, group/institutional structure, and religious/spiritual orientation.

Define current degree of personal control, decision making, and independence.

Consider the impact of surgery/hospitalization and possible effects on lifestyle.

CONCERNS WITH THE UNKNOWN

Identify the client's specific areas of concern.

Identify the client's expectations of surgery, changes in current health status, and effect on daily living.

CONCERNS WITH BODY IMAGE

Identify the client's current roles or relationships and view of self.

Determine perceived or potential changes in role or relationships and impact on body image.

PAST EXPERIENCES

Review the client's previous surgical experiences, hospitalizations, and treatments.

Determine the client's response to those experiences (positive and negative).

Identify the client's current perceptions of surgical procedure in relation to the above and information from others (e.g., a neighbor's view of a personal surgical experience).

KNOWLEDGE DEFICIT

Identify the client's understanding of the surgical procedure, including preparation, care, interventions, activities, restrictions, and expected outcomes.

Identify the accuracy of information the client has received from others, including health team, family, friends, and neighbors.

and/or the presence of a support person for the assessment interview.[10-12]

Table 11-4 provides ideas on how to enhance cognitive functions for the ambulatory surgical client. These suggestions are particularly applicable for the older client.

The extremely anxious client also needs additional consideration during the assessment process. The nurse must try to avoid introducing new concepts or terms that may increase the anxiety level and further impair thought processes and cognitive ability. A nursing care plan related to the psychosocial aspects of the preoperative client is presented in Table 11-5.

Assessment of the outpatient surgical client. Assessment for the outpatient surgical (OpSu) client is usually completed in two phases. A self-assessment form is completed by the client at home and then reviewed with the staff of the OpSu unit during a presurgical visit (Fig. 11-1). This interview is usually conducted 2 to 3 days before

Table 11-4   Enhancing Cognitive Functions in Geriatric Ambulatory Surgery Clients

PREOPERATIVE

Schedule procedures well in advance.

Provide written instructions (use large type).

Provide a checklist instruction (use large type).

Telephone the client the day before surgery and confirm instructions, reinforce priority items, and identify the caretaker.

Have the client bring a list of current medications, including name, dose, and frequency of administration (check for use of over-the-counter drugs).

Provide a map and instructions for locating the ambulatory surgery unit.

DAY OF SURGERY

Allow the client adequate time to undress.

Permit the client to keep clothing and sensory aids as long as possible.

Talk slowly, use nonmedical terms, and stress one point at a time.

Have the same nurse admit and discharge the client.

INTRAOPERATIVE

Keep the client warm and control the amount of exposure of the operative site.

Decrease anxiety-producing stimuli.

Get the client's attention before speaking; speak slowly, clearly, and loud enough to be heard.

Adapted with permission from Kupferer SS and others: Geriatric ambulatory surgery patients: assessing cognitive functions, AORN J 47:755, 1988. Copyright @ AORN Inc., 10170 East Mississippi Avenue, Denver, Co 80231.

Table 11-5

 NURSING CARE PLAN FOR THE PREOPERATIVE CLIENT*

Defining Characteristics	Nursing Interventions	Evaluation Criteria
NURSING DIAGNOSIS: Anxiety related to lack of knowledge about preoperative routines, physical preparation for surgery, postoperative care, and potential body image change		
Signs of anxiety ranging from mild to high, such as verbal expression of concern, restlessness, irritability, agitation, and crying; repeated questioning about impending surgery	For lack of knowledge about preoperative routines, encourage client to verbalize concerns; provide information as client requests it; instruct client about time of surgery, food or fluid restrictions, informed consent, physical preparation required, operating room environment, intravenous lines, other likely drains, anesthesia; instruct client about role and responsibility during the preoperative phase. For lack of knowledge about physical preparation for surgery, explain the purpose of the particular bowel or skin preparation ordered, if any. For lack of knowledge about postoperative care, describe awakening in the recovery room; explain why fluids may be restricted; explain the purpose of frequent vital signs assessment; teach how to turn, cough, and deep breathe; explain pain control and other comfort measures that may be used. For lack of knowledge about potential body image changes related specifically to the expected bodily changes associated with the respective surgery, assess client's areas of concern (e.g., use of blood, presence of scar, change in body structure or function); identify impact on roles—economic, occupational, emotional; identify support services; make referrals as needed; ensure privacy; use open communication, active listening, and nonjudgmental responses; observe verbal and nonverbal cues; notify physician if fear of death is overwhelming.	Anxiety relieved or maintained at tolerable level; relaxed facial expression and body movements; expression of feeling less anxious; expression of an understanding of preoperative routine, surgery, and postoperative routine; vital signs within normal limits; informed consent given

*This general preoperative care plan is used in conjunction with a surgical care plan specific to the type of surgery being performed.

SURGICAL OUTPATIENT DEPARTMENT

SHORT STAY DATA BASE
Surgical Outpatient/Inpatient with anticipated stay of 48 hours or less

Dear Patient:

  Please complete this side of the form, labeled A, and the top half of the reverse side. If you are a surgical outpatient or are being admitted to the hospital the morning of your surgery, please be sure to bring this form with you when you visit for preoperative testing.

A. Patient _____ Dr. _____ Date of Surgery _____

Age _____ Have you been a patient here previously? _____ If so, when? _____

Responsible party to accompany you home _____ Phone _____

Date of last ECG _____ Where? _____

Have you had previous surgery? No _____ If Yes, please list the following:

Surgery	Date	Where hospitalized
_____	_____	_____
_____	_____	_____
_____	_____	_____

Have you had any serious illness or infections requiring hospitalization (e.g., pneumonia, urinary tract infections)? No _____ If Yes, please state:

Illness/infection	Date	Where hospitalized
_____	_____	_____
_____	_____	_____

Have you had any complications or ill effects related to any anesthesia? No _____ If Yes, please explain: _____
_____
_____

Do you have any blood relatives that have had any complications related to anesthesia? No _____ If Yes, please explain: _____

Do you have any allergies? No _____ If Yes, please list and state reaction:

Medication	Reaction
_____	_____

Other:

Do you take any medications (e.g., aspirin, birth control pills)? No _____ If Yes, please state: _____
_____

(over)

Fig. 11-1 Short stay data base. (Courtesy Elliot Hospital, Manchester, NH.)

A. Health history continued:

Have you had any of the following? Please answer *Yes* or *No*.

_____ **Problems with your lungs**
_____ Wheezing
_____ Asthma
_____ Bronchitis
_____ Shortness of breath
_____ Pneumonia
_____ Emphysema

Other medical problems

_____ Diabetes
_____ Hepatitis
_____ Liver problems
_____ Yellow jaundice
_____ Anemia
_____ Weakness
_____ Frequent muscle cramps

_____ Persistent cough
_____ Other

_____ **Problems with your heart**
_____ Heart attack
_____ Rheumatic fever
_____ Fluttering heart

_____ Numbness
_____ Back problems/pain
_____ Kidney problems
_____ Bladder problems
_____ Frequent infections
_____ Frequent colds
_____ History of high fevers

_____ Chest pain
_____ Angina
_____ High blood pressure
_____ Palpitations
_____ Racing heartbeat
_____ Heart murmur
_____ Other problems

_____ Treatment for emotional problems
_____ Epilepsy
_____ Bleeding tendencies
_____ Fainting spells
_____ Blood tranfusions— any complications _____

Other problems you think we should know about _____

Drinking habits: Alcohol? No _____ Yes _____ Frequency _____ Amount _____

Smoking habits: Nonsmoker _____ Cigarettes _____ Cigars _____ Other _____

No./day _____ x _____ years   Ever smoked _____

Reminder: PLEASE BRING THIS COMPLETED FORM WITH YOU WHEN YOU VISIT THE HOSPITAL FOR YOUR PREOPERATIVE TESTS.

_____
Patient (age 18 and over)

_____   _____
Parent or Guardian   Nurse Signature

B. TO BE COMPLETED BY HOSPITAL PERSONNEL PRIOR TO SURGERY OR PROCEDURE

Scheduled Surgery or Procedure _____

NPO _____

Have you taken medications today? _____ If Yes, what? _____

_____ What time? _____

Date _____ Time _____

T _____ P _____ R _____ BP _____ HEIGHT _____ WEIGHT _____

General appearance _____

Behavior _____

Dentures? No _____ Yes _____   Loose teeth? No _____ Yes _____

Glasses? No _____ Yes _____   Contact lenses? No _____ Yes _____

Other prosthetic devices? No _____ Yes _____

COMMENTS: PROBLEM LIST:

_____   _____

_____   _____

_____   _____
                                                         Nurse Signature

Table 11-6 Common Preoperative Laboratory
Tests

Test	Area Assessed
Urinalysis	Renal status, hydration, urinary tract infection/disease
Chest x-ray film	Pulmonary disorders, cardiac enlargement
Blood studies: RBC, Hb, Hct, WBC, WBC differential	Anemia, immune status, infection
Electrolytes	Acid-base balance
ABGs, oximetry	Pulmonary and metabolic function
Prothrombin or partial thromboplastin time	Bleeding tendencies
Fasting blood sugar	Metabolic status, diabetes
Creatinine	Renal function
Blood urea nitrogen	Renal function
Electrocardiogram	Cardiac disease, electrolyte abnormalities
Pulmonary function studies	Pulmonary status
Type and cross-match	Blood availability for replacement (elective surgery clients may have own blood available)

RBC, Red blood count; *Hb*, hemoglobin; *Hct*, hematocrit; *WBC*, white blood cell count; *ABGs*, arterial blood gases.

the scheduled surgery, usually at the same time that preoperative laboratory studies are done. In some instances an initial introductory phone contact is made with the client.

Physiological Assessment

The preoperative period is used by both the physician and the nurse to do the following:
1. Determine the adequacy of the client's health status to undergo the proposed surgery
2. Identify and correct (if possible) any operative risk factors
3. Establish baseline data for comparison in the postoperative period

Table 11-6 lists the diagnostic tests that are commonly performed on preoperative clients. In some hospitals, the fasting blood sugar (FBS), blood urea nitrogen (BUN) determination, and electrocardiogram (ECG) are done only when the client is over 40 years of age. Additional tests may be done as indicated by the client's health status or for the planned surgical procedure. For example, an electrolyte profile will be done for the client who is taking diuretics or potassium supplements.

Many physiological stressors may put the client at risk for surgical complications, whether the surgery is an elective or an emergency procedure. However, risk is particularly influenced by the client's age, nutrition, body system status (respiratory, cardiovascular, renal, and hepatic), and current drug therapy. A physiological assessment of the preoperative client is presented in Table 11-7.

Older adult client. In general, the older the client, the greater the risk of complications developing after surgery. The nurse must be particularly alert when assessing and caring for the older adult surgical client. An event that has little affect on a younger client may be overwhelming to the older client. The surgical risk in older adults is related to normal physiological aging changes (see Chapter 4 and Table 4-8), which compromise organ function, reduce reserve capacity, and limit the body's ability to adapt to stress. This decreased ability to cope with stress, compounded by the additional burden of one or more chronic illnesses, anxiety, and the surgery itself, increases the risk of complications.[13-24]

Nutritional status. Assessment of nutritional status includes recognition of two problems that can increase operative risk: obesity and nutritional deficiencies. Obesity makes access to the surgical site more difficult and thus prolongs the surgery. It predisposes the client to wound dehiscence, wound infection, and incisional herniation because adipose tissue impairs approximation of the wound edges and is less vascular than other tissues. The inhalation anesthesic is absorbed and stored by adipose tissue and then released postoperatively. Therefore, the obese client requires more anesthetic and recovers more slowly from its effects. Nutritional deficiencies of protein and vitamins A, C, and B complex are particularly significant, since each of these substances is essential for wound healing. Older adults are often at high risk of malnutrition and fluid volume deficits associated with poor eating habits, dentition, and absorption changes as well as economic restrictions. Nutritional deficiencies impair the ability to withstand surgery. Surgery may be postponed until weight is gained or reduced and deficiencies are corrected.

Respiratory status. Assessment of respiratory status includes detection of acute and chronic problems. The presence of an upper respiratory infection usually results in postponement of surgery. A history of respiratory allergies should be communicated to the anesthesiologist because it may increase the risks associated with inhalation anesthesia. Chronic obstructive lung disease and senile emphysema, which are often present in the older adult client as a result of normal aging changes of the respiratory system, impair the client's gas exchange during and after surgery and also predispose to pulmonary infection and obstruction. The client who smokes should be encouraged to abstain preoperatively but may find this difficult during a time of heightened anxiety. Clients who smoke and those with chronic lung disease may receive preoperative pulmonary therapy, including intermittent positive pressure breathing (IPPB) and chest physiotherapy in addition to the usual breathing and coughing instruction.

Cardiovascular status. Assessment of cardiovascular status is particularly focused on detection of angina, recent myocardial infarction, hypertension, and congestive heart failure. The older adult client's cardiovascular system is subject to many age-related changes. The overall effect of these physiological changes is a diminished cardiac reserve and a reduced ability to adapt successfully to emotional and physiological stressors.

Any of these conditions may increase operative risk. Clients with recognized dysrhythmias may be monitored

Table 11-7 Physiological Assessment of the Preoperative Client*

NUTRITIONAL STATUS

Weigh client.

Determine recent weight loss through a diet history (e.g., a negative nitrogen balance may lead to postoperative complications of delayed or impaired wound healing, fluid imbalances, and infection).

Assess food and fluid intake pattern (older adults frequently have a preexisting nutritional deficit).

Identify any drug therapies that may affect electrolyte balance. Consider prescribed and over-the-counter medications (e.g., potassium-depleting diuretics, excessive use of laxatives or antacids).

Assess for the use of dentures and bridges (loose dentures or teeth may be dislodged during intubation).

RESPIRATORY STATUS

Identify acute or chronic problems; note the presence of infection or chronic obstructive lung disease.

Note the history of smoking, including the time interval since the last cigarette and the number of cigarettes smoked per day. (Remember that although smoking should be discouraged preoperatively, it may be difficult for clients to stop during this time of anxiety.)

Assess breath sounds for clarity, and determine baseline respiratory rate, pattern, and the use of accessory muscles of respiration.

CARDIOVASCULAR STATUS

Identify acute or chronic problems; focus on the presence of angina, hypertension, congestive heart failure, and recent history of myocardial infarction.

Assess baseline pulses: apical, radial, and pedal for rate and characteristics (compare one side to the other).

Assess for the presence of edema (including dependent areas), noting location and severity.

Assess neck veins for distention.

INTEGUMENTARY AND MUSCULOSKELETAL STATUS

Assess the mucous membranes for dryness and intactness.

Determine skin status; note drying, bruising, or breaks in integrity of surface.

Note any limitations in range of motion, weakness, or impairments to ambulation.

*See related body system chapters for more specific assessments and related laboratory studies.

---

electrocardiographically during and after surgery. Those receiving digitalis therapy will have serum potassium levels carefully monitored to avoid the adverse and toxic effects of anesthetic agents. Dehydration may require correction with fluid therapy preoperatively. Although a preoperative fluid balance assessment should be completed for all clients, it is especially critical for the older adult because the reduced adaptive capacity leaves only a narrow margin of safety between overhydration and underhydration. If anemia is present, a blood transfusion may be given preoperatively. Blood typing and crossmatching are done on many clients so that compatible blood will be available for transfusion if necessary during or after surgery. Autologous (self) blood donations are also frequently done.

Renal and hepatic status. Renal and hepatic status are of concern for health care workers because many anesthetics and adjunctive drugs are detoxified by the liver and excreted by the kidneys. The kidneys also regulate fluid and electrolyte balance and eliminate metabolic wastes during the postoperative period. Chronic liver disease may be accompanied by bleeding tendencies as well as poor wound healing and increased susceptibility to infection. Renal and hepatic function is also affected by physiological changes of aging that give rise to altered metabolism and excretion of drugs and potential fluid and electrolyte imbalances.

Use of medications. A careful history of medication use is essential to preoperative assessment. This should include drugs used for recreational as well as therapeutic purposes. Regular use of many prescription or nonprescription drugs may result in an increased operative risk:

1. *Steroids* may impair the body's ability to respond to the stress of anesthesia and surgery, mask symptoms of postoperative infection, and interfere with the body's normal immune function.
2. *Anticoagulants* and *salicylates* may increase bleeding during surgery.
3. *Antibiotics* may be incompatible with or potentiate anesthetic agents.
4. *Tranquilizers* potentiate the effect of narcotics and barbiturates (agents used for anesthesia), and cause hypotension.
5. *Antihypertensives* may predispose to shock by the combined effect of blood pressure reduction and anesthetic vasodilation.
6. *Diuretics* may increase the potassium loss already begun by the body's response to stress.
7. *Alcohol* will place the surgical client at risk when used chronically (see Chapter 60). When liver function is affected, metabolism of anesthetic agents is prolonged, nutritional status is altered, and the potential for postoperative complications is increased.

PREOPERATIVE ASSESSMENT

<u>Directions:</u> Form should be completed 1 to 24 hours before surgery by a registered professional nurse and become part of the client's permanent nursing record. Fill in the blanks, circle the appropriate descriptors, and add comments as necessary.

<u>General information</u>

Client _Gwendolyn Abbamonto_ Rm. # _361_ Hosp. # _000-000_ Date _8-1-91_

Age _42_ Ht _5'2"_ Wt _140_ Sex _♀_ Religion _Methodist_ Occupation _Teacher_

Surgeon _Dr. Jones_ Anesth. _General_ Surgical prodecure _Cholecystectomy_

Previous surgery _T & A_ Previous hospitalizations _3 (2 children)_ Recent illness &/or infection _None_

Allergies _None_ Medications _None_ Family support _Husband_

Preadmission testing done _X_ Abnormal lab results _None_

Permits OR _X_ Special _____ Blood _X_ Ordered _X_ # of units _2 — autologous_

<u>Assessment factors</u>

Blood pressure - Rt arm _130/80_ Lt arm _126/78_ Sitting _128/76_ Standing _118/82_ Lying _124/78_
Temperature _98⁸_ (po) rectal, axillary
Apical/radial pulse _80_ (equal) unequal, regular, irregular, bounding, feeble
Respiration _20_ (normal) noisy, orthopneic, dyspneic, irregular
Cough (none) occasional, frequent, dry, productive, comments_____
Smoker (yes) no, pks/day _____ years _Was a smoker until 1 year ago_
Peripheral pulses absent, (present) quality (normal) bounding thready
Jugular venous distention (none) present, describe_____
Edema (none) present, describe location and extent_____
Skin color (pink) pale, cyanosis, dusky, jaundiced, comments_____
Skin condition rash, bruises, redness, turgor, wound, comments _intact, elastic, smooth_
Paralysis/weakness (none) present, describe_____
Deformities (none) present, describe_____
Mobility (no impairment) impairment, describe_____
Consciousness (conscious) semiconscious, comatose
Mental status (oriented) disoriented, to person, place, time
Anxiety low, (moderate) high _excessive concern about post-op pain_
Comprehension (understands) does not understand, forgetful
Vision (normal) decreased (Rt, Lt), blind (Rt, Lt), glasses, contacts
Hearing (normal) decreased (Rt, Lt), deaf (Rt, Lt), hearing aid (Rt, Lt)
Speech (clear) slurred
Language (speaks English,) speaks _Spanish as a second language_

<u>Comments</u>

Summary of visit: _Very receptive to nurse, attentive, asks questions freely_

Information given: _Reinforced techniques for pain control and availability of medications_

Client's reception to information: _Eager to have surgical procedure_

Other: _Demonstrated effective coughing, deep breathing, and incisional splinting techniques_

Signed: _ME Walker, RN_

Fig. 11-2 Preoperative assessment.

8. *Insulin or antidiabetic agents* used in the management of the diabetic client may require dose or agent adjustment during the surgical hospitalization because of increased body metabolism, stress, and anesthesia (see Chapter 43).

9. *Cardiac-specific medications,* such as digoxin and nitroglycerin, may also require adjustment of dose or agent because of increased body system demands and the anesthetic agents used.

10. *Eyedrops* or *inhalers* may interact negatively with anesthetic agents. Clients may need to be questioned directly about these drugs because they often do not think of these agents as medications.

Recording of baseline nursing data. In addition to participating in the assessment of the client's health status and operative risk, the nurse records preoperative baseline data about the client to be used for comparison during the intraoperative and postoperative periods. Observations may be recorded on a form designed for the purpose (Fig. 11-2) or in the nursing notes.

This information, along with that obtained in the admission nursing interview, is extremely important for the nurses in the recovery room and on the postoperative nursing unit. The data enable them to more accurately evaluate the client's postoperative status and to individualize postoperative care. These data include a record of vital signs, including a full-minute apical and radial pulse; peripheral pulses; and sitting, standing, and lying blood pressures in both arms. Allergies, nutritional and integumentary status, neurological status, vision, hearing, and speech and language should also be noted.

■ Nursing Management of the Preoperative Client

Legal preparation

Before nonemergency surgery can be legally performed, the client must sign a *voluntary* and *informed consent* in the presence of a witness.[25] This document protects not only the client but also the surgeon, the hospital, and its employees. While the responsibility for obtaining consent is ultimately the surgeon's, it is often the nurse who obtains and witnesses the client's signature on a permit such as the one shown in Fig. 11-3.

For consent to be voluntary, the client must not be persuaded or coerced in any way in deciding to undergo the procedure. The nurse who stands at the bedside while the client reads the permit or who offers a pen along with the permit may inadvertently be applying pressure for the client to hurry and sign it. A far better approach is to leave the client alone to read the permit in an unhurried manner. The nurse can return after a brief time and ask if the client understands the permit or has any questions before signing. The client may be asked to state what the permit is about to determine if the document is understood. The nurse may have to read the contents of the form to the older adult client who has difficulty reading standard-sized printed material.

The client must also be mentally clear and competent at the time the consent is obtained. This includes freedom from the influence of any drugs that may affect rational thinking. Therefore, the permit should be signed before the client is given either analgesic or preanesthetic medication.

For consent to be informed, two criteria must be met. First, the client must understand the nature of the surgery (including what, if any, organs are to be removed). Second, the client must be informed of the risks and benefits of the surgery, including possible complications as well as changes in body function. The client must be aware of available alternatives to the proposed surgery for a truly informed choice to be made. Adequate time must be provided for the client to ask any questions before consenting. Even after signing the permit, the client must be made aware that permission may be withdrawn at any time. Although the physician is responsible for providing these explanations to the client, the nurse should determine that the client has received and understood them fully. If any confusion or doubt exists, the nurse should ask the physician to clarify further before having the client sign the permit.

The nurse plays a vital role as client advocate in ensuring that the consent for surgery is truly voluntary and informed. Fulfilling this role may present a difficult challenge. However, the added effort is necessary and worthwhile.

If the client is a minor or if the client is unconscious or mentally incapable of signing the permit, the written permission may be signed by a responsible family member. In surgical procedures involving sterilization (e.g., vasectomy, tubal ligation) the spouse as well as the client may be required to sign the operative permit. Local hospital policies should be checked for further clarification on this matter.

In the case of the mentally incapable, the client must be judged to be incompetent by a court of law before a relative or guardian may give consent.[26] Advanced age alone does *not* signify incompetence.

In an emergency when the client is unable to sign the consent form, consent may be obtained from the relative or guardian by telephone. In that case, two physicians or both a physician and a nurse need to be on the telephone line, one to act as a witness. Consent may also be received by telegram. In extreme emergencies, two or more physicians may sign the chart documenting the need for surgery. When the next of kin refuses to sign a consent form and the physician believes the client's life is endangered without surgery, the court may intervene and give consent.

Procedures for obtaining consent vary among states and institutions. The nurse should be aware of the state's nurse practice act and the institutional or agency policies that apply to a personal situation.

Psychological preparation

In preparing clients psychologically for surgery, nurses must strike a balance between telling so little that clients are unprepared and telling so much that they are overwhelmed. Nurses who observe carefully and listen sensitively to clients can usually determine how much information is enough in each instance.

A number of health team members participate in providing a client with information and instruction during the preoperative period. The admitting physician or surgeon is

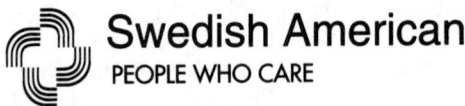

Swedish American
PEOPLE WHO CARE

<u>CONSENT TO OPERATION, ANESTHETICS, OBSTETRICAL PROCEDURES,
AND OTHER MEDICAL SERVICES</u>

Date_____ Time_____ AM
                                                 PM

1) I authorize the performance on _____
                                        (Name of Patient)

   of the following operation_____

   to be performed under the direction of Dr. _____

2) I consent to the performance of operations and procedures in
   addition to or different from those now contemplated whether or
   not arising from presently unforeseen conditions, which the above
   named doctor or associates or assistants may consider necessary
   or advisable in the course of the operation.

3) I consent to the administration of such anesthetics as may be
   considered necessary or advisable by the physician for this service'
   with the exception of _____.
                          (State "None," "Spinal Anesthesia," etc.)

4) I consent to the photographing or televising of the operation or
   procedures to be performed, including appropriate portions of my
   body for medical, scientific, or educational purposes, provided my
   identity is not revealed by the pictures or by descriptive texts
   accompanying them.

5) For the purpose of advancing medical education, I consent to the
   admittance of observers to the operating room.

6) I consent to the disposal by hospital authorities of any tissues
   or parts that may be removed.

7) I am aware that sterility may result from this operation. I know
   that a sterile person is not capable of becoming a parent.

8) The nature and purpose of the operation, possible alternative
   methods of treatment, the risks involved, and the possibility
   of complications have been fully explained to me. No guarantee
   or assurance has been given by anyone as to the results that
   may be obtained.

_____
(Signature of Patient or Authorized Person to Consent for Patient)

_____
(Witness)

*Note: Cross out any paragraphs above that do not apply.

Fig. 11-3   Operative permit. (Courtesy Swedish American Hospital, Rockford, Ill.)

responsible for explaining the need for surgery and its nature during office visits before admission. In some instances, a client has not met the surgeon before hospitalization. The anesthesiologist or anesthetist visits the client on the day or evening before surgery. At this time, premedication orders are written, and an explanation of anesthesia is given to the client.

In some hospitals, the operating room nurse also makes a preoperative visit to offer information, assurance, and support to the client. During this visit the nurse also completes a preoperative assessment of the client, identifies actual and potential problems, and formulates nursing diagnoses that will guide the perioperative plan of care. In addition, the visit by the perioperative nurse gives the client someone to recognize on arrival at the surgical suite. The client may also be visited by a member of the clergy or by a spiritual counselor employed by the hospital.

The major responsibility for preparing the client for surgery generally falls to the staff nurse on the unit. This nurse offers support and explanations, verifies that the client has understood information provided by other health team members, and instructs the client in specific activities to be done postoperatively.

Instructional preparation

The positive values of preoperative teaching include an increased satisfaction with nursing care by clients and nurses and a reduction of (1) fear and anxiety, (2) postoperative vomiting, (3) use of pain medication, (4) number of complications, (5) duration of hospitalization, and (6) recovery time following discharge.[27-34] In addition, the client has a right to know what to expect and how to participate effectively during the surgical experience.

The principles of teaching and learning (see Chapter 6) are applicable to the instruction of the surgical client. The nurse should be particularly aware of the effect of anxiety on learning and should allow time for repetition and reinforcement, as well as for verification of the client's understanding.

Preoperative instruction may be given to the client alone, in a group, or both. The nurse should consider choice of words carefully, stressing the positive whenever possible. The explanation that elastic stockings will be used to assist circulation during reduced activity is just as accurate as and less alarming than saying that they are used to prevent formation of blood clots. It is helpful to involve family members in teaching as well. This technique relieves their own concerns and anxieties, improves their attitudes toward hospitalization and surgery, and engages their assistance in supporting and encouraging the client throughout the experience.

Three types of preoperative teaching should be included: cognitive, sensory, and participatory. Cognitive information provides the client with factual information about schedules, procedures, and protocols. Sensory information provides the client with a description of physical sensations, what is to be felt, seen, heard, tasted, and smelled during a procedure. Participatory teaching includes demonstrations of the aspects of postoperative care in which the client is actively involved, such as turning, coughing, and deep breathing.

The areas to be covered in preoperative teaching are outlined in Fig. 11-4. In general, the client should be made aware of what will happen, when it will happen, why it is necessary, and how to participate most therapeutically. When teaching the following postoperative preventive techniques, the nurse should first describe and demonstrate each technique and then observe the client's return demonstration.

Documentation of preoperative instruction is vital. A checklist (Fig. 11-5) is used by many institutions to ensure that all areas of instruction are covered and that documentation is completed. Documentation may also be made in the nurses' notes.

Deep-breathing and coughing techniques. Deep-breathing and coughing techniques in the postoperative period help the client to eliminate inhalation anesthetics, prevent alveolar collapse, and move respiratory secretions to larger airway passages for expectoration. They should be done several times each hour during the immediate postoperative period.

The client should be instructed to practice deep breathing and coughing in a similar position that would be assumed after surgery (semi-Fowler's, with knees bent and flat in bed). Because the sitting and standing positions allow maximum lung expansion, the client should also be encouraged to practice these breathing techniques when sitting at the side of the bed or ambulating.

Diaphragmatic or abdominal breathing is accomplished by inhaling slowly and deeply through the nose, holding the breath for a few seconds, and then exhaling slowly but completely through the mouth. The client's hands should be placed lightly over the lower ribs and upper abdomen. This allows the client to feel the abdomen rise during inspiration and fall during expiration.

Following four to six deep breaths, the client should cough deeply from the lungs rather than the throat. If secretions are present in the respiratory passages, deep breathing often will move them up to stimulate the cough reflex without any voluntary effort by the client, and they can then be expectorated.

The client who is to have a thoracic or abdominal incision should also be shown how to splint it while deep breathing and coughing. This technique minimizes discomfort and increases willingness to carry out the respiratory exercises. Splinting may be accomplished in several ways by the nurse or client (Fig. 11-6). If incentive spirometry or other mechanical devices are to be used postoperatively, the client should be taught the proper method of using the device most effectively.

Leg exercises. Leg exercises by the postoperative client help to facilitate venous return and prevent venous stasis. Although any number of leg movements may be helpful, it is most important that the client rhythmically contract and relax the calf (gastrocnemius) and thigh (quadriceps) muscles to create a pumping action along the veins where thrombus formation is likely to occur. Gastrocnemius pumping is accomplished when the client alternately flexes and extends the ankle by pressing the feet against a footboard or the nurse's hands. Quadriceps setting is accomplished by pressing the back of the knee against the bed

PREOPERATIVE TEACHING OUTLINE

TOPIC			CLIENT KNOWLEDGE	DATE RN SIG
Client verbalizes or demonstrates Knowledge and understanding of:	Yes	No	Comments (goal accomplished, needs reinforcement)	
Surgery/anesthesia				
Nature and duration of surgery				
Type of anesthesia				
Time surgery scheduled				
What to ask surgeon/anesthesiologist				
Permits				
Expectations day before surgery				
Skin prep				
Enemas, laxative, douche, etc.				
Food, fluid, smoking restrictions				
Bedtime sedation				
Diagnostic measures				
Expectations day of surgery				
Hygienic measures				
Removal of cosmetics, dentures, etc.				
Hospital attire				
Care of possessions				
Insertion of tubes (e.g., urinary, nasogastric)				
Preoperative medications				
Time to go to surgery				
Transport to surgery (transfer to cart, side rails up)				
Surgical holding area				
Surgical climate (noise, lights, temperature, dress)				
When family can visit				
Where family can wait during surgery				
Expectations after surgery				
Recovery room stay (and intensive care unit if necessary)				
Availability of analgesic				
Equipment in use postoperatively (e.g., IV, oxygen, tubes, catheters, elastic stockings, dressings)				
Unusual sensations				
Vital signs				
Dietary changes				
Postoperative preventive techniques				
Deep breathing and coughing				
Incisional splinting				
Leg and foot exercises				
Turning in bed, getting out of bed, ambulating				

Fig. 11-4   Preoperative teaching outline checklist.

PREOPERATIVE CHECK LIST

Date _____ 19 _____ N/A, Not applicable
Initial appropriate space

PATIENT PREPARATION ON CLINICAL	Yes	No
1. Preoperative teaching documented _____		
2. Vital signs prior to properative medication		
BP _____ T _____ P _____ R _____ _____		
3. AM Care _____ Bath or shower _____		
4. Voided Amount ____ Time _____ Catheter ____		
5. All nail polish & makeup removed _____		
6. Preop medications given _____ Time _____		
7. Side rails up _____		
8. Family here _____		
9. _____		
10. _____		

Please note pertinent information prior to surgery (e.g., deafness, anxiety level, physical limitations, language barriers, level of consciousness, colostomy, family) _____
_____
_____
_____
_____
_____
_____
_____

List allergies

PREOPERATIVE PREPARATION	UNIT Yes	UNIT No	UNIT N/A	OR Yes	OR No
1. Master card numbers & Identiband numbers are the same _____					
2. Medication profile on chart _____					
3. Allergies (inquire /list) _____					
4. NPO status _____ Time _____					
5. Elastic hose ordered and applied _____					
6. Dentures &/or partial plate _____					
7. Contact lenses _____ Glasses _____					
8. Hairpins _____ Hairpiece _____					
9. Prosthesis _____					
10. Jewelry, medals _____					
11. Wedding rings taped _____					
12. Operative permit _____					
a. Identification of site _____					
Right _____ Left _____					
b. Operative procedure _____					
13. Special permit(s) _____					
14. Blood permit _____					
a. Type & crossmatch # of units _____					
b. Type & screen and hold # of units _____					
c. Blood ready _____					
15. LABORATORY					
a. CBC _____ b. Urinalysis _____					
c. SMA 12/60 Done _____ On chart _____					
d. Electrolytes Done _____ On chart _____					
16. Culture Done _____ Report on chart _____					
17. ECG Done _____ Report on chart _____					
18. Pulmonary function screening Done _____ On chart _____					
19. Chest x-ray Done _____ On chart _____					
20. History & physical					

Removed Placed
Removed Placed
Removed Placed
Removed Placed
Removed Placed

SPECIAL ORDER(S):

NURSING UNIT	OPERATING ROOM

Ready for surgery _____
Time _____
Signature _____   Signature _____
Date _____ 19 _____   Date _____ 19 _____

Fig. 11-5 Preoperative checklist. (Courtesy Rockford Memorial Hospital, Rockford, Ill.)

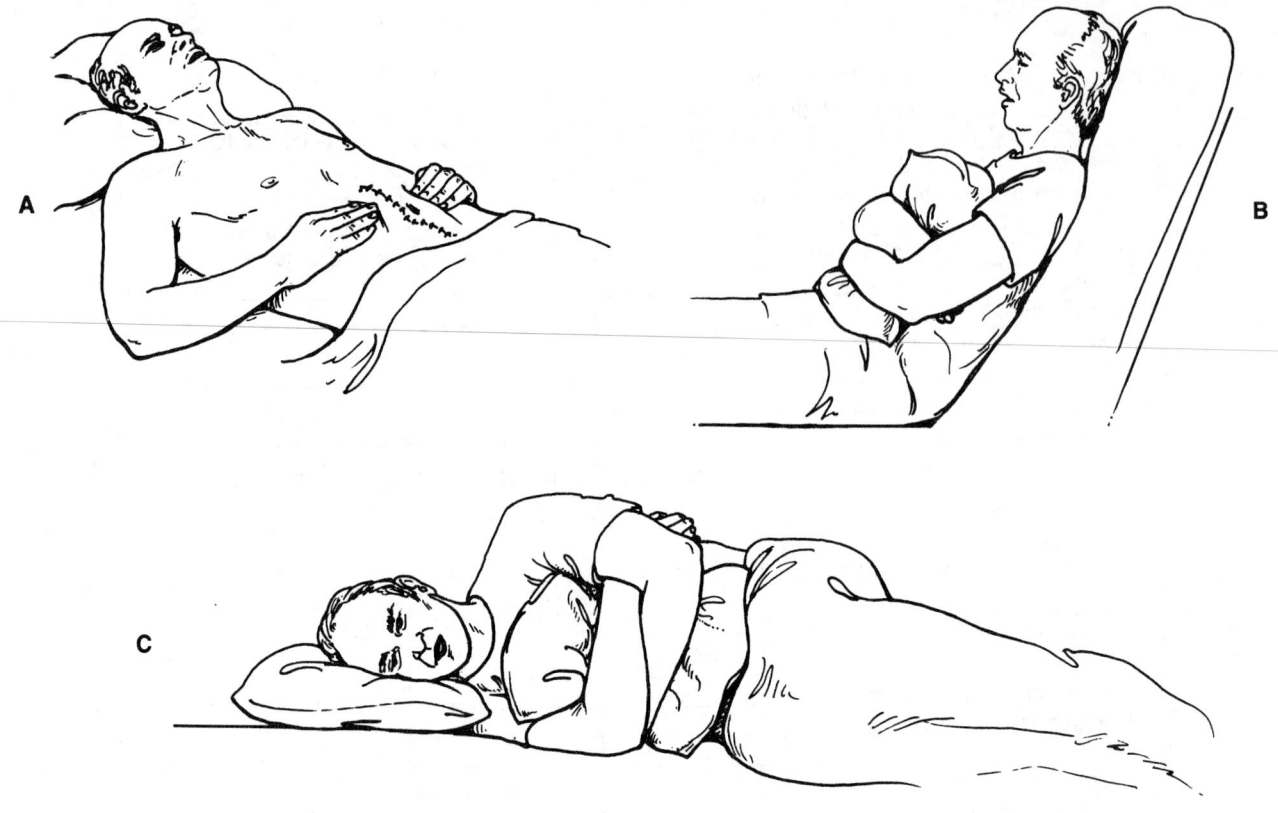

Fig. 11-6 Techniques for splinting wound when coughing.

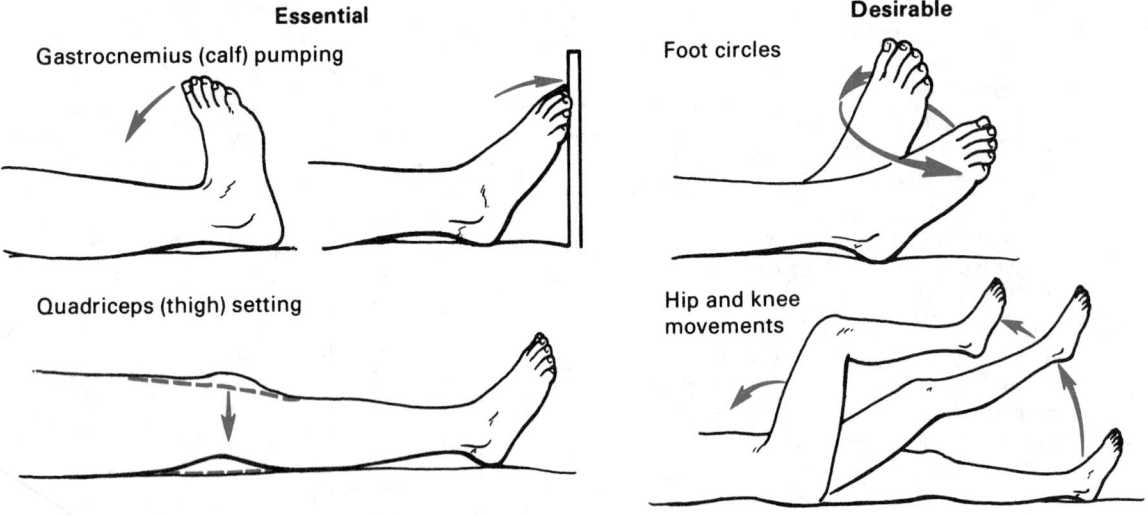

Fig. 11-7 Postoperative leg exercises.

and then relaxing it. These should each be done about 10 to 12 times each hour.

Additional exercises that may be helpful, especially if the client is not allowed to ambulate immediately, are foot circles and hip and knee movements. The latter may prove too painful for the client who has an abdominal incision. These exercises are illustrated in Fig. 11-7.

Movement in bed and ambulation. The client will be expected to turn (usually from side to back to side or in a side, side, back cycle) every 1 to 2 hours postoperatively to prevent respiratory and circulatory complications. Preoperative practice using the side rails for assistance in turning is helpful. The client should also practice getting out of bed to ambulate in a manner that minimizes strain on the incision and discomfort. One helpful technique is to turn on the side and then push up to a sitting position. Another technique is to raise the head of the bed until the client is sitting erect and can then pivot the legs over the side of the bed.

The client should also be informed of anticipated activity postoperatively. The trend is to ambulate clients on the day of surgery or the first postoperative day. If this will not be the plan, the client should know the reason.

Physical preparation

The evening before surgery. Physical preparation of the client for surgery is designed to minimize operative and postoperative risks and complications. Specific preoperative orders are written by the surgeon for each client. In many hospitals these orders automatically cancel any previous orders. The nurse needs to be alert for the inadvertent cancellation of therapies (e.g., drugs such as corticosteroids and antidysrhythmics) that should be continued throughout the surgical experience. If such an omission occurs, the physician should be notified.

For the outpatient surgical client, specific instructions for preparation are reviewed at the time of the preadmission assessment, and written directions are given. As with the hospitalized client, the nurse must be attentive to directions for continuing prescription medications.

BOWEL ELIMINATION. Cleansing or small-volume hypertonic enemas or suppositories are not routinely ordered for the surgical client. However, bowel elimination status and patterns should be assessed. This is particularly essential for the client who must avoid straining postoperatively (e.g., after rectal, prostate, or eye surgery). It is also important for the client whose mobility will be affected postoperatively (e.g., after orthopedic, neurological, and vascular procedures). Bowel-elimination measures, if ordered, should be carried out well before bedtime so that they will not interfere with needed rest.

SKIN PREPARATION. Preparation of the skin at and around the incisional site is designed to reduce the number of microorganisms present, control wound contamination, and reduce the risk of wound infection. The skin of the presurgical client should be intact and in a healthy condition, particularly at the incisional site.

Cleansing may involve simple washing with soap and water or more prolonged scrubbing with an antiseptic solution such as Betadine. The amount of hair removal is variable and generally depends on the surgeon's preference. Hair removal is generally done by shaving with a safety or electric razor and is usually completed immediately before the area is cleansed and the incision is made. In some instances a depilatory cream may be used. Shaving is accompanied by the hazard of nicking the skin. Depilatories may produce skin irritation or rash, particularly when used in sensitive areas such as the groin or axilla. Any disruption of skin integrity is to be avoided. If a cut or skin irritation occurs, it should be recorded and reported. In some instances, hair removal is omitted entirely in the belief that unshaven but clean skin is less likely to be associated with sepsis.

Skin preparation may be ordered the evening before or on the morning of surgery. It then becomes the responsibility of the staff nurse, who should always be careful to assess the client for allergies or sensitivities, particularly to iodine, since it is a constituent of the agents frequently used as antiseptics.

HYGIENIC MEASURES. A bath or shower the evening before surgery cleanses the skin and may also help the client to relax and sleep throughout the night. A shampoo is advisable at this time. It may be several days to a week before the client can again easily wash the hair. Depending on the client's preference and the scheduled time of surgery, these activities may be deferred until the morning of the surgery.

REST AND SLEEP. A restful night's sleep before surgery is important so that the client will be in the best condition to withstand the surgical trauma and its aftermath. The nurse should use all necessary comfort measures to ensure that the client falls asleep and stays asleep throughout the night. A hypnotic is usually ordered and given at bedtime for this reason. It is often considered the beginning of the anesthetic preparation of the surgical client.

FOOD AND FLUIDS. The client is usually kept on NPO ("nothing by mouth") status after midnight before surgery to ensure that the upper gastrointestinal tract will be empty. However, if surgery is scheduled late in the day, food or fluid restrictions may be started after a clear liquid breakfast. In either instance, the possibility of vomiting and the risk of aspiration during the anesthetic and postoperative periods are reduced. Solid food must be withheld for a minimum of 6 hours before general anesthesia. Variations do occur; water is sometimes given up until 4 hours before surgery, and some prescription medications (e.g., cardiac and respiratory drugs) may also be taken during this time.

The client should be informed of these restrictions, encouraged to eat a nourishing supper, and encouraged to maintain a good fluid intake during the evening. Older adult or dehydrated clients may have an intravenous line started to avoid a period without fluid intake. An NPO sign should be posted in a conspicuous place, and all personnel should be informed of the restriction. Oral intake during the time of restriction may result in delay of surgery.

The day of surgery. The nursing responsibility immediately before surgery includes final preparation of the client, as well as checking to determine that all orders have been carried out and that records are complete and ready to accompany the client to the operating room. The preoperative checklist (Fig. 11-5) provides an efficient and visible means of ensuring that no detail has been forgotten.

HYGIENE AND ATTIRE. The client should be awakened in time to complete morning care, including any hygienic measures not carried out the evening before. Cosmetics and nail polish should be removed, since the color of the lips and nail beds is frequently observed. However, the adequacy of oxygenation is more accurately monitored with oximetry (see Chapter 21). All prostheses, including dentures, wigs, and contact lenses, are generally removed to avoid loss or damage to them. However, consideration should be given to the individual self-esteem needs of the client. Some anesthesiologists may prefer that dentures remain in place. Hairpins or clips are removed so that they will not accidentally injure the client's scalp or face. A hospital gown is worn both for ease of access to the surgical site and to avoid staining or damaging the client's clothing. The addition of client headcaps and boots may also be required in some hospitals.

CARE OF VALUABLES. All valuables, including jewelry and money, should be taken by the client's family or locked up securely according to agency policy. Their disposition should be recorded clearly. If the client prefers not to remove a wedding ring, it may be securely tied with gauze and then wrapped and fastened around the wrist. Tape should not be used for this purpose since it may remove stones from their settings. Specific agency policy regarding this process should be followed.

COMPLETING THE CHART. The nurse should determine that all orders and procedures have been completed and recorded in the client's chart before giving the preanesthetic medication. This includes checking for the presence of a signed consent for surgery, other necessary consents such as transfusion permit, the history and physical examination reports, a record of all consultations, baseline vital signs, diagnostic test results, and nurses' notes complete to that point.

URINARY ELIMINATION. The client should urinate immediately before being given preanesthetic medication. This prevents involuntary elimination under anesthesia, lessens the chance of accidental nicking of the bladder during surgery, and reduces the possibility of urinary retention during early postoperative recovery. When surgery is in the area of the bladder, as in gynecological procedures, an indwelling catheter may be inserted either preoperatively, in the holding room, or in the operating room.

PREANESTHETIC MEDICATION. Preanesthetic medications are given at a prescribed time 30 to 60 minutes before surgery or "on call" when notified by the operating room. The on-call procedure is used when many surgeries are planned in sequence in the same operating suite. The operating room usually calls the unit about 30 to 60 minutes before the client's surgery is expected to begin.

With the use of surgical holding rooms, many preoperative and on-call medications are given intravenously in this area and not on the general unit. In either case, the nurse or anesthetist needs to give the preanesthetic medication as soon as notified so that the medication can achieve the expected results. Preanesthetic drugs are designed to facilitate the administration of the anesthetic, to reduce risks, and to calm the client (Table 11-8). The client may receive a single drug or a combination of drugs.

Sedatives and hypnotics are most frequently used alone but may be combined with other central nervous system depressants, such as tranquilizers and narcotics. Anticholinergics may be added to reduce secretions, although their preoperative use is decreasing. For the OpSu and same-day-admit surgical client, medications that provide sedation are the premedications of choice. These are frequently given intravenously rather than intramuscularly to facilitate faster recovery of the client.

Premedication should be administered to the client in bed after all other preoperative preparation has been com-

Table 11-8 Frequently Used Preoperative Medications

Drug	Purpose and Effects
NARCOTICS	
Morphine, meperidine (Demerol), butorphanol (Stadol), nalbuphine (Nubain)	Induces euphoria, facilitates anesthesia induction, requires less anesthetic
SEDATIVE-HYPNOTIC-ANTIANXIETY AGENTS	
Flurazepam (Dalmane)	Promotes relaxation and sleep
Diazepam (Valium), hydroxyzine (Vistaril, Atarax), midazolam (Versed)	Produces drowsiness and sedation, reduces anxiety and apprehension, potentiates action of narcotics, facilitates anesthesia induction, has antiemetic effect
ANTICHOLINERGICS	
Atropine, glycopyrrolate (Robinul), scopolamine	Reduces salivary and bronchial secretions, keeps respiratory passages clear and dry, reduces hazard of atelectasis, blocks heart-slowing impulses from vagus nerve, blocks memory of pain or discomfort (scopolamine only)

pleted. The client should be told that the medications will help with relaxation and that drowsiness may occur without the loss of consciousness. The client needs to know that although the mouth will feel dry if an anticholinergic is used, no fluids should be taken. The client should also be instructed not to smoke or to get out of bed. Side rails should be raised, with the bed level in a low position, and the call light should be placed within reach. Family members may remain until the client is transferred. A quiet environment, conducive to rest, should be provided.

TRANSPORTATION TO THE OPERATING ROOM. When operating room personnel arrive on the unit, the nurse assists in the movement of the client to a transfer cart, using a blanket for cover, modesty, and warmth. The side rails of the cart are raised, and the safety belts are secured. The nurse reports on the client's status, indicating any special needs or concerns. Documentation of the time and mode of transfer is made in the clinical record. The record, including the preoperative checklist and any other required forms such as the medication profile sheet, is sent to the operating room with the client.

In many institutions the family may accompany the client to the holding area/operating room area. The nurse should ensure that any family members who are present at this time know where to wait during surgery and what to expect when the client returns.

During the client's absence or before the client's return from surgery, the nurse prepares the room by making up a surgical bed. Included are a washable blanket for warmth, additional disposable pads for any expected drainage, folded draw sheets or bath blankets to assist with lifting and movement, and added pillows for positioning. Daily care equipment such as bedpans, urinals, emesis basins, and tissue should also be available. Any additional equipment, such as IV poles or an overhead trapeze, should also be brought to the room. Additional items (e.g., oxygen/suction setups, IV pumps) may be indicated at the time of the pretransfer from the recovery room/postanesthesia unit.

Postoperative flow sheets used for documentation may be placed at the bedside. The furniture should be arranged so that the transfer cart may easily be brought alongside the bed when the client is brought to the room.

C ase *Study*

ELECTIVE SURGERY

Mrs. Gwendolyn Abbamonto, a 42-year-old elementary school teacher, is admitted to the hospital for an elective cholecystectomy. After several episodes of epigastric distress during the year, she consulted her family physician. X-rays revealed gallstones, and she was referred to a surgeon, who recommended surgery within a few months. She has chosen to have her surgery in June to allow time for full recuperation before returning to work in the fall. Her husband is taking 2 weeks' vacation to care for their children, aged 7 and 12. Mrs. Abbamonto's previous hospitalizations were for a tonsillectomy at age 10 with open-drip ether anesthesic and for delivery of her two children by the Lamaze psychoprophylactic method of childbirth. She smoked one pack of cigarettes a day until a year ago, when she stopped entirely.

Discussion Questions

1. What factors in Mrs. Abbamonto's background or personal situation may influence her emotional and physical reactions to this hospitalization and surgery?
2. What should she know if her consent to surgery is to be truly informed? How would you approach her to obtain her written consent?
3. In teaching her breathing exercises preoperatively, what are the best techniques to use?
4. What measures would you expect to carry out on the evening before surgery? Why?
5. What measures would you expect to carry out on the morning of surgery? Why?

R eview *Questions*

The number of the question corresponds to the same-numbered objective at the beginning of the chapter.

1. Which of these surgical procedures involves removal of a body organ?
   a. herniorrhaphy
   b. cholecystectomy
   c. mammoplasty
   d. colostomy
2. A nursing intervention to assist the client in coping with fear of pain would be to
   a. describe the degree of pain expected
   b. explain the availability of pain medication
   c. inform the client of the frequency of pain medication
   d. divert the client when talking about pain
3. More anesthesic may be required by the client who is
   a. dehydrated
   b. a smoker
   c. obese
   d. an older adult
4. The range of preoperative vital signs should be recorded
   a. for all clients
   b. when a general anesthesic is to be used
   c. if client has a history of cardiovascular disease
   d. when the client is an older adult
5. Mr. Jensen, an alert man of 75 years of age, is to undergo elective hip surgery. The operative permit must be signed in the presence of a witness by
   a. Mr. Jensen
   b. Mr. and Mrs. Jensen
   c. either Mr. or Mrs. Jensen
   d. Mr. Jensen and the surgeon
6. When teaching the preoperative client deep-breathing techniques, the nurse should have the client
   a. sit in a comfortable chair at the bedside
   b. keep abdominal muscles tight and flat while inhaling
   c. inhale through the nose and exhale through the mouth
   d. cough from the throat rather than from the lungs
7. Which measure should be done last on the morning of surgery?
   a. administer preanesthetic medication
   b. ask client to void in the bathroom
   c. remove jewelry and lock up securely
   d. check chart for signed consent form
8. The preoperative client is kept NPO after midnight to prevent
   a. overhydration or fluid overload postoperatively
   b. urinary incontinence in the operating room
   c. nicking of stomach or intestine during surgery
   d. vomiting and aspiration during anesthesia
9. A primary consideration in the instruction of the older preoperative client is
   a. using large-print material
   b. planning for additional time for teaching
   c. using touch to aid communication
   d. recognizing that cognitive function is decreased

REFERENCES

1. LeMaitre GD and Finnegan JA: The patient in surgery: a guide for nurses, ed 4, Philadelphia, 1980, WB Saunders Co, p 3.
2. Brooks SM: Fundamentals of operating room nursing, ed 2, St Louis, 1979, The CV Mosby Co, p 5.

3. Wetchler BV: Ambulatory surgery: patient selection criteria 1987, AORN J 45:30-38, 1987.

4. Nathanson SN: Ambulatory surgery: characteristics of a successful ambulatory surgery program, AORN J 47:592-598, 1988.

5. Berger S and King E: Elder care, designing services for the elderly, AORN J 51:448-454, 1990.

6. Janis IL: Stress attitudes and decisions: selected papers, New York, 1982, Praeger Publishers, pp 193-213, 259-285.

7. Nyamathi A and Kashewabara A: Preoperative anxiety: its effects on cognitive thinking, AORN J 47:164-170, 1988.

8. Phippen ML: Patient shame: implications for perioperative nursing, AORN J 46:88-94, 1987.

9. Wheeler BR: Crisis intervention: recognizing and helping patients overcome anxiety, AORN J 47:1242-1248, 1988.

10. Kupferer DD, Uebele JA, and Levin DF: Geriatric ambulatory surgery patients: assessing cognitive functions, AORN J 47:752-766, 1988.

11. Santo-Novak DA: Seven keys to assessing the elderly, Nursing 18:60-63, 1988.

12. Williams MA and others: Predictors of acute confusional states in hospitalized elderly patients, Res Nurs Health 8:31-40, 1988.

13. Adams F: Fluid intake: how much do elders drink? Geriatr Nurs 4:218-221, 1988.

14. Farnella-Reedy D: Fluid intake: how can you prevent dehydration? Geriatr Nurs 4:224-226, 1988.

15. Felver L and Pendarvis JH: Electrolyte imbalances: intraoperative risk factors, AORN J 49:992-1008, 1989.

16. Iverson-Carpenter MS and others: Fulfilling nutritional requirements, J Gerontol Nurs 14:16-24, 1988.

17. Johnson ME: High-risk surgical patients, J Gerontol Nurs 14:8-15, 1988.

18. Latz PA and Wyble SJ: Elderly patients: perioperative nursing implications, AORN J 46:238-253, 1987.

19. Ford AB: Health function in the old and very old, J Am Gerontol Soc 3:187-197, 1988.

20. Metheny N: Preoperative fluid balance assessment, AORN J 33:51-54, 1981.

21. Meyer-Gaspar P: Fluid intake: what determines how much patients drink? Geriatr Nurs 4:221-224, 1988.

22. Walker ML: Growing old: increased surgical risks in the elderly, AORN J 43:887-890, 1986.

23. Wysock AB: Surgical wound healing: a review for perioperative nurses, AORN J 49:502-518, 1989.

24. Murphy EK: OR nursing law: informed consent, part I, AORN J 47:1009-1116, 1988.

25. Haddad AM: Determining competency, J Gerontol Nurs 14:19-22, 1988.

26. Aasen N: Interventions to facilitate personal control, J Gerontol Nurs 13:21-28, 1987.

27. Clement JM: Touch research findings and use in perioperative care, AORN J 45:1429-1438, 1987.

28. Pothrock JC: Perioperative nursing research, part 1: preoperative psychoeducational interventions, AORN J 49:597-616, 1989.

29. Doyle D: Health teaching strategies in a day hospital, J Gerontol Nurs 14:12, 1988.

30. Yount ST, Edgell J, and Jakovek V: Perioperative teaching; a study of nurses' perceptions, AORN J 51:572-579, 1990.

31. King I and Tarsitano B: The effect of structured and unstructed preoperative teaching: a replication, Nurs Res 31:324-329, 1982.

32. Pease RA: Praise elders to help them learn, J Gerontol Nurs 11:16-20, 1985.

33. Moss RC: Overcoming fear: a review of research on patient family instruction, AORN J 43:107-112, 1986.

34. Rice VH and Johnson JE: Preadmission self-instruction booklet, post-admission exercise performance and teaching time, Nurs Res 32:147-151, 1984.

CHAPTER

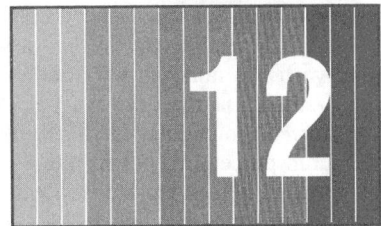

12

Nursing Role in Management
Client During Surgery

Patricia Robertson Hercules
M. Kent Powell

L

1. *Describe the physical environment of the operating room and the preoperative holding area.*
2. *Describe the functions of the members of the surgical team.*
3. *Explain the nursing role during the preoperative, intraoperative, and postoperative phases of a surgical intervention.*
4. *Describe basic principles of aseptic technique used in the operating room.*

5. *Differentiate between general and regional or local anesthesia, including advantages, disadvantages, and rationale for choice of the anesthetic technique.*
6. *Identify the basic characteristics of the techniques and drugs used to induce and maintain general anesthesia.*
7. *Discuss techniques for administering local and regional anesthetics.*
8. *Discuss the characteristics of adjunct agents used with general anesthesia and their implications to the postoperative care nurse.*

Nursing care of the surgical client requires understanding of the intraoperative phase of surgical care. This knowledge allows the nurse to monitor the client's response to the stressors related to the surgical experience. Use of the nursing process during the intraoperative phase is necessary as a framework for the delivery of care.

PHYSICAL ENVIRONMENT
Operating Room

The surgical environment is a unique acute-care setting removed from other hospital clinical units (Fig. 12-1). It is controlled geographically, environmentally, and bacteriologically and is restricted in terms of the inflow and outflow of personnel. Its physical location is preferably adjacent to the postanesthesia recovery area and the surgical intensive care unit. This allows for close collaboration for postanesthesia recovery. Careful consideration of design, location, and control of the physical environment assists

Reviewed by Brenda M. Robinson, CRNA, M.A.E., Staff Nurse Anesthetist, University of New Mexico Hospital, Albuquerque, N.M., and John Duvall, M.D. (deceased), Anesthesiology, The Methodist Hospital, Houston, Texas.

with the prevention of infection and provides physical safety and comfort for the client and the operating room team.

Several methods are used to prevent the transmission of infection. Filters and controlled airflow in the ventilating systems provide dust control. Positive air pressure in the rooms prevents air from entering the operating rooms from the halls and corridors. Dust-collecting surfaces such as open shelves, windows, and ledges are omitted. Materials that are resistant to the corroding effects of strong disinfectants are used. The functional design lends ease to the practice of aseptic technique by the operating room team.

Physical safety and comfort are aided by the use of operating room furniture that is conductive, adjustable, easy to clean, and easy to move. Overhead and ancillary lighting and electrical plugs are explosion proof. All equipment is checked frequently to ensure electrical safety. Line isolation monitors are installed to assess proper function of all electrical equipment devices. The lighting is designed to provide a low- to high-intensity range for precise view of the surgical site. A communication system provides a means for the delivery of routine and emergency messages.[1]

261

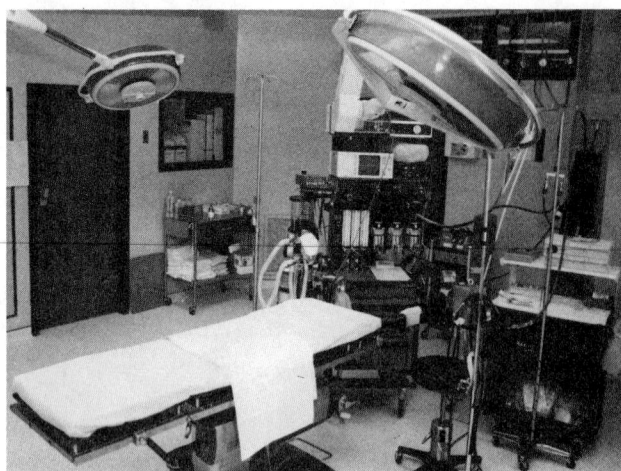

Fig. 12-1 A modern operating room. (Courtesy Lovelace Medical Center, Albuquerque, NM.)

The temperature is controlled at from 20° C to 24° C (68° F to 75° F) and the humidity is regulated at a minimum of 50% to facilitate client comfort under the surgical drapes, team comfort during the procedure, and an environment that is unfavorable to bacterial incubation and growth.[1]

The privacy of the client is achieved by restriction of the influx of hospital personnel and visitors. Special permission must be obtained to enter the suite during the surgical procedure.

Preoperative Holding Area

The preoperative holding area is a special waiting area inside or outside the surgical suite. The size varies according to hospital design and can range from a centralized holding area to accommodate numerous clients to a small designated area immediately outside the actual room scheduled for the surgical procedure. In this area the perioperative nurse makes the final identification and assessment before the client is transferred into the operating room for surgery.

Many institutions permit the family or a friend to accompany and wait with the client until it is time to be transferred to the operating room. Separation from loved ones just before surgery can produce anxiety.

THE SURGICAL TEAM

When the client awaiting surgery is transported from the nonsurgical area to the preoperative holding area, the perioperative nurse is usually the first member of the surgical team encountered. Along with the final assessment and necessary tasks before the surgery, the nurse provides physical comfort measures and assists in reducing the client's anxiety.

Registered Nurse

The perioperative nurse is a registered nurse who implements client care based on the nursing process. Two different roles may be assumed by the perioperative nurse.

Intraoperative responsibilities may involve either *sterile* or *nonsterile* activities, depending on the role assumed for a particular surgery. If the nurse is not scrubbed, gowned, and gloved and remains in the unsterile field, the role of the *circulating nurse* is implemented. If the nurse follows the designated scrub procedure, gowns and gloves in sterile attire, and remains within the sterile field, the role of the *scrub nurse* is implemented. Specific task-oriented duties of each of these functions are outlined in Table 12-1.

The function of the perioperative nurse is not limited to task-oriented duties. The perioperative nurse actively implements nursing care in the preoperative, intraoperative, and postoperative phases of the surgical client's care. These three phases of client care are presented in the scope of practice developed by the Association of Operating Room Nurses (Fig. 12-2). The nursing activities that characterize each of these phases are presented in Table 12-2. The *preoperative phase* begins with the decision to have surgery and ends when the client is transferred to the operating table. The *intraoperative phase* begins when the client is transferred to the operating table and ends with admittance to the postanesthesia care area. The *postoperative phase* begins when the client is admitted to the postanesthesia care area and ends with a home or clinic evaluation.[2]

Licensed Vocational Nurse and Technician

In some institutions, the scrub nurse is a technically trained operating technician or a licensed practical nurse. Scrub nurses assist the surgeon by passing instruments and implementing other technical functions during the surgical procedure. This role is supervised by and can also be assumed by a registered nurse.

Surgeon and Assistant

The surgeon is the physician who assumes responsibility for the surgical procedure. The surgeon may be the client's primary physician or one who was selected by the client's physician to collaborate with the primary physician. The surgeon is primarily responsible for the following:

1. Preoperative client assessment, including need for surgical intervention, choice of surgical procedures, and management of preoperative workup
2. Client safety and management in the operating room
3. Postoperative management of the client

The surgeon's assistant is a physician who functions in an assisting role during the surgical procedure. The assistant usually holds retractors to expose surgical areas and assists with hemostasis and suturing. In some instances, especially in educational settings, the assistant may perform some portions of the operative procedure under the direct supervision of the surgeon.

In some institutions the surgeon's assistant is a nonphysician who is permitted to function in the role of the assistant under the direct supervision of the physician. The assistant may be a resident, an intern, a physician's assistant, a nurse practitioner, or a registered nurse. Hospital policies define this role and physician responsibility when the assistant's position is filled by a nonphysician.

Table 12-1 Duties of the Perioperative Nurse

CIRCULATING ROLE

Reviews anatomy, physiology, and the surgical procedure.
Assists with preparing the room:
  Practices aseptic technique.
  Monitors the activities of others.
  Ensures that needed items are available and sterile (if required).
  Checks mechanical and electrical equipment and environmental factors.
  Arranges the furniture in workable order.
Identifies and assesses the client.
Checks the chart and relates pertinent data.
Admits the client to the operating room suite.
Assists with transferring the client to the operating table.
Participates in insertion and application of monitoring devices.
Protects the client during induction of anesthesia.
Positions the client.
Prepares the client's skin for the surgical incision.
Monitors the draping procedure and all activities requiring asepsis.
Completes the intraoperative record.
Records, labels, and sends to proper locations tissue specimens and cultures.
Evaluates blood and fluid loss.
Records amount of drugs and medications used during local anesthesia.

CIRCULATING ROLE—cont'd

Coordinates all activities in the room with team members and other health-related personnel and departments.
Counts sponges, needles, and instruments.
Monitors practices of aseptic technique in self and others.
Accompanies the client to the postanesthesia recovery area.
Reports pertinent information to the recovery area nurses.

SCRUB ROLE

Reviews anatomy, physiology, and the surgical procedure.
Assists with preparation of the room.
Scrubs, gowns, and gloves self and other members of the surgical team.
Prepares the instrument table and organizes sterile equipment for functional use.
Assists with the draping procedure.
Passes instruments to the surgeon and assistants by anticipating their needs.
Counts sponges, needles, and instruments.
Monitors practices of aseptic technique in self and others.
Keeps track of irrigation solutions used for calculation of blood loss.
Reports amounts of local anesthetics and epinephrine solutions used by anesthetist.

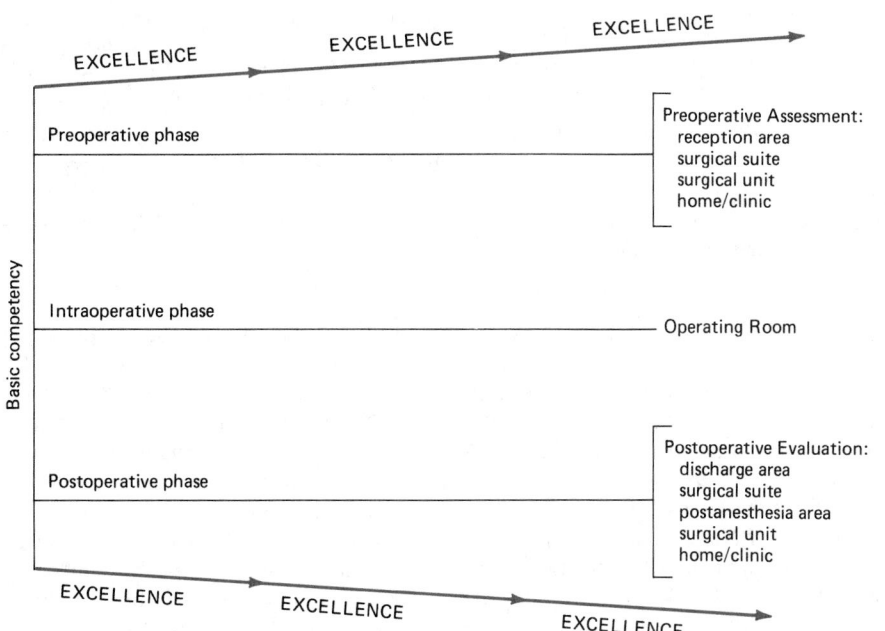

Fig. 12-2 Perioperative practice: a continuum. (From A model for perioperative nursing practice, AORN J 41:190, 1985.)

Table 12-2 Nursing Activities in Perioperative Nursing Practice

Preoperative Phase	Intraoperative Phase	Postoperative Phase
ASSESSMENT	**MAINTENANCE OF SAFETY**	**COMMUNICATION OF INTRAOPERATIVE INFORMATION**

Home/clinic
  Initiates initial preoperative assessment
  Plans teaching methods appropriate to client's needs
  Involves family in interview
Surgical unit
  Completes preoperative assessment
  Coordinates client teaching with other nursing staff
  Explains phases in perioperative period and expectations
  Develops a plan of care
Surgical suite
  Assesses client's level of consciousness
  Reviews chart
  Identifies client
  Verifies surgical site
	Ensures that the sponge, needle, and instrument counts are correct
	Positions the client
	  Functional alignment
	  Exposure of surgical site
	  Maintenance of position throughout procedure
	Applies grounding device to client
	Provides physical support
		Gives client's name
		States type of surgery performed
		Provides contributing intraoperative factors (e.g., drain, catheters)
		States physical limitations
		States impairments resulting from surgery
		Reports client's preoperative level of consciousness
		Communicates necessary equipment needs

PLANNING	**PHYSIOLOGICAL MONITORING**	**POSTOPERATIVE EVALUATION**

Determines a plan of care	Calculates effects on client of excessive fluid loss
	Distinguishes normal from abnormal cardiopulmonary data
	Reports changes in client's pulse, respirations, temperature, and blood pressure
		Recovery area
		  Determines client's immediate response to surgical intervention
		Surgical unit
		  Evaluates effectiveness of nursing care in the OR
		  Determines client's level of satisfaction with care given during perioperative period
		  Evaluates products used on client in the OR
		  Determines client's psychological status
		  Assists with discharge planning
		Home/clinic
		  Seeks client's perception of surgery in terms of the effects of anesthetic agents, impact on body image, distortion, immobilization
		  Determines family's perceptions of surgery

PSYCHOLOGICAL SUPPORT	**PSYCHOLOGICAL MONITORING***	
Tells client what is happening Determines psychological status Gives prior warning of noxious stimuli Communicates client's emotional status to other appropriate members of the health care team	Provides emotional support to client Stands near or touches client during procedures and induction Continues to assess client's emotional status Communicates client's emotional status to other appropriate members of the health care team	
	NURSING MANAGEMENT	
	Provides physical safety for the client Maintains aseptic, controlled environment Effectively manages human resources	

Modified from Association of Operating Room Nurses: A model for perioperative nursing practice, AORN J 41:192-193, 1985.
*Done before induction and if the client is conscious.

Anesthetist*

The term *anesthetist* may be defined as "one who administers anesthesia," and can refer to an anesthesiologist or a nurse anesthetist. An anesthesiologist is a medical doctor who has specialized in the field of anesthesia. A nurse anesthetist is a registered nurse who has graduated from a school accredited by the Council on Accreditation of the American Association of Nurse Anesthetists and has passed national certification examinations to become a certified registered nurse anesthetist (CRNA). Both the anesthesiologist and the nurse anesthetist are qualified to administer anesthetics to the client and to assume responsi-

bility for the maintenance of physiological homeostatis and management of physiological complications throughout the intraoperative period. Regardless of whether the role is filled by an anesthesiologist or a nurse anesthetist, each is responsible for the quality of the practice.

Anesthesia may be provided by anesthesiologists or nurse anesthetists working alone or in combination. The latter is often referred to as the *anesthesia team* approach. When working in the team approach the anesthesiologist assumes the responsibility of supervision of the nurse anesthetist, but the nurse anesthetist is fully responsible for the care personally delivered. When the nurse anesthetist is practicing alone, the surgeon assumes the responsibility for medical supervision. Anesthetists are also governed by the policies of the hospital where they are practicing.

*The terms *anesthesiologist* and *anesthetist* (certified registered nurse anesthetist or CRNA) are used interchangeably in the chapter.

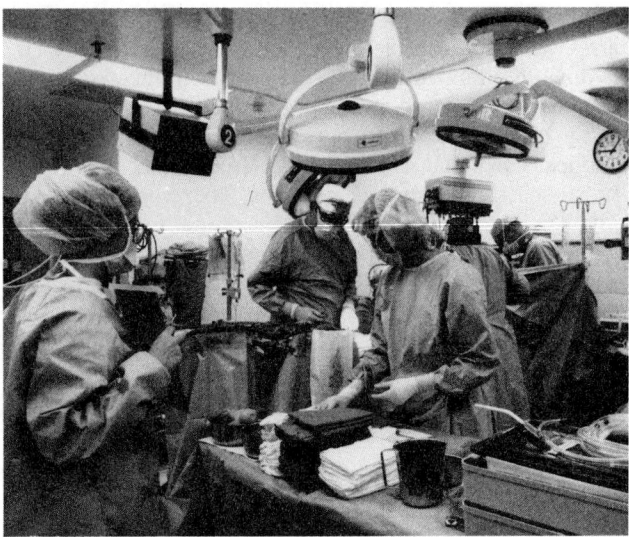

Fig. 12-3 An operative procedure in progress. (Courtesy The Methodist Hospital, Texas Medical Center, Houston, Tex.)

The responsibilities generally accepted for the anesthetist are the following:

1. Assessing the client preoperatively to determine the safest anesthetic for the particular needs and operative procedure
2. Prescribing preoperative medications
3. Administering the anesthetic during the surgical procedure and informing the surgeon if difficulties arise in the client's stability
4. Administering fluids and electrolytes, medications, and blood products throughout the surgical procedure
5. Supervising the postanesthesia recovery of the client

In preparation for and carrying out of the surgical procedure, members of the surgical team (the circulating nurse, the scrub nurse, the surgeon, the assistant, and the anesthetist) collaborate to ensure that the client is receiving the best possible care (Fig. 12-3).

▪ Nursing Management of the Surgical Client

Preoperative phase

Assessment. The preoperative assessment of the surgical client establishes safe intraoperative and postoperative nursing care. Assessment data gathered by the nurse on the surgical unit is pertinent to the nursing care implemented by the perioperative nurse (see Chapter 11). Collaboration between the two nursing units is important so that continuity of client care is ensured.

It is the perioperative nurse's responsibility to participate in the assessment process. When the data cannot be gathered on the surgical unit, they are acquired in the preoperative holding area of the surgical suite (see Table 12-2).

PSYCHOSOCIAL ASSESSMENT. The nurse who regularly provides nursing care in the operating room is knowledgeable about the activities that occur when the client is transferred into the surgical suite. This knowledge allows informative and reassuring explanations, especially to the frightened client.

Fear of the surgical procedure or anesthesia can be alleviated by the perioperative nurse. Specific questions relating to details of the surgical procedure and anesthesia are referred to the surgeon or anesthetist. However, general questions regarding surgery or anesthesia should be answered by the perioperative nurse. Examples of these questions include: "When will I go to sleep?" "Who will be in the room?" "When will my doctor arrive?" "How much of my body will be exposed and to whom?" "Will I be cold?" "When will I wake up?" Knowledge of hospital intraoperative routine provides the data on which to answer such general questions.

It is especially important that the perioperative nurse has knowledge of the client's spiritual and cultural habits and beliefs. Care must be taken that infringement on the client's rights and privileges is not made without prior consent.

PHYSICAL ASSESSMENT. Physical assessment data that are specifically important to intraoperative nursing care include baseline data such as vital signs, height, weight, age, allergic reactions, condition and cleanliness of skin, skeletal and muscle impairments, perceptual difficulties, level of consciousness, and any sources of pain or discomfort. Baseline vital signs are important when drugs and anesthetics are administered. These data provide a means to evaluate the effects of intraoperative medications. Height and weight of the client guide the nurse regarding the placement of the client within the parameters of width and length of the operating table. Age can indicate the need for extra warmth or cooling, since it can reflect the rate of basal metabolism. Some allergic reactions may be avoided with such simple measures as a change in "prepping" solutions or the type of tape used with dressings. The condition and cleanliness of the skin guide the nurse in determining the amount and type of intraoperative skin preparation solutions, as well as alerting the team to the potential for infections because of open or closed skin lesions. A knowledge of skeletal and muscle impairments helps to prevent injury to the client during positioning. Perception difficulty, such as vision or hearing impairments, will guide the nurse to adapt communication techniques to individual needs. An altered level of consciousness necessitates increased safety and protection techniques. Communicating identified sources of pain to other health team members prevents subjecting the client to unnecessary discomfort.

CHART ASSESSMENT. Chart data required vary with hospital policy, client condition, and planned surgical procedure. Examples of data that should be gathered during the preoperative assessment include the following:

1. History and physical examination
2. Urinalysis
3. Complete blood count
4. Signed operative permit
5. Serum electrolyte values
6. Chest x-ray film
7. Electrocardiogram
8. Special diagnostic tests

A knowledge of these chart data will contribute to an understanding of the client's past and present history, cardiopulmonary status, and potential for infection. The chart should be read carefully, since other data pertinent for a particular client will be documented.

Admitting the client. Hospital policy designates the exact procedure that should be followed when admitting the client to the operating room suite. A general routine includes initial greeting, extension of human contact and warmth, and proper identification. The identification process includes asking the client to state name, the surgeon's name, and the operative procedure and location and comparing the hospital identification numbers with the client's identification band and the chart. The client is further identified by the surgeon before the induction of anesthesia. In some institutions this is done in the holding area and in others in the operating room.

The admitting procedure is continued with reassessment of the client and time for last-minute questions. The nurse continues to review the chart for the previously mentioned data and notes any abnormalities. The client is questioned concerning valuables, prostheses, and last intake of food and fluid. Validation is made that the correct preoperative medication was given if ordered, and a warm blanket, pillow, or position adjustment is provided if the client is uncomfortable. Most hospitals require the client's hair to be covered just before transfer.

Intraoperative phase

Transferring the client. Once the client has been properly identified and the operating room has been adequately prepared, the client is transferred into the room for the surgery. Anytime a client is transferred from one bed to another, the wheels of the stretcher should be locked, and a sufficient number of personnel should be available to lift, guide, and prevent accidental falling. Once the client is on the operating table, a safety strap should be snugly placed across the client's thighs. If monitor leads (e.g., electrocardiograph leads) or the intravenous catheter has not been inserted in the preoperative holding area, these are usually applied at this time.

Room preparation. Before transferring the client into the specific operating room, the nurses spend significant time preparing the room to ensure privacy, safety, and prevention of infection. Surgical attire (specially designed pants or dresses, masks, caps or hoods, and shoe covers) is worn by all persons entering the operating room suite. All electrical and mechanical equipment is checked for proper functioning. Aseptic technique is practiced as each surgical item is opened and placed systematically on the instrument table for use. Sponges, needles, and instruments are counted to ensure accurate retrieval at the close of the procedure.

During this time and during the procedure, the roles of the nurses are delineated. The scrub nurse scrubs hands and arms, gowns and gloves in sterile surgical attire, and touches only those items within the sterile field. The circulating nurse remains in the unsterile field and implements those activities that permit touching all unsterile items and the client.

SCRUBBING, GOWNING, AND GLOVING. All sterile members of the surgical team (scrub nurse, surgeon, technician, and assistant) are required to mechanically cleanse their hands and arms with detergent before entering the sterile field. This is done to eliminate dirt and skin oil from the skin and to decrease the microbial count as much as possible. The scrub helps prevent the growth of microbes beneath the surgical gown and gloves. The detergent used should be a broad-spectrum microbicidal agent. The procedure should involve a minimum of 5 minutes of mechanical friction with a specially designed sterile surgical brush. During the actual procedure of scrubbing, the team members' fingers and hands should be scrubbed first with progression to the arms and elbows. The hands should be held higher than the elbows at all times to prevent detergent suds and water from draining from the unclean (above elbows) to the clean and previously scrubbed areas (hands and fingers)[3] (Fig. 12-4).

Once the scrub procedure is completed, the team members enter the room to clothe themselves in the surgical gowns and gloves (Fig. 12-5). Because the gowns and gloves are sterile, it is permissible for the scrubbed person to manipulate and organize all sterile items for use during the procedure.

BASIC ASEPTIC TECHNIQUE. Aseptic technique is practiced in the operating room to prevent the entrance of microorganisms into the surgical wound and thus prevent infections. This is implemented through the creation and maintenance of a sterile field. The center of the sterile field is the site of the surgical incision. Inanimate items in the sterile field include surgical items and equipment that have been sterilized by appropriate sterilization methods.

There are specific principles that the team members should understand to practice aseptic technique. Unless

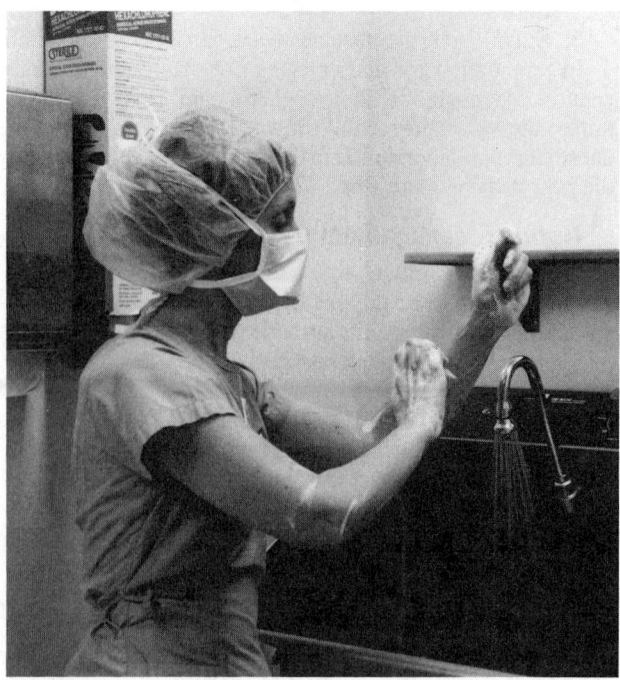

Fig. 12-4 Surgical scrub. (Courtesy The Methodist Hospital, Texas Medical Center, Houston, Tex.)

these principles are followed, the safety of the client is compromised and the potential for postoperative infection is increased. Table 12-3 presents basic principles of aseptic technique.[1,4]

Assisting the anesthesia team. During the time the nurse checks the operating room to complete its preparation, the anesthesia team is preparing the client for the administration of the anesthetic. The nurse must understand the mechanism of anesthetic administration as well as the pharmacological effects of the agents. The nurse should know the location of all emergency drugs and equipment in the operating room area.

The circulating nurse is involved in placing monitoring

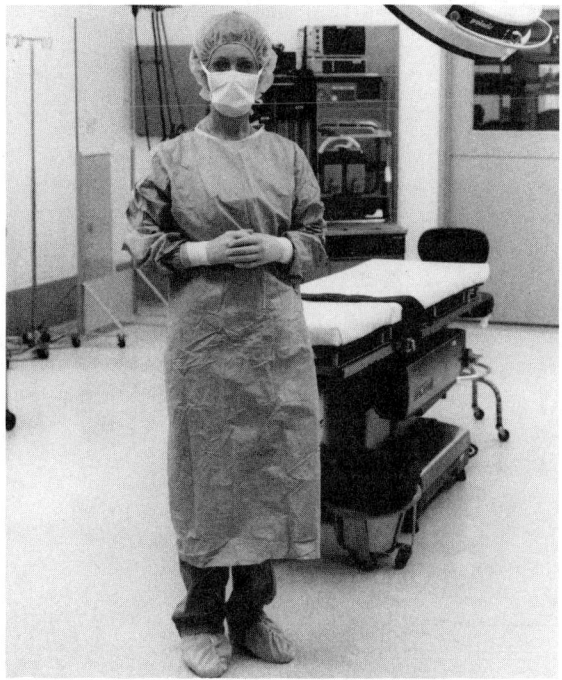

Fig. 12-5 Sterile surgical attire. (Courtesy The Methodist Hospital, Texas Medical Center, Houston, Tex.)

devices to be used during the surgical procedure (e.g., urinary catheter, ECG leads), as well as the electrical grounding pad.

If the client is to have a general anesthetic, the nurse remains at the client's side to ensure safety and assist the anesthetist if needed. These responsibilities may include protecting the client from falling, obtaining blood pressure measurements, and starting an intravenous line.

Positioning the client. Positioning the client usually follows induction of a general anesthetic, or if a different anesthetic technique is used, the anesthetist will indicate when to begin positioning of the client. At this time, relaxation and surgical exposure can best be facilitated. When positioning for the surgical procedure, care must be used to (1) provide correct skeletal alignment, (2) prevent undue pressure on bony prominences and skin, (3) provide for adequate thoracic excursion, (4) prevent occlusion of arteries and veins, (5) avoid stretching and compression of nerve tissue, (6) provide modesty in exposure, and (7) recognize and respect individual needs such as previously assessed aches, pains, or deformities. It is a nursing responsibility to secure the extremities, provide adequate padding and support, and obtain sufficient physical or mechanical help to avoid unnecessary straining on self or the client.

Various positions in which the client may be positioned include supine, prone, Trendelenburg, lateral, kidney, lithotomy, jackknife (Kraske), and sitting (Fig. 12-6). The supine is the most common position used. It is suited for surgery involving the gastrointestinal tract, heart, and breast. The prone position allows easy access for back surgeries (e.g., laminectomies). The lithotomy position is used for some pelvic organ surgery (e.g., vaginal hysterectomy). The sitting position is used for craniotomies.[5]

Preparing the surgical site. The goal of skin preparation (prepping) is to reduce the number of organisms available to migrate to the surgical wound. The preoperative skin preparation discussed in Chapter 11 is vital. However, intraoperatively another skin preparation is done immediately before the incision is made. The task of prepping is usually the responsibility of the circulating nurse.

The skin is prepared by mechanically scrubbing or cleansing with antimicrobial agents identified as being

---

Table 12-3 Principles of Basic Aseptic Technique in the Operating Room

1. All materials that enter the sterile field must be sterile.
2. Sterilization is the only means by which an item can be considered sterile; if it comes in contact with an unsterile item, it becomes contaminated.
3. Contaminated items should be removed immediately from the sterile field.
4. Sterile team members must wear only sterile gowns; once dressed for the procedure, they should recognize that all parts of the gown are considered *unsterile* except the front from chest to table level and the sleeves to 2 inches above the elbow.
5. A wide margin of safety must be maintained between the sterile and unsterile fields.
6. Team members' motions should be from sterile to sterile or from unsterile to unsterile.
7. Tables are considered sterile only at tabletop level, and items extending beneath this level are considered contaminated.
8. The edges of a sterile package are considered contaminated once the package has been opened.
9. Bacteria travel on airborne particles and will enter the sterile field with excessive air movements and currents.
10. Bacteria travel with moisture and liquids by capillary action from surface to surface.
11. Bacteria harbor on the client's and the team members' hair, skin, and respiratory tracts.

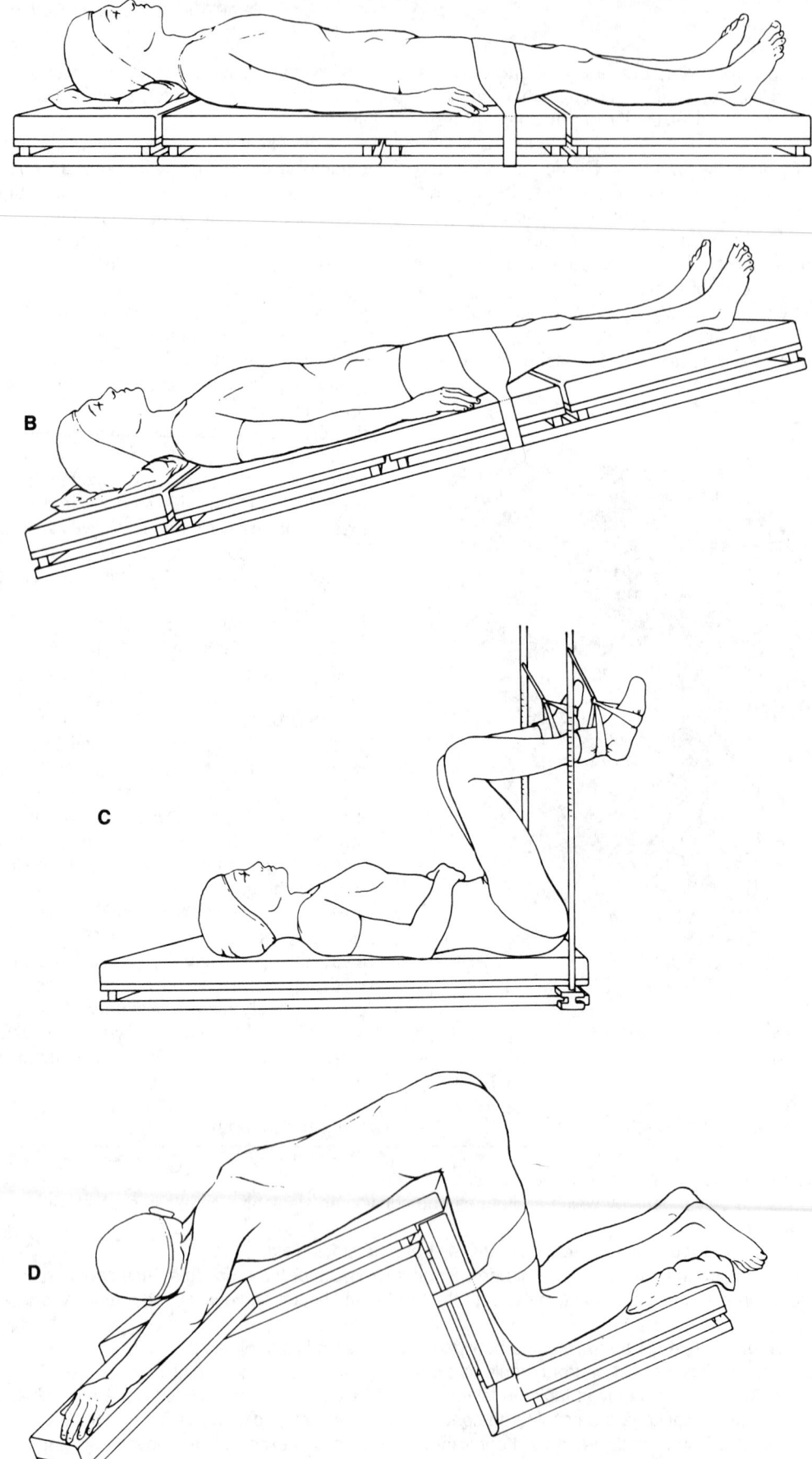

Fig. 12-6 Positioning the client in surgery. **A,** Dorsal recumbent (supine) position. **B,** Trendelenburg's position. **C,** Lithotomy position for vaginal and rectal operations. **D,** Jackknife position for proctological operation.

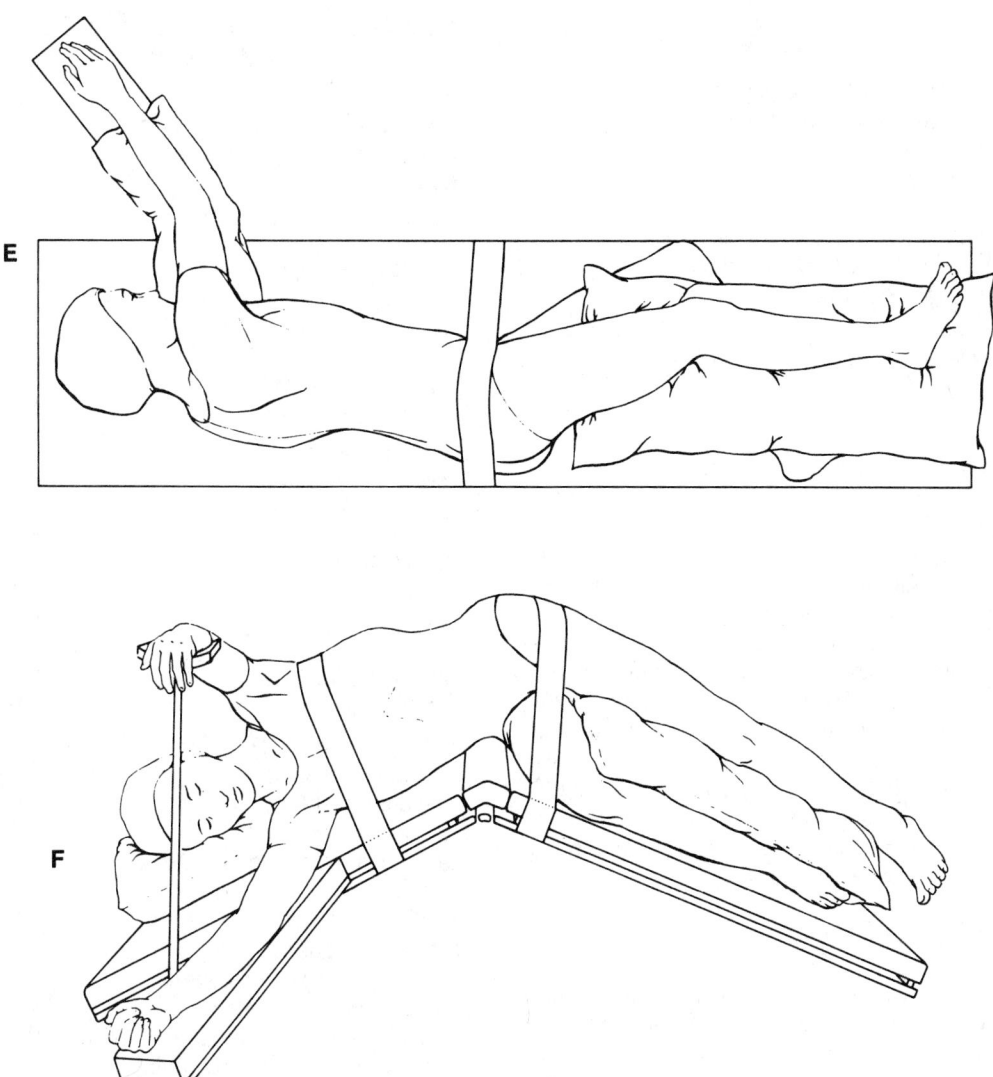

Fig. 12-6—cont'd **E,** Lateral position for chest operations. **F,** Lateral position for kidney operations. (From Meeker MH and Rothrock JC: Alexander's care of the patient in surgery, ed 9, St Louis, 1991, Mosby—Year Book, Inc, pp 107-112.)

nonallergic to the client. The nurse first ensures that excess hair has been removed from the area around the surgical site (if indicated). This area is then scrubbed in a circular motion. The principle of scrubbing from the clean area (site of the incision) to the dirty area (periphery) is observed at all times. A liberal area is cleansed to allow for added protection and unexpected occurrences during the procedure.

After preparation of the client's skin, the sterile members of the surgical team drape the area. Only the site to be incised is left exposed.

Postoperative phase

Toward the end of the surgical procedure the anesthetist begins to reverse the effects of the anesthetic agents so that the client will emerge more rapidly. This not only allows more physiological control of the client during the transfer to the postanesthesia area but also encourages more rapid and safer recovery.

The anesthetist and the surgeon or another member of the surgical team accompany the client to the postanesthesia care area or recovery room. A report of the client's status and the procedure is communicated (see Chapter 13).

During this portion of the intraoperative and postoperative phases of client care the perioperative nurse initiates evaluation of the client's response to nursing care. Evaluation of client care is most effectively determined when the nurse addresses outcome criteria, which are found in Table 12-4.[6]

CLASSIFICATION OF ANESTHESIA

The anesthetic method and agent are selected by the anesthetist in collaboration with the surgeon and the client. Factors contributing to the decision include the client's current health status and history, emotional stability, and factors relating to the operative procedure (e.g., length, position, site, use of electrocautery). The anesthetist vali-

Table 12-4 Outcome Criteria for the Surgical Client

Demonstration of knowledge of the physiological and psychological responses to surgical intervention
Freedom from infection
Maintenance of skin integrity
Freedom from injury related to positioning, extraneous objects, or chemical, physical, and electrical hazards
Maintenance of fluid and electrolyte balance
Participation in the rehabilitative process

Modified from Association of Operating Room Nurses: Patient outcome standards for perioperative nursing, AORN J 39:40, 1984.

dates this information during the preoperative assessment, makes the final decision, and writes the order for the preoperative medication.

Anesthesia is classified according to the effect that it has on the client's sensorium (central nervous system) and pain perception. *General anesthesia* is defined as the loss of sensation with a loss of consciousness and reflexes. *Local anesthesia* is defined as loss of sensation without loss of consciousness and generally refers to infiltration of a local anesthetic agent in a limited area. *Regional anesthesia* is defined as the loss of sensation to a region of the body without loss of consciousness (e.g., spinal or epidural blocks). That is, general anesthesia has a direct effect on the central nervous system, and local anesthesia interrupts nerve impulses along the nerve fiber cells.

General Anesthesia

General anesthesia is usually the category of choice for clients who (1) are having surgical procedures that require significant skeletal muscle relaxation, last for long periods of time, or require awkward positions because of the location of the incisional site; (2) are extremely anxious; and (3) refuse local or regional anesthetic techniques. General anesthetics can be administered by four different methods: *intravenous, inhalation, rectal,* and *intramuscular* (Table 12-5).

Intravenous induction agents. Virtually all routine adult general anesthetics begin with an intravenous induction agent. These agents have a smooth and rapid action that clients find very desirable, but they do not maintain the unconscious state more than a few minutes if given alone. These agents can be separated into barbiturates and nonbarbiturate hypnotics.

Barbiturates. The most frequently administered intravenous agents to induce general anesthesia are the short-acting barbiturates. Of those available, the two most frequently used are thiopental sodium (Pentothal) and sodium methohexital (Brevital).

Induction with both agents is rapid. In higher doses, these agents can cause cardiovascular depression, hypotension, tachycardia, and respiratory depression and/or apnea that may last into the postoperative period and require close observation or even mechanical ventilation. Leakage of the barbiturates into the tissue surrounding the vein can cause severe pain and damage because of the alkalinity of

Table 12-5 General Anesthesia Drugs and Methods

INTRAVENOUS AGENTS
Barbiturates

Thiopental sodium (Pentothal)
Sodium methohexital (Brevital)

Nonbarbiturate hypnotic

Etomidate (Amidate)
Propofol (Diprivan)

INHALATION AGENTS
Volatile liquids

Halothane (Fluothane)
Enflurane (Ethrane)
Isoflurane (Forane)

Gaseous agents

Nitrous oxide
Compressed air

ANESTHESIA ADJUNCTS
Narcotics

Fentanyl (Sublimaze)
Sufentanil (Sufenta)
Alfentanil (Alfenta)
Morphine sulfate
Meperidine hydrochloride (Demerol)

Muscle relaxants

Depolarizing agents
   Succinylcholine (Anectine)
Nondepolarizing agents
   Vecuronium bromide (Norcuron)
   Atacurium besylate (Tracrium)
   Pancuronium bromide (Pavulon)
   Tubocurarine (Curare)
   Metocurarine (Metubine)
   Gallamine triethiodide (Flaxedil)

Hypnotic-sedatives

Midazolam (Versed)
Diazepam (Valium)

Antiemetics

Droperidol (Inapsine)
Dissociative anesthetics
Ketamine hydrochloride (Ketalar)

the drugs. If they are injected into an artery, arterial spasms may occur.[7]

Rectal administration of short-acting barbiturates is used only occasionally today because of individual differences in absorption rate in the colon. This type of anesthetic is most frequently administered to children to produce a sleep state before the use of other anesthetics.

Nonbarbiturate hypnotics. Etomidate (Amidate) and propofol (Diprivan) are nonbarbiturate hypnotic agents. Etomidate produces little or no cardiovascular or respiratory depression. These features make it preferable to the barbiturates in potentially unstable clients. Cardiovascular and respiratory depression is dose related with propofol. An annoying side effect common to both agents is pain on injection. Etomidate also can cause myoclonia and postoperative nausea and vomiting. Propofol can be used as an induction agent and to maintain general anesthetic levels. Its extremely rapid elimination may favor its use in short (less than 2 hours) outpatient procedures in which shortened recovery time and early discharge are important. Propofol also causes less nausea and vomiting than many other anesthetic agents.[7]

Inhalation agents. The inhalation agents use for general anesthesia may be *volatile liquids* (liquid at room temperature) or *gases* (gas at room temperature). Volatile liquids are vaporized into a gaseous state together with a carrier gas such as oxygen. The oxygen and anesthetic vapor are passed through a precalibrated vaporizer on the anesthesia machine. The gaseous agents are stored in pressurized tanks and their delivery is controlled by calibrated flowmeters on the anesthesia machine. All inhalation agents are administered with oxygen to prevent hypoxic mixtures being delivered to the client.

Inhalation agents enter the body through the alveoli in the respiratory tract. This makes them desirable because their depth can be quickly altered through changes in the respiratory exchange. However, an undesirable characteristic is their irritating effect on the respiratory passages. Complications that may arise are coughing, laryngospasm (muscular spasms of the larynx), increased secretions, and, at deep planes of anesthesia, respiratory depression and obstruction. In addition, some of the agents stimulate the vomiting center of the brain, leading to the potential for postoperative aspiration of secretions.[8]

Inhalation agents may be administered through a mask, a tracheal tube, or an endotracheal tube. They may also be used to induce the general anesthetic (usually through a mask) in a technique known as an *inhalation induction*. Exhaled gases from the client pass through the anesthesia machine and through a system that allows for reabsorption of the carbon dioxide before it is mixed with more fresh gases and vaporized volatile agent. These agents are also used to maintain the anesthetic state. The safest means of delivery of these anesthetic gas mixtures is through a cuffed endotracheal tube. Proper positioning of the endotracheal tube must be ensured by auscultation of the chest immediately after intubation to detect (1) endobronchial intubation (the tube is inserted too far and only one lung is ventilated) or (2) esophageal intubation. If these are detected immediately, the problem can be corrected quickly without catastrophic results. The endotracheal tube with an inflated cuff permits mechanical ventilation, control of respiration with an open airway, easy access to the tracheobronchial tree for suctioning, and less chance for regurgitation of stomach contents and aspirated secretions. In emergency surgical procedures in which the client has not been on NPO status, the circulating nurse will frequently be responsible for applying pressure on the anterior neck over the cricoid cartilage (Sellick's maneuver). This compresses the esophagus to prevent aspiration of stomach contents before inflation of the protective cuff. The nurse must be certain that suction is readily available to the anesthetist at the time of induction and throughout the intraoperative period.

Complications of endotracheal intubation include those primarily associated with its insertion and removal. These include damage to teeth, laryngospasm, laryngeal edema, postoperative sore throat, and/or hoarseness due to injury or irritation of the vocal cords or surrounding tissues.[9]

After the endotracheal tube is removed, the nurse should observe for respiratory complications. Oxygen, suction apparatus, emergency drugs, and equipment for reinsertion of the endotracheal tube must be readily available.

Volatile Liquids. Diethyl ether was introduced during the nineteenth century and was accepted as the first useful general anesthetic agent. Certain signs were identified as stages of anesthesia as the client passed from altered consciousness (stage 1) to excitement (stage 2) to surgical relaxation (stage 3). If an overdose had occurred, the client would have progressed to stage 4 (circulatory and respiratory failure). These stages were readily identified because the induction of the anesthetic progressed very slowly with ether. Today, the client passes through these stages very quickly, since induction with the newer agents is much more rapid. Although the nurse should be aware that these stages do occur, priority is not placed on being able to identify them.[9]

Agents such as diethyl ether, cyclopropane, ethylene, and divinyl ether are considered obsolete because of their inflammability. The only agents that should be used in operating rooms are those that meet all recommendations of the National Fire Protection Association.

Methoxyflurane (Penthrane), a nonexplosive agent, is the strongest of the volatile agents but the least often administered because of the occurrence of nephrotoxicity.[7] For this reason, it is now not used clinically when there are better agents available.

Halothane (Fluothane) is a halogenated hydrocarbon that is nonexplosive and nonirritating to the respiratory tract. In appropriate doses it is a strong anesthetic and bronchodilator, and it has a low incidence of postoperative nausea and vomiting. During its administration, cardiac depression and peripheral vasodilation resulting in hypotension may occur. Although hepatic inflammation and damage have occurred after the use of halothane anesthetics, halothane has never been fully implicated to be the causative agent. Because halothane has a documented history of hepatotoxcity, its use has decreased dramatically as better agents have become available. It is now rarely used for adults. Pediatric clients have never been shown to have the hepatic problems with halothane, so use of this agent is still very prevalent in inhalation inductions in children because its odor is less pungent than the other inhalation agents in current use.[10]

Halothane sensitizes the myocardium to the presence of catecholamines, which increases the incidence of ventricular dysrhythmias. The nurse should make careful calculations of the dose of epinephrine injected during surgical procedures. The anesthetist needs to be informed of its use before injection.

Enflurane (Ethrane) is a halogenated ether that is nonexplosive and rapid acting. It allows ready management of cardiovascular status and produces minimal respiratory secretions. It is also a good muscle relaxant and provides for rapid postoperative recovery with minimal nausea and vomiting. Seizure activity has been seen during enflurane anesthesia at high concentrations. Enflurane can cause renal damage in some situations. Because recovery is rapid and there is little residual analgesia, the nurse should realistically evaluate the occurrence of pain in the postoperative period.

Isoflurane (Forane) is also a halogenated ether that is an isomer of enflurane but with very different properties. It is also nonexplosive and even more rapid acting than enflurane. Its metabolism by the body is minimal, and it has not been found to be toxic to any organs of the body. Isoflurane also causes much less cardiovascular depression than either halothane or enflurane and is preferable in potentially unstable clients. Higher concentrations of isoflurane do produce tachycardias at times, but this is generally diminished by the other anesthesia adjuncts. As with all inhalation agents, analgesia leaves the client very rapidly, so the nurse must be ready to evaluate the occurrence of pain in the postoperative period. Isoflurane is used more than any other inhalation agent in the United States at this time.

Gaseous Agents. Nitrous oxide is a gaseous agent that provides more analgesia than unconsciousness. It is the most widely administered gas because of its favorable qualities. Nitrous oxide use speeds the passage of the volatile anesthetics into the client. Because it is a weak anesthetic, nitrous oxide is administered as a single agent only in minor procedures requiring little anesthesia and muscular relaxation. When it is administered in combination with other anesthetic agents, its potentiating effects allow smaller amounts of the accompanying drugs. Its primary harmful effect results from administration without a sufficient amount of oxygen. This can lead to varying degrees of hypoxia and respiratory depression. Its effects are readily reversible by its discontinuation. The major concern with the use of nitrous oxide is that recent clinical studies have shown significant cardiac depression with its use.[7] This can cause problems if the client has existing cardiac disease or dysfunction. Nitrous oxide has also been shown to cause an increased incidence of nausea and vomiting because of its effects on the middle and inner ear. Nitrous oxide also diffuses into existing air spaces in the body and can cause problems if the increase in pressure cannot be equalized.

Compressed air may be used with oxygen in the client in whom nitrous oxide use would be precluded. These situations may include (1) severe cardiac disease, (2) history of nausea and/or vomiting with nitrous oxide use, (3) existing bowel obstruction, and (4) surgery of the middle or inner ear.

Helium is another gas that is used occasionally. It has limited use because the gas is very expensive.

Adjuncts to general anesthesia. As mentioned previously, general anesthesia is rarely limited to one agent. Agents added to the anesthetic (other than intravenous induction agents or inhalation agents) are called *adjuncts*. These agents are added to the anesthetic for several reasons, which may include pain relief, amnesia, and muscle relaxation. Adjuncts include opiates, neuromuscular blocking agents (muscle relaxants), and hypnotics. Generally, the reasons for adding these agents are varied and combined. Most often, a goal of the anesthetist is rapid awaking of a comfortable and pain-free client. Combinations of these adjuncts may be added to accomplish this goal. Opiates decrease the concentrations of inhalation agents used and allow for analgesia to continue into the postoperative period. Use of muscle relaxants also decreases the concentrations of the inhalation agents used by ensuring that the client will be relaxed for an optimal surgical situation and will not move. Using lesser concentrations of inhalation agents may sometimes allow recall of events under anesthesia, but addition of the hypnotic agents can ensure that the amnestic state will be intact.

Opiates. Opiates are also called *narcotics*. The most common opiates in use in anesthesia today are fentanyl (Sublimaze), sufentanil (Sufenta), and alfentanil (Alfenta). These are all synthetic opiates, and sufentanil and alfentanil are analogs of fentanyl. These agents are all extremely potent but, at the same time, short acting. Sufentanil is the most potent of these opiates and provides the most cardiovascular stability of any of the opiates. For this reason, it is used as a sole agent in most cardiovascular surgery. Narcotics in very high doses, combined with muscle relaxants, can serve in an anesthetic capacity, but recall has been observed. For this reason, hypnotic agents are also added in this technique. Alfentanil is less potent than fentanyl or sufentanil, but its length of action is also much shorter, so its use is seen frequently in anesthetics for short outpatient procedures. Morphine sulfate and occasionally meperidine hydrochloride (Demerol) are used, but they tend to have more undesirable side effects. The use of morphine sulfate and meperidine hydrochloride is seen much more in the postoperative period.

The primary disadvantage of all opiates is respiratory depression by slowing of the respiratory rate. These effects should be closely monitored by the nurse in the postanesthesia period.

Neuromuscular Blocking Agents. Neuromuscular blocking agents (muscle relaxants) are a group of agents given to the client to produce paralysis. These agents can produce deep muscle relaxation with relatively light levels of anesthesia. This stage of surgical relaxation is very important, since adequate surgical exposure and relaxation are essential in many types of surgical procedures. The nurse should know that client awareness occasionally occurs under deep-relaxation, light anesthesia techniques. Therefore care should be taken to keep the operating room as quiet as possible.

The two categories of muscle relaxants or neuromuscular blocking agents are *depolarizing agents* and *nondepolarizing agents*. Depolarizing agents such as succinylcholine (Anectine) depolarize the motor end plate and prevent further depolarization. This yields paralysis until uptake and metabolism of the agent occurs and allows nerve conduction to return to normal function, usually within 10 minutes. Nondepolarizing agents such as vecuronium bromide (Norcuron), atracurium besylate (Tracrium), tubocurarine (Tubarine), pancuronium bromide (Pavulon), metocurine (Metubine), and gallamine triethiodide (Flaxedil), interfere with nerve impulse transmission at the myoneural junction by competing at the motor end plate with acetylcholine. As with the depolarizing agents, the end result is paralysis, with the effects lasting much longer than with the depolarizing agents.[11]

Disadvantages involving the administration of muscle relaxants are of special concern to the postanesthesia nurse. The duration of their action may be longer than the surgical procedure, or reversal agents may not be effective in completely eliminating the residual effects. The client must be carefully observed for airway patency and respiratory muscle movement. Lack of movement and return of reflexes and strength may indicate the need for an artificial airway and ventilator. If the client is intubated, the endotracheal tube should not be removed without careful assessment of return of muscular strength and tidal volume. A good test of the client's strength is the ability to lift the head off the bed and hold it up for a few seconds.

Hypnotics. Hypnotics are agents that cause amnesia and sedation. Their use in anesthesia is varied and may be for induction of general anesthesia or as sedatives and hypnotics for the supplementation of local and regional anesthesia. Their use for induction of general anesthesia involves use of higher doses than would be used in the awake client. When administered, these agents should be given in small incremental doses until the desired effect is reached. Administration in this manner allows the nurse to observe the client closely for the side effects of these agents, which are mainly respiratory depression, airway obstruction, apnea, and cardiovascular depression. Respiratory depression is the most frequent side effect but is generally not seen unless the agents are administered too rapidly or in doses that are too high. The nurse must be aware that these agents will potentiate any narcotics, sedatives, or sedative side effects from any other medications administered.

The most commonly used hypnotics are in the benzodiazapine class: diazepam (Valium) and midazolam (Versed). Because of its superior amnestic properties and lighter sedation, midazolam is presently the most frequently used hypnotic in anesthesia.

Antiemetics. Antiemetics are medications that reduce or eliminate the incidence of nausea and vomiting. The most commonly used agent for this purpose in anesthesia is droperidol (Inapsine). This agent has antiemetic properties at all doses and heavy sedation and tranquilization properties at higher doses. As with the hypnotics, droperidol will potentiate the depressant effect of any other medications given to the client.

Dissociative Anesthetics. Dissociative anesthetics interrupt associative brain pathways while blocking sensory pathways. The client may appear awake but is actually asleep. The agent administered as a dissociative anesthetic is ketamine hydrochloride (Ketalar). It is particularly ad-

vantageous in that it does not relax upper airway muscles and tissues. Therefore the probability of airway obstruction is minimal. In spite of this advantage, ketamine should never be administered without resuscitative equipment immediately available. Since ketamine has no cardiac-depressant effect, it is a suitable agent in clients who are poor surgical risks.

Ketamine's principal disadvantage is the hallucinogenic state it produces in the postoperative period. The likelihood of this is reduced by keeping the total dose of the drug as low as possible and by using adjunct drugs. The nurse should approach the client slowly and quietly, since startling touch and loud sounds may elicit hallucinatory reactions. Ketamine may be administered intravenously or intramuscularly.[8] Ketamine's hallucinations flashbacks (recurrence of bad dreams) preclude its use in adults and adolescents, but it is still useful in pediatric and geriatric clients in whom the hallucinogenic incidence is much less. Intramuscular administration of ketamine is occasionally used in children who are uncooperative or who need painful procedures before an inhalation anesthetic. This produces a sleepy, cooperative state before the use of other anesthetic agents.

Local Anesthesia

Local anesthetics allow an operative procedure to be performed on a part of the body without loss of consciousness. All local anesthetics act by blocking the conduction of nerve impulses through altering nerve cell permeability to sodium, resulting in a decrease in the degree of membrane depolarization to prevent the development of a propagated action potential.[12]

Local anesthetics frequently administered are cocaine, procaine hydrochloride, tetracaine hydrochloride (Pontocaine), dibucaine hydrochloride (Nupercaine), lidocaine hydrochloride (Xylocaine), mepivacaine hydrochloride (Carbocaine), and bupivacaine hydrochloride (Marcaine).

Advantages. Advantages of local anesthesia are numerous for the client who is assessed as a suitable recipient. A suitable client is one who is not allergic to the drug, who is having a surgical procedure that does not require an unconscious state, and whose anxiety or apprehension is not excessive. Because loss of consciousness does not occur, the induction and recovery hazards of a general anesthetic do not exist. Minimum equipment is needed, and the cost is lower. Local anesthesia is especially beneficial for persons who have taken in liquids or solid food before surgery or who are having minor procedures performed on an outpatient basis.

Disadvantages. Disadvantages of local anesthesia include (1) lack of client acceptance because of awareness during the procedure, (2) lack of feasibility of localizing some anatomical sites, and (3) unanticipated rapid absorption of the agent into the bloodstream in unsuspected circumstances. Manifestations of overdose and/or rapid absorption include lightheadedness, dizziness, ringing in ears, loss of consciousness, and seizure activity.[5]

Methods of administration. There are a variety of methods for administering local anesthetics (Table 12-6). *Topical application* is application of the agent directly to

Table 12-6 Methods for Administering Local Anesthesics

Regional application	Topical application
Nerve block	Local infiltration
Intravenous regional block	
Field block	
Central nerve blocks	
Spinal block	
Epidural block	
Lumbar-peridural block	
Caudal-sacral block	

the skin, mucous membrane, or open surface. *Local infiltration* is injection of the agent into the tissues through which the surgical incision will pass. *Regional application* is injection of the agent at some location along the conductive nerve pathway to and from the region selected to be anesthetized. Regional application is achieved away from the surgical field.

There are several types of regional anesthesia. The *nerve block* is the injection of a specific nerve at a given point, as an intercostal, median, or axillary nerve block. The *intravenous regional block* with a tourniquet (Bier's block) is the injection of the agent intravenously into an extremity after a tourniquet has been applied and the extremity exsanguinated. The tourniquet should always remain inflated a minimum of 30 minutes. The nurse should observe the client when the tourniquet is released. It is possible to have symptoms of local anesthetic overdose when the tourniquet is released. Therefore, the nurse should observe the client closely at that time. The *field block* is a type of infiltration anesthesia in which the anesthetic is injected around the area of the surgical procedure by a series of injections. *Central nerve blocks* are those that anesthetize the spinal cord nerves (motor and sensory) near their origin. The *spinal block* affects the nerves in the subarachnoid space, and the *epidural block* affects those nerve roots passing through the epidural space. The epidural block may use a lumbar or a sacral approach.[13]

Epidural and spinal anesthesia. Spinal or epidural anesthesia is achieved by injection of a local anesthetic agent into the spinal fluid (subarachnoid) or the epidural space between two lumbar vertebrae. Once injected, sensory and motor sympathetic routes of the nerve cell are anesthetized. Anesthesia spreads to the uppermost desired level as additional fibers are gradually affected.

Epidural or spinal anesthesia is administered primarily for surgery of the lower abdomen and lower extremities. The client can remain conscious during the surgical procedure or can be sedated. The onset of spinal anesthesia is faster than that of epidural anesthesia because the spinal nerves are uncovered in the subarachnoid space and absorb the drug more rapidly. The effects are usually more pronounced with the spinal anesthetic, although profound sympathetic blockade can be seen with either technique.

The client must be closely observed for manifestations induced by blockage of the sympathetic nervous system. These include hypotension, bradycardia, and nausea and vomiting. If the block extends upward, the client may experience respiratory depression. The level of the sensory and sympathetic block is controlled by the amount of drug used, the rapidity of injection, and the position of the operating table.

An advantage of epidural over spinal anesthesia is lack of postanesthesia headache. The headache experienced after spinal anesthesia is thought to occur from leakage of spinal fluid at the site of injection. The incidence of headaches is seen much less now with the common use of smaller-gauge spinal needles (22 gauge or smaller). A headache is possible after an epidural anesthetic if the needle is advanced too far and punctures the dura. This "wet tap" is done with a 17- or 18-gauge epidural needle and almost always produces a headache. All clients who have spinal anesthesia should be encouraged to force fluids postoperatively to help prevent this complication.

Additional Anesthesia Mechanisms

Controlled hypotension is a technique used during the administration of anesthetics to decrease the amount of expected blood loss by lowering the blood pressure. *Hypothermia* is the deliberate lowering of the body temperature to decrease body metabolism and thus reduce the need for oxygen. *Cryoanesthesia* involves cooling or freezing a localized area to block pain impulses of localized nerve impulses. *Hypnoanesthesia* uses hypnosis to produce an alteration in pain consciousness. *Acupuncture* achieves loss of sensation by the use of intense local stimulation with fine-gauge needles at meridian points throughout the body.[5]

Intraoperative Implications of Age Extremes

Although anesthetic agents have become safer over the years, pediatric and older adult clients demonstrate varying and unique responses to the anesthetizing process. Several physiological alterations may occur because of immature metabolic processes or the aging process.

The older adult client experiences a decrease in the respiratory protective reflexes. There are decreased ability to cough, increased mucosal secretions, decreased thoracic compliance, and degeneration in lung parenchymal tissue. This series of alterations in pulmonary status may lead to a decrease in ventilation and perfusion. These changes, in combination with the geriatric client's decreased ability to readily eliminate pharmacological agents, have many implications for before, during, and after surgery. Reactions to anesthetic agents need to be carefully monitored and their postoperative elimination assessed before the client is left without one-to-one nursing supervision.[14]

Circulatory function in the older adult is altered because of thickened elastic fibers in the vasculature. As a result, compensatory responses to changes in blood pressure and volume are decreased. There is a decreased circulating blood volume, and blood pressure is usually increased. Circulatory parameters need to be closely monitored throughout surgery and into the postanesthesia period.

Renal perfusion in the older adult usually decreases,

and there is a decrease in the ability of the client to excrete those drugs that are normally excreted by the kidney. Because the glomerular filtration rate decreases, renal cortical vascular deterioration occurs. This increases the client's susceptibility to renal failure. Signs of renal failure are carefully assessed intraoperatively as well as in the postoperative phase of the client's care.

Many older adult clients experience a decrease in their ability to communicate because of presbyopia and presbycusis. This poses a special need for clear and concise communication in the operating room, especially when preoperative sedation is superimposed on the existing sensory deficit. Skin elasticity in the older adult is decreased because of atrophy and loss of collagen. This makes the skin very sensitive to injury from tape, electrodes, warming and cooling blankets, and certain types of dressing. In addition, the older adult client often has fragile bones and osteoarthritis. These factors reinforce the need for careful transferring, lifting, and positioning techniques.[15]

R eview Questions

The number of the question corresponds to the same-numbered objective at the beginning of the chapter.

1. Which of the following characteristics of the operating room environment facilitates the prevention of infection in the surgical client?
   a. conductive furniture
   b. filters in the ventilating system
   c. explosion-proof electrical plugs
   d. adjustable lighting
2. Select from the following the activity that is *not* a function of the registered nurse in the operating room.
   a. administering local anesthetic
   b. checking electrical equipment
   c. implementing the nursing process
   d. scrubbing for the surgical procedure
3. Preoperative assessment by the perioperative nurse is initiated in a variety of settings. Which setting is inappropriate for preoperative client assessment?
   a. home or clinic setting
   b. clinical unit
   c. postanesthesia care unit
   d. preoperative holding areas
4. When scrubbing at the scrub sink, the surgical team members should
   a. hold hands higher than the elbows
   b. scrub from elbows to hands
   c. scrub for a minimum of 10 minutes
   d. scrub without mechanical friction
5. Mrs. Jones is scheduled for an abdominal hysterectomy. She is extremely anxious and has a tendency to hyperventilate when upset. Which type of anes-

thetic would probably be most appropriate for Mrs. Jones?
   a. general anesthetic
   b. local anesthetic
6. Clients having general anesthesia usually prefer induction with intravenous agents because
   a. they are nonexplosive agents
   b. induction is rapid and pleasant
   c. the client is not intubated
   d. the odor of the agent is not offensive
7. The injection of the local anesthetic into the tissues through which the surgical incision will pass is the technique of
   a. topical application
   b. nerve block
   c. regional application
   d. local infiltration
8. Deliberate lowering of the body temperature to decrease body metabolism is known as
   a. controlled hypotension
   b. hypothermia
   c. hypnoanesthesia
   d. none of the above

REFERENCES

1. Gruendemann BJ and Meeker MJ: Alexander's care of the patient in surgery, St Louis, 1987, The CV Mosby Co.
2. Association of Operating Room Nurses: A model of perioperative nursing practice, AORN J 41:188-194, 1985.
3. Association of Operating Room Nurses: Recommended practices for surgical hand scrubs, AORN J 39:1084-1085, 1984.
4. Association of Operating Room Nurses: Recommended practices for basic aseptic technique. In AORN standards of practice, Denver, 1987, Association of Operating Room Nurses.
5. Atkinson LJ and Kohn ML: Berry and Kohn's introduction to operating room techniques, ed 6, New York, 1986, McGraw-Hill Book Co.
6. Association of Operating Room Nurses: Patient outcome standards for perioperative nursing, AORN J 39:400, 1984.
7. Wood M and Wood AJ: Drugs and anesthesia: pharmacology for anesthesiologists, ed 2, Baltimore, 1990, Williams & Wilkins.
8. Barash PG, Cullen BF, and Stoelting RK: Clinical anesthesia, Philadelphia, 1989, JB Lippincott Co.
9. Miller RD: Anesthesia, ed 2, vol 1, New York, 1986, Churchill Livingstone.
10. Miller RD: Anesthesia, ed 2, vol 2, New York, 1981, Churchill Livingstone.
11. Katz RL: Muscle relaxants: basic and clinical aspects, New York, 1985, Grune & Stratton.
12. Scott DB: Techniques of regional anaesthesia, Norwalk, Conn, 1989, Appleton & Lange/Mediglobe.
13. Miller RD: Anesthesia, ed 2, vol 2, New York, 1986, Churchill Livingstone.
14. Blitt CD: Monitoring in anesthesia and critical care medicine, ed 2, New York, 1990, Churchill Livingstone.
15. Katz J, Benumot JL, and Kadis LB: Anesthesia and uncommon diseases, ed 3, Philadelphia, 1990, WB Saunders Co.

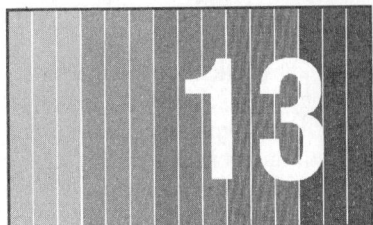

CHAPTER 13

Nursing Role in Management
Postoperative Client

JoAnn Fett Allison
Carol Wikoff Love

L earning Objectives

1. *Identify the nursing responsibilities in admitting the postoperative client to the recovery room.*
2. *Explain the etiological factors and nursing assessment and management of potential problems during the postanesthesia recovery period.*
3. *Describe the initial nursing assessment and nursing management of the postoperative client immediately after transfer from the recovery room to the general care unit.*
4. *Explain etiological factors and nursing assessment and management of potential problems during the postoperative period.*
5. *Identify the information needed by the postoperative client in preparation for discharge.*
6. *Identify the specific postoperative needs of both the older adult and the ambulatory surgery client.*

The postoperative period begins after surgery and continues until the client is discharged from medical care. This chapter focuses on the common features of postoperative nursing care for the client undergoing surgery. The problems and nursing care related to specific surgical procedures are discussed in the appropriate chapters of this text.

POSTOPERATIVE CLIENT IN THE RECOVERY ROOM
Receiving the Client From the Operating Room

The client's immediate recovery period is supervised by the recovery room nurse, an educated specialist working in a specially equipped environment. The recovery room (RR) or postanesthesia recovery room (PAR) is located close to the operating suite. In the event of an emergency, the anesthesiologist and the surgeon are nearby.

The goal of the recovery room nurse is to promote an uneventful recovery from anesthesia and the immediate effects of surgery. This requires that the nurse prevent complications when possible, recognize complications and intervene early when they do occur, and protect the client from injury during recovery.

The anesthesiologist* and the operating room nurse (in some agencies) accompany the client to the recovery room and report to the recovery room nurse. This report includes a review of the anesthesia and operative record with emphasis on the following information:

1. Client's name and age
2. Nature and outcomes of the planned or actual surgery performed
3. Special client conditions (e.g., allergies, chronic illnesses) existing preoperatively
4. Type of anesthesia and agents used
5. Drugs administered during surgery
6. Complications (such as hemorrhage or cardiac irregularity) during surgery and specific interventions
7. Estimated blood loss, blood replacement, and intravenous (IV) fluid intake
8. Amount of urine output during the surgery
9. Placement, type of drains, tubes, or suction devices and the nature and amount of drainage
10. Overall evaluation of client's intraoperative response, vital signs, and general condition at the conclusion of surgery and a comparison with preoperative status
11. Review of the postoperative orders with emphasis on immediate needs such as positioning, care restrictions, laboratory testing, and medication administration.

A written record (Fig. 13-1) of all observations and treatment measures during the postanesthesia recovery pe-

Reviewed by Judith A. Paice, R.N., M.S., Practitioner-Teacher, Department of OR and Surgical Nursing, Rush-Presbyterian-St. Luke's Medical Center; Assistant Professor, Rush University, Chicago, Illinois.

*The terms *anesthesiologist* and *anesthetist* (certified registered nurse anesthetist or CRNA) are used interchangeably in this chapter.

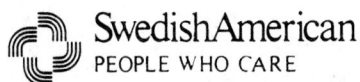
SwedishAmerican
PEOPLE WHO CARE

RECOVERY ROOM RECORD

DATE:
OPERATION:
SURGEON:
ANESTHESIOLOGIST:
ANESTHESIA:

R E C O V E R Y S C O R E

			IN						OUT	
Able to move 4 extremities	2	ACTIVITY								
Able to move 2 extremities	1									
Able to move 0 extremities	0									
Able to deep breathe and cough	2	RESPIRATION								
Dyspnea or limited breathing	1									
Apneic	0									
BP ± 20% of Preanesthetic level	2	CIRCULATION								
BP ± 20-50% of Preanesthetic level	1									
BP ± 50% of Preanesthetic level	0									
Awake	2	CONSCIOUSNESS								
Arousable	1									
Not responding	0									
Pink	2	COLOR								
Pale, dusky, other	1									
Cyanotic	0									
		TOTAL								

AIRWAY: ORAL ☐   NASAL ☐   ENDO ☐

O₂: MASK ☐   T-TUBE ☐   CANN/CATH ☐

SPECIAL REMARKS: _____

_____

_____

_____

CUFF BP ☒   (EXTREM_____)   PULSE ●   RESP ○   ART BP X

TIME

```
200                                          200
180                                          180
160                                          160
140                                          140
120                                          120
100                                          100
 80                                           80
 60                                           60
 40                                           40
 20                                           20
  0
TEMP
```

IV FLUIDS

ADMISSION_____   FOLEY ☐ _____

_____   _____

_____   _____

_____   NG TUBE _____

_____   _____

DISMISSAL _____   _____

_____   DRAINAGE TUBES __

_____   _____

INTAKE			OUTPUT		
	OR	RR		OR	RR
IV			URINE		
BLOOD			EBL		
TOTAL			TOTAL		

TIME:	MEDICATIONS/PROCEDURES	NURSING NOTES
ADMISSION		

REPORT GIVEN TO:_____ RECOVERY ROOM NURSE(S)_____

TIME:_____

RR665-001 10/83 REV.

Fig. 13-1   Recovery room record. (Courtesy Swedish American Hospital, Rockford, Ill.)

Table 13-1 Client Assessment on Admission
to Recovery Room

Time of arrival in recovery room
Patency of airway
Presence of artificial airway devices
    Pharyngeal airway
    Endotracheal tube
    Tracheostomy tube
Vital signs
    Temperature, pulse, and respirations
    Blood pressure
Color of skin, nail beds, and lips
Appearance of skin (moist or dry, warm or cool)
Level of consciousness
Presence or absence of reflexes
    Eyelid
    Pharyngeal
    Cough
    Gag and swallowing
Intravenous infusion
    Type of solution
    Amount in bottle or bag
    Flow rate
    Appearance and location of IV site
Dressings, drains, and tubes
    Intactness and function
    Connection to drainage
    Amount and character of drainage
Oxygen in use
    Mode of administration
    Flow rate
Presence or absence of urge to void
    Bladder distention

riod is essential. Many recovery rooms have a special form for this purpose, which includes a recovery score for the client. Measurements of the client's recovery and vital signs are generally done every 15 minutes until the client is stable and then every 30 minutes until the client's discharge from the PAR.

The initial nursing assessment of a client on admission to the recovery room is listed in Table 13-1. Assessments are made of respiratory, cardiovascular, and central nervous system (CNS) function, fluid volume status, and safety needs. Factors considered by the nurse during this initial assessment are the client's preoperative status, the surgery performed, and the anesthetic and adjunctive drugs used.

Potential Alterations in Respiratory Function

Etiology. In the postanesthesia period the related etiological factors may be airway obstruction, hypoventilation, aspiration of foreign material into the lung, or a combination of these and other factors (Table 13-2). The client who is an older adult, who smokes heavily, or who has a chronic lung disease is at particular risk. However, respiratory complications may occur with any client who has been anesthetized.

Airway obstruction is most frequently caused by blockage of the oral airway by the client's tongue.[1] The base of the tongue falls backward against the soft palate and occludes the pharynx. This is most pronounced in the supine position (Fig. 13-2).

Hypoventilation is the inadequate gas exchange of CO_2 and O_2 at the alveolar level. Respirations may be shallow, with frequent alterations in pattern, rate, and tidal volume. This is most likely due to the effects of anesthetic and/or narcotic depression of the respiratory center. The immediate dangers of hypoventilation are hypoxia and hypercapnia, as well as the hazards of atelectasis and hypostatic pneumonia.

Aspiration of material such as stomach contents, airway secretions, bloody drainage, and foreign bodies into the lungs can also contribute to airway obstruction and altered breathing patterns. Later complications of aspiration are atelectasis and pneumonia. Loss or depression of reflexes due to the effects of anesthesia and narcotics is the primary cause. However, persons who are obese and immobile, have had head or neck surgery, or must be maintained in a supine position are at particular risk.

■ Nursing Management of Respiratory Function

Nursing assessment

For an adequate respiratory assessment, the nurse needs to evaluate airway patency, chest symmetry, and the depth, rate, and character of respirations. The nurse should place a cupped hand over the client's nose and mouth to evaluate the forcefulness of exhaled air.

The chest wall should be observed for symmetry of movement with a hand placed lightly over the xyphoid process. It should also be determined whether abdominal and/or accessory muscles are being used for breathing. If they are moving excessively, it may indicate respiratory distress.

Breath sounds should be auscultated anteriorly, laterally, and posteriorly. Decrease or absence of breath sounds will be detected when airflow is diminished or obstructed. The presence of crackles or wheezes may indicate the need for suctioning of secretions.

The regular monitoring of vital signs permits the nurse to recognize early signs of respiratory distress. The presence of hypoxia from any cause may be reflected by rapid breathing, gasping, apprehension, restlessness, and a rapid or thready pulse. Impaired ventilation may initially be detected by the observation of slowed breathing or diminished chest and abdominal movement during the respiratory cycle.

The characteristics of sputum or mucus should be noted and recorded. Mucus from the trachea and throat is colorless and thin in consistency. Sputum from the lungs and bronchi is thick with a slight yellow tinge.

Nursing diagnoses

Nursing diagnoses related to potential alterations of respiratory function for the client in the recovery room may include, but are not limited to, the following:

Ineffective airway clearance
Ineffective breathing pattern
Impaired gas exchange
High risk for aspiration

Table 13-2 Common Immediate Postoperative Respiratory Complications

Complications and Causes	Mechanisms	Nursing Observations	Intervention
Airway obstruction			
Tongue falling back	Muscular flaccidity associated with ↓ consciousness and muscle relaxants	Snoring respirations Decreased air movement	Neck hyperextension Pulling of mandible forward Mechanical airway
Retained thick secretions	Secretion stimulation by anesthetic agents Dehydration of secretions from anticholinergic medication	Noisy respirations Rhonchi	Suctioning Deep breathing and coughing IV hydration IPPB with mucolytic agent Bronchoscopy
Laryngospasm	Irritation from endotracheal tube or anesthetic gases Most likely to occur after removal of endotracheal tube	Inspiratory stridor (crowing respiration) Sternal retraction	Oxygen Pulling of mandible forward IV atropine or muscle relaxant Intubation
Laryngeal edema	Allergic drug reaction Mechanical irritation from intubation Fluid overload	Similar to laryngospasm	Oxygen Antihistamines or steroids Sedatives Possible intubation
Bronchospasm	Preexisting asthma Irritation from anesthetic gases	Expiratory wheezing	IPPB IV bronchodilators (isoproterenol [Isuprel] or aminophylline)
Hypoventilation			
Drug-induced CNS depression	Prolonged effect of anesthesia and adjunct drugs Excessive pain medication	↓ Respiratory rate Shallow respirations Apnea	Deep breathing and coughing Mechanical ventilation Narcotic antagonists
Drug-induced peripheral muscle paralysis	Excessive use of muscle relaxants	Similar to drug-induced peripheral muscle paralysis	Deep breathing and coughing Mechanical ventilation Anticholinesterase drugs
Mechanical restriction	Tight casts or dressings Abdominal distention Position preventing lung expansion	Shallow respirations	Deep breathing and coughing Repositioning Loosening of cast or dressing Nasogastric intubation
Pain	Shallow breathing to prevent incisional pain (especially with chest and abdominal surgery)	Similar to mechanical restriction	Analgesic in reduced dose
Aspiration of vomitus			
Retention of food or fluid in stomach	Gastric secretions (may accumulate even in fasting client)	Vomitus (may or may not be expelled by mouth)	Turning on side or turning of head to side Suctioning
Delayed gastric emptying	Pain, fear, narcotics, anticholinergic medications delaying gastric emptying		Nasogastric intubation Coughing Antiemetic
Position change after narcotics	Narcotics and movement stimulating chemoreceptor trigger zone in medulla		

IPPB, Intermittent positive pressure breathing.

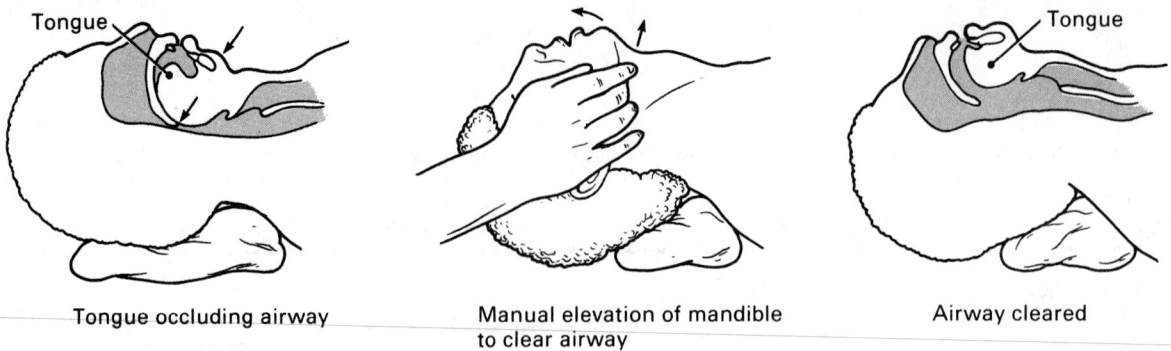

Tongue occluding airway   Manual elevation of mandible to clear airway   Airway cleared

Fig. 13-2 Etiology and relief of airway obstruction due to client's tongue.

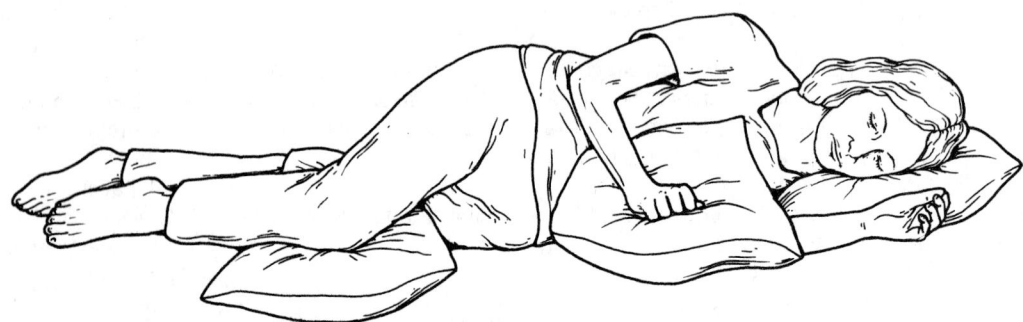

Fig. 13-3 Positioning of client during recovery from general anesthesia.

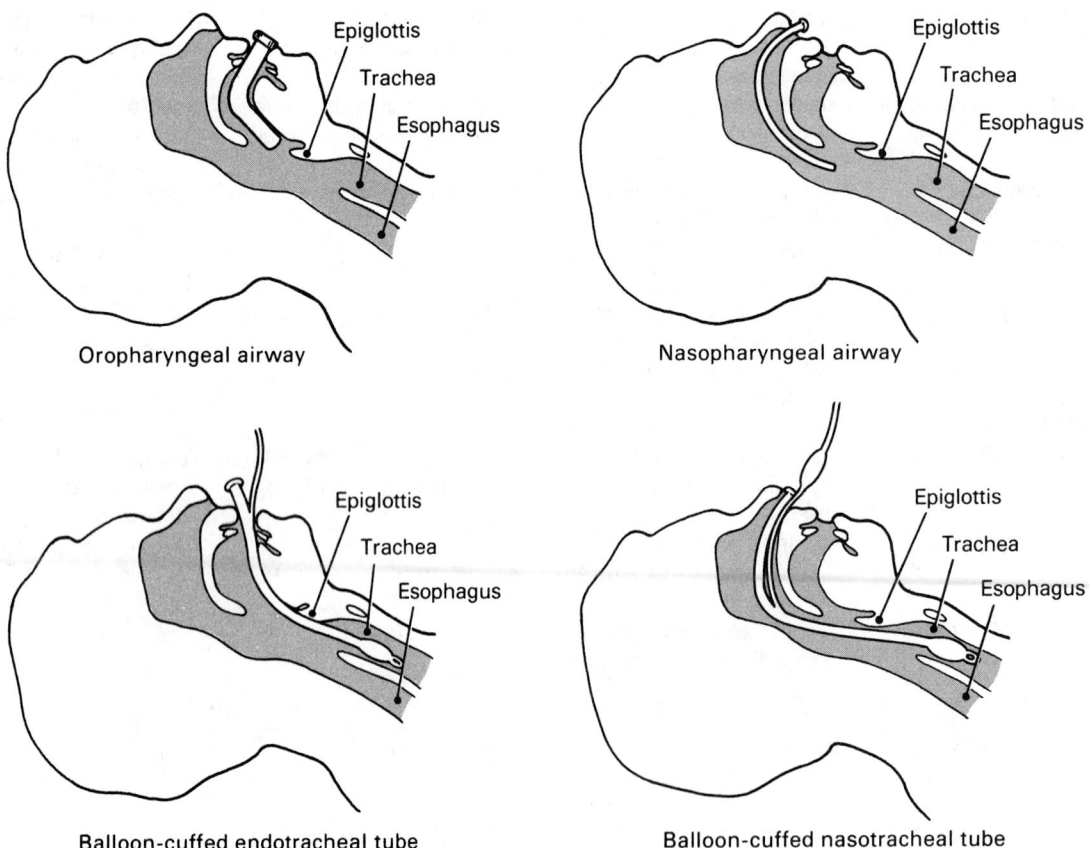

Oropharyngeal airway   Nasopharyngeal airway

Balloon-cuffed endotracheal tube   Balloon-cuffed nasotracheal tube

Fig. 13-4 Mechanical devices to prevent airway obstruction during recovery from anesthesia.

Nursing interventions

During the postanesthesia recovery period, the nurse routinely carries out measures aimed at prevention or detection of possible respiratory problems.

Proper positioning to facilitate respirations or breathing is essential. Unless contraindicated by the surgical procedure, the unconscious or semiconscious client should be in a side-lying or semiprone position (Fig. 13-3). If the client must be supine, the head should be turned to the side to avoid aspiration. The client should be turned from side to side hourly to allow for bilateral lung expansion. The supine position should be avoided until protective pharyngeal reflexes have returned. The client's uppermost arm should rest on a pillow rather than on the chest wall to permit full chest movement. Dressings or binders on the chest or abdomen should be inspected to ensure that they are not constricting.

As soon as possible after surgery, the older adult should be placed in a low Fowler's position. This position maximizes expansion of the thorax by decreasing the pressure of the abdomen on the diaphragm. In addition, every older adult who has had general anesthesia should receive oxygen, preferably by nasal cannula, until fully conscious.

Patency of the airway is an ever-present concern in the unconscious client. If the upper respiratory tract appears to be obstructed, it may often be cleared simply by moving the client's lower jaw forward and upward (Fig. 13-2). If secretions are present, they may be removed by suctioning. Several mechanical devices are available to prevent airway obstruction in the anesthetized client (Fig. 13-4). *Pharyngeal airways* are usually removed by the client when reflexes have recovered sufficiently to gag or push the device out with the tongue. *Endotracheal extubation* has traditionally been the responsibility of the anesthesiologist but is beginning to be done by nurses in some areas. Criteria for safe extubation include (1) adequate ventilation and movement of air evidenced by observation and auscultation and (2) client can lift head off stretcher and hold it up for 30 seconds.

Deep breathing and coughing should be initiated as soon as the client enters the recovery room. Even while semiconscious, the client who has been instructed in these techniques preoperatively will respond to a verbal reminder. Deep breathing helps to clear inhalation anesthetic agents from the body and hasten recovery, prevent pooling of secretions, and decrease the tendency to hypoventilate. The client who is left alone tends to drift back to sleep and breathe shallowly or even become apneic. Verbal stimuli must be provided by the nurse until the respiratory center recovers sufficiently to respond to the usual stimulant of increased carbon dioxide concentration in the blood.

Potential Alterations in Cardiovascular Function

Etiology. *Transient hypotension* is relatively common in the recovery room. However, if hypotension is persistent and severe, it may indicate shock. Hypotension and shock postoperatively are most commonly related to hypovolemia, residual effects of anesthesia, and severe pain. Other possible causes are adrenal insufficiency and cardiac failure (Table 13-3).

Table 13-3 Common Immediate Postoperative Cardiovascular Complications

Contributing Factors	Intervention
Hypovolemia	
Blood loss	Leg elevation
Hemorrhage	Oxygen
Preoperative dehydration	IV fluids or blood
Inadequate fluid or blood replacement	Accurate intake and output
GI drainage	
Effects of anesthesia and drugs	
Conduction anesthesia (vasomotor depression)	Leg elevation
	Oxygen
	IV fluids
	Vasopressors
General anesthesia	Leg elevation
	Oxygen
	IV fluids
	Vasopressors
	Stimulation to regain consciousness
Excessive narcotic dosage	Oxygen
	Narcotic antagonists (Nalline, Lorfan, Narcan)
Pain	
Withholding of narcotics	IV or IM analgesic in reduced dosage
Incisional discomfort	Assessment for complicating factors
Adrenal insufficiency	
Chronic steroid use	IV hydrocortisone
Prolonged or excessive stress	IM cortisone or hydrocortisone
Cardiac failure	
Preexisting cardiac disease	Digitalization
Circulatory overload from excessive fluid replacement	Diuretics
	ECG monitoring

GI, Gastrointestinal; *IM*, intramuscular.

Hypovolemia results from inadequate blood or fluid replacement after surgical losses (intraoperative and postoperative). Blood loss during most surgical procedures ranges between 100 and 500 ml but may be greater if surgery involves highly vascular areas or if bleeding is difficult to control. Blood transfusions are generally given only if the estimated blood loss exceeds 500 ml. With the dangers inherent in blood transfusion, replacement of one unit of blood is avoided if at all possible. Serious hypovolemic shock does not usually develop in the adult until 1.5 to 2 L of blood volume has been lost.[2]

Residual effects of anesthesia may produce mild hypotension during the period of recovery from any general anesthetic. A fall in blood pressure may also accompany the use of spinal or epidural anesthesia. This can be caused by arteriolar dilatation due to paralysis of the preganglionic sympathetic nerves and a fall in cardiac output due to reduced venous return. As the effects of anesthesia decrease, the client's blood pressure usually returns to preoperative levels. Since narcotic analgesics may also lower blood pressure, their administration before the effects of anesthesia subside may further lower the client's blood pressure.

While moderate pain tends to produce an increase in blood pressure, more severe pain may cause hypotension because of autonomic reflexes mediated by norepinephrine release. The release of norepinephrine results in a decrease in heart rate and cardiac output. This response may be great enough to produce shock, particularly when pain occurs in combination with the vasodilating effects of anesthesia and depleted fluid volume.[3]

■ Nursing Management of Cardiovascular Function

Nursing assessment

The most important aspect of the cardiovascular assessment is frequent monitoring of vital signs. They are usually monitored every 15 minutes or more often until stabilized, and then at less frequent intervals. A common schedule is every 15 minutes × 4, every 30 minutes × 4, every 1 hour × 4, and then every 4 hours (the 4 × 4 rule). Postoperative vital signs should be compared with preoperative as well as with intraoperative readings to determine when they are stabilizing at a normal level for the client's situation. The anesthesiologist or surgeon should be notified if the following occur:

1. Systolic blood pressure is less than 90 mm Hg or greater than 160 mm Hg.
2. Pulse rate is less than 60 beats per minute (bpm) or greater than 120 bpm.
3. A narrowing of the pulse pressure occurs.
4. A gradual decrease in blood pressure over several consecutive readings occurs.
5. An irregular cardiac rhythm develops.

Cardiac monitoring is recommended for any client who has a history of cardiac disease and for all older adult clients who have undergone major surgery, regardless of whether they have cardiac problems.[4] An apical/radial pulse should be assessed carefully and any irregularities or deficits should be reported.

Assessment of skin color, temperature, and moisture provides valuable information in detecting cardiovascular problems. Hypotension accompanied by a normal pulse and warm, dry, pink skin usually represents the residual vasodilating effects of anesthesia and suggests only a need for continued observation. Hypotension accompanied by a rapid pulse and cold, clammy, pale skin may be due to impending hypovolemic shock and requires immediate treatment.

Nursing diagnoses

Nursing diagnoses related to potential alterations in cardiovascular function for the client in the recovery room may include, but are not limited to, the following:

Decreased cardiac output
Fluid volume deficit
Altered tissue perfusion
Potential complication: hypovolemic shock

Nursing interventions

During postanesthesia recovery, many of the nurse's actions are directed at prevention or early detection of hypotension, shock, and other cardiovascular problems (Table 13-3). (The nursing role in assessment and management of hypotension and shock is described in Chapter 27.)

If shock develops, the client's legs should be elevated enough to maintain a downward slope toward the trunk of the body. The head should not be lowered past the flat position. If a person has had spinal anesthesia or cranial surgery, these measures should not be taken. This positioning can cause impairment of the diaphragm or increase intracranial pressure. It is better to position this client with the head elevated 30 degrees and a pillow placed under each leg.

Pain and Discomfort

As the effects of anesthesia wear off, the client begins to perceive incisional pain as well as discomforts associated with the presence of dressings, drains, tubes, and other equipment. Pain or discomfort may also be associated with a distended bladder, uncomfortable positions during the operative procedure, or a serious complication such as myocardial infarction.

Analgesic drugs are frequently administered in the recovery room for relief of pain. Sometimes the medical order is written that the dose may be reduced by one third to one half. A full dose of pain medication, along with the residual effect of preanesthetic medication and intraoperative agents, can cause respiratory depression and decreased blood pressure.

Although hypotension alone is not an indication to withhold pain medication, it does require nursing judgment based on sound client assessment when the medication is administered. Continued monitoring of the client's response is essential after the administration of pain medication.

■ Nursing Management of Recovery from Anesthesia

Nursing assessment

General anesthesia. Recovery from general anesthesia occurs in the reverse sequence from the events of induction. Hearing is the first sensation to return. There is considerable variation in the mode of emergence experienced by clients, depending on the type and dose of anesthetic agents used, the client's physical status, and individual idiosyncratic responses. Advances in the technique of anesthesia administration and monitoring, along with the development of new agents, have made the reversal process more rapid. Clients are frequently extubated and responsive when admitted to the PAR.

The nurse should always be alert to the possibility of unexpected deepening of anesthesia, particularly the rebound effect of neuromuscular blocking agents. This effect is seen in a change in the level of consciousness and a decline in reflexes. Neuromuscular function is checked by the client's ability to hold the head up for 10 seconds and initiate a firm hand grasp.[5] Additional measurements may be made of inspiratory and expiratory flow rates. Change in the level of consciousness or a decline in reflexes presents a special danger to the client whose artificial airway has already been removed.

Regional anesthesia. Recovery from regional anesthesia (spinal and epidural) also occurs in a reverse sequence from induction. Position sense returns first, then motion, then sensation, and finally autonomic (sympathetic) vasomotor function.[6] The nurse should note the time of recovery of both motion and sensation. The regional anesthetic client may be transferred from the PAR to the general care unit when vital signs are stable and the effects of anesthesia are regressing.

Some clients have spinal or postpuncture headaches when their heads are raised after regional anesthesia. This type of headache, involving postural pain and throbbing occipital or frontal discomfort and sometimes nuchal rigidity, may develop within an hour to 2 or 3 days after surgery. It may last for a day, a week, or even longer. The postural headache is believed to be caused by a decrease in cerebrospinal fluid pressure due to leakage at the puncture site. This results in compensatory intracranial vasodilation, "sagging" of the brain, and tension on its pain-sensitive supporting structures. It is more frequent in young adults, in female clients during the preovulation phase of the menstrual cycle, and in those clients who expect it to happen. Spinal headache is less likely to occur if a small-gauge needle is used for injection and if postoperative hydration of the client is adequate.[7,8] Keeping the client flat for 12 to 24 hours after surgery to prevent a headache is generally considered outdated but may still be practiced.

Nursing diagnoses

Nursing diagnoses related to recovery from anesthesia for the client in the recovery room include, but are not limited to, the following:

Sensory/perceptual alterations
High risk for injury
Altered thought processes
Impaired verbal communication
High risk for altered hypothermia

Nursing interventions

Safety and comfort. The client must be turned and positioned carefully during recovery from anesthesia to avoid damage to eyes, skin, muscles, nerves, and blood vessels. Before lid reflexes return, the cornea may inadvertently be scratched by personnel, equipment, or the client. Before sensation and motion return, the client may remain in a position that places pressure on skin or nerves or that obstructs circulation. Flaccid muscles may easily be overstretched and injured during turning if adequate support is not provided. The use of side rails and safety straps on the recovery stretcher prevents injury during this period.

The client should be kept warm by the use of heated or reflective blankets and reduced exposure of body surfaces. Anesthetic agents, adjunctive drugs, the cool environment of the operating room, and intraoperative body exposure will all lower the body temperature. The client may enter the recovery room with a body temperature as low as 36.5°

C. The nurse must take appropriate measures to prevent further chilling until the body temperature has stabilized.[9-11] The client with a low body temperature has many altered physiological responses including slowed circulation, which delays the elimination of the anesthetic and therefore prolongs recovery time.

Decreases in muscle mass, mobility, and the thermoregulating mechanism all place the older adult client at risk of hypothermia during the intraoperative and postoperative phases of the surgical experience. Consequences for these clients are increased risk of cardiac failure and thrombosis.

Communication. Even the client who has been told what to expect in the recovery room may be frightened or confused on awakening in the strange environment. Since hearing is the first sense to return in the unconscious client, the nurse should explain all activities from the moment of admission to the PAR. Orientation includes telling the client the following:

1. The surgery is completed.
2. The client is in the recovery room.
3. The family or significant other has been notified.
4. Who is caring for the client and what is being done.
5. What time it is.

When possible, the family should be contacted by the recovery room nurse and a brief status report regarding the client should be given.

Discharge from the Recovery Room

The surgeon or anesthesiologist authorizes the client's release from the recovery room and transfer to the clinical unit or intensive care unit. A scoring system is used to determine the client's general condition and readiness for discharge. The most common system is a modification of the APGAR score, which includes the parameters of activity, respiration, circulation, consciousness, and color (Fig. 13-1). A maximum score of 10 indicates a client in the best condition for transfer. A client with a score of less than 7 is not transferred or is admitted to an intensive care unit (ICU).[3]

A newer system of assessment, REACT, uses the parameters of respiration, energy, alertness, circulation, and temperature (Table 13-4). With this system the data assessed give a more objective measurement of the client's status and responsiveness. A score of 10 indicates a fully recovered client, safe for discharge.

The client is usually evaluated as ready for discharge to the general unit when the following criteria are met:

1. Vital signs are stabilized.
2. Respirations and circulation are adequate.
3. Anesthetic effects have been reversed (with regional anesthesia, movement is present).
4. The client is oriented and easily arousable (or at the preoperative state of consciousness).
5. Complications are not present or are under control.

The recovery room nurse accompanies the client to the clinical unit and assists in settling the client into bed. A report is given to the unit nurse, detailing the client's response to the intraoperative and immediate postoperative events. Written orders are reviewed with the nurse admitting the client to the unit, and special care needs are iden-

Table 13-4 REACT Scoring System

Category	Findings	Score
Respiration	Needs ventilator	0
	Spontaneous respiration present but needs artificial airway	1
	Spontaneous respiration present and needs no support; respiratory rate is at least 10/min	2
Energy	Does not move legs, even with stimulation	0
	Moves legs; cannot keep head up	1
	Moves legs; can keep head up	2
Alertness	Awakens only when vigorously stimulated	0
	Awakens only when gently stimulated	1
	Seldom dozes, usually awake	2
Circulation	Systolic blood pressure is less than 80 mm Hg *or* either the radial or ulnar pulse is weak	0
	Systolic blood pressure is between 80 mm Hg and preoperative resting level *and* the radial and ulnar pulses are strong	1
	Systolic blood pressure is at preoperative resting level or higher *and* the radial and ulnar pulses are strong	2
Temperature	Axillary temperature is less than 95° F (35° C)	0
	Axillary temperature is 95° F to 96° F (35° C to 35.5° C)	1
	Axillary temperature is higher than 96° F (35.5° C)	2

Interpreting a REACT score:

A score of 10 indicates the client is fully recovered from the anesthesia and can return to the room.

A score of 9 indicates the client is experiencing residual anesthetic effects, such as mild drowsiness or moderate hypotension. The client should be transferred cautiously.

A score of 8 or below indicates the client should remain in the recovery room, unless being transferred to an intensive care unit.

Adapted from Frauline K and Murphy P: R.E.A.C.T.—a new system for measuring postanesthesia recovery, Nursing 14:102, 1984.

Table 13-5 Postoperative Care and Follow-Up for Geriatric Ambulatory Surgical Clients

PHASE I

Return sensory aids to client as soon as possible

Repeat information to help reorient client

Review intraoperative medications before giving additional medications

Use reality-distorting medications sparingly

PHASE II

Give instructions for home care to client and caretaker; use demonstrations when appropriate

Provide written instructions (enlarged print) concerning home care for reference

Transcribe any verbal instructions from surgeon on home care instruction sheet

Encourage client to postpone making any important decisions for 24 hours

Confirm availability of adult support for home care

DAY AFTER SURGERY FOLLOW-UP CALL

Assess for complications

Review home care instructions

Answer questions

Modified from Kupferer SS and others: Geriatric ambulatory surgery patients: assessing cognitive functions, AORN J 47:755, 1988.

tified. After giving a verbal report to the unit nurse regarding the client's status on admission to the unit, the recovery room nurse's responsibility for care ends.

Ambulatory surgery. The recovery of a client in an ambulatory surgery setting may occur in two phases. Phase I applies to the client who has had general anesthesia. The assessments and interventions for the general PAR are also used in the care of this client. Overall depth of anesthesia and recovery may be less, since the client is at low risk physically and the surgical procedure is less involved and of shorter duration. When recovered, the client moves to phase II of recovery and is transferred to the outpatient surgical unit (OpSu) for further monitoring and care. Ambulation is initiated and specific preparation for discharge is begun.

A client not requiring general anesthesia or sedation moves directly into phase II of recovery and is transferred directly to the OpSu from the operating room. Vital signs are monitored, usually every 30 minutes, and gradual preparation for ambulation and discharge is started. The needs specific to the older adult client during phases I and II of recovery are listed in Table 13-5.[12]

POSTOPERATIVE CLIENT ON THE CLINICAL UNIT

The nurse who receives the client on the clinical unit from the RR or PAR assesses the baseline vital signs and completes a brief but complete assessment of the client

Table 13-6 Nursing Assessment and Care of Client on Admission to Clinical Unit

Record time of client's return to unit
Take baseline vital signs
   Assess airway and breath sounds
Assess neurological status, including level of consciousness
   and movement of extremities
Assess wound, dressing, drainage tubes
   Note type and amount of drainage
   Connect tubing to gravity or suction drainage
Assess color and appearance of skin
Assess urinary status
   Note time of voiding
   Note presence of catheter and total output (report if output
     <30 ml/hr)
   Check for bladder distention or urge to void
   Note catheter patency
Assess pain and discomfort
   Note last dose and type of pain control
   Note current pain intensity

Position for airway maintenance, comfort, safety (bed in low
   position, side rails up)
Check IV infusion
   Note type of solution
   Note amount of fluid remaining
   Note flow rate
   Check integrity of insertion site and size of needle
Receive report from the recovery room nurse and compare
   with admission status
Attach call light within reach and reorient client to use of call
   light
Ensure that emesis basin and tissues are available
Determine emotional condition and support
   Check for presence of family member or significant other
Check and carry out postoperative orders

(Table 13-6). When the recovery room nurse accompanies the client, the client's status on admission to the unit can be evaluated and compared with the status on discharge from the recovery room. Documentation of the transfer is then completed, a more in-depth assessment is done, and postoperative orders and nursing care are implemented (Fig. 13-5).

Potential Problems During the Postoperative Period

The nurse is aware that the potential for the possible problems of the immediate postanesthetic period continues into this early postoperative period. As recovery continues, however, these early concerns are replaced by different potential problems during subsequent postoperative days (Fig. 13-6). Nursing assessment and management are based on knowledge of the potential complications (and associated manifestations) from surgery in general, as well as those associated with specific surgical procedures (Table 13-7). A general nursing care plan for the postoperative client is presented in Table 13-8.

Early ambulation is the most significant general nursing measure to prevent postoperative complications. Since it was first advocated nearly 40 years ago, the value of early ambulation has been obvious.[13] The exercise associated with walking (1) increases smooth muscle tone; (2) improves gastrointestinal (GI) and urinary tract function; (3) stimulates circulation, which prevents venous stasis and speeds wound healing; and (4) increases vital capacity and maintains normal respiratory function. Ambulation is especially important for the older adult client because hazards of immobility develop earlier, last longer, and may have more lasting effects in the older adult.[14,15]

Potential Alterations in Respiratory Function

Etiology. Atelectasis and pneumonitis (hypostatic pneumonia) can occur in the postoperative surgical client and are particularly common after abdominal and thoracic surgery.[16] *Atelectasis* (alveolar collapse) occurs when mucus blocks bronchioles or when the amount of alveolar surfactant (the substance that holds the alveoli open) is reduced (Fig. 13-7). As air becomes trapped beyond the plug and is eventually absorbed, the alveoli collapse. Atelectasis may affect a portion or an entire lobe of the lung.

The postoperative development of mucous plugs and/or decreased surfactant production is directly related to hypoventilation, a constant recumbent position, ineffective coughing, and smoking. Increased bronchial secretions occur when the respiratory passages are irritated by heavy smoking, acute or chronic pulmonary infection or disease, and the drying of mucous membranes that occurs with intubation, inhalation anesthesia, and dehydration. Without intervention, atelectasis can progress to *pneumonitis* when a secondary infection develops in the stagnant mucus.

▪ Nursing Management of Respiratory Function
Nursing assessment
Nursing assessment of the client's respiratory rate, patterns, and breath sounds is essential to identify potential respiratory problems (see p. 278).
Nursing diagnoses
Nursing diagnoses related to potential alterations in respiratory function for the postoperative client include, but are not limited to, the following:
Ineffective airway clearance
Altered breathing patterns
Altered gas exchange
Potential complication: pneumonia
Potential complication: atelectasis
High risk for aspiration
Nursing interventions
The client should be assisted to breathe deeply several times every hour, as demonstrated preoperatively. Splinting the incision with a pillow or a rolled blanket provides
Text continued on p. 291.

POST-OP/FREQUENT VITAL SIGN SHEET

Date_____

Time returned
to floor_____

Addressograph plate

Procedure done:_____

Vital signs BP_____ Temp_____ Pulse_____ Respirations_____

Level of consciousness Alert_____ Lethargic_____ Stuporous_____ Semi-comatose_____ Comatose_____

Integumentary assessment   Skin   Cool_____   Clammy_____   Warm_____   Dry_____
Color   Pink_____   Pale_____   Cyanotic_____

Description and location of surgical site and/or dressing:_____

_____

_____

EBL_____

Tubes or drains Type_____   Location_____

Emptied Yes_____   No_____

Suction Yes_____   No_____   Type LCS_____   GOMCO_____

Urinary drainage devices Yes_____   No_____

Oxygen Yes_____   No_____   Cannula_____   Ventimask_____   # of liters_____

IV Yes_____   No_____

Blood infusing   Yes_____   No_____

PCA pump Yes_____   No_____

Medications received in Recovery Room:_____

_____

Additional information:

Date	Time	Temp	Pulse	Resp	BP	Comments

Signature

Fig. 13-5   Postop/frequent vital sign sheet. (Courtesy Elliot Hospital, Manchester, NH.)

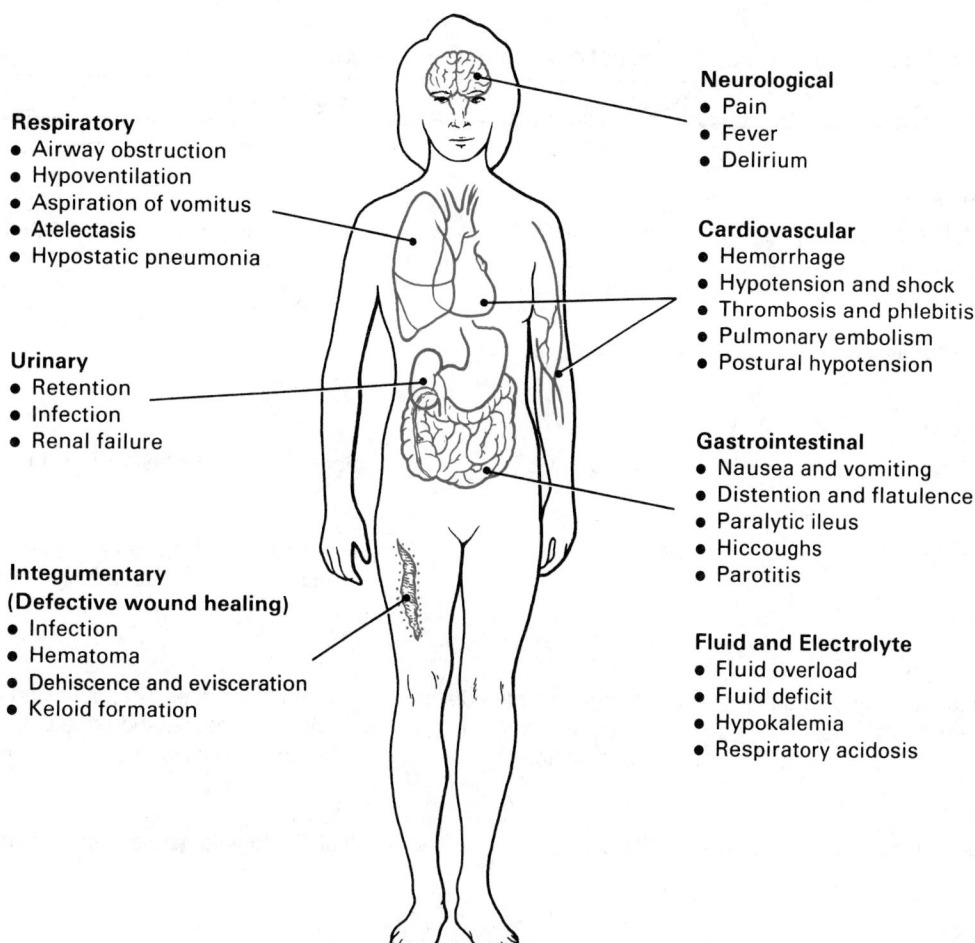

Neurological
- Pain
- Fever
- Delirium

Respiratory
- Airway obstruction
- Hypoventilation
- Aspiration of vomitus
- Atelectasis
- Hypostatic pneumonia

Cardiovascular
- Hemorrhage
- Hypotension and shock
- Thrombosis and phlebitis
- Pulmonary embolism
- Postural hypotension

Urinary
- Retention
- Infection
- Renal failure

Gastrointestinal
- Nausea and vomiting
- Distention and flatulence
- Paralytic ileus
- Hiccoughs
- Parotitis

**Integumentary
(Defective wound healing)**
- Infection
- Hematoma
- Dehiscence and evisceration
- Keloid formation

Fluid and Electrolyte
- Fluid overload
- Fluid deficit
- Hypokalemia
- Respiratory acidosis

Fig. 13-6   Potential problems in the postoperative period.

Table 13-7 Common Postoperative Complications in the Clinical Unit

Common Cause	Occurrence	Manifestations
EARLY COMPLICATIONS		
Abdominal distention		
Surgical manipulation of bowel, swallowed air	Within 48 hr	Increased abdominal girth, tympanic percussion, complaints of "gas pains" or "fullness"
Atelectasis		
Mucus, shallow respirations	Within 48 hr	Fever, increased pulse and respirations, dyspnea, cyanosis
Hypostatic pneumonia		
Shallow respirations	Within 48 hr	Same as in atelectasis; purulent, bloody sputum
Hypoxia		
Respiratory depression, mucus, pain, poor positioning	Within 48 hr	Increased blood pressure, bounding pulse, restlessness, difficult breathing
Shock		
Loss of fluids and electrolytes, trauma, medications, sepsis	Most common immediately postop but may occur anytime	Drop in blood pressure; bounding pulse; clammy, cool skin; decreased urine output; restlessness; lethargy; marked increase in temperature
Urinary retention		
Medication, local edema, positioning	6-8 hr postop	Inability to void, restlessness, bladder distention
Wound hemorrhage		
Slipped suture, dislodged clot, wound evisceration	Within 48 hr	Same as in shock, profuse drainage
LATER COMPLICATIONS		
Thrombophlebitis		
Venous stasis, IV irritation	Variable	Skin warm to touch, red, tender; calf pain with dorsiflexion; firmness
Wound infection		
Poor technique	3-6 days postop	Skin warm to touch, red, and tender; fever; chills; malaise; purulent drainage
Wound dehiscence		
Old age, malnutrition, unusual strain	6-8 days postop	Separation of wound edges; sudden, profuse pink drainage
Wound evisceration		
Same as in wound dehiscence	6-8 days postop	Dehiscence with protrusion of abdominal viscera through incision

Adapted from Croushore T: Postoperative assessment: the key to avoiding the most common nursing mistakes, Nursing 9:47-50, 1979.

Table 13-8

NURSING CARE PLAN FOR THE POSTOPERATIVE CLIENT*

Defining Characteristics	Nursing Interventions	Evaluation Criteria
NURSING DIAGNOSIS: Pain related to surgical incision and reflex muscle spasm		
Tense and guarded body posture, facial grimacing, tachycardia, restlessness, irritability, hypertension or hypotension, moaning, diaphoresis, complaints of pain	Assess pain for character, location, and effectiveness of relief measures. Position to relieve pain. Assure client of your efforts to reduce pain. Administer analgesics as ordered. Assess effectiveness. Convey accepting attitude. Plan nonpharmacological pain relievers such as distraction, massage, and imagery.	Expression of satisfaction with pain relief, pain not interfering with postoperative recovery
NURSING DIAGNOSIS: Nausea and vomiting related to gastrointestinal distention, medication and anesthesia effects, and stimulation of vomiting center or chemoreceptor trigger zone		
Complaints of nausea, refusal to take fluids and/or solids, observed or reported vomiting	Assess precipitating factors and eliminate when possible (e.g., unpleasant smells, sights). Control pain. Maintain patency of nasogastric tube if present. Advance diet only as tolerated. Monitor gastrointestinal effects of medications, especially narcotics. Administer antiemetics as indicated. Assess bowel sounds.	Reduction or prevention of nausea and vomiting
NURSING DIAGNOSIS: High risk for infection related to surgical incision, inadequate nutrition and fluid intake, presence of environmental pathogens, invasive catheters, and immobility		
Elevated body temperature; red, swollen, warm area surrounding incision or indwelling catheters; elevated white blood cell count; elevated pulse and respiratory rate; purulent drainage from wound	Monitor for and report any significant change in temperature, appearance of wound, or drainage. Use strict aseptic technique in providing wound care, including hand washing, sterile dressing technique. Monitor daily caloric intake. Ensure a minimum of 2000 calories and 2500 ml/day (greater if there metabolic demands are increased). Weigh daily and notify physician if greater than 5% weight loss from baseline. Minimize exposure to environmental pathogens by avoiding contact between client and others with infection. Maintain aseptic technique in care of invasive lines. Monitor daily for any changes indicative of infection. Report to physician. Help client turn, cough, and breathe deeply every 1 to 2 hours while awake.	No evidence of infection
NURSING DIAGNOSIS: Ineffective airway clearance related to inadequate cough and tenacious secretions		
Abnormal breath sounds, shallow respirations, nonproductive cough	Provide for pain relief before having the client cough and breathe deeply. Provide a minimum of 2500 ml/day of fluids unless contraindicated. Provide preoperative teaching of proper coughing and deep-breathing techniques. Assist client with turning, coughing, and deep breathing every 1 to 2 hours while awake. Monitor use of incentive spirometer. Discourage smoking. Suction if necessary. Monitor breath sounds and temperature.	Normal breath sounds, effective cough

*This general postoperative care plan should be used in conjunction with a nursing care plan specific to the type of surgery being performed.

Continued.

Table 13-8

 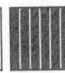

NURSING CARE PLAN FOR THE POSTOPERATIVE CLIENT*—cont'd

Defining Characteristics	Nursing Interventions	Evaluation Criteria

NURSING DIAGNOSIS: Potential complication: hemorrhage related to ineffective vascular closure

Decreasing blood pressure; rapid pulse and respirations; cool, clammy skin; pallor; bright red blood on dressing	Observe surgical site and dressings regularly (q hr for 4 hr, then q 4 hr) for signs of bleeding, including dependent sites. Monitor vital signs regularly from q 15 minutes in RR to q 2-4 hr as indicated in postoperative unit. Report abnormalities. Monitor for changes in mental status, such as restlessness and sense of impending doom. Monitor hematocrit and hemoglobin levels as ordered.	Early detection and implementation of treatment of hemorrhage

NURSING DIAGNOSIS: Potential complication: thromboembolism related to dehydration, immobility, vascular manipulation, or injury

Redness, swelling, pain; increased warmth along path of vein; positive Homans' signs; edema or pain in extremity; chest pain; hemoptysis; tachypnea; dyspnea; restlessness	Assess every shift for signs of thromboembolism. Teach or perform range of motion to lower extremities. Encourage early ambulation. Avoid pressure under knees from bed or pillows. Apply antiembolism stockings, if ordered. Remove every shift for 1 hour. Maintain adequate hydration.	No thromboembolic event

NURSING DIAGNOSIS: Potential complication: urinary retention related to horizontal positioning, pain, fear, or analgesic and anesthetic medications

Inability to void, distended bladder	Monitor intake and output. Percuss bladder routinely for 48 hours postoperatively. Notify physician if no urine output within 6 hours after surgery. Position client in as normal position as possible for voiding. Provide privacy. Apply pain measures. Relieve client's fears by providing explanations and encouragement. Monitor urinary effects of analgesic and anesthetic medications.	Urine output of at least 30-50 ml/hour without complaints of urgency or bladder fullness

NURSING DIAGNOSIS: Potential complication: paralytic ileus related to bowel manipulation, immobility, pain medication, and anesthestics

Absence of bowel sounds and flatus, abdominal distention, nausea and vomiting	Assess every shift for abdominal distention, presence of flatus, and/or stool. Maintain NPO status until peristalsis returns, and ensure patency of nasogastric tube. Insert rectal tube as needed to expel flatus. Provide frequent oral hygiene.	Early detection and treatment of paralytic ileus

NURSING DIAGNOSIS: Impaired home management related to lack of knowledge about follow-up care

Frequent questioning about self-care at home, expression of difficulty in performing any part of self-care at home, absence of assistance at home	Teach client and family about signs and symptoms of infection to observe and report, nutritional needs of client, activity restrictions, wound care, medication requirements. Ensure client's or family member's skills in performing self-care before discharge or arrange for referral for home care. Allow sufficient practice in technical skills such as dressing change for client and/or family member to become confident. Together with client, identify aspects of self-care with which assistance may be needed. Make appropriate referrals. Assist client to plan follow-up care with surgeon.	Expression of satisfaction with own knowledge and skill level or with plan made for home care

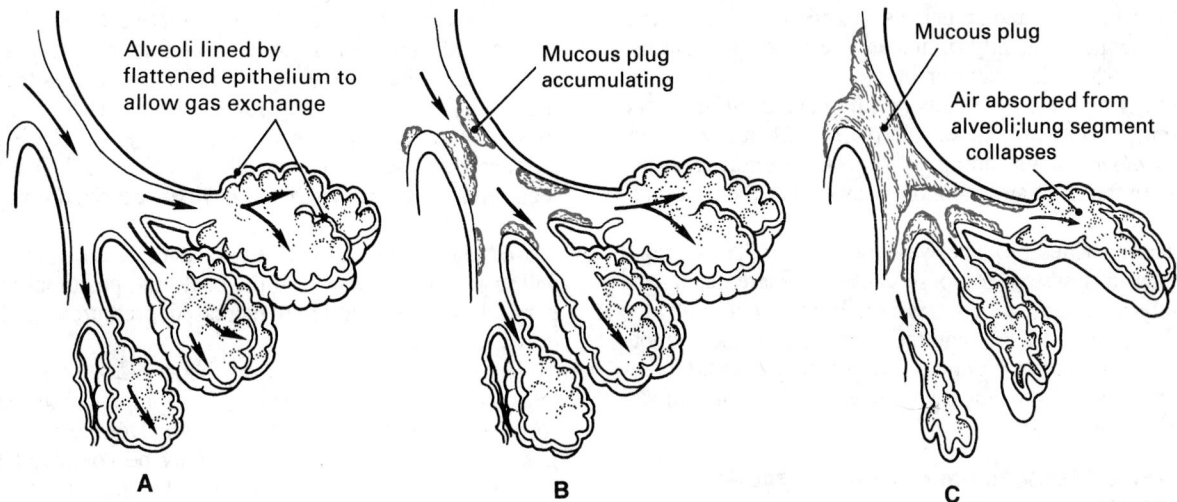

Fig. 13-7 Postoperative atelectasis. **A,** Normal bronchiole and alveoli. **B,** Mucous plug in bronchiole. **C,** Collapse of alveoli due to atelectasis following absorption of air.

support to weakened muscles and also aids in coughing and expectoration of secretions. Incentive spirometry is increasingly used as an adjunct to traditional deep breathing and coughing techniques.[17]

The client's position should be changed every 1 to 2 hours to allow full chest expansion and increase perfusion of both lungs. Ambulation, not just sitting in a chair, should be aggressively carried out as soon as physician approval is given. Adequate and regular analgesic medication should be provided, since incisional pain often is the greatest deterrent to client participation in effective ventilation and ambulation. The client should also be reassured that these activities will not cause the incision to separate. Adequate hydration, either parenteral or oral, is essential to maintain the integrity of mucous membranes and to keep secretions thin and loose for easy expectoration.

Potential Alterations in Cardiovascular Function

Etiology. Postoperative fluid and electrolyte imbalances are contributing factors to alterations in cardiovascular function. They may develop as a result of a combination of the body's normal response to the stress of surgery, excessive fluid losses, and improper IV replacement. The body's fluid status directly affects cardiac output. Fluid retention during the first 2 to 5 postoperative days is a result of the stress response. This body response serves to maintain both blood volume and blood pressure (see Chapter 5). Fluid retention results from the secretion and release of two hormones by the anterior pituitary: adrenocorticotropic hormone (ACTH) and antidiuretic hormone (ADH). ACTH stimulates the adrenal cortex to secrete aldosterone and cortisol. These adrenal cortical hormones promote sodium and water retention, which increases blood volume. ADH release leads to a decrease in urinary output, which ultimately increases blood volume.

Fluid overload may occur during this period of fluid retention when intravenous fluids are administered too rapidly, when chronic disease (e.g., cardiac or renal disease)

exists, or when the client is an older adult. Conversely, *fluid deficit* may be related to slow or inadequate fluid replacement, which leads to decreases in cardiac output and tissue perfusion. Untreated preoperative dehydration or intraoperative or postoperative losses from vomiting, bleeding, or drainage from drain tubes may be contributing factors in fluid deficits.

Hypokalemia is an added consequence of urinary and GI losses and results when potassium is not replaced in IV fluids. The loss of potassium directly affects the contraction and pumping ability of the heart and thus may also contribute to decreased cardiac output and overall body tissue perfusion. Adequate replacement of potassium is usually 40 mEq/day. However, it should not be given until adequate renal function has been established. A urine output of at least 30 ml/hour is generally considered reflective of adequate renal function.

Cardiovascular status is also affected by the state of *tissue perfusion* or blood flow. The stress response contributes to an increase in clotting tendencies in the postoperative client by increasing platelet production and circulating levels of glucocorticoids. *Blood clots* may form in leg veins as a result of inactivity, body position, and pressure, all of which lead to venous stasis and decreased perfusion. *Deep vein thrombosis,* especially common in older adults and immobilized clients, is a potentially life-threatening complication because it may lead to *pulmonary embolism.*[18,19] *Superficial thrombophlebitis* is an uncomfortable but less ominous complication that may develop in a leg vein as a result of venous stasis or in the arm veins as a result of irritation from IV needles or solutions. Clots may also form in pelvic veins after gynecological surgery when retractors or other instruments have injured the vein wall. If a piece of a clot becomes dislodged, it can cause a pulmonary infarction of a size proportionate to the vessel in which it lodges.

Syncope (fainting) is another factor that reflects the cardiovascular status. It may indicate decreased cardiac output, fluid deficits, and/or defects in cerebral tissue perfusion. Syncope frequently occurs as a result of postural hypotension when the client ambulates. It is more common in clients who are older adults or who have been immobile for long periods of time. Normally, when the client quickly moves to a standing position, the arterial pressoreceptors in the neck and the thorax respond to the accompanying fall in blood pressure with sympathetic nervous stimulation, which produces vasoconstriction. This sympathetic nervous system response causes an increase in, and therefore maintains, blood pressure. In the older adult, the immobile, and the postanesthetic clients, these sympathetic and vasomotor functions may be diminished. Consequently, syncope develops when the client sits up rapidly or during ambulation.

■ Nursing Management of Cardiovascular Function

Nursing assessment

Specific assessment of cardiovascular function includes the regular monitoring of the client's blood pressure, heart rate, pulses, and skin temperature and color. Results should be compared with preoperative status and the immediate postoperative/intraoperative findings.

Nursing diagnoses

Nursing diagnoses related to potential altered cardiovascular function in the postoperative client include, but are not limited to, the following:

Altered cardiac output: decreased

Fluid volume deficit

Altered tissue perfusion

Activity intolerance

Potential complication: thromboembolism

Nursing interventions

An accurate intake and output record should be kept during the postoperative period, and laboratory findings (e.g., electrolytes, hematocrit, osmolarity/specific gravity) should be monitored. Nursing responsibilities relating to IV management are critical during this period. In particular, the nurse should be alert for symptoms of too slow or too rapid a rate of fluid replacement. Assessment should also be made of the infusion site for discomfort and the hazards associated with the intravenous administration of potassium (see Chapter 10). *Thirst* is one of the most annoying discomforts with which the postoperative client must contend. This may be related to the drying effects of anticholinergic drugs, anesthetic gases, and fluid deficits. Adequate and regular mouth care is helpful while the client is in an NPO status.

Leg exercises, as demonstrated preoperatively, should be encouraged 10 to 12 times every 1 to 2 hours. The muscular contraction produced by these exercises and by ambulation facilitates venous return from the lower extremities. The ambulating client should pick up the feet rather than shuffling them so that muscular contraction is maximized. When confined to bed, the client should alternately flex and extend the legs. When the client is sitting in a chair or lying in bed, there should be no pressure to impede venous flow through the popliteal space. Crossed legs, pillows behind the knees, and elevation of the bed knee gatch must be avoided.

Some surgeons routinely prescribe elastic stockings or mechanical aids such as sequential stockings to stimulate and enhance the massaging/milking action that is transmitted to the veins when leg muscles contract.[19] The nurse must remember that these aids are useless if the legs are not exercised and may actually impair circulation if the legs remain inactive or if the devices are sized or applied improperly. When in use, these stockings must be removed and reapplied at least once every shift for skin care and inspection. The skin of the heels and posttibial areas is particularly susceptible to increased pressure and breakdown.

The use of low-dose heparin therapy (5000 units subcutaneously every 8 to 12 hours) is a prophylactic measure for venous thrombosis and embolism. Dosage may be begun 2 hours before surgery and may be continued for as long as 7 days postoperatively or until the client is fully ambulatory. This low-dose heparin does not significantly increase the risk of bleeding during surgery or in the postoperative period. However, this prophylactic measure is not routine and remains controversial.[20]

The nurse may prevent syncope by slowly making changes in the client's position. Progression to ambulation can be achieved by first raising the head of the client's bed for 1 to 2 minutes, then assisting the client to stand beside the bed, at the same time monitoring the radial pulse for rate and quality. If no changes or complaints are noted, ambulation can be started. If faintness occurs, the nurse can help the client sit on the edge of the bed while continuing to monitor the pulse. If changes occur or if the client complains of feeling faint during ambulation, the nurse should provide assistance to a nearby chair or ease the client to the floor. The client should remain in either location until recovered and then helped to walk back to the bed. If faintness occurs, it is often frightening for the client (and for the unprepared nurse), but syncope poses no real physiological danger, although injury can result from a fall.

Potential Alterations in Urinary Function

Etiology. Low urine output (800 to 1500 ml) in the first 24 hours may be expected, regardless of fluid intake. This is due to increased aldosterone and ADH secretion resulting from the stress of surgery, fluid restriction before surgery, loss of fluids due to evaporation during surgery, drainage, and diaphoresis. By the second or third day, the client will diurese after fluid has been mobilized and the immediate stress reaction subsides.

Actual urinary retention can occur in the postoperative period for a variety of reasons. Anesthesia depresses the nervous system, including the micturition reflex arc and the higher centers that influence it. This allows the bladder to fill more completely than normal before the urge to void is felt. It also impedes voluntary micturition. Anticholinergic and narcotic drugs may also interfere with the ability to initiate voiding or to empty the bladder completely.

Retention is more likely to occur after lower abdominal or pelvic surgery because spasm or guarding of the abdominal and pelvic muscles interferes with their normal function in micturition. Pain may clutter perception centers and interfere with the client's awareness of the less intense and more familiar sensation arising as the bladder fills. Voiding ability is probably impaired to the greatest extent by immobility and the recumbent position in bed. Lack of skeletal muscle activity decreases smooth muscle (bladder detrusor) tone, and the supine position reduces the ability to relax the perineal muscles and external sphincter.

Oliguria, the diminished output of urine related to intake, is associated with acute renal failure and is a less common although more serious problem after surgery. It may result from renal ischemia caused by inadequate renal perfusion secondary to a hemolytic reaction due to the transfusion of incompatible blood or altered cardiovascular function.

■ Nursing Management of Urinary Function

Nursing assessment

The urine of the postoperative client should be examined for both quantity and quality. The color, amount, consistency, and odor of the urine should be noted. Indwelling catheters should be assessed for patency, and urine output should be at least 30 ml/hr. If a catheter is not present, the client should be able to void about 200 ml of urine at the first voiding after surgery. Most people urinate within 6 to 8 hours after surgery. If no voiding occurs, the bladder should be inspected, palpated, and percussed for distention.

Nursing diagnoses

Nursing diagnoses related to potential altered urinary function in the postoperative client include, but are not limited to, the following:

Altered patterns of urinary elimination
Urinary retention: acute
High risk for urinary infection

Nursing interventions

The nurse may facilitate voiding by normal positioning of the client: sitting for females and standing for males. Providing reassurance to the client regarding the ability to void and the use of techniques such as running water or drinking water, blowing bubbles through a straw, or pouring warm water over the perineum, may also be of assistance. Ambulation, preferably to the bathroom, and the use of a bedside commode are additional helpful measures to assist in voiding.

The surgeon often leaves an order to catheterize the client in 8 to 12 hours if voiding has not occurred. Because of the possibility of infection associated with catheterization, the nurse should first try other measures to induce voiding and validate that the bladder is actually full. If the bladder becomes overdistended, it is traumatized and more susceptible to infection if catheterization becomes necessary. In assessing the need for catheterization, the nurse should consider fluid intake during and after surgery and evidence of bladder fullness (e.g., palpable fullness above the symphysis pubis, discomfort when pressure is applied over the bladder, or the presence of the urge to void). Because of the possibility of infection associated with an indwelling catheter, straight catheterization is preferred.

Potential Alterations in Gastrointestinal Function

Etiology. Slowed GI function and altered patterns of food intake may lead to the development of several distressing postoperative symptoms that are most pronounced after abdominal surgery. Nausea and vomiting may be caused by the action of anesthetics or narcotics, by slowed peristalsis resulting from the handling of the bowel during surgery, and by resumption of oral intake too soon after surgery.

Abdominal distention is another common problem caused by decreased peristalsis due to handling of the intestine during surgery and to limited dietary intake after surgery. Motility of the large intestine may be reduced for 3 to 5 days, although motility in the small intestine resumes within 24 hours. Swallowed air and GI secretions may accumulate in the colon, producing flatulence and gas pains.

Hiccoughs (singultus) are intermittent spasms of the diaphragm caused by irritation of the phrenic nerve, which innervates the diaphragm. Postoperative sources of direct irritation of the phrenic nerve may be gastric distention, intestinal obstruction, intraabdominal bleeding, and a subphrenic abscess. Indirect irritation of the phrenic nerve may be produced by acid-base and electrolyte imbalances. Reflex irritation may come from drinking very hot or cold liquids or from the presence of a nasogastric tube. Hiccoughs usually last only a short time and subside spontaneously. Occasionally they may be persistent but are rarely debilitating.

Parotitis is an inflammation of the parotid glands (also referred to as *surgical mumps*) that occurs when the normal stimulation of salivary secretion provided by eating is absent and the salivary ducts become blocked. It is uncomfortable for the client, producing considerable pain, swelling, and fever. It is also dangerous because a secondary staphylococcal infection can develop.

■ Nursing Management of Gastrointestinal Function

Nursing assessment

The assessment of bowel sounds is begun in the PAR and is continued routinely in the postoperative period. The abdomen should be auscultated in all four quadrants to determine the presence, frequency, and characteristics of the sounds. Bowel sounds are frequently absent or diminished in the immediate postoperative period when peristalsis is decreased.

Nursing diagnoses

Nursing diagnoses related to potential alterations in GI function in the postoperative client may include, but are not limited to, the following:

Nausea and vomiting
Pain related to hiccoughs
Altered nutrition: less than body requirements
Potential complication: paralytic ileus

Nursing interventions

Depending on the nature of the surgery, the client may resume oral intake as soon as the gag reflex returns. Sometimes the client is kept on NPO status for several days until bowel sounds are heard. While the client is receiving nothing by mouth, intravenous infusions are given to maintain fluid and electrolyte balance. A nasogastric tube may be used to decompress the stomach to prevent nausea, vomiting, and abdominal distention. When oral intake is allowed after the return of bowel sounds, clear liquids are begun and the IV infusion is continued. If oral intake is well tolerated by the client, the IV is discontinued and the diet is advanced until a regular diet is tolerated.

While the client is on NPO status, regular mouth care is essential for comfort and stimulation of salivary glands. Nausea and vomiting may be prevented or relieved by the administration of an antiemetic drug (usually of the phenothiazine type) given IV, intramuscularly, or by rectal suppository. In some instances, a nasogastric tube is inserted when symptoms persist.

Abdominal distention may be prevented or minimized by early and frequent ambulation and by resumption of a normal diet, both of which stimulate intestinal peristalsis. The nurse should assess the client regularly to detect the resumption of normal intestinal peristalsis as evidenced by the return of bowel sounds and the passage of flatus.

The client may need to be encouraged to expel flatus and to be assured that this is necessary and desirable. Gas pains, which tend to become pronounced on the second or third postoperative day, may be relieved by ambulation and frequent repositioning. Positioning the client on the right side permits gas to rise along the transverse colon and facilitates release. Bisacodyl (Dulcolax) suppositories may also be ordered to stimulate peristalsis and expulsion of flatus. Less used interventions include the placement of a rectal tube or the use of rectal lavage with right-sided positioning.

The postoperative client who is hiccoughing should first be assessed in an attempt to determine the cause. In many instances, simple irrigation of the nasogastric tube to restore patency will solve the problem. Techniques such as holding the breath while drinking water, swallowing 1 or 2 teaspoons of sugar, and rebreathing carbon dioxide from a paper bag may help. Drug therapy may include administration of atropine or phenothiazine. For intractable cases, a phrenic nerve block or phrenic nerve crush may be employed.

Parotitis may be prevented primarily by meticulous mouth care. Although chewing gum and sucking on hard candy are sometimes recommended to stimulate salivation, these activities may lead to increased swallowing of air and abdominal distention in the postoperative client. Antibiotic intervention as well as incision and drainage of the involved gland is sometimes necessary.

Potential Alterations of the Integument

Etiology. Surgery generally involves an incision through the skin and underlying tissues. This means disruption of the protective skin barrier and a need for wound healing, which is one of the major concerns of the postoperative period.

An adequate nutritional state is essential for wound healing. Amino acids are readily available for the healing process because of the catabolic effects of the stress response. The client who was well nourished preoperatively can tolerate the postoperative delay in nutritional intake. However, clients with preexisting nutritional deficits, such as those with chronic metabolic diseases (e.g., diabetes, ulcerative colitis, alcoholism), are more prone to problems of wound healing. Wound healing is also a concern for the older client and is affected by multiple factors.[21]

Wound infection may result from contamination of the wound from three major sources: exogenous flora (present in the environment and on the skin), oral flora, and intestinal flora. The incidence of wound sepsis is higher among clients who are malnourished, immunosuppressed, or aged or those who have prolonged hospital stays or lengthy surgical procedures (lasting more than 3 hours). Infection may involve the entire incision and may extend downward through the deeper tissue layers. An abscess may form locally, or the infection may penetrate entire body cavities, as is the case in peritonitis. Evidence of wound infection usually does not become apparent before the third to the fifth postoperative day. The signs include local manifestations of redness, swelling, and increasing pain and tenderness at the site. Systemic signs are fever and leukocytosis.

An accumulation of fluid within a wound may create pressure, impair circulation and wound healing, and predispose to infection. These are the reasons the surgeon may place a drain in the incision or make a stab wound adjacent to the incision to allow for drainage. These drains may be of soft rubber and drain into a dressing, or they may be firm catheters attached to a Hemovac or other source of gentle suction. (Wound healing and complications are discussed in Chapter 7.)

■ Nursing Management of Surgical Wounds
Nursing assessment

Nursing assessment of the wound and dressing requires knowledge of the type of wound, drains inserted, and expected drainage related to the specific type of surgery. A small amount of serous drainage is common from any type of wound. If a drain is in place, a moderate to large amount of drainage may be expected. For example, a cholecystectomy incision with accompanying Penrose drain is expected to have a moderate amount of serosanguineous drainage with some bile drainage within the first 24 hours. In contrast, an inguinal herniorrhaphy should have only minimal serous drainage during the postoperative period.

In general, drainage is expected to change from sanguineous (red) to serosanguineous (pink) to serous (straw-colored) over a period of hours and days. Bloody drainage may be normal after certain types of surgery (e.g., chest surgery). However, it should not last more than a few hours and should decrease in volume over time. Continuation of bleeding or an increase in drainage after it has once subsided often signals a problem. Wound infection may be accompanied by purulent drainage. Wound dehiscence (separation and disruption of previously joined wound edges) may be preceded by a sudden discharge of brown, pink, or clear drainage (Table 13-7).

Nursing diagnoses

Nursing diagnoses related to potential alterations in the integumentary system of the postoperative client include, but are not limited to, the following:

Impaired tissue integrity

High risk for infection

Nursing interventions

When drainage occurs on the dressing, it should be circled with a pen and marked with the date and time. The type, amount, color, consistency, and odor of drainage

Table 13-9 Expected Drainage from Tubes and Catheters

Substance	Daily Amount	Color	Odor	Consistency
INDWELLING CATHETER				
Urine	500-700 ml, 1-2 days postop; 1500-2500 ml thereafter	Clear, yellow	Ammonia	Watery
GASTROSTOMY TUBE				
Gastric contents	Up to 1500 ml/day	Pale, yellow-green	Sour	Watery
HEMOVAC				
Wound drainage	Variable with procedure	Variable with procedure	Same as wound dressing	Variable
T TUBE				
Bile	500 ml	Bright yellow to dark green	Acid	Thick
NASOGASTRIC TUBE				
Gastric contents	Up to 1500 ml	Pale yellow-green	Sour	Watery
MILLER-ABBOTT TUBE				
Intestinal contents	Up to 3000 ml	Dark green or brown	Neutral acid, fecal	Thick

Adapted from Croushore T: Postoperative assessment: the key to avoiding the most common nursing mistakes, Nursing 9:47, 1979.

should be noted and recorded. (Expected drainage from tubes is outlined in Table 13-9.) The effect of position changes on drainage should also be assessed. The surgeon should be notified of any excessive or abnormal drainage and significant changes in vital signs.

The surgical incision may or may not be covered with a dressing after the first few hours. The incision may be covered with a transparent, impermeable, adherent dressing immediately after surgery, but 24 to 48 hours later it may be opened to the air if there are no drains or drainage. Agency policy determines whether the nurse may change the initial operative dressing or simply reinforce it when the dressing is saturated.

When a dressing is changed, the number and type of drains present should be noted. Care should be taken to avoid dislodging drains during dressing removal. When the dressing is changed, the incision site should be examined carefully. The area around the sutures may be slightly reddened and swollen, an expected inflammatory response. However, the skin around the incision should be of normal color and temperature. Abnormal findings include unusually warm skin around the incision, purple hard areas in the site (possibly from hemorrhage into the tissue), and other signs of infection. The nurse should wear gloves when removing a dressing. The gloves should be sterile if the nurse expects to handle the drain or palpate the wound. Sterile technique should be used when any new dressing is applied. If healing is by primary intention, little or no drainage is present, and no drains are in place. A single-layer dressing is sufficient. When drains are in place, when moderate to heavy drainage is occurring, or when healing occurs other than by primary intention, a multiple-layer dressing is needed. (Wound care is discussed in Chapter 7.)

Potential Alterations in Neurological Function

Etiology. Pain and fever are two clinical manifestations mediated by the CNS that may present problems for the postoperative client. (The assessment and management of the client in pain are discussed in Chapter 51.)

Postoperative pain is produced by the interaction of a number of physiological and psychological factors. The skin and underlying tissues have been traumatized by the incision and retraction during surgery. In addition, there may be reflex muscle spasms around the incision. Anxiety and fear, sometimes related to the anticipation of pain, create tension and further increase muscle tone and spasm. The effort and movement associated with deep breathing, coughing, and changing position may aggravate pain by creating tension or pull on the incisional area.

When the internal viscera is cut, no pain is felt. However, pressure within the internal viscera elicits pain. Therefore deep visceral pain may signal the presence of a complication such as intestinal distention, bleeding, or abscess formation.

Postoperative pain is usually most severe within the first 48 hours and subsides thereafter. Variation is considerable, according to the procedure performed and the client's individual pain tolerance or perception.

Temperature variation in the postoperative period provides valuable information about the client's status. Hypothermia may be present for a few hours while the client is recovering from the effects of anesthesia and body heat loss during surgery. Fever may occur at any time during

Table 13-10 Significance of Postoperative
Temperature Changes

Time After Surgery	Temperature	Possible Causes
Up to 12 hr	Hypothermia to 34.5° C (94° F)	Effects of anesthesia Body heat loss in surgical exposure
First 24-48 hr	Elevation to 38° C (100.4° F)	Inflammatory response to surgical stress
	Above 38° C (100.4° F)	Lung congestion, atelectasis Dehydration
Third day and later	Elevation above 37.7° C (100° F)	Wound infection Urinary infection Respiratory infection Phlebitis Parotitis (rare)

the postoperative period (Table 13-10). A mild elevation (up to 38° C, 100.4° F) during the first 48 hours usually reflects the surgical stress response. A moderate elevation (above 38° C) is caused most frequently by respiratory congestion or atelectasis and less frequently by dehydration. After the first 48 hours, a moderate to marked elevation (above 37.7° C, 99.9° F) is usually caused by infection.

Wound infection, particularly from aerobic organisms, is often accompanied by a fever that spikes in the afternoon or evening and returns to near normal levels in the morning. The respiratory tract may be infected secondary to stasis of secretions in an atelectatic region. The urinary tract may be infected secondary to catheterization. Superficial thrombophlebitis may occur at the IV site or in the leg veins. The latter may produce a temperature elevation between 7 and 10 days after surgery.

Intermittent high fever accompanied by shaking chills and diaphoresis suggests septicemia. This may occur at any time during the postoperative period because microorganisms may have been introduced into the bloodstream during surgery (especially in GI or genitourinary [GU] procedures) or picked up later from the site of a wound or a urinary or vein infection.

It is important to know what the client's normal temperature is when the significance of postoperative temperatures is being assessed. Studies of older adult clients report that normal mean temperatures are lower than in younger subjects and are more variable.

■ Nursing Management of Neurological Function

Nursing assessment
The initial aspect of the neurological assessment is determination of the level of consciousness. Anesthetized cli-

ents resume consciousness in a predictable pattern. By the time clients return to the clinical unit, they are usually awake or easily arousable. The nurse always needs to be alert for possible deepening of anesthesia effects, especially when administering pain medication in the early postoperative period.

Pain assessment may be difficult in the early postoperative period. The client may not be able to verbalize the presence or severity of pain. The nurse should observe for clues of pain such as a wrinkling face or brow, a clenched fist, moaning, diaphoresis, and an increased pulse rate.

Nursing diagnoses
Nursing diagnoses related to potential alterations in neurological function of the postoperative client may include, but are not limited to, the following:

Sensory/perceptual alterations
Pain
Ineffective thermoregulation
High risk for altered body temperature
Sleep pattern disturbance

Nursing interventions
Postoperative pain relief is essentially a nursing responsibility, since the surgeon's orders for analgesic medication and other comfort measures are usually written on an as needed basis.[22,23] During the first 48 hours or longer, narcotic analgesics (e.g., morphine or meperidine) are required to relieve the moderate to severe pain. After that time, nonnarcotic analgesics may be sufficient as pain intensity decreases.

Nurses must examine their own attitudes toward pain and suffering. Too often nurses undermedicate their clients in an attempt to protect them from addiction, an imagined hazard that simply does not exist during the few days of extreme postoperative discomfort. Studies have shown that nurses tend to give less pain medication to older adults and female clients.[24-27]

During the first 24 to 48 hours, the client should be medicated freely every 3 to 4 hours if necessary because (1) the greatest relief is obtained when an analgesic is administered as pain is beginning rather than when it has become more severe and (2) relative freedom from pain is essential to gain the client's cooperation in activities of deep breathing, coughing, turning, and ambulating. When the client does request pain medication, it should be given promptly because minutes can seem like hours to a person in pain.

Analgesic administration should be timed so that it is in effect during activities that may be painful for the client, such as ambulating. Although narcotic analgesics are often essential for the postoperative client's well-being, they are not without undesirable side effects. These side effects (slowed intestinal peristalsis and spasms of the sphincter of Oddi, nausea and vomiting, respiratory and cough depression, and hypotension) are most common with the opiates.

Before administering any analgesic, the nurse should first assess the nature of the client's pain, including location, quality, and intensity. If it is incisional pain, the analgesic is appropriate. If it is remote chest or leg pain, medication may simply mask a complication that must be reported and documented. If it is gas pain, narcotic medication can aggravate it. The nurse should notify the physician and request a change in the order if the analgesic either fails to relieve the pain or makes the client excessively lethargic or somnolent.

Patient-controlled analgesia (PCA) and epidural analgesia are two alternative approaches for pain control. The goals of PCA are to provide immediate analgesia and to maintain a constant, steady serum level of the analgesic agent. It involves self-administration of predetermined doses of analgesia by the client. The route of delivery may be IV or oral.[28,29]

Epidural analgesia is the infusion of pain-relieving medications through a catheter placed into the epidural space surrounding the spinal cord. The goal of epidural analgesia is delivery of medication directly to opiate receptors in the spinal cord, thus preventing some of the systemic side effects of IV and IM narcotic analgesia. However, it is not self-administered. The administration may be intermittent or constant and is monitored by the nurse. The overall effectiveness and the technique of administration result in a constant circulating level and a total reduced dose of medication. Medication is delivered before pain is severe.[30-32]

A number of other measures may be helpful in preventing or relieving postoperative pain. If abdominal surgery has been performed, the client should be instructed to use the limbs rather than the abdominal muscles in turning and getting out of bed. Techniques of controlled breathing or relaxation may be used for pain relief. Both methods have a similar rationale, which includes anxiety reduction, attention distraction, muscle relaxation, and provision of a sense of control over the pain experience.[33-36] Transcutaneous electrical nerve stimulation (TENS) has also been effective in decreasing pain perception in postoperative clients.[37]

The nurse's role with respect to postoperative fever may be preventive, diagnostic, and therapeutic. Meticulous asepsis is a preventive measure that should be maintained with regard to the wound and IV site, as well as frequent observation for early signs of inflammation.

The client's temperature is usually measured every 4 hours for the first 48 hours postoperatively and then less frequently if no problems develop. If fever develops, chest x-rays may be taken, along with cultures of the wound, urine, or blood, depending on the suspected cause. If infection is the source of the fever, antibiotics are started IM or by IV piggyback as soon as cultures have been obtained. If the fever is extreme (>41° C, 105.8° F), antipyretic drugs and body-cooling measures may be employed.

Potential Alterations in Psychological Function

Etiology. Anxiety and depression may occur in the postoperative client for many reasons (see Chapter 11). These states may be more pronounced in the client who has had radical surgery (e.g., colostomy) or amputation or whose findings suggest a poor prognosis (e.g., inoperable tumor). A history of a neurotic or psychotic disorder should alert the nurse to the possibility of postoperative anxiety and depression. However, these responses may develop in any client as part of the grief response to loss of a body organ or disturbance in body image and may be exacerbated by a lowered response to stress.

Confusion or delirium may arise from a variety of psychological and physiological sources, including fluid and electrolyte imbalance, hypoxia, drug toxicity, sleep deprivation, and sensory alteration, deprivation, or overload. Delirium tremens due to alcohol withdrawal may be responsible for as much as 25% of all postoperative delirium.[6] It is characterized by restlessness, insomnia and nightmares, tachycardia, apprehension, confusion and disorientation, irritability, and auditory or visual hallucinations, and it may be treated by the administration of alcohol (see Chapter 60).

■ Nursing Management of Psychological Function

Nursing diagnoses

Nursing diagnoses related to potential alterations in psychological function in the postoperative client include, but are not limited to, the following:

Anxiety
Ineffective individual coping
Self-care deficit: partial to total
Altered health maintenance
Sensory/perceptual alterations

Nursing interventions

The nurse attempts to prevent psychological problems in the postoperative period by providing adequate support for the client. Supportive measures include taking time to listen and talk with the client, offering explanations and genuine reassurance, and encouraging the presence and assistance of significant others. The nurse must observe and evaluate the client's behavior to distinguish a normal reaction to the stress situation from one that is becoming abnormal or excessive. The recognition of the alcohol withdrawal syndrome in a client not previously known to be an alcoholic presents a particular challenge. Any unusual or disturbed behavior should be reported immediately so that diagnosis and treatment may be instituted.

Planning for Discharge and Follow-Up Care

Preparation for the client's discharge is an ongoing process throughout the surgical experience that begins during the preoperative period. The informed client is therefore prepared as events unfold and gradually assumes greater responsibility for self-care during the postoperative period.

As the day of discharge approaches, the nurse should be certain that the client has the following information:

1. Care of wound site and any dressings
2. Action and possible side effects of any medications; when and how to take them
3. Activities allowed and prohibited; when various physical activities can be resumed safely (e.g., driving a car, returning to work, sexual intercourse, leisure activities)
4. Dietary restrictions or modifications
5. Symptoms to be reported (e.g., development of incisional tenderness or increased drainage, discomfort in other parts of the body)
6. Where and when to return for follow-up care

DISCHARGE SUMMARY/INSTRUCTIONS

Date of discharge_____
Time of discharge_____

Addressograph plate

Discharge to: Home_____   Nursing home_____   Hospital_____   AMA_____
                Group Home_____   DRG exempt_____   Expired_____   Other_____

Transfer papers completed: Yes_____   N/A_____

Follow-up instructions to client or significant other
    ADL:_____
_____

    Wound care/dressing/appliances:_____
_____

    Special teaching:_____
_____

    Diet:_____
_____

Medication card given to client   Yes_____   N/A_____

Prescriptions given to client   Yes_____   N/A_____

Medications reviewed with client/significant other   Yes_____   N/A_____

Potential fookd/drug interactions with_____   Discussed and literature provided   Yes_____   N/A_____

Next physician appointment_____

Telephone number_____

Outpatient appointment   Date_____   Time_____   Place_____

Valuables returned   Date and person_____   Yes_____   N/A_____

Medications returned to client   Date and person_____   Yes_____   N/A_____

I acknowledge receipt and understanding of the above instructions. I also understand that if I have any problems or questions regarding the use of medications or changes in my condition, I should contact my physician.

_____   _____
Signature of client /significant other   Signature of nurse   Date

Fig. 13-8   Discharge summary/instructions. (Courtesy Elliot Hospital, Manchester, NH.)

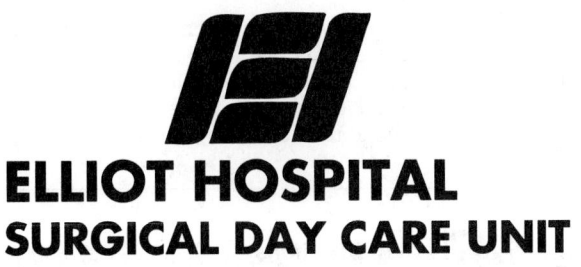

ELLIOT HOSPITAL
SURGICAL DAY CARE UNIT ▬▬▬▬▬

955 AUBURN STREET, MANCHESTER, NH 03104   (603) 669-5300 EXT. 2183, 2143

Although you will not be discharged until you are considered "street fit," that is, have minimal nausea, have had oral liquids, and are able to stand and walk, the effects of the anesthetics used for your surgery may be longer lasting than you might realize. Therefore, for a safe recovery from anesthesia, please observe the following instructions.

1. You must be accompanied by a responsible adult to drive you home at the time of discharge.

2. Do not attempt to return to work on the day of your surgery.

3. Do not drink alcoholic beverages for 24 hours.

4. Do not drive any vehicle or operate any dangerous equipment for at least 24 hours (e.g. tractors, snowblowers, lawn mowers, chain saws).

5. You should not make any important business or personal decisions for a least 24 hours.

6. For your diet, start with small amounts of food that you tolerate easily, such as liquids and soup. If you have nausea or vomiting, don't eat or drink for two hours, then progress slowly with liquids. It may be several hours or even the next morning before you feel like eating.

7. You should make arrangements for someone to be with you during the first 24 hours after discharge from the hospital.

8. Limit physical activity for 24 hours.

9. Dizziness, blurred vision, or nausea may occur, but these side effects usually disappear completely within 24 hours. Many people don't experience any side effects at all. Sore throat and muscle aches occur occasionally, but seldom require treatment.

10. If you received a nerve block anesthetic or IV regional, be especially careful not to burn or otherwise injure yourself, since your sensation of pain may be impaired for 1 or more hours.

Special instructions:_____

_____

_____

_____

_____

You may have one friend or one family member stay with you in the Surgical Day Care Unit.

I UNDERSTAND AND AGREE TO FOLLOW THE ABOVE INSTRUCTIONS.

_____
Client/Family Guardian

_____ Date _____
Nurse

Fig. 13-9   Discharge instructions from a surgical day care center. (Courtesy Elliot Hospital, Manchester, NH.)

7. Answers to any individual questions or concerns

If the physician has not provided information about particular diet or activity prescriptions or restrictions, the nurse should either obtain this or encourage the client to do so. Attention to complete discharge instruction may prevent needless distress for the client. Written instructions are important for reinforcing the information given to the client. The nurse should specifically document in the record the discharge instructions provided the client and the family (Fig. 13-8). For the client the postoperative phase of care continues and extends into the recuperative period. Assessment and evaluation of the client after discharge may be accomplished by a follow-up call.[38]

Ambulatory surgery discharge. The client leaving the OpSu must be able to provide a degree of self-care and must be mobile and alert. Postoperative pain, nausea, and vomiting must be controlled. The body functions for the general postoperative client must also be evaluated in the OpSu client. Overall, the client must be stable and near the level of preoperative functioning for discharge from the unit. On discharge, both specific and general instructions are given to the client verbally and reinforced with written directions (Fig. 13-9). The client may not drive and must be accompanied by a responsible adult at the time of discharge. A follow-up evaluation of the client's status is made by telephone, and any specific questions and concerns are addressed.

C ase Study

ELECTIVE SURGERY

Mrs. Gwendolyn Abbamonto, a 42-year-old elementary school teacher who is married and the mother of two children, has undergone an elective cholecystectomy for gallstones. The surgery under general anesthesia was uncomplicated. A Penrose drain was placed in the gallbladder bed and brought out through a stab wound adjacent to the right upper quadrant abdominal incision. Her surgeon has written these postoperative orders:

Nasogastric tube to low intermittent suction; irrigate prn.
IV: Follow present 1000 ml D_5W with 1000 mL Ringer's lactate q 8 hr and 1000 ml D_5W with 40 mEq KCl q 8 hr
Turn, cough, and deep breathe every hour
Ambulate this PM and then qid
Vital signs per routine
Morphine sulfate 10 mg IM q 4 hr prn
Change dressing over drain prn

Discussion Questions

1. What nursing measures should be taken in the recovery room to protect Mrs. Abbamonto from hazards during postanesthesia recovery?
2. How should it be determined that she is sufficiently recovered from general anesthesia to be transferred to her room?
3. What is the purpose of ambulating this client on the evening of surgery?
4. What factors may particularly predispose Mrs. Abbamonto to the following postoperative problems: atelectasis, wound infection, abdominal distention, and hyponatremia?
5. What type of drainage is expected from the incision and Penrose drain during the first three postoperative days?
6. What nursing observations indicate to the surgeon that her nasogastric tube can be removed and oral intake resumed? Describe how to implement the following doctor's orders:

removal of nasogastric tube; sips of water to diet as tolerated; and D/C IV.

7. If Mrs. Abbamonto complains of cramping abdominal pain on the third postoperative day, what measures should be used to relieve it? Why?

R eview Questions

The number of the question corresponds to the same-numbered objective at the beginning of the chapter.

1. As soon as the client enters the recovery room, the nurse routinely
   a. initiates range of motion to extremities
   b. assesses level of consciousness and presence of reflexes
   c. starts a unit of whole blood
   d. removes the oropharyngeal airway
2. Which of these nursing actions is *not* desirable during recovery from general anesthesia?
   a. encouraging deep breathing and coughing
   b. placing the client in a supine position
   c. suctioning to remove excess respiratory secretions
   d. auscultating the client's chest bilaterally
3. During the first 24 to 48 hours postoperatively, analgesic medication should be given
   a. every 3 hours, even if pain is not present
   b. every 3 to 4 hours as soon as pain begins
   c. every 4 to 6 hours when pain becomes fairly severe
   d. as infrequently as possible to avoid addiction
4. A mild temperature elevation (up to 38° C) in the first 48 hours postoperatively usually reflects
   a. surgical stress response
   b. respiratory congestion
   c. wound infection
   d. urinary infection
5. Which of the following should the client have in preparation for discharge?
   a. rationale for abstinence from sexual intercourse for 4 to 6 weeks
   b. need to call hospital clinical unit to report any abnormal signs or symptoms
   c. time frame for when various physical activities can be resumed
   d. referral to nutritional center for management of dietary restrictions
6. A consideration in planning the discharge of an ambulatory surgical client is
   a. discharge with a responsible adult
   b. provision of written instruction
   c. ambulation as soon as possible
   d. sufficient pain control

REFERENCES

1. Borchardt A and Fraulini KE: A guide to solving postanesthesia problems, Nursing 18:66-86, 1988.
2. Hardy JD: Surgical complications. In Sabiston DC, ed: Davis Christopher textbook of surgery, ed 12, Philadelphia, 1981, WB Saunders Co, p 422.

3. Fraulinei KE: After anesthesia: a guide for PACU, ICU, and medical-surgical nurses, Norwalk, Conn, 1987, Appleton & Lange, p 221.

4. Steinberg FU, ed: General surgery in care of the geriatric in the tradition of E.V. Cowdry, ed 6, St Louis, 1983, The CV Mosby Co, p 317.

5. Chitwood L: Unveiling the mysteries of anesthesia, Nursing 17:52, 1987.

6. Drain CE and Christopher SS: The recovery room: a critical care approach to post anesthesia nursing, ed 2, Philadelphia, 1987, WB Saunders Co, p 214.

7. Kalbach LR: Spinal headache: cause and care, Orthop Nurs 8:51, 1989.

8. Lachman VD: Is spinal anesthesia as bad as it sounds? Nursing 16:42, 1986.

9. Richards M: Perioperative nursing research: part VI: postoperative phase, AORN J 50:120, 1989.

10. Crayne HL and Miner DG: Thermo resuscitation for postoperative hypothemia using reflective blankets, AORN J 47:222, 1988.

11. Burkle NL: Inadvertent hypothermia, J Gerontol Nurs 14:26, 1988.

12. Kitz DS and others: Discharging outpatients: factors nurses consider to determine readiness, AORN J 48:87, 1988.

13. Slotman GJ, Jed EH, and Burchard KW: Adverse effects of hypothermia in postoperative patients, Am J Surg 149:495, 1985.

14. Jackson MR: Elder care: implication of surgery in very elderly patients, AORN J 50:859, 1989.

15. Gioella EC and Bevil CW: Nursing care of the aging client: promoting healthy adaptation, Norwalk, Conn, 1985, Appleton-Century-Crofts, p 482.

16. Howie J: How and when should I respond to postoperative fever? Am J Nurs 89:984, 1989.

17. Spearing C: Incentive spirometry: inspiring your patient to breathe deeply, Nursing 17:50, 1987.

18. Dickinson SP and Bury GM: Pulmonary embolism: anatomy of a crisis, Nursing 19:39, 1989.

19. Fahey VA: An in-depth look at deep vein thrombosis, Nursing 19:86, 1989.

20. Nurses' drug alert, Am J Nurs 87:1192, 1987.

21. Wysocki AB: Surgical wound healing, AORN J 49:502, 1989.

22. McCaffery M: Giving meperidine for pain: should it be so mechanical? Nursing 17:60, 1987.

23. McCaffery M: Giving narcotics for pain: a problem solver handbook, Nursing 19:161, 1989.

24. Infante MC and Mooney NE: Interactive aspects of pain assessment, Orthop Nurs 6:31, 1987.

25. Faherty BS and Grier MR: Analgesic medication for elderly people post surgery, Nurs Res 33:369, 1989.

26. Eliopoulos C: A guide to the nursing of the aging, Baltimore, 1987, Williams & Wilkins Co, pp 41, 216.

27. Eland JM: Pain management and comfort, J Gerontol Nurs 14:11, 1988.

28. Jones L: Patient controlled oral analgesia, Orthop Nurs 6:38, 1987.

29. Schulte-Kresl JL: Patient controlled analgesia: a new system for pain management, AORN J 48:481, 1988.

30. Haight IC: What you should know about epidural analgesia, Nursing 17:58, 1987.

31. Genge ML: Epidural analgesia in the orthopaedic patient, Orthop Nurs 7:11, 1988.

32. Eaton JA: Continuous meperidine infusion for postoperative pain, Orthop Nurs 7:29, 1988.

33. Moss VA: Music and the surgical patient: the effect of music on anxiety, AORN J 48:64, 1988.

34. Bowers ME: Self-regulation techniques in the elderly, J Gerontol Nurs 15:15, 1989.

35. Tovar KM and Cassmeyer VL: Touch: the beneficial effects for the surgical patient, AORN J 49:1356, 1989.

36. McGuire L: Administering analgesics: which drugs are right for your patient, Nursing 20:34, 1990.

37. Hargraves A and Lander J: Use of transcutaneous electric nerve stimulation for postoperative pain, Nurs Res 38:159, 1989.

38. Cave LA: Follow-up phone calls after hospital discharge, Am J Nurs 89:942, 1989.

SECTION III REFERENCES

BOOKS

Breslow MJ, Miller CF, and Rogers MC: Perioperative management, St Louis, 1990, Mosby–Year Book, Inc.

Brooks SM: Fundamentals of operating room nursing, ed 2, St Louis, 1979, The CV Mosby Co.

Carrollm LJ: A nurses' guide to caring for elders, New York, 1988, Springer Publishing Co.

Eliopoulos C: A guide to the nursing of the aging, Baltimore, 1987, Williams & Wilkins.

Gerontological nursing: concepts and practice, Philadelphia, 1988, WB Saunders Co.

Groah LK: Operating room nursing: perioperative practice, ed 2, Norwalk Conn, 1990, Appleton & Lange.

Tighe SMB: Instrumentation for the operating room: a photographic manual, ed 3, St Louis, 1989, The CV Mosby Co.

JOURNALS

Burden N: Post anesthesia while the patient is unconscious, RN, Apr 1988, p 34.

Burton-Maree N: Outpatient anesthesia for orthopaedic procedures, Orthop Nurs 6:2, 1987.

Fillette MK and Caruso CC: Intraoperative tissue injury: major causes and preventive measures, AORN J 50:1, 1989.

Kam BW and Werner PW: Self-care theory. Application to perioperative nursing, AORN J 51:1365, 1990.

Kleinbeck SVM: Developing nursing diagnosis for a perioperative care plan: a classroom project, AORN J 49:6, 1989.

MacKenzie P and Beresford LA: Planning and documentation: addressing patient needs in a day surgery setting, AORN J 47:2, 1988.

Reeder JM: Ethical dilemmas in perioperative nursing practice, Nurs Clin North Am 24:999, 1989.

Schafer WG: Malignant hyperthermia: potential crisis in patient care, AORN J 50:2, 1989.

Takahaski JJ and others: Project alpha: designing courses that recruit and retain OR nurses, AORN J 51:497, 1990.

Tolley RG and others: Perioperative nursing: designing, implementing a baccalaureate elective, AORN J 52:105, 1990.

Tovar MK and Cassmeyer VL: Touch: the beneficial effects for the surgical patient, AORN J 49:5, 1989.

Wahl SC: Septic shock, Nursing 19:1, 1989.

William M and Brett SP: Discharge surveys: a quality assurance method for ambulatory surgery, AORN J 49:5, 1989.

Wiseman SJ: Patient advocacy: the essence of perioperative nursing in ambulatory surgery, AORN J 51:754, 1990.

Wombwell ME: The nursing elective experience—one strategy to promote perioperative nursing, Todays OR Nurse 12:22, 1990.

ORGANIZATIONS

American Association of Nurse Anesthetists
216 Higgins Road
Park Ridge, IL 60068

American Society of Post Anesthesia Nurses

Association of Operating Room Nurses
10170 East Mississippi Avenue
Denver, CO 80231

Intravenous Nurses Society
2 Brighton Street
Belmont, MA 02178

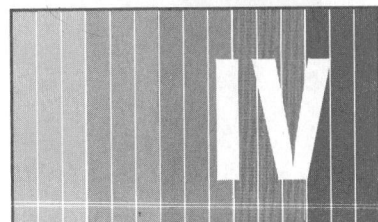
PROBLEMS RELATED TO ALTERED SENSORY INPUT

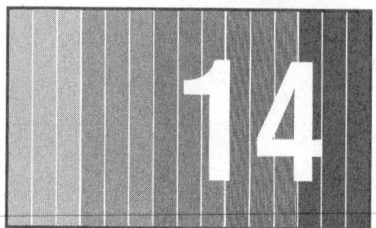

CHAPTER

14

Nursing Assessment
Vision and Hearing

Pamela S. Schremp
Mary E. Means

The importance of vision and hearing to well-being and communication cannot be overestimated. Not only do the eyes and ears sense nearby stimuli, they also provide information about the world away from the immediate environment of a person. Impairment of either of these two senses causes many changes in the client's mobility and ability to interact with others.

The visual system consists of internal and external structures. The internal structures are the iris, lens, ciliary body, choroid, and retina. The external structures are the eyelids, eyelashes, conjunctiva, cornea, sclera, and external ocular muscles.

STRUCTURES AND FUNCTIONS OF THE VISUAL SYSTEM
Ocular Structures

External structures and functions. The external structures serve a very important role in protecting the eye. The eyelids, or palpebrae, and eyelashes protect the eye from dust and foreign particles (Fig. 14-1). The eye is further protected by the surrounding bony orbit as well as by fat

pads located inferiorly (below) and posteriorly (behind) the globe (eyeball). The upper eyelid blinks spontaneously approximately 15 times a minute, distributing tears over the anterior surface of the eyeball.

The eyelids open and close through the action of muscles innervated by cranial nerves (CNs). Muscular action also helps hold the eyelids against the eyeball. The *tarsal plate,* a tough sheet of connective tissue within the lids, maintains the shape of the eyelids. When open, the upper eyelid rests just below the *limbus,* where the cornea and sclera meet.

The inner surface of the eyelids is covered by a transparent mucous membrane, the palpebral conjunctiva. This structure takes on the pink color of the underlying tissue while forming a pocket. The bulbar conjunctiva is located over the sclera. It contains tiny blood vessels that are most visible in the periphery. The bulbar conjunctiva terminates at the corneal-scleral limbus.

The *sclera* comprises the posterior five sixths of the external eye. It is referred to as *the white of the eye* because it is composed of collagen fibers meshed together into an opaque structure. It encircles the globe and joins the cornea at the limbus.

The transparent *cornea* comprises the anterior one sixth

Reviewed by Tana Durnbaugh, R.N., Ed.D., Professor, College of Lake County, Grayslake, Illinois.

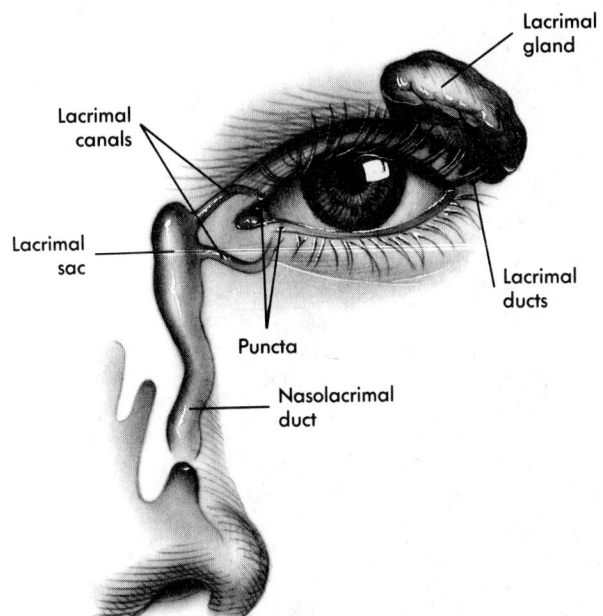

Fig. 14-1   External eye and lacrimal apparatus. (Adapted from Seeley R, Stephens T, and Tate P: Anatomy and physiology, St Louis, 1989, Times Mirror/Mosby College Publishing, p 469.)

of the globe. It is one of the most sensitive tissues in the body and is innervated by the trigeminal nerve (CN V). The avascular cornea obtains oxygen through the epithelial or external layer and through a pump mechanism in the endothelial or internal layer. When the cornea receives a decreased oxygen supply or is affected by trauma or disease, it becomes edematous and cloudy. The resultant cloudy state impedes transmission of light and can be very painful. The cornea also has refractive powers. Its curvature bends (refracts) light rays to help bring the light rays into focus on the retina.

Many glands provide secretions to make up the tear film that covers the anterior surface of the globe. The tear film moistens the cornea and provides oxygen and nourishment. Tears, moved over the anterior surface of the eye by blinking and eye movements, are drained by the lacrimal punctum through the lacrimal sac and into the nose (Fig. 14-1). The amount of tears produced decreases with sleeping, aging, and some diseases such as Sjögren's syndrome and rheumatoid arthritis. Increased production of tears occurs with trauma, presence of a foreign body, and diseases of the conjunctiva, cornea, eyelids, and nasal mucosa.

Each eye is moved by extraocular muscles. Neuromuscular coordination produces simultaneous movement of the eyes in the same direction (*conjugate movement*).

The eyeball. The eyeball is composed of three layers and is filled with fluid (Fig. 14-2). The tough outer layer is composed of the sclera and the transparent cornea. The middle layer or uveal tract includes the iris, choroid, and ciliary body. The *iris*, known for providing color to the eye, functions with the pupil to regulate the amount of light entering the eye. The *pupil*, located in the center of the iris, is a small round opening through which light

passes to enter the eye. When the iris contracts, it uses constrictor muscles located at the pupillary margin and parasympathetic innervation to make the pupil become smaller. The amount of light entering the eye is then limited. The sympathetic nervous system, along with dilator muscles, controls iris dilatation. When stimulated, the dilator muscles pull the iris away from the center opening of the pupil, allowing the pupil to expand and light to enter.

The highly vascular *choroid*, or middle layer, nourishes the retina and the posterior segment (back part) of the eye. Many of the blood vessels responsible for the nutrition of the retina are located in the choroid.

The ciliary body extends from the iris to the peripheral retina. It contains ciliary processes that secrete aqueous humor, a clear fluid located in the anterior and posterior chambers.

The *retina*, the light-sensitive layer, is the innermost layer. It is responsible for converting images into a form the brain can understand and process as vision. The retina is composed of two types of photoreceptor cells, rods and cones. Rods are stimulated in dim or darkened environments, and the cones are receptive to colors and bright environments. There are approximately 110 to 125 million rods and 6.5 million cones in each retina.[1] The *macula*, a centrally located area, has a high concentration of cones and is relatively free of blood vessels. Within the macula is the *fovea centralis*, a pinpoint depression composed solely of cones. This is the area of sharpest vision and central focus. Nourishment to the macula comes from two sources: the choroid and the underlying pigment epithelium, the lowest layer of the retina.

With the exception of the macula, the retina is nourished by retinal arterioles and veins. This blood supply enters the eye through the optic disc. These vessels are very important because they can be easily inspected with an ophthalmoscope. The condition of the retinal arteries is a good indicator of the vascular system in general.

The optic disc is located nasally from the macula and has a depression within it called the *physiological cup*. The optic disc is the optic nerve (CN I) and carries the visual impulses toward the brain.

Refractive media. For light to reach the retina, it must pass through a number of structures: the cornea, aqueous humor, lens, and vitreous. Each structure has a different density and plays a role in helping the image fall focused on the retina. The transparent cornea is the first structure through which light passes. It is responsible for the majority of light bending or refracting necessary for clear vision.[2]

Aqueous humor, a clear watery fluid, fills the anterior and posterior chambers of the anterior cavity of the eye. The anterior chamber is located between the cornea and the iris, and the posterior chamber is located between the iris and lens (Fig. 14-2). Aqueous humor is produced by the ciliary process. It passes through the pupil from the posterior chamber into the anterior chamber (Fig. 14-3). It drains through the trabecular meshwork located in the angle formed by the cornea and iris, and into the canal of Schlemm. This circular canal conveys fluid into scleral veins, which enter the circulation of the body. The aqueous humor bathes and nourishes the lens and the endothe-

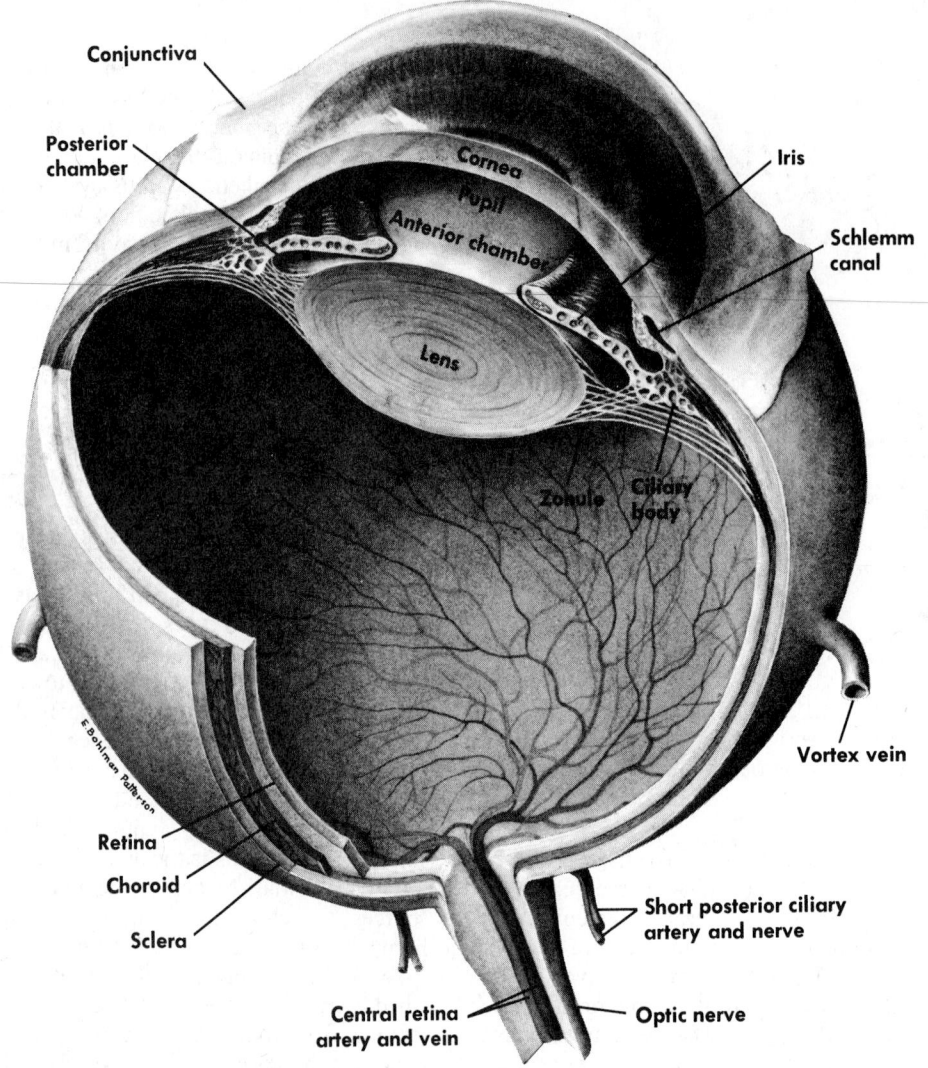

Conjunctiva

Posterior chamber

Cornea

Pupil

Anterior chamber

Iris

Schlemm canal

Lens

Zonule

Ciliary body

E Bohlman Patterson

Retina

Choroid

Sclera

Vortex vein

Short posterior ciliary artery and nerve

Central retina artery and vein

Optic nerve

Fig. 14-2 The human eye. (From F Newell: Ophthalmology: principles and concepts, ed 6, St Louis, 1986, The CV Mosby Co.)

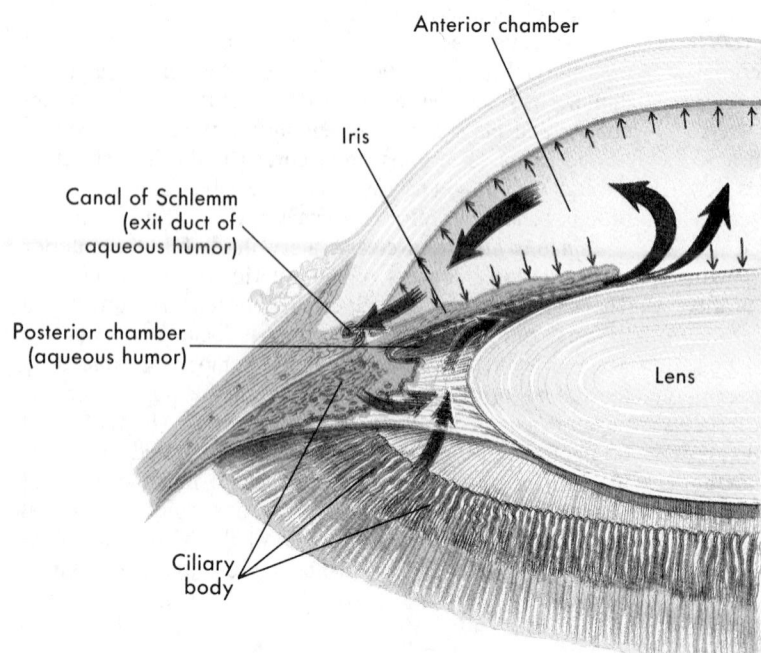

Anterior chamber

Iris

Canal of Schlemm (exit duct of aqueous humor)

Posterior chamber (aqueous humor)

Lens

Ciliary body

Fig. 14-3 Aqueous humor *(heavy arrows)* is believed to be formed mainly by secretion by the ciliary body into the posterior chamber. It passes into the anterior chamber through the pupil, from which it is drained away by the ring-shaped canal of Schlemm and finally into the anterior ciliary veins. *Small arrows* indicate pressure of the aqueous humor. (From Anthony C and Thibodeau G: Textbook of anatomy and physiology, St Louis, 1987, Times Mirror/Mosby College Publishing, p 327.)

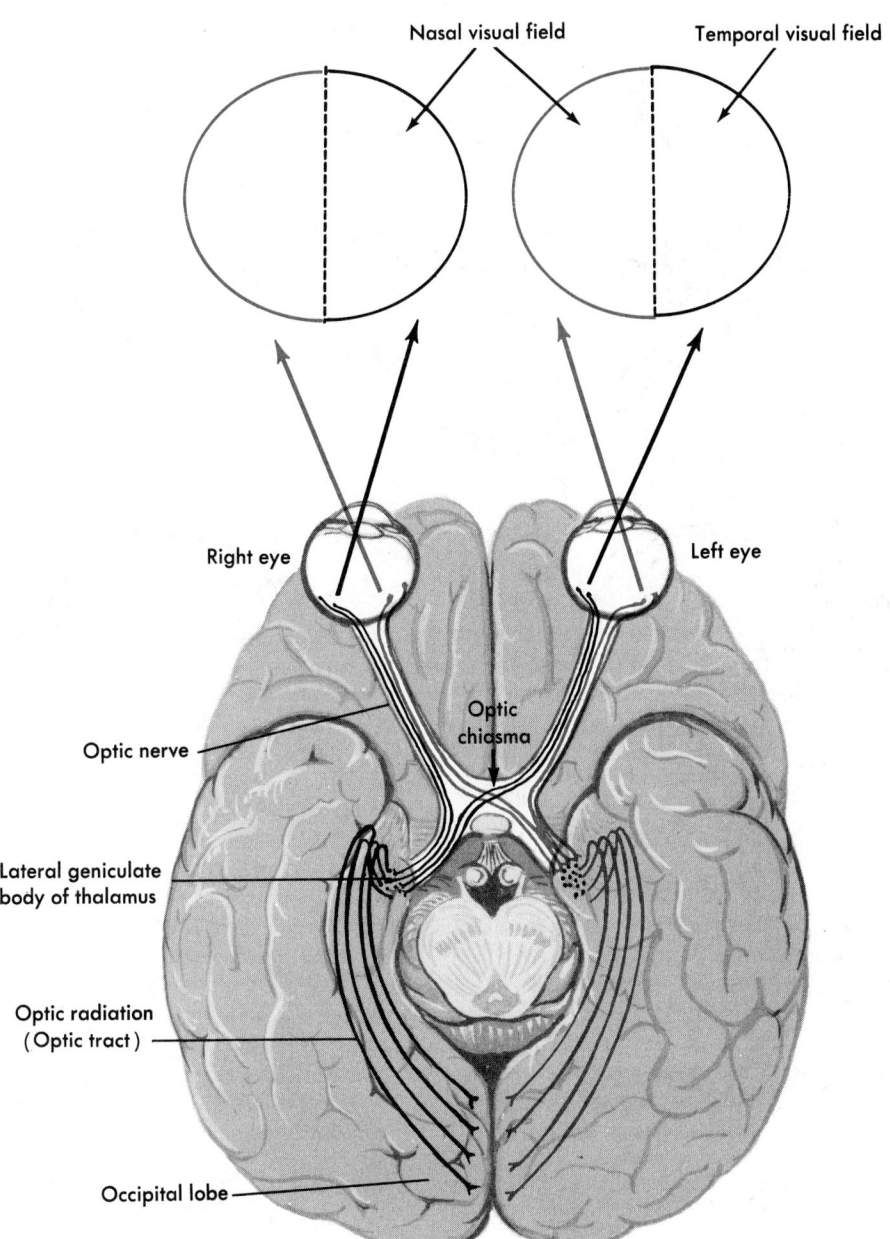

Fig. 14-4   Visual pathways. Fibers from nasal portion of each retina cross over to opposite side of optic chiasma, terminating in lateral geniculate body of opposite side. Location of a lesion in the visual pathway determines the resulting visual defect. (From Anthony C and Thibodeau G: Textbook of anatomy and physiology, St Louis, 1987, Times Mirror/Mosby College Publishing, p 337.)

lium of the cornea. Excess production or decreased outflow can elevate intraocular pressure above the normal 10 to 21 mm Hg, a condition known as *glaucoma.*

The lens is a biconvex structure located behind the iris and supported in place by small fibers called *zonules.* The primary function of the lens is to bend light rays, allowing the rays to fall onto the retina. Contraction and relaxation of the zonules alter the shape of the lens, which affects its focusing ability. Since light rays pass through the lens, it must remain clear. Anything altering the clarity of the lens affects light transmission. The lens contains a thick gelati-

nous material enclosed in a clear capsule. Degenerative changes and disease cause the lens to become thicker, cloudy, or opaque. This condition is called a *cataract.*

Vitreous humor is located in the posterior cavity, the large area behind the lens and in front of the retina (Fig. 14-2). The gelatinous consistency of the vitreous helps to hold the retina in place and gives shape to the eye. With aging the vitreous becomes more liquid.[2]

Visual pathways. Once the image travels through the refractive media, it is focused on the retina inverted and reversed left to right (Fig. 14-4). For example, if the ob-

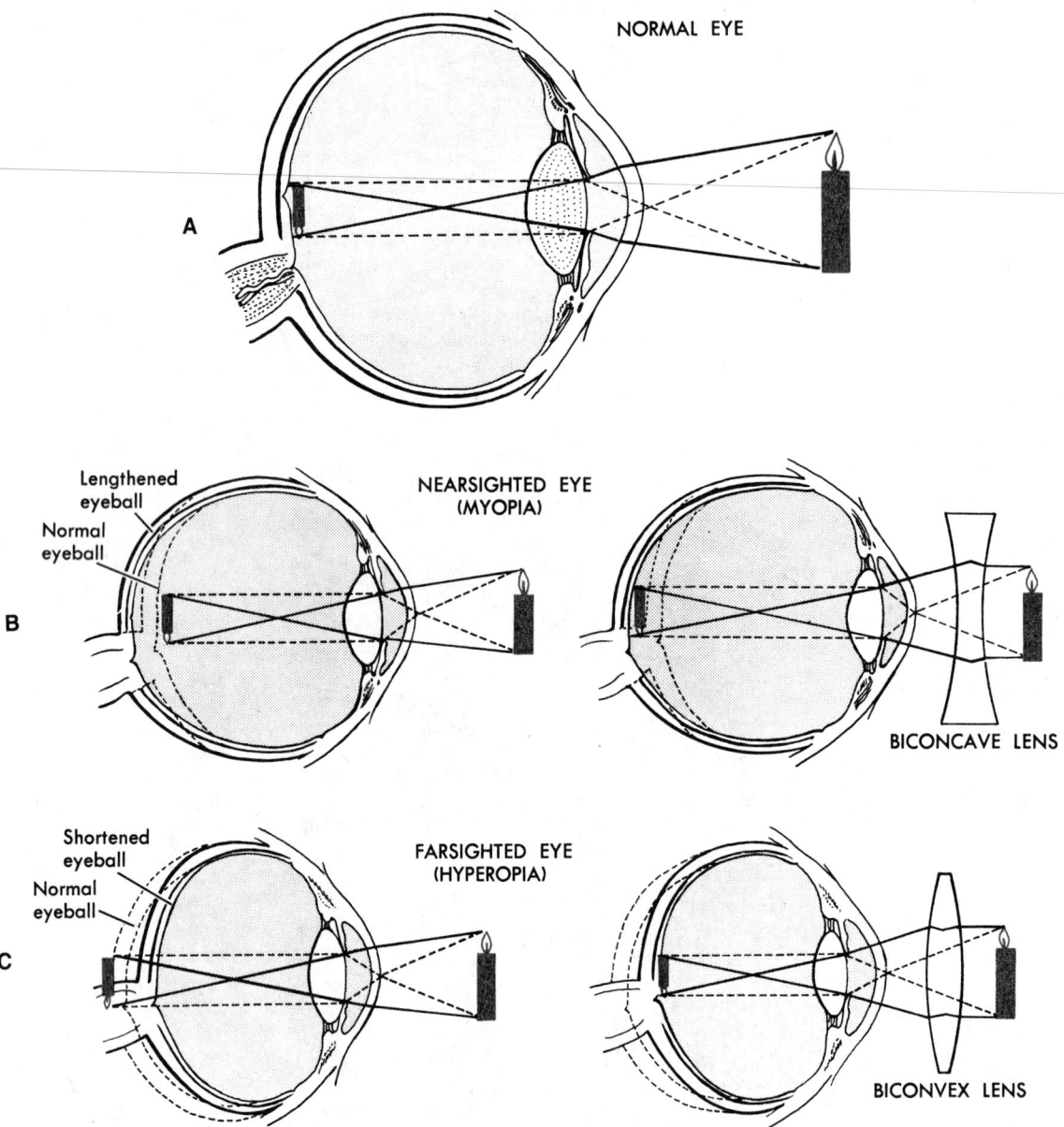

Fig. 14-5 **A,** In the normal eye, light rays from an object are refracted by the cornea, aqueous humor, lens, and vitreous humor and converge on the fovea of the retina, where an inverted image is clearly formed. **B,** Myopic eye focuses the image in front of the retina. This may occur when the eyeball is too long or the lens is too thick. Correction is by concave lens. **C,** Hyperopic eye can only focus the image at a hypothetical distance behind the retina. This may occur when the eyeball is too short or the lens is too thin. Correction is by convex lens. (From Anthony C and Thibodeau G: Textbook of anatomy and physiology, St Louis, 1987, Times Mirror/Mosby College Publishing, p 333.)

ject is seen in the left upper temporal field, it will be focused upside down and in the lower nasal area of the retina. From the retina, the impulses travel through the optic nerve back to the optic chiasm, where the nasal fibers of each eye cross over to the other side. Fibers from the left field of both eyes form the left optic tract and travel to the left occipital cortex. The fibers from the right field of both eyes form the right optic tract and travel to the right occipital cortex.

Refractive errors. *Refraction* is the ability of the eye to bend light rays so that they fall on the retina. In the emmetropic (normal) eye, parallel light rays are focused through the lens into a sharp image on the retina from a distance of approximately 20 feet (Fig. 14-5, *A*).

Myopia, or nearsightedness, occurs when the refracting ability of the eye is too great for its length. As a result, the image falls in front of the retina. The discrepancy occurs from a short anteroposterior diameter or excessive refract-

Table 14-1   Age-Related Changes in the Visual System

Smaller pupil (senile miosis) with decreased efficiency to constrict and dilate
Shallow anterior chamber (from thickening of lens); less efficient reabsorption of intraocular fluid
Accumulation of yellow substances on lens
Decreased elasticity of lens
Loss of elasticity of eyelids (senile ptosis)
Decreased visual field
Altered lens transparency
Decreased lacrimal secretion
Milky or yellow ring encircling periphery of iris
Alterations in lens and vitreous humor
Sclerotic and blood vessel changes in macula

---

ing power. A concave lens is used to facilitate correct refraction (Fig. 14-5, *B*).

Hyperopia, or farsightedness, occurs when objects are focused behind the eye. Contributing factors include a small anteroposterior diameter and insufficient refracting power. In this state, distance vision is fine, but close-up objects cannot be seen clearly. In hyperopia, a convex lens is used to correct the refraction (Fig. 14-5, *C*).

Astigmatism is caused by an unevenness in the corneal curvature, causing horizontal and vertical rays to be focused at two different points on the retina, which results in visual distortion. It can be myopic or hyperopic in nature in relation to where the image falls.

Presbyopia occurs as a normal process of aging. As the lens ages and becomes less elastic, it loses the ability to bulge and accommodate for near vision. Convex lenses for reading and near vision become necessary.

Effects of Aging

There are many age-related changes of the visual system. These changes can have serious consequences for the older adult because severely compromised vision or blindness can result. Table 14-1 outlines normal age-related changes of the visual system.

ASSESSMENT OF THE VISUAL SYSTEM
Subjective Data

Health history. The health history is used to obtain information that will guide the direction of the ophthalmic examination. It also gives the client an opportunity to get to know the examiner. This period of familiarity is critical, since many aspects of the ophthalmic examination are performed in very close proximity to the client.

Demographic data. The nurse notes the client's age. Cataracts, retinal detachments, dry eye, entropion, ectropion, and glaucoma develop with increasing frequency as the client ages. The nurse should be alert for clients who live alone, since these clients are at greater risk of vision-related accidents.

The sex of the client is important because deficiencies in color vision occur more frequently in males. Hereditary color defects are relatively common. About 1 in 12 males

and 1 in 200 females have anomalous color vision of the red-green type commonly referred to as *color blindness.* Anomalous blue-green vision is much less common.[3]

Current health problem. The nurse gathers data regarding the reason the client is seeking health care at this time. The following questions should be asked:
1. *Chief complaint* (using the client's own words if possible)
2. *Location:* Does the problem involve one eye or both?
3. *Quality:* What does it feel like? Is the eye itchy? Or does the sensation feel like a foreign body?
4. *Quantity:* How bad is it? If pain is involved, the nurse can ask the client to rate the pain on a 1 to 10 scale. The nurse can also ask the client to describe how much impact the problem has. For example, a client may reply, "The glare is so bad at night, I've had to quit driving after dark."
5. *Setting:* When does the problem happen? Some clients may notice itching and tearing when they are around certain fumes or animals.
6. *Timing:* When did the problem begin? Any client who complains of sudden or persistent loss of vision that began in the previous 48 hours should be seen immediately.
7. *Aggravating and relieving factors:* What makes the problem better or worse? Does the client notice that the burning goes away with the application of cool compresses?
8. *Associated manifestations:* Does anything unusual happen at about the same time as the problem? For example, the vision loss may be preceded by a headache.

Past health history. The eye not only reflects ocular diseases; it often indicates systemic diseases. In addition to asking questions about diseases known to cause visual problems, the nurse should ask the client about preexisting conditions, since their presence can complicate the treatment of ocular disorders. For example, certain β-blocking eyedrops must be used with caution or avoided in the client with asthma.[4] The nurse should question the client regarding the presence of the following:
1. Pediatric and adult diseases with possible ocular complications, including diabetes, hypertension, cancer, hypothyroidism or hyperthyroidism, rheumatoid arthritis, syphilis and other sexually transmitted diseases (STDs), acquired immunodeficiency syndrome (AIDS), muscular dystrophy, myasthenia gravis, and multiple sclerosis
2. Ocular diseases, including strabismus, amblyopia, the use of glasses, refractive errors in childhood, glaucoma, cataracts, retinal detachment, and refractive error (noting last examination and change in lenses) in adulthood
3. Immunizations, including measles (especially in women of childbearing years)
4. Hospitalizations, surgical procedures related to eye problems, any surgical procedure involving the eye or brain, injuries such as automobile accidents and blows to the head or eye, and laser procedures performed

5. Medications, including use of current prescription and over-the-counter (OTC) drugs

When discussing medications, clients may not mention OTC drug use. However, many of these drugs have ocular effects. For example, cold preparations contain a form of epinephrine that can affect pupil size. The nurse should specifically ask whether the client uses any prescription drugs such as corticosteroids, thyroid medications, or agents such as oral hypoglycemics and insulin to lower blood glucose levels. Cortisone preparations may contribute to the development of glaucoma or cataracts. The nurse should also note the use of any antihistamines or decongestants, since these drugs are known to cause dryness of the eyes.

Each drug reported by the client should correspond with a disease or disorder previously described by the client. If a medication cannot be correlated with the list, the nurse should ask the client to explain the reason the drug is used.

It is also important for the nurse to question about use of ophthalmic medications, specifically eyedrops. Many clients do not consider eyedrops, even prescription ones, a medication. It is important to note the name, strength, and schedule of administration for each ocular medication. This information is very important, since it affects findings such as the intraocular pressure reading.

Allergies to medications and other substances should be noted. The nurse also needs to determine whether the client has any allergies related to eye medications or that result in symptoms such as ocular redness, itching, or tearing. Allergies to cosmetics should also be noted.

Family history. Refractive errors and many eye problems are hereditary, and a careful family history is necessary. Questions about systemic diseases, such as arteriosclerosis, diabetes, thyroid disease, hypertension, arthritis, and cancer, should be asked. The nurse should also ask for information about eye diseases such as cataracts, ocular tumors, glaucoma, refractive errors (especially myopia and hyperopia), and retinal degenerative conditions (e.g., macular degeneration, retinal detachment, retinitis pigmentosa).

Social and personal history. A full field of vision and a minimum visual acuity may be required for certain occupations. The nurse should ask the client about the workplace and type of work. The client should be asked whether fumes, smoke, or eye irritants are present in the workplace. Many occupations place workers in conditions in which eye injuries may occur. For example, factory workers may be at risk from flying metal debris. Information should be obtained about eye safety practices, such as the use of goggles or safety glasses. Workers can also be exposed to eyestrain in the office. Video display terminals are often introduced without alterations of the workplace. Existing lighting and a horizontal gaze can result in screen reflection. Dazzling glare can also be a problem if the terminal faces a window or some other bright light source.

The nurse should inquire about leisure activities, such as participation in sports. Injuries to the globe can occur after blows to the head during sports such as racquetball and baseball. Cross-country skiers may have fungal ulcers after an abrasion caused by low-hanging tree limbs. Darts can cause penetrating eye injuries.

Lifestyle of the client should also be explored. Questions regarding health practices, care of contact lenses, and dexterity to insert contact lenses are of concern. Dexterity is of the utmost importance if contact lenses are being considered for an older adult. Type of contact lenses used and wearing time may provide information for health teaching. Information should be obtained regarding use of sunglasses in bright light, since prolonged exposure to ultraviolet light can affect the retina. Night-driving habits and any problems encountered should be noted.

If the client has diabetes, it is important to determine adherence to a diabetic regimen and the amount of blood sugar control achieved. An increased blood glucose level triggers a series of events within the lens that causes it to take on additional fluid, leading to visual changes.

Review of systems. Symptoms related to other systems can mimic eye problems. It is necessary to question the client about possible sinusitis and neurological problems such as headaches. Clinical manifestations related to the visual system include the following:

1. *Pain or discomfort:* Foreign body sensation that is lessened with lid closure; photophobia; irritation or itching; and severe, sharp, throbbing pain
2. *Changes in vision:* Progression, blurriness, diplopia (images side by side or above one another), blind spots or scotomas, spots or floaters in front of the eye, loss of all or part of vision, decreased color perception, halos around light, and flashes of light in the eye
3. *Redness:* Eyelids, parts of eyelids, and conjunctivae
4. *Swelling:* Certain times of day, area of eyelid, and periorbital changes
5. *Drainage:* Increased or decreased tearing, purulent drainage, crusting of eyelids or eyelashes, and blood or purulent material in anterior chamber

Objective Data

Physical examination. Most objective data regarding the eyes are obtained by inspection. Since many parts of the visual system are available for inspection, the nurse must have a thorough understanding of the eye. Correct documentation of a normal physical examination is noted in Table 14-2. Age-related changes and physical assessment findings are listed in Table 14-3.

Table 14-2 Normal Physical Assessment of the Visual System

Eyes bilaterally symmetrical; eyebrows, lids, and lashes intact without deformity; conjunctiva and cornea clear; sclera white without redness
Visual acuity 20/20 in both eyes, without glasses
Extraocular movements intact without nystagmus
No ptosis or lid lag
PERRLA
Parallel corneal light reflex
Ability to read newsprint at 35 cm (14 inches) without corrective lenses

PERRLA, Pupils equal, round, reactive to light and accomodation.

Table 14-3

Age-Related Changes of the Visual System and Differences in Assessment Findings

Changes	Differences in Assessment Findings
INTERNAL	
Opaque and yellowed lens, loss of ability to increase thickness and curvature secondary to protein changes	Presbyopia, decreased color discrimination of blue spectrum, cataracts (opaque lens)
Changes in retinal vasculature	Narrowed, pale, straighter arterioles that branch more acutely
Macular degeneration	Loss of central vision
Detachment or liquification of vitreous humor	Complaints of "floaters"
EXTERNAL	
Fatty deposits in corneal margin	Arcus senilis
Flattened and cloudy cornea	Cloudy appearance of cornea
More rigid iris	Decrease in pupil size, slower response to light
Loss of orbital fat, decreased muscle tone, changes in elastic tissue of eyelids	Entropion, ectropion, mild ptosis
Altered or decreased tear secretion	Irritated eyes

Initial observation. The examination begins as the nurse enters the room. As the nurse approaches the client, notation is made of how the client is dressed. Unusual color combinations may indicate a color vision deficit. Any unusual head position should be noted. Clients experiencing diplopia may hold their heads in a skewed position in an attempt to relieve the problem. Clients with a corneal abrasion or who are photophobic will cover their eyes with their hands to try to block out room light.

The nurse extends a hand as the client is approached. By shaking hands with the client, the nurse can make a crude estimate of depth perception.

Visual acuity. Visual acuity is the first assessment conducted for medical and legal reasons. The nurse must be able to prove what the acuity was before rendering care.

The client sits or stands 20 feet from the Snellen chart. Glasses or contact lenses should be left in place unless they are used solely for reading. The client is asked to cover the left eye and then read the smallest line that can be comfortably read. If that line is read with two or fewer errors, the examiner instructs the client to read the next lower line. The nurse notes the smallest line the client reads with two or fewer errors. The standard of 20 feet is recorded and then the distance in feet on the line of the Snellen chart that the client read successfully. For example, for the client who can read down to the 30-foot line the acuity is recorded as 20/30 OD (oculus dexter). (OD is the ophthalmic abbreviation for right eye.) OS (oculus sinister) means left eye. OU (oculus uterque) refers to both eyes. A reading of 20/30 OD means that the client can read at 20 feet what the person with normal vision can read at 30 feet with the right eye. The client is asked to cover the right eye, and the process is repeated.

If the client cannot read letters, a picture eye chart can be used. A second option is the use of an eye chart that presents the letter E in four different directions. The client is asked to point in the direction the E faces.

Nurses may need to evaluate visual acuity when the client is unable to see the 20/400 letter. For persons with low vision, the nurse holds a number of fingers up in front of the client and asks whether or not they can be seen. If the client can see the fingers, the nurse asks for the left eye to be covered. A random number of fingers are held up in front of the client, who is asked to state how many fingers are raised. This procedure is repeated 5 times. If the client correctly identifies the number of fingers 3 of the 5 times, the vision is recorded as "counts fingers at ___feet." The distance the nurse stood from the client is also recorded. Vision in the left eye is examined after the client covers the right eye.

If the nurse must assess visual acuity without access to an eye chart, an accurate assessment is still possible. Examples of other stimuli acceptable for use include newsprint or the label on a container. The acuity is recorded as "reads newspaper headline at ___inches."

Visual fields. Peripheral vision is assessed by testing visual fields. A simple but gross method of determining visual fields is the confrontation test. The client and nurse are seated facing each other 2 to 3 feet apart. The client and the examiner cover opposite eyes. For example, the nurse occludes the left eye, while the client covers the right eye. Covering eyes in this manner helps the nurse and the client have approximately the same visual fields. A pencil or other small but visible object is held equidistant between the client and the nurse. Without moving the eyes to the left or right, the client reports when able to view the object. The object is brought in from the periphery from six different directions. For example, the object can be brought in from the periphery from the 2, 4, and 6 o'clock positions. Any difference from the examiner's field is noted. Use of the examiner's field as the standard is acceptable only if the examiner's field of vision is normal. The test is then performed for the other eye. Test results for the normal eye are described as "confrontation fields full." A note is made as to the use of corrective lenses during the test. If a defect is noted in the client's field, its location is described as thoroughly as possible. Common descriptors used for this purpose include location (nasal or temporal) and position (superior or inferior). A visual field with an observed deficit may be documented as follows: "Confrontation fields full with decrease noted in the inferior nasal quadrant." Any client with a defect in visual fields should be referred to an ophthalmologist.

Perimetry testing is another method for assessing the visual field. A semicircular instrument, marked in degrees, can be used to obtain a more accurate account and a written diagram of the field. Computerized fields can also be obtained. When computerized fields are used, a record of response to a consistent and controlled stimulus is available for comparison.

Extraocular muscle functions. The corneal light reflex is used to evaluate the position of the eyes. In a darkened room, the client is asked to look straight ahead while a penlight is shone directly on the cornea. The light reflection should be located in the center of both corneas as the client faces the light source. Deviation of the light source reflection can indicate esodeviation (turning in) or exodeviation (turning outward) of the eye.

The cover-uncover test will also detect faulty alignment of the eyes. While the client looks at an object held by the examiner, one eye is covered. The examiner observes for movement of the uncovered eye. If the uncovered eye moves to look at the object, it was deviated before the straight eye was covered. The covered eye is observed for movement to focus when uncovered. Both eyes are tested. Movement of either eye indicates strabismus (crossing of the eyes). If no movement occurs, the alignment of the eyes is termed *straight.*

The extraocular movements of the eyes are tested to determine neuromuscular balance. The client is asked to follow the examiner's index finger through the six cardinal fields of gaze (Fig. 14-6). The examiner shows an object and asks the client to follow the object with the eyes while keeping the head facing forward. The eyes should follow equally with parallel and coordinated movements. While the client looks at each field of gaze, the nurse observes for *nystagmus,* which is a rhythmic jerking motion of the eyes. It is a normal finding on far lateral gaze but not when the eye is in other positions.

Corneal reflex. The corneal reflex tests the functioning of the trigeminal nerve (CN V). This test is performed only when there is strong suspicion of a defect. It is frequently performed in cases of known or suspected brain death. This test should not be performed in clients who are wearing contact lenses or in whom a corneal abrasion is suspected. A wisp of cotton is brought in laterally and lightly touched against the cornea. The client should blink with both eyes when the cornea is touched if the reflex is intact. Tearing may be observed as a response to the irritation.

Inspection of extraocular structures. Inspection of the external ocular structures includes observation of both eyes. For the examination, the client is seated at eye level with the examiner. The physical characteristics of the eyes should be similar unless a history of ocular surgery or an eye problem exists. The nurse looks to see whether the client's eyes are spaced equally (i.e., one eye is not laterally or medially displaced). Placement of the eyes in the orbit is also noted. Any bulging of the eye is noted.

Eyebrows, eyelashes, and eyelids. The eyebrows and eyelashes should be examined for hair distribution, color, position, and presence of lesions. Any absence of hair is carefully noted. If the history reveals recent exposure to lice, the eyebrows should be examined for evidence of nits. The nurse also observes for any crusting or scales in the eyebrow area. Ability to raise and lower the eyebrow should be observed.

Direction of the eyelashes should be documented. The lashes should be extending outward, away from the eyelid margin. There should be no areas where eyelashes are missing unless a client has recently undergone chemotherapy.

The eyelids are examined for position as well as for the presence of edema, redness, and tenderness. The upper eyelid should rest at or just below the superior limbus. No white sclera should be visible between the eyelid and the

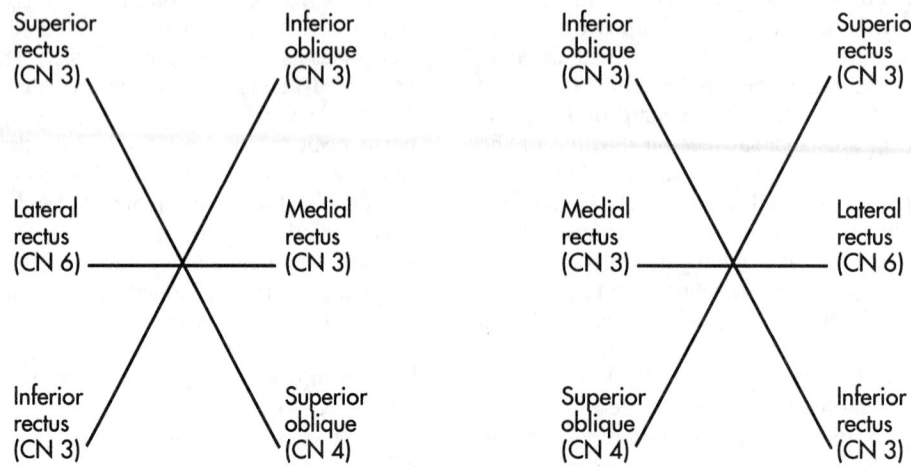

Fig. 14-6   Cardinal fields of gaze with corresponding muscles and nerves.

superior limbus. The lower eyelid rests just below the inferior limbus. Edema can cause the eyelid to droop below its normal resting position. Redness and tenderness along the eyelid-eyelash margin may indicate the presence of a stye (hordeolum) or chalazion.

The eyelids should be in close proximity to the globe with the eyelashes directed away from the eye. When the eyes are closed, the eyelids should just touch one another or approximate. Inward turning of the eyelid is called an *entropion*. If the eyelid turns too far inward, the eyelashes can brush up against the surface of the eye, causing pain. The outward turning of the eyelid (an *ectropion)* is frequently associated with older persons and can cause problems related to irritation and placement of eyedrops.

If the nurse suspects a foreign body or if direct examination of the posterior surface of the eyelid is needed, the upper eyelid must be everted. The client is instructed to look downward while the nurse gently grasps the eyelid near the insertion of the eyelashes. A cotton-tipped applicator is placed horizontally against the midsection of the upper eyelid. The nurse gently flips the eyelid over the applicator while exerting gentle pressure against the eyelid. The client continues to look down while the everted eyelid and exposed palpebral conjunctiva are examined for color, texture, and the presence of redness, lesions, or foreign bodies. The conjunctiva is normally pink, smooth, and free from lesions or foreign bodies. To reposition the eyelid, the client looks up then blinks normally. The eyelid then falls into place.

Conjunctiva and sclera. The examiner's hands are washed before beginning the assessment. The conjunctiva and sclera are easily examined at the same time. The structures are evaluated for color, smoothness, and presence of lesions. To examine the palpebral conjunctiva, the examiner places a forefinger over the cheekbone and gently pulls down. This maneuver will expose the palpebral conjunctiva of the lower lid. It is assessed for color (normally pale pink), texture (normally smooth), and the presence of lesions or foreign bodies and lesions.

The bulbar conjunctiva covering the sclera is normally clear, with fine blood vessels visible. These blood vessels are more common in the periphery.

The sclera is normally white. A pale blue cast due to scleral thinning may be found in older adults. The blue cast is actually the vascular choroid showing through. A slight yellow cast may be found in dark-pigmented persons from some groups, such as blacks and American Indians.

Cornea. A light is shone obliquely on the cornea while the nurse observes the surface for smoothness, clarity, and foreign bodies. The surface should be smooth and without irregularities. The cornea should be clear, transparent, and shiny. In an older client, a white ring at the limbus, called *arcus senilis,* is normal. A fluorescein test strip can be used to determine the presence of abrasions or irregularities. The test strip is moistened with a drop of sterile saline solution and touched to the lower conjunctival sac. The client is instructed to blink several times to distribute the solution across the cornea. Any irregularities of the cornea will stain a brilliant green.

Anterior chamber. Oblique light is used for inspection of the anterior chamber. The iris should appear flat and not bulging toward the cornea. The area between the cornea and the iris should be clear. No blood or purulent material should be observed. Since blood and purulent material have a viscosity greater than aqueous humor, they will settle to the lower portion of the chamber.

Iris. Both irides should be of similar color and shape. However, a color difference between the irides occurs in a small portion of the population. The iris should be inspected with the upper lid raised. Any area of missing iris tissue will be evident, since the colored iris tissue will be missing. Round or notched areas of missing iris tissue are probably the result of cataract or glaucoma surgery. The cause of these areas should be documented.

Pupil. The pupil is examined for size, shape, and reactivity. The pupils are also compared to each other with respect to symmetry. In a small percentage of the population the pupils are unequal in size. This normal variation is called *anisocoria.* Pupil size varies with age. Infants and older adults have a miotic or small pupil. Normal range for pupil size is 3 to 7 mm.[5]

Pupils are usually round in shape. Persons who have had sections of the iris removed during eye surgery may have keyhole-shaped pupils.

Pupils are tested for accommodative response. The client is asked to focus on a distant object while the nurse places an object 10 to 12 cm into the client's central vision. The client is asked to focus on the near object. Normal response is for the pupils to converge and constrict symmetrically. This response is slower in older persons.

The room is darkened to check pupillary response. A penlight is brought in laterally and shone on the right pupil. The pupil of the illuminated eye constricts in what is called the *direct response. Consensual response* occurs when the pupil of the other eye (left eye) constricts when the light is on the right eye. The other eye is then tested for direct response with the light shining onto the left eye. The consensual response of the right eye is also observed. This test is more difficult to interpret in dark-eyed persons.

Normal characteristics and responses of the pupil are documented as *PERRLA.* This abbreviation represents *pu*pils *e*qual, *r*ound, *r*eactive to *l*ight and *a*ccommodation.

Palpation. The eyelids are gently palpated to detect irregularities, nodules, and discomfort. Intraocular pressure can be roughly estimated by gently placing the tips of the index and second fingers over the closed eyelid with the client looking down. With experience, the examiner will be able to detect an increase in the intraocular pressure. This test should not be done if the client has recently had ocular surgery or if injury to the globe is suspected.

Finally, the lacrimal system is evaluated. The lacrimal sac is palpated first. The index finger is pressed below the inner canthus against the orbital rim to detect the presence of nodules, swelling, drainage, or pain. The puncta can be observed if the examiner gently pulls the lower eyelid down against the cheek. To expose the lacrimal gland, the nurse asks the client to look down while the upper lid is being retracted. The lacrimal gland is examined for evidence of swelling (Fig. 14-1). Common assessment abnormalities of the eye are presented in Table 14-4.

Table 14-4

Common Assessment Abnormalities of the Eye

Findings	Description	Possible Etiology and Significance
SUBJECTIVE DATA		
Pain	Foreign body sensation	Superficial corneal erosions from wearing of contact lenses (hard), foreign body on conjunctiva, cornea
	Lessened with lid closure	Corneal abrasion
	Severe, deep, throbbing	Iritis, acute glaucoma, infection of the eye
Photophobia (sudden and persistent)	Abnormal intolerance to light	Inflammation of cornea, iris, conjunctiva
Blurred vision	Gradual or sudden inability to see clearly	Refractive errors, corneal opacities, cataracts, retinal changes such as detachment, macular degeneration; optic neuritis or atrophy, central retinal vein or artery thrombosis, changes related to control of diabetes
Scotoma	Blind spot or area of vision loss within visual field	Glaucoma, chorioretinitis, injury, migraine headache
Scotoma (central)	Blind spot involving central vision	Macular degeneration, occlusion of vessels of eye or brain
Spots or floaters	Sudden appearance of spots, spiderwebs, curtain, or floaters within field of vision	Hemorrhage into the vitreous humor, impending retinal detachment, intraocular hemorrhage, chorioretinitis
Dryness	Decreased tear formation or changes in tear composition; decrease in amount of fluid bathing the eye	Changes in cornea, sleep, age, certain diseases
Halo around lights	Presence of halo when looking at lights	Glaucoma
Excessive glare	Light reflection onto periphery of retina	Cataract formation and aging
Diplopia	Double vision	Involvement of CNs, extraocular muscles
OBJECTIVE DATA		
Eyelids		
Allergic reactions	Redness with watering and itching along lashes	Many allergens, eye trauma resulting from rubbing eye because of itching
Hordeolum or stye	Small abscesses along lid edge	Bacterial invasion of lids and glands of eyelids
Chalazion	Infection of meibomian glands within the tarsal framework of the lids	Bacterial invasion of sebaceous glands (meibomian) of eyelid
Marginal blepharitis	Reddened lid margins, crusting of lashes	Instruction in care of eyelids needed to prevent spread of infection
Dacryocystitis	Inflammation of lacrimal sac resulting in raised area near nose and medial lower lid	Blockage of the nasolacrimal duct and subsequent infection
Xanthelasma	Raised, yellowish plaques that are circumscribed along nasal portion of each lid	Normal observation or accompanying symptom of lipid disorders
Conjunctiva		
Conjunctivitis	Reddened, swollen mucous membrane	Conjunctivitis (pinkeye), trauma, edema, iritis, bacterial infection
Sclera		
Jaundice	Yellow color to all of sclera	Jaundice
Cornea		
Corneal abrasion	Irregularity of epithelium of cornea, usually causing much pain	Trauma, overwearing of contact lens, improper fit of contact lens
Corneal opacity	Whitish part or all of normally transparent cornea	Scar tissue formation due to inflammation, infection; blocking of visual stimuli, causing blindness; referral necessary if recent
Pterygium	Triangular thickening of bulbar conjunctiva that grows over the cornea	Distortion of vision, surgical removal necessary if progression to central cornea

Table 14-4

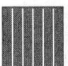

Common Assessment Abnormalities of the Eye—cont'd

Findings	Description	Possible Etiology and Significance
OBJECTIVE DATA—cont'd		
Lid position		
Ptosis	Drooping of upper lid margin over pupil when eyes are open, unilateral or bilateral	CN III involvement, myasthenia gravis, congenital, trauma, edema
Ectropion	Outward turning of lower lid and lashes	Relaxation of framework of eyelid associated with aging, paralysis of facial nerve; edema of palpebral conjunctiva; maceration of skin possible
Entropion	Inward turning of lower lid and lashes	Contraction of scar on conjunctiva or tarsus, muscle contraction; irritation of conjunctiva, cornea possible
Lid lag	Slower closing of one lid and/or jerky movements	Possible involvement of cranial nerve VII
Blepharospasm	Inability to open lids	Inflammation, involvement of CN V, VII
Blinking		
Decreased; monocular, bilateral	Decreased closure of upper palpebral fissure	Possible involvement of CN VII, dryness and damage to cornea
Eyeball		
Monocular, bilateral exophthalmos	Protrusion of eyeball, incomplete closure of lids possible, visible white sclera above iris when eyelids open	Possible thyroid disease, tumor behind eye, possible frontal sinus enlargement; dryness of cornea
Pupils		
Irregular, square		Intraocular lens that clips onto iris, normal
Asymmetrical in reaction to light and accommodation		Involvement of cranial nerves or extraocular muscles
Constricted	Smaller than 3 mm, miosis	Miotic medication for glaucoma, normal for older adults; damage to sympathetic nerve supply; narcotic use
Asymmetrical corneal light reflex		Weakness of intraocular muscles, strabismus; involvement of extraocular muscles, CN III, IV, VI
Cloudiness/gray		Formation of cataract
Iris		
Change in color		Iritis, uveitis
Extraocular muscles		
Strabismus	Deviation of extraocular movements in one or more positions	Neuromuscular involvement; involvement of CN III, IV, VI or extraocular muscle
Visual field defect		
Peripheral	Partial or complete loss of peripheral vision	Glaucoma, complete or partial interruption along vision pathway
Central	Loss of central vision	Macular disease, possible nuclear cataract
Lens		
Cataract	Opacification of lens leading to progressive loss of vision	Diabetes, aging, congenital, trauma

Table 14-5

Diagnostic Studies of the Visual System

Study	Description and Purpose	Nursing Responsibility
Perimetry	Semicircular instrument marked in degrees that is an accurate map of peripheral vision, visual fields. It is noninvasive and painless.	Explain procedure to client.
Refraction	Refractor: Instrument containing a large number of lenses mounted on rotating wheels is used with the client in a sitting position. Client identifies lens that increases visual acuity. Cycloplegic drugs are usually used to block accommodation. Determines refractive error and aids in prescription of eye glasses, contact lenses.	Explain procedure to client. Administer ordered cycloplegic drug in correct eye or eyes. Assess dilatation of pupil. Protect pupil from light while dilated; instruct client to wear sunglasses. Explain temporary difficulty in reading because of dilatation.
	Retinoscope: Instrument held by physician at distance of 2 feet that directs focused light into the eye. A specific refractive error will distort the focused light, aiding the identification of refractive error. It can be easily used on infants.	Explain procedure to client. If cycloplegic drugs are used, follow same nursing actions as above.
Ophthalmoscopy (fundoscopy)	An ophthalmoscope magnifies and lights the fundus (inner layer) of the eye, thus allowing visualization of optic disc, four main pairs of vessels, and macular area. Direct ophthalmoscopy is used for diagnosis of abnormalities of these areas and requires dilated pupil to examine peripheral retina.	Explain procedure to client. Darken room. Administer ordered cycloplegic drug.
Indirect	An indirect ophthalmoscope is worn on the head of the examiner and a hand-held magnifying lens is used to observe the retina for holes or detachment. The stereoscopic view is larger and has more illumination. Better observation of peripheral retina can be attained.	Place client in seated or supine position.
Biomicroscopy (slit-lamp examination)*	A binocular microscope is capable of ×50 magnification. Assesses anterior eye for abnormalities of the cornea, iris, lens, and depth of anterior chamber angle.	Position client in chair, chin on chin rest.

*See Fig. 14-8.

DIAGNOSTIC STUDIES

Diagnostic tests are available to provide specific information about the internal parts of the eye, especially the anterior chamber and vessels. Many are done with special equipment in the physician's office and outpatient clinic (Table 14-5). Similar tests are often ordered for ophthalmic and neurological problems.

Direct ophthalmoscopy. Direct ophthalmoscopy, a technique that uses a hand-held instrument called an *ophthalmoscope,* is used to bring ocular structures into crisp focus. The eye is the only part of the body in which blood vessels and nerves can be visualized.

When using the ophthalmoscope, the nurse directs the beam of light obliquely into the client's pupil. The red reflex should then be visible. This reflex results from the light reflecting off the pink color of the retina. Any dense areas in the lens, such as a cataract, will decrease the red reflex. The reflex is followed inward until the fundus, or back of the eye, comes into view. Both arterioles and veins can be seen. Arterioles are smaller, thinner, and

Table 14-5

Diagnostic Studies of the Visual System—cont'd		

Study	Description and Purpose	Nursing Responsibility
Tonometry		
Schiotz	Instrument indents or flattens cornea by slight pressure to measure intraocular pressure.	Position client in chair, head back, or in the supine position with the head facing upward. Cornea is anesthetized with one drop of 0.5% proparacaine. Caution client not to rub eyes for 15 minutes after drops are instilled.
Applanation with biomicroscope	Instrument applies force to flatten an area of cornea (more accurate than Schiotz tonometry).	Seat client as for biomicroscopy. Administer topical anesthesia as above.
Gonioscopy (direct or indirect)	Special lens and instruments observe anterior chamber of eye, especially in glaucoma and inflammation of anterior eye.	Explain procedure to client.
Ultrasonography	Technique is used to determine tissue masses when unable to view the fundus because of hemorrhage and to determine tumor within eye or orbit. It should be performed before vitrectomy for diabetic retinopathy to determine status of retina.	Explain procedure to client.
Fluorescein angiography	Fluorescein 5 ml is given IV in hand or arm. Serial pictures are made at time of injection, 5 min, and 20 min. Allows microscopic visualization and slides of the flow of blood through the vessels of the pigment epithelium and the retina for diagnosis of abnormalities of vessels and retina.	Administer cycloplegic drugs for dilatation of pupil. Seat client in front of camera with chin on chin rest. The flashing bright-blue light used for camera may cause client discomfort, blinking, and difficulty seeing 1 to 2 minutes after test. Use caution if client is epileptic. Explain that client may notice yellow coloration of face for 6 to 24 hr; urine will be greenish-yellow for 24 to 36 hr. Observe for extravasation at IV site and manifestations of allergy to dye.
Electroretinography	Study measures the electrical response of the retina to flash of light. Contact lens electrode is placed over camera. Component parts include a recorder with pick up, amplifier, and readout. It is a helpful diagnostic aid in clients with diffuse retinal damage, with or without ophthalmoscopic changes.	Explain procedure to client. Darken room. Administer topical anesthetic eyedrop before placement of contact lens electrode.

lighter red and reflect light better than veins. Areas where arterioles and veins cross are examined for nicking or narrowing. These changes are indicators of blood vessel pathology associated with diabetes and hypertension.

A blood vessel is followed toward the optic nerve. The optic nerve, or disc, is examined for size, color, and abnormalities. The disc is creamy yellow with distinct margins. A slight blurring of the nasal margin is common.

A central depression in the disc, called the *physiologi-cal cup,* may be seen. This area is the exit site for the optic nerve. The cup should be less than one half of the diameter of the disc. The presence of any unusual rings or crescents surrounding the disc should be documented.

The background of the eye is then examined for color and the presence of hemorrhage or exudate. The fundus, or retinal background, should also be evaluated for any hemorrhage, hole, tear, or lesion. Small hemorrhages can be associated with diabetes or hypertension. Hemorrhages can appear in various shapes, such as dots or flames.

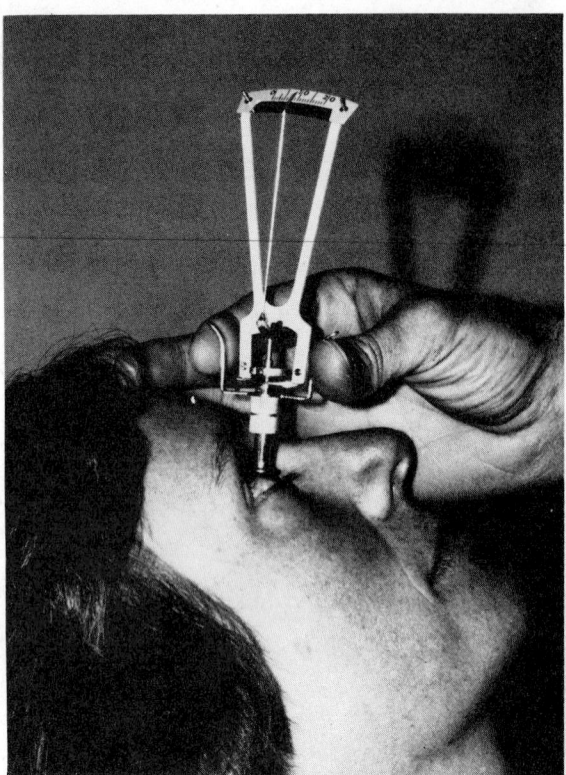

Fig. 14-7 Schiotz tonometer. The sterile footplace is resting on the anesthetized cornea. One hand of the examiner is stabilizing the tonometer. Although not shown, the lids can be held apart with the other hand. (Courtesy Ophthalmic Photography, Department of Ophthalmology, Ohio State University, Columbus.)

Finally, the macula is examined for shape and appearance. This area of high reflectivity is devoid of any blood vessels.

Important information regarding the health of the body's vascular system can be obtained through direct visualization with an ophthalmoscope. Practice is needed to become skilled in the use of this instrument. Frustration is frequently encountered when the nurse begins using the ophthalmoscope.

Slit lamp. The slit lamp permits examination of the eye under great magnification. A narrow beam (slit) of light is directed onto the eye to brightly illuminate a small section. The client's chin is positioned in a chin rest to stabilize the head. No pain or discomfort is associated with this examination. Attachments to the slit lamp are used for testing intraocular pressure.

Tonometry. One of the most frequently used diagnostic tests is the tonometry test with either the Schiotz tonometer (Fig. 14-7) or the applanation tonometer. In the former test the intraocular pressure of the eye is measured with the Schiotz tonometer resting on the anesthetized cornea. The client, lying flat or seated with the head turned upward, is directed to look at a spot overhead and to hold both eyes wide open. The tonometer is brought in from the side and the footplate is placed on the cornea in a perpen-

dicular position. The tonometer is stabilized and the pressure is read and converted in terms of the weight used.[6] A chart is available for this conversion. Normal intraocular pressure is 12 to 22 mm Hg. An applanation tonometer applied to the cornea during examination with a biomicroscope provides a more accurate reading of intraocular pressure (Fig. 14-8). The client must be cautioned not to rub the eyes for 15 minutes so that the anesthetized cornea is not scratched. Elevations in intraocular pressure may indicate glaucoma. Other tests are used to confirm the diagnosis.

Noncontact tonometry is another type of tonometry that uses a puff of air against the cornea to cause indentation. No anesthetic is necessary, since nothing comes in contact with the eye except the puff of air. Air striking the cornea may startle the client, so prior warning is necessary. The speed with which the test can be performed and the absence of anesthetic use make it an ideal method for screening.

Color vision testing. Color vision enables people to most accurately perceive the environment and be alert to indications of danger, and it is critical for certain occupations. A congenital color defect is present in 8% of men and 0.5% of women.[5] Several methods for assessing color vision exist. The Ishihara color plates test for color vision is based on the client's ability to trace patterns in a series of multicolored charts. This test is sensitive for diagnosing red-green defects but is not sensitive for diagnosing blue defects.

STRUCTURES AND FUNCTIONS OF THE AUDITORY SYSTEM

The auditory system is composed of the peripheral auditory system and the central auditory system. The *peripheral system* includes the structures of the ear itself—the external, middle, and inner ear (Fig. 14-9). This system is concerned with the reception and perception of sound. The inner ear functions in hearing and balance. The *central system* (the brain and its pathways) integrates and assigns meaning to what is heard.

External Ear

The external ear is composed of the auricle or pinna and the auditory canal. The *auricle* is composed of cartilage and connective tissue covered with epithelium, which also lines the external auditory canal (Fig. 14-9). The external auditory canal in the adult is approximately 2.5 cm long and has a slight S shape. Sebaceous and other glands in the outer half of the canal secrete cerumen, or wax. By waterproofing the ear canal, cerumen functions to protect the epithelium from maceration.[6]

Hair is present in the outer half of the canal. This hair may be profuse and coarse, especially in the older male client. The inner half of the ear canal is quite sensitive. The function of the external ear and canal is to collect and transmit sound waves to the *eardrum,* or *tympanic membrane.* This shiny, translucent, pearl-gray membrane is composed of skin, connective tissue, and mucous membrane. It is obliquely positioned at the medial end of the canal.

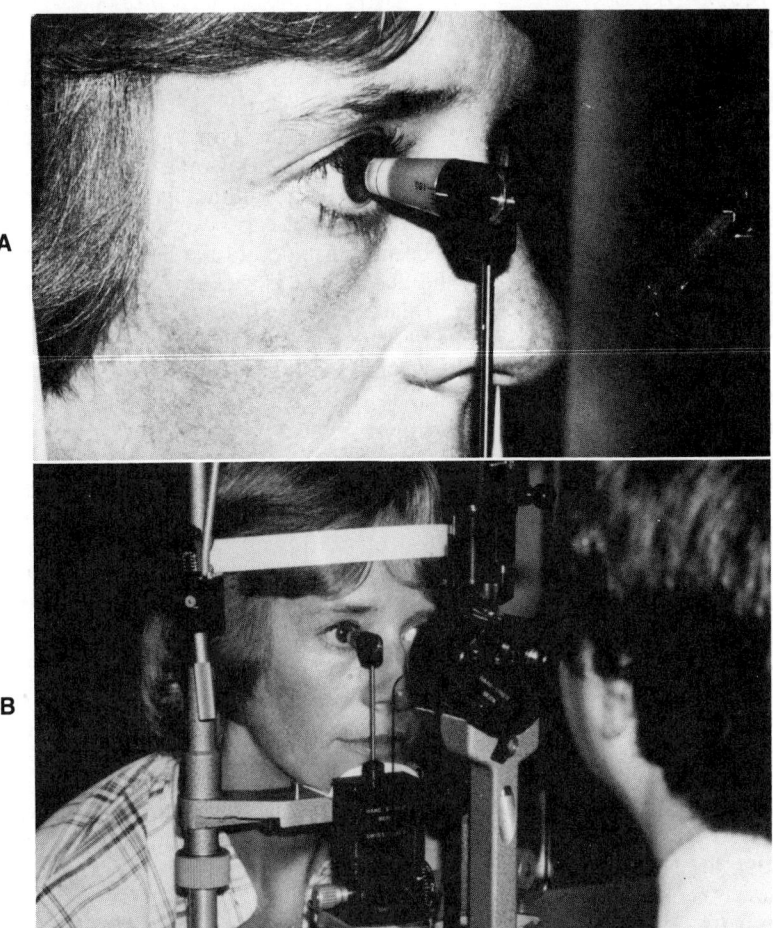

Fig. 14-8 **A,** Applanation tonometry with biomicroscopy. (Courtesy Ophthalmic Photography, Department of Ophthalmology, Ohio State University, Columbus.) **B,** The client's head is positioned with the chin resting on the chin rest. The examiner adjusts the biomicroscope to measure intraocular pressure as shown and also to view the cornea and internal eye. The applanation tonometer is only part of the instrument.

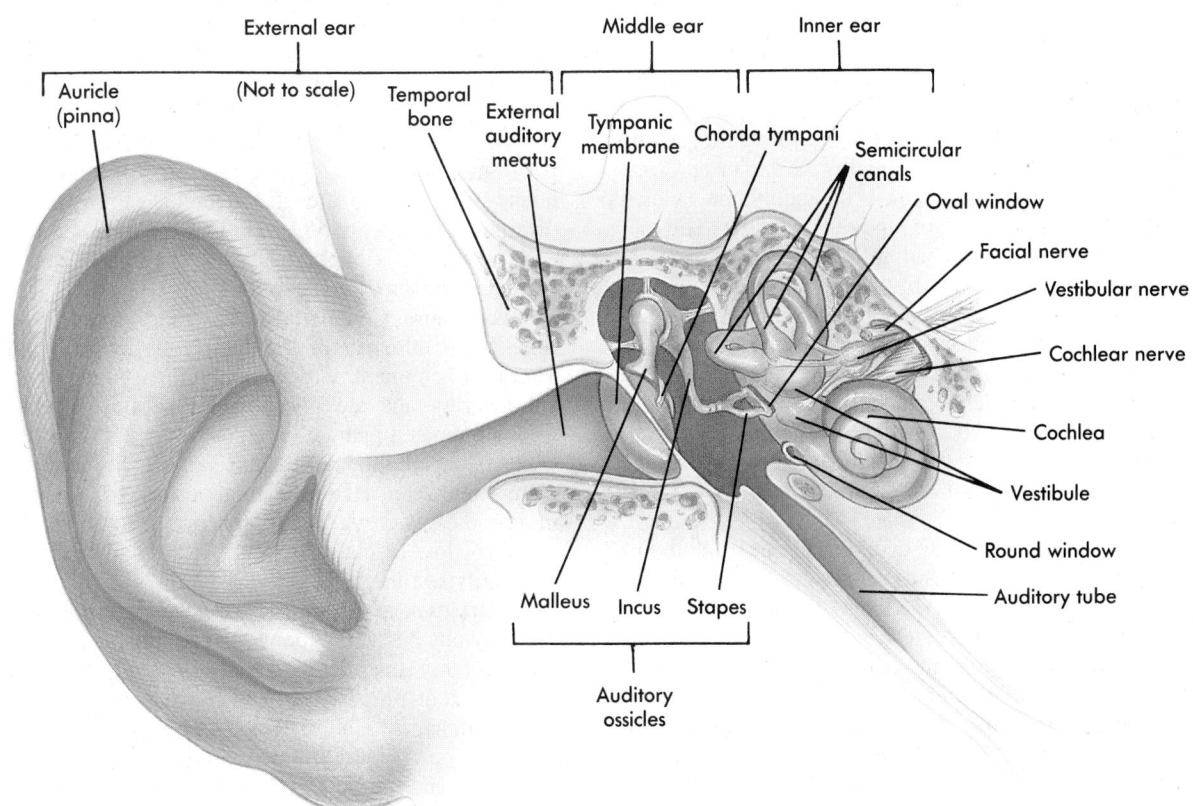

Fig. 14-9 External, middle, and inner ears. (From Seeley R, Stephens T, and Tate P: Anatomy and physiology, St Louis, 1989, Times Mirror/Mosby College Publishing, p 481.)

Middle Ear

Mucous membrane lines the middle ear and is continuous from the nasal pharynx via the eustachian tube. The middle ear cavity, which is located in the temporal bone, contains the *malleus, incus,* and *stapes* bones (collectively called the *ossicular chain*). The malleus articulates with the incus, which articulates with the head of the stapes. These articulations are freely movable synovial joints. The footplate of the stapes is positioned in the oval window and vibrates, causing the fluid in the inner ear to be set in motion. The round window covered with mucous membrane also opens into the inner ear and allows for dissipation of the fluid disturbances. The superior part of the middle ear is called the *epitympanum,* or the attic, and also communicates with air cells within the mastoid bone. The air cells are lined with the same mucous membrane as the middle ear.

The *middle ear* cavity is filled with air, and equalization of atmospheric air pressure is accomplished by the auditory tube. This tube is opened during yawning or swallowing. Blockage of the tube can occur with allergies, nasopharyngeal infections, and enlarged adenoids. Of clinical significance is the fact that the facial nerve (CN VII) traverses above the oval window of the middle ear. The thin bony covering of the facial nerve (CN VII) can become eroded or traumatized by chronic ear infection or trauma during ear surgery.

The external and middle portions of the ear function to conduct and magnify sound waves from the environment. This is called *air conduction.* Problems in these two parts of the ear may cause conductive hearing loss, resulting in the client not hearing normal or loud sounds.

Inner Ear

The inner ear, composed of the bony labyrinth and the membranous labyrinth, houses the end organ receptors for hearing and balance. The receptor organ for hearing is the *cochlea,* a coiled structure. It contains the organ of Corti, whose tiny hair cells are bathed in endolymph, which transmits the sound waves from the oval window. The mechanical stimulus is converted into an electric chemical impulse and then transmitted by CN VIII to the brain.

The *vestibular apparatus,* the organ of balance, is composed of the three semicircular canals and the utricle. The vestibular apparatus is bathed by the same endolymph fluid. Surrounding the endolymph is the perilymph fluid, which cushions these two sensitive organs and communicates with the brain and the subarachnoid spaces of the brain. The nervous stimuli are communicated by the vestibular portion of CN VIII.

Pathology of the inner ear or along the nerve pathway from the inner ear to the brain can result in sensorineural hearing loss. This causes the client to hear high-pitched tones as muffled and distorted but not necessarily decreased in loudness. Problems within the central auditory system from the cochlear nuclei to the cortex cause central hearing loss. This type of hearing loss causes difficulty in understanding the meaning of the words heard. (Types of hearing loss are discussed in Chapter 15.)

Transmission of sound. Sound waves are conducted by air and picked up by the auricles and auditory canal.

The taut tympanic membrane is struck by the sound waves, causing it to vibrate. The ossicles are joined to amplify sound waves received by the tympanic membrane and transmit the waves to the inner ear by a lever action. The footplate of the stapes vibrates in the oval window to conduct sound waves to the inner ear.[7]

Once sound has been transmitted to the liquid medium of the inner ear, the disturbance is picked up by the tiny sensory hair cells of the cochlea, which initiate nerve impulses. These impulses are carried by nerve fibers to the main branch of the acoustic portion of CN VIII (acoustic) and then to the brain.

Effects of Aging

Age-related changes of the auditory system can result in impaired hearing. Decreased efficiency of the cochlea and hair cells of the organ of Corti result in presbycusis, the loss of ability to hear high-frequency sounds. Impairment of the otic nerve can result in tinnitus, a ringing in the ear. Hearing loss can have serious consequences on the lifestyle of a person. Particularly in the frail older adult, hearing loss can lead to isolation and deterioration.

ASSESSMENT OF THE AUDITORY SYSTEM
Subjective Data

Health history. Many problems related to the ear are sequelae of childhood illnesses or result from problems of adjacent organs. Consequently, a careful assessment of past medical problems is important.

Past health history

PEDIATRIC AND ADULT ILLNESSES. The client needs to be questioned regarding previous problems regarding the left and right ears, especially problems experienced during childhood. The frequency of acute middle ear infections (otitis media), perforations of the eardrum, drainage, complications, and history of mumps and measles should be recorded. Data concerning residual or chronic otitis media, perforation of the eardrum, pain, and amounts and frequency of drainage are also obtained. Problems such as dizziness, tinnitus, and hearing loss are recorded in the client's words. It is important to ask the client to describe a complaint of dizziness in detail.

IMMUNIZATIONS. Congenital hearing losses can result from rubella or influenza in the first trimester of pregnancy. Therefore pregnant women and other young women of childbearing age are questioned regarding whether they were vaccinated against rubella or ever had rubella. If the client is uncertain about having had rubella, a hemagglutination inhibition (HI) test can be performed. A titer of 8 or more indicates previous exposure to the antibody. The absence (or low levels) of rubella HI antibody indicates susceptibility to rubella.[8]

HOSPITALIZATIONS, TRAUMA, AND MEDICATION. Information regarding previous hospitalizations for ear surgery as well as for tonsillectomy and adenoidectomy is obtained. Information about current or past medications that are ototoxic (i.e., cause damage to CN VIII) and can produce hearing loss, tinnitus, and disequilibrium is obtained. The amount of aspirin used and the frequency of its use are important, since tinnitus can result from high aspirin intake. Aminoglycosides, salicylates, antiprotozoal agents, and analgesics are the most important drug groups that are potentially oto-toxic.[9] Careful monitoring is essential. Many drugs produce inner ear damage that is reversible with cessation of treatment and substitution of an alternate medication. Information about allergies is important because the eustachian tube can become edematous and prevent aeration of the middle ear. This occurs more frequently in children.

Since prematurity can cause hearing problems, information about the client's birth is important. Head injury is a frequent cause of decreased or lost hearing and should be investigated.

Family history. Information regarding family members with hearing loss and the type of hearing loss is important, especially in the assessment of congenital and sensorineural hearing loss in the aging client (presbycusis).

Social and personal history. The client should be questioned regarding employment or contact with environments that have excessive noise levels, such as work with jet engines and machinery, contact with the firing of firearms, and electromagnified music. Use of preventive devices worn in noisy environments is recorded. Information about swimming habits, especially in contaminated waters, is also obtained. If hearing loss has occurred, the client should be asked about the related effects on daily life.

Review of systems. Symptoms related to the auditory system are similar to many of the symptoms of the upper respiratory and neurological systems. Information to be obtained regarding each ear and its function includes the following:

Hearing loss: Onset (e.g., sudden or gradual over hours or months); type; ability to hear certain words, sounds, or muffled sounds; effect of environmental noise

Pain: Feelings (e.g., discomfort, fullness); effect of movement of auricle (e.g., increased); type (e.g., referred from throat, requiring determination of throat problems or dental disease)

Drainage from external ear: Type (e.g., serosanguineous, bloody, purulent, clear); odor (e.g., putrid)

Tinnitus: Type and pitch (low, high); noise heard (e.g., roaring, humming, hissing); time of day

Dizziness: Onset, duration, frequency, precipitating factor

Nausea and vomiting: Present with dizziness

Objective Data

Physical examination. The nurse can collect valuable objective data regarding the client's ability to hear during the health history interview. Clues such as posturing of the head and appropriateness of responses should be noted. Does the client ask to have certain words repeated? Does the client intently watch the examiner but miss comments when not looking at the examiner? Such observations are significant and should be recorded. This is also important because the client is often not aware of hearing losses or does not admit to decreases until moderate losses have occurred. A normal assessment of the ear is recorded as shown in Table 14-6. Age-related changes of the auditory system and related differences in assessment findings are listed in Table 14-7.

External ear. The external ear is observed and palpated before inspection of the external canal and tympanum. The auricle, preauricular area, and mastoid area are inspected for equality of conformation of both ears, color of skin, nodules, swelling, redness, and lesions. The auricle and mastoid areas are then palpated for tenderness and nodules. Grasping the auricle may elicit pain, especially if inflammation of the external ear and/or canal is present.

External auditory canal and tympanum. Before insert-

Table 14-6 Normal Physical Assessment of the Auditory System

Ears symmetrical in location and shape
Auricles without lesions or discharge
Canal clear, tympanic membrane intact, landmarks and light reflex intact
Ability to hear low whisper at 30 cm; Rinne results: AC > BC; Weber results: lateralization equal

Table 14-7

 Age-Related Changes of the Auditory System and Differences in Assessment Findings

Changes	Differences in Assessment Findings
EXTERNAL EAR	
Increased production of and drier cerumen	Occlusion of canal with earwax; potential hearing loss
Increased hair growth	Visible hair
MIDDLE EAR	
Atrophic changes of tympanic membrane	Conductive hearing loss
INNER EAR	
Hair cell degeneration, neuron degeneration in auditory nerve and central pathways, reduced blood supply to cochlea	Presbycusis, diminished sensitivity to high-pitched sounds, impaired speech reception, tinnitus
Less effective vestibular apparatus in semicircular canals	Alterations in balance and body orientation

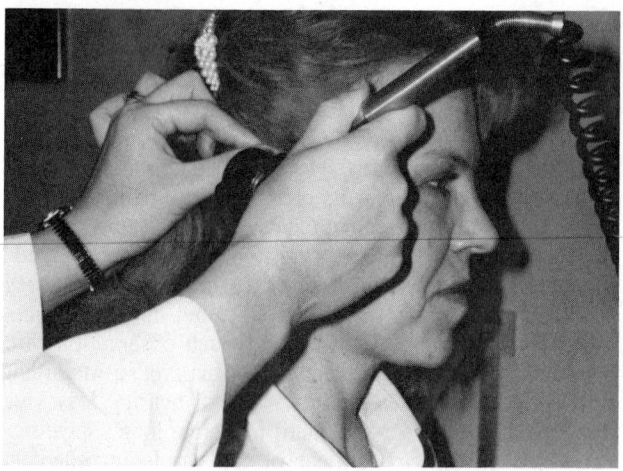

Fig. 14-10 Otoscopic examination of the adult ear. Auricle is pulled up and back. Otoscope is stabilized with right hand on client's face.

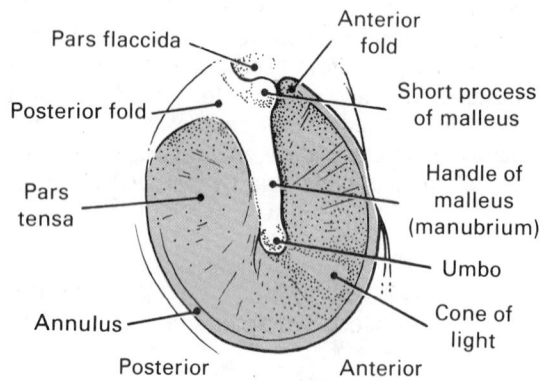

Fig. 14-11 Normal landmarks of the right tympanic membrane as seen through an otoscope.

ing an otoscope, the nurse should inspect the canal opening for patency, palpate the tragus, and move the ear about to check for discomfort. After inspecting the canal opening for patency, an otoscopic examination is performed. A speculum slightly smaller than the size of the canal is selected. The client's head is tipped to the opposite shoulder. In the adult client the top of the auricle is grasped and gently pulled up and back to straighten the canal. The otoscope, held in the examiner's right hand and stabilized on the client's head by the fingers, is inserted slowly (Fig. 14-10). The canal is observed for the color and amount of cerumen. If a large amount of cerumen is present, the tympanum may not be visible. The tympanum is observed for color, landmarks, contour, and intactness (Fig. 14-11).

The tympanic membrane separates the external ear from the middle ear. It is pearl-gray, white, or pink; shiny; and translucent. The anteroinferior quadrant is situated obliquely in the ear canal and is farthest from the examiner. The major landmarks are formed by the short process of the malleus superiorly, the handle or manubrium, and the umbo. From the innermost part of the tympanum a light reflex or cone of light is formed with the point directed to-

ward the umbo. The circumference of the tympanum is surrounded by a dense, whitish, fibrous ring, or annulus, except in the superior area. The tympanum within the annulus is taut and is referred to as the *pars tensa*. Superior to the short process of the malleus is the *pars flaccida*, or flaccid part of the tympanum. The malleolar folds are anterior and posterior to the short process of the malleus. Changes to observe in the tympanum include color, landmarks, and effect of light. Table 14-8 summarizes common assessment abnormalities of the auditory system. The middle and inner ear cannot be examined directly with the otoscope because of the tympanic membrane.

Tests for hearing acuity. Tests involving the whispered and spoken voice can provide gross screening information about the client's ability to hear. Audiometry provides more specific information that can be used for diagnosis and treatment.

In the whispered test the examiner stands 30 to 60 cm to the side of the client and, after exhaling, speaks using a low whisper. A louder whisper is used if the client does not respond correctly. Spoken voice, increasing in loudness, is similarly used. The client is asked to repeat numbers or words or answer questions. Each ear is tested. The ear not being tested is masked with the client occluding the ear or with the examiner moving a finger rapidly, close to the ear canal.

In another test a ticking watch is placed 2 to 5 cm from the ear being tested and the opposite ear is masked. The client with normal hearing should be able to hear the ticking. However, the variation among watches makes this test a very gross one for assessing hearing acuity. Clients with sensorineural loss cannot hear the high-pitched tones of a ticking watch.

TUNING FORK TESTS. Tuning fork tests aid in differentiating between conductive and sensorineural hearing loss. Tuning forks of 500 and 1000 Hz are used. Both skill and experience are necessary to ensure accurate results. If a problem is suspected, further evaluation by pure-tone audiometry is essential. The most common tuning fork tests are the Rinne and the Weber tests.

For the Rinne test the base of an activated tuning fork is held on the mastoid bone until the client signals that the tone can no longer be heard. The fork is then moved to 2.5 cm from the ear canal. The client reports whether the sound can be heard and for how long. The examiner times each response. The Rinne test is positive when the client reports that air conduction is heard longer than bone conduction. This can indicate normal hearing or a sensorineural loss. If the client hears the tuning fork better by bone conduction, the Rinne test is negative and indicates that a conductive hearing loss is present.

For the Weber test an activated tuning fork is placed on the midline of the skull, the forehead, or the teeth. The client is asked to indicate where the sound is heard best. The normal response is perception of equal loudness bilaterally. If a client has a conductive hearing loss in one ear, sound is heard louder (lateralizes) in that ear. If a sensorineural loss is present, sound is louder in the good ear. Other diagnostic tests may reveal a mixed hearing loss.

Vestibular system. Nystagmus, an abnormal rhythmic jerking motion of the eyes within the field of binocular vi-

Table 14-8

Common Assessment Abnormalities of the Ear

Finding	Description	Possible Etiology and Significance
EXTERNAL EAR AND CANAL		
Sebaceous cyst behind ear	Usually within skin, possible presence of black dot (opening to sebaceous gland)	Removal or incision and drainage if painful
Tophi	Hard nodules in the helix or antihelix consisting of uric acid crystals	Associated with gout, metabolic disorder; further diagnosis needed
Impacted cerumen	Wax that has not normally been excreted from the ear, no visualization of eardrum	Decreased hearing possible, sensation of fullness in auditory canal, removal necessary before otoscopic examination
Discharge in canal	Infection of external ear, usually painful	Swimmer's ear, infection of external ear; possible causes of ruptured eardrum and otitis media
Swelling of pinna, pain	Infection of glands of skin, hematoma due to trauma	Aspiration (for hematoma)
Scaling or lesions	Change in usual appearance of skin	Seborrheic dermatitis, squamous cell carcinoma
Exostosis	Bony growth extending into canal causing narrowing of canal	Possible interference with visualization of tympanum, usually asymptomatic
TYMPANUM		
Retracted eardrum	Appearance of shorter, more horizontal malleus; absent or bent cone of light	Absorption of air from middle ear, blockage of eustachian tube, negative pressure in middle ear
Hairline fluid level, yellow-amber bubbles above fluid level	Due to transudate of blood and serum, meniscus of fluid producing hairline appearance	Serous otitis media
Bulging red or blue eardrum, lack of landmarks	Fluid-filled middle ear, pus, blood	Acute otitis media, perforation possible
Early stage hyperemic vessels	Complaint of severe pain	Usually in children
Perforation of eardrum (central or marginal)	Previous perforations of the eardrum that have failed to heal (in adults); thin, transparent layer of epithelium surrounding eardrum	Chronic otitis media, referral necessary
Recruitment	Disproportionate loudness of sound from malfunction of inner ear	Hearing aid difficult to use

sion, can be caused by disturbances in the endolymph fluid. The movement of the endolymph fluid stimulates receptor cells and causes nystagmus. Lesions in the central nervous system and drug toxicity can also cause nystagmus. In a test for nystagmus the client looks straight ahead and then follows the examiner's finger to an extreme lateral gaze. Quick jerking movement along the way, except on extreme lateral gaze, is considered abnormal. Caloric testing and electronystagmography also test the function of the vestibular system.

DIAGNOSTIC STUDIES
Audiometry

Audiometry is useful as a screening test for hearing acuity and as a diagnostic test for determining the degree and type of hearing loss. The audiometer produces pure tone of simple sound waves. Sound is described according to the number of vibrations that take place each second. Cycles per second (cps) or hertz (Hz) follow the number representing the vibrations (e.g., 2000 cps or Hz).

The frequency of sound is determined by how fast a sound source vibrates. The higher the frequency, the higher the pitch. Hearing loss can affect specific sound frequencies and influences the success of a hearing aid. The intensity or strength of a sound wave is expressed in terms of decibels (dB), ranging from 0 dB to 140 dB, with 0 being the softest. The intensity of a sound required to make any frequency barely audible to the average normal ear is 0 dB. *Threshold* refers to the signal level at which pure tones are detected (pure tone thresholds) or the signal level at which the client correctly hears 50% of the signals (speech reception thresholds).

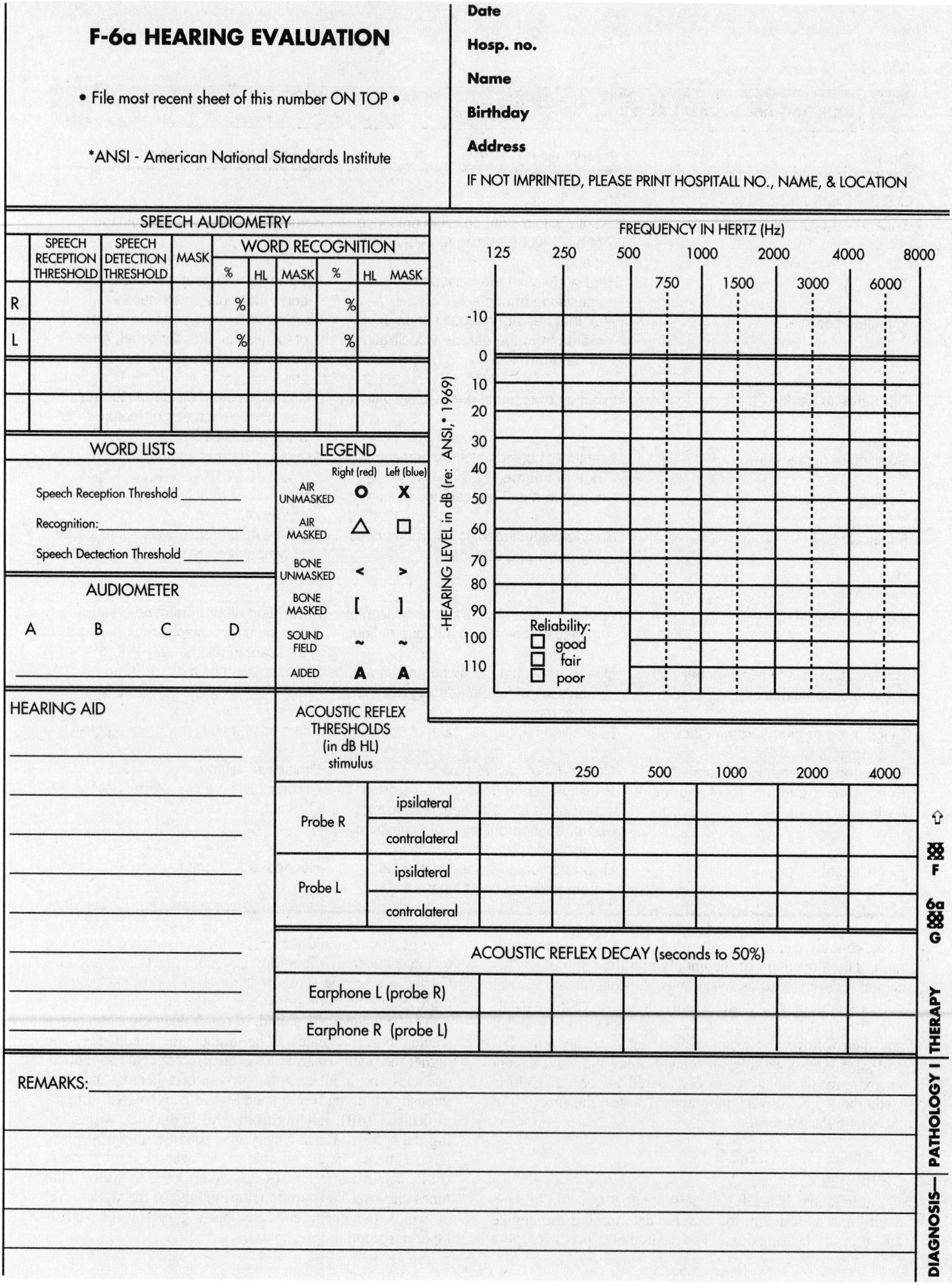

F-6a HEARING EVALUATION

• File most recent sheet of this number ON TOP •

*ANSI - American National Standards Institute

Date

Hosp. no.

Name

Birthday

Address

IF NOT IMPRINTED, PLEASE PRINT HOSPITALL NO., NAME, & LOCATION

SPEECH AUDIOMETRY

	SPEECH RECEPTION THRESHOLD	SPEECH DETECTION THRESHOLD	MASK	WORD RECOGNITION					
				%	HL	MASK	%	HL	MASK
R				%			%		
L				%			%		

WORD LISTS

Speech Reception Threshold _____

Recognition: _____

Speech Dectection Threshold _____

LEGEND

	Right (red)	Left (blue)
AIR UNMASKED	O	X
AIR MASKED	△	□
BONE UNMASKED	<	>
BONE MASKED	[	]
SOUND FIELD	~	~
AIDED	A	A

AUDIOMETER

A   B   C   D

_____

HEARING AID

_____

_____

_____

_____

_____

_____

_____

_____

FREQUENCY IN HERTZ (Hz)

125 250 500 1000 2000 4000 8000

750 1500 3000 6000

-HEARING LEVEL in dB (re: ANSI,* 1969)

-10 0 10 20 30 40 50 60 70 80 90 100 110

Reliability:
☐ good
☐ fair
☐ poor

ACOUSTIC REFLEX THRESHOLDS (in dB HL) stimulus

		250	500	1000	2000	4000
Probe R	ipsilateral					
	contralateral					
Probe L	ipsilateral					
	contralateral					

ACOUSTIC REFLEX DECAY (seconds to 50%)

Earphone L (probe R)					
Earphone R (probe L)					

REMARKS: _____

⇧

✖ F

6a

G ✖

DIAGNOSIS— PATHOLOGY I THERAPY

Fig. 14-12 The client's hearing level is plotted on the audiogram. (Courtesy Medical Records Subcommittee of The University of Iowa Hospitals and Clinics, Iowa City, Ia.)

Table 14-9

Diagnostic Studies of the Auditory System

Study	Description and Purpose	Nursing Responsibility
AUDITORY		
Pure-tone audiometry	Sounds are presented through earphones in soundproof room. Client responds nonverbally when sound is heard. Response is recorded on an audiogram. Purpose is to determine hearing range of client in terms of dB and Hz for diagnosing conductive and sensorineural hearing loss.	Nurse does not usually participate in examination.
Bone conduction	Vibrator is placed on mastoid process and hearing by bone conduction is recorded. Diagnoses conductive hearing loss.	
One-syllable word-lists	Words are presented and recorded at comfortable level of hearing to determine percentage correct and word understanding.	
High-frequency pure tones of 12,000 to 15,000 Hz	Normally, client can hear pure tone for 1 minute. Those with pressure on CN VIII will not hear pure tones. Levels of intensity are increased, which client cannot hear. Higher frequencies are used. If tones used before administration of ototoxic drug, decrease at this level during drug administration indicates cochlear damage and need to discontinue use of drug.	Nurse does not usually participate in examination.

Continued.

Normal speech presented comfortably loud is approximately 40 to 65 dB; a soft whisper is 20 dB. Normally, a child and a young adult can hear frequencies of about 16 to 20,000 Hz, but hearing is most sensitive from 500 to 4000 Hz. This is similar to the frequencies used in speech. A 40 to 45 dB loss in all frequencies causes moderate difficulty in hearing normal speech. A hearing aid is helpful because it magnifies sound. A client with a 15 to 20 dB loss in only the higher frequencies, such as 4000 Hz, has difficulty hearing the high-pitched consonants. Words such as *cheese, thin,* and *fin* are not perceived accurately but sound muffled or distorted. A hearing aid is not as helpful because it causes the sound to be louder but not clearer.

Screening audiometry. Screening audiometry is the testing of large numbers of persons with a fast, simple test to detect possible hearing problems. A pass-fail criterion is used to screen out persons who will or will not be given additional diagnostic testing. Persons who fail the screening should be referred for threshold audiometry.

In screening audiometry, the audiometer is usually set at a hearing level of 10 to 20 dB. The client wears earphones as the tester sweeps across the available signal frequencies. The client is directed to raise a hand when a sound is heard. Responses to air-conducted tones are checked at each frequency setting.

Pure-tone audiometry. A pure-tone audiometer produces pure tones at varied frequencies and intensities. Threshold audiometry generally determines detection thresholds for seven frequencies from 250 to 8000 Hz. The intensity is plotted against the frequency on an audiogram (Fig. 14-12). The right ear is represented by a red circle and the left ear by a blue X on the audiogram.

In a quiet setting a tone loud enough to be clearly heard by the client is presented. The threshold level for frequency is then determined. A person with thresholds at 25 dB hearing loss has significant problems in everyday communication situations. Usually the lower limit used for acceptable hearing for children is 15 to 20 dB. The 26 dB hearing loss is used as a guideline for further action. A hearing aid or surgery is rarely recommended for a hearing loss of less than 26 dB.[10]

Specialized Tests

The audiologist can perform many additional tests since the advent of newer audiometers and computers that record pressures of electric impulses from the middle ear, inner ear, and brain (Table 14-9). The most common test per-

Table 14-9

Diagnostic Studies of the Auditory System—cont'd		
Study	**Description and Purpose**	**Nursing Responsibility**
AUDITORY—cont'd		
Evoked response audiometry or audiometric brainstem response	Procedure is similar to electroencephalogram. Electrodes are attached to client in a darkened room. A computer is used to isolate the auditory from other electrical activity of the brain. Test is useful for uncooperative client or clients who cannot volunteer useful information.	Explain procedure to client. Do not leave client alone in darkened room.
Cortical (stimulus, pure tone, or broadband)	Test focuses on electrical activity at cerebral cortex level.	
Brainstem (stimulus, pure tone, or broadband)	Study measures electrical peaks along auditory pathway of inner ear to brain and gives possible diagnosis of acoustical neuromas, brainstem problems, or vascular accident.	
VESTIBULAR		
Caloric test stimulus	Endolymph of the semicircular canals is stimulated by irrigation of cold (20° C) or warm (36° C) solution into ear. Client is seated or in supine position. Observation of type of nystagmus, nausea and vomiting, falling, and vertigo produced is helpful in diagnosing disease of labyrinth. Decreased function is indicated by decreased response and indicates disease of vestibular system. Other ear is tested similarly and results are compared.	Observe client for vomiting. Assist if necessary. Ensure client safety.
Electronystagmography	Electrodes are placed near client's eyes and movement of eyes (nystagmus) is recorded on graph during specific eye movements and when ear is irrigated. Study diagnoses diseases of vestibular system.	

formed by the audiologist is pure-tone audiometry done under ideal testing conditions. A soundproof room is used for greater accuracy of results. The audiologist can also test bone conduction by audiometry to diagnose conductive hearing loss. The more specialized tests of the auditory system are most often performed in an outpatient setting by an audiologist. There is seldom any nursing responsibility involved.

Test for vestibular function. The caloric test is done to determine the function of the vestibular system. The external ear is irrigated with cold or warm water, which causes disturbances in the endolymph. The client's reaction is observed for type of eye movements (opposite to stimulated ear) and falling toward the stimulated ear. Drugs that may affect the test include alcohol, central nervous system depressants, and barbiturates. The client's use of them should be known to the physician before testing.

R *eview Questions*

The number of the question corresponds to the same-numbered objective at the beginning of the chapter.
1. The third, fourth, and sixth cranial nerves control
   a. visual fields
   b. extraocular movement
   c. nystagmus
   d. pupil size

2. The parts of the eye that refract light rays are the
   a. anterior and posterior chambers
   b. cornea and pupil
   c. bulbar conjunctiva and lens
   d. cornea and lens
3. A history of a high intake of aspirin can result in
   a. tinnitus
   b. vertigo
   c. sensorineural hearing loss
   d. conductive hearing loss
4. The abbreviation used to designate both eyes is
   a. OU
   b. OD
   c. OS
5. Which of the following is a normal finding in assessing the ear?
   a. absent cone of light
   b. pearl-gray tympanic membrane
   c. BC > AC
   d. retracted tympanum
6. Presbyopia is caused by
   a. decreased lacrimal secretion
   b. decreased visual field
   c. shallow anterior chamber
   d. decreased elasticity of lens
7. The purpose of tonometry is to determine
   a. refractive error
   b. corneal curvature
   c. intraocular pressure
   d. sensitivity of the cornea

REFERENCES

1. Seeley R, Stephens T, and Tate P: Anatomy and physiology, St Louis, 1989, The CV Mosby Co, p 475.
2. Newell F: Ophthalmology: principles and concepts, ed 6, St Louis, 1986, The CV Mosby Co.
3. Amos J, ed: Diagnosis and management in vision care, Boston, 1987, Butterworths, p 673.
4. Walsh J, Gold A, and Charles H: Physician's desk reference for ophthalmology, ed 18, Oradell, NJ, 1990, Medical Economics Books.
5. Boyd-Monk H and Steinmetz C: Nursing care of the eye, Norwalk, Conn, 1987, Appleton & Lange, p 65.
6. Upchurch DT, ed: Otolaryngology, Oradell, NJ, 1989, Medical Economics Books, p 3.
7. Thompson JM and others: Mosby's manual of clinical nursing, ed 2, St Louis, 1989, The CV Mosby Co, p 663.
8. Bryant N: Laboratory immunology and serology, Philadelphia, 1986, WB Saunders Co, p 181.
9. Booth JB, ed: Scott-Brown's otolaryngology-otology, ed 5, London, 1987, Butterworths, p 465.
10. Templer J and others, eds: Otolaryngology—head and neck surgery: principles and concepts, St Louis, 1987, Ishiyaku EuroAmerica, p 16.

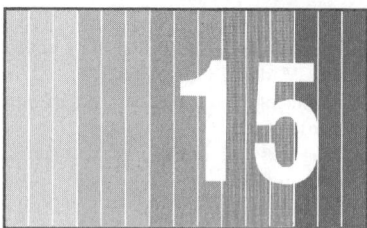

CHAPTER

15

Nursing Role in Management

Problems of Vision and Hearing

Pam Schremp
Mary Means

L earning Objectives

1. *Describe the types of refractive errors and appropriate corrections.*
2. *Describe the etiology and management of external ocular disorders.*
3. *Explain the pathophysiology, clinical manifestations, and therapeutic and nursing management for the client with selected intraocular disorders.*
4. *Describe nursing measures to promote health of the eyes and ears.*
5. *Explain the general preoperative and postoperative care of the client undergoing surgery of the eye or ear.*
6. *Describe the action and uses of common pharmacological agents used in treating problems of the eyes and ears.*

7. *Explain the pathophysiology, clinical manifestations, and therapeutic and nursing management of common eye and ear problems.*
8. *Compare the cause, management, and rehabilitative potential of conductive and sensorineural hearing loss.*
9. *Explain the use, care, and client education related to assistive devices for eye and ear problems.*
10. *Describe the common causes and assistive measures for blindness and deafness.*
11. *Describe the psychological nursing measures used to assist the client in adapting to decreased vision and hearing.*

VISUAL PROBLEMS
HEALTH PROMOTION AND MAINTENANCE

The nurse must be aware of the great potential for preventing problems of vision through appropriate nursing interventions. Early recognition of conditions that can cause blindness is a major nursing responsibility. Conditions or situations that should alert the nurse to potential visual problems include the following:

1. Congenital blindness can be due to a rubella infection in the mother during the first trimester of pregnancy. This condition can be prevented by the use of rubella (German measles) vaccine to maintain normal rubella titers in women of childbearing age. Those who come in contact with this group of women, especially those who work in health care agencies, must also be immunized.

2. Monitoring the arterial blood gas values and the levels of oxygen delivered to premature and newborn infants is very important to prevent retinopathy of prematurity (ROP). Administration of excessive oxygen to newborn infants results in fibrovascular growths within the eye, causing blindness.

3. Community education is an important nursing responsibility. Teaching the need for eye examinations, especially for adults over 40 years of age, is essential. Glaucoma can cause blindness if not recognized early and treated. Open-angle glaucoma is often first identified by measurement of intraocular pressure with a tonometer. The nurse can support and assist with community glaucoma screening programs. Clients with diabetes should have yearly ophthalmic examinations to ensure early treatment of retinopathy.[1] It is also essential that children who have strabismus or suppression amblyopia be identified early.

Reviewed by Tana H. Durnbaugh, R.N., Ed.D., Professor, College of Lake County, Grayslake, Illinois.

4. Eye injuries can lead to blindness. It is estimated that 95% of eye injuries can be prevented.[1] Potential sources of eye injuries need to be identified and corrected. Many eye injuries are caused by flying metal pieces in home workshops and in the use of welding equipment. Use of safety glasses greatly reduces these injuries.

5. Incorrect wearing of contact lenses is also a common source of trauma to the eye.[4] Correct wearing and proper cleaning techniques reduce many of the problems that are potential causes of impaired vision or blindness.

6. The correct use of safety equipment, such as seat belts and shoulder harnesses in cars and goggles and helmets by those riding motorcycles, needs to be encouraged and made mandatory.

7. Correct handling of cleaning solutions containing alkali or acid that can cause chemical burns needs to be emphasized. Many home products contain lye, which can cause blindness if splashed in the eye. It is important to teach consumers that immediate, thorough irrigation of the eye while seeking medical care is critical emergency home care management.

8. As more information becomes known about the causes of congenital blindness and inherited eye problems, genetic counseling will be helpful in reducing visual problems.

9. Nurses should take leading roles in educating athletes regarding the potential for sports-related eye injuries from small, fast-moving balls in sports such as tennis and racquetball. Skiers should be advised of the danger of exposure to ultraviolet light and the potential for corneal abrasions from low-hanging tree branches. Nurses should be aware of sports-specific risks to eye health if they are to provide appropriate education to specific groups.

REFRACTIVE ERROR

The most common visual problem is refractive error. This defect of the refracting media of the eye prevents light rays from converging into a single focus on the retina. Defects are due to irregularities of the corneal curvature, the focusing power of the lens, and the length of the eye. The major symptoms are blurred vision and discomfort. Corrective lenses are used to improve the focus of light rays on the retina (Fig. 15-1). Approximately 143 million Americans require some form of visual correction.[2]

Myopia

The myopic eye causes light rays to be focused anterior to the retina. When a myopic person looks at a distant object, light rays from near objects focus on the retina. Myopia requires fairly frequent changes of glasses during childhood and especially during adolescence, when the eyeball lengthens excessively. This excessive lengthening is generally attributed to genetic factors.

Other causes of myopia involve the excessive bending of light rays by the cornea and the lens. A minus lens (concave) is required for better focus (Table 15-1).

Recently, some persons with mild to moderate myopia have been able to discontinue the use of glasses or contact lenses as a result of a somewhat controversial surgical procedure called *radial keratotomy*. Following local anesthesia, 8 to 16 radial cuts are made in the periphery of the cornea. Placement of these partial-thickness cuts weakens the cornea, allowing it to change shape and flatten. Light rays can then be better focused on the retina. Either undercorrection or overcorrection of the client's refractive error is possible. Complications include infection and corneal scarring. In some clients, sensitivity to glare may result. Long-term data on the efficacy of this surgical treatment are currently being collected.

Astigmatism

Astigmatism is caused by the unequal curvature of the cornea and causes the light rays to be bent unequally and not come to a single focus on the retina. Correction of the unequal curvature of the cornea is through the use of a cylinder lens. Myopia or hyperopia can coexist with astigmatism.

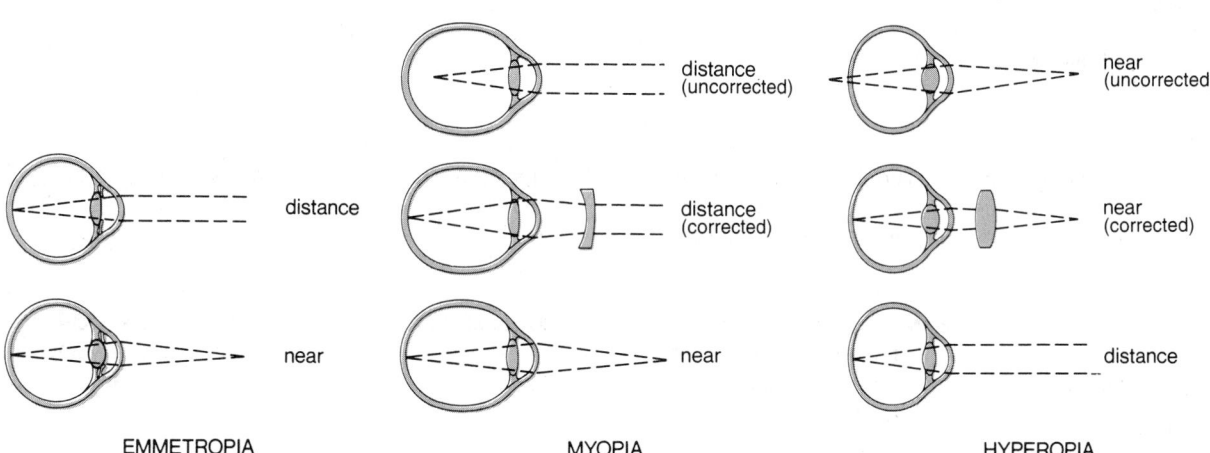

Fig. 15-1 Emmetropic, myopic, and hyperopic eye with corrected and uncorrected vision.

Table 15-1 Correction of Refractive Errors

Description	Symptoms	Type of Spectacle Correction	Type of Contact Lenses
EMMETROPIA			
Focus of light on retina, distance vision without accommodation, near vision with accommodation	Normal vision	Not indicated	Not indicated
MYOPIA			
Elongated eyeball or excessive refractive power of cornea and lens (e.g., when viewing distant object, light rays focused in front of retina; with near object, focus of light rays on retina); accommodation for closer objects	Blurred distance vision (evident in early school years); squinting to narrow amount of light entering eye and improve focus	Biconcave (minus)	Hard, soft, gas permeable
HYPEROPIA			
Short eyeball with insufficient refractive power to focus light rays on the retina without accommodation (e.g., when viewing new object light rays focused behind retina); focus of light on retina for far and near vision by accommodation; earlier experience with presbyopia than those with emmetropia	Ocular fatigue	Convex (plus)	Hard, soft, gas permeable
ASTIGMATISM			
Unequal curvature of cornea causing light to focus at no clear point, associated with any of the above refractions	Blurred vision, ocular fatigue	Cylinder	Hard, soft (if Toric lens)
PRESBYOPIA			
Larger and harder aging lens that cannot flatten or accommodate for near vision	Blurred near vision, holding of fine print more than 10 inches away from eye	Reading, bifocals, convex for near vision	Monovision, hard, soft, blended
APHAKIA			
Absence of lens due to congenital defect, trauma, or surgery (cataract extraction)	No near vision; if one eye involved, image on retina one-third larger than with normal eye	Thick, concave; asperial	Soft, extended wear; intraocular (surgically implanted)

Presbyopia

Presbyopia is the loss of accommodation due to age. As the eye ages, the ocular lens becomes larger, firmer, and less elastic. The accommodative ability decreases. After the age of 60 the lens has become so inelastic that accommodation is not possible.[3] Initially, the client experiences difficulty in reading newsprint unless held at arm's length. Vision is best corrected by reading glasses if no other refractive error is present. Bifocal glasses are prescribed for those with other refractive errors. Trifocals are prescribed when the client requires correction for middistance of 68 to 137 cm (27 to 50 inches).

Hyperopia

Hyperopia (farsightedness) causes the light rays to focus behind the retina and requires the use of accommodation to focus the light rays on the retina for near and far objects. The treatment of hyperopia uses a convex or plus lens to facilitate focusing.

APHAKIA

By definition, *aphakia* is the absence of the lens. The lens is removed during cataract surgery or can be dislocated by trauma. Once the lens is removed, the refracting power of the eye is reduced by 20% to 30%. Without the focusing ability of the lens, images are projected behind the retina. A strong convex lens is used to improve the eye's refracting power.

A second surgical treatment for aphakia is called *epikeratophakia*. In this procedure, donor corneal tissue is frozen and reshaped on a lathe to the strength and shape needed. During surgery, the donor tissue is sutured over the client's cornea. Sutures are left in place for several weeks or until the epithelium has regenerated. Candidates for epikeratophakia include clients who have contact lens intolerance, severe myopia, or keratoconus (noninflammatory protrusion of the central part of the cornea).

STRABISMUS

The deviation of one eye from the other in an outward, inward, upward, or downward direction when the client is fixing on an object is called *strabismus*. In children, strabismus requires early medical intervention to prevent development of suppression amblyopia. Suppression amblyopia is reduced vision in an eye caused by cerebral blockage of the visual stimulus. However, the eye is normal on examination.

If strabismus develops in the adult client, diplopia (double vision) is the chief complaint. Strabismus in the adult may be due to thyroid disease, neuromuscular problems of the eye muscles, and cerebral lesions.

CORRECTION
Glasses

Glasses are one way to correct refractive errors. Many styles and colors are available to meet individual needs and preferences. Table 15-1 outlines the specific corrections of glasses for different refractive problems. In cleaning glasses care must be taken to prevent scratching of the lens.

Contact Lenses

Contact lenses are another way to correct refractive errors (Table 15-1). The contact lens, riding on the tear film of the cornea, usually provides better vision without the distortion of glasses and their frames. The contact lens is held in place by surface tension. Blinking causes the tear film to move under and over the contact lens. The tear film is very important because it provides oxygen for the cornea. If the oxygen is depleted, the corneal epithelium becomes swollen, visual acuity decreases, and the client experiences severe discomfort.

Altered or decreased tear formation can make the wearing of contact lenses difficult. Tear production can be disturbed by antihistamines, decongestants, diuretics, birth control pills, and the hormones produced by pregnancy. Conjunctivitis caused by allergies can also affect the wearing of contact lenses.

The types of contact lenses and their advantages and disadvantages are presented in Table 15-2. In general, the nurse needs to know whether the client wears contact lenses, the frequency of medical supervision, pattern of wear (daily versus extended) and care practices (Fig. 15-2). The nurse must be able to identify the presence of contacts and know how to remove them in an emergency situation. Shining a light obliquely on the eyeball can help identify the presence of a contact lens. If necessary, the nurse can remove hard contact lenses by means of a small suction cup. If the client can sit upright, the contact lens can be removed as follows: (1) wash hands; (2) stand beside client, placing nondominant hand against client's cheek; (3) place index finger of nondominant hand near lateral canthus; (4) pull tissue gently upward and outward; and (5) instruct client to blink. The lens will fall into the nurse's hand and should be stored in a case filled with the appropriate solution and labeled with the client's name.

Soft contact lenses can be removed as follows: (1) Place the client upright (if possible); (2) wash hands; (3) place the middle finger of the dominant hand against the lower eyelid; (4) gently pull the lower eyelid down against the cheekbone; (5) slide the lens down off the cornea and onto the sclera; (6) with the thumb and index finger, pinch the lens off the eye; and (7) store the lens in a case filled with normal saline solution and label with the client's name.

The client should be instructed regarding the signs and symptoms of possible contact lens problems that indicate the need for medical consultation. These include (1) a red and painful eye; (2) a sudden change in vision; (3) repeated irritation of the eye; (4) excess secretions from the eye; and (5) "spectacle blur" (hazy vision) that lasts more than 24 hours after the wearing of hard contact lenses.

EXTERNAL OCULAR DISEASE
Infections

One of the most common conditions encountered by the ophthalmologist is infection of the external eye. Many microorganisms affect the lids and conjunctiva and can involve the avascular cornea. Conditions that predispose to infection of the cornea are irritation of the cornea, decreased tear film, and decreased blinking. The client who has decreased resistance or is immunosuppressed is more

Table 15-2 Types of Contact Lenses

Type	Description	Advantages	Disadvantages
HARD			
Polymethylmethacrylate (PMMA)	Rigid plastic; 8-10 mm in diameter (incomplete coverage of cornea); specific wetting, cleansing, soaking solutions necessary	Can be tinted, polished, and reground. Lasts 4-7 years. Is least expensive in terms of cost, equipment, follow-up care. Can correct greatest range of visual problems.	Requires gradually increased wearing time up to 14 hr. If wearing schedule disrupted, wearing schedule should be restarted. Dust particles under lens cause discomfort. Painful corneal edema results with overwearing. Spectacle blur occurs when glasses are used after contact use. Direct impact injury may shatter lens and injure eye.
GAS-PERMEABLE			
Cellulose acetate butyrate or 65% PMMA with silicone	Rigid plastic allowing oxygen and other gases to pass through and nourish cornea; same size as hard contacts	Fit is more comfortable than hard contact lenses. Requires less adaptation time and less problem with corneal edema. Provides better correction of astigmatism than soft lenses.	Cost is greater than for hard contact lenses.
SOFT			
Hydrophilic plastic (30%-40% water)	Consistency of cornflake until immersed in sterile water or normal saline solution (to soft, gelatinlike material); larger than hard lenses (12.5-16 mm in diameter, complete coverage of cornea and small portion of sclera); conscientious cleaning necessary*; enzymatic cleaner weekly	Fits snugly on cornea, prevents particles entering under lens. Little adaptation is needed. Reduces glare. Can be worn intermittently and up to 18 hr/day.	Is fragile and lasts approximately 2 years. Cannot be tinted. Can shrink in dry environments or deficient tear film (will tighten and blur vision). Visual acuity is less than with hard contacts. Easily absorbs dust, smoke, protein from tears, aerosol sprays, oil from makeup, and microorganisms. Correction of astigmatism is poor.
EXTENDED WEAR			
Hydrophilic plastic, 60%-80% water	Similar to soft lens; follow-up care, good personal hygiene, and cooperative client necessary	Can be worn for several weeks or longer without removal (although weekly removal is recommended). Used after cataract extraction; reduces distortion of cataract glasses and image size difference if only one cataract removed. Is useful for clients with decreased manual dexterity.	Is more fragile than soft lenses and splits easily. Requires close medical supervision. Cost is greatest of all lenses. Complications of infections and vascularization of cornea can occur. Lens deposits occur. Lens life is about 6 months.
Disposable extended wear	Multipack dispenser package with six lenses; each lens immersed in sterile, buffered saline solution with shelf-life of 4 years	Does not require use of lens care solutions; can be worn for up to 7 days. Deposit buildup is minimal.	Long-term data on what, if any, problems can occur are not available.

PMMA, Polymethylmethacrylate.
*See Fig. 15-2.

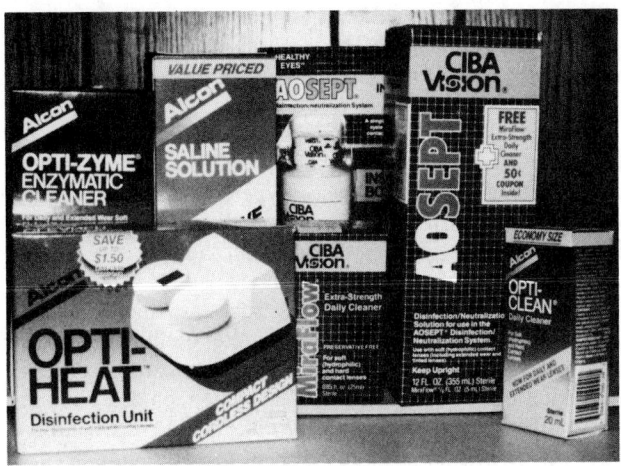

Fig. 15-2 Commonly used contact lens care products.

prone to ocular infections. Infection of the cornea can cause corneal ulceration with a potential for perforation, scarring, and blindness. Many eye infections are treated on an outpatient basis. It is a nursing responsibility to teach the client appropriate interventions related to the specific infection.

Lids. *Hordeolum* (stye), a staphylococcal infection of the lid margin, is fairly common. A red, swollen, circumscribed, and acutely tender area develops rapidly. If there is a tendency for recurrence, appropriate antibiotic ointments are indicated. A search for other possible sources of staphylococcal infection elsewhere on the body is indicated. Warm, moist compresses are applied at least three to four times a day until the lesion opens and purulent material drains.

Chalazion, an inflammation of the meibomian glands within the lids, usually develops slowly over a period of weeks. The blocked gland enlarges and becomes tender. Redness of the palpebral conjunctiva may be noted when the eyelid is everted. The client may also experience eye fatigue, photophobia, and epiphora (overflow of tears due to excessive secretion or obstruction of the ducts). Management includes warm compresses and antibiotics if there is infection. If the chalazion becomes chronic, excision of the gland may be necessary.

Marginal blepharitis is a common chronic bilateral inflammation of the lid margins. The lids are red rimmed with many scales or crusts on the lid margins and lashes. The client complains of burning, itching, irritation, and photophobia. Small ulcers may occur at the lid margins. Conjunctivitis may also occur.

If the blepharitis is caused by a staphylococcal infection, therapeutic management includes the use of an appropriate ophthalmic antibiotic ointment. Seborrheic blepharitis, related to seborrhea of the scalp and eyebrows, is treated with an antiseborrheic shampoo for the scalp and eyebrows. Often blepharitis is due to both staphylococcal and seborrheal microorganisms, and the treatment must be more vigorous to avoid hordeolum, keratitis (inflammation of the cornea), and other eye infections. Conscientious hy-

gienic practices involving skin and scalp need to be emphasized. Gentle cleansing of the lid margins with baby shampoo can effectively soften and remove crusting.

Conjunctiva

Bacterial infections. Acute conjunctivitis (pinkeye) is a common bacterial infection that is most often seen in children. It is usually caused by the *Staphylococcus aureus* organism and can become epidemic. If it is caused by *Pneumococcus* or *Haemophilus* microorganisms, the conjunctiva rapidly becomes red and a discharge develops. The discharge changes from watery to mucopurulent. Small breaks in the corneal epithelium may be noted. The client complains of mild irritation. The condition is usually self-limiting, but prevention of spread by careful hand-washing and use of individual or disposable towels and washcloths is important. Topical antibiotics are prescribed.

Viral infection. Viral infections are caused by herpesvirus type 1, herpes zoster virus, and adenoviruses. Viral infections of the conjunctiva produce redness, a watery discharge, and follicles of the conjunctiva. Follicles are avascular white or gray, round, raised areas. Viral infections produce disease that may be mild and self-limiting or severe and debilitating.

Herpes simplex virus keratitis is one of the most common severe ocular infections found in the United States today. It is a growing problem, especially with immunosuppressed clients such as those receiving chemotherapy and corticosteroids. Small, clear vesicles surrounded by erythema appear on the palpebral conjunctiva and spread to the cornea. The resulting corneal ulcer has a characteristic dendritic (tree-branching) appearance. Vesicular skin lesions can also appear on the skin of the lids and the lid margins. Pain and photophobia are common. Usually self-limiting, the disease may last 2 to 3 weeks. Therapeutic management is with idoxuridine ointment (Stoxil, IDU). Corticosteroids are contraindicated because they contribute to a longer course, possible deeper ulceration of the cornea, and systemic complications. If the ulcer is not responsive to IDU after 7 to 10 days, vidarabine (Vira-A) or trifluorothymidine is prescribed for topical administration. Newer drugs are also used, including acyclovir (Zovirax). Recurrent dendritic keratitis may be a problem.

Herpes zoster or varicella is caused by a single member of the herpesvirus group, herpesvirus varicellae (varicella zoster virus [VZV]). Varicella (chickenpox) occurs most often in childhood. Herpes zoster (shingles) occurs most frequently in older adults and in immunosuppressed persons. Herpes zoster appears to represent an activation of an endogenous infection that has persisted in latent form after an earlier attack of varicella. The VZV spreads via the dorsal root or cranial nerve ganglion. Involvement of superficial branches of the ophthalmic division of the trigeminal nerve (CN V) includes the forehead, eyelid, and eyes. The first symptom is pain in the ocular area, followed by erythema over the nerve root distribution and a fine, fluid-filled papular rash. The papules become turbid and yellow, break open, and form crusts with eventual scarring. Unilateral involvement occurs most frequently, with symptoms seldom crossing the midline.[4] In 40% of clients with ocular VZV, lesions will develop on the cornea and the cornea will eventually lose its sensation. Involvement of the inner eye also occurs, most frequently when the nasociliary branch of the trigeminal nerve is involved, which is seen as lesions on the tip of the nose. The disease process lasts 5 to 6 weeks or longer. Therapeutic management includes analgesia for the pain, topical and systemic corticosteroids to reduce the inflammatory process, antiviral agents such as acyclovir (Zovirax) to reduce viral replication, mydriatic agents to dilate the pupil and relieve pain, and topical antibiotics to combat secondary infection. Warm moist compresses are applied to the eyes to promote comfort.

Careful assessment and diagnosis of herpes zoster is important because the lesions may be similar to those of herpesvirus type 1, but the therapeutic management is quite different.

The adenoviruses are the most frequent cause of epidemic ocular disease. Several of the adenoviruses are resistant to chlorine and are spread during the swimming season. They are also spread by hands and by ophthalmic equipment such as tonometers.

Chlamydial infections. Although rare in the United States, the chlamydial infection trachoma is the leading cause of blindness in the world. It is especially prevalent in the Middle East, Africa, and South America. Trachoma affects only isolated groups in the southwestern United States. Progressing through several stages, trachoma eventually causes blindness as a result of corneal scarring. The World Health Organization advocates treatment with systemic and topical antibiotics such as tetracycline and erythromycin. It is a preventable cause of blindness, and trachoma control requires better health delivery systems, sanitation, and education of the underdeveloped populations affected.

Fungal infections. Fungal infections are on the increase in developed countries and are more prevalent in the temperate zone. Ocular fungal infections are more common in southern and southwestern parts of the United States. Fungal organisms that infect the lids, conjunctiva, and cornea include *Candida albicans, Fusarium,* and *Aspergillus* species. Fungal infections are often associated with corneal abrasions caused by branches and bushes.

No characteristic corneal lesion occurs. At first the lesion may resemble a staphylococcal infection. Therapeutic management of fungal infections includes pimaricin (Natamycin), amphotericin B (Fungizone), and miconazole. When used as topical agents, these drugs can be very irritating to the eye. Amphotericin B (Fungizone) can be nephrotoxic, causing an elevated blood urea nitrogen concentration, nausea, chills, fever, and phlebitis.

Fungal infections within the eye involving the uveal tract and retina are common in certain areas. Histoplasmosis is endemic in the Ohio River valley and eastern United States and produces a chorioretinitis resulting in decreased vision and retinal detachment.

Allergies and Irritants

Common manifestations of allergic reactions include a milky, edematous appearance of the conjunctiva (chemosis); tearing; stringy secretions; and complaints of itchiness. Although there are limitless possibilities for allergens to the eyes, grasses, pollens, and animal dander are common offenders. Antihistamines may be useful in reducing symptoms.

Contact allergies caused by topical medication such as atropine, neomycin, contact lens solutions, and broad-spectrum antibiotics produce hyperemia and irritation. Management involves removal of the offending agent. Topical corticosteroids provide relief but should not be continued over a long period of time.

Common irritants to the eye such as smoke, smog, chemicals, makeup, and silver nitrate ophthalmic drops can cause swelling of the conjunctiva, tearing, redness, and irritation. Therapeutic management includes elimination of the source. Redness and discomfort may continue for a period of time after removal of the offending agents. Cool compresses may promote comfort.

■ Nursing Management of Extraocular Problems

Careful asepsis and frequent, thorough hand washing are essential to prevent spread of organisms from one eye to the other, to other clients, and to the nurse. Specific procedures, including body substance isolation, must be carried out conscientiously. Warm compresses may be ordered. The material used for the compress should be disposed of appropriately to prevent cross-contamination.

The medication regimen may be complicated and involve the use of several eye medications at frequent intervals. Careful administration and recording of medications is essential. If eye medications are used at home, the nurse should instruct the client on their proper administration as well as on the importance of hand washing.

Clients may require eyedrops as frequently as every hour. When several eyedrops are used, administration times should be staggered. For example, if two different eyedrops are ordered hourly, one drop should be administered on the hour and one on the half-hour. This staggered schedule promotes maximum absorption.

Clients who need frequent administration of eyedrops may experience sleep deprivation. Common symptoms include short attention span, irritability, confusion, and disorientation. Grouping necessary activities together and allowing periods of rest, in addition to providing a quiet environment, may be of benefit. Clients with sleep deprivation can usually tell that they are behaving in a manner different from their baseline. This change can cause feelings of concern. Clients need reassurance that this behavior change is normal and is caused by a lack of sleep.

The nurse must assess and record changes in the eye, such as edema, redness, decreasing visual acuity, and increasing discomfort. If indicated by this assessment, analgesia may be given. Often a darkened room may increase client comfort. If vision is decreased, the nurse should attempt to provide stability in the environment.

Trauma

Although the eyes are well protected by a bony orbit and by fat pads, many sources of trauma to the eye are associated with everyday activities. In the United States, an estimated 1.3 million eye injuries occur each year. Of

Table 15-3

Prehospital Emergency Care of the Client With an Eye Injury*

Possible etiologies: Foreign bodies (e.g., glass, metal, wood), direct trauma to the eye, burns to the eye

CLINICAL MANIFESTATIONS

Extreme pain
Photophobia
Protruding foreign body
Redness, swelling
Increased flow of tears
Paralysis of eye movement
Bleeding
Double or decreased vision
Loss of sensation above eye or over cheek
Excessive nasal discharge

MANAGEMENT

Determine mechanism of injury
Do not wash injured eye except when chemical or detergent injury has occurred
Do not attempt to treat injury; cover both eyes with dry sterile eye patches
Assess for other associated injuries (especially to globe of eye)
Do not put any medicines or solutions into eye
Do not remove any blood clots or blood from eye
Apply cold compresses to forehead

*See Chapter 59 for a general discussion on measures related to prehospital emergency care.

these injuries, 40,000 result in permanent visual impairment.[5] Prehospital care of the client with an eye injury is covered in Table 15-3. Inflammation and infection are frequently occurring complications of trauma. The avascular central cornea and intraocular contents provide a supportive base for pathogens. In addition, the relatively limited access of the eye to the body's immune defenses makes infection after eye injury a serious possibility.

Entropion, the turning in of the lower lid margin, can easily traumatize the cornea by movement of the eye against the lid and lashes. It can be caused by spasm of the eyelid muscles, burns, inflammation, and loss of tissue support due to aging. The client will complain of irritation that may be accompanied by redness of the conjunctiva. Temporary management includes taping the lower lid to the face or pulling the lid away from the globe, but surgical correction is necessary.

Alteration in the Corneal Tear Film

Decrease or alteration in the tear film can cause drying or irritation of the cornea. Decreased tear formation and lack of the mucoid layer occur with aging, with arthritis, and with other connective tissue diseases.[6]

Ectropion is the turning out and sagging of the lower lid as a result of aging, injury, paralysis to the CN VII,

trauma, or burns. Tears spill out onto the cheeks, causing irritation and drying of the conjunctiva and cornea. Plastic surgery is necessary to correct the lid position.

Decreased blinking or closure of the eyelid leads to drying of the cornea. Injury to the facial nerve (CN VII) prevents closure of the eyelid on the affected side. Clients with *exophthalmos* (abnormal forward displacement of the eye usually associated with hyperthyroidism) may be unable to completely close their lids.

Therapeutic management. Management to prevent drying of the cornea is aimed at treatment of the cause. Application of topical lubricants such as methylcellulose (Ultra Tears) every 1 to 2 hours provides symptomatic relief. Lacri-Lube, a bland ointment, can be used at night or when drops cannot be applied frequently. If topical medication fails to relieve the irritation, an eye pad taped with enough pressure to keep the lid closed can be used. This can also be used during sleep. A plastic shield without holes or plastic wrap can provide increased humidity and moisture. Surgical treatment to suture the lids together (tarsorrhaphy) may be necessary to protect the cornea, especially in unconscious clients.

Nurses play an important role in observing the affected eye or eyes, noting the client's complaints, and reporting changes. Administration of eye medications at the frequency needed is especially important. If plastic tape or pressure eye pads are used, the lids must remain closed so that no further irritation of the cornea can occur. Increasing the amount of liquid consumed as well as the humidity of the environment may decrease the discomfort of the nonblinking eye. If able, the client may manually close the lid to moisten the cornea and to decrease discomfort.

Cornea

Many problems affect the cornea. More than 2 million persons in the United States experience corneal disorders each year. Corneal disease accounts for only 6% of legal blindness in the United States.[7] This percentage is probably low because most corneal problems cause severe pain, requiring the client to seek early medical treatment. Early treatment is essential for inflammations and infections of the cornea.

Keratitis. Keratitis is caused by bacterial, viral, and fungal microorganisms, as well as chemical and mechanical injuries to the epithelium of the cornea. A recent increase in the incidence of keratitis has been related to the *Acanthamoeba* organism. This problem is associated with the use of saline solution prepared from distilled water for use in contact lens care. Keratitis is painful and reduces visual acuity. Once the epithelium is denuded, the area is open to the possibility of infection. Clients with decreased resistance, vitamin A deficiency, malnutrition, diabetes, and inability to close the eyelid and those taking systemic corticosteroids are more susceptible to a variety of microorganisms. Infection of the cornea will not produce drainage because the cornea is avascular. The inflammatory reaction can extend to the iris and ciliary body, and pus or a hypopyon can form in the anterior chamber. Depending on the depth of the corneal ulcer and virulence of the disease, corneal perforation can occur with loss of eye contents if the eye is rubbed or pressure is applied. After many infections, scarring and opacities result, causing decreased visual acuity.

Diagnosis of exposure keratitis is based on the presence of redness and/or elevation of the conjunctiva in the exposed areas. When a fluorescein dye is instilled, small corneal erosions are noted.

In nonexposure forms of keratitis, the infecting agent is diagnosed from scrapings of the corneal layer, which are sent for cultures and sensitivity studies. Biomicroscopic and ophthalmoscopic examinations aid in diagnosis.

Therapeutic management includes immediate use of topical antibiotics every 1 to 2 hours. Parenteral antibiotics are administered after sensitivity studies are done. However, systemic administration of antibiotics does not reach high levels in the anterior chamber and cornea. Deep ulcerations can be treated by subconjunctival injections of antibiotic every 12 to 24 hours. Corticosteroids are not advocated systemically but are used topically to decrease the inflammatory response and scarring of the cornea. Topical anesthetics are also avoided, since they can result in further corneal damage secondary to rubbing. Eye pads may be contraindicated; organism growth is increased in dark environments. Exposure keratitis is treated by provision of adequate corneal moisture (Lacri-lube, Refresh PM). Pressure patching may be required to keep the eyelid closed.

Corneal scarring and opacities. If corneal scarring causes opacities of the cornea and decreased visual acuity, a corneal transplant *(keratoplasty)* can be performed to replace the cloudy cornea.

Keratoconus is a bilateral degenerative disease that is inherited as an autosomal recessive trait. It is associated with Down syndrome, asthma, atopic dermatitis, and retinitis pigmentosa.

The anterior cornea thins and protrudes forward, taking on a cone shape. Keratoconus appears during adolescence and is slowly progressive between the ages of 20 and 60 years. The only symptom is blurred vision caused by the

Table 15-4   Common Eye Medications for Pupil Dilatation

Drug	Action	Uses	Implications
Mydriatics and cycloplegics	Dilatation of pupil by contracting radial muscle of iris, constriction of conjunctival blood vessels	Pupil dilatation	Systemic tachycardia and ↑ BP, trembling, sweating, pallor
Sympathomimetics Phenylephrine HCl (Neo-Synephrine)	Very potent mydriatic without cycloplegic action	Adjunct of cycloplegic agents, preoperative agent	Caution necessary for clients with hypertensive cardiovascular disease
Parasympatholytics Cycloplegics	Blocking of acetylcholine and radial muscles of iris → dilatation → mydriasis; paralysis of ciliary muscle and blockage of accommodation for near vision	Treatment of inflammation (uveitis and keratitis)	Contraindicated in glaucoma, narrowing of iridocorneal angle resulting
Atropine sulfate (Atropisol, Isopto Atropine)	Most potent cycloplegic, long duration (2-4 weeks), production of mydriasis in 30 min	Examination of inner parts of eye, intraocular surgery (preoperative and postoperative use)	Side effects, including dryness of mouth; sensitivity to light; difficulty in focusing; fever, ↑ pulse, hot, flushed, dry skin (in infants, children); storage out of reach of children necessary
Scopolamine hydrobromide (Isopto Hyoscine)	Faster action than atropine, shorter duration	Inflammatory conditions of the uveal tract	Lesser response in heavily pigmented (dark brown or black) irises
Homatropine hydrobromide (Isopto Homatropine)	Shorter action than atropine and scopolamine	Preoperative agent	Noting of allergies necessary, dimming of lights for comfort
Cyclopentolate hydrochloride (Cyclogyl)		Mydriatic agent, diagnostic studies (with phenylephrine)	
Tropicamide (Mydriacyl)	Fast onset, short duration	Examination (not in inflammatory conditions)	

variable astigmatism associated with the altered corneal shape. Hard contact lenses are used to correct the refractive error as well as to decrease the pointedness of the cornea early in the process. The cornea can perforate as the thinning of the central cornea progresses. Keratoplasty is indicated prior to perforation.

Therapeutic management. Keratoplasty is indicated for clients who experience corneal degeneration and dystrophies, scarring, opacities, chemical burns, and trauma. Although corneal problems leading to blindness are not common, a corneal transplant can restore vision that otherwise would be lost. The clients may be young, including infants, and many are still in the work force when a corneal transplant is performed. Approximately 37,000 transplants were performed in 1987.[8] The success rate has increased, making corneal transplantation the most successful transplant operation.[7] A second transplant can be performed if rejection occurs. Healthy donor eyes are procured as soon as possible after death, placed in a special nutritive solution, and refrigerated until used. Tissue typing, better instruments, finer sutures, postoperative use of topical corticosteroids, and careful follow-up have decreased rejection of the donor graft.

The most commonly used corneal transplant is the penetrating keratoplasty, a technique in which the full thickness of the recipient's diseased cornea is removed and replaced with donor tissue. If a cataract is present, it can be removed at the time of the corneal transplant.

Previously the client was "on call" for a corneal transplant for days, months, or longer. Surgery was performed as soon as possible or up to 48 hours after a donor cornea was obtained unless the cornea had been cryopreserved. With newer methods of preservation and more donors, the surgery is presently usually done on an elective basis. The surgery is usually performed with the aid of local anesthesia. Besides the routine preoperative preparation for a penetrating keratoplasty, specific medications may be ordered. The client's eyes may be treated with a miotic to constrict the pupil and prevent trauma to the lens. A mydriatic (Table 15-4) may be used if the lens is to be removed because of a cataract.

The donor cornea is prepared after determination of the size required. The host's diseased cornea is removed and the donor cornea, or "button," is sutured into place. The anterior chamber is re-formed with a balanced saline solution, and the wound is sutured closed. An eye pad and a metal shield are applied to the treated eye after an antibiotic ointment is instilled. The shield is left in place until eyedrops are started. It should not be removed earlier without a specific order. The main concerns after surgery are that the corneal grafts remain intact, that rejection is minimal or recognized early, and that complications such as infection do not occur. Healing is prolonged because the cornea is avascular and the corticosteroid eyedrops used reduce the inflammatory process. The sutures remain in place 5 to 6 months or longer. Progress of the eye is monitored by biomicroscopic examination and tonometry. Topical medications are ordered accordingly. Clients are usually discharged with corticosteroids and antibiotic eyedrops. The postoperative nursing care is similar to the care

of the client after any eye surgery. The client must be kept comfortable and the incision protected from external pressure. An increase in intraocular pressure should be prevented.

INTRAOCULAR DISEASES
Cataract

Cataract formation is the development of an opacity within the lens. It may occur in both eyes, but there may be asymmetry related to the stage of involvement. It is not a "growth over the eye," as many people believe.

Significance. Opacities of the lens are the leading cause of self-declared vision impairment and the third-leading cause of preventable blindness.[9] The incidence of cataracts increases with age. Of persons 85 years of age or older, 95% have developed lens opacities. Cataracts impair the vision of approximately 3.3 million Americans.[7] Approximately 1.25 million cataract extractions are performed each year, making it the leading surgical procedure performed on Americans over 65 years of age.[9]

Etiology. The lens enlarges with age and cataracts develop as a result of alterations in the metabolism and transport of nutrients within the lens. The most common type of cataract is degenerative or related to advancing age. Degenerative cataracts develop over a period of 3 to 20 years. Among clients with age-related cataract, 10% to 15% have diabetes or blood sugar abnormalities. Clients with diabetes tend to be younger than other clients when cataracts develop. Accumulation of sorbitol from sustained high levels of glucose leads to a high osmotic gradient within the lens fibers.[10] Other etiological factors in the development of opacities of the lens are presented in Table 15-5.

Clinical manifestations. The clinical manifestations of cataracts include gradual decrease in vision, blurry vision,

Table 15-5 Etiological Factors of Cataract Formation

Degenerative (age-related)
Trauma
    Contusion
    Penetrating injury
Congenital
    Maternal rubella
    Inborn errors of metabolism
    Chromosomal defects
Radiation induced
    Environmental
    Therapeutic
Ultraviolet light
Drug induced
    Systemic corticosteroids
    Prolonged use of topical corticosteroids
    Echothiophate (miotic)
    Chlorpromazine (Thorazine)
Secondary
    Ocular infections (uveitis)

glare caused by the scattering of light by the opacities, and decreased color perception. If only one lens is involved, the client may be unaware of the changes until the unaffected eye is accidentally covered and a "sudden" loss of vision is experienced. One type of cataract (age related) in which there is rapid enlargement of the lens causes the client to become more myopic. This condition requires frequent eyeglass correction before surgery. At present, no approved treatment for cataracts other than surgical removal is available. If the cataract is not removed, the client's vision will progressively deteriorate. Secondary glaucoma can also occur if the enlarging lens causes increased intraocular pressure.

Diagnostic studies. Diagnosis is based on decreased visual acuity. Examination by ophthalmoscope and slit-lamp biomicroscope demonstrates the presence of the opacity. The fundus may become totally obscured by the opacity, creating a white pupil. Excessive enlargement of the lens can also be detected by these methods. Tonometry may indicate increased intraocular pressure caused by the enlarged lens.

Therapeutic management. Most surgery is performed when the client's decreasing vision interferes with normal activities such as driving, reading, and watching television. Occupational needs and lifestyle changes must also be considered. Extraction is usually not recommended until vision in the eye is 20/50 or worse. The goals of cataract surgery are to remove the source of visual impairment and to restore vision. Preoperative preparation is similar to the preparation of the client for corneal transplant. Since the client is usually an older adult, chronic diseases need to be assessed and controlled. Antibiotic eyedrops are frequently ordered for use the day before the surgery. Table 15-6 presents the therapeutic management of cataracts.

The pupil is dilated by mydriatic and cycloplegic medications (see Table 15-4). Some clients may require a reduction in intraocular pressure by hyperosmolar drugs. Local anesthesia is used for most cataract extractions. Almost all clients have cataract extraction done on the day of admission (same-day surgery), and do not stay in the hospital overnight unless complications occur.

Intraoperative phase. Surgical removal of the lens is an intraocular procedure. If the whole lens is removed, it is an intracapsular extraction. If the lens material is removed, leaving the posterior lens capsule in place, it is an extracapsular extraction. In the intracapsular cataract extraction, a cryoprobe freezes and adheres to the lens. With the use of α-chymotrypsin, an enzyme, the zonule fibers are softened and break as the frozen lens is removed by withdrawing the cryoprobe. A peripheral iridectomy may be performed through a V-shaped opening made at the periphery of the iris to prevent pupil block. Without the lens in the eye, the vitreous humor can block the flow of aqueous humor through the pupil and cause secondary glaucoma; however, the iridectomy allows aqueous humor to flow into the anterior chamber via this new route. The extracapsular cataract extraction procedure allows placement of certain types of intraocular lens in the posterior chamber between the iris and the remaining posterior lens capsule. A much smaller incision is made when phacoemulsifica-

Table 15-6

Diagnostic and Therapeutic Management: Cataract

DIAGNOSTIC

Measurement of visual acuity, glare testing
Ophthalmoscopy, direct and indirect
Biomicroscopy
Tonometry
Perimetry
Keratometry (measurement of curves of cornea)

THERAPEUTIC

Preoperative
  Mydriatic, cycloplegic
  Antibiotic (topical)
  Osmotic diuretics; carbonic anhydrase inhibitors
Surgery
  Removal of lens
    Intracapsular extraction
    Extracapsular extraction
    Phacoemulsification
  Correction
    Intraocular lens implant
    Epikeratophakia
    Contact lenses
    Eyeglasses
Postoperative
  Analgesia
  Mydriatic
  Corticosteroids, topical
  Antibiotic, topical
  Eye shield
  Compresses

tion is used. A special instrument inserted into the anterior chamber delivers ultrasonic vibrations and breaks up the lens content. The lens particles are then irrigated and aspirated through this same instrument.

At the end of the procedure a subconjunctival antibiotic is administered, and an antibiotic/steroid ointment is instilled. The eye is covered with a pressure patch and a protective shield to promote rapid healing of the epithelium.

Intraocular lens insertion. Intraocular lenses are tiny plastic lenses that are inserted into the anterior or posterior chamber in front of or behind the iris. They provide the least distorting optical correction. The choice of lens depends on the type of cataract extraction performed, the size of the eye, and the ophthalmologist's preference. Clients considered for an intraocular lens are usually over 50 years of age. The older person has more difficulty adjusting to the thick glasses or contact lenses required after cataract surgery. More complications occur after lens implantation. These include vitreous loss, intraocular infection, glaucoma, and postoperative inflammation. Most complications are temporary and can be treated successfully.[11] Clients with recurrent ocular diseases such as glaucoma or inflammatory disease do not do as well with an intraocular lens implant.

If clients are unable to have an intraocular lens implant and have had difficulty with corrective lenses, an epikeratophakia procedure may be performed. A frozen cornea from a donor eye is cut on a lathe to a specific dimension and applied to the anterior surface of the cornea to increase its refracting ability. Light rays can be better focused on the retina with this "living lens."

Postoperative phase. Most clients have day surgery and are discharged as soon as the effects of sedative agents have ceased. Careful verbal and written instructions must be given to the client regarding activity restrictions, medications, eye care, safety, and follow-up. The client who remains overnight in the hospital is usually out of bed with assistance on the day of surgery. At the first examination the surgeon will carefully check the anterior chamber for depth and intraocular pressure of the eyeball. A flat chamber may cause adhesions of the iris and cornea. Warm or cold compresses may be ordered to decrease the conjunctival and lid edema and to remove secretions from the lid and lashes. The eye shield must be worn during sleep for 1 month or more to prevent the client from inadvertently rubbing or bumping the eye, causing damage. The eye shield is usually removed during the day so that the client can wear glasses for serviceable vision. The lower layer of the cornea heals over in 48 hours, but it will take approximately 6 weeks for all layers of the corneal incision to heal.

■ Nursing Management Following Eye Surgery

The nursing care plan for the client after eye surgery is shown in Table 15-7.

Nursing interventions

Acute intervention. Preoperatively, the nurse must assess the client's visual acuity, especially in the untreated eye. With the treated eye patched after surgery, the client will need special consideration if sight is limited in the other eye. Clients fear eye surgery and need an opportunity to voice their fears. Postoperatively, the nurse's main concerns are the comfort and safety of the client, the avoidance of external pressure to and increased intraocular pressure within the eye, and the prevention of complications. The client usually experiences minimal pain and scratchiness of the eye. Mild analgesics are usually sufficient to relieve these problems. Cyclopegic eyedrops and compresses will also decrease the pain, as will refrigerating the eyedrops (if appropriate). If pain increases, the surgeon must be notified, since this may indicate complications of hemorrhage and/or increased intraocular pressure.

Ophthalmologists differ as to amount of postoperative activity and restrictions they advise. Avoidance of activity that increases intraocular pressure, such as squeezing the eyelids, bending over to put on slippers, and straining for lifting or defecating is usually recommended. Activities permitted include climbing steps, reading, riding in but not driving a car, walking, watching television, and performing light housekeeping tasks such as washing dishes and dusting. A laxative of the client's choice is usually allowed. Vomiting also increases intraocular pressure and

should be prevented whenever possible. The nurse must maintain a safe environment to prevent trauma to the client as a result of falling or bumping the eye. Fewer restrictions are needed when phacoemulsification is used. Many of these clients drive several days after surgery.

Rehabilitative management. Before discharge the client must be instructed in the care of the eye. Information should include activity restrictions, medications, follow-up care, complications, and self-care activities. The client's family should be included in the instruction, since many clients will be unable to administer their own medications because of poor vision. Opportunity for return demonstration of care requiring skilled techniques must be planned. Written directions and schedules are valuable teaching aids related to medication and activity restrictions.

The client's aphakic eye after surgery will require refractive error correction. If only one lens has been removed, images will be 33% larger than the vision perceived by the normal eye. Glasses reduce the difference to 20% to 25%, but the brain may not fuse to this difference. Glasses can provide good central vision but distort peripheral vision. Objects suddenly pop into view. Walls and steps appear curved and distorted, and the client will underreach for objects. The newer aspheric plastic lenses decrease some of the peripheral distortion and are lighter, but the cost is greater. A contact lens can be fitted at 1 month.

Most clients can wear an extended-wear lens for at least 7 to 14 days. The magnifying effect is reduced to 8%. If the lens becomes uncomfortable or if tearing, redness, or decreased vision develops, the ophthalmologist must be contacted. If discomfort develops, the lens should be removed and examined for coating, deposit, and damage. Abrasions, ulceration, infection, or irritation should also be reported. The wearer of an extended-wear lens should avoid swimming and irritating or noxious fumes when the lens is in place.

Retinal Tear and Detachment

Retinal detachment is a separation of the two layers of the retina, the neural retina and the underlying pigment epithelium. Once the layers are separated, fluid can enter between them, causing permanent loss of vision unless corrected surgically. Each year, 1 of every 10,000 Americans experiences a retinal detachment.[12]

Etiology. There are many causes of retinal detachment. The most common cause of separation is formation of a hole or tear in the retina. Retinal tears can be caused by vitreous traction as the vitreous humor shrinks with age. The liquid vitreous humor enters the hole and separates the retina layers. As the eye moves, more separation can occur in minutes or over a period of years. As the retina separates, the corresponding field of vision becomes distorted. This type of detachment is called a *rhegmatogenous* retinal detachment. Contributing factors of rhegmatogenous retinal detachment include the myopic and aphakic eye that has a larger posterior cavity. This causes more force to be exerted on the retina as the eye moves. Diseases such as lattice degeneration, which develops a firm vitreoretinal adhesion, cause approximately one third of tear-induced detachments. Severe diabetic retinopathy can cause shrink-

Table 15-7

 NURSING CARE PLAN FOR THE CLIENT AFTER EYE SURGERY

Defining Characteristics	Nursing Interventions	Evaluation Criteria

NURSING DIAGNOSIS: Anxiety related to actual or possible loss of vision

Anxiety and restlessness, frequent questions about outcome	Encourage verbalization. Give careful explanations of all treatments and activities. Include family in planning and teaching. Reassure client about quality of care being received.	Optimistic attitude toward positive outcome

NURSING DIAGNOSIS: High risk for fall related to poor vision, possible presence of eyepatch

Tentative, hesitant gait; groping for supports when ambulating; hitting or tripping on objects in path	Stabilize environment. Advise use of side rails. Assist with ambulation and activities of daily living.	No incidence of falls

NURSING DIAGNOSIS: Pain related to surgical manipulation of tissue and eyelid edema

Expression of pain and pressure in affected eye, withdrawal	Apply warm or cold compresses as ordered, using clean washcloth. Teach client and family to do this after thorough hand washing. Administer analgesic as ordered.	Expression of satisfaction with pain control

NURSING DIAGNOSIS: Altered health maintenance related to lack of knowledge regarding eye care complications, medications, and activity restrictions after discharge

Frequent questions about postdischarge care	Review written directions with client and family. Return demonstration on compresses, instillation of eyedrops, and eye pads. Review activity and reading restrictions.	Knowledge of complications to report, restrictions, and follow-up care

NURSING DIAGNOSIS: Potential complication: increased intraocular pressure

Blurred vision, headache, decreasing visual acuity	Instruct client to avoid activities that increase intraocular pressure, such as bending, coughing, squeezing eyelids. Reinforce need to comply with eye medication routine.	No increase in intraocular pressure

NURSING DIAGNOSIS: High risk for self-care deficit related to impaired vision and activity restrictions

Inability to perform part or all of activities of daily living	Assess current ability related to personal hygiene, dressing, mobility, eating, and toileting. Assist client with activities of daily living as needed or requested. Contact an occupational therapist if needed for adaptive equipment such as long-handled sponges or reachers.	Achievement of activities of daily living, with or without assistance

NURSING DIAGNOSIS: Impaired home maintenance related to poor vision and postsurgical activity restrictions

Expression of concern over ability to manage independently in home environment	Determine assistance client will need to maintain home environment. Assess client's functional abilities and appropriateness of preferred environment for postsurgical recovery. Assist client and family with planning for assistance after discharge. Assess client's support system.	Return to preferred environment after surgery with assistance from appropriate resources

age of the vitreous humor as a result of retinal vessel hemorrhage into it.

Traction detachments can also result when the retina is pulled away from the epithelium by fibrous tissue. Although a less common cause, trauma to the head or eye may precipitate a detachment, especially in an eye with degenerative changes. The majority of retinal tears, however, do not develop into detachments. It is difficult to determine which tears will eventually detach. Both eyes can be involved. Nonrhegmatogenous retinal detachments are caused by fluid accumulating between the choroid and retinal layers as a result of a tumor or an inflammatory disease of these layers.

Clinical manifestations and complications. A common symptom of retinal detachment is the appearance of flashing lights, lasting only a few seconds, followed by the sudden presence of many moving spots or floaters. Retinal detachment causes the release of blood cells that become suspended in the vitreous humor and can be seen by the client. Another manifestation is a visual field loss, which is often described as a curtain coming across the field of vision. The visual field loss is reversed from the area of retinal involvement. A visual field loss in the inferior temporal area is due to a detachment in the superior nasal retina. On ophthalmoscopy, the retina appears pale, translucent, in folds, and tremulous as the eye moves.

Retinal detachment can result in the loss of vision in the area of detachment. If the detachment involves the macular area, permanent loss of central vision occurs and affects the client's ability to read, write, do close work, and see faces. However, some peripheral vision can be restored if treated early.

Therapeutic management. Direct and indirect ophthalmoscopy is used to identify the site of the tear or detachment (Table 15-8). Once the problem is diagnosed, the client will usually be referred to an ophthalmologist who specializes in retinal surgery. The client may need to be transported with the head down and/or with the eyes bilaterally patched to avoid further detachment. The principles of treatment include sealing the hole by creation of an inflammatory reaction that will cause a chorioretinal adhesion or scar and approximation of the detached retina against the underlying layer.

Photocoagulation is the use of an intense, precisely focused light beam, such as the argon laser or a xenon light, to create an inflammatory reaction. The light is directed at the area of the retinal hole or tear, producing a scar to seal edges of the tear and preventing fluid from collecting in the subretinal space and causing a detachment. Photocoagulation is used when there is only a small tear with little or no detachment. It is usually performed on an outpatient basis. After the treatment the client will experience marked blurring of vision because of the flashing bright lights, but vision should return to the previous level within 12 hours.

Cryopexy or *diathermy* is the application of extreme cold or heat to create an inflammatory reaction and produce a scar similar to that produced by the laser. A cryoprobe or diathermy instrument is applied to the external globe over the tear. Cryotherapy is used more frequently

Table 15-8

Diagnostic and Therapeutic Management: Detached Retina

DIAGNOSTIC

Measurement of visual acuity
Ophthalmoscopy, direct and indirect
Biomicroscopy
Ultrasound

THERAPEUTIC

Eye pads (as ordered)
Positioning of client with retinal hole area lowermost
Photocoagulation
Surgery
    Cryotherapy (cryoretinopexy) ⎫ Stimulation of
    Diathermy   ⎭ scar
    Silicone explant   ⎫
    Encircling procedure fascia, ⎪ Approximation of retinal
       silicone   ⎬ layers against choroid
    Release of subretinal fluid ⎪
    Intraocular air/gas   ⎭
Postoperative
    Analgesia
    Positioning (as ordered)
    Eye pads
    Mydriatics
    Antiinflammatory, antiinfective agents
    Compresses

today because less tissue reaction occurs. It is often performed on an outpatient basis with the aid of local anesthesia. Approximation of the detached retina can also be accomplished by indenting the eyeball, causing the pigment epithelium, choroid, and sclera to move toward the detached retina. This is accomplished by a surgical procedure. A silicone explant can be sutured against the sclera for localized detachments. A scleral buckling procedure, in which an encircling band is used to keep the choroid in contact with the retina to promote attachment, can also be used (Fig. 15-3). Materials used are silicone, Teflon, or fascia from the client or from a cadaver. Folds and wrinkles in the retina are repaired to facilitate reattachment. A large accumulation of fluid between the retinal layers is released by insertion of a needle and performance of a subretinal tap to facilitate approximation of the retinal layers. New techniques use oil or gas with a specific gravity less than that of the vitreous to enhance attachment.[13] These agents float up against the repaired hole or tear, holding it in place. General anesthesia is usually used.

Surgery is 90% successful. Additional procedures may be necessary for some clients. Retinal detachment can involve one or both eyes. Other areas of detachment can occur later. The treated eye may not regain maximum vision for 3 months.

Preoperatively, the client is often kept on bed rest and restricted position, occasionally with bilateral eye pads.

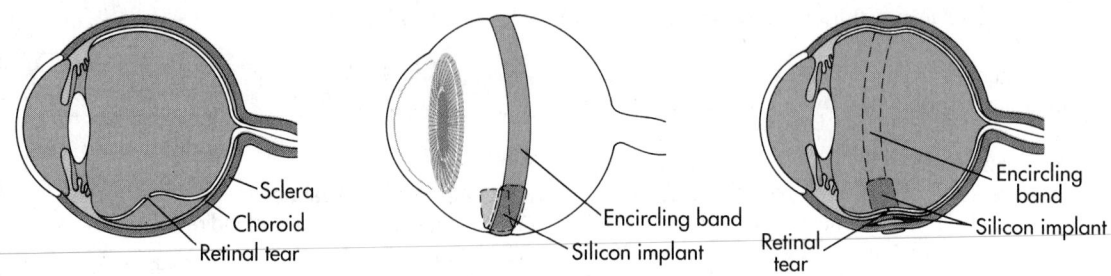

Labels: Sclera, Choroid, Retinal tear; Encircling band, Silicon implant; Retinal tear, Encircling band, Silicon implant

Fig. 15-3   Retinal detachment: examples of surgical repair.

The rationale for positioning a client with a retinal detachment preoperatively or immediately postoperatively is to keep the retinal tear lowermost (dependent position) within the eye, allowing the retina to fall back against the pigment epithelium. Preoperatively, this position is used to prevent further detachment, especially if the macular area is endangered. Bilateral patches may be used to reduce quick eye movements that could cause further detachment. Most ophthalmologists patch only the operative eye.

Postoperatively, the client may be kept on bed rest for a day or may be up and about, depending on the position of the repair and the surgeon's preference. A position with the detachment area lowermost may be indicated to assist in approximation of the two layers, allowing the adhesion scar to form. Clients can be assisted to assume the head-down position when lying in bed or sitting up with the head turned to the side and placed on an overbed table.

When oil or gas is used, the client is positioned to allow the bubble to float up next to the detachment. Care must be taken to prevent these agents from coming in contact with the lens. Mydriatics, analgesics, and compresses are ordered. The conjunctiva and lids are red and swollen.

■ Nursing Management of Retinal Detachment
Nursing interventions
Acute intervention. Since retinal detachment is an emergency situation, the client is often extremely anxious. Emotional needs and fear of blindness must not be overlooked as preparations for surgery progress. Information regarding past experience with retinal surgery is helpful in planning care. Specific nursing interventions are similar to the postoperative nursing care for the client undergoing any type of eye surgery and are discussed in Table 15-7.

The client is usually hospitalized for 1 to 2 days after surgical repair. Ambulation is permitted on the first day. Discharge planning should be started as soon as possible to allow supervised practice of eyedrop instillation and compress application.

Rehabilitation. Reading, writing, close work, and watching television may be restricted in the immediate postoperative period, since the rapid eye movements associated with these activities may cause further detachment. An eye pad is worn for comfort as needed. Some clients may be restricted from certain activities, such as combing or shampooing hair and shaving. Before discharge, the client must be able to identify the signs of retinal detachment and the action to take if it occurs again. The client is seen

by the ophthalmologist every few days for the first several weeks after surgery.

Diabetic Retinopathy

Diabetic retinopathy is a complication of diabetes mellitus that affects the ocular arterioles and capillaries. It is the leading cause of legal blindness among adults between the ages of 20 and 74.[14]

Most diabetic clients develop some retinopathy over 10 to 15 years. Control of diabetes does not appear to affect the course of retinal disease. Rather, the occurrence of diabetic retinopathy seems to be correlated with the duration of the diabetes; the longer the person has had diabetes, the more likely the presence of retinopathy is.

The two types of vessel changes are background and proliferative retinopathy. The *background* type causes dilatation and microaneurysms of the retinal vessels, which can allow fluid and fatty deposits to leak into the retina. Dot-shaped hemorrhages in the retinal layers may be noted. Fluid can collect in the macular area, causing blurring and distortion of central vision. *Proliferative retinopathy* involves the formation of many new vessels (neovascularization) on the surface of the retina and optic nerve; these vessels are weak and bleed into the vitreous humor.

As the disease progresses, capillaries can gradually become occluded, decreasing blood supply to the retina. Retinal hypoxia occurs. In response to the ischemia, the body develops new blood vessel networks. The development of these new vessels, usually on the optic nerve and surface of the retina, indicates advancement of the retinopathy to the proliferative state. These new fragile blood vessels bleed easily into the vitreous. The bloodstained vitreous humor develops adhesions and contracts, causing tears and detachments of the retina. Visual acuity decreases as the bloodstained vitreous makes light transmission to the retina difficult. Severe loss of sight is possible. Blindness may even result.

Diagnostic studies. The changes in vessels are visible on ophthalmoscopic examination unless the vitreous humor is opaque. Fluorescein angiography readily identifies the vascular changes in the subretinal and retinal areas by leakage of dye. Ultrasonography helps identify detached retinal areas, especially if the vitreous humor is opaque. Electroretinography is used to elicit retinal response by use of a very bright light transmitted through the opaque vitreous humor. Examination by an ophthalmologist at regular intervals is critical.

Table 15-9

Diagnostic and Therapeutic Management: Diabetic Retinopathy

DIAGNOSTIC

Measurement of visual acuity
Ophthalmoscopy
Biomicroscopy
Tonometry
Fluorescein angiography
Ultrasonography
Electroretinopathy (ERG)

THERAPEUTIC

Photocoagulation
Surgery
   Vitrectomy
   Repair of retinal detachment*

*See Table 15-8.

Therapeutic management. Until recently, little could be done to treat diabetic retinopathy. Currently, photocoagulation is used early in the disease process (Table 15-9). If bleeding into the vitreous humor occurs, a vitrectomy can be performed.

Photocoagulation with the argon laser is used to coagulate the microaneurysms and new growth of vessels in and on the retina. This procedure may require several treatments. Photocoagulation may prevent severe bleeding within the eye. Simply destroying the newly formed vessels does not eliminate the underlying hypoxic state. Other treatments are necessary to prevent their recurrence. In panretinal photocoagulation (PRP), scattered laser burns are placed in the periphery of the retina to destroy the tissue. Oxygen requirement of the retina is reduced, and the stimulus for new blood vessel growth is eliminated. Some loss of peripheral and night vision occurs, but central vision and color vision are spared.[15]

Since 1970, surgery involving removal of the vitreous humor by entering the posterior cavity of the eye (vitrectomy) has been developed. *Vitrectomy* has provided a means of removing the bloodstained vitreous humor and allows restoration of vision in clients who previously had no hope of visual improvement. It is performed when the body is unable to absorb the blood from the vitreous. The vision of the client who has had a vitrectomy will not clear immediately and may be poorer for a short time after surgery than it was preoperatively. It may take up to 6 months for vision to reach its maximum.

Further bleeding of the vessels during surgery is a complication of a vitrectomy. If bleeding occurs after surgery, the blood is no longer trapped in the vitreous humor to block vision but will be absorbed over a period of a week or more. Secondary glaucoma can occur as a result of bleeding. Severe infection within the eye (endophthalmitis) can occur and requires immediate treatment.

Approximately 75% of the clients who undergo vitrec-

tomy experience improved vision. These procedures treat only the manifestations of diabetic retinopathy. They do not halt either the disease or the progress of the retinopathy.

▪ Nursing Management of Diabetic Retinopathy

Preoperatively, the client should understand the purpose of the planned surgery and the expected results. The diabetes should be well controlled. Postoperatively, antibiotics are injected subconjunctivally, and an eye patch and shield are applied. Vital signs are monitored closely because an elevation of blood pressure may cause hemorrhage within the eye. Increased or sharp pain in the eye is significant and must be reported. Sleeping with the head of the bed elevated can decrease pressure in the retinal capillaries. The client should be instructed not to bend over or to engage in activities that increase intraocular pressure. The client's understanding of diabetes should be assessed during the hospitalization. A teaching plan is initiated in areas where a knowledge deficit regarding diabetes and health care of the eye has been identified.

Intraocular Hemorrhage

Retinal hemorrhage. Arteries or arterioles are present throughout the retina and choroid in addition to those that are visible on the surface of the retina on ophthalmoscopic examination. Bleeding from any of these vessels can occur in the choroid, between the choroid and the pigment epithelium of the retina, in the subretinal layers, and on the surface of the retina. These hemorrhages may be small to large, staining a large area of tissue. Fluorescein angiography is used to determine the source of bleeding.

Vitreous hemorrhage. Vitreous hemorrhage may vary from a small number of red blood cells within the vitreous humor (floaters) to a mass of blood within the vitreous gel that blocks perception of light. The blood is usually from the superficial vessels of the retina.

The cause of the hemorrhage includes changes within the arterial walls due to hypertension, arteriosclerosis, and diabetes. Blood disorders such as leukemia can also cause bleeding of the retinal and choroidal vessels. Vitreous hemorrhage is often caused by traction on the retina by vitreous contraction and changes due to diabetes.

Treatment depends on the cause. Photocoagulation can be used to stop bleeding vessels early in the disease process.

Anterior chamber hemorrhage. Anterior chamber hemorrhage *(hyphema)* can occur as a result of direct or indirect trauma to the eye or, rarely, iridocyclitis (inflammation of the iris and the ciliary body) associated with rheumatoid arthritis, especially in young persons. The blood is visible in the anterior chamber. Since the blood has a viscosity greater than that of aqueous humor, it will settle to the lower portion of the anterior chamber. If the hemorrhage is the result of trauma, the client's eye will need to be immobilized with bed rest and eye patches until the bleeding stops. Clients are usually hospitalized, since rebleeding may occur up to several days later. Hemolyzation of the blood occurs. If the hemolyzed blood obstructs the trabecular meshwork, intraocular pressure may rise.

Glaucoma

Glaucoma comprises a number of problems within the eye that are characterized by increased intraocular pressure. Increased intraocular pressure initially causes damage to the optic disc and nerve cells of the retina. At this point the client has no signs or symptoms. If not recognized and treated, glaucoma causes blindness that could have been prevented in most clients.

Significance. Glaucoma is the second-leading cause of permanent blindness in America and the leading cause of blindness among black Americans. At least 2 million persons have glaucoma, and of these, more than 50% are unaware that they have the disease.[16]

Pathophysiology. Although the visual problem of glaucoma occurs in the optic disc and retina of the eye, the mechanism that causes increased intraocular pressure is in the anterior part of the eye. The ciliary body secretes approximately 4 to 5 ml of aqueous humor a day. This bathes the lens with nutrients and then flows through the pupil into the anterior chamber, where it bathes the corneal endothelium. Aqueous humor exits the eye through the trabecular meshwork and the canal of Schlemm in the iridocorneal angle of the anterior chamber (see Fig. 14-3). This outflow of aqueous humor can be decreased by several mechanisms.

Primary open-angle glaucoma (chronic simple glaucoma) is the most common form of glaucoma. It is hereditary and involves degenerative changes in the trabecular meshwork or aqueous outflow. Commonly, the aqueous outflow is constantly subnormal and tends to worsen over time. In other cases the adequacy of outflow may be normal but is accompanied by excessive production of aqueous humor. Because the aqueous humor cannot leave the eye at the same rate at which it is produced, it remains in the eye and increases the pressure. The increased pressure affects the sensitive nerve tissue of the optic disc, causing ischemia. As ischemia of the optic nerve tissue occurs, peripheral vision is lost. Vision loss can progress toward blindness if the intraocular pressure is not controlled.

Primary angle-closure glaucoma (acute glaucoma) is caused by blockage of the trabecular meshwork. Although rare, it occurs suddenly and constitutes an emergency. In this condition the iris is pushed forward, blocking the outflow channels, thus increasing pressure. This may be precipitated by several conditions: (1) The lens blocks the flow of aqueous humor into the anterior chamber, and increased pressure quickly builds up in the posterior part of the eye, causing the iris to fall forward and block outflow channels and (2) narrowing of the peripheral angle of the anterior chamber occurs secondary to aging. Dilatation of the pupil pushes the iris forward and blocks the outflow mechanism. Dilatation of the pupil can be caused by a mydriatic drug, excitement, or darkness. Mydriatic ophthalmic medications should *not* be given to a person with a narrow anterior chamber angle.

Secondary glaucoma is caused by other ocular diseases that block the outflow channels, cause a narrow angle, or increase the volume of fluid within the eye. Increased cells produced by hemorrhage in the eye, inflammatory processes such as uveitis, and trauma can block the outflow channels. Poor wound healing after cataract surgery with aqueous loss can cause a flat anterior chamber. Tumors within the eye increase the volume, and intraocular pressure rises.

Clinical manifestations and complications. Primary open-angle glaucoma develops slowly and without symptoms. The gradual visual field defects are usually not identified by the client until much peripheral vision is lost. Vague signs may include experiencing brow area headaches, seeing halos around bright lights, and needing frequent changes of glasses in the client over 40 years of age.

Acute angle-closure glaucoma causes definite symptoms, including sudden, excruciating pain about the eyes and/or headache. Associated nausea, vomiting, and abdominal pain may cause the clinician to suspect an abdominal problem. Colored halos about lights and sudden blurred vision with decreased light perception are other symptoms. The eye may be reddened, and the cornea may be steamy in appearance.

Manifestations of subacute or chronic angle-closure glaucoma appear gradually and include transient blurred vision, halos around lights, and slight pain about the eyes. Manifestations of secondary glaucoma include increasing pain, increased intraocular pressure, and other specific symptoms depending on the causative ocular disease.

Depending on the type of glaucoma, the result is decreased visual fields due to the pressure and resultant ischemia of the nervous tissue. If not treated, blindness can occur.

Diagnostic studies. Intraocular pressure as measured by tonometry is elevated in glaucoma. The normal intraocular pressure is 10 to 21 mm Hg. If the client has an elevated reading, several readings need to be taken over a period of time and at various times of the day to determine a pattern. In open-angle glaucoma, the tonometry reading is between 22 and 32 mm Hg. In acute angle-closure glaucoma, the tonometry reading may be 50 mm Hg or higher. Biomicroscopic examination demonstrates a normal angle for open-angle glaucoma. In angle-closure glaucoma, a markedly narrow or flat anterior chamber angle, an edematous cornea, a fixed and moderately dilated pupil, and ciliary injection may be noted. Gonioscopic examination reveals specifics of the iridocorneal angle. The visual fields initially show a small, football-shaped defect gradually progressing to a nasal and superior field defect in chronic open-angle glaucoma. In acute angle-closure glaucoma the visual fields may be markedly decreased. Central vision may be 20/20 OU in both eyes. As the glaucoma progresses, the optic disc becomes wider, deeper, and paler (light gray or white). This finding, called *cupping,* may be one of the first signs of chronic open-angle glaucoma. Photographs taken of the optic disc for comparison over time demonstrate an increase in the cup-to-disc ratio and progressive blanching. On examination, secondary glaucoma reveals causative factors such as inflammation, tumor, and hemorrhage.

Therapeutic management

Chronic open-angle glaucoma. Initially, the treatment of chronic open-angle glaucoma is pharmacological (Table 15-10). Surgery is performed if control of intraocular pressure cannot be achieved. Miotic medications that increase the outflow of aqueous humor and constrict the pupil are

Table 15-10 Common Medications Used for Glaucoma

Types/Drug	Mechanisms of Action	Indications for Use and Side Effects
MIOTICS		
Cholinergic action (parasympathomimetics)	Direct acting, lowering of intraocular pressure, induction of contraction of iris sphincter muscle leading to pupil constriction, dilatation of vessels where aqueous humor leaves eye, increase in outflow of aqueous humor	Toxicity, causing headache, salivation, sweating, nausea and vomiting, diarrhea, bronchial spasm; 6 months to develop
Carbachol (Isoptocarbachol)	Longer duration of action than pilocarpine	Open-angle or angle-closure glaucoma
Pilocarpine (Isopto Carpine, Pilocar)	Safest and most widely used miotic; induction of miosis in 15 min, with maximum effect in 30-60 min; induction of spasms of accommodation with fixation of lens for near vision for 2 hr	Decrease in visual acuity; administration 3-4 times daily necessary; stinging on administration; resistance to action possible; titrating of dosage to client necessary; brow ache and myopia common; used in Ocusert-reservoir placed in upper or lower conjunctival cul-de-sac for continuous delivery; available as gel for night use
Anticholinesterase agents	Indirect acting, inhibition of destruction of acetylcholine, promotion of iris sphincter actions of constricting pupil and allowing ciliary muscle to be in spasm	Side effects of headache, eye pain, blurred vision, dilated vessels of conjunctiva
Physostigmine (Eserine)	Moderate action, reversal of atropine mydriasis	Aging changes, including oxidation and turning pink or brown, indicating need for discarding Open-angle glaucoma, conjunctivitis, allergic reaction possible
Echothiophate iodide (Phospholine Iodide)	Slow onset of action	Open-angle glaucoma, aphakic glaucoma, and congenital glaucoma; loss of potency at room temperature; refrigerator storage
ADRENERGIC AGENTS		
Sympathomimetics, mydriatics	↓ Formation of aqueous and ↑ outflow, leading to ↓ intraocular pressure (IOP), constriction of conjunctival blood vessels	Wide-angle glaucoma, glaucoma secondary to uveitis; precipitator of attack of acute glaucoma possible; local reactions of hyperemia, corneal edema, allergic reaction, brow ache; stinging on administration; systemic tachycardia and ↑ BP; staining of soft contact lenses
Epinephrine (Epifrin, Glaucon, Epitrate, Epinal, Eppy)		
Dipivefrin (Propine)	Conversion to epinephrine on entering the eye	Less frequent administration, used with other antiglaucoma drugs, fewer systemic side effects
β-Adrenergic receptor blocking agent (nonspecific) Timolol maleate (Timoptic) Levobunolol (Betagan) Betaxolol (Betoptic)	Reduction of IOP by unknown mechanisms	Used with caution in clients with history of cardiac or pulmonary disease; used with miotics and carbonic anhydrase inhibitors, if necessary; slowing of pulse rate possible; additive effect with systemic β-blocking agents (e.g., propranolol [Inderal], metoprolol [Lopressor]); long duration; given once or twice daily; no significant effect on heart rate
Carbonic anhydrase inhibitors Methazolamide (Neptazane) Acetazolamide (Diamox)	Slowing of production of aqueous humor by inhibiting carbonic anhydrase	Potassium depletion possible; side effects of lethargy, anorexia, numbness and tingling of face and extremities Monitoring of electrolytes necessary Contraindicated in Addison's disease and adrenal insufficiency

Table 15-11

Diagnostic and Therapeutic Management: Glaucoma

DIAGNOSTIC

Visual acuity
Tonometry
Biomicroscopy
Ophthalmoscopy
Perimetry
Gonioscopy
Fundus photographs

THERAPEUTIC

Chronic open-angle
  Cholinergic agents (miotics), topical
  Adrenergic agent (epinephrine, Propine), topical
  Carbonic anhydrase inhibitors
  β-Adrenergic blocker, topical
  Surgery
    Argon laser trabeculoplasty
    Filtering procedures
      Trabeculectomy
      Other (sclerectomy, thermal sclerotomy)
    Reduction of aqueous production by cyclotherapy
      Cyclocryotherapy
      Cyclodiathermy
  Avoidance of corticosteroids, topical, systemic
Acute angle-closure
  Cholinergic, topical (pilocarpine)
  Hyperosmotic agents, PO or IV
  Analgesia—narcotic
  Surgery (for ophthalmic emergency)
  Laser (peripheral iridotomy)

used. A carbonic anhydrase inhibitor and a β-adrenergic blocking agent may also be used to reduce the secretion of aqueous humor. The diagnostic and therapeutic management of glaucoma is shown in Table 15-11.

If pharmacological control of intraocular pressure is not successful, a laser trabeculoplasty is performed with the aid of local anesthesia, often on an outpatient basis. Approximately 50 to 100 laser "spots" are evenly spaced around the trabecular meshwork. After the laser procedure, scarring develops and places tension on the trabecular meshwork, pulling open the drainage channels. The pressure drops over time; topical corticosteroids are used to reduce intraocular inflammation. Medications used to lower intraocular pressure should be continued until the client is seen in 1 week by the surgeon. Further follow-up is necessary to determine the need for continuation of medications. Approximately 50% to 75% of clients show improvement.[17] If this procedure does not lower pressure, a filtering procedure to create a bypass of the trabecular meshwork and the canal of Schlemm is performed. Currently, the trabeculectomy procedure is used. A channel is made by an incision into the conjunctiva and sclera for the creation of a scleral flap and removal of part of the iris and trabecular meshwork. The scleral flap is closed loosely, but the conjunctival incision is tightly sutured. Aqueous humor drains under the conjunctiva, where it is absorbed into the systemic circulation.

Success rate with these procedures is 70% to 80%.[18] If the filtering procedure is not effective, cyclocryotherapy is used. A cryoprobe is touched to the sclera external to the ciliary body, freezing parts of the ciliary body. Freezing causes local destruction of the ciliary tissue and decreased production of aqueous humor. The procedure may be repeated. It can also be used in the treatment of acute glaucoma.

A second type of operation for the treatment of glaucoma is a shunting procedure. This involves the surgical placement of a small tube and reservoir to shunt aqueous humor from the anterior chamber to the implanted reservoir. A bubble of aqueous humor develops over the reservoir and is absorbed into the systemic circulation, thus bypassing the scarred or obstructed trabecular meshwork. Intraocular pressure is therefore reduced. Positioning the reservoir posteriorly allows the surgeon to use tissue not damaged from previous filtering surgery, thus decreasing the chance for scar tissue formation. Complications include ocular hypotony due to rapid reduction in intraocular pressure, hyphema, blockage of the shunt, excessive scar tissue formation, and the progression of cataracts.

Acute angle-closure glaucoma. Acute angle-closure glaucoma is an ocular emergency that requires immediate interventions to lower intraocular pressure by administration of miotics and oral glycerin (glycerol) medications. If this treatment is not successful, intravenous (IV) mannitol is used. Meperidine or another narcotic is given for relief of severe pain. If the pressure has not been reduced, an emergency outpatient procedure is done. A peripheral laser iridotomy is performed, allowing the aqueous humor to flow through a newly created opening in the iris and into normal outflow channels. This same procedure may be performed on the other eye as a precaution, since a large number of clients have an acute attack in the other eye.

The surgical procedure of peripheral iridectomy may be indicated if the peripheral laser iridotomy is not effective. These procedures are considered curative for acute angle-closure glaucoma.

Secondary glaucoma. Secondary glaucoma is managed by treatment of the underlying problem and by use of antiglaucoma drugs. If treatment fails, glaucoma can progress to absolute glaucoma, resulting in a hard, sightless, and usually painful eye requiring *enucleation* (surgical removal of the eye).

Pharmacological management. One of the most common miotics used is pilocarpine 1% to 4%. Carbachol may be used if pilocarpine is not effective. Epinephrine, 0.5% to 2%, or Propine, 0.1%, instilled 1 to 2 times a day, decreases formation of aqueous humor and increases aqueous humor outflow. This drug may be prescribed by some ophthalmologists before a miotic medication. A carbonic anhydrase inhibitor such as acetazolamide (Diamox) may be used to reduce production of aqueous humor and maintain a low intraocular pressure.

One of the newer drug groups for the treatment of glaucoma consists of the β-adrenergic blocking agents. Timolol maleate (Timoptic) reduces aqueous humor secretions without pupil constriction. It is a nonspecific β-blocking agent that can affect the $β_1$ and $β_2$ receptors in the heart and lungs. Nonspecific β-blockers must be used with caution for clients with known pulmonary or cardiac problems. Betaxotol (Betoptic) is a cardioselective β-blocker that does not affect heart rate and causes milder pulmonary effects.[19] It can be used in combination with other β-adrenergic blocking agents. The client requires continued supervision, since these drugs control but do not cure glaucoma. With maintenance of normal intraocular pressures, the optic nerve theoretically receives a better blood supply and oxygen.

Corticosteroids may be used postoperatively with the filtering or shunting procedure to delay scar tissue formation associated with wound healing and to keep the fistula open. A possible side effect of corticosteroids is increased intraocular pressure and prolonged wound healing, which contributes to the formation of wound leaks.

■ Nursing Management of Glaucoma

Acute open-angle glaucoma

Nursing intervention for the client with acute primary open-angle glaucoma involves education and support, as well as preoperative and postoperative care. The procedure to be performed should be explained to the client. Appropriate medications should be administered and recorded. Time should be allowed for the client to verbalize fears and for the nurse to clarify information before surgery. The client's fear of blindness should be recognized by the nurse.

Postoperatively, meticulous attention to accurate administration of eye medication is critical. The operative eye may be receiving a mydriatic, an antibiotic, and corticosteroids. The untreated eye may be receiving a miotic and a β-blocking agent. An error in drug administration could result in serious consequences.

Planning for discharge must be very specific in terms of medications, their purpose and frequency, and the eye in which each medication is to be used. Vague symptoms indicating increased intraocular pressure, such as aching around the eye and change in vision, should be reported and follow-up care sought. Compliance with medication for chronic conditions is known to be as low as 50%. Therefore every effort must be made to make sure the client continues to take antiglaucoma medications. Often the side effects may be the reason for noncompliance. A client with open-angle glaucoma must always take medication.

Clients must be encouraged to regard eyedrops as a sight-saving measure. Adjusting the administration time of medications to a format compatible with the client's lifestyle will decrease side effects and improve adherence to the prescribed regimen. The nurse must stress the need for supervised follow-up care.

Acute angle-closure glaucoma

Because of the suddenness of symptoms and the presence of pain and nausea, the client with acute angle-closure glaucoma is usually very frightened. Every effort should be made to reduce stress and to provide a quiet, dark environment. The need for frequent administration of pilocarpine drops and tonometry readings should be explained. Administration of osmotic diuretics requires accurate intake and output records and monitoring of the cardiovascular system. Nausea is a frequent side effect of oral osmotic agents. Administering them over crushed ice or with lemon juice may decrease the associated nausea. Since laser treatment or surgery is usually necessary, preparations should be explained to the client and significant others. Postoperatively, the client should experience relief of the severe pain. Plans for similar surgery in the other eye are usually made. Preparation for use of postoperative eye medications at home should be included. This client will not usually need antiglaucoma medications, but the need for follow-up care should be stressed.

Macular Degeneration

Age-related macular degeneration (AMD) is the most common cause of legal blindness in Americans over 60 years of age. Its prevalence increases with age, affecting 28% of persons between the ages of 75 and 85.[20] Other associations include race (usually white), sex (slight female preponderance), positive family history, and a history of cigarette smoking. Capillaries are responsible for providing nourishment to the macula sclerose. Without an adequate blood supply, cells responsible for vision wear out and central vision is reduced. The client experiences blurry vision, which may partially resolve, only to occur again.

Clients with *exudative macular degeneration,* the more severe form that accounts for approximately 90% of legal blindness due to AMD, notice a sudden decrease in central visual acuity.[20] The underlying layers of the retina detach, allowing the ingrowth of blood vessels (neovascularization) into the macular area. Typically, these blood vessels create a blistered macular appearance. Laser photocoagulation may decrease the bleeding and slow the process if neovascularization is present. The client eventually loses central vision of the affected eye, but peripheral vision remains. Even when the condition is successfully treated, subretinal neovascular membranes can recur at new sites in the same eye or the other eye. Mobility without assistance is usually possible, but the client is unable to read, drive, or recognize faces and details. This results in a very frustrating handicap. Once both foveae have been damaged, the only helpful measures are low-vision aids and magnifiers.

Intraocular Inflammation

Uveitis includes a variety of diseases that affect part or all of the uveal layer and the adjacent retina. Besides microorganisms, the uveal tract is affected by collagen diseases, such as arthritis (with accompanying iritis and sclerouveitis), and autoimmune reactions, such as sympathetic uveitis. Pain and photophobia are common symptoms. Therapeutic management is determined by the causative agent and the tissue affected and often involves extended treatment.

Endophthalmitis is an extensive intraocular infection involving the posterior cavity or the anterior parts of the eye. Although rare, it can be a devastating complication of intraocular surgery and penetrating eye injuries. Causative organisms include fungi and gram-positive and gram-negative bacteria with an increasing incidence of the latter group of organisms. Manifestations include ocular pain, photophobia, decreased visual acuity, headaches, upper lid edema, reddened and swollen conjunctiva, and corneal edema.

Panophthalmitis is an extension of the infectious process to the extraocular muscles and the orbit. There are pain on movement of the eye and involvement of the trigeminal nerve (CN V), which can cause exquisite but diffuse pain when certain activities such as combing the hair are performed. Therapeutic management includes appropriate antibiotics given systemically, subconjunctivally, and/or intravitreally (into the vitreous humor). Corticosteroids may be given to decrease the inflammatory reaction and the destruction of tissue. If the infection is not controlled, enucleation may be necessary.

Clients with intraocular inflammation are noticeably anxious and frightened. They fear sudden and total loss of vision as well as the inability to regain their eyesight. The provision of accurate information and support is an important role for the nurse.

Enucleation

Enucleation is the removal of the eye as a result of injury, infection, absolute glaucoma, pain, sympathetic ophthalmia, and malignancy of the eye. Fewer enucleations are being done for malignancy of the eye because of current management with cryotherapy, radiation, and chemotherapy. Surgery includes severing the extraocular muscles close to the globe. A round implant is inserted to provide shape. The conjunctiva is closed over the implant. The resultant area has an appearance similar to that of the oral mucosa. The sutured muscles over the globe provide some movement to the prosthesis and help fill the cavity. A plastic shell or conformer is placed over the tissue until the prosthesis is fitted. A pressure dressing is applied for at least 24 hours.

Postoperative nursing observations that indicate development of complications include excessive bleeding on the dressing, increased pain, and temperature elevation. Instruction in care of the orbit includes instillation of topical antibiotics and ointment or drops and cleansing of the wound.

In approximately 1 month the prosthesis is designed by an ocularist to closely resemble the remaining eye. The client is taught how to remove, cleanse, and insert the prosthesis. Special polishing is periodically required to remove dried protein secretions. The nurse may need to remove the prosthesis when the client is unconscious or unable to do it. The procedure is as follows: After thorough hand washing, the lower lid is pulled down and toward the cheekbone. The prosthesis will usually slip out. A special small suction tip can also be used (Fig. 15-4). The prosthesis is cleaned with a mild soap and rinsed well. It is stored in a container lined with a soft cloth or 4 × 4 inch bandage to prevent scratches and damages. The container should be labeled with the client's name. For reinsertion of the prosthesis, the upper lid is opened by pressure on the upper bony orbit, the top of the prosthesis (usually marked) is placed under the upper lid, and the lower lid is pulled down. The lower edge of the prosthesis slips under the lid with a little pressure on the prosthesis (Fig. 15-5).

Blindness

Blindness does not necessarily imply total inability to see (Table 15-12). Many persons who are classified as legally blind have light perception and some limited acuity. Those persons who are legally blind are eligible for federal and state assistance, income tax exemptions, and state service programs for rehabilitation. Another group, defined as *visually impaired,* includes those with monocular vision and some who cannot read newsprint but have better than 20/200 OU vision. This group also qualifies for some state assistance.

Incidence and etiology. In the United States, it is estimated that 10 million persons are visually impaired, of whom 1.5 million have extreme vision loss to the point of being unable to read newsprint.

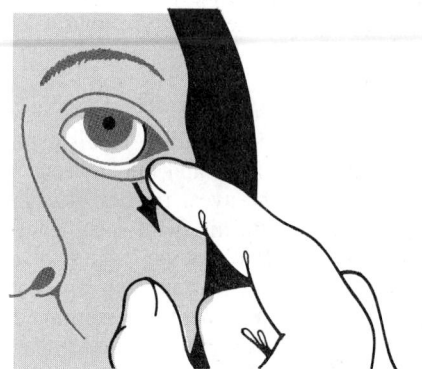
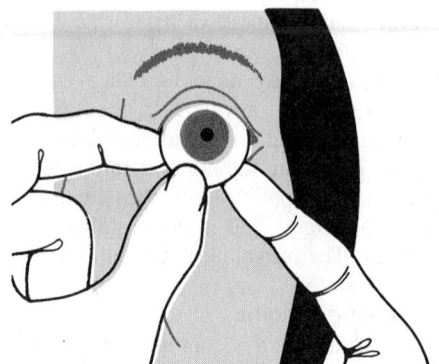

Fig. 15-4 Removal of ocular prosthesis.

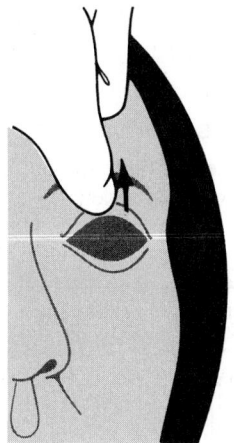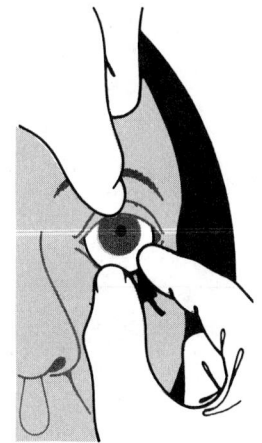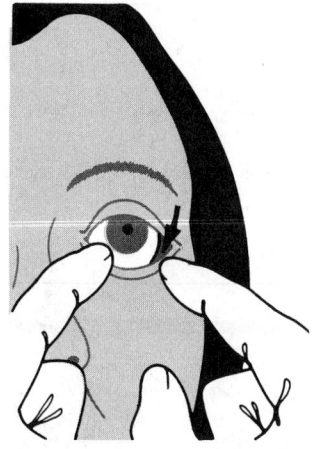

Fig. 15-5 Insertion of ocular prosthesis.

Table 15-12 Definition of Legal Blindness in the United States

Persons who have a central visual acuity for distance of 20/200 or poorer in the better eye with correction; or a visual acuity of better than 20/200, but with a field of vision no greater than 20 degrees in its widest diameter

From Operational Research Department, National Society to Prevent Blindness: Data analysis, vision problems in the U.S., 1980, p 3.

■ Nursing Management of Blindness

Acute intervention

Emotional support of the client depends on the time frame associated with the blindness. Sudden blindness allows no time to arrive at acceptance or to learn compensatory skills. The loss of vision affects all parts of the personality, often leading to a poor self-concept and disorganization in the client's lifestyle, relationships with others, and sexuality. The nurse must be perceptive, convey respect and gentleness, and use strategies to help the client cope with the losses and gain a better self-concept.

If vision fails gradually, the client and the nurse have an opportunity to plan and work through many of the emotional aspects of this situation. Both the nurse and the client need to reflect on their attitudes toward this catastrophic occurrence. The client must be allowed to express anger and depression and to work through the grieving process. The nurse must validate with the client when teaching can be best implemented. The client's family needs to be included in discussions and encouraged to express concerns.

Those persons who have been blind since birth or early life are usually easily identified by their manner and their use of assistive devices.

In caring for the blind in the hospital or other health care settings, the nurse needs to be aware of certain factors to facilitate communication and provide a safe environment for the blind client. In approaching the client, nurses should call the name before touching the client, introduce themselves, and provide information regarding the purpose of the interaction. Eye contact and facial response are very important to validate whether the message has been received. The nurse must be aware of these aspects of communication with the blind to determine responses to interventions.

The client should be informed when the nurse leaves the room. The family should not be questioned about the client if the client is present. Activity and noise surrounding the client should be described to assist the client with orientation and validation of the environment. The nurse should speak normally and not be hesitant about using such words as "see." Often people raise their voices when talking to the visually impaired or blind, which does not help the communication.

The client should be encouraged to be as independent as possible. Independence is facilitated by a stable environment. When orienting the blind client to a room, the nurse should identify one object as the focal point and describe the location of other objects in relation to it. For example, "The bed is straight ahead, about 10 steps. To the left is the chair. To the right is the nightstand." The client should be led to each major structure in the room. Many clients will prefer to touch each object. The nurse should never leave a blind client alone in the middle of an unfamiliar area because or the absence of a reference point can provoke great anxiety.

Once the visually impaired or blind person has placed an object such as clothing or furniture in a certain position, it should not be rearranged. Doors should be fully open or shut but never left half-open. Items on a meal tray can be described in terms of a clock superimposed over the plate, such as "eggs are at 6 o'clock and bacon is at 12 o'clock." When the nurse is uncertain whether help is needed, the client should be consulted. Such openness is usually appreciated by the blind person and avoids misunderstanding and dependency.

When ambulating in an unfamiliar place, the blind client usually appreciates assistance. The client should place

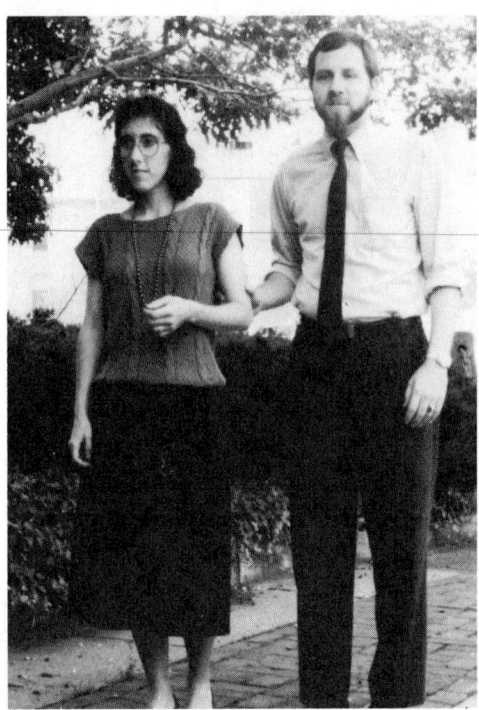

Fig. 15-6 Sighted guide technique for assisting blind person to ambulate. Note how the client holds the arm of the guide.

a hand on the assistant's arm. The assistant should walk a half-step ahead of the blind person, describing objects that are approaching as "on your left is an open door" (Fig. 15-6). The blind person should never be pushed ahead of the assistant.

Other senses of the blind person should be stimulated in meaningful ways. A radio or television may be quite relaxing to some, and others prefer that someone read or talk to them. The use of touch can be a source of security and comfort to the blind person in an unfamiliar environment.

Rehabilitation

Clients who are legally blind are eligible for mobility, braille, and rehabilitative training funded by state and federal agencies. The client or family should contact Services for the Blind and Rehabilitation Services of their state.* Pilot dogs are available to a certain group of clients who can care for them and need assistance with travel. Often young blind persons prefer a dog. Although costly, a variety of electronic and computer devices are available. Talking books are available through some libraries.

For those with impaired vision, a large number of low-vision aids are available, ranging from magnifying glasses to small cameras incorporated into eyeglasses. Clients should be encouraged to seek help and information about available aids. Referral to a low-vision center is appropri-

---

*A list of agencies that service the blind can be obtained from the American Foundation for the Blind, Incorporated, 15 West 16th Street, New York, NY 10011. Many of these agencies are listed after the bibliography.

ate. Specific devices are available to help in measuring and injecting insulin for the visually impaired or blind diabetic client.

Ocular Manifestations of AIDS

Ocular effects are seen in three of four clients with acquired immunodeficiency syndrome (AIDS).[21] These manifestations can be classified by location and pathophysiology.

External manifestations. The most common lesion in the anterior segment of the eye is Kaposi's sarcoma. These nontender red-purple lesions are plaquelike and are prone to ulceration. They appear most frequently in the lower fornix or on the eyelid, but they can also appear on the conjunctivae. The client may experience discomfort from lesions that press against ocular structures or disturb function.

Diagnosis of Kaposi's sarcoma can be made by biopsy or based on presentation. Treatment is aimed at removing the sarcoma with the smallest possible degree of structural and functional alteration. Conjunctival lesions can be easily excised. Local recurrence is possible if the lesion is not completely removed. Appropriate caution in body substance isolation must be taken during surgery to avoid exposing personnel to the human immunodeficiency (HIV) virus. Prompt hemostasis of bleeding vessels decreases blood in the surgical field. Bleeding frequently occurs because of the vascular nature of the lesion. All microsurgical needles and other supplies contaminated with secretions must be handled in accordance with organizational policy.

If excision of the lesion will possibly cause a defect in lid function, radiation therapy is another treatment option.[22] Careful attention must be directed toward protecting ocular structures that are not being radiated.

Other external manifestations common in clients with AIDS are related to the compromised immune system, which increases the client's susceptibility to opportunistic organisms. Two common organisms affecting this population include the herpes zoster virus and various fungi.

Internal manifestations. Several retinal changes occur in clients with AIDS. The condition most commonly appears as cotton-wool spots, retinal hemorrhages, and retinitis. Cotton-wool spots suggest focal retinal ischemia and appear as fluffy white patches. The ischemia involves the nerve fiber layer of the retina and is caused by the occlusion of arterioles and capillaries.[23] Dot- , blot- , and flame-shaped hemorrhages are noted in multiple layers of the retina. Hemorrhages with a central white area, called *Roth's spots,* have also been observed.

Cytomegalovirus (CMV) retinitis is a common opportunistic infection occurring in persons with AIDS. The cytomegalovirus is a member of the herpes family. Damage and necrosis of retinal cells result from direct invasion of the organism. Granular white dots on the retina are an early finding. Occurring in proximity to blood vessels, the lesions extend into patches of opacification. If not treated, the patches expand and blood vessel occlusion occurs. Optic nerve atrophy and papilledema can also occur. The diagnosis of CMV retinitis is based on discovery of characteristic clinical findings.

One treatment for CMV retinitis involves use of ganciclovir. This drug is similar to acyclovir (Zovirax). Research has shown that it stops the prolific and sight-threatening nature of this disease.[24] Once the retinitis is controlled, maintenance doses of the drug are required.

Left untreated, the CMV retinitis can evolve to acute retinal necrosis. Retinal tissues appear white and flake off into the vitreous. Ocular pain, marked changes in vision, and retinal edema are other signs and symptoms of this disorder. (See Chapter 8 for an additional discussion of AIDS.)

HEARING PROBLEMS
HEALTH PROMOTION AND MAINTENANCE

The nurse has an important role in the preservation of hearing. To fulfill this role, the nurse should do the following:

1. Instruct clients to keep objects out of the ear. Ears should be cleaned only with a washcloth and finger. Bobby pins and cotton-tipped applicators should especially be avoided. A quick movement can cause a perforated eardrum.
2. Support environmental noise control. Sensorineural hearing loss due to increased and prolonged environmental noise, such as amplified sound, is occurring in young adults at an increasing rate. Health teaching regarding avoidance of continued exposure to noise levels greater than 85 to 95 dB is essential. Continued exposure to noise causes some persons to be more irritable and tense. Nurses should monitor noise levels in hospitals and at home to promote rest and recovery from illness. Interventions such as seeking different and less noisy equipment or a different time to use noisy equipment are possible solutions. In work environments known to have high noise levels (over 90 dB), ear protectors must be worn. A variety of protectors are available. They are worn over the ears or in the ears to prevent hearing loss. Periodic audiometric screening should be part of the health maintenance policies of industry. This provides baseline data on hearing to measure subsequent hearing loss. Ear protectors should be worn during skeet shooting and other recreational pursuits with high noise levels. Young adults should be encouraged to keep amplified music to a reasonable level. Hearing loss caused by noise is not medically correctable.
3. Promote use of childhood immunizations, including MMR (measles, mumps, rubella). Various viruses can cause deafness as a result of fetal damage and malformations affecting the ear. Children of mothers who had rubella in the first trimester of pregnancy are especially vulnerable, although infection in the second or third trimester can also cause deafness.[25]
4. Monitor the client's reaction to drugs that cause ototoxicity. Clients who are receiving ototoxic drugs, such as aspirin and certain antibiotics, should be assessed for tinnitus and decreased hearing. When these symptoms develop, immediate withdrawal of the offending drug may prevent further damage and may cause the symptoms to disappear.
5. Identify clients who have a potential for hearing loss. Children who are chronic mouth breathers need referral. Enlarged adenoids can block the nasal passages as well as the eustachian tube, preventing aeration of the middle ear. This also predisposes to serous otitis media. Children who have acute otitis media frequently need to be watched for signs of chronic otitis media. It is important that children complete the full course of antibiotics prescribed for the acute episode.
6. Be observant of symptoms that indicate hearing loss at all ages. These symptoms include asking others to speak up, answering questions inappropriately, not responding when not looking at the speaker, straining to hear, cupping hands around ear, showing irritability with others who do not speak up, and increasing sensitivity to slight increases in noise level. Often the client is not aware of minimal hearing loss or may compensate by using these mannerisms. Children will often be inattentive, bored, or uncooperative when they have decreased hearing caused by a middle ear infection (conductive type of loss) or an inner ear problem (sensorineural loss).

EXTERNAL EAR AND CANAL
Trauma

Trauma to the ear can cause injury to the subcutaneous tissue that may result in a hematoma. If the hematoma is not aspirated, an inflammation of membranes of the ear cartilage (perichondritis) can result. Antibiotics are given to prevent infection. Blows to the ear also cause hearing loss if there is dislocation of the ossicles of the middle ear. It is important to obtain a very careful history of the accident and to assess the hearing of a client who has had a blow to the ear.

External Otitis

External otitis involves inflammation or infection of the epithelium of the ear auricle and canal. It is more common in the summer. Swimming in contaminated waters is frequently implicated and is called *swimmer's ear*. Trauma caused by picking the ear or use of sharp objects such as hairpins frequently causes the initial break in the skin.

Etiology. External otitis may be caused by infections, dermatitis, or both. Bacteria or fungi may be the cause. The bacteria most commonly cultured are *Pseudomonas aeruginosa, Proteus vulgaris, Escherichia coli,* and *Staphylococcus aureus.* The most common fungi are *Candida albicans* and *Aspergillus* organisms.[26] Fungi are often the causative agents of external otitis, especially in warm, moist climates. The warm, dark environment of the ear canal provides a good medium for the growth of microorganisms.

Clinical manifestations and complications. Pain is one of the first signs of external otitis. It is caused by stretching of the tight epithelium of the ear canal by the inflammatory process. Pain is especially noted on movement of the auricle or an application of pressure to the tragus (directly in front of the ear). Drainage from the ear may be serosanguineous or purulent. If it is the result of an infection caused by a *Pseudomonas* organism, the drainage

Table 15-13

Diagnostic and Therapeutic Management: External Otitis

DIAGNOSTIC

Otoscopic examination
Culture and sensitivity

THERAPEUTIC

Analgesics (depending on severity)
Warm compresses
Cleansing of canal
Ear wick
Antibiotic otic drops
Systemic antibiotics

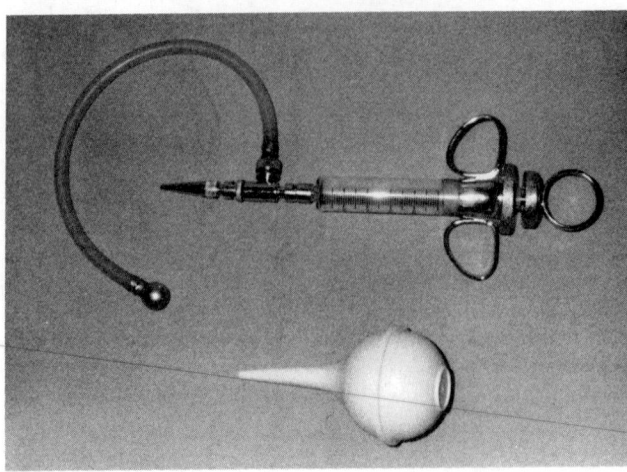

Fig. 15-7 Types of equipment used to irrigate the external ear canal. A bulb syringe *(below)* and an ear irrigation apparatus used in doctors' offices and clinics *(above)* are shown.

will be green and have a musty smell. Temperature elevations occur when there is extensive involvement of the tissue. The swelling of the ear canal can block hearing and cause dizziness.

Therapeutic and Nursing Management of External Otitis

Diagnosis is made by observation with the otoscope light and the largest speculum the ear will accommodate. The eardrum may be normal if it can be visualized. Culture and sensitivity studies of the drainage may be done. Aspirin or codeine will usually control the pain. After the ear canal is cleansed, a wick of cotton is placed in the ear canal to help deliver the antibiotic eardrops. Wicking should be used with caution in clients such as the very young and confused or psychotic clients, who might push it farther into the ear. Topical antibiotics include polymyxin B, colistin, neomycin, and chloromycetin. Nystatin is used for fungal infections. Corticosteroids may also be used. If the surrounding tissue is involved, systemic antibiotics are prescribed. Warm, moist compresses or heat may be prescribed. Improvement should occur in 48 hours, but more time is required for resolution.

Careful handling and disposal of material saturated with drainage are important. Otic (ear) drops should be administered at room temperature. The tip of the dropper should not touch the auricle during administration. The ear is positioned so that the drops can run down the canal. This position should be maintained for 2 minutes after eardrop administration to allow absorption of drops. The diagnostic and therapeutic management of external otitis is shown in Table 15-13.

Cerumen and Foreign Bodies in the External Ear Canal

Impacted cerumen can cause discomfort and decreased hearing, which is often described as a hollow sensation. In older persons, the earwax becomes drier and is not easily removed from the canal. Water that enters the canal during a shower or swimming may cause swelling of the cerumen, resulting in blockage of the canal. Management involves irrigation of the canal with body-temperature solutions. Special syringes can be used and vary from the simple bulb syringe to special irrigating equipment used in the physician's office or clinic (Fig. 15-7). The client is placed in a sitting position with an emesis basin under the ear. The auricle is pulled up and back. The flow of solution is directed to the top of the canal. It is important that the ear canal not be completely occluded with the syringe tip. If this irrigation does not remove the wax, a special cerumen spoon can be used. Mild lubricant drops may be used to soften the earwax, and irrigation may then be effective in removing the impacted cerumen.

If an insect enters the ear canal, the best action is to drown it with mineral oil or olive oil and then flush it out. If a wood tick has become attached to the tissue, it is removed with ear forceps.

Malignancy

Malignancy of the external ear and canal is common. The predominant signs include a chronic ulcer of the auricle and persistent drainage from the canal. This drainage is tinged with blood and does not diminish with treatment. Therapeutic management includes biopsy and other diagnostic studies to determine invasion of underlying tissue and bone. Treatment involves surgery. If the malignancy involves the ear canal and temporal bone, radical surgery of the middle and inner ear with resection of the facial nerve (CN VII), auditory nerve (CN VIII), and part of the temporal bone may be necessary.

MIDDLE EAR AND MASTOID

The most common problem of the middle ear is acute otitis media, usually a childhood disease associated with colds, sore throats, and blockage of the eustachian tube. Pain, fever, malaise, headache, and reduced hearing are clinical manifestations of acute otitis media. Therapeutic management involves antibiotics and, if necessary, a myr-

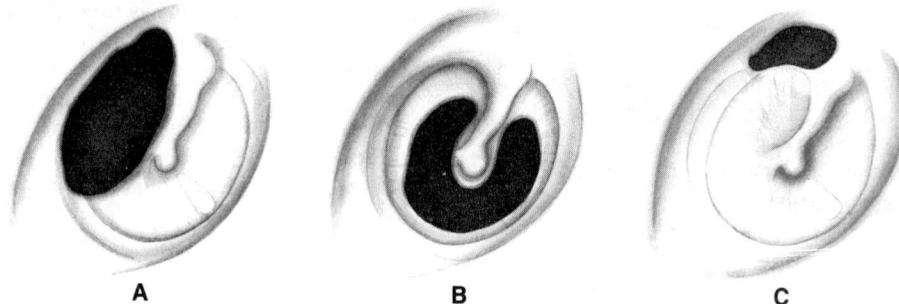

Fig. 15-8 Three common tympanic perforations. **A,** Small central perforation (hearing is usually good). **B,** Large central perforation around the handle of the malleus (hearing is usually poor). **C,** Marginal perforation of Shrapnell's membrane (hearing is usually good). Cholesteatomas commonly occur in patients with a marginal perforation and are always present with attic perforation. (From DeWeese DD and others: Otolaryngology: head and neck surgery, ed 7, St Louis, 1988, The CV Mosby Co.)

ingotomy. This surgical procedure involves an incision in the tympanum to release the increased pressure and exudate in the ear. Since the advent of treatment with antibiotics, the incidence of severe and prolonged infections of the middle ear and mastoid has been greatly reduced except in areas where health care is inadequate or people have limited access to health care.

Chronic Otitis Media and Mastoiditis

Significance and etiology. Chronic infection of the middle ear is more common in persons who experienced episodes of acute otitis media in early childhood. Organisms involved in chronic otitis media include *Staphylococcus, Streptococcus, Proteus, Pseudomonas,* and *E. coli.* Because the mucous membrane is continuous, both the middle ear and the air cells of the mastoid are usually involved in the chronic infectious process.

Clinical manifestations. In chronic otitis media, there is a continuous or intermittent ear drainage that may be thin and mucoid or thick, white, yellow, or green with a foul odor. The client's main complaint is of hearing loss due to destruction of the ossicles from the purulent discharge. Occasionally, a facial palsy or an attack of vertigo may alert the client to this condition. Chronic otitis media is usually painless, but if pain is present, it indicates drainage under pressure and possible extension of the infection to the brain.

The eardrum is usually perforated. If the perforation is marginal, the epithelium of the external ear can grow into the middle ear. The skin sheds, and debris and drainage form a ball or growth called a cholesteatoma. This can cause pressure and erode the thin bony covering over the facial nerves (CN VII), resulting in decreased motor function of the same side of the face. A labyrinth fistula can also result, causing vertigo.

Diagnostic studies. Otoscopic examination reveals a marginal or central perforation of the eardrum (Fig. 15-8). A central perforation has tympanum remaining around all points of the circumference. Some eardrums may be healed but have an area that is more flaccid and thinner,

Table 15-14

Diagnostic and Therapeutic Management: Chronic Otitis Media

DIAGNOSTIC

Otoscopic examination
Culture and sensitivity
Mastoid x-ray films

THERAPEUTIC

Ear irrigations
    Acetic acid (equal amounts of white vinegar and warm water)
Otic drops, powders
Antibiotics, systemic
Surgery
    Tympanoplasty*
    Mastoidectomy (modified)
    Analgesic
    Antiemetic

*See Table 15-15.

indicative of a previous perforation. Cultures and sensitivity tests are necessary to identify the organisms involved and the appropriate antibiotic to use. The audiogram may demonstrate no loss in hearing or a loss as great as 50 to 60 dB if the ossicles have been partially destroyed or disarticulated (separated).

X-ray films, polytomography, or a CT scan of the temporal bone may demonstrate bone destruction, absence of ossicular tissue, or the presence of a mass.

Therapeutic management. The aim of treatment is to rid the middle ear of infection (Table 15-14). Systemic antibiotic therapy based on the sensitivity study is initiated. In addition, ear irrigations with sterile normal saline solution at body temperature is used to remove the drainage and debris. Antibiotic eardrops and 2% acetic acid drops

Table 15-15 Types of Tympanoplasty

I	Absorbable Gelfoam sponge placed in middle ear to support fascia or vein graft under the tympanic membrane
II	Fascia or perichondrium grafted over remnant of malleus to correct ossicular defect
III	Removal of necrosed ossicles except for stapes, with fascia or perichondrium graft placed over stapes
IV	Removal of necrosed ossicles except for footplate of the stapes, with fascia or perichondrium graft placed over footplate
V	Fenestration made into horizontal semicircular canal and then closed with fascia or perichondrium graft

are also used to reduce infection. If there is a recurrence, the client may need to be hospitalized for parenteral administration of antibiotics, such as the cephalosporins (gentamicin, carbenicillin), if the offending organisms are gram-negative bacteria.

Often the perforation will not heal in response to conservative treatment and surgery is necessary. Surgery to restore the conductive hearing by reconstruction of the middle ear is called a *tympanoplasty*. Diseased tissue and ossicles are removed, and a graft is used to make an intact tympanum. The incision may be endaural (incision around the tympanum) or postauricular (behind the auricle or ear). The type of tympanoplasty depends on the amount of involvement (Table 15-15). Less hearing is restored with types IV and V.

A mastoidectomy is often performed concurrently with tympanoplasty to remove diseased tissue and the source of infection. A modified mastoidectomy aims at preserving function by removing as little tissue as possible. Removal of tissue stops short of the middle ear structures that appear capable of survival. A radical mastoidectomy is required when disease is extensive, requiring complete removal of all middle ear structures, or when complete exposure is necessary. No attempt is made to restore conductive hearing. The middle ear and mastoid become one large cavity. This surgery is rarely done today but was used before ear infections were treated with antibiotics.

■ Nursing Management Following Tympanoplasty

Routine preoperative care is provided before tympanoplasty and includes teaching postoperative expectations (Table 15-16). Postoperative concerns are the avoidance of complications such as hemorrhage and facial nerve paralysis and of increased pressure in the middle ear. The client is instructed to avoid blowing the nose because this causes increased pressure in the eustachian tube and the middle ear cavity and could dislodge the graft to the tympanum. Coughing and sneezing can cause similar disruption and are to be avoided if possible. If the client must cough or sneeze, leaving the mouth open will reduce the pressure increase. It is essential that the client be helped when getting up the first time, since dizziness, loss of balance, and a fall may occur.

A cotton ball dressing is used for an endaural incision. If a postauricular incision is used and a drain is in place, a mastoid dressing is used. A 4 × 4 inch dressing is cut to fit behind the ear and fluffs are applied over the ear to prevent the outer circular head dressing from placing pressure on the auricle. It is necessary to monitor the tightness of the dressing and the amount of drainage postoperatively.

Serous Otitis Media

Serous otitis media (effusion of the middle ear) is an accumulation of sterile fluid in the middle ear. The middle ear fluid may become very thick and mucoid (called *glue* ear) and may be bloody. It may occur at any age but is more frequent in children. Causes of serous otitis media include an obstruction of the eustachian tube and failure of the eustachian tube to open. If the eustachian tube does not open and allow equalization of atmospheric pressure, negative pressure within the middle ear pulls (effuses) fluid from the tissues and capillaries. Allergic reaction of the mucosa can also cause blockage of the eustachian tube and/or cause fluid within the ear. Overgrowth of nasopharyngeal lymphoid tissue and chronic sinusitis are also factors that may contribute to middle ear effusion.

Complaints include a feeling of fullness of the ear and decreased hearing. Clients do not experience pain, fever, or discharge from the ear. Otoscopic examination may reveal a normal tympanic membrane or minimal dullness and retraction. Tympanometry and pneumotoscopy may demonstrate limited tympanic membrane motion.

Decongestants and antihistamine medication, decongestant nasal spray, and exercises such as swallowing and gum chewing are used to open the eustachian tube. If the effusion is not relieved in a few days or a week, a *myringotomy* is performed. A ventilating tube is frequently used for children who have recurrent serous otitis media or others with dysfunction of the eustachian tube. The client who has a ventilating tube in the eardrum must be instructed not to swim or get water in the ear.

Otosclerosis

Otosclerosis, an autosomal dominant disease, is the fixation of the footplate of the stapes in the oval window by a bony growth. It is a common cause of conductive hearing loss in young adults, especially women, and may be accelerated during pregnancy. It involves both ears but at different rates. This condition is rare in blacks. Spongy bone develops from the bony labyrinth, causing immobilization of the footplate of the stapes. Approximately 10% of the population has this condition, but not all have symptoms.[27] Hearing loss is typically bilateral, although one ear frequently shows a greater hearing loss. The client is often unaware of the problem until the loss becomes so severe that difficulty is encountered in communication. Loss of hearing usually becomes increasingly severe.

Otoscopic examination may reveal a pinkish orange discoloration of the tympanum (Schwartz's sign) caused by the vascular and bony changes within the middle ear. The Rinne test, using the 512 Hz tuning fork, favors bone conduction. Bone conduction is equal to or greater than air conduction (BC ≥ AC). This is a negative Rinne test. The Weber test lateralizes to the poor ear or to the ear with the

Table 15-16

NURSING CARE PLAN FOR THE CLIENT AFTER MIDDLE EAR SURGERY

Defining Characteristics	Nursing Interventions	Evaluation Criteria

NURSING DIAGNOSIS: Pain related to surgical incision and localized pressure and edema

Verbalization of pain, isolation, withdrawal	Assess degree of pain. Report excessive ear pain immediately. Administer analgesics as needed; assess and document effectiveness. Encourage client to avoid sudden movements. Do not position client on operative side.	Satisfaction with pain relief

NURSING DIAGNOSIS: Potential complication: bleeding from operative site

Bright red drainage from operative ear or on dressing	Assess, record, and report unusual bleeding or drainage from operative site. Elevate head of bed 30 degrees.	Early detection and reporting of postoperative bleeding

NURSING DIAGNOSIS: High risk for injury related to decreased hearing acuity and dizziness

Decreased hearing, lack of awareness of environmental warning sounds, dizziness when upright	Determine client's hearing level. Assist with assessing environment to identify and alter injury risk factors. Assess and monitor dizziness. Assist with ambulation as needed.	Identification of factors that increase risk of injury, formulation of plan to alter environment to reduce risk, no incidence of injury

NURSING DIAGNOSIS: Potential complication: facial nerve paralysis

Inability to perform activities controlled by facial nerve (e.g., wrinkle eyebrows)	Assess facial nerve function (e.g., client able to wrinkle eyebrows, close lids, wrinkle nose, smile, bare teeth symmetrically). Notify physician if problem observed.	Early detection of facial nerve involvement

NURSING DIAGNOSIS: Impaired verbal communication related to hearing loss

Unawareness of being addressed, no tracking of sound, inappropriate response when addressed, verbalization of inability to hear part or all of spoken communication, inattentive, use of loud speaking voice	Assess ability to receive verbal messages. Use techniques to increase ability to hear, such as slowed speech, lip reading. Attempt to determine whether a message has been received accurately.	Expression of satisfaction with communication pattern, use of alternative method to communicate (if indicated)

NURSING DIAGNOSIS: Social isolation related to inability to make meaningful contact with another secondary to hearing deficit

Most often alone; few, if any, visitors or phone calls; verbalization of feelings of aloneness	Assess client preference for relationships. Try to introduce to person with similar disability. Include client in group activities.	Expression of satisfaction with level of assistance available

NURSING DIAGNOSIS: Altered health maintenance related to lack of knowledge of self-care and signs and symptoms of complications

Frequent questioning related to self-care and complications, inability to answer or incorrect responses regarding self-care and possible complications	Instruct client not to blow nose or cough and to sneeze with mouth open to prevent fluctuation of air pressure in middle ear. Give written instructions. Teach self-care and signs and symptoms of complications.	Adequate knowledge base to take care of self and identify complications

Table 15-17

Diagnostic and Therapeutic Management: Otosclerosis

DIAGNOSTIC

Otoscopic examination
Rinne test (512 Hz tuning fork)
Weber test
Audiometry

THERAPEUTIC

Hearing aid
Surgery (stapedectomy)
  Analgesia
  Antiemetic
  Antibiotic
  Antimotion drugs

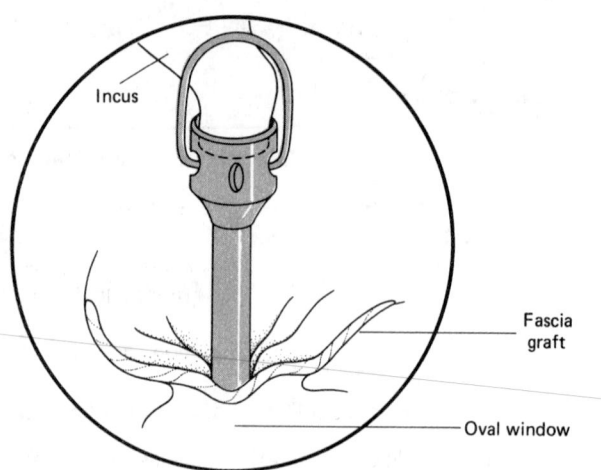

Fig. 15-9 A commonly used stapedectomy technique. A stainless steel prosthesis replaces the stapes. The fascia graft over the oval window thins out and becomes contiguous with the adjacent mucoperiosteum.

greatest conductive hearing loss. An audiogram demonstrates good hearing by bone conduction, but poor hearing is shown by air conduction or an "air-bone" gap audiogram. Usually a 20 to 25 dB difference between air-conduction and bone-conduction levels of hearing is seen.

Therapeutic management. The stapedectomy surgical procedure is the operation of choice today and is usually performed with the client under local anesthesia. The poorer ear is repaired first and the other ear is operated on later. (The therapeutic management of otosclerosis is shown in Table 15-17.)

In stapedectomy, an endaural incision is made, and the operating microscope is used for visualization. The two most common procedures performed are a total stapedectomy, with perichondrium or fascia grafting over the oval window and placement of a prosthesis with attachment to the incus (Fig. 15-9), or a stapedectomy, with fenestration into the footplate for insertion of a wire and piston. The prosthesis or wire and piston completes the ossicular chain, and movement initiated by sound waves can occur and be transmitted to the perilymph. The tympanum is replaced, and packing is placed in the external ear canal. A cotton ball dressing is placed over the auricle. During surgery, the client will often report the increased ability to hear in the operative ear. Because of the accumulation of blood and fluid in the middle ear, the hearing level decreases but does return to near-normal levels. In 90% to 95% of clients, normal hearing is restored.

A perilymph fistula (incomplete closure of the oval window) can occur with symptoms of widely fluctuating hearing levels, tinnitus, and dizziness. A few clients (6%) may develop a sensorineural hearing loss. An audiogram is repeated when the ear is healed.

Similar care is provided for the client after a stapedectomy and for the client who had a tympanoplasty. Postoperatively, the client may experience dizziness, nausea, and vomiting because of the proximity of the surgery to the labyrinth. Some clients will demonstrate nystagmus on lateral gaze because of disturbance of the perilymph.

INNER EAR PROBLEMS

Three symptoms that indicate disease of the inner ear are vertigo (whirling), sensorineural hearing loss, and tinnitus (ringing). Vertigo arises from the vestibular labyrinth, whereas hearing loss and tinnitus arise from the auditory labyrinth. There is much overlap between manifestations of inner ear problems and central nervous system disorders.

Ménière's Disease

Ménière's disease is characterized by the triad of symptoms caused by inner ear disease—vertigo, tinnitus, and hearing loss. It incapacitates clients because of sudden, severe attacks of vertigo. Symptoms usually begin around 40 years of age. Usually one ear is involved; however, 20% to 28% of clients have bilateral involvement.

The cause of the disease is unknown, but hydrops (dilatation due to fluid physiology) of the endolymphatic system occurs. Attacks of *vertigo* are sudden and occur without warning. Before attacks clients may experience intraear fullness. They complain that the environment is whirling wildly and that they must lie down or they will fall. Some clients report that they are whirling in space. The duration may be hours or days, and attacks may occur several times a year. Nausea and vomiting accompany the vertigo.

Tinnitus of a low pitch may be present in the affected ear all the time or be newly present or intensified during an attack. Hearing loss fluctuates but over a period of years may worsen until no functional hearing remains.

Therapeutic management (Table 15-18) includes diagnostic tests to rule out central nervous system disease. The audiogram demonstrates a hearing loss in the low tones. Vestibular tests indicate decreased function.

The glycerol test may suggest the diagnosis of Ménière's disease. An oral dose of glycerol is given, and hearing threshold and speech discrimination are tested 1 to

Table 15-18

Diagnostic and Therapeutic Management: Ménière's Disease

DIAGNOSTIC

History
Audiometric studies, including speech discrimination, tone decay
Vestibular tests, including caloric test, positional tests
Electronystagmography
Neurological examination
Glycerol test

THERAPEUTIC

Acute (one or more)
  Sedative (diazepam)
  Anticholinergic (atropine)
  Vasodilator (histamine)
  Antihistamine (Benadryl)
Chronic (one or more)
  Diuretics
  Antihistamines
  Vasodilators
  Neuroleptics
  Vitamins
  Diazepam (Valium)
  Low-salt diet
  Restriction of caffeine, nicotine, or alcohol intake
Conservative surgical intervention
  Endolymphatic shunt
  Vestibular nerve section
Destructive surgical intervention
  Labyrinthotomy
  Labyrinthectomy

3 hours after administration. Improvement in hearing or speech discrimination supports a diagnosis of Ménière's disease. The improvement is attributed to the osmotic effect of glycerol that pulls fluid from the inner ear.

During the acute attack, atropine may be given to decrease the autonomic nervous system function. Diazepam (Valium) is often used instead of atropine. Reassurance that the problem is not due to a major cerebral dysfunction is very important. Management between attacks may include vasodilation, diuretics, antihistamines, a low-sodium diet, and other interventions. Diazepam (Valium) and Antivert (Bonamine plus nicotinic acid) are commonly used to reduce the dizziness. Over a period of time, most clients respond to the prescribed medications but must learn to live with the unpredictability of the attacks. Approximately 80% of clients experience improvement with therapeutic management.[28] Conservation of hearing is a main concern for clients who have repeated attacks. Surgical decompression of the endolymphatic sac is performed to reduce the pressure on the cochlear hair cells and to prevent further damage and sensorineural hearing loss. If relief is not achieved with endolymphatic shunt surgery and hearing remains good, vestibular nerve section may be performed to alleviate vertigo and preserve hearing. When involvement is unilateral, surgical destruction of the labyrinth, causing loss of the vestibular and cochlear function, is performed. Careful therapeutic management can decrease the possibility of progressive sensorineural loss in many clients.

During the acute attack, the client is kept in a quiet, darkened room in a comfortable position. Since motion aggravates the whirling and roaring sensations, the client is moved only for essential care; bathing may not be essential. An emesis basin should be available, since vomiting is common. Medications and fluids are administered parenterally, and intake and output are monitored. When the attack subsides, the client is assisted with ambulation because unsteadiness may remain. Similar care is provided after surgical destruction of the labyrinth; the client will have severe tinnitus and vertigo, which decrease over a period of days.

Labyrinthitis

Infection or inflammation of the inner ear may affect the cochlear or vestibular portion of the labyrinth or both areas. Infection can enter from the meninges, the middle ear, or the bloodstream. Symptoms of vertigo, tinnitus, and sensorineural hearing loss are due to problems in the labyrinth. Nystagmus, an abnormal rhythmic, jerking movement of the eye, accompanies the vertigo and has a horizontal beat. Nystagmus is caused by abnormal currents in the endolymph fluid, causing the eyes to have a rhythmic jerking movement with a quick and a slow component.

The direction of the nystagmus is designated by the fast component (e.g., right-beating nystagmus). Nystagmus is also caused by dysfunction of the brainstem and cerebellum. Central nystagmus is not usually accompanied by vertigo.

Suppurative labyrinthitis due to infection causes severe vertigo similar to that of an attack of Ménière's disease. It lasts for days to weeks, progressing until the vestibular function is destroyed. Complete destruction of the cochlear portion occurs, causing deafness. Eventually the client learns to walk without support. Vestibular neuronitis causes vertigo, nausea, vomiting, and nystagmus. A viral infection may be the etiological factor. The client recovers after a week or more. Tinnitus is not present, and hearing loss does not occur. Toxic labyrinthitis is caused by ototoxic drugs that may cause vertigo. However, most ototoxic drugs affect the cochlea, resulting in tinnitus and eventually hearing loss.

Acoustic Neuroma

An acoustic neuroma is a benign tumor that occurs where the acoustic nerve (CN VIII) enters the internal auditory canal or the temporal bone from the brain. It is important that early diagnosis be made because the neuroma can compress the facial nerve and arteries within the internal auditory canal. It can expand into the cerebellopontine angle and involve other cranial nerves and the brain by compression.

Early symptoms are unilateral, progressive, sensorineural hearing loss, unilateral tinnitus, and intermittent vertigo. Diagnostic tests include neurological, audiometric, and vestibular tests, and tomograms (CT scans) and magnetic resonance imaging (MRI).

Surgery to remove small tumors is performed through the middle cranial fossa. A translabyrinthine approach is usually used for medium-sized tumors. Although hearing is destroyed by this approach, advantages include good access to the tumor and preservation of the facial nerve. Posterior cranial fossa or retrolabyrinthine approaches are used for large tumors (greater than 3 cm in size).

Hearing Impairment and Deafness

Incidence. Communication disorders are the primary handicapping disability in the United States. In the United States, 20 million persons have impaired hearing in one or both ears. Hearing impairment is common among older adults. Nearly half of the persons who need assistance with hearing disorders are 65 years of age or older. Between 2% and 4% of children have a hearing loss, with 3 million school-age children affected.[29]

Etiology and types of hearing loss. Conductive loss occurs in the outer and middle ear and impairs the sound being conducted from the outer to the inner ear. It is caused by conditions interfering with air conduction, such as impacted cerumen, middle ear disease, and otosclerosis. Antibiotics, tubes in the eardrum, and surgery usually correct the problem. The audiogram demonstrates an air-bone gap of at least 15 dB.

An air-bone gap occurs when hearing sensitivity by bone conduction is significantly better than by air conduction. Clients may speak softly because they hear their voice, which is conducted by bone, as loud. This client hears better in a noisy environment. A hearing aid is quite helpful for a client with a 40 to 50 dB loss or more, although the device often is not necessary because of the excellent results of treatment.

Sensorineural hearing loss is caused by impairment of function of the inner ear or its central connections. Congenital and hereditary factors, noise trauma over a period of time, aging (presbycusis), Ménière's disease, and ototoxicity can cause sensorineural hearing loss. Systemic diseases, such as certain collagen diseases, diabetes, syphilis, and Paget's disease, can also cause sensorineural deafness. The two main problems associated with sensorineural loss are the ability to hear sound but not understand speech and lack of understanding of the problem by others. The ability to hear high-pitched sounds diminishes. The consonants are high-pitched sounds and give intelligibility to speech. Words are difficult to distinguish, and sound is muffled. An audiogram demonstrates a loss in dB levels of the 4000 Hz range, which can progress to the 2000 Hz range. A hearing aid may help some who have a 30 dB loss or more by reducing the strain of trying to hear, but the sounds will still be muffled. *Presbycusis,* degenerative change of the inner ear, is a major cause of sensorineural hearing loss, especially in older adults. It is a progressive problem that results in many social and emotional problems for the affected older adult. The control of inner

ear diseases such as Ménière's disease can prevent further hearing loss. If the sensorineural loss is due to an ototoxic drug, further loss should not occur if the drug is discontinued.

Mixed hearing loss is caused by a combination of conductive and sensorineural losses. Careful evaluation is needed before corrective surgery for conductive loss is planned because the cause of the sensorineural loss will still remain.

Central hearing loss is caused by problems in the central nervous system from the auditory nucleus to the cortex. The client is unable to understand or to put meaning to the incoming sound. Functional hearing loss may be due to an emotional or psychological factor. The client does not seem to hear or respond to pure-tone hearing tests, but no organic cause can be identified. A careful history is helpful, since there is usually a reference to deafness within the family. Psychological counseling may help. Referral to qualified hearing and speech services is indicated.

Hearing loss can also be classified by the decibel (dB) level or loss as recorded on the audiogram. Normal hearing is in the 0 to 25 dB range. A mild impairment is present at the 30 dB hearing level. A moderate impairment is in the 31 to 55 dB range.

A *moderate to severe impairment* is in the 56 to 70 dB range. The *severely impaired* have a loss in the 70 to 90 dB range. The *profoundly deaf* have a loss greater than 90 dB. Many in this last group are the congenitally deaf.

Manifestations of hearing loss. If the hearing loss is congenital and profound, the great difficulty in learning speech and conceptual thinking is quite evident. Rehabilitation must be started early.

Deafness is often called the "unseen handicap" because it is not until conversation is initiated with a deaf adult that the difficulty in communication is realized. It is important that the health professional be aware of the need for thorough validation of the deaf person's understanding of health teaching. Descriptive visual aids can be helpful. Because of the difficulty in communication, deaf persons often seek relationships with other deaf persons. Those who develop hearing loss later in life vary in the amount of loss and the reactions to it.

Interference in communication and interaction with others can be the source of many problems for client and family. Often the client refuses to admit or may be unaware of impaired hearing. Irritability is common because of the intentness with which the client must listen to understand speech. The loss of clarity of speech in clients with sensorineural hearing loss is most frustrating. The client may hear what is said but not understand it. Withdrawal, suspicion, loss of self-esteem, and insecurity are common reactions to hearing loss.

Rehabilitation of the client with impaired hearing. It is important that the client with a suspected hearing loss have a hearing assessment by a qualified audiologist. If a hearing aid is indicated, it should be fitted by an audiologist or a speech and hearing specialist. There are many types of aids available—the body-worn aid, the eyeglasses style, the behind-the-ear style, and the in-the-ear style—each with advantages and disadvantages. A very small in-the-ear type is also available (Fig. 15-10). Client acceptance of a hearing aid may present a real problem. The nurse needs to be prepared to give careful instruction on its use and maintenance and to assist the client during the period of adjustment.

Initially, use of the hearing aid should be restricted to quiet situations in the home. The client needs to first adjust to voices (including the client's own) and household sounds. The client should also experiment by increasing and decreasing the volume as situations require. As adjustment to the increase in sounds and background noise occurs, the client will be ready to try a different listening environment, such as a small party where several people will be talking simultaneously. Next the environment can be expanded to the outdoors. After adapting to controlled situations, the client will be ready to encounter environments such as the shopping mall or grocery store. Adjustment to different environments occurs gradually over weeks to months, depending on the individual client.

When the hearing aid is not being worn, it should be placed in a dry cool area where it will not be inadvertently damaged or lost. The battery should be disconnected or removed. Battery life averages 1 week, and clients should be advised to purchase only a month's supply at a time. Earmolds should be cleaned weekly or as needed. Toothpicks or pipe cleaners may be used to clear a clogged eartip.

Speech reading can be helpful in increasing communication. It allows for approximately 40% understanding of the spoken word. In speech reading, many words will look alike to the client (e.g., *rabbit* and *woman*). If the client wears glasses, they should be used to facilitate speech reading. The nurse can help the client by using and teaching verbal and nonverbal communication techniques (Table 15-19). The hearing aid should be readily available to the client at all times.

The cochlear implant is being used as a hearing device for the profoundly deaf. The system consists of a surgically embedded coil beneath the skin behind the ear and an electrode wire placed in the cochlea. The implanted parts interface with externally worn components. The system stimulates the auditory nerve by an electric current. The implant is intended for use with clients whose inner ear hair cells are damaged, resulting in a sensory impairment. The implant offers the profoundly deaf the ability to hear environmental sounds, such as a telephone, doorbell, garbage disposal, footsteps, and fire alarms. Clients with cochlear implants have limited understanding of speech. Speech sounds are muffled and distorted. Clients impaired by a hearing loss after language has been acquired benefit most from cochlear implants. The positive aspects of a cochlear implant include providing sound to persons who heard none, improved lipreading, monitoring the loudness of their own speech, an improved sense of security, and decreased feelings of isolation. With continued research, the cochlear implant may offer the possibility of aural rehabilitation for a range of hearing problems.

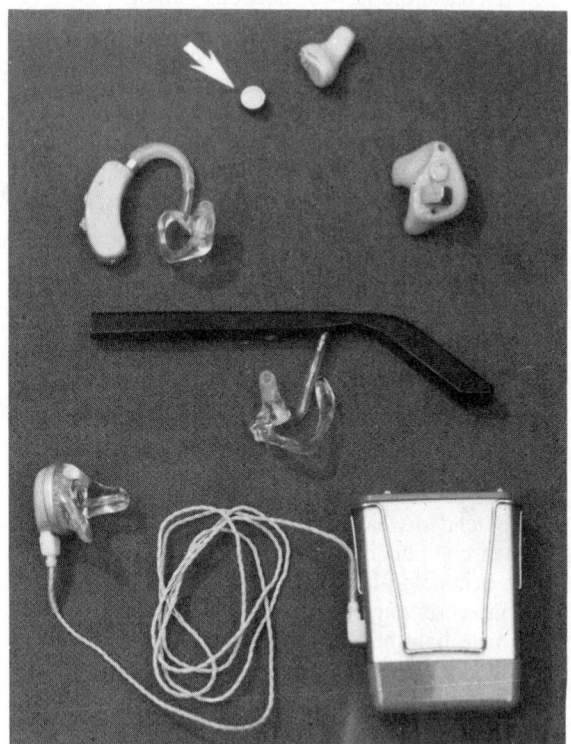

Fig. 15-10 Types of hearing aids. Below is the older aid with a battery pack worn on the body and a wire connected to the ear mold. Next is the earpiece containing battery and mold worn in the ear canal. Above to the left is the behind-the-ear battery with ear mold. To the right is a small ear canal mold with battery. Above is the newer, smaller mold worn in the ear canal. *Arrow* identifies the small battery used for the newer hearing aids.

Table 15-19   Communicating with the Client with Impaired Hearing

NONVERBAL AIDS

Draw attention by hand movements
Have light on face
Avoid covering mouth or face with hands
Avoid chewing, eating, smoking while talking
Maintain eye contact
Avoid distracting environments
Avoid careless expression that the client may misinterpret
Use touch
Move close to better ear
Avoid light behind speaker

VERBAL AIDS

Speak normally, slowly
Do not overexaggerate facial expression
Do not overenunciate
Use simple sentences
Rephrase sentence; use different words
Write name or difficult words
Avoid shouting

C ase Study

CATARACT EXTRACTION

Mr. O., a 62-year-old man, was admitted to the hospital for extraction of a cataract in his left eye. He had been noticing a gradual decrease in visual acuity OS and complained of glare, especially when in bright lights.

   Visual acuity 20/80 OS; 20/40 OD with correction (bifocal lens); biomicroscopic examination revealing a nuclear cataract OS and small cataract OD.

   Preoperative orders: Atropine 1% gtts i̇ OS, h.s. and in am

   Neosporin ophthalmic gtts i̇ OS, h.s. and in am

   Phenylephrine 10% gtts i̇ OS; cyclopentolate 2% gtts i̇ OS; preoperatively q 15 min × 3

   Valium 10 mg PO with small amount of water on call to surgery

   NPO after midnight

The surgery was performed under local anesthesia. The lens was removed by extracapsular extraction. An intraocular lens was inserted in the posterior chamber. Mr. O. returned to his room with an eye pad and a metal shield on the treated eye.

Discussion Questions

1. Explain the reasons for Mr. O.'s symptoms.
2. Why were the preoperative eye medications given? What are the actions of each?
3. Would Mr. O. be able to fill out his menu after surgery without his glasses?
4. What precautions need to be taken with the operative eye?
5. What will vision of the left eye be when the patch is removed?
6. If Mr. O. had not had an intraocular lens implant, he would have glasses or an extended-wear contact lens. Which would provide the best vision for him?
7. What signs that indicate complications should the client be aware of?

R eview Questions

The number of the question corresponds to the same-numbered objective at the beginning of the chapter.

1. Causes of myopia include
   a. short eyeball
   b. flat cornea
   c. excessive refractive power of lens
   d. increased intraocular pressure
2. All the following actions may be helpful for the client who has decreased blinking because of non-function of a facial nerve (CN VII) *except*
   a. bilateral patches
   b. lubricant eyedrops instilled frequently
   c. increased moisture in the environment
   d. securely placed eye pad to close eyelid during sleep
   e. closing lid manually when eye feels dry
3. The client who is experiencing a retinal detachment may complain of all the following *except*

a. curtain over part of field
b. increase of floaters
c. halo around bright lights
d. flashing lights for a short period of time
e. unable to wipe away dark spots in visual field

4. Health maintenance and promotion of the ear include all *except*
   a. encouraging immunization against childhood measles, mumps, and rubella
   b. wearing ear protectors with noise levels above 70 dB
   c. monitoring environmental noise levels
   d. monitoring hearing on clients receiving ototoxic drugs
5. Postoperatively, the client who has had cataract extraction will need to
   a. stay in bed for several days
   b. wear an eye shield for 1 month, especially at night
   c. receive narcotics for 24 to 48 hours for pain
   d. have an immediate fitting with prescription glasses
6. Pilocarpine eyedrops
   a. dilate the pupil
   b. constrict the pupil
   c. decrease the flow of aqueous humor
   d. relax iris sphincter muscle
7. Characteristics of serous otitis media may include
   a. thick, mucoid middle ear fluid
   b. eustachian tube obstruction
   c. perforated eardrum
   d. retracted eardrum
8. The client who has a sensorineural hearing loss will
   a. have difficulty understanding speech
   b. hear high-pitched sounds better
   c. be directed to discontinue ototoxic drugs
   d. not experience muffled sounds with a hearing aid
9. The least expensive contact lens as far as cost, equipment, and follow-up care are concerned is the
   a. soft lens
   b. hard lens
   c. gas-permeable lens
   d. extended-wear lens
10. When communicating with a hearing-impaired client, it is helpful to
    a. increase voice pitch
    b. have light behind the speaker
    c. increase enunciation
    d. avoid hands to face
11. An important nursing responsibility in aiding a client to adapt to a loss of vision is to
    a. relieve the client of the need to make decisions
    b. teach the family to care for the client
    c. encourage the client to be as independent as possible
    d. see to the client's physical needs

REFERENCES

1. Public Information Committee: Eye injuries: prevention and first aid, American Academy of Ophthalmology, 1987, p 1.

2. InVision, Bausch and Lomb, Quincy, Mass, 1987, InVision Institute, p 1.

3. Moses R: Accommodation. In Moses RA, ed: Adler's physiology of the eye: clinical application, ed 8, St Louis, 1987, The CV Mosby Co, p 309.

4. Pederson K and Nulty G: Nursing grand rounds: herpes zoster ophthalmicus, J Ophthal Nurs Technol 6:153, 1987.

5. Parke D and Hamill BM: Injury to the eye. In Mattox K, Moore E, and Feliciano D, eds: Trauma, Norwalk, Conn, 1988, Appleton & Lange, p 289.

6. Tarail J: Sjogren's syndrome, Am J Nurs 87:325, 1987.

7. National Advisory Eye Council: Vision research: a national plan executive summary, 1983-1987, Pub No 82-2469, Washington, DC, Public Health Service, National Institutes of Health—Department of Health Education and Welfare, US Government Printing Office, p 7.

8. Eye Bank Associations of America: The 1988 report of eyebanking activity, Eye Bank Associations of America, Washington, DC, p 2.

9. Anterior Segment Panel Quality of Care Committee: Cataract in the otherwise healthy eye, San Francisco, 1990, American Academy of Ophthalmology, p 2.

10. Newell F: Ophthalmic surgery: principles and concepts, ed 4, St Louis, 1987, The CV Mosby Co, p 86.

11. Jaffe N: Cataract surgery and its complications, ed 4, St Louis, 1987, The CV Mosby Co, p 327.

12. Public Information Committee: Detached and torn retina, San Francisco, 1987, American Academy of Ophthalmology, p 1.

13. Hosein A: Use of silicone oil in vitreo-retinal surgery, J Ophthal Nurs Technol 7:127, 1988.

14. Retinal Panel Quality of Care Committee: Diabetic retinopathy, San Francisco, 1989, American Academy of Ophthalmology, p 2.

15. Burlew J: Diabetic retinopathy: the path to blindness can be blocked, J Ophthal Nurs Technol 4:12, 1989.

16. Anterior Segment Panel Quality of Care Committee: Glaucoma, San Francisco, 1989, American Academy of Ophthalmology, p 7.

17. Vaughan D and Asbury T: General ophthalmology, ed 11, Los Altos, Calif, 1986, Lange Medical, p 172.

18. Sherwood M: The Schocket procedure: anterior chamber shunt to an encircling band, J Ophthal Nurs Technol 5:187, 1986.

19. Chan P: Ocular pharmacology review. Paper presented at meeting of the American Society of Ophthalmic Registered Nurses Association, Philadelphia, July 1989.

20. Vaughan D and Asbury T: General ophthalmology, ed 12, Norwalk, Conn, 1989, Lange Medical Publications, p 178.

21. Mines J and Kaplan H: Acquired immunodeficiency syndrome, Int Ophthalmol Clin 26:75, 1986.

22. Parrish C, O'Day D, and Hoge T: Spontaneous fungal ulcers as ocular manifestation of acquired immunodeficiency syndrome, Am J Ophthalmol 303:104, 1987.

23. Pomerantz R and others: Infection of the retina by human immunodeficiency virus type I, N Engl J Med 317:1645, 1989.

24. Henderly M and others: Cytomegalovirus retinitis as the initial manifestation of the acquired immune deficiency syndrome, Am J Ophthalmol 103:316, 1987.

25. Booth JB, ed: Scott-Brown's otolaryngology—otology, ed 5, London, 1987, Butterworths, p 102.

26. DeWeese DD and others: Otolaryngology—head and neck surgery, ed 7, St Louis, 1988, The CV Mosby Co, p 396.

27. DeWeese DD and others: Otolaryngology—head and neck surgery, ed 7, St Louis, 1988, The CV Mosby Co, p 457.

28. Templer J and others, eds: Otolaryngology—head and neck surgery: principles and concepts, St Louis, 1987, Ishiyaku EuroAmerican, p 49.

29. DeWeese DD and others: Otolaryngology—head and neck surgery, ed 7, St Louis, 1988, The CV Mosby Co, p 444.

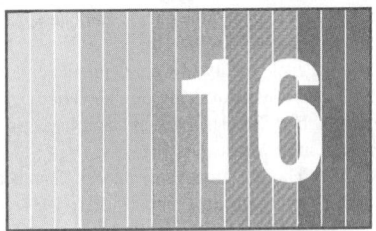

CHAPTER

16

Nursing Assessment
Integumentary System

Idolia Cox Collier

L *earning Objectives*

1. *Describe the structures and functions of the integumentary system.*
2. *Describe age-related changes in the integumentary system and differences in assessment findings.*
3. *Describe the significant subjective and objective data related to the integumentary system that should be obtained from a client.*
4. *Describe specific assessments to be made during the physical examination of the skin and appendages.*
5. *Explain the critical components for describing a lesion.*

6. *Describe the appropriate techniques used in the physical assessment of the integumentary system.*
7. *Explain the structural and assessment differences in black skin.*
8. *Differentiate normal from common abnormal findings of a physical assessment of the integumentary system.*
9. *Describe the purpose, the significance of results, and the nursing responsibilities of diagnostic studies of the integumentary system.*

The integumentary system is composed of the skin, hair, nails, and glands (sebaceous, apocrine, and eccrine). The skin is further divided into three layers: the epidermis, dermis, and subcutaneous layers (Fig. 16-1).

STRUCTURES OF THE SKIN AND APPENDAGES
Epidermis

The *epidermis* is the thin (0.06 mm to 0.1 mm), avascular outermost layer of the skin. It is nourished by diffusion from blood vessels in the dermis and returns waste products in the same way. The two types of cells of the epidermis are melanocytes (5%) and keratinocytes (95%).

Melanocytes are scattered throughout the basal layer of the epidermis. They produce melanin, a pigment that shields the deeper structures of the skin from sunlight. All races have basically the same number of melanocytes. The wide range of skin colors is due to the size and distribution of the melanosomes produced by the melanocytes. Sunlight and hormones stimulate melanin production.

Keratinocytes develop from cells in the basal layer of the epidermis. After division, one cell remains in the basal

cell layer and is called a *basal cell*. The other keratinocyte makes its way to the skin surface (stratum corneum of the epidermis), where it flattens, dehydrates, and becomes keratinized.[1] The upward movement of keratinocytes from the basement membrane to the stratum corneum takes about 14 days. The sloughing of the stratum corneum takes an additional 14 to 30 days. If dead cells slough off too rapidly, the skin will appear thin, eroded, or atrophic. If new cells are forming faster than old cells are shed, the skin becomes scaly and thickened. Deviations in this cycle account for many dermatological problems. Keratinocytes produce a specialized protein (keratin), which is vital to the protective barrier function of the skin.

Dermis

The *dermis* (1 to 4 mm thick) is the layer beneath the epidermis and the principal mass of the skin. It gives the skin substance, provides support, and functions to absorb and reduce environmental stress and strain. It is composed primarily of fibrils of collagen. In addition, there are blood vessels, nerves, lymphatic vessels, hair follicles, and sebaceous and sweat glands. Collagen, water, and a gel-like ground substance serve to support the structures of the epidermis and dermis. Collagen is responsible for the mechanical strength of the skin.

Reviewed by Sandra J. Somma, R.N., B.S.N., Yale New Haven Hospital, Yale University School of Medicine, Department of Dermatology, New Haven, Connecticut.

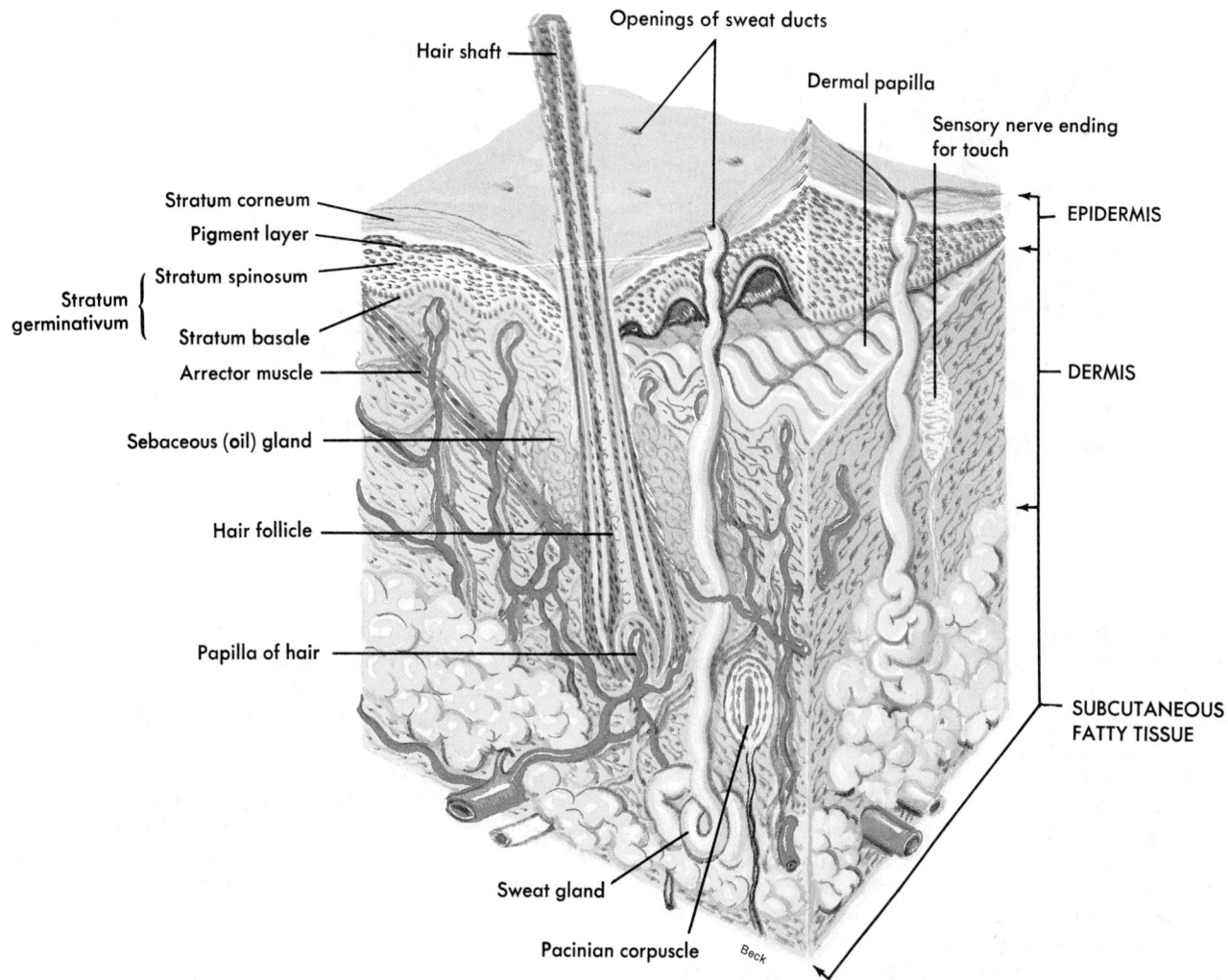

Hair shaft

Openings of sweat ducts

Dermal papilla

Sensory nerve ending for touch

Stratum corneum

Pigment layer

Stratum spinosum

Stratum germinativum {

Stratum basale

Arrector muscle

Sebaceous (oil) gland

Hair follicle

Papilla of hair

Sweat gland

Pacinian corpuscle

EPIDERMIS

DERMIS

SUBCUTANEOUS FATTY TISSUE

Beck

Fig. 16-1 Microscopic view of the skin in longitudinal section. The epidermis is shown raised at one corner to reveal the dermal papillae. (From Anthony C and Thibodeau G: Textbook of anatomy and physiology, ed 12, St Louis, 1987, The CV Mosby Co, p 77.)

Subcutaneous Layer

The *subcutaneous layer,* or hypodermis, is constructed of loose connective tissue and fat cells. This layer gives substance to the skin and is similar to the dermis except for the presence of fat cells. The anatomical distribution of the subcutaneous layer is a secondary sex characteristic and is also controlled by heredity, age, and eating habits. The subcutaneous layer acts as a shock absorber and insulator for the body.

Epidermal Appendages

Appendages of the skin include the hair, nails, and glands (apocrine, eccrine, and sebaceous). These originate from the epidermal layer, although they are anatomically located in both the epidermis and the dermis. They receive nutrients, electrolytes, fluids, and innervation from the dermis. Hair and nails are specialized keratin that becomes dry and firm. The growth of hair (Fig. 16-1) occurs in sev-

eral phases. Each hair goes through a resting (telogen), a growth (anagen), and transitional (catagen) phase. A scattered pattern of phases keeps the numbers of hairs relatively constant. Chemical, mechanical, or psychological factors can convert all hair to the atrophy phase, resulting in baldness. There are no hair follicles on the palms or soles. No new hair-producing structures develop after birth. Scalp hair grows about 1 cm per month, and 50 to 100 hairs are lost each day.

Nails grow from the nail matrix, which is usually hidden by skin at the base of the nail (Fig. 16-2). Nails grow at one third the rate of hair. Fingernails grow faster (0.1 mm/day) than toenails (0.05 mm/day). Nails can be injured by direct trauma and are subject to the same problems as the skin. Abnormal nails (e.g., Beau's lines, psoriatic pits) result from an epidermal problem affecting the nail matrix that gives rise to the nail plate.

Sebaceous, apocrine, and eccrine glands complete the

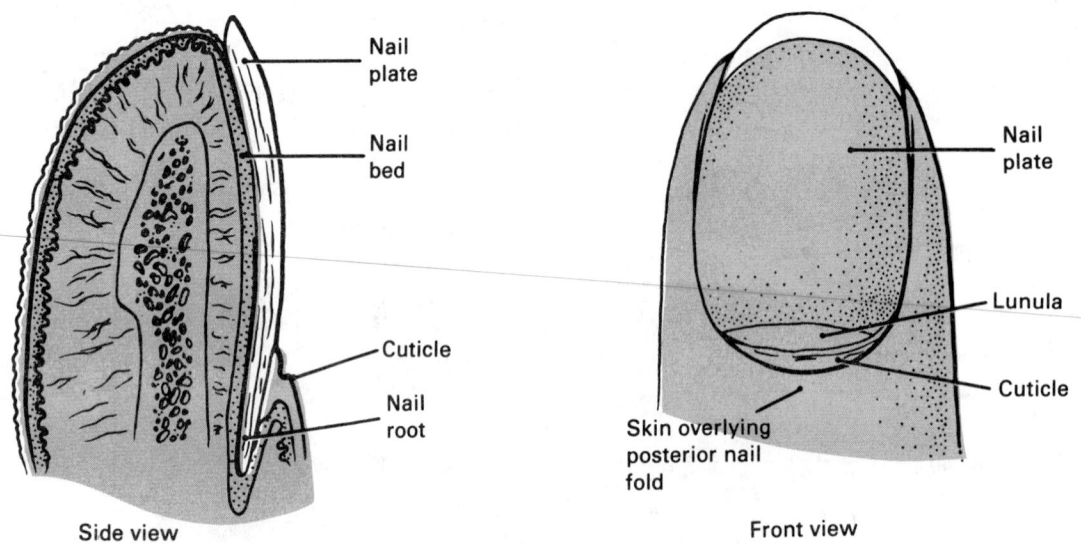

Side view   Front view

Fig. 16-2   Structure of a nail.

epidermal or accessory appendages. The *sebaceous glands* secrete sebum, a complex lipid mixture that is emptied into the hair shaft. These glands depend on the male hormone androgen to initiate and continue production. Sebaceous glands are present on all areas of the skin except the palms and soles. They are most numerous and largest on the face, scalp, upper chest, and back. The activity of sebaceous glands is under hormonal control.

Apocrine gland secretion serves no known function in human beings.[2] These glands secrete an odorless fluid from the hair shaft that produces a distinctive body odor when acted on by bacteria normally present on the skin. These glands are found in the axillae, the anogenital and periumbilical areas, the areolae, the external auditory canal (ceruminous glands), and the eyelids (glands of Moll).[3] Apocrine glands become functional at puberty, atrophy with age, and are mediated by adrenergic innervation and by the circulating catecholamines epinephrine and norepinephrine.

Eccrine (sweat) glands are mediated by cholinergic innervation. Heat is the primary stimulus, but other physiological stimuli, including stress, are important. They are located all over the body, especially on the forehead, palms, and soles. Eccrine glands secrete sweat to the surface of the body by sweat ducts. Increased sweat production in response to heat is part of the thermoregulatory system.

FUNCTIONS OF THE SKIN

The skin is the largest organ of the body, and its primary function is to protect the underlying tissue by acting as a surface barrier to the external environment. The skin also protects by preventing excessive loss of water and mechanical trauma and by inhibiting bacterial invasion.

The skin is the major receptor for general sensation. The nerve endings within the skin supply information to the brain related to pain, touch, pressure, and temperature. The skin controls heat regulation by its ability to respond to internal and external temperature variations by vasoconstriction or vasodilation. Coincidental to heat regulation is the skin's function of excretion. Between 600 and 900 ml of water is lost daily through insensible perspiration. Endogenous production of vitamin D_3, which is critical to bone metabolism, occurs in the epidermis.

The fat of the subcutaneous layer insulates the body. The aesthetic functions of the skin include the mirroring of emotions as well as displaying the individual identity of a person. Since it is almost a complete barrier, the skin plays a minimal role in absorption.

EFFECTS OF AGING

The rate of age-related skin changes is influenced by the person's history of sun exposure, hygiene practices, heredity, nutrition, and general state of health. Exposure to ultraviolet rays is the major contributor to the look of aging skin. Wrinkling of sun-exposed areas such as the face is worse than on sun-shielded areas such as the buttocks. In addition, a decrease in the level of sex hormones and atrophy of the skin and epidermal appendages correlate with the look of aging.

Dry, thin skin, graying hair, lax skin, increased capillary permeability, the presence of lentigines (brown spots), and seborrheic keratoses all confirm advancing age. A variety of neoplasms appear on the skin as a part of the aging process. These benign growths include seborrheic keratoses, cherry angiomas, and skin tags.[4] A common premalignant lesion is the actinic keratosis, which appears on areas of chronic sun exposure. In older adults, two less common findings that are directly related to sun exposure are squamous cell carcinoma and basal cell carcinoma.

Poor nutrition contributes to aging of the skin through a decrease in protein, calories, and vitamins. The collagen stiffens, elastic fibers degenerate, and the amount of subcutaneous tissue decreases. These changes, with the added effects of gravity, lead to wrinkling (Fig. 16-3). Blood vessels close to the skin give a ruddy appearance. Sweat-

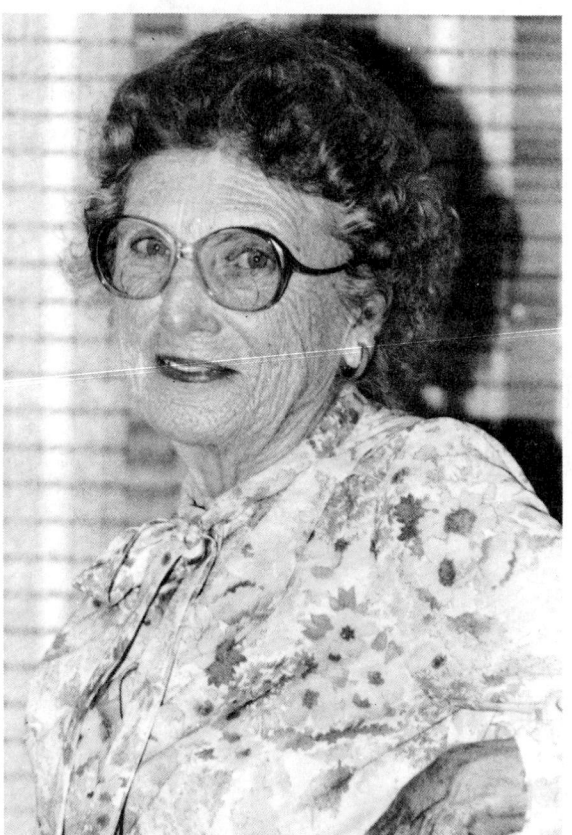

Fig. 16-3   A lifetime of high sun exposure in a dry south-western state resulted in deep wrinkling in this older woman.

Table 16-1   Normal Physical Assessment of the Integumentary System

Skin pink and warm; good turgor; no petechiae, purpura, lesions, or excoriations
Nails pink, round, and mobile with 160-degree angle
Hair shiny and full
Amount and distribution of hair appropriate for age and sex
No flaking of the scalp, forehead, or pinna

Table 16-2   Questions to Ask When a Skin Problem Is Present

When did it start?
Where did it start?
Are you still getting new outbreaks?
Has the lesion/rash/problem changed from its initial appearance?
Has it spread? How?
Does it itch or hurt you?
Was there any change in your health, hygiene, or environment before the outbreak?
Does anything make it better? Worse?
Have you treated it in any way? Any previous medical interventions?

ing diminishes as eccrine glands become less active. The rate of hair and nail production decreases as a result of atrophy of the involved structures. Vitamin deficiencies can cause dry, thin hair that has a tendency to fall out. (See Table 16-3 for age-related changes in the skin.)

ASSESSMENT OF THE INTEGUMENTARY SYSTEM

The assessment of the skin begins at the initial contact with the client and continues throughout the examination. Specific areas of the skin are examined during examination of other areas of the body unless the chief complaint is that of a dermatological problem. A general statement about the skin should be recorded (Table 16-1) and specific problems should be noted under the appropriate system. In addition to the usual procedure performed in investigation of a problem (see Chapter 3), questions presented in Table 16-2 should also be asked when a skin problem is noted.

Subjective Data

Health history

Past health history. Past health history will indicate the reasons for scars related to trauma or surgery. Specific major illnesses that could have dermatological implications include collagen, renal, and hepatic diseases and certain immune disorders. A careful medication history is impor-

tant, especially in relation to vitamins, steroids, hormones, and antimetabolites. Any food, drug, or contact allergy and the specific pattern of allergic reaction should be recorded.

Family history. The client should be questioned about a family history of diabetes, blood dyscrasias, allergic disorders, cancer (specifically skin cancers such as melanoma), and specific dermatological problems. Many congenital or familial problems, such as neurofibromatosis, have skin manifestations as the primary or secondary problem. Often these conditions are rare. The client should be asked whether such problems are present in any member of the family.

Social and personal history. The unique identity and lifestyle of a client often affect the skin. Advancing age brings anticipated changes to the skin. Wrinkling and coolness result from a loss of subcutaneous fat. Decreased blood flow to the skin produces a thickening of fingernails and toenails and a loss of hair. Dry skin can result from local climate conditions, excessive exposure to sun, and poor nutrition and hydration.

Hygiene practices and use of cosmetics should be investigated carefully. Specific brand names of preparations that are used should be recorded. A diet history will reveal the adequacy of nutrients essential to healthy skin, such as vitamins A, D, E, and C; dietary fat; and protein. Food allergies should be elicited. The client should be questioned regarding the influence of environmental factors such as exposure to irritants, the sun, unusual cold, or unhygienic conditions related to recreation or occupation. Skin rashes

MACULE

A circumscribed, flat discoloration, which may be brown, blue, red, or hypopigmented

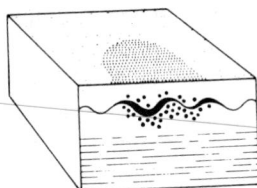

PLAQUE

A circumscribed, elevated, superficial, solid lesion more than 0.5 cm in diameter, often formed by the confluence of papules

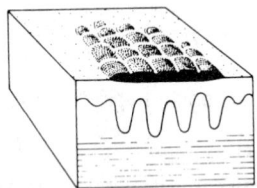

WHEAL

A firm edematous plaque resulting from infiltration of the dermis with fluid; wheals are transient and may last only a few hours

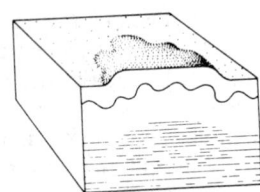

VESICLE

A circumscribed collection of free fluid up to 0.5 cm in diameter

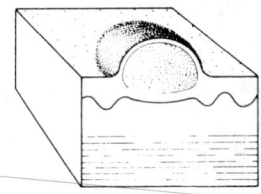

PAPULE

An elevated solid lesion up to 0.5 cm in diameter; color varies; papules may become confluent and form plaques

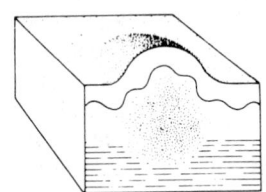

NODULE

A circumscribed, elevated, solid lesion more than 0.5 cm in diameter; a large nodule is referred to as a tumor

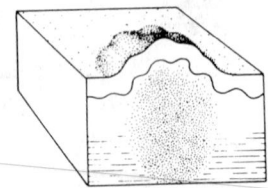

PUSTULE

A circumscribed collection of leukocytes and free fluid that varies in size

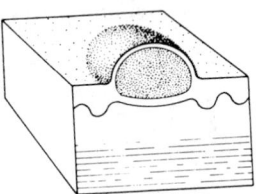

Fig. 16-4 Characteristics of primary skin lesions. (From Habif T: Clinical dermatology: a color guide to diagnosis and therapy, ed 2, St Louis, 1990, Mosby–Year Book, Inc.)

due to allergies and irritants are among the most common occupational problems. Exercise and sleep practices should be investigated. The client should be encouraged to express the personal and emotional implications of the dermatological problem.

Review of systems. It is important to obtain a history of cutaneous changes. The client should be specifically questioned about any past problems, such as rashes, lumps, itching, dryness, lesions, ecchymoses, and masses. The nurse should also ask about specific changes in the skin, hair, and nails and a change in a specific lesion such as a mole that has changed in its size, color, or texture. If the client admits to any of these problems, specific characteristics of the symptom should be obtained.

Objective Data

Physical examination. Characteristics of primary (basic) skin lesions are shown in Fig. 16-4. Secondary skin lesions are shown in Fig. 16-5.

General principles of the assessment of the skin are as follows:

1. Have a good source of light, preferably daylight.
2. See that the client is undressed for an adequate skin examination.
3. Be systematic and proceed from head to toe.
4. Compare symmetrical parts.
5. Perform general inspection and then lesion-specific examination.
6. Use the metric system for measurements.

SCALES

Excess dead epidermal cells that are produced by abnormal keratinization and shedding

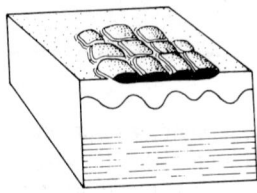

EROSIONS

A focal loss of epidermis; erosions do not penetrate below the dermoepidermal junction and therefore heal without scarring

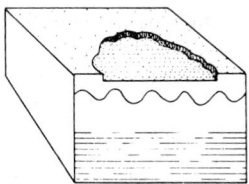

FISSURE

A linear loss of epidermis and dermis with sharply defined, nearly vertical walls

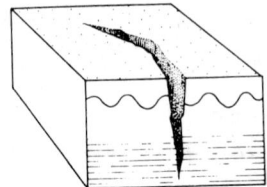

CRUSTS

A collection of dried serum and cellular debris; a scab

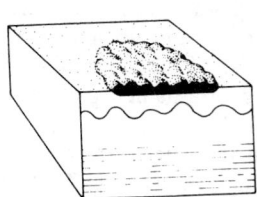

SCAR

An abnormal formation of connective tissue implying dermal damage; after injury or surgery scars are initially thick and pink but with time become white and atrophic

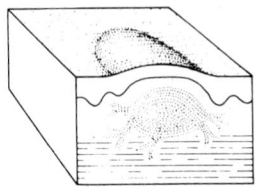

ULCERS

A focal loss of epidermis and dermis; ulcers heal with scarring

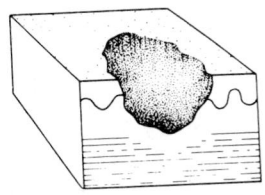

ATROPHY

A depression in the skin resulting from thinning of the epidermis or dermis

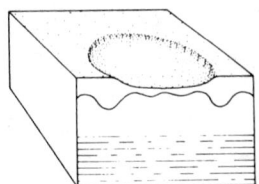

Fig. 16-5　Characteristics of secondary skin lesions. (From Habif T: Clinical dermatology: a color guide to diagnosis and therapy, ed 2, St Louis, 1990, Mosby–Year Book, Inc.)

7. Use appropriate terminology and nomenclature when reporting or recording. Photographs are useful to document findings.

Inspection

COLOR. The skin is inspected for color, vascularity, and the presence of lesions. The critical factor in assessment of skin color is change. Many skin colors that are normal for a particular client are signs of a pathophysiological condition in another client. The color of the skin depends on the amount of melanin (brown), carotene (yellow), oxyhemoglobin (red), and reduced hemoglobin (bluish-red) present at a particular time. The most reliable areas in which to assess color are the areas of least pigmentation, such as the sclera, conjunctiva, nail beds, lips, and buccal mucosa.

Table 16-3

Age-Related Changes of the Integumentary System and Differences in Assessment Findings

Changes	Differences in Assessment Findings
SKIN	
Decreased subcutaneous fat, muscle laxity, degeneration of elastic fibers, collagen stiffening	Increased wrinkling, sagging breasts, redundant flesh around eyes, slowness of skin to flatten when pinched together (tenting)
Decreased extracellular water, surface lipids, and sebaceous gland activity	Dry, flaking skin with possible signs of excoriation due to pruritus
Less active apocrine and sebaceous gland activity	Dry skin with minimal to no perspiration
Increased capillary fragility and permeability	Evidence of bruising
Increased melanocytes in basal layer with pigment accumulation	Senile lentigines on face and back of hands
Diminished blood supply	Decrease in rosy appearance of skin and mucous membrane; cool to touch; diminished awareness of pain, touch, temperature, and peripheral vibration
Decrease in proliferative capacity	Diminished rate of wound healing
HAIR	
Decreased melanin and melanocytes	Graying hair
Decreased oil	Dry, coarse hair; scaly scalp
Decrease in density of hair follicles	Thinning and loss of hair, loss of hair in outer one half or one third of eyebrow
Cumulative androgen effect, decreasing estrogen levels	Facial hirsutism; baldness
NAILS	
Decreased peripheral blood supply	Thick, brittle nails with diminished growth
Increased keratin	Ridging
Decreased circulation	Prolonged return of blood to nails on blanching

Activity, emotions, cigarette smoking, and edema as well as respiratory, cardiovascular, and hepatic problems can all directly affect the color of the skin.

VASCULARITY. The skin is examined for problems related to vascularity, such as areas of bruising, and vascular and purpuric lesions, such as angioma, petechiae, or purpura. Reaction to direct pressure should be noted. If a lesion blanches on direct pressure and then refills, the redness is due to dilated blood vessels. If the discoloration remains, it is the result of subcutaneous or intradermal bleeding that may be due to vasculitis. This examination technique, called *diascopy*, uses a magnifying glass, microscope slide, or clear plastic plate.

LESIONS. If a lesion is found on inspection of the skin, a detailed examination must follow. Type, color, size, distribution and grouping, location, and consistency should be recorded. Characteristics of common skin lesions are described in Figs. 16-4 and 16-5. Lesions should be measured with a transparent ruler. If more than one lesion is present, the range of sizes should be recorded. Distribution refers to the localized or generalized occurrence of the lesion. Many skin diseases have characteristic distribution. For example, acne affects the face, upper chest, and back; psoriasis affects the knees and elbows (among other areas); and *Monilia* infections affect intertriginous areas. Group-

ing or configuration is identified as annular (circular), linear (in a line), or clustered (a group of lesions located close together). The location of the lesion should be carefully described. A full-body diagram is often useful for this purpose. Accurate description and documentation of this information are the key. Use of the appropriate terms to describe the lesion should give a mental picture of the lesion.

Age-related changes in the integumentary system and differences in assessment findings are listed in Table 16-3. Common assessment abnormalities of the skin are described in Table 16-4.

Palpation. Palpation of the skin provides information about temperature, turgor and mobility, moisture, and texture. Temperature of the skin is best assessed by palpating the upper lip, palms, or forehead with the backs of the hands. The temperature of the skin increases when blood flow to the dermis is increased. There will be a localized increase with burns and local inflammation. A generalized increase in temperature will result from fever. A decreased body temperature will be noted when there is shock, chilling, or emotional trauma.

Turgor and mobility refer to the elasticity of the skin. There is a loss of turgor with dehydration and aging. Emotional tension increases muscle tension and consequently

Table 16-4

Common Assessment Abnormalities of the Skin

Finding	Description	Possible Etiology and Significance
Alopecia	Loss of hair (localized or general)	Heredity, friction, rubbing, traction, trauma, infection, inflammation, chemotherapy, pregnancy, stress, emotional shock, tinea capitis, immunological factors
Angioma	Tumor consisting of blood or lymph vessels	Normal increase with aging, liver disease, pregnancy, varicose veins
Carotenemia (carotenosis)	Yellow discoloration of skin, no yellowing of sclerae, most noticeable on palms and soles	Vegetables containing carotene (e.g., carrots, squash), hypothyroidism
Comedo (blackheads and whiteheads)	Keratin, sebum, microorganism, and epithelial debris within a dilated follicular opening	Acne vulgaris
Cyanosis	Slightly bluish gray or dark purple discoloration of the skin and mucous membranes due to presence of excessive amounts of reduced hemoglobin in capillaries	Cardiorespiratory problems; vasoconstriction, asphyxiation, anemia, leukemia, and malignancies
Cyst	Sac containing fluid or semisolid material	Obstruction of a duct or gland, parasitic infection
Depigmentation (vitiligo)	Congenital or acquired loss of melanin resulting in white, depigmented areas	Genetic, chemical and pharmacological agents, nutritional and endocrine factors, burns and trauma, inflammation and infection
Ecchymosis	Large, bruiselike lesion caused by collection of extravascular blood in dermis and subcutaneous tissue	Trauma, bleeding disorders
Erythema	Redness occurring in patches of variable size and shape	Heat, certain drugs, alcohol, ultraviolet rays, any problem that causes dilatation of blood vessels to the skin
Excoriation	Superficial excavations of epidermis	Pruritus, trauma
Hematoma	Extravasation of blood of sufficient size to cause visible swelling	Trauma, bleeding disorders
Hirsutism	Male distribution of hair in women and children	Abnormality of gonads or adrenal glands, decrease in estrogen levels, familial trait
Intertrigo	Dermatitis of apposing surfaces of the skin	Moisture, obesity, *Monilia* infections
Jaundice	Yellow (in whites) or yellowish-brown (in blacks) discoloration of the skin, best observed in the sclera secondary to increased bilirubin in the blood	Liver disease, red blood cell hemolysis; pancreatic cancer, common bile duct obstruction
Keloid	Hypertrophied scar beyond margin of incision or trauma	Predisposition more common in blacks
Lichenification	Thickening of the skin with accentuated skin markings	Repeated scratching and irritation
Mole (melanocytic nevus)	Benign overgrowth of melanocytes	Defects of development; excessive numbers and large, irregular moles often familial
Petechiae	Pinpoint, discrete deposit of blood less than 1 to 2 mm in the extravascular tissues and visible through the skin or mucous membrane	Inflammation, marked dilatation, blood vessel trauma, blood dyscrasias that result in bleeding tendencies (e.g., thrombocytopenia)
Telangiectasia	Visibly dilated, superficial, cutaneous small blood vessels, commonly found on face and thighs	Aging, acne, sun exposure, alcohol, liver failure, steroid medication, irradiation, certain systemic diseases, and skin tumors; normal variant
Tenting	Failure of skin to return immediately to normal position after gentle pinching	Aging, dehydration, cachexia
Varicosity	Increased prominence of superficial veins	Interruption of venous return (e.g., from tumor, incompetent valves, inflammation)

increases skin turgor. The examiner assesses turgor by gently pinching an area of skin together. The best area to use for assessing turgor is the skin over the sternum. Skin with good turgor will immediately return to its original position.

Moisture of the skin is the dampness or dryness of the skin. Moisture increases in intertriginous (two approximate surfaces) areas. The amount of moisture present on the skin varies with the temperature of the environment, muscular activity, and body temperature. Skin dries with age as a result of a decrease in the activity of the sebaceous glands and a decrease in surface lipids, which allows for greater evaporation. Decreased humidity also causes dry skin.

Texture refers to the fineness or coarseness of the skin. Extremes of either type of texture can reflect local trauma or systemic disease. For example, in hyperthyroidism the skin is fine, and in hypothyroidism the skin is coarse. Increased thickness is often work-related and should not be mistaken for a pathophysiological condition. It may be the result of repeated injury through rubbing or itching (lichenification) and may indicate an underlying problem.

Assessment of Black Skin

The degree of color of black-skinned persons is genetically determined. The dark skin color results from the reflection of light as it strikes the underlying skin pigment. Increased activity of melanocytes resulting in large

Table 16-5

Diagnostic Studies of the Integumentary System		
Study	Description and Purpose	Nursing Responsibility
BIOPSY		
Punch, excisional or incisional, shave	Small sample of skin is removed for microscopic examination to determine diagnosis of a specific problem.	Verify that consent form is signed. Inform client that local anesthetic may be used. Assist with procedure. Instruct client to keep biopsy area dry until healed and to contact physician for biopsy result. Ensure that specimen is tagged properly for superior, inferior, medial, and lateral edges.
MICROSCOPIC TESTS		
Potassium hydroxide	Hair, scales, or nails are examined for hyphae of fungus infection. Specimen is put on glass slide and 10% to 40% concentration of potassium hydroxide is added.	Instruct client regarding purpose of test. Prepare slide.
Tzanck test (Wright's, Giemsa's, and Papanicolaou stain)	Fluid and cells from vesicles or bullae are examined to diagnose herpes virus. Specimen is put on slide, stained, and examined microscopically for multinucleated giant cells.	Inform client of purpose of test. Use sterile technique for collection of fluid.
Culture	The test will identify fungal, bacterial, and viral organisms. For fungi, scraping is performed if the fungus is superficial; biopsy is performed if the fungus is systemic involving the skin. For bacteria, material is obtained from intact pustules, bullae, or abscesses. For viruses, bullae are scraped and exudate is taken from center of lesion.	Instruct client regarding purpose and specific procedure. Refrigerate specimen if not sent to laboratory immediately.
MISCELLANEOUS		
Wood's light	Examination of skin with long-wave ultraviolet light causes specific substances to fluoresce (e.g., *Pseudomonas* organisms, erythrasma, fungal infections, vitiligo).	Explain purpose of examination. Inform client it is not painful.

amounts of melanin production accounts for the darker skin color. This increased melanin forms a natural sun shield for black skin.

The structures and functions of black skin are basically no different than those of white skin, but they are more difficult to assess. Practice and comparison are necessary. Less pigmented areas such as the buccal mucosa, tongue, lips, and nail beds are areas that best indicate color changes such as cyanosis and pallor.[5] Rashes are often difficult to observe and may need to be palpated.

Black skin is predisposed to certain skin conditions. These include pseudofolliculitis, keloids, and mongolian spots. Because of the darkness of the skin of some black persons, color often cannot be used as an indicator of systemic conditions (e.g., flushed skin with fever).

DIAGNOSTIC STUDIES

The main diagnostic technique related to skin problems is inspection of an individual lesion and a careful history related to the problem. If a definitive diagnosis cannot be made by inspection alone, other tests may be indicated (Table 16-5).

A biopsy of a characteristic skin lesion is a common diagnostic aid. Early lesions are usually selected for biopsy because they are most typical. A biopsy is indicated in all conditions in which malignancy is suspected or a specific diagnosis is questionable.

Incisional, excisional, and scrape or shave biopsies can be both therapeutic and diagnostic. A punch biopsy is performed with a small tubular knife that looks much like a cookie cutter. This tool cuts out a small piece of tissue for microscopic examination. The size of the biopsy specimen is determined by the location of the biopsy. If the site is normally visible, such as on the face, the smallest possible piece of tissue that will still yield an accurate diagnosis is taken. Immunofluorescence, a special technique used on the biopsy specimen, may be indicated in certain conditions, such as bullous diseases and lupus erythematosus.

R eview Questions

The number of the question corresponds to the same-numbered objective at the beginning of the chapter.
1. The main component of the dermis is
   a. keratin
   b. fat cells
   c. blood vessels
   d. collagen
2. The most important factor in aging of skin relates to
   a. nutrition
   b. sun exposure
   c. heredity
   d. use of makeup
3. The best area to assess skin color is the
   a. conjunctivae
   b. buttocks
   c. hands
   d. cheeks
4. When a lesion blanches on direct pressure, the redness is due to a
   a. vasculitis
   b. dilated blood vessel
   c. intradermal hemorrhage
   d. ecchymosis
5. Lesions that are in a circle are referred to as
   a. clustered
   b. linear
   c. annular
6. The most important assessment technique related to the skin is
   a. inspection
   b. palpation
   c. percussion
   d. auscultation
7. Black skin is less susceptible to sunburn than lighter skin because of the presence of increased amounts of
   a. melanin
   b. keratin
   c. stratum corneum
   d. follicles
8. The most common cause of an excoriation is
   a. vasoconstriction
   b. pruritus
   c. moisture
   d. hemolysis
9. Herpesvirus diseases are diagnosed by the use of
   a. Tzanck test
   b. Wood's light
   c. potassium hydroxide
   d. punch biopsy

REFERENCES

1. Hill MJ: The skin: anatomy and physiology, Dermatol Nurs 2:13, 1990.
2. Arnold HL, Odom RB, and James WD, eds: Andrews' diseases of the skin, ed 8, Philadelphia, 1990, WB Saunders Co, p 9.
3. Lever WF and Schaumburg G: Histopathology of the skin, ed 7, Philadelphia, 1990, JB Lippincott Co, p 24.
4. Fenske NA, Gravson LD, and Newcomer VD: Common problems of aging skin, Patient Care 23:225, 1989.
5. Fitzpatrick TB and others: Dermatology in general medicine, ed 3, New York, 1987, McGraw-Hill Book Co, p 24.

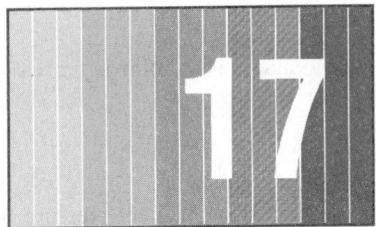

CHAPTER

17

Nursing Role in Management

Problems of the Integumentary System

Idolia Cox Collier

Learning Objectives

1. Describe health promotion and maintenance practices related to the skin.
2. Explain the etiology, clinical manifestations, and therapeutic and nursing management of common acute dermatological problems.
3. Describe the psychological and physiological effects of chronic dermatological conditions.
4. Explain the etiology, clinical manifestations, and management of malignant dermatological disorders.
5. Explain the etiology, clinical manifestations, and management of bacterial, viral, and fungal infections of the integument.
6. Explain the etiology, clinical manifestations, and management of infestations and bites.

7. Explain the etiology, clinical manifestations, and management of dermatological disorders related to allergies.
8. Explain the etiology, clinical manifestations, and management related to benign dermatological disorders.
9. Describe the dermatological manifestations of common systemic diseases.
10. Explain the indications and nursing management related to plastic surgery and skin grafts.
11. Explain the etiology, clinical manifestations, and management of pressure sores.

Problems of the skin are often difficult to manage because of the visibility of this organ. Although clothing and cosmetics can disguise or cover some skin problems, many problems cannot be hidden so easily. The emotional impact of skin problems often is more serious than the skin problem itself. For instance, acne is little more than a nuisance disease in relation to systemic health. However, to the adolescent attempting to establish personal identity, it can be a barrier to establishment of a peer group and pleasant social outlets.

A dichotomy often exists between the actual seriousness of a skin problem and the emotional impact of the problem. The therapeutic and nursing management of integumentary problems is presented before specific problems are discussed. These general considerations common to many dermatological problems apply to many specific diseases as well.

Reviewed by Sandra Somma, R.N., B.S.N., Yale New Haven Hospital, Yale University School of Medicine, Department of Dermatology, New Haven, Connecticut.

◼ Therapeutic and Nursing Management of the Integumentary System

Health promotion and maintenance

Health promotion and maintenance practices related to problems of the skin often parallel health practices appropriate for general good health. The skin reflects both physical and psychological well-being. Specific health promotion and maintenance activities appropriate to good skin health include avoidance of environmental hazards, adequate rest and exercise, proper hygiene and nutrition, and cautious use of self-treatment.

Environmental hazards

SUN. Many people are unaware that the effects of years of exposure to the sun are cumulative and damaging. The ultraviolet (UV) rays of the sun cause degenerative changes in the dermis, which result in premature aging due to loss of elasticity and to thinning, wrinkling, and drying of the skin. Prolonged and repeated sun exposure is a major factor in precancerous and cancerous lesions. Actinic damage, actinic keratoses, basal cell epithelioma, squamous cell epithelioma, and malignant melanoma are dermatological problems associated directly or indirectly with sun exposure.[1]

Nurses should be strong advocates of moderation in sun exposure. Vitamin D_3 is produced in the skin and is necessary for vitamin D synthesis. However, only a few minutes of sun on small areas of the body is adequate to meet this need. Specific wavelengths of the sun (Table 17-1) have different effects on the skin. Tanning is the body's defense against further sunburn and is caused by increased production of melanin. The turnover time of the skin is shortened and results in peeling. Fair-skinned persons should be especially cautious about excessive sun exposure since they have smaller amounts of the natural protection afforded by melanin.

Sunscreens can block out ultraviolet A (UVA) and ultraviolet B (UVB) wavelengths. There are two types of sunscreen—chemical and physical. *Chemical sunscreens* are more frequently used, as they are more aesthetically acceptable. Chemical sunscreens work by absorbing and scattering the rays of sun on the skin. *Physical sunscreens* are thick and opaque and work by reflecting UV radiation. They block all UVA and UVB radiation, as well as visible light. They are most effective and affordable but, when applied, are thick, messy, and cosmetically unacceptable.

The Food and Drug Administration has rated popular sunscreen products. The higher the *sun protective factor (SPF)*, the greater the screening effect up to 15. SPF 15 indicates 93% protection and SPF 30 indicates 97%. Doubling the SPF does not double the protection. A summary of the various types of sunscreens is presented in Table 17-2. Para-aminobenzoic acid (PABA) has been removed from many sunscreen products because it stains clothing and can cause contact dermatitis.[2] Consumers need to select the sunscreen most appropriate for their needs (Table 17-3). Reapplication is necessary after swimming and every 1 to 2 hours if one is exercising or perspiring. Direc-

Table 17-1 Wavelengths of the Sun and Effect on Skin

Wavelength	Nanometer Rating	Effect
Short (UVC)	Below 290	Does not reach earth; blocked by atmosphere
Middle (UVB)	280-320	Causes sunburn and cumulative effect of sun damage
Long (UVA)	320-400	Can produce elastic tissue damage and actinic skin damage; contributes to formation of skin cancer

Table 17-2 Skin Types and Recommended SPF

Skin Type	Sensitivity to UV Light	Sunburn and Tanning History	Recommended Sun Protection Factor
I	Very sensitive	Always burns easily; never tans	15 or more
II	Very sensitive	Always burns easily; tans minimally	15 or more
III	Sensitive	Burns moderately; tans gradually and uniformly (light brown)	10 to 15
IV	Moderately sensitive	Burns minimally; always tans well (moderate brown)	6 to 15
V	Minimally sensitive	Rarely burns; tans profusely (dark brown)	6 to 15
VI	Insensitive	Never burns; deeply pigmented (black)	None indicated

From Pathak MA: Sunscreens and their use in the preventive treatment of sunlight-induced skin damage, J Dermatol Surg Oncol 13:739-750, 1987.

Table 17-3 Types of Sunscreens

Chemical Ingredients	UVA/UVB Protection	Comments
PABA and PABA esters	UVB	Can cause contact dermatitis; implicated in cross-sensitivity reactions in persons allergic to benzocaine, procaine, paraphenylenediamine, and sulfonamides; may cross-react with antihypertensives or diuretics to produce eczematous dermatitis
Non-PABA sunscreens: benzophenones, cinnamates	UVA, UVB (weakly)	Use if allergic to PABA
Broad-spectrum sunscreens: combination of PABA or PABA esters and benzophenones or cinnamates	UVA, UVB	Provides maximum prevention of skin damage secondary to sun exposure

From Lawler P and Schreiber S: Cutaneous malignant melanoma: nursing's role in prevention and early detection, Oncol Nurs Forum 16:349, 1989.

tions accompanying specific products should be followed as application time before exposure varies according to the product.

The nurse can also inform the client about other means of protection from the damaging effects of the sun, such as wearing a large-brimmed hat and a long-sleeved shirt or carrying an umbrella. Clients need to know that the rays of the sun are most dangerous between 10 AM and 2 PM standard time or 11 AM and 3 PM daylight time, regardless of the latitude. Even on overcast days a serious sunburn can occur, since up to 80% of UV rays can penetrate through the clouds. Other factors that increase the possibility of a sunburn include being in a hot environment, at high altitudes and in the mountains, in wind, and in or near water, which reflects 100% of the sun's rays.[3]

Certain topical and systemic medications potentiate the effect of the sun, even with brief exposure. These photosensitizing medications include the tetracyclines, tretinoin (Retin-A), some diuretics, some nonsteroidal antiinflammatory drugs, antimicrobials, hypoglycemic agents, birth control pills, sulfonamides, some antipsychotics and antidepressants, certain topical anesthetics, perfumes, and psoralens. The chemicals in these medications absorb light and release energy that harms cells and tissues. Nurses have a role in educating clients who are taking these medications about their photosensitizing ability.

IRRITANTS AND ALLERGENS. The nurse needs to reinforce the need to avoid exposure to known irritants (e.g., ammonia, harsh detergents). In addition, allergens that have troubled the client in the past or that are known to produce problems on exposure (e.g., poison ivy) should be avoided. Many irritants and allergens have a cumulative effect, producing more serious dermatoses on repeated exposure. Aside from costly and time-consuming desensitization, the most obvious strategy is avoidance.

Drugs used to treat a variety of conditions may cause dermatological reactions. In fact, drugs are the most frequently identified cause of urticaria and should always be suspected when this condition occurs. The eruption will usually occur within 1 week of exposure to the offending drug.[3]

RADIATION. Although most radiology departments are extremely cautious in protecting both themselves and their clients from the effects of excessive radiation, the nurse should help the client make intelligent decisions about radiologic procedures. X-rays can be invaluable in both diagnosis and therapy, but indiscriminate use can cause serious side effects to the skin, as well as other body processes. In the past (30 years ago), cystic acne was treated with radiation. This information is important, since the clients who were thus treated have an increased incidence of basal cell carcinoma.

Rest and sleep. Rest and sleep are important health-promotion considerations in relation to the skin. Although the exact effects of sleep are not known, it is thought to be restorative.[4] Slow-wave sleep is believed to have physically restorative functions.[5] Rest reduces the threshold of itching and protects the skin from the effects of scratching.[6]

Exercise. Exercise increases circulation and dilates the blood vessels. In addition to the healthy glow produced by

exercise, the psychological effects can also improve one's appearance and mental outlook. However, caution needs to be used to avoid or protect oneself from overexposure to heat, cold, and sun during outdoor exercise.

Hygiene. Hygienic practices should match the skin type, lifestyle, and culture of the client. The person with oily skin will need to cleanse the skin with a drying agent more often than the person with dry skin. Dry skin might benefit from superfatted soaps and measures to increase moisture, such as the application of moisturizers to the skin.

The normally acidic skin (pH 4.2 to 5.6) and perspiration protect against bacterial overgrowth. Most soaps are alkaline with degreasing power and cause a neutralization of the skin surface and loss of protection. The use of more neutral soaps and avoiding hot water and vigorous rubbing can noticeably decrease local irritation and inflammation.

In general, the skin and hair should be washed often enough to remove excess oil and excretions as well as to prevent odor. Older persons should avoid the use of harsh soaps and shampoos and should decrease the frequency of bathing because of the increasing dryness of their skin. Moisturizers should be used after bath or shower, while the skin is still damp, to seal in moisture.

Nutrition. A well-balanced diet adequate in the basic four food groups can produce healthy skin, hair, and nails. Certain elements are particularly essential to good skin health, however. These include the following:

1. *Vitamin A*—essential for maintenance of normal cell structure in epithelial surfaces.
2. *Vitamin B complex*—essential to complex metabolic functions. Deficiencies of niacin and pyridoxine manifest as dermatological symptoms such as erythema, bullae, and seborrhea-like lesions.
3. *Vitamin C (ascorbic acid)*—essential for connective tissue formation and normal wound healing. Absence causes damage to the dermis.
4. *Vitamin K*—deficiency interferes with normal prothrombin synthesis in the liver and can lead to cutaneous purpura.
5. *Protein*—adequate supply of protein is necessary for cell synthesis.
6. *Unsaturated fatty acids*—specifically linoleic and arachidonic acids. Necessary to maintain the function and integrity of cellular and subcellular membranes in tissue metabolism.

Obesity has an adverse effect on the skin. The increased subcutaneous fat deposits can lead to stretching and overheating. Overheating causes an increase in sweating, which has an adverse effect on normal or inflamed skin. Obesity also has an influence on the development of type II diabetes with its concomitant skin complications (see Chapter 43).

Self-treatment. The nurse needs to increase the client's awareness of the dangers of self-diagnosis and treatment. The wide variety of over-the-counter skin preparations can indeed confuse the consumer. General instructions that the nurse can discuss with the client would stress the duration of the treatment and the need to follow package directions closely. Skin problems are generally slow to produce symptoms and slow to resolve. If the package insert of an over-the-counter drug says its use should not exceed 7 days, this warning should be heeded. If the directions say to apply twice daily, the urge to double the dose and hasten the cure must be avoided. If any systemic signs of inflammation or extension of the skin problem (e.g., an increased number of lesions or increased erythema or swelling) develop, self-care should be stopped and the help of a professional should be enlisted.

General Measures to Treat Acute Dermatological Problems

Diagnostic studies. A careful history is of prime importance in the diagnosis of skin problems. The clinician must be skilled at detecting any evidence that could lead to the cause of the extraordinary number of skin problems. After a careful history and examination, individual lesions are inspected. On the basis of the history, physical examination, and appropriate diagnostic tests, either medical, surgical, or combination therapy will be planned.

Therapeutic and pharmacological management. Many different treatment methods are used in dermatology. Some are disease-specific, whereas others work for unknown reasons. Advances in this field have brought relief to many previously chronic, untreatable conditions. Many of the specific therapeutic treatments require specialized equipment and are usually reserved for use by the dermatologist. Pharmacological treatments are prescribed by many clinicians. Their effectiveness can often be related to the base (or vehicle) in which the medication is prepared. Table 17-4 summarizes the common agents used as bases for topical preparations and their therapeutic considerations.

Phototherapy. The use of the sun as a source of UV wavelengths causes erythema, desquamation, and pigmentation. It also has bactericidal effects. UV light (UVL) causes a temporary suppression of basal cell mitosis followed by a rebound increase in cell turnover.

Two types of light, or a combination of the two (UVA, UVB), are used to treat many dermatological conditions. Psoralen plus UVA light (PUVA) is a form of phototherapy. The photosensitizing drug psoralen is given to clients 90 minutes before exposure to UVA to enhance the effect of UVL in the UVA spectrum (Table 17-1). Usually petroleum jelly or a tar preparation is applied to the affected area in a thin layer before exposure to UVB. Conditions that are responsive to effective wavelengths with or without drugs include atopic dermatitis, cutaneous T-cell lymphoma, pruritus, psoriasis, and vitiligo.[5]

UVL in the specific wavelengths can be produced artificially. Therapeutic doses of UVA and UVB can be measured and used to treat spectrum-specific diseases (Fig. 17-1). Prolonged exposure to UVL can result in basal or squamous cell carcinoma. Frequent skin assessments must be performed on all clients receiving phototherapy. Clients should be cautioned about the potential hazards of using photosensitizing chemicals and further exposure to UV rays from sunlight or high-intensity artificial light during the course of phototherapy. Protective eye wear that blocks 100% of ultraviolet light is prescribed for clients receiving PUVA to protect their eyes, since psoralen is absorbed by the lens of the eye. This is to prevent cataract formation. Clients are instructed to use the eyewear for 24 hours after taking the medication when outdoors or near a bright window because UVA penetrates glass. The recent evidence of immunosuppressive effects of PUVA requires careful ongoing monitoring of clients.

Radiation. The use of radiation for the treatment of dermatological conditions varies greatly according to local custom and availability. Better treatments are now available for most benign conditions. However, radiation remains useful in the treatment of cutaneous malignancies. Even if radiotherapy is planned, a biopsy must first be performed to obtain a pathological diagnosis, since melanoma does not respond well to radiotherapy.[7]

Radiation to malignant cutaneous lesions is a painless treatment that is similar in cost to surgery. It produces minimal damage to surrounding tissue. It is a particularly effective treatment for the older adult or debilitated client who cannot tolerate even a minor surgical procedure and for such areas as the nose, eyelids, and canthal areas, where preservation of the surrounding tissue is of prime consideration. Careful shielding is necessary to prevent ocular lens damage if the irradiated area is around the eyes.

Radiation therapy usually requires multiple visits. It is most effective on lesions above the neck. However, it produces permanent alopecia of the irradiated areas. Adverse effects include telangiectasia, atrophy, hyperpigmentation, depigmentation, ulceration, chronic radiodermatitis, and squamous cell carcinoma. (Radiation therapy is discussed in Chapter 9.)

Total-body skin irradiation (electron beam) may be the treatment of choice or adjunctive therapy for cutaneous T-cell lymphoma. Treatment follows a lengthy course, and toxicity to internal organs must be avoided. Clients experience transient loss of hair and radiation dermatitis with

Table 17-4 Common Bases for Topical Medications

Agent	Therapeutic Considerations
Powder	Promotion of dryness, increase in evaporation, absorbing of moisture by area possible, common base for antifungal preparations
Lotion	Suspension of insoluble powders in water; cooling and drying, with residual powder film after evaporation of water; useful in subacute pruritic eruptions
Cream	Emulsions of oil and water, most common base for topical medications, lubrication and protection
Ointment	Oil with differing amounts of water added in suspension, lubrication and prevention of dehydration, petrolatum most common
Paste	Mixture of powder and ointment, use when drying effect necessary because moisture is absorbed

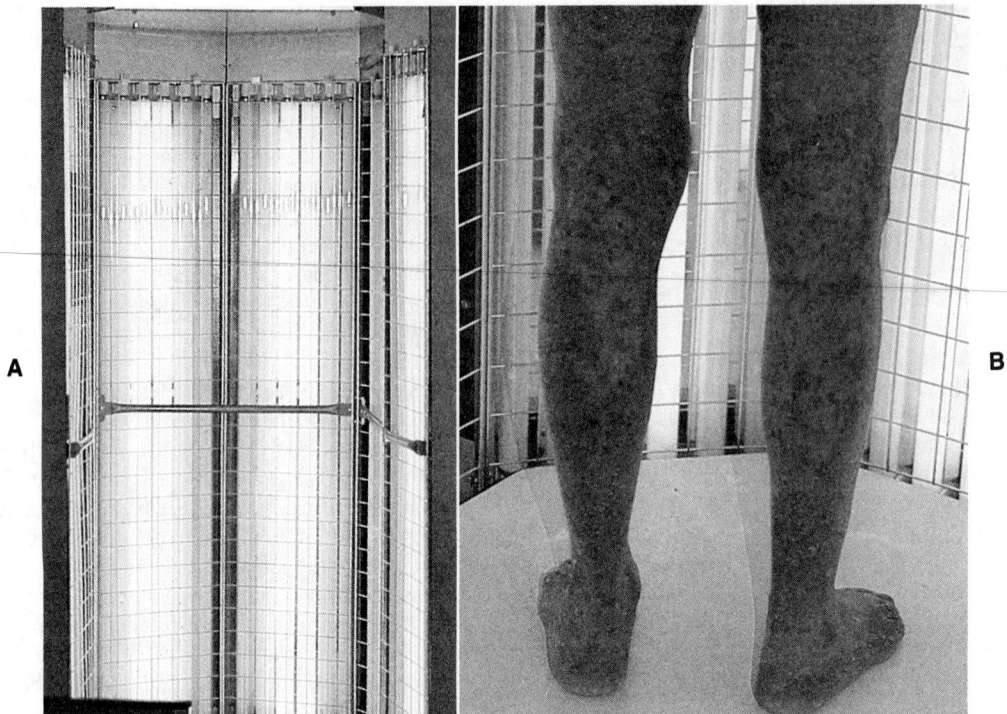

Fig. 17-1 Phototherapy is a method for treating spectrum-specific diseases. The client's eyes must be protected during the phototherapy session. **A,** PUVA unit. **B,** Client with psoriasis undergoing PUVA therapy. (Courtesy William Chapman, Albuquerque, New Mexico.)

transient loss of sweat gland function. This treatment ages the skin about 20 years.

Antibiotics. Antibiotics are used both topically and systemically to treat dermatological problems and are often used in combination. The use of topical antibiotics is controversial and reflects the philosophy of the care provider as to their efficacy. If used, topical antibiotics should be applied to clean debrided skin. Occlusive dressings should not be used. Common topical antibiotics include bacitracin (used for gram-positive organisms), neomycin and gentamicin (used for *Staphylococcus* and most gram-negative organisms), and erythromycin (used for gram-positive cocci—staphylococci and streptococci—and gram-negative cocci and bacilli). Topical erythromycin and clindamycin (solutions or gels) are used in the treatment of acne vulgaris.

If there are signs of systemic infection, a systemic antibiotic should be used. Systemic antibiotics (most often synthetic penicillins, erythromycin, and tetracycline) are useful in the treatment of bacterial infections and acne vulgaris. They are particularly useful for erysipelas, cellulitis, carbuncles, and severe infected eczema. Culture of the lesion should guide the choice of antibiotic. Many of the more popular systemic antibiotics are not used topically because of the danger of allergic contact dermatitis. Clients require drug-specific instructions on the proper technique of taking or applying antibiotics. For instance, oral tetracycline must be taken on an empty stomach and never

with a dairy product, which would interfere with absorption.

Corticosteroids. More than one half of the prescriptions written by dermatologists are for glucocorticoids. Glucocorticoids are amazingly effective in treating a wide variety of dermatological conditions and can be used topically, intralesionally, or systemically.

Topical glucocorticoids are used for their local antiinflammatory action, as well as for their antipruritic effects. Attempts to diagnose a lesion should be made before a steroid preparation is applied, since steroids will mask the clinical picture. Steroids are useful in the treatment of most dermatoses. Once a sufficient amount of medication is dispensed, limits should be set on the duration and frequency of application. With prolonged use the more potent steroid formulations can cause adrenal suppression, especially if occlusion is used. Recovery is rapid when treatment is discontinued. Fluoridated corticosteroids are more effective than nonfluoridated corticosteroids. However, fluoridated corticosteroids produce side effects, including atrophy of the skin due to impaired cell mitosis and collagen production from capillary fragility, striae, and susceptibility to bruising when their use is prolonged. Rosacea eruptions, severe exacerbations of acne vulgaris, and dermatophyte infections may also occur. Rebound dermatitis is not uncommon when therapy is ceased. Nonfluoridated corticosteroids such as hydrocortisone and desonide (Tridesilon) act more slowly but can be used for a longer period of time without producing serious side effects. Nonfluoridated corticosteroids are used on the face and intertriginous areas. The potency of a particular preparation is related to the concentration of active drug in the preparation. The ointment form represents the most efficient delivery system. Creams and ointments should be applied in thin layers and slowly massaged into the site one to four times a day as prescribed by the physician. The nurse must stress that only a small amount of medication is necessary—more is *not* better.

Intralesional glucocorticoids are injected directly into or just beneath the lesion. This method provides a reservoir of medication whose effect will last several weeks to months. Intralesional injection is particularly useful in the treatment of psoriasis, lupus erythematosus, cystic acne, eczema, hypertrophic scars, and keloids. A 2.5 to 10 mg/ml suspension of triamcinolone acetonide (Kenalog) is the most common dose range for intralesional injection. A small amount is injected into the site of each lesion.

Systemic glucocorticoids can have remarkable results in the treatment of dermatological conditions. However, they often have undesirable systemic effects (Chapter 44). Steroids can be administered in short-term therapy for such acute conditions as poison ivy. They may also be used for life-threatening situations, such as anaphylaxis. Long-term steroid therapy for dermatological conditions is reserved for chronic bullous diseases, severe systemic effects of collagen and immunological responses, and as a last resort when other therapies have failed.

Antihistamines. The use of antihistamines should be limited to conditions that exhibit urticaria; angioedema; pruritus associated with many dermatological problems such as atopic dermatitis, psoriasis, and contact dermatitis; and other allergic cutaneous reactions. Antihistamines compete with histamine for the receptor site, thus preventing its pharmacological response. Antihistamines have anticholinergic, antipruritic, and sedative effects. Several different antihistamines may have to be tried before the satisfactory therapeutic effect is achieved. A major side effect of antihistamine use is sedation. The client must be warned about sedative effects, a particular problem when one is driving or operating heavy machinery. Antihistamines should be used with particular caution in the older adult because of their long half-life.

Topical fluorouracil. Fluorouracil (5-FU) is a topical cytotoxic agent with selective toxicity for sun-damaged cells. Not only does it remove the majority of premalignant and superficial malignant lesions that can be seen; it will also uncover and destroy clinically undetectable lesions of this type.[8] It does not damage normal tissue. 5-FU is effective in treating actinic (sun-damaged) areas on the face but it is less effective on the hands and treatment must be modified. 5-FU is available in three strengths—1%, 2%, 5%—as a solution or a cream. It is not adequate for the treatment of diagnosed skin cancers. If treatment is not effective, biopsy of the suspicious areas should be performed.

Client compliance is the major problem with the use of 5-FU. The medication produces painful, eroded areas over the damaged skin within 4 days. Treatment must continue

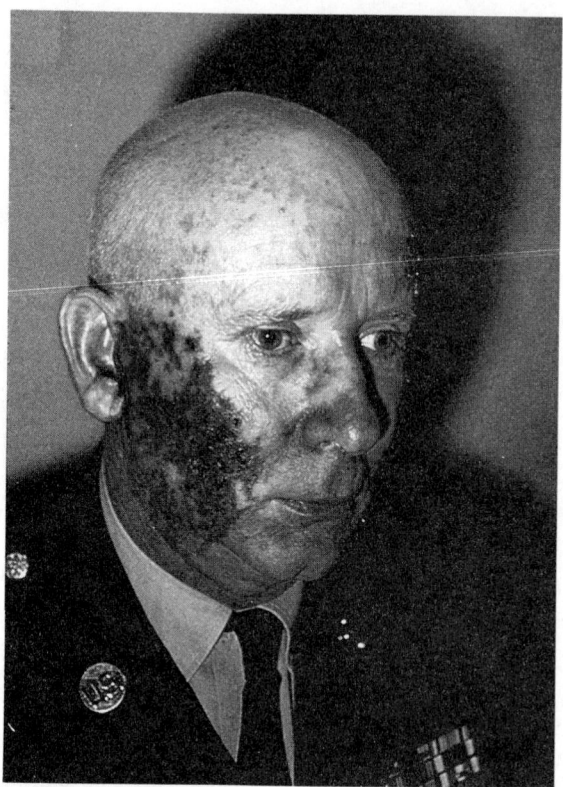

Fig. 17-2 Client being treated with 5-FU. (Courtesy Larry Becker.)

with applications one to two times a day for 2 to 4 weeks. Healing may take up to 3 weeks after medication is stopped (Fig. 17-2). Since fluorouracil is a photosensitizing drug, the client must be instructed to avoid sunlight during treatment. Clients need to be educated about the effect of the medication and should be warned that they will look worse before they look better. Medication causes the dermatitis, so clients can plan their social activities accordingly. After effective treatment, treated skin is smooth and free of actinic keratoses, although sometimes a second course is prescribed.

Disease-specific drugs. Many dermatological conditions are treated by specific drug preparations, which are outlined in tables throughout this chapter.

Surgical interventions. Certain dermatological conditions are best treated by surgical methods.

Electrodesiccation and electrocoagulation. Electrical energy can be converted to heat by the tip of an electrode. This results in tissue being destroyed by burning. The major uses of this type of therapy are point coagulation of bleeding vessels and destruction of small telangiectasias. Electrodesiccation usually involves more superficial destruction, and a monopolar electrode is used. Electrocoagulation has a deeper effect, with better hemostasis and an increased possibility of scarring. A dipolar electrode is used for electrocoagulation.

The major disadvantages of electrodesiccation and electrocoagulation are scarring, inability to control depth of burning, and lack of a biopsy specimen.

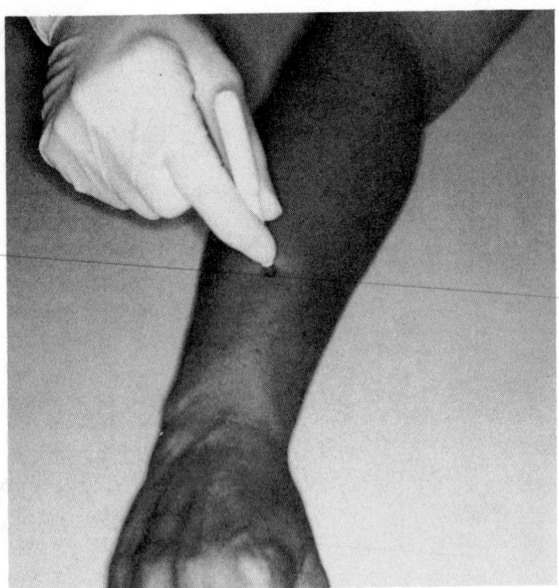

Fig. 17-3 Punch biopsy for pathology specimen.

Curettage. Curettage is the removal of tissue by means of an instrument with a circular cutting edge attached to a handle. The tissue is scooped away. Although the curette is not strong enough to cut normal skin, it is useful for removing many types of small skin tumor, such as warts, molluscum contagiosum, seborrheic keratoses, and small basal and squamous cell cancers. The area to be curetted is anesthetized before the procedure. Hemostasis is obtained with the use of ferric subsulfate (Monsel's solution) gelatin foam, aluminum chloride in alcohol (Drysol), or gauze pressure. A small scar may form. The specimen may be sent for biopsy.

Punch biopsy. Punch biopsy is a common dermatological procedure used to obtain a tissue sample for histological study or to remove small lesions. Its use is generally reserved for lesions of less than 0.5 cm. Before the induction of local anesthesia, the biopsy area is outlined so that landmarks will not be obscured by the anesthetizing agent. The biopsy punch cores out a small cylinder of skin when its sharp edge is twirled between the fingers. The core of skin is snipped from the subcutaneous fat and appropriately preserved for examination (Fig. 17-3). Hemostasis is usually achieved by gelatin foam packing to reduce scarring. All punch biopsy sites will heal without sutures, but sites of 3 mm or larger are often closed with sutures, especially if the scar is to be minimized. Multiple small biopsy specimens can help delineate the borders of a basal cell carcinoma.

Cryosurgery. Skin lesions are destroyed by freezing. Topical or intralesional liquid nitrogen is the agent most commonly used for cryosurgery. Although the exact mechanism is not clearly understood, the use of liquid nitrogen causes death or destruction of the treated skin. Probably ice crystals rupture the cell membrane.

Liquid nitrogen is a cold, liquefied gas with a temperature of $-196°$ C ($-320.8°$ F). For cells to be destroyed, the agent used must go to at least $-20°$ C ($-4°$ F). Liquid nitrogen can explode if kept in an air-tight container.

Liquid nitrogen can be applied topically (directly onto the benign or precancerous lesion) with a cotton swab or with the appropriate container (Cry-AC) for several freeze-and-thaw cycles. Clients are informed that they will feel a cold sensation. The lesion will first become swollen and red. It may blister. Next, a scab will form and fall off in 1 to 3 weeks. The skin lesion will be sloughed along with the scab. Growth of new skin will follow. Cryosurgery is a useful treatment for common and genital warts, cutaneous tags, seborrheic keratoses, actinic keratoses, and many other less common skin conditions.

When used for treatment of a neoplasm, a microthermocouple needle is inserted to measure tissue temperature at placed depth. Liquid nitrogen is then applied topically until the desired temperature is measured. Neoplastic cells require a much deeper, prolonged freeze for destruction. When cancer cells are destroyed, a copious clear drainage is produced, and the site will drain significantly large amounts for 1 to 3 weeks after the freezing. Local anesthesia is usually required. Cyrosurgery is inexpensive, rapid, and leaves minimal scarring. The major disadvantage of this treatment is lack of a tissue specimen.

Excision. Excision should be considered if the lesion involves the dermis. Complete closure of the excised area usually results in good cosmetic results. Fair cosmetic results can be obtained with partial closure, but cosmetic reconstruction may be required. This method is particularly suited to problems on the face. To minimize scarring, hemostasis can be obtained by direct pressure or by packing with absorbable material.

Healing by second intention on areas such as the nose, oral lips, cheek, and chin may heal with a depression if the wound is deep. Closure by means of plastic surgery may yield more desirable results. The specimen is usually sent for biopsy.

Another type of excision is the Mohs procedure, which is a microscopically controlled excision of tissue suspected of harboring a malignancy. This procedure sections the surgical specimen horizontally, so that 100% of the surgical margin can be examined. Any residual tumor not removed by the first surgical excision can be removed in serial excisions performed the same day. This is the treatment of choice for the majority of skin cancers. The procedure is done on an outpatient basis.

■ Nursing Management of Dermatological Problems

Acute interventions

Dermatological conditions are not common reasons for hospitalization. Although it may not be the primary reason for hospitalization, many hospitalized clients will exhibit concurrent skin problems that warrant nursing intervention and client education.

If the nursing care is in an acute-care setting, the nurse will be both administering and teaching the appropriate treatments. If the client is in an outpatient setting, the nursing focus will be on client education, with opportunities provided for demonstration and redemonstration. Subsequent visits provide the opportunity to evaluate client understanding and treatment effectiveness.

Nursing interventions related to dermatological condi-

Table 17-5

NURSING CARE PLAN FOR THE CLIENT WITH CHRONIC SKIN LESIONS

Defining Characteristics	Nursing Interventions	Evaluation Criteria
NURSING DIAGNOSIS: Pain: pruritus related to presence of skin lesions		
Pruritus, areas of excoriated skin, agitation and anxiety over itching sensation	Decrease environmental irritants (e.g., heat, scratchy coverings). Use topical and systemic antiinflammatory medications. Provide a cool environment. Use cool, wet dressings, soaks, and baths. Administer antihistamines as necessary. Keep client's nails trimmed short. Provide diversional activities.	Satisfactory control of pruritus
NURSING DIAGNOSIS: High risk for infection related to open lesion, presence of environmental pathogens and exudate		
Open draining lesions; redness, swelling, and pain at lesion sites; lymphadenopathy and fever; indications of scratching	Teach client measures to prevent scratching, such as tepid baths and a cool environment. Practice and teach careful hand washing and proper disposal of dressings and contaminated linens. Inform client of dangers of scratching.	No evidence of secondary infection
NURSING DIAGNOSIS: Pain: dry skin related to inadequate fluid intake, too frequent cleansing, dryness from treatment medications		
Dry, flaking skin	Use nonirritating moisturizing agents. Provide adequate fluid (2000 to 3000 ml/day) and fat intake. Avoid frequent bathing. Encourage use of superfatted soap.	Moist, well-lubricated skin
NURSING DIAGNOSIS: Self-esteem disturbance related to presence of unsightly lesions		
Verbalization of self-disgust and despair over appearance of lesions, isolation, reluctance to look at lesions or participate in self-care	Discuss situation with client in open, accepting manner. Do not show shock or disgust at the sight of lesions. Touch the client, if appropriate to the situation. Provide counseling, if indicated.	Realistic hope for resolution of open lesions, maintenance of normal social relationships

Continued.

tions fall into broad categories. They are applicable to many skin problems in both inpatient and outpatient settings. Table 17-5 discusses nursing care for a client with chronic lesions.

Wet dressings. The use of wet dressings is a common dermatological procedure used to dry exudative lesions, relieve itching, suppress inflammation, and debride a wound. In addition, wet dressings will increase penetration of topical medications, promote sleep by relieving discomfort, and enhance removal of scales, crusts, and exudate.[10] Such materials as thin sheeting or gauze sponges can be used for dressings. Ingenuity is sometimes required when odd-shaped parts of the body must be covered.

The prescribed dressing is put into fresh solution, held until it is no longer dripping, and applied to the affected area (Fig. 17-4)). Occlusion of the dressing with plastic or additional material is rarely done because of the likelihood of maceration (wrinkling) of the skin. The dressing should be left in place 15 to 30 minutes. The compress is then removed and replaced with a new one. This treatment may be used two to four times a day or continuously. If the skin appears macerated, the dressings should be discontinued for 2 to 3 hours. The client should be protected from discomfort and chilling by protection of linens and bedclothes with pads or plastic.

Common solutions used for wet dressings are listed in Table 17-6. Tap water, at room temperature, is the most common solution. Potassium permanganate must be completely dissolved before use since the crystals may burn the skin. This solution must be freshly prepared to maintain its oxidative properties. If potassium permanganate solution turns brown, it should be discarded and fresh solution made. Boric acid is not recommended as a wet dressing solution because of potential systemic toxicity due to percutaneous absorption, especially on open skin. The best solution to use on the eyes is plain cool water.

Table 17-5

NURSING CARE PLAN FOR THE CLIENT WITH CHRONIC SKIN LESIONS—cont'd

Defining Characteristics	Nursing Interventions	Evaluation Criteria

NURSING DIAGNOSIS: Altered health maintenance related to lack of knowledge of disease process, management plan, prevention of scarring, care of lesions, possible cosmetic surgery, and use of OTC medications

Questions on self-care activities and possibilities for surgery to improve appearance, lack of understanding of disease process or management plan	Answer questions completely. Teach client about disease process, management plan, care of lesions. Discuss possible cosmetic surgery options. Advise client to carefully follow guidelines for OTC medication. Inform client of signs indicating a worsening of condition, such as increase in number of lesions, increase in erythema and swelling, and fever.	Verbalization of confidence in ability to care for self and explore surgical options, understanding of disease process and management plan, seeking medical help (if self-medication ineffective or condition worsens)

NURSING DIAGNOSIS: Anxiety related to chronicity of problem and personal appearance

Verbalization of anxiety and frustration over chronicity of problem and appearance of skin from scarring and lichenification, information needed on suitable cover-up techniques	Encourage client to continue with medical regimen. Counsel client regarding healthy life practices. Advise client on skilled use of cosmetics. Involve family members for support.	Hope regarding cessation of new lesions, improved appearance with use of cosmetics

NURSING DIAGNOSIS: Social isolation related to decreased activities secondary to poor self-image, fear of rejection, and lack of knowledge related to cover-up techniques

Isolation, lack of social activities, verbalization of dissatisfaction with social life	Encourage socialization in client's interest areas. Arrange psychiatric referral, if indicated. Teach skillful use of cosmetics, cover-up agents, and clothing. Encourage use of related support groups, if needed.	Satisfactory social life

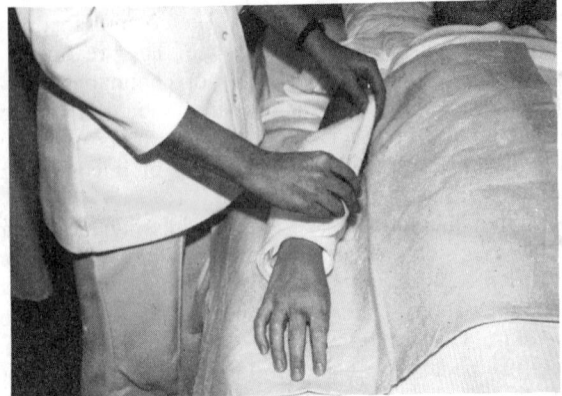

Fig. 17-4 Wet dressings are a common dermatological procedure. They are particularly effective in drying moist, oozing wounds.

Wet dressings do not need to be sterile. They should be cool when an antiinflammatory effect is desired and tepid when the purpose is to debride an infected, crusted lesion. These treatments are excellent ways to remove the scabs left by the collection of debris at a wound site. Although a scab initially is protective, it later retards healing and feeds bacteria.

Baths. Baths are appropriate when large body areas need to be treated. They also have sedative and antipruritic effects. Some medications, such as oilated oatmeal, potassium permanganate, and sodium bicarbonate, can be added directly to the bath water. One cup of the mixture can be added to 2 cups of water and then added to the bath water. The tub should be half-full of water. Both the bath water and the prescribed solution should be at a temperature that is comfortable for the client. The client can soak for 15 to 20 minutes three to four times a day, depending on the severity of the dermatitis and the client's discomfort. It is

Table 17-6 Wet Dressing Solutions

Agent	Preparation	Use
Acetic acid	Vinegar is 5% acetic acid; make 1% solution by adding ½ cup of vinegar (white or brown) to 1 pint of water	Bactericidal
Burow's solution (aluminum sulfate and calcium acetate)	One packet or tablet in 1 pint of water produces a modified 1:40 Burow's solution	Mildly antiseptic for acute inflammation
Magnesium sulfate (Epsom salt)	8 tsp to 1 L of water	Debridement, cleansing
Potassium permanganate	1 crushed 65 mg tablet to 250 ml of water	Antiseptic, disinfectant
Silver nitrate	1 tsp of 50% stock to 1 L of water	Antiseptic, disinfectant
Sodium bicarbonate	8 tsp to 1 L of water	Antipruritic
Sodium chloride	2 tsp to 1 L of water	Antipruritic, cleansing, debridement
Water	Tap water, does not need to be sterile	Debridement, cleansing, antiinflammatory

important to stress to the client that the skin not be towel-dried but allowed to air-dry when possible. If this is too chilling for the client, the skin should be gently patted to prevent increasing irritation and inflammation. The addition of oils makes the bathtub extremely slippery and should be avoided. If oils are used in the tub, the utmost caution must be used in transferring clients to prevent disastrous accidents. An equally effective means of lubricating the skin is to apply a moisturizer to gently dried skin directly after the bath. This helps to retain the moisture in the hydrated cells.

Topical medications. Generally, topical medications are best applied with the ungloved hand. This method allows the nurse to palpate the lesion and assess progress of the treatment. A thin layer of ointment and cream should be applied to clean skin and spread evenly in a downward motion. An alternate method is to apply the medication directly onto the dressings. However, pastes are designed to protect the affected area. They should be applied thickly with a tongue blade or a gloved hand. Draining lesions and lesions with greasy medication can be covered with a light dressing to prevent soiling clothes. Clients need specific directions on proper application technique of prescribed topical medications.

Control of pruritus. Pruritus (itching) can be caused by almost any physical or chemical stimulus to the skin, such as drugs, insects, and dry skin. The annoying sensation of itching is probably an automatic attempt to remove the offending agent from the skin and thus relieve the itch. The itch sensation is carried by the same nonmyelinated nerve fibers as pain. If the epidermis is damaged or absent, the sensation will be felt as pain rather than an itch.

The itch-scratch-itch cycle needs to be broken to prevent excoriation and eventual lichenification. Control of pruritus is important also because it is difficult to diagnose a lesion that is excoriated and inflamed.

Certain circumstances make itching worse. Anything that causes vasodilation, such as heat or rubbing, should be avoided. Dryness of the skin lowers the itch threshold

and increases the itch sensation. Any internal or external factors that increase blood flow to an area increase itching.

Measures that the nurse can use or teach the client to use to break the itch cycle should be attempted. A cool to cold environment or dressings cause vasoconstriction and decrease itching. The use of topical corticosteroids reduces inflammation and causes vasoconstriction. Menthol, camphor, or phenol can be used to numb the itch receptors or to cool the skin from evaporation of these volatile compounds. Systemic antihistamines can be used if necessary to provide relief to a miserable client while the underlying cause of the pruritus is diagnosed and treated.

Wet dressings can be used effectively to relieve pruritus. Thin, old sheets are placed in warm water, wrung out, and placed over the pruritic area. After 10 to 15 minutes the dressing is removed and the skin is allowed to air-dry. A lubricant is then applied to the skin. This procedure can be repeated as necessary for comfort. Topical antipruritic medications should be applied as directed by the physician.

Prevention of spread. Most skin problems are not contagious. The unnecessary use of gloves can be demoralizing to an already sensitive client. However, if in doubt, the nurse should wear gloves until a definite diagnosis has been established. The most common contagious lesions that should be easily recognized by nurses include impetigo, staphylococcis, pyoderma, primary chancre and secondary syphilis lesions, scabies, and pediculosis. Careful hand washing and safe disposal of soiled dressings are the best means of preventing spread of skin problems. Universal precautions appropriate for use with all clients are discussed in Chapter 8.

Prevention of secondary infections. Open lesions on the skin are susceptible to invasion by other organisms. Meticulous hygiene, hand washing, and dressing changes are important to prevent secondary infections. Also, the client should be warned about scratching lesions, which can cause excoriations and create a portal of entry for pathogens. The client's nails should be trimmed short to minimize trauma from scratching. Previously mentioned measures to decrease pruritus should be employed.

Specific skin care. Nurses are often in a position to advise clients regarding care of the skin following simple dermatological surgical procedures, such as excision and cryosurgery. Client follow-up should be individualized. Poor follow-up and wound care can ruin the best surgical result.[9] In general, the healing process would include care of oozing wounds, scabs, and stitched wounds.

Oozing wounds are best treated with wet to dry dressings for debridement and an antibiotic ointment, such as polymyxin B (Polysporin) or bacitracin. The ointment will inhibit infection and keep the bandage from sticking. If the bandage gets wet, both ointment and bandage need to be reapplied.

Initially, a scab should be left alone to be a protective coating for the damaged skin beneath it. Scabs should be kept dry. They can be covered during the day for cosmetic purposes but should be exposed at night. If a scab gets wet, it should be dried gently. After a while, the scab should be removed gently, after soaking, to encourage healing and remove a site for bacterial growth.

A wound that required stitches is handled much like an oozing wound. The area should be covered with a pressure bandage and an antibiotic ointment should be used. Stitches will generally be removed in 4 to 10 days, although facial stitches may be removed earlier to prevent scarring. Sometimes every other stitch will be removed after the third day. The primary dressing may be removed after 24 to 48 hours so the incision can be exposed to air.[10] Incision lines require daily cleansing, usually with hydrogen peroxide. A topical antibiotic, such as bacitracin or Polysporin, is then applied and the wound is either covered with a dry sterile dressing or left open to air. The client can expect some swelling and discomfort in the first 24 hours. Mild analgesics such as acetaminophen should control the discomfort. The client needs to know the manifestations of inflammation such as redness, fever, or increased pain or swelling and signs of infection, such as purulent drainage. If these manifestations occur, they should be reported to the care giver.

Chronic management

Psychological effects of chronic dermatological problems. The emotional toll is indeed heavy for persons who suffer from chronic skin problems such as eczema, psoriasis, and atopic and seborrheic dermatitis. The sequelae of chronic skin problems could result in employment problems with subsequent financial implications, a frail and easily damaged body image, problems with sexuality, and increasing and progressive frustration. The usual lack of systemic overt illness coupled with the visibility of the skin lesions presents a real problem to the client.

The nurse must continue to be optimistic and help the client comply with the prescribed regimen. The client must be allowed to verbalize the "why me?" question, even though there is no ready answer. Reinforcement of the prescribed hygiene and treatment measures is an important part of the nursing management.

Many lesions can be camouflaged with the skillful use of cosmetics. Individual sensitivity to product ingredients must always be considered in the selection of a cosmetic product. Oil-free, hypoallergenic cosmetics are available and could be beneficial to the allergic client. Rehabilitative cosmetics are available to help camouflage and deemphasize such lesions as vitiligo or melasma or postoperative wound sites. These products are opaque, smudge resistant, and water resistant.

In addition to specific skin conditions that tend to chronicity, other factors affecting the outcome of long-term dermatological problems include skin type, history of previous attacks, family history, complications, intolerance to therapy, environmental factors, lack of adherence to the prescribed regimen, endocrine factors, and psychological factors. Lesions that follow a chronic pattern often are associated with lichenification and scarring.

Physiological effects of chronic dermatological problems. Scarring of old lesions may take place concurrently with continuing exudation in a chronic skin condition. When a lesion is large and deep, the edges cannot approximate and excessive numbers of keratinocytes are destroyed. The defect is filled with granulation tissue, which is replaced with dense bundles of collagen. The resulting scar is permanent, with loss of hair or sweat glands and decreased innervation.

Scars are pink and vascular at first. As they age they become avascular and white with increasing strength. An old scar will have 85% of the strength of the undamaged skin.[11] Different parts of the body scar differently. Other than the face and neck, which heal fairly well because of a good blood supply, scars usually remain conspicuous.

Although there are methods of reducing or removing scars, these are usually not practical for use with chronic skin conditions. Since acute lesions are often present concurrently with the chronic lesions, the scarring would simply repeat itself. Obviously, the location of the scar is the determining factor with respect to its cosmetic implications. Facial scars are the most damaging psychologically since they are so visible. Again, creative use of cosmetics can do much to mask the scarring of chronic skin conditions. The best treatment is prevention of scarring by control of the problem in the acute phase.

Lichenification is another consequence of chronic skin problems. It is the thickening of skin due to proliferation of keratinocytes with accentuation of the normal markings of the skin. The resulting plaque may be uniform or irregular. Lichenification is caused by scratching or rubbing of the skin and is often associated with atopic dermatoses and pruritic conditions. Although any area of the body may be affected, the hands and forearms are common sites. Treatment of the cause of the itching is the key to prevention of lichenification. Excoriations are often evident in the thickened skin as a result of the pruritus.

The side effects of both topical and systemic long-term steroid therapy must always be considered when such therapy used to treat chronic skin conditions. The dangers of prolonged use of topical glucocorticoids are discussed earlier in this chapter. (Systemic steroid therapy is discussed in Chapter 44.)

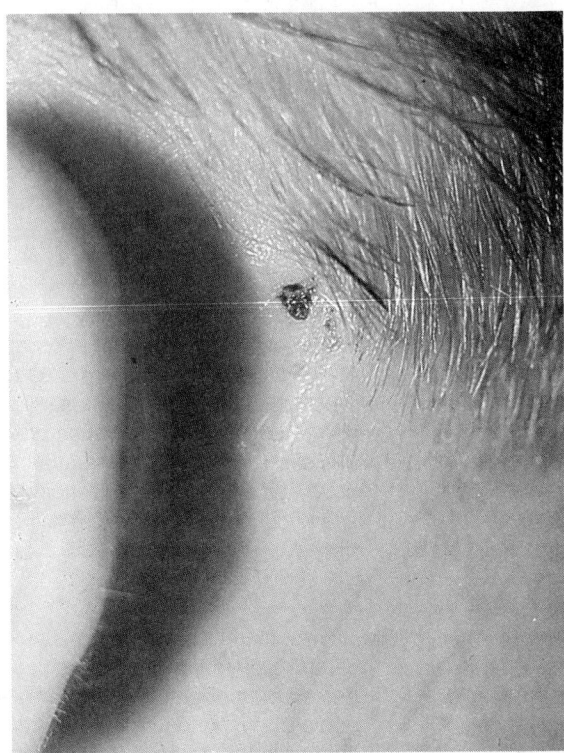

Fig. 17-5 Basal cell epithelioma. Note the typical pearly border. (Courtesy Larry Becker, Albuquerque, New Mexico.)

DERMATOLOGICAL DISORDERS
Malignant Conditions

Nonmelanoma skin cancer accounts for at least 50% of all malignancies reported yearly in the United States.[1] Malignant neoplasms of the skin exhibit the characteristics of all malignant conditions (Chapter 10). However, skin malignancies generally grow slowly (Fig. 17-5). Adequate and early treatment can lead to complete cure. The fact that skin lesions are so very visible increases the likelihood of early detection and diagnoses. The presence of a lesion that persists and does not heal is highly suspicious. Evidence from the client's history related to skin type, history of sun exposure, outdoor versus indoor occupation, and history of genetic diseases characterized by intolerance to sunlight (e.g., albinism), exposure to tar and systemic arsenicals, in addition to the persistent lesion is an indication for a biopsy of the lesion. Two different patterns of sun exposure are associated with skin cancer. In the first, solar exposure alone causes skin cancer in a manner modulated by individual differences in sensitivity and in total exposure. In the second type, intense intermittent exposure and the presence of precursors and lesions are risk factors. More than 90% of all skin cancers occur on parts of the body that are exposed to the sun's radiation, such as the face, neck, scalp, and ears.[4] A biopsy should be performed to confirm the diagnosis before specific treatment is started.

Many types of skin cancer are preventable. Although the number of deaths attributable to nonmelanoma skin cancer is small, the tumors have an inherent potential for severe local destruction, permanent disfigurement, and disability. The most common etiological factor, chronic sun exposure, should be consciously avoided by the use of sunscreens and protective clothing. The incidence of skin cancer increases with age in persons who have accumulated substantial sun exposure. Dark-skinned persons are less susceptible to skin cancers because of the naturally occurring increase in melanin, the most effective sunscreen. The incidence of skin cancer increases with proximity to the equator and high altitude because of the increased intensity of UV exposure.[12] Depletion of the stratosphere ozone layer has also been implicated in the recent increase of skin cancer. It is estimated that a 1% depletion of the ozone layer would result in a 3% to 6% increase in skin cancer.[13]

Malignant melanoma and lung cancer in women are the two malignancies that are increasing most rapidly in the United States. Melanoma has doubled every 10 years in the last 30 years. Risk factors that may contribute to this increase include UV radiation; lack of skin pigmentation; genetic, hormonal, and immunological factors; and societal and lifestyle changes that lead to greater skin exposure.[14]

Recent research has shown that approximately 2% to 5% of the white population has an abnormal mole pattern called *dysplastic nevus syndrome* (DNS), which marks persons as being at increased risk of melanoma. There are two subtypes of DNS. In familial DNS, in which two or more first-degree family members have melanoma and dysplastic nevi, the lifetime risk of melanoma developing in family members is 100%. Persons with sporadic DNS and no family history of malignant melanoma have an 18% lifetime risk of malignant melanoma. When compared with the general public, whose estimated risk is 0.7%, a positive family history significantly increases a person's lifetime risk.[15]

The earliest clinically detectable abnormality associated with this syndrome is an increase in the number of morphologically normal-looking nevi at around the age of 5 or 6 years. Another proliferation occurs around adolescence, and some of the nevi become morphologically atypical. Generally, family members who have clinically normal skin in their mid-twenties will remain normal. The inability to tan has been identified as an important risk factor for malignant melanoma. Obtaining a detailed family history related to DNS and melanoma is an important epidemiological responsibility of the clinician. A family's tendency to sunburn easily and a positive family history of skin cancer are significant risk factors for the development of malignant melanoma. Fig. 17-6 presents the *ABCDs* of melanoma detection. Table 17-7 compares DNS and other common types of skin cancer.

Infections

Bacterial infections. The skin is covered with great numbers of microorganisms, especially bacteria. *Staphylococcus epidermidis* and diphtheroids are the most common

Table 17-7 Malignant Conditions of the Skin

Etiology and Pathophysiology	Clinical Manifestations	Treatment and Prognosis
ACTINIC KERATOSES		
Actinic (sun) damage	Flat or slightly elevated, dry, hyperkeratotic scaly papule; possibly flat, rough, or verrucous; adherent scale, which returns when removed; often multiple; rough scale on red base; often on erythematous sun-exposed areas; increase in number with age	Curettage, electrosurgery, cryosurgery, chemical caustics, topical application of 5-fluorouracil over entire area for 14-21 days; no effect on healthy skin and other lesions; recurrence possible, even with adequate treatment; untreated lesion possibly leading to squamous cell carcinoma (1% incidence)
DYSPLASTIC NEVUS SYNDROME		
Morphologically between common acquired nevi and melanoma; formal histogenetic precursor of cutaneous malignant melanoma	Often larger than 5 mm; irregular border, possibly notched; variegated color mixture of tan, brown, black, red, and pink within single mole; presence of at least one flat portion, often at edge of mole; frequently multiple; uncommon before puberty; most common site on back, but possible in uncommon mole sites such as scalp or buttocks	Marker of increased risk for melanoma; careful monitoring of persons suspected of familial tendency to melanoma or dysplastic nevus syndrome necessary to increase likelihood of early diagnosis of melanoma; indication for excisional biopsy for suspicious lesions
BASAL CELL EPITHELIOMA	**Nodular/ulcerative**	
Change in basal cell; no maturation or normal keratinization; continuing division as basal cells and formation of enlarging mass; from excessive sun exposure, genetic skin type, arsenicals, x-ray irradiation, scars, and some types of nevi; basal cells possibly pigmented but absent in nevi	Small, slowly enlarging papule; borders semitranslucent or "pearly," with overlying telangiectasia; erosion, ulceration, and depression of center; normal skin markings lost **Superficial** Erythematous, sharply defined, barely elevated multinodular plaques with varying scaling and crusting; similar to eczema but not pruritic	Excisional surgery, chemosurgery, electrosurgery, cryosurgery, x-ray therapy; 95% cure rate; slow-growing tumor that invades local tissue; metastasis rare
SQUAMOUS CELL CARCINOMA	**Early**	
Frequent occurrence on previously damaged skin (e.g., from sun, irradiation, scar); malignant tumor of squamous (prickle) cell of epidermis; invasion of dermis, surrounding skin; metastasis possible	Firm nodules with indistinct borders with scaling and ulceration; opaque **Late** Covering of lesion with scale or horn from keratinization; most common on sun-exposed areas such as face and hands	Surgical removal, cryosurgery, radiation therapy, chemosurgery, Mohs procedure or microscopically controlled excision, electrodesiccation, and curettage; untreated lesion possibly metastasizing to regional lymph nodes; high cure rate with early detection and treatment

Table 17-7 Malignant Conditions of the Skin—cont'd

Etiology and Pathophysiology	Clinical Manifestations	Treatment and Prognosis
CUTANEOUS T-CELL LYMPHOMA		
Origination in skin; chronic, slowly progressing disease with grave prognosis; possible etiologies of environmental toxins and chemical exposure	Prevalent in twice as many men as women in United States; classic presentation involving three stages—patch, plaque, and tumor; history of persistent macular eruption followed by gradual appearance of indurated plaques	Topical nitrogen mustard, radiation therapy, systemic chemotherapy, PUVA, and photopheresis; 5-year life expectancy with only skin manifestations and no treatment; greatly decreased survival rate with generalized erythroderma with exfoliation and abnormal cells in bloodstream
MALIGNANT MELANOMA		
Neoplastic growth of melanocytes anywhere on skin, eyes, or mucous membranes; classification according to major histological mode of spread; potential invasion and widespread metastases	Irregular color, irregular surface, irregular border; variegated color including red, white, blue, black, gray, brown; flat or elevated, eroded or ulcerated; often under 1 cm in size; most common sites in males and females on back; in females on chest and lower legs	Wide excision, full-thickness surgical removal; correlation of survival rate with depth of invasion; poor prognosis unless diagnosis and treatment early; spreading by local extension, regional lymphatic vessels, and bloodstream; adjuvant therapy after surgery possibly necessary if lesions greater than 1.5 mm in depth

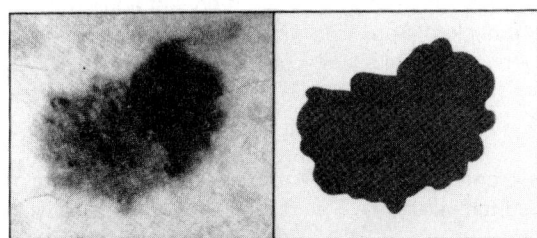

A **Asymmetry** one half unlike the other half

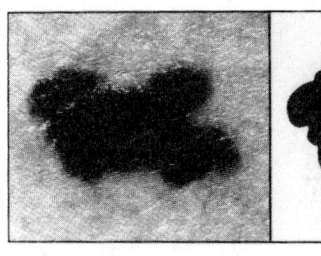

B **Border irregular** scalloped or poorly circumscribed border

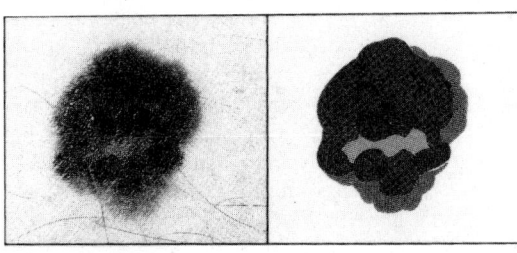

C **Color varied** from one area to another; shades of tan and brown; black; sometimes white, red, or blue

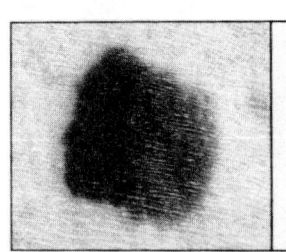

D **Diameter larger** than 6 mm as a rule (diameter of a pencil eraser)

Fig. 17-6 The ABCDs of melanoma. (From Stop: Look for danger signs, Evanston, Ill, American Academy of Dermatology, Inc.)

Table 17-8 Common Bacterial Infections of the Skin

Etiology and Pathophysiology	Clinical Manifestations	Treatment and Prognosis
IMPETIGO Group A β-hemolytic streptococci, staphylococci, or combination of both; associated with poor hygiene and low socioeconomic status; primary or secondary infection; contagious	Vesiculopustular lesions that develop thick, honey-colored crust surrounded by erythema; pruritic; most common on face	**Systemic antibiotics** 400,000 units oral penicillin qid × 10 days, 600,000 units of benzathine penicillin IM in single injection, or 250 mg erythromycin qid × 10 days **Local antibiotics** Warm saline or aluminum acetate soaks followed by soap-and-water removal of crusts; topical antibiotic cream; with no treatment, glomerulonephritis possible when streptococcal strain nephritogenic; meticulous hygiene essential
FOLLICULITIS Usually staphylococci; present in areas subjected to friction, moisture, oil, or grease	Small pustule at hair follicle opening with minimal erythema; development of crusting; most common on scalp, beard, extremities in men; tender to touch	Soap (e.g., Hibiclens) and water cleansing; topical antibiotics (e.g., Bactroban); warm compresses of water or aluminum acetate solution; healing usually without scarring; if lesions extensive and deep, possible scarring and loss of involved hair follicles
FURUNCLE Deep infection with staphylococci around hair follicle, often associated with severe acne or seborrheic dermatitis	Tender erythematous area around hair follicle; draining of pus and core of necrotic debris on rupture; most common on face, back of neck, axillae, breasts, buttocks, perineum, thighs; painful	Incision and drainage, occasionally antibiotics, meticulous care of involved skin, frequent application of warm, moist compresses
FURUNCULOSIS Increased incidence in clients who are obese, chronically ill, or regularly exposed to grease or oils or who have diabetes mellitus	Lesions as above, malaise, regional adenopathy, elevated temperature	Warm compresses; systemic antibiotic after culture and sensitivity study of drainage (usually semisynthetic, penicillinase-resistant, oral penicillin such as cloxacillin and oxacillin); measures to reduce surface staphylococci, including antimicrobial cream to nares, armpits, and groin and antiseptic to entire skin; often recurrent with scarring; incision and drainage of soft lesions; prevention or correction of predisposing factors; meticulous personal hygiene
CARBUNCLE Multiple, interconnecting furuncles	Many pustules appearing in erythematous area, most common on nape of neck	Treatment same as furuncles, often recurrent despite production of antibodies, healing slow with scar formation

Table 17-8 Common Bacterial Infections of the Skin—cont'd

Etiology and Pathophysiology	Clinical Manifestations	Treatment and Prognosis
CELLULITIS		
Inflammation of subcutaneous tissues; possibly secondary complication or primary infection; often following break in skin; *S. aureus* and streptococci usual causative agents; deep inflammation of subcutaneous tissue from enzymes produced by bacteria	Hot, tender, erythematous, and edematous area with diffuse borders; malaise and fever	Moist heat, immobilization and elevation, systemic antibiotic therapy, hospitalization if severe; progression to gangrene possible if untreated
ERYSIPELAS		
Superficial cellulitis primarily involving the dermis; group A β-hemolytic streptococci	Red, hot, sharply demarcated plaque, which is indurated and painful; bacteremia possible; most common on face and extremities; toxic signs, such as fever, elevated white blood cell count, headache, malaise	Systemic antibiotics—usually penicillin, hospitalization (often required)

Table 17-9

 Prehospital Emergency Care of the Client with a Surface Skin Wound*

Possible etiologies: Penetrating objects, avulsions, contusions, incised wounds, abrasions

CLINICAL MANIFESTATIONS

Redness, swelling
Bleeding
Pain
Surrounding nerve and vascular impairment
Discoloration of skin
Fear and anxiety

MANAGEMENT

Assess for bleeding areas; rule out other injuries.
Check wound for impaled objects, pieces of glass, or debris.
Do not attempt to remove any penetrating object. Stabilize for removal under controlled environment.
Cleanse wound with isotonic solution.
For an avulsed wound, fold the skin flap back into normal position and then control bleeding.
Apply bulky sterile dressing to area and immobilize injured part.

*See Chapter 59 for a general discussion of measures related to prehospital emergency care.

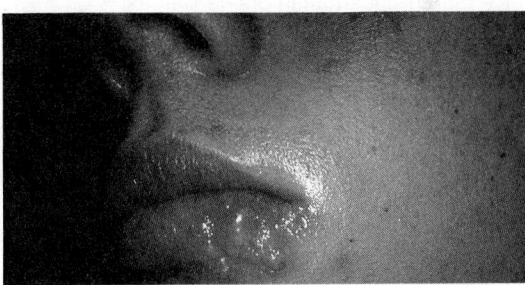

Fig. 17-7 Herpesvirus on the lips. (Courtesy Larry Becker, Albuquerque, New Mexico.)

bacteria present on the skin. The skin provides the ideal environment for bacterial growth, with abundant supplies of warmth, food, and water.

Bacterial infection *(pyoderma)* occurs when the balance between the host and the microorganisms is upset (Table 17-8). This can occur as a primary infection following a break in the skin. It can also occur as a secondary infection to already damaged skin or as a sign of a systemic disease.

Healthy persons can develop bacterial skin infections. Predisposing factors such as moisture, obesity, skin disease, systemic steroids and antibiotics, chronic disease, and diabetes mellitus all increase the likelihood of infection. Good hygienic practices and general good health inhibit bacterial infections. If an infection is present, the resulting drainage is infectious. Meticulous skin hygiene is necessary to prevent spread of the infection.

Trauma is a common source of skin infection. Table 17-9 outlines the prehospital care of a client with a surface skin wound.

Viral infections. Viral infections of the skin are as difficult to treat as viral infections anywhere in the body. A virus is an ultramicroscopic organism that is an obligatory parasite. That is, it requires living cells to survive. Viruses must go to the lower layers of the epidermis to replicate, since the outer layers are dead cells. The stratum corneum, hair, and nails cannot be affected by viruses.

The body attempts to destroy the protein coat surrounding the core of the genetic material of the virus. The affected cell can become injured in this attempt and a lesion can result (Fig. 17-7). Lesions can also result from an in-

Table 17-10   Common Viral Infections of the Skin

Etiology and Pathophysiology	Clinical Manifestations	Treatment and Prognosis
HERPES SIMPLEX VIRUS TYPE 1 Generally oral infections; virus remaining in nerve root ganglion and possibly returning to skin to produce recurrence when exacerbated by sunlight, trauma, menses, stress, and systemic infection; contagious to those not previously infected; increase in severity with age; transmission by respiratory droplets or virus-containing fluid, such as saliva or cervical secretions; no protection against subsequent infection in other areas with episodes of infection in one area	**First episode** Symptoms occurring 3-7 days or more after contact; painful local reaction; grouped vesicles on erythematous base; systemic symptoms, such as fever and malaise possible or asymptomatic presentation possible **Recurrent** Small; recurrence in similar spot; characteristic grouped vesicles on erythematous base	Symptomatic medication; soothing, moist compresses; petrolatum to lesions; scarring not usual result; antiviral agents such as acyclovir (Zovirax) and idoxuridine (Stoxil)
HERPES SIMPLEX VIRUS TYPE 2 Generally genital infections; recurrence more frequent than oral-labial infections		
HERPES ZOSTER Activation of the varicella-zoster virus; frequent occurrence in immunosuppressed clients; potentially contagious to anyone who has not had varicella or who is immunosuppressed	Linear patches along dermatome of grouped vesicles on erythematous base; usually unilateral and on trunk; burning, pain, and neuralgia preceding outbreak; mild to severe pain during outbreak	Symptomatic; wet compresses, white petrolatum to lesions; analgesia; mild sedation at bedtime; systemic corticosteroids to shorten course and decrease likelihood of postherpetic neuralgia (controversial); usual healing without complications but scarring possible; postherpetic neuralgia possible; idoxuridine or acyclovir possible agents if eye involvement
HUMAN IMMUNODEFICIENCY VIRUS Retrovirus; serious defect in cell-mediated immunity; selective attack of helper/inducer lymphocytes, decreasing number and interfering with function; progression from initial infection to AIDS-related complex to AIDS*	Markers for AIDS; commonly caused by infections; common dermatopathies occurring more readily on exposed skin on head, neck, and upper trunk; common cutaneous manifestations, including herpes simplex, herpes zoster, molluscum contagiosum, warts/condyloma, hairy leukoplakia (viral); *Candida albicans, Tinea versicolor,* dermatophytes (fungal); *S. aureus* (bacterial); seborrheic dermatitis, xeroderma, papular eruptions (proliferative); thrombocytopenic purpura (vascular); Kaposi's sarcoma (34%) (neoplastic); and pruritus, yellow or dark blue nails, premature graying of hair	Disease-specific treatment; for Kaposi's sarcoma, radiation for individual lesions for palliation; vinblastine, vincristine, etoposide; chemotherapeutic agents possibly aggravating immunosuppression

*See Chapter 8.

Table 17-10 Common Viral Infections of the Skin—cont'd

Etiology and Pathophysiology	Clinical Manifestations	Treatment and Prognosis
VERRUCA VULGARIS		
Caused by human papillomavirus; spontaneous disappearance in 1-2 years possible; mildly contagious by autoinoculation; specific response dependent on body part affected	Circumscribed hypertrophic, flesh-colored papule limited to epidermis; painful on lateral compression	Multiple treatments, including surgery—scoop removal with scissors and currette; liquid nitrogen therapy; blistering agents—cantharidin; keratolytic agents—salicylic acid; treatment rather than primary lesion possibly resulting in scarring
PLANTAR WARTS		
Caused by human papillomavirus	Wart on bottom surface of foot, growing inward because of pressure of walking or standing; painful when pressure applied; interrupted skin markings; cone-shaped with black dots (thrombosed vessels) when pared	Usual treatment with frequent paring followed by application of patches of impregnated chemicals to continue to decrease regrowth; overaggressive destruction possibly resulting in painful, hypertrophic scar

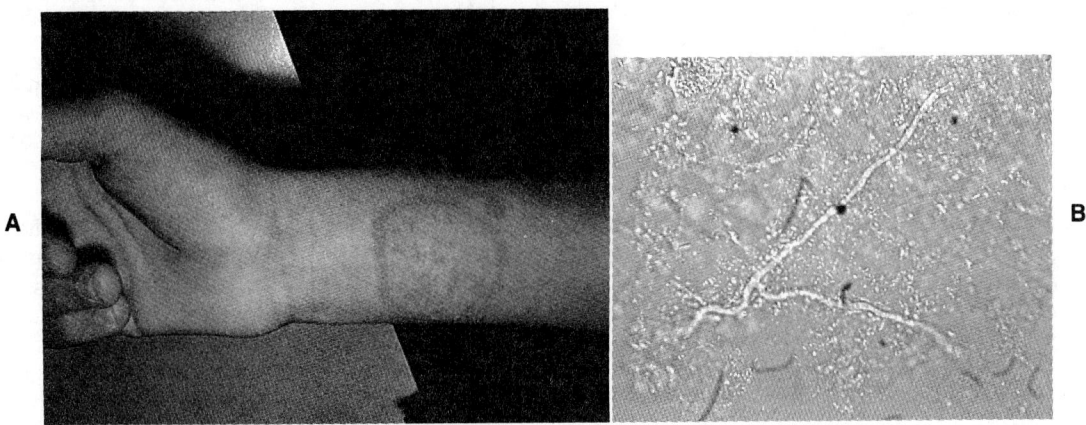

Fig. 17-8 **A,** Tinea corporis (ringworm). **B,** Hyphae on slide prepared with potassium hydroxide. (Courtesy Larry Becker, Albuquerque, New Mexico.)

flammatory response to the viral interference with cell function and morphology (Table 17-10). Herpes simplex, herpes zoster, and warts are the most common viral infections affecting the skin.

Fungal infections. Because of the huge number of identified fungi, it is almost impossible to avoid exposure to some pathological varieties. Many fungi have valuable functions in modern society, as in food preparation (e.g., molds, cheese) and drug synthesis (e.g., penicillin). Many fungi have serious deleterious effects as well.

Microscopic examination of the scraping of suspicious lesions in 10% to 20% potassium hydroxide is an easy, inexpensive diagnostic aid. The appearance of hyphae (threadlike structures) is indicative of a fungal infection

(Fig. 17-8, *A* and *B*). The clinical characteristics of fungal infections are easily recognized (Table 17-11).

Dermatophytes are the fungi that cause ringworm. These are referred to as *tinea,* followed by a word designating the location of the lesion (e.g., tinea capitis occurs on the head).

Infestations and Insect Bites

The possibilities for exposure related to insect bites and infestations are almost limitless. In many instances, an allergy to the venom plays a major role in the reaction. In other cases, the clinical manifestations are due to a reaction to the eggs, feces, or body parts of the invaders (Fig. 17-9). Certain persons will react with a severe hypersensi-

Table 17-11 Common Fungal Infections of the Skin and Mucous Membranes

Etiology and Pathophysiology	Clinical Manifestations	Treatment and Prognosis
CANDIDIASIS		
Caused by yeastlike fungus of *Candida albicans;* also known as moniliasis; 50% of adults symptom-free carriers; presenting in warm, moist areas such as crural area, oral mucosa, and submammary folds; AIDS, chemotherapy, radiation, and organ transplantation related to depression of cell-mediated immunity that allow yeast to become pathogenic; production of symptoms by imbalance between host and normal inhabitant of gastrointestinal tract, mouth, vagina	**Mouth** White, cheeselike patches leaving erosions when removed **Vagina** Vaginitis, with red, edematous, painful vaginal wall, white patches; vaginal discharge; pruritus; pain on urination and intercourse **Skin** Diffuse papular erythematous rash with pinpoint satellite lesions around edges of affected area	Microscopic examination and culture; nystatin or other specific medication as vaginal suppository or oral lozenge; abstinence or use of condom; eradication of infection with appropriate medication; skin hygiene to keep it clean and dry; mycostatin powder effective on skin lesions; avoidance of lubricants
TINEA CORPORIS		
Various dermatophytes, commonly referred to as ringworm	Typical annular appearance, well-defined margins with fine cigarette paper scale; erythematous	Cool compresses; topical antifungals for isolated patches; clotrimazole, miconazole, tolnaftate, and haloprogin creams or solutions
TINEA CRURIS		
Various dermatophytes, commonly referred to as "jock itch"	Well-defined border in groin area	Topical antifungals, including clotrimazole, miconazole, tolnaftate, and haloprogin cream or solution
TINEA UNGUIUM		
Various dermatophytes	Only few nails on one hand affected; nails on toes possibly affected; fungal scale close to outer margin of lesion; brittle, thickened, broken nails with white or yellow discoloration	Topical antifungals, including clotrimazole, miconazole, tolnaftate, and haloprogin cream or solution; griseofulvin moderately successful on fingernails; poor response on toenails; debridement of toenails to normal contour if problematic
TINEA PEDIS		
Various dermatophytes, commonly referred to as athletes foot	Interdigital scaling and maceration; erythema and blistering; pruritus; painful	Topical antifungals, including clotrimazole, miconazole, tolnaftate, and haloprogin cream or solution

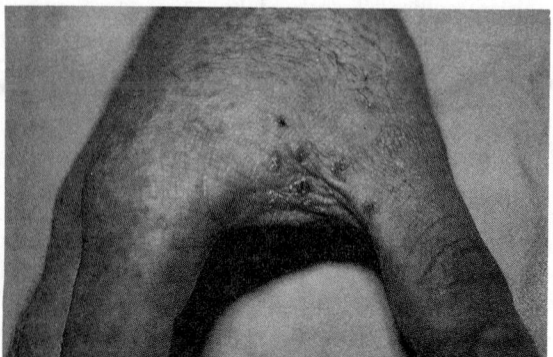

Fig. 17-9 Scabies on a hand. (Courtesy Larry Becker, Albuquerque, New Mexico.)

Table 17-12   Common Infestations and Insect Bites

Name	Etiology and Pathophysiology	Clinical Manifestations	Treatment and Prognosis
Bees and wasps	Hymenoptera	Intense, burning, local pain; swelling and itching; severe hypersensitivity possibly leading to anaphylaxis	Cool compresses; local application of antipruritic lotion; antihistamines if indicated; usually uneventful recovery; quick relief from pain by rubbing area with dilute solutions of meat tenderizer (papain); application of pulverized aspirin to moistened site
Bedbugs	Cimicidae; feeding periodic, usually at night; present in furniture, walls during day	Wheal surrounded by vivid flare; firm urticaria transforming into persistent lesion; severe pruritus; often grouped in threes appearing on noncovered parts of body	Bedbug controlled by chlorocyclohexane; lesions usually requiring no treatment; severe itching possibly requiring use of antihistamines or topical steroids

Pediculosis
  Head lice
  Body lice and pubic lice
	Pediculus humanus var. *capitis*
	Pediculus humanus var. *corporis; Phthirius pubis;* obligate parasites that suck blood, leave excrement and eggs on skin, live in seams of clothing (if body lice) and in hair as nits; reaction due to delayed hypersensitivity to saliva and feces acting on antigen; transmission of pubic lice often by sexual contact
		Minute, red, noninflammatory; points flush with skin; progression to papular wheal-like lesions; pruritus; secondary excoriation, especially parallel linear excoriations in intrascapular region; firmly attached to hair shaft in head and body lice	γ-Benzene hexachloride or pyrethrins to treat various parts of body; application as directed; contact screening with bed partners, playmates, shared head gear

Scabies	*Sarcoptes scabiei;* penetration of stratum corneum; depositing of eggs; allergic reaction due to presence of eggs, feces, mite parts; transmission by direct physical contact, only occasionally by shared personal items	Severe itching, especially at night, usually not on face; presence of burrows, especially in interdigital webs, flexor surface of wrists, and anterior axillary folds; redness, swelling, vesiculation	10% crotamiton, γ-benzene hexachloride, benzyl benzoate 12%-25%; complete eradication possible; recurrence possible; treatment of sexual partner in positively diagnosed scabies; antibiotics if dermatitis and secondary infections present
Tick	*Borrelia burgdorferi;* spirochete transmitted by ticks in certain areas at any time during 2-year life cycle, most commonly during nymphal stage; endemic areas that include Northeast, Mid-Atlantic states, parts of Midwest and West	Spreading, ringlike rash 3 to 4 weeks after bite; commonly in groin, buttocks, axillae, trunk, and upper arms and legs; warm, itchy, or painful rash; flulike symptoms; cardiac, arthritic, and neurological manifestations possible; unreliable laboratory test; no acquired immunity	Oral antibiotics, such as doxycycline (Vibramycin), tetracycline (Achromycin); IV antibiotics for arthritic, neurological, and cardiac symptoms; rest and healthy diet

Table 17-13 Common Allergic Conditions of the Skin

Etiology and Pathophysiology	Clinical Manifestations	Treatment and Prognosis
CONTACT DERMATITIS		
Manifestation of delayed hypersensitivity, absorbed agent acting as antigen, sensitization after several exposures, appearance of lesions 12 to 48 hours after contact with allergen	Red, hivelike papules and plaques; sharply circumscribed with occasional vesicles; exposed areas more common; usually pruritic; relation of area of dermatitis to causative agent (e.g., metal allergy and dermatitis on ring finger)	Topical corticosteroids, antihistamines; skin lubrication; elimination of contact allergen; avoidance of irritating affected area; systemic steroids if sensitivity severe
URTICARIA		
Usually allergic phenomena presence of edema in upper dermis due to local increase in permeability of capillaries, usually due to histamine	Spontaneously occurring and rounded elevations, varying size, usually multiple	Removal of source, antihistamine therapy
DRUG REACTION		
Any drug that acts as antigen and causes hypersensitive reaction possible cause, certain drugs more prone to reactions (e.g., penicillin, mediated by circulating antibodies)	Rash of any morphology; often red, macular and papular, semiconfluent, generalized rash with abrupt onset; appearance as late as 14 days after cessation of drug; possibly pruritic	Withdrawal of drug if possible, antihistamines, local or systemic corticosteroids possibly necessary
ATOPIC DERMATITIS		
Exact cause unknown, often beginning in infancy and clearing with age, association with allergic conditions, elevation of IgE levels common, genetically determined often family history, decreased itch threshold, stress and increased water contact (e.g., frequent hand washing, thumb sucking) other possible agents	Scaly, red to red-brown, circumscribed lesions; accentuation of skin markings; pruritic; symmetrical eruptions common in antecubital and popliteal space in adults	Topical corticosteroids, coal tar therapy, intralesional steroids, lubrication of dry skin, systemic steroids if severe, reduction of stress, antibiotics for secondary infection

tivity (anaphylaxis), which can be life-threatening (Chapter 8).

Prevention of insect bites by avoidance or by the use of repellants is somewhat effective. Meticulous hygiene related to personal articles, clothing, bedding, examination and care of pets, as well as careful selection of sexual partners, can reduce the incidence of infestations. A rash on only exposed body parts is highly suggestive of an insect bite. Routine inspection is necessary where there is a risk of tick bites and Lyme disease (Table 17-12).

Allergic Dermatological Problems

Dermatological problems associated with allergies and hypersensitivity reactions present a real challenge to the clinician (Table 17-13). The pathophysiology related to allergic and contact dermatitis is covered in Chapter 8. Often only the most careful family history and discussion of exposure to possible offending agents will yield valuable data. Patch testing involves the application of allergens to the client's skin (usually on the back) for 48 to 72 hours,

after which the test sites are examined for erythema, vesicles, or both. Patch testing is used by dermatologists to determine possible causative agents. This information is valuable to the client. The best treatment of allergic dermatitis is avoidance. The extreme pruritus of contact dermatitis and its potential for chronicity make it a frustrating problem for the client, the nurse, and the dermatologist.

Benign Dermatological Problems

Although the list of benign dermatoses is extensive, some of the most commonly seen and distressing problems are summarized in Table 17-14.

DERMATOLOGICAL MANIFESTATIONS OF SYSTEMIC DISEASES

Dermatological manifestations of systemic disease may be either specific or nonspecific. Specific conditions display the same pathophysiological process in relation to the skin as the internal disease process. Nonspecific conditions do not resemble the internal problem but are helpful in es-

Table 17-14 Common Benign Conditions of the Skin

Etiology and Pathophysiology	Clinical Manifestations	Treatment and Prognosis
ACNE		
Inflammatory disorder of sebaceous glands; more common in teenagers but possible development in adulthood; persistence into adulthood possible; secondary result of iodides, bromides, corticosteroids, androgen-dominant birth control pills	Noninflammatory lesions, including comedones (blackheads) and closed comedones (whiteheads); inflammatory lesions, including papules and pustules; most common on face, neck, and upper back	Mechanical removal of multiple lesions with comedo extractor after comedo opened with fine needle or blade; topical application of benzoyl peroxide as antibacterial and peeling agent; use of peeling and irritating agents such as retinoic acid; long-term antibiotic therapy—topical or systemic; phototherapy: aim of treatment to suppress new lesions; spontaneous remission possible; often improvement with exposure to summer sun; use of isotretenoin (Accutane) for severe cystic acne to possibly provide lasting remission; contraindicated in pregnant women or women intending to become pregnant while on drug; monitoring of liver function tests, cholesterol, and triglycerides essential
MOLES		
Grouping of normal cells derived from melanocytelike precursor cells; hereditary determination possible	Hyperpigmented areas that vary in form and color; flat, slightly elevated, haloid, verrucoid, polypoid, dome-shaped, sessile, or papillomatous; preservation of normal skin markings; hair growth possible	No treatment necessary except for cosmetic reasons, skin biopsy for diagnostic decisions
PSORIASIS		
Chronic dermatitis, which involves excessively rapid turnover of epidermal cells; family predisposition	Sharply demarcated scaling plaques of the scalp, elbows, and knees; palms, soles, and fingernails possibly affected; localized or general, intermittent or continuous	Aim of retarding growth of epidermal cells; difficult to medicate; usually topical corticosteroids, tar, anthralin; intralesional injection of corticosteroids for chronic plaques; sunlight; ultraviolet light; alone or with topical or systemic potentiation; no cure; control possible; wrapping of affected areas often indicated; antimetabolites (especially methotrexate) for difficult cases
SEBORRHEIC KERATOSES		
Benign, genetically determined growths; found in increasing number with age; no association with sun exposure	Irregularly round or oval, flat-topped papules or plaques; surface often warty; appearance of being stuck on; increase in pigmentation with age of lesion; usually multiple and possibly itchy	Removal by curettage or cryosurgery for cosmetic reasons or to eliminate source of irritation; minimal scarring

Continued.

Table 17-14 Common Benign Conditions of the Skin—cont'd

Etiology and Pathophysiology	Clinical Manifestations	Treatment and Prognosis
SKIN TAGS		
Common after midlife; appearance on neck, axillae, and upper trunk; association with colonic adenomatous polyps	Small, skin-colored, soft, pedunculated papules	No treatment unless for cosmetic reasons or because of repeated trauma; surgical removal possible (if requested); usually just "clipping off" without anesthesia; occult blood testing and flexible sigmoidoscopy necessary
LIPOMA		
Benign tumor of adipose tissue, often encapsulated, most common in 40- to 60-year-old age group	Rubbery, compressible, round mass of adipose tissue; single or multiple; variable in size, possibly extremely large; most common on trunk, back of neck, and forearms	Usually no treatment, biopsy to differentiate from liposarcoma, excision usual treatment (when indicated)
VITILIGO		
Unknown cause; genetically influenced, most noticeable in dark-skinned persons and those with summer tan; complete absence of melanocytes; noncontagious	Focal amelanosis (complete loss of pigment); macular; variation in size and location; usually symmetrical and permanent	Attempts at repigmentation with sunlight and psoralens; depigmentation of pigmented skin with extensive disease (>50% of body involved); cosmetics and stains for camouflage and to deemphasize vitiliginous areas
LENTIGO		
Increased number of normal melanocytes in basal layer of epidermis, senile lentigos ("liver spots") related to aging and sun exposure	Hyperpigmented, brown to black, flat lesion; usually on sun-exposed areas	Treatment only for cosmetic purposes, liquid nitrogen, possible recurrence in 1 to 2 years

tablishing a diagnosis. The skilled clinician should always consider the possibility that a particular dermatosis is a clue to an internal, less obvious problem.

Certain neoplasms that arise at various internal sites are sometimes associated with both specific and nonspecific cutaneous manifestations. Although there is generally no relationship between morphology of the lesion and site of origin, certain types of malignancies do seem to metastasize to certain anatomical sites. For instance, lung cancers usually metastasize to the chest or scalp, while metastasis from the breast commonly appears on the anterior part of the chest.[16]

Certain life changes have recognized associated dermatoses. At *puberty*, male- or female-pattern hair growth will be evident as a secondary sex characteristic. Increased apocrine gland activity can lead to body odor. The increased sebaceous gland activity stimulated by androgens can result in seborrhea and acne.

Pregnancy is characterized by physiological skin changes, including hyperpigmentation and increased perspiration. *Menopause* is often accompanied by hot flashes, increased perspiration, facial hair growth, and varying de-

grees of scalp hair loss. Old age often presents skin problems related to dryness, wrinkling, hyperpigmentation, and actinic changes. System-specific dermatological manifestations of internal disorders are presented in Table 17-15.

PLASTIC SURGERY
Elective Cosmetic Surgery

The possible cosmetic changes that can be made surgically are almost limitless. Cosmetic surgery includes such techniques as breast enlargement; breast reduction; chemical, mechanical, and surgical face-lift; eyelid lift; hair transplant; nose corrections; removal of double chin; correction of receding or prominent chin; abdomen lift; buttocks reduction; thigh lift; correction of elephant ears; and liposuction of many body areas.

The reasons for the surgery are as varied as the techniques. The most common reason that people suffer the discomfort and financial expense (most are not covered by insurance) of cosmetic surgery is to improve their body image. People project their personal image of themselves. If they feel better about themselves as a result of cosmetic

Table 17-15 Dermatological Manifestations of Systemic Problems*

Systemic Problem	Dermatological Manifestations
ENDOCRINE	
Increased growth hormone	Hyperplasia and thickening of dermis, hair, nails
Hyperthyroidism	Increased sweating, warm skin with persistent flush, thin nails, vitiligo and alopecia, fine, soft hair
Hypothyroidism	Cold, dry, pale to yellow skin; slightly hyperkeratotic epidermis with follicular plugging; generalized nonpitting edema; dry, coarse, brittle hair; brittle, slow-growing nails
Glucocorticoid excess (Cushing's syndrome), induced endogenously or exogenously	Atrophy; striae; epidermal thinning; telangiectasia; acne; decreased subcutaneous fat over extremities; thin, loose dermis; impaired wound healing; increased vascular fragility; mild hirsutism; excessive collection of fat over clavicles, back of neck, abdomen, and face; increased incidence of pyodermas
Addison's disease	Loss of body hair (especially axillary), generalized hyperpigmentation (especially in folds)
Androgen excess	Enlarged facial pores, male sex characteristics, acne, acceleration of coarse hair growth
Androgen deficiency—postpuberty	Development of sparse hair; marked reduction in sebum production
Hypoparathyroidism	Opaque, brittle nails with transverse ridges; coarse, sparse hair with patchy alopecia; eczematous and exfoliative dermatitis; hyperkeratotic and maculopapular eruptions
Hyperpituitarism (acromegaly)	Coarsened skin, deepened lines; increased oiliness and sweating; acne; increased number of nevi, hyperpigmentation; hypertrichosis
Hypopituitarism (Froëlich's syndrome)	Smooth skin; scant hair growth; obesity; small, thin fingernails
Diabetes mellitus	Increased xanthomas and carotene, shin spots, necrobiosis lipoidica diabeticorum, delayed wound healing
GASTROINTESTINAL	
Ulcerative colitis, Crohn's disease	Pyoderma gangrenosum, mouth ulcers
Liver disease	Jaundice, itching, pigmentary abnormalities, alterations in nails and hair, spider angiomas, telangiectasia
Biliary tract obstruction	
Deficiency of essential fatty acids	Scaly skin
Malabsorption syndrome	Acquired ichthyosis
Cystic fibrosis	Abnormal sweat gland function resulting in failure to conserve sodium
MUSCULOSKELETAL AND CONNECTIVE TISSUE	
Systemic lupus erythematosus	Maculopapular semiconfluent rash (butterfly rash)
Scleroderma	Leathery hardening and stiffness of skin
Dermatomyositis	Edema; purplish-red upper eyelids; butterfly rash; scaly, macular erythema over knuckles; linear telangiectasia of posterior nail fold
METABOLIC	
Lipidoses	Xanthomas
Vitamin A deficiency	Generalized dry hyperkeratoses (phrynoderma)
Hypervitaminosis A	Hair loss, dry skin
Vitamin B_1 (thiamine) deficiency	Edema, redness of soles of feet
Vitamin B_2 (riboflavin) deficiency	Red fissures at corner of mouth, glossitis
Nicotinic acid (niacin) deficiency	Pellagra; redness of exposed areas of hand/feet, face/neck; infected dermatitis
IMMUNE	
Drug sensitivity	Rash of any morphology
Serum sickness	Pruritus
Cancer of breast, stomach, lung, uterus, kidney, ovary, colon, bladder	Metastasis to skin
Hodgkin's disease	Pruritus and nonspecific erythemas
Lymphomas	Papules, nodules, plaques, pruritus

*Refer to the systemic disease for specific information.

Continued.

Table 17-15 Dermatological Manifestations of Systemic Problems*—cont'd

Systemic Problem	Dermatological Manifestations
CARDIOVASCULAR	
Arteriosclerosis	Venous thrombosis, decreased oxygenation leading to gangrene
Rheumatic heart disease	Petechiae, urticaria, rheumatic nodules, erythema nodosum and multiforme
Periarteritis nodosa	Periarteritis nodules
Thromboangiitis obliterans (Buerger's disease)	Superficial migrating thrombophlebitis, pallor or cyanosis, gangrene, ulceration
RESPIRATORY	
Inadequate oxygenation secondary to respiratory disease	Cyanosis
HEMATOLOGICAL	
Anemia	Pallor, hyperpigmentation, pale mucous membranes, hair loss, nail dystrophy
Clotting disorders	Purpura, petechiae, ecchymosis
RENAL	
Chronic renal failure	Dry skin, pruritus, uremic frost, pallor, dry skin, bruises, petechiae
REPRODUCTIVE	
Primary syphilis	Chancre
Secondary syphilis	Generalized skin lesions
Late benign syphilis	Gummas
Paget's disease	Eczematous patch of nipple and areola
NEUROLOGICAL	
Syringomyelia, chronic sensory polyneuropathies, spinal cord trauma	Trophic changes in skin due to sensory denervation, decubitus ulcers, anesthesia, paresthesias

*Refer to the systemic disease for specific information.

surgery, they will often act more confident and self-assured. Often social position and economic considerations are part of the decision. The youth-oriented society often feels uncomfortable doing business with someone who appears to be aging. Also, increased longevity provides a larger population to whom cosmetic surgery is especially appealing.

Regardless of the reason the client elects to have cosmetic surgery, the nurse should maintain a supportive, nonjudgmental attitude. If the client wishes to change a body feature perceived as unattractive, then it is a personal decision to undergo cosmetic surgery and the nurse should support this decision.

Chemical face-lift or peel. A *chemical face peel* uses a cauterant to the skin to cause a controlled burn. This results in superficial destruction of the upper layers of the skin and a tightening of the deep layers. The most common indications for a chemical peel include pigmentation problems, skin damage due to radiation, freckles, superficial acne scarring, and actinic and seborrheic keratoses.

After the client is sedated, a solution (buffered phenol, trichloroacetic acid, or 20% resorcinol) is painted on the skin, with care taken to avoid the eyes. Postoperative care is prescribed specifically by the physician. It may include refraining from activities, talking, and chewing, and it may involve the application of compresses (vinegar) and topical ointments. There will be moderate swelling and crusting for 1 week. Within 7 to 8 days new skin will appear, and healing will be complete by 10 days. Redness will persist for 6 to 8 weeks. A pink tone will be apparent for several months. Once healing is complete, the skin will have a more youthful appearance because of a new superficial layer of skin.

Since there is a reduction of melanin as a result of this procedure, the client must be instructed to absolutely avoid the sun for 6 months to prevent unsightly hyperpigmentation. Aside from the fact that it is relatively painful, chemical peeling results in the new skin being lighter than the old skin. This can cause a disparity in the color between the treated and untreated areas. There is a possibility that this procedure can cause scarring. Chemical peeling is considered the better treatment for wrinkles and certain types of hyperpigmentation.

Topical tretinoin. Topical application of tretinoin (Retin-A) provides some reversal of photodamaged skin. Fine and coarse wrinkling improves. There is a reduction in the number of lentigines (age spots) and in the color of freckles. Actinic keratoses decrease in number. Deep wrinkles and expression lines are usually not affected by tretinoin.[17] The main adverse effect is a cutaneous reaction characterized by erythema, swelling, and scaling, which generally improves when treated with emollients or when application of tretinoin is stopped or decreased to every other day.

The response to tretinoin appears to be dose related. The usual dose is 0.025%, 0.05%, or 0.1% in a cream base. Gradual introduction to tretinoin begins with application every other day, aiming for nightly application as tolerated. Treatment is not usually stopped when inflammation occurs unless the inflammation is severe. Maximum response occurs after 8 to 12 months of treatment. Thereafter application three to four times a week should maintain improvement.

A sunscreen must be used in combination with tretinoin to prevent further sun damage and to protect against the greater photosensitivity that clients experience during tretinoin therapy.[18] Sun-sensitizing substances such as products containing sulfur, resorcinol, salicylic acid, or benzoyl peroxide should be avoided.

Dermabrasion. *Dermabrasion* is the removal of epidermis and a portion of the superficial layer of the dermis with preservation of sufficient epidermal adnexa to allow for spontaneous reepithelialization of the abraded surface.[19] Dermabrasion is used to treat acne scars, hypertrophic scars, and sun-damaged and wrinkled skin and to correct pigmentary abnormalities, usually on the face.

There has been marked improvement in the tools used for this procedure. Dermabrasion uses an electrically driven waterproof carbide abrasive paper cylinder and diamond-impregnated burrs. Dermabrasion is most often performed in office surgical suites.

After the formation of a coagulum from the serum, there is a proliferation of squamous epithelium from the adnexal elements. By the third to the fourth postoperative day, a thin epidermis begins to regenerate and collagen is laid down. Pigmentation does not begin until 3 to 4 weeks after abrasion. Exposure to the sun must be strictly avoided for 2 to 4 months to prevent hyperpigmentation.

In general, the instructions to dermabrasion clients are focused on prevention of drying. Petroleum jelly, Polysporin ointment, and wet soaks are included in the instructions and are to be applied at varying times on particular postoperative days. Clients are instructed to use a heavy layer of ointment when not soaking. Instructions for postoperative wound care vary widely among practitioners. Specific care needs to be well understood by the client. Sunscreens (SPF 30) should be used if the client is outdoors. The most common complications include hyperpigmentation, hypopigmentation, keloids, herpes simplex, milia, persistent erythema, telangiectasia, and infection.

Face-lift. A *face-lift* (rhytidectomy) is the lifting and repositioning of the lower two thirds of the face and neck to improve appearance (Fig. 17-10).[20] Indications for this procedure include the following:

1. Redundant soft tissue resulting from dermatitis (e.g., smallpox or acne scarring)
2. Asymmetrical redundancy of soft tissues (e.g., facial palsy)

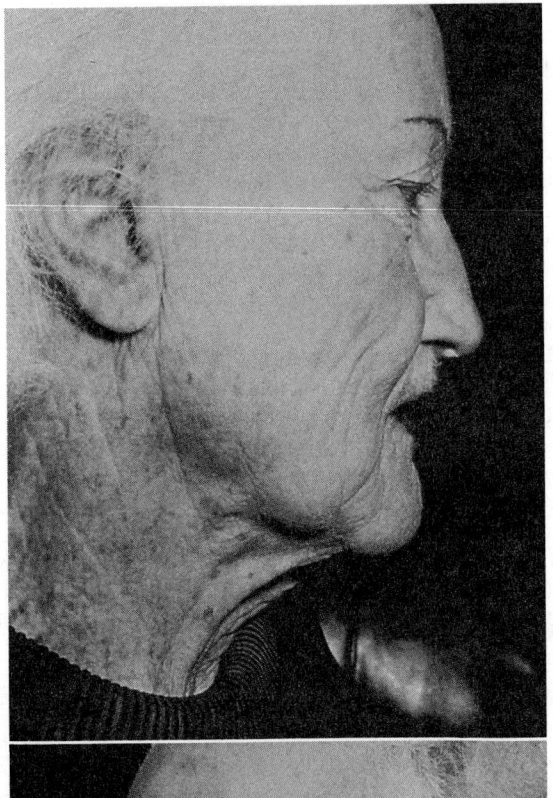

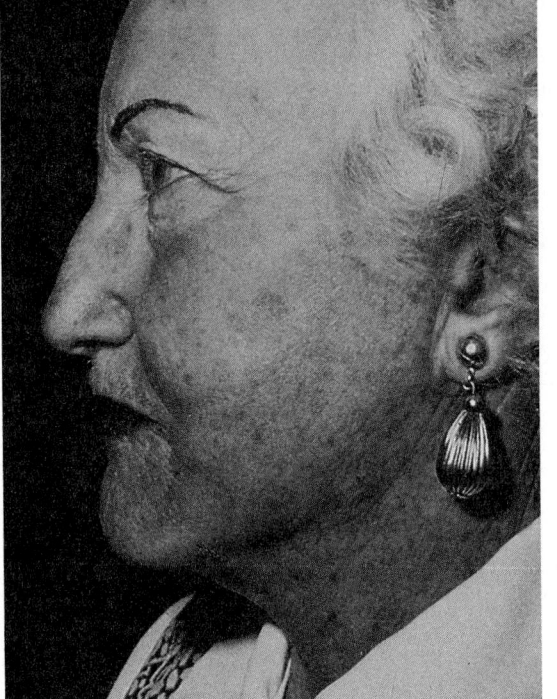

Fig. 17-10 **A,** Before face-lift. **B,** After face-lift. (Courtesy Richard Gooding, Albuquerque, New Mexico.)

3. Redundant soft tissues resulting from trauma
4. Preauricular lesions
5. Redundant soft tissues resulting from solar elastosis, changes in body weight, and gravitation
6. Restoration of body image

The surgical approach and lines of incisions vary according to the nature of the deformity and the position of the hairline. Prevention of hematoma formation is the most important postoperative consideration. A pressure dressing is usually used the first 24 to 48 hours to reduce the possibility of hematoma formation. Once the dressing is removed, there is little pain. The sutures are removed from the fifth to the tenth postoperative day. Antibiotics are used at the discretion of the surgeon. Infection is not a common problem.

Liposuction. *Liposuction* is a technique for removing subcutaneous fat to improve facial and body contours. Although not a substitute for diet and exercise, it can be successful in removing areas of fat that are resistant to other techniques from virtually any body area.

Although relatively free of complications, possible contraindications for the procedure include use of anticoagulants, history of inflammatory fat disease, uncontrolled hypertension, diabetes mellitus, and poor cardiovascular status. Persons under 40 years of age with good skin elasticity are the best candidates. However, clients ranging in age from 16 to 70 years can be treated successfully.[21]

The procedure is usually performed, with the aid of local anesthesia, on an outpatient basis. One or more sessions may be necessary, depending on the size of the area to be treated. A blunt-tipped cannula is inserted through a ½-inch incision and pushed into the fat to break it loose from the fibrous stroma. Multiple repeated thrusts disrupt

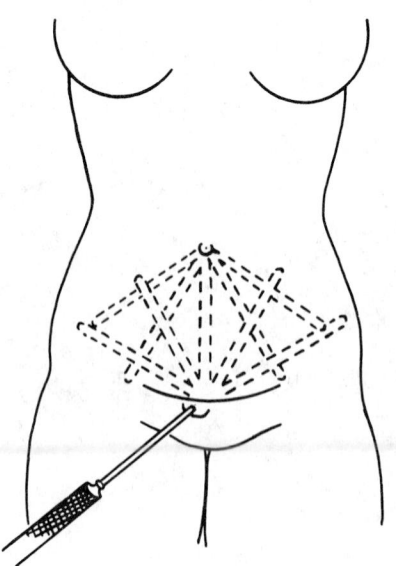

Fig. 17-11 Liposuction. Site of incision and tunneling pattern for abdominal liposuction procedure. (From Habif TF: Clinical dermatology: a color guide to diagnosis and therapy, St Louis, 1990, Mosby–Year Book, Inc, p 690.)

the fat and create tunnels (Fig. 17-11). The loosened fat is removed with a very powerful suction. The area is taped. Firm bandaging helps to contour the skin and reduce the chance of postoperative bleeding and serum accumulation. It may take several months for the final results to be evident.

■ Nursing Management of Cosmetic Surgery

Many cosmetic surgical procedures are being performed in well-equipped day surgeries or in plastic surgeons' office surgery suites. Several interventions related to cosmetic surgery are appropriate, regardless of where or how the nurse-client relationship develops.

Preoperative management

A major consideration relates to informed consent and realistic expectations of what cosmetic surgery can accomplish. Although this information is usually provided by the surgeon, the nurse can and should reinforce this dialogue and answer questions and concerns. For instance, a facelift has little or no effect on deep wrinkling of the forehead and temples, deep nasolabial grooves, or vertical lip wrinkles. Before and after treatment photographs of similar cases are often useful in helping the client to set realistic expectations.

The client also needs to understand the time frame for healing. The fullest results cannot, in some instances, be expected for as long as 1 year after the procedure. The oozing, crusting phase of the abrasive procedures must be explained so the client can plan time off from work if this seems necessary. The final results of the cosmetic procedures are affected by age, general state of health, and general skin type. Should a health problem be apparent, efforts should be made to correct or control the problem before the procedure.

Postoperative management

Most of the cosmetic procedures are not exceptionally painful. Usually mild analgesics are sufficient to keep the patient comfortable.

Even though infection is not a common problem after cosmetic surgery, the nurse needs to assess the surgical sites for signs of infection. Systemic signs of infection such as fever and increased respirations should also be carefully monitored. The client should be aware of signs of infection and told to report any such signs immediately so that appropriate antibiotic intervention can be started.

If the surgery involved alteration in the circulation to the skin, such as the undermining done in a face-lift, a careful monitoring of adequate circulation is necessary. Warm, pink skin that blanches on pressure indicates that adequate circulation is present in the surgical area.

Skin Grafts

Uses. Skin grafts may be necessary to provide protection to underlying structures or to reconstruct areas for cosmetic or functional purposes. Ideally, wounds heal by primary intention. However, large, surgically created wounds, trauma, and chronic wounds can cause extensive tissue destruction, making primary intention healing impossible. In these cases, skin grafting may be necessary. Improved surgical techniques make it possible to graft skin, bone, cartilage, fat, fascia, muscles, and nerves. For cosmetically pleasing results, the color, thickness, texture, and hair-bearing nature of skin used for grafting must be chosen to match the recipient site.[22]

Types. The two types of skin grafts are *free grafts* and *skin flaps*. Free grafts are further differentiated according to the method of providing a blood supply to the grafted skin. One method is to transfer the graft (epidermis and part or all of the dermis) to the recipient site from the donor site. If the graft is an autograft (from the client's own body) or an isograft (from an identical twin), it will revascularize and become fixed to the new site. Chapter 18 discusses full and split skin grafts in detail.

Another method of free skin grafting is by reconstructive microsurgery. With the use of an operating microscope, circulation is immediately established in the free flap by anastomosis of the blood vessels from the skin flap to the vessels in the recipient site. This highly technical and time-consuming surgery is being used in many situations that were previously treated with the use of skin flaps.[22]

Skin flaps involve moving a section of skin and subcutaneous tissue from one part of the body to another without terminating the vascular attachment. The vascular attachment is called a pedicle. Skin flaps are used to cover wounds with a poor vascular bed, when padding is needed, and to cover wounds over cartilage and bone. There may be a need for intermediate flap placement if the recipient site is far removed from the donor.

The flap is advanced to the recipient site when circulation is well established at the intermediate site. The type of flap and the route of transfer are individually determined according to the needs of the client and the nature of the defect to be repaired.

Soft tissue expansion is a relatively new technique for providing skin for resurfacing a defect, such as a burn scar, or for removing a disfiguring mark, such as a tattoo.[17]

A subcutaneous tissue expander of an appropriate size and shape is placed under the skin. The expander is kept in place for the length of time it takes for the skin needed for the procedure to grow. This may be from several weeks to 3 to 4 months. Then the old incision is opened, the expander is removed, and the soft tissue is ready to be used as an advancement flap. The tissue expander next to a defect retains the primary tissue characteristics such as color and texture.

The placement of the expander is usually done on an outpatient basis. Weekly expansion with saline solution can be done in a health care setting or by the client at home.

∎ Nursing Management of Skin Grafts

After a skin graft, several areas need to be assessed. The most critical assessment is related to the vascular supply to the grafted site. If the area is not dressed, it should be regularly assessed for color, warmth, capillary refill, and turgor. If the grafted area has a dressing, it is usually left in place until removed by the surgeon. Systemic signs of infection, such as fever and pain must be monitored.

After a skin graft the client may often have to assume unnatural positions that lead to pain, stiffness, and frustration. The nurse is challenged to assist the client to divert attention from this awkward situation. Often tranquilizers or sedatives are necessary to assist the client through this period. Appropriate nursing intervention related to altered mobility must also be considered.

Although pain is not usually a major problem, the nurse should provide pain relief when necessary. Conversation, diversion, and massage, as well as medication, should be used to maintain client comfort. The immobility enforced by certain grafting procedures presents the expected potential complications of pneumonia, pulmonary emboli, and decubital ulcers. Aggressive measures by the nursing staff should be instituted to prevent such complications.

Skin grafting may involve long periods of hospitalization, with the constant threat of graft death. Since this is a particularly difficult time emotionally for the client, the nurse needs to be supportive and understanding. Expectations of the results of the graft must be realistic if the client is not to suffer depression as the result of unfulfilled expectations. The family and friends of the client need consideration and explanation of procedures and restrictions imposed by the grafting procedures.

Pressure Sores

Prevention and treatment of pressure sores are usually the responsibility of the nurse. Therefore it is important that the nurse be aware of the latest issues related to pressure sore management. The current trend is to keep a pressure sore slightly moist, rather than dry, to enhance epithelialization.[23] In addition to the nurse, other members of the health team, such as the plastic surgeon, the nutritionist, the physical therapist, and the occupational therapist, can provide valuable input into complex treatment necessary to prevent and treat pressure sores.

Etiology and Pathophysiology. Direct pressure is the primary cause of tissue ischemia and ulcer formation. Simple erythema or hyperemia around the edges of the involved area is the first event in ulcer formation. If pressure is unrelieved, ischemia will follow, leading to cutaneous, subcutaneous, and muscle necrosis, and clinically obvious ulceration.

Another cause of pressure sore development is *shearing*. Shearing occurs when tissue layers slide over each other, causing the subcutaneous blood vessels to kink or stretch, interrupting blood flow. When the client slides down in bed or is raised in bed without the use of a draw sheet, this type of tissue injury can result.

Pressure in excess of arterial capillary pressure (32 mm Hg), sustained for a period of 1 to 2 hours, will occlude the tissue capillaries and result in ischemia. Pressure is most severe in body areas over bony prominences. The most common skin sites affected by pressure sores are over the ischium, sacrum, and trochanter (60%) and the pretibial area, malleolus, and heel (17%).[24]

In addition to pressure and shearing force, other factors that predispose to the development of pressure sores include impaired circulation, anemia, contractures, mental deterioration, physical dependence, immobility, inconti-

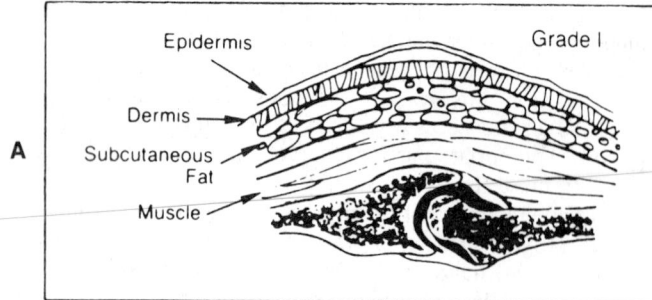
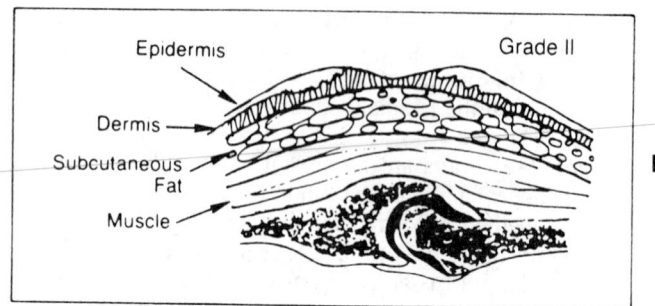
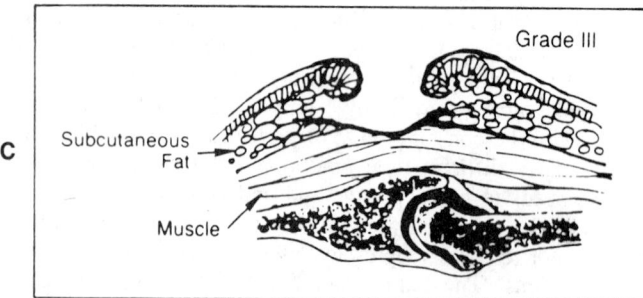
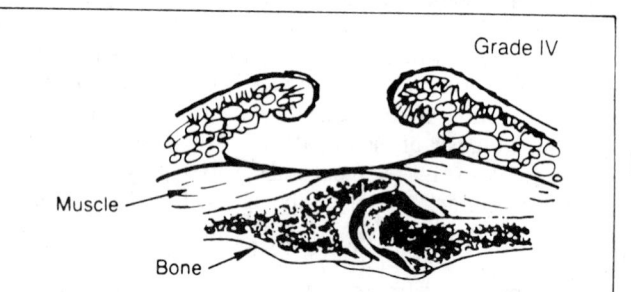

Fig. 17-12 Staging of pressure sores. **A,** Stage I. Erythema not resolving within 30 minutes of pressure relief. Epidermis remains intact. *Reversible with intervention.* **B,** Stage II. Partial-thickness loss of skin layers involving epidermis and possibly penetrating into but not through dermis. May present as blistering with erythema and/or induration; wound base is moist and pink, painful, and free of necrotic tissue. **C,** Stage III. Full-thickness tissue loss extending through dermis to involve subcutaneous tissue. Presents as shallow crater unless covered by eschar. (If wound involves necrotic tissue, staging cannot be confirmed until wound base is visible.) May include necrotic tissue; undermining, sinus tract formation; exudate; and/or infection. Wound base is usually not painful. **D,** Stage IV. Deep tissue destruction extending through subcutaneous tissue to fascia and possibly involving muscle layers, joint, and/or bone. Presents as a deep crater. May include necrotic tissue; undermining, sinus tract formation; exudate; and/or infection. Wound base is usually not painful. (From International Association for Enterostomal Therapy: Standards of care: dermal wounds: pressure sores, Irvine, Calif, 1987.)

nence, old age, hyperglycemia, and poor nutritional status.

Clinical manifestations. The clinical manifestations of pressure sores depend on the stage of the ulcer. Figure 17-12 describes the four stages of pressure sore development. If the ulcer becomes infected, the client may display signs of infection, such as leukocytosis and fever. In addition, the pressure sore may increase in size, odor, and drainage, have necrotic tissue, and be indurated, warm, and painful. The most common complication of a pressure sore is recurrence.[24]

■ Therapeutic and Nursing Management of Pressure Sores

Both conservative and surgical management strategies are used in the treatment of pressure sores, depending on the stage and condition of the ulcer. Therapeutic and nursing management will be discussed together, since the activities are interrelated.

Nursing assessment

Subjective and objective data that should be obtained from a person with a pressure sore are presented in Table 17-16.

Nursing diagnoses

Nursing diagnoses are determined when the problem and etiological factors are supported by clinical data. Nursing diagnoses related to pressure sores may include, but are not limited to, those presented in Table 17-17.

Nursing interventions

Health maintenance and promotion. A primary nursing responsibility is the identification of clients at risk for the development of pressure sores. Factors that put a client at risk for the development of pressure sores include impaired circulation, anemia, contractures, mental deterioration, physical dependence, immobility, incontinence, and old age. Systemic illnesses such as diabetes, collagen disease, vascular diseases, leprosy, and neurological disorders that affect sensation result in greater risk of ulcer formation. Both obesity and emaciation put clients at higher risk. Prevention remains the best treatment for pressure sores.

Pressure reduction devices, such as alternating pressure mattresses, egg-crate-like matresses, wheelchair cushions, padded commode seats, foam boots, and lift sheets are useful in preventing pressure and shearing force. How-

Table 17-16

Nursing Assessment of the Client With Pressure Sores

SUBJECTIVE DATA

History
Stroke; spinal cord injury; prolonged bed rest or immobility; circulatory impairment; altered level of consciousness; advanced age; diabetes; recent trauma or surgery; nutritional status, obesity, or emaciation; anemia; incontinence; dehydration

Medications
Use of narcotics, spinal and general anesthesia, hypnotics, muscle paralyzers, corticosteroids

Pain
Pressure sore area

Neurological
Altered sensation in area of pressure sore

OBJECTIVE DATA

General
Fever

Integumentary
Diaphoresis, edema, and redness, especially over bony areas, such as sacrum, hips, elbows, heels, knees, ankles, shoulders, and ear rims; staging*

Possible findings
Leukocytosis, positive cultures from pressure sore

*See Fig. 17-12.

Table 17-17

NURSING CARE PLAN FOR THE CLIENT WITH A PRESSURE SORE

Defining Characteristics	Nursing Interventions	Evaluation Criteria
NURSING DIAGNOSIS: Impaired skin integrity related to pressure and inadequate circulation		
Evidence of pressure sore from grade I to grade IV; complaints of pain or discomfort in affected area; presence of risk factors such as immobility, old age, debilitation, diminished mental status, poor nutrition, pronounced bony prominences, incontinence, altered cutaneous sensation	Assess causative factors such as activity, mobility, presence or absence of sensory deficits, nutrition and hydration status, circulation and oxygenation, skin moisture status. Assess and document wound in relation to location, size, granulation tissue visible and/or epithelialization, necrotic tissue, local or systemic infection, presence and character of exudate, including volume, color, consistency, and odor. Classify wound. Use pressure relief device if indicated. Institute position change schedule. Keep head of bed at or below 30-degree angle and flat when not contraindicated. Use assistive devices to aid client movement (e.g., trapeze, turning sheets, lifts). Protect client's skin from excess moisture. Institute 2000 to 3000 calories/ day (more if increased metabolic demands), 2000 ml/day of fluid. Initiate prescribed treatment based on stage of the pressure sore. Monitor progress of wound on a regular basis. Educate client and family relative to cause, prevention, and treatment of pressure sore. Refer if indicated.	Intact skin
NURSING DIAGNOSIS: Self-esteem disturbance related to pressure sores		
Poor self-care, negative attitude and remarks, social isolation, inadequate support system, use of ineffective coping strategies such as anger and blaming	Assess values attached to body, coping styles and strategies, lifestyle and social activities, personal support systems, and evidence of negative self-concept. Encourage verbalization about pressure sore. Provide realistic, honest feedback. Reinforce and teach appropriate coping strategies. Provide support, counseling, and appropriate information about pressure sore prevention and treatment to client and family. Refer for counseling, if appropriate.	Positive self-concept evidenced by active participation and compliance with treatment plan, if possible; resumption of role-related responsibilities and relationships, if possible

Adapted from Standards of Care: Dermal wounds: pressure sores, Irvine, Calif, 1987 International Association for Enterostomal Therapy.

ever, they are not adequate substitutes for frequent repositioning.

Acute intervention. Once a pressure sore has developed, the nurse should initiate interventions based on the grade, size, and presence of infection. Careful documentation should be made of the size of the pressure sore. A plastic ruler or lesion-measuring card can be used to note the sores' maximum length and width in centimeters. The area, in square centimeters, can be determined by multiplying half the length times half the width times 3.14 (pi).[23] To find the depth of the sore, gently probe it with a sterile cotton-tipped applicator. Then measure the length of the portion of the applicator that probed the sore. If possible, pictures of the pressure sore should be taken initially and at regular intervals during the course of treatment.

A *stage I pressure sore* will usually heal completely once the pressure on the affected area is relieved. The affected area should not be massaged because this action may increase tissue trauma.[25] The involved area can be covered with a transparent dressing, which is an adhesive, sterile dressing that is impermeable to water and bacteria but permeable to moisture vapor and oxygen. This dressing can be left in place for the 1 to 2 weeks that it takes for the area to heal.

A *stage II pressure sore* is reversible if detected early. After irrigation with the prescribed solution, a transparent dressing with a pouch to collect exudate can be applied. The dressing should be reapplied if the edges become loose. This sore takes 2 to 4 months to heal.

A *stage III pressure sore* is usually irrigated daily, and a transparent dressing with a pouch or a hydrocolloid dressing is applied. A hydrocolloid dressing interacts with exudate to form a hydrated gel over the wound. The gel protects the new tissue from being damaged. These dressings are relatively impermeable to oxygen. Both the transparent and the hydrocolloid dressings are contraindicated for an infected pressure sore or one with exposed muscles, tendons, or bones (grade IV).[26]

A *stage IV pressure sore* is treated by debridement, intravenous fluids, and antibiotics. The sores may take months or even years to heal (Fig. 17-13). A wet-to-dry gauze dressing is applied daily after irrigation of the wound with a prescribed solution. Enzymes may be used to liquefy necrotic tissue. With the use of a sterile technique, the affected area should have a saline-soaked gauze dressing gently packed into the wound. Once the wound is clean, surgical debridement may be necessary. Reconstruction of the pressure sore site by such measures as split-thickness grafts and free skin flap procedures may be necessary.

The maintenance of adequate nutrition is an important nursing responsibility for the client with a pressure sore. Often, the client is debilitated and has a poor appetite secondary to inactivity. The caloric intake needed to correct and maintain a nutritional balance may be as high as 4200 calories a day. Oral feedings should be high in calories and proteins and should be supplemented with vitamins. Nasogastric feedings can be used to supplement the oral feedings, if necessary. Intravenous hyperalimentation of

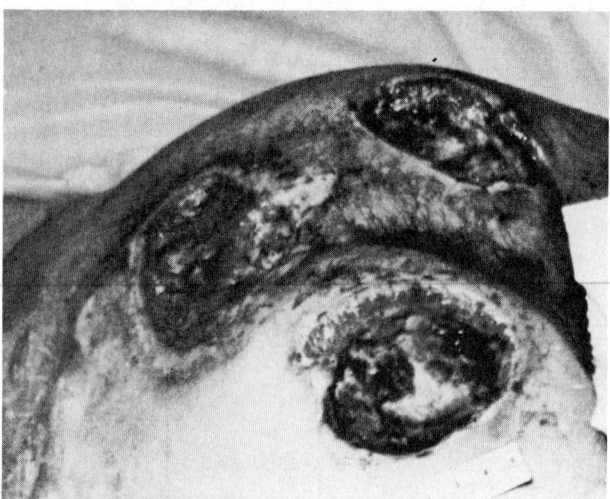

Fig. 17-13 Stage IV pressure sore.

amino acid–glucose solutions is used when oral and nasogastric feedings are inadequate. A nursing care plan for the client with a pressure sore is presented in Table 17-17.

Chronic management. Since recurrence of pressure sores is common, the education of both the client and the care provider in prevention techniques is extremely important. The care provider needs to know the etiology of pressure sores, prevention techniques, early signs, nutritional support, and care techniques for active pressure sores. Since the client with a pressure sore often requires extensive care for other health problems, it is important that the nurse support the caregiver through the added responsibility of pressure sore treatment.

C *ase Study*

BASAL CELL EPITHELIOMA

John Martin, 67 years of age, is a fair-skinned, balding, retired construction worker. He comes to the dermatology clinic with a papule of 6 months' duration behind his right ear. He states that a scab forms, falls off, and re-forms. On inspection, the lesion has semitranslucent borders with absence of normal skin marking. A diagnosis of basal cell epithelioma is made on biopsy.

Discussion Questions

1. What facts about this client support the diagnosis?
2. What are the usual clinical characteristics of a basal cell carcinoma?
3. How was a definitive diagnosis made?
4. What treatment options are available for a basal cell epithelioma?
5. What is the likelihood of metastatic spread with this lesion?
6. What are the nursing responsibilities related to client education for Mr. Martin?

Review Questions

The number of the question corresponds to the same-numbered objective at the beginning of the chapter.

1. Sunscreens primarily block out
   a. UVA wavelengths
   b. UVB wavelengths
   c. UVC wavelengths
2. The most common medications used to treat dermatological problems are
   a. topical corticosteroids
   b. antibiotics
   c. keratolytics
   d. antipruritics
3. Scars from deep injury to the dermis result in
   a. increased innervation
   b. increased sweating
   c. decreased collagen
   d. loss of hair
4. The most common etiological factor related to skin cancer is
   a. chronic sun exposure
   b. hereditary predisposition
   c. prolonged irritation
   d. inadequate vitamin C intake
5. The pathogen involved in impetigo is
   a. *Escherichia coli*
   b. *Pseudomonas aeruginosa*
   c. *Proteus*
   d. group A β-hemolytic streptococci
6. Scabies is spread by
   a. systemic involvement
   b. contaminated articles
   c. direct physical contact
   d. airborne transfer
7. A common site for the lesions associated with atopic dermatitis is the
   a. palmar surface of the feet
   b. antecubital space
   c. temporal area
   d. buttocks
8. A common benign skin problem associated with aging is
   a. psoriasis
   b. skin tags
   c. vitiligo
   d. lipomas
9. A systemic respiratory problem would most commonly affect the skin by
   a. increased pruritus
   b. pallor
   c. changes in color
   d. increased perspiration
10. An important client instruction after a chemical peel or dermabrasion is
    a. increased fatty acids in the diet
    b. use of superfatted soaps
    c. avoidance of sun exposure
    d. keep the treated areas moist
11. At stages III and IV of pressure sore treatment the specific goal is to
    a. debride and clean the wound environment
    b. prevent skin maceration from incontinence
    c. promote good nutrition
    d. promote hydration

REFERENCES

1. Frankel DH: Mohs micrographic surgery for nonmelanoma skin cancer, Hosp Pract 2:16, 1990.
2. Draelos ZK: Cosmetics in dermatology, London, 1990, Churchill Livingstone, p 165.
3. Habif TF: Clinical dermatology: a color guide to diagnosis and therapy, ed 2, St. Louis, 1990, The CV Mosby Co, p 363.
4. American Academy of Dermatology: The sun and your skin, Evanston, Ill, 1987, The Academy, p 1.
5. Habif TF: Clinical dermatology: a color guide to diagnosis and therapy, ed 2, Philadelphia, 1985, WB Saunders Co, p 490.
6. Moschella SL and Hurley H: Dermatology, vol 1, ed 2, Philadelphia, 1985, WB Saunders Co, p 423.
7. Mackie RM: Skin cancer, Chicago, 1989, Year Book Medical Publishers, p 24.
8. Moschella SL and Hurley H: Dermatology, vol 1, ed 2, Philadelphia, 1985, WB Saunders Co, p 393.
9. Roenigk R and Roenigk H: Dermatologic surgery: principles and practice, New York, 1989, BC Decker, Inc, p 169.
10. Neuberger GB: Wound care: what's clear, what's not, Nursing 17:34, 1987.
11. Bickley HC: Practical concepts in human disease, Baltimore, 1975, Williams & Wilkins Co, p 49.
12. Fenske NA, Grayson LD, and Newcomer VD: Common problems of aging skin, Patient Care 23:228, 1989.
13. Krepke A: Impact of ozone depletion in skin cancer, Skin Cancer Foundation Journal 6:7, 1988.
14. Lawler PE and Schreiber S: Cutaneous malignant melanoma: nursing's role in prevention and early detection, Oncol Nurs Forum 16:345, 1989.
15. Greene MH and others: Acquired precursors of cutaneous nevus syndrome: the familial dysplastic nevus syndrome, N Engl J Med 312:91, 1986.
16. Caughman SW, May RJ, and Russo G: Cutaneous signs of internal cancer, Patient Care 23:30, 1989.
17. Strohecker BA and others: Soft tissue expansion, Am J Nurs 88:668, 1988.
18. Gilchrest B: Skin aging and photoaging, Dermatol Nurs 2:79, 1990.
19. Roenigk R and Roenigk H: Dermatologic surgery: principles and practice, New York, 1989, BC Decker, Inc, p 959.
20. Tardy ME and Klingensmith M: Face-lift surgery: principles and variations. In Roenigk R and Roenigk H: Dermatologic surgery: principles and practice, New York, 1989, BC Decker, Inc, p 1239.
21. Habif TF: Clinical dermatology: a color guide to diagnosis and therapy, ed 2, St. Louis, 1990, The CV Mosby Co., p 690.
22. Goodman T: Grafts and flaps in plastic surgery, AORN 48:652, 1988.
23. Sebern M: Home-team strategies for treating pressure sores, Nursing 17:51, 1987.
24. Goodman T, Thomas C, and Rappaport N: Skin ulcers: overview, nursing implications, AORN J 52:24, 1990.
25. Iverson-Carpenter M: Impaired skin integrity, J Gerontol Nurs 14:25, 1988.
26. Conforti C: Dressed for successful healing, Nursing 19:59, 1989.

Nursing Role in Management
Burn Client

Kerry A. Dalen
Sue E. Elster

L earning Objectives

1. Describe the causes and prevention of burn injuries.
2. Describe the burn injury classification system.
3. Differentiate between the involved structures and the clinical appearance of partial- and full-thickness burns.
4. Identify the parameters used to determine the severity of burns.
5. Describe the pathophysiological changes, clinical manifestations, and therapeutic and nursing management of each burn phase.
6. Explain fluid and electrolyte shifts during the emergent and acute burn phases.

7. Differentiate among the nutritional needs of the burn client during the three burn phases.
8. Explain the physiological and psychosocial aspects of burn rehabilitation.
9. Describe the therapeutic and nursing management of the emotional needs of the burn client and family.
10. Describe special needs of nursing staff caring for the burn client and possible ways to meet those needs.
11. Discuss the issues involved and rationale of preparing the client to return home.
12. Describe interventions the nurse may use in the management of pain in the burn client.

SIGNIFICANCE

An estimated 2.5 million Americans seek medical care each year for burns. Approximately 100,000 are hospitalized and 70,000 require intensive care services. An estimated 12,000 of these people die annually as a direct result of their burns. Children (especially preschoolers) and older adults account for over two thirds of all burn fatalities.[1]

The major cause of fires in the home is carelessness with cigarettes. Major causes of burns include hot water from water heaters set above 140° F (60° C), cooking accidents, space heaters, combustibles such as gasoline and charcoal lighter fluid, steam from radiators, and chemicals.

Health Promotion and Maintenance

Most burn injuries can be prevented. The nurse as a citizen and health care provider is in a good position to do home safety assessments and to educate clients before accidents occur. Home safety measures include the use of

smoke alarms and fire extinguishers. Families should have fire drills, and each family member should know where to go and what to do in case of fire. Local fire departments can inform the public of regional fire codes as well as perform home safety checks.

Knowledge of potential sources for burn injury allows problem solving for burn prevention (Tables 18-1 and 18-2). Teaching people proper use of appliances such as space heaters, electrical cords, wiring, outlets, outdoor grills, and hot water heaters can do much to prevent burn injury. Nurses can be instrumental in teaching home care of minor burns to the public. Industrial nurses should teach burn prevention in the work setting.

TYPES OF BURN INJURY
Thermal Injury

The most common type of burn is thermal injury, which can be caused by flame, flash, scald, or contact with hot objects[2] (Table 18-2 and Fig. 18-1).

Although the corneal reflex generally protects the eyes from burn injury, corneal burns and abrasions can occur under circumstances similar to inhalation injuries. Intense

---

Reviewed by Nancy C. Molter, R.N., M.N., C.C.R.N., Lieutenant Colonel, Army Nurse Corps, Chief Nurse, U.S. Army Institute of Surgical Research, Fort Sam Houston, Texas.

Table 18-1 Common Places and Causes of Burn
Injury

Occupational Hazards	Home and Recreational Hazards
Steam pipes	Hot water heaters set higher than
Chemicals	60° C (140° F)
Hot metals	Multiple extension cords per out-
Tar	let
Electricity from power	Frazzled or defective wiring
lines	Pressure cookers
Combustible fuels	Radiators
	Open space heaters
	Carelessness with cigarettes or
	matches
	Improper use of outdoor grills
	Improper use of flammables (e.g.,
	starter fluid, gasoline, kero-
	sene)
	Household cleaning agents
	Hot grease or liquids from cook-
	ing
	Excessive exposure to sunlight
	Electrical storms

Table 18-2 Causes of Thermal Burn Injury

Cause	Examples
Flame	Clothing ignited with fire
Flash	Flame burn associated with explosion (combusti-
	ble fuels)
Scald	Too-hot bath water
	Spilled hot beverages
	Hot grease or liquids from cooking
	Steam burns (pressure cookers, automobile radi-
	ators)
Contact	Hot metal (outdoor grill)
	Hot, sticky tar

heat or noxious chemical byproducts can damage delicate corneal tissue. When corneal burns are suspected, an ophthalmologist should see the client as soon as possible. Because of the rapid facial edema that can occur with burns, an immediate nursing assessment of possible eye injury is needed because the eyelids may become swollen shut within the first few hours after injury, making examination difficult. In addition, contact lenses should be removed if they are present.

Chemical Injury

Chemical injuries are the result of tissue injury and destruction from necrotizing substances (Fig. 18-1, *B*). With chemical injuries, it is important to remove the person from the burning agent, or vice versa. The latter is accomplished by lavaging the affected area with copious amounts

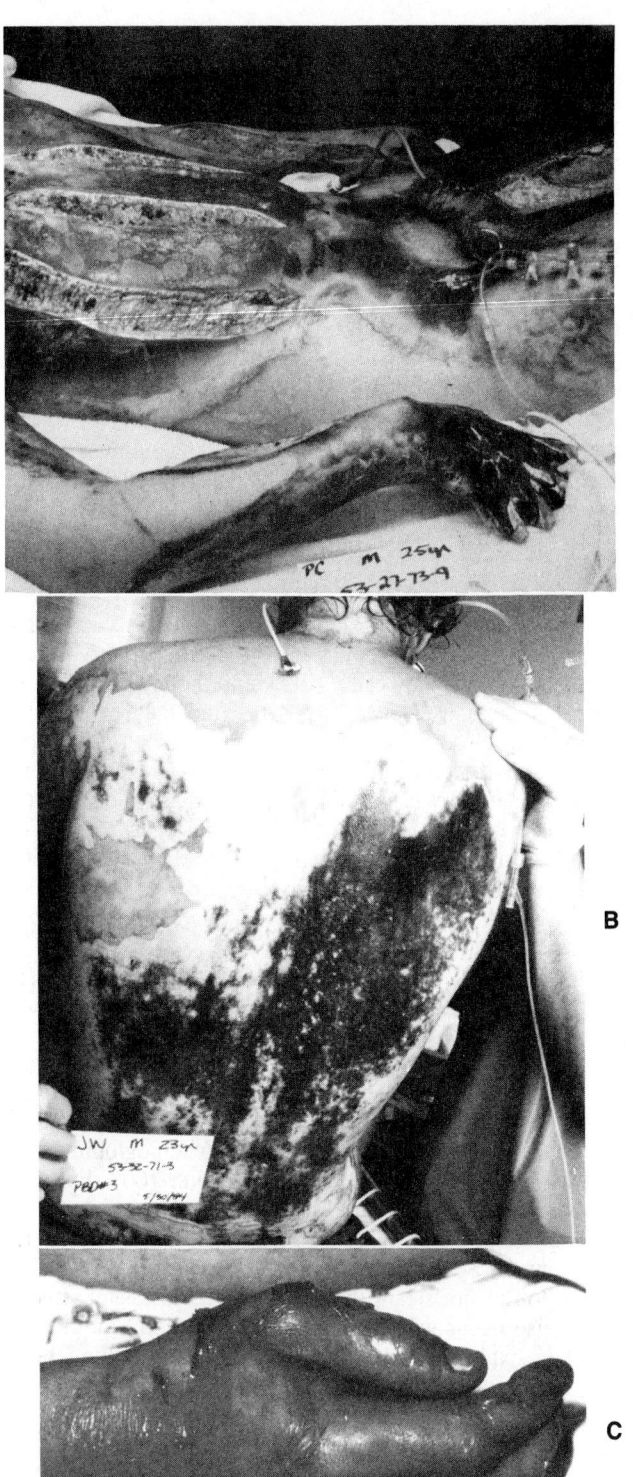

Fig. 18-1 Types of burn injury. **A,** Client with full-thickness flame burns. Blackened fingertips are burned to bone. **B,** Full-thickness chemical burns with characteristic discoloration. **C,** Partial-thickness hand burn with thin-walled, fluid-filled blisters.

of water. Any clothing containing the chemical should be removed. Otherwise the burning process will continue as long as the chemical is in contact with the skin.

Chemicals can produce respiratory injuries as well as skin or eye injuries. When chlorine is inhaled, toxic gas produces respiratory distress. Byproducts of burning substances (e.g., carbon) are toxic to the sensitive respiratory mucosa. Tissue destruction may continue for up to 72 hours after a chemical injury.

Chemical burns are most commonly caused by acids. However, alkali burns also occur, and they are more difficult to manage than acid burns. Alkaline substances are not neutralized by tissue fluids as readily as acid substances are. Alkalies adhere to tissue, causing protein hydrolysis and liquefaction. This damage continues even when the alkali is neutralized. Examples of alkalies that cause burn injury are cleansing agents, drain cleaners, and lyes.

Smoke and Inhalation Injury

Smoke and inhalation of hot air or noxious chemicals can cause damage to the tissues of the respiratory tract. Breathing hot air may cause damage to the respiratory mucosa, although it rarely happens because the vocal cords and glottis close as a protective mechanism. Gases are cooled to body temperature by the time they reach the lung parenchyma. Smoke inhalation injuries usually account for damage to respiratory mucosa in the first 5 days after injury. It is an important determinant of mortality in fire victims. Inhalation injuries are present in 20% to 30% of the clients admitted to burn centers and 60% to 70% of clients who die in burn centers.[3]

There are three types of smoke and inhalation injuries:

1. *Carbon monoxide poisoning:* Carbon monoxide poisoning and asphyxiation account for the majority of deaths at the fire scene. Often the survivors of fires, especially those who have been trapped in a closed space, will have elevated carboxyhemoglobin levels. The client should have a carboxyhemoglobin level obtained and be treated quickly with 100% humidified oxygen.
2. *Inhalation injury above the glottis:* This type of injury is very rare and usually occurs with the inhalation of hot steam that is under high pressure. It can also occur with the aspiration of scalding liquids or in explosions in which a victim is breathing high concentrations of very hot air under pressure. If there is heat damage to the upper airway, it is usually severe enough to cause a mechanical obstruction as a result of swelling. Inhalation injury above the glottis is a medical emergency.
3. *Inhalation injury below the glottis:* A general principle to remember is that inhalation injury above the glottis is thermally produced, and below the glottis it is chemically produced. The tissue injury to the lower respiratory tract is related to the length of exposure to smoke or toxic fumes.

These clients must be observed closely for signs of respiratory distress or compromise and must be treated quickly and efficiently if they are to survive. Respiratory tract

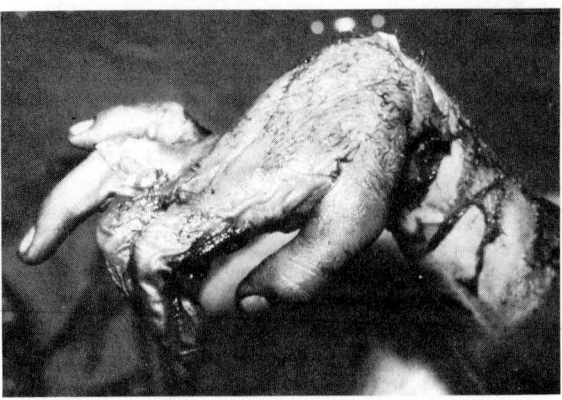

Fig. 18-2 Electrical injury produces heat coagulation of blood supply and contact area as electric current passes through the skin.

complications from burn injury are discussed in greater detail later in this chapter.

Electrical Injury

Electrical injury results from coagulation necrosis that is due to intense heat generated from an electric current (Fig. 18-2). It can also result from direct damage to nerves and vessels causing tissue anoxia and death. The severity of the electrical injury depends on the amount of voltage, tissue resistance, current pathways, and surface area in contact with the current and on the length of time current flow was sustained. Tissue densities offer various amounts of resistance to electric current. For example, fat and bone offer the most resistance, whereas nerves and blood vessels offer the least resistance. Current that passes through vital organs (brain, heart, kidneys) will produce more profound damage than current that passes through other tissue. In addition, electrical sparks may have ignited the client's clothing, causing a combination of thermal and electrical injury.

Nursing assessment of the client with electrical injury should be thorough. Often the wounds of electric current entry and exit are all that are visible, masking the possibility of extensive, underlying tissue damage. Noting the client's position when the injury was sustained in conjunction with identifying the entry and exit wounds can help the nurse to assess which underlying organ structures may have been affected. Contact with electric current can cause tetanic muscle contractions strong enough to fracture the long bones and vertebrae. Another reason to suspect long bone or spinal fractures is a fall from a height. Most electrical injuries occur when the victim is elevated above the ground (e.g., during the work of a utility pole lineman) and comes in contact with a current source. For this reason all clients with electrical burns should be treated for a potential cervical spine injury. This includes cervical spine injury precautions during transport and a spinal x-ray to rule out any injury.

Electrical injury puts the client at risk for cardiac arrest or dysrhythmias, severe metabolic acidosis, and myoglobinuria, which can lead to acute renal tubular necrosis. The

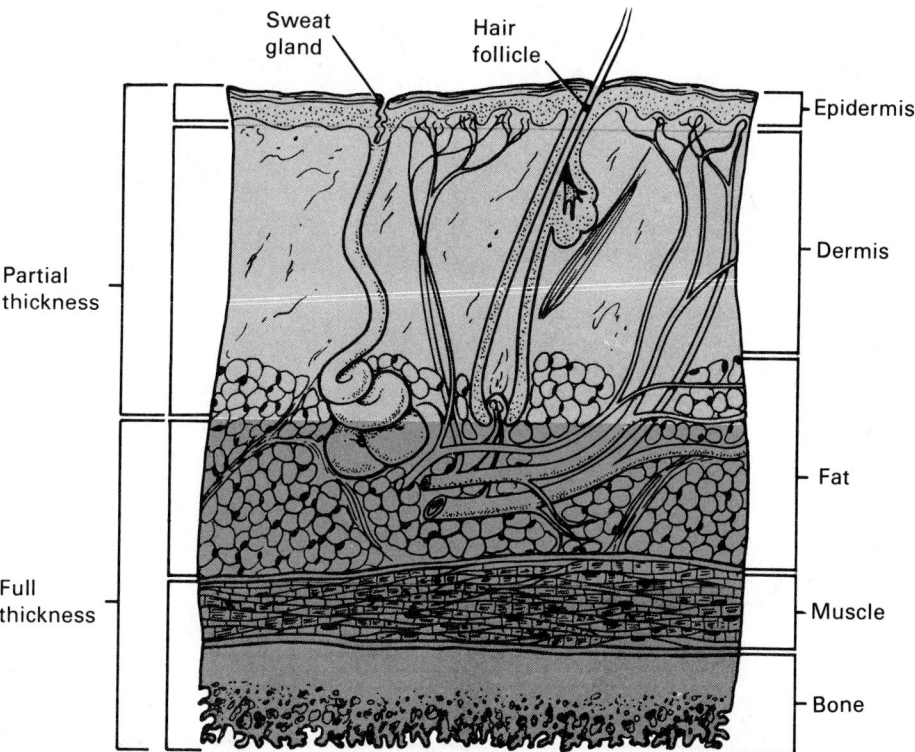

Fig. 18-3 Cross section of skin indicating the degree of burn and structures involved.

electrical shock event can cause immediate cardiac stand-still or fibrillation. If this occurs, cardiopulmonary resuscitation (CPR) should be initiated immediately. Delayed cardiac dysrhythmias or arrest may also occur without warning during the first 24 to 48 hours after injury. Therefore the client should be monitored continuously. Because of extensive tissue destruction and cell rupture, severe metabolic acidosis develops within minutes after the injury, even in the absence of cardiac arrest. Arterial blood gas analysis should be performed to assess the acid-base balance. Sodium bicarbonate may be administered in amounts sufficient to maintain the serum pH at near-normal levels. The problem persists for about 24 hours after injury; therefore, sodium bicarbonate is often added to each bottle of intravenous (IV) fluid administered to maintain a normal acid-base balance.

Myoglobin is released from muscle tissue into the circulation whenever massive muscle damage occurs. It is then transported to the kidneys where it can mechanically block the renal tubules because of its large size. This process can result in acute tubular necrosis (ATN) and eventual acute renal failure if not appropriately treated (see Chapter 41). Treatment consists of infusing Ringer's lactate solution at a rate to maintain urine output at 75 to 100 ml/hr until urine samples indicate that the myoglobin has been flushed from the circulatory system. In addition, an osmotic diuretic (e.g., mannitol) may be given to maintain urine output. (Radiation burn injury is discussed in Chapter 9, and cold thermal [frostbite] injury is discussed in Chapter 60.)

CLASSIFICATION OF BURN INJURY

The treatment of burns is related to the severity of the injury. Severity is determined by (1) depth of burn, (2) extent of burn calculated in percent of total body surface area (TBSA), (3) location of burn, (4) age of victim, (5) concomitant injury, and (6) past health history indicating poor-risk factors for recovery.

Depth

Burn injury involves the destruction of the integumentary system (see Chapter 16). The skin is divided into three layers including the epidermis, dermis, and subcutaneous tissue (Fig. 18-3). The *epidermis,* or nonvascular outer layer of the skin, is about the thickness of a sheet of paper. It is composed of many layers of nonliving epithelial cells that provide a protective barrier to the skin, hold in fluids and electrolytes, regulate heat, and keep harmful agents in the external environment from injuring or invading the body. The *dermis,* which lies below the epidermis, is about 30 to 45 times thicker than the epidermis. The dermis contains connective tissues with blood vessels and highly specialized structures consisting of hair follicles, nerve endings, sweat glands, and sebaceous glands. Under the dermis lies the *subcutaneous tissue,* which contains major vascular networks, fat, nerves, and lymphatics. The subcutaneous tissue acts as shock absorber and heat insulator for the underlying structures—muscles, tendons, bones, and internal organs.

In the past, burns were defined by degrees: first-degree,

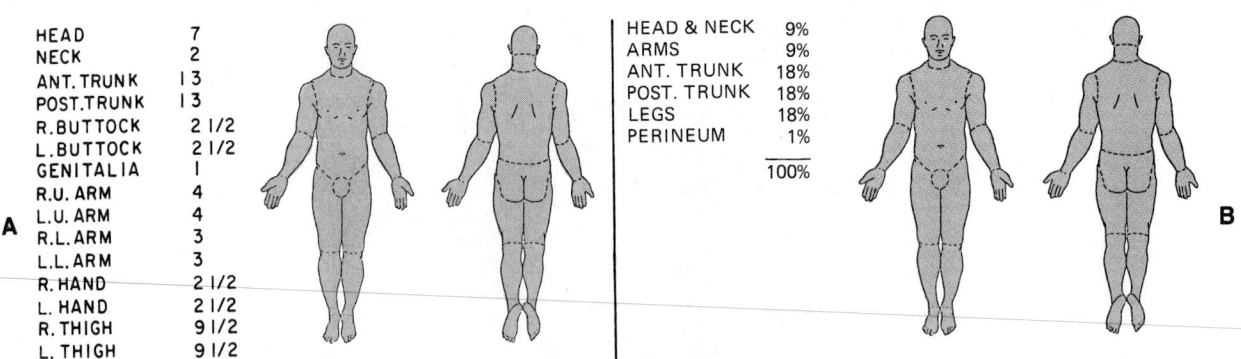

HEAD	7
NECK	2
ANT. TRUNK	13
POST. TRUNK	13
R. BUTTOCK	2 1/2
L. BUTTOCK	2 1/2
GENITALIA	1
R.U. ARM	4
L.U. ARM	4
R.L. ARM	3
L.L. ARM	3
R. HAND	2 1/2
L. HAND	2 1/2
R. THIGH	9 1/2
L. THIGH	9 1/2
R. LEG	7
L. LEG	7
R. FOOT	3 1/2
L. FOOT	3 1/2
	100 %

HEAD & NECK	9%
ARMS	9%
ANT. TRUNK	18%
POST. TRUNK	18%
LEGS	18%
PERINEUM	1%
	100%

Fig. 18-4 **A,** Lund and Browder chart. By convention, areas of partial-thickness injury are colored in blue and areas of full-thickness injury in red. First-degree burns are not calculated. **B,** Rule of Nines chart.

Table 18-3 Classification of Burn Injury Depth

Classification	Clinical Appearance and Cause	Cause	Structure*
Partial-thickness skin destruction			
Superficial	Erythema, blanching on pressure, pain and mild swelling, no vesicles or blisters (although after 24 hr skin may blister and peel)	Superficial sunburn or quick heat flash	Only superficial devitalization with hyperemia is present. Tactile and pain sensation is intact.
Deep	Fluid-filled vesicles that are red, shiny, wet (if vesicles have ruptured); severe pain due to nerve injury; mild-to-moderate edema	Flame, flash, scald, or contact burns	Epidermis and dermis are involved to varying depth. Some skin elements, from which epithelial regeneration can occur, remain viable.
Full-thickness skin destruction	Dry, waxy white, leathery, or hard skin; visible thrombosed vessels; insensitivity to pain and pressure because of nerve destruction; possible involvement of muscles, tendons, and bones	Flame, scald, chemicals, tar, or electric current	All skin elements and nerve endings are destroyed. Coagulation necrosis is present.

*See Fig. 18-3.

second-degree, and third-degree burns. The American Burn Association now advocates a more explicit definition categorizing the burn according to depth of skin destruction: partial-thickness and full-thickness burns. Table 18-3 reflects the comparison of the depth of injury.

Extent

Two commonly used guides for determining the extent of a burn wound are the Lund and Browder chart (Fig. 18-4, *A*) and the Rule of Nines (Fig. 18-4, *B*). (Only partial- and full-thickness burns are included in calculating TBSA.) The Lund and Browder chart is considered to be more accurate because the client's age in proportion to relative body-part size is taken into account. The Rule of Nines is easy to remember and is considered very adequate for initial assessment. For irregular or odd-shaped burns, the palmar surface of the client's hand is considered to be about 1% of the TBSA. The extent of a burn is often re-

Table 18-4 American Burn Association Adult Burn Classification

Magnitude of Burn Injury	Partial Thickness* (Second Degree)	Full Thickness* (Third Degree)	Other Factors
Minor	<15%	<2%	Does not involve special care areas (eyes, ears, face, hands, feet, perineum); excludes electrical injury, inhalation injury, complicated injury (fractures), all poor-risk clients (extremes of age, concomitant disease)
Moderate uncomplicated	15%-25%	<10%	Excludes electrical injury, inhalation injury, complicated injury, all poor-risk clients; does not involve special care areas
Major	>25%	>10%	Includes all burns involving hands, face, eyes, ears, feet, or perineum; includes inhalation injury, electrical injury, complicated burn injury, and all poor-risk clients

*Figures indicate percentage of TBSA involved.

vised after edema has subsided and demarcations of zones of injury are clearer.

Location

The location of the burn wound has a direct relationship to the severity of the burn injury. Burns of the face and neck and circumferential burns of the chest may inhibit respiratory function. These injuries may also indicate the possibility of inhalation injury and respiratory mucosal damage. Edema of the face and neck may cause mechanical obstruction of the airway.

Burns of the hands, feet, joints, and eyes are of major concern because they make self-care impossible and jeopardize later function. Hands and feet are very difficult to manage medically because of superficial vascular and nerve-supply systems.

The ears and nose, composed mainly of cartilage, are susceptible to infection because of poor blood supply to the cartilage. Burns of the buttocks or genitalia are susceptible to infection and may be the source of emotional conflict because of the pain involved and possible disfigurement. Circumferential burns of the extremities can cause circulation compromise distal to the burn with later neurological impairment of the affected extremity.

Age

Because of an immature immune system and generally poor body defense mechanisms, infants are less able to cope with burn injuries. Older adults heal more slowly and have more difficulty with rehabilitation than children or younger adults. Infection of the burn wound and pneumonia are common complications in burn clients who are older adults.

Poor-Risk Factors

Any person with preexisting cardiovascular, pulmonary, or renal disease has a poorer prognosis for recovery because of the tremendous demands placed on the body by a burn injury. Clients with diabetes or peripheral vascular disease are at high risk for gangrene and poor healing, especially with foot and leg burns. General physical debilitation from any chronic disease, including alcoholism, drug abuse, and malnutrition, renders the client less physiologically competent to deal with a burn injury. In addition, clients who concurrently sustained fractures, other trauma, or head injuries have a poorer prognosis for recovery from the burn injury.

Major Versus Minor Burns

The American Burn Association classifies burns into major, moderate uncomplicated, and minor injuries by depth, extent, location, and poor-risk factors (Table 18-4). The American Burn Association recommends that major burn injuries be treated at burn centers or burn units that have optimal facilities and personnel for handling such severe trauma.

PHASES OF BURN MANAGEMENT

Burn management can be classified into three phases: *emergent* (resuscitative), *acute,* and *rehabilitative.*

Prehospital Care

The initial consideration in aiding burn victims is to remove them from the source of burn and/or stop the burning process. If a burn is small (10% or less of TBSA) it may be covered with a clean, cool, tap water–dampened towel for the client's comfort and protection until definitive medical care is instituted. It is believed that cooling of the injured area (if small) within 1 minute minimizes the depth of injury. Tap water is acceptable for flushing. Time should not be wasted trying to find sterile water or saline solution.

If the burn is large, primary considerations are focused on the "ABCs" (see Chapter 30) (1) *airway:* check for patency, soot around nares, or singed nasal hair; (2) *breathing:* check for adequacy of ventilation; and (3) *circulation:* check for presence and regularity of pulses.[4] If the burn is large, it is not advisable to immerse the burned body part in cool water because doing so would lead to extensive heat and electrolyte loss. The burn should never be packed in ice. As much clothing as possible should be removed. The client should be wrapped in a dry, clean sheet or blanket to prevent further contamination of the wound and to provide warmth.

Table 18-5

Prehospital Emergency Care of the Client with Chemical Burns*

Etiology: Exposure to strong acids or alkali or corrosive materials

CLINICAL MANIFESTATIONS

Burning, degeneration of tissue-exposed materials
Discoloration of injured exposed skin
Localized pain
Edema of surrounding tissue

MANAGEMENT

Remove the chemical from contact with client's body.
Flush chemical from wound and surrounding area with saline solution or water. Brush powders off before flushing.
Remove shoes, watches, and jewelry.
Blot skin dry with clean towels. *Do not* rub dry.
Cover all burned area with dry, sterile dressing or clean, dry sheet.
Attempt to determine offending agent to direct later treatment (i.e., whether it is acid or alkaline).

*See Chapter 59 for a general discussion on measures related to prehospital emergency care.

Table 18-6

Prehospital Emergency Care of the Client with Inhalation Injury*

Etiology: Exposure of respiratory tract to intense heat or flames, inhalation of noxious chemicals or smoke, inhalation of carbon monoxide gas

CLINICAL MANIFESTATIONS

Rapid, shallow respirations
Increasing hoarseness
Coughing
Sooty, smoky smell on client's breath
Productive cough of grayish sputum
Irritation of upper airways or burning pain in throat or chest
Difficulty swallowing
Bluish skin color
Restlessness, anxiety

MANAGEMENT

Remove client from toxic environment.
Establish and maintain airway. Administer humidified oxygen at 100% by mask.
Be prepared to intubate if respiratory distress occurs.
Remove all clothing that may restrict breathing.
Establish IV line with large-gauge needle.
Monitor vital signs.
Place client in high Fowler's position.
Assess for facial and neck burns or other signs of trauma.
Prepare for emergency endotracheal intubation if indicated.

*See Chapter 59 for a general discussion on measures related to prehospital emergency care.

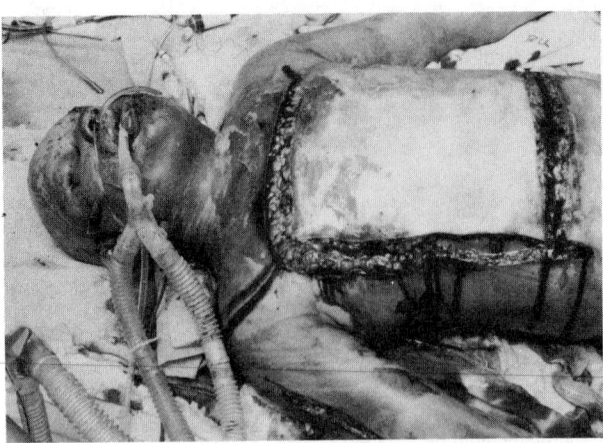

Fig. 18-5 Massive total body edema occurs during the emergent phase of major burn injury. Escharotomy of the chest facilitates lung expansion.

Table 18-7

Prehospital Emergency Care of the Client with Electrical Burns*

Etiology: Exposure to any source that carries electric current (e.g., lightning, electric wires, utility wires)

CLINICAL MANIFESTATIONS

Leathery, white, charred black thrombosed vessels
Burn odor
Impaired sensation to touch
Lack of blanching of skin
Minimal or absence of pain
Depth of wound, which can include epidermis, dermis, subcutaneous fat, muscle, and bone

MANAGEMENT

Remove client from contact with current source.
Avoid contact with electric current during rescue.
Assess for patent airway, breathing, and circulation; provide for support if necessary; assess for cervical spine injury.
Assess burn areas, especially the entrance and exit sites.
Check pulses distal to burns.
Assess for any fractures; splint if necessary.
Cover burn sites with dry, sterile dressing or clean, dry sheet.
Treat for shock and establish an IV line.

*See Chapter 59 for a general discussion on measures related to prehospital emergency care.

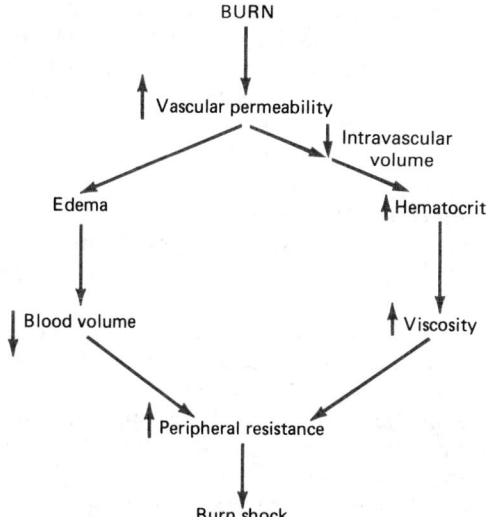

BURN

↑ Vascular permeability

↑ Intravascular volume

Edema

↑ Hematocrit

↓ Blood volume

↑ Viscosity

↑ Peripheral resistance

Burn shock

Fig. 18-6 At the time of major burn injury, the capillaries increase in permeability. All fluid components of the blood begin to leak into the interstitium, casing edema and a decreased blood volume. The red blood cells and white blood cells do not leak. Therefore the hematocrit increases and the blood becomes viscous. The combination of decreased blood volume and increased viscosity produces increased peripheral resistance. Burn shock, a type of hypovolemic shock, rapidly ensues and continues for about 24 hours.

The burn client may also be a trauma client. Often the burn is accompanied by other life-threatening injuries that may take priority over the burn wound.[5]

Prehospital care of the client with various types of burns is presented in tables that describe chemical burns (Table 18-5), inhalation injury (Table 18-6), electrical burns (Table 18-7), and thermal burns (Table 18-8).

Emergent Phase

Definition. The *emergent* (resuscitative) *phase* is the period of time required to resolve the immediate problems resulting from burn injury. This time period may last from burn onset to 5 or more days but usually lasts 24 to 48 hours. This phase begins with fluid loss and edema formation and continues until fluid mobilization and diuresis begin (Fig. 18-5).

Pathophysiological changes

Fluid and electrolyte shifts. The greatest initial threat to a major burn victim is hypovolemic shock. It is caused by a massive shift of fluids out of blood vessels as a result of increased capillary permeability. As the capillary walls become more permeable, water, sodium, and later plasma proteins (especially albumin) move into the interstitial spaces and other surrounding tissue (Fig. 18-6). The colloidal osmotic pressure decreases with progressive loss of protein from the vascular space. This results in more fluid shifting out of the vascular space into the interstitial spaces. (Fluid accumulation in the interstitium is called *second spacing.*) Fluid also moves to areas that normally have minimal to no fluid, a phenomenon called *third spacing.* Examples of third spacing in burn injury are exudate and blister formation.

Table 18-8

Prehospital Emergency Care of the Client with Thermal Burns

Possible etiologies: Contact with hot liquids or hot solids, flash flame, open flame, steam, or ultraviolet rays

CLINICAL MANIFESTATIONS
Partial-thickness (superficial) burns

Redness
Pain
Moderate to severe tenderness
Minimal edema
Blanching on pressure

Partial-thickness (deep) burns

Moist blebs, blisters
Mottled white, pink to cherry red
Hypersensitive to touch or air
Moderate to severe pain
Blanching on pressure

Full-thickness burns

Dry, leathery eschar
White, waxy, dark brown, or charred appearance
Charred or thrombosed blood vessels visible under eschar
Strong burn odor
Impaired sensation when touched
Absence of pain
Lack of blanching on pressure
Easy removal of hair from burn area

MANAGEMENT
Eliminate the cause of the burn.
Ensure adequate airway; inspect the face and neck; assess for singed nasal hair, hoarseness of voice, stridor, soot in the sputum.
Administer humidified oxygen; be ready to intubate if necessary.
Ensure adequate breathing; know mechanism of injury (e.g., an explosion, car accident); check for rib fracture, pneumothorax, or hemothorax.
Ensure adequate circulation; start IV line with large-gauge needle wherever possible.
Note client's general appearance.
Assess vital signs.
Remove all potentially constricting items (e.g., shoes, rings, jewelry, clothes).
Examine and treat for other associated injuries.
Determine depth, extent, and severity of burn.
Provide pain relief.
Debride obviously dead tissue, dirt, and twigs from the wound and rinse with warm water.
Apply cold compresses or immerse in cold water for minor injuries only (less than 10% TBSA burn); monitor for hypothermia closely; use only if unable to control pain by other means.
If blisters form, do not rupture; cover the wounds with a clean, dry sheet; sterile dressings are not necessary.
Transport as soon as possible to a burn center.

The net result of the fluid shift is volume depletion within the vasculature. Edema, decreased blood pressure, increased pulse, and other manifestations of hypovolemic shock are clinically detectable manifestations (see Chapter 27). If not corrected, these events can lead to irreversible hypovolemic shock and death.

Another source of fluid loss is the result of insensible loss by evaporation from large, denuded body surfaces. The normal insensible loss of 30 to 50 ml/hr may increase to as much as 200 to 400 ml/hr in the severely burned client.

The circulatory status is also impaired because of hemolysis of red blood cells. The red blood cells are hemolyzed by a circulating factor that is released at the time of the burn as well as by the direct insult of the burn injury. Thrombosis in the capillaries of burned tissue causes an additional loss of red blood cells. An elevated hematocrit is commonly due to hemoconcentration. After fluid balance has been restored, lowered hematocrit levels are found, and an anemic state is more readily detectable.

Sodium and potassium are involved in electrolyte shifts. Sodium is rapidly shifted to the interstitial spaces and remains there until edema formation ceases (Fig. 18-7). A potassium shift develops initially because injured cells and hemolyzed red blood cells release potassium into the extracellular spaces.

Toward the end of the emergent phase, if fluid replacement is adequate, capillary membrane permeability will be restored. Fluid loss and edema formation will cease. Interstitial fluid will gradually return to the vascular space (Fig. 18-7). Clinically, diuresis will be noted with very low urine specific gravities. Serum potassium levels will be markedly elevated initially as fluid mobilization brings potassium from the interstitium to the vascular space. Hypokalemia may occur at this time or in a few days as a result of the loss of potassium from diuresis and potassium movement back into cells. Serum sodium levels will increase as sodium returns to the vascular space. Later, normal serum sodium values are found with loss of sodium in urine.

Inflammation and healing. Burn injury causes coagulation necrosis whereby tissues and vessels are damaged or destroyed. Polymorphonuclear leukocytes and monocytes accumulate at the site of injury. Fibroblasts and newly formed collagen fibrils appear and begin wound repair within the first 6 to 12 hours after injury. (The inflammatory response is discussed in Chapter 7.)

Immunological changes. Burn injury causes widespread impairment of the immune system.[6] The skin barrier to invading organisms is destroyed, circulating levels of immunoglobulins are decreased, and many changes in white blood cells (WBCs)—both quantitative and qualitative—occur. Depression of neutrophil chemotactic, phagocytic, and bactericidal activity is found after burn injury. Burn size–related alterations of lymphocyte populations include a depression of T-helper cells and increased T-suppressor cells. In addition, decreased levels of interleukin-1 (produced by macrophages) and interleukin-2 (produced by lymphocytes) are also found in some persons with burn injury. All of these changes in the immune system can make the burn client more susceptible to infection.

Clinical manifestations. The burn client may be in shock from pain and hypovolemia. Areas of full-thickness and deep partial-thickness burns are anesthetic because the nerve endings are destroyed. Superficial partial-thickness burns are very painful. Blisters filled with fluid and protein may occur in partial-thickness burns. The client will experience an intense thirst because of the relative fluid loss. The fluid is not actually lost from the body as much as it is sequestered in the interstitial spaces and third spaces. It is hard to visualize severe dehydration in someone who is so obviously edematous (Fig. 18-5). Unconsciousness in a burn client is usually not due to the burn. The most common reason is hypoxia associated with smoke inhalation. Other possibilities include head trauma and an overdose of sedative or pain medication.

The client may be disoriented and have difficulty recalling the sequence of events that led up to the burn injury. The client will have minimal urine output and will have signs of adynamic ileus as a result of the body's response to massive trauma and potassium shifts. Shivering may occur as a result of chilling that is due to heat loss, anxiety, or pain.

Complications. The three major organ systems most susceptible to complications during the emergent phase of burn injury are the cardiovascular, respiratory, and renal systems.

Cardiovascular system. Cardiovascular system complications include dysrhythmias and hypovolemic shock, which may progress to irreversible shock.[7] Circulation to the extremities can be severely impaired by circumferential burns and subsequent edema formation. These processes occlude the blood supply causing ischemia, necrosis, and eventually gangrene. *Escharotomies* (incisions through the

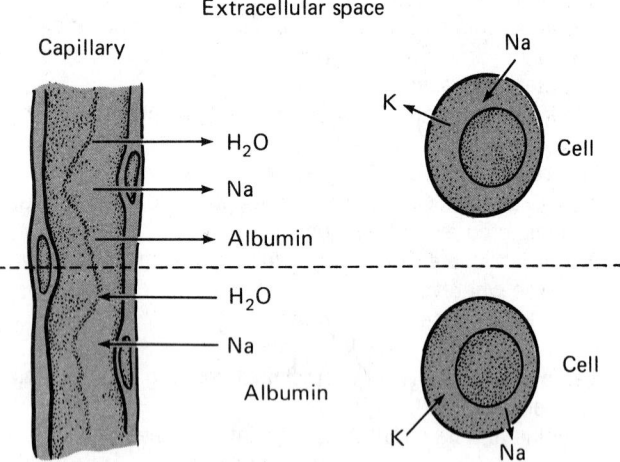

Extracellular space

Fig. 18-7 The effects of burn shock during the first 24 hours are shown *(above the dotted line)*. As the capillary seal is lost, the interstitial edema fluid is formed. The cellular integrity is also altered, with sodium moving into the cell in abnormal amounts and potassium leaving the cell. The shifts after the first 24 hours are shown *(below the dotted line)*. The water and sodium move back into the circulating volume through the capillary. The albumin remains in the interstitium. Potassium is transported into the cell and sodium is transported out as the cellular integrity returns.

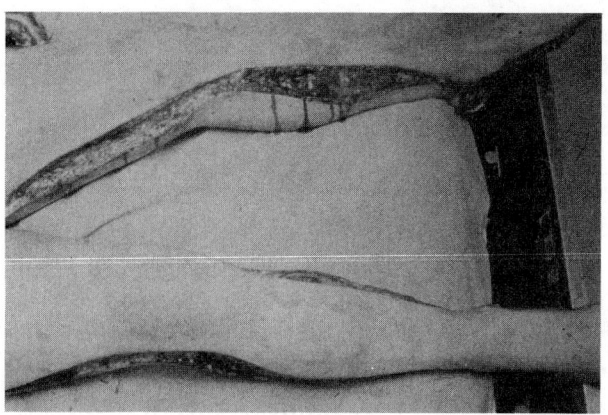

Fig. 18-8 Circumferential full-thickness burns can tighten into tourniquets as edema forms. An escharotomy was performed medially and laterally on this client's legs. The blood flow to the left leg remained inadequate, and a fasciotomy was performed.

Table 18-9 Clinical Manifestations of Respiratory Injury Associated with Burns

UPPER RESPIRATORY TRACT INJURY

Edema, hoarseness, difficulty swallowing, copious secretions, stridor, substernal and/or intercostal retractions, total airway obstruction

INHALATION INJURY

Initial absence of manifestations possible; high degree of suspicion if client was trapped in fire and/or has facial burns, singed nasal or facial hair; dyspnea, carbonaceous sputum, wheezing, hoarseness, altered mental status

eschar) are frequently performed to restore circulation to compromised extremities (Fig. 18-8). Another method that has been used in recent years is enzymatic debridement. Travase is a topical enzymatic debrider that can work well without the scar surgical escharotomies leave. When used, it does require more fluid than calculated by the resuscitation formula in the initial 24 hours. There is also a fair amount of bleeding that occurs, and blood transfusions may be required. In recent years, enzymatic debridement has been primarily used for small burn areas.

Initially, there is an increase in blood viscosity with burn injuries because of the fluid loss that occurs in the emergent period. Microcirculation is impaired because of the damage to skin structures that contain small capillary systems. These two events result in a phenomenon called *sludging*. Sludging can be corrected by adequate fluid replacement, which is calculated with one of the burn resuscitation formulas (see Table 18-11).

Respiratory system. The respiratory system is especially vulnerable to two types of respiratory injury: (1) upper airway burns that cause edema formation and obstruction of the airway and (2) inhalation injury (Table 18-9). Upper airway distress may occur with or without smoke inhalation.

Upper respiratory tract injury results from direct heat injury and/or edema formation and can lead to mechanical airway obstruction and asphyxia. The edema associated with upper respiratory tract burn injury is massive and occurs in most clients with major burn injuries (Fig. 18-3). Mechanical obstruction of the airway is not limited to clients with flame burns of the upper airway, since the edema that accompanies scald burns to the face and neck can be equally lethal when the pressure of the accumulated edema compresses the airway externally.[8] Flame burns to the neck and chest may contribute to respiratory difficulty because the inelastic eschar becomes tight and constricting from the underlying edema.

Management involves early nasotracheal or endotracheal intubation before the airway is actually compromised (Fig. 18-9, *A*). Early intubation eliminates the necessity

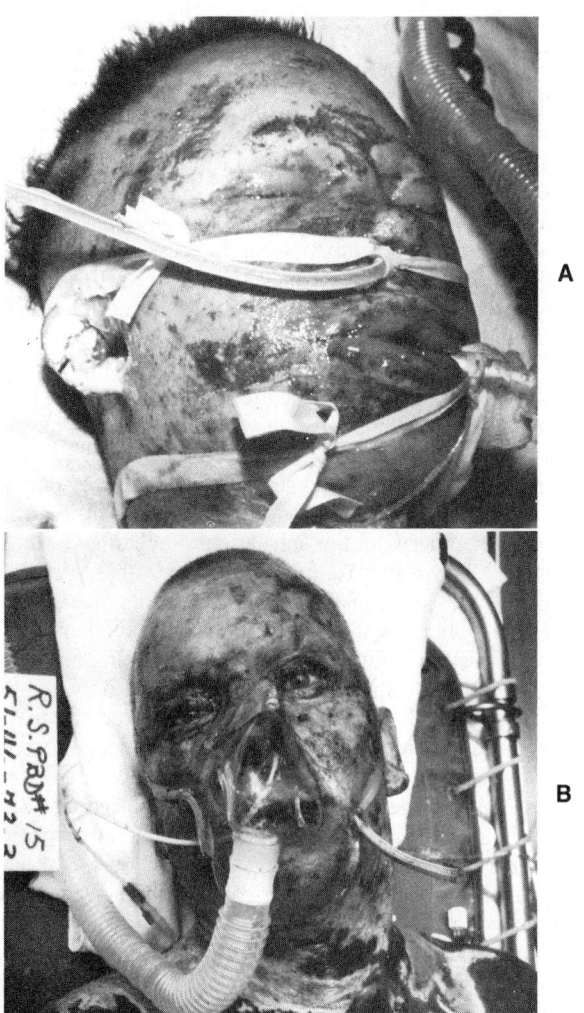

Fig. 18-9 **A,** Massive upper airway edema requires intubation to prevent mechanical airway obstruction. **B,** Edema subsides in 3 to 6 days.

Table 18-10

Therapeutic Management: Burn Client		
Emergency Phase	**Acute Phase**	**Rehabilitation Phase**

Fluid therapy
  Assess fluid needs.*
  Begin IV fluid replacement.
  Insert indwelling catheter.
  Monitor urine output.
Wound care
  Start hydrotherapy or cleansing.
  Debride as necessary.
  Assess extent and depth of burns.
  Initiate topical antibiotic therapy.
  Administer tetanus toxoid or tetanus
    antitoxin.
	Fluid therapy
	  Replace fluids, depending on individ-
	    ual client needs.
	  Administer red blood cells (if neces-
	    sary).
	Wound care
	  Assess wound daily.
	  Observe for complications.
	  Continue hydrotherapy.
	  Continue debridement (if necessary).
	Early excision and grafting
	  Provide homografts.
	  Provide autografts.
	  Care for donor site.
		Counsel and teach client and family.
		Encourage and assist client in resuming
		  self-care.
		Begin physical therapy for maintenance
		  and rehabilitation of motion.
		Correct contractures and scarring (sur-
		  gery, physical therapy, or splinting).
		Discuss possible cosmetic or recon-
		  structive surgery.

*See Table 18-11.

for emergency tracheostomy after respiratory problems have become apparent. In general, clients with major injuries involving burns to the face and neck will require intubation within 1 to 2 hours after burn injury. (Nasotracheal and endotracheal intubations are discussed in Chapter 20.) After intubation, clients may be placed on ventilatory assistance, and the delivered oxygen concentration is determined by assessing arterial blood gas values (see Chapter 23). Extubation may be indicated when the edema resolves, usually 3 to 6 days after burn injury (Fig. 18-9,*B*), unless severe inhalation injury is involved. Escharotomies may be needed to relieve respiratory distress secondary to circumferential, full-thickness burns of the neck and trunk.

Inhalation injury refers to a direct insult at the alveolar level secondary to the inhalation of chemical fumes or smoke. The result is interstitial edema that prevents the diffusion of oxygen from the alveoli into the circulatory system. Clients with smoke inhalation frequently exhibit *no* physical manifestations of injury during the first 24 hours after sustaining a major burn. The only diagnostic indicator may be a history of prolonged exposure to smoke or fumes. Therefore the nurse must be especially sensitive to signs of respiratory distress such as increased agitation or change in the rate or character of respirations. Sputum that contains carbon may be present. Generally, there is no correlation between the extent of TBSA burn and severity of inhalation injury, since inhalation injury is a factor of time exposure plus the type and density of the material inhaled. The initial chest x-ray film may appear normal, and the arterial blood gas values may be within the normal range.

Within 6 to 12 hours after injury in which smoke inhalation is probable, the client should have a fiberoptic bronchoscopy to assess the lower respiratory tract. Significant findings include the extramucosal appearance of carbon-

aceous material, mucosal edema, vesicles, erythema, hemorrhage, and ulceration. A radioactive xenon 133 ventilation-perfusion scan may be used to assess the ventilatory removal of gases that are normally expelled. Clients with inhalation injury have delayed clearance of gas. The results of the scan may also demonstrate areas containing no gas or areas in which the gas remains for many minutes. A disadvantage of this test is that the client must be transported to the special radiology unit of the hospital.

Impaired gas exchange related to carbon monoxide poisoning often accompanies smoke inhalation. Inhalation of carbon monoxide can produce significant hypoxemia. The carbon monoxide, produced by incomplete combustion of carbon-containing materials, has an affinity for hemoglobin 200 times that of oxygen. Carboxyhemoglobin concentration should be measured as soon as the client reaches the hospital. The presence of increased concentrations of carboxyhemoglobin suggests that the client has inhaled a significant amount of smoke. The characteristic cherry-red skin associated with carbon monoxide poisoning may not be present in clients with burn shock because of the decrease in blood flow to the skin.

Treatment of inhalation injury includes administration of humidified air and 100% oxygen as required. The client should be placed in a high Fowler position, encouraged to cough and deep breathe every hour, repositioned every 1 to 2 hours, given chest physiotherapy, and suctioned as necessary. If respiratory failure is impending, nasotracheal or endotracheal intubation should be performed and the client should be supported with mechanical ventilation. Positive end-expiratory pressure (PEEP) may be used to prevent collapse of the alveoli and progressive respiratory failure (see Chapter 23). Bronchodilators may be administered by IV to treat severe bronchospasm. Carbon monoxide poisoning is treated by administering a 100% concen-

Table 18-11 Formulas for Estimating Fluid Replacement of an Adult Burn Client

| Formula | First 24 Hours | Second 24 Hours | |
	Crystalloids	Colloids	Glucose in Water
Brooke (modified)	Lactated Ringer's solution: 2.0 ml/kg/% burn; ½ given over first 8 hr; ½ given over next 16 hr	0.3 to 0.5 ml/kg/% burn	Amount to replace estimated evaporative losses
Parkland (Baxter)	Lactated Ringer's solution: 4 ml/kg/% burn; ½ given first 8 hr; ¼ given each next 8 hr	20% to 60% of calculated plasma volume	Amount to replace estimated evaporative losses

trate of oxygen until the carboxyhemoglobin levels return to normal.

Clients with preexisting pulmonary problems (e.g., chronic obstructive pulmonary disease) are more likely to sustain respiratory infection. Pneumonia is a common complication of major burns (especially in older adults) due to debilitation, abundant microbial flora, and the relative immobility of clients. If fluid replacement is too vigorous, clients can succumb to pulmonary edema.

Renal system. The most common renal complication of a burn in the emergent phase is *acute tubular necrosis (ATN)*. Because of the hypovolemic state, blood flow to the kidneys is decreased, causing renal ischemia. If this continues, acute renal failure may develop.

With full-thickness and electrical burns, myoglobin (from muscle cell breakdown) and hemoglobin (from red blood cell breakdown) are released into the bloodstream and occlude renal tubules. Adequate fluid replacement and diuretics can counteract myoglobin and hemoglobin obstruction of the tubules.

Therapeutic management. From the onset of the burn event until the client is stabilized, medical therapy predominantly consists of airway management, fluid therapy, and wound care (Table 18-10). As soon as the client arrives at a health care facility, a fluid replacement line is secured in a large vein, preferably by percutaneous puncture. If this is not feasible, a jugular or subclavian line is inserted through unburned or even burned tissue. A cutdown is a final measure but is rarely used because of the high incidence of infection and sepsis. It is critical to establish access to a large vein that can accommodate large volumes of fluid. Peripheral veins, especially those in the feet or legs, are not generally used.

Fluid therapy. Intravenous fluid therapy is usually instituted in clients with burns greater than 20% of TBSA. The type of fluid replacement is determined by size and depth of burn, age of the client, and individual considerations such as dehydration in the preburn state or preexisting chronic illness. Each burn unit has a preference for a single replacement regime, which is used almost exclusively. Fluid replacement is accomplished with either crystalloid solutions (physiological saline, lactated Ringer's, or 5% dextrose and saline) and/or colloids (albumin, dextran, or fresh frozen plasma).

Of the many formulas that are used for fluid replace-

Table 18-12 Fluid Resuscitation with the Parkland (Baxter) Formula*

FORMULA

4 ml lactated Ringer's solution
    per
% TBSA burn
    per
kg body weight
= total fluid requirement for first 24 hr after burn

APPLICATION

½ of total in first 8 hr
¼ of total in second 8 hr
¼ of total in third 8 hr

EXAMPLE

For a 70 kg client with a 50% TBSA burn:
4 ml × 70 kg × 50% TBSA burn = 14,000 ml
                                = 14 L in 24 hr
½ of total in first 8 hr = 7000 ml (875 ml/hr)
¼ of total in second 8 hr = 3500 ml (436 ml/hr)
¼ of total in third 8 hr = 3500 ml (436 ml/hr)

*Formulas are guidelines. Fluid is administered at a rate to produce 30 to 50 ml of urine output per hour.

ment the Brooke formula and the Parkland (Baxter) formula are commonly employed (Table 18-11). All formulas are estimates. The Parkland formula has been widely used because it is easy to calculate and monitor and because it provides a reliable method of fluid replacement for most clients.

As noted in Table 18-12, the Parkland formula gives fluid in the following manner: 4 ml lactated Ringer's solution per kilogram of body weight per percent TBSA burned. This quantity is calculated for the first 24 hours, with one half of the total quantity given in the first 8 hours after injury because it is during that period that fluid loss is greatest. (*Note:* This 24 hours is not calculated from time of arrival to hospital but from the time of injury.) One quarter of the total quantity is then given in the second 8-hour period, and the final quarter is given in the last 8-hour period (Table 18-12).

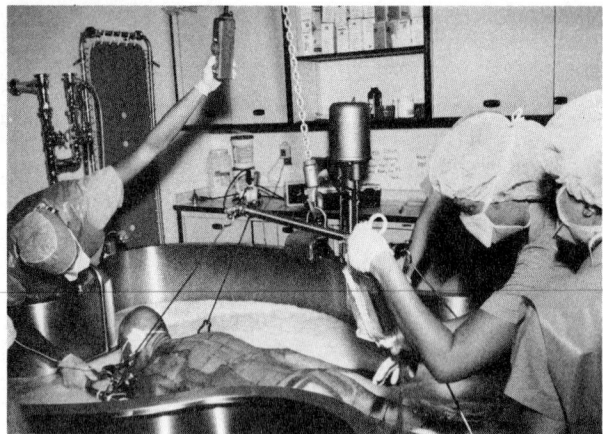

Fig. 18-10 Client is being bathed in a Hubbard tank.

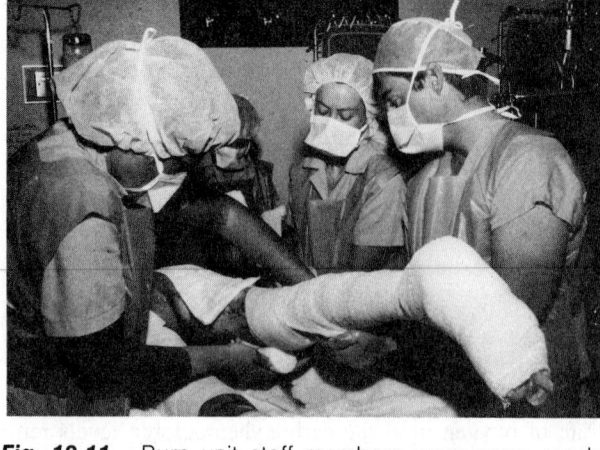

Fig. 18-11 Burn unit staff members wear caps, masks, plastic aprons, and sterile gloves when changing dressings.

The second 24 hours of fluid replacement consists of ensuring adequate dextrose in water replacement to maintain a serum sodium level below 140 mEq/L. Colloidal solutions (e.g., Plasmanate, albumin) are also routinely given. The amount is calculated with a formula and the client's body weight, which predicts the replacement volume. Colloidal solutions are not given until the second 24 hours, when capillary permeability begins to return to normal, because premature infusion of plasma would result in leakage out of the vascular space as a result of increased capillary permeability. After this time, the plasma remains in the vascular space and expands the circulating volume.

Assessment of the adequacy of fluid replacement is best made by use of more than one parameter, and urinary output is the most commonly used. Assessment parameters include the following:

1. Urine output: 30 to 50 ml/hr in an adult
2. Cardiopulmonary factors: blood pressure* (systolic ≥90 to 100 mm Hg), pulse rate (≤100), respiration (16 to 20 breaths per minute)
3. Sensorium: alert and oriented to time, place, and person

Wound care. Wound care may be delayed until a patent airway, adequate circulation, and adequate fluid replacement have been established. Goals of wound care are to *(1)* cleanse and debride the area of necrotic tissue and debris that would promote bacterial growth; *(2)* minimize further destruction to viable skin; *(3)* promote client comfort.

Cleansing and debridement can be done in a Hubbard tank (Fig. 18-10), in a shower, or in bed. During these procedures, loose, necrotic skin is removed. Large blisters may be opened to eliminate media for bacterial growth. All burned areas with hair (except eyebrows) should be shaved, including the head and perineum. Thereafter,

daily shaving is required to minimize pathogen accumulation. Care should be taken to accomplish this procedure as quickly and deftly as possible. Immersion in a Hubbard tank for longer than 20 to 30 minutes can cause electrolyte loss from open burned areas. Prolonged immersion can lead to chilling after the bath and cross-contamination of wounds from one area of the body to another. Because of these factors, some institutions do not submerge the client. The water does not need to be sterile, and tap water not exceeding 40° C (104° F) is acceptable. Because pathogenic organisms are present on the burn wound, a surgical detergent, disinfectant, or cleansing agent is used. The client may be bathed 2 times daily to limit the amount of bacterial growth.

Infection is the most serious threat to further tissue injury and possible sepsis. The source of infection in burn wounds is the client's own residual flora, predominately from the skin, respiratory tract, and gastrointestinal tract. The prevention of cross-contamination from one client to another is a priority for nursing care. Two methods of wound treatment used to control infection are the *open method* and the *closed method.*[9] In the open method the client's burn is covered with a topical antibiotic and has no dressing. The closed method uses sterile gauze dressings impregnated with or laid over a topical antibiotic. These dressings are changed 2 to 3 times every 24 hours.

When wounds are exposed, staff must wear hats, masks, gowns, and plastic aprons (Fig. 18-11). When removing dressings and washing the wound the nurse should use nonsterile disposable gloves. Sterile gloves are used when applying ointments and sterile dressings. In addition, the room must be kept warm (about 29.4° C [85° F] and humid [60%]). All attire is changed before the nurse treats another client. Careful hand washing is also required to prevent cross-contamination. After the client has been treated in the tub, the tank and agitators are disinfected with a chemical preparation.

Coverage is the primary goal for burn wounds. Survival is directly related to prevention of wound contamination.

---

*Blood pressure is most appropriately measured by an arterial line. Peripheral measurement is often invalid due to early vasoconstriction and edema.

Table 18-13 Sources of Grafts

Source	Graft Name	Coverage
Client's own skin	Autograft	Permanent
Cadaveric skin	Homograft or allograft (same species)	Temporary (3 days to 2 weeks)
Porcine skin	Heterograft or xenograft (different species)	Temporary (3 days to 2 weeks)

Since there is rarely enough unburned skin in the major burn victim for immediate skin grafting, other temporary wound closure methods are used. Allograft or homograft skin (usually from cadavers) is commonly used for wound closure (Table 18-13). However, rejection occurs because the host's immune system acts against the foreign substance.

Other measures. Routine lab tests are performed initially and serially to monitor electrolyte balance. Blood for measurement of arterial blood gases may be drawn to determine adequacy of ventilation and perfusion. Physical therapy is begun immediately, sometimes in the Hubbard tank. Early range-of-motion (ROM) exercises are necessary to facilitate mobilization of the extravasated fluid back to the vascular bed. Exercise of body parts also maintains function and reassures the client that movement is still possible.

Pharmacological intervention. Tetanus toxoid is given routinely to all burn victims because of the likelihood of anaerobic burn-wound contamination. In the absence of active immunization within 10 years before the burn injury, tetanus immunoglobulin should be administered at another site, with a different syringe and needle to prevent inactivation of the immunoglobulin by tetanus toxoid.

Analgesics are ordered to promote client comfort. Early in the postburn period, IV pain medications should be given because (1) gastrointestinal function is slowed or impaired because of shock or paralytic ileus, and (2) intramuscular (IM) injections will not be absorbed adequately in burned or edematous areas. Pooling of medications will occur in the tissues because of poor circulation. When fluid mobilization begins, the client can be overdosed from the interstitial accumulation of previous IM medications.

Common narcotics used for pain control are listed in Table 18-14. The need for analgesia should be evaluated early relative to the burn injury. The drug of choice for pain control is morphine, but meperidine and methadone may also be used. These drugs provide adequate pain control and a sedative effect. The client is in great pain with large burns (especially those that are predominantly partial-thickness). Withholding pain medication in the emergent and acute phases of burn recuperation is not only inhumane but also unethical.

After the wound is cleansed, topical antibacterial agents are applied and may be covered with a light dressing or left open to air (Fig. 18-12). Systemic antibiotics are not

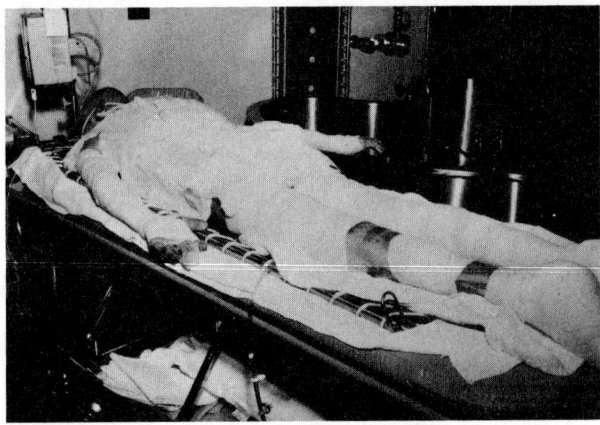

Fig. 18-12 Client being treated with silver sulfadiazine burn cream. The light Kerlix gauze dressings allow active range of motion.

Table 18-14 Drugs Commonly Used in Burn Treatment

Types and Names of Drugs	Purpose
NUTRITIONAL SUPPORT	
Vitamins A, C, E, and multivitamins	Promotes wound healing
Minerals: zinc, folate, iron (ferrous sulfate, ferrous gluconate)	Promotes cellular integrity and hemoglobin formation
ANALGESIA AND SEDATIVE	
Morphine	Diminishes pain perception
Meperidine (Demerol)	Diminishes pain perception
Methadone	Relieves pain, elevates mood
Secobarbital (Seconal)	Induces sleep
Haloperidol (Haldol)	Produces antipsychotic and sedative effects, promotes sleep
Midazolam (Versed)	Has short-acting amnestic properties
GASTROINTESTINAL SUPPORT	
Cimetidine (Tagamet)	Decreases incidence of Curling's ulcer
Nystatin (Mycostatin)	Prevents overgrowth of *Candida albicans* in oral mucosa
Mylanta, Maalox	Neutralizes stomach acid

usually used in controlling burn wound flora, especially after 48 hours, because there is little to no blood supply to the burn eschar, and consequently, there is little delivery of the antibiotic to the wound. Some burn centers prophylactically administer IV penicillin for the first 3 to 4 days to reduce the proliferation of gram-positive organisms.

Table 18-15 Topical Antibiotic Therapy Used in Burn Wound Therapy

Drug	Indications for Use	Advantages	Disadvantages
Silver sulfadiazine (Silvadene)	Gram-positive and gram-negative organisms, *Candida albicans*	Wide-spectrum antibacterial action; no limit to motion because of light or no dressing; fast, painless, easy to apply	Possible depression of granulocyte formation; possible allergic reaction to sulfa component in susceptible clients
Silver nitrate	Most gram-positive organisms and some *Pseudomonas species*	Wide-spectrum antibacterial action; effectiveness against fungal organisms; inexpensive	Possible severe electrolyte depletion (primarily sodium and chloride); severe limited motion because of bulky dressing; grayish-black staining of everything it touches; limited penetration of deeper tissues
Mafenide acetate (Sulfamylon)	Gram-positive and gram-negative organisms, most anaerobes	Wide-spectrum antibacterial action; most effective of all topical antibiotics; penetration of eschar better than other agents; open treatment of burn wound possible; good treatment for electrical burns	Pain on application for 15-30 minutes; acid-base derangements because it is a carbonic anhydrase inhibitor; allergic reaction to sulfa component in susceptible clients

Topical burn agents penetrate the eschar, thereby inhibiting bacterial invasion of the wound (Table 18-15). Silver sulfadiazine is commonly used because it is effective, and unlike mafenide (Sulfamylon), it is painless. Systemic sepsis remains a leading cause of death in clients with major burns because resistant organisms develop with exposure of bacteria to topical agents over time. Most burn units use one topical agent almost exclusively and change to another at the first sign of organism resistance. Systemic antibiotic therapy is initiated when the clinical diagnosis of invasive burn wound sepsis is made or when some other source of sepsis is identified (e.g., pneumonia).

A variety of drugs may be administered to the burn client (Table 18-15). Frequently, superinfections develop in the client's mucous membranes (mouth and genitalia) as a result of antibiotic therapy and low resistance in the host. The offending organism is usually *Candida albicans*. This is treated with nystatin (Mycostatin) mouthwash. When a normal diet is resumed, yogurt or lactobacillus (Lactinex) may be given by mouth to reintroduce the normal intestinal flora that have been destroyed by antibiotic therapy. Supplemental vitamins and iron may be given as early as the emergent phase. However, the need for these supplements usually does not occur until the acute phase.

Nutritional considerations. Fluid replacement takes priority over nutritional needs in the initial emergent phase. Clients with large burns frequently develop paralytic ileus within a few hours as a result of the body's response to major trauma. A nasogastric tube is inserted and connected to low intermittent suction for decompression. When bowel sounds return at 48 to 72 hours after injury, alimentation can be initiated beginning with clear liquids and progressing to a diet high in protein and calories.

A hypermetabolic response proportional to the size of the wound is observed. Resting metabolic expenditure may be increased by 50% to 100% above normal for major burns. Core temperature is elevated. Plasma catecholamines, which stimulate heat production, and substrate mobilization are increased. Massive catabolism is characterized by protein mobilization and increased gluconeogenesis. Caloric needs are often in the 5000 kcal/day range. Failure to supply adequate calories and protein actually leads to malnutrition. Clients are not given water to drink ad libitum, but rather calorie-containing liquids because of the great need for calories and the potential for water intoxication.

Major advances have been made in the area of liquid nutritional supplementation (see Chapter 35). Nutritional formulas have been developed that provide adequate protein and calories without excessive water.[10] Another recent discovery has been the ability to advance a very thin latex feeding tube by fluoroscopic guidance into the duodenum, bypassing the stomach. This allows for quicker absorption of nutrients and a decrease in the nausea and vomiting associated with high-volume tube feedings into the stomach. These clients can be maintained on a more continuous feeding schedule, which does not have to be interrupted by surgical interventions. Since the liquid goes past the pyloric sphincter, the client does not have to remain NPO for extended periods before surgery, as is required when the tube is in the stomach.

■ Nursing Management of Burns

In the emergent phase, client survival depends on quick and thorough assessment and intervention. It may be the nurse who makes the initial assessment of depth, degree, and percent of burn and who coordinates the actions of the burn team. The nurse assesses the adequacy of fluid replacement, provides wound care, and offers support to the client and family (Table 18-16).

Text continued on p. 423.

Table 18-16

NURSING CARE PLAN FOR THE BURN CLIENT

Defining Characteristics	Nursing Interventions			Evaluation Criteria
	Emergent Phase	**Acute Phase**	**Rehabilitative Phase**	

NURSING DIAGNOSIS: High risk for fluid volume deficit related to evaporative loss, plasma loss, and shift of fluid into interstitium secondary to burn injury

Urine output > intake, output <30 ml/hr, decreased blood pressure, altered mental status, drainage from burn wounds	Assess pulses, blood pressure, circulation, and sensation to all extremities every 1 to 2 hr. Assess mental status. Assess intake and output hourly. Check daily weights. Assess pulmonary function. Monitor serial laboratory tests. Give fluids according to client needs.	Use emergent phase interventions as necessary. Monitor electrolyte levels regularly. Provide oral fluids if client is able to drink.	No intervention is required.	Urine output >30 to 50 ml/hr, stable vital signs, clear sensorium, sodium and potassium levels within acceptable range, systolic blood pressure >90 mm Hg

NURSING DIAGNOSIS: Pain related to burn injury, treatments, and shearing injuries

Demonstration of discomfort and pain	Give IV analgesia as needed. Keep client warm. Elevate burned arms on pillows. Administer medication for pain 30 min before interventions. Provide emotional support. Reposition client carefully using lifting sheet as necessary.	Plan adequate rest periods. Administer medication before interventions. Plan diversional activities.	Be aware that client's pain is replaced by itching. Keep skin lubricated. Teach client to watch for injuries to new skin.	No pain or tolerable level of pain

NURSING DIAGNOSIS: Total self-care deficit related to pain, immobility, and perceived helplessness

Inability or unwillingness to participate in self-care	Assess client's ability to perform self-care activities. Assist or intervene as appropriate. Assist client in remaining in emotional control.	Increase client's self-care activities as appropriate. Ensure that client participates in planning care as able.	Assess and arrange for needed adaptations in living arrangements and lifestyle to accommodate optimal self-care.	Optimal performance of self-care

Continued.

Table 18-16

 NURSING CARE PLAN FOR THE BURN CLIENT—cont'd

Defining Characteristics	Nursing Interventions			Evaluation Criteria
	Emergent Phase	Acute Phase	Rehabilitative Phase	

NURSING DIAGNOSIS: High risk for impaired physical mobility related to joint contractures secondary to pain and immobility

Difficulty in performing active ROM, pain on movement; assumption of position of comfort that may be dysfunctional; reluctance to ambulate and participate in self-care; fear of activities that involve joint movement	Initiate and encourage passive and active ROM during hydrotherapy and during waking hours. Maintain neck, arms, legs in extension positions. Keep hands in functional position. Help client to ambulate four times a day if possible.	Increase mobility and activity as tolerated. Teach ways to avoid contractures. Have client assume as much self-care as possible. Use anticipatory guidance and teaching to alleviate anxiety.	Plan daily program with client and/or appropriate resources for continuing activity program as needed.	Maximum potential ROM of all extremities, absence of contractures

NURSING DIAGNOSIS: Altered nutrition: less than body requirements related to increased caloric demands and inability to ingest increased requirements

Weight loss, low serum albumin level, inability or unwillingness to ingest food	Chart caloric intake. Maintain client NPO with nasogastric tube to low intermittent suction. Assess return of bowel sounds. Initiate hyperalimentation and IV fluid replacement. Institute progressive diet to meet nutritional needs if bowel sounds are present.	Continue to monitor peristalsis. Offer high-protein, high-carbohydrate diet. Assess client food preferences and offer food when client is able to eat. Monitor duodenal tube feedings, titrating to client's tolerance.	Continue to meet nutritional needs. Once skin coverage is achieved, reduce calories to prevent excess weight gain (if necessary).	Positive nitrogen balance, weight loss not >10% of body weight

Table 18-16

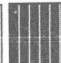

NURSING CARE PLAN FOR THE BURN CLIENT—cont'd

Defining Characteristics	Nursing Interventions			Evaluation Criteria
	Emergent Phase	Acute Phase	Rehabilitative Phase	

NURSING DIAGNOSIS: High risk for infection related to impaired skin integrity, endogenous flora, and suppressed immune response

| Fever, purulent drainage, edema, redness, leukocytosis | Use good hand-washing technique. Use sterile technique during topical antibiotic application and dressing changes. Ensure that hydrotherapy and debridement last for no longer than 30 min per session. Shave appropriate areas. Evacuate blisters and remove devitalized tissue. Cleanse area around eyes with normal saline solution (if burned). Perform perineal care every 2 hr (while client is catheterized). Apply topical antibiotic or sterile dressings as indicated. Start systemic antibiotics intravenously. Give tetanus vaccine if necessary. Observe wound daily for separation of eschar; check wound margins for cellulitis. | Monitor burn wound margins for signs of infection. Note any change in behavior or sensorium as a possible precursor to sepsis. Perform hydrotherapy and debridement carefully. Monitor body temperature and urine output. Monitor donor sites for possible infection. | Instruct client and family about signs and symptoms of infection. Teach family how to perform dressing changes. | Wound free of debris and loose necrotic tissue, minimum infection, rapid infection control |

Continued.

Table 18-16

NURSING CARE PLAN FOR THE BURN CLIENT—cont'd

Defining Characteristics	Nursing Interventions			Evaluation Criteria
	Emergent Phase	Acute Phase	Rehabilitative Phase	

NURSING DIAGNOSIS: Anxiety related to pain, separation from family, guilt associated with injury, lack of knowledge about treatment and outcome, financial needs, and appearance

| Questions about treatment and prognosis, withdrawn or overtly angry, expression of concerns about scarring | Administer medication for pain before interventions. Encourage family visits and participation in care. Be open to client's expressions of feelings about burn event. Provide information or explanation as assessment indicates. Describe burn process, signs and symptoms to client and family on admission. Explain therapeutic interventions, precautionary measures, gowning, hand washing, and visiting policy on admission. | Assist client and family in realistic expectations of near and distant future (anticipatory guidance). | Provide avenues for client and family to maintain contact with hospital personnel after discharge. Plan counseling if needed. | Verbalization of reduction of anxiety, body language indication of rest and comfort, verbalization of change in self-image |

NURSING DIAGNOSIS: Dysfunctional grieving (family, individual) related to change in body image, actual or perceived impact of injury on lifestyle, role relationships, and occupation

| Crying, withdrawal, unwillingness to look at self or participate in self-care, expression of concern about impact of injury on lifestyle | Reassure client that swelling will subside in 2 to 4 days. | Plan for family interaction. Assist client to progress through stages of grief and acceptance at own pace. Be realistic and positive during interventions. Set goals within limitations. | Assess need for and provide means of professional counseling if appropriate. | Verbalization of realistic goals regarding future lifestyle, acceptance of altered body image |

Care of special areas is initiated by the nurse. The face is very vascular and subject to a greater amount of edema. The face is treated by the open method because facial dressings cause disorientation and confusion. Eye care for corneal burns or edema is done with slightly warmed physiological saline rinses as often as every hour. Periorbital edema can prevent opening of the eyes. This can be very frightening to clients; the nurse must assure them that the swelling is not permanent and that vision will soon be restored. Instillation of methylcellulose drops or artificial tears into the eyes for moisture provides additional client comfort and prevents corneal abrasions.

Hands and arms should be extended and elevated on pillows or in slings to minimize edema. Ears should be kept free of pressure because of their poor vascularization and predisposition to infection. Clients with ear burns are not allowed to use pillows because of the danger of the burned ear sticking to the pillow case, thereby causing bleeding, pain, or infection of the ear cartilage.

The perineum must be kept clean and as dry as possible. In addition to providing hourly urine outputs, an indwelling catheter prevents urine contamination of the perineal area. Frequent perineal and catheter care is essential.

Acute Phase

The acute phase begins with the mobilization of extracellular fluid and subsequent diuresis. The acute phase is concluded when the burned area is completely covered or when the wounds are healed. This may take weeks or many months.

Pathophysiological changes. Burn injury involves pathophysiological changes in many body systems. Diuresis from fluid mobilization occurs, and the client is no longer grossly edematous. Areas that are full- or partial-thickness burns are more evident. Bowel sounds return. The client is now aware of the enormity of body changes and the presence of pain. Healing begins when WBCs have surrounded the burn wound and phagocytosis begins. Necrotic tissue begins to slough. Fibroblasts lay down matrices of the collagen precursors that eventually form granulation tissue. Kept free from infection, a partial-thickness burn wound will heal from the edges and from below. However, full-thickness burn wounds must be covered by skin grafts. Often, healing time and length of hospitalization are decreased by early excision and grafting.

Clinical manifestations. Full-thickness wounds will be dry and waxy white to dark brown and will have no sensation because nerve endings have been destroyed. Partial-thickness wounds are pink to cherry red and wet and shiny with serous exudate. These wounds may or may not have intact blisters and are very painful when touched or exposed to air (Fig. 18-13).

Over time, the margins of full-thickness eschar will begin to separate, allowing for debridement of the wound. Usually full-thickness wounds will require surgical debridement and skin grafting to speed the healing process.

Partial-thickness wounds will also form eschar but will not be as thick, so they will begin separating sooner and healing more quickly. Once partial-thickness eschar is removed, epithelialization begins at the wound margins and appears as red or pink scar tissue. The epithelial buds eventually close in the wound, and the wound heals spontaneously without surgical intervention.

Laboratory values. Because the body is attempting to reestablish fluid and electrolyte homeostasis in the initial acute phase, it is important to follow serum values closely.

Sodium. *Hyponatremia* can occur with silver nitrate topical antibiotic therapy as a result of sodium loss through the eschar. If hydrotherapy is too lengthy (usually longer than 20 to 30 minutes), the hypotonicity of the bath water pulls sodium from the open burn areas. Other causes of hyponatremia include excessive gastrointestinal drainage, diarrhea, and excessive water intake. Symptoms of hyponatremia include weakness, dizziness, muscle cramps, fatigue, headache, tachycardia, and confusion. Burn clients may also develop a dilutional hyponatremia referred to as *water intoxication*. To avoid this condition, the client should drink fluids other than water, such as juices or soft drinks.

Hypernatremia may be seen after successful fluid replacement if copious amounts of hypertonic solutions were required. Other causes of hypernatremia include improper tube feeding therapy or improper fluid administration. Manifestations of hypernatremia include thirst; dried, furry tongue; lethargy; confusion; and, possibly, convulsions.

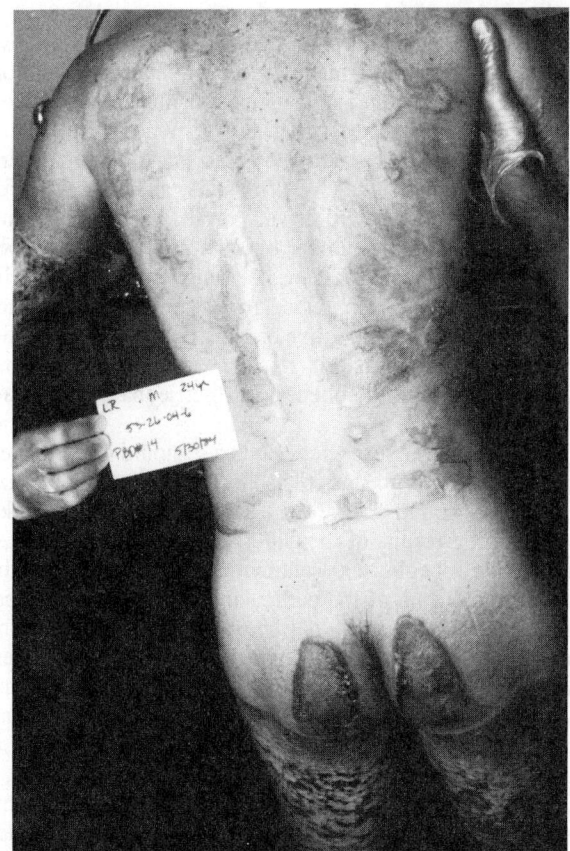

Fig. 18-13 On postburn day 14, this client has an almost healed partial-thickness burn to the back. Areas of full-thickness injury remain on legs.

Potassium. *Hyperkalemia* is noted if the client has renal failure, adrenocortical insufficiency, or massive deep muscle injury with large amounts of potassium released from damaged cells. Cardiac dysrhythmias and ventricular failure can occur with excessive elevations (potassium level >7 mEq/L). Muscle weakness and electrocardiographic changes are observed clinically (see Chapter 10).

Hypokalemia is observed with silver nitrate therapy and lengthy hydrotherapy. Other causes of this deficit include vomiting, diarrhea, prolonged gastrointestinal suction, and prolonged IV therapy without potassium supplementation. Constant potassium losses occur through the burn wound.

Complications

Infection. The course of recovery from major burn injury is never smooth. The body's first line of defense, the skin, has been destroyed by burn injury. Pathogens often proliferate before phagocytosis has begun. The media for pathogenic growth are quite favorable. If bacterial density at the junction of the eschar with underlying viable tissue rises to >10^5/g, the client has a wound infection. In the presence of an infection, localized inflammation, induration, and suppuration will be seen at the burn wound margins. Partial-thickness burns can convert to full-thickness burns in the presence of infection. A histological examination of a burn-wound biopsy is the most reliable means of differentiating colonization of nonviable tissue from invasive infection of viable tissue.

Wound infection may progress to transient bacteremia from wound manipulation (e.g., after debridement and hydrotherapy). The client may develop an invasive infection or sepsis. Manifestations of sepsis include an elevated temperature, increased pulse and respiratory rate, decreased blood pressure, and decreased urine output. There may be mild confusion, chills, malaise, and loss of appetite. The WBC count will usually be between 10,000 and 20,000/μl. This high number of WBCs is misleading because the cells themselves are not functional, and the client remains immunosuppressed for a period of time after the burn injury. The causative organisms of sepsis are usually gram-negative bacteria (e.g., *Pseudomonas, Proteus* organisms), putting the client in further jeopardy of possible septic shock.

When sepsis is suspected, cultures should be obtained immediately from all possible sources: urine, oropharynx, IV site, and wound. However, treatment should not be delayed pending results of the culture and sensitivity studies. Therapy will begin with antibiotics appropriate for the usual residual flora of the particular burn unit. The topical antibiotic that is used may be continued or may be changed to another agent. Although their use is controversial, steroids may be given to stabilize cell membranes and minimize endotoxin release. At this stage, the client's condition is critical, requiring very close monitoring of vital signs.

Cardiovascular and respiratory systems. The same cardiovascular and respiratory system complications may be present in the acute phase as in the emergent phase.

Neurological system. Neurologically, the client usually has no physically based problems unless severe hypoxia from respiratory injuries or complications from electrical injuries occur. However, a poorly understood phenomenon is likely to be seen. The client can become extremely disoriented, may withdraw or become combative, and has hallucinations and frequent nightmare-like episodes. Delirium is more acute at night and occurs more often in older clients. This is a transient state lasting from a day or two to several weeks. Various causes have been considered, including electrolyte imbalance, massive stress, cerebral edema, sepsis, and intensive care unit psychosis syndrome.

Musculoskeletal system. The musculoskeletal system takes center stage for complications during the acute phase. As the burns begin to heal and scar tissue forms, the skin is less supple and pliant. ROM may be limited and contractures can occur. Rigorous physical therapy is imperative to maintain optimal joint function. A good time for exercise is during and after hydrotherapy when the skin is softer. Passive and active ROM should be done to all joints. Clients with neck burns should sleep without pillows or with their heads hanging slightly over the top of the mattress to encourage hyperextension. Splints may be applied to keep joints in functional positions.

Gastrointestinal system. The gastrointestinal system also exhibits complications. Adynamic ileus results from sepsis. However, diarrhea is more commonly present than ileus and is caused by the use of rich supplemental feedings. Constipation can occur as a side effect of narcotic analgesics and decreased mobility. *Curling's ulcer,* a type of gastroduodenal ulcer characterized by diffuse superficial lesions including mucosal erosion, is caused by a generalized stress response resulting in decreased production of mucus and increased gastric acid secretion. The best treatment for Curling's ulcer is the prophylactic use of antacids and cimetidine (Tagamet), which prevent histamine stimulation. Many major burn clients also have occult blood in their stools during the acute phase.

Endocrine system. *Stress diabetes* may be seen transiently because of increased mobilization of glycogen stores and subsequent conversion to glucose. There is also an increase in insulin production and release. However, insulin's effectiveness is decreased, leading to an elevated blood sugar level. Later, hyperglycemia can be caused by the supranormal caloric intake necessary to meet the metabolic requirements. When this occurs, the treatment is supplemental insulin, not decreased feeding. Urine glucose is checked hourly and an appropriate amount of insulin is given if glycosuria is present. Glucometers may also be used to assess blood glucose; serum glucose samples are more accurate than urine samples, since the urine tested may have been in the bladder for hours. As the client's metabolic demands are met and less stress is placed on the entire system, this stress-induced condition is reversed.

Therapeutic management. The three predominant therapeutic interventions in the acute phase are (1) fluid replacement, (2) wound care, and (3) early excision and grafting.

Fluid replacement. Fluid replacement continues from the emergent phase into the acute phase on the basis of client needs. IV therapy is provided to replace fluid losses, administer medications, and administer transfusions of plasma or blood products. The type of fluid replacement depends on the client's specific needs. Common types of

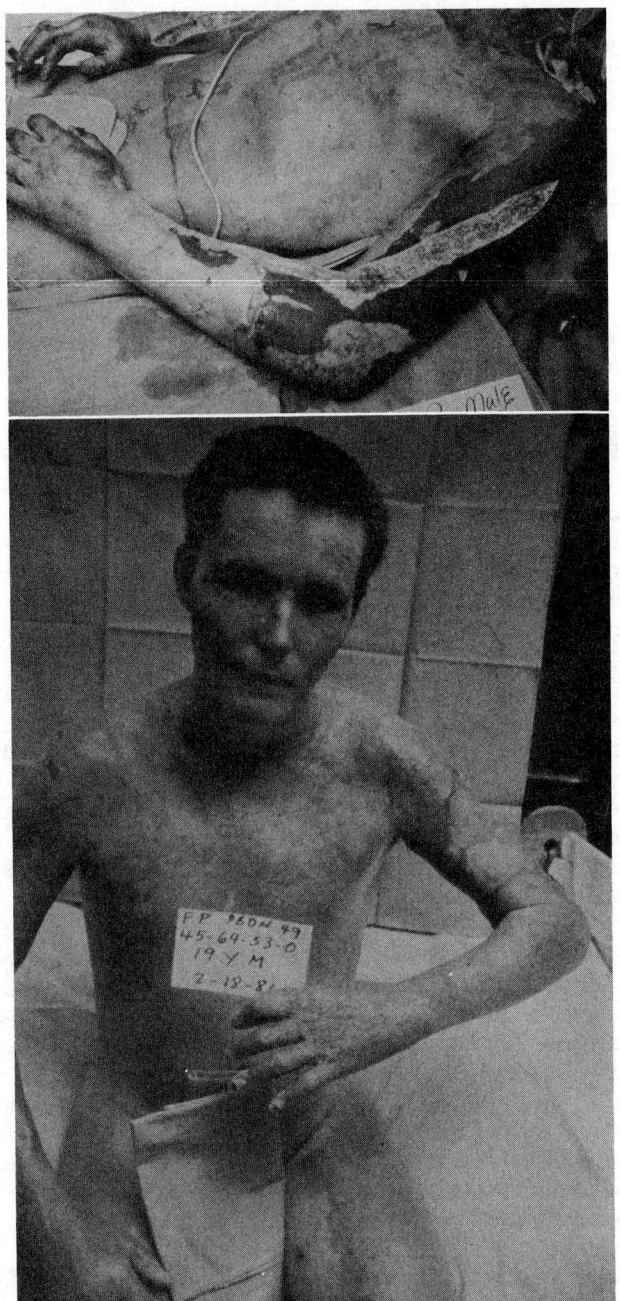

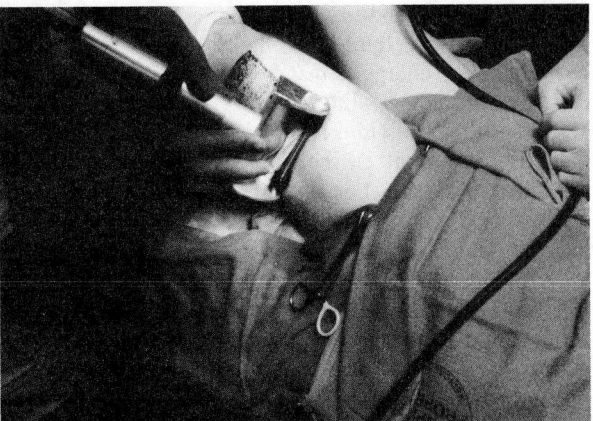

Fig. 18-15 The surgeon harvests skin from a client's thigh using a dermatome.

Fig. 18-14 A, Client with full-thickness arm and torso burns before skin grafting. **B,** Client on postburn day 49 after skin grafting is accomplished.

replacement are normal saline solution, Ringer's lactate solution, and various concentrations of glucose in saline solution or water. Packed red blood cells, fresh frozen plasma, and Plasmanate are also commonly given at this time.

Wound care. Wound care consists of daily observation, assessment, and debridement. Wound care is usually done by nursing staff and involves active debridement of the wound with scalpels, forceps, and scissors. If the eschar is thick and hard as in full-thickness burns, a grid escharotomy may be necessary. This procedure involves cross-

hatching the eschar with a scalpel. This is painless for the client because nerve endings have been damaged by the burning process. The grid eschar allows more of the burn surface to be "an edge," thus promoting eschar separation from viable tissue. A grid eschar has been less commonly performed in recent years because the preferred treatment is early excision of the eschar.

Excision and grafting. Current therapeutic management of burn wounds involves early removal of the necrotic tissue followed by application of split-thickness autograft skin (Fig. 18-14). This remarkable therapy has changed the management of burn care in the last 10 years. In the past, major burn clients had low rates of survival because healing and wound coverage took so long that the client usually succumbed first to infection or malnutrition. Now, mortality rates can be greatly reduced and morbidity can be decreased by early intervention. Candidates for early excision and grafting are those with stable cardiovascular systems after initial fluid resuscitation.

Eschar is removed down to subcutaneous tissue or fascia, depending on the degree of injury. The graft must be placed on clean, viable tissue to achieve good adherence. Hemostasis is achieved by pressure and application of topical thrombin or epinephrine, after which the wound is covered with autograft or allograft skin (see Table 18-9). With early excision, function is restored and scar tissue formation is lessened. Since the dead tissue is planed off until viable tissue is reached, extensive bleeding is expected to occur, which poses a problem when grafting is performed. Clots between the graft and the wound keep the graft from adhering to the wound. One method of managing the clotting problem is to excise the wound on one day and to graft it on the next day. The excised wounds are soaked every 4 hours with an antibiotic solution between the surgeries. This will also ensure that the wound has been excised to viable tissue, since it can be visualized with a clear field to check the depth.

Donor skin is taken from the client for grafting by means of a dermatome, which removes a thin layer (split-thickness) of skin from an unburned site (Fig. 18-15). The donor skin can be meshed to allow for greater wound coverage, or it may be applied as a sheet graft for a better cosmetic result in grafting of face, neck, and hands.

Nutritional considerations. The goals of nutritional management of the burn client during the acute phase are to (1) minimize energy demands and (2) provide adequate calories to promote healing.

The burn client is in a hypermetabolic and highly catabolic state as a result of the burn injury. Decreasing catecholamine release by minimizing pain, fear, anxiety, and cold can maximize client comfort and conserve energy. Infection also consumes a great deal of energy.

Daily caloric intake is crucial. Estimated caloric needs per 24 hours for the adult with burns of greater than 20% TBSA can be calculated by the following formula:

$$(25 \text{ kcal} \times \text{kg of body weight})$$
$$+ (40 \text{ kcal} \times \% \text{ TBSA burn})$$

Caloric needs are often 5000 kcal/day. By the end of the first week after burn injury, the client's caloric and nutritional requirements should be met. Encourage the client to eat high-protein, high-carbohydrate foods to meet increased caloric needs. Ideally, the client should not lose more than 10% of preburn weight.

Optimally, the client should take a normal diet by mouth as soon as bowel function returns. If this is not possible, a feeding tube can be placed and a complete liquid diet administered. Diet supplements can be given by mouth or intravenously in the form of total parenteral nutrition (see Chapter 35).

If family members wish to bring in the client's favorite foods, this should be encouraged. The client's appetite is usually diminished, and constant encouragement is necessary to achieve adequate intake.

■ Nursing Management of the Acute Phase

During this phase, wound care consumes most of the nursing care hours. Yet this should not negate the importance of supportive care, comfort and hygiene measures, and physical therapy.

Pain assessment and management

One of the most critical functions a nurse performs during this phase is pain assessment and management. It becomes very difficult in burn nursing to separate empathy from sympathy and to act appropriately when clients are so vulnerable and ill. Almost every intervention that is performed for clients causes pain in spite of the fact that helping to cure is the goal. Clients may experience rare moments of relative comfort, but they know that these moments will not last. The nurse must understand the physiological as well as the psychological bases of pain (see Chapter 51). Allowing clients to ventilate feelings of anger, hostility, and frustration serves to assist them in expression of their pain.

There are several interventions that nurses may try to help clients deal with pain.[11] These interventions can also help the nurses cope with interventions that cause pain. First, it is helpful to get an order for a dosage range of a narcotic (e.g., morphine sulfate 5 to 10 mg IV every 1 to 3 hours for pain). When the order is written this way, it allows the nurse some freedom to try medicating clients according to responses to the medication. That is, the nurse

may find that giving 5 mg every hour works better than giving 10 mg every 3 hours. This method can include clients' input if they are alert and also gives them some control over their pain. If clients are unable to participate, the nurse will have to assess response to medication by physiological parameters (i.e., heart rate, blood pressure, and respiratory rate).

The second intervention is the use of several drugs in combination. This includes the use of morphine with diazepam (Valium) or midazolam (Versed). The effect of midazolam is short-term memory loss, so if it is given 15 to 20 minutes before a dressing change, clients will not recall the event. Midazolam lasts about 30 to 60 minutes after it is administered. Buprenorphine (Buprenex) is another drug that has come into use recently. The mechanism of action is not entirely understood, but it is proposed that it exerts its analgesic effect via high-affinity binding to opiate receptors in the central nervous system. It is a narcotic antagonist so it cannot be used in combination with other narcotic analgesics. Buprenorphine works well for those clients who are unable to be relieved from pain with high doses of narcotics.

A third method of managing pain is an alternative manner in which the nurse and client work together to find a way to cope with pain. It involves the use of relaxation tapes, visualization, guided imagery, biofeedback, and meditation. These techniques are used as adjuncts to traditional narcotic treatment of pain. They are not meant to be used exclusively to control pain in the burn client.

The nurse explores with the client what the best way is to manage the pain with one or more of these techniques. Visualization and guided imagery can be helpful to the nurse as well as the client. These two techniques can take several forms but the easiest method is for the nurse to ask questions about a favorite hobby or recent vacation destinations. The nurse can then search these areas further by asking questions that make clients visualize and describe their most recent vacation. When using this method, both the nurse and the client have to think of other things besides the task at hand (e.g., a dressing change) to keep the conversation flowing. It is up to the nurse to maintain the exchange. Relaxation tapes can also be helpful, especially when played at night to help the client fall asleep. The use of these techniques involves a more in-depth nurse/client relationship and can leave both with a sense of accomplishment.

The most important point to remember about pain management is that the more control that clients have in managing their own pain, the more successful it will be. There has been a recent trend toward the use of patient controlled analgesic (PCA) pumps. An IV solution is made up to contain a certain dose of a narcotic per milliliter (e.g., morphine 2 mg/ml). Clients have a control that they can operate to deliver a preset dose of the IV narcotic. The machine is locked onto this dose, so there is no possibility of clients getting more than what is prescribed. Results of this method are promising and may be a way in which burn centers can help to manage pain in their clients in the future. (PCA is discussed in Chapters 14 and 51.)

The acute pain that occurs during surgical procedures to

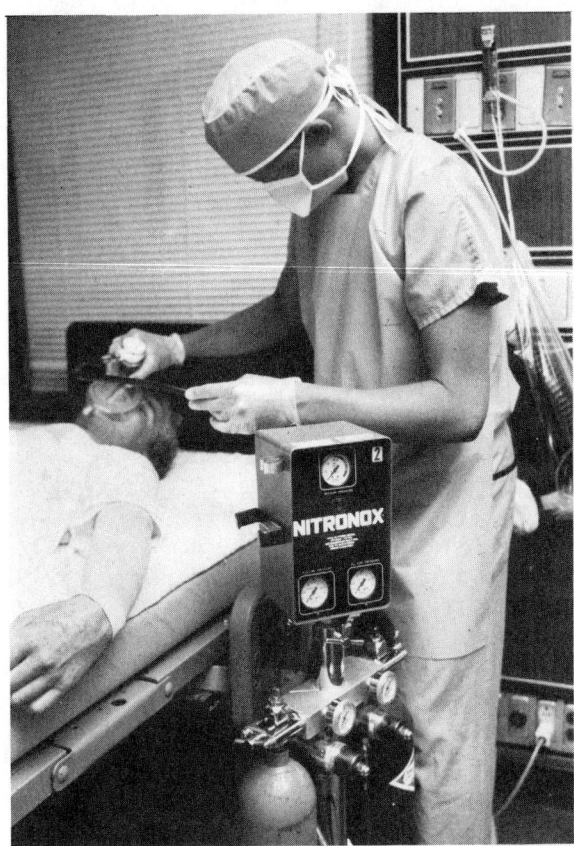

Fig. 18-16 Client using the Nitronox delivery system. The treatment is started about 5 minutes before the procedure.

achieve wound coverage has been diminished with the use of the *Nitronox System*. This system delivers a preset mixture of oxygen and nitrous oxide. There are two mixture systems: one for administration at sea level altitudes (50% oxygen, 50% nitrous oxide), and one for high altitude use (35% oxygen, 65% nitrous oxide). The client breathes the gas through a demand-valve system by either mask or a mouthpiece (Fig. 18-16). The system is generally limited to use once a day for 3 to 4 days after excision and grafting. The effects of prolonged nitrous oxide use have not been studied. Therefore, its use is currently limited to only the most painful situations.

Wound care

Debridement, dressing changes, topical antibiotic therapy, graft care, and/or donor site care are done 2 to 3 times daily. Appropriate coverage of the graft (if it is not kept open to air) should include fine-mesh gauze in closest proximity to the graft before other dressings are applied. Xeroform dressing, a fine mesh, absorbent gauze impregnated with 3% bismuth tribromophenate, may be used over grafted areas. It has a petrolatum base that keeps the gauze from adhering to graft sites, and it also has mild antibacterial properties.

Sheet skin grafts must be free of serous blebs. Blebs prevent the graft from interfacing and growing to the wound itself. Evacuation of blebs is done by aspiration with a tuberculin syringe or by pricking or cutting the peripheral margin of the bleb and rolling (with a sterile swab) the fluid from the center of the bleb to the exit site. Never roll the bleb to the edge of the graft. This only serves to separate adherent graft from the wound.

Donor site care methods have been controversial over the years. Although heat lamps promote drying of donor sites covered with mesh gauze dressings, new types of dressings are being evaluated with the goal of shortening healing time. (The average healing time is 10 to 14 days.) By decreasing this time, donor site skin can be reharvested earlier to cover wounds in clients with major burns.

Research has shown that reepithelialization occurs more rapidly in a moist environment that is relatively free of bacteria. One new method of treatment involves the use of Xeroform gauze, which is placed over the new donor site after hemostasis is achieved. The wound is covered with a bulky dressing for 24 hours. The dressing is changed, and usually the Xeroform gauze has adhered to the donor site wound. The areas are rewrapped with fine mesh gauze impregnated with mycitracin ointment over the donor site that is covered by Xeroform gauze, and a bulky dressing is applied over the whole area. The dressings are changed every 12 hours. This type of donor site care allows for a moist environment with topical antibiotic coverage to prevent infection. Healing time is about 7 to 10 days. With this method of care, the donor sites remain supple, which can make ambulation easier for the client.

Another method currently under investigation involves the use of Biobrane synthetic skin substitute. It is a type of fabric with collagen fibers on one side, which adhere to a superficial wound. It can be removed along with the healed scar in 7 to 10 days. Some centers are also trying a transparent type of membrane that adheres to the good skin around a donor site but not to the wound. This keeps the wound moist with the goal of facilitating reepithelialization. Silver-impregnated porcine xenograft has also been tried on donor sites. Healing time averaged 9 days, and clients reported less discomfort and blood seepage from the wound during healing. The porcine xenograft sloughs off as healing occurs.

Scarlet-red gauze is another type of dressing that can be used on donor sites. It is a fine mesh gauze impregnated with a blend of lanolin, olive oil, and petroleum. A possible advantage of this treatment is acceleration of wound reepithelialization. It has the disadvantage of causing red stains on clothing and linens. It can also cause discomfort related to the way the material dries, hardens, and pulls underlying skin.

Emotional support

Since the nurse has the most prolonged contact with the client and family, it is natural for them to see the nurse as an important source of emotional support. The nurse must assist the client in maintaining personal worth and reestablishing a satisfactory body image. The nurse must have an almost unlimited supply of patience and understanding. Often health care workers are the target for anger and hostility from clients who have no other focus or method of expressing these feelings.

Working with the family is a challenge for the nurse.

Loved ones need to see the importance of reestablishment of a client's independence. Family members will be confused by all the changes they see in the various burn phases. It is helpful for the family to view the burned areas frequently so that they can see the progress of healing. The nurse should involve the family as team members during the client's hospitalization.

The stress of the burn injury occasionally precipitates a psychiatric crisis. Treatment by a psychiatrist who can prescribe psychotropic drugs is indicated when this occurs. Early psychiatric intervention is also crucial if the client has been previously treated for a psychiatric disorder or if the burn incident was a suicide attempt.

Rehabilitation Phase

The *rehabilitation phase* is defined as beginning when the client's burn wound is covered with skin or healed and the client is capable of assuming some self-care activity. This can occur as early as 2 weeks to as long as 2 or 3 months after the burn injury. Goals for this period are to assist the client in resuming a functional role in society and to accomplish functional and cosmetic reconstruction.

Pathophysiological changes and clinical manifestations. The burn wound heals either by primary intention or by grafting. Layers of epithelialization begin rebuilding the tissue structure destroyed by the burn injury. Collagen fibers present in the new scar tissue help healing and add strength to weakened areas. After healing, the new skin appears flat and pink. In approximately 4 to 6 weeks the area becomes raised and hyperemic. If adequate ROM is not instituted, the new tissue will shorten, causing contracture. Mature healing is reached in 6 months to 1 year when suppleness has returned and the pink or red color has faded to a slightly lighter hue than the surrounding unburned tissue. It takes longer for black skin to regain its dark color, since many of the melanocytes are destroyed. Often the skin never regains its original color.

Scarring has two components: the first is discoloration, and the second is contour. The discoloration of scars fades with time. However, scar tissue tends to develop altered contours; that is, it is no longer flat or slightly raised but becomes elevated and enlarged above the original burn injury area. Pressure can help to keep a scar flat. Gentle capillary pressure is maintained on the healed burn with pressure garments (Fig. 18-17). These garments are worn 24 hours a day for up to 1 year after burn injury. They may be removed for short periods for bathing.

The client will experience discomfort from itching where healing is occurring. Nivea cream and diphenhydramine (Benadryl) serve to ease the itching. As "old" epithelium is replaced by new cells, flaking will occur. The newly formed skin is extremely sensitive to trauma. Blisters are likely to form from very slight pressure or friction. Additionally, these newly healed areas can be hypersensitive or hyposensitive to cold, heat, and touch. Grafted areas are more likely to be hyposensitive until peripheral nerve regeneration occurs. Healed burn areas must be protected from direct sunlight for 1 year to prevent hyperpigmentation and sunburn injury.

Complications. The most common complications of burn injury are skin and joint contractures and hyper-

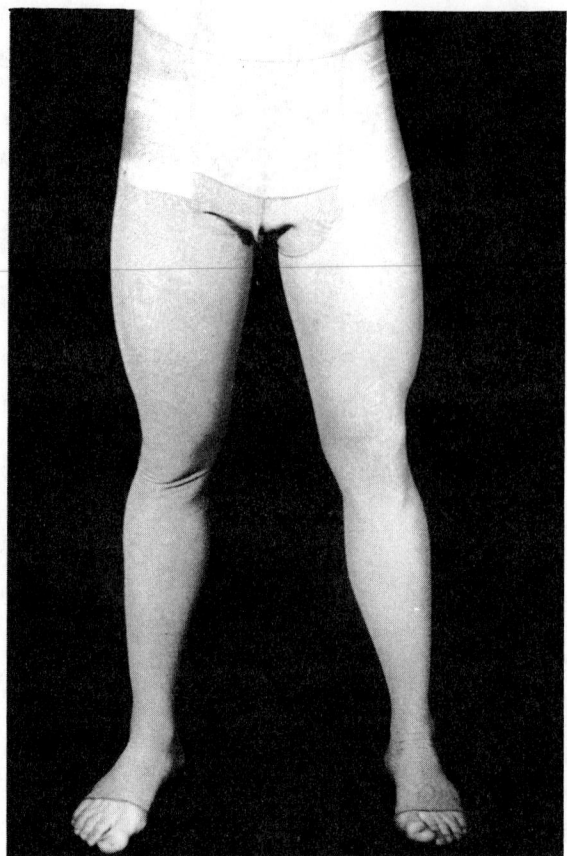

Fig. 18-17 Jobst pressure garments are worn 24 hours a day over burn scars for about 1 year after injury. The compression from these stretchy appliances helps compress the scar.

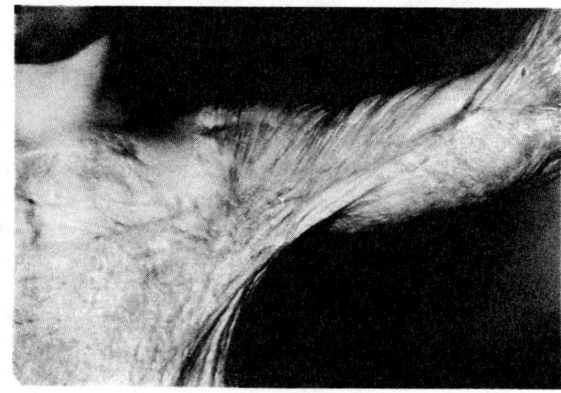

Fig. 18-18 Contracture of axilla. (Courtesy Medcom.)

trophic scarring (Fig. 18-18). Because of pain, the client will prefer to assume a flexed position for comfort. This position predisposes the wounds to contracture formation. Positioning, splinting, and exercise should be instituted on admission to minimize this complication. These procedures should be continued until the skin matures.

Areas that are most subject to contracture formation include the anterior and lateral neck areas, axillae, antecubital fossae, fingers, groin areas, popliteal fossae, and ankles. These areas encompass major joints. Not only does the skin over these areas develop contractures, but the underlying tissues such as the ligaments and tendons also have a tendency to shorten in the healing process. Therapy is aimed at extension of body parts because the flexors are stronger than the extensors. Legs should be wrapped before ambulation after grafting and donor site healing. This pressure prevents blister formation. Once the skin is completely healed, pressure garments can replace leg wraps to grafted areas.

■ Therapeutic and Nursing Management of Rehabilitation

Members of the health care team share responsibilities for assisting the client in returning to optimal function during the rehabilitation phase. Because of the severe psychological impact of burn injury, health care providers must be sensitive and attuned to the clients' feelings. They must assist clients to adjust emotionally by encouraging them to ventilate their fears regarding loss of function, deformity, disfigurement, and financial burdens. Having expressed these fears, clients can then be assisted in a realistic appraisal of their particular situations, emphasizing what they *can* do, not what they *cannot* do. Self-esteem is usually low for burn clients. An overwhelming fear is loss of relationships because of perceived or actual physical disfigurement. In a society and culture in which physical beauty is highly valued, alterations in body image usually result in psychological distress. Allowing appropriate independence and encouraging clients to assist in the care of others with burn trauma will involve them in activities that may help to restore self-esteem. Counseling continues when clients go home. Clients need reassurance that their feelings during this period of adjustment are normal and that frustration is to be expected as they attempt to resume their normal lifestyles.

During the rehabilitation phase, both client and family are actively learning how to care for the treated and healing wounds. Since the client may go home with unhealed open areas, instruction will be needed in dressing changes and wound care. An emollient cream (e.g., Nivea) should be used routinely on healed areas to keep the skin supple and to decrease itching and flaking. The client and family will need anticipatory guidance to know what to expect physiologically as well as psychologically during recovery.

Cosmetic or reconstructive surgery is often needed for major burns. It is important that the client understand the need or possibility of reconstructive surgery before leaving the hospital.

The role of exercise and appropriate physical therapy cannot be overemphasized. The progression of physical therapy from hydrotherapy to passive ROM, to active ROM, to stretching, ambulation, and ultimate restoration of function is a lengthy and painful process that lasts for at least 1 year after burn injury. Constant encouragement and reassurance are necessary to maintain clients' spirits and morale. Clients soon regard physical therapy as an integral part of their treatment.

Nutritional considerations. By this time in the client's recovery, the negative nitrogen balance should have been corrected. However, it is still important to maintain a high-calorie, high-protein diet. The problem with anorexia decreases at this time. As the client's oral intake increases, the tube feedings are gradually tapered and discontinued. The client with a functional problem in eating (especially burn injury to the hands) may need assistance from occupational therapy to obtain devices to correct or lessen the problem. Often, all that is necessary is padding the handle of a fork or spoon with several layers of gauze so that grip is better established.

Toward the end of hospitalization, clients occasionally need assistance from a dietitian. Because they have been encouraged to eat for such a long period of time while their burn wounds were acute, clients have difficulty, as healing approaches completion, in controlling their appetite and in avoiding unwanted weight gain.

EMOTIONAL NEEDS OF THE CLIENT AND FAMILY

Because of the suddenness and severity of burn trauma, the client and family are plunged into physical and emotional crises.[12] Health care providers must be prepared to assess psychoemotional cues from the client and family and to provide appropriate intervention throughout the client's course of recovery.

Clients will experience thoughts and feelings that are very frightening and disturbing to them, such as guilt over the burn accident, reliving of the experience, fear of death, and concern about future therapy and the concomitant pain. Families may share any or all of these feelings. At times they will feel helpless in trying to assist their loved ones. During this period of adjustment, the nurse should provide time for clients and their families to be alone. Allow family members (if they indicate a desire) to assist clients with position changes and eating. It is important that families be kept informed of the client's progress.

For nurses to adequately deal with the enormous range of emotional response that the burn client may exhibit, it is important to have an understanding of the circumstances of the burn, past family interactions, and past coping experiences with stressful stimuli. At any time the various emotional responses of fear, anxiety, anger, guilt, and depression may be experienced (Table 18-17). Another commonly seen emotional response is *regression*. Clients will revert to behavior that helped them cope with stressful past situations. Frank psychosis can also be observed. Unless the client had a psychiatric condition before the burn injury, this psychosis is usually transient.

Therapeutic intervention for the client at this point does not necessarily indicate the care of a psychiatrist. Nurses, physicians, social workers, or anyone else who has a rapport with the client and a good understanding of personal feelings in such situations can be therapeutic. The client can best convey some of these negative but normal emotions to a health care provider who can interact without the client sensing retaliation. Acknowledgment that the feelings are real and valid does much to help the client. The nurse should not belittle or scorn a client's regression but should be firm and consistent in assisting the client to cope.

Table 18-17 Emotional Responses of Burn Clients

Emotion	Possible Verbal Expression
Fear	Will I die?
	What will happen next?
	Will I be disfigured?
	Will my spouse or friend still love me?
Anxiety	I feel out of control.
	What's happening to me?
	When will it end?
Anger	Why did this happen to me?
	Those nurses enjoy hurting me.
Guilt	If only I'd been more careful.
	I was punished because I was bad.
Depression	It's no use going on like this.
	I don't care what happens to me.
	I wish people would leave me alone.

Major emotional tasks confront clients and their families. As more and more independence is expected from clients, they must confront new fears: "Can I do it?" "Am I a desirable partner, father?" Open communication must exist in clients' environments during this phase of recovery.

The difficult issue of *sexuality* must be met with honesty. Physical attractiveness will be altered in the client who has sustained a major burn. Acceptance of this alteration is very difficult at first for the client and family. The nature of skin injury in itself causes modifications in processing sexual stimuli. Since touch is such an important part of sexuality, the client's need for it may be altered. Immature scar tissue may make the sensation of touch unpleasant or may dull it. The normal pleasure response is altered, and the client's sexuality is affected. This is usually transient, but the client and family need to know that it is normal and receive anticipatory guidance from health care personnel to avoid undue emotional strain.

Family and client support groups may be beneficial in meeting the challenge of emotional needs. Speaking with others who have experienced burn trauma can be beneficial.

SPECIAL NEEDS OF THE NURSING STAFF
Psychoemotionally Demanding Role

A logical extension of the emotional trauma of the client includes the emotional trauma of the nurse.[13] The nurse must deal with unpleasant, rejective, hostile clients and with the fact that burn therapy is almost always painful. The nurse will sometimes see many hours of client care suddenly obliterated by sepsis and death. Because of long hospitalizations and intense contact, the relationships between caregivers and care receivers can result in very strong bonds that can be either healthy and healing or destructive and draining. Burn clients can develop demanding or punitive attitudes, which cause the nurse to be reluctant to care for them. Nurses and clients can also develop warm, trusting relationships that provide a mutually satisfying network not only during hospitalization but also

during long-term rehabilitation. Sometimes the bond can be so strong that clients have difficulty separating from the hospital and staff. The frequency of family contact can be rewarding as well as draining to nurses. Newcomers to burn nursing often find it difficult to deal with not only the deformities caused by burn injury but also the odor, the unpleasant sight of the wound, and the reality of the pain that accompanies the burn.

Many nurses feel that the care they give makes the critical difference in helping the clients survive and cope with the severe injury. This type of reward keeps nurses caring for burn clients.

Intensive Care Milieu

Most victims of major burns are treated in an intensive care unit. This requires critical and frequent assessments, as well as frequent changes in therapy as the client's condition changes. Highly stressful environments tend to result in a rapid staff turnover. Thus, new personnel are continuously being trained to function in this complex environment. Concern over whether to resuscitate a severely burned victim causes much internal stress. Ethical dilemmas confront nurses and other health care providers. Many institutions are using the supportive services of ethics committees. Included among the various environmental stimuli that can be overwhelming to the nurse is the variety of sophisticated equipment used in burn units. Tension and intense emotions are ever present in this intensive care environment.

Support services for burn nurses in the form of group meetings led by a psychiatrist, psychologist, psychiatric clinical nurse specialist, or social worker are often organized. Such meetings help the nursing staff deal with difficult feelings they experience in caring for the burn client. Nurses need the opportunity to ventilate their feelings of anger and hostility to a nonretaliatory listener. This therapeutic communication process often distinguishes truly fine burn nursing from mere custodial burn nursing.

INNOVATIONS IN BURN RESEARCH

A major focus of burn research continues to be the study of burn shock. Although the process is well described, its causes remain obscure. A recent development in burn therapy is the use of plasma exchange to reverse burn shock in selected groups of clients. Several immunology studies are under way to describe the causes of the almost total immunosuppression that occurs after a burn injury. The problem of pain is being studied by several burn units to explore the body's own reserves for dealing with pain such as the beta endorphins or prostaglandins. Nutrition is being redefined in terms of the ideal calorie-to-nitrogen ratio and the role of branch-chain amino acids. Topical agents are being expanded to include semipermeable membranes saturated with active antimicrobial agents. (Several new topical antibiotic products are now being studied, including agents used in other countries.) Attempts are being made to grow usable permanent skin from a small sample of the client's own skin or from other species or to grow synthetic skin artificially.

BURN DIAGRAM

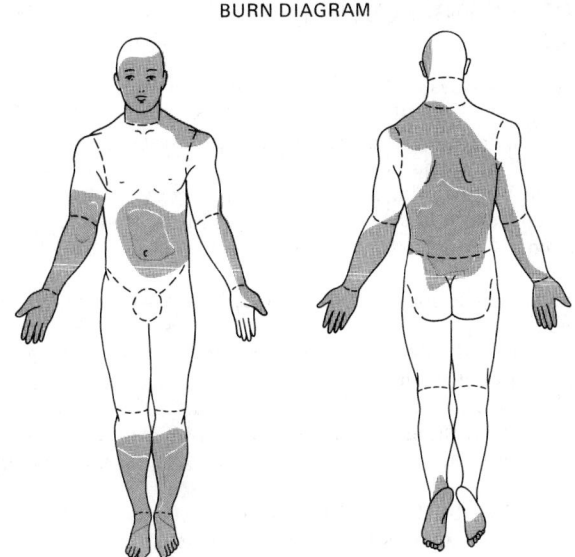

Fig. 18-19 Estimation of Mac's burns. *Pink areas* are third-degree, full-thickness burns. *Gray areas* are second-degree, partial-thickness burns.

C ase Study

SEVERE BURN CLIENT

Mac, a 57-year-old man, was admitted to the emergency room by ambulance with severe full- and partial-thickness burns over his body (Fig. 18-19). He had good health before an explosion from a gas heater in his small apartment. His injury was sustained 3 hours before admission. A physical examination reveals a 70 kg male in acute distress. His pulse is 128 and slightly irregular. His blood pressure is 106/80. An IV is started, and an indwelling catheter inserted into his bladder.

Discussion Questions

1. Estimate from the Lund and Browder diagram the client's percentage of burn. Is the client critical? Why?
2. Calculate the first 24 hours of fluid replacement for Mac according to the Parkland (Baxter) formula.
3. What fluid and electrolyte changes would Mac encounter during the first 48 hours? Explain their pathophysiological bases.
4. Is Mac's injury one in which inhalation injury is expected? Why?
5. After fluid replacement is begun, Mac's urine output is 25 ml/hr. What is the significance of this finding?
6. What physical changes that will occur in the first few days after his burn injury does the nurse need to inform Mac about?
7. Mac has had return of bowel sounds but has no appetite. What should the nurse do and in what order of priority?
8. Mac is reluctant to move his arms. What specific tasks of daily living can be encouraged for Mac to receive the supplemental physical therapy he needs?

R eview Questions

The number of the question corresponds to the same-numbered objective at the beginning of the chapter.

1. Extent of electrical injury can be difficult to assess because
   a. victims are often in shock
   b. the entry and exit wounds are very deep
   c. internal damage is not readily apparent
   d. electrical injury is usually smaller than thermal injury
2. Which of the following is least likely to result in a full-thickness burn injury?
   a. scald injury
   b. sunburn
   c. chemical burn
   d. electrical injury
3. A partial-thickness burn has which of the following characteristics?
   a. red, shiny, wet appearance
   b. generalized erythema with no vesicles
   c. exposed fascia
   d. dry, waxy appearance
4. The extent of burns is assessed by
   a. looking at which body parts are involved
   b. determining preexisting risk factors
   c. using guides to indicate burn location relative to total body surface
   d. estimating what is a full-thickness as opposed to what is partial-thickness burn
5. Silver sulfadiazine is the topical antibiotic of choice because it
   a. is rapidly absorbed by blood
   b. is effective against bacterial growth with few side effects
   c. is a carbonic anhydrase inhibitor
   d. maintains adequate pH of the newly forming skin buds
6. Which of the following events occurs during the early emergent phase?
   a. large proteins adhere to vascular walls
   b. potassium moves into the cell
   c. sodium and water are sequestered in interstitial fluid
   d. red blood cells hemolyze from large volumes of rapidly administered fluid
7. To maintain a positive nitrogen balance in a major burn, the client must
   a. eat at least 500 calories 3 times per day
   b. eat rice and whole wheat for the chemical effect on nitrogen balance
   c. increase normal adult caloric intake by 3 times
   d. eat a high-protein, low-carbohydrate diet
8. A burn client is said to be in the rehabilitative phase when
   a. the burn wound is healed or closed
   b. physical therapy is no longer needed
   c. scars have faded and skin looks normal
   d. the client can return to work

9. It is important for the burn client and family to
   a. see the burn wound 3 times per day
   b. talk frequently with the nurse about the client's progress
   c. allow nurses to do total care for the client to prevent infection
   d. avoid discussion of the client's progress to minimize false hope
10. The burn nurse needs
   a. special psychological training
   b. to be sensitive to the needs of the client and family
   c. much physical strength because of the client's debilitation
   d. to hide all personal feelings for the client and family
11. Discharge planning begins
   a. after the emergent phase
   b. after grafting
   c. at least 1 week before discharge
   d. on admission
12. Pain management of the burn client involves
   a. giving set doses of medications at scheduled times
   b. sympathizing with the client
   c. using traditional and alternative methods of pain control
   d. having the nurse maintain control of the client's medication

REFERENCES

1. Advanced Burn Life Support (ABLS) Curriculum, Lincoln, Neb, 1989.
2. Dyer C and Roberts D: Thermal trauma, Nurs Clin North Am 25:85-117, 1990.
3. Wilding PA: Care of respiratory burns—hard work can bring spectacular results, Prof Nurse 5:412-420, 1990.
4. Robertson C and Fenton O: ABC of major trauma: management of severe burns, Br Med J 301:282-286, 1990.
5. Smith G and Savinski-Bozinko G: Giving emergency care for burns, Nursing 19:55-62, 1989.
6. Robins EV: Immunosuppression of the burned patient, Crit Care Nurs Clin North Am 1:767-774, 1989.
7. Robins EV: Burn shock, Crit Care Nurs Clin North Am 2:299-307, 1990.
8. Jarlsberg CR: Action stat! Neck and chest burns, Nursing 20:33, 1990.
9. Bayley EW: Wound healing in the patient with burns, Nurs Clin North Am 25:205-222, 1990.
10. Marvin JA: Nutritional support of the critically injured patient, Crit Care Nurs Q 11:21-34, 1988.
11. van der Does W: Pain and anxiety ratings during burn care, Nurs Times 86:53, 1990.
12. Roberts D and Appleton V: Psychosocial care of burn-injured patients, Plast Surg Nurs 9:62-65, 1989.
13. Lewis KF and others: Survey of perceived stressors and coping strategies among burn unit nurses, Burns 16:109-112, 1990.

SECTION IV REFERENCES
BOOKS

Bartlett JD and Jaanus SD, eds: Clinical ocular pharmacology, ed 2, Boston, 1989, Butterworth Publishers.
Callen JP: Dermatological signs of internal disease, Philadelphia, 1988, WB Saunders Co.
Coleman WP and others: Cosmetic skin surgery: principles and techniques, St Louis, 1990, Mosby–Year Book, Inc.
Cummings CW and others: Otolaryngology—head and neck surgery, St Louis, 1989, The CV Mosby Co.
Davson H: Physiology of the eye, ed 5, New York, 1990, Pergamon Press.
Dolecek R and others, eds: Endocrinology of thermal burns: pathophysiologic mechanisms and clinical interpretation, Philadelphia, 1990, Lea & Febiger.
Geefand SA: Hearing: an introduction to psychological and physiological acoustics, ed 2, New York, 1990, Marcel Dekker, Inc.
Glasscock III ME, Jackson CG, and Josey AF: Handbook of audiology, St Louis, 1990, Mosby–Year Book, Inc.
Gold D and Weingeist TA, eds: The eye in systemic disease, Philadelphia, 1990, JB Lippincott Co.
Habif TP: Clinical dermatology: a color guide to diagnosis and therapy, ed 2, St Louis, 1990, Mosby–Year Book, Inc.
Jordan RE, ed: Immunologic diseases of the skin, Norwalk, Conn, 1991, Appleton & Lange.
Jurkiewicz MJ and others: Plastic and reconstructive surgery: principles and practices, St Louis, 1990, Mosby–Year Book, Inc.
Leibovic KN, ed: Science of vision, New York, 1990, Springer-Verlag.
Marsh JL: Current therapy in plastic and reconstructive surgery, St Louis, 1989, The CV Mosby Co.
Musiek FE: Contemporary issues in clinical audiology, St Louis, 1989, The CV Mosby Co.
Proctor B: Surgical anatomy of the ear and temporal bone, New York, 1989, Thieme Medical Publishers, Inc.

JOURNALS

Alderman C: Psoriasis: whose skin is it anyway, Nurs Stand 4:26, 1990.
Allen MN: The meaning of visual impairment to visually impaired adults, J Adv Nurs 14:640, 1989.
Andrews J and Gunnlaugsdottir V: Eye diseases: vision of the future, Geriatr Nurs Home Care 8:18, 1988.
Bayley EW: Wound healing in the patient with burns, Nurs Clin North Am 25:205, 1990.
Bayley EW and others: Standards for burn nursing practice, J Burn Care Rehabil 10:362, 1989.
Black M and others: Criteria map: potential for skin breakdown—a quality assurance tool for use in any setting, QRB 15:340, 1989.
Brechtelsbauer DA: Adult hearing loss, Prim Care 17:249, 1990.
Cleary ME and Fahy C: Lighting a lamp for persons who are visually challenged, Diabetes Educ 15:331, 1989.
Cobb N, Maxwell G, and Silverstein P: Patient perception of quality of life after burn injury: results of an eleven-year survey, J Burn Care Rehabil 11:330, 1990.
Crow R: Wound care: the challenge of pressure sores, Nurs Times 84:68, 1988.
DeWitt S: Nursing assessment of the skin and dermatologic lesions, Nurs Clin North Am 25:235, 1990.
Dolinger RD: Pressure sores and optimum skin care, J Palliat Care 6:50, 1990.

Edmonds SE: Resources for the visually impaired, J Ophthalmic Nurs Technol 9:14, 1990.

French S: Understanding partial sight, Nurs Times 84:32, 1988.

Gosnell DJ and Pontius C: A model for quality assurance for decubitus ulcer monitoring, Decubitus 1:24, 1988.

Guidelines for preventing pressure sores, Nurs Stand 4:26, 1989.

Hardy MA: A pilot study of the diagnosis and treatment of impaired skin integrity: dry skin in older persons, Nurs Diagn 1:57, 1990.

Hinchcliffe S: Benign and malignant skin conditions, Nursing 4:28, 1990.

Hinchcliffe S: Skin lesions 2: a study involving pigmented areas, Nursing 4:30, 1990.

Hoff J: Effecting a change in nursing practice: pressure ulcer prevention, J Nurs Qual Assur 3:56, 1989.

Hotter AN: Wound healing and immunocompromise, Nurs Clin North Am 25:193, 1990.

Jones PL and Millman A: Wound healing and the aged patient, Nurs Clin North Am 25:263, 1990.

Kamenir S and Nahwegezhic R: Skin assessment: a tool for nursing staff, Perspectives 13:4, 1989.

Kee CC: Sensory impairment: factor x in providing nursing care to the older adult, J Community Health Nurs 7:45, 1990.

Knight DB and Scott H: Contracture and pressure necrosis, Ostomy Wound Manage 26:60, 1990.

Lawlor MC: Common ocular injuries and disorders: part I: acute loss of vision, JEN 15:32, 1989.

McConnell EA: Clinical do's and don'ts: placing your patient in the lateral position, Nursing 20:65, 1990.

Nicol NH: Actinic keratosis: preventable and treatable like other precancerous and cancerous skin lesions, Plast Surg Nurs 9:49, 1989.

Norris RM: Common sense tips for working with blind patients, Am J Nurs 89:360, 1989.

Norwicki CR and Sprenger CK: Temporary skin substitutes for burn patients: a nursing perspective, J Burn Care Rehabil 9:209, 1988.

Payne RL and Martin ML: The epidemiology and management of skin tears in older adults, Ostomy Wound Manage 26:26, 1990.

Scott M: Eye care: visions of the future, Nurs Stand 3:36, 1989.

Smalley PJ: Lasers in otolaryngology, Nurs Clin North Am 25:645, 1990.

Tenpas DM: Multidisciplinary team approach to skin care, Ostomy Wound Manage 26:50, 1990.

VanEtten NK, Sexton P, and Smith R: Development and implementation of a skin care program, Ostomy Wound Manage 27:40, 1990.

Van Ness C: The implementation of a quality assurance study and program to reduce the incidence of hospital-acquired pressure ulcers, J Enterostomal Ther 16:61, 1989.

Ward RS and others: Prosthetic use in patients with burns and associated limb amputations, J Burn Care Rehabil 11:361, 1990.

ORGANIZATIONS

American Academy of Facial, Plastic and Reconstructive Surgery
1110 Vermont Avenue, NW
Washington, DC 20005

American Council of the Blind
1010 Vermont Avenue, NW, Suite 1100
Washington, DC 20005

The American Foundation for the Blind
15 West 16th Street
New York, NY 10011

American Society of Ophthalmic Registered Nurses, Inc.
P.O. Box 3030
San Francisco, CA 94119

American Society of Plastic and Reconstructive Surgical Nurses, Inc.
North Woodbury Road, Box 56
Pitman, NJ 08071

American Speech-Language-Hearing Association
10801 Rockville Pike
Rockville, MD 20852

Associated Services for the Blind
919 Walnut Street
Philadelphia, PA 19107

Association for Education and Rehabilitation of the Blind and Visually Impaired
206 North Washington Street, Suite 320
Alexandria, VA 22314

Dermatology Nurses Association
North Woodbury Road
Box 56
Pitman, NJ 08071

Fight for Sight
160 East 56th Street, Eighth floor
New York, NY 10022

Guide Dogs for the Blind, Inc.
P.O. Box 1200
San Raphael, CA 94915

International Association of Laryngectomees
c/o American Cancer Society
1599 Clifton Road, NE
Atlanta, GA 30329

Library of Congress National Library Service for the Blind and Physically Handicapped
1291 Taylor Street, NW
Washington, DC 20543

National Association for the Deaf
814 Thayer Avenue
Silver Spring, MD 20910

National Association for the Visually Handicapped
22 West 21st Street
New York, NY 10010

National Eye Institute/National Institutes of Health
US Department of Health and Human Services
9000 Rockville Pike
Bethesda, MD 20892

National Institutes of Health/National Eye Institute
US Department of Health and Human Services
9000 Rockville Pike
Bethesda, MD 10892

National Psoriasis Foundation
6443 Southwest Beaverton Highway, Suite 210
Portland, OR 97221

National Society to Prevent Blindness, Inc.
500 East Remington Rd.
Schaumberg, IL 60173

Recording for the Blind, Inc.
20 Roszel Road
Princeton, NJ 08540

The Seeing Eye
P.O. Box 375
Morristown, NJ 07960-0375

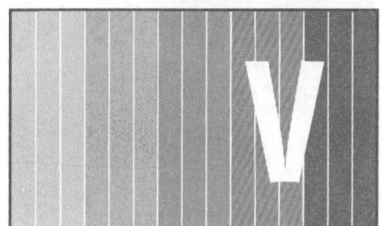

PROBLEMS OF OXYGENATION

CHAPTER

19

Nursing Assessment

Respiratory System

Leslie A. Hoffman
Jan D. Manzetti

L *earning Objectives*

1. *Describe the structures and functions of the upper respiratory tract, the lower respiratory tract, and the chest wall.*
2. *Describe the process that initiates and controls inspiration and expiration.*
3. *Describe the process of gaseous diffusion within the lungs.*
4. *Identify the functions of the respiratory defense mechanisms.*
5. *Describe the significance of arterial blood gas values and the oxyhemoglobin dissociation curve in relation to respiratory function.*

6. *Identify significant subjective and objective data related to the respiratory system that should be obtained from a client.*
7. *Describe the techniques used in physical assessment of the respiratory system.*
8. *Differentiate normal from common abnormal findings on physical assessment of the respiratory system.*
9. *Describe the purpose, nursing responsibilities, and significance of results related to diagnostic studies of the respiratory system.*
10. *Identify the significance of data obtained from common pulmonary function test*

The respiratory system includes the respiratory tract, the lungs, and supporting structures. Its primary purpose is to obtain oxygen from atmospheric air. Oxygen is necessary for normal cellular function within the body. The respiratory system also performs an excretory function by ridding the body of some of the end products of metabolism (e.g., carbon dioxide).

STRUCTURES AND FUNCTIONS

The respiratory system is continuous but is often divided into two portions for discussion and study. These portions are the *upper respiratory tract,* or upper airway, and the *lower respiratory tract,* or lower airway (Fig. 19-1). The upper airway structures are the nose, pharynx, adenoids, tonsils, epiglottis, larynx, and trachea. The lower airway structures are the bronchi, bronchioles, alveolar ducts, and alveoli. With the exception of the right and left mainstem bronchi, all lower airway structures are contained within the lungs. The right lung is divided into three

lobes (upper, middle, and lower) and the left lung into two lobes (upper and lower) (Fig. 19-2). The structures of the chest wall are also essential to respiration. These include the rib cage, the pleura, and the muscles of respiration.

Upper Respiratory Tract

The nose is made of bone and cartilage. Internally, the nose is divided into two passages, or nares, by the septum. The interior of the nose is shaped into many rolling projections called *turbinates.* These increase the surface area for warming and moistening air. The nose, like the rest of the respiratory tract, is lined with mucous membrane. It is also lined with very small hairs. The internal nose opens directly into the sinuses. The nasal cavity connects with the pharynx, a tubular passageway that is subdivided from above downward into three parts: the nasopharynx, the oropharynx, and the laryngopharynx.

As air enters the nose, it is conditioned for use in the lower airway by being warmed, moistened, and filtered. This conditioning serves a protective function. Most large foreign particles that are inhaled are removed in the nose or in the nasopharynx. They either are caught by the nasal

---

Reviewed by Frances Jackson, R.N., Ph.D., Assistant Professor of Nursing, Oakland University School of Nursing, Rochester, Michigan.

436

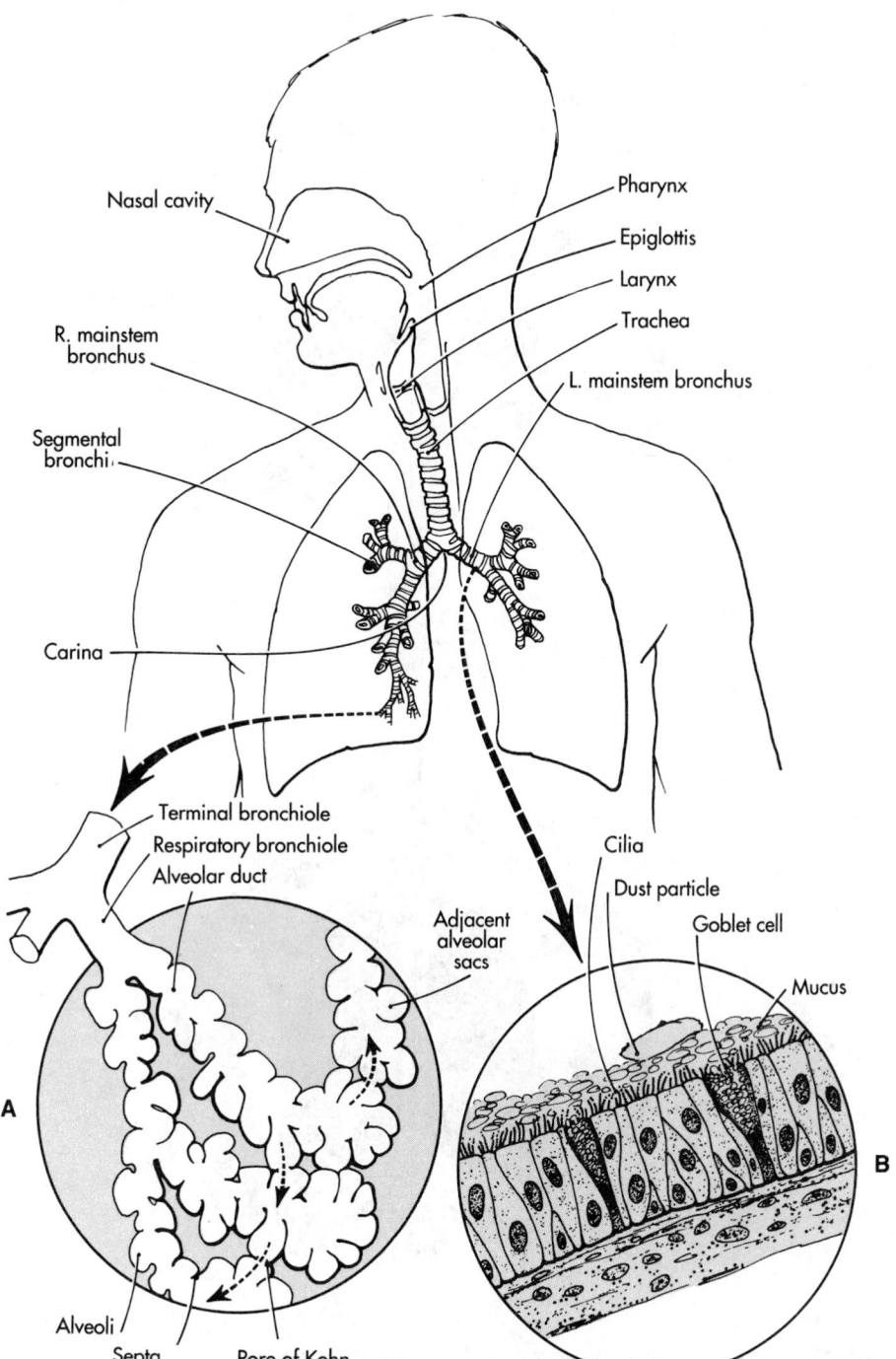

Fig. 19-1 Structures of the respiratory tract. **A,** Pulmonary functional unit. **B,** Ciliated mucous membrane. (From Price S and Wilson L: Pathophysiology: clinical concepts of disease processes, ed 4, St Louis, 1991, Mosby–Year Book, Inc.)

hairs or strike the mucosa where they are removed by the cilia.[1]

The olfactory nerve endings (receptors for the sense of smell) are located in the roof of the nose. The *adenoids* and *tonsils,* which are small masses of lymphatic tissue, are found in the nasopharynx and the oropharynx, respectively.

Air passes through the nose to the oropharynx. Air may also enter the oropharynx through the mouth. However, the mouth breather loses the protective and conditioning functions of the nose.

The epiglottis is a small flap at the base of the tongue. During swallowing, the larynx elevates so that a small cartilage tips against the epiglottis, closing off the trachea.

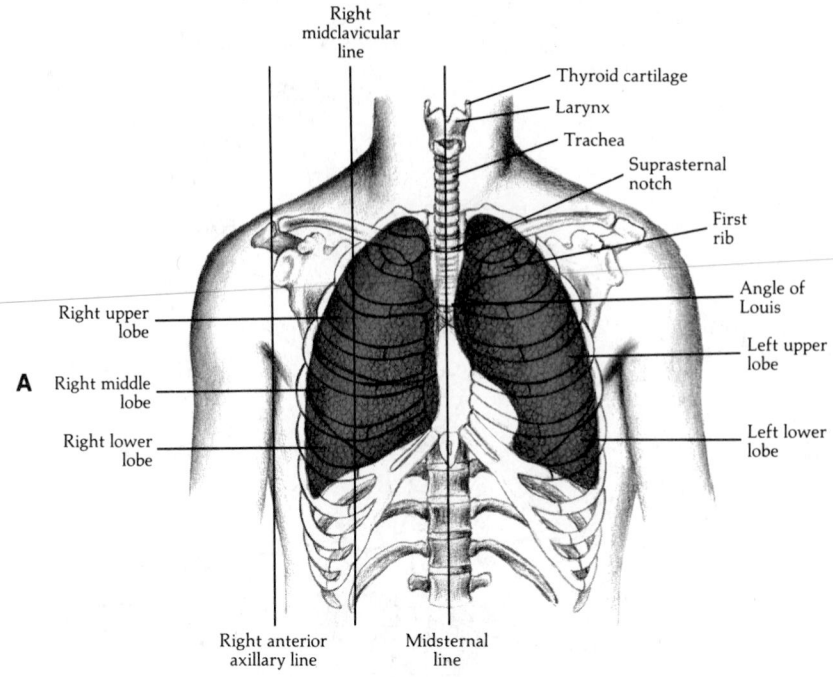

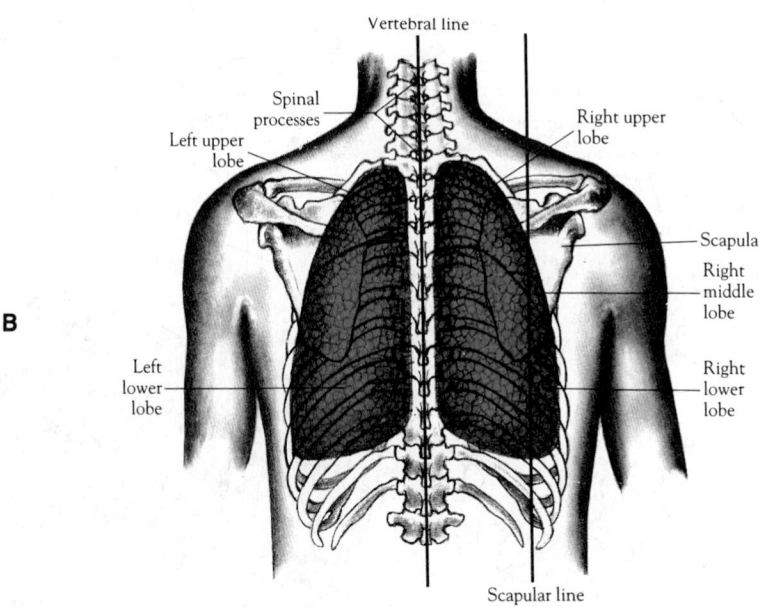

Fig. 19-2 Anatomical landmarks and structures of the chest. **A,** Anterior chest. **B,** Posterior chest. (From Thompson J and others: Clinical nursing, ed 2, St Louis, 1990, The CV Mosby Co, p 138.)

This movement serves a protective function and prevents the entrance of food into the lower respiratory tract, which could result in severe coughing or aspiration.

Air moves from the oropharynx through the laryngopharynx and the larynx, where the vocal cords are located, and then down into the trachea. The trachea is a cylindrical tube about 11 cm long and 1.5 cm in diameter in the adult. It is supported by U-shaped cartilages, which are incomplete at the posterior surface. The cartilage keeps the trachea from collapsing. On the posterior surface, the car-

tilages of the trachea are bridged by connective tissue and smooth muscle. This design allows the esophagus to expand when a bolus of food is swallowed. The cartilages of the trachea are connected by elastic ligaments. The trachea bifurcates into the right and left mainstem bronchi at a point called the *carina*. The carina is located at the level of the manubriosternal junction. The manubriosternal junction is sometimes called the *angle of Louis*. The carina is very sensitive, and touching it, as might occur during insertion of a suction catheter, elicits vigorous coughing.

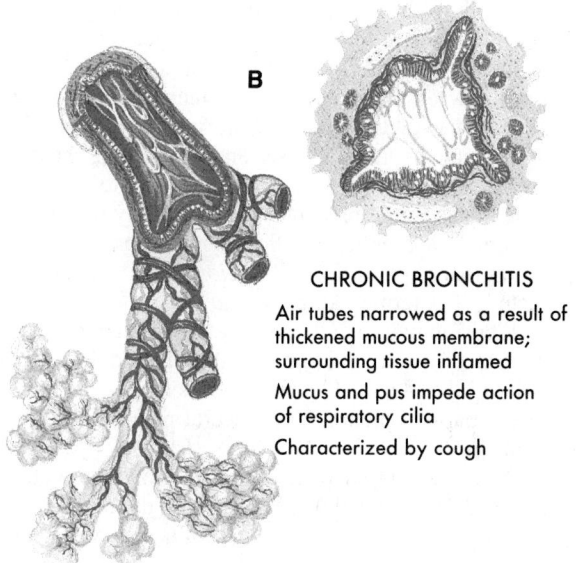

Fig. 19-3 Appearance of terminal bronchiole and air sacs in **A,** emphysema, **B,** chronic bronchitis, and **C,** bronchial asthma. (From Thibodeau G: Structure and function of the body, ed 8, St Louis, 1988, The CV Mosby Co, p 354.)

EMPHYSEMA

Walls of individual air sacs torn; repair not possible

Small air tubes collapse, trapping air; exhalation difficult

Lung tissue becomes inelastic; lungs enlarged, resulting in barrel-chest appearance

CHRONIC BRONCHITIS

Air tubes narrowed as a result of thickened mucous membrane; surrounding tissue inflamed

Mucus and pus impede action of respiratory cilia

Characterized by cough

BRONCHIAL ASTHMA

Swollen mucous membranes of air tubes and surrounding tissue

Muscles of air tubes become spastic, causing narrowing

Thick mucus fills air tubes and sacs; breathing becomes labored; expiration difficult

Lower Respiratory Tract

Once air passes the carina, it is in the lower respiratory tract. The mainstem bronchi enter the lungs through a slit called the *hilus*. The right mainstem bronchus is shorter, wider, and straighter than the left mainstem bronchus. Because of these characteristics, aspiration of foreign objects is more likely to occur in the right lung than in the left lung.

Each mainstem bronchus subdivides several times to form the lobar, segmental, and subsegmental bronchi. Further divisions form the bronchioles. The most distant bronchioles are called the *terminal* and *respiratory bronchioles*. Beyond these lie the alveolar ducts and sacs. The bronchioles are encircled by smooth muscles that constrict and dilate in response to various stimuli. The terms *bronchoconstriction* and *bronchodilatation* are used to refer to a decrease or an increase in diameter of the airways caused by contraction of these muscles. The different appearances of bronchioles and air sacs related to several pathological processes are illustrated in Fig. 19-3.

No exchange of oxygen or carbon dioxide takes place until air enters the respiratory bronchioles. The area of the respiratory tract from the nose to the respiratory bronchioles serves only as a conducting pathway and is therefore termed the *anatomical dead space* (V_D) or *conducting zone*. This space must be filled with every breath, but the air that fills it is not available for gas exchange. In adults, a normal tidal volume (V_T), or volume of air exchanged with each breath, is about 500 ml. Of each 500 ml inhaled, about 150 ml remains in the V_D.

After moving through the conducting zone, air reaches the respiratory zone, composed of the respiratory bronchioles and alveoli. Although most gas exchange occurs in the alveoli, some also occurs in the respiratory bronchioles. Respiratory bronchioles have alveoli that open directly into the lumina of the bronchioles.

Alveoli are small compartments that form the functional unit of the lungs. The alveoli are interconnected by pores of Kohn, which allow movement of air from alveolus to alveolus (Fig. 19-1). Bacteria can also move through these pores, resulting in an extension of respiratory infection to previously noninfected areas. The 300 million alveoli in the adult have a total volume of about 2500 ml and a surface area for gas exchange that is about the size of a tennis court. The alveoli are separated from the capillaries by the interstitial space. The alveolar-capillary membrane is very thin (less than 1 μm or $\frac{1}{1000}$ mm) and is the site of gaseous exchange. In emphysema the walls of the alveoli are dilated and enlarged. This markedly impairs gas exchange (Fig. 19-3).

Surfactant. The lung can be conceptualized as a collection of 300 million bubbles (alveoli), each 0.3 mm in diameter. Such a structure is inherently unstable and, as a consequence, the alveoli have a natural tendency to collapse. The alveolar surface is composed of two kinds of cells, type I and type II cells. Type II cells secrete a phospholipid, surfactant, which performs the essential function of preventing alveolar collapse. Surfactant lowers surface tension in the alveoli. This decreases the tendency of the alveoli to collapse and reduces the amount of pressure needed to inflate the alveoli. Surfactant is rapidly destroyed and thus must be continually replaced. Normally, each person takes a slightly larger breath, termed a *sigh*, after every five to six breaths. The sigh breath stretches the alveoli and causes surfactant to be secreted by type II cells.

When there is a deficiency of surfactant in the alveolar lining, the lungs become stiff as a result of decreased compliance and there is widespread *atelectasis* (collapsed, airless alveoli). Surfactant is not formed until relatively late in fetal life. In infants born without sufficient amounts of surfactant, respiratory distress syndrome (RDS), a condition that is often fatal, develops. The pathophysiology resulting in adult respiratory distress syndrome (ARDS) also causes a surfactant deficiency (see Chapter 23).

Blood supply. The lungs have two different types of circulation, pulmonary and bronchial. The pulmonary circulation provides the lungs with blood for gas exchange. The pulmonary artery receives deoxygenated blood from the right ventricle of the heart and branches so that each pulmonary capillary is directly connected with many alveoli. Oxygen and carbon dioxide exchange occurs at this point. The pulmonary venous system returns oxygenated blood to the left atrium of the heart.

The bronchial circulation starts with the bronchial arteries, which arise from the thoracic aorta. It provides oxygen to the structures of the airways and other pulmonary tissues. Most of this blood is carried away from the lungs by the pulmonary veins.[2]

When blood from the bronchial circulation enters the pulmonary veins, it is oxygen depleted, having given up oxygen to nourish the bronchi. This oxygen-depleted blood is mixed with oxygen-rich blood from the pulmonary circulation. This creates a condition termed *venous admixture* (i.e., mixing of unventilated, deoxygenated blood with ventilated, oxygenated blood). Venous admixture occurs in two situations: when there is an anatomical shunt and when there is a physiological shunt. *Shunt* refers to blood that has entered the arterial system without traveling through ventilated lung areas. *Anatomical shunt* occurs

as a result of anatomical conditions within the respiratory system (i.e., deoxygenated blood from the bronchial circulation mixing with oxygenated blood). *Physiological shunt* occurs as a result of pathophysiological changes that allow the alveoli to fill with fluid. This can occur in pulmonary edema, pneumonia, and ARDS.

Chest Wall

The structures of the chest wall include the rib cage, the intercostal muscles, and the diaphragm. The chest cavity is lined with a membrane called the *parietal pleura* and the lungs with a membrane called the *visceral pleura* (Fig. 19-4). The parietal and visceral pleurae are joined and form a closed, double-walled sac. The space between the pleural layers, termed the *pleural cavity* or *intrapleural space,* is a potential space. In the normal adult, this space is filled with a thin film of fluid, which serves two purposes: (1) It provides lubrication, allowing the layers of pleura to slide over each other during breathing, and (2) it increases cohesion between the pleural layers, thereby facilitating expansion of the pleura and lung during inspiration. In conditions such as lung cancer and congestive heart failure, larger amounts of fluid may accumulate in the pleural space because there is blockage of the lymphatic drainage system or a change in colloid osmotic pressure. This condition is termed a *pleural effusion*. If the fluid becomes infected, it is termed an *empyema*.

Pleuritic pain may be associated with conditions such as pleural effusion, pulmonary emboli, and lung cancer involving the pleura. Pleuritic pain is caused by involvement of the parietal pleura. The visceral pleura does not contain pain fibers.

The chest is shaped, supported, and protected by 24 ribs (12 on each side). The ribs and the sternum make up the thorax. Several muscles are attached to the ribs. The

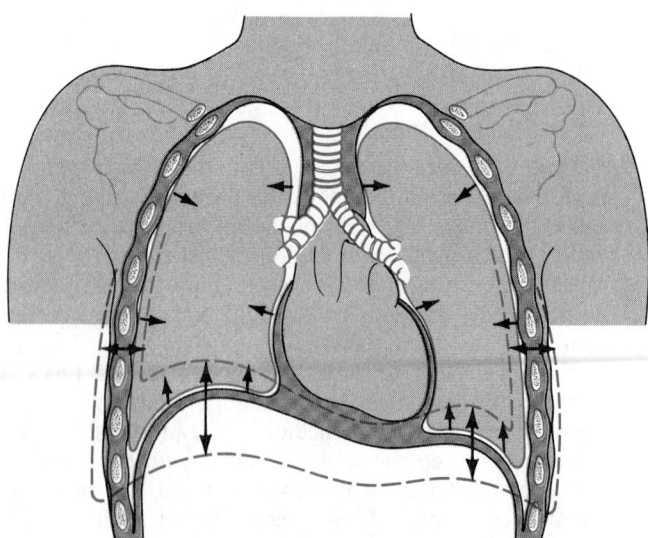

Fig. 19-4 Frontal section of chest and lung showing pleural space. *Single arrows* indicate the retractive force; *double arrows* show the excursions of the lung bases and periphery between deep inspiration and expiration.

external intercostal muscles and parasternal muscles function to raise the rib cage and thereby help to increase the size of the thoracic cavity. The scalene muscles and sternocleidomastoid muscles assist with this function during labored respirations. However, the diaphragm is the major muscle of respiration. When the diaphragm contracts, it descends, pushing the abdominal contents downward and increasing the size of the thoracic cavity.

The intercostal muscles are innervated by nerves coming from the spinal cord between vertebrae T1 and T11. The diaphragm is innervated by the phrenic nerve, which comes from the spinal cord between C3 and C5. All nerves are linked to the respiratory center in the medulla via the spinal cord. This pattern of innervation is significant in relation to the effect of spinal cord injuries. Lesions at C6 and C7 do not affect the phrenic nerve, and diaphragm function remains normal. Although function of the intercostal muscles is lost, these clients can move sufficient volumes of air with their diaphragms to breathe without the use of a ventilator. Injuries at the C3 to C5 level cause partial or total diaphragm paralysis, which markedly limits air movement. These clients typically have tidal volumes of 50 to 100 ml (normal is 500 ml) and are dependent on a ventilator.

Physiology of Respiration

Ventilation. Ventilation involves *inspiration* (movement of air into the lungs) and *expiration* (movement of air out of the lungs). The physical process of ventilation is accomplished by the changing intrathoracic pressure in relation to atmospheric pressure. Since gas flows from an area of higher pressure to one of lower pressure, the pressure within the lungs and thorax must be less than atmospheric pressure for inspiration to occur. This is accomplished by the contraction of the diaphragm and external intercostal muscles and the enlargement of the thoracic cavity (see Fig. 19-4). As the thoracic cavity enlarges, intrathoracic pressure becomes less than the atmospheric pressure and air moves into the lungs. With deep inspiration, the diaphragm moves 3 to 5 cm or from the level of the tenth to the twelfth rib. Some conditions (e.g., postoperative pain, neuromuscular disease) may limit thoracic movement and cause clients to breathe with smaller tidal volumes. As a result, they do not fully inflate their lungs and are prone to atelectasis.

In contrast to the active efforts of inspiration, expiration is passive. As the muscles relax, the thoracic cavity becomes smaller by the process of elastic recoil. Intrathoracic pressure rises, causing air to move out of the lungs. Expiration is an active process if the internal intercostal and abdominal muscles are involved. Examples of active expiration include severe dyspnea seen in an attack of asthma or exacerbation of chronic obstructive pulmonary disease (COPD) (see Chapter 22).

Compliance and elastic recoil. Compliance (distensibility) is a measure of the elasticity of the lungs and thorax. Compliance is decreased in restrictive lung diseases, such as idiopathic pulmonary fibrosis and pleural effusion. Compliance is also decreased when there is a deficiency of surfactant. Increased compliance is found when there is

destruction of alveolar walls and loss of tissue elasticity, as in emphysema.

Elastic recoil is the tendency for the lungs to recoil after being stretched or expanded. The elasticity of lung tissue is due to the elastin fibers found in the alveolar walls and surrounding the bronchioles and capillaries.

Diffusion. When a person inhales normally, the alveoli fill with air. This causes the alveolar oxygen concentration to become higher than the concentration of oxygen in the blood. At the same time the alveolar concentration of carbon dioxide is less than the carbon dioxide concentration of the blood in the pulmonary capillary.[3] Therefore oxygen diffuses across the alveolar-capillary membrane into the blood, and carbon dioxide diffuses into the alveoli until equilibrium is reached (Fig. 19-5).

The ability of the lungs to adequately oxygenate arterial blood is assessed by examination of the Pao_2 and arterial oxygen saturation (Sao_2). Oxygen is carried in the blood in two forms, dissolved oxygen and oxygen in chemical combination with hemoglobin. The Pao_2 represents the amount of oxygen dissolved in the plasma. The Pao_2 is expressed in millimeters of mercury (mm Hg). The Sao_2 is the amount of oxygen being carried by the hemoglobin in comparison with the amount of oxygen the hemoglobin can carry. The Sao_2 is expressed as a percentage. For example, if the Sao_2 is 90%, then 90% of the hemoglobin attachments for oxygen have oxygen attached to them.

Oxygen-hemoglobin dissociation curve. The affinity of hemoglobin for oxygen is described by the oxygen-hemoglobin dissociation curve (Fig. 19-6). Oxygen delivery to the tissues depends on the amount of oxygen transported to the tissues and the ease with which hemoglobin gives up oxygen once it reaches the tissues. In the upper flat portion of the curve, fairly large changes in the Pao_2 cause a small change in hemoglobin saturation. For this reason, if the Pao_2 drops from 100 to 60 mm Hg, the saturation of hemoglobin changes by only 7% (from the normal of 97% to 90%). Thus, the hemoglobin remains 90% saturated despite a 40 mm Hg drop in the Pao_2. This portion of the curve also explains the reason most clients are considered adequately oxygenated when their Pao_2 is greater than 60 mm Hg. Increasing the value above this level causes little change in hemoglobin saturation, and if high concentrations of oxygen can be avoided there is less risk of oxygen toxicity.

The lower portion of the curve indicates a different type of protection. As the hemoglobin becomes further desaturated, larger amounts of oxygen are released for tissue use. This is an important method of maintaining the pressure gradient between the blood and the tissues. It also ensures an adequate oxygen supply to peripheral tissues, even if oxygen delivery is compromised.

Many factors alter the affinity of hemoglobin for oxygen. When the oxygen dissociation curve shifts to the left, blood picks up oxygen more readily in the lungs but delivers oxygen less readily to the tissues. This is seen in alkalosis, in hypothermia, and when the $Paco_2$ is decreased. When the curve shifts to the right, the opposite occurs. Blood picks up oxygen less rapidly in the lungs but delivers oxygen more readily to the tissues. This is seen in aci-

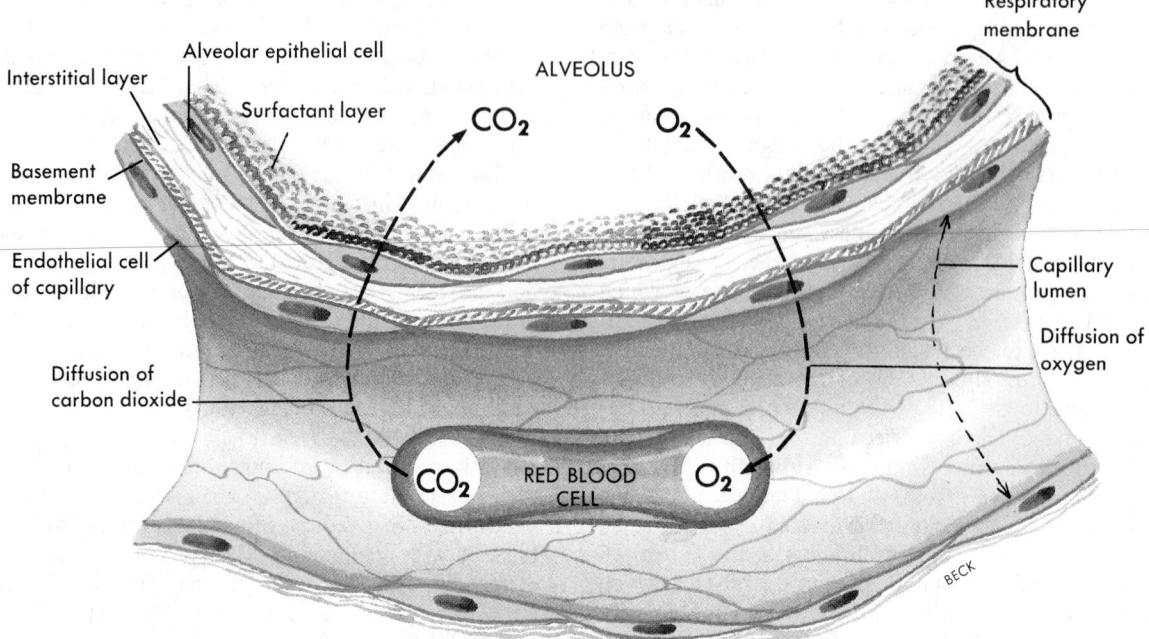

Fig. 19-5 A small portion of the respiratory membrane greatly magnified. An extremely thin interstitial layer of tissue separates the endothelial cell and basement membrane on the capillary side from the epithelial cell and surfactant layer on the alveolar side of the respiratory membrane. The total thickness of the respiratory membrane is less than 1 μm. (From Thibodeau G: *Structure and function of the body*, ed 8, St Louis, 1988, The CV Mosby Co, p 337.)

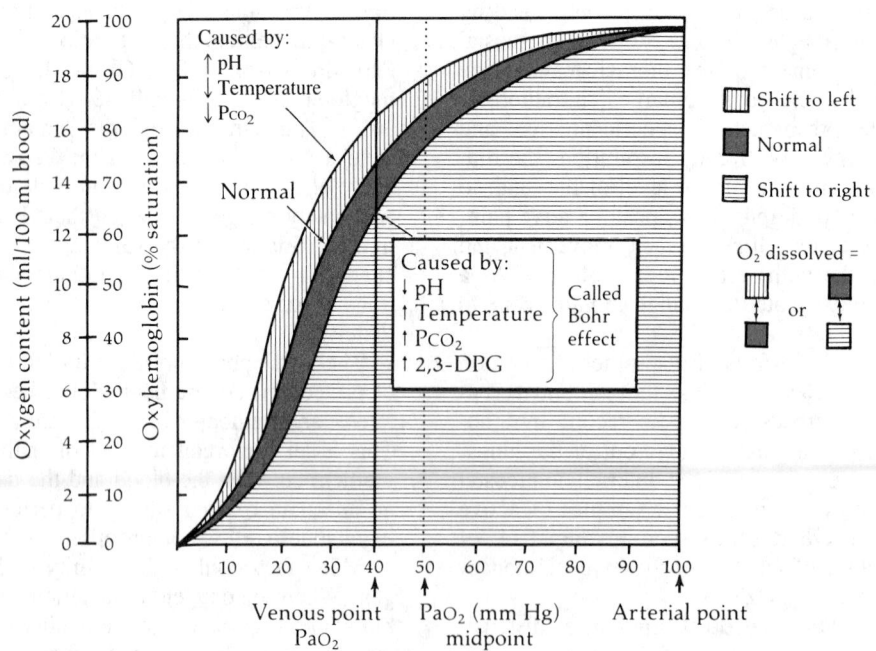

Fig. 19-6 Oxygen-hemoglobin dissociation curve. *Insets* show the effects of acidity and temperature changes.

dosis, in hyperthermia, and when the $Paco_2$ is increased.[4]

Clients with conditions that cause a leftward shift of the curve, such as the hypothermia that follows open heart surgery, may be given higher concentrations of oxygen until their temperature normalizes. This helps to compensate for decreased oxygen unloading in the tissues.

Two methods are used to assess the efficiency of gas transfer in the lung: analysis of arterial blood gases and oximetry. These measurements provide important data for making clinical decisions about oxygen therapy, mechanical ventilation, and effectiveness of the management regimen.

Arterial blood gases. Arterial blood gases (ABGs) are measured to determine oxygenation status and acid-base balance. ABG analysis includes measurement of the partial pressure of oxygen (Pao_2) and carbon dioxide ($Paco_2$), acidity (pH), and bicarbonate (HCO_3) in arterial blood. The Sao_2 is also calculated during this analysis.[5]

Blood for ABG analysis is obtained by means of an arterial puncture (typically the radial or femoral artery) or by insertion of a plastic cannula, termed an *arterial line,* into one of these arteries. The latter approach permits ABG sampling without repeated punctures.

Normal values for ABGs are given in Table 19-1. The normal Pao_2 decreases with advancing age. The normal Pao_2 also varies in relation to the distance above sea level. At higher altitudes, the barometric pressure is lower, resulting in a lower inspired oxygen pressure (Pio_2) and a lower Pao_2 (Table 19-1).

Clients with such conditions as COPD will experience symptoms of impaired gas exchange earlier in the disease process if they live at high altitudes. This change in Pao_2 also affects those who travel by airplane. Most airplanes are pressurized to approximate an altitude of 5000 to 6000 feet. For this reason, clients with COPD may need to avoid this form of travel.

A special type of catheter, called a *pulmonary artery catheter,* can also be used to obtain blood for analysis. Blood obtained from the pulmonary artery is called *mixed venous blood* because it consists of blood that has returned from the superior and inferior venae cavae and is "mixed"

in the right ventricle. Because blood in the pulmonary artery has not yet passed through the pulmonary capillary bed, it is lower in oxygen and higher in carbon dioxide than blood that has just left the lungs and entered the arterial system. Normal values for mixed venous blood are given in Table 19-1.

Oximetry. ABG values provide accurate information about oxygenation and acid-base balance. However, they are invasive, require laboratory analysis, and expose the client to the risk of bleeding from the arterial puncture. It is also possible to monitor oxygenation without drawing blood samples. The technique involves use of oximetry.[6]

An oximeter emits two wavelengths of light, one red and one infrared (Fig. 19-7, *A*). Blood that is well oxygenated (red) absorbs light differently than blood that is deoxygenated (blue). The oximeter transmits a beam of light through the vascular bed of the ear or finger and determines how much light is absorbed by oxygenated and deoxygenated blood. The Sao_2 is calculated from this information and displayed as a digital reading. When a pulse oximeter is used, the heart rate is also displayed. Oximetry is particularly valuable in intensive care units (ICUs) and during exercise testing. Changes in Sao_2 can be quickly detected and appropriate changes made in the plan of care (Table 19-2). The normal Sao_2 is greater than 95%.

Values obtained by oximetry become less accurate if the Sao_2 is less than 80%. At this level, oxygenated blood is darker, making it more difficult for the oximeter to distinguish between oxygenated and deoxygenated blood. The Sao_2 will be falsely elevated if the client is exposed to carbon monoxide, such as occurs with smoking. Carboxyhemoglobin is cherry red. The oximeter cannot distinguish between the colors of oxygenated hemoglobin and carboxyhemoglobin.

Venous oxygen saturation ($S\bar{v}o_2$) can also be monitored with the use of oximetry.[7] When the $S\bar{v}o_2$ is monitored, the light-emitting probe is placed in one lumen of a pulmonary artery catheter (Fig. 19-7, *B*). A decrease in $S\bar{v}o_2$ suggests that less oxygen is being delivered to the tissues or that more oxygen is being consumed. Changes in $S\bar{v}o_2$ provide an early warning of a change in cardiac output and

Table 19-1 Normal Arterial and Venous Blood Gas Values*

Laboratory Value	Arterial Blood Gases		Venous Blood Gases*	
	Sea Level (Atmospheric Pressure 760 mm Hg)	1-Mile Elevation (Atmospheric Pressure 629 mm Hg)	Mixed Venous Blood	
pH	7.35-7.45	7.35-7.45	pH	7.34-7.37
Pao_2	80-100 mm Hg	65-75 mm Hg	Pvo_2	38-42 mm Hg
Sao_2	> 95%†	> 95%†	Svo_2	60%-80%†
$Paco_2$	35-45 mm Hg	35-45 mm Hg	$Pvco_2$	44-46 mm Hg
HCO_3	22-26 mEq/L	22-26 mEq/L	HCO_3	24-30 mEq/L

Pvo_2, Partial pressure of oxygen in venous blood; $S\bar{v}o_2$, venous oxygen saturation.

*Assumes client is ≤ 60 years of age and breathing room air. Room air has a fractional inspired oxygen concentration (Fio_2) of 0.21.

†The same normal values apply when Sao_2 and $S\bar{v}o_2$ are obtained by oximetry.

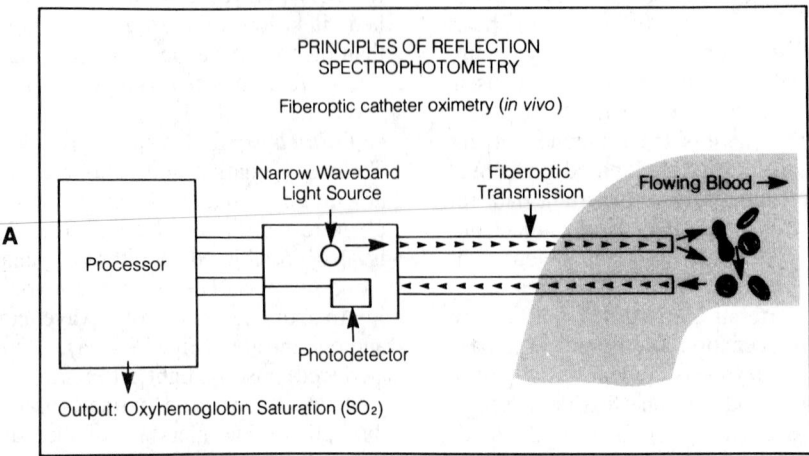

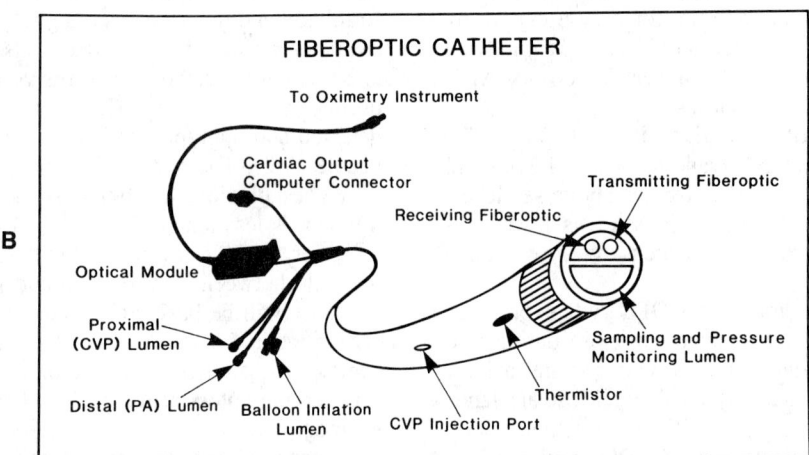

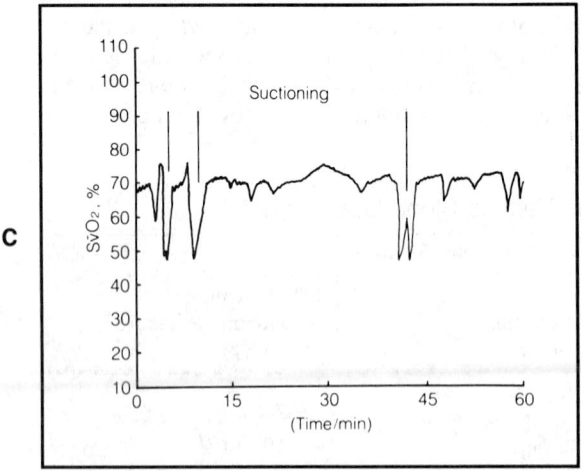

Fig. 19-7 With oximetry, oxygen saturation can be monitored without the need for blood sampling. **A,** Light from the photodetector is reflected from flowing blood. **B,** The pulmonary artery catheter used to monitor $S\bar{v}O_2$. **C,** Decline in $S\bar{v}O_2$ during endotracheal suctioning. (From Fahey PJ: Continuous measurement of blood oxygen saturation in the high-risk patient, vol 2, San Diego, 1985, Beach International, pp 18, 61, 71.)

Table 19-2 Critical Values for $\bar{P}ao_2$ and Sao_2

Pao₂ (%)	Sao₂ (%)	Considerations
≥70	≥94	Adequate unless client is hemodynamically unstable or has oxygen-unloading problem: With a low cardiac output, dysrhythmias, a leftward shift of the oxyhemoglobin dissociation curve, or carbon monoxide inhalation, higher values may be desired. Benefits of a higher blood oxygen value need to be balanced against the risk of oxygen toxicity.
60	90	Adequate in almost all clients: Values are at steep part of oxygen-hemoglobin dissociation curve. Provides adequate oxygenation but with lesser margin of error than above.
55	88	Adequate for clients with chronic hypoxemia if no cardiac problems occur: These values are also used as criteria for prescription of continuous oxygen therapy.
40	75	Inadequate but may be acceptable on a short-term basis if the client also has carbon dioxide retention: A high Paco₂ may cause CO_2 narcosis. In this situation, respirations are stimulated by a low Pao₂. Thus the Pao₂ cannot be raised rapidly. The nurse may use low-flow, low-concentration oxygen therapy to gradually increase the Pao₂. Monitoring for dysrhythmias is necessary.
<40	<75	Inadequate: Tissue hypoxia and cardiac dysrhythmias can be expected.

Modified from Wesmiller SW and Hoffman LA: Interpreting your patient's oxygenation status, Orthop Nurs 8:56-60, 1989.

tissue oxygen delivery. Clinicians can immediately assess the effect of treatment or routine interventions such as suctioning (Fig. 19-7). The normal S$\bar{v}$o₂ is 60% to 80%.

Oxygen delivery. Several questions need to be asked to determine whether the client is receiving adequate oxygen:

1. What is the client's Pao₂ or Sao₂ compared to expected normal values? (Normal values are given in Table 19-1.)
2. What is the trend? Has there been a rapid decline in Pao₂ or Sao₂? An acute drop in the Pao₂ can be life threatening. A gradual decline, such as that seen in COPD, is tolerated with fewer symptoms.
3. What is the degree of hypoxemia? Because of the shape of the oxygen-hemoglobin dissociation curve, clients with a Pao₂ above 60 mm Hg or a Sao₂ greater than 90% are at less risk than those with lower values (see Table 19-2).
4. Are there clues that suggest hypoxia? Although the terms *hypoxia* and *hypoxemia* are often interchanged, they have different meanings. Hypoxia refers to a deficiency in tissue oxygenation and is associated with symptoms that reflect inadequate oxygen delivery to vital organs, such as the heart and the brain (Table 19-3). Clients who are hypoxic are not adequately oxygenated. Hypoxemia refers to a blood oxygen level that is lower than normal (i.e., less than 80 mm Hg). Depending on the extent of change, hypoxemia may or may not be associated with symptoms. If there are symptoms that suggest inadequate tissue oxygenation, a change in oxygen therapy may be indicated.

Cardiac output (see Chapter 26) and hemoglobin level (see Chapter 24) also need to be assessed. The Pao₂ and Sao₂ are important in determining whether the tissues are receiving sufficient oxygen. However, if there is an alteration in cardiac output or hemoglobin level, a client may have a normal Pao₂ and Sao₂ and inadequate tissue oxygen delivery. For

Table 19-3 Signs and Symptoms of Hypoxia

RESPIRATORY

Tachypnea
Dyspnea

CARDIOVASCULAR

Tachycardia
Dysrhythmias, such as premature ventricular contractions
Increased pulmonary vascular resistance
Cyanosis (late sign)

CENTRAL NERVOUS SYSTEM

Restlessness
Disorientation
Personality change
Combativeness
Coma

OTHER

Fatigue
Decreased urinary output

From Wesmiller SW and Hoffman LA: Interpreting your patient's oxygenation status, Orthop Nurs 8:56-60, 1989.

this reason, an assessment that considers only the Pao₂ or Sao₂ is insufficient.

Control of Respiration

The respiratory center is composed of cell clusters in the medulla. These cells respond to chemical and mechanical signals from the body. Impulses are sent from the medulla to the respiratory muscles through the spinal cord and phrenic nerves. Respirations are controlled by chemoreceptors and mechanical sensors.

Chemoreceptors. A chemoreceptor is a receptor that responds to a change in the chemical composition ($Paco_2$ and pH) of the fluid around it. Central chemoreceptors are located in the medulla and respond to changes in the hydrogen ion (H^+) concentration. An increase in the H^+ ion concentration (acidosis) causes the medulla to increase the respiratory rate and tidal volume. A decrease in H^+ ion concentration (alkalosis) has the opposite effect. Changes in $Paco_2$ regulate ventilation primarily by their effect on the pH of the cerebrospinal fluid. When the $Paco_2$ level is increased, more CO_2 is available to combine with H_2O and form carbonic acid (H_2CO_3). This lowers the cerebrospinal fluid pH and stimulates an increase in respiratory rate. The opposite process occurs with a decrease in $Paco_2$ level. Conditions such as COPD may alter lung function and result in chronically elevated $Paco_2$ levels (see Chapter 22).

Peripheral chemoreceptors are located in the carotid bodies at the bifurcation of the common carotid arteries and in the aortic bodies above and below the aortic arch. The peripheral chemoreceptors respond to decreases in Pao_2 and pH and to increases in $Paco_2$. These changes also cause stimulation of the respiratory center.

In a healthy person an increase in $Paco_2$ or a decrease in pH causes an immediate increase in the respiratory rate. The process is very precise. The $Paco_2$ does not vary more than about 3 mm Hg when lung function is normal.

When the $Paco_2$ is chronically elevated, the medulla may become insensitive and not respond by increasing the respiratory rate. This condition is termed *carbon dioxide narcosis.* Hypoxemia becomes the most important stimulus for respiration. This stimulus, referred to as *hypoxic drive,* allows respiration to continue despite decreased sensitivity of the medulla. Client management involves giving oxygen in low concentrations (24% to 28% or 1 to 2 L/min), with the goal of slowly decreasing the $Paco_2$ and slowly increasing the Pao_2 (see Table 19-2). Slow changes are important. The hypoxic stimulus to breathe must be maintained until the $Paco_2$ reaches a more normal level and the medulla again functions normally (see Chapter 22).

Mechanical receptors. Mechanical receptors are located in the lungs, upper airways, chest wall, and diaphragm. They are stimulated by a variety of physiological factors, such as irritants, muscle stretching, and alveolar wall distortion. Signals from the stretch receptors aid in the control of respiration. As the lungs inflate, pulmonary stretch receptors activate the inspiratory center to inhibit further lung expansion. This is called the *Hering-Breuer reflex.* It prevents overdistention of the lungs. Impulses from the mechanical sensors are sent through the vagus nerve to the brain. Juxtacapillary (J) receptors are believed to cause the rapid respiration (tachypnea) seen in pulmonary edema. These receptors are stimulated by fluid entering the pulmonary interstitial space.

Respiratory Defense Mechanisms

Respiratory defense mechanisms are very efficient in protecting the lungs from inhaled particles, microorganisms, and toxic gases. The defense mechanisms include (1) filtration of air, (2) the mucociliary clearance system, (3) the cough reflex, (4) reflex bronchoconstriction, and (5) alveolar macrophages.

Filtration of air. Nasal hairs filter the inspired air. In addition, the abrupt changes in direction of airflow that occur as air moves through the nasopharynx and larynx increase air turbulence. This causes particles and bacteria to impact on the mucosa lining these structures. Most large particles (greater than 5 μm in diameter) are removed in this manner.

The velocity of airflow slows greatly after it passes the larynx, facilitating the deposition of smaller particles (1 to 5 μm in size). They settle out like sand in a river, a process referred to as *sedimentation.* Particles less than 1 μm in size are too small to settle in this manner. They are deposited by diffusion in the alveoli. Particle size is very important. Large particles (greater than 5 μm) are less dangerous because they are removed in the nasopharynx and do not reach the alveoli.

Mucociliary clearance system. Below the larynx, movement of mucus is accomplished by the *mucociliary clearance system.* This term is used to indicate the interrelationship between the secretion of mucus and the ciliary activity. Mucus is continually secreted at a rate of about 100 ml/day by goblet cells and submucosal glands. It forms a mucous blanket that contains the impacted particles and debris from distal lung areas (see Fig. 19-1). The small amount of mucus normally secreted is swallowed without being noticed. Secretory immunoglobulin A (IgA) in the mucus contributes to protection against bacteria and viruses.

Cilia cover the airways from the level of the trachea to the respiratory bronchioles (Fig. 19-8). Each ciliated cell contains about 200 cilia. Cilia beat rhythmically about 1000 times per minute in the large airways, moving mucus toward the mouth. The ciliary beat is slower farther down the tracheobronchial tree. As a consequence, particles that penetrate more deeply into the airways are removed less rapidly. Ciliary action is impaired by dehydration, smoking, inhalation of high oxygen concentrations, infection, and ingestion of drugs such as atropine, alcohol, and anesthetics. Clients with chronic bronchitis often have repeated upper respiratory infections. Cilia are often destroyed during these infections, resulting in impaired secretion clearance, a chronic productive cough, and frequent respiratory infections (see Fig. 19-3).

Cough reflex. The cough is a protective reflex action that clears the airway by a high-pressure, high-velocity flow of air. It is a backup for mucociliary clearance, especially when this clearance mechanism is overwhelmed or ineffective. Coughing is effective in removing only secretions that are above the subsegmental level. Secretions below this level need to be moved upward by the mucociliary mechanism or by interventions such as postural drainage before they can be removed by coughing.

Reflex bronchoconstriction. Another defense mechanism is reflex bronchoconstriction. In response to the inhalation of large amounts of irritant substances (e.g., dusts, aerosols), the bronchi constrict in an effort to prevent entry of the irritants. Some clients, such as those with asthma, have hyperactive airways and may experience bronchocon-

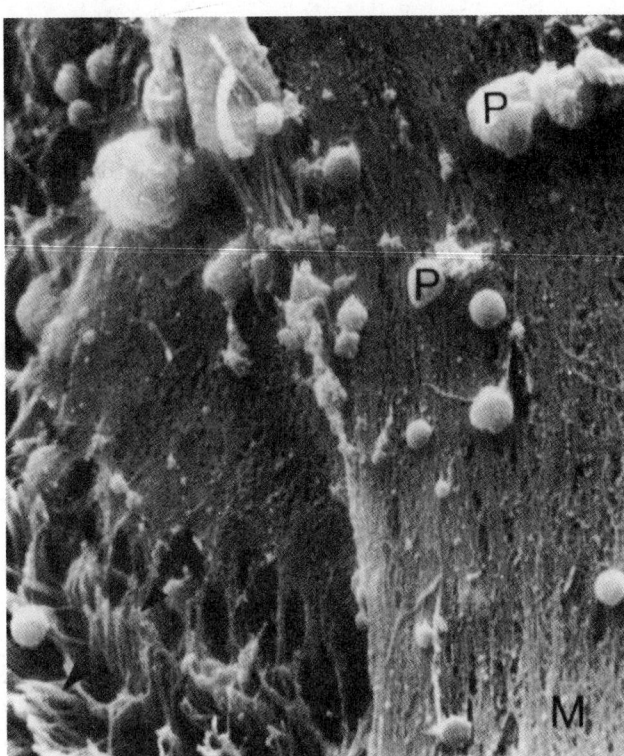

Fig. 19-8 Extracellular mucus *(M)* lining the luminal surface of the airway mucosa. Inhaled particles *(P)* and cellular debris are trapped on the mucous layer and transported along the airway surface by the underlying cilia *(arrows)*. The mucous layer is situated at the tips of the cilia, separated from the cell surfaces by a fluid or sol layer. (From Sturgess JM: Structure of the human airway mucosa: control of airway secretions, Semin Respir Med 5:302, 1984. Reprinted by permission.)

striction after inhalation of cold air, perfume, or other strong odors.

Alveolar macrophages. Ciliated cells are not found below the level of the respiratory bronchioles. The primary defense mechanism at the alveolar level is alveolar macrophages. Alveolar macrophages rapidly phagocytize inhaled foreign particles such as bacteria. The debris is moved to the level of the bronchioles for removal by the cilia, or it is removed from the lungs by the lymphatic system. Alveolar macrophage activity can be impaired by cigarette and marijuana smoking, viral infections, prolonged corticosteroid therapy, and a number of chronic diseases.

Particles that cannot be adequately phagocytized tend to remain in the lungs for indefinite periods and can stimulate inflammatory or fibrogenic responses. Coal dust and silica can stimulate a fibrous reaction (see Chapter 21).

Effects of Aging

The structures of the respiratory system change as a result of the aging process (see Table 19-7). The respiratory center becomes less responsive to increases in $Paco_2$ or decreases in Pao_2. Older adults do not react to a change in Pao_2 or $Paco_2$ with the marked increase in respiratory rate and tidal volume seen in younger clients. In conditions of increased metabolic demand, such as stress and illness, this diminished response may place the older client at greater risk of tissue hypoxia. The chest wall stiffens and the pressure a client can achieve during a maximal inspiration or expiration decreases. These changes decrease the client's ability to generate the high airflows required for effective coughing. Because cough effectiveness is decreased, older clients are at a greater risk of pulmonary complications after surgery. Small airways in the lung bases also close earlier in the expiratory process, a change referred to as a *decrease in closing volume*. As a consequence, more inspired air is distributed to the lung apices, where ventilation is less well matched to perfusion. Therefore, Pao_2 decreases. The Pao_2 associated with a given age can be calculated by means of the following equation:

$$Pao_2 \text{ (mm Hg)} = 103.5 - (0.42 \times \text{age [yr]})$$

For example, the normal Pao_2 for a client 80 years of age is $103.5 - (0.42 \times 80) = 70$ mm Hg, as compared to a Pao_2 of 93 mm Hg for a 25-year-old person.

ASSESSMENT OF THE RESPIRATORY SYSTEM
Subjective Data

Health history. The goal of the health history is to determine the client's health status, symptoms, and risk factors. Because of the chronic nature of respiratory problems, many clients will relate a change in symptoms rather than the development of new symptoms when describing the present illness.[8] Such changes should be carefully documented because they often suggest the cause of the illness. For example, a change in the volume, tenacity (thickness), or color of sputum suggests onset of a lower respiratory tract infection.

While obtaining the history, it is also important to make pertinent observations related to the client's respiratory status. Does the client speak in complete sentences or pause for breath between words or sentences? Is any hoarseness noted? Does the client have a productive cough?

Past health history

PEDIATRIC AND ADULT ILLNESSES. The upper and lower respiratory systems are common sites of minor and major health problems. The nurse should determine the frequency of upper respiratory problems (e.g., colds, sore throats, sinus problems). The nurse should ask whether changes in the weather affect these problems. A history of lower respiratory problems such as asthma, COPD, pneumonia, and tuberculosis, should also be elicited. The nurse needs to investigate problems related to other systems that affect the respiratory system. For example, clients with acquired immunodeficiency syndrome (AIDS) frequently experience respiratory infections because function of their immune system is compromised. Clients with cardiac dysfunction may experience dyspnea as a consequence of decreased cardiac output.

IMMUNIZATIONS. The dates of immunization against pneumonia (Pneumovax) and influenza should be recorded. Pneumovax confers lifelong immunity against pneumococcal pneumonia. Vaccination against influenza is needed yearly in the fall.

HOSPITALIZATIONS. The nurse should determine whether the client has been hospitalized for a respiratory problem. If so, the dates, chief complaint, therapy (including surgery), and current status of the problem should be recorded, as well as whether a chest x-ray film was taken. This x-ray film may provide valuable baseline data if a respiratory problem is identified.

INJURIES. The client should be questioned about trauma to structures of the respiratory system, such as a broken nose, fractured ribs, or pneumothorax (collapsed lung).

MEDICATION HISTORY. It is important to obtain a medication history with particular reference to drugs prescribed for respiratory problems, such as antibiotics, bronchodilators, and steroids. Over-the-counter drugs and prescription drugs should be included. The reason for taking the medication, as well as the name of the drug, dose, frequency, duration of use, effect, and side effects, should be determined. Past and present usage should be elicited.

RESPIRATORY EQUIPMENT. Use and frequency of use of a nebulizer, oxygen therapy, negative-pressure ventilator, or other equipment should be documented. Questions should be asked about the use of postural drainage and percussion.

ALLERGIES. The nurse should determine whether the client has allergies. If so, the client should be questioned about precipitating factors such as medications, foods, pollen, and strong odors. Dusts or fumes found in the workplace may also cause an allergic response. The nurse should also ask about humidifiers in the home. Water in the air conditioner and in furnace humidifiers may be a source of molds, which can cause an allergic reaction when inhaled. The characteristics of the allergic reaction, such as runny nose, wheezing, scratchy throat, or tightness in the chest; the severity of the reaction; and the client's age when it first occurred should be documented.

Family history. The client should be questioned about a family history of respiratory problems such as allergies, asthma, COPD, and cystic fibrosis. The smoking history of household members should be noted.

Personal and social history. Almost all components of a person's life can influence respiratory status. The following areas are of particular importance:

OCCUPATION. Dusts or substances used in the workplace may cause respiratory problems. The nurse should document the nature of the client's work and the frequency and intensity of exposure to fumes, toxins, asbestos, coal dust, or silica. Such hobbies as woodworking (sawdust) or pottery (silica) and exposure to animals (allergies) may also cause respiratory problems.

GEOGRAPHICAL LOCATION. The nurse should ask where the client has lived and traveled. Fungal infections of the lung are most common among persons living or traveling in the southwest (coccidioidomycosis) and the Mississippi River Valley (histoplasmosis). (Other fungal lung infections and their common geographical locations are presented in Chapter 21.)

ENVIRONMENT. The nurse should determine the extent of the client's mobility within the home and neighborhood.

The nurse should also note whether the client's housing (e.g., number of steps, levels) poses an environmental problem that may increase isolation.

NUTRITION. Weight loss is associated with increased airflow obstruction and decreased survival in COPD. The nurse should compare actual weight to ideal body weight. A body weight less than 90% of ideal body weight is considered significant because it suggests protein depletion. The nurse should determine whether food intake is altered by anorexia (from medications), fatigue (from hypoxemia, increased work of breathing), early satiety (from lung hyperinflation), or social isolation. Anorexia and weight loss are also common symptoms in clients with lung cancer, tuberculosis, and AIDS.

SMOKING. A careful smoking history is a critical part of the health history. The risk of lung cancer rises in direct proportion to the number of cigarettes smoked. Smoking increases the risk of COPD and lung cancer and may exacerbate existing symptoms. The nurse should ask the client about current and past smoking habits and determine the number of pack-years. This is done by multiplying the number of packs smoked per day by the number of years smoked. For example, a person who smoked 1½ packs per day for 10 years has a 15 pack-year history. Pulmonary function tests may reveal damage to the small airways with less smoke exposure.

SUBSTANCE ABUSE. If a problem is confirmed, information about community agencies providing counseling should be offered. Alcohol decreases ciliary action, which reduces mucociliary clearance. Heavy alcohol consumption depresses the cough reflex and predisposes to aspiration of secretions and pneumonia. The risk of tuberculosis and cancer of the head and neck region is also increased.

Narcotic addiction may involve the sharing of needles contaminated with blood containing the human immunodeficiency virus (HIV). Clients who test positive for HIV are predisposed to developing AIDS. Clients at risk for becoming infected with HIV should be questioned about symptoms of respiratory infection (e.g., dyspnea, cough, and fever).

ACTIVITY LEVEL. Information related to the lifelong activity pattern of the client should be obtained. The nurse should ask, "As a child, did you miss school frequently because of colds and respiratory problems? Could you keep up with your peers and participate in physical education? As an adult, can you keep up with your peers in their activities? Compare your present activity level to that of the last 6 months, 1 year, and 5 years."

SEXUALITY. The dyspnea associated with many respiratory problems may cause sexual problems. However, clients can continue to have good sexual relationships despite marked physical limitations. The nurse needs to determine whether breathing difficulties have caused alterations in sexual activity.

Clients who engage in homosexual relationships, relationships with intravenous (IV) drug abusers, or relationships with multiple sexual partners increase their risk of becoming HIV positive and of developing AIDS.

SELF-CARE STRATEGIES. The nurse should determine the client's usual self-care strategies. Does the client understand the respiratory problem and how to appropriately manage care? If a self-care deficit exists, the nurse should develop a plan for health teaching.[9]

Review of systems. The nurse should specifically question the client about the signs and symptoms of respiratory problems. These include cardinal signs and symptoms (which include cough, sputum, hemoptysis, wheezing, breathlessness, and chest pain) as well as constitutional signs and symptoms (which include fever, hoarseness, anorexia, weight loss, and dependent edema). The nurse should inquire about problems of the nose and sinuses, such as colds, discharge, epistaxis, sinus pain, and swelling. The date of the last x-ray examination of the chest should be recorded. If the client responds positively to any of the problems asked in the review of systems, detailed information should be obtained (see Chapter 3).

Because hypoxia can cause neurological symptoms, the nurse should ask about restlessness, personality change, and disorientation, which can indicate inadequate tissue oxygenation. Cardiac manifestations, such as tachycardia, may accompany respiratory problems. Gastrointestinal (GI) manifestations, such as anorexia and weight loss, may also result from a respiratory problem.

Objective Data

Physical examination. Vital signs, including temperature, pulse, respirations, and blood pressure as well as weight, are important data to collect before examination of the respiratory system.

Nose. The nose is inspected for inflammation, deformities, and symmetry. The nurse tilts the client's head backward and pushes the tip of the nose upward gently. With a nasal speculum and a good light, the interior of the nose is inspected (Fig. 19-9). The mucous membrane should be pink and moist, with no evidence of edema (bogginess),

exudate, or bleeding. The nasal septum should be observed for deviation, perforations, and bleeding. Some nasal deviation is normal in adults. The turbinates should be observed for polyps, which are abnormal, fingerlike projections of swollen nasal mucosa. Polyps may result from long-term irritation of the mucosa, as from allergies.

Mouth and pharynx. Using a good light source, the nurse inspects the interior of the mouth for color, lesions, masses, gum retraction, bleeding, and poor dentition. The tongue is inspected for symmetry and presence of lesions. The nurse observes the pharynx by pressing a tongue blade against the middle of the back of the tongue. The pharynx should be smooth and moist, with no evidence of exudate, ulcerations, or swelling. The color, symmetry, and any enlargement of the tonsils is noted (Fig 19-9). The nurse stimulates the gag reflex by placing a tongue blade on the back of the tongue. A normal response indicates that the ninth and tenth cranial nerves are intact and that the airway is protected.

Neck. The nurse inspects the neck for symmetry and presence of tender or swollen areas. The lymph nodes are palpated while the client is sitting erect with the neck slightly flexed. Progress is front to back from the nodes around the ears, to the nodes at the base of the skull, and then to those located under the angles of the mandible to the midline. Some clients have small, mobile, nontender individual nodes *(shotty nodes)*, which are the result of previous infection and are not considered signs of pathology. However, tender, hard, or fixed nodes are indicative of disease. The location and characteristics of any nodes that are palpated are described. (Lymph node palpation is described in more detail in Chapter 24.)

Heart. Findings that reflect respiratory health include heart rate, location of the point of maximal impulse, jugular venous distention, and dependent edema. (Cardiac assessment is discussed in Chapter 26.)

Thorax and lungs. Imaginary lines can be drawn on the chest to help in identifying abnormalities (Fig. 19-2). Abnormalities can be described in relation to their location to these lines (e.g., 2 cm from the right midclavicular line).

Chest examination is best performed in a well-lighted, warm room with measures taken to ensure the client's privacy. Either the anterior or the posterior of the chest may be examined first, depending on clinician preference.

INSPECTION. The client undresses to the waist. If able, the client should be sitting upright or leaning on the bedside table. The nurse observes client's overall appearance and notes any evidence of respiratory distress, such as nasal flaring, use of accessory muscles, and intercostal retraction or bulging. The nurse also notes whether the shoulders are at the same level. Surgical procedures (e.g., pneumonectomy, lobectomy) and congenital deformities (e.g., kyphoscoliosis) alter lung volume and may cause unequal height of the shoulders. The shape of the ribs is determined. Normally, the ribs slope at a 45-degree angle in relation to the spine. In chronic airflow limitation (e.g., in COPD and cystic fibrosis), the ribs become more horizontal. The nurse observes for abnormalities in the sternum that may inhibit normal respiratory excursion. These are *pectus carinatum* or "pigeon chest," which is a prominent protrusion

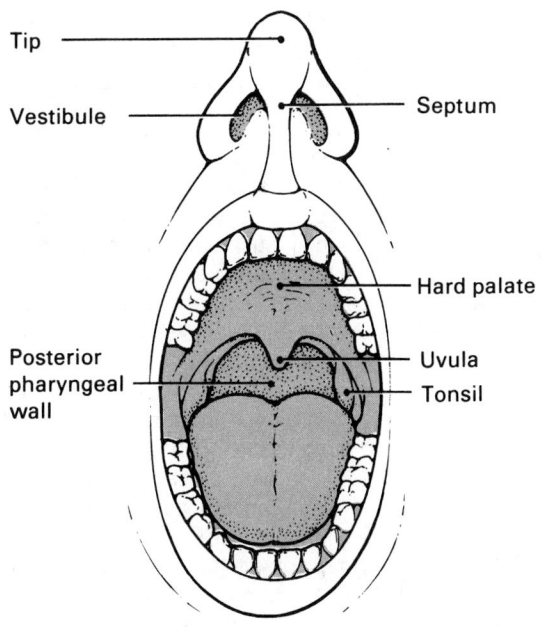

Fig. 19-9 Structures of the nose and mouth.

of the sternum, and *pectus excavatum* or "funnel chest," an indentation of the lower sternum above the xiphoid process. An increased anteroposterior diameter (from front to back) is "barrel chest." The chest should move over all lung areas. This is best checked by the nurse's moving the eyes clockwise (or counterclockwise) and observing each portion of the chest sequentially while standing directly in front of the client.[10] Respiratory rate, depth, and rhythm are observed. The normal rate is 10 to 20 respirations per minute. Expiration should be twice as long as inspiration. The nurse notes whether respirations are costal (from the upper chest) or abdominal.

In addition, the nurse observes for cyanosis of the lips, buccal mucosa, or nail beds. Causes of cyanosis include inadequate oxygenation, decreased cardiac output, vasoconstriction, and vascular obstruction. The use of pursed-lips breathing is noted, and the skin is inspected for diaphoresis, cyanosis, swelling, nodules, lesions, bruises, scars, and abnormal superficial venous patterns that may be signs of vascular or cardiac disorders. In dark-skinned clients, cyanosis is difficult to assess and may appear as a gray rather than blue color. Cyanosis is best observed in dark-skinned clients in the conjunctivae, lips, palms, and soles of the feet. The fingers are inspected for tobacco stains or evidence of clubbing (an increase in the angle between the base of the nail and the fingernail to 180 degrees or more, usually accompanied by an increase in the depth, bulk, and sponginess of the end of the finger).

When inspecting the posterior part of the chest, the nurse has the client lean forward. This position moves the scapula away from the spine, so there is more exposure of the area to be examined. The same sequence of observations are performed. In addition, any spinal curvature is noted. Common abnormalities of the spine that can affect breathing include kyphosis, scoliosis, and kyphoscoliosis.

PALPATION. The nurse determines tracheal position by gently placing the index fingers on either side of the trachea just above the suprasternal notch and gently pressing back-ward. Normal tracheal position is midline; deviation to the left or right is abnormal. The mobility of the trachea is noted. Tracheal deviation occurs with pneumothorax (toward the collapsed lung), pneumonectomy (toward the surgical side), and lobar atelectasis (toward the collapsed lobe).

The nurse determines symmetry of chest movement or expansion at the level of the diaphragm. The nurse places the hands over the lower anterior chest wall and moves them inward until the thumbs meet at midline. "Extra" skin should be raised between the thumbs to allow for easy movement when the client inhales. The client is asked to breathe deeply to determine equality and extent of movement. The space between the thumbs on inspiration is a rough measurement of expansion. Normal expansion is 1 inch. To determine movement of the lower lobes on the posterior part of the chest, the nurse places the hands under the axillae and moves the thumbs until they meet over the spine (Fig. 19-10).

Normal chest movement is equal. Unequal expansion occurs when air entry is limited by conditions involving the lung (e.g., atelectasis, pneumothorax), the chest wall (e.g., incisional pain), or the pleura (e.g., pleural effusion). Equal but diminished expansion occurs in conditions that produce a hyperinflated or barrel chest or in neuromuscular disease (e.g., amyotrophic lateral sclerosis, spinal cord lesions).[11] Movement may be absent or unequal over a pleural effusion, atelectasis, or pneumothorax.

Tactile fremitus is vibration of the vocal cords on phonation. To elicit this, the nurse places the palms or the ulnar surfaces of the hands against the client's chest and asks the client to repeat a phrase such as "ninety-nine." The nurses moves the hands from side to side from either top to bottom or bottom to top of the chest. All areas of the anterior and posterior parts of the chest are palpated, and

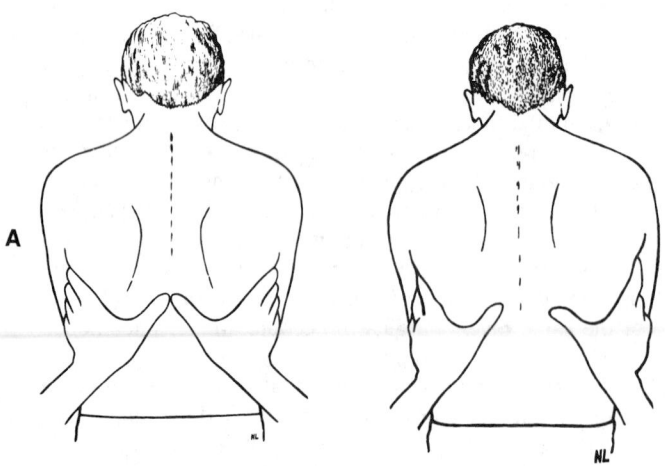

Fig. 19-10 Estimation of thoracic expansion. **A,** Exhalation. **B,** Maximal inhalation. (From Wilkins RL and others: Clinical assessment in respiratory care, ed 2, St Louis, 1990, Mosby–Year Book, Inc, p 63.)

Table 19-4 Percussion Sounds

Sound	Description
Resonance	Low-pitched sound heard over normal lungs
Hyperresonance	Loud, lower-pitched sound than normal resonance heard over hyperinflated lungs, such as in chronic obstructive lung disease and acute asthma
Tympany	Drumlike, loud, empty quality heard over gas-filled stomach or intestine or pneumothorax
Dull	Medium-intensity pitch and duration heard over areas of "mixed" solid and lung tissue, such as over the top area of the liver, partially consolidated lung tissue (pneumonia), or fluid-filled pleural space
Flat	Soft, high-pitched sound of short duration heard over very dense tissue where air is not present

vibrations from similar areas are compared. Tactile fremitus is most intense in the first and second interspace lateral to the sternum and between the scapulae because these areas are closest to the major bronchi. Fremitus is less intense farther away from these areas.[12]

Increase, decrease, or absence of fremitus should be noted. Increased fremitus occurs when the lung becomes filled with fluid or more dense. This is noted in pneumonia, above a pleural effusion (the lung is compressed upward), and over a tumor. Fremitus is decreased if the nurse's hand is farther from the lung or the lung is hyperinflated. This is noted over a pleural effusion, in pneumothorax, and in barrel chest. Absent fremitus may be present with lung tumors and atelectasis. The anterior chest is more difficult to palpate for fremitus due to the presence of large muscles and breast tissue.

Rhonchal fremitus is a palpable vibration caused by air traveling past thick mucus. It can be felt with the hand on the chest and may change or clear with coughing.

PERCUSSION. Percussion is done to assess density or aeration of the lungs. Percussion sounds are described in Table 19-4. (The technique for percussion is described in Chapter 3.)

The anterior part of the chest is usually percussed with the client in a semisitting or supine position. Starting below the clavicles, the nurse percusses downward, interspace by interspace. The entire thorax should be resonant, with the exception of the area of cardiac dullness (Fig. 19-11). For percussion of the posterior chest, the client should sit leaning forward with the arms folded. Percussion should begin across the top of the shoulder to identify the apices of the lungs and progress from side to side. The entire posterior chest should be resonant to the level of the diaphragm.

Diaphragmatic excursion (the amount of downward movement of the diaphragm with a full inspiration following a full expiration) may be assessed by percussion. The client is instructed to breathe normally while the nurse percusses down the back. When the percussion note changes from resonance to dullness, the location is noted. The client is asked to inspire and hold a breath. Starting at the previous area of dullness, the nurse percusses down until dullness is again noted. The difference between the two areas of dullness is the diaphragmatic excursion. Normal movement is 3 to 5 cm (1 to 2 inches) or from the level of the tenth to the twelfth rib. The diaphragm moves upward in conditions that increase intra-abdominal pressure (e.g., pregnancy, ascites) and downward in conditions that cause lung hyperinflation (e.g., COPD).

AUSCULTATION. The diaphragm of the stethoscope is used for auscultation because it transmits the higher-pitched sounds more common in respirations. The diaphragm is pressed firmly against the skin to eliminate outside sounds. The client is instructed to breathe slowly and deeply

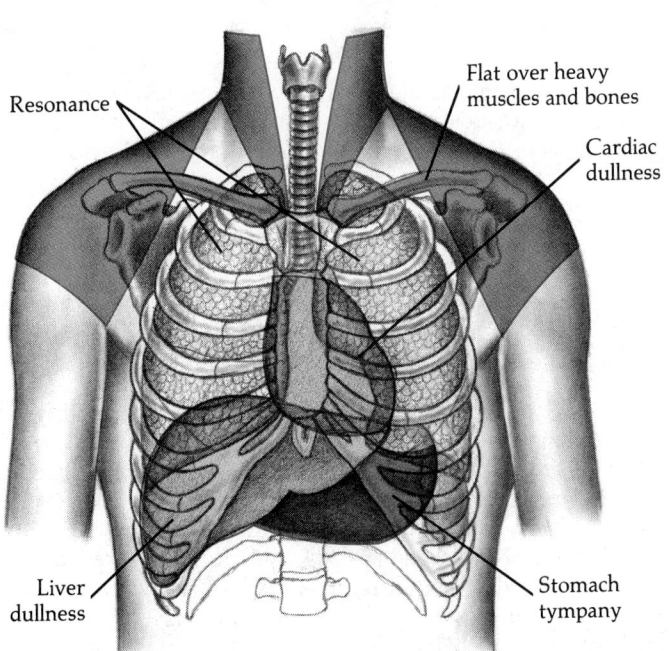

Fig. 19-11 Diagram of percussion areas and sounds in the anterior chest. (Modified from Thompson J and others: Clinical nursing, ed 2, St Louis, 1990, Mosby–Year Book, Inc, p 139.)

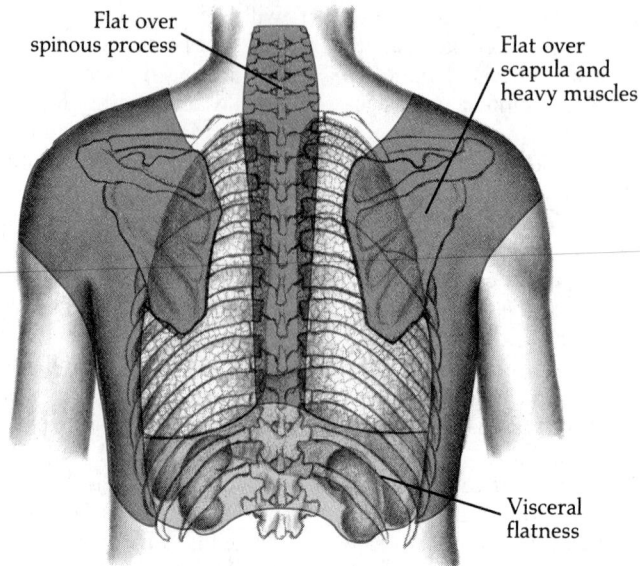

Flat over
spinous process

Flat over
scapula and
heavy muscles

Visceral
flatness

Fig. 19-12   Diagram of auscultation areas in the posterior chest. Auscultation may proceed from the lung bases to the apices or vice versa, comparing opposite areas of the chest. (Modified from Thompson J and others: Clinical nursing, ed 2, St Louis, 1989, The CV Mosby Co, p 139.)

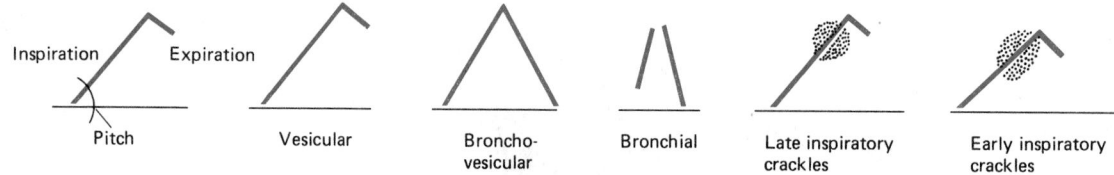

Inspiration   Expiration

Pitch   Vesicular   Broncho-vesicular   Bronchial   Late inspiratory crackles   Early inspiratory crackles

Fig. 19-13   Diagrammatic model of breath sounds. Inspiration is shown by the upstroke and expiration by the downstroke. Vesicular sounds have a 3:1 ratio, with inspiration lasting longer than expiration. Bronchovesicular sounds have a 1:1 ratio, with inspiration and expiration equal in duration, and bronchial sounds have a 2:3 ratio, with a gap between inspiration and expiration. Fine and coarse crackles are typically heard at points marked by the dots.

through the mouth. The sequence and positioning of percussion is also used in this procedure (Fig. 19-12). At each placement of the stethoscope, the nurse listens to one respiratory cycle of inspiration and expiration and notes the pitch (e.g., high, low), intensity, duration, and the presence of adventitious and abnormal sounds. Normal and adventitious sounds are more easily identified by visualization of a diagrammatic model (Fig. 19-13).

There are three normal breath sounds: *vesicular, bronchovesicular,* and *bronchial.* Vesicular sounds are relatively soft, low-pitched, gentle, rustling sounds. They are heard over all lung areas except the major bronchi. Bronchovesicular sounds have a medium pitch and intensity and are heard anteriorly over the mainstem bronchi on either side of the sternum and posteriorly between the scapulae. Inspiration is equal to expiration. Bronchial sounds are louder and higher-pitched and resemble air blowing through a hollow pipe. There is a gap between inspiration and expiration, reflecting the short pause between these respiratory cycles. Bronchial sounds are heard over the manubrium.

The term *abnormal breath sounds* is used to describe bronchial or bronchovesicular sounds heard in the peripheral lung fields. Adventitious sounds include *crackles (rales), rhonchi, wheezes,* and *pleural friction rubs.* Table 19-5 describes these sounds and gives possible etiologies.

Table 19-5

Common Assessment Abnormalities of the Thorax and Lungs

Finding	Description	Possible Etiology and Significance*
INSPECTION		
Inspiratory flaring of nares	Outward movement of nares on inspiration in an attempt to increase air intake	Severe respiratory distress
Use of accessory muscles, tripod position	Leaning forward on arms and elbows and active use of neck and shoulder muscles to assist breathing	Moderate-to-severe respiratory distress, COPD, asthma
Intercostal retractions	Pulling of muscles between ribs, indicating obstruction to free inflow of air	Possible airway obstruction (if sudden onset), COPD in exacerbation, asthma in exacerbation
Intercostal bulging	Outward protrusion of spaces between ribs	Forced expiration in COPD, asthma; tension pneumothorax; massive pleural effusion
Pursed lips on exhalation	Exhalation through mouth with lips pursed together to slow exhalation	COPD, asthma
Splinting	Rigid holding of chest to avoid increasing pain when breathing	Recent thoracic or abdominal incision, chest trauma, pleurisy
Pectus excavatum	Depression of lower end of sternum	Congenital
Pectus carinatum	Forward projection of sternum	Congenital
Increased anteroposterior diameter	Chest abnormally wide from front to back, ribs nearly horizontal rather than normal 45-degree slope	COPD, asthma, cystic fibrosis
Kyphosis	Convex curvature of thoracic spine	Degenerative osteoarthritis (aging); chronic steroid administration; tuberculous osteomyelitis (Pott's disease)
Scoliosis	Lateral curvature of spine	Poor posture, uneven leg length, idiopathic
Kyphoscoliosis	Combination of kyphosis and scoliosis resulting in compression of one lung and overdistention of the other	Tuberculous osteomyelitis (Pott's disease), congenital cause, idiopathic
PALPATION		
Altered chest movement	Unequal or equal but diminished movement of two sides of chest with respiration	Unequal movement caused by atelectasis, pneumothorax, pleural effusion; Equal, but diminished movement caused by barrel chest, restrictive disease
Altered tactile fremitus	Increase or decrease in vibrations	Decrease in pleural effusion, pneumothorax; increase in pneumonia, atelectasis
PERCUSSION		
Hyperresonance	Loud, lower-pitched sound over areas that normally produce a resonant sound	Lung hyperinflation (COPD), lung collapse (pneumothorax)
Dullness	Medium-pitched sound over areas that normally produce a resonant sound	Pneumonia, pleural effusion, large area of atelectasis

*Limited to common etiological factors. (Further discussion of conditions listed may be found in Chapters 21 to 23.)

Continued.

Table 19-5

Common Assessement Abnormalities of the Thorax and Lungs—cont'd

Findings	Description	Possible Etiology and Signifance
AUSCULTATION		
Fine crackles	Series of short, explosive, high-pitched sounds heard just before the end of inspiration; result of rapid equalization of gas pressure when collapsed alveoli or terminal bronchioles suddenly snap open; similar sound to that made by rolling hair between fingers just behind ear	Interstitial fibrosis (asbestosis), interstitial edema (early pulmonary edema), alveolar filling (pneumonia), loss of lung volume (atelectasis)
Coarse crackles	Series of short, low-pitched sounds caused by air passing through airway intermittently occluded by mucus, unstable bronchial wall, or fold of mucosa; evident on inspiration and, at times, expiration; similar sound to blowing through straw under water; increase in bubbling quality with more fluid	Congestive heart failure, pulmonary edema, pneumonia with severe congestion, COPD
Rhonchi	Continuous rumbling, snoring, or rattling sounds due to obstruction of large airways with secretions; most prominent on expiration; change often evident after coughing or suctioning	COPD, cystic fibrosis, pneumonia
Wheezes	Continuous high-pitched squeaking sound caused by rapid vibration of bronchial walls; first evident on expiration but possibly evident on inspiration as obstruction of airway increases; possibly audible without stethoscope	Bronchospasm (caused by asthma), airway obstruction (caused by foreign body, tumor)
Stridor	Continuous musical sound of constant pitch; result of partial obstruction of larynx or trachea	Croup, epiglottitis, vocal cord edema after extubation, foreign body
Absent breath sounds	No sound evident over entire lung or area of lung	Pleural effusion, mainstem bronchi obstruction, large atelectasis
Pleural friction rub	Creaking or grating sound due to roughened, inflamed surfaces of the pleura rubbing together; evident during inspiration and expiration and no change with coughing; usually uncomfortable, especially on deep inspiration	Pleurisy, pneumonia, pulmonary infarct
Bronchophony, whispered pectoriloquy	Spoken or whispered syllable more distinct than normal on auscultation	Pneumonia
Egophony	Spoken "e" similar to "a" on auscultation, due to altered transmission of voice sounds	Pneumonia, pleural effusion

*Limited to common etiological factors. (Further discussion of conditions listed may be found in Chapter 21 to 23.)

A record of the normal physical assessment of the respiratory system is shown in Table 19-6. Common assessment abnormalities are presented in Table 19-5. Age-related changes in the respiratory system and differences in assessment findings are presented in Table 19-7.

DIAGNOSTIC STUDIES
Blood Studies

Common blood studies used to assess the respiratory system are the hemoglobin (Hb or Hgb), hematocrit (Hct), and ABG determinations (see Tables 19-1 and 19-2). Other studies that may be done include electrolyte and enzyme analyses. Table 19-8 describes nursing responsibilities associated with these tests.

Oximetry

Oximetry is used to noninvasively monitor SaO_2 and SvO_2 (see Tables 19-1 and 19-2). Nursing care associated with this monitoring is discussed in Table 19-8 (see also Chapter 21).

Sputum Studies

Single sputum specimens are examined for culture and sensitivity and for cytological assessment. Appropriate antibiotic therapy is determined by analysis of organisms grown from the culture. A 24-hour specimen is used to test

for tuberculous bacilli. Nursing responsibilities for collection of these specimens are given in Table 19-8. Regardless of whether specimens are ordered, it is important to observe the sputum for color, hemoptysis, volume, and viscosity.

Table 19-6 Normal Physical Assessment of the Respiratory System

Nose is symmetrical with no deformities. Nasal mucosa is pink and moist with no edema, exudate, or blood. Nasal septum is straight, without perforations. No polyps are evident. Oral mucosa is light pink and moist, with no exudate or ulcerations. Tonsils are present and not inflamed or enlarged. Pharynx is smooth, moist, and pink. Neck is symmetrical and trachea is in the midline. No nodes are palpable. Chest has a normal configuration, with no evidence of injury. Respirations are normal, at the rate of 14/min. Excursion is equal bilaterally, with no increase in tactile fremitus. Percussion is resonant throughout. Breath sounds are normal throughout, without crackles, rhonchi, or wheezes. No axillary nodes are palpable.

Table 19-7

 Age-Related Changes of the Respiratory System and Differences in Assessment Findings

Changes	Differences in Assessment Findings
PHARYNX AND LARYNX	
Muscle atrophy, slackening of vocal cords, loss of elasticity of laryngeal muscles and cartilages	Soft voice and more difficult to understand, rise in pitch
TRACHEA	
Upper dorsal scoliosis	Tracheal deviation
CHEST WALL, RIB CAGE, AND RESPIRATORY MUSCLES	
Atrophy of respiratory muscles, progressive kyphosis, more rigid rib cage, calcification of costal margins, flattening of diaphragm, osteoporosis	Increased anteroposterior diameter and barrel chest appearance, possible alteration of thoracic anatomical landmarks, reduced chest movement and respiratory excursion, decreased cough effectiveness, increased work of breathing, less tolerance for exercise and stress, distant breath sounds
LUNGS	
Loss of lung elasticity (decreased elastic recoil), enlargement of bronchioles and alveolar ducts, decrease in number of alveoli, increase in diameter of alveoli	Decreased vital capacity, tidal volume, inspiratory and expiratory reserve volume; increased residual and functional residual volume; hyperresonance on percussion; decreased breath sounds
Atrophy of epithelium and reduced ciliary movement in lower airways	Ineffective cough, slowed cough reflex
Thickening of alveolar membrane and decreased capillary network; increase in residual volume, leading to less efficient oxygen–carbon dioxide exchange	Progressive decrease in PaO_2 to approximately 70-85 mm Hg, decrease in oxygen saturation

Table 19-8

Diagnostic Studies of the Respiratory System

Study	Description and Purpose	Nursing Responsibility
BLOOD STUDIES		
Hemoglobin	This test reflects amount of hemoglobin available for combination with oxygen. Venous blood is used. *Normal level* for adult male is 13-16 g/dl; *normal level* for adult female is 12-14 g/dl.	Explain procedure and its purpose.
Hematocrit	This test reflects ratio of red blood cells to plasma. Increased hematocrit (polycythemia) found in chronic hypoxia. Venous blood is used. *Normal* for adult man is 42%-50%; *normal* for adult woman is 40%-48%.	Explain procedure and its purpose.
ABG	Arterial blood is obtained through puncture of radial or femoral artery or through arterial line. This test is performed to assess need for oxygen therapy, change in oxygen therapy or change in ventilator settings.*	Indicate whether client is using oxygen (percentage, L/min). Avoid change in oxygen therapy or interventions (e.g., suctioning, position change) for 20 minutes before obtaining sample. Cleanse skin with alcohol swab and assist with positioning (palm up, wrist slightly hyperextended). Collect blood into heparinized syringe. To ensure accurate results, expel all air bubbles, sheath needle, and place sample in ice, unless it will be analyzed in less than 1 minute. Apply pressure to artery for 5 minutes or longer if client has clotting disorder.
Oximetry	This test monitors arterial or venous oxygen saturation. Device attaches to the earlobe, finger, forehead, or nose for Sao_2 monitoring or is contained in a pulmonary artery catheter for $S\bar{v}o_2$ monitoring. This study is used for continuous monitoring in ICUs, inpatient and outpatient settings, and exercise testing.*	Apply monitoring probe to finger, earlobe, bridge of nose, or forehead. Record values at ordered intervals; institute changes as needed if values are not within expected range.
SPUTUM STUDIES		
Culture and sensitivity	Single sputum specimen is collected in a sterile container. Purpose is to diagnose bacterial infection and to select effective antibiotic. Specimen may also be collected to evaluate treatment.	Collect specimen to be cultured before giving antibiotics, unless purpose is to evaluate treatment.
Gram stain	Staining of sputum permits classification of bacteria into gram-negative and gram-positive types. The results guide therapy until culture and sensitivity results are obtained.	Instruct client to expectorate sputum into the container after coughing deeply. Obtain sputum (mucoidlike), not saliva. Obtain specimen in early morning because secretions collect during night. If unsuccessful, try increasing oral fluid intake unless fluids are restricted. Also collect sputum in sterile container (sputum trap) during suctioning or by aspirating secretions from the trachea. Send specimen to laboratory promptly.

*For normal values, see Table 19-1.
†Also known as ventilation/perfusion ($\dot{V}/\dot{Q}$). See Fig. 19-15.
‡See Fig. 19-16.

Table 19-8

Diagnostic Studies of the Respiratory System—cont'd

Study	Description and Purpose	Nursing Responsibility
SPUTUM STUDIES—cont'd		
Acid-fast stain	This test is performed to collect sputum for acid-fast bacilli (tuberculosis). Typical time for collection is 3 days.	Instruct client in importance of saving all sputum. Cover all sputum specimens. Remove container when specimen is obtained or when container is full. Replace with fresh container to decrease spread of infection and maintain esthetics.
Cytology	Single sputum specimen is collected in special container with fixative solution. Purpose is to determine presence of abnormal cells that may indicate malignant condition.	Send specimen to laboratory promptly.
RADIOLOGY		
Chest x-ray study	This test is used to screen, diagnose, and evaluate change. Most common views are posteroanterior and lateral.	Instruct client to undress to waist, put on gown, and remove any metal between neck and waist. Stay out of range of or shielded from radiation.
Computerized axial tomography	This test is performed for diagnosis of lesions difficult to assess by conventional x-ray studies, such as those in the hilum and mediastinum. Images obtained show body structures in cross-section.	Same as for chest x-ray study.
Lung scan†	This test used to identify areas of the lung not receiving airflow (ventilation) or blood flow (perfusion). It involves injection of radioisotope and inhalation of small amount of radioactive gas (xenon). A γ-detecting device is used to record radioactivity. Ventilation without perfusion suggests pulmonary embolus.	Same as for chest x-ray study. Also check for dye allergy. Know that no precautions are needed afterward because the gas and isotope transmit radioactivity for only a brief interval.
Pulmonary angiogram	This study is used to visualize pulmonary vasculature and locate obstruction or pathological conditions such as pulmonary embolus. A radiopaque dye is injected, usually through a catheter, into the pulmonary artery or right side of the heart.	Same as for chest x-ray study. Know that dye injection may cause flushing, warm sensation, and cough. Apply pressure dressing to injection site after procedure. Monitor blood pressure, pulse rate, and circulation distal to injection site closely. Report and record significant changes.
ENDOSCOPIC EXAMINATIONS		
Bronchoscopy	This study is typically performed in pulmonary procedure room. Flexible fiberoptic scope is used for diagnosis, biopsy, specimen collection, or assessment of changes. It may also be done to suction mucous plugs or to remove foreign objects.	Instruct client to be on NPO status for 6-12 hours.‡ Obtain signed permit. Give diazepam if ordered by physician before procedure to aid relaxation. After procedure, keep client NPO until gag reflex returns and monitor for laryngeal edema. If biopsy was done, monitor for hemorrhage and pneumothorax.
Mediastinoscopy	This test is used for inspection and biopsy of lymph nodes in mediastinal area.	Prepare client for surgical intervention. Obtain signed permit. Afterward, monitor as for bronchoscopy.

Continued.

Table 19-8

Diagnostic Studies of the Respiratory System—cont'd		
Study	**Description and Purpose**	**Nursing Responsibility**
BIOPSY		
Lung biopsy§	Specimens may be obtained by transbronchial, percutaneous, or open-lung biopsy. This test is used to obtain specimens for laboratory analysis.	Same as bronchoscopy if procedure done with bronchoscope; same as thoracentesis if done percutaneously; and same as thoracotomy if open-lung biopsy done.‖ Obtain signed permit.
OTHER		
Thoracentesis	This test is used to obtain specimen of pleural fluid for diagnosis, to remove pleural fluid, or to instill medication. The physician inserts a large-bore needle through the chest wall into pleural space. Chest x-ray film is always obtained after procedure to check for pneumothorax and other changes.‖	Explain procedure to client and obtain signed permit before procedure. Position client upright, instruct not to talk or cough, and assist physician during procedure. Apply dressing after procedure. Observe for signs of pneumothorax after procedure. If large volume of fluid is removed, monitor for decrease in shortness of breath. Send labeled specimens to laboratory.
Pulmonary function tests	This test is used to evaluate lung function. It involves use of a spirometer to diagram air movement as client performs prescribed respiratory maneuvers.¶	Avoid scheduling immediately after mealtime. Explain procedure to client. Provide rest after the procedure.

§See Fig. 19-17.
‖See Chapter 21.
¶For normal values, see Tables 19-10 and 19-11.

Table 19-9   Skin Tests Used in Respiratory Disorders

Test	Purpose and Description
Purified protein derivative (PPD)	Positive result indicates that client's immune system has reacted to tubercle bacillus. The results do not differentiate between active and dormant infections. The test involves intradermal injection of 0.1 ml of intermediate-strength purified protein derivative into inner aspect of the forearm. Test is read 48-72 hr after injection. Results are interpreted as follows: *Positive reaction:* 10 mm or more of induration; interpretation as positive for past or present infection with *Mycobacterium tuberculosis* *Doubtful reaction:* 5-9 mm of induration; probable infection with *M. tuberculosis* for person known to have been in close contact with infectious person (i.e., subject with infectious sputum or person with radiographical or clinical evidence of disease compatible with tuberculosis) *Negative reaction:* 0-4 mm of induration; no repeat test necessary unless evidence of clinical tuberculosis
Coccidioidomycosis test	Positive results indicate active or previous coccidioidomycosis infection. Test involves intradermal injection of coccidioidin or spherulin. It is read at 24-72 hr. Positive findings are reddened area and induration of 5 mm or more. Immediate reaction is nonspecific.
Histoplasmosis test	Positive results indicate active or previous histoplasmosis infection. Test involves intradermal injection of histoplasmin. It is read at 24-48 hr. Positive findings are reddened area and induration of 5 mm or more. Previous histoplasmosis tests may also cause positive reaction.

Skin Tests

In persons who have suspected or diagnosed respiratory disease, skin tests for allergies or for an immune reaction to a fungal or viral disease may be performed. Skin tests involve the intradermal injection of an antigen. A positive reaction is seen as an inflammatory response consisting of redness and induration (a raised, hardened area). Table 19-9 describes commonly used skin tests.

Nursing responsibilities are similar for all skin tests. First, to prevent a false-negative reaction, the nurse should be certain that the injection is intradermal and not subcutaneous. After the injection, the sites should be circled and the client instructed not to remove the marks. When charting administration of the antigen, the nurse should draw a diagram of the forearm and hand and label the injection sites. The diagram is especially helpful when more than one test is administered.

When reading the test results, the nurse should use a good light. If induration is present, a marking pen should be brought in from the periphery on all four sides of the induration. As the pen touches the raised area, a mark should be made. The nurse then determines the diameter of the induration in millimeters. Reddened, flat areas should not be measured.

Radiographic Studies

Chest x-ray examination. A chest x-ray study is probably the most commonly used test for respiratory screening and diagnosis. It is also used to assess progression of disease and response to treatment. The most common views used are the posteroanterior (PA) and lateral. The anteroposterior (AP) view is used when a portable bedside chest x-ray machine is necessary. In a PA view the ray passes from back to front, and in an AP view it passes from front to back. The results of the final product are slightly different. The heart size appears larger in the AP view. (See Table 19-8 for nursing responsibilities related to chest x-ray studies.)

Computerized axial tomography. A computerized axial tomography (CAT) scan is used to examine cross-sections of the entire body. X-ray signals are fed into a computer, which synthesizes them into a plane of the domain. CAT scans are used for evaluating areas difficult to assess by conventional x ray, such as the mediastinum, hilum, and pleura.

Lung scan. A lung scan or ventilation-perfusion ($\dot{V}/\dot{Q}$) scan is used primarily to check for the presence of a pulmonary embolus. There is no specific preparation or aftercare for the procedure. An IV radioisotope is given, and the pulmonary vasculature is outlined and photographed. The client inhales a radioactive gas, which outlines the alveoli, and another photograph is taken. The two photographs of the lung are compared. If areas are ventilated but not perfused, the presence of an embolus should be suspected (Fig. 19-14).

Pulmonary angiography. Pulmonary angiography is used to confirm the diagnosis of an embolus if findings of the lung scan are inconclusive. A series of x-ray films is taken after radiopaque dye is injected into the pulmonary

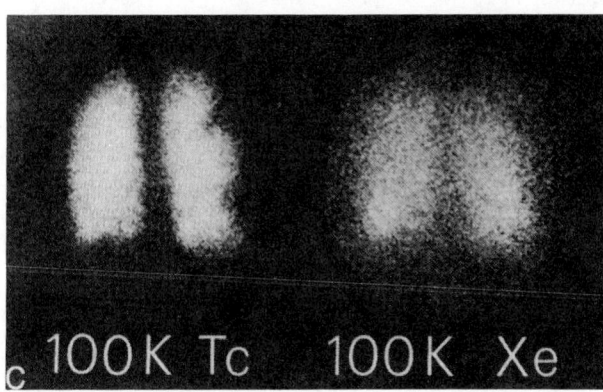

Fig. 19-14 Ventilation-perfusion scan. Normal perfusion image is labeled *100K Tc*. Normal ventilation scan is labeled *100K Xe*. (From Goldhaber SZ: Pulmonary embolism and deep venous thrombosis, Philadelphia, 1985, WB Saunders Co, p 46.)

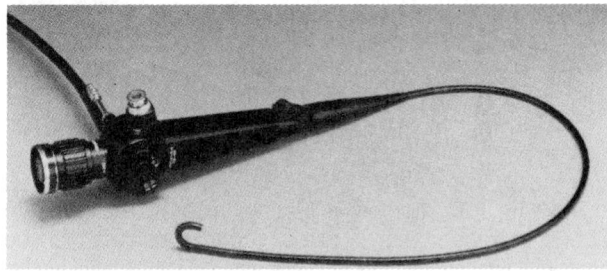

Fig. 19-15 Fiberoptic bronchoscope. (From Pentax Precision Instrument Corp, Orangeburg, NY.)

artery. This test also detects congenital and acquired lesions of the pulmonary vessels.

Endoscopic Examinations

Bronchoscopy. Bronchoscopy is a procedure in which the bronchi are visualized through a fiberoptic tube (Fig. 19-15). It may be used for biopsy specimen collection, assessment of changes due to treatment, and removal of mucous plugs or foreign bodies. The procedure can be performed in a pulmonary procedure room, with the client either lying down or seated. After the nasal pharynx and the oral pharynx have been anesthetized with local anesthetic, the bronchoscope is coated with lidocaine (Xylocaine) and inserted, usually through the nose, and threaded down into the airways. Bronchoscopy can also be done on mechanically ventilated clients. The scope is inserted through the endotracheal tube. The nursing care for this procedure is described in Table 19-8.

Mediastinoscopy. For mediastinoscopy a scope is inserted through a small incision in the suprasternal notch and advanced into the mediastinum. This procedure is used for inspection and biopsy of lymph nodes in the mediastinal area. It is useful in diagnosing carcinoma, granulomatous infections, and sarcoidosis. The procedure is per-

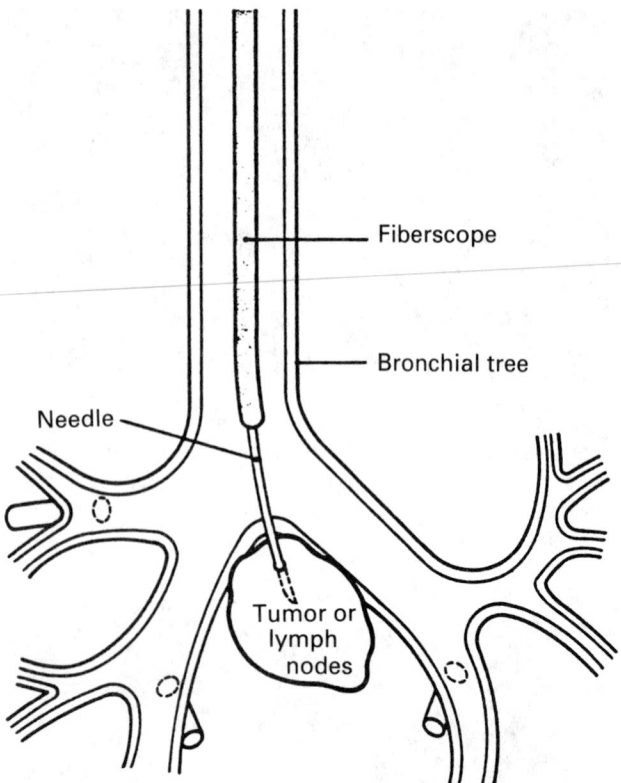

Fig. 19-16 Transbronchial needle biopsy. The diagram shows a transbronchial biopsy needle penetrating the bronchial wall and entering a mass of subcarinal lymph nodes or tumor. (From du Bois RM and Clarke SW: Fiberoptic bronchoscopy in diagnosis and management, New York, 1987, Harper & Row–Gower Medical Publishing, Ltd, p 3.5.)

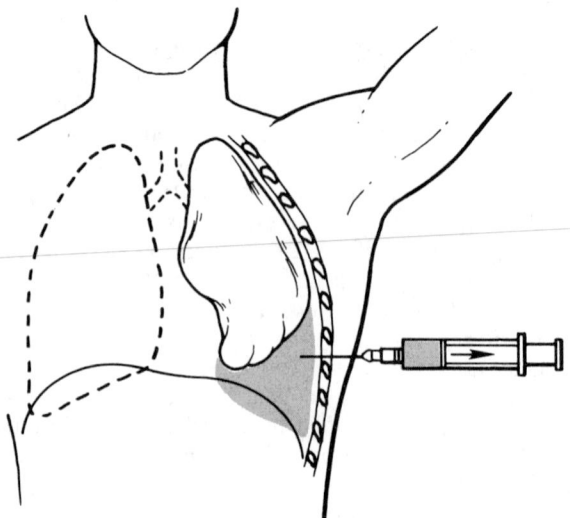

Fig. 19-17 Thoracentesis. The needle has penetrated the fluid-filled pleural space to remove fluid.

formed in the operating room, and the client is given a general anesthetic.

Lung Biopsy

Lung biopsy may be done in one of several ways. The purpose of all techniques is to obtain tissue, cells, or secretions for evaluation.

Transbronchial lung biopsy involves passing a forceps or needle through the bronchoscope. A specimen is obtained with forceps or aspirated through a needle (Fig. 19-16). Specimens can be cultured or examined for malignant cells. A combination of transbronchial lung biopsy and bronchoalveolar lavage (BAL) is used to differentiate infection and rejection in lung transplant recipients and to diagnose AIDS. BAL involves alternately injecting and aspirating small amounts (50 ml) of fluid. Nursing care is the same as for fiberoptic bronchoscopy.

Percutaneous needle biopsy involves aspiration of cells from a lesion through an 18- to 20-gauge needle inserted through the skin. Fluoroscopy is used to guide insertion of the needle.

Open lung biopsy is used when pulmonary disease cannot be diagnosed by other procedures. The client is anes-

thetized, and the chest is opened with a standard thoracotomy incision. The chest wall and lung are inspected and a biopsy specimen is removed. The nursing care for the procedure is the same as for any client who has anesthesia for a surgical procedure. (For detailed nursing care see operative procedures in Chapter 21.) The client may have a chest tube inserted.

Thoracentesis

Thoracentesis is the insertion of a needle through the chest wall into the pleural space to obtain specimens for diagnostic evaluation, remove pleural fluid, and instill medication into the pleural space (Fig. 19-17). The client is positioned upright, usually sitting on a chair and leaning with elbows on the bed or the overbed table. Feet and legs should be well supported. The back and lateral areas of the chest are exposed. The skin is cleansed and prepared at the site of choice. A local anesthetic (1% Xylocaine) is instilled subcutaneously before insertion of the thoracentesis needle. (The nursing care is described in Table 19-8.)

Pulmonary Function Tests

Pulmonary function tests (PFTs) measure lung volumes and airflow. The results of PFTs are used to diagnose pulmonary disease, monitor disease progression, evaluate the extent of disability, and evaluate response to bronchodilators. PFTs are performed with the use of a spirometer, an instrument that measures and diagrams airflow across time.

It is helpful to look at the way airflow and lung volume can be measured to understand PFTs. PFTs involve asking the client to inhale and exhale while various measurements are taken. When a PFT is performed, the client's age, sex, height, and weight are first obtained. This information is entered into a computer. For the test, the client is asked to insert the mouthpiece, to take as deep a breath as possible, and to blow as hard, as fast, and as long as possible. Ver-

Table 19-10 Lung Volumes and Capacities

Parameter	Definition	Normal Values
VOLUMES		
Tidal volume (V_T)	Volume of air inhaled and exhaled with each breath, only a small proportion of total capacity of lungs	0.5 L
Expiratory reserve volume (ERV)	Additional air that can be forcefully exhaled after normal exhalation is complete, no complete emptying of lungs	1.5 L
Residual volume (RV)	Amount of air remaining in lungs after forced expiration, air available in lungs for gas exchange between breaths	1.5 L
Inspiratory reserve volume (IRV)	Maximum volume of air that can be inhaled forcefully after normal inhalation	2.5 L
CAPACITIES		
Total lung capacity (TLC)	Maximum volume of air that lungs can contain (TLC = IRV + V_T + ERV + RV)	6.0 L
Functional residual capacity (FRC)	Volume of air remaining in lungs at end of normal exhalation (FRC = ERV + RV), increase or decrease possible with lung disease	3.0 L
Vital capacity (VC)	Maximum volume of air that can be exhaled after maximum inspiration (VC = IRV + V_T + ERV), higher VC for men (generally)	4.5 L
Inspiratory capacity (IC)	Maximum volume of air that can be inhaled after normal expiration (IC = V_T + IRV)	3.5 L

Table 19-11 Common Measures of Pulmonary Function

Measure	Description	Normal Value*
Forced vital capacity (FVC)	Amount of air that can be quickly and forcefully exhaled after maximum inspiration	Over 80% of predicted
Forced expiratory volume in first second of expiration (FEV_1)	Amount of air exhaled in first second of FVC, valuable clue to severity of airway obstruction	Over 80% of predicted
FEV_1/FVC	Dividing of value for FEV_1 by value for FVC, useful in differentiating obstructive and restrictive pulmonary dysfunction	Over 80% of predicted
Forced midexpiratory flow rate ($FEF_{25\%-75\%}$)	Measurement of airflow rate in middle half of forced expiration, early indicator of disease of small airways	Over 80% of predicted
Maximal voluntary ventilation (MVV)	Deep breathing as rapidly as possible for specified period; test for airflow, muscle strength, coordination, airway resistance; important factor in exercise tolerance	About 170 L/min
Peak expiratory flow rate (PEFR)	Maximum airflow rate during forced expiration, aid in monitoring bronchoconstriction in asthma	Up to 600 L/min
Maximum inspiratory pressure (MIP)	Amount of negative pressure generated on inspiration, indication of ability to breathe deeply and cough	−25 cm H_2O minimum

*Normal values vary with height, weight, age, and sex of client.

bal encouragement is given to ensure that the client continues blowing out until exhalation is complete. The computer determines the actual value, the predicted (normal) value, and the percentage of the predicted value for each test. A normal value is greater than 80% of the predicted value. Normal values for PFTs are shown in Tables 19-10 and 19-11 and in Figs. 19-18 and 19-19.

Interpretation of PFT involves first looking at the forced expiratory volume in the first second of expiration (FEV_1), which tells how much air was expelled in the first second of testing. The percentage predicted should be noted. If this value is greater than 80%, the test is normal. If it is less than 80%, two possibilities may exist: less air than normal entered the lungs or air left the lungs more slowly

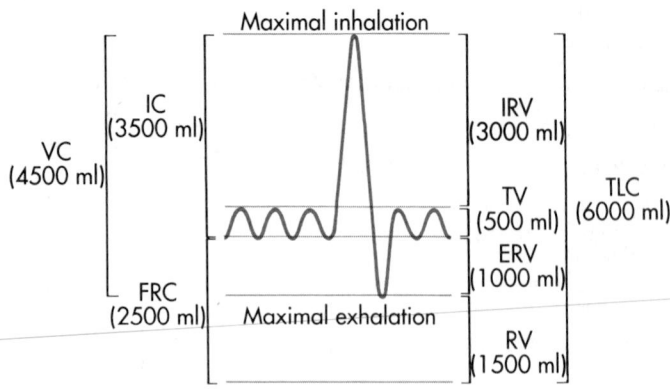

Fig. 19-18 Relationship of lung volumes and capacities.

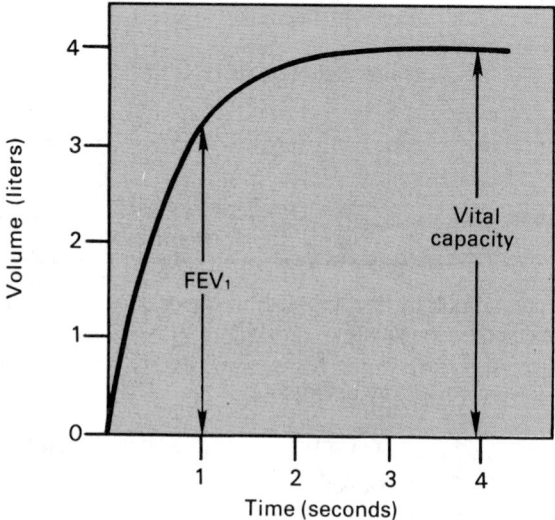

Fig. 19-19 The normal forced expirogram. Volume in the spirometer is plotted against time. The vital capacity *(VC)* is represented by the total volume expired. The *FEV₁* is the volume of air expired during the first second.

than normal. The ratio of FEV_1 to forced vital capacity (FVC) is then checked. This value tells how much air left the lungs in relation to the amount inhaled. The FEV_1/FVC is interpreted as follows: greater than 80%, normal; 60% to 79%, mild airflow obstruction; 40% to 59%, moderate airflow obstruction; and less than 40%, severe airflow obstruction. Clients with severe airflow obstruction commonly have COPD.

Pulmonary function parameters can also be used to determine the need for mechanical ventilation or the readiness to be weaned from ventilatory support. Measurements of vital capacity, negative inspiratory force (NIF), and respiratory rate are used to make this determination (see Chapter 23).

Exercise Testing

Clients who enter a pulmonary rehabilitation program often undergo exercise testing to determine the amount of activity that can be tolerated. Exercise testing is also used in disability evaluations. Measurements are made of maximal oxygen consumption (Vo_{2max}) and other parameters. A complete exercise test involves walking on a treadmill while expired oxygen and carbon dioxide, respiratory rate, heart rate, and rhythm are monitored. A modified test (desaturation test) may also be used. In this case the goal is to determine Sao_2 during exercise.

▢R eview Questions

The number of the question corresponds to the same-numbered objective at the beginning of the chapter.

1. What is the function of surfactant?
   a. It facilitates oxygen transport across the alveolar membrane.
   b. It provides a continuous nutrient supply to the alveoli.
   c. It decreases resistance to expansion and prevents collapse of the alveoli.
   d. It allows air exchange between alveolar sacs.
2. The primary regulators of respirations are
   a. decreased carbon dioxide and increased pH
   b. decreased pH and increased carbon dioxide
   c. decreased oxygen and increased pH
   d. increased oxygen and increased carbon dioxide
3. The partial pressure of oxygen in the atmosphere depends on the
   a. partial pressure of carbon dioxide
   b. barometric pressure
   c. pressures of other gases in the air
   d. moisture in the air
4. The most important respiratory defense mechanism distal to the respiratory bronchioles is the
   a. alveolar macrophage
   b. reflex bronchoconstriction
   c. mucociliary clearance mechanism
   d. impaction of particles
5. A rightward shift of the oxygen-hemoglobin dissociation curve
   a. interferes with release of oxygen at the tissue level
   b. causes oxygen to have a greater affinity for hemoglobin
   c. facilitates release of oxygen at the tissue level
   d. is caused by metabolic alkalosis
6. To determine a client's smoking history in pack-years, the nurse first determines the number of packs smoked per day and the number of years the client smoked. These values are then
   a. divided
   b. subtracted
   c. added
   d. multiplied
7. When auscultating the chest, the nurse should use which part of the stethoscope?

a. diaphragm
b. bell
c. both diaphragm and bell
d. whatever part is preferred

8. Which of the following is the normal percussion sound for examination of the lungs?
   a. dull
   b. flat
   c. resonant
   d. tympany

9. Which of the following nursing measures related to ABG collection is not accurate?
   a. Stabilize the client for 20 minutes before the procedure on the ordered oxygen flow.
   b. Collect blood in a heparinized syringe.
   c. Place the specimen immediately on ice after it is withdrawn.
   d. Apply pressure to the puncture site for 1 minute.

10. The amount of air left in the lungs after a forced exhalation is called the
    a. dead space volume
    b. functional residual volume
    c. residual volume
    d. expiratory reserve volume

REFERENCES

1. Thibodeau G and Anthony CP: Structure and function of the body, ed 8, St Louis, 1988, The CV Mosby Co, pp 337-354.
2. Price S and Wilson L: Pathophysiology: clinical concepts of disease processes, ed 3, New York, 1986, McGraw-Hill Book Co.
3. West JB: Respiratory physiology: the essentials, ed 3, Baltimore, 1985, Williams & Wilkins, pp 1-30.
4. Martin L: Pulmonary physiology in clinical practice: the essentials for patient care and evaluation, St Louis, 1987, The CV Mosby Co, pp 112-128.
5. Lindell KO and Wesmiller SW: Using arterial blood gases to interpret acid-base balance, Orthop Nurs 8:31-34, 1989.
6. Schroeder CH: Pulse oximetry: a nursing care plan, Crit Care Nurs 8:50-68, 1988.
7. Hardy GR: SvO_2 continuous monitoring techniques, Dimens Crit Care Nurs 7:8-17, 1988.
8. Wilkins RL, Sheldon RL, and Krider SJ: Clinical assessment in respiratory care, St Louis, 1986, The CV Mosby Co, pp 43-86.
9. Kersten LD: Comprehensive respiratory nursing: a decision-making approach, Philadelphia, 1989, WB Saunders Co, pp 181-211, 252-335.
10. Freedberg PD, Hoffman LA, and Cagno JA: Physical examination of the chest, Philadelphia, 1988, WB Saunders Co.
11. Hoffman LA: Ineffective airway clearance related to neuromuscular dysfunction, Nurs Clin North Am 22:151-166, 1987.
12. Seidel HM and others: Mosby's guide to physical examination, St Louis, 1987, The CV Mosby Co, pp 245-275.

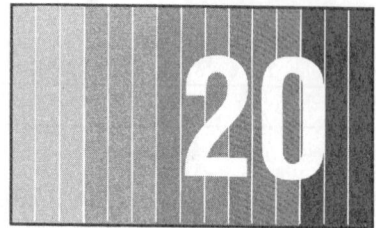

CHAPTER

20

Nursing Role in Management

Upper Respiratory Problems

Jan D. Manzetti
Leslie A. Hoffman

L earning Objectives

1. Describe the clinical manifestations and nursing management of problems of the nose.
2. Describe the clinical manifestations and nursing management of problems of the paranasal sinuses.
3. Describe the clinical manifestations and nursing management of inflammatory problems of the pharynx and larynx.
4. Discuss the nursing management of a client requiring endotracheal intubation or a tracheostomy.
5. Identify steps involved in suctioning an airway and performing tracheostomy care.
6. Describe the risk factors and warning symptoms associated with oral cancer and cancer of the larynx.
7. Discuss the nursing management of the client with a laryngectomy.
8. Describe methods used in voice restoration for clients with temporary or permanent loss of speech.

The structures that make up the upper respiratory tract are the nose, paranasal sinuses, pharynx, larynx, and trachea. During the process of breathing these structures are subject to repeated exposure to microorganisms, fumes, gases, and carcinogens. For this reason, disorders involving the upper respiratory tract are very common.

STRUCTURAL AND TRAUMATIC DISORDERS OF THE NOSE
Deviated Septum

Deviated septum occurs as a result of nasal trauma, thumb-sucking, nose-picking, or congenital factors. Deviation causes the septum to protrude into the air passage of one nostril, obstructing air entry. On inspection, the septum is bent to one side with the air passage reduced. Minor septal deviations cause no symptoms. Major deviations may cause postnasal discharge, sinusitis, facial pain (due to sinus obstruction or infection), cosmetic deformity, or nosebleeds. Discomfort from nasal obstruction is variable and is not always related to the amount of nasal blockage.

A *submucous resection* (SMR) or a *septoplasty* may be

performed to surgically correct the deformity when major symptoms or discomfort occur. If a septoplasty is performed, the deviated septum is reconstructed, aligned, and straightened with minimal cartilage and bone removal. An SMR involves removal of the deviated section of cartilage and bone. Although an SMR typically results in a better airway, clients can experience deformities later if excessive tissue is removed. Complications are rare. Meningitis can occur if either surgical procedure is performed when the client has a nasal or sinus infection.

Nursing management is similar to that for rhinoplasty (see p. 467). Health promotion is aimed at prevention of precipitating factors, such as accidental falls sustained in childhood.

Nasal Fracture

Nasal fracture is most often caused by trauma sustained as a result of an athletic injury. Complications of the fracture are airway obstruction and cosmetic deformity. The type of fracture can be classified as *unilateral, bilateral,* or *complex.* A unilateral fracture typically produces little or no displacement. Bilateral fractures, the most common, give the nose a flattened look. Powerful frontal blows cause complex fractures, which may also shatter frontal bones. Diagnosis of nasal fracture is based on client his-

---

Reviewed by Regina M. Maibusch, R.N., M.S., Respiratory Clinical Nurse Specialist, St. Michael Hospital, Milwaukee, Wisconsin.

464

tory, direct observation of internal and external nasal structures, and x-ray findings.

On inspection, the client's nose may be deviated to one side or depressed, with epistaxis and a positive history of trauma. The nurse should note the presence of edema or hematoma and the ability to breathe through each side of the nose. The nose is inspected internally for septal deviation, hemorrhage, and leakage of cerebrospinal fluid. If clear drainage is observed, a test for glucose is performed. A positive reaction for glucose indicates that the nasal discharge is cerebrospinal fluid. Injury of sufficient force to fracture nasal bones causes considerable swelling of soft tissues. With extensive swelling, it may be difficult or impossible to verify the presence of a fracture or deformity until reexamination several days after the injury when edema is subsiding.

Ice may be gently applied to the face and nose to reduce edema and bleeding. When a fracture is confirmed, the goal of therapeutic management is to reduce the fracture by open or closed reduction. This will reestablish the cosmetic appearance and proper function of the nose and provide an adequate airway.

The goals of nursing management are reduction of edema, prevention of complications, client education, and emotional support. If the injury cannot be reduced, open reduction (septoplasty or rhinoplasty) may be required.

Rhinoplasty

Rhinoplasty is surgical reconstruction of the nose. It is performed to improve airway function when trauma or developmental deformities result in nasal obstruction or when desired for aesthetic reasons.[1]

Assessment of expectations is a critical aspect of the client's preparation for rhinoplasty. Body image is multidimensional and includes the self-perception of the body as a physical, psychological, and social entity. For this reason any actual or perceived alteration, such as a deformed or enlarged nose, can affect self-esteem and interactions with others. The client's expectations concerning the results of surgery should be assessed with regard to expected physical, psychological, and social change. Photographs made to precise life-size measurements can be prepared to simulate the client's probable appearance after reconstruction.[2] Use of these photographs may help clients decide whether to undergo rhinoplasty. Expected results of surgery should be explained frankly and truthfully to avoid disappointment.

Procedure. Rhinoplasty is performed with the use of regional anesthesia. The entire nose is anesthetized by injection of lidocaine at points that block involved nerve pathways and thus pain transmission. Lidocaine is not injected directly into the operative area so that distortion of the nasal bridge or the tip of the nose is prevented. The client is given preoperative sedation and additional sedation in the operating room just before the lidocaine injection. Incisions are made internally and externally. Tissue may be added or removed, and the nose may be lengthened or shortened. A variety of plastic prosthetic implants may be used to reshape the nose. Postoperatively, Steri-Strips are placed to hold the skin against the septal carti-

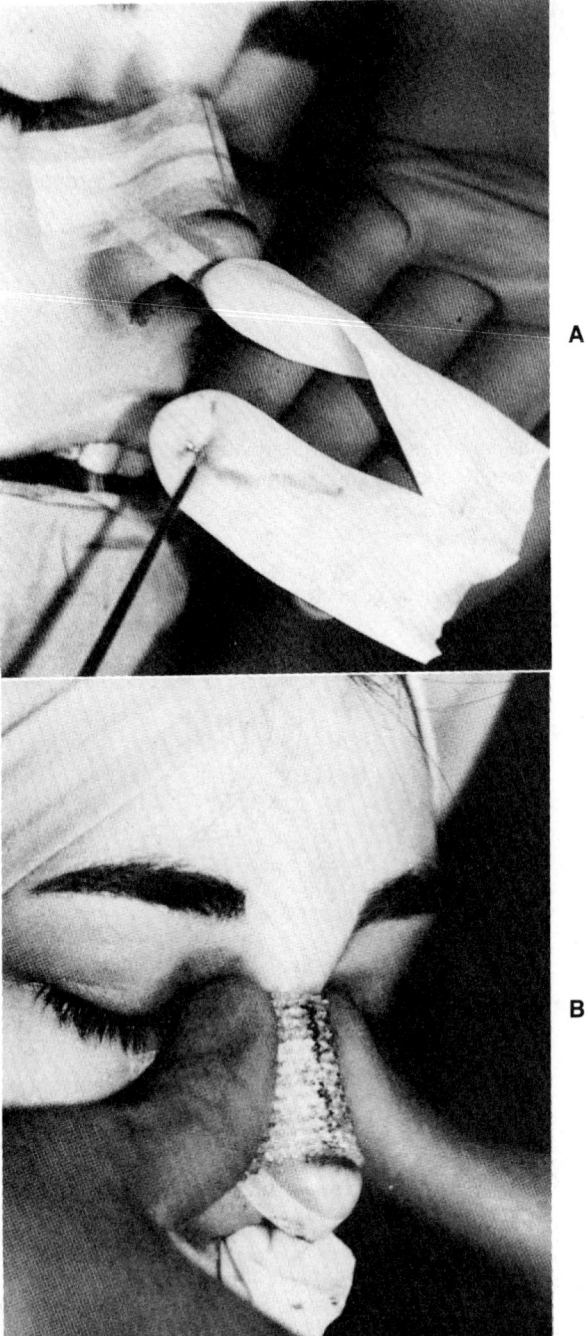

Fig. 20-1 Basic rhinoplasty dressing. **A,** Application of tape. **B,** Molding of a plastic splint . (From McKinney P and Cunningham BL: Rhinoplasty, New York, 1989, Churchill Livingstone, p 66.)

lage, and a drain is inserted to divert bleeding and prevent crusting in the incisional area. One technique uses trimmed fingers of a surgical glove as the drain (Fig. 20-1). A plastic splint is molded to the new shape of the nose. The drain is removed on the day after surgery. The splint is removed in 3 to 5 days, depending on the amount of edema.

Table 20-1

NURSING CARE PLAN FOR THE CLIENT WITH A RHINOPLASTY

Defining Characteristics	Nursing Interventions	Evaluation Criteria

NURSING DIAGNOSIS: Altered health maintenance related to lack of knowledge of postoperative course, pain management, and prevention of complications

Questioning about care, anxiety	Explain surgical procedure, expected postoperative course, and required self-care. Answer questions as needed.	Verbalization of information about expected routine and self-care

NURSING DIAGNOSIS: Ineffective airway clearance related to presence of packing, nasal edema, and mouth breathing

Abnormal respiratory rate, rhythm, or depth; snoring sound during inspiration	Check rate and character of respirations q 4 hr for 24 hr. Instruct client to not blow nose, to sneeze with mouth open, to avoid coughing, and to use mouth breathing.	Normal respiratory rate, rhythm, and depth; successful adaptation to mouth breathing
Mucosal swelling, ecchymosis	Instruct client to maintain semi-Fowler's position and bed rest with bathroom privileges for 24 hr and to minimize facial movement for 48 hr (excessive body or face movement may promote increase in facial edema). Apply 4 × 4 inch pads dipped in ice water to incisional area prn. Avoid excessive pressure on surgical area.	Minimal to no swelling or bruising

NURSING DIAGNOSIS: Potential complication: nasal hemorrhage related to surgical hemorrhage

Hypotension, tachycardia; continued drainage of serosanguineous fluid from operative site	Check blood pressure, pulse rate q 4 hr for 24 hr. Give no aspirin or aspirin-containing drugs. Note correct placement of exterior dressing. Change dressing prn. Report to physician any fresh bleeding or displacement of the drain.*	Stable vital signs, no bleeding

NURSING DIAGNOSIS: Pain related to incisional edema, dry mucous membranes, or inadequate comfort measures

Report of pain, facial mask of pain, dry mucous membranes	Describe to client the amount of pain expected. Include client in planning rest periods. Administer analgesics and teach client to apply iced 4 × 4 inch pads prn. Teach client gentle cleaning techniques (e.g., use of Q-tips and water-soluble jelly or hydrogen peroxide when drain has been removed).	Report of minimal or no pain; satisfaction with pain control; moist, intact mucous membranes

NURSING DIAGNOSIS: Body-image disturbance related to postoperative edema and changed facial appearance

Verbalization of concern about appearance, anxiety	Inform client that most facial edema subsides gradually over a period of 1 month. (It may take up to 8 months for all edema to subside.) Help client to remain realistic regarding surgical results.	Report of client feeling less anxious and optimistic about positive surgical outcome

*See Fig. 20-1.

■ Nursing Management of Rhinoplasty

To reduce the risk of bleeding, clients should be instructed to refrain from taking aspirin or aspirin-containing drugs for 2 weeks before surgery. Nursing diagnoses specific to the client undergoing a rhinoplasty include, but are not limited to, those presented in Table 20-1. Nursing intervention during the postoperative period includes assessment of respiratory status and observation of the surgical site for hemorrhage, edema, and discoloration. Interventions are directed toward pain control, reduction of edema, and prevention of infection. The outcome of rhinoplasty is most often satisfactory and pleasing to the client. The client's self-esteem may be enhanced as a result of the cosmetic change.

Epistaxis

Epistaxis (nosebleed) occurs as a result of bleeding from a rich network of veins in the nares, most commonly originating from Kiesselbach's plexus in the anterior part of the nose. Causes of epistaxis include external trauma, nose picking (usually termed idiopathic), hypertension, tumor growth, blood dyscrasias, and inflammation. Most nosebleeds can be stopped with first aid measures. First aid interventions are (1) to keep the client quiet; (2) to place the client in a sitting position, leaning forward, or when that is not possible, to place the client in a reclining position with head and shoulders elevated; (3) to apply direct pressure by pressing on the bleeding nostril; (4) to apply cold compresses to the forehead and have the client suck on ice; (5) to partially insert a small gauze pad (not cotton) into the bleeding nostril and again apply pressure (if bleeding continues); and (6) to obtain medical assistance (if bleeding still does not stop).

Therapeutic management. Therapeutic management of epistaxis involves accurate localization of the bleeding site and cauterization or ligation of the problem vessel.[3] In addition, the nose may be packed. Local packing may consist of nasal petrolatum gauze, ribbon gauze that has been soaked in a vasoconstricting solution, or a cotton ball wedged firmly in the desired location (Fig. 20-2). When posterior nasal packing is used, strings attached to the packing are brought to the outside and taped to the cheek for ease of removal. After a postnasal pack is in place, the anterior part of the involved nostril is packed with gauze (Fig. 20-2). Inflatable balloons can also be used as a nasal pack. Antibiotics are typically prescribed to prevent infection.

■ Nursing Management of Epistaxis

If bleeding can be controlled with the use of a vasoconstrictive agent or cauterization, the client can be discharged after being taught about home care. Cauterization produces a crust (scab), which must remain in place until the mucosa has healed. Clients should be instructed to avoid activities that may dislodge the crust, such as blowing the nose, athletic activities, heavy lifting, or bending. When sneezing, the client should open the mouth.

Clients with posterior packing require hospitalization, since the large pack may obstruct the airway. The client should be observed for signs of airway obstruction or more bleeding. Mouth care should be provided, and a call bell should be placed within easy reach. Nasal dryness can be decreased by breathing high humidity oxygen delivered by face tent. A nasal sling (a folded 2 × 2 inch gauze pad) should be taped over the nares to absorb drainage. The nurse reminds the client not to bend over, sneeze, cough,

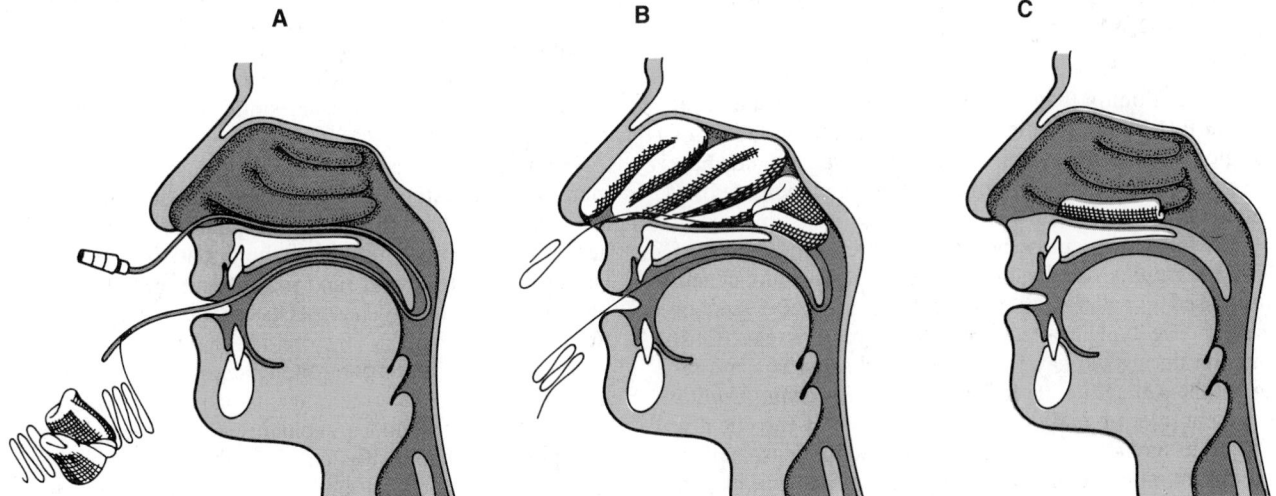

A   **B**   **C**

Fig. 20-2 Method for placing local and postnasal packing. **A,** For a postnasal pack a catheter is passed through the bleeding side of the nose and pulled out through the mouth with a hemostat. Strings are tied to the catheter and the pack is pulled into the mouth and up behind the soft palate into the nasopharynx. **B,** After the postnasal pack is in place, the anterior part of the involved nares is packed with gauze. **C,** For a local pack a small piece of gauze or small cotton ball is wedged in place at the bleeding site. (Modified from DeWeese DD and others: Otolaryngology—head and neck surgery, ed 7, St Louis, 1988, The CV Mosby Co, pp 120-122.)

or blow the nose. The presence of packing is charted. Posterior packs are usually kept in place for 4 to 5 days. Before removal, the packing may be saturated with hydrogen peroxide. After removal of the nasal packing, the nares may be gently cleaned and lubricated with petroleum jelly.

Facial Trauma

Fractures of the maxilla, zygoma, mandible, and nose usually result from severe direct trauma, such as a blow with a fist, a fall, or an automobile accident. Facial injury rarely threatens life, but the consequences of this injury can be life threatening. The skull is similar to a closed box. It is a rigid sphere filled with contents that are noncompressible. Normally, the volume of the skull is constant. If the volume of contents within the skull increases (e.g., from intracranial hemorrhage), intracranial pressure will increase, potentially impairing brain function. For this reason, clients who experience facial trauma should be assessed immediately. General principles applicable for all facial injuries are to (1) ensure an adequate airway, (2) stop the hemorrhage, (3) assess level of consciousness, (4) prevent increasing the injury, and (5) protect the wound. Any obstruction by dentures, vomitus, or broken teeth must be removed promptly. Hemorrhage in the facial area (e.g., the cheek) is usually treated with direct pressure. Impaled foreign bodies should not be removed until medical assistance is available, since removal may cause hemorrhage by removing pressure from an otherwise tamponaded vessel. Assessment of the extent of injury is based on the history, findings on physical assessment, and x-ray examination. Facial fractures are managed by various techniques of open reduction and immobilization. (Fractures of the mandible are discussed in Chapter 34).

INFLAMMATION AND INFECTION OF THE NOSE AND PARANASAL SINUSES
Allergic Rhinitis

Allergic rhinitis (hay fever) is the reaction of the nasal mucosa to a specific antigen (allergen). Manifestations of allergic rhinitis are nasal obstruction (due to edema), sneezing, itching and tearing of the eyes, and increased secretion of mucus.[4]

Two forms are seen, seasonal and perennial. Attacks of *seasonal rhinitis* usually occur in the spring and fall and are caused by allergy to pollens from trees, flowers, or grasses. The typical attack lasts for several weeks (most common during the hay fever season), disappears, and recurs at the same time the following year. *Perennial rhinitis* is present intermittently or constantly. Usually the client is allergic to environmental contacts such as pollens, molds, house dust mites, animal epithelia such as feathers, or particular foods. Since symptoms of perennial rhinitis resemble those of the common cold, clients may believe they have continuous or repeated "colds."

Allergic rhinitis is usually mediated by IgE antibody fixed to the surface of mast cells in the tissues lining the respiratory tract (Fig. 8-5). When an allergen diffuses across the mucous membrane, there is a resultant release of substances, including histamine, bradykinin, serotonin, prostaglandins, eosinophil chemotactic factor, and leuko-

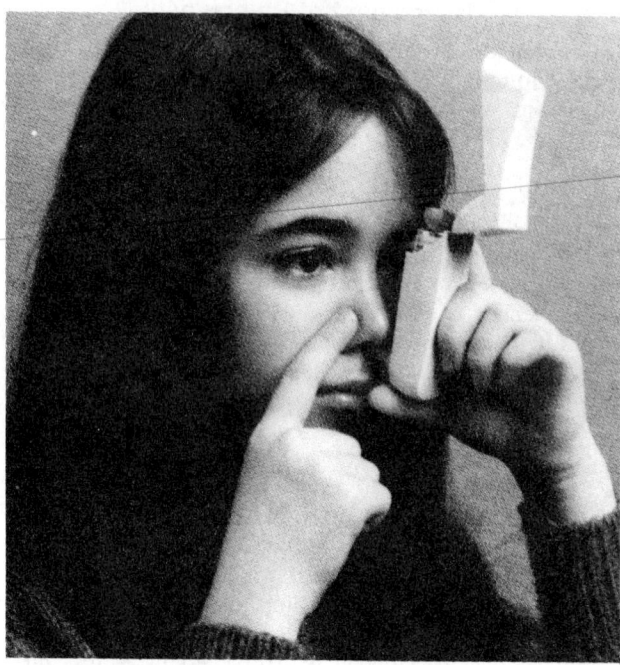

Fig. 20-3 Use of an inhaler to administer nasally inhaled steroids. (Courtesy Allen Hansburys, Division of Glaxo, Inc.)

trienes (Table 8-9). Some of these substances increase capillary permeability, whereas others cause erythema, bronchoconstriction, and swelling of the nasal mucosa.

Clinical manifestations. The client may have coldlike symptoms, including nasal congestion, paroxysmal sneezing, itching, and clear, watery secretions. The nasal turbinates will appear pale, boggy, and swollen. The turbinates may fill the air space and press against the nasal septum. The posterior ends of the turbinates can become so enlarged that they obstruct sinus aeration or drainage, resulting in sinusitis.

With chronic exposure to allergens, responses include increased congestion, a sensation of pressure, and postnasal drip. The client may also complain of cough, hoarseness, or recurrent need to clear the throat. Congestion may be sufficient to cause snoring. Nasal polyps may be present if the allergy has persisted for a long period of time.

Therapeutic management. Diagnostic studies include allergy testing to determine agents causing the allergic reaction. Therapy includes avoidance of antigens, immunotherapy (see Chapter 8), and drug therapy. Drug therapy may involve the use of antihistamines, decongestants, nasally inhaled cromolyn, or nasally inhaled steroids (Fig. 20-3). Typically, an antihistamine or decongestant is used first. If this therapy is not effective, steroids or cromolyn may be used.

■ Nursing Management of Allergic Rhinitis

Clients receiving drug therapy need careful instructions about proper use (Table 20-2). Antihistamines cause vasoconstriction and decreased capillary permeability. How-

Table 20-2 Drug Therapy for Allergic Rhinitis

Preparation*	Mechanisms of Action	Side Effects	Nursing Actions
ANTIHISTAMINES			
Chlorpheniramine (Comtrex, Triaminic), diphenhydramine (Benadryl), astemizole (Hismanal), terfenadine (Seldane)	Competitive inhibitors of histamine; result in vasoconstriction and decreased capillary permeability	Drowsiness, headache, fatigue, dry mouth, central nervous system agitation; less drowsiness with non-sedating antihistamines (astemizole, terfenadine)	Warn client that operating machinery and driving may be dangerous because of sedative effect. Explain that CNS effect can be potentiated by use of depressants, alcohol, hypnotics, and antianxiety agents.
DECONGESTANTS **Inhaled long acting**			
Oxymetaxoline (Dristan long-lasting spray), xylometazoline (4-Way long-acting spray) **Oral** Pseudoephedrine (Actifed, Sine-Aid), phenylephrine (Dimetapp, Dristan), phenylpropanolamine (Alka-Seltzer Plus)	Stimulation of α receptors of adrenergic nervous system, causing vasoconstriction of nasal arterioles and decreased turbinate swelling	Rhinitis medicamentosa (rebound nasal congestion), occasional hypertensive reactions	Advise client of adverse reactions. Teach that these drugs should not be used for more than 3 days or more than 3 or 4 times per day. Teach client to discard inhalers when no longer needed and to not allow another person to use the same applicator. Advise that some preparations are contraindicated for clients with hypertension, diabetes mellitus, or thyroid disease.
CORTICOSTEROIDS **Inhaled**			
Beclomethasone (Vancenase-AQ, Beconase-AQ), flunisolide (Nasalide)	Reduction of nasal edema by direct action of inhaled steroid on nasal mucosa†	Sneezing, nasal bleeding, dryness and stinging; minimal of systemic absorption with use of nasal route	Advise client to clear nostril before inhaling drug and to inhale through nose. Teach client to report viral, bacterial, and sinus infections. Tell client to report any conditions that develop (client may need to discontinue steroids because they suppress immune response and may potentiate infection).
MAST CELL INHIBITOR			
Cromolyn sodium (Nasalcrom)	Inhibition of release of chemical mediators from mast cells, preventing allergic reaction; initial treatment before allergy season begins	Sneezing, nasal stinging, burning	Advise client to clear nostril before inhaling spray and to inhale through nose. Teach client that drug prevents but does not reverse symptoms after they develop. For seasonal rhinitis, teach client to administer before expected contact and use 3 or 4 times a day until exposure ends. For perennial rhinitis, teach that treatment may be required for 3 to 4 weeks before drug begins to be effective.

*Partial listing of available medications.
†See Fig. 20-3.

ever, the client may experience drowsiness as a side effect. If this occurs, a nonsedating antihistamine (terfenadine [Seldane], astemizole [Hismanal]) can be substituted. Decongestant sprays may be effective initially in decreasing congestion. However, they cause marked vasoconstriction of the arterioles of the nasal mucosa, have no effect on nasal response to the antigen, and should not be used for more than 3 days. If their use is prolonged, clients may experience *rhinitis medicamentosa* (rebound nasal congestion). Vessels initially constrict and then dilate, causing chronic nasal obstruction. This outcome may cause the client to use more of the drug with less effect.

If decongestants are prescribed, clients should be taught appropriate precautions. Inhaled steroids should not be used if a nasal infection is present. Because nasal cromolyn prevents but does not relieve symptoms, administration must begin before exposure to allergens. Best relief is often obtained with the combination of an intranasal corticosteroid with a nonsedating antihistamine. The nurse should also teach the client about ways to prevent or reduce exposure to allergens.[5] Examples include removal of down-filled pillows, diligent dusting and vacuuming, and removal of pets from the home. Immunotherapy is most effective against symptoms caused by pollen. However, it may also reduce symptoms caused by other allergens (see Chapter 8).

Acute Viral Rhinitis

Acute viral rhinitis (common cold or acute coryza) is caused by viruses that invade the upper respiratory tract. It is the most prevalent infectious disease. Common causative agents are rhinoviruses, respiratory syncytial virus, and adenoviruses.[6] These organisms are spread by airborne droplet sprays emitted by the infected person while breathing, talking, sneezing, and coughing, or by direct hand contact.

Colds occur frequently because of multiple infections with many antigenically unrelated viruses. Frequency increases in the winter months, when staying indoors and overcrowding are more common. Other factors, such as chilling, fatigue, physical and emotional stress, and the immune status of the client, may increase susceptibility.

The client with acute viral rhinitis has a group of symptoms that includes rhinorrhea, sneezing, nasal congestion, sore throat, lethargy, and fatigue. Knowledge of the symptom complex that is "going around" and the client's history of recent exposure to the contaminant are the usual methods of diagnosis. The client is contagious during the first 3 days. The cold is self-limiting within 2 to 14 days.[7]

Therapeutic management. Rest, fluids, proper diet, isolation, antipyretics, and analgesics are recommended. Complications include pharyngitis, sinusitis, otitis media, tonsillitis, and chest infections. Unless symptoms of these complications are present, antibiotic therapy is not indicated. Antibiotics have no effect on viruses and, if taken injudiciously, may produce resistant organisms.

■ Nursing Management of Acute Viral Rhinitis

During the cold season, clients with chronic illnesses or compromised immune status should be advised to avoid crowded, close situations and persons with obvious cold symptoms. The nurse should recommend that the client get adequate rest. If the client cannot avoid contact with a person who has a cold, frequent hand washing may prevent contamination through direct spread.

Nursing diagnoses specific to the client with an upper respiratory infection include, but are not limited to, those presented in Table 20-3. Interventions are directed toward relieving annoying symptoms, promoting comfort, and instructing the client in prevention of secondary bacterial invasion. The client should be encouraged to take increased amounts of fluids, which serve to liquefy secretions in the lungs, ensure hydration, and compensate for evaporative loss due to fever. Antihistamine-decongestant therapy reduces postnasal drip and significantly decreases the severity of cough, nasal obstruction, and nasal discharge.

The client should be taught to recognize the symptoms of secondary bacterial infection, such as a temperature higher than 38° C (100.4° F), exudate on the tongue, tender glands, and a sore, red throat. In clients with pulmonary disease, signs of infection include a change in sputum from mucoid to purulent. Because infection can progress rapidly, many clients with chronic respiratory disease are taught to inspect their sputum and to begin a 10- to 14-day course of antibiotic therapy on their own if this change occurs. Clients with pulmonary disease who have not been taught to begin antibiotics should call their physician if they notice a change in sputum character.

Influenza

Influenza (flu) is an acute, contagious viral infection of the respiratory tract. About 48 million cases of influenza occur in the United States every winter, accounting for about 3.9 million hospitalizations and 20,000 deaths. Many persons who contract influenza are under 5 or over 65 years of age or have chronic cardiac or pulmonary disease. Influenza virus has a remarkable ability to change over time, which accounts for its ability to cause widespread illness. Minor changes in the virus, called *antigenic drifts,* develop each winter. Because the change is minor, most clients will have some previous immunity. Major changes, called *antigenic shifts,* occur every 10 to 30 years. Few clients will have immunity to these changes and pandemics may occur. Influenza virus occurs in three strains—A, B, and C. Subtypes are named by the strain, site of isolation, and year (e.g., A/Taiwan/89).

Influenza is spread by direct or indirect contact with small-particle droplets generated during coughing. These aerosols remain suspended in the air for hours. Only one infectious unit (presumably one virus) is required to infect a susceptible person.

Clinical manifestations. The onset of flu is typically abrupt with respiratory symptoms of a dry cough, sore throat, sneezing, and watery nasal discharge usually lasting 3 to 7 days. Systemic symptoms, including headache, fatigue, chills, anorexia, muscle aches, and prostration, last 2 to 4 days. Recovery may require 2 to 3 weeks. The convalescent phase may be marked by hyperreactive airways and a chronic cough. Factors that are most important in making a diagnosis of the flu are the client's history,

Table 20-3

 NURSING CARE PLAN FOR THE CLIENT WITH UPPER RESPIRATORY INFECTIONS

Defining Characteristics	Nursing Interventions	Evaluation Criteria

NURSING DIAGNOSIS: **Altered respiratory function related to mucosal edema, excessive secretion production, airway irritability, and cough**

Cough, tachypnea, increased nasal and respiratory secretions, inability to tolerate breathing of cold air	Check rate and character of respirations q 4 hr for 24 hr to detect respiratory distress. Humidify air as needed. Encourage intake of fluids. Administer antihistamine-decongestant prn. Administer throat lozenges or antitussive prn. Instruct client to place a scarf or mask over the nose and mouth when breathing cold air.	Cough decreased or absent, normal respiratory rate, normal secretion production

NURSING DIAGNOSIS: **High risk for ineffective thermoregulation related to infection**

Temperature greater than 38° C (100.4° F), chills, diaphoresis	Check temperature q 4 hr. Give antipyretic medications prn. Use cooling sponge bath or alcohol rub prn. Keep client dry and lightly covered to avoid chilling. Reduce room temperature. Encourage increased fluid intake. Monitor intake and output.	Temperature less than or equal to 38° C, absence of chills and diaphoresis, adequate state of hydration

NURSING DIAGNOSIS: **Activity intolerance related to physical discomfort, fatigue, and inadequate comfort measures**

Complaints of aches, pains; sense of weakness	Encourage bed rest or reduction of physical activity. Give analgesics (e.g., aspirin, acetaminophen) prn.	Absence of aches, pain, fatigue

NURSING DIAGNOSIS: **Potential complication: viral/bacterial pneumonitis**

Acute respiratory distress with marked dyspnea, hypoxemia, diffuse crackles, purulent sputum; tongue exudate; tender glands; red, sore throat	Instruct client about proper diet, rest, and activity. Teach client to report symptoms that do not resolve, such as increase in fever, dyspnea, or secretion production, tender glands, tongue exudate. Administer antibiotics as prescribed if bacterial infection develops.	Normal white blood cell count; absence of fever, dyspnea, or sputum production; normal respiratory rate, rhythm, and depth; no evidence of sore throat, tender glands, tongue exudate

Continued.

clinical findings, and knowledge of other cases of influenza in the community.

Although most clients recover with no ill effects, some experience complications. The main complications of flu include tracheobronchitis, viral pneumonia, and bacterial pneumonia. Tracheobronchitis may persist for up to 3 weeks but is not a serious health risk. Viral pneumonia typically develops within 48 hours of the onset of influenza and may be fatal. Persons who have a preexisting pulmonary disease or cardiac valvular disease are particularly predisposed. Bacterial pneumonia may occur in older adults and those with cardiopulmonary disease, but it also affects otherwise healthy adults. Manifestations include a "relapse" 1 to 4 days after convalescence from influenza, a productive cough, and evidence of pneumonia on a radiograph of the chest. On rare occasions, extrapulmonary complications involve the heart and liver. Because of this risk for complications, clients should be cautioned against continuing an aerobic exercise schedule when they are ill with the flu.

Table 20-3

NURSING CARE PLAN FOR THE CLIENT WITH UPPER RESPIRATORY INFECTIONS—cont'd

Defining Characteristics	Nursing Interventions	Evaluation Criteria
NURSING DIAGNOSIS: Altered health maintenance related to lack of knowledge of measures to prevent cold or influenza		
No annual flu shot, no precautions with regard to exposure to persons with flu or cold symptoms, absence of use of measures to avoid spreading virus	Encourage client to seek yearly influenza immunization in the fall, especially if in a high-risk group.* Instruct client to avoid crowds during cold and influenza season and to avoid contact with persons known to have viral infections. Recommend measures to decrease fatigue and increase hand washing. Advise taking amantadine if in a high-risk group, exposed to flu, and not immunized. Teach importance of balance between rest, activity, and good nutrition.	Yearly flu shot (if indicated), avoidance of crowds and maintenance of balance of rest and activity, frequent hand washing, prescription for amantadine obtained if in a high-risk group and exposed to flu without immunization
NURSING DIAGNOSIS: Self-care deficit related to malaise, fever, and immobility		
Inability to perform part or all of activities of daily living, bedfast	Assess support system. Assist client to make arrangements for assistance during acute phase of illness. Ensure provision of adequate fluids, food, and rest.	Meeting of client's basic needs by others until resumption of ability for self-care

*See Table 20-4.

Table 20-4 Recommendations for Influenza Immunization

HIGHEST PRIORITY

Adults and children with chronic disorders of the cardiopulmonary system that are severe enough to have required regular medical follow-up or hospitalization during the preceding year

Residents of nursing homes or other facilities that care for clients of any age with chronic medical conditions (at least 80% of residents should be immunized)

HIGHER PRIORITY

Physicians, nurses, and other health care personnel who have extensive contact with high-risk clients (e.g., primary care personnel, staff of intensive care units, and neonatal intensive care units)

HIGH PRIORITY

Otherwise healthy persons over the age of 65

Adults and children with chronic metabolic diseases (including diabetes mellitus), renal disease, anemia, immunosuppression, or asthma who have required regular follow-up or hospitalization in preceding year

Modified from Morbid Mortal Weekly Reports 38:297-311 1989.

■ Therapeutic and Nursing Management of Influenza

Nursing diagnoses specific to the client with an influenza include, but are not limited to, those presented in Table 20-3. Most clients with influenza require only symptomatic therapy. Older adults and those who have a chronic illness may require hospitalization. Antibiotics are not indicated unless secondary bacterial infection occurs. The primary goals in nursing management are supportive measures directed toward relief of symptoms and prevention of secondary infection.

Because of the morbidity and mortality associated with influenza, prevention is of utmost importance. Yearly vaccination is the single most important measure for preventing or minimizing influenza symptoms.[8] To be effective, the vaccine must be given in the fall before exposure to the flu virus occurs. The nurse should advocate that high-risk clients receive vaccination during routine office visits or, if hospitalized, at the time of discharge. Those at highest risk are adults and children with chronic cardiovascular or pulmonary problems and residents of nursing homes. High priority should also be given to vaccination of all health care professionals in contact with high-risk clients (Table 20-4). By being vaccinated, the nurse can decrease the risk of transmitting influenza to those with less ability to cope with the effects of this illness. Families of high-risk clients

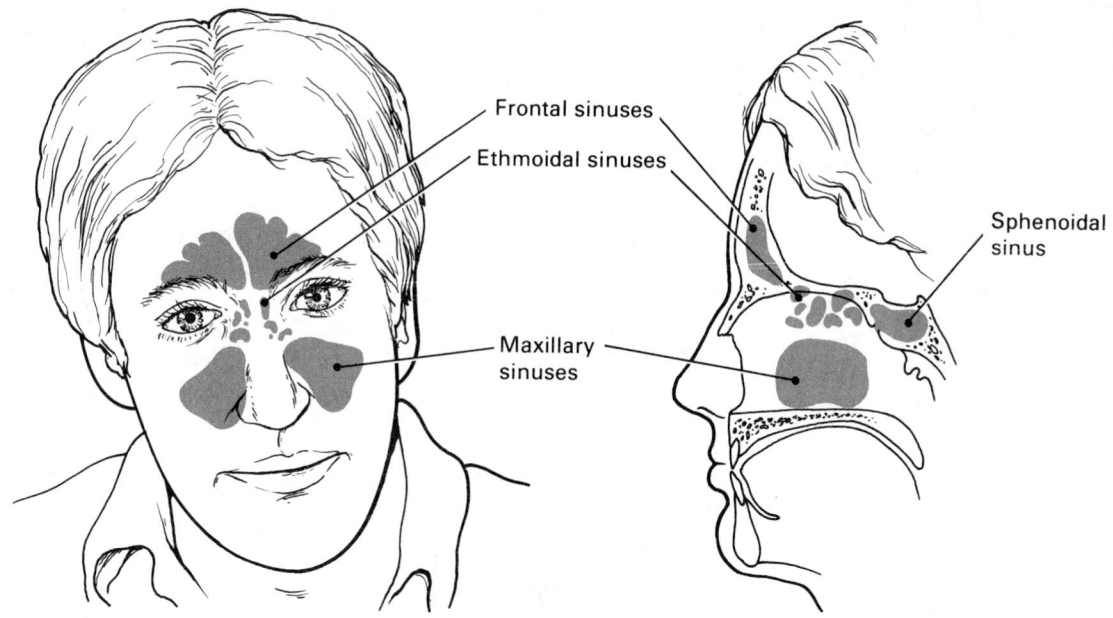

Fig. 20-4 Location of the sinuses.

should also be vaccinated to decrease the client's risk of exposure.

Despite the availability of this simple preventive measure, only about 30% of high-risk clients are vaccinated every year. Many avoid vaccination out of fear of a reaction. Changes in methods of vaccine preparation make this highly unlikely. Since the 1970s, vaccines have been highly purified and reactions are rare. About 5% of those vaccinated experience a low-grade fever, malaise, or myalgia for 8 to 24 hours after vaccination. Since the vaccine is produced in eggs, persons with hypersensitivity to egg protein should not be given influenza vaccine.

Amantadine (Symmetrel) may prevent development of influenza or decrease severity of symptoms if given before or within 48 hours of exposure. The drug is presumed to act by inhibiting virus shedding and must be taken daily for the duration of the outbreak. High-risk clients who are exposed to persons with influenza or who have influenza (with no prior vaccination) may benefit from taking amantadine.

Sinusitis

Acute sinusitis. Acute sinusitis is an inflammation of one or more of the sinus cavities (Fig. 20-4). The most common predisposing factor is a viral infection of the upper respiratory tract, resulting in obstruction of sinus drainage and bacterial invasion. Other causes include rhinitis, a tooth abscess, swimming and diving trauma, and nasal surgery. Predisposing factors include anatomical abnormalities such as a deviated nasal septum and nasal polyps. Because the nasal and sinus mucous membranes are continuous, infections spread rapidly from the nasal passages to the sinuses. Gram-positive cocci (*Streptococcus pneumoniae, Staphylococcus pyogenes,* and *Haemophilus influenzae)* are the most common causative organisms.

Clinical manifestations. Symptoms of acute sinusitis include acute severe pain across the infected sinuses associated with fever and malaise. The client looks and feels sick. Sinus pain is caused by the accumulation of pus and absorption of air behind a blocked ostium. In some instances, location of the pain marks the site of infection. Clients may also experience recurrent headaches that change in intensity with position and disappear after arising after secretions drain.

Major complications are the result of erosion of bone and spread of infection to adjacent structures (e.g., orbital cellulitis, orbital abscess). Severe local pain, headache, vomiting, high fever, shaking chills, and obvious systemic illness suggest the onset of this problem. Urgent admission to the hospital is required for accurate diagnosis.

Physical assessment involves inspection of the nasal mucosa, palpation of the sinus points for pain, and transillumination (shining a bright light in the client's mouth to light the sinus). X-rays of the sinus should also be taken. Findings indicative of acute sinusitis include a hyperemic and edematous mucosa, enlarged turbinates, tenderness over the frontal and maxillary sinuses, and decreased translucency. Normally the sinuses are translucent because they are filled with air. Fluid accumulation interferes with light transmission and decreases translucency. X-ray films may show the sinuses to be opaque (filled with fluid) or partially opaque (filled with air and fluid). Any exudate from the involved sinus should be examined for culture and sensitivity.

■ Therapeutic and Nursing Management of Acute Sinusitis

Nursing diagnoses specific to the client with acute sinusitis include, but are not limited to, those presented in Table 20-5. Therapeutic goals for acute sinusitis are pain

Table 20-5

NURSING CARE PLAN FOR THE CLIENT WITH ACUTE OR CHRONIC SINUSITIS

Defining Characteristics	Nursing Interventions	Evaluation Criteria

NURSING DIAGNOSIS: Pain related to sinus obstruction, inflammation or infection, and inadequate comfort measures

Pain over involved sinuses, infected nasal discharge	Encourage increased fluid intake (8 to 10 glasses of water daily) and use of steam inhalations (15-minute vaporization of boiled water) to promote secretion drainage. Instruct client to maintain semi-Fowler's position (head of bed elevated 30 degrees) to promote sinus drainage. Administer analgesics and vasoconstrictors prn. Teach client proper use of vasoconstrictor medications. Discourage smoking. Administer antibiotics as indicated.	No pain when pressure applied over involved sinus, drainage of secretions, correct technique when using vasoconstrictors, normal temperature

NURSING DIAGNOSIS: Altered nutrition: less than body requirements related to decreased appetite and altered taste sensation

Inadequate food intake, less than recommended daily allowance	Encourage frequent oral hygiene. Provide nutritious, attractive foods.	Usual appetite, maintenance of normal body weight

NURSING DIAGNOSIS: Altered health maintenance related to lack of knowledge of self-care, pain management, and prevention of chronic sinusitis

Anxiety, questioning about care, continued purulent nasal discharge, sinus pain, cough	Instruct client on use of pain and antibiotic medications, local hydration techniques, and nutrition and hydration issues. Answer questions completely about self-care responsibilities. Instruct client to follow interventions for acute sinusitis. Teach client to avoid factors that predispose to exacerbations, such as swimming and diving. If allergy is cause, follow instructions regarding environmental control, drug therapy, and immunotherapy.	Absence of nasal discharge, cough, sinus pressure; accurate description of self-care requirements related to hydration, infection control, pain management

NURSING DIAGNOSIS: High risk for infection related to impaired skin and mucosal integrity

Fever (38° C, 100.4° F)	Check temperature q 4 hr for 24 hr. Administer antibiotics as ordered. Administer mouth care after meals if oral incision present. Monitor white blood cell count. Report any signs of infection to physician.	Absence of inflammation, normal temperature and white blood cell count

NURSING DIAGNOSIS: Pain related to surgical procedure

Report of pain, facial mask of pain	Instruct client to maintain semi-Fowler's position (head of bed elevated 30 degrees) to promote sinus drainage. Place ice bag on operative site. Administer analgesics as needed. Report severe pain to physician because it may indicate infection or inadequate drainage.	Minimal to no pain

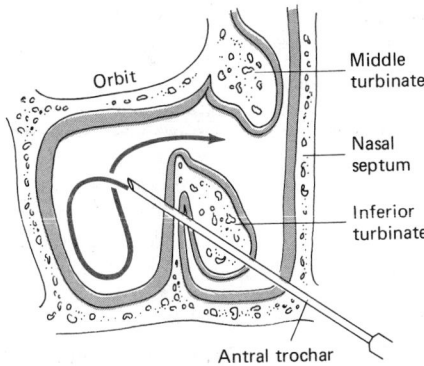

Fig. 20-5 Antral puncture. A trochar is inserted under the inferior turbinate (through the medial wall of the antrum). Contents of the sinus can be washed into the nose through the natural ostium. (From DeWeese DD and others: Otolaryngology—head and neck surgery, ed 7, St Louis, 1988, The CV Mosby Co, p 96.)

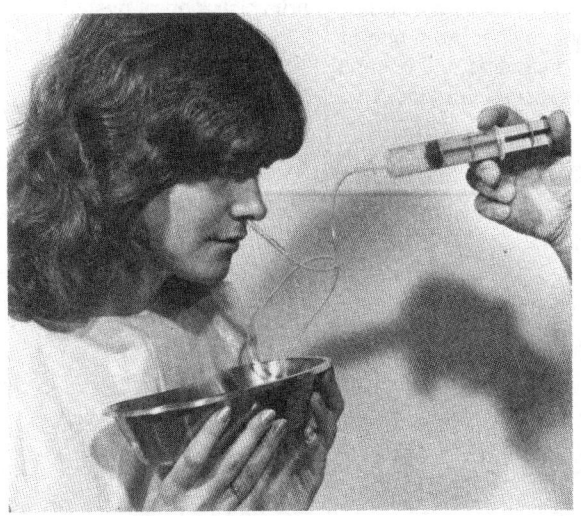

Fig. 20-6 Antral lavage. With the head tipped forward, solution returns through the natural ostium and out the anterior nose for examination and/or culture. (From DeWeese DD and others: Otolaryngology—head and neck surgery, ed 7, St Louis, 1988, The CV Mosby Co, p 96.)

relief, infection control, and promotion of sinus drainage. Vasoconstricting nose drops (e.g., ephedrine 1%) and antibiotics improve natural sinus drainage by reducing mucosal swelling. Analgesics relieve symptoms. In some clients the condition persists as a subacute infection. Most often, operative drainage of sinuses is not done until after the acute infection has subsided, but there are exceptions. When pain remains severe and pus fails to drain, surgery (antral puncture) may be required (Fig. 20-5).

Chronic sinusitis. Chronic sinusitis occurs when no treatment or inadequate treatment is received in the acute or subacute stage or when recurrent bacterial attacks damage the sinus mucosa, causing irreversible tissue damage. Many clients who complain of headaches, nasal obstruction, and tenderness over the sinuses have symptoms

caused by allergies rather than sinusitis. Therefore, a diagnosis is typically not made unless the client has recurrent episodes of acute infection with purulent drainage.

When chronic sinusitis becomes prolonged or complications develop, surgical intervention is indicated. Goals are to remove all diseased tissue and bone, restore drainage, and eradicate the infection. Surgical procedures may involve drainage of the maxillary, frontal, ethmoid, or sphenoid sinuses. Antral puncture and lavage may open the sinus temporarily and remove mucopurulent material (Fig. 20-6). Intranasal antrostomy is a procedure used to create a nasal window to open the sinus and allow pus and other secretions to drain. The Caldwell-Luc radical antrostomy procedure is a more radical type of surgery performed when the maxillary mucosa is irreversibly damaged. An incision is made under the upper lip above the roots of the teeth to enter the maxillary sinus. Diseased mucosa and periosteum are removed. Nursing diagnoses specific to the client with chronic sinusitis include, but are not limited to, those presented in Table 20-5.

OBSTRUCTION OF THE NOSE AND PARANASAL SINUSES
Polyps

Nasal polyps are benign projections of edematous mucous membrane that form slowly in response to repeated swelling of the sinus or nasal mucosa. Allergic rhinitis is the most common predisposing factor. Once nasal polyps are present, they enlarge, partly by growing and partly by swelling from increased edema, until they protrude into the airway or occlude the nose. Polyps are typically classified as *edematous, gray-white, fibrous,* or *vascular.* They may be multiple or bilateral, and they can exceed the size of a grape. Polyps can cause great anxiety for the client who fears they are malignant. Polyps tend to recur if the underlying allergy is not well controlled.

Clinical manifestations are nasal obstruction, nasal discharge (usually clear mucus), and speech distortion. Nasal polyps are removed surgically with a wire snare or forceps after induction of local anesthesia.

Foreign Bodies

Foreign bodies are any objects or substances located in any tissue or body cavity that are foreign to the location in which they are found. Inorganic foreign bodies (e.g., buttons, beads) may cause no symptoms, may lie undetected for weeks, and may be accidentally discovered on routine examination as a calcium deposit called a *rhinolith.* Organic foreign bodies (e.g., wood, cotton, paper) produce a local inflammatory reaction and nasal discharge, which may become purulent and foul smelling. A unilateral, foul-smelling discharge should alert the nurse or the physician to this problem. The client may have no pain.

All foreign bodies should be removed from the nose through the route of entry. Sneezing with the opposite nostril closed may be effective. Sneezing can be elicited by having clients smell pepper. Irrigation of the nose or pushing the object backward should not be attempted, since either could cause airway obstruction and death. If the object cannot be removed by sneezing or blowing the nose, the client should be seen by a physician.

Table 20-6 Common Upper Respiratory Problems Involving the Pharynx

| Organism | Manifestations | | Management |
	Local	Systemic	
VIRAL			
Adenoviruses 4 and 7 ECHO viruses Coxsackie virus	Red, sore throat; dysphagia	Slight fever (38° C)	Symptomatic treatment, including rest, warm gargles, aspirin
BACTERIAL			
Group A *Streptococcus pyogenes*	Tonsillar cover of white or yellow patches, dysphagia	Fever (39° C)	Penicillin, erythromycin, bed rest, increase in fluids
H. influenzae, H. parainfluenzae, C. diphtheriae, C. hemolyticum, S. pneumoniae (rare)	Patchy, nonadherent exudate	Anorexia, malaise, fever (39° C)	Increase in fluids, administration of antipyretics analgesics as needed Measurement of temperature qid
FUNGAL			
Candidiasis	White, irregular patches overlying shallow ulcers; possible lack of symptoms	Cutaneous or disseminated infections, evident with use of inhaled steroids and in immunosuppressed persons	Administration of nystatin
SEXUALLY TRANSMITTED **Gonococcal**			
Neisseria gonorrhoeae	Sore throat, possibly similar symptoms that appear with other conditions causing sore throat	Possible lack of symptoms	Penicillin, tetracycline, probenecid; follow-up cultures after 10 to 14 days of treatment; use of condoms or abstinence until completion of treatment
Herpes			
Herpes simplex virus type I, type II	Punched-out ulcerations, multiple vesicles	Cutaneous or disseminated lesions, erythema of gingivae, excessive salivation, fever	Administration of acyclovir

PROBLEMS RELATED TO THE PHARYNX
Acute Pharyngitis

Acute pharyngitis can be caused by a bacterial, viral, or fungal infection. Acute follicular pharyngitis ("strep throat") results from bacterial invasion by *S. pyogenes.* Such organisms as gonorrhea and herpes simplex can also cause pharyngitis as a result of transmission during orogenital contact. Acquired immunodeficiency syndrome (AIDS) must be considered as a potential diagnosis in any at-risk client who has symptoms of pharyngitis, tonsillitis, and cervical lymphadenopathy. AIDS is characterized by a profound defect in cell-mediated immunity that leads to opportunistic infections. Because of this, normal ability to resist infection is compromised. (Management of the client with AIDS is discussed in Chapter 8.) Symptoms and management of pharyngitis are summarized in Table 20-6.

Clinical manifestations. Symptoms may range in severity from complaints of a "scratchy throat" to pain so severe that swallowing is difficult. The pharynx should be carefully inspected in an effort to determine the cause. In viral infections the throat may appear mildly red with some congestion of blood vessels. In severe strep throat, the throat is typically an intense red-purple with patchy yellow exudate and hypertrophy of lymphoid tissue. If the pharyngitis is due to diphtheria, a gray-white false membrane, termed a *pseudomembrane,* is seen covering the oropharynx, nasopharynx, and laryngopharynx and sometimes extending to the trachea. White irregular patches suggest infection with *Candida albicans.* However, appearance is not always diagnostic. Exudate and involvement of the tonsils may be present in either bacterial or viral infection. Cultures of the pharyngeal mucosa, tonsils, or exudate are done to establish the cause and direct appropriate management. Even with severe infection, the culture may be negative.

■ Therapeutic and Nursing Management of Acute Pharyngitis

The goals of nursing management are infection control, symptomatic relief, and prevention of secondary complications. Because cultures can be negative even when infection is present, clients suspected of having strep throat are often treated with antibiotics. Fungal infections are treated with nystatin, an antifungal antibiotic. The preparation should be held in the mouth as long as possible before it is swallowed. Treatment should continue until symptoms are gone and cultures are negative. Gonorrhea is treated with antibiotics. In addition, rapid epidemiological tracing and compliance with the treatment regimen are essential to prevent further transmission and emergence of antimicrobial-resistant strains.

Nursing interventions include encouraging bed rest, alleviating the sore throat with warm saline gargles and an ice collar, using a steam vaporizor to soothe inflamed mucous membranes, and administering analgesics for pain and antipyretics to reduce fever. The client's temperature should be checked frequently. The client should be encouraged to increase fluid intake and to take cool, bland liquids and gelatin that will not irritate the pharynx. Citrus juices should be avoided, since they irritate the mucous membrane.

Peritonsillar Abscess

Peritonsillar abscess (quinsy) typically occurs as a complication of acute pharyngitis. Bacterial infection results in invasion of one or both tonsils. The tonsils may enlarge sufficiently to threaten airway patency. The client will experience a high fever, leukocytosis, and chills.

After culture and sensitivity testing, treatment consists of antibiotic therapy with penicillin. Early detection and treatment with antibiotics may clear the infection and prevent abscess development. If an abscess develops, antibiotics alone will not clear the infection. Incision and drainage of the infected tonsil or tonsils are required. Once the acute process subsides, the nurse should teach the client careful oral hygiene.

Sleep Apnea Syndrome

Sleep apnea syndrome is a condition in which airflow is temporarily obstructed during sleep.[9] Airflow obstruction occurs when the tongue and the soft palate fall backward and partially or completely obstruct the pharynx (Fig. 20-7). The obstruction may last from 10 seconds to as long as 2 minutes. During the apneic period, the client experiences severe hypoxemia (decreased PaO_2), hypercapnia (increased $PaCO_2$), and acidosis. These changes interrupt sleep and cause the client to partially awaken. When the client begins to awaken, the tone of the muscles of the upper airway increases. The tongue and soft palate move forward and the airway opens. Apnea and arousals occur repeatedly during the night separated by several normal breaths. The cause of sleep apnea is not definitely known. However, three factors appear to be involved: (1) shape of the upper airway, (2) neural control of the respiratory muscles, and (3) hormonal balance. In *obstructive*

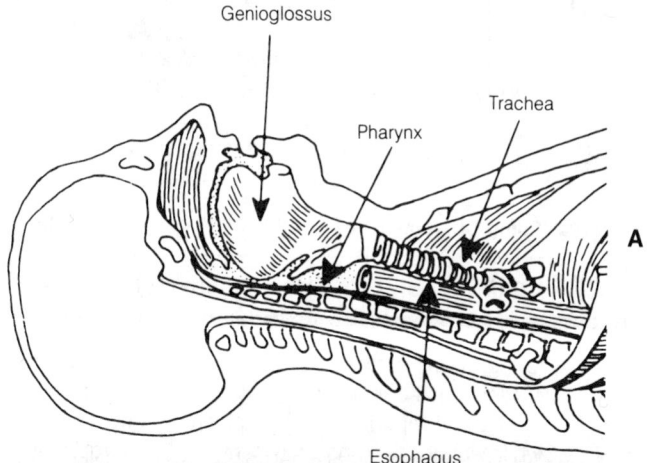

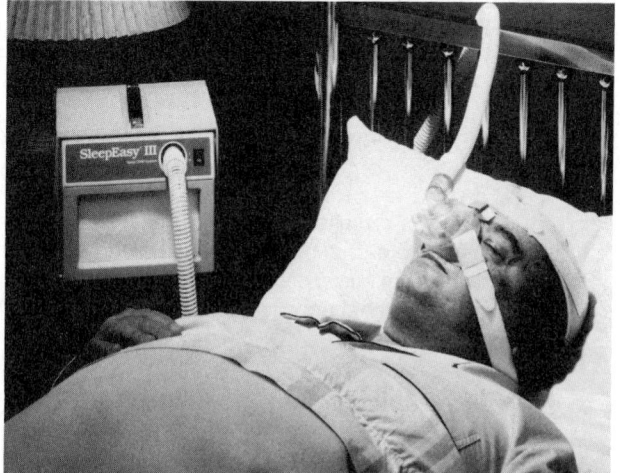

Fig. 20-7 Obstructive sleep apnea. **A,** During sleep, the tongue (genioglossus) falls backward obstructing the airway. Snoring is caused by air moving through the obstructed airway. (From Millman RP and Fishman AP: Sleep apnea syndromes. In Fishman AP, ed: Pulmonary diseases and disorders, vol 2, ed 2, New York, 1988, McGraw-Hill Book Co, p 1349.) **B,** Management of sleep apnea often involves sleeping with a nasal mask in place. The pressure supplied by air coming from the compressor opens the oropharynx and nasopharynx, thereby preventing occlusion of the airway. (Courtesy Respironics, Inc, Monroeville, Penn.)

sleep apnea, respiratory efforts continue despite airflow obstruction. In *central sleep apnea,* respiratory effort and airflow are absent. *Mixed sleep apnea* occurs when there are symptoms of both disorders. Greater than 95% of clients with sleep apnea have obstructive sleep apnea.[10]

Clinical manifestations. Clinical manifestations of sleep apnea include frequent awakening at night, insomnia, and excessive daytime sleepiness. The client's bed partner may complain about loud snoring. The snoring may be so loud that both persons cannot sleep in the same room. Other symptoms include morning headaches (from carbon dioxide retention), personality changes, and irrita-

Table 20-7

 NURSING CARE PLAN FOR THE CLIENT WITH SLEEP APNEA

Defining Characteristics	Nursing Interventions	Evaluation Criteria
NURSING DIAGNOSIS: Sleep pattern disturbance related to inability to sleep normally because of airflow obstruction during sleep		
Snoring; tremors of hands and feet; restlessness during sleep; morning headache; reports of falling asleep while eating, carrying on a conversation, driving	Assist client to recognize that breathing problems may be cause of symptoms. Assess severity of symptoms. Teach client and spouse that problems are result of airflow obstruction and should respond to treatment. Teach need to avoid driving until management is effective.	Recognition of relationship between sleep and breathing problem, seeking of treatment, avoidance of driving until symptoms resolve
NURSING DIAGNOSIS: Self-esteem disturbance related to changes in body image, role performance, and personal identity		
Unwillingness to discuss symptoms, refusal to take part in own care, withdrawal from social contacts, change in usual pattern of responsibility	Assess client's ability to understand and cope with symptoms experienced. Inform client and spouse about support groups. Assess client for symptoms of depression.	Attendance at support groups such as Alert, Well and Keeping Energetic (AWAKE); expression of positive feelings about self
NURSING DIAGNOSIS: Altered nutrition: greater than body requirements related to increased appetite and inadequate exercise		
Inability to regulate caloric intake to reduce, maintain normal weight	Assist client to recognize that obesity is contributing to present illness. Educate client about weight-loss methods.	Initiation of weight-loss program, achievement of weight goal
NURSING DIAGNOSIS: Impaired home maintenance management related to knowledge deficit regarding use of equipment to modify breathing pattern		
Anxiety; questioning about care; noncompliance with use of nasal CPAP; complaints of nasal dryness, burning, congestion; presence of epistaxis, conjunctivitis	Teach client how to apply CPAP device. Instruct client that device will create a positive pressure, which will help to hold airway open during sleep.* Teach that therapy must be used for several weeks to determine effectiveness. Teach client that these symptoms result from dry air blowing into nose and eyes. Instruct client to use room humidifier or humidifier incorporated in airway circuit. For traveling, humidifier can be replaced by use of chin strap. A corticosteroid or saline nasal spray may also be used. Check mask to determine correct fit.	Knowledge of purpose and demonstration of proper use of mask; adherence to plan of care; resolution of conjunctivitis, epistaxis; correct fit of mask

*See Figs. 20-7

bility. Symptoms of sleep apnea may result in impotence. Family life and the client's ability to maintain employment are also often compromised. As a result, the client may experience severe depression. The client should be assessed to determine psychological adjustment, and appropriate referral should be made if problems are identified.

Diagnosis of sleep apnea is made during an overnight sleep study with the use of polysomnography. The client's sleep stages, ventilation, respiratory effort, gas exchange, and heart rate are monitored. A diagnosis of sleep apnea requires documentation of 5 or more apneas per hour or 30 or more apneas per night.

Therapeutic management. Therapeutic management may involve use of (1) general measures such as weight loss and avoidance of alcohol, (2) drugs that stimulate the respiratory system (e.g., medroxyprogesterone) or reduce daytime drowsiness (e.g., protriptylline), (3) positive pressure applied to the nasopharynx, termed *nasal continuous positive airway pressure* (CPAP), or (4) surgery. Surgical treatment may involve a nasal septal repair, a tracheostomy, or a uvulopalatopharyngoplasty (UVPP). UVPP involves excision of the tissues of the soft palate, uvula, and posterior lateral pharyngeal wall. The goal is to remove obstructing tissue.

General measures such as drug therapy and surgery are often not successful. Most clients find weight loss difficult. Medications are usually not effective. Tracheostomy may relieve symptoms because the tracheal opening is below the site of airflow obstruction. However, meticulous care is required to prevent infection. The most effective management for sleep apnea involves use of nasal CPAP applied by means of a mask that fits tightly over the nose (Fig. 20-7). Positive pressure is created by an air compressor connected to the mask by wide-bore tubing. The pressure supplied by air from the compressor opens the oropharynx and nasopharynx, preventing occlusion of the airway. As a result of the continuous airflow, some clients using nasal CPAP experience nasal dryness, burning, or congestion. Interventions to relieve these symptoms include use of a room humidifier or a humidifier incorporated in the airway circuit.[11] When the client is traveling, the humidifier can be replaced by use of a chin strap. A corticosteroid or saline nasal spray may also be used to treat dryness and congestion.

Another problem associated with use of nasal CPAP is discomfort from the high pressure and difficulty in exhaling, especially if the compressor is set to provide an airway pressure greater than 12 cm H_2O. A new device, the BiPaP ventilator, may resolve this problem. It delivers a higher airway pressure during inspiration (when the airway is most likely to be occluded) and a lower airway pressure during expiration (so that the client exhales against less resistance).

■ Nursing Management of Sleep Apnea

Nursing diagnoses specific to the client with sleep apnea include, but are not limited to, those presented in Table 20-7. Teaching will vary, depending on the type of interventions selected.[12] Referral to a support group may be very beneficial. The client can share concerns and feelings with others who have the same problems and discuss strategies for resolving these problems.

PROBLEMS RELATED TO THE TRACHEA AND LARYNX
Airway Obstruction

Airway obstruction may be complete or partial. Complete airway obstruction is a medical emergency (see Chapter 30). Partial airway obstruction may occur as a result of aspiration of food or a foreign body. The most common symptoms are choking, gagging, and coughing. In addition, partial airway obstruction may result from laryngeal edema, a tumor, tracheal stenosis, and neurological depression. Common symptoms are stridor, use of accessory muscles, suprasternal and intercostal retractions, wheezing, restlessness, and tachycardia. Breath sounds may be diminished. Prompt assessment and treatment are essential because partial obstruction may quickly progress to complete obstruction.[13] Interventions that may be required to maintain a patent airway include cricothyroidotomy (see Chapter 30), endotracheal intubation, and tracheostomy. Clients may have few or no symptoms if the obstruction is minor. Unexplained or recurrent symptoms indicate the need for additional tests, such as a chest x-ray, pulmonary function tests, and bronchoscopy.

Endotracheal Intubation

Endotracheal intubation is the insertion and placement of a tube into the trachea through the mouth (*oral intubation*) or nose (*nasal intubation*) (Fig. 20-8). Clients requiring intubation are often unconscious or hemodynamically unstable. Indications for endotracheal intubation are to (1) maintain a patent airway, (2) facilitate or control breathing when mechanical ventilation is required, (3) remove tracheobronchial secretions, (4) provide high concentrations of oxygen, and (5) prevent aspiration of secretions.[14]

■ Nursing Management of Endotracheal Intubation

Tubes used for intubation vary in design and related nursing care (Figs. 20-8 and 20-9 and Table 20-8). Teaching will vary depending on the illness of the client and the device selected.

Before intubation, if the client is conscious, the nurse should explain the need for endotracheal intubation, the procedure involved, and sensations (gagging and a feeling of suffocation) that may be experienced during the procedure. The nurse should explain that because of the inflated cuff, it will not be possible to talk after the tube is in place but that normal speech will be possible after the tube is removed. The need for the procedure and the approximate duration of intubation should also be explained.

Before intubation, the nurse should ensure that the client is properly oxygenated, assemble and check the equipment to be used during the procedure, remove any dentures or partial plates the client may have, and administer medication as ordered.[15] Premedication varies, depending on the client's health status. In the operating room, intubation is preceded by administration of IV barbiturates (to induce sleep) and a muscle relaxant. In ICUs a topical anes-

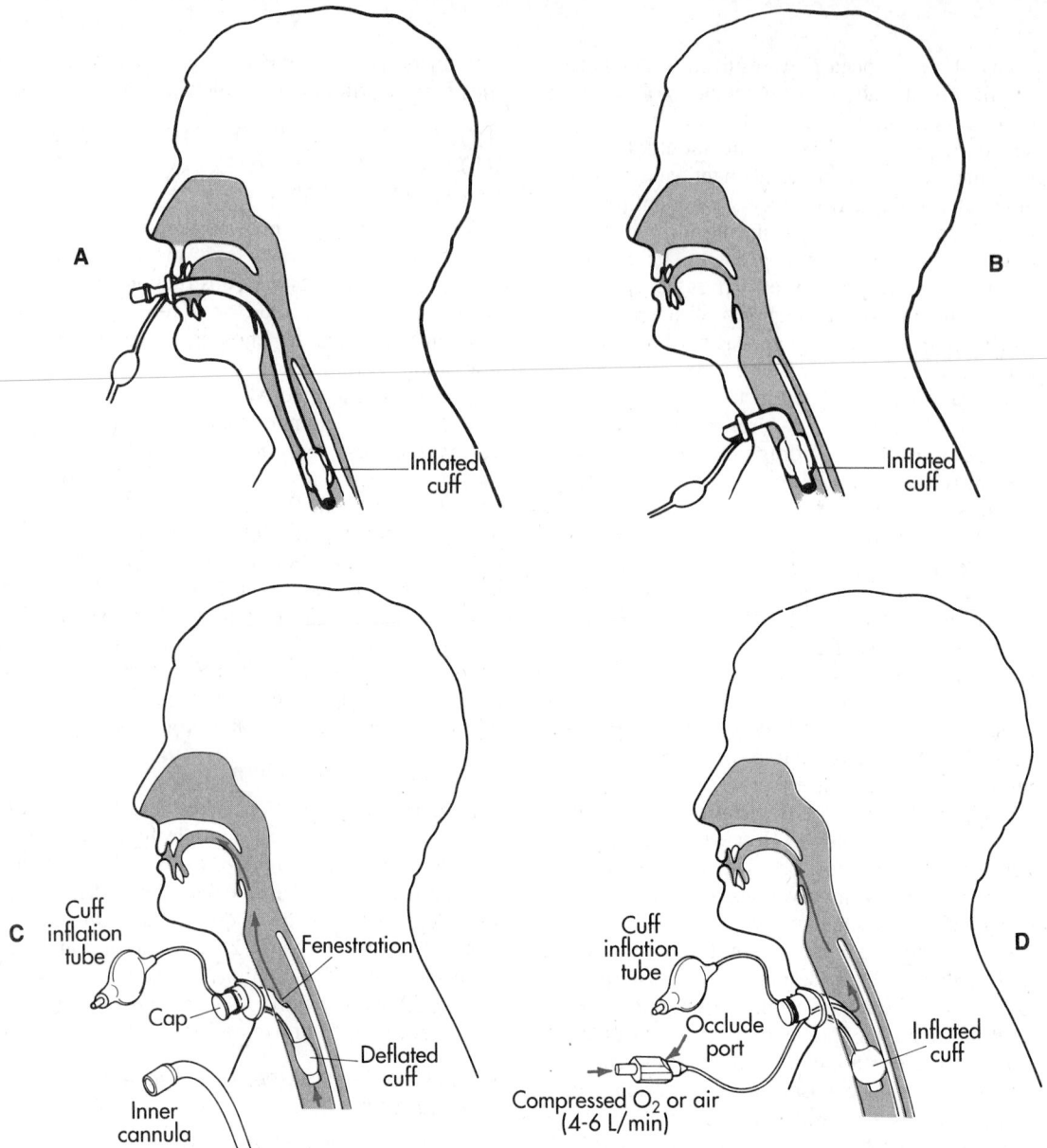

Fig. 20-8 **A,** Placement of endotracheal tube. **B,** Placement of tracheostomy tube. Both tubes have inflated cuffs. **C,** Fenestrated tracheostomy tube with cuff deflated, inner cannula removed, and tracheostomy tube capped to allow air to pass over the vocal cords. **D,** Speaking tracheostomy tube. One tubing is used for cuff inflation. The second tubing is connected to a source of compressed air or oxygen. When the port on the second tubing is occluded, air flows up over the vocal cords, allowing speech with an inflated cuff. (See Tables 20-8 and 20-10 for related nursing management.)

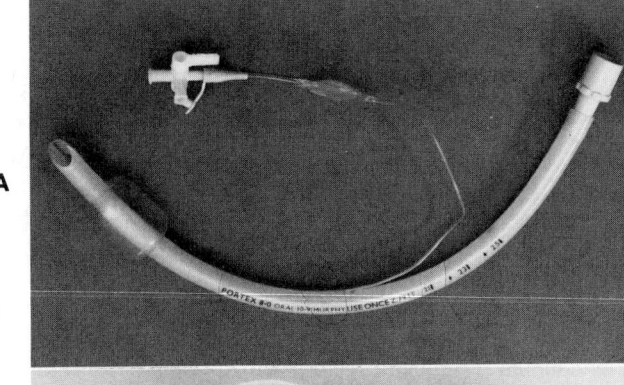

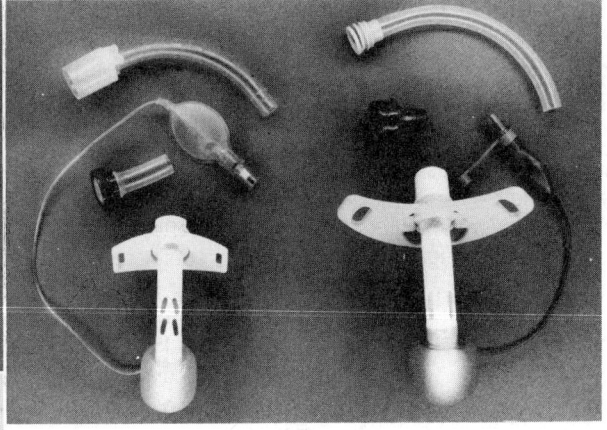

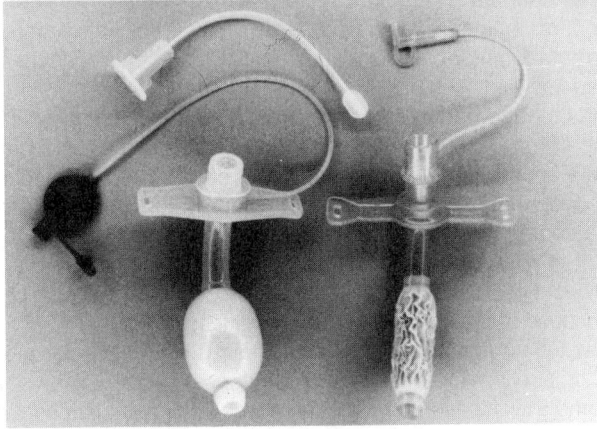

Fig. 20-9 Types of endotracheal and tracheostomy tubes. **A,** Disposable oral/nasal tube with cuff, stopcock and pilot balloon. **B,** Shiley and Portex fenestrated tracheostomy tube with cuff, inner cannula, decannulation plug, and pilot balloon. **C,** Bivona (Fome-Cuf) tracheostomy tube with foam cuff and obturator (one cuff is deflated on tracheostomy tube). (See Tables 20-8 and 20-10 for related nursing management.)

Table 20-8   Characteristics and Nursing Management of Artificial Airways

Tube	Characteristics	Nursing Management
Disposable oral or nasal endotracheal tube with cuff, pilot balloon, stopcock*	Low-pressure, high-volume cuff distributes cuff pressure over large area and minimizes pressure on tracheal wall when properly inflated.	Inflate cuff to minimal occluding volume. Place stethoscope over the neck and auscultate.† Listen for air leak while slowly injecting air into cuff. Continue until no leak is heard. If the client does not require mechanical ventilation, auscultate while ventilating with manual resuscitation bag. Alternatively, inflate cuff by minimal leak technique. To inflate using this technique, first determine minimal occluding volume. Then withdraw 0.1 ml of air, allowing a small leak. (This technique places less pressure on tracheal mucosa than minimal occluding volume. However, the client is at greater risk of aspiration because the seal is not complete.) Monitor and record cuff pressure q 8 hr: Attach a pressure-recording manometer to the pilot balloon port with a stopcock and attached syringe.† Pressurize the tubing leading to the manometer by injecting a small amount of air into the tubing. Close stopcock to the syringe. Measure cuff pressure at peak inspiratory pressure if client is on ventilator, or if client is breathing spontaneously, measure cuff pressure after a deep inspiration or after a breath, using a manual resuscitation bag. Cuff pressure should be <20 mm Hg or <25 cm H_2O to prevent tracheal necrosis. To add or remove air (1) close stopcock to the manometer and inflate or deflate the cuff; (2) close stopcock to the syringe and measure pressure again. Record the pressure and amount of air added or removed. Report inability to keep cuff inflated or need to use progressively larger air volumes to keep cuff inflated. (If the cuff requires progressively larger air volumes, tracheal dilatation may be present. If the cuff will not hold air, the tube must be replaced.)

*See Fig. 20-8.
†See Fig. 20-10.

Continued.

Table 20-8 Characteristics and Nursing Management of Artificial Airways—cont'd

Tube	Characteristics	Nursing Management
Fenestrated tracheostomy tube (Shiley, Portex) with cuff, inner cannula, decannulation plug‡	When inner cannula is removed, cuff deflated, and plug inserted, fenestration in outer cannula allows air to pass over vocal cords. Client can then speak. Low-pressure cuff distributes cuff pressure over large area.	Assess risk of aspiration before removing inner cannula. Deflate cuff. Have client swallow small amount of clear liquid or 30 ml of water colored with methylene blue dye. Note any coughing. Suction trachea to check for the presence of colored secretions. If no aspiration is noted, a fenestrated tube may be used. *Never* insert plug in tracheostomy tube until cuff is deflated and inner cannula is removed. (Prior insertion will prevent client from breathing [no air inflow], which may precipitate cardiac arrest.) Monitor cuff pressure q 8 hr. Clean inner cannula as needed.§
Speaking tracheostomy tube (Portex, National) with cuff, two external tubings*	This tube has two external tubings, one leading to the cuff and the second to an opening above the cuff. When above-cuff tubing is connected to air source, air flows out this opening and up over the vocal cords, allowing the client to speak when the cuff is inflated. Low-pressure cuff distributes cuff pressure over large area.	Once the tube has been inserted, wait 2 days before instructing the client in its use so that the stoma can close around the tube and prevent leaks. When client desires to speak, connect above-cuff tubing to a source of compressed air (or oxygen). Be certain to identify the correct tubing. (If gas flow enters the cuff, it will rupture, requiring an emergency tube change.) Use lowest flow (typically 4 to 6 L/min) that will result in speech because high flows dehydrate the mucosa. Cover tubing adaptor, which will cause the air to flow upward. Instruct client to speak in short sentences, since voice will become a whisper with long sentences. To prevent mucosal dehydration, disconnect air inflow system when client does not want to speak. If desired, use system to monitor aspiration risk. Give the client ice chips with 5 or 6 drops of methylene blue with the cuff inflated. Suction via the talk port. (If dye is suctioned, the client has aspirated). Estimate the volume of aspirate by collecting secretions in a sputum trap. Monitor cuff pressure q 8 hr.
Tracheostomy tube (Bivona Fome-Cuf) with foam-filled cuff‖	This tube has cuff filled with plastic foam. Cuff is deflated *before* insertion and allowed to passively inflate after insertion. Pilot balloon tubing is not capped, and no cuff pressure monitoring is required. Low-pressure cuff distributes cuff pressure over large area.	When inserting tube, withdraw all air with a 20 ml syringe; then cap pilot balloon tubing to prevent air entry. After tube is inserted, remove cap from pilot balloon tubing, allowing cuff to reinflate. Do not inject air into tubing or cap tubing while it is in client because air will flow in and out in response to pressure changes (head turning) and thereby maintain minimal occluding volume.
Tracheostomy button (Olympic) with spacers, outer cannula, plug¶	This tube maintains stoma patency and ability to talk with plug in place. With plug removed, it allows suctioning and access for emergency ventilation. It can be individualized to client's stoma size with spacers provided with kit.	Do not insert button before assessing aspiration risk. Measure stoma size; add spacers as needed. Insert lubricated button in stoma. Insert plug in button, which causes petals at the back of button to flare and hold button in stoma. After insertion, rotate button 180 degrees to ensure that it is not adhering to tracheal tissue. Instruct client to clean area around stoma daily with hydrogen peroxide and to remove and clean button at least twice a week. Be aware that if button is not removed, tissue may granulate around petals, predisposing to bleeding.

‡See Figs. 20-8 and 20-9.
§See Table 20-11.
‖See Fig. 20-9.
¶See Fig. 20-14.

thetic spray is typically used. Hypnotics, muscle relaxants, and deep sedation are avoided, since these decrease the client's ability to cough and to breathe deeply. In emergency situations, intubation may be done without premedication.

If oral intubation is selected, intubation will be accomplished with the aid of a laryngoscope. The client is placed in a supine position with the head extended, the neck fully flexed, and the jaw pulled forward. The endotracheal tube is then passed through the mouth and vocal cords and into the trachea. With nasal intubation, insertion is accomplished by manipulating the endotracheal tube via the nose through the nasopharynx and vocal cords and into the trachea. Both techniques have advantages and disadvantages. An oral endotracheal tube is easier to insert and easier to suction. However, orally placed tubes are more easily dislodged, can be occluded if the client bites on the tube, may be poorly tolerated, and may make oral hygiene difficult. Nasal tubes are more easily secured, allow for easier oral hygiene, and may be better tolerated by the client. However, their use is associated with serious complications, including sinusitis, otitis media, and epistaxis after removal.

After intubation, nursing responsibilities include (1) inflating the cuff, (2) assessing correct tube placement by auscultating bilateral breath sounds (sounds in both lungs), (3) assessing oxygenation status and acid-base balance and reporting untoward changes, (4) suctioning to remove secretions, (3) providing mouth care at least once per shift, (4) alternating placement of oral tubes to prevent pressure necrosis, (5) preventing accidental disconnection from the ventilator or extubation, and (6) preventing cuff overinflation.

After the tube is in position, the cuff should be *immediately* inflated to prevent aspiration of mouth or stomach contents. The lungs should be ventilated with the manual resuscitation bag to check correct placement of the tube. Bilateral breath sounds should be present. If sounds cannot be heard in both lungs, the physician should be notified. The tube may have been inserted too far, resulting in the tip being in the right mainstem bronchus rather than above the carina. The cuff must be deflated, the tube withdrawn 2 to 3 cm, the cuff reinflated, and the lungs auscultated again to correct tube placement. A bite block may be placed in the client's mouth to prevent biting on the tube.

The endotracheal tube is connected to oxygen by means of a T tube or to a mechanical ventilator. The client should also be suctioned (Table 20-9). Arterial blood gases (ABG) should be assessed 10 to 20 minutes after intubation to determine oxygenation status and acid-base bal-

---

Table 20-9 Suctioning an Endotracheal Tube or Tracheostomy

1. Assess need for suctioning q 2 hr. (Indications include coarse rales or rhonchi, coughing, and increasing peak inspiratory pressure if client is receiving mechanical ventilation.) Do not suction routinely.
2. If suctioning is indicated, explain procedure to client.
3. Collect necessary equipment (usually available in disposable set): sterile suction catheter, sterile gloves, sterile water, sterile cup or basin, sterile towel, goggles.
4. Check suction source and regulator. Adjust suction pressure until dial reads −120 mm Hg with tubing occluded.
5. Check equipment used for preoxygenation, which may be provided by a reservoir-equipped manual resuscitation bag connected to 100% oxygen at 12 to 15 L/min or adjustment of the ventilator oxygen concentration to 100%.
6. Wash hands. Put on goggles.
7. Use sterile technique to open sterile package, fill cup (or basin) with water, put on sterile gloves, and connect catheter to suction source. Designate one hand as contaminated for disconnecting, bagging, and operating the suction control.
8. Assess client's heart rate and rhythm to provide a baseline for detection of changes during suctioning.
9. Preoxygenate. (Methods include 4 to 5 breaths of 100% oxygen using manual resuscitation bag or 4 to 5 ventilator breaths at 100% oxygen.[18,19])
10. Lubricate catheter tip with water and gently insert catheter until obstruction is met. Do *not* apply suction during insertion.
11. After catheter is inserted, withdraw 1 cm. Apply suction intermittently while withdrawing catheter in a rotating manner. If secretion volume is large, apply suction continuously.
12. Limit suction time to 10 seconds. Discontinue suctioning if heart rate decreases from baseline by 20 bpm, increases from baseline by 40 bpm, or a dysrhythmia occurs.
13. After suctioning , oxygenate with 4 to 5 breaths by manual resuscitation bag or ventilator.
14. Rinse catheter with sterile water.
15. If secretions are tenacious, instill 5 ml normal saline solution into the airway. Oxygenate and ventilate after instillation.
16. Limit insertions of suction catheter to three passes.
17. Oxygenate client with 4 or 5 breaths by manual resuscitation bag or ventilator after the last suction pass.
18. Return inspired oxygen concentration to previous setting.
19. Rinse catheter and suction the oropharynx or use mouth suction.
20. Dispose of catheter by wrapping it around fingers of gloved hand and pulling glove over catheter. Discard all equipment in proper waste container.
21. Auscultate to assess changes in lung sounds; record time, amount, and character of secretions and client's response to suctioning.

---

bpm, Beats per minute.

ance. These values are used to evaluate need for change in mechanical ventilator settings. In addition, oximetry is used to provide continuous monitoring of oxygenation status (see Chapter 19).

The endotracheal tube must be secured in position. If not, it can be accidentally pulled out by the client or by traction on the tubing when the client is turned. The tube may also move down into the right mainstem bronchus, causing all inspired air to go into one lung.

Two approaches are used to maintain tube position: endotracheal tube holders and adhesive tape. If adhesive tape is used, the tube will be taped securely to the face. If a tube holder is used, straps will be placed around the client's head and a device (e.g., plastic, Velcro strip) positioned to hold the tube in place.[16]

Some clients experience skin excoriation, pressure sores, or tissue necrosis as a consequence of excessive or prolonged pressure from the tube, tube-holder straps, or adhesive tape. This problem can be prevented by removing the tape once each day and moving the tube to another position. If a tube holder is used, the straps can be loosened, the area under the straps massaged, and the straps reapplied. Mouth care and shaving can be done at this time. This procedure must be performed by two nurses. One nurse holds the tube and the second performs the remaining care. Because tube position may change during repositioning or when tube-holder straps are adjusted, presence of bilateral breath sounds should always be confirmed by auscultation after the procedure has been completed. Some clinicians do not advocate routine retaping because this increases the risk of tube movement within the trachea or extubation.

After the tube is taped in position, a chest x-ray film is taken to confirm correct placement. The tip of the endotracheal tube should be 3 to 5 cm above the carina. The carina is the site where the trachea branches into the right and left bronchi. After correct tube placement is con-

firmed, the number of centimeters the tube extends beyond the teeth or gingivae should be recorded on the client's chart. Correct placement should be verified each shift in one or more of the following ways: (1) auscultate breath sounds in both lungs, (2) measure tube protrusion in comparison to the previous measurement, and/or (3) note position of the tip of the tube on chest x-ray film.

Appropriate cuff inflation should be documented after placement is confirmed and once each shift. Cuffs are plastic balloons that encircle the endotracheal tube; they are inflated to form a seal between the tube and the trachea (Fig. 20-10). The cuff is inflated by injection of air into the fine-bore tubing leading to the balloon. The cuff should be inflated with the least amount of air that will adequately seal the trachea.[17] The amount of air will vary according the size of the client's trachea and the tube size. Cuffs are required during endotracheal intubation because the tube passes through the epiglottis, splinting it open. Consequently, the client cannot protect the airway from aspiration.

Cuff overinflation predisposes the client to tracheal necrosis because excessive pressure prevents the flow of blood through tracheal capillaries. A tracheoesophageal fistula may then result. Such fistulas rarely, if ever, heal unless the client can be extubated. Normal capillary perfusion is 30 mm Hg. For normal tracheal capillary blood flow, the volume of air instilled to achieve a seal should not cause pressure that exceeds 20 mm Hg or 25 cm H_2O. (A pressure of 20 mm Hg is equal to 27 cm H_2O.)

The balloon should be inflated to *minimal occluding volume* (MOV) to minimize cuff damage to the trachea. MOV can be determined by inflating the cuff until no leak (sound) is heard on ventilator inspiration when a stethoscope is placed over the trachea (Fig. 20-10). Alternatively, some clinicians advocate using the *minimal leak technique* (MLT). With MLT, the cuff is inflated in the same manner and 0.1 ml of air is withdrawn, allowing a

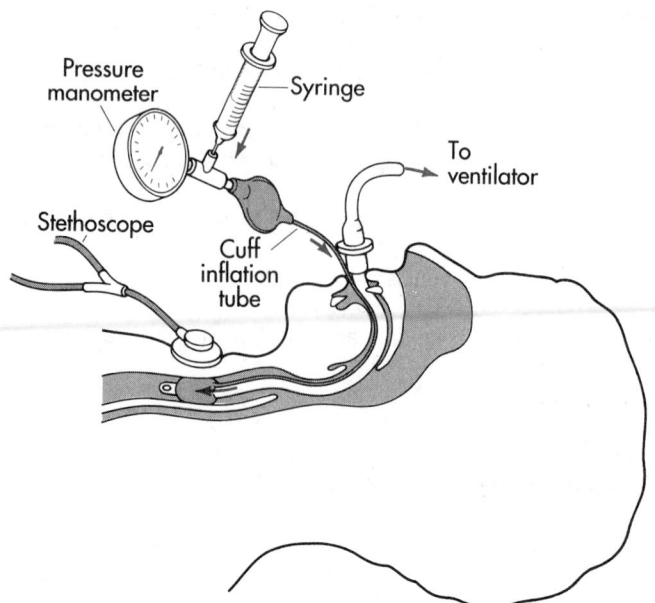

Pressure manometer

Syringe

Stethoscope

Cuff inflation tube

To ventilator

Fig. 20-10 Technique for determining inflation to minimal occluding volume and cuff pressure. The cuff is inflated until no leak is heard on inspiration when a stethoscope is placed over the trachea. Air is injected using a syringe connected to a stopcock and pressure manometer. (See Tables 20-8 and 20-10 for related nursing management.)

small leak. MLT places less pressure on tracheal mucosa than MOV. With MLT, however, there is greater risk of aspiration because the seal is not complete.

Cuff pressure must be measured to verify that it does not exceed 20 mm Hg or 25 cm H_2O. For mechanically ventilated clients, cuff pressure should be measured at the end of the ventilator inspiration (peak inspiratory pressure). For spontaneously breathing clients, cuff pressure should be measured with the use of a manual resuscitation bag after a deep inhalation or after a breath. (See Table 20-8 for additional care required in monitoring of cuff pressure.)

Extubation (tube removal) should be done as early as possible. The health care team should assess the client's status each day to determine whether (1) goals for ABG can be maintained without mechanical ventilation, (2) the underlying condition has improved so that intubation is no longer required, (3) spontaneous respiration can be maintained without the ventilator, and (4) the client can cough, clear secretions, and protect the airway. In addition, the client's vital capacity, tidal volume, maximum inspiratory pressure, and respiratory rate are evaluated (see Chapter 23).

If assessment indicates that these criteria have been met, extubation can be planned. Extubation should be attempted *only* by trained persons and when persons trained in reintubation are present. The nurse selects a time when the client is rested, explains the procedure, and places the client in a sitting position. The endotracheal tube and the area above the cuff (oropharynx) are suctioned. The tape or tube holder is loosened, the cuff is deflated, and while the client takes deep breath, the tube is removed at peak inspiration. Once the tube is removed, the client coughs to clear secretions. The mouth is suctioned, and humidified oxygen is administered through a face mask. The client is observed for signs of laryngospasm (e.g., stridor, dyspnea) and respiratory distress (e.g., restlessness, irritability, tachycardia, tachypnea). An oximeter should be used to monitor SaO_2. If the client cannot tolerate extubation, reintubation may be necessary.

Tracheostomy

A *tracheotomy* is a surgical incision into the trachea for the purpose of establishing an airway. A *tracheostomy* is the tracheal stoma or opening that results from tracheotomy (see Fig. 20-8). Correct placement of the tube requires careful dissection. For this reason a tracheotomy is not performed as an emergency procedure. The procedure can be performed at the bedside, but it is most frequently done in an operating room with the client under local anesthesia.

Indications for tracheostomy are to (1) bypass an upper airway obstruction, (2) facilitate the removal of respiratory tract secretions, (3) facilitate weaning from a respirator by reducing anatomical dead space, and (5) permit long-term mechanical ventilation.[20,21] A tracheostomy has several advantages over endotracheal intubation. Client comfort may be increased because no tube is present in the mouth. The client can swallow and eat with the tube in place. The client can speak if the tracheostomy cuff can be deflated.

In addition, there is less chance of accidental tube displacement, since the tube is shorter and cannot enter the right mainstem bronchus.

If extubation is not possible after 7 to 10 days of endotracheal intubation, most clinicians believe a tracheostomy should be performed. Others elect to extend endotracheal intubation as long as 2 to 3 weeks. In making this decision, the risks and complications associated with endotracheal intubation (e.g., laryngeal and vocal cord damage) must be balanced against the risks and complications of a tracheostomy (e.g., tracheal stenosis, pulmonary infection).

Insertion of a tracheostomy tube is done with the use of an obturator. This device fits snugly in the tube and has a smooth, tapered end that protrudes just beyond the tip (Fig. 20-9) and facilitates insertion. After the tracheostomy tube is placed in the airway, the physician immediately removes the obturator so that air can flow through the tube.

▪ Nursing Management of Tracheostomy

Nursing diagnoses specific to the client with a tracheostomy include, but are not limited to, those presented in Table 20-10. Teaching will vary, depending on the illness of the client and the device selected.

Before the tracheostomy, the nurse should explain to the client and the family the purpose of the procedure and inform them that the client will not be able to speak after the tube is in place if an inflated cuff is used. The client and the family should be told that normal speech will be possible as soon as the cuff can be deflated. A magic slate or pad and pencil should be provided.

Some tracheostomy tubes have two cannulas—an outer cannula, which remains in place, and an inner cannula, which can be removed for cleaning (Table 20-11). The cleaning procedure removes mucus that has accumulated on the inside of the tube. If airway humidification is adequate, this accumulation of mucus should not occur and a tube without an inner cannula can be used.

A tracheostomy tube is held in place with twill tapes (Fig. 20-11). Because the tube is not sutured in place, several precautions are required: (1) The tapes should not be changed for at least 24 hours after the insertion procedure; (2) a replacement tube of equal or smaller size should be kept at the bedside, where it is readily available for emergency reinsertion; and (3) the tube should not be changed for a minimum of 7 days after insertion. Retention sutures are often placed in the tracheal cartilage when the tracheostomy is performed. They should be taped to the skin in a place and manner that leaves them accessible if the tube is dislodged.

If a tracheostomy tube becomes dislodged, the nurse should immediately attempt to replace it. For emergency tube insertion, the retention sutures are grasped and the opening is spread. The obturator is inserted in the replacement tube, a water-soluble lubricant is applied to the tip, and the tube is inserted in the stoma at a 45-degree angle to the neck. If insertion is successful, the obturator is removed immediately so that air can flow through the tube. If the tube cannot be replaced, the client's level of respira-

Table 20-10

NURSING CARE PLAN FOR THE CLIENT WITH A TRACHEOSTOMY*

Defining Characteristics	Nursing Interventions	Evaluation Criteria

NURSING DIAGNOSIS: Impaired verbal communication related to use of artificial airway and cuff

Defining Characteristics	Nursing Interventions	Evaluation Criteria
Anxiety, inability to communicate, signs of frustration	Assess client's level of consciousness. If client is alert, provide call bell within easy reach, magic slate, pad and pencil, artificial larynx, or communication board with illustrations of requests. Reassure client that speech will return when cuff can be deflated (if laryngectomy has not been performed). Read lips for cues. Provide for continuity of care. Suggest use of tubes (fenestrated, speaking tracheostomy tube, valve) that permit speech.†	Communication of wants and needs in manner appropriate to level of consciousness

NURSING DIAGNOSIS: Potential complication: hypoxemia related to misplaced or improperly functioning tube

Defining Characteristics	Nursing Interventions	Evaluation Criteria
Restlessness, agitation, confusion, tachycardia, bradycardia, dysrhythmias; SaO_2 less than 90%; accidental expulsion of tube from airway	Elevate head of bed if tolerated. Auscultate chest. If coarse rales, rhonchi are present, suction airway. Check tube position and function.‡ If tube is misplaced from airway, grasp the retention sutures and spread opening. Insert tube with obturator in place at 45-degree angle to neck. If successful, remove obturator immediately. If not, assess the level of respiratory distress to determine whether client can breathe without tube for a short interval. Notify the physician. If distress is severe, ventilate with bag-mask or bag-stoma (laryngectomy) until assistance arrives.	Absence of restlessness, agitation, confusion; normal vital signs; Sao_2 greater than 90%; correct tube replacement; no respiratory distress

NURSING DIAGNOSIS: Ineffective airway clearance related to difficulty expectorating sputum

Defining Characteristics	Nursing Interventions	Evaluation Criteria
Coarse rales, rhonchi on auscultation; tenacious secretions; increase in restlessness; change in mentation; ineffective or absent cough	Assess for respiratory distress. Assist client to semi-Fowler's position, if tolerated. Suction airway. Monitor humidification system to ensure provision of adequate humidity. Instill normal saline solution during suctioning procedure. Teach client to inhale 4 or 5 times through nose, breathe out through airway, and then cough, if not on ventilator. Encourage oral fluids, if tolerated.	Maintenance of patent airway, secretions expectorated without need to suction airway, chest clear to auscultation

*Specific nursing interventions for the intubated client who is on a ventilator are discussed in Chapter 23 and Table 23-14.
†See Figs. 20-8 and 20-9 and Table 20-8.
‡See Table 20-8.
§See Tables 20-9 and 20-11.
‖See Fig. 20-12.

Table 20-10

NURSING CARE PLAN FOR THE CLIENT WITH A TRACHEOSTOMY—cont'd

Defining Characteristics	Nursing Interventions	Evaluation Criteria

NURSING DIAGNOSIS: **High risk for infection related to bypass of airway defense mechanisms and impaired skin integrity**

Defining Characteristics	Nursing Interventions	Evaluation Criteria
Elevated white blood cell count and temperature, change in color of secretions, purulent secretions	Use strict aseptic technique for suctioning tracheostomy during hospitalization. Wash hands before touching equipment. Change oxygen-delivery equipment q 48 hr. Empty condensate into waste receptacle, not into humidifier or nebulizer. Keep stoma clean and dry with frequent tracheostomy care. Report to physician any elevation in temperature or white blood cell count, change in secretion color, and purulent drainage from stoma.§	Normal white blood cell count and temperature, white secretions, no erythema or purulent secretions

NURSING DIAGNOSIS: **Altered nutrition: less than body requirements related to decreased oral intake, altered taste sensation, and swallowing difficulty**

Defining Characteristics	Nursing Interventions	Evaluation Criteria
Inadequate caloric intake, weight loss	Provide ongoing caloric count. Monitor weight. Provide food, beverages that client prefers. Perform mouth care q 8 hr.	Usual appetite, maintenance of normal body weight

NURSING DIAGNOSIS: **Impaired swallowing related to tracheostomy tube**

Defining Characteristics	Nursing Interventions	Evaluation Criteria
Inability to swallow without difficulty with cuff inflated	Assess swallow and gag reflexes by deflating cuff, asking client to swallow small amount of clear liquid or 30 ml water colored with methylene blue dye. Note coughing. Suction trachea and check for colored secretions. (If none present, client may tolerate eating with cuff deflated.)	Normal swallowing function with cuff deflated or with cuff inflated (if former not tolerated)

NURSING DIAGNOSIS: **Impaired home maintenance management related to lack of knowledge about care of tracheostomy at home**

Defining Characteristics	Nursing Interventions	Evaluation Criteria
Questioning about care (client, family), anxiety	Assess ability of client and significant other to provide care at home, including airway care, ability to respond appropriately to emergencies. Teach clean suction technique, good hand washing, home preparation of sterile saline solution, use of one catheter for 24 hr, methods of cleaning and reusing catheters, clean technique for tracheostomy care.‖ Make referral for visiting nurse or home care.	Demonstration of techniques by client and significant other for suctioning, care of equipment, tracheostomy care; verbalization of expected outcomes and time to contact health care professionals (if problems arise) by client and significant other

Table 20-11   Tracheostomy Care

1. Explain procedure to client.
2. Gather necessary sterile equipment (often available as a prepackaged kit), including sterile suction catheter, sterile water, basin, towel, gloves, drape, tube brush or pipe cleaners, hydrogen peroxide (3%), 4 × 4 inch pads, tracheostomy ties, and tracheostomy dressing (optional).
3. Position client in semi-Fowler's position.
4. Assemble needed materials on bedside table next to client.
5. Suction and oxygenate client.*
6. Unlock and remove inner cannula.†
7. If disposable inner cannula is used, replace with new cannula. If nondisposable cannula is used, do the following:
   a. Immerse inner cannula in 3% hydrogen peroxide and clean inside and outside of cannula with tube brush or pipe cleaners.
   b. Drain hydrogen peroxide from cannula; immerse cannula in sterile water; remove from sterile water and shake to dry.
   c. Insert inner cannula into outer cannula with curved part downward and lock in place.
8. Remove dried secretions from around stoma with 4 × 4 inch gauze pad soaked in hydrogen peroxide. Rinse with sterile water and another 4 × 4 inch gauze pad. Gently pat area around stoma dry.
9. Unless excessive amounts of exudate are present, avoid using tracheostomy dressing. If drainage is excessive, place dressing around tube.‡ Change the dressing frequently because wet dressings promote infection and stoma irritation.
10. Change tracheostomy ties.§ Prepare two twill tapes about 16 inches in length. Cut a slit in each tape 1 inch from the end.‡ Remove old ties. To prevent accidental tube removal, secure tracheostomy tube by gently applying pressure to flange of tube. Place slit end into opening of outer cannula and loop it through the other end of tape. Tie tapes together with double knot at side of the neck. (An alternative to cutting slits is to thread twill tape through openings in the outer cannula and tie tape on both sides of the neck.) Ensure that tapes are loose enough to allow one finger to be inserted under them.

---

*See Table 20-9.
†Many tracheostomy tubes do not have inner cannulas. Care for these tubes includes all steps except those for inner cannula care.
‡See Fig. 20-11.
§Tracheostomy ties should not be changed for 24 hours postoperatively.

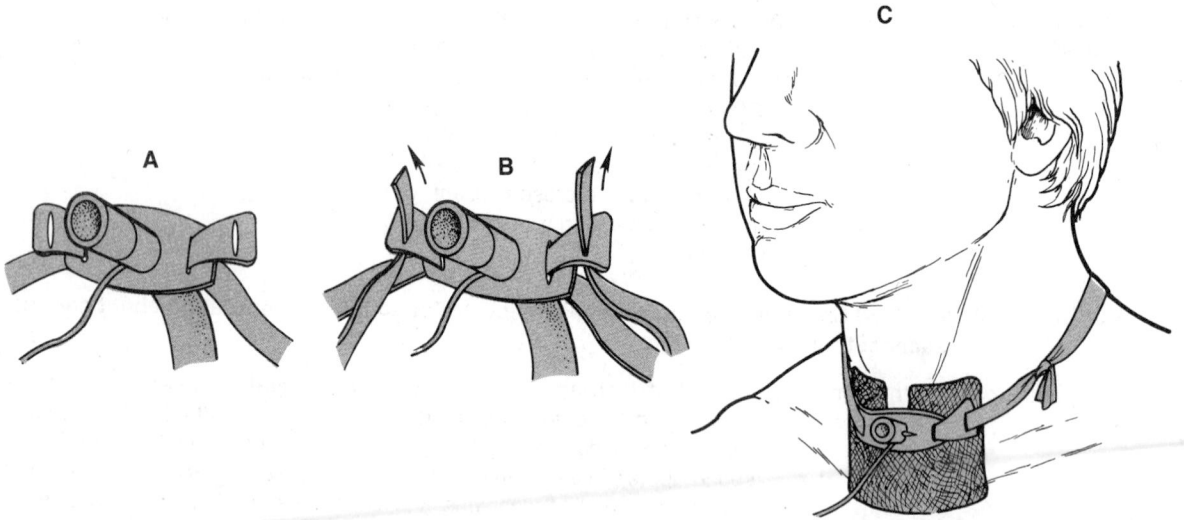

Fig. 20-11   Changing tracheostomy ties. **A,** A slit is cut about 1 inch from the end. The slit end is put into the opening of the cannula. **B,** A loop is made with the other end of the tape. **C,** The tapes are tied together with a double knot on the side of the neck.

tory distress is assessed. Minor dyspnea may be alleviated by use of semi-Fowler's position until assistance arrives. Severe dyspnea may progress to respiratory arrest. If this situation occurs, the stoma should be covered with a sterile dressing and the client ventilated with bag-mask ventilation until help arrives. Postlaryngectomy clients need to be ventilated with mouth-to-stoma ventilation, since there is

no communication between the tracheal and upper airways.

After 7 days, the tracheostomy tube is more easily reinserted because of tract formation. Because healing is variable, the first tracheostomy tube change should be performed by a physician, with equipment for ventilation and reintubation available. Afterward, the tube should be

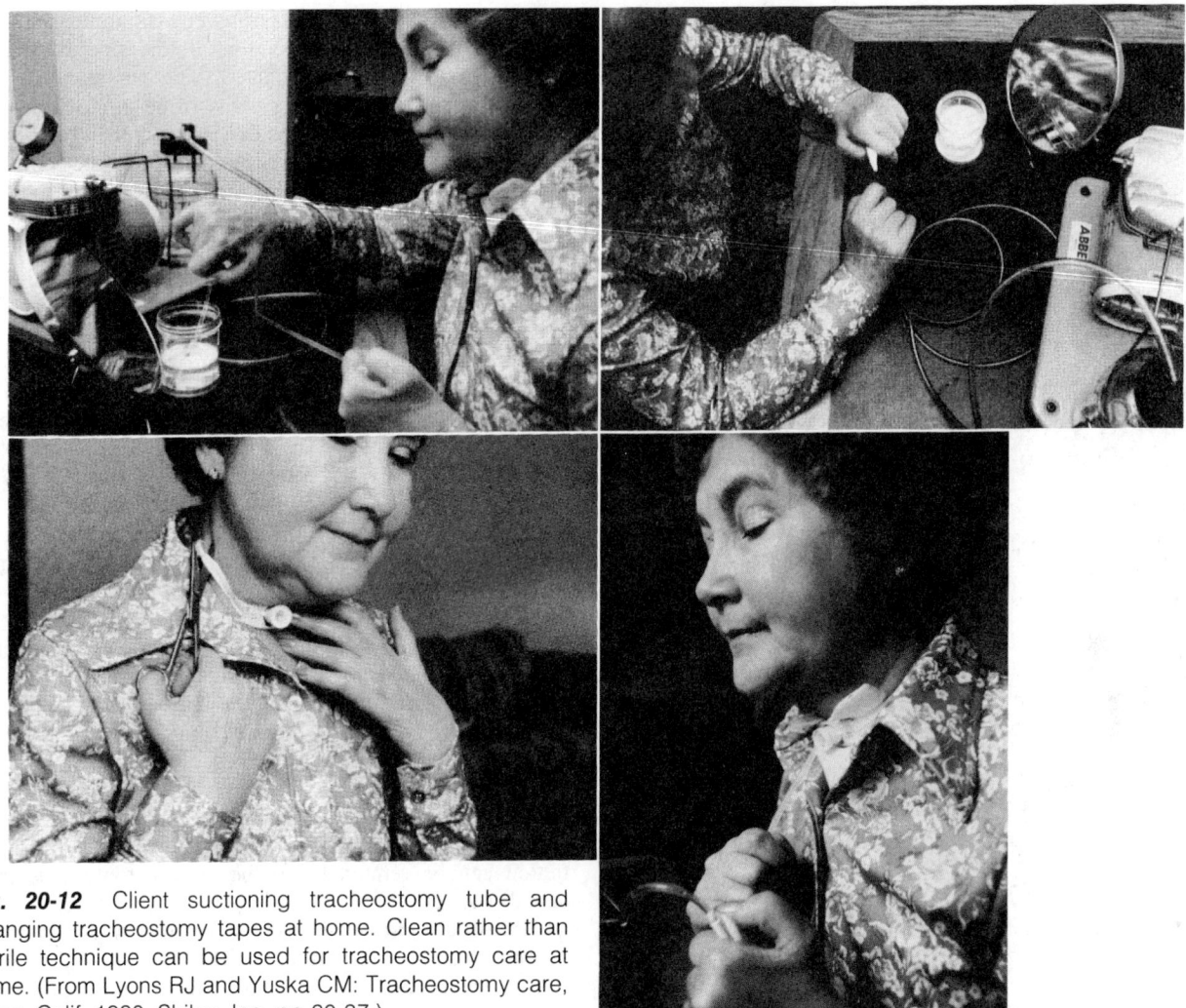

Fig. 20-12 Client suctioning tracheostomy tube and changing tracheostomy tapes at home. Clean rather than sterile technique can be used for tracheostomy care at home. (From Lyons RJ and Yuska CM: Tracheostomy care, Irvine, Calif, 1980, Shiley, Inc, pp 30-37.)

changed approximately once a month. When a tracheostomy has been in place for several months, the tract will be well formed. Clients can then be taught to perform this procedure and suction the tracheostomy at home (Fig. 20-12).

Both cuffed and uncuffed tracheostomy tubes are available. Because a tracheostomy tube enters the airway below the glottis, a cuff is not required on a tracheostomy tube. A tracheostomy tube with an inflated cuff should always be used if the client is at risk of aspiration. Procedures for care of a cuffed tracheostomy tube are the same as for a cuffed endotracheal tube.

Speech with a tracheostomy tube. Several tracheostomy tubes and valves have been designed to facilitate speech when a tracheostomy tube is in place. The nurse can be an advocate in promoting use of these specialized devices. Their use can provide great psychological benefit and facilitate self-care for the client with a tracheostomy.

A *speaking tracheostomy tube* has two tubings. One connects to the cuff and is used for cuff inflation. The second tubing connects to an opening just above the cuff (Fig. 20-8). When the second tubing is connected to a low-flow (4 to 6 L/min) air or oxygen source, sufficient air moves up over the vocal cords to permit speech. This client can then speak, even though the cuff is inflated.

A *fenestrated tube* is typically used in clients who can swallow without risk of aspiration but who still require suctioning for removal of secretions. It may also be used in clients who require mechanical ventilation for less than 24 hours a day. Assessment of a client's ability to tolerate the use of this tube begins with assessment of gag and swallow reflexes. The cuff is first deflated and the client is instructed to swallow a small amount of clear liquid or 30 ml of water colored with methylene blue dye. Any coughing is noted. Next, the trachea is suctioned to check for the presence of blue-colored secretions. If there is no indication of aspiration, the client is judged to have competent epiglottic function. A fenestrated tube may then be used.

A fenestrated tube has one or more openings on the surface of the outer cannula that permit air from the lungs to flow over the vocal cords (Figs. 20-8 and 20-9). Several steps are involved in the use of this device. First, the inner cannula is removed, the cuff is deflated, and a cap is placed in the tracheostomy tube. It is important to perform

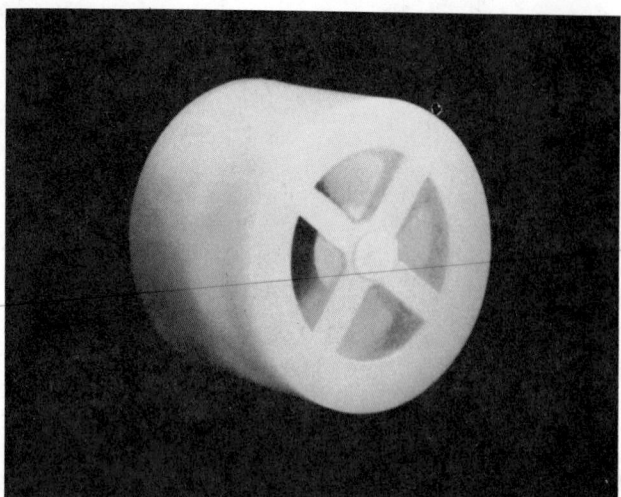

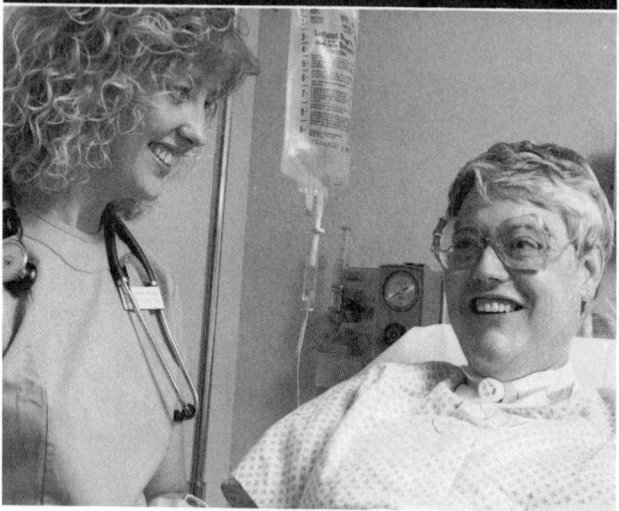

Fig. 20-13 Passy-Muir speaking tracheostomy valve. The valve is placed over the tracheostomy opening after cuff deflation. The device is used for clients who require an inflated cuff for mechanical ventilation or sleep apnea management at night but who can breathe spontaneously without problems with the cuff deflated during the day. (Courtesy Passy & Passy, Inc, Irvine, Calif.)

the steps in this order because severe respiratory distress may result if the tube is capped before the inner cannula is removed and the cuff is deflated. The nurse should frequently assess the client for signs of respiratory distress when a fenestrated cannula is first used. If the client is not able to tolerate the procedure, the cap should be removed, the inner cannula replaced, and the cuff reinflated.

When a fenestrated tube is used, the client can breathe spontaneously through the larynx, speak, and cough up secretions. However, the tracheostomy tube remains in place. Suctioning can still be done. The tube can also be connected to a mechanical ventilator.

Speaking tracheostomy valves are an alternative to the use of a fenestrated tube. When these valves are used, the cuff is deflated and the valve is placed over the tracheostomy tube (Fig. 20-13). The speaking valve contains a thin plastic diaphragm that opens on inspiration and closes on expiration. During inhalation, air flows in through the valve. During expiration, the diaphragm moves against the plastic cover and air flows upward over the vocal cords. Ability to tolerate cuff deflation must be evaluated in clients using this device.

A *tracheostomy button* is a short outer tube that extends from the skin to the anterior tracheal wall. No tube is present in the airway. The button is used for short periods (e.g., several weeks) to evaluate ability to tolerate tube removal. The tube can be plugged, permitting normal speech and coughing. However, the plug can be quickly removed if suctioning is needed. The tube maintains a patent tract. If withdrawal of the tracheostomy tube is not tolerated, the button can be removed and the tracheostomy tube reinserted (Fig. 20-14).

Decannulation. When the client is able to cough up secretions and maintain ABG without mechanical ventilation, the tracheostomy tube can be removed. The stoma is covered with a dressing and tape. Epithelial tissue will begin to form in 24 to 48 hours and the opening will close in several days. Surgical intervention is not required.

Laryngeal Polyps

Laryngeal polyps may develop on the vocal cords from vocal abuse (e.g., excessive talking, singing) or irritation

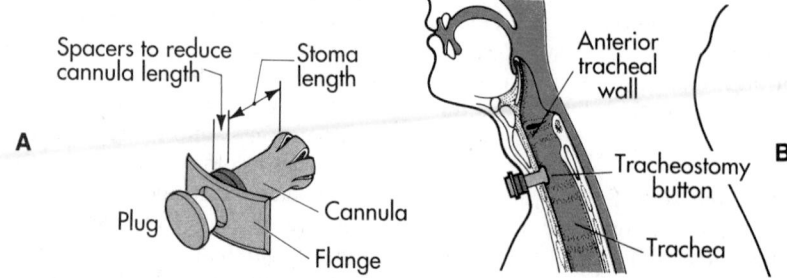

Fig. 20-14 Olympic tracheostomy button. **A,** Tracheostomy button inserted into the stoma. The button extends from the stoma opening to the anterior tracheal wall. **B,** Parts of the tracheostomy button. The button consists of a cannula, spacers that adapt the button to the length of the stoma, and a plug that fits into the cannula. The plug is removed for suctioning.

(e.g., cigarette smoking). The most common symptom is hoarseness. Very large polyps may cause dyspnea and stridor. Polyps may be treated conservatively with voice rest. Surgical removal is often advocated because seemingly benign polyps are sometimes later found to be malignant.

Cancer of the Head and Neck

The estimated number of new cases of cancer involving the head and neck (excluding skin cancer) is about 42,000. This number represents 4.3% of total new cancer cases.[22] Approximately 4 times as many men as women have head and neck cancer. The usual time of diagnosis is after the age of 40. Although the number of persons who have this cancer is relatively small, disability is great because of the potential loss of voice, disfigurement, and social consequences.

The nurse is in a key position to detect early signs of head and neck cancer. Early detection is especially important for these clients. If the cancer is localized, extensive surgical resection is necessary, and the cancer is more likely to be curable. However, many clients do not report symptoms because they do not know their significance or because they fear the consequences. Subjective and objective data that should be obtained from a person at risk of head and neck cancer are presented in Table 20-12.

Table 20-12

**Nursing Assessment of the
Client with Laryngeal Cancer**

SUBJECTIVE DATA

History
Positive family history; heavy tobacco use (smoking, chewing, snuff); chronic and heavy alcohol abuse; excessive use of voice; exposure to fumes, pollution, or radiation; chronic laryngitis

Medications
Use of over-the-counter medications for sore throat

Pain
Throat pain or soreness for more than 2 weeks; referred ear pain

Respiratory
Sensation of a lump in the throat; cough; hemoptysis; dyspnea (late symptom)

Gastrointestinal
Dysphagia (late symptom)

OBJECTIVE DATA

General
Cervical lymphadenopathy

Respiratory
Hoarseness; palpable neck mass (tender, hard, fixed); tracheal deviation; stridor (late symptom)

Possible findings
Mass on direct and indirect laryngoscopy; tumor on soft tissue x-ray films of the neck, barium swallow, CT scan or contrast laryngography; positive biopsy

Oral cancer. Early signs of oral cancer include a white or raised patch, termed *leukoplakia,* on the lips or within the mouth or an ulcer that fails to heal. Pain is typically not present in early lesions. Clients at high risk include those who are cigar or pipe smokers or who use snuff. The client should be taught to inspect the mouth and to report any lesions. The entire mouth should be inspected, including the area under the tongue and dentures. The importance of early detection should be stressed. With early detection, a cure is often possible. Both leukoplakia and carcinoma in situ (localized to a defined area) may precede invasive carcinoma by many years. The 5-year survival rate is greater than 90% in clients who have lesions smaller than 3 cm and no evidence of metastases.

Laryngeal cancer. The larynx consists of three areas: the supraglottis, which includes the epiglottis; the glottis, which includes the vocal cords; and the subglottis, which is located below the vocal cords and ends at the first tracheal ring. Signs and symptoms of cancer of the larynx vary with the region affected.

When cancer involves the vocal cords, hoarseness is the most frequent symptom. If this symptom persists longer than 2 weeks, a medical evaluation is indicated. Pain and sore throat occur late and suggest extension of the cancer.

When the supraglottic region is involved, hoarseness is not a common symptom. The most frequent early symptom is mild pain on swallowing. The client may complain of a mild persistent irritation or sore throat, which is localized in one area. Symptoms may be confused with those of a cold. Unlike a cold, however, they persist for months and are not relieved by treatment for cold symptoms. Mild difficulty in swallowing is also a common symptom. Some clients experience a sensation of a "lump in the throat" or a change in voice quality.

Diagnostic studies. Diagnosis is based on the client's history, physical examination, and the results of tests to evaluate the presence and extent of the lesion. A laryngeal mirror is used to visualize the laryngeal area and determine mobility of the larynx and vocal cords. The presence of a tumor restricts tissue mobility. Computerized tomographic (CT) scans and a chest x-ray film are used to further evaluate extent of the lesion and the presence of metastasis. Neoplastic tissue is identifiable on the CT scan because it contains tissue of greater density or because it distorts, displaces, or destroys normal anatomical structures. If the presence of a lesion is confirmed, a barium swallow is usually done to evaluate swallowing ability, detect encroachment of the tumor into the esophageal area, and determine whether there is a second primary tumor in the esophagus. If testing suggests metastasis beyond the chest area, additional tests will be ordered. The final phase of the diagnostic evaluation involves biopsy of areas that may contain tumor.

Therapeutic management. On the basis of the information obtained, a decision will be made about the stage of the disease by means of the tumor, nodes, metastasis (TNM) system. This system identifies the extent of the disease and guides principles of treatment. Most small lesions can be treated by either radiation therapy or surgical intervention. Choice of treatment is based on such factors as

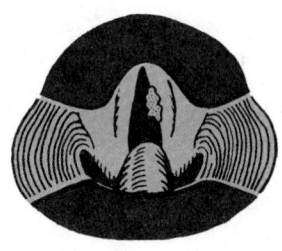

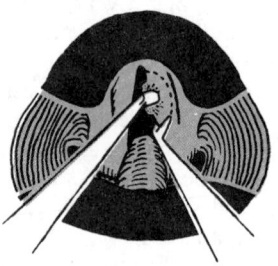

Fig. 20-15 Excision of laryngeal cancer. This cancer of the right vocal cord meets criteria for resection by transoral cordectomy. The cord is fully mobile and the lesion can be fully exposed. It does not approach or cross the anterior commissure. (From Donald PJ: Head and neck cancer: management of the difficult case, Philadelphia, 1984, WB Saunders Co, p 102.)

extent of disease, cosmetic considerations, and urgency of treatment. More advanced disease is managed with combinations of surgical interventions and radiation therapy or surgical interventions, radiation therapy, and chemotherapy. Radiation therapy and surgical interventions are the only curative modalities for cancer of the head and neck.

If there is no evidence of metastasis, lesions of the lip and oral cavity can be managed with local resection. Margins of the resected tissue are examined for tumor cells, and radiation therapy is given if the results are positive. Since subclinical metastasis (metastasis not detected by testing), is always possible, a combined management regimen consisting of surgical intervention and postoperative radiation therapy may be used. If the lesion is widespread, more extensive dissection is required.

Early vocal cord lesions are typically managed by radiation therapy. This therapy is usually successful in eliminating the tumor and preserving the quality of the voice. If treatment is not successful, surgical intervention will be performed. This may involve a cordectomy, which involves excision of the vocal cord, or a hemilaryngectomy, which is a partial laryngectomy (Fig. 20-15). Both procedures allow the voice to be preserved, but it usually remains hoarse. Advanced lesions are managed by total laryngectomy. In this procedure the entire larynx and preepiglottic region are removed and a permanent tracheostomy is performed. Radical neck dissection (see Chapter 34) frequently accompanies total laryngectomy. Depending on the extent of involvement, extensive dissection and reconstruction may be performed. In some types of surgical in-

tervention, dissection is so extensive that primary closure of the entire wound may not be possible. A combination of primary closure of skin edges, skin grafts, and regional or distant flaps may be used. Skin grafts are usually taken from the anterior portion of the thigh. Postoperative radiation therapy is used to control metastasis. Some clients refuse surgical intervention or are judged to be at too high a risk for the procedure. Radiation therapy may be used as the sole treatment in this circumstance.

Brachytherapy, a concentrated form of radiation therapy, involves placement of a radioactive source directly into or near the tumor. The goal is to deliver high doses of radiation to the target area and to limit exposure of surrounding tissues. Thin hollow plastic needles are inserted into the tumor area. A radioactive source (iridium seeds) is placed in the needles. The seeds emit continuous radiation. Brachytherapy can be used alone or combined with external radiation or surgical intervention.

Cancerous nodes in the neck that resist radiation treatments sometimes respond if heat is added to the treatment regimen. When hyperthermia is used, these nodes are exposed to temperatures of 46° C to 49° C (115° F to 120° F) for an hour before and after radiation treatments.

■ Nursing Management of Cancer of the Head and Neck

Health maintenance and promotion

Development of head and neck cancer is closely related to personal habits, primarily cigarette smoking. Cigarette smokers have an increased risk of lung cancer as well as head and neck cancer. Alcohol has been implicated as a causative factor for some head and neck cancers. The effects of alcohol and tobacco seem to be additive. Head and neck cancer may also be associated with the use of chewing tobacco. Snuff dipping, or the placement and retention of tobacco in the cheek, is a common practice in some areas of the United States. Long-term snuff users are at increased risk of oral cancer. The nurse should include information about these risk factors in health teaching.

Acute intervention

Nursing diagnoses specific to the client with a laryngectomy include, but are not limited to, those presented in Table 20-13. A diagnosis of cancer involving the facial area produces anxiety and is traumatizing and frightening. The client and the significant other need to deal with the psychological impact of the diagnosis of cancer in addition to possible altered modes of communication and change in body image. Assessment of the client's concerns is integral to the plan of care. It is vital to implement a consistent team approach as well as to include the client and the significant other in all aspects of teaching and care.[23]

The client and the significant other must be taught about the type of procedure to be performed and the care required. This information includes (1) changes that will occur as a result of radiation therapy or surgical intervention, (2) duration of these changes, (3) changes in the voice and ability to eat, (4) alternate methods of speech, (5) self-help groups and community resources, and (6) emotional adjustments to be anticipated by the client and the significant other.

Table 20-13

NURSING CARE PLAN FOR THE CLIENT HAVING RADICAL NECK SURGERY OR A PERMANENT LARYNGECTOMY*

Defining Characteristics	Nursing Interventions	Evaluation Criteria

NURSING DIAGNOSIS: Anxiety related to lack of knowledge regarding surgical procedure, postoperative course, pain management, and prevention of complications

Questioning about impending surgery, anxiety	Assess knowledge desired by client to allay fears and answer questions. Facilitate discussion of expected alterations in physical appearance. Encourage sharing of feelings and concerns. Provide information about what to expect after surgery (e.g., pain management, tracheostomy, nasogastric tube, drainage tubes). Establish means of communication preoperatively.	Decrease in anxiety about surgery, calm appearance

NURSING DIAGNOSIS: Ineffective airway clearance related to difficulty expectorating sputum and presence of tracheostomy

Ineffective or absent cough; rhonchi or coarse rales on auscultation; abnormal rate, pattern of breathing	Auscultate chest and monitor respiratory rate, pattern q 4 hr for 24 hr. Monitor Sao_2 or ABGs. Encourage deep breathing and coughing to clear secretions. Suction prn. Administer supplemental humidification as prescribed.	Secretions cleared with coughing, lungs clear on auscultation, normal respiratory rate and pattern

NURSING DIAGNOSIS: Altered tissue perfusion related to tissue edema and disruption of vascular and lymphatic drainage

Swollen and tense skin, serous drainage from wound drainage tubes	Maintain head of bed at 30 to 40 degrees to decrease tissue edema. Monitor heart rate, blood pressure, hemoglobin, and hematocrit to detect excessive bleeding. Monitor patency of drainage tubes, amount, color of drainage. Assess skin flap integrity q 4 hr (for warmth, swelling, color). Clean incision as prescribed.	Decrease in tissue edema; serous drainage with decreased volume; no swelling, tenseness, or warmth in area over skin flaps; stable vital signs

NURSING DIAGNOSIS: Altered nutrition: less than body requirements related to pain and edema at surgical site

Inability to tolerate oral feedings	Provide frequent oral hygiene. Instill tube feedings as ordered. When oral feedings begin (usually allow several days for wound healing), give clear liquids and advance as tolerated. Stay with client during meals and observe for swallowing difficulty. Deflate cuff during meals as soon as tolerated. Teach specialized swallowing techniques (e.g., Valsalva maneuver with supraglottic laryngectomy).	Resumption of normal oral intake, swallowing without coughing or aspiration, weight maintenance or weight gain (if appropriate)

Modified from Sawyer DL and Bruya MA: Care of the patient having radical neck surgery or permanent laryngostomy: a nursing diagnostic approach, Focus Crit Care 17:166-173, 1990.
*See Table 20-10.

Continued.

Table 20-13

NURSING CARE PLAN FOR THE CLIENT HAVING RADICAL NECK SURGERY OR A PERMANENT LARYNGECTOMY*—cont'd

Defining Characteristics	Nursing Interventions	Evaluation Criteria
NURSING DIAGNOSIS: Pain related to surgical procedure		
Report of pain, facial mask of pain	Assess client manifestations of pain (e.g., facial expression, reluctance to cough or move). Administer pain medication as prescribed. Monitor edema at incision site. Logroll head and chest to prevent strain on sutures. Teach self-support of head and neck when up (interlock hands behind head to provide support when moving to sitting position).	Verbalization that pain is controlled, expression of comfort
NURSING DIAGNOSIS: Body-image disturbance related to altered facial appearance		
Unwillingness to participate in self-care, view self in mirror, or visit with others	Assess preoperative body image. Assess client's readiness to view and touch reconstructed area; assist and encourage client to do so. Encourage support from family members. Refer to a support group. Encourage client to verbalize feelings about body image and to participate in self-care. Prepare visitors to prevent shocked response.	Participation in self-care; willingness to view self in mirror, visit with others
NURSING DIAGNOSIS: Impaired verbal communication related to removal of vocal cords		
Inability and/or unwillingness to use voice rehabilitation methods	Anticipate needs. Answer call bell immediately. Communicate to staff that client cannot speak. Instruct in alternate methods of communication (e.g., magic slate, communication board). Refer client to speech therapist to learn use of voice prosthesis, electrolarynx, or esophageal speech.	Ability to communicate clearly using method of choice

Modified form Sawyer DL and Bruya MA: CAre of the patient having radical neck surgery or permanent larygostomy: a nursing diagnostic approach, Focus Crit Care 17:166-173, 1990.
*See Table 20-10.

The care plan should include assessment of the client's support system to facilitate discharge planning. As a result of the association between head and neck cancer and excessive alcohol consumption, the client may not have a significant other to provide assistance after discharge. The client may not be employed or may be employed in a job that cannot be continued.

The client's nutritional status may be poor as a result of a delay in seeking health care until after a substantial weight loss had occurred. The dietician and the social worker should be consulted if problems are identified.

Radiation therapy. The nurse can suggest interventions to reduce side effects of radiation therapy.[24] Dry mouth, the most frequent and annoying problem, typically begins within a few weeks of treatment. The client's saliva decreases in volume and becomes very thick. The change may be temporary or permanent. The volume of secretions can be increased with the use of sugarless gum, candy, and artificial saliva. Good oral hygiene, peroxide mouth rinses, and increased fluid intake may help relieve symptoms. Additional side effects of radiation therapy include taste changes and stomatitis. Stomatitis is most common if the oral cavity is in the field of therapy. Irritation, ulceration, and pain are common complaints. Rinses of half-strength peroxide or of baking soda and water can be used to clean and soothe irritated tissues. Commercial mouth-

Table 20-13

NURSING CARE PLAN FOR THE CLIENT HAVING RADICAL NECK SURGERY OR A PERMANENT LARYNGECTOMY*—cont'd

Defining Characteristics	Nursing Interventions	Evaluation Criteria
NURSING DIAGNOSIS: Impaired home maintenance management related to lack of knowledge about home care after discharge		
Anxiety, questioning about care	Assess ability of client to learn information. Provide written instructions for client and significant other. Teach client to perform suction in front of mirror and provide positive reinforcement. Teach cleansing of tracheostomy or laryngectomy tube, voice prosthesis. Supervise care until client and significant other are comfortable with techniques. Teach client to cover stoma before performing activities that may lead to inhalation of foreign materials (e.g., shaving, application of makeup). Teach client to report changes, such as stoma narrowing, difficulty in swallowing, lump in throat (possible recurrence of tumor or tracheal stenosis). Make referral for home health care visit to evaluate self-care.	Verbalization of steps and rationale for self-care, demonstration of steps to be used in carrying out self-care, knowledge of when to contact health care professionals for problem solving

washes and hot or spicy foods should be avoided because they are irritating. If the problem is severe, a mixture of equal parts of antacid, diphenhydramine (Benadryl), topical lidocaine, and glycerine can be used. The client may also have tenacious secretions and increased crusting at the tracheostomy site. Interventions include use of a humidifier and instillation of normal saline solution into the tracheostomy during suctioning (Table 20-9).

Good nutrition is important because calories and protein are needed for tissue repair. Antiemetics or analgesics may be given before meals to reduce nausea and mouth pain. Bland foods may be better tolerated. Caloric intake may be increased by adding dry milk or Polycose to foods during preparation, selecting foods high in calories, and using oral supplements. If adequate intake cannot be maintained, nasogastric feedings may be used.

Current techniques do not produce radiation "burns." However, skin over the field often becomes reddened and sensitive to touch. All exposure to the sun should be avoided to reduce discomfort. Corticosteroid sprays may be used to provide symptomatic relief.

Preoperative teaching. Preoperatively, some clients find relief from anxiety by learning more about what to anticipate after the surgical intervention. Others may want to receive only limited amounts of information. Most teaching will then need to be done in the postoperative period.

One teaching method involves use of a "teaching tray" containing equipment that will be used after the procedure.

Items in the tray include a tracheostomy tube, a nasogastric tube, and diagrams of the anatomical structures of the airway. The client and the significant other handle the equipment while explanations are given about its purpose.

Teaching must include information about changes in speech after surgical intervention. If a hemilaryngectomy is performed, the client will have a temporary tracheostomy. If a total laryngectomy is performed, the tracheostomy will be permanent. Airflow patterns before and after a total laryngectomy are shown in Fig. 20-16. Means of communicating without being able to speak should be demonstrated by the nurse or a speech pathologist. If the client will not be returning to the preoperative area after surgery, nurses from the postoperative unit should be encouraged to participate in preoperative teaching.

Postoperative management. After surgical intervention has been performed, airway management is the primary concern. The client will be placed in a semi-Fowler's position to decrease edema and place less tension on the suture lines. Vital signs should be monitored frequently because of the risk of hemorrhage.

More frequent suctioning of the mouth is required after head and neck surgery because the client cannot swallow secretions or saliva. After edema subsides and aspiration is no longer a risk, the cuff may remain deflated. Procedures for care of the client with a tracheostomy are discussed in Tables 20-10 and 20-11.

Wound management is also a priority. Pressure dress-

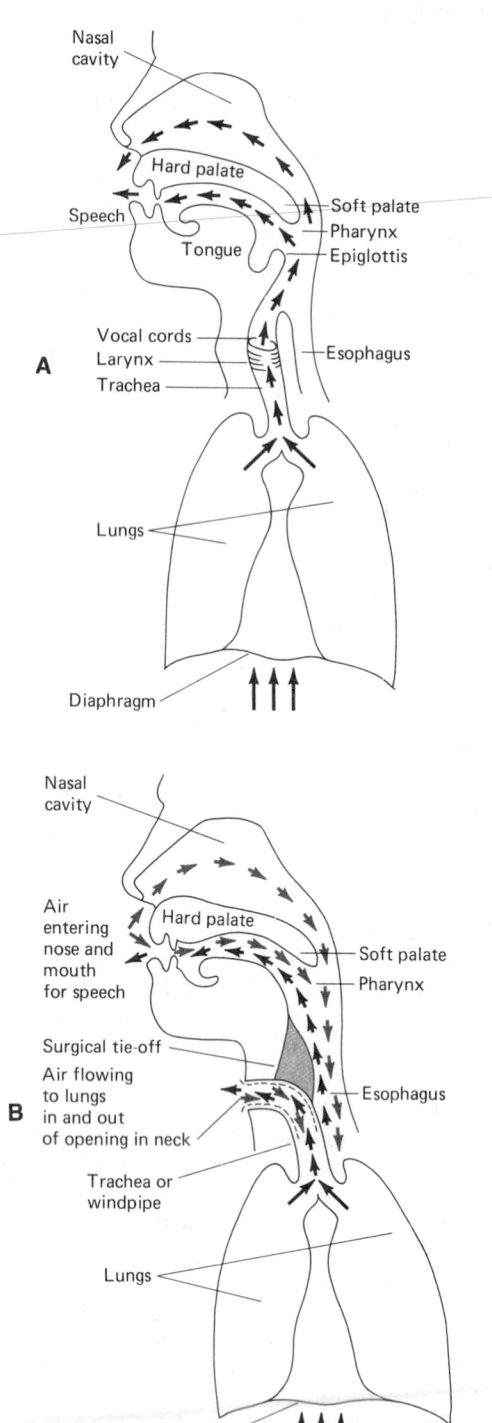

Fig. 20-16 **A,** Normal airflow in and out of the lungs. **B,** Airflow in and out of the lungs after total laryngectomy. Clients using esophageal speech trap air in the esophagus and release it to create sound. (From the American Cancer Society.)

ings, packing, or drainage tubes may be used, depending on the type of surgical procedure. If skin flaps are employed, dressings are typically not used. This allows better visualization of the incision and avoids excessive pressure on the tissue. Function of drainage tubes should be monitored every 4 hours for 24 hours to ensure that they are functioning properly. If the tubing obstructs, fluid will accumulate under the skin flap and predispose the client to impaired wound healing and infection. After the drainage tubes are removed, the area should be closely monitored to detect any swelling. If fluid continues to accumulate, aspiration may be necessary.

Nutritional considerations. Most clients return from the operating room with a nasogastric tube. It is the responsibility of the nurse to assess correct placement and function of the tube (see Chapter 35). Correct tube function is important. Gastric distention may lead to vomiting, aspiration, stress on the suture line, or wound contamination. Clients who undergo extensive surgical procedures may require tube feedings to maintain nutrition until healing is sufficient to permit oral intake.

Changes in swallowing after surgery can be anticipated. The type and degree of difficulty will vary, depending on type of surgical procedure. When a supraglottic laryngectomy is performed, the surgeon excises the upper portion of the larynx, including the epiglottis and the false vocal cords. The true vocal cords, which are used for speech, are not removed, and a permanent tracheostomy is avoided. The client can speak because the true vocal cords remain intact. However, new swallowing techniques must be learned to compensate for removal of the epiglottis. To swallow after surgery, the client must perform a Valsalva maneuver (forced exhalation against a closed glottis). The Valsalva maneuver exaggerates the normal swallowing process and tightly closes the vocal cords, facilitating passage of food into the stomach.

Voice rehabilitation. A speech therapist or speech pathologist should meet with the client to discuss voice restoration. The International Association of Laryngectomees is an association of laryngectomy clients that focuses on assisting clients to reestablish speech. Local groups, called "Lost Cord Clubs," identify members who can visit the client, preferably preoperatively.

Several options are available to restore speech. These include use of a voice prosthesis, an Electrolarynx, and esophageal speech. The most commonly used voice prosthesis is the Blom-Singer prosthesis (Fig. 20-17). This soft plastic device is inserted into a fistula made between the esophagus and the trachea. The puncture may be created at the time of surgery or afterward, depending on the preference of the surgeon. The prosthesis allows air from the lungs to enter the esophagus but prevents aspiration. To speak, the client blocks the stoma with the finger. Air moves from the lungs, through the prosthesis, into the esophagus, and out the mouth. Speech is produced the same way as before surgery, by moving the tongue and lips to form sound into words. A tracheostoma valve is also available for use with this prosthesis. With the valve in place, the client does not need to close off the stoma to speak.

Clients using this prosthesis should be instructed to avoid eating foods (cheese, pasta, beans) that may clog the

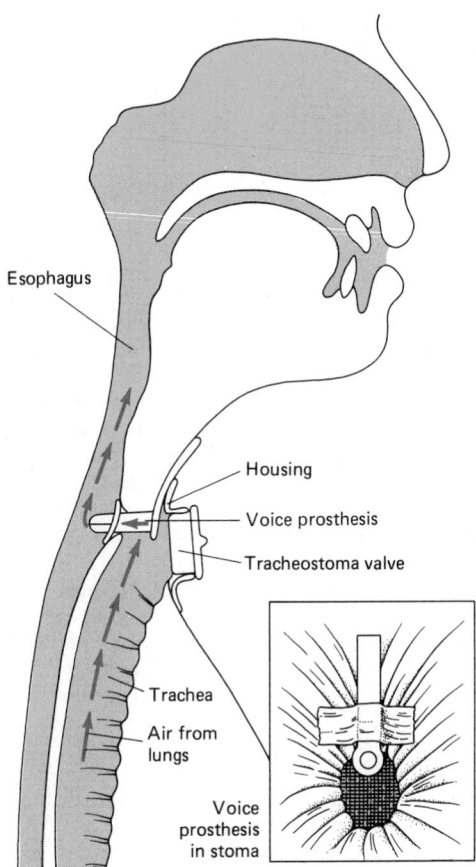

Fig. 20-17 Blom-Singer voice prosthesis and tracheostoma valve. With this prosthesis and valve, clients with a laryngectomy can speak normally. Insert *(lower right)* shows laryngectomy stoma and voice prosthesis with tracheostoma valve removed.

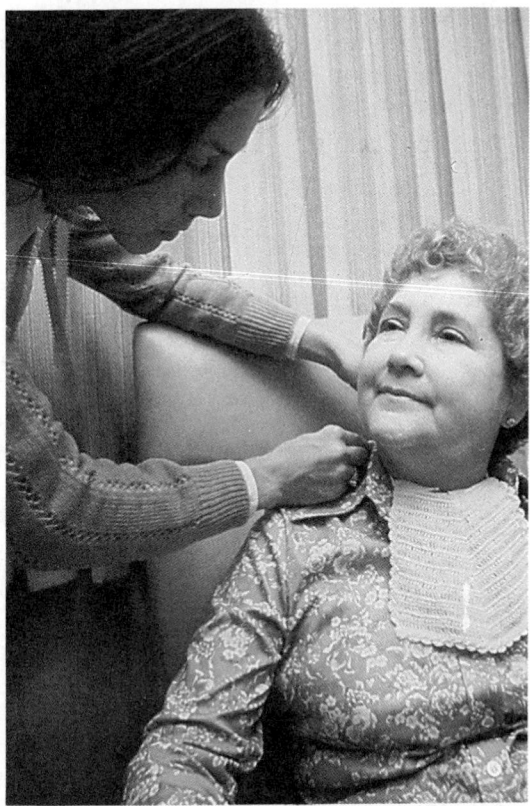

Fig. 20-18 Laryngectomee with stoma guard. (From Lyons RJ and Yuska CM: Tracheostomy care, Irvine, Calif, 1980, Shiley, Inc, p 42.)

device. They need to wear a rubber shower collar when taking a shower. Swimming is contraindicated. The prosthesis needs to be cleaned and should be replaced with a new one when it becomes blocked with mucus.

The electrolarynx is a hand-held battery-powered device that creates speech with the use of sound waves. One device, the Cooper-Rand Electrolarynx, uses a plastic tube placed in the corner of the roof of the mouth to create vibrations. To create the most normal sound when using the Cooper-Rand Electrolarynx, the client should (1) avoid trying to use the tongue to hold the tube in place; (2) compress the tone generator for short intervals and speak in phrases, rather than full sentences; (3) speak using large movements of the lips, tongue, and jaw, rather than keeping the mouth partially closed; (4) talk face-to-face with the listener; and (5) practice, since development of skills takes time. Another type of artificial larynx is placed against the neck rather than in the mouth. With experience the client can learn to move the lips in ways that create normal-sounding speech. With both devices, voice pitch is low and the sound resembles that of a robot or machine.

Esophageal speech is a method of swallowing air, trapping it in the esophagus, and releasing it to create sound. The air causes vibration of the pharyngoesophageal seg-ment and sound (initially, similar to a belch). With practice, 50% of clients will develop some speech skills, but only 10% will develop fluent speech.

Stoma care. Before discharge, the client should be instructed in the care of the laryngectomy stoma.[25] The area around the stoma should be washed daily with a moist cloth. If a laryngectomy tube is in place, the tube will need to be removed every 4 to 5 days and cleaned in the same manner as a tracheostomy tube (see Table 20-11). If dried secretions form around the stoma, they may be removed with Q-Tips. A scarf, a loose shirt, or a crocheted stoma shield can be used to shield the stoma (Fig. 20-18). The client should cover the stoma with a loose dressing or with the hand when coughing, since mucus may be expectorated. Also, the stoma should be covered during any activity that might lead to inhalation of foreign materials (e.g., shaving, application of makeup). Since water can easily enter the stoma, the client should wear a plastic collar when taking a shower. Swimming is contraindicated. Initially after surgery, humidification will be supplied by oxygen mist through the tracheostomy adaptor. Later, a bedside humidifier can be substituted. Oral fluid intake must be maintained, especially in dry weather. The client should be told of the importance of wearing a Medic-Alert bracelet or other identification that alerts others in an emergency situation of the use of neck breathing (Fig. 20-19).

Since the client no longer breathes through the nose, the ability to smell smoke and food may be lost. Advise the client to install smoke detectors in the home. It is impor-

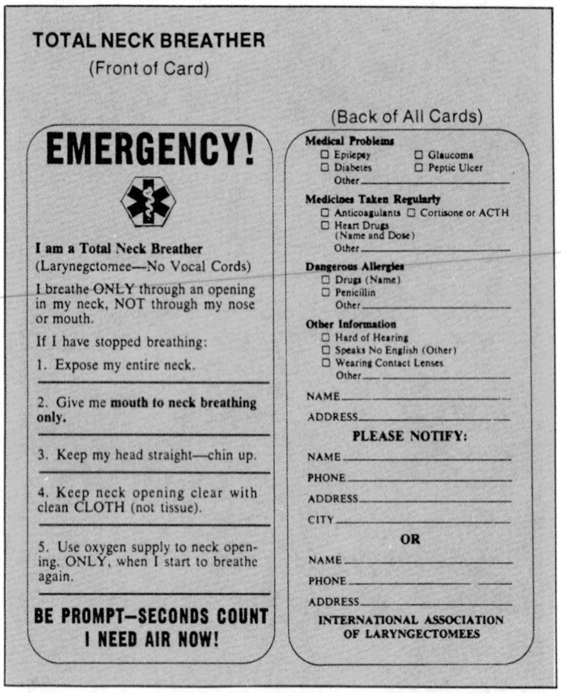

Fig. 20-19 Emergency identification of a neck breather.

tant for food to be colorful, attractively prepared, and nutritious, since taste may also be diminished.

The client can resume exercise, recreation, and sexual activity when able. Most clients can return to work 1 to 2 months after laryngectomy. However, as many as 50% never return to full-time employment. The changes that follow laryngectomy are upsetting. Loss of speech, loss of the ability to taste and smell, inability to produce audible sounds (including laughing and weeping), and the presence of a permanent tracheal stoma that produces undesirable mucus are often overwhelming to the client.

Although changes in body image resulting from the surgical procedure are discussed before surgery, the client may not be prepared for the reality of the changes. Clients with a strong self-image typically make an easier adjustment. Many clients who have head and neck cancer also have a substance abuse problem, an altered self-image, and problems in expressing feelings before surgery. These problems make adjustment even more difficult. Reaction of the significant other is important. Acceptance by another person can promote an improved self-image. Encouraging the client to participate in self-care activities is another important part of rehabilitation.

Palliative treatment. Despite the use of surgical interventions and radiation therapy, the cure rate is disappointingly low for advanced head and neck cancer. The 5-year survival rate is less than 30%. Reasons include a high death rate from causes that are not related to cancer (e.g., cirrhosis, chronic obstructive lung disease, cardiovascular disease), discovery of a second primary tumor, and failure to control local or regional disease.

Uncontrolled metastatic cancer of the larynx is often painful, leaving the affected person in a severely debili-

tated state. When a lesion with disabling metastasis becomes ulcerated, fungated, or infected, the ulcer should be removed surgically. Palliative radiotherapy may also be used.

C ase Study

CANCER OF THE LARYNX

Mr. C., a 60-year-old man, was admitted for evaluation of mild pain on swallowing and a sore throat that had persisted over the past year. The symptoms had worsened in the last 2 months. The client had used various cold remedies to relieve the symptoms without relief. His weight was 160 pounds, 5 pounds less than usual. He attributed his weight loss to "no appetite and trouble swallowing certain foods." Although he had stopped smoking 2 months ago, he had smoked three packs of cigarettes a day for 40 years. He also consumes a six-pack of beer a day. He was accompanied to the clinic by his daughter. Examination by laryngoscopy showed enlarged cervical lymph nodes and an epiglottic lesion. A tumor was located just above the vocal cords. No evidence of metastasis was found. A supraglottic laryngectomy was performed. After the procedure, Mr. C. returned to his room with a tracheostomy tube with inflated cuff, a nasogastric tube, and four small neck drains connected to low suction. His vital signs were stable, and he complained of little pain.

Discussion Questions

1. What information in the assessment suggests that Mr. C. might be at risk of cancer of the larynx?
2. What diagnostic tests are typically performed to evaluate the extent of this problem?
3. What teaching is needed before and after laryngectomy?
4. Discuss the nursing diagnoses and nursing interventions involved in the management of the client who requires a laryngectomy.
5. Discuss methods used to restore the voice after laryngectomy. How do these methods differ in regard to the techniques used to produce speech after removal of the vocal cords?
6. What teaching is required to assist this client to assume self-care after his surgery? What precautions should the client take because of his stoma?
7. What steps would you take to assess the support system available for this client? How would you plan to incorporate his daughter in the plan of care?

R eview Questions

1. "Rebound nasal congestion" or rhinitis medicamentosa is the result of
   a. chronic sinusitis
   b. frequent nasal infections
   c. an antigen-antibody interaction
   d. prolonged use of vasoconstrictor agents
2. The client with acute sinusitis may have all of the following symptoms *except*
   a. decreased translucency
   b. hyperemic and edematous mucosa
   c. recurrent episodes of purulent infection
   d. tenderness when pressure is applied over the sinuses

3. All of the following groups should receive yearly influenza vaccination *except*
   a. persons with an allergic reaction to egg protein
   b. residents of nursing homes
   c. adults with chronic pulmonary or cardiovascular problems
   d. health care professionals in contact with high-risk clients
4. The cuff on an endotracheal tube or tracheostomy should be inflated
   a. with 5 ml of air
   b. with 10 ml air
   c. until the pilot balloon is tense
   d. until minimal occluding volume is reached
5. Suctioning should be performed
   a. every 2 hours even if the chest is clear to auscultation
   b. when rhonchi or coarse rales are heard on auscultation
   c. when the cuff is deflated
   d. after completion of the nasogastric feeding
6. Symptoms of laryngeal cancer include all of the following *except:*
   a. hoarseness
   b. sore throat
   c. leukoplakia
   d. mild pain on swallowing
7. Nursing management of the client immediately after a laryngectomy includes all of the following *except*
   a. changing the surgical dressing
   b. ensuring that the nasogastric tube is patent
   c. placing the client in semi-Fowler's position
   d. monitoring vital signs
8. When using a voice prosthesis, the client
   a. swallows air using a Valsalva maneuver
   b. places a vibrating device in the mouth or on the neck
   c. inhales through the stoma and breathes out through the mouth
   d. inhales through the mouth and breathes out through the stoma

REFERENCES

1. McKinney P and Cunningham BL: Rhinoplasty, New York, 1989, Churchill Livingstone.
2. Guyuron B: Precision rhinoplasty, part I: the role of size photographs and soft-tissue cephalometric analysis, Plast Reconstr Surg 81:489-499, 1988.
3. Petruzzelli GJ and Johnson JT: How to stop a nosebleed, Postgrad Med 86:44-56, Sept 15, 1989.
4. Lieberman P: Rhinitis allergic and nonallergic, Hosp Pract Jun 15, pp 117-145, 1988.
5. O'Hollaren MT and Bardana EJ: Successfully managing chronic rhinitis, J Respir Dis 11:565-573, 1990.
6. Douglas RG and Edelson PJ: Respiratory viral infections. In Fishman AP, ed: Pulmonary diseases and disorders, vol 2, ed 2, New York, 1988, McGraw-Hill Book Co.
7. Curley FJ and others: Cough and the common cold, Am Rev Respir Dis 138:305-311, 1988.
8. Recommendations of the Immunization Practices Advisory Committee: Prevention and control of influenza, part 1: vaccines, Morbid Mortal Weekly Rep 38:297-311, 1989.
9. Martin L: Obstructive sleep apnea: preventing complications, Dimens Crit Care Nurs 8:83-91, 1989.
10. Millman RP and Fishman AP: Sleep apnea syndromes. In Fishman AP, ed: Pulmonary diseases and disorders, vol 2, ed 2, New York, 1988, McGraw-Hill Book Co.
11. Strumpf DA and others: Alternative methods of humidification during use of nasal CPAP, Respir Care 35:217-222, 1990.
12. Mishoe SC: Diagnosis and treatment of sleep apnea syndrome, Respir Care 32:183-201, 1987.
13. Dennison RD: Managing the patient with upper airway obstruction, Nursing '87 17:34-41, 1987.
14. Wilson DJ: Airway appliances and management. In Kacmarek RM and Stoller JK: Current respiratory care, Philadelphia, 1988, BC Decker, Inc.
15. Hoffman LA and Maszkiewicz RC: Airway management for the critically ill patient, Am J Nurs 87:39-53, 1987.
16. Tasota FJ and others: Evaluation of two methods used to stabilize oral endotracheal tubes, Heart Lung 16:140-146, 1987.
17. Snowberger P: Decreasing tracheal tissue damage due to excessive cuff pressures, Dimens Crit Care Nurs 5:136-142, 1986.
18. Chulay M and Graeber G: Efficacy of hyperinflation and hyperoxygenation suctioning interventions, Heart Lung 17:15-22, 1988.
19. Stone KS and others: Effects of lung hyperinflation on mean arterial pressure and postsuctioning hypoxemia, Heart Lung 18:377-385, 1989.
20. March HM and others: Timing of tracheostomy in the critically ill patient, Chest 96:190-193, 1989.
21. Heffner JE: Medical indications for tracheotomy, Chest 96:186-190, 1989.
22. Million RR, Cassisi NJ, and Clark JR: Cancer of the head and neck. In DeVita VT, Hellman S, and Rosenberg SA, eds: Cancer: principles and practice of oncology, vol 1, ed 3, Philadelphia, 1989, JB Lippincott Co.
23. Sawyer DL and Bruya MA: Care of the patient having radical neck surgery or permanent laryngostomy: a nursing diagnostic approach, Focus Crit Care 17:166-173, 1990.
24. Brandt B: What you should know about radiation implant therapy to the head and neck, Oncol Nurs Forum 16:579-582, 1989.
25. Siegler BA: Nursing care for head and neck tumor patients. In Thawley SE and Panje W: Comprehensive management of head and neck tumors, Philadelphia, 1987, WB Saunders Co.
26. Hall IS and Coman BH: Diseases of the nose, throat and ear, ed 13, London, 1987, Churchill Livingstone.

CLIENT RESOURCES

Alert, Well and Keeping Energetic (AWAKE)

This is a health awareness group for clients with sleep disordered breathing and is sponsored by the Association of Polysomnographic Technologists. For information, contact Lucy Seger, Presbyterian-University Hospital, Pittsburgh, PA 15213.

Sleeping Problems: What Can You Do?

This patient-teaching booklet is provided by Respironics, Inc., 530 Seco Rd., Monroeville, PA 15146.

Lung Line

Clients who have a question about lung disease can call 1-800-222-LUNG, a toll-free information service staffed by registered nurses who have received special education in respiratory care. The Lung Line is offered by the National Jewish Center for Immunology and Respiratory Medicine, Denver, CO, and operates Monday through Friday, 10:30 AM to 7 PM (EST). In Denver, the number is 398-1477.

Laryngectomy Clients

An organization for laryngectomy clients is International Association of Laryngectomees, American Cancer Society, 777 Third Ave, New York, NY 10017.

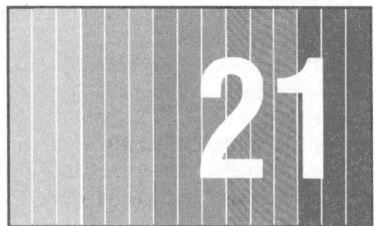

CHAPTER

21

Nursing Role in Management

Lower Respiratory Problems

Joyce Tremper Mitchell

L earning Objectives

1. Describe the pathogenesis, types, clinical manifestations, and therapeutic and pharmacological management of pneumonia.
2. Explain the nursing role in management of the client with pneumonia.
3. Describe the pathogenesis, classification, clinical manifestations, complications, diagnostic abnormalities, and therapeutic, pharmacological, and nursing management of tuberculosis.
4. Identify the causes, clinical manifestations, and therapeutic and nursing management of pulmonary fungal infections.
5. Explain the pathophysiology, clinical manifestations, therapeutic and nursing management of bronchiectasis and lung abscess.
6. Identify the indications for oxygen therapy, methods of delivery, and complications of oxygen administration.
7. Identify the clinical features and management of occupational lung diseases.

8. Describe the causes, risk factors, pathogenesis, clinical manifestations, and therapeutic and nursing management of lung cancer.
9. Describe risks associated with cigarette smoking and the role of nurses in assisting clients to stop smoking.
10. Identify the mechanisms involved and the clinical manifestations of pneumothorax, fractured ribs, and flail chest.
11. Describe the purpose, methods, and nursing responsibilities related to chest tubes.
12. Explain the types of chest surgery and appropriate preoperative and postoperative care.
13. Compare and contrast extrapulmonary and intrapulmonary restrictive lung disorders in terms of causes, clinical manifestations, and management.
14. Describe the pathophysiology, clinical manifestations, and management of pulmonary hypertension and cor pulmonale.
15. Discuss the use of heart-lung transplantation as an alternative treatment for end-stage pulmonary hypertension.

There is a wide variety of problems that affect the lower respiratory system. Lung diseases that are characterized primarily by an obstructive disorder, such as asthma, emphysema, chronic bronchitis, and cystic fibrosis, are discussed in Chapter 22. All other lower respiratory problems are discussed in this chapter.

PULMONARY INFECTIONS

Pulmonary infections annually rank among the top 10 causes of death in the United States. Bacterial pneumonias

remain the leading infectious cause of death in spite of the availability of antimicrobial agents.[1] Tuberculosis, although potentially curable and preventable, is still a significant public health problem in the United States and the rest of the world.

Acute Bronchitis

Acute bronchitis is a common pulmonary infection that occurs most frequently in clients with chronic obstructive pulmonary disease (COPD) but also in other clients, usually as a sequela to an upper respiratory tract infection. Clients present with fever, cough, tachypnea, purulent sputum, and occasionally pleuritic chest pain. On ausculta-

---

Reviewed by Frances Jackson, R.N., Ph.D., Assistant Professor, Oakland University School of Nursing, Oakland, Michigan.

tion, diffuse rhonchi and crackles (rales) may be heard. Chest radiograph differentiates acute bronchitis from pneumonia, since there is usually no evidence of consolidation or infiltrates with bronchitis. The origin of most cases of acute bronchitis is viral, but bacterial causes (*Streptococcus pneumoniae* or *Haemophilus influenzae*) are also common.

Acute bronchitis does not require hospitalization unless the client shows symptoms of dehydration. Treatment is generally with a broad-spectrum antibiotic (e.g., ampicillin, tetracycline, or erythromycin) for 7 to 10 days. Clients with COPD who present with symptoms of acute bronchitis are usually treated empirically with broad-spectrum antibiotics, and modifications in therapy are made if they prove ineffective. Often, clients with COPD are taught to recognize symptoms of acute bronchitis and to begin a course of antibiotics when symptoms occur. Many clinicians believe that the delay that may occur if the client waits to be examined by a physician and then begins to take antibiotics often results in a more severe infection. This delay may cause serious consequences for clients with severe chronic disease.

In the education of clients on the use of antibiotics, it is important to stress that the full course of the drug must be taken to minimize development of resistant organisms. Additionally, timing of drug dosing related to food intake and avoidance of certain foods taken concurrently with certain medications (e.g., milk and antacids with tetracycline) should be discussed with the client.

Pneumonia

Significance. Pneumonia, or pneumonitis, is an acute inflammation of the lung parenchyma. Until 1936, pneumonia was the leading cause of death in the United States. Then sulfa drugs and penicillin were discovered and used in the treatment of pneumonia. However, in spite of antibiotics, pneumonia is still quite common, and some types of the disease have a very high mortality rate. About 1% of the American population will have pneumonia at some time in their lives. Pneumonia is the sixth leading cause of death in the United States.

Pathophysiology

Normal defense mechanisms. Normally, the airway distal to the larynx is sterile because of protective defense mechanisms. These mechanisms include the following (see Chapter 19):

1. Filtration and humidification of air
2. Warming of inspired air
3. Epiglottis closure over the trachea
4. Cough reflex
5. Mucociliary escalator mechanism
6. Secretion of immunoglobulin A
7. Alveolar macrophage
8. Serum immunoglobulin G

Factors predisposing to pneumonia. Pneumonia is more likely to result when the defense mechanisms become incompetent or are overwhelmed by the virulence or quantity of infectious agents. Altered consciousness depresses the cough and epiglottal reflexes, which may allow aspiration of oropharyngeal contents into the lungs. Tra-

Table 21-1 Factors Predisposing to Pneumonia

Smoking
Air pollution
Altered consciousness: alcoholism, head injury, seizures, anesthesia, drug overdose
Tracheal intubation (endotracheal intubation, tracheostomy)
URI
Chronic diseases: chronic lung disease, diabetes mellitus, heart disease, uremia, cancer
Immunosuppression
  Drugs (corticosteroids, cancer chemotherapy, immunosuppressive therapy after organ transplant)
  Acquired immunodeficiency syndrome (AIDS)
Malnutrition
Inhalation or aspiration of noxious substances
Debilitating illness
Bed rest and prolonged immobility
Altered oropharyngeal flora

cheal intubation interferes with the normal cough reflex and the mucociliary escalator mechanism. It also bypasses the upper airways in which filtration and humidification of air normally take place. The mucociliary escalator mechanism is impaired by air pollution, cigarette smoking, viral upper respiratory tract infections (URIs), and normal changes of aging. In cases of malnutrition the formation and activity of lymphocytes and polymorphonuclear leukocytes are altered. Certain diseases such as leukemia, alcoholism, and diabetes mellitus are associated with an increased frequency of gram-negative bacilli in the oropharynx.[2] (Gram-negative bacilli are not normal flora.) Altered oropharyngeal flora can also occur secondary to antibiotic therapy given for an infection elsewhere in the body. (The factors predisposing to pneumonia are shown in Table 21-1.)

Acquisition of organisms. Organisms that cause pneumonia reach the lung by three methods:

1. Aspiration from the nasopharynx or oropharynx: Many of the organisms that cause pneumonia are normal inhabitants of the pharynx in healthy adults.
2. Inhalation of microbes present in the air: Examples include *Mycoplasma pneumoniae* and fungal pneumonias.
3. Hematogenous spread from a primary infections elsewhere in the body.

Types of pneumonia. Pneumonia can be caused by bacteria, viruses, Mycoplasma organisms, fungi, *Pneumocystis carinii,* chemicals, dust, gases, and a variety of other organisms and materials (Table 21-2). Pneumonia is usually classified according to the causative organism. Sometimes pneumonia is classified on the basis of areas and type of lung involvement (Fig. 21-1).

Gram-positive bacterial pneumonias. Gram-positive bacteria (*S. pneumoniae, Staphylococcus aureus,* and group A β-hemolytic streptococci) account for most bacterial pneumonias acquired in the community. Recently, *S. aureus* has become an increasingly common cause of

Table 21-2 Comparison of Types of Pneumonia

Causative Agent	Characteristics	Clinical Manifestations and Complications
GRAM-POSITIVE BACTERIAL PNEUMONIAS		
Pneumococcal pneumonia (*Streptococcus pneumoniae*)	URI usually preceding, usual involvement of one or more lobes, incubation period of 1 to 3 days, peak incidence in winter and spring, damage to host by overwhelming growth of organism, necrosis of lung tissue (unusual), chest x-ray film showing lobar infiltration,* nasopharyngeal carriers, frequent finding of herpes labialis in association with pneumonia, persons with chronic heart or lung disease, diabetes mellitus, cirrhosis at risk	Abrupt onset, elevated temperature, tachypnea, chills and rigor, productive cough (often bloody, rusty, or green), nausea and vomiting, malaise, myalgia, weakness, pleuritic chest pain, atelectasis, lung abscess (rare), pleural effusions (25%-50%), empyema, metastatic infection (meninges, joints, heart valves), bacteremia (25%)
Staphylococcal pneumonia (*Staphylococcus aureus*)	Acquisition via hematogenous route or via aspiration into lungs; nasopharyngeal carriers (35%-50% of population); necrotizing infection causing destruction of lung tissue; chest x-ray film showing bronchopneumonia*; risk factors of chronic lung disease, leukemia, other debilitating diseases; influenza infection (10 to 14 days earlier) often preceding; drug abusers, diabetics, clients on long-term hemodialysis at risk as carriers; occurrence more frequent in hospitalized clients than in persons in community; prolonged antibiotic therapy usually necessary; high mortality rate in chronically debilitated clients, newborns	Abrupt onset, chills, high fever, productive cough with sputum (often bloody and purulent), tachypnea, progressive dyspnea, pleuritic chest pain, empyema, pleural effusions, lung abscess
Streptococcal pneumonia (*Streptococcus pyogenes*)	Occurrence in military populations after influenza epidemics and sporadically in community, strep throat often associated, occurrence most frequent in winter, transmission to lung by inhalation or aspiration, destruction of lung tissue, chest x-ray film showing bronchopneumonia	Fever (usually >39° C [102.2° F]), chills, cough, pharyngitis, hemoptysis, pleuritic chest pain, dyspnea, myalgia, empyema (common), pleural effusions, bacteremia, mediastinitis, pneumothorax, bronchiectasis
Anthrax pneumonia (*Bacillus anthracis*)	Association with agricultural or industrial exposure (e.g., individuals working with animal hair or contaminated animal hides or bones), transmission to lung via inhalation, formation of spores, ingestion and transport of spores to hilar lymph nodes (site of multiplication of bacteria) by alveolar macrophages, hemorrhagic pneumonitis possible	Early manifestations: insidious onset (2 to 4 days), mild fever, myalgia, malaise, fatigue, nonproductive cough Later manifestations: dyspnea, profuse diaphoresis, cyanosis
Friedländer's pneumonia (*Klebsiella pneumoniae*)	Most common gram-negative pneumonias acquired outside hospital; alcoholics, diabetics, persons with chronic lung disease, and postoperative clients at risk; transmission to lung via aspiration of oropharyngeal organisms; chest x-ray film showing lobar consolidation*; rapid progression to lung abscess possible; high mortality and morbidity rates	Sudden onset, fever, cough, purulent sputum, hemoptysis, malaise, pleuritic chest pain, extensive lung necrosis, lung abscess, empyema, pericarditis, meningitis

*See Fig. 21-1.
†Organism has characteristics of both bacteria and viruses.

Table 21-2 Comparison of Types of Pneumonia—cont'd

Causative Agent	Characteristics	Clinical Manifestations and Complications
GRAM-NEGATIVE BACTERIAL PNEUMONIAS—cont'd		
Pseudomonas pneumonia (*Pseudomonas aeruginosa*)	Most common gram-negative hospital-acquired pneumonia; predisposition from endotracheal intubation, intermittent positive-pressure breathing treatments, suctioning, respiratory therapy equipment; high mortality rate in critically ill clients; chest x-ray film showing nodular bronchopneumonia*; persons with chronic lung disease, debilitating diseases, tracheostomies, cancer, and kidney transplants or those taking immunosuppressive drugs or broad-spectrum antibiotics at risk; high mortality rate (50%-90%)	High fever, cough, copious sputum, hypoxia, cyanosis, lung abscess
Influenza pneumonia (*Haemophilus influenzae*)	Increase in incidence; transmission to lung by endogenous aspiration; chest x-ray films showing bronchopneumonia in multiple lobes or lobar consolidation; alcoholics and persons with chronic lung disease, recent viral infections, and immune deficiencies at risk; high mortality rate, especially in older adult clients	Usual gradual onset, sometimes abrupt; fever; chills; cough; purulent sputum; hemoptysis; sore throat; dyspnea; nausea and vomiting; pleuritic chest pain; pleural effusions; lung abscess (common); empyema (common)
Legionnaires' disease (*Legionella pneumophila*)	Occurrence in outbreaks or sporadic, transmission to lung from airborne organisms, proliferation of organisms in water reservoirs (e.g., air-conditioning cooling towers), cigarette smokers and persons with serious underlying diseases (e.g., chronic lung or heart conditions) at increased risk, erythromycin effective	Myalgia (initially), headache (initially), fever, chills, nonproductive cough, pleuritic chest pain, nausea and vomiting, diarrhea, mental confusion, respiratory failure (major complication), healing with fibrosis common
ANAEROBIC BACTERIAL PNEUMONIAS		
Anaerobic streptococci, fusobacteria, *Bacteroides* species	Transmission to lung usually by aspiration of oropharyngeal secretions but occasionally via blood from gastrointestinal or genitourinary tract or wound infections; three or four anaerobes usually causing infections; persons with poor dental hygiene, periodontal disease, and history of altered consciousness at risk; chest x-ray film often showing lung abscess, empyema, necrotizing pneumonia	Similar to pneumococcal pneumonia, except for insidious onset; foul-smelling sputum; necrotizing pneumonitis (aspiration induced); lung abscess; empyema
MYCOPLASMA PNEUMONIA		
Mycoplasma pneumonia (*Mycoplasma pneumoniae*)†	Transmission from person to person by respiratory droplets; incubation period of 9 to 21 days; involvement of epithelial lining of respiratory system; common in children, military populations, college-age groups; increase in cold agglutinin titer in serum or complement fixation with negative bacterial culture; chest x-ray film showing interstitial pneumonia, often bilaterally*	Gradual onset; URI, including fever (low-grade), nasal congestion, pharyngitis; lower respiratory tract involvement (e.g., bronchitis, bronchiolitis); headache; malaise; cough (initially usually nonproductive); maculopapular rashes

Continued.

Table 21-2 Comparison of Types of Pneumonia—cont'd

Causative Agent	Characteristics	Clinical Manifestations and Complications
VIRAL PNEUMONIAS		
Influenza viruses; adenovirus; parainfluenza viruses; respiratory syncytial virus	Influenza A most common in civilian adults; responsible for about one half of all pneumonias; peak incidence in winter; transmission from person to person by respiratory droplets; usually self-limiting; symptomatic treatment; adverse effect on many respiratory defense mechanisms, predisposing clients to secondary bacterial pneumonia; chest x-ray film showing interstitial pneumonia*	Fever, chills, headache, myalgia, anorexia, sneezing, nasal congestion, cough (initially nonproductive)
PROTOZOAN PNEUMONIA		
Interstitial plasma cell pneumonia *(Pneumocystis carinii)*	Opportunistic infection; persons with immunosuppression (e.g., recipients of organ transplants, clients with AIDS, and those with hematological malignancies) at highest risk; presentation similar to other atypical pneumonias	Cough (usually nonproductive), fever, night sweats, dyspnea (may be only with exertion)

*See Fig. 21-1.

nosocomial pneumonia. The most common type of pneumonia is pneumococcal pneumonia caused by *S. pneumoniae*.

Gram-negative bacterial pneumonias. There has been an increasing incidence of aerobic gram-negative bacterial pneumonias. They account for 20% of community-acquired pneumonias and 40% to 60% of hospital-acquired pneumonias.[1] Organisms that cause gram-negative pneumonias include *Klebsiella, Pseudomonas, Haemophilus, Serratia, Escherichia coli,* and *Proteus*. Most of these organisms enter the lung after aspiration of particles from the client's own pharynx. Immunosuppressive therapy, general debility, endotracheal intubation, and prolonged antibiotic therapy may be predisposing factors. Respiratory therapy equipment that is not cleaned is a potential source of infection.

Anaerobic bacterial pneumonias. Most anaerobic pneumonias are caused by aspiration of oropharyngeal secretions. Infections usually involve multiple organisms, and aerobic organisms are also found in many cases of anaerobic pneumonia.

Mycoplasma pneumonia. The transmission of mycoplasma pneumonia is from person to person by respiratory droplets. Intrafamily or intragroup (e.g., the military) spread is common. Mycoplasma pneumonia is usually treated with antibiotics.

Viral pneumonias. Viruses are the most common cause of pneumonia in infants and children. In adults, viruses account for a small number of lower respiratory tract infections.

The initial manifestations of viral pneumonia are highly variable but are usually similar to those of influenza and include fever, myalgia, headache, rhinorrhea, and dry cough. On chest x-ray film there is usually an interstitial pattern of lung involvement. The x-ray study may demonstrate extensive pulmonary involvement, although there are minimal physical findings on examination. These types of pneumonias are typically mild and self-limiting and result in no permanent lung damage in previously healthy individuals. Treatment is usually for relief of symptoms, since antibiotics are not effective. Occasionally, viral pneumonias set the stage for bacterial involvement. The client may have concurrent viral and bacterial pneumonia.[3]

Primary influenza viral pneumonia syndrome, although rare, is severe and may be fatal. It occurs primarily in clients who are older adults or who are debilitated or who have chronic lung or heart disease. The alveoli fill with fibrin, fluid, red blood cells (RBCs), and macrophages. These individuals have severe hypoxemia, tachycardia, and tachypnea. The mortality rate is extremely high in spite of ventilatory support. If the individual survives, pulmonary fibrosis is a common complication.

Viral pneumonia is also found in association with systemic viral diseases such as measles, varicella-zoster virus, and herpes simplex. Varicella pneumonia is more common in adults with chicken pox than in children.

Two antiviral drugs, amantadine and rimantadine, are approved for parenteral use in treatment of viral respiratory infections, and they have been shown to have therapeutic benefit in uncomplicated cases of influenza infections in adults.[4] Vaccines against adenovirus and influenza are currently available. Since adenovirus pneumonia is not common in the general population, the use of adenovirus

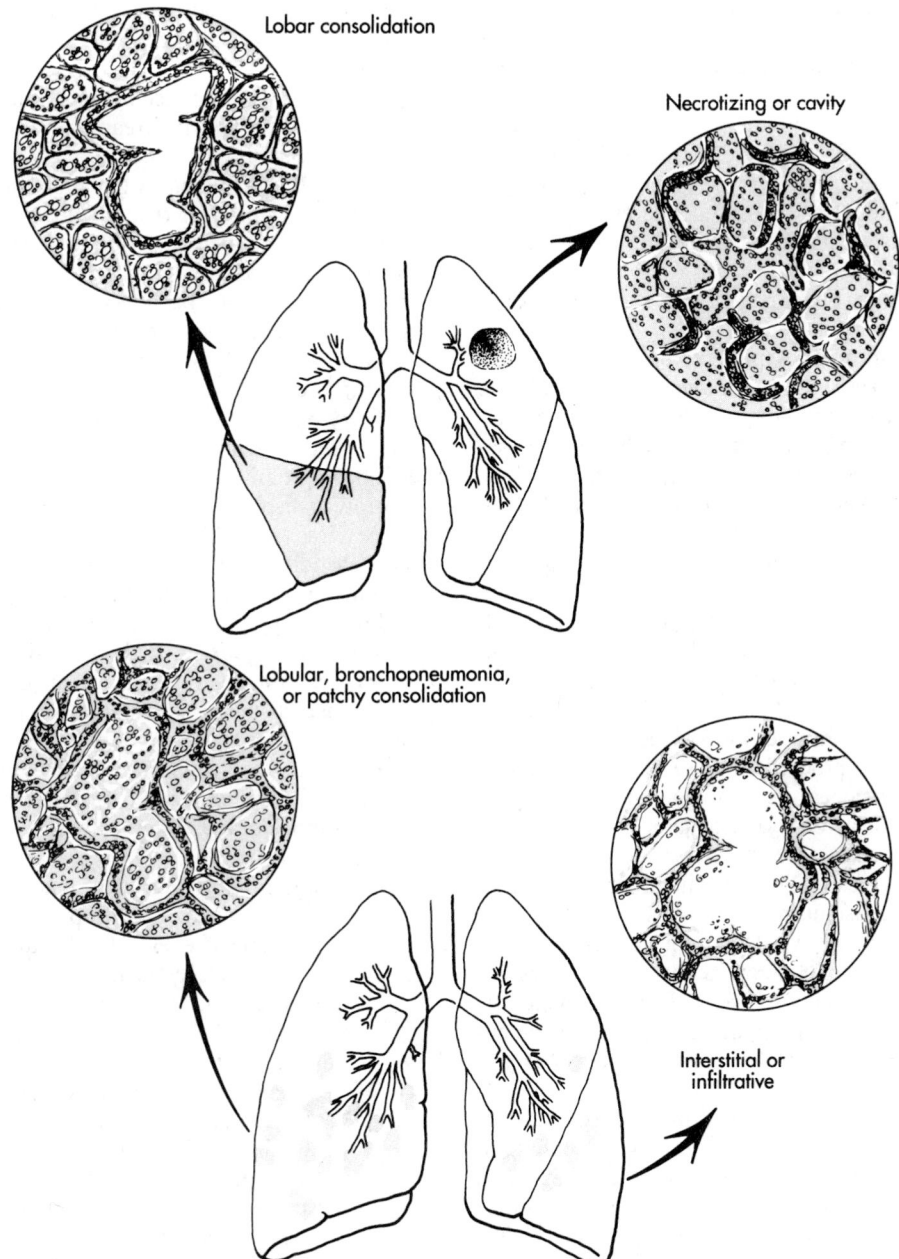

Fig. 21-1 Forms of pneumonia. *Lobar:* Entire lobe is consolidated. Exudate chiefly intraalveolar *(inset). Pneumococcus* and *Klebsiella* are common infecting organisms. *Necrotizing:* Granuloma may undergo caseous necrosis and form a cavity. Fungi and tubercle bacillus are common infecting organisms. *Lobular:* Patchy distribution displayed. Fibrinous exudate is chiefly in bronchioles. *Staphylococcus* and *Streptococcus* are common infecting organisms. *Interstitial:* Perivascular exudate and edema found between the alveoli, caused by virus or mycoplasmal infection. (From Price S and Wilson L: Pathophysiology: clinical concepts of disease processes, ed 4, St Louis, 1991, Mosby–Year Book, Inc.)

vaccine has been limited to high-risk groups such as military recruits. Influenza vaccine is considered a mainstay of prevention and is recommended annually for use in individuals considered to be at high risk of serious influenza (see Table 20-4).

Amantadine has also been used as a chemoprophylactic agent against influenza A virus infections. It acts by preventing the penetration of the virus into the host cell. It is used primarily in outbreaks of the virus and in high-risk individuals. Amantadine needs to be given daily throughout the period of influenza exposure. Side effects are uncommon and consist primarily of reversible minor central nervous system (CNS) effects.

Fungal pneumonia. Fungi may also be a cause of pneumonia (see pp. 518-519).

Aspiration pneumonia. Aspiration pneumonia is frequently called *necrotizing pneumonia* because of the pathological changes in the lungs. It usually follows aspiration of material in the mouth into the trachea and subsequently the lungs. The aspirated material—food, water, vomitus—is the triggering mechanism for the pathology of pneumonia.

If the aspirated material is an inert substance (e.g., barium or nonacid stomach contents), the initial manifestation is usually due to obstruction of airways. When the aspirated materials contain gastric acid, there is chemical injury to the lung parenchyma with infection as a secondary event usually 48 to 72 hours later. The infecting organism is usually one of the normal oropharyngeal flora, and the clinical manifestations proceed as those of a classic pneumococcal or streptococcal pneumonia. Multiple organisms, including both aerobes and anaerobes, are isolated from the sputum of these individuals.

Persons who have aspiration pneumonia usually have a history of loss of consciousness (e.g., as a result of seizure, anesthesia, head injury, alcohol intake). With loss of consciousness, the gag and cough reflexes are depressed, and aspiration is more likely to occur. The dependent portions of the lung are most often affected, primarily the superior segments of the lower lobes, which are dependent in the supine position.

Pneumonia in the compromised host. Certain clients with an altered immune response are highly susceptible to respiratory infections. Individuals considered at high risk are those with severe protein-calorie malnutrition, immune deficiencies, clients who have had transplants, and clients who are being treated with radiation therapy, cancer chemotherapy drugs, and corticosteroids (especially for a prolonged period). These individuals have a variety of altered conditions, including suppressed B- and T-lymphocyte function, depressed bone marrow function, and decreased levels of neutrophils and macrophages. In addition to the causative agents (especially gram-negative bacteria), other agents that cause pneumonia in immunosuppressed clients are *Pneumocystis carinii* (a protozoan), cytomegalovirus, and fungi.

Pneumocystis carinii, a protozoan organism, rarely causes pneumonia in healthy individuals. The chest x-ray usually shows a diffuse bilateral alveolar pattern of infiltration. In widespread disease, the lungs are massively consolidated. Clinical manifestations are insidious and include fever, tachypnea, tachycardia, dyspnea, nonproductive cough, and hypoxemia. Pulmonary physical findings are minimal in proportion to the serious nature of the disease. Treatment consists of a 14-day course of trimethoprim-sulfamethoxazole (Bactrim) as the primary agent and pentamidine isethionate, which was recently approved by the FDA for treatment of pneumocystis pneumonia. The mortality rate for *P. carinii* pneumonia (PCP) is about 50%. Untreated, the mortality rate is 100%. In populations with high risk for development of *P. carinii* pneumonitis (e.g., clients with hematological malignancies or AIDS), secondary prophylaxis with trimethoprim-sulfamethoxazole may be advocated. Aerosols of pentamadine isethionate have shown promising results as a treatment option for *P. carinii* pneumonia and as a prophylactic measure.[5]

Cytomegalovirus, also called *cytomegalic inclusion virus,* is the most important type of viral pneumonia in immunocompromised clients, particularly in renal or bone marrow transplant recipients. Cytomegalovirus, a type of herpesvirus, gives rise to latent infections and reactivation with shedding of infectious virus. This type of interstitial pneumonia can be a mild disease or it can be fulminant and produce pulmonary insufficiency and death. Often, cytomegalovirus coexists with other opportunistic bacterial, fungal, or protozoan agents in causing pneumonia. There is no specific therapy available for this type of pneumonia.[4]

Pneumococcal pneumonia. Pneumococcal pneumonia is the most common cause of bacterial pneumonia.

Pathophysiology. There are four characteristic stages of the disease process:

1. *Congestion:* After the pneumococcus organisms reach the alveoli via droplets or saliva, there is an outpouring of edema fluid into the alveoli. The organisms multiply in the serous fluid and the infection is spread. The pneumococci damage the host by their overwhelming growth and interference with lung function.
2. *Red hepatization:* There is massive dilatation of the capillaries, and alveoli are filled with organisms, neutrophils, RBCs, and fibrin (Fig. 21-2). The lung appears red and granular, or liverlike, which is why the process is called *hepatization.*
3. *Gray hepatization:* Blood flow decreases, and leukocytes and fibrin consolidate in the affected part of the lung.
4. *Resolution:* Complete resolution and healing occur if there are no complications. The exudate becomes lysed and is processed by the macrophages. The normal lung tissue is restored, and the person's gas-exchange ability returns to normal.

Clinical manifestations. Typically an upper respiratory tract infection precedes a case of pneumococcal pneumonia. The incubation period is 1 to 14 days. Presenting manifestations include an acute onset of fever, chills, productive cough with greenish, bloody, or rusty sputum, and pleuritic chest pain. Nausea and vomiting are also observed, and systemic manifestations such as malaise, my-

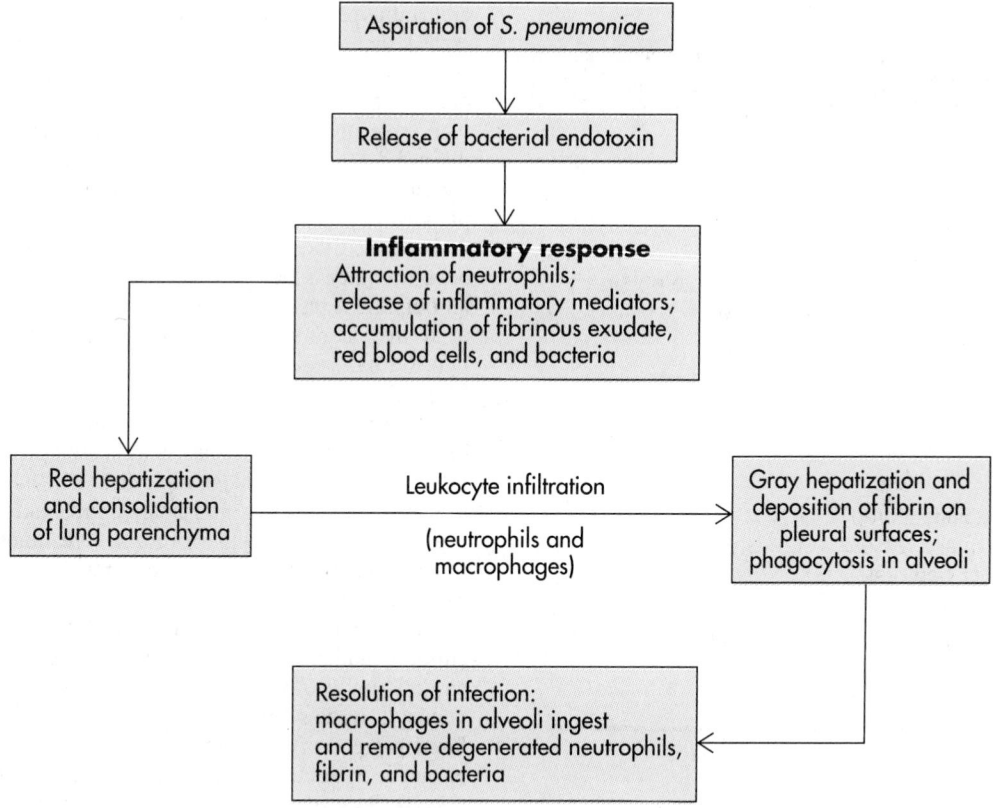

Fig. 21-2 Pathophysiological course of pneumococcal pneumonia. (From McCance KL and Huether SE: Pathophysiology: the biological basis for disease in adults and children, St Louis, 1990, Mosby–Year Book, Inc, p 1078.)

algia, and weakness are common. Tachycardia, tachypnea, and chest splinting are commonly found. Findings on physical examination of the chest may include dullness to percussion, diminished or bronchial breath sounds in the affected part of the lung, crackles (rales), and a pleural friction rub. The client's skin may have a dusky appearance because of hypoxemia. If the lower lobes are involved, the client may experience mild to severe abdominal pain.

Complications. Pneumococcal pneumonia generally runs an uncomplicated course. The associated mortality rate is about 10%. Complications that do develop are more frequently found in individuals with underlying chronic diseases. Complications may include the following:

1. *Pleurisy* (inflammation of the pleura) is a relatively common accompanying problem of pneumonia. Pain develops when the parietal and visceral pleurae rub together.

2. *Pleural effusion* occurs in many clients. Usually, the effusion is sterile and is reabsorbed in 1 to 2 weeks. Occasionally, it requires aspiration by means of thoracentesis.

3. *Atelectasis* (collapsed, airless alveoli) of one or part of one lobe may occur. These areas usually clear with effective coughing and deep breathing or vigorous tracheal suctioning.

4. *Delayed resolution* results from persistent infection and is seen on x-ray film as residual consolidation. Usually, the physical findings return to normal within 2 to 4 weeks.

5. *Lung abscess* is *not* a common complication of pneumococcal pneumonia. It is seen more frequently with other types of pneumonia, such as staphylococcal and gram-negative pneumonias (see pp. 501, 504).

6. *Empyema* (accumulation of purulent exudate in the pleural cavity) is relatively infrequent but requires antibiotic therapy and drainage of the exudate by a chest tube or open surgical drainage.

7. *Pericarditis* results from spread of the infecting organism from an infected pleura or via a hematogenous route to the pericardium (the fibroserous sac around the heart).

8. *Arthritis* results from systemic spread of the organism. The affected joint is swollen, red, and painful, and a purulent exudate can be aspirated.

9. *Meningitis* caused by pneumococcus is second only to meningococcus as a cause of purulent meningitis. Any client with pneumococcal pneumonia who is disoriented, confused, or somnolent should have a lumbar puncture to evaluate the possibility of pneumococcal meningitis.

10. *Endocarditis* can develop when the organisms attack the endocardium and the valves of the heart.

Table 21-3

Diagnostic and Therapeutic Management: Bacterial Pneumonia

DIAGNOSTIC

History and physical examination
Gram stain of sputum
Sputum culture and sensitivity test (transtracheal aspiration or bronchoscopy with aspiration if unable to obtain via cough or induced production of sputum)
Chest x-ray study
ABGs (if indicated)
Complete blood count
Blood cultures

THERAPEUTIC

Appropriate antibiotic therapy*
Increased fluid intake (at least 3 L every 24 hr)
Limited activity or bed rest
Antipyretics
Analgesics
Oxygen therapy (if indicated)
Aerosol therapy

---

*See Table 21-4.

The clinical manifestations are similar to those of acute bacterial endocarditis (see Chapter 31).

Diagnostic studies. The common diagnostic measures for pneumonia are presented in Table 21-3. Immediate identification of the organism is critical in order to institute appropriate antimicrobial therapy. Blood and sputum cultures may take 24 to 72 hours. Therefore a Gram stain of the sputum provides the information on which the initial therapy is based. Usually, the predominant organism can be identified on a Gram stain. If the client cannot voluntarily produce a sputum specimen (see techniques presented in Table 19-8), procedures such as transtracheal aspiration and fiberoptic bronchoscopy may be used. Transtracheal aspiration involves inserting a catheter into the trachea through the cricothyroid membrane and withdrawing secretions for testing.

Chest x-ray films often show a typical pattern characteristic of the infecting organism (see Table 21-2). Arterial blood gases (ABGs), if obtained, usually reveal hypoxemia. Leukocytosis is found in about 80% of clients with pneumonia, usually with a leukocyte count greater than 15,000 with a shift to the left.[2]

Therapeutic management. Prompt treatment with the appropriate antibiotic almost always cures bacterial and mycoplasma pneumonia. Currently, there is no effective treatment for viral pneumonia. In uncomplicated cases, the client responds to drug therapy within 1 to 2 days. Indications of improvement include decreased temperature, improved breathing, and reduced chest pain.

In addition to antibiotic therapy, supportive measures may be used, including oxygen therapy to treat hypoxemia, analgesics such as codeine to relieve the chest pain,

and antipyretics such as aspirin or acetaminophen to decrease the temperature. Chest physiotherapy to mobilize secretions has been widely used. However, evidence from one recent study suggests that it is of no benefit to clients who have uncomplicated pneumonia without chronic lung disease.[6] During the acute febrile phase, clients' activity should be restricted, and rest should be encouraged and planned.

Most individuals with mild to moderate illness who have no other underlying disease process can be treated on an outpatient basis. If there is a serious underlying disease or if the pneumonia is accompanied by severe dyspnea, hypoxemia, or other complications, the client should be hospitalized.

Pneumococcal vaccine. Pneumococcal vaccine has been developed, and its use is indicated primarily for those individuals considered at high risk who (1) have chronic illnesses such as lung and heart disease and diabetes mellitus, (2) are recovering from a severe illness, (3) are age 65 or older, or (4) are in nursing homes or other long-term care facilities.

The vaccine is not recommended for pregnant women, children under 2 years of age, or those with febrile disease. Usually 0.5 ml is given intramuscularly or subcutaneously. It was previously believed that the vaccine offered protection for 5 years. The current recommendation is that it is good for the person's lifetime. However, it is not 100% effective in prevention of pneumococcal pneumonia, since it contains only 15% to 18% of the 80 or more serotypes.[2]

Pharmacological management. The introduction of sulfonamides in the 1930s and penicillin in the 1940s revolutionized the treatment of pneumonia. Today penicillin is still the drug of choice for a great number of bacterial pneumonias. The main problems with the use of antibiotics in pneumonia are (1) the development of resistant strains of organisms and (2) the client's hypersensitivity or allergic reaction to certain antibiotics. Table 21-4 outlines the major antimicrobial agents used in the treatment of pneumonia and respiratory infections. It is extremely important to identify accurately the infecting organism so that the appropriate drug therapy can be instituted. Initial antimicrobial therapy is based in large part on the results of the Gram-stain smear analysis. More definitive information may later be obtained from the sputum culture and sensitivity test, and the antibiotic can be changed if indicated.

In acute cases, antibiotics are usually given parenterally for the first few days and then administered orally. In mild cases, oral administration is adequate for the duration of the illness. It is extremely important that the client continue taking the antibiotics for the prescribed period (usually at least 10 days) to prevent a relapse of pneumonia and the development of resistant strains of the organism. Before antibiotics are given, it is necessary to obtain the client's history regarding possible drug allergies.

Nutritional considerations. Fluid intake of at least 3 liters per day is very important in the supportive treatment of pneumonia. If oral intake cannot be maintained, intravenous (IV) administration of fluids and electrolytes may

Table 21-4   Antibiotic Drug Therapy Used for Pneumonia

Drug	Common Side Effects	Comments
PENICILLINS		
Penicillin G (Bicillin), penicillin G with procaine, penicillin V, ampicillin, amoxicillin, carbenicillin (Geopen), methicillin, nafcillin, oxacillin, cloxacillin, dicloxacillin, piperacillin (Pipracil), azlocillin (Axlin), ticarcillin (Ticar), bacampicillin (Spectrobid), amoxicillin and potassium clavulanate (Augmentin)	Low incidence of side effects, hypersensitivity reactions (15%), neurotoxicity (from procaine penicillin), hepatotoxicity, neutropenia, interstitial nephritis (especially from methicillin)	Frequently drug of choice in treatment of bacterial and anaerobic pneumonias, broad-spectrum activity, monitoring for superinfection necessary
CEPHALOSPORINS		
Cephalothin (Keflin),* cephapirin (Cefadyl),* cefazolin (Ancef, Kefsol),* cephradine (Anspor),* cephalexin (Keflex), cefotaxime (Claforan),‡ moxalactam (Moxam),‡ cefoperazone (Cefobid),‡ cefamandole (Mandol),† cefaclor (Ceclor),† cefotetan disodium (Cefotan),‡ cefoxitin sodium (Mefoxin)†	Gastrointestinal disturbances, phlebitis (from IV administration), nephrotoxicity, hypersensitivity reactions (2%-5%)	Primary therapy in *Klebsiella* pneumonia, along with an aminoglycoside; useful for therapy when mixed infection present; broad-spectrum activity; use when client has known hypersensitivity to penicillins; rapid absorption from gastrointestinal tract
AMINOGLYCOSIDES		
Kanamycin (Kantrex), gentamicin (Garamycin), tobramycin (Nebcin), amikacin (Amikin), neomycin (Neobiotic)	Nephrotoxicity, audiotoxicity, hypersensitivity reactions, neuromuscular blockade	Particularly effective against gram-negative bacilli, poor absorption after oral administration, monitoring of blood urea nitrogen and serum creatinine necessary, assessment of hearing before and during therapy necessary
MISCELLANEOUS DRUGS		
Erythromycin	Gastrointestinal disturbances, infrequent hypersensitivity reactions, reversible hepatotoxicity, phlebitis (with IV administration)	Primary therapy for Legionnaires' disease, drug of choice for treatment of mycoplasma pneumonia
Tetracycline	Gastrointestinal disturbances, photosensitivity, hypersensitivity	Primarily effective against gram-positive bacilli, alteration of gastrointestinal absorption with antacid or milk ingestion
Clindamycin	Gastrointestinal disturbances, hypersensitivity reactions	Particularly effective against anaerobic bacteria, also effective against gram-positive bacteria
Chloramphenicol	Bone marrow suppression, optic neuritis	Broad-spectrum antibiotic, not for treatment of minor infections
Vancomycin	Nephrotoxicity, audiotoxicity, phlebitis	IV administration necessary, infrequent use for pulmonary infections, effective against gram-positive organisms
Lincomycin	Gastrointestinal disturbances, hypersensitivity reactions	Not a first choice drug but useful for clients allergic to penicillin
Aztreonam (Azactam)	Gastrointestinal disturbances, CNS disturbances	Bactericidal against gram-negative aerobic pathogens
Ciprofloxacin (Cipro)	Gastrointestinal disturbances, CNS disturbances	Broad-spectrum activity

*First generation.
†Second generation.
‡Third generation; increased activity against gram-negative and resistant organisms and less activity against gram-positive organisms than first-generation agents.

be necessary for the acutely ill client. A blenderized or processed liquid diet may be tolerated better than solid food by the client in the acute phase of pneumonia. An intake of at least 1500 calories per day should be maintained to provide energy for the increased metabolic processes in the client. Small, frequent meals are tolerated better by the dyspneic client.

Table 21-5

Nursing Assessment of the Client with Pneumonia

SUBJECTIVE DATA

History
Recent: URI, hospitalization, especially with loss of consciousness or abdominal or thoracic surgery; lung cancer; COPD; cigarette smoking; alcoholism; prolonged bed rest or immobility; diabetes; chronic debilitating disease; AIDS; exposure to chemical toxins, dust, allergens, pollutants; poor nutritional status; splenectomy
Medications
Use of antibiotics, antipyretics; steroids; chemotherapy or any other immunosuppressants
General
Fever, chills, anorexia, malaise, fatigue, weakness
Pain
Pain with breathing, chest pain, headache, myalgia
Respiratory
Dyspnea, cough (productive or dry)
Gastrointestinal
Nausea and vomiting; diarrhea

OBJECTIVE DATA

General
Restlessness or lethargy; splinting of affected area
Integumentary
Diaphoresis or dry skin with poor turgor; pallor, flushing, or circumoral and nail-bed cyanosis
Respiratory
Tachypnea; pharyngitis; asymmetric chest movements or retraction; decreased excursion; nasal flaring; use of accessory muscles (neck, abdomen); grunting; crackles, rhonchi, bronchial or absent breath sounds, pleural friction rub on auscultation; dull over consolidated areas, tactile fremitus; pink, rusty, purulent, green, yellow, or white sputum (amount may be scant to copious) on percussion
Cardiovascular
Tachycardia
Neurological
Changes in mental status; confusion to delirium
Possible findings
Leukocytosis; abnormal ABGs with decreased or normal P_{O_2}, decreased P_{CO_2}, and increased pH initially, and later decreased P_{O_2}, increased P_{CO_2}, and decreased pH; positive sputum gram stain and culture; nonsegmental consolidation with air bronchograms and/or patchy or diffuse infiltrates on chest x-ray film

■ Nursing Management of the Client with Pneumonia

Nursing assessment

Subjective and objective data that should be obtained from an individual with pneumonia are presented in Table 21-5.

Nursing diagnoses

Nursing diagnoses are determined when the problem and etiological factors are supported by clinical data. Nursing diagnoses related to pneumonia may include, but are not limited to, those presented in Table 21-6.

Nursing interventions

Health promotion and maintenance. There are many nursing interventions to help prevent the occurrence as well as the morbidity associated with pneumonia. Teaching individuals to practice good health habits such as proper diet and hygiene, adequate rest, and regular exercise can maintain their natural resistance to infecting organisms. If possible, exposure to URIs should be avoided. If a URI occurs, it should be treated promptly with supportive measures (e.g., rest, fluids, antipyretics). If symptoms persist for more than 3 or 4 days, the person should obtain medical care. Individuals at high risk for pneumonia (e.g., the chronically ill and older adults) should be encouraged to obtain both influenza and pneumococcal vaccines.

In the hospital, the nursing role involves identifying clients at risk (see Table 21-1) and taking measures to prevent the development of pneumonia. Clients with altered consciousness should be placed in positions (e.g., side-lying, upright) that will prevent them from aspirating. They should be turned and repositioned at least every 2 hours to facilitate adequate lung expansion and to discourage pooling of secretions.

Clients who have a feeding tube generally require attention to positioning of the tube to prevent aspiration (see Chapter 35). Although the distal end of the feeding tube is usually in the small intestine and the tube is very small, an interruption in the integrity of the cardiac sphincter of the stomach still exists, which can allow reflux of the intestinal contents.

Clients who have difficulty swallowing (e.g., stroke clients) need assistance in eating, drinking, and taking medication to prevent aspiration. Clients who have recently had surgery and others who are immobile need assistance with turning, coughing, and deep-breathing measures at frequent intervals (see Chapter 13). The nurse must be careful to avoid overmedication with narcotics or sedatives, which can cause a depressed cough reflex and accumulation of fluid in the lungs. The gag reflex should be present in individuals who have had local anesthesia to the throat before the administration of fluids or food.

Strict medical asepsis and adherence to universal precautions should be practiced by the nurse to reduce the incidence of nosocomial infections. The client with an infection should not be placed in the same room with a client who is recovering from surgery or one with chronic lung disease. Respiratory therapy equipment should be properly cleaned and changed, and disposable equipment should be used as much as possible. Strict sterile aseptic technique should be used when suctioning a client.

Table 21-6

NURSING CARE PLAN FOR THE CLIENT WITH PNEUMONIA

Defining Characteristics	Nursing Interventions	Evaluation Criteria
NURSING DIAGNOSIS: Ineffective breathing pattern related to pneumonia, anxiety, positioning, and pain		
Rapid respirations, dyspnea, tachypnea, nasal flaring, altered chest excursion, inability to lie down	Assess degree of pain and anxiety. Take vital signs and auscultate lungs every 2-4 hr. Monitor arterial blood gases if ordered. Administer oxygen as indicated. Assess its effectiveness. Decrease anxiety (e.g., with relaxation techniques, diversion) and provide a quiet, restful environment. Position client in semi-Fowler's or other comfortable position for breathing (may use reclining chairs).	Respiratory rate of 12-18 breaths/min, expression of feeling of comfort
NURSING DIAGNOSIS: Ineffective airway clearance related to pain, positioning, fatigue, and thick secretions		
Ineffective cough or thick, tenacious sputum; abnormal breath sounds; dyspnea	Assist client to cough by splinting chest and teaching client how to cough effectively (inhale slowly through nose, exhale, and cough). Provide receptacle and tissues for disposal of sputum. Provide means of oral hygiene after production of sputum. Give expectorants and cough suppressants as ordered. Provide humidification of inhaled air. Maintain fluid intake of 3 L daily. Use chest physiotherapy, if indicated, to mobilize secretions. Observe characteristics of sputum and report any significant changes (e.g., from mucoid to grossly purulent).	Clear breath sounds, effective cough with expectoration of sputum, normal chest x-ray film or evidence of resolution
NURSING DIAGNOSIS: Pain related to pleuritis, positioning, and ineffective pain reduction and/or comfort measures		
Pleuritic chest pain, pleural friction rub, shallow respirations, decreased breath sounds	Administer analgesics as ordered. Position client comfortably. Premedicate with analgesics before uncomfortable therapies are given. Assist with intercostal nerve block if necessary. Observe for possible complications (e.g., pleural effusion, empyema) if pain persists.	Alleviation of pain, normal lung excursion
NURSING DIAGNOSIS: High risk for transmission of infection related to lack of knowledge of preventive measures		
Nose and/or mouth not covered during sneeze or cough, no hand washing	Teach client to use tissues when coughing and expectorating sputum. Place used tissues in wax-lined paper bag and dispose of properly. Wash hands thoroughly after contact with infected client. Teach client to practice these techniques at home as well as in hospital. Do not put infectious client in same room with client at high risk for pneumonia (e.g., client who is recovering from surgery, has chronic lung disease, is immunosuppressed, or is older adult).	No spread of infection
NURSING DIAGNOSIS: High risk for health maintenance deficit related to lack of knowledge regarding treatment regimen after discharge		
Frequent questioning about disease and its management	Assess ability to continue self-care at home. Encourage client to continue on full course of antibiotic therapy. Instruct client on the importance of rest and limited activity. Encourage client to obtain adequate rest, good nutrition, and fresh air. If indicated, encourage client to stop or decrease cigarette smoking. Teach client to continue coughing and deep breathing exercises. Teach client the importance of follow-up care and the need to seek medical attention for symptoms related to respiratory infections. Encourage client to obtain vaccinations (pneumococcal and influenza) if at high risk for pneumonia.	Following of regimen, including medications, fluid therapy, activity schedule

Continued.

Table 21-6

NURSING CARE PLAN FOR THE CLIENT WITH PNEUMONIA—cont'd

Defining Characteristics	Nursing Interventions	Evaluation Criteria

NURSING DIAGNOSIS: Altered nutrition: less than body requirements related to fatigue, anorexia, nausea, vomiting, and environmental stimuli

Defining Characteristics	Nursing Interventions	Evaluation Criteria
Weight loss, anorexia, nausea, vomiting	Assist with meals. Determine client's food preferences and provide when possible. Provide means of oral hygiene before meals. Provide frequent small meals. Monitor environment to reduce negative stimuli. Monitor client's weight and caloric intake.	Maintenance of normal body weight and adequate strength to perform activities of daily living

NURSING DIAGNOSIS: Potential complication: hypoxemia related to impaired gas exchange in lungs

Defining Characteristics	Nursing Interventions	Evaluation Criteria
Restlessness, anxiety, confusion, combative reactions, cyanosis; changes in respiratory rate	Administer oxygen and antibiotics as ordered. Monitor vital signs as indicated. Assess and monitor mental status and respiratory status. Report changes from baseline values.	Absence or early detection of signs of hypoxemia

NURSING DIAGNOSIS: Ineffective thermoregulation related to pneumonia and ineffective comfort measures

Defining Characteristics	Nursing Interventions	Evaluation Criteria
Diaphoresis, chills, flushing, thirst, headache, malaise	Administer antibiotics as prescribed. Observe for side effects and toxicity associated with antibiotic therapy. Administer antipyretics as ordered. Take temperature every 2-4 hr. Observe for continuing or recurring fever and report finding to physician. Provide fluid intake (at least 3 L/day). Provide frequent clothing and linen changes if diaphoresis occurs. Keep client comfortable and dry.	Expression of increased comfort as fever subsides

NURSING DIAGNOSIS: Activity intolerance related to fatigue, treatment regimen, interrupted sleep/wake cycle, hypoxia, and weakness

Defining Characteristics	Nursing Interventions	Evaluation Criteria
Fatigue, unwillingness or inability to exert self, dyspnea, increased pulse and respiration, dizziness on exertion	Provide bed rest and limited physical activity. Assess response to activity and plan changes accordingly. Limit visitors and long conversations. Plan nursing care in blocks to ensure periods of rest. Maintain a pleasant, calm environment. Place needed items (e.g., tissues, call bell) within easy reach. Plan for uninterrupted sleep periods.	Verbalization of feeling of being rested; cooperation during ambulation, required activities

Acute intervention. Although many clients with pneumonia are treated on an outpatient basis, the nursing care plan presented in Table 21-6 is applicable to both these individuals and in-hospital clients. It is important for the nurse to remember that pneumonia is an acute, infectious disease. Although most cases of pneumonia are potentially completely curable, complications can result. Nurses must be aware of these complications and their manifestations.

Chronic management. Clients need to be reassured that complete recovery from pneumonia is possible. It is extremely important to emphasize the need to take all of the prescribed medication and to return for follow-up medical care and evaluation. Adequate rest is needed to maintain progress toward recovery and to prevent a relapse. Clients need to be told that it may be weeks before they feel their usual vigor and sense of well-being. A prolonged period of convalescence may be necessary for older adults or chronically ill clients.

Clients considered to be at high risk for pneumonia should be told about available vaccines and should discuss them with the health care worker. Deep-breathing and coughing exercises should be practiced for 6 to 8 weeks after the clients are discharged from the hospital.

Tuberculosis

Tuberculosis (TB) is a bacterial infectious disease transmitted by *Mycobacterium tuberculosis*. It usually involves the lungs, but it also occurs in the kidneys, bones, lymph nodes, and meninges and can be disseminated throughout the body.

Significance. Since the introduction of chemotherapy in the late 1940s and early 1950s, there has been a dramatic decrease in the prevalence of TB. Ten to 15 million people are infected with or harbor the tubercle bacillus. The majority of these individuals have healed or dormant TB. It is estimated that about 25,000 cases of active TB will be reported each year. About 10% of these cases represent relapses. These statistics indicate that TB, in spite of being potentially curable and preventable, is still a major public health problem in the United States. Recently, the Centers for Disease Control has launched a plan to eliminate TB in the United States by the year 2000.[7] The emphasis will be on collaboration with state and local health departments to improve their individual-case surveillance, their monitoring of compliance with completion of therapy, and their provision of preventative therapy for appropriate individuals.

The tubercle bacillus may remain dormant for many years and then reactivate and produce clinical TB. Infection with *M. tuberculosis* involves a lifelong relationship between humans and the tubercle bacillus; dormant organisms may remain alive in the host for life. The infected host has been referred to as a "walking time bomb" in whom TB may develop and who may serve as a source of infection for others.

High-risk individuals for TB include residents of inner-city neighborhoods, foreign-born persons, older adults, and the socioeconomically disadvantaged of all races. TB is found in high incidence in a few areas of the United States where there is a large population of Native Americans such as Arizona and New Mexico, and in counties near the Mexican border. Hawaii has had the highest rate of new cases in the past few years.

Pathophysiology. *M. tuberculosis,* a gram-positive, acid-fast bacillus, is usually spread via airborne droplet nuclei, which are produced when infected individuals cough, sneeze, or speak. Once released into a room, the organisms are dispersed and can be inhaled by a susceptible host. Brief exposure to a few tubercle bacilli rarely causes an infection. Rather, it is more commonly spread to individuals who have had repeated close contact with an infected person. TB is not highly infectious, and transmission usually requires close, frequent, or prolonged exposure. The disease cannot be spread by hands, books, glasses, dishes, or other fomites.

When the bacilli are inhaled, they pass down the bronchial system and implant themselves on the respiratory bronchioles or alveoli. The lower parts of the lungs are usually the site of initial bacterial implantation. After implantation, the bacilli multiply with no initial resistance from the host. The organisms are engulfed by phagocytes (initially neutrophils and later macrophages) and may continue to multiply within the phagocytes.

While a cellular immune response is being activated, the bacilli can be spread through the lymphatic channels to regional lymph nodes and via the thoracic duct to the circulating blood. Thus organisms may be spread throughout the body before sufficient activation of the cell-mediated immune response is available to bring the infection under control. The organisms find favorable environments for growth primarily in the upper lobes of the lungs, kidneys, epiphyseal lines of the bone, and cerebral cortex.

Eventually, the acquired cellular immunity limits further multiplication and spread of the infection. A characteristic tissue reaction called an *epithelioid cell granuloma* results after the cellular immune system is activated. This granuloma (also called an *epithelioid cell tubercle*) is due to fusion of the infiltrating macrophages. The granuloma is surrounded by lymphocytes. This reaction usually takes 10 to 20 days.

The central portion of the lesion (called a *Ghon tubercle*) undergoes necrosis characterized by a cheesy appearance and hence is named *caseous necrosis.* The lesion may also undergo liquefactive necrosis in which the liquid sloughs into connecting bronchi and produces a cavity. Tubercular material may enter the tracheobronchial system, allowing airborne transmission of infectious particles.

Healing of the primary lesion usually takes place by resolution, fibrosis, and calcification. The granulation tissue surrounding the lesion may become more fibrous and form a collagenous scar around the tubercle. A *Ghon complex* is formed, consisting of the Ghon tubercle and regional lymph nodes. Calcified Ghon complexes may be seen on chest x-rays films.

When a tuberculous lesion regresses and heals, the infection enters a latent period in which it may persist without producing a clinical illness. The infection may remain dormant for life, or it may develop into clinical disease if the persisting organisms begin to multiply rapidly.

If the initial immune response is not adequate, control of the organisms is not maintained and clinical disease results. Certain individuals are at a higher risk for clinical disease, including those who are immunosuppressed for any reason (e.g., clients with AIDS, those receiving cancer chemotherapy or long-term prednisone therapy), have diabetes mellitus, are less than 2 years old, or are adolescents.

About 5% of individuals are incapable of containing the initial infective process. An additional 5% of those who do produce an effective immune response later lose this capability; dormant bacilli then begin to multiply, and the disease is reactivated. The reasons for reactivation are not well understood, but they are related to decreased resistance found in older adults, individuals with concomitant diseases, and those who are receiving immunosuppressive therapy.

Classification. In 1974 the American Thoracic Association and American Lung Association adopted a classification system that covers the entire population. This classification system has since been revised (Table 21-7).

Clinical manifestations. In the early stages of TB, the person is usually free of symptoms. Many cases are found incidentally when routine chest x-rays are done, especially in older adults.

Systemic manifestations may initially consist of fatigue, malaise, anorexia, weight loss, low-grade fevers (especially in the late afternoon), and night sweats. These manifestations are related to the lymphokine production that is stimulated by the immune response to the tubercle bacilli. The weight loss may not be excessive until late in the dis-

Table 21-7 Classification of TB

CLASS 0

No TB exposure, not infected (no history of exposure, negative tuberculin skin test)

CLASS 1

TB exposure, no evidence of infection (history of exposure, negative tuberculin skin test)

CLASS 2

TB infection without disease (significant reaction to tuberculin skin test, negative bacteriological studies, no roentgenographic findings compatible with tuberculosis, no clinical evidence of tuberculosis)

CLASS 3

TB infection with disease (positive bacteriological studies or both a significant reaction to tuberculin skin test and clinical and/or roentgenographic evidence of current disease)

CLASS 4

No current disease (history of previous episode of TB or abnormal, stable roentgenographic findings in a person with a significant reaction to tuberculin skin test; negative bacteriological studies if done; no clinical and/or roentgenographic evidence of current disease)

CLASS 5

TB suspect (diagnosis pending)

Adapted from Diagnostic standards and classification of tuberculosis and other mycobacterial diseases, New York, 1981, American Lung Association.

ease and is often attributed to overwork or other factors. Irregular menses may also be present in premenopausal women.

A characteristic pulmonary manifestation is a cough that becomes frequent and produces mucoid or mucopurulent sputum. Chest pain characterized as dull or tight may also be present. Hemoptysis is not a common finding and is usually associated with more advanced cases. Sometimes TB has more acute, sudden manifestations; the client presents with high fever, chills, generalized flulike symptoms, pleuritic pain, and a productive cough.

Complications

Miliary TB. If a necrotic Ghon complex erodes through a blood vessel, large numbers of organisms invade the bloodstream and are spread to all body organs. This is called *miliary* or *hematogenous TB*. The client may be either acutely ill with fever, dyspnea, and cyanosis or chronically ill with systemic manifestations of weight loss, fever, and gastrointestinal (GI) disturbance. Hepatomegaly, splenomegaly, and generalized lymphadenopathy may be present.

Pleural effusion. A pleural effusion is caused by the release of caseous material into the pleural space. The bacteria-containing material triggers an inflammatory reaction and a pleural exudate of protein-rich fluid.

A form of pleurisy called *dry pleurisy* may result from a superficial tuberculous lesion involving the pleura. It appears as localized pleuritic pain on deep inspiration.

Tuberculous pneumonia. Acute pneumonia may result when large amounts of tubercle bacilli are discharged from the liquefied necrotic lesion into the lung or lymph nodes. The clinical manifestations are similar to those of bacterial pneumonia, including chills, fever, productive cough, pleuritic pain, and leukocytosis.

Other organ involvement. Although the lungs are the primary site of tuberculosis, other body organs may also be involved. The meninges may become infected after rupture of a caseous tubercle into the subarachnoid space. Bone and joint tissue may be involved in the infectious disease process. The kidneys, lymph nodes, and both female and male genital tracts may also be infected.

Diagnostic studies

Tuberculin skin testing. The body's immune response can be demonstrated by hypersensitivity to a tuberculin skin test. A positive reaction occurs 3 to 10 weeks after the initial infection, corresponding to the time needed to mount an immune response.

Purified protein derivative (PPD) of tuberculin is used primarily to detect the delayed hypersensitivity response. (The procedure for performing the tuberculin skin test is described in Chapter 19.) Once acquired, sensitivity to tuberculin tends to persist throughout life. A positive reaction indicates the presence of a tuberculous infection, but it does not show whether the infection is dormant or causing a clinical illness.

Chest x-ray study. Although the findings on chest x-ray examination are extremely important, it is not possible to make a diagnosis of TB solely on the basis of this examination. This is because other diseases can mimic the appearance of TB.

The abnormality most commonly found in TB is multinodular lymph node involvement with cavitation in the upper lobes of the lungs. This is often referred to as the *parenchymal lymph node complex*. Calcification of the lung lesions generally occurs within several years of the infection.

Bacteriological studies. The demonstration of tubercle bacilli bacteriologically is essential for establishing a diagnosis. Microscopic examination of stained sputum smears for acid-fast bacilli is usually the first bacteriological evidence of the presence of tubercle bacilli. It is a quick, easy examination and provides the physician with valuable information. A major disadvantage is that over 10,000 bacteria per milliliter of specimen are required to produce a positive smear. In addition to sputum, material for examination can be obtained from gastric washings, cerebrospinal fluid, or pus from an abscess.

The most accurate means of diagnosis is a culture technique. The major disadvantage of this method is that it takes 2 weeks or more for the mycobacterium to grow.

Table 21-8

 Diagnostic and Therapeutic Management: Tuberculosis

DIAGNOSTIC

History and physical examination
Tuberculin skin test
Chest x-ray study
Bacteriological studies
    Sputum smear
    Sputum culture

THERAPEUTIC

Long-term treatment with antimicrobial drugs*
Follow-up bacteriological studies

---

*See Table 21-9.

The advantage is that it can detect small quantities (10 bacteria per milliliter of specimen).

Therapeutic management. The treatment of TB rarely requires in-hospital treatment. Most clients are treated on an outpatient basis, and many can continue to work and maintain their lifestyles with few changes (Table 21-8). Hospitalization may be used for diagnostic evaluation, for the severely ill or debilitated, and for those who experience adverse drug reactions or treatment failures.

The mainstay of TB treatment is pharmacological. Drug therapy is used to treat individuals with clinical disease as well as to prevent disease in an infected person. Drugs are usually administered as a single dose before breakfast to ensure adequate GI absorption.

Pharmacological management

Active disease. Treatment of TB usually consists of a combination of at least two drugs. The reason for combination therapy is to increase the therapeutic effectiveness and decrease the development of resistant strains of *M. tuberculosis*. It has been shown that single-drug therapy can result in rapid development of resistant strains.

The four primary drugs used are isoniazid, rifampin, streptomycin, and ethambutol (Table 21-9). Other drugs are primarily used for treatment of resistant strains or if the client develops toxicity to the primary drugs.

A problem with anti-TB therapy is the length of time medication must be taken. In the past, 18 to 24 months was the usual period of time required for individuals to adhere to the medical regimen. Recent studies have indicated that a shorter course of therapy may be effective. Although there are variations, protocol consists of using isoniazid and rifampin for a minimum of 9 months. After a period of time (2 weeks to 2 months), daily administration may be changed to twice weekly.[8]

The recommendation of the American Thoracic Society is that treatment continues for at least 9 months and longer if necessary (until at least 6 months have elapsed from conversion of a positive sputum to negative).[9] If the case of TB is complicated, these guidelines need to be individualized.

In follow-up care for clients on long-term therapy, it is very important to monitor for (1) effectiveness of drugs and (2) development of toxic side effects. Usually, sputum specimens are initially obtained weekly and then monthly to assess the effectiveness of the medication. The regimen is considered to be effective if the client converts to a negative sputum status. Over 90% of clients convert to negative sputum status within 3 months.[9]

An important reason for follow-up care is to ensure adherence to the treatment regimen. Many individuals do not adhere to the treatment program in spite of understanding the disease process and the value of treatment.

The client needs to be followed up for 12 months after completion of therapy to check for the development of resistant strains. The major causes of treatment failure are poor client adherence and an inappropriately prescribed drug regimen. Retreatment regimens are more complicated, require the use of at least two new drugs, and are more expensive.

Preventive treatment. Pharmacological management can be used to prevent a TB infection from developing into a clinical disease. The indications for preventive therapy (chemoprophylaxis) are presented in Table 21-10. Close contacts of individuals with infectious clinical TB should be examined with tuberculin skin tests. Close contacts who are less than 4 years of age should be given treatment even if the tuberculin skin test is negative.

Some individuals carry dormant TB infections, which may develop into active disease in some situations. Examples of this include positive reactors who (1) demonstrate some degree of immunosuppression, such as persons who are on prolonged steroid therapy; (2) have a malignant condition such as Hodgkin's disease; (3) have diabetes mellitus; or (4) have had a gastrectomy. These individuals will benefit from prophylactic treatment for TB.

The drug generally used in prophylactic chemotherapy is isoniazid. It is effective and inexpensive and can be administered orally. It is usually administered once daily for 12 months.

Bacille Calmette-Guérin vaccine. Bacille Calmette-Guérin (BCG) is a live attenuated vaccine that has limited usefulness in the United States because of the low rate of infection. It is recommended for persons who have negative tuberculin skin tests but who are repeatedly exposed to pulmonary tuberculosis (e.g., individuals assigned to work in countries with a high prevalence rate). It is also used for young children in countries with a high rate of TB. The vaccine does not reduce the chance of natural infection but may decrease the seriousness of clinical TB when it does occur.

▪ Nursing Management of the Client with Tuberculosis

Nursing assessment

It is important to determine whether the client was ever exposed to a person with TB. The client should be assessed for productive cough, night sweats, afternoon tem-

Table 21-9 Drug Therapy Used in Tuberculosis

Drug	Mechanisms of Action	Side Effects	Comments
FIRST-LINE DRUGS			
Isoniazid (INH)	Interferes with DNA metabolism of tubercle bacillus	Peripheral neuritis, hepatotoxicity, hypersensitivity (skin rash, arthralgia, fever), optic neuritis, vitamin B_6 neuritis	Metabolism primarily by liver and excretion by kidneys, pyridoxine (vitamin B_6) administration during high-dose therapy as prophylactic measure, use as single prophylactic agent for active TB in individuals whose PPD converts to positive, ability to cross blood-brain barrier
Rifampin	Has broad-spectrum effects, inhibits RNA polymerase of tubercle bacillus	Hepatitis, febrile reaction, GI disturbance, peripheral neuropathy, hypersensitivity	Most common use with isoniazid, low incidence of side effects, suppression of effect of birth control pills, possible orange urine
Ethambutol (Myambutol)	Inhibits RNA synthesis and is bacteriostatic for the tubercle bacillus	Skin rash, GI disturbance, malaise, peripheral neuritis, optic neuritis	Side effects uncommon and reversible with discontinuation of drug, most common use as substitute drug when toxicity occurs with isoniazid or rifampin
Streptomycin	Inhibits protein synthesis and is bactericidal	Audiotoxicity (eighth cranial nerve), nephrotoxicity, hypersensitivity	Cautious use in older adults, those with renal disease, and pregnant women
SECOND-LINE DRUGS			
Ethionamide	Inhibits protein synthesis	GI disturbance, hepatotoxicity, hypersensitivity	Valuable retreatment of resistant organisms Contraindication in pregnancy
Capreomycin	Inhibits protein synthesis and is bactericidal	Audiotoxicity, nephrotoxicity	Cautious use in older adults
Kanamycin	Interferes with protein synthesis	Audiotoxicity, nephrotoxicity	Use in selected cases for retreatment of resistant strains
Pyrazinamide	Has bactericidal effect (exact mechanism is unknown)	Jaundice (rare), fever, skin rash, hyperuricemia	High rate of effectiveness when used with streptomycin or capreomycin
Para-aminosalicylic acid (PAS)	Interferes with metabolism of tubercle bacillus	GI disturbance (frequent), hypersensitivity, hepatotoxicity	Interference with absorption of rifampin, infrequent use
Cycloserine	Inhibits cell-wall synthesis	Personality changes, psychosis, rash	Contraindication in individuals with a history of psychosis, use in retreatment of resistant strains

Table 21-10 Indications for Preventive TB Therapy

Exposure of household members and other close associates to newly diagnosed client

Newly infected client

Significant tuberculin skin test reactors with abnormal chest x-ray study

Significant tuberculin skin test reactors in special clinical situations (taking steroids, having diabetes mellitus, silicosis, gastrectomy)

Other significant tuberculin skin test reactors in persons up to age 35

Other significant tuberculin skin test reactors in persons over age 35 (only in special epidemiological situations)

Modified from Joint Statement of the American Thoracic Society and the Centers for Disease Control: Treatment of tuberculosis and tuberculosis infection in adults and children, Am Rev Respir Dis 134:355-363, 1986.

perature elevation, weight loss, pleuritic chest pain, and crackles over the apex of the lung.

If the client has a productive cough, an early morning sputum specimen will be required for an acid-fast bacillus (AFB) smear to detect the presence of mycobacteria.

Nursing diagnoses

Nursing diagnoses that are specific to the client with TB include, but are not limited to, the following:

1. Ineffective breathing pattern related to decreased lung capacity
2. Altered nutrition: less than body requirements related to chronic poor appetite, fatigue, and productive cough
3. High risk for noncompliance related to lack of knowledge of disease process, lack of motivation, and long-term nature of treatment
4. Altered health maintenance related to lack of knowledge about the disease process and therapeutic regimen
5. Activity intolerance related to fatigue, decreased nutritional status, and chronic febrile episodes

Nursing interventions

Health promotion and maintenance. The ultimate goal related to TB in the United States is eradication. The public health nurse and clinical nurse have especially important responsibilities. Selective screening programs in known high-risk groups may be of value in detecting individuals with TB. Persons with positive tuberculin skin tests should have chest x-rays to assess for the presence of TB. Another important measure is to identify the contacts of individuals who have TB. These contacts should be assessed for the possibility of infection and the need for chemoprophylactic treatment.

When an individual has respiratory symptoms such as cough, dyspnea, or productive sputum, especially if accompanied by a history of night sweats and/or unexplained weight loss, the nurse should assess for the presence of TB. Even if the suspected respiratory problem is something else, such as emphysema, pneumonia, or lung cancer, it is possible that the client may also have TB.

Acute intervention. Acute in-hospital care is seldom required for clients with TB. If hospitalization is needed, it is usually for a brief period of time. Respiratory isolation is generally indicated until the client responds to chemotherapy (usually within days to a few weeks). Clients who are unlikely to transmit tubercle bacilli (i.e., those without a cough) do not need to be placed in respiratory isolation. Masks are of limited value unless they are made of fabric designed to filter out droplet nuclei. They also need to be molded to fit tightly around the nose and mouth. Adequate ventilation of room air is important. Ultraviolet radiation in client rooms or air ducts that vent the air in the room to outside of the hospital enhance the effect of normal ventilation. From 1 to 2 hours of direct sunlight may kill the bacillus.

Clients should be taught to cover their noses and mouths with paper tissue every time they cough, sneeze, or produce sputum. The tissues should be thrown into a paper bag and disposed of with the trash, burned, or flushed down the toilet. Masks are necessary only during face-to-face contacts. It is preferable that clients wear the masks. Clients should also be taught careful hand-washing techniques after handling sputum and soiled tissues.

Most treatment failures occur because clients neglect to take the medication, discontinue it prematurely, or take it irregularly. It is important for the nurse to develop a therapeutic, consistent relationship with each client. The nurse needs to understand the client's lifestyle and to provide flexibility in planning a program that facilitates the client's participation in and completion of therapy. The nurse should educate clients so that they fully understand the need for dedication to the prescribed regimen. Ongoing reassurance helps clients understand that faithfulness can mean cure. If clients cannot or will not adhere to a self-administered medication regimen, medication may have to be given by a responsible person on a daily or intermittent basis.

Some clients may feel that there is a social stigma attached to TB. These feelings need to be discussed, and clients need to be reassured that individuals with TB can be cured if they follow the prescribed regimen. Many people still remember when TB victims were sent away to TB sanitoriums and isolated from society. The health care worker's attitude toward individuals with TB should be no different from the attitude toward those with pneumonia. Both diseases are infectious and potentially curable. The American Lung Association provides excellent literature for teaching about the disease as well as providing emotional support to the client and family.

Chronic management. When the chemotherapy regimen has been completed, most individuals can be considered adequately treated. Follow-up care may be indicated during the subsequent 12 months, including bacteriological studies and chest x-ray films. Because about 5% of individuals experience relapse, clients should be taught to recognize the symptoms that indicate recurrence of TB. If these symptoms occur, they should seek immediate medical attention.

Clients need to be instructed about certain factors that could reactivate TB, such as immunosuppressive therapy, malignancy, and prolonged debilitating illness. If clients

Table 21-11 Fungal Infections of the Lung

Organism	Characteristics
HISTOPLASMOSIS	
Histoplasma capsulatum	Indigenous to soil of North American river valleys, inhalation of mycelia into lungs, infected individuals often free of symptoms, generally self-limiting, chronic disease similar to TB
COCCIDIOIDOMYCOSIS	
Coccidioides immitis	Indigenous to semiarid regions of southwestern United States, inhalation of arthrospores into lungs, suppurative and granulomatous reaction in lungs, symptomatic infection in one third of individuals
BLASTOMYCOSIS	
Blastomyces dermatitidis	Indigenous to southeastern and midwestern United States, inhalation of fungus into lungs, progression of disease often insidious, possible involvement of skin
CRYPTOCOCCOSIS	
Crytococcus neoformans	True yeast, indigenous worldwide in soil and pigeon excreta, inhalation of fungus into lungs, possible meningitis
ASPERGILLOSIS	
Aspergillus niger or *Aspergillus fumigatus*	True mold inhabiting mouth, widely distributed, invasion of lung tissue resulting in possible necrotizing pneumonia possible allergic bronchopulmonary aspergillosis requiring corticosteroid therapy in individuals with asthma
CANDIDIASIS	
Candida albicans	Leading cause of mycotic infections in hospitalized and immunocompromised hosts, ubiquitous and frequent colonization of upper respiratory and GI tracts, infections often following broad-spectrum antibiotic therapy (systemic or inhaled), possible development of localized pulmonary infiltrate to widespread bilateral consolidation with hypoxemia
ACTINOMYCOSIS	
Actinomyces israeli	Not a true fungus, pseudohyphae present; anaerobic, gram-positive, higher bacteria with branching hyphae; presence of necrotizing pneumonia after aspiration; pneumonitis, commonly in lower lobes with abscess or empyema formation
NOCARDIOSIS	
Nocardia asteroides	Not a true fungus; aerobic, higher bacteria with branching hyphae; soil saprophyte widely distributed in nature; acquisition of infection from nature; rarely present in sputum without accompanying disease

experience any of these events, they need to tell their health care providers so that they can be closely monitored for reactivation of TB. In some situations, it may be necessary to put clients on anti-TB chemotherapy.

Atypical mycobacteria. Pulmonary disease that closely resembles TB may be caused by atypical acid-fast mycobacteria. This type of pulmonary disease is indistinguishable from TB clinically and radiologically but can be differentiated by bacteriological culture. These organisms are not believed to be airborne and thus are not transmitted by droplet nuclei.

Atypical mycobacteria that affect the lung include *M. kansasii*, *M. scrofulaceum*, *M. intracellularis*, and *M. xenopi*. These bacteria (especially *M. avium-intracellulare* and *M. scrofulaceum*) may also invade the cervical lymph nodes, causing lymphadenitis. This type of pulmonary disease typically occurs in white men with a history of COPD or silicosis.

Treatment depends on identification of the causative agent and determination of drug sensitivity. Many of the drugs used in treating TB are employed in combating infections from atypical mycobacteria.

Pulmonary Fungal Infections

Pulmonary fungal infections are increasing in incidence. They are found most frequently in seriously ill clients who are being treated with corticosteroids, antineoplastic and immunosuppressive drugs, or multiple antibiotics; they are also found in clients with AIDS.[10] Types of fungal infections are presented in Table 21-11. These infections are not transmitted from person to person, and clients do not have to be placed in isolation. The clinical

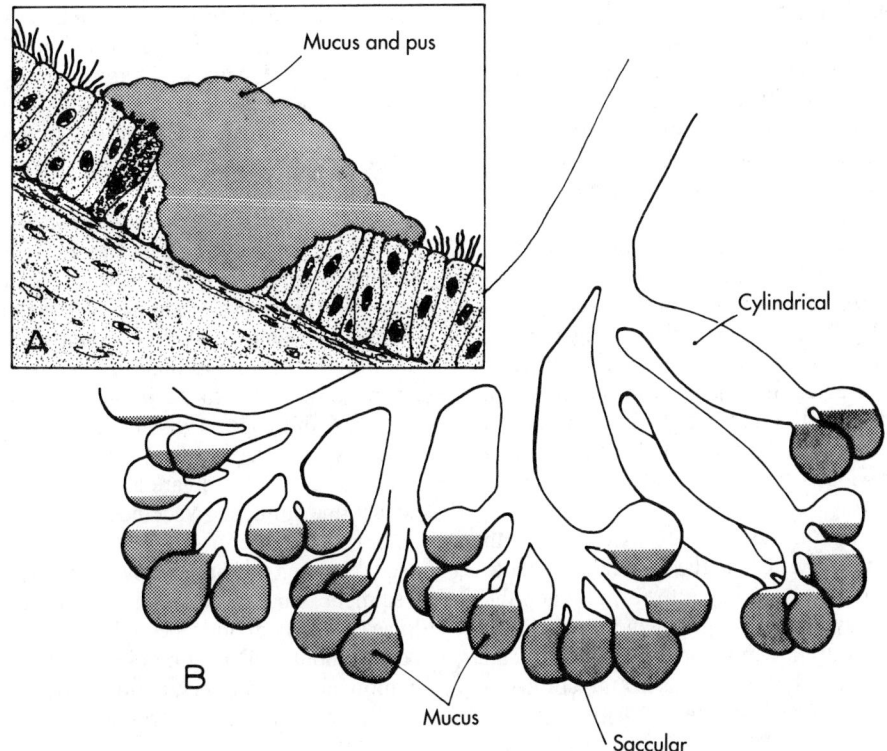

Fig. 21-3 Pathological changes in bronchiectasis. **A,** Longitudinal section of bronchial wall where chronic infection has caused damage. **B,** Collection of purulent material in dilated bronchioles, leading to persistent infection. (From Price S and Wilson L: Pathophysiology: clinical concepts of disease processes, ed 4, St Louis, 1991, Mosby–Year Book, Inc.)

manifestations are similar to those of bacterial pneumonia. Skin and serology tests are available to assist in identifying the infecting organism.[11] However, identification of the organism in a sputum specimen or in other body fluids is the best diagnostic indicator.

Amphotericin B is the drug most widely used in treating systemic fungal infections. It must be given intravenously to achieve adequate blood and tissue levels because it is poorly absorbed from the GI tract. Amphotericin B is considered a toxic drug with many possible side effects, including hypersensitivity reactions, fever, chills, malaise, nausea and vomiting, thrombophlebitis at the injection site, and abnormal renal function. Many of the side effects during infusion can be avoided by medication with aspirin or diphenhydramine (Benadryl) 1 hour before the infusion. Additionally, the infusion is best tolerated if given in less than 1 hour. Inclusion of a small amount of hydrocortisone hemisuccinate in the infusion helps to decrease the irritation of the veins, which is important because infusions are given 2 to 3 times weekly. Monitoring of renal function is critical while a person is receiving this drug. Renal changes are at least partially reversible. Amphotericin infusions are incompatible with most other drugs. Amphotericin is frequently administered every other day after an initial period of several weeks of daily therapy. Total treatment with the drug may range from 4 to 10 weeks.

Ketoconazole is an oral imidazole compound with anti-fungal activity that is successful in treatment of coccidioidomycosis in clinical trials, especially in disease that affects skin and soft tissue. Its usefulness in serious systemic disease as a first-line drug remains controversial. Its action is primarily to control the fungal infection and localize it rather than to cure it.

5-Fluorocytosine has also been used in selected types of pulmonary fungal infections. It is given orally and becomes widely distributed in the body. Adverse reactions include abdominal discomfort, diarrhea, hepatotoxicity, and bone marrow suppression.

Bronchiectasis

Pathophysiology. *Bronchiectasis* is a disorder characterized by permanent, abnormal dilatation of one or more large bronchi. The pathophysiological change that results in dilatation is destruction of the elastic and muscular structures of the bronchial wall. There are two types of bronchiectasis: saccular and cylindrical (Fig. 21-3). *Saccular* bronchiectasis occurs mainly in large bronchi and is characterized by cavitylike dilatations. The affected bronchi end in large sacs. *Cylindrical* bronchiectasis involves medium-sized bronchi that are mildly to moderately dilated.

The most common cause of bronchiectasis is bacterial infection, but other conditions such as congenital factors and obstruction predispose persons to the development of infection. Congenital factors include altered bronchial structures such as cysts and cul-de-sacs, which lead to pooling of secretion. A defect in cilia causing them to be immobile is also associated with the development of bronchiectasis. In cystic fibrosis, there is retention and thickening of mucus that may plug the airways. A variety of immunodeficiency diseases are associated with recurrent bacterial pneumonias. Some inhalation exposures, particularly to irritant gases such as oxides of sulfur and nitrogen, have been noted as causes of bronchiectasis.

Obstructive processes of any kind can predispose individuals to bronchiectasis. Examples include lung tumors, tumor masses in the chest cavity, aspirated foreign objects, and thick, tenacious secretions such as those found in chronic bronchitis. The obstruction causes the bronchi and bronchioles to distend and balloon out below the level of obstruction. This provides a good place for organisms to proliferate.

Almost all forms of bronchiectasis are associated with bacterial infections. Infections cause the bronchial walls to weaken, and pockets of infection begin to form. When the walls of the bronchial system are injured, the mucociliary mechanism is damaged, allowing bacteria, mucus, and dust to accumulate within the pockets. The infection becomes worse and results in bronchiectasis.

The disease process is often believed to start in childhood as an acquired disorder, beginning with respiratory complications secondary to influenza, measles, or whooping cough. Recurring lower respiratory tract infections are another pattern of disease in childhood that may predispose individuals to bronchiectasis. This pattern is typically seen in individuals with cystic fibrosis, asthma, α-1 antitrypsin deficiency, and immunodeficiency diseases.

Clinical manifestations. The primary manifestations of bronchiectasis vary considerably depending on the extent and location of the disease process. They include chronic cough with production of mucopurulent sputum, hemoptysis, and recurrent pneumonia. The cough is paroxysmal and is often stimulated with position changes. Other manifestations include exertional dyspnea, fatigue, weight loss, anorexia, and fetid breath. Sinusitis frequently accompanies diffuse bronchiectasis. The manifestations of advanced, widespread bronchiectasis are generalized wheezing, digital clubbing, and cor pulmonale.

Diagnostic studies. An individual with a chronic productive cough with increased sputum (which may be blood streaked) should be suspected of having bronchiectasis. Characteristic findings in the health history such as childhood diseases complicated by respiratory infections or chronic bronchitis are very significant. Chest x-rays are usually done and may show streaky infiltrates. Bronchography involves instilling liquid radiopaque material into the bronchial system via a catheter or bronchoscope and is useful in evaluating individuals with moderate to severe cases of bronchiectasis. Bronchoscopy may be useful in identifying the source of secretions or sites of hemoptysis in individuals with chronic productive coughs.

Collection of sputum to evaluate its quantity, characteristics, and microbial content may provide additional information regarding the severity of impairment and the presence of active infection. Pulmonary function studies may be abnormal in advanced bronchiectasis, showing a decrease in vital capacity, expiratory flow, and maximum voluntary ventilation and an increase in ventilation-perfusion mismatching with resultant hypoxemia. A complete blood count may be normal or show evidence of anemia and leukocytosis.

Therapeutic management. Bronchiectasis is difficult to treat. Antibiotics are the major form of treatment and should be given on the basis of sputum culture results. Other forms of drug therapy may include bronchodilators, mucolytic agents, and expectorants. Maintaining good hydration is very important to liquefy secretions. Postural drainage is vital to facilitate expectoration of sputum. (Postural drainage is discussed in Chapter 22.) The individual should reduce exposure to excessive air pollutants and irritants, avoid cigarette smoking, and obtain pneumococcal and influenza vaccines.

Surgical resection of parts of the lungs, although not used as often as previously, may be done if therapeutic treatment is not effective. Surgical resection of an affected lobe or segment may be indicated for the client with repeated bouts of pneumonia, hemoptysis, and disabling complications. Surgery is not advisable when there is diffuse or widespread involvement.

■ Nursing Management of Bronchiectasis

Health promotion and maintenance

The incidence of bronchiectasis has shown a decline in recent years. This is partially due to the administration of measles and pertussis vaccines, which decreases the incidence of bronchiectasis caused by these diseases. Early detection and treatment of lower respiratory tract infections prevent them from developing into complications such as bronchiectasis. Any obstructing lesion or foreign body should be removed promptly. Other measures to decrease the occurrence or progression of bronchiectasis include avoiding cigarette smoking and decreasing exposure to pollution. Children with persistent coughs should receive evaluations to determine the source of the problem.

Acute and chronic interventions

An important nursing goal is to promote drainage and removal of bronchial mucus. The client should be taught effective deep-breathing exercises and effective ways to cough (Table 22-12). Postural drainage should be done on affected parts of the lung (see Fig. 22-16). Some individuals require elevation of the foot of the bed by 4 to 6 inches to facilitate drainage. Pillows may be used in the hospital as well as the home to help clients assume postural drainage positions. Administration of the prescribed antibiotics, bronchodilators, or expectorants is important. Clients need to understand the importance of taking the prescribed regimen of drugs to obtain maximum effectiveness. Clients should be aware of possible side or adverse effects that must be reported to the physician.

Rest is important to prevent overexertion. Bed rest may be indicated during the acute phase of the illness. Chilling and excess fatigue should be avoided.

Good nutrition is important and may be difficult to maintain because clients are often anorexic. Oral hygiene to cleanse the mouth and remove dried sputum crusts may improve clients' appetites. Offering foods that are appealing may also increase the desire to eat. Adequate hydration to help liquefy secretions and thus make it easier to remove them is extremely important. Unless there are contraindications such as concomitant congestive heart failure or renal disease, clients should be instructed to drink at least 3 L of fluid daily. To accomplish this, they should be advised to increase fluid consumption from their baselines by increasing intake by one glass per day until the goal is reached. Generally, they should be counseled to use low-sodium fluids to avoid systemic retention.

Direct hydration of the respiratory system may also prove beneficial to ease expectoration of secretions. Usually, a bland aerosol with normal saline solution delivered by a jet-type nebulizer is used. Clients with bronchiectasis should avoid ultrasonic nebulizers because they often induce bronchospasm. At home, a steamy shower can prove effective; expensive equipment that requires frequent cleaning is often unnecessary. It is important that clients take an inhaled bronchodilator 10 to 15 minutes before the use of a bland aerosol to prevent bronchoconstriction.

Clients and families should be taught to recognize significant manifestations to be reported to the health care provider. These manifestations include increased sputum production, grossly bloody sputum, increasing dyspnea, fever, chills, and chest pain.

Lung Abscess

Pathophysiology. *Lung abscess* is a pus-containing lesion of the lung parenchyma that gives rise to a cavity. The cavity is formed by necrosis of the lung tissue. In many cases the causes and pathogenesis of lung abscess are similar to those of pneumonia. The most common etiological factor of a lung abscess is aspiration of material into the lungs (Table 21-12). In addition to producing infection, the organisms involved cause necrosis of the lung tissue. Examples include enteric gram-negative organisms such as *Klebsiella, S. aureus,* and anaerobic bacilli. Lung abscess can also result from hematogenously spread lung infarct secondary to pulmonary embolus, malignant growth, TB, and various parasitic and fungal diseases of the lung.

The areas of the lung most commonly affected are the apical segments of the lower lobes and the posterior segments of the upper lobes. Fibrous tissue usually forms around the abscess in an attempt to wall it off. The abscess may erode into the bronchial system, causing the production of foul-smelling sputum. It may grow toward the pleura and cause pleuritic pain. Multiple small abscesses can occur within the lung.

Clinical manifestations and complications. The onset of a lung abscess is usually insidious, especially if anaerobic organisms are the primary cause. A more acute onset occurs with aerobic organisms. The most common manifestation is cough producing purulent sputum (often dark brown) that is foul smelling and foul tasting. Hemoptysis is common, especially at the time that an abscess ruptures into a bronchus. Other common manifestations are fever, chills, prostration, pleuritic pain, dyspnea, cough, and

Table 21-12 Common Causes of Lung Abscess

Type of Abscess	Cause
Aspiration abscess	Alcoholism, postanesthesia, oversedation, coma (e.g., diabetic, epileptic, drug overdose, cerebrovascular accident), oral infection, food or foreign body, laryngeal palsy, carcinoma of esophagus ("spill-over" aspiration)
Malignant abscess	Necrotic bronchial carcinoma, secondary to bronchial obstruction and stasis of secretions, head and neck malignancies
Pulmonary embolus	Pulmonary infarct infection, septic emboli, fragments from bacterial endarteritis
Infection	Pneumonia, pyogenic bacteria (notably *S. aureus*), defective ciliary action, ineffective expectoration, infected cysts, necrotic lesions, subdiaphragmatic infections (usually liver), open chest wounds

From Kinney M and others: AACN's clinical reference for critical-care nursing, ed 2, New York, 1988, McGraw-Hill Book Co, p 796.

weight loss. The history may reveal a predisposing condition such as alcoholism, pneumonia, or oral infection.

Physical examination of the lungs indicates dullness to percussion and decreased breath sounds on auscultation over the segment of lung involved. There may be transmission of bronchial breath sounds to the periphery if the communicating bronchus becomes patent and drainage of the segment begins. Crackles (rales) may also be present in the later stages as the abscess drains. Oral examination often reveals dental caries, gingivitis, and periodontal infection.

Complications that can occur include chronic pulmonary abscess, hemorrhage from abscess erosion into blood vessels, brain abscess as a result of the spread of infection, bronchopleural fistula, and empyema from abscess perforation into the pleural cavity.

Diagnostic studies. A chest x-ray before drainage of the abscess reveals a circumscribed area of infiltration. After the abscess is drained, a chest x-ray will show an area of consolidation with a wall around a lucent zone. Sputum culture and Gram stain are necessary to identify the infecting organism. Bronchoscopy may be used in cases of abscess in which drainage is delayed or in which there are factors that suggest an underlying malignancy. Leukocytosis is usually present.

Therapeutic management. Antibiotics given for a prolonged period (up to 6 weeks) are usually the primary method of treatment. Penicillin is generally the drug of choice because of the frequent presence of anaerobic organisms. Chest physiotherapy and postural drainage are sometimes used to drain abscesses located in the lower or posterior portions of the lung. Surgery is rarely indicated but occasionally may be indicated when reinfection of a large cavitary lesion occurs or to establish a diagnosis when there is evidence of an underlying neoplasm or chronic associated disease. The use of bronchoscopy for drainage of an abscess is controversial. Some clinicians believe that this procedure may spread the infection to other parts of the lung. If used, bronchoscopy should not be performed until after 24 to 48 hours of antimicrobial therapy.

■ Nursing Management of Lung Abscess

Drainage of the abscess and treatment of the infection are the primary goals. The client should be taught how to cough effectively. Chest physiotherapy will help to loosen secretions. Postural drainage according to the lung area involved will aid the removal of secretions (see Fig. 22-8). Frequent (every 2 to 3 hours) mouth care is needed to relieve the putrid odor from the foul-smelling sputum. Diluted hydrogen peroxide and mouthwash are often effective.

Because of the need for prolonged antibiotic therapy, the client must be aware of the importance of continuing the medication for the prescribed period. The client needs to know about untoward side effects to be reported to the health care provider. Sometimes the client is asked to return periodically during the course of antibiotic therapy for repeat cultures and sensitivity tests to ensure that the infecting organism is not becoming resistant to the antibiotic. When antibiotic therapy is completed, the client is reevaluated.

Rest, good nutrition, and adequate fluid intake are all supportive measures to facilitate recovery. If dentition is poor and dental hygiene is not adequate, the client should be encouraged to obtain dental care.

OXYGEN THERAPY

Oxygen therapy is frequently used in the treatment of respiratory problems. Oxygen (O_2) is a colorless, odorless, tasteless gas that constitutes 20.95% of the atmosphere. Used clinically it is considered a drug. Administering supplemental O_2 raises the partial pressure of O_2 (Po_2) in inspired air.

Indications

Oxygen is usually administered to treat hypoxemia caused by (1) *respiratory disorders* such as COPD, pneumonia, atelectasis, lung cancer, and pulmonary emboli; (2) *cardiovascular disorders* such as myocardial infarction, dysrhythmias, angina pectoris, and cardiogenic shock; and (3) *CNS disorders* such as overdose of narcotics, anesthesia, head injury, and disordered sleep (sleep apnea).

Methods

The goal of O_2 administration is to supply the client with adequate O_2 to maximize the O_2-carrying ability of the blood. There are various methods of O_2 administration

(Table 21-13 and Figs. 21-4, 21-5, and 21-6). The method selected depends on factors such as the fraction of inspiratory O_2 (Fio_2) and humidification required, client cooperation, and comfort.

Most methods of O_2 administration are low-flow devices that deliver O_2 in concentrations that vary with the person's breathing. In contrast, the Venturi mask is a high-flow device that delivers fixed concentrations of O_2. With the Venturi mask, O_2 is delivered to a small jet (Venturi device) in the center of a wide-based cone (Fig. 21-7). Air is *entrained* (pulled through) openings in the cone as O_2 flows through the small jet. The mask has large vents through which exhaled air can escape. The degree of restriction or narrowness of the jet determines the amount of entrainment and dilution of pure O_2 with room air and thus the concentration of O_2.

Humidification and Nebulizers

Oxygen obtained from cylinders or wall systems is dry. Dry oxygen has an irritating effect on mucous membranes and dries secretions. Therefore it is important that O_2 be humidified when administered, either by humidification or nebulization. A common device used for humidification when the client has a catheter, cannula, or low-flow mask is a *bubble humidifier*. It is a small plastic jar filled with sterile distilled water. It is attached to the O_2 source by means of a flowmeter. O_2 passes into the jar, bubbles through the water, and then goes through tubing to the client's catheter, cannula, or mask. The purpose of the bubble humidifier is to restore the humidity conditions of room air. However, the need for bubble humidifiers at flow rates between 1 and 4 L/min is controversial when humidity in the environment is adequate.[12]

Another means of administering humidified O_2 is via a *nebulizer*. It delivers particulate water mist (aerosols) with a high degree of humidity. The humidity can be raised by heating the water, which increases the ability of the gas to hold moisture. Heated (37° C, 98.6° F) and humidified (100%) gas is required when the upper airway is bypassed. When nebulizers are used, large-size tubing should be employed to connect the device to a face mask or T bar. If small-size tubing is used, condensation can occlude the flow of O_2.

Complications

Combustion. Oxygen supports combustion and increases the rate of burning. This is why it is so important that smoking be prohibited in the area in which O_2 is being used. A "No Smoking" sign should be prominently displayed on the client's door. The client should also be cautioned against smoking cigarettes with O_2 prongs or a catheter in place.

Carbon dioxide narcosis. In some cases of respiratory distress, increasing the O_2 flow rate may be quite harmful. Normally, carbon dioxide (CO_2) accumulation is a major stimulant of the respiratory center. However, individuals with a long-standing history of COPD or who are heavily sedated have a tendency to hypoventilate and to retain CO_2. Gradually, the respiratory center loses its sensitivity to the elevated CO_2 level. For these individuals, the major

Text continued on p. 527.

Table 21-13 Methods of Oxygen Administration

Advantages	Disadvantages	Nursing Interventions
NASAL CATHETER		
Catheter allows continuous, uninterrupted O_2 therapy. Client receives O_2 even if a mouth breather. Catheter does not interfere with client care.	Catheter must be inserted into nasopharynx through a nostril and can produce excoriation of the nares. High-flow rates (>6 L/min) can cause drying of nasal membranes. Inadvertent gas flow distends the stomach. Cannula does not permit a high degree of humidification and must be taped to client's face.	Catheter should be changed every 8 hr, alternate the nostrils. Distance that catheter is to be inserted is measured from distance between tip of nose and earlobe. A flow rate of 5-6 L/min gives an O_2 concentration of about 30%. Method is best used for short-term therapy.
NASAL CANNULA		
Cannula may be used by a restless client. It is a safe and simple method that is relatively comfortable and acceptable. It is useful for a client requiring low O_2 concentrations (e.g., those with COPD). It allows client to move about in bed. Client can eat, talk, or cough while wearing device.	Cannula is difficult to maintain in position and can be easily dislodged. Client must be alert and cooperative to keep cannula in proper place. High-flow rates (>5 L/min) dry nasal membranes and may cause pain in frontal sinuses.	Nasal cannula should be stabilized when caring for a restless client. A flow rate of 2 L/min gives an O_2 concentration of about 28%. Amount of O_2 inhaled depends on room air and client's breathing pattern. Most clients with COPD can tolerate 2 L/min via cannula.
SIMPLE FACE MASK		
O_2 can be given quickly for short periods of time. O_2 concentrations of 35%-50% can be achieved with flow rates of 6-12 L/min. Mask provides adequate humidification of inspired air.	Lack of client tolerance results in inadequate therapy. Mask may be uncomfortable because tight seal must be maintained between face and mask. Mask may produce pressure necrosis of the skin and confines heat radiating from the face about nose and mouth. It must be removed to eat or drink.	Wash and dry under mask every 2 hr. Mask needs to fit snugly. Nasal cannula may be provided while client is eating. Watch for pressure necrosis at the top of ears from elastic straps. (Gauze or other padding may be used to alleviate this problem.) Method requires at least 5 L/min flow to prevent accumulation of expired air in the mask.
VENTURI MASK*		
Mask can deliver precise, high-flow rates of O_2. Lightweight plastic, cone-shaped device is fitted to face. Masks are available for delivery of 24%, 28%, 31%, 35%, and 40% O_2. Adaptors can be applied to increase humidification.	Mask is uncomfortable and must be removed when client eats. Client can talk but voice may be muffled.	Mask must be changed to deliver higher concentrations of O_2. Method is especially helpful for administering low, constant O_2 concentrations to clients with COPD. Air entrainment ports must not be occluded.
PARTIAL REBREATHING MASK		
Mask is lightweight and easy to use. Reservoir bag conserves O_2. Concentrations of 40%-60% can be achieved using flow rates of 6-10 L/min.	Mask cannot be used with a high degree of humidity.	Method is useful when blood O_2 concentrations must be raised. It is not recommended for client with COPD and should never be used with a nebulizer. Bag should not be allowed to deflate.

*See Fig. 21-7.

Continued.

Table 21-13 Methods of Oxygen Administration—cont'd

Advantages	Disadvantages	Nursing Interventions
NONBREATHING MASK		
High concentrations of O_2 can be delivered accurately. O_2 flows into bag and mask during inhalation. Valve prevents expired air from flowing back into bag. Concentrations of 60%-90% can be achieved.	Mask cannot be used with a high degree of humidity.	Mask should fit snugly. Flow rate must be sufficient to keep bag from collapsing during inspiration.
OXYGEN-CONSERVING CANNULA		
Cannula has a built-in reservoir that increases O_2 concentration delivered and allows client to use lower flow, which increases comfort and lowers cost. It is reportedly more comfortable than standard cannulas.	Cannula cannot be cleaned: manufacturer recommends changing cannula every week. It is more expensive than standard cannulas and requires evaluation with ABGs and oximetry to determine correct flow for client. Cannula is highly visible.	Method is generally indicated for clients requiring long-term O_2 therapy at home versus during hospitalization. It may be "moustache" or "pendant" type.
TRANSTRACHEAL CATHETER†		
Catheter is less visible. Flow requirement may be reduced 60%-80%, which greatly increases amount of time available from portable source of O_2. Less nasal irritation occurs.	Client and/or family must learn care for tracheostoma and how to replace catheter. Procedure is invasive. Procedure and replacement adds costs to O_2 therapy.	Method may not be appropriate for clients with excessive mucus production from "clogging."
FACE TENT		
Tent is ideal for providing moderate to high-density aerosol. O_2 concentration administered varies with O_2 flow rate.	Face tent is less reliable than face mask for maintaining high inspiration of O_2 concentration.	Open plastic mask fits under chin. Temperature of aerosol needs to be checked to prevent burning the client. It is rarely used.
TENT OR INCUBATOR		
Tent or incubator has ability to control temperature and humidity.	Tent or incubator has limited usefulness. It is difficult to maintain adequate concentrations of O_2. Method isolates client from environment.	Tent should be flushed with O_2 every time it is opened. Nurse should assess for leaks around canopy.
TRACHEOSTOMY COLLAR		
Collar can deliver high humidity and O_2 via tracheostomy.	Condensed fluid in tubing may drain into tracheostomy. Secretions collect inside collar and around tracheostomy. O_2 concentration is lost into atmosphere because collar does not fit tightly.	Collar attaches to neck with elastic strap and should be removed and cleaned at least every 4 hr to prevent aspiration of fluid and infection.
TRACHEOSTOMY T BAR		
Tight fit allows better O_2 and humidity delivery than tracheostomy collar.	Condensed fluid in tubing may drain into tracheostomy.	T bar needs to be removed for suctioning. Mörch swivel may be used to eliminate the need for removal. It should be emptied as necessary.

†See Fig. 21-9.

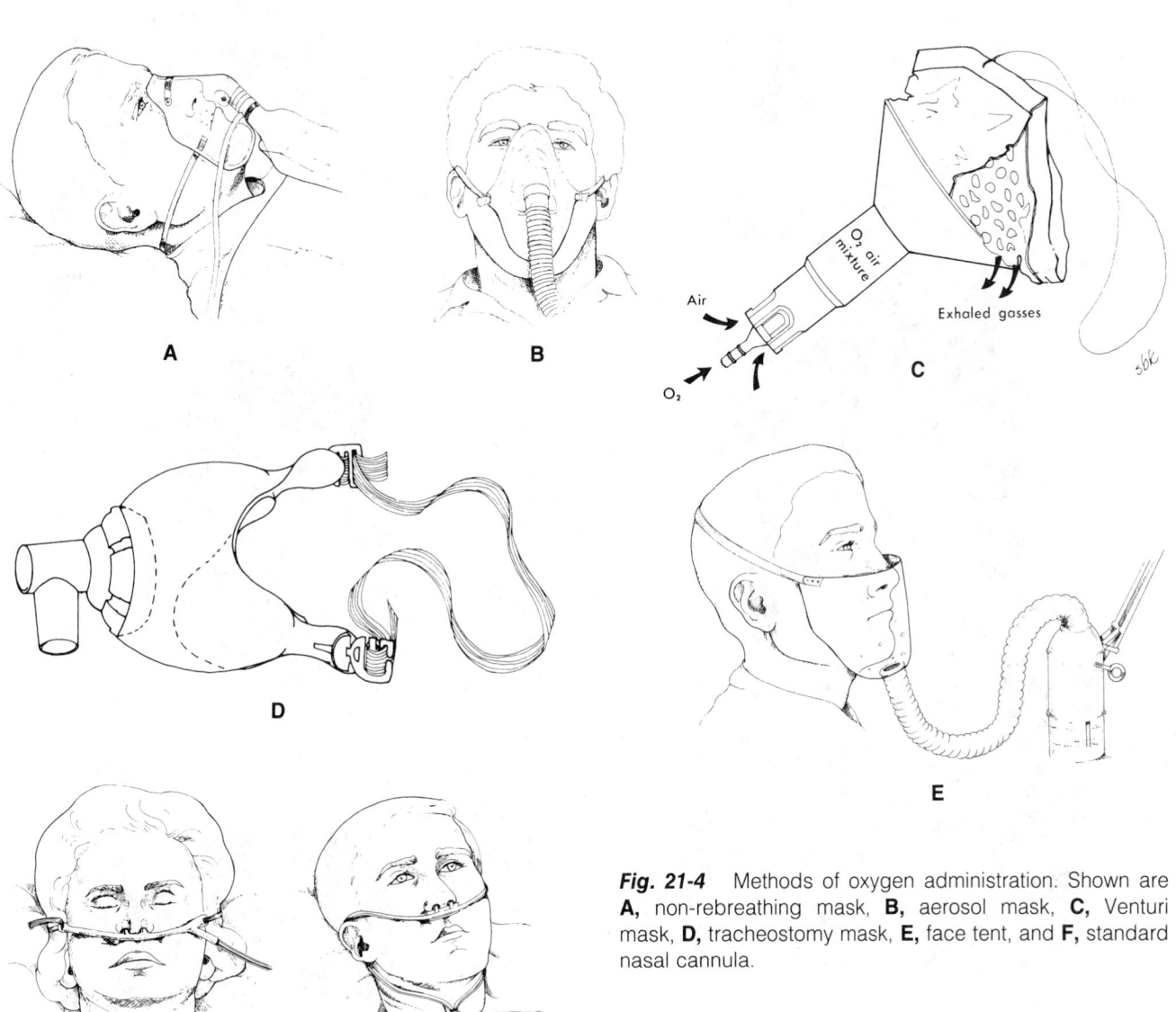

A

B

Air

O_2 air mixture

O_2

Exhaled gasses

C

D

E

F

Fig. 21-4 Methods of oxygen administration. Shown are **A,** non-rebreathing mask, **B,** aerosol mask, **C,** Venturi mask, **D,** tracheostomy mask, **E,** face tent, and **F,** standard nasal cannula.

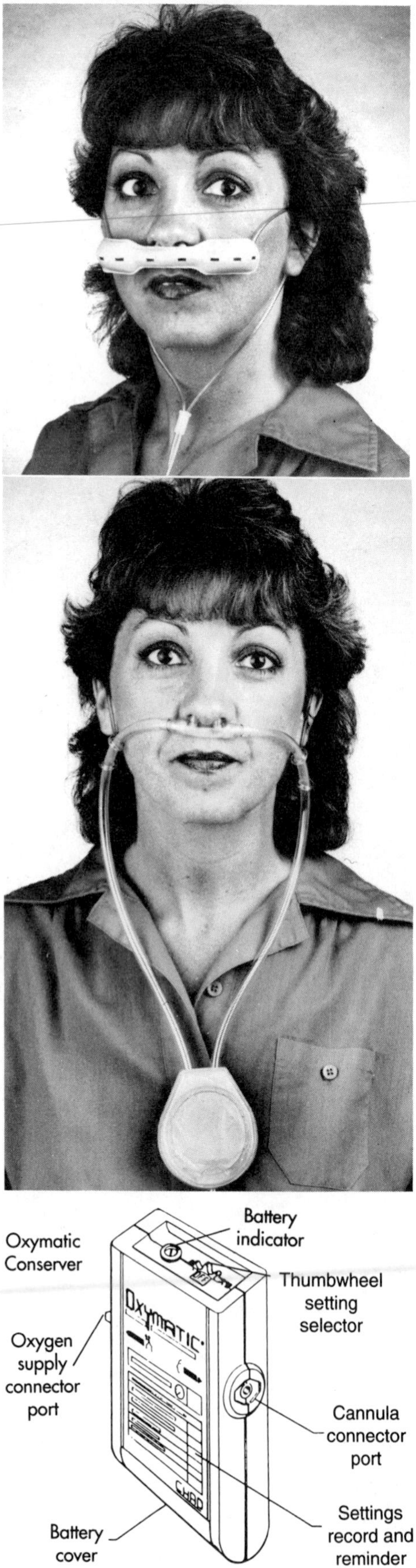

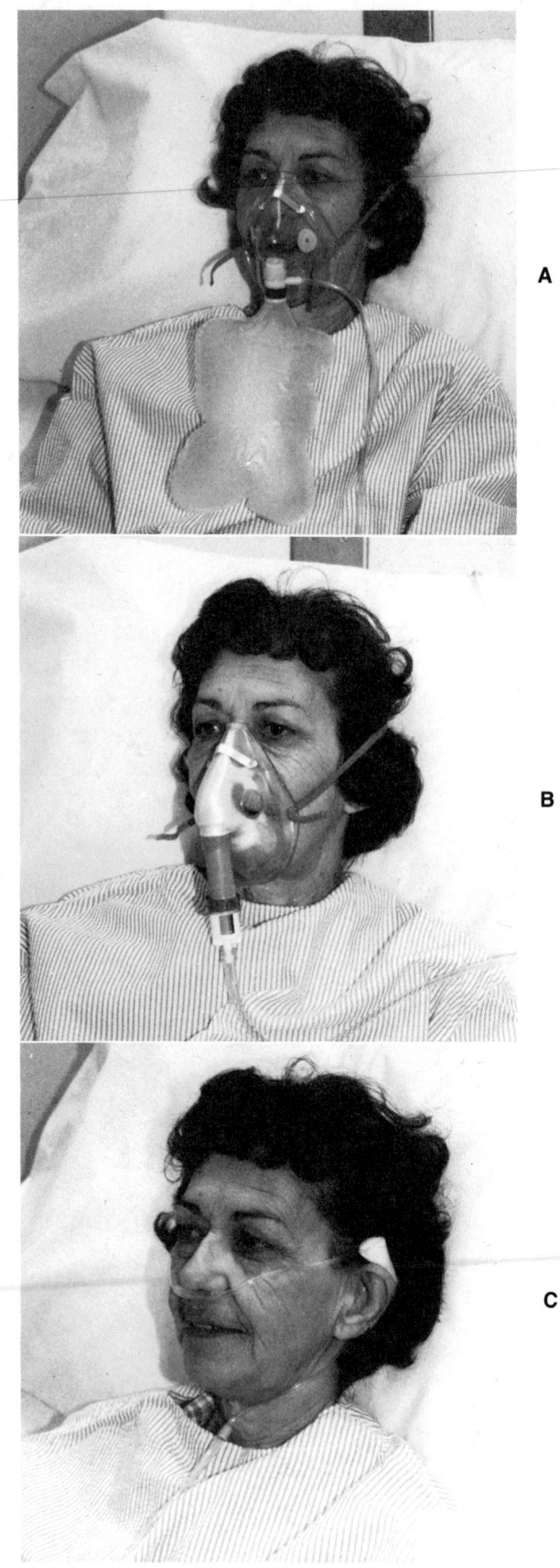

Oxymatic
Conserver

Battery
indicator

Thumbwheel
setting
selector

Oxygen
supply
connector
port

Cannula
connector
port

Battery
cover

Settings
record and
reminder

Fig. 21-5 Oxygen-conserving devices. Moustache-type oxygen-conserving cannula, pendant type conserving cannula, and demand-pulse delivery unit.

Fig. 21-6 **A,** Nonrebreathing mask in place. **B,** Venturi mask in place. **C,** Standard cannula with ears padded.

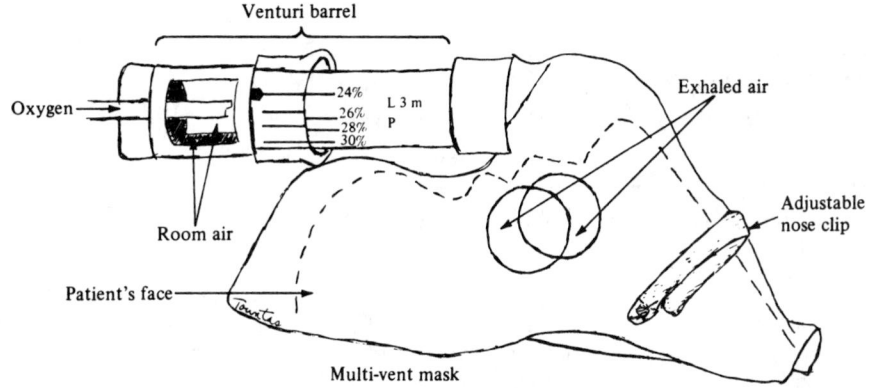

Fig. 21-7 Venturi mask mixes room air with oxygen at preset ratios. (From Shortridge LM and Lee EJ: Introductory skills for nursing practice, New York, 1980, McGraw-Hill Book Co, p 311.)

stimulant of respiration becomes hypoxemia. When O_2 is administered in high concentrations, the hypoxic stimulus is eliminated and the rate and depth of ventilation will decrease. The client will subsequently develop hypercapnia and eventually CO_2 narcosis.

It is critical to start O_2 at low flow rates until ABGs can be obtained. ABGs are used as a guide to determine what Fio_2 level is sufficient and can be tolerated. The client's mental status and vital signs should be assessed before starting O_2 therapy and frequently thereafter.

Oxygen toxicity. Pulmonary O_2 toxicity may result from prolonged exposure to a high Pao_2. The development of O_2 toxicity is determined by client tolerance, exposure time, and effective dose. It is believed that high concentrations of O_2 may inactivate pulmonary surfactant and lead to the development of the adult respiratory distress syndrome (ARDS). The lungs from individuals who die after prolonged administration of 100% O_2 show some or all of the following abnormalities on autopsy[13]:

1. Lungs are heavy, "beefy," and edematous.
2. Hyaline membranes cover many alveoli, alveolar ducts, and respiratory bronchioles.
3. Many alveoli are filled with hemorrhagic exudate.
4. Alveolar septa are markedly increased.

Early manifestations of O_2 toxicity are reduced vital capacity, cough, substernal chest pain, nausea and vomiting, paresthesia, nasal stuffiness, sore throat, and malaise. The later stages of O_2 toxicity affect the alveolar-capillary gas exchange unit, causing edema and production of copious sputum. The end stage of O_2 toxicity is progressive fibrosis of the lungs.

Prevention of O_2 toxicity is very important for the client who is receiving O_2. The amount of O_2 administered should be just enough to maintain the Pao_2 within a normal or acceptable range for the client. ABGs should be monitored frequently to evaluate the effectiveness of therapy as well as to guide the tapering of supplemental O_2. A safe limit of O_2 concentrations has not yet been established. All levels above 50% to 60% should be considered potentially toxic. Levels of 40% and below may be regarded as relatively nontoxic and may not result in devel-

opment of significant O_2 toxicity if the exposure period is short.

Absorption atelectasis. Normally nitrogen, which constitutes 79% of the air we breathe, is not absorbed into the bloodstream, and it prevents alveolar collapse. When high concentrations of O_2 are given, nitrogen is washed out of the alveoli and replaced with O_2. If airway obstruction occurs, the O_2 is absorbed into the bloodstream and the alveoli collapse. This process is called *absorption atelectasis*.

Infection. Infection can be a major hazard of O_2 administration. Heated nebulizers present the highest risk. The constant use of humidity supports bacterial growth: the most common infecting organism is *Pseudomonas aeruginosa*. Disposable equipment should be used and changed every 48 hours to prevent infection. A hospital policy of frequent changes of disposable equipment should be instituted. Both equipment and respiratory secretions should be gram stained and cultured frequently. (Nursing care of the client who is receiving O_2 therapy is presented in Table 21-14.)

Chronic Oxygen Therapy at Home

Data that suggest effectiveness of chronic supplemental O_2 have been gathered only on clients with underlying COPD. However, most clinicians believe that data apply to other chronic hypoxemic pulmonary disorders. Improved prognosis has been noted in clients with COPD who receive nocturnal or continuous O_2 to treat hypoxemia. The longer that the continuous daily use of O_2 is maintained, the greater the improvement.[14] This improved prognosis results from preventing progression of the disease and subsequent cor pulmonale, thus decreasing the development of fatal dysrhythmias.

The potential benefit of long-term O_2 therapy should be evaluated when the client's condition has stabilized. There should be an accurate, current diagnosis and an optimal medical regimen prescribed by a physician knowledgeable in treatment of chest disease. Short-term home O_2 therapy (1 to 30 days) may be indicated for clients in whom hypoxemia persists to discharge such clients safely. For example, clients with underlying COPD who develop serious

Table 21-14

 NURSING CARE PLAN FOR THE CLIENT RECEIVING OXYGEN

Defining Characteristics	Nursing Interventions	Evaluation Criteria
NURSING DIAGNOSIS: High risk for impaired skin integrity related to the O_2 administration device and humidity		
Redness at contact of O_2 mask or cannula and skin, tenderness at contact points, disruption of skin surface	Do not fit strap too tightly if mask is used. Remove it every 2 hr and wash and dry skin. Pad any pressure points. Observe tops of ears for skin breakdown of pressure points.	No skin breakdown from cannula
NURSING DIAGNOSIS: Altered oral mucous membranes related to O_2 therapy		
Drying, redness, cracking of nasal mucosa, possibly bleeding	Use water-based jelly on lips and nasal mucosa. Do not obstruct cannula outlets with jelly. Provide frequent oral hygiene. Provide humidification via humidifier or nebulizing device.	No evidence or complaints of mucosal discomfort
NURSING DIAGNOSIS: High risk for infection related to presence of environmental pathogens and bacterial contamination of equipment		
Moisture from mask on face, large amount of expectorated sputum in/on delivery device	Remove mask or collar and cleanse with water every 4-8 hr. Cleanse skin carefully at this time and as necessary. Change disposable equipment frequently. Remove secretions that are coughed out. Empty container using universal precautions.	No evidence of infection
NURSING DIAGNOSIS: High risk for injury related to fire hazard secondary to O_2-enriched environment		
Continuous O_2 use, positive smoking history	Post "No Smoking" warning sign prominently. Do not use electric razors, portable radios, open flames, wool blankets, or mineral oils. Do not allow smoking in room. Teach client about precautions related to home O_2 therapy.	No incidence of fire
NURSING DIAGNOSIS: Potential complication: CO_2 narcosis in client with COPD		
ABGs showing CO_2 above normal (>45 mm Hg) with or without abnormal pH, history of COPD	Identify clients at risk for CO_2 narcosis. Administer O_2 at ordered level only. Monitor results of ABGs. Do not increase the O_2 at low flow rates (1-3 L/min) until ABGs can be obtained. Assess baseline level of consciousness, respiratory rate, and pulse rate and monitor frequently. Teach client and family not to increase O_2 flow rate unless directed to do so by a physician or nurse.	No CO_2 narcosis as evidenced by a rising P_{CO_2} and/or decreased level of consciousness
NURSING DIAGNOSIS: Potential complication: O_2 toxicity related to enriched O_2 environment		
O_2 at Fi_{O_2} $>50\%$; complaints of sore throat, substernal aching, cough, confusion	Administer O_2 at the lowest level that produces acceptable ABGs. Monitor ABGs frequently. Monitor client for manifestations of substernal discomfort, cough, nasal congestion, sore throat, and confusion. Do not attempt to use Fi_{O_2} over 50% for more than 24 hr unless specifically indicated.	Minimal O_2 therapy to maintain P_{O_2} at adequate level necessary

Table 21-14

 NURSING CARE PLAN FOR THE CLIENT RECEIVING OXYGEN—cont'd

Defining Characteristics	Nursing Interventions	Evaluation Criteria

NURSING DIAGNOSIS: Impaired home maintenance management related to lack of knowledge regarding O_2 therapy

Continuous O_2 therapy, mask O_2 or home O_2, concern about ability to maintain satisfactory O_2 therapy at home	Administer O_2 continuously unless it is specifically ordered only for exercise or sleep. Encourage client to wear the O_2-delivery device properly. If a mask is used, provide a nasal cannula during meals. Take rectal temperature if mask is being used. Provide enough tubing to reach from O_2 source to bathroom (if client is ambulatory) or to move around house (if client is at home). Provide portable O_2 for ambulation outside hospital room or home. Wean client from O_2 in increments when ABG values indicate that this can be done safely. Provide client with information on home O_2 delivery.	No interruptions in O_2 therapy, maintenance of adequate oxygenation

respiratory infections may continue to have clearing of the infection after completion of antibiotic therapy and discharge from the hospital. These patients may demonstrate continued hypoxemia for 4 to 6 weeks after discharge.

At sea level, a resting room air Po_2 of less than 55 mm Hg is generally considered to be a fundamental criteria that indicates potential benefit to be gained from long-term O_2 therapy. Clients who demonstrate Pao_2 greater than 55 mm Hg but who also have evidence of hypoxia and organ dysfunction such as secondary pulmonary hypertension, secondary erythrocytosis, impaired mental status, and CNS dysfunction are considered candidates for chronic O_2 therapy.[15]

The need for O_2 during exercise may be demonstrated by showing significant desaturation with exertion and an increased tolerance for exercise when using supplemental O_2. The necessity for O_2 therapy during sleep to control sleep-induced hypoxemia is not well delineated. Significant nocturnal desaturation with associated sleep disturbance, cardiac dysrhythmias, or pulmonary hypertension should be demonstrated. Preferably these effects should be abolished by the use of O_2.

Technology for evaluation and monitoring clients for O_2 therapy consists primarily of two modalities: arterial puncture for ABGs and ear oximetry. Another method, transcutaneous monitoring, has been developed and is useful in neonatal intensive care unit (ICU) settings, but its reliability in adults is quite variable and thus not beneficial.[16]

ABGs provide the full range of gas values necessary to evaluate acid-base and oxygenation status of a client. However, technical errors that can decrease their validity are possible (e.g., too much heparin, failure to properly ice the sample, or improper calibration of the ABG equipment). Ear oximetry should be used to avoid excessive invasive techniques during evaluation studies. An ear oximeter is a machine that measures light transmission through the ear and reports O_2 saturation of the arterial blood, giving a constant digital display.[17] It can be used to monitor saturation continuously during sleep, changes in position, and exertion to determine an individualized prescription for O_2 use. In addition, oximetry is useful in determination of O_2 requirements during hospitalization and during the weaning process from ventilatory support.

Periodic reevaluations are necessary for clients who are using chronic supplemental O_2. Generally the recommendation is that they should be reevaluated every 6 months during the first year of therapy and annually after that, as long as they remain stable.

Nasal cannulas, either regular or the O_2-conserving type (see Table 21-13), are usually used to deliver O_2 from a central source in the home. The source may be a liquid O_2 storage system, compressed O_2 in tanks, or an O_2 concentrator or extractor, depending on the client's home environment, activity level, and proximity to an O_2 supply company (Table 21-15). The client can use extension tubing (up to 50 feet) without adversely affecting the O_2 flow delivery to increase mobility in the home, provided that the flowmeter is the back pressure–compensated type. Small portable systems may be provided for clients who remain active outside the home (Fig. 21-8).

Reservoir cannulas have been on the market for several years. They operate on the principle of storing O_2 in a small reservoir during exhalation. The O_2 is then delivered to the client during the subsequent inhalation, almost like a bolus effect. The reservoir cannulas can reduce flow requirements by approximately 50%. Newer reservoir cannulas are available, and they may be less visible than the original moustache type. One is the pendant type, and another fits onto the frame of eyeglasses (Fig. 21-5).

Table 21-15   Home Oxygen Delivery Systems

System	Advantages	Disadvantages	Comments
Liquid oxygen (reservoir/portable unit)	Portable unit that can be refilled by client from reservoir, duration approximately 1 week to 10 days, shoulder-pack portable unit giving 6-8 hr supply at 2 L/min	Liquid system slightly more expensive, depending on location; not available everywhere; generally limited to urban areas	As liquid warms to gas, some is vented from the system. In summer, evaporation is accelerated and may decrease supply to less than 1 week.
Compressed tank O_2 (H or J tank/E or A cylinder for portable)	Good availability	Duration of H or J tank at 2 L/min flow about 50 hr; storage of 4-5 large cylinders in the home necessary to have 1-week to 10-day supply; portable cylinder on cart; cumbersome and heavy	Some even smaller tanks (D or M) may be used; these can be refilled from large cylinders, which are at least half full and weigh about 10 lb. Tank can be carried on shoulder strap.
Concentrator or extractor (E or A cylinder for portable)	On wheels, movable from room to room; weekly delivery of supply not necessary; compact, excellent system for rural or homebound clients	Noisy; increase in electricity bill by $20-$30 per month (not reimbursable by insurance); greater than 3 L flow resulting in significant decrease in concentration	Concentrator should be kept in room other than bedroom, and extension tubing should be used if noise disturbs sleep.
Demand delivery system	Simple to use, change in rate of delivery with respiratory rate	Mechanically complex; only safe use with portable system when client is awake (unless presence of alarm for disconnection) oxygenation possibly less efficient with exertion	System may be separate unit that can be used with liquid or cylinder. Method uses sources (Oxymatic) or is "built in" to liquid system.

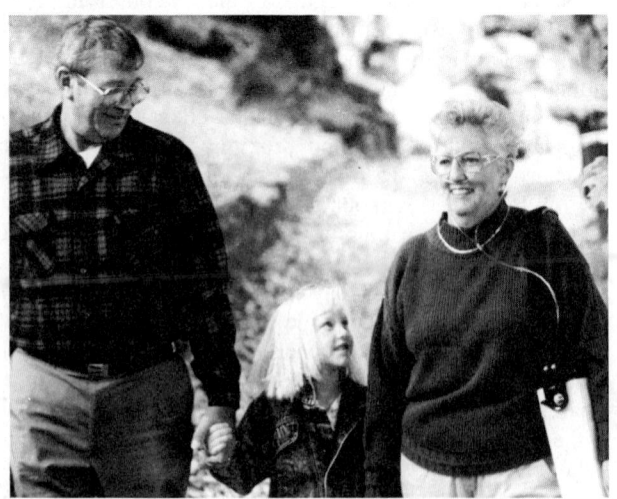

Fig. 21-8   Portable liquid oxygen system. (Courtesy Cryogenics—Minnesota Valley Engineering, New Prague, Minn.)

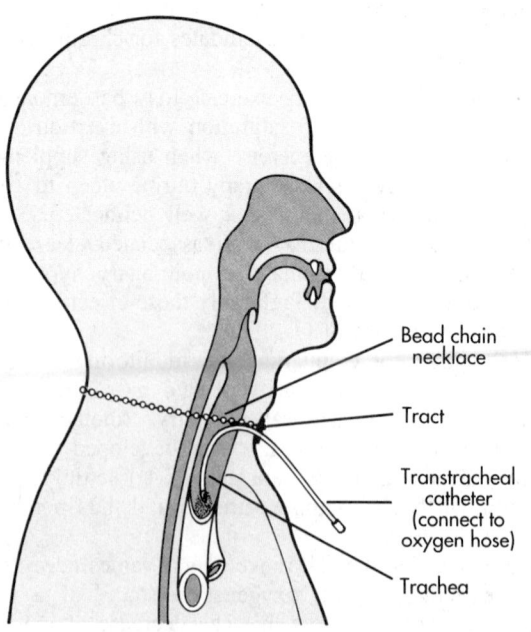

Fig. 21-9   Transtracheal catheter for oxygen administration.

Recent technological advances in the delivery of chronic O_2 therapy include transtracheal O_2 delivery and intermittent-demand O_2 delivery systems. The greatest stimulus for these advances has been the increasingly high cost of home O_2 therapy. However, other benefits in addition to less waste of O_2 and therefore lower cost include the potential for less nasal irritation, prolonged availability of portable O_2 stores, and in the case of transtracheal O_2, less visibility of the O_2 delivery device.[18]

Transtracheal O_2 delivery requires a surgical procedure to insert the small O_2 catheter into the client's trachea (Fig. 21-9). Nursing care involves teaching the client and family how to care for the tracheostoma as well as how to clean and change the transtracheal catheter. Delivery of supplemental O_2 transtracheally reduces the flow requirement by 30% to 50%.[18]

Intermittent-demand delivery systems are mechanically complex devices. They deliver "pulses" of O_2 to the client, usually during inspiration, and thus eliminate wasted flow during exhalation as is experienced during continuous flow. There are intermittent-demand units that operate independently of a particular system as well as units that are built into the delivery device itself.

Home O_2 systems are usually rented from a company that sends a respiratory therapist or pulmonary nurse specialist to the client's home. The therapist teaches the client how to use the O_2 system, how to care for it, and how to recognize when the supply is running low and needs to be reordered.

Clients who use home O_2 should be encouraged to remain active and to travel normally. If travel is by automobile, arrangements can be made for O_2 to be available at the destination point. O_2 supply companies can often assist in these arrangements. If a client wishes to travel by airplane, the airlines require notification of the need for O_2 during the flight when reservations are made. Since the cabins are pressurized to an elevation of 7000 or 8000 feet, clients who use supplemental O_2 should have O_2 provided during flight. The plane's O_2 system must be used. Clients may not use their O_2 systems during flight, since they are not properly pressurized. Most airlines will allow portable reservoirs (liquid or tank) to be carried in the baggage compartment for use at the point of destination as long as they are empty and the valves are left open. Generally, clients should be encouraged to avoid prolonged exposure to high elevations during travel unless they are instructed by their physician regarding adjustments in their O_2 flow to attempt to compensate for altitude.

OCCUPATIONAL LUNG DISEASES

Occupational lung diseases result from inhaled dust or chemicals.[19] The duration of exposure and the amount of inhalant have a major influence on whether exposed individuals will have lung damage. Another factor is the susceptibility of the host.

Pneumoconiosis is a general term for lung diseases caused by inhalation and retention of dust particles. The literal meaning of pneumoconiosis is "dust in the lungs." Examples of this condition are silicosis, asbestosis, and berylliosis. The classic response to the inhaled substance is diffuse parenchymal infiltration with phagocytic cells. This eventually results in *diffuse pulmonary fibrosis* (excess connective tissue). Fibrosis is the result of tissue repair after inflammation. Pneumoconiosis and other occupational lung diseases are presented in Table 21-16.

Clinical Manifestations

Symptoms of occupational lung disease usually do not occur until at least 10 to 15 years after the initial exposure to the inhaled irritant. Dyspnea and cough are often the earliest manifestations. Chest pain and productive sputum usually occur later. Complications that often result are pneumonia, chronic bronchitis, emphysema, and lung cancer. Manifestations of these complications can be the reason the client seeks health care.

Pulmonary function studies show reduced vital capacity. A chest x-ray film will often reveal lung involvement specific to the primary problem. Cor pulmonale is a late complication, especially in conditions characterized by diffuse pulmonary fibrosis.

Occupational asthma refers to the development of symptoms of shortness of breath, wheezing, cough, and chest tightness as a result of exposure to fumes or dust that trigger an allergic response. The obstruction may initially be reversible or intermittent, but continued exposure results in permanent obstructive changes. The best-known causative agent in occupational asthma is toluene diiocyanate (TDI), which is used in the production of rigid polyurethane foam.[20]

Therapeutic Management

The best approach to management is to try to prevent or decrease occupational risks. Well-designed, effective ventilation systems can reduce exposure to irritants. Wearing masks is appropriate in some occupations. Mining and industrial commissions are planning ways to decrease exposure to dusts and other irritants. New materials that are developed need to be studied in terms of their potential risks. Cigarette smoking adds increased insult to the lungs, and persons at risk for occupational lung disease should not smoke.

Early diagnosis is essential if the disease process is to be halted. The best treatment is to decrease or stop exposure to the harmful agent. Some places of employment at which there is a known risk of lung disease may require periodic chest x-rays and pulmonary function studies for exposed employees. These measures can detect pulmonary changes before symptoms develop.

There is no specific treatment for most occupational lung diseases. Treatment is directed toward providing symptomatic relief. If there are coexisting problems such as pneumonia, chronic bronchitis, emphysema, or reversible airway obstruction (asthma), they are treated.

LOWER RESPIRATORY TRACT MALIGNANCIES
Lung Cancer

Significance. Primary lung cancer is the leading cause of death in men and women who have malignant disease in

Table 21-16 Occupational Lung Diseases

Disease	Agents/Industries	Description	Complications
Asbestosis	Asbestos fibers present in insulation, construction material (roof tiling, cement products), shipyards, textiles (for fireproofing), automobile clutch and brake linings	Disease appears 15-35 yr after first exposure. Interstitial fibrosis develops. Pleural plaques, which are calcified lesions, develop on pleura. Dyspnea, basal rales, and decreased vital capacity are early manifestations.	Bronchogenic carcinoma, especially in cigarette smokers; mesothelioma (rare type of cancer affecting pleura and peritoneal membrane)
Berylliosis	Beryllium dust present in aircraft manufacturing, metallurgy, rocket fuels	Noncaseating granulomas form. Acute pneumonitis occurs after heavy exposure. Interstitial fibrosis can also occur.	Progress of disease possible after removal of stimulating inhalant
Bird fancier's, breeder's, or handler's lung	Bird droppings or feathers	Hypersensitivity pneumonitis is present.	Progressive fibrosis of lung
Byssinosis	Cotton, flax, and hemp dust (textile industry)	Airway obstruction is caused by contraction of smooth muscles. Chronic disease results from severe airway obstruction and decreased elastic recoil.	Progression of chronic disease after cessation of dust exposure
Coal worker's pneumoconiosis (black lung)	Coal dust	Incidence is high (20%-30%) in coal workers. Deposits of carbon dust cause lesions to develop along respiratory bronchioles. Bronchioles dilate because of loss of wall structure. Chronic airway obstruction and bronchitis develop. Dyspnea and cough are common early symptoms.	Progressive, massive lung fibrosis; increased risk of chronic bronchitis and emphysema with smoking
Farmer's lung	Inhalation of airborne material from moldy hay or similar matter	Hypersensitivity pneumonitis occurs. *Acute* form is similar to pneumonia, with manifestations of chills, fever, and malaise. *Chronic*, insidious form is type of pulmonary fibrosis.	Progressive fibrosis of lung
Siderosis	Iron oxide present in welding materials, foundries, iron ore mining	Dust deposits are found in lung.	
Silicosis	Silica dust present in quartz rock in mining of gold, copper, tin, coal, lead; also present in sandblasting, foundries, quarries, pottery making, masonry	In *chronic* disease, dust is engulfed by macrophages and may be destroyed, resulting in fibrotic nodules. *Acute* disease results from intense exposure in short time period. Within 5 yr, it progresses to severe disability from lung fibrosis.	Increased susceptibility to TB; progressive, massive fibrosis; high incidence of chronic bronchitis
Silo filler's disease	Nitrogen oxides from fermentation of vegetation in freshly filled silo	Chemical pneumonitis occurs.	Progressive bronchiolitis obliterans

the United States. Until recently, more cases of lung cancer were found in men than in women. That situation is changing, probably because cigarette smoking has become socially acceptable for women since the 1930s and 1940s. Beginning in 1986, deaths from lung cancer in women exceeded deaths from all other cancers and are expected to continue to increase.[21]

The mortality rate from lung cancer has increased over the past 50 years. In the past decade the death rate has escalated sharply for men and women. In 1989 there were 140,000 lung cancer deaths, and deaths of men were roughly double those of women.[22] The overall 5-year survival rate is 13%, which is the poorest prognosis for any cancer other than cancers of the pancreas, liver, and esophagus.

Lung cancer occurs most commonly in an individual more than 50 years old with a long history of cigarette smoking. The disease is found most frequently in persons 40 to 75 years of age.

Causes and risk factors. Cigarette smoking is by far the major risk factor in the development of lung cancer. Smoking is responsible for approximately 80% to 90% of all lung cancers.[21] About 1 of every 10 heavy smokers eventually develops lung cancer. Cigarette smoking causes a change in the bronchial epithelium, which usually returns to normal when smoking is discontinued. The risk of lung cancer is gradually lowered and continues to decline with time.[23]

The risk of developing lung cancer is directly related to total exposure to cigarette smoke measured by total number of cigarettes smoked in a lifetime, depth of inhalation, and tar and nicotine content of the cigarettes smoked. Studies are also beginning to show that there is a risk from secondhand or "sidestream" smoke; that is, the nonsmoking spouse or child of a smoker has a higher risk of developing lung cancer than the nonsmoking spouse or child of a nonsmoker. One study reports that nonsmoking wives of smokers have a 34% higher rate of lung cancer than nonsmoking wives of nonsmokers.[23] Heredity may play a role in both the tendency to smoke and the predisposition to develop lung cancer. Since only a few persons (1 of 10) who are at high risk actually develop lung cancer, there must be a difference in the host's ability to deal with the repeated insult of smoking.

Those who smoke pipes and cigars have also been shown to have an increased risk of developing lung cancer, which is slightly higher than that of nonsmokers. Cigar smokers are at higher rate for lung cancer than are pipe smokers. However, heavy smoking of small cigars and inhalation of smoke from small cigars have been shown to correlate with the rates of lung cancer observed in cigarette smokers.

Another major risk factor for lung cancer is inhaled carcinogens. These include asbestos, nickel, iron and iron oxides, uranium, polycyclic aromatic hydrocarbons, chromates, arsenic, and air pollution. Exposure to these substances is common for employees of industries involved in paper, chemical, or petroleum manufacturing.[24] The cigarette smoker who is also exposed to one or more of these chemicals or to high amounts of air pollution is at significantly higher risk for lung cancer.

Lung cancer does occur in individuals who have never smoked or worked with carcinogens. The reasons for this are not known but heredity may play a part. The host's response to environmental insults is important.

Another possible risk factor is preexisting pulmonary diseases such as TB, pulmonary fibrosis, bronchiectasis, and COPD. Chronic inflammatory conditions often precede cancer. The incidence of lung cancer correlates with the degree of urbanization and population density. One reason for this may be increased exposure to irritants and pollutants.

Pathophysiology. The pathogenesis of primary lung cancer is not well understood. Over 90% of cancers originate from the epithelium of the bronchus (bronchogenic). They grow slowly; it takes 8 to 10 years for a tumor to reach 1 cm in size, which is the smallest detectable lesion on an x-ray film. Lung cancers occur primarily in the segmental bronchi or beyond and have a preference for the upper lobes of the lungs. Pathological changes in the bronchial system show nonspecific inflammatory changes with hypersecretion of mucus, desquamation of cells, reactive hyperplasia of the basal cells, and metaplasia of normal respiratory epithelium to stratified squamous cells.

Primary lung cancers are often categorized into histological types (Table 21-17). They metastasize primarily by direct extension and via the blood circulation and the lymph system. The common sites for metastatic growth are the liver, brain, bones, scalene lymph nodes, and adrenal glands (Fig. 21-10).

Paraneoplastic syndrome. Certain lung cancers cause the *paraneoplastic syndrome,* which is characterized by various manifestations caused by certain substances (e.g., hormones, enzymes, antigens) produced by the tumor cells. Small cell carcinomas are most commonly associated with the paraneoplastic syndrome. The systemic manifestations are the following:

1. *Hormonal* (Table 21-18)
2. *Dermatological,* including dermatomyositis and acanthosis nigricans
3. *Neuromuscular,* including peripheral neuropathy, cortical cerebellar degeneration, and a syndrome similar to myasthenia gravis
4. *Vascular and hematological,* including thrombocytopenic purpura, anemia, leukemialike reaction, thrombophlebitis, and nonbacterial endocarditis
5. *Connective tissue,* including nonspecific arthralgias, hypertrophic pulmonary osteoarthropathy, and digital clubbing.

Clinical manifestations. The clinical manifestations of lung cancer are usually nonspecific and present late in the disease process. Manifestations depend on the type of primary lung cancer. Often there is extensive metastasis before symptoms become apparent. Persistent pneumonitis that is due to obstructed bronchi may be one of the earliest manifestations, causing fever, chills, and cough.

One of the most significant symptoms, and often the one reported first, is a persistent cough that may be productive of sputum. Blood-tinged sputum may be produced because of bleeding caused by malignancy, but hemoptysis is not a common early presenting symptom. Chest pain

Table 21-17   Comparison of the Types of Primary Lung Cancer

Cell Type	Risk Factors	Characteristics	Response to Therapy
NONSMALL CELL LUNG CANCER			
Squamous cell (epidermoid) carcinoma	Almost always associated with cigarette smoking, is associated with exposure to environmental carcinogens (e.g., uranium, asbestos).	Accounts for 40%-50% of lung cancers, is more common in men, arises from the bronchial epithelium, produces earlier symptoms because of bronchial obstructive characteristics, does not have a strong tendency to metastasize, metastasizes locally by direct extension, causes cavitating pulmonary lesions	Surgical resection is often attempted, life expectancy is better than for undifferentiated (anaplastic) carcinoma
Adenocarcinoma	Has been associated with lung scarring and chronic interstitial fibrosis, is not related to cigarette smoking	Accounts for 25% of lung cancers, is more common in women, often has no clinical manifestations until widespread metastasis is present, metastasizes via bloodstream, is most commonly located in peripheral portions of lungs*	Surgical resection is often attempted, cancer does not respond well to chemotherapy
Large cell undifferentiated	Has high correlation with cigarette smoking and exposure to environmental carcinogens	Accounts for 5%-15% of lung cancers, commonly causes cavitation, is highly metastatic via lymphatics and blood	Surgery is not usually attempted because of high rate of metastases, tumor may be radiosensitive but often recurs
SMALL CELL LUNG CANCER			
Small cell anaplastic undifferentiated (includes oat cell)	Is associated with cigarette smoking, exposure to environmental carcinogens	Accounts for 25% of lung cancers, is most malignant form, tends to spread early via lymphatics and bloodstream, is frequently associated with endocrine disturbances	Cancer has poorest prognosis; however, recent chemotherapy gains have been substantial: 70% response rate with chemotherapy; radiation is used as adjuvant therapy, as well as palliative measure; average median survival is less than 1 year

*See Fig. 21-10.

may be present and localized or unilateral, ranging from mild to severe. Dyspnea and an auscultatory wheeze may be present if there is bronchial obstruction.

Later manifestations may include nonspecific systemic symptoms such as anorexia, fatigue, weight loss, and nausea and vomiting. Hoarseness may be present as a result of involvement of the recurrent laryngeal nerve. Unilateral paralysis of the diaphragm, dysphagia, and superior vena cava obstruction may occur because of intrathoracic spread of the malignancy. There may be palpable lymph nodes in the neck or axilla. Mediastinal involvement may lead to pericardial effusion, cardiac tamponade, and dysrhythmias.

Diagnostic studies. Chest x-ray films are widely used in the diagnosis of lung cancer. Anyone who has had a cough or a change in a cough for more than 2 to 3 weeks should be evaluated by chest x-ray examination. The findings may show the presence of the tumor and/or abnormalities related to the obstructive features of the tumor such as atelectasis and pneumonitis. The x-ray film can also show evidence of metastasis to the ribs or vertebrae and the presence of pleural effusion. Lung tomograms may be used to locate the tumor and to estimate the extent of involvement of nearby structures.

Computed tomography (CT) is also used in the diagnosis of lung cancer. With CT scans, the location and extent

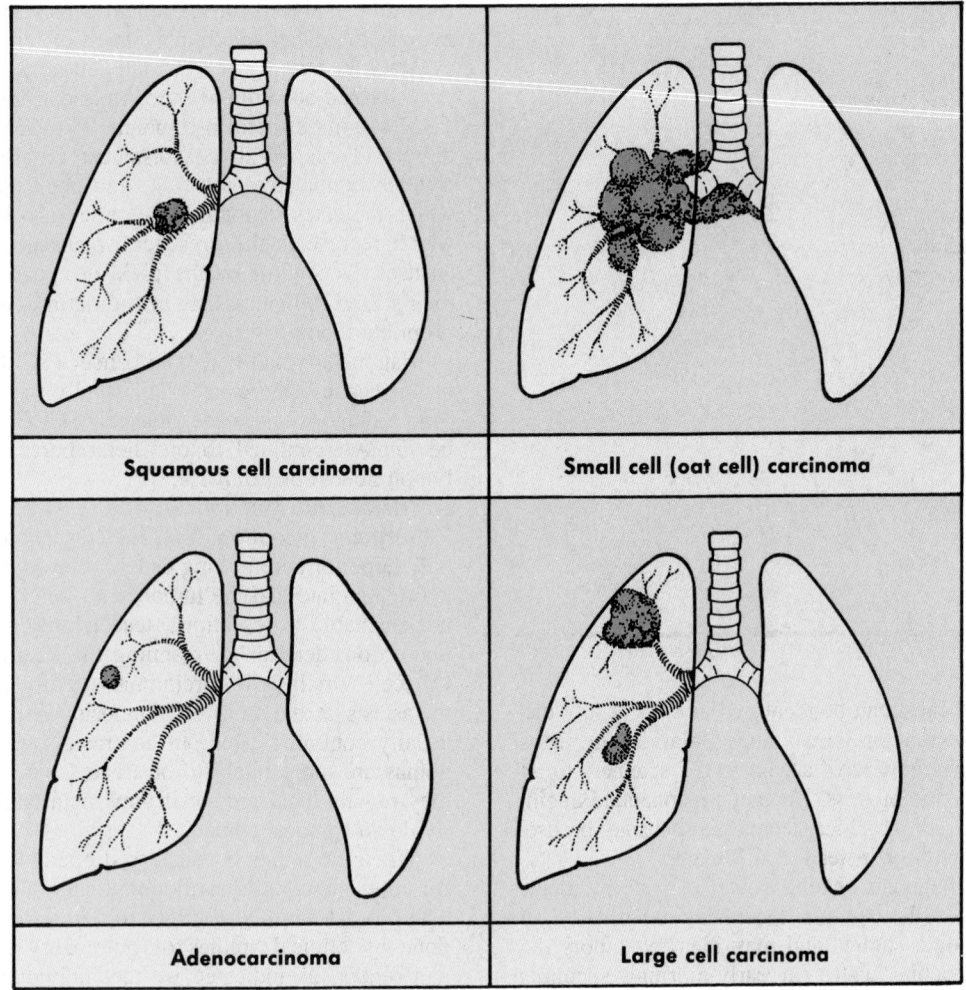

Squamous cell carcinoma

Small cell (oat cell) carcinoma

Adenocarcinoma

Large cell carcinoma

Fig. 21-10 Predominant sites of types of lung cancer. (From McCance KL and Huether SE: Pathophysiology: the biological basis for disease in adults and children, St Louis, 1990, Mosby–Year Book, Inc, p 1086.)

Table 21-18 Ectopic Hormone Syndromes of Lung Cancer

Syndrome	Ectopic Hormone	Most Common Cell Type
Cushing's syndrome	ACTH	Oat cell (small cell)
Syndrome of inappropriate antidiuretic hormone	Antidiuretic hormone	Oat cell (small cell)
Hypercalcemia	Parathyroid hormone	Squamous cell
Gynecomastia	Follicle-stimulating hormone	Large cell
Carcinoid syndrome	5-hydroxyacetic acid from serotonin breakdown	Oat cell (small cell) Bronchial adenoma (adenocarcinoma)

From Murray JF and Nadel JA: Textbook of respiratory medicine, Philadelphia, 1988, WB Saunders Co, p 418.

Table 21-19

Diagnostic and Therapeutic Management: Lung Cancer

DIAGNOSTIC

History and physical examination
Chest x-ray study
Sputum for cytological study
Bronchoscopy
Mediastinoscopy
Scalene node biopsy
Pulmonary angiography
Lung scan
CT scan
FNA
MRI

THERAPEUTIC

Surgery
Radiation therapy
Chemotherapy
Immunotherapy
Laser surgery

of masses in the chest can be identified as well as any mediastinal involvement or lymph node enlargement. Most large communities now have access to CT scanners to assist in the diagnostic process. Magnetic resonance imaging (MRI) is a new radiographical technique that may be used in combination with or instead of CT scans.

A definitive diagnosis of lung cancer is made by identifying malignant cells. Sputum specimens are usually obtained for cytologic studies and may identify tumors that involve the bronchial wall. An early-morning specimen that has been obtained by having the client cough deeply provides the most accurate results. However, malignant cells may not be obtained even in the presence of a lung cancer.

The use of the fiberoptic bronchoscope is very important in the diagnosis of lung cancer, particularly when the lesions are endobronchial or are in close proximity to an airway. It provides direct visualization and allows biopsy specimens to be obtained. A biopsy is usually the best method for establishing the presence of a malignant tumor.

Mediastinoscopy involves the insertion of a scope via a small anterior chest incision into the mediastinum to examine for metastasis in the anterior mediastinum or hilum or extrapleurally in the chest. It is also used to determine the stage of the lung cancer, which is important in determining the treatment plan.

Other diagnostic studies include radionuclide scans of the liver, spleen, bone, or brain and scalene lymph node biopsy to determine metastatic spread (Table 21-19). Pulmonary angiography and lung scans may be performed to assess overall pulmonary status. Fine-needle aspiration (FNA) may be used to obtain a tissue sample to determine tumor histology. FNA is most useful in cases involving a

peripheral lesion near the chest wall, and it is usually attempted in an effort to avoid a thoracotomy.[25] If a thoracentesis is performed to relieve a pleural effusion, the fluid should be analyzed for malignant cells. (Table 21-19 summarizes the diagnostic management of lung cancer.)

Staging. Staging of nonsmall cell lung cancer (NSCLC) is performed according to the American Joint Committee's TNM staging system in a manner similar to that for other tumors (Table 21-20). Assessment criteria are *T,* which denotes tumor size, location, and degree of invasion; *N,* which indicates regional lymph node involvement; and *M,* which represents the presence or absence of distant metastases. Depending on the TNM designation, the tumor is then staged, which assists in estimating prognosis and appropriate therapy.

Staging of small-cell lung cancer (SCLC) has not been useful because the cancer has usually metastasized by the time a diagnosis is made. Instead, SCLC is determined to be *limited* (confined to one hemothorax and to regional lymph nodes) or *extensive.*[26]

Therapeutic management

Surgical resection. Surgical resection is usually the only hope for cure in lung cancer. Unfortunately, detection is often so late that the tumor is no longer localized and is not amenable to resection. Resectability of the tumor is a major consideration in planning the surgical intervention. Oat cell (small cell) carcinomas usually have widespread metastasis at the time of diagnosis. Therefore surgery is usually contraindicated. In contrast, squamous cell carcinomas are more likely to be treated with surgery because they remain localized, or if they metastasize, they primarily do so by local spread.

When the tumor is considered operable with a potential for cure, the client's cardiopulmonary status must be evaluated to determine the ability to withstand surgery. This is done by clinical studies of pulmonary function, ABGs, and others, as indicated by the individual's status. Contraindications for thoracotomy include hypercapnia, pulmonary hypertension, cor pulmonale, and markedly reduced lung function. Coexisting conditions such as cardiac, renal, and liver disease are also contraindications for surgery.

A tumor may be potentially resectable, but because it is located in a critical area such as the trachea or too close to the heart, it may be considered inoperable. The type of surgery performed is usually a *lobectomy* (removal of one or more lobes of the lung) and less often a *pneumonectomy* (removal of one entire lung).

Radiation therapy. Radiation therapy is used as a curative approach in individuals who have resectable tumors but who are considered poor surgical risks. Adenocarcinomas are the most radioresistant type of cancer cell. Although small-cell carcinomas are very radiosensitive, radiation (even when used in combination with chemotherapy) does not significantly improve the mortality rate because of the early metastases of this type of cancer.

Radiation therapy is also done as a palliative procedure to reduce distressing symptoms such as cough, hemoptysis, bronchial obstruction, and superior vena cava syndrome. It can be used to treat pain that is due to metastatic

Table 21-20 Lung Cancer TNM Classifications

TUMOR DEFINITIONS

T_x Tumor proved by cytologic studies but not visualized by radiograph or bronchoscopically

T_0 No evidence of tumor

T_{is} Carcinoma in situ

T_1 Tumor 3 cm or less in greatest dimension, surrounded by lung or visceral pleura, without invasion proximal to lobar bronchus

T_2 Tumor greater than 3 cm in diameter or invading visceral pleura or with atelectasis or obstructive pneumonitis extending to the hilum; proximal extent of tumor at least 2 cm from carina

T_3 Tumor with direct extension into chest wall, diaphragm, mediastinal pleura, or pericardium without involvement of mediastinal viscera; tumor within 2 cm of carina but not involving carina

T_4 Tumor invading mediastinal viscera or carina or with malignant pleural effusion

NODAL INVOLVEMENT

N_0 No nodal metastasis

N_1 Metastasis to peribronchial or ipsilateral hilar lymph nodes

N_2 Metastasis to ipsilateral mediastinal or subcarinal lymph nodes

N_3 Metastasis to contralateral mediastinal or hilar lymph nodes or any scalene or supraclavicular node

DISTANT METASTASES

M_0 No known metastasis

M_1 Presence of distant metastasis

STAGE GROUPING

Occult Carcinoma	T_x	N_0	M_0
Stage 0	T_{is}	Carcinoma in situ	M_0
Stage I	T_1	N_0	M_0
	T_2	N_0	M_0
Stage II	T_1	N_1	M_0
	T_2	N_1	M_0
Stage IIIA	T_3	N_0	M_0
	T_3	N_1	M_0
	T_{1-3}	N_2	M_0
Stage IIIB	Any T	N_3	M_0
	T_4	Any N	M_0
Stage IV	Any T	Any N	M_1

Modified from Mountain CF: A new international staging system for lung cancer, Chest 89:2255-2335, 1986.

bone lesions or cerebral metastasis. Radiation used as a preoperative or postoperative adjuvant measure has not been found to significantly increase survival in the client with lung cancer.[27]

Chemotherapy. Chemotherapy may be used in the treatment of nonresectable tumors or as adjuvant therapy to surgery in NSCLC with distant metastases. Multiple drug regimens (i.e., protocols including combination chemotherapy) using cyclophosphamide, methotrexate, methyl CCNU, and vincristine have increased the survival rate in clients with oat cell carcinomas. Most persons with SCLC enjoy partial or complete responses to combination chemotherapy. However, they need to be aware that a cure or long-term survival is rarely a reality.

Chemotherapy has not shown any significant results when used for treatment of squamous cell carcinoma and adenocarcinoma. Symptomatic improvement and tumor regression will usually last for only a period of months.

Immunotherapy. Immunotherapy as adjuvant therapy has been used in individuals with cancer including malignant lung tumors. (Immunotherapy is discussed in Chapter 9.)

Laser surgery. Laser surgery, with the use of the Nd-YAG laser via a fiberoptic bronchoscope, makes it possible to remove bronchial lesions up to 2 cm in depth.[28] It is a complicated procedure, often requiring general anesthesia to control the client's cough reflex. Relief of the symptoms from airway obstruction can be dramatic. However, it is not a curative therapy for cancer.

■ Nursing Management of the Client with Lung Cancer

Nursing assessment

It is important to determine the understanding of the client and the family concerning the diagnostic tests (those completed as well as those planned), the diagnosis or potential diagnosis, the treatment options, and the prognosis. At the same time, the nurse can assess the level of anxiety

Table 21-21

Nursing Assessment of the Client with Lung Cancer

SUBJECTIVE DATA

History
Positive family history; smoking history (number of cigarettes smoked per day, years of smoking, depth of inhalation, amount of tar and nicotine in cigarettes); exposure to secondhand smoke; airborne carcinogens (e.g., asbestos, nickel, uranium, chromates, iron, hydrocarbons, arsenic) or other pollutants; urban living environment; chronic lung disease, including TB, COPD, bronchiectasis

Medications
Use of cough medicines or other respiratory medications

General
Fever, chills, anorexia, fatigue, weight loss (late symptoms)

Pain
Chest pain or tightness (mild to severe), shoulder and arm pain, headache, bone pain (late symptoms and bone and brain metastasis)

Respiratory
Persistent cough (productive or nonproductive); frequent respiratory infections; dyspnea, hemoptysis (late)

Gastrointestinal
Nausea and/or vomiting, dysphagia (late); jaundice (liver metastasis)

OBJECTIVE DATA

General
Neck and axillary lymphadenopathy, paraneoplastic syndromes (syndrome of inappropriate antidiuretic hormone; ACTH secretion; hypercalcemia; vascular, neuromuscular, dermatological, and connective tissue disorders)

Respiratory
Wheezing, hoarseness, stridor, unilateral diaphragm paralysis, pleural effusions (late signs)

Cardiovascular
Edema of neck and face (superior vena cava syndrome), finger clubbing, pericardial effusion, cardiac tamponade, dysrhythmias (late signs)

Neurological
Unsteady gait (brain metastasis)

Musculoskeletal
Pathological fractures, muscle wasting (late)

Possible findings
Low serum sodium and hypercalcemia (paraneoplastic syndrome); observance of lesion on chest x-ray film, CT scan, or lung scan; positive sputum or bronchial washings for cytological studies; positive fiberoptic bronchoscopy and biopsy findings

experienced by the client and the support provided and needed by the client's significant others. Subjective and objective data that should be obtained from a client with lung cancer are presented in Table 21-21.

Nursing diagnoses

Nursing diagnoses specific to the client with lung cancer include, but are not limited to, the following:

1. Ineffective airway clearance secondary to increased tracheobronchial secretions
2. Anxiety related to lack of knowledge of diagnosis or unknown prognosis/treatments
3. Pain from pressure of tumor on surrounding structures and erosion of tissues
4. Altered nutrition: less than body requirements related to increased metabolic demands, increased secretions, weakness, and anorexia
5. Altered health maintenance related to lack of knowledge about the disease process and therapeutic regimen
6. Ineffective breathing pattern related to decreased lung capacity

Nursing interventions

Health promotion and maintenance. The best way to halt the epidemic of lung cancer is to stop persons from smoking. In agreement with this primary prevention goal, the U.S. Surgeon General has set forth the objective of achieving a smokeless society by the year 2000. Important nursing activities to assist in the progress toward this goal include promoting smoking cessation programs and actively supporting education and policy changes deterring social, economic, and political patterns that have, in the past, encouraged smoking. Some recent important changes that have occurred as the result of nonsmokers' assertions that sidestream smoke is a health hazard are laws requiring designation of nonsmoking areas in most public places and a ban on smoking on most domestic airline flights. These are examples of beginning steps toward the goal of a smokeless society. Other strategies may be to ban cigarettes and other tobacco products or to tax them heavily to prevent many people, such as adolescents, from taking up the habit or continuing it. Despite the small advances being made, strong political influences by tobacco-producing states remain to maintain low taxes on the sale of cigarettes and to actually obtain subsidies for tobacco growers.[23]

For those individuals who do have a tobacco habit, efforts should be made to assist them to stop smoking. Nicotine is described as being 6 to 8 times more addictive than alcohol, so quitting is not an easy task and requires much support. Research into smoking behaviors is in the early stages. However, many factors are recognized as being important in the initiation and continuation of smoking, such as peer pressure, rebelliousness, curiosity, self-image, environmental cues, and psychological needs. Programs designed to assist individuals to stop smoking use strategies such as education, environmental control, social support, and slow nicotine withdrawal with varying degrees of success. Other methods offered in smoking cessation programs may involve hypnosis, behavioral interventions, nicotine weaning (with products such as Nicorette gum), and aversion therapy. Group support programs, individual therapy, and self-help options are also available.

It is estimated that approximately 1 million smokers quit each year and that 2 of every 5 smokers have made three or more unsuccessful attempts to quit.[29] The nurse needs to be aware of resources in the community to assist individuals who are interested in quitting. Local chapters of the American Lung Association and the American Cancer Society have information on available programs.

An important part of concentrated efforts to prevent smoking-related health problems is recognizing what influences people, particularly children and adolescents, to begin smoking. Programs developed to help children explore the external influences (e.g., peer pressure) to start smoking and that help them identify alternative behaviors make it less likely for these children to start smoking. An emphasis on the health hazards of smoking, as well as on those of other addictive behaviors, should be part of the total curriculum beginning in elementary schools.

Nurses who smoke are in a difficult position to help clients change their smoking habits. A study in 1986 showed nurses to have a higher rate of smoking than the general female population.[30] Nurses as role models can do much to facilitate or harm educational attempts with persons in the community as well as in the hospital. Therefore if nurses smoke, they must try to stop before they can serve as role models for clients. A smoker turned nonsmoker may be in a good position to suggest strategies for success.

Screening chest x-ray films every 6 to 12 months may be of value for individuals who are considered at high risk for lung cancer. This consideration applies to persons employed in uranium mining, asbestos-related industries, iron foundries, and other industries with known respiratory carcinogens, as well as to those who are heavy cigarette smokers.

When a nurse is obtaining a history from a client (even one with nonrespiratory problems), it is important to get information related to respiratory carcinogens. The client should be asked about occupational exposure to asbestos, uranium, arsenic, nickel, iron and iron oxides, and excessive exposure to air pollution. In addition, a detailed history of cigarette smoking should be obtained. This information should be used to evaluate the client's risk of developing lung cancer and also to teach the client about early recognition of symptoms. Anyone with a history of exposure to respiratory carcinogens who has pneumonitis that persists for longer than 2 weeks in spite of antibiotic therapy should be evaluated for the possibility of lung cancer.

Individuals with a chronic cough or a change in the character of a cough should be encouraged to obtain care. In addition, persons with chronic or recurring respiratory infections should be carefully evaluated, especially if they are cigarette smokers.

Acute intervention. Care of the client with lung cancer will initially involve support and reassurance during the diagnostic evaluation. (Specific nursing measures related to the diagnostic studies are outlined in Chapter 19.)

Another major responsibility of the nurse is to help clients and their families deal with the diagnosis of lung can-

cer. Clients may feel guilty about their cigarette smoking having caused the cancer and need to discuss this feeling with someone who has a nonjudgmental attitude. Questions regarding each client's condition should be answered honestly. Additional counseling from a social worker, psychologist, or member of the clergy may be needed.

Specific care of the client will depend on the treatment plan. (Care of the client undergoing radiation therapy and chemotherapy is discussed in Chapter 9.) The nurse has a major role in providing client comfort, in teaching methods to reduce pain, and in assessing indications for hospitalization (see Chapter 9).

Chronic management. The client who has had a surgical resection with intent to cure should be followed up carefully for manifestations of metastasis. The client and family should be told to contact the physician if symptoms such as hemoptysis, dysphagia, chest pain, and hoarseness develop.

For many individuals who have lung cancer, very little can be done to significantly prolong their lives. Radiation therapy and chemotherapy can be used to provide palliative relief from distressing symptoms. Constant pain becomes a major problem. (Measures used to relieve pain are discussed in Chapter 51; care of the client with cancer is discussed in Chapter 9.)

Other Types of Lung Tumors

Other types of primary lung tumors include sarcomas, lymphomas, and bronchial adenomas. Bronchial adenomas are small tumors that arise from the lower trachea or major bronchi and are considered malignant because they are locally invasive and frequently metastasize. Clinical manifestations of bronchial adenomas include hemoptysis, persistent cough, localized obstructive wheezing, and purulent bronchitis. There may be secondary bronchiectasis in longstanding cases. Bronchial adenomas frequently cause endocrine paraneoplastic manifestations. They can usually be treated successfully with surgical resection.

The lungs are a common site for secondary metastases and are more often affected by metastatic growth than by primary lung tumors. The pulmonary capillaries, with their extensive network, are ideal sites for tumor emboli. In addition, the lungs have an extensive lymphatic network. The primary malignancies that spread to the lungs often originate in the GI or genitourinary (GU) tracts and in the breast. General symptoms of lung metastases are chest pain and nonproductive cough.

Benign tumors of the lung are generally classified as *mesenchymal.* Their occurrence is rare, and they have the potential to become malignant. The most common mesenchymal tumors are chondromas, which arise in the bronchial cartilage, and leiomyomas, which are myomas of smooth, nonstriated muscle fibers.

Hamartomas of the lung are mixtures of fibrous tissue, fat, and blood vessels. They are congenital malformations of the connective tissue of the bronchiolar walls.

CHEST TRAUMA AND THORACIC INJURIES

Traumatic injuries fall into two major categories: (1) blunt trauma and (2) penetrating trauma. *Blunt trauma*

Table 21-22   Common Traumatic Chest Injuries and Mechanisms of Injury

Mechanism of Injury	Common Related Injury
BLUNT TRAUMA	
Blunt steering-wheel injury to chest	Rib fractures, flail chest, pneumothorax, hemopneumothorax, cardiac contusion, pulmonary contusion, cardiac tamponade, great vessel tears
Shoulder-harness seat belt injury	Fractured clavicle, dislocated shoulder, rib fractures, pulmonary contusion, pericardial contusion, cardiac tamponade
Crush injury (e.g., heavy equipment crushing thorax)	Pneumothorax and hemopneumothorax, flail chest, great vessel tears and rupture, decreased blood return to heart with decreased cardiac output
PENETRATING TRAUMA	
Gunshot or stab wound to chest	Open pneumothorax, tension pneumothorax, hemopneumothorax, cardiac tamponade, esophageal damage, tracheal tear, great vessel tears

Table 21-23

Prehospital Emergency Care of the Client with a Chest Injury*

Possible etiologies: Blunt or penetrating trauma from a fall, being struck by an object, structural collapse, or a steering-wheel injury

CLINICAL MANIFESTATIONS

Obvious trauma to the chest wall (e.g., bruising)
Chest pain
Dyspnea, shortness of breath, difficulty in breathing
Cough
Asymmetrical movement of chest wall
Marked cyanosis of mouth, face, nail beds, mucous membranes
Rapid, weak pulse
Decreased blood pressure
Deviation of trachea
Distended neck veins
Bloodshot or bulging eyes

MANAGEMENT

Remove all clothing to assess injury sites.
Assess for airway obstruction. Monitor and assist with respirations if necessary.
Monitor vital signs and level of consciousness.
Give high flow O_2 via nasal cannula.
Assess for tension pneumothorax.
Seal any open chest wound with an airtight dressing and tape.
Do not remove impaled objects; stabilize them with bulky dressings.
Assess for other injuries such as bleeding and treat appropriately.
Observe for signs of shock.
Put client in a semi-Fowler's position or lay client on the injured side if breathing is easier.
Be prepared for nausea and vomiting. Have suction equipment ready.

*See Chapter 59 for a general discussion on measures related to prehospital emergency care.

occurs when the body is struck by a blunt object such as a steering wheel. The external injury may appear minor, but the impact may cause severe, life-threatening internal injuries such as a ruptured spleen. *Contrecoup trauma,* a type of blunt trauma, is caused by the impact of parts of the body against other objects. This type of injury differs from blunt trauma primarily in the velocity of the impact. Internal organs are rapidly forced back and forth within the bony structures that surround them, so that internal injury is sustained not only on the side of the impact but also on the opposite side where the organ or organs hit bony structures. If the velocity of impact is great enough, organs and blood vessels can literally be torn from their points of origin. Many head injuries are caused by contrecoup trauma.

Penetrating trauma occurs when a foreign body impales or passes through the body tissues (e.g., as in gunshot wounds and stabbings). Table 21-22 describes selective traumatic injuries as they relate to the categories of trauma and the mechanism of injury. Prehospital care of the client with a chest injury is presented in Table 21-23.

Thoracic injuries range from simple rib fractures to life-threatening tears of the aorta, vena cava, and other major vessels. The most common thoracic emergencies are described in Table 21-24. Clients with major vessel tears require immediate fluid replacement and surgery (see Chapter 32).

Pneumothorax

A *pneumothorax* is a complete or partial collapse of a lung as a result of an accumulation of air in the intrapleural space. Pneumothorax should be suspected after any blunt trauma to the chest wall. Pneumothorax may be closed or open. Pneumothorax associated with trauma may be accompanied by hemothorax, a condition called *hemopneumothorax.*

Closed pneumothorax. Closed pneumothorax has no associated external wound. The most common form is a *spontaneous pneumothorax,* which is caused by rupture of small blebs on the visceral pleural space. The cause of the blebs is unknown. This condition occurs most commonly in otherwise healthy individuals between 20 and 40 years of age, usually in male cigarette smokers. There is a tendency for this condition to recur.

Table 21-24 Clinical Manifestations and Emergency Management of Thoracic Injuries

Injury	Definition	Clinical Manifestation	Emergency Management
Pneumothorax	Collection of air between chest wall and lung	Dyspnea, pain, decreased movement of involved chest wall, diminished breath sounds on injured side	Insertion of large-bore needle with attached one-way valve to release air from pleural cavity, chest tube insertion to underwater seal or one-way valve, application of vented dressing
Hemothorax	Collection of blood between chest wall and lung, usually occurring with pneumothorax	Same as pneumothorax	Insertion of chest tube and aspiration of pleural cavity, treatment of hypovolemic shock if present
Tension pneumothorax	Collection of air between chest wall and lung; no escape of air during expiration; rapid increase of air in pleural cavity, causing shifting of intrathoracic organs and increased intrathoracic pressure	Cyanosis, air hunger, violent agitation, trachea deviated to side opposite injury, subcutaneous emphysema	Insertion of chest tube or large-bore needle to relieve air pressure in thorax, treatment of hypoxia
Flail chest	Fracture of two or more adjacent ribs in two or more places, causing loss of stability of chest wall; possibly occurring with pneumothorax, hemothorax, and/or tension pneumothorax	Paradoxical movement of chest wall and respiratory distress	Humidified O_2 therapy, reexpansion of the lung, IV fluids (some situations requiring intubation and mechanical ventilation), intercostal nerve blocks to relieve pain, judicious use of systemic analgesics, rapid administration of IV fluids
Cardiac tamponade	Rapid collection of blood in pericardial sac from laceration of blood vessels, pericardium's inelasticity preventing heart from pumping blood	Muffled and distant heart sounds, failing or absent blood pressure or pulses, steadily increasing central venous pressure; distention of neck veins possible	Cardiopulmonary resuscitation if no pulses present, immediate aspiration of blood from pericardium with needle and syringe by physician, surgery to repair torn vessel

Other causes of closed pneumothorax include the following:

1. Injury to the lungs from mechanical ventilation
2. Injury to the lungs from insertion of a subclavian catheter
3. Perforation of the esophagus
4. Injury to the lungs from broken ribs
5. Ruptured blebs or bullae in a client with COPD

Open pneumothorax. Open pneumothorax occurs when air enters the pleural space through an opening in the chest wall (Fig. 21-11, *B*). Examples include stab or gunshot wounds and surgical thoracotomies. A penetrating chest wound is often referred to as a *sucking chest wound.*

An open pneumothorax should be covered with a vented dressing. This allows air to escape from the vent and decreases the likelihood of tension pneumothorax developing. (A vented dressing is one secured on three sides, with the fourth side left untaped.) If the object that caused the open chest wound is still in place, it should not be removed until a physician is present.

Tension pneumothorax. Tension pneumothorax may result from either an open or a closed pneumothorax. In an open chest wound, a flap may act as a one-way valve; thus, air can enter on inspiration but cannot escape. Intrathoracic pressure increases, the lung collapses, and the mediastinum is shifted toward the unaffected side, which is subsequently compressed. As the intrathoracic pressure increases, cardiac output is altered because there is decreased venous return and compression of the great vessels. Tension pneumothorax is a medical emergency because both the respiratory and circulatory systems are affected. Nurses and paramedics are now being trained to insert large-bore needles and chest tubes into the chest wall to release the trapped air. Tension pneumothorax may also occur when chest tubes are clamped or become blocked in a client after insertion for treatment of pneumothorax;

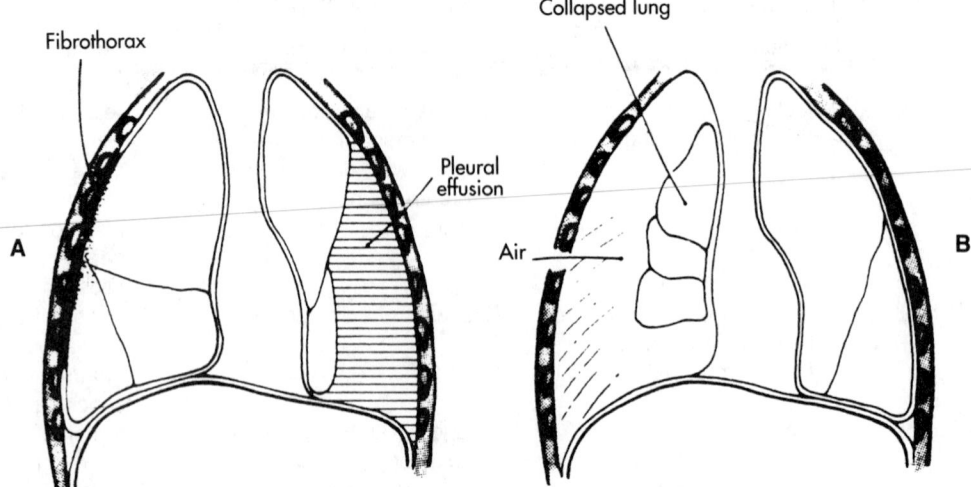

Fig. 21-11 Disorders of the pleura. **A,** Fibrothorax resulting from an organization of inflammatory exudate and pleural effusion. **B,** Collapse of lung due to an open pneumothorax. (From Price S and Wilson L: Pathophysiology: clinical concepts of disease processes, ed 4, St Louis, 1991, Mosby–Year Book, Inc.)

Table 21-25

 Prehospital Emergency Care of the Client with Pneumothorax*

Possible etiologies: Presence of air in pleural space either from rupture or laceration of the lungs or external chest wound (e.g., fractured ribs)

CLINICAL MANIFESTATIONS

Sudden, sharp chest pain
Shallow, rapid respirations
Dyspnea
Decreased or absent breath sounds; hyperresonnance on affected side
Cough with or without hemoptysis
Tachycardia and decreased blood pressure (in tension pneumothorax)

MANAGEMENT

Ensure patent airway to support ventilations.
Administer O_2
Monitor vital signs.
In extreme conditions, know that a needle thoracentesis may be used under physician's direction to release pressure in pleural space.

*See Chapter 59 for a general discussion on measures related to prehospital emergency care.

unclamping the tube or relief of the obstruction will remedy this situation.

Hemothorax. Hemothorax is an accumulation of blood in the intrapleural space. It is frequently found in association with open pneumothorax and is then called a *hemopneumothorax*. Causes of hemothorax include chest trauma, lung malignancy, complication of anticoagulant therapy, pulmonary embolus, and tearing of pleural adhesions.

Clinical manifestations. The client with a pneumothorax has respiratory distress including shallow, rapid respirations, dyspnea, and air hunger. Chest pain and a cough with or without hemoptysis may be present. On auscultation there are no breath sounds over the affected area, and hyperresonance may be heard. A chest x-ray shows the presence of pneumothorax.

If a tension pneumothorax develops, severe respiratory distress, tachycardia, and cyanosis occur. The trachea and point of maximal impulse (PMI) shift to the unaffected side. Prehospital emergency care of the client with a pneumothorax is presented in Table 21-25.

Therapeutic management. If the amount of air or fluid accumulated in the intrapleural space is minimal, no treatment is needed because it will gradually be absorbed. If the amount of air or fluid is minimal, the pleural space can be aspirated with a large-bore needle. Needle aspiration is often a lifesaving measure. The most definitive and common form of treatment of pneumothorax and hemothorax is to insert a chest tube and connect it to water-seal drainage. Repeated spontaneous pneumothorax may need to be treated surgically by a partial pleurectomy or by application of an irritating agent such as tetracycline to the pleural surfaces via a pleural catheter to promote adherence of the pleurae to one another—a procedure called *pleurodesis* or *sclerosing*. Pleurodesis is a painful procedure. Clients should be prepared to expect the discomfort, and analgesics should be administered before the instillation of the sclerosing agent.[31]

Fractured Ribs

Rib fractures are the most common type of chest injury resulting from trauma. Ribs 4 to 9 are most commonly fractured because they are least protected by chest mus-

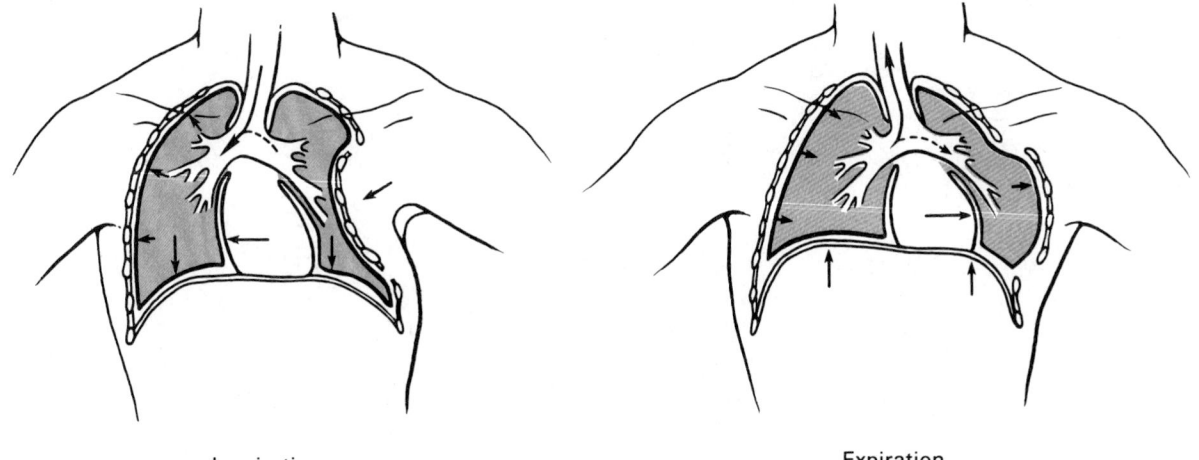

Inspiration

Expiration

Fig. 21-12 Flail chest produces paradoxical respiration. On inspiration the flail section sinks in with the mediastinal shift to the uninjured side. On expiration the flail section bulges outward with the mediastinal shift to the injured side.

cles. If the fractured rib is splintered or displaced, it may damage the pleura and lungs.

Clinical manifestations of fractured ribs include pain (especially on inspiration) at the site of injury. The individual splints the affected area and takes shallow breaths to try to decrease the pain. Because the individual is reluctant to take deep breaths and cough, atelectasis may develop because of decreased ventilation.

The main goal in treatment is to decrease pain so that the client can breathe adequately to promote good chest expansion. Intercostal nerve blocks with local anesthesia are most frequently used to provide pain relief. The nerves of the affected ribs and the two intercostal nerves above and below the injured rib are also blocked. The effect of the anesthesia lasts for a period of hours to days. It needs to be repeated as necessary to provide pain relief. Strapping the chest with tape or using a binder is not common practice. Most physicians believe that these measures should be avoided because they reduce lung expansion and predispose the individual to atelectasis. Narcotic drug therapy must be individualized and used with caution because these drugs can depress respirations.

Flail Chest

Flail chest results from multiple rib fractures, causing instability of the chest wall (Fig. 21-12). The chest wall cannot provide the bony structure necessary to maintain bellows action and ventilation. The affected (flail) area will move paradoxically to the intact portion of the chest during respiration. During inspiration the affected portion is sucked in, and during expiration it bulges out. This paradoxical chest movement prevents adequate ventilation of the lung in the injured area. This defect itself does not cause hypoxia. The major difficulty in flail chest is that the underlying lung has been injured. Associated pain and this lung injury, giving rise to loss of compliance, will contribute to the alteration in the respiratory pattern and lead to hypoxia.

A flail chest is usually apparent on visual examination

of the unconscious client. The client manifests rapid, shallow respirations, cyanosis, and tachycardia. A flail chest may not be initially apparent in the conscious client due to splinting of the chest wall. The client moves air poorly, and movement of the thorax is asymmetrical and uncoordinated. Palpation of abnormal respiratory movements, crepitus of the rib, chest x-ray, and ABGs assist in the diagnosis.

Initial therapy consists of adequate ventilation, humidified O_2, and careful administration of crystalloid IV solutions. The definitive therapy is to reexpand the lung and ensure adequate oxygenation. Although many clients can be managed without the use of mechanical ventilation, a short period of intubation and ventilation may be necessary until the diagnosis of the lung injury is complete.

Positive end-expiratory pressure (PEEP) used with mechanical ventilation to improve oxygenation will maintain positive pressure in the lungs throughout the respiratory cycle. (Mechanical ventilation is discussed in Chapter 23.) The lung parenchyma and fractured ribs will heal with time.

Chest Tubes and Pleural Drainage

Under normal conditions, intrapleural pressure is below atmospheric pressure (about 4 to 5 cm H_2O below atmospheric pressure during expiration and about 8 to 10 cm H_2O below atmospheric pressure during inspiration). (Intrapleural pressure and the intrapleural space are described in Chapter 19.) If intrapleural pressure becomes equal to atmospheric pressure, the lungs will collapse (pneumothorax). Air can enter the intrapleural space by a variety of mechanisms including traumatic chest injury (e.g., gunshot wound, fractured rib), thoracotomy, and spontaneous pneumothorax. Excess fluid accumulation can occur in the pleural space as a result of impaired lymphatic drainage (e.g., from malignancy) or changes in the colloid osmotic pressure (e.g., congestive heart failure). Empyema is purulent pleural fluid, which may be associated with lung abscesses or pneumonia.

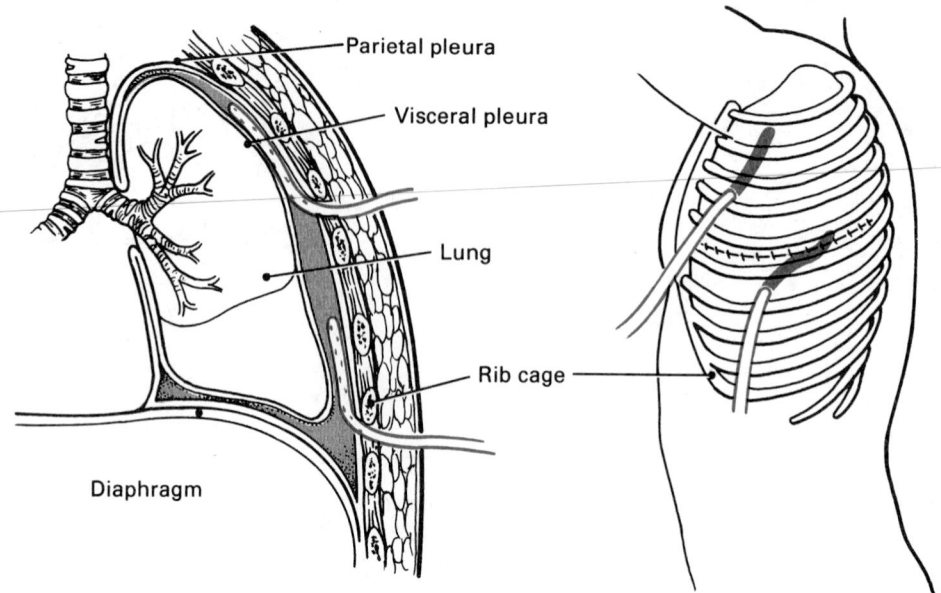

Fig. 21-13 Placement of chest tubes.

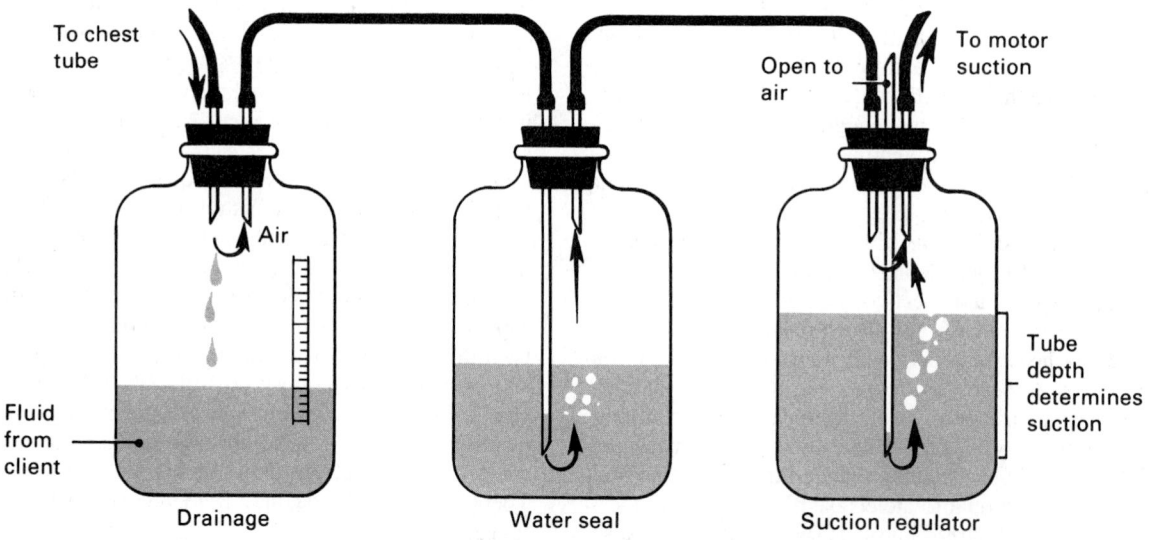

Fig. 21-14 Three-bottle water-seal suction. *Bottle I* is the drainage bottle. A vertical piece of tape should be applied to the outer surface of the drainage bottle. The time and the fluid level should be marked hourly on the tape. *Bottle II* is the water-seal bottle. *Bottle III* is the suction control bottle. The length of glass tube below the water surface determines the amount of suction.

Small accumulations of air or fluid in the pleural space may not require removal by thoracentesis or chest-tube insertion. Instead it may be reabsorbed over a period of time. The purposes of chest tubes and pleural drainage are to remove the air and fluid and to restore normal intrapleural pressure so that the lungs can reexpand.

Chest tube insertion. A physician can insert a chest tube in the emergency room, at the client's bedside, or in the operating room, depending on the situation. In the operating room, the chest tube is inserted via the thoracotomy incision. In the emergency room or at the bedside, the client is placed in a sitting position or is lying down with the affected side elevated. The area is prepared with antiseptic solution, and the site is infiltrated with a local anesthetic agent. After a small incision is made, one or two chest tubes are inserted into the pleural space. One catheter is placed anteriorly through the second intercostal space to remove air (Fig. 21-13). The other is placed posteriorly through the eighth or ninth intercostal space to drain fluid and blood. The tubes are sutured to the chest wall, and the puncture wound is covered with an airtight dressing. During insertion, the tubes are kept clamped. After the tubes are in place in the pleural space, they are connected to drainage tubing and pleural drainage. Each tube

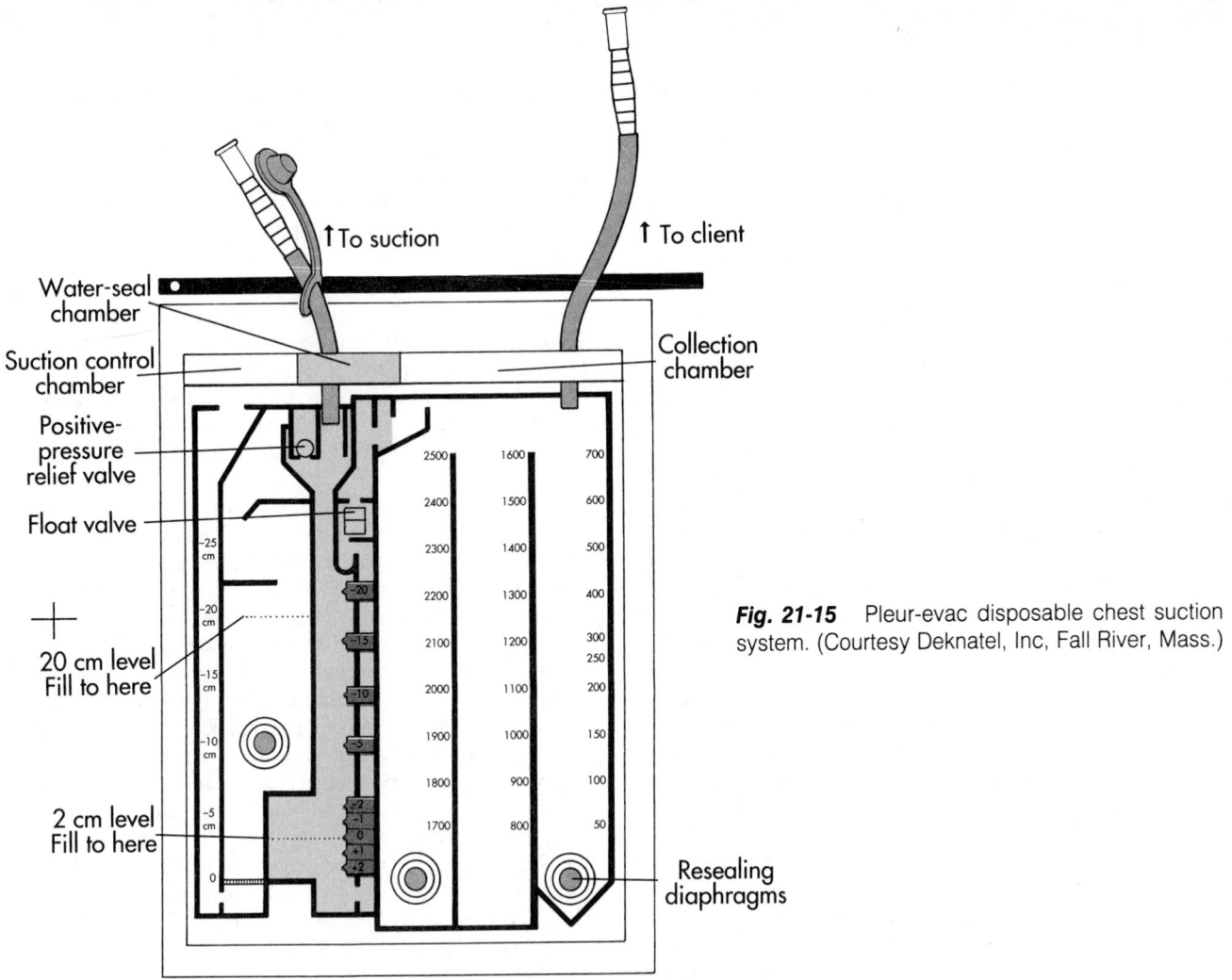

Water-seal
chamber

Suction control
chamber

Positive-
pressure
relief valve

Float valve

20 cm level
Fill to here

2 cm level
Fill to here

↑ To suction   ↑ To client

Collection
chamber

Resealing
diaphragms

Fig. 21-15 Pleur-evac disposable chest suction system. (Courtesy Deknatel, Inc, Fall River, Mass.)

may be connected to a separate drainage system and suction. More commonly, a Y connector is used to attach both chest tubes to the same drainage system.

Pleural drainage. Most pleural drainage systems have three basic compartments, each with its own separate function. The three compartments were bottles in early drainage systems and were known as the *three-bottle system* (Fig. 21-14).

The first compartment, or *collection chamber,* receives fluid and air from the chest cavity. The air in the chamber is vented to the second compartment called the *water-seal chamber,* which acts as a one-way valve. Air enters from the collection chamber via a connector that enters under water in the second compartment. The air bubbles up through the water, and no air can reenter the collection chamber because of the water seal.

A third compartment, which is used to apply controlled suction to the system, is called the *suction control chamber.* The suction control bottle uses a tubing partially submerged in a column of water, which is also vented to the atmosphere (see Fig. 21-14). Suction is applied to the bottle through a separate opening. The amount of suction applied is regulated by the depth of the tubing in the water, not by the amount of suction applied to the system. An increase in suction does not result in an increase in negative pressure applied to the system. Instead, excess suction merely draws in air through the vented tubing.

The removal of air from the pleural space is facilitated during periods when the client's intrathoracic pressure is increased, such as during exhalation, coughing, or sneezing. As a result, more air bubbles are noted in the water-seal chamber during these activities. A lack of bubbling during exhalation or coughing may indicate a blockage in the chest tube (e.g., kinking or clotting) or expansion of the lung with no further air in the pleural space.

A variety of commercial disposable plastic chest drainage systems are available. Most operate on the same principle as the three-bottle system. One popular system is the Pleur-evac, which is shown in Fig. 21-15. (Note the correspondence of the chambers to the bottles shown in the three-bottle system in Fig. 21-14.)

These units can be used only for collection or for collection and water seal. The manufacturer's suggestions for use are included with the equipment. The plastic units allow the client mobility and decrease the risk of breaking or spilling the drainage system.

Heimlich valves. Another device that may be used to evacuate air from the pleural space is the Heimlich valve. This valve is a collapsible rubber tube that is attached to the external end of the chest tube. The valve opens whenever the pressure is greater than atmospheric pressure and closes when the reverse occurs. The Heimlich valve functions like a water seal and is usually used for emergency transport or in special home care situations.[32]

■ Nursing Management of Chest Tubes

Some general guidelines for nursing care of clients with chest tubes and water-seal drainage systems include the following:

1. Keep all tubing as straight as possible and coiled loosely, and do not let the client lie on it.
2. Keep all connections between chest tubes, drainage tubing, and the drainage collector tight. Taping at connections and at the top of the bottle helps prevent air leaks.
3. Keep the water seal and suction control chamber at the appropriate water levels by adding sterile water as needed, since water loss by evaporation may occur.
4. Place a piece of tape on the outside of the drainage bottle. The time of measurement and the fluid level should be marked according to the prescribed orders. Marking intervals may range from once per hour to every 8 hours. Any change in the quantity or characteristics of drainage (e.g., clear yellow to bloody) should be reported to the physician and recorded.
5. Observe for air bubbles in the water-seal chamber and fluctuations in the glass tube or chest tubes. Air should be bubbling out from the glass tube. If no fluctuations are observed (rising with inspiration and falling with expiration in spontaneously breathing clients; the opposite occurs during positive-pressure mechanical ventilation), the drainage system is blocked or the lungs are reexpanded. If bubbling increases, there may be an air leak.
6. Check for bubbling in the water seal. Normally, this is intermittent. When bubbling is continuous and constant, the nurse may determine the source of the air leak by *momentarily* clamping the tubing at successively distal points away from the client until the bubbling ceases. Retaping tubing connections or replacing the drainage apparatus may be necessary to prevent the air leak.
7. Monitor the client's clinical status. Vital signs should be taken frequently, lungs auscultated, and the chest wall observed for any abnormal chest movements.
8. Never elevate the drainage system to the level of the client's chest. Secure the bottles to the metal drainage stand or racks. The drainage bottles should not be emptied unless they are in danger of overflowing.
9. Encourage the client to cough and deep breathe periodically to facilitate lung expansion.
10. Check the position of the bottle. If the bottle is overturned and the water seal is disrupted, return the bottle to an upright position and encourage the client to take a few deep breaths, followed by forced exhalations and/or cough maneuvers.

Milking and stripping of chest tubes may briefly increase the amount of negative pressure applied to the pleural space. The increased negative pressure should enhance the evacuation of fluid in chest tubes and prevent the development of clots and obstruction from the stagnation of fluids. Although further study is still needed to evaluate the effects of routine stripping of pleural and mediastinal tubes on the lung and mediastinal tissue, present practice advocates the use of these procedures when there is bloody drainage or when the fluid in the collection bottle tends to clot. When chest tubes are used for air collection alone, stripping and milking is not usually performed.[33] Each clinical situation should be evaluated individually, and unit protocol and physician preferences should be ascertained before initiation of stripping and milking. Nurses should keep in mind that these procedures can cause the client to experience pain and that dislodgement of the tube may occur if the tube is not stabilized above the area that is being stripped. Clamping of chest tubes is no longer advocated as routine clinical practice unless they become disconnected.[34]

The danger of a rapid accumulation of air in the pleural space causing tension pneumothorax is far greater than that of a small amount of atmospheric air entering the pleural space. Chest tubes are *momentarily* clamped to change the drainage apparatus or to check for air leaks. Continuous clamping may be ordered by the physician before discontinuing the use of the chest tube once it has been determined that normal pleural pressures have been reestablished and the lung has been reexpanded. The most important intervention to perform when a chest tube becomes disconnected is to reestablish a water-seal system immediately. In some hospitals, when disconnection occurs, the chest tube is immersed in sterile water (about 2 cm) until the system can be reestablished. It is important for the nurse to know the unit protocol, individual clinical situation (whether an air leak exists), and physician preference before resorting to prolonged chest tube clamping.

Chest tube removal

Clients with chest tubes may have daily chest x-ray studies to follow the course of lung reexpansion. The chest tubes are removed when the lungs are reexpanded and fluid drainage has ceased. Sometimes the amount of suction is decreased or the tubes are clamped off for a period of time before they are removed. If the tubing is clamped, clients must be observed closely for signs and symptoms of tension pneumothorax. The tube is removed by cutting the sutures, applying a sterile petroleum jelly gauze dressing, having the client take a deep breath, exhale, and bear down (Valsalva maneuver), and then removing the tube. The site is covered with an airtight dressing, the pleura seals itself off, and in several days the wound is healed. The wound should be observed for drainage and should be reinforced if necessary. The client should be observed for any manifestations of respiratory distress, which may signify a recurrent or new pneumothorax.

CHEST SURGERY

Chest surgery is performed for a variety of reasons, some of which unrelated to primary lung problems. For example, a thoracotomy is performed for heart and esophageal surgery. The types of chest surgery are compared in Table 21-26.

Preoperative Care

Before chest surgery, baseline data are obtained on the respiratory and cardiovascular systems. Diagnostic studies

Table 21-26 Chest Surgeries

Type	Description	Indication	Comments
Lobectomy	Removal of one lobe of lung	Lung cancer, bronchiectasis, TB, emphysematous bullae, benign lung tumors, fungal infections	Most common lung surgery, postoperative insertion of two chest tubes, expansion of remaining lung tissue to fill up space
Pneumonectomy	Removal of entire lung	Lung cancer (most common), extensive TB, bronchiectasis, lung abscess	Performance of surgery only when lobectomy or segmental resection will not remove all diseased lung, no drainage tubes (generally), fluid gradually filling space where lung has been removed, turning of client with unaffected side dependent contraindicated, position of client on back or operative side with head elevated
Segmental resection	Removal of one or more lung segments	Bronchiectasis, TB	Technically difficult, purpose of removal of lung segment, insertion of chest tubes, expansion of remaining lung tissue to fill space
Wedge resection	Removal of small, localized lesion that occupies only part of a segment	Lung biopsy, excision of small nodules	Need for chest tubes postoperatively
Decortication	Removal or stripping of thick, fibrous membrane from visceral pleura	Empyema	Use of chest tubes and drainage postoperatively
Exploratory thoracotomy	Incision into thorax to look for injured or bleeding tissues	Chest trauma	Use of chest tubes and drainage postoperatively
Thoracotomy not involving lungs*	Incision into thorax for surgery on other organs	Hiatal hernia repair, open heart surgery, esophageal surgery, tracheal resection, aortic aneurysm repair	—
Thoracoplasty	Removal of ribs without entering pleura	Reduction of size of chest cavity	Historical importance in treating TB, possible use to decrease lung size in area of chronic empyema, use before resectional surgery (rarely)

*For comments on thoracotomy not involving the lungs, see discussion of individual diseases in text.

usually performed are pulmonary function studies, chest x-ray film, lung scans, electrocardiograph (ECG), ABGs, blood urea nitrogen (BUN), serum creatinine, blood glucose, serum electrolytes, and complete blood count. Additional studies of cardiac function such as cardiac catheterization may be done for the client who is to undergo a pneumonectomy.

A careful physical assessment of the lungs, including percussion and auscultation, should be done. This will allow the nurse to compare preoperative and postoperative findings.

The client should be encouraged to stop smoking before surgery to decrease secretions and increase O_2 saturation. In the anxious period before surgery, this is not an easy thing for the habitual smoker to do.

Postural drainage may be indicated to help drain the lungs of accumulated secretions. This is especially indicated for the client with a lung abscess or bronchiectasis.

Some preoperative teaching focuses on effective deep breathing and coughing or incentive spirometry (see Table 22-12). If the client practices these techniques before surgery, they will be easier to perform postoperatively. The client should be told that adequate medication will be given to reduce the pain, and the client is helped to splint the incision with a pillow to facilitate deep breathing and coughing.

For most types of chest surgery, chest tubes are inserted and connected to water-sealed drainage systems. The purpose of these tubes should be explained to the client. In addition, O_2 is frequently given the first day after surgery. Range-of-motion exercises on the surgical side similar to those for the mastectomy client (see Chapter 46) should be taught to the client.

The thought of losing part of a vital organ is frequently frightening. The client should be reassured that the lungs have a large degree of functional reserve. Even after the

Table 21-27

 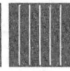

NURSING CARE PLAN FOR THE CLIENT AFTER THORACOTOMY

Defining Characteristics	Nursing Interventions	Evaluation Criteria
NURSING DIAGNOSIS: Ineffective airway clearance related to inability to cough secondary to pain from surgical procedure and positioning		
Rhonchi, wheezes, complaints of pain, inability to cough or deep breathe, temperature elevation, atelectasis on chest x-ray film	Place client in semi-Fowler's position. Assist client to turn, deep breathe, and cough every 1-2 hr initially. Splint chest incision when breathing exercises and coughing are performed. Plan coughing exercises after pain relief is obtained. Auscultate lungs before and after deep-breathing and coughing regimens. If secretions are not being removed, perform suctioning if necessary. Observe the color and characteristics of sputum.	Lungs clear to auscultation, ability to clear secretions
NURSING DIAGNOSIS: Impaired gas exchange related to air and fluid collections in pleural space		
Chest tube or tubes with drainage, decreased breath sounds on surgical side, abnormal ABGs	Monitor chest drainage system (see text).	Full expansion of lung, normal breath sounds bilaterally, normal ABGs
NURSING DIAGNOSIS: Ineffective breathing pattern related to pain, position, and possible complications on affected side		
Shortness of breath, shallow respirations, use of accessory muscles	Administer O$_2$ via nasal prongs or mask (if ordered). Assess respiratory rate every 1-2 hr. Auscultate lungs every 2-3 hr. Monitor the results of ABGs. Observe for manifestations of complications such as pneumothorax or hemothorax. Assist client with deep breathing. Position client for comfort and ease of breathing. Encourage use of incentive spirometer every 2-3 hr.	Respiratory rate 12-18 breaths/min, ease of respiration
NURSING DIAGNOSIS: Anxiety related to feelings of dyspnea and pain		
Anxious facial expression, inability to cooperate with instructions to breathe slowly	Stay with client during procedures, providing encouragement and explanations. Evaluate chest tubes to validate proper functioning. Provide feedback about effective breathing. Administer pain medication as ordered. Monitor the effectiveness. Use nonpharmacological measures such as distraction and relaxation techniques.	Relief from anxiety

removal of one lung, there is enough lung tissue to maintain adequate oxygenation. However, the client should be instructed to include adequate rest periods to allow compensation for the decreased diffusion capacity that occurs.

The nurse should be available to deal with the questions asked by the client and the family. Questions should be answered honestly. The nurse should try to facilitate the expression of concerns, feelings, and questions. (General preoperative care and preoperative teaching are discussed in Chapter 11.)

Surgical Interventions

Thoracotomy surgery is considered major surgery because the incision is large, cutting into bone, muscle, and cartilage. The two types of thoracic incisions are (1) *median sternotomy*, performed by splitting the sternum, and (2) *lateral thoracotomy*. The median sternotomy is primarily used for surgery involving the heart.

The two types of lateral thoracotomy are posterolateral and anterolateral. The posterolateral thoracotomy is used for most surgeries involving the lung. The incision is made from the anterior axillary line below the nipple level posteriorly at the fourth, fifth, or sixth intercostal space. It is rarely necessary to remove the ribs. Strong mechanical retractors are used to gain access to the lung. The anterolateral incision is made in the fourth or fifth intercostal space from the sternal border to the midaxillary line. This procedure is commonly used for surgery or trauma victims, mediastinal operations, and wedge resections of the upper and middle lobes of the lung.

Table 21-28 Relationship of Lung Volumes to Type of Ventilatory Impairment

Interpretation	FVC	FEV$_1$	FEV$_1$/FVC	RV	TLC
Normal	Normal	Normal	Normal	Normal	Normal
Airway obstruction	Normal or low	Low	Low	High	High
Lung restriction	Low	Normal or low	Normal or high	Normal or low	Low
Obstruction and restriction	Low	Low	Low	Variable	Variable

From American Lung Association: Chronic obstructive pulmonary disease, ed 5, New York, 1977, American Lung Association.

The extensiveness of the thoracotomy incision often results in severe pain for the client after surgery. Because muscles have been severed, the client is reluctant to move the shoulder and arm on the surgical side. Chest tubes are placed in the pleural space except in pneumonectomy surgery. In a pneumonectomy, the space from which the lung was removed gradually fills with serosanguineous fluid.

Postoperative Care

Specific measures related to the care after a thoracotomy are presented in Table 21-27. The specific follow-up care depends on the type of surgical procedure. (General postoperative care is discussed in Chapter 13).

RESTRICTIVE RESPIRATORY DISORDERS

Restrictive respiratory disorders are characterized by decreased compliance of the lungs or chest wall or both. This is in contrast to obstructive disorders, which are characterized by increased resistance to airflow. Pulmonary function tests are the best means to use in differentiating between restrictive and obstructive respiratory disorders (Table 21-28). Restrictive disorders are characterized by reduced vital capacity (VC) and reduced total lung capacity, with a normal or reduced functional residual capacity (FRC) and residual volume (RV). Obstructive disorders are characterized by normal or decreased VC, increased total lung capacity (TLC), reduced ratio of forced air expiration volume in the first second of expiration (FEV$_1$) to functional vital capacity (FVC), increased FRC, and increased RV. Mixed obstructive and restrictive disorders are often manifested. For example, a client may have both chronic bronchitis (an obstructive problem) and pulmonary fibrosis (a restrictive problem).

Restrictive problems are generally categorized into *extrapulmonary* and *intrapulmonary* disorders. Extrapulmonary causes of restrictive lung disease include disorders involving the CNS, neuromuscular system, and chest wall (Table 21-29). In these disorders, the lung tissue is normal. Intrapulmonary causes of restrictive lung disease involve the pleura or the lung tissue (Table 21-30).

Pleural Effusion

Types. Pleural effusion is a collection of fluid in the pleural space (see Fig. 21-11, *A*). It is not a disease but rather a sign of a serious disease. It is frequently classified as *transudative* or *exudative* according to whether the protein content of the effusion is low or high, respectively. A transudate occurs primarily in noninflammatory conditions and is an accumulation of protein-poor, cell-poor fluid. Transudative pleural effusions (also called *hydrothorax*) are caused by (1) increased hydrostatic pressure found in congestive heart failure or (2) decreased oncotic pressure (from hypoalbuminemia) found in chronic liver or renal disease. In these situations, fluid movement is facilitated out of the capillaries and into the pleural space.

An exudate is an accumulation of fluid and cells in an area of inflammation. An exudative pleural effusion results from increased capillary permeability characteristic of the inflammatory reaction. Examples of this effusion occur secondary to pulmonary inflammations or malignancies.

The type of pleural effusion can be determined by a sample of pleural fluid obtained via thoracentesis (a procedure done to remove fluid from the pleural space). Exudates have a specific gravity above 1.015 and a high protein content, and the fluid is clear or pale yellow. Transudates have a lower specific gravity and low to no protein content. The fluid is dark yellow or amber. The fluid can also be analyzed for red and white blood cells, malignant cells, bacteria, glucose, pH, and lactic dehydrogenase.

An *empyema* is a pleural effusion that contains pus. It is caused by conditions such as pneumonia, TB, and lung abscess. A complication of empyema is *fibrothorax*, in which there is fibrous fusion of the visceral and parietal pleurae (see Fig. 21-11, *A*).

Clinical manifestations. Common clinical manifestations of pleural effusion are progressive dyspnea and decreased movement of the chest wall on the affected side. There may be pleuritic pain from the underlying disease. Physical examination of the chest will indicate dullness to percussion and absent or decreased breath sounds over the affected area. The chest x-ray will indicate an abnormality if the effusion is greater than 250 ml.

Manifestations of empyema include the manifestations of pleural effusion as well as fever, night sweats, cough, and weight loss. A thoracentesis reveals an exudate containing thick, purulent material.

Thoracentesis. If the cause of the pleural effusion is not known, a diagnostic thoracentesis is needed to obtain pleural fluid for analysis (see Fig. 19-17). If the degree of pleural effusion is severe enough to impair breathing, a therapeutic thoracentesis is done to remove fluid.

A thoracentesis is performed by having the client sit on the edge of a bed and lean forward over a bedside table. The puncture site is determined by chest x-ray and percussion of the chest to determine the maximum degree of dullness. The skin is cleaned with an antiseptic solution and anesthetized locally. The physician inserts the thoracentesis needle into the intercostal space. Fluid can be aspirated with a syringe, or tubing can be connected to allow fluid to drain into a sterile collecting bottle. After the fluid is removed, the needle is withdrawn, and a bandage is applied over the insertion site.

Table 21-29   Extrapulmonary Causes of Restrictive Lung Disease

Disease or Alteration	Description	Comments
CENTRAL NERVOUS SYSTEM		
Head injury, CNS lesion (e.g., tumor, cerebrovascular accident)	Injury to or impingement on respiratory center, causing hypoventilation or hyperventilation; relationship of manifestations to increased intracranial pressure*	Management is directed toward treating the underlying cause, maintaining the airway, using mechanical ventilation for supportive care, and assessing for manifestations of increased intracranial pressure.
Narcotic and barbiturate use	Depression of respiratory center, respiratory rate of <12 breaths/min	Respiratory depression is caused by drug overdose or inadvertent administration of drugs to a person with respiratory difficulty. These drugs should not be administered to a person with a respiratory rate of <12 breaths/min.
NEUROMUSCULAR SYSTEM		
Guillain-Barré syndrome	Acute inflammation of peripheral nerves and ganglia; paralysis of intercostal nerves leading to diaphragmatic breathing; paralysis of vagal preganglionic and postganglionic fibers leading to reduced ability of bronchioles to constrict, dilate, and respond to irritants	Client often has to be put on mechanical ventilation for supportive care.†
Amyotrophic lateral sclerosis‡	Progressive degenerative disorder of the motor neurons in the spinal cord, brain stem, and motor cortex; respiratory system involvement as a result of interruption of nerve transmission to respiratory muscles, especially diaphragm	—
Myasthenia gravis‡	Defect in neuromuscular junction, respiratory system involvement as a result of interruption of nerve transmission to respiratory muscles	—
Muscular dystrophy	Hereditary disease; eventual involvement of all skeletal muscles; paralysis of respiratory muscles, including intercostals, diaphragm, and accessory muscles	Pulmonary problems develop late in disease process.
CHEST WALL		
Chest-wall trauma (e.g., flail chest, fractured rib)	Rib fracture causing inspiratory pain; voluntary splinting of chest, resulting in shallow, rapid breathing; impaired ventilatory ability due to paradoxical breathing (see text)§	—
Pickwickian syndrome (extreme obesity)	Excess adipose tissue interfering with chest-wall and diaphragmatic excursion, somnolence from hypoxemia and CO_2 retention, polycythemia from chronic hypoxia	Weight loss generally causes reversal of symptoms. Prevention and prompt treatment of respiratory infections are important. Condition is worsened in supine position.
Kyphoscoliosis	Posterior and lateral angulation of the spine; restriction of ventilation as a result of alteration in thoracic excursion; increase in work of breathing; pattern of rapid, shallow breathing; reduction of lung volume; compression of alveoli and blood vessels	Only small number of persons with condition develop severe respiratory problems.

*See Chapter 52.
†See Chapter 55 for clinical manifestations and management.
‡See Chapter 54 for clinical manifestations and management.
§See Fig. 21-12.

Table 21-30 Intrapulmonary Causes of Restrictive Lung Disease

Disease or Alteration	Description
PLEURAL DISORDERS	
Pleural effusion	Accumulation of fluid in pleural space secondary to altered hydrostatic or oncotic pressure, fluid collection greater than 250 ml, showing up on chest x-ray study
Pleurisy	Inflammation of pleura, classification as fibrinous (dry) or serofibrinous (wet), wet pleurisy accompanied by an increase in pleural fluid and possibly resulting in pleural effusion
Pneumothorax	Accumulation of air in pleural space with accompanying lung collapse
PARENCHYMAL DISORDERS	
Atelectasis	Condition of lung characterized by collapsed, airless alveoli; possibly acute (e.g., in postoperative client) or chronic (e.g., in client with malignant tumor)
Pneumonia	Acute inflammation of lung tissue caused by bacteria, viruses, fungi, chemicals, dusts, and other factors
Pulmonary fibrosis	Excessive connective tissue in the lungs resulting from healing and tissue repair after inflammation, possible localized fibrosis (e.g., from lung abscess, TB, pneumonia) or diffuse (e.g., from pneumoconiosis, sarcoidosis, cystic fibrosis, Hamman-Rich syndrome), progressive dyspnea on exertion as a result of decreased compliance of lungs and increased work of breathing, progressive disabling and frequently fatal in diffuse pulmonary fibrosis
ARDS*	Atelectasis, pulmonary edema, congestion, and hyaline membrane lining the alveolar wall; result of variety of conditions, including shock lung, O_2 toxicity, gram-negative sepsis, cardiopulmonary bypass, and aspiration pneumonia

*See Chapter 23 for clinical manifestations and management.

Usually only 1000 to 1200 ml of pleural fluid is removed at one time to prevent mediastinal shift and compromised venous return. A follow-up chest x-ray should be done to detect a possible pneumothorax that could have been induced by perforation of the pleura. After the procedure the client should be observed for any manifestations of respiratory distress.

Therapeutic management. The main goal of management of pleural effusions is to treat the underlying cause. For example, adequate treatment of congestive heart failure with diuretics and sodium restriction will result in decreased pleural effusions. The treatment of pleural effusions secondary to malignant disease represents a more difficult problem. These types of pleural effusions are frequently recurrent and accumulate quickly after thoracentesis. Infusions of cancer chemotherapeutic agents directly into the pleural space are used to decrease the number of recurrent effusions.

Treatment of empyema is directed at drainage of the pleural space via thoracentesis or a closed thoracotomy tube. Appropriate antibiotic therapy is also needed to eradicate the causative organism. If a fibrothorax results from the empyema and causes severe pulmonary restriction, a decortication surgical procedure is done in which the pleural membranes are separated.

Pleurisy

Pleurisy (also called *pleuritis*) is an inflammation of the pleura. The most common causes are pneumonia, TB, chest trauma, pulmonary infarctions, and neoplasms. The inflammation usually subsides with adequate treatment of the primary disease. Pleurisy can be classified as *fibrinous* (dry), with fibrinous deposits on the pleural surface, or *se-* *rofibrinous* (wet), with increased production of pleural fluid that may result in pleural effusion.

The pain of pleurisy is typically abrupt and sharp in onset and is aggravated by inspiration. The client's breathing is shallow and rapid to avoid unnecessary movement of the pleura and chest wall. A pleural friction rub may be heard 1 to 2 days after the onset of symptoms.[35]

Treatment of pleurisy is aimed at treating the underlying disease and providing pain relief. Taking analgesics as well as lying on or splinting the affected side may provide some relief. The client should be taught to splint the rib cage when coughing. Intercostal nerve blocks may be done if the pain is severe.

Atelectasis

Atelectasis is a condition of the lungs characterized by collapsed, airless alveoli. The most common cause of atelectasis is airway obstruction that is due to retained exudates and secretions. This is frequently observed in the postoperative client. Normally, the pores of Kohn provide for collateral passage of air from one alveolus to another. Deep inspiration is necessary to open the pores effectively. For this reason, coughing and deep-breathing exercises are important in preventing atelectasis in high-risk clients (e.g., postoperative, immobilized clients). Pulmonary fibrosis can occur as a complication of chronic atelectasis. (The prevention and treatment of atelectasis are discussed in Chapter 13.)

Pulmonary Fibrosis

A common cause of diffuse pulmonary fibrosis is occupational inhalation of organic and inorganic substances. Other causes of diffuse pulmonary fibrosis include the

Hamman-Rich syndrome (an unusual form of interstitial pneumonia) and sarcoidosis.

Sarcoidosis is the presence of granulomatous lesions and proliferation of lymph tissue, which can involve any body organ including the lungs. The disease is most common in American blacks between the ages of 20 and 35. The clinical course of the disease varies from self-limiting to progressive, widespread granulomatous inflammation and fibrosis. Marked pulmonary fibrosis can be present with severe restrictive lung disease. Cor pulmonale can develop in the advanced stages. There is no specific treatment for sarcoidosis. Often the disease is self-limiting, and the client gets well without treatment. Corticosteroids have been used to relieve symptoms and suppress the acute inflammation.

VASCULAR LUNG DISORDERS
Pulmonary Edema

Pulmonary edema is an abnormal accumulation of fluid in the alveoli and interstitial spaces of the lungs. It is a complication of various heart and lung diseases (Table 21-31). It is considered a medical emergency and may be life threatening.

Normally, there is a balance between the hydrostatic and oncotic pressures in the pulmonary capillaries. If the hydrostatic pressure increases or the colloid oncotic pressure decreases, the net effect will be fluid leaving the pulmonary capillaries and entering the interstitial space. This stage is referred to as *interstitial edema*. At this stage the lymphatics can usually drain away the excess fluid. If fluid continues to leak from the pulmonary capillaries, it will enter the alveoli. This stage is referred to as *alveolar edema*. Pulmonary edema interferes with gas exchange by causing an alteration in the diffusing pathway between the alveoli and the pulmonary capillaries.

The most common cause of pulmonary edema is left-sided congestive heart failure. (The clinical manifestations and management of pulmonary edema are described in Chapter 29.)

Chronic forms of pulmonary edema are not common. This condition can be asymptomatic for a long period of time while structural changes such as pulmonary fibrosis result. An early manifestation of this condition may be

Table 21-31 Causes of Pulmonary Edema

Congestive heart failure
Overhydration with IV fluids
Hypoalbuminemia: nephrotic syndrome, hepatic disease, nutritional disorders
Altered capillary permeability of lungs: inhaled toxins, inflammation (e.g., pneumonia), severe hypoxia, near drowning
Mechanical ventilation
Lymph malignancies
Respiratory distress syndrome (e.g., O_2 toxicity)
Unknown causes: neurogenic condition, narcotic overdose, high altitude

---

paroxysmal nocturnal dyspnea as a result of increased hydrostatic pressure in the lungs in the recumbent position.

Pulmonary Embolism

Pulmonary embolism is the most frequently encountered pulmonary illness in a general hospital and is responsible for more than 50,000 deaths annually in the United States.[36] A pulmonary embolism is caused by thrombotic occlusion of the pulmonary arterial system. The most common source of the thrombus is the deep veins of the legs. The thrombus breaks loose and travels as an embolus until it lodges in the pulmonary vasculature.

The result of the thromboembolic occlusion is complete or partial occlusion of the pulmonary arterial blood flow to parts of the lung. Thus the lung is ventilated but not perfused. As the pressure increases in the pulmonary vasculature, pulmonary hypertension may result. (Pulmonary embolism is described in detail in Chapter 32.)

Pulmonary Hypertension

Pathophysiology. Normally, the pulmonary circulation is characterized by low resistance and low pressure. Cardiac output can increase significantly with no increase in the pressure in the pulmonary vasculature. In pulmonary hypertension the pulmonary pressure is elevated because of an increase in pulmonary vascular resistance to blood flow through small arteries and arterioles.

A 60% to 70% reduction in the vascular bed is required before pulmonary hypertension develops. The increase in vascular resistance may be anatomical or vasomotor related in origin.

The reasons for an anatomical increase in vascular resistance include (1) loss of capillaries as a result of alveolar wall damage, as found in COPD, (2) stiffening of the pulmonary vasculature, as found in pulmonary fibrosis, and (3) obstruction of blood flow, as found with pulmonary emboli.

Vasomotor increase in pulmonary vascular resistance is found in conditions characterized by alveolar hypoxia and hypercapnia. These conditions cause localized vasoconstriction and shunting of blood away from poorly ventilated alveoli. Alveolar hypoxia and hypercapnia can be caused by a wide variety of conditions, including the Pickwickian syndrome, kyphoscoliosis, neuromuscular diseases, and other conditions characterized by alveolar hypoventilation with normal lungs.

It is possible to have a combination of anatomical restriction and vasomotor constriction. This is found in the client with long-standing chronic bronchitis who has chronic hypoxia in addition to loss of lung tissue.

Pulmonary hypertension is almost always caused by pulmonary or cardiac disorders. One type, called *primary pulmonary hypertension,* is not associated with either pulmonary or cardiac disease. The person with this disorder is typically a woman between the ages of 20 and 40. The basic cause of the problem is unknown. No definitive therapy is available, and the course is often one of slow downhill progression.

Clinical manifestations. The most common manifestations of pulmonary hypertension are dyspnea and weakness. These symptoms initially present only when there is an increased cardiac output (e.g., during exercise or with fever) or during hypoxia (e.g., with pulmonary infection). Eventually, the condition occurs even during rest. Pulmonary hypertension increases the work load of the right ventricle and causes right ventricular hypertrophy, a condition called *cor pulmonale.*

Cor Pulmonale

Cor pulmonale is characterized by hypertrophy of the right ventricle secondary to a respiratory disorder. Pulmonary hypertension is usually a preexisting condition in individuals with cor pulmonale. Cor pulmonale may be present with or without overt cardiac failure.

The most common cause of acute cor pulmonale is a massive pulmonary embolism. In general, however, cor pulmonale is chronic, resulting from alveolar hypoxia in COPD. Almost any disorder that affects the respiratory system can cause cor pulmonale. The etiology and pathogenesis of pulmonary hypertension and cor pulmonale are outlined in Fig. 21-16.

Clinical manifestations. Clinical manifestations of cor pulmonale include dyspnea, cough, retrosternal or substernal pain, and fatigue. Chronic hypoxia leads to polycythemia and increased total blood volume and viscosity

of the blood. Thus compensatory mechanisms that are due to hypoxemia can aggravate the pulmonary hypertension. Attacks of cor pulmonale in a person with underlying chronic respiratory problems are frequently triggered by an acute respiratory tract infection.

If heart failure accompanies cor pulmonale, additional manifestations such as peripheral edema, weight gain, distended neck veins, full, bounding pulse, and enlarged liver will also be found. (Heart failure is discussed in Chapter 29.) A chest x-ray will show an enlarged right ventricle and pulmonary artery.

Therapeutic management. The primary management of cor pulmonale is directed at treating the underlying pulmonary problem that precipitated the heart problem (Table 21-32). Low-flow O_2 therapy is used to correct the hypoxemia and reduce vasoconstriction in chronic states of respiratory disorders. In acute states (e.g., those that are due to pulmonary emboli), higher concentrations of O_2 may be required. If fluid and electrolyte and acid-base imbalances are present, they need to be corrected. Diuretics and a low-sodium diet will help to decrease the plasma volume and the load on the heart. Bronchodilator therapy is indicated if the underlying respiratory problem is due to an obstructive disorder. Antibiotic therapy is indicated if the cor pulmonale was precipitated by an infection. The use of digitalis may be necessary to treat the accompanying heart failure. If digitalis is used, smaller doses than usual are recommended because hypoxemia predisposes clients to digitalis toxicity. Antidysrhythmic drugs are given if indicated. Phlebotomies may be needed in clients with hematocrits over 60 g/dl to reduce the hematocrit and blood volume.

Chronic management of cor pulmonale that results from COPD is similar to that described for COPD (see Chapter 22). Continuous low-flow O_2 during sleep, exercise, and small, frequent meals may allow the client to feel better and be more active. Vasodilator therapy has been

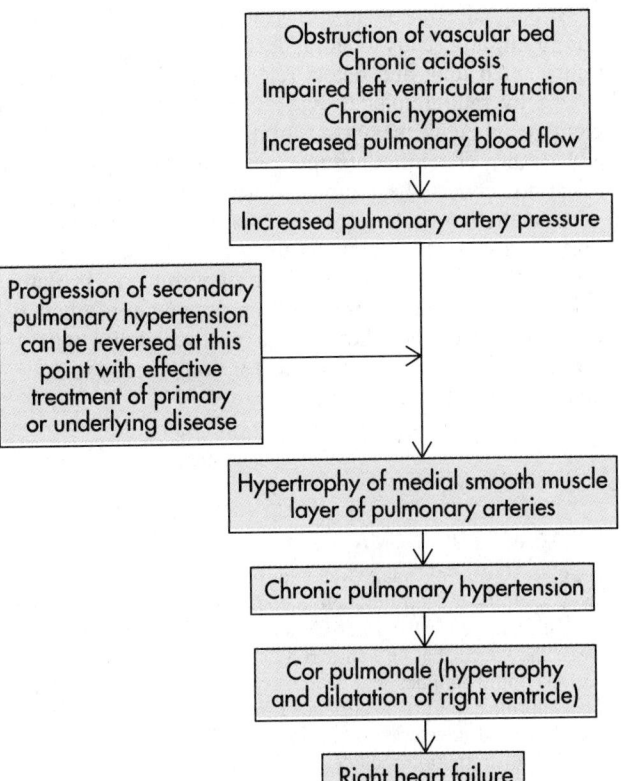

Fig. 21-16 Pathogenesis of pulmonary hypertension and cor pulmonale. (From McCance KL and Huether SE: Pathophysiology: the biological basis for disease in adults and children, St Louis, 1990, Mosby–Year Book, Inc.)

Table 21-32

Diagnostic and Therapeutic Management: Cor Pulmonale

DIAGNOSTIC

History and physical examination
ABGs
Serum and urine electrolytes
Continual monitoring with ECG

THERAPEUTIC

Bed rest
O_2 therapy
Bronchodilators
Diuretics (e.g., furosemide)
Low-sodium diet
Fluid restriction
Antibiotics
Digitalis (if left-sided heart failure)

evaluated as a possible treatment for pulmonary hypertension, both primary hypertension and that accompanying COPD. The results have been contradictory. However, recent studies have not supported the use of such drugs in the treatment of pulmonary hypertension and resultant cor pulmonale.[37]

LUNG TRANSPLANTATION

In 1968 the first clinical lung transplant was performed in the United States. Early failures were encountered because of technical problems (e.g., bronchial disruption, respiratory insufficiency) related to transplantation of a unilateral lung as well as those related to immunosuppression (e.g., pneumonia, graft rejection). A breakthrough came with the introduction of cyclosporine, a T-lymphocyte immunosuppressive agent, for use in other transplantations. (Cyclosporine is discussed in Chapter 41.) Currently, through the technical advance of performing heart and lung transplants simultaneously and the use of cyclosporine, the results have been more favorable. Since 1981, more than 300 clients have undergone heart-lung transplants. The current 1-year survival rate is approximately 60% to 70%.[38]

The candidates for heart-lung transplantation are generally young (less than 50 years of age) and suffer from severe, irreversible pulmonary hypertension (e.g., Eisenmenger's syndrome as a result of severe left-to-right shunts secondary to a congenital pathophysiological condition or primary pulmonary hypertension). Other disorders that may be indicators for heart-lung transplantation include end-stage COPD, cystic fibrosis, fibrosing alveolitis, and pulmonary fibrosis secondary to irradiation or medication or idiopathic pulmonary fibrosis. To be considered for transplantation, the client must be evaluated by cardiologists and cardiac surgeons and must be shown to have severe disease, poor functional ability, and an estimated life expectancy of less than 6 to 12 months.

Single-lung transplantation has become an increasingly viable option with improvements in surgical and organ preservation techniques, immunosuppressive protocols, and availability of donor lungs. The advantages of maximizing the use of donor organs is apparent if both heart and lungs can be used from a single donor. Candidates for single-lung transplantation differ from those for heart-lung transplantation in that they must have no serious cardiac disease, especially no left ventricular dysfunction. Additionally, potential recipients of single-lung transplants should have a poor 6-month prognosis or be dependent on mechanical ventilation to maintain adequate gas exchange.

Candidates for heart-lung or single-lung transplantation should not have any significant psychiatric disorders or systemic disease. Candidates and their families undergo thorough psychological screening to determine their ability to cope with a postoperative regimen that requires strict adherence to immunosuppressive therapy, continuous monitoring for early signs of infection, and prompt reporting of manifestations of infection for medical evaluation.

Early pulmonary postoperative complications of heart-lung transplantation include respiratory dysfunction, the "implantation response," and infection. Initially, clients experience a shallow breathing pattern and difficulty in clearing secretions secondary to denervation of the lung below the trachea, with a resultant decrease in mucociliary clearance and lymphatic drainage. Aggressive pulmonary clearance measures—including aerosolized bronchodilators, chest physiotherapy, and deep-breathing and cough techniques—are mandatory to minimize potential complications.

The implantation response, commonly encountered between 4 and 21 days after surgery, is a reversible phenomenon that presents with fever, impaired gas exchange, tachypnea, and diffuse pulmonary infiltrates. The causes are believed to be denervation, lymphatic disruption, ischemia, and surgical trauma. Treatment consists of aggressive chest physiotherapy, administration of diuretics, and supportive mechanical ventilation as needed on a short-term basis.

Rejection of lung transplants is believed to be a long-term rather than a short-term problem, particularly since the use of excellent immunosuppressive therapy with cyclosporine, azathioprine, and prednisone has become standard practice. Signs of rejection include an increase in pulmonary artery pressure, worsening of hypoxemia, new alveolar infiltrates, and an increase in polymorphonuclear neutrophils (PMNs) in the tracheal secretions. Treatment of rejection consists of administration of high-dose IV methylprednisolone and sometimes antilymphocyte globulin.

Bronchoalveolar lavage may be used as well as technetium 99m lung scans to show decreased arterial flow to the transplanted lung and detect rejection earlier than demonstrable by radiographical evidence. Infection in the transplant recipient is the most significant cause of morbidity and death. The immunosuppression necessary to prevent rejection renders the recipient susceptible to many pathogens, including bacterial, fungal, viral, nocardial, and protozoal organisms. Infections are primarily pulmonary and are usually either nosocomial or opportunistic in nature. As the area of heart-lung and single-lung transplantation continues to evolve, hope for a prolonged life with improved quality may be realistic for some individuals with end-stage heart and lung disease.

C *ase Study*

BACTERIAL PNEUMONIA

Greg, a 31-year-old man, was admitted to the hospital with cold sweats; chills; a deep productive cough with thick, rust-colored sputum; and generalized muscle and joint pain. For the past week, he stated that he had had a "chest cold" and was taking various antihistamines and decongestants that brought no relief. That morning, he had experienced increased difficulty in breathing and developed intermittent chills. Results of a physical examination included dusky nail beds and mucous membranes and shallow respirations. Greg's vital signs showed a temperature of 40° C (104° F), pulse 114, respiration 28; blood pressure 140/88. Lung sounds were barely audible in the lower lobes of the lungs, and crackles were heard. A chest x-ray film showed bilateral lobar pneumonia of the lower lobes.

Laboratory Results

White blood cell count	28,000/μl
Differential	76% segmented neutrophils, 6% band neutrophils
Culture of sputum	*S. pneumoniae*

ABG Results
(room air)

pH	7.55
$Paco_2$	30 mm Hg
Pao_2	50 mm Hg
O_2 saturation	80%
Bicarbonate	26 mEq/L

Treatment

Procaine penicillin, 600,000 units intramuscularly immediately and every 12 hr
Force fluids to 3 L/24 hr
Chest x-ray film every other day
O_2 administration at 4 L/min

Discussion Questions

1. What are the main classifications of pneumonia and their characteristics? What is the most common type of pneumonia?
2. What predisposing factors contribute to the development of pneumonia?
3. What are the typical manifestations of acute bacterial pneumonia? Which ones did Greg exhibit? What are the pathophysiological bases for the various clinical manifestations?
4. Explain the bases for each of the medical treatments that were prescribed for Greg.
5. What complications may result from bacterial pneumonia? Compare these complications to those characteristic of viral pneumonia.
6. Explain the results of the chest x-ray film and the laboratory studies.

R eview Questions

The number of the question corresponds to the same-numbered objective at the beginning of the chapter.

1. Which of the following statements characterize pneumococcal pneumonia?
   a. generally causes an interstitial type of pneumonia
   b. usually self-limiting and treated symptomatically
   c. characterized by productive cough with rust-colored sputum
   d. most common complication is pneumothorax
2. Which of the following would *not* be considered an appropriate nursing intervention for the client with pneumonia?
   a. assisting with postural drainage every 2 to 3 hours
   b. teaching the client proper disposal of soiled tissues
   c. allowing the client to sleep in the semi-Fowler's position
   d. administering analgesics for chest pain
3. Clinical manifestations of TB include
   a. chest pain and morning sweats
   b. productive cough and high-grade fevers
   c. night sweats and cough
   d. hemoptysis and rust-colored sputum
4. All of the following are types of fungal infections *except*
   a. histoplasmosis
   b. coccidioidomycosis
   c. aspergillosis
   d. mycoplasmosis
5. Bronchiectasis is characterized by
   a. bronchoconstriction and mucosal edema
   b. hypersensitivity of small bronchioles
   c. chronic dilatation of the bronchi
   d. rupture of bronchi secondary to fibrosis
6. The major advantage of a Venturi mask is that it can
   a. deliver precise, high-flow rates of O_2
   b. provide continuous 100% humidity
   c. be used while a client eats and sleeps
   d. deliver up to 80% O_2
7. A common pathophysiological characteristic of many types of pneumoconiosis is
   a. diffuse airway obstruction
   b. diffuse pulmonary fibrosis
   c. benign tumor growth
   d. liquefactive necrosis
8. The type of lung cancer generally associated with the best prognosis because it is potentially surgically resectable is
   a. squamous cell carcinoma
   b. small cell carcinoma
   c. adenocarcinoma
   d. undifferentiated large cell carcinoma
9. Which of the following would probably *not* be considered a risk associated with the development of lung cancer?
   a. living in rural environment
   b. heredity
   c. cigar smoking
   d. preexisting pulmonary disease
10. A common cause of flail chest is
    a. multiple rib fractures
    b. spontaneous pneumothorax
    c. kyphoscoliosis
    d. atelectasis
11. The purpose of closed chest-tube drainage is to
    a. prevent the escape of air from the pleural space
    b. produce additional negative alveolar pressure
    c. equalize the pressure in the chest cavity
    d. remove air and fluid from the pleural space
12. Nursing measures that should be instituted after a thoracotomy include all the following *except*
    a. range-of-motion exercises on the affected upper extremity
    b. keeping the client off the unaffected side after a pneumonectomy
    c. monitoring chest-tube drainage and functioning
    d. using a shoulder sling to immobilize the affected upper extremity

13. The Guillain-Barré syndrome causes respiratory problems primarily by
    a. depressing the CNS
    b. paralyzing the diaphragm secondary to trauma
    c. interrupting nerve transmission to respiratory muscles
    d. deforming chest-wall muscles
14. Which of the following descriptions best characterizes cor pulmonale?
    a. right ventricular hypertrophy secondary to increased pulmonary vascular resistance
    b. right ventricular hypertrophy secondary to congenital heart disease
    c. pulmonary congestion secondary to left ventricular failure
    d. excess serous fluid collection in the alveoli secondary to heart failure
15. Heart-lung transplantation is advocated to be useful for which of the following conditions?
    a. end-stage COPD
    b. primary pulmonary hypertension
    c. cystic fibrosis
    d. adenocarcinoma

REFERENCES

1. National Center for Health Statistics: Monthly statistics report, 33:1-44, 1984.
2. Johnson CC and Finegold SM: Pyogenic bacterial pneumonia, lung abscess, and empyema. In Murray JF and Nadel JA: Textbook of respiratory medicine, Philadelphia, 1988, WB Saunders Co, pp 803-855.
3. Rytel MW: Influenza and its complications, recognition and prevention, Hosp Pract 22:102A-102V, 1987.
4. Hayden FG and Gwaltney JM: Viral infections. In Murray JF and Nadel JA: Textbook of respiratory medicine, Philadelphia, 1988, WB Saunders Co, pp 748-802.
5. Petersen C, Slutkin G, and Mills J: Parasitic infections. In Murray JF and Nadel JA: Textbook of respiratory medicine, Philadelphia, 1988, WB Saunders Co, pp 950-986.
6. Graham WGB and Bradley DA: Efficacy of chest physiotherapy and intermittent positive-pressure breathing in the resolution of pneumonia, N Engl J Med 299:624-627, 1978.
7. Update: tuberculosis elimination—United States, Morbidity and Mortality Weekly Report 39:153-156, 1990.
8. Sutton FD: TB and its fellow travelers, Hosp Pract 22:75-93, 1987.
9. American Thoracic Society and Centers for Disease Control: Treatment of tuberculosis and tuberculosis infection in adults and children, Am Rev Respir Dis 134:355-366, 1986.
10. Sarosi GA and Davies SF: Fungal infections. In Murray JF and Nadel JA: Textbook of respiratory medicine, Philadelphia, 1988, WB Saunders Co, pp 916-949.
11. Hammarsten JE and Hammarsten JF: Histoplasmosis: recognition and treatment, Hosp Pract 25:95-126, 1990.
12. Fulmer JD and Snider GL: ACCP-NHLBI National Conference on Oxygen Therapy, Chest 86:234-237, 1984.
13. Massaro D: Oxygen: toxicity and tolerance, Hosp Pract 21:95-101, 1986.
14. Openbrier DR, Hoffman LA, and Wesmiller SW: Home oxygen therapy: evaluation and prescription, Am J Nurs 88:192-197, 1988.
15. Openbrier DR, Fuoss C, and Mall CC: What patients on home oxygen therapy want to know, Am J Nurs 88:198-202, 1988.
16. Birdsall C: How do you measure transcutaneous oxygen? Am J Nurs 87:1273-1274, 1987.
17. Ehrhardt BS and Graham M: Pulse oximetry, Nursing 20:50-54, 1990.
18. Hoffman LA and Wesmiller SW: Home oxygen: transtracheal and other options, Am J Nurs 88:464-469, 1988.
19. Mandel JH, Baker BA: Recognizing occupational lung disease, Hosp Pract 24:21-30, 1989.
20. Chan-Yeung M and Malo JL: Occupational asthma, Chest 91(suppl):130S, 1987.
21. McNaull FW: Lung cancer. What are the odds? Am J Nurs 87:1428-1429, 1987.
22. American Cancer Society: Cancer statistics 1989, Cancer 39:3-20, 1989.
23. McNaull FW: Lung cancer: tobaccoism in America, Am J Nurs 87:1430-1433, 1987.
24. US National Research Council: Environmental tobacco smoke: measuring exposures and assessing health effects, Washington, DC, 1986, National Academy Press.
25. Armstrong DA: Lung cancer: the diagnostic workup, Am J Nurs 87:1433, 1987.
26. Engelking C: Lung cancer: the language of staging, Am J Nurs 17:1434-1437, 1987.
27. Haylock PJ: Lung cancer: radiation therapy, Am J Nurs 87:1441-1445, 1987.
28. Maran JN and Gray MA: Pulmonary laser therapy, Am J Nurs 88:828-831, 1988.
29. Pollin W: The role of the addictive process as a key step in causation of all tobacco-related diseases, JAMA 252:2874, 1984.
30. Dalton JA and Swenson I: Nurses and smoking: role modeling and counseling behaviors, Oncol Nurs Forum 76:1449-1451, 1986.
31. Waxman KS: Pleural disorders. In Shoemaker W and others: Textbook of critical care, Philadelphia, 1989, WB Saunders Co.
32. Connor PA: When and how do you use a Heimlich flutter valve? Am J Nurs 87:288-290, 1987.
33. Erickson RS: Mastering the ins and outs of chest drainage, part 1, Nursing 19:37-44, 1989.
34. Erickson RS: Mastering the ins and outs of chest drainage, part 2, Nursing 19:46-49, 1989.
35. Davis NB: Danger signs: pleural fricton rub, Nursing 18:70-71, 1988.
36. Moser K: Pulmonary embolism. In Murray JF and Nadel JA: Textbook of respiratory medicine, Philadelphia, 1988, WB Saunders Co, pp 1299-1327.
37. Niederman MS and Matthay RA: Cardiovascular function in secondary pulmonary hypertension, Heart Lung 15:341-351, 1986.
38. Muirhead J: Heart and heart-lung transplantation, Nurs Clin North Am 24:865-880, 1989.

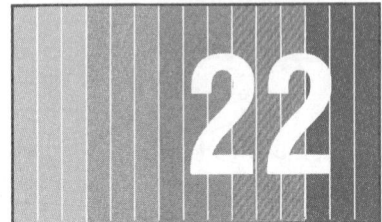

CHAPTER

22

Nursing Role in Management
Obstructive Pulmonary Diseases

Terri E. Weaver
Trisch Van Sciver

L earning Objectives

1. *Describe the types, etiology, pathophysiology, clinical manifestations, and therapeutic and pharmacological management of asthma.*
2. *Describe the nursing role in management of the client with asthma.*
3. *Differentiate among the etiology, pathogenesis, clinical manifestations, complications, and therapeutic management of chronic bronchitis and pulmonary emphysema.*
4. *Describe the effects of cigarette smoking on the lungs.*
5. *Explain the respiratory therapy and nursing management of the client with chronic bronchitis and pulmonary emphysema.*
6. *Describe the pathophysiology, clinical manifestations, and therapeutic and nursing management of the client with cystic fibrosis.*

Chronic obstructive airway disease (COPD) is a de-scriptive term for diseases characterized by obstruction of the small airways (Fig. 22-1). Included in this grouping are asthma, pulmonary emphysema, chronic bronchitis, and asthmatic bronchitis. Clients with asthma have varia-tions in airflow over time, whereas the limitation in expi-ratory airflow in clients with emphysema or chronic bron-chitis is generally more constant.[1] The client with a diag-nosis of COPD may have distinguishing features of two or even all three diseases. Asthma is discussed as a separate entity. Emphysema and chronic bronchitis are considered together, and their differences are indicated where appro-priate. Cystic fibrosis is a genetic disorder that pro-duces airway obstruction because of changes in the secre-tory glands. Although it resembles chronic bronchitis, its pathogenesis is different.

Fig. 22-1 Relationships among emphysema, chronic bronchitis, and asthma. Type A individuals with severe em-physema and little bronchitis are often labeled "pink puff-ers." Type B individuals are often labeled "blue bloaters." Clients with mixed syndromes are depicted by the *x* area.

ASTHMA

As defined by the American Thoracic Society, *asthma* is a clinical syndrome characterized by increased respon-siveness of the tracheobronchial tree to a variety of stim-uli.[2] The hyperresponsiveness of the airways is variable, producing spontaneous fluctuations in the severity of ob-struction. Its clinical course is unpredictable, and it varies from person to person ranging from paroxysms of dysp-nea, wheezing, and cough, which may be mild and diffi-cult to detect, to severe and unremitting symptoms such as in status asthmaticus. Asthma differs from other obstruc-tive disorders such as emphysema and chronic bronchitis because it is currently considered more a disease of in-flammation than of obstruction.

Significance

Asthma affects up to 5% of the population in the United States, and the total prevalence of asthma has increased 61% since 1970.[3] There are an estimated 9.9 million cases of asthma, with 3.2 million of these in children less than

Reviewed by Sr. Regina Maibusch, R.N., M.S., Respiratory Clinical Nurse Specialist, St. Michael Hospital, Milwaukee, Wisconsin.

557

Table 22-1   Triggers of Acute Asthma Attacks

Antigen inhalation	Occupational exposure
Animal danders	Metal salts
House dust mite	Wood and vegetable dusts
Pollens	Industrial chemicals and
Molds	plastics
Air pollutants	Pharmaceutical agents
Exhaust fumes	Food additives
Perfumes	Sulfites (bisulfites and met-
Oxidants	abisulfites)
Sulfur dioxides	Tartrazine
Cigarette smoke	Menses
Aerosol sprays	Esophageal reflux
Viral upper respiratory	Emotional stress
infection	
Paranasal sinusitis	
Exercise and cold, dry air	
Drugs	
Aspirin	
Nonsteroidal antiinflamma-	
tory drugs	
Acetaminophen	
β-Adrenergic blockers	

18 years of age.[4] The morbidity associated with the disease is dramatic. It affects school attendance, occupational choices, physical activity, and many other aspects of life.

The mortality rate for asthma has been increasing since 1977, with a 31% increase during the past decade. In 1987 more than 4000 deaths were related to asthma. These findings may be related to an increase of allergens in the environment, increased death rate among blacks and lower socioeconomic groups, delay in seeking help, inadequate medical treatment, and client noncompliance with prescribed therapy.[5]

Etiology

In the past, asthma was classified as allergic (extrinsic) and nonallergic (intrinsic) asthma. *Allergic asthma* is associated with a personal and/or family history of allergies such as allergic rhinitis, urticaria, and eczema. In these persons, exposure to allergens such as pollens, animal dander, or certain foods triggers an asthma attack. However, pure extrinsic asthma is found in only a minority of persons with asthma. *Nonallergic* (intrinsic or idiosyncratic) *asthma* is not related to specific precipitating allergens and is not associated with a family history of allergies.[6] Nonspecific factors such as a common cold, respiratory tract infection, and environmental pollutants may trigger an asthma attack.

Unfortunately, most clients do not fit clearly into either category but fall into a mixed group with features of each. In general, those clients whose onset of the disease is early in life (childhood or adolescence) will have a strong allergic component, whereas those whose onset is later in life (after 35 years of age) tend to be nonallergic or to have mixed causes.

The most common denominator underlying asthma is

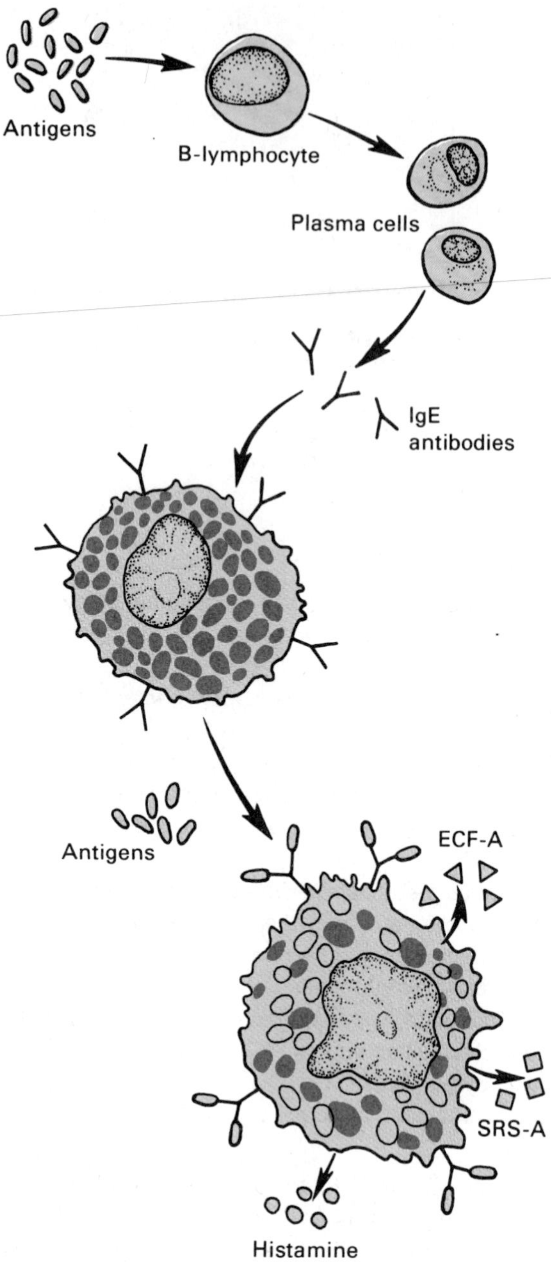

Fig. 22-2   Mechanism of mediator release in an asthma attack.

nonspecific *hyperirritability* or *hyperresponsiveness* of the tracheobronchial tree. Although a number of causes of increased airway reactivity in asthma have been postulated, the basic mechanism remains unknown. The most popular hypothesis is that of *airway inflammation*. After exposure to an initiating stimulus, mast cells are activated to release a variety of mediators (see p. 128). The *stimuli* or *triggers* that increase airway responsiveness and incite acute episodes of asthma can be grouped into various categories (Table 22-1). Rather than discussing asthma as an allergic or nonallergic disease, it is preferable to focus on the triggers or precipitating factors for asthma.

Antigen inhalation. Allergic asthma is an example of a Type I hypersensitivity reaction (see Chapter 8). In some persons with asthma an exaggerated IgE response develops to certain antigens (allergens), such as dust, pollens, grasses, and animal danders. IgE antibodies attach to mast cells found beneath the basement membrane in the bronchial wall (Fig. 22-2). Reexposure to even minute amounts of the antigen results in antigen binding to the antibody. The IgE–mast cell complexes remain for long periods of time, so the second exposure will trigger mast cell release even years after the initial exposure to the antigen. When IgE-sensitized mast cells are reexposed to the antigen, two processes occur: degranulation of mast cells with subsequent release of granules (Table 8-9) and disruption of the phospholipid cell membrane. Both processes result in the release of histamine, bradykinin, leukotrienes, prostaglandins, platelet-activating factor, and chemotactic factors. These mediators cause an intense inflammatory reaction associated with the classic immediate allergic reaction of asthma, which consists of bronchial smooth muscle contraction (bronchospasm), vascular congestion and edema formation, and increase in the amount and character (tenacious) of sputum (Figs. 22-3 and 22-4). This immediate response occurs within 5 to 30 minutes of exposure to an allergen and subsides in another 30 to 90 minutes. Clinically, the client has wheezing, chest tightness, and dyspnea.

The *delayed* or *late-phase reaction* begins 2 to 8 hours after exposure to an allergen and may last for several hours and sometimes for days or months.[7] The late-phase response is primarily characterized by inflammation and inflammatory cells. The chemotactic factors that are elaborated, such as eosinophil and neutrophil chemotactic factors of anaphylaxis and leukotriene B_4, bring neutrophils and eosinophils to the site of the reaction. These cells can subsequently release mediators that cause mast cells to release histamine and other mediators that eventually set up a self-sustaining cycle. In addition, mononuclear cells (lymphocytes and monocytes) are attracted to influx into the area.[8]

These series of reactions known as the late-phase reaction heighten airway reactivity, which in turn worsens the symptoms of future asthma attacks (Fig. 22-5). The person becomes hyperresponsive not only to specific allergens, but also to nonspecific stimuli such as air pollution, cold air, and dust. At this point, identifying the original allergen may be difficult, and less stimulation is required to produce a reaction. The airway hyperreactivity may be related to the exposure of sensory nerves as a result of epithelial injury caused by the repeated late-phase reactions. Ultimately these processes cause increased airway resistance, which causes air trapping in the alveoli and hyperinflation of the lungs.[9]

Respiratory infections. Respiratory infections are the most common precipitating factors of an acute asthma attack. Well-controlled studies have demonstrated that respiratory viruses and not bacteria or allergy are the major etiological factors.[10] Bacterial respiratory infections, with the exception of sinusitis, do not have a major role in exacerbations of asthma. Infections cause inflammatory changes in the tracheobronchial system and alter the mucociliary mechanism. Therefore they increase the hyperresponsiveness of the bronchial system. Increased airway responsiveness can last from 2 to 8 weeks after the infection in both

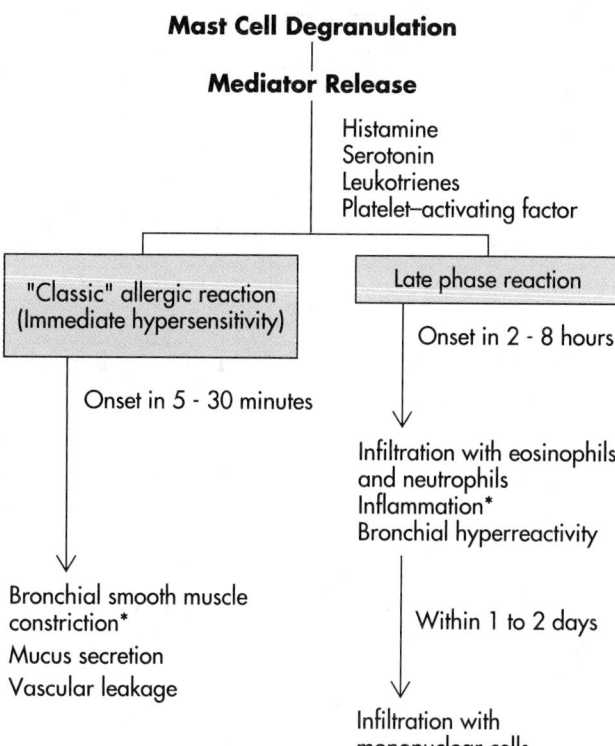

Fig. 22-3 Immediate hypersensitivity and late phase reactions of asthma. Items with an *asterisk* are primary processes.

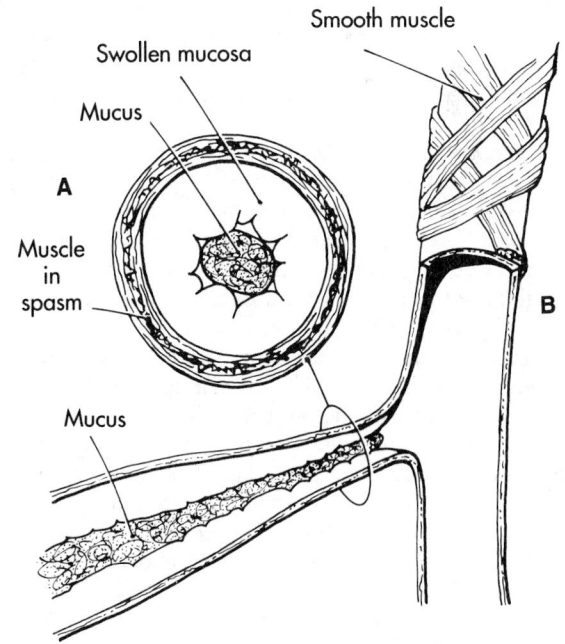

Fig. 22-4 Factors causing expiratory obstruction in bronchial asthma. **A,** Cross section of a bronchiole occluded by muscle spasm, swollen mucosa, and mucus in the lumen. **B,** Longitudinal section of a bronchiole. (From Price S and Wilson L: Pathophysiology: clinical concepts of disease processes, ed 4, St Louis, 1991, Mosby–Year Book, Inc.)

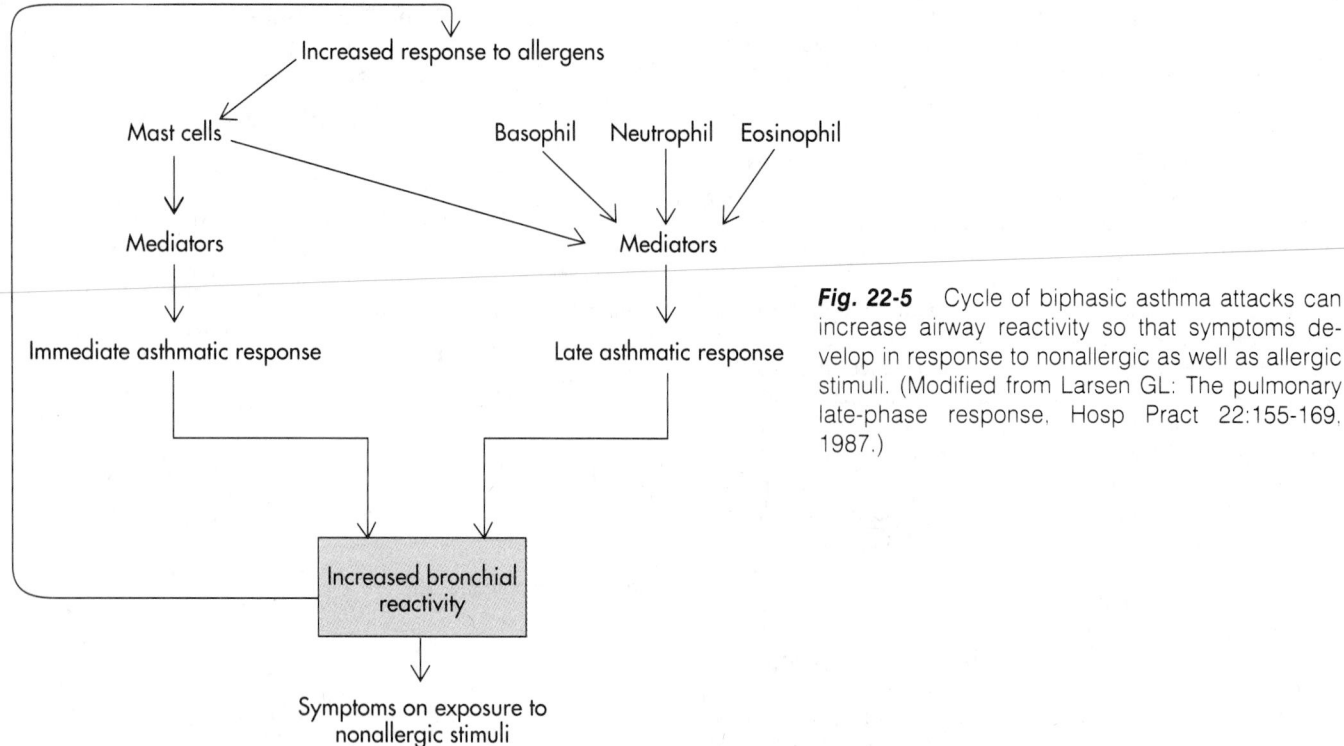

Fig. 22-5 Cycle of biphasic asthma attacks can increase airway reactivity so that symptoms develop in response to nonallergic as well as allergic stimuli. (Modified from Larsen GL: The pulmonary late-phase response, Hosp Pract 22:155-169, 1987.)

normal and asthmatic persons. Asthma may develop after an influenzalike illness in infants or young children and adults more than 30 years of age. Three outcomes are possible after a viral respiratory tract infection. (1) It may resolve and not cause asthma; (2) it may trigger airway inflammation and cause a transient asthmalike syndrome that subsides in 2 to 3 weeks, continue for several months, and then subside spontaneously or after medical intervention; or (3) it may go on to become chronic nonallergic asthma.[6]

Exercise. Asthma can be induced or made worse by physical exertion. Provocation of bronchospasm by exercise is probably operative to some extent in every person with asthma, and in some it may be the only trigger mechanism that will produce symptoms. Thus it is called exercise-induced asthma (EIA). Typically, it occurs after several minutes of vigorous exercise (e.g., jogging) and is characterized by bronchospasm. Cromolyn sodium or β_2 inhalants may be of value in helping these persons to maintain bronchodilatation during exercise. By causing obligatory mouth breathing of cold, dry air, physical exertion may induce bronchospasm. This is probably why physical exertion is a contributing factor to an attack in many persons with asthma. The client should perform a brief warmup of stretching for 2 to 3 minutes before exercise. During exercise in cold or dry climate conditions, breathing through a scarf or mask may decrease the likelihood of symptoms.

Drugs and food additives. Intolerance to drugs is present in some asthmatic persons. If these sensitized persons ingest aspirin or nonsteroidal antiinflammatory agents (e.g., indomethacin), approximately 2 hours later wheezing will develop. Salicylates are also found in many foods, beverages, and flavorings. Other agents that may precipitate asthma in susceptible clients are tartrazine (yellow dye No. 5, found in many foods), vitamins, and sodium metabisulfate (a food preservative commonly found in fruits, beer, and wine and used extensively in salad bars to protect vegetables from oxidation).

These agents are thought to interfere with prostaglandin metabolic pathways, leading to enhanced production of leukotrienes, some of which are potent bronchoconstrictors. The onset of a typical reaction occurs 15 to 180 minutes after ingestion and is marked by profuse rhinorrhea, often accompanied by macular erythema and/or nausea, vomiting, intestinal cramps, and diarrhea. Acute asthma begins after the nasal symptoms appear. Pretreatment with steroids or cromolyn does not prevent the reaction. Usually epinephrine and theophylline, given shortly after the onset, will control the symptoms.

Although sensitivity to salicylates persists for many years, the nature and severity of the reaction can change over time. Dietary restrictions of tartrazine (if applicable) and avoidance of aspirin and nonsteroidal antiinflammatory medications are required.

Emotional stress. Another factor often discussed in relationship to the etiology of asthma is psychological or emotional stimuli. Rarely are these factors the sole cause of asthma. Contrary to the thinking of some persons, asthma is not a psychosomatic disease. However, psychological or emotional factors may aggravate symptoms of asthma and on occasion initiate an asthma attack. An asthma attack is a frightening experience. It is possible that the emotional components develop as a result of the client's feelings and reactions to the diagnosis of asthma.

In depressed clients with asthma, an imbalance between cholinergic and adrenergic systems may cause a transient increased cholinergic response of bronchoconstriction.[11]

The extent to which psychological factors participate in the induction and/or continuation of an attack is unknown but probably varies from client to client and, in the same client, from episode to episode.

Pathophysiology

The prominent pathophysiological features of asthma are a reduction in airway diameter and increased airway resistance related to (1) mucosal inflammation, (2) constriction of bronchial smooth muscles, and (3) excess production of mucus (Fig. 22-6). Accompanying these changes are bronchial muscle hypertrophy; basement membrane thickening; mucous gland hypertrophy; thick, tenacious sputum; hyperinflation and air trapping in the alveoli; increased work of breathing; alterations in respiratory muscle function; abnormal distribution of both ventilation and perfusion; and altered arterial blood gases (ABGs). Although asthma is considered a disease of the airways, eventually all aspects of pulmonary function are compromised during an asthma attack. In addition to the inflammatory aspects of asthma, alterations in the autonomic nervous system have also been noted.

The autonomic nervous system, consisting of the parasympathetic and sympathetic systems, innervates the lungs. Bronchial muscle tone is regulated by vagal nerve impulses through the parasympathetic system. Afferent and efferent impulses are conducted through the vagus nerve to the medulla and back to the lungs. When airway nerve endings are stimulated by mechanical or chemical stimuli (e.g., air pollution, cold air, dust), increased release of acetylcholine causes reflex bronchoconstriction that is intensified by decreased mast cell stability with an increase in mediators causing bronchospasm.

Both α- and β-adrenergic receptors of the sympathetic nervous system are located in the bronchi. When the α receptors are stimulated, bronchoconstriction occurs. When the β receptors (β_2 receptors are primarily located in the bronchi) are stimulated, bronchodilatation occurs.

Increased permeability of airway epithelium may allow greater access of inhaled irritants to airway smooth muscle and to sensory nerve endings that stimulate bronchoconstriction by reflex mechanisms. The balance between α and β receptors is mediated primarily by cyclic adenosine monophosphate (cAMP). α-Adrenergic stimulation results in decreased levels of cAMP, leading to (1) increased mast cell release of chemical mediators and (2) bronchoconstriction. β-Adrenergic stimulation results in increased levels of cAMP, which (1) inhibits release of chemical mediators and (2) promotes bronchodilatation. Epinephrine and β_2-adrenergic drugs act primarily on β receptors.

Clinical Manifestations

Asthma is characterized by an unpredictable and variable course. An attack of asthma may have an abrupt onset but is usually more gradual. Attacks often occur at night. Most last for a few minutes to several hours, and then the client recovers. Between attacks the client may be asymptomatic with normal pulmonary function. However, in some persons, compromised pulmonary function may result in a state of continuous asthma and chronic debilitation.

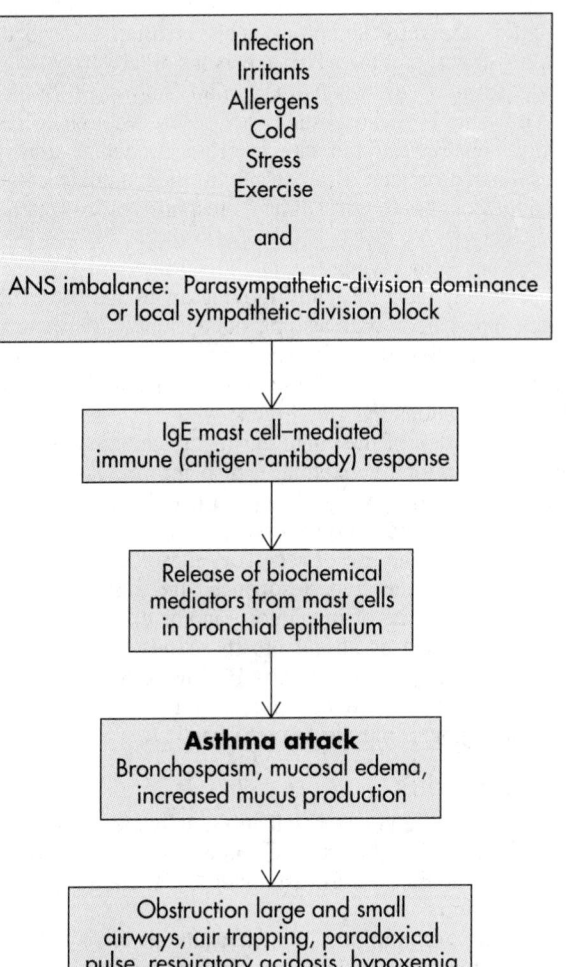

Fig. 22-6 Pathophysiology of asthma. (From McCance KL and Huether SE: Pathophysiology: the biological basis for disease in adults and children, St Louis, 1990, Mosby–Year Book, Inc, p 1071.)

The characteristic clinical manifestations of asthma are wheezing, cough, dyspnea, and chest tightness after exposure to a precipitating factor or trigger. Expiration may be prolonged. Instead of a normal inspiratory/expiratory ratio of 1:2, it may be prolonged to 1:3 or 1:4. Normally the bronchioles constrict during expiration. However, because of the bronchospasm that occurs in addition to the edema and mucus in the bronchioles, the airways become more narrow than usual. Therefore it takes more time for the air to move out of the bronchioles. This produces the characteristic prolonged, wheezing expirations.

Wheezing is an unreliable sign to gauge the severity of an attack. Many clients with minor attacks wheeze loudly, whereas others with severe attacks do not wheeze. Wheezing occurs first on exhalation, but as asthma progresses the client wheezes during inspiration and expiration. Severely diminished breath sounds are an ominous sign, indicating severe obstruction and impending respiratory failure.

The cough may be nonproductive, or mobilization of secretions may be difficult, indicating widespread bronchiolar mucus plugging or production of thick, tenacious, white, gelatinous mucus. In some clients with asthma, cough is the only symptom. This is often described as *cough-variant* asthma. These persons likely have a low-grade form of asthma with a mild degree of bronchospasm. This bronchospasm is not severe enough to cause airflow obstruction but can increase bronchial tone and cause irritation and stimulation of the cough receptors. Usually cough-variant asthma is responsive to bronchodilator therapy.

Persons with asthma feel as though they are suffocating because they have difficulty moving air in and out of their lungs. The person with asthma sits upright and uses the accessory muscles of respiration during an acute attack to try to get enough air. The more difficult breathing becomes, the more anxious the client feels.

Examination of the client during an acute attack usually reveals signs of hypoxemia, which may include restlessness, increased anxiety, inappropriate behavior, and increased pulse and blood pressure. The respiratory rate is increased with the use of accessory muscles. Percussion of the lungs indicates hyperresonance, and auscultation indicates the presence of inspiratory and/or expiratory wheezing. Diminished or absent breath sounds are an ominous sign and may indicate significant decrease in air movement resulting from the client's exhaustion and an inability to generate enough muscle force to ventilate.

Complications

Chronic asthma can result in complications such as rib fractures, pneumothorax, pneumomediastinum, atelectasis, and pneumonia. Status asthmaticus is another possible complication.

Status asthmaticus. Status asthmaticus is a severe, life-threatening complication of asthma that may be refractory to the usual treatment of asthma. An axiom describes status asthmaticus: "The longer it lasts, the worse it gets, and the worse it gets, the longer it lasts." Acute asthmatic

attacks account for nearly 1 million emergency room visits per year in the United States, with hundreds of thousands of hospital admissions per year.[1] Of the persons with asthma admitted to the hospital, approximately 10% will require intensive care unit (ICU) monitoring or ventilatory assistance for status asthmaticus.

Causes of status asthmaticus include viral illnesses, ingestion of aspirin or other nonsteroidal antiinflammatory drugs, emotional stress, increases in environmental pollutant or other antigen exposure, abrupt discontinuation of drug therapy (especially corticosteroids), abuse of aerosol medication, and ingestion of β-adrenergic blocking agents.[12]

The client has clinical manifestations similar to those of asthma, but they are more severe and more prolonged. Extreme anxiety, fear of suffocation, severely increased work of breathing, and diaphoresis are common. The absence of diaphoresis may indicate significant dehydration. Sternocleidomastoid, intercostal, and supraclavicular muscle retractions reflect increased respiratory work.

Although wheezing is often audible without a stethoscope, auscultation may not always be reliable because the airflow obstruction may be so severe in some clients that airflow is not sufficient to produce audible wheezing or other abnormal lung sounds.[1] The chest appears fixed in a hyperinflated position and is often described as "tight," indicating severely decreased movement of air through the constricted bronchial airways. A peak expiratory flow rate (PEFR) of less than 150 ml indicates severe obstruction.[1]

Forced exhalation with the use of the abdominal musculature can result in increased intrathoracic pressure transmitted to the great vessels and heart. Neck vein distention and a pulsus paradoxus of as much as 40 mm Hg may result. (Pulsus paradoxus is described in Chapter 31.) Hypertension, sinus tachycardia, and frequently ventricular ectopy occur. These three conditions are related to hypox-

Table 22-2 Arterial Blood Gas Results Correlated with Clinical Manifestations during an Acute Asthmatic Attack

Time Frame	pH	PaCO_2	PaO_2	Physiological Event	Clinical Manifestations
Early in attack	↑	↓	↓	Alveolar hyperventilation → hypocarbia	Use of all accessory muscles of ventilation to overcome increased airway resistance
				Hypoxemia secondary to ventilation-perfusion mismatch	Increased heart rate, diaphoresis, chest tightness, cough, wheezing
				Adequate alveolar ventilation	
Progressive attack	N	N	↓	CO_2 not being eliminated as well	Tiring of client and difficulty with increased work of breathing
				Decrease in effective alveolar ventilation	
Prolonged attack status asthmaticus	↓	↑	↓	Hypercarbia indicating that ventilation is no longer adequate	Exhaustion, diminished breath sounds, intubation and mechanical ventilation necessary
				Alveolar hypoventilation → respiratory acidosis	
				Worsening hypoxemia as result of hypoventilation and ventilation-perfusion mismatch	

PaO_2, Arterial oxygen pressure.

emia, catecholamine administration, and underlying coronary artery disease in the older adult population. Electrocardiogram (ECG) results may show sinus tachycardia or signs of strain on the right side of the heart secondary to pulmonary vasoconstriction, which may be seen as P-pulmonale and a right axis deviation. Hypoxemia with hypocapnia usually occurs initially as the client attempts to hyperventilate and maintain adequate oxygenation and ventilation. As the severity of the attack increases, the work of breathing increases, making it more difficult for the client to overcome the increased resistance to breathing. The client begins to fatigue, causing more carbon dioxide (CO_2) retention. ABGs deteriorate to normocapnia (normal arterial CO_2 pressure) and then ultimately to hypercapnia and hypoxemia (Table 22-2). A moderate elevation in $Paco_2$ may be tolerated without intubation and mechanical ventilation if the client remains alert and cooperative and continues to improve during the first 2 to 3 hours of treatment.

Complications of status asthmaticus include pneumothorax, pneumomediastinum, acute cor pulmonale with right ventricular failure, and severe respiratory muscle fatigue leading to respiratory arrest. Repeated attacks of status asthmaticus can lead to irreversible emphysema. Death from status asthmaticus is usually due to respiratory arrest or cardiac failure.

Diagnostic Studies

Wheezing and respiratory distress characterize a variety of disorders, including asthma, chronic bronchitis, emphysema, cystic fibrosis, pulmonary edema, upper airway and bronchial obstruction, tracheobronchitis, bronchiolitis, aspiration, and pulmonary embolism. Certain diagnostic studies must be performed to determine whether these symptoms are caused primarily by asthma. The severity of the clinical manifestations of asthma determines the appropriate diagnostic studies.

In the client who is not in distress, a detailed history may indicate previous attacks of a similar nature, often precipitated by a known cause. Pulmonary function tests are usually within normal limits between attacks if the client has no other underlying pulmonary disease. Pulmonary function tests are frequently used to diagnose asthma and are important for an objective measurement of airflow obstruction. The client with asthma usually has a reduction in forced expiratory volume (FEV) in one second (FEV_1), PEFR, and FEV as compared with forced vital capacity (FVC) ratio (FEV_1/FVC), and forced expiratory flow rate during the middle of a FVC ($FEF_{25\%-75\%}$), with the degree of obstruction depending on the values obtained. (The normal values for pulmonary function tests are discussed in Chapter 19.)

These parameters will be decreased from their baseline levels during an exacerbation and in some clients may be within normal limits during a remission. Confirmation of the diagnosis can be made by inducing bronchospasm with bronchial provocation testing with known quantities of such bronchial irritants as histamine, methacholine, cold air, and specific antigens known to be tolerated by the normal person. An increase of 15% or more in the FEV_1 in response to a bronchodilator when the client is not having an exacerbation is another diagnostic indicator of asthma.[2]

Sputum and serum eosinophilia (5% of the total white blood cell [WBC] count) and elevated serum IgE levels may also occur in asthma. A chest radiograph in an asymptomatic client with asthma is usually normal. In a mild asthma attack, ABGs usually indicate a respiratory alkalosis with an arterial oxygen pressure (Pao_2) near normal. Hypercapnia and respiratory acidosis indicate severe disease with a FEV_1 of less than 15% predicted value.[2]

Allergy skin testing may be of some value in trying to determine sensitivity to specific antigens. However, a positive skin test does not necessarily mean that the allergen (antigen) is causing the asthma attack. On the other hand, a negative allergy test does not mean that the asthma is not allergy related. A radioallergosorbent test (RAST) is used in some centers to identify allergic causes in certain clients who show negative skin tests and in those who should not be tested (e.g., severely eczematoid clients).

If the client has wheezing and acute distress, it is not feasible to obtain a detailed history (although a family member may supply some pertinent information). During an acute attack of asthma, bedside spirometry (specifically FEV_1, FVC, and PEFR) may be used to monitor pulmonary function test results. Serial spirometic parameters, oximetry, and/or measurement of ABGs help to provide information about the severity of the attack as well as the response to therapy. ABG changes during the stages of an asthmatic attack are listed in Table 22-2. A complete blood cell count (CBC) and serum electrolytes are also obtained to help direct the course of therapy.

A sputum specimen for Gram stain and culture may be obtained to rule out the presence of bacterial infection, especially if the client has purulent sputum, has a history of upper respiratory tract infection, is febrile, or has an elevated WBC count. A chest x-ray film obtained during an acute attack may show findings resembling emphysema with the presence of hyperinflation. Occasionally the chest radiograph reveals complications of asthma such as mucoid impaction, atelectasis, and pneumomediastinum.

Therapeutic Management

The initial treatment of asthma is aimed at alleviating bronchoconstriction with bronchodilator therapy. In the past, theophylline was the first-line drug for asthma but has now been replaced by other bronchodilators and anti-inflammatory agents. Currently β_2-adrenergic agonists are the most effective bronchodilators in use. Therapy for acute asthma, status asthmaticus, and chronic asthma is shown in Table 22-3.

Acute asthma. A client frequently comes to the emergency room or a physician's office in acute respiratory distress. The choice of treatment of acute asthma depends on the severity of the attack and response to initial therapy. Severity can be measured objectively by measuring FEV_1 or PEFR. Oxygen (O_2) therapy should be started immediately, and its administration should be monitored by pulse oximetry and in more severe cases by measurement of ABGs. Initial therapy should include inhaled β_2-adrenergic agonist drugs administered by metered-dose inhaler (MDI) or nebulizer. They are given every 20 minutes to 4 hours as necessary.

Although recent studies have questioned the value of

Table 22-3

Diagnostic and Therapeutic Management: Asthma

DIAGNOSTIC

History and physical examination
Pulmonary function studies including response to bronchodilator therapy
Chest x-ray film
Measurement of ABGs and oximetry
Allergy skin testing (if indicated)
Sputum specimen for Gram stain and culture (if indicated)
Blood level of eosinophils

THERAPEUTIC

Acute asthma

Inhaled β-adrenergic drugs
Nasal or mask O_2
IV aminophylline
IV or oral corticosteroids
Inhaled or nebulized anticholinergic agents
Fluid intake of 3 L/day

THERAPEUTIC—cont'd

Status asthmaticus

Inhaled β-adrenergic drugs and/or anticholinergic agents
IV aminophylline
O_2 by mask or nasal prongs
IV corticosteroids
IV fluids
IV magnesium
Intubation and assisted ventilation (if indicated)

Chronic asthma

Elimination of causative factors or triggers (if known)
Desensitization (immunotherapy) (if indicated)
β-Adrenergic drugs (inhaled or oral)
Theophylline compound (oral) (if indicated)
Corticosteroids (inhaled or oral)
Cromolyn sodium (inhaled)

Table 22-4   Drugs Used in the Treatment of Asthma and COPD

Drug	Route of Administration	Mechanisms of Action
Metaproterenol (Alupent, Metaprel)	Nebulizer, oral tablets, elixir, MDI	Selectively stimulates β_2-adrenergic receptors, producing bronchodilatation. Increases mucociliary clearance.
Albuterol (Proventil, Ventolin)	Nebulizer, MDI, oral tablets, rotahaler	Same as above.
Pirbuterol (Maxair)	MDI	Same as above.
Isoetharine (Bronkometer, Bronkosol)	Nebulizer, MDI	Same as above.
Terbutaline (Bicanyl, Brethine, Brethaire)	Oral tablets, nebulizer,* subcutaneous, MDI	Same as above.
Bitolterol (Tornalate)	MDI	Same as above.
Epinephrine (Adrenalin)	Subcutaneous, MDI, nebulizer	Stimulates α, β_1, and β_2 receptors.† Stimulates β_2 receptors, producing bronchodilatation.
Isoproterenol (Isuprel)	MDI, subcutaneous, nebulizer, IV (rarely used)	Stimulates β_1 and β_2 receptors. Primarily affects β_2 receptors. Acts quickly.

*Not currently FDA approved for use as bronchodilator.
†Cardiac stimulant effects are discussed in Chapters 26 and 28.

administering aminophylline in the treatment of acute asthma, intravenous (IV) aminophylline should be considered if the asthma attack is severe or there is minimal or no response to inhaled β agonists. A loading dose is usually administered and then is followed by continuous infusion. Corticosteroids are indicated if the initial response is insufficient (e.g., no response within 30 to 60 minutes), if the client has had several recent asthma attacks, or if the client is receiving steroid therapy. The choice of oral or IV administration of corticosteroids depends on the severity of the attack. Nebulized ipratropium or glycopyrrolate may be administered every 4 to 6 hours if the acute attack does not respond to these measures. Therapy should be continued until the client is breathing comfortably, wheezing has disappeared, and pulmonary function study results are near the client's normal values.

Status asthmaticus. Clients with status asthmaticus require most of the therapeutic measures discussed previously, but there may be increased frequency and dose of inhaled bronchodilators. When an MDI is used, the typical dose is two to six puffs every 3 to 4 or 4 to 6 hours, depending on the medication selected (Table 22-4). Therapy with inhaled agents is usually initiated despite prior home use, since drug delivery at home may have been submaximal and higher doses given under supervision may be beneficial.

Continuous monitoring of the client is critical. Bedside spirometric FEV_1 and PEFR are easy to do and provide objective data on lung function. FEV_1 requires a full and sustained exhalation, whereas PEFR requires only a forceful huff. Therefore PEFR is less tiring and easier to obtain.

IV aminophylline may be added to the treatment regimen if the client does not respond to β-adrenergic drugs. Venous access is initiated, and a loading dose of aminophylline is given during at least a 20-minute period IV piggyback (provided the client has not been taking oral aminophylline preparations before coming to the emergency room). If the client has been taking methylxanthines at home (see Table 22-4), a serum theophylline level should be obtained and a reduced dose of aminophylline may be given. The loading dose is followed by a continuous-maintenance aminophylline infusion.

IV corticosteroids are usually administered, although their peak effect is not apparent for 6 to 12 hours. IV methylprednisolone is administered every 6 hours. Anticholinergic drugs such as ipratropium (Atrovent) are used if the client is taking a β-adrenergic antagonist such as propranolol (Inderal), has serious cardiac dysrhythmias or angina, or is having side effects from β-adrenergic drugs. An anticholinergic drug may also be added to the treatment regimen if severe obstruction persists. The usual dose of ipratropium (Atrovent) is two to four puffs every 4 to 6

Side Effects	Comments
Tachycardia, BP changes, nervousness, palpitations, muscle tremors, nausea, vomiting, vertigo, insomnia, drying oropharynx, headache, hypokalemia	Should not be used in clients with angina or other cardiac disorders. Has fairly rapid onset of action (5-10 min). Duration of action is 3-4 hr. Oral lasts up to 8 hr.
Same as above	Has slow onset of action (15 min). Duration of action is 4-8 hr, extended-release, 8-12 hr.
Same as above	Oral lasts up to 8 hr.
Same as above	Pink appearance of sputum may result. Has fast onset of action (5 min) but short duration of 2-3 hr.
Same as above	Has slow onset of action (except nebulized and subcutaneous route). Duration of action is 4-6 hr.
Same as above	Duration of action is 4-8 hr.
Headache, dizziness, palpitations, tremors, restlessness, hypertension, dysrhythmias, tachycardia	Is used primarily to treat bronchial asthma attacks. Should not be used in client with dysrhythmias or hypertension. Instruct client regarding self-administration of inhalants. Abuse can lead to excessive cardiac side effects. Duration of action is 1-2 hr.
Tachycardia, headache, nausea, palpitations, tremor, insomnia, dysrhythmias	Instruct client regarding self-administration of inhalants. Abuse can lead to excessive cardiac side effects. Duration of action is 1-2 hr. Used today for pulmonary functions testing only.

Continued.

Table 22-4   Drugs Used in the Treatment of Asthma and COPD—cont'd

Drug	Route of Administration	Mechanisms of Action
ANTIINFLAMMATORY AGENTS		
Corticosteroids		
Hydrocortisone (Solu-Cortef)	IV	Have antiinflammatory and immunosuppressive effects. Decrease edema in bronchial airways. Act synergistically with β_2 agonists. Decrease mucus secretion. Are effective in late-phase reaction of asthma.
Methylprednisolone (Medrol)	Oral	
(Solu Medrol)	IV	
Prednisone	Oral	
Beclomethasone (Vanceril, Beclovent)	MDI, nasal spray, ophthalmic solution	Same as above. Acts locally in respiratory tract with relatively little systemic absorption.
Triamcinolone acetonide (Azmacort)	MDI	Same as above.
Flunisolide (Aerobid)	MDI	Same as above.
Mast cell stabilizer		
Cromolyn sodium (Aarane, Intal)	Nebulizer, spin inhaler, MDI, nasal spray, ophthalmic solution	Inhibits release of histamine and SRS-A by acting directly on mast cell. May act by interference with calcium ion influx across cell membrane.
ANTICHOLINERGICS		
Atropine sulfate, ipratropium (Atrovent), atropine, methonitrate, glycopyrrolate, (Robinul)	Nebulizer, MDI	Blocks action of acetylcholine, resulting in bronchodilatation.
METHYLXANTHINE DERIVATIVES		
Slow-acting agents: Slo-Phyllin, Aminophylline, Theolair, Choledyl, Somophyllin; *intravenous agent:* Aminophylline; *sustained-release agents:* Aminodur, Dura-tabs, Choledyl SA, Constant-T, Theo-Dur, Theolair-SR, Elixophyllin, Slo-Bid Gyrocaps, Theo-Dur Sprinkles; *24 hr agents:* Theo-24, Uniphyl	Oral tablets, IV, elixir, rectal suppositories (rarely used)	Major effects are relaxation of bronchial smooth muscles, and improved contractility of fatigued diaphragm. Other effects are mild diuresis, increased gastric acid secretion, stimulation of mucociliary clearance, stimulation of CNS and respiration, pulmonary vasodilatation, improved exercise tolerance.
MUCOLYTICS		
Acetylcysteine (Mucomyst) (10% and 20%)	Nebulizer	Enzyme breaks down mucoproteins. Decreases viscosity of mucus and enhances mobilization of secretions.
Iodinated glycerol (Organidin)	Oral tablets, elixir	Increases output of thin respiratory tract fluid. Liquefies mucus.

SRS-A, Slow-reacting substance of anaphylaxis.

Side Effects	Comments
Cushingoid appearance, skin changes (acne, striae, bruising), osteoporosis, increased appetite, obesity; peptic ulcer, hypertension, hypokalemia, cataracts, menstrual irregularities, muscle weakness, immunosuppression, catabolic, dysphonia, growth retardation	Alternate-day therapy minimizes side effects. Oral dose should be taken in morning with food or milk. When given in high doses, client must be observed for epigastric distress. H_2 blockers (ranitidine, cimetidine) and antacids may help minimize GI effects. Clients taking long-term steroids may be given vitamin D and calcium to prevent osteoporosis. Should never be abruptly discontinued but tapered gradually over time to prevent adrenal insufficiency. If during tapering client has recurrence of symptoms, physician should be notified. Are usually used concomitantly with bronchodilator.
Oral thrush infections, hoarseness, irritated throat, dry mouth, cough, few systemic effects	Is not recommended for acute asthma attack. Rinse mouth with water or mouthwash after use to prevent oral fungal infections. Use after MDI bronchodilator. MDI steroids should be discontinued during acute asthma attack. Nasal spray and eye drops are used for allergic rhinitis.
Same as above	Same as above.
Same as above	Requires only twice-a-day use.
Irritation of throat, relatively nontoxic effects, bronchospasm	Not a bronchodilator. Used for asthma (e.g., before exercise) prophylactically if allergen is causative agent. May use bronchodilator inhaler 5-10 min before cromolyn inhaler is used. Instruct client in correct use of inhaler. May follow treatment with glass of water to reduce pharyngeal irritation. May take 4-6 wk before clinical response occurs. Nasal spray and eye drops used for allergic rhinitis and conjunctivitis.
Drying of oral mucosa, cough, flushing of skin, bad taste, fewer systemic effects with glycopyrrolate	Atropine is contraindicated in clients with glaucoma and bladder neck obstruction. Ipratropium bromide can be used in clients with glaucoma and bladder neck obstruction. Half-life of ipratropium is 3-4 hr. Its duration is longer than that of atropine. Atropine's duration of action is longer than that of β_2-agents. These drugs can be used alone or in conjunction with β agonists in nebulizers. Alternating schedules of β-adrenergic and atropine administration may be helpful in some clients. Temporary blurred vision will occur if sprayed in eyes.
Tachycardia, blood pressure changes, dysrhythmias, anorexia, nausea, vomiting, nervousness, irritability, headache, muscle twitching, flushing, epigastric pain, diarrhea, insomnia, palpitations	Wide variety of response to drug metabolism exists. Therapeutic theophylline level should be 10-20 μg. Half-life is decreased by smoking and is increased by heart failure and liver disease. Cimetidine, ciprofloxacin, and erythromycin may rapidly increase theophylline levels. Gastrointestinal side effects may be alleviated by taking drug with food or antacids. Client should be instructed to lie down if dizziness is experienced. Client must be encouraged to take drugs even when feeling well. Extra doses should not be taken when symptoms are present unless prescribed by physician. Side effects should be reported but medication not stopped unless symptoms are severe. Sustained-release tablets should be taken whole and not chewed or crushed. If client has difficulty swallowing, bead-filled preparations may be used, and they can be emptied onto food but should not be chewed.
Bronchospasm, hemoptysis, nausea, vomiting	After administration of mucolytics, secretions may become profuse. Use of mucolytic agents may not be necessary if client is kept well hydrated and humidified. Usually combined with bronchodilator when administered.
Gastrointestinal irritation, rash, thyroid gland enlargement	Same as above, except agent is not usually combined with a bronchodilator.

hours. Magnesium has been used in certain situations to treat status asthmaticus. It acts by relaxing the bronchial smooth muscle.

Supplemental O_2 is given by Venturi mask or nasal prongs (typically 2 L/min) to achieve a Pao_2 of at least 60 mm Hg. An arterial catheter may be inserted to facilitate frequent ABG monitoring. Because the client's insensible loss of fluids is increased and the metabolic rate is increased, IV fluids are given to provide optimal hydration. Sodium bicarbonate administration is usually limited to treatment of severe metabolic or respiratory acidosis (pH <7.29), since effective bronchodilatation by adrenergic agents is not possible if the client has extreme acidosis. Bronchoscopy, although rarely performed during an acute attack, may be necessary to remove thick mucous plugs.

Occasionally, asthma attacks are so severe that the client requires mechanical ventilation if there is no response to treatment. Indications for mechanical ventilation are persistence or progressive CO_2 retention and respiratory acidosis, clinical deterioration indicated by fatigue and hypersomnolence, and cardiopulmonary arrest. In status asthmaticus the goals of initiating mechanical ventilation are to achieve a Pao_2 equal to or greater than 60 mm Hg and a normal pH.

Louder wheezing may actually occur in the airways that are responding to the therapy as airflow in the airways increases. As improvement continues and airflow increases, breath sounds increase and wheezing decreases. As the client begins to respond to therapy and symptoms begin to subside, it is important to remember that despite the disappearance of most of the bronchospasm, the edema and cellular infiltration of the airway mucosa and the viscid mucous plugs may take several days to improve. Thus intensive therapy must be continued even after clinical improvement has occurred. Steroid dosage is usually tapered rapidly, and the client is given oral steroids for several weeks. IV aminophylline and frequent airway care with aerosolized medications and chest physiotherapy is continued for several days after clinical improvement is noted. The client's cough often becomes productive of mucous plugs, and chest sounds improve. If the client is asked to perform a forced expiratory maneuver, a faint wheeze may still be heard. Finally, the client can be switched to oral bronchodilators and can use a β_2-adrenergic MDI before discharge.

Chronic asthma. Clients who have persistent airflow obstruction and frequent attacks of asthma should be taught to avoid asthma attacks by avoiding triggers of acute attacks and treating themselves before exercise. The choice of drug therapy for chronic asthma depends on the severity of symptoms. Most require inhaled β-adrenergic drugs on a regular basis (e.g., two puffs every 4 to 6 hours). The client with mild asthma or EIA should use inhaled β_2-adrenergic agents before engaging in exercise or when anticipating exposure to antigens known to cause asthma. For more severe asthma, inhaled corticosteroids, oral sustained-release theophylline drugs, inhaled cromolyn, and/or inhaled ipratropium can be used to alleviate symptoms. Some persons require continuous oral corticosteroids, which should be maintained at as low a dosage as

possible and administered on alternate days (if possible) to reduce systemic side effects. Methotrexate and troleandomycin (TAO) may be used in clients with chronic steroid-dependent asthma or COPD who have required very high doses of oral prednisone. Methotrexate and TAO are used in combination with methylprednisolone (Medrol) to decrease the dose of this drug required by prolonging its half-life.

Pharmacological Management

Bronchodilators. Three classes of bronchodilator drugs currently used in asthma therapy are β-adrenergic agonists, methylxanthine derivatives, and anticholinergics (see Table 22-4).

β-Adrenergic agonist drugs. β Agonists are by far the most effective bronchodilators currently in use.[13] Activation of β_2-adrenergic receptors on airway smooth muscle leads to activation of adenylate cyclase and to an increase in intracellular cAMP and subsequent bronchodilatation (Fig. 22-7). β Agonists relax the smooth muscle of all airways from the trachea to the terminal bronchioles. There is also evidence that β adrenergics increase mucociliary clearance.

Inhaled selective β_2 agonists (e.g., metaproterenol, albuterol, terbutaline, fenoterol) have a rapid onset of action (within minutes) and are effective for 3 to 6 hours when asthma is not severe. Inhaled β agonists are indicated for the short-term relief of bronchoconstriction and are the treatment of choice for acute exacerbations of asthma. They are also useful in prevention of bronchospasm precipitated by exercise and other stimuli because they prevent mediator release from mast cells and neurotransmitter release from cholinergic nerves. They do not inhibit either the late-phase reaction or the subsequent bronchial hyperresponsiveness.

Longer-acting β_2 agonists that are inhaled, such as formoterol and salmeterol, are currently undergoing clinical trials. There is no indication for the administration of nonselective β-adrenergic agonists (e.g., isoproterenol), which are associated with a high incidence of cardiovascular side effects (e.g., tachycardia, palpitations) because of their stimulation of β_1-adrenergic receptors.

Orally administered β agonists are less useful because of the increased incidence of side effects from these preparations. The most common side effects are tremor, tachycardia, and palpitations.

Methylxanthine derivatives. Methylxanthine derivative (theophylline) preparations are less effective bronchodilators than β agonists.[13] Although historically they have been the first-choice therapy for asthma, there is now a trend toward introducing theophylline as an additional bronchodilator later in the therapeutic regimen. Theophylline may have a synergistic effect with β agonists. Theophylline is not effective as an inhalant and must be given orally or intravenously as aminophylline. The therapeutic plasma concentration is 10 to 20 μg/ml.

The main therapeutic action of methylxanthine derivatives on the respiratory system is bronchodilatation. Traditionally, theophylline was thought to exert bronchodilatation by inhibiting the production of phosphodiesterase,

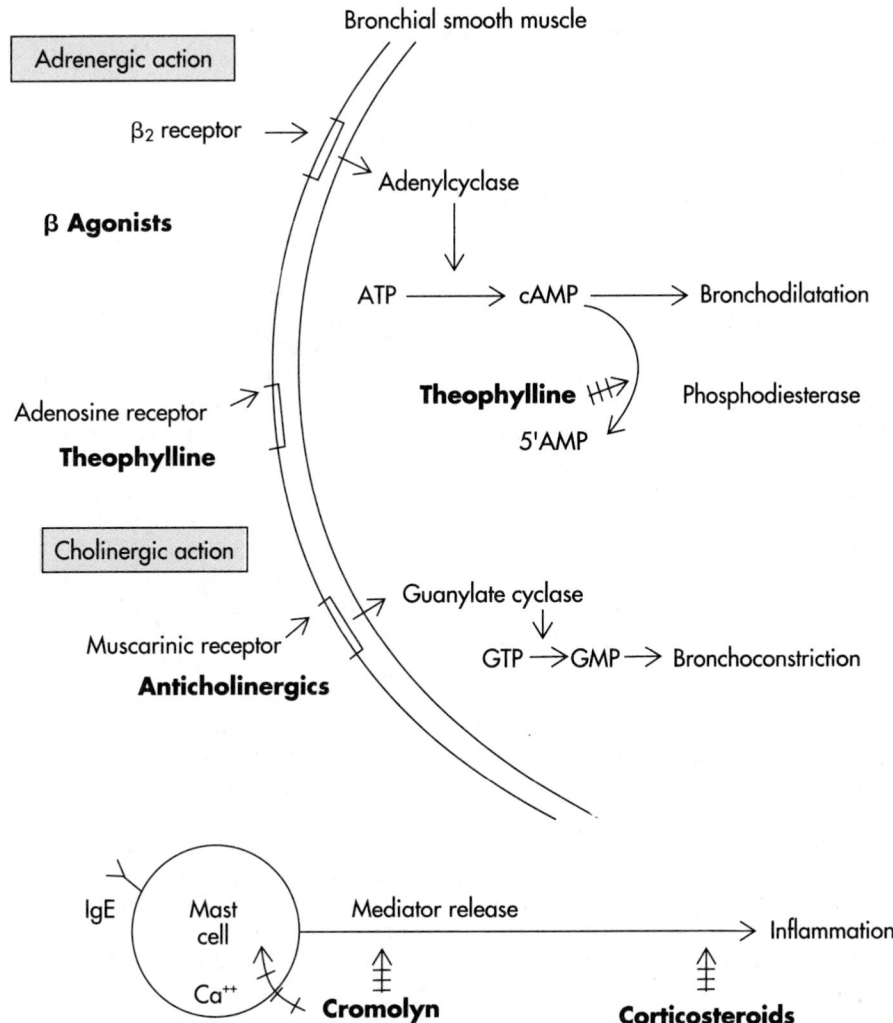

Fig. 22-7 Mechanism of action of drugs used in asthma and COPD. Bronchodilatation can occur from stimulation of β_2 receptors, blocking of cholinergic receptors, and inhibition of phosphodiesterase. Cromolyn may prevent the influx of calcium and stabilize mast cells, preventing mediator release. Theophylline may also act by antagonizing the adenosine receptor on the smooth muscle cell. Corticosteroids act to suppress the inflammatory response.

thus preventing the breakdown of cAMP (Fig. 22-7). However, current research has shown that bronchodilatation occurs only minimally at therapeutic theophylline concentrations. It is now theorized that theophylline's bronchodilatory effect occurs secondarily to its effect on calcium ion influx into cell membranes and/or its inhibition of certain prostaglandins that cause bronchoconstriction.

Theophylline inhibits the late-phase reaction, implying that it has antiinflammatory action. However, it does not prevent bronchial hyperresponsiveness. Long-acting theophylline products administered at bedtime are used to treat clients with nocturnal asthma. The main problem with theophylline is the relatively high incidence of side effects, which include nausea, headache, gastrointestinal (GI) distress, cardiac dysrhythmias, and seizures.

Anticholinergic drugs. Airway diameter is predominantly controlled by the parasympathetic division of the autonomic nervous system. The effects of acetylcholine on the airways are increased mucus secretion and smooth muscle contraction, resulting in bronchoconstriction. Anticholinergic agents (e.g., ipratropium) inhibit only the component of bronchoconstriction caused by cholinergic nerves. Thus they are less effective than β agonists and are usually used in combination with other bronchodilators.

The onset of action of anticholinergics is slower than β agonists, peaking at 1 hour and lasting longer, usually up to 8 hours. Systemic side effects of anticholinergics are uncommon with ipratropium because it is poorly absorbed.

Antiinflammatory drugs. Because chronic inflammation is a primary component of asthma, agents such as corticosteroids and cromolyn, which suppress the inflammatory response, are important therapeutic agents in the treatment of asthma. These drugs do not have an immediate effect and may be regarded as prophylactic therapy.

Corticosteroids. Although corticosteroids are remarkably effective in suppressing the inflammation induced by asthma, they are still greatly underused.[14] Steroids do not block the classic immediate response to allergens but do block the late-phase reaction and subsequent bronchial hyperresponsiveness. The onset of action occurs about 3 to 6 hours after administration. They act by inhibiting the release of mediators from macrophages and eosinophils, reducing the microvascular leakage in the airways, inhibiting the influx of inflammatory cells into the reactive site, and decreasing peripheral blood eosinophilia.

Steroids given by inhalation (e.g., beclomethasone, flunisolide, triamcinolone) are active topically and can control the disease without systemic side effects. Steroids are effective when used twice a day in stable asthma or four times a day if asthma becomes unstable.

Short courses of orally administered steroids are indicated for acute exacerbations of asthma, particularly after viral infections. Maintenance dosages of oral corticosteroids may be necessary to control asthma in a minority of clients. A single dose in the morning to coincide with endogenous cortisol production is associated with fewer side effects. In addition, alternate-day dosing is associated with fewer side effects.

Cromolyn sodium. Cromolyn sodium (Intal) is thought to inhibit the release of mediators from mast cells, thus inhibiting the immediate response from exercise and allergens. It also prevents the late-phase response and bronchial hyperresponsiveness by acting on macrophages and eosinophils. Cromolyn also prevents the bronchoconstriction induced by sulfur dioxide and bradykinin. It is not effective in all clients, and there is no way to predict who is most likely to respond. It is the antiinflammatory drug of first choice in children, but it can also be used with success in adults for EIA and seasonal allergen asthma. Client education, which emphasizes rationale for use and correct method of administration, is important for effective client compliance.

Client teaching related to drug therapy. Information about medications should include the name, dosage, method of administration, schedule (in relation to meals and activities of daily living), purpose, side effects, appropriate action if side effects occur, consequences of improper use, and the importance of refilling the prescription before the medication runs out. A sample medication instruction sheet for clients is presented in Fig. 22-8.

Inhalation of drugs is often preferred to oral administration because a lower dose is needed and systemic side effects are reduced. In bronchodilators the onset of action is faster. Inhalation devices include nebulizers and MDIs (Fig. 22-9). Nebulizers, which deliver a large dose with tidal breathing, are usually used for severe asthma and in children. MDIs are usually effective, but some persons, particularly children and older adults, may have problems with the coordination needed to activate and inhale.

Clients should be given the following instructions on the use of MDIs:

1. Assemble inhaler and briefly shake contents.
2. Exhale completely.
3. Hold inhaler approximately 1 to 1½ inches from opened mouth (this helps to prevent impaction of the medication in the mouth and pharynx).
4. Inhale deeply while activating the inhaler so that the medication is sucked into the lungs with inspiration.
5. Immediately close mouth and hold a deep inspiration for 5 to 10 seconds.
6. Wait 1 to 2 minutes and repeat from step 1.
7. Rinse inhaler and mouth with water (this reduces the chance of an oral infection developing).

Steps 2 and 3 are the most difficult to coordinate. Tube spacers or reservoirs (Fig. 22-9, *C*) can be used for clients with poor coordination. These allow for slow inhalation of the particles without worry of timing of the propellant with the inhalation cycle. Although it is not the preferred or recommended way, step 3 can be modified so that the inhaler is placed in the open mouth but with the lips not sealed around the mouthpiece. With this method, room air is entrained to help accelerate the movement of the medication into the lungs.

One of the major problems with metered-dose adrenergic drugs is the potential for abuse (i.e., using them much more frequently than prescribed rather than seeking needed medical care). Therefore the client must receive explicit instructions in the correct therapeutic use of these drugs.

Poor compliance with asthma therapy remains a major problem in the long-term management of chronic asthma. Clients will use β-agonist inhalers because they provide immediate relief of symptoms. However, they often do not take prophylactic therapy (inhaled steroids or cromolyn) regularly because they see no immediate benefit. It is important to explain to the client the importance and purpose of taking regularly inhaled steroid therapy and to emphasize that the maximal improvement may take weeks to months.

Nonprescription combination drugs. Several nonprescription combination products are available as over-the-counter (OTC) drugs. They are usually combinations of a bronchodilator, an expectorant, and a sedative. (Some of these drugs are listed in Table 22-5.) These agents are advertised as drugs to relieve bronchospasm. In general, they should be avoided by persons with obstructive lung disease. Many persons consider these drugs safe because they can be obtained without a prescription.

Some of the dangers of these drugs are as follows[13]:

1. Epinephrine acts for only a short period of time, and rebound bronchospasm may occur.
2. Clients seeking relief have a tendency to overuse the agent.
3. A combination of ephedrine and theophylline can enhance the adverse side effects of each of these drugs.
4. Phenobarbital interferes with the action of steroids

MEDICATION INSTRUCTIONS FOR PULMONARY PATIENTS

Name: _____

Your diagnosis is: ☐ Chronic Obstructive Pulmonary Disease (COPD)   ☐ Chronic Bronchitis
☐ Emphysema   ☐ Asthma
☐ _____
Your medications are checked and the dosage is written.

☐ OXYGEN at _____ liters per minute for _____ hours a day.

☐ Oxygen is prescribed to decrease the strain on your heart and to keep your oxygen in your blood (PaO$_2$) normal.

☐ BRONCHODILATOR MEDICINES

These medications relax the muscles around your air tubes (bronchial tubes) and keep your air tubes open (dilated) so that you can breathe easier.

Important: Bronchodilator medications may have other effects that you'll notice. These include upset stomach, heartburn, and palpitations and feeling jittery or nervous and muscle tremors. Taking the pills with food or an antacid can help. If these side effects are bothersome, please let us know. Also, it is important not to overuse your bronchodilator inhaler or nebulizer treatment. Only use it every 2-3 hours for shortness of breath. If you find that you need it more often, contact us.

☐ PILLS

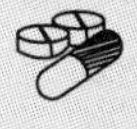

☐ Theodur _____ milligram (mg.) tablets, take _____ tablets every _____ hours.
☐ Brethine/bricanyl (Terbutaline) _____ mg. tablets, take _____ tablets every _____ hours.
☐ Alupent (Metaproterenol) _____ mg. tablets, take _____ tablets every _____ hours.
☐ Ventolin (Albuterol) _____ mg. tablets, take _____ tablets every _____ hours.

_____

☐ INHALERS

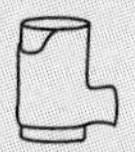

☐ Alupent (Metaproterenol) – White   ☐ Brethair (Terbutaline) – Yellow and white
☐ Ventolin (Albuterol) – Blue   ☐ Maxair (Pirbuterol) – Blue and white
☐ Proventil (Albuterol) – Yellow
Use _____ puff (s) of your inhaler:
   ☐ 4 times a day (e.g. with meals and at bedtime) and every 2-3 hours as needed for increased shortness of breath

_____

☐ Atrovent (Ipatropium) Green and white
A bronchodilator with a different mode of action that those above, it is frequently used in combination with above inhalers. Use _____ puff(s) of Atrovent 4 times a day.

_____

☐ Rotohaler (Ventolin or Proventol)

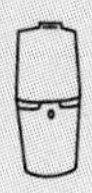

Use _____ capsule(s) 4 times a day (e.g. with meals and at bedtime) and every 2-3 hours as needed for shortness of breath.

☐ NEBULIZER TREATMENTS

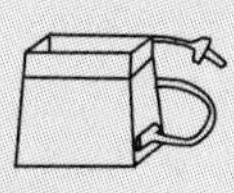

☐ Alupent (Metaproterenol) use _____ cc in _____ cc of saline, take _____ times a day, and every 2-3 hours as needed for shortness of breath.
☐ Ventolin/proventil (Albuterol) use _____ cc in _____ cc of saline, take _____ times a day, and every 2-3 hours as needed for shortness of breath.
☐ Atropine (20 cc bottle with 0.4 mg/cc) use _____ cc _____ times a day. Do not dilute further with saline.

_____

Fig. 22-8 Medication instructions for pulmonary patients. (Courtesy Lovelace Medical Center, Albuquerque, NM.)   *Continued.*

☐ CORTICOSTEROIDS (Steroids)

These medications are all relatives of the hormone cortisol, which is normally produced by your body. They help to dilate the bronchial tubes, decrease the swelling of the bronchial tube lining, and decrease lung inflammation. All steroids must be taken on a regular schedule because they do not give immediate effects; rather, they prevent wheezing, so they are *not* to be used as you "need" them, but regularly to prevent symptoms. They must never be discontinued suddenly, and they should be taken only as directed by your physician.

☐ Prednisone _____ milligram (mg) tablets, take _____ tablets every morning _____ tablets every other morning as listed in the following schedule:

_____

_____

_____

Note: Always take your prednisone in the morning (if it is only once a day) and with milk or food always.

☐ STEROID INHALERS

    ☐ Vanceril (Beclomethasone) – Pink   ☐ Beclovent (Beclomethasone) – Brown

    ☐ Azmacort (Triamcinolone acetonide) – White   ☐ Aerobid (Flunisolide) – Purple and gray

Take _____ puffs _____ times a day (1-2 minutes) after you take your bronchodilator inhaler or nebulizer treatment. Eat food or rinse your mouth with water after using.

☐ INTAL (Cromolyn sodium)

This is a medication that is used to prevet asthma (wheezing). Since it only works to prevent asthma, it must be taken regularly. Take _____ puffs of Intal Inhaler _____ times a day. Take _____ mg liquid medication in your nebulizer _____ times a day. Cromolyn may be taken about 1-2 minutes after your bronchodilator inhaler of nebulizer treatment.

☐ OTHER MEDICATIONS

☐ Diuretics (water pills): _____

☐ Antibiotics (fight infection): Please complete your entire prescription of antibiotics. _____

☐ Antihypertensives (lower blood pressure and decrease the work of your heart): _____

☐ Potassium supplements (replace potassium that is lost with certain diuretics and with prednisone): _____

☐ Stomach medications (decrease stomach acid secretion or relieve heart burn): _____

☐ Other medications: _____

_____

_____

_____

Fig. 22-8—cont'd   Medication instructions for pulmonary patients. (Courtesy Lovelace Medical Center, Albuquerque, NM.)

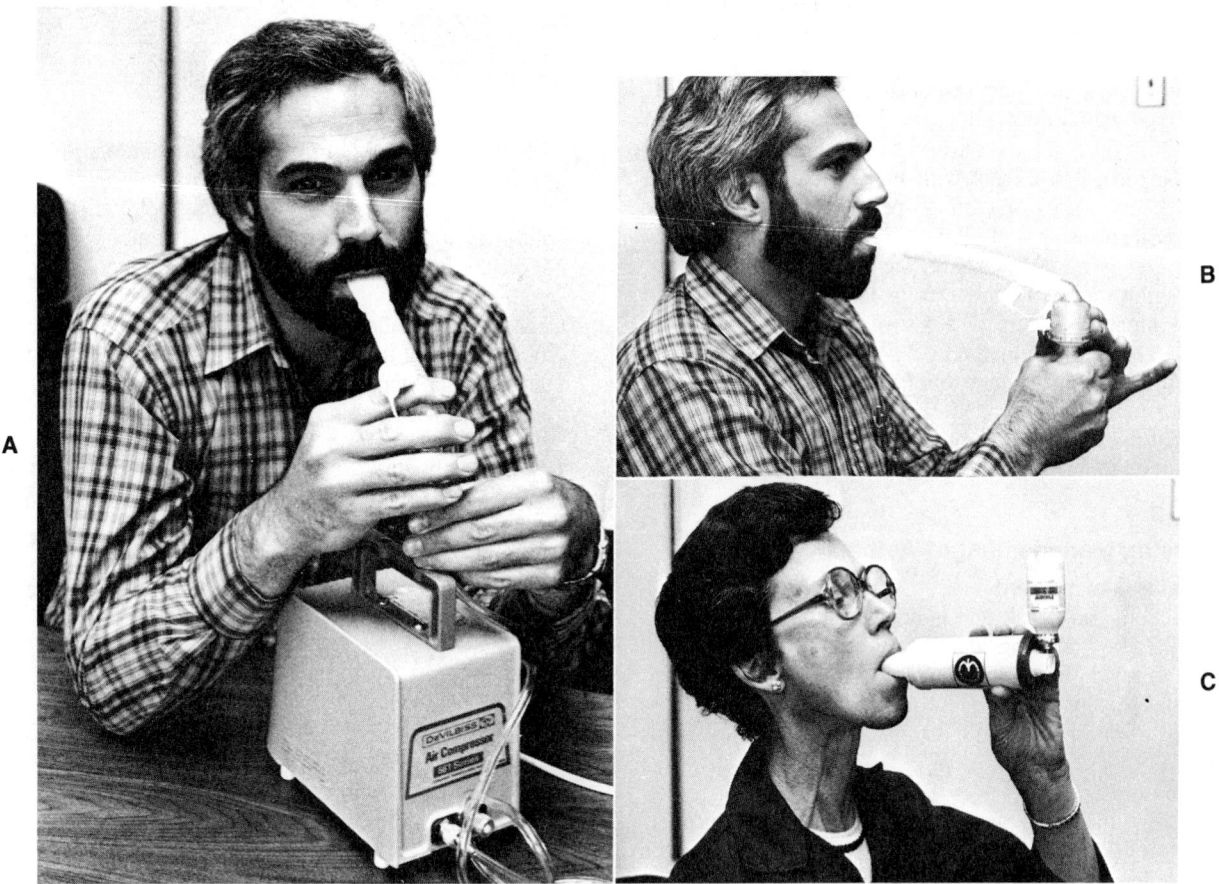

Fig. 22-9 Methods of administering inhaled respiratory treatments. **A,** Solution can be administered by inhalation with a nebulizer powered by a compressor. **B,** Solution can be administered with a hand-bulb nebulizer. **C,** An MDI with a spacer. (From Wiener M and Pepper G: Clinical pharmacology and therapeutics in nursing, ed 2, New York, 1985, Mc-Graw-Hill Book Co, p 435.)

Table 22-5   Nonprescription Combination Asthma Drugs

Drug Product	Ingredients		
	Sympathomimetic	**Xanthine**	**Other**
Amodrine	Ephedrine	Aminophylline	Phenobarbital
Asthma Nefrin inhalant	Epinephrine	—	Chlorobutanol
Bronkaid tablets	Ephedrine	Theophylline	Guaifenesin
Bronkaid mist	Epinephrine	—	Ascorbic acid, alcohol
Bronkotabs	Ephedrine	Theophylline	Guaifenesin, phenobarbital
Primatene M tablets	Ephedrine	Theophylline	Pyrilamine
Primatene P tablets	Ephedrine	Theophylline	Phenobarbital
Primatene Mist	Epinephrine	—	Ascorbic acid, alcohol
Tedral	Ephedrine	Theophylline	Phenobarbital
Vaponefrin inhalant	Epinephrine	—	Chlorobutanol
Verquad	Ephedrine	Theophylline	Guaifenesin, phenobarbital

and thus is contraindicated in asthma clients receiving steroid therapy.

5. Freon is a gas used to propel some inhalant medications. It can cause bronchospasm and possibly cardiac dysrhythmias.

An important teaching responsibility of health professionals is to warn clients about the dangers associated with nonprescription combination drugs. These drugs are especially dangerous to clients with underlying cardiac problems. Clients who insist on or persist in taking one of these medications should be cautioned to read and follow the accompanying directions on the label. Another way of discouraging the use of these drugs is to monitor carefully and reevaluate the effectiveness of the prescribed drug therapy. The drug regimen may have to be adjusted to help the client obtain maximum relief from bronchospasm. An attitude of understanding and caring will often reassure the client that the health care workers are concerned. This may prevent the client from attempting to find relief at the local drugstore.

■ Nursing Management of Asthma

Nursing assessment

If a client can speak and is not in acute distress, a detailed history, including identification of any precipitating factors and what has helped to alleviate attacks in the past, can be taken. Subjective and objective data that should be obtained from a person with asthma are presented in Table 22-6.

Nursing diagnoses

Nursing diagnoses are determined when the problem and etiological factors are supported by clinical data. Nursing diagnoses related to asthma may include, but are not limited to, those presented in Table 22-7.

Nursing interventions

Health promotion and maintenance. The nursing role in preventing asthma attacks or decreasing their severity focuses primarily on teaching the client and family. The client should be taught to avoid, if possible, known potential allergens (e.g., cigarette smoke) and precipitating factors (e.g., excess exercise, cold air, aspirin). Staying indoors when there is a high degree of air pollution may be helpful. If cold air cannot be avoided, dressing properly with scarves or using a mask may prevent an asthma attack. Aspirin and nonsteroidal antiinflammatory drugs such as indomethacin should be avoided if they are known to precipitate an attack. Many OTC drugs contain aspirin, and the client should be instructed to read the labels carefully. Desensitization (immunotherapy) may be partially effective in decreasing the client's sensitivity to known allergens (see Chapter 8).

Prompt diagnosis and treatment of upper respiratory tract infections may prevent an exacerbation of asthma. If occupational irritants are involved as etiological factors, the client may need to consider changing jobs. β-Blocking agents such as propranolol are contraindicated. (These drugs and their indications for use are discussed in Chapters 28 and 29.)

The client should be encouraged to maintain a fluid intake of 2 to 3 L/day, good nutrition, and adequate rest. If

Table 22-6

Nursing Assessment of the Client with Asthma

SUBJECTIVE DATA

History
Positive family history of allergies or respiratory disease; allergic rhinitis; relationship of symptoms to seasons, exposure to pollen, danders, feathers, mold, dust, foods and milk, inhaled irritants, infection, weather changes, exercise, emotion, smoking; number of attacks per week

Medications
Use and discontinuance of steroids, bronchodilators, cromolyn sodium; medications that may precipitate an attack such as aspirin, nonsteroidal antiinflammatory agents, β blockers, indomethacin, cholinergics, antibiotics

General
Decreased exercise tolerance, insomnia, fear, fatigue, emotional or physical stress

Respiratory
Dyspnea, cough, sputum production (amount, character, color), chest tightness, feelings of suffocation, air hunger

OBJECTIVE DATA

General
Anxiety, restlessness or exhaustion, confusion, appearance, body position

Integumentary
Diaphoresis, cyanosis (circumoral, nailbed)

Respiratory
Wheezing, crackles, diminished or absent breath sounds, and rhonchi on auscultation; sputum (thick, white, tenacious), increased work of breathing with use of accessory muscles; intercostal and supraclavicular retractions; tachypnea with hyperventilation; prolonged expiration

Cardiovascular
Tachycardia, pulsus paradoxus, jugular venous distention, hypertension or hypotension, premature ventricular contractions

Possible findings
Abnormal ABGs during attacks, elevated serum IgE, positive skin tests for allergens, chest x-ray film demonstrating hyperinflation with attacks, abnormal pulmonary function tests showing decreased flow rates, FVC, FEV_1, PEFR, and FEV_1/FVC ratio that improve between attacks and with bronchodilators

exercise is planned, administering cromolyn sodium 15 to 30 minutes before should prevent bronchospasm.

Acute intervention. An important nursing goal during an acute attack is to decrease the client's sense of panic. A calm, quiet, reassuring attitude may help the client to relax. The client should be positioned comfortably (usually sitting) to maximize chest expansion. Staying with the client and being available provide additional comfort. It is important to monitor the client's respiratory and cardiovas-

Table 22-7

NURSING CARE PLAN FOR THE CLIENT WITH ASTHMA

Defining Characteristics	Nursing Interventions	Evaluation Criteria

NURSING DIAGNOSIS: Ineffective breathing pattern related to increased airway resistance caused by bronchospasm, mucosal edema, and mucus production

Defining Characteristics	Nursing Interventions	Evaluation Criteria
Dyspnea, wheezing, rapid respiratory rate, use of accessory muscles	Provide comfortable position (e.g., bed rest in high Fowler's position or recliner chair). Administer bronchodilators as ordered. Administer humidified O_2. Auscultate breath sounds q 1-2 hr. Monitor ABGs and/or pulse oximetry. Assess blood pressure, heart rate, respiratory rate, and level of consciousness q 15 min until stable and then q 2-4 hr. Premedicate with bronchodilators before doing deep-breathing and coughing exercises or chest physiotherapy. Evaluate effectiveness of nebulizer treatments and assess need for increase or decrease in frequency of treatments. Teach client to slow respiratory rate, breathing in deeply through the nose and exhaling 2-3 times (as long as inspiration) through pursed lips. Assess and document breathing pattern including respiratory rate, depth, relationship of inspiration to exhalation, use of accessory muscles, presence of chest discomfort. If ordered, assist with pulmonary function tests.	Absence of wheezing and chest tightness, return of breath sounds indicating better airflow, respiratory rate of 12-24/min, ABGs, oximetry, and pulmonary function tests within normal limits

NURSING DIAGNOSIS: Ineffective airway clearance related to bronchospasm, ineffective cough, excessive mucus production, tenacious secretions, and fatigue

Defining Characteristics	Nursing Interventions	Evaluation Criteria
Ineffective cough, inability to raise airway secretions, adventitious breath sounds	Monitor and control environment for possible allergens (e.g., dust, smoke, flowers). Auscultate, percuss, and palpate lungs to assess sounds. Assess client's ability to cough effectively. Teach effective coughing techniques.* If client is unable to cough and/or expectorate secretions, evaluate possible causes (e.g., respiratory muscle fatigue, thick secretions, severe bronchospasm, decreased level of consciousness). As ordered, assist in and evaluate administration of bronchodilator drugs, steroid therapy, chest physiotherapy. Observe and note character and quantity of coughed or suctioned sputum and secretions. If ordered, send sputum for Gram stain and culture and sensitivity.	No bronchospasm, breath sounds indicating good air movement, effective and productive cough of clear or white secretions

NURSING DIAGNOSIS: Activity intolerance related to fatigue secondary to exertion and inadequate oxygenation

Defining Characteristics	Nursing Interventions	Evaluation Criteria
Inability or unwillingness to ambulate, increase in pulse and respirations on exertion	Evaluate fatigue in relationship to work of breathing (signs of hypercarbia, hypoxemia). Have extension tubing hooked to O_2. Plan 1-2 hr rest periods. Provide total care for client at onset with progressive self-care as tolerated. Provide small amounts of liquid, progressing to soft diet.	Feeling of being rested, increased energy to do self-care activities

*See Table 22-12.

Continued.

Table 22-7

 NURSING CARE PLAN FOR THE CLIENT WITH ASTHMA—cont'd

Defining Characteristics	Nursing Interventions	Evaluation Criteria
NURSING DIAGNOSIS: Sleep pattern disturbance related to dyspnea, anxiety, frequent assessments and treatments, and side effects of some medications		
Dyspnea, inability to sleep or sleep for short intervals only, inability to fall asleep, not rested on awakening	Administer O_2 as ordered. Plan nursing care so that uninterrupted periods of sleep are possible. If possible, administer medications that increase heart rate several hours before bedtime. Observe for signs and symptoms of sleep apnea syndrome.	Sleeping for several hours at a time, feeling rested on awakening
NURSING DIAGNOSIS: Anxiety related to difficulty breathing, perceived or actual loss of control, and fear of suffocation		
Anxiety over condition, restlessness, elevated vital signs	Interact with client in a calm, unhurried, supportive manner. Explanations should be simple and concise. Directions may need to be repeated several times. Do *not* sedate. Stay with client. Encourage and demonstrate slow, deep breathing. Promptly treat any exacerbations of an attack. Anticipate client's needs. Provide anticipatory guidance for client to prevent exacerbations. Place in room near nurses' station or where client can be frequently observed. Teach relaxation techniques.	Calm feeling, reduction of anxiety over asthma
NURSING DIAGNOSIS: High risk for respiratory infection related to decreased pulmonary function, ineffective airway clearance, and possible steroid therapy		
Elevated temperature, pulse, and respiration; productive cough; adventitious breath sounds	If sputum is mucopurulent, obtain sputum Gram stain and culture and sensitivity. Administer antibiotic as ordered. Monitor temperature q 4 hr and prn, sputum character and quantity. Monitor for localized decrease in breath sounds, decreased Pao_2, inability to raise secretions. Provide deep-breathing and coughing exercises. Monitor all respiratory treatments that are administered.	No sputum or clear to white sputum, normal temperature, clear chest x-ray film
NURSING DIAGNOSIS: High risk for fluid volume deficit related to inadequate intake secondary to fatigue, excessive loss resulting from tachypnea, and diaphoresis		
Thick sputum, dry mucous membranes and skin, decreased urinary output	Administer IV fluids as ordered. Later, encourage oral fluids to 3000 ml/day. Provide for oral hygiene. Monitor intake and output and body weight. May use *humidified* O_2 equipment. Assess viscosity and ease of expectorating sputum. Monitor vital signs at least q 2-4 hr.	Moist mucous membranes and thin, easily expectorated sputum

cular systems. This includes auscultating lung sounds; taking the pulse rate, respiratory rate, and blood pressure; and monitoring ABGs or pulse oximetry and PEFR rates if used. The client's work of breathing (i.e., use of accessory muscles, degree of fatigue) and response to therapy should also be evaluated.

When the acute attack subsides, the nurse should provide rest and a quiet, calm environment for the client. When the client has recovered from exhaustion, the nurse should attempt to obtain information about the client's history and pattern of asthma. A thorough assessment should be done (see Table 22-6). This information is important in

Table 22-7

NURSING CARE PLAN FOR THE CLIENT WITH ASTHMA—cont'd

Defining Characteristics	Nursing Interventions	Evaluation Criteria

NURSING DIAGNOSIS: Altered health maintenance related to lack of knowledge about management of bronchospasms, medications, use of nebulizer, role of proper rest and activity, adequate hydration, signs and symptoms of respiratory infection, and factors that may precipitate an asthma attack

Defining Characteristics	Nursing Interventions	Evaluation Criteria
Frequent questioning regarding all aspects of long-term management	Administer bronchodilators as prescribed. Increase activity as tolerated. Assess client's response to bronchodilators, hydration, and increased activity. Assess client's understanding and develop a teaching plan for home care including proper balance of rest and activity; names, actions, side effects, frequency, and dose of prescribed medications; use of nebulizer and inhaler; use of inhaled bronchodilator before strenuous activity to prevent attack; and avoidance of allergens and irritants. Explain effect of dehydration on sputum production and consequent effect on bronchospasm. Assist in planning client's self-administered adequate fluid intake. Explain factors that may contribute to infections and assist in planning preventive measures. Explain method to evaluate color, character, and amount of sputum on regular basis. Review physician's orders with regard to infection and acute attack (take medications as ordered or seek medical attention). Assist in identifying factors that have precipitated attacks and develop plans to prevent them. Stress importance of taking medications regularly as ordered. Teach client to seek medical attention if medicine does not relieve attack or if dyspnea occurs at night. Teach client how to slow respiratory rate by breathing in through nose and out through pursed lips, 2-3 times, as long as inspiration. Inform client about American Lung Association and its services and literature such as *Living with Asthma*.	Elimination of symptoms of bronchospasm, respiratory rate of 12-20/min, knowledge of home management program and importance of adequate fluid intake, knowledge of evidence of infection and appropriate actions for prevention or management

NURSING DIAGNOSIS: Impaired gas exchange: hypoxemia related to alveolar hypoventilation and bronchospasm†

NURSING DIAGNOSIS: Dyspnea related to increase in airway resistance (bronchospasm)†

†See Table 22-15.

planning an individualized nursing care plan for the client. Well-thought-out written plans involving the client and significant others increase the client's control over the situation and (ideally) increase confidence and compliance.

Chronic management. It is important to remember that asthma is potentially controllable and that every effort should be made to keep the client free of symptoms. The client with asthma usually takes several medications with different routes of administration and time frames for dosage (e.g., tapering steroid schedules, using several different inhalers with different indications). The drug regimen itself can be confusing and complex. Clients with asthma need to learn about their numerous medications and to develop self-management strategies. The client and the health professionals need to monitor the client's responsiveness to medication. It is very easy to undermedicate or overmedicate a client with asthma unless careful monitoring is ongoing. Some clients may benefit from keeping a diary to record the medication used, the presence of wheezing or coughing, the drug's side effects, and the activity level. This information will be valuable in helping the physician adjust the medication. The client needs to understand the importance of continuing the medication even when symptoms are not present. If worsening bronchospasm or severe side effects of the drugs occur, the client needs to seek medical attention.

The client should be taught to maintain a fluid intake of 2 to 3 L/day. Good nutrition and avoidance of overeating are other important measures. Physical exercise (e.g., swimming) within the client's limit of toleration is also beneficial. If dyspnea occurs on exertion, it can be prevented with cromolyn sodium or the use of a β-adrenergic MDI.

Clients need to be instructed in recognizing triggers of an acute exacerbation so that they can medicate early, continue medication according to individually predetermined protocols until symptoms improve, or seek emergency care at a predetermined place. Many persons with asthma have peak flow meters at home with which they can monitor their PEFRs, use a decrease in PEFR to adjust medications, seek medical advice early, and perhaps prevent severe exacerbations. It is most helpful for the physician or nurse to write out a detailed individual protocol of what to do with medications once early warning signs of an acute exacerbation occur.

Counseling may be indicated to help clients and their families resolve personal, family, social, and occupational problems that have resulted from asthma. Relaxation therapies (e.g., yoga, meditation, and breathing techniques) may be of value in helping a client relax respiratory muscles and decrease respiratory rate. A healthy emotional outlook can also be very important in preventing future asthma attacks. One resource that can be used when teaching clients about asthma is the American Lung Association, which has educational materials about asthma, including the *Asthma Handbook*.

PULMONARY EMPHYSEMA AND CHRONIC BRONCHITIS

The clinical use of the terms *chronic obstructive pulmonary disease (COPD)* and *chronic obstructive lung disease (COLD)* is common. COPD may be defined "as the process characterized by the presence of chronic bronchitis and/or emphysema that may lead to the development of obstructed airways; the airway obstruction may be partially reversible and is often accompanied by airway hyperreactivity."[15] Although the preferred term is *predominant emphysema* or *predominant chronic bronchitis*, there is actually usually some overlap between them. The disease spectrum of COPD includes asthmatic bronchitis, chronic bronchitis, and emphysema. Acute intermittent and totally reversible asthma are not included in the COPD designation.

Significance

At least 16 million people in the United States have emphysema and chronic bronchitis.[4] This number probably represents only the more advanced cases, and the true number of cases may be twice that figure. It accounts for almost 4% of all the deaths in the United States.[16] The death rate for emphysema and chronic bronchitis is more than 18,000 per year, making COPD the fifth leading cause of death. White males account for more than one third of the deaths.[17]

COPD is related primarily to cigarette smoking. There seems to be a 20-year lag between taking up smoking and developing the disease. Currently COPD is found primarily in men more than 45 years of age. However, the incidence in women is now steadily increasing, perhaps because women began smoking in large numbers in the 1930s and 1940s. Disability allowances paid by Social Security for COPD rank second after heart disease.[4]

Etiology

Chronic irritation of the lungs is the primary etiological mechanism in COPD. There are three major irritants—cigarette smoking, infection, and inhaled irritants. The development of COPD in a person is extremely variable and depends on the inherent host susceptibility and on the nature and severity of exposure to the irritant. The host susceptibility factors that cause some people to develop pathological lung changes and others to remain free of symptoms are unclear and still under investigation. One known host susceptibility is α_1-antitrypsin (AAT) deficiency.

Cigarette smoking. Cigarette smoking is the most common cause of COPD in the United States. Airway obstruction develops in 15% of smokers, and 80% to 90% of cases of COPD in the United States are related to cigarette smoking.[18] Cigarette smoking is responsible for 82% of COPD deaths.[4] In addition to being linked with emphysema, chronic bronchitis, and lung cancer, cigarette smoking has also been implicated as a factor in cancers of the mouth, pharynx, larynx, esophagus, pancreas, and bladder. Approximately 142,000 deaths were attributed to lung cancer in 1989. Cigarette smoking is responsible for about 87% of lung cancer deaths.[4]

When cigarettes are smoked, thousands of chemicals and gases are inhaled into the lungs. Many carcinogens have been isolated from cigarette smoke; 3,4-benzpyrene has been shown to be the most dangerous. At least 23 other components of the tar fraction of cigarette smoke have been identified as carcinogens, cocarcinogens, tumor promoters, tumor initiators, and mutagens. Nicotine is probably not a carcinogen, but it has other important effects. It acts by stimulating the sympathetic nervous system, resulting in increased heart rate, increased peripheral vasoconstriction, increased blood pressure, and increased cardiac work load. These effects of nicotine compound the problems in a person with coronary artery disease.

Cigarette smoke has a number of direct effects on respiratory tract tissue (Table 22-8). The irritating effect of the smoke causes hyperplasia of cells, including goblet cells, which subsequently results in increased production of mucus. Hyperplasia reduces airway diameter and increases the difficulty of clearing secretions. Smoking reduces the ciliary activity and may cause actual loss of ciliated cells. Smoking also produces abnormal dilatation of the distal air

Table 22-8   Effects of Tobacco Smoke on the Respiratory System

Area of Defect	Acute Effects	Chronic Effects
Respiratory mucosa		
Nasopharyngeal	↓ Sense of smell	Cancer
Tongue	↓ Sense of taste	Cancer
Vocal cords	Hoarseness	Chronic cough, cancer
Bronchus/bronchioles	Bronchospasm, cough	Chronic bronchitis, asthma, cancer
Cilia	Paralysis, sputum accumulation, cough	Chronic bronchitis, cancer
Mucous glands	↑ Secretions, ↑ cough	Hyperplasia and hypertrophy of glands, chronic bronchitis
Alveolar macrophages	↓ Function	Increased incidence of infection
Elastin and collagen fibers	↑ Destruction by proteases, ↓ function of antiproteases (α_1-antitrypsin), ↓ synthesis and repair of elastin	Emphysema

Modified from US Public Health Service: The health consequences of smoking—healthy people, Rockville, Md, 1979, US Department of Health and Human Services. Office of Smoking and Health.

space, with destruction of alveolar walls.[18] Many cells develop large, atypical nuclei; this phenomenon is considered a precancerous condition.

Carbon monoxide (CO) is a component of tobacco smoke. It has a high affinity for hemoglobin and combines with it more readily than does O_2. Therefore the smoker's O_2-carrying capacity is reduced. In addition, when inhaling the smoke, the smoker is inhaling a lower percentage of O_2 than normal. Therefore there is less O_2 available at the alveolar level. The heart's need for O_2 is increased because of the sympathetic stimulation of nicotine. Because the blood's O_2-carrying capacity is reduced, the heart must pump more rapidly to supply tissues adequately with O_2. CO also seems to impair psychomotor performance and judgment and may cause psychological stress.

Exposed nonsmokers are affected by involuntary exposure to smoke *(passive smoking)*. The effects in children are an increased incidence of respiratory illnesses and pulmonary function abnormalities. Nonsmoking spouses who live with a spouse who smokes have decreased pulmonary function and an increased risk for lung cancer. In addition, nonsmokers who remain in the presence of smokers have increased levels of CO, which indicate that they are significantly exposed to smoke.[19]

Fortunately, only 30% of adults in the United States now smoke as compared to 42% in 1964.[17] This decrease can be related to the widespread publicity of the harmful effects of smoking and the vocal response of nonsmokers who are concerned about the effects of passive smoking.

A major theory regarding the relationship between cigarette smoking and emphysema is that cigarette smoke may cause an imbalance between proteolytic enzymes that digest lung connective tissue and protease inhibitors, one of which is AAT. Other evidence indicates that oxidants in tobacco smoke can activate AAT and that in the presence of cigarette smoke, neutrophils and macrophages in the lung liberate proteases, resulting in digestion of lung tissue. There is also evidence to indicate that other chemicals in cigarettes may interfere with normal repair and synthesis of lung elastic fibers.[18]

Infection. No viral or bacterial agent has been identified as the sole cause of COPD. However, recurring respiratory tract infections are a major contributing factor to the aggravation and progression of COPD. Recurring infections impair normal defense mechanisms, making the bronchioles and alveoli more susceptible to injury. In addition, persons with COPD are more prone to respiratory infections, which subsequently intensify the pathological destruction of lung tissue and the progression of COPD. The most common causative organisms are *Haemophilus influenzae* and *Streptococcus pneumoniae*. Retained secretions provide a good medium for their proliferation.

Inhaled irritants. The incidence of COPD is higher in urban than in rural areas. This may partially be explained by the air pollution and occupational irritants to which persons are exposed. Inhaled irritants cause a nonspecific inflammatory response. More macrophages and neutrophils are found in the lungs. Proteases in these cells can destroy alveoli, and this process has been implicated in the pathogenesis of COPD.

Exposure to occupational gases and dusts can cause lung fibrosis and focal areas of emphysema. Exposure to air pollution and occupational irritants worsens the dyspnea of COPD by causing bronchospasm and mucosal edema.

Heredity. A form of familial primary emphysema is related to a deficiency of AAT, a glycoprotein that normally has an inhibitory effect on proteolytic enzymes. The level of AAT is controlled by a pair of autosomal codominant genes. Low levels of AAT are related to homozygosity for the deficiency gene (ZZ), intermediate levels to heterozygosity (MZ), and normal values to homozygosity for the normal gene (MM). The incidence of ZZ homozygotes ranges from 1 out of 3500 persons to 1 out of 1670 persons,[20] and 5% to 10% of persons are heterozygous.[21] In the homozygous group, onset of symptoms often occurs before the age of 40 and as frequently in women as in men. Although somewhat controversial, some evidence suggests that persons with the heterozygous condition may also be predisposed to emphysema.

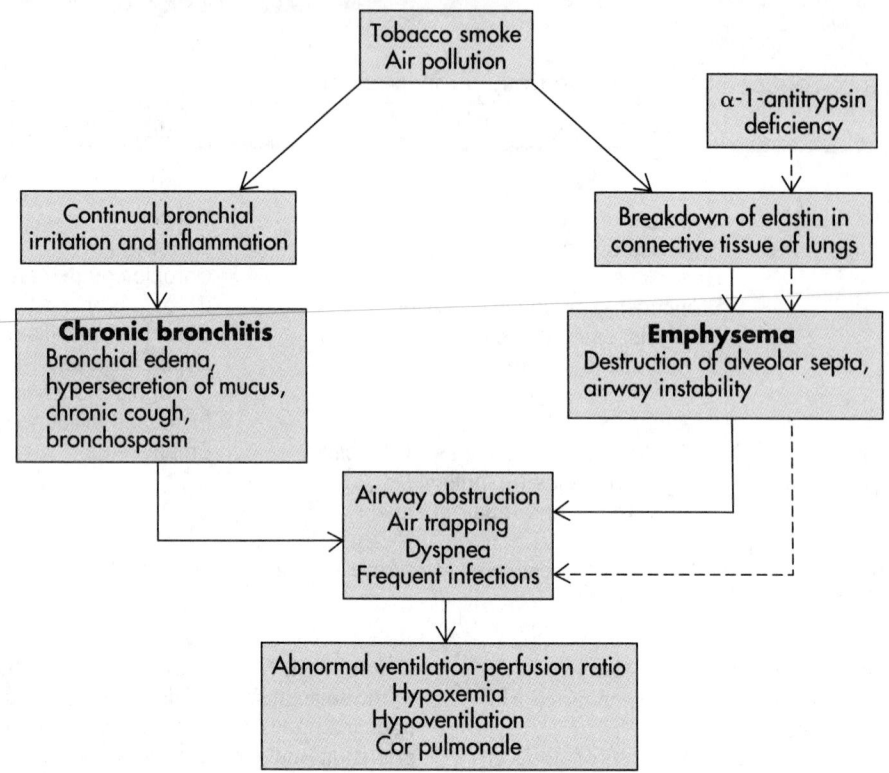

Fig. 22-10 Pathophysiology of chronic bronchitis and emphysema. *Dashed arrows* indicate role of α_1-antitrypsin deficiency, if present. (From McCance KL and Huether SE: Pathophysiology: the biological basis for disease in adults and children, St Louis, 1990, Mosby–Year Book, Inc, p 1072.)

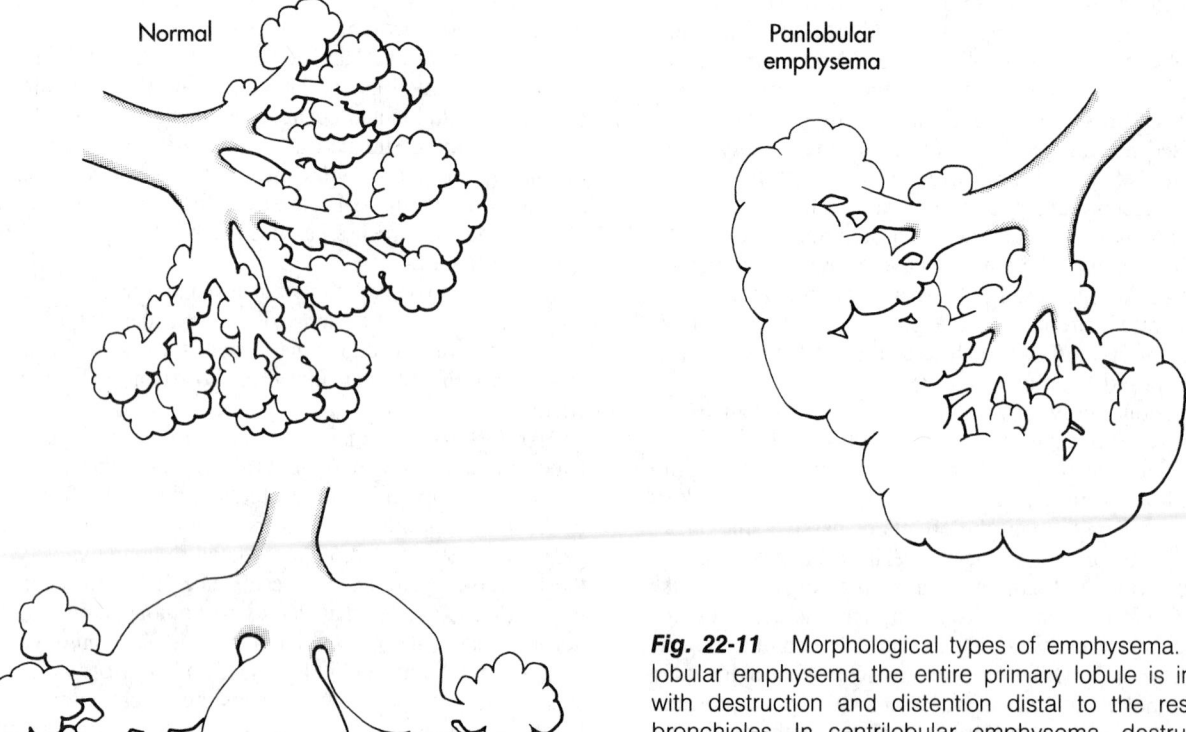

Fig. 22-11 Morphological types of emphysema. In panlobular emphysema the entire primary lobule is involved, with destruction and distention distal to the respiratory bronchioles. In centrilobular emphysema, destruction is central, involving primarily the respiratory bronchioles. (From Price S and Wilson L: Pathophysiology: clinical concepts of disease processes, ed 4, St Louis, 1991, Mosby–Year Book, Inc.)

Emphysema results when lysis of lung tissues by proteolytic enzymes from neutrophils and macrophages occurs because of the AAT deficiency. Normally, AAT inhibits the action of these enzymes. Therefore lower levels of AAT result in insufficient inactivation and subsequent destruction of lung tissue. The effect of smoking is greatly exacerbated in these clients. IV or nebulizer-administered AAT (Prolastin) augmentation therapy is available for certain persons with AAT deficiency. The infusions are administered weekly.[22] Its effectiveness in slowing the progression of the disease needs to be evaluated.

Aging. Some degree of emphysema is common in the lungs of older persons, even nonsmokers, and is often referred to as *senile emphysema*. With aging there is dilatation of the air spaces, decreased elasticity of lung tissue, and increased rigidity of the chest wall. However, clinically significant emphysema is usually not caused by aging alone.

Pathophysiology

It is very common clinically to find in the same person a combination of emphysema and chronic bronchitis, often with one condition predominating (Fig. 22-10).

Pulmonary emphysema. Pulmonary emphysema is a condition of the lung characterized by abnormal, permanent enlargement of the air spaces distal to the terminal bronchioles, accompanied by destruction of their walls, and without obvious fibrosis. Structural changes include (1) hyperinflation of alveoli; (2) destruction of alveolar walls; (3) destruction of alveolar capillary walls; (4) narrowed, tortuous, small airways; and (5) loss of lung elasticity.

There are two major types of emphysema, *centrilobular* and *panlobular* (Fig. 22-11). In centrilobar emphysema the primary area of involvement is the central part of the lobule. Respiratory bronchioles enlarge, the walls are destroyed, and the bronchioles become confluent. Chronic bronchitis is often associated with centrilobular emphysema. It is more common than panlobular emphysema.

In contrast, panlobular emphysema involves distention and destruction of the whole lobule. Respiratory bronchioles, alveolar ducts and sacs, and alveoli are all affected. There is progressive loss of lung tissue and a decreased alveolar-capillary surface area. Severe panlobular emphysema is usually found in persons with AAT deficiency. In some clients with emphysema, bullae (large cystic areas) develop. When emphysema is severe, it is difficult to distinguish the two types, which may coexist in the same lung.

The pathophysiological mechanisms involved in emphysema are not totally understood. Small bronchioles become obstructed as a result of mucus, smooth muscle spasm, the inflammatory process, collapse of bronchiolar walls, and other causes. Recurrent infectious processes lead to increased production and stimulation of neutrophils and macrophages. These cells release proteolytic enzymes that can destroy alveolar tissue. This process results in more inflammation, more edema, and exudate formation.

In a healthy person there is a balance between elastases and proteases and antiproteases. In smokers there are increased numbers of polymorphonuclear neutrophils and macrophages. Release of their elastases/proteases may overwhelm the normal antiprotease defense. In addition, smoking inactivates AAT (antiprotease). In familial emphysema, AAT activity is greatly diminished and may be overwhelmed by normal proteinase activity.

In emphysema there is destruction of elastin and collagen, which are the supporting structures of the lung. Because of this, there is no pull or traction on the walls of the bronchioles (Fig. 22-12). Like air being blown into a paper bag, air goes into the lungs easily but is unable to come out on its own and remains in the lung. Thus the bronchioles tend to collapse (especially on expiration), and air is trapped in the distal alveoli, resulting in hyperinflation and overdistention of the alveoli. This trapped air in the lungs gives the client the typical barrel-chested appearance. In emphysema the lungs can be inflated easily but can deflate only partially. As more alveoli are destroyed and alveoli coalesce, larger air spaces called *blebs* (in the visceral pleura) and *bullae* (in the lung parenchyma) may develop (Fig. 22-13).

Because of the loss of alveolar walls and the capillaries surrounding them, there is a decrease in the amount of surface available for diffusion of O_2 in the blood. Clients with emphysema compensate for this by increasing their respiratory rate to increase alveolar ventilation. Typically, the client with pure emphysema does not have difficulty with hypoxemia at rest until late in the disease. However, hypoxemia may develop during exercise, and the client may benefit from O_2. Hypercapnia and respiratory acidosis do not develop until late in the disease process.

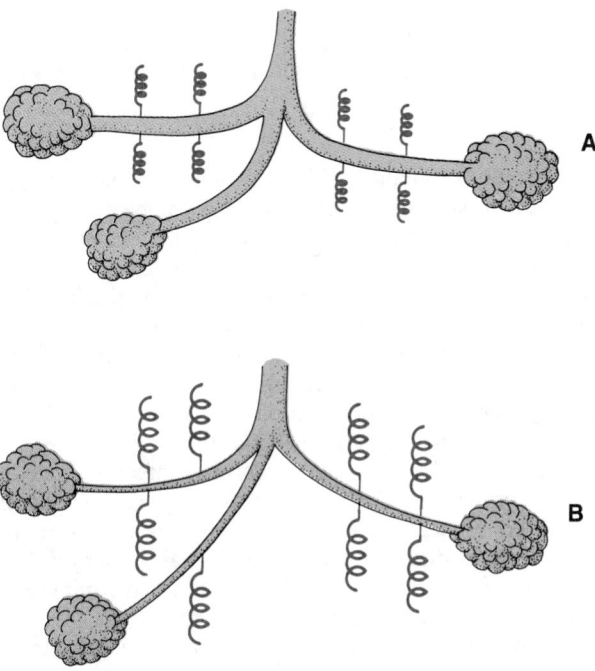

Fig. 22-12 **A,** Normal elastic support of airways resulting in normal airway size. **B,** Reduced elastic support resulting in reduced airway size.

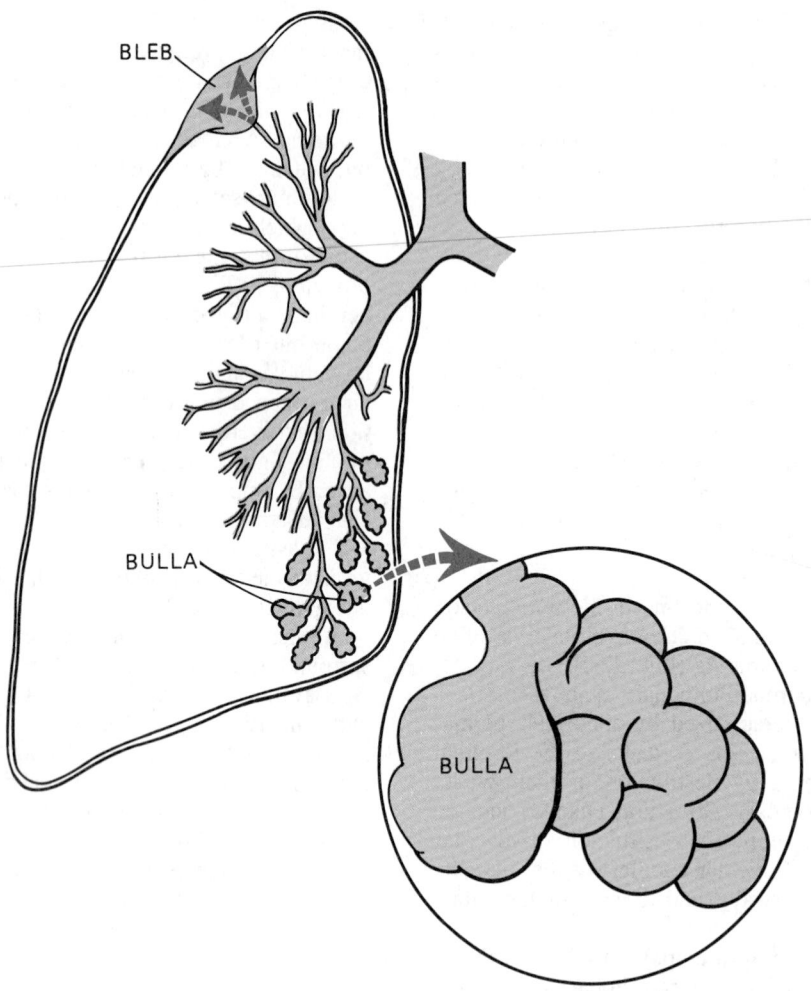

Fig. 22-13 Pulmonary blebs and bullae. (From Price S and Wilson L: Pathophysiology: clinical concepts of disease processes, ed 4, St Louis, 1991, Mosby–Year Book, Inc.)

Chronic bronchitis. Chronic bronchitis is excessive production of mucus in the bronchi accompanied by a recurrent cough that persists for at least 3 months of the year during at least 2 successive years. Pathological changes in the lung consist of (1) hypertrophy and hyperplasia or mucous-secreting glands in the trachea and bronchi (Fig. 22-14); (2) increase in goblet cells; (3) disappearance of cilia; (4) chronic inflammatory changes and narrowing of small airways; and (5) altered function of alveolar macrophages, leading to increased bronchial infections. Frequently, the airways are colonized with organisms. Infections can occur when the number of organisms increases. Excess amounts of mucus are found in the airways and sometimes may occlude small bronchioles. Eventually, there may be scarring of the bronchial wall. In contrast to emphysema, the alveolar structure and capillaries are normal.

Chronic inflammation is the primary pathological mechanism involved in causing the changes characteristic of chronic bronchitis. The inflammatory response causes vasodilatation, congestion, and mucosal edema. The mucous glands are stimulated to hypertrophy and become hyper-plastic. This hyperplasia, inflammatory swelling, and excess, thick mucus cause narrowing of the airway lumen and result in diminished airflow.[23] Greater resistance to airflow increases the work of breathing. Hypoxemia and hypercarbia develop more frequently in chronic bronchitis than in emphysema because there is a tendency for hypoventilation as well as ventilation-perfusion mismatch (i.e., a disproportionate relationship between ventilation and perfusion). Because the constricted bronchioles are clogged with mucus, there is a physical barrier to ventilation. In addition, there is a diminished respiratory drive, with a tendency to hypoventilate and retain CO_2. The result is that many areas of the lung are not ventilated and O_2 diffusion cannot occur. Frequently, clients with chronic bronchitis require O_2 both at rest and during exercise as their disease progresses. Peribronchial fibrosis may also result from the healing process secondary to inflammatory changes.

Coughing is stimulated by retained mucus that cannot adequately be removed as a result of decreased cilia and lessened mucociliary activity. The cough is often ineffec-

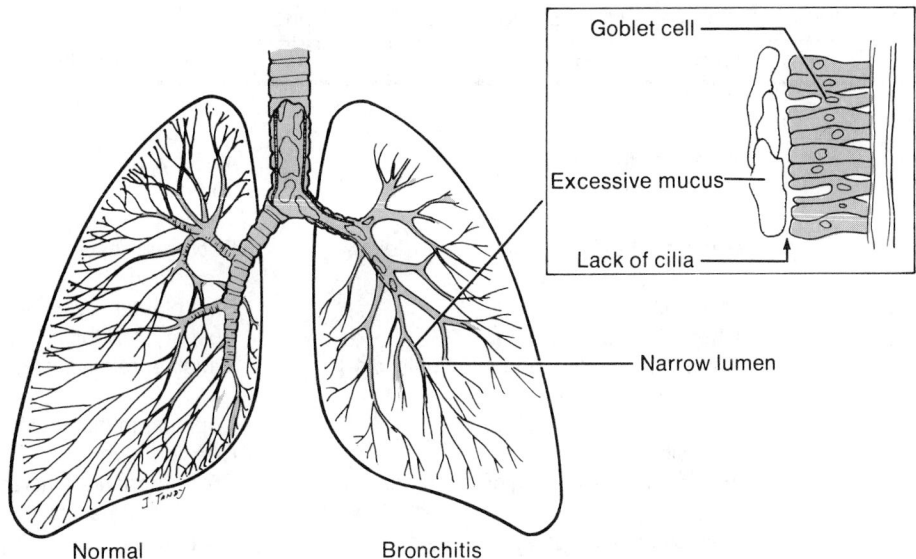

Fig. 22-14 Characteristic defect of bronchitis is hyperplasia and overactivity of mucus-secreting bronchial glands, causing airway lumen to be significantly narrowed. (From Groer MW and Shekleton ME: Basic pathophysiology: a conceptual approach, ed 3, St Louis, 1989, The CV Mosby Co, p 604.)

tive to remove secretions adequately because the person cannot inspire deeply enough to cause air to flow distal to retained secretions. Frequently, bronchospasm (asthma) will develop in clients with chronic bronchitis. This is frequently called *asthmatic bronchitis*. Bronchospasm is usually more common in those with a history of cigarette smoking. The bronchospasm adds to the already increased airway resistance, resulting in further increased work of breathing and impaired gas exchange.

Clinical Manifestations

The clinical manifestations of COPD vary from those of pure emphysema ("pink puffers") to those of pure chronic bronchitis ("blue bloaters"). Most clients with COPD have features of both (Table 22-9).

Pulmonary emphysema. In emphysema an early symptom is dyspnea which becomes progressively more severe. Minimal coughing is present, with no sputum or small amounts of mucoid sputum. As more alveoli become overdistended, increasing amounts of air are trapped. This causes a flattened diaphragm and an increased anteroposterior diameter of the chest, forming the typical barrel chest. Effective abdominal breathing is decreased because of the flattened diaphragm from the overdistended lungs. The person becomes more of a chest breather, relying on the intercostal and accessory muscles. However, this type of breathing is not very effective because the ribs become fixed in an inspiratory position.

Hypoxemia (especially during exercise) may be present, but hypercapnia does not develop until late in the disease. The term pink puffer is used because with hyperventilation there is adequate oxygenation of tissues and no cyanosis is present. The person is characteristically thin and under-

weight, but the exact cause for this is not well understood. One possibility is that the pink puffer is in a hypermetabolic state with increased energy requirements that are partly due to the increased work of breathing. It seems that even when these people have adequate calorie intake, they still experience weight loss. Pink puffers have protein-calorie malnutrition with loss of lean muscle mass and subcutaneous fat. (Malnutrition is discussed in Chapter 35.)

Later in the course of the disease, secondary chronic bronchitis may develop. In advanced stages, finger clubbing may be present in both emphysema and chronic bronchitis. Other characteristics are presented in Table 22-9.

Chronic bronchitis. In chronic bronchitis the earliest symptom is usually a frequent, productive cough during most winter months. It is often exacerbated by respiratory irritants and cold, damp air, and bronchospasm can occur at the end of paroxysms of coughing.[21] Frequent respiratory infections are another common manifestation. Somewhat later, dyspnea on exertion may develop. A history of cigarette smoking for many years is almost always present. Unfortunately, clients often attribute their chronic cough to smoking.

Hypoxemia and hypercapnia result from hypoventilation caused by increased airway resistance. These persons are referred to as blue bloaters because their skin is often reddish blue. This color results from polycythemia and cyanosis. Polycythemia develops as a result of increased production of red blood cells (RBCs) secondary to the body's attempt to compensate for chronic hypoxemia. Hemoglobin concentrations may reach 20 g/dl or more. Cyanosis develops because there is at least 5 g/dl of unoxygenated hemoglobin.

People with chronic bronchitis are usually of normal

Table 22-9 Comparison of Pulmonary Emphysema and Chronic Bronchitis*

	Pulmonary Emphysema	Chronic Bronchitis
CLINICAL FEATURES		
Age	60-70 yr (disabling)	40-50 yr (disabling)
	30-40 yr (onset)	20-30 yr (onset)
Body build	Thin	Tendency toward obesity
Health history	Generally healthy, occasional insidious dyspnea, smoking	Recurrent respiratory tract infections, smoking
General appearance	Pink puffer	Blue bloater, cyanosis
Weight loss	Often marked	Absent or slight
Dyspnea	Slowly progressive and eventually disabling	Variable, relatively late
Sputum	Scanty, mucoid	Copious, mucopurulent
Cough	Negligible	Considerable
Chest examination	Marked increase in anteroposterior diameter, quiet or diminished breath sounds, limited diaphragmatic excursion	Slight to marked increase in anteroposterior diameter, scattered rales, rhonchi, wheezing
Cor pulmonale	Occasional	Common
DIAGNOSTIC STUDY RESULTS		
ABGs	Near normal, mild ↓ Pa_{O_2}	↓ Pa_{O_2}, ↑ Pa_{CO_2}
Chest x-ray film	Hyperinflation, flat diaphragm, attenuated peripheral vessels, small or normal heart, widened intercostal margins	Cardiac enlargement, normal or flattened diaphragm, evidence of chronic inflammation, congested lung fields
Lung volumes		
Total lung capacity	Increased	Normal or slightly increased
Residual volume	Increased	Increased
Vital capacity	Decreased	Decreased
FEV_1	Decreased	Decreased
FEV_1/FVC	Decreased <70%	Decreased <70%
Hematocrit and hemoglobin	Normal until late in disease	Increased
PATHOLOGY		
	Widespread emphysema, usually panlobular type	Some centrilobular emphysema possible Airway changes

*Most persons with COPD have features of both pulmonary emphysema and chronic bronchitis.

weight or heavyset, with a robust appearance. Emphysema of the centrilobular type frequently develops.

Complications

Cor pulmonale. Cor pulmonale is hypertrophy of the right side of the heart, with or without heart failure, resulting from pulmonary hypertension. In COPD, pulmonary hypertension is caused primarily by constriction of the pulmonary vessels in response to alveolar hypoxia, with acidosis further potentiating the vasoconstriction (Fig. 22-15). Chronic alveolar hypoxia also causes arteriolar muscle hypertrophy. Chronic hypoxia also stimulates erythropoiesis, which increases the viscosity of the blood. Failure of the right side of the heart results as the right ventricle tries to pump the thickened blood through the narrowed lumen of the pulmonary vessels. Because pulmonary vascular constriction may be reversed if the alveolar Pa_{O_2} is increased, the primary treatment of cor pulmonale is low-flow O_2.

The clinical manifestations of cor pulmonale are related to dilatation and failure of the right ventricle with subsequent intravascular volume expansion and systemic venous congestion. Heart sound changes include accentuation of the pulmonic component of the second heart sound, right-sided ventricular diastolic S_3 gallop, and early systolic ejection click along the left sternal border. ECG changes include increased P-wave amplitude (P-pulmonale) in leads II, III, and aV_F; a tendency for right axis deviation; and incomplete right bundle branch block. Overt manifestations of right-sided heart failure may develop, which include distended neck veins (jugular venous distention or JVD), hepatomegaly, epigastric distress, peripheral edema, and weight gain.

Therapeutic management of cor pulmonale is continuous low-flow O_2. Use of digitalis is controversial. Dietary salt restriction is sometimes recommended, especially if overt congestive heart failure is present. Although diuretics are usually used, they should be used cautiously be-

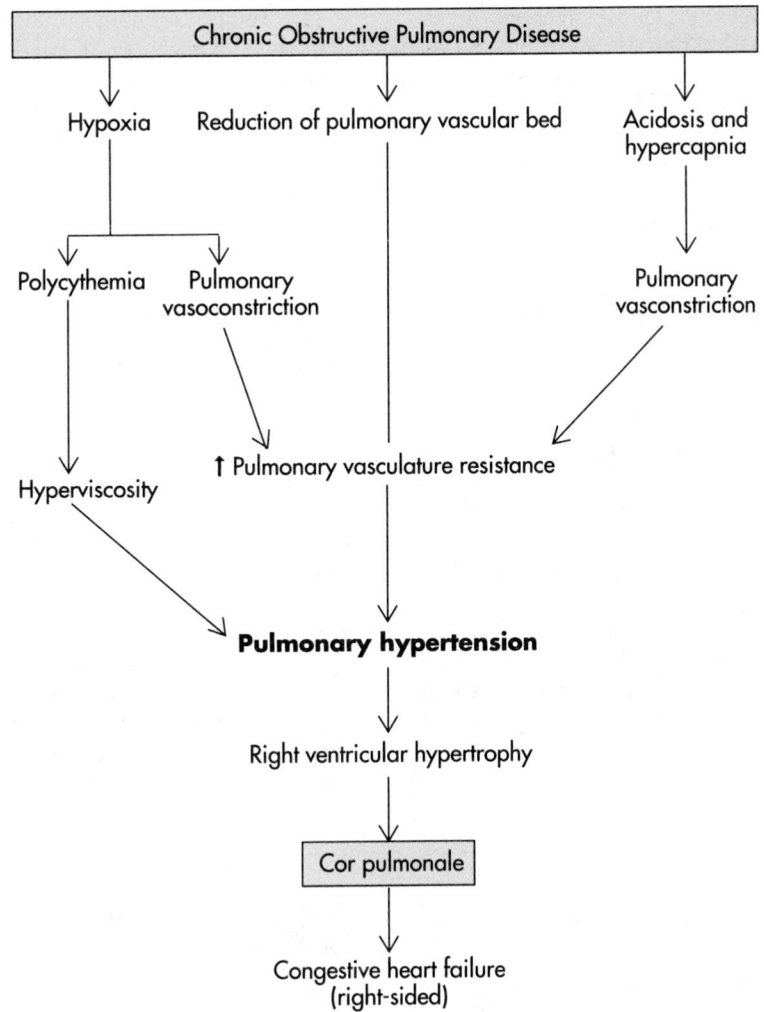

Fig. 22-15   Mechanisms involved in the pathophysiology of cor pulmonale secondary to COPD.

cause of their tendency to deplete potassium and chloride and reduce intravascular volume and cardiac output. (Cor pulmonale is discussed further in Chapter 21.)

Acute respiratory failure. The most common event leading to acute respiratory failure in COPD is acute respiratory tract infection (usually viral) or acute bronchitis. An exacerbation of cor pulmonale either alone or occurring simultaneously with other etiological causes of acute respiratory failure may lead to acute respiratory failure. Discontinuance of bronchodilator or steroid medication may also precipitate respiratory failure. The use of β-blocker medications (e.g., propranolol [Inderal]) may also exacerbate acute respiratory failure in the client with an asthmatic component to the COPD. The indiscriminate use of sedatives and/or narcotics especially in the preoperative or postoperative client who retains CO_2 may suppress ventilatory drive and lead to ventilatory failure. The hypercapnia (elevated CO_2) presents a serious problem when O_2 therapy is being given. Because of the persistent elevation of CO_2, the respiratory center no longer responds to increases in CO_2. Therefore hypoxemia is the primary respiratory stimulant. If too much O_2 is administered, the hypoxic

drive is removed and breathing slows or stops. Persons with COPD who are CO_2 retainers should be treated with low flow rates of O_2 with careful monitoring of ABGs. Surgery or severe, painful illness involving the chest or abdominal organs may lead to splinting and ineffective ventilation and respiratory failure. Careful preoperative screening, which includes pulmonary function tests and ABG monitoring, is important in clients with a heavy smoking history and COPD to prevent postoperative pulmonary complications. (Respiratory failure is defined and discussed in Chapter 23.)

Peptic ulcer and esophageal reflux. The incidence of peptic ulcer disease is increased in persons with COPD. The reason for this occurrence is not known. Possibly it is due to side effects from the long-term use of bronchodilator or steroid drugs.[24] Another factor may be the stressful nature of the disease. It is important to test gastric aspirates and feces for occult blood.

Esophageal reflux, which may or may not be associated with a hiatal hernia, occurs frequently in clients with COPD and may aggravate respiratory symptoms. The reflux and accompanying heartburn may be aggravated or even precipitated by theophylline or β-adrenergic drugs. As a result of esophageal irritation or aspiration into the tracheobronchial tree, reflux airway constriction and obstruction may occur. (The treatment of hiatal hernia and esophageal reflux is discussed in Chapter 34.)

Pneumonia. Pneumonia is a frequent complication of COPD. The most common causative agents are *S. pneumoniae, H. influenzae, Mycoplasma* organisms, and viruses. The most common manifestation is purulent sputum. Systemic manifestations such as fever, chills, and leukocytosis may not be present. (The treatment of pneumonia is discussed in Chapter 21.)

Diagnostic Studies

An important goal of the diagnostic workup is to determine the major disease component of COPD (e.g., emphysema, asthma, or asthmatic or chronic bronchitis) and the severity of progression. This enables the physician to design an individualized treatment plan.

Chest x-ray films taken early in the disease may show no abnormalities. Later in the disease the findings presented in Table 22-9 may be present.

Pulmonary function studies are useful in diagnosing and assessing the severity of COPD. The most significant findings are related to increased resistance to expiratory airflow. Typical findings are as follows:
1. Reduced FEV_1
2. Reduced $FEF_{25\%-75\%}$
3. Reduced maximum voluntary ventilation (MVV)
4. Reduced vital capacity (VC)
5. Reduced FEV_1/FVC ratio
6. Reduced diffusing capacity for carbon monoxide (D_LCO)
7. Increased residual volume (RV)
8. Increased total lung capacity (TLC)
9. Increased functional residual capacity (FRC)

When the FEV_1/FVC ratio is less than 70%, it suggests the presence of obstructive lung disease. The value of FEV_1 in milliliters can serve as a rough guideline to determine the severity of the client's lung disease and the degree of disease progression. When compared with previous values, it can also give a fair estimate of the level of expected activity tolerance for the client (Table 22-10).

ABGs are usually monitored. In the later stages of COPD, typical findings are low Pao_2, elevated $Paco_2$, decreased pH, and increased bicarbonate levels. In the early stages there may be a normal or only slightly decreased Pao_2 and a normal $Paco_2$.

Table 22-10 Correlation of FEV_1 with Probable Clinical Manifestations

Approximate FEV_1 (ml)	Probable Clinical Manifestation
1500	Shortness of breath just beginning to be noticed
1000	Shortness of breath with activity
500	Shortness of breath at rest

An exercise test to determine O_2 saturation in the blood with pulse oximetry or an arterial line with ABGs may be done to evaluate whether there is desaturation with exercise. An ECG may be normal or show signs indicative of right ventricular failure (e.g., low voltage, right axis deviation, P-pulmonale). Echocardiogram or gated pool nuclear blood studies can be used to evaluate right-sided as well as left ventricular function.

Therapeutic Management

In general, COPD is an irreversible process. Reversibility depends on the extent of asthma or bronchospasm present. Certain clients with COPD have emphysema that may be described as fixed airway disease, meaning that there is no reversibility. The primary goals of therapeutic management are to (1) improve ventilation, (2) promote secretion removal, (3) prevent complications and progression of symptoms, and (4) promote client comfort and participation in care (Table 22-11). The majority of these clients are treated on an outpatient basis. They are hospitalized for acute exacerbations and complications such as respiratory failure, pneumonia, and congestive heart failure.

Cessation of cigarette smoking in the early stages is probably the most significant factor in slowing the progression of the disease. After discontinuation of smoking, the accelerated decline in pulmonary function slows and returns to the more normal level of nonsmokers. Thus the

Table 22-11

Diagnostic and Therapeutic Management: COPD

DIAGNOSTIC

History and physical examination
Chest x-ray film
Pulmonary function tests
Sputum specimen for Gram stain and culture (if indicated)
ABG monitoring
ECG
Exercise testing with oximetry or ABG monitoring
Echocardiogram or cardiac nuclear scans

THERAPEUTIC

Treatment of respiratory infections
Bronchodilator therapy
    β-Adrenergic agonists
    Anticholinergic agents (ipratropium)
    Long-acting theophylline preparations
    Corticosteroids
Chest physiotherapy and postural drainage (if indicated)
Breathing exercises
Hydration of 3 L/day
Cessation of cigarette smoking
Appropriate rest periods and exercise
Client and family education
Influenza immunization yearly
Pneumovax immunization ($\times$1)
Low flow rate O_2 (if indicated)

sooner the smoker stops, the less pulmonary function is lost and the sooner the symptoms decrease, particularly cough and sputum production. Health care providers have a responsibility to inform each smoking client about the effects of smoking, offer suggestions and guidelines on how to quit, and refer the client to a smoking cessation program. The physician may prescribe Nicorette, a chewing gum that contains 2 mg of nicotine per piece. This gum is merely an adjunct to smoking cessation and may help to lessen nicotine withdrawal symptoms, but the client must be committed to stopping. Other environmental or occupational irritants should be evaluated for their possible negative effect, and ways to control or avoid them should be determined. For example, aerosol hair sprays and smoke-filled rooms can be avoided. The client with COPD should have vaccinations with influenza virus vaccine yearly and with pneumococcal vaccine once in a lifetime. Clients with COPD are extremely susceptible to pulmonary infections. Respiratory infections should be treated as soon as possible. Often the best indication of their presence is the increasing quantity, viscosity, or purulence of sputum. Clients are sometimes given a 7- to 10-day supply of antibiotics and told to begin taking them at the first signs of change in sputum. The most common antibiotics given are ampicillin, amoxicillin, amoxicillin with clavulanate (Augmentin), tetracycline, erythromycin, and trimethoprim-sulfamethoxazole.[2]

Bronchodilator drug therapy is often helpful in relieving symptoms (see p. 568). Although clients with COPD do not respond as dramatically as those with asthma to bronchodilator therapy, a reduction in dyspnea and increase in FEV_1 are usually achieved. Many physicians believe that bronchodilator therapy is best given as maintenance therapy rather than just as a treatment for acute symptoms. However, the routine use of bronchodilator therapy in all clients with COPD is controversial, especially in people with pure emphysema.

β-Adrenergic agonists are considered the mainstay therapy by many for treatment of COPD. The preferred route of administration is by MDI or nebulizer. Anticholinergic agents, specifically ipratropium by inhaler, are effective bronchodilators in clients with COPD. Because it is poorly absorbed systemically, it has almost no side effects. This drug is best taken on a regular basis. Long-acting theophylline may be of some value in the treatment of COPD. Although it has some action as a mild bronchodilator in clients with partial reversibility of airflow obstruction, its principal value may relate to improving contractility of the diaphragm and decreasing diaphragmatic fatigue.

The use of corticosteroid therapy in COPD remains controversial. The persons most likely to benefit from these drugs are those who have a background of asthma in childhood, experience asthmatic bronchitis, have a relatively short duration of disease, or frequently experience exacerbations that do not respond to therapy with β agonists and theophylline.

Mucolytic expectorants (e.g., iodinated glycerol, glycerol guiacolate) may be effective as adjuvant therapy in treating mucus-complicated COPD. These agents may decrease cough frequency, cough severity, and chest discomfort.

Home O_2 therapy is used in certain COPD clients who have significant hypoxemia. O_2 may be prescribed for continuous use, only at night, or with exercise. Long-term administration of O_2 is probably the most effective therapy for the prevention and treatment of cor pulmonale. (O_2 therapy is discussed in Chapter 21.)

Respiratory Therapy

Respiratory care is a collaborative effort involving respiratory therapists and nurses. The client with COPD develops a rapid respiratory rate to try to compensate for dyspnea. In addition, the accessory muscles of breathing in the neck and upper part of the chest are used excessively to promote chest wall movement. Breathing exercises can assist the client during rest and activity (e.g., lifting, walking, stair climbing). The main types of breathing exercises are (1) pursed-lip breathing and (2) diaphragmatic breathing.

The purpose of using *pursed-lip breathing* is to prolong exhalation and thereby prevent bronchiolar collapse and air trapping. Clients are taught to inhale slowly through the nose and then to exhale slowly through pursed lips almost as if they wanted to whistle. Exhalation should be at least twice as long as inhalation. It is helpful to have the nurse demonstrate the breathing exercises so that the client can imitate the action. Various techniques can be used to teach pursed-lip breathing, such as the following:

1. Blowing through a straw in a glass of water with the intent of forming small bubbles
2. Blowing at a lit candle enough to bend the flame without blowing it out
3. Steadily blowing a table-tennis ball across a table.

Diaphragmatic (abdominal) breathing focuses on using the diaphragm instead of the accessory muscles to achieve maximum inhalation and to slow the respiratory rate. The client should be made aware of the difference between chest breathing and abdominal breathing. This can be done by having the client lie down or assume a semi-Fowler's position and by placing one hand on the chest and the other on the abdomen. The client should observe which hand moves during inspiration. The abdomen should protrude on inhalation with diaphragmatic breathing. The value of diaphragmatic movement in increasing lung expansion should be stressed by the nurse.

In the setting of extreme acute dyspnea when the client is hospitalized for infection and/or heart failure, it is more important to focus on helping the client to slow the respiratory rate by using the principles of pursed-lip breathing. Diaphragmatic (abdominal) breathing requires more energy and thus should be taught only when the client has achieved a stable rehabilitative state such as before discharge or in a home care rehabilitation program.

To practice diaphragmatic breathing, the client should keep the hand on the abdomen and concentrate on filling up the abdomen by inhaling slowly through the nose. Another technique is to wrap a towel gently around the abdomen and to pull it tight during exhalation. The client then attempts to stretch the towel with slow inhalation by diaphragmatic breathing. On exhalation the client uses pursed-lip breathing and draws the towel tighter to promote effective expiration.

Table 22-12   Guidelines for Effective Coughing

1. Client assumes a sitting position with head slightly flexed, shoulders relaxed, knees flexed, and forearms supported by pillow.
2. Client then drops head and bends forward while using slow, pursed-lip breathing to exhale.
3. Sitting up again, client uses diaphragmatic breathing to inhale slowly and deeply.
4. Client repeats steps 2 and 3 three to four times to facilitate mobilization of secretions.
5. Before initiating a cough, client should take a deep abdominal breath, bend slightly forward, and then huff cough (cough three to four times on exhalation). Client may need to support or splint thorax or abdomen to achieve a maximum cough.

Another technique to assist in diaphragmatic breathing is to place a small pillow, magazine, or book on the abdomen. This provides tactile stimulation and visual feedback. If the object rises on inspiration, the person is given positive feedback that diaphragmatic breathing is taking place.

Pursed-lip breathing and diaphragmatic breathing should be practiced together for 8 to 10 repetitions three or four times per day. These techniques give the client more control over breathing, especially during dyspnea.

Effective coughing. Many persons with COPD have developed ineffective coughing patterns that cannot clear their airways adequately or raise sputum. In addition, they fear that they may develop spastic coughing resulting in dyspnea. Guidelines for effective coughing are presented in Table 22-12. The main goals of effective coughing are to conserve energy, reduce fatigue, and facilitate removal of secretions.

Chest physiotherapy. Chest physical therapy is indicated in clients who produce large amounts (greater than 30 ml) of sputum daily, such as those with chronic bronchitis, bronchiectasis, and cystic fibrosis; those who have retained secretions as indicated on chest x-ray film or by auscultation, or those who have lobar atelectasis not related to open-heart surgery. Clients who produce small amounts (less than 30 ml) of sputum or have asthma or lobar atelectasis following open-heart surgery would not benefit from chest physical therapy.[25]

Chest physiotherapy consists of percussion, vibration, and postural drainage (Table 22-13). Percussion and vibration are manual or mechanical techniques used to augment postural drainage. Postural drainage uses the principle of gravity to assist in bronchial drainage. Percussion and vibration are used after the person has assumed a postural drainage position to assist in loosening the mobilized secretions. Percussion, vibration, and postural drainage may assist in bringing secretions into larger, more central airways. However, effective coughing is then necessary to help raise these secretions. Therefore, after each drainage position change, the client should be given time to cough and deep breathe. Sometimes it takes several hours after chest physiotherapy for secretions to be expectorated. It is important that chest physiotherapy be evaluated in light of relief of the client's symptoms. It is very important that

Table 22-13   Steps in Chest Physiotherapy

1. Perform procedure 1 hr before meals or 1-3 hr following meals.
2. Administer bronchodilator (if nebulized or MDI is ordered) about 15 min before procedure.
3. Collect needed equipment such as tissues, emesis basin, paper bag, and pillows.
4. Help client assume correct position for postural drainage based on findings from x-ray film, auscultation, palpation, and percussion of chest. Position should be maintained for 5-15 min to mobilize secretions via gravity.
5. Observe client during treatment to assess tolerance. Particularly observe breathing and color changes, especially duskiness in face.
6. Have client take several deep abdominal breaths.
7. Percuss appropriate area for 1-2 min.
8. Vibrate the same area while the client exhales 4-5 deep breaths.
9. Assist client to cough while assuming same position. Splinting with towel or hands may be necessary to aid in effective coughing. Client may have to assume sitting position to generate enough airflow to expel secretions. (Coughing productively may be a long waiting process that may occur 30 min after procedure.) Suction may be necessary if coughing is not effective.
10. Repeat percussion, vibration, and coughing until client no longer expectorates mucus.
11. Repeat same procedure in all necessary positions.
12. After procedure, help client assume a comfortable position, assist with oral hygiene, and discard used tissues.
13. Evaluate and chart effectiveness of treatment by amount of sputum produced and the results of auscultation. Also chart client tolerance.

these procedures be performed by a trained person.[25]

Postural drainage. The lungs are divided into five lobes, three on the right side and two on the left. There are 18 segments in the lungs. The purpose of various positions in postural drainage is to drain each segment toward the larger airways from which sputum can be coughed up. The postural drainage positions are determined by the areas of involved lung, which are assessed by chest x-ray film, percussion, palpation, and auscultation (Fig. 22-16). Bronchodilator aerosol drug and/or hydration therapy is frequently administered before postural drainage. The chosen postural drainage position is maintained for a designated period of time (usually 5 to 15 minutes). The degree of slope can be obtained with pillows, blocks, books, or a tilt board.

The frequency and choice of postural drainage depends on the location of retained secretions and client tolerance to dependent positions. A common order is for 2 to 4 times per day. In acute situations, postural drainage may be done as frequently as every 1 to 2 hours. The procedure should be planned to occur and be completed at least 1 hour before meals and 3 hours after meals.

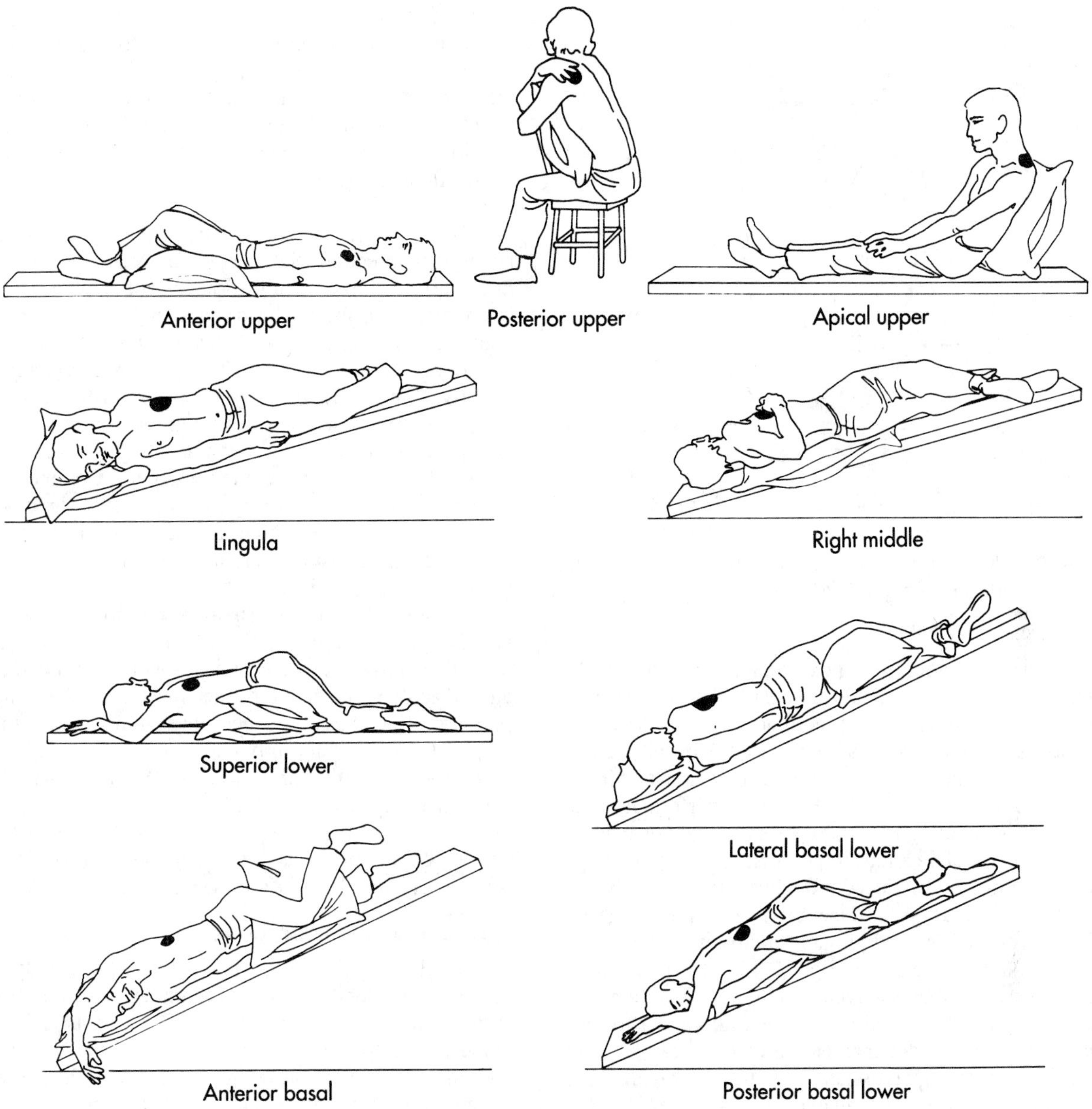

Anterior upper

Posterior upper

Apical upper

Lingula

Right middle

Superior lower

Lateral basal lower

Anterior basal

Posterior basal lower

Fig. 22-16 Representative positions for postural drainage. The *shaded area* in each drawing indicates the segment of the lung in which drainage is promoted. (Modified from Eubanks DH and Bone RC: Comprehensive respiratory care: a learning system, ed 2, St Louis, 1990, Mosby—Year Book, Inc.)

If a client has difficulty in assuming various positions, adaptations will need to be made. The angle can be reduced or the time decreased. A side-lying position can be used for those persons who cannot tolerate a head-down position. Some positions for postural drainage (e.g., Trendelenburg) should not be performed on clients with chest trauma, hemoptysis, heart disease, or head injury and in other situations where the client's condition is not stable.

Percussion. Percussion is performed in the appropriate postural drainage position with the hands in a cuplike position (Fig. 22-17). The hands are cupped, and the fingers and thumbs closed. The cupped hand should create an air pocket between the client's chest and the hand. Both hands may be cupped and used in an alternating rhythmic fash-

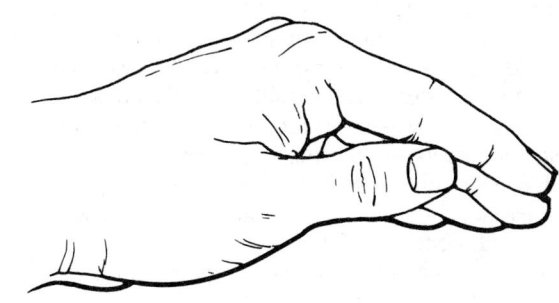

Fig. 22-17 Cupped-hand position for percussion. The hand should be cupped as though scooping up water.

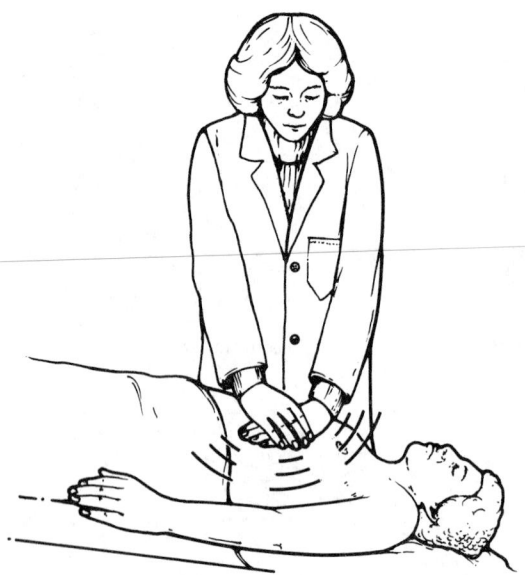

Fig. 22-18 Vibration is rhythmic, rapid massage with the flat of the hand during a long exhalation.

ion. Percussion is done with flexion and extension of the wrists. A hollow sound should be heard if it is done correctly. The air-cushion impact facilitates the movement of thick mucus. A thin towel may be placed over the area to be percussed, or the client may choose to wear a T-shirt or hospital gown. Percussion should not be performed over the kidneys, sternum, spinal cord, or any tender or painful area. Other contraindications to percussion include hemoptysis, carcinoma, and induced bronchospasm.

Vibration. Vibration is done by repeated tensing the hand and arm muscles and pressing mildly with the flat of the hand on the affected area (Fig. 22-18). It is done while the client slowly exhales a deep breath. The vibrations facilitate movement of secretions to larger airways. Mild vibration is tolerated better than percussion and can be used in situations where percussion may be contraindicated. Commercial vibrators are available for home use.

Aerosol-nebulization therapy. Devices that deliver a suspension of very fine particles of liquid in a gas are commonly used to deliver medications to the COPD client. Nebulizers are usually powered by a compressed air or O_2 generator (see Fig. 22-8). At home the client may have an air-powered compressor. In the hospital, wall O_2 or compressed air is used to power the nebulizer. Medication is nebulized or reduced to a fine spray, and depending on several factors (including droplet size), it can be breathed into the client's tracheobronchial tree. Several medications can be administered via aerosol form, the advantage being that this is a rapid-acting form of administration with few systemic effects. Medications that are routinely nebulized include several bronchodilators (e.g., metaproterenol, isoetharine, isoproterenol, terbutaline, atropine), Mucomyst, and cromolyn sodium.

The client should be placed in a position that allows for most efficient breathing (preferably upright) to ensure adequate penetration and deposition of the aerosolized medi-

cation. The client must breathe slowly and deeply through the mouth and hold inspiration for 2 to 3 seconds. Deep diaphragmatic breathing will help to ensure deposition of the medication. After the treatment the client should be instructed to cough effectively. Postural drainage and chest physiotherapy are ideally administered after bronchodilator medications are given.

A disadvantage of the use of nebulizer equipment is the possibility that the nebulizer unit will serve as a source of respiratory infection. Since there has been a recent upsurge in the use of home nebulization for clients with COPD, it is important for the health professional in the hospital and home care setting to review cleaning procedures for home respiratory equipment with the client. A frequently used, effective home-cleaning method is to wash the nebulizer daily in soap and water, rinse it with water, and soak it for 20 to 30 minutes in a 1:1 white vinegar–water solution followed by a water rinse and air drying. Commercial respiratory cleaning agents may also be used if directions are followed carefully. Cleaning the nebulizer in the top shelf of an automatic dishwasher saves time, and the hot water destroys most organisms.

Intermittent positive-pressure breathing. Intermittent positive-pressure breathing (IPPB) is the use of a pressure-limited ventilator to deliver a gas volume with humidity and/or aerosol medication. The machine applies positive pressure, thus forcing a certain volume of air into the lungs. IPPB can transiently decrease the work of breathing and improve ventilation. Although this modality of treatment is rarely used in COPD, it can be used for clients with severe end-stage respiratory muscle failure to improve ventilation. It is more commonly used in clients with restrictive lung disease (see Chapter 21).

Nutritional Considerations

The client with COPD should try to keep body weight for height in standard range. Eating becomes an effort, especially in the later stages of COPD. It is difficult for some clients to hold their breath while swallowing; therefore inadequate amounts of food are eaten. Other proposed reasons for malnutrition include loss of appetite related to a decreased sense of taste and smell and GI disturbances. To decrease dyspnea and conserve energy, clients should rest at least 30 minutes before eating and select foods that they can prepare in advance. Exercise and treatments should be avoided at least 1 hour before and after eating. The exertion involved in the preparation and eating of food is often very fatiguing. The use of a microwave oven may help to conserve client energy in food preparation. Many clients with COPD have feelings of bloating and early satiety when eating. This can be attributed to swallowing air while eating, side effects of medication (especially theophylline), and the abnormal position of the diaphragm relative to the stomach in association with hyperinflation. A full stomach puts pressure on the diaphragm and decreases lung movement. Liquid, blenderized, or commercial diets may be helpful. Foods that require a great deal of chewing should be avoided or served in another manner (e.g., grated, pureed).[26] Cold foods may give less of a sense of fullness than hot foods.

Clients with pink puffer COPD have a greater than normal nutritional requirement for protein and calories. A high-calorie, high-protein diet is recommended and can be divided into five to six small meals per day. High-protein, high-calorie nutritional supplements can be offered between meals. Ice cream added to these supplements can help to increase calories. (Nutritional supplements are discussed in Chapter 35 and Tables 35-14 and 35-15). Gas-forming foods should be avoided. If the client has O_2 prescribed, use of supplemental O_2 by nasal prongs while eating may also be beneficial. Fluid intake should be at least 3 L/day unless contraindicated for other medical conditions such as heart failure. Fluids should be taken between meals (rather than with them) to prevent excess stomach distention and to decrease pressure on the diaphragm. Sodium restriction may be indicated if there is accompanying heart failure. Loss of appetite and nausea may also occur as a result of increased production of mucus and as an effect of some of the prescribed medications. If anorexia is a problem, various strategies can be used, including having the client eat high-calorie food first, having favorite foods available, and adding butter, mayonnaise, or sauces to supply additional calories. Taking medicines with milk or meals and performing bronchial drainage procedures about 1 hour before meals may help.

■ Nursing Management of Emphysema and Chronic Bronchitis

Nursing assessment

Subjective and objective data that should be obtained from a person with emphysema or chronic bronchitis are presented in Table 22-14.

Nursing diagnoses

Nursing diagnoses are determined when the problem and etiological factors are supported by clinical data. The nursing diagnoses related to emphysema and chronic bronchitis are presented in Table 22-15.

Nursing interventions

Health promotion and maintenance. The incidence of COPD will decrease if more persons choose not to start smoking or will stop smoking. Avoiding or controlling exposure to occupational and environmental pollutants is another preventive measure to maintain healthy lungs. (These factors are discussed in the section on nursing management of lung cancer in Chapter 21.)

Early detection of small-airway disease is important. Persons who have smoked for only a few years may have early evidence of obstructive airways. Often, these changes cannot be detected from pulmonary function studies until extensive damage is present. It is extremely important for these people to stop smoking and avoid inhaling irritants while their disease is still reversible. Failure to follow this advice will inevitably lead to irreversible COPD.

As health professionals, nurses who smoke should reevaluate their smoking behavior and its relationship to their health. It is also important for nurses to counsel clients and peers regarding the harmful effects of smoking and to encourage them to quit. Referring them to self-help groups in the community may be especially valuable.

Text continued on p. 596.

Table 22-14

 Nursing Assessment of the Client with Emphysema or Bronchitis

SUBJECTIVE DATA

History
Positive family history of respiratory disease, AAT deficiency; smoking (including passive smoking); pack-years; long-term exposure to chemical pollution, respiratory irritants, occupational fumes, dust; recurrent respiratory infections

Medications
Use of O_2, bronchodilators, steroids, antibiotics, anticholinergics, over-the-counter drugs

General
Fatigue, anorexia, weight loss (emphysema) or gain (chronic bronchitis); inability to carry out activities of daily living; insomnia; sitting-up position for sleeping

Pain
Chest and abdominal muscle soreness, headache

Respiratory
Dyspnea (progressive), especially on exertion; recurrent cough; sputum production (color, odor, viscosity, amount); orthopnea; paroxysmal nocturnal dyspnea

Cardiovascular
Palpitations, swelling of feet

OBJECTIVE DATA

General
Debilitation, anxiety, restlessness, position assumed

Integumentary
Cyanosis (bronchitis), pallor or ruddy color, poor skin turgor, clubbing, easy bruising

Respiratory
Respiratory distress; rapid, shallow breathing; inability to speak; prolonged expiratory phase; pursed-lip breathing; wheezing; rhonchi, crackles, diminished or bronchial breath sounds; decreased chest excursion and diaphragm movement; use of accessory muscles; hyperresonant or dull chest sounds on percussion

Cardiovascular
Tachycardia, dysrhythmias (especially multifocal atrial tachycardia), edema of lower extremities, pulsus paradoxus, JVD, distant heart tones, right-sided S_3

Musculoskeletal
Muscle atrophy, increased anteroposterior diameter (barrel-chest)

Possible findings
Abnormal ABGs, polycythemia, pulmonary function tests showing expiratory airflow obstruction (e.g., low FEV_1, low FEV_1/VC, large residual volume, decreased expiratory flow rate), chest x-ray film showing flattened diaphragm and hyperinflation (emphysema) or infiltrates (bronchitis), ECG showing dysrhythmias

Table 22-15

NURSING CARE PLAN FOR THE CLIENT WITH COPD

Defining Characteristics	Nursing Interventions	Evaluation Criteria

NURSING DIAGNOSIS: Ineffective airway clearance related to expiratory airflow obstruction, ineffective cough, environmental irritants leading to hypersecretion and/or decreased mucociliary transport, decreased airway humidity, and infection in airways

Difficulty in expectorating sputum, presence of abnormal breath sounds, ineffective or absent cough, no audible breath sounds	Evaluate cough pattern and encourage cough. Facilitate deep breathing by elevating head or sitting client up. Position to facilitate cough and prevent aspiration. Ensure hydration (oral intake approximately 2 L/day, humidified ambient air). Provide bronchial drainage treatments (positioning, percussion, and vibration) when indicated. Coordinate inhaled bronchodilator administration to facilitate clearance. Minimize exposure to environmental irritants and/or pathogenic organisms. Promote smoking cessation. Teach alternative cough techniques (e.g., quad, huff),* signs and symptoms of infection, and airway clearance techniques.	Expectoration of sputum without difficulty, normal breath sounds, effective coughing

NURSING DIAGNOSIS: Ineffective breathing pattern related to obstruction to airflow, increased work of breathing, respiratory muscle fatigue or failure, and anxiety

Respiratory rate <11 or >24 breaths/min, inspiratory/expiratory ratio >1:1, irregular breathing rhythm (e.g., use of accessory muscles of breathing inappropriate to level of activity), discoordinated abdominal thoracic muscle motion	Evaluate breathing patterns. Position client to maximize respiratory effect (i.e., sitting with stabilization of shoulders). Administer O_2 if appropriate. Initiate energy conservation techniques. Provide relaxation training (e.g., biofeedback, progressive muscle relaxation, imagery). Use airway clearance techniques. Teach and demonstrate pursed-lip and abdominal breathing.	Reported decrease in dyspnea; respiratory rate, rhythm, depth, and timing within normal limits; use of accessory muscles appropriate to activity level

NURSING DIAGNOSIS: Impaired gas exchange: hypercapnia related to alveolar hypoventilation

$Paco_2$ more than 45 mm Hg and abnormal for client's baseline, headache on awakening	Ensure adequate alveolar ventilation by providing frequent stimulation (e.g., talking, turning, and positioning), teaching pursed-lip breathing to prolong expiratory phase and slow rate, avoiding use of respiratory depressants. Administer and teach appropriate use of bronchodilator. Teach potential hazard of excessive levels of inspired O_2 to clients with blunted CO_2 drive to breathe. Teach signs, symptoms, and consequences of hypercapnia (e.g., confusion, somnolence, headache, irritability, decrease in mental acuity, increase in respiration, facial flush, diaphoresis). Teach avoidance of central nervous system depressants. Administer and teach appropriate use of bronchodilators.	$Paco_2$ of 40 mm Hg or client's usual compensated baseline value, demonstration of correct techniques to normalize $Paco_2$ (e.g., secretion clearance and bronchodilator therapies), improved mental status

Modified from a care plan developed by the American Thoracic Society.
*See Table 22-12.

Table 22-15

 NURSING CARE PLAN FOR THE CLIENT WITH COPD—cont'd

Defining Characteristics	Nursing Interventions	Evaluation Criteria

NURSING DIAGNOSIS: **Impaired gas exchange: hypoxemia related to alveolar hypoventilation, intrapulmonary shunting, low ventilation to perfusion ratio, diffusion impairment, decreased ambient O_2, and decreased barometric pressure (high altitude)**

Defining Characteristics	Nursing Interventions	Evaluation Criteria
Pao_2 <60 mm Hg or Sao_2 < 90% at rest (for acute COPD at sea level), Pao_2 <60 mm Hg or Sao_2 < 90% during exercise (for chronic COPD at sea level)	Administer O_2 if appropriate. Teach and monitor proper placement of supplementary O_2 devices (e.g., nasal cannula). Select O_2 supply systems and devices (e.g., nasal cannulas, mask) that are appropriate to client activities of daily living (rest, sleep, exercise). Avoid unnecessary activity and provide assistance with activities of daily living. Teach and encourage deep breathing and pursed-lip breathing. Implement airway clearance techniques, if appropriate. Teach client and family early signs and symptoms of impaired gas exchange (e.g., increased respiratory rate, irritability, anxiety, restlessness, dyspnea). Administer and teach appropriate use of bronchodilator. Counsel client about management of hypoxemia associated with air travel and/or increased altitude. Advise avoidance of respiratory depressants.	Return of Pao_2 to normal range for client, increased independence in activities of daily living, improved mental status

NURSING DIAGNOSIS: **Dyspnea related to increased airways resistance (bronchospasm and/or retained secretions), psychological stress provoking and worsening dyspnea (anxiety, depression, fear), noxious environmental stimuli, and air trapping**

Defining Characteristics	Nursing Interventions	Evaluation Criteria
Unpleasant breathing sensation (shortness of breath, breathlessness), gasping, truncated speech patterns, abnormal use of accessory muscles at rest	Administer and/or teach effective use of drugs and equipment (e.g., bronchodilators, diuretics, antibiotics, analgesics, mood elevators). Schedule rest and activity. Provide relaxation training (e.g., biofeedback, imagery, progressive muscle relaxation). Provide psychomotor distraction techniques to desensitize dyspnea (e.g., progressive exercise with coaching). Assist client to assume position of comfort (e.g., tripod position, elevated backrest, supported upper extremities to fix shoulder girdle). Remove or limit noxious environmental stimuli. Teach, encourage, and demonstrate pursed-lip breathing.	Diminished sensation of unpleasant breathing, less anxiety

NURSING DIAGNOSIS: **Self-care deficit related to lowered energy level, hypoxemia, and depression**

Defining Characteristics	Nursing Interventions	Evaluation Criteria
Dependency, fatigue, weakness, muscle wasting, shortness of breath on exertion or rest, inadequate intake, poor personal hygiene	Assess type of self-care deficits. Teach energy conservation measures, including lifting on exhalation, modifying house, using assistive devices, transferring techniques, pacing activities, and planning periods of rest. Refer for occupational therapy when appropriate. Administer O_2, if appropriate. Teach appropriate physical conditioning exercises. Investigate need for personal assistance in home. Refer to agencies that provide necessary assistance.	Achievement of activities of daily living by client or with partial or total assistance, decrease in shortness of breath on exertion

Continued.

Table 22-15

NURSING CARE PLAN FOR THE CLIENT WITH COPD—cont'd

Defining Characteristics	Nursing Interventions	Evaluation Criteria

NURSING DIAGNOSIS: Altered nutrition: less than body requirements related to poor appetite, lowered energy level, shortness of breath, gastric distention, sputum production, and depression

Weight loss >10% of ideal body weight, serum albumin level below normal laboratory values, weight loss, weakness, muscle wasting, dehydration, decreased muscle tone, poor skin integrity	Assess dietary preferences and dental status. Monitor daily caloric intake. Identify foods that require little work to prepare or eat. Plan periods of rest after food intake. Provide menu suggestions for high-protein, high-calorie foods. Provide high-protein, high-calorie liquid supplements if necessary. Teach client to avoid gas-producing foods. Provide O_2 supplement during meals as required and prescribed. Refer to agency for financial or nutritional assistance as necessary (e.g., Meals-on-Wheels, food stamps). Be aware that client may benefit from six small meals throughout day.	Maintenance of body weight within normal range for height and age

NURSING DIAGNOSIS: Fluid volume excess related to fluid retention secondary to cor pulmonale or steroid use

Peripheral and/or sacral edema; increased dyspnea; abnormal breath sounds (rales, crackles, wheezes); weight gain >3 lb in 1 wk or 2 lb on consecutive days; JVD; taut, shiny skin; pedal edema	Auscultate chest and heart for abnormal sounds. Continually assess change in activity level; JVD; edema and amount of pitting; electrolyte, hemoglobin, and hematocrit levels. Monitor input and output and daily weights. Teach positions to enhance venous return. Teach client to weigh self daily and report weight gain >3 lb/wk or 2 lb on consecutive days without evidence of other cause. Elevate head of bed if client is dyspneic. Teach client to report increase in dyspnea. Administer O_2, if appropriate. Provide bed or chair rest during acute phase. Monitor and teach effectiveness of drug therapy (e.g., diuretics and potassium supplement, digoxin). Restrict sodium intake, if prescribed.	No evidence of fluid retention, baseline weight for client

NURSING DIAGNOSIS: Sleep pattern disturbance related to anxiety, depression, hypoxemia and/or hypercapnia, and shortness of breath

Insomnia, lethargy, fatigue, restlessness, irritability; decreased level of activities of daily living; morning headaches; decreased Pa_{O_2} with or without increased Pa_{CO_2}; orthopnea, paroxysmal nocturnal dyspnea	Identify usual sleep habits. Assist client to identify sources of discomfort and wakefulness. Observe for signs and symptoms of sleep apnea syndrome. Identify client-specific methods of relaxation, and teach client relaxation methods. Encourage exercise and activity during daylight hours. Instruct client regarding position for easier breathing. Instruct client to eat small evening meals. Administer O_2, if appropriate. Encourage verbalization of feelings. Assist client to identify source of help during night. Instruct client in maintaining an environment conducive to rest (e.g., clothing, temperature, position, noise level). Teach potential dangers in use of respiratory depressants. Teach avoidance of alcoholic beverages, caffeine products, or other stimulants before bedtime. Teach signs and symptoms of early hypoxemia and/or hypercapnia. Administer sedatives as prescribed.	Verbalization of feeling of being rested, improvement in sleep pattern

Modified from a care plan developed by the American Thoracic Society.

Table 22-15

Defining Characteristics	Nursing Interventions	Evaluation Criteria

NURSING DIAGNOSIS: Sexual dysfunction related to physiological alterations, hypoxemia, shortness of breath, effect of medications, and psychological factors

Decrease in desire for or interest in sex; decrease in social interactions with actual or potential sexual partners; avoidance of discussion of subject; inappropriate verbal or physical sexual behaviors; decrease in sexual activity; report of impotence; divorce or breakup of relationships; decrease in interest in appearance; increase in passivity; increase in feelings of hopelessness	Determine basis for dysfunction—physical or psychological. Teach use of O_2 during sexual activities, if appropriate. Provide opportunity for client and significant other to discuss feelings regarding problem. Help partner to understand change. Teach effects of medication and recommend modification, if necessary. Encourage client and partner to explore other means of sexual expression and planning of sexual activity in terms of energy levels during the day. Counsel client and partner on sexual positions to conserve energy. Refer for counseling, if indicated.	Verbalization of satisfaction with sexual functioning

NURSING DIAGNOSIS: High risk for disturbance in self-concept, body image, self-esteem, role performance related to changes in body appearances, function, personal and societal role, and increased physical and psychological dependence

Carelessness in dress and grooming; expression of depression and/or anxiety; difficulty in decision making; withdrawal from social situations, family interactions and work-related responsibilities; ineffectual social interactions; verbal and nonverbal expression of decrease in self-worth; increase in dependent behaviors	Determine basis for disturbance in self-concept. Help client identify and optimize physical and psychological strengths. Help client maintain social interaction by participation in family and social activities. Help family or significant others to understand client's limitations and need for acceptance. Help family understand client's need for independence and feeling of significant worth.	Maintenance of social contacts, expression of positive feelings about self

NURSING DIAGNOSIS: High risk for infection related to decreased pulmonary function, possible steroid therapy, ineffective airway clearance, and lack of knowledge regarding signs and symptoms of infection and preventive measures

Change in color, quantity, odor, and viscosity of sputum; difficulty in mobilizing secretions; foul oral odor; increase in cough; increase in dyspnea; fever; chills; diaphoresis; increase in respiratory rate; abnormal breath sounds (gurgles, wheezing); hypoxemia and/or hypercapnia; excessive fatigue	Teach client to avoid contact (whenever possible) with persons with respiratory infections. Encourage client to obtain vaccines for influenza and pneumococcal pneumonia. Teach proper care and cleaning of home respiratory equipment. Instruct client to seek medical attention for manifestations of infection, such as changes in sputum characteristics, excessive fatigue, increased cough, increased shortness of breath, fever, chills, diaphoresis, chest discomfort, and wheezing. Teach client to initiate plan of care previously discussed with physician when infections occur (e.g., increase fluid intake, begin antibiotics, increase steroid dosage).	Demonstration of behaviors designed to minimize risk of infection, seeking of medical attention for appropriate interventions, absence of infection

These groups are sponsored by such organizations as the American Lung Association, American Cancer Society, and American Heart Association. These groups also have literature available that provides helpful guidelines, encouragement, and support. Nurses need to participate actively in developing policies establishing smoke-free working environments for themselves and others, controlling smoking in public places, requiring self-extinguishing cigarettes to prevent fire deaths and injuries, prohibiting advertising and tobacco promotions, and mandating health warning labels on cigarette packages.

Early diagnosis and treatment of respiratory tract infections are another way to decrease the incidence of COPD. Avoiding exposure to large crowds in the peak periods for influenza may be necessary, especially for older adults and persons with a history of respiratory problems. Influenza (given yearly) and pneumococcal pneumonia (given once in a lifetime) vaccines are recommended for clients with COPD.

Families with a history of AAT deficiency need to be aware of the genetic nature of the disease. Genetic counseling may be appropriate for clients who are planning to have children.

Acute intervention. Clients with COPD will require acute intervention for complications such as pneumonia, cor pulmonale, and acute respiratory failure. (The nursing care for these conditions are discussed in Chapters 21 and 23.) Once the crisis in these situations has been resolved, the nurse can assess the degree and severity of the underlying respiratory problem. (The section on assessment in Chapter 19 provides a beginning tool to use in obtaining information from the client.) The information obtained will help to plan the nursing care (Table 22-15).

When a client with COPD is first diagnosed or when a client has complications that require hospitalization, the nurse should expect a variety of emotional responses from the person ranging from denial and guilt to depression. Guilt may be due to the realization that the disease was caused largely by cigarette smoking. Depression may be experienced as the severity and chronicity of the disease are realized. Denial may exist if the disease is not yet severe enough to cause much physical limitation. The nurse needs to convey a sense of understanding and caring to the client.

Chronic management. By far the most important aspect in the long-term care of the client with COPD is education (Table 22-16). Because COPD is a chronic, debilitating disease, the client will benefit by being able to exert some control over the disease. Because each COPD client has different learning expectations, motivations, and needs, teaching must be adapted individually. Therefore it is important before beginning to teach or develop a teaching plan to first assess the client's level of knowledge, motivations, and goals. The nurse should help the client understand that it is possible to plan treatment aimed at preserving lung function and slowing the progression of the disease. Client and family participation in the treatment plan is essential. Respiratory care, as well as other related approaches, (see Table 22-15) will be ongoing.

The health professional usually finds that it is not real-

Table 22-16 Components of a Teaching Plan for the Client with Obstructive Pulmonary Disease

Basic understanding of drug, O_2, respiratory, and other therapies
Knowledge of the signs and symptoms of respiratory infection, heart failure, and bronchospasm
Knowledge of good nutrition
Knowledge of energy conservation techniques
Demonstration of abdominal breathing and pursed-lip breathing
Demonstration of chest physiotherapy including vibration, percussion, and postural drainage, when indicated
Steps for healthy psychological coping
Basic understanding of lung function and pathophysiology

istic to teach everything at one time. For example, if the client has recently been hospitalized for acute respiratory failure resulting from a respiratory infection, the focus of teaching may be on helping the client identify the signs and symptoms of a respiratory infection (e.g., fever, increased dyspnea, purulent sputum, increased use of inhalers or nebulizer treatments without relief) and writing down with input from the client a plan that may be used if these symptoms recur. The plan may include the following: notify the physician, increase fluid intake, with the physician's order increase bronchial drainage and nebulizer treatments (e.g., from twice a day to four times per day), begin taking prescribed antibiotics, monitor for decrease or increase in symptoms, and notify the physician of the effects of these interventions.

ACTIVITY CONSIDERATIONS. Energy conservation is another important component in COPD rehabilitation. These clients are typically upper thoracic and neck breathers, using accessory muscles rather than the diaphragm. Thus they have difficulty performing upper-extremity activities, particularly those activities that require arm elevation above the head. Frequently the client has already adapted alternative energy-saving practices for activities of daily living. Alternative methods of hair care, shaving, showering, and reaching may need to be explored. An occupational therapist may help with ideas in these areas. Assuming a tripod posture (elbows supported on a table, chest in fixed position) and a mirror placed on the table during use of an electric razor or hair dryer conserves much more energy than when the client stands in front of a mirror to shave or blow-dry hair. The client should be encouraged to make a schedule and plan daily and weekly activities so as to leave plenty of time for rest periods. The client should also try to sit as much as possible when performing activities. Another energy-saving tip is to exhale when pushing, pulling, or exerting effort during an activity.

Walking is by far the best physical exercise for the COPD client. Coordinated walking with slow, pursed-lip breathing without breath holding is a difficult task that requires conscious effort and frequent reinforcement. During coordinated walking and breathing, the client is taught to breathe through the nose while taking one step, then to breathe through pursed lips while taking two to four steps (the number depends on the client's tolerance). Walking should occur at a slow pace with rest periods as necessary so that the client can lean on a tree, post, or O_2 tank. Once the client is able to successfully perform coordinated walking with pursed-lip breathing, diaphragmatic breathing may also be incorporated if the client has practiced and mastered this at rest. The nurse should walk with the client, giving verbal reminders as necessary regarding breathing (inhalation and exhalation) and steps. Walking with the client helps to decrease anxiety and to maintain a slow pace; it also enables the nurse to observe the client's actions and physiological responses to the activity. Many clients with moderate or severe COPD are anxious and fearful of walking or performing exercise. These clients and their families require much support while they build the confidence they need to walk or to perform daily exercises.

Clients should be encouraged to walk 15 to 20 minutes per day with gradual increases. Severely disabled clients can begin at a slow pace by walking for 2 to 5 minutes three times per day and slowly building up to 20 minutes a day, if possible. Adequate rest periods should be allowed. Parameters to monitor are resting pulse and pulse rate after walking. Pulse rate after walking should not exceed 75% to 80% of the maximum heart rate (maximum heart rate is $220 -$ age in years). In clients with COPD and without significant heart disease, it is usually dyspnea and the limitation in breathing rather than increased heart rate that limits the exercise. Clients should be told that their shortness of breath will probably increase during exercise (as it does for healthy individuals) but that they are not overdoing the activity if this increased shortness of breath returns to baseline within 3 to 5 minutes after the cessation of exercise. Clients may benefit from keeping a diary or log of their exercise program. The diary can help provide a realistic evaluation of the client's progress. In addition, the diary can help motivate the client and add to the client's sense of accomplishment. Stationary cycling can also be used either alone or with walking. Cycles are particularly valuable when weather prevents walking outside.

Modifying but not abstaining from sexual activity can also contribute to a healthy psychological well-being. Using an inhaled bronchodilator before lovemaking can help ventilation. Also, clients with COPD will use less energy if they plan sexual activity during the part of the day when their breathing is best, use slow pursed-lip breathing, refrain from lovemaking after eating or other strenuous activity, do not assume a dominant position, and do not prolong foreplay. These aspects of lovemaking require open communication between partners regarding their needs and expectations.

Adequate sleep is extremely important. Getting adequate amounts of sleep can be difficult for COPD clients. Medications may cause irritability and insomnia. Many clients with COPD have postnasal drip or nasal congestion that may cause coughing and wheezing at night. Nasal saline douches before sleep and in the morning may help. The physician may also prescribe a nasal decongestant that

may be used at bedtime. Long-acting theophylline preparations frequently aid in promoting sleep by decreasing bronchospasm and airway obstruction.

Long-term use of O_2 therapy has improved the quality of life for many clients with COPD. The use of controlled, low-flow O_2 at home can improve the client's exercise tolerance and appetite and alleviate pulmonary hypertension. (Increased pulmonary vascular resistance is associated with alveolar hypoxia.) If pulmonary hypertension is reduced, the risk of cor pulmonale decreases. In addition, chronic hypoxia is partially corrected, and secondary polycythemia is less likely to develop. One of the major benefits of O_2 use at home is that clients have a sense of well-being and gain more freedom in their choice of activities. Because hypoxemia worsens during sleep in some clients with hypoxemic COPD, supplemental O_2 during the night is definitely indicated for them. (O_2 therapy is discussed in Chapter 21.)

PSYCHOSOCIAL CONSIDERATIONS. Healthy psychological coping is often the most difficult task to master. People with COPD frequently have to deal with many lifestyle changes that may involve decreased ability to care for themselves, decreased energy for social activities, and loss of a job. Emotions frequently encountered include anxiety, depression, social isolation, denial, and dependence. The expression of these emotions becomes complicated because of the relationship of emotional expression to breathing. For example, anxiety normally produces an increase in respiratory rate, and depression usually goes along with inactivity, which in the COPD client can translate into decreased exercise tolerance, increased dyspnea, increased dependence, and ultimately, worsening of depression. A vicious circle of emotional entrapment can occur. Learning new ways to express emotions with the use of relaxation techniques involving breathing can be helpful. Slowing their pace with frequent rest periods, open and honest communication with supportive significant others, and avoidance of anxiety-producing situations (if necessary) may need to be learned.

The client with COPD may benefit from several relaxation techniques. One is the use of a progressive relaxation technique in which the client listens either to a tape or to the client's own or another voice and gradually begins to tighten and relax muscle groups. Relaxation may begin in the head and neck area and end in the legs. Self-hypnosis, meditation, and massage (self-massage or massage from others) are other alternative relaxation therapies.

Clients frequently ask whether moving to a warmer or drier climate will help. In general, such a move is not significantly beneficial. Moving to places with an elevation of 4000 feet or more should be discouraged because of the lower partial pressure of O_2 found in the air at higher elevations. A disadvantage of moving may be that a person leaves an occupation, friends, and familiar environment, which could be psychologically stressful. Any advantage gained from a different climate may be outweighed by the psychological effects of the move.

Pulmonary rehabilitation. Pulmonary rehabilitation should be considered for clients with symptomatic COPD. According to the American Thoracic Society, the objectives of pulmonary rehabilitation are to (1) control and alleviate as much as possible the symptoms and pathophysiological complications of respiratory impairment and (2) teach the client how to achieve optimal capability for carrying out activities of daily living. The overall goal is to increase the quality of life. The components of pulmonary rehabilitation include physical therapy (e.g., bronchial hygiene, exercise conditioning, breathing retraining, energy conservation), nutrition, and education and other topics such as smoking cessation, environmental factors, health promotion, psychological counseling, and vocational rehabilitation. Although much of this intervention should be routinely included in the comprehensive approach to the client with COPD, the referral of clients to a structured pulmonary rehabilitation program should also be considered.[27]

CYSTIC FIBROSIS

Cystic fibrosis (CF) is an autosomal recessive multisystem disease characterized by altered function of the exocrine glands involving primarily the lungs, pancreas, and sweat glands. Abnormally thick, abundant secretions from mucous glands can lead to a chronic, diffuse, obstructive pulmonary disorder in almost all clients. Exocrine pancreatic insufficiency is associated with about 85% to 90% of the cases of CF. Sweat glands excrete increased amounts of sodium and chloride.

Significance

The disease occurs primarily in white persons, with a frequency of 1 in 2000 births among whites and 1 in 17,000 births among blacks. Both sexes are equally affected. According to the Cystic Fibrosis Foundation Center, at least 30,000 people in the United States had CF in 1990. About 20% of these are young adults.[28]

CF was once exclusively a pediatric disease. However, because of improved and aggressive treatment, the median survival of clients with CF has increased from less than 2 years in 1950 to almost 25 years of age currently; many survive to their thirties and forties.[28] Each person has an individual spectrum of the disease and time course of deterioration.

Pathophysiology

CF is transmitted as an autosomal recessive trait. The carrier rate in the white population is 1 in 20. Recently the CF gene was identified on chromosome 7, permitting antenatal diagnosis and carrier detection. There is evidence of defective ionic transport of sodium and chloride across epithelial surfaces. The defect has been located in the chloride channel.[29] The high concentrations of sodium and chloride in the sweat of clients with CF results from the impermeability of chloride reabsorption in the sweat duct. The basic pathophysiological mechanism is obstruction of exocrine gland ducts with thick, viscous secretions that adhere to the lumen of the ducts (Fig. 22-19). The glands distal to the duct eventually undergo fibrosis.

In the respiratory system, both upper and lower respiratory tracts can be affected. Upper respiratory tract manifestations may be present and include nasal polyposis. The hallmark of respiratory involvement in CF is its effect on the airways. The disease progresses from being a disease of the small airways (chronic bronchiolitis) to an entity that eventually involves the larger airways and finally causes destruction of lung parenchyma. Thick secretions obstruct bronchioles and lead to air trapping and hyperinflation of the lungs. The stasis of mucus provides an excellent growth medium for bacteria. The most common organisms cultured from the sputum of clients with CF are *S. aureus, H. influenzae,* and *Pseudomonas aeruginosa.*[28,29]

Lung disorders that can result include pneumonia, bronchiolitis, bronchitis, bronchiectasis, atelectasis, and emphysema. There is progressive loss of lung tissue from inflammation and scarring, and the resultant chronic hypoxia leads to pulmonary hypertension and cor pulmonale. Blebs and large cysts in the lung are also severe manifestations of lung destruction. Other pulmonary complications include hemoptysis (which can sometimes be fatal) and pneumothorax.

Initially, CF is an obstructive lung disease caused by the overall obstruction of the airways with mucus. Later, CF also progresses to a restrictive lung disease because of the fibrosis, lung destruction, and thoracic wall changes. Death is usually due to extensive respiratory infection. Cor pulmonale is a common late complication caused by extensive loss of lung tissue and chronic hypoxia.

Pancreatic insufficiency is due primarily to mucus plugging the pancreatic duct and its branches, which results in fibrosis of the acinar glands of the pancreas. The exocrine function of the pancreas is altered and may completely stop. Pancreatic enzymes such as trypsinogen, lipase, and amylase do not reach the intestine to digest ingested nutrients. There is malabsorption of fat, protein, and fat-soluble vitamins (e.g., A, D, E, K). Fat malabsorption results in steatorrhea, and protein malabsorption results in failure to grow and gain weight. In advanced pancreatic insufficiency, diabetes mellitus may occur if the islets of Langerhans become fibrotic.

The sweat glands excrete four times the normal amount of sodium and chloride. This abnormality does not seem to affect the general health of the person. However, this finding is useful as a diagnostic indicator.

The liver may become involved. Biliary cirrhosis may not be recognized until late in the disease. Hepatobiliary disease is common in older clients. Chronic cholestasis, inflammation, fibrosis, and cirrhosis are present. Portal hypertension can also occur.

The function of the reproductive system is altered. This finding is important because more persons with CF are living to adulthood. The adult male is usually sterile (although not impotent) as a result of structural changes in the vas deferens, seminal vesicles, and epididymis. The female usually has delayed menarche and may develop secondary amenorrhea. She may be unable to become pregnant because of the increased viscosity of the cervical mucus. However, women with CF do become pregnant, but the fertility rate is lower than in healthy women. The baby is heterozygous (and hence a carrier) for CF if the father is not a carrier. If the father is a carrier, there is a 50% chance that the baby will have CF.

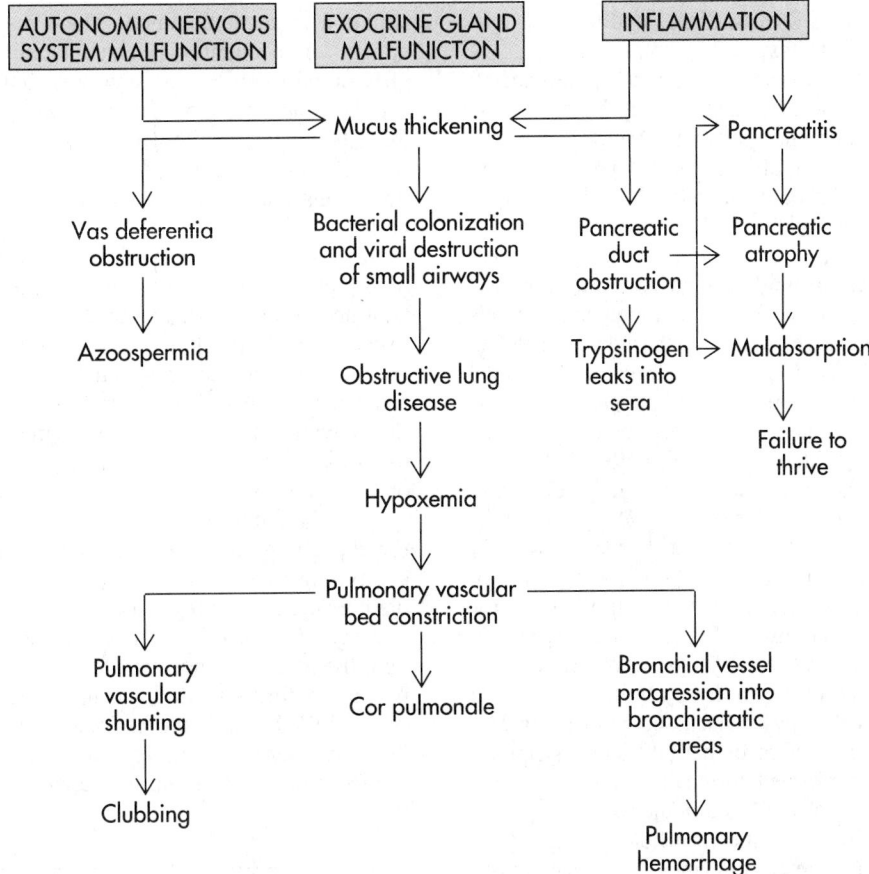

Fig. 22-19 Progression of cystic fibrosis. (Modified from Cherniack RM: Current therapy of respiratory disease, ed 3, St Louis, 1989, The CV Mosby Co, p 187.)

Clinical Manifestations and Complications

The clinical manifestations of CF vary depending on the severity of the disease. An initial finding of meconium ileus in the newborn infant is present in 10% of persons with CF. Early manifestations in childhood are failure to grow, clubbing, persistent cough with mucus production, tachypnea, and large, frequent bowel movements. A large, protuberant abdomen may develop with an emaciated appearance of the extremities. Other respiratory problems that may be indicative of CF are recurring lung infections such as bronchiolitis, bronchitis, and pneumonia.

The severity and progression of the disease vary from person to person. In the past decade, it has been shown that with early diagnosis and immediate institution of intensive care, the prognosis can be significantly improved.

Diagnostic Studies

The main diagnostic test for CF is the sweat chloride test with the pilocarpine iontophoresis method. Pilocarpine carried by a small electric current is used to stimulate sweat production. The sweat is collected on filter paper or gauze and then analyzed for sodium and chloride concentrations. The test takes about 40 minutes. Values greater than 65 mEq/L for both sodium and chloride are suggestive of CF, especially in a person who has other clinical features of the disease. The degree of sodium and chloride elevation does not necessarily correlate with the severity of the disease. Fetal diagnosis can now be made by analyzing gene markers from the chorionic villus tissue. Other diagnostic studies that may be done include chest x-ray film, pulmonary function tests, fecal analysis for fat, and duodenoscopy for quantitative determination of enzymes.

Therapeutic Management

No specific therapy exists for this disease. The management of pulmonary problems in CF is aimed at relief of airway obstruction and control of infection. Drainage of thick bronchial mucus is assisted by aerosol and nebulization treatments of medications used to liquefy mucus and to facilitate coughing. Aerosolized decongestants (e.g., phenylephrine hydrochloride), Mucomyst, and bronchodilators (e.g., β$_2$ agonists, theophylline) may be used. Chest physiotherapy (e.g., postural drainage, vibration, and percussion) has been the mainstay of treatment for some time.

Aerobic exercise seems to be effective in clearing the airways. Important needs to consider in planning an aerobic exercise program for the client with CF are that frequent rest periods should be interspersed throughout the exercise regimen, that increased nutritional demands of exercise should be met, and that the client should learn to observe for manifestations of heat illness and to drink lots of fluid and replace salt losses.

Antimicrobial treatment is initiated for the treatment of infection. Prolonged high-dose therapy may be necessary because many drugs are abnormally metabolized and rapidly excreted in clients with CF. Pharmacokinetic and kidney function studies should therefore be monitored closely. Oral agents commonly used are trimethoprim-sulfamethoxazole, tetracycline, chloramphenicol, cephalosporins, antistaphylococcal penicillins, and new oral quinolones, especially ciprofloxacin. Newer compounds that show promise with gram-negative spectrums include cefsulodin, ceftazidime, nalidixic acid, and thienamycin. Although oral and aerosolized antimicrobial therapy provided 20% to 80% of the time is usually adequate, some clients require a 10- to 20-day course of IV antimicrobial therapy. If home facilities are adequate, CF clients and their families may choose to continue parenteral therapy at home. The usual treatment for acute infectious exacerbations is aminoglycosides, penicillin, or third-generation cephalosporins. Aerosolized bronchodilators and antiinflammatory agents (e.g., cromolyn) are used in selected clients, particularly before chest physical therapy (see Table 22-4). Clients who have cor pulmonale or hypoxemia may require home O_2 therapy (O_2 therapy is discussed in Chapter 21). Sclerosing of the pleural space or partial pleural stripping and pleural abrasion performed surgically are usually indicated for recurrent episodes of pneumothorax.

The management of pancreatic insufficiency includes a drug preparation of pancreatic enzymes (e.g., pancrease, Cotazym-S, and Creon), high-calorie intake, and multivitamins. Fat restriction is usually not necessary. Improvement in nutritional status has been shown with the use of short-term caloric supplements. However, no long-term benefit in nutritional or pulmonary status has been demonstrated.[29] Added dietary salt is indicated whenever sweating is excessive, such as during hot weather, in the presence of fever, or from intense physical activity.

■ Nursing Management of Cystic Fibrosis

Nursing diagnoses related to CF may include, but are not limited to, ineffective airway clearance, ineffective breathing pattern, impaired gas exchange, altered nutrition, and altered growth and development (see Table 22-15). Chest physical therapy is the mainstay of intervention for ineffective airway clearance in this population (see p. 588). The family or person with CF has a great financial and emotional burden. The cost of drugs, special equipment, and continual care is often a great financial hardship. Emotionally, the burden of living with a chronic disease at a young age can be overwhelming. Community resources are often available to help the family. In addition, in many areas the Cystic Fibrosis Foundation can be of assistance.

The nurse and other health professionals can assist young adults to gain independence by helping them assume responsibility for their care and for their vocational or school goals. A major problem that needs to be discussed at this time is sexuality. Delayed or irregular menstruation is not uncommon. There may be delayed development of secondary sex characteristics such as breasts in girls or prolonged short stature in boys. The person may use the illness to avoid certain events or relationships. On the other hand, healthy persons may be hesitant to make friends with someone who is sick. Other crises and life transitions that must be dealt with in the young adult include building confidence and self-respect on the basis of achievements, persevering with employment goals, developing motivation to achieve, learning to cope with the treatment program, and adjusting to the need for dependence if health fails.

The issue of marrying and having children is difficult. Most men with CF are sterile. Women with the disease may have difficulty becoming pregnant. An additional factor is that any child produced will either be a carrier of CF or have the disease. Another concern is the shortened life span of the parent with CF and that parent's ability to care for the child must be taken into consideration. Genetic counseling may be an appropriate suggestion for the couple considering having children.

Regardless of how well the person is coping with living with the disease, a normal life span is not possible. As the person continues toward and into adulthood, the nurse and other skilled health professionals need to be available to help the client and family cope with complications resulting from the disease and to prepare for dying.

C ase Study

ACUTE ASTHMATIC ATTACK

Fred, a 20-year-old man, was seen in the emergency room for an asthma attack. He stated that he had had a history of asthma since childhood and had positive reactions to various allergens including house dust and grasses. He was not aware of what precipitated his current attack, but it occurred while he was trying out for the college football team.

Fred uses an Alupent inhaler at home. During the past 24 hours, he has increased his Alupent inhalations every 2 hours without relief. At present, he is not receiving steroid therapy.

On physical examination, he was in acute respiratory distress. Vital signs revealed a temperature of 39° C (102.2° F), pulse 126 beats/min, respirations 32 breaths/min, and blood pressure 140/88 mm Hg. He was sitting upright using his accessory muscles for ventilation, was audibly wheezing, and was diaphoretic. Auscultation of the chest revealed diffuse expiratory and inspiratory wheezing.

Discussion Questions

1. Explain the pathophysiology of asthma.
2. How does asthma differ from chronic bronchitis and pulmonary emphysema?
3. What could be the precipitating factors in Fred's asthma attack?
4. What are the clinical manifestations of a asthma attack? Which of these did Fred manifest?
5. What can a nurse do to alleviate his acute respiratory distress?

R *eview Questions*

The number of the question corresponds to the same-numbered objective at the beginning of the chapter.

1. Asthma is best characterized as
   a. an obstructive disease with loss of alveolar walls
   b. an inflammatory disease
   c. a steady progression of bronchoconstriction
   d. an obstructive disease characterized by mucus production

2. The teaching plan for the asthmatic client includes all of the following *except*
   a. preventing or limiting exposure of the client to antigens
   b. isolating the client to prevent respiratory infections
   c. preventing psychological invalidism
   d. deep-breathing and coughing exercises to clear the airway

3. COPD is characterized by all of the following *except*
   a. increased airway resistance on expiration
   b. fibrosis of the alveolar capillary surface
   c. an excessive amount and retention of secretions
   d. decreased residual volume

4. Which of the following effects does cigarette smoking have on the respiratory system?
   a. hyperplasia of goblet cells and increased production of mucus
   b. increased proliferation of ciliated cells
   c. hypertrophy of the alveolar membrane
   d. destruction of all alveolar macrophages

5. One of the most important things a nurse can teach a client with COPD is to
   a. obtain adequate rest in the supine position
   b. move to a hot, dry climate
   c. know the signs of infection
   d. perform chest physical therapy

6. Diagnostic studies that would probably be abnormal in a person with CF are
   a. pancreatic enzymes and hormones
   b. pulmonary function study and sweat test
   c. sweat test and vitamin B tolerance test
   d. insulin tolerance and blood sugars

REFERENCES

1. Dean NC and Brown JK: Status asthmaticus, Postgrad Med 84:103-114, 1988.
2. American Thoracic Society: Standards for the diagnosis care of patients with chronic obstructive pulmonary disease and asthma, Am Rev Respir Dis 136:225-244, 1987.
3. American Lung Association: Public policy briefing kit, New York, 1989.
4. American Lung Association: ALA memo, update details XIII, New York, 1990, pp 1-17.
5. Weiss KB and others: Changing patterns of asthma mortality: identifying target populations at high risk, JAMA 264:1683-1687, 1990.
6. Newhouse MT: Etiology of intrinsic asthma, Agents Actions Suppl 28:17-25, 1989.
7. Kaliner MA: The late-phase reaction and its clinical implications, Hosp Pract 22:73-83, 1987.
8. Larsen GL: The pulmonary late-phase response, Hosp Pract 22:155-159, 1987.
9. Norn S and Clementsen P: Bronchial asthma: pathophysiological mechanisms and corticosteroids, Allergy 43:401-405, 1988.
10. Frick WE and Bussie W: Respiratory infections: their role in airway responsiveness and pathogenesis of asthma, Clin Chest Med 9:539-549, 1988.
11. Miller BD: Depression and asthma: a potentially lethal mixture, J Allergy Clin Immunol 80:481, 1987.
12. Bjerklie SJ: Status asthmaticus, Am J Nurs 90:52-55, 1990.
13. Barnes PJ: A new approach to the treatment of asthma, N Engl J Med 321:1517-1527, 1989.
14. Barnes PJ: Chronic asthma. In Cherniak RM: Current therapy of respiratory disease, ed 3, Philadelphia, 1989, BC Decker, pp 132-136.
15. Snider GL: Chronic obstructive pulmonary disease: risk factors, pathophysiology and pathogenesis, Ann Rev Med 40:411-429, 1989.
16. Feinleib M and others: Trends in COPD morbidity and mortality in the United States, Am Rev Respir Dis 140:S9-S18, 1989.
17. Davis RN and Novotny TE: The epidemiology of cigarette smoking and its impact on chronic obstructive pulmonary disease, Am Rev Respir Dis 140:S82-S84, 1989.
18. The health consequences of smoking: chronic obstructive lung disease—a report of the Surgeon General, Rockville, Md, 1985, US Department of Health and Human Services.
19. Jackson FN and Holle RHO: Smoking: perspectives, Primary Care 12:197-216, 1985.
20. Buist AS: Alpha-1-antitrypsin deficiency in lung and liver disease, Hosp Pract 24:51-59, 1989.
21. Dines DE: Chronic bronchitis: managing the disease and related infections, Postgrad Med 79:235-237, 1986.
22. American Thoracic Society: Guidelines for the approach to the patient with severe hereditary alpha-1-antitrypsin deficiency, Am Rev Respir Dis 140:1491-1497, 1989.
23. Kutty K and Varkey B: Chronic obstructive pulmonary disease, Postgrad Med 84:60-80, 1988.
24. Petty TL: COPD in the setting of "multidimensional" illness, Hosp Pract 23:39-50, 1988.
25. Hoffman LA, Mazzocco MC, and Roth JE: Fine tuning your chest PT, Am J Nurs 87:1566-1572, 1987.
26. Openbrier DR and Covey M: Ineffective breathing pattern related to malnutrition, Nurs Clin North Am 22:225-247, 1987.
27. Make BJ and Paine R: Pulmonary rehabilitation for COPD patients, Hosp Pract 22:26-34, 1987.
28. Welsh MJ and Fick RB: Cystic fibrosis, J Clin Invest 80:1523-1526, 1987.
29. Stern RC: Cystic fibrosis: recent developments in diagnosis and treatment, Pediatr Rev 7:276-286, 1986.

CHAPTER 23

Nursing Role in Management
Respiratory Failure

Trisch Van Sciver
Terri E. Weaver

Respiratory intensive care may be administered in a specialized respiratory intensive care unit (ICU) or in a medical, surgical, coronary, or trauma unit. Respiratory intensive care of the critically ill client with a respiratory problem requires an organized team approach to provide a continuous, well-defined management program. The intensive care nurse is an integral member of this health team. Respiratory intensive care nursing is based on understanding cardiopulmonary anatomy and physiology and the pathophysiology of acute respiratory failure. Essential nursing skills include the ability to monitor clients closely, with an understanding of physiological parameters, and to anticipate and detect complications and initiate measures to correct them immediately. Adept performance of technical skills involved in airway care and respiratory management of the client is essential. The nurse is also responsible for the regulation and coordination of the emotional and physical aspects of care for the totally dependent client.

Reviewed by Sr. Regina Maibusch, R.N., M.S., Respiratory Clinical Nurse Specialist, St. Michael Hospital, Milwaukee, Wisconsin.

Nurses working in specialized respiratory ICUs may share with the respiratory therapist a variety of skills unique to this setting, including intubation, extubation, changing of tracheostomy tubes, performance of pulmonary function tests, use of the oximeter, administration of aerosolized bronchodilators and mucolytic agents, and use of long-term arterial blood gas (ABG) monitoring equipment.

The goal of this chapter is to provide an introduction to the knowledge and skills involved in the care of the client with acute respiratory failure. Four general areas are discussed:

1. Pathophysiology of acute respiratory failure and related nursing management
2. Adult respiratory distress syndrome, a type of acute respiratory failure
3. Care of the client with an artificial airway
4. Physiological principles, types, modes, hazards, and nursing care of the client receiving mechanical ventilation

Psychological support measures for the client in acute respiratory distress and the family affected are discussed throughout the chapter.

ACUTE RESPIRATORY FAILURE

Acute respiratory failure is present when alveolar ventilation is inadequate to meet the body's needs. The lungs can no longer adequately oxygenate the blood. Although no universal definition exists, the most common definition used is an arterial oxygen pressure (Pao_2) of less than 50 mm Hg and/or an arterial carbon dioxide pressure ($Paco_2$) of greater than 50 mm Hg at sea level.[1]

Acute respiratory failure in a client with chronic restrictive or obstructive lung disease cannot be defined according to the criteria used for the client with normal lungs. Clients with chronic pulmonary diseases are able to tolerate and compensate for a significant degree of hypoxemia and/or hypercapnia. Many stable, ambulatory clients with chronic pulmonary disease maintain Pao_2 levels as low as 60 mm Hg or $Paco_2$ levels as high as 50 mm Hg with a normal pH. In chronic lung disease, acute respiratory failure can be defined as alveolar ventilation inadequate to oxygenate the blood sufficiently, as evidenced by an acute decrease in Pao_2 and/or an increase in $Paco_2$ (with an acidic pH) from the client's baseline parameters.

Risk Factors

All critically ill clients are at risk for respiratory distress and/or acute respiratory failure. These clients have already sustained significant injury to one or more body organ systems. Because there are so many functional systemic interrelationships in the body, disequilibrium in one body system frequently leads to disequilibrium in other systems.

Clients who have undergone recent abdominal or thoracic surgery are at risk for respiratory failure as a result of splinting of their incision, abdominal distention, restrictive bandages, tubes, and reduced ventilation as a result of pain. Extremely obese clients may also be at an increased risk of respiratory failure because of the restriction of ventilation. Comatose clients or those with decreased levels of consciousness and depression of respiratory control center (e.g., after anesthesia, narcotics use, or head injury) are prone to aspiration pneumonia and respiratory failure. Clients who have sustained thoracic or spinal injuries are predisposed to ineffective ventilation. Because of a loss of normal respiratory or protective mechanisms and decreased ventilatory reserve, clients who show evidence of lung disease or who are heavy smokers are at high risk for acute respiratory failure. These clients are especially vulnerable when an infection develops, when the person has surgery, or when other diseases develop. Immunosuppressed clients are also prone to acute respiratory failure for similar reasons. Finally, because of the reduction in ventilatory capacity that accompanies aging, older adults are also at risk for acute respiratory failure, especially when other risk factors are present.

Prevention

Measures to help prevent respiratory failure include preoperative screening and evaluation of all high-risk clients. Pulmonary function tests should be performed and ABG levels assessed preoperatively in high-risk clients to determine the operative risk and to establish baseline parameters for postoperative care. Measures to optimize ventilation such as using parenteral and aerosolized bronchodilators, using incentive spirometry, and teaching effective coughing and deep-breathing techniques are important to prepare the client for surgery. Preoperative teaching of all surgical clients is essential, especially for clients preparing for thoracic or abdominal surgery, so that they will be familiar with what is necessary and expected postoperatively. Cessation of smoking, even 24 hours before surgery, improves mucociliary function, mucous clearance, and oxygenation as a result of decreased carbon monoxide (CO) levels. Early postoperative ambulation and assuming an upright position beginning on the first postoperative day for at least several times during each day are important.

Frequent monitoring of the respiratory status of clients who are critically ill or comatose is imperative. ABG analysis is often an initial part of the workup during admission to the ICU. Astute observation and measurement of the

Table 23-1   Causes of Hypercapnic Acute Respiratory Failure

Alveolar hypoventilation
   Decreased ventilatory drive
      Sedative and narcotic overdosage
      Postoperative anesthetic depression
      Excessive O_2 tensions (especially in the presence of chronic hypercapnia)
      Sleep apnea
   Decreased ventilatory response
      Neuromuscular diseases
         Guillain-Barré syndrome
         Myasthenia gravis
         Bulbar poliomyelitis
         Multiple sclerosis
         Amyotrophic lateral sclerosis
      Spinal cord trauma
      Weakness of respiratory muscles
         Muscular dystrophy
         Severe COPD
      Restrictions to ventilation
         Obesity
         Kyphoscoliosis
         Postoperative pain and splinting
         Pleurisy
         Rib fracture
         Pleural effusions and fibrosis
         Pneumothorax
      Airway obstruction
      Sleep apnea
   Increased CO_2 production
      Increased work of breathing
      Fever, infection
$\dot{V}/\dot{Q}$ mismatch*

*See Table 23-2.

client's respiratory status will assist in early detection of respiratory problems. These measurements include the breathing rate, pattern, and depth; frequent assessment of breath sounds; vital signs and level of consciousness; and pulse oximetry and/or ABGs. Subjective client evaluation is also important. Early recognition of the clinical symptoms of respiratory distress and immediate implementation of corrective measures may prevent further deterioration and failure of the client's respiratory mechanisms.

Pathophysiology

The mechanisms involved in acute respiratory failure result in an increase of carbon dioxide (CO_2) and/or a decrease of oxygen (O_2) in the blood. Mechanisms that contribute to or cause the development of *hypercapnic ventilatory failure* (also called *hypoxemic-hypercapnic respiratory failure* and *Type II respiratory failure*) characterized by elevated $Paco_2$ and decreased Pao_2 are alveolar hypoventilation and ventilation-perfusion ratio ($\dot{V}/\dot{Q}$) mismatch (Table 23-1). Mechanisms that contribute to or cause the development of *hypoxemic respiratory failure* (also called *nonventilatory respiratory failure* and *Type I respiratory*

Table 23-2 Causes of Hypoxemic Acute Respiratory Failure

Alveolar hypoventilation*
$\dot{V}/\dot{Q}$ mismatch
  Decreased ventilation
    Pneumonia
    Atelectasis
    Asthma
    Chronic and acute bronchitis
    Emphysema
    Cystic fibrosis
  Decreased perfusion
    Severe emphysema
    Pulmonary embolus
Diffusion abnormalities
  Diffuse interstitial fibrosis
  Collagen diseases of the lung
    Scleroderma
    Systemic lupus erythematosus
    Rheumatoid lung
  Asbestosis
  Sarcoidosis
  Interstitial pneumonia
  Pulmonary edema
Shunts
  Consolidated pneumonias
  Acute respiratory distress syndrome
  Pulmonary embolus
  Severe hypoxemia
  Hypoalbuminemia
  Sepsis

---

*See Table 23-1.

failure) characterized by normal or decreased Pa_{CO_2} and decreased Pa_{O_2} are alveolar hypoventilation, $\dot{V}/\dot{Q}$ mismatch, shunts, and diffusion abnormalities (Table 23-2).[1]

Mechanisms of hypercapnic ventilatory failure

Alveolar hypoventilation. Alveolar or effective ventilation is the volume of gas per breath that is available for gas exchange in functioning alveoli or terminal respiratory units. When an adult takes a normal breath (tidal volume or V_T) of 500 ml, approximately 150 ml of this gas never reaches the alveoli to be involved in gas exchange. This 150 ml is called the *anatomical dead space* (V_D) and is approximately equal in number to a person's weight in pounds (a 150-pound person has approximately 150 ml of V_D). The remaining 350 ml is the gas available for alveolar ventilation per breath.

Adequate alveolar ventilation is necessary to exchange O_2 for CO_2 in the alveoli. The Pa_{CO_2} is related directly to the amount of CO_2 produced metabolically and inversely to the effective alveolar ventilation. Therefore increased Pa_{CO_2} indicates decreased alveolar ventilation (hypoventilation) and accumulation of CO_2 produced metabolically. Decreased Pa_{CO_2} indicates increased alveolar ventilation (hyperventilation). For the Pa_{CO_2} to remain constant, alveolar ventilation must increase or decrease in proportion to the CO_2 produced metabolically.

Alveolar hypoventilation exists when effective ventilation of the alveoli is no longer adequate for the body's metabolic rate. Less O_2 is supplied, and less CO_2 is removed. Consequently, alveolar and arterial CO_2 levels increase and O_2 levels decrease. Alveolar hypoventilation is commonly caused by diseases outside the lungs, and often the lungs are normal (see Table 23-1).

PHYSIOLOGICAL EFFECTS OF HYPOVENTILATION. The main physiological feature of hypoventilation is hypercapnia (elevated Pa_{CO_2} greater than 50 mm Hg). This occurs because ventilation is inadequate to remove the CO_2 produced by cellular metabolism. A subsequent physiological effect of increased Pa_{CO_2} is a decrease in Pa_{O_2}. In the lungs, the blood extracts more O_2 from the alveolar gas for delivery to the tissues than it gives up CO_2 to the lungs, so a one-to-one relationship does not exist for exchange of O_2 and CO_2 in the blood. When the Pa_{CO_2} increases by 8 mm Hg, the Pa_{O_2} falls by about 10 mm Hg in the presence of pure hypoventilation. As the level of CO_2 increases in the blood (Pa_{CO_2}), the level of CO_2 in the alveoli also increases. Less space is left in the alveoli for O_2. This results in a decrease in Pa_{O_2} that is proportional to the rise in Pa_{CO_2}. Pa_{O_2} cannot fall to very low levels from pure hypoventilation because even if Pa_{CO_2} increases from 35 to 75 mm Hg, Pa_{O_2} decreases from 100 to 50 mm Hg. If hypoxemia exists before the hypoventilation, Pa_{O_2} may be decreased significantly (i.e., a Pa_{O_2} of 60 mm Hg would drop to 50 mm Hg, with a Pa_{CO_2} increase of 10 mm Hg). In clients with normal lungs an increase in Pa_{CO_2} causes an increase in minute ventilation (minute ventilation is $V_T \times$ respiratory rate $\times$ 60 seconds). In normal persons, when Pa_{CO_2} is greater than 70 mm Hg, ventilation can be depressed and eventually lead to coma and death.[2]

A second physiological effect of increased Pa_{CO_2} is decreased pH. Respiratory acidemia results as CO_2 accumulates in the plasma ($CO_2 + H_2O \rightleftharpoons H_2CO_3 \rightleftharpoons H^+ + HCO_3^-$). No significant increase in plasma bicarbonate occurs in acute hypercapnia because it takes the kidney 48 to 72 hours to retain enough bicarbonate to compensate for the acidemia. In contrast, in chronic hypercapnia the plasma bicarbonate is elevated enough to bring the pH of the blood within the normal range. In chronic hypercapnia, metabolic alkalosis compensates for the respiratory acidosis.

A low serum chloride level occurs in acute respiratory failure. The mechanism for this is as follows: As bicarbonate ions (HCO_3^-) move from the cells to the plasma to buffer the H_2CO_3, the chloride ions move into the cell to maintain electroneutrality. This is called the *chloride shift*. As the CO_2 accumulates, and with it hydrogen ions (H^+), the serum becomes more acidic. H^+ enters the cells and potassium ions (K^+) flow from the cells to the plasma in an attempt to achieve electroneutrality. Initially, serum K^+ may be increased, but as the acidemia becomes prolonged or more pronounced, total body K^+ (both intracellular and extracellular) is depleted as the excess K^+ is excreted by the kidneys. Thus the client can demonstrate both hypokalemia and hypochloremia as a result of respiratory failure.

Hypoxemia alone can cause vasoconstriction of the pulmonary circulation, resulting in pulmonary hypertension and shunting of blood away from the alveoli. Respiratory

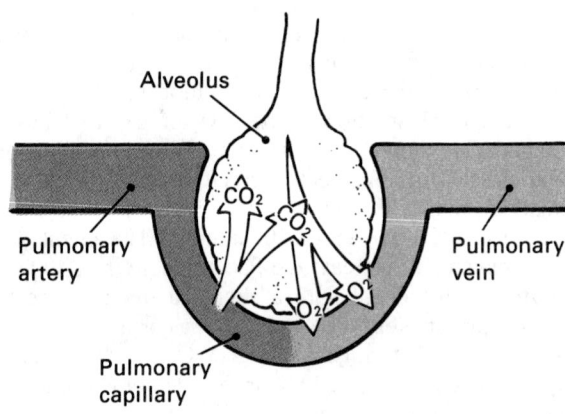

Fig. 23-1 Normal gas exchange unit in the lung.

acidemia seems to potentiate this effect. Therefore as CO_2 rises, with the subsequent development of acidosis, the elevation of the pulmonary artery pressure increases relative to the level of hypoxemia.

Central nervous system (CNS) alterations may occur as a result of the combination of hypoxemia, increased $Paco_2$, and acidemia. The client has a headache because increased CO_2 causes vasodilatation of cerebral blood vessels and increased cerebral blood flow. Cerebrospinal pressure may be elevated, and the client may exhibit papilledema, drowsiness, convulsions, tremors, confusion, slurred speech, restlessness, decreased deep tendon reflexes, fluctuations of mood, and *asterixis* (flapping tremor).

Ventilation-perfusion mismatch. $\dot{V}/\dot{Q}$ mismatch can cause an elevated $Paco_2$ and a decreased Pao_2.

Mechanisms of hypoxemic respiratory failure. *Hypoxemia,* or *low O_2 tension* in the arterial blood (Pao_2 <50 to 60 mm Hg), can contribute to the development of hypoxia or lack of tissue O_2 and acute respiratory failure. Arterial O_2 levels are not solely responsible for effective tissue oxygenation. The hemoglobin (Hb) level, Hb O_2-carrying capacity, cardiac output, and distribution of blood flow to the tissues are all involved in the delivery of O_2 to the tissues and thus determine the state of tissue oxygenation. Respiratory mechanisms that may cause hypoxemia and subsequent acute hypoxemic respiratory failure are (1) alveolar hypoventilation, (2) $\dot{V}/\dot{Q}$ mismatch, (3) shunts, and (4) diffusion abnormalities.

Alveolar hypoventilation. Alveolar hypoventilation, although manifested predominantly by increased CO_2, causes hypoxemia.

Ventilation-perfusion mismatch. Altered $\dot{V}/\dot{Q}$ relationships in the lungs, or $\dot{V}/\dot{Q}$ mismatch, are the most common cause of hypoxemia. The $\dot{V}/\dot{Q}$ relationship means that where there is ventilation or O_2 in the lung, there must be matching blood perfusion to that area for efficient gas exchange to occur (Fig. 23-1). In the normal lung the overall $\dot{V}/\dot{Q}$ is 0.8. Normal resting alveolar ventilation is approximately 4 L/min [($V_T - V_D$) × respiratory rate = 4 L], and cardiac output is approximately 5 L/min in an adult. Therefore the $\dot{V}/\dot{Q}$ is 4:5, or 0.8. An alteration or mismatch will occur if there is blood flow to underventilated areas or ventilation to areas where blood flow is decreased

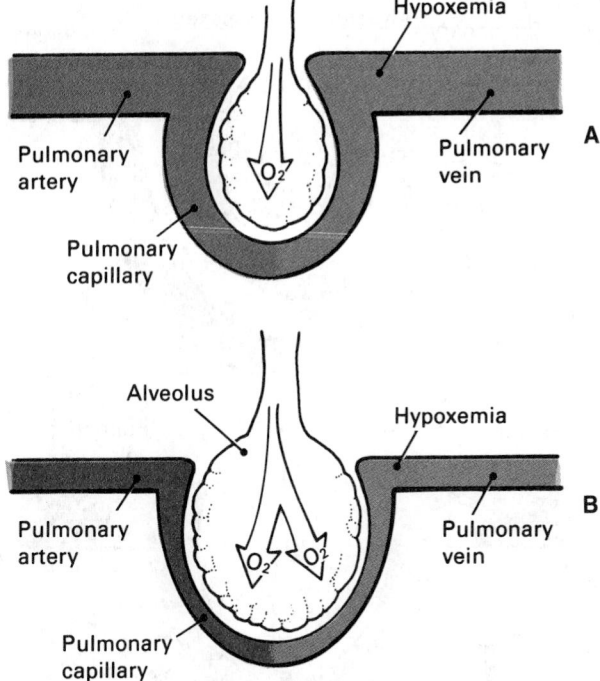

Fig. 23-2 Gas exchange unit illustrating $\dot{V}/\dot{Q}$ mismatch. **A,** $\dot{V}/\dot{Q}$ mismatch with decreased ventilation and normal perfusion. **B,** $\dot{V}/\dot{Q}$ mismatch with normal ventilation and decreased perfusion. Note the narrowing of the blood vessel.

or absent (Fig. 23-2). Changes in resistance, compliance, and blood flow cause different $\dot{V}/\dot{Q}$ in different areas of the lungs.

Hypoventilation (generalized decreased alveolar ventilation) is usually not classified as $\dot{V}/\dot{Q}$ mismatch. CO_2 retention and hypoventilation may occur as a result of $\dot{V}/\dot{Q}$ mismatch if a client is unable to compensate by increasing the ventilation in the presence of airway obstruction. Regional alterations in ventilation and perfusion are more frequently classified as $\dot{V}/\dot{Q}$ mismatch.

Examples of processes that cause $\dot{V}/\dot{Q}$ mismatch are pneumonia, atelectasis, chronic and acute bronchitis, severe emphysema, asthma, and pulmonary embolism. In pulmonary embolism (depending on the size of the vessel blocked), ventilation is sustained in an area that is perfused either poorly or not at all. The other examples are processes in which there is sustained perfusion of poorly ventilated zones of the lung.

Sometimes $\dot{V}/\dot{Q}$ mismatch or imbalance is referred to as *physiological shunting.* This term implies that blood does not become well oxygenated despite contact with alveoli.

Shunts. Shunting is also a cause of hypoxemia (Fig. 23-3). A shunt occurs when blood enters the arterial system from the venous system without going through or being exposed to ventilated areas of the lung. Essentially, the blood is shunted from the right to the left side of the heart without participating in gas exchange. Blood that has a Pao_2 similar to venous blood is then mixed with arterial blood as it enters the left atrium. The overall O_2 level of this blood that will be pumped to the tissues is then lower than blood that has engaged in gas exchange.

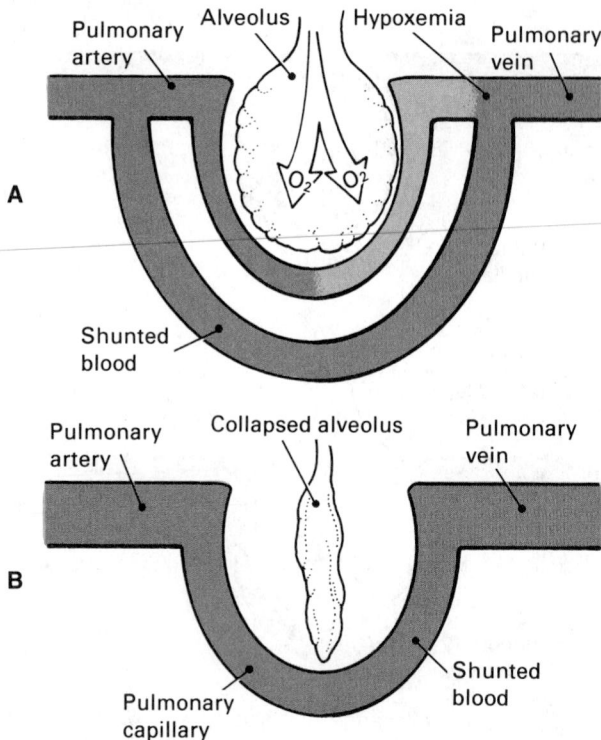

Fig. 23-3 Two types of shunts. **A,** Anatomical shunt. The vessel that receives no ventilation has shunted blood mixing with oxygenated blood. **B,** Anatomical-like shunt. Perfusion continues in the absence of ventilation, and blood cannot be oxygenated.

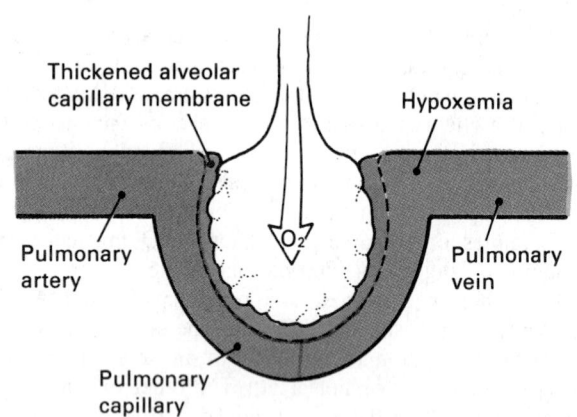

Fig. 23-4 Diffusion abnormality. Exchange of CO_2 and O_2 cannot occur because of the thickened alveolar-capillary membrane.

A shunt can be viewed as an extreme $\dot{V}/\dot{Q}$ disturbance. Shunting can occur in situations in which the blood perfuses large areas of nonventilated or underventilated alveoli (as in consolidated pneumonia) or the blood bypasses alveoli (as in pulmonary emboli). The most common shunts are extrapulmonary and include those that occur in congenital heart disease through atrial or septal defects or a patent ductus arteriosus. These represent an anatomical shunt of blood from the right to the left side of the heart, bypassing gas exchange in the lung.

Intrapulmonary anatomical shunts are associated with arteriovenous fistulas in congenital defects and in hepatic cirrhosis. Anatomicallike or intrapulmonary shunts exist when there is obstruction to the flow of gas to lobes or segments of the lung, as in pneumonia with consolidation.

The classic difference between $\dot{V}/\dot{Q}$ mismatch and anatomicallike shunts is demonstrated by having the client breathe 100% O_2 for 15 to 30 minutes. The client with $\dot{V}/\dot{Q}$ mismatch will increase the Pao_2 to more than 400 mm Hg, whereas the client with a shunt cannot increase the Pao_2 to approximately the level seen in normal persons or in those with a $\dot{V}/\dot{Q}$ mismatch. In $\dot{V}/\dot{Q}$ mismatch the increased fraction of inspired O_2 or the fractional concentration of O_2 delivered to the client (Fio_2) in poorly or intermittently ventilated areas provides enough O_2 to correct the ventilation problem by increasing the Pao_2 and saturating the Hb. However, in a client with shunting the increased Fio_2 does not correct the oxygenation problem because mixed venous blood continues to flow through the shunted area and mixes with blood that has perfused normal alveoli. The poorly oxygenated blood from the shunt area lowers the Pao_2 of the blood with which it is mixed, resulting in no increase or a limited increase in Pao_2.

Diffusion abnormalities. Diffusion abnormalities are also a cause of hypoxemia. These abnormalities indicate an impairment in the equilibration between the oxygen pressure (Pao_2) in the alveoli and in the pulmonary capillaries (Fig. 23-4). Diffusion does not occur normally for the following reasons:

1. The contact time for the red blood cells (RBCs) at the capillary membrane is decreased (e.g., intense physical exercise increases blood flow).
2. Pulmonary capillary blood is reduced as the result of obstruction or destruction of vessels (e.g., in severe emphysema).
3. There is a thickened blood-gas membrane, also classified as alveolar-capillary block (e.g., in fibrosis, pulmonary edema).

A combination of these effects may also disrupt diffusion.

Hypoxemia caused by diffusion impairment can be corrected by the administration of 100% O_2. The rate of movement of O_2 across the blood-brain barrier is proportional to the Pao_2 difference between the alveolar gas and capillary blood. As Fio_2 in the alveoli increases, Pao_2 increases. Thus O_2 transfer is facilitated by increases in the pressure of O_2, with the result of improved oxygenation. O_2 (100%) administration is not usually done in the client with long-term CO_2 retention, such as in chronic obstructive pulmonary disease (COPD), since CO_2 narcosis may develop (see Chapter 22).

Severe diffusion problems must be present to cause a clinical decrease in the Pao_2. Usually, clients have concurrent $\dot{V}/\dot{Q}$ abnormalities or shunt problems. Hypercapnia is usually not present because CO_2 is 20 times more permeable than O_2 across the respiratory membrane. Diseases in which a diffusion abnormality may contribute to hypoxemia include diffuse interstitial fibrosis, collagen-vascular disease of the lung (e.g., scleroderma, systemic lupus erythematosus), asbestosis, sarcoidosis, interstitial pneumonia, and cardiogenic pulmonary edema.

Interrelationship of mechanisms. Hypoxemic respiratory failure frequently is caused by a combination of hypoventilation, diffusion impairment, shunting, and/or $\dot{V}/\dot{Q}$ mismatch. The client with acute respiratory failure secondary to acute pneumonia has a $\dot{V}/\dot{Q}$ imbalance because the inflammation, edema, and hypersecretion of exudate within the bronchioles and terminal respiratory units obstruct airways and impair ventilation in the alveoli. Hypoventilation can result from pain from pleuritic inflammation and subsequent shallow breathing. Interstitial edema caused by secretion and fluid accumulation can cause diffusion abnormalities. Consolidation of lung lobules as a result of secretion accumulation and alveolar collapse can cause shuntlike effects.

PHYSIOLOGICAL EFFECTS OF HYPOXEMIA. Arterial O_2 levels are not solely responsible for effective tissue oxygenation. The Hb level, Hb O_2-carrying capacity, cardiac output, and distribution of blood flow to the tissues are all involved in the delivery of O_2 to the tissues and thus determine the state of tissue oxygenation.

Hypoxia (decreased oxygenation of the tissues) occurs when the amount of O_2 in the blood is not adequate to support aerobic metabolism. Aerobic metabolism provides the energy for cellular activities in which O_2 is used. CO_2 is the waste product of aerobic metabolism. When O_2 insufficiency persists, the cells must shift from aerobic to anaerobic metabolism. Anaerobic metabolism, using more fuel and producing less energy, is less efficient than aerobic metabolism. The waste product of anaerobic metabolism is lactic acid. This is more difficult than CO_2 to remove from the body because it has to be buffered with sodium bicarbonate. When the body does not have adequate amounts of sodium bicarbonate to buffer the lactic acid produced by anaerobic metabolism, metabolic acidosis and cell death occur.

The hypoxemia and metabolic acidosis have an adverse effect on the vital organs, especially the heart and CNS. It causes a depressant effect on the brain, and permanent brain damage may occur. The heart tries to compensate for the decreased O_2 level in the blood by increasing heart rate and cardiac output. However, as the oxygenation decreases and acidosis increases, the heart muscle is unable to function and a slowing and eventual cessation of cardiac activity occurs, resulting in systemic shock. Renal function is also impaired, and sodium retention, proteinuria, edema formation, tubular necrosis, and uremia may occur. Gastrointestinal (GI) function alterations include abnormal liver function, abdominal pain, and bowel infarction.

Clinical Manifestations

Clinical manifestations of respiratory failure are related either to the accumulation of CO_2 and/or to the decrease in O_2 in the bloodstream (Table 23-3). The rapid onset of symptoms is related to the rate of buildup of CO_2, the loss of O_2, and the ability of the client's compensatory mechanisms to overcome these changes. When the client's compensatory mechanisms fail to facilitate removal of CO_2 and the conservation of O_2, symptoms of tissue hypoxia and/or hypercapnia in the vital organs appear. The client may have rapid, shallow respirations because the lungs contain fluid and are noncompliant and stiff. The client may increase the respiratory rate in an effort to blow off accumu-

Table 23-3 Clinical Manifestations of Acute Respiratory Failure Related to Hypoxemia and Hypercapnia

Manifestations	Findings
HYPOXEMIA	
Restlessness, agitation, disorientation, confusion, delirium, loss of consciousness, dyspnea	Cardiac dysrhythmias; tachycardia; hypertension; cyanosis (may not be present until hypoxemia is severe); pale, cool, clammy skin
HYPERCAPNIA	
Headache, somnolence, dizziness, coma	Hypertension; tachycardia; asterixis; warm, flushed skin; diaphoresis; bounding pulse; papilledema; decreased deep tendon reflexes

lated CO_2. As CO_2 continues to increase, a slower respiratory rate may indicate that the client is no longer able to eliminate accumulated CO_2.

Acceptable ABG values may be present, but the client may be working extremely hard to attain them. Accessory muscles may be used during inspiration and/or expiration. During normal tidal breathing, the diaphragm moves about 3 to 5 cm. However, with forced inspiration or expiration, diaphragmatic excursion may be as much as 10 cm. Accessory muscles of inspiration that may be used are the scalene muscles, which elevate the first two ribs, and the sternocleidomastoids, which raise the sternum. Small muscles of the neck, head, and face play a minor role as accessory inspiratory muscles. Normally, expiration is passive. When expiration becomes active during distress or increased exercise, the abdominal muscles and internal intercostals are used. Intercostal and supraclavicular retractions are an indication that these muscles are working hard to aid in ventilation.

Clients with advanced COPD with inspiratory muscle fatigue may exhibit asynchronous respirations. Normally, the thorax and abdomen move synchronously outward on inspiration and inward on exhalation. During asynchronous breathing an outward movement of the abdomen occurs during exhalation and an inward movement occurs during inspiration. Asynchronous breathing probably results from inefficient diaphragm position and maximal use of accessory muscles of respiration.

The length of inspiration compared with that of expiration (I/E ratio), which is normally 1:1.5 or 1:2, may be decreased (e.g., 1:5). The expiratory time is usually prolonged in airway obstruction. The pattern of respiratory response to activity may be altered. The client may use few accessory muscles at rest but may activate more muscle groups with increased activity.

The position the client assumes is also a clue to the effort associated with breathing. The client may prefer to sit straight up or lean forward, resting on the elbows, or to lie partially on one side or the other depending on the location of the pulmonary disease. Asymmetrical chest expansion may occur from (1) splinting an incision or trauma site, (2) pleural effusion, (3) pneumothorax, or (4) a paralyzed hemidiaphragm. Pursed-lip or open-mouth breathing may be used. The client who is working hard to breathe may become extremely diaphoretic and may be able to speak only two or three words at a time between breaths.

Because of the increased work of breathing, there may be wide swings in intrathoracic pressure during inspiration and expiration. Thus the nurse may be able to detect a pulsus paradoxus of greater than 10 mm Hg during inspiration. (The physiology of pulsus paradoxus is described in Chapter 31.) The degree of paradox can aid in assessing the degree of respiratory distress. A paradox of as much as 50 mm Hg can be present in severe respiratory distress. Improvement in paradox usually correlates with clinical improvement, except in severe respiratory distress, when the client becomes exhausted and is unable to generate enough respiratory effort to produce intrathoracic pressure changes of the magnitude necessary for a paradox to occur.

In mild hypoxemia the sympathetic nervous system is stimulated, producing an increased heart rate and cardiac output. Peripheral vasoconstriction also occurs to shunt blood to vital organs and to increase blood pressure (BP). The skin may become pale, cool, and clammy. In pure hypercapnic ventilatory failure, vasodilatation is peripheral. Thus the client may have warm, flushed skin and a bounding pulse.

Clinical manifestations related to the cardiovascular system include tachycardia, mild hypertension (partly due to the release of catecholamines), increased cardiac output, cardiac dysrhythmias, and deleterious effects on cardiac function with subsequent failure. These manifestations are especially evident in the presence of coronary artery disease and pulmonary hypertension (secondary to alveolar hypoxia) and are further aggravated by respiratory acidosis (if present). With severe, prolonged hypoxemia, bradycardia and hypotension may result.

The CNS is particularly prone to low O_2 and high CO_2 levels. The client may have a headache because increased CO_2 causes vasodilatation of cerebral blood vessels and increased cerebral blood flow. Cerebrospinal pressure may be elevated, and the client may exhibit papilledema, drowsiness, convulsions, tremors, confusion, slurred speech, restlessness, fluctuations of mood, clouding of consciousness, poor concentration, Cheyne-Stokes respirations, electroencephalogram abnormalities, decreased deep tendon reflexes, and asterixis (flapping tremor). As hypoxemia progresses and becomes more severe, convulsions, retinal hemorrhages, and permanent brain damage may occur.

As the level of Pao_2 decreases, further cyanosis may occur. However, this is a very late sign of hypoxemia. Cyanosis occurs when there is more than 5 g of unsaturated Hb per deciliter of blood and therefore is another late sign of hypoxemia. Central cyanosis occurs when the Hb is desaturated of O_2. It is best observed as a dusky gray and then purplish color in the mucous membranes (especially buccal mucosa), lips, tongue, and face. Peripheral cyanosis reflects decreased blood flow through the capillary bed, usually caused by decreased cardiac output or vasoconstriction. This is most often observed in the nail beds. Cyanosis may not occur in the anemic client despite decreased Pao_2 because Hb is decreased. In contrast, a client with polycythemia may appear cyanotic even though the O_2 content is normal (e.g., "blue bloater" COPD client with chronic bronchitis). Cyanosis by itself is not a reliable indicator of oxygenation status; it must be evaluated together with other clinical parameters.

Clients with chronic pulmonary disease may be able to tolerate a significant degree of hypoxemia and hypercarbia. Clinical signs of hypercapnia (e.g., tachycardia, papilledema, decreased deep tendon reflexes, confusion) may be apparent if the CO_2 retention is of rapid onset. However, these clinical signs are often absent or subtle if chronic hypercapnia has been a feature of the client's disease. Only when the condition progresses to coma, with slow or gasping respirations or even apnea, may the diagnosis of respiratory failure be clinically obvious. For this reason it is important to observe the client with chronic pulmonary disease closely for subtle changes in respiratory pattern and mental status.

Diagnostic Studies

The most specific diagnostic study used to determine respiratory failure is assessment of ABGs. These levels are monitored as indicated by the client's respiratory status to detect changes, trends, and response to therapy. Pulse oximetry is frequently used for continuous monitoring, but in respiratory failure, ABGs provide more useful information. Other routine studies performed are chest x-ray film, complete blood cell count, serum electrolytes, urinalysis, and electrocardiogram (ECG). Cultures of the sputum and blood are obtained as necessary to determine sources of possible infection. If pulmonary embolus is suspected, a $\dot{V}/\dot{Q}$ lung scan or pulmonary angiography may be done. Pulmonary function tests may be used to determine respiratory function.

In severe respiratory failure, measurement of cardiac output and mixed venous blood gases by a thermodilution pulmonary artery catheter (see Chapter 28) is an important aid in determining the amount of blood flow to tissues and the response to treatment. Monitoring of pulmonary artery, pulmonary wedge, and left atrial pressures is done to determine whether the cause of lung fluid accumulation is cardiac or pulmonary. These parameters are also monitored to determine the response of the lung and heart to hypoxemia, their state of compliance, and the client's response to therapeutic regimens. (Pulmonary artery catheters and monitoring are discussed in detail in Chapter 28.)

Blood from the pulmonary artery port (mixed venous blood) of the pulmonary artery catheter can be sampled. Mixed venous blood O_2 tension ($P\bar{v}o_2$) is an indication of the state of tissue oxygenation. The normal Po_2 of mixed venous blood is 35 to 40 mm Hg with an average O_2 saturation ($S\bar{v}o_2$) of 75% (acceptable range of 60% to 80%).[3] An increase in $P\bar{v}o_2$ of more than 60 mm Hg indicates that the tissues are not extracting and using O_2 or are not being perfused (e.g., in cyanide poisoning). A decrease in $P\overline{v}o_2$ (to less than 35 mm Hg) indicates that the tissues are using more O_2 than they would normally. It is possible to monitor directly the $S\overline{v}o_2$ of mixed venous blood with a pulmonary artery catheter known as the *pulmonary artery oximetrix*. Continuous $S\overline{v}o_2$ monitoring can decrease the need for frequent ABG determinations. Clinically, a decreased Pao_2 and $S\overline{v}o_2$ is evident in severe hypoxemia caused by decreased Pao_2, decreased O_2-carrying capacity of Hb, or decreased cardiac output.[3]

Another method of monitoring O_2 saturation is with a pulse oximeter. A pulse oximeter monitors the O_2 saturation by electronically measuring the (optical) density of light absorbed by the arterial blood. The oxisensor is placed on either the ear, finger, toe, foot, or nose (Fig. 23-5). A beam of light passes through the tissue and measures the absorption of light by oxygen-hemoglobin. Accurate O_2 saturation measurement depends on adequate tissue perfusion to the skin.[4] Oximetry is used in critically ill clients to provide continuous assessment of oxygenation status and to monitor clients receiving ventilation as adjustments are made.

The pulse oximeter is accurate within two digits at arterial O_2 saturation (Sao_2) levels of 70% to 100%. When the Pao_2 is approximately 60 mm Hg, the Hb is 90% saturated with O_2 (Sao_2 is 90%) (see Fig. 19-6). Thus 90% Sao_2 represents the lower end of the spectrum and a minimum level of Sao_2, whereas 97% to 98% saturation is consistent with Pao_2 in the range of 85 to 100 mm Hg (depending on altitude). Therefore marked changes in Pao_2 from 60 to 100 mm Hg can occur with only modest changes in saturation if the Sao_2 is greater than 90%.

Another method of assessing oxygenation is by monitoring transcutaneous O_2 ($P_{tc}o_2$) by an electrode applied to the skin surface. $P_{tc}o_2$ is usually 6 to 10 mm Hg less than Pao_2 because of a loss of O_2 through the skin and blood. Monitoring of $P_{tc}o_2$ is rarely used in adults, although it is used frequently in pediatric critical care areas.

Monitoring of transcutaneous CO_2 ($P_{tc}co_2$) is done in some centers. $P_{tc}co_2$ is a measure of the effectiveness of alveolar ventilation. It is measured the same way as $P_{tc}o_2$.

The value for $P_{tc}co_2$ is 4 to 6 mm Hg higher than that for $Paco_2$ because of local production of CO_2 at the skin.

Calculation of the shunt fraction ($\dot{Q}_S/\dot{Q}_T$), by $P\overline{v}o_2$ in the client receiving 100% O_2, is useful in diagnosing the presence and degree of intrapulmonary shunt. The $\dot{Q}_S/\dot{Q}_T$ is expressed as a fraction or percentage of the cardiac output that does not become oxygenated in the lungs. A $\dot{Q}_S/\dot{Q}_T$ of more than 30% indicates that more than 30% of the cardiac output is unoxygenated blood. This reduced oxygenation of the tissues is an ominous sign and signifies significant cardiopulmonary deterioration and hypoxemia.

Calculation of the difference between the alveolar and the arterial tensions [$D(A - a)o_2$ or $P(A - a)o_2$] aids in determining whether the cause of hypoxemia is secondary to hypoventilation. $D(A - a)o_2$ also assesses the difficulty with which O_2 moves from the alveolus across the alveolar-capillary membrane and into the arterial blood.

Normal young subjects 21 to 30 years of age breathing room air have a $D(A - a)o_2$ of 5 to 10 mm Hg.[5] With normal aging, as more lung units with unequal ventilation and perfusion accumulate, the gradient increases. The gradient may increase to a mean of 16 mm Hg in the 61- to 75-year age group of healthy adults.[6] In the presence of alveolar hypoventilation, when an extrapulmonary factor affects the lungs (e.g., CNS depression resulting from drugs or paralysis of respiratory muscles), the alveolar ventilation rate decreases. Consequently, the amount of O_2 reaching the alveolus (PAo_2) will decrease, with a subsequent but proportional decrease in Pao_2. Thus the $D(A - a)o_2$ will remain constant. However, if an intrapulmonary defect is present (e.g., $\dot{V}/\dot{Q}$ mismatch, shunt), the alveolar ventilation rate is not usually affected adversely until the later stages of the disease, and the PAo_2 remains constant or increases slightly. The amount of O_2 reaching the alveolus from the air is not affected. However, the Pao_2 will decrease disproportionately, depending on the exchange defect at the alveolar-capillary membrane. Consequently, the $D(A - a)o_2$ will be widened.

For calculation of $D(A - a)o_2$, the partial pressure of O_2 in the alveolus (PAo_2) is first calculated, and then the Pao_2, which is given in the ABG, is subtracted. The following equation, known as the alveolar air equation, is used to calculate PAo_2:

$$PAo_2 = Fio_2 \times (P_B - 47 \text{ mm Hg}) - \frac{Paco_2}{R}$$

In this equation, P_B is the barometric pressure (i.e., at sea level $P_B = 760$ mm Hg and 47 mm Hg is the partial pressure of water vapor in the trachea). Thus $Fio_2 \times (P_B - 47)$ is equal to the partial pressure of inspired O_2 (Pio_2). The CO_2 gas is then subtracted. The amount of CO_2 will depend on R, the respiratory exchange ratio of CO_2 produced to O_2 consumed. For most calculations, R is assumed to be 0.8, the respiratory quotient ratio of CO_2 produced to O_2 consumed. Therefore the PAo_2 is the following:

$$PAo_2 = Pio_2 - \frac{Paco_2}{0.8}$$

Calculation of the $D(A - a)o_2$ at an Fio_2 greater than 0.21 may also be performed, but it requires different

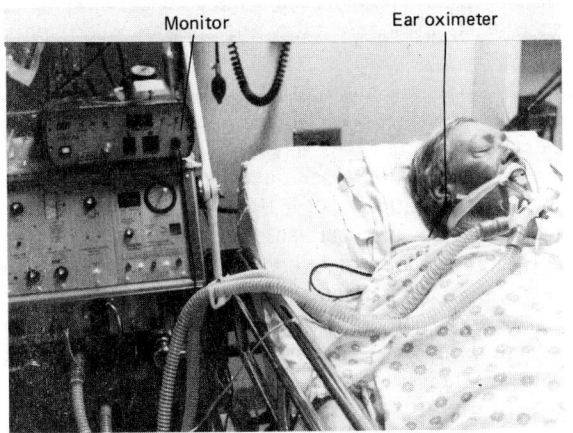

Monitor   Ear oximeter

Fig. 23-5 Client on an Emerson ventilator being monitored via an ear oximeter.

guidelines. Calculation of the $D(A - a)o_2$ at which the client is breathing 100% O_2 will also give an indication of the extent of the shunt. At an Fio_2 of 100%, for each 100 mm Hg difference between PAo_2 and Pao_2 ($D[A - a]o_2$), there is approximately a 5% shunt. $D(A - a)o_2$ determination is also helpful in assessing the effects of positive end-expiratory pressure (PEEP), chest physiotherapy, fluid administration, diuretics, and dialysis.

Intrapulmonary shunting can also be evaluated by the a/A ratio (the ratio of Pao_2 to PAo_2). With the a/A ratio the extent of intrapulmonary shunting is determined by comparing the Pao_2 with the PAo_2. For determination of the a/A ratio, the PAo_2 is calculated with the alveolar air equation described previously. The Pao_2 is divided by the PAo_2. As the a/A ratio decreases, the degree of shunting increases. Normally, a/A ratios exceed 0.75. Ratios less than this indicate the presence of intrapulmonary shunting beyond the normal value of 5% to 6%.[5]

■ Therapeutic and Nursing Management of Acute Respiratory Failure

Nursing assessment

Subjective and objective data that should be obtained from an person with acute respiratory failure are presented in Table 23-4.

Nursing diagnoses

Nursing diagnoses are determined when the problem and etiological factors are supported by clinical data. Nursing diagnoses related to acute respiratory failure may include, but are not limited to, those in Table 23-5.

Nursing interventions

Management of acute respiratory failure depends on the underlying disease process (Table 23-6). However, several aspects of management are common to many types of respiratory failure. The therapeutic and nursing management of acute respiratory failure are strongly interdependent and contiguous.

Maintenance of adequate oxygenation

OXYGEN ADMINISTRATION. If hypoxemia is secondary to hypoventilation, provision and maintenance of adequate ventilation will usually overcome the problem of gas exchange. Hypoxemia secondary to $\dot{V}/\dot{Q}$ mismatch usually responds favorably to the lowest concentration of O_2 necessary to maintain the Pao_2—at least 55 to 60 mm Hg administered by mask or cannula. Hypoxemia secondary to shunting is usually refractory (refractory hypoxemia) to the administration of high concentrations of O_2 by mask and ultimately requires mechanical ventilation. The client with chronic pulmonary disease requiring O_2 should receive low-flow O_2 (1 to 3 L/min) through a nasal cannula or Venturi mask. The Venturi mask provides an exact concentration of O_2. In contrast, low flow through a nasal cannula delivers O_2 concentrations that vary with the client's minute ventilation. Both low-flow O_2 and the Venturi mask generally correct severe arterial hypoxemia in chronically ill clients without unduly suppressing respiration by reducing the hypoxic drive. (Other methods of O_2 administration are discussed in Chapter 21.)

MAINTENANCE OF HEMOGLOBIN CONCENTRATION AND CARDIAC OUTPUT. To ensure adequate O_2 delivery to the tissues, adequate Hb saturation can be provided by keeping the client's Pao_2

Table 23-4

Nursing Assessment of the Client with Acute Respiratory Failure

SUBJECTIVE DATA

History
Smoking, drug abuse, human immunodeficiency virus infection with respiratory complications, generalized trauma, sepsis, shock, recent thoracoabdominal surgery, respiratory disease (e.g., COPD, asthma, pneumonia), disseminated intravascular coagulation, precipitating factors in persons with lung disease (e.g., infection, surgery), cancer, immunosuppressed clients, previous lung surgeries (e.g., pneumonectomy)

General
Fatigue, headaches

Respiratory
Dyspnea, wheezing, coughing (productive or nonproductive)

OBJECTIVE DATA

General
Appearance (e.g., indications of anxiety, body appearance), speech pattern

Respiratory
Use of accessory respiratory muscles; breathing pattern (during rest, exercise, sleep), including rate, rhythm, I/E ratio, asymmetric chest movement, retractions, and splinting on inspection; tactile fremitus, crepitus, and deviated trachea on palpation; thoracoabdominal resonance on percussion; absent or diminished breath sounds, rales, rhonchi, wheezes, pleural friction rub, inspiratory stridor, bronchial or bronchovesicular sounds in abnormal location on auscultation

Cardiovascular
Peripheral edema (extremities, sacral, periorbital), jugular venous distention, cyanosis

Neurological
Change in level of consciousness, alertness, memory

Diagnostic findings
Abnormal ABG and/or oximetry findings; decreased peak expiratory flow rate; altered values of serum electrolytes, Hb, hematocrit; abnormal findings on chest x-ray film, CT scan, MRI, pulmonary artery and capillary wedge pressures

greater than 60 mm Hg. When the Pao_2 is 60 mm Hg or greater, the Hb is 90% saturated (see Fig. 19-6). An adequate Hb concentration of 10 g/dl or greater and maintenance of an adequate cardiac output are also important in ensuring adequate O_2 delivery.

BP should be maintained at the most efficient level for each client. Usually, a systolic BP of at least 90 mm Hg is adequate to maintain perfusion to the vital organs. A urine output of 30 ml/hr or more is an indication of adequate renal perfusion. If the systolic BP is maintained at at least 90 mm Hg, changes in mental status may be attributed to the levels of O_2 and CO_2 in the blood rather than to decreased perfusion to the brain.

Table 23-5

NURSING CARE PLAN FOR THE CLIENT WITH ACUTE RESPIRATORY FAILURE

Defining Characteristics	Nursing Interventions	Evaluation Criteria

NURSING DIAGNOSIS: Potential complication: hypoxemia related to alveolar hypoventilation, intrapulmonary shunting, $\dot{V}/\dot{Q}$ mismatch, diffusion impairment*

Pao_2 <60 mm Hg or Sao_2 <90% at rest (for acute clients at sea level), Pao_2 <60 mm Hg or Sao_2 <85% during exercise (for chronic clients at sea level), dyspnea on exertion, lethargy, fatigue, cyanosis	Position client to promote optimal gas exchange (e.g., elevate head of bed 45 degrees, use tripod position). Assist with ventilatory support measures (e.g., mechanical ventilation).	Return of Pao_2 to baseline normal

NURSING DIAGNOSIS: Potential complication: hypercapnia related to alveolar hypoventilation and low $\dot{V}/\dot{Q}$ mismatch*

$Paco_2$ >50 mm Hg with pH <7.35, headache on awakening, somnolence	Administer drugs prescribed to reverse respiratory depression (e.g., Narcan). Monitor vital capacity in clients with neuromuscular weakness. Monitor ventilatory parameters for changes that suggest possible increase in $Paco_2$, such as MIP $\leq$−20 cm H_2O, vital capacity $\leq$10-15 ml/kg, respiratory rate >35 breaths/min, increasing lethargy or drowsiness. Assist with ventilatory support measures (e.g., mechanical ventilation, mask ventilation), if required.	$Paco_2$ <40 mm Hg or client's baseline value, pH 7.35 to 7.45

NURSING DIAGNOSIS: Ineffective airway clearance related to infection in airways, decreased level of consciousness, presence of an artificial airway, thoracic and/or abdominal neuromuscular dysfunction, pain, and expiratory airflow obstruction*

Difficulty in expectoration of sputum, presence of abnormal breath sounds (e.g., rhonchi, rales), cough ineffective or absent	Humidify inspired air if upper airway is bypassed or O_2 is being used at >4 L/min. Perform tracheobronchial suctioning if coughing ineffective or if artificial airway is present. Perform chest physiotherapy. Splint chest or abdominal incision with pillow or hand. Turn q 2 hr. Stabilize artificial airway. Ensure adequate fluid intake of 2-3L/24 hr as indicated.	Absence of abnormal breath sounds (e.g., rhonchi, rales), presence of effective cough, easy expectoration of sputum, ability to perform airway clearance modalities

NURSING DIAGNOSIS: Ineffective breathing pattern related to neuromuscular impairment, pain, musculoskeletal impairment, anxiety, CNS depression, respiratory muscle fatigue or failure, increased work of breathing, expiratory obstruction to airflow, and weaning attempt*

Respiratory rate <11 or >24 breaths/min, alteration of I/E ratio, irregular breathing rhythm (e.g., use of accessory muscles of breathing inappropriate to level of activity)	Provide comfort measures (e.g., positioning, analgesics). Provide mechanical support, if indicated. Evaluate ability to meet criteria to wean from mechanical ventilation.	Respiratory rate, depth, timing within normal limits; respiratory rhythm within normal limits for age; synchronous thoracoabdominal movement; use of accessory muscles appropriate to level of activity

*See Table 22-15 for additional nursing interventions.

Continued.

Table 23-5

 NURSING CARE PLAN FOR THE CLIENT WITH ACUTE RESPIRATORY FAILURE—cont'd

Defining Characteristics	Nursing Interventions	Evaluation Criteria

NURSING DIAGNOSIS: High risk for fluid volume excess related to increases in peripheral or pulmonary fluid secondary to cor pulmonale, heart failure, or acute respiratory distress syndrome*

Pao_2 <60 mm Hg; peripheral and/or sacral edema; increasing dyspnea; abnormal breath sounds (rales); weight gain >2-3 lb on consecutive days; jugular venous distention; taut, shiny skin; peripheral or sacral edema	Monitor fluid status assessed by intake and output, daily weights, jugular venous distention, pulmonary artery, or pulmonary capillary wedge pressures (when appropriate). Assist with ventilatory support measures (e.g., mechanical ventilation) when appropriate. Restrict fluid intake if prescribed.	Decrease in weight toward normal range, return of Pao_2 to normal range, absence of abnormal breath sounds (rales), diminished sensation of distressed breathing, decrease in or absence of signs of peripheral edema; output $\geq$ intake; diminished pulmonary artery and/or pulmonary capillary wedge pressure

NURSING DIAGNOSIS: Altered nutrition: less than body requirements related to poor appetite, lowered energy level, shortness of breath, sputum production, presence of an artificial airway, and increased caloric requirements*

Less than 10% ideal body weight, serum albumin level below normal laboratory values, weight loss, weakness, muscle wasting, dehydration, decreased muscle tone, poor skin integrity, presence of artificial airway and/or mechanical ventilation	Provide high-protein, high-calorie, low-carbohydrate, enteral or parenteral nutrition as prescribed. Monitor serum albumin and transferrin levels. Take appropriate measures to prevent aspiration (e.g. positioning, use of small-bore feeding tube). Monitor fluid status (intake and output, weight) with use of parenteral nutrition. With parenteral nutrition, monitor for signs of CO_2 increase during weaning as result of carbohydrate load.	Within 10% of ideal body weight, serum albumin level within normal laboratory values, stabilized or increasing weight without increase as result of fluid

NURSING DIAGNOSIS: Anxiety related to dyspnea, intubation, severity of illness, and uncertain outcome

Increased pulse, respiratory rate, BP; agitation, restlessness; verbalization of anxiety over health situation	Perform interventions in a calm, assured manner. Reassure client of competence of caregivers. Answer questions simply and honestly.	Decrease in anxiety, relaxed demeanor, verbalization of hopeful attitude toward outcome

NURSING DIAGNOSIS: Dyspnea related to increased airway resistance, air trapping or hyperinflation, decreased lung compliance, and decreased chest wall compliance*

*See Table 22-15 for additional nursing interventions.

Table 23-6   Therapeutic Management of Acute Respiratory Failure

Maintenance of adequate oxygenation
  O_2 administration to keep Pao_2 >60 mm Hg
  Maintenance of adequate Hb concentration
  Maintenance of adequate cardiac output
  Prevention and assessment of tissue hypoxia
  Measures to decrease stress and anxiety and promote
    comfort
Improvement of alveolar ventilation
  Maintenance of patent airway
    Effective coughing
    Suctioning
    Positioning
  Measures to assist in liquefaction and movement of
    secretions
    Humidification
    Adequate hydration
    Chest physiotherapy (if indicated)
    Bland aerosols and ultrasonic nebulization
  Relief of bronchospasm
    Bronchodilators
    Aerosolized bronchodilators
    Corticosteroids (when indicated)
  Reduction of pulmonary congestion
    Diuretics
  Mechanical ventilation
Treatment of underlying cause of failure
Continuous monitoring and evaluation of treatment

PREVENTION AND ASSESSMENT OF TISSUE HYPOXIA. Close observation for clinical manifestations of vital organ hypoxia is needed, including frequent assessment of the client's mental and neurological status for cloudiness of sensorium, poor concentration, restlessness, stupor, lethargy, somnolence, tremors, slurred speech, depressed tendon reflexes, and asterixis. Cardiovascular status assessment includes direct or indirect BP monitoring; monitoring of cardiac output, pulmonary artery and wedge pressures and cardiac rate and rhythm; and assessment for symptoms of right- and left-sided heart failure. Older clients and clients with coronary artery disease are susceptible to the effects of decreased tissue O_2 on the myocardium. Fluid and electrolyte levels should be carefully assessed in relation to renal and cardiac response. Serial evaluations of serum electrolytes are made to determine the existence of anion or cation excesses or deficiencies. Incremental replacement of potassium and bicarbonate may be indicated in the presence of hypokalemia and severe acidemia. Continuous and serial monitoring of O_2 saturation, ABGs, $P_{tc}O_2$ and $P_{tc}CO_2$, and $S\bar{v}O_2$ by oximeter or pulmonary artery catheter can be helpful in assessing oxygenation.

MEASURES TO DECREASE STRESS AND PROMOTE COMFORT. The client should be maintained in an atmosphere as quiet and relaxed as possible. Rising levels of stress and anxiety can further increase O_2 demands. The respiratory rate can also be increased. In clients with COPD, this results in decreased time for exhalation, increased air trapping, and

therefore an enhanced sensation of dyspnea. Fear of suffocation or death is not uncommon, and the client must be supported emotionally as well as physically at this time. Providing reassurance, spending as much time as possible with the client at the bedside, and ensuring that help can be received immediately (e.g., by making a call light readily available) may help to decrease the client's anxiety level. Anxiety may also be reduced through the use of relaxation techniques. Frequently a family member or friend will have a soothing effect on the client. It is important to evaluate the effect of visitors on the client's anxiety level.

Often clients in respiratory distress (especially those with chronic lung disease) prefer to be in an open area without curtains or with a door or window open. Activity should be kept to a minimum within reason. Positioning the client for comfort and for the most efficient ventilation is important. Frequent rest periods need to be provided, and efficient scheduling of care, treatments, assessments, and diagnostic studies is important.

The client with pronounced acute hypercapnia is often sleepy. In this case it is important to keep the client awake and breathing at regular intervals because sleeping will result in further hypoventilation. Patting the client on the back, keeping the lights on, and giving frequent reminders to breathe can help. Interpreting facial expressions and body language, using questions that require short yes-and-no answers or head nodding, or using a word board for communication will help to limit the amount of energy the client expends for communication.

Measures to increase physical comfort are also important. A cool cloth placed on the forehead to remove perspiration and to refresh the face is usually appreciated. Sips of cool water or ice chips (if tolerated) can also be offered with assistance. Mouth care is especially important for the client who is a mouth breather because of the drying effects of inspired air on the mucous membranes. Removing a perspiration-soaked gown, lightly sponging the client's upper torso, and helping the client into a dry gown will often suffice for a daily bath.

Improvement of alveolar ventilation. In respiratory failure the work of breathing is increased, and often the CO_2 production is excessive in relation to the amount of alveolar ventilation that is occurring. Reduction of both CO_2 production and the work of breathing, with subsequent improvement in alveolar ventilation, can be accomplished by instituting therapy to relieve airway obstruction or pulmonary congestion. If these intensive measures fail, mechanical ventilation may be required to assist or control the ventilation.

MAINTENANCE OF A PATENT AIRWAY. Maintenance of a patent airway is essential. Obstruction of the airway caused by the accumulation of secretions and/or bronchospasm occurs frequently. If secretions are obstructing the airway, the client should be encouraged to cough if possible. Effective coughing requires a deep inhalation, effective glottic closure, and high expiratory flows (see Table 22-12). These abilities need to be evaluated in the client to determine whether the cough is effective.

Clients with neuromuscular weakness may have a flow limitation as a result of decreased volume and an inability to produce adequately high pleural pressures. Augmented coughing may be helpful in these clients or in an exhausted client. Augmented coughing is performed by placing the flat palm of the hand or hands on the thorax (rib springing) in the area where the presence of secretions has been detected by auscultation or on the abdominal musculature below the xiphoid process. As the client ends the deep inspiration and begins expiration, the hands should be moved forcefully downward, facilitating chest compression or increased abdominal pressure. This measure helps to produce muscle movement, increases pleural pressure and expiratory flows, and augments or assists the cough. Coughing at the end of expiration is helpful in clients with severe airway obstruction because it can cause compression of the more distal or peripheral airways and may help "milk" or move secretions into the proximal airways. Frequently, having the client breathe as deeply as possible (if able) may stimulate the cough. "Huff" coughing with the glottis open may be used for clients who have problems with glottic closure, such as those with endotracheal or tracheal tubes in place.

Positioning the client either by elevating the head of the bed to at least 45 degrees (if tolerated) or by using a reclining chair bed may maximize thoracic expansion. Clients with a unilateral pulmonary process should be positioned with the unaffected lung in the dependent position. This is important in preventing hypoxemia because the "down" lung gets more perfusion. If the diseased lung were down, more $\dot{V}/\dot{Q}$ mismatch would occur. Recording and noting the client's position when drawing ABGs in unilateral lung disease is helpful in evaluating the results. The client should be placed on the side if there is any possibility that the tongue will obstruct the airway or that aspiration may occur. An oral or nasal airway should be kept at the bedside and used when necessary.

If the client's cough is ineffective in removing secretions, nasopharyngeal or nasotracheal suctioning is indicated. Adequate oxygenation and monitoring of the client are essential during these procedures. Although rarely indicated, bronchoscopy may be employed to remove secretions, especially if they are extremely thick and tenacious. Intermittent positive-pressure breathing (IPPB) may also be helpful in certain cases of respiratory muscle weakness to aid in volume expansion and to increase ventilation.

MEASURES TO LIQUEFY AND MOBILIZE SECRETIONS. If bronchial secretions are thick, viscid, and difficult to raise, efforts to thin them should be made. Adequate hydration is necessary to keep secretions thin and easy to remove.

Bland aerosols of sterile normal saline solutions or water administered by a nebulizer may be used to liquefy secretions. Occasionally, ultrasonic nebulization treatments of sterile water or saline solution may be used. The client's response to aerosol therapy must be assessed. Aerosol therapy may induce bronchospasm, severe bouts of coughing, and decreased Pao_2. Nebulized acetylcysteine (e.g., Mucomyst) or other mucolytic agents have been used to thin secretions. These agents are usually mixed together with a bronchodilator. However, the value of these agents is questionable, and they are often irritating. In some clients they induce bronchospasm. They have not proved to be more effective than bland mists or adequate hydration.

Chest physiotherapy in certain situations (e.g., sputum production greater than 30 ml/day) can be an effective means of improving the removal of retained secretions (see Fig. 22-16). If tolerated, postural drainage, percussion, and vibration performed manually or by a mechanical vibrator to the affected lung segments may assist in moving secretions to larger airways where they can be removed by effective coughing or suctioning. If nasotracheal suctioning and other measures to liquefy and mobilize secretions are ineffective, it may become necessary to insert an endotracheal (ET) or tracheostomy tube to facilitate suctioning of secretions.

RELIEF OF BRONCHOSPASM. Relief of bronchospasm (if present) will aid in maximal bronchodilatation and increase effective alveolar ventilation. An intravenous (IV) loading dose of aminophylline is infused initially in an acute attack of bronchospasm. If the client has not recently been taking oral aminophylline preparations, the loading dose is followed by a continuous infusion sufficient to maintain theophylline blood levels of 10 to 20 μg/ml. Aerosolized β_2-agonist bronchodilators such as metaproterenol (Alupent), albuterol (Ventolin), and isoetharine (Bronkosol) (see Table 22-4) diluted with sterile water or normal saline solution may also be administered at regular intervals depending on the client's response. These bronchodilators can be administered by a hand-held nebulizer. IPPB administration of these drugs is sometimes used in severe end-stage COPD and in restrictive lung diseases (e.g., quadriplegia, myasthenia gravis) that prevent the client from taking a deep breath. In some centers cases of severe bronchospasm are treated with IV infusions of isoproterenol (Isuprel) or terbutaline as a final effort to prevent intubation and mechanical ventilation.

The client's response to the effects of these β-adrenergic bronchodilators should be monitored. In some clients bronchodilator administration results in an initial worsening of arterial hypoxemia. This is due to redistribution of the inspired gas away from areas that continue to be perfused to areas with decreased perfusion caused by localized hypoxia. Administration of an O_2-enriched gas mixture simultaneously with the bronchodilator may help to alleviate the subsequent hypoxemia. (Side effects and nursing management related to bronchodilators are discussed in Chapter 22 and Table 22-4).

Corticosteroids are frequently used in conjunction with bronchodilating agents when bronchospasm and inflammation are present. The dose of steroids depends on the severity of bronchospasm and the client's clinical status (see Chapter 22).

REDUCTION OF PULMONARY CONGESTION. Pulmonary congestion precipitating acute respiratory failure can occur as a result of right- or left-sided heart failure or leakage of fluid into the pulmonary interstitial space because of a defective capillary-alveolar membrane as in pulmonary edema (either cardiac or noncardiac in etiology). The accumulation of lung water can further aggravate and inhibit alveolar ventilation. Therefore it is important for the nurse to monitor for signs and symptoms of heart failure and to be able to interpret the pressures obtained by the pulmonary artery catheter.

Diuretics may be used to treat pulmonary congestion.

Digitalization is not usually recommended unless left ventricular failure or cardiac tachyatrial dysrhythmias are present. If digitalis is used, ABGs, ECG, and serum electrolytes are monitored closely, since digitalis in the presence of hypoxemia, hypokalemia, and acidemia can increase cardiac irritability. Close monitoring of edema, daily weights, and intake and output are imperative.

MECHANICAL VENTILATION. If intensive measures fail to improve alveolar ventilation and the client continues to deteriorate clinically, mechanical ventilation may be instituted to assist or control ventilation. (See Table 23-15 for guidelines for determining the need for mechanical ventilation for clients without chronic lung disease.) Clinical observation of the client is important in making a decision to institute mechanical ventilation.

Clients with chronic lung disease need to be evaluated on the basis of their limited pulmonary function. Baseline values for clients with chronic disease obtained when respiratory distress is not present often meet the criteria for mechanical ventilation. Clients need to be evaluated relative to the clinical manifestations and the response to therapy. For example, a client with an acute exacerbation of asthma usually demonstrates hypocapnia and respiratory alkalemia with hypoxemia in the early stages rather than hypercapnia and respiratory acidemia with hypoxemia. In these clients a rise in $Paco_2$, even into the normal range, is an ominous sign because it signifies exhaustion and impending respiratory failure. Ventilatory support is imperative.

Treatment of the underlying cause of respiratory failure. In clients with absolute hypoventilation the primary problem can usually be diagnosed rapidly, and appropriate therapy can be initiated. When the problem is drug overdose, dialysis or other methods to promote excretion of the drug are undertaken. Specific measures are available for clients with myasthenia gravis, whereas clients with Guillain-Barré syndrome often require long-term ventilatory support until the disease process runs its course. Infection is often the primary cause of acute respiratory failure in the immunosuppressed client. Appropriate cultures must be obtained and antibiotic therapy begun as soon as possible. Bronchoscopy or lung biopsy may need to be performed to obtain specimens for determining the underlying respiratory disease.

Continuous monitoring of the effects of treatment. A flowchart that shows the client's ABG measurements and results of other laboratory and clinical studies, including vital signs, pulmonary artery and wedge pressures, weights, intake and output, medications and dosage, electrolytes, complete blood cell count, and respiratory parameters, is extremely helpful. Accurate, clear documentation of objective and subjective assessments on the client's flowchart is an important aspect of care. Management of the client should be evaluated regularly, and the therapeutic regimen should be altered as indicated by the client's response.

ADULT RESPIRATORY DISTRESS SYNDROME

Adult respiratory distress syndrome (ARDS) is a sudden, progressive disorder consisting of pulmonary edema of noncardiac origin, severe dyspnea, hypoxemia refrac-

Table 23-7 Terms Synonymous with Adult Respiratory Distress Syndrome

Shock lung	Acute respiratory failure
Traumatic wet lung	Low-flow lung syndrome
Wet lung	Noncardiogenic pulmonary
Septic lung	edema
Congestive atelectasis	Adult hyaline membrane
Hemorrhagic atelectasis	disease
Capillary leak syndrome	White lung
Postperfusion (pump) lung	Progressive pulmonary con-
Posttraumatic pulmonary	solidation
insufficiency	Da Nang lung

tory to supplemental O_2, reduced lung compliance, and diffuse pulmonary infiltrates.[7] ARDS has also been defined as respiratory failure with severe refractory hypoxemia that arises from diffuse alveolar, epithelial, and endothelial damage in the lung. ARDS is not a disease with a single cause but represents the final stage in a common pathway of acute lung injury. This syndrome is more commonly encountered in adults with previously normal lungs than in those with preexisting lung disease. ARDS is known by several clinical terms (Table 23-7). Frequently the general term *adult respiratory distress syndrome* is used with reference to suspected cause, such as ARDS secondary to sepsis.

Many clinical disorders are associated with the development of ARDS (Table 23-8). Sepsis and gastric aspiration have been identified as the clinical disorders most frequently associated with an increased risk of ARDS. ARDS develops in approximately 20% to 40% of clients with sepsis.[8] The risk of ARDS increases with the number of high-risk disorders in the same client.

It is estimated that ARDS develops in approximately 150,000 people each year.[9] Despite many years of research and improved therapy since it was first described in 1967, ARDS continues to have a bleak prognosis. The mortality rate remains high at 50% to 70%.[9] Death from ARDS is seldom caused by progressive, irreversible respiratory failure. Rather, people with ARDS die of multiple organ systems failure and uncontrolled or recurrent infection. The mortality rate from ARDS secondary to sepsis ranges from 60% to 90%.[9]

In recent years the understanding of ARDS has dramatically improved with the recognition that ARDS is one manifestation of multiple organ injury, especially when caused by sepsis or trauma. Ongoing research continues into the etiological mechanisms of ARDS, identification of a marker or markers that may indicate the onset of lung injury, and new therapies. It is hoped that new and continuous research will answer these questions, improve therapy, and increase survival in the future. The outcome can be improved only by early recognition and intervention.

Pathophysiology

The initial trauma to the lungs in ARDS occurs in clients with a variety of disorders (Table 23-8). Because ARDS does not develop in all clients with these types of

Table 23-8 Conditions Predisposing to ARDS

INFECTIOUS CAUSES	INHALED TOXIC AGENTS
Gram-negative sepsis	O_2
Bacterial pneumonia	Smoke
Viral pneumonia	Toxic gases
Pneumocystis carinii	
ASPIRATION	**HEMATOLOGICAL DISORDERS**
Gastric	Massive blood transfusion
Fresh and salt water	Disseminated intravascular
(drowning)	coagulation
Ethylene glycol	Transfusion reaction
Hydrocarbon fluids	Postcardiopulmonary bypass
	or resuscitation
SHOCK	**IMMUNOLOGICAL REACTIONS**
Traumatic	Drug allergy
Hemorrhagic	Anaphylaxis
Septic	
TRAUMA	**OTHER**
Generalized	Radiation pneumonitis
Fat embolism	Amniotic fluid emboli
Lung contusion	Increased intracranial pres-
Multiple major fractures	sure
Head injury	High altitude
	Fluid overload
METABOLIC DISORDERS	Eclampsia
Pancreatitis	Goodpasture's syndrome
Uremia	Drug overdose

Table 23-9 Mediators of Acute Lung Injury

Complement component C5a
Neutrophil products, including proteases and O_2 radicals
Monocyte and macrophage products, including tumor ne-
crosis factors, interleukin-1, and granulocyte colony–
stimulating factor
Arachidonic acid metabolites, including prostaglandins and
leukotrienes
Coagulation products, including kallikreins, kinins, fibrin
degradation products, and plasminogen-activating factor
Histamine
Serotonin
Endotoxin

clinical disorders, it is assumed that there is a disturbance in normal protective mechanisms. Despite the heterogeneity of the disorders that cause ARDS, the common abnormal finding is diffuse alveolar-capillary membrane damage with subsequent leakage of fluid from the vascular space into the interstitium and alveoli.

An exact cause for the damage to the alveolar-capillary membrane is not known. However, many cellular and humoral mediators are thought to be involved[10] (Table 23-9

and Fig. 23-6). (These mediators are discussed in Chapters 7 and 8.) The results of the release of these inflammatory mediators are structural damage to the lungs, increased vascular permeability, development of microemboli of platelets and fibrin within pulmonary vasculature, vasoconstriction leading to increased vascular resistance, and bronchoconstriction.

The pathophysiological changes in ARDS are divided into three phases, which correlate with clinicopathophysiological alterations and include (1) injury or exudative phase, (2) reparative or proliferative phase, and (3) fibrotic phase.

Injury or exudative phase. This phase occurs approximately 1 to 7 days (usually 24 to 48 hours) after the initial lung trauma. It is characterized by alveolar capillary and endothelial cell injury, increased vascular permeability, and edema. Because of the disruption of the normal alveolar capillary membrane in ARDS, there is an accumulation of alveolar fluid (pulmonary edema) (Fig. 23-7). Normally the force tending to push fluid out of the capillary is the capillary hydrostatic pressure (also known in the lungs as *pulmonary capillary wedge pressure*). The force tending to pull fluid into the capillaries is the colloidal osmotic pressure in the blood. The net balance of these forces results in a normal continuous filtration of fluid from the pulmonary capillaries into the interstitial space. Alveolar type I cells that line the alveolar wall make the alveolus virtually impermeable to fluid and solute flow from the interstitium. As fluid in the interstitium accumulates, equilibrium is maintained by flow of fluid into peribronchial and perivascular spaces and thus into the lymphatics. However, with excessive fluid accumulation, lymph channels become compressed by the fluid, and the fluid flows from the interstitium into the alveolus, ultimately producing alveolar or pulmonary edema.

The earliest form of pulmonary edema is characterized by engorgement of the peribronchial and perivascular interstitial spaces and is known as *interstitial edema*. When fluid crosses the alveolar epithelium into the alveolar spaces, the alveoli fill with fluid, and because the alveoli are unventilated, oxygenation of the blood passing through them is not possible. In ARDS, alveolar type I and type II cells are damaged. The result is further fluid and protein accumulation, which inactivates surfactant. Surfactant normally lowers the surface tension of the alveolar lining fluid and maintains alveolar stability by preventing alveolar collapse, increasing lung compliance, and decreasing the work of breathing. As a consequence of the damage to the alveolar type II cells and inactivation of existing surfactant, the alveoli become increasingly unstable and tend to collapse unless filled with interstitial fluid.[11,12]

During this stage, hyaline membranes begin to line the alveoli. These membranes are thought to result from the exudation of high-molecular-weight substances (particularly fibrinogen) in the edema fluid. Hyaline membranes contribute to the development of fibrosis and atelectasis, leading to a decrease in gas exchange capability and lung compliance.

The essential disturbances that characterize the injury or exudative phase of ARDS are interstitial and alveolar

Injury to Alveolar-Capillary Membrane

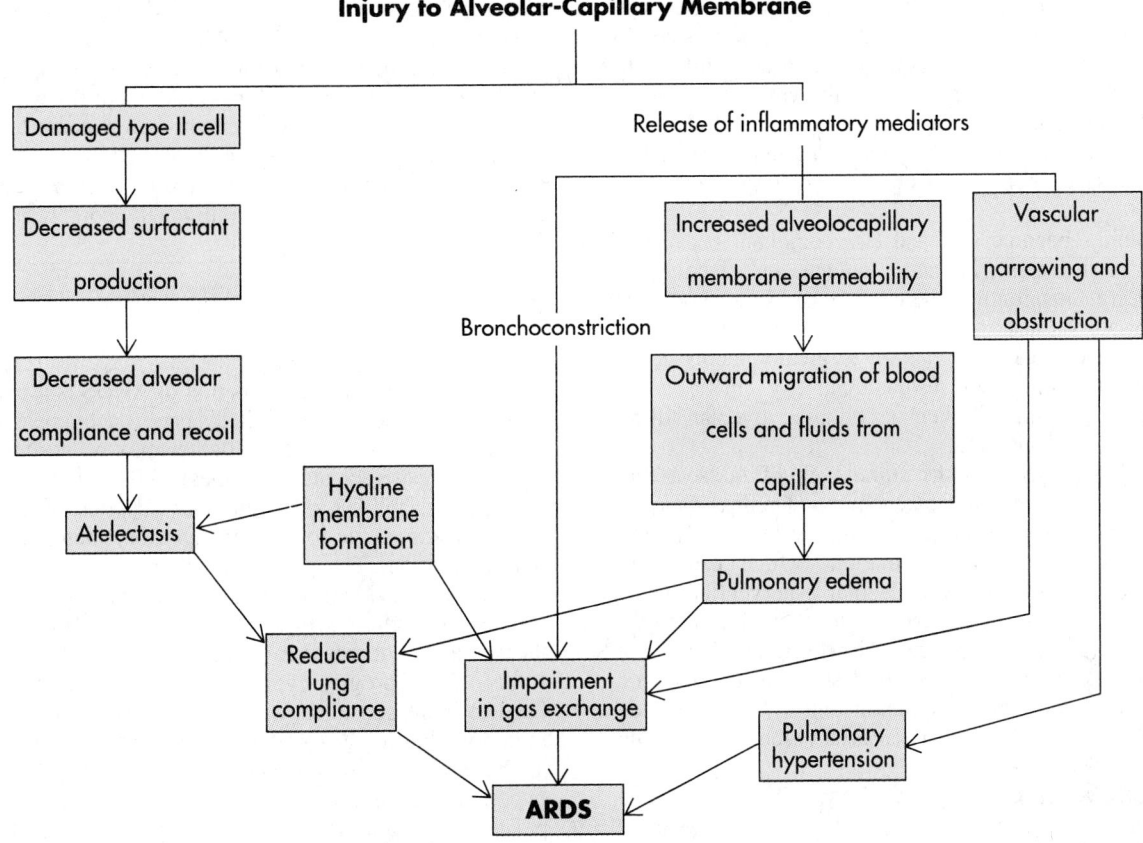

Fig. 23-6 Pathophysiology of ARDS.

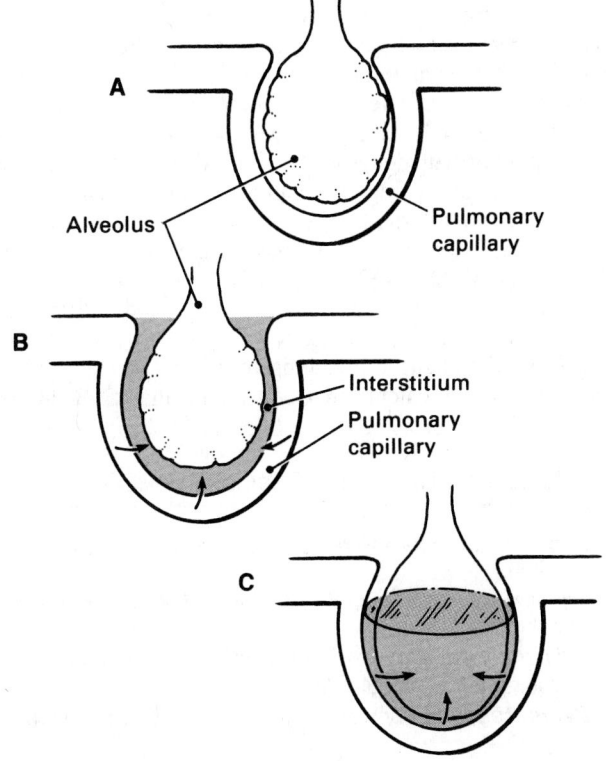

Fig. 23-7 Stages of edema formation in ARDS. **A,** Normal alveolus and pulmonary capillary. **B,** Interstitial edema occurs with increased flow of fluid into the interstitial space. **C,** Alveolar edema occurs when the fluid crosses the blood-gas barrier.

edema (noncardiogenic pulmonary edema) and atelectasis. Severe $\dot{V}/\dot{Q}$ mismatch and shunting of blood occur as blood flows through alveoli that are collapsed or filled with fluid. Diffusion limitations and impairment may occur because of thickening of alveolar-capillary interfaces. Hypoxia and subsequent severe hypoxemia that is refractory to increasing concentrations of O_2 (refractory hypoxemia) develop.

The lungs become stiff and less compliant because of the loss of surfactant, interstitial edema, and alveolar collapse. Large inspiratory pressures must be generated by the respiratory muscles to inflate the noncompliant lungs. Therefore the work of breathing is greatly increased. In addition, the functional residual capacity (FRC) is decreased as a result of alveolar collapse, alveolar filling, and interstitial thickening.

Both hypoxemia and the stimulation of juxtacapillary receptors in the stiff lung parenchyma (J reflex) cause an increase in respiratory frequency and decreased VT. This results in alveolar hyperventilation, which causes increased removal of CO_2. The alveolar hyperventilation and a reflexive increase in cardiac output attempt to compensate for the severe hypoxemia. However, as alveoli collapse and fill with fluid, increased shunting of blood occurs, and alveolar hypoventilation and symptoms of decreased cardiac output and decreased tissue perfusion develop.

Reparative or proliferative phase. The reparative or proliferative phase begins 1 to 3 weeks after the initial lung injury. During this phase, there is an influx of granulocytes and mononuclear cells and fibroblast proliferation as part of the inflammatory response. The injured lung has an immense regenerative capacity after acute lung injury. One mechanism that results in repair of the alveolar capillary membrane is the proliferation of type II pneumocytes that differentiate into type I alveolar epithelium.

The proliferative phase is complete when the diseased lung becomes characterized by dense, fibrous tissue. Lung compliance continues to decrease as a result of interstitial fibrosis. Hypoxemia worsens because of the thickened alveolar membrane, causing diffusion defects and shunting. If the reparative phase persists, widespread fibrosis results. If the proliferative phase is arrested, the lesions resolve.

Fibrotic phase. The fibrotic phase occurs approximately 3 to 4 weeks after the initial lung injury. This phase is also called the *chronic* or *late phase* of ARDS. By this time the lung is completely remodeled by sparsely collagenous and fibrous tissues. There is diffuse scarring and fibrosis, resulting in decreased lung compliance. In addition, the surface area for gas exchange is significantly reduced because the interstitium is fibrotic, and hypoxemia therefore continues. Pulmonary hypertension results from pulmonary vascular obliteration and fibrosis.

Clinical Progression

The progression of ARDS varies from client to client. Some persons survive the acute phase of lung injury with the pulmonary edema resolving and completely recover in a few days. This is called ARDS with *rapid reversal*. Others go on to the fibrotic (late or chronic) stage requiring long-term mechanical ventilation, and their chance of survival is poor. This is called ARDS with *delayed* or *sustained reversal*. It is not known why some clients successfully repair their injured lungs and recover, whereas in others, ARDS progresses.[9] Several factors seem to be important in determining the course of ARDS, including the nature of the initial injury, extent and severity of coexisting organ diseases, and the pulmonary complications related to intensive care.[13]

Clinical Manifestations

At the time of the initial injury and for several hours to 1 to 2 days afterward, the client may have no respiratory symptoms. The initial presentation of ARDS is often insidious. The client may exhibit dyspnea, tachypnea, cough, and restlessness. Chest auscultation may be normal or reveal fine, scattered rales (crackles). ABG analyses usually demonstrate mild hypoxemia and respiratory alkalosis. The alkalosis is due to the compensatory increase in alveolar ventilation. The chest x-ray film may be normal, or there may be evidence of minimal scattered interstitial infiltrates. The chest x-ray film may not show edema until there is a 30% increase in lung water content.[9]

As ARDS progresses, symptoms develop that are related to increased lung water accumulation and decreased lung compliance. Respiratory discomfort becomes evident as the work of breathing increases. Noisy tachypneic and hyperpneic respirations as well as intercostal and suprasternal retractions may be present. Pulmonary function tests reveal decreased static and effective compliance and decreased lung volumes, particularly FRC (although it is not measured). Tachycardia, diaphoresis, changes in sensorium with decreased mentation, cyanosis, and pallor may be present. Chest auscultation usually reveals scattered to diffuse rales and rhonchi. The chest x-ray film usually demonstrates diffuse and extensive bilateral interstitial and alveolar infiltrates. Usually a pulmonary artery catheter will be inserted to determine whether the cause of the pulmonary edema is cardiogenic. ARDS or noncardiogenic pulmonary edema is the usual diagnosis if the pulmonary capillary wedge pressure is within normal limits.

Progressive arterial hypoxemia despite the increased O_2 tension of air inspired by the mask, cannula, or ET tube is a *hallmark* of ARDS (Table 23-10). This is referred to as *refractory hypoxemia*. The $D(A - a)O_2$, or the difference between PAO_2 and PaO_2, can be as high as 200 to 500 mm Hg when the client is breathing room air (normal <15 to 20 mm Hg). A calculated $\dot{Q}_S/\dot{Q}_T$ more than 30% of the

---

Table 23-10 Diagnostic Findings in ARDS

Hypoxemia: Severe refractory hypoxemia (a/A ratio of <0.3)

Chest x-ray film: Diffuse bilateral interstitial and alveolar infiltrates

Pulmonary capillary wedge pressure: <18 cm H_2O (excluding left ventricular failure)

Decreased lung compliance: High ventilatory pressures

---

cardiac output and an a/A ratio of less than 0.3 are other signs. ABG values may demonstrate a normal $Paco_2$ despite severe dyspnea and hypoxemia. An elevated $Paco_2$ signifies that the client is no longer able to compensate and is increasing the alveolar ventilation in response to hypoxemia and other stimuli.

As ARDS progresses it is associated with profound respiratory distress requiring ET intubation and assisted ventilation. Bronchial breath sounds are frequently associated with this stage. The chest x-ray film is often termed "white out" or "white lung," since consolidation and coalescing infiltrates pervade the lungs, leaving few recognizable air spaces. Severe hypoxemia, hypercapnia, and metabolic acidosis with symptoms of end organ or tissue hypoxia may ensue if prompt therapy is not instituted.

Complications

Complications (Table 23-11) may develop as a result of ARDS itself or treatment. The major cause of death in ARDS is nonpulmonary major organ failure (MOF), often accompanied by sepsis. It is not known yet whether ARDS is chiefly a lung disorder or a more generalized disorder of the entire microvasculature from generalized endothelial injury. The organs most commonly involved are the kidneys, liver, and heart, and the CNS and hematological and GI systems are also involved.

Nosocomial pneumonia as a complication of ARDS is associated with a 90% mortality rate.[14] Risk factors predisposing to nosocomial infections include impaired host defenses, contaminated support equipment, contaminated invasive monitoring devices, and colonization of the respiratory tract, in addition to organisms transmitted by health care providers in contact with the client. Frequent monitoring of sputum smears and cultures and assessment of the quality, quantity, and consistency of sputum should be done. The presence of fever warrants a workup to determine the source of infection. Serial chest x-ray films and blood cell counts with a white blood cell (WBC) differential must be closely monitored. Observing and changing cannula sites as necessary may prevent sepsis. All stopcocks should be capped or covered and old blood flushed from them to prevent bacterial contamination and growth.

Excessively high inflation pressures may be required to inflate the stiff, noncompliant lungs in ARDS. *Barotrauma* (e.g., pneumothorax, pneumomediastinum, tension pneumothorax) may result from these high pressures. Therefore monitoring of peak inflation pressures and breath sounds is essential.

Stress ulcers are common, and prophylactic use of antacids every 1 to 2 hours (to keep the gastric pH >5) and/or IV cimetidine (Tagamet) or ranitidine (Zantac) may prevent GI hemorrhage. Guaiac testing of stools and emesis and monitoring of hematocrit values are important to detect occult bleeding.

Disseminated intravascular coagulation (DIC) may occur with ARDS. (The pathophysiology of DIC is discussed in Chapter 25.) Frequent monitoring of platelet counts, fibrinogen level, and partial thromboplastin and prothrombin times is helpful in the early detection of DIC. Observation and assessment of bleeding from venipuncture sites and mucous membranes and during ET suction are important. The client should also be observed for the presence of bruises and petechiae.

Renal failure can occur because of the effects of hypoxemia or hypercapnia on kidney function and mechanical ventilation on the renal system and through management of problems associated with ARDS such as hypotension, shock, and aminoglycoside nephrotoxicity. The adequacy of renal function should be continually assessed by monitoring urinary output and specific gravity, urine composition, blood urea nitrogen (BUN), and serum creatinine levels.

■ Therapeutic and Nursing Management of ARDS

Nursing assessment

Because ARDS is a cause of acute respiratory failure, the subjective and objective data that should be obtained from a person with ARDS are the same as for acute respiratory failure and are presented in Table 23-5.

Nursing diagnoses

Nursing diagnoses are determined when the problem and etiological factors are supported by clinical data. Nursing diagnoses related to ARDS may include, but are not limited to, those described for acute respiratory failure and are presented in Table 23-6.

Nursing interventions

Preventive measures for ARDS include those for acute respiratory failure. Astute observation of the respiratory status of high-risk clients is especially important. Judicious fluid administration and monitoring of the fluid status by intake and output records, weights, clinical manifestations of increased lung water (e.g., rales, deteriorating ABGs, increased work of breathing), and body fluid accumulation (e.g., jugular venous distention; sacral, periorbital, or pe-

---

Table 23-11 Complications Associated with ARDS

Infection	Renal complications
Nosocomial pneumonia	Cardiac complications
Catheter-related infection	Decreased cardiac output
Sepsis (bacteremia)	Dysrhythmias
Respiratory complications	Hematological complications
Pulmonary emboli	Anemia
Pulmonary barotrauma	Thrombocytopenia
(e.g., pneumothorax,	DIC
pneumomediastinum,	CNS complications
subcutaneous emphy-	ET intubation complications
sema)	Laryngeal ulceration
O_2 toxicity	Tracheal ulceration
Pulmonary fibrosis	Tracheal malacia
Gastrointestinal complications	Tracheal stenosis
Stress ulceration and	
hemorrhage	
Ileus	
Pneumoperitoneum	

Modified from Mitchell RS and others: Synopsis of clinical pulmonary disease, ed 4, St Louis, 1989, The CV Mosby Co, p 269.

Table 23-12 Principles of Therapeutic
Management for ARDS

Identify and treat underlying condition.
Establish an airway (usually ET tube).
Institute mechanical ventilation:
1. Volume-cycled ventilator
2. PEEP
Maintain oxygenation:
1. O$_2$ administration
2. Packed RBCs
Increase cardiac output:
1. Dolbutamine
2. Dobutamine
Monitor oxygenation and cardiac output:
1. Arterial line
2. Pulmonary artery catheter
3. Oximetry
Maintain fluid balance:
1. Colloids, crystalloids
2. Diuretics
3. Ultrafiltration
Treat infections.

ripheral edema; hepatomegaly; splenomegaly) are important. Expeditious treatment of the initial disorder (e.g., prompt treatment with antibiotics or surgery to remove the source of infection in sepsis and maintenance of BP and urine flow in shock) is necessary and may prevent further deterioration of the client and the development of ARDS.

At the time of the initial lung injury and for as long as 12 to 48 hours thereafter, the client may be free of respiratory symptoms or signs of distress. Usually, abnormal findings on physical examination are indications that ARDS has progressed beyond the initial stages. Prompt recognition of clinical manifestations and treatment may help to prevent the development of severe forms of ARDS.

Management of ARDS includes many of the therapeutic and nursing regimens used in acute respiratory failure. Measures to improve alveolar ventilation and maintain adequate PaO$_2$ in the management of acute respiratory failure also apply to ARDS. However, many therapeutic and nursing therapies are unique to ARDS (Table 23-12).

Treatment of the underlying disorder. Sepsis is often an initiating mechanism of ARDS. Prompt culturing of exudates, secretions, and blood and surgical debridement (if indicated) of an infected area are necessary. Antibiotic therapy should be instituted as soon as possible. For clients already receiving antibiotics, blood cultures with antibiotic removal device should be ordered.

If severe arterial hypotension and shock are the initiating factors, restoration of adequate BP is essential. Frequently, overzealous administration of fluids in the attempt to restore BP leads to circulatory overload and pulmonary edema. Other conditions contributing to ARDS are presented in Table 23-9.

Maintenance of adequate oxygenation. O$_2$ administration through a face mask or cannula (prongs) is usually in-

adequate to treat the refractory hypoxemia of ARDS. The rule of thumb for O$_2$ administration is to give the client the lowest concentration of O$_2$ in inspired air that suffices to maintain a PaO$_2$ of approximately 60 mm Hg. When the FiO$_2$ concentration exceeds 0.5 for more than a few days, O$_2$ toxicity is virtually inevitable.

ET intubation with subsequent mechanical ventilation is almost always required. When the client receives mechanical ventilation, a large V$_T$ (10 to 15 ml/kg) is usually used to reverse microatelectasis and shunting. The respiratory rate of the ventilator is set to keep the pH at 7.35 to 7.45 and to prevent alkalosis, which may impair O$_2$ unloading at the tissue level, depress cardiac output, and initiate dysrhythmias.

When adequate oxygenation is not achieved by mechanical ventilation of the client at high lung volumes or when the PaO$_2$ remains less than 60 mm Hg with an FiO$_2$ of more than 0.5 to 0.6, the use of PEEP is indicated. PEEP is a ventilatory maneuver that applies positive pressure to the airway and lungs at the end of exhalation. Expiration normally occurs when the pressure in the chest becomes equal to atmospheric pressure or zero. When positive pressure is applied to the lung at the end of expiration, the lung is kept partially expanded and the alveoli are prevented from totally collapsing. The mechanism of action of PEEP is related to its ability to recruit or open up collapsed alveoli and increase the FRC. It also acts in this way to decrease shunting and improve oxygenation and lung compliance. Inverse ratio ventilation (IRV) is another ventilatory mode that is currently used to increase oxygenation.

Maintenance of cardiac output and hemoglobin concentration. There is a need for continuous hemodynamic monitoring of the client with ARDS who is receiving ventilator and PEEP therapy. An arterial line should be inserted to obtain continuous recording of BP and to make it easier to obtain frequent ABG measurements. (Specific nursing measures for the client with an indwelling arterial cannula are discussed in Chapter 28.)

Cardiac output can be assessed by the thermodilution port of the pulmonary artery catheter. Mixed venous O$_2$ samples can also be obtained from the distal part of the catheter. Calculation of the arterial venous oxygen (A − V)o$_2$ difference can be performed by determining P$\bar{v}$o$_2$. The (A − V)o$_2$ is the difference in the O$_2$ content of arterial and mixed venous blood. This value gives an indication of cardiac output if thermodilution is not available. The normal (A − V)o$_2$ difference is 4.5 vol% to 6 vol%, and an (A − V)o$_2$ difference of more than 6 vol% suggests impaired O$_2$ delivery. It is important to be able to assess cardiac output accurately by using one of these methods to determine the effects of PEEP and other therapies on the client's cardiopulmonary status.

If cardiac output falls, it may be necessary to administer fluids or colloid solutions or to lower PEEP. Use of inotropic drugs such as dolbutamine (Dolbutrex), dopamine (Intropin), or dobutamine (Dobutrex) may also be necessary.

Hb is usually kept at levels of more than 10 g/dl with an adequate saturation of more than 90% (when PaO$_2$ is more than 50 to 60 mm Hg). Packed RBCs may be administered to increase the O$_2$-carrying capacity of the blood.

Maintenance of fluid balance. Maintenance of fluid balance is precarious in the client with ARDS. Leaky capillaries increase lung water and cause pulmonary edema; however, the client may be volume depleted and prone to hypotension and decreased cardiac output from mechanical ventilation and PEEP.

Generally, the client is kept dry with the use of diuretics. The pulmonary capillary wedge pressure (which indicates the fluid status of the left side of the heart) is kept as low as possible without impairing cardiac output. The client is usually placed on mild fluid restriction, and diuretics are used as necessary. The client is maintained with strict intake and output and daily weights. Electrolytes and the fluid status are monitored.

Continuous arteriovenous hemofiltration (CAVH) is another approach to managing some cases of ARDS that are refractory to conventional measures. (CAVH is discussed in Chapter 41.) The use of CAVH in ARDS removes large quantities of plasma water, thus increasing colloid osmotic pressure, decreasing lung work, and causing improvement in gas exchange. Although CAVH has been used successfully in some cases of severe ARDS, it is not routinely used.

Other management considerations. The use of corticosteroids in the management of ARDS has been controversial for many years. Their use in sepsis and ARDS have not been shown to have any effect or to alter the outcome of ARDS.[15] Nonsteroidal antiinflammatory agents, antiendotoxin antibodies, and surfactant are being investigated as therapeutic agents in the treatment of ARDS. Sedation and neuromuscular blocking agents are often used in clients with ARDS who are restless and tachypneic and who breathe out of phase with the ventilator.

ARTIFICIAL AIRWAY

An artificial airway is created by inserting a tube into the trachea that bypasses the upper airway and laryngeal structures. *Intubation* is the process of tube insertion, and *extubation* is the process of its removal. Artificial airways are required for persons receiving mechanical ventilation. Other indications for their use include relief of airway obstruction, airway protection (e.g., after general anesthesia until the cough and other protective mechanisms return), and facilitation of secretion removal.

There are two basic types of artificial airways, *endotracheal* (ET) *tube* and *tracheostomy*. An ET tube may be inserted into the mouth (orotracheal) or nose (nasotracheal). (The types of tubes and indications for use are discussed in Chapter 20.)

Complications of Endotracheal Intubation

The major complications of ET intubation result from injury to the hypopharynx, larynx, and trachea and are related to the pressure exerted on upper airway structures by the tube and cuff. Improper tube placement, aspiration, oral and nasal pressure sores, and accidental extubation are also potential problems.[16]

Oral, nasal, and pharyngeal damage. Nasotracheal intubation may cause erosion and necrosis of the nasal septum and turbinates and sinusitis by blockage of the ostia.

Injury to the lips, teeth, tongue, and posterior pharynx may occur when the oral intubation route is used. Measures to prevent these complications include proper positioning and stabilization of the ET tube so that it does not put pressure on the sides of the nose or mouth, as well as daily changes in the position of the oral ET tube from one side of the mouth to the other. The mouth and nose should be inspected frequently for evidence of pressure areas and ulceration.

The mouth should be inspected daily to assess the condition of the mucosa, gums, and teeth. Because the client's mouth is always open when an ET tube is in place, the lips and mouth should be moistened with saline or water swabs to prevent drying of the mucosa. Mouth care, including cleaning of the teeth and gums, should be performed daily to prevent injury to the gums and loss of dentition resulting from the accumulation of plaque in the mouth. Mouthwash containing alcohol should not be used to clean the mouth because these preparations dry the mucosa, predisposing it to crack and thus creating sites for infection.

Laryngeal and tracheal damage. Laryngeal injury from ET tubes and cuffs is common. Movement of the client and the tube during the ventilatory cycle contributes to laryngeal and tracheal injury. The development of vocal cord congestion or a membranous glottis even when the client is intubated for less than 30 hours is common. Clients with laryngeal damage can exhibit stridor or symptoms of upper airway obstruction, which may be indicative of laryngospasm. Pulmonary edema can be produced by laryngospasm. Postextubation symptoms of laryngeal damage include hoarseness, sore throat, cough, sputum production, and hemoptysis. Paranasal sinusitis has been found in many nasally intubated clients. Sinusitis should be suspected when there is an unexplained fever, purulent nasal drainage, sinus tenderness, or unexplained sepsis.[17] Although the upper airway is damaged with intubation, the site of injury usually heals rapidly, with complete resolution of symptoms in most clients within 3 to 6 months. The incidence of more serious laryngeal and tracheal damage increases with the duration of intubation. Ulceration of the tracheal mucosa and problems with tracheal stenosis, tracheomalacia, tracheoesophageal fistulas, and tracheainnominate bleeding have greatly decreased in incidence and severity with the use of low-pressure cuffs.

Tracheal stenosis is a stricture or narrowing of the airway caused by the healing process, resulting in scarring of the trachea. *Tracheomalacia,* a destruction or softening of the tracheal cartilages, results in collapse of the trachea during inspiration. Stenosis may occur alone, although malacia and stenosis often occur together.

Development of a tracheoesophageal fistula may occur with prolonged use of both ET and hard plastic, large-bore nasogastric tubes. A hard plastic nasogastric tube resting against the posterior esophageal wall and an ET tube resting in the trachea may also exert pressure on the anterior part of the esophagus. This continuous pressure may lead to weakness in the posterior tracheal and anterior esophageal wall with development of a fistula. Thus tube feedings for the long-term ventilatory client should be administered by a small-diameter soft feeding tube that can be aspirated to check for gastric residual (see Chapter 35 for a discussion of tube feedings).

Tracheomalacia may be present if increasing volumes of air are required to seal the cuff or if a large air leak persists around the cuff. An increase in the cuff/tube width ratio seen on a chest x-ray film may also be a clue to the presence of tracheomalacia. Tracheal stenosis should be suspected if decreasing volumes of air are required to seal the ET tube cuff. Tracheoesophageal fistulas may be detected or tested for by adding food coloring to tube feeding and observing for the coloring in suctioned secretions. Suctioned secretions can be tested with a dipstick for the presence of glucose. Normally, tracheal secretions should be negative for glucose.

If symptoms of laryngeal and tracheal problems occur, they usually become evident after extubation. Clients need to be observed closely for manifestations of airway obstruction after extubation, including hoarseness, cough, aspiration, swallowing difficulties, sore throat, inspiratory stridor, and respiratory distress.

Inspiratory stridor can be assessed by placing the diaphragm of the stethoscope at the neck and listening for a high-pitched musical sound on inspiration. Inspiratory stridor is a cardinal clinical manifestation of glottic edema. If it is heard immediately after extubation, the client should be treated aggressively with racemic epinephrine nebulization and steroids. Usually, hoarseness, cough, and sore throat end after a period of time. If these manifestations persist, they must be investigated. An intubation and tracheostomy tray should be kept nearby in case reintubation becomes necessary.

An exceedingly rare complication of an artificial airway is rupture of the innominate artery from erosion of the ET tube or cuff into the anterior part of the tracheal wall. This is usually a fatal event and is heralded by blood gushing from the ET tube. Rapidly overinflating the cuff on the ET tube may help to tamponade the bleeding vessel until more definitive treatment is obtained.

Laryngeal and tracheal injuries may be minimized by the following procedures:

1. Use of the smallest-diameter ET tube that permits efficient ventilation without undue added resistance to ventilation
2. Use of swivel connectors and flexible tubing to connect the client's tube to the ventilator (which minimizes traction on the airway)
3. Stabilization of the airway
4. Support of the client's head and tubes when turning and avoidance of undue head motion
5. Use of proper cuff inflation and low-pressure cuffs
6. Use of a small-bore, soft, flexible, and easily aspirated feeding tube when prolonged enteral feedings are required on an intubated client

Improper tube placement and accidental extubation. Improper tube placement is another potential hazard of ET intubation. It is possible for the tube to be inserted into the esophagus or to slip so that it extends into the right mainstem bronchus and ventilates only the right lung.[18] Positioning of the distal tube orifice against the carina or tracheal wall may cause airway obstruction. Kinking of the ET tube when the client moves the head may occur and cause airway obstruction. The use of a bite block or placement of an oral airway will prevent the client from biting on the ET tube. There are also ready-made orotracheal tube holders that help to stabilize the tube.

A chest x-ray film should be taken immediately after intubation or at any time if there is ever a question of tube placement so that the tube may be repositioned as needed. The tip of the ET tube should be seen on chest x-ray film at least 2 cm above the carina. Chest auscultation should also be done immediately after intubation and before securing the tube to determine the presence of bilateral equal breath sounds. Auscultation of breath sounds is performed regularly, at least every 4 hours. The tube must be well secured to prevent slipping or accidental extubation. Accidental extubation can be prevented in the client who is not fully mentally alert (e.g., after anesthesia, during heavy sedation) by the use of soft wrist restraints. It is wise to mark the tube with india ink at the lip or nose level or to note the centimeter mark closest to the lip or nose level and chart it on the care plan or flowchart. This mark provides a quick reference point to check proper tube placement.

The ET tube should not extend more than 1½ to 3 inches out of the client's nose or mouth because this can add to pressure exerted on these structures. Once ET position has been verified by chest x-ray film, the ET tube can be cut and the adapter reapplied. It is important to chart that the tube has been cut. In some centers the cut portion is taped on the wall at the head of the bed as another reminder.

Aspiration. Aspiration is a potential hazard because oral secretions can accumulate above the cuff; when the cuff is deflated, the secretions may move into the lungs. For this reason the posterior of the pharynx should be suctioned before cuff deflation. Oral intubation increases salivation, so the mouth should be suctioned frequently. Clients themselves can use a Yankauer or tonsil suction. Other factors that may cause aspiration include cuff leak, tracheal distention, and tracheoesophageal fistula.

Tracheostomy tubes. Tracheostomy tubes are currently the preferred artificial airway for long-term intubation (see Chapter 20). Upper airway damage is minimized and the client's comfort is maximized if a tracheostomy is performed early in the course of treatment. The client may be able to eat normally and to speak if a tracheostomy tube that allows speech is used.

There is much debate on the subject of when to perform a tracheotomy in the client with an oral or nasotracheal ET tube. With the use of ET tube cuffs that are designed to minimize the pressure against the tracheal mucosa and the use of techniques to maintain low cuff pressures, ET tubes can be left in place longer. Presently there is no consensus on the length a time an ET tube should be left in place. The situation varies with the client, physician, and institution. The span of time ranges from 72 hours to 2 to 3 weeks; some institutions use ET intubation in clients for up to 6 weeks without harmful sequelae. Nasotracheal intubation can usually be tolerated by the client for longer periods of time than oral intubation. However, the disadvantage of the possible development of sinusitis and increased airway resistance due to the smaller tube must be considered.

Care of the Artificial Airway

Types of cuffs. ET and tracheostomy tubes may have either hard (high-pressure, low-volume) or soft (low-pressure, high-volume) cuffs. The purpose of the cuff is to create a seal between the airway and the tube so that gas from the ventilator will go into the lung instead of escaping around the tube. A secondary purpose of the cuff is to minimize aspiration of gastric contents into the lungs.

Hard cuffs have high intracuff pressures and a narrow area of tracheal wall contact. These are used mostly for short-term intubation, usually in the operating room. Soft cuffs are made of soft, pliable material that tends to inflate evenly and conforms to the tracheal contour. Soft cuffs are also known as *low-pressure cuffs*. Lower cuff pressures are diffused over a wider area of the trachea, minimizing tracheal and laryngeal damage. Soft cuffs are preferred and are used almost exclusively today.

There are several different types of low-pressure cuffs, varying in composition and in the inflation methods used. The Bivona Fome cuff, the Lanz tube, the Portex, and the Shiley PRV tubes are examples of the many types of cuffed tracheal tubes available.

Cuff problems. A common problem that may occur in all cuffs inflated with air is overinflation of the cuff, particularly during inspiration when positive-pressure ventilation is used. A cuff inflated to seal during the peak inspiratory phase is overinflated during the exhalation phase. This overinflation of the cuff results in tracheal dilatation. The cuff is reinflated with additional air and the cycle is repeated as tracheal dilatation progresses to ensure no-leak ventilation. Tracheal dilatation may lead to esophageal compression, causing aspiration and difficulty in swallowing. This problem is prevented by the minimal occlusive volume or the minimal leak technique of cuff inflation and maintenance of intracuff pressures at less than 25 cm H_2O or less than 18 to 20 mm Hg.

Another rare problem peculiar to some low-pressure cuffs is ballooning of the cuff over the tube lumen, resulting in airway obstruction. This can occur if the cuff is overinflated. Conditions that may indicate this problem are an increase in peak airway pressure, decrease in exhaled V_T, increased resistance during bag ventilation of the client, difficulty in passing a suction catheter, and an abnormal musical sound associated with inhalation. If this problem is suspected, the cuff should be totally deflated, the airway patency checked, and the cuff slowly reinflated.

Ineffective sealing of the artificial airway because of cuff rupture and inadequate cuff inflation are other cuff problems that may be encountered. A decrease in exhaled V_T; inadequately maintained PEEP level; noisy gurgling heard on inspiration; and aspiration of saliva, vomitus, or ingested materials may signal these events. The quickest and easiest method to verify a leak in the cuff is to withdraw the air in the cuff with a syringe. If air cannot be withdrawn by this method, a cuff leak or rupture is proba-

bly present. The cuff should be reinflated, the number of cubic centimeters of air needed to be injected should be noted, and the air should be withdrawn.

The amount of air previously needed to inflate the cuff and the amount of air withdrawn should be compared with the amount of air instilled. Differences in these amounts can indicate a leak in the cuff. An attempt to aspirate air from the cuff should always be made before air is instilled into the cuff. This will prevent overinflation of the cuff. Leaks in the sideport balloon line or balloon-port connection valve can sometimes be corrected by using a small angiocath or intracath attached to a three-way stopcock. If the balloon is defective, a new tube is indicated.

Cuff care. Three popular techniques recommended for cuff inflation and maintenance are (1) the *minimal leak technique*, (2) *minimal occlusive volume* (MOV), and (3) *intracuff pressure measurement*. The minimal leak technique and intracuff pressure measurement are frequently used together. MOV and intracuff pressure measurement should be used together.

In the minimal leak technique, a minimal leak should be present in the cuff at the moment in the ventilatory cycle when the tracheal diameter is maximum (peak inspiration). The back of the oropharynx is first suctioned to prevent aspiration of secretions that may lodge on top of the cuff. Next, the cuff is deflated totally to prevent accidental overinflation. With the diaphragm of the stethoscope placed in the neck area (approximately where the cuff is situated), air is slowly injected into the cuff by a syringe at end inspiration on a ventilator-delivered breath until no gurgling is heard. Enough air is withdrawn into the syringe until a slight leak is auscultated at the peak of inspiration on a ventilator-delivered breath. The nurse or respiratory therapist should record the amount of air necessary for the minimal leak and the amount of air in milliliters on the flowchart or nurse's notes at least once a day and as needed (some hospitals perform this every shift).

The same procedure as for the minimal leak technique is followed to obtain an MOV except that the minimal leak procedure is omitted. Air should be injected into the cuff until no gurgling is auscultated at the neck. The cuff port is connected by a three- or four-way stopcock to an aneroid pressure gauge and the pressure is read at end exhalation to measure the intracuff pressure (see Fig. 20-8, *E*). The cuff pressure should not exceed 25 cm H_2O or 18 to 20 mm Hg. This is considered the maximum amount of pressure that will permit maximum capillary flow under normal BP conditions. The volume of air in the cuff and the intracuff pressure should be checked every day or every shift, depending on hospital policy, and recorded on the flowchart or nurse's notes. When MOV is used, it is essential to check cuff pressures to ensure that the cuff is not overinflated, thus increasing pressure on the tracheal wall. Intracuff pressures may also be used to check the pressure attained in the cuff when the minimal leak technique is used. This ensures double protection for the airway structures.

When PEEP is used, MOV and intracuff pressure measurements are necessary because use of a minimal leak may allow air to escape from the lungs during end exhala-

Table 23-13 Suctioning Procedure for a Client on a Mechanical Ventilator

GENERAL MEASURES

1. Wash hands.
2. Explain procedure, purpose, and sensations to client.
3. Prepare all equipment:
   Check negative suction pressure (usual range between -80 and -120 mm Hg).
   Pour sterile normal saline solution into sterile container.
   Turn on O_2 flow to bag ventilator to 15 L.
   Place bag ventilator on bed.
   Open suction catheter and glove packages. Suction catheter should be no wider than half the diameter of artificial airway.

One-person method

1. Disconnect client from ventilator (instill 5-10 ml sterile normal saline solution by needleless syringe into artificial airway during inspiration *if secretions are thick*).
2. Preoxygenate with 100% O_2* and hyperventilate client with resuscitation bag or ventilator breaths 3-6 times (done before and after suctioning).
3. Connect client to ventilator.
4. Put on sterile glove and pick up catheter with sterile hand.
5. Connect catheter to suction tubing, using sterile hand for catheter and nonsterile hand for suction tubing.
6. Disconnect client from ventilator.
7. Using nonsterile hand, stabilize artificial airway and hold catheter suction regulator (client may turn head to right with chin up to attempt to place catheter in left mainstem bronchus).
8. Insert catheter gently, swiftly, and without suction with sterile hand.
9. When resistance is met, pull back catheter 1-2 cm without suction.
10. Begin depressing suction vacuum regulator in an on-off (intermittent) fashion with nonsterile hand while rotating catheter in sterile hand between thumb and forefinger.
11. Swiftly remove catheter. Each suctioning pass should not exceed 15 sec.
12. Rinse catheter in sterile saline between suctioning passes as necessary.
13. With nonsterile hand, reconnect client to ventilator.
14. Depress manual breath or sigh button (if activated) on ventilator to hyperventilate or ventilate client.†
15. Let client equilibrate for 30 sec to 1 min or as needed.
16. Rinse catheter with sterile normal saline solution.
17. Repeat procedure as needed.
18. Place client back on ventilator.
19. Suction oropharynx.
20. Discard catheter.
21. Hyperventilate and oxygenate via resuscitation bag or ventilator for three to six breaths.
22. Assess client's tolerance to suctioning (continuous observation of the client during entire suctioning procedure is necessary).

Two-person method

1. First person instills normal saline solution as necessary; hyperventilates and preoxygenates before, between, and after suctions; stabilizes airway.
2. Second person suctions as in one-person method.

---

*Use O_2 concentration of 60% or less for clients with chronic hypercapnia who are breathing spontaneously.
†As nurse becomes more adept at suctioning, bag ventilation may be done with nonsterile hand between suctioning passes. Ideally, it is better for two persons to hyperventilate the client with two hands. (One nurse with one hand on the bag ventilator can generate up to 800 ml, and with two hands up to 1000 ml.)

tion. In addition, PEEP may be slightly decreased. Changes in head and neck position can also cause pressure and volume variations in the cuff. For these reasons, cuff pressure and volume measurements should be obtained with the client in a consistent position, preferably with the head of the bed elevated to 30 degrees. Adjustments in cuff volume and/or pressure may have to be made with

changes in the client's position. Clients who receive general anesthesia can experience increased cuff pressures caused by diffusion of anesthetic gases into the air-inflated tube cuff.[17]

Suctioning. Suctioning of the client's ET or tracheostomy tube should be performed as needed, not just routinely. Signs that may indicate the presence of secretions

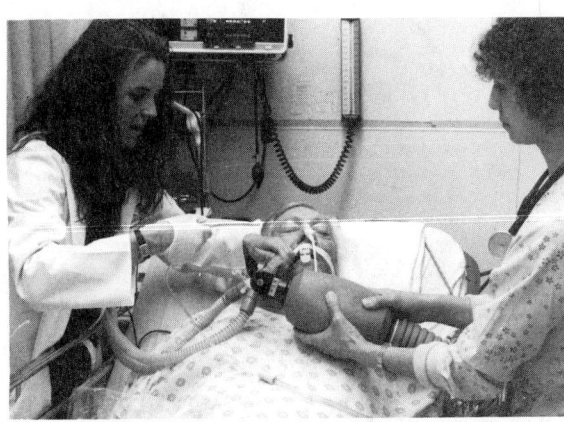

Fig. 23-8 The two-person suctioning method.

in the airways include dyspnea, increased ventilator peak-inspiratory pressures, activation of the ventilator pressure alarm, noisy or gurgling respirations, coarse rales, and rhonchi. The recommended procedure for suctioning is presented in Table 23-13.

Complications associated with suctioning include hypoxemia, cardiac dysrhythmias, damage to the mucosal membrane, pneumothorax, contamination and infection, retained secretions, and anxiety. Hypoxemia occurs when O_2-enriched gas is sucked out of the lungs with the secretions and replaced by room air that enters around the catheter. Other causes of hypoxemia may be bronchospasm caused by airway irritation and microatelectasis resulting from aspiration of intrapulmonary air. The Pao_2 may be reduced by 10 to 39 mm Hg with ET suctioning.[19]

Measures to prevent hypoxemia include (1) preoxygenation and postoxygenation and hyperinflation of the client's lungs with 100% O_2, preferably from a volume ventilator with a manual sigh or breath, or by a bag ventilator for three to six breaths; (2) limiting each suction pass to 10 to 15 seconds; and (3) returning the client to the ventilator or continuing to use the bag ventilator (Ambu) at the client's own respiratory rate between suctioning passes. Spontaneously breathing clients with chronic hypercapnia (e.g., clients with COPD) should not receive bag ventilation with 100% O_2. Instead, bag ventilators with 35% to 60% O_2 should be used, and the client should be assessed for spontaneous ventilatory activity after the suctioning procedure.

Ideally, two persons should perform the suctioning procedure so that one person can use both hands to bag ventilate the client (Fig. 23-8). This is important because hyperinflation with volumes 1½ times the Vt ensures adequate preoxygenation. One-handed bagging may not ensure this volume. The use of a volume-controlled ventilator to hyperinflate the client is an alternative method but introduces the risk of an unknown lag time between O_2 adjustment and delivery because there is a delay of 1 to 2 minutes before the ventilator actually delivers the increased concentration of 95% to 100% O_2. If the O_2 concentration is increased, it should be returned to the presuctioning level after suctioning. The Bennett 7200 Micropro-

cessor ventilator has a button to depress for increasing O_2 to 100%. The ventilator will automatically decrease the O_2 to the preset O_2 level after 2 minutes.

During the suctioning procedure, the client must be observed for tachycardia, dysrhythmias, hypertension, diaphoresis, and pallor or graying of mucous membranes. If any of these manifestations occur, the client should be bag ventilated or placed back on the ventilator until equilibration occurs before another suction pass is attempted.

Three causes of cardiac dysrhythmias during suctioning are (1) arterial hypoxemia, producing myocardial hypoxia; (2) vagal stimulation secondary to tracheal irritation; and (3) sympathetic nervous system stimulation caused by anxiety. Specific dysrhythmias that may occur include tachycardia; premature atrial, junctional, and ventricular beats; bradycardia; and possibly asystole. A suctioning pass should be limited to 5 to 10 seconds in clients with hypoxemia or bradycardia. Suctioning should be terminated if serious dysrhythmias develop, and the client should be bag ventilated slowly with 100% O_2 until the dysrhythmias subside. Excessive suctioning should be avoided in clients with hypoxemia or bradycardia.

Mucosal damage to tracheal structures may occur because of excessive negative suction pressures, too-vigorous insertion of the catheter, and the characteristics of the suction catheter itself. The presence of blood streaks and/or tissue shreds in aspirated mucus indicates that mucosal damage has occurred. Trauma to the mucosa can be prevented by the following:

1. The use of blunt or ring-tipped catheters with side holes
2. Limiting negative suction pressure to −80 to −120 mm Hg
3. Insertion of the catheter without suction
4. Withdrawal of the catheter 1 to 2 cm before applying suction to prevent the catheter from adhering to the mucosa
5. Lubrication of the catheter tip with sterile saline solution
6. Application of intermittent suction as the catheter is removed
7. Insertion of the catheter as gently and quickly as possible
8. Stabilization of the ET tube
9. Gentle rotation of the catheter and swift removal

The client is prone to infection for several reasons, including loss of upper airway protective mechanisms, disease, poor host defenses, and cross-contamination. Specific measures involved with suctioning that may help to prevent infection are frequent hand washing, using disposable one-time fluid reservoirs and catheters, covering the end of the T piece or ventilator tubing in a catheter wrapper to limit contamination from bedclothes, using meticulous sterile technique, and never suctioning the trachea with a catheter contaminated from the pharynx.

Although rare, pneumothorax may occur when a client is suctioned with a large catheter inserted into a small-diameter artificial airway. There is inadequate space for air to move in or out around the catheter, so when a vacuum is applied, the lung may collapse (microatelectasis may also occur). For prevention of lung collapse, the suction catheter should not occupy more than half the internal diameter of the tube being suctioned, negative suction pressures should be maintained at -80 to -120 mm Hg, and on-off suction pressure should be used when removing the catheter to prevent excessive buildup of negative pressure.

Secretions may be thick and difficult to suction due to inadequate hydration, inadequate humidification, or inaccessibility of the left mainstem bronchus or lower airways. Chest physiotherapy and having the client turn and cough before suctioning may help to move secretions into larger airways.[20] Instillation of 5 to 10 ml of sterile saline solution into the artificial airway during inspiration will cleanse the tube and stimulate coughing and the removal of thick secretions. The use of angle-tipped, directional tip, or coudé catheters while the client's head is tilted up and to the right may increase the possibility of entering the left mainstem bronchus. Turning the client's head to the right may make access to the left mainstem bronchus easier if angle-tipped, directional tip, or coudé catheters are not available.

Feelings of anxiety may arise during suctioning because the client feels unable to breathe or has a feeling of choking or because the client has never undergone suctioning before and does not know what to expect. A simple explanation should precede each suctioning procedure. Clients should be made aware that they will not be able to breathe for a short period but that they will soon be connected to O_2 and receive ventilation.

The client should also know that suctioning often stimulates coughing. If the client has a severe coughing spell during suctioning, bag ventilation with slow, small-volume breaths may help to alleviate the cough. Large volumes of air are not recommended because they may distend the lungs and stimulate further coughing episodes by reflex. The nurse should assume a calm, assured manner and allow clients to participate by bag ventilating themselves if possible. The client who has received ventilation immediately may need to be disconnected and bag ventilated until the coughing spell diminishes.

Suctioning a client with a PEEP greater than 10 cm H_2O must be carefully performed with the use of the hyperventilation and preoxygenation procedure that is best tolerated by the client. Hyperventilation and preoxygenation may be performed with special ventilator bags with PEEP attachments. These bags may be somewhat difficult to maneuver and may require the two-person suctioning method. A special pop-off port between the ventilator and the artificial airway used in some institutions allows suctioning through the port. Immediate closure of the port after each suctioning pass may help to maintain PEEP and oxygenation. In the latter case the Fio_2 may be increased to 1.0 for 2 minutes before suctioning if time is available. If a PEEP bag ventilator or a pop-off port is not available, turning up the Fio_2 to 1.0 and reconnecting the client to the ventilator between suctioning passes (without sighing) is superior to bag ventilating the client with a bag without a PEEP attachment.

A suction catheter system (Ballard system) in which a suction catheter is enclosed in a plastic sleeve connected

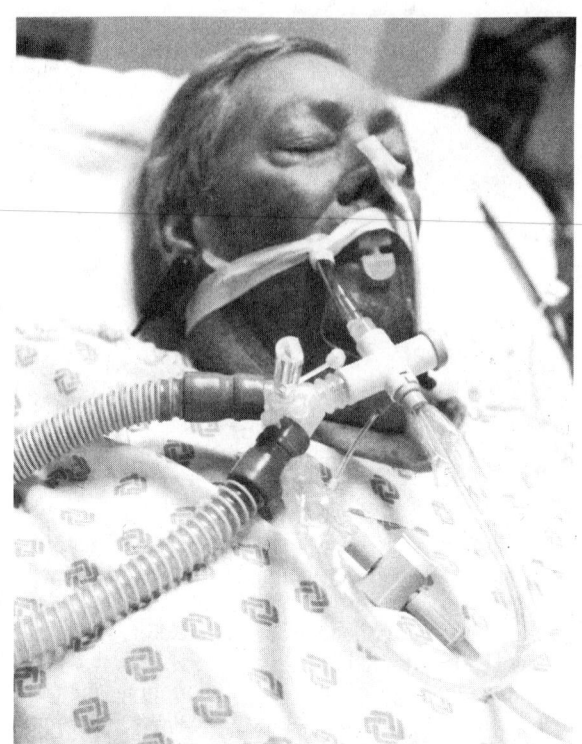

Fig. 23-9 Ballard suctioning catheter setup on a client with an oral ET tube and oral airway. A small-diameter feeding tube is also in place.

directly to the client's artificial airway and ventilator is being used in many critical care units (Fig. 23-9). With this system it is not necessary to use sterile gloves, thus contributing to increased efficiency and ease in suctioning. The entire system is changed every 24 hours, and it has been determined that this closed system reduces cross-contamination and autocontamination. Some drawbacks to the system are that the connection at the client's airway is somewhat heavy and tends to cause extra pulling on the airway. Another problem with the system is the difficulty in assessing how far down the catheter is when suctioning. When a nurse or respiratory therapist is adept in the system's use, the feeling of control over the catheter placement increases. The Ballard system allows the client to stay connected to the ventilator during the entire suctioning procedure. Manual sighs or breaths may be given. Nursing care of the client with an artificial airway is summarized in Table 23-14.

MECHANICAL VENTILATION

Mechanical ventilation is the process in which ventilation (the movement of air or O_2-enriched air into and out of the lungs) is performed by a mechanical ventilator (Fig. 23-10). Mechanical ventilation is not a curative measure; it is a supportive technique that assists in ventilating and oxygenating the client while therapeutic and nursing treatments enable recovery of the underlying disease process. For a summary of general guidelines on the need for mechanical ventilation, see Table 23-15.

Text continued on p. 632.

Table 23-14

 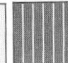

NURSING CARE PLAN FOR THE CLIENT WITH AN ARTIFICIAL AIRWAY*

Defining Characteristics	Nursing Interventions	Evaluation Criteria

NURSING DIAGNOSIS: Ineffective airway clearance related to accumulation of secretions in lungs, inability to mobilize secretions, drying of mucous membranes, and prolonged immobility

Defining Characteristics	Nursing Interventions	Evaluation Criteria
Presence of abnormal breath sounds (rhonchi, rales), frequent or absent cough, presence of thick or copious secretions, high peak inspiratory pressures on ventilator or frequent high-pressure alarm sounds on ventilator	Use effective suctioning technique.† Observe for blood streaks or tissue particles in suctioning aspirate. Use blunt ring-tipped catheters. Use catheter with diameter <½ tube diameter. Use negative suction pressure (−80 to −120 mm Hg). Instill 5-10 ml sterile saline solution by needleless syringe if secretions are thick. Use postural drainage, vibration, and percussion maneuvers when indicated.‡ Change client's position every 2 hr as tolerated. Suction before position change if clinical signs warrant. Keep ventilator tubing cleared of condensed water. Empty ventilator tubings before client position changes and as needed. Assess need for other measures to facilitate secretion mobilization. Administer aerosolized bronchodilators (if indicated).	Absence of abnormal breath sounds, thin and easily removed secretions, lungs clear to auscultation

NURSING DIAGNOSIS: High risk for respiratory infection related to exposure to environmental pathogens, removal of normal protective barrier to infection with use of artificial airway, and decreased resistance secondary to debilitated state, prolonged immobility, and inadequate nutrition

Defining Characteristics	Nursing Interventions	Evaluation Criteria
Change in color, quantity, odor, and viscosity of sputum; difficulty in suctioning secretions; increase in cough; fever; chills; diaphoresis; increase in respiratory rate with spontaneous ventilation; abnormal breath sounds (e.g., rales, rhonchi, wheezing); tachycardia; worsening of ABGs; flushing of skin; elevated WBC count; evidence of infiltrate or atelectasis on chest x-ray film; positive sputum cultures; decrease in lung compliance	Observe sputum for changes. Obtain sputum culture and order sensitivity test if secretions become purulent or tenacious, change color, or become odorous. Ensure that ventilator tubing is changed at least every 24-48 hr. Periodically clean and change bedside bag ventilator and tubing. Use sterile technique with suctioning.† Provide mouth care. Provide adequate nutritional and fluid intake.	No evidence of infection, negative sputum cultures

*Nursing care for a client with a tracheostomy is presented in Table 20-10.
†See Table 23-13.
‡See Chapter 22.

Continued.

Table 23-14

NURSING CARE OF THE CLIENT WITH AN ARTIFICIAL AIRWAY*—cont'd

Defining Characteristics	Nursing Interventions	Evaluation Criteria

NURSING DIAGNOSIS: High risk of injury related to improper suctioning, potential for aspiration of gastric secretions, right mainstem intubation, esophageal intubation, accidental extubation, mechanical obstruction or kinking of ET tube, cuff herniation over tip of ET tube, and irritation secondary to presence of artificial airway

Defining Characteristics	Nursing Interventions	Evaluation Criteria
Progressive hypoxemia, tachycardia, tachypnea, increase in BP, cyanosis, absent or unilateral breath sounds, dyspnea, inability to ventilate client with ventilation bag, inability to introduce suction catheter into ET tube, misplacement of ET tube on chest x-ray film, high peak airway pressures and frequent high airway pressure alarms, aspiration of gastric contents, positive methylene blue test, frequent suctioning	Use bite block or oral airway if client bites on tube. Stabilize and/or secure tube. Move client with care if connected to ventilator. Avoid traction on ET tube from ventilator tubing. Support client's head and airway. Mark tube with india ink or indelible marker at lip or nose insertion point. Cut off excess ET tube beyond 1-3 in from oral insertion point once in correct position. Note on chart that tube has been cut. Use rolled towel or sheet to support ET tube/mechanical ventilator manifold connection. Auscultate breath sounds immediately after intubation, q 4 hr, and as needed. Ensure that chest x-ray film is done immediately after intubation and whenever serious question of tube position arises.	Proper alignment of tube, no accidental extubation, no aspiration, no evidence of gastric contents in tracheal aspirate, no evidence of tracheal trauma
	If there is question of mechanical obstruction, place client in sniffing position (hyperextend head) and attempt to pass catheter. If catheter will not pass, deflate cuff totally and try again. Oxygenate and ventilate client after cuff has been slowly reinflated. Suction posterior pharynx and mouth before cuff deflation.	
	Elevate head of bed and inflate cuff during tube feedings. Use small-bore feeding tubes for enteral nutrition. Check for aspiration of tube-feeding by observing consistency of suctioned tracheal aspirate. Add food coloring to feedings to make identification easier. If suspicious of esophageal fistula, perform methylene blue test. Inject methylene blue diluted in water into feeding tube. If blue secretions suctioned, test is positive. Test secretions with dipstick for glucose. If positive, aspiration or regurgitation may have occurred. If client is eating, encourage anteflexion of head to open esophagus wider. Keep cuff inflated and elevate head of bed while client is eating. Insert nasogastric tube if client feels nauseated and is apt to vomit. Position client in side-lying position (never flat on back) if danger of aspiration is high.	

*Nursing care for a client with a tracheostomy is presented in Table 20-10.
§Modified from Kersten LD: *Comprehensive respiratory nursing*, Philadelphia, 1989, WB Saunders Co, pp 693-696.

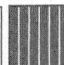

Table 23-14

NURSING CARE PLAN FOR THE CLIENT WITH AN ARTIFICIAL AIRWAY*—cont'd

Defining Characteristics	Nursing Interventions	Evaluation Criteria

NURSING DIAGNOSIS: Altered oral mucous membrane and impaired skin integrity related to tissue trauma caused by presence of artificial airway, open mouth, dryness of mouth; dehydration; decreased salivary flow as result of decreased jaw movements; and increased oral secretions, frequent mechanical stimulation with suction catheter, and lack of humidity§

| Presence of red, shiny, edematous mucosa of mouth; bleeding tendency of gingivoe or mucosa of mouth; presence of stomatitis; coated or encrusted oral ulcers; red, dry, swollen tongue with white or brownish coating | With bite block or oral airway removed, gently brush mouth and teeth with toothbrush, toothette, or swab with equal mixture of saline solution and hydrogen peroxide every 4-8 hr and as needed. Rinse with saline solution. Brush tongue as tolerated. Clean mouth and teeth, and provide mouth care every 1-2 hr. Clean bite block or oral airway with equal amounts of saline solution and hydrogen peroxide solution and replace in mouth. Apply lip lubricant to lips with cotton applicators or gloved hands. Check temperature on ventilator thermostat or feel temperature of ventilator gas with hand to ensure that adequate humidity and warmth are being applied by mechanical ventilator or O_2 source. Check cascade water level on ventilator. Discard water in cascade before refilling with distilled water. | Pink, moist, intact mucous membranes; absence of lesions, crusts, hard debris |

NURSING DIAGNOSIS: High risk for ineffective breathing pattern related to possible upper airway damage secondary to cuffed ET tube

| Tachypnea, tachycardia, decreased breath sounds, inspiratory stridor, use of accessory muscles, inability to phonate, hoarseness, sore throat, cough, swallowing difficulties after extubation | Use smallest-diameter ET tube that will support effective ventilation. Use only low-pressure cuffs for intubation. Use minimal leak or MOV technique and cuff pressures of <15-18 mm Hg (or 25 cm H_2O). Stabilize tube, tubing, and client's head when turning. Limit client's head movements. Use swivel adaptor connection between client and ventilator. Provide frequent care of mouth and nares. Inspect nares with flashlight and sides of mouth around oral ET tube for areas of pressure or ulceration. Change positions of oral ET tube at least once a day. Secure tube firmly with tape or tube holder. Assess chest x-ray films for tracheal size and relationship to tube. Observe for clinical signs of aspiration. Record amount of air and pressure in cuff q 8-24 hr. Assess for cuff leak (e.g., hissing or gurgling at mouth, decreased V_T). Deflate cuff when mechanical ventilation not required for ventilation. Immediately after extubation, monitor client closely for signs of respiratory distress secondary to laryngeal edema and other signs of upper airway damage. | Maintenance of normal integrity of upper airway structures, ability of client to phonate and swallow adequately within 1 wk after extubation |

Continued.

Table 23-14

NURSING CARE PLAN FOR THE CLIENT WITH AN ARTIFICIAL AIRWAY*—cont'd

Defining Characteristics	Nursing Interventions	Evaluation Criteria
NURSING DIAGNOSIS: Impaired verbal communication related to inability to speak secondary to intubation		
Inability to speak	Provide client with paper and pencil, magic slate, alphabet board, or talking device for artificial airways. Learn to read client's body language, facial expression, and signals. Attempt to anticipate client's needs. Provide easily accessible call light or bell. Explain temporary nature of problem and that client will be hoarse after intubation. Acknowledge that inability to speak can be frustrating.	Provision of effective method of communication, ability of client to communicate needs
NURSING DIAGNOSIS: Altered nutrition: less than body requirements related to possible inability to take nourishment orally, increased caloric demands secondary to clinical condition, and need for mechanical ventilation‖		

*Nursing care for a client with a tracheostomy is presented in Table 20-10.
‖See Table 23-5 for nursing interventions related to this nursing diagnosis.

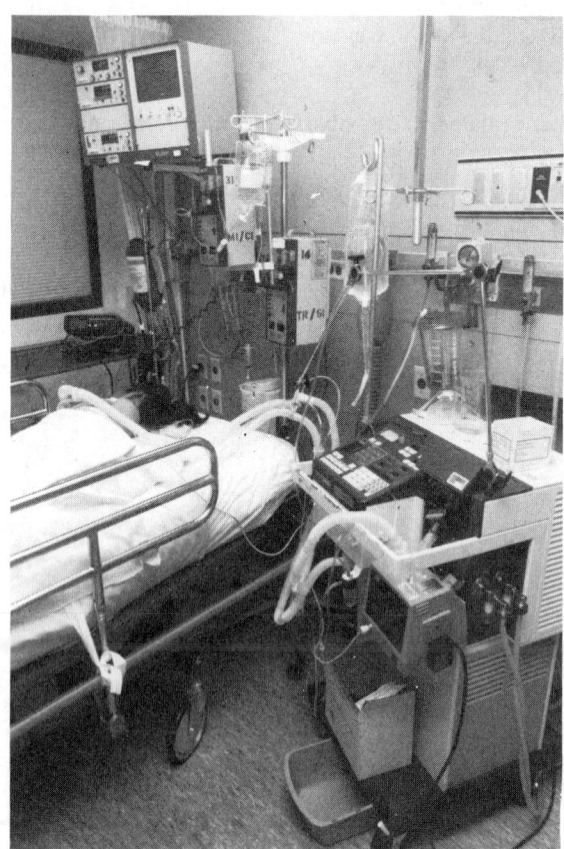

Fig. 23-10 Client being maintained on a Bennett 7200 Microprocessor ventilator.

Table 23-15   Indications for Mechanical Ventilation and Weaning

	Measurement and Significance	Normal Values*	Mechanical Ventilation Indicated*	Weaning Feasible*
TESTS OF VENTILATORY RESERVE OR MECHANICAL ABILITY				
V_T	Amount of air exchanged during normal breathing at rest	7-9 ml/kg	<5 ml/kg	>5 ml/kg
Respiratory rate per minute		12-20	<10 or >35	12-20
Forced vital capacity	Maximal inspiration and then measurement of air during maximal forced expiration; determination of whether client can sigh deeply enough to avoid atelectasis; best indicator of ventilatory reserve; client's cooperation necessary	65-75 ml/kg	<10-15 ml/kg	>10-15 ml/kg
Peak inspiratory pressure, negative inspiratory force	Complete occlusion of anaeroid manometer attached to airway or mouth for 10-20 sec while negative inspiratory efforts of client noted; useful index of neuromuscular strength; less client cooperation necessary	−75-100 cm H_2O	>−25 cm H_2O	<−20 cm H_2O
Forced expiratory volume in 1 sec	Volume of air measured in first second of exhalation of forced vital capacity maneuver; use in clients with COPD to determine degree of obstruction	50-60 ml/kg	<10 ml/kg	>16 ml/kg
Resting minute ventilation	Multiplication of tidal volume by respiratory rate for 1 minute, general indication of client's total ventilation	5-10 L/min	>10 L/min	<10 L/min
V_D/V_T	Estimation from V_T; accurate calculation requiring $Paco_2$ and partial pressure of CO_2 in mixed expired gas; measurement of portion of each breath that actually does not participate in gas exchange; indication of lungs' efficiency in removing CO_2	0.25-0.40	>0.6	<0.5-0.6
$Paco_2$	Indication of lungs' efficiency in removing CO_2 and reflection of body's acid-base status	35-45 mm Hg	>55 mm Hg	<45 mm Hg
TESTS OF OXYGENATION CAPABILITY				
$\dot{Q}_S/\dot{Q}_T$	Determination of amount of cardiac output shunted ($\dot{Q}_S$) in relation to amount of total cardiac output ($\dot{Q}_T$); indication of extent of shunt expressed as a percentage of cardiac output	<5%	>30%	<20%
$D(A - a)o_2$, $P(A - a)o_2$	Calculation from Pao_2, PAo_2, and respiratory quotient on Fio_2 of 1.0; indication of lung's ability to oxygenate blood; index of extent of $\dot{V}/\dot{Q}$ mismatch, diffusion defect, or shunt	25-65 mm Hg	>450 mm Hg	<300-350 mm Hg
Pao_2	Provision of evidence of lung's ability to oxygenate arterial blood; Pao_2 of 60 mm Hg necessary to saturate Hb by 90% for adequate tissue oxygenation	80-110 mm Hg (altitude dependent)	<60 mm Hg with Fio_2 >0.6	>70-80 mm Hg with Fio_2 ≤0.5

*These parameters are only guidelines and must be related to the individual client's status (e.g., clients with severe COPD may have a normal $Paco_2$ of 60 mm Hg and values lower than normal for FEV_1, VC, MV, and maximal voluntary ventilation).

Mechanical ventilation is not indicated in cases in which disease reversibility is not possible (e.g., end-stage respiratory failure in clients with severe COPD). Clients with chronic pulmonary disease and their families who are managed by pulmonary health care specialists on a continuous, long-term basis frequently have the opportunity to decide the issue of mechanical ventilation long before terminal respiratory disease develops. Other clients with chronic disease never discuss the subject, and the decision to use mechanical ventilation should be made by the physician, client, and family at the onset of clinical deterioration in any illness. It is much easier for the physician, client, and family to decide not to institute ventilatory support initially than it is to remove the support system once it has been initiated. The decision to use mechanical ventilation must be made carefully.

Types of Mechanical Ventilators

Mechanical ventilators are divided into two major categories: negative-pressure and positive-pressure ventilators.

Negative-pressure ventilators. *Negative-pressure ventilators* are chambers that encase the chest or body and produce a subatmospheric, or negative, pressure around it. The negative pressure surrounding the chest wall causes the chest wall to be pulled outward. This reduces intrathoracic pressure and causes air to rush in through the upper airway, which is outside the sealed chamber. Expiration is passive because the machine cycles off and allows the chest to relax. This type of ventilation is similar to the normal mode of ventilation because inspiration is normally produced by decreasing the pleural and intrathoracic pressures and because expiration is normally passive.

The iron lung formerly used to treat poliomyelitis is an example of a negative-pressure ventilator. Another type of negative-pressure ventilator is the cuirass, which is a rigid shell fitted to the thorax and connected by a flexible hose to a pump that generates negative pressure. Disadvantages to this type of negative-pressure ventilator are that the rigid shell can cause skin irritation in those areas that come in contact with the shell and that it has to be individually fitted. Other negative-pressure ventilators include the Poncho ventilator (Puritan Bennett, Emerson) and the Pulmowrap (Lifecare). These ventilators are made of a flexible nylon cover that fits over the head and ties with drawstrings at the neck and fastens to the arms or wrists and upper legs with elastic (Fig. 23-11). The Poncho and Pulmowrap are more comfortable than the cuirass and less likely to cause skin breakdown caused by pressure areas. New developments in negative-pressure ventilation now enable not only controlled ventilation but an assist-control mode in which the client can initiate a breath and be assisted by the ventilator.

These lightweight, portable negative-pressure ventilators are used extensively in the home for clients with neuromuscular diseases, CNS disorders, diseases and fractures of the spinal cord, and severe COPD for nighttime ventilation. Negative-pressure ventilators are not indicated for use in acutely ill clients. With the use of these ventilators, observation of the client is limited and the negative intrapleural pressure must not be interrupted.

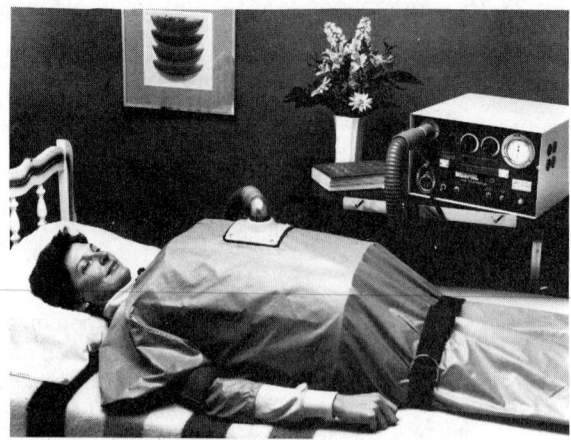

Fig. 23-11 Negative-pressure ventilator. (Courtesy LIFE-CARE Pulmo-Wrap.)

Positive-pressure ventilators. *Positive-pressure ventilation* is the primary method of mechanical ventilation used with acutely ill clients. The inspiratory cycle of ventilation is accomplished when the ventilator forces air into the lungs under positive pressure. Intrathoracic pressure is raised by the inflation of the lungs with positive pressure rather than lowered, as it is normally on inspiration. Expiration occurs by passive relaxation of the diaphragm, just as in normal expiration. Positive pressure can also be added to the lungs during expiration.

The three types of positive-pressure ventilators are (1) time-cycled or time-limited, (2) pressure-cycled or pressure-limited, and (3) volume-cycled or volume-limited. Each type is classified by the physical parameter that ends the inspiratory cycle.

Time-cycled or time-limited ventilators. Time-cycled or time-limited ventilators terminate inspiration and switch to expiration at a definite preset time. The VT is regulated by adjusting the length of inspiration and the flow rate of the pressurized gas. The VT and inspiratory pressure delivered to the client may vary somewhat from one breath to the next. Time-cycled ventilators such as the Baby Bird, Air Shields, and Veriflo CV 200 are used primarily for neonates and infants. The Emerson postoperative ventilator, Emerson IMV, Engstrom ER 500, Engstrom ECS 2000, and Veriflo CV 2000 are time-cycled ventilators used for adults. Time-cycled ventilators also have fail-safe pressure limits beyond which the ventilator ceases to push gas into the lungs to prevent overdistention of the lung and barotrauma.

Pressure-cycled or pressure-limited ventilators. Pressure-cycled or pressure-limited ventilators terminate the inspiratory phase or the VT delivered to the client when a preselected airway pressure is achieved. The volume of gas delivered to the client and the duration of delivery vary according to airway resistance, pulmonary compliance, and integrity of the ventilator circuit. For example, increased resistance (pressure) in the airway as a result of secretions or decreased chest compliance causes the pressure-limited ventilator to cease delivering gas before an

Table 23-16 Settings of Mechanical Ventilation

Tidal volume: V_T is amount of air exchanged with each ventilator-delivered breath. Usual volume is 10-15 ml/kg. For clients of average weight, amount of air is usually 500-1000 ml.

Respiratory rate: Respiratory rate is number of breaths per minute the ventilator delivers and depends on mode of ventilation.* Rate is usually set to keep pH and $Paco_2$ within normal range. Rate can be as low as 1 breath/min (e.g., on IMV) to 20-30 breaths/min.

Inspiratory/expiratory ratio: I/E is ratio of time involved in inspiration to time in expiration. During normal spontaneous breathing, expiration takes twice as long as inspiration. Usually 1 to 2 ratio is set unless inverse-ratio ventilation is in use.

Fraction of inspired O_2: Fio_2 varies depending on ABG results. It can range from 0.21 (ambient air) to 1.0 (100% O_2). Many ventilators have in-line O_2 analyzers with digital displays.

Sensitivity: Sensitivity is control that adjusts ventilatory response to client's respiratory effort. When sensitivity is off, machine controls breathing and does not respond to client effort. Can be adjusted to allow client to initiate ventilator (assist-control) breath or to breathe spontaneously (IMV mode).

Sighs: Sighs are periodic breaths that are larger than normal V_T (usually 1-2 times). They inflate more alveoli and prevent atelectasis. Ventilators can be set to deliver sighs at preset rate.

Spirometer: Spirometer measures expired V_T and is usually built into machine and has digital readout. V_T and/or minute volume can be read from spirometer. Alarm sounds when exhaled V_T is less than preset volume on spirometer. Alarm can be activated by spirometer malfunction (e.g., sticking of bellows, disconnection or leakage of tubing within ventilator, and disconnection of ventilator from client).

Pressure limit dial: Pressure limit dial is adjustable setting to regulate maximal pressure that ventilator can generate to deliver V_T. It is usually set about 10 cm H_2O pressure above pressure needed to deliver desired V_T. Pressure alarm can also be activated by coughing, secretion accumulation, decreased lung compliance, development of pneumothorax, resistance to machine, and occlusion of ET or tracheostomy tube.

System pressure gauge: Gauge has dial that fluctuates with pressure in client's airway during ventilatory cycle. When preset volume of gas is delivered, amount of positive pressure in airways at maximal inspiration is recorded. During exhalation, dial stylus returns to 0 unless PEEP is used. With 10 cm PEEP, stylus falls to 10 cm above 0 point, but as inspiration begins, stylus may fall 1 or 2 cm as client initiates own breath. Lung compliance is inversely related to peak inspiratory pressures.

*See Table 23-17.

adequate volume is reached. In addition, unless each breath delivered to the client is measured, there is no way to know the exact gas volume delivered.

Pressure-limited ventilators usually lack a system to deliver precisely controlled levels of O_2 and a means for administering PEEP. Pressure-cycled ventilators are not used as frequently as time-cycled or volume-cycled ventilators for acutely ill clients. They are used predominantly for IPPB treatments, home therapy, short-term ventilation, or in a client whose lungs are relatively free of resistance and compliance disease. Examples of pressure-cycled ventilators are the Bennett PR-1 and PR-2 and the Bird Mark 7. These may be used with a mask, mouthpiece, or artificial airway.

Volume-cycled or volume-limited ventilators. The most commonly used mechanical ventilators for intubated adults and older children are the volume-cycled or volume-limited ventilators. Volume-cycled ventilators terminate the inspiratory phase or flow of gas into the lung when a designated, preset volume of gas is delivered into the ventilator circuit (e.g., after the client has received the inspiratory gas). Volume-cycled ventilators also have built-in, pressure-limiting valves that prevent excessive pressure from building up in the lungs so that the preset volume is achieved. Once the pressure limit is reached, the remainder of the tidal volume is vented to the air.

The major advantages of volume-cycled ventilators are

that a readily measurable volume of gas is delivered to the client, volume delivery remains constant despite resistance and compliance changes in the lungs (unlike the situation with pressure-cycled ventilators), and a consistent inspired O_2 concentration can easily be maintained. The disadvantages are that these ventilators are often bulky and expensive. Examples of volume-cycled ventilators are the Bennett MA I, Bennett MA II, Bournes Bear I, Ohio 560, Monaghan 225, and Foregger 210. Also included are the following microprocessors: Bear 5 CRT, Puritan-Bennett 7200 A (Fig. 23-10) or 7200 SP, Bird 6400 ST, Siemens Servo 900, Land E, PPG IRISA, and Hamilton Amadpus (Infrasonics Adult Star Ventilator). Some ventilators, such as the Monoghan 225, can be adapted to function as pressure, time, or volume cycled.

Settings of Mechanical Ventilators

The various functions and settings of the mechanical ventilator are presented in Table 23-16. These settings are chosen by the physician after carefully evaluating the client's status (e.g., ABGs, body weight, level of consciousness) and after consulting with the respiratory therapist and nurse who are caring for the client. The mechanical ventilator must be as finely tuned as possible to the client's ventilatory pattern. Therefore the settings must be frequently evaluated and adjusted until the client achieves optimal ventilation.

It is especially important to ensure that all ventilator alarms are turned on at all times. Alarms can alert the nurse and respiratory therapist to potentially dangerous situations of mechanical malfunction or client asynchrony with the ventilator. On many ventilators the alarms can be temporarily bypassed or silenced for up to 2 minutes for suctioning. After that period of time, the alarm system automatically becomes functional again.

Modes of Volume-Cycled Ventilation

The volume-cycled ventilator may be set to operate in a number of modes (Fig. 23-12). *Mode* refers to the manner in which the ventilator delivers breaths to the client. The mode chosen usually depends on current institutional practice. Another factor influencing the choice of mode is the

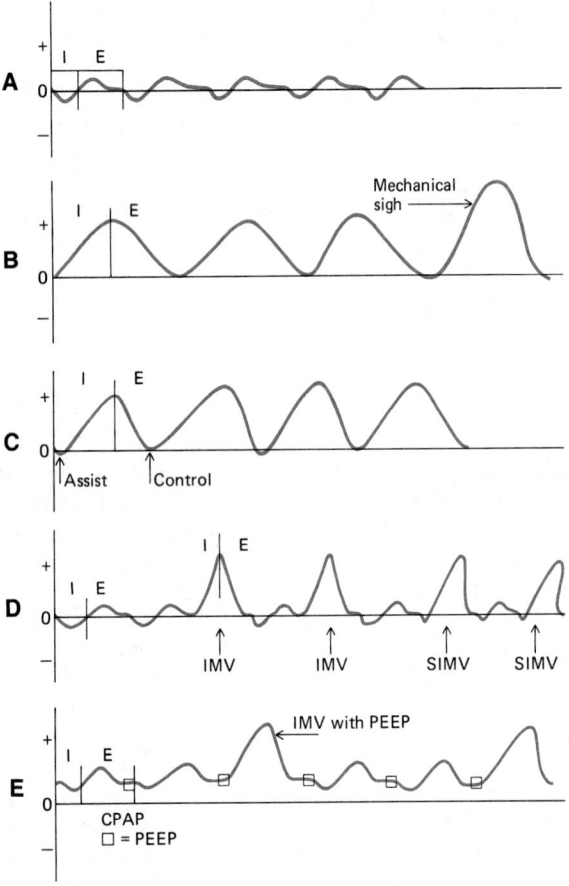

Fig. 23-12 Airway pressures with the use of different ventilatory modes. **A,** Normal spontaneous breathing. Inspirations occurring during negative intrapleural pressure. Exhalation occurring with slight positive intrapleural pressure and returning to 0 (atmospheric pressure). **B,** Controlled positive-pressure ventilation. Inspiration with positive-pressure exhalation back to atmospheric pressure. **C,** Assist-control positive-pressure ventilation. Inspiration initiated by client pulling negative; ventilator continues inspiration with positive pressure. Exhalation back to atmospheric pressure. **D,** IMV and SIMV breaths interspersed with spontaneous breaths. **E,** IMV with PEEP and CPAP breaths.

ventilatory status of the client, as evidenced by the respiratory drive and pattern and ABG analysis. The three basic modes of mechanical ventilation are (1) controlled ventilation, (2) assist-control ventilation, and (3) intermittent mandatory ventilation (IMV). These modes are compared in Table 23-17.

Controlled mechanical ventilation. Controlled mechanical ventilation (CMV) is usually used when the client has no drive to breathe or is unable to spontaneously breathe. Clients receiving controlled ventilation who do not have apnea usually require some type of sedation or paralyzing agent to facilitate optimal oxygenation and ventilation.

Neuromuscular blocking agents. Long-term neuromuscular blocking medications that can be used include pancuronium (Pavulon), vercuronium (Norcuron), and atracurium (Tracurium). They can be administered as continuous IV infusions or IV bolus. Before the initiation of neuromuscular blockade in the extremely agitated client, it is important to assess the client for other causes of agitation, including ET tube position, pain, hypoxemia, pulmonary embolism, drug reaction, and emotional distress. Before using a paralyzing agent, the client should be educated about this type of drug, including the effect of the client being unable to move and the reasons for this effect. The client should also be told that sedative and pain medications will be administered. Usually when clients are paralyzed, they are also given some form of sedation such as diazepam to help relieve the anxiety that might accompany this type of experience. Even though completely paralyzed, the client can be awake and able to hear, see, and think.

In clients with suppressed spontaneous ventilation, close monitoring is essential. The nurse is responsible for monitoring the effects of neuromuscular blockade on the client. The drugs can be titrated to client movement but are more accurately and safely monitored by the use of a peripheral nerve stimulator. An electrode is applied to the ulnar nerve near the wrist, and supramaximal stimuli are applied. Muscle contraction (twitching) in the fingers is an indicator of paralysis.

Intermittent mandatory ventilation. IMV is a primary mode of ventilatory support in most centers. It is used both to provide continuous ventilation and to wean the client from the ventilator. The potential benefits of IMV as a primary mode of ventilatory support include avoidance of respiratory alkalosis, prevention of the client "fighting" the ventilator, lower mean airway pressure, more uniform intrapulmonary gas distribution, and prevention of muscle atrophy.[21]

There are major differences between the cardiopulmonary effects of IMV and those of controlled or assisted ventilation. Spontaneous inspiration decreases intrathoracic pressure, reduces mean intrathoracic pressure, and enhances venous return. Cardiac output and venous return are more normal than with the other modes of mechanical ventilation. Because of the lower mean intrathoracic pressure, higher levels of PEEP may be used with IMV than with assisted or controlled ventilation.

Weaning clients from ventilators can be accomplished

by a more physiologically sound method. Instead of abruptly removing clients from ventilators and letting them breathe totally on their own, IMV may be used. IMV allows a smooth transition from controlled to spontaneous ventilation by gradually decreasing the IMV or ventilator rate as clients assume an increasing percentage of the total work of breathing.

The disadvantages of IMV are not as great as the advantages. One disadvantage occurs when the client receiving IMV at a very low rate (receiving one to four breaths/min) ceases active, spontaneous breathing. In this situation, ventilation is not adequately supported. IMV at low rates should be used only in clients who have regular, spontaneous breathing. Weaning with or without IMV demands close clinical assessment of the client. Weaning with IMV may take a longer time because each IMV breath is gradually removed. Another disadvantage of IMV is that during weaning from mechanical ventilation, clients are often left at low IMV rates rather than being rested, and they often become overly fatigued. This is a concern for the client, especially during the night.

There are two methods of delivering IMV breaths to the

Table 23-17 Modes of Mechanical Ventilation

Description	Advantages	Disadvantages	Uses
CONTROLLED MECHANICAL VENTILATION			
Machine delivers preset number of breaths/min at preset volume. Client cannot trigger breathing.	Work of breathing is totally controlled by ventilator.	Does not allow client to initiate breathing or respiratory rate to change with varying client needs. Airway pressure always positive during inspiration, compromising venous return. Provides limited use of respiratory muscles.	Apnea secondary to brain damage, respiratory muscle paralysis, drug overdose, sedation
ASSIST-CONTROL VENTILATION			
Delivery of a breath is triggered by inspiratory effort of client after preselected time interval has elapsed. If client fails to initiate breathing, ventilator cycles as in controlled ventilation.	Client can initiate own breathing, use respiratory muscles, and alter respiratory rate according to need. Intrathoracic pressure decreases transiently before inspiratory phase to allow for venous return and enhanced cardiac output.	Problems of overventilation and underventilation are possible and can occur in anxious clients or in those with low lung compliance.	Wide range of situations in which clients are spontaneously breathing but have ventilatory failure or gas exchange inefficiency
INTERMITTENT MANDATORY VENTILATION			
Client breathes spontaneously at own V_T and rate. At preset frequency, ventilator delivers a breath.	Ventilator breaths are not synchronized to client's respiratory pattern. Machine breath can be given during client's exhalation or peak inhalation.	Allows maintenance of even minor spontaneous excursions. Respiratory muscles remain in use. Ventilator augments client's own efforts.	Wide range of situations in which clients need ventilatory support, method of weaning
SYNCHRONIZED INTERMITTENT MANDATORY VENTILATION			
Ventilation method is modification of IMV. Ventilator is synchronized to client's ventilatory rate. Machine set to give certain number of breaths and is triggered by client's inspiration.	Ventilator does not compete with client's own breathing.	At low rate levels, client may not be adequately ventilated. Low volume and rate alarms need to be set when low levels are used.	Same as above

client: continuous-flow IMV and demand-flow IMV. The demand-flow IMV system (e.g., MA-2, Bear I, Servo 900C) requires that the client generate sufficient negative inspiratory pressure to open up or activate a demand valve for spontaneous breathing. In some cases the client must generate as much as 3 to 6 cm of negative pressure to breathe spontaneously. This can increase the work of breathing, O_2 consumption, and CO_2 production in some clients. With continuous-flow IMV (Emerson) the client does not need to activate a demand valve to breathe spontaneously because there is a continuous flow of O_2-enriched gas through the system. A modified continuous-flow system (flow-by) in the Puritan-Bennett 7200a also decreases the work of breathing in a manner similar to that of continuous flow. Because of the increased work of breathing associated with demand-flow IMV, some centers use continuous-flow IMV or T piece (Briggs' adapter) for weaning clients from the ventilator.

Other Ventilatory Maneuvers

Positive end-expiratory pressure. PEEP is a ventilatory maneuver in which positive (greater than atmospheric) pressure is applied to the client's airway at end exhalation. Normally, expiration is passive, and the airway pressure on the ventilator system pressure dial would drop to zero. With PEEP a preset level of pressure is selected so that the pressure falls to the level of positive pressure at end exhalation.

The lungs are partially inflated even during end exhalation. Therefore PEEP increases the functional residual capacity (FRC) (or the amount of gas in the lung after normal exhalation), and consequently improves oxygenation of the client. The mechanisms by which PEEP increases FRC and oxygenation include increased distention of already patent alveoli, prevention of alveolar collapse during end exhalation, and the recruitment of previously collapsed alveoli.[21] PEEP often allows the Fio_2 to be reduced to less than 0.50, which prevents the hazard of O_2 toxicity. As an example of how PEEP works, a client may need an Fio_2 of 0.7 to maintain a Pao_2 of 60 mm Hg. With a PEEP of 5 to 10 cm H_2O, the Fio_2 can be reduced to 0.5 while a Pao_2 of 60 mm Hg is maintained.

Because PEEP is a unit of pressure, it is measured in centimeters of water. PEEP is prescribed in increments of 2 to 5 cm H_2O. The amount of PEEP selected is determined by the amount that improves oxygenation without decreasing BP and cardiac output. This is called *best* or *optimal* PEEP. In some centers, PEEP is also regulated by monitoring changes in static and effective lung compliance curves as well as oxygenation and cardiac output. In critically ill clients receiving ventilation to prevent atelectasis, 5 cm H_2O of PEEP is sometimes used prophylactically. According to this concept, 5 cm H_2O of PEEP in the intubated client will replace the glottic mechanism and help maintain a normal FRC by preventing alveolar collapse. Clinical studies vary regarding the benefits of physiological PEEP.

PEEP of 5 cm H_2O is also used for clients who have a history of alveolar collapse during weaning. PEEP has demonstrated an improvement in gas exchange, vital capacity, and inspiratory force when used during weaning.

When PEEP is used during mechanical ventilation, the maximal inspiratory pressure increases in relation to the amount of PEEP added. For example, if a client is receiving a ventilator breath and the maximal inspiratory pressure recorded on the ventilator pressure gauge is 30 cm H_2O and the expiratory pressure is zero, the client's maximal inspiratory pressure will be 40 cm H_2O and the end-expiratory pressure will be 10 cm H_2O when 10 cm H_2O of PEEP is added. Thus the level of positive pressure achieved during mechanical ventilation with PEEP is often relatively high. When PEEP is applied during controlled or assist-control ventilation, the term *continuous positive-pressure ventilation* may be used. Ventilator terminology is confusing and usually varies from institution to institution. However, by understanding the basic concepts of the different modes and maneuvers of ventilatory assistance, it becomes easy to apply the terms used by the individual institution.

The use of IMV with PEEP is now the most common method to administer PEEP. The decreased mean airway pressure that occurs during spontaneous breathing is enough to prevent some of the adverse effects produced by the increased pressures.

In general, it is believed that the major purpose of PEEP is maintaining adequate tissue oxygenation and gas exchange while trying to prevent O_2 toxicity. Its secondary role in the prevention of atelectasis is also important. Some practitioners think that PEEP may assist in healing damaged lungs by maintaining airway stability and accelerating the production of surfactant. This belief is not yet supported in clinical studies.

PEEP is indicated in lungs that are characterized by diffuse disease, severe hypoxemia unresponsive to Fio_2 greater than 0.5, and loss of compliance or stiffness. The classic example of indications for PEEP therapy is in ARDS.

PEEP is generally contraindicated or must be used with extreme caution in clients with highly compliant lungs, unilateral or nonuniform disease, hypovolemia, and low cardiac output. In these situations the adverse effects of PEEP may outweigh any benefits obtained.

Continuous positive airway pressure. Continuous positive airway pressure (CPAP) is the use of PEEP in a client who is breathing spontaneously. With CPAP there is a constant flow of gas at a rate that is greater than the client's spontaneous inspiratory flow rate. Therefore the client's airway pressure never falls to zero, and there is always some degree of positive pressure (perhaps 1 to 2 cm during inspiration) on the airway at all times. For example, if CPAP of 5 cm H_2O is applied to the client's airway at end exhalation, when the client inspires, 1 to 2 cm H_2O is pulled down from the 5 cm CPAP to inhale. At exhalation the airway pressure is 5 cm H_2O. The client who is receiving IMV with PEEP receives CPAP when breathing spontaneously. In the past the client receiving CPAP was usually an infant, but currently CPAP is being used more in adults, especially for the treatment of obstructive sleep apnea syndrome. CPAP can be administered by a tight-fitting mask or an ET or tracheal tube. The latter two methods are preferred. One problem associated with CPAP in adults is that unless the person can cooperate (and not fight and attempt to exhale the air down to atmospheric pressure), the work of breathing may be increased.

Pressure support ventilation. Pressure support ventilation (PSV) is similar to CPAP with the exception that the positive pressure occurs only during inspiration. Like CPAP, PSV is used in conjunction with the client's spontaneous respirations. A preset level of positive airway pressure is selected so that the flow of gas is at a rate greater than the client's spontaneous inspiratory flow rate. As the client initiates a breath, the machine senses this spontaneous effort and supplies a rapid flow of gas, supporting the client's inspiratory efforts. The preset level of pressure is supplied throughout the inspiratory cycle until the flow of gas decreases to a minimum level specific to each ventilator. With positive-pressure ventilation, the length of inspiration, inspiratory flow, and respiratory rate are determined by the client. The achieved V_T depends on the level of pressure support and the compliance of the airway and chest wall. PSV can be used as a mode of mechanical ventilation or a method for weaning the client from the ventilator. The use of PSV as a sole ventilatory support during acute respiratory failure in clients with unstable respiratory drive, bronchospasm, secretions, pain, or anxiety is ill advised unless backed up by volume-cycled breaths at a frequency sufficient to provide for the client's total minute-ventilation needs.[21] IMV can also be used with PSV as a means of providing a backup rate in clients whose ventilatory efforts are uncertain. Suggested advantages to pressure support are that it increases client comfort, decreases the work of breathing because the client's inspiratory efforts are augmented, decreases O_2 consumption because the client does not have to work as hard to inspire, and increases endurance conditioning because the client is exercising the muscles when breathing spontaneously.[22] Pressure support is delivered in increments of 2 up to 20 to 30 cm H_2O to ensure an adequate total volume. It is important to monitor the client during PSV breaths to ensure that tidal and minute volumes are adequate.

Inverse-ratio ventilation. Inverse-ratio ventilation (IRV) is a ventilatory strategy in which inspiration is prolonged and expiration shortened so that the I/E ratio exceeds 1 (e.g., 2:1, 3:1). With IRV a prolonged positive pressure is applied during inspiration to progressively expand collapsed alveoli. The short expiratory time causes *intrinsic* or *auto-PEEP,* which prevents alveoli from recollapsing and promotes stabilization. An IRV peak airway pressure is lower than with controlled or assist-control positive-pressure ventilation with PEEP. However, mean airway pressure is higher. Because IRV imposes a nonphysiological breathing pattern, the client requires sedation and/or paralysis. IRV is indicated for clients with ARDS who continue to have refractory hypoxemia despite a PEEP of 15 cm H_2O or more. Not all clients with poor oxygenation respond to IRV.

Nocturnal nasal positive-pressure ventilation. In clients who require mechanical ventilation but in whom intubation is undesirable, nocturnal nasal positive-pressure ventilation (NNPPV) with a nasal mask, or in some instances an oral mouthpiece, and volume ventilator can be used to provide mechanical ventilation. Similar to home negative-pressure ventilators, NNPPV is noninvasive and can provide mechanical ventilation at night in clients with increasing respiratory failure, chronic hypoventilation, increasing fatigue, or significant O_2 desaturation at night. NNPPV can also be used in clients who have decreased pulmonary muscle strength as a result of CNS or neuromuscular diseases (e.g., poliomyelitis, muscular dystrophy) and those with chest wall deformities (e.g., kyphoscoliosis). However, unlike negative-pressure ventilators, NNPPV prevents airway collapse because of the positive nasal pressure and provides greater mobility and comfort and better synchronization. By preventing nocturnal desaturation, NNPPV can also improve daytime ABG values. This type of mechanical ventilation uses a soft nasal mask that fits well and has soft padding around the outside. The mask can usually be applied by the client and is secured with Velcro straps. Because drying of nasal passages can sometimes be a problem with NNPPV, humidification or nasal decongestant nasal drops may be used.[22]

High-frequency ventilation. High-frequency ventilation (HFV) is another method of mechanical ventilation used in some institutions for the care of high-risk and severely ill clients. HFV seems to minimize many of the complications attributed to conventional mechanical ventilation because of its lower mean airway pressures. HFV refers to a group of ventilatory techniques that have small V_Ts (usually 1 to 5 ml/kg of body weight) and rapid respiratory rates (100 to 300 breaths/min). The three types of HFV are high-frequency positive-pressure ventilation, high-frequency jet ventilation (HFJV), and high-frequency oscillation. Currently, HFJV is used mainly in clients with bronchopleural fistulas because lower peak airway pressures are required to prevent worsening of this condition. Some clients with ARDS with acute respiratory failure and bronchopleural fistulas may also benefit from HFJV, although results of trials do not indicate many advantages or improvement in mortality rates over conventional forms of mechanical ventilation.[23]

Adverse Effects of Mechanical Ventilation

Although mechanical ventilation may improve the client's alveolar ventilation and oxygenation, it can also cause adverse effects. Sometimes it is difficult to sort out complications of mechanical ventilation from the underlying disease. The nursing measures related to these problems are presented in Table 23-18.

Cardiovascular system. Circulatory problems can result from positive-pressure mechanical ventilation caused by transmission of the increased mean airway pressure, thus increasing intrathoracic pressure and causing compression of thoracic vessels during inspiration. This results in a decreased venous return to the heart, decreased left ventricular end-diastolic volume (preload), decreased cardiac output, and lowered blood pressure. Mean airway pressure may be further increased with higher increments of PEEP. Maintenance of an I/E ratio of 1:1.5 or 1:2 allows a longer period of time in the low-pressure exhalation cycle. Other methods to decrease mean airway pressures include avoiding large V_Ts and minimizing the level of PEEP. These measures enhance venous return.

If the lungs are stiff and noncompliant (as in ARDS), airway pressures will not be easily transmitted to the heart

Table 23-18

NURSING CARE PLAN FOR THE CLIENT ON MECHANICAL VENTILATION

Defining Characteristics	Nursing Interventions	Evaluation Criteria

NURSING DIAGNOSIS: High risk for injury related to possible machine malfunction, accidental disconnection, inability to breathe unassisted, asynchrony with ventilator, and settings unsuitable to maintain adequate ventilation

Hypoxemia and/or hypercapnia, tachycardia, tachypnea, increase in BP, agitation, confusion, headache, lethargy, cyanosis; respiratory pattern asynchronous with machine's pattern of ventilation; machine malfunction or disconnection	Begin mechanical ventilation slowly (especially in clients with COPD). Lower $Paco_2$ only to client's baseline level. Monitor ABGs, $P\overline{v}o_2$, and $D(A - a)o_2$. ABGs should be drawn approximately 20 min after each ventilator change, serially thereafter, and whenever there are changes in client's clinical status. Assess client for other possible causes of hyperventilation (e.g., retained secretions, hypoxemia, pain, fear, and anxiety). Check ventilator settings (Fio_2, respiratory rate, V_T, O_2 flow rate, PEEP, airway pressure, thermistor temperature, and I/E ratio) and evaluate if appropriate to clinical situation. Keep bag ventilator connected to O_2 source at bedside. Clients fighting ventilator may be slowly bag ventilated for 3 to 6 breaths to help synchronize them with ventilator. Determine cause of asynchrony. Try verbally coaching client to breathe with ventilator. Sedation (with morphine, diazepam, or haloperidol) may be necessary if pain or anxiety is identified as the cause. Observe client for complications of alkalemia (e.g., hypokalemia, cardiac dysrhythmias, poor tissue oxygenation, neuromuscular irritability, seizures, coma). Client receiving PEEP should not be pulling subatmospheric or negative airway pressures on inspiration. Turn all alarms on. If audible alarms are turned off during suctioning, turn them on immediately after. Respond immediately to alarm. One person should bag ventilate client while another person checks ventilator tubing for disconnections, leaks, and sticky bellows. When connecting ventilator circuit to artificial airway (especially tracheostomy), twist connection rather than pushing it together. Check cuff for leaks. Monitor weaning of client carefully. Monitor ventilator tubing q 1-2 hr for condensed water and drain when water present.	ABGs within normal range for client; maintenance of pH at 7.35-7.45; early detection of signs and symptoms of decreased Pao_2 and increased $Paco_2$; synchronous breathing with ventilator; early detection, correction, or prevention of complications associated with mechanical malfunction or disconnection

NURSING DIAGNOSIS: Altered tissue perfusion related to decreased cardiac output secondary to positive-pressure ventilation

Decrease in BP, cardiac output, $P\overline{v}o_2$, urine output, tissue O_2 delivery; increase in pulse, pulmonary capillary wedge pressure, central venous pressure; presence of dysrhythmias, mental confusion	Monitor vital signs q 2-4 hr. Observe for clinical manifestations of decreased cardiac output (e.g., restlessness, decreasing levels of consciousness, low urine output, weak peripheral pulses, narrowed pulse pressure, slow capillary refill, pallor, fatigue, and chest pain). Monitor direct measurement of cardiac output by thermodilution, $P\overline{v}o_2$, or $(A - V)o_2$ difference, especially when >10 cm H_2O PEEP is used. Administer plasma expanders, vasopressors as ordered.	BP within client's normal range, no evidence of decreased tissue perfusion, adequate urinary output

Sections of this nursing care plan were modified from Kersten LD: Comprehensive respiratory nursing, Philadelphia, 1989, WB Saunders Co, pp 720-726.
PCWP, Pulmonary capillary wedge pressure; *PAS,* pulmonary artery pressure—systolic, *PAD,* pulmonary artery pressure—diastolic.
*See Table 23-14.

Table 23-18

 NURSING CARE PLAN FOR THE CLIENT ON MECHANICAL VENTILATION—cont'd

Defining Characteristics	Nursing Interventions	Evaluation Criteria

NURSING DIAGNOSIS: **Fluid volume excess related to excess fluid intake from IV therapy, blockage of insensible water loss by respiration, and decreased renal perfusion secondary to positive-pressure ventilation**

Increase in body weight or failure to lose weight with starvation; fluid intake greater than output; low hematocrit and serum sodium from hemodilution; presence of peripheral edema, jugular venous distention, rales, decreased breath sounds	Maintain strict intake and output. Consider blockage of insensible water loss through respiration and closed humidification system of mechanical ventilator for accurate intake and output. Weigh client daily. Observe client for clinical manifestations of fluid overload (e.g., weight gain or failure to lose weight if only nutrition is maintenance IV solutions), hemodilution (low hematocrit, low serum sodium), edema, and rales. Take readings of PCWP, PAS, PAD at end exhalation, preferably by strip chart recorder or from waveform.	No signs of peripheral or pulmonary edema, balanced intake and output, no evidence of hemodilution, weight gain appropriate for nutritional intake

NURSING DIAGNOSIS: **Ineffective airway clearance related to presence of artificial airway, problems with positioning, accumulation of secretions, and immobility**

Presence of abnormal breath sounds, frequent or absent cough, presence of thick or copious secretions with suctioning, high peak airway pressures or frequent high-pressure alarm sounds on ventilator	Use large V$_{TS}$ (12-15 ml/kg). Change client's position q 2 hr. Have client cough and, if feasible, deep breathe q 2 hr. Auscultate breath sounds q 2-4 hr.*	Absence of abnormal breath sounds, secretions thin and easily removed

NURSING DIAGNOSIS: **High risk for respiratory infection related to exposure to environmental pathogens, presence of artificial airway, decreased resistance secondary to debilitated state, prolonged immobility, and inadequate nutrition***

NURSING DIAGNOSIS: **Potential complication: gastric distention related to improper tube placement, GI bleeding, or ileus**

Presence of abdominal distention, large gastric air bubble on chest x-ray film or on percussion over stomach, decrease in spontaneous V$_T$ and increase in respiratory rate, tender abdomen on palpation, complaints of stomach uneasiness, sudden decrease in amount of gastric drainage, guaiac-positive stools or nasogastric aspirate, dark red or bloody stools or nasogastric aspirate decrease in hematocrit	Take daily measurements of abdominal girth at umbilicus. Assess for abdominal distention, tympany, and bowel sounds. Test stools and gastric drainage for occult blood. Monitor hematocrit. Assess client's complaints of pain, fullness, bloated feeling, or need for laxative. Maintain adequate bowel evacuation program. Check for gastric air on chest x-ray film. Administer antacids, cimetidine, or ranitidine and tube feedings as ordered. If abdominal distention present, elevate head of bed to allow for optimal diaphragmatic excursion. Confirm correct position of nasogastric tube.	Maintenance of GI integrity, normal bowel sounds, no evidence of GI bleeding, no abdominal distention

Continued.

Table 23-18

 NURSING CARE PLAN FOR THE CLIENT ON MECHANICAL VENTILATION—cont'd

Defining Characteristics	Nursing Interventions	Evaluation Criteria

NURSING DIAGNOSIS: Altered nutrition: less than body requirements related to inability to take in nourishment orally and increased caloric demands secondary to clinical condition and need for mechanical ventilation†

NURSING DIAGNOSIS: Impaired physical mobility related to restricted movement secondary to prolonged mechanical ventilation and clinical condition

Defining Characteristics	Nursing Interventions	Evaluation Criteria
Inability to perform active range-of-motion exercises, presence of signs of pressure areas	Provide progressive ambulation for clients receiving long-term ventilation. Periodically walk client while pushing ventilator or bag ventilate with O_2. Perform active and passive range-of-motion exercises (e.g., leg lifts, knee bends, quadriceps setting, arm circles). Prevent contractures and external rotation of hips by proper positioning. Observe for pressure areas. Prevent decubitus ulcers by frequent turning, massaging pressure points, maintaining good nutrition, and using special mattress. Prevent foot drop with use of footboard, high-top sneakers, having client flex foot several times. As soon as medically stable, client should sit in chair. Use pneumatic anti-embolism stockings and prophylactic heparin as ordered.	Normal range of motion of joints, no evidence of pressure sores or thromboemboli, ability to get out of bed for short periods of time

NURSING DIAGNOSIS: Anxiety related to clinical condition, possible machine malfunction or disconnection, inability to communicate, environmental factors, possibility of death, and fear of suffocation and choking related to oral airway

Defining Characteristics	Nursing Interventions	Evaluation Criteria
Expression of feelings of anxiety, anxious appearance	Assess client's behavior for clues of handling stressful situation. Be available to family and offer support and help. Assure client of continuous monitoring by well-trained staff. Give simple, honest explanations regarding care and progress. Offer positive reinforcement for client behaviors that demonstrate improvement. Allow client to make decisions regarding care (e.g., which side to turn on, when to bathe, when to eat). Provide periods of privacy for client and significant others. Converse with client and family members about client and family interests. Provide for diversion and occupational therapy as needed and tolerated. Schedule care to allow frequent rest periods. Encourage family to bring client's personal items to bedside. Provide calendar and clock. Refer to psychiatric liaison clinical nurse specialist, psychiatrist, or hospital chaplain when appropriate.	Communication by client and family of feelings and anxieties, absent or manageable anxiety level

Sections of this nursing care plan were modified from Kersten LD: Comprehensive respiratory nursing, Philadelphia, 1989, WB Saunders Co, pp 720-726.
†See Tables 23-5 and 23-14.
‡This assessment is especially important in clients receiving PEEP because they are at more risk of barotrauma.

Table 23-18

NURSING CARE PLAN FOR THE CLIENT ON MECHANICAL VENTILATION—cont'd

Defining Characteristics	Nursing Interventions	Evaluation Criteria

NURSING DIAGNOSIS: Sleep pattern disturbance related to anxiety, depression, hypoxemia and/or hypercapnia, environmental factors, and possibility of death

Insomnia, restlessness, irritability, disorientation, morning headaches; psychotic behavior; awake frequently	Perform bedtime preparations (e.g., wash client's face and hands, rub back, provide oral care). Turn off lights at night. Provide pharmacological intervention as ordered. Move client to room with window (if available) to help with orientation to day and night. Orient client to person, place, and time. Provide relaxation techniques and tapes to promote relaxation. Schedule activities so that client gets at least 2 hr uninterrupted time to sleep.	Indication of feeling rested on awakening, no evidence of sleep disturbance, need to awaken for treatments minimal

NURSING DIAGNOSIS: Potential complication: pneumothorax or pneumomediastinum secondary to barotrauma caused by positive-pressure ventilation

Sudden increase in peak inspiratory pressure (>5 cm H_2O more than client's usual), sudden client agitation or coughing with frequent activation of high-pressure alarm, decrease in static and effective compliance, palpable subcutaneous emphysema over neck and anterior chest areas, deterioration in ABGs and BP, decrease or absence of breath sounds hyperresonance on percussion; pneumomediastinum, pneumothorax on chest x-ray film	Observe for manifestations of pneumothorax (see text). If pneumothorax is suspected, obtain chest x-ray film. Observe for symptoms of tension pneumothorax (see text). Bag ventilate with O_2 source or use lower V_T. Notify physician and set up for chest tube insertion immediately. Check ventilator settings every shift. Record level of peak inspiratory pressure to establish baseline data to evaluate changes in lung compliance.‡	Normal breath sounds on auscultation on both lungs, peak airway pressure of <30 cm H_2O, no subcutaneous emphysema

and blood vessels. Therefore the effects of mechanical ventilation on cardiac output are reduced. However, the danger of transmission of high airway pressures with very compliant lungs (e.g., in emphysema) is increased, and cardiac output may decrease.

The hemodynamic complications of decreased venous return that are induced by positive-pressure ventilation are exaggerated by hypovolemia (e.g., hemorrhage, multiple trauma) and decreased venous tone (e.g., sepsis, hypoglycemia, spinal shock). IMV reduces the cardiovascular effects of mechanical ventilation.

Some studies have found an improvement in cardiac performance after the institution of mechanical ventilation in clients with poor left ventricular function.[24] It is postulated that positive-pressure ventilation decreases right-sided heart preload by its increase in intrathoracic pressure. Also, the increased airway pressure may restrict left ventricular filling by mechanical compression of the alveo-

lar capillaries. The last two effects may improve the failing left ventricle by optimizing ventricular end-diastolic volume. Further research is needed on the effects of mechanical positive-pressure ventilation on the failing left ventricle.

Weaning hemodynamically unstable clients with heart failure or noncardiogenic pulmonary edema from positive-pressure ventilation can lead to further hemodynamic deterioration. Cardiac output must be monitored carefully. Direct measurement by pulmonary artery thermodilution, measurement of Pao_2, or calculation of the $(A - V)o_2$ difference is extremely important in clients receiving 10 cm H_2O or more of PEEP. If cardiac output falls, vasopressors, plasma expanders, and increased IV fluids may be required. Also, clients with hypovolemia or who have decreased cardiac output may be volume loaded before the institution of increased levels of PEEP. This decreases the problems associated with a drop in cardiac output. As positive airway pressure is removed and venous return is increased, the client must be observed for symptoms of cardiac overload and pulmonary edema.

Renal system. After 48 to 72 hours of mechanical ventilation, progressive fluid retention often occurs. This fluid retention can lead to pulmonary edema without evidence of cardiac failure, particularly when the level of mean airway pressure on the ventilator is increased (e.g., in PEEP therapy). Positive-pressure ventilation, especially with PEEP, causes a decreased urinary output and sodium retention. These findings are primarily caused by a decreased cardiac output, which leads to decreased renal blood and subsequent decreased urinary excretion of sodium. The decreased renal blood flow stimulates renin release (see Fig. 39-6), which results in increased aldosterone secretion and subsequent sodium and water retention. Fluid retention may also be related to an increased secretion of aldosterone.[25]

Another mechanism contributing to fluid retention is the prevention of the normal insensible loss of water (300 to 500 ml/day) from the client's respiratory system by the closed humidification system on the ventilator. In addition, the inspired air is saturated with humidity before the client inhales it. A net water gain of 300 to 500 ml/day or more may occur. Fluid restriction and diuretic therapy may be needed to promote water loss.

Pulmonary system

Barotrauma. As higher inflation pressures are required to inflate the lungs, the risk of pneumothorax, pneumomediastinum, and subcutaneous emphysema increases. Clients with highly compliant or floppy lungs (e.g., in emphysema) are at greater risk because the increased airway pressure readily distends the lungs and may rupture alveoli or emphysematous blebs. Clients with stiff lungs, such as those with ARDS, who require high inspiratory pressures and high levels of PEEP and clients with suppurative lung abscesses resulting from necrotizing organisms such as staphylococci or gram-negative bacteria are also susceptible to barotrauma.

Air can escape from the alveoli or interstitium into the pleural space, accumulate, and become trapped. This buildup of air increases pleural pressure and collapses the lung under it. This condition is called *pneumothorax* (see Fig. 21-11). "Ball-valving" is a common cause of pneumothorax. This phenomenon occurs in an area of the lung that can accept air during inspiration but cannot expel it during expiration. Because respiratory bronchioles are larger on inspiration than on expiration, they may close on expiration, thus contributing to the buildup of gas in the lung.[25] Because positive-pressure breathing can rapidly convert a simple pneumothorax into a life-threatening tension pneumothorax, a chest tube must be rapidly inserted. In tension pneumothorax the mediastinum and contralateral lung are compressed, with development of extremely compromised cardiac output.

Fortunately, this is a rare occurrence. If a tension pneumothorax develops, the client should be removed from the ventilator and ventilated with a bag ventilator connected to an O_2 source, or the V_T on the ventilator can be decreased to reduce airway pressures until a chest tube can be inserted.

Clinical manifestations that may indicate the development or presence of a pneumothorax include tachypnea, asymmetrical chest expansion, decreased or absent breath sounds and/or hyperresonance to percussion on the affected side, subcutaneous emphysema with crepitus (crackly edema), particularly in the neck area, sharply increased peak inspiratory pressures on the system pressure gauge, and absence of lung markings at affected sites demonstrated on chest x-ray film. The client may not get enough air or may have chest pain on the affected side.

Clinical manifestations of tension pneumothorax are more severe and may include all the signs of pneumothorax in addition to tracheal deviation to the unaffected side, neck vein distention, thready pulse, hypotension, mediastinal and tracheal shift, and compression of the contralateral lung visualized on chest x-ray film.

Pneumomediastinum usually begins with the rupture of alveoli into the interstitium of the lung, followed by progressive movement of air into the mediastinum and the subcutaneous tissues of the neck. This is commonly followed by the development of a pneumothorax. The presence of new, unexplained subcutaneous air should indicate the need for immediate chest x-ray film. Frequently pneumomediastinum and subcutaneous emphysema in the neck are too small to be detected radiographically or clinically before the development of a pneumothorax.

Subcutaneous emphysema may occur after a tracheotomy as a result of leakage of air from the surgical site, or it may occur around the site and area of the chest where a chest tube has been placed for a pneumothorax. In the latter case, subcutaneous emphysema is usually caused by the passage of gas from the pleural space into the tube wound, indicating that the space is not being adequately drained. The patency of the chest tube must be determined frequently to prevent a further increase in the pneumothorax.

Alveolar hypoventilation. The pressurized gas of the mechanical ventilator tends to flow to the areas of least resistance and high compliance. Therefore some of the alveoli that are collapsed may not be ventilated, producing hypoventilated lung areas and atelectasis. The use of large V_T, small increments of PEEP, and/or sighing of the client lessens the likelihood of the development of atelectasis. Frequent position changes and suctioning also help. The major clinical indicators of atelectasis are decreased breath sounds over the area and a drop in the Pa_{O_2}. Increased secretions in the lungs can also cause hypoventilation. This can be prevented by turning the client every 1 to 2 hours, providing chest physiotherapy in areas of the lung with increased secretions, encouraging deep breathing and coughing, and performing suctioning as needed.

A V_T or respiratory rate set too low on the ventilator can decrease minute ventilation and lead to hypoventilation. A cuff that leaks or tubings that are not securely attached may cause leakage of air and may lower the delivered V_T. Too low an IMV rate in a client who is unable to produce adequate spontaneous ventilation can also lead to hypoventilation.

Alveolar hyperventilation. Respiratory alkalosis may occur in clients with chronic respiratory acidosis (chronic alveolar hypoventilation and CO_2 retention, such as found in clients with COPD) in whom compensatory renal retention of bicarbonate has restored the pH toward normal. The mechanical ventilator removes CO_2, whereas the serum bicarbonate level stays elevated. (Normally, the kidneys require 2 to 3 days to alter the bicarbonate level.) Therefore the ventilator can move the client from a state of compensated acidosis to one of severe alkalosis.

Alkalemia, especially if induced abruptly, can have serious consequences. As the bicarbonate level increases in the blood, H^+ and K^+ decrease. The resulting hypokalemia predisposes the client with oxygenation or cardiac problems to dysrhythmias. Alkalemia also shifts the oxygen-hemoglobin dissociation curve to the left, making O_2 release to the tissues more difficult (see Fig. 19-6). Neuromuscular irritability, seizures, coma, and death can also occur.

Mechanical ventilation should begin slowly and remain at a level that will not dramatically lower the arterial $Paco_2$ to prevent the occurrence of alkalosis in the client with compensated respiratory acidosis. The client's ABGs must be assessed 15 to 30 minutes after mechanical ventilation begins and after each ventilator change, serially thereafter, and whenever changes in the client's clinical status occur. The $Paco_2$ should be gradually lowered only to the client's baseline (before acute illness) level. Usually clients with COPD on the ventilator do better with a short inspiratory and longer expiratory time because of the nature of their obstructive disease.

Respiratory alkalosis can also occur if the rate or V_T is set too high (mechanical overventilation) or if the client receiving assisted ventilation with IMV is hyperventilating. Hyperventilation means that the $Paco_2$ is less than 35 mm Hg because the client or the ventilator is blowing off CO_2 too rapidly. Decreasing the respiratory rate or V_T can help correct the respiratory alkalosis. However, if the current rate and volume are necessary to provide adequate ventilation and prevent atelectasis, mechanical dead space may be added.

It is important to determine the cause of the hyperventilation or decreased $Paco_2$. Hyperventilation can be caused by retained secretions, hypoxemia, pain, fear, and anxiety, or it can be a compensatory mechanism for metabolic acidosis. The ABG levels need to be analyzed to determine whether the respiratory alkalosis or hyperventilation is compensating for a primary problem of metabolic acidosis (e.g., diabetic acidosis). In the client with diabetic acidosis as an underlying problem, the diabetes must be controlled (see Chapter 43). Sedation and the addition of dead space as treatments for this problem can block the one compensatory mechanism available to the client.

Clients who fight the ventilator or breathe out of synchrony with it may be very anxious and/or in pain. Secretion accumulation and movement or kinking of the ET tube in the airway may also cause this problem. If the client is anxious and fearful, sitting and providing body contact by touching the client's hand or arm and verbally coaching the client to breathe with the ventilator will help. If these measures fail, manually bagging the client slowly with the bag ventilator connected to an O_2 source may help to slow the breathing enough to bring it in synchrony with the ventilator. The client may require morphine, diaz-epam, or other prescribed sedatives if pain or extreme anxiety occurs. However, sedation must be administered with extreme caution in clients on IMV at low rates because the respiratory drive may be significantly depressed.

Intrinsic or auto-PEEP. Intrinsic or auto-PEEP, which occurs as a result of inadvertent air trapping, is a consequence of high minute ventilation. It can be seen in clients with ARDS and obstructive diseases such as COPD. Auto-PEEP causes the same hemodynamic effects as regular or extrinsic PEEP.

Pulmonary infection. Pulmonary infection is a common complication of mechanical ventilation. Because the normal defenses of the upper airway have been bypassed by the ET or tracheostomy tube, the client is at increased risk of infection. In addition, a poor nutritional state, immobility, and the underlying disease process (e.g., immunosuppression, organ failure) make the client more prone to infections.

In clients receiving prolonged mechanical ventilation, sputum cultures invariably grow organisms that are usually gram-negative.[26] Gram-negative bacteria such as *Pseudomonas, Serratia,* and *Klebsiella* are abundant in both the hospital environment and the client's digestive tract. Organisms can be spread in a number of ways, including contaminated respiratory equipment, inadequate hand washing, prolonged close contact with clients, adverse environmental factors such as poor room ventilation and high traffic flow, and decreased client ability to cough and clear secretions.[26] Colonization of the upper respiratory tract by aspiration of gram-negative organisms is a predisposing factor in the development of gram-negative pneumonia. (Gram-negative pneumonia is discussed in Chapter 21.)

The risk of infection can be minimized by using strict aseptic technique while suctioning or handling the artificial airway. Frequent hand washing is imperative. The humidifier and tubing on the ventilator provide a warm, moist environment conducive to the growth of organisms. Ventilator tubing is changed at least every 24 to 48 hours. When water has condensed in the tubing, it should be drained out of the system, especially before turning or repositioning the client. This measure will prevent the client from aspirating the water. Corrugated ventilator tubings must be pulled gently to remove water that has condensed in the folds. Chest physiotherapy, adequate humidification of inspired gases, and sterile suctioning may help to prevent infection by eliminating secretion accumulation. The manual ventilator bag (e.g., Ambu bag) and O_2 tubing kept at the client's bedside also need to be replaced and cleaned periodically (at least every 24 to 48 hours).

Clinical evidence suggesting pulmonary infection includes fever, an elevated WBC count, increasing purulence of sputum, sputum odor, auscultation that reveals rales or rhonchi, and evidence of pulmonary infiltrates on chest x-ray film. The client is treated with antibiotics only after appropriate cultures are taken by tracheal suctioning or bronchoscopy and when infection is evident. Antibiotics should not be used prophylactically.

Neurological system. In clients with head injury, positive-pressure ventilation, especially with PEEP, can impair cerebral blood flow. The basis for this is related to increased intrathoracic positive pressure impeding venous drainage from the head, as evidenced by jugular venous distention and decreased cardiac output.

Gastrointestinal system. The process of mechanical ventilation is stressful and increases the client's risk of developing stress ulcers and GI bleeding. Clients who have a preexisting ulcer or who are receiving corticosteroid therapy are at an especially increased risk. Gastroscopy evidence demonstrates that gastric mucosal changes occur in many critically ill clients. It is also believed that PEEP may contribute to ischemia of the gastric mucosa by increasing resistance in splanchnic blood vessels.

Prophylactic administration of antacids to maintain a gastric pH of more than 5 has dramatically reduced the occurrence of GI bleeding. Early and frequent nasogastric feedings have also been successfully used to decrease gastric ulcers and bleeding. Prophylactic use of cimetidine (Tagamet) and ranitidine (Zantac), administered intravenously or orally, decreases the acidity of gastric secretions and prevents stress ulcer formation and hemorrhage. Cimetidine and ranitidine have been used alone or in combination with antacid therapy.

Gastric and bowel dilatation, although rare, may occur as a result of the accumulation of gas in the stomach. Gas may escape from around the cuff of the ET tube and may be swallowed or aspirated into the stomach. The irritation of an artificial airway may cause excessive air swallowing and subsequent gastric dilatation. Gastric or bowel dilatation may put pressure on the vena cava, decrease cardiac output, and prohibit adequate diaphragmatic excursion during spontaneous breathing. Elevation of the diaphragm as a result of ileus or bowel dilatation leads to compression of the lower lungs, which may cause atelectasis and compromise respiratory function. Large amounts of ascites may have a similar effect. Decompression of the stomach can be accomplished by the insertion of a nasogastric tube. Some physicians routinely insert nasogastric tubes prophylactically when mechanical ventilation is initiated. It is especially important to insert a nasogastric tube to prevent aspiration if the client is in danger of vomiting.

Immobility, sedation, and stress contribute to decreased peristalsis. The inability to exhale against a closed glottis may make defecation difficult. Therefore the client is predisposed to the development of paralytic ileus and constipation.

Nutritional considerations. Mechanical ventilation, immobility, and the physical and emotional stresses associated with critical illness contribute to the poor nutritional status of the client. The presence of an ET tube eliminates the normal route for eating. Clients with a nasotracheal tube are allowed liquid and semiliquid feedings orally if test feedings indicate lack of aspiration. It is difficult for the client to swallow and to ingest sufficient calories, protein, and fat. A client with a tracheostomy can eat normally once the wound has healed. When the client is eating with a tracheostomy tube, the cuff is usually inflated and the client should tilt the head slightly forward to facilitate swallowing and to prevent aspiration. Often, soft foods (e.g., puddings, ice cream) are more easily swallowed than liquids.

Clients who have been without food for 3 to 5 days and who are unlikely to eat within a week should have some type of nutritional program initiated. Inadequate nutrition makes the client receiving prolonged mechanical ventilation more prone to poor O_2 transport secondary to anemia and to poor tolerance of minimal exercise. Disuse of respiratory muscles and poor nutrition result in decreased respiratory muscle strength. In addition, caloric expenditure is elevated in the presence of fever, anxiety, pain, and the increased work of breathing. Serum albumin and transferrin levels are usually decreased. Inadequate nutrition can delay weaning, decrease the speed of recovery from illness, and decrease resistance to infection.

Total parenteral nutrition supplemented with IV fat emulsion (Intralipid) fulfills the nutritional requirements for many clients. Nasogastric or gastric feedings of high-protein liquids (e.g., Ensure, Pulmocare, Ensure Plus, Isocal, Vivonex, Enrich, Osmolyte) are another method of attaining adequate nutrition. Pulmocare is a nutritional enteral feeding that is high in protein and fat and low in carbohydrates. Its use may be beneficial in clients who retain CO_2 because the carbohydrate load is less than that in conventional enteral feedings. Decreasing carbohydrate content in the diet can help to lower CO_2 levels in the client with hypercapnia. Vitamin and mineral replacements, as well as water, are also important. A dietitian must be involved in this aspect of the client's care. (Nutritional considerations are discussed in Chapter 35.)

The intubated client receiving nasogastric feedings should have the ET cuff inflated and the head of the bed elevated. A soft, flexible, small-bore, and easily positioned feeding tube should be inserted. Care must be taken when suctioning the mouth with a tonsil (Yankauer) apparatus; it may catch on to the small feeding tube and cause it to be displaced from the stomach. Position of the feeding tube should be verified by chest x-ray film.

Tube feedings are given as a slow, continuous drip because rapid infusion can cause diarrhea and absorption problems. Usually feedings are begun in small quantities and increased according to client tolerance. If the client is not tolerating tube feedings at a certain concentration (e.g., diarrhea develops), discontinuing the feedings for several hours and then beginning at a lower concentration may help. Problems with malabsorption and decreased gastric emptying can be assessed by discontinuing the tube feeding for 30 to 60 minutes and checking for the amount of residual tube feeding in the stomach by aspirating with a syringe. Metoclopramide (Reglan) is sometimes used to increase GI motility and decrease problems with absorption.

If more than half the amount of the tube feeding given per hour is aspirated, the aspirate should be reintroduced slowly into the stomach and the tube should be clamped for another 30 minutes to 1 hour and rechecked for residual. The gastric emptying time varies from person to person. The feedings should be administered in an amount and at an infusion rate best tolerated by the client.

Tube feedings should be temporarily stopped if the client is in a head-down postural drainage position (for at least 30 minutes before treatment), if bowel sounds are absent, or if regurgitation occurs. The client must be observed closely for signs of hypoglycemia if the tube feedings are rapidly discontinued for long periods of time. Food coloring in the feedings can help to identify the presence of feedings in material suctioned from the trachea. The presence of a positive glucose reaction on a dipstick of tracheal secretions may indicate insufflation of feedings into the trachea. If there is evidence that aspiration may have occurred, the tube feeding should be discontinued immediately and the physician notified. (Nursing care related to tube feedings is discussed in Chapter 35.)

Musculoskeletal system. Improvement or maintenance of muscle strength and prevention of the problems of immobility are important. Exercise tolerance is enhanced by adequate analgesia for pain and adequate nutritional intake. Progressive ambulation of clients receiving long-term ventilation can be attained while the client is receiving ventilation. This is done by pushing the ventilator with the client or by ambulating with an oxygenized bag ventilator (e.g., Ambu bag) while giving periodic hyperinflations. Passive and active exercises, consisting of movements to maintain muscle tone in the upper and lower extremities, should be done in bed. Simple maneuvers such as leg lifts, knee bends, quadriceps setting, or arm circles are always possible and appropriate. Prevention of contractures, pressure areas, decubitus ulcers, foot drop, external rotation of the hip and legs, and other deformities by proper positioning is also important.

Psychological effects. The client who is receiving mechanical ventilation is often under a great deal of physical and emotional stress. Vital functions have been altered. The client is unable to speak, eat, or breathe normally and is restricted in activity. Often the client is in the center of a maze of tubes and machines that create fear and anxiety. Ordinary functions such as having a bowel movement or coughing are complicated. Death may seem inevitable. The client's productive role in society and in the family is temporarily suspended. Being unable to participate fully in family matters may cause feelings of inadequacy, overwhelming helplessness, and frustration.

These problems are further compounded by the sensory overload and deprivation in the ICU. Ringing alarms, flickering lights, frequent interruptions by personnel (often without warning), and lack of meaningful input are examples of such experiences. The passage of time loses its meaning when lights are on constantly or when noises prevent sleep. Sleep and waking cycles are disturbed. Problems caused by sleep deprivation add to the client's stress.

It is the responsibility of the nurse to ensure that the client's needs are met. The nurse should be able to pick up behavioral clues to determine whether the client is coping effectively with the stressful situation. If coping is not effective, the health team needs to be alerted and supportive measures must be sought. For example, the client may be distressed because of a family problem that can be solved through consultation with family members and the health team. Effective coping mechanisms require positive reinforcement and sustained strengthening. The need for psychological support cannot be overemphasized.

The client must be given a means to communicate. Signals, paper and pencil, alphabet boards, word boards, magic slates, and in some instances tracheostomy tubes that allow speech can be used. Touching the client's arm or hand and being able to read body language and facial expressions are also important.

Measures to make the client's environment more restful include (1) efficient scheduling of care to reduce interruptions, (2) simulation of a night-day environment by turning the lights off at night, (3) a calendar and clock near the bed, (4) personal articles and pictures of loved ones, and (5) a calm, reassuring approach. Tape-recorded relaxation tapes of soothing music may also help the client to relax. Sedation may be required to enhance sleep. The client receiving long-term ventilation should be moved to an area where there is a window to appreciate better both night and day and the outside world. Even though the client is unable to converse, the client will still appreciate being addressed. The nurse should discuss the client's interests and, most of all, explain in simple terms what the different tubes and equipment are and what progress is being made. Reassuring the client honestly about progress and allowing the client as much control as possible over care may ease the frustration of dependence. Deciding when to bathe or wash hair, which direction to turn, or what to eat may be the client's only way of maintaining control in an overwhelming situation.

The client's family needs emotional support as well. The first time family members visit the client, it may be important for the nurse to go with them. The family members should be told briefly what the tubes are for, and they should be encouraged to touch, hug, and speak to the client. A chair should be provided and the siderail lowered so that they can have contact with their loved one. Privacy should be provided as much as possible. The effect of the client's visitors should be assessed. Occasionally, significant others have a difficult time dealing with a sick loved one and may need help and support. The family should be included in the plan of care. If a family member expresses a wish to participate in physical care such as shaving or oral hygiene, the nurse should encourage such activity.

Many institutions have family support systems. Chaplains, social workers, and psychologists are often members of the health team. These support personnel may assist the family and client to adjust to problems resulting from the client's hospitalization.

Machine malfunction or disconnection. It is possible for mechanical ventilators to malfunction or to become disconnected from the client. When turned on and operative, alarm systems can alert the nurse and therapist to problems. A study on accidental ventilator disconnections found that most fatalities occur while the alarm is turned off, even though most accidental disconnections in critical care settings are discovered by alarm activation.[27] This study also found that by far the most frequent site for disconnections is between the tracheal tube and the adapter (client-machine interface). Disconnection was also found to be more likely at a tracheostomy tube than at a nasal or oral ET tube because it is physically more difficult to exert pressure on the tracheostomy tube connector and because the pressure may be painful for the client. Suggestions

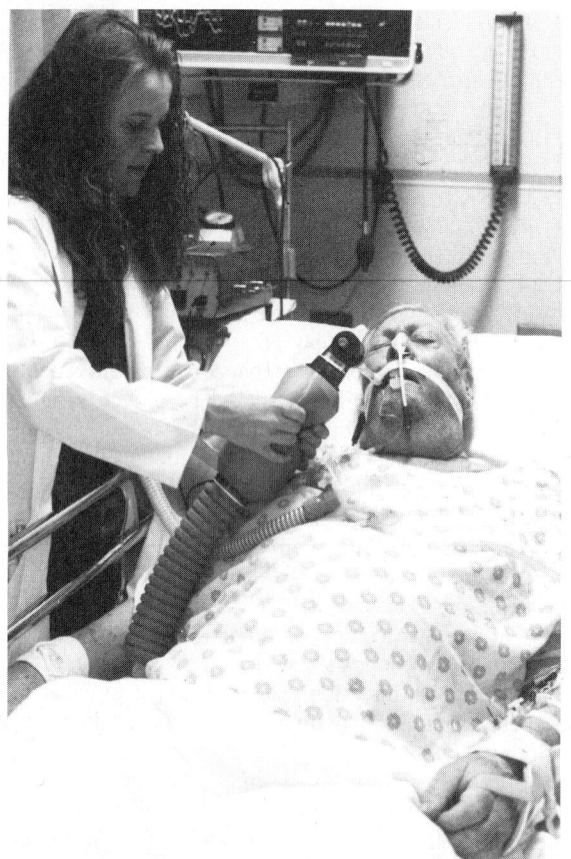

Fig. 23-13 If a ventilator malfunctions, the client should be maintained by bag ventilation.

from the study are (1) to respond immediately to alarms and (2) once at the client's bedside, to evaluate the entire breathing circuit while ventilating the client with an Ambu bag (Fig. 23-13). Twisting the ventilator-tracheostomy connection rather than pushing these together is safer. Other important factors are that (1) alarms should be kept on during suctioning if there is no silencer button and (2) if turned off, alarms must be immediately turned on after suctioning.

Manual resuscitation bag. Although the Ambu (air mask bag unit) is not the only example of a manual resuscitation bag or bag ventilator, it is the best known. This unit consists of a bag that is fitted to either a face mask or an attachment fitting the client's tracheostomy or ET tube. There are two basic types of bags, the *anesthesia bag* and the *self-inflatable bag*. The anesthesia bag is used by the anesthesiologist in surgery to ventilate the client; it delivers 100% O_2 with its source. Adaptations of this bag have been made to produce PEEP bags for clients receiving more than 10 cm H_2O PEEP.

Several kinds of self-inflatable bags are used for resuscitation and kept at the bedside for clients receiving mechanical ventilation. If a mask is used in resuscitation, it is important first to insert an oral or nasopharyngeal airway to maintain airway patency. The mask must then be tightly fitted to the face (first placed on the chin and then over the nose) and the neck hyperextended to keep the airway

patent. The nurse should use a regular rate of about 10 breaths/min and watch the rise and fall of the client's chest for confirmation that ventilation is adequate.

Self-inflatable bags vary in the concentration of O_2 delivered. All bags require flows of 15 L/min. Bags that usually contain reservoir tubings and other devices to entrain O_2 deliver O_2 concentrations of 90% to 95%. The slower the bag is deflated and inflated, the higher the O_2 concentration that will be delivered. Both the Hope II and old Hope bag with reservoir tubing and adaptor deliver an Fio_2 of 0.90 to 0.95. The Laerdal bag (clear green) delivers an Fio_2 of 0.5 to 0.6 and with reservoir tubing, 0.75 to 0.8. The Bennett Puritan bag (brown) delivers an Fio_2 of 0.35 to 0.40.

Weaning from Mechanical Ventilation

Weaning is the process of gradually reducing ventilator support until the client is able to perform self-ventilation. Clients who require mechanical ventilation are weaned from the ventilator and the ET tube promptly (e.g., in drug overdose and postoperative open heart surgery without complications) or require prolonged ventilatory assistance through a tracheostomy or ET tube (e.g., in clients with ARDS or COPD). Clients likely to require prolonged mechanical ventilation can generally be identified as those who have underlying lung disease and develop respiratory failure because of surgical procedures, trauma, or infection. Preparations for the weaning process begin when the client initially receives ventilation. These preparations include the optimization of nutritional status, exercise tolerance, fluid electrolyte and acid-base balance, cardiac output and status, level of consciousness, pulmonary status, and psychological status.

Data to determine the weaning ability of clients should be compiled from many sources (see Table 23-15). Criteria also vary among clients depending on previous lung status and ventilatory reserve. For weaning to be successful, the client should be as clinically stable as possible. Respiratory parameters should demonstrate that the client has a patent effective airway, adequate ventilatory muscle strength, and an effective cough. The lung's ability to oxygenate the arterial blood adequately is evident when stable ABGs (with a Pao_2 of at least 60 mm Hg) can be achieved with an Fio_2 of less than 0.5. The lungs should be reasonably clear on chest x-ray film and on auscultation. It is important to have an alert, well-rested client relatively free from pain who will readily take deep breaths to obtain optimum alveolar ventilation and to prevent atelectasis. This does not mean complete withdrawal from sedatives or analgesics. Instead, an intelligent approach to titration of medications to achieve pain relief and decreased anxiety without excessive drowsiness is indicated.

Basically, three weaning methods are in clinical use. A common method is to give the client IMV and to gradually reduce the frequency of ventilation breaths as the client's ventilatory status permits. In another method in which pressure-support ventilation is used as a method of weaning, the amount of pressure is slowly decreased (5 cm/hr to 5 cm/shift or longer) until the client is able to breathe spontaneously without pressure support. In a third method the client is transferred from assisted mechanical ventilation or IMV to humidified O_2 through a T piece or Briggs' adapter. Clients usually require an Fio_2 of 10% higher without ventilation to maintain adequate Pao_2 and saturation levels because the V_T frequently drops with spontaneous respiration and $Paco_2$ increases. The time off the ventilator is usually limited to 5 to 10 min/hr, increasing by increments of 5 to 10 min/hr if tolerated. The weaning procedure is carried out during the day, and the client is given ventilation at night until the client is able to breathe all day with only periodic sighing. Allowing the client to rest at night is important, regardless of the weaning technique used.

Before weaning, the client should be prepared psychologically, and continued psychological support should be maintained. The nurse should explain the weaning process and report the client's progress. The client should be placed in a sitting or semirecumbent position and should be as comfortable as possible. Before weaning, respiratory parameters are measured (see Table 23-15) to provide a baseline with which frequent serial determinations can be compared. The V_T, negative inspiratory force, and vital capacity are most frequently measured. ABGs are drawn at specified periods during the weaning procedure. The cuff may be deflated totally or partially during weaning unless it is needed to prevent aspiration, since tracheal tubes add to airway resistance.

The client must be monitored closely for signs of respiratory distress, restlessness, tiring, somnolence, shallow breathing, use of accessory muscles of ventilation, tachycardia, decrease or increase in BP, tachypnea or bradypnea, ECG changes, pallor or graying of mucous membranes, and excessive secretion buildup with a need for frequent suctioning. Statements from the client regarding weaning tolerance must also be considered. Continuous oximetry is a helpful tool while weaning clients.

When the client is extubated, the airway should be thoroughly suctioned and the cuff deflated. An O_2 mask or cannula should be set up at the bedside and be ready for use. Care of the mouth or nares is also given after extubation once the client has been stabilized with O_2 delivered by mask or cannula. ABGs are obtained 20 to 30 minutes after extubation. The client must be monitored continuously for the presence of respiratory distress, not only because of previous lung problems but also because laryngeal and/or tracheal edema may develop and symptoms of acute upper airway obstruction may occur. Measures to ensure pulmonary toilet, coughing, deep breathing, turning, and suctioning (if necessary) must be continued.

Home Mechanical Ventilation

Mechanical ventilators are no longer limited to the intensive care unit but are now a part of home health care. Families and friends can be taught to give responsible care to a person receiving mechanical ventilation, making home mechanical ventilation an alternative to prolonged hospitalization.[28] The emphasis on controlling hospital health care costs has increased the early discharge of clients and the need to provide highly technical care such as mechanical ventilation in home settings.

Home mechanical ventilation has several advantages. Having the client in the home eliminates the strain that the hospital setting may impose on family dynamics. The feeling of helplessness by family members when they first hear about the necessity for long-term mechanical ventilation is frequently countered by the ability of the family to participate fully in the client's care in the home setting.[29] At home the client may be able to participate more in the activities of daily living around a more individualized schedule and, because of the smaller size of the home ventilator, be more mobile.[30] Another advantage of home mechanical ventilation is the reduction in the client's risk of nosocomial infection.

Several disadvantages related to home mechanical ventilation include reimbursement, equipment, caregiving, and the complex needs of these clients.[31] In addition to the need for extensive nursing care, nonreimbursable care and products can make home mechanical ventilation a disadvantage. Financial resources need to be carefully assessed when the decision to arrange for home mechanical ventilation is being made. Another disadvantage of home mechanical ventilation is its potential impact on the family. Family members may seem enthusiastic about caring for their loved one in the home but may be motivated by guilt or lack of understanding of the potential sacrifices they may have to make financially and in time and commitment.

Both negative- and positive-pressure (volume) ventilators can be used in the home. Negative-pressure ventilators are frequently the ventilator of choice because they do not require an artificial airway and are less complicated to use. Small, portable volume ventilators that can be attached to a wheelchair or placed on a bedside table, such as the Puritan Bennett Companion 2801 and Lifecare PLV 102, are available. The settings and alarms on these ventilators are similar to the larger ones used in ICUs, and some ventilators have IMV capability.

R eview Questions

The number of the question corresponds to the same-numbered objective at the beginning of the chapter.

1. Which of the following is *not* a cause of hypoxemic respiratory failure?
   a. $\dot{V}/\dot{Q}$ mismatch
   b. shunting
   c. diffusion abnormalities
   d. alveolar hyperventilation
2. Which of the following may enhance ventilation in the client with expiratory wheezing and prolonged exhalation?
   a. bronchodilator administration (IV, aerosol)
   b. ultrasonic nebulization with normal saline solution
   c. aerosolized Mucomyst
   d. administration of a large volume of IV fluids
3. The most common early manifestations of ARDS that the nurse may observe are
   a. cyanosis and apprehension
   b. dyspnea and tachypnea
   c. respiratory distress and frothy sputum
   d. hypotension and tachycardia

4. Which of the following is true concerning fluid management in the stable ARDS client?
   a. pulmonary capillary wedge pressure is maintained at high levels (<10 mm Hg)
   b. pulmonary capillary wedge pressure is kept as low as possible without impairing cardiac output
   c. diuretics and fluid restriction are rarely used
   d. frequent and vigorous administration of salt-poor albumin is used

5. The nurse can reduce the danger of hypoxemia induced by suctioning the lungs of the ventilated client by
   a. preoxygenating and hyperventilating the client before and after suctioning
   b. suctioning only once per hour
   c. asking the client to take deep breaths before and after suctioning
   d. asking the client to cough during suctioning

6. A volume-cycled ventilator does which of the following?
   a. delivers gas flow for a preset period of time
   b. delivers gas flow until a preset pressure is reached
   c. delivers gas flow until a preset volume is reached
   d. any of the above depending on the settings used

7. Maintenance of client safety is extremely important for the client receiving mechanical ventilation. Which of the following is imperative to ensure this?
   a. maintain an oral airway on all intubated clients
   b. restrain all clients receiving mechanical ventilation
   c. decrease the sound of ventilator alarms to avoid startling the client
   d. keep a bag ventilator with an O_2 source at the bedside at all times

REFERENCES

1. Hanley ME and Bone RC: Acute respiratory failure: pathophysiology, causes and clinical manifestations, Postgrad Med 79:166-176, 1986.
2. Bates D: Respiratory function in disease, ed 3, Philadelphia, 1989, WB Saunders Co.
3. White KM and others: The physiologic basis for continuous mixed venous oxygen saturation monitoring, Heart Lung 19:548-551, 1990.
4. Birdsall C: How and when do you use pulse oximetry? Am J Nurs 87:158-165, 1987.
5. Bennett DA and Bleck TP: Diagnosis and treatment of neuromuscular causes of acute respiratory failure, Clin Neuropharmacol 11:303-347, 1988.
6. George R: Alveolar ventilation, gas transfer, and oxygen delivery. In George R and others: Chest medicine essentials of pulmonary medicine, ed 2, New York, 1990, Williams & Wilkins, pp 57-90.
7. Pecty T: Adult respiratory distress syndrome. In Mitchell RS and others: Synopsis of clinical pulmonary disease, ed 4, St Louis, 1989, The CV Mosby Co, pp 257-271.
8. Matthay MA: The adult respiratory distress syndrome, Clin Chest Med 11:575-580, 1990.
9. George R and others: Chest medicine: essentials of pulmonary and critical care medicine, ed 2, New York, 1990, Williams & Wilkins, pp 441-452.
10. Rinaldo J and Christman J: Mechanisms and mediators of the adult respiratory distress syndrome, Clin Chest Med 11:621-632, 1990.
11. Raffin TA: ARDS: mechanisms and management, Hosp Pract 22:65-80, 1987.
12. Bradley RB: Adult respiratory distress syndrome, Focus Crit Care 14:48-59, 1987.
13. Hansen FA and others: Adult respiratory distress syndrome: clinical features and pathogenesis. In Fishman A: Pulmonary diseases and disorders, ed 2, New York, 1988, McGraw-Hill Book Co, pp 2201-2213.
14. Niederman M and Fein A: Sepsis syndrome, the adult respiratory distress syndrome, and nosocomial pneumonia: a common clinical sequence, Clin Chest Med 11:633-656, 1990.
15. Goldstein G and Luce JM: Pharmacologic treatment of the adult respiratory distress syndrome, Clin Chest Med 11:773-787, 1990.
16. Pingleton SK: Complications of acute respiratory failure, Am Rev Respir Dis 137:1463-1493, 1988.
17. Heffner J: Airway management in the critically ill patient, Crit Care Clin 6:533-550, 1990.
18. Adriani J, Naraghi M, and Ward M: Complications of endotracheal intubation, South Med J 81:739-744, 1988.
19. Goodnough SKC: The effects of oxygen and hyperinflation on arterial oxygen tension after endotracheal suctioning, Heart Lung 14:11-17, 1985.
20. Panacek EA and others: Selective left endobronchial suctioning in the intubated patient, Chest 95:885-887, 1989.
21. Sassoon G and others: Ventilatory modes: old and new, Crit Care Clin 6:605-634, 1990.
22. Burns SM: Advances in ventilator therapy, Focus Crit Care 17:227-237, 1990.
23. Villar J and others: Nonconventional techniques of ventilatory support, Crit Care Clin 6:579-603, 1990.
24. Rasanen J and others: Acute myocardial infarction complicated by respiratory failure: the effects of mechanical ventilation, Chest 85:21-28, 1984.
25. Dolan JT: Critical care nursing: clinical management through the nursing process, Philadelphia, 1991, FA Davis Co, p 633.
26. Kersten LD: Comprehensive respiratory nursing, Philadelphia, 1989, WB Saunders Co, p 727.
27. Janowski MJ: Accidental disconnections from breathing systems: what the FDA found—and what you can do about it, Am J Nurs 84:241-244, 1984.
28. Make BJ: Long-term management of ventilator-assisted individuals: the Boston University experience, Resp Care 31:303-310, 1986.
29. Donohue WJ and others: Long-term mechanical ventilation: guidelines for management in the home and at alternate community sites, Chest 90:1S-37S, 1986.
30. Frace RM: Home ventilation: an alternative to institutionalization, Focus Crit Care 13:28-34, 1986.
31. Plummer AL, O'Donohue WJ, and Petty TL: Consensus conference on problems in home mechanical ventilation, Am Rev Respir Dis 140:555-560, 1989.

CHAPTER

24

Nursing Assessment
Hematological System

Bonnie Mowinski Jennings

Bonnie Mowinski Jennings

L earning Objectives

1. *Describe the structures and functions of the hematological system.*
2. *Differentiate among the types of blood cells and their functions.*
3. *Explain the normal clotting mechanism.*
4. *Identify the significant subjective and objective assessment data related to the hematological system that should be obtained from a client.*
5. *Describe the appropriate techniques used in the physical assessment of the lymphatic system.*
6. *Differentiate normal from common abnormal findings of a physical assessment of the hematological system.*
7. *Describe the purpose, the significance of results, and the nursing responsibilities related to diagnostic studies of the hematological system.*

Hematology is the study of blood and blood-forming tissues. This includes the blood cells, the bone marrow, the spleen, and the lymph system. A basic knowledge of hematology is useful in clinical settings to evaluate the client's ability to transport oxygen and carbon dioxide, coagulate blood, and combat infections. The study of the blood often includes the *mononuclear phagocyte system*. In the past, this system was known as the *reticuloendothelial system*. Monocytes and macrophages are involved in phagocytosis and the immune response (see Chapters 7 and 8).

Reviewed by Hilary Sigmon, R.N., Ph.D., Nurse Science Administrator, National Center for Nursing Research, National Institutes of Health, Bethesda, Maryland.

The opinions and assertions in this chapter are the views of the author and are not to be construed as official or as reflecting the views of the Department of the Army or the Department of Defense.

STRUCTURES AND FUNCTIONS OF THE HEMATOLOGICAL SYSTEM
Bone Marrow

Bone marrow is the soft material that fills the central core of bones. It is the blood-forming tissue that produces the three major cell components of the blood: *erythrocytes* (red blood cells or RBCs), *leukocytes* (white blood cells or WBCs), and *platelets*. The blood components develop from a common stem cell, but as they mature, several different, distinct cells evolve (Fig. 24-1). An understanding of the function of particular blood cell types enhances the nurse's ability to interpret laboratory data.

In the fetus, most of the bone marrow actively produces blood cells. In the adult, however, active production of marrow is generally limited to the ends of long bones, vertebrae, flat cranial bones, sternum, ribs, scapulae, clavicles, pelvis, and sacrum.

Blood Cells

Erythrocytes. *Erythropoiesis* (production of erythrocytes, or RBCs) is largely regulated by cellular oxygen requirements and general metabolic activity. The process of erythropoiesis is stimulated by hypoxia and controlled hormonally by *erythropoietin*, a hormone synthesized and released by the kidney. Erythropoietin stimulates the bone marrow to increase erythrocyte production. Erythropoiesis is also influenced by nutritional requirements, with iron, vitamin B_{12}, and folic acid being essential nutrients for erythropoiesis.[1]

Hemolysis (destruction of erythrocytes) by macrophages removes abnormal, defective, damaged, and old RBCs from circulation. It takes place in the bone marrow, liver, and spleen. Hemolysis increases bilirubin production. The normal life span of an erythrocyte is 120 days.

Several distinct cell types evolve during erythrocyte maturation (Fig. 24-1). The *reticulocyte* is an immature erythrocyte. The reticulocyte count measures the rate at which new RBCs appear in the circulation. Reticulocytes are capable of maturing within 48 hours of release into circulation. Therefore assessing the number of reticulocytes

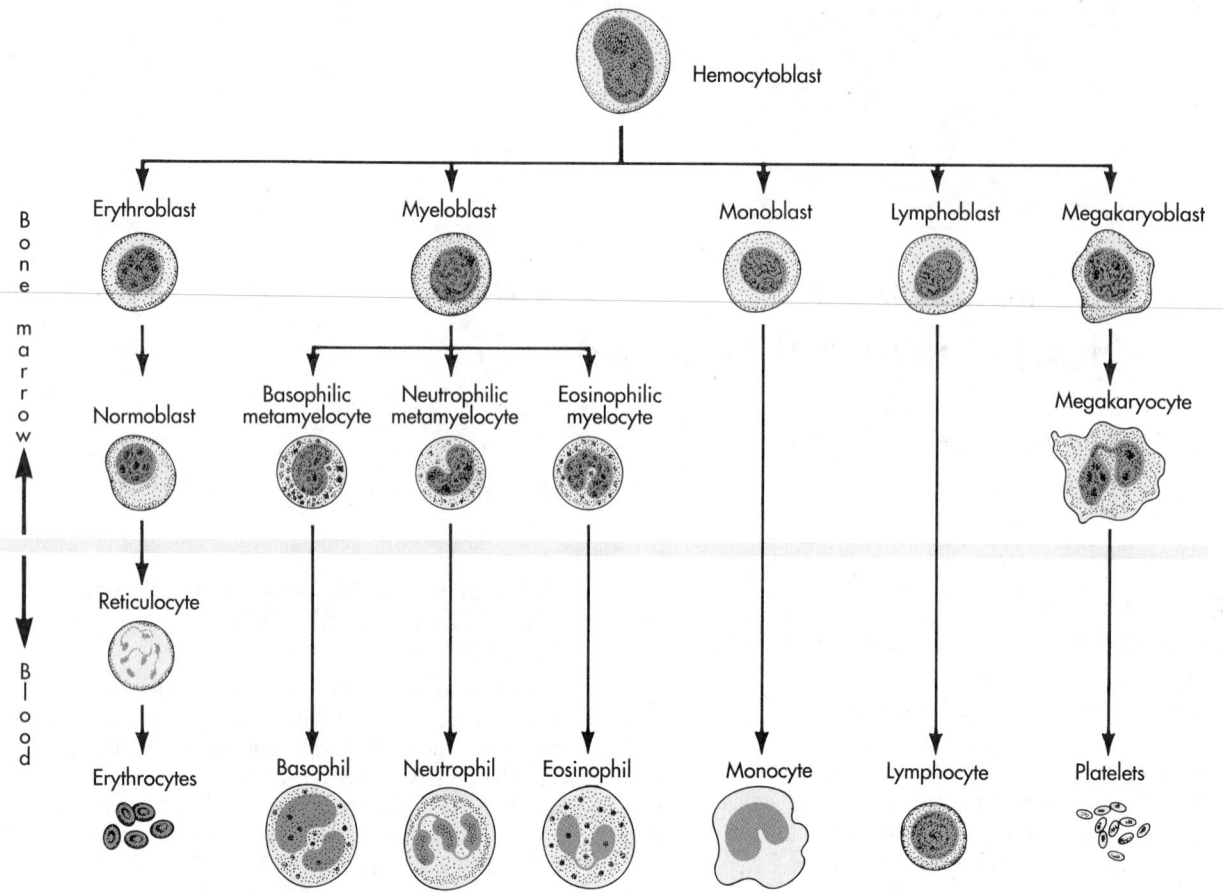

Fig. 24-1 Development of blood cells.

is a useful means of evaluating the adequacy of erythrocyte production. The functions of erythrocytes include transport of gases (both oxygen and carbon dioxide) and assistance in maintaining the acid-base balance through the buffering capability of hemoglobin.

Hemoglobin, the major component of erythrocytes, gives them their characteristic red color when combined with oxygen. Iron and protein form the molecular structure of hemoglobin. The function of hemoglobin is to transport oxygen. Therefore, although adequate oxygen may be inspired into the lungs, it may not reach the tissues unless there is an adequate amount of hemoglobin to carry it. Consequently, the significance of any type of anemia is its effect on tissue oxygenation.

Leukocytes. Leukocytes, the white cells of the blood, also develop in a series of cell types that vary in maturity (Fig. 24-1). The three kinds of mature leukocytes are *granulocytes, lymphocytes,* and *monocytes.* The main function of the granulocytes and monocytes is *phagocytosis* of bacteria and foreign particles that invade the body. Phagocytosis is a process by which cells ingest or engulf any unwanted organism and then digest and kill it. The main function of lymphocytes is related to the immune response (see Chapter 8).

Granulocytes. Granulocytes are so named because they contain granules in their cytoplasm. Granulocytes (also

known as *polymorphonuclear leukocytes,* or PMNs) consist of *neutrophils, eosinophils,* and *basophils.*

Neutrophils, also called *polys* or *segs,* have strong phagocytic activity. They are the primary phagocytic cells involved in acute inflammatory responses. Eosinophils have a similar but reduced ability for phagocytosis. One of their primary functions is to engulf antigen-antibody complexes formed during an allergic response. They also are able to defend against parasitic infections. Basophils have a limited role in phagocytosis. Their granules in the cytoplasm contain heparin, serotonin, and histamine. If a basophil is stimulated by an antigen or by tissue injury, it will respond by releasing its granules. This is part of the response seen in allergic and inflammatory reactions.

Lymphocytes. Lymphocytes are produced in the bone marrow and form the basis of the cellular and humoral immune responses. There are two lymphocyte cell types: B cells and T cells. B cells, produced in the bone marrow, mediate the humoral immune response. When B cells are stimulated by antigens, they are activated to plasma cells. Plasma cells produce antibodies (also known as *immunoglobulins*) that mediate humoral immunity.

T-cell precursors originate in the bone marrow and then migrate to the thymus gland for further differentiation. They mediate cellular immunity. T cells are involved in the cellular immune response against intracellular viruses, tuberculosis, contact irritants (e.g., poison ivy), cancer, parasites, fungi, and transplant antigens that provoke rejection of organs. Various subtypes of T cells have been identified. Among these are the T-helper cells and the T-suppressor cells. (The details of lymphocyte function are presented in Chapter 8.)

Monocytes. Monocytes are produced in the bone marrow and circulate briefly in the blood. They are large, slow-moving, potent phagocytic cells that can ingest small or large masses of matter, such as bacteria, dead cells, tissue debris, and old or defective RBCs. Monocytes are the second type of WBC to arrive at the scene of an injury (neutrophils are the first). When monocytes leave the blood and enter tissues, they differentiate into *macrophages*, which are more phagocytic than monocytes. Macrophages also interact with lymphocytes to facilitate the humoral and cellular immune responses.

Platelets. Platelets, or *thrombocytes,* are derived from megakaryocytes (Fig. 24-1). The primary function of platelets relates to blood clotting. Platelet performance depends on both quantitative and qualitative features.[2] Platelets must be available in sufficient numbers (quantitatively sufficient) and must be structurally sound to work properly (qualitatively adequate). Platelets are also involved in homeostasis by maintaining capillary integrity by working as "plugs" to close any openings in the capillary wall. At the site of any damage, platelet activation is initiated. Increasing numbers of platelets accumulate to form a platelet plug. Platelets are also important to the process of clot shrinkage and retraction.

Spleen

Another component of the hematological system is the spleen, which is located in the upper left quadrant of the abdomen.

The functions of the spleen can be classified into four general groups:

1. *Hematopoietic function:* The spleen produces RBCs during fetal development.
2. *Filter function:* The splenic structure provides an ideal filter mechanism. For example, the spleen removes old and defective erythrocytes from the circulation by the mononuclear phagocyte system. Another example of filtering involves the reuse of iron. The spleen is able to catabolize hemoglobin released by hemolysis and return the iron component of the hemoglobin to the bone marrow for reuse.
3. *Immune function:* The spleen contains a rich supply of lymphocytes and monocytes.
4. *Storage function:* About 30% of the platelet mass is stored in the spleen.

Lymph System

The *lymph system,* consisting of lymphatic capillaries, ducts, and lymph nodes, carries fluid from the interstitial spaces to the blood. It is by means of the lymph that proteins, fat from the gastrointestinal (GI) tract, and certain hormones are able to return to the blood. The lymph system also returns excess interstitial fluid to the blood, which is important in preventing the development of edema.

Lymph fluid is pale yellow interstitial fluid that has diffused through lymphatic capillary walls. It circulates through a special vasculature, much as blood moves through blood vessels. The formation of lymph fluid increases when interstitial fluid pressure rises, thereby forcing more fluid into the lymph system. When too much interstitial pressure develops or when something interferes with the reabsorption of lymph, *lymphedema* develops. The lymphedema that may occur as a complication of a radical mastectomy is often caused by the obstruction of lymph flow resulting from by the removal of nodes.

The lymphatic capillaries are thin-walled, endothelium-lined vessels that have an irregular diameter. They are somewhat larger than blood capillaries and do not contain valves. Lymphatic capillaries unite to form lymphatic vessels, which carry all lymph to either the right lymphatic duct or the thoracic duct. These large lymphatic ducts drain into subclavian veins in the neck.

The lymph nodes are also a part of the lymphatic system. Structurally, the nodes are small, round to bean-shaped organs of varying sizes. A primary function of lymph nodes is filtration of bacteria and foreign particles carried by lymph. Lymph nodes are distributed throughout the body along lymph vessels. They are situated both superficially and deep. The superficial nodes can be palpated, but the deep nodes must be visualized radiographically (see Fig. 24-4).

Normal Clotting Mechanisms

Hemostasis is a normal homeostatic process of blood clotting and blood lysing.[3] Blood clotting minimizes blood loss when various body structures are injured. Three components contribute to normal clotting: *vascular response, platelet response,* and *plasma clotting factors.*

Vascular response. When a blood vessel is injured, an immediate local vasoconstrictive response occurs. Vasoconstriction reduces the leakage of blood from the vessel not only by restricting the vessel size but also by pressing the endothelial surfaces together. The latter reaction enhances vessel wall stickiness and maintains closure of the vessel even after the vasoconstriction subsides. Vascular spasm may last for 20 to 30 minutes, thus allowing time for the platelet response and plasma clotting factors to be activated.

Platelet response. Platelets are activated when they are exposed to interstitial collagen from an injured blood vessel. Platelets stick to one another and form clumps. The stickiness is known as *adhesiveness,* and the formation of clumps is called *aggregation* or *agglutination.* When a blood vessel is injured, the circulating platelets are exposed to the collagen from the inner lining of the vessel. This interaction causes the platelets to release substances such as platelet factor 3 (PF3), serotonin, and epinephrine, which facilitate coagulation.

At the same time, platelets release adenosine diphosphate (ADP), which increases platelet adhesiveness and aggregation, thereby enhancing the formation of a platelet plug.

In addition to their independent contribution to clotting, platelets also facilitate the reactions of the plasma clotting

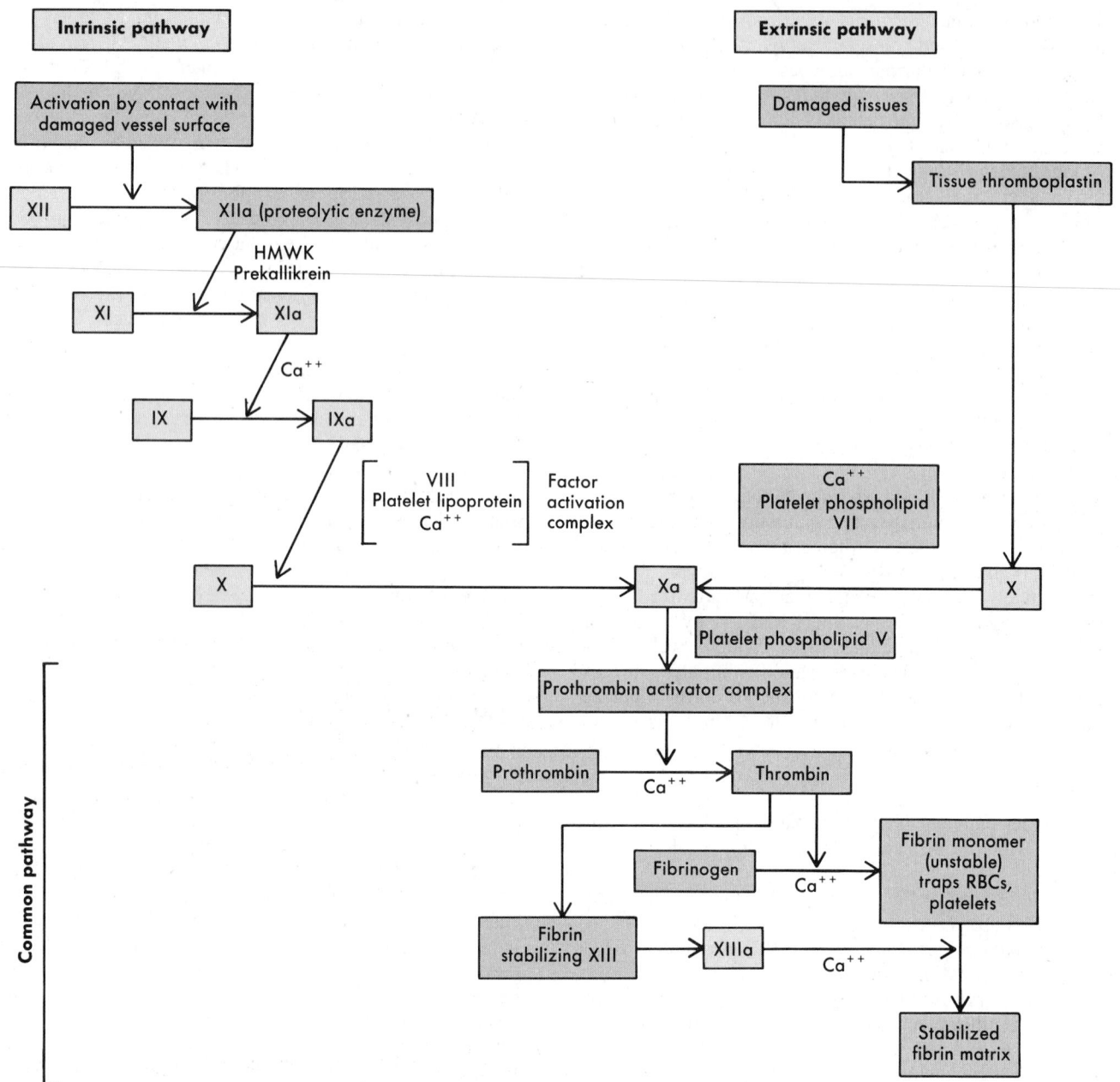

Fig. 24-2 Coagulation mechanism showing steps in the intrinsic pathway and extrinsic pathway. (From McCance KL: Pathophysiology, St Louis, 1989, The CV Mosby Co, p 775.)

factors. As depicted in Fig. 24-2, platelet lipoproteins stimulate necessary conversions in the clotting process.

Plasma clotting factors. The plasma clotting factors are labeled in various ways to include the use of both names and Roman numerals (Table 24-1). Plasma proteins circulate in inactive forms until stimulated to initiate clotting through one of two pathways, *intrinsic* or *extrinsic*. The intrinsic pathway is activated by collagen exposure from endothelial injury when the blood vessel is damaged. The extrinsic pathway is initiated when tissue thromboplastin is released extravascularly from injured tissues.

Regardless of whether clotting is initiated by substances internal or external to the blood vessel, coagulation ultimately follows the same final common pathway of the clotting cascade. *Thrombin* in the common pathway is the most powerful enzyme in the coagulation process (Fig. 24-2). It converts fibrinogen to fibrin, which is an essential component of a blood clot.

Anticoagulants. Just as some blood elements (procoagulants) foster coagulation, others (anticoagulants) interfere with clotting. This countermechanism to blood clotting serves to keep blood in its fluid state. Anticoagulation may

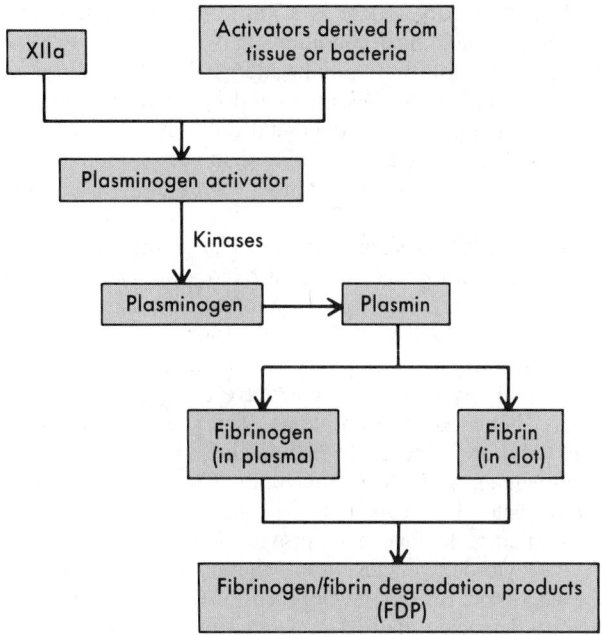

Fig. 24-3 Fibrinolytic system. (From McCance KL: Pathophysiology, St Louis, 1989, The CV Mosby Co, p 776.)

Table 24-1 Coagulation Factors

Factor	Name or Synonym
I	Fibrinogen
II	Prothrombin
III	Thromboplastin
	Tissue factor
IV	Calcium
V	Proaccelerin
	Labile factor
	Ac globulin
VI	Not assigned
VII	Stable factor
	Convertin
	Serum prothrombin conversion accelerator
VIII	Antihemophilic globulin
	Antihemophilic factor
IX	Plasma thromboplastin component
	Antihemophilic factor B
X	Stuart-Prower factor
	Stuart factor
XI	Plasma thromboplastin antecedent
	Antihemophilic factor C
XII	Hageman factor
XIII	Fibrin-stabilizing factor

be achieved by two means, antithrombins and fibrinolysis. As the name implies, *antithrombins* keep blood fluid by antagonizing thrombin, a powerful coagulant. Endogenous heparin is an example of an anticoagulant.

The second means of maintaining blood in its fluid form

is *fibrinolysis*. The fibrinolytic system is initiated when plasminogen is activated to plasmin (Fig. 24-3). Thrombin is one of the substances that can activate the conversion of plasminogen to plasmin, thereby propagating fibrinolysis.[5] The plasmin attacks either fibrin or fibrinogen by splitting the molecules into smaller elements known as fibrin split products (FSPs) or fibrin degradation products (FDPs). (More information about FSPs can be found in Table 24-6 and in the discussion of disseminated intravascular coagulation in Chapter 25.)

If fibrinolysis is excessive, clients will be predisposed to bleeding. In such a situation, bleeding results from the destruction of fibrin in platelet plugs or from the effects of increased FSPs, which include impaired platelet aggregation, reduced prothrombin, and an inability to stabilize fibrin.

Effects of Aging

There seem to be no changes in basal hematopoiesis that occur with aging. However, there may be a diminished reserve capacity of the bone marrow that will result in a diminished ability of an older adult to compensate for an acute or chronic illness.[4] In older adults, the total number and differential count of WBCs show no major changes with aging. However, in response to an infection, the WBC count does not rise as high as it would in a younger adult. Often the primary manifestation of the leukocyte response is an increase in the number of band (immature) forms in an otherwise normal WBC count. These findings suggest a diminished marrow granulocyte reserve in older adults.

The hemoglobin level decreases with aging. Iron deficiency has usually been responsible for the low hemoglobin levels. Iron absorption is not impaired in the older client, but use of orally administered iron for hemoglobin production is reduced. The osmotic fragility of RBCs is increased in older persons, and this may account for the increased mean corpuscular volume (MCV) and the decreased mean corpuscular hemoglobin concentration (MCHC) of RBCs of older persons.

The erythrocyte sedimentation rate (ESR) increases significantly with age. Therefore the ESR is of limited value in detecting disease in older adults. (The effects of aging on hematological studies are presented in Table 24-5.)

ASSESSMENT OF THE HEMATOLOGICAL SYSTEM
Subjective Data

Health history. Much of the evaluation of the hematological system is based on a thorough health history. Consequently, the nurse must be knowledgeable about the items to include in the nursing history so that questions may be phrased in a manner eliciting the most information related to the hematological problem.[5]

Past health history. It is important to learn whether the client has had prior hematological problems. A previous laboratory determination of anemia must be explored, as should diagnoses of mononucleosis, malabsorption, liver disorders such as hepatitis or cirrhosis, and spleen disorders. Specific past surgical procedures to ask about include splenectomy, tumor removal, prosthetic heart valve placement, surgical excision of the duodenum (which is responsible for iron absorption), and partial or total gastrectomy (which removes parietal cells), thus reducing intrinsic factor and the absorption of vitamin B_{12}. The nurse should also ascertain how wound healing progressed postoperatively and if and when any bleeding problems occurred in relation to the surgery. Wound healing and bleeding should be discussed as responses to past injuries (including minor trauma) and to dental extractions. The nurse should also ask about any recurring infections and problems with blood clotting.

Known allergies and allergic reactions, including anaphylaxis, must be addressed. The number of previous blood transfusions and possible complications during the blood administration must also be evaluated. The nurse should ask whether the client has had any abnormal bleeding or bruising in the past.

Current medications. There are many drugs that may interfere with normal hematological function (Table 24-2). In addition to these drugs, many antineoplastic agents used to treat malignant disorders cause depression of the bone marrow (see Chapter 9).

Family history. There is a known genetic influence in certain hematological conditions as well as in other blood diseases that follow familial patterns. When a family history is taken, the following should be explored: jaundice, anemia, malignancies, congenital RBC dyscrasias such as sickle cell disease, and bleeding disorders (the predisposition to bleed, as in hemophilia, or to clot, as in polycythemia).

Social and personal history. The significant areas of data that need to be gathered in relation to social and personal history are exposure to radiation, exposure to chemicals, dietary history, and sexual history. It is known that persons who have been exposed to radiation, as a treatment modality or by accident, have a higher incidence of certain hematological problems. The same is true of persons who are exposed to chemicals (e.g., benzene, lead, naphthalene, and phenylbutazone). Chemical exposure is often related to occupation.

A dietary history may provide clues to the cause of erythrocyte deficiencies. Iron, vitamin B_{12}, and folic acid are necessary for the development of RBCs. Iron and folic acid deficiencies may be prevented by adequate intake of foodstuffs such as liver, meat, eggs, whole-grain and en-

Table 24-2 Drugs Affecting Hematological Function and Laboratory Values

Drug	Clinical Use	Hematological Effect
Aminosalicylic acid (Pamisyl, PAS)	Antituberculin	Leukocytosis secondary to hypersensitivity
Amphotericin B (Fungizone)	Antifungal	Anemia
Acetylsalicylic acid (aspirin) and aspirin-containing compounds (e.g., Empirin, Percodan)	Analgesic, antipyretic, antiinflammatory	Reduced platelet aggregation, prolonged bleeding time
Azathioprine (Imuran)	Immunosuppression	Anemia, leukopenia
Carbamazepine (Tegretol)	Pain of trigeminal neuralgia	Anemia, leukopenia, thrombocytopenia
Chloramphenicol (Chloromycetin)	Antibiotic	Anemia, neutropenia, thrombocytopenia
Chlorothiazide (Diuril)	Diuretic	Thrombocytopenia (occasional)
Oral contraceptives and diethylstilbestrol	Birth control, menopausal symptoms, functional uterine bleeding, cancer of prostate, postmenopausal cancer of the breast	Increase in factors II, V, VII, VIII, IX, X; increase in fibrinogen; increase in thrombin; decrease in prothrombin and partial thromboplastin times; increase in coagulation and thromboemboli formation (overall)
Diphenylhydantoin (Dilantin)	Anticonvulsant, antidysrhythmic	Anemia
Epinephrine (Adrenalin)	Sympathomimetic	Leukocytosis
Glucocorticoids (ACTH, prednisone)	Antiinflammatory	Lymphopenia, neutrophilia
Isoniazid (INH)	Antituberculin	Neutropenia
Methyldopa (Aldomet)	Antihypertensive	Hemolytic anemia
Phenacetin (APC, Empirin compound)	Analgesic, antipyretic	Anemia
Phenylbutazone (Butazolidin)	Antiinflammatory	Anemia, leukopenia, neutropenia, thrombocytopenia
Procainamide hydrochloride (Pronestyl)	Antidysrhythmic	Agranulocytosis
Quinidine sulfate	Antidysrhythmic	Agranulocytosis, anemia, thrombocytopenia
Trimethoprim-sulfamethoxazole (Bactrim, Septrim)	Antibacterial	Anemia, leukopenia, neutropenia, thrombocytopenia

riched breads and cereals, potatoes, leafy green vegetables, dried fruits, legumes, and citrus fruits. Inadequate vitamin B_{12} ingestion may be due to poor dietary intake (especially lack of liver, milk, and eggs). Folic acid deficiencies may be offset by a diet including foods that are also high in iron.

Alcohol abuse must be tactfully explored. Chronic alcohol abusers frequently have vitamin deficiencies. Alcohol also exerts a damaging effect on the liver, where several clotting factors are produced. Consequently, bleeding problems can develop and should be anticipated in cases of known alcohol abuse.

Review of systems. Many of the symptoms related to hematological dysfunction are more generalized than specific. General complaints that should alert the nurse to the possibility of a hematological disorder include fatigue, apathy, lethargy, malaise, weakness, chills, fever, night sweats, weight loss, heat intolerance, and poor wound healing. Specifics of the chief complaint should be evaluated and a methodical review of systems should be completed. A general complaint (e.g., a bruise on the thigh) indicates a need to assess the skin and musculoskeletal system of the involved area.

The client should be questioned about anemia, unusual or excessive bleeding or bruising, and lymph node swelling, as well as poor wound healing and other indicators of infection. Past blood transfusions and possible reactions should be recorded. If there is a positive response, a history of the system involved should be obtained.

Questions that evaluate hematological problems should be posed to avoid missing critical information. Symptoms of anemia may be manifest through excessive fatigue, dyspnea with activity, or palpitations. Indications of WBC function may be ascertained by determining whether the client has experienced swelling in glands or lymph nodes, how long node enlargement has been present, and whether there is any associated tenderness. Incidents of fever should also be explored fully. Bleeding and bruising, as manifestations of clotting deficiencies, can be evaluated by determining how often the client discovers new bruises, whether bleeding is spontaneous or the result of trauma, and whether bruises develop regularly at sites of immunizations, parenteral injections, or venipunctures.

Objective Data

Physical examination. A complete physical examination is necessary to examine accurately all systems that affect or are affected by the hematological system (see Chapter 3). For example, a decreasing level of consciousness may be due to an intracranial hemorrhage and indicates the need for a neurological examination. Absent bowel sounds may be due to abdominal hemorrhage and indicate the need for a complete GI examination. The nurse must keep in mind that signs and symptoms can be due to hematological problems, even though these are not the obvious cause (Table 24-3).

Lymph nodes are distributed throughout the body. The superficial nodes can be evaluated by light palpation (Fig. 24-4). Deep nodes are detected radiographically. Lymph nodes should be assessed symmetrically with regard to (1) location, (2) size (in centimeters), (3) degree of fixation (e.g., movable, fixed), (4) tenderness, and (5) texture.

The examiner should lightly palpate lymph nodes over the appropriate areas.[6] The pads of the index and third fingers are most often used. The examiner should gently roll the skin over the area and concentrate on feeling for possible lymph node enlargement. When not specifically examined for their status, lymph nodes are usually palpated during the examination of the region where the nodes are located. For example, the axillary lymph nodes are examined at the completion of a breast examination.

It is important to develop a sequence when examining the lymph nodes. The lymph nodes of the head and neck drain areas of the mouth, throat, abdomen, breast, thorax, and arm. A convenient sequence for examination is preauricular, posterior auricular, occipital, tonsillar, submaxillary, submental, superficial cervical, posterior cervical chain, deep cervical chain, and supraclavicular (Fig. 24-4). This portion of the lymph node examination is usually done while the examiner is standing behind the client.

The axillary lymph nodes drain lymph from the chest wall, breasts, arms, and hands. The pectoral, subscapular, and lateral groups of nodes are palpated next. The epitrochlear nodes, located in the antecubital fossa between the biceps and triceps muscles, are then examined. These nodes drain specific areas of the forearm and hand. The inguinal lymph nodes are palpated last. These nodes drain the lower extremities.

Lymph nodes are generally not palpable unless there is residual enlargement from a previous or current infection. It may be normal to find small (0.5 to 1.0 cm), mobile, discrete, firm, nontender nodes, known as *shotty nodes.* Tender nodes are usually due to inflammation, whereas hard or fixed nodes are suggestive of malignancy.

Additional hematological data can also be acquired from other body systems. It is important to include careful inspection of the skin (see Chapter 16) and palpation of the liver and spleen (see Chapter 33) in a hematological assessment. The most direct means of evaluating the hematological system is through laboratory analysis and other diagnostic studies.

DIAGNOSTIC STUDIES

The nurse should recognize the need to thoroughly explain any diagnostic procedures to the client. It is common for clients to be anxious when faced with illness. Therefore instructions must be simple, clear, and repeated when necessary to decrease anxiety and ensure the client's compliance with preparatory protocols. Whether studies are performed on an outpatient or an inpatient basis, written instructions regarding the procedures facilitate compliance. If a diverse ethnic population is served, it is helpful to have instructions translated into the dominant language.

The repeated acquisition of blood specimens may be very disconcerting for the client. Some clients as well as staff members become concerned that the amount of blood withdrawn for tests could lead to adverse effects. Although multiple blood studies may be uncomfortable, it is only in rare situations that diagnostic blood withdrawal predisposes clients to significant volume loss.[7]

Table 24-3

Common Assessment Abnormalities of the Hematological System

Finding	Possible Etiology and Significance
SKIN	
Pallor of skin or nail beds	Decrease in quantity of hemoglobin (anemia)
Flushing	Increase in hemoglobin (polycythemia)
Jaundice	Accumulation of bile pigment due to rapid or excessive hemolysis
Purpura, petechiae, and ecchymoses	Hemostatic deficiency of platelets or clotting factors resulting in hemorrhage into the skin
Excoriation and pruritus	Scratching from intense pruritus secondary to disorders such as Hodgkin's disease
Leg ulcers	Common in sickle cell disease, especially prominent on the malleoli
Brownish discoloration	Hemosiderin and melanin from the breakdown of erythrocytes
Cyanosis	Increase in amounts of reduced hemoglobin (secondary polycythemia)
EYES	
Jaundiced sclera	Accumulation of bile pigment due to rapid or excessive hemolysis
Conjunctival pallor	Reduction in quantity of hemoglobin (anemia)
Retinal hemorrhages	More frequent in concurrent states of thrombocytopenia and anemia than with thrombocytopenia alone
MOUTH	
Pallor	Reduction in quantity of hemoglobin (anemia)
Gingival and mucosal ulceration	Neutropenia
Gingival infiltration (swelling, reddening, bleeding)	Leukemia due to impeded movement of granulocytes and monocytes through gingiva-tooth attachment into mucous membrane or to inability of impaired leukocytes to combat oral infections
Gingival or mucosal bleeding	Hemorrhagic diseases, thrombocytopenia
Smooth tongue texture	Pernicious and iron deficiency anemia
LYMPH NODES	
Lymphadenopathy, tenderness	Normal response to infection in infants and children; cancerous invasion causative factor in adults; enlargement due to infection, foreign infiltrates, or metabolic disturbances, especially with lipids
CHEST	
Widened mediastinum	Enlarged lymph nodes
Generalized sternal tenderness	Leukemia resulting from increased bone marrow cellularity, causing increase in pressure and bone erosion
Localized sternal tenderness	Multiple myeloma due to stretching of periosteum
Tachycardia	Compensatory mechanism in anemia to increase cardiac output
Widened pulse pressure	Compensatory mechanism in anemia to increase cardiac output by increasing stroke volume
Murmurs	Usually systolic murmur in anemia due to increased quantity and speed of low-viscosity blood going through pulmonic valve
Bruits (especially carotid bruits)	Anemia due to increased flow of low-viscosity blood swirling through blood vessels
ABDOMEN	
Hepatomegaly	Leukemia
Splenomegaly	Leukemia, lymphomas, mononucleosis
Splenic bruits and rubs	Splenic infarction

Table 24-3

 | **Common Assessment Abnormalities of the Hematological System—cont'd** |

Finding	Possible Etiology and Significance
NERVOUS SYSTEM	
Pain and touch, position and vibratory sensation, tendon reflexes	Impaired nervous system function due to vitamin B_{12} deficiency or compression of nerves by masses
BACK AND EXTREMITIES	
Back pain	Acute hemolytic reaction from flank pain due to renal involvement with hemolysis; multiple myeloma from enlarged tumors that stretch periosteum or weaken supportive tissue, causing ligament strain and muscle spasm
Arthralgia	Leukemia due to aching in bones that contain marrow, sickle cell disease from hemarthrosis
Bone pain	Bone invasion by leukemia cells, bone demineralization resulting from various hematopoietic malignancies enhancing possibility of pathophysiological fractures

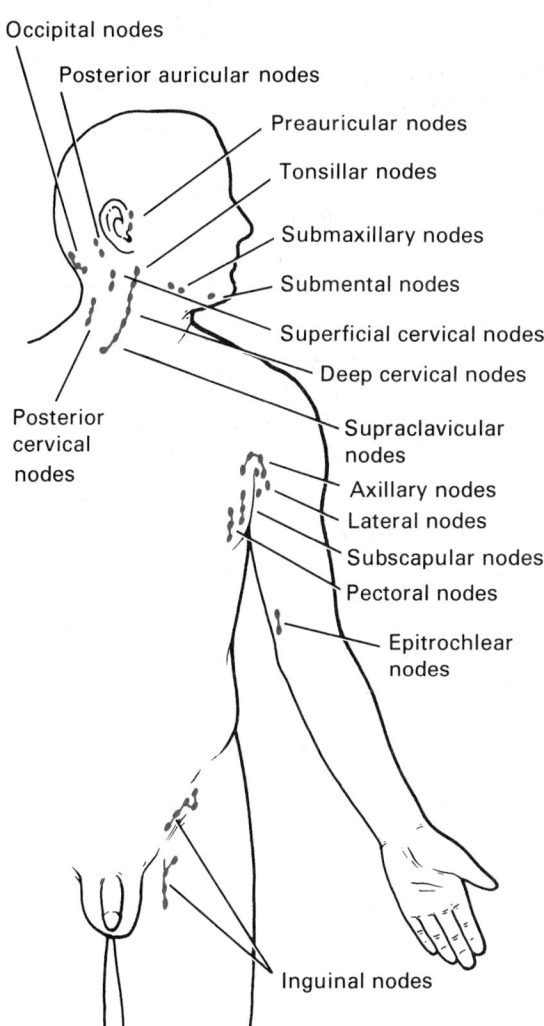

Fig. 24-4 Palpable superficial lymph nodes.

Table 24-4   CBC Studies

Study	Description and Purpose	Normal Values
Hb	Measurement of gas-carrying capacity of RBC	Women: 12-16 g/dl Men: 13.5-18 g/dl
Hct	Comparison of volume of RBC to volume of plasma as percent of total blood volume	Women: 38%-47% Men: 40%-54%
Total RBC count	Count of number of circulating RBCs	Women: $4.0\text{-}5.0 \times 10^6/\mu l$ Men: $4.5\text{-}6.0 \times 10^6/\mu l$
Red cell indices		
Mean corpuscular volume (MCV) $= \dfrac{\text{Hct} \times 10}{\text{RBC} \times 10^6}$	Determination of relative size of RBC; low MCV reflection of microcytosis, high MCV reflection of macrocytosis	82-98 fl
Mean corpuscular hemoglobin (MCH) $= \dfrac{\text{Hb} \times 10}{\text{RBC} \times 10^6}$	Measurement of average weight of Hb/RBC; low MCH indication of microcytosis or hypochromia, high MCH indication of macrocytosis	27-33 pg
Mean corpuscular hemoglobin concentration (MCHC) $= \dfrac{\text{Hb}}{\text{Hct}} \times 100$	Evaluation of RBC saturation with Hb; low MCHC indication of hypochromia, high MCHC evident in spherocytosis	32%-36%
WBC count	Measurement of total number of leukocytes	5000-10,000/μl
WBC differential	Determination of whether each kind of WBC is present in proper proportion, determination of absolute value by multiplying percentage of cell type by total WBC count and dividing by 100	Neutrophils: 50%-70% Eosinophils: 2-4% Basophils: 0%-2% Lymphocytes: 20%-40% Monocytes: 4%-8%
Platelet count	Measurement of number of platelets available to maintain platelet clotting functions (not measurement of quality of platelet function)	150,000-400,000/μl

Table 24-5   Effects of Aging on Hematological Studies

Study	Changes
CBC studies	
Hb	Decreased
MCV	Increased
MCHC	Decreased
WBC count	Diminished response to infection
Platelets	Unchanged
Clotting studies	
Partial thrombo-plastin time	Reduced
Fibrinogen	May be elevated
Factors V, VII, VIII, IX	May be elevated
ESR	Increased significantly
Iron studies	
Serum iron	Reduced
Total iron-binding capacity	Reduced

ESR, Erythrocyte sedimentation rate.

Finally, the nurse must capitalize on all appropriate opportunities to use independent nursing assessment and clinical judgment. For example, when there is a suspicion of bleeding, it is important to perform guaiac tests of the stool, nasogastric secretions, or emesis and a Hematest of the urine.

Laboratory Studies

Complete blood count. The complete blood count (CBC) involves several laboratory tests (Table 24-4), each of which serves to assess the three major blood cells formed in the bone marrow. Although the status of each cell type is important, the entire system may be disrupted by diseases as well as by treatments of diseases. When the entire CBC is suppressed, a condition known as *pancytopenia* exists. In such cases, clients need care directed toward the management of anemia, infection, and hemorrhage (see Chapter 25). The effects of aging on hematological studies are presented in Table 24-5.

Red blood cells. Normal values of some RBC tests are reported separately for men and for women because normal values are based on body mass and men usually have a larger body mass than women.

The *hemoglobin (Hb)* value is reduced in cases of anemia, hemorrhage, and states of hemodilution, such as

Table 24-6 Clotting Studies

Study	Description and Purpose	Normal Values
Prothrombin time	Assessment of extrinsic coagulation by measurement of factors I, II, V, VII, X	12-15 sec
Activated partial thromboplastin time	Assessment of intrinsic coagulation by measuring factors I, II, V, VIII, IX, X, XI, XII; longer with use of heparin	30-45 sec
Bleeding time	Measurement of time small skin incision bleeds, reflection of ability of small blood vessels to constrict	1-6 min
Thrombin time	Reflection of adequacy of thrombin, prolonged thrombin time indication that coagulation is inadequate secondary to decreased thrombin activity	8-12 sec
Fibrinogen	Reflection of level of fibrinogen; increase in fibrinogen possible indication of enhancement of fibrin formation, making client hypercoagulable; decrease in fibrinogen indication that client possibly predisposed to bleeding	200-400 mg/dl
Fibrin split products	Reflection of degree of fibrinolysis, reflection of excessive fibrinolysis and predisposition to bleed (if present), possible indication of disseminated intravascular coagulation	<10 mg/l
Protamine sulfate tests	Reflection of presence of fibrin monomer (portion of fibrin remaining after elements that polymerize and stabilize clot detach), positive test indication of predisposition to bleed and possible presence of disseminated intravascular coagulation	Negative

those that occur when the fluid volume is excessive. Increases in hemoglobin are found in polycythemia or in states of hemoconcentration, which can develop from volume depletion.

The *hematocrit (Hct)* value is determined by spinning blood in a centrifuge, which causes erythrocytes and plasma to separate. The erythrocytes, being the heavier elements, settle to the bottom. Reductions and elevations of hematocrit value are seen in the same conditions that raise and lower the hemoglobin value. The hematocrit value generally equals 3 times the hemoglobin value.

The *total RBC count* is reported as RBC $\times$ 10^6 (million). However, total RBC count is not always reliable in determining the adequacy of RBC function. Consequently, other data, such as hemoglobin, hematocrit, and RBC indices, must also be evaluated. The RBC count is altered by the same conditions that raise and lower the hemoglobin and hematocrit values.[8]

RBC indices are special indicators that reflect RBC volume, color, and saturation. These parameters may provide insight into the cause of anemia. (The significance of these parameters is discussed further in Chapter 25.)

White blood cells. The *white blood cell differential* is of considerable significance because it is possible for the total WBC count to remain essentially normal despite a marked change in one type of leukocyte. For example, a client may have a normal WBC count of 8800/μl while the differential count may show a relative proportion of lymphocytes to be 10%. This is an abnormal finding that warrants further investigation.

An important concept related to neutrophil counts is the shift to the left. When infections are severe, more granulo-cytes are released from the bone marrow as a compensatory mechanism. To meet the increased demand, many young, immature PMNs or bands are seen. The usual laboratory procedure is to report the WBCs in order of maturity (see Fig. 24-1), with the less mature forms on the left side of the written report. Consequently, the existence of many immature cells is referred to as a *shift to the left*.

Platelet count. Bleeding may occur when platelet counts are depressed, a condition known as *thrombocytopenia*. If platelets are functioning properly, most hematologists believe that clients can undergo necessary surgery with platelet counts as low as 50,000/μl (normal count is 150,000 to 400,000/μl). Once platelet counts drop to between 20,000 and 30,000/μl, spontaneous hemorrhage is probable. When platelets are depressed to 10,000/μl, the possibility of intracerebral hemorrhage is significantly increased. Clotting studies are presented in Table 24-6.

Erythrocyte sedimentation rate. Increased erythrocyte sedimentation rates (ESR, or sed rate) are common during acute and chronic inflammatory reactions when cell destruction is increased. They are also found in persons with malignancy, myocardial infarction, and end-stage renal disease. Although the sedimentation rate is a very nonspecific test, it is often used as a routine screening procedure.

Blood typing and Rh factor. Blood group antigens (A and B) are found on RBC membranes and form the basis for the ABO blood typing system. The presence or absence of one or both of the two inherited antigens is the basis for the four blood groups: A, B, AB, and O. Blood group A has A antigens, group B has B antigens, group AB has both antigens, and group O has neither A nor B antigens. Each person has antibodies in the serum called *anti-A* and *anti-B* that react with A or B antigens. These antibodies are found when the corresponding antigen is absent from the RBC surface. For example, B antibodies are found in persons with blood group A (Table 24-7).

Blood reactions based on ABO incompatibilities result from intravascular hemolysis of the RBCs. Erythrocytes agglutinate when a serum antibody is present to react with the antigens on the RBC membrane. Therefore agglutination occurs in group A blood when B antigens are introduced. The anti-B antibodies will react with the B antigen, thus initiating the process that results in RBC hemolysis.

The Rh system is based on a third antigen, D, which is also found on the RBC membrane. Rh-positive persons have the D antigen, whereas Rh-negative persons do not. About 85% of persons are Rh positive and 15% are Rh negative. As a result of transfusion therapy or during childbirth, an Rh-negative person may be exposed to Rh-positive blood. Such exposure results in formation of an antibody, anti-D, which acts against Rh antigens. (Rh-positive persons normally have no anti-D.) The person is then sensitized to Rh-positive blood, and a second exposure to Rh-positive blood will cause a severe hemolytic reaction. A Coombs' test can be used to evaluate the person's Rh status (Table 24-8).

Lymphangiography

Lymphangiography is radiological visualization of the lymph system after the injection of dye. The purpose of this procedure is to assess deep lymph nodes. It is particularly useful in detecting lymph node involvement in malignant conditions.

The procedure begins with the intracutaneous injection of a blue dye into the webs of the toes. (It is less commonly done through the hands.) The dye is absorbed by the lymph vessels, making them visible through the skin on the dorsum of the foot. Once visible, the dorsum of

Table 24-7 ABO Blood Group Names and Compatibilities*

Blood Group	RBC Agglutinogen(s)	Serum Agglutinin(s)	Compatible Donor Blood Groups	Incompatible Donor Blood Groups
A	A	Anti-B	A and O	B and AB
B	B	Anti-A	B and O	A and AB
AB	A and B	Neither	A, B, AB, and O	None
O	Neither (universal donor)	Anti-A and anti-B	O	A, B, and AB

*ABO blood groups are named for the antigen found in the RBCs. Compatibility is based on the antibodies present in the serum.

Table 24-8 Miscellaneous Laboratory Blood Studies

Study	Description and Purpose	Normal Values
ESR	Measurement of RBCs that settle to bottom of test tube in 1 hr; certain blood elements, especially protein, possibly affecting results	Women: 1-20 mm in 1 hr Men: 1-15 mm in 1 hr
Reticulocyte count	Measurement of immature RBCs, reflection of bone marrow activity in producing RBCs	0.5%-1.5% of RBC count
Bilirubin	Measurement of degree of RBC hemolysis or liver's inability to excrete normal quantities of bilirubin, increase in indirect bilirubin with hemolytic problems	Total: 0.3-1.3 mg/dl Direct: 0.1-0.3 mg/dl Indirect: 0.1-1.0 mg/dl
Iron		
Serum iron	Reflection of amount of iron combined with proteins in serum, accurate indication of status of iron storage and use	50-150 µg/dl
Total iron-binding capacity	Measurement of percentage of saturation of transferrin, a protein that binds iron; evaluation of amount of extra iron that can be carried	250-410 µg/dl
Coombs' test	Differentiation among types of hemolytic anemias, detection of immune antibodies	
Direct	Detection of antibodies that are attached to RBCs	Negative
Indirect	Detection of antibodies in serum	Negative

each foot is injected with a local anesthetic agent, and a small superficial incision is made over the lymph vessels. The lymph vessel is then cannulated with a very small needle. Once the needle is inserted, it is important that clients not move their feet to avoid the possibility of dislodging the needle. When the lymph vessels are cannulated, a radiopaque oil is injected very slowly by means of an automated pump. The usual dose of oil for adults is 7 ml in each foot administered over 45 to 60 minutes. Fluoroscopy may be used during the injection to watch the filling of the lymph vessels. Immediately after the dye has been injected, several radiographs will be taken from various angles. A second set of radiographs will be taken the next day when the lymph channels are emptied. The incisions on the feet are sutured closed when the procedure is complete.

The lymph nodes can also be seen by means of isotopic (technetium 99m) lymphangiography. Compared with radiographical lymphangiography, isotopic lymphangiography is less invasive and does not require dye injection. However, the isotope's short life prevents serial studies.

Nursing responsibilities related to lymphangiography and other common studies of the hematological system are presented in Table 24-9.

Biopsies

Biopsy procedures specific to hematological assessment are bone marrow examination and lymph node biopsy. In

Table 24-9

Diagnostic Studies of the Hematological System

Study	Description and Purpose	Nursing Responsibility
URINE STUDIES		
Bence Jones protein	An electrophoretic measurement is used to detect the presence of the Bence Jones protein, which is found in most cases of multiple myeloma. Negative finding indicates that client is normal.	Acquire random urine specimen.
RADIOISOTOPE STUDIES		
Spleen scan	Radioactive isotope is injected intravenously. Images from the radioactive emissions are used to evaluate the structure of the spleen. Client is not source of radioactivity.	No specific nursing responsibilities.
Bone scan	Same procedure as for the spleen scan, except used for the purpose of evaluating the structure of the bones.	No specific nursing responsibilities.
Isotopic lymphangiography	Radionuclide study is used to assess lymph nodes and lymph system. Technetium 99m is used. Technique is less invasive than radiographic lymphangiography.	No specific nursing responsibilities.
RADIOLOGICAL STUDIES		
Lymphangiography	Purpose is to evaluate deep lymph nodes. Radiopaque oil-based dye is infused slowly into the lymph vessels via small needles in the dorsum of each foot. Radiographs are taken immediately and on next day.	Inform the client about what to anticipate. Obtain consent form. Assess for iodine sensitivity. Give preoperative sedation, if indicated. Instruct client that urine will be blue from the dye excretion for 1-2 days. Inform client that transient fever, general malaise, and diffuse muscle aches may be experienced for 12 to 24 hr. Watch for signs of oil embolus to lungs (hacking cough, dyspnea, pleuritic pain, and hemoptysis).

Continued.

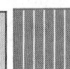

Table 24-9

Diagnostic Studies of the Hematological System—cont'd		
Study	**Description and Purpose**	**Nursing Responsibility**
RADIOLOGICAL STUDIES—cont'd		
Computerized tomography	Noninvasive radiological examination using computer-assisted x-ray study evaluates the spleen, liver, or lymph nodes.	No specific nursing responsibilities.
Magnetic resonance imaging	Noninvasive procedure produces sensitive images of soft tissue without using contrast dyes. No ionizing radiation is required. Technique is used to evaluate spleen, liver, and lymph nodes.	Instruct client to remove all metal objects and ask about any history of surgical insertion of staples, plates, or other medical appliances.
BIOPSIES		
Bone marrow	Technique involves removal of bone marrow through a locally anesthetized site to evaluate the status of the blood-forming tissue. It is indicated in diagnosis of multiple myeloma, all types of leukemia, and some lymphomas. It is also done to assess efficacy of leukemic therapy.*	Explain procedure to client. Obtain signed consent form. Consider pre-procedure analgesic administration to enhance client comfort and cooperation. Apply pressure dressing after procedure. Assess biopsy site for bleeding.
Lymph node biopsy	Purpose is to obtain lymph tissue for histological examination to determine diagnosis and therapy.	Explain procedure to client. Obtain signed consent form. Use sterile technique in dressing changes after procedure. Carefully evaluate wound for healing. Assess client for complications, especially bleeding.
Open	Test is performed in operating room with direct visualization of the area.	
Closed (needle)	Test is performed at bedside.	
BLOOD STUDIES†	—	—

*See Chapter 25.
†See Tables 24-4, 24-6, and 24-8.

general, these procedures are done when a diagnosis cannot be established from a peripheral blood smear or when more information about the possible hematological problem is needed.

Bone marrow examination. Bone marrow examination is important in the evaluation of many hematological disorders. It involves the aspiration and/or biopsy of bone marrow with a syringe and needle. The aspirate is made into smears that are useful for cytological diagnosis.

The site of bone marrow aspiration is determined by the age of the client and the skill of the physician or specially credentialed nurse. In adults, the sites most easily aspirated are the anterior and posterior iliac crests. The tibia may provide an additional site in young children. Although hazards of bone marrow aspiration are minimal, there is a possibility of penetrating the bone and damaging underlying structures.

The skin over the puncture site is cleansed with a bactericidal agent. The skin, subcutaneous tissue, and periosteum are infiltrated with a local anesthetic agent. The client may be uncomfortable when the periosteum is infiltrated. Once the area is anesthetized, the special marrow needle is inserted through the cortex of the bone. The stylet of the needle is then removed, the hub is attached to a 10 ml syringe, and 0.2 to 0.5 ml of the fluid marrow is aspirated. The aspiration is experienced by the client as a suction pain, which may be quite uncomfortable but lasts for only a few seconds.

After the marrow aspiration, the needle is removed. Pressure is applied over the aspiration site to ensure hemostasis. If the client is thrombocytopenic, pressure may be required for 5 to 10 minutes or longer.

If a bone biopsy is required, the preparatory procedure remains the same, but a different needle is used. The needle has a cutting blade that allows a specimen of the bone to be removed. When either a marrow aspirate or a biopsy specimen is acquired, a glass slide is carefully prepared with a thin film of the marrow.

Lymph node biopsy. Lymph node biopsy involves obtaining lymph tissue for histological examination to determine the diagnosis and therapy. This may be accomplished by either an open biopsy or a needle (closed) biopsy. In the open biopsy procedure an incision is made and the lymph node and surrounding tissue are dissected whenever possible. Care must be taken because neoplastic cells can be disseminated during the biopsy procedure if the knife passes through tissues containing cancerous cells. An open biopsy may be performed with local or general anesthesia in the operating room.

A needle or closed biopsy may also be performed to analyze lymph tissue. This bedside technique is performed by a skilled physician. Sterile technique is essential throughout the procedure. Nursing personnel must recognize the possibility of insidious bleeding, and direct pressure should be applied after the biopsy procedure to achieve hemostasis. Personnel should continue to observe the site for bleeding, and vital signs should be monitored. The sterile dressing should be changed as ordered and the wound inspected for healing. It is important to recognize that if a needle biopsy is negative, it may signify only that the cancer cells were not a part of the tissue in the biopsy specimen. However, a positive finding is sufficient evidence for confirming a diagnosis.

R eview Questions

The number of the question corresponds to the same-numbered objective at the beginning of the chapter.

1. An important function of the spleen in the adult is
   a. RBC production
   b. monocyte production
   c. removal of defective erythrocytes
   d. platelet production
2. Which of the following are both types of granulocytes?
   a. basophils and neutrophils
   b. monocytes and eosinophils
   c. thrombocytes and lymphocytes
   d. erythrocytes and eosinophils
3. Which of the following substances are necessary for converting prothrombin to thrombin?
   a. fibrinogen and factor IX
   b. thromboplastin and calcium
   c. platelet factor III and factor V

d. fibrin-stabilizing factor and sodium
4. Which of the following information obtained from the health history has a significant relationship to the hematological system?
   a. multiple pregnancies
   b. early menopause
   c. jaundice
   d. bladder surgery
5. Which of the following statements accurately describes the technique to palpate lymph nodes?
   a. gentle, firm pressure should be applied to deep lymph nodes
   b. normally, superficial lymph nodes are not palpable
   c. the index and third fingers should lightly palpate superficial lymph nodes
   d. the tips of the second, third, and fourth fingers should apply firm pressure for palpation
6. Which of the following is considered a normal finding of the lymph node examination?
   a. shotty nodes
   b. firm, tender nodes
   c. hard, fixed nodes
   d. mobile, hard nodes
7. Which of the following is an important nursing responsibility following lymphangiography?
   a. apply pressure dressing to biopsy site
   b. take precautions for isotope elimination
   c. immobilize lower extremities for 24 hours
   d. instruct client that urine may be blue

REFERENCES

1. McKenzie SB, ed: Textbook of hematology, Philadelphia, 1988, Lea & Febiger.
2. Thorup OA, ed: Leavell and Thorup's fundamentals of clinical hematology, Philadelphia, 1987, WB Saunders Co.
3. Pittiglio DH and Sacher RA, eds: Clinical hematology and fundamentals of hemostasis, Philadelphia, 1987, FA Davis Co.
4. Williams WJ, ed: Hematology in the aged, New York, 1990, McGraw-Hill Book Co, pp 112-114.
5. Griffin JP: Hematology and immunology: concepts for nursing, Norwalk, Conn, 1986, Appleton-Century-Crofts, pp 19-23.
6. McConnell EA: Getting the feel of lymph node assessment, Nursing 18:54-57, 1988.
7. Powers LW: Diagnostic hematology: clinical and technical principles, St Louis, 1989, The CV Mosby Co.
8. Tilkian SM, Conover MB, and Tilkian AG: Clinical implications of laboratory tests, St Louis, 1987, The CV Mosby Co, pp 396-440.

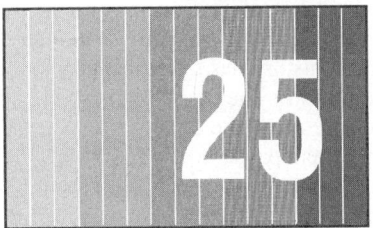

CHAPTER

25

Nursing Role in Management

Hematological Problems

Bonnie Mowinski Jennings

L *earning Objectives*

1. *Describe the general clinical manifestations and complications of anemia.*
2. *Differentiate between the etiological and morphological classifications of anemia.*
3. *Describe the causes, specific clinical manifestations, diagnostic findings, and therapeutic and pharmacological management of iron-deficiency anemia, pernicious anemia, and sickle cell anemia.*
4. *Explain the nursing management of anemia.*
5. *Describe the pathophysiology, clinical manifestations, and therapeutic and nursing management of polycythemia vera.*
6. *Compare and contrast the pathophysiology, clinical manifestations, and therapeutic management for idiopathic thrombocytopenic purpura and acquired thrombocytopenia.*
7. *Explain the nursing management of thrombocytopenia.*
8. *Describe the types, clinical manifestations, diagnostic findings, and therapeutic and nursing management of hemophilia.*
9. *Explain the pathophysiology, diagnostic findings, and therapeutic and nursing management of disseminated intravascular coagulation.*

10. *Describe the common causes, clinical manifestations, and therapeutic and nursing management of granulocytopenia.*
11. *Compare and contrast the major types of leukemia in regard to age at onset and distinguishing clinical and laboratory findings.*
12. *Explain the rationales for induction and maintenance chemotherapy and combination chemotherapy.*
13. *Describe the nursing management of the client with leukemia.*
14. *Differentiate between Hodgkin's and non-Hodgkin's lymphomas in terms of clinical manifestations, staging, and therapeutic and nursing management.*
15. *Describe the pathophysiology, clinical manifestations, and therapeutic and nursing management of multiple myeloma and mononucleosis.*
16. *Differentiate between splenomegaly and hypersplenism in terms of etiology and therapeutic management.*
17. *Describe the nursing management of the client receiving blood transfusions.*

The purpose of this chapter is to provide information on red blood cell abnormalities, clotting disorders, white blood cell abnormalities, lymph system disturbances, and spleen disorders.

The opinions and assertions in this chapter are the views of the author and are not to be construed as official or as reflecting the views of the Department of the Army or the Department of Defense.
Reviewed by Carol S. Dolan, R.N., M.S.N., O.C.N., Manager and Director, Nursing Services, University of New Mexico Cancer Center, Albuquerque, New Mexico.

664

ANEMIA
Definition and Classification

Anemia is a reduction below normal in the number of erythrocytes, the quantity of hemoglobin, and the volume of packed red cells (hematocrit) caused by rapid loss, impaired production of erythrocytes, and increased destruction of erythrocytes. Because red blood cells (RBCs) transport oxygen (O_2), a deficit in erythrocytes leads to tissue hypoxia. This hypoxia accounts for most of the clinical manifestations of anemia. Anemia is not a specific disease but a manifestation of a pathological process. Anemia is

Table 25-1 Etiological Classification of Anemia

DECREASED ERYTHROCYTE PRODUCTION

Decreased hemoglobin synthesis
    Iron deficiency
    Thalassemias (decreased globin synthesis)
    Sideroblastic anemia (decreased porphyrin)
Nuclear cytoplasmic defects (DNA)
    Vitamin B_{12} deficiency (pernicious anemia)
    Folic acid deficiency
Decreased number of erythrocyte precursors
    Hypoplastic anemia
    Marrow infiltration (leukemia, lymphoma, myelofibrosis)
    Chronic disease

BLOOD LOSS

Acute
    Trauma
    Blood vessel rupture
Chronic
    Gastrointestinal
    Menstrual flow

INCREASED ERYTHROCYTE DESTRUCTION*

Intrinsic
    Abnormal hemoglobin (HbS—sickle cell anemia)
    Defective glycolysis with enzyme involvement
    Membrane abnormalities (paroxysmal nocturnal hemo-
        globinuria)
Extrinsic
    Physical trauma (prosthetic heart valves, extracorpo-
        real circulation)
    Antibodies (isoimmune and autoimmune)
    Infectious agents and toxins (malaria)

---

*Hemolytic anemias.

Table 25-2 Relationship of Morphological Classification and Etiologies of Anemia

Morphology	Etiology
Normocytic, normochromic	Acute blood loss, hemolysis, chronic renal disease, cancers, sideroblastic anemia, refractory anemia, diseases of endocrine dysfunction, hypoplastic anemia, pregnancy
Macrocytic, normochromic	Pernicious anemia, folic acid deficiency, liver disease (including effects of alcohol abuse), postsplenectomy
Microcytic, normochromic	Chronic disease
Microcytic, hypochromic	Iron-deficiency anemia, thalassemia, lead poisoning

identified by laboratory evaluation. In addition, further investigation must be done to determine its cause.[1]

Anemia may result from primary hematological problems or may develop as a secondary consequence of defects in other body systems. The many kinds of anemia can be grouped according to either a *morphological* or an *etiological classification*. Morphological classification is based on descriptive, objective laboratory information about erythrocyte size and color. (The terms used in this classification system are explained in Chapter 24.) Etiological classification is related to the clinical conditions causing the anemia, such as decreased erythrocyte production, blood loss, and increased erythrocyte destruction (Table 25-1). Although the morphological system is the most accurate means of classifying anemias, it is easier to discuss client care by focusing on the etiological problem. Table 25-2 states morphological classifications to various etiologies.

Mechanisms to Compensate for Hypoxia

Regardless of the source of anemia, the deficit in erythrocytes reduces the blood's O_2-carrying capacity, which leads to tissue hypoxia. The physiological effects of anemia are stimulated by tissue hypoxia and activation of physiological compensatory mechanisms that attempt to meet cellular O_2 needs.

The four major compensatory responses for anemia include the following:

1. A shift of the oxygen-hemoglobin dissociation curve to the right, thereby facilitating removal of more O_2 by the tissues at the same partial pressure of O_2 (Fig. 25-1)
2. Redistribution of blood by an automatic physiological process that diverts the blood away from tissues that have an abundant blood supply but a low O_2 requirement (e.g., skin) to tissues that have higher O_2 needs (e.g., brain, muscle, myocardium)
3. Increased cardiac output achieved by increased heart rate or increased stroke volume to meet O_2 demands of the tissues as the severity of the anemia increases
4. Increased rate of erythrocyte production within 4 to 5 days after erythropoietin production has increased in response to tissue hypoxia

Clinical Manifestations

The clinical manifestations of anemia are primarily due to the body's response to hypoxia. The intensity of the manifestations varies depending on the severity of the anemia and the presence of coexisting diseases. The severity of anemia may be determined by the hemoglobin (Hb) levels. *Mild* states of anemia (Hb 10 to 14 g/dl) may exist without causing symptoms. If symptoms develop, they are usually attributed to an underlying disease or a compensatory response to heavy exercise. Cardiopulmonary adaptations to exercise include palpitations, dyspnea, and diaphoresis. In cases of *moderate* anemia (Hb 6 to 10 g/dl), the cardiopulmonary symptoms are increased with chronic fatigue during rest as well as activity. Clients with *severe* anemia (Hb less than 6 g/dl) display many clinical manifestations involving multiple body systems (Table 25-5).

Table 25-3   Clinical Manifestations of Anemia

Body System	Severity of Anemia		
	Mild (Hb 10-14 g/dl)	**Moderate (Hb 6-10 g/dl)**	**Severe (Hb < 6 g/dl)**
Integument	None	None	Pallor, jaundice, pruritus
Eyes	None	None	Icteric conjunctiva and sclera, retinal hemorrhage, blurred vision
Mouth	None	None	Glossitis, smooth tongue
Cardiovascular	Palpitations	Increased palpitations	Tachycardia, increased pulse pressure, systolic murmurs, intermittent claudication, angina, congestive heart failure, myocardial infarction
Pulmonary	Exertional dyspnea	Dyspnea	Tachypnea, orthopnea, dyspnea at rest
Neurological	None	None	Headache, vertigo, irritability, depression, impaired thought processes
Gastrointestinal	None	None	Anorexia, hepatomegaly, splenomegaly
Musculoskeletal	None	None	Bone pain
General	None	Fatigue	Sensitivity to cold, weight loss, lethargy

Hb, Hemoglobin.

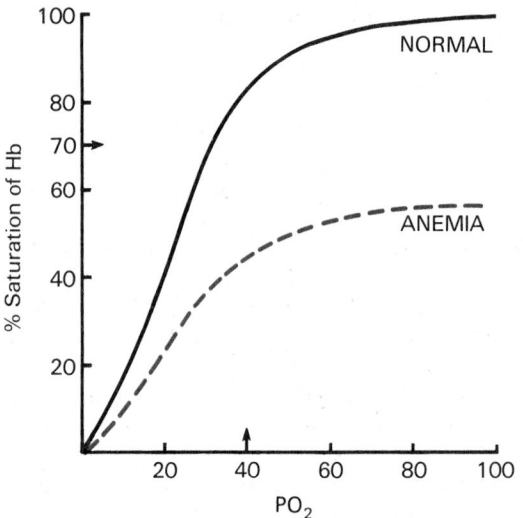

Fig. 25-1   Oxygen-hemoglobin dissociation curve. The oxygen-hemoglobin curve of a normal person *(solid line)* with hemoglobin of 15 g/dl compared to that of a person with anemia *(dashed line)* with hemoglobin of 6 g/dl. The shift to the right seen with the anemic person is a compensatory mechanism. While the O_2 transport capability of hemoglobin is decreased with the shift to the right, hemoglobin release of O_2 to the tissues is facilitated; that is, hemoglobin gives up O_2 more readily when the curve shifts to the right.

Integumentary changes. Integumentary changes may be reflected as pallor, jaundice, and pruritus. The pallor results from reduced amounts of hemoglobin and reduced blood flow to the skin. Jaundice occurs when the skin is stained by bile pigment, which increases from hemolysis of RBCs. Pruritus occurs because of increased serum and skin bile salt concentrations. In addition to the skin, the sclera of the eyes and mucous membranes should be evaluated for jaundice because they reflect the integumentary changes more accurately.

Cardiopulmonary manifestations. Cardiopulmonary manifestations of severe anemia result from additional attempts by the heart and lungs to bring adequate amounts of oxygen to the tissues. Cardiac output is maintained by increasing the pulse rate. The low viscosity of the blood contributes to the development of systolic murmurs and bruits. In extreme cases or when concomitant heart disease is present, angina pectoris and high output failure may occur if myocardial O_2 needs cannot be met. Myocardial infarction (MI) may also occur. Cardiomegaly, pulmonary and systemic congestion, ascites, and peripheral edema may develop as the heart is overworked. The dyspnea of severe anemia demonstrated by the presence of orthopnea and tachypnea is an inappropriate response of the body to hypoxia or hypercapnia. It is inappropriate because the available hemoglobin is already fully saturated with O_2.

■ Nursing Management of Anemia

Nursing assessment
Subjective and objective data that should be obtained from an individual with anemia are presented in Table 25-4.

Nursing diagnoses
Nursing diagnoses specific to the client with anemia include, but are not limited to, those presented in Table 25-5.

Nursing interventions
The numerous causes of anemia necessitate different nursing interventions specific to the needs of the client. Nevertheless, there are certain general components of care that may be required by all clients with anemia. These are stated in the nursing care plan presented in Table 25-4.

Table 25-4

 Nursing Assessment of the Client with Anemia

SUBJECTIVE DATA	OBJECTIVE DATA

SUBJECTIVE DATA

History

Positive family history, race, ethnicity, nutritional status; recent blood loss, surgery, or trauma; chronic liver, endocrine, or renal disease (including dialysis); GI disease (gastrectomy, small bowel resection, malabsorption syndrome, ulcers, gastritis, or hemorrhoids); inflammatory disorders; heavy menses or pregnancy; prosthetic heart valves; exposure to radiation or chemical toxins (arsenic, lead, benzenes, copper)

Medications

Use of vitamin and iron supplements; aspirin, anticoagulants, oral contraceptives, phenobarbital, penicillins, indomethacin, phenacetin, quinine, quinidine, phenytoin (Dilantin), methyldopa (Aldomet), sulfonamides

General

Fatigue, weakness, malaise, vertigo, anorexia, weight loss, night sweats, cold intolerance, depression, frequent infection

Pain

Headache; abdominal, chest, and bone pain; painful tongue

Respiratory

Dyspnea, orthopnea, cough, hemoptysis

Cardiovascular

Palpitations

Gastrointestinal

Nausea and vomiting, flatulence, diarrhea or constipation, dysphagia, dyspepsia, heartburn, tarry stools, pica

Urinary

Hematuria, decreased urinary output

Neurological

Paresthesias of feet and hands; disturbances in vision, taste, or hearing

Musculoskeletal

Muscle weakness and decreased strength

OBJECTIVE DATA

General

Lethargy, apathy, general lymphadenopathy, fever

Integumentary

Pale skin and mucous membranes; blue or pale white sclera; poor skin turgor; brittle, spoon-shaped fingernails; jaundice; petechiae; ecchymoses; nose or gingival bleeding; poor healing; dry, brittle, thinning hair

Respiratory

Tachypnea

Cardiovascular

Tachycardia, systolic murmur, intermittent claudication, ankle edema, dysrhythmias, postural hypotension

Gastrointestinal

Hepatosplenomegaly; glossitis; beefy, red tongue; stomatitis; abdominal distention

Neurological

Confusion, impaired judgment, irritability, ataxia, unsteady gait, paralysis

Possible findings

↓ Hb; ↓ Hct; ↓ serum iron, ferritin, folate, or vitamin B_{12}; guaiac positive stools

ANEMIA DUE TO DECREASED ERYTHROCYTE PRODUCTION

Normally, RBC production is in equilibrium with RBC destruction and loss. This balance is necessary to ensure that an adequate number of erythrocytes are available. RBCs must be replenished because they are viable for only 120 days. Three significant alterations in erythropoiesis may occur that decrease RBC production: (1) decreased hemoglobin synthesis may lead to iron-deficiency anemia, thalassemia, and sideroblastic anemia; (2) defective nuclear cytoplasm of the RBCs may lead to pernicious anemia and folic acid deficiency; and (3) diminished availability of erythrocyte precursors may result in hypoplastic anemias and chronic disease anemias (Table 25-1).

Iron-Deficiency Anemia

Iron-deficiency anemia is one of the most common chronic disorders found in human beings. It is present in 10% to 30% of the population in the United States. This type of anemia is prevalent among the poor and in areas of the world where dietary intake of iron is inadequate. Regardless of economics or geography, iron-deficiency anemia is most common in infants, children, and women who are premenopausal or pregnant.

Iron is present in the body as heme in hemoglobin and in a stored form. The heme in hemoglobin accounts for two thirds of the iron. The other one third of iron is stored as ferritin and hemosiderin in the bone marrow, spleen, and liver. Normally, 1 mg of iron is lost daily through the

Table 25-5

NURSING CARE PLAN FOR THE CLIENT WITH ANEMIA

Defining Characteristics	Nursing Interventions	Evaluation Criteria
NURSING DIAGNOSIS: Activity intolerance related to decreased hemoglobin and imbalance between oxygen supply and demand		
Difficulty in tolerating increased activity subjectively and objectively (increased blood pressure, pulse, respiration), statement of feeling fatigued with minimal exertion	Plan care to alternate periods of rest and activity; strive for a 1:3 rest/activity ratio; assist client with activities of daily living as needed. Place objects within client's reach to reduce physiological demands brought on by exertion. Reduce demands placed on client by limiting visitors, phone calls, noise, interruptions by hospital staff. Monitor vital signs to evaluate activity tolerance (e.g., pulse < 100, respirations ≤ 20).	Feeling of being rested, participation in activities of daily living (e.g., bathing, dressing, grooming, feeding) to greatest extent possible, vital signs within acceptable range
NURSING DIAGNOSIS: Potential complication: hypoxemia related to decreased hemoglobin		
Dyspnea; decrease in O_2 saturation, increase in Pa_{CO_2}, cyanosis	Administer O_2 as ordered. Transfuse with blood products as ordered. Change client's position slowly; evaluate dizziness as sign of cerebral hypoxia. Monitor hemoglobin.	Normal hemoglobin values, resolution of hypoxemia, heart and respiratory rates within normal limits
NURSING DIAGNOSIS: Altered nutrition: less than body requirements related to disease, treatment, and lack of knowledge of adequate nutrition		
Weight loss, low serum albumin, weight below normal for height, weakness, poor color and skin turgor, inadequate diet	With input from client, establish range of optimal weight outcomes as well as dietary plan. Teach and monitor use of a food diary. Encourage oral hygiene four times a day or after meals to enhance taste. Precede meals with antacids or other agents as ordered to reduce gastric distress. Teach basics of good nutrition, especially importance of including nutrients needed for RBC production. Provide opportunity for client to make supervised food selections.	Maintenance of weight, then gradual increase within range of ideal; consumption of well-balanced, high-caloric diet; adequate intake of nutrients necessary for RBC production

Table 25-5

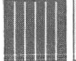

NURSING CARE PLAN FOR THE CLIENT WITH ANEMIA—cont'd

Defining Characteristics	Nursing Interventions	Evaluation Criteria
NURSING DIAGNOSIS: Self-care deficit: partial to total related to weakness and fatigue		
Inability to accomplish part or all of activities of daily living	Assess client's ability to perform activities of daily living. Assist with deficits in self-care. Pace activities and intersperse periods of rest.	Satisfactory completion of activities of daily living independently or with assistance
NURSING DIAGNOSIS: Impaired physical mobility related to immobility and weakness		
Inability to ambulate independently, reluctance to self-mobilize	Assess client's ability to ambulate. Maintain bed rest or assist with ambulation as appropriate. Promote active or passive range of motion as indicated.	Maintenance of joint functioning, increase in mobility as disease resolves
NURSING DIAGNOSIS: Anxiety related to inability to care for self and lack of knowledge of cause of weakness and prognosis		
Frequent questioning about reason for weakness and outcome of disease; restlessness, apathy; concern about ability for self-care	Teach client about causes of weakness and course of disease. Include family in teaching. Answer questions accurately and honestly. Assess need for assistance and help client make realistic plans.	Acceptance of condition, cooperation with plan of care, expression of confidence that needs will be met
NURSING DIAGNOSIS: Altered health maintenance related to lack of knowledge about lifestyle adjustments, appropriate nutrition, and medication regimen		
Questioning about lifestyle adjustments, diet, medication prescriptions	Review and teach client about lifestyle changes and nutrition and medication information. Teach about and monitor response to supplemental drugs that aid in RBC production.	Demonstration of knowledge about lifestyle changes, nutrition and medication regimens
NURSING DIAGNOSIS: High risk of injury: falls related to weakness and dizziness		
Unsteady gait, dizziness when changing positions or ambulating	Teach client to change position slowly. Discourage client from ambulating alone. Assess vital signs before ambulating.	No injuries from falling

Table 25-6 Nutrients Needed for Erythropoiesis

Nutrient	Role in Erythropoiesis	Food Sources
Vitamin B$_{12}$	RBC maturation	Organ and muscle meats, especially liver
Folic acid	RBC maturation	Green leafy vegetables, liver, meat, fish, legumes, whole grains
Iron	Hemoglobin synthesis	Liver and muscle meats, eggs, dried fruits, legumes, dark green leafy vegetables, whole-grain and enriched bread and cereals, potatoes
Vitamin B$_6$	Hemoglobin synthesis	Meats (especially pork and liver), wheat germ, legumes, potatoes, cornmeal, bananas
Amino acids	Synthesis of nucleoproteins	Eggs, meat, milk and milk products (cheese, ice cream), poultry, fish, legumes, nuts
Vitamin C	Conversion of folic acid to its active forms, aid in iron absorption	Citrus fruits, leafy green vegetables, strawberries, cantaloupe

GI tract, sweat, and urine. When the stored supplies of iron are depleted, hemoglobin production is reduced.

Causes. Iron deficiency may develop from inadequate dietary intake, malabsorption, blood loss, chronic fever, or hemolysis. Iron is obtained from foods in our diet. Approximately 1 mg of iron is absorbed from every 10 to 20 mg of iron ingested. Therefore, only about 5% to 10% of the ingested iron is absorbed. This amount of iron is adequate to meet the needs of men and older women, but it is inadequate for those individuals who have higher iron needs (e.g., pregnant women). Table 25-6 lists nutrients needed for erythropoiesis.

Malabsorption of iron is common after certain forms of GI surgery and in malabsorption syndromes. Surgical procedures such as subtotal gastric resection often involve the removal of the duodenum. Iron absorption primarily occurs in the duodenum. Malabsorption syndromes commonly involve disease of the upper small intestine. The absorption of iron is impeded in malabsorption states because the absorptive surface is lost.

Blood loss is a major cause of iron deficiency in adults because 2 ml of blood contain 1 mg of iron. The three major sources of chronic blood loss are GI, genitourinary (GU), and respiratory. GI bleeds are often occult and therefore may exist for a considerable time before the diagnosis is made. From 50 to 75 ml of blood from the upper GI tract is required to cause stools to appear as *melena*. The black color of melena results from the action of intestinal enzymes on the blood. This condition must be differentiated from other causes of black stools, such as excessive iron intake. Common causes of GI blood loss in the adult are peptic ulcer, hiatal hernia, neoplasia, and gastritis. GU blood loss occurs primarily from menstrual bleeding. The average monthly menstrual blood loss is about 45 ml and causes the loss of about 22 mg of iron. Hemoptysis may account for significant blood loss from the respiratory tract. Although hemoptysis may be overt in most clients, individuals can swallow bloody sputum in quantities large enough to show up as occult blood in stools.

Pregnancy contributes to iron deficiency because of the diversion of iron to the fetus for erythropoiesis, blood loss at delivery, and lactation. Iron-deficiency anemia may also develop from intravascular hemolysis of RBCs that may develop from the mechanical trauma of prosthetic heart valves. In addition, dialysis for treatment of chronic renal failure may induce iron-deficiency anemia because of the blood trapped in the equipment used in dialysis.

Clinical manifestations. In the early course of iron-deficiency anemia, the client may be free of symptoms. As the disease becomes chronic, any of the general manifestations of anemia may develop (Table 25-3). There are also some specific clinical symptoms that typify iron-deficiency anemia. Pallor is the most common finding, and *glossitis* (inflammation of the tongue) is the second most general feature in iron-deficiency anemia. Other findings include *cheilitis* (inflammation of the lips) and splenomegaly. In addition, the client may report headache, paresthesias, and a burning sensation of the tongue, all of which are caused by lack of iron in the tissues.

Diagnostic studies. Laboratory abnormalities characteristic of iron-deficiency anemia are presented in Table 25-7. Other diagnostic studies are done to determine the cause of the iron deficiency. For example, endoscopy and radiography may be used to detect GI bleeding.

Therapeutic management. Because anemia is a symptom, the main goal of therapeutic treatment for iron-deficiency anemia is to treat the underlying disease. In addition, efforts are directed toward replacing iron (Table 25-8). This may be done through increasing the intake of iron. If nutrition is adequate, increasing iron intake by dietary means may not be reasonable, since it is difficult for nutritional intake to exceed 7 mg of iron per 1000 kcal without the use of dietary supplements. (A half pound of steak supplies 8 mg of iron.) Consequently, oral or occasionally parenteral iron supplements are generally used. If the iron deficiency is from significant acute blood loss, transfusion of packed RBCs may be required (see p. 708).

Pharmacological management. Oral iron should be used whenever possible because it is inexpensive and con-

Table 25-7 Laboratory Study Findings in Anemias

	Iron Deficiency	Thalassemia Major	Pernicious Anemia	Folic Acid Deficiency	Hypoplastic Anemia	Chronic Disease	Acute Blood Loss	Chronic Blood Loss	Sickle Cell Anemia	G6PD Deficiency	Hemolytic Anemia
Hb	↓	↓	↓	↓	↓	↓	↓	↓	↓	↓	↓
Hct	↓	↓	↓	↓	↓	↓	↓	↓	↓	↓	↓
RBC	↓	↓	↓	↓	↓	↓	↓	↓	↓	↓	↓
MCV	↓	N	↑	↑	N	N	N	↓	N	N	N
MCH	↓	N	N or slight ↓	N or slight ↓	N	N	N	↓	N	N	N
MCHC	↓	N	↑	↑	N	N	N	↓	N	N	N
Retic	N or ↓	↑	↓	N	↓	N	N	N or ↑	↑	↑	↑
Serum iron	↓	↑	N	N	±N	↓	N	↓	N to ↑	N to ↑	↑
TIBC	↑	↑	N	N	±N	↓	N	↓	N to ↓	N to ↓	↓
Bilirubin	N to ↓	↑	N	N	N	±N	N	N to ↓	↑	N to ↑	N to ↑
Sed rate	N or slight ↑	—	—	—	—	↑	—	N or slight ↑	Very ↓	—	—
Platelets	N or ↑	—	↓	—	↓	↑	—	↑	↑	—	—
Other findings	—	—	↓ vitamin B₁₂, positive Schilling's test, achlorhydria	↓ folate	↓ WBC	—	—	—	*	—	—

G6PD, Glucose-6-phosphate dehydrogenase; *Hb*, hemoglobin; *Hct*, hematocrit; *MCV*, mean corpuscular volume; *N*, normal; *MCH*, mean corpuscular hemoglobin; *MCHC*, mean corpuscular hemoglobin concentration; *retic*, reticulocytes; *TIBC*, total iron-binding capacity; *sed rate*, erythrocyte sedimentation rate.
*See Table 25-10.

venient. Many iron preparations are available. Four factors that should be considered in the administration of iron are the following:

1. The dosage should provide 150 to 200 mg elemental iron daily. This can be ingested in three or four daily doses, with each tablet or capsule of the iron preparation containing between 50 and 100 mg of iron. (For example, a 300-mg tablet of ferrous sulfate contains 65 mg of elemental iron.)
2. Iron is best absorbed in an acidic environment. For this reason and to avoid binding the iron with food, iron should be taken about an hour before meals when the duodenal mucosa is most acidic. (Taking iron with orange juice, a form of ascorbic acid, also enhances iron absorption.) Gastric side effects, however, may necessitate ingesting the iron with meals. Enteric coated iron may prove ineffective because the iron may not be released in an area in the intestine that facilitates absorption.
3. Undiluted liquid iron may stain the client's teeth. Therefore it should be diluted and ingested through a straw.
4. Mild GI side effects of iron administration may occur, including pyrosis (heartburn), constipation, and diarrhea. If side effects develop, the dose and type of iron supplement may be adjusted. For example, many individuals who need supplemental iron cannot tolerate ferrous sulfate because of the effects of the sulfate base. However, ferrous gluconate may be

Table 25-8

Diagnostic and Therapeutic Management: Iron-Deficiency Anemia

DIAGNOSTIC

History and physical examination
RBC count, including morphology
Reticulocyte count
Hematocrit and hemoglobin levels
Serum iron
Total iron-binding capacity
Fecal examination for occult blood

THERAPEUTIC

Identification and treatment of underlying cause
Administration of ferrous sulfate 300 mg 3 to 4 times per day
Administration of iron dextran IM or IV
Diet rich in foods containing iron
Transfusion of packed RBC

an acceptable substitute. All clients should know that the use of iron preparations will cause their stools to become black because excess iron is excreted by the GI tract.

In some situations, it may be necessary to administer iron parenterally. Parenteral use of iron is indicated for malabsorption, intolerance of oral iron, a need for iron beyond oral limits, or poor client compliance in taking the oral preparations of iron. Parenteral iron can be given intramuscularly (IM) or intravenously (IV).

Because IM iron solutions may stain the skin, separate needles should be used for withdrawing the solution and for injecting the medication. About 0.4 to 0.5 ml of air should be left in the syringe to clear the iron completely from the syringe.

Iron should be given deep IM in the upper outer quadrant of the buttocks, with a 2- to 3-inch needle with a 19 to 20 gauge. Preferably, no more than 2 ml of iron is given in a single injection. A Z-track technique should be used for injection to prevent leakage of the iron solution to the subcutaneous (SC) tissue. The site should not be massaged after the injection is given.

Nutritional considerations. The client should be taught which foods are good sources of iron (Table 25-6).

■ Nursing Management of Iron-Deficiency Anemia

It is important to recognize groups of individuals who are at an increased risk for the development of iron-deficiency anemia. These include infants, teenage girls, premenopausal and pregnant women, persons from low socioeconomic backgrounds, and individuals suffering from blood loss. Diet teaching, with an emphasis on foods high in iron, is very important for these groups. Supplemental iron is especially important for the pregnant woman.

If anemia is present, it is important to discuss with the client the need for diagnostic studies to identify the cause. Appropriate nursing measures for the client with anemia are presented in Table 25-5. Compliance with dietary and drug therapy needs to be emphasized. The hemoglobin level and RBC count should be reassessed to evaluate the response to therapy. To replenish the body's iron stores, the client should take iron therapy for 2 to 3 months after the hemoglobin level returns to normal. If the hemoglobin level remains low, the client should be reevaluated for the cause of anemia.

Thalassemia

Another cause of decreased erythrocyte production is known as *thalassemia*. As in iron deficiency, it is a disease of inadequate production of normal hemoglobin. (Hemolysis also occurs in thalassemia, but insufficient production of normal hemoglobin is the predominant problem.) In contrast to iron-deficiency anemia in which heme synthesis is the problem, thalassemia involves a problem with the globin protein. Therefore the basic defect of thalassemia is abnormal hemoglobin synthesis.

Etiology. Thalassemias are a group of autosomal recessive genetic disorders commonly found in members of ethnic groups whose origins are near the Mediterranean Sea. Individuals with thalassemia may have a heterozygous or homozygous form of the disease. Persons who are heterozygous have one thalassemic gene and one normal gene. They are said to have *thalassemia minor* or the *thalassemic trait,* which is a mild form of the disease. Homozygous persons have two thalassemic genes, causing a severe condition known as *thalassemia major.*

Clinical manifestations. Clients with thalassemia minor are frequently asymptomatic because they adjust to their gradually acquired chronic state of anemia. Occasionally, splenomegaly may develop in these clients, and mild jaundice may be manifested if malformed erythrocytes are rapidly hemolyzed. Persons who have thalassemia major are pale and display other general symptoms of anemia (see Table 25-3). In addition, they have marked splenomegaly and hepatomegaly. Jaundice from RBC hemolysis is prominent. Chronic bone marrow hypertrophy may cause thickening of the cranium, leading to an appearance resembling Down syndrome. Thalassemia major is a life-threatening disease in which growth, both physical and mental, is often retarded.

Therapeutic management. The diagnostic findings of thalassemia major are summarized in Table 25-7. Thalassemia minor requires no treatment because the body adapts to the reduction of normal hemoglobin. Thalassemia major is usually treated with blood transfusions and folic acid supplementation. There is no medication or diet therapy to treat thalassemia. Transfusions are administered often enough to keep the hemoglobin level at about 10 g/dl. This level is low enough to foster the client's own erythropoiesis without enlarging the spleen. Because RBCs are sequestered in the enlarged spleen, thalassemia may be treated by splenectomy. However, even with therapeutic management, the person with thalassemia major will gradually progress to a fatal outcome.

Pernicious Anemia

Normally, a protein known as *intrinsic factor* is secreted by the parietal cells of the gastric mucosa. Intrinsic factor is required for vitamin B_{12} (extrinsic factor) absorption. Therefore if intrinsic factor is not secreted, vitamin B_{12} cannot be absorbed. (Vitamin B_{12} is normally absorbed in the distal ileum.) In pernicious anemia, gastric secretion of intrinsic factor is defective, thus inhibiting vitamin B_{12} absorption. Although once fatal, pernicious anemia is now very treatable with modern therapy. Currently the term is often used inappropriately for any vitamin B_{12} deficiency. Pernicious anemia is only one cause of vitamin B_{12} deficiency, and the term should be used only to describe the situations in which the gastric mucosa is clearly not secreting intrinsic factor.

One of the functions of vitamin B_{12} is related to deoxyribonucleic acid (DNA) synthesis, which affects erythrocyte production. When DNA synthesis is impaired, defective RBC maturation results. The RBCs are large (macrocytic) and abnormal and are referred to as *megaloblasts*. These RBCs are easily destroyed because of their fragile membranes. Another common cause of megaloblastic anemia is folic acid deficiency (see p. 673).

Etiology. Pernicious anemia is predominantly manifested in persons more than 60 years of age. This condition is always seen in clients who have undergone either total gastrectomy or small bowel resection involving the ileum. It is due to the loss of the mucosal surface that secretes intrinsic factor, either by surgery or because of malabsorption syndromes. Individuals in whom pernicious anemia develops are believed to be genetically predisposed. Currently, the mechanism of converting a genetic predisposition to fully developed pernicious anemia is unknown. An autoimmune reaction against gastric parietal cells has been suggested to account for the gastric atrophy that leads to the development of pernicious anemia. Relatives of persons with pernicious disease show an increased incidence of the disease.

Clinical manifestations. General symptoms of anemia develop because of tissue hypoxia (Table 25-3). A megaloblastic anemia is seen. GI manifestations occur as a result of gastric mucosal changes. These include a sore tongue, anorexia, nausea, vomiting, and abdominal pain. Neurological symptoms may present when the nervous system needs more vitamin B_{12} to function properly. Typical neurological manifestations of the disease involve paresthesias of the feet and hands, reduced vibratory and position senses, muscle weakness, and impaired thought processes. These neurological manifestations help differentiate anemia due to B_{12} deficiency from anemia due to folate deficiency. Because pernicious anemia has an insidious onset, it may take several months for these manifestations to develop.

Diagnostic studies. Pernicious anemia yields laboratory data reflective of megaloblastic anemia (Table 25-7). The erythrocytes appear large (macrocytic) and have abnormal shapes. This structure contributes to the ease of erythrocyte destruction because the cell membrane is very fragile.

When pernicious anemia is suspected, several additional studies are conducted. Serum vitamin B_{12} levels will be reduced below 100 μg. A gastric analysis is done to ascertain the cause of the vitamin B_{12} deficiency. A nasogastric tube is inserted, the client is injected with histamine to stimulate gastric juice secretion, and the gastric juice is aspirated by the nasogastric tube over a period of time. If analysis of the gastric juice reveals achlorhydria (the absence of free hydrochloric acid in a pH never less than 3.5), depressed parietal cell function can be determined. This finding is diagnostic of pernicious anemia.

Another means of assessing parietal cell function is by a Schilling's test. After radioactive vitamin B_{12} is administered to the client, the amount of B_{12} excreted in the urine is measured. Individuals who cannot absorb vitamin B_{12} excrete only a small amount of this radioactive form. The same procedure may be followed with the addition of intrinsic factor parenterally. Absorption of vitamin B_{12} when intrinsic factor is added is diagnostic of pernicious anemia.

Therapeutic and pharmacological management. In addition to identifying and treating the underlying disorder, the treatment of pernicious anemia is based on replacing vitamin B_{12}. Without vitamin B_{12} administration, these persons will die in 1 to 3 years. However, as long as supplemental vitamin B_{12} is used, pernicious anemia will remain in remission.

Parenteral use of vitamin B_{12} (cyanocobalamin or hydroxycobalamin) is the treatment of choice for pernicious anemia. The efficacy of vitamin B_{12} injections in altering the otherwise fatal course of pernicious anemia cannot be overemphasized. The dosage and frequency of vitamin B_{12} administration may vary. A typical administration pattern may be as follows: 200 μg IM daily for 2 weeks, 200 μg IM twice a week for 4 weeks, and 200 μg IM monthly for life.

Nutritional considerations. Regardless of how much vitamin B_{12} is ingested, the client is not able to absorb it due to the lack of intrinsic factor. Therefore dietary management is not a reasonable approach for vitamin B_{12} replacement in pernicious anemia. However the client should be instructed on adequate dietary intake to maintain good nutrition (Table 25-6).

■ Nursing Management of Pernicious Anemia

Because of the familial predisposition involved in pernicious anemia, clients who have a positive family history should be evaluated for symptoms of anemia. Although disease development cannot be prevented, early detection and treatment can lead to reversal of symptoms.

The nursing measures presented in Table 25-5 are appropriate for the client with pernicious anemia. In addition to these measures, the nurse should ensure that injuries are not sustained because of the diminished sensations to heat and pain resulting from the neurological impairment. The client must be protected from burns and trauma. If heat therapy is required, the client's skin must be evaluated at frequent intervals to detect reddening. Irritation from nasogastric tubes and restrictive clothing may not be perceived by the client due to reduced pain sensations.

Ongoing care for the person with pernicious anemia is primarily related to ensuring good client compliance in returning for monthly vitamin B_{12} injections. There must also be careful follow-up to assess for neurological problems. Neurological problems may not be fully corrected even by adequate therapy. Because the potential for gastric carcinoma is increased in pernicious anemia, clients should have frequent and careful follow-up care.

Folic Acid Deficiency

Folic acid deficiency also causes megaloblastic anemia. Folic acid is required for DNA synthesis leading to RBC formation and maturation. Four common causes of folic acid deficiency are the following:

1. Poor nutrition, especially a lack of leafy green vegetables, liver, citrus fruits, yeast, dried beans, nuts, and grains
2. Malabsorption syndromes, particularly small bowel disorders
3. Drugs that impede the absorption and use of folic acid such as methotrexate and oral contraceptives as well as anticonvulsants such as phenobarbital and diphenylhydantoin
4. Alcohol abuse and anorexia

The clinical manifestations of folic acid deficiency are similar to those of pernicious anemia. The disease develops insidiously, and the client's symptoms may be attributed to other coexisting problems such as cirrhosis or esophageal varices. GI disturbances include dyspepsia and a smooth, beefy red tongue. The absence of neurological problems is an important diagnostic finding. This lack of neurological involvement differentiates folic acid deficiency from pernicious anemia.

The diagnostic analysis for folic acid deficiency reveals the laboratory data reflective of megaloblastic anemia (see

Table 25-7). In addition, the serum folate level is less than 4 ng (normal is 7 to 20 ng), the serum vitamin B_{12} level is normal, and the gastric analysis is positive for hydrochloric acid.

Folic acid deficiency is treated by replacement therapy. The usual dose is 1 mg/day by mouth. In malabsorption states, up to 5 mg/day may be required. The duration of treatment depends on the reason for the deficiency. The client should be encouraged to eat foods containing large amounts of folic acid (see Table 25-6).

Hypoplastic Anemia

Hypoplastic (aplastic) anemia is a life-threatening stem cell disorder resulting in a hypoplastic, fatty bone marrow that causes a pancytopenia. Therefore hypoplastic anemia is somewhat of a misnomer in that all marrow elements— erythrocytes, leukocytes, and platelets—are quantitatively decreased, although they are qualitatively normal.

The incidence of hypoplastic anemia is quite low, affecting about 4 persons per 1 million. There are various etiological classifications for hypoplastic anemia, but overall there are three major contributing factors:

1. Idiopathic or unknown reasons for development, which account for about half the cases of hypoplastic anemia
2. Congenital origin due to chromosomal alterations
3. Acquired as a result of exposure to ionizing radiation, chemical agents (e.g., benzene, insecticides, arsenic), viral and bacterial infections (e.g., hepatitis and miliary tuberculosis, respectively), and prescribed medications (e.g., alkylating agents, analgesics, anticonvulsants, antimetabolites, antimicrobials)

Clinical manifestations. Hypoplastic anemia usually develops very insidiously. Clinically, the client may be seen with symptoms caused by suppression of any or all bone marrow elements. General manifestations of anemia such as fatigue and dyspnea as well as cardiovascular and cerebral responses may be seen (see Table 25-3). Clients with granulocytopenia have fever and are susceptible to infection. Thrombocytopenia is manifested by a predisposition to bleed (e.g., petechiae, ecchymoses, nosebleeds).

Diagnostic studies. The diagnosis is confirmed by laboratory studies. Because all marrow elements are affected, hemoglobin, white blood cell (WBC), and platelet values are often decreased in hypoplastic anemia (Table 25-7). However, the RBC indices are normal. The condition is therefore classified as a normocytic, normochromic anemia. The reticulocyte count is low. Other test findings of platelet function, such as the bleeding time, are prolonged.

Hypoplastic anemia can be further evaluated by assessing various iron studies. The serum iron and total iron-binding capacity (TIBC) are elevated as initial signs of erythroid suppression. Bone marrow examination may be done for any anemic state. However, the findings are especially important in hypoplastic anemia because the marrow is hypocellular with increased yellow marrow (fat content), a finding referred to as a *dry tap*.

■ Therapeutic and Nursing Management of Hypoplastic Anemia

Management of hypoplastic anemia is based on identifying and removing the causative agent (when possible) and offering supportive care until the pancytopenia can be treated. Nursing interventions appropriate for the client with anemia are presented in Table 25-5. Nursing care plans for clients with thrombocytopenia and neutropenia are presented in Tables 25-16 and 25-24, respectively. Generally, every effort must be made to prevent complications from infection and hemorrhage.

Although the prognosis of untreated hypoplastic anemia remains poor, advances in medical management have improved client survival. In the past, the disease was fatal in about 75% of clients. Current treatments of choice include bone marrow transplantation and/or immunosuppressive therapy with antithymocyte globulin (ATG).

The treatment of choice for adults under the age of 30 who have human leukocyte antigen (HLA)–matched siblings is allogeneic bone marrow transplantation. The best results occur in younger clients who have not had previous transfusions.[2] Prior transfusions increase the risk of graft rejection.

For adults more than 40 years of age or those without HLA-matched siblings, the treatment of choice is ATG, which is a horse serum containing polyclonal antibodies against human T cells. The rationale for this therapy is that aplastic anemia is an immune-mediated disease. Responses to ATG are usually only partial, but the blood counts are high enough to give the clients a transfusion-free life.[3]

Anemia of Chronic Disease

Anemia may develop in several chronic conditions. In renal disease there is a relationship between the degree of anemia and the severity of uremia. Although several mechanisms may be involved in the development of anemia with renal disease, the primary factor is decreased erythropoietin, which is a hormone made in the kidneys that is necessary for erythropoiesis. With decreased renal function, decreased levels of erythropoietin are produced (see Chapter 41).

Chronic liver disease may also contribute to the development of anemia. Anemia may result from the folic acid deficiencies caused by inadequate nutrition in abusers of alcohol or from blood loss due to chronic gastritis. The use of alcohol itself may reduce erythropoiesis. Anemia may also result from splenomegaly, which is commonly found in advanced stages of cirrhosis (see Chapter 38).

Chronic inflammations and malignant tumors are other conditions in which anemia may be present. The mechanisms involved include increased RBC destruction accompanied by a failure to augment erythropoiesis to compensate for the rise in destruction.

Chronic endocrine diseases may also lead to anemia. Hypopituitary and hypothyroid states both lead to reduced tissue metabolism. Therefore tissue oxygen needs are diminished, leading to a reduced production of erythropoietin by the kidneys. Adrenal hypofunction caused by either adrenalectomy or Addison's disease also evokes an anemic response. This is also believed to result from lowered metabolic requirements and decreased O_2 needs.

ANEMIA DUE TO BLOOD LOSS

Anemia resulting from blood loss may be caused by either acute or chronic problems.

Acute Blood Loss

Acute blood loss occurs as a result of sudden hemorrhage. Causes of acute blood loss include trauma, complications of surgery, and diseases that disrupt vascular integrity. There are two major clinical concerns in such situations. First, there is a sudden reduction in the total blood volume that may lead to hypovolemic shock. Second, if the acute loss is more gradual, the body maintains its blood volume by slowly increasing the plasma volume. Consequently, the circulating fluid volume is preserved, but the number of erythrocytes available to carry O_2 is significantly diminished. For example, there is loss of 25% of the blood volume before the hematocrit level drops below 30.

Clinical manifestations. The clinical manifestations of anemia from acute blood loss are caused by the body's attempts to maintain an adequate blood volume and meet O_2 requirements. Table 25-9 summarizes the clinical manifestations of clients with varying degrees of blood volume loss. It is essential to understand that clinical symptoms are valuable indicators of the degree of blood loss because laboratory data may not accurately reflect the severity of hemorrhage for 2 to 3 days.

The nurse should be alert to the client's expression (verbal or nonverbal) of pain. Internal hemorrhage may cause pain because of tissue distention, organ displacement, and nerve compression. Pain may be localized or referred. In the case of retroperitoneal bleeding, clients may not experience abdominal pain. Instead, they may have numbness and pain in a lower extremity secondary to compression of the lateral cutaneous nerve, which is located in the region

Table 25-9 Clinical Manifestations of Acute Blood Loss

Total Body Volume Lost (%)	Clinical Manifestations
10	None
20	No detectable signs or symptoms at rest, tachycardia and slight postural hypotension with exercise
30	Normal supine blood pressure and pulse at rest, postural hypotension and tachycardia with exercise
40	Blood pressure, central venous pressure, and cardiac output below normal at rest; rapid, thready pulse and cold, clammy skin
50	Shock and potential death

of the first to third lumbar vertebrae. The major complication of acute blood loss is irreversible shock (see Chapter 27).

Diagnostic studies. When blood volume loss is sudden, the body reacts by constricting the vascular space. Also, because plasma volume has not yet had a chance to increase, the loss of RBC mass is not reflected in laboratory data, and the results may seem normal or high for 2 to 3 days. However, once the plasma is replaced by endogenous and exogenous means, the RBC mass is less concentrated. At this time, erythrocytes, hemoglobin, and hematocrit levels are usually low and reflect the blood loss.

Therapeutic management. Therapeutic management is initially concerned with (1) replacing blood volume to prevent shock, and (2) identifying the source of the hemorrhage and stopping the blood loss. IV fluids used in emergencies may be dextran, Hetastarch, albumin, or crystalloid electrolyte solutions such as Ringer's lactate. The amount of infusion varies with the solution used. (Management of shock is discussed in Chapter 27.)

Once volume replacement is established, attention can be directed to correcting RBC loss. The body needs 2 to 5 days to manufacture more RBCs in response to increased erythropoietin. Consequently, blood transfusions may be necessary to achieve an immediate effect. Although whole blood replaces blood volume at the rate of 500 ml/U, 12 to 24 hours must elapse before stable hemoglobin and hematocrit changes are seen. Packed RBCs provide half the volume of whole blood and replace about two times as much hemoglobin as 1 U of whole blood.

The client may also need supplemental iron because the iron supply affects the marrow production of erythrocytes. When anemia exists after acute blood loss, dietary sources of iron will probably not be adequate to maintain iron pools. For every 2 ml of blood lost, 1 mg of iron is also lost. Therefore, oral or parenteral iron preparations are administered.

■ Nursing Management of Acute Blood Loss

In the case of trauma, it may be impossible to prevent the situation leading to the blood loss. For postoperative clients, exact evaluation of blood loss by various drainage tubes and dressings facilitates early assessment of the source of hemorrhage and appropriate treatment.

The nursing care plan in Table 25-5 is relevant to the anemia resulting from acute blood loss. In this situation, blood product replacement is almost certainly necessary (see pp. 707, 709).

Once the source of hemorrhage is identified, blood loss is controlled, and fluid and blood volume are replaced, the anemia should begin to correct itself. There should be no need for long-term treatment of this type of anemia.

Chronic Blood Loss

The sources of chronic blood loss are similar to those of iron-deficiency anemia (e.g., bleeding ulcer, hemorrhoids, menstrual blood loss). The effects of chronic blood loss are usually related to the depletion of iron stores and are usually considered as iron-deficiency anemia.

Management of chronic blood loss anemia involves identifying the source and stopping the bleeding. Supplemental iron may be required. The nursing measures correlate with those presented in Table 25-5 depending on the severity of the anemia.

ANEMIA DUE TO INCREASED ERYTHROCYTE DESTRUCTION

The third major cause of anemia is the destruction or *hemolysis* of RBCs at a rate that exceeds production. Hemolysis may occur because of problems intrinsic or extrinsic to the RBCs. Intrinsic hemolytic anemias result from defects in the RBCs themselves caused by abnormal hemoglobin (e.g., sickle cells), enzyme deficiencies that alter glycolysis (glucose-6-phosphate dehydrogenase [G6PD] deficiency), or RBC membrane abnormalities. Intrinsic hemolytic anemias are usually hereditary. Because defective RBCs are hemolyzed, these clients may benefit from the administration of normal erythrocytes. Extrinsic hemolytic anemias are acquired. The client's RBCs are normal, but damage is caused by external factors such as antibodies, toxins, or mechanical injury (e.g., prosthetic heart valves).

The two sites of hemolysis are classified as *intravascular* or *extravascular*. Intravascular destruction occurs within the circulation; extravascular hemolysis takes place in the macrophages of the spleen, liver, and bone marrow. The spleen is the primary site of the destruction of RBCs that are moderately damaged. Fig. 25-2 indicates the sequence of events involved in extravascular hemolysis.

The client with hemolytic anemia manifests the general symptoms of anemia (see Table 25-3) as well as manifestations specific to this type of anemia. Jaundice is likely because the increased destruction of RBCs causes an elevation in bilirubin levels. The spleen and liver may enlarge because of their hyperactivity, which is related to phagocytosis of the defective erythrocytes. Cholelithiasis may also develop because the excessive bilirubin forms pigmented stones in the gallbladder.

In all causes of hemolysis a major concern of treatment is to maintain renal function. When a RBC is hemolyzed, the hemoglobin molecule is released and cleared by the kidneys. The hemoglobin molecule can obstruct the renal tubule and lead to acute tubular necrosis (see Chapter 41). In addition, excessive amounts of urobilinogen develop from the RBC breakdown and must be cleared by the kidneys.

Sickle Cell Anemia

Sickle cell disease is a very serious disorder that occurs when an abnormal hemoglobin, hemoglobin S (HbS), develops in place of the normal hemoglobin A (HbA). The disease is predominant in blacks, affecting 1 person in 12. It is an incurable type of anemia that is often fatal by middle age.[4] The difficulty with sickle cell anemia is that when deprived of O_2, the HbS assumes various crescent or sickle shapes. Erythrostasis develops when sickled red cells are trapped in small blood vessels. The erythrostasis causes further O_2 deprivation, which potentiates more sickling. The increased concentration of sickle cells makes the circulation more sluggish, thus exerting a profound effect on all major organs. The abnormal shape of the hemoglobin is recognized by the body, and the cell is hemolyzed. Initially the sickling is reversible on reoxygenation but eventually becomes irreversible with cells being hemolyzed.

Etiology. Sickle cell anemia is an autosomal recessive genetic disorder in which the person is homozygous for HbS. Some persons may have *sickle cell trait*, a mild condition that may be asymptomatic. Persons with sickle cell trait are heterozygous, with about one fourth of their hemoglobin in the abnormal S form and three fourths as normal A (Fig. 25-3). *Sickle cell crises* (exacerbations of sickling) develop only if clients become extremely hypoxic.

The mutation that causes HbS to develop involves one amino acid. One valine amino acid is substituted for a glutamic acid. This substitution leads to an abnormal linking reaction that causes the development of deformed crescent-shaped cells when O_2 tension is lowered (Fig. 25-4).

Clinical manifestations. Infants do not manifest symptoms until 6 months of age, at which time most of the fetal hemoglobin (HbF) has been replaced by HbS. Children

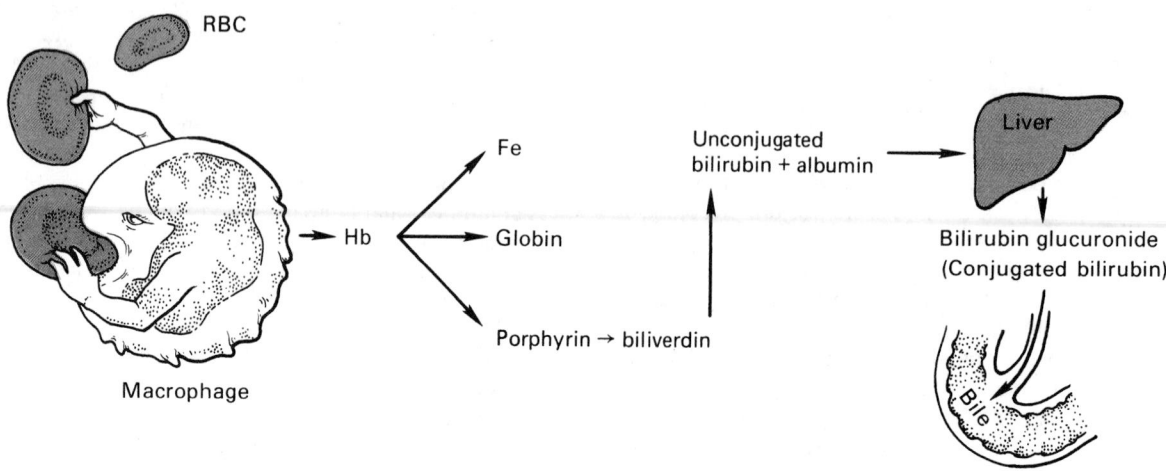

Fig. 25-2 Sequence of events in extravascular hemolysis.

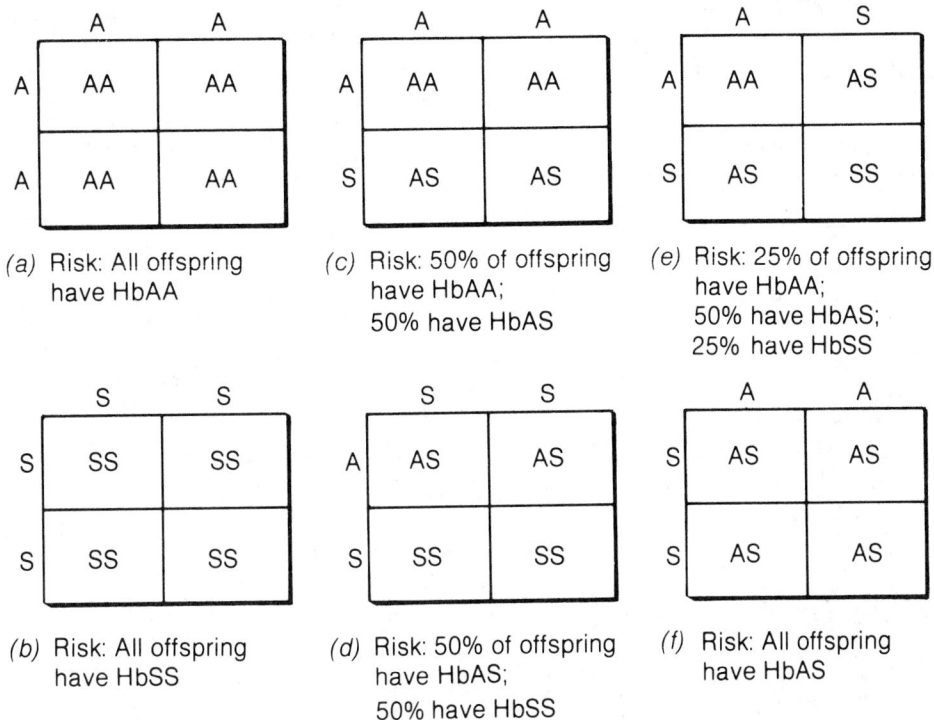

(a) Risk: All offspring have HbAA

(c) Risk: 50% of offspring have HbAA; 50% have HbAS

(e) Risk: 25% of offspring have HbAA; 50% have HbAS; 25% have HbSS

(b) Risk: All offspring have HbSS

(d) Risk: 50% of offspring have HbAS; 50% have HbSS

(f) Risk: All offspring have HbAS

Fig. 25-3 Inheritance patterns of sickle cell disease. The *boxes* represent the possible genetic make-up of children from parents with various genotypes.

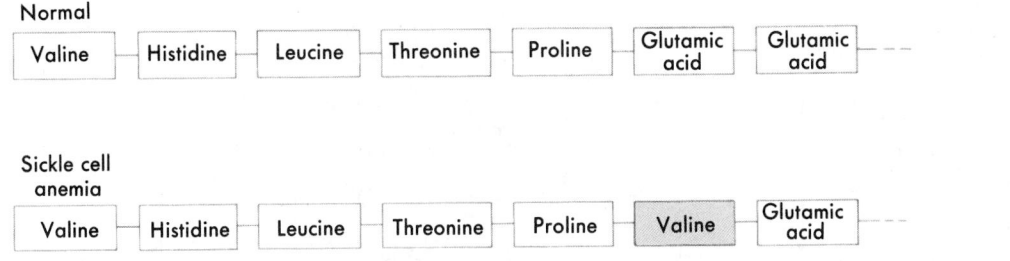

First seven amino acids in normal and sickle cell hemoglobin

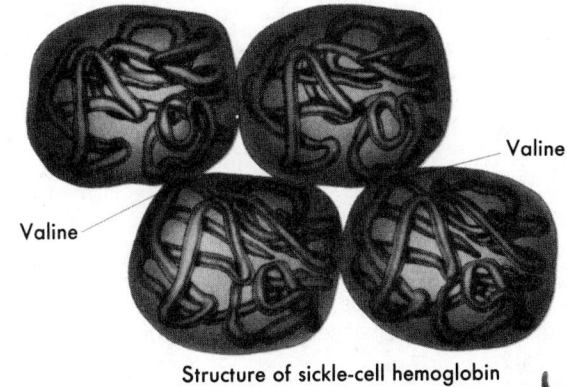

Structure of sickle-cell hemoglobin

Fig. 25-4 Sickle cell hemoglobin is produced by a recessive allele of the gene encoding the β chain of hemoglobin. It represents a single amino acid change from glutamic acid to valine at the sixth position in the chain. In the folded β chain molecule the sixth position contacts the α chain, and the amino acid change causes the hemoglobins to aggregate into long chains, altering the shape of the cell. (From Raven PH and Johnson GB: Biology, ed 2, St Louis, 1989, Times Mirror/Mosby College Publishing.)

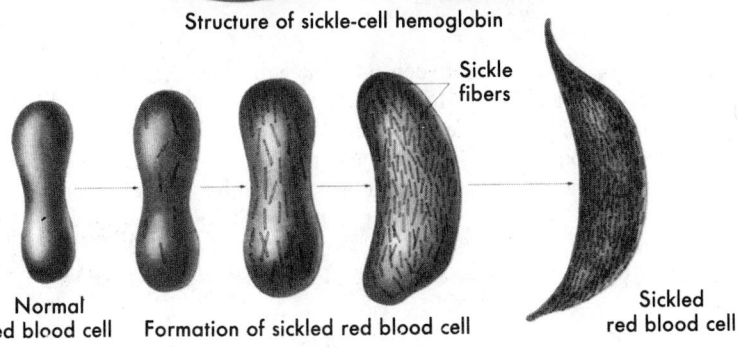

Normal red blood cell   Formation of sickled red blood cell   Sickled red blood cell

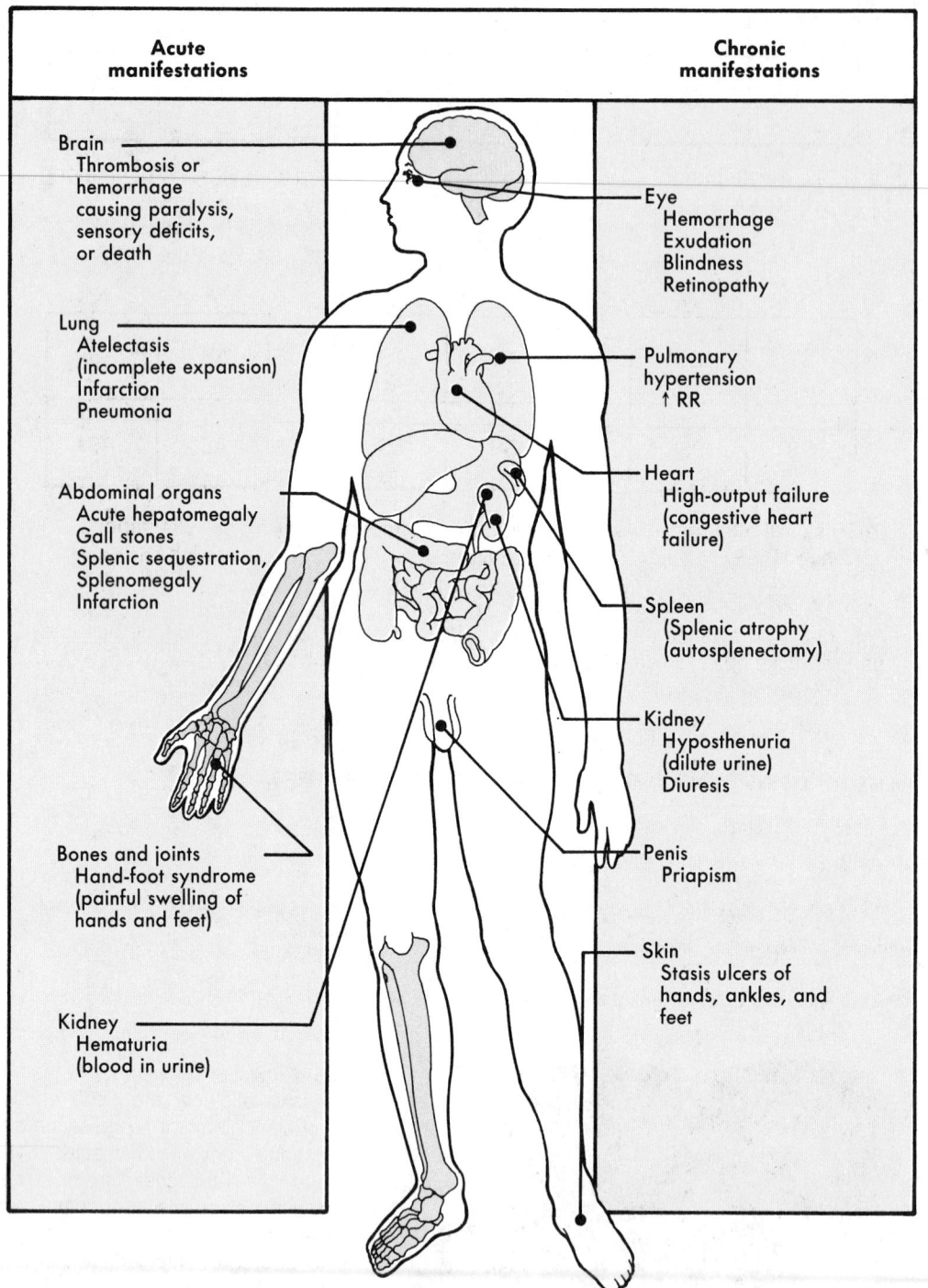

Acute manifestations	Chronic manifestations

Brain
Thrombosis or hemorrhage causing paralysis, sensory deficits, or death

Lung
Atelectasis (incomplete expansion)
Infarction
Pneumonia

Abdominal organs
Acute hepatomegaly
Gall stones
Splenic sequestration,
Splenomegaly
Infarction

Bones and joints
Hand-foot syndrome (painful swelling of hands and feet)

Kidney
Hematuria (blood in urine)

Eye
Hemorrhage
Exudation
Blindness
Retinopathy

Pulmonary hypertension
↑RR

Heart
High-output failure (congestive heart failure)

Spleen
(Splenic atrophy (autosplenectomy)

Kidney
Hyposthenuria (dilute urine)
Diuresis

Penis
Priapism

Skin
Stasis ulcers of hands, ankles, and feet

Fig. 25-5 Clinical manifestations of sickle cell disease. (From McCance KL and Huether SE: Pathophysiology: the biological basis for disease in adults and children, St Louis, 1990, Mosby–Year Book, Inc, p 839.)

manifest a general impairment of growth and development and a failure to thrive (Fig. 25-5). In general, they have an increased susceptibility to infection. One reason for this increased susceptibility is the failure of the spleen to phagocytize foreign substances because of marked impairment of splenic function from fibrosis.

Persons with sickle cell anemia have a severe form of hemolytic anemia. The hemoglobin level usually ranges between 6 and 8 g/dl. The mean RBC survival time is 10 to 15 days. As a result of the accelerated RBC breakdown, the client has characteristic clinical findings of hemolysis (jaundice, elevated serum bilirubin levels, hepatomegaly) and laboratory test results (Table 25-7).

Sickle cell crisis. Sickle cell crisis refers to a syndrome that develops rapidly. The painful crisis is due to an increased rate of sickling. On deoxygenation, the RBC con-

Table 25-10 Laboratory Assessment of Sickle Cell Trait and Sickle Cell Anemia

Study	Description	Sickle Cell Trait	Sickle Cell Anemia
Peripheral smear	Small amount of peripheral blood specimen is smeared on a slide.	Normal	Partially or completely sickled cells
Sickle cell preparation	Blood specimen reaction is observed in hypoxic setting.	Sickle cells	Sickle cells
Sickledex	Blood is mixed with a solution that deoxygenates HbS; this becomes insoluble and causes turbidity. Development of cloudiness is positive for presence of HbS.	Positive	Positive
Hemoglobin electrophoresis	Blood specimen is exposed to electric field and types of hemoglobin are separated.	HbS and HbA	HbS

taining HbS changes from a biconcave disc to an elongated, crescent or sickle cell. These sickling cells clog the small capillaries. The resulting hemostasis promotes a self-perpetuating cycle of local hypoxia, deoxygenation of more erythrocytes, and more sickling. As blood vessels become occluded, thrombosis occurs. This can ultimately lead to necrosis of the infarcted tissue from lack of O_2.

Precipitating factors include conditions that cause hypoxia or deoxygenation of the RBCs, such as viral or bacterial infections, high altitudes, emotional or physical stress, surgery, and blood loss. Crises can also be precipitated by elevated blood viscosity, which may result from dehydration due to vomiting, diarrhea, or diaphoresis. Sometimes the crisis occurs spontaneously, with no apparent precipitating event. The frequency of sickle cell crisis varies. Crises may occur frequently and then may not recur for months or years. The attack may last for 4 to 6 days.

These attacks may appear suddenly and affect various parts of the body, especially the chest, abdomen, bones, and joints. Organs that have a high need for O_2 are most immediately affected and form the basis for many of the complications of sickle cell disease. The heart may become ischemic and enlarged, leading to electrocardiographic changes. Pulmonary infarctions may cause chest pain and ultimately lead to cor pulmonale. The kidneys may be injured from the increased blood viscosity as well as the lack of O_2. Splenic enlargement is not common in adults because the spleen is usually fibrosed from prior episodes of thrombosis. However, hepatomegaly is a frequent finding. Bone changes may include osteoporosis and, after infarction, osteosclerosis. Aching in the joints, especially those of the hands and feet, is a common complaint. Chronic leg ulcers may result from the hypoxia and are especially prevalent around the ankles.

Sickle cell crises may occasionally involve the central nervous system (CNS). Clients may present with seizures or impaired consciousness. Although these crises may be fatal, they are usually reversible.

Additional symptoms may develop during the crises that complicate sickle cell anemia. These symptoms are related to pain and aplasia. The pain may occur spontaneously or may be precipitated by infection and cold intolerance. The pain usually begins in the extremities and lasts for 4 to 6 days. Aplastic crises occur when a stressor significantly decreases erythropoiesis. The anemia is therefore exacerbated as hemolysis continues.

Shock is also a possible development in sickle cell crisis. Capillary hypoxia may result in changes in membrane permeability, leading to plasma loss, hemoconcentration, and further circulatory stagnation, causing an increased reduction of the circulating fluid volume.

Diagnostic studies. Differentiating sickle cell trait from sickle cell anemia is essential during the diagnostic workup. Tables 25-7 and 25-10 indicate the significant distinguishing laboratory features. In addition, an IV pyelogram may be done to evaluate the kidneys, and radiographs of the bones may show skeletal changes.

Therapeutic management. Therapeutic care for clients with sickle cell anemia is essentially supportive. There is no treatment specific for the disease. Therapy is usually directed toward alleviating the symptoms due to complications of the disease. For example, chronic leg ulcers may be treated with bed rest, antibiotics, warm saline soaks, mechanical or enzyme debridement, and sterile dressings.

Sickle cell crises usually require hospitalization. O_2 may be administered to alter hypoxia and control sickling. Rest is instituted to reduce metabolic requirements, and fluids and electrolytes are administered to reduce blood viscosity and maintain renal function. Sedatives and analgesics are used to treat pain. Transfusion therapy is indicated when an aplastic crisis occurs.[5]

Because these clients have an increased need for folic acid, it is important for them to obtain daily supplements. Blood transfusions should be used judiciously to treat a crisis. They have little if any role in the treatment between crises. In general, iron therapy is not indicated.

■ Nursing Management of Sickle Cell Anemia

Because of the hereditary nature of sickle cell disease, genetic counseling is the only form of prevention. For genetic counseling to be effective, screening must be done to detect those persons who have sickle cell trait. Otherwise, its mild effects may go unrecognized.

The basic care for clients with sickle cell anemia is discussed in Table 25-5. Long-term care for these clients is also of great importance. Long-term management is based mostly on client education. Clients and their families must understand the basis of the disease and the reasons for supportive care. Clients must be taught ways to avoid crises. These include taking steps to reduce the chance of developing hypoxia, such as avoiding high altitudes, and seeking medical attention quickly to counteract problems such as upper respiratory tract infections.[6] Education on pain control is also needed, since the pain during a crisis may be severe and often requires considerable analgesia.

G6PD Deficiency

G6PD is an RBC enzyme that acts as the initial catalyst in glycolysis. G6PD deficiency is a sex-linked disorder and directly affects the erythrocyte's ability to resist oxidative damage. Consequently, when G6PD is reduced, there is a decrease in glucose use by the RBCs. If erythrocytes are exposed to oxidative foods and drugs, the metabolic needs of RBCs increase. However, the G6PD deficiency interferes with glucose metabolism and leads to damage of older RBCs, which are then destroyed by hemolysis in 7 to 12 days.

G6PD deficiency is relatively common, especially in blacks and in persons with Mediterranean heritage. Hemolytic episodes are triggered by viral and bacterial infections. Drugs and toxins also cause hemolysis in persons deficient in G6PD. Drugs that may cause oxidative problems are antimalarial drugs, sulfonamides, nitrofurantoins, analgesics (e.g., phenacetin), and chloramphenicol.

Generally, the only clinical manifestation and laboratory indication of G6PD deficiency is hemolytic anemia (see Table 25-7). A definitive diagnosis can be made by doing serum assays of the G6PD level.

Managing the hemolysis seen in G6PD deficiency is relatively easy. Because only older RBCs are destroyed by the oxidative agent, the younger cells survive. The cause of the hemolytic reaction must be removed. During the period of acute hemolysis, the client will require rest, adequate hydration, and assessment of kidney function. Attention should be focused on preventing the hemolytic disorders by treating infections promptly and screening black clients for G6PD deficiency before giving an oxidant drug.

Acquired Hemolytic Anemia

Extrinsic causes of hemolysis can be separated into three categories: (1) physical factors, (2) antibodies, and (3) infectious agents and toxins. Physical destruction of RBCs results from the exertion of extreme force on the cells. Traumatic events causing disruption of the RBC membrane include hemodialysis, extracorporeal circulation used in heart-lung bypass, and prosthetic heart valves. In addition, the force needed to push blood through abnormal vessels, such as those that have been burned or affected by angiopathic disease (e.g., diabetes mellitus), may also physically damage RBCs.

Antibodies may destroy RBCs by the mechanisms involved in antigen-antibody reactions. The reactions may be of an *isoimmune* or *autoimmune* type. Isoimmune reactions occur when antibodies develop against antigens from another person of the same species. Blood transfusion reactions typify this response, especially when donor cells are hemolyzed by the recipient's antibodies due to an ABO mismatch. Another isoimmune reaction is known as *hemolytic disease of the newborn* (HDN). In the past this disorder was referred to as *erythroblastosis fetalis*. In this situation, maternal antibodies that have been previously sensitized either through previous pregnancy or transfusion destroy the RBCs of the fetus, resulting in a hemolytic anemia.

Autoimmune reactions result when individuals develop antibodies against their own erythrocytes. Autoimmune hemolytic reactions may be idiopathic, developing with no prior hemolytic history as a result of the immunoglobulin IgG covering the red cells, or *secondary* to other autoimmune diseases (systemic lupus erythematosus, leukemia, lymphoma) or drugs (penicillin, indomethacin, phenylbutazone, phenacetin, quinidine, quinine, and methyldopa).

The third category of acquired hemolytic disorders is caused by infectious agents and toxins. Infectious agents may foster hemolysis in four ways: (1) by invading the red cell and destroying its contents (e.g., parasites such as in malaria); (2) by releasing hemolytic substances (e.g., *Clostridium perfringens*); (3) by generating an antigen-antibody reaction; and (4) by contributing to splenic hypertrophy as a means of increasing the removal of damaged erythrocytes from the circulation.

Various agents may be toxic to RBCs and cause hemolysis. These hemolytic toxins involve chemicals such as oxidative drugs, arsenic, lead, copper, and snake venom.

Treatment and management of acquired hemolytic anemias involve general supportive care until the causative agent can be eliminated or at least rendered less injurious to the erythrocytes. Supportive care may include administering corticosteroids and blood products or removing the spleen. (To compare and contrast the laboratory findings in the various types of anemia, refer to Table 25-7.)

POLYCYTHEMIA

Polycythemia involves the production and presence of increased numbers of circulating erythrocytes. There is usually an associated increase in the blood's hemoglobin concentration. The increase in erythrocytes is so great that blood circulation is impaired as a result of the increased blood viscosity and volume.

Etiology

The two types of polycythemia are polycythemia vera and secondary polycythemia. Their etiologies and pathogenesis differ, although their complications and clinical manifestations are similar. *Polycythemia vera,* also known as *primary polycythemia,* is a neoplastic disease arising from an intrinsic cell defect.[7] The cell defect affects not only erythrocytes but also granulocytes and platelets, leading to increased production of each of these blood elements. The disease develops insidiously and follows a chronic, vacillating course. It develops in clients who are usually more than 50 years of age. From this myeloproliferative disorder, clients experience enhanced blood viscosity and blood volume, as well as congestion of organs and tissues with blood.

The other main type of polycythemia, *secondary polycythemia,* is caused by hypoxia rather than a defect in the RBC itself. Hypoxia stimulates erythropoietin production in the kidney to stimulate erythrocyte production. The need for O_2 may be caused by high altitude, pulmonary disease, cardiovascular disease, alveolar hypoventilation, defective O_2 transport, or tissue hypoxia. Consequently, secondary polycythemia is a physiological response in which the body tries to compensate for a problem rather than a pathological response. (Secondary polycythemia is discussed in Chapter 22.)

Clinical Manifestations and Complications

Circulatory manifestations of polycythemia vera are due to the hypertension caused by the increased blood volume and viscosity. They are often the first symptoms and include subjective complaints of headache, vertigo, dizziness, tinnitus, and visual disturbances. In addition, the client may experience angina, congestive heart failure, intermittent claudication, and thrombophlebitis, which may be complicated by embolization. These manifestations are caused by blood vessel distention, impaired blood flow, circulatory stasis, thrombosis, and tissue hypoxia caused by the hypervolemia and hyperviscosity. Generalized pruritus may be a striking symptom and is related to histamine release from an increased number of basophils.

Hemorrhagic phenomena caused by either vessel rupture from overdistention or inadequate platelet function may be displayed by petechiae, ecchymoses, epistaxis, or GI bleeding. Hemorrhage can be acute and catastrophic.

Hepatomegaly and splenomegaly, which develop from organ engorgement, may contribute to client complaints of satiety and fullness. The client may also experience pain due to peptic ulcer caused by the increased gastric secretions or the liver and spleen engorgement. Skin manifestations include severe pruritus, which is believed to be due to altered histamine metabolism, and plethora (ruddy complexion).

Hyperuricemia is caused by the increase in cell destruction that accompanies the excessive cell production. Uric acid is one of the products of cell destruction. As cell destruction increases, uric acid production also increases, thus leading to hyperuricemia. This problem may cause a secondary form of gout.

Diagnostic Studies

The following laboratory manifestations are seen in clients with polycythemia vera: (1) elevated hemoglobin and RBC count; (2) elevated WBC count with basophilia; (3) elevated platelets; and (4) elevated leukocyte alkaline phosphates, uric acid, and vitamin B_{12}.

If a bone marrow examination is used in establishing the diagnosis, it will show a hypercellularity of RBCs, WBCs, and platelets. Splenomegaly will be found in 75% of clients with polycythemia.

Therapeutic Management

Once the diagnosis of polycythemia vera is made, treatment is directed toward reducing blood volume and viscosity as well as bone marrow activity. Phlebotomy may be done to diminish blood volume until the desired hematocrit level is achieved. The aim of phlebotomy is to reduce and keep the hematocrit to less than 45% to 48%. Generally at the time of diagnosis 300 to 500 ml of blood may be removed every other day until the hematocrit is reduced to normal levels. Individuals managed with repeated phlebotomies eventually become deficient in iron, although this effect is rarely symptomatic. Iron supplementation should be avoided. Hydration therapy is used to reduce the blood's viscosity. Myelosuppressive agents such as melphalan, busulfan, hydroxyurea, cyclophosphamide, and radioactive phosphorus may be given to inhibit bone marrow activity. Allopurinol may reduce the number of acute gouty attacks. Antiplatelet agents such as aspirin and dipyridamole used to prevent thrombotic complications are controversial because of increased GI symptoms, including bleeding.

■ Nursing Management of Polycythemia Vera

Because the exact etiology of polycythemia vera is unclear, preventing it may not be possible. However, because secondary polycythemia is generated by any source of hypoxia, problems may be prevented by maintaining adequate oxygenation. Therefore, controlling chronic pulmonary disease and avoiding high altitudes may be important.

When acute exacerbations of polycythemia vera develop, the nurse has several responsibilities. Depending on the institution's policies, the nurse may either assist with or perform the phlebotomy. Fluid intake and output must be judiciously evaluated during hydration therapy to avoid fluid overload (which further complicates the circulatory congestion) and underhydration (which can cause the blood to become even more viscous). If myelosuppressive agents are used, the nurse must administer the drugs as ordered and observe the client for side effects.

Assessment of the client's nutritional status and collaboration with the dietitian may be necessary to offset the inadequate food intake that can result from GI symptoms of fullness, pain, and dyspepsia. Activities must be instituted to decrease thrombus formation. The immobility normally imposed by hospitalization may rapidly compromise the client. Active or passive leg exercises, and ambulation when possible, should be initiated.

Because of its chronic nature, polycythemia vera requires ongoing evaluation. Phlebotomy may need to be done every 2 to 3 months, reducing the blood volume by about 500 ml each time. The nurse must evaluate the client for the development of complications. Although the incidence is small, leukemia and lymphomas develop in some clients with polycythemia. These occurrences may be due to the chemotherapeutic drugs used to treat the disease. However, in some clients with polycythemia these malignant disorders have developed without chemotherapy treatment. The major cause of morbidity and mortality from polycythemia vera is arterial thrombosis. Over time, it

Table 25-11 Causes of Acquired Thrombocytopenia

BONE MARROW DISORDERS

Aplastic anemia
Megaloblastic anemia
Hematological malignant disorders
Chronic alcoholism

NONMARROW DISORDERS

Immune disorders
   Idiopathic thrombocytopenic purpura
   Drug induced
   Systemic lupus erythematosus
Hypersplenism
Disseminated intravascular coagulation
Thrombotic thrombocytopenic purpura
Viral infections (e.g., infectious mononucleosis)
Acquired immunodeficiency syndrome
Deficiencies of vitamin B_{12}, folic acid, and iron
Exposure to ionizing radiation

Table 25-12 Drugs Causing Thrombocytopenia

SUPPRESSION OF PLATELET PRODUCTION

Thiazide diuretics, alcohol, estrogen hormones

IMMUNE-MEDIATED PLATELET DESTRUCTION

Analgesics

Acetaminophen, aspirin and aspirin-containing drugs,* phenylbutazone, morphine

Antibiotics

Cephalothin, penicillin, streptomycin, sulfonamides, para-aminosalicylate, rifampicin

Cinchona alkaloids

Quinidine, quinine

Nonsteroidal antiinflammatory agents

Ibuprofen (Motrin, Advil), indomethacin (Indocin), naproxen (Naprosyn)

Miscellaneous agents

Diphenylhydantoin (Dilantin), phenobarbital, meprobamate, cimetidine, digitalis derivatives, anesthetics, β-blocking agents

*See Table 25-14.

may progress or convert to acute or chronic myelocytic leukemia.

CLOTTING PROBLEMS

Clotting disorders may be caused by a disturbance in any component of the hemostatic process, which includes platelets and clotting factors. Three major clotting problems are (1) thrombocytopenia (platelet deficiency), (2) hemophilia (a particular clotting factor deficiency), and (3) disseminated intravascular coagulation (a syndrome that affects all components of the hemostatic system).

Thrombocytopenia

Etiology. Thrombocytopenia is a reduction of platelets below the normal range of 150,000 to 400,000/µl. The two primary etiological types are idiopathic and acquired. *Idiopathic thrombocytopenic purpura* (ITP) was originally named because its cause was unknown. However, it is now known that ITP is an autoimmune disease. In ITP, platelets are coated with antibodies. Although these platelets function normally, when they reach the spleen, macrophages sequester the platelets and destroy them because of their altered structures. This platelet destruction results in the extravasation of small amounts of blood into tissues and mucous membranes, forming bruises. Platelets normally survive 8 to 10 days, but in ITP, survival is only 1 to 3 days. Acute ITP is seen predominantly in children following a viral illness. Chronic ITP occurs most commonly in women between 20 and 40 years of age. Chronic ITP has a gradual onset, and transient remissions occur.

Whereas ITP is the result of increased platelet destruction, *acquired thrombocytopenia* is due to diminished or defective platelet production. Acquired thrombocytopenia may result from many conditions (Tables 25-11 and 25-12). It is important for the nurse to become aware of the numerous conditions that may affect platelet production and destruction.

Clinical manifestations. Thrombocytopenia may be manifested by the appearance of bruises known as *purpura*. Small, flat, pinpoint red or reddish-brown purpura is known as *petechiae*, and larger purplish lesions caused by hemorrhage are called *ecchymoses* (Fig. 25-6). Ecchymoses may be flat or raised; on occasion pain and tenderness are present. Either type of purpura results from blood loss into the tissues. Petechiae result from intradermal bleeding caused by vascular or platelet abnormalities. Ecchymoses develop from subcutaneous bleeding caused by trauma or clotting disorders.

Prolonged bleeding after routine procedures such as venipuncture or IM injection may also indicate thrombocytopenia. Because the bleeding may be internal, the nurse must also be aware of manifestations that reflect this type of blood loss. Internal bleeding may be manifested as weakness, fainting, dizziness, tachycardia, abdominal pain, and hypotension.

The major complication of thrombocytopenia is hemorrhage. The hemorrhage may be insidious or acute, internal or external. It may occur in any area of the body, including joints, retina, and brain. Cerebral hemorrhage is fatal in about 5% of persons with ITP.[8] Insidious hemorrhage may first be detected by discovering the anemia that accompanies blood loss.

Diagnostic studies. The platelet count is decreased in cases of thrombocytopenia. Any reduction below 150,000/µl may be termed *thrombocytopenia*. However, spontaneous bleeding does not usually occur until platelet counts are less than 50,000/µl. When the count drops below 20,000/µl, life-threatening hemorrhages (e.g., intracranial bleeding) are a major problem.

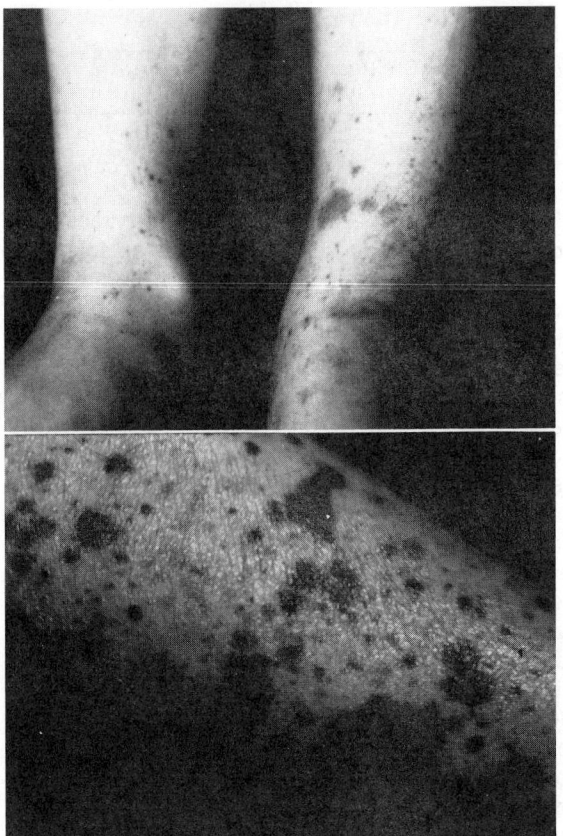

Fig. 25-6 Examples of ecchymoses.

Table 25-13

 Diagnostic and Therapeutic Management: Thrombocytopenia

DIAGNOSTIC

History and physical examination
Platelet count
Bleeding time
Bone marrow biopsy
Hematocrit and hemoglobin levels

THERAPEUTIC

Idiopathic
   Corticosteroids
   Platelet transfusion
   γ-Globulin IV
   Immunosuppressives (cyclophosphamide, azathioprine)
   Splenectomy
Acquired
   Identification and treatment of cause
   Corticosteroids
   Platelet transfusions
Thrombotic
   Plasma infusions
   Plasmapheresis
   Corticosteroids

The bleeding time, a reflection of platelet function, is prolonged. Test results that assess other clotting mechanisms, such as the clotting time, prothrombin time, and partial thromboplastin time, are normal. Bone marrow analysis shows megakaryocytes (precursors of platelets) to be normal or increased, but platelets are reduced. Bone marrow examination is done to rule out possible causes such as leukemia and other myeloproliferative disorders.

Anemia is present in proportion to the amount of blood lost. Therefore, it is important to monitor hemoglobin and hematocrit values as well as to observe the client for cardiopulmonary distress and other manifestations of anemia.

Therapeutic management. Therapeutic management of thrombocytopenia is based on differentiating the etiology of ITP from that of acquired thrombocytopenia, since each requires a different treatment plan (Table 25-13).

Idiopathic thrombocytopenic purpura. The three main therapies used to manage the client with ITP are corticosteroids, splenectomy, and platelet transfusions. Adrenal corticosteroids are used to treat ITP because of their ability to suppress the phagocytic response of splenic macrophages. This alters the spleen's recognition of platelets and increases their life spans. In addition, corticosteroids depress antibody formation. Initial treatment is with prednisone, which reduces the binding of antibody to the platelet surface. Corticosteroids also reduce capillary fragility and bleeding time. The mechanism that causes these events is poorly understood.

Splenectomy is indicated if clients do not respond to prednisone initially or require unacceptably high doses to maintain an adequate platelet count. Approximately 80% of clients benefit from splenectomy, resulting in a complete or partial remission. The effectiveness of splenectomy is based on four factors. First, the spleen contains an abundance of the macrophages that sequester and destroy platelets. Second, structural features of the spleen enhance antibody-coated platelets and macrophage interaction. Third, some antibody synthesis occurs in the spleen; thus antiplatelet antibodies decrease after splenectomy. Fourth, the spleen normally sequesters about one third of the platelets, so its removal increases the number in circulation.

Treatment may also include high doses of γ-globulin in clients who are unresponsive to splenectomy and corticosteroids. It works by competing with the platelet antibodies for macrophage receptors. γ-Globulin effectively raises the platelet count, but the beneficial effects only last from 1 to 2 weeks.

Recently danazol, an attenuated androgen, has been used with success in some clients. Immunosuppressive therapy used in refractory cases includes vincristine, vinblastine, azathioprine, and cyclophosphamide. Platelet transfusions may be used to elevate platelet counts in cases of life-threatening hemorrhage. Platelets should not be administered prophylactically because of the possibility of antibody formation. ABO compatibility is not a necessary prerequisite for platelet transfusions. However, it has been discovered that after multiple platelet transfusions from more than 20 donors, isoimmunization develops. The immunity is caused by the presence of HLA on the platelet membrane. Therefore, by using lymphocyte typing to de-

Table 25-14   Commonly Used Aspirin-Containing
Medications

ANALGESICS
Narcotic

Ascriptin with codeine	Fiorinal with codeine
Aspirin with codeine	Percodan
Darvon compound with ASA	Percodan-Demi
Empirin compound with codeine	

Nonnarcotic

Ascriptin	Excedrin PM
Ascriptin A/D	Fiorinal
Bufferin	Midol
Empirin compound	Trigesic
Equagesic	Vanquish
Excedrin	

OTHER

Alka-Seltzer

---

termine that the HLA types of the donor and the recipient are identical, multiple platelet transfusions can be used more effectively. In addition, clients may be premedicated with benadryl and hydrocortisone to decrease the possibility of reacting to platelet transfusions. Sometimes meperidine (Demerol) is used with the antihistamine and corticosteroid. Aspirin and aspirin-containing compounds (see Table 25-14) should be avoided in clients with thrombocytopenia.

Acquired thrombocytopenia. The therapeutic management of acquired thrombocytopenia is based on identifying and removing the causative agent. While the precipitating factor is being investigated, the client may receive corticosteroids to enhance capillary integrity and platelet transfusions if life-threatening hemorrhage develops. Splenectomy is not used because the spleen is not contributing to the thrombocytopenia.

In some situations, acquired thrombocytopenia may be caused by the therapy used to treat another problem. For example, in leukemia the client may receive certain chemotherapeutic drugs that will cause bone marrow suppression. Therefore the client must be supported throughout the course of thrombocytopenia to give the chemotherapy treatment an opportunity to be effective.

■ **Nursing Management of Thrombocytopenia**

Nursing assessment

Subjective and objective data that should be obtained from a client with thrombocytopenia are presented in Table 25-15.

Nursing diagnoses

Nursing diagnoses related to a client with thrombocytopenia include, but are not limited to, those presented in Table 25-16.

Table 25-15

**Nursing Assessment of the
Client with Thrombocytopenia**

SUBJECTIVE DATA

History
Recent hemorrhage, excessive bleeding, or viral illness; cancer (especially leukemia or lymphoma); aplastic anemia; systemic lupus erythematosus; alcoholism; cirrhosis; chronic renal failure; exposure to radiation or toxic chemicals
Medications
Use of thiazide diuretics, furosemide (Lasix), aspirin, acetaminophen, estrogens, gold salts, indomethacin (Indocin), phenylbutazone, penicillins, cephalothin, streptomycin, sulfonamides, quinidine, quinine, phenobarbital, methyldopa, phenytoin (Dilantin), diabinese, meprobamate, antineoplastic drugs
General
Weakness, fainting, malaise, fatigue
Pain
Pain and tenderness in bleeding areas (e.g., abdomen, head, extremities)
Integumentary
Easy bruising
Respiratory
Epistaxis, hemoptysis, dyspnea
Gastrointestinal
Bleeding gingivae, coffee ground or bloody vomitus
Urinary
Hematuria
Reproductive
Menorrhagia, metrorrhagia

OBJECTIVE DATA

General
Fever, lethargy
Integumentary
Petechiae, ecchymoses, purpura
Cardiovascular
Tachycardia, hypotension (significant bleeding)
Gastrointestinal
Blood-filled bullae in mouth, splenomegaly, abdominal distention, guaiac positive stools
Neurological
Slurred speech, decreased level of consciousness (CNS bleeding)
Possible findings
Platelet count <150,000/μl, prolonged bleeding time

Nursing interventions

Health promotion and maintenance. It is important for the nurse to discourage excessive use of over-the-counter (OTC) medications known to be possible causes of acquired thrombocytopenia. Many medications contain aspirin as an ingredient. Aspirin reduces platelet adhesiveness, thus potentially contributing to thrombocytopenia.

Table 25-16

NURSING CARE PLAN FOR THE CLIENT WITH THROMBOCYTOPENIA

Defining Characteristics	Nursing Interventions	Evaluation Criteria

NURSING DIAGNOSIS: Altered cardiopulmonary, cerebral, and/or renal tissue perfusion related to bleeding

Prolonged bleeding from venipuncture site or injection site, epistaxis, gingival bleeding, GI and genitourinary bleeding, ecchymoses, petechiae; bleeding within CNS (headache, confusion, disorientation, changes in level of consciousness)	Evaluate mucous membranes and skin each shift or more often for epistaxis, petechiae, ecchymoses, hematomas. Hematest all excretions and observe for blood in emesis, sputum, feces, urine, nasogastric secretions, wound secretions. Assess CBC and platelet count daily or more often if warranted. Measure all blood loss; weigh linen and dressings saturated with blood, count sanitary napkins. Assess for retinal hemorrhage (visual impairment). *Do not* administer aspirin or aspirin-containing products because of their effects on platelet adhesiveness. Teach client to avoid OTC medications that contain aspirin. Control active bleeding with ice, packing, or direct pressure. Reduce chance of CNS bleed by preventing increased intracranial pressure by teaching client to avoid Valsalva maneuver (e.g., straining at stool); administering stool softeners as ordered; avoiding rectal temperatures, suppositories, and enemas; teaching client to cough, sneeze, and blow nose gently; administering medications to suppress vomiting and coughing; preventing shivering; evaluating mental status for alterations (e.g., headaches, vertigo, irritability, confusion). If client is receiving therapeutic agents that are toxic to the bladder, force fluids to 3000 ml/day if not contraindicated by cardiovascular problems, avoid ingestion of substances that may irritate bladder epithelium (e.g., coffee, tea, alcohol, tobacco, spices such as pepper and curry), encourage frequent voiding (about q 2 hr). Administer blood products as ordered. Understand various purposes of transfusion therapy, differentiate various types of blood products, administer and monitor blood products properly, intervene with transfusion reactions.	Maintenance of pulse, respirations, blood pressure within acceptable range of client's normal; no evidence of gross or occult bleeding, including absence of CNS bleeding; administration of required blood products with appropriate intervention if transfusion reaction occurs; maintenance of adequate urine output (>30 ml/hr)

NURSING DIAGNOSIS: High risk for altered oral mucous membrane related to treatment, disease, or blood-filled bullae

Presence of blood-filled bullae in mouth; bleeding, tender gingivae and lips	Assess oral mucosa daily. Remove dentures daily and assess oral cavity. Provide oral hygiene with minimal friction: use soft bristle toothbrush, cotton swabs, mild mouthwash, or irrigating syringe to cleanse mouth. Evaluate integrity of nares, especially if nasogastric tube, endotracheal tube, or nasal O_2 is in use.	Pink, moist, lesion-free oral mucosa, tongue, and lips; no irritation or injury to mucous membrane; adequate nutritional intake

Continued.

Table 25-16

NURSING CARE PLAN FOR THE CLIENT WITH THROMBOCYTOPENIA—cont'd

Defining Characteristics	Nursing Interventions	Evaluation Criteria
NURSING DIAGNOSIS: High risk for impaired tissue integrity related to interventions and tissue sensitivity to trauma		
Multiple skin punctures, bruising after even minor pressure or trauma events	Reduce number of venipunctures and initiate IV therapy judiciously. Consider use of alternate venous access devices. Avoid IM and SC injections—if used, apply local pressure with dry, sterile 2 × 2 inch gauze for 5-10 min after needle is removed. Use electric razor for shaving to reduce cuts. Reduce frequency of cuff blood pressures and alternate extremities used for readings. Pad rails and other firm surfaces, especially if client is combative or at risk for seizures. Be very gentle when turning client, changing dressings.	Maintenance of tissue integrity, no evidence of petechiae, ecchymoses, purpura, hematoma
NURSING DIAGNOSIS: Anxiety related to lack of knowledge of disease process, activity, nutrition, and medication		
Frequent questioning about disease management; anxiety, restlessness; inability to answer or incorrect answering of disease-related questions	Assess learning needs related to disease management. Discuss complications and signs that should be reported such as trauma prevention, need for high fluid intake, medication management, and need for periods of rest and exercise. Provide opportunities for client to verbalize concerns. Foster care decisions and planning by client.	Verbalization and/or demonstration by client or family of required knowledge and skills to manage home care

It is also important for the nurse to encourage persons to have a complete medical evaluation if manifestations of bleeding tendencies (e.g., prolonged epistaxis, petechiae) develop. In addition, the nurse must be observant for early signs of thrombocytopenia in clients receiving cancer chemotherapy drugs.

Acute intervention. The goal during acute episodes of thrombocytopenia is to prevent or control hemorrhage (Table 25-16). In clients with thrombocytopenia, bleeding is usually from superficial sites; deep bleeding (into muscles, joints, abdomen) occurs only when clotting factors are diminished. It is important to emphasize that a seemingly minor nosebleed may lead to hemorrhage in a client with severe thrombocytopenia. Bleeding from the posterior nasopharynx may be difficult to detect because the blood may be swallowed. If an IM or SC injection is unavoidable, the use of a small-gauge needle and application of direct pressure for at least 5 to 10 minutes after injection is indicated.

In women with thrombocytopenia, menstrual blood loss may exceed the usual amount and duration. Counting sanitary napkins used during menses is another important intervention to detect excess blood loss. Fifty milliliters of blood will completely soak a sanitary napkin.

The proper administration of platelets is an important nursing responsibility.[9] Platelet concentrate is administered because it is not practical to give the client the amount of fresh blood needed to increase the platelet level effectively. Platelet concentrate is a yellow liquid that contains only plasma and platelets. It contains 30 to 50 ml per unit of platelets. One unit of platelets, usually 30 to 50 ml in volume, can be derived by centrifuging 500 ml of whole blood.

One unit of platelets will increase the platelet count by about $10,000/\mu l$. Therefore several units of platelets are usually transfused. Once acquired from a donor, platelets can be stored at room temperature for 1 to 5 days. Gentle agitation of the bag is useful to prevent the platelets from adhering to the plastic. The actual infusion procedure may vary among institutions, but an IV infusion is needed. A filter tubing is always used.

Chronic management. Clients with ITP who are receiving glucocorticosteroids should be monitored frequently for their response to therapy. If the ITP is treated by splenectomy, there is usually no recurrence. Persons with acquired thrombocytopenia must be taught to avoid causative agents when possible (see Table 25-11). If the causative agents cannot be avoided, clients should learn to detect the development of thrombocytopenic problems.

Clients with either ITP or acquired thrombocytopenia should have planned periodic medical evaluations to assess the client's status and to intercede in situations in which exacerbations and bleeding are likely to occur. The client must be cautioned to avoid trauma if platelet counts are below normal levels. Contact sports such as football should be avoided.

Thrombotic thrombocytopenia purpura. Thrombotic thrombocytopenia purpura (TTP) is an uncommon syndrome characterized by microangiopathic hemolytic anemia, thrombocytopenia, neurological abnormalities, fever (in the absence of infection), and renal abnormalities. The disease is associated with enhanced agglutination and platelets, which form microthrombi that deposit in arterioles and capillaries. The cause of the platelet agglutination is unknown. TTP is seen primarily in adults between the ages of 20 and 50 with a slight female predominance. The syndrome is occasionally precipitated by the use of estrogen or pregnancy.

Anemia is universal and may be very severe. RBC morphology indicates fragmented cells with marked reticulocytosis. Thrombocytopenia is present and may be severe, but coagulation studies are normal. TTP is treated with plasma infusion and/or plasmapheresis (see Chapter 8). The mechanism for the therapeutic response is not fully understood. Treatment should be continued daily until the client is in complete remission. Splenectomy, corticosteroids, and dextran have also been used with success.

Hemophilias

Hemophilias are hereditary bleeding disorders caused by reduced clotting activity of specific coagulation factors. The three major forms of hemophilia are *hemophilia A* (classic hemophilia), *hemophilia B* (Christmas disease), and *von Willebrand's disease.* Hemophilia A is the most common form of hemophilia, comprising about 80% of all cases. The incidence of hemophilia A is about 1 in 10,000 males; hemophilia B is seen in 1 in 100,000 males. The deficiency and inheritance patterns of the three forms of hemophilia are compared in Table 25-17.

Clinical manifestations and complications. Clinical manifestations and complications related to hemophilia include (1) slow, persistent, prolonged bleeding from minor trauma and small cuts; (2) delayed bleeding after minor injuries (the delay may be several hours or days); (3) uncontrollable hemorrhage after dental extractions or irritation of the gingiva with a hardbristle toothbrush (Fig. 25-7); (4) epistaxis, especially after a blow to the face; (5) GI bleeding from ulcers and gastritis; (6) hematuria from GU trauma and splenic rupture resulting from falls or abdominal trauma; (7) ecchymoses and SC hematomas (common); (8) neurological signs such as pain, anesthesia, and paralysis, which may develop from nerve compression caused by hematoma formation; and (9) *hemarthrosis* (bleeding into the joints), which may lead to joint deformity severe enough to cause unresolvable crippling (most commonly in the knees, elbow, and ankles).

These manifestations are especially important when seen in children because the disease may not yet be diagnosed. In adults, these developments are also significant because they suggest that the hemophilia is poorly controlled. All clinical manifestations relate to bleeding, and any bleeding episode in persons with hemophilia may result in death from hemorrhage.

Hemophilia had been considered primarily a disease of childhood because of early death from the complications. Advances in its treatment now enable persons with hemo-

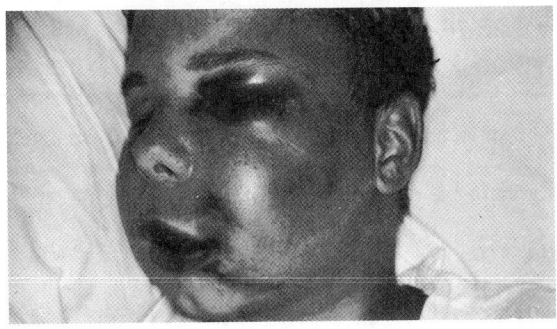

Fig. 25-7 Hematoma that developed in a hemophiliac after dental treatment. (From Williams WJ and others, eds: Hematology, ed 2, New York, 1977, McGraw-Hill Book Co.)

Table 25-17 Comparison of Hemophilic States

Disorder	Deficiency	Inheritance Pattern
Hemophilia A	Factor VIII	Recessive sex-linked (transmitted by female carriers, displayed almost exclusively in males)
Hemophilia B	Factor IX	Recessive sex-linked (transmitted by female carriers, displayed almost exclusively in males)
von Willebrand's disease	Factor VIII and platelet dysfunction	Autosomal dominant, seen in both sexes

philia to live into adulthood. Although it is now possible to control the complications, hemarthroses and severe hemorrhage are the most common difficulties to be managed. In addition, because of the repeated use of blood components, the development of hepatitis is common. Unfortunately many persons with hemophilia are seropositive for human immunodeficiency virus (HIV) infection transmitted via cryoprecipitates and factor VIII concentrates, and acquired immunodeficiency syndrome (AIDS) has already developed in many clients. Before 1986, donated blood and blood products were not tested for HIV antibody. Routine testing is now used, all factor concentrates are prepared from plasma obtained from HIV-seronegative donors, and the product is heat-treated to further reduce the likelihood of virus transmission.

Therapeutic and pharmacological management. Laboratory studies are used to determine the type of hemophilia present. Any factor deficiency within the intrinsic system (factors VIII, IX, XI, or XII) will yield the laboratory results presented in Table 25-18.

The goals of therapeutic management are to prevent and treat bleeding. The therapeutic regimen for a person with hemophilia focuses on maintaining adequate blood levels of the deficient clotting factors. This goal is achieved by

Table 25-18 Laboratory Results in Hemophilia

Test	Comments
Prothrombin time	No involvement of extrinsic system
Thrombin time	No impairment of thrombin-fibrinogen reaction
Platelet count	Adequate platelet production
Partial thromboplastin time	Prolonged finding due to deficiency in any intrinsic clotting system factor
Bleeding time	Prolonged finding in von Willebrand's disease because of structurally defective platelets, normal in hemophilia A and B because platelets not affected
Factor assays	Reduction of factor VIII in hemophilia A and von Willebrand's disease, reduction of factor IX in hemophilia B

Table 25-19 Antihemophilic Factor Preparations

Name	Factor Replacement	Source
Fresh-frozen plasma	Replacement of all clotting factors except platelets, frequent use until diagnosis is confirmed because it replaces both factor VIII and factor IX	Blood bank
Cryoprecipitates	Replacement of factor VIII and fibrinogen	Blood bank
Concentrates*	Factor VIII (e.g., Factorate, Hemofil, Koate, Profilate), factor IX (e.g., Konyne, Profilnine, Proplex)	Commercially prepared lyophilized products

*None of these preparations can be used to treat von Willebrand's disease because the factor for platelet adhesion is removed during the manufacturing process.

assessing clinical manifestations, determining blood levels of the factors concerned, and administering the necessary clotting component.

Replacement of deficient clotting factors is the primary means of supporting clients with hemophilia. In addition to treating acute crises, replacement therapy may be given before surgery and dental care as a prophylactic measure. The standard therapeutic products are cryoprecipitate and factor VIII or IX concentrates (Table 25-19). Cryoprecipitate, which contains primarily factor VIII and fibrinogen, is prepared from plasma, frozen rapidly, and kept frozen until used. Before administration, the cryoprecipitate is thawed slowly and should be used within 6 hours.

Factor VIII concentrates are prepared from multiple donors and supplied as a lyophilized powder. It can be refrigerated and reconstituted just before use. Three developments have increased the safety of factor VIII therapy: First, heat treating the lyophilized concentrates can inactivate HIV. Second, highly purified factor VIII can be purified from plasma using monoclonal antibody elution columns. Third, genetic cloning techniques have resulted in the availability of recombinant factor VIII, which is equivalent to the plasma product. Use of this product should avoid infectious complications.

Factor IX deficiency can be treated with fresh-frozen plasma or a plasma fraction enriched in prothrombin complex proteins (factor IX concentrate). Factor IX concentrate is available as a lyophilized concentrate and also contains prothrombin and factors VII and X.

For mild hemophilia, desmopressin acetate may be used to cause an increase in factor VIII. The mechanism of action of this drug is unknown. However, its effect is relatively short-lived, and it is an appropriate therapy only for procedures such as dental extractions or care.

Complications of treatment include development of inhibitors to factors VIII or IX, transfusion-transmitted infectious disorders, allergic reactions (more commonly seen with the use of cryoprecipitate), and thrombotic complications with the use of factor IX because it contains activated coagulation factors. Because of the exposure to many blood donors, the risk of transfusion infection is high. Most clients with hemophilia who have received treatment demonstrate evidence of exposure to hepatitis B and non-A–non-B hepatitis. Before 1986, many clients with hemophilia were given products contaminated with HIV.

The most common difficulties with therapeutic management are starting therapy too late and stopping it too soon. Generally, minor bleeding episodes should be treated for at least 72 hours; surgery and traumatic injuries may dictate support for 10 to 14 days.

■ Nursing Management of Hemophilia
Health promotion and maintenance

Because of the hereditary nature of hemophilia, referral for genetic counseling is essential when considering preventive measures. This is especially important today because persons with hemophilia are living longer and reaching an age when reproduction is possible.

Acute interventions

Nursing interventions are related primarily to controlling bleeding and include the following:

1. The nurse should stop the topical bleeding as quickly as possible by applying direct pressure or ice, packing the area with Gelfoam or fibrin foam, and applying topical hemostatic agents such as thrombin.
2. The nurse should administer the blood component ordered to raise the client's level of the deficient coagulation factor.
3. The nurse should prevent crippling deformities from hemarthrosis. When joint bleeding occurs, it is important to rest the involved joint totally, in addition to administering antihemophilic factors (AHFs). The

joint may be packed in ice. Analgesics are needed to reduce the severe pain. However, aspirin should *never* be used. As soon as bleeding ceases, it is important to encourage mobilization of the affected area through range-of-motion (ROM) exercises and physical therapy. Actual weight bearing should be avoided until all swelling has resolved and muscle strength has returned.

4. The nurse should manage any life-threatening complication that may develop as a result of hemorrhage. Examples include nursing interventions to prevent or treat airway obstruction from hemorrhage into the neck and pharynx, as well as early assessment and treatment of intracranial bleeding.

Chronic management

Chronic management is a primary consideration for clients with hemophilia because the disease follows a progressive, chronic course. The quality as well as the length of life may be significantly affected by the client's knowledge of the illness and how to live with it. The client and family can be referred to the local chapter of the National Hemophilia Society to encourage associations with other individuals who are dealing with the problems of hemophilia. The nurse must provide ongoing assessment of the client's adaptation to the illness. Psychosocial support and assistance should be readily available as needed.

Most of the long-term care measures are related to client education. Clients with hemophilia must be taught to recognize disease-related problems and to learn which can be resolved at home and which require hospitalization. Immediate medical attention is required for severe pain or swelling of a muscle or joint that restricts movement or inhibits sleep and for a head injury, a swelling in the neck or mouth, abdominal pain, hematuria, melena, and skin wounds in need of suturing.

Daily oral hygiene must be performed without causing trauma (see Table 25-16 for techniques). Understanding how to prevent injuries is another consideration. This is no easy task with all the potential sources of trauma. Clients can learn to participate in noncontact sports (e.g., golf) and wear gloves when doing household chores to prevent cuts or abrasions from knives, hammers, and other tools. The client should wear a Medic-Alert tag to ensure that health care providers know about the hemophilia in case of an accident.

Clients need information about routine follow-up care and their compliance with scheduled visits must be assessed. Reliable persons can be taught to administer AHF at home. This requires instructions regarding venipuncture and infusion techniques.

Disseminated Intravascular Coagulation

Disseminated intravascular coagulation (DIC) is a serious bleeding disorder resulting from acceleration of normal clotting with a subsequent decrease in clotting factors and platelets. These changes may lead to uncontrollable hemorrhage. The name of the problem may be misleading because it suggests that the blood is clotting, which is only partially true. The disorder is a paradoxical condition characterized by profuse bleeding and thrombosis. DIC is al-

Table 25-20 Predisposing Conditions to DIC Development

THROMBOPLASTIC SUBSTANCES
Obstetrical conditions

Abruptio placentae
Retained dead fetus
Amniotic fluid embolus
Septic abortion

Neoplasias

Prostate cancer

Acute leukemias

Giant cavernous hemangioma
Bronchogenic cancer

ACTIVATION OF FACTOR XII
Hemolytic processes

Transfusion of mismatched blood
Acute hemolysis from infection or immunological disorders

Tissue damage

Extensive burns and trauma
Heat stroke
Severe head injury
Transplant rejections
Postoperative damage, especially after extracorporeal membrane oxygenation
Fat and pulmonary emboli
Snake bites

POORLY DEFINED MECHANISMS

Shock
Acute bacterial infections, especially those leading to septicemia
Glomerulonephritis
Thrombotic thrombocytopenia purpura
Cirrhosis
Acute fulminant hepatitis

---

ways caused by an underlying disease. The underlying disease must be treated for the DIC to resolve.

Etiology. DIC is not a disease but rather an abnormal syndrome caused by another process. The disorders known to predispose clients to DIC are listed in Table 25-20. DIC is most frequently associated with obstetrical catastrophes, metastatic malignant tumors, massive trauma, and sepsis. In each case, a tentative triggering mechanism of coagulation has been identified (Table 25-20).

Initially in DIC, the normal coagulation mechanisms are enhanced. Abundant intravascular thrombin, the most powerful coagulant, is produced (Fig. 25-8). It catalyzes the conversion of fibrinogen to fibrin and enhances platelet aggregation. There is widespread fibrin and platelet deposition in capillaries and arterioles, resulting in thrombosis. Excessive clotting activates the fibrinolytic system to produce fibrin-split (fibrin-degradation) products. These prod-

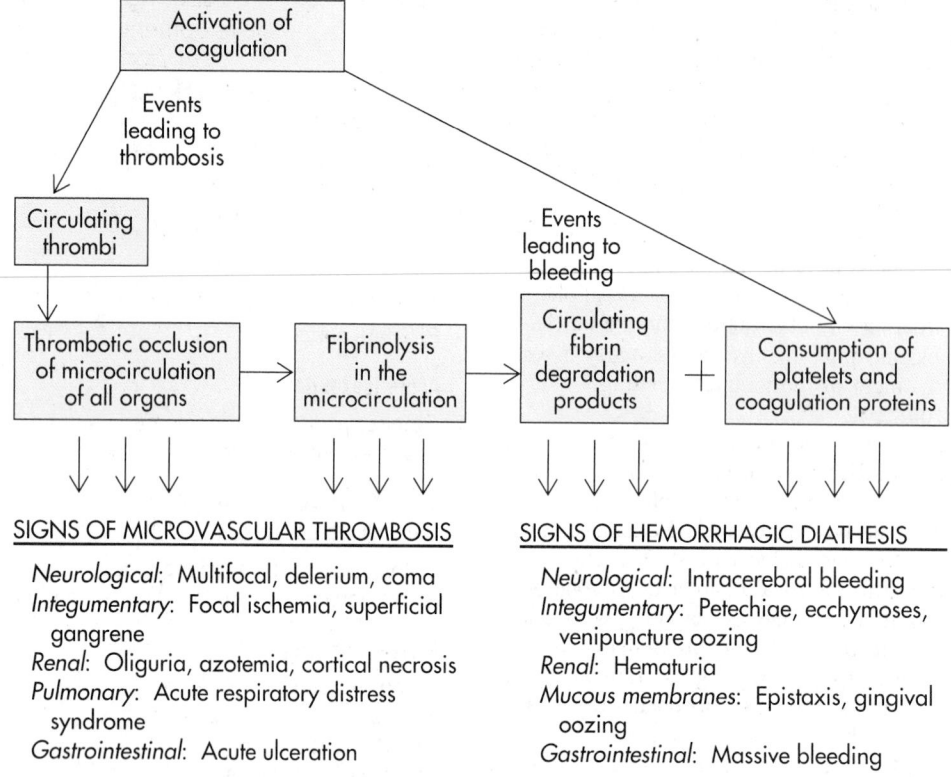

Fig. 25-8 The sequence of events that occurs during disseminated intravascular coagulation, leading to the clinical appearance of thrombotic and hemorrhagic phenomena. (From Marder VJ: Microvascular thrombosis. In Dietchy JM, ed: Science and practice of clinical medicine, vol 6, New York, 1980, Grune & Stratton, p 230.)

ucts inhibit the clotting of normal blood by acting as anti-coagulants. Ultimately, with clots being lysed and clotting factors being depleted, the blood loses its ability to clot. Therefore a stable clot cannot be formed at injury sites. This situation predisposes the client to hemorrhage.

Chronic DIC is most commonly seen in clients with long-standing illnesses such as malignant disorders or autoimmune diseases.[10] These clients may have subclinical disease manifested only by laboratory abnormalities. Although easy bruising or hemorrhage may occur, many of these persons have signs of venous thrombosis.

Clinical manifestations. There is no well-defined sequence of events in acute DIC. Bleeding in a person with no previous history or obvious cause should be questioned because it may be one of the first manifestations of acute DIC. General manifestations include weakness, malaise, and fever. Bleeding manifestations of DIC are multifactorial (Fig. 25-8) and include consumption and depletion of platelets and coagulation factors as well as formation of fibrin split products that have anticoagulant properties. Bleeding manifestations may present as *integumentary changes,* including pallor, petechiae, oozing blood, venipuncture site bleeding, hematomas, and occult hemorrhage; as *respiratory changes,* such as tachypnea, hemoptysis, and orthopnea; as *cardiovascular changes,* such as tachycardia and hypotension; as *GI changes,* including abdominal distention and bloody stools; as *urinary changes,* such

as hematuria; as *neurological changes,* such as vision changes, dizziness, headache, changes in mental status, and irritability; and as *musculoskeletal changes,* including bone and joint pain.

Thrombotic manifestations are a result of fibrin and/or platelet deposition in the microvasculature (Fig. 25-8) and may present as *integumentary changes,* including acral cyanosis, electrocardiogram (ECG) changes, ischemic tissue necrosis (e.g., gangrene), and hemorrhagic necrosis; as *respiratory changes,* such as tachypnea, dyspnea, pulmonary emboli, and acute respiratory distress syndrome; as *cardiovascular changes,* including ECG changes and venous distention; as *GI changes,* such as abdominal pain and paralytic ileus; and as *urinary changes,* such as and oliguria.

Diagnostic studies. As more clots are made in the body, more breakdown products from fibrinogen and fibrin are also formed. These are called *fibrin-split* (fibrin-degradation) *products* (FSPs), and they work in three ways to interfere with blood coagulation. First, they coat the platelets and interfere with platelet function. Second, they interfere with thrombin and thereby disrupt coagulation. Third, the FSPs attach to fibrinogen, which interferes with the polymerization process necessary to form a stable clot.

The protamine sulfate test is another diagnostic test of active DIC. Protamine sulfate can bind with fibrin-split products and free the fibrin monomer so that it can be po-

Table 25-21 Laboratory Abnormalities of DIC

Test	Finding
SCREENING TESTS	
Prothrombin time (PT)	Prolonged
Partial thromboplastin time (PTT)	Prolonged
Activated partial thromboplastin time (APTT)	Prolonged
Thrombin time (TT)	Prolonged
Fibrinogen	Reduced
Platelets	Reduced
SPECIAL TESTS	
Fibrin-split products (FSP)*	Elevated
Protamine sulfate	Strongly positive
Factor assays (for factors V, VII, VIII, X, XIII)	Reduced
D-Dimers (cross-linked fibrin fragments)	Elevated
Antithrombin III	Reduced

*Fibrin-degradation products (FDP).

lymerized and form a stable clot. A weakly positive test may occur after surgery, with liver disease, or with thrombosis. A strongly positive protamine sulfate test is highly indicative of DIC. Fragmented erythrocytes (schistocytes), indicative of partial occlusion of small vessels by fibrin thrombi, may be found on blood smears. Tests used to diagnose DIC and their findings are listed in Table 25-21.

Therapeutic management. It is important to diagnose DIC quickly, institute therapy that will resolve the underlying causative disease or problem, and then treat the DIC itself. Establishing that DIC is occurring and investigating potential causes are considerably easier than knowing what therapy should be used to counteract the condition. The treatment of DIC is currently under investigation as researchers attempt to validate the most suitable means of managing this dangerous syndrome. Consequently, it is imperative that the nurse maintain an ongoing awareness of current modes of therapy.

Treating the disease that causes DIC may entail supportive measures for those entities. Other causes of DIC may require highly specific therapeutic intervention. Regardless of the etiology, treating the primary disease process is essential to the resolution of DIC.

Depending on its severity, DIC may be treated by one of the following methods (Fig. 25-9). First, if DIC is diagnosed in a client who is not bleeding, no therapy for DIC is necessary. Treatment of the underlying disease may be sufficient to reverse the DIC. Second, when the client is bleeding, therapy is directed toward providing support with necessary blood products while treating the primary disorder. The blood products are administered on the basis of specific component deficiencies. Platelets are given to correct thrombocytopenia, cryoprecipitate replaces factor VIII and fibrinogen, and fresh-frozen plasma (FFP) re-places all clotting factors except platelets and provides a source of antithrombin.

Clients with manifestations of thrombosis need immediate anticoagulation with IV heparin. The use of heparin in the treatment of DIC is still controversial. It should be reserved for persons with thrombosis or those who continue to bleed in spite of vigorous treatment with plasma and platelets.[11] If heparin is used to treat DIC, it must be used in conjunction with blood product support and must be administered by continuous, low-dose, IV infusion.

Another treatment that has been used is epsilon aminocaproic acid (EACA, Amicar) because of its ability to inhibit fibrinolysis. The use of EACA is controversial because it can enhance thrombosis. Generally it is only used as adjunctive therapy to heparin.

Antithrombin III (AT-III) is a coagulation factor that inhibits the action of thrombin during heparin therapy. It is indicated only when the underlying cause of DIC cannot be eliminated and AT-III levels are low. Chronic DIC does not respond to oral anticoagulants, but it can be controlled with long-term, low-dose SC or IV heparin.

■ Nursing Management of DIC

Nursing diagnoses

Nursing diagnoses for DIC include, but are not limited to, the following:

1. High risk of injury related to altered clotting mechanisms
2. Altered cerebral, cardiopulmonary, renal, GI, and peripheral tissue perfusion related to bleeding and sluggish or diminished blood flow secondary to thrombosis
3. Pain related to bleeding into tissues and diagnostic procedures
4. Anxiety related to fear of the unknown, disease process, diagnostic procedures, and therapy
5. Ineffective individual coping related to the stress of serious illness
6. High risk for decreased cardiac output related to fluid volume deficit and hypotension

Nursing interventions

Nurses must be alert to the possible development of DIC and especially to the precipitating factors listed in Table 25-20. This may be difficult because these clients are usually extremely ill due to the primary problems that precipitated the DIC. It is important to recognize which illnesses predispose clients to this potentially lethal problem. The nurse must also remember that because DIC is secondary to an underlying disease, additional care is required as appropriate for managing the causative problem. Correcting the primary disease also helps resolve the DIC.

Appropriate nursing interventions are essential to the survival of clients with DIC.[12] Astute, ongoing assessment, active attention to manifestations of the syndrome, and institution of appropriate treatment measures are challenging nursing responsibilities. Early detection of bleeding, both occult and overt, must be a primary goal. The client should be thoroughly assessed for external signs of bleeding (e.g. petechiae, oozing at IV sites or injection sites) as well as internal signs of bleeding (e.g., changes in

THERAPY

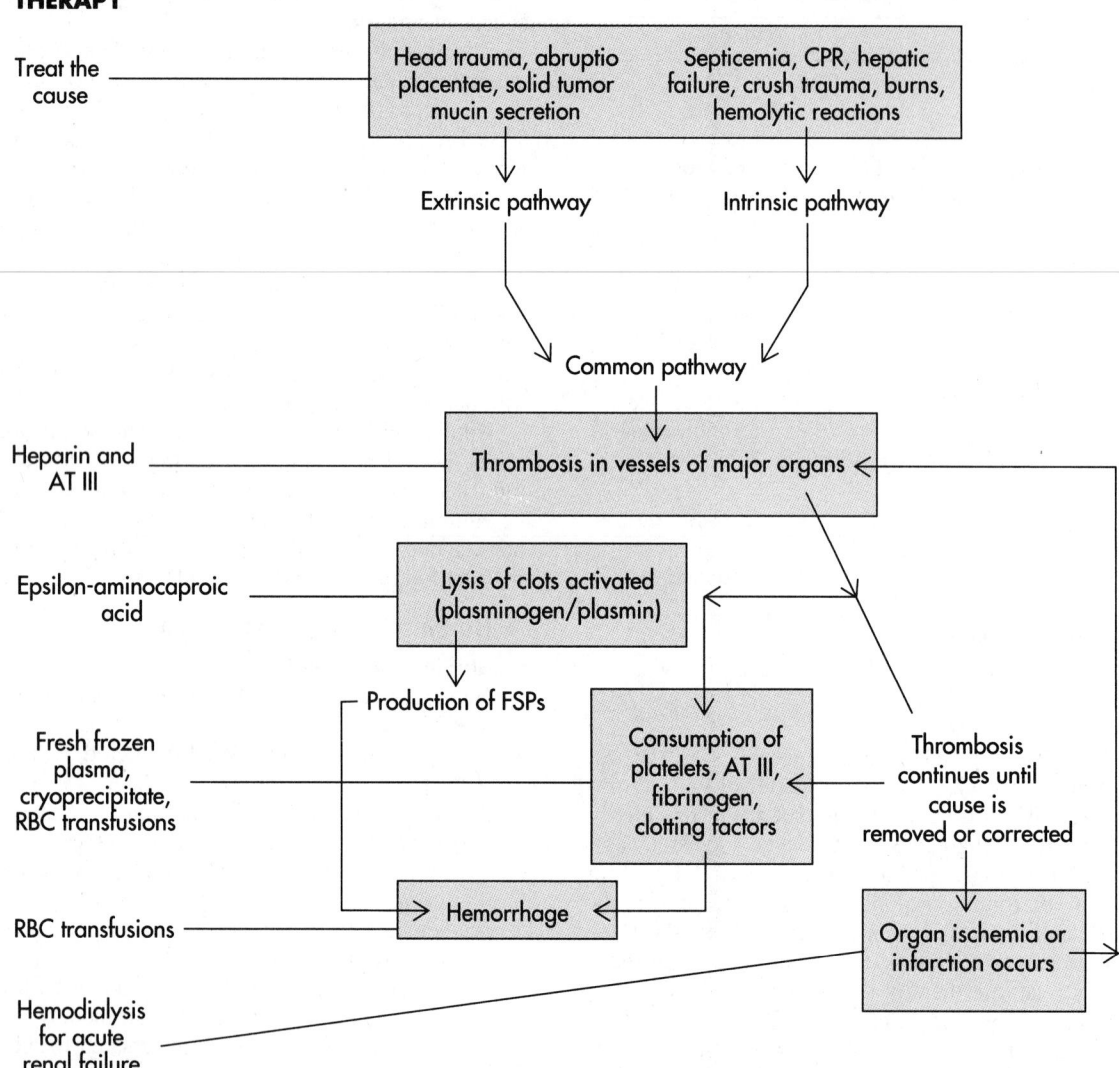

Treat the cause —————— | Head trauma, abruptio placentae, solid tumor mucin secretion | Septicemia, CPR, hepatic failure, crush trauma, burns, hemolytic reactions |

Extrinsic pathway — Intrinsic pathway

Common pathway

Heparin and AT III ————— Thrombosis in vessels of major organs

Epsilon-aminocaproic acid ————— Lysis of clots activated (plasminogen/plasmin)

Production of FSPs

Fresh frozen plasma, cryoprecipitate, RBC transfusions ————— Consumption of platelets, AT III, fibrinogen, clotting factors

Thrombosis continues until cause is removed or corrected

RBC transfusions ————— Hemorrhage

Organ ischemia or infarction occurs

Hemodialysis for acute renal failure

Fig. 25-9 Intended sites of action for therapies in DIC. (From Thelan LA and others: Textbook of critical care nursing: diagnosis and management, St Louis, 1990, Mosby–Year Book, Inc, p 823.)

mental status, increasing abdominal girth, pain). Any sites of bleeding should be carefully monitored to assess progression of the disease. Tissue damage should be minimized and the client protected from additional foci of bleeding. (Table 25-16 discusses nursing care for clients with thrombocytopenia, and nursing measures related to anemia are presented in Table 25-5.)

An additional responsibility is to administer blood products properly if they are ordered. Infusing cryoprecipitate or FFP is similar to giving any other blood product (see p. 709). Cryoprecipitate comes in bags of 10 to 20 ml each. When it is used to treat DIC, up to 30 bags of cryoprecipitate may be required to support the client. Fresh plasma is also frozen to preserve factors V and VIII. It takes about 20 minutes to thaw a unit that contains 200 to 250 ml.

Neutropenia, Granulocytopenia, and Agranulocytosis

Leukopenia refers to a decrease in the total WBC count (granulocytes, lymphocytes, and monocytes). *Granulocytopenia* is a deficiency of granulocytic cells, including neutrophils, eosinophils, and basophils. Traditionally granulocytopenia actually refers to *neutropenia* (an insufficient amount of neutrophils). Neutropenia in adults is defined as a neutrophil count of less than 1000 to 1500/μl. The term *agranulocytosis* is actually a synonym for severe neutropenia. Neutrophil counts below 500/μl constitute agranulocytosis. Regardless of the terminology, it is important to recognize that a leukopenic state can develop in many diseases, but it is not a disease itself. Neutropenia is a concern because of the neutrophil's role in phagocytosis.

Table 25-22 Clinical Conditions Associated with
Neutropenia

HEMATOLOGICAL

Idiopathic neutropenias
Leukemia
Aplastic anemia
HIV infection

NUTRITIONAL DEFICIENCIES

Vitamin B_{12}
Folic acid

DRUG INDUCED

Alkylating agents (e.g., chlorambucil, cyclophosphamide)
Antimetabolites (e.g., methotrexate, 6-mercaptopurine)
Phenothiazines (e.g., chlorpromazine)*
Anticonvulsants (e.g., diphenylhydantoin)*
Antimicrobials (e.g., chloramphenicol, penicillin, sulfonamides)*
Antitumor antibiotics (e.g., daunorubicin, doxorubicin)
Vinca alkaloids (e.g., vincristine, vinblastine)

SECONDARY TO OTHER DISEASES

Severe sepsis
Malignant tumors with bone marrow infiltration
Diseases with splenomegaly

*Infrequently causes neutropenia.

The major causes of granulocytopenia or neutropenia are summarized in Table 25-22.

Clinical manifestations. Clients with granulocytopenia are predisposed to infection. The most common infections are pneumonia, cellulitis, and septicemia. When the WBC count is depressed or immature WBCs are present, the usual phagocytic mechanisms are impaired. Because of the diminished phagocytic response, the classic signs of infection—redness, heat, and swelling—are not manifested. Therefore, the presence of fever is of great significance.[13]

When fever is associated with granulocytopenia, it is generally assumed to be a result of infection. Other manifestations of granulocytopenia may include fatigue and weakness. The mucous membranes of the throat and mouth are particularly susceptible to bacterial invasion. If an infection develops in these areas, the client may complain of sore throat and dysphagia. Other manifestations of granulocytopenia may include ulcerative lesions of the pharyngeal and buccal mucosa, tachycardia, and severe chills. The client with pneumonia often presents only with shortness of breath or nonproductive cough.

Diagnostic studies. The main methods for assessing neutropenia are peripheral blood and bone marrow examinations (Table 25-23). A total WBC count of less than 5000/μl reflects leukopenia. Only a differential count can confirm the presence of neutropenia (neutrophil count <1000 to 1500/μl). If the differential WBC count reflects an absolute neutropenia of 500 to 1000/μl, the client is at

Table 25-23

 Diagnostic and Therapeutic Management: Neutropenia

DIAGNOSTIC

History and physical examination
WBC count with differential count
Peripheral blood smear
Hematocrit and hemoglobin values
Reticulocyte and platelet count
Bone marrow aspiration and/or biopsy
Cultures of nose, throat, sputum, urine, obvious lesions (as indicated)
Chest x-ray film

THERAPEUTIC

Identification of cause
Identification of source of infection (if present)
Antibiotic therapy
Granulocyte transfusions
Laminar airflow isolation

moderate risk for a bacterial infection; an absolute neutropenia of less than 500/μl places the client at severe risk. If the monocyte count is 400 to 600/μl or greater, the client with neutropenia has some intrinsic resistance to infection.

A peripheral blood smear is used to assess for immature forms of granulocytes. The hematocrit level, reticulocyte count, and platelet count are done to evaluate general bone marrow function. Bone marrow aspirations and biopsies are done to examine cellularity and cell morphology. Additional studies may be done as indicated to assess spleen and liver function.

Therapeutic management. The factors involved in therapeutic management for neutropenia include (1) determining the cause of the neutropenia, (2) identifying the offending organisms if infection has developed, (3) instituting antibiotic therapy, (4) determining the need for granulocyte transfusions, and (5) assessing the usefulness of special isolation such as laminar airflow (Table 25-23).

The cause of the granulocytopenia may be easily removed (e.g., by termination of phenothiazines), or it may be recognized but not altered (e.g., the need to continue chemotherapy to treat leukemia). In some situations the neutropenia resolves when the primary disease is treated (e.g., folic acid deficiency).

Systemic infections caused by bacterial and fungal septicemias are common in clients with granulocytopenia. Pneumonias of bacterial and fungal origins are also prevalent. *Pneumocystis carinii* is an especially severe cause of pneumonia. Organisms that are known to be common sources of infection include *Staphylococcus aureus* and gram-negative organisms such as *Escherichia coli*, *Pseudomonas aeruginosa,* and *Klebsiella pneumoniae*. Fungi and the client's own bacteria have been identified as contributing significantly to life-threatening infection. The fungi that are involved include *Candida* (usually *C. albicans*) and *Aspergillus*. Viral infections caused by varicella-zoster and herpes simplex may also prove difficult to treat.

The therapeutic approach to identifying the infective organism depends on acquiring cultures from various sites. Serial blood cultures (at least two) are essential, along with cultures of sputum, the throat, lesions, wounds, urine, and feces. It may also be necessary to do a tracheal aspiration, bronchoscopy with bronchial brushings, or lung biopsy to diagnose the cause of pneumonic infiltrates.

Once cultures are obtained, antibiotic therapy must be initiated if fever is present. The use of antibiotics prophylactically is not usually recommended. However, in clients with AIDS, pentamidine is used prophylactically to prevent *P. carinii*. The life-threatening nature of granulocytopenia necessitates the institution of broad-spectrum antibiotics until culture results are returned. Administration of antibiotics must be via IV due to the rapidly lethal effects of infection. Oral antibiotics are not sufficiently potent and do not act as rapidly. In addition, antibiotics are often used in combination for clients with neutropenia to capitalize on their synergistic effects. Usually an aminoglycoside is used with an antipseudomonal penicillin or cephalosporin. Regardless of the combination, the nurse must watch for side effects. Side effects common to aminoglycosides include nephrotoxicity and ototoxicity, and side effects common to cephalosporins include rashes, fever, and pruritus.

Granulocyte transfusions remain a controversial issue. However, they may be used when the client with granulocytopenia remains febrile in spite of antibiotic therapy. Just as RBC and platelet transfusions are used to treat anemia and thrombocytopenia, respectively, granulocyte transfusions in conjunction with antibiotics improve survival for clients with severe granulocytopenia. Granulocyte transfusions have been associated with lethal pulmonary reactions characterized by diffuse intraalveolar hemorrhages when combined with the use of amphotericin B.

Not all health care facilities have the capability to prepare granulocyte transfusions because a technique known as *leukapheresis* is required. WBCs are often obtained by cell separation. Donors are connected to the leukapheresis machine, and WBCs are separated from other blood elements. The remaining blood elements are returned to the donor.

Once the decision is made to administer granulocytes, one or two donors should be obtained. The donor needs to be ABO and Rh compatible with the client because some RBCs are present in the WBC concentrate. In addition, HLA compatibility may also be necessary.

A final consideration is to assess the best means to protect the client whose own defenses against infection are compromised. Hand washing and laminar airflow isolation are the two primary interventions. The use of protective (reverse) isolation is a controversial matter. Many clinicians believe that its use is of little value, whereas others support its use in certain clients.[14] The Centers for Disease Control (CDC) has eliminated reverse isolation as a category. The CDC advocates hand washing before, during, and after care. This seemingly routine technique has a significant effect in reducing infection. It must be emphasized and enforced despite its seeming simplicity. The CDC also encourages separating immunocompromised clients from those who are infected or who have conditions that increase the probability of transmitting infections. Private rooms are useful whenever possible.

Laminar airflow rooms (LAFRs) are controversial, extremely expensive, and warranted for only the most severely compromised clients. However, they are very useful in preventing infection in clients whose treatment will lead to granulocytopenia (e.g., clients with leukemia who are receiving chemotherapy or waiting for bone marrow recovery). These rooms provide a virtually sterile environment by filtering the air through extremely efficient air filters and using a blower system that provides a laminar flow of air free from convection and conduction currents. There are two reasons for using LAFRs for clients with granulocytopenia. First, they reduce the incidence of hospital-acquired infections in these persons. Second, they provide an environment in which the client's own flora, also a potential source of infection, may be reduced to a minimum through the use of prophylactic topical and oral antibiotics.

■ Nursing Management of Neutropenia

The nursing measures presented in Table 25-24 are critical to the survival of clients with neutropenia. The value of good nursing care in reducing the development of infection or limiting its extent cannot be overemphasized.

The nurse is usually responsible for administering granulocyte transfusions. Granulocytes are given through standard blood filter tubing with normal saline solution to minimize cell lysis. Microaggregate filters are not used because they eliminate infusion of platelets present in the granulocyte suspension.

Granulocytes are usually administered over a 2- to 4-hour period. There are about 200 to 300 ml per granulocyte suspension. Granulocytes can be stored for only 48 hours. RBCs, platelets, and other WBCs may also be in the suspension. Consequently, transfusion reactions may occur. Therefore the initial 50 to 75 ml of the granulocyte infusion should be administered over 1 hour, and the client should be monitored closely for any manifestations of a reaction.

The nurse must also monitor the client for unwanted developments during granulocyte transfusion. These include fever and shaking chills, allergic reactions, hypotension, respiratory changes, hemolytic reactions, and graft-versus-host reaction.

Fever and shaking chills occur commonly and are more frequent if the client is febrile at the time the transfusion begins. Therefore transfusion may be postponed until the client's temperature is less than 38.7° C (101.7° F). The source of this febrile response is not clear, but as with platelet administration, prophylactic premedication with steroids, antihistamines, and meperidine reduces febrile episodes.

The nursing role in dealing with the febrile state is important. There is no need to stop the granulocyte transfusion, but the febrile reaction may be minimized by slowing the infusion so that it takes 4 hours.

Table 25-24

 NURSING CARE PLAN FOR THE CLIENT WITH NEUTROPENIA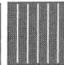

Defining Characteristics	Nursing Interventions	Evaluation Criteria

NURSING DIAGNOSIS: **High risk for infection related to decreased resistance and presence of environmental pathogens and ineffective hygiene of self or caregivers**

Defining Characteristics	Nursing Interventions	Evaluation Criteria
Fever without evidence of redness, heat, swelling; neutrophil count < 1500/μl	Recognize signs of infection. Evaluate oral temperature q 4 hr; report elevations >100.4° F to physician. Administer acetaminophen as an antipyretic *after* evaluating fever. Avoid using aspirin if client is thrombocytopenic. Assess cause of local and systemic manifestations of infection (chills, complaints of being cold when environment is warm, sore throat, persistent cough, chest pain, burning on urination, rectal pain). Use proper skin preparation technique for initiating and maintaining IVs or obtaining blood culture specimens. Evaluate fluid status during febrile episodes. Assess intake and output to include fluid lost through perspiration. Assess skin turgor and mucous membranes. Institute antibiotic therapy as ordered. Dilute medication adequately to diminish vein irritation. Establish administration schedule to maximize pharmacological effects and minimize side effects of drugs. Assess for superinfections that may develop with extended use of antibiotics. Recognize that oral antibiotics are often not effective to the extent needed by these clients. Institute good hand washing technique with antiseptic solution for all persons in contact with client. Place client in private room. Limit visitors. Screen visitors and hospital staff members with colds or potentially communicable illnesses. Routinely culture common sources of contamination (e.g., bathtubs or shower heads, respiratory therapy equipment). Provide meticulous perianal care to prevent perirectal abscess. Avoid invasive procedures to the greatest extent possible (e.g., venipunctures, urinary catheters, enemas, rectal suppositories). Teach client necessary personal hygiene techniques (e.g., hand washing, pulmonary hygiene). Administer granulocytes as ordered.	Free from signs and symptoms of infection, minimal exposure to environmental pathogens

Continued.

Table 25-24

NURSING CARE PLAN FOR THE CLIENT WITH NEUTROPENIA—cont'd

Defining Characteristics	Nursing Interventions	Evaluation Criteria

NURSING DIAGNOSIS: **High risk for altered oral mucous membrane related to treatment, disease, nausea, vomiting, or anorexia**

Defining Characteristics	Nursing Interventions	Evaluation Criteria
Sore throat, dysphagia, oral or pharyngeal ulcerations, stomatitis, oral infections	Remove dentures daily and evaluate fit. Assess oral mucosa daily for defining features. Distinguish stomatitis (inflammation of oral mucosa) from candidiasis (which is also known as moniliasis or *thrush*). Subacute candidiasis shows soft white patches on mucosa. Chronic candidiasis shows dry, red, buccal mucosa. Administer nystatin (Mycostatin), an antifungal, as ordered. Encourage client to use mouthwash q 2 hr for comfort (e.g., baking soda, hydrogen peroxide, normal saline solution, diphenhydramine [Benadryl] elixir). Use soft bristle toothbrushes, toothettes, or an irrigating syringe to cleanse mouth; avoid lemon and glycerin swabs. Apply topical anesthetics for discomfort (viscous lidocaine [Xylocaine], oral antiseptic [Chloraseptic], oxethazaine). Apply petroleum jelly to lips to moisten.	Pink, moist, lesion-free oral mucosa, tongue, lips; no inflammation, lesions, crusts, or hardened debris; no evidence of infection; no discomfort with talking or swallowing

NURSING DIAGNOSIS: **Activity intolerance related to weakness and fatigue**

Defining Characteristics	Nursing Interventions	Evaluation Criteria
Difficulty in ambulation and self-care, expression of feeling weak on exertion	Assess client's activity capabilities. Assist with ambulation and self-care as needed. Assure client of willingness to be of assistance. Plan schedule to allow for periods of uninterrupted rest.	Ability to ambulate and perform self-care without feelings of fatigue or discomfort

With allergic reactions manifested by urticaria, hives, wheezing, or hypotension, the transfusion must be stopped and the physician notified. As with reactions to other blood products, the IV line should be kept open with normal saline solution. The physician determines whether the granulocyte transfusion can proceed.

Two situations that require the granulocyte infusion to be discontinued are hypotensive responses and respiratory reactions. Hypotensive responses occur infrequently. A moderate reaction reduces blood pressure (BP) by 10 mm Hg; more severe reactions may involve symptoms of shock. With moderate reactions, the transfusion can continue, but severe hypotension dictates discontinuing the transfusion, keeping the IV site open with normal saline solution, and notifying the physician. Respiratory reactions manifested by dyspnea and cyanosis are rare. The occurrence of these reactions is more frequent when pulmonary infections are present. It is believed that the reaction results from the migration of the leukocytes to the pulmonary microvasculature. In this situation, intervention follows the pattern used with severe hypotension.

Hemolytic reactions may occur as a result of the presence of erythrocytes in the granulocyte suspension. These may be immediate or delayed for up to 3 days. Graft-versus-host disease (GVHD) may develop from lymphocytes in the granulocyte suspension if the client is immunosuppressed. In this type of reaction, the donated transfused lymphocytes mount an immune response against the recipient's cells. (GVHD is discussed in Chapter 8.)

LEUKEMIA

Leukemia is the general term used to describe a malignant disorder affecting the blood and blood-forming tissues of the bone marrow, lymph system, and spleen. It is a disease that, in differing forms, may affect all age groups. Leukemia results in an accumulation of dysfunctional cells because of a loss of cell division regulation. It follows a progressive course that is eventually fatal if untreated. Leukemias comprise 8% of all cancers, and an estimated 27,000 new cases were diagnosed in 1989.[15]

Pathophysiology

Regardless of the specific type of leukemia involved, the etiology is not fully understood. Like many cancers, it is thought to result from a combination of factors. Several predisposing factors have been identified, including various chemical agents such as benzene, genetic factors such as chromosomal alterations, viruses, immunological deficiencies, the prior use of certain antineoplastic drugs, and exposure to large doses of radiation. There is an increased incidence of leukemia in radiologists, persons living near areas where radiation testing is conducted, persons previously treated with radiotherapy or chemotherapy, and survivors of the bombing of Nagasaki and Hiroshima.

As leukemia progresses, fewer normal blood cells are produced. The abnormal leukocytes continue to multiply. They infiltrate and damage the bone marrow, lymph nodes, spleen, and other organs, including the CNS. Because of crowding of the bone marrow by leukemic cells, bone marrow suppression occurs. The client is predisposed to anemia from the lack of RBCs, thrombocytopenia from reduced platelets, and granulocytopenia from the deficiency of functional WBCs.

Classification

The two major categories of leukemia are acute and chronic. In the past, these designations had significant prognostic implications related to the duration of the illness. However, current therapeutic measures have increased the survival of clients with certain forms of acute leukemia beyond that of clients with certain forms of chronic leukemia. Although the terms *acute* and *chronic* are still used, they refer primarily to cell maturity and the nature of the disease onset. In acute leukemia, the bone marrow is infiltrated with young, undifferentiated, immature cells, often referred to as *blasts*. The disease has a rapid onset and requires immediate and aggressive intervention. The bone marrow in individuals with chronic leukemia consists primarily of differentiated mature WBCs, and the disease onset is more gradual.

Additional classification of leukemia is done by identifying the type of leukocyte involved, whether a granulocyte (myelocyte) or a lymphocyte. By combining the acute and chronic categories with the cell type involved, specific types of leukemia can be identified. Four major kinds of leukemia are acute lymphoblastic leukemia (ALL), acute myeloblastic leukemia (AML) (also called acute nonlymphoblastic leukemia [ANLL]), chronic myelocytic (granulocytic) leukemia (CML), and chronic lymphocytic leukemia (CLL). These forms of leukemia are compared in Table 25-25.

The nomenclature allows for general discussion of leukemia but does not differentiate the many subtypes of acute leukemia. A French-American-British (FAB) classification system was developed to better differentiate acute myeloid and lymphoid forms of leukemia (Table 25-26). It refers to three types of acute lymphoblastic leukemia (L_1, L_2, and L_3) that are distinguished by certain cytological features and the degree of heterogeneity of the leukemic cell population. The FAB system divides acute myeloid leukemia into six subtypes (M_1, M_2, M_3, M_4, M_5, and M_6) according to the direction of differentiation along one or more cell lines and the degree of cellular maturation. The traditional AML (ANLL) and ALL labels are used in conjunction with the FAB nomenclature. Additional work is being done to use monoclonal antibodies to differentiate types of WBCs and their precursors to facilitate diagnosis and classification of the leukemia. (Monoclonal antibodies are discussed in Chapter 8.)

Acute myeloblastic leukemia. AML is also referred to as acute nonlymphoblastic leukemia (ANLL). Approximately 85% of the acute leukemias in adults are the my-

eloid type.[15] Its onset may be abrupt and dramatic. Clients have serious infections and abnormal bleeding.

AML is characterized by uncontrolled proliferation of myeloblasts, the precursors of granulocytes. There is hyperplasia of the bone marrow and spleen. The clinical manifestations are usually related to replacement of normal hematopoietic cells in the marrow by leukemic cells and, to a lesser extent, to infiltration of other organs (see Table 25-25).

Acute lymphoblastic leukemia. ALL is most common in children and accounts for 15% of acute leukemia in adults. In ALL, immature lymphocytes proliferate in the bone marrow. Fever is present in the majority of clients at the time of diagnosis. Symptoms may appear abruptly with bleeding or fever, or they may be insidious with progressive weakness, fatigue, and bleeding tendencies. CNS manifestations are especially common in ALL and represent a serious problem. Leukemic meningitis due to arachnoid infiltration occurs in many clients with ALL.

Chronic myelocytic leukemia. CML is also referred to as chronic granulocytic leukemia (CGL). CML is caused by excessive development of neoplastic granulocytes in the bone marrow. The excess neoplastic granulocytes move into the peripheral blood in massive numbers and ultimately infiltrate the liver and spleen. Immature and mature granulocytes are found in the bone marrow and peripheral blood, but mature cells are dominant peripherally.

The chromosomal abnormality found in 90% of individuals with CML is an exchange of genetic information between chromosome pairs 9 and 22 and is called the *Philadelphia chromosome*. This alteration is directly attributed to the disease process.[16] Complications of CML are related to blastic crises that change chronic leukemia to acute disease (infiltration of more immature cells). Increased numbers of myeloblasts are found in both bone marrow and blood. The chronic phase of CML persists for 2 to 4 years and can usually be well controlled by treatment (see Table 25-28). The blastic phase of CML is refractory to therapy, and the client lives for only a few months.

Chronic lymphocytic leukemia. CLL is characterized by the production and accumulation of functionally inactive but long-lived, mature-appearing lymphocytes. In the United States the type of lymphocyte involved is usually the B cell. The lymphocytes infiltrate the bone marrow, spleen, and liver. Lymph node enlargement throughout the body is commonly found (Fig. 25-10). There is an increased incidence of infection. CLL tends to cluster in families. Complications from CLL are uncommon initially but may develop as the disease advances. Pressure on nerves from enlarged lymph nodes can cause pain and even paralysis. Mediastinal node enlargement can lead to pulmonary symptoms. Because CLL is a disease of older clients, treatment decisions must be made by considering the progression of the disease and side effects of treatment. Many individuals in the early stages of CLL require no treatment. As the disease progresses, various treatments can be used to control symptoms (see Table 25-28).

Uncommon leukemias. In addition to the four major types of leukemia, there are other kinds of leukemia that are seen infrequently. One of these affects the monocytes

Table 25-25 Types of Leukemia

Type	Age of Onset	Clinical Manifestations	Diagnostic Findings	Prognosis
Acute myeloblastic leukemia	Increase in incidence with advancing age, peak incidence between ages 60 and 70	Fatigue and weakness, headache, mouth sores, minimal hepatosplenomegaly and lymphadenopathy, anemia, bleeding, fever, infection, sternal tenderness	Low RBCs, Hb, Hct; very low platelet count; low to high WBC count with myeloblasts; markedly hypercellular bone marrow with myeloblasts	High mortality from infection and hemorrhage, remission in about 45%-75% of clients, survival after 2 years only 15%-20%
Acute lymphoblastic leukemia	Before age 14, peak incidence between ages 2 and 9 and in older adults	Fever; pallor; bleeding; anorexia; fatigue and weakness; bone, joint, and abdominal pain; generalized lymphadenopathy; infections; weight loss; hepatosplenomegaly; headache; mouth sores; neurological manifestations, including CNS metastases, increased intracranial pressure, secondary to meningeal infiltration	Low RBC, Hb, Hct; low platelet count; low, normal, or high WBC count; transverse lines of rarefaction at ends of metaphysis of long bones on x-ray film; hypercellular bone marrow with lymphoblasts; lymphoblasts also possible in cerebral spinal fluid	Good response to treatment (95% initial remission), 50% long-term survival in adults, children between ages 2 and 10 with best prognosis, good prognosis with WBC count of <20,000-30,000/μl at presentation
Chronic myelocytic leukemia	25 to 60 years of age, peak incidence around 45 years of age	No symptoms early in disease, fatigue and weakness, fever, sternal tenderness, weight loss, bone pain, massive splenomegaly, increase in sweating	Low RBCs, Hb, Hct; high platelet count early, lower count later; increase in polymorphonuclear neutrophils, normal number of lymphocytes, and normal or low number of monocytes in WBC differential; low leukocyte alkaline phosphatase; presence of Philadelphia chromosome in 90% of clients (only manifested in this disease)	Death usually from infection and hemorrhage; after diagnosis, 2-4 years usual survival
Chronic lymphocytic leukemia	50 to 70 years of age, rare below age 30, predominance in males	No symptoms usually, detection of disease often during examination for unrelated condition, chronic fatigue, anorexia, splenomegaly and lymphadenopathy, hepatomegaly	Mild anemia and thrombocytopenia with disease progression; increase in lymphocytes in WBC count; increase in presence of lymphocytes in bone marrow	Prognosis related to extent of organ infiltration, usual survival from 2-10 years, 4-6 years median survival

Hb, Hemoglobin; *Hct,* hematocrit.

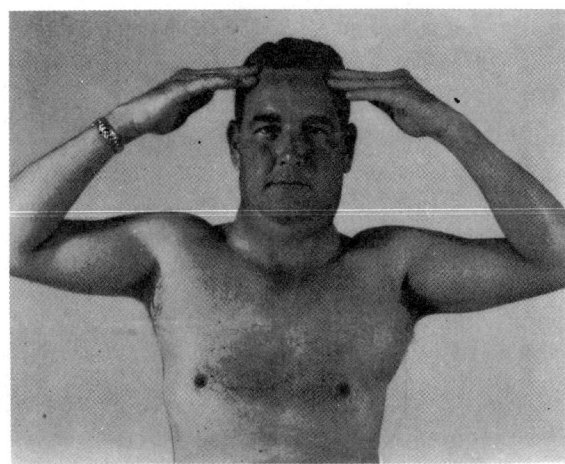

Fig. 25-10 Axillary and cervical lymph node enlargement in a person with CLL. (From Williams WJ and others, eds: Hematology, ed 2, New York, 1977, McGraw-Hill Book Co.)

Table 25-26 FAB Classification of Acute Leukemia

Acute lymphoblastic leukemia
   L1—Common childhood leukemia
   L2—Adult ALL
   L3—Rare subtype, blasts resembling those in Burkitt's
      lymphoma
Acute myeloblastic leukemia
  Granulocytic
    M1—Myeloblastic leukemia without maturation
    M2—Myeloblastic leukemia with maturation
    M3—Hypergranular promyelocytic leukemia
  Monocytic
    M4—Myelomonocytic leukemia
    M5—Monocytic
  Erythroid
    M6—Erythroleukemia

---

and is therefore known as *monocytic leukemia.* Clients with acute monocytic leukemia have weakness and fatigue progressing to exhaustion, anorexia, pallor, chills, and fever. Chronic monocytic leukemia is typified by a more insidious onset. In both types of monocytic leukemia, common findings are gingival hyperplasia, inflammation, bleeding, and infection. The second rare form of leukemia affects RBCs and is known as *erythroleukemia* or *DiGugliemo's syndrome.* It is considered a WBC disorder because ultimately the disease progresses to affect granulocytes.

Hairy cell leukemia represents about 2% of all adult leukemias. It is a chronic disease of lymphoproliferation predominantly involving B lymphocytes. There is an overproduction of hairy cells that infiltrate the bone marrow and spleen. In addition, the spleen sequesters increasing numbers of normal hematopoietic cells. α-Interferon is very effective in the treatment of this type of leukemia. Although its mechanism of action is not known, α-interferon may have a direct antigrowth effect and stimulate the immune system.

Clinical Manifestations

The manifestations of leukemia are varied (see Table 25-25). Essentially, they relate to problems caused by bone marrow failure and the formation of masses composed of leukemic infiltrates. Bone marrow failure results from inadequate production of normal marrow elements; therefore clinical manifestations of anemia, thrombocytopenia, and neutropenia are found. Leukemic infiltration leads to such findings as splenomegaly, hepatomegaly, lymphadenopathy, bone pain, meningeal irritation, and oral lesions.

Diagnostic Studies

Peripheral blood evaluation and bone marrow examination are the primary methods of diagnosing leukemia. (See Table 25-25 for the usual findings.) Monoclonal antibodies reactive to WBCs have been used to identify cell types and stage of development of leukemic cell populations. The identification of WBC subtypes improves the reliability of diagnosis and classification.

Therapeutic and Pharmacological Management

Once diagnosis of leukemia has been made, therapeutic management consists of ordering chemotherapeutic drugs and sometimes radiation therapy, examining clients on an ongoing basis to evaluate their progress, and intervening to prevent complications of the disease and the therapy (e.g., hemorrhage and infection). It is necessary to know the principles of cancer chemotherapy, including cellular kinetics, the use of multiple drugs rather than single agents, and the cell cycle. To understand the aggressive medical approach needed by clients with leukemia (see Chapter 9).

Remission is the goal of treatment for leukemia. Although the disease is not considered curable at this time, it can be brought under control. In complete remission there is no evidence of overt disease on physical examination, and the bone marrow and peripheral blood appear normal. A lesser state of control is known as partial remission. Partial remission is characterized by no overt clinical disease and a normal peripheral blood smear, but the disease remains in the bone marrow.

Although curing leukemia is not currently possible, the survival period after diagnosis is increasing as a result of attaining and maintaining remissions.[17] However, each time clients have a relapse, the succeeding remission will be much more difficult to achieve. Consequently, clients' compliance during therapy is of paramount importance.

The usual chemotherapy protocol is divided into three stages: induction, consolidation, and maintenance.[18] A fourth stage, intensification, may also be used. *Induction* therapy is the attempt to induce or bring about a remission. Induction is aggressive treatment that seeks to destroy leukemic cells in the tissues, peripheral blood, and bone marrow. During induction therapy a client may become devastatingly ill and predisposed to complications because the bone marrow is severely depressed by the drugs. Throughout induction, therapeutic and nursing interventions to combat anemia, thrombocytopenia, and leukopenia may significantly affect the client's survival.

Terms used to describe postremission chemotherapy include *intensification, consolidation,* and *maintenance.* Intensification, or high-dose therapy, may be given after induction therapy or several months later. This therapy may use the same drugs at higher dosages used during induction or other drugs that are thought to be non-cross-resistant to the induction drugs. Consolidation therapy is started after a remission is achieved with induction therapy. It may consist of one or two additional courses of the same drugs used during induction or high-dose therapy (intensive consolidation). The purpose of consolidation therapy is to eliminate remaining leukemic cells.

Maintenance therapy is treatment with lower doses of the same drugs used in induction or other drugs given every 3 to 4 weeks for a prolonged period. The goal is to maintain the remission once it is achieved, thereby keeping the body free of leukemic cells. Consequently it leads to fewer complications and is usually better tolerated.

In addition to chemotherapy, radiotherapy may be ordered for clients with chronic leukemia. Total body radiation may be used, or fields may be restricted to the liver and spleen or other organs affected by infiltrates. In acute leukemia, cranial irradiation and intrathecal methotrexate are used prophylactically to decrease the chance of CNS involvement. The use of immunotherapy in the treatment of leukemia is being investigated (see Chapter 9).

Chemotherapy regimens. The chemotherapeutic agents used to treat leukemia vary. The choice of drugs and the sequence of therapy depend on the preference of the cancer specialist as well as on current research findings. Therefore there are no definitive protocols of treatment for the various types of leukemias. Table 25-27 lists chemotherapeutic agents used to treat leukemia. Table 25-28 gives examples of treatment regimens used in various types of leukemia.

Table 25-27 Chemotherapeutic Agents Used to Treat Leukemia

Drug Classification	Drug Name
Alkylating agents	Busulfan (Myleran), chlorambucil (Leukeran), cyclophosphamide (Cytoxan)
Antitumor antibiotics	Daunorubicin (Cerubidine), doxorubicin (Adriamycin), mitoxantrone (Novantrone)
Antimetabolites	Cytarabine/cytosine arabinoside (Cytosar/Ara-C), 6-mercaptopurine (Purinethol), methotrexate (Folex, Mexate), 6-thioguanine (6-TG)
Corticosteroid	Prednisone
Nitrosoureas	Carmustine (BCNU)
Plant alkaloid	Vincristine (Oncovin), vinblastine (Velban)
Miscellaneous	L-Asparaginase (Elspar), hydroxyurea (Hydrea), etoposide (VP-16)

Table 25-28 Treatments Used in Leukemia

Drug Therapy	Other Therapy
ACUTE MYELOBLASTIC LEUKEMIA	
Daunorubicin, cytosine arabinoside, doxorubicin, 6-thioguanine, mitoxantrone, combination chemotherapy of antitumor antibiotic and cytosine arabinoside or antitumor antibiotic and cytosine arabinoside and thioguanine	Bone marrow transplant
ACUTE LYMPHOBLASTIC LEUKEMIA	
Daunorubicin, doxorubicin, vincristine, prednisone, L-asparaginase, cyclophosphamide, methotrexate, 6-mercaptopurine, cytosine arabinoside, combination chemotherapy of cyclophosphamide and vincristine and prednisone and antitumor antibiotic and L-asparaginase, combination chemotherapy of daunorubicin and cytosine arabinoside and 6-mercaptopurine and vincristine and prednisone	Cranial radiation therapy, intrathecal methotrexate
CHRONIC MYELOCYTIC LEUKEMIA	
Busulfan (Myleran); hydroxyurea (Hydrea); combination chemotherapy including any of the following: cytosine arabinoside, thioguanine, daunorubicin, methotrexate, prednisone, vincristine, L-asparaginase, carmustine, 6-mercaptopurine	Radiation (total body or spleen), bone marrow transplant, interferon, leukapheresis
CHRONIC LYMPHOCYTIC LEUKEMIA	
Chorambucil (Leukeran), cyclophosphamide (Cytoxan), prednisone, CVP protocol (cyclophosphamide, vincristine, and prednisone)	Radiation (total body, lymph nodes, or spleen), splenectomy, colony-stimulating factors, interferon

Combination chemotherapy is the mainstay of treatment for leukemia. The three purposes for using multiple drugs are to (1) decrease drug resistance, (2) minimize the toxicity of high doses of single agents by using multiple drugs with varying toxicities, and (3) interrupt cell growth at multiple points in the cell cycle.

Acronyms made from the letters of the drugs used in the combination may be used to identify the regimen. For example, *COAP* stands for cyclophosphamide, Oncovin, arabinoside, and prednisone. This combination of drugs is used in the treatment of acute leukemia.

Bone marrow transplantation. Bone marrow transplantation (BMT) is another mode of treatment for acute leukemia. The transplant may be allogeneic (from an HLA-matched donor) or autologous (from the individual's own bone marrow harvested during remission).[19] Common indications for bone marrow transplants include ALL, AML, CML, Hodgkin's disease, non-Hodgkin's lymphoma, breast cancer, aplastic anemia, and congenital immunodeficiencies.

Allogeneic BMT. In allogeneic BMT, high doses of chemotherapy and usually total body irradiation are given to suppress a person's immune system so that new marrow can engraft and eliminate malignant cell populations in recipients with malignancies. Possible donors are evaluated for histocompatibility with the recipient. (Histocompatibility antigen testing is discussed in Chapters 8 and 41.) Donor bone marrow is aspirated from the bone, usually from the iliac crest, but it can also be obtained from the sternum or ribs. It is then prepared and infused intravenously into the recipient. The marrow stem cells reconstitute the recipient's marrow. Usually 2 to 4 weeks are required for the transplanted marrow to start producing peripheral blood elements.[20] During this pancytopenic period it is critical for the client to be in a protective isolation environment receiving supportive care. Granulocyte, RBC, and platelet transfusions may be necessary to maintain circulating blood cells during this time.

The primary complications of clients with allogeneic BMT are GVHD, relapse of leukemia (especially ALL), and infection (especially interstitial pneumonia). GVHD is mediated by competent T cells infused with the donor marrow that mount an attack against the recipient's immune system (see Chapter 8). Interstitial pneumonia is most often caused by cytomegalovirus.

Autologous BMT. Bone marrow can be harvested from the person during remission and treated to remove residual neoplastic cells using monoclonal antibodies or chemical agents. The bone marrow is then cryopreserved (frozen) and stored until it is used for transplant. Autologous BMT is often called *bone marrow rescue* because it is given to the client following high-dose chemotherapy and/or radiation. The increased doses of chemotherapy and radiation made possible by bone marrow rescue have produced favorable outcomes in some neoplasms, particularly solid tumors.

■ Nursing Management of Leukemia
Nursing assessment

Subjective and objective data that should be obtained from a client with leukemia are presented in Table 25-29.

Table 25-29

Nursing Assessment of the Client with Leukemia

SUBJECTIVE DATA

History
Positive family history; exposure to chemical toxins (e.g., benzene, arsenic), radiation, or viruses (Epstein-Barr, HTLV-1); chromosome abnormalities (e.g., in clients with Down syndrome, Klinefelter's syndrome, Fanconi's syndrome)

Medications
Use of phenylbutazone, chloramphenicol, chemotherapy or radiation for treatment

General
Chills, fever, bleeding tendencies, progressive weakness, syncope, malaise, fatigue, anorexia, night sweats, irritability, weight loss, frequent infections

Pain
Headache; bone tenderness; muscle cramps; sore throat; bone, joint, abdominal pain

Integumentary
Easy bruising

Respiratory
Dyspnea, epistaxis, cough

Gastrointestinal
Dysphagia, nausea and vomiting, mouth sores, diarrhea, dark stools

Urinary
Hematuria, decreased urine output

Reproductive
Prolonged menses, menorrhagia, impotence

Neurological
Paresthesias, numbness, tingling, visual disturbances

OBJECTIVE DATA

General
Generalized lymphadenopathy, lethargy

Integumentary
Pallor or jaundice; petechiae, ecchymoses, purpura, reddish-brown to purple cutaneous infiltrates, purple skin tumors, macules, and papules

Cardiovascular
Tachycardia, systolic murmurs

Neurological
Seizures, disorientation, confusion, decreased coordination, cranial nerve palsies, papilledema

Musculoskeletal
Muscle wasting

Possible findings
Low, normal, or high WBC count with shift to the left (↑ blast cells); anemia, decreased hematocrit and hemoglobin, thrombocytopenia, Philadelphia chromosome; hypercellular bone marrow aspirate or biopsy with myeloblasts, lymphoblasts, markedly reduced normal cells

Nursing diagnoses

Nursing diagnoses related to leukemia include those appropriate for anemia (Table 25-5), thrombocytopenia (Table 25-16), and neutropenia (Table 25-24).

Nursing interventions

Acute intervention. The nursing role during acute phases of leukemia is extremely challenging because the client will have many physical and psychosocial needs. Because it is a form of cancer, the diagnosis of leukemia often evokes great fear. It may be viewed as a hopeless, horrible disease with many painful and undesirable consequences. Leukemia is often equated with death. The diagnosis of leukemia elicits many emotional responses based on the realization that life is finite. The nurse has a special responsibility in helping clients and families deal with these feelings. The nurse must help clients realize that although their future may be uncertain, they can learn to live in spite of their illness. Families may need help in adjusting to the chronic effects of illness (e.g., dependence, withdrawal, changes in role responsibilities, and alterations in body image) and the losses imposed by the sick role.

The nurse must develop skills to help clients resolve their problems. A positive outlook by the client may increase the efficacy of therapy and will affect the quality of the client's life. It must also be recognized that human compassion is greatly needed but may be less available because chronically ill clients are often deserted and isolated. Because nurses have contact with clients 24 hours a day, they can help reverse feelings of abandonment and loneliness. However, more technical needs often take priority over talking with clients. Therefore nurses face a special challenge in learning how to meet the intense psychosocial needs of clients with leukemia while continuing to offer the complex physical care that is usually required. Consulting with other health professionals (e.g., psychiatric clinical specialists, oncology clinical specialists, social workers) may help the nurse develop the skills required to meet the many needs of clients with leukemia.

From a physical care perspective, the nurse is challenged to make astute assessments and plan care to help the client survive the severe side effects of chemotherapy. The life-threatening results of bone marrow suppression (anemia, thrombocytopenia, neutropenia) require aggressive nursing interventions (see Tables 25-5, 25-16, and 25-24). Additional complications of chemotherapy may affect the client's GI tract, nutritional status, skin and mucosa, cardiopulmonary status, hepatorenal system, and neuromuscular system. (Nursing interventions to reduce discomfort related to these problems are discussed in Chapter 9.)

The nurse must be knowledgeable about all drugs being administered. This includes the mechanism of action, purpose, routes of administration, usual doses, potential side effects, and toxic effects of the drugs. In addition, the nurse must know how to assess laboratory data reflecting the effects of the drugs. Client survival and comfort during aggressive chemotherapy are significantly affected by the quality of nursing care.

Chronic management. Ongoing care for the client with leukemia is necessary to ensure that the disease remains in remission or under control. Client compliance with maintenance chemotherapy regimens is very important. Therefore clients and their significant others must be educated to understand the nature of leukemia and the rationale for treatment. They must also be taught about the drugs and when to seek medical attention.

Rehabilitation also aims to provide psychological support to the client and family as they deal with the negative connotations of the diagnosis of leukemia. Assistance may be needed to reestablish the various relationships that are a part of the client's life. Friends and family may not know how to interact with the client. All the individuals involved may need help to focus on reality and living as opposed to being obsessed with death. Involving the client in groups such as CanSurmount and Make Today Count may help the client adapt to living with illness by learning from others with similar problems. Exploring resources in the community (e.g., American Cancer Society, Meals-on-Wheels, wheelchair taxis) may reduce the financial burden and the feelings of dependence. Spiritual support may give the client inner strength and peace.

It is expected that the client will need support in adapting to any physical limitations or changes imposed by the illness. Clients may feel more positive if emphasis is placed on what they can do rather than on the restrictions that now exist. The nurse may involve other health care providers in meeting the client's needs, but the nurse must recognize the obligation to identify these needs and initiate a referral or consultation. For example, physical therapy personnel may be asked to develop an exercise program to prevent posttreatment deficits caused by drug-induced peripheral neuropathy.

The nurse's approach to the long-term management of leukemia affects the quality of the client's life. It is a responsibility that cannot be minimized. This is especially true because leukemia has a cyclical course of remissions and exacerbations that constantly impinges on and affects the client's relationships and ability to function.

LYMPHOMAS

Lymphomas are malignant neoplasms that affect lymphatic structures and involve proliferation of histiocytes and lymphocytes. There are two major types of lymphoma—Hodgkin's disease and non-Hodgkin's lymphoma.

Hodgkin's Disease

Hodgkin's disease, comprising 33% of all lymphomas, is a malignant condition characterized by proliferation of abnormal histiocytes called *Reed-Sternberg cells*. The disease has a bimodal age-specific incidence, occurring most frequently in persons from ages 15 to 35 and above age 50. In adults, it is twice as prevalent in men as in women.

Pathophysiology. The cause of Hodgkin's disease remains unknown. It is possible that genetic, immunological, and viral factors interact to cause it. Nevertheless, treatment is impressively successful.

Normally, the lymph nodes are composed of connective tissues that surround a fine mesh of reticular fibers and cells. In Hodgkin's disease the normal structure of lymph nodes is destroyed by hyperplasia of the monocytes/macrophages. The disease is believed to arise in a single location (it originates in lymph nodes in 90% of clients) and then spreads along adjacent lymphatics. It eventually infiltrates other organs, especially the lungs, spleen, and liver. In about two thirds of clients, the cervical lymph nodes are the first to be affected. When the disease begins above the diaphragm, it remains confined to lymph nodes for a variable period of time. Disease originating below the diaphragm frequently spreads to extralymphoid sites such as the liver.

A diagnostic feature of Hodgkin's disease is the presence of Reed-Sternberg cells. They are malignant histiocytes with large, multinucleated cells. These cells are often seen in lymph node biopsy material before they appear in the bone marrow or peripheral blood.

Clinical manifestations. The onset of symptoms in Hodgkin's disease is usually insidious. The initial development is most often enlargement of cervical, axillary, or inguinal lymph nodes. This lymphadenopathy affects discrete nodes that remain movable and nontender. The enlarged nodes are not painful unless nerves are involved.

Client complaints may include weight loss, fatigue, weakness, fever, chills, tachycardia, and night sweats. The findings of fever, night sweats, and weight loss (referred to as *B symptoms*) correlate with a poor prognosis. After the ingestion of even small amounts of alcohol, individuals with Hodgkin's disease complain of rapid onset of pain at the site of disease. The cause for the alcohol-induced pain is unknown. Generalized pruritus without skin lesions may develop. Cough, dyspnea, stridor, and dysphagia may all reflect mediastinal node involvement.

Other physical findings may include hepatomegaly and splenomegaly, but they are usually not present unless the disease is advanced. Anemia results from increased destruction as well as decreased production of erythrocytes. Other physical signs vary depending on where the disease has spread. For example, intrathoracic involvement may lead to superior vena cava syndrome, enlarged retroperitoneal nodes may cause palpable abdominal masses, jaundice may occur from liver involvement, and spinal cord compression leading to paraplegia may occur with extradural involvement. Bone pain occurs as a result of osteoblastic bone lesions.

Diagnostic studies. Peripheral blood analysis, lymph node biopsy, bone marrow examination, and radiological evaluation are important means of evaluating Hodgkin's disease. Peripheral blood analysis often reveals a hypochromic microcytic anemia, neutrophilic leukocytosis (15,000 to 25,000/μl) that may be associated with lymphopenia, and an increased platelet count. Leukopenia and thrombocytopenia may develop, but they are usually a consequence of treatment or superimposed hypersplenism. In addition to evaluating marrow elements, other blood studies may show hypoferremia caused by excessive iron uptake by the liver and spleen, elevated leukocyte alkaline phosphatase from liver and bone involvement, hypercalcemia from bone involvement, and hypoalbuminemia.

Excisional lymph node biopsy offers a definitive means of diagnosis. If removed, an enlarged peripheral lymph node can be examined histologically for the presence of the diagnostic Reed-Sternberg cells.

Bone marrow biopsy is rarely helpful because there are no characteristic findings. In Hodgkin's disease there may be indications of granulocytic and megakaryocytic hyperplasia, but these findings are not unique to Hodgkin's disease. Reed-Sternberg cells may be found in the bone marrow of clients with advanced disease.

Radiological evaluation can help to localize the disease. Chest radiographs may show mediastinal lymphadenopathy, and an IV pyelogram may show renal displacement caused by retroperitoneal node enlargement. Radioisotope studies may assist in evaluating the liver, bone, and brain. Computerized tomography (CT) scans may help in detecting abdominal lymph node enlargement. Lymphangiography is especially useful because it allows assessment of lymph nodes and lymph vessels, especially the retroperitoneal structures, which are difficult to visualize.

Therapeutic management. For treatment to be as precise as possible, Hodgkin's disease needs to be staged. Staging involves determining the extent and involvement of the disease. This is important because Hodgkin's disease may be very localized or very diffuse. Treatment depends on the nature of the disease. The nomenclature used in staging involves an A or B classification, depending on whether symptoms are present when the disease is found, and a Roman numeral (I to IV) that reflects the location and extent of the disease (Table 25-30).

Diagnostic studies are conducted to assess the stage of Hodgkin's disease. However, there may also be a need to demonstrate the actual extent of abdominal involvement.

In the past, surgical staging that included laparotomy and splenectomy was standard procedure. The purpose of surgical staging is to establish the extent of abdominal involvement that is critical to guiding therapy based on the stage of the disease. Technological advances such as CT scanning have augmented the array of techniques available for noninvasive evaluation. Although the method is controversial at present, many institutions continue to use surgical staging to ensure accurate diagnosis.

Once the stage of Hodgkin's disease is established, therapeutic management focuses on selecting a treatment plan. Treatment for Hodgkin's disease has improved considerably. Radiation therapy can cure 95% of clients with stage I or stage II disease. Radiation given over 4 to 6 weeks may permanently cure Hodgkin's disease. Stage IIIA disease is treated with both radiotherapy and chemotherapy. The role of radiation as a supplement to chemotherapy in stages III and IV is controversial. Advances in treatment now enable some stage IIIB and stage IV diseases to be cured with chemotherapy. (Cure is defined as an absence of disease for more than 5 years.) (Chapter 9 reviews the principles of radiotherapy and chemotherapy.)

Pharmacological management. Chemotherapy is the treatment of choice for disseminated Hodgkin's disease (stages IIIB and IV). Chemotherapeutic agents used in Hodgkin's disease are listed in Table 25-31. Combination chemotherapy works well because, as in leukemia, drugs are used that have an additive antitumor effect without increasing side effects. As with leukemia, therapy must be aggressive. Therefore potentially life-threatening problems

Table 25-30 Staging Classification for Lymphomas

Stage	Definition
I	Involvement of single lymph node region (I) or single extralymphatic organ or site (I_E)
II	Involvement of two or more lymph node regions on same side of diaphragm (II) or localized involvement of extra-lymphatic organ or site and one or more lymph node regions on same side of diaphragm (II_E)
III	Involvement of lymph node regions on both sides of diaphragm (III), which may also be accompanied by involvement of the spleen (III_s) or by localized involvement of an extralymphatic organ or site (III_E), or both (III_{sE})
IV*	Diffuse or disseminated involvement of one or more extralymphatic organs or tissues, with or without associated lymph node involvement
A	No general symptoms
B	Presence of one of the following symptoms: (1) unexplained weight loss of more than 10% of body weight in 6 mo before admission, (2) unexplained fever with temperatures above 38° C (100.4° F), (3) night sweats

*Biopsy-documented involvement of stage IV sites is also denoted by letter suffixes: *M*+, marrow; *L*+, lung; *H*+, liver; *P*+, pleura; *O*+, bone; *D*+, skin and subcutaneous tissue.

Table 25-31 Chemotherapeutic Agents Used in Hodgkin's Disease

ALKYLATING AGENTS

Nitrogen mustard, mechlorethamine (Mustargen)
Cyclophosphamide (Cytoxan)
Chlorambucil (Leukeran)
Procarbazine (Matulane)
Carmustine (BCNU)
Dacarbazine (DTIC)

ANTITUMOR ANTIBIOTICS

Doxorubicin (Adriamycin)
Bleomycin (Blenoxane)
Mitoxantrone (Novantrone)

PLANT ALKALOIDS

Vinblastine (Velban)
Vincristine (Oncovin)

CORTICOSTEROIDS

Prednisone

MISCELLANEOUS

Etoposide (VP-16)

Table 25-32 Combination Chemotherapy Used in Hodgkin's Disease

MOPP: Nitrogen mustard, vincristine (Oncovin), procarbazine, prednisone
MVPP: Nitrogen mustard, vinblastine, procarbazine, prednisone
CVPP: Cyclophosphamide, vinblastine, procarbazine, prednisone
ABVD: Adriamycin, bleomycin, vinblastine (Velban), dacarbazine (DTIC)

are encountered in an attempt to achieve a remission.

The most widely known chemotherapy regimen is called *MOPP*, which stands for the four drugs composing it: *M*, mechlorethamine (nitrogen mustard); *O*, Oncovin (vincristine); *P*, procarbazine (Matulane); and *P*, prednisone. Other chemotherapeutic regimens have been designed and used with good success (Table 25-32).

Maintenance chemotherapy does not contribute to increased survival once a complete remission is achieved. Occasionally, single drugs may be administered palliatively to clients who cannot tolerate intensive combination therapy. The most serious consequence of treatment for Hodgkin's disease is the emergence of secondary malignancies (see Chapter 9).

■ Nursing Management of Hodgkin's Disease

The nursing care for Hodgkin's disease is largely based on managing pancytopenia and other side effects of therapy. Because the survival of clients with Hodgkin's disease depends on their response to treatment, supporting the client through the myelosuppressive state is extremely important (see Tables 25-5, 25-16, and 25-24). Psychosocial considerations are just as important as they are with leukemia (see p. 702). Because the prognosis for Hodgkin's disease is better than that for many forms of leukemia, clients must be helped to deal with their disease realistically even though they know it is a malignant disorder.

The client undergoing radiotherapy will need special nursing consideration. In addition to the side effects, which are similar to those of chemotherapy, the skin in the radiation field requires special attention. Also, the nurse must understand the concepts related to administration of radiotherapy (see Chapter 9).

Once the client is in remission, ongoing maintenance treatment is not needed. However, it is imperative that the client learn the importance of returning for subsequent examinations as scheduled.

Non-Hodgkin's Lymphoma

Non-Hodgkin's lymphomas (NHL) are a heterogenous group of malignant neoplasms of the immune system.

Table 25-33 Classification of Non-Hodgkin's Lymphomas

LOW GRADE

Small lymphocytic
Follicular, small cleaved cell
Follicular, mixed small cleaved and large cell

INTERMEDIATE GRADE

Follicular, large cell
Diffuse, small cleaved cell
Diffuse, mixed; small and large
Diffuse, large cell

HIGH GRADE

Large cell, immunoblastic
Lymphoblastic
Small noncleaved cell

Table 25-34 Hodgkin's and Non-Hodgkin's Lymphomas

Parameter	Hodgkin's Disease	Non-Hodgkin's Lymphomas
Age	Younger	Older
Degree of debilitation	Less	More
Presence of B symptoms	More likely	Less likely
Spread at presentation	Local to regional	Advanced
Histopathological classification	Singular	Many different classifications

They are classified by a variety of schemes. The most common one is presented in Table 25-33. The disorders are variable in clinical presentation and course, varying from indolent disease to rapidly progressive disease. Common names for different types of NHL include *Burkitt's lymphoma, reticulum cell sarcoma,* and *lymphosarcoma.* There is no hallmark feature in NHLs that parallels the Reed-Sternberg cell of Hodgkin's disease. However, almost all NHLs involve lymphocytes arrested in various stages of development.[21] Table 25-34 presents a comparison of Hodgkin's disease and NHL.

NHLs usually originate outside the lymph nodes, the method of spread cannot be anticipated, and the majority of clients have widely disseminated disease at the time of diagnosis. The primary clinical manifestation is painless lymph node enlargement. Because the disease is usually disseminated when it is diagnosed, other symptoms will be present depending on where the disease has spread (e.g., hepatomegaly with liver involvement).

Clients with high-grade lymphomas may have lymphadenopathy and constitutional symptoms such as fever, night sweats, and weight loss. The peripheral blood is usually normal, but some lymphomas may present in a "leukemic" phase.

Diagnostic studies used for NHL resemble those used for Hodgkin's disease. Lymph node biopsy establishes the cell type and pattern. Staging, as described for Hodgkin's disease, is used to guide therapy. The prognosis for NHL is not as good as that for Hodgkin's disease. Treatment for NHL involves radiotherapy and chemotherapy. Radiotherapy alone may be effective for treatment of stage I disease, but combination radiation therapy and chemotherapy are used for other stages. Initial chemotherapy uses alkylating agents such as cyclophosphamide and chlorambucil. Combination chemotherapy such as CVP (cyclophosphamide, vincristine, and prednisone) or CHOP (CVP and adrimycin) are also used. Biological response modifiers (BRMs) such as interferons, interleukin-2, and tumor necrosis factor are also being investigated for treatment of NHL. (BRMs are discussed in Chapter 9.)

MULTIPLE MYELOMA

Multiple myeloma, or plasma cell myeloma, is a condition in which neoplastic plasma cells infiltrate bone marrow and destroy bone. Clients usually live for about 2 years after diagnosis if untreated. The incidence of multiple myeloma approximates that of Hodgkin's disease. The disease is twice as common in men as in women and usually develops after the age of 40, with a peak incidence around the age of 55.

Pathophysiology

There are many hypotheses regarding the etiology of multiple myeloma (e.g., chronic inflammation, chronic hypersensitivity reactions, viral influences), but no actual cause has been identified. The disease process involves excessive production of plasma cells. Plasma cells are activated B cells and thus produce immunoglobulins that serve to protect the body (see Chapter 8). However, in multiple myeloma the plasma cells are neoplastic and infiltrate the bone marrow and develop into tumors. Ultimately, the plasma cells destroy bone and invade the lymph nodes, liver, spleen, and kidneys. The neoplastic plasma cells produce an abnormal immunoglobulin that cannot develop into antibodies. This abnormal immunoglobulin is known as a *myeloma protein.* As myeloma protein increases, normal plasma cells are reduced, which further compromises the body's normal immune response.

Clinical Manifestations

Multiple myeloma develops slowly and insidiously. Clients remain relatively free of symptoms until the disease is advanced, at which time skeletal pain is the major manifestation. Pain in the pelvis, spine, and ribs is particularly common. Diffuse osteoporosis develops as the myeloma protein destroys more bone. Osteolytic lesions are seen in the skull, vertebrae, and ribs. Vertebral destruction can lead to collapse of vertebrae with ensuing compression of the spinal cord, requiring emergency laminectomy to prevent paraplegia. Loss of bone integrity can lead to the development of pathophysiological fractures. Bony degeneration also causes calcium to be lost from bones. It enters the serum, causing hypercalcemia.

Hypercalcemia may be reflected by renal, GI, or neurological changes such as polyuria, anorexia, and confusion. In addition, cell destruction contributes to the development of hyperuricemia, which, along with the high protein levels caused by the presence of the myeloma protein, can result in renal failure from renal tubular obstruction and interstitial nephritis from the uric acid precipitates. The client may display symptoms of anemia, thrombocytopenia, and granulocytopenia, all of which are related to the replacement of normal bone marrow elements with plasma cells.

Diagnostic Studies

Evaluating multiple myeloma involves laboratory, radiological, and bone marrow examination. Pancytopenia may be found on laboratory assessment. High serum protein may be present. Hyperuricemia, hypercalcemia, and elevated creatinine may also be found by laboratory tests. In addition to serum tests, a special urine study can be done. An abnormal globulin known as *Bence Jones protein* is found in the urine in cases of multiple myeloma.

Radiological studies involve normal radiographs and isotope scans to establish the degree of bone involvement. The studies document the presence of diffuse bony lesions, demineralization, and osteoporosis in areas of the affected skeleton.

Bone marrow analysis shows significantly increased numbers of plasma cells in the bone marrow. Other components of the marrow are normal.

Therapeutic Management

The therapeutic approach involves managing both the disease and its symptoms, since the chronic phase of multiple myeloma may last for more than 10 years. Ambulation and adequate hydration are ordered to offset hypercalcemia, hyperuricemia, and dehydration. Weight bearing helps the bones reabsorb some calcium, and fluids dilute the calcium load and prevent protein precipitates from causing renal tubular obstruction.

Control of pain is another goal of therapeutic management. Analgesics, orthopedic supports, and localized radiation help to reduce the skeletal pain. Chemotherapy is used to reduce the number of plasma cells. The agents most frequently used are the alkylating drugs, including melphalan (Alkeran), cyclophosphamide (Cytoxan), chlorambucil (Leukeran), and carmustine (BCNU). Adrenocorticosteroids may be added because they exert an antitumor effect in some clients. Radiotherapy is another important component of treatment, primarily because of its palliative effect on localized lesions.

Drugs may also be used to counteract complications. For example, allopurinol (Zyloprim) may be given to reduce hyperuricemia, and IV sodium chloride and furosemide help to promote renal excretion of calcium.

■ Nursing Management of Multiple Myeloma

Maintaining adequate hydration is a primary nursing consideration to minimize problems from hypercalcemia.

Fluids are administered to attain an output of 1.5 to 2 L per day. This may require an intake of 3 to 4 L. In addition, weight bearing helps bones to reabsorb some of the calcium, and steroids may augment the excretion of calcium. Once chemotherapy is initiated, the uric acid levels rise because of the increased cell destruction. Hyperuricemia must be resolved by ensuring adequate hydration and using allopurinol.

Because of the potential for pathophysiological fractures, the nurse must use careful planning and methods to move and ambulate clients. A slight twist or strain in the wrong area (e.g., a weak area in the client's bones) may be sufficient to cause fracture.

Pain management requires innovative and knowledgeable nursing intervention. If radiotherapy is used to diminish pain from localized myeloma lesions, appropriate skin care techniques must be used. Mild analgesics such as acetaminophen or acetaminophen and codeine may be more effective than potent analgesics in diminishing bone pain. Braces, especially for the spine, may also help control pain. As in any pain management situation, the nurse is responsible for assessing the client and for implementing necessary nursing measures to reduce if not alleviate the pain (see Chapter 51).

Chemotherapy must be given properly, with attention to side effects developed by the client. Pancytopenia in particular requires nursing intervention.

The client's psychosocial needs require sensitive, skilled management. As with leukemia, it is important to help the client and significant others adapt to changes fostered by chronic sickness, to deal with reality rather than create fantasies, and to adjust to losses of various magnitudes. The symptoms of multiple myeloma remit and exacerbate. Consequently, hospital care is needed at various times during the course of the illness. The final, acute phase is unresponsive to treatment and usually short. The ways clients and families deal with confronting death may be affected by the manner in which they learned to accept and live with the chronic nature of the disease.

MONONUCLEOSIS

Mononucleosis, often referred to as "mono" or the "kissing disease," is a benign, self-limiting disease characterized by lymph node enlargement, lymphocytosis, and elevated temperature. It occurs most commonly among children of ages 3 to 5 and adolescents and young adults of ages 15 to 25. It may occur in isolated cases or epidemics. Although benign, the disease may incapacitate clients because of the extreme fatigue associated with it.

Etiology

Mononucleosis is caused by the Epstein-Barr virus, a type of herpesvirus. The exact mode of transmission is not known, but secretions from mucous membranes of the mouth, GI tract, and respiratory tract, are believed to be involved. Mononucleosis does not develop in persons who have antibodies to the Epstein-Barr virus; those who are deficient in these antibodies acquire the disease when infected by the Epstein-Barr virus. Once exposed, susceptible clients manifest symptoms of disease after a 30- to 40-day incubation period. Symptoms evolve gradually, intensifying as the disease becomes apparent. After causing mononucleosis, the Epstein-Barr virus may lie dormant in lymphocytes and other lymphatic tissue, thus contributing to the development of immunity.

Clinical Manifestations

General complaints before the actual onset of mononucleosis are rather vague. A severe headache, fatigue, malaise, chills, puffy eyelids, anorexia, and a distaste for smoking cigarettes may develop early in the illness. As the disease becomes more acute, more than 80% of clients have a triad of symptoms, including fever, painful lymph node enlargement (especially cervical, axillary, and groin nodes), and sore throat. The sore throat may be severe enough to cause dysphagia. If the spleen is enlarged by massive lymphocyte infiltration, pain will occur in the left upper quadrant.

It is rare for significant complications to develop from mononucleosis. The problems that may occur include pneumonia, neurological changes, splenic rupture, thrombocytopenia, hemolytic anemia, airway obstruction, and cardiac involvement.

Diagnostic Studies

Initially, the WBC and differential cell counts are normal, but within a week a leukocytosis (WBC greater than 20,000/μl) will occur. There is a rise in lymphocytes and monocytes to over 50%, with 10% to 20% atypical lymphocytes. Other laboratory studies evaluate the presence of heterophil antibody and measure the Epstein-Barr virus antibody. When positive, the test is indicative of mononucleosis. Because the viral level fluctuates, a negative finding does not totally rule out the presence of mononucleosis. Liver function studies may be used to ascertain whether any liver involvement exists. Throat cultures may be positive for β-hemolytic streptococci in one third of clients.

▪ Therapeutic and Nursing Management of Mononucleosis

There is no specific therapeutic protocol for clients with mononucleosis. Clients may need to be hospitalized for 2 to 3 weeks to ensure that they get adequate rest, nutrition, and fluids and that fever is properly managed. Isolation procedures are not required because mononucleosis is minimally contagious in adults. Antibiotics have not proved useful unless the throat culture is positive for β-hemolytic streptococci. Analgesics may alleviate discomfort, and steroids may reduce pharyngeal swelling and fever.

Nursing interventions are most appropriate when the disease is actually present. Helping the client to comply with the physician's orders, especially bed rest, may prove challenging if fatigue is negligible. The nurse may suggest the use of a saline solution gargle to ease sore throat pain. The nurse must also detect the development of complications. For the client with splenomegaly, the nurse must emphasize the need to avoid any possible activities that can lead to splenic rupture. For example, the client should avoid the Valsalva maneuver with bowel movements, and abdominal trauma from lifting or sports must be avoided until resolution of the splenic enlargement.

The need for ongoing care after mononucleosis is un-

common. After 2 to 3 weeks, the client can usually return to a normal lifestyle. If the mononucleosis is seen in older adults, complications may be more common and complete disease resolution may take longer.

DISORDERS OF THE SPLEEN

The spleen performs many functions (see Chapter 24). The spleen is affected by many illnesses. Splenomegaly occurs in neoplastic diseases such as lymphoma and leukemia, as well as in nonneoplastic disorders such as infections, collagen vascular diseases, anemias, thrombocytopenic purpura, hypersensitivity reactions, and cirrhosis. When the spleen enlarges, its normal filtering capacity increases. Consequently, there is often a reduction in the number of circulating blood cells.

Hypersplenism is a spleen disorder in which destructive spleen functions are exaggerated, leading to decreased peripheral blood elements and increased bone marrow cellularity. Splenomegaly usually develops, but it is not always present. Hypersplenism may be a primary condition, such as with ITP, or it may develop secondary to another illness, such as with lymphomas, leukemia, or any problem leading to portal hypertension.

Splenectomy is the treatment of choice for primary hypersplenism because it eliminates the problem. Spleen removal or radiotherapy to the spleen may be done in cases of secondary hypersplenism in an attempt to increase platelet counts. Another major indication for splenectomy is splenic rupture. The spleen may rupture from trauma, inadvertent tearing during other surgical procedures, and diseases such as mononucleosis.

Nursing responsibilities for clients with spleen disorders vary depending on the nature of the problem. Splenomegaly may be painful and may require analgesic administration; care in moving, turning, and positioning; and evaluation of lung expansion, since spleen enlargement may impair diaphragmatic excursion. If anemia, thrombocytopenia, or leukopenia develops from splenomegaly or hypersplenism, nursing measures must be instituted to support the client and prevent life-threatening complications. If splenectomy is performed, the nurse must provide the meticulous care warranted after any surgery. In addition, there must be special observation for hemorrhage, which could lead to shock, fever, and abdominal distention.

After splenectomy, immunological deficiencies may develop. IgM levels are reduced, and IgG and IgA values remain within normal limits. Postsplenectomy clients are especially vulnerable to infection. Younger clients are at significantly greater risk than older clients, but the risk is present for all ages. These clients are highly susceptible to infection from encapsulated organisms such as pneumococcus. This complication is prevented by immunization with polyvalent pneumococcal vaccine. Although the mechanism of action governing the efficacy of this intervention is unknown, the treatment protocol suggests immunization before the splenectomy and every 3 years thereafter.

BLOOD COMPONENT THERAPY

Blood component therapy is frequently used in managing hematological diseases. Many therapeutic and surgical

Table 25-35 Blood Products

Description	Special Considerations	Indications for Use
WHOLE BLOOD		
Whole blood contains normal constituents of whole blood. Coagulation is prevented by collecting blood with citrate-phosphate-dextrose or acid-citrate-dextrose, with citrate complexing calcium and dextrose providing energy source for RBCs. Donor unit contains 450 ml of whole blood and 60 ml of preservative.	Whole blood should not be stored for more than 21 days, at which time 70%-80% of RBCs are viable. WBCs and platelets are nonviable. Hyperkalemia develops when in storage from death of RBCs. Large volume necessary is drawback, especially in clients with cardiovascular disease. It takes 12-24 hr before Hb and Hct rise. After 24 hr, Hb increases 1 g/dl/U and Hct 2%-3%/U as extra fluid volume is eliminated via kidneys.	Acute, rapid bleeding; hypovolemia caused by hemorrhage
FRESH WHOLE BLOOD		
Whole blood is used less than 12 hr after donation.	Use of fresh blood has been replaced by component therapy.	Rare use unless RBCs, platelets, factors V and VIII necessary (e.g., in client requiring massive transfusion)
PACKED RBCs		
Packed RBCs are prepared from whole blood by sedimentation or centrifugation. Hct is about 80%. One unit contains 250-300 ml.	Use of RBCs for treatment allows remaining components of blood (e.g., platelets, albumin, plasma) to be used for other purposes. Fresh packed cells needed if hyperkalemia is consideration. There is less danger of fluid overload. It is preferred RBC source because it is more component specific.	Anemia, high risk of fluid overload (e.g., renal and cardiac disease), acute bleeding
FROZEN RBCs		
Frozen RBCs are prepared from RBCs using glycerol for protection and frozen. They can be stored for 3 yr at −87° C (−188.6° F).	They must be used 24 hr after thawing. During thawing process, successive washings with saline solution remove majority of WBCs and plasma proteins.	Autotransfusion, clients with previous febrile reactions to transfusions
PLATELETS		
Platelets are prepared from fresh whole blood within 4 hr after collection. One unit contains 30-60 mL of platelet concentrate; should have yellow tinge.	Multiple units of platelets can be obtained from one donor by platelet plateletpheresis pheresis. They can be kept at room temperature for 1-5 days depending on type of collection and storage bag used. Bag should be agitated periodically. Expected increase is 10,000/μl/U. Failure to rise may be due to fever, sepsis, splenomegaly, or DIC. Alloimmunization prevents increases in platelets. Donor compatibility may be necessary.	Bleeding due to thrombocytopenia

Hct, Hematocrit.
*See Table 25-19 for special considerations.

Table 25-35 Blood Products—cont'd

Description	Special Considerations	Indications for Use
FRESH-FROZEN PLASMA		
Liquid portion of whole blood is separated from cells and frozen. One unit contains 200-250 ml. Plasma is rich in clotting factors but contains no platelets. It may be stored for 1 yr. It must be used within 2 hr after thawing.	Use of plasma in treating hypovolemic shock is being replaced by pure preparations such as albumin and by plasma expanders.	Bleeding due to liver disease, hypovolemia due to burns, multiple transfusions, clotting defects
ALBUMIN		
Albumin is prepared from plasma. It can be stored for 5 yr. It is available in 5% or 25% solution. It does not transmit hepatitis.	Albumin 25 g/100 ml is osmotically equal to 500 ml of plasma. Hyperosmolar solution acts by moving water from extravascular to intravascular space.	Hypovolemic shock, albuminemia, liver failure
CRYOPRECIPITATES* AND COMMERCIAL CONCENTRATES		
Cryoprecipitate is prepared from fresh-frozen plasma, with 10-20 ml/bag. It can be stored for 1 yr. Once thawed, it needs to be used.	—	Bleeding due to hemophilia or DIC
WBCs		
WBCs are prepared by continuous-flow centrifugation or filtration leukapheresis, with 200-500 ml/bag.	Neutrophils have very short life span in circulation. They are administered slowly over 2-4 hr. Administration does not cause rise in WBC count but increases marginal pool. Occurrence of fever and shaking chills during infusion is common and may not require cessation of transfusion. Prophylactic premedication with steroids, meperidine, and antihistamines may reduce febrile response.	Neutropenia (e.g., in clients with BMTs, chemotherapy with resultant bone marrow suppression)

[handwritten: see alot to replace clotting factors]

[handwritten: Rarely see because of Rx.]

procedures depend on blood and blood product therapy. However, blood component therapy only temporarily supports the client until the underlying problem is resolved. Because transfusions are not free from hazards, they should be used sparingly or avoided unless absolutely necessary. Nurses must be careful to avoid developing a complacent attitude about this common but potentially dangerous therapy.

Traditionally, the term *blood transfusion* meant the administration of whole blood. Blood transfusion now has a broader meaning because of the ability to administer specific components of blood such as platelets, RBCs, and plasma (Table 25-35).[22] Blood component therapy allows a single unit of donated whole blood to be given to three or four recipients. Component therapy is also a means to diminish complications associated with transfusion therapy.

Administration Procedure

An IV line using an 18- or 19-gauge needle is started. (Smaller-size needles may be used for platelets, albumin, and cryoprecipitates, and when blood is not administered under pressure.) The blood administration tubing with a filter should have a stopcock or other means to develop a closed system, with blood open to one port and isotonic saline solution infusing through the other. Glucose solutions should not be used because they induce RBC aggregation, which can cause plugging of the filter and tubing. Glucose also causes hemolysis of the RBCs. Lactated Ringer's solutions should also be avoided because they cause agglutination.[23] The tubing should be flushed with isotonic saline solution before as well as after administering blood. No other additives (including medications) should be given via the same tubing as the blood unless the tubing is cleared with saline solution.

When the blood or blood components have been obtained from the blood bank, positive identification of the donor blood and recipient must be made. Improper product to client identification causes 90% of transfusion reactions, thus placing a great responsibility on nursing personnel to carry out the identification procedure appropriately. Nurses should check the local hospital policy for the exact procedure. The blood bank is responsible for typing and cross matching the donor's blood with the recipient's blood. (These procedures are discussed in Chapter 24.)

The blood should be administered as soon as it is brought to the client. It should not be refrigerated on the unit because the refrigeration will not be controlled. If the blood is not used right away, it should be returned to the blood bank.

During the first 15 minutes of blood infusion, the nurse should stay with the client. If there are any unwanted reactions, they are most likely to occur at this time. The rate of infusion during this period should be no more than 2 ml/min. Blood should not be infused quickly unless an emergency exists. Rapid infusion of cold blood causes the client to become chilled. If rapid replacement of large amounts of blood is necessary, a blood-warming device should be used.

After the first 15 minutes, the rate of infusion is governed by the clinical condition of the client and the product being infused. Most clients not in danger of fluid overload, such as those in congestive heart failure, can tolerate the infusion of one unit of blood over 2 hours. The transfusion should not take more than 4 hours to administer. Blood remaining after 4 hours should not be infused because of the length of time it has been removed from refrigeration.[24]

If a transfusion reaction occurs, the following steps should be taken: (1) discontinue the transfusion; (2) maintain a patent IV line with dextrose or saline solution; (3) notify the physician; (4) save the blood bag and tubing and send them to the blood bank for examination; (5) notify the blood bank; (6) complete transfusion reaction reports; (7) collect required blood and urine specimens at intervals stipulated by hospital policy to evaluate for free hemoglobin; and (8) carefully monitor the client, with special attention directed to vital signs, particularly blood pressure, and urine output.

The blood bank or laboratory identifies the cause of the reaction by repeating the type and cross match or by doing other studies such as direct and indirect Coombs' tests.

Autotransfusion

Autotransfusion, or autologous transfusion, consists of removing whole blood from a person and transfusing that blood into the same person. The problems of incompatibility, allergic reactions, and transmission of disease can be avoided. There are various methods of autotransfusion. These include the following:

1. *Elective phlebotomy (predeposit transfusion):* A person donates blood before a planned surgical procedure. The blood can be frozen and stored for up to 3 years. Usually the blood is stored without being frozen and is given to the person within a few weeks of donation. This technique is especially beneficial to the client with a rare blood type.

2. *Autotransfusion:* Blood that was lost during major surgical procedures or traumatic injury is collected and filtered. Anticoagulants are added, and the blood is reinfused into the person. There are now commercially available autotransfusion systems, such as the Sorenson autotransfusion system and the Haemonetic Cell Saver, that prepare the blood for reinfusion.

Blood Transfusion Reactions

The complications of transfusion therapy are significant and necessitate judicious evaluation of the client. Blood transfusion reactions can be classified as immunological and nonimmunological (Table 25-36).

Immunological reactions

Hemolytic reactions. The most common cause of hemolytic reactions is transfusion of ABO-incompatible blood. This is an example of a type II cytotoxic hypersensitivity reaction (see Chapter 8). Severe hemolytic reactions are rare. Most mistakes are due to mislabeling specimens and administering blood to the wrong individual.

When a hemolytic reaction occurs, antibodies in the recipient's serum react with antigens on the donor's RBCs. This results in agglutination of cells, which can obstruct capillaries and block blood flow. Hemolysis of the RBCs releases free hemoglobin into the plasma. The hemoglobin is filtered by the kidney and is found in the urine (hemoglobinuria). Hemoglobin may obstruct the renal tubules, leading to acute renal failure (see Chapter 41).

The clinical manifestations of the hemolytic reaction may be mild or severe and usually develop within the first 15 minutes of transfusion. Infrequently, delayed transfusion reactions occur 2 to 14 days after the administration of blood. (The clinical manifestations and nursing management for the client with a hemolytic reaction are presented in Table 25-36.)

Allergic reactions. Allergic reactions result from the recipient's sensitivity to a component of the donor's blood. These reactions are more common in individuals with a history of allergies. Antihistamines may be used to prevent allergic reactions. Epinephrine or corticosteroids may be used to treat a severe reaction. Clients in whom allergic reactions develop often have fewer problems with washed or leukocyte-depleted RBCs.

Febrile reactions. Febrile reactions are most commonly caused by the presence of leukocyte or thrombocyte incompatibility (e.g., the donor's platelets versus the recipient's antibodies) induced by previous transfusions. Many individuals who receive five or more transfusions develop circulating antibodies to WBCs. Febrile reactions are less likely to occur as a result of contaminated tubing or equipment. These reactions can often be prevented by using washed RBCs from which the WBCs and plasma proteins have been removed.

Nonimmunological reactions. Nonimmunological reactions include circulatory overload, infections, diverse effects of massive blood transfusion, and air embolism.

Circulatory overload. Individuals with cardiac or renal insufficiency are at risk to develop congestive heart failure from circulatory overload. This is especially true if a large quantity of blood is infused in a short period of time.

Table 25-36   Transfusion Reactions

Reaction	Prevention	Clinical Manifestation	Nursing Management
Hemolytic transfusion reaction	Identify client and blood product to ensure proper match. Double-check all blood products with another nurse or health professional. Begin infusion at slow rate, and remain with client for first 15 min. Severe reactions tend to begin soon after initiation of transfusion.	Usually immediate onset; delayed onset when Rh incompatibility involved; burning sensation along the vein; facial flushing; fever, chills; temperature 40° C (104° F) or higher; chest pain; rapid, labored respirations; headache; low back pain; shock	Stop transfusion immediately to reduce further risk. Severity of reaction is related to amount transfused. Treat shock if present. Administer oxygen, fluids, epinephrine as ordered by physician. Recheck blood slip with unit of blood and client's blood to determine if error was made. Obtain two blood samples from vein distant from infusion site. Send one specimen for centrifugation (pink or red plasma indicates hemolysis), the other to blood bank with remainder of transfusion. Obtain first voided urine to test for hemoglobinuria. Specimen may be red or black, indicating potential renal damage. With suspected renal involvement, prompt treatment with mannitol is ordered to promote diuresis and prevent renal tubular damage. Monitor fluid and electrolyte balance as soon as diuresis begins.
Allergic reaction	Determine whether client has a history of allergy, particularly a previous allergic reaction to transfused blood products. Administer antihistamine (e.g., diphenhydramine [Benadryl]) or corticosteroids orally or parenterally 15-20 min before starting infusion.	Urticaria (hives), pruritus; facial and/or glottal edema (rare); asthma (rare); pulmonary edema with infiltrates (rare); anaphylaxis	Stop transfusion immediately. Treat life-threatening reactions (e.g., edema, anaphylaxis) immediately. Administer antihistamine parenterally.
Febrile reaction	Keep client covered and warm during transfusion. Administer antipyretic medication to persons known to have this reaction. Transfusion with leukycyte-poor RBCs or frozen washed packed cells may prevent this reaction in persons susceptible to it.	Chills and fever, with onset usually about 1 hr after start of infusion; headache, flushing, tachycardia, general discomfort; possible persistence of symptoms for 8-10 hr; most symptoms more transient	Stop transfusion immediately. Treat symptoms. Take vital signs as needed.
Bacterial reaction	Maintain aseptic collection techniques. Change transfusion equipment frequently. Do not allow blood to stand at room temperature unnecessarily, even while infusing. Do not use blood that has been heated to above room temperature. Do not prewarm infusions. Inspect all blood for evidence of hemolysis.	Shaking, fever; severe hypotension; dry, flushed skin; pain in abdomen and extremities; vomiting and bloody diarrhea	Stop transfusion immediately. Administer broad-spectrum antibiotics immediately by the most rapid route as ordered. Treat shock aggressively. Monitor vital signs, fluid, and electrolyte balance.

Continued.

Table 25-36 Transfusion Reactions—cont'd

Reaction	Prevention	Clinical Manifestation	Nursing Management
Circulatory overload	Give packed cells to clients susceptible to circulatory overload (e.g., older adults, infants, persons with cardiac or respiratory disorders). Administer infusion slowly, with client in a sitting position.	Tightness in chest, labored breathing; dry cough; rales at base of lungs; pulmonary edema	Stop or slow transfusion, depending on severity of symptoms. Have client sit up. Monitor vital signs. Treat severe overload with rotating tourniquets or phlebotomy. Administer diuretics as ordered.
Air embolism	Avoid introducing air into system. If air is introduced, stop infusion.	Cyanosis, dyspnea, shock, cardiac arrest	Lower client's head and turn client on left side. Air will collect in right atrium, where it can be released gradually to lungs. Treat shock and/or cardiac arrest immediately if these conditions occur.

When possible, these individuals should be given packed RBCs instead of whole blood. When blood is needed, it should be infused as slowly as possible and monitored with central venous pressure readings. Central venous pressure readings above 15 cm H_2O usually indicate circulatory overload. If a pulmonary artery catheter is in place, wedge pressure readings above 18 mm Hg indicate elevated left atrial pressure and impending failure.

Infection. Many infections can be transmitted by blood transfusion, including hepatitis, malaria, and cytomegalovirus. In addition, blood can become infected from improper handling and storage. However, with careful handling, bacterial contamination and growth rarely occur.

Hepatitis is the most common infection transmitted, although its incidence has been decreasing. Hepatitis B virus can be detected in the blood by the presence of hepatitis B surface antigen (HBsAg). It is now becoming more apparent that hepatitis non-A, non-B viruses are responsible for a large number of hepatitis cases (see Chapter 38). A new test for hepatitis C (a type of non-A, non-B hepatitis) antibodies in donor blood is reducing this risk.

In the past, HIV was transmitted by contaminated blood and blood products. This posed a serious problem for individuals who needed multiple or repeated transfusions, especially persons with hemophilia who required antihemophiliac factor, which may be prepared from pooled plasma of 2000 to 5000 donors. Presently, donor education, donor screening, and HIV-antibody testing have virtually eliminated the transmission of HIV by blood transfusion or blood product therapy.

Massive blood transfusion. *Massive blood transfusion reaction* is defined as replacement that exceeds the total blood volume within 24 hours. In this situation, blood component therapy is still the preferred intervention if there is some degree of control in the situation. However, in cases of extremely rapid exsanguination, the simpler approach may be to use only whole blood as replacement.

In stored whole blood, platelets and RBCs deteriorate, clotting factors become deficient, and hyperkalemia and acidosis develop. For prevention of problems from excessive use of stored blood, 1 unit of fresh blood should be used for every 5 to 6 units of stored blood. If fresh blood is not available, platelet concentrate and fresh frozen plasma can also be given.

Two additional problems, hypothermia and hypocalcemia, may occur when massive blood transfusions are needed. Hypothermia with cardiac dysrhythmias can result from rapid infusion of large quantities of cold blood. Blood-warming equipment should be used to prevent this problem. Hypocalcemia can occur from the use of large quantities of citrated blood (i.e., calcium binds to the citrate). Calcium gluconate should be administered IV after the infusion of every 2 units of blood. Calcium should never be added directly to the blood.

Air embolism. The incidence of air embolism has been decreased by the use of plastic blood bags. However, air may be introduced if the tubing is changed during the transfusion procedure.

C ase Study

ANEMIA

Clare, a 20-year-old black woman who lives in New York City, was brought to a Denver emergency room with severe joint and abdominal pain. She complained of frequent urination during the past 2 nights and knee joint swelling. Two days previously, she had gone hiking in the Rocky Mountains with her brother, whom she was visiting in Denver.

Clare's history included one other similar episode when she had acute pneumonia at the age of 11. She stated that she usually felt fatigued but thought it was due to her active social life. Physical assessment demonstrated the presence of splenomegaly and an enlarged, inflamed knee joint. Laboratory results included the following:

Hct	30%
Hb	10 g/dl
WBC	20,000/μl

Discussion Questions

1. What components of the laboratory results suggest anemia?
2. What is the pathophysiological basis of Clare's anemia? Why might symptoms have developed in Denver?
3. What precipitates a crisis of this type of anemia?
4. How is an anemic crisis with this etiology treated?
5. What are the pathophysiological bases of pain related to this type of anemia?
6. What measures should Clare take to prevent further crises?

R eview Questions

The number of the question corresponds to the same-numbered objective at the beginning of the chapter.

1. Which of the following are clinical manifestations of anemia?
   a. muscle twitching and petechiae
   b. pallor and bleeding tendencies
   c. headaches and tachycardia
   d. polyphagia and purpura
2. A normocytic, normochromic anemia may be caused by
   a. bone marrow suppression
   b. folic acid deficiency
   c. vitamin B_{12} deficiency
   d. chronic infection
3. The clinical manifestations of sickle cell crisis develop primarily as a result of
   a. capillary permeability
   b. erythrostasis
   c. hemorrhage
   d. transfusions
4. Which of the following is an important nursing intervention to provide warmth for a client with anemia who complains of being cold?
   a. hot-water bottle
   b. hyperthermia blanket
   c. heating pad
   d. socks and blankets
5. The vascular problems in polycythemia result from
   a. hyperviscosity and hypovolemia
   b. hypoviscosity and hypervolemia
   c. hyperviscosity and hypervolemia
   d. hypoviscosity and hypovolemia
6. The etiologies of ITP and acquired thrombocytopenia, respectively, are
   a. increased platelet destruction for both
   b. decreased platelet production for both
   c. increased platelet destruction; decreased platelet production
   d. decreased platelet production; increased platelet destruction
7. When providing care for a client with thrombocytopenia, the nurse must avoid administering aspirin or aspirin-containing products because they
   a. disguise fevers
   b. destroy RBCs
   c. increase intracranial pressure
   d. interfere with platelet aggregation
8. Which blood elements do the three major types of hemophilia affect?
   a. factor VIII, factor IX, platelets
   b. factor VII, factor IX, red cells
   c. factor VI, factor X, fibrinogen
   d. factor VIII, factor IX, thrombin
9. DIC is
   a. a hereditary disorder that may lead to diffuse hemorrhage
   b. an acquired disorder that may lead to diffuse hemorrhage
   c. a hereditary disorder that may lead to localized hemorrhage
   d. an acquired disorder that may lead to localized hemorrhage
10. Which sign of infection is the client with granulocytopenia most likely to display?
    a. redness
    b. pus
    c. heat
    d. fever
11. A 65-year-old woman has enlarged cervical lymph nodes, an elevated lymphocyte count, and severe anemia. Which of the following types of leukemia does this description most likely characterize?
    a. acute lymphocytic leukemia
    b. acute myelocytic leukemia
    c. chronic lymphocytic leukemia
    d. chronic granulocytic leukemia
12. Multiple drugs are used in predetermined combinations to treat leukemia and lymphomas because
    a. the chance that one drug will be effective is increased
    b. they are more effective without having exacerbating side effects
    c. no one knows what drugs help clients with lymphoma
    d. they can interrupt cell growth at multiple points in the cell cycle
13. An important nursing measure in the management of a client with chronic leukemia is to
    a. reassure the client that most chemotherapeutic agents induce remission
    b. tell the client that induction chemotherapy is less toxic than maintenance chemotherapy
    c. discuss the client's feelings about the disease
    d. discuss with the family the client's need to maintain a dependent role
14. Stage IA Hodgkin's disease means that the
    a. disease is on one side of the diaphragm and symptoms are present
    b. disease is on one side of the diaphragm and symptoms are absent
    c. disease is on both sides of the diaphragm and symptoms are present
    d. disease is on both sides of the diaphragm and symptoms are absent
15. As mononucleosis becomes more acute, a common triad of symptoms develops, including

a. fatigue, cough, and headache
b. chills, anorexia, and vomiting
c. fever, painful lymphadenopathy, and sore throat
d. weight loss, night sweats, and splenomegaly

16. Clients with mononucleosis who have splenomegaly are at risk for
a. infection
b. RBC abnormalities
c. splenic rupture
d. renal failure

17. Clinical manifestations of a hemolytic transfusion reaction include
a. chills and back pain
b. vomiting and urticaria
c. tachycardia and asthmatic attack
d. severe hypotension and petechiae

REFERENCES

1. Powers LW: Diagnostic hematology, St Louis, 1990, The CV Mosby Co.
2. Young NS: Aplastic anemia, Curr Ther Hematol Oncol 3:1-4, 1988.
3. Rappeport JM and Bunn HF: Bone marrow failure, aplastic anemia. In Wilson JD and others, eds: Harrison's principles of internal medicine, New York, 1990, McGraw-Hill Book Co, pp 1567-1569.
4. Rivers R and Williamson N: Sickle cell anemia: complex disease, nursing challenge, RN 53:24-29, 1990.
5. Pavel JN: Red blood cell transfusions for anemia, Semin Oncol Nurs 6:117-122, 1990.
6. London F: Nursing diagnoses and caring for patients with sickle cell disease, Adv Clin Care 5:12-16, 1990.
7. Schroeder SA and others: Current medical diagnosis and treatment, Norwalk, Conn, 1990, Appleton & Lange, pp 346-349.
8. Schneiderman E: Thrombocytopenia in the critically ill patient, Crit Care Nurs Q 13:1-6, 1990.
9. Fuller AK: Platelet transfusion therapy for thrombocytopenia, Semin Oncol Nurs 6:123-128, 1990.
10. Wolfe DW: Hematologic complications of malignancy, Top Emerg Med 8:13-24, 1986.
11. Esparaz B: Disseminated intravascular coagulation, Crit Care Nurs Q 13:7-13, 1990.
12. Suchak BA and Barbon CB: Disseminated intravascular coagulation: a nursing challenge, Orthop Nurs 8:61-69, 1989.
13. Oniboni AC: Infection in the neutropenic patient, Semin Oncol Nurs 6:50-60, 1990.
14. Pizzo PA: Combating infections in neutropenic patients, Hosp Pract 24:93-98, 1989.
15. Maguire-Eisen M: Diagnosis and treatment of adult acute leukemia, Semin Oncol Nurs 6:17-24, 1990.
16. Collins PM: Diagnosis and treatment of chronic leukemia, Semin Oncol Nurs 6:31-43, 1990.
17. Konradi D and Stockert P: A close-up look at leukemia, Nursing 17:34-41, 1989.
18. Gale RP and Quinn SJ: The management of acute leukemias, Clin Adv Oncol Nurs 1:1-7, 1989.
19. Wikle T and others: Bone marrow transplant: today and tomorrow, Am J Nurs 90:48-58, 1990.
20. Romond EH and others: Bone marrow transplantation, Hosp Pract 24:169-184, 1989.
21. Rahr VA and Tucker R: Non-Hodgkin's lymphoma: understanding the disease, Cancer Nurs 13:56-61, 1990.
22. McGuire DB and Braine HG: Blood component therapy, Semin Oncol Nurs 6:91-171, 1990.
23. Querin JJ and Stahl LD: Twelve simple steps for successful blood transfusions, Nursing 20:68-81, 1990.
24. Freedman S and others: Nursing considerations in the administration of blood component therapy, Semin Oncol Nurs 6:155-162, 1990.

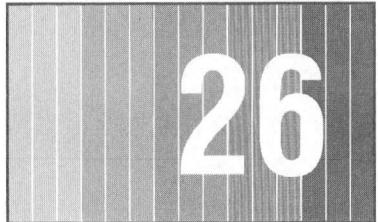

CHAPTER 26

Nursing Assessment
Cardiovascular System

Dina D'Addio Wilson
Carol E. Smith

---

1. Describe the anatomical location and function of the following cardiac structures: pericardial layers, atria, ventricles, semilunar valves, and atrioventricular valves.
2. Describe coronary circulation and the areas of heart muscle supplied by each blood vessel.
3. Explain the normal sequence of events involved in the conduction pathway of the heart.
4. Describe the structure and function of arteries, capillaries, and veins.
5. Define blood pressure and the mechanisms involved in its regulation.

6. Identify the significant subjective and objective assessment data related to the cardiovascular system that should be obtained from a client.
7. Describe the appropriate techniques used in the physical assessment of the cardiovascular system.
8. Differentiate normal from common abnormal findings of a physical assessment of the cardiovascular system.
9. Describe the purpose, significance of results, and nursing responsibilities of invasive and noninvasive diagnostic studies of the cardiovascular system.
10. Identify waveforms of a normal electrocardiogram and components of the normal sinus rhythm.

The cardiovascular system consists of the heart, the arteries, the veins, and the capillaries. The function of this system is to circulate the blood, enabling oxygen, nutrients, and hormones to reach cells of the body and waste products of cells to be eliminated.

STRUCTURES AND FUNCTIONS OF THE CARDIOVASCULAR SYSTEM
Heart

Structure. The heart is a four-chambered muscular organ about the size of a fist. It is the pump of the cardiovascular system. The heart lies within the thorax between the lungs. Its beating is often palpable at the fifth intercostal space about 2 inches left of the midline (Fig. 26-1). This pulsation, arising at the apex of the heart, is known as the *point of maximum impulse* (PMI).

The heart wall is composed of three layers. The *en-*

docardium is the thin inner lining, the *myocardium* is the middle muscular layer, and the *epicardium* is the outer serous membrane. Around the heart is the *pericardial sac,* enclosing the heart the way a glove encloses a fist. This sac consists of a visceral (inner) layer and a parietal (outer) layer. The visceral layer is in contact with the epicardium. Between the visceral and parietal layers is the *pericardial space.* A small amount of fluid in this space acts as a lubricant for the movement of the layers with each heartbeat.

The heart's four chambers are separated by a septum, with two chambers on the right side and two on the left. The upper chambers on each side are the *atria*, and the lower chambers are the *ventricles*. The atrial myocardium is thinner than that of the ventricles, and the left ventricular wall is much thicker than the right ventricular wall. Its added thickness is needed to allow the chamber to pump blood into the systemic circulation.

Blood flow through the heart
Cardiac valves. The right atrium receives venous blood from the inferior and superior venae cavae and the coronary sinus. The blood then passes through the *tricuspid*

Reviewed by Linda Griego. R.N.. M.S.N.. C.C.R.N.. Clinical Nurse Specialist. M/CICU. University of New Mexico Hospital. Albuquerque. New Mexico.

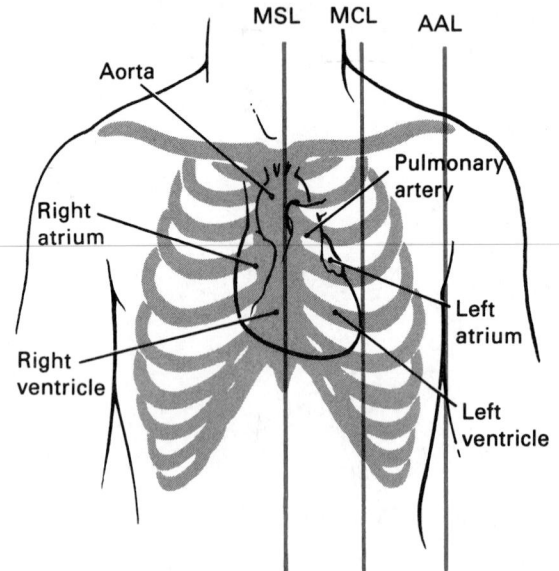

Fig. 26-1 Orientation of the heart within the thorax. Red lines indicate the midsternal line (MSL), midclavicular line (MCL), and anterior axillary line (AAL). (Modified from Price S and Wilson L: Pathophysiology: clinical concepts of disease processes, ed 4, St Louis, 1991, Mosby–Year Book, Inc.)

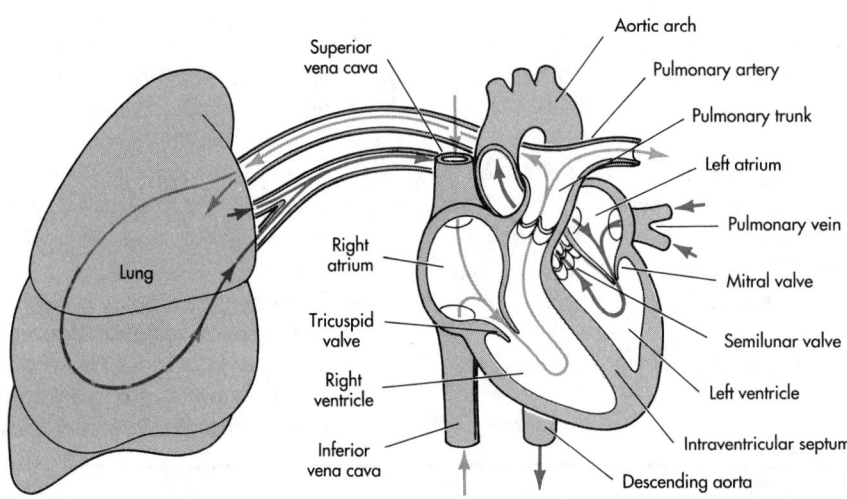

Fig. 26-2 Schematic representation of blood flow through the heart. *Arrows* indicate direction of flow.

valve into the right ventricle. With each contraction, the right ventricle pumps blood into the pulmonary artery. At the entrance to the pulmonary artery is the *pulmonic valve.*

Blood from the lungs flows into the left atrium by way of the pulmonary veins. It then passes through the *mitral valve* and into the left ventricle. As the heart contracts, blood is ejected through the aortic valve into the aorta and thus enters the systemic circulation (Fig. 26-2).

The four valves of the heart serve to keep blood flowing in one direction. The atrioventricular (AV) valves (tricuspid and mitral) prevent backflow into the atria at the start of each contraction of the ventricles. The cusps of the valves are attached to thin strands of fibrous tissue called *chordae tendineae* (Fig. 26-3). These are anchored in papillary muscles projecting from the walls of the ventricles. The pulmonic and aortic valves prevent blood from regurgitating into the ventricles at the end of each ventricular

contraction. These valves have three cusps. They are also known as *semilunar valves.*

Blood supply to the myocardium. The myocardium has its own coronary circulation, allowing for constant nourishment by blood so that contraction can continue. Immediately above the cusps of the aortic valve are the sinuses of Valsalva, with openings to the right and left coronary arteries. Blood flow into the coronary arteries occurs primarily during diastole. The branches of the coronary arteries carry blood to different areas of the myocardium (Fig. 26-4). The right coronary artery and its branches usually supply the right atrium, the right ventricle, and a portion of the posterior wall of the left ventricle. The left coronary artery and its branches supply the left atrium and the massive walls of the left ventricle. In 90% of all persons, the atrioventricular node, part of the cardiac conduction system (see p. 718), receives its nourishment from

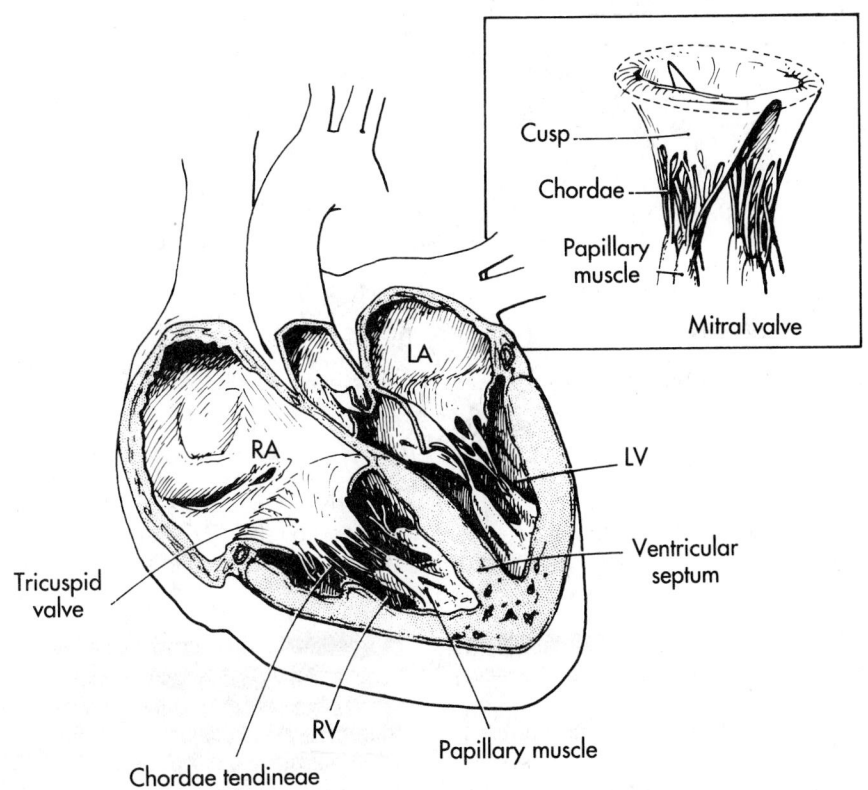

Fig. 26-3 Anatomical structures of the AV valves. (From Price S and Wilson L: Pathophysiology: clinical concepts of disease processes, ed 4, St Louis, 1991, Mosby–Year Book, Inc.)

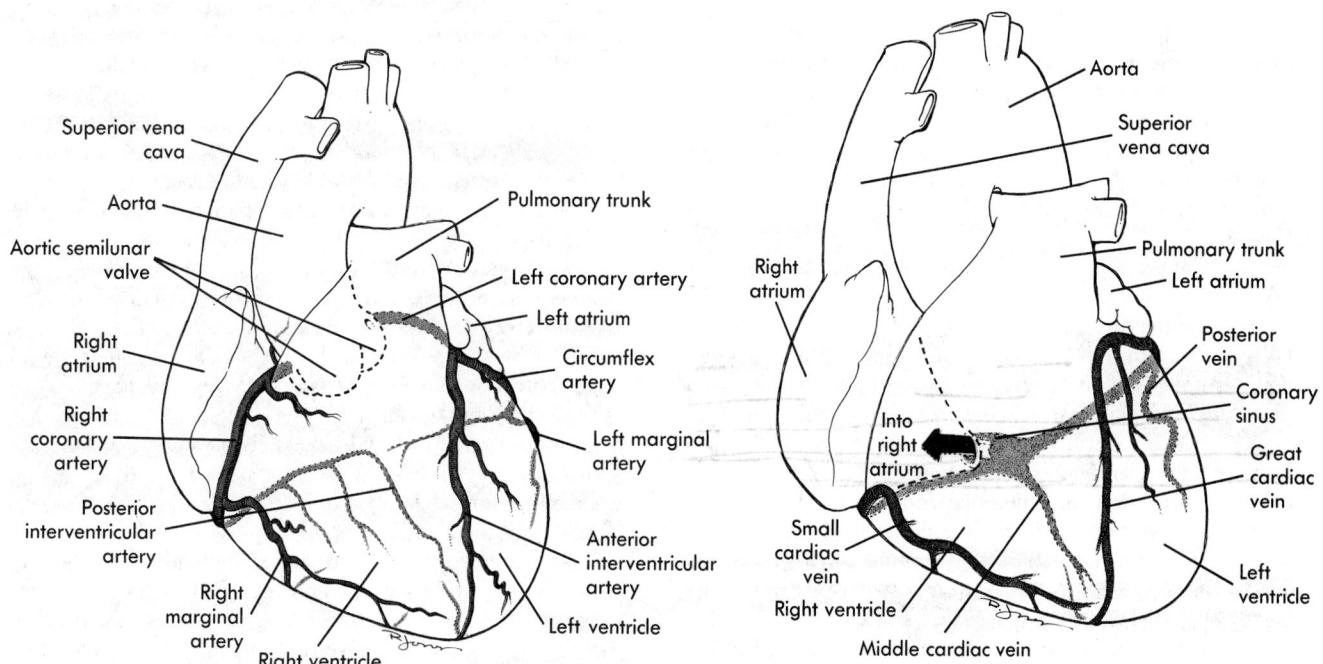

Fig. 26-4 Coronary arteries.

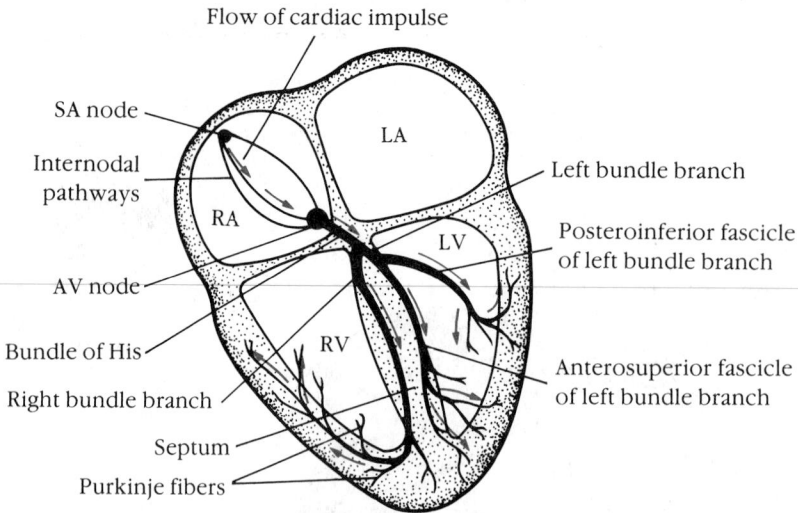

Fig. 26-5 Conduction system of the heart. (Modified from Kinney M and others: Comprehensive cardiac care, ed 7, St Louis, 1991, Mosby—Year Book, Inc.)

the right coronary artery. For this reason, obstruction of this artery often causes serious defects in cardiac conduction.

If blood flow through any part of the coronary arterial system is interrupted, some of the myocardium loses its ability to function. The effect on the heart as a whole depends on the size of the area deprived of oxygen (O_2). If blood flow is reduced gradually, alternate routes may develop in time to nourish the endangered myocardium. These alternate routes are called *collateral circulation* and may be compared to a detour for a road blocked with traffic.

The divisions of coronary veins essentially parallel the coronary arteries. Most of the blood from the coronary system drains into the coronary sinus, which empties into the right atrium near the entrance to the inferior vena cava.

Conduction system. In the heart wall are pathways of special myocardial tissue for the wave of excitation or action potential that triggers each contraction of the heart muscle. This conduction system starts at the *sinoatrial (SA) node,* a tiny knob of tissue in the wall of the right atrium near the entrance of the superior vena cava (Fig. 26-5).

Because the normal heartbeat begins as an action potential generated in the SA node, this node is called the *pacemaker of the heart.* The action potential is the consequence of a sudden change in the membrane potential of node cells that occurs because of the rapid influx of sodium ions into the cells and the outflux of potassium ions. This shift in electrolytes abolishes the polarized condition that exists when node cells are at rest (i.e., electrically negative inside, positive outside); the cell membranes become *depolarized.* The action potential created at that instant moves in concentric waves throughout the atria.

The mechanical contraction of the heart muscle follows the depolarization of the cells. Contraction occurs when the actin and myosin filaments of the contractile units of the heart come together. Calcium, which enters the contractile units, initiates this contraction. Calcium flows into the cell following depolarization. Thus the shift in the sodium ions, which leads to changes in the polarized condition in the conduction system tissue, is also associated with muscle contraction initiated by calcium ion influx. Because the muscle fibers are in contact with one another, the walls of the atria contract almost as one unit. The action potential travels through the atria to the *atrioventricular (AV) node,* located in the right atrium near the ventricle. The action potential pauses briefly in the AV node, which allows contraction and emptying of the atria to proceed before contraction of the ventricles begins. The excitation then moves through the *bundle of His* and along the interventricular septum by way of the *left and right bundle branches.* The left bundle branch has two fascicles, an anterior one and a posterior one. From there, the action potential diffuses widely through the walls of both ventricles by means of *Purkinje fibers.* The conduction system allows coordinated contraction of the heart chambers.

The cardiac cycle starts with depolarization of the SA node. Its climax is ejection of blood into the pulmonary and systemic circulations. It ends with *repolarization,* when the contractile fiber cells and the conduction pathway cells regain their resting polarized condition. Cardiac muscle cells have a compensatory mechanism that makes them unresponsive or *refractory* to restimulation during the action potential. During systole there is an *absolute refractory period* during which cardiac muscle does not respond to any stimuli. After this period, cardiac muscle gradually recovers its excitability and a *relative refractory period* occurs by early diastole.

Electrocardiogram. The action potential can be detected on the body surface and recorded as an electrocardiogram (ECG). The letters *P, QRS,* and *T* are used to identify the separate waveforms (Fig. 26-6). The first wave (P) begins with the firing of the SA node and represents depolarization of the fibers of the atria. The QRS wave represents depolarization from the AV node through-

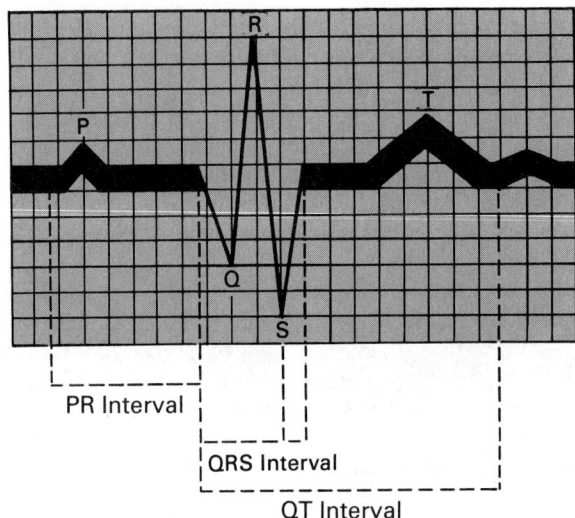

Fig. 26-6 The normal ECG pattern. The P wave represents depolarization of the atria. The QRS complex indicates depolarization of the ventricles. The T wave represents repolarization of the ventricles. The PR interval is a measure of the time required for the impulse to spread from the SA node to the ventricles.

Table 26-1   ECG Waves

Normal Waveforms and Intervals	Normal Timing	Normal Sinus Rhythm*
P	0.06-0.12 sec	Precedes QRS-T waves
QRS	0.06-0.10 sec	Follows each P wave
T	0.16 sec	Follows each QRS wave
PR interval	0.12-0.20 sec	Should not vary from one complex to another
QT interval	Varies with pulse rate (0.31-0.38 sec at heart rate of 72 bpm)	Should not vary from one complex to another; should not be more than half the RR interval
RR interval	Timing varies with pulse rate	Should be equidistant, with slight variations on respiration

bpm, Beats per minute.
*At 60-100 bpm.

out the ventricles. There is a delay of impulse transmission through the AV node that accounts for the time sequence between the end of the P wave and the beginning of the QRS wave. The last component of the cardiac cycle (the T wave) represents repolarization of the ventricles.

Intervals between these waves reflect the length of time it takes for the impulse to travel from one area of the heart to the other. These time intervals can be measured (Table 26-1). Deviations from these time references can indicate pathology.

Cardiac output. *Cardiac output* (CO) is the amount of blood pumped by each ventricle in 1 minute. It is calculated by multiplying the *stroke volume* (SV) (the amount of blood ejected from one ventricle with one heartbeat) by the *heart rate* per minute (HR):

$$CO = SV \times HR$$

For the normal adult at rest, cardiac output is maintained at approximately 5 L/min.

Factors affecting cardiac output. There are numerous factors that can affect either the heart rate or the stroke volume. The heart rate is regulated primarily by the autonomic nervous system. The factors affecting the stroke volume are *preload, contractility,* and *afterload.*[2]

Starling's law states that the more fibers are stretched, the greater their force of contraction. The volume of blood in the ventricles at the end of diastole, before the next contraction, is referred to as *preload.* Preload determines the amount of stretch placed on myocardial fibers. The greater the amount of stretch placed on myocardial fibers, the greater the force of the next contraction; thus stroke volume is increased. Oral nitrate drugs (e.g., nitroglycerin, isosorbide [Isordil]) are commonly used as medications to decrease preload because they primarily dilate veins. Venous return indirectly determines the stroke volume.

Contractility, another factor affecting stroke volume, can be influenced by the sympathetic nervous system as well as by epinephrine, whether produced endogenously by the body or administered as a drug. Increasing contractility raises the stroke volume by increasing ventricular emptying. Digitalis is one of the medications that increase contractility of heart muscle.

Afterload is the amount of force the ventricle must exert to open the semilunar valves and eject blood. Afterload is affected by the size of the ventricles, wall tension, and arterial pressure. If the arterial pressure is elevated, the ventricles will meet increased resistance to ejection of blood. Eventually, this can result in ventricular hypertrophy. Thus increased afterload results from increased arterial pressure or ventricular hypertrophy. Certain classes of drugs, such as arterial vasodilators and angiotensin-converting enzyme (ACE) inhibitor agents (e.g., hydralazine [Apresoline] and captopril [Capoten]), decrease afterload, thus increasing stroke volume and cardiac output. Such drugs are used in the treatment of conditions in which afterload is increased (e.g., congestive heart failure, hypertension).

Cardiac reserve. Considering the numerous factors affecting cardiac output, the fact that the cardiovascular system is able to adjust to the body's demands is a marvel. For example, the demand for increased output occurs with hypovolemia, exercise, and stress. The ability to respond to these demands and increase cardiac output threefold or fourfold is referred to as *cardiac reserve.*

The increase in cardiac output results from an increase in heart rate or stroke volume. The heart rate can increase to as high as 180 beats per minute (bpm) for short periods without deleterious effects. The stroke volume can be increased by increasing either preload or contractility.

Vascular System

Blood vessels. The three major types of blood vessel in the vascular system are the *arteries,* the *veins,* and the *capillaries.* Arteries travel away from the heart and, except for the pulmonary artery, carry oxygenated blood. Veins travel toward the heart and, except for the pulmonary veins, carry deoxygenated blood. Small arteries are called *arterioles,* and small veins are called *venules.* Blood circulates from the heart into arteries, arterioles, capillaries, venules, veins, and back to the heart.

Arteries and arterioles. The arterial system differs from the venous system by the amount or type of tissue that makes up arterial walls (Fig. 26-7). The large arteries have thick walls that are composed mainly of elastic tissue. This elastic property creates a low-resistance reservoir for blood as well as a recoil that propels blood forward into the circulation. Large arteries also contain some smooth muscle. Examples of large arteries are the aorta and the pulmonary artery.

Arterioles have relatively little elastic tissue but much smooth muscle. They respond readily to autonomic nervous control by dilating or constricting. The amount of blood flow to each organ and various tissues is directly related to the degree of constriction of the arteriole lumen. Arterioles serve as the major control of arterial blood pressure and distribution of blood flow.

Capillaries. The thin capillary wall is made up of endothelial cells, with no elastic or muscle tissue present (Fig. 26-7). There are an estimated 25,000 miles of capillaries in an adult.[1] The exchange of cellular nutrients and metabolic end products takes place through these many thin-walled vessels.

Veins and venules. Veins are large-diameter, thin-walled vessels that return blood to the right atrium (Fig. 26-7). The larger veins contain semilunar valves at intervals to maintain the blood flow toward the heart and to prevent backward flow. The amount of blood in the venous system is affected by a number of factors, including arterial flow, compression of veins by skeletal muscles, alterations in thoracic and abdominal pressures, and right atrial pressure.

The largest veins are the *superior vena cava,* which returns blood to the heart from the head, neck, and arms, and the *inferior vena cava,* which returns blood to the heart from the lower part of the body. These large-diameter vessels are affected by the pressure in the right side of the heart. Elevated right atrial pressure can cause distended neck veins or liver engorgement as a result of resistance of blood flow.

Venules are relatively small tubules made up of a small amount of muscle and connective tissue. Venules serve to collect blood from various capillary beds and channel it to the larger veins.

Regulation of the Cardiovascular System

Autonomic nervous system. The autonomic nervous system consists of the *sympathetic system* and the *parasympathetic system.*

Effect on the heart. Stimulation of the sympathetic system increases the heart rate, the speed of impulse conduction through the AV node, and the force of atrial and ventricular contractions. This effect is mediated by specific sites in the heart called β *receptors,* which respond to sympathetic release of norepinephrine.

In contrast, stimulation of the parasympathetic system (mediated by the vagus nerve) causes a decrease in heart rate by the action on the SA node and slows conduction through the AV node. Other factors that affect the heart, such as exercise, emotion, temperature, and medications, may also be mediated through this autonomic receptor system.

Effect on blood vessels. The source of neural control of blood vessels is also the autonomic nervous system. Sympathetic fibers extend to the peripheral vasculature. It has been postulated that vessels contain two types of receptors in the smooth muscle and that these respond differently to sympathetic nerve stimulation. These are the α and β receptors. When the α receptors are stimulated, vasoconstriction occurs. When the β receptors are stimulated, vasodilatation occurs. The parasympathetic system does not have a major influence on the peripheral vasculature.

Baroreceptors. Baroreceptors in the aortic arch, carotid sinus (at the origin of the internal carotid artery), vena cava, atria, and pulmonary arteries are sensitive to stretch or pressure within the arterial system. Stimulation of these receptors sends information to the vasomotor center in the brainstem. This results in inhibition of the sympathetic nervous system and enhancement of the parasympathetic influence, causing a decreased heart rate and peripheral vasodilatation.

Decreased arterial pressure causes the opposite effect.

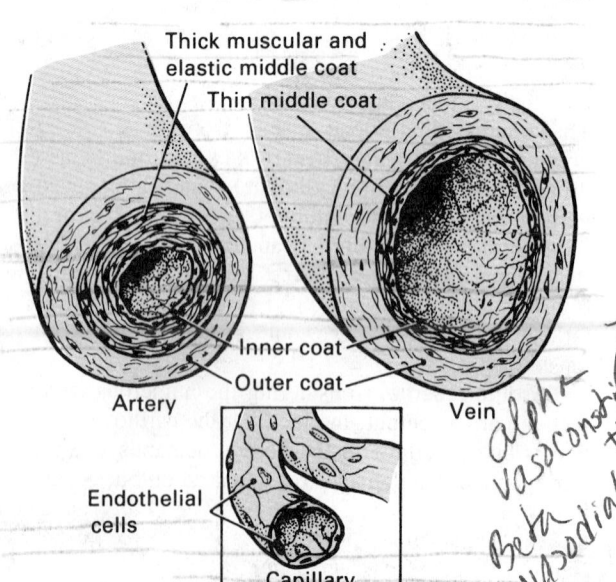

Fig. 26-7 Comparative thickness of layers of the artery, vein, and capillary.

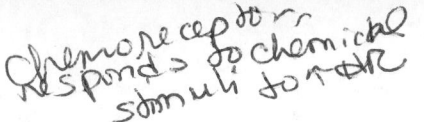

Baroreceptors control only temporary changes, such as changes in position.

Chemoreceptors. Chemoreceptors are located in the aortic arch and carotid body. They are capable of initiating changes in heart rate and arterial pressure in response to chemical stimulation. They are stimulated by decreased O_2 pressure (Po_2), increased carbon dioxide (CO_2) pressure (Pco_2), and decreased plasma pH. When the chemoreceptor reflexes are stimulated, they subsequently stimulate the vasomotor center to increase cardiac activity.

Blood Pressure

The arterial blood pressure (BP) is a measure of the pressure exerted by blood against the walls of the arterial system. The *systolic* pressure is the peak pressure exerted against the arteries when the heart contracts. The *diastolic* pressure is the residual pressure of the arterial system during cardiac relaxation. BP is usually expressed as the ratio of systolic to diastolic pressure.

The two main factors influencing BP are CO and peripheral vascular resistance (PR):

$$BP = CO \times PR$$

Peripheral resistance is the force opposing the movement of blood. This force is created primarily in small arteries and arterioles.

The arterial BP is influenced by changes in either cardiac output or peripheral resistance. (These factors are discussed in Chapter 27.)

Measurement of arterial blood pressure. BP can be measured by invasive and noninvasive techniques. The invasive technique consists of catheter insertion into an artery. The catheter is attached to a recording device and the pressure is measured directly (see Chapter 28).

However, the easiest technique is the noninvasive, indirect measurement of BP with a sphygmomanometer and a stethoscope. The sphygmomanometer consists of an inflatable cuff and a pressure gauge. The blood pressure is measured externally by listening for sounds, called *Korotkoff sounds,* produced over an artery when it is constricted. The brachial artery is the usual site for taking BP.

The balloon cuff is inflated to a pressure in excess of the systolic pressure. This causes blood flow in the artery to cease. As the pressure in the cuff is lowered, Korotkoff sounds are heard. The Korotkoff sounds are divided into five phases. The *first phase* is a tapping sound caused by the spurt of blood into the constricted artery as the pressure in the cuff is gradually deflated. This sound is considered the *systolic measurement.* The *second phase* begins with a murmur, usually 10 to 15 mm Hg below the systolic tap. The *third phase* begins 14 to 20 mm Hg below the second phase and begins when the murmur changes again to a tapping sound. The *fourth phase* begins when this tapping sound becomes muffled and less intense. The *fifth phase* occurs when the sound disappears.

The true diastolic pressure lies between the fourth and fifth phases. For greatest accuracy, the diastolic pressure should be recorded as both the muffled sound and the disappearance of sound (e.g., 120/84/80).[3] Occasionally, the sounds will be heard all the way to 0. In this case, the

blood pressure should be recorded as 120/80/0. In actual practice, BP is often recorded as two numbers. The first number indicates the appearance of sound, and the second number represents the cessation of sound. Another noninvasive way to measure blood pressure indirectly is to use an automatic cyling device. These automated BP monitors have been found to correlate closely with the results obtained by auscultating BP.

Pulse pressure and mean arterial pressure. *Pulse pressure* is the difference between the systolic and diastolic pressures. It is normally about one third of the systolic pressure. If the blood pressure is 120/80, the pulse pressure is 40. An increased pulse pressure may occur in exercise or in arteriosclerosis of the larger arteries. A decreased pulse pressure may be found in cardiac failure or hypovolemia.

Another measurement related to blood pressure is *mean arterial pressure*. It is not the average of the diastolic and systolic pressures because the duration of diastole exceeds that of systole at normal heart rates. Mean arterial pressure is calculated by adding the diastolic pressure to one third of the pulse pressure:

Mean arterial pressure = diastolic pressure + ⅓ pulse pressure

A person with a blood pressure of 120/60/0 has a mean arterial pressure of 80.

Effects of Aging

There is some controversy related to the effects of aging on the cardiovascular system. This is partly due to the presence of atherosclerosis in many older adults, which makes it difficult to separate physiological from pathological alterations. (Age-related changes are presented in Table 26-5.)

The most important molecular change in cardiac structure is related to collagen, which is a major component of valves, endocardium, and epicardium. With increased age, the amount of collagen in the heart increases. Collagen stiffens, affecting the contractile and distensile properties of the myocardium. In addition to collagen degeneration, heart valves also undergo lipid accumulation and calcification. The aortic valve is usually more involved than the mitral valve. The deposition of lipofuscin (brown lipid) is the most specific cellular age-related change. However, it does not appear to have any effect on myocardial function.

The resting heart rate is not markedly affected by aging. However, one of the major age-associated alterations in the cardiovascular response to exercise is a striking decrease in the cardiac response (e.g., decreased stroke volume, cardiac output, and heart rate).

The number of pacemaker cells in the SA node decreases with age, which can result in sinus node dysfunction (e.g., sustained sinus bradycardia). There is also fibrosis and increased microcalcification of the conduction system. A normal ECG shows little change with aging. However, there are small, inconspicuous increases in PR, QRS, and QT intervals. There is also a decrease in the amplitude of QRS complex (probably a result of left ventricular thickening).

The number and function of β-adrenergic receptors in

the heart decrease with age. Therefore older adults are less sensitive to β-adrenergic agonists and antagonist drugs.

With aging, the amount of elastin in arterial walls decreases, apparently as a result of destruction. In the arteries, thickening and fibrosis lead to increasing stiffness. There is an increase in pulse pressure in older adults because of an increase in systolic pressure and a lower rate of increase in the diastolic pressure. These changes are related to loss of vascular distensibility and elastic recoil.

Despite the changes associated with aging, under normal circumstances the heart is able to function adequately. However, cardiovascular reserve is markedly diminished by the aging process.

ASSESSMENT OF THE CARDIOVASCULAR SYSTEM
Subjective Data

Health history. A careful health history and physical examination of the cardiovascular system provide critical assessment data. Common chief complaints that should alert the nurse to the possibility of underlying cardiac or vascular disease must be explored and documented (Table 26-2).

Past health history

PEDIATRIC AND ADULT ILLNESSES. The client should be questioned about the existence or history of the following conditions, which may have an influence on the current cardiovascular status:

Alcoholism or excessive drinking	Kidney disease
Anemia	Pneumonia
Asthma	Rheumatic fever
Bleeding disorders	Rubella
Bronchitis	Scarlet fever
Collagen diseases	Streptococcal sore throat
Diabetes mellitus	Stroke
Gout	Syncope
Hypertension	Thrombophlebitis
Intermittent claudication	Varicosities
	Influenza

HOSPITALIZATIONS. The client should also be asked about specific treatments or hospitalizations experienced. Any hospitalizations for diagnostic workups or cardiovascular symptoms should be explored. It should be noted whether an ECG or a chest x-ray film was taken for baseline data.

CURRENT MEDICATIONS. An assessment of the client's current and past use of medication should be made. This includes over-the-counter (OTC) drugs as well as prescription drugs. For example, aspirin, which prolongs the blood-clotting time, is contained in many drugs used for alleviation of cold symptoms.

A medication assessment should list the name of the drug and the client's understanding of its purpose, side effects, and self-administration. Specific categories of drugs frequently used in clients with cardiovascular problems include antihypertensives, anticoagulants, diuretics, glycosides, and nitrates. Drugs that may adversely affect the cardiovascular system should also be assessed. Some of these, and examples of their effect on the cardiovascular system, are as follows:

Tricyclic antidepressants: Dysrhythmias
Phenothiazines: Dysrhythmias and hypotension
Oral contraceptives: Thrombophlebitis
Doxorubicin (Adriamycin): Cardiomyopathy
Lithium: Dysrhythmias
Corticosteroids: Sodium and fluid retention
Theophylline preparations: Tachycardia and dysrhythmias
Recreational or abused drugs: Tachycardia and dysrhythmias

ALLERGIES. A question about the client's allergies is appropriate. The nurse should determine whether a drug reaction or allergy was ever experienced. If the client has been treated for allergies, understanding of this therapy should be ascertained. The client should also be asked whether an anaphylactic reaction has ever been experienced.

OBSTETRICAL AND GYNECOLOGICAL PROBLEMS. The obstetrical or gynecological background, such as water weight gain, use of oral contraceptives, and venereal disease, should be noted.

Family history. Confirmed illnesses of blood relatives can highlight any hereditary or familial tendencies toward coronary artery disease, peripheral vascular disease, hypertension, bleeding, cardiac disorders, diabetes mellitus, atherosclerosis, and stroke. In addition, disorders affecting the vascular system, such as intermittent claudication and varicosities, may be familial. Finally, a family history of

Table 26-2 Cues to Cardiovascular Problems

Symptom	Description
Fatigue	No energy, more rest than normal necessary, normal activities resulting in tiring
Fluid retention	Weight gain, bloated feeling; swelling; tightening of clothing; shoes no longer fitting comfortably; marks or indentations left from constricting garments
Irregular heartbeat	Sensation of heart in throat or skipped beats, racing heart; dizziness
Dyspnea	Air hunger, especially after exertion; pillows necessary for sleep or use of chair
Pain	Indigestion, burning, numbness, tightness, or pressure in midchest; epigastric or substernal pain, radiating to shoulder, neck, arms
Tenderness in calf of leg	Inability to bear weight; swelling of the involved extremity; inflamed, warm skin over vein
Aching in calves	Distended, discolored, tortuous veins in calves of legs; ache in lower extremities after standing for short periods

noncardiac conditions, such as asthma, renal disease, and obesity, should be assessed.

Social and personal history

BACKGROUND INFORMATION. The client's sex, race, and age are all related to cardiovascular health. Discussing the client's marital status, role in the household, age and number of children, living environment, significant others, spiritual orientation, and coping mechanisms may assist the nurse in identifying stressors or strengths and support systems in the client's life.

The strong correlation between components of a client's lifestyle and cardiovascular health supports the need for a careful scrutiny of stressors, exercise, diet, sleep, and habits.

STRESSORS. The client should be asked to identify areas that cause stress or anxiety. Potentially stressful areas include marital relationships, family, job, church, friends, finances, and housing. Although many persons enjoy certain activities, they can be stressful at the same time that they are rewarding. The usual methods of coping with stress should be investigated. Behaviors such as explosive, rapid speech and emotions such as anger and hostility have been associated with risk of cardiac disease. The client and the family should be asked about the frequency of these types of behavior.

EXERCISE. The benefit of exercise to cardiovascular health is indisputable. Sustained aerobic exercise is the most beneficial. The nurse should carefully inquire about the types of exercise done, the duration and frequency of each, and the occurrence of any unwanted effects. The length of time the exercise program has been practiced should be recorded. Participation in individual or group sports should also be noted, along with frequency and duration. Any symptoms indicative of cardiovascular problems during exercise should be recorded.

DIET. The client's weight in relation to height and build should be determined. Problems of being underweight or overweight should be noted. The amount of salt, saturated fats, and triglycerides in the diet should be determined. A typical day's diet should be examined for its adequacy in relation to the client's lifestyle. In addition to actual food habits, the client's attitudes and plans in relation to diet should be investigated. Food intake and exercise patterns should be complementary. The "big eater" should be the disciplined exerciser. Conversely, the sedentary person should adjust caloric intake accordingly to avoid overtaxing the heart by increasing the work load due to excessive weight.

SLEEP. The client should be asked specific questions related to sleep habits: "How many pillows do you sleep on at night? How big are the pillows? How many times a night do you awaken to urinate? Do you ever wake up suddenly and feel as if you cannot catch your breath? What do you do when this happens?" A healthy, content person should fall asleep easily, sleep soundly without awakening, and wake up feeling refreshed and ready to face the day. Although there are many possible causes, cardiovascular problems are often to blame for interrupted sleep patterns.

HABITS. The most critical question to ask about habits is whether the client smokes. The number of pack-years of smoking (number of packs per day times the number of years the client has smoked) should be computed. The client's attitude toward smoking, as well as attempts to stop, should be discussed. Alcohol use should also be recorded. This information should include type of beverage, amount, frequency, and any changes in the reaction to it. The use of habit-forming drugs (including recreational drugs) should also be noted.

Review of systems.

The client should be questioned about past problems with the cardiovascular system. Specific inquiry should be made about the following conditions:

Hypertension	Chest pain
Rheumatic fever	Palpitations
Murmurs	Wheezing
Weight gain	Fainting
Shortness of breath	Leg cramps
Orthopnea	Claudication
Edema	Varicose veins
Fatigue	Cold or blue feet

When a cardiovascular problem is present, it affects other body systems, especially the pulmonary, renal, and neurological systems. Questions should be asked about these systems. This includes an appraisal of manifestations such as the following:

Wheezing	Dark, concentrated
Productive cough	urine
Shortness of breath	Leg edema or
Asymmetrical	numbness
weakness	Dizzy spells
Loss of memory	

Objective Data

Physical examination

Blood pressure.

After the client's general appearance has been observed, vital signs, including BP, heart and respiratory rate, and temperature, are taken. The blood pressure should be measured while the client is sitting, lying, and standing. An appropriate cuff size should be used for accurate readings. Normally, there is a reduction of up to 15 mm Hg in the systolic blood pressure and 3 to 5 mm Hg in the diastolic blood pressure in the standing position. BP measurements should be taken in both arms. These readings may vary from 5 to 15 mm Hg. A greater variance indicates pathology. BP in the lower extremities is expected to be 10 mm Hg higher than in the upper extremities.

Peripheral vascular system

INSPECTION. Inspection of the skin color, hair distribution, and venous blood flow provides information about arterial blood flow and venous return. The extremities should also be inspected for conditions such as edema, thrombophlebitis, varicose veins, and lesions such as stasis ulcers. Edema in the extremities can be caused by gravity, interruption of venous return, or elevation of right atrial pressure.

A measure used for assessing arterial flow to the extremities is the *capillary filling time*. The client's nail beds are squeezed to produce blanching and observed for the re-

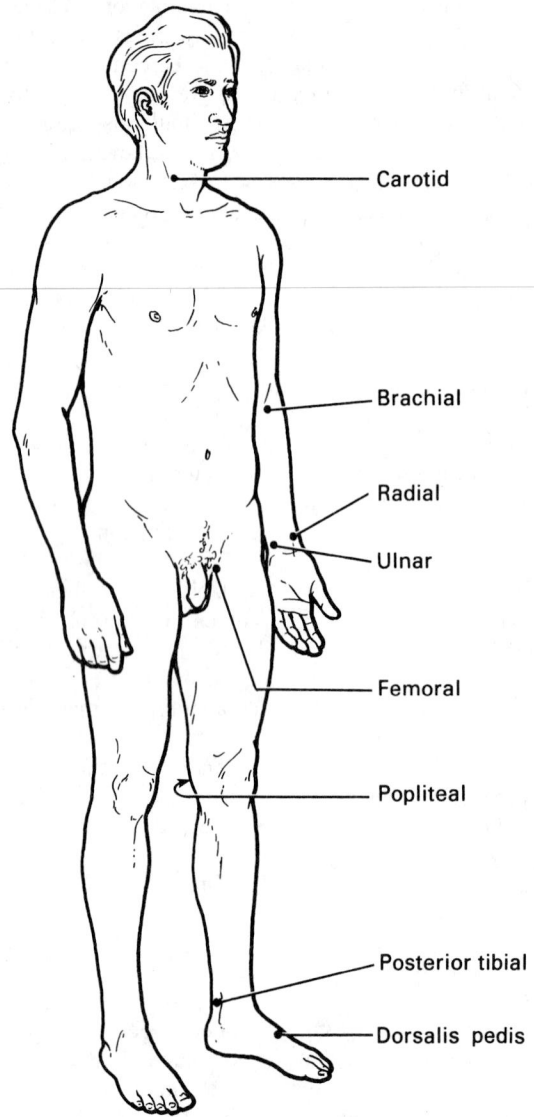

Fig. 26-8 Common sites for palpating arteries.

turn of color. With normal arterial capillary perfusion, the color will return within 3 seconds.

The large veins in the neck (*internal* and *external* jugulars) should be inspected while the client is gradually elevated to an upright position. Distention and prominent pulsations of these neck veins can be caused by right atrial pressure elevation.

PALPATION. Palpation of the pulses in the neck and extremities also provides information on arterial blood flow. The pulses should be palpated to assess the volume and pressure within each vessel, as well as the condition of the arterial walls. Characteristics of the arteries on the right and left sides of the body are also compared. It is important to palpate each carotid pulse separately to avoid vagal stimulation and subsequent dysrhythmias.

When palpating the arteries identified in Fig. 26-8, the assessor should note the pressure of the pulse wave or how far the vessel wall distends when the pulse occurs. This

judgment of the pulsation volume is recorded as *normal, bounding, thready,* or *absent.* A scale may be used to document pulse volume or amplitude[4]:

0— Absent
1+—Barely palpable
2+—Decreased
3+—Full (normal)
4+—Bounding

The *rigidity* (hardness) of the vessel should also be noted. The normal pulse will feel like a tap, whereas a vessel wall that is narrowed or bulging will vibrate. A term for a palpable vibration is *thrill.*

AUSCULTATION. An artery that has a narrowed or bulging wall may also create an abnormal buzzing or humming called a *bruit.* It can be heard through a stethoscope placed over the vessel. Auscultation of major arteries such as the abdominal aorta, carotids, and femorals should be part of the initial cardiovascular assessment. Abnormalities of the vascular system are described in Table 26-3.

Thorax

INSPECTION AND PALPATION. An overall inspection of the bony structures of the thorax, such as the sternoclavicular joints, the manubrium, and the upper part of the sternum, is the initial step in the examination. Pulsations of the aortic arch or the innominate arteries may be observed or palpated in this area in some normal persons. Thrills caused by abnormalities of these vessels may also be detected.

The next step in examining the thorax is to inspect the areas where the cardiac valves project their sounds by identifying the *intercostal spaces* (ICSs). The raised notch *(angle of Louis)* that is created where the manubrium and the body of the sternum are joined is readily palpable in the midline of the sternum. The angle of Louis is at the level of the second rib and can therefore be used to distinguish the ICSs.

The following auscultatory areas can be located (Fig. 26-9); the *aortic area* in the second right ICS near the sternum, the *pulmonic area* in the second left ICS near the sternum, the *tricuspid area* in the fifth left ICS close to the sternum, and the *mitral area* in the left midclavicular line at the level of the fifth ICS. A fifth auscultatory area is *Erb's point,* located at the third left ICS near the sternum.

Normally, no pulsations are found in these areas unless the client has a very thin chest wall. Valvular disorder may be suspected if abnormal pulsations or thrills are felt. Next, the epigastric area, which lies on either side of the midline just below the xyphoid process, is inspected and palpated. The pulsation of the abdominal aorta may be visible and can normally be palpated here. Next, the precordium, which is located between the apex and the sternum, is inspected for heaves. *Heaves* are sustained lifts of the chest wall in the precordial area that can be seen or palpated. They may be caused by left ventricular enlargement. Normally, no pulsations are seen or felt here.

The mitral area is inspected for the PMI while the client is recumbent. This pulsation or ventricular thrust normally has a short duration and lies within the midclavicular line in the fifth ICS (apex). If the PMI is not visible, the area should be palpated by placing the palm of the right hand in the apical area and feeling for the thrust. If the PMI is pal-

Table 26-3

Common Assessment Abnormalities of the Cardiovascular System

Finding	Description	Possible Etiology and Significance
PULSE		
Pulse volume		
Bounding	Sharp, brisk, rapidly rising pulse	Bradycardia, anemia, aortic valve incompetency
Thready	Weak, slowly rising pulse	Blood loss, mitral stenosis
Absent	Lack of pulse	Atherosclerosis, thrombus, trauma
Thrill	Vibration of vessel or chest wall	Aneurysms, aortic regurgitation
Rigidity	Stiffness or inflexibility of vessel wall	Hardening or thickening of wall, atherosclerosis
Bruit	Humming through stethoscope held over vessel	Narrowing of vessel, atherosclerosis, or aneurysms
Tachycardia	Heart rate over 100 bpm	Exercise, anxiety, shock, need for increased cardiac output
Bradycardia	Heart rate less than 60 bpm	Rest, SA node (pacemaker) damage, athletic conditioning, side effect of drugs (e.g., β-blocker medications)
Dysrhythmia	Irregular heart rate, skipped heartbeats	Damage to cardiac conduction pathway, ischemia, side effect of drugs
VENOUS ABNORMALITIES		
Distended neck veins	Vertical distance between intersection of angle of Louis and level of jugular distention greater than 3 cm with client sitting at 45 degree angle	Elevated right atrial pressure
Pitting edema of lower extremities or sacral area	Visible finger indentation after application of firm pressure	Interruption of venous return to heart, fluid in tissues
Thrombophlebitis	Red, warm, tender, hard vein; edema, pain, tenderness of extremity	Venous stasis, damage to endothelial layer of vein, hypercoagulability of blood
Positive Homans' sign	Presence of calf pain during sharp dorsiflexion of foot	Thrombophlebitis
SKIN		
Unusually warm hands or feet	Warmer than normal	Possible thyrotoxicosis and severe anemia
Cold hands or feet	Cold to touch, external covering necessary for comfort	Intermittent claudication, peripheral arterial obstruction, low cardiac output
Central cyanosis	Bluish or purplish tinge in central areas such as tongue, conjunctivae, inner surface of lips	Incomplete O_2 saturation of arterial blood due to pulmonary or cardiac disorders (e.g., congenital defects)
Peripheral cyanosis	Bluish or purplish tinge in extremities or in nose and ears	Reduced blood flow due to heart failure, vasoconstriction, cold environment
Color changes in extremities with postural change	Pallor, cyanosis, mottling of skin after limb elevation; glossy skin	Chronic decreased arterial perfusion
Stasis ulcers	Darkly pigmented, edematous areas of skin; open or oozing fluid	Poor venous return, varicose veins, incompetent venous valves

Continued.

Table 26-3

Common Assessment Abnormalities of the Cardiovascular System—cont'd

Findings	Description	Possible Etiology and Significance
EXTREMITIES		
Clubbing of nail beds	Obliteration of normal angle between base of nail and skin	Endocarditis, congenital defects, prolonged O_2 deficiency
Splinter hemorrhages	Small red to black streaks under fingernails	Infective endocarditis (infection of endocardium, usually in area of cardiac valves)
Abnormal capillary filling time	Blanching of nail bed for more than 3 sec after release of pressure	Reduced arterial capillary perfusion, anemia
Varicose veins	Visible dilated, tortuous vessels in lower extremities	Incompetent valves in vein
Asymmetry in limb circumference	Measurable swelling of involved limb	Thrombophlebitis, varicose veins
CARDIAC AUSCULTATORY ABNORMALITIES		
Third heart sound (S_3)	Extra heart sound, low pitched, ending in early diastole, similar to sound of a gallop	Left ventricular failure; mitral regurgitation, volume overload, hypertension (possible)
Fourth heart sound (S_4)	Extra heart sound, low pitched, ending in late diastole, similar to sound of a gallop	Forceful atrial contraction from resistance to ventricular filling (e.g., in left ventricular hypertrophy, pulmonary stenosis, hypertension, coronary artery disease, aortic stenosis)
Cardiac murmurs	Swishing between normal heart sounds; characterization by loudness, pitch, shape, quality, duration, timing	Cardiac valve disorder, abnormal blood flow patterns

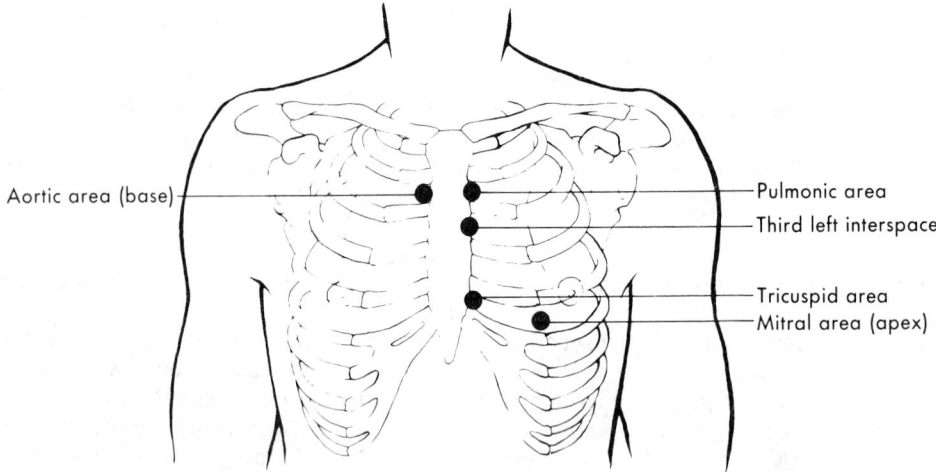

Fig. 26-9 Cardiac auscultatory areas. (From Kinney M and others: Comprehensive cardiac care, ed 7, St Louis, 1991, Mosby–Year Book, Inc.)

pable, its position is recorded in relation to the midclavicular line and ICSs. When the PMI is left of the midclavicular line, the heart may be enlarged.

PERCUSSION. The borders of the right and left sides of the heart can be estimated by percussion. The examiner stands to the right of the recumbent client and percusses along the curve of the rib in the fourth and fifth ICSs, starting at the midaxillary line. The percussion note over the heart is dull in comparison with the resonance over the lung and is recorded in relation to the midclavicular line.

AUSCULTATION. The movement of the cardiac valves creates some turbulence in the blood flow. The vibration of the blood causes normal heart sounds (Fig. 26-10). These sounds can be heard through a stethoscope placed on the

Pulmonic and aortic areas (Base)

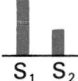

$$S_1 \quad S_2$$

Tricuspid and mitral areas (Apex)

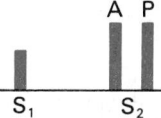

$$S_1 \quad S_2$$

Normal physiological splitting of S_2
(best heard at pulmonic area during inspiration)

A P

$$S_1 \qquad S_2$$

Fig. 26-10   Heart sounds. *A,* Aortic; *P,* pulmonic.

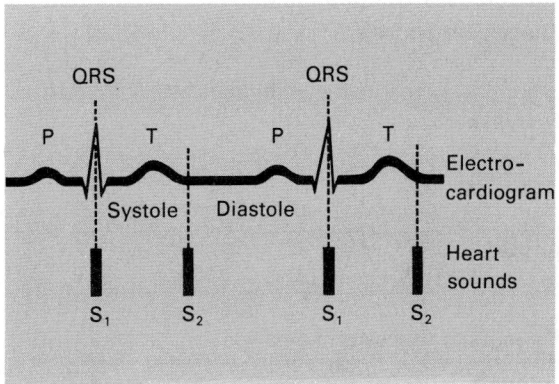

Fig. 26-11   Relationship of ECG, cardiac cycle, and heart sounds.

chest wall. The first heart sound (S_1), which is associated with the closure of the tricuspid and mitral (AV) valves, has a soft *lub* sound. The second heart sound (S_2), which is associated with the closure of the aortic and pulmonic (semilunar) valves, has a sharp *dub* sound. S_1 signals the beginning of systole, the period of ventricular contraction. S_2 signals the beginning of diastole, the period of ventricular relaxation (Fig. 26-11). The examiner should listen to the auscultatory areas in sequence with both the diaphragm and bell of the stethoscope.

The first and second heart sounds are heard best with the diaphragm of the stethoscope because they are high-pitched. Extra heart sounds (S_3 or S_4), if present, are heard best with the bell of the stethoscope because they are low pitched. It is important to explain that the nurse will be listening to the heart while the client is sitting leaning forward and in the left lateral decubitus position. Leaning forward while sitting accentuates sounds from the second ICSs (aortic and pulmonic areas). The left lateral decubitus position accentuates sounds produced at the mitral area.

Initially, the nurse will listen at the apical area with the diaphragm of the stethoscope while simultaneously palpating the radial pulse. If fewer radial than apical pulses are counted, a *pulse deficit* is present. A client with a pulse deficit should have the apical and radial pulse taken often to monitor this abnormality. A judgment about the rhythm (regular or irregular) is also made when listening at the apex.

Palpating the carotid artery while auscultating is also important because it allows differentiation of S_1 from S_2 and systole from diastole. Because S_1 (lub) occurs almost simultaneously with ventricular ejection, it is heard when the carotid pulse is felt. When listening at the other valvular areas, the examiner should always concentrate on the periods of systole and diastole as well as on the first and second heart sounds.

Normally, no sound is heard between S_1 and S_2 during the periods of systole and diastole. Sounds that are heard during these periods probably represent abnormalities and should be described. An exception to this is a normal splitting of S_2, which is best heard at the pulmonic area during inspiration. Splitting of this heart sound can be abnormal if it is heard during expiration or if it is constant (fixed) during the respiratory cycle.

Murmurs are sounds produced by turbulent blood flow through the heart or the walls of large arteries. Most murmurs are the result of cardiac abnormalities, but some occur in normal cardiac structures. Murmurs are graded on a six-point scale of loudness and recorded as a Roman numeral ratio; the numerator is the intensity of the murmur and the denominator is always VI, which indicates that the six-point scale is being used. Number *I* indicates a very soft, faint murmur; number *VI* indicates that the murmur can be heard without a stethoscope.[4]

If an abnormal sound is heard, it should be recorded. This description should include the timing (during systole or diastole), location (the site on the chest where it is heard the loudest), pitch (heard best with the diaphragm or the bell of the stethoscope), position (heard best when client is recumbent, sitting and leaning forward, or in the left lateral decubitus position), characteristic (harsh, musical, soft, short, long), and any other abnormal findings (irregular cardiac rhythms or palpable chest wall heaves) associated with the sound.

The abnormal sounds occurring during systole and diastole are classified as either murmurs or extra sounds. The most common abnormal sounds and abnormal assessment findings are described in Table 26-3. The data from inspection, palpation, percussion, and auscultation are presented in Table 26-4. Table 26-5 lists the cardiovascular assessment changes associated with aging.

DIAGNOSTIC STUDIES

There are numerous diagnostic techniques that add to the information obtained from the history and physical examination of the cardiovascular system. These procedures are usually classified as noninvasive or invasive. If only needle insertion for withdrawal of blood or injection of dye is used, these studies are usually considered noninvasive. Catheter insertion for angiography is considered an invasive procedure. The most common studies used to as-

Table 26-4 Normal Physical Assessment of the Cardiovascular System

Inspection	Normal skin color and capillary filling time, symmetrical thorax, no visible PMI, no jugular venous distention with client at a 45 degree angle
Palpation	Palpable PMI in fifth ICS at midclavicular line; no forceful pulsations, thrills, or heaves; slight palpable pulsations of abdominal aorta in epigastric area; equal carotid pulses bilaterally; equal pulses of extremities bilaterally; no evidence of impaired arterial flow or venous return in lower extremities
Percussion	Dull to percussion 10 cm to left on mid-sternal line, indistinguishable right-sided heart border by percussion
Auscultation	Readily heard heart sounds across four valvular areas, heart rate regular at 72 bpm, no murmurs or extra heart sounds, louder apical pulse when client is in left lateral decubitus position

sess the cardiovascular system are presented in Table 26-6.

Certain responsibilities of the nurse remain the same, whether the client is to undergo an invasive or a noninvasive procedure. First, the nurse must see that the procedure is scheduled and that any necessary preliminaries (e.g., special diets or changes in medication) are completed. Appropriate safety measures, such as use of bedside rails after administration of preprocedure medications or identification of client allergies, should be instituted. Comfort measures, such as oral care before the procedure, are important. The nurse must also check to see that the client's permission for the procedure has been obtained if it is required. It is important that the client understand the procedure. The client may have inaccurate information that causes unnecessary anxiety regarding the diagnostic study.

Noninvasive Studies

Chest x-ray film. A radiographical picture can depict cardiac contours, heart size and configuration, and anatomical changes in individual chambers (Fig. 26-12). The radiographical image records any displacement or enlargement of the heart. It is more accurate than percussion in determining the size of the heart.

Electrocardiogram. The basic P, QRS, and T waveforms are used to assess cardiac function. Deviations from the normal sinus rhythm can indicate abnormalities in heart function.

Table 26-5

 Age-Related Changes of the Cardiovascular System and Differences in Assessment Findings

Changes	Differences in Assessment Findings
CHEST WALL	
Senile kyphosis	Altered chest landmarks for palpation, percussion, and auscultation
HEART	
Myocardial hypertrophy, increase in collagen and scarring, decrease in elasticity	Decrease in cardiac reserve, slight decrease in heart rate
Downward displacement	Difficulty in isolating apical pulse
Decrease in cardiac output, heart rate, stroke volume in response to exercise or stress	Slowed, decreased response to stress; slowed recovery
Cellular aging changes and fibrosis of conduction system	Decrease in amplitude of QRS complex and lengthening of PR, QRS, and QT intervals; left axis deviation; irregular cardiac rhythms
Valvular rigidity from calcification, sclerosis, or fibrosis, impeding complete closure of valves	Systolic murmur (aortic or mitral) possible without being indication of cardiovascular complications
BLOOD VESSELS	
Arterial stiffening due to loss of elastin in arterial walls, thickening of intima of arteries and progressive fibrosis of media	Elevation in systolic and possibly diastolic blood pressure (e.g., 160/90); possible widened pulse pressures; more pronounced arterial pulses; pedal pulses often not detectable; color and temperature changes in extremities; loss of hair on lower legs
Increase in tortuosity and varicosities of veins	Ulcerated, inflamed, painful, or cordlike varicosities

Table 26-6

 Diagnostic Studies of the Cardiovascular System

Study	Description and Purpose	Nursing Responsibility
NONINVASIVE		
Radiological		
Chest x-ray	Client is placed in three or four upright positions so that the size of the heart and any calcifications can be noted. Normal heart size and contour for the individual's age, sex, and size are noted. No calcifications are seen in coronary arteries or valves.	Inquire about frequency of recent x-ray examinations and possibility of pregnancy. Provide lead shield for unexposed areas.
ECG	Small electrodes are placed on surface of the chest and extremities while leads are changed to detect conduction patterns as the direction of current varies. Technique can detect rhythm of heart, site of pacemaker, position of heart, size of ventricles, and presence of injury.*	Observe for electrical safety hazards. Inform client that no discomfort is involved.
Echocardiogram M mode Two dimensional	Small transducer that emits ultrasonic sound waves is moved across the client's chest wall above the heart. Transducer records sound waves that are bounced off the heart.	Place client supine on bed or examining table. Instruct client and family about the procedure and sensations (pressure and rubbing from the movement of the transducer across the chest). No contraindications to procedure exist.
Phonocardiogram	Graphic recording of heart sounds is performed by placing microphone on surface of body. Method is better than stethoscope for recording low-frequency sounds (gallop sounds). It provides information on murmurs and timing of various sounds.	Explain procedure to client.
Nuclear cardiology	Study involves intravenous injection of radioactive isotope. Radioactive uptake is counted over the heart by γ-scintillation camera. It supplies information about myocardial contractility, myocardial perfusion, and acute cell injury.	Explain procedure to client. Explain that radioactive isotope used is a small, diagnostic amount and will lose most of its radioactivity in a few hours. Inform client that camera is positioned over heart and that ECG electrode patches are placed on chest.
Thallium imaging	Thallium 201 is injected intravenously and used to evaluate blood flow in different parts of heart. Cold spots correlate with areas of infarction. For stress testing, intravenous thallium is given after client reaches maximum heart stress on bicycle or treadmill. Primary use is to evaluate coronary artery disease and early detection of acute MI. Waiting period after injection is 10-15 min. It can be done on an outpatient basis.	Explain procedure to client.
Technetium pyrophosphate scanning	Technetium 99m pyrophosphate is injected intravenously and taken up in areas of MI, producing hot spots. Maximum results are produced when performed 1 to 6 days after suspected MI. Waiting period after injection is 1½-2 hr. Scan is usually done in nuclear medicine department. It can be done in critical care unit in some hospitals.	Explain procedure to client.
Blood pool imaging	Technetium 99m pertechnetate is injected intravenously. Single injection allows sequential evaluation of heart for several hours. Study is indicated for clients with recent MI or congestive heart failure, especially if not recovering well. It can be used to measure effectiveness of various cardiac medications and can be done at client's bedside.	Explain procedure to client. Inform client that procedure involves little or no risk.

*For normal findings, see Table 26-1.

Continued.

Table 26-6

Study	Description and Purpose	Nursing Responsibility
NONINVASIVE—cont'd		
Magnetic resonance imaging	This noninvasive imaging technique obtains information about cardiac tissue integrity, aneurysms, ejection fraction, cardiac output, and patency of proximal coronary arteries. It does not involve ionizing radiation and is extremely safe procedure. It provides images in multiple planes with uniformly good resolution, but has limited use in critical care clients because of access and equipment problems. It cannot be used in persons with any implanted metallic devices.	Explain procedure to client.
Serum enzymes CPK	CPK enzymes are found in heart, skeletal muscle, and brain cells. Within 6 hr of MI, CPK is elevated. It returns to *normal* within 48-72 hr, which is <160 units/ml in men and <130 units/ml in women.	Avoid CPK elevation created by intramuscular injections that damage muscle cells.
CPK-MB fraction SGOT or AST	This isoenzyme is cardiospecific. Within 6-8 hr after cardiac infarction, SGOT rises. It peaks within 24-48 hr and returns to *normal* (7-40 units/ml) in 4-8 days. It is not specific to cardiac muscle damage.	Because SGOT can be elevated by other disorders such as liver damage, elicit a thorough history.
LDH	LDH has five different isoenzymes. Pattern of elevation is similar to that of SGOT after cardiac infarction except that LDH remains elevated for 5-7 days. *Normal* is 95-200 units/L.	When drawing blood, be sure that it is not hemolyzed because hemolysis will falsely raise LDH level.
LDH$_1$ and LDH$_2$	LDH isoenzyme subgroups are contained in heart muscle. Test determines LDH$_1$/LDH$_2$ ratio. If LDH$_1$/LDH$_2$ >1, it is indicative of MI.	
Serum lipids Cholesterol	Cholesterol is a blood lipid. Elevated cholesterol is considered a risk factor for atherosclerotic heart disease. *Normal level* is 140-220 mg/dl (varies with age and sex). Level can be measured at any time of the day in the nonfasting state.	Explain procedure to client. Inform client that fasting state is necessary for at least 12 hr (except for water) and that no alcohol intake is allowed for 24 hr before testing.
Triglycerides	Triglycerides are mixtures of two or three fatty acids. Elevations are associated with cardiovascular disease. *Normal* is 40-190 mg/dl (varies with age).	
Lipoproteins	Electrophoresis is done to separate lipoproteins into HDL, LDL, VLDL, and chylomicrons (see text). There are marked day-to-day fluctuations in serum lipid levels. More than one determination is needed for accurate diagnosis and treatment. *Normal values* for plasma lipoproteins vary with age. Desirable LDL is <130 mg/dl.	

Table 26-6

Diagnostic Studies of the Cardiovascular System—cont'd

Study	Description and Purpose	Nursing Responsibility
NONINVASIVE—cont'd		
Drug levels	Blood tests are done to determine therapeutic and toxic levels of drugs in the body.	Ensure appropriate timing of test with medication schedule.
Digoxin	Therapeutic level is 1-2 ng/ml; toxic level is >3 ng/ml.	
Quinidine	Therapeutic level is 2.5-5 μg/ml; toxic level is >5 μg/ml.	
Propranolol (Inderal)	Therapeutic level is 20-85 ng/ml; toxic level is >150 ng/ml.	
INVASIVE		
Cardiac catheterization	Study involves insertion of catheter into heart. Information can be obtained about O₂ saturation and pressure readings within chambers. Dye can be injected to assist in examining structure and motion of heart. Procedure is done by insertion of catheter into a vein (for right side of heart) or an artery (for left side of heart) (see text).	Before the procedure, obtain written permission. Withhold food and fluids for 6-18 hr before procedure. Give sedative, if ordered. Inform client about use of local anesthesia, insertion of catheter, and feeling of warmth and fluttering sensation of heart as catheter is passed. Note that client may cough when catheter is inserted into pulmonary artery and that client is monitored by ECG throughout procedure. After the procedure, assess circulation to extremity used for catheter insertion after procedure. Check peripheral pulses, color, and sensation of extremity every 15 min for 4 hr and then with decreasing frequency. Observe injection site for swelling and bleeding. Place sandbag over arterial site, if indicated. Monitor vital signs. Assess for abnormal heart rates, dysrhythmias, and signs of pulmonary emboli (respiratory difficulty).
Coronary angiography	Study involves injection of radiopaque dye directly into coronary arteries by same procedure as for cardiac catheterization. It is used to evaluate patency of coronary arteries and collateral circulation.	Same as for cardiac catheterization.
Peripheral arteriography and venography†	Study involves injection of radiopaque dye into either arteries or veins. Serial x-ray films are taken to detect and visualize any atherosclerotic plaques, occlusions, aneurysms, or traumatic injury.	Carefully explain procedure to client. Give mild sedative, if ordered. Check extremity with puncture site for pulsation, warmth, color, and motion after procedure. Inspect insertion site for bleeding or swelling. Observe client for allergic reactions to dye.
Digital subtraction angiography	This type of arteriography involves intravenous injection of contrast media. Catheter is threaded into superior vena cava. When contrast media circulate through arteries, computerized subtraction technique "subtracts" structures that block clear view of arteries. Most portions of cardiovascular system (except coronary arteries) can be studied by this technique. It can be performed on an outpatient basis and has many fewer complications than arteriography. Fluoroscopy used to help position catheter.	Keep client NPO 2 hr before test. Inform client that slight feeling of warmth may be experienced as contrast medium is injected and that ECG monitoring is done throughout procedure. Explain to client that test takes about 1 hr.

†Additional venous diagnostic studies are found in Table 32-9.

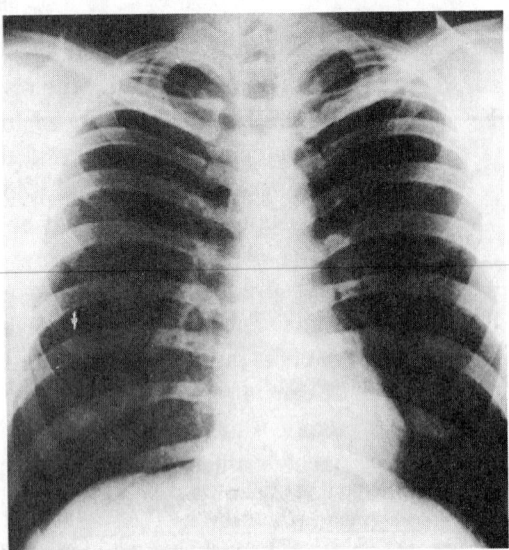

Fig. 26-12 Chest x-ray film showing outline of the heart. (From Kinney M and others: Comprehensive cardiac care, ed 7, St Louis, 1991, Mosby–Year Book, Inc.)

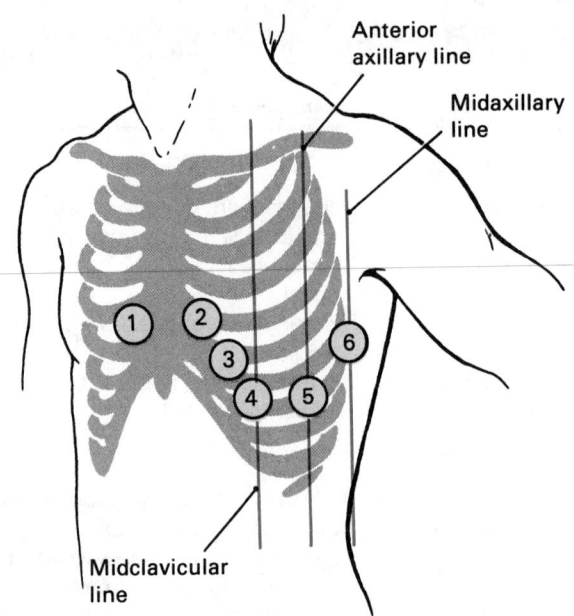

Fig. 26-14 Placement of chest leads for a 12-lead ECG.

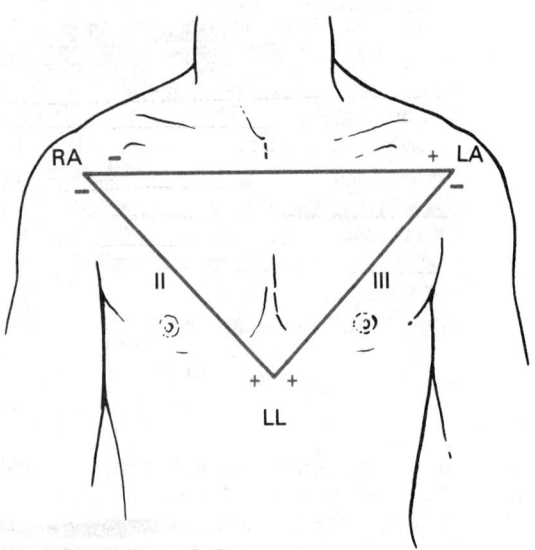

Fig. 26-13 Conventional polarity of the three standard leads is indicated by + and −. (From Price S and Wilson L: Pathophysiology: clinical concepts of disease processes, ed 4, St Louis, 1991, Mosby–Year Book, Inc.)

There are numerous types of electrographical monitoring, including *resting, exercise* or *stress testing,* and *continuous ambulatory monitoring.*[5] A resting ECG helps to identify primary conduction abnormalities, cardiac dysrhythmias, cardiac hypertrophy, pericarditis, site and extent of MI, pacemaker performance, and effectiveness of drug therapy and is used to monitor recovery from an MI.

In an exercise or stress ECG the person pedals a stationary bicycle or walks on a treadmill while ECG and BP measurements are taken to evaluate the heart's response to physical stress. This test is valuable in assessing asymptomatic cardiac disease and helping to define limits for exercise programs.

Continuous ambulatory ECG can provide more diagnostic information than a standard resting ECG, which records less than 1 minute of the heart's activity. In this test a portable Holter monitor is attached and the ECG is recorded over a 24- to 36-hour period while the person performs daily activities. The person records these activities in a log book.

ECG leads. Recording of an ECG involves the use of five electrodes. An electrode is placed on each of the four limbs. The right-leg electrode is used as an inactive ground electrode. The fifth electrode is used for various placements on the precordium.

Electrical impulses generated by the heart are picked up by the electrodes, magnified by an amplifier, and recorded. The recording is done by machines that produce a direct tracing by a stylus on paper. The paper contains a graphic background, which permits rapid interpretation of the waveforms.

Each combination of electrodes used in standard electrocardiography is called a *lead.* Each lead gives a continuous recording of changes in potential (or voltage) during the cardiac cycle between any two of the electrodes or between one electrode and a combination of others.

In a standard 12-lead ECG, five electrodes attached to the arms, legs, and chest measure current from 12 different views or leads. The three limb leads are I, II, and III (Fig. 26-13). Lead I records the direction of electric current and voltage detected between the right- and left-arm electrodes. Lead II is a right-arm and left-leg combination. Lead III records the electrical activity using the left-arm and left-leg electrodes. The unipolar augmented limb leads (aV_R, aV_L, and aV_F) measure electrical potential between one augmented limb lead and the electrical midpoint of the remaining two leads. The fifth electrode is placed in various locations, starting at the right sternal border in the

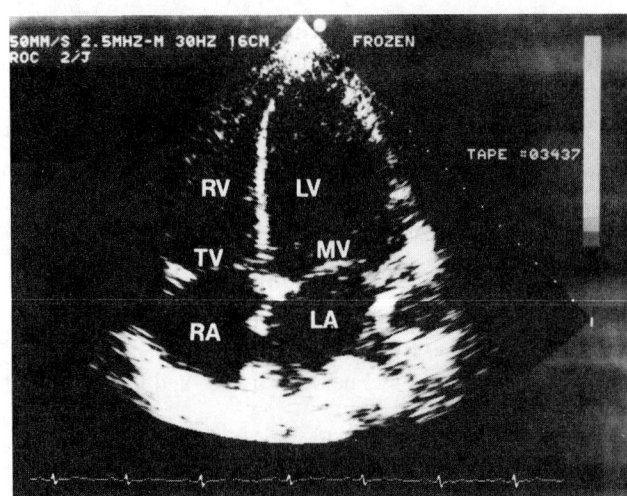

Fig. 26-15 Apical four-chamber two-dimensional echocardiographic view in a normal client. *LA*, Left atrium; *RA*, right atrium; *TV*, tricuspid valve; *LV*, left ventricle; *RV*, right ventricle; *MV*, mitral valve. (From Kinney M and others: Comprehensive cardiac care, ed 7, St Louis, 1991, Mosby–Year Book, Inc.)

fourth ICS (V_1) and moving across the chest (V_1 through V_6), as indicated in Fig. 26-14. These are known as *chest* or *V* leads.

Echocardiogram. The *echocardiogram* (ultrasound cardiogram) uses ultrasound waves (high-frequency sound waves) to record the movement of the structures of the heart. In the normal heart, ultrasonic sound waves directed at the heart are reflected back in typical configurations (Fig. 26-15). The echocardiogram provides information about abnormalities of (1) valvular structure and motion, (2) cardiac chamber size and contents, (3) ventricular muscle and septal motion and thickness, and (4) pericardial sac.

Two commonly used types are the *M-mode* (motion-mode) and the *two-dimensional* (2-D, real-time, cross-sectional) echocardiogram. In the M-mode a single ultrasound beam is directed toward the heart, recording the motion of the intracardiac structures. The 2-D echocardiogram sweeps the ultrasound beam through an arc, producing a cross-sectional view in real time, and shows correct spatial relationships among the structures.

An additional measurement used in conjunction with the echocardiogram is the *Cardiac Doppler*. Like the echocardiogram, it is based on the Doppler effect, which refers to a change in frequency of sound, light, or other waves caused by the motion of the source of the observer. The classic example is the change in the pitch of a train whistle as it moves past a stationary observer. The Cardiac Doppler adds quantitative and qualitative information on valvular abnormalities, congenital cardiac defects, and cardiac function. The characteristics of the measured blood flow can be evaluated by means of the audio and graphical display of the spectral analysis that is seen along with the echocardiographical imaging.[6]

One of the newest developments in cardiac ultrasound is *Doppler color flow imaging* (CFI). The CFI display includes information about direction and velocity of blood flow. The different colors seen on the echo image correlate with abnormal flow seen in cardiac shunts and diseased valves. The advantage of CFI is that it is a combination of Doppler flow information and 2-D echo imaging, which can shorten the examination time by simultaneously locating abnormal blood flow with color-coded images of its spatial extent.[7]

A new procedure called *stress echocardiography* adds only 10 to 15 minutes to a routine treadmill test and is a relatively low-cost and noninvasive procedure compared with the traditional cardiac radionuclide diagnostic examinations.[8]

Nuclear cardiology. Radioactive tracer studies are being used with increasing frequency to diagnose cardiovascular problems. Small amounts of radioactive isotopes are injected intravenously (IV), and recordings are made of the radioactivity emitted over a specific area of the body. The total radiation exposure is minimal. The circulation of this tagged material can be used to detect coronary artery blood flow, intracardiac shunts, motion of ventricles, and size of the heart chambers. This procedure is also used in evaluating the site and extent of myocardial ischemia or infarction. The most commonly used nuclear imaging tests include thallium imaging, technetium pyrophosphate scanning, and blood pool imaging.[9]

Thallium imaging. *Thallium imaging* (also called *myocardial perfusion imaging*) involves the injection of thallium 201, an analogue of potassium. After IV injection, it accumulates in various regions of the myocardium in direct proportion to myocardial blood flow. Then it is subsequently taken up by healthy, viable myocardial cells. In the presence of severe coronary artery narrowing and decreased blood flow to an area, the accumulation of thallium in that area is decreased. This is referred to as a *perfusion defect*. Areas that do not take up thallium are often referred to as *cold spots* on the scan. Perfusion defects usually correlate with the degree of the myocardial ischemia or infarction.

Perfusion imaging with thallium is also used with exercise testing to determine whether the coronary blood flow changes with increased activity. Stress exercising imaging may show an abnormality even when a resting image is normal. This procedure is indicated to diagnose coronary artery disease, determine the prognosis in already diagnosed coronary disease, assess the physiological significance of a known coronary lesion, and assess the effectiveness of various therapeutic modalities such as bypass surgery or angioplasty.[10]

Technetium pyrophosphate scanning. This technique involves injection of the radionuclide technetium 99m pyrophosphate. In contrast to thallium, this radioisotope accumulates in ischemic or damaged myocardial tissue, thus forming a *hot spot* on the scan. This test can be used to detect and define the location and size of an acute MI, but it does not indicate old areas of infarction. It is most reliable when performed between 24 and 72 hours after the onset of symptoms. Clients with unstable angina pectoris may undergo these studies to differentiate their chest pain from an acute MI. It is also valuable in diagnosing an acute MI when ECG or cardiac enzymes tests are inconclusive.

Blood pool imaging. *Blood pool imaging* (also called *radionuclide angiocardiography*) involves the IV injection of technetium 99m pertechnate. It differs from the previous two tests in that the isotope stays in the bloodstream and is not picked up by myocardial tissue. In first-pass imaging the radioactivity is followed through the circulatory system with a scintillation camera. The size, shape, and sequence of filling of the various chambers of the heart can be studied. This allows for evaluation of right and left ventricular function, wall motion of both ventricles, and calculation of the ejection fraction (portion of isotope ejected during each heartbeat).

After the first-pass imaging, images of the blood pool of the heart throughout the cardiac cycle *(gated cardiac blood pool studies)* can be done. The radioisotope is tagged in vivo or in vitro to red blood cells, and a scan of the heart then simultaneously reveals all the cardiac chambers and great blood vessels.[10] The client's ECG provides a gate, or physiological marker, of when end diastole and end systole occur within the cardiac cycle. Multiple-gated acquisition (MUGA) scanning can be used to record 16 to 32 points of a single cardiac cycle, yielding sequential images that can be studied like motion picture films. These studies can also be combined with exercise to evaluate cardiac reserve and function.[9]

Positron emission tomography (PET) is a new imaging technique used for the assessment of myocardial blood flow and myocardial metabolism. Radionuclides specific to a variety of metabolic pathways can be synthesized with positron-emitted radiolabels and injected into the client. The radionuclides most frequently used are oxygen-15, carbon-11, and nitrogen-13. These substances can be incorporated into intracellular compounds without altering their biological activity. For example, oxygen-15 is extracted for substrate metabolism by the heart muscle and therefore can be used to image overall myocardial metabolism. The positron camera is similar in size to a computerized tomography (CT) scanner. Currently, this diagnostic procedure is experimental because the costs of these studies are great, instrumentation is expensive, and (because of the short-lived nature of the radionuclides used) on-site cyclotrons or accelerators are a necessity.[9]

Blood tests. There are numerous blood studies that contribute information about the cardiovascular system. For example, studies of the blood itself reflect the O_2-carrying capacity (red blood cell count and hemoglobin) and coagulation properties (clotting times). (See Chapter 24 for hematology studies.)

Enzymes. *Enzymes* are found in all cells, with each cell type having its own specific enzymes. When cells are injured, they release their enzymes into the circulation. The enzymes characteristic of cardiac injury are creatine phosphokinase (CPK), lactic dehydrogenase (LDH), and serum glutamic-oxaloacetic acid (SGOT)—also called *serum aspartate aminotransferase* (AST). Because these enzymes are found in a variety of body tissues, they can be elevated as a result of injury to the muscles, liver, and other organs. For example, an elevation of LDH can mean heart, liver, skeletal muscle, lung, or kidney damage. For this reason, *isoenzymes,* multiple forms of an enzyme that have the same function, can be identified by electrophoresis and are organ specific. Their determination is a better indicator of cardiac injury than assessment of the total enzymes.

There are five isoenzymes of LDH, with LDH_1 and LDH_2 primarily found in the heart, RBCs, and kidneys; LDH_3 in the lungs; and LDH_4 and LDH_5 in the liver and skeletal muscle. Usually LDH_1 and LDH_2 levels rise 8 to 12 hours after an acute MI. An elevated LDH level in which LDH_1 levels exceed LDH_2 levels (the reversal of their normal pattern) is a reliable indication of acute MI.

CPK is present in heart muscle, skeletal muscle, and brain tissue. CPK-MB is found primarily in heart muscle, CPK-BB in the brain and nervous tissue, and CPK-MM in skeletal muscle.

SGOT is present in the heart, liver, skeletal muscles, kidneys, pancreas, and RBCs. Although a high correlation exists between an MI and elevated SGOT levels, no heart-specific isoenzymes exist to assist in identifying the specific organ damaged. Therefore, testing for SGOT in assessment of myocardial injury is often considered superfluous.

Blood lipids. Blood lipids consist of triglycerides, cholesterol, and phospholipids. They circulate in the blood bound to protein. Thus, they are often referred to as *lipoproteins.*

Triglycerides are the main storage form of lipids and constitute about 95% of fatty tissue. *Cholesterol,* a structural component of cell membranes and plasma lipoproteins, is a precursor of glucocorticoids, sex hormones, and bile salts. In addition to being absorbed from food in the gastrointestinal (GI) tract, cholesterol can also be synthesized in the liver. *Phospholipids* contain glycerol, fatty acids, phosphates, and a nitrogenous compound. Although formed in most cells, phospholipids usually enter the circulation as lipoproteins synthesized by the liver. *Apoproteins* are water-soluble proteins that combine with most lipids to form lipoproteins.

Different classes of lipoproteins contain varying amounts of the naturally occurring lipids (see Fig. 28-7). Electrophoresis is done to separate lipoproteins into the following groups[11]:

1. *Chylomicrons:* Primarily exogenous triglycerides from dietary fat
2. *Very low-density lipoproteins* (VLDL): Primarily endogenous triglycerides with moderate amounts of phospholipids and cholesterol
3. *Low-density lipoproteins* (LDL): Mostly cholesterol with moderate amounts of phospholipids
4. *High-density lipoproteins* (HDL): About one-half protein and one-half phospholipids and cholesterol

An elevation in LDL has a strong and direct association with coronary artery disease; increased HDL has been inversely associated with the risk of coronary artery disease. High levels of HDL serve a protective role by mobilizing cholesterol from tissues. Although the association between elevated serum cholesterol levels and coronary artery disease exists, determination of total cholesterol level is not sufficient for the assessment of coronary risk. It is important to determine whether elevated cholesterol levels are related to increased LDL or HDL.

Two important considerations in the measurement of blood lipid levels are that the client has to be fasting (12 to 14 hours) for useful information to be obtained and that there can be marked fluctuations from day to day in the same person. Therefore several measurements should be made before a definite diagnosis is made and dietary or drug therapy is implemented.

Recent evidence indicates that levels of plasma apoprotein A-1 (the major HDL protein) and apolipoprotein B (the major LDL protein) are better predictors of coronary artery disease than HDL or LDL. Therefore measurements of these lipoproteins may replace cholesterol-lipoprotein determinations in assessing the risk of coronary artery disease. (Blood lipids and their relationship to coronary artery disease are discussed in Chapter 28.)

Invasive Studies

Cardiac catheterization. Cardiac catheterization is a definitive means of obtaining information about cardiac disorders. This procedure can be used to measure intracardiac pressures and O_2 levels in various parts of the heart, as well as cardiac output. With injection of dye and x-ray visualization, the chambers of the heart can be outlined.

Cardiac catheterization is performed by insertion of a radiopaque catheter into the right or left side of the heart. For the right side of the heart, a catheter is inserted through an arm vein (basilic or cephalic) or a femoral leg vein. The catheter is advanced into the vena cava, the right atrium, and the right ventricle. The catheter is further inserted into the pulmonary artery, where it can be wedged or lodged in position. This position is called the *pulmo-*

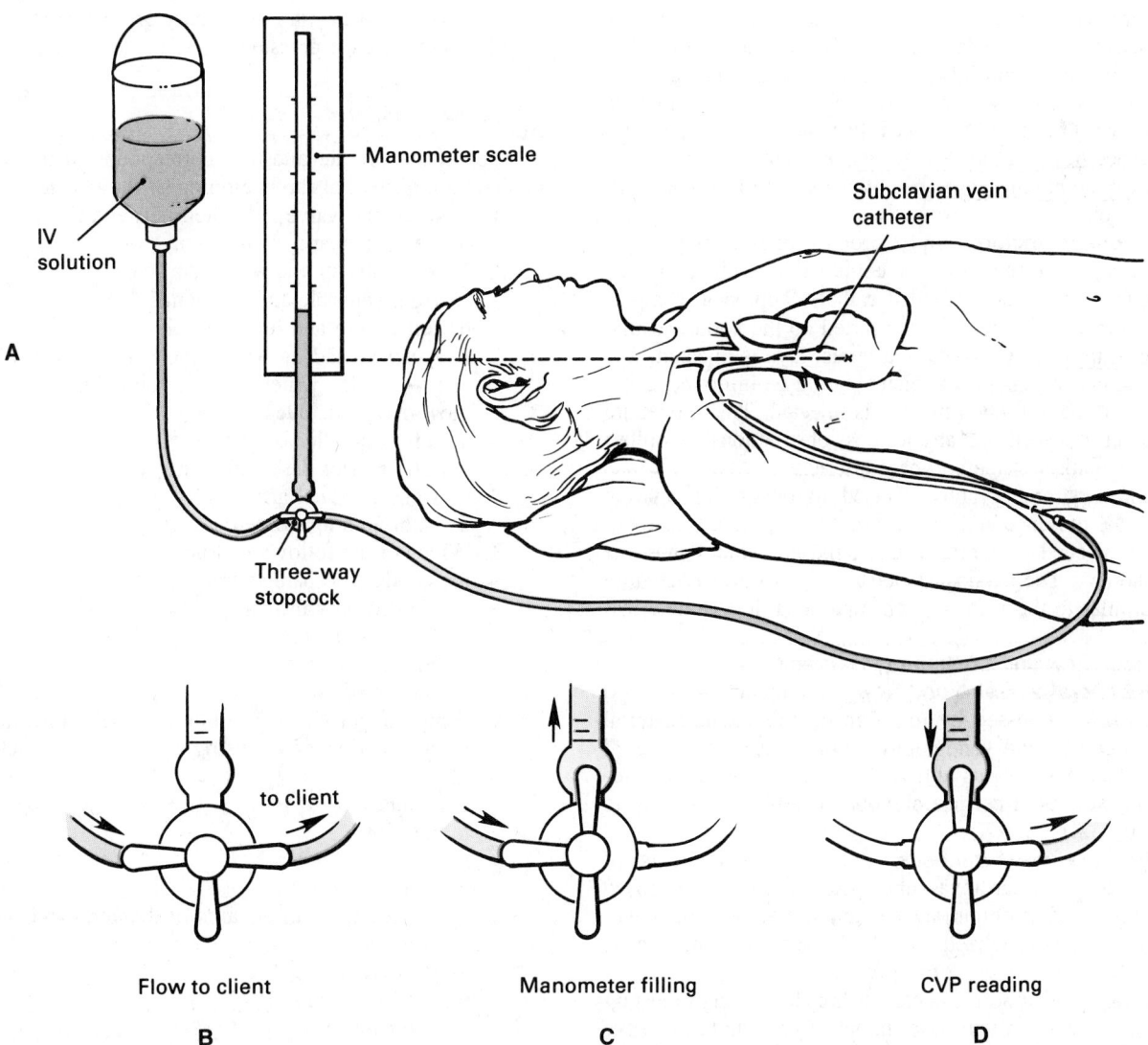

Fig. 26-16   CVP measurement. **A,** Placement of the manometer in relationship to the client. **B,** Stopcock is turned for intravenous flow to the client. **C,** Stopcock is turned so that manometer fills with fluid. **D,** Stopcock is turned so that fluid in manometer flows to the client. A CVP reading is obtained when the fluid level stabilizes.

nary capillary wedge position and can be used to measure pressures reflecting the function of the left side of the heart.

The left-sided approach is performed by insertion of a catheter into the brachial artery or the femoral artery. The catheter is passed in a retrograde manner up the aorta, across the aortic valve, and into the left ventricle.

Blood is taken from various chambers and analyzed for its O_2 content. Pressures in the various chambers are recorded. With the use of dye injections, the structures of the heart can be visualized and the size of the chambers determined.

Complications of cardiac catheterization include looping, kinking, or breaking off of the catheter, blood loss, allergic reaction to the dye, infection, thrombus formation, air or blood embolism, dysrhythmias, MI, cerebrovascular accident, and puncture of the ventricles, cardiac septum, or lung tissue.

Nurses have preprocedure and postprocedure responsibilities for clients undergoing cardiac catheterization. The client should be told how long (2 to 3 hours) the catheterization procedure will take, as well as where it will take place. Most hospitals have a cardiac catheterization laboratory specifically designed for the procedure. (See Table 26-6 for the nursing responsibilities related to cardiac catheterization.)

Coronary angiography. Coronary angiography (arteriography) is often done in conjunction with a cardiac catheterization. The left-sided catheter approach is modified so that the catheters are inserted up the aorta and into the openings of the coronary arteries. Dye is injected, and x-ray films are taken. The client should be informed that a flush may be felt when the dye is injected. This procedure is useful in identifying any lesions, obstructions, or collateral circulation of the coronary arteries.

Coronary angiography is used to obtain information about the presence and severity of coronary artery disease. This is needed to confirm the diagnosis and to determine the therapy. The nursing responsibilities for this procedure are similar to those for a client with a cardiac catheterization.

Blood flow and pressure measurements

Peripheral vessel blood flow. Peripheral vessel blood flow can be assessed by injection of radiopaque material (arteriography and venography). With these tests, arterial occlusions and venous abnormalities can be located. (Additional studies of peripheral blood vessels are discussed in Chapter 32.)

Pressure measurements. Bedside measurements of pressures in the cardiovascular system are frequently used to assess cardiac output and the appropriate fluid management of the hospitalized client. One such measurement is the *central venous pressure* (CVP).

In this procedure a catheter is threaded through the jugular or subclavian vein into the superior vena cava to the right atrium. The end of the catheter is connected to a three-way stopcock, a fluid system, and a water manometer (Fig. 26-16). An IV solution is maintained at a slow drip rate into the vein. The stopcock is opened to the manometer, which is then filled with IV solution. The stop-

cock is then turned to allow the fluid in the manometer to flow through to the client.

When the fluid level reaches a point that is equal to pressure in the superior vena cava or right atria, the fluid level stabilizes and a reading is taken. Then the stopcock is returned to the original position so that the IV solution can flow to the client.

For an accurate reading, the base of the manometer should be at the level of the right atrium. The pressure readings directly reflect the right ventricular filling and diastolic pressure. The CVP reading is influenced by the function of the left side of the heart, pressures in the pulmonary vessels, venous return to the heart, and the position of the client when the reading is taken. The last factor must be kept in mind to obtain an accurate reading. The CVP reading is used less frequently since the introduction of pulmonary artery pressures.

Other pressure readings taken at the bedside include the mean arterial pressure, the pulmonary artery pressure, and the pulmonary wedge pressure (see Chapter 28).

R eview Questions

The number of the question corresponds to the same-numbered objective at the beginning of the chapter.

1. A semilunar valve is located between the
   a. vena cava and right atrium
   b. right atrium and right ventricle
   c. right ventricle and pulmonary artery
   d. left atrium and left ventricle
2. If a person had an MI of the anterior wall of the left ventricle, which of the following arteries is most likely occluded?
   a. left circumflex artery
   b. left anterior descending artery
   c. right marginal artery
   d. right anterior descending artery
3. Which of the following structures is *not* involved in the conduction pathway of the heart?
   a. sinuses of Valsalva
   b. Purkinje fibers
   c. bundle branches
   d. bundle of His
4. Which of the following blood vessels has the primary function of diffusing nutrients and metabolites?
   a. venules
   b. arterioles
   c. arteries
   d. capillaries
5. Chemoreceptors in the arch of the aorta and carotid body are stimulated by
   a. decreased P_{CO_2}
   b. increased pH
   c. decreased P_{O_2}
   d. increased arterial pressure
6. The purpose of testing for capillary filling time is to assess
   a. arterial flow to the extremities
   b. venous circulation to the hands

c. lymphatic obstruction of venous return

d. thrombus formation in veins

7. The auscultatory area in the left midclavicular line at the level of the fifth ICS is the
   a. tricuspid area
   b. mitral area
   c. aortic area
   d. pulmonic area

8. Palpable precordial thrills may be caused by
   a. heart murmurs
   b. pulmonary edema
   c. gallop rhythms
   d. right ventricular hypertrophy

9. Which of the following is an important nursing responsibility for a client having an invasive cardiovascular diagnostic study?
   a. Tell client that general anesthesia will be given.
   b. Instruct client to do a surgical scrub of the insertion site.
   c. Check the peripheral pulses and percutaneous site.
   d. Instruct client about radioactive isotope injection.

10. A P wave on an ECG represents an impulse
    a. arising at the AV node and spreading to the bundle of His
    b. arising at the AV node and depolarizing the atria
    c. arising at the SA node and repolarizing the atria
    d. arising at the SA node and depolarizing the atria

REFERENCES

1. Vander AJ, Sherman JH, and Luciano DS: Human physiology—the mechanisms of body function, ed 4, New York, 1985, McGraw-Hill Book Co, pp 326, 341.
2. Kleinhenz TJ: The inside story on preload and afterload, Nursing 15:50-55, 1984.
3. Ravin A: The clinical significance of the sounds of Korotkoff, West Point, Pa, Merck, Sharp & Dohme, pp 1-29.
4. Thelan L, Davie J, and Arden L: Textbook of critical care nursing, ed 1, St Louis, 1990, Mosby–Year Book Inc, pp 167-168.
5. Andreoli K and others: Comprehensive cardiac care, ed 6, St Louis, 1987, The CV Mosby Co, pp 64-66.
6. DeMaria A, ed: Cardiac Doppler: abnormal flow patterns, Andover, Mass, 1985, Hewlett-Packard Medical Products Group, p 35.
7. Color flow imaging: the newest modality for cardiac ultrasound, Andover, Mass, 1987, Hewlett-Packard Medical Products Group.
8. Crouse I: Identification of coronary artery disease with stress echocardiography, Adv Medicine 10:1-6, 1989.
9. Lyons K: Cardiovascular nuclear medicine, Norwalk, Conn, 1985, Appleton & Lange, pp 9, 18, 293.
10. Miller D and others: Clinical cardiac imaging, New York, 1985, McGraw-Hill Book Co, p 28.
11. Schell M: Cholesterol, lipoproteins, lipid profiles: a challenge in patient education, Focus Crit Care 17:203-211, 1989.

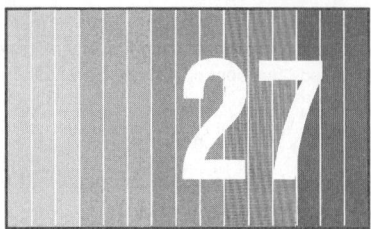

Nursing Role in Management
Blood Pressure Disturbances

Judith J. Barrows

Reviewed by Sharon Walker, R.N., M.S.N., C.C.R.N., C.N.R.N., Critical Care Staff Nurse, Albuquerque, New Mexico, and Beth Pulliam, R.N., M.S.N., Clinical Nurse Specialist, Vanderbilt University Medical Center, Nashville, Tennessee.

L earning Objectives

1. Describe the mechanisms involved in the regulation of normal blood pressure.
2. Define the shock syndrome.
3. Differentiate among the three classifications of the causes and mechanisms of shock.
4. Describe the pathophysiology and clinical manifestations of the three stages of the shock syndrome.
5. Describe the effects of shock on the major body systems.
6. Compare the therapeutic and pharmacological management of the client with each of the different types of shock.
7. Discuss the nursing management for the client in shock.
8. Identify the risk factors associated with essential hypertension.
9. Describe the clinical manifestations and complications of hypertension.
10. Describe the therapeutic, pharmacological, and dietary management of hypertension.
11. Discuss the management of the older adult client with hypertension.
12. Describe the nursing management for the client with hypertension, emphasizing client education.
13. Describe the differences between clinical manifestations and management of hypertensive emergencies and hypertensive urgencies.

Adequate systemic arterial blood pressure is essential for circulation of blood to all body tissues. This chapter discusses the regulation of blood pressure and focuses on two disturbances in blood pressure—shock and hypertension.

REGULATION OF SYSTEMIC ARTERIAL PRESSURE

For the review of the regulatory mechanisms of systemic arterial pressure, it is important to consider the following equation:

Arterial blood pressure (BP) = Cardiac output (CO) × Systemic vascular resistance (SVR)

Cardiac output is defined as the *stroke volume* (amount of blood pumped from one ventricle per beat, approximately 70 ml) multiplied by the heart rate (HR) for 1 minute. *Systemic vascular resistance* (SVR) refers primarily to the vasomotor tone of the blood vessels in the peripheral vascular system. SVR is the force opposing the movement of blood. This force is created primarily in the small arteries and arterioles. A small change in the diameter of the arterioles creates a major change in the SVR. The venules can hold large amounts of the blood volume. If SVR is increased, a greater amount of pressure is needed to force the blood around the circulatory pathways and the work load of the heart is increased.

The mechanisms that regulate BP have an effect on either CO or SVR. Regulation of normal systemic arterial pressure is a complex process involving the nervous, renal, and endocrine systems (Fig. 27-1).

Nervous System

Sympathetic nervous system. The nervous system, which reacts within seconds to minutes after a decrease in

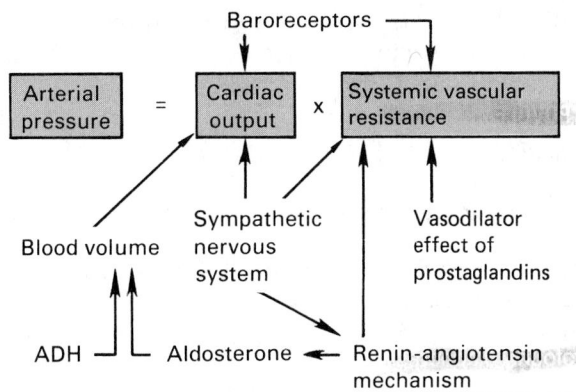

Fig. 27-1 Mechanisms involved in regulation of BP

Table 27-1 Sympathetic Nervous System Receptors

Receptor	Location	Action When Stimulated
α_1	Smooth muscles of peripheral blood vessels	Vasoconstriction of peripheral arterioles
α_2	Smooth muscles of peripheral blood vessels and gastrointestinal tract	Constriction of selected vascular beds and relaxation of smooth muscle of gastrointestinal tract
β_1	Myocardium	Increase in contractility (positive inotropic effect), increase in HR (positive chronotropic effect), increase in conduction through atria and ventricles (positive dromotropic effect)
β_2	Smooth muscles of peripheral blood vessels and lungs	Mild vasodilatation of peripheral arterioles, bronchodilation
Dopaminergic receptors	Primarily renal and mesenteric blood vessels	Vasodilatation

CO, increases arterial pressure primarily by activation of the sympathetic nervous system. When BP falls to below-normal levels, activation of the sympathetic nervous system results in secretion of epinephrine and norepinephrine from sympathetic nerve endings and the adrenal medulla. Sympathetic stimulation accelerates the HR and the force of myocardial contraction. This results in increased CO and sustains perfusion to vital organs, primarily the brain and heart.

When the sympathetic nervous system is stimulated, it stimulates the peripheral vasculature to constrict. This vasoconstriction causes an increase in SVR. Sympathetic control is the most important factor related to increasing SVR.

Sympathetic nervous system receptors are classified as alpha$_1$ (α_1), alpha$_2$ (α_2), beta$_1$ (β_1), and beta$_2$ (β_2) receptors. β_1-Receptors in the heart respond to sympathetic stimulation with increased HR, increased force of contraction, and increased speed of conduction. α_1-Receptors are located in the peripheral vasculature and cause vasoconstriction when stimulated. The smooth muscles of the blood vessels have both α and β_2 receptors (Table 27-1).

The sympathetic vasomotor center is located in the medulla of the brain. During exercise the motor area of the cortex is activated, and this activates the vasomotor center and therefore the sympathetic nervous system. During postural changes from lying to standing, the vasomotor center is stimulated to activate the sympathetic nervous system, causing peripheral vasoconstriction and an increased venous return to the heart. If this did not happen, there would be inadequate blood flow to the brain. BP may be reduced by stimulation of the parasympathetic system, which decreases the HR (via the vagus nerve) and thereby decreases CO.

Baroreceptors. *Baroreceptors (pressoreceptors)* are specialized nerve receptors located in the carotid arteries and arch of the aorta. When BP rises to above-normal levels, the baroreceptors are stimulated. They are sensitive to stretching and, when stimulated, send inhibitory impulses to the sympathetic vasomotor center in the brain and stimulate the vagus nerve. This results in dilatation of peripheral arterioles, a reduced HR, and decreased contractility of the heart.

A fall in BP leads to activation of the sympathetic system because the inhibitory effect of the baroreceptors has been removed. The result is constriction of the peripheral arterioles, increased HR, and increased contractility of the heart. The baroreceptors control only temporary changes in BP. In the presence of long-standing hypertension, the baroreceptors become adjusted to elevated levels of BP and recognize this level as "normal."

Renal System

The kidneys assist in regulating blood pressure by controlling sodium and extracellular fluid (ECF) volume (see Chapter 39). The retention of sodium results in increased water retention, which causes an increased ECF volume. This increased ECF volume increases the venous return to the heart and therefore elevates the stroke volume, which elevates the BP.

Another important mechanism related to the renal system is the renin-angiotensin mechanism. In response to sympathetic stimulation or decreased blood flow through the kidneys, renin is secreted from the juxtaglomerular apparatus in the afferent arterioles of the kidney. Renin activates angiotensinogen to angiotensin I; this is converted by the lungs into angiotensin II, which can increase BP by two different mechanisms. First, it is a potent vasoconstrictor, which increases vascular resistance, resulting in an immediate increase in BP. Second, angiotensin II indi-

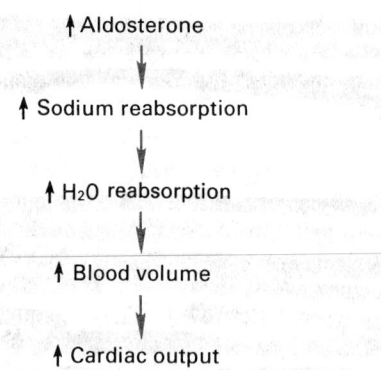

↑Aldosterone

↓

↑ Sodium reabsorption

↓

↑ H₂O reabsorption

↓

↑ Blood volume

↓

↑ Cardiac output

Fig. 27-2 Mechanisms of action of aldosterone.

rectly increases BP by stimulating the adrenal cortex secretion of aldosterone, which causes sodium retention by the kidneys (see Fig. 39-6). Increased sodium levels result in increased blood volume and increased CO (Fig. 27-2).

Prostaglandins secreted by the renal medulla have a vasodilator effect on the systemic circulation. This results in decreased vascular resistance and lowering of BP. One type of prostaglandin increases renal blood flow and promotes sodium excretion, which also helps to maintain BP within normal limits. (Prostaglandins are discussed in Chapter 7.)

Endocrine System

When the sympathetic nervous system is stimulated, it stimulates the adrenal medulla to release epinephrine and norepinephrine. These hormones raise the BP by causing vasoconstriction, which increases SVR. They also increase CO by increasing HR and myocardial contractility.

The adrenal cortex is stimulated by angiotensin to release aldosterone. (Release of aldosterone is also regulated by other factors, such as low sodium levels; see Chapters 10 and 42.) Aldosterone stimulates the kidneys to retain sodium and therefore water. This increases BP by increasing CO (Fig. 27-2).

The increased sodium in the blood stimulates the release of antidiuretic hormone (ADH) by the pituitary gland. ADH increases the ECF volume by stimulating the kidneys to retain water. Therefore, the increased blood volume can cause an elevation in BP.

In the healthy person, these regulatory mechanisms function in response to the demands of the body. When either shock or hypertension develops, the BP-regulating mechanisms become defective. Therapeutic and nursing management is directed toward changing the CO or vascular resistance of the client so that the BP can return to normal.

THE SHOCK SYNDROME

Shock is a clinical syndrome representing an extreme state of circulatory failure. Regardless of the cause of shock, the end result is the same: *impaired tissue perfusion* leading to cellular dysfunction. Unless the client receives prompt therapeutic intervention to interrupt the cardiovascular collapse, death will occur.[1] Shock is a complex

Table 27-2 Classifications and Precipitating Factors of Shock

HYPOVOLEMIC SHOCK

Hemorrhage
Burns
Loss of gastrointestinal fluid (vomiting, diarrhea)
Excessive use of diuretics
Internal sequestration of fluids (ascites, peritonitis)
Diabetes insipidus
Diabetic ketoacidosis
Profound diaphoresis

CARDIOGENIC SHOCK

Myocardial infarction (most common cause)
Cardiac dysrhythmias
Cardiomyopathy
Obstructive causes, including cardiac tamponade, tension pneumothorax, acute valvular damage, pulmonary embolism

DISTRIBUTIVE SHOCK
Neurogenic shock

Spinal cord injury
Spinal anesthesia or deep general anesthesia
Vasomotor center depression (e.g., severe pain, drugs, hypoglycemia)

Septic shock

Infection caused by invasive procedures (especially urological procedures)
Infection caused by indwelling lines and catheters
Postabortion and postpartum infection
Compromised clients, including older adults and infants, clients with a chronic disease (e.g., diabetes, cancer, acquired immunodeficiency syndrome), clients receiving immunosuppressive therapy, malnourished and/or debilitated clients

Anaphylactic shock

Insect bites/stings
Drugs
Contrast media
Blood transfusions
Anesthetic agents
Foods
Vaccines

group of signs and symptoms that may be precipitated by a variety of etiological factors. It is important to note that shock cannot be defined in terms of hypotension, since the shock syndrome may be manifested in the absence of hypotension. Conversely, hypotension may occur in the absence of shock.

Significance

The morbidity and mortality associated with shock are extremely difficult to determine. Some estimates have

Table 27-3 Hemodynamic Effects of Shock

Type of Shock	Cardiac Output	Central Venous Pressure	Systemic Vascular Resistance	Pulmonary Artery Pressure*	Pulmonary Capillary Wedge Pressure*
Distributive	↑ or ↓	↑ or ↓	Early: ↓ late: ↑	↑ or ↓	↑ or ↓
Hypovolemic	↓	↓	↑	↓	↓
Cardiogenic	↓	↑	↑	↑	↑

*Pulmonary artery pressures are explained in Chapter 28.

been reported. For example, cardiogenic shock occurs in approximately 10% to 15% of clients hospitalized with acute myocardial infarction (MI).[2] Despite current therapeutic measures, most studies indicate at least an 80% mortality rate for cardiogenic shock as a result of an acute MI.[2] Septic shock caused by gram-negative bacteria (endotoxic shock) has increased tenfold in the past 25 years, with mortality rates ranging from 30% to 70%.[3] Fatal anaphylactic reactions to penicillin are estimated to occur after 1 of every 100,000 injections and constitute 75% of all fatal anaphylactic reactions.[4] Death of trauma victims is often due to complications of shock.

Etiology and Pathophysiology

Although there have been many attempts to classify shock, none have been totally satisfactory. Table 27-2 presents one classification system, listing common types of shock and precipitating factors. This classification is based on a consideration of defects in the three primary mechanisms responsible for adequate circulation: (1) vascular tone (distributive shock), (2) intravascular volume (hypovolemic shock), and (3) the ability of the heart to act as a pump (cardiogenic shock). Table 27-3 compares the hemodynamic effects of the three types of shock.

Distributive shock. *Distributive shock* includes three types of shock: neurogenic, septic, and anaphylactic. In this shock state, relative hypovolemia occurs when vasodilatation increases the size of the vascular space and results in altered distribution of the blood volume rather than actual loss of the volume. This type of shock is often complicated by loss of intravascular fluid from increased capillary permeability. In distributive shock, there is no change in the ability of the heart to pump blood or in the blood volume but rather a decrease in the vascular tone.

Neurogenic shock. Neurogenic shock, an uncommon occurrence, is caused by massive vasodilatation as a result of loss of sympathetic vasoconstrictor tone in the vascular smooth muscles. The massive vasodilatation causes pooling of blood, decreased venous return to the heart, decreased CO, and eventually inadequate tissue perfusion. There are several precipitating factors that can lead to neurogenic shock (see Table 27-2). Disease or injury to the spinal cord can interrupt transmission of sympathetic nerve impulses to peripheral blood vessels, resulting in spinal shock. Spinal anesthesia can also block the transmission of impulses from the sympathetic nervous system. Depression of the vasomotor center of the medulla as a result of

drugs, fear, severe pain, or hypoglycemia can also decrease vasoconstrictor tone of peripheral blood vessels.

Septic shock. Septic shock occurs primarily in hospitalized clients as a result of overwhelming infection and is more common in infants, in older adults, and in persons with compromised immune systems. Bacterial endotoxins released from gram-negative bacteria are the primary cause of death from septicemia. Septic shock can also occur secondary to staphylococcal, streptococcal, fungal, and protozoan (e.g., *Pneumocystis carinii*) infections. The clinical presentation of this type of shock is often very subtle, especially in the older, debilitated, or malnourished client. Often, septic shock has two distinct clinical pictures: *warm shock* and *cold shock*. In the early stages, warm shock (or high-output or hyperdynamic shock) occurs. In this stage, vasodilatation occurs, resulting in decreased SVR and high or normal CO because of the decreased peripheral resistance. The BP is usually low, but the skin is warm, pink, and dry, and there is a good urinary output. In the more advanced stages of shock, cold shock (or low-output or hypodynamic shock) occurs. In this stage, increased sympathetic stimulation and vasoconstriction occur, resulting in increased SVR, decreased CO, decreased urinary output, decreased BP, and metabolic acidosis. Myocardial depression, often global and severe, is believed to be the result of circulating myocardial depressants. In addition, endotoxins cause the release of histamine, which results in increased capillary permeability and further decreases circulating blood volume (relative hypovolemia). The client's skin becomes cold and clammy.

Anaphylactic shock. Anaphylaxis is an acute and potentially life-threatening allergic reaction. (Table 27-2 lists common precipitating factors.) It is an immediate hypersensitivity reaction characterized by dilatation of arterioles and capillaries and increased capillary permeability throughout the body. Anaphylactic shock can result in respiratory and circulatory failure. (Refer to Chapter 8 for discussion of anaphylactic shock.)

Hypovolemic shock. *Hypovolemic shock* occurs when there is an actual loss of intravascular fluid volume. This loss results in decreased venous return to the heart, decreased stroke volume, decreased CO, circulatory insufficiency, and eventually inadequate tissue perfusion. In this situation, there is no decrease in the pumping ability of the heart or dilatation of the vascular space. The fluid that is lost may be either whole blood, plasma, or water and electrolytes. Common causes of actual hypovolemia include hemorrhage, burns, and gastrointestinal (GI) fluid losses. (Other causes are listed in Table 27-2.)

Hemorrhage. Hemorrhage refers to an excessive loss of whole blood. The amount of blood loss that results in the shock syndrome depends on the efficiency of a person's compensatory mechanisms. A blood deficit of 15% to 25% (750 to 1300 ml) in an adult with normal circulating volume is indicative of hemorrhagic shock.[5] Hemorrhagic shock frequently occurs after trauma and is secondary to such problems as bleeding esophageal varices or ruptured aortic aneurysms. It can also occur as a result of a surgical procedure, delivery of a baby, or coagulation disorders.

Burns. Plasma is the primary fluid lost from the vascular space in burn injuries (see Chapter 18). Because of increased vascular permeability, there is a rapid shift of plasma from the vascular space to the interstitial space. The greater the burn area, the greater the quantity of plasma lost. This loss of plasma from the intravascular space causes increased viscosity of the blood and sludging of blood components. The latter also contributes to increased SVR and decreased tissue perfusion.

Gastrointestinal fluid losses. GI fluid losses usually occur secondary to severe vomiting, diarrhea, or excessive drainage from a nasogastric tube or fistula and result in a loss of water and electrolytes. Susceptibility to shock due to these factors is generally age related. Infants and older adults are at highest risk because of the decreased efficiency of their physiological compensatory mechanisms.

Cardiogenic shock. *Cardiogenic shock,* often referred to as *pump failure,* occurs when the heart can no longer pump blood efficiently to all parts of the body and CO is decreased. There is no decreased intravascular volume or increased vascular space. The major cause of this type of shock is extensive myocardial necrosis due to MI.

Cardiogenic shock occurs when at least 45% of the left ventricular muscle mass has been damaged by infarction and ischemia.[6] Other causes of pump failure include cardiac dysrhythmias, which impair the efficiency of myocardial contractions, and end-stage congestive heart failure (see Chapters 28 and 29).

Structural changes in the heart, such as ventricular septal defect and ventricular rupture, can result in shock.[7] Cardiogenic shock can also occur when there is sudden obstruction to blood flow as a result of such factors as cardiac tamponade, tension pneumothorax, acute valvular dysfunction, and pulmonary embolism.

Clinical Manifestations

Clinical manifestations of the shock syndrome are directly related to the pathophysiological mechanisms involved. The progression of shock is variable and depends on several factors: (1) the client's age and state of health before the initial incident, (2) duration of the shock state, (3) responses to therapy, and (4) correction of treatable causes or precipitating factors of persistent shock (e.g., inadequate volume replacement, inadequate ventilation, acid-base abnormalities, adrenal insufficiency, and hypothermia).[8]

Shock is a dynamic event in which several different processes may be occurring at any one point in time. In addition, a client may progress toward death or toward normal homeostatic functioning over widely varying time periods. The shock syndrome is commonly divided into three stages: (1) early or compensatory shock, (2) intermediate or progressive shock, and (3) late or irreversible shock.

Early or compensatory shock. *Early* or *compensatory shock* is the initial, reversible stage in which compensatory mechanisms are effective in maintaining a normal or near-normal BP. In this stage, most of the metabolic needs of the body continue to be met. The pathophysiological sequence of events occurring during this stage is detailed in Fig. 27-3.

Pathophysiology. Regardless of the cause, the body attempts to compensate for the decreased arterial pressure in a variety of ways. First, a decrease in arterial pressure causes a similar decrease in capillary hydrostatic pressure. When the hydrostatic pressure no longer exceeds the colloidal osmotic pressure, fluid moves from the interstitial space to the intravascular space. This process is sometimes called *autotransfusion*. It may add sufficient volume to the vascular space to maintain normal arterial pressure without the aid of other compensatory mechanisms.

In addition to autotransfusion, baroreceptors sense a fall in arterial pressure. This results in increased sympathetic nervous system activity in the form of α- and β-adrenergic receptor stimulation (Table 27-1). Stimulation of $α_1$-adrenergic receptors causes selective peripheral vasoconstriction. Blood flow to the heart and brain is maintained, whereas blood flow to the kidneys, GI tract, and skin is decreased.

The decrease in blood flow to the kidneys stimulates the adrenal cortex to release aldosterone, which stimulates the kidneys to reabsorb sodium (Fig. 27-2). The increased sodium reabsorption raises the osmolarity of the blood and stimulates the release of ADH. This results in increased water reabsorption by the kidneys, increased blood volume, and increased venous return to the heart. Thus venous return is increased by the combination of autotransfusion, vasoconstriction, and hormonal changes. Increased venous return, as well as the increased HR and myocardial contractility caused by β-adrenergic receptor stimulation, results in increased CO, maintenance of BP, and adequate tissue perfusion.

Clinical manifestations. The clinical manifestations of early or compensatory shock are subtle and are often overlooked (Table 27-4). One of the most reliable signs of early or compensatory shock is the client's level of consciousness. Subtle changes in sensorium, usually in the form of restlessness, irritability, or apprehension, are frequently observed and are primarily caused by hypoxia of brain cells. Sedation at this time is contraindicated because it will mask important neurological signs. Pupil size may not be an accurate indicator of the degree of shock because drugs such as atropine and morphine will cause dilatation of the pupil.

During this stage the resting supine BP may be slightly elevated, slightly decreased, or normal for the client. For this reason, the BP may not be a useful indicator of early shock. Orthostatic hypotension (a decrease in systolic BP

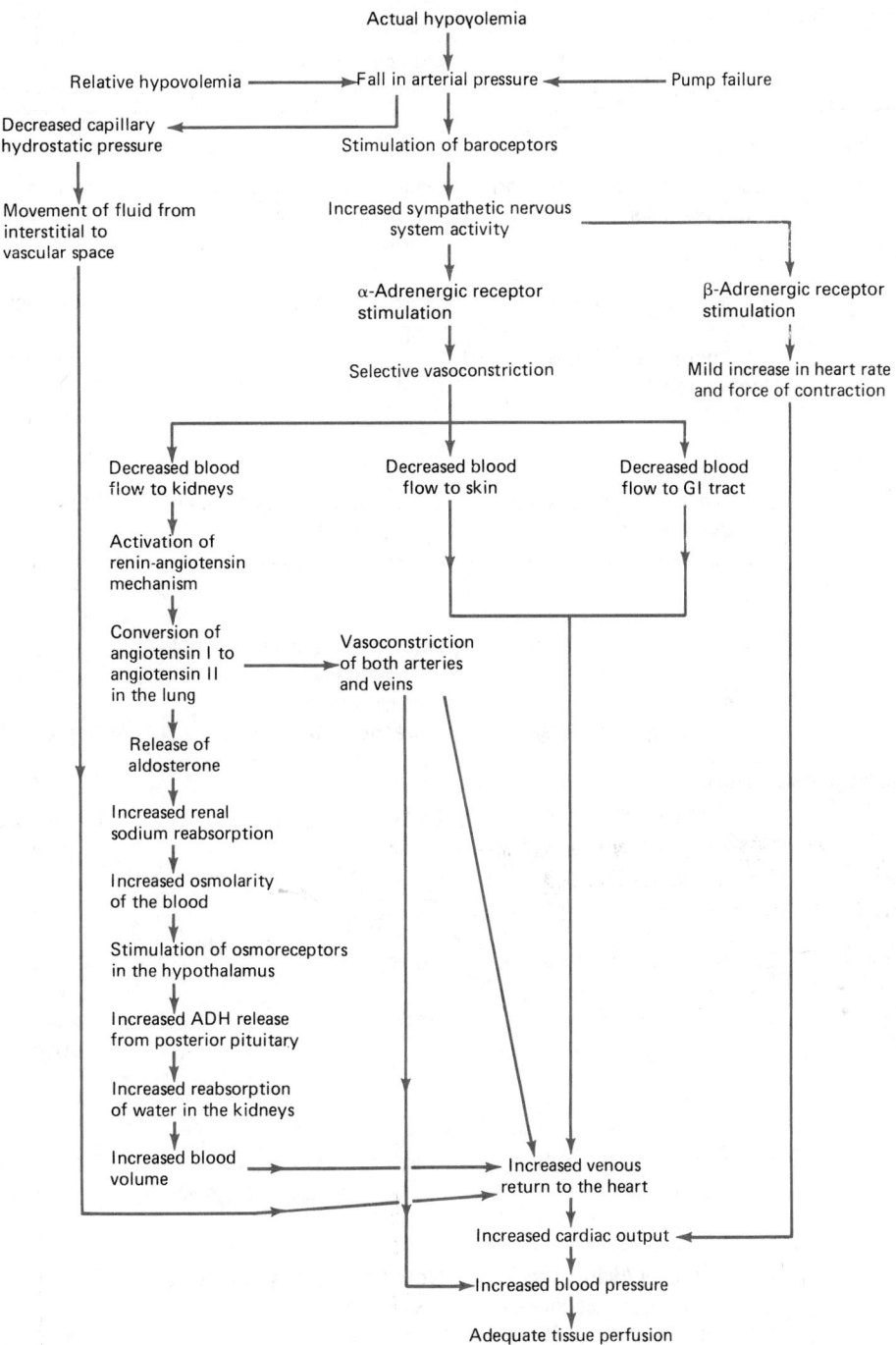

Fig. 27-3 Early or compensatory shock: initial reversible stage during which compensatory mechanisms are effective.

of at least 15 mm Hg when a client is raised from a flat position to an elevation of 45 degrees) is significant and indicates absolute or relative volume depletion. Normally a person is able to compensate by peripheral vasoconstriction for the increased flow of blood to the vessels in the lower extremities when changing from a supine to an elevated position. Volume-depleted clients are unable to compensate because they are already vasoconstricted or a condition exists that is causing their vessels to remain dilated (e.g., distributive shock).[9]

The HR in early shock is slightly increased. The pulse may be bounding or thready, depending on the stroke volume and the degree of peripheral vasoconstriction. Respirations increase in rate and depth in an attempt to compensate for tissue hypoxia, resulting in respiratory alkalosis. Urine output in early shock may decrease somewhat but

Table 27-4 Clinical Manifestations Correlated With Severity of Shock

Clinical Manifestations	Early or Compensatory Shock	Intermediate or Progressive Shock	Late or Irreversible Shock
NEUROLOGICAL STATUS			
Level of consciousness	Restlessness, irritability, and apprehension	Listlessness or agitation; apathy, confusion, alteration or decrease in response to painful stimuli	Unconsciousness, absent reflexes possible
Orientation	Maintenance of orientation, few slightly slurred words but normal sentences	Orientation possible, slowed speech	Confusion and disorientation with slurred, incoherent speech
Pupils	Normal size (2-4 mm) or dilated	Normal size or dilated	Dilating to dilated, slowly constricting or nonreactive
CARDIOVASCULAR STATUS			
HR	Slight increase (20 beats/min above client's normal)	Tachycardia (rate of 100-150 beats/min)	Slow and irregular
Amplitude of pulse	Bounding or thready	Weak and thready	Thready, often pulse deficit
BP			
Systolic	Normal or slight elevation	Decrease, usually 25% below usual BP with decrease in pulse pressure	Falling
Diastolic	Normal or slight increase	Increase or beginning to fall	Approaching 0
Assessment for orthostatic hypotension			
BP	15-25 mm Hg decrease (systolic)	25-50 mm Hg decrease (systolic)	Marked decrease to unobtainable
Symptoms	No light headedness	Light headedness	Inability to sit up
RESPIRATORY STATUS			
Rate	Greater than client's normal rate	Rapid, >20/min	Slow
Depth	Deeper than normal	Shallow	Shallow with irregular rhythm such as Cheyne-Stokes or Biot's respirations
RENAL STATUS			
Urine output	Slight decrease but within normal limits	Oliguria (<20 ml/hr) with increase in specific gravity	18 ml/hr or less, progressing to anuria with proteinuria
GENERAL STATUS			
Appearance of skin	Pale and cool (warm and flushed in septic shock)	Cold and clammy, cyanosis possible	Cold, clammy, and cyanotic
Body temperature	Decrease, normal, or increase	Usually subnormal (subnormal or elevation in sepsis)	Significant decrease
Degree of thirst	Normal or slight increase	Marked increase	Severe increase if client conscious

usually remains within normal limits. Because of extravascular volume depletion, the client may complain of thirst. In addition, thirst may be due to decreased secretion of saliva secondary to peripheral vasoconstriction. The skin may feel cool but not cold or clammy. An exception is septic shock, in which the skin will feel warm and dry. The body temperature at this stage will be slightly decreased except in septic shock, in which it is likely to be elevated.

Intermediate or progressive shock. *Intermediate or progressive shock* is the stage during which compensatory mechanisms are becoming ineffective and may even be

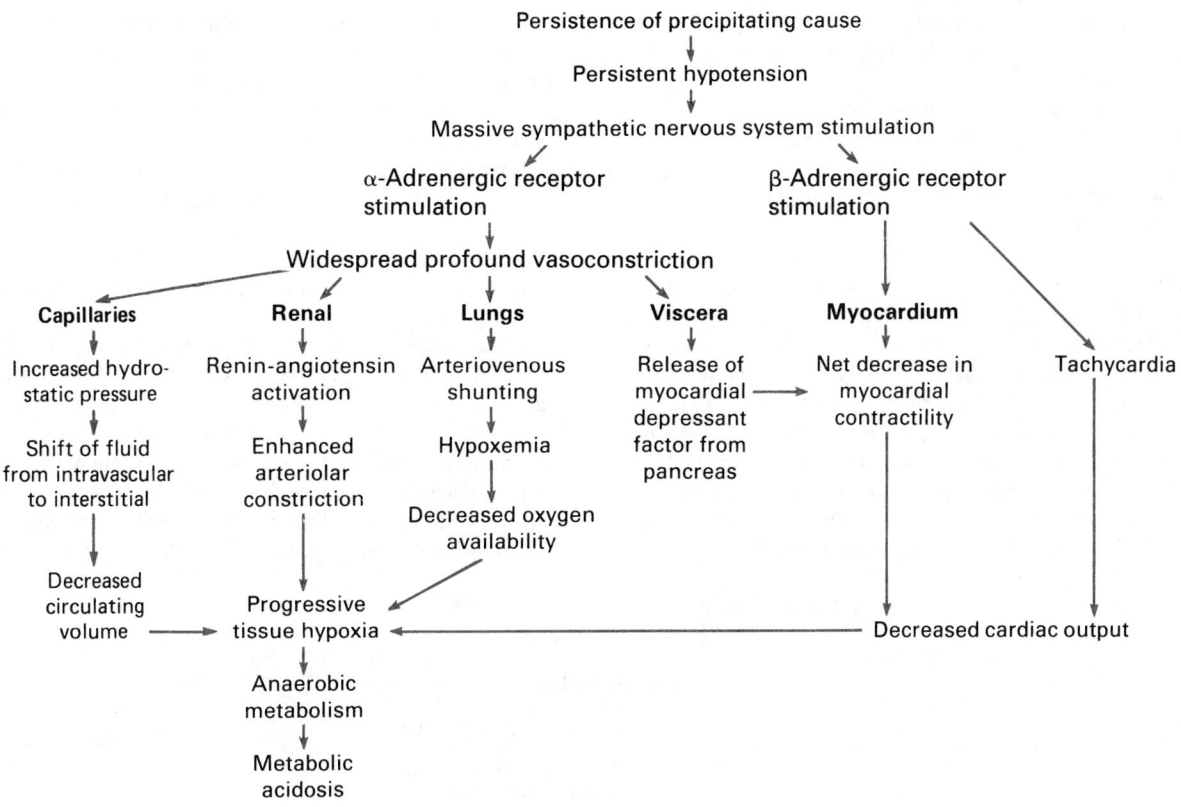

Persistence of precipitating cause

↓

Persistent hypotension

↓

Massive sympathetic nervous system stimulation

α-Adrenergic receptor stimulation   β-Adrenergic receptor stimulation

Widespread profound vasoconstriction

Capillaries	**Renal**	**Lungs**	**Viscera**	**Myocardium**	
Increased hydro-static pressure	Renin-angiotensin activation	Arteriovenous shunting	Release of myocardial depressant factor from pancreas →	Net decrease in myocardial contractility	Tachycardia
Shift of fluid from intravascular to interstitial	Enhanced arteriolar constriction	Hypoxemia			
		Decreased oxygen availability			
Decreased circulating volume →	Progressive tissue hypoxia ←			← Decreased cardiac output	

Anaerobic metabolism

↓

Metabolic acidosis

Fig. 27-4   Intermediate or progressive shock: Compensatory mechanisms are becoming ineffective.

detrimental to the client. The pathophysiological sequence of events occurring during this stage is outlined in Fig. 27-4. Aggressive management is necessary at this stage to reverse the shock state.

Pathophysiology. When shock is not detected and the precipitating cause is not corrected during the early stage, a massive sympathetic nervous system response occurs. α-Adrenergic responses continue, causing profound constriction of most vascular beds. Prolonged, severe vasoconstriction and decreased CO adversely affect cellular function, capillary dynamics, systemic circulation, and specific organ systems.[10] Renal ischemia leads to activation of the renin-angiotensin mechanism, causing even more pronounced vasoconstriction (see Fig. 39-6). Despite the attempt of the body to increase CO by increasing the HR and myocardial contractility, there is a net decrease in CO. This decreased output and profound peripheral vasoconstriction lead to tissue hypoxia, which causes the cells to undergo anaerobic metabolism. A by-product of anaerobic cellular metabolism is lactic acid production. The accumulation of lactic acid leads to metabolic acidosis.

Associated with the sympathetic response is the secretion of large amounts of catecholamines from the adrenal medulla. These augment the α- and β-receptor effects. In addition, catecholamines facilitate the cellular metabolism of the brain and heart. They cause the release of lipids that can be readily metabolized by the heart. Catecholamines also cause the liver to release its glycogen stores in the form of glucose. In addition, the pancreatic release of insulin is suppressed. Therefore the brain, which does not require insulin for glucose utilization, has large quantities of glucose available for metabolism.

Clinical manifestations. The manifestations of the intermediate or progressive stage of shock are presented in Table 27-4. The client demonstrates listlessness, apathy, and confusion. In addition, a decreased response to painful stimuli may be observed.

When the BP begins to fall, the client is no longer in early shock. Regardless of the previous normal BP, a systolic pressure below 80 mm Hg should be regarded as a danger signal. It is important to remember that a hypertensive client does not often initially display a pressure this low. A good guide for determining hypotension is a reduction in BP greater than 25% of the baseline level for the client. In addition to hypotension, a narrowed pulse pressure is often present. This finding is indicative of decreased stroke volume, as evidenced by decreased systolic pressure, and sustained vasoconstriction, as demonstrated by the elevated or normal diastolic pressure.[11]

Since cuff pressures may be inaccurate during this stage of shock because of the peripheral vasoconstriction, intraarterial monitoring or the use of a Doppler apparatus provides more reliable pressure readings (Chapter 28). If this equipment is unavailable, it may be necessary to take a palpated BP. This is done by palpating the brachial or radial pulse rather than listening for the first Korotkoff sound. The point at which the pulse is first felt is the systolic reading. It is not possible to obtain a diastolic reading with this procedure.

Tachycardia is evident during this stage of shock, and the pulse is weak and thready. Older adults and clients who are receiving β-adrenergic blocking drugs may be an exception and show little change in their HRs. Other cardiovascular effects of shock during the intermediate or progressive stage are shown in Table 27-4.

Respirations increase in rate in an attempt to compensate for tissue hypoxia and metabolic acidosis. However, the respirations become more shallow as the client begins to tire and becomes weaker. Urine output decreases and may fall below 20 ml/hr, indicating inadequate renal perfusion, which can lead to renal failure. The lips and mucosa are dry, and the client may continue to complain of thirst. The skin is cold, pale, and clammy, with slow capillary refill noted. There may be cyanosis due to tissue hypoxia. Body temperature is usually subnormal.

Late or irreversible shock. *Late* or *irreversible shock* is the stage during which compensatory mechanisms are either nonfunctioning or totally ineffective. Cellular necrosis and multiple organ failure occur. Attempts to restore the BP have failed, and death is imminent.

Pathophysiology. As shock progresses, there is little or no evidence of sympathetic nervous system activity. Thus one of the major compensatory mechanisms has failed. There is pooling and sludging of blood because of the lack of vasomotor tone. Thrombosis of the small blood vessels also occurs.

Tissue hypoxia resulting from peripheral vasoconstriction and decreased CO makes it necessary for cells to metabolize anaerobically (Fig. 27-5). The accumulation of lactic acid and other acid metabolites in the body's tissues contributes to cell death. The acid environment also causes increased capillary permeability and dilatation of the precapillary sphincters. Increased capillary permeability allows fluid and plasma proteins to leave the vascular space.

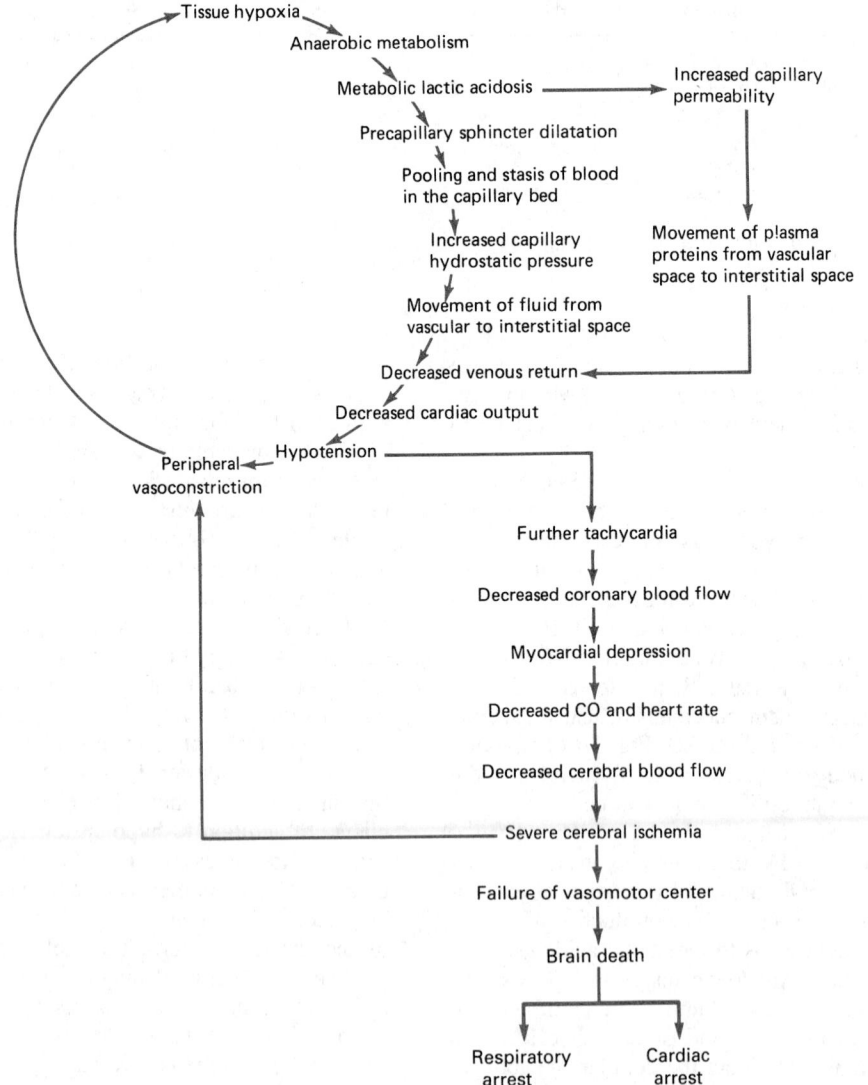

Fig. 27-5 Late or irreversible shock: Compensatory mechanisms are not functioning or are totally ineffective.

Because the venous end of the capillaries remains constricted while the arterial end is dilated, blood pools in the capillary bed. This also causes fluid to move out of the vascular space. The loss of fluid from the vascular space leads to hypotension, which causes further peripheral vasoconstriction, and a vicious cycle of decompensation ensues.

As shock progresses, hypotension and the resulting tachycardia decrease coronary blood flow leading to myocardial depression, which further decreases CO and results in bradycardia. Cerebral blood flow can no longer be maintained and severe cerebral ischemia occurs, resulting in a last effort by the sympathetic nervous system to cause peripheral vasoconstriction. The body cannot maintain vasoconstriction for long with the vicious cycle repeating itself. Failure of the vasomotor center then occurs, which results in loss of sympathetic tone. The result is brain anoxia and brain death, resulting in respiratory or cardiac arrest and death.[10]

Clinical manifestations. During the late or irreversible stage of shock, all body systems, especially the cardiovascular system, show evidence of decompensation (Table 27-4). The client is usually unconscious and may be unresponsive to all stimuli. Reflex responses may also be absent. The systolic BP continues to fall and may not respond to therapeutic measures to raise it. The diastolic blood pressure falls toward 0. The HR becomes progressively slower. The pulse is weak, and a pulse deficit may be present. Cardiac dysrhythmias may develop because of (1) an ischemic myocardium and (2) increased serum potassium levels from the release of potassium from the dead cells.

Because of respiratory center depression, there are likely to be slow, shallow respirations with an irregular rhythm and sometimes Cheyne-Stokes respirations. Urine output is minimal, and there may be a progressive rise in serum creatinine and blood urea nitrogen (BUN) levels, indicating some degree of renal failure. The skin is cold and clammy, with a significant decrease in temperature. (In septic shock, the client's body temperature may be either elevated or subnormal, depending on the age and clinical condition of the client.) Cyanosis may be present and is usually observed in the lips, mucous membranes, and nail beds. However, it may be more obvious in the palms, soles, and palpebral conjunctiva (inside the eyelid) of dark-skinned clients.

Complications

Infection may be a complication of shock as well as a potential cause of the shock syndrome. The shunting of blood to the vital organs results in a decreased supply to the various parts of the mononuclear phagocyte system. This may decrease the body's ability to remove bacteria and their endotoxins from the blood. The vascular changes resulting in hypoxia to the intestine, in combination with the depressed monocytes/macrophages, cause clients to be particularly susceptible to septicemia due to *Escherichia coli.*

A variety of other complications may result from prolonged or severe shock. Acute tubular necrosis may occur when impaired renal perfusion causes destruction of tubular epithelial cells (see Chapter 41). *Adult respiratory distress syndrome* (ARDS) is frequently associated with shock syndrome. Although no one specific factor has been known to cause ARDS, a period of hypoperfusion to the lungs with resulting pulmonary hypotension is common in this syndrome (see Chapter 23). Stasis of blood in capillary beds, as well as other factors present during shock, predisposes to a disorder called *disseminated intravascular coagulation* (DIC), particularly in clients with septic shock (see Chapter 25). Finally, shock may end in death.

Diagnostic Studies

No single laboratory test can diagnose the presence of the shock syndrome, yet a variety of diagnostic studies may assist in monitoring the progression and severity of shock. These studies are detailed in Table 27-5.

Therapeutic Management

For both the physician and the nurse, the critical factor in management of the shock syndrome is early recognition and treatment before irreversible cell damage occurs (Table 27-6). Successful management of shock depends on the ability to do the following:
1. Identify clients at high risk for shock
2. Diagnose the shock syndrome swiftly and accurately
3. Control or alleviate the primary cause
4. Implement appropriate therapeutic measures to correct pathological changes and enhance tissue perfusion

Prehospital care. Prehospital care of the client in shock is extremely important and may greatly increase the client's chance of survival. Table 27-7 outlines the prehospital care of acute traumatic shock.

Diagnosis. The history and physical examination provide initial clues leading to a diagnosis of shock as well as identifying persons at high risk for shock. A history of a recent event that may be associated with shock (e.g., trauma, infection, crushing chest pain) is significant. Changes in sensorium and decreased levels of consciousness reported by others are also important considerations.

During the physical examination, it is important to observe for the clinical manifestations of shock. Of particular importance is the immediate overall impression of central nervous system (CNS) function, which is a measure of cerebral perfusion. Also, the status of the cutaneous vascular bed is noted because it may be indicative of impaired peripheral tissue perfusion.

In addition to the history and physical examination, various diagnostic studies are ordered to corroborate the diagnosis and assist in identifying the cause of the shock. A central venous pressure (CVP) catheter (see Chapter 26), a pulmonary artery catheter (see Chapter 28), or both are placed for accurate, ongoing hemodynamic monitoring. A chest x-ray film may reveal thoracic trauma or pulmonary changes consistent with shock. A 12-lead electrocardiogram or cardiac monitor may indicate alterations in cardiac electrical activity, which can be an effect of the shock syndrome. Arterial blood gases (ABGs) are important to detect any acid-base abnormalities and to assess the oxygen-

Table 27-5 Diagnostic Study Abnormalities in Shock Syndrome

Diagnostic Study	Abnormal Finding	Significance of Abnormality
BLOOD		
Red blood cell count, hematocrit, hemoglobin	Normal	Remains within normal limits in shock because of relative hypovolemia and pump failure and in hemorrhagic shock before fluid restoration
	Decrease	Decreases in hemorrhagic shock after fluid resuscitation when fluids other than blood are used
	Increase	Increases in nonhemorrhagic shock due to actual hypovolemia because fluid lost does not contain erythrocytes
White blood cell count with differential	Leukopenia	Occurs in severe shock, especially when caused by gram-negative sepsis
	Leukocytosis with increased neutrophils	Is common in all forms of shock, especially hemorrhagic shock; neutrophils increase in response to tissue injury
Erythrocyte sedimentation rate	Increase	Is nonspecific, increases are in response to tissue injury
BUN	Increase	Usually indicates impaired kidney function due to hypoperfusion as a result of severe vasoconstriction
Serum creatinine	Increase	Usually indicates impaired kidney function due to hypoperfusion as a result of severe vasoconstriction, is more sensitive indicator of renal function than BUN
Blood sugar	Increase	Occurs in early shock because of release of liver glycogen stores in response to catecholamines
	Decrease	Occurs because of depleted glycogen stores with hepatocellular dysfunction possible as shock progresses
Serum electrolytes		
Sodium	Increase	Occurs early in shock because of increased secretion of aldosterone, causing renal retention of sodium
	Decrease	May occur iatrogenically when excess hypotonic fluid is administered after fluid loss
Potassium	Increase	Occurs when cellular death liberates intracellular potassium; also occurs in acute renal failure, after red blood cell hemolysis in transfusion reactions, and in the presence of acidosis
	Decrease	Occurs early in shock because of increased secretion of aldosterone, causing renal excretion of potassium
Calcium	Decrease	Sometimes occurs after rapid infusion of large amounts of citrated blood, also occurs secondary to respiratory alkalosis of early shock
	Increase	Occurs secondary to lactic acidosis, permitting increased ionization of calcium
Arterial blood gases	Respiratory alkalosis	Occurs early in shock secondary to hyperventilation
	Metabolic acidosis	Occurs later in shock when organic acids, such as lactic acid, accumulate in blood from anaerobic metabolism
Blood cultures	Growth of one organism (usually)	Grow gram-negative organisms most frequently in clients who are in septic shock
URINE		
Specific gravity	Increase	Occurs secondary to the action of ADH
	Fixed at 1.010	Occurs in acute tubular necrosis

Table 27-6

Diagnostic and Therapeutic Management: Shock Syndrome

DIAGNOSTIC

History and physical examination
Diagnostic studies*
Placement of CVP or pulmonary artery catheter, if indicated
Chest x-ray film
Twelve-lead ECG or cardiac monitor
Identification of cause of shock (if possible)

THERAPEUTIC

General measures

Establishment of a patent airway and administration of oxygen (ventilatory assistance with endotracheal intubation, if indicated)
Placement of at least two large, peripheral intravenous lines
Fluid resuscitation
  Typing and cross matching for whole blood or packed cells and administration of blood or blood components as indicated
Crystalloids (balanced electrolyte solutions)
  Plasma volume expanders
  Autotransfusion
Stabilization of BP (vasopressor agents and fluids, if indicated)
Placement of indwelling urinary catheter
Correction of acid-base imbalance as indicated by arterial blood gases
Pharmacological therapy†
Treatment of cardiac dysrhythmias
Emotional support of client and family

Specific measures

Hypovolemic shock
  Control of bleeding (if indicated)
  Use of MAST suit (if necessary)
  Surgery (if indicated)
  Reduction of fluid loss from vomiting and diarrhea
  Volume replacement and blood (if necessary)

THERAPEUTIC—cont'd
Specific measures—cont'd

Cardiogenic shock‡
  Administration of inotropic agents to increase cardiac contractility
  Careful fluid administration if client volume depleted
  Reduction of work load of heart by decreasing afterload with vasodilator drugs
  Reduction of work load of heart by decreasing preload with diuretics
  Intraaortic balloon pump to increase coronary perfusion and decrease afterload (if indicated)
  Thrombolytic therapy and/or coronary angioplasty (if indicated)
  Emergency cardiac surgery (e.g., coronary artery revascularization, valve replacement, repair of ventricular aneurysm, if indicated)
Distributive shock
  Septic shock
    Collection of cultures to identify organism
    Administration of appropriate antibiotics
    Administration of fluid
    Administration of steroids (if indicated)
    Use of MAST suit (if indicated)
  Anaphylactic shock
    Maintenance of open airway
    Administration of epinephrine for vasoconstriction and bronchodilatation
    Administration of diphenhydramine to counteract effects of histamine
    Administration of aminophylline for bronchodilatation
    Administration of fluid
    Administration of steroids (if indicated)
    Use of MAST suit (if indicated)
  Neurogenic shock
    Treatment according to cause
    Correction of underlying cause (if possible)
    Administration of fluid
    Use of MAST suit (if indicated)

*See Table 27-5.
†See Table 27-8.
‡See Chapter 28.

Table 27-7

Prehospital Emergency Care of the Client in Acute Traumatic Shock*

Etiology: Major trauma resulting in multiple injuries that are associated with blood loss

CLINICAL MANIFESTATIONS

Restlessness, anxiety, weakness, disorientation, glassy-eyed look, dull affect
Weak, rapid pulse
Decrease in BP
Cold, clammy skin
Shallow, irregular breathing
Extreme thirst
Nausea and vomiting
Chills
Feeling of impending death

MANAGEMENT

Establish and maintain airway. Monitor breathing and administer oxygen.
Monitor vital signs, level of consciousness, and cardiac rhythm.
Administer intravenous fluids using large-bore needle.
Examine all body areas for body alignment, lacerations, and bleeding sites.
Stop all bleeding and oozing of fluid. Use gentle, firm, direct pressure with sterile gauze compresses. If there is arterial bleeding, dressing should be thick and bulky with direct compression over site. Be prepared to use MAST suit.
Maintain good physiological body position. *Do not* put client in Trendelenburg position.
Avoid any excessive handling. Always stabilize head, neck, and back.
Maintain normal body temperature.

---

*See Chapter 59 for a general discussion of measures related to prehospital emergency care.

---

ation status of the client. An indwelling catheter is placed in the bladder to measure urine output, which is an indicator of renal perfusion.

General therapeutic management

Oxygen and ventilatory assistance. Management of shock begins by ensuring that the client has an adequate airway (see Table 27-6). This may be accomplished solely by hyperextension of the neck (unless contraindicated by possibility of spinal cord injury). Placement of an oral airway or endotracheal (ET) intubation may be necessary. Clients who are not breathing spontaneously require mechanical ventilatory assistance. In addition, all clients in shock must receive sufficient supplemental oxygen (usually via nasal prongs or a mask) to maintain an arterial oxygen pressure (Pao_2) of 60 mm Hg or higher and to avoid hypoxemia.

Client position. In terms of the client's cardiovascular status, the recommended position for the treatment of shock is supine, with the legs elevated to an angle of 45 degrees. The trunk should be horizontal, the head at the level of the chest, and the knees straight. However, a client in cardiogenic shock with accompanying pulmonary edema and respiratory distress will not tolerate the supine position. This client should be allowed to sit in the upright position if that is the position of greatest comfort. The Trendelenburg (head-down) position should be avoided in shock because it may do the following:
1. Initiate aortic and carotid sinus reflexes, causing impaired cerebral blood flow
2. Cause the abdominal organs to press against the diaphragm, thus limiting respiratory excursion
3. Decrease filling of the coronary arteries, causing myocardial ischemia
4. Cause an increase in intracranial pressure in the presence of a head injury

Fluid resuscitation. Because shock (with the possible exception of cardiogenic shock) almost always involves a decreased effective circulating blood volume, the cornerstone of shock therapy is expansion of that volume by the intravenous (IV) administration of appropriate fluids. At least two large-gauge IV needles should be inserted immediately before severe vasoconstriction occurs and intravenous access becomes difficult. A central venous line is preferred. The choice of fluid for volume expansion remains controversial. However, it is generally accepted that balanced electrolyte solutions (e.g., lactated Ringer's solution) are used in the initial resuscitation from shock due to hemorrhage. However, approximately two thirds of the volume will diffuse out of the vascular space. Therefore, three times the estimated fluid loss needs to be administered in volume resuscitation.[5] If needed, whole blood or packed cells are administered as soon as they are available, after typing and cross matching. The client's hematocrit value can be used as a guide for blood administration, since one unit of whole blood or packed cells will raise the hematocrit level 2 to 4 points. (Blood transfusions are discussed in Chapter 25.)

Balanced electrolyte solutions may be the only fluid used in volume replacement when neither blood nor serum proteins have been lost, as in shock due to GI fluid loss or cardiogenic shock. Plasma volume expanders (fluids with large molecules that can be retained in the blood vessels) are used in the treatment of shock when plasma protein loss is excessive, as in burn shock and peritonitis (Table 27-8).

The amount and type of fluid given depend on the client's need. This can be assessed by observing BP, pulse rate, urine output, skin perfusion, and presence and location of rales (crackles). The fluid challenge is one of the most popular methods of fluid administration. This procedure involves delivering a specific amount of fluid within a designated period of time. If the CVP and the pulmonary capillary wedge pressure (PCWP) remain low or normal during fluid challenge, the need for more fluid is indicated. However, it must be emphasized that physical assessment of the client is an extremely important indicator of the cli-

Table 27-8   Drugs Used in the Treatment of Shock

Drug	Mechanism of Action	Type of Shock	Nursing Implications
SYMPATHOMIMETICS*			
Dobutamine (Dobutrex)	Primarily stimulates β₁ receptors with minimal α-adrenergic effect. Increases myocardial contractility without inducing marked tachycardia.	Cardiogenic shock in absence of profound hypotension	Do not give with sodium bicarbonate. Observe for hypotension, dysrhythmias, and tachycardia at higher doses.
Dopamine (Intropin)	Is precursor of epinephrine and norepinephrine; has dose-dependent actions. Stimulates α- and β-adrenergic receptors, causing peripheral vasoconstriction and positive inotropic effect. Increases renal perfusion at low doses only.	All types of shock, especially in clients with oliguria (low dose) or with decreased SVR; often with nitroprusside for cardiogenic shock	Administer drug through central venous catheter or large peripheral vein (infiltration may cause tissue damage). Monitor client for hypotension, tachycardia, and dysrhythmias. Be aware that intravascular volume should be adequate.
Epinephrine (Adrenalin)	Stimulates α and β receptors. Counteracts effects of histamine. Causes bronchodilatation and peripheral vasoconstriction, elevating BP. Also stimulates electrical activity during cardiac arrest.	Drug of choice for anaphylactic shock, treatment in cardiac arrest (IV push) for asystole and ventricular fibrillation and to increase mean BP	Observe for cardiac dysrhythmias, dyspnea, pulmonary edema, and severe headaches. In emergencies, give drug through ET tube.
Isoproterenol (Isuprel)	Stimulates β-adrenergic receptors, causing vasodilatation and marked inotropic and chronotropic effects.	Shock with accompanying bradycardia unresponsive to atropine, not appropriate for cardiac arrest	Observe for ventricular dysrhythmias and extreme tachycardia (increased rate increases oxygen demands).
Levarterenol (Levophed)	Stimulates α- and β-adrenergic receptors, causing marked vasoconstriction as well as inotropic and chronotropic effects.	All types, especially shock due to decreased SVR; usually second-line drug after dopamine	Be aware that drug is best administered through a central venous line and is sometimes given with phentolamine to prevent excessive vasoconstriction and tissue sloughing if infiltration occurs. Closely monitor rapid fluctuations in BP. Closely monitor urine output (severe decrease in renal perfusion may occur). Be aware that drug may also cause reflex bradycardia.
Metaraminol (Aramine)	Stimulates α and β receptors, causing marked vasoconstriction. Causes inotropic effects in some clients.	Shock due to relative or actual hypovolemia	Observe for reflex bradycardia, oliguria, and decreased level of consciousness. Do not use in hypertensive clients.
Methoxamine (Vasoxyl)	Simulates α-adrenergic receptors, causing vasoconstriction.	Shock due to relative or actual hypovolemia	Observe for cardiac dysrhythmias, especially bradycardia.
Phenylephrine (Neo-Synephrine)	Predominately stimulates α receptors, causing vasoconstriction.	Shock due to relative or actual hypovolemia	Observe for reflex bradycardia and ventricular ectopy.

*All sympathomimetic drugs are incompatible with sodium bicarbonate.

Continued.

Table 27-8 Drugs Used in the Treatment of Shock—cont'd

Drug	Mechanism of Action	Type of Shock	Nursing Implications
VASODILATORS			
Nitroglycerin (Tridil)	Primarily acts as venous vasodilator. Dilates veins and arteries at higher doses.	Cardiogenic shock, usually with inotropic agent	Monitor BP carefully. Observe for reflex tachycardia. Be aware that headache is common. Use non-PVC tubing and glass bottle to prevent drug absorption.
Sodium nitroprusside (Nipride)	Acts as a potent vasodilator on veins and arteries. May increase or decrease CO depending on the extent of preload and afterload reduction.	Primarily cardiogenic shock with increased SVR and preload and afterload and decreased CO, often with inotropic drug such as dopamine	Closely monitor for hypotension and reflex tachycardia. Administer only with D_5W and protect solution from light. Be aware that thiocyanate toxicity and cyanide poisoning may occur when used for more than 72 hours.
Morphine sulfate	Is narcotic analgesic and acts as potent venodilator (decreases preload) with some arterial dilatation (decreases afterload).	Primarily cardiogenic shock (to decrease preload)	Monitor carefully for hypotension and respiratory depression. Have Narcan at bedside.
CORTICOSTEROIDS			
Dexamethasone (Decadron), hydrocortisone (Solu-Cortef), methylprednisolone (Solu-Medrol)	Inhibits inflammatory process, stabilizes lysosomal membranes, reduces capillary permeability, reduces release of chemical mediators in the septic process, and promotes sodium retention.	Septic shock (controversial), serious cases of anaphylactic shock	Monitor client for GI bleeding and hypotension. Be aware that these drugs may make control of diabetes difficult and slow wound healing.
COLLOID THERAPY			
Albumin 5%	Promotes volume expansion, with capability reported to be approximately 1:1 with a duration of 4 to 24 hr.	All types of shock	Be aware that minimal side effects of chills, fever, and urticaria may develop.
Dextran (Dextran 40, Dextran 70).	Has similar degrees of volume expansion with Dextran 40 and Dextran 70. Have longer duration of action with Dextran 70.	Limited use because of potentially serious side effects With Dextran 40 and Dextran 70	Note that agent alters clotting factors and has antiplatelet effect. Also need to monitor closely for hypersensitivity reactions and acute renal failure.
Plasma protein fraction	Has albumin as primary component, and similar action to that of albumin.	All types of shock	Be aware that drug may cause greater hypersensitivity reactions than albumin.
Hetastarch	Acts as volume expander and is at least as effective as albumin.	All types of shock	Be aware that drug may be 50% less costly than albumin. Use cautiously with clients with congestive heart failure, renal failure, or bleeding disorder (due to anticoagulant effect).

ent's fluid status. Often the other parameters, such as CVP and PCWP, are not available and thus assessment is essential. Complications of excessive volume replacement, such as pulmonary edema and postresuscitation hypertension (sustained systolic BP above 150 mm Hg and diastolic BP[12] above 100 mm Hg for at least 6 hours after fluid resuscitation) should be noted.[12] Both conditions can be treated with diuretics.

Acid-base imbalance. Frequent monitoring of ABGs allows the physician to prescribe therapy to correct acid-base imbalances. This may be accomplished through the IV infusion of sodium bicarbonate or through the use of ventilatory assistance. When a mechanical ventilator is used to correct acid-base imbalances, it is sometimes necessary to administer a paralyzing drug such as pancuronium bromide (Pavulon), especially if the client is competing with the ventilator. This allows better control of the rate and depth of respirations by the ventilator.

Cardiac dysrhythmias. Methods of treating cardiac dysrhythmias are detailed in Chapter 30.

Specific therapeutic management. In addition to general management of shock, each type of shock has specific interventions (see Table 27-6). A major priority for most types of shock is volume replacement. Blood and blood products are needed for hemorrhagic shock. Since control of bleeding is essential, surgical intervention may be required. The military antishock trousers (MAST) suit is helpful in controlling internal and external hemorrhage while it helps to increase CO and enhance tissue perfusion (see Fig. 27-6). The MAST suit should not be deflated until the client is either in the operating room or in a con-

trolled situation with experienced personnel. Volume replacement is administered to maintain the BP as the pressure in the MAST suit is gradually relieved over 30 to 60 minutes.

Cardiogenic shock may require careful fluid replacement guided by hemodynamic monitoring if the client is volume depleted. The goal of therapy is to increase cardiac contractility while decreasing afterload and thus the work load of the heart. Inotropic and vasodilator agents (Table 27-8) are commonly used. In addition, diuretics to decrease preload (venous return) are indicated if the client is volume overloaded.

Drug therapy alone has not significantly decreased the mortality of cardiogenic shock. The intraaortic balloon pump, drug therapy, and cardiac surgery, if indicated, are currently the most accepted treatment modalities.[6] The intraaortic balloon pump is a counterpulsation device that is inserted into the aorta near the aortic arch (see Chapter 28). The goal of this intervention is to decrease the left ventricular afterload while increasing diastolic pressure and thus coronary blood flow.

In all types of distributive shock, fluid administration is essential to support the BP because of the vasodilated circulatory system. Once intravascular volume has been restored, vasopressors may be indicated to help support the BP through peripheral vasoconstriction.[1] In septic shock, antibiotic administration should be initiated as soon as cultures have been obtained. Steroids may or may not be used (see p. 754). Assessment is very important because subtle changes can rapidly occur and the client's condition can quickly deteriorate. Also, the client is often an older per-

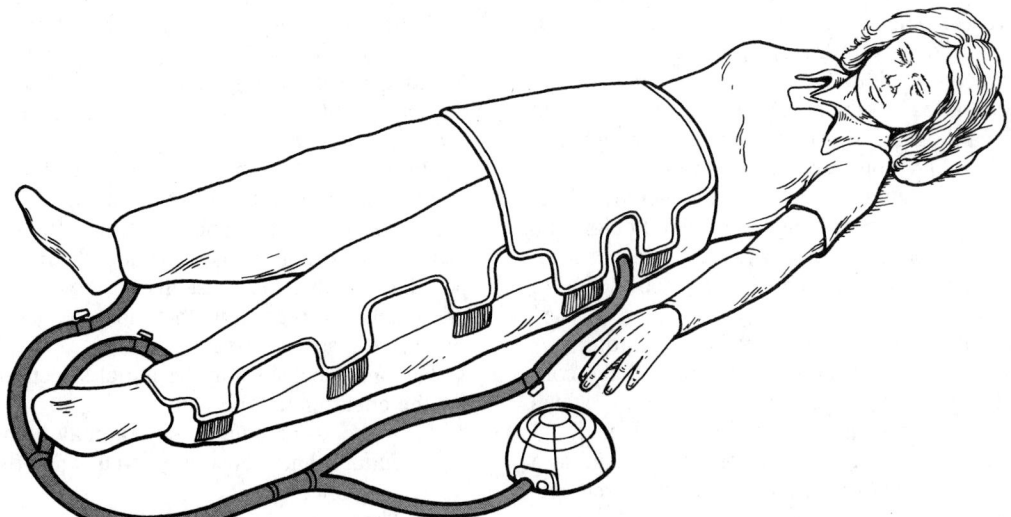

Fig. 27-6 MAST or pneumatic antishock garment is a one-piece garment placed over the client's legs and abdomen. When inflated, the vessels in the legs and abdomen are compressed, transferring blood from the lower body to the heart, brain, and other vital organs. The MAST suit also controls hemorrhage, stabilizes pelvic and femoral fractures, and distends arm veins to facilitate IV insertion. The MAST suit is indicated for life-threatening hypotension due to absolute or relative hypovolemia. The major complication results from rapid deflation before restoration of adequate intravascular volume. The MAST suit should be removed only if a physician is present, IV fluids are infusing, and the client is prepped and in the operating room if surgery is indicated.

son or has other underlying medical problems that make management more difficult. Full-blown anaphylactic shock is very dramatic, and immediate drug intervention is required. The primary drug is epinephrine, which causes peripheral vasoconstriction and bronchodilatation. Aminophylline is also used when bronchoconstriction is severe. Diphenhydramine (Benadryl) is used to counteract the effects of histamine. However, it is not effective for the life-threatening vasodilatation or bronchoconstriction. Steroids may also be administered, but their effect is not immediate. Neurogenic shock has multiple causes, and therefore the treatment varies. Fluid replacement for BP maintenance and tissue perfusion continues to be extremely important.

The MAST suit may be indicated for all types of distributive shock if hypotension continues despite the use of fluids and drugs.

Pharmacological Management

The primary purpose of drugs used in the treatment of shock is correction of the poor tissue perfusion. These drugs are usually administered IV. Drugs used in the treatment of shock are presented in Table 27-8.

Sympathomimetic drugs. Many of the drugs used in the treatment of shock have an effect on the sympathetic nervous system. Drugs that mimic the action of the sympathetic nervous system are called *sympathomimetic drugs*. The primary goal of sympathomimetic therapy in shock is to support BP to maintain perfusion of vital organs with a minimum of adverse effects.[13]

Many of these drugs cause peripheral vasoconstriction and are referred to as *vasopressor drugs*. These vasopressor drugs have the potential of causing severe peripheral vasoconstriction and may further jeopardize tissue perfusion, either directly or indirectly. The increased SVR also increases the work load of the heart and can be detrimental to a client in cardiogenic shock, causing further myocardial damage. Use of vasopressor drugs is reserved for clients who have been unresponsive to other therapy. Adequate volume replacement must be administered before the use of any vasopressor drug, since peripheral vasoconstrictor effects in low-volume states can be very detrimental to tissue perfusion.

These drugs often have an effect on the myocardium. A positive *inotropic* effect occurs when the force of the contraction is strengthened. A *chronotropic* effect occurs when the rate or timing of the contractions is affected.

It is generally agreed that vasopressors can be used as a temporary adjunctive measure to increase cerebral and coronary blood flow.

The goal of vasopressor therapy is to achieve and maintain a *mean* arterial BP of 70 to 80 mm Hg and improved tissue perfusion. This ensures adequate blood flow to the heart and brain to prevent an MI (or extension of an infarction in cardiogenic shock) or a cerebrovascular accident.

Vasodilator drugs. Vasodilator drugs have commonly been used in cardiogenic shock to decrease preload and afterload, thus reducing the work load of the heart. The use of vasodilator drugs in other types of shock has recently achieved popularity. These drugs are administered on the assumption that inhibition of peripheral vasoconstriction allows redistribution of pooled blood, which enhances capillary flow and tissue perfusion, especially of the kidneys and splanchnic area. A major concern prior to the use of vasodilators is ensuring adequate plasma volume and myocardial tone to fill the dilated vessels. Therefore vasodilators are often used in conjunction with plasma volume expanders and inotropic drugs. The goal in vasodilator therapy, as in vasopressor therapy, is to maintain a mean BP of 70 to 80 mm Hg. It is also important to closely monitor CVP, pulmonary artery pressures, and arterial pressure so that fluid administration can be increased or the dose of the vasodilator drug decreased if a precipitous fall in pressure occurs.

Corticosteroids. Corticosteroids are recommended for all serious cases of anaphylaxis, although they are not indicated for the initial treatment.[14] Steroids may prevent the delayed symptoms that are thought to be caused by basophil release of chemical mediators. Corticosteroids stabilize the basophil membranes, minimizing degranulation and the release of chemical mediators; these drugs do not affect the mast cells (see Table 27-8).

There continues to be controversy regarding the usefulness of corticosteroids in the treatment of septic shock.[13] When steroids are administered in the high-dose range, as used in septic shock, they may cause a variety of problems for the client, such as immunosuppression, GI bleeding, psychosis, and increased incidence of death as a result of secondary infection. Because of the lack of evidence of beneficial effects and the seriousness of the side effects, high-dose steroids are not indicated for the treatment of severe sepsis and septic shock.[15-17]

Antibiotics. Susceptibility to infection is increased in all clients with prolonged shock of nonseptic etiology. Broad-spectrum prophylactic antibiotic therapy may be indicated. Antibiotics are always used in the treatment of septic shock.

Before antibiotic therapy is begun, specimens of blood, urine, wound exudate, and sputum should be obtained for bacteriological culture and sensitivity studies. The anatomical sites of origin of the infection should be identified, if possible, so that the most likely etiological agent can be predicted. The organisms that most frequently cause septic shock are gram-negative.

Factors to consider in the initial selection of antibiotics for the client are as follows:

1. A broad-spectrum antibiotic may be needed because culture and sensitivity study reports are not yet available.
2. The serum half-life of drugs may be increased because of renal or hepatic insufficiency.
3. Some antibiotics are nephrotoxic or hepatotoxic.

■ Nursing Management of Shock

Nursing assessment

Subjective and objective data that should be obtained from a person with shock are presented in Table 27-9.

Nursing diagnoses

Nursing diagnoses are determined when the problem and etiological factors are supported by the clinical data.

Nursing diagnoses related to shock may include, but are not limited to, those presented in Table 27-10.

Nursing interventions

Health promotion and maintenance. Prevention of the shock state is an essential nursing responsibility. To prevent shock, the nurse must first identify persons who are at risk. In general terms, the very old, the very young, and persons who have chronic, debilitating diseases have increased susceptibility to shock. More specifically, any person who sustains surgical or accidental trauma is at high risk of shock due to hemorrhage, spinal cord injury, burn injuries, and the conditions listed in Table 27-2. Older adults who take barbiturates, as well as persons with diabetes whose disease is not well controlled or who do not adhere to therapy, may go into shock. Persons who experience angina or who have a history of MI are potential candidates for cardiogenic shock. All clients with symptoms of angina or MI should be encouraged to seek medical attention immediately. Persons with a severe allergy to such substances as drugs, shellfish, and insect bites and persons who use diuretics or who have diabetes insipidus may also develop shock.

After identification of susceptible persons, implementation of the nursing process is essential to help prevent shock. A thorough baseline nursing assessment with frequent ongoing assessments to monitor and detect changes in the client's condition are the initial nursing actions. Identification of pertinent nursing diagnoses, implementation of appropriate nursing interventions, and evaluation of these actions should follow. Clients who have an acute MI, especially of the anterior portion of the left ventricle, are at greater risk of cardiogenic shock. The focus of prevention is to decrease the work load of the heart and thus reduce the extent of myocardial damage through rest and drug therapy. Careful monitoring of fluid balance can help prevent hypovolemic shock. Intake and output, weights, and drainage from wounds and tubes must be carefully calculated and documented. Immediate control of hemorrhage is essential. A client who is at risk of sepsis must be carefully monitored. Limitation of portals of entry into the body, including IVs and indwelling catheters, is important. Aseptic technique must be used with all procedures.

Clients who have severe allergies should be cautioned to wear a Medic-Alert tag and to report their allergies to health care providers. These clients may also be instructed about the availability of special kits that contain equipment and medication for the treatment of acute hypersensitivity reactions. The risk of anaphylactic shock can be decreased if clients are carefully questioned about allergies before administration of a new drug or antibiotics (even if the client has received this drug in the past) or before undergoing a diagnostic procedure involving the use of an IV dye. Early immobilization of spinal cord injuries can help prevent neurogenic shock. In addition, health education is important to prevent the onset of disease that may result in shock. For example, cessation of smoking and exercising regularly may help decrease the risk of MI.

Acute intervention. The nursing role in the acute stages of shock involves (1) monitoring the client's ongoing physical and emotional status to detect subtle changes in

Table 27-9

 Nursing Assessment of the Client in Shock

SUBJECTIVE DATA

History
Recent: MI, pulmonary embolism, infection, surgery, spinal cord injury, hemorrhage, trauma, or burns
Severe: Diabetes, dehydration, congestive heart failure, valvular dysfunction, pancreatitis, intestinal obstruction, use of tampons, severe reaction to insect bites or stings or blood products
Medications
Severe reaction to any drugs, vaccines, contrast dye, general anesthesia; drug overdose (including insulin)
General
Weakness, dizziness, restlessness, fainting, thirst
Cardiovascular
Palpitations, chest pain
Respiratory
Dyspnea, feeling of tightness, productive or nonproductive cough
Gastrointestinal
Nausea, vomiting, abdominal cramps
Urinary
Decreased urine output
Integumentary
Urticaria and pruritus (anaphylactic shock), chills, diaphoresis

OBJECTIVE DATA

General
Fever (septic), normal or subnormal temperature (other types of shock)
Integumentary
Pale, cool, moist skin or warm, flushed skin (septic and anaphylatic shock); cyanosis (later shock); urticaria, rash, and angioedema (anaphylaxis)
Respiratory
Tachypnea; wheezing, choking, coughing (anaphylaxis)
Cardiovascular
Tachycardia; hypotension; weak, thready pulse; flat neck veins (except in cardiogenic shock); abnormal heart sounds; dysrhythmias
Gastrointestinal
Vomiting, hyperactive or diminished bowel sounds
Urinary
Decreased urinary output
Neurological
Initially: Restlessness, anxiety
Later: Altered mentation, lethargy, stupor, coma
Possible findings
Altered serum electrolytes, decreased hemoglobin and hematocrit, leukocytosis, hypoxemia, and hypocapnia; respiratory alkalosis and metabolic acidosis; elevated BUN and cardiac enzymes (cardiogenic); positive wound, blood, and body fluid cultures; abnormal chest and abdominal x-ray films and ECG

Table 27-10

 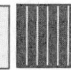

Defining Characteristics	Nursing Interventions	Evaluation Criteria

NURSING DIAGNOSIS: Potential complication: Organ ischemia/dysfunction related to decreased tissue perfusion

Neurological ischemia/dysfunction

Changes in mentation or level of consciousness; *early:* restlessness, apprehension, agitation; *late:* apathy, confusion, lethargy, stupor, coma, paresthesias, headache, hyporeflexia, decreased pupillary reaction, seizures	Perform neurological assessment every hour, including orientation, level of consciousness, pupillary response, motor response, presence or absence of reflexes. Record and report any changes. Question about headache and paresthesias. Avoid sedation and narcotics. Monitor for seizure activity and initiate precautions as needed. Protect confused client from injury with soft restraints as needed and close observation. Keep side rails up at all times.	Normal orientation and level of consciousness as evidenced by alertness, ability to follow commands, and normal pupillary and motor responses; no headache, paresthesias, or seizures; no injury

Renal ischemia/dysfunction

Urine output <20 ml/hr, increase in urine specific gravity, elevation in serum BUN and creatinine, abnormal serum electrolytes, low urine sodium, protein and blood in urine, metabolic acidosis	Insert indwelling catheter. Accurately measure intake and output. Monitor laboratory values and specific gravity. Check urine for blood, protein. Take daily weights. Administer fluids and sympathomimetics as ordered and assess results. Watch for fluid overload.	Normal urine output ≥30 ml/hr and normal laboratory values, no signs of hypervolemia or hypovolemia

Gastrointestinal ischemia/dysfunction

Abdominal pain, distention, nausea, vomiting, anorexia, diarrhea, thirst, constipation, absent or diminished bowel sounds	Keep client on NPO status. Insert nasogastric tube as needed. Monitor bowel sounds every 2 to 4 hr. Check stools and emesis for blood. Assess abdominal distention. Measure intake and output. Maintain adequate hydration.	No abdominal pain or distention; active bowel sounds, normal stools; adequate hydration; no nausea or vomiting

Peripheral vascular ischemia/dysfunction

Cool, pale, or cyanotic extremities; diminished or absent peripheral pulses; pain, tingling, or numbness in extremities; necrotic or gangrenous extremities; poor capillary refill	Monitor peripheral pulses. Assess for color, warmth, and size of extremities. Watch for pressure sores. Keep client warm and dry. Report any changes in perfusion. Avoid restrictive clothing and stockings.	Palpable peripheral pulses; normal color, temperature, and size of extremities; capillary refill ≤2 sec; no pain or paresthesias in extremities

Respiratory ischemia/dysfunction

Early: Rapid (>20/min), deep respirations; *late:* rapid (30-40/min), shallow respirations, dyspnea, use of accessory muscles, cyanosis, adventitious breath sounds and cough, abnormal chest x-ray film; *early:* respiratory alkalosis ($\downarrow Pco_2$, $\uparrow pH$), normal or low Pao_2; *late:* metabolic acidosis ($\downarrow pH$, $\downarrow HCO_3$) and hypoxemia ($\downarrow Pao_2$)	Initiate oxygen and maintain $Sao_2 \geq 90\%$. Monitor ABGs. Auscultate breath sounds every 1-2 hr. Record and report rales, wheezes, and decreased or unequal breath sounds. Assist client to cough and deep breathe. Suction as needed. Keep head of bed slightly elevated. Obtain chest x-ray films as ordered. Monitor skin color, mucous membranes for cyanosis. Assess respiratory rate, depth, and pattern. Maintain patent airway and prepare for mechanical ventilation.	Normal breathing and chest x-ray film, adequate oxygenation, normal or baseline ABGs within normal limits, breath sounds at baseline, good skin color, patent airway without retained secretions

bpm, Beats per minute.

Table 27-10

NURSING CARE PLAN FOR THE CLIENT IN SHOCK—cont'd

Defining Characteristics	Nursing Interventions	Evaluation Criteria

NURSING DIAGNOSIS: Decreased cardiac output related to absolute or relative hypovolemia

Increased diastolic, decreased systolic BP; postural hypotension; tachycardia; weak, thready pulse; flat neck veins; low CVP and PCWP; thirst and dry mucous membranes; falling urinary output <30 ml/hr; altered mentation; dysrhythmias; tachypnea; hypoxemia; pallor or cyanosis; cool, clammy skin	Monitor vital signs, CVP, pulmonary artery pressures every 15 min to 1 hr. Administer crystalloid, colloids, sympathomimetics as ordered and assess response. Maintain two IV lines. Record accurate intake and output and daily weight. Monitor laboratory and x-ray findings. Keep client warm. Administer oxygen to keep $Sao_2 \geq 90\%$.	Normal BP (for client); HR 60-110 bpm; strong peripheral pulses; normal CVP (1-8 mm Hg) and PCWP (6-12 mm Hg); warm, dry, pink skin; urinary output ≥30 ml/hr; normal mentation; no dysrhythmias; respiratory rate >12 and <20; return of laboratory findings and x-ray films to baseline; $Sao_2 \geq 90\%$

NURSING DIAGNOSIS: Fear and anxiety related to severity of condition, perceived threat of death, and family distress

Verbalization of anxiety about condition, fear of death to family, staff, or withdrawal with no communication; facial, muscle tension; restlessness; voice and hand tremors; sleeplessness; tense, narrowed focus of attention; diaphoresis; increase in heart and respiratory rate	Acknowledge expressed fear and anxiety. Demonstrate concern, respect for client. Try to draw out client if withdrawn. Seek out significant other's perception of situation and enlist help. Maintain calm and reassuring demeanor and environment. Explain interventions, client status, and equipment simply and honestly. Assess level of understanding. Keep call bell within easy reach. Teach simple relaxation techniques. Check on client and family frequently. Use humor if appropriate.	Open verbalization of anxieties and fears by client and significant others; more relaxed appearance; verbalization of reduced anxiety; asking of appropriate questions; reduction in heart and respiratory rate; ability to relax, sleep; return of sense of humor; less tense appearance

the client's condition, (2) planning and implementing nursing interventions and therapy, (3) evaluating the client's response to therapy, and (4) providing emotional support to the client and significant others. Nursing responsibilities also include judging when it is necessary to alert other health team members to changes in the client's status that may warrant reevaluation of treatment. (Nursing care of the client in shock is described in Table 27-10.)

As care is begun, it is essential for the nurse to obtain the following brief history from the client or another knowledgeable person:

1. Description of the events leading to the shock condition
2. Time of onset and duration of symptoms
3. Past health history, especially medications and allergies
4. Care received before hospital admission
5. Date of last tetanus immunization if shock is due to trauma
6. Client's religious faith
7. Presence of Medic-Alert tag

NEUROLOGICAL STATUS. Neurological checks, including pupillary response, orientation, and level of consciousness, should be performed at least every hour. The client's neurological status is the best indicator of cerebral blood flow. The nurse should be alert to clinical manifestations that may indicate neurological involvement, such as blurred vision, agitation, confusion, overalertness, and paresthesias.

Attempts should be made to orient the client to time, place, and person. If the client is in an intensive care unit (ICU), orientation to the environment is particularly important. Measures such as minimizing noise and light levels should be taken to control sensory input. A day-night cycle of activity and rest should be maintained as much as possible. Sensory overload and disruption of the client's diurnal cycle may contribute to an altered neurological status.

CARDIOVASCULAR STATUS. Much of the therapy for shock is based on information about the client's cardiovascular status. Until the client is stable, BP, CVP, and pulmonary artery pressures (if available) should be determined every 5 minutes. (Pulmonary artery pressures are discussed in

Chapter 28.) Once the client is stable, the PCWP should be obtained only as often as needed to avoid complications associated with balloon inflation. Pulmonary artery pressure provides more information about left ventricular function than does the CVP. The PCWP most accurately reflects left ventricular function, especially in the presence of lung problems (e.g., pulmonary embolism, chronic lung disease) when the pulmonary artery pressure is often inaccurate. Trends in pulmonary artery pressures are more important than the individual numbers themselves. In addition, care should be taken to avoid dependence on these numbers, since direct physical assessment of the client is extremely valuable.

The client's electrocardiogram (ECG) should be monitored continuously to detect dysrhythmias that may result from the shock itself or from medications used in treatment. The rate and quality of peripheral and apical pulses should be compared every 5 to 10 minutes, and heart sounds should be assessed for quality and the presence of gallops or murmurs. The latter may indicate early heart failure. The frequency of this monitoring is decreased as the client's condition improves.

In addition to carrying out these measures, which are necessary to monitor the client's cardiovascular status, the nurse must administer the prescribed therapy, which is designed to correct the client's impaired cardiovascular status.

RESPIRATORY STATUS. The respiratory status of the client in shock must be assessed frequently to ensure adequate oxygenation and early detection of respiratory complications, as well as to provide data regarding the client's acid-base status. The rate, depth, and rhythm of respirations are initially monitored every 10 minutes. Increased rate and depth provide information regarding the client's attempts to correct metabolic acidosis. Alterations in respiratory rhythm may indicate cerebral complications. Chest sounds should be assessed every hour for the development of rales (crackles), which indicate the presence of fluid buildup in the lungs.

ABGs are often measured as frequently as every 30 minutes. The nurse generally withdraws the blood specimen with a heparinized syringe from an arterial line. Initial interpretation of blood gases is often the responsibility of the nurse. A Pao_2 below 60 mm Hg (in the absence of chronic lung disease) indicates the presence of hypoxemia and the need for administration of higher oxygen concentrations or for a different method of oxygen administration. A low $Paco_2$ in the presence of a low pH and a low or normal bicarbonate level indicates that the client's hyperventilation is compensating for the metabolic acidosis. A rising $Paco_2$ in the presence of a persistently low pH indicates the need for intubation and ventilatory assistance.

RENAL STATUS. Hourly measurements of urinary output are essential in assessment of the adequacy of renal perfusion. An indwelling catheter is inserted to facilitate measurements. Urine output of less than 20 ml/hr indicates inadequate perfusion of the kidneys. Measurement of urinary specific gravity every hour is also important to detect the onset of acute tubular necrosis. The nurse should be sure that blood is drawn daily for serum BUN and creatinine determinations and should alert the physician if elevations in these values occur.

BODY TEMPERATURE AND SKIN CHANGES. In the presence of an elevated or subnormal temperature, rectal temperatures should be obtained hourly. If normal, the temperature needs to be monitored only every 4 hours. The client should be kept comfortably warm with the use of light covers and the control of environmental temperature. If the client's temperature rises, this condition may be treated with medication such as acetaminophen suppositories, tepid sponge baths, removal of some covers, or a hypothermia blanket. It is important to avoid extremes of temperature because they cause an increased metabolic need for oxygen and increased carbon dioxide production.

Skin color should be assessed for pallor, flushing, and cyanosis. Diaphoresis or piloerection should be noted. In addition, the rapidity of capillary refill should be assessed as an indicator of peripheral vasoconstriction.

GASTROINTESTINAL STATUS. Bowel sounds should be auscultated every 8 hours, and abdominal distention should be assessed through percussion and serial measurements of abdominal girth. If bowel sounds are not present, a nasogastric tube may have to be inserted. Decompression by suction should continue until bowel sounds return. The nasogastric drainage should be measured as part of the fluid output and tested for occult blood. If the client has a bowel movement, the stool should also be checked for occult blood.

NUTRITIONAL CONSIDERATIONS. During the acute phase of the shock syndrome, the client receives nothing by mouth. As recovery begins, nutrition plays an important role in limiting morbidity. Since anorexia is almost universally present, parenteral or enteral feeding is often used. Enteral tube feeding via a feeding pump is commonly the initial method of supplying nutrition. Contraindications to this type of feeding include absence of bowel sounds, peritonitis, and intestinal anastomosis. Parenteral feeding is generally adopted only if tube feedings are contraindicated or if they fail to meet the client's caloric requirements. (Total parenteral nutrition and enteral tube feedings are discussed in Chapter 35.)

Clients in shock should be weighed daily to determine whether their caloric needs are being met. If the client experiences a significant weight loss, dehydration should be ruled out before additional calories are provided parenterally. Measurements of serum BUN levels also provide pertinent data, since falling levels may indicate overhydration.

Oral care for the client in shock is essential. A water-soluble lubricant applied to the lips prevents drying and cracking. Moist swabbing of the tongue and oral mucosa with saline solution, diluted mouthwash, or half-strength peroxide is also helpful. Lemon and glycerin swabs should not be used because they can cause drying of the mucosa.

PERSONAL HYGIENE. Hygiene is especially important to clients in shock because their impaired tissue perfusion predisposes to infection and skin breakdown. Oral and perineal hygiene, as well as a complete bath, should be provided when necessary and not according to a schedule. Since clients will fatigue easily, activities must be carefully planned to allow rest periods. If the client is able to perform some self-care, the nurse should allow independent action and assist only when necessary. Using an alternating-pressure or egg-crate mattress, turning the client every 2 hours, and positioning the client in good body alignment help prevent decubitus ulcer formation.

EMOTIONAL SUPPORT. The effects of the client's anxiety and fear in the face of this critical, life-threatening situation are frequently overlooked or underestimated. Anxiety and fear may aggravate respiratory distress and increase cathecholamine secretion. It is important for the nurse to remember that compassionate understanding is as essential as scientific and technical expertise in the total care of a client in shock.

In planning and implementing the nursing care of the client in shock, the nurse should assess the client's anxiety. Medication to decrease anxiety may seem to be the simplest mode of therapy, but much more can be accomplished by nonpharmacological interventions. In many shock situations, sedation is contraindicated.

The nurse should always talk to clients, including those who are intubated or appear comatose. If the intubated client is capable of writing, a magic slate or a pencil and paper should be provided. The client should also receive simple explanations of procedures *before* they are carried out, as well as information regarding the current plan of care and its rationale. If the client asks questions about progress and prognosis, simple and honest answers should be given.

Privacy should be provided as much as possible, but the client should be assured that assistance is readily available should it be required. The call bell should be within reach. In addition, joking, teasing, and "kidding around" among health care personnel should be kept to a minimum or carried out where the client cannot hear it. This sort of behavior can often lead the client to believe that staff members are having too much fun to be able to provide adequate care. Furthermore, conversations about the client should not take place where the client can overhear them. Such conversations can constitute a violation of the client's confidence or may be misinterpreted in a way that causes the client unnecessary distress.

Finally, many clients desire the comfort of a priest, rabbi, or minister at this time. The nurse should offer to call a member of the clergy rather than wait for the client or the family to express a wish for spiritual comfort.

The client's family and significant others also need support and comfort at this time. They should be kept informed of the client's status and prognosis and of the current plan of care and its rationale. Insofar as possible the same person should continue to serve as liaison nurse to decrease anxiety and avoid confusing contradictions. Family members and friends should be shown where they can wait and where a telephone can be found. Directions to the restrooms and to the hospital cafeteria are also appropriate.

Visits with the client should be facilitated rather than hindered. The nurse should explain in simple terms the purpose of the tubes and machines surrounding the client, and the family should be informed of what they may and may not touch. Privacy should be ensured as much as possible. The family should also be instructed to avoid tiring the client.

Chronic management. Rehabilitation of the client in shock necessitates prevention or early treatment of complications and correction of the precipitating cause. The nurse should continue to assess the client for indications of complications throughout the recovery period. These include such problems as chronic renal failure after acute tubular necrosis or the development of fibrotic lung disease as a result of ARDS (see Chapters 41 and 23).

HYPERTENSION

Hypertension, commonly called *high blood pressure,* is sustained high mean arterial pressure. The diagnosis of hypertension is confirmed in adults when the average of two or more BP measurements on at least two visits reveals a diastolic pressure of 90 mm Hg or higher or a systolic pressure of 140 mm Hg or higher.[18]

The status of hypertension control has improved considerably over the past 15 years. Large-scale education programs provided by various organizations have increased the awareness of hypertension. Although detection efforts should continue, mass screening for hypertension is now rarely indicated. Instead, the focus should be threefold: (1) controlling BP in persons already identified as having hypertension, (2) detecting the groups at high risk of getting hypertension, and (3) reaching those with limited access to the health care system.[18]

Significance

Hypertension is often asymptomatic, which is the crux of the problem. Many times there are no symptoms to motivate persons to seek treatment. When symptoms do occur, they are often ignored by the person, who believes that they are probably insignificant.

In the United States, 58 million people either have elevated BP (systolic BP of 150 mm Hg or greater and/or diastolic BP of 85 mm Hg or greater) or are taking antihypertensive medication.[18] The incidence of hypertension increases with age, is higher in blacks (38%) than in whites (29%), and is more prevalent in men (33%) than in women (27%) until the age of 55.[19]

Classification

Table 27-11 defines the BP classification for people 18 years of age and older. The diastolic range of 85 to 89 mm Hg is classified as high-normal; it requires more frequent BP checks than diastolic readings of less than 85 mm Hg.

Severe hypertension is defined as a diastolic reading of 115 mm Hg or greater. Accelerated hypertension means the client has a diastolic pressure usually above 120 mm Hg and a grade III retinopathy (see Table 27-13). The etiology of hypertension can be classified as either primary or secondary.

Essential hypertension. Essential (primary) hypertension accounts for 90% of all cases of hypertension. The onset of essential hypertension is usually between the ages of 30 and 50 years. Although there is a family tendency, the exact cause remains unknown, and therefore there are no definite measures for preventing essential hypertension.

Table 27-11 Classification of Blood Pressure*

Range (mm Hg)	Category†
DIASTOLIC	
<85	Normal BP
85-89	High-normal BP
90-104	Mild hypertension
105-114	Moderate hypertension
≥115	Severe hypertension
SYSTOLIC‡	
<140	Normal BP
140-159	Borderline isolated systolic hypertension
≥160	Isolated systolic hypertension

US Department of Health and Human Services: The 1988 report of the Joint National Committee on Detection, Evaluation, and Treatment of High Blood Pressure, Washington, DC, 1988, Public Health Service, National Institutes of Health.
*Classification based on the average of two or more readings on two or more occasions in adults 18 years of age or older.
†A classification of borderline isolated systolic hypertension or isolated systolic hypertension takes precedence over high-normal BP when both occur in the same person. High-normal BP takes precedence over a classification of normal BP when both occur in the same person.
‡Diastolic BP is <90.

Pathophysiology. For arterial pressure to rise, there must be an increase in either CO or SVR (see p. 738). If SVR is increased, a greater amount of pressure is required to pump blood throughout the body. The concept of SVR is so important in understanding arterial BP that some clinicians have defined hypertension as increased SVR. Most persons with hypertension have a normal CO.

Although the cause of essential hypertension is not known, several risk factors are known to be related to the development of essential hypertension or contribute to the disease. These are presented in Table 27-12.

Excess sodium intake. Excessive salt intake is considered responsible for initiation of hypertension in some persons. Studies on populations with a high sodium intake in their diets (e.g., blacks who eat many foods that are high in sodium and persons living on islands who cook fish in ocean water) show that hypertension develops at an early age. In addition, an excessive amount of sodium has been found in the arteriolar walls of some hypertensive persons. Sodium causes water retention, which causes the walls to swell with resulting constriction of the lumen and increased SVR. Therefore both actions (increased CO and increased SVR) may result in increased BP.

Altered renin-angiotensin mechanism. In some persons with essential hypertension, excess quantities of renin are secreted by the kidney. This results in the conversion of angiotensinogen to angiotensin (see Fig. 39-6). The angiotensin causes direct arteriolar constriction and a secondary increase in aldosterone. This is followed by retention of water and electrolytes, with resultant hypertension. In most clients with essential hypertension, the plasma renin

Table 27-12 Risk Factors in Essential Hypertension

Age	Condition develops between 30 and 50 yr of age. Peak incidence is 35 yr of age.
Sex	It primarily affects men over 35 yr of age and women over 45 yr of age.
Race	The incidence of hypertension is twice as great in blacks as in whites.
Family history	Multifactorial genetic factors account for an estimated one third of cases of essential hypertension.
Obesity	Weight gain is associated with increased frequency of hypertension. There is a high correlation of obesity and physical inactivity with hypertension.
Stress	Stress results in increased sympathetic nervous system activity.
Cigarette smoking	Nicotine in cigarettes causes vasoconstriction and increased catecholamine release, resulting in increased HR.
Excess sodium intake	High sodium intake can maintain elevated BP in some hypertensive clients and can decrease the efficacy of certain antihypertensives.
Elevated serum lipids	Elevated levels of cholesterol and triglycerides are primary risk factors in atherosclerosis, which is a contributing factor to hypertension.
Alcohol intake	Alcohol consumption (more than 1 oz of ethanol a day) may lead to elevated BP, poor compliance with antihypertensive therapy, and possibly refractory hypertension.
Sedentary lifestyle	A regular exercise program can help control weight and may decrease BP.

level is normal, but in 10% to 17% of clients, the plasma level has been found to be elevated. These clients are said to have *high-renin essential hypertension.*

Excessive mineralocorticoids. With elevated renin levels, aldosterone is increased. However, hypertensive clients with normal or low renin levels have also been found with elevated aldosterone levels. Some of these clients also have an elevation of other mineralocorticoids.

Stress and increased sympathetic activity. It has long been recognized that arterial pressure is influenced by factors such as anger, fear, pain, and exercise. Physiological responses to stress, which are normally protective, may persist to a pathological degree, resulting in increased sympathetic nervous activity. Increased sympathetic stimulation results in increased systemic vascular vasoconstriction and an increased HR. Renin release is stimulated by increased sympathetic nervous activity. This results in activation of the angiotensin mechanism and increased aldosterone secretion, both leading to elevated BP.

Secondary hypertension. Secondary hypertension is elevated BP with an identified cause that often can be corrected by surgery or medication. This type of hypertension accounts for less than 5% of hypertension in adults and 75% to 80% of hypertension in young children.[20]

Causes of secondary hypertension include the following:

1. Coarctation of the aorta
2. Renal disease, such as renal artery stenosis, and parenchymal disease (see Chapters 40 and 41)
3. Endocrine disorders, such as pheochromocytoma, Cushing's syndrome, and hyperaldosteronism (see Chapter 44)

Hypertension in the Older Adult

In the United States, 45% of persons over 65 years of age have hypertension (systolic BP of 160 mm Hg or greater or a diastolic BP of 95 mm Hg or greater).[21] Isolated systolic hypertension affects 30% of persons 80 years of age or older.[22] Atherosclerotic changes in older adults cause increased rigidity of the aortic wall and peripheral arteries. These changes cause increased SVR and increased systolic BP with a wide pulse pressure because the diastolic pressure usually remains relatively normal.

Treatment for most older adults with isolated systolic hypertension initially involves nonpharmacological therapy.[18] Drug therapy is usually reserved for older persons with elevations of both systolic and diastolic pressures. A general guideline for treatment is to lower the BP slowly. A BP of 160/95 is acceptable for persons over 65 years of age, rather than a pressure of 140/90, which is the goal for persons under the age of 50.

Because of varying degrees of impaired cardiovascular reflex mechanisms, postural or orthostatic hypotension occurs often in older adults, especially in those with systolic hypertension. Postural hypotension in this age group is often associated with volume depletion or chronic disease states, such as adrenal insufficiency or electrolyte imbalance.[23] Antihypertensive drugs should be started at low doses and given at bedtime when the client is supine to help prevent or minimize orthostatic hypotension. Careful monitoring of the client's postural vital signs is essential until the BP and intravascular volume have been stabilized.[22]

β-blocking drugs in older adults may not be as effective as other agents because of reduced β-receptor activity. Loop diuretics such as furosemide and ethacrynic acid may cause hypovolemia. Members of this age group are more likely to have symptoms from the hypovolemia, especially if they are taking digitalis. Potassium replacement is important. (Foods high in potassium are listed in Table 41-8).

Clinical Manifestations

Hypertension is often called the "silent killer" because symptoms do not usually develop until the disease is advanced. If symptoms develop as a late manifestation, they are usually secondary to effects on blood vessels in the various organs and tissues or to the increased work load of the heart. The most common complaint is a headache, which occurs frequently in the morning and disappears as the day goes on. It is usually in the occipital region and may be no more than a feeling of stiffness or tightness. Headache is characteristic of severe hypertension and is thought to be due to changes in cerebrospinal fluid (CSF). In the supine position, CSF pressure increases, resulting in headache. When the person stands upright, the CSF pressure decreases and the headache disappears.

Other possible manifestations are easy fatigability, dizziness, and palpitations. Blurring of vision and epistaxis (nosebleed) may also occur as a result of vascular disease. Epistaxis is not a common manifestation and is associated with severe hypertension.

Complications

The most common complications are target organ damage occurring in the heart (hypertensive heart disease), brain (cerebrovascular disease), kidney (nephrosclerosis), and eyes (retinal damage).

Hypertensive heart disease

Coronary artery disease. Hypertension is the primary cause of stroke and cardiac failure in the United States and is the major treatable risk factor for coronary artery disease.[24] In addition to increasing the rate of atherosclerosis, elevated BP causes the entire inner lining of the arteriole to become thickened as a reaction to the high pressure. This characteristic change results from hyperplasia of connective tissues in the intima of the arteriole. These arteriolar changes account for a high incidence of coronary artery disease and the resulting problems of angina pectoris and MI.

Congestive heart failure. Congestive heart failure (CHF) occurs when the heart can no longer pump effectively against the increasing resistance. The increased resistance to blood flow increases the cardiac work load. To generate greater pressure, the myocardium of the left ventricle first hypertrophies. When the hypertrophied ventricle can no longer function effectively, the left ventricle dilates (Fig. 27-7). Heart failure can result from excess dilatation (see Chapter 29). The client may complain of shortness of breath on exertion and of paroxysmal nocturnal dyspnea. A chest x-ray film will show an enlarged heart, and an ECG will show left ventricular hypertrophy.

Cerebrovascular disease. As a result of hypertension, the blood vessels become more rigid because of thickening of vessel walls and replacement of smooth muscle tissue with fibrous tissue. The vessel is weakened by this process and tends to rupture more easily. Because of these abnormal processes, changes in cerebral circulation include the following:

1. Intense constriction of cerebral arterioles
2. Microaneurysms of small cerebral arteries
3. Progressive atherosclerotic changes
4. Increase in intracranial pressure

As a result of these changes, the client may experience transient ischemic attacks (TIA) or a cerebrovascular accident (CVA) as a result of thrombosis of cerebral vessels, intracerebral hemorrhage, or emboli.

Hypertensive encephalopathy may occur after a marked rise in BP if the cerebral blood flow is not decreased by autoregulation. With the increase in BP the cerebral vessels dilate and cerebral edema develops and produces a

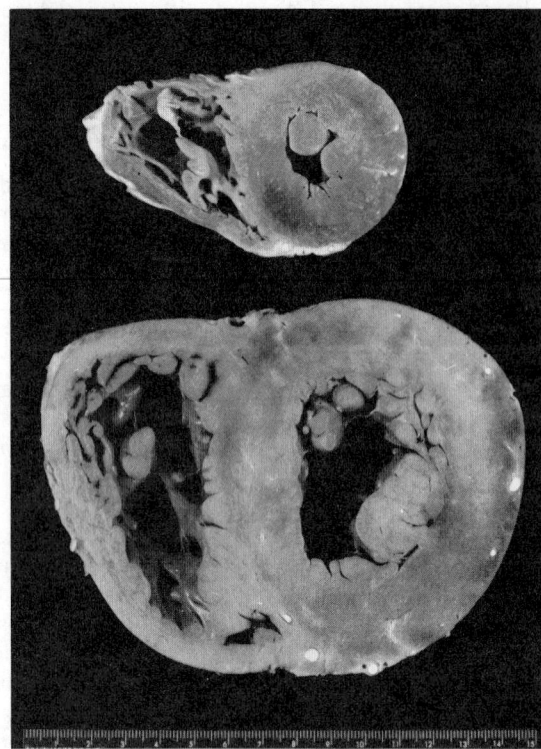

Fig. 27-7 Massively enlarged heart caused by hypertrophy of both ventricles. The normal heart weighs 325 g. The heart with biventricular hypertrophy weighs 1100 g. The client had suffered from severe systemic hypertension. (From Kissane JM: Anderson's pathology, ed 9, St Louis, 1990, Mosby–Year Book, Inc, p 681.)

rise in intracranial pressure. The increased intracranial pressure may be sufficient to decrease or halt blood flow to the brain.

Nephrosclerosis. In the kidney, nephrosclerosis results from longstanding hypertension. This disorder is the direct result of ischemia due to the narrowed lumen of the intrarenal blood vessels. Gradual closure of the arteries and arterioles leads to destruction of the glomeruli, atrophy of the tubules, and eventual death of nephrons. These changes eventually lead to renal failure. Common laboratory abnormalities are proteinuria, elevated BUN and serum creatinine levels, and microscopic hematuria.

Renal complications are prevalent and severe in malignant hypertension. There is rapid deterioration in renal function because of necrotizing arteriolitis.

Retinal damage. An ophthalmoscope is used to visualize the blood vessels of the eye. The appearance of the retina provides important information about the severity and prognosis of the hypertensive process. The retina is the only place in the body where the blood vessels can be directly visualized. Therefore, retinal damage provides an indication of vessel damage in the heart, brain, and kidney. Manifestations of retinal damage include blurring of vision, retinal hemorrhage, and loss of vision.

Retinal changes are graded according to severity of damage. The Keith-Wagener classification of retinal

Table 27-13 Keith-Wagener Classification of Retinal Changes

Grade I	Vascular spasm and arteriolar narrowing in terminal branches of vessels
Grade II	Definite arteriovenous nicking (arterioles cross vein and compress it)
Grade III	Flame-shaped hemorrhages and fluffy cotton-wool exudates
Grade IV	Any of the above and papilledema (swelling of optic disk)

Table 27-14

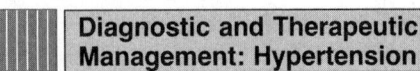

Diagnostic and Therapeutic Management: Hypertension

DIAGNOSTIC

History and physical examination
Routine urinalysis
Serum electrolytes and uric acid
BUN and serum creatinine
Blood glucose (preferably 2 hr postprandial)
Complete blood count
Serum lipid profile, cholesterol, and triglycerides
Chest x-ray film
ECG

THERAPEUTIC

Diet
  Restriction of sodium
  Reduction of weight (if indicated)
  Restriction of cholesterol and saturated fats
Restriction of alcohol
Cessation of smoking
Reduction of stress—biofeedback and relaxation
Exercise program
Antihypertensive drugs*
Periodic monitoring of BP
  Weekly monitoring if diastolic BP > 105 mm Hg
  Every 4 mo if no symptoms and stable diastolic BP < 105 mm Hg

*See Table 27-15.

changes is presented in Table 27-13. Grade IV findings of papilledema are characteristic of malignant hypertension.

Diagnostic Studies

The client's BP measurements in both arms should be carefully evaluated to detect hypertension. The average of at least two BP measurements (taken 5 minutes apart while the client is seated) should be used to determine which clients should return for subsequent evaluation.[25]

There is some controversy as to how extensive a diagnostic workup should be performed on a person with hypertension. Because most hypertension is essential, how much testing should be done to detect secondary hypertension?

Table 27-14 lists basic laboratory studies that are performed in persons with sustained hypertension. Routine urinalysis, BUN, and serum creatinine tests are used to screen for renal involvement. Measurement of serum electrolytes, especially potassium levels, is important to detect aldosteronism. Blood glucose levels are important because they can assist in identifying endocrine causes of hypertension, such as diabetes mellitus and Cushing's syndrome. Urinary catecholamine levels are used to diagnose pheochromocytoma. Serum cholesterol and triglyceride levels may provide an indication of risk factors that predispose to atherogenesis. Uric acid levels are determined to establish a baseline, since the levels often rise with diuretic therapy. A chest x-ray film provides baseline information regarding heart size, as well as aortic dilatation and rib notching, which occur in coarctation of the aorta. An ECG provides baseline information regarding the cardiac status.

Therapeutic Management

The goal in treating hypertensive clients is to prevent the morbidity and mortality associated with high BP (see Table 27-14). The decision to initiate therapy depends on two major factors: (1) the severity of the BP elevation and (2) the presence of other complications.[18] Decisions about treatment are usually based on BP measurements taken over two to three visits. If the diastolic BP is consistently greater than 105 mm Hg, antihypertensive drug therapy is indicated. In clients with diastolic pressures between 90 and 105 mm Hg, age, sex, race, and other controllable risk factors are considered before drug therapy is begun.

Follow-up monitoring of the BP is very important. Weekly recordings are indicated for clients with a diastolic BP above 105 mm Hg. After the BP has stabilized, it should be monitored every 4 months to ensure control and to assess for target organ damage.

Nondrug therapeutic interventions are indicated in all persons with either borderline or sustained hypertension. These measures include diet management, regular exercise, stress reduction, and smoking cessation. (Management of risk factors is discussed in Chapter 28 and Table 28-4.)

Regular exercise. Regular isotonic exercise, such as walking, jogging, and swimming, can help control BP, promote relaxation, and control body weight. A moderate amount of exercise at regular intervals is better than vigorous exercise at irregular intervals. The type of exercise that is done is very important. *Isometric* exercises, such as pushing heavy weights or tightening muscles against fixed objects, can raise the BP significantly and should be avoided in persons known to have hypertension. Health professionals should advise clients with hypertension to seek medical advice before beginning any exercise program and to initiate the exercise gradually.

Stress reduction and management. Stress reduction and management will help reduce BP and will help control other aspects of the client's life. The person should learn to identify the events and agents that act as stressors in life

and develop and implement methods to cope with them. Relaxation techniques represent one means of dealing with stress. These techniques include yoga, transcendental meditation, and physical relaxation. Relaxation techniques have been used successfully in mitigating stress and decreasing sympathetic activity, thereby lowering BP, especially in clients with mild hypertension. Relaxation techniques have also been used effectively in combination with drug therapy for clients with more severe hypertension.

One simple relaxation exercise is walking. Another is to stand still and breathe slowly through the nose, let the breath rise from the diaphragm (not the stomach), and concentrate on exhalation.

Psychotherapy has been used as a method of lowering BP, with successful results reported. It can help clients deal with anxiety and deal constructively with hostile and aggressive impulses. Counseling has always been advocated as a method of increasing client adherence to the therapeutic regimen.

Biofeedback uses equipment that gives the client continuous feedback so that bodily processes regulated by the autonomic nervous system (but not consciously perceived and controlled) can be self-regulated. Decreases in BP as the result of biofeedback have been reported, although there are no data that demonstrate its long-term effectiveness.

Avoidance of cigarette smoking. Although there is a lack of definitive evidence linking smoking to hypertension, the benefits of tobacco avoidance have been conclusively proven. Therefore smoking cessation is strongly recommended.[18]

Pharmacological Management

The general goals of pharmacological management of hypertension are to (1) reduce and maintain the diastolic BP at less than 90 mm Hg (95 mm Hg if over age 65) and (2) keep uncomfortable or disabling side effects to a minimum (Table 27-15). The drugs currently available for treating hypertension have two main actions: (1) reduction of SVR and/or (2) decrease in the volume of circulating blood. The drugs used in the treatment of hypertension include diuretics, adrenergic (sympathetic) inhibiting agents, vasodilators, angiotensin-converting enzyme–inhibiting agents, and calcium antagonists (Fig. 27-8).

Although the precise action of diuretics in the reduction of BP is unclear, they do produce a negative sodium balance in the arteriolar walls, release water for excretion, reduce plasma volume, and reduce the vascular response to catecholamines. Adrenergic-inhibiting agents act by diminishing the sympathetic reflexes that increase BP. Vasodilators decrease the BP by dilating the arterioles. Angiotensin-converting enzyme–inhibiting agents decrease BP by blocking the renin-angiotensin-aldosterone system, decreasing fluid volume, and decreasing SVR. Calcium antagonists cause vasodilatation of peripheral arterioles by blocking the movement of extracellular calcium into cells (see Chapter 28).

The individualized step-care therapy for hypertension is based on stepwise additions of various antihypertensive drugs until adequate control is achieved (Fig. 27-9). How-

Text continued on p. 769.

Table 27-15 Antihypertensive Drug Therapy*

Agent	Mechanisms of Action	Side Effects and Adverse Effects	Nursing Considerations
DIURETICS			
Thiazides and related sulfonamide diuretics			
Bendroflumethiazide (Naturetin), benzthiazide (Aquatag, Exna), chlorothiazide (Diuril), chlorthalidone (Hygroton), cyclothiazide (Anhydron), hydrochlorothiazide (Esidrix, Hydrodiuril, Oretic), hydroflumethiazide (Saluron), indapamide (Lozol), methyclothiazide (Enduron), metolazone (Zaroxolyn), polythiazide (Renese), quinethazone (Hydromox), trichlormethiazide (Metahydrin, Naqua)	Act on ascending loop of Henle and distal tubule; prevent reabsorption of sodium and chloride; reduce ECF and CO, causing initial effect; reduce SVR, causing long-term effect; usually lower blood pressure moderately within 3-4 days; higher than normal doses rarely add to effect on BP and can worsen adverse effects	Electrolyte imbalances, including hypercalcemia, hypochloremia, hypokalemia, hypomagnesemia, hyponatremia; orthostatic hypotension; hypercholesteremia; hyperglycemia; hypertriglyceridemia; hyperuricemia; GI manifestations, including anorexia, vomiting, diarrhea, pancreatitis; central nervous system effects, including dizziness, vertigo, headache; hematological effects, including leukopenia, agranulocytosis, thrombocytopenia; hypersensitivity effects, including photosensitivity, purpura, rash; sexual dysfunction; weakness	Monitor for hypokalemia and alkalosis. Be aware that thiazides potentiate cardiotoxicity of digitalis by producing hypokalemia and that nonsteroidal antiinflammatory drugs can decrease diuretic and antihypertensive effects of thiazide type of diuretics. Advise client to supplement diet with potassium-rich foods.† If potassium solution supplement needed, advise client to drink it with fruit juice or water to minimize unpleasant taste.
Loop diuretics			
Bumetanide (Bumex), ethacrynic acid (Edecrin), furosemide (Lasix)	Act on ascending loop of Henle to prevent reabsorption of chloride and sodium; are more potent than thiazide diuretics; have shorter duration of action than thiazide type of diuretics and may be less effective for treatment of hypertension; furosemide reserved for clients with fluid retention that cannot be controlled with thiazides or for clients with impaired renal function	Same as thiazides, including fluid and electrolyte depletion and, in severe cases, cardiovascular collapse; also reversible hearing loss, metabolic alkalosis, GI upset (most common with ethacrynic acid)	Monitor for hypokalemia and alkalosis. Measure fluid intake and output and weigh client daily. Be aware that effect of drug increases with dosage.
Potassium-sparing diuretics			
Amiloride (Midamor), spironolactone (Aldactone), triamterene (Dyrenium)	Used mainly with thiazide diuretics to prevent or correct hypokalemia; block sodium-potassium exchange mechanism in the distal portion of tubule; prevent sodium from being reabsorbed and retain potassium; triamterene and amiloride act on distal tubule to block potassium secretion independently of aldosterone; spironolactone blocks effect of aldosterone on kidney tubule	Renal insufficiency, hyperkalemia, GI disturbances, skin eruptions, hirsutism, headache, urticaria, drug fever, photosensitivity, gynecomastia in males, inability to achieve or maintain erection, menstrual irregularities, ataxia with spironolactone, and blood dyscrasias with triamterene	Monitor for hyperkalemia, especially in clients with renal impairment or diabetes, in older adults, and those receiving other drugs that can lower aldosterone secretion, such as captopril and nonsteroidal antiinflammatory drugs. Do not use potassium supplements.

*All drugs are normally given orally unless otherwise indicated.
†See Table 41-8.

Table 27-15 Antihypertensive Drug Therapy*—cont'd

Agent	Mechanisms of Action	Side Effects and Adverse Effects	Nursing Considerations
ADRENERGIC INHIBITORS			
β-Adrenergic blockers			
Acebutolol (Sectral), atenolol (Tenormin), metoprolol (Lopressor), nadolol (Corgard), pindolol (Visken), propranolol (Inderal), timolol (Blocadren)	Reduce BP by decreasing CO, sympathetic stimulation, and renin secretion by kidney; reduce SVR (with long-term use)	Bronchospasm, heart failure, bradycardia, arterioventricular conduction block, impaired peripheral circulation, nightmares, depression, weakness, GI disturbances, insomnia, decreased exercise tolerance, sexual dysfunction masking hypoglycemic symptoms	Assess client for manifestations of heart failure and heart block. Check pulse regularly. Be aware that drugs are contraindicated with a history of CHF, chronic obstructive pulmonary disease, heart block, asthma, or diabetes mellitus and that sudden withdrawal can be hazardous in clients with heart disease.
Centrally acting α blockers			
Clonidine (Catapres)	Inhibits impulse through sympathetic nerve pathways; causes central α-receptor stimulation, decreasing sympathetic tone peripherally; results in dilatation of arterioles and veins; does not inhibit reflex responses as completely as drugs that act peripherally	Dry mouth, sedation, impotence, constipation, allergic reaction, dizziness, headache, fatigue, anxiety, severe rebound hypertension (if drug abruptly discontinued)	Suggest chewing gum or hard candy to relieve dry mouth. Be aware that alcohol and sedatives increase central nervous system depression. Use for hypertensive urgencies.
Guanabenz (Wytensin)	Same as clonidine	Same as clonidine	Same as clonidine.
Guanfacine hydrochloride (Tenex)	Same as clonidine	Same as clonidine	Same as clonidine.
Methyldopa (Aldomet)	Same as clonidine	Sedation, fatigue, orthostatic hypotension, decreased libido, impotence, dry mouth, hemolytic anemia, hepatotoxicity, GI disturbances, sodium and water retention, psychic depression	Instruct client about daytime sedation and avoidance of hazardous activities. Be aware that activities requiring mental work may be an indication not to use drug. Give IV for hypertensive emergencies.
Peripheral-acting adrenergic inhibitors			
Guanethidine (Ismelin)	Prevents release of norepinephrine, resulting in peripheral vasodilatation; usually lowers CO and reduces systolic BP more than diastolic; produces greatest effects in standing position	Marked orthostatic hypotension, diarrhea, cramps, bradycardia, retrograde ejaculation, sodium and water retention; cumulative effects (over several weeks)	Because of adverse effects, drug is reserved for severe hypertension unresponsive to other drugs. It is not recommended for persons with cerebral vascular insufficiency or coronary artery disease or in older adults because of orthostatic hypotension. The hypotensive effect is delayed for 2-3 days and lasts 7-10 days after withdrawal. Severe postural hypotension is aggravated by anything that stimulates vasodilatation (e.g., hot environment, alcohol, or hot shower). Use diuretic.

Continued.

Table 27-15 Antihypertensive Drug Therapy*—cont'd

Agent	Mechanisms of Action	Side Effects and Adverse Effects	Nursing Considerations
ADRENERGIC INHIBITORS—cont'd			
Peripheral acting adrenergic inhibitors—cont'd			
Guanadrel sulfate (Hylorel)	Same as guanethidine, except with shorter duration of action	Same as guanethidine	Same as guanethidine.
Reserpine (Serpasil)	Acts both peripherally and centrally to deplete norepinephrine stores; results in peripheral vasodilatation	Nasal congestion, drowsiness, GI distress, mental depression, bizarre dreams, bradycardia, syncope, impotence	Be aware that history of depression is a contraindication. Monitor for depression and personality changes. Advise client to eliminate barbiturates, alcohol, and narcotics.
α-Adrenergic blockers			
Phentolamine (Regitine)	Blocks α-adrenergic receptors, resulting in peripheral vascular dilatation	Acute prolonged hypotension, cardiac dysrhythmias, tachycardia, weakness, flushing	Use for pheochromocytoma.
Prazosin hydrochloride (Minipress), terazosin hydrochloride (Hytrin)	Blocks peripheral vascular α-adrenergic receptors, resulting in dilatation of arterioles and veins	Profound orthostatic hypotension with syncope (1-3 hr after first dose), disappearing with continued use; headache; drowsiness; paresthesias; blurred vision; impotence; frequent urination; fluid retention	Prevent hypotension and syncope by giving small initial dose at bedtime and advising client not to get up for 3 hr. Use cautiously in older adults because of orthostatic hypotension.
Combined α- and β-adrenergic blockers			
Labetalol (Normodyne, Trandate)	Has nonselective action, resulting in α-adrenergic blocking properties	Orthostatic hypotension, sexual dysfunction (more than other β-adrenergic blocking drugs); bronchospasm, peripheral vascular insufficiency	Same as β-blockers. Give IV for hypertensive emergencies.
VASODILATORS			
Diazoxide (Hyperstat)	Has direct action (used only in hypertensive emergencies)	Sodium and water retention, hyperglycemia, hypotension, skin rash, fever, dysrhythmias, nausea, vomiting, chest pain, hyperuricemia	Inject via IV push within 30 sec. Administer diuretic because of sodium retention. Use cautiously in clients with diabetes and cerebrovascular insufficiency.
Hydralazine (Apresoline)	Acts primarily on smooth muscle of arterioles to cause vasodilatation and reduce SVR; usually decreases diastolic and systolic pressure proportionally and causes little orthostatic hypotension; acts more on arterioles than veins and is less potent than minoxidil	Tachycardia, fluid retention, nasal congestion, flushing, headache, palpitations, GI symptoms, hepatitis, CHF, angina exacerbation, lupuslike syndrome.	Be aware that headaches sometimes occur when drug is started or when dosage is increased. Discontinue drug if lupuslike syndrome occurs. Give drug IM or IV for hypertensive emergencies.

*All drugs are normally given orally unless otherwise indicated

Table 27-15 Antihypertensive Drug Therapy*—cont;d

Agent	Mechanisms of Action	Side Effects and Adverse Effects	Nursing Considerations
VASODILATORS—cont'd			
Minoxidil (Loniten)	Produces arterial vasodilatation with no venous effect	Reflex tachycardia, marked sodium and water retention (often not controllable with large doses of furosemide), CHF, weakness, hirsutism, aggravation of angina	Be aware that major disadvantage is reflex-increased sympathetic activity. Use only for treatment of severe hypertension resistant to other therapy. Use for hypertensive urgencies.
Nitroglycerin (Tridil)	Acts primarily as venous vasodilator; is effective in hypertensive emergencies, especially in clients with myocardial ischemia	Hypotension, headache	Closely monitor BP. Observe for drug tolerance, which may occur with repeated and prolonged use.
Sodium nitroprusside (Nipride)	Has direct action (used in hypertensive emergencies); is administered by continuous IV infusion with immediate effect	Hypotension, nausea, sweating, headache, restlessness, confusion, twitching, thiocyanate toxicity	Carefully titrate dosage to client's response. Use intraarterial monitoring system. Be aware that drug is light sensitive and stable for 24 hr. Monitor thiocyanate levels.
GANGLIONIC BLOCKERS			
Trimethaphan (Arfonad)	Blocks neural transmission at autonomic ganglia (used in hypertensive emergencies); is drug of choice for treatment of aortic dissection	Dry mouth, urinary retention, constipation, orthostatic hypotension, weakness, dilated pupils	Administer IV for rapid onset of action. Carefully titrate drug. Continually monitor BP after administration.
ANGIOTENSIN-CONVERTING ENZYME INHIBITORS			
Captopril (Capoten), enalapril maleate (Vasotec), lisinopril (Prinivil, Zestril)	Inhibit angiotensin-converting enzyme, lowering SVR; is effective for essential hypertension and renovascular hypertension and in severe refractory hypertension; may be more effective than some three-drug regimens	Loss of taste (leading to severe anorexia), cough, fatal bone marrow depression, transient maculopapular rash, hyperkalemia, membranous glomerulopathy, nephrotic syndrome, tachycardia, orthostatic hypotension	Use aspirin substitute because aspirin can decrease drug's effectiveness. Be aware that diuretics may not be required for effective therapy, but combination of diuretic and captopril is more effective than either drug alone. Use captopril for hypertensive urgencies.
CALCIUM ANTAGONISTS			
Diltiazem hydrochloride (Cardizem), nifedipine (Procardia), verapamil (Isoptin), verapamil SR (long-acting)	Cause vasodilatation of peripheral arterioles by blocking movement of extracellular calcium into cells, resulting in decreased SVR	Nausea, headache, hypotension, peripheral edema; reflex increase in HR (with nifedipine); reflex decrease in HR (with diltiazem); minimal change in HR (with verapamil); constipation (with verapamil and diltiazem)	Use with caution in clients with CHF; contraindicated with second- and third-degree heart block. Give nifedipine sublingually or have client chew drug for hypertensive urgencies. Be aware that the higher the BP, the more significant the decrease in BP is once drug therapy is initiated.

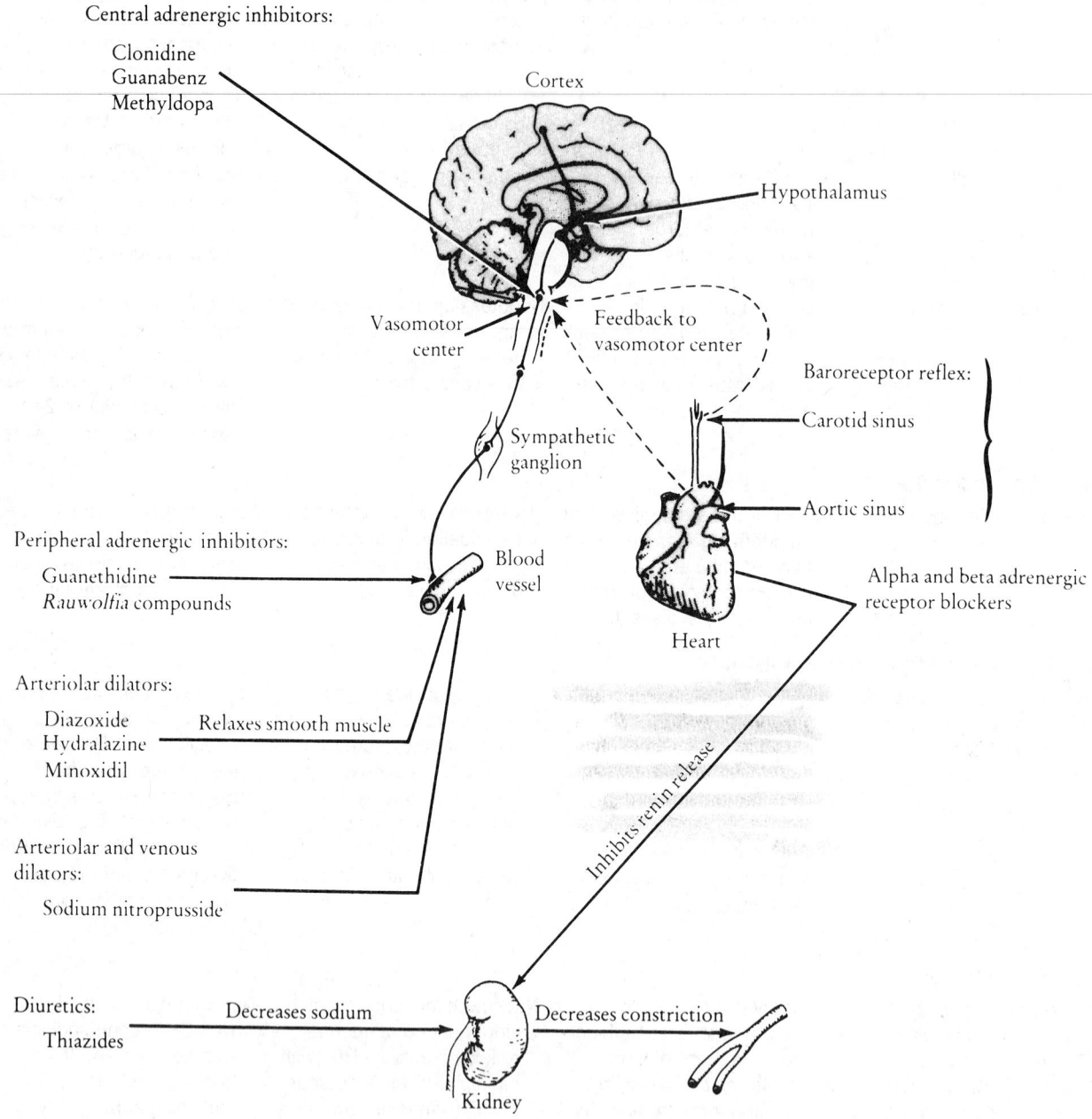

Fig. 27-8 Site and method of action of various antihypertensive drugs. (Modified from McHenry LM and Salerno E: Pharmacology in nursing, ed 17, St Louis, 1989, The CV Mosby Co, p 494.)

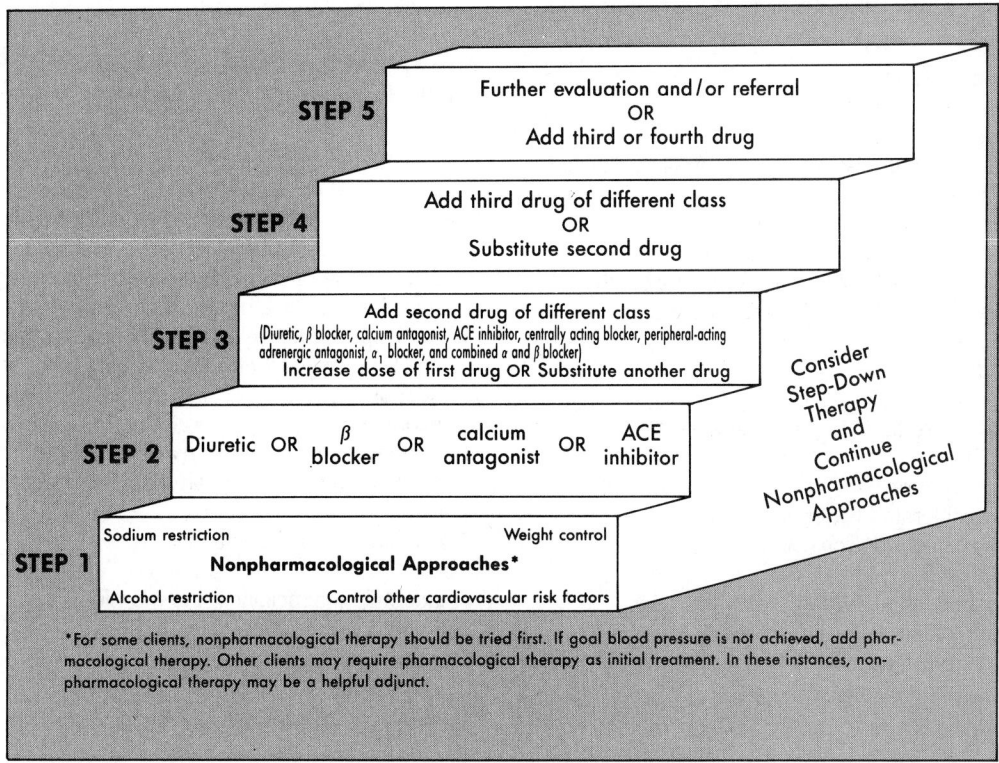

Fig. 27-9   Individualized step-care therapy for hypertension. (From US Department of Health and Human Services: The 1988 report of the Joint National Committee on Detection, Evaluation, and Treatment of High Blood Pressure, Washington, DC, 1988, Public Health Service, National Institutes of Health.)

ever, this is only one suggested approach to the treatment of hypertension. Because of the large numbers of effective antihypertensive drugs, there are many excellent therapeutic options for lowering BP effectively with minimal side effects.[18] In the individualized step-care approach, *step one* involves nonpharmacological approaches. Some clients may require pharmacological therapy as a first step in addition to the nonpharmacological approaches.

In *step two,* initial drug therapy may be a thiazide type of diuretic, a β blocker, a calcium antagonist, or an ACE inhibitor. *Step three* involves three options: adding a second drug of a different class, increasing the dose of the first drug, or substituting another drug. The optional other classes of drugs include α_1 blockers, centrally acting α blockers, peripheral-acting adrenergic antagonists, combined α and β blockers, and vasodilators. The use of the adrenergic-inhibiting drugs with diuretic therapy prevents the sodium and water retention that occurs when the adrenergic-inhibiting drugs are used alone. Vasodilator drugs cause a compensatory increase in sympathetic nervous system activity, resulting in tachycardia and increased CO. If vasodilators are used with sympathetic inhibitors, reflex activation of the sympathetic nervous system does not occur.

Step four involves addition of a third drug of a different class or substitution of a second drug. *Step five* includes further evaluation, referral, or addition of a third or fourth drug.

Adverse effects of the drugs may be so severe or undesirable that the client does not comply with therapy. Table 27-15 describes the major effects for each drug. Hyperuricemia, hyperglycemia, and hypovolemia are common complications with both thiazide and loop diuretics. Hyperkalemia can be a serious side effect of the potassium-sparing diuretics. Impotence may occur with many of the diuretics. Orthostatic hypotension and sexual dysfunction are two undesirable effects of adrenergic-inhibiting agents. Tachycardia and orthostatic hypotension are potentially adverse effects of both vasodilators and angiotensin-converting enzyme–inhibiting agents.

If a client does not respond to antihypertensive therapy, possible causes of refractory hypertension should be considered (Table 27-16).

Nutritional Considerations

Dietary management of hypertension consists of sodium restriction, caloric restriction if the client is overweight, and restriction of cholesterol, fat, and alcohol intake.

Sodium restriction. Although only certain clients with hypertension may respond to sodium limitations, there is no hazard from moderate dietary sodium restriction. A high sodium intake may also limit the effectiveness of cer-

Table 27-16 Causes of Refractory Hypertension

Nonadherence to therapy
Drug-related causes
  Too low dosage
  Inappropriate combinations (e.g., two centrally acting adrenergic inhibitors)
  Rapid inactivation (e.g., hydralazine)
  Effects of other drugs, including sympathomimetics, antidepressants, corticosteroids, nonsteroidal antiinflammatory drugs, nasal decongestants, and oral contraceptives
Associated conditions
  Increasing obesity
  Alcohol intake (more than 1 oz of ethanol a day)
  Renal insufficiency
  Renovascular hypertension
  Malignant or accelerated hypertension
  Other causes of hypertension
Volume overload
  Inadequate diuretic therapy
  Excess sodium intake
  Fluid retention from reduction of BP
  Progressive renal damage

Modified from US Department of Health and Human Services: The 1988 report of the Joint National Committee on Detection, Evaluation, and Treatment of High Blood Pressure, Washington, DC, Public Health Service, National Institutes of Health, p 20.

Table 27-17

Nursing Assessment for the Client with Elevated Blood Pressure

SUBJECTIVE DATA

History
Family history of hypertension or cardiovascular disease; history of cardiovascular, cerebrovascular, renal, or thyroid disease or diabetes mellitus; race; pregnancy; congenital aortic constriction; acromegaly, salt and fat intake, psychosocial and environmental factors influencing BP; activity level; recent weight gain; smoking and alcohol use

Medications
Use of any prescription or over-the-counter medications, previous use of antihypertensive drug therapy

General
Dizziness, fatigue, epistaxis

Pain
Headaches (especially in the morning)

Respiratory
Dyspnea on exertion

Cardiovascular
Palpitations on exertion

Urinary
Nocturia

Neurological
Blurred vision, paresthesias, headaches

OBJECTIVE DATA

Cardiovascular
BP consistently above 140 mm Hg systolic and 90 mm Hg diastolic, peripheral edema, retinal vessel changes, abnormal heart sounds, diminished or absent peripheral arterial pulses, bruits

Musculoskeletal
Muscle cramps

Possible findings
Abnormal serum electrolytes (especially potassium); elevated BUN, creatinine, glucose, cholesterol, and triglyceride levels; abnormal urinalysis; abnormal chest x-ray film showing cardiomegaly, aortic dilatation, or rib notching; abnormal ECG demonstrating left ventricular hypertrophy

---

tain antihypertensive drugs.[18] The mechanism by which the BP is lowered by restriction of sodium is not fully understood. However, it is known that restricting sodium reduces the ECF volume and the circulating plasma volume, thus decreasing the work of the heart.

A common recommended restriction is 2 g of sodium per day or 5 g of salt per day. This involves not adding salt in the preparation of foods or at meals and avoiding foods known to be high in sodium (see Table 29-8).

Caloric restriction. Obesity has a high correlation with hypertension. Weight reduction has a significant effect on lowering BP in many persons, especially young to middle-aged adults. The amount of caloric restriction depends on the degree of obesity. When a person decreases caloric intake, sodium intake is also usually reduced. Therefore an additional benefit is achieved with a weight-reduction diet.

Modification of dietary fats. Lipid restriction should include limiting the intake of cholesterol as well as dietary saturated fats. This practice may retard the progress of atherosclerosis (see Chapter 28).

Modification in alcohol consumption. Alcohol consumption needs to be assessed in clients with hypertension. The exact mechanism by which alcohol raises BP is not known. It is possible that alcohol increases renin or aldosterone. Chronic alcohol abuse elevates cortisol. Available studies suggest that the consumption of three or more alcoholic drinks daily is a definite risk factor in hypertension.[26] Therefore alcohol consumption needs to be evaluated, and the client should be advised to reduce intake if

drinking is heavy. The client with hypertension should limit the use of alcohol to less than 1 oz per day.

■ Nursing Management of Hypertension
Nursing assessment
Subjective and objective data that should be obtained from a client with hypertension are presented in Table 27-17.

Nursing diagnoses
Nursing diagnoses are determined when the problem and the etiological factors are supported by the clinical data. Nursing diagnoses related to a client with an elevated

Table 27-18 Nursing Diagnoses Related to a Client with Elevated Blood Pressure

Health management deficit related to lack of knowledge of basic physiology, complications, medications, stress modification, diet, exercise, and home monitoring of BP

Anxiety related to complications of management regimen, potential complications, and necessary lifestyle changes

Pain related to vascular headache

High risk for sexual dysfunction related to use of antihypertensive medications

High risk for noncompliance with prescribed treatment regimen related to inadequate instruction, unpleasant side effects of the medications, subsiding of symptoms, return of BP to normal range while on medications, lack of motivation, high cost of some medications, inconvenient schedule for taking medications, and lack of a trusting relationship between client and health care provider

High risk for complications of high BP and its treatment regimen related to advanced age

High risk for failure to identify those clients with elevated BP related to lack of screening areas or client's lack of knowledge or interest to obtain baseline BP reading

Table 27-19 Appropriate Technique for Measuring Blood Pressure

1. Client should be seated with the arm bared, supported, and positioned at heart level. The client should not have smoked or ingested caffeine within 30 minutes before measurement.
2. Blood pressure should be taken in both arms initially.
3. Measurement should begin after 5 minutes of quiet rest.
4. The appropriate cuff size must be used to ensure an accurate measurement. The rubber bladder should encircle at least two thirds of the arm. Several sizes of cuffs (e.g., child, adult, and large adult) should be available.
5. Measurements should be taken with a mercury sphygmomanometer, a recently calibrated aneroid manometer, or a validated electronic device.
6. Both systolic and diastolic pressures should be recorded. The disappearance of sound should be used for the diastolic reading.
7. Two or more readings (taken at least 5 minutes apart) should be averaged. If the first two readings differ by more than 5 mm Hg, additional readings should be obtained.
8. The client should be informed of the reading and advised of the need for periodic remeasurement.

From 1988 Report of the Joint National Committee on Detection, Evaluation and Treatment of High Blood Pressure, Washington, DC, Public Health Service, National Institutes of Health, p 20.

BP may include, but are not limited to, those presented in Table 27-18.

Nursing interventions
Health promotion and maintenance

INDIVIDUAL CLIENT EVALUATION. The majority of cases of hypertension are identified through routine screening procedures such as insurance, preemployment, and military physical examinations. Nurses in these settings, as well as in most other practice settings, are in an ideal position to (1) assess for the presence of hypertension, (2) identify the risk factors for hypertension and coronary artery disease, and (3) educate clients regarding this disease. In addition to BP determination, a complete health assessment should include such factors as age, sex, race, diet history (including sodium and alcohol intake), weight patterns, and identification of physical and psychosocial stressors. Another factor to include in the health history is a family history of heart disease, stroke, renal disease, and diabetes mellitus. Medications taken, both prescribed and over-the-counter, should be noted. The client should be asked about any previous documentation of high BP and the results of treatment (if any).

Initially, the BP is taken two or three times, at least 1 or 2 minutes apart, with the average pressure recorded as the value for that visit. Waiting for 1 or 2 minutes between readings allows the venous blood to drain from the arm and prevents inaccurate readings. The BP is assessed most accurately if readings are taken when the client is in either the supine or the sitting position and then the standing position. Usually the systolic pressure decreases on standing, whereas the diastolic pressure increases.

BP measurements should be done under standardized conditions and with accurate equipment (Table 27-19). BP measurements of both arms should be performed initially to detect any differences between arms. The BP should not be obtained immediately after a stressful event, such as walking up stairs. In the procedure the client's arm is uncovered and placed at the level of the heart. The cuff should be inflated until no pulse is felt in the brachial artery located in the antecubital fossa of the arm being used. The cuff is then inflated an additional 10 to 20 mm Hg to ensure vascular occlusion. In obese persons, a cuff larger than the normal 12 to 14 cm cuff should be used to obtain accurate readings. The pressure is released at 2 mm Hg per second. Releasing any slower or faster may create inaccurate readings. Both systolic and diastolic pressures should be recorded, with the diastolic pressure recorded as the disappearance of sound.

SCREENING PROGRAMS. Mass screening for detection of hypertension is seldom necessary. Effort and resources should be focused on the following factors: (1) controlling BP in persons already identified as having hypertension; (2) identifying and controlling BP in high-risk groups, such as blacks, obese persons, and blood relatives of persons with hypertension; and (3) screening those persons with limited access to the health care system.[18] Nurses involved in screening programs should be aware of general guidelines for BP detection and evaluation (Table 27-20). At the time of the BP measurement, each client should be informed in writing of the numerical value of the reading and, if necessary, why further evaluation is important.

RISK FACTORS. Client education regarding risk factors is

Table 27-20 Follow-Up Criteria for Initial Blood Pressure Measurement*

Range (mm Hg)	Recommended Follow-Up†
DIASTOLIC	
<85	Recheck within 2 yr
85-89	Recheck within 1 yr
90-104	Confirm within 2 mo
105-114	Evaluate or refer promptly to source of care within 2 wk
≥115	Evaluate or refer immediately to source of care
SYSTOLIC‡	
<140	Recheck within 2 yr
140-199	Confirm within 2 mo
≥200	Evaluate or refer promptly to source of care within 2 wk

With permission of the 1988 Joint National Committee on Detection, Evaluation, and Treatment of High Blood Pressure, Washington, DC, Public Health Service, National Institutes of Health, p 2.

*The average of two or more measurements should be taken on two or more occasions. The criteria are applicable to adults 18 years of age or older.

†If recommendations for follow-up of diastolic and systolic BP are different, the shorter recommended time for recheck and referral should take precedence.

‡Diastolic BP is <90 mm Hg.

appropriate for individual and mass screening programs. Risk factors can easily be identified and their modification discussed with the client. Groups at high risk of having hypertension (e.g., children of hypertensive clients) may also benefit from identification of risk factors. (Health-promoting behaviors for risk factors related to coronary artery disease are discussed in Table 28-4.)

Acute intervention. The majority of clients with mild to moderate hypertension are managed on an outpatient basis. Clients with severe hypertension, either newly diagnosed or uncontrolled, are frequently hospitalized. The purpose of hospitalization is to lower the BP, determine the underlying cause of the hypertension, and treat the cause if it is secondary hypertension. The primary goal of the nurse at this stage of intervention is to assist in reducing BP and to begin client education.

For the client with severe hypertension, the nurse needs to monitor the BP every 1 to 2 hours and then with decreasing frequency as the pressure stabilizes. Antihypertensive drug therapy at this time may be given parenterally. This requires very frequent (every 2 to 5 minutes) BP checks, which can be done with an automated BP monitoring machine. Careful monitoring of vital signs provides information regarding the effectiveness of these drugs and the client's response to therapy.

Client assessment is essential to evaluate the client with severe hypertension. Frequent neurological checks, including level of consciousness, pupillary size and reaction, movement of extremities, and reactions to stimuli, help to detect any changes in the client's condition. Cardiac, pul-

monary, and renal systems should be monitored for decompensation due to the severe elevation in BP (e.g., pulmonary edema, CHF, angina, and renal failure).

If the client has headaches, the nurse should assess when they occur and what precipitating factors are present. In addition to lowering the BP, nursing interventions for headache include the modification of factors that may cause stress. Appropriate interventions include encouraging the client to verbalize fears, answering questions concerning the hypertension, and eliminating excess noise in the client's environment.

The client with fatigue and anxiety should be provided with a schedule that alternates long rest periods with periods of activity. It is important to plan for emotional as well as physical rest. The nurse should discuss with the client measures to reduce stress and decrease tension. In some situations, it may be appropriate to administer tranquilizers if ordered.

Chronic management. The primary nursing responsibilities for long-term management of the client with hypertension are to assist in reducing BP and to begin or continue client education (Table 27-21). Client education includes the following:

1. Diet therapy
2. Drug therapy
3. Stress modification
4. Exercise
5. Home monitoring of BP (if appropriate)
6. Smoking cessation (if applicable)

DIET THERAPY. The client and family usually need to be educated about sodium-restricted diets. The client needs to be instructed on reading the labels of over-the-counter drugs as well as packaged foods to identify hidden sources of sodium. It is helpful to review the client's normal diet and to have the client identify foods high in sodium. (Weight-reduction diets are discussed in Chapter 35, and diets low in cholesterol and saturated fats are discussed in Chapter 28.)

DRUG THERAPY. Side effects of antihypertensive drug therapy are common. Sometimes the number or degree of side effects is related to the dosage and may decrease with long-term use of the drug. In certain cases, it is necessary to change the drug or decrease the dosage. With some drugs, side effects can be alleviated by arranging a convenient schedule. For example, diuretics work best if taken early in the morning rather than at night when frequent urination interrupts sleep. Side effects of vasodilators and adrenergic inhibitors decrease if the drugs are given in the evening. With some drugs, side effects can be decreased if the drugs are given with meals. Dry mouth and frequent voiding are common side effects of diuretics. Chewing sugarless gum or candy may relieve the dry mouth.

A common side effect of several of these drugs is orthostatic hypotension. This condition is due to an alteration of the nervous system's mechanisms for regulating pressure, which are required for positional changes. Consequently, the client may feel dizzy, weak, and faint when assuming an upright position after sitting or lying down. Specific measures to control or decrease orthostatic hypotension are presented in Table 27-21.

Sexual dysfunction may occur with many of the antihy-

Table 27-21 Teaching Plan for the Client with Hypertension

When presenting information to the client, the nurse should do the following:

1. Provide the numerical value of the client's BP and explain that it exceeds normal limits.
2. Inform client that hypertension is usually asymptomatic and symptoms do not reliably indicate BP levels.
3. Explain that long-term follow-up and therapy are necessary.
4. Explain that therapy will not cure, but should control hypertension.
5. Tell client that hypertension control is usually compatible with an excellent prognosis and a normal lifestyle.
6. Explain the potential dangers of uncontrolled hypertension.
7. Be specific about the names, actions, dosages, and side effects of prescribed medications.
8. Tell client to plan regular and convenient times for taking medications.
9. Tell client to not discontinue drugs or decrease the dosage if side effects develop but to consult first with the health care provider.
10. Tell client to not abruptly discontinue drugs because withdrawal may cause a severe hypertensive reaction.
11. Tell client to not double up on doses when a dose is missed.
12. Inform client that if BP increases, do not take an increased dosage before consulting with the health care provider.
13. Tell client to not take a medication belonging to someone else.
14. Inform client that side effects often diminish with time.
15. Tell client to consult with the health care provider about changing drugs or dosages if impotence or other sexual problems develop.
16. Tell client to supplement diet with foods high in potassium (e.g., citrus fruits and green leafy vegetables) if taking potassium-losing diuretics.
17. Tell client to avoid hot baths, excessive amounts of alcohol, and strenuous exercise within 3 hr of taking medications that promote vasodilatation.
18. Explain that to decrease orthostatic hypotension, the client should arise slowly from bed, sit on side of bed for a few minutes, stand slowly, not stand still for prolonged periods of time, do leg exercises to increase venous return, sleep with head of bed raised or on pillows, and lie or sit down when dizziness occurs.

pertensive drugs (see Table 27-15) and can be a major reason that a male client does not adhere to his treatment regimen. Rather than discussing a personal sexual problem with a health professional, the client often finds it easier to discontinue the drug on his own. Often the nurse must approach the client on this sensitive subject and encourage discussion of any sexual dysfunction he may be experiencing. The sex problems are likely to be easier for the client to discuss and handle once he realizes the drug may be the source of his problem and the side effects can be decreased or eliminated by changing to another antihypertensive drug.

STRESS MODIFICATION. The first approach to stress modification is identification of areas or factors that produce stress for a particular client. The client needs to understand the relationship between stress and hypertension. The nurse and the client should plan ways for the client to handle stress more effectively (see Chapter 5).

EXERCISE. The client needs assistance in developing a graduated exercise program. Isometric exercises should be discouraged. An isotonic exercise program based on the client's current exercise activities can be planned.

HOME MONITORING. Clients should be assessed individually about the feasibility of teaching them and/or a family member to take BP readings at home. For most clients, home BP measurement gives a more valid indication of the BP because the client is more relaxed. It is important to emphasize to the client that a single reading is not as important as a series of readings over a period of time. The client should be instructed to take BP readings weekly (unless otherwise instructed) once the BP has stabilized. A log of the BP measurements should be maintained by the client.

Home BP readings may help to achieve client compliance by reinforcing the need to remain on therapy. Some clients may become excessively concerned with their BP readings when using home monitoring. Generally, however, this practice should reassure the client that the treatment is effective.[27]

CLIENT NONCOMPLIANCE. A major problem in the long-term management of clients with hypertension is poor compliance with the prescribed treatment regimen. The reasons are many and include (1) inadequate client instruction, (2) unpleasant side effects of drugs, (3) subsiding of symptoms so that the client feels "cured," (4) return of BP to normal range while on medication, (5) lack of motivation, (6) high cost of drugs, and (7) lack of a trusting relationship between the client and the health care provider.

Individual assessment to determine the reasons the client is not complying with the treatment regimen and development of an individual plan with the client's assistance are essential. The plan needs to be compatible with the client's personality, habits, and lifestyle. Active client participation increases the likelihood of adherence to the treatment plan. Measures such as involving the client in medication scheduling convenient to a daily routine, helping the client link pill-taking with another daily activity, and involving family members (if necessary) help increase client compliance. Substituting combination tablets for multiple drugs once the BP is stabilized may also facilitate compliance, since the client has to take fewer drugs each day and the cost is less. It is important to help the client and the family understand that hypertension is a chronic condition that cannot be cured but can be controlled with drug therapy, diet therapy, reduction of stress, an exercise program, periodic evaluation, and other relevant lifestyle changes.

Hypertensive Emergencies and Urgencies

Hypertensive emergencies are not as common today as in the past.[18] When they do occur, however, prompt recognition and management are essential to decrease the threat to organ function and life. Hypertensive emergency is a situation in which a client's BP needs to be lowered within 1 hour to avoid worsening of complications. Possible complications include hypertensive encephalopathy, intracranial hemorrhage, acute left ventricular failure with pulmonary edema, dissecting aortic aneurysm, severe hypertension associated with pregnancy, head trauma, extensive burns, unstable angina, and acute MI.[18] *Hypertensive urgency* is a situation in which a client's BP needs to be reduced within a few hours to 24 hours. Examples include accelerated hypertension without immediate complications and severe perioperative hypertension.[20]

Clinical manifestations. A hypertensive emergency is often manifested as *hypertensive encephalopathy,* a syndrome in which a sudden rise in arterial pressure is associated with headache, nausea, vomiting, convulsions, confusion, stupor, and coma. Other common manifestations are blurred vision and transient blindness. The manifestations of encephalopathy are probably due to cerebral edema and spasms of cerebral vessels.

Renal insufficiency ranging from minor impairment to complete renal shutdown may occur. Rapid cardiac decompensation with developing pulmonary edema is also possible.

Client assessment is extremely important, especially monitoring for signs of neurological dysfunction, retinal damage, CHF, pulmonary edema, and renal failure. The neurological manifestations are often similar to the presentation of a CVA. However, a CVA may show focal or lateralizing signs.

Therapeutic management. BP measurement alone is a poor indicator of the seriousness of the client's condition and is not the major factor in deciding the treatment for a hypertensive crisis. The association between elevated BP and signs of new or progressive end-organ damage (e.g., central nervous system, cardiac, or renal damage) determines the seriousness of the situation. Initially, the treatment goal is a 25% decrease in mean arterial pressure with a minimum diastolic pressure of 100 mm Hg.[28] Clients who have aortic dissection may need lower pressures.

True hypertensive emergencies require hospitalization, parenteral administration of antihypertensive drugs, and intensive-care monitoring.[29] However, oral agents may be administered in addition to the parenteral drugs as a more effective means of lowering BP and to help make an earlier transition to long-term therapy. The IV drugs used for hypertensive emergencies are (1) vasodilators such as sodium nitroprusside, nitroglycerin, diazoxide, and hydrala-

zine and (2) adrenergic inhibitors such as phentolamine, trimethaphan, labetalol, and methyldopa.

Sodium nitroprusside is the most effective parenteral drug for the treatment of hypertensive emergencies.[30] The mechanisms of action and the adverse effects of these drugs are presented in Table 27-15. The drugs are administered IV and have a rapid (within seconds to minutes) onset of action. The client's BP and pulse should be taken every 2 to 3 minutes during the initial administration of these drugs. The use of an intraarterial line (see Chapter 28) or an automated BP monitoring machine (e.g., Dynamap) to monitor the BP is ideal, with the cuff pressure being a double check. The rate of administration is titrated according to the level of BP. It is important to prevent hypotension and its effects in a person whose body has adjusted to hypertension. An excessive reduction in BP may cause stroke, MI, or visual changes.[28] Continual ECG monitoring is frequently done to observe for cardiac dysrhythmias. Extreme caution is needed in clients with coronary artery disease or cerebral vascular insufficiency. Hourly urinary output should be measured to assess renal perfusion, which reflects CO.

Hypertensive urgencies usually do not require emergency IV medications but can be managed with oral agents. These clients may not need admission to an ICU.[30] The oral drugs used for hypertensive urgencies, described in Table 27-15, are captopril, clonidine, minoxidil, and nifedipine. Sublingual or oral nifedipine is widely used for hypertensive urgencies, although it has not yet been approved for the treatment of hypertension by the U.S. Food and Drug Administration.[28] Nifedipine has been shown to lower the BP within 10 to 15 minutes, with the maximal reduction in BP occurring within 30 minutes to 1 hour.[29] Biting a nifedipine capsule and swallowing its contents with water, rather than taking the drug sublingually, is recommended in hypertensive urgencies to achieve rapid therapeutic plasma levels of nifedipine, since absorption from the oral cavity is slow and incomplete.[31] However, the disadvantage of oral medications such as nifedipine is the inability to regulate the dosage moment to moment, as can be done with IV medications.

Lowering the BP with the antihypertensive drugs may reverse the crisis in a day or two. If the hypertension cannot be controlled, the prognosis is very poor.

Once the hypertensive crisis is resolved, it is important to determine the cause of the hypertension. The client will need appropriate management and extensive education to avoid future crises.

C *ase Study*

ESSENTIAL HYPERTENSION

Mr. K. is a 49-year-old black man with a strong family history of hypertension. He has not seen a doctor or had his BP checked in many years. Mr. K. was first admitted to the hospital in June with gross hematuria of unknown etiology and hypertension with grade I retinopathy in both eyes. On admission, his BP was 234/134. Physical examination revealed no abnormalities. A laboratory workup was within normal limits except for a urinalysis that revealed occult blood and proteinuria.

He was placed on a low-sodium diet, methyldopa (Aldomet), and chlorothiazide (Diuril). His hematuria cleared up in 1 week, his BP was 180/105, and he was discharged with instructions to continue with his medication.

One year later he was readmitted to the hospital with BP of 170/120. He complained of severe chest pains with syncope, sharp occipital headaches, and dyspnea. An ECG showed an inferior wall MI with ischemic ST changes. Eye examination revealed grade II retinopathy in the left eye and grade I retinopathy in the right eye. Mr. K. admitted to taking his medication rarely and missing several of his clinic appointments for BP checks.

Discussion Questions

1. What risk factors related to hypertension were present in Mr. K.'s situation? What are other possible risk factors?
2. What evidence of target organ damage was present on the first admission?
3. Explain the rationale for his therapy.
4. What client-teaching measures should have been included in Mr. K.'s nursing care on his first admission?
5. What further evidence of target organ damage was present on his second admission?
6. What nursing interventions may help this client become more consistent in following the recommended treatment regimen?

R eview Questions

The number of the question corresponds to the same-numbered objective at the beginning of the chapter.

1. Mechanisms that regulate normal BP include all the following *except*
   a. parathormone feedback
   b. CO
   c. SVR
   d. renin-angiotensin mechanism
2. Shock is best defined as
   a. cardiovascular collapse
   b. vasodilatation
   c. inadequate tissue perfusion
   d. acute pump failure
3. A type of shock that results from vasodilatation is
   a. diabetic shock
   b. septic shock
   c. cardiogenic shock
   d. hemorrhagic shock
4. Which of the following events occurs during intermediate or progressive shock?
   a. massive sympathetic nervous system stimulation
   b. stimulation of aortic and carotid sinus baroreceptors
   c. severe brain anoxia
   d. movement of fluid into the intravascular space
5. Which one of the following organs is adversely affected first by arterial vasoconstriction, resulting in shunting of blood?
   a. heart
   b. lung
   c. brain
   d. kidney
6. Which of the following fluids is generally used in the initial resuscitation of hemorrhagic shock?
   a. Ringer's lactate
   b. packed red cells
   c. dextran
   d. plasma
7. If tolerable, the appropriate position for the client in shock is
   a. Trendelenburg
   b. high Fowler's
   c. reverse Trendelenburg
   d. supine with legs elevated
8. Which of the following is *not* considered a risk factor in hypertension?
   a. rural living
   b. family history of hypertension
   c. being a black male
   d. increasing age
9. Complications of hypertension include
   a. rheumatic heart disease and renal disease
   b. retinal damage and MI
   c. CHF and diabetes
   d. stroke and pheochromocytoma
10. What is the most common problem in the management of hypertension?
    a. The disease is too complicated to treat adequately.
    b. Clients fail to adhere to the treatment regimen.
    c. Hypertensive drugs are seldom effective.
    d. There is a sudden onset of retinal complications.
11. What condition occurs more commonly in the older adult population?
    a. increased elasticity of the peripheral arteries
    b. decreased sensitivity to most drugs
    c. increased renal excretion and/or hepatic metabolism
    d. postural hypotension
12. Many of the antihypertensive drugs have which adverse effect in common?
    a. bradycardia
    b. orthostatic hypotension
    c. sexual dysfunction
    d. hypokalemia
13. Which of the following is *not* a true statement regarding hypertensive emergencies?
    a. Sodium nitroprusside is the most effective parenteral drug for treating this condition.
    b. True hypertensive emergencies require hospitalization and intensive-care monitoring.
    c. Examples of hypertensive emergencies include hypertensive encephalopathy and intracranial hemorrhage.
    d. There are situations in which BP should be reduced within 3 to 24 hours.

REFERENCES

1. Peters J and Utset O: Vasopressors in shock management: choosing and using wisely, J Crit Illness 4:62-68, 1989.
2. Andreoli K and others: Comprehensive cardiac care, ed 6, St Louis, 1987, The CV Mosby Co, p 124.
3. Wahl S: Septic shock: how to detect it early, Nursing 19:52-59, 1989.
4. Wasserman S: Anaphylaxis. In Middleton E, Reed CE, and Ellis EF, eds: Allergy: principles and practices, ed 2, St Louis, 1983, The CV Mosby Co, p 689.
5. Meyers K and Hickey M: Nursing management of hypovolemic shock, Crit Care Nurse 11:57-67, 1988.
6. Reskenov L: Cardiogenic shock, Chest 83:893-898, 1983.
7. Mayberry-Toth B and Landron S: Complications associated with acute myocardial infarction, Crit Care Nurse Q 12:49-63, 1989.
8. Perry A: Shock complications: recognition and management, Crit Care Nurse Q 11:1-8, 1988.
9. Memmer M: Acute orthostatic hypotension, Heart Lung 17:134-140, 1988.
10. Thompson J and others: Cardiogenic shock: causes, diagnosis, and management, J Crit Illness 2:22-36, 1987.
11. Rice V: Shock management, part II: pharmacologic intervention, Crit Care Nurse Q 5:42-57, 1985.
12. Rice V: Shock management, part I: fluid volume replacement, Crit Care Nurse Q 4:69-82, 1984.
13. Hancock B and Eberhard N: The pharmacologic management of shock, Crit Care Nurse Q 11:19-29, 1988.
14. Soto-Aguilar M: Anaphylaxis: why it happens and what to do about it, Postgrad Med 82:154-170, 1987.
15. Luce J: Pathogenesis and management of septic shock, Chest 91:883-888, 1987.
16. Bone R and others: A controlled clinical trial of high-dose methylprednisolone in the treatment of severe sepsis and septic shock, N Eng J Med 317:653-665, 1987.
17. Hinshaw L and others: Effect of high-dose glucocorticoid therapy on mortality in patients with clinical signs of systemic sepsis, N Engl J Med 317:659-665, 1987.
18. US Department of Health and Human Services: The 1988 report of the Joint National Committee on Detection, Evaluation, and Treatment of High Blood Pressure, Washington, DC, 1988, Public Health Service, National Institutes of Health, p 5.
19. Subcommittee on Definition and Prevalence of the 1984 Joint National Committee: Hypertension prevalence and the status of awareness, treatment, and control in the United States, Hypertension 7:457-468, 1985.
20. Hill M and Cunningham S: The latest words for high BP, Am J Nurs 89:504-508, 1989.
21. US Department of Health and Human Services: The 1988 Report of the Joint National Committee on Detection, Evaluation, and Treatment of High Blood Pressure, Washington, DC, 1988, Public Health Service, National Institutes of Health, p 36.
22. Lipsitz L: Hypertension in the elderly, Hosp Pract 24:119-141, 1989.
23. Valle B and Lemberg L: Syncope in the elderly, Heart Lung 18:426-429, 1989.
24. Frolich E: Calcium antagonists for initial therapy of hypertension, Heart Lung 18:370-375, 1989.
25. Frolich E and others: Recommendations for human blood pressure determination by sphygmomanometers: report of a special task force appointed by the steering committee, American Heart Association, Hypertension 11:210A-222A, 1988.
26. MacMahon S and Norton R: Alcohol and hypertension: implications for prevention and treatment, Ann Intern Med 5:124-125, 1986.
27. Hunt J and others: Devices used for self-measurement of blood pressure, Arch Intern Med 145:2231-2234, 1985.
28. Drugs for hypertensive emergencies, Med Letter, pp 32-34, May 1989.
29. Gonzales D and Ram V: New approaches for the treatment of hypertensive urgencies and emergencies, Chest 93:193-195, 1988.
30. Dequattro V: Treating hypertensive crisis: which drug for which patient? J Crit Illness 2:24-35, 1987.
31. VanHarten J and others: Negligible sublingual absorption of nifedipine, Lancet 2:1363-1364, 1987.

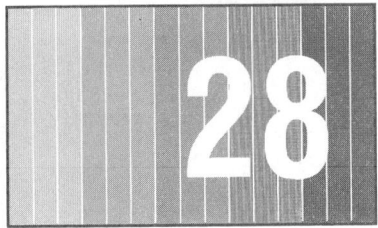

Nursing Role in Management

Coronary Artery Disease

Mary Ann Cammarano House
Linda Griego

---

*L*earning Objectives

1. Describe the etiology and pathophysiology of coronary artery disease.
2. Explain the nursing role in health promotion and maintenance related to risk factors for coronary artery disease.
3. Describe the precipitating factors, types, clinical presentation, and therapeutic, pharmacological, and surgical management of sudden cardiac death.
4. Describe the precipitating factors, types, clinical manifestations, and therapeutic and pharmacological management of angina pectoris.
5. Explain the nursing role in the management of the client with angina pectoris.
6. Describe the pathophysiology of myocardial infarction from the onset of injury through the healing process.

7. Describe the clinical manifestations, complications, diagnostic study abnormalities, and therapeutic management of myocardial infarction.
8. Describe the nursing role in the rehabilitative management of the client following myocardial infarction.
9. Identify the emotional and behavioral reactions to myocardial infarction.
10. Explain the significance of an exercise program following myocardial infarction.
11. Describe the principles of hemodynamic monitoring and related nursing management.
12. Describe the purpose and function of the intraaortic balloon pump.
13. Describe the management of cardiogenic shock.

CORONARY ARTERY DISEASE

Coronary artery disease (CAD) is a type of blood vessel disorder that is included in the general category of atherosclerosis. *Atherosclerosis* is derived from two Greek words: *athere,* meaning "fatty mush," and *skleros,* meaning "hard." This word combination indicates that atherosclerosis begins as soft deposits of fat that harden with age. Atherosclerosis is often referred to as "hardening of the arteries." Although this condition can occur in any artery in the body, the atheromas (fatty deposits) have a preference for the coronary arteries. Arteriosclerotic heart disease (ASHD), cardiovascular heart disease (CVHD), ischemic heart disease (IHD), coronary heart disease (CHD), and CAD are synonymous terms used to describe the disease process. Other terms used to describe the disease mechanisms involved in CAD are *plaque formation, atheromatous deposits,* and *coronary occlusions.*

Significance

CAD is the major cause of death in the United States (Fig. 28-1). The American Heart Association reports that almost 514,000 persons die yearly of heart attacks. Although this has decreased by 85,000 deaths per year since 1980, heart attacks, or myocardial infarctions (MIs), are still the leading cause of all cardiovascular disease deaths and deaths in general. An estimated 66,890,000 persons have one or more forms of heart disease. The estimated prevalence of the major cardiovascular diseases is presented in Fig. 28-2.

Etiology and Pathophysiology

Atherosclerosis is the major cause of CAD. It is characterized by a focal deposit of cholesterol and lipids, primarily within the intimal wall of the artery. The genesis of plaque formation is the result of complex interactions between the components of the blood and the elements forming the vascular wall.[1] The concept of endothelial injury is central to current theories of atherogenesis. Table 28-1

Reviewed by Beverly Hydo, R.N., M.S.N., Clinical Nurse Specialist, Medical Nursing, William Beaumont Hospital, Royal Oak, Michigan.

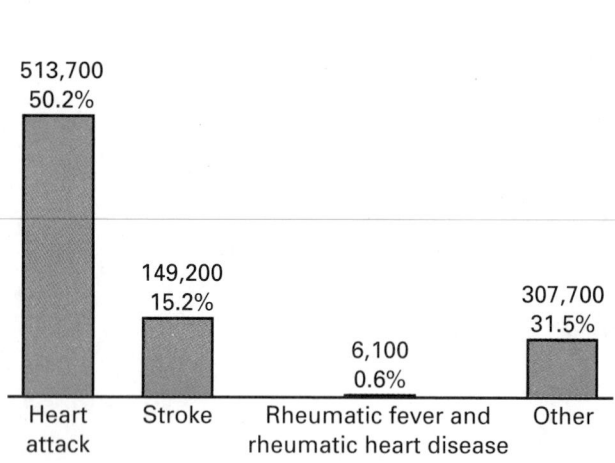

Fig. 28-1 Deaths due to cardiovascular diseases. (From American Heart Association, Heart Facts, National Center, Dallas, 1990.)

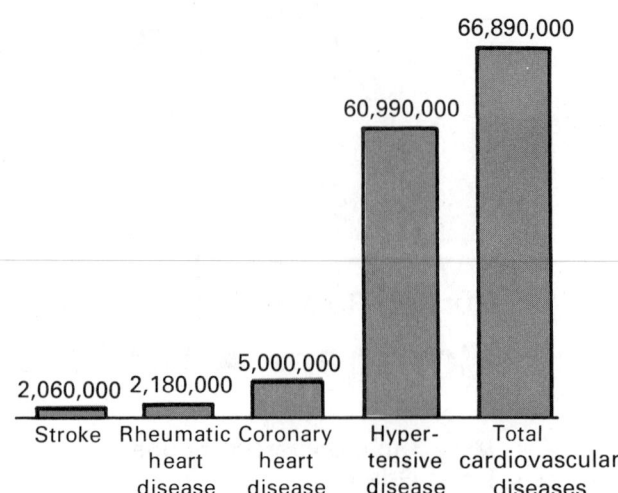

Fig. 28-2 Estimated prevalence of the major cardiovascular diseases. (From American Heart Association, Heart Facts, National Center, Dallas, 1990.)

Table 28-1 Theories of Atherogenesis

ENDOTHELIAL INJURY

Endothelium is "injured" by hyperlipidemia, hypertension, or other chemical irritants. Factors are released into the subendothelium and induce the migration of smooth muscle cells into the intima. Smooth muscle cells initiate synthesis of collagen, elastic fiber proteins, and proteoglycans (a substance that tends to provide a nonthrombogenic surface). Intracellular and extracellular lipids begin to accumulate, as well as platelets and other clotting factors, and a lesion-associated superimposed thrombus is formed.

LIPID INFILTRATION

Lipids from the circulation enter the endothelium and accumulate in smooth muscle in response to mechanical or inflammatory trauma. Lipoproteins become trapped and damage occurs. Endothelial permeability is altered.

AGING

Atherosclerotic changes occur in everyone and become more evident as aging progresses.

THROMBOGENIC

Red blood cells, platelets, and lipids accumulate along the intima of arteries. Microthrombi form. Platelets aggregate, releasing substances that alter endothelial permeability. The thrombus extends and reactivates the cycle.

VASCULAR DYNAMICS

Mechanical factors (e.g., hypertension) increase intraluminal pressure, which leads to altered membrane permeability, resulting in increased lipid infiltration.

CAPILLARY HEMORRHAGE

Lipids accumulate in plaques as a result of capillary hemorrhage.

LIPID METABOLIC

Low-density lipoproteins migrate into the arterial wall, accumulating in the intimal and medial layers of the artery. Cholesterol is deposited by the low-density lipoproteins.

---

summarizes theories of atherogenesis, with endothelial injury being the leading theory for the cause of atherosclerotic disease.

Intact normal endothelium is nonreactive to platelets and leukocytes as well as coagulation, fibrinolytic, and complement factors. However, the endothelial lining can be altered as a result of chemical injuries, such as hyperlipidemia (nondenuding), or high-shear stress, such as hypertension (denuding). With either type of endothelial alteration, platelets are activated and release a growth factor that stimulates smooth muscle proliferation. The smooth muscle cell proliferation entraps lipids, which are calcified over time and form an irritant to the endothelium upon which platelets adhere and aggregate. Thrombin is generated, and fibrin formation and thrombi occur (Fig. 28-3). Endothelial replication is normally very slow in adults, but in the presence of hypertension and hyperlipidemia, increased cell turnover leads to transient repeated denuding of the endothelium.

Development stages. CAD takes many years to develop. When it becomes symptomatic, the disease process is usually well advanced. The stages of development in

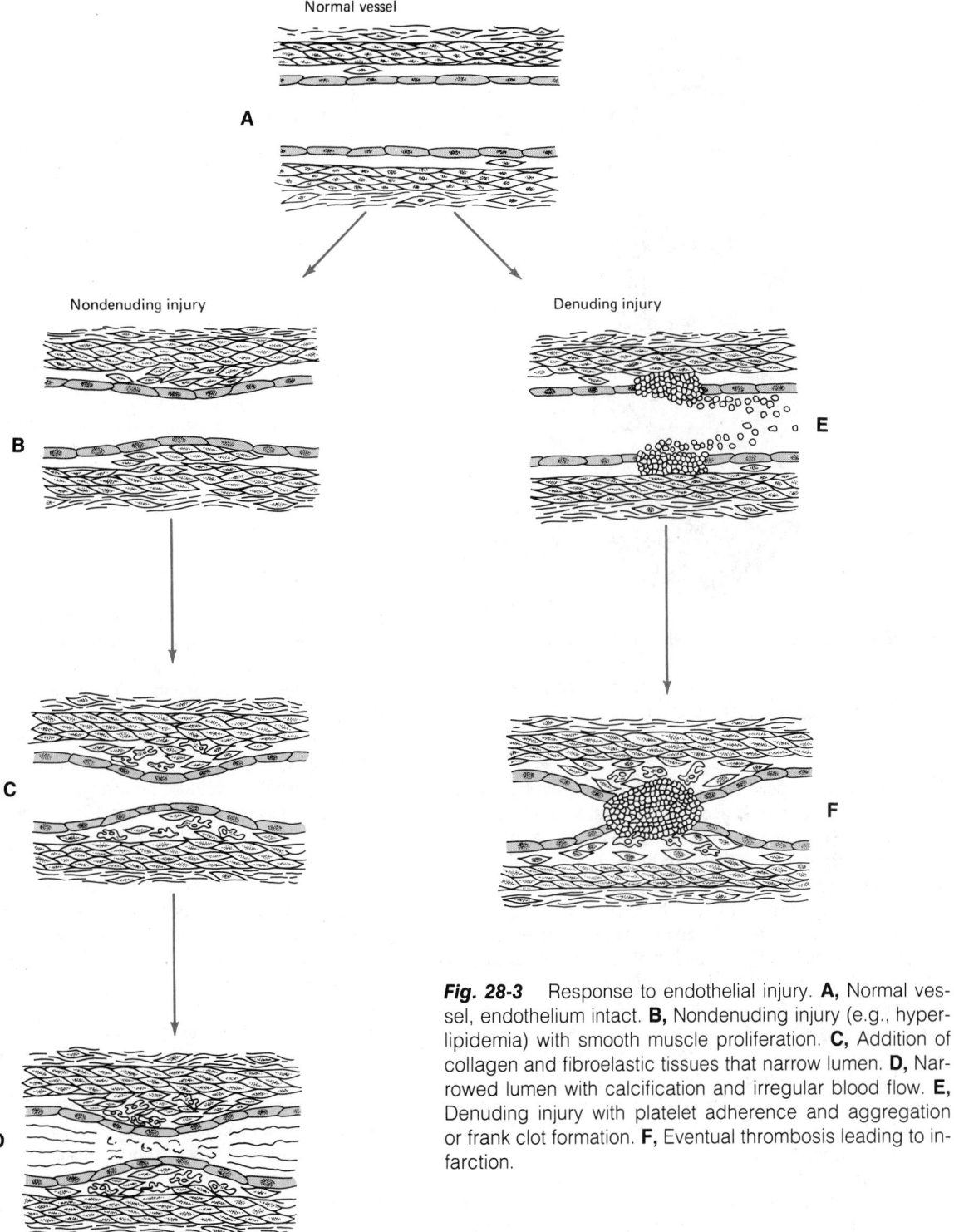

Normal vessel

A

Nondenuding injury

B

C

D

Denuding injury

E

F

Fig. 28-3 Response to endothelial injury. **A,** Normal vessel, endothelium intact. **B,** Nondenuding injury (e.g., hyperlipidemia) with smooth muscle proliferation. **C,** Addition of collagen and fibroelastic tissues that narrow lumen. **D,** Narrowed lumen with calcification and irregular blood flow. **E,** Denuding injury with platelet adherence and aggregation or frank clot formation. **F,** Eventual thrombosis leading to infarction.

atherosclerosis are (1) fatty streak; (2) smooth muscle cell proliferation, which creates a raised fibrous plaque; and (3) complicated lesion (Fig. 28-4).

Fatty streak. Fatty streaks are the earliest lesions of atherosclerosis and are characterized by lipid-filled smooth muscle cells. As streaks of fat develop within the smooth muscle cells, a yellow tinge appears. Fatty streaks are usually observed in the coronary arteries by age 15 and involve an increasing amount of surface area as the client ages. It is generally believed that they are reversible.

Raised fibrous plaque. The raised fibrous plaque stage is the beginning of progressive changes in the arterial wall.

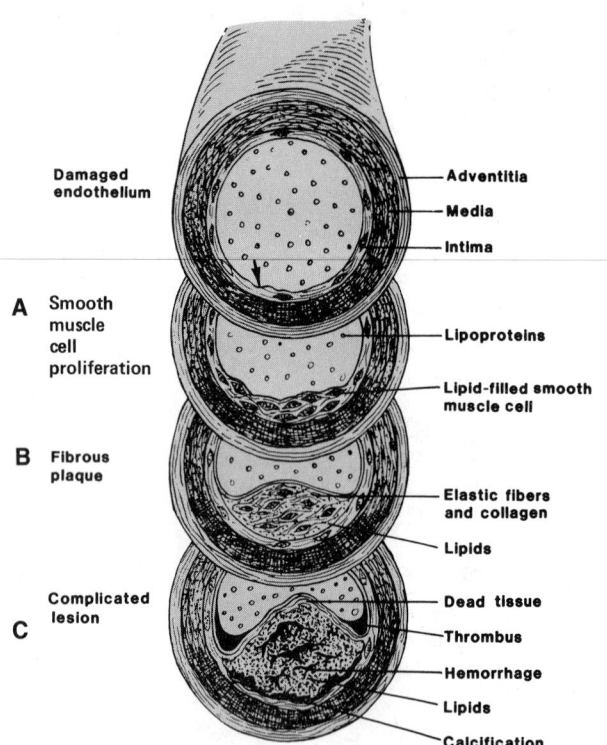

Fig. 28-4 The stages of development in the progression of atherosclerosis include, **A,** smooth muscle cell proliferation, which creates, **B,** a raised fibrous plaque and, **C,** a complicated lesion. (After Herb Smith.)

These changes appear in the coronary arteries by the age of 30 and increase with age. The arterial wall changes are initiated by chronic endothelial injury that results from many factors, including elevated blood pressure (BP), high blood cholesterol, heredity, carbon monoxide produced by smoking, and possibly toxic substances within the blood. Normally the endothelium repairs itself immediately, but in persons with CAD the endothelium is *not* rapidly replaced, allowing low-density lipoproteins and growth factor from platelets to stimulate smooth muscle proliferation and thickening of the arterial wall. Once endothelial injury has occurred, lipoproteins (the carrier substances within the bloodstream) transport cholesterol and other lipids into the arterial intima (Fig. 28-4). Lipids may cause smooth muscle damage as well as contribute to plaque thickening and instability. As these lipids and other substances pass through the vessels, they adhere to the roughened, damaged wall, thereby causing the lesion buildup or structural abnormality. Collagen tissue, elastic fibers, and smooth cells filled with fat cover the lesion. The fibrous plaque looks grayish or whitish.

Platelets also play a part in the overgrowth of smooth muscle cells. Once the artery's inner wall has become damaged, platelets may accumulate in large numbers, leading to a thrombus. The thrombus may adhere to the wall of the artery, leading to narrowing or total occlusion of the artery.

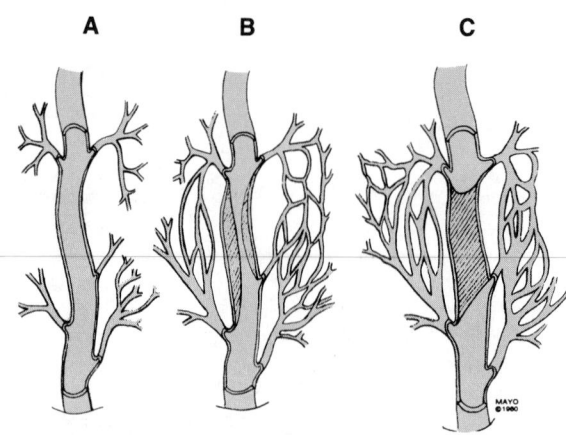

Fig. 28-5 Vessel occlusion with collateral circulation. **A,** Open, functioning coronary artery. **B,** Partial coronary artery closure with collateral circulation being established. **C,** Total coronary artery occlusion with collateral circulation bypassing the occlusion to supply the myocardium. (Courtesy Mayo Clinic, Rochester, Minn.)

Complicated lesion. The final stage in the development of the atherosclerotic lesion is the most dangerous. The plaque consists of a core of lipid materials (mainly cholesterol) within an area of dead tissue. With the incorporation of lipids, thrombi, damaged tissue, and some accumulation of calcium, the growing lesion becomes complex. As the lesion continues to grow and becomes complex, dark, hardened, necrotic tissue appears within the arteries, causing rigidity and hardening. This complex lesion may totally or partially occlude the artery.

Collateral circulation. Normally, some arterial branching (called *collateral circulation*) exists within the coronary circulation. The growth of collateral circulation is attributed to two factors: (1) the inherited predisposition to develop angioblastic properties and (2) the presence of chronic ischemia. When an atherosclerotic plaque occludes the normal flow of blood through a coronary artery and ischemia is chronic, increased collateral circulation develops (Fig. 28-5). When occlusion of the coronary arteries occurs slowly over a long period of time, there is a greater chance of adequate collateral circulation developing, and the myocardium may still receive an adequate amount of oxygen. However, with rapid-onset CAD or coronary spasm, the time is inadequate for collateral development, and a diminished arterial flow results in a more severe ischemia or infarction. Clinically, the younger person is frequently seen to have the more severe infarction as a result of inadequate collateral formation.

Risk Factors

Risk factors are characteristics or conditions that are statistically associated with a high incidence of a disease. Many risk factors have been associated with atherosclerosis; the three most significant ones are elevated serum lipids, hypertension, and cigarette smoking.[2]

These correlations are derived from studies of very

Table 28-2 Risk Factors in Coronary Artery Disease

Unmodifiable	Modifiable
Age	**Major**
Gender (men > women until 60 yr of age)	Elevated serum lipids
	Hypertension
Race (blacks < whites)	Cigarette smoking
Genetic predisposition and family history of heart disease	Diabetes mellitus*
	Minor
	Obesity (>30% overweight)
	Sedentary lifestyle
	Stressful lifestyle

*May be hereditary.

large populations. Risk factors in different populations may vary in prominence. For example, glucose intolerance has been found to be a major risk factor in European populations but only a minor one in United States populations. Major risk factors in the United States, such as high serum cholesterol and hypertension, are less prevalent in Japanese, Puerto Rican, and Hawaiian populations.

Risk factors can be categorized as unmodifiable and modifiable (Table 28-2). *Unmodifiable* risk factors are age, gender, race, and genetic inheritance. *Modifiable* risk factors include elevated serum lipids, hypertension, smoking, obesity, sedentary lifestyle, and stress in daily living. Although control of diabetes is recommended, it has not been proven to decrease the incidence of CAD.

Data on risk factors have been obtained in several major studies. In the Framingham study (one of the most widely known), 5209 men and women were observed for 20 years.[2] Over time, it was noted that elevated serum cholesterol (> 240 mg/dl), elevated systolic BP (≥ 160 mm Hg), and cigarette smoking (one or more packs a day) were correlated with an increased incidence of CAD. The younger the subject at the time of induction to the study, the more predictive were the values. Other implicated risk factors and indicators included altered carbohydrate tolerance, sedentary lifestyle, electrocardiographic (ECG) abnormalities, and reduced lung vital capacity.

The Evans County, Georgia, longitudinal study looked at differences in risk factors between blacks and whites.[3] Blacks manifested a lower incidence of risk in all categories. Occupation seemed to be the only clue to the differences. Blacks engaged in more activity and physical labor than the more sedentary whites. Blacks are known to be at higher risk of hypertension (see Chapter 27).

The Western Collaborative Group longitudinal study addressed psychosocial issues of behavior in relation to risk factors.[4] Personal characteristics such as competitiveness, high-achievement orientation, impatience, time urgency, excessive drive and hostility, and abrupt speech and gestures are described as type A behaviors (see p. 784).

Unmodifiable risk factors

Age, gender, and race. The incidence of the first MI is greater for the white, middle-aged man. After the age of 60, the incidence in men and women equalizes, although there is early evidence to suggest that more women are being seen with CAD earlier because of increased stress, increased cigarette smoking, presence of hypertension, and use of birth control pills. Blacks, although more prone to hypertension, are at less risk of CAD than whites of the same age. MIs in the Oriental population in the United States are less frequent than in whites, but the rates are higher than in the countries of origin.

Family history and heredity. Genetic predisposition is an important factor in the occurrence of CAD, although the exact mechanism of inheritance is not fully understood. Some congenital defects in coronary artery walls predispose to the formation of plaques. Familial hyperlipoproteinemia, an autosomal dominant trait, has been strongly associated with CAD at early ages. In most cases of angina or MI, the client can name a close family member who has died either suddenly of an unknown cause or of a documented heart attack.

Diabetes mellitus. The incidence of CAD is greater among persons who have diabetes, even those with well-controlled blood sugars, than the general population. Clients with diabetes manifest CAD not only more frequently but also at earlier ages. There is no age difference between diabetic men and women for the onset of manifestations of CAD. Diabetes virtually eliminates the lower incidence of cardiovascular disease in women. Latent diabetes is frequently diagnosed at the time of infarction. Because persons with diabetes have an increased tendency toward connective tissue degeneration, it is thought that this condition may account for the tendency toward atheroma development seen in the diabetic population.

Modifiable risk factors

Elevated serum lipids. An elevated serum lipid level is one of the three most firmly established risk factors in CAD.[5] The various types of serum lipids are presented in Fig. 28-6. More specifically, the risk of CAD is associated with a serum cholesterol level of more than 200 mg/dl or a fasting triglyceride level of more than 150 mg/dl. The liver is capable of producing cholesterol from saturated fats, even when the dietary intake of fats is severely limited. A high correlation between cholesterol and triglyceride levels has been found. Elevated triglyceride levels are correlated with obesity and a sedentary lifestyle.

For lipids to be used and transported by the body, they need to become soluble in blood by combining with proteins. Lipids combine with protein to form macromolecules called *lipoproteins*. Lipoproteins are vehicles for fat mobilization and transport. The different types of lipoprotein vary in composition and are classified as high-density lipoproteins (HDLs), low-density lipoproteins (LDLs), and very-low-density lipoproteins (VLDLs) (see Fig. 28-7 and Chapter 26).

HDLs contain more protein by weight and less lipid than any other lipoprotein. HDLs carry lipids away from arteries and to the liver for metabolism (Fig. 28-8). There-

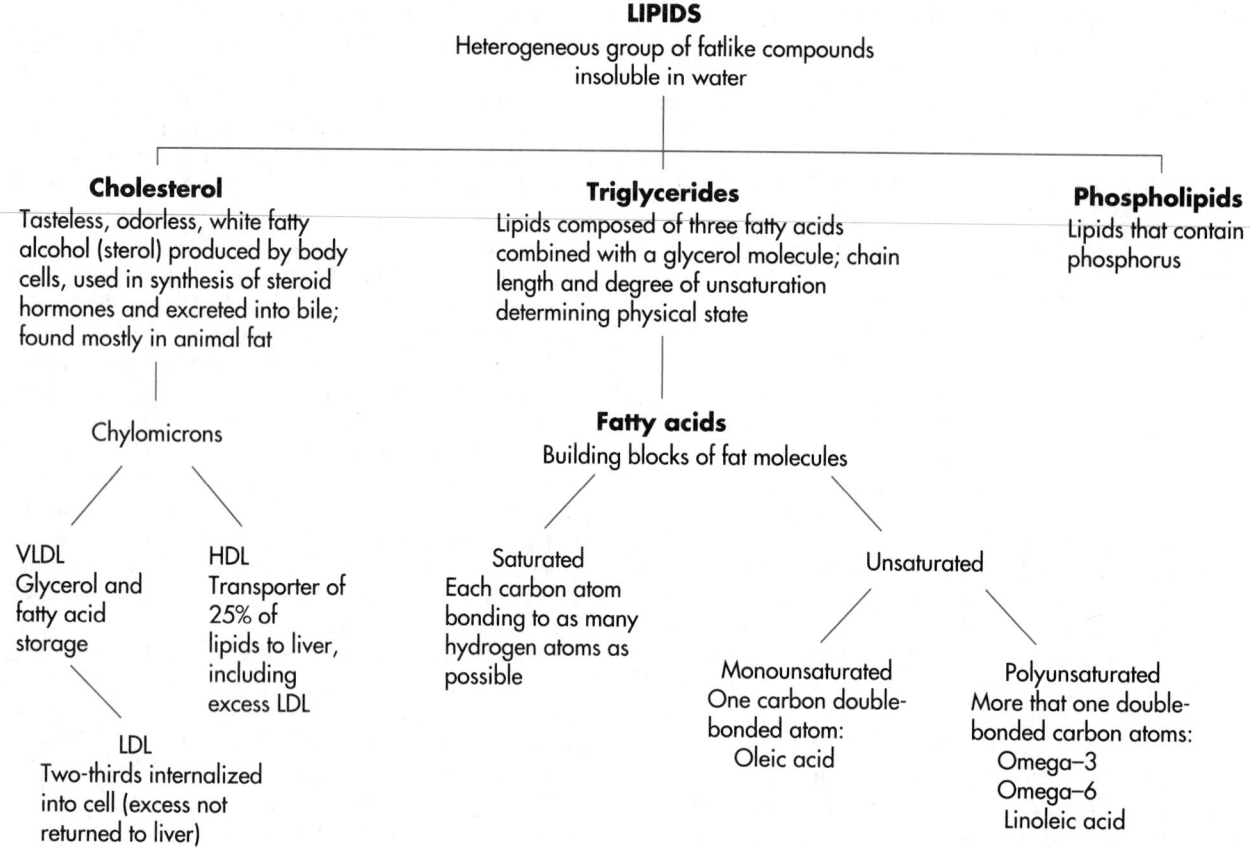

Fig. 28-6 Types of serum lipids. (Modified from Schell M: Cholesterol, lipoproteins, lipid profiles: a challenge in patient education, Focus Crit Care 17:204, 1990.)

fore high serum HDL levels are desirable. This process of HDL transport prevents lipid accumulation within the arterial walls. The higher the HDL levels in the blood, the lower the risk of CAD. HDL levels are generally higher in women than in men and are increased by physical activity. Persons who have had an MI have lower concentrations of HDL than matched controls. In general, HDL levels are high in children and women, decrease with age, and are lowest in persons with CAD. Current research on drug and dietary therapy is concentrating on ways to elevate HDL levels.

HDLs are broken down into HDL_2 and HDL_3. HDL_2 seems to protect the arteries from developing atherosclerosis. Exercise significantly raises HDL_2, which helps to clear out the fat load from the blood plasma. It is also interesting to note that premenopausal women have roughly three times greater HDL levels than men. After menopause their HDL_2 levels quickly approximate those of men.

LDLs contain more cholesterol than any of the other lipoproteins and have an affinity for arterial walls.[6] Elevated LDL levels correlate most closely with an increased incidence of atherosclerosis. Therefore low serum LDL levels are desirable.

VLDLs contain most of the triglycerides. The direct correlation of VLDLs with heart disease is uncertain. High VLDL concentrations may increase the risk of premature atherosclerosis when associated with other factors such as diabetes, hypertension, and cigarette smoking.

Hypertension. The second primary risk factor in CAD is hypertension, which is defined as a BP greater than or equal to 140/90 mm Hg. In the Framingham study a three-fold increase in the incidence of CAD was reported for middle-aged men with arterial pressures exceeding 160/95 mm Hg compared with those with BPs of 140/90 mm Hg or less. The cause of hypertension in 90% of those affected is unknown, but it is usually controllable with diet or medication.

The stress of a constantly elevated BP increases the rate of atherosclerotic development. This is related to the shearing stress, causing denuding injury of the endothelial lining. Atherosclerosis, in turn, causes narrowed, thickened arterial walls and decreases the distensibility and elasticity of vessels. More force is required to pump blood through diseased arterial vasculature, and this increased force is reflected in a higher BP. This increased work load is also manifested by an enlarged heart (cardiac hypertrophy) and/or a loss of efficiency with each contraction. Salt intake is positively correlated with elevated BP because of fluid retention, adding volume and increasing systemic vascular resistance (SVR) to the cardiac work load.

Smoking. The third primary risk factor in CAD is cigarette smoking. Pipe and cigar smokers have not been

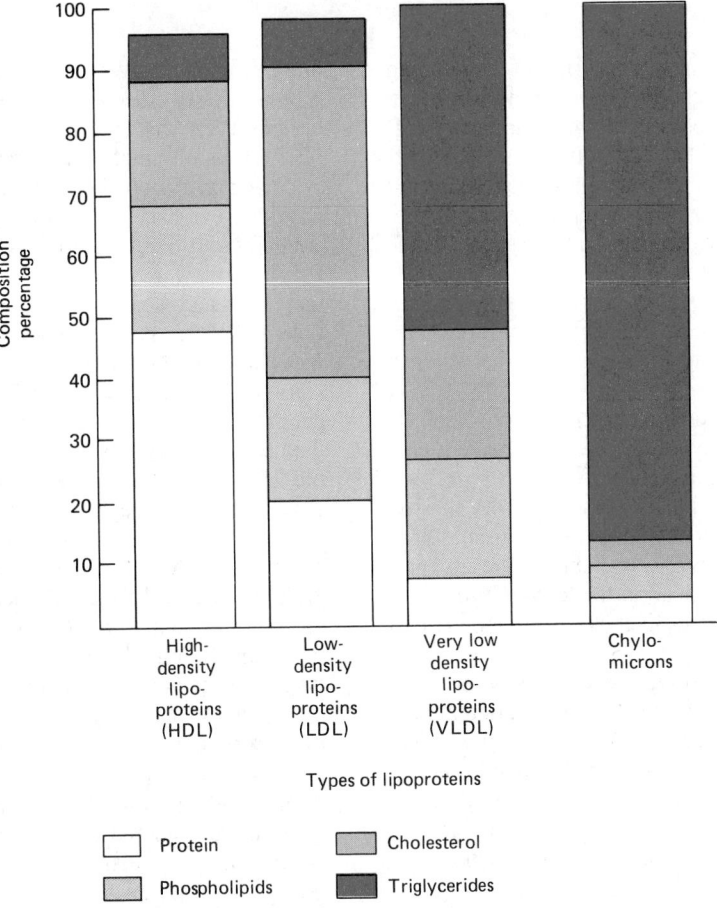

Fig. 28-7 Composition of various types of lipoproteins.

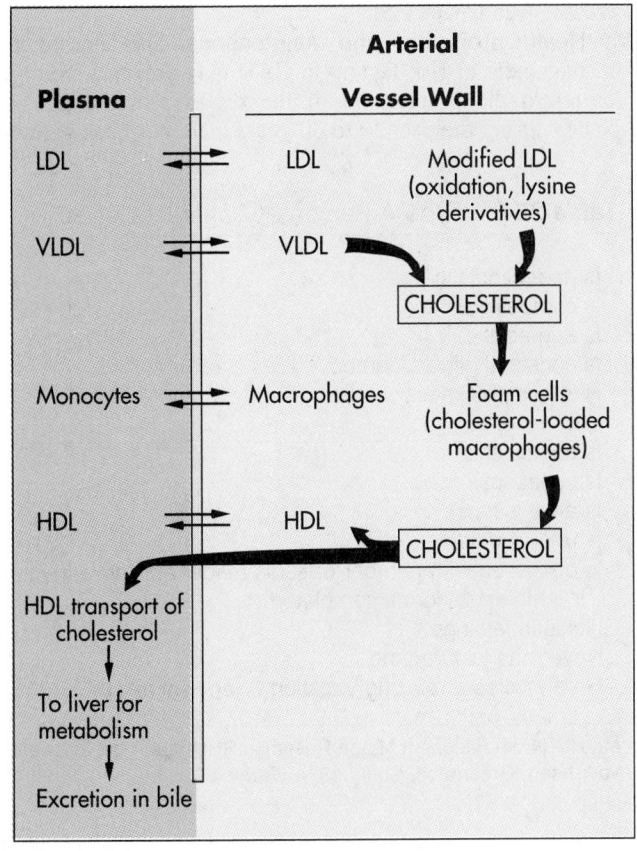

Fig. 28-8 Specific types of plasma lipoproteins *(LDL and VLDL)* deliver cholesterol to cells of the blood vessel wall, mostly to macrophages that become cholesterol foam cells. These are predominant early features of atherosclerotic lesions. *HDL* is an important cholesterol-transporting carrier, delivering cholesterol to the liver to be excreted in the bile.

found to have an increased risk. The risk of developing CAD is two to six times higher in cigarette smokers than in nonsmokers.[7] Risk is proportional to the number of cigarettes smoked. Changing to lower nicotine or a filter does not affect risk. Cessation of smoking has been shown to reduce the risk to nonsmoker levels after a period of time.

Nicotine in the cigarette smoke causes catecholamine (epinephrine, norepinephrine) release. These hormones cause an increased heart rate (HR), increased BP, and peripheral vasoconstriction. These changes increase the cardiac work load, necessitating greater myocardial oxygen consumption.

Carbon monoxide, a by-product of combustion, affects the oxygen-carrying capacity of hemoglobin by reducing the sites available for oxygen transport. Thus, the effects of an increased cardiac work load, combined with the oxygen-depleting effect of carbon monoxide from smoking, significantly decrease the oxygen available to the myocardium. There is also some indication that carbon monoxide may be a chemical irritant as well, thus causing nondenuding injury to the endothelium.

Obesity. *Obesity* is defined as a weight 30% or more than that considered standard for a person's height and body build. The mortality from CAD is statistically higher in obese persons than in those of normal weight. The increased risk is proportional to the degree of obesity. However, obesity in the absence of other high-risk factors probably subjects a person to only a modest increase in risk. Obese persons are thought to produce increased levels of LDL, which are strongly implicated in atherosclerosis. Obesity is often associated with hypertension. Hypertension is three times more likely to develop in obese persons than in those with normal weight. Obesity does not lead to hypertension, but hypertension is present in 60% of obese clients. As obesity increases, the heart size grows, causing increased myocardial oxygen consumption.

Sedentary lifestyle. A sedentary lifestyle implies a lack of adequate physical exercise on a regular basis. Some practitioners define regular physical exercise as exercise that occurs at least three times a week for at least 30 minutes, causing perspiration and an increase in the HR by 30 to 50 beats per minute (bpm). The role of physical activity, or the lack of it, as a cardiac risk factor is complex and the study of this factor is only beginning. There is evidence to suggest that physically inactive persons are more prone to develop CAD. Some occupational studies have indicated that jobs involving heavy physical activity are associated with a lower risk than sedentary jobs, but a confounding variable is socioeconomic status, which may be responsible for some of the risk association.

The mechanism by which a sedentary lifestyle predisposes to CAD is still unknown. It is thought that (1) physically active people have increased HDL levels and that (2) exercise enhances fibrinolytic activity, thus reducing the risk of clot formation. The theory that exercise encourages the development of collateral circulation has not been effectively demonstrated in human beings.

Exercise training for those who are physically inactive is thought to decrease the risk of CAD through more efficient lipid metabolism, increased HDL_2 production, and more efficient oxygen extraction from the working muscle groups, thereby decreasing the cardiac work load. It may be observed that physically active persons are seldom obese, thus eliminating two risk factors in CAD.

Stress and behavior patterns. The Framingham study provided evidence that certain behaviors and lifestyles are conducive to the development of CAD.[8] Type A and type B behaviors were described by Friedman and Rosenman in the 1960s and were further elaborated in the 1970s by Jenkins and Zyzanski. Type A behaviors include perfectionism and a hardworking, driving personality. Type A persons suppress anger and hostility, have a sense of time urgency, are impatient, and create stress and tension within themselves, often when a situation does not warrant it (Table 28-3). They are more prone to heart attacks than type B persons, who are more easygoing, take upsets in stride, know their limitations, take time to relax, are not overachievers, and are able to keep priorities in perspective. Although not all characteristics are present in one person all the time, people *tend* to be type A or type B.

In the Framingham study, type A women manifested twice the incidence of CAD and three times the incidence of angina seen in type B women. Among type A men, there was a twofold risk of angina, MI, and CAD compared with type B men.[8]

Sympathetic stimulation and its effect on the heart is generally considered to be the physiological mechanism by which stress predisposes to the development of CAD. Sympathetic stimulation causes an increased release of epinephrine and norepinephrine from the adrenal medulla. This stimulation influences the heart by increasing the HR and intensifying the force of myocardial contraction. Therefore the demand for oxygen consumption greatly increases (see Chapter 5).

Health promotion and maintenance. The appropriate management of risk factors in CAD may prevent, modify, or retard the progression of the disease. In the United States during the past 20 to 30 years there has been a grad-

Table 28-3 Type A Personality Characteristics

Is perfectionistic
Is competitive
Is aggressive
Is constantly time oriented
Has hurry sickness
Can never say "no"
Is compulsive
Is impatient
Is always tense
Is unduly irritable
Is obsessed with number of sales made, articles written, clients seen, forms completed
Holds in feelings
Never has leisure time
Rarely takes a relaxing vacation or any vacation

Modified from Friedman M and Roseman RH: Type A behavior and your heart, Greenwich, Conn, 1974, Fawcett.

ual and persistent decline in coronary deaths. The decline can be attributed to the efforts of consumers to become generally healthier and individual initiatives to alter hazardous lifestyles. Emphasis on prevention and early treatment of heart disease must be ongoing.

Identification of high-risk persons. In both the acute-care setting and the community, the nurse needs to identify persons at high risk of CAD. Screening for high risk involves obtaining personal and family histories. Clients are questioned about a family history of heart disease in parents, grandparents, or siblings. The presence of any cardiovascular symptoms should be noted. Environmental factors, such as eating habits, type of diet, and level of exercise, are assessed to elicit lifestyle patterns. A psychosocial history is included to determine smoking habits, alcohol ingestion, type A behaviors, recent life stresses (events), sleeping habits, and the presence of anxiety or depression. The place of work and the type of work can yield important information on the kind of activity performed; exposure to pollutants, allergens, or noxious chemicals; and the degree of emotional stress associated with employment.

The interviewer seeks to identify the client's attitudes and beliefs about health and illness. This information can give some indication of how disease and lifestyle changes may affect the client and can reveal possible misconceptions about heart disease. Knowledge of the client's educa-

tional background is frequently helpful in deciding at what level to begin teaching. If the client is taking medications, it is important to know what they are, when they are taken, and what the client's attitude is regarding the taking of medications.

Management of high-risk persons. Once high-risk persons are identified, preventive measures can be taken. Risk factors such as age, gender, and genetic inheritance cannot be modified. However, the person with any of these risk factors can modify the risk of CAD by controlling or changing the additive effects of modifiable risk factors. For example, a young man with a family history of heart disease can decrease the risk of an MI by maintaining an ideal weight, getting adequate physical exercise, reducing intake of saturated fats, and not smoking.

Persons who have modifiable risk factors need to be encouraged and motivated to make changes in their lifestyle to reduce the risk of heart disease. The nurse can play a major role in teaching health-promoting behaviors to persons at risk of CAD (Table 28-4). For highly motivated persons, knowing *how* to reduce this risk may be the only information needed to get them make changes.

For those who are less motivated to assume responsibility for their health, the idea of risk factor reduction may be so remote that they are unable to bring the threat of CAD into their real world. Especially in the absence of symptoms, few desire to make lifestyle changes. The nurse

Table 28-4 Management of Risk Factors in Coronary Artery Disease

Risk Factor	Health-Promoting Behaviors	Risk Factor	Health-Promoting Behaviors
Hypertension	Have regular blood pressure checkups; take prescribed medications for blood pressure control; reduce salt intake; stop smoking; control or reduce weight	Elevated serum lipids	Reduce animal (saturated) fat intake; reduce total fat intake; adjust total caloric intake to achieve and maintain ideal body weight; engage in regular exercise program; increase amount of complex carbohydrates and vegetable proteins in diet
Smoking	Enroll in structured program to stop smoking if support system is needed; change daily routines associated with smoking to reduce desire to smoke; substitute other activities for smoking; ask family members to support efforts to stop smoking	Sedentary lifestyle	Develop and maintain routine for physical activity that is done at least three times a week; increase activities to a fitness level
Obesity	Change eating patterns and habits; reduce caloric intake; exercise regularly to increase caloric expenditure; avoid fad and crash diets, which are not effective in the long run; avoid large, heavy meals	Stressful lifestyle	Increase awareness of behaviors that are detrimental to health; alter patterns that are conducive to stress and rushing (e.g., get up 30 min earlier so breakfast is not eaten on way to work; take 20 min day to meditate); set realistic goals for self; reassess priorities in light of health needs; learn to cope with unavoidable stress; avoid excessive and prolonged stress; plan time for adequate rest and sleep
Diabetes mellitus*	Follow the recommended diet; reduce weight and control diet; monitor blood glucose levels regularly		

*See Chapter 43 for additional health-promoting behaviors.

PRINCIPLES OF LOW-FAT DIET

Visible fat (e.g., butter, cream, margarine, salad dressing, cooking oil) is restricted to 1 tsp per meal.
Only lean meats, skim milk, and no more than 7 eggs per week are used.
Foods high in fat content (e.g., avocados, fat, meat, olives, nuts) are avoided.
Foods are not prepared with added fat for cooking.

PRINCIPLES OF LOW-CHOLESTEROL, LOW-SATURATED-FAT DIET

The fat content of the diet is modified to increase the ratio of polyunsaturated fatty acids to saturated fatty acids.
Organ meats are restricted because they are high in cholesterol although low in total fat.
Only 2 whole eggs per week are used because egg yolk is high in cholesterol. Egg white may be used as desired.
Vegetable oils are used in cooking and food preparation. Coconut and palm oils are not allowed because of their high content of saturated fats.
If weight reduction is desired, caloric level should be specified.

	Low-Fat Diet			Low-Cholesterol, Low-Saturated-Fat Diet		
SAMPLE MENUS						
Breakfast						
1 fruit	½ cup orange juice	1 banana	¼ cantaloupe	½ cup orange juice	1 banana	¼ cantaloupe
1 starch	¾ cup dry cereal	½ cup oatmeal	½ cup corn meal mush	¾ cup dry cereal	½ cup oatmeal	½ cup corn meal mush
1 egg	1 poached egg	1 hard-boiled egg	1 scrambled egg	Low-cholesterol egg	1 corn tortilla with 1 tsp special vegetable oil margarine	1 slice toast with 1 tsp special vegetable oil margarine
1 starch	1 slice toast with 1 tsp butter or margarine	1 flour tortilla	1 slice toast with 1 tsp butter or margarine	1 slice toast with 1 tsp special vegetable oil margarine	1 cup skim milk	1 cup skim milk
1 fat	1 cup skim milk	1 skim milk	1 cup skim milk	1 cup skim milk	Coffee with sugar	Coffee with sugar
1 skim milk	Coffee with sugar	Coffee with 1 tsp cream	Coffee with sugar	Coffee with sugar		

	Low-Fat Diet			Low-Cholesterol, Low-Saturated-Fat Diet		
Lunch						
2 meat	2 oz baked chicken	2 oz lean hamburger	2 oz baked fish	Baked chicken (skinless)	¾ cup dry cottage cheese with peach slices	Fried fish (scale fish only, cooked with allowed oils)
1 starch	Mashed potato	Hamburger bun	Baked potato	Mashed potato with 1 tsp special vegetable oil margarine	Saltine crackers	Fried potatoes (cooked with allowed oils)
1 vegetable	Tossed salad with vinegar, lemon juice	Lettuce, tomato, pickle	Zucchini	Tossed salad with vinegar, vegetable oil margarine	Cucumber and tomato slices	Zucchini
1 starch	Bread with 1 tsp margarine or butter	1 tsp mayonnaise	Bread with 1 tsp butter or margarine	Angel food cake	1 tsp special vegetable oil margarine	Cornbread (made with allowed oils)
1 fat	Angel food cake	Sherbet	Gelatin dessert	Iced tea with sugar and lemon	Sherbet	Gelatin dessert
1 dessert	Iced tea with sugar and lemon	Carbonated beverage	Lemonade		Carbonated beverage	Lemonade

	Low-Fat Diet			Low-Cholesterol, Low-Saturated-Fat Diet		
Dinner						
2 meat	2 oz lean roast beef	Green chili stew (made with 2 oz lean beef cubes, potato slices, tomato, chili)	2 oz lean pork chop	Lean roast beef	Green chili stew (made with lean beef cubes, potato slices, tomato, chili)	Breaded lean pork chop
1 starch	Rice	1 flour tortilla	Corn on the cob	Rice with 1 tsp special vegetable oil margarine	1 corn tortilla with 1 tsp special vegetable oil margarine	Corn on the cob with 1 tsp special vegetable oil margarine
1 vegetable	Green beans	Pudding (made from skim milk and egg whites)	Okra	Green beans	Pudding (made from skim milk and egg whites)	Okra
1 starch	Dinner roll with 1 tsp butter or margarine	Fruit punch	Bread with 1 tsp margarine or butter	Dinner roll with 1 tsp special vegetable oil margarine	Fruit punch	Biscuit (made with allowed oils)
1 fat	Canned peach		Watermelon slice	Canned peach		Watermelon slice
1 fruit	1 cup skim milk		Buttermilk	1 cup skim milk		Buttermilk
1 skim milk						

should first assist these persons in clarifying their personal values. Then, by explaining the risk factors and having them identify their own vulnerability to various risks, the nurse may help them to recognize their susceptibility to CAD. Some persons will prove recalcitrant until they begin to manifest overt symptoms or actually suffer an infarction. Others, having suffered a heart attack, may find the idea of changing lifelong habits totally unacceptable. The nurse must be able to identify such attitudes and respect them as human rights.

Physical fitness. The last two decades have seen a surge of interest in attaining and maintaining health. Physical fitness has become a field of major importance. A 1984 Harris poll determined that 59% of the people in the United States engage in regular exercise, a 24% increase since 1961.[9] Communities are developing exercise programs for persons of all ages and with all health needs, ranging from "Slimnastic" aerobic exercise classes to cardiac walking-jogging programs. Local YMCAs often sponsor exercise classes, jogging courses, bicycling courses, and related offerings. Jogging has become a science. Many shopping malls open their doors in the early morning to allow people to walk indoors. The American Heart Association takes pride in its annual "Run for Your Life" race as well as other events dramatizing the need for physical activity to promote health. Many large corporations provide gymnasiums where their employees can exercise. For many people, running may be inadvisable; these people should be encouraged to pursue walking, swimming, or whatever exercise will accommodate their individual physical abilities.

Health education in schools. The recent awareness of the body and physical health is also seen in school systems. School nurses have an important role in teaching good health practices. Besides teaching physical fitness topics, the school nurse can inform students on how the body functions and responds to daily living. Lifestyle habits can be positively influenced at early ages to decrease the need for drastic changes later in life that confront the students' parents. The school nurse must take advantage of the social climate that promotes health and health practices and find innovative ways to present these values to a receptive, youthful audience before the habits of that audience become inflexible. Health awareness programs have been initiated as early as preschool to try to establish health patterns for life. Follow-up on the effectiveness of early childhood health education will not yield data on cardiac risk for many years to come, yet the energy and effort to change lifestyle patterns cannot be left until adulthood when habits are set. Nurses can provide valuable consultation to schools and the educational process at all levels.

Nutritional considerations. Clients with elevated serum cholesterol and triglyceride levels should first achieve a normal weight.[10] Then they should be maintained on a diet that emphasizes a decreased intake of saturated fat and cholesterol (Table 28-5). Red meats, eggs, and milk products are major sources of saturated fat and cholesterol. If the serum triglyceride level is elevated, alcohol intake should be reduced or eliminated. Although there is no conclusive relationship between sodium intake and hypertension, the client at risk of CAD should avoid excessive sodium intake.

The role of dietary management is not yet well defined. None of the current dietary regimens used to treat hyperlipidemia have demonstrated a significant reduction in morbidity and mortality from CAD.

Pharmacological management. Persons with serum cholesterol levels above 200 mg/dl are at high risk of CAD and should be treated. Treatment usually begins with diet restriction, decreased dietary fat content, lower cholesterol intake, and exercise instruction. Serum cholesterol levels are redrawn after 3 months of diet therapy. If they remain elevated, drug therapy may be started (Table 28-6). Various pharmacological agents are available to treat hyperlipidemia[11] (Table 28-7).

Drugs that increase lipoprotein removal. The major route of elimination of cholesterol is via conversion to bile acids in the liver. Two bile acid–sequestering agents are currently available. These resins primarily lower LDL cholesterol and also cause an increase in HDL. The resins are nonabsorbable compounds that interfere with the enterohepatic circulation of bile acids. There is increased conversion of cholesterol to bile acids and decreased hepatic cholesterol content, resulting in an increased number of LDL receptors.

The two resins that are available are cholestyramine (Questran) and colestipol (Colestid). Recently a new preparation of cholestyramine (Colybar), containing 4 g of cholestyramine in a bar form, has become available for clients. Administration of these drugs can be associated with complaints related to palatability and with a variety of upper and lower gastrointestinal (GI) complaints, including constipation, abdominal pain, belching, heartburn, and nausea.

The resins have been known to interfere with absorption of other drugs, such as warfarin, thiazides, thyroid hormones, and β blockers. Separating the time of administra-

Table 28-6 Guidelines for Treatment of High Blood Cholesterol in Adults

Decision	Basis	Cholesterol, mmol/l (mg/dl)		
		Desirable	Borderline-High	High
LDL estimation	Total C	<5.2 (200)	5.2-6.1 (200-239)*	>6.2 (240)
Treatment				
Diet	LDL	<3.4 (130)	3.4-4.1 (130-159)*	>4.2 (160)
Drug†	LDL			>5.1 (190) or >4.2 (160)*

From National Cholesterol Education Program, Dallas, American Heart Association.
*Becomes high-risk if definite CAD or more than two risk factors are present.
†After a trial of diet alone.

Table 28-7 Drugs Used to Treat Hyperlipoproteinemia

Name	Mechanisms of Action	Side Effects	Nursing Considerations
Cholestyramine (Questran, Colybar)	Is bile acid–binding resin, increases production of LDL receptors in liver, increases synthesis of cholesterol for use by liver as bile acids	Unpleasant gritty quality to taste, GI disturbances (e.g., nausea, dyspepsia, constipation), skin rash	Be aware that drug is effective and safe for long-term use, that side effects diminish with time, and that drug interferes with absorption of digoxin, thiazides, β blockers, fat-soluble vitamins, folic acid.
Colestipol (Colestid)	Same as cholestyramine	Same as cholestyramine	Same as cholestyramine.
Nicotinic acid (niacin, Nicobid, Niac, Nicospan)	Inhibits synthesis and secretion of VLDL and LDL from liver, increases HDL levels	Hot flashes and pruritus in upper torso and face, GI disturbances (e.g., nausea and vomiting, dyspepsia, diarrhea)	Be aware that most side effects subside with time and that decreased liver function and dysrhythmias may occur with high doses. Have client take aspirin ½ hour before drug to prevent flushing and take drug with meal.
Clofibrate (Atromid)	Promotes lipolysis of VLDL and reduces hepatic VLDL synthesis, reduces triglyceride levels	Nausea, diarrhea, weight gain, increased liver enzymes	Monitor liver function tests.
Gemfibrozil (Lopid)	Reduces hepatic VLDL synthesis and inhibits VLDL secretion, reduces triglyceride levels	Mild GI disturbances (e.g., nausea and diarrhea)	Be aware that drug is generally well tolerated.
Lovastatin (Mevacor)	Increases liver rate of LDL removal from plasma, decreases liver synthesis of LDL	Rash, mild GI disturbances, insomnia, elevated liver enzymes, lens opacities	Be aware that drug is well tolerated with few side effects. Monitor client with liver function tests and eye examinations.
Probucol (Lorelco)	Inhibits oxidation and tissue deposition of LDL, promotes clearance of LDLs, decreases cholesterol synthesis	Nausea, diarrhea, flatulence, abdominal pain, prolonged QT interval	Monitor ECG at intervals. Be aware that taking drug with meals may decrease side effects.

tion of the resins from that of other drugs may decrease this side effect.

Drugs that restrict lipoprotein production. *Nicotinic acid* (niacin) is a B vitamin that has been used in conjunction with diet therapy. Nicotinic acid is highly effective in lowering cholesterol and triglyceride levels by interfering with their synthesis. Side effects of this drug may include severe flushing, pruritus, and GI distress.

Clofibrate (Atromid) is effective primarily in lowering serum triglyceride levels and has some cholesterol-lowering activity as well. It appears to act by decreasing the synthesis of lipids. Side effects include malaise, nausea, diarrhea, and occasional increases in liver enzymes.

Gemfibrozil (Lopid) is primarily effective in lowering VLDL levels and triglycerides, and it also increases HDL cholesterol. Most clients tolerate the drug well. Complaints may include GI irritability.

Lovastatin (Mevacor) is a new type of drug. It is a competitive inhibitor of the biosynthesis of cholesterol. Most clients may be successfully treated with either 20 mg or 40 mg per day. Side effects include rash, GI symptoms, insomnia, elevated liver enzymes, and possible opacities of eye lenses. A baseline eye examination may be required before administration of this drug is started.

Drug therapy for hyperlipidemia is likely to be prolonged, perhaps continuing for a lifetime. It is essential that diet modification be used with the greatest effect to minimize the need for drug therapy. Clients must fully understand the rationale and goals of treatment as well as the safety and side effects of drugs.[12]

Coronary Artery Disease in Older Adults

The incidence of cardiac disease is markedly increased in older adults and is the leading cause of death in older persons. Angina can be disabling in this population, and affected persons must place increased reliance on health care services to remain independent.[13,14]

The nurse caring for the older adult with CAD must be aware of the physiological changes that occur in the cardiovascular system. Structural changes in the myocardium include (1) increased collagen and fat deposition, (2) myofibrillar degeneration, and (3) endocardial thickening.[13,15] Calcification of the heart valves and degeneration of the conduction system can also occur. The majority of pacemakers are placed in persons more than 65 years of age. Also, resting HR decreases with age, and maximum HR with exercise decreases with age.

In older adults, loss of elastic fiber and increased collagen in the arterial media diminish elasticity and distensibility of arteries.[15] These changes cause an increase in systolic BP and increased SVR. These combined changes lead to a decrease in cardiac output (CO) by 1% per year. This is probably secondary to decreased contractility of the myocardium and increased afterload caused by the increase in SVR. Decreased arterial wall elasticity blunts the responsiveness to baroreceptors in the aortic arch as well.[15] Circulating norepinephrine levels are also increased with age. However, receptors may be less responsive to catecholamines.

The nurse must be aware of these changes in older adults and must keep in mind the effect they could have on the care of these clients. Because older adults have decreased responsiveness to catecholamines, their response to stress may be blunted; HR may not rise as quickly in response to pain or to declining CO. They may have atypical symptoms when experiencing an acute MI. The sudden occurrence of symptoms such as profound weakness and dyspnea should be investigated. In addition, many of the antianginal agents that cause postural hypotension may not be well tolerated secondary to the decreased responsiveness of the baroreceptors. The client who has been on bed rest should sit for 3 to 5 minutes before ambulating. Also, antianginal agents that can slow HR must be used with caution in these clients, who may have degeneration of the conduction system. These clients may be at increased risk of drug toxicity because of declining hepatic and renal function.

The older client should be included in any cardiac rehabilitation program. Up to 50% of diminished function in older adults can be attributed to inactivity.[13] Activity performance, endurance, and ability to tolerate stress can be improved in the older adult with physical training. Positive psychological benefits can be derived from a planned exercise program and can include increased self-esteem, heightened emotional well-being, and improved body image.[16] The endurance type of aerobic exercise rather than strength-building isometric exercise should be encouraged.

When planning an exercise program for the older adult, nurses should remember the following: (1) longer warm-up periods are needed, (2) longer periods of low-level activity or longer rest periods between sessions are advisable, and (3) heat intolerance may be caused by decreased ability to sweat efficiently. Clients should be taught to avoid exercising in extremes of temperature and to maintain a moderate pace. Target HR for older adults is 60% to 75% of the maximum HR. They should exercise a minimum of 30 minutes three times a week, with no more than 2 days between activities.[13]

By knowing the changes that can occur in the older adult's cardiovascular system, the nurse can assist clients with CAD to live with their disease and to maximize their activity.

CLINICAL MANIFESTATIONS

There are three major clinical manifestations of CAD: sudden cardiac death, angina pectoris, and acute MI.

Sudden Cardiac Death

Sudden cardiac death is the unexpected collapse and cardiopulmonary arrest of a previously well-appearing person within minutes to 1 hour after the onset of acute symptoms. It occurs secondary to natural (not accidental or traumatic) causes.[17] The afflicted person may or may not have a documented prior history of cardiovascular disease.

Significance. Sudden cardiac death accounts for approximately 400,000 deaths per year in the United States or, roughly, one death per minute. It is the leading cause of death in industrialized nations.[18] A study conducted by Sharma and Wyeth[19] found that of 1070 persons who experienced sudden cardiac death, 325 survived the initial cardiopulmonary arrest. Only 120 of these sudden cardiac death survivors were discharged from the hospital without neurological impairment. Long-term follow-up of this survivor group revealed that only 44% were still alive after 6 years and that the vast majority of deaths in the survivor group were due to recurrent sudden cardiac death. Other studies indicate that of those persons who survive sudden cardiac death, 25% die in the first year after the event and 36% die within 2 years.[20,21]

Etiology. In most instances, sudden cardiac death occurs as a primary manifestation of CAD, and victims usually have multivessel coronary atherosclerosis. Many of these persons, however, have no known history of cardiovascular disease. Less commonly, sudden cardiac death may occur as a result of a primary left ventricular outflow obstruction. These obstructions may be secondary to such diseases as aortic stenosis, idiopathic hypertrophic subaortic stenosis (IHSS), and coarctation of the aorta.

Persons who experience sudden cardiac death as a result of CAD fall into two groups: (1) those who had an acute MI and (2) those who did not have an acute MI. The latter group accounts for the majority of cases (approximately 75%) of sudden cardiac death.[21] In this instance, victims usually offer no warning signs or have no known precedent symptoms. Typically, death is a result of dysrhythmia formation, usually ventricular tachycardia, ventricular fibrillation, or both. These clients are at risk of recurrence of sudden death, probably because of continued electrical instability of the myocardium that caused the initial event to occur.

The second, smaller group of clients includes those who have had acute MI and have suffered sudden cardiac death. In these cases the clients usually do have prodromal symptoms, such as chest pain and dyspnea, and they have less chance of recurrent sudden cardiac death than those who have not had MI.

Risk factors. Persons at increased risk of sudden cardiac death include those with the following risk factors:

1. Male gender
2. Family history of premature atherosclerosis
3. Cigarette smoking
4. Diabetes
5. Hypercholesterolemia

Therapeutic management. Survivors of sudden cardiac death generally require a diagnostic workup to determine whether they have had an acute MI. Thus serial cardiac isoenzymes and ECGs must be obtained, and the client must be treated accordingly (see pp. 798-801). In addition, since most persons with sudden cardiac death have CAD secondary to multivessel coronary atherosclerosis, cardiac catheterization is indicated to determine the possible location and extent of coronary artery occlusion. Percutaneous transluminal cutaneous angiography or coronary artery bypass graft surgery may be indicated (see Chapter 29).

Most sudden cardiac death clients have a lethal dysrhythmia that is associated with a high incidence of recurrence. Thus it is useful to know when those persons are most likely to have a recurrence and what pharmacological regimen is the most effective treatment. Around-the-clock Holter monitoring and exercise stress testing may help elicit this information. An *electrophysiology study (EPS)* is most useful in aiding in this determination. This examination is performed under fluoroscopy; pacing electrodes are placed in selected intracardiac areas, and stimuli are selectively used to attempt to evoke dysrhythmias. The client's response to various antidysrhythmic medications can thus be determined and monitored in a controlled environment.

Most commonly, clients who have experienced sudden cardiac death can be treated with antidysrhythmic medications such as procainamide, quinidine, flecainide, and amiodarone. Some selected clients, however, are largely refractory to pharmacological therapy and may require the surgical implantation of a ventricular defibrillator (see Chapter 30).

The nurse caring for a survivor of sudden cardiac death needs to be attuned to the client's psychosocial adaptation to this sudden "brush with death." Many of these clients develop a "time bomb" mentality. They fear the recurrence of cardiopulmonary arrest and may become anxious, angry, and depressed. Their families are likely to experience the same feelings. The grief response varies among persons and families. The nurse should be attuned to the specific needs of the client and the family and educate them accordingly while providing appropriate emotional support.

Angina Pectoris

Angina pectoris is literally translated as pain (angina) in the chest (pectoris). Myocardial ischemia is expressed symptomatically as angina. More specifically, angina pectoris is transient chest pain due to myocardial ischemia. It usually lasts for only a few minutes (3 to 5) and commonly subsides when the precipitating factor (usually exertion) is relieved. Typical exertional angina should not persist

Table 28-8 Factors Determining Myocardial Oxygen Needs

Decreased Oxygen Supply	Increased Oxygen Demand or Consumption
↓ Hematocrit	↑ Heart rate
↓ Hemoglobin-binding capacity	↑ Contractility
↓ Coronary blood flow	↑ Left ventricular wall tension
↑ Diastolic pressure	↑ Systolic BP
↑ Coronary vascular resistance	↑ Ventricular volume
Coronary spasm	↑ Myocardial wall thickness
↓ Blood volume	

longer than 20 minutes after rest and/or administration of nitroglycerin.

Pathophysiology. Myocardial ischemia develops when the demand for myocardial oxygen exceeds the ability of the coronary arteries to supply it (Table 28-8). The primary reason for insufficient flow is narrowing of coronary arteries by atherosclerosis. Although skeletal muscle extracts only 20% of available oxygen and maintains a reserve, the myocardium (at rest) extracts 75% to 85% of the available oxygen. If myocardial oxygen needs are not met from this near-maximum extraction, coronary blood flow is increased through vasodilatation and increased rate of flow.

In persons with CAD, the coronary arteries are unable to dilate to meet increased metabolic needs because they are already chronically dilated beyond the obstructed area. For ischemia due to atherosclerosis to occur, the artery is usually 75% or more stenosed. In addition, the diseased heart has difficulty increasing the rate of flow. This creates an oxygen deficit. In addition to atherosclerotic stenosis, oxygen deficit is caused by coronary artery spasm and coronary thrombosis. In coronary artery spasm the constriction is transient and reversible and causes either subtotal or total narrowing of the coronary artery. The coronary artery spasm is usually associated with an underlying atherosclerotic plaque, although spasms do occur in arteries without significant stenosis. The duration of the spasm determines whether the myocardium will sustain ischemia (not resulting in cell death) or actual infarction (resulting in cell death).

Coronary thrombosis resulting from ulceration of a plaque with subsequent fibrin and platelet aggregation leading to clot formation was thought to be the cause of coronary occlusion. It is now known that thrombosis, stenosis, and spasm are all causes of coronary occlusion and the resulting angina pectoris.

Other factors responsible for a discrepancy between myocardial oxygen needs and oxygen supply include low BP, low blood volume, drugs causing vasoconstriction, valvular disorders, stenosis of the coronary ostia (either congenital or secondary to syphilis), and aortic stenosis. Excessive catecholamine stimulation (e.g., from cocaine intoxication and overdose), anemia, oxygen-hemoglobin disorders, and chronic lung disease may also contribute to myocardial ischemia.

The left ventricle is most susceptible to ischemia and injury because of its higher myocardial oxygen demand, larger mass, higher wall tension, and higher systemic pressures. Ischemia causes transient left ventricular dysfunction resulting in an increased left ventricular diastolic pressure. Ischemia also causes elevated pulmonary capillary wedge pressure (PCWP) and elevated right-sided heart pressure. These three factors eventually increase the oxygen deficit of the myocardium. Dysrhythmias may occur in the presence of myocardial ischemia because of cellular irritability. Dysrhythmias decrease the efficiency of the cardiac pump and thereby increase the need for myocardial oxygen while decreasing the available supply.

Research indicates that up to 90% of ischemia is asymptomatic. This type of ischemia is referred to as *silent ischemia*. This phenomenon occurs in clients with and without diabetes mellitis–related neuropathy. This creates an iceberg phenomenon, in which the angina is merely the tip of the iceberg. Ischemia with pain (angina) or without pain has the same prognosis. Diabetes mellitus and hypertension are associated with an increased prevalence of silent ischemia. It is imperative to remember that when ischemia is present, whether it is asymptomatic or manifest as angina, the myocardium is at risk.

On the cellular level, the myocardium becomes cyanotic within the first 10 seconds of coronary occlusion. ECG changes appear. With total occlusion of the coronary arteries, contractility ceases after several minutes, depriving the myocardial cells of glucose for aerobic metabolism. Anaerobic metabolism begins and lactic acid accumulates. Myocardial nerve fibers are irritated by the increased lactic acid and transmit a pain message to the cardiac nerves and upper thoracic posterior roots (the reason for referred cardiac pain to the left shoulder and arm). Under ischemic conditions, cardiac cells are viable for about 20 minutes. With restoration of blood flow, aerobic metabolism resumes and contractility is restored. Cellular repair also begins.

Precipitating factors. Extracardiac factors may precipitate myocardial ischemia and anginal pain. These include the following:

1. Physical exertion, which increases the HR: Increasing the HR decreases the time the heart spends in diastole, which is the time of greatest coronary blood flow. Walking outdoors is the most common form of exertion that produces an attack. Isometric exertion of the arms, as in raking leaves, painting, or lifting heavy objects, also causes exertional angina.
2. Strong emotions, which stimulate the sympathetic nervous system and increase the work of the heart: This results in an increase in HR, BP, and myocardial contractility.
3. Consumption of a heavy meal (especially if the person exerts afterward), which can increase the work of the heart: During the digestive process, blood is diverted to the GI system, causing a low flow rate in the coronary arteries.
4. Temperature extremes, either hot or cold, which increase the work load of the heart (blood vessels constrict in response to a cold stimulus; blood vessels dilate and blood pools in the skin in response to a hot stimulus): Cold weather also causes increased metabolism to maintain internal temperature regulation.
5. Cigarette smoking, which causes vasoconstriction and an increased HR because of nicotine's stimulation of catecholamine release: It also diminishes available oxygen by increasing the level of carbon monoxide.
6. Sexual activity, which increases the cardiac work load and sympathetic stimulation: In a person with severe CAD, the resulting extra work load of the heart may precipitate angina.
7. Stimulants, such as cocaine or caffeine, which cause increased HR and subsequent myocardial oxygen demand: Stimulation of catecholamine release is the precipitating factor.

Types

Stable angina. *Stable angina (classic)* refers to chest pain occurring intermittently over a long period of time with the same pattern of onset, duration, and intensity of symptoms. Stable angina is usually exercise induced. Pain at rest is unusual. An ECG usually reveals ST segment depression, indicating subendocardial ischemia. The discomfort may be mild or severe and disabling, but it is usually infrequent because the person restricts activities so that pain is not precipitated.

Unstable angina. *Unstable angina (progressive, crescendo,* or *preinfarctional angina)* is different from stable angina. Unlike stable anginas, it is unpredictable. It is easily provoked by minimal or no exercise, during sleep, or even at total rest. Unstable angina is associated with increased stenosis of vessels and multivessel involvement. Recent findings associate unstable angina with deterioration of a once stable atherosclerotic plaque. This lesion can progress to an MI, or it can heal. The frequency, duration, and intensity of symptoms of unstable angina increase dramatically (usually over a 3-month period) as the disease in the vessels rapidly progresses, culminating in infarction within 18 months after its onset. It is believed that unstable angina may have a spasm component to it and is frequently treated with calcium channel blockers (see p. 796). An unstable lesion is believed to be at increased risk of thrombosis, which is why aspirin or systemic anticoagulation is the treatment of choice.

Prinzmetal's angina. *Prinzmetal's angina* (variant angina) often occurs at rest, usually in response to spasm of a major coronary artery. The spasm may occur in the absence of atherosclerotic disease, as well as with documented disease. Prinzmetal's angina is not usually precipitated by increased physical demand. Coronary spasm can be described as a strong contraction of smooth muscle in the coronary artery caused by an increase in intracellular calcium ions. Factors that may precipitate coronary artery spasm include increased myocardial oxygen demand and increased levels of a variety of substances (e.g., histamine, angiotensin, epinephrine, norepinephrine, and pros-

Table 28-9 Comparison of the Pain of Angina Pectoris and Myocardial Infarction

Angina	Myocardial Infarction
PRECIPITATING FACTORS	
Stress, either physiological (exertion) or psychological	Exertion or at rest
Digestion of a heavy meal	Physical or emotional stress
Valsalva maneuvers during micturition or defecation	Often no precipitating factors or any factor associated with angina
Extremes of weather	
Hot baths or showers	
Sexual excitation	
LOCATION	
Midanterior chest	Midanterior chest
Substernal	Substernal
Abdominal with radiation to neck, back, arms, fingers	Subscapular, midscapular
Diffuse, not easily located	Diffuse
	Radiation to neck and jaw or down arm or arms to fingers
DESCRIPTION	
Deep sensation of tightness or a squeezing feeling	Severe pressure, squeezing, or heaviness with a crushing, oppressive quality
Mild to moderate in severity or pressure	
Similar attacks each time	Report of such severe pain that client would rather die than experience pain again
Twinges or dullness in thoracic area	Residual "soreness" for several days following MI
ONSET AND DURATION	
Gradual or sudden onset	Sudden onset
Usual duration of 15 min or less (usually no more than 30 min)	Duration of 30 min to 2 hr
	No relief from rest or nitroglycerin
ASSOCIATED CLINICAL MANIFESTATIONS	
Apprehension	Apprehension
Dyspnea	Nausea and vomiting
Diaphoresis	Dyspnea
Nausea	Diaphoresis
Desire to void	Extreme fatigue
Belching	Dizziness or faintness (after abatement of pain)

taglandins). When spasm occurs, the client experiences pain and marked, transient ST segment elevation. The pain may occur during rapid eye movement (REM) sleep when myocardial oxygen consumption increases; it may be relieved by some form of exercise or it may disappear spontaneously. Cyclical, short bursts of pain at a usual time each day may also occur with this type of angina.

Nocturnal angina and angina decubitus. *Nocturnal angina* occurs only at night but not necessarily when the person is in the recumbent position or during sleep. Angina decubitus is chest pain that occurs only while the person is lying down and is usually relieved by standing or sitting.

Clinical manifestations. The most common initial symptom of a client with angina is *chest pain* or discomfort (Table 28-9). The exact cause of the pain is unknown, but neurogenic pain at the site of ischemia is most likely. On direct questioning, some clients may deny feeling pain but will refer to a vague sensation, a strange feeling, pres-

sure, or ache in the chest. It is an unpleasant feeling, often described as a constrictive, squeezing, heavy, choking, or suffocating sensation. Many persons complain of severe indigestion or burning. Although most of the discomfort experienced by persons with angina appears substernally, the sensation may occur in the neck or radiate to the shoulders and down the arms (Fig. 28-9). Often people will complain of pain between the shoulder blades and dismiss it as not being heart pain. Depending on the severity of the anginal attack, the person may remain motionless or may clench a fist over the sternal area. Persons experiencing angina often refer to a feeling of anxiety and impending doom. Relief of classic angina pectoris is usually obtained with rest or cessation of activity. Prinzmetal's angina differs from stable or unstable angina in that it is longer in duration and may wake people from sleep.

Complications. Dysrhythmias, such as premature contractions or fibrillations, may occur in a person with angina. The cells deprived of oxygen and nutrients may be-

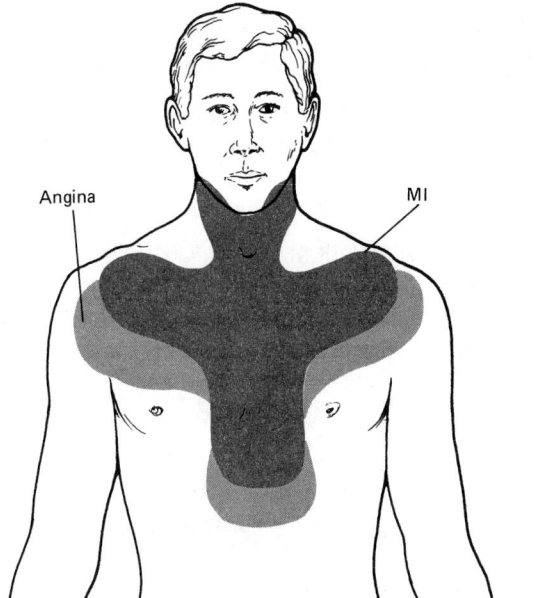

Fig. 28-9   Location of chest pain during angina or MI.

Table 28-10

 Diagnostic and Therapeutic Management: Angina Pectoris

DIAGNOSTIC

History and physical examination
Chest x-ray film
ECG
Serum enzyme level tests
Serum lipid level tests
Exercise stress tests
Nuclear imaging studies
Angiography studies
Stress echocardiography

THERAPEUTIC
Acute angina attacks

Nitroglycerin (sublingual)

Chronic anginal prophylaxis

Nitroglycerin ointment (e.g., Nitrol)
Transdermal controlled-release nitrates
Long-acting nitrates (e.g., Isordil, Sorbitrate)
β-Adrenergic blocking agents
Calcium-blocking agents
Antithrombotic therapy (e.g., aspirin, dipyridamole)

come irritable and develop into sites for ectopic pacemaker cells. Decreased myocardial contractility also occurs in persons experiencing angina.

Because some anginal pains may be vague, the client may not perceive the discomfort as important, dismiss its occurrence, proceed with an activity, and sustain an MI. (If ischemia persists in the presence of an increased myocardial oxygen demand, an MI will occur.) When chest pain is reported to a health care provider, the diagnosis of angina may not be the first consideration, since many problems can mimic midthoracic discomfort. All clients complaining of chest pain should be evaluated to rule out angina and MI.

Diagnostic studies. When a client has a history indicating CAD, the physician may take several courses of action (Table 28-10). After a detailed history and physical examination, a chest x-ray film is usually taken to look for cardiac enlargement, cardiac calcifications, and pulmonary congestion. Laboratory tests may be done to ascertain serum lipid and cardiac enzyme values. Serum lipid levels are assessed to screen for positive risk factors, and enzyme levels are checked to rule out the occurrence of infarction. An ECG is obtained and compared to an earlier tracing when possible.

Frequently, treadmill exercise testing is done for clients with stable angina to examine ST segment changes during exercise as an indirect assessment of coronary artery perfusion. (Unstable angina is a contraindication for use of the treadmill.) Severely abnormal ECGs on exercise testing, indicating gross disease processes, may show the need for

angiography. Unfortunately, the ECG stress test is not always conclusive for CAD. A false-positive reaction may be found (especially in women), and a false-negative reaction may be seen if the client is exercised submaximally. Ambulatory ECG testing with client-recorded activity may be effective in identifying silent ischemia. It is also helpful in differentiating Prinzmetal's angina because the incidence of spasm occurs more commonly in the early hours (5 to 6 AM).

Nuclear imaging is being widely used as a noninvasive measurement of myocardial perfusion. Thallium 201 is the isotope of choice to detect ischemia, and technetium 99m stannous pyrophosphate is used to detect the "hot spots" of actual infarcted tissue. Thallium stress tests are also frequently performed. The client is injected with thallium and proceeds with exercise on a treadmill, with scanning done at peak exercise and 2 to 4 hours after exercise. Positron emission tomography (PET), a noninvasive technique, is also useful in identifying and quantifying ischemia and infarction (see Chapter 26).

The physician may propose coronary angiography. This study allows visualization of the coronary arteries for obstruction and helps to determine the treatment and prognosis. Clients with unstable angina should undergo coronary angiography to evaluate the extent of the disease and to determine the most appropriate therapeutic modality. Coronary angiography is the only way to confirm the diagnosis of Prinzmetal's angina. This is often possible only with the intracoronary injection of ergonovine maleate to provoke a spasm.

Other new techniques for diagnosing coronary artery stenosis include use of echocardiography with exercise. Stress echocardiograms may be used when clients have an abnormal baseline ECG. The client has a baseline echocardiogram before exercise stress testing and then proceeds with the treadmill exercise test. Immediately after the conclusion of the test, another echocardiogram is performed to detect any new regional abnormal wall motion. This increases the sensitivity of the treadmill test.

Another technique using an echocardiogram can be used for clients who are unable to exercise. In these clients, a dobutamine stress echocardiogram can be performed. Echocardiography is done during a step-wise infusion of dobutamine, which causes a progressive increase in HR just as occurs with exercise. That is, the heart is being exercised chemically. Again, new abnormality of the regional wall motion is determined. The test is stopped if a wall motion abnormality or angina develops or the client reaches the target HR or the peak dobutamine dose of 30 μg/kg/min.

Therapeutic management. The most common initial therapeutic intervention for angina is the use of nitrate therapy to enhance coronary blood flow (Table 28-10). Prehospital emergency care of the client with chest pain is presented in Table 28-11.

Two advances in the treatment of CAD are *laser angioplasty* and *percutaneous transluminal coronary angioplasty* (PTCA). In laser angioplasty a catheter is introduced through a peripheral artery into the diseased coronary artery. A small laser on the tip of the catheter vaporizes the plaqued areas of the artery, thereby facilitating blood flow. A disadvantage of this procedure is that the technique needs refinement so that the proper laser strength for a given thickness of atherosclerotic plaque will be known. Current research is perfecting this technique to move it from experimentation to therapeutic practice. The laser may also be used in the future to make a small opening in completely occlusive lesions, making them more amenable to angioplasty.[22]

A more common intervention has been PTCA.[23] In a catheterization laboratory a catheter equipped with a balloon tip (which can be inflated) is inserted into the appropriate coronary artery. When the lesion is located, the catheter is passed through and just past the lesion, the balloon is inflated, and the atherosclerotic plaque is compressed, resulting in vessel dilatation.

The advantages of PTCA are that (1) it provides an alternative to therapeutic and usual surgical intervention; (2) it is performed with local anesthesia; (3) it eliminates the recovery from thoracotomy required for bypass surgery and its complications; (4) the client is ambulatory 24 hours after the procedure; (5) the length of hospital stay is approximately 4 days compared with the 10- to 14-day stay of someone having open heart surgery with a coronary artery bypass graft (CABG), thus reducing hospital costs; and (6) there is rapid return to work (approximately 2 weeks after PTCA) instead of a 3-month convalescence after CABG.

However, there are many disadvantages to PTCA. First, not all persons with CAD are candidates for PTCA.

Table 28-11

 Prehospital Emergency Care of the Client with Chest Pain*

Possible etiologies: Chest trauma, CAD, pleurisy, pneumonia, pneumothorax, pericarditis, pulmonary edema, pulmonary emboli, stress, strenuous exercise, drugs, shock, aortic aneurysms, hiatal hernia

CLINICAL MANIFESTATIONS

Pain located in neck, breast bone, left arm, left shoulder
Cold, clammy skin
Profuse diaphoresis
Nausea and vomiting
Difficulty in breathing
Weakness
Pallor
Anxiety—feeling of impending doom
Tachycardia, irregular HR, palpitations
Decreased BP
Fainting, loss of consciousness

MANAGEMENT

Place in semi-Fowler's position.
Assess severity and location of pain; medicate for pain as ordered.
Monitor cardiac rhythm and vital signs.
Administer oxygen by face mask or nasal cannula at 4 to 6 L.
Loosen any constrictive clothing; comfort and reassure client.
Be prepared to perform cardiopulmonary resuscitation or defibrillation.
Start intravenous line with large-gauge needle.
Determine client's cardiac history.
Maintain calm environment.

*See Chapter 59 for a general discussion on measures related to prehospital emergency care.

Good candidacy requirements include documented ischemia from an ECG or a thallium scan, less than a 1-year history of disabling angina so that the likelihood is high that the atheromas are not yet calcified, potential candidacy for CABG, preferably single-vessel disease not at vessel branches, good ventricular function, and good collateral blood flow. Preferably the lesions are not extensively calcified and are less than 2 cm in length. Dilatation may also be done for stenotic grafts from a previous CABG, although these vessels usually require repeated dilatation. The other major disadvantage of PTCA is the number of complications that can result. The most serious complication is dissection of the dilated artery where the intimal lesion is pushed farther up or down the intimal lining instead of being compressed. If the damage is extensive, the coronary artery could rupture, causing cardiac tamponade (see Chapter 31), ischemia and infarction, a fall in CO, and possible death. There is also danger from infarction should the lesion be calcified and a portion of the plaque dislodge and occlude the vessel distal to the catheter. The chance of coronary spasm from the mechanical irritation of the catheter is present, as well as chemical irritation from the contrast dye injection used to visualize the artery and catheter/balloon. Blood flow distal to the lesion can also be compromised when the balloon is inflated.

A catheter has been developed with an additional lumen for a small amount of blood flow distal to the inflation area if a large amount of myocardium is at risk. The possibility of dysrhythmias is always present. The risk of restenosis after PTCA is about 30% in the first 6 months.[24]

Generally, coronary artery bypass surgery is recommended if the client is under the age of 65 and has (1) significant left main coronary artery obstruction or (2) triple-vessel disease. Bypass surgery is usually recommended for persons with unstable angina who demonstrate a poor response to therapy, requiring repeat angioplasty. The success of such treatment varies (see Chapter 29).

Pharmacological management

Antiplatelet aggregation therapy. Antiplatelet aggregation therapy is the first line of pharmacological intervention in the treatment of angina. Aspirin is the drug of choice. Recent studies indicate that up to a 50% reduction in unstable angina progression to MI occurs with the use of aspirin.[25] Dipyridamole (Persantine) is also used as an antiplatelet-aggregation agent.

Nitrates. Nitrates, which are commonly classified as vasodilators, are the next step in the treatment of angina. Nitrates produce their principal effects by the following:

1. Dilating peripheral blood vessels: This results in decreased SVR, venous pooling, and decreased venous blood return to the heart. Therefore myocardial oxygen requirements are lessened because of the reduced cardiac work load.
2. Dilating coronary arteries and/or collateral vessels: This may increase blood flow to the ischemic areas of the heart. When the coronary arteries are severely atherosclerotic, however, coronary dilatation is difficult to achieve.

NITROGLYCERIN. Nitroglycerin given sublingually (SL) will usually relieve pain in about 3 minutes and has a duration of approximately 45 minutes. The usual recommended dose is one tablet taken sublingually, which can be followed at 5-minute intervals with two more doses. If nitroglycerin tablets have been necessary and relief from anginal pain has not been obtained after 3 tablets and 15 minutes, the client should be instructed to seek medical attention.

Nitroglycerin can be used prophylactically before undertaking an activity that the client knows may precipitate an anginal attack. In these instances the client can take a tablet 5 to 10 minutes before beginning the activity. Any changes in the usual pattern of pain, especially increasing frequency or nocturnal angina, should be reported to the physician.

Nitroglycerin tablets are marketed in light-resistant bottles closed with metal caps. Since they tend to lose potency, the client should be advised to purchase a new supply every 6 to 9 months.

NITROGLYCERIN OINTMENT. Nitroglycerin (Nitrol and Nitro-paste) is a 2% nitroglycerin topical ointment dosed by the inch. It is placed on the skin (preferably the trunk of the body), where it is absorbed slowly, producing anginal prophylaxis for 3 to 6 hours. It has been found to be especially useful for nocturnal and unstable angina because it acts for a longer period of time than SL nitroglycerin. Its disadvantages include its messiness and its rapid absorption, necessitating repeated application.[26]

TRANSDERMAL CONTROLLED–RELEASE NITRATES. Currently there are two types of systems available for transdermal drug administration: reservoir and matrix. Transderm-Nitro is the reservoir type, in which the drug migrates to the absorption site through a rate-controlled permeable membrane. Nitro-Dur and Nitro-Disc are the matrix type, in which the drug is slowly dispersed through a polymer matrix to the skin absorption site. Both reservoir and matrix delivery systems offer the advantages of steady plasma levels within the therapeutic range over 24 hours, thus making only one application per day necessary. The reservoir system offers the disadvantage of dose dumping if the reservoir seal is punctured or broken. An advantage of the matrix system is that there can be no dose dumping. Both systems achieve plasma steady states by 2 hours.

LONG-ACTING NITRATES. Long-acting nitrates such as isosorbide dinitrate (Isordil, Sorbitrate) are longer acting than SL nitroglycerin and, when used in adequate doses, are effective in reducing the incidence of anginal attacks. Their mechanisms of action and side effects are similar to those of nitroglycerin. The effects of oral isosorbide dinitrate may last for up to 8 hours.

Because of the vasodilating properties of nitrates, the predominant side effect of nitrate drugs is headache from the dilatation of cerebral blood vessels. This problem can be alleviated by reducing the dosage. Sometimes the body can build up a tolerance for the drug so that the headaches abate but the principal antianginal effect is still present. However, the body has a tendency to develop a tolerance to the effects of nitrates.[27] A strategy found effective to combat this tolerance is providing a nitrate-free period within each 24-hour period. Other complications of the vasodilator drugs are orthostatic hypotension (nitrate syncope) and an aggravation of cerebral vascular insufficiency.

INTRAVENOUS NITROGLYCERIN. Intravenous (IV) nitroglycerin (Nitrol IV, Nitrostat IV, Nitro-Bid IV, Tridil) has been used in treating hospitalized clients with unstable angina refractory to standard therapeutic treatment. It has an immediate onset of action and can be titrated to prevent, treat, and stop acute attacks of angina. IV nitroglycerin has also been used in MI. The rationale for use in MI has been to increase the collateral blood flow to the ischemic area and reduce myocardial oxygen demand because of decreasing preload and afterload. Tolerance is also a side effect of IV nitrate therapy. An effective strategy for this phenomenon is titrating down the dose at night (during sleep) and titrating the dose up during the day.

β-Adrenergic blocking agents. β-Blocking agents available for the prophylaxis of angina are propranolol (Inderal), metoprolol (Lopressor), nadolol (Corgard), atenolol

(Tenormin), oxyprendol (Trasicor), pindolol (Visken), and timolol (Blocadren). These drugs produce a direct decrease in myocardial contractility, HR, SVR, and BP, all of which reduce the myocardial oxygen demand. Side effects of the β blockers may include bradycardia, hypotension, wheezing, and GI complaints. Many clients also complain of weight gain, depression, and sexual dysfunction. The β blockers should not be discontinued abruptly without medical supervision.

Calcium-blocking agents. Calcium-blocking agents such as nifedipine (Procardia), verapamil (Calan, Isoptin), diltiazem (Cardizem), and nicardipine (Cardene) are the next step in the management of angina. Most of these agents now have sustained-release versions for longer action with hope of increased client compliance. The three primary effects of calcium channel blockers are (1) systemic vasodilatation with decreased SVR, (2) decreased myocardial contractility, and (3) coronary vasodilatation.

Each drug manifests these effects to a different degree. It is important to understand action potentials in cardiac muscle cells to comprehend the mechanisms of action of the calcium channel blockers. Briefly, cardiac cells are surrounded by a protein lipid layer called the *sarcolemma*, which is a semipermeable membrane that separates net positive (extracellular surface) and net negative (intracellular surface) charges by excluding sodium ions (Na^+) and calcium ions (Ca^{2+}) and retaining potassium ions (K^+).

The two types of fiber in the heart are fast-response fibers, which include all contractile tissue of atria and ventricles, the conduction system, and the distal atrioventricular (AV) nodal regions, and slow-response fibers of the sinoatrial (SA) node, the automatic cells of the proximal AV node regions, and AV ring fibers. The action potential for the slow-response fibers has slowly rising action potentials and slower conduction rates. Therefore these spontaneously depolarizing action potentials depend greatly on the slow inward Ca^{2+} current. Therefore a calcium channel blocker has a depressant effect on the SA node rate of discharge, and the conduction velocity through the AV node is decreased, thus slowing the HR.

Cardiac muscle and vascular smooth muscle cells are more dependent on extracellular calcium than skeletal muscles and are therefore more sensitive to calcium channel-blocking agents. The effect of calcium channel blockers on smooth muscle of both coronary and systemic arteries is to cause relaxation and relative vasodilatation, thus increasing blood flow. Verapamil has antidysrhythmic properties (see Chapter 30). Myocardial work load is decreased with calcium channel blockers by increased coronary blood flow through vasodilatation and reduction in myocardial oxygen demand mediated through a decrease in HR and afterload. Calcium channel-blocking agents have also been effective in controlling angina from either "fixed" atherosclerotic lesions or vasospasm. Verapamil, nifedipine, and diltiazem have also been shown to consistently decrease systemic BP in the hypertensive client (see Table 27-15).

Calcium channel blockers potentiate the action of digoxin by increasing serum digoxin levels during the early part (first week) of therapy. Therefore serum digoxin levels should be closely monitored upon institution of this therapy, and the client should be taught the signs and symptoms of digoxin toxicity.

■ Nursing Management of Angina
Nursing assessment
Subjective and objective data that should be obtained from a client with angina are presented in Table 28-12.
Nursing diagnoses
Nursing diagnoses specific to the client with angina include, but are not limited to, the following:
1. Pain (chest pain or discomfort) related to ischemic myocardium
2. Anxiety related to diagnosis and awareness of being a victim of heart disease, pain and limited activity tolerance, uncertainties about the future, diagnostic tests, and pending surgery
3. Altered cardiopulmonary tissue perfusion related to decreased cardiac output and abnormalities of left heart function
4. Decreased cardiac output related to myocardial ischemia affecting contractility
5. Activity intolerance related to myocardial ischemia

Nursing interventions
Acute intervention. Some of the main nursing objectives for the client with angina are pain assessment, evaluation of treatment, and reinforcement of appropriate therapy. Because chest pain can be due to many factors other than ischemia (e.g., pericarditis, valvular disease, pulmonary artery stenosis, MI, and congestive cardiomyopathy), it is important to have a clear understanding of the client's chest pain. The questions a nurse asks may elicit a history of anginal pain. The nurse should determine whether breathing in or out or changing positions makes the client's chest pain better or worse. Anginal pain does not vary with body position or respirations. In contrast, the pain of pericarditis does. It should be ascertained whether the pain is deep or superficial, mild or intense. Cardiac pain is usually described as deep and intense, but occasionally it may be characterized as a dull ache. Very few persons can successfully ignore cardiac pain.

The client should be asked whether the pain is diffuse or well localized. Cardiac pain is usually diffuse. The client may rub the entire chest to explain where the pain is occurring. The nurse should instruct the client to quantify each pain experience by rating the pain on a scale from 1 to 10, with 10 being excruciating pain and 1 being barely noticeable. By doing this, the nurse can assess the effectiveness of treatment during a pain experience as well as discriminate between subsequent pain experiences.

If a nurse is present during an anginal attack, the following measures should be instituted: (1) administration of oxygen, (2) prompt pain relief with a nitrate or a narcotic analgesic, (3) determination of vital signs, (4) ECG, (5) physical assessment of the chest, and (6) comfortable positioning of the client. The client will most likely appear distressed and have pale, cool, clammy skin. The BP and pulse rate will probably be elevated and an atrial gallop

Table 28-12

Nursing Assessment of the Client with Angina Pectoris

SUBJECTIVE DATA

History
Positive family history of heart disease; previous history of MI, angina, aortic stenosis, or cardiomyopathy; hypertension, diabetes, anemia, lung disease; relationship of pain to activity (including sexual), meals, emotional arousal, exposure to cold; smoking; fat and sodium intake

Medications
Use of nitrates, calcium antagonists, cocaine, α blockers, oxytocin, hydralazine, propranolol

General
Feelings of impending doom, lightheadedness

Pain
Substernal chest pain or pressure (squeezing, constricting, aching, sharp, tingling) lasting <20 minutes; referral to arms (especially left), jaw, neck, shoulders, back; relief with rest and/or nitroglycerin

Respiratory
Dyspnea

Cardiovascular
Palpitations

Gastrointestinal
Indigestion, heartburn, nausea, belching

OBJECTIVE DATA

General
Anxiety

Integumentary
Diaphoresis, pallor

Cardiovascular
Tachycardia, pulsus alterans, dysrhythmias (especially ventricular), ventricular gallop, atrial gallop

Possible findings
Negative cardiac enzymes, elevated serum lipids; positive exercise stress test and thallium scans; demonstration of ST and T wave abnormalities on ECG; positive coronary angiography

---

(S_4) sound may be heard. If a ventricular gallop (S_3) is heard, it may indicate left ventricular decompensation. A murmur may be heard during an anginal attack secondary to ischemia of a papillary muscle. The murmur is likely to be transient and abates with the cessation of symptoms. Supportive and realistic assurance as well as a calm, soothing manner helps to reduce the client's anxiety.

The client needs to be instructed in the proper use of nitroglycerin. It should be easily accessible to the client at all times. For protection from degradation, it should be kept in a tightly closed dark glass bottle. The client should be instructed to place a nitroglycerin tablet beneath the tongue and allow it to dissolve. This should cause a fizzing or slightly warm feeling locally. The client should be warned that HR may increase and a pounding headache, dizziness, or flushing may occur. The client should be cautioned against rising to a standing position quickly because postural hypotension may occur after nitroglycerin ingestion. If the pain has not been relieved after 5 minutes, the client should be told to take another nitroglycerin tablet. This procedure may be repeated for pain relief every 5 minutes, not to exceed the ingestion of three tablets. If pain persists after three doses, the client should seek immediate medical attention.

Chronic management. The client needs to be reassured that a long, productive life is possible, even with angina. Prevention of angina is preferable to its treatment, and this is where instruction is important. The client needs to be educated regarding coronary artery disease and angina, precipitating factors, risk factors, and medications.

Client teaching can be handled in a variety of ways. One-to-one contact between nurse and client is often the most effective procedure. The time spent in providing daily care is often an ideal teaching period. Teaching tools, such as pamphlets, films at the bedside, a heart model, and especially written information, are necessary components of client and family education (see Chapter 6).

Clients need to be assisted in identifying factors that precipitate angina (see p. 791). They should be given instruction on how to avoid or control precipitating factors. For example, they should be cautioned to avoid exposures to extremes of weather and taught not to eat large, heavy meals. If a heavy meal is ingested, adequate rest should be planned for 1 to 2 hours after eating because blood is pooled in the GI tract to aid digestion.

The client needs to be assisted in identifying personal risk factors in CAD. Once these risk factors are known, various methods of decreasing them should be discussed (see Table 28-4).

Educating the client and the family about diets that are low in sodium and reduced in saturated fats may be appropriate. Maintaining ideal body weight is most important in controlling angina, since weight above this level increases the myocardial work load and may cause pain. Eating large meals also contributes to angina, and clients may need to eat several small meals in place of three moderate to large meals each day.

Adhering to a regular, individualized exercise program that conditions the heart rather than overstressing the myocardium is most important. Nurses should consult with a physician or a physical therapist in instructing the client regarding an exercise program (see pp. 812-813).

It is important to educate the client and the family in the use of nitroglycerin. Nitroglycerin tablets or ointments may be used prophylactically before an emotionally stressful situation, sexual intercourse, or physical exertion (e.g., climbing a long flight of stairs).

Counseling should be provided to assess the psychological adjustment of the client and the family to the diagnosis of CAD and the resulting angina pectoris. Many clients feel a threat to their identity and self-esteem and are unable to fill their roles in society. These emotions are normal and very real.

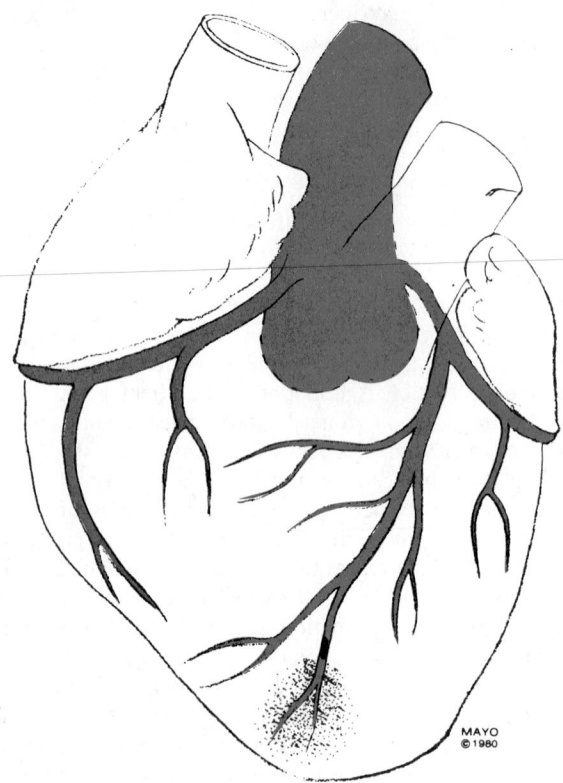

Fig. 28-10 Occlusion of coronary artery, causing MI. (Courtesy Mayo Clinic, Rochester, Minn.)

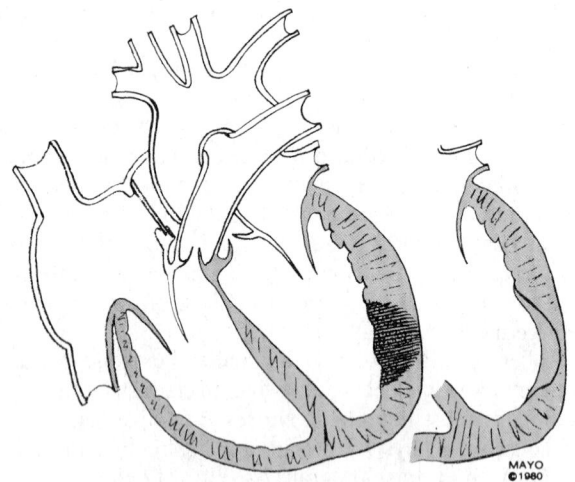

Fig. 28-11 Transmural MI involving the thickness of the total wall. (Courtesy Mayo Clinic, Rochester, Minn.)

Myocardial Infarction

An MI occurs when ischemic intracellular changes become irreversible and necrosis results. Angina due to ischemia causes reversible cellular injury, and infarction is the result of sustained ischemia, causing irreversible cellular death (Fig. 28-10).

Prehospital mortality in clients with acute MI is approximately 30% to 50%. A substantial number of these deaths

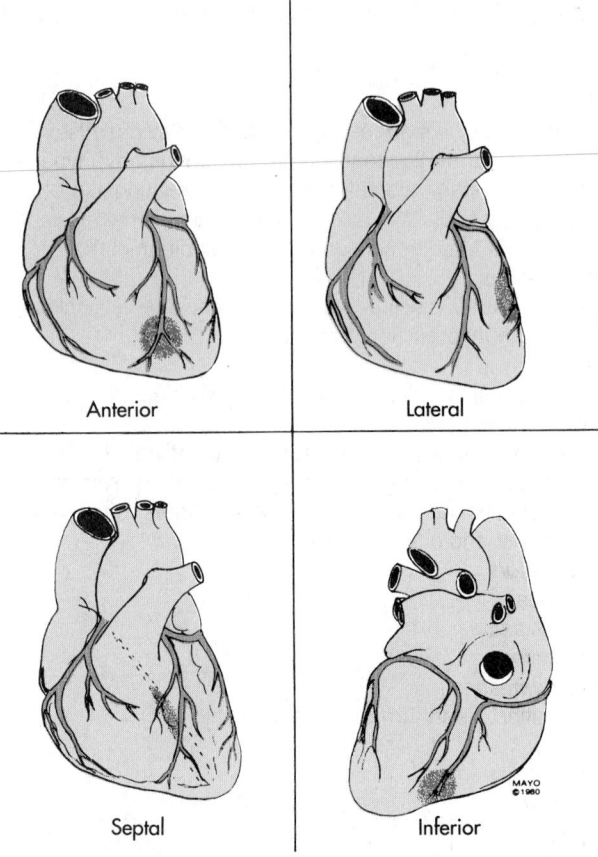

Fig. 28-12 Four common locations where MI occurs. (Courtesy Mayo Clinic, Rochester, Minn.)

occur before hospitalization. Mortality among clients who reach the hospital is about 5%. Most of these deaths occur within the first 3 to 4 days.[28]

Pathophysiology. Cardiac cells can withstand ischemic conditions for about 20 minutes before cellular death (necrosis) begins. Contractile function of the heart stops in the areas of myocardial necrosis. The degree of altered function depends on the area of the heart involved and the size of the infarct. Most infarcts involve the left ventricle. A transmural MI occurs when the entire thickness of the myocardium in a region is involved (Fig. 28-11). A subendocardial MI (nontransmural) exists when the damage has not penetrated through the entire thickness of the myocardial wall.

Infarctions are described by area of occurrence as anterior, inferior, lateral, or posterior wall infarctions. Common combinations of areas are the anterolateral or anteroseptal MI. An inferior MI is also called a *diaphragmatic MI* (DMI) (Fig. 28-12).

The location and area of the infarct correlate with the part of the coronary circulation involved. For example, inferior wall infarctions are usually the result of right coronary artery lesions. Anterior wall infarctions are usually due to lesions in the left anterior descending artery. Lesions in the left circumflex artery usually cause posterior or inferior MIs.

The degree of preestablished collateral circulation also determines the severity of infarction. In individuals with a history of heart disease, adequate collateral channels may have been established that provide the area surrounding the infarction site with some blood supply and oxygen. This is one explanation of why the younger person who has a severe MI is often more likely to have a more serious impairment than an older person with the same degree of occlusion.

Healing process. The body's response to cell death is the inflammatory process (see Chapter 7). Within 24 hours, leukocytes infiltrate the area. Enzymes are released from the dead cardiac cells and are important diagnostic indicators (see p. 802). The proteolytic enzymes of the neutrophils and macrophages remove all necrotic tissue by the second or third day. During this time, the necrotic muscle wall is thin. The development of collateral circulation improves areas of poor perfusion and may limit the zones of injury and infarction. Once infarction takes place, catecholamine-mediated lipolysis and glycogenolysis occur. These processes allow the increased plasma glucose and free fatty acids to be used by the oxygen-depleted myocardium for anaerobic metabolism. For this reason, serum glucose levels are frequently elevated after MI and may be the reason for a pseudodiabetic state.

The necrotic zone is clearly identifiable by ECG changes within 4 to 10 days and by technetium scanning 24 to 72 hours after the onset of symptoms. At this point, the phagocytes (neutrophils and monocytes) have cleared the necrotic debris from the injured area, and the collagen matrix that will eventually form scar tissue is laid down.

At 10 to 14 days after MI the beginning scar tissue is still weak. The myocardium is considered to be especially vulnerable to increased stress because of the unstable state of the healing heart wall. (It is also at this time that the client's activity level may be increasing so special caution and assessment is necessary.) By 6 weeks after MI, scar tissue has replaced necrotic tissue. At this time, the injured area is said to be healed. The scarred area is often less compliant than the surrounding fibers. This condition may be manifested by uncoordinated wall motion, ventricular dysfunction, and/or pump failure.

Clinical manifestations

Pain. Severe, immobilizing chest pain not relieved by rest or nitrate administration is the hallmark of MI (see Table 28-6). The pain is due to the inadequate oxygen supply to the myocardium. Persistent and unlike any other pain, it is usually described as a heaviness, tightness, or constriction. Common locations are substernal or retrosternal, radiating to the neck, jaw, and arms or to the back. It may occur while the client is active or at rest, asleep or awake. It usually lasts for 20 minutes or more and is described as more severe than anginal pain. The pain may be located atypically in the epigastric area. The client may have taken antacids without relief. Some clients may not experience pain but may have "discomfort," weakness, or shortness of breath.

Nausea and vomiting. The client may be nauseated and vomit. Nausea and vomiting can result from reflex stimulation of the vomiting center by the severe pain (see Chapter 36). These symptoms can also result from vasovagal reflexes from the area of the infarcted myocardium that affect the GI tract.

Sympathetic stimulation. During the initial phases of MI, increased catecholamines (norepinephrine and epinephrine) are released. The increased sympathetic response results in diaphoresis and vasoconstriction of peripheral blood vessels. On physical examination, the client's skin will be ashen, clammy, and cool. This condition is often referred to as a "cold sweat."

Fever. The temperature may increase within the first 24 hours up to 38° C (100.4° F) and occasionally to 39° C (102.2° F). The temperature elevation may last for as long as 1 week. This increase in temperature is a systemic manifestation of the inflammatory process caused by the infarcted myocardium.

Cardiovascular manifestations. The BP and pulse rate may be elevated initially. Later, the BP may drop because of decreased CO. Urine output may be decreased. Rales (crackles) may be noted in the lungs, persisting for several hours to several days. Hepatic engorgement and peripheral edema may indicate overt cardiac failure. Jugular veins may be distended and may have obvious pulsations, indicating early right ventricular dysfunction and pulmonary congestion.

Cardiac examination may reveal abnormal precordial movements suggestive of ventricular aneurysm. Heart sounds may seem distant, but close auscultation may reveal splitting of heart sounds, indicating left ventricular dysfunction. Other abnormal sounds suggesting ventricular dysfunction are S_4 and S_3. In addition, the presence of murmurs may indicate valve incompetency. A loud holosystolic apical murmur may be due to papillary muscle rupture.

Complications

Dysrhythmias. The most common complications after an MI are dysrhythmias, found in 80% of MI clients. Dysrhythmias are caused by any condition that affects the myocardial cell's sensitivity to nerve impulses, such as ischemia, electrolyte imbalances, and sympathetic nervous system stimulation. The intrinsic rhythm of the heartbeat is disrupted, causing either a very fast HR (tachycardia), a very slow HR (bradycardia), or an irregular beat, all of which adversely affect the ischemic myocardium.

Life-threatening dysrhythmias occur most often with anterior wall infarction, pump failure, and shock. Complete heart block is seen in massive infarction. Ventricular fibrillation, a common cause of sudden death, is a lethal dysrhythmia that most often occurs within the first 4 hours after the onset of pain. Premature ventricular contractions (PVCs) may precede ventricular tachycardia and fibrillation. Ventricular dysrhythmias need immediate treatment. (See Chapter 30 for a detailed description of dysrhythmias and their management.)

Congestive heart failure. Congestive heart failure (CHF) is a complication that occurs when the pumping power of the heart has diminished. In the client with an acute MI it is common to see some degree of left ventricular dysfunction in the first 24 hours. Depending on the severity and extent of the injury, CHF occurs initially with subtle signs such as slight dyspnea, restlessness, agitation, or slight tachycardia. Jugular vein distention from right-sided heart failure, crackles heard in the lungs, distention of upper lobe veins on an upright chest x-ray film, and the presence of an S_3 or S_4 heart sound may indicate the onset of heart failure. (The treatment of acute CHF is discussed in Chapter 29.)

Cardiogenic shock. Cardiogenic shock occurs when inadequate oxygen and nutrients are supplied to the tissues because of left ventricular failure. It occurs when there is dysfunction of much of the left ventricle due to infarction. Cardiogenic shock occurs in 10% to 15% of clients hospitalized with acute MI (see p. 820).

Papillary muscle dysfunction. Papillary muscle dysfunction may occur if the infarcted area includes or is adjacent to these structures. Papillary muscle dysfunction causes mitral regurgitation, which increases the volume of blood in the left atrium. This condition aggravates an already compromised left ventricle. It is detected by a systolic murmur at the cardiac apex radiating toward the axilla. Papillary muscle rupture is a severe complication causing massive mitral regurgitation, which results in dyspnea, gross pulmonary edema, and decreased CO. Treatment consists of (1) rapid afterload reduction with nitroprusside or intraaortic balloon pumping and (2) immediate open heart surgery with mitral valve replacement.

Ventricular aneurysm. Ventricular aneurysm results when the infarcted myocardial wall becomes thinned and bulges out during contraction (Fig. 28-13). In the acute stage after MI this is called an *ischemic bulge*. If the aneurysm still exists after scar tissue is laid down, it is called a *ventricular aneurysm*. Ventricular aneurysms are identified by palpation of ectopic impulses; bulges seen on x-ray film, echocardiogram, or fluoroscopy; or persistent, long-term ST segment changes on an ECG. Ventricular angiography can definitively diagnose ventricular aneurysm.

The client with a ventricular aneurysm may experience intractable CHF, dysrhythmias, and angina. Besides ventricular rupture, which is fatal, ventricular aneurysms harbor thrombi, cause dysrhythmias, and promote left ventricular dysfunction. Surgical excision is the treatment for ventricular aneurysms severe enough to cause dysfunction.

Pericarditis. Acute pericarditis, an inflammation of the visceral or parietal pericardium, or both, may result in cardiac compression, lowered ventricular filling and emptying, and cardiac failure.[29] It may occur 2 to 3 days after an acute MI as a common complication of the infarction. Chest pain, which may vary from mild to severe, is aggravated by inspiration, coughing, and movement of the upper body and usually accompanies acute pericarditis. The pain may radiate to the back and down to the left arm, making it difficult to differentiate from acute myocardial ischemia. The pain may be relieved by sitting in a forward position.

Assessment of the client with pericarditis may reveal a

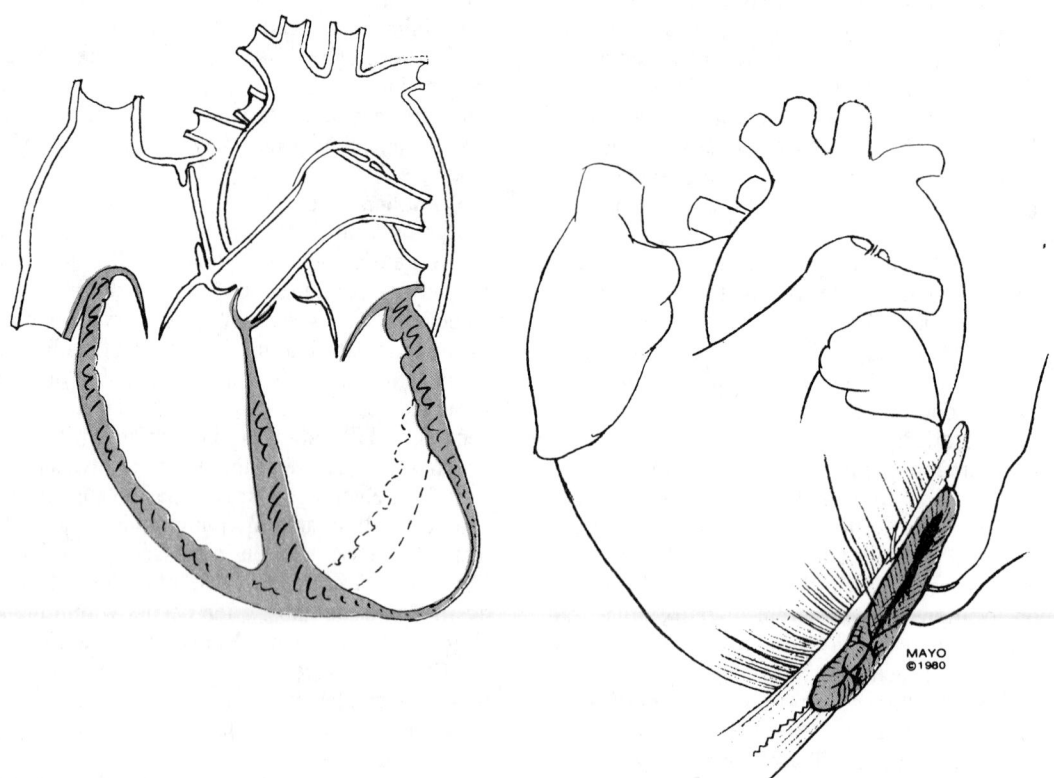

Fig. 28-13 Ventricular aneurysm and surgical repair. (Courtesy Mayo Clinic, Rochester, Minn.)

friction rub over the pericardium. The sound may be best heard with the diaphragm of the stethoscope at the mid to lower sternal border. It may be persistent or intermittent. Fever may also be present.

Diagnosis of pericarditis can be made with serial 12-lead ECGs. ECG changes reflect the inflammation and may produce characteristic ST-T segment elevations, which are persistent. Treatment may include pain relief by aspirin, steroids, or indomethacin.

Dressler syndrome. Dressler syndrome (post-MI syndrome) is characterized by pericarditis with effusion and fever that develops 1 to 4 weeks after MI. It may also occur after open heart surgery. It is thought to be due to an antigen-antibody reaction to the necrotic myocardium. The client experiences pericardial pain, fever, a friction rub, left pleural effusion, and arthralgia. Laboratory findings include an elevated white blood cell (WBC) count and an elevated sedimentation rate. Steroids are used to treat this condition.

Pulmonary embolism. Pulmonary embolism may be seen in the client with acute MI who has had bouts of CHF or dysrhythmias or has been extremely immobile because of prolonged bed rest. The source of the thrombus may be the roughened endocardium or leg veins. Early detection of emboli is accomplished by observing for pallor or cyanosis, heart failure unresponsive to treatment, and an unexplained pleural effusion. Acute massive pulmonary embolism causes sudden, severe dyspnea and is usually fatal. (Pulmonary emboli are discussed in more detail in Chapter 32.)

Diagnostic studies. Three noninvasive diagnostic parameters are used to determine whether a person has sustained an acute MI: (1) the client's history of pain, risk factors, and health history, (2) 12-lead ECG consistent with acute MI (ST-T wave elevations of greater than 1 mm in more than two contiguous leads), and (3) measurement of serial myocardial serum enzymes.

Clinical presentation. The client's clinical presentation is important; however, many clients do not have the classic unrelenting chest pain characteristic of acute MI. Clients may complain of a feeling of weakness, severe indigestion, shortness of breath, or chest discomfort. Risk factor analysis may indicate the client's propensity for an acute event. Any client's presentation that is suggestive of an acute MI should be treated as quickly as possible to rule out an infarction.

ECG findings. Serial ECGs are approximately 80% specific for diagnosing an acute MI and represent a leading diagnostic criterion. Areas of ischemia or infarction may be noted on the ECG. Changes in rate and rhythm of the heart may also be diagnostic for abnormalities. Since the acute infarction is a dynamic process that occurs over time, the ECG may reveal the time sequence of ischemia, injury, infarction, and resolution of the infarction (Table 28-13).

The 12-lead ECG may be normal when the client comes to an emergency room with a complaint of pain typical of ischemic chest pain, but within a few hours it may have changed to show the infarction process. These changes take place when cellular damage has occurred, interrupting the normal electrical depolarization. Fig. 28-14 correlates

Table 28-13 ECG Changes with Myocardial Infarction*

Phase I	Phase II	Phase III	Phase IV
Abnormal Q waves Elevated ST segment Inverted T waves	Gradual return of ST segment to baseline	Return of T waves to normal or near-normal configuration	Remnant Q wave

*Inferior wall infarction shows ST elevation, T inversion, and pathophysiological Q wave in leads II, III, and aV_F; inferolateral and posterolateral wall infarction shows reduced R and T inversion, with or without ST elevation in V_5, V_6, and aV_L; posterior wall infarction shows mirror image of normal ECG; anterior wall infarction shows typical infarction pattern in leads I, aV_L, V_2-V_6.

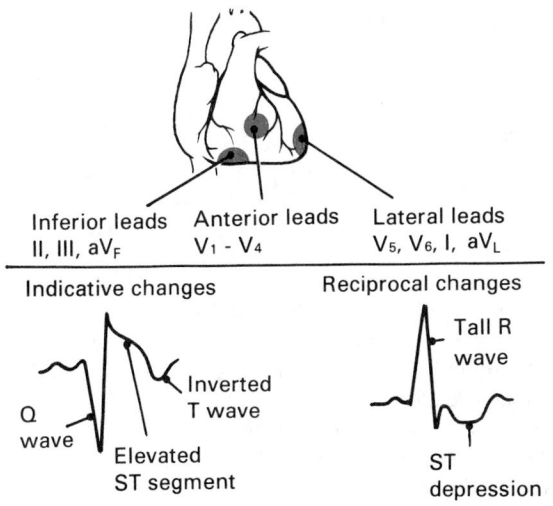

Fig. 28-14 Indicative changes occur in leads that examine the area of infarction. Reciprocal changes occur in leads opposite the area of infarction.

the anatomy with areas of infarction and with changes that occur on the 12-lead ECG. Changes that are present in the leads that examine infarcted areas of the heart are called indicative changes (i.e., they are indicative of infarction). Changes in the leads opposite infarcted areas are called reciprocal changes.

In general, the area of infarction correlates more closely with side effects and complications than with mortality rates. With inferior wall damage, AV blocks are commonly seen, since the right coronary artery perfuses the SA and AV node tissue in 80% to 90% of people. CHF, left ventricular aneurysms, cardiogenic shock, and complete heart block are more frequently seen with anterior MI, since the front surface of the left ventricle and part of the septum are damaged. An inferior wall MI may also cause CHF, dysrhythmias, and cardiogenic shock. Acute MI occasionally occurs in the right ventricle. It is manifested by pain, signs of increased venous pressure (distended neck veins, low PCWP but high central venous pressure), and low CO.

Cardiac enzymes. An important diagnostic criterion for acute MI is laboratory assessment of serial cardiac serum enzymes. The cardiac enzymes are lactic dehydrogenase (LDH) and creatine phosphokinase (CPK). When cardiac cells die, their cellular enzymes are released into circulation. The increase in serum enzymes after cellular death occurs can demonstrate whether cardiac damage has occurred and may indicate the approximate extent or severity of the damage. (Fig. 28-15 indicates the peak level and duration of these enzymes in the presence of MI.) Other causes of increased serum enzymes may make the differential diagnosis more difficult. These include pulmonary embolism, intramuscular damage, seizure activity, cardiopulmonary resuscitation (CPR), and other muscle-damaging events.

CPK levels begin to rise about 6 hours after an acute MI and return to normal within 2 to 3 days. The CPK enzymes may be fractionated into bands, including the MB band. The MB band is specific to the myocardial cell and may more specifically quantify myocardial damage. Depending on the individual laboratory, MB bands greater than 3% indicate MI.

Although cardiac enzymes are excellent diagnostic indicators of the acute MI, they are not immediately available to the physician or nurse because the laboratory needs time to develop the results. Today there are three new potential noninvasive markers for the diagnosis of acute MI. They include CK-MM isoforms, myoglobin, and RP-30 isonitrile scanning, which may make a diagnosis of acute MI almost immediately in the emergency department. With serum testing, these markers aid in the rapid diagnosis of acute MI. These tests are not yet available in every clinical facility.

Other measures. For the assessment of cardiac size and pulmonary congestion, an initial chest x-ray film is helpful but not diagnostic of the acute MI. The appearance of distended upper lobe veins may indicate early left ventricular dysfunction. The WBC count may rise to 12,000 to 14,000/μl or higher. Increases in fasting blood glucose level to 300 mg/dl may also occur secondary to the body's stress response to injury.

Radionuclide imaging has become increasingly important in establishing the diagnosis in MI. Nuclear imaging is considered an extremely sensitive indicator of myocardial damage. Myocardial nuclear scans, done by injecting IV radioactive isotopes, can help make the diagnosis of acute MI when other data are inconclusive. After an IV injection of thallium, the amount of thallium present in each myocardial region is determined by two factors: the amount of coronary blood flow to that region and the degree of viable myocardium. Ischemia or infarcted myocardial regions receiving little or no coronary blood flow ac-

Table 28-14

Diagnostic and Therapeutic Management: Myocardial Infarction

DIAGNOSTIC

History and physical examination
Serum enzyme level tests (e.g., CPK, LDH)
12-lead ECG
Chest x-ray film
Complete blood count, thyroid profile
Nuclear imaging studies
Echocardiogram

THERAPEUTIC

IV therapy
Continual ECG monitoring
Morphine sulfate IV 2-4 mg/hr prn (meperidine if client is allergic to morphine)
Oxygen therapy
Monitoring of vital signs every 1-4 hr
Lidocaine IV drip infusion (if ordered)
Bed rest with progressive activity
Recording of intake and output every hour
Thrombolytic therapy (as indicated)
Anticoagulant therapy (e.g., heparin IV)
Antithrombotic therapy (e.g., ASA)
Nitroglycerin IV

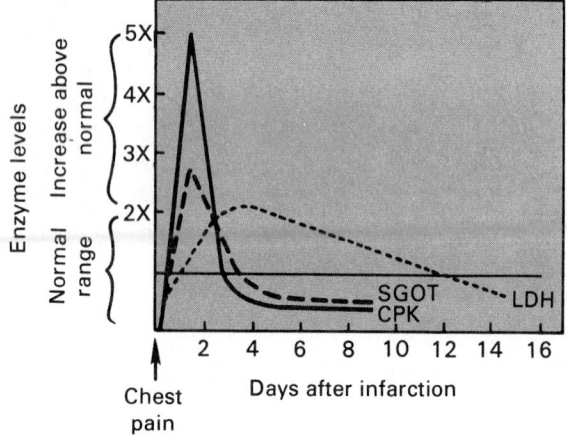

Fig. 28-15 Heart muscle enzyme levels in the blood after MI.

cumulate little or no IV thallium. Such regions appear as cold spots on the scan and thus indicate an area of ischemia or infarct. However, this technique does not differentiate old from new infarcts. Technetium pyrophosphate scanning can localize areas of acute necrosis. When given IV to the client, technetium complexes with calcium in irreversible, ischemic myocardial tissue. An area of infarct is visualized as a zone of increased radionuclide uptake and thus derives the name *hot spot*. Optimum time for imaging after an acute MI is 24 to 48 hours, but the scan may remain positive for up to 10 days. (Nuclear imaging is also described in Chapter 26 and Table 26-6.)

Therapeutic management. Initial management of the client with MI is best accomplished in a cardiac care unit (CCU), where constant monitoring is available. Dysrhyth-mias may be detected by nurses trained in continuous ECG monitoring techniques, and appropriate treatment can be instituted. An IV route is established to provide an accessible means for emergency drug therapy. Morphine sulfate or meperidine may be given IV for relief of pain. Oxygen is usually administered by nasal cannula at a rate of 2 to 6 L/min. The diagnostic and therapeutic management of MI is presented in Table 28-14, and typical admission orders containing diagnosis and treatment orders are shown in Table 28-15.

A continuous IV infusion of prophylactic lidocaine may be given to prevent ventricular fibrillation—the greatest threat to life immediately after MI. In many persons, episodes of fibrillation are preceded by premature ventricular contractions. The incidence of ventricular fibrillation has

---

Table 28-15 CCU Admission Orders

ADMISSION

Continuous monitor, rhythm strips, and dysrhythmia analysis
Vital signs q 2 hr for first 8 hr, then q 4 hr from 0600 to 2400 or as needed
Intake and output hourly
IV infusion of 500 ml 5% dextrose and water to keep vein open
Diet: Determined by condition of client _____
Daily weight____ ✔ _____
(Must be checked if wish to have done)
Oxygen 3 L/min by cannula or 5-8 L/min by mask
Absolute bed rest with bathroom privileges for 24 hr

CPR*

Defibrillation with 200 joules for ventricular fibrillation
Epinephrine 1 mg IV push
Type of resuscitation:
DNR _____ EPS (treatment of dysrhythmias and defibrillation only—no CPR to be done) _____ Dr. Heart Stat✔
Open Chest _____ (if none of above checked, open chest massage performed)

DYSRHYTHMIAS

Lidocaine 75-100 mg bolus, then IV drip (500 ml 5% dextrose in water with 2 g lidocaine) of 2-4 mg/min for PVCs more than
   6/min, R-on-T, multifocal or sequential
Atropine 0.5-1.0 mg IV for ventricular rate <50 with BP <90 and/or symptoms of poor cerebral perfusion

MEDICATION

Pain
   Severe _Morphine Sulfate 3mg. IV every 5 min. until relief_
   Mild _Acetaminophen 600 mg PO every 3-4 hr._
Hypnotic _Dalmane 15 mg PO hs MR x1_
Laxative _MOM 30 cc q hs prn_
Stool softener _Colace 100 mg PO bid_
Antiemetic _____
Antithrombotic _ASA every day_
Anticoagulant _(5% dextrose in water) Heparin 20,000 ul/500 ml to run at 1000 ul/hr_

LABORATORY

Cardiac profile on admittance and q 8 hr × 3
ECG Dates _4/5, 4/6, 4/7_ _____
Serum K+ every other day while in CCU
Routine lab UA, CBC, serum electrolytes, PTT
Other_Chest x-ray examination on admittance (if not done in ER)_

---

*By certified personnel only.

decreased to about 1% to 2%. Thus the use of prophylactic lidocaine is an area of much controversy. If the client is past the first 4 to 6 hours, when ventricular fibrillation is greatest, or if the client does not display premature ventricular contractions, prophylactic lidocaine may not be prescribed.

Vital signs are taken frequently during the first few hours after admission and monitored closely thereafter. Bed rest and limitation of activity are usual initially, with a gradual increase in activity.

A pulmonary artery (PA) catheter and intraarterial line may be used to accurately monitor intracardiac, pulmonary artery, and systolic arterial pressures so that the most effective mode of treatment in the acute phase can be determined. In the presence of severe left ventricular dysfunction, an intraaortic balloon pump (IABP) may be used to assist ventricular ejection and promote coronary artery perfusion.

Cardiac catheterization. Although the treatment for acute MI is to lyse the thrombus and reperfuse the myocardium, some clients may not be candidates for thrombolytic therapy or may have a complicated course necessitating an emergent cardiac catheterization. Clients with acute MI may have a catheterization early in the treatment phase to locate the exact lesion (or lesions) and to assess the severity, the presence of collateral circulation, and left ventricular function.

With actual visualization of the coronary artery system and left ventricular function, the physician can prescribe a treatment modality most beneficial to the client. Direct intracoronary thrombolytic therapy may be tried, PTCA may be performed, IABP insertion may be done, or the determination that CABG should be done can be made.

Percutaneous transluminal coronary angioplasty. If a proximal to midproximal, well-defined lesion is located during the cardiac catheterization, PTCA may be performed. Although it may be done during the acute phase, this technique is usually instituted 7 to 10 days after the initial catheterization. PTCA is a nonoperative alternative to surgery for clients who have coronary artery narrowing. Transluminal dilatation can increase the diameter of the artery with the use of percutaneous, fluoroscopically guided catheters to relieve stenotic or occlusive lesions in the proximal to midproximal, coronary artery circulation.

The technique is similar to cardiac catheterization. A double-lumen polyvinyl balloon catheter is guided into the coronary artery to the site of the occlusion. The balloon is inflated at the site of stenosis, thereby directly increasing the diameter of the artery. After PTCA, regional coronary blood flow is increased and myocardial metabolism is restored. PTCA is therefore indicated for the relief of myocardial ischemia in clients with noncalcified, occlusive, compressible coronary artery lesions.

Thrombolytic therapy. Thrombolytic therapy is the standard of practice in the treatment of acute MI. The goal in the treatment of acute MI is to salvage as much myocardial muscle as possible. Historically, treatment of acute MI had been directed at the client's symptoms only (i.e., dysrhythmia and CHF), and nothing was done for the acute process of infarction. This treatment modality de-

Table 28-16 Thrombolytic Agents Used to Treat Myocardial Infarctions

Streptokinase
Urokinase
Tissue plasminogen activator
Anisoylated plasminogen–streptokinase activator complex (APSAC, Eminase)
Prourokinase (scu-PA)

creased mortality from 30% to approximately 15% in the 1970s. With the advent of thrombolytic therapy, treatment has progressed to actually stopping the infarction process instead of just treating symptoms. In the 1990s mortality rates have decreased to 5% with thrombolytic treatment.[30]

It is now known that 80% to 90% of all acute MIs are secondary to thrombus formation.[30] Perfusion to the myocardium distal to the occlusion is halted causing progressive ischemia, cell death, necrosis, and acute MI.

The acute MI process therefore takes time. The earliest tissue to become ischemic is the subendocardium (the innermost layer of tissue in the cardiac muscle). Necrosis spreads toward the epicardium in a phenomenon known as the *wave front of necrosis*.[31] Myocardial cells do not die instantly; it takes approximately 4 to 6 hours for the entire thickness of the muscle to become necrosed in the majority of clients, and this is known as a *transmural infarction*.

Treatment of the acute MI is geared to quickly dissolving the thrombus in the coronary artery and reperfusing the myocardium before cellular death occurs. To be of most benefit, thrombolytics must be given within that first 6 hours after the onset of pain. If reperfusion occurs within that time, a 25% reduction in mortality has been shown.[30]

INDICATIONS AND CONTRAINDICATIONS. The commonly used thrombolytics (Table 28-16) can be given by the intracoronary or IV route. IV thrombolytic therapy is preferred because it can be given quickly, with excellent results in opening the artery. Although these drugs have different mechanisms of action and different pharmacokinetics, they all produce an open artery by lysis of the thrombus in the coronary artery.

Since all the thrombolytics produce lysis of the pathological clot, they may also lyse homeostatic clots (such as in the stomach or over a postoperative site). Therefore client selection is very important because persons receiving thrombolytic therapy may have a minor or major bleeding episode as a consequence of therapy. Not all clients who have an acute MI are candidates for thrombolytic therapy (Table 28-17). Inclusion criteria to receive an IV thrombolytic agent are (1) chest pain typical of acute MI less than or equal to 6 hours in duration, (2) chest pain for more than 6 hours if intermittent with ongoing ischemia, and (3) 12-lead ECG findings consistent with acute MI, irrespective of location.[31,32]

PROCEDURE. Once the client has been assessed for risk factors of possible side effects of the therapy and is considered a candidate, IV thrombolysis can begin. An agent is selected according to the client's profile and the physi-

Table 28-17 Contraindications for Thrombolytic Therapy

ABSOLUTE CONTRAINDICATIONS

Any history of stroke
Uncontrolled hypertension
    Systolic BP > 180
    Diastolic BP > 110
Recent surgery or trauma (within 2 weeks)
Active internal bleeding
Known bleeding disorder

MAJOR CONTRAINDICATIONS

Acute, poorly controlled hypertension (BP > 180/110)
Malignancy
Recent, prolonged CPR
Acute pericarditis
Pregnancy

MINOR CONTRAINDICATIONS

Age greater than 75 yr
Endocarditis
Advanced illness
Diabetic retinopathy
Atrial fibrillation

cian's preference. Each hospital has a protocol to follow for administration of thrombolytic agents. However there are several common factors. Blood is drawn, three lines for IV therapy are started, and all other invasive procedures done before the thrombolytic agent are given, reducing the possibility of bleeding in the client.

The time therapy begins is noted, and the client is monitored frequently during the dose and maintenance protocol. ECG, vital signs, and heart and lung assessments are completed as often as every 5 minutes to ensure the client's response to therapy. When reperfusion occurs (i.e., the coronary artery that was occluded is patent and blood flow is reestablished to the myocardium), several clinical markers may occur. These include chest pain resolution; return of ST segment to baseline on the ECG; the presence of reperfusion dysrhythmias; and marked, rapid rise of the CPK enzyme within 3 hours of therapy, peaking within 12 hours.[33,34]

The nurse must closely monitor these clients for signs of reperfusion dysrhythmias, including (1) increase in premature ventricular contractions, (2) ventricular tachycardia, (3) ventricular fibrillation, and (4) accelerated idioventricular rhythm. Sometimes bradycardia, AV blocks, and asystole can occur, depending on the location of the infarction. Unfortunately, these clinical markers do not always occur when the artery opens. If they do occur, the nurse should document their presence and have another ECG done.

Another major concern with therapy is reocclusion of the artery. In this situation the client seems to have a reperfused artery and is stable. However, since the area around the thrombus is unstable, another clot may form or spasm of the artery may occur. Because of this possibility, most physicians begin heparin therapy. An IV bolus is given, followed by a heparin drip to maintain the client's partial thromboplastin time (PTT) at one-and-one-half times normal. This prevents another clot from forming in the coronary artery. Despite this therapy, in about 12% to 15% of the clients in whom reperfusion occurs, another clot will develop. If another clot develops, the client has similar complaints of chest pain, ECG changes, and hemodynamic compromise. The physician is notified and further action is taken to determine the cause of the reocclusion. The client may go to the cardiac catheterization laboratory for further invasive diagnostic procedures.

The major complication with thrombolytic therapy is bleeding. The client is receiving an agent that causes clot dissolution and that may cause the client to go into a lytic state. Minor bleeding is expected in these persons. Prevention of bleeding is essential, and proper client selection and screening are imperative. Ongoing nursing assessment is also essential. If minor bleeding does occur (such as surface bleeding from IV sites or gingival bleeding), it can be controlled and thrombolytic therapy should not be stopped. If, however, there is a major bleeding episode, such as massive GI or genitourinary (GU) bleeding, the physician should be notified and the thrombolytic therapy should be stopped. The nurse must pay particular attention to signs and symptoms of bleeding, such as a drop in BP, an increase in HR, positive guaiac from the NG aspirate or stool, hematuria, a sudden change in the client's level of consciousness, and oozing of blood from IV or catheter sites.

Coronary artery bypass graft surgery. CABG surgery may be a treatment choice in a select group of patients with acute MI (see Chapter 29).

Experimental treatment. Experimental research is now being conducted on the use of laser therapy combined with cardiac catheterization to lyse thrombus formation and clear obstructed vessels. Although research is being conducted on types of laser technology, research centers are using this approach to vaporize and evacuate thrombus material later in the course of acute MI.[22] Although laser therapy appears promising in the treatment of chronic atherosclerosis, it does not appear to be the treatment of choice for acute MI.

Pharmacological management

IV nitroglycerin. IV nitroglycerin (NTG) may be used in the initial therapeutic treatment of the client with an acute MI. NTG given IV may reduce pain and decrease preload and afterload while increasing the myocardial oxygen supply. Its action may also increase collateral circulation to the ischemic areas of the myocardium. The dose of NTG is titrated higher to a dose that decreases the client's pain while maintaining an adequate BP. The major side effect of IV NTG is hypotension accompanied by diaphoresis, nausea, vomiting, and occasionally rate dysrhythmias.

Antidysrhythmic drugs. Dysrhythmias are the most common complications after an MI. (The drugs used in the treatment of dysrhythmias are discussed in Chapter 30.)

Morphine. Morphine sulfate is given for acute cardiac pain relief because it reduces anxiety and decreases the cardiac work load by lowering myocardial oxygen consumption, reducing contractility, lowering BP, and slowing the HR. Morphine is given IV because (1) after infarction there may be poor peripheral perfusion, which may cause pooling of medication, rendering the medication ineffective until the circulation is restored, at which time drug overdose may occur, and (2) serum enzymes are affected by an intramuscular (IM) injection.

Meperidine (Demerol) may be given, but it is given less frequently than morphine because it is more likely to induce vomiting and to initiate a vasovagal response. Both drugs can depress respirations, which may cause hypoxia, a condition to be avoided in myocardial ischemia and infarction.

Positive inotropic drugs. Positive inotropic drugs that increase the heart's contractility may be used in the client with AMI. However, caution should be used. This group of drugs increases the heart's demand for oxygen (increased myocardial oxygen consumption [MV_{O_2}]) at a time when therapy is used to decrease the demand and increase the heart's supply of oxygen (increased flow). Digitalis, amrinone (Inocor), and dobutamine (Dobutrex) are examples of drugs that increase the heart's pumping action (contractility). Their use is indicated when left ventricular failure is present. Nursing interventions during the use of inotropics should include frequent vital signs and heart and lung assessment for evidence of further left ventricular failure or ischemia.

β *Blockers.* The use of β blockers early in the acute phase of the MI and during a 1-year follow-up regimen has decreased morbidity. Clients who had β blockers for the acute MI and for 1 year following the infarction had less chance of reinfarction and increased survival.[30]

Drug choice and dose depend on the physician. Nursing interventions during the use of acute β blockers in acute MI should include frequent vital signs and heart and lung assessment. Bradycardia and hypotension may result. The client's physiological response to bradycardia dictates the treatment.

Stool softeners. After MI the client is predisposed to constipation as a result of bed rest and narcotic administration. Stool softeners such as dioctyl sodium sulfosuccinate (Colace) are given to facilitate and promote the comfort of bowel evacuation. This prevents straining and the resultant vagal stimulation from the Valsalva maneuver. (The Valsalva maneuver is explained in Chapter 37.) Vagal stimulation produces bradycardia and can provoke dysrhythmias. Another real danger of straining is that when the action is stopped, venous return to the heart is suddenly increased. This may result in overloading of a weakened heart.

Nutritional considerations. During the first 5 days after MI a soft, bland, low-sodium diet is usually given in multiple feedings. Because an increased coronary output is needed for digestion, this type of diet decreases energy expenditures. The diet may be restricted in saturated fats or cholesterol and is usually low in sodium to prevent fluid retention. The client may have a clear liquid diet the first day when there may still be nausea.

■ Nursing Management of Myocardial Infarction
Nursing assessment
Subjective and objective data that should be obtained from a client with an MI are presented in Table 28-18.
Nursing diagnoses
Nursing diagnoses specific to a client with an MI include, but are not limited to, those presented in Table 28-19.

Table 28-18

Nursing Assessment of the Client with Myocardial Infarction

SUBJECTIVE DATA

History
Positive family history for CAD; previous angina or MI; hypertension, diabetes, chronic obstructive pulmonary disease; relationship of pain to activity; salt, fat, and nicotine intake; activity level, stress

Medications
Use of nitrates, calcium antagonists, cocaine, propranolol

General
Profound weakness, dizziness, syncope, apprehension, feelings of impending doom

Pain
Severe substernal or precordial pain, described as heavy or crushing, lasting more than 30 minutes and not relieved by rest or nitrates; radiation to neck, back, or arms possible

Integumentary
Profuse sweating

Respiratory
Dyspnea

Cardiovascular
Palpitations

Gastrointestinal
Nausea and vomiting, indigestion, heartburn

OBJECTIVE DATA

General
Fever, anxiety, restlessness

Integumentary
Cold, clammy skin

Respiratory
Tachypnea, rales

Cardiovascular
Tachycardia or bradycardia; dysrhythmias (especially ventricular); elevated BP (initially); S_4, possible S_3; murmur and/or rub and diminished heart tones

Urinary
Decreased urinary output

Possible findings
Positive serum cardiac enzymes, leukocytosis; normal chest x-ray film or signs of pulmonary congestion, cardiomegaly; positive radionuclide scan, coronary arteriography

Table 28-19

NURSING CARE PLAN FOR THE CLIENT WITH MYOCARDIAL INFARCTION

Defining Characteristics	Nursing Interventions	Evaluation Criteria

NURSING DIAGNOSIS: **Acute pain related to lactic acid production from myocardial ischemia and altered myocardial oxygen supply**

Severe chest pain, tightness or constriction, radiation of pain to neck, arms, or back	Administer oxygen through nasal cannula. Administer morphine sulfate IV as needed. Monitor vital signs q 1-2 hr. Assess mental status frequently. Continue to evaluate client's level of comfort. Explain the importance of reporting and rating any pain so that it can be evaluated and treated.	Comfortable, ability to rest

NURSING DIAGNOSIS: **Altered cardiac tissue perfusion related to myocardial damage, ineffective CO, and potential pulmonary congestion**

Decrease in BP and urine output, rales in lungs, hepatic engorgement and peripheral edema, splitting of heart sounds, presence of S_4 and S_3	Minimize cardiac work load during healing. Explain necessity for bed rest and decreased activity. Allow rest periods between concentrated nursing care times. Provide long, uninterrupted rest periods. Monitor oxygen administration. Assess comfort level (try to keep client free of pain). Assess urine output to determine adequacy of renal blood flow. Assess vital signs q 1-2 hr. Auscultate heart and lung sounds q 2-3 hr.	BP and pulse within normal limits for individual, respiratory rate of 12-18/min

NURSING DIAGNOSIS: **Impaired gas exchange related to ineffective breathing pattern and decreased systemic tissue perfusion secondary to decreased CO**

Confusion, somnolence, cyanosis, restlessness, irritability	Treat pain. Elevate head of bed. Relieve anxiety. Monitor effects of medications. Hold medication and notify physician if respiratory rate less than 12/min. Maintain oxygen therapy as ordered. Monitor blood gases and oximetry; report abnormalities.	Improvement in blood gases, improvement in cerebral function (i.e., return of usual mental status), no evidence of cyanosis

NURSING DIAGNOSIS: **Anxiety related to present status and unknown future, possible lifestyle changes, pain, and perceived threat of death**

Restlessness, anxiety; verbalization of concern over many health-related aspects such as lifestyle changes and prognosis	Assess anxiety with regard to stressors affecting client. Determine client's past coping mechanisms and effectiveness. If client needs information, provide it clearly and simply at client's level of understanding. Administer diazepam as needed. Assess support systems and incorporate into plan of care if effective (i.e., family may be most effective in reducing client's stress).	Physical and emotional comfort, sense of well-being

NURSING DIAGNOSIS: **Activity intolerance related to fatigue secondary to decreased CO and poor lung and tissue perfusion**

Fatigue with minimal activity, inability to care for self without dyspnea and increase in pulse rate	Meet client's needs quickly and efficiently. Encourage client to maintain bed rest until instructed otherwise. Have articles client may want or need within easy reach. Monitor response to activity (BP, pulse, respiration, color).	Minimal expenditure of energy in the first few days after MI

Continued.

Table 28-19

| | NURSING CARE PLAN FOR THE CLIENT WITH MYOCARDIAL INFARCTION—cont'd | |

Defining Characteristics	Nursing Interventions	Evaluation Criteria

NURSING DIAGNOSIS: Self-esteem disturbance related to lack of control, illness event, and perceived or actual role changes

| Expression of feelings of helplessness and low self-esteem, minimal participation in self-care | Allow client as much autonomy as possible by giving necessary information that will provide feeling of control. Allow client to assist in planning care. Inform client of what to expect in hospital. Demonstrate method to take pulse so that client can determine what limits are during recovery. | Visualization of recovery from MI as time-limited curtailment of normal activities, understanding of importance of limited activity at this time, realistic visualization of future activities |

NURSING DIAGNOSIS: Constipation related to immobility, change in diet, possible fluid restriction, and medications

| Difficulty passing stool, dry and hard stool | Administer stool softeners as ordered. Provide bedside commode. Instruct client to avoid straining. Provide foods high in bulk. If client is unsuccessful, obtain laxative order from physician. | Normal bowel evacuation pattern |

NURSING DIAGNOSIS: Sleep pattern disturbance related to complex treatment regimen, stressful environment, and frequent interruptions

| Report of feeling tired on awakening, frequent napping, fitful sleep with frequent interruptions | Monitor flow of people into client's room. Plan nursing care to provide optimal rest. Provide calm, restful environment. Attempt to maintain client's sleep-wake cycle. If client's condition is stable, do not awaken for vital signs. | Feeling of being rested, minimum interruptions |

NURSING DIAGNOSIS: Altered health maintenance related to lack of knowledge of disease process, rehabilitation, home activities, diet, and medications

| Frequent questioning about illness, management, and aftercare | Teach at client's level of understanding. Provide guidelines with rationale for recommended actions to be taken. Make recommendations to client in a realistic manner so that client can see self carrying them out. Include family when information is given, especially regarding homecoming. Be specific when giving discharge instructions; write them down for client to take home. | Knowledge of causes of heart attack, appropriate response for future symptoms, recommended lifestyle changes, immediate plan of care, appropriate expectations after discharge, activity and diet guidelines |

NURSING DIAGNOSIS: Grieving related to actual or perceived losses secondary to cardiac condition

| Losses, such as occupation, role, status, and previous lifestyle; denial of need to alter lifestyle | Assess potential losses and changes that client will need to make. Encourage discussion of ways to alter lifestyle to client's satisfaction. Assure client of self-worth. Assist client to plan realistic lifestyle adjustments. | Beginning of resolution of grief over losses and changes, positive planning for future |

Nursing interventions

Acute intervention. Acute nursing interventions for the client with MI are best done in a specialized care unit such as a CCU. Since the advent of CCUs in the early 1960s, medical and nursing care has improved dramatically, and countless lives have been saved.

Acute nursing intervention includes the initial intensive care unit (ICU) stay (2 to 3 days) and the rest of hospitalization (5 to 7 days). Priorities for client care in the initial phase of recovery after MI include (1) pain assessment and relief, (2) physiological monitoring, (3) promotion of rest and comfort, (4) alleviation of stress and anxiety, and (5) understanding of the client's emotional and behavioral reactions. Proper management of these priorities decreases the oxygen needs of a compromised myocardium. In addition, the nurse needs to institute measures to avoid the hazards of immobility while encouraging rest.

PAIN. Morphine should be given as needed to eliminate or reduce chest pain. The nurse should instruct the client to rate the pain on a scale of 1 to 10 to assist in the assessment and treatment of pain. In addition to relieving pain, morphine acts as a sedative to relieve anxiety. Since clients do not always verbalize their pain, the nurse must be attuned to other manifestations of pain, such as restlessness, elevated pulse rate or BP, clutching of the bedclothes, or other nonverbal cues. NTG IV, if given, should be titrated. Once pain is relieved, the nurse may have to deal with denial in a client who interprets the absence of pain as an absence of cardiac damage. After the pain medication has been administered, the efficacy of the drug and the client's response should be assessed.

MONITORING. Clients have continuous ECG monitoring while in the CCU and usually after transfer to a step-down or general unit. The nurse should be trained in ECG interpretation so that dysrhythmias causing further deterioration of the cardiovascular status can be identified and eliminated. During the initial period after MI, ventricular fibrillation is the most common dangerous dysrhythmia. In many clients, this dysrhythmia is preceded by premature ventricular contractions and/or ventricular tachycardia.

In addition to frequent vital signs, intake and output should be evaluated at least once a shift, and physical assessment should be carried out to detect deviations from the client's baseline parameters. Included is the assessment of lung sounds and heart sounds and inspection for evidence of fluid retention (e.g., distended neck veins, hepatic engorgement, presacral or anterior tibial edema). Since clients are frequently on strict bed rest initially, dorsiflexion of the feet (Homans' sign) to elicit deep calf pain should also be done to evaluate the presence of deep-vein thrombosis.

Assessment of the client's oxygenation status is helpful, especially if the client is receiving oxygen. Also, the nares should be checked for irritation or dryness, which can cause considerable discomfort if the nasal route is used for oxygen administration.

REST AND COMFORT. With a severe insult to the myocardium, as in the case of infarction, it is important for the nurse to promote rest and comfort. Bed rest may be ordered for the first 2 to 3 days in a severe MI. Clients with

---

Table 28-20 Phases of Rehabilitation

Phase I—Time when client is in the CCU: Activity level depends on severity of MI; client may rest in bed or chair; attention focuses on management of pain, anxiety, dysrhythmias, and cardiogenic shock

Phase II—Time from transfer from the CCU to discharge from hospital: Resumption of activities begins to the point of self-care at the time of discharge; information giving and teaching are appropriate at this time

Phase III—Time of convalescence at home: Client and family examine and possibly restructure lifestyles and roles; exercise program begins, commonly a walking program, which progresses daily during first week and then weekly; client undergoes exercise treadmill test at about 8 wk to determine work load of recovering myocardium

Phase IV—Time of recovery and maintenance: Involvement with the community rehabilitation program for physical training and fitness continues

---

an uncomplicated MI may rest for periods of time in a chair.

When sleeping or resting, the body requires less work from the heart than it does when active. It is important to plan nursing and therapeutic actions to ensure adequate rest periods free from interruption. Comfort measures that can promote rest are smooth bedclothes, frequent oral care, adequate warmth, dim lighting, a quiet atmosphere, and assurance that personnel are nearby and responsive to the client's needs.

It is important that the client understand the reasons activity is limited. In spite of this limitation, however, the client is not immobilized. Gradually, the cardiac work load is increased through more demanding physical tasks so that the client can achieve a discharge activity level for home care. Phases of rehabilitation are outlined in Table 28-20.

ANXIETY. Anxiety is present in all clients in various degrees. The nurse's role is to identify the source of anxiety and assist the client in reducing it. If the client is afraid of being alone, a family member should be allowed to sit quietly by the bedside or to check in with the client frequently. If a source of anxiety is fear of the unknown, the nurse should explore these concerns with the client and help with appropriate reality testing.

If anxiety is due to lack of information, the nurse should provide teaching appropriate to the client's stated need and level. This does not mean that the nurse initiates the cardiac education protocol. Instead, the nurse answers the client's questions with clear, simple explanations sufficient to reduce the client's anxiety.

It is very important to start teaching at the client's level rather than to present a prepackaged protocol. Usually, clients are not yet ready to hear about the pathogenesis of heart disease. The earliest questions usually relate to how the disease affects their perceived control and independence. These questions usually include the following:

When will I leave the CCU?

When can I be out of bed?
When will I be discharged?
When can I return to work?
How much change will I have to make in my life?
Will this happen again?

The nurse should advise that a more complete teaching program begins once the client is feeling stronger. Frequently, the client may not be able to consciously examine the most pervasive concern of all MI victims: Am I going to die? Even if a client denies this concern, it is helpful for the nurse to initiate conversation by remarking that fear of dying is a common concern reported by most clients who have suffered an MI. This gives the client "permission" to talk about an uncomfortable and fearful topic.

EMOTIONAL AND BEHAVIORAL REACTIONS. The emotional and behavioral reactions of a client are varied and frequently follow a predictable response pattern (Table 28-21). The role of the nurse in intervention is to understand what the client is currently experiencing, to assist the client in testing reality, and to support the use of constructive coping styles. Denial may be a positive coping style in the early phase of recovery from MI.

Table 28-21 Emotional and Behavioral Responses to Acute Myocardial Infarction

Denial
May have history of ignoring symptoms related to heart disease
Minimizes severity of medical condition
Ignores activity restrictions
Avoids discussing MI or its significance

Anger
Is commonly expressed as "why did this happen to me?"
May be directed at family, staff, or medical regimen

Anxiety and fear
Fears death and long-term disability
Overtly manifests apprehension, restlessness, insomnia, tachycardia
Less overtly manifests increased verbalization, projection of feelings to others, hypochondriasis
Fears activity, recurrent heart attacks, and sudden death

Dependency
Is totally reliant on staff
Is unwilling to perform tasks or activities unless approved by physician
Wants to be monitored by ECG at all times
Is hesitant to leave CCU or hospital

Depression
Experiences mourning period over loss of health, altered body function, and changes in lifestyle
Realizes seriousness of situation
Begins to worry about future implications of health problem
Shows manifestations of withdrawal, crying, anorexia, apathy
May be more evident after discharge

Realistic acceptance
Focuses on optimum rehabilitation
Plans changes compatible with altered cardiac function

The nurse has an obligation to maximize and enhance the client's support systems. This entails assessing the support structure of the client and family and allowing it to function. Often clients are separated from their most significant support systems at the time of hospitalization. The nurse's role can include talking with the family, informing them of the client's progress, allowing the client and the family to interact as necessary, and supporting the family members who will be able to provide the necessary support to the client. Open visitation is helpful in decreasing anxiety and increasing support for the client with an MI.

Chronic management. *Rehabilitation* may be defined as the process of helping the client adjust to a disability by teaching integration of all resources and concentrating more on existing abilities than on permanent disabilities. Cardiac rehabilitation is the restoration of a person to an optimal state of function in six areas: physiological, psychological, mental, spiritual, economic, and vocational. Many persons recover from an MI physically, yet they may never attain psychological well-being because of misconceptions about the illness or a need to practice illness behaviors. Returning to work and resuming all activities have long been outcome measures of cardiac rehabilitation and are important in terms of the cost effectiveness of cardiac care and rehabilitation. A sample rehabilitation program is presented in Table 28-22.

In considering rehabilitation, nurses and clients must recognize that CAD is a chronic disease. It will not be cured, nor will it disappear by itself. Therefore basic changes in lifestyle must be made to promote recovery and health. These changes must frequently be made at a time when a person is middle-aged and is already dealing with aging and all its associated stresses. The client must also realize that recovery takes time. Resumption of physical activity after MI is slow and gradual. With appropriate and adequate supportive care, however, recovery is more likely to occur.

CLIENT EDUCATION. Once the acute stage of MI has passed, the client is transferred to a step-down, intermediate-care, or regular hospital unit. The goals of nursing care are ongoing. In addition, a very important nursing goal is client and family education. This teaching begins with the CCU nurse and progresses through the staff nurse to the community health nurse. The purpose of education is to give the client and family the tools they need to make informed decisions about attainment of health. For teaching to be meaningful, the client must have a need to learn. Careful assessment of the client's learning needs helps the nurse to set goals and objectives that are realistic. (Guidelines for client teaching are discussed in Chapter 6.)

The timing of the teaching is important. When clients or families are in crisis (either physiological or psychological), they may not have learning needs. It is important to remember that (1) early questions should be answered initially in simple, brief terms, without detailed elaboration and that (2) the answers to these questions require repetition and follow-up (elaboration) as the shock and disbelief accompanying a crisis subside and the client and the family are better able to focus on new information.

In addition to teaching the client and the family what they wish to know, there are several types of information

Table 28-22 Inpatient Rehabilitation: Seven-Step Myocardial Infarction Program

	Step	Date	M.D. Initials	Nurse/ PT Notes	Supervised Exercise	CCU/Ward Activity	Educational-Recreational Activity
CCU	1	_____			Active and passive ROM of all extremities, in bed, teaching of ankle plantar and dorsiflexion—repeated hourly when awake	Partial self-care, self-feeding, dangling legs on side of bed, using bedside commode, sitting in chair 15 min 1-2 times a day	Orientation to CCU; personal emergencies, social service aid as needed; answering of client questions as needed
	2	_____			Active ROM all extremities with client sitting on side of bed	Sitting in chair 15-30 min 2-3 times a day, complete self-care in bed	Orientation to rehabilitation team, program; smoking cessation; provision of educational literature if requested; planning of transfer from CCU
Ward	3	_____			Warm-up exercises, 2 METs of stretching, calisthenics; walking for 50 ft and back at slow pace	Sitting in chair ad lib, transport to ward class in wheelchair, walking in room	Normal cardiac anatomy and function, development of atherosclerosis, education about effects of MI, 1-2 METs craft activity
	4	_____			ROM and calisthenics, 2.5 METs; walking length of hall (75 ft) and back at average pace; teaching of pulse counting	OOB as tolerated, walking to bathroom, walking to ward class with supervision	Coronary risk factors and their control
	5	_____			ROM and calisthenics, 3 METs; checking of pulse counting; walking few stairsteps; walking 300 ft bid	Walking to waiting room or telephone, walking in ward corridor prn	Diet, energy conservation, work simplification techniques (as needed), 2-3 METs craft activity
	6	_____			Continuation of earlier activities, walking down flight of steps (return by elevator), walking 500 ft bid, instruction on home exercise	Tepid shower or tub bath with supervision, to OT, cardiac clinic teaching room with supervision	Heart attack management, including medications, exercise, surgery, response to symptoms, family and community adjustments on return home; craft activity prn
	7	_____			Continuation of earlier activities; walking up flight of steps; walking 500 ft bid; continuation of home exercise instruction, presentation of information regarding outpatient exercise program	Continuing all previous ward activities	Discharge planning, including medications, diet, activity, return appointments, scheduled tests, return to work, community resources; educational literature; medication cards; craft activity prn

Modified from Wenger N: Rehabilitation of the patient with symptomatic atherosclerotic coronary heart disease. In Hurst JW and others, eds: The heart, ed 7, 1990, New York, McGraw-Hill Book Co, p 1110.
ROM, Range of motion; *MET,* metabolic equivalent; *OOB,* out of bed; *OT,* occupational therapy.

that are considered necessary in achieving health. A teaching plan for the client with MI should include the following:

1. Anatomy and physiology of the heart and vessels
2. Cause and effect of atherosclerosis
3. Definition of terms (e.g., CAD, angina, MI, sudden death, CHF)
4. Signs and symptoms of angina and MI and reasons they occur
5. Healing after infarction
6. Identification of risk factors
7. Rationale for tests and treatment, including ECG, blood tests, and angiography and monitoring, rest, diet, and medications
8. Appropriate expectations about recovery and rehabilitation (anticipatory guidance)
9. Measures to take to promote recovery and health
10. Importance of the gradual, progressive resumption of activity

Some nurses have found that an algorithm sheet listing these categories and who gave the information is helpful in documenting information given to the client and family.

When medical terminology is used, its meaning should be explained in lay terms. For example, it can be explained that (1) the heart, a four-chambered pump, is a muscle that needs oxygen like all other muscles and (2) when vessels become narrowed by atherosclerosis, the process is similar to a buildup of mineral deposits inside water pipes, which causes less water to flow through at a higher pressure. It is a good idea for the nurse to have a model of the heart or to use a pad and pencil to sketch what is being explained. This can even be done as informally as on the back of a tissue box. It is critically important not to lose timing because the appropriate materials are not available. Literature written for a lay audience is available through the American Heart Association.

Anticipatory guidance involves preparing the client and the family for what to expect in the course of recovery and rehabilitation. By learning what to expect during treatment and recovery, the client gains a sense of control over life. This sense of perceived control allows the client to consciously consider stressors and thus possibly to promote recovery. The idea of perceived control is operationalized as the process by which the client exercises choice and makes decisions by cutting back. Cutting back is one way of minimizing the psychophysiological losses after MI (or any other life-changing event). The client considers what must be cut back (changed), weighs this against what should be cut back, and finally determines what will be cut back. For example, a middle-aged man who smokes two packs of cigarettes a day, is 20 pounds overweight, and gets no physical exercise has a seemingly overwhelming task. He may decide that he *can* live with a weight-reduction diet and will get more exercise (although perhaps not daily) but that it is not possible for him to quit smoking. He reasons that because he is modifying two of the three risk factors, he will be safe if he cuts back on smoking. Ideally the smoking risk factors should be a priority for this client, but if information regarding risks and effects of smoking is not accepted, the nurse must respect the client's need for control.

PHYSICAL EXERCISE. Exercise is an integral part of the rehabilitation program. It is necessary for optimal physiological functioning and psychological well-being. It has a direct, positive effect on maximal oxygen uptake, increasing CO, decreasing blood lipids, decreasing BP, increasing blood flow through the coronary arteries, increasing muscle mass and flexibility, improving the psychological state, and assisting in weight loss and control. A regular schedule of moderate exercise, even after many years of sedentary living, is very beneficial.

One method used to identify levels of physical activities is through metabolic equivalent (MET) units: 1 MET is the amount of oxygen needed by the body at rest—3.5 ml of oxygen per kilogram per minute or 1.4 calories/kg of body weight per minute. The MET is used to determine the energy costs of various exercises (Table 28-23).

In the hospital, the activity level is gradually increased so that by the time of discharge the client can tolerate moderate-energy activities of 3 to 5 METs. Many clients with an uncomplicated MI are in the hospital only about 7 days. By day 4 or 5 they can stand in the room, perhaps even ambulate in the hallway. Many physicians order low-level treadmill tests before discharge to assess readiness for discharge, accurate HR for an exercise prescription, and potential for reinfarction. If tests are positive (i.e., ischemia at a low level of energy expenditure), the client is evaluated for cardiac catheterization before discharge and possible bypass grafting. If the test is negative, a catheterization may be suggested for 1 month after discharge. Because of the short hospitalization, it is critical to give the client specific guidelines for activity and exercise so that overexertion will not occur. It is helpful to stress that when the client "listens to what the body is saying"—the most important facet of recovery—uncomplicated recovery should proceed.

Teaching clients to check their own pulse rate is a nursing responsibility. Clients should be taught the parameters within which to exercise. They should be told the maximum HR that they should have at any point. If the HR exceeds this level or does not return to the rate of the resting pulse, they should stop. Clients should be instructed to stop exercising if pain or dyspnea occurs.

In normal, healthy persons the minimum threshold for improving cardiorespiratory fitness is 60% of the age-predicted maximum HR. The ideal training target HR is 80% of maximum HR. The client who has been physically inactive and is just beginning an exercise program should do so under supervision whenever possible. The more important factor is the client's response to exercise in terms of symptoms rather than absolute HR. This is a point that cannot be overstressed in teaching of the MI client. In addition, cardiac clients on medications (especially β blockers) may not be able to increase HR to any degree and should have a treadmill test to determine an individual target HR.

The basics for cardiac conditioning within the cardiac population include the following:

1. *Type of exercise:* Exercise should be regular, rhythmic, and repetitive, using large muscles to build up endurance (e.g., walking, cycling, swimming, rowing).

2. *Intensity:* Exercise intensity should be determined by the client's HR. If a treadmill test has not been performed, the person recovering from MI should not exceed 20 bpm over the resting pulse rate.
3. *Duration:* Exercise can be from 20 to 30 minutes. It is important to begin slowly at personal tolerance (perhaps only 5 to 10 minutes) and build up to 30 minutes.
4. *Frequency:* Client should exercise three times a week. If done at low duration (5 to 10 minutes), exercise can be done daily but is best done on nonconsecutive days.

In addition, it is helpful to teach these clients about "warm up" and "cool down" with exercise. Mild stretching for 3 to 5 minutes before the exercise activity and 5 minutes after the activity is sufficient. Activity should not be started or stopped abruptly.

The basic categories of exercise are static *(isometric)* and dynamic *(isotonic)*. Most daily activities are a mixture of the two. Static exercise involves the development of tension during muscular contraction but produces little or no change in muscle length or joint movement. Lifting, carrying, and pushing heavy objects are primarily isometric activities. Since the HR and BP increase very rapidly during isometric work, exercise programs involving isometric exercises should be limited.

Isotonic exercises involve changes in muscle length and joint movement with rhythmic contractions at relatively low muscular tension. Walking, jogging, swimming, bicycling, and jumping rope are examples of activities that are predominantly isotonic. Isotonic exercise can put a safe, steady load on the heart and lungs and may also improve the circulation in many organs.

RESUMPTION OF SEXUAL ACTIVITY. It is important to include sexual counseling for cardiac clients and their partners. This often-neglected area of discussion may be difficult for both clients and health care providers to approach. However, the cardiac client's concern about resumption of sexual activity after MI often produces more stress than the physiological act itself. It is reported that most cardiac clients, especially women, do not resume sexual activity after MI.[35] The majority of these clients changed their sexual behavior not because of cardiac inability but because they were concerned about sexual inadequacy, death during coitus, and impotence. The misconceptions held by these persons could have been clarified with specific counseling by a concerned health care provider.

Before the nurse provides guidelines on resumption of sexual activity, it is important to know the physiological status of the client, the physiological effects of sexual activity, and the psychological effects of having a heart attack. One study concluded that sexual activity for middle-aged men with their usual partners is no more strenuous than climbing two flights of stairs.

Most nurses are unsure of how and when to begin counseling about resumption of sex. It is helpful to consider sex as a physical activity and to discuss or explore feelings in this area when other physical activities are discussed. One helpful approach is: "Many people who have had a heart attack wonder when they will be able to resume sexual activity. Has this been of concern to you?" or "If this

Table 28-23 Energy Expenditure in METs

Low-energy activities (less than 3 METs or less than 3 cal/min)	
Activities in hospital:	
Resting supine	1.0
Sitting	1.2
Eating	1.4
Conversing	1.4
Washing hands, face	2.5
Activities outside hospital:	
Sewing by hand	1.4
Sweeping floor	1.7
Painting, sitting	2.5
Driving car	2.8
Assembling radio	2.7
Sewing by machine	2.9
Moderate-energy activities (3-6 METs or 3-6 cal/min)	
Activities in hospital	
Sitting on bedside commode	3.6
Walking at 2.5 mph	3.6
Showering	4.2
Using bedpan	4.7
Walking at 3.75 mph	5.6
Activities outside hospital	
Bricklaying	4.0
Tractor plowing	4.2
Ironing, standing	4.2
Mopping	4.2
Bowling	4.4
Cycling at 5.5 mph on level ground	4.5
Golfing	5.0
Dancing	5.5
High-energy activities (6-8 METs or 6-8 cal/min)	
Ambulating with braces and crutches	8.0
Performing carpentry	6.8
Mowing lawn by hand	7.7
Playing singles tennis	7.1
Riding on trotting horse	8.0
Walking at 5 mph	6.5
Ascending stairs	7.0
Very high energy activities (8-10 METs or 8-10 cal/min)	
Skiing	9.9
Jogging at 5 mph	8.0
Shoveling snow	8.5
Ascending stairs with a 17 lb load	9.0
Extremely high-energy activities (more than 10 METs or more than 11 cal/min)	
Playing handball	
Cycling at 13 mph	
Ascending stairs with a 22 lb load	

has been of concern to you, this information should be helpful." This type of nonthreatening statement (1) brings up the topic, (2) allows the client to explore personal feelings, and (3) gives the client an opportunity to raise questions with the nurse or another health care provider. Common guidelines are presented in Table 28-24.

Clients need to know that the inability to perform sexually after MI is common and that impotence usually disappears after several attempts. The nurse should reinforce the idea that patience and understanding usually solve the problem. Clients may assume the position of choice.

It is not uncommon for clients who experience chest pain on physical exertion to have some angina during sexual stimulation or intercourse. Clients should be instructed to take nitroglycerin prophylactically. It is also helpful to have clients avoid sex soon after a heavy meal or after excessive ingestion of alcohol, when extremely tired or stressed, or with unfamiliar partners. Anal intercourse is to be avoided because of the likelihood of eliciting a vasovagal response.

Clients should be counseled that resumption of sex depends on personal desires and on the physician's assessment of the extent of recovery. It is usually recommended that clients refrain from sex until 4 to 8 weeks after MI. Some physicians believe that clients should decide when they are ready to resume sex. Others say that clients must be able to climb two flights of stairs briskly without dyspnea or angina before sexual activity can be resumed. There are medical practitioners whose experience leads them to believe that when the client and the partner are ready emotionally, they are most likely ready physiologically.

Reading material on resumption of sexual activity may be presented to the client to facilitate discussion. The nurse should return to clarify and explain as necessary. Calmly and matter-of-factly introducing the subject of resumption of sexual activity during teaching about physical activity has positive effects of eliciting questions and concerns that might not have otherwise surfaced. For example, the nurse might begin, "Sexual activity is like other forms of activity and should be gradually resumed after MI. If your ability to perform sexually is concerning you, the energy expenditure has been found to be no more than walking briskly or climbing two flights of stairs." This forms a factual basis for clients to begin to seek information and explore their own feelings about resuming sex.

HEMODYNAMIC MONITORING

Hemodynamic monitoring refers to the monitoring of blood flow and pressure within the cardiovascular system. *Indirect monitoring* involves a noninvasive procedure. A common example is taking an arterial BP with a sphygmomanometer and stethoscope. (The steps involved in taking an accurate blood pressure reading are presented in Chapter 26.)

Direct or invasive monitoring allows for the ongoing assessment of critical BPs in and around the heart. It is commonly used in ICUs because direct monitoring provides the quickest and most accurate physiological data.

Basic Pressure System

The three basic components of pressure monitoring include a catheter, a transducer, and a monitor. Direct monitoring requires transformation of physiological pressures into an electrical event that can be displayed, recorded, and quantified. This transformation is accomplished with a transducer. The transducer connects with the catheter system from the client to provide the data to be viewed on the oscilloscope. A diaphragm within the transducer detects pressure changes and allows for accurate data collection, evaluation, and documentation.

A specialized catheter or line (depending on the purpose of the monitoring) is inserted into the area where monitoring is to be measured: radial, femoral, or dorsalis pedis artery for arterial pressure or pulmonary artery for pulmonary artery pressure. The catheter system is connected to an IV solution, such as dextrose and water with heparin or normal saline solution with heparin. Within the transducer is a flush device that allows for a continuous movement of solution (at a rate of 3 to 5 ml/hr) into the catheter to maintain line patency. This flush system is maintained under pressure to prevent backup of blood into the pressure line.

Table 28-24 Guidelines for Resumption of Sexual Activity After Myocardial Infarction

Planning of resumption of sexual activity should correspond to sexual activity before the heart attack.

Physical training (exercise) seems to improve the physiological response to coitus; therefore daily exercise during recovery should be encouraged.

Consumption of food and alcohol should be reduced before intercourse is anticipated (e.g., waiting 3-4 hr after ingesting a large meal before engaging in sexual activity).

Familiar surroundings and a familiar partner reduce anxiety.

Masturbation may be a useful sexual outlet and may reassure the client that sexual activity is still possible.

Temperature should be comfortable, not extreme. Hot or cold showers should be avoided just before and just after intercourse.

Foreplay is desirable because it allows a gradual increase in heart rate before orgasm.

Positions during intercourse are a matter of individual choice.

Orogenital sex places no undue strain on the heart. This form of sexual expression depends entirely on the individuals involved.

A relaxed atmosphere free of fatigue is optimal.

Prophylactic use of nitrates is effective in decreasing angina during sexual activity.

Anal intercourse may cause undue cardiac stress because of the possibility of inducing a vasovagal response.

■ Nursing Management of Pressure Lines

There are certain basic principles of nursing care in clients with pressure lines. Each ICU has a specific protocol to follow. Nurses should familiarize themselves with the procedures designed to reduce the three major risks: (1) hemorrhage, (2) thrombosis with emboli, and (3) infection.

The flush solution is kept in a closed system under a pressure greater than the client's systolic pressure to prevent hemorrhage (from bleeding back into the line, which could quickly decrease blood volume if left unchecked). This is done by means of a specialized type of pump on the IV solution bag. It is important to tape all connections to maintain a closed system. If a stopcock became loose, blood can easily move back up the tubing and out the stopcock, quickly reducing blood volume in the client. Alarms on monitoring equipment should always be preset to note changes in pressure and therefore alert the nurse of pressure changes. Pressure on the flush bag must also be kept at a preset level to prevent backup of blood into the tubing.

A preset heparin solution is continuously flushed through the line to prevent thrombus formation. If a thrombus begins to form, a dampening of the waveform may appear. A dampened waveform is one in which the waves have a decreased amplitude, creating a falsely decreased pressure reading. In such cases the line should be flushed with the fast-flush valve on the tubing. If the wave is still dampened, the nurse should attempt to aspirate the clot with a syringe. Aspirated blood should not be injected back into the client.

A careful technique for insertion and maintenance of the line is mandatory to prevent infections. Lines are inserted under aseptic conditions whenever possible, since they are potential direct routes by which bacteria can enter the vascular system. The skin is cleaned according to hospital procedure, usually with an iodine preparation. A cutdown or a percutaneous stick is performed with the aid of local anesthesia. All lines are sutured to the skin and covered with an occlusive dressing. Insertion sites should be covered with an occlusive dressing. The line should be removed if there is any sign of infection at the insertion site or if there are systemic signs of an infection. Lines should not be left in any longer than necessary because they increase the client's susceptibility to infection.

Another important nursing procedure is balancing and calibration of the transducers. Since physiological pressures are related to atmospheric pressures, the transducer must be balanced at atmospheric pressure. Once the transducer is balanced, the monitor is calibrated to show the desired pressure. The procedures for balancing and calibrating the transducer are specified by the type of equipment used and the unit protocol. After calibration is completed, pressure tracing readings are taken with the client in the same position (flat or with the head of the bed elevated) as when the transducer was calibrated. The transducer should be maintained at the level of the right atrium at all times to ensure proper readings.

Arterial Blood Pressure

Continuous monitoring of the arterial BP is indicated for critically ill clients who (1) have hypotension with peripheral vasoconstriction; (2) are receiving potent vasoactive drugs, such as nitroprusside or dopamine; (3) require frequent blood samples, as for arterial blood gases (ABGs); or (4) have increased intracranial pressure.

An arterial line is commonly inserted in the radial or femoral artery. It is important that the site of insertion be stabilized so that the line is not being moved back and forth. This may be done by means of an arm board.

Fig. 28-16 illustrates a typical arterial waveform for a normal BP. The sharp ascent during systole is correlated with the depolarization and contraction of the ventricles. Diastole is represented by a slower descent, starting with the dicrotic notch, which indicates the closing of the aortic valve.

Pulmonary Artery Flow–Directed Catheter

A pulmonary artery (PA) flow–directed catheter (the Swan-Ganz is the most common of these catheters) is used for measuring the pulmonary artery pressure (PAP) and the mean pulmonary capillary wedge pressure (PCWP). These pressures are an indirect reflection of the left ventricular end diastolic pressure (LVEDP). In the absence of acute mitral valve incompetence (insufficiency), the PCWP is a good indicator of left ventricular function.

The original PA catheters had a double lumen, with one lumen terminating at the tip of the catheter and the other, smaller one in the balloon near the tip. The balloon can be inflated near the tip without occluding it. Newer quadruple-lumen PA catheters have a third lumen for measuring the right atrial pressure and a thermistor tip for measuring blood temperature, which is used in determining CO. Some catheters are also equipped with an atrial electrode or pacing wire. The electrode may be used to record atrial electrograms or to pace the atrium, as well as to perform the functions of any other triple-lumen catheter. Another flow-directed catheter is equipped with a fiberoptic tip, enabling the measurement of mixed venous oxygen saturation in the pulmonary artery. This arrangement is of great

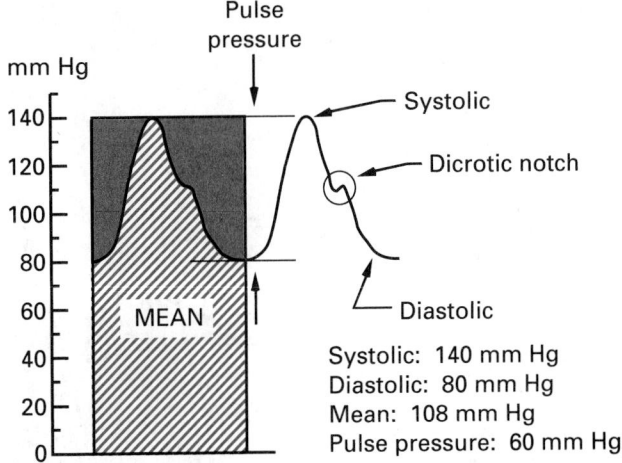

Fig. 28-16 Typical arterial pressure waveform. (From Kinney M and others: AACN's clinical reference for critical care nursing, New York, 1981, McGraw-Hill Book Co, p 1010.)

Systolic: 140 mm Hg
Diastolic: 80 mm Hg
Mean: 108 mm Hg
Pulse pressure: 60 mm Hg

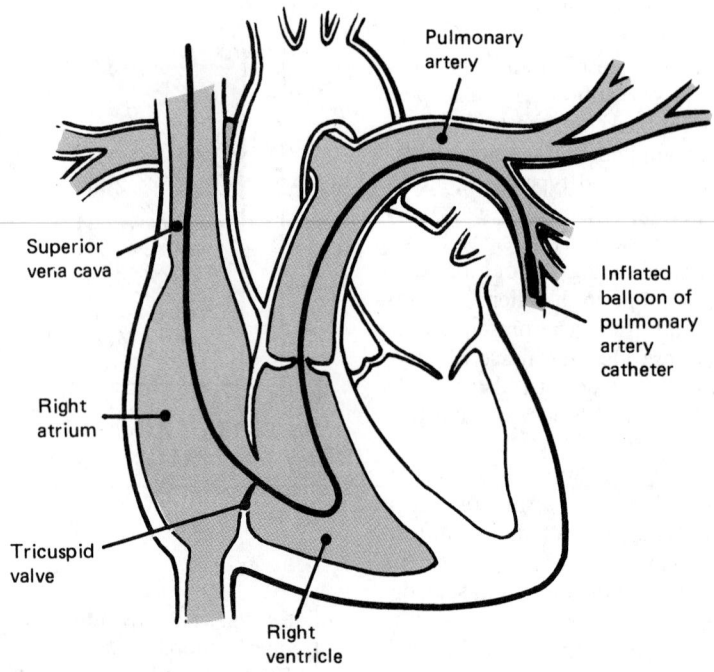

Fig. 28-17 Insertion of a PA catheter through the right side of the heart to the pulmonary artery.

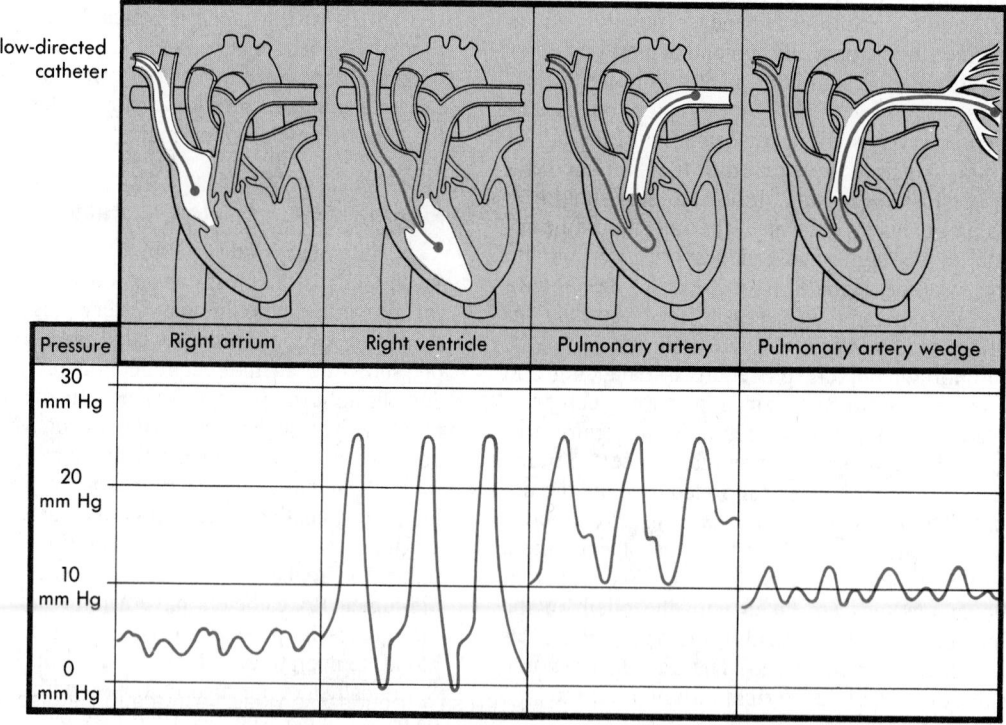

Fig. 28-18 PA catheter insertion with corresponding waveforms. (From Thelan LA and others: Textbook of critical care nursing: diagnosis and management, St Louis, 1990, Mosby–Year Book, Inc, p 243.)

benefit to the client, since only one catheter is passed to serve multiple functions.

After the catheter is attached to the transducer (set up similarly to an arterial line), it is inserted through the internal or external jugular, subclavian, antecubital, or femoral vein and advanced into the right atrium (Fig. 28-17). In the right atrium or ventricle the balloon is fully inflated and allowed to float into the PA until it wedges in a pulmonary arteriole and the pressures are documented. Right atrial pressure is normally 0 to 5 mm Hg and is expressed as a mean pressure. Right ventricular pressure is normally 20 to 25/0 to 5 mm Hg. PAP is normally 25/6 to 12 mm Hg, with a normal PCWP of 4-12 mm Hg. During the insertion procedure, the monitor is observed for changes in pressure waves, which aids in determining the location of the catheter tip (Fig. 28-18).

Once the catheter is in the PA, as evidenced by the characteristic wedge wave, the balloon is deflated and an x-ray film is taken to confirm the proper placement. The catheter is then sutured in place. An occlusive dressing is applied and changed every 24 to 48 hours, depending on unit protocol. The PA systolic pressure (top of the wave) represents contraction of the right ventricle and reflects right ventricular function in a person with normal lungs. The PA end diastolic pressure (bottom of the wave) represents the pressure in the pulmonary arterioles and capillaries to the flow of blood.

When the balloon is inflated, pressures from the right side of the heart are blocked so that the catheter tip measures pressure in the pulmonary capillaries during diastole. The PCWP is usually lower or equal to the PA diastolic pressure and indirectly measures left-atrial filling pressure. Left-atrial filling pressure reflects LVEDP, a measurement used to evaluate therapeutic treatment of the client. By using LVEDP, the nurse can titrate vasoactive drips to maximize the client's CO.

As soon as the PCWP reading is taken, the balloon must be deflated to prevent pulmonary infarction. Another potential risk associated with taking the PCWP reading is rupture of the balloon due to overinflation.

The PA catheter gives the nursing and medical team data regarding myocardial functioning. Data obtained from direct measurements may then be calculated to determine cardiac function. These data may include CO, ventricular contractility, left ventricular stroke work and index, LVEDP, and afterload. These data then determine treatment protocols and medicine regimens.

There are hazards associated with the PA catheter that are not found with arterial lines. In addition to thrombosis and embolus formation, there may be air emboli as a result of the injection of air into the ports or rupture of the balloon. Fragments from balloon rupture may embolize. The PA catheter may also advance into a wedge position on its own. This can be seen by the change in waveform, underlining the need for continuous monitoring. If the catheter is left in a wedge position, a small pulmonary infarction may occur. Changing a client's position or withdrawing the catheter 1 to 2 cm should alleviate the problem.

Ventricular dysrhythmias may occur during insertion or removal of the catheter or if the catheter dislodges and mi-

Table 28-25 Determinants of Cardiac Output

Factors affecting stroke volume	Factors affecting HR
Afterload	Autonomic nervous system
Preload	Effects of exercise
Contractility of left ventricle	

grates back to the right ventricle. This may be noted by changes in the pressure waveform (Fig. 28-18) as well as on the ECG. The physician should be notified if this occurs.

Cardiac Output

CO (which is calculated by multiplying stroke volume and HR) is another measure of cardiac function. Table 28-25 summarizes the determinants of CO. Any change in the stroke volume or heart rate must be balanced by a change in the other value to maintain CO.[36] If the stroke volume is decreased because a massive hemorrhage has reduced the circulating blood volume, the HR increases to compensate. If the HR increases, the stroke volume decreases (e.g., in tachydysrhythmias, diastolic filling time is shortened).

Most types of PA catheters allow direct CO determinations by the thermodilution method. The catheter allows iced solution or room temperature solution (depending on the unit protocol) to be injected at a specified rate into the proximal port of the catheter or into the right atrium. A thermistor at the tip of the catheter senses the temperature of the blood as it passes, and a special computer calculates the CO on the basis of time and of changes in the temperature of the blood. Normal CO is 4 to 8 L/min. Although CO gives information regarding left ventricular function, it varies among persons according to body size. A more accurate indicator of left ventricular function is the cardiac index (CI). CO divided by body surface area yields the CI. The normal CI is 2.4 to 4.8 $L/min/m^2$.

Other Pressures

Other pressures that are monitored are central venous pressure (CVP) (see Chapter 26) and left atrial pressure (LAP). LAP measurement requires that a catheter be inserted directly into the left atrium during a surgical procedure. Thus it is associated with cardiovascular surgery. This pressure is used in determining the LVEDP, since the LAP directly indicates left ventricular filling pressures. It is especially critical in preventing the entrance of air into this line because of the high risk of an air embolus to the coronary arteries or brain.

INTRAAORTIC BALLOON PUMP
Description

The intraaortic balloon pump (IABP) is a mechanical device that provides circulatory assistance to the compromised heart by reducing afterload (the amount of tension the ventricle must develop during contraction to eject

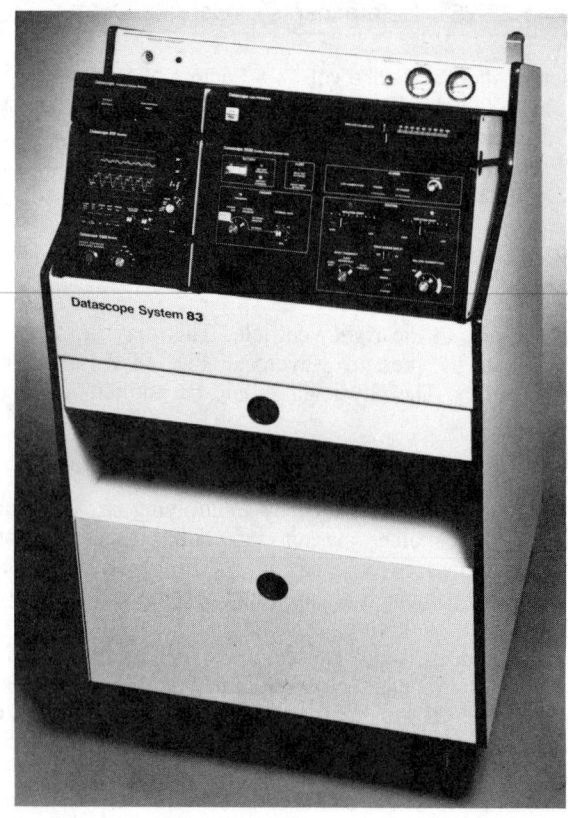

Fig. 28-19 Intraaortic balloon pump. (Courtesy Datascope System, Montvale, NJ.)

Table 28-26 Uses for the Intraaortic Balloon Pump

INDICATIONS

Preinfarction, accelerating, or crescendo angina (when conventional modes of therapy, such as bed rest, nitrates, β blockers, and calcium blockers have failed)

Severe cardiac disease (when client is undergoing cardiac catheterization or noncardiac surgery)

Acute MI with any of the following:

Ventricular aneurysm accompanied by ventricular dysrhythmias Acute ventricular septal defect Acute mitral regurgitation Cardiogenic shock Continuing chest pain	Allows time for emergency angiography and corrective cardiac surgery to be performed

Preoperative, intraoperative, and postoperative open heart surgery (e.g., aneurysectomy, revascularization, or valve replacement); cardiogenic shock associated with any of the above conditions

CONTRAINDICATIONS

Irreversible brain damage

Terminal or untreatable diseases of any major organ system

Ruptured or dissecting aortic or thoracic aneurysm

Generalized peripheral vascular disease (may prevent placement of balloon)

Insufficient aortic valve (considered an *absolute* contraindication)

blood) and augmenting the aortic diastolic pressure (see Figure 28-19).[37] Table 28-26 lists the various clinical conditions for which an IABP is used.

The sausage-shaped balloon is inserted into the common femoral artery with the aid of local anesthesia and advanced upward until it is in the descending thoracic aorta just below the left subclavian artery and above the renal arteries. The balloon is timed to inflate and deflate in synchrony with the client's heart action. Usually, the ECG is used initially to time deflation of the balloon on the R wave and inflation on the T wave. The arterial wave is used to adjust the timing precisely so that balloon inflation occurs at the dicrotic notch on the arterial tracing and deflation occurs just before systole. The balloon pump con-

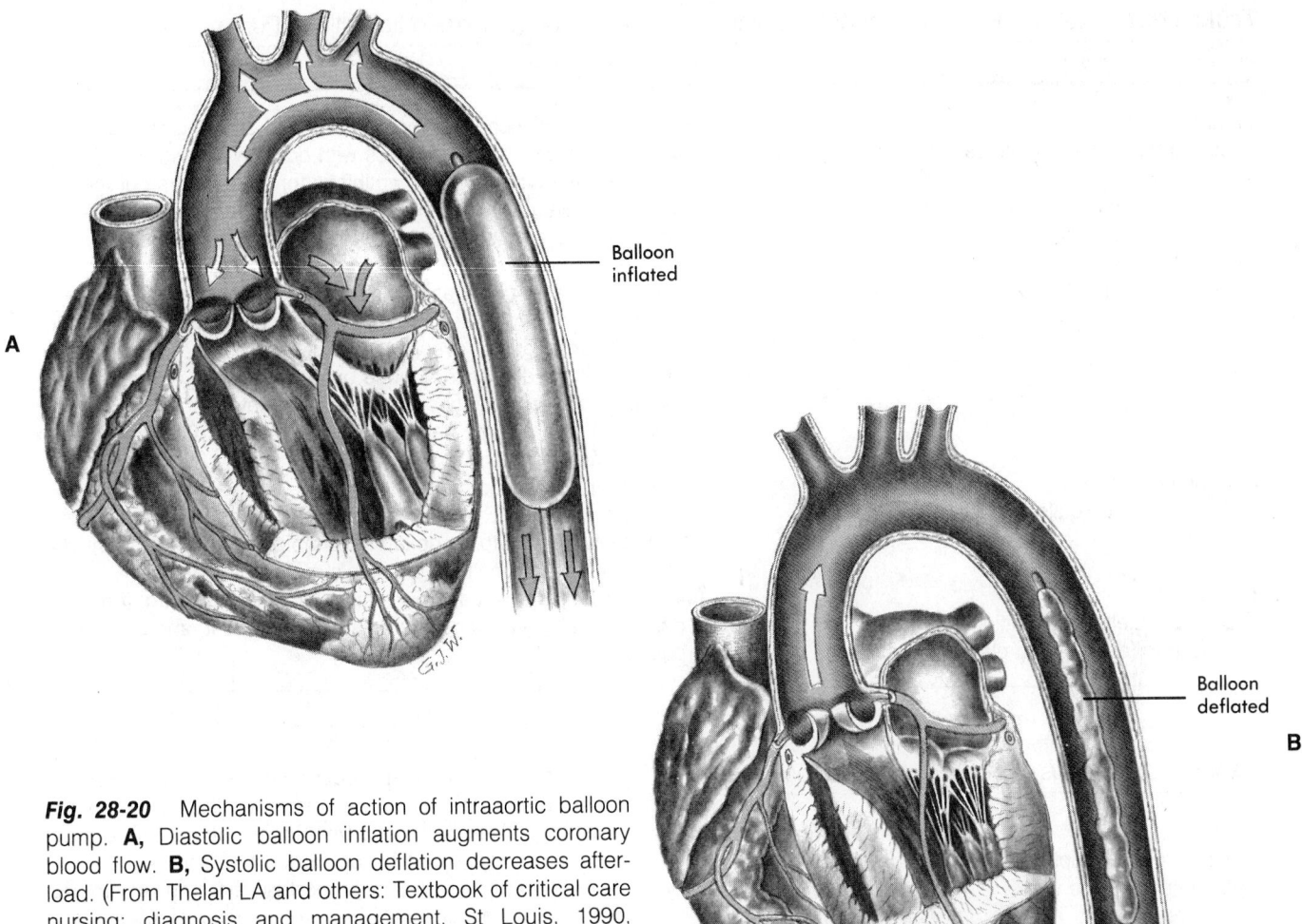

Fig. 28-20 Mechanisms of action of intraaortic balloon pump. **A,** Diastolic balloon inflation augments coronary blood flow. **B,** Systolic balloon deflation decreases afterload. (From Thelan LA and others: Textbook of critical care nursing: diagnosis and management, St Louis, 1990, Mosby—Year Book, Inc, p 323.)

sole contains the controls and alarms for inflation and deflation of the balloon. The balloon action is referred to as *counterpulsation* because the timing of the balloon inflations is the opposite of the ventricular contractions.

Effects of Counterpulsation

The effects of counterpulsation are seen with inflation and deflation of the balloon. The balloon is rapidly inflated at the beginning of diastole immediately after the aortic valve has closed, partially occluding the aorta (Fig. 28-20). Displaced blood is forced downward into the extremities and upward into the coronary arteries and the main branches of the aortic arch. The diastolic arterial pressure rises (diastolic augmentation), increasing perfusion of the vital organs and perfusion pressure for the coronary arteries. The rise in coronary artery perfusion pressure usually causes an increase in the total blood flow to the myocardium and may also increase the development of coronary artery collateral circulation.

The balloon is rapidly deflated just before systole (Fig. 28-20). The suddenly created void causes the pressure in the aorta to drop below the pressure that would exist if no balloon were in place. With the aortic resistance to left ventricular ejection reduced (reduced afterload), the left ventricle empties more easily and completely. As a result, the oxygen consumption of the myocardium decreases.

■ Nursing Management of the Intraaortic Balloon Pump

Beginning, maintaining, and terminating the IABP require nurses who are highly skilled and who work closely with skilled physicians. Clients being treated with the IABP are prone to infections and to arterial, thromboembolic, and hematological complications. Complications are rarely caused by malfunction of the balloon or console because of the fail-safe alarm systems and the automatic unit shutdown safety features that take over when an unsafe pumping condition develops. Nursing management of the complications is covered in Table 28-27. In addition, the nurse monitors the ECG, hemodynamic parameters, and clinical condition of the client every 15 to 60 minutes to determine the effectiveness of the balloon pump.

Table 28-27 Nursing Management of Potential Complications of the Intraaortic Balloon Pump

Potential Complication	Nursing Management
Wound infection Due to multiple lines into cardiovascular system	Use strict aseptic technique for insertion and dressing changes for all lines. Cover all insertion sites with occlusive dressings. Administer prescribed prophylactic antibiotic for entire course of therapy.
Respiratory infection Due to immobilization	Reposition client q 2 hr, being careful not to displace balloon. Avoid causing ECG artifact during physical therapy of chest.
Arterial trauma Due to insertion or displacement of balloon	Evaluate and mark peripheral pulses before insertion of balloon to use as baseline for assessing pulses after insertion. After insertion of balloon, evaluate perfusion to both extremities every hour. Measure urine output every hour (occlusion of renal arteries causes severe decrease in urine output). Observe arterial waveforms for sudden changes. Restrain cannulated leg to prevent flexion. Do not elevate head of bed higher than 30 degrees or flex cannulated leg at the hip.
Thromboembolism Due to trauma, balloon obstruction of blood flow distal to catheter	Administer prophylactic heparin if ordered. Evaluate pulses, urine output every hour. Evaluate level of consciousness every hour. Do not allow balloon to be deflated for more than 30 min. Manually inflate and deflate balloon if console malfunctions.
Hematological Due to platelet aggregation along the balloon (decrease in platelets possible)	Administer Rheomacrodex (low-molecular-weight dextran) if ordered. Monitor anticoagulation status, hematocrit, and platelet count.

Table 28-28 Causes of Cardiogenic Shock

Acute MI	Severe valvular dysfunction
Papillary muscle rupture	
Left ventricular free wall rupture	Myocardial contusion
Acute ventricular septal defect	Cardiac tamponade
	Massive pulmonary embolus
End-stage cardiomyopathy	

CARDIOGENIC SHOCK

Cardiogenic shock is the shock syndrome due to primary cardiac dysfunction. It is also called *pump failure* and has replaced dysrhythmias as the most frequent fatal complication of acute MI. The most common cause of cardiogenic shock is extensive left ventricular dysfunction resulting from acute MI (Table 28-28). Cardiogenic shock occurs in approximately 20% of clients with acute MI and is responsible for 70% of in-hospital deaths after acute MI. The mortality rate from cardiogenic shock after acute MI in any setting is as high as 80% to 95%. It is more likely to occur when there has been previous infarction or when the current infarction is so massive that at least 40% of the myocardium is destroyed.

Pathophysiology and Clinical Manifestations

The primary mechanism of cardiogenic shock is a significant reduction in the size of the contracting myocardium. Pump failure causes a decrease in tissue perfusion and eventually involves all body organs (Fig. 28-21).

In MI the process is initiated by an obstruction of a major coronary artery, which results in myocardial ischemia and infarction. With the infarction there is a decrease in myocardial compliance and therefore a decrease in contractility. Thus decreased functioning of the left ventricle occurs, as evidenced by decreased CO and BP. There is then less arterial pressure to perfuse the coronary arteries. This continued decrease in coronary perfusion causes increased ischemia of the myocardium leading to a larger infarction, less contractility, dysrhythmias, and metabolic acidosis. These conditions further reduce the effective functioning of the left ventricle.

Hemodynamic studies on clients with cardiogenic shock demonstrate a high LVEDP, which will be reflected as a high PWCP, low CO, a low CI, severe hypotension, and no evidence of hypovolemia. The cycle continues to repeat until it is reversed or death occurs. This process may be enhanced by production of a myocardial depressant factor (MDF). A severe decrease in CO is thought to stimulate production of MDF by activating splanchnic lysosomes. This MDF is circulated in the serum and further depresses myocardial function.

The following criteria have been established to define cardiogenic shock:
1. Systolic pressure $\leq$ 90 mm Hg, which has shown a decrease of approximately 30 mm Hg
2. Peripheral circulation insufficient to maintain tissue perfusion; massive vasoconstriction due to sympathetic stimuli (e.g., cool, moist skin)
3. Change in mentation and level of consciousness
4. Urinary output $\leq$ 20 ml/hour for a 2-hour period; administration of diuretics causing little or no effect
5. CI $\leq$ 2.0 L/min/m^2
6. No relief of symptoms with pain relief and oxygen administration
7. PCWP $\geq$ 18 mm Hg

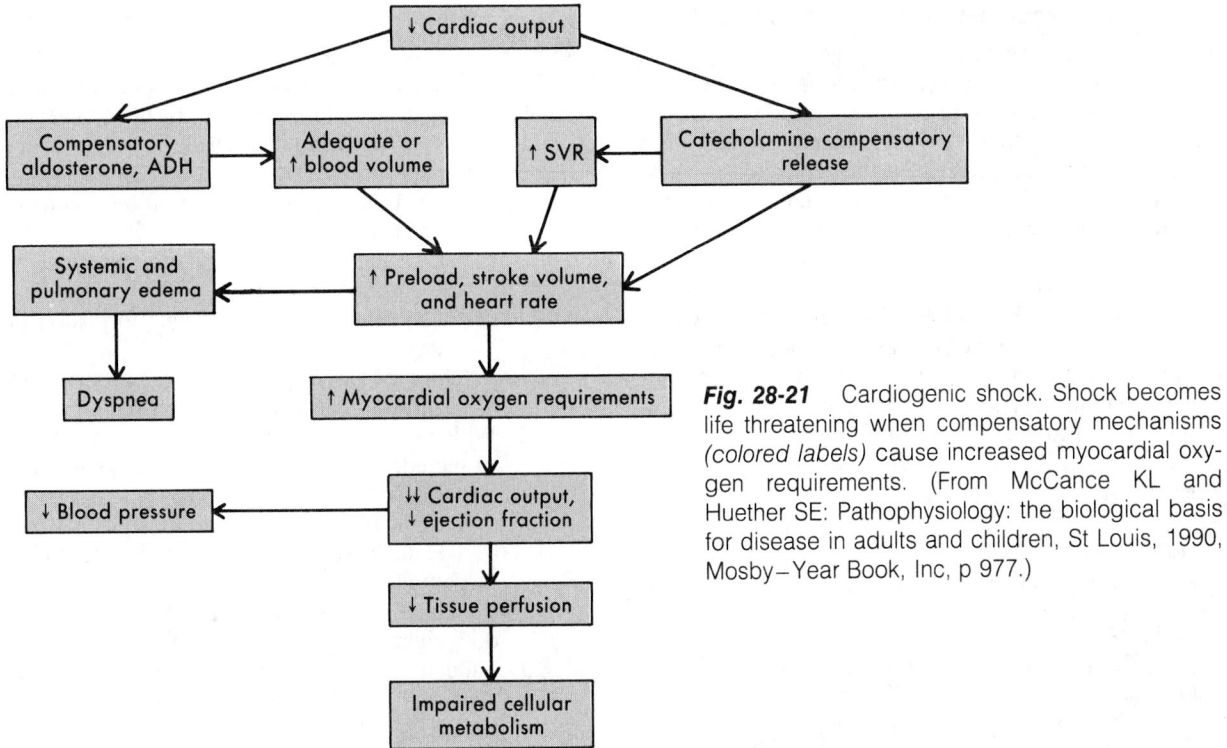

Fig. 28-21 Cardiogenic shock. Shock becomes life threatening when compensatory mechanisms *(colored labels)* cause increased myocardial oxygen requirements. (From McCance KL and Huether SE: Pathophysiology: the biological basis for disease in adults and children, St Louis, 1990, Mosby–Year Book, Inc, p 977.)

Diagnostic Studies

The client in cardiogenic shock is usually already in the CCU, although some clients are admitted to the hospital in shock. Diagnostic management involves the use of various hemodynamic monitoring devices to determine the extent of pump failure and the response to treatment (see Table 28-29). These monitoring devices include arterial pressure lines, a PA catheter, and ECG monitoring. Diagnostic management may also include emergency cardiac catheterization with possible PTCA.

Therapeutic Management

The goal of therapy is to interrupt the vicious circle of pump failure (i.e., to increase coronary circulation, increase contractility, decrease the coronary work load, and increase systemic BP). Since cardiogenic shock results from massive myocardial damage, the prognosis is poor even with aggressive therapy.

Pharmacological Management

The major drugs currently being used are dobutamine and nitroprusside. Dobutamine has been chosen because of its ability to increase the force of myocardial contraction without increasing the HR while increasing arterial BP. Nitroprusside is also combined with either dopamine or dobutamine for its vasodilating effect and the reduction in afterload to help improve CO.

In recent years the IABP has been used to improve the hemodynamic status of clients with cardiogenic shock. If use of the IABP is instituted early in the occurrence of cardiogenic shock, the prognosis is somewhat improved. The IABP is a temporary device used to stabilize the hemodynamics before PTCA or revascularization can be done.

However, overall 1- to 2-year survival rates are poor

Table 28-29

Diagnostic and Therapeutic Management: Cardiogenic Shock

DIAGNOSTIC

Placement of arterial pressure line in peripheral artery and frequent readings (at least every 15 min)
Placement of catheter in PA and hourly readings of PCWP
Continuous ECG monitoring
Determination of CO
Measurement of urine output q1hr
Cardiac catheterization

THERAPEUTIC

Administration of oxygen
Administration of IV fluids to raise left ventricular filling pressure to 16-18 mm Hg if client is hypovolemic
Administration of inotropic agent IV (titrating to systolic BP of 90 mm Hg)
Administration of IV vasodilator to maintain PCWP of 16-18 mm Hg
Placement on IABP
Emergency PTCA if indicated
Emergency coronary artery bypass if indicated

because of the severity of underlying myocardial disease. Some clients do respond well and live long enough to have revascularization surgery. (Cardiac surgery is discussed in Chapter 29.) Cardiac transplantation and artificial heart insertion are alternatives in the treatment of progressive shock.

■ Nursing Management of Cardiogenic Shock

The nursing management of cardiogenic shock begins with the recognition of its onset through observation of vital signs, urinary output, skin condition, and level of consciousness and lung and heart assessment. Circulation is supported as much as possible with medications. These clients are monitored closely and often have arterial and PA monitoring devices. The client is often in respiratory distress and may have to be intubated and placed on a mechanical ventilator. (The nursing care of clients on ventilators is discussed in Chapter 23.) The care of the client in shock is supportive and includes assessment and monitoring of the cardiovascular, respiratory, urinary, neurological, and integumentary systems. Drugs are regulated carefully and titrated to obtain the desired effect.

C ase Study

MYOCARDIAL INFARCTION

Chester T., a 47-year-old successful businessman, was rushed to the hospital by a rescue squad after experiencing crushing substernal pain radiating down his left arm. He also had dizziness, nausea, diaphoresis, and shortness of breath. He revealed a history of angina pectoris, hypertension, and obesity (although he had just lost 10 pounds). He has three teenage children, who were causing problems for him, and his business partner had just died of cancer.

After an ECG was taken, a diagnosis of inferolateral wall MI was made. The client's ECG also showed premature ventricular contractions and tachycardia.

Laboratory results indicated that all the following were significantly elevated:

Triglycerides	220 mg/dl
Cholesterol	350 mg/dl
CPK	730 units/L

Therapeutic treatment:
Hydrochlorothiazide, 50 mg twice a day
Oxygen at 3 L/min
Bed rest
Vital signs every hour
1500-calorie, 3 g-sodium, low-cholesterol diet
IV at keep-open rate
Lidocaine drip for PVCs
Morphine prn

Discussion Questions

1. Which coronary artery was most likely occluded in Chester's coronary circulation?
2. Explain the pathogenesis of CAD. What risk factors may contribute to its development? What risk factors were present in Chester's life?
3. What is angina pectoris? How does angina differ from MI?
4. What happens to the infarcted muscle of the heart after the initial injury?
5. List the clinical manifestations that Chester exhibited and explain the pathophysiological bases.
6. Explain the significance of the results of the ECG and the laboratory tests.
7. For each treatment measure Chester received, explain the physiological reason for its use.
8. What complications may result from an MI?
9. Would Chester be a candidate for thrombolytic therapy?

R eview Questions

The number of the question corresponds to the same-numbered objective at the beginning of the chapter.

1. Which of the following changes occurs in the development of CAD?
   a. formation of fibrous tissue around coronary artery orifices
   b. accumulation of lipid and fibrous tissue within the coronary arteries
   c. diffuse involvement of plaque formation in coronary veins
   d. chronic vasoconstriction of coronary arteries leading to permanent vasospasm
2. Which of the following measures is not appropriate to include in a teaching plan to decrease risk factors for CAD?
   a. modification of a stressful lifestyle
   b. weight reduction and decreased dietary intake of saturated fats
   c. reduction and control of hypertension
   d. weight lifting to increase CO
3. Sudden cardiac death is a primary manifestation of
   a. mitral valve disease
   b. CHF
   c. IHD
   d. cardiomyopathy condition
4. Which of the following describes the pain associated with angina pectoris?
   a. pain that is not relieved by nitroglycerin or rest
   b. substernal chest pain precipitated by activity
   c. crushing, heavy pain lasting 15-20 minutes
   d. substernal pain penetrating to and radiating down the back
5. Which of the following should be included in a teaching plan for a client with angina?
   a. prophylactic use of nitroglycerin
   b. behavior modification to prevent recurrent MI
   c. symptoms of digitalis toxicity
   d. knowledge of foods that are high in potassium
6. Healing following MI is well established
   a. within 3 weeks after the infarction
   b. when chest pain and dyspnea are not present
   c. about 6 to 8 weeks after the infarction
   d. at 4 to 6 days after the infarction
7. The most common complication in the first week after MI is
   a. ventricular rupture
   b. Dressler syndrome
   c. cardiogenic shock
   d. dysrhythmias
8. A client 5 days after MI is very restless and apprehensive. The nurse can help by
   a. structuring the environment and routine so that the client can rest
   b. encouraging the family to provide for client's physical care and emotional support
   c. allowing client to participate in planning and carrying out activities
   d. providing all care by doing everything for client

9. Three days after MI, a client states that he does not understand what the alarm is about because his problem is just bad indigestion. His reaction is an example of
   a. anger
   b. projection
   c. depression
   d. denial

10. A post-MI client being prepared for discharge should be instructed to
   a. take it easy until healing is complete
   b. stay at home and avoid exposure to the environment
   c. begin a graduated, progressive exercise program
   d. do isometric exercises in a relaxed environment

11. Major risks associated with hemodynamic monitoring include all the following *except*
   a. hemorrhage
   b. thrombosis with emboli
   c. infection
   d. hepatitis

12. The purpose of an IABP is to mechanically assist left ventricular function by
   a. reducing afterload and increasing diastolic pressure
   b. increasing afterload and augmenting systolic pressure
   c. increasing preload and decreasing diastolic pressure
   d. reducing preload and decreasing systolic pressure

13. Cardiogenic shock may be managed by all the following measures *except*
   a. dopamine or dobutamine
   b. mechanical ventilation
   c. IABP
   d. rotating tourniquets

REFERENCES

1. Rifkind BM: Lowering plasma cholesterol—a contemporary view, Cardiol Board Rev 6:4-9, 1989.
2. Kannel WB: CHD risk factors: a Framingham study update, Hosp Pract 25:119-130, 1990.
3. Cassel JC: Summary of major findings of the Evans County cardiovascular studies, Arch Intern Med 128:887-889, 1971.
4. Jenkins CD and others: Prediction of clinical coronary heart disease by a test for coronary-prone behavior pattern, N Engl J Med 290:1271-1275, 1974.
5. Memmer MK: Hypercholesterolemia: causes, significance, and diagnoses, Progr Cardiovasc Nurs 4:33-48, 1989.
6. Dietschy JM: LDL cholesterol: its regulation and manipulation, Hosp Pract 25:67-78, 1990.
7. Kannell WB: Update on the role of cigarette smoking in coronary artery disease, Am Heart J 101:319-328, 1989.
8. Haynes SG and others: The relationship of psychosocial factors to coronary heart disease in the Framingham study, Am J Epidemiol 111:37-58, 1980.
9. Hartley L: The role of exercise in the primary and secondary prevention of atherosclerotic coronary artery disease, Cardiovasc Clin 15:1-18, 1985.
10. Stoy DB: Controlling cholesterol with diet, Am J Nurs 89:1625-1627, 1989.
11. Stoy DB: Controlling cholesterol with drugs, Am J Nurs 89:1628-1633, 1989.
12. Scheel M: Cholesterol, lipoproteins, lipid profiles: a challenge in patient education, Focus Crit Care 17:203-211, 1990.
13. Laudin RJ and others: Exercise testing and training of the elderly patient, Cardiovasc Clin 15:201-218, 1984.
14. Vetter NJ and Ford D: Angina among elderly people and its relationship with disability, Age Ageing 19:159-163, 1990.
15. Stanley M: Cardiovascular physiology in the elderly, Crit Care Nurs Q 5:69-71, 1985.
16. Morrissey MJ and Baldwin J: Exercise and chronic heart disease? Geriatr Nurs 8:138-140, 1987.
17. Stone JH: Sudden death. In Schwartz GR and others, eds: Principles and practice of emergency medicine, Philadelphia, 1986, WB Saunders Co, pp 828-836.
18. Melendez LJ: Acute chest pain. In Sibbald W, ed: Synopsis of critical care, ed 3, Baltimore, 1988, Williams & Wilkins Co, pp 7-10.
19. Sharma B and Wyeth RP: Six-year survival of patients with and without painless myocardial ischemia and out of hospital ventricular fibrillation, Am J Cardiol 61:10F-15F, 1988.
20. Miccolo MA: Management of patients with sudden cardiac death caused by ventricular arrhythmias, J Cardiovasc Nurs 3:1-13, 1988.
21. Lonegrave T and Thompson P: The role acute myocardial infarction in sudden cardiac death: a statistician's nightmare, Am Heart J 96:711-720, 1978.
22. Hall LT: Cardiovascular lasers: a look into the future, Am J Nurs 90:27-30, 1990.
23. Topol EJ: Coronary angioplasty in myocardial infarction, Hosp Pract 25:73-79, 1990.
24. Galen K and Hallman J: Recurrence of stenosis after angioplasty, Heart Lung 15:585-587, 1986.
25. Vetrovec G: Left ventricular function in ischemia: therapies and diagnosis implications. Paper presented at Controversies in Cardiology, Bradenton, Fla, Oct 1989.
26. McConnell EA: Applying nitroglycerin ointment correctly, Nursing 20:70, 1990.
27. Kalman JM: Nitrate tolerance: a new look at an old problem, Focus Crit Care 17:407-409, 1990.
28. Pasternak RC and Braunwald E: Acute myocardial infarction. In Wilson and others, eds: Harrison's principles of internal medicine, New York, 1990, McGraw-Hill Book Co.
29. Rodgers ML: Pericarditis, Nursing 20:52-58, 1990.
30. Antman EM and Braunwald E: Acute MI management in the 1990's, Hosp Pract 25:65-82, 1990.
31. Misinski M: Pathophysiology of acute myocardial infarction: a rationale for thrombolytic therapy, Heart Lung 17:743-750, 1988.
32. Kline EM: Recombinant tissue-type plasminogen activator in acute myocardial infarction: role of the critical care nurse, Heart Lung 16:779-786, 1987.
33. Henderson E: Assessment of successful reperfusion after thrombolysis, Heart Lung 17:761-770, 1988.
34. Kleven MR: The critical care nurse's role in the noninvasive assessment of myocardial reperfusion. In Clochesy JM and Ward CR, eds: AACN clinical issues in critical care nursing, Philadelphia, 1990, JB Lippincott Co, p 1.
35. McCann ME: Sexual healing after heart attack, Am J Nurs 89:1133-1140, 1989.
36. Dennison RD: Understanding the four determinants of cardiac output, Am J Nurs 90:35-41, 1990.
37. Joseph DL and Bate S: Intraaortic balloon pumping: how to stay on course, Am J Nurs 90:42-47, 1990.

Nursing Role in Management
Congestive Heart Failure and Cardiac Surgery

Mary Ann Cammarano House
Linda Griego

Table 29-1 Common Causes of Congestive Heart Failure

CHRONIC	ACUTE
Coronary artery disease	Acute myocardial infarction
Hypertensive heart disease	Dysrhythmias
Rheumatic heart disease	Pulmonary emboli
Congenital heart disease	Thyrotoxicosis
Cor pulmonale	Hypertensive crises
Cardiomyopathy	Rupture of papillary muscle
Anemia	Ventricular septal defect
Bacterial endocarditis	

CONGESTIVE HEART FAILURE

Congestive heart failure (CHF) is a cardiovascular state in which the heart is unable to pump an adequate amount of blood to meet the metabolic needs of the tissues. CHF is not a disease but a syndrome caused by a variety of pathophysiological processes (Table 29-1).

Pathophysiology

CHF is usually manifested by biventricular failure, although one ventricle may precede the other in dysfunction.[1] Normally, the pumping actions of the left and right sides of the heart complement each other, producing a continuous flow of blood. However, as a result of pathological conditions, one side may fail while the other side continues to function normally for a period of time. Because of the prolonged strain, the functioning side of the heart will eventually fail, resulting in biventricular failure.

The most common form of initial heart failure is left-sided failure. CHF occurs in a retrograde fashion, progressing from the left ventricle (LV) to the pulmonary system to the right ventricle (RV) (Fig. 29-1). This will usually lead to and is the main cause of right-sided failure. Right-sided failure can occur without preceding left ventricular failure as a result of right ventricular myocardial infarction or cor pulmonale (see Fig. 22-15) CHF will eventually develop in the majority of persons with moderate-to-severe cardiac disease.

Left-sided failure. Left-sided failure results from left ventricular dysfunction, which causes blood to back up through the left atrium and into the pulmonary veins. The increased pressure causes fluid extravasation from the pulmonary capillary bed into the interstitium and then the alveoli, which is manifested as pulmonary congestion and edema. The most common causes of left-sided failure are diseases of the coronary arteries, hypertension, cardiomyopathy, and rheumatic heart disease.

When a myocardial infarction (MI) occurs, myocardial tissue is damaged and replaced by scar tissue. The scar tissue is less elastic and has poorer contractility than undamaged myocardium. The loss of myocardial mass increases

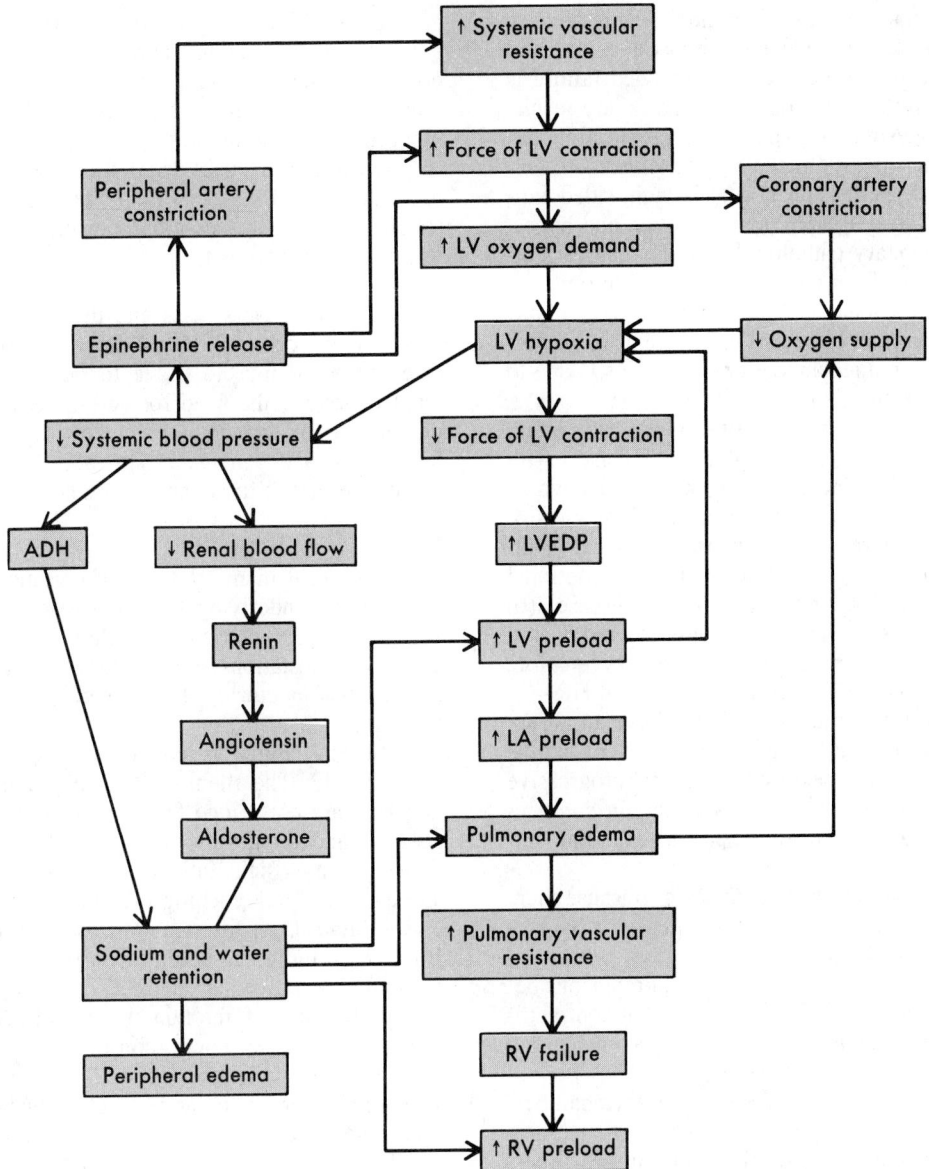

Fig. 29-1 Left heart failure (congestive heart failure) from elevated systemic vascular resistance. Left heart failure leads to right heart failure. Systemic vascular resistance and preload are exacerbated by renal and adrenal mechanisms. *LV,* Left ventricular; *LVEDP,* left ventricular end-diastolic pressure; *LA,* left atrial; *ADH,* antidiuretic hormone. (From McCance KL and Huether SE: Pathophysiology: the biological basis for disease in adults and children, St Louis, 1990, Mosby–Year Book, Inc, p 972.)

the work load on the remaining functional tissue. If the functioning myocardium cannot compensate for this loss, the volume of blood ejected from the ventricle is decreased and heart failure results. This failure may have a rapid onset (acute CHF) or a more insidious onset (chronic CHF).

When hypertension is present, the heart must pump blood against a high arterial pressure. Eventually, this can lead to left ventricular hypertrophy. Hypertrophic muscle has poor contractility and over time will result in failure. Cardiomyopathy (CMP) is the third leading cause of CHF. There are different types of CMP, but the end result is a

LV that has lost the ability to maintain adequate cardiac output resulting in CHF.

In aortic valvular heart disease, the LV must contract forcefully to pump blood through the stenotic aortic valve. Over time, this results in left ventricular failure. This requires an increased amount of pressure that must be generated by the LV. In addition, the valve often fails to close completely and blood is regurgitated into the LV. In mitral valve disease, a similar process involving the left atrium occurs.

Right-sided failure. Right-sided failure from a weakened RV causes venous congestion in the systemic circulation and results in peripheral edema, hepatomegaly, and splenomegaly. The primary cause of right-sided failure is left-sided failure. In this situation, left-sided failure results in pulmonary congestion and increased pressure in the blood vessels of the lung (pulmonary hypertension). Eventually, pulmonary hypertension results in right-sided failure. Cor pulmonale (right ventricular dilatation and hypertrophy due to pulmonary pathology) can also cause right-sided failure. Causes of cor pulmonale include chronic obstructive pulmonary disease and pulmonary emboli. Distended neck veins can be seen when a client with right-sided failure is in a semirecumbent position. This is due to increased pressure in the right atria.

Factors precipitating heart failure. There are certain factors that can precipitate heart failure in a person with heart disease. Examples include (1) dysrhythmias, which lead to ineffective mechanical pumping; (2) reduction or cessation of cardiac therapy, either pharmacological or dietary; (3) infections, either viral or bacterial; (4) emotional or physical stress; (5) second type of heart disease; (6) anemia, which causes an increased heart rate (HR) as a compensatory mechanism to maintain tissue oxygenation; and (7) thyrotoxicosis, which causes an increased HR.

Compensatory mechanisms. CHF can have an abrupt onset as with acute myocardial infarction (AMI) or can be an insidious process and the result of slow, progressive changes. The overloaded heart resorts to certain compensatory mechanisms to try to maintain adequate cardiac output (CO).

Sympathetic nervous system activation. Because there is inadequate stroke volume and CO, baroreceptor reflexes cause sympathetic nervous system activation, which increases the release of epinephrine and norepinephrine. This results in an increased HR and myocardial contractility to raise CO. This response also increases myocardial oxygen demands.

Dilatation. Dilatation is an enlargement of the chambers of the heart. It occurs when pressure in the heart chambers (usually the LV) is elevated over time. The muscle fibers of the heart stretch and thereby increase their contractile force. However, this increased contractility produces greater wall tension, and more myocardial oxygen is required for contraction. Therefore, dilatation is a mechanism developed to cope with increasing blood volume. After maximum hypertrophy, dilatation becomes the primary compensatory mechanism. Eventually, it becomes inadequate because the elastic elements of the muscle fibers are overstrained. Dilatation can progress to mitral valve incompetence and regurgitation, which further increase the cardiac work load.

Renal response to heart failure. As CO falls, blood flow to the kidneys decreases, causing decreased glomerular filtration. This is interpreted by the juxtaglomerular apparatus in the kidneys as *decreased volume.* A complex reaction begins. The kidneys release renin, which reacts with angiotensinogen to form angiotensin (see Fig. 39-6). Angiotensin causes (1) the adrenal cortex to release aldosterone, which causes sodium retention, and (2) increased vasoconstriction, which increases the arterial pressure.

The posterior pituitary senses the increased osmotic pressure due to sodium retention and secretes antidiuretic hormone (ADH). ADH increases water reabsorption in the renal tubules, causing water retention. The decreased renal blood flow also stimulates the secretion of ADH.

The cycle previously detailed is a repeating cycle creating a downward spiral of the client's condition, since vasoconstriction increases afterload and causes an increased work load on the heart.

Hypertrophy. In chronic CHF, hypertrophy is an increase in the muscle mass and the cardiac wall thickness due to overwork and strain. It occurs slowly because it takes time for muscle tissue to develop. As myocardial mass increases, the need for additional blood and oxygen grows. The oxygen requirement of the myocardium is referred to as *MVo₂ demand.* This additional demand cannot always be met in the client with heart disease.

Clinical Manifestations

The clinical manifestations of chronic CHF depend on age, on the underlying type and extent of heart disease, and on which ventricle is failing to pump effectively. These manifestations include fatigue, dyspnea, tachycardia, edema, nocturia, skin changes, behavioral changes, and chest pain.

Fatigue. Fatigue is one of the earliest symptoms of chronic CHF. The client notices fatigue after activities that normally are not tiring. The fatigue is due to impaired circulation and oxygenation of the tissues. It is sometimes described as "sick fatigue" because of the decreased amounts of blood reaching the musculoskeletal system.

Dyspnea. Dyspnea is a common sign of chronic CHF. It is caused by increased pulmonary pressures secondary to interstitial and alveolar edema. This results in poor gas exchange because of fluid in the alveoli. The shortness of breath makes the client conscious of air hunger that prompts rapid, shallow respirations. Dyspnea can occur with mild exertion or at rest. *Orthopnea* is shortness of breath that occurs when the client is in a recumbent position.

Paroxysmal nocturnal dyspnea (PND) occurs when clients are asleep. It is probably caused by the reabsorption of fluid from dependent body areas when the people lie down. Clients awaken in a panic, feel that they are suffocating, and have a strong desire to sit up to seek respiratory relief. Careful questioning of clients will reveal adaptive behavior such as sleeping with two or more pillows to aid breathing.

Tachycardia. Because CO is diminished, there is an increased sympathetic nervous system stimulation to compensate for low output. (It is important to remember that CO equals stroke volume multiplied by HR.) If the stroke volume decreases, the HR increases to maintain the CO.

Edema. Edema is a common sign of CHF. It may occur in the legs (peripheral edema), liver (hepatomegaly), abdominal cavity (ascites), lungs (pulmonary edema and pleural effusion), and other parts of the body. If the client is bedfast, sacral edema will most likely develop. Pressing the edematous skin with the finger may leave a transient indentation *(pitting edema).* The development of dependent edema and/or a sudden weight gain of 2 kg or more is often indicative of exacerbated CHF.

Nocturia. A person with chronic CHF will have decreased cardiac output, impaired renal perfusion, and decreased urinary output during the day. However, when the person lies down at night, fluid movement from interstitial spaces back into the circulatory system is enhanced. This causes increased renal blood flow and diuresis. The client may complain of having to void 6 or 7 times during the night.

Skin changes. Because tissue capillary oxygen extraction is increased in a person with chronic CHF, the skin appears dusky. It is also cold and diaphoretic to the touch. The peripheral vasoconstriction that occurs to shunt blood to vital organs is a minor compensatory mechanism in chronic CHF.

Behavioral changes. Cerebral circulation may be impaired with chronic CHF, especially in the presence of more widespread atherosclerosis. The client or family may report unusual behavior including restlessness, confusion, and decreased attention span or memory. These behavioral changes occur most often at night, possibly because the client is experiencing less stimulation than during the day.

Chest pain. In the presence of atherosclerosis, CHF can precipitate chest pain because of decreased coronary perfusion from decreased CO and increased myocardial work. Anginal type pain may accompany CHF whether it is acute or chronic.

Table 29-2 lists the physical manifestations of left and right ventricular failure. The client with chronic CHF will probably have manifestations of biventricular failure.

Complications

Pulmonary edema. *Pulmonary edema* is a term used to refer to an acute, life-threatening situation in which the

lung alveoli become filled with serous or serosanguineous fluid (Fig. 29-2). The most common factor in the onset of pulmonary edema is left ventricular failure due to coronary artery disease. (Other etiological factors are listed in Table 21-31.) Distinctive histories aid in differentiating pulmonary edema from adult respiratory distress syndrome (see Chapter 23).

The mechanisms of all the conditions resulting in pulmonary edema are not fully understood. Pulmonary edema may occur when compensatory mechanisms fail to effectively handle additional stress on the heart.

In most cases of left-sided heart failure, there is an increase in the pulmonary venous pressure due to decreased efficiency of the left ventricle. This results in engorgement of the pulmonary vascular system (veins, capillaries, and arteries). As a result, the lungs become less compliant (stiff), and there is increased resistance in the small airways. In addition, the lymphatic system increases its flow to help maintain a constant volume of the pulmonary extravascular fluid. This early stage is clinically associated with a mild increase in the respiratory rate and a decrease in both arterial Pao_2 and $Paco_2$.

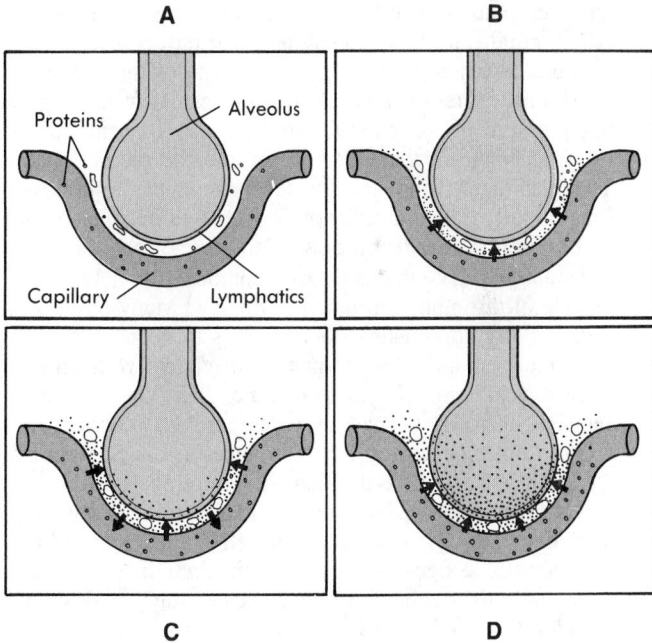

Fig. 29-2 As pulmonary edema progresses, it inhibits oxygen and carbon dioxide exchange at the alveolar capillary interface. **A,** Normal relationship. **B,** Increased pulmonary capillary hydrostatic pressure causes fluid to move from the vascular space into the pulmonary interstitial space. **C,** Lymphatic flow increases in an attempt to pull fluid back into the vascular or lymphatic space. **D,** Failure of lymphatic flow and worsening of left heart failure result in further movement of fluid into the interstitial space and into the alveoli. (From Thelan LA and others: Textbook of critical care nursing: diagnosis and management, St Louis, 1990, Mosby–Year Book, Inc, p 279.)

Table 29-2 Clinical Manifestations of Heart Failure

Right-Sided Heart Failure	Left-Sided Heart Failure
Peripheral edema	Increased heart rate
Weight gain	Left ventricular hypertrophy (PMI displaced inferiorly and posteriorly)
Edema of dependent body parts (sacrum, anterior tibias, pedal edema)	Poor oxygen exchange (arterial blood gases: ↓ Pao_2, slight ↑ $Paco_2$)
Ascites	Pulmonary edema (rales)
Anasarca (massive generalized body edema)	Dyspnea (shallow respirations up to 32-40/min)
Jugular vein distention	Orthopnea, paroxysmal nocturnal dyspnea
Liver engorgement (hepatomegaly)	Cough (dry hacking caused by alveolar irritation from fluid accumulation)
Splenomegaly	S_3 heart sound (from vibrations of ventricle wall due to resistance to ventricular filling)

If pulmonary venous pressure continues to increase, the increase in intravascular pressure causes more fluid to move into the interstitial space than the lymphatics can handle. The edema is interstitial at this point. At this stage, there is more severe tachypnea, the blood gases worsen, and radiographic changes can be noted. If the pulmonary venous pressure increases further, the tight alveoli lining cells are disrupted and a fluid containing red blood cells (RBCs) and large molecules moves into the alveoli *(alveolar edema)* because the pulmonary hydrostatic pressure exceeds normal. As the disruption becomes worse due to further increases in the pulmonary venous pressure, the alveoli and airways are flooded with fluid (see Fig. 29-2). This is accompanied by a worsening of the blood gases (i.e., lower Pao_2 and possible increased $Paco_2$ and progressive acidemia).

Clinical manifestations of pulmonary edema are unmistakable. The client may be agitated, pale, and possibly cyanotic. The skin is clammy and cold due to increased sympathetic nervous system stimuli. The client has severe dyspnea, as evidenced by the obvious use of accessory muscles of respirations, a respiratory rate greater than 30 per minute, and orthopnea. There may be wheezing and coughing with the production of frothy, blood-tinged sputum. Auscultation of the lungs may reveal bubbling rales, wheezes, and rhonchi throughout the lungs. The client's HR is rapid, and blood pressure (BP) may be elevated or at shock levels depending on the severity of the edema.

Pleural effusion. Pleural effusion results from increasing pressure in the pleural capillaries. A transudation of fluid occurs from these capillaries into the pleural space. The pleural effusion usually develops in the right lower lobe initially. (Pleural effusion is discussed in Chapter 21.)

Left ventricular thrombus. With acute or chronic CHF, the enlarged LV and poor CO combine to increase the chance of thrombus formation in the LV. Many physicians will initially administer anticoagulants to decrease the development of thrombus formation in clients with chronic CHF and in some clients with acute CHF. Once a thrombus has formed, it may also decrease LV contractility, CO, and further worsen the client's perfusion. Susceptibility to emboli from the thrombus is also a possibility.

Hepatomegaly. CHF can lead to severe hepatomegaly. The liver lobules become congested with venous blood. The hepatic congestion leads to impaired liver function. Eventually liver cells die, fibrosis occurs, and cirrhosis can develop (see Chapter 38).

Weight changes. There are many factors that contribute to weight changes. Initially, there may be a progressive weight gain due to fluid retention. The client with CHF has an increased metabolic rate. At the same time, decreased oxygen and nutrients are transported to the tissues. Often, the client is too sick to eat. Abdominal fullness from ascites and hepatomegaly frequently causes anorexia and nausea. In many cases, the muscle and fat loss is masked by the client's edematous condition. The actual weight loss may not be apparent until after the edema subsides.

Decompensated heart failure. When the compensatory mechanisms of dilatation, hypertrophy, and tachycardia

---

Table 29-3

 Diagnostic and Therapeutic Management: Chronic Congestive Heart Failure

DIAGNOSTIC

History and physical examination
Determination of underlying cause
Chest x-ray film
ECG
Exercise-stress testing
Echocardiography
Hemodynamic monitoring

THERAPEUTIC

Treatment of underlying cause
Oxygen therapy at 2-6 L/min
Rest
Digitalis preparations
Diuretics*
Vasodilator drugs
   ACE inhibitors
   Nitrates
   Hydralazine (Apresoline)
   Calcium channel blockers
Inotropic therapy
   Amrinone (Inocor)
   Dopamine
   Dobutamine
Daily weights
Sodium-restricted diet

*See Table 29-6.

---

function to provide adequate CO to maintain tissue oxygenation, the client has *compensated heart failure.* When these mechanisms can no longer assist the heart in maintaining CO, the client has *decompensated heart failure.* Without treatment, this state is fatal. Even with treatment, the prognosis is not good.

Diagnostic Studies

The primary goal in diagnosis is to determine the underlying cause of heart failure. Diagnostic measures to assess the degree of heart failure include physical examination, chest x-ray film, electrocardiogram (ECG), hemodynamic assessment, and echocardiogram (Table 29-3).

The chest x-ray film is an important diagnostic measure for assessing and monitoring heart failure. Initial abnormalities in CHF, such as prominent, congested upper lobe pulmonary veins, can be seen on x-ray studies. Later changes, such as interstitial pulmonary edema and pulmonary effusion, can also be visualized. The degree of cardiac enlargement is also readily observed.

An ECG is of value in detecting chronic heart failure. Atrial enlargement is seen by P wave changes in the early phases of CHF. Left ventricular hypertrophy can also be detected by high voltage, especially in V_5 and V_6, and deep S waves in V_1 and V_2. It can also be used to detect

Table 29-4 New York Heart Association Functional Classification of Persons with Congestive Heart Failure

Class 1

No limitation on physical activity; ordinary physical activity not resulting in symptoms

Class 2

Slight limitation on physical activity; no symptoms at rest, but symptoms possible with ordinary physical activity

Class 3

More severe limitations; client usually comfortable at rest; clinical manifestations with unusual physical activities

Class 4

Inability to carry on any physical activity without producing symptoms; symptoms possible at rest

Table 29-5 Manifestations of Digitalis Toxicity

CARDIOVASCULAR

Bradycardia; tachycardia; pulse deficit; dysrhythmias, including premature ventricular contractions, first-degree AV blocks, atrial fibrillation

GASTROINTESTINAL

Anorexia, nausea, vomiting, diarrhea, abdominal pain

NEUROLOGICAL

Headache, drowsiness, confusion, insomnia, muscle weakness

VISUAL

Double vision, blurred vision, colored vision (usually green or yellow), visual halos

cardiac dysrhythmias and changes due to myocardial ischemia or MI. Exercise-stress testing may provide more valuable information than an ECG taken with the client at rest.

Echocardiography can be used to measure the size of the cardiac chambers and to assess ventricular function. Cardiac catheterization and angiocardiography are useful in detecting underlying heart disease. Hemodynamic monitoring via a pulmonary artery catheter (right-sided heart catheterization) provides a means of directly assessing cardiac function. Determination of preload, afterload, contractility, CO, cardiac index, systemic vascular resistance, and work index can be made.

The New York Heart Association has developed functional guidelines for classifying people with CHF. The classification is based on the person's tolerance to physical activity (Table 29-4).

Therapeutic Management

One of the most important goals of treatment for CHF is to treat the underlying cause. If dysrhythmias have precipitated the failure, they should be treated accordingly (see Chapter 30). If the underlying cause is hypertension, antihypertensives should help (see Chapter 27). Valvular defects can be treated with surgery (see Chapter 31). If the cardiac dysfunction is a result of ischemic heart disease, specific interventions such as thrombolytic therapy and percutaneous transluminal coronary angiography (PTCA) may be warranted.

In a person with CHF, oxygen saturation of the blood is reduced because the blood is not adequately oxygenated in the lungs. Administration of oxygen improves saturation and assists greatly in meeting tissue oxygen needs. Thus oxygen therapy helps to relieve dyspnea and fatigue. Optimally, either arterial blood gases (ABGs) or pulse oximetry is used to monitor the effectiveness of oxygen therapy.

Physical and emotional rest allows the client to conserve energy and decreases the need for additional oxygen. The degree of rest recommended depends on the severity of heart failure. A client with severe CHF needs to be on bed rest with limited activity. A client with mild CHF can be ambulatory with a restriction of strenuous activity. The client should be instructed to group activities with adequate recovery periods in between.

Pharmacological Management

Pharmacological therapy for CHF includes the use of digitalis preparations, diuretics, and vasodilator drugs.[2]

Digitalis preparations. Digitalis preparations (cardiac glycosides) have been the mainstay in the treatment of CHF. However, the use of digitalis preparations has recently become controversial, and they are used more judiciously. It is particularly useful in the treatment of heart failure accompanied by atrial flutter and fibrillation and a rapid ventricular rate. Digitalis preparations increase the force or strength of cardiac contraction (*inotropic action*). They also decrease the conduction speed within the myocardium and slow the HR (*chronotropic action*). This action provides more complete emptying of the ventricles, thus diminishing the volume remaining in the ventricles during diastole. CO increases because of an increased stroke volume from improved contractility.

With digitalis preparations, a digitalizing dose much higher than the maintenance dose is given to achieve adequate blood levels rapidly. The maintenance dosage varies from person to person.

The range between therapeutic and toxic effects is narrow and can be affected by other drugs or concurrent disease processes. Monitoring the blood levels of digoxin is vital. The normal therapeutic range for digoxin is 1 to 2 ng/ml.

All persons receiving digitalis preparations are subject to digitalis toxicity (Table 29-5). Some of the earliest symptoms of toxicity are anorexia, nausea, and vomiting. Dysrhythmias are a common indication of digitalis toxicity. Although almost any dysrhythmia can occur, the types most frequently found are premature beats, atrial fibrillation, and first-degree heart block.

Hypokalemia is one of the most common causes of digitalis toxicity resulting in dysrhythmias because low serum potassium levels enhance ectopic pacemaker activity. Monitoring the serum potassium levels of clients receiving both digitalis preparations and potassium-losing diuretics (e.g., thiazides, loop diuretics) is essential. Other electrolyte imbalances, such as hypercalcemia and hypomagnesemia, can also precipitate toxicity.

Diseases of the kidney and liver increase the susceptibility of digitalis toxicity because most of the preparations are metabolized and eliminated by these organs. Older adults are prone to digitalis toxicity because digitalis has more time to accumulate with the slowed body metabolism that occurs with aging.

The usual treatment of toxicity consists of withholding the drug until the symptoms subside. In the case of life-threatening toxicity, digoxin immune Fab (ovine) (Digibind) is an antidote that can be given. The treatment of life-threatening dysrhythmias is instituted as needed (see Chapter 30).

Diuretics. Diuretics are used in heart failure to mobilize edematous fluid, reduce pulmonary venous pressure, and reduce preload (Table 29-6). If excess vascular volume is excreted, blood volume returning to the heart can be reduced and cardiac function improved.

Diuretics act on the kidney by promoting excretion of sodium and water. Many varieties of diuretics are available, and some have specific indications for use. Thiazide diuretics are usually the first choice because of their convenience, safety, and effectiveness. They are particularly useful in treating edema secondary to CHF as well as in controlling hypertension. The thiazides inhibit sodium reabsorption in the distal tubule, thus promoting excretion of sodium and water.

Three potent diuretics, all classified as loop diuretics, are furosemide (Lasix), ethacrynic acid (Edecrin), and bumetanide (Bumex). These drugs act powerfully on the ascending loop of Henle to promote sodium and water excretion. Furosemide is more commonly used because it is slightly more predictable in its response. Bumetanide is a short-acting diuretic with a rapid onset and a half life of 1 to 1.5 hours. It is used when furosemide has not produced diuresis or when a client is allergic to furosemide. Problems in using bumetadine include decreased potassium, ototoxicity, and possible allergic reaction in clients who are sensitive to sulfa type drugs.

Table 29-6 Diuretic Therapy Used in Congestive Heart Failure*

Drugs	Mechanism of Action	Side Effects and Adverse Effects
THIAZIDES		
Chlorothiazide (Diuril), hydrochlorothiazide (HydroDiuril, Oretic, Esidrix), chlorthalidone (Hygroton	Increase in sodium, chloride, and water excretion by inhibiting reabsorption of sodium and chloride in the distal tubule; excretion of potassium in conjunction with sodium	Hypokalemia, increased uric acid, hypercalcemia, hyperglycemia, dermatological reactions
LOOP DIURETICS		
Furosemide (Lasix), ethacrynic acid (Edecrin), bumetanide (Bumex)	Very potent diuretics that increase urine output by preventing sodium and water reabsorption in the loop of Henle and distal tubule	Hypokalemia, hyperglycemia, hyperuricemia
POTASSIUM-SPARING AGENTS		
Spironolactone (Aldactone)	Inhibition of action of aldosterone in distal tubule; increased sodium excretion and potassium retention	Hyperkalemia, gynecomastia, amenorrhea, gastrointestinal disturbances
Triamterene (Dyrenium)	Unkown mechanism of action; action on distal tubule to cause sodium excretion and potassium retention	Hyperkalemia, nausea and vomiting, leg cramps
COMBINATION AGENTS		
Aldactazide (spironolactone and hydrochlorothiazide)	More potent diuretic effect than single agents alone	Gastrointestinal disturbances, dizziness, dry mouth, avoidance of hypokalemia possible
Dyazide (triamterene and hydrochlorothiazide)	Potassium-sparing effects	

*For more information on diuretic therapy, see Table 27-15.

Spironolactone (Aldactone) and triamterene (Dyrenium) are potassium-sparing diuretics that promote sodium and water excretion but block potassium excretion. These are milder diuretics because of their potassium-sparing property. A combination of diuretics may be administered for maximum potential (Table 29-6).

Vasodilator drugs. Vasodilator therapy is replacing digitalis therapy as the primary treatment for clients with CHF who also have normal sinus rhythm.[3] These drugs reduce systematic vascular resistance (a factor affecting afterload) and pulmonary and peripheral venous pressure. Reducing peripheral resistance increases left ventricular stroke volume and CO. Reducing pulmonary and peripheral venous pressure causes a reduction in left ventricular preload. Thus myocardial function is enhanced and myocardial oxygen demand is lessened.

Vasodilator drugs include angiotensin-converting enzyme (ACE) inhibitors, nitrates, calcium channel blockers, hydralazine (Apresoline), and prazosin (Minipress). The ACE inhibitors (captopril [Capoten], enalapril [Vasotec], and lisinopril [Prinivil, Zestril]) are effective drugs in the treatment of CHF. They block the conversion of angiotensin I to angiotensin II (see Figure 39-6), which is a potent vasoconstrictor and also stimulates aldosterone secretion. In CHF the ACE inhibitors increase CO by lowering preload and afterload through promoting salt and water excretion. They also decrease sodium and water retention by suppressing the secondary aldosteronism of decompensated heart failure. The benefits of ACE inhibitors are enhanced with use of a diuretic. The most significant side effects of ACE inhibitors are hypotension, potassium retention, functional renal insufficiency with high doses, and cough.

Nitrates are primarily preload reducing agents. They are particularly beneficial in the management of myocardial ischemia related to CHF because they promote vasodilatation of coronary arteries. The use of nitrates plus hydralazine and ACE inhibitors plus diuretics prolongs survival in clients with severe heart failure.[4] Some problems with vasodilator therapy occur over time. Clients may develop a tolerance to nitrates and prazosin. Calcium channel blockers may not be tolerated long term because they are negative inotropic agents. (Vasodilator drugs are discussed in more detail in Chapter 30 and Table 30-20.)

Nutritional Considerations

The edema of chronic CHF is often treated by dietary restriction of sodium. The degree of sodium restriction depends on the severity of the heart failure and the effectiveness of diuretic therapy. Diets that are severely restricted in sodium are rarely prescribed because they are unpalatable and client compliance is very low.

The normal daily dietary intake of sodium ranges from 3000 to 7000 mg. A commonly prescribed diet for a client with mild CHF is a 2 g sodium diet (Table 29-7). All foods high in sodium should be eliminated (Table 29-8). For more severe CHF, sodium intake is restricted to 500 to 1000 mg. On this diet, milk, cheese, bread, cereals, and canned soups and some canned vegetables must be eliminated.

Fluid restrictions are not commonly prescribed for clients with mild-to-moderate CHF. Diuretic therapy and digitalis preparations act as effective diuretics to promote fluid excretion. However, in moderate-to-severe CHF, fluid restrictions are necessarily implemented.

The client and family need to be told which foods are high in sodium. Salt substitutes frequently contain potassium and their use should be approved by the physician. The client needs to be instructed how to read labels to look for sodium as an ingredient.

■ Nursing Management of Congestive Heart Failure

Nursing assessment

Subjective and objective data that should be obtained from a client with CHF include those presented in Table 29-9.

Nursing diagnoses

Nursing diagnoses specific to the client with CHF include, but are not limited to, those presented in Table 29-10.

Nursing interventions

Health promotion and maintenance. An important measure used to prevent heart failure is the treatment or control of the underlying heart disease. In rheumatic valvular disease, valve replacement should be planned before lung congestion develops in the client. Prophylactic antibiotics should be given to people with a known history of rheumatic heart disease when they undergo surgery or procedures involving instrumentation (e.g., cystoscopy, tooth extraction).

Another important preventive measure concerns early and continued treatment of hypertension. Hyperlipidemic states in persons with coronary artery disease (CAD) need to be managed with diet, exercise, and medication. The use of antidysrhythmic agents or pacemakers is indicated for people with serious dysrhythmias or conduction disturbances.

Acute intervention. Many persons with CHF do not experience an acute episode. If they do, they are usually initially managed in a critical care unit and later transferred to a general unit when their condition has stabilized. The nursing care plan in Table 29-10 applies to the client with stabilized acute or chronic CHF.

Chronic management. CHF may be a chronic illness for most persons. Important nursing responsibilities are (1) educating the client about the physiological changes that have occurred and (2) assisting the client to adapt to both the physiological and psychological changes. It must be emphasized to the client that it is possible to live productively with this health problem.

DIET AND WEIGHT MANAGEMENT. Diet education and weight management are critical to the client's control of chronic CHF. The nurse or dietitian should obtain a detailed diet history, determining not only what foods the client eats and when but also the sociocultural value of food. The nurse can use this data base to assist the client in solving problems. The client should be taught what foods are low and high in sodium and ways to enhance food flavors without the use of salt (e.g., substituting lemon juice and vari-

Table 29-7 Low-Sodium Diets

GENERAL PRINCIPLES

Do not add salt or seasonings containing sodium when preparing foods.
Do not use salt at the table.
Avoid high-sodium foods.*
Limit milk products to 2 cups daily.

SAMPLE MENU PLANS FOR 2 g SODIUM DIET*

Breakfast

1 cup milk	½ cup milk	½ cup milk
¾ cup Puffed Wheat	½ cup Cream of Wheat	½ cup grits
Sugar	Sugar	Boiled egg
Toast	Tortilla	2 tsp butter
Margarine	Fried egg	1 biscuit made with low-sodium baking powder
Scrambled egg	Coffee	
Coffee		Coffee

Lunch

½ cup chicken salad sandwich with 1 tsp mayonnaise	½ cup pinto beans	2 oz fried fish
Fresh fruit	½ cup chili with meat	Creamed carrots
1 cup milk	Tossed salad with oil and vinegar	Roll and butter
Iced tea	Tortilla	Canned fruit
	½ cup gelatin dessert	Soda
	Coffee	

Dinner

3 oz roast beef	3 oz fried steak	3 oz pork chop
1 baked potato	½ cup fried potatoes	½ cup boiled potatoes
2 tsp sour cream	½ cup zucchini or corn	½ cup greens cooked without salt pork
2 tsp margarine	1 cup chocolate pudding	1 cup ice cream
½ cup green beans	Bread and butter or margarine	Sugar cookies
1 dinner roll	Coffee	Coffee
½ cup sherbet		
Coffee		

MODIFICATIONS FOR OTHER LOW-SODIUM DIETS

500 mg sodium diet

Restrict milk products to 1 cup daily.
Limit meat to 4 oz daily.
Use salt-free butter, bread, vegetables, and starches.

1000 mg sodium diet

Restrict milk products to 1 cup daily.
Use salt-free butter and vegetables.

4 g sodium diet

Allow cooking with small amounts of salt.
Allow 3 cups milk products daily.

*See Table 29-8.

Table 29-8 High-Sodium Foods

Beverages	Mineral water, club soda, Dutch-processed cocoa
Breads	Saltines, baking powder biscuits, muffins, Bisquick, pretzels, salted snack crackers and chips; quick breads such as cornbread, nut bread; pancakes, waffles (including mixes)
Cereals	Instant cooked cereal, processed bran cereals, commercial granola
Dairy	Commercial buttermilk, regular cheese
Desserts	Commercial baked products, baked products and puddings made from mixes
Fats	Bacon fat, salted nuts or seeds, commercial dips (e.g., containing sour cream), regular salad dressings, mayonnaise
Juices	Tomato juice, V-8 juice, Clamato, Bloody Mary mixes
Meat	Smoked or cured products—bacon, ham, sausage, salt pork, hot dogs, lunch meat, corned or chipped beef, organ meats, shellfish, sardines, herring, anchovies, caviar, kosher meats, canned tuna fish and salmon, mackerel
Potato or substitute	Salted potato chips, salted french fries, instant potatoes, rice, noodle mixes
Seasonings	Salt, excessive amounts of baking powder, baking soda; celery, onion, and garlic salt and other seasoned salt and peppers; meat tenderizers, AćCent, MSG, worcestershire, soy sauce, mustard, catsup, horseradish, chili sauce, tomato sauce, barbeque sauce, steak sauce
Soup	Commercial soups, bouillon cubes, powdered dehydrated soups
Vegetables	Sauerkraut, tomato juice, V-8 juice, vegetables in creamed or seasoned sauces, frozen vegetables processed with salt or sodium
Miscellaneous	Olives, pickles, salted popcorn, commercially prepared, frozen or canned entrees (e.g., pot pies, TV dinners); Mexican, Italian, Oriental dishes as ordinarily prepared

Table 29-9

 Nursing Assessment of the Client with Congestive Heart Failure

SUBJECTIVE DATA

History
Coronary artery disease (including recent myocardial infarction), hypertension, cardiomyopathy, valvular or congenital heart disease, thyroid or lung disease, rapid or irregular heart beat, sodium intake, anemia, pregnancy, recent weight gain, number of pillows used for sleeping
Medications
Use of and compliance with anti-CHF medications; use of estrogens, steroids, phenylbutazone, indomethacin, verapamil, minoxidil, propranolol
General
Fatigue, dizziness, syncope, anorexia, weight gain
Pain
Chest pain and/or heaviness
Respiratory
Dyspnea, orthopnea, cough, paroxysmal nocturnal dyspnea
Cardiovascular
Palpitations
Gastrointestinal
Nausea or vomiting
Urinary
Decreased urine output (daytime), nocturia
Neurological
Behavioral changes

OBJECTIVE DATA

Integumentary
Cool, diaphoretic skin; cyanosis or pallor
Respiratory
Tachypnea, rales, wheezes; frothy, blood-tinged sputum
Cardiovascular
Tachycardia, S_3; distended neck veins; peripheral edema (right-sided heart failure)
Gastrointestinal
Abdominal distention, hepatosplenomegaly, ascites
Neurological
Restlessness, confusion, decreased attention or memory
Possible findings
Altered serum electrolytes (especially hyponatremia), hypoxemia, elevated BUN, creatinine, and liver function tests; chest x-ray film demonstrating cardiomegaly, pulmonary congestion, and interstitial pulmonary edema; echocardiogram showing increased chamber size and decreased wall motion
ECG—atrial and ventricular enlargement

ous spices). Low-sodium, potassium-rich diets are usually prescribed for clients with chronic CHF. However, low-sodium diets are not palatable and require a strong dedication on the part of the client and family to make necessary changes.

When weight reduction is indicated to decrease the cardiac work load, the nurse and dietitian can assist the client and family in menu planning. Instructing clients to weigh themselves daily is important for monitoring fluid retention as well as weight reduction. Clients should be instructed to weigh themselves at the same time each day, preferably before breakfast, with the same type of clothing. This helps to ensure valid comparisons from day to day and to identify early signs of fluid retention.

DRUG THERAPY. Clients with CHF are usually required to take medication for the rest of their lives. This often becomes difficult because clients may be asymptomatic when

Table 29-10

 NURSING CARE PLAN FOR THE CLIENT WITH CONGESTIVE HEART FAILURE

Defining Characteristics	Nursing Interventions	Evaluation Criteria
NURSING DIAGNOSIS: Activity intolerance related to fatigue secondary to cardiac insufficiency, pulmonary congestion, and inadequate nutrition		
Dyspnea, shortness of breath (SOB), weakness, fatigue, increase/decrease in pulse or exertion	Have client rest in bed or chair when tired. Provide emotional and physical rest. If client is in bed, teach leg exercises to prevent phlebothrombosis. Assess client daily for dyspnea, fatigue, and pulse rate to determine level of activity that can be performed. Provide frequent small feedings instead of three large meals per day. Teach client about expenditure of energy on various activities.*	Achievement of needs by client or care provider
NURSING DIAGNOSIS: Sleep pattern disturbance related to nocturnal dyspnea and inability to assume favored sleep position		
Inability to sleep through night	Explain etiology of nocturnal dyspnea. Explore with client alternative positions of comfort to relieve dyspnea.	Feeling of being rested after sleep
NURSING DIAGNOSIS: Fluid volume excess related to pump failure		
Edema, dyspnea on exertion, SOB	Evaluate degree of peripheral edema and measure abdominal girth daily. Administer digitalis agents and diuretics as prescribed. Assess intake and output q 8 hr. Weigh client daily. Observe manifestations of hypokalemia. Provide sodium-restricted diet as ordered.	Reduction or elimination of hypervolemia
NURSING DIAGNOSIS: High risk for impaired skin integrity related to edema or immobility		
Edema; taut, shiny skin; impaired mobility	Handle edematous skin gently. Pad bony prominences. Assess edematous areas every shift for skin breakdown. Perform passive ROM to extremities q 4 hr.	No breakdown of skin at edematous areas
NURSING DIAGNOSIS: Impaired gas exchange related to excessive preload, mechanical failure, or immobility		
Increased respiratory rate, SOB, dyspnea on exertion	Elevate head of bed to Fowler's position. Support client's arms with pillows; use footboard. Administer oxygen by nasal cannula. Auscultate for lung and heart sounds q 4 hr.	Respiratory rate of 12-18/min
NURSING DIAGNOSIS: Anxiety related to dyspnea or perceived threat of death		
Restlessness, irritability, expression of feelings of life threat	Assess facial expression and behavior for feeling of apprehension. Allow client to ask questions. Promote sense of security by answering call light promptly, explaining all procedures. Assess past methods of coping and assist in adapting these methods to present lifestyle limitations. Demonstrate calm behavior with client. Use measures to decrease dyspnea (e.g., rest, elevation of head of bed).	Expression of feeling less apprehensive about condition and prognosis

*See Table 28-23.

Table 29-10

NURSING CARE PLAN FOR THE CLIENT WITH CONGESTIVE HEART FAILURE—cont'd

Defining Characteristics	Nursing Interventions	Evaluation Criteria
NURSING DIAGNOSIS: Ineffective individual coping related to alterations in lifestyle, possible inability to use past coping methods, or perceived loss of control		
Use of ineffective coping behaviors such as shouting, blaming, anger; withdrawal, social isolation, increased dependency	Teach client about disease process and altered physiological function. Encourage client to adopt lifestyle compatible with degree of heart impairment. Assist client and family in planning necessary changes. Encourage the client who seems discouraged or hopeless to plan and participate in own plan of care. Question client regarding concerns. Support positive coping strategies. Suggest alternate strategies to replace ineffective ones.	Expression of satisfaction with self-participation in care and use of positive coping strategies
NURSING DIAGNOSIS: Self-care deficit (total) related to dyspnea and fatigue		
Inability to perform part or all of activities of daily living	Assist client with all activities of daily living as needed. Assure client of your willingness to assist with personal care. Advise family of client's fluctuating abilities regarding self-care activities.	Achievement of activities of daily living by client with assistance as necessary from health care provider
NURSING DIAGNOSIS: Altered health maintenance related to lack of knowledge regarding signs and symptoms of CHF, proper diet, and medications		
Lack of adherence to low-sodium diet, questioning of disease, diet, and medications	Teach client manifestations to report, including shortness of breath at rest; swelling of ankles, feet, or abdomen; loss of appetite, nausea, or vomiting; weight gain of 1 to 2 kg in a 2-day period; frequent urination; persistent cough; changes in HR ± 20 beats different from usual. Instruct client on dietary restrictions (e.g., low sodium, possible weight reduction) and medication regimen.	Expression of confidence regarding knowledge of disease process and dietary and medication regimen

CHF is under control. It must be stressed that the disease is chronic and that medication must be continued to keep the heart failure under control. Clients need to understand the importance of maintaining adequate drug levels as well as the danger of omitting or making up missed doses. In some situations, it is helpful to work out a system that helps clients to remember to take the medication.

Clients need to evaluate the action of the prescribed medication. They should be taught to recognize the manifestations of digitalis toxicity (see Table 29-5). Clients should also be taught how to take their pulse rate and to know under what circumstances drugs, especially digitalis preparations, should be held and a physician consulted. The pulse rate should always be taken for a full minute. A pulse rate lower than 60 beats per minute (bpm) may be a contraindication to taking a digitalis preparation unless specified otherwise by the physician. A slow pulse rate may indicate a need to alter the digitalis therapy. However, in the absence of primary heart block or the development of ventricular ectopy, a pulse rate of 60 beats/min or less is not a contraindication to taking digitalis. A pulse rate of 50 bpm (especially in a client who is also taking β-blocking drugs) may be acceptable.

Clients should also be taught the symptoms of hypokalemia if they are taking diuretics that cause potassium excretion. (Manifestations of hypokalemia are discussed in Chapter 10.) Hypokalemia sensitizes the myocardium to digitalis. Consequently, toxicity may develop from an ordinary dose of digitalis. Frequently, clients who are taking thiazide or loop diuretics are given supplemental potassium.

REST. The nurse can instruct the client in energy-saving and energy-efficient behaviors after an evaluation of daily activities has been done. For example, once the nurse understands the client's daily routine, suggestions can be made for simplification of work or modification of an activity. Frequently, the client needs a prescription for rest after an activity. Many hard-driving persons need that "permission" to not feel lazy. Sometimes an activity that the client enjoys may need to be eliminated. In such situations the client should be helped to explore alternative activities that cause less physical and cardiac stress. The physical environment may require modification in situations in which there is an increased cardiac work load demand (e.g., frequent climbing of stairs, inaccessibility to shopping areas). The nurse can help the client identify areas where outside assistance can be obtained.

Nurses are also responsible for encouraging clients who are discouraged and for motivating those who feel that their situation is unmanageable. This may require that the nurse assist the client and family in making lifestyle changes that they can accept and comply with. Often the nurse can begin this process by establishing small, achievable goals with the client. Continuous support by the family and health care providers is important. If the client does not adhere to the prescribed regimen, it is important to determine the reasons. After this evaluation process, it may be necessary to plan an alternative therapeutic regimen that is more compatible with the client's lifestyle.

■ Therapeutic and Nursing Management of Acute Congestive Heart Failure and Pulmonary Edema

The goal of therapy is to improve left ventricular function by decreasing intravascular volume, decreasing venous return, improving gas exchange and oxygenation, increasing CO, and reducing anxiety. Many of the measures may be done simultaneously. Table 29-11 lists the major components of the therapeutic approach.

Decreasing intravascular volume

Decreasing intravascular volume with the use of diuretics improves left ventricular function by reducing venous return to the failing LV. A loop diuretic (e.g., furosemide, bumetanide) is the drug of choice for decreasing volume, since it may be administered quickly by IV push and its action within the kidney occurs rapidly.

By decreasing venous return to the LV and thereby reducing preload, the overfilled LV contracts more efficiently and CO will improve. This measure increases LV function, decreases pulmonary vascular pressures, and improves gas exchange.

Intravenous (IV) nitroglycerin (NTG) is a vasodilator used in the treatment of acute and chronic CHF. NTG reduces circulating volume by decreasing preload and also increases coronary artery circulation by dilating the coronary arteries. Therefore, NTG reduces preload, slightly reduces afterload (in high doses), and increases myocardial oxygen supply.

Another method of decreasing intravascular volume (although seldom used today) is phlebotomy, which involves the removal of 300 to 500 ml of whole blood. Rotating tourniquets are a form of phlebotomy and are usually tried before a phlebotomy is done.

Decreasing venous return

Decreasing venous return reduces the amount of volume returned to the LV during diastole. This can be accomplished in several ways. Placing the client in a high Fowler's position with the feet dangling at the bedside helps to

Table 29-11

Diagnostic and Therapeutic Management: Acute Congestive Heart Failure and Pulmonary Edema

DIAGNOSTIC

History and physical examination
ABGs
Chest x-ray film
Insertion of pulmonary artery catheter and peripheral arterial line
Twelve-lead ECG and monitor
Echocardiogram

THERAPEUTIC

Maintenance of client in high Fowler's position with legs dangling
Oxygen by mask or nasal catheter
Morphine IV
Diuretics IV (furosemide or bumetanide)
Nitroglycerin IV
Nitroprusside IV
ACE-inhibitor IV
Aminophylline IV (if wheezing)
Inotropic therapy (dobutamine, amrinone, digitalis)
IPPB (if indicated)
BP, HR, RR, PCWP, urinary output at least q 1 hr
Daily weights
Possible cardioversion
Endotracheal intubation and mechanical ventilation
Treatment of underlying cause

IPPB, Intermittent positive-pressure breathing; *BP*, blood pressure; *HR*, heart rate; *RR*, respiratory rate; *PCWP*, pulmonary capillary wedge pressure.

decrease venous return because of the pooling of blood in the extremities. This position also increases the thoracic capacity, allowing for improved ventilation.

Decreasing afterload

Afterload is the amount of wall tension the LV must develop during systole to eject blood into the aorta, that is, the amount of work the LV has to produce to eject blood to the systemic circulation. Systemic vascular resistance is a determinant of afterload, as is LV filling. If afterload is reduced, the CO of LV improves and thereby decreases pulmonary congestion.

IV nitroprusside is a potent vasodilator that reduces preload and afterload. Because of its potent effects on the vascular system, it is the drug of choice for the client with pulmonary edema. By reducing both preload and afterload (by arteriolar and venous dilatation), myocardial contraction improves, increasing CO and reducing pulmonary congestion. Complications of IV nitroprusside include hypotension, which may require dobutamine IV to maintain a mean arterial BP of 80 mm Hg and thiocyanate toxicity that can develop after 48 hours of use. Morphine is also a drug that reduces preload and afterload. It dilates both the pulmonary and systemic blood vessels, a goal in decreasing pulmonary pressures and improving the exchange of gases.

Improving gaseous exchange and oxygenation

Gaseous exchange may be improved by several measures. IV morphine helps to decrease oxygen demands that may be raised as a result of anxiety and the subsequent increased musculoskeletal and respiratory activity. Administration of oxygen helps increase the percentage of oxygen in inspired air. (Oxygen therapy is discussed in Chapter 21.) Aminophylline may be ordered to dilate the bronchioles and to prevent or decrease bronchospasm. In addition, an arterial line may be used to assess arterial pressure as well as to provide a site for withdrawal of specimens for blood gases. In severe pulmonary edema the client may need to be intubated and placed on a mechanical ventilator.

Improving cardiac function

Although digitalis improves LV function by its positive inotropic action, there is still controversy over its use in the presence of LV failure. Digitalis will increase contractility but will also increase myocardial oxygen consumption. Newer inotropic drugs (e.g., dobutamine and amrinone) that increase contractility without increasing oxygen consumption are more effective drugs. Dobutamine and amrinone cause increased myocardial contractility and peripheral vasodilatation. Whatever increase in MVO_2 is induced by these agents is counteracted by subsequent vasodilatation. However, these drugs are very potent vasoactive substances and the client requires close observation and monitoring.

Reducing anxiety

Reduction of anxiety is facilitated by the sedative action of morphine administered IV. When morphine is used, the client needs to be watched closely for respiratory depression. In addition, a calm approach in providing care helps to reduce anxiety.

CARDIOMYOPATHY

Cardiomyopathy (CMP) is a term used to describe cardiovascular disease resulting from a primary dysfunction of the cardiac muscle that is not associated with CAD, hypertension, valvular, vascular, or pulmonary disease. (End-stage CAD may be referred to as *ischemic cardiomyopathy*, but it is included in this section.) Diagnosis of CMP is made by the client's clinical manifestations and the noninvasive and invasive cardiac procedures performed to rule out other causes of dysfunction.

Clients with CMP present three general types of problems: First, CMP can produce severe heart failure that is usually treated on an outpatient, chronic basis. However, exacerbations occur and are commonly treated in an acute care setting. Thus, acute heart failure complicating chronic dysfunction may represent one clinical presentation of the client with CMP. Another important factor that may develop in this type of client is an acute unrelated (or drug therapy–related) illness necessitating acute care. Third, these clients may present to an intensive care unit (ICU) after surviving a sudden death experience or after a syncopal episode. Most often these episodes are secondary to

malignant ventricular dysrhythmias. This client presents a particular challenge to the nurse and often has unique management needs that should be individualized for each person.

The World Health Organization has classified the cardiomyopathic conditions into three general types: *dilated* (congestive), *hypertrophic,* and *restrictive* (Fig. 29-3).[5,6] Each of these types has its own pathogenesis, clinical presentation, and treatment protocols. The use of myocardial biopsy to make a specific diagnosis in clients with cardiomyopathies is increasing.

Dilated Cardiomyopathy

Pathophysiology. Dilated (congestive) cardiomyopathy is the most common type of CMP, accounting for greater than 90% of all cases, and is characterized by ventricular dilatation and impaired systolic function. What makes this disorder unique from chronic CHF is that the walls of the ventricle do not become hypertrophic. This is thought to be due to the rapid destruction of cells that leaves the ventricles with little time to develop extra muscle.[6] Deterioration is rapid after the development of symptoms, and as many as 20% to 50% of clients are expected to die within a year.

There is no specific cause that has been identified, although dilated CMP often follows an infectious myocarditis. Thyrotoxicosis, diabetes mellitus, toxins (especially alcohol), chemotherapeutic agents, nutritional deficiencies, peripartum, and drugs causing a hypersensitivity reaction have all been associated with the development of dilated CMP[7] (see Table 29-12). Regardless of the initial cause, it results in a diffuse inflammation and rapid degeneration of myocardial fibers that decreases contractile function.

Clinical manifestations. Clinically, the client may present with signs and symptoms of CHF. These symptoms can include fatigue, dry cough, dyspnea, orthopnea, palpitations, and anorexia. Signs can include edema, weak peripheral pulses, pallor, hepatomegaly, and jugular venous distention.[8] The client may also present with dysrhythmias or systemic embolism. The diagnosis of dilated CMP is made on the basis of the client's history and by ruling out other conditions that cause CHF.

■ Therapeutic and Nursing Management of Dilated Cardiomyopathy

Interventions focus on controlling the CHF by enhancing myocardial contractility and unloading the LV much the same way as in the treatment of chronic CHF (Table 29-13). Digitalis is definitely used in the presence of atrial fibrillation, diuretics are used for preload reduction, and vasodilators such as the ACE inhibitors (see p. 831) are used to reduce afterload.[9]

Unfortunately, dilated CMP does not respond well to therapy. Intermittent dobutamine infusions or "pulse inotropic therapy" is a new therapy used in the treatment of dilated cardiomyopathy. Clients are admitted to the hospital for a 72-hour infusion of dobutamine. After infusion, many clients experience an improvement in symptoms that lasts several weeks after therapy. Other therapy includes administration of antidysrhythmic agents and anticoagula-

Table 29-12   Characteristics of Cardiomyopathies

Dilated	Hypertrophic	Restrictive
ETIOLOGY		
Idiopathic condition, alcoholism, pregnancy, myocarditis, nutritional deficiency (vitamin B_1), exposure to toxins and drugs, genetic disease	Inherited disorder (autosomal dominant), possible chronic hypertension	Amyloidosis, postradiation, post–open heart surgery, diabetes
MAJOR MANIFESTATIONS		
Fatigue, weakness, palpitations, dyspnea, dry cough	Exertional dyspnea, fatigue, angina, syncope, palpitations	Dyspnea, fatigue, palpitations
CARDIOMEGALY		
Moderate to marked	Mild	Mild to moderate
CONTRACTILITY		
Decreased	Increased or decreased	Normal or decreased
VALVULAR INCOMPETENCE		
Atrioventricular valves, particularly mitral	Mitral valve	Mitral valve
DYSRHYTHMIAS		
Sinoatrial tachycardia, atrial and ventricular dysrhythmias	Tachydysrhythmias	Atrial and ventricular dysrhythmias
CARDIAC OUTPUT		
Decreased	Decreased	Normal or decreased
STROKE VOLUME		
Decreased	Normal or increased	Decreased
EJECTION FRACTION		
Decreased	Increased	Normal or decreased
OUTFLOW TRACT OBSTRUCTION		
None	Increased	None

tion agents to prevent systemic embolization from mural thrombi that can form in the dilated ventricles. Since the cause of dilated CMP remains unclear, intervention is often unsatisfactory in producing a cure.

Clients with terminal end-stage cardiomyopathy may go on to require cardiac transplantation. At the present time about 47% of heart transplants are performed for treatment of cardiomyopathic conditions. Cardiac transplantation has a good prognosis as far as survival rate. However, donor hearts are difficult to obtain, and the surgical procedure is expensive. Many clients with dilated CMP die while awaiting heart transplantation.

Clients with dilated cardiomyopathy are very ill people with a grave prognosis who need expert nursing care. Nursing care should focus on monitoring the response to medications, monitoring for dysrhythmias, and preventing or rapidly detecting systemic emboli. The nurse should also educate the client about the disease process and assist the client in spacing daily activities to allow for periods of rest. These clients are in great need of emotional support. Information regarding candidacy for heart transplantation and their grave prognosis must be given honestly and empathically. Survivors of sudden cardiac death must be allowed to talk about their experience and express their fears in an open atmosphere. Nurses should include family members and other support systems when planning the client's care.

Hypertrophic Cardiomyopathy

Pathophysiology.   Hypertrophic cardiomyopathy (HCM) produces asymmetrical myocardial hypertrophy (Fig. 29-4) without ventricular dilatation and appears to be an autosomal dominant disease. Another name for this disorder is *idiopathic hypertrophic subaortic stenosis* (IHSS). The four main characteristics of HCM are massive ventricular hypertrophy; rapid, forceful contraction of the LV; im-

Hypertrophic	Restrictive	Dilated (congestive)	Normal

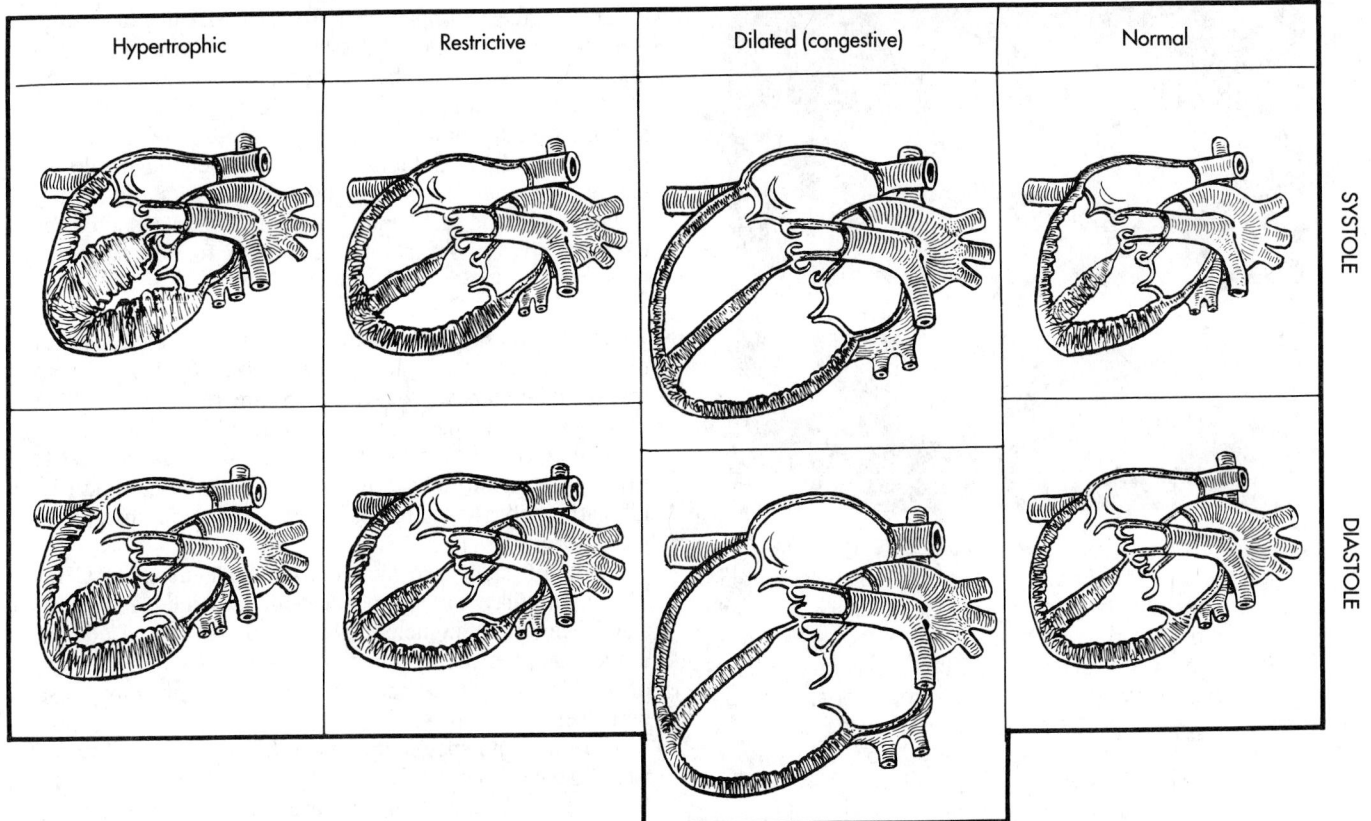

Fig. 29-3 Types of cardiomyopathies. (From Thelan LA and others: Textbook of critical care nursing: diagnosis and management, St Louis, 1990, Mosby–Year Book, Inc, p 386.)

paired relaxation; and obstruction to aortic outflow (may not be present in all clients). The primary defect of HCM is diastolic dysfunction. Impaired ventricular relaxation inhibits adequate filling of the ventricles during diastole. Decreased ventricular filling and obstruction to outflow can result in decreased cardiac output, especially during exertion when increased cardiac output is needed (see Table 29-12).

Clinical manifestations. Client manifestations may include exertional dyspnea because of elevated left ventricular end-diastolic pressure that occurs when an increase in CO during exercise cannot be obtained. Angina can occur and is most often due to the increased left ventricular muscle mass or compression of the small coronary arteries by the hypercontractile ventricular myocardium. These clients may also present with syncope, or near syncope, especially during exertion. Syncope in this population is most often due to an increase in obstruction to aortic outflow during increased activity, but it can also be caused by dysrhythmias. Palpitations are also common in these clients and are most often due to dysrhythmias.[10] Common dysrhythmias include supraventricular tachycardia, atrial fibrillation, ventricular tachycardia, and ventricular fibrillation. Any of these dysrhythmias may lead to loss of consciousness or sudden cardiac death of the client, which is the most common cause of death in this population.[11]

Table 29-13

Diagnostic and Therapeutic Management: Cardiomyopathies

DIAGNOSTIC

History and physical examination
ECG
Chest x-ray film
Echocardiogram
Nuclear studies
Cardiac catheterization

THERAPEUTIC

Treatment of underlying cause
Digitalis (except in hypertrophic CMP in normal sinus rhythm)
Diuretics
ACE inhibitors
Bed rest (if indicated)
Anticoagulants (if indicated)
Antidysrhythmics (if indicated)
β-Adrenergic blocking agents (for hypertrophic CMP)
Intermittent infusions of dobutamine (investigational)
Heart transplant

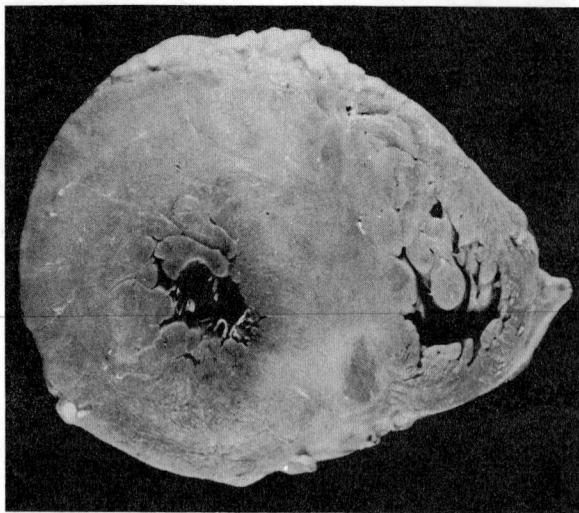

Fig. 29-4 Hypertrophic cardiomyopathy. Cross section through the ventricles is viewed from the base with the anterior surface at the bottom. Notice that the cavity of the left ventricle is unusually small, that the wall of the left ventricle is circumferentially thickened, and that the interventricular septum, especially anteriorly, is disproportionately thickened even more than the free wall (asymmetric septal hypertrophy). This individual was a 59-year-old woman who had hypertrophic cardiomyopathy complicated by mitral regurgitation and CHF; she died of ventricular fibrillation. Her heart weighed 500 g. (From Kissane JM: Anderson's pathology, ed 9, St Louis, 1990, Mosby–Year Book, Inc, p 683.)

■ Therapeutic and Nursing Management of Hypertrophic Cardiomyopathy

Goals of intervention are to improve ventricular filling by reducing ventricular contractility and relieving left ventricular outflow obstruction. This can be accomplished with β blockers or calcium channel blockers. Digitalis preparations are contraindicated in these clients unless they are used to treat atrial fibrillation. CHF may also be present in various degrees but is usually not present until later stages. Antidysrhythmics are also used to control dysrhythmias; however, their use has not proven to prevent sudden death in this group.

Some clients may be candidates for surgical treatment of their hypertrophied septum. The indications for surgery include severe symptoms refractory to therapy with marked obstruction to aortic outflow. The surgery is called a *ventriculomyotomy* and *myectomy*. It involves incision of the hypertrophied septal muscle and/or resection of some of the hypertrophied muscle. Most clients have good symptomatic improvement after surgery and improved exercise tolerance. However, about 12% do not improve after surgery, and operative mortality has been reported to be as high as 7% to 26%.[7]

The degree of impairment from HCM can range from mild to severe. Some clients have an abnormal ECG and know the disease is in their family but have no symptoms. Nursing interventions focus on relieving symptoms, observing for and preventing complications, and providing emotional and psychological support. Education should focus on teaching clients to adjust lifestyle to avoid strenuous activity and dehydration. Again, clients should be taught to space their activities and allow for rest periods.

Restrictive Cardiomyopathy

Restrictive cardiomyopathy is the rarest of the cardiomyopathic conditions. It is characterized by loss of ventricular compliance. The ventricles are resistant to filling and therefore demand high diastolic filling pressures to maintain CO. Systolic function is normal or near normal.[12] Etiology is again unknown but may include amyloidosis, idiopathic fibrosis, sarcoidosis, and radiation therapy to the thorax.[12]

Common signs and symptoms include those of CHF. The client may have signs of both left-sided and right-sided heart failure, including dyspnea, peripheral edema, ascites, and hepatic dysfunction. *Kussmaul's sign* (bulging of the internal jugular neck veins on inspiration) may also be present.

Currently, no specific treatment for restrictive CMP exists. Interventions are again aimed at improving diastolic filling and the underlying disease process. Treatment includes conventional therapy for CHF and dysrhythmias. Heart transplant may also be a consideration. Nursing care is very similar to the care of a client with CHF. As in the treatment of clients with HCM, the clients should be taught to avoid situations that impair ventricular filling, such as strenuous activity and dehydration.

Crack Heart

Illicit drug abuse is a growing concern in the United States. Cocaine use has dramatically increased, and cocaine-related emergency room visits have increased 200% in the last 5 years. With the advent of crack cocaine, the smokable form of cocaine, the incidence of fatal outcomes has also increased. Diagnosis such as AMI in a 22-year-old person who uses cocaine is not uncommon. Every nurse should be aware of the drug problem and look for drug abuse.

One significant problem is the increase in cardiomyopathies in young, previously healthy persons who have used cocaine. The cocaine causes increased MVo_2 and decreased oxygen supply and can cause ischemia and infarction. This may lead to an AMI or ischemic cardiomyopathy. The CMP produced is difficult to treat. Interventions deal mainly with the CHF that ensues. These clients have a very poor prognosis.

CARDIAC SURGERY

CCUs or ICUs are often used as the immediate recovery or postrecovery site for clients undergoing cardiac surgery. Close monitoring and management of these clients require the specialized skills and knowledge of the nurse. Because clients requiring cardiac surgery need similar types of pre-

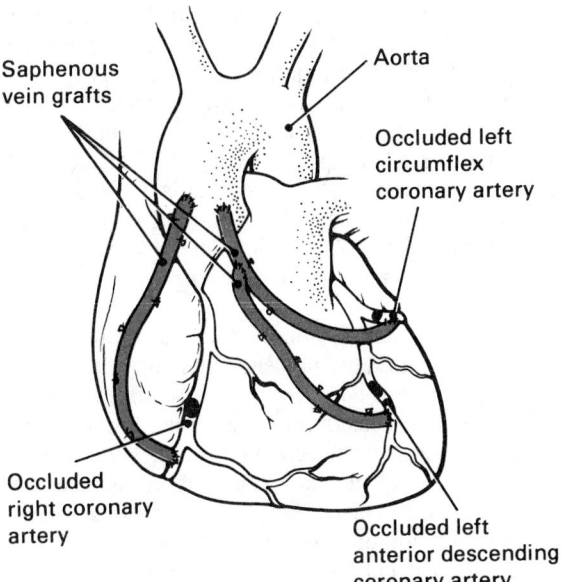

Fig. 29-5 Saphenous aortocoronary artery bypass or revascularization involves taking a piece of saphenous vein from the leg and creating a conduit for blood from the aorta to the area below the blockage in the coronary artery. A triple bypass is illustrated. (Courtesy Mayo Clinic, Rochester, Minn.)

operative and postoperative care, their general management is described.

Cardiac Surgeries in the Adult

Myocardial revascularization. Myocardial revascularization, or coronary artery bypass grafting, is the main surgical treatment for coronary artery disease (Fig. 29-5). It usually involves a graft from the saphenous vein or the internal mammary artery for aortocoronary bypass. In the former procedure, the saphenous vein from one of the client's legs is removed and reversed (so that the valves will not obstruct the blood flow). Segments are then sutured in place so that blood may flow from the aorta to a distal segment of the obstructed coronary artery to establish perfusion of the myocardium. The coronary artery is considered obstructed if its diameter is narrowed by more than 75% to 80%. Revascularization surgery has a mortality rate of about 1% to 2%, with an 85% rate of functional improvement (80% of clients have their anginal pain completely eliminated). Revascularization has been shown to decrease mortality rates for those clients with severe left main stem stenosis and/or severe three-vessel disease. Possible indications for cardiac surgery are shown in Table 29-14.

Nursing care for these clients involves caring for two surgical sites: the chest and the leg. The care of the leg wound is similar to the postoperative care after the stripping of varicose veins (see Chapter 32). The management of the chest wound, which involves a thoracotomy, is similar to that of other chest surgeries. (The nursing management of the client with a thoracotomy is presented in Table 21-27.)

Table 29-14 Indications for Cardiac Surgery

Aneurysm of sinus of Valsalva
Aortic stenosis and regurgitation
Atherosclerotic coronary artery disease
Constrictive pericarditis
Dissecting aortic aneurysm
Mitral stenosis and regurgitation
Myocardial trauma or rupture
Tricuspid insufficiency or stenosis
Ventricular aneurysm
Ventricular septal defect
Ventricular dysrhythmias

Valvular surgeries. Almost all cardiac valvular surgeries require cardiopulmonary bypass. A closed mitral commissurotomy is the only possible exception. It involves incising the fused leaflets of the mitral valves if there is no significant calcification of the valve. (Chapter 31 describes the causes, therapeutic management, and surgical interventions of various valvular diseases.)

Both mitral valve disease and aortic valve disease may require valvular replacement when therapeutic management is no longer effective in the presence of increasing heart failure. Over the last 20 years, a wide variety of valves has been introduced in an attempt to find the most suitable prosthesis. The type of valve used depends on individual client data such as cardiac anatomical structure, age, past health history, and lifestyle. The major types of valves are mechanical, biological heterografts (from a species other than human beings), and homografts (from human beings).

Ventricular septal defects. Ventricular septal rupture occasionally occurs as a complication of acute MI. Since this defect has a high mortality rate with therapeutic treatment alone, surgical repair is indicated and may be performed on an emergency basis. The septal defect may be sutured or patched depending on the size of the rupture.

Ventricular aneurysmectomy. Ventricular aneurysms located on the anterolateral or apical part of the LV may also be excised. These are large, noncontracting areas that interfere significantly with adequate cardiac contraction and CO. They are often a site for the development of mural thrombi within the ventricle. The ventricle is opened and allowed to collapse so that the thinned scar tissue is cut away and any thrombotic material removed before the ventricle is closed (see Fig. 28-13).

Cardiac transplantation. The first heart transplant was performed in 1967. Since that time, heart transplantation has developed into a viable option for clients with terminal cardiac disease. The approximate 2-year survival rates are 80%.[13] Clients with end-stage heart disease with no other therapeutic or surgical options and a poor prognosis for more than 6 months' survival are considered for transplantation. Table 29-15 lists indications and contraindications for this surgical procedure.

In pairing donor and recipient there must be ABO blood

Table 29-15 Indications and Contraindications for Cardiac Transplantation

INDICATIONS

Under 55 years of age*
Functional class IV status (NYHA)
Vigorous and healthy individual (except for end-stage cardiac disease) who would benefit from procedure
Compliance with medical regimens
Demonstrated emotional stability
Financial resources available

CONTRAINDICATIONS†

Systemic disease
Active infection
Pneumonia
Recent or unresolved pulmonary infarction
Severe pulmonary hypertension
Moderate to severe azotemia and/or hepatic abnormalities
Obesity
History of drug or alcohol abuse or mental illness

NYHA, New York Heart Association.
*Age criteria may vary at different institutions.
†Contraindications may vary at different cardiac transplant centers.

---

group compatibility, negative lymphocyte cross-match, and avoidance of transplantation from a CMV-positive donor to a CMV-negative recipient. HLA matching (as discussed in Chapters 8 and 41) is not usually done in cardiac transplantation. This is because of the limited number of donors, time constraints (less than 4 hours required from removal from donor to surgical implantation), and lack of proven value of HLA matching on survival.

The recipient is prepared for surgery and cardiopulmonary bypass using a median sternotomy incision. The usual surgical procedure involves removing the recipient's heart, except for the posterior right and left atrial walls and their venous connections. The recipient's heart is then replaced with the donor heart, which has been trimmed to match. Care is taken to preserve the integrity of the donor SA node so that a sinus rhythm may be achieved postoperatively.

Immunosuppressive therapy usually includes azathioprine (Imuran), corticosteroids, and cyclosporine, an antifungal immunosuppressant.[14] (The mechanisms of action and side effects of these immunosuppressants are discussed in Chapter 41.) Cyclosporine was first used in heart transplantation in 1980. Currently, it is usually used with corticosteroids for maintenance immunosuppression. Its use has resulted not only in reduced rejection but also in slowing the rejection process so that early treatment can be instituted. As a result, rejection episodes have been less dangerous and both client survival and rehabilitation have improved. Another immunosuppressant is OKT3, a monoclonal antibody specifically designed to react with T cells.[15,16] It is primarily used to treat acute rejection episodes. (OKT3 is discussed in Chapter 41.) OKT3 and antithymocytic globulin may also be used early as a prophylactic agent after transplantation.

The postoperative care is similar to that of other open heart surgeries (see p. 844). The amplitude and electrical activity of the ECG are monitored very closely to evaluate the function of the donor heart and to detect early rejection. Endomyocardial biopsies via the right internal jugular vein are performed at repeated intervals to detect rejection. In addition, T-lymphocyte monitoring is done to assess the recipient's immune status. With the use of cyclosporine, the usual parameters of rejection such as change in ECG voltage are less valid, and monitoring requires more frequent endomyocardial biopsies to detect rejection.

Because the client is immunosuppressed, nursing management should involve prevention of infection, which is the leading cause of death in this population. Many deaths due to infection occur during augmented immunosuppressive therapy for acute rejection episodes. Nursing care involves a great deal of emotional support and teaching of both the client and the family, since transplantation is a last resort. In addition, often these clients are long distances from their homes and significant others.

■ Therapeutic and Nursing Management of Clients Requiring Cardiac Surgery

Preoperative management

The preoperative period may vary from a few hours to a month or more depending on the client's physical condition. Some conditions, such as a stab wound to the heart, require immediate surgical intervention. With other conditions, such as heart failure associated with mitral stenosis or regurgitation, the client must be stabilized and prepared for surgery. It is desirable that the client's cardiac and physical condition be stabilized before surgery. For example, dysrhythmias should be controlled, CHF treated, and anginal pain relieved.

Extensive diagnostic studies are usually done before cardiac surgery. Most clients have a cardiac catheterization to measure changes in pressure and blood gases in cardiac chambers and across valves. This is performed to look for structural abnormalities or to confirm the diagnosis and to assess the left ventricular function. Coronary arteriography is also done to observe the coronary perfusion of the myocardium. Other diagnostic studies include echocardiograms, phonocardiograms, stress testing, and nuclear scanning.

In addition, baseline data is obtained just before surgery. These include a chest x-ray film, ECG, coagulation studies (e.g. clotting time, prothrombin time, fibrinogen, and platelets), complete blood count (CBC), urinalysis, serum electrolytes, blood urea nitrogen, serum creatinine levels, and cardiac enzymes. Pulmonary function studies may be performed on clients with pulmonary disease or a history of smoking. Clients also have their blood typed and cross-matched.

Other baseline data obtained shortly before surgery include an accurate body weight to aid in fluid management and vital signs, including temperature, since an elevated temperature is an indication for postponement of surgery.

To improve their respiratory status, clients who smoke must stop smoking at least 1 week and preferably a month or more before surgery. This helps decrease the amount of bronchial secretions and thus reduces the postoperative risk of atelectasis and pneumonia. However, it may be difficult for many clients to stop smoking because of their anxiety about the surgery.

It may be necessary to modify the client's medications to prevent adverse reactions. Digoxin should be discontinued 24 to 36 hours before surgery. This is usually done because digitalis toxicity is common in the early postoperative period. (Digitalis preparations are usually not stopped in clients with atrial fibrillation with a rapid ventricular response.) Propranolol (Inderal) may be tapered 24 hours to 2 weeks before surgery if the client tolerates weaning (i.e., has no anginal or hypertensive episodes). Since propranolol has both negative chronotropic and inotropic effects, it should be weaned before surgery. However, clients who require propranolol may be given positive inotropic agents or glucagon in the early postoperative period to counteract the effects of propranolol.

If the client's heart failure is compensated for, diuretics may be discontinued 24 to 48 hours before surgery. This will help reduce potassium loss and hypovolemia. Clients receiving long-acting insulins will be switched to regular insulin on a sliding-scale basis the day before surgery. They remain on the sliding scale into the postoperative period. Other drugs that may need modification include corticosteroids, anticoagulants, antihypertensives, and phenothiazines. The nurse should check with the physician concerning changes in any drug that is questionable.

To prevent incisional infections, the client should be instructed to shower several times using a bacteriostatic soap such as Betadine or hexachlorophene. In addition, the client is usually started on parenteral antibiotics within 12 hours of surgery. The physician discusses at length with the client and significant others the nature of the surgery including the procedures, expected outcomes, possible complications, and postsurgical care.

Nursing management complements the various aspects of therapeutic management. Extensive preoperative teaching is a major responsibility of the nurse. It deals with general postoperative concerns (see Chapters 1 and 13), in addition to the specialized concerns related to cardiovascular surgery. A high level of anxiety is common because of the client's perception of the central role of the heart in maintaining life. The purpose of the teaching is to help reduce anxiety. The teaching may be more helpful to clients if the sensations that may be experienced are described in addition to the procedures to be performed. Table 29-16 outlines the topics that should be included. Clients should be encouraged to ask questions and discuss their concerns. It is essential that the nurse report significant concerns to the physician so that a coordinated approach can be developed to deal with the client's anxiety.

Family members should also be involved in the preoperative teaching. This will help to alleviate their anxiety so that they can support the client more effectively during this period. It is important that the family know about the various tubes, lines, monitoring devices, and postoperative routines to be aware that these are normal procedures and that they are not an indication of trouble. The family may also be able to help provide comfort for the client and identify idiosyncrasies of the client, such as routines and habits.

Table 29-16 Preoperative Teaching List for Cardiovascular Surgery

Operating room	Provide trip to operating room to see area and meet staff.
	Provide trip to waiting room for family.
	Inform client that conversations and events from the operating room experience may be remembered.
CCU or ICU	Provide trip to see area and meet staff (if desired).
Early postoperative period in CCU or ICU	Explain that client may lose track of time and place and may have hallucinations (visual, auditory, taste).
	Explain ECG monitoring leads.
	Discuss location and purpose of tube and when it will be removed.
	Discuss endotracheal tube; since client cannot talk, devise method of calling a nurse.
	Explain nasogastric tube; inform that ice chips are provided and that client may eat when tube is removed.
	Explain that arterial lines are used for pressure measurements.
	Explain that venous lines are used for fluid or medication administration.
	Explain that bloody red drainage will occur from the chest tubes and that a pulling sensation is felt when the tubes are removed.
	Explain that retention catheter is used for input and output and ease of urine elimination.
	Inform client that thirst may be felt.
Postoperative routine	Explain mechanical ventilation.
	Explain suctioning.
	Explain the importance of coughing and turning.
	Discuss frequent monitoring of vital signs and continuous cardiac monitoring.
Pain medications	Explain that client can ask for pain medication to be comfortable for coughing and moving.
	Inform client that the body will be achy and sore for first week postoperatively.
IPPB (if used)	Provide demonstration and ask for return demonstration.
Post-CCU or ICU routines	Provide overview of discharge regimens.
Emotional reaction	Explain that depression is common.

Intraoperative management

Many cardiovascular surgeries are being performed with the client on a heart-lung machine or a *cardiopulmonary bypass*. This allows the surgeon to work on the heart that has been put into asystole or a slowly contracting state. The heart-lung machine serves as a pump to circulate and oxygenate blood. The machine receives blood from catheters in the venae cavae or right atrium, oxygenates it, and returns the blood to the client through a catheter in the aorta. This is usually done in conjunction with hypothermia (about 25° C to 28° C for bypass and valvular surgeries). The time on the heart-lung machine is closely monitored and kept to a minimum because the longer the client is on it, the more complications may develop. In addition, careful anesthesia and precise monitoring of the cardiac rhythm, vital signs, blood gases, electrolytes, and coagulation status are components of the procedure. Often clients are placed on the intraaortic balloon pump (IABP) and a left atrial pressure (LAP) line and a left ventricular pacing wire are inserted during the surgery.

Postoperative management

Complications that may occur as a result of cardiac surgery are outlined in Table 29-17. Much of the postoperative management is directed toward the prevention or early detection of these complications. Postoperative assessment is outlined in Table 29-18. The physician and nurses work very closely during this time with much overlapping of functions, depending on the policies of the institution.

Table 29-17 Complications of Cardiac Surgery

EARLY POSTOPERATIVE PERIOD

Low cardiac output syndrome due to hypovolemia, acidosis, acute MI, CHF, drugs such as propranolol, mediastinal tamponade, pulmonary embolism, or incomplete or faulty surgical repair
Acute MI, especially with aortocoronary bypass surgery
Cardiac dysrhythmias
Hemorrhage
Pulmonary embolism, especially with saphenous vein aortocoronary bypass
Low-grade fever
Depression
Wound infection
Electrolyte disturbances
Systemic arterial hypertension
Cerebral infarcts due to air or thrombus emboli
Confusion, agitation, and disorientation
Disseminated intravascular coagulation
Adult respiratory distress syndrome
Renal failure

LATE POSTOPERATIVE PERIOD

Wound infection
Hepatitis
Postpericardiotomy syndrome
Systemic arterial emboli and infective endocarditis, with valvular surgeries

On completion of cardiac surgery, the client is transferred immediately to a CCU or ICU. (Some hospitals have separate heart recovery rooms because the CCU and the operating room are not close together.) The nursing staff should have been notified of the client's estimated time of arrival and status so that all the equipment is ready to provide care.

On arrival the client should already be lying on the postoperative bed. The client should be transferred directly from the surgical table to the postoperative bed to save time and energy. Usually a team of two nurses admits the client on arrival to the unit. This is a crucial time for the client, since complications may occur early and during transport. When the client arrives, the nurse team will connect the monitoring devices (e.g., ECG, arterial lines) and suction equipment (e.g., chest tubes, nasogastric tubes) so

Table 29-18 Postoperative Assessment

NERVOUS SYSTEM

Pupil size and reaction
Orientation/level of consciousness
Motor functioning

RESPIRATORY SYSTEM

Placement of endotracheal tube
Settings on mechanical ventilator
Character of respirations
Breath sounds and secretions
Arterial blood gases

CARDIOVASCULAR AND HEMATOLOGICAL SYSTEMS

Cardiac rhythm
Peripheral pulses
Blood pressure
Venous or pulmonary artery pressures
Temperature
Fluid status
Chest tubes
Coagulation status
Cardiac output

RENAL SYSTEM

Urinary output
Urine character, color, specific gravity
Electrolytes

GASTROINTESTINAL SYSTEM

Nasogastric secretions
Bowel sounds

INTEGUMENTARY SYSTEM

Skin breakdown
Incisional healing and drainage

PAIN

Quality or intensity
Location

that the client's hemodynamic parameters can be assessed immediately. The endotracheal tube is checked, and the client is attached immediately to a preset mechanical ventilator. As soon as the equipment is properly connected and calibrated, the nurse should immediately assess the client's neurological, respiratory, and cardiac status to determine the level of anesthesia as well as the ventilation and perfusion status. Reports from the anesthesiologist and surgeon are often given during this initial assessment period. Baseline laboratory data are collected, including ABGs, serum electrolytes, CBC, clotting profile, and cardiac enzymes.

The nurse also collects baseline data on the cardiovascular status by checking the arterial blood pressure, PAP, PCWP, LAP (if a line was inserted during surgery), heart sounds, cardiac rhythm, and peripheral pulses. The client's monitoring devices (e.g., pulmonary artery catheter, left atrial line) depend on the client's preoperative condition, the intraoperative procedures and findings, the surgeon's preference, and the unit's protocol. Many clients return from surgery intubated with only a CVP line; others may require a pulmonary artery catheter, an LAP line, and a pacing wire and may be on the IAPB. These variations are of primary importance in preparing for the client and in planning for care.

Once the initial assessment is made, the client is placed on frequent vital signs (e.g., BP and HR initially every 15 minutes for the first 4 hours, then every 30 minutes for 4 hours, and later every hour). Other indicators may be measured at least every hour, such as urinary output, PCWP or PAP, temperature, breath sounds, and respiratory parameters. In addition, the wave patterns for the arterial pressure, PA catheter, LAP, and ECG are constantly monitored for significant changes. Peripheral pulses also need to be checked every 1 to 2 hours.

Care of the client's chest tubes is indicated by the surgeon's preference and the unit's protocol. Chest tubes must be kept patent so that blood from the mediastinum and pericardium can drain adequately. Plugging or clotting in the chest tube may obstruct the drainage and severely compromise the client. Chest tube drainage (amount and character) is also assessed and recorded frequently (every 15 minutes for the first few hours postoperatively).

The client also needs care to prevent problems associated with immobility. This includes turning from side to side. The head of the bed may be elevated 30 degrees when vital signs are stable. The client may have antiembolic stockings in place. While on the ventilator, the client needs to be suctioned (see Chapter 24). When the endotracheal tube is removed, the client needs to cough and deep breathe. Clients can also sit in a chair, usually by the end of the first day postoperatively. Progressive ambulation is then encouraged.

Most tubes and lines are removed within 3 days of surgery. Because rest periods are important, care must be planned to allow for uninterrupted sleep, especially during the early period of intensive care. Pain medications are also very important because they allow the client to be active and to participate in coughing and deep-breathing exercises. The client and the family need many explanations

and much support. They should be allowed to spend as much time together as the client's condition allows.

After a short period in the CCU the client is moved to a step-down area if further ECG monitoring or care is necessary, or sometimes if the client's condition is stable, the client may be moved to a general surgical unit. After transfer, the clients' activity levels are gradually increased and nutritional patterns are resumed. Medication regimens are adjusted. The client is prepared for discharge, and referrals are made to appropriate community resources. Home regimens and medications are discussed, and the client should be given written instructions. Wound care, diet, and activity levels should be discussed in specific terms with the client and the family. Evaluation should be made of their level of knowledge and of the need for further teaching before discharge.

Postoperative Complications

The possible complications resulting from cardiac surgery are summarized in Table 29-17.

Hypovolemia. The most common complication in the early postoperative period is low CO syndrome, usually due to hypovolemia. It is evidenced by hypotension, oliguria, and cutaneous vasoconstriction. If it is due to hypovolemia, the central venous pressure (CVP), left atrial pressure (LAP), and pulmonary capillary wedge pressure (PCWP) will be low.

The treatment for hypovolemia is blood replacement in the form of packed RBCs (see Chapter 25). Blood is often transfused according to the measured loss in the chest tube drainage to prevent hypovolemia. Sometimes clients can be autotransfused. A special chest tube drainage set can be used to reinfuse blood into the client. If the client cannot be stabilized with transfusions, the client may need to be returned to surgery for hemostasis. Careful recording of all intake and output (IVs, IV flush fluids, chest drainage, gastrointestinal drainage, blood, urine, and medications) is essential to monitor fluid balance.

Cardiac tamponade. Mediastinal or cardiac tamponade may be a cause of low output syndrome. Cardiac tamponade is pressure on the heart caused by the accumulation of fluid, such as blood, in the pericardium. Clinical manifestations include a decrease in chest tube drainage, decrease in the precordial pulsation, quiet heart sounds, and increased size of the heart on percussion. A chest x-ray film shows an enlarged heart and a widened mediastinum. The ECG may show a decrease in the amplitude of the waves. The PCWP, LAP, and CVP are increased. Pulsus paradoxus—the abnormal (more than 10 mm Hg) fall in systolic BP on inspiration—may be present. It can be determined by taking BP with a cuff. As the cuff is deflated, it is stopped at the first Korotkoff sound while the client is breathing normally. If the Korotkoff sound is heard during both inspiration and expiration, no pulsus paradoxus exists. However, if the sound is heard only on expiration, the cuff is deflated slowly until the first Korotkoff sound is heard on both inspiration and expiration. If the difference in pressure between inspiration and expiration is greater than 10 mm Hg, the client has pulsus paradoxus.

Since the post–heart surgery client already has a mediastinal tube in place, the treatment for cardiac tamponade is one of the following:

1. Disconnect other chest tubes and clean out the mediastinal tube with a catheter.
2. Remove the tube and break up the clot by inserting a gloved finger into the stoma, then reinsert the chest tube.
3. Return the client to the operating room, where bleeding can be further assessed and treated.

The other treatment for cardiac tamponade in clients who do not have mediastinal tubes in place is pericardiocentesis. This procedure involves the insertion of a needle into the pericardium to remove fluid (see Fig. 31-6).

Dysrhythmias. Dysrhythmias are common postoperatively. A common cause of dysrhythmias is serum potassium imbalance (i.e., hyperkalemia or hypokalemia), necessitating frequent evaluation of serum potassium levels. Frequent PVCs and ventricular tachycardia are managed. Atrial dysrhythmias are common with mitral and aortic valve replacements. Atrial flutter or fibrillation may occur about 36 hours after aortocoronary bypass or about 6 or 7 days postoperatively with pulmonary embolism (see Chapter 30 for treatment of dysrhythmias).

Emboli. Pulmonary embolism occurs most often after the third postoperative day. It is common in clients with saphenous aortocoronary bypass surgery. Because the clinical manifestations of pulmonary emboli are not always overt, the nurse should report to the physician any client who has transient weakness, dyspnea, or faintness. Lung scans are often used in the diagnosis. Anticoagulation is the usual method of treatment. (The prevention and treatment of pulmonary emboli are discussed in Chapter 32.)

Arterial embolism may occur after aortic or mitral valve surgery. These clients are frequently placed on long-term anticoagulant therapy. The client needs to be observed for evidence of a cerebral embolism such as a sudden change in the level of consciousness, slurring of speech, or one-sided weakness.

Fever. Fever is a very common complication of cardiac surgery and may be the result of pericarditis, which commonly occurs. An elevated temperature increases the work load of the heart because it increases metabolism. The nurse is involved in preventing potential problems that cause fever as well as assisting in collecting information to assess the cause. The client's body temperature is taken at least every 4 hours. Causes of a fever may be atelectasis, urinary tract infection, pneumonia, thrombophlebitis, drug reaction, transfusion reaction, and wound infection. Treatment is directed toward curing the infection and reducing the fever.

Another possible cause of fever is endocarditis. It rarely occurs in the first weeks postoperatively, probably because

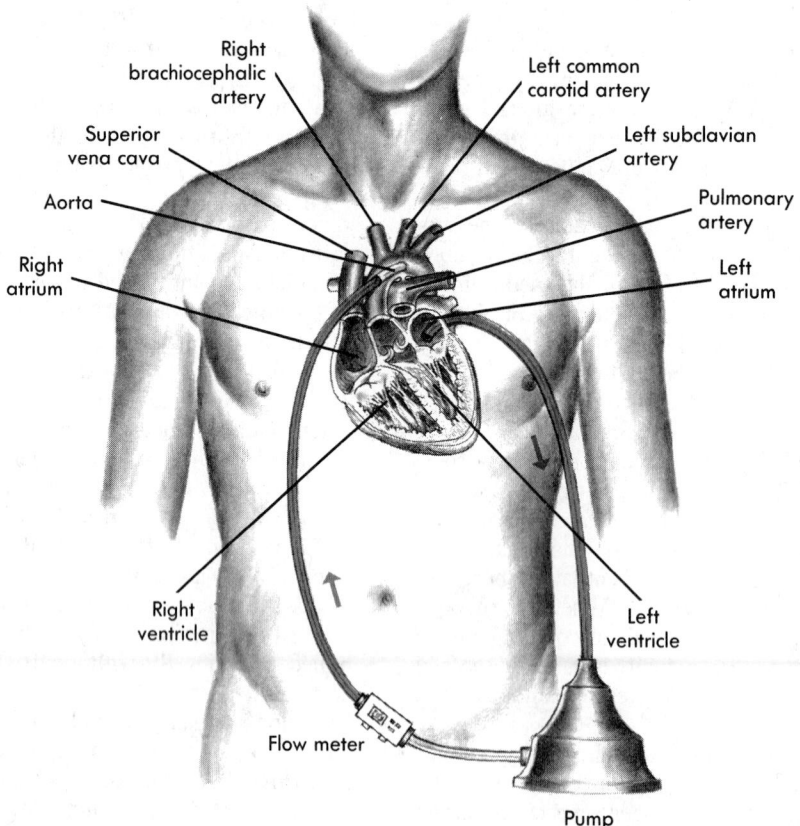

Fig. 29-6 Left ventricular assist device. (From Thelan LA and others: Textbook of critical care nursing: diagnosis and management, St Louis, 1990, Mosby–Year Book, Inc, p 326.)

of the widespread use of prophylactic antibiotics. However, it can occur with valvular replacements. (Endocarditis is discussed in Chapter 31.)

Intraoperative myocardial infarction. Of primary importance in all cardiovascular surgery, especially in bypass grafts, is the preservation of myocardial tissue. The incidence of intraoperative and perioperative MI may be as high as 25%. Several methods of preserving myocardial tissue during surgery have been developed, primarily cold cardioplegia. Immediately after the aorta is cross-clamped, a cold solution high in potassium is infused around the heart and into the aortic root. This process is repeated whenever the myocardial temperature rises to approximately 19° C. This technique lowers the myocardial oxygen consumption and the metabolic rate to prevent ischemia.

During the immediate postoperative period, serial ECGs are taken and cardiac enzymes are assessed to detect intraoperative infarction. It is sometimes difficult to assess if an intraoperative MI has occurred, since enzymes may be elevated because of the surgical procedure itself and an ECG may be difficult to evaluate (as with complete left bundle branch block). Preoperative and postoperative radionuclide scanning gives the best evaluation of coronary perfusion. If an infarct has occurred, the prognosis is worsened and the hospital stay is lengthened.

Mechanical Assist Devices

Mechanical assistance devices, either a left ventricular assist (VAD) (Fig. 29-6) or a totally implantable device, have been used to maintain a client until a suitable donor heart can be found.[17] The VAD is also used for the client who cannot be weaned from cardiopulmonary bypass because of persistent ventricular failure with cardiogenic shock. The use of VAD after an acute MI or after cardiac surgery will divert 25% to 50% of systemic blood flow around the heart and allow the heart to rest and recover.

When the VAD is used, surgically placed cannulas in the left atrium and aorta are attached to an external pump device (Fig. 29-6). Blood is diverted from the left atrium into the pumping device, which then pumps blood out of the systemic circulation by way of the aortic cannula.

C ase Study

CONGESTIVE HEART FAILURE

Elena, a 62-year-old Spanish-American woman, complained of increasing dyspnea on exertion. She could not walk two blocks without becoming short of breath, and she had to sleep with her head elevated on three pillows.

Her past health history showed that Elena had a severe MI at the age of 58. She recovered without serious complications. She was discharged with instructions to take furosemide on alternate days. Over the last 2 months, she has had increasing dyspnea on exertion. About 2 weeks ago she saw her doctor for treatment of a respiratory tract infection, frequent cough, and some edema in her legs. She told her physician that she did not always remember to take her pills.

Her present physical examination showed an older adult female in respiratory distress. A diastolic heart murmur, moist rales in both lungs, and cyanotic lips and extremities were noted. Her ankles were noticeably edematous and her neck veins distended. Her vital signs were noted:

Height	5'3"
Weight	140 lb
BP	130/90
Pulse	98
Respirations	30 and shallow

The results of a chest x-ray film showed an enlarged heart with both right and left ventricular hypertrophy and fluid in the lower lobes of the lungs. Therapeutic treatment consisted of Lasix 40 mg twice a day; a 2-g sodium diet; oxygen 6 L/min, and daily weights.

Discussion Questions

1. Explain the pathogenesis of Elena's heart disease.
2. What clinical manifestations of congestive heart failure did Elena exhibit? Which ones reflect left-sided heart failure? Which ones reflect right-sided heart failure?
3. What is the significance of the findings of the chest X-ray film?
4. Explain the rationale for each of the medical orders prescribed for Elena.
5. What are appropriate nursing orders?
6. What is the priority in the nursing care plan? Why?
7. What teaching measures should be instituted to prevent recurrence of an acute episode of CHF?

R eview Questions

1. Manifestations of left-sided heart failure include
   a. peripheral edema, jugular vein distention, and varicose veins
   b. dyspnea on exertion, rales, and S_3 heart sound
   c. fatigue, cyanosis, and hepatomegaly
   d. substernal soreness, hypertension, and diplopia
2. The nutritional considerations of a client with CHF emphasize primarily a
   a. reduction in dietary sodium
   b. decreased fluid intake
   c. low-cholesterol, low-saturated-fat diet
   d. reduction in dietary potassium
3. For managing a client with acute pulmonary edema, which medication will serve to reduce anxiety and improve oxygenation?
   a. morphine sulfate
   b. aminophylline
   c. nitroprusside
   d. furosemide
4. Which of the following is *not* characteristic of dilated cardiomyopathy?
   a. accounts for the majority of cases of cardiomyopathic conditions
   b. intraventricular septum is disproportionately hypertrophied
   c. etiological factors may include alcohol abuse and pregnancy
   d. prognosis is poor and client may need cardiac transplant
5. Which of the following does *not* accurately describe cardiac transplantation?

a. most common complications are rejection and infection
b. HLA-tissue typing is not important to decrease rejection episodes
c. surgical procedure involves removing all of recipient's own heart
d. endomyocardial biopsies are an important method to monitor possible rejection

6. Preoperative teaching for the prospective cardiac surgical client should include all the following *except*
   a. routines in the CCU that will be experienced
   b. steps of myocardial cellular metabolism
   c. probability of experiencing hallucinations and of depression postoperatively
   d. sensations that may be experienced postoperatively

REFERENCES

1. Braunwald E: Heart failure. In Wilson JD and others, eds: Harrison's principles of internal medicine, ed 12, New York, 1991, McGraw-Hill Book Co, pp 890-898.
2. Keller KB and Lamberg L: Changing concepts in the management of congestive heart failure, Heart Lung 19:425-429, 1990.
3. Galvao M: Role of angiotensin-converting enzyme inhibitors in congestive heart failure, Heart Lung 19:505-512, 1990.
4. CONSENSUS Trial Study Group: Effects of enalapril on mortality in severe congestive heart failure, N Engl J Med 316:1429-1435, 1987.
5. Purcell JA: Advances in the treatment of dilated cardiomyopathy. In G Wlody, CR Ward, and JM Clochesy, eds: AACN clinical issues in critical care nursing, Philadelphia, 1990, JB Lippincott Co.
6. Purcell JA and Holder CK: Cardiomyopathy, understanding the problem, Am J Nurs 89:59-75, 1989.
7. Giles TD and Sander GE: Cardiomyopathy, Littleton, Mass, 1988, PSG Publishing Co.
8. Rahko PS and Orie JE: The clinical presentation and laboratory evaluation of congestive and ischemic cardiomyopathies, Cardiovasc Clin 19:75-119, 1988.
9. Leier CV and Unverferth DV: Medical therapy of end-stage congestive and ischemic cardiomyopathy, Cardiovasc Clin 19:243-251, 1988.
10. Shaver JA and others: Clinical presentation and noninvasive evaluation of the patient with hypertrophic cardiomyopathy, Cardiovasc Clin 19:149-192, 1988.
11. Mirade VA: Idiopathic hypertrophic subaortic stenosis, Crit Care Nur 8:102-111, 1988.
12. Shabetai R: Pathophysiology and differential diagnosis of restrictive cardiomyopathy, Cardiovasc Clin 19:123-132, 1988.
13. Hunt SA and Schroeder JS: Managing patient after cardiac transplantation, Hosp Pract 24:83-100, 1989.
14. Metzger JT and Hoffman LA: Cardiac transplantation: the changing faces of immunosuppression, Heart Lung 17:414-425, 1988.
15. Rogers KR and others: Using OKT3 to reverse cardiac allograft rejection, Heart Lung 18:490-496, 1989.
16. Dault LA and others: Reversing cardiac transplant rejection with Orthoclone OKT3, Am J Nurs 89:953-955, 1989.
17. Oaks TE and others: Results of mechanical circulatory assistance before heart transplantation, J Heart Transplantation 8:113-116, 1989.

CHAPTER

30

Nursing Role in Management

Dysrhythmias

Carolyn I. Johns

Table 30-1 Properties of Cardiac Tissue

Automaticity	Ability to initiate an impulse spontane-ously and continuously
Contractility	Ability to respond mechanically to an im-pulse
Conductivity	Ability to transmit an impulse along a membrane in an orderly manner
Excitability	Ability to be electrically stimulated

L earning Objectives

1. *Identify the clinical characteristics and electrocardiographic patterns of common dysrhythmias.*
2. *Describe the therapeutic and nursing management of common dysrhythmias.*
3. *Differentiate between defibrillation and cardioversion regarding the indications for use and physiological effects.*
4. *Describe the management of clients with pacemakers, including both temporary and permanent pacemakers.*
5. *Explain the essential elements of basic cardiac life support.*
6. *Describe the subdiaphragmatic abdominal thrust (Heimlich maneuver) and indications for use.*

DYSRHYTHMIA IDENTIFICATION AND TREATMENT

The ability to recognize dysrhythmias is an essential skill for the nurse. Prompt assessment of an abnormal cardiac rhythm and the client's response to the rhythm is a critical function. This chapter describes basic principles of common dysrhythmias (abnormal cardiac rhythms). For more information on dysrhythmias, the reader is referred to detailed texts on electrocardiographic (ECG) interpretation. (The normal function of the electrical system of the heart is discussed in Chapter 26.) Therapeutic and nursing management of dysrhythmias is described in this chapter, and included are drug therapy, pacemaker therapy, and principles of basic and advanced cardiac life support.

Conduction System

There are four properties of cardiac tissue enabling the conduction system to initiate an electrical impulse, which

Reviewed by Sandi Martin, R.N., B.S.N., C.C.R.N., Head Nurse, Intensive Coronary Care, The Methodist Hospital, Houston, Texas.

is transmitted through the cardiac tissue and stimulates muscle contraction (Table 30-1). The conduction system of the heart consists of specialized neuromuscular tissue located throughout the heart (Fig. 26-5). Initiation of a normal cardiac impulse begins in the *sinoatrial* (SA) *node* in the upper right atrium and is transmitted over the atrial myocardium via Bachmann's bundle and internodal pathways to the atrioventricular (AV) node. From the AV node, the impulse spreads through the bundle of His and down the left and right bundle branches, emerging in the Purkinje fibers, which distribute the impulse to the ventricles.

Conduction to the point just before the impulse leaves the Purkinje fibers takes place within the time of the PR interval of the ECG. When the impulse emerges from the Purkinje fibers, ventricular depolarization occurs, producing mechanical contraction of the ventricles and the QRS complex on the ECG. The electrical activity of the heart is illustrated in Fig. 26-6.

Nervous Control of the Heart

The autonomic nervous system plays an important role in the rate of impulse formation, the speed of conduction, and the strength of cardiac contraction. The specific components of the autonomic nervous system that affect the heart are the right and left vagus nerve fibers of the parasympathetic fibers and the sympathetic nerves.

Stimulation of the vagus nerve causes a decreased rate

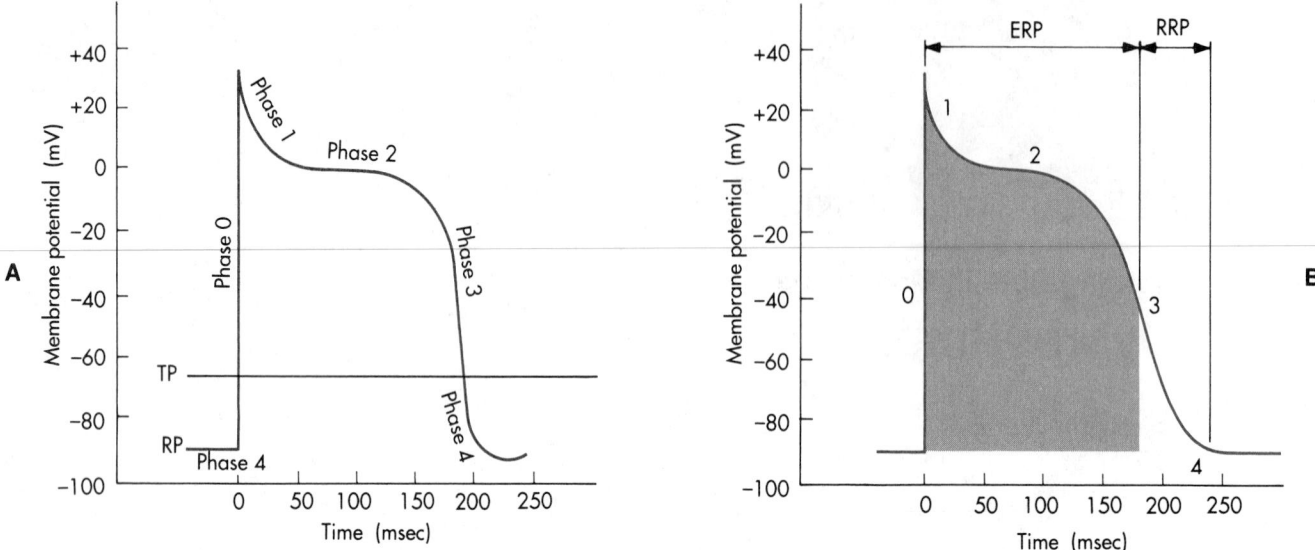

Fig. 30-1 A, Phases of the cardiac action potential. The electrical potential. measured in *mV*, is indicated along the vertical axis of the graph. Time, measured in milliseconds *(ms)*, is indicated along the horizontal axis. The action potential consists of three to five phases, labeled as phase *0* through phase *4*. Each phase represents a particular electrical event or combination of electrical events. The events, the duration of the events and action potential, and the transmembrane potential vary with the type of cardiac cell being measured. **B,** Two parts of the refractory period. The effective refractory period extends from phase 0 to approximately −60 mV in phase 3. The remainder of the action potential is the relative refractory period. *TP,* Threshold potential; *RP,* resting potential.

of firing of the SA node, slowed impulse conduction of the AV node, and a decreased force of cardiac muscle contraction. Stimulation of the sympathetic nerves that supply the heart has, essentially, the opposite effect on the heart.

ECG Monitoring

The ECG is a graphic tracing of the electrical impulses produced in the heart. The deflections on the ECG are produced by the movement of charged ions across the membranes of myocardial cells, representing depolarization and repolarization.

The membrane of a cardiac cell is semipermeable and maintains a high concentration of potassium and a low concentration of sodium inside the cell. A high concentration of sodium and a low concentration of potassium are maintained outside the cell. The inside of the cell at rest, or in the *polarized* state, is negative compared to the outside. When a cell or groups of cells are stimulated, each cell membrane changes its permeability and allows sodium to migrate rapidly into the cell, making the cell positive compared to the outside *(depolarization)*. A slower movement of ions across the membrane restores the cell to the polarized state, and this is called *repolarization*. In Fig. 30-1, the phases are as follows: phase 4 is a polarized state; phase 0 is the upstroke of rapid depolarization; and phase(s) 1, 2, and 3 represent repolarization. When antidysrhythmic drugs are used in a clinical setting, a nurse's understanding of the ionic shifts in the cardiac cell and the action potential mechanism is important. Antidysrhythmic drugs have a direct effect on the action potential.

Conventionally, there are 12 recording leads in the ECG. Six of the 12 ECG leads measure electrical forces in the frontal plane (leads I, II, III, aV$_R$, aV$_L$, and aV$_F$) (Fig. 30-2), and the remaining six leads (V$_1$ through V$_6$) measure the electrical forces in the horizontal plane (precordial lead sites). The 12-lead ECG may demonstrate structural changes, which may be indicative of ischemia, infarction, enlarged cardiac chambers, electrolyte imbalance, or drug toxicity.[2] Obtaining 12 views of the heart that show cardiac rhythm is also helpful in the assessment of dysrhythmias. An example of a normal 12-lead ECG appears in Fig. 30-3.

When a client's ECG is being continuously monitored, one or two single ECG leads are used. The most common leads used are lead II and lead MCL$_1$, which corresponds to V$_1$ in the standard 12-lead ECG (Fig. 30-4). These leads most clearly demonstrate the P wave and QRS complexes.

The ECG can be visualized continuously on a monitor oscilloscope. A recording of the ECG "strip" is done on ECG paper attached to the monitor. This provides documentation of the client's rhythms and a means for thoroughly assessing and documenting dysrhythmias.[3]

It is essential to know how to measure time and voltage on the ECG paper to correctly interpret an ECG. ECG paper consists of large (heavy lines) and small (light lines) squares (Fig. 30-5). Each large square incorporates 25 smaller squares (5 horizontal and 5 vertical). Each small square represents 0.04 second horizontally and 0.1 mV vertically. This means that the large square equals 0.20

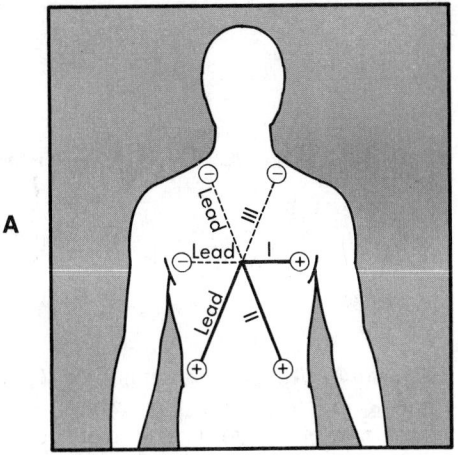

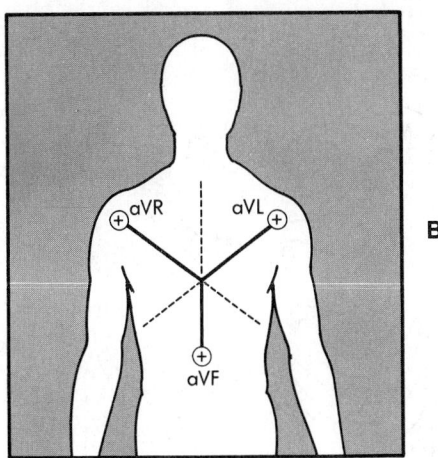

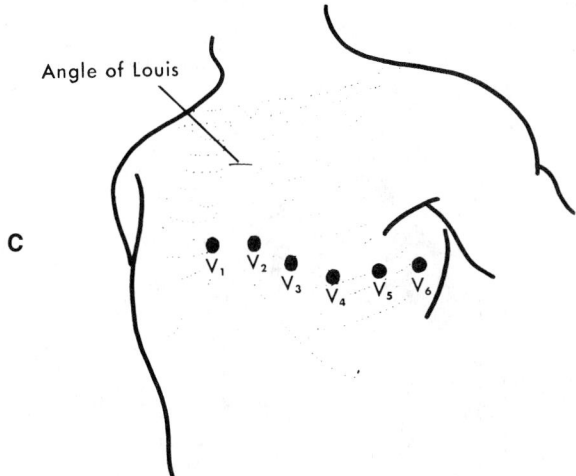

Fig. 30-2 **A,** Limb leads I, II, and III. Leads are located on the extremities. Illustrated are the angles from which these leads view the heart. **B,** Lead placement for augmented limb leads aV_R, aV_L, and aV_F. These unipolar leads use the calculated center of the heart as their negative electrode. (From Thelan LA and others: Textbook of critical care nursing: diagnosis and management, St Louis, 1990, Mosby–Year Book, Inc, p 182.) **C,** Lead placement for the chest electrodes: V_1, fourth intercostal space at the right sternal border; V_2, fourth intercostal space at the left sternal border; V_3, equidistant between V_2 and V_4; V_4, fifth intercostal space at the left midclavicular line; V_5, anterior axillary line and same horizontal level as V_4; V_6, midaxillary line and same horizontal level as V_4. (From Goldberger AL and Goldberger E: Clinical electrocardiography: a simplified approach, ed 3, St Louis, 1986, The CV Mosby Co.)

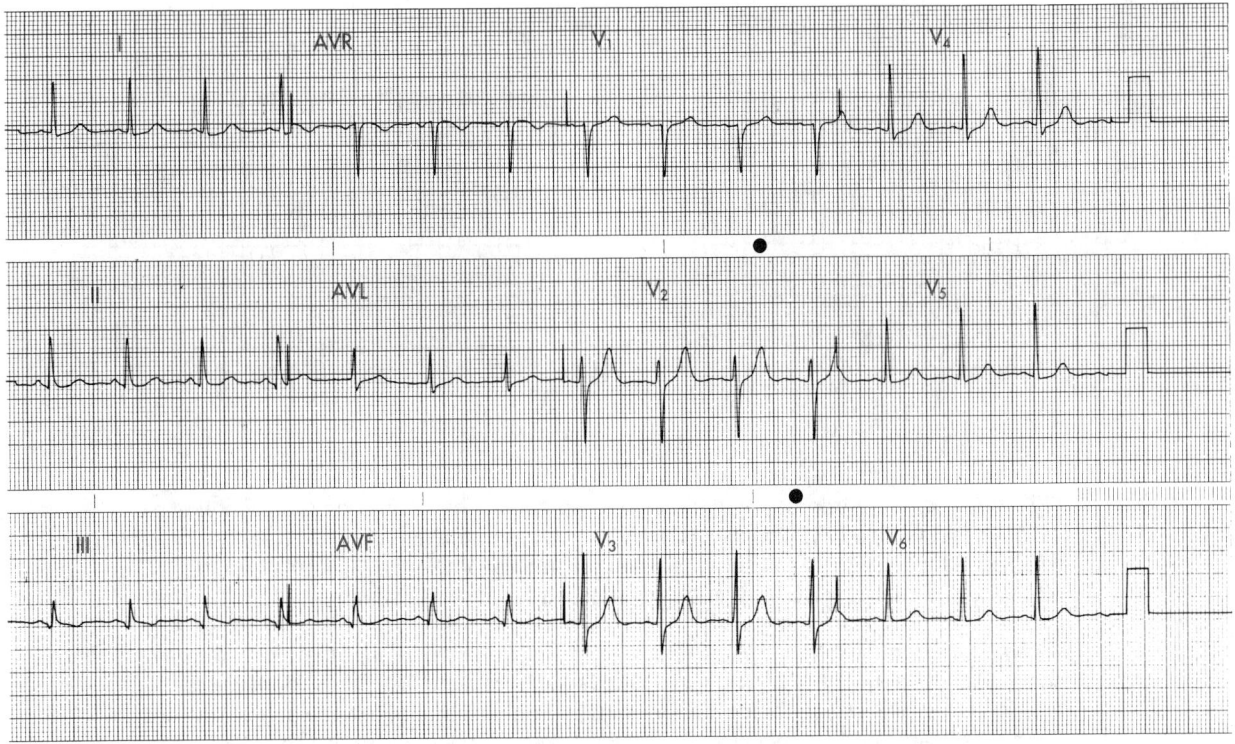

Fig. 30-3 Twelve-lead ECG showing a normal sinus rhythm.

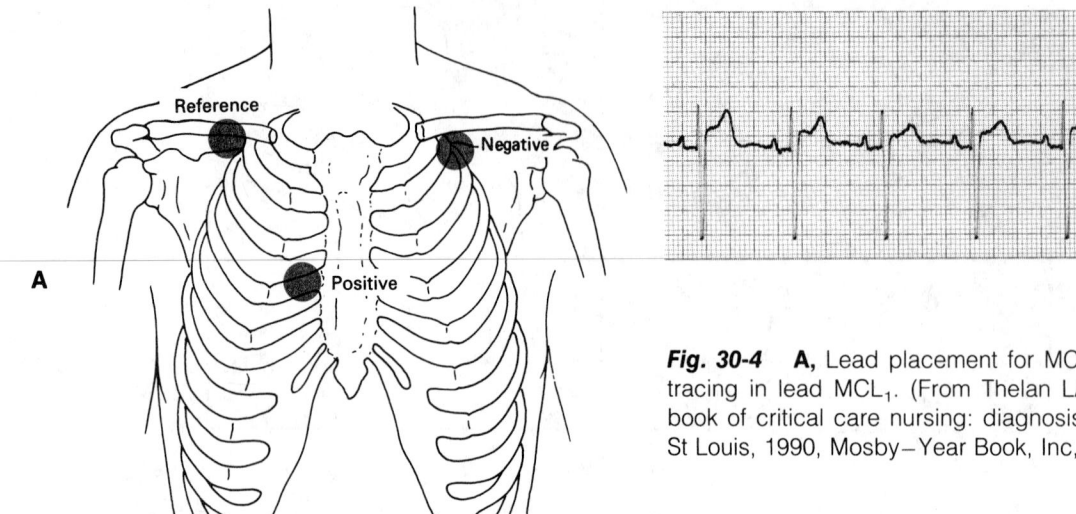

Fig. 30-4 **A,** Lead placement for MCL₁. **B,** Typical ECG tracing in lead MCL₁. (From Thelan LA and others: Textbook of critical care nursing: diagnosis and management, St Louis, 1990, Mosby–Year Book, Inc, p 188.)

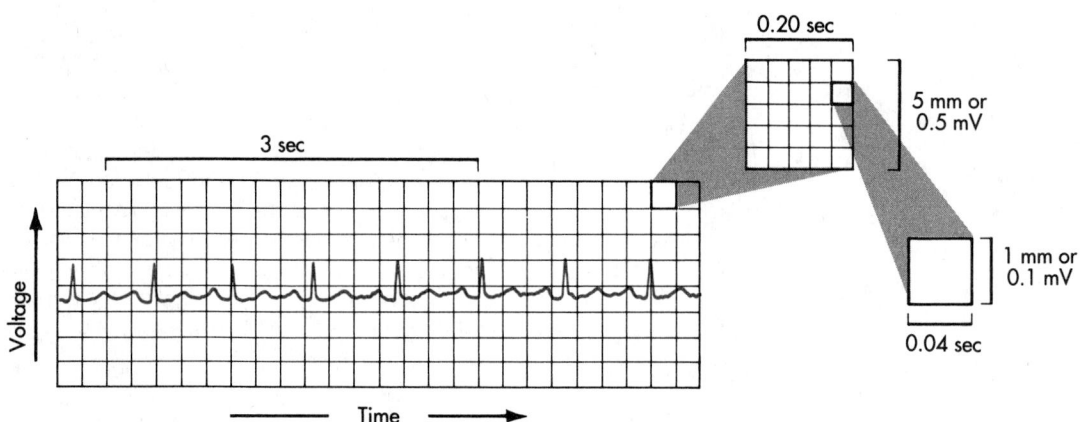

Fig. 30-5 Time and voltage on the ECG.

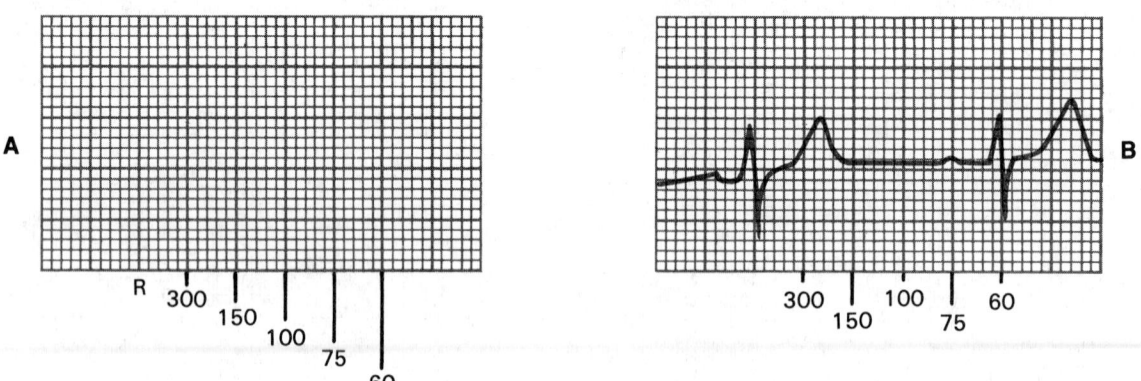

Fig. 30-6 **A,** The *R* represents the first QRS complex. The *underlines* represent the location of the second QRS complex (R to R interval), and the number indicates the HR. *5 small squares = 300,* 6 small squares = 250, 7 small squares = 214, 8 small squares = 187, 9 small squares = 167, *10 small squares = 150,* 11 small squares = 136, 12 small squares = 125, 13 small squares = 115, 14 small squares = 107, *15 small squares = 100, 20 small squares = 75.* **B,** A rate of 60 bpm, determined with the estimated rate scale: 300-150-100-75-60-50. The scale always starts with the first heavy, dark line to the right of the R or S wave, *not* the heavy, dark line on which the R or S wave is located. (From Passman J and Drummond CD: The EKG: basic techniques for interpretation, New York, 1976, McGraw-Hill Book Co, p 199.)

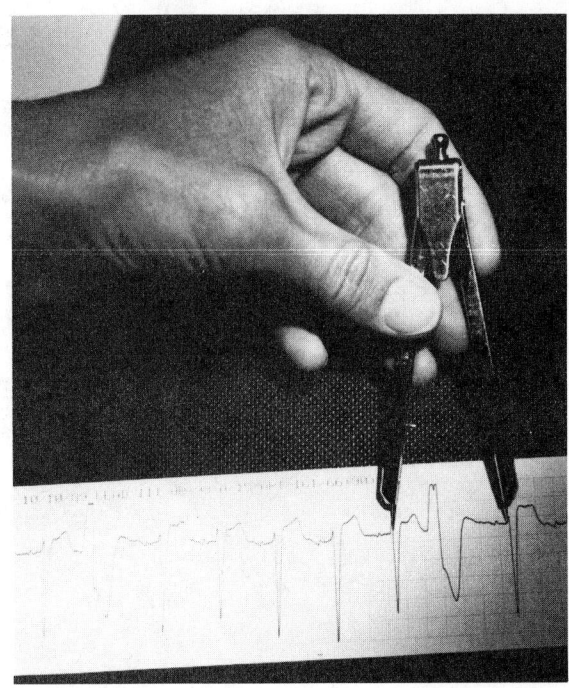

Fig. 30-7 Calipers used to help make wave and baseline determinations. (Courtesy Pam Brown, Albuquerque.)

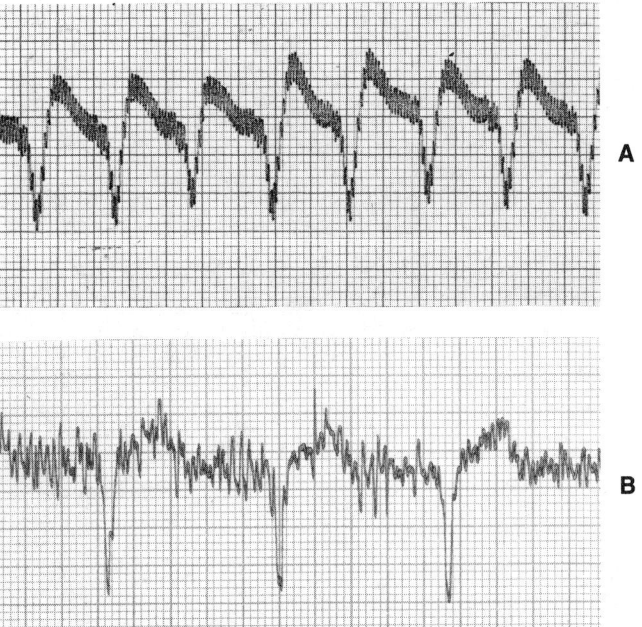

Fig. 30-8 **A,** Artifact—60-cycle interference. **B,** Artifact—muscular movement. (From Thelan LA and others: Textbook of critical care nursing: diagnosis and management, St Louis, 1990, Mosby–Year Book, Inc, p 183.)

second and that 300 large squares equal 1.0 minute. Vertically, one large square is equal to 0.5 mV. These squares are used to calculate the heart rate (HR) and intervals between different ECG complexes.

A variety of ways can be used to calculate the HR from an ECG. Probably the most accurate way is to count the number of QRS complexes in a 1-minute time interval. However, this method is cumbersome and time consuming. If the rhythm is regular, a simpler process can be used. Every 3 seconds, a marker appears on the ECG paper. The nurse can count the number of QRS complexes in a 6-second interval and multiply that number by 10. This will yield the number of complexes or beats per minute (bpm).

Another rapid method for calculating the HR when a regular rhythm is present is to count the number of small squares between two QRS complexes (R-R interval). An R wave is the first upward deflection of the QRS complex. The nurse divides 1500 by the number of small squares to get the precise HR. Tables that show these calculations are available (Fig. 30-6, *A*). This method can also be used by locating an R wave that falls on a heavy vertical line (Fig. 30-6, *B*) or by memorizing the landmarks at increments of large squares. After finding the R wave that falls on a heavy vertical line, the nurse goes from one heavy line to the next counting "300, 150, 100, etc." to the next QRS complex.

An additional way to measure distances on the ECG grid is to use calipers (Fig. 30-7). Calipers are used for fine measurements, especially for those components of a specific wave. Many times a P or R wave will not fall directly on a light or heavy line. The fine points of the cali-

pers can be placed exactly on the components to be measured and then moved to another part of the grid for time measurement, which is accurate to 0.04 second.

ECG leads are attached to the client's chest wall via an electrode pad fixed with electrical conductive paste. For best contact, hair on the chest wall should be shaved and skin should be prepared with acetone to remove excess oil and debris. In the case of a diaphoretic client, benzoin may be applied to the skin before electrode placement. If leads and electrodes are not firmly placed or if there is muscle activity or electrical interference from an outside source, an artifact may be seen on the monitor. An *artifact* is a distortion of the baseline and waveforms seen on the ECG (Fig. 30-8) and makes it almost impossible to accurately identify the cardiac rhythm.

Assessment of Cardiac Rhythm

In assessing the cardiac rhythm, the nurse must make an accurate interpretation of a dysrhythmia and immediately proceed to evaluate the consequences of that dysrhythmia for the individual client. Assessment of the client's hemodynamic response to a dysrhythmia provides guidance in therapeutic intervention. If possible, a determination of the cause of the dysrhythmia should be made. Tachycardias can cause a decrease in cardiac output (CO) and possible hypotension. Certain dysrhythmias may precipitate more life-threatening dysrhythmias.[4] It is clear that the client, not just the dysrhythmia, must be treated.

Normal sinus rhythm refers to the normal conduction pattern of the cardiac cycle, which originates in the SA node (Fig. 30-9). Fig. 30-10 shows the normal electrical pattern of the cardiac cycle. Table 30-2 provides a descrip-

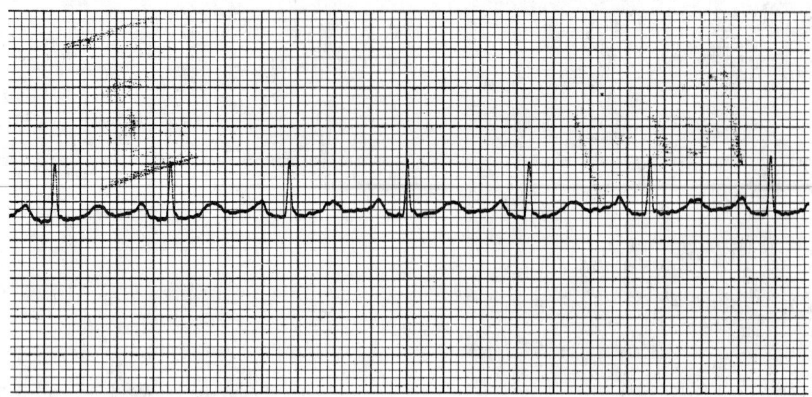

Fig. 30-9 Normal sinus rhythm in lead II.

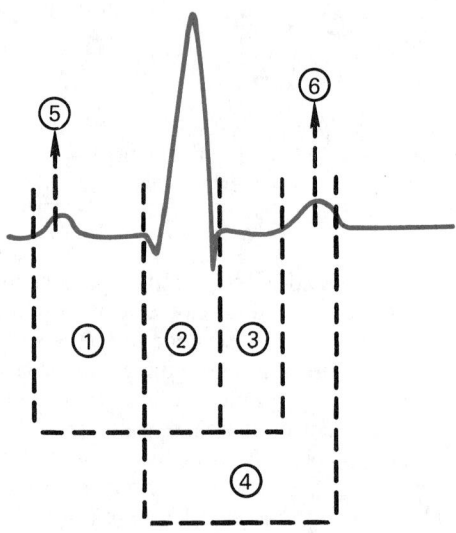

Fig. 30-10 The ECG complex as seen in a normal sinus rhythm. *1*, PR interval (normal is 0.12-0.20 sec); *2*, QRS complex (normal is 0.60-0.10 sec); *3*, ST segment (normal is 0.12 sec); *4*, QT interval (normal is 0.34-0.43 sec); *5*, P wave (normal is 0.06-0.12 sec); *6*, T wave (normal is 0.16 sec).

Table 30-2 Definition and Significance of ECG Intervals*

Description	Duration (sec)	Significance of Disturbance
PR interval: From beginning of P wave to beginning of QRS complex; represents time taken for impulse to spread through the atria, AV node and His bundle, the bundle branches and Purkinje fibers, to a point immediately preceding ventricular activation	0.12 to 0.20	Disturbance in conduction usually in AV node, His bundle, or bundle branches but can be in atria as well
QRS interval: From beginning to end of QRS complex; represents time taken for depolarization of both ventricles	0.06 to 0.10	Disturbance in conduction in bundle branches and/or in ventricles
QT interval: From beginning of QRS to end of T wave; represents time taken for entire electrical depolarization and repolarization of the ventricles	0.34 to 0.43	Disturbances usually affecting repolarization more than depolarization such as drug effects, electrolyte disturbances, and rate changes

From Andreoli KG and others: Comprehensive cardiac care, ed 7, St Louis, 1991, Mosby–Year Book, Inc.
*HR influences the duration of these intervals, especially those of the PR and QT intervals.

tion of ECG intervals and significance of disturbances. The P wave represents the depolarization of the atrium (passage of an electrical impulse through the atrial muscle), resulting in atrial contraction. The QRS complex represents depolarization of the ventricles, resulting in ventricular contraction. The T wave represents repolarization of the ventricles, or the time at which the ventricles return to the prestimulated state. The PR interval represents the period during which the impulse spreads through the atria, AV node, His bundle, and Purkinje fibers. The QRS interval represents the time it takes for depolarization of both ventricles. The QT interval represents the time it takes for complete depolarization and repolarization of the ventricles.

Electrophysiological Mechanisms of Dysrhythmias

Disorders of impulse formation can initiate dysrhythmias. The heart has specialized cells found in the sinus node, parts of the atria, the AV node, and the His-Purkinje system, which are able to discharge spontaneously. This is called *automaticity*. Normally, the main pacemaker of the heart is the sinus node, which spontaneously discharges at 60 to 100 times per minute (Table 30-3). A pacemaker from another site may be discharged in two ways: If the SA node discharges more slowly than a secondary or latent pacemaker, the electrical discharges from the secondary pacemaker may passively *escape* and discharge automatically at their intrinsic rates. These secondary pacemakers may originate from the AV node or the His-Purkinje system at rates of 40 to 60 times per minute and 30 to 40 times per minute, respectively. A second means by which latent pacemakers can originate occurs when the discharge rate is accelerated abnormally, and other "pacemakers" take control of the sinus node. A premature beat or a series of premature beats can then occur (tachycardia) from ectopic foci in the atria, ventricles, or AV junction.

The impulse initiated by a pacemaker focus must be conducted to the entire heart chamber. The property of myocardial tissue that enables it to be depolarized by a stimulus is called *excitability*. This is an important part of the propagation of the impulse from one fiber to another. The level of excitability is determined by the length of time after depolarization during which the tissues can be restimulated. The recovery period after stimulation is called the *refractory phase* or *period*. The *absolute refractory phase* or *period* occurs when excitability is zero and heart tissue cannot be stimulated. The *relative refractory period* occurs slightly later in the cycle, and excitability improves. In states of full excitability, the heart is completely recovered. Fig. 30-11 shows the relationship between the refractory period and the ECG.

Table 30-3 Rates of the Conduction System

SA node	60-100 times/min
AV junction	40-60 times/min
Purkinje fibers	20-40 times/min

If conduction is depressed and if some areas of the heart are blocked, the unblocked areas are activated earlier than the blocked areas. When the block is unidirectional, this uneven conduction may allow the initial impulse to *reenter* areas that were previously not excitable but have recovered. The reentering impulse may be able to depolarize the atria and/or ventricles, causing a premature beat. If the *reentrant excitation* continues, tachycardia occurs.

Dysrhythmias occur as the result of various abnormalities and disease states.[9] The cause of a dysrhythmia influences the treatment of the client. Common causes of dysrhythmias are presented in Table 30-4.

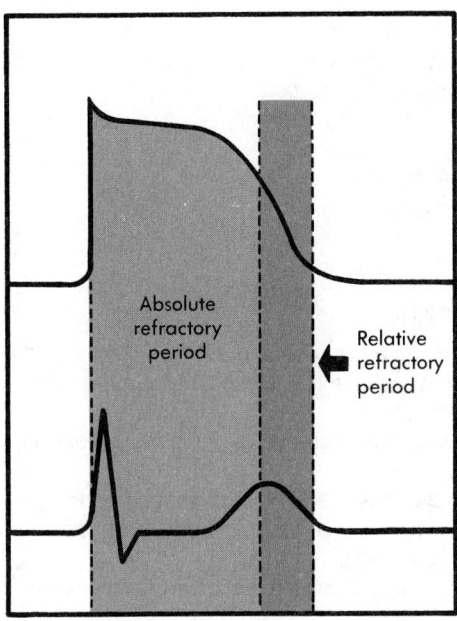

Fig. 30-11 Absolute and relative refractory periods correlated with the cardiac muscle's action potential and with an ECG tracing. (From Thelan LA and others: Textbook of critical care nursing: diagnosis and management, St Louis, 1990, Mosby–Year Book, Inc, p 185.)

Table 30-4 Common Causes of Dysrhythmias

Drug effects or toxicity
Myocardial cell degeneration
Hypertrophy of cardiac muscle with strain
Emotional crisis
Connective tissue disorders
Alcohol
Coffee, tea, tobacco
Electrolyte imbalance
Cellular hypoxia
Stretched cardiac tissue
Edema
Acid-base imbalances
Myocardial ischemia
Degeneration of the conduction system

Table 30-5

Prehospital Emergency Care of the Client with a Dysrhythmia*

Possible etiologies: Poisoning, acute myocardial infarction, congestive heart failure, pulmonary disorders, drownings, electrolyte imbalances, shock, stress, drugs

CLINICAL MANIFESTATIONS

Irregular HR and rhythm
Chest pain
Dizziness, syncope
Fainting
Extreme restlessness
Decreased level of consciousness
Feeling of impending doom
Numbness, tingling of arms
Weakness and fatigue
Cold, clammy skin
Diaphoresis
Pallor
Nausea and vomiting

MANAGEMENT

Apply cardiac electrodes and monitor client's cardiac rhythm. Calculate HR. Determine whether rhythm is regular or irregular.
Assess airway and breathing. Support with oxygen at 4-6 L via cannula.
Start intravenous line with large-gauge needle.
If cardiac rhythm is abnormal, report to physician and await drug orders.
Reassure client. Provide calm environment.

*See Chapter 59 for a general discussion on measures related to prehospital emergency care.

Dysrhythmias occurring in out-of-hospital settings present problems of management. Clinical manifestations are varied and occur in a variety of situations. Determination of the rhythm by cardiac monitoring is a high priority. Prehospital care of the client with a dysrhythmia is outlined in Table 30-5. The emergency medical system is activated if indicated after the client has been assessed.

Evaluation of Dysrhythmias

In addition to continuous ECG monitoring during hospitalization, several other methods are used to evaluate cardiac dysrhythmias and the efficacy of antidysrhythmic drug therapy. An *electrophysiology test* (an invasive method) and *Holter monitoring* and *exercise treadmill testing* (noninvasive methods) are performed on both an inpatient and an outpatient basis.

Electrophysiological testing is performed to identify different mechanisms of tachydysrhythmias as well as heart blocks, bradydysrhythmias, and dysrhythmic causes of syncope.[5] It is often used to determine the effectiveness of antidysrhythmic drugs. It involves introducing several electrode catheters transvenously to the right side of the heart with fluoroscopic guidance. Electrical stimulation to various areas of the atrium and ventricle is performed, and the inducibility of dysrhythmias is determined. This is a fairly unpleasant experience for most clients, since ventricular tachycardia or ventricular fibrillation is often induced, and cardioversion and defibrillation are performed to convert the rhythm. Some types of "near death" experiences have been reported by some clients. Emotional support to these clients by nurses is important. Nursing care before and after the procedure is similar to that for cardiac catheterization.

The Holter monitor is a device that records the ECG while clients are ambulatory.[6,7] The device can record heart rhythm for 24 hours while clients go about their daily activities. A diary is maintained by each client, recording activities and any symptoms. Events in the diary can later be correlated with any dysrhythmias observed on the recording by the evaluator. It is generally a useful device for detecting significant dysrhythmias and evaluating drug efficacy during a client's normal activities. It can also be used for detecting ischemia by analyzing ST segments. A weakness of the device is that clients who have frequent ventricular dysrhythmias, some of which may be lethal, may not happen to have these dysrhythmias during the 24 hours that they are monitored. Many physicians believe that electrophysiological testing is more reliable for the determination of malignant dysrhythmias.

Exercise treadmill testing is used for evaluation of cardiac rhythm response to exercise. Exercise-induced dysrhythmias can be reproduced and analyzed, and drug therapy can be evaluated.[8] These tests are performed with routine treadmill testing protocols.

Types of Dysrhythmias

When assessing cardiac rhythm, a systematic approach must be used. The recommended approach is to note the rate, the rhythm, P wave, QRS complex, relationship of P wave to QRS complex, the PR interval, QRS interval, and QT interval. Questions to consider are: Are premature ventricular complexes present? Are escape beats present? What is the dominant rhythm? What is the clinical significance of the dysrhythmia? What is the treatment for the particular dysrhythmia? Examples of the ECG tracings of common dysrhythmias are presented in Figs. 30-12 through 30-20. Descriptive characteristics of common dysrhythmias are presented in Table 30-6.

Sinus bradycardia. In sinus bradycardia, the conduction pathway is the same as that in sinus rhythm, but the sinus node discharges at a rate of less than 60 bpm (Fig. 30-12, *A*).

Clinical associations. Sinus bradycardia is a normal sinus rhythm in aerobically trained athletes and in other individuals as well, during sleep. It occurs in response to carotid sinus massage, the Valsalva maneuver, hypothermia, increased intraocular pressure, increased vagal tone, and the administration of parasympathomimetic drugs. Disease states associated with sinus bradycardia are hypothyroidism, increased intracranial pressure, obstructive jaundice, and inferior wall myocardial infarction (MI).

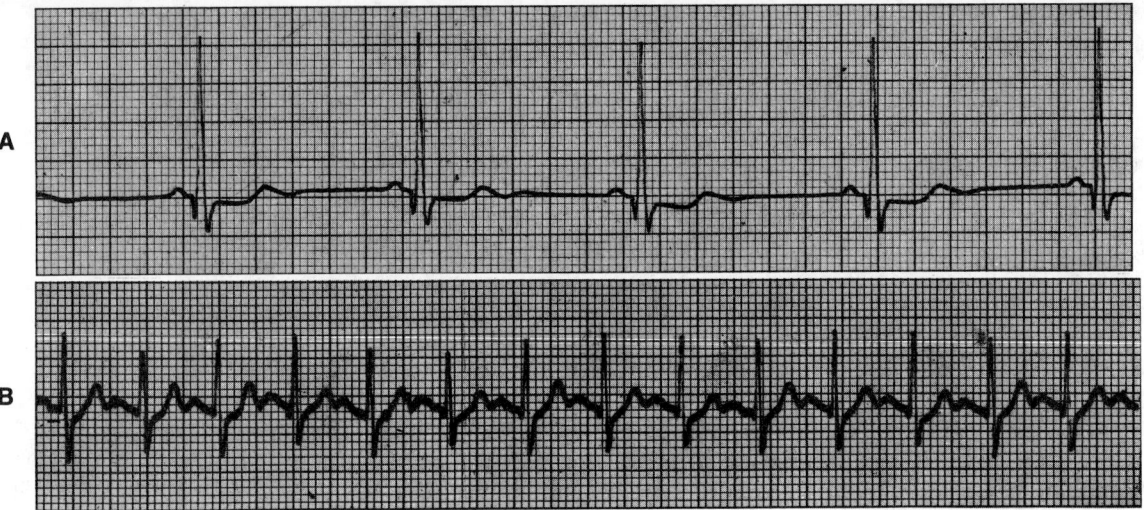

Fig. 30-12 **A,** Sinus bradycardia of 50 bpm. **B,** Sinus tachycardia of 140 bpm. (From Conover MB: Understanding electrocardiography: arrhythmias and the 12-lead ECG, ed 5, St Louis, 1988, The CV Mosby Co, p 86.)

Table 30-6 Characteristics of Common Dysrhythmias

Pattern	Rate and Rhythm	P Wave	PR Interval	QRS Complex
NSR	60-100 bpm and regular	Normal	Normal	Normal
PVC	60-100 bpm and irregular	Not usually present	Not measurable	Wide and distorted
Ventricular tachycardia	100-250 bpm and regular or irregular	Not usually present	Not measurable	Wide and distorted
Ventricular fibrillation	Not measurable and irregular	Absent	Not measurable	Not measurable
Sinus bradycardia	<60 bpm and regular	Normal	Normal	Normal
Sinus tachycardia	>100 bpm and regular	Normal	Normal	Normal
PAC	Usually 60-100 bpm and irregular	Abnormal shape	Normal or variable	Normal (usually)
PSVT	100-300 bpm and regular	Abnormal shape, may be hidden	Variable	Normal (usually)
Atrial flutter	*Atrial:* 250-350 bpm and regular *Ventricular:* >100 bpm and irregular	Sawtooth	Variable	Normal (usually)
Atrial fibrillation	*Atrial:* 350-600 bpm and irregular *Ventricular:* >100 bpm and irregular or possibly any rate	Chaotic	Not measurable	Normal (usually)
Junctional rhythms	40-140 bpm and regular	Abnormal (may be hidden)	Variable	Normal (usually)
First-degree heart block	Normal and regular	Normal	>0.20 sec	Normal
Second-degree heart block				
Type I (Mobitz I)	*Atrial:* Normal and regular *Ventricular:* Slower and irregular	Normal	Progressively lengthened	Normal
Type II (Mobitz II)	*Atrial:* Usually normal and regular or irregular *Ventricular:* Slower and regular or irregular	Normal	Normal or prolonged	Normal or preceded by widened wave, two or more P waves
Third-degree heart block	Ventricular rate 20-40 bpm and regular	Normal, but no connection with QRS complex	Variable	Normal or widened, no connection with P waves

ECG characteristics. In sinus bradycardia, **HR** is less than 60 bpm, and **rhythm** is regular. The **P wave** precedes each QRS complex and has a normal contour and a fixed interval. The **PR interval** is normal, and the **QRS interval** has a normal contour and normal length.

Significance. The clinical significance of sinus bradycardia depends on how the client tolerates it hemodynamically. Hypotension with decreased CO may occur in some circumstances. An acute MI may predispose the heart to escape dysrhythmias and premature beats.

Treatment. Treatment consists of administration of atropine and isoproterenol for clients with symptoms. Pacemaker therapy may be required.

Sinus tachycardia. The conduction pathway is the same in sinus tachycardia as that in normal sinus rhythm. The discharge rate from the sinus node is increased as a result of vagal inhibition or sympathetic stimulation. The sinus rate is greater than 100 bpm (Fig. 30-12, *B*).

Clinical associations. Sinus tachycardia is associated with physiological stresses such as exercise, fever, pain, hypotension, hypovolemia, anxiety, anemia, hypoxia, hypoglycemia, myocardial ischemia, congestive heart failure (CHF), and thyrotoxicosis. It can also be an effect of

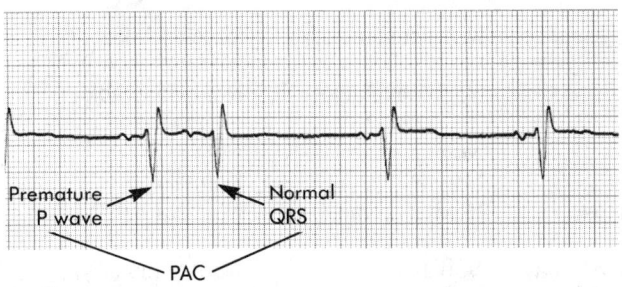

Fig. 30-13 Normally conducted PAC. The early P wave is indicated by the *arrow,* and the QRS that follows is of normal shape and duration. (From Thelan LA and others: Textbook of critical care nursing: diagnosis and management, St Louis, 1990, Mosby–Year Book, Inc, p 196.)

drugs such as epinephrine, norepinephrine, caffeine, atropine, theophylline, nifedipine, or hydralazine.

ECG characteristics. In sinus tachycardia, **HR** is greater than 100 bpm, and **rhythm** is regular. The **P wave** is normal, precedes each QRS complex, and has a normal contour and fixed interval, the **PR interval** is normal, and the **QRS interval** has a normal contour.

Significance. The clinical significance of sinus tachycardia depends on the client's tolerance of the increased HR. The client may have symptoms of dizziness, and hypotension may occur. Increased myocardial oxygen consumption is associated with increased HR. Angina or an increase in infarct size may accompany persistent sinus tachycardia in the setting of acute MI.

Treatment. Treatment is determined by underlying causes. In certain settings, β-blocker therapy is used to reduce HR and decrease myocardial oxygen consumption.

Premature atrial contraction. A premature atrial contraction (PAC) is a contraction originating from an ectopic focus in the atrium in a location other than the sinus node. It originates in the left or right atrium and travels across the atria by an abnormal pathway, creating a distorted P wave (Fig. 30-13). At the AV node it is stopped (nonconducted PAC), delayed (lengthened PR interval), or conducted normally. It moves through the AV node and in most cases is conducted normally through the ventricles.

Clinical associations. In a normal heart, a PAC can result from emotional stress or the use of caffeine, tobacco, or alcohol. A PAC can also result from disease states such as infection, inflammation, thyrotoxicosis, chronic obstructive pulmonary disease, heart disease (including atherosclerotic heart disease), valvular disease, and other diseases; a PAC can also be caused by enlarged atria.

ECG characteristics. **HR** varies with the underlying rate and frequency of the PAC, and **rhythm** is irregular. The **P wave** has a different contour from that of a normal P wave. It may be notched or have negative deflection, or it may be hidden in the preceding T wave. The **PR interval** may be shorter or longer than a normal PR interval originating from the sinus node, but it is within normal

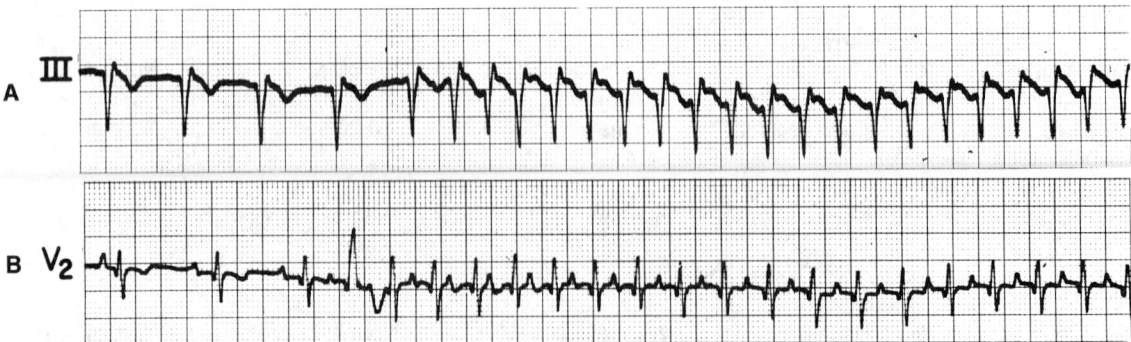

Fig. 30-14 Paroxysmal supraventricular tachycardia. **A,** Sudden onset of supraventricular tachycardia (215 bpm). The P waves cannot be identified. **B,** Supraventricular tachycardia (172 bpm) initiated by a PAC. The first beat of the tachycardia indicates aberration; subsequent beats show normal conduction. (From Wenger N, Hurst JW, and McIntyre MC, eds: Cardiology for nurses, New York, 1980, McGraw-Hill Book Co, p 235.)

limits. The **QRS complex** is usually normal. If it is 0.10 second or longer, abnormal conduction through the ventricles is present.

Significance. A PAC may be a prelude to supraventricular tachycardias.

Treatment. Treatment depends on the client's symptoms. Withdrawal of sources of stimulation such as caffeine may be warranted. Drugs such as digoxin, quinidine, procainamide, flecainide, and β blockers can be used.

Paroxysmal supraventricular tachycardia. Paroxysmal supraventricular tachycardia (PSVT) is a dysrhythmia originating in an ectopic focus anywhere above the bifurcation of the bundle of His (Fig. 30-14). Identification of the ectopic focus is sometimes quite difficult with a 12-lead ECG. It occurs with the reentrant phenomenon (reexcitation of the atria when there is a one-way block). A run of repeated premature beats is initiated and is usually heralded by a PAC. *Paroxysmal* refers to an abrupt onset and termination. Termination is sometimes followed by a brief period of asystole. Some degree of AV block may be present.

Clinical associations. In normal hearts, PSVT is associated with overexertion, emotional stress, changes of position, deep inspiration, and stimulants such as caffeine and tobacco. In disease states, PSVT is associated with rheumatic heart disease, Wolff-Parkinson-White (WPW) syndrome, digitalis intoxication, coronary artery disease, or cor pulmonale.

ECG characteristics. In PSVT, **HR** is 100 to 300 bpm, and **rhythm** is regular. The **P wave** is often hidden in the preceding T wave and has an abnormal contour. The **PR interval** may be prolonged, shortened, or normal, and the **QRS complex** may have a normal or abnormal contour.

Significance. The clinical significance of PSVT depends on symptoms and HR. A prolonged episode and HRs greater than 180 bpm may precipitate a decreased CO with hypotension and myocardial ischemia.

Treatment. Treatment includes vagal stimulation as well as pharmacological therapy. Vagal stimulation induced by carotid massage or the Valsalva maneuver may be used to treat PSVT. The drug of choice is verapamil, a calcium channel blocker. Digitalis and propranolol can also be used. However, exceptions are made in WPW syndrome. Adenosine is a drug with a very short half-life that has recently been proven to be effective in restoring normal sinus rhythm in clients with PSVT.

Atrial flutter. Atrial flutter is an atrial tachydysrhythmia identified by recurring, regular, sawtooth-shaped flutter waves (Fig. 30-15, *A*) and is best visualized in leads II, III, aV$_F$, and V$_1$ on the 12-lead ECG. It is usually associated with a slower ventricular response. Because of the refractoriness of the AV node, there is usually some AV block in a fixed ratio of flutter waves to QRS responses (e.g., 2:1, 3:1). It is a relatively rare dysrhythmia.

Clinical associations. Atrial flutter rarely occurs in a normal heart. In disease states, it is associated with coronary artery disease, hypertension, mitral valve disorders, pulmonary embolus, hyperthyroidism, and drugs such as digitalis, quinidine, and epinephrine.

ECG characteristics. **Atrial rate** is 250 to 350 bpm. The **ventricular rate** varies according to the conduction ratio. In 2:1 conduction, the ventricular rate is typically about 150 bpm. **Atrial rhythm** is regular, and **ventricular rhythm** is usually regular. The **P wave** is represented by sawtooth waves or F waves, the **PR interval** is variable, and the **QRS complex** is normal in contour.

Significance. High ventricular rates associated with atrial flutter can decrease CO and cause serious consequences such as heart failure, especially in clients with underlying heart disease.

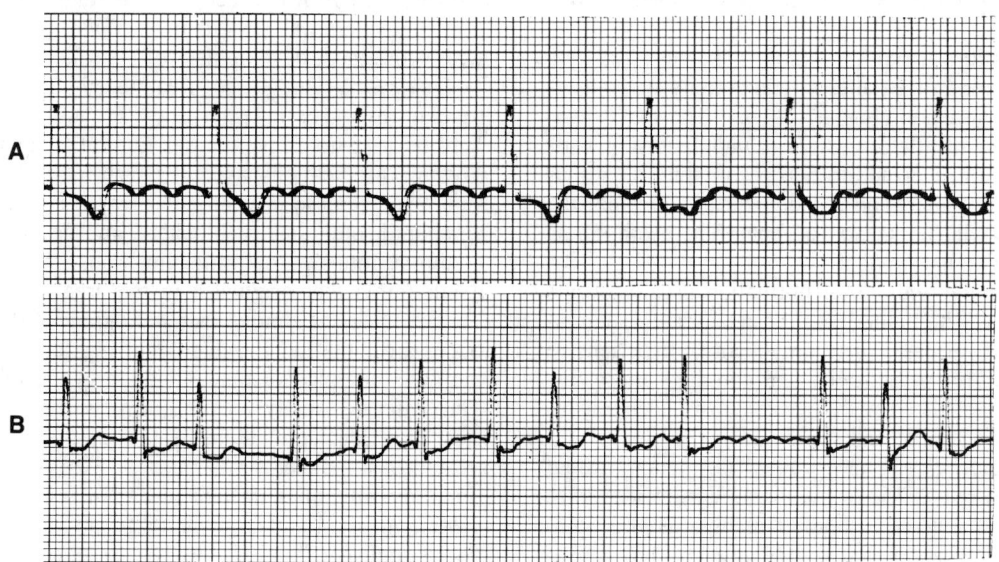

Fig. 30-15 **A,** Atrial flutter with two to three P waves before the QRS complex. **B,** Atrial fibrillation. Note the jagged, irregular baseline between the QRS complexes.

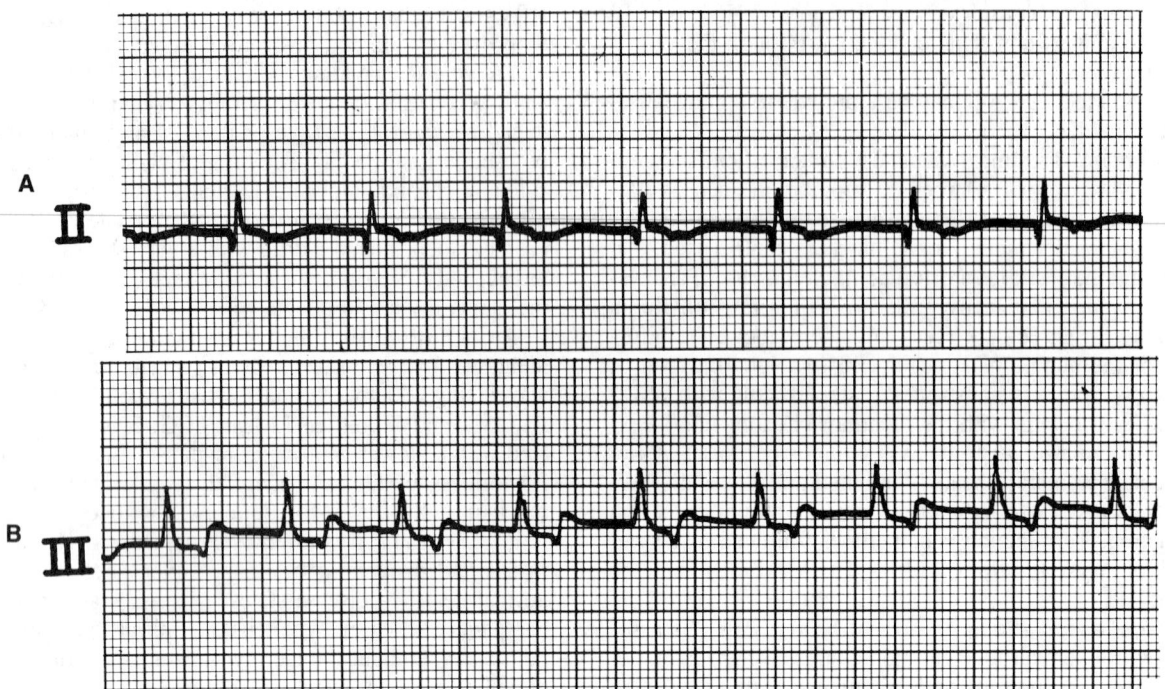

Fig. 30-16 **A,** Accelerated junction rhythm (88 bpm). **B,** Junctional tachycardia (100 bpm). Inverted P waves occur on the ST segment and are produced by a 1:1 retrograde atrial activation. (From Wenger N, Hurst JW, and McIntyre MC, eds: Cardiology for nurses, New York, 1980, McGraw-Hill Book Co, p 241.)

Treatment. The primary goal in treatment of atrial flutter is to slow the ventricular response by increasing AV block. Electrical cardioversion may be used to convert the atrial flutter to sinus rhythm in an emergency situation. Drugs used include verapamil, digoxin, quinidine, procainamide, and β blockers, as well as other antidysrhythmics.

Atrial fibrillation. Atrial fibrillation is characterized by a total disorganization of atrial electrical activity without effective atrial contraction (Fig. 30-15, *B*). The ECG demonstrates baseline fibrillatory waves or undulations of variable contour at a rate of 300 to 600 per minute. Ventricular response is irregular, and if the client is untreated, the ventricular rate will be 100 to 160 bpm. The dysrhythmia may be chronic or intermittent.

Clinical associations. Atrial fibrillation usually occurs in those clients with underlying heart disease, such as rheumatic heart disease, cardiomyopathy, hypertensive heart disease, CHF, pericarditis, and coronary artery disease. It is also associated with thyrotoxicosis, alcoholism, infection, gastroenteritis, and stress.

ECG characteristics. During atrial fibrillation, **atrial rate** may be as high as 350 to 600 bpm. **Ventricular rate** can vary from as low as 50 bpm to as high as 180 bpm. **Atrial rhythm** is chaotic, and **ventricular rhythm** is usually irregular. Ventricular rhythm may be regular if there is complete AV block *(ventricular escape rhythm)*. The **P wave** shows fibrillatory waves, but no definite P wave can

be observed. The **PR interval** is not measurable, and the **QRS complex** usually has a normal contour.

Significance. Atrial fibrillation can often result in a decrease in CO because of ineffective atrial contractions and a rapid ventricular response. Thrombi may form in the atria as a result of ineffective atrial contraction. Embolization to the arterial system may occur as a complication with subsequent development of a stroke.

Treatment. The goal of treatment is a decrease in ventricular response. In emergency situations, cardioversion may be used to convert atrial fibrillation to normal sinus rhythm. Medications used for pharmaceutical cardioversion or a decrease in ventricular response include digoxin, verapamil, quinidine, β blockers, and flecainide.

Junctional dysrhythmia. Junctional rhythm refers to a dysrhythmia that originates in the area of the AV node. The impulse may move in a retrograde fashion that produces an abnormal P wave occurring just before or after the QRS complex or that is hidden in the QRS complex. The impulse usually moves normally through the ventricles. Junctional premature beats may occur, and they are treated in a manner similar to that for PACs. Other junctional dysrhythmias include *junctional escape rhythm, accelerated junctional rhythm* (Fig. 30-16, *A*), and *junctional tachycardia* (Fig. 30-16, *B*). These dysrhythmias are treated according to the client's tolerance of the rhythm and the circumstances.

Clinical associations. Junctional escape rhythm is often

associated with aerobically trained individuals who have sinus bradycardia. It may occur with acute MI, especially inferior MI, and disease of the sinus node. Accelerated junctional rhythm and junctional tachycardia are observed with acute inferior MI, digitoxicity, and acute rheumatic fever and during open heart surgery.

ECG characteristics. In junctional escape rhythm, **HR** is 40 to 60 bpm, in accelerated junctional rhythm it is 60 to 100 bpm, and in junctional tachycardia it is 100 to 140 bpm. **Rhythm** is regular. The **P wave** is abnormal in contour and inverted, or it may be hidden in the QRS complex. The **PR interval** is less than 0.12 second when the P wave precedes the QRS complex. The **QRS complex** is usually normal.

Significance. Junctional escape rhythm serves as a safety mechanism occurring when the primary pacemaker has not been activated. Escape rhythms such as this should not be suppressed. Accelerated junctional rhythm and junctional tachycardia indicate a problem with the sinus node. If these rhythms are rapid, they may result in a reduction of CO and possible heart failure.

Treatment. Treatment varies according to the type of junctional dysrhythmia. If a client has symptoms with an escape junctional rhythm, atropine can be used. In accelerated junctional rhythm and junctional tachycardia that are due to digoxin toxicity, digoxin is withheld. In the absence of digitoxicity, propranolol, phenytoin, or verapamil may be used.

First-degree AV block. First-degree AV block is a type of AV block in which every impulse is conducted to the ventricles but the duration of AV conduction is prolonged (Fig. 30-17). This is manifested by a PR interval greater than 0.20 second. After the impulse moves through the AV node, it is usually conducted normally through the ventricles.

Clinical associations. First-degree AV block is associated with MI, chronic ischemic heart disease, rheumatic fever, hyperthyroidism, vagal stimulation, and drugs such as digitalis, β blockers, flecainide, encainide, and IV verapamil.

ECG characteristics. In first-degree AV block, **HR** is normal, and **rhythm** is regular. The **P wave** is normal, the **PR interval** is prolonged for more than 0.20 second, and the **QRS complex** usually has a normal contour.

Significance. First-degree AV block may be a precursor of higher degrees of AV block.

Treatment. There is no treatment for first-degree AV block.

Second-degree AV block, type I. Type I AV block (Mobitz I, Wenckebach phenomenon) includes a gradual lengthening of the PR interval, which occurs because of the AV conduction time that is prolonged until an atrial impulse is nonconducted and a QRS complex is dropped (Fig. 30-17). Once a ventricular beat is dropped, the cycle repeats itself with progressive lengthening of the PR intervals until another QRS complex is dropped. The rhythm appears on the ECG in a pattern of grouped beats. The duration of the QRS complex is normal or prolonged. Type I AV block most commonly occurs in the AV node, but it can also occur in the His-Purkinje system.

Clinical associations. Type I AV block may result from use of drugs such as digoxin or β blockers. It may also be associated with ischemic cardiac disease and other diseases that can slow AV conduction.

Treatment. **Atrial rate** is normal, but **ventricular rate** may be slower as a result of dropped QRS complexes. **Ventricular rhythm** is irregular. The **PR interval** progressively lengthens before the nonconducted P wave occurs. The **P wave** has a normal contour. The **PR interval** lengthens progressively until a P wave is nonconducted and a QRS complex is dropped. The **QRS complex** has a normal contour.

Significance. Type I AV block is usually a result of myocardial ischemia in inferior MI. It is almost always transient and is usually well tolerated. However, it may be a warning signal of an impending significant AV conduction disturbance.

Treatment. If the client is free of symptoms, atropine is used to increase HR. A temporary pacemaker may be needed for a client with acute MI.

Second-degree heart block, type II. In type II second-degree AV block (Mobitz II) a P wave is nonconducted without progressive antecedent PR lengthening, and this almost always occurs in a setting of bundle branch block (Fig. 30-17). On conducted beats, the PR interval is constant. Second-degree heart block is a more serious type of block in which a certain number of impulses from the sinus node are not conducted to the ventricles. This occurs in ratios of 2:1, 3:1, and so on when there are two P waves to one QRS complex, three P waves to one QRS complex, and so on. It may occur with varying ratios. Type II AV block almost always occurs in the His-Purkinje system.

Clinical associations. Type II AV block is associated with rheumatic and atherosclerotic heart disease, acute anterior MI, digitoxicity, and Lenegre's disease and Lev's disease.

ECG characteristics. **Atrial rate** is usually normal; **ventricular rate** depends on the intrinsic rate and the degree of AV block. **Sinus rhythm** is regular, but **ventricular rhythm** may be irregular. The **P wave** has a normal contour. The **PR interval** may be normal or prolonged but remains fixed on conducted beats. The **QRS complex** widens to more than 0.12 second because of bundle branch block.

Significance. Type II AV block usually progresses to third-degree AV block and is associated with a poor prognosis. The reduced HR may result in decreased CO with subsequent hypotension and myocardial ischemia. Type II AV block is an indication for therapy with a permanent pacemaker.

Treatment. Temporary treatment before the insertion of a permanent pacemaker involves the use of a temporary pacemaker. Drugs including atropine and isoproterenol (Isuprel) can be tried as temporary measures to increase HR until pacemaker therapy is available.

Third-degree AV heart block. Third-degree AV heart block (complete heart block) constitutes one form of AV dissociation in which no impulses from the atria are conducted to the ventricles (Fig. 30-17). The atria are stimu-

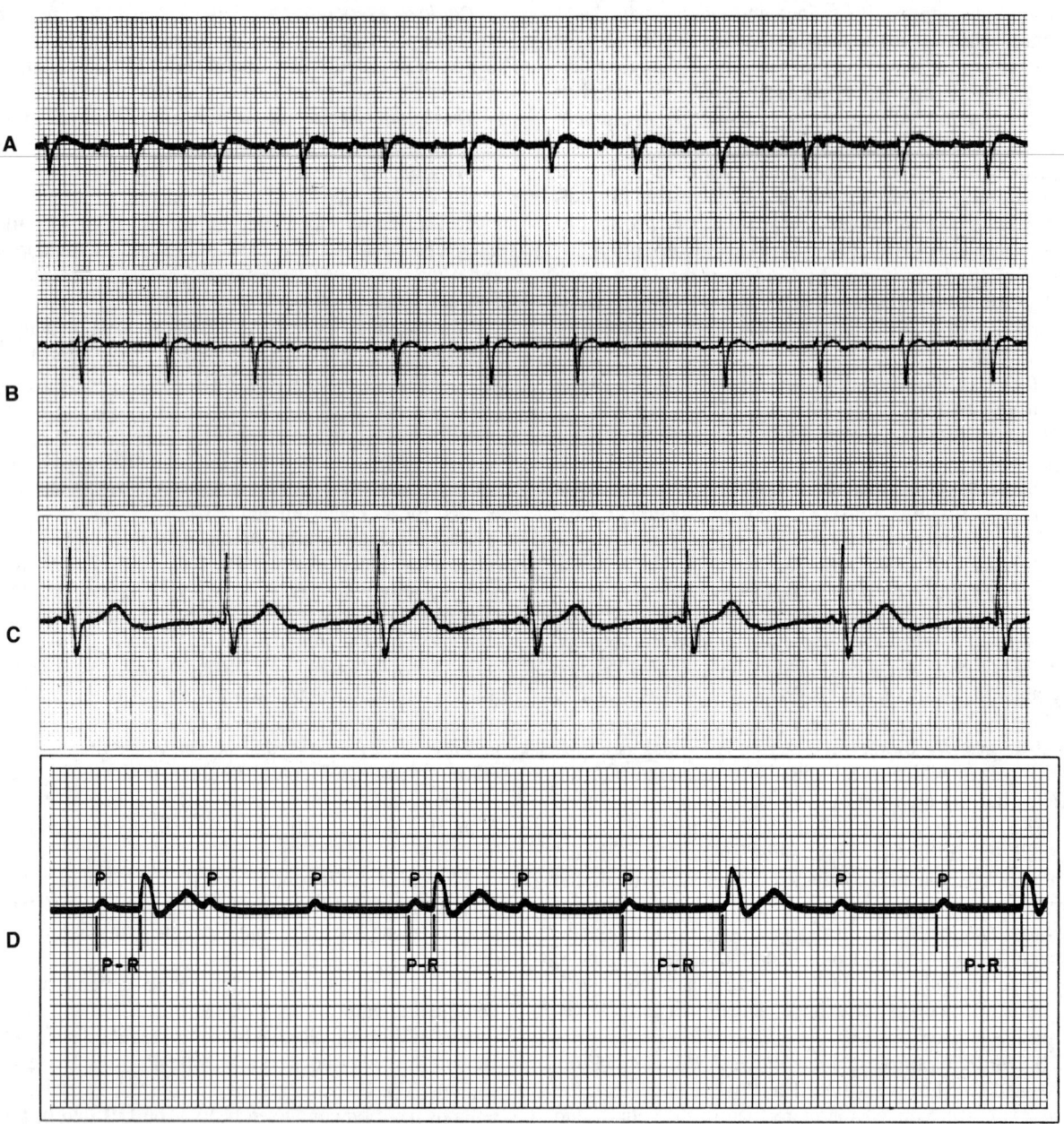

Fig. 30-17 Heart block. **A,** First-degree heart block. Note the delayed PR interval. **B,** Second-degree heart block, type I (Mobitz I, Wenckebach). **C,** Second-degree heart block, type II (Mobitz II). **D,** Complete heart block (third degree). The irregular PR intervals indicate the presence of a complete heart block.

lated and contract independently of the ventricles. The ventricular rhythm is an escape rhythm, and the focus may be above or below the bifurcation of the His bundle.

Clinical associations. Third-degree heart block is associated with fibrosis or calcification of the cardiac conduction system, coronary artery disease, myocarditis, cardiomyopathy, open heart surgery, Lev's disease, Lenegre's disease, and some systemic diseases such as amyloidosis and scleroderma.

ECG characteristics. The **atrial rate** is usually a sinus rate of 60 to 100 bpm. The **ventricular rate** depends on

the site of the block. If it is in the AV node, the rate is 40 to 60 bpm, and if it is in the Purkinje system, it is 20 to 40 bpm. **Atrial** and **ventricular rhythms** are regular but asynchronous. The **P wave** has a normal contour. The **PR interval** is variable, and there is no time relationship between the P wave and the QRS complex. The **QRS complex** is normal if escape rhythm is initiated in the His bundle or above. It is widened if escape rhythm is initiated below the His bundle.

Significance. Third-degree AV block almost always results in reduced CO with subsequent ischemia and heart

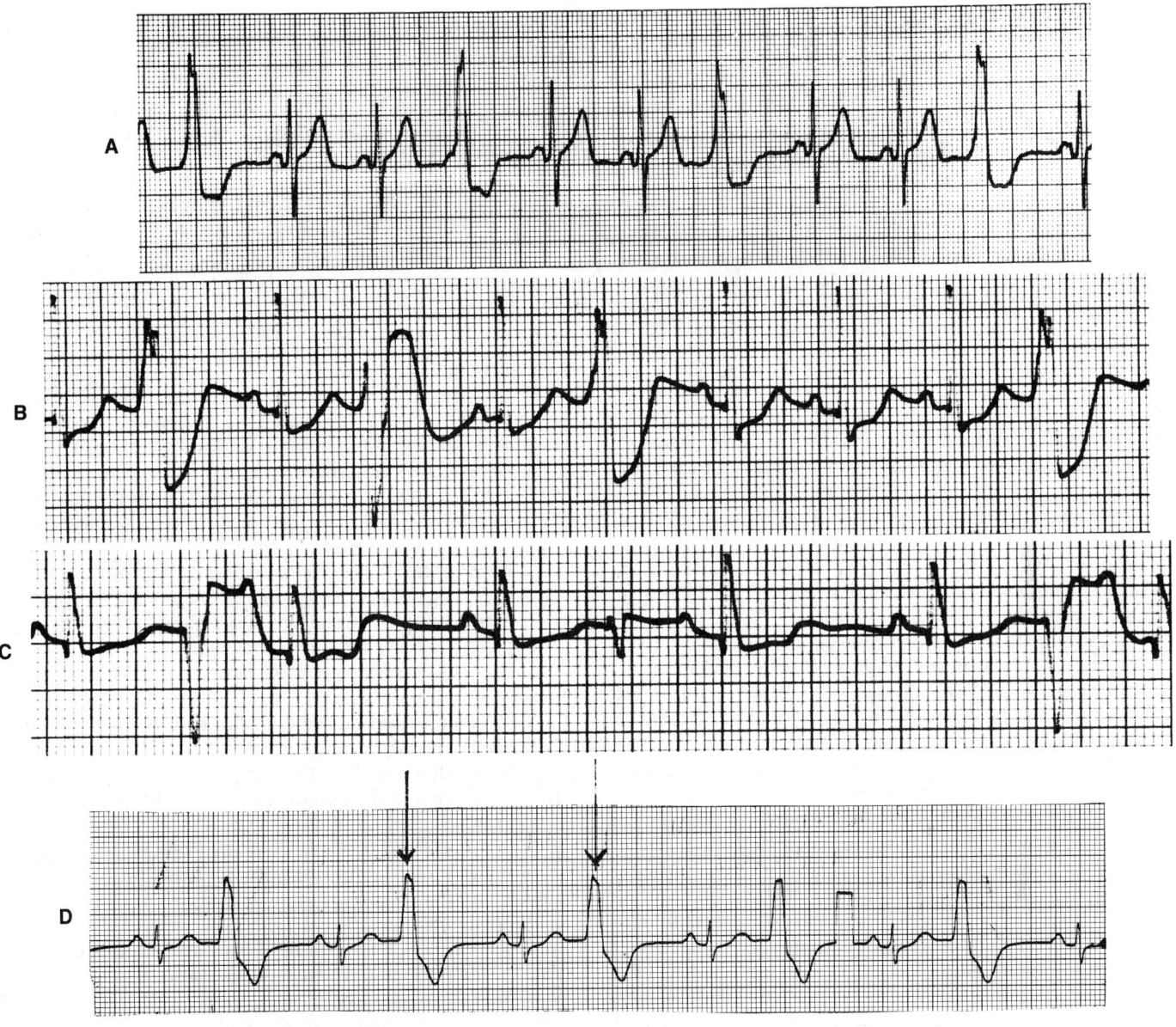

Fig. 30-18 PVCs. **A,** Ventricular trigeminy. **B,** Multifocal PVC. **C,** Fusion (interpolated) PVCs. **D,** Ventricle bigeminy.

failure. Syncope from an AV block such as this (Stokes-Adams syndrome) may result from severe bradycardia or even periods of asystole.

Treatment. A temporary pacemaker may be inserted on an emergency basis in a client with acute MI. The use of drugs such as atropine and isoproterenol is a temporary treatment to increase HR before pacemaker insertion.

Premature ventricular contractions. A premature ventricular contraction (PVC) is a contraction originating in an ectopic focus in the ventricles. It is the premature occurrence of a QRS complex, which is wide and distorted in shape, compared to a QRS complex initiated from the supraventricular tissue (Fig. 30-18). The QRS complex is usually wider than 0.12 second, and the T wave is generally large and opposite in direction to the major deflection of the QRS complex. Retrograde conduction may occur,

and the P wave may be seen following the ectopic beat. PVCs that are initiated from different foci appear different in contour from each other and are termed *multifocal PVCs*. When every other beat is a PVC, it is called *ventricular bigeminy*. When every third beat is a PVC, it is called *ventricular trigeminy*. Two consecutive PVCs are called *couplets*. Three consecutive PVCs are called *triplets*. *Ventricular tachycardia* occurs when there are three or more consecutive PVCs. When a PVC falls on the T wave of a preceding beat, the *R on T phenomenon* occurs and is considered to be quite dangerous, since it may precipitate ventricular tachycardia or ventricular fibrillation.

Clinical associations. PVCs are associated with stimulants such as caffeine, alcohol, aminophylline, epinephrine, isoproterenol, and digoxin. They are also associated with hypokalemia, hypoxia, fever, exercise, and emotional

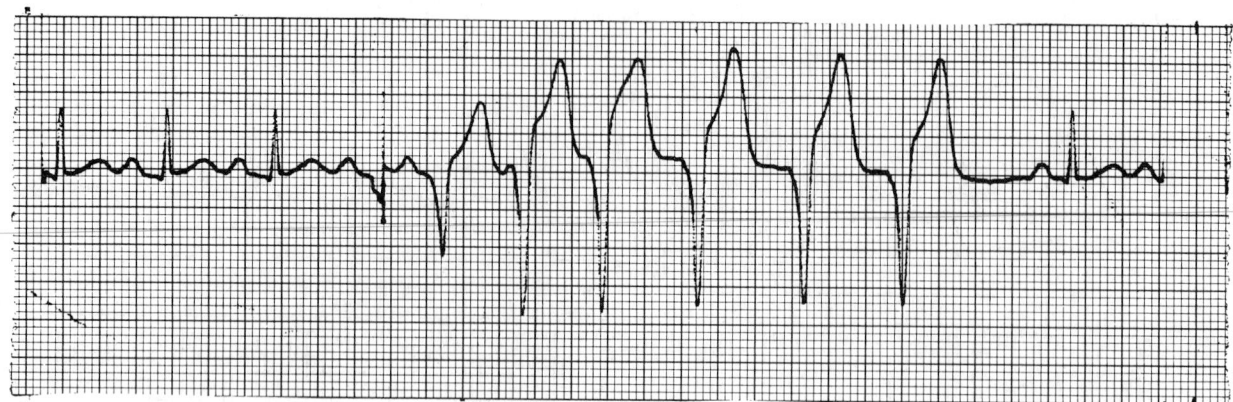

Fig. 30-19 Ventricular tachycardia.

stress. Disease states associated with PVCs include MI, mitral valve prolapse, CHF, and coronary artery disease.

ECG characteristics. HR varies according to intrinsic rate and number of PVCs. **Rhythm** is irregular because of premature beats. A **retrograde P wave** is possible; the **P wave** is rarely visible and is usually lost in the QRS complex of PVC. The **PR interval** is not measurable. The **QRS complex** is wide and distorted in shape, more than 0.10 second.

Significance. PVCs are usually a benign finding in clients with normal hearts. In heart disease, depending on frequency, PVCs may reduce the CO and precipitate angina and heart failure. PVCs in ischemic heart disease or acute MI represent ventricular irritability. They may also occur as *reperfusion dysrhythmias* after lysis of a coronary artery clot with thrombolytic therapy in acute MI.

Treatment. Indications for treatment in an appropriate clinical setting include (1) six or more PVCs occurring per minute, (2) ventricular couplets and triplets, (3) multifocal PVCs, and (4) R on T phenomenon. If these symptoms are not treated, ventricular tachycardia or ventricular fibrillation may occur. For treating PVCs, lidocaine is the drug of choice, with an initial IV bolus of 1 mg/kg followed by a second bolus of 0.5 mg/kg and continuous lidocaine infusion of 2 to 4 mg/min. Procainamide is the second drug of choice if lidocaine is ineffective.

Ventricular tachycardia. The ECG diagnosis of ventricular tachycardia is made when a run of three or more PVCs occurs. The QRS complex is distorted in appearance, with a duration exceeding 0.12 second and with the ST-T direction pointing opposite to the major QRS deflection (Fig. 30-19). It occurs when an ectopic focus or foci fire repetitively and the ventricle takes control as the pacemaker. The ventricular rate is 110 to 250 bpm, and the R-R interval may be irregular or regular. AV dissociation may be present, with P waves occurring independently of the QRS complex. The atria may also be depolarized by the ventricles in a retrograde fashion.

Ventricular tachycardia may be *sustained* (lasting longer than 30 seconds) or *nonsustained* (lasting 30 seconds or less). *Torsades de pointes* is a type of ventricular tachycardia characterized by a QRS contour that gradually changes its polarity over a series of beats. It usually occurs when QT prolongation is present.

The appearance of ventricular tachycardia is an ominous sign because it usually indicates the presence of cardiac disease. It is considered to be a life-threatening dysrhythmia because of decreased CO and the possibility of deterioration of ventricular tachycardia to ventricular fibrillation, which is a lethal dysrhythmia.

Clinical associations. Ventricular tachycardia is associated with acute MI, coronary artery disease, cardiomyopathy, mitral valve prolapse, long QT syndrome, and coronary reperfusion after thrombolytic therapy. The dysrhythmia has also been observed in clients who have no evidence of cardiac disease.

ECG characteristics. **Ventricular rate** is 110 to 250 bpm. **Rhythm** may be regular or irregular. The **P wave** may be noted to "march through" the ventricular rhythm in AV dissociation, or it may occur after the QRS complex in a regular pattern of retrograde conduction.

The **PR interval** is not measurable. The **QRS complex** is prolonged for more than 0.10 second, and its contour is distorted.

Significance. Ventricular tachycardia may cause a severe decrease in CO as a result of decreased ventricular diastolic filling times and loss of atrial contraction. The result may be pulmonary edema, shock, and insufficient blood flow to the brain. The dysrhythmia must be treated quickly, even if it occurs only briefly and stops abruptly.[10] The episodes may recur if prophylactic treatment is not begun.[11] Ventricular fibrillation may also develop.

Treatment. If the client is hemodynamically stable, treatment consists of administration of a lidocaine bolus of 1 mg/kg/min with subsequent boluses of 0.5 mg/kg/min up to 3 mg/kg body weight. If this abolishes the tachycardia, a continuous lidocaine infusion of 2 to 4 mg/min should be started. If lidocaine is ineffective, IV procainamide may be tried. Up to 100 mg/min IV may be given until tachycardia is terminated or until the QRS complex widens; if hypotension occurs, up to 750 to 1000 mg may be administered. If this treatment is successful, a continuous procainamide infusion of 2 to 4 mg/min should be started. A third drug of choice is bretylium, given IV at a dose of 5 mg/kg over several minutes and increased to 10 mg/kg at 15 to 30 minutes (not to exceed 40 mg/kg). A continuous infusion of bretylium 1 to 2 mg/min may be started.

If a client is unconscious or hemodynamically unstable,

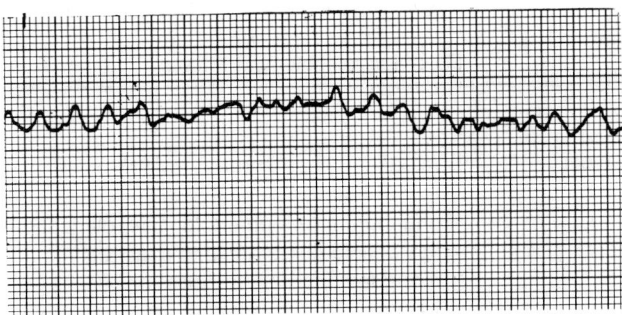

Fig. 30-20 Ventricular fibrillation.

immediate cardioversion, starting initially with 50 joules, is the recommended treatment. A defibrillator is used in the synchronized mode for cardioversion. The machine is timed to discharge on an R wave in order to effectively convert the ventricular tachycardia to a sinus rhythm. If a client is awake before cardioversion, a sedative may be given before delivery of the electrical discharge.

Ventricular fibrillation. Ventricular fibrillation is a severe derangement of the heart rhythm characterized on the ECG by irregular undulations of varying contour and amplitude (Fig. 30-20). This represents the firing of multiple ectopic foci in the ventricle. Mechanically, the ventricle is simply "quivering," and no effective contraction or CO occurs.

Clinical associations. Ventricular fibrillation occurs in acute MI and myocardial ischemia and in chronic diseases such as coronary artery disease and cardiomyopathy. It may occur during cardiac pacing or cardiac catheterization procedures as a result of catheter stimulation of the ventricle. It may also occur with coronary reperfusion after thrombolytic therapy. Other clinical associations are accidental electrical shock, hyperkalemia, and hypoxemia.

ECG characteristics. **HR** is not measurable. **Rhythm** is irregular and chaotic. The **P wave** is not visible, and the **PR interval** and the **QRS complex** are not measurable.

Significance. Ventricular fibrillation results in unconsciousness, absence of pulse, apnea, and seizures. If left untreated, the client with this condition will die.

Treatment. Treatment consists of immediate initiation of cardiopulmonary resuscitation (CPR) and initiation of advanced cardiac life support measures with use of defibrillation and definitive drug therapy. If a defibrillator is immediately available, there should be no delay in using it.

Asystole. Asystole represents the total absence of ventricular electrical activity. Occasionally, P waves can be seen. No ventricular contraction occurs, since depolarization does not occur. This is a lethal dysrhythmia and requires immediate treatment. Ventricular fibrillation may masquerade as asystole. Thus the rhythm should be assessed in more than one lead. The prognosis of a client with asystole is poor.

Clinical associations. Asystole is usually due to advanced cardiac disease, a severe cardiac conduction system disturbance, or end-stage CHF.

Significance. Generally, clients with asystole have end-

stage cardiac function or have a prolonged arrest and cannot be resuscitated.

Treatment. Treatment consists of CPR with initiation of advanced cardiac life support measures, which include intubation and IV therapy with epinephrine and atropine.

Electromechanical dissociation. Electromechanical dissociation (EMD) is a situation in which electrical activity can be observed on the ECG, but there is no mechanical activity of the ventricles and the client has no pulse. Prognosis is poor unless the underlying cause can be identified and corrected. The most common correctable causes of EMD are hypovolemia, cardiac tamponade, tension pneumothorax, hypoxemia, and acidosis. Other less correctable causes of EMD include massive myocardial damage from infarction, prolonged ischemia during resuscitation, and pulmonary embolism. Treatment begins with CPR followed by intubation and IV therapy with epinephrine. Treatment is directed toward correction of the underlying cause.

Antidysrhythmic Drugs

An increasing number of antidysrhythmic drugs have become available.[12-17] The Vaughn-Williams table of drug classifications separates the drugs by primary effects on the cardiac intracellular action potential (Table 30-7). Table 30-8 includes pertinent data pertaining to the most commonly used drugs in each class.

Table 30-7 Vaughn-Williams Classification of Antidysrhythmic Drugs

CLASSIFICATION I: DRUGS THAT DEPRESS UPSTROKE OF ACTION POTENTIAL

Prolong repolarization

Quinidine
Procainamide (Pronestyl)
Disopyramide (Norpace)

Accelerate repolarization

Lidocaine
Tocainide (Tonocard)
Mexilitine (Mexitil)

Have little or no effect on repolarization

Flecainide (Tambocor)
Encainide (Enkaid)

CLASSIFICATION II: β BLOCKERS

Propanolol (Inderal)
Nadolol (Corgard)

CLASSIFICATION III: DRUGS THAT PROLONG REPOLARIZATION

Bretylium (Bretylate, Bretylol)
Amiodarone (Cordarone)

CLASSIFICATION IV: CALCIUM CHANNEL BLOCKERS

Dittiazem (Cardizem)
Verapamil (Calan, Isoptin)

Table 30-8   Antidysrhythmic Drugs*

Drug	Indications	Major Pharmacological Effects
CLASSIFICATION IA		
Quinidine	Symptomatic PVCs, ventricular tachycardia, atrial fibrillation, atrial flutter, PSVT	Decreases phase zero of rapid depolarization of action potential (rapid sodium channel); slows phase four depolarization in Purkinje fibers; inhibits conduction along fast limb of AV nodal or bypass tract reentrant dysrhythmias
Procainamide (Pronestyl, Procan)	Ventricular and supraventricular dysrhythmias	Has similar effects as quinidine but does not prolong QT interval
Disopyramide (Norpace)	Ventricular and supraventricular dysrhythmias	Has similar effects as quinidine and procainamide but with significant anticholinergic or atropinelike effects
CLASSIFICATION IB		
Tocainide (Tonocard)	Ventricular dysrhythmias	Is a primary amine analog of lidocaine; has similar effects as lidocaine; inhibits fast sodium current while shortening action potential duration (i.e., shortening of QT interval)
Mexilitine (Mexitil)	Ventricular dysrhythmias	Has similar effects as lidocaine; depresses inward sodium current, with a decrease in rate of rise of action potential; does not prolong QT interval
CLASSIFICATION IC		
Flecainide (Tambocor)	Recurrent ventricular dysrhythmias, supraventricular dysrhythmias (effective in WPW syndrome)	Inhibits fast sodium current (Class I agent) and powerfully inhibits His-Purkinje conduction; prolongs PR and QRS intervals, causing prolongation of QT; inhibits AV nodal pathway in some AV nodal reentrant dysrhythmias
Encainide (Enkaid)	Ventricular and supraventricular dysrhythmias, including those of WPW syndrome	Has similar electrophysiological effects as flecainide but has little negative inotropic effect
CLASSIFICATION II **β-Blockers**		
Nonselective Propanolol (Inderal) Nadolol (Corgard) Timolol (Blocadren) Pindolol (Visken) Cardioselective Metoprolol (Lopressor) Atenolol (Tenormin) Acebutalol (Bectral)	Inappropriate sinus tachycardia, PSVT provoked by emotion or exercise, dysrhythmias of pheochromocytoma, exercise-induced ventricular dysrhythmias, dysrhythmias of mitral valve prolapse, acute myocardial ischemia and infarction	Induces β-adrenergic blockade; inhibits increases in HR, AV nodal conduction, myocardial contractility; shows cardioselective effect in some (i.e., predominant effect on β_1 receptors in heart, less effect on β_2 receptors in bronchial tree and peripheral vasculature)

*Classified according to Vaughn-Williams classification of antidysrhythmic drugs.

Adverse Effects	Nursing Considerations
Limiting side effects in at least 30% of clients, including nausea, diarrhea, headache, dizziness, tinnitus, fever, rash, thrombocytopenia, hemolytic anemia, anaphylaxis, and prolongation of QT interval with possible development of ventricular dysrhythmias including torsades de pointes (i.e., polymorphic ventricular tachycardia), representing prodysrhythmic effect (i.e., worsening of initial rhythm)	Assess carefully for side effects. Ensure continuous ECG monitoring at drug initiation. Reduce digoxin dose when quinidine therapy is started because quinidine increases blood digoxin levels.
Gastrointestinal intolerance, rash, agranulocytosis, drug-induced lupus syndrome, torsades de pointes, bundle branch block, AV block	Be aware that long-term therapy is not recommended because of risk of development of lupuslike syndrome and that procainamide does not affect digoxin levels.
Negative inotropic effects that may worsen heart failure; anticholinergic effects, including dry mouth, urinary hesitancy or retention, constipation; QRS and QT prolongation, producing torsades de pointes and other dysrhythmias	Be aware that the presence of heart failure is absolute contraindication to use of drug.
Neurological effects, including dizziness, tremor, paresthesias; gastrointestinal effects, including nausea, vomiting, diarrhea; severe effects, including leukopenia, thrombocytopenia, pulmonary fibrosis	Be aware that tocainide does not have negative inotropic effect and can be used safely in CHF.
Neurological effects, including tremor, dysarthria, dizziness, paresthesias, diplopia, nystagmus, confusion, anxiety; gastrointestinal effects, including nausea and vomiting	Be aware that mexilitine has a narrow therapeutic-toxic margin. Closely observe clients for side effects. Be aware that drug is important antidysrhythmic for clients with CHF and that it does not have negative inotropic properties.
Prodysrhythmic effect (aggravation of ventricular dysrhythmias in 5%-12% of clients), decreased myocardial contractility (possibly exacerbating heart failure), dizziness, blurred vision, tremor, constipation, pruritus	Ensure continuous ECG monitoring after initiation of therapy. Frequently measure PR and QRS intervals. Be alert to any increase in ventricular dysrhythmias. Observe clients for any worsening of symptoms of CHF.
Prolongation of PR, QRS, and QT interval, significant exacerbation of ventricular dysrhythmias (prodysrhythmic effect) in 10%-15% of clients, dizziness, diplopia, vertigo, paresthesias, leg cramps, headache, metallic taste in mouth	Be aware that may be given safely to clients with CHF and reduced left ventricular function.
Decreased myocardial contractility with possible development of CHF, sinus bradycardia, asystole, AV block, bronchospasm, fatigue, impotence, insomnia, nightmares, hypoglycemia in clients with diabetes	Inform clients that abrupt discontinuation of β-blocking drugs can cause "rebound" syndrome.

Continued.

Table 30-8 Antidysrhythmic Drugs*—cont'd

Drug	Indications	Major Pharmacological Effects
CLASSIFICATION III		
Amiodarone (Cordarone)	Recurrent atrial fibrillation, supraventricular tachydysrhythmias associated with WPW syndrome, recurrent ventricular tachycardia, recurrent ventricular fibrillation	Prolongs action potential duration without significantly effective depolarization; increases refractor period of atrium, AV node, and ventricle; increases refractory period and slows conduction in accessory pathways in WPW syndrome; prolongs QT interval
Bretylium (Bretylol, Bretylate)†	—	—
CLASSIFICATION) IV		
Diltiazem,‡ verapamil†	—	—

*Classified according to Vaughn-Williams classification of antidysrhythmic drugs.
†See Table 30-19.
‡Not available in IV form in the United States.

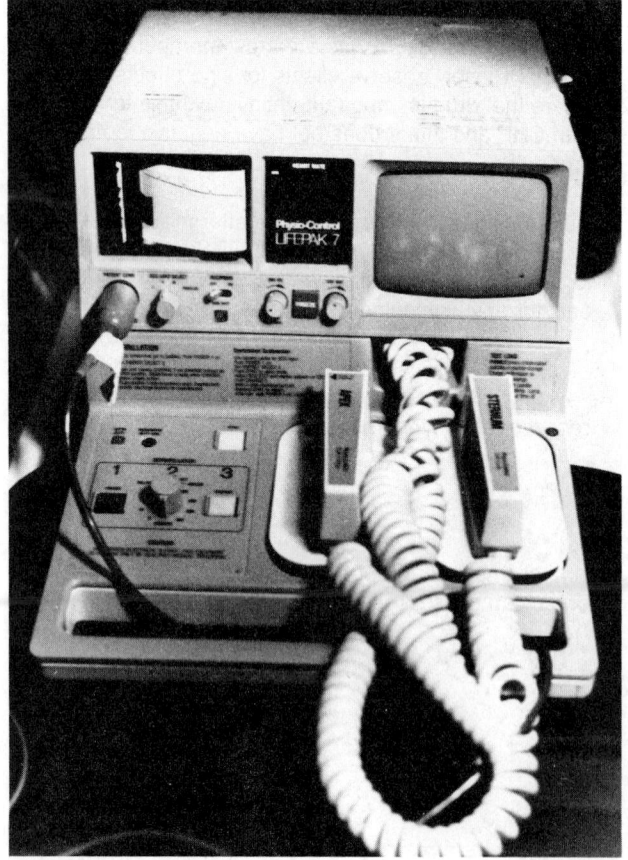

Fig. 30-21 Life-Pak. A lightweight, battery-powered defibrillator with monitoring capabilities. (Courtesy Pam Brown, Albuquerque.)

Defibrillation

Defibrillation is the most effective method of terminating ventricular fibrillation. It is most effective when the myocardial cells are not anoxic or acidotic. Therefore defibrillation should ideally be performed within 15 to 20 seconds of the onset of the dysrhythmia. Defibrillation is accomplished by the passage of a direct current (DC) electrical shock through the heart that is sufficient to depolarize the cells of the myocardium. The intent is that subsequent repolarization of myocardial cells will allow the SA node to resume the role of pacemaker.[18] The output of a defibrillator is quantified in *joules* or *watts per second*. The recommended energy for initial shock in defibrillation is 200 joules with a second shock of 200 to 300 joules as needed and a third shock of 360 joules if defibrillation is unsuccessful. High doses of electricity during defibrillation have been found to cause myocardial damage; thus, the lowest effective electrical output is the one with which to start.

A defibrillator is one part of standard emergency equipment available (Fig. 30-21). There are many different models of defibrillators. Nurses should be very familiar with the operation of the type of defibrillator that is used on his or her unit. Proficiency verification in use of the defibrillator is recommended annually for nursing staff members who use it.

The following steps are to be taken for defibrillation: (1) CPR should be in progress if the defibrillator is not immediately available; (2) the defibrillator should be turned on and the proper energy level should be selected, and (3) someone should verify that the synchronizer switch is turned off. Conductive materials in the form of saline pads, electrode gel, or defibrillator gel pads are applied to the chest where defibrillator paddles will be placed. This decreases electrical impedance and helps to prevent burns. The paddles are charged by means of a button on the defibrillator or a button on the paddles themselves. The paddles are placed on the chest wall (Figs. 30-22 and 30-23);

Adverse Effects	Nursing Considerations
Nausea, anorexia, insomnia, weakness, fatigue, microdeposits in cornea, thyroid dysfunction, pulmonary toxicity, hepatic toxicity, bluish discoloration of skin, exacerbation of ventricular dysrhythmias with torsades de pointes, worsening SA node dysfunction and abnormal AV node conduction; very long half-life (possibly several weeks); weeks of therapy necessary for development of therapeutic level	Inform clients of potential toxicity. Ensure regular follow-up care to determine the best dosage and to check for toxicity with chest x-ray film, pulmonary examinations, thyroid tests, and retinal examinations. Emphasize potential for bluish discoloration of skin. Educate clients about protecting themselves from sun exposure with skin barriers of clothing and lotions. Caution clients about concomitant use with digoxin and/or coumadin.

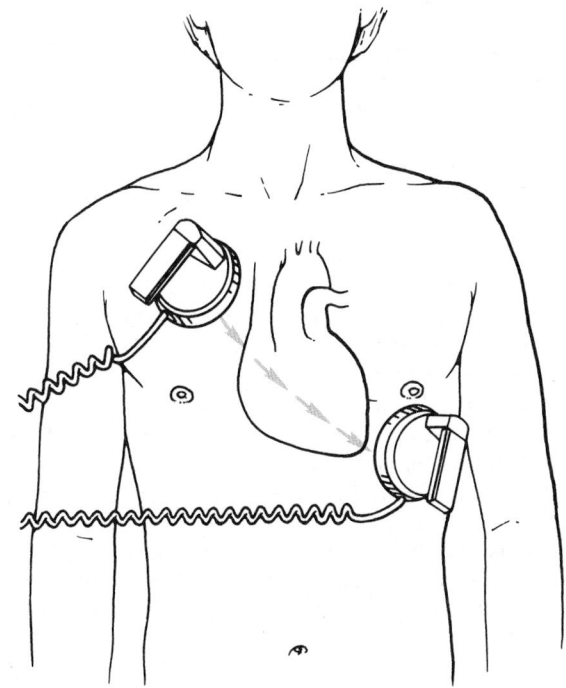

Fig. 30-22 Paddle placement and current flow in defibrillation.

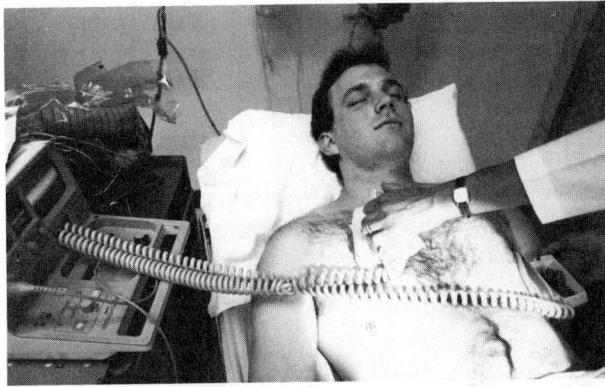

Fig. 30-23 Placement of defibrillator paddles. (Courtesy Pam Brown, Albuquerque.)

one is placed to the right of the sternum just below the clavicle, and the other is placed to the left of the precordium. The operator applies 20 to 25 pounds of pressure to the paddles. The operator calls "all clear" to ensure that personnel are not touching the client or the bed at the time of discharge. The defibrillator is then discharged by depressing buttons on both paddles simultaneously.

Electrical cardioversion is the therapy of choice for hemodynamically unstable ventricular or supraventricular tachydysrhythmias. A synchronized circuit in the defibrilla-tor is used to deliver a countershock that is programmed to occur during the QRS complex of the ECG.

The procedure for cardioversion is the same as for defibrillation with the following exceptions: If synchronized cardioversion is done on a nonemergency basis when the client is awake and hemodynamically stable, clients may be sedated with diazepam or anesthetized with a short-acting barbiturate before the procedure. Strict attention to maintenance of a patent airway is important in this situation. When a client with supraventricular tachycardia or ventricular tachycardia is hemodynamically unstable, cardioversion is performed as quickly as possible.

Automatic implantable cardioverter-defibrillator. In the past several years the automatic implantable cardioverter-defibrillator (AICD) has been developed as an acceptable treatment for those clients who have malignant ventricular dysrhythmias.[19-21] Clients who qualify for this device have been shown by electrophysiological studies to be prone to lethal tachydysrhythmias in spite of drug therapy. This new modality appears to significantly decrease

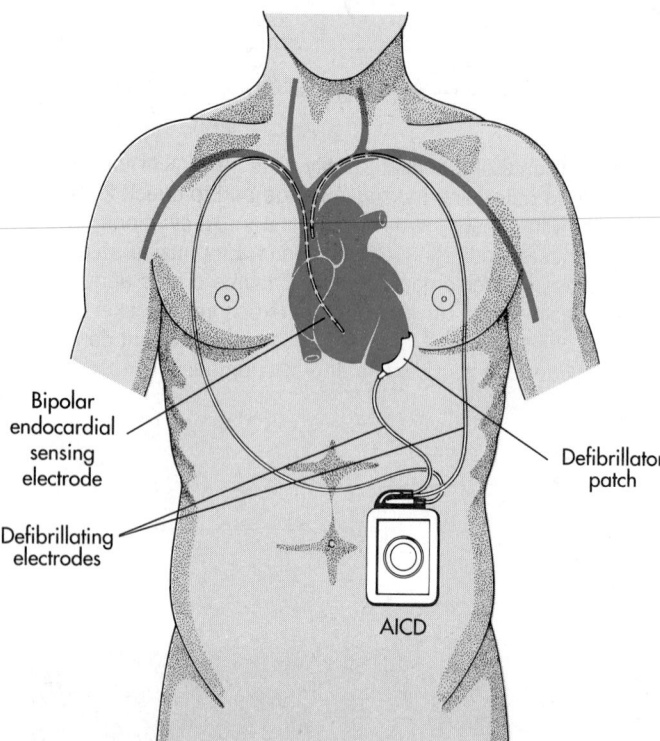

Fig. 30-24 The AICD pulse generator is placed in a subcutaneous pocket in the abdomen. Bipolar endocardial sensing electrode is placed in the right ventricular apex. Defibrillating electrodes are positioned in the superior vena cava (spring lead) and over the apex of the heart (mesh patch covered with silicone and rubber).

Table 30-9 Discharge Instructions for Client and Family after AICD Implantation

When the AICD fires:
  The client should lie down.
  One person should stay with the client while another contacts the physician.
  Someone should call an ambulance if client loses consciousness. CPR should be delayed until device fires unsuccessfully four times or fails to fire after 30 seconds.
  If someone is touching the client when the AICD fires, that person may feel a slight but harmless shock.
  If alone, the client should call an ambulance immediately and then lie down.
The AICD battery must be checked every 2 months.
A "Medic-Alert" bracelet should be worn at all times.
An information card about the AICD should be easily accessible in the client's wallet.
The manual for clients provided by the AICD manufacturer should be read.
Family members should learn CPR.
The nurse should assist client with the development of positive coping strategies to reduce stress.

cardiac mortality rates and has added a new dimension to the management of lethal dysrhythmias and the prevention of sudden cardiac death.

The AICD consists of a lithium battery–powered pulse generator with three wires (Fig. 30-24). The generator box is implanted subcutaneously in the abdomen. The AICD sensing system monitors the HR and rhythm and identifies ventricular tachycardia or ventricular fibrillation. About 25 seconds after the sensing system detects a lethal dysrhythmia, the defibrillating mechanism delivers a 25-joule shock to the client's heart muscle. If the first shock is unsuccessful, the generator recycles up to three times, delivering a maximum of 30 joules.

The postoperative recovery period after implantation of an AICD is usually a prolonged hospitalization with careful observation for appropriate AICD response to dysrhythmias. The implantation procedure itself carries a low risk, and possible complications that the nurse should be aware of are similar to those for permanent pacemaker implantation. Occasionally, an AICD is implanted during open heart surgery, which results in a different risk and complication profile.

Education of the client who is receiving an AICD is of extreme importance. The client experiences a variety of emotions including fear of body image change, fear of recurrent dysrhythmias, expectation of pain with AICD discharge (described as a feeling of a blow to the chest), and anxiety about going home. Table 30-9 describes the discharge instructions for clients with AICDs and their families.

Pacemakers

The artificial cardiac pacemaker is an electronic device used in place of the SA node, the natural cardiac pacemaker of the heart. Implantable pacemakers were first developed in the 1950s. The artificial cardiac pacemaker is an electrical circuit in which the battery provides electricity that travels through a conducting wire to the myocardium, and the myocardium stimulates the heart to beat (i.e., it "captures" the heart).

Approximately 1 million persons in the world have implanted pacemakers. Recent advances in technology have been applied extensively to pacemakers. This has resulted in sophisticated noninvasively programmable single- and dual-chambered pacemakers with specialized circuits that weigh only 40 to 50 g. Pacemakers have been developed that are more physiologically accurate, pacing both the atrium and the ventricle, as well as increasing HR when appropriate.

Permanent pacemakers are those that are implanted totally within the body (Fig. 30-25), and *temporary pacemakers* are those with the power source outside the body (Fig. 30-26). The permanent pacemaker power source is implanted subcutaneously in the chest (Fig. 30-25, *B*) or abdomen and is attached to pacer electrodes, which are threaded transvenously to the right ventricle and/or the right atrium (Fig. 30-25, *A*). Indications for insertion of permanent pacemaker are listed in Table 30-10.

Temporary pacemakers are usually used with a lead or wire threaded transvenously to the right ventricle and with

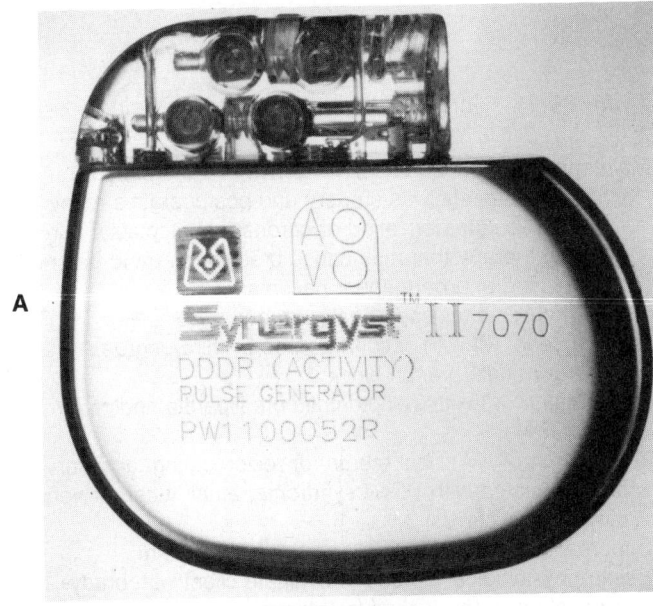

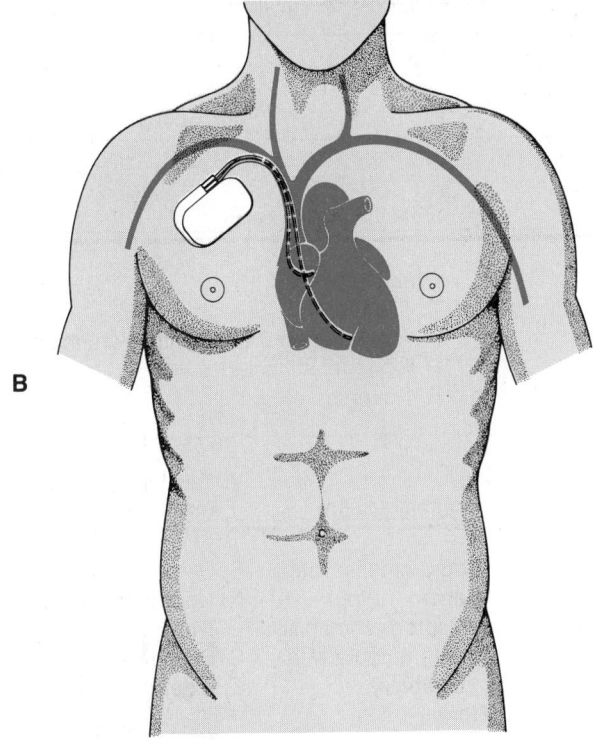

Fig. 30-25 **A,** Synergyst II, a new dual-chamber, rate-responsive pacemaker from Medtronic, Inc, is designed to detect body movement and automatically increase or decrease paced HRs based on the level of physical activity. **B,** Cardiac leads in both the atrium and ventricle enable a dual-chamber pacemaker to sense and pace in both heart chambers.

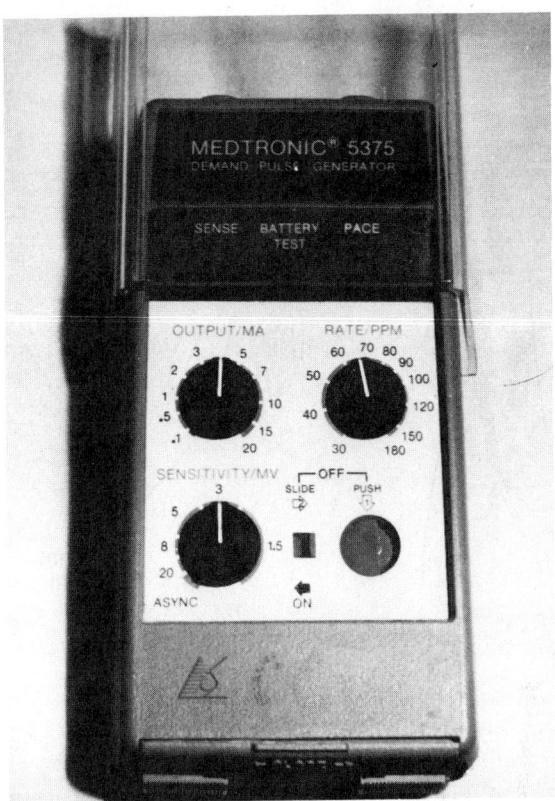

Fig. 30-26 Temporary external demand pacemaker. (Courtesy Medtronic, Inc, Minneapolis.)

Table 30-10 Indications for Permanent Pacemaker Therapy

Sinus node dysfunction
Third-degree AV block
Fibrosis or sclerotic changes of cardiac conduction system
Sick sinus syndrome
Mobitz II second-degree AV block
Hypersensitive carotid sinus syndrome
Chronic atrial fibrillation with slow ventricular response
Tachydysrhythmias
Bifascicular block

a wire attached to a power source externally (Fig. 30-27). They are inserted in cardiac care units in emergency situations. Indications for temporary pacing are listed in Table 30-11.

The Intersociety Commission for Heart Disease (ICHD) has established pacemaker terminology to describe different types of pacemakers. A code of three letters was introduced in 1974 to provide a shorthand description of the many pacing modes. The three letters denote the chamber paced, the chamber sensed, and the pacemaker's response to the stimulus. Table 30-12 gives the code key. Using the ICHD code, the physician and nurse team can precisely determine the characteristics of the pacemaker used.

In the early 1980s the ICHD code was expanded to a more descriptive five-letter system for a more appropriate description of the more sophisticated pacing units that are used today (Table 30-12). If only the rate and/or output of

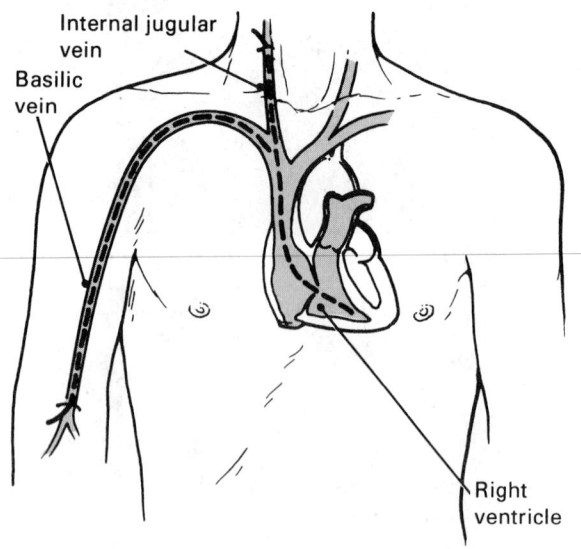

Fig. 30-27 Temporary pacemaker catheter insertion.

Table 30-11 Indications for Temporary Pacing

Maintenance of adequate HR and rhythm during special circumstances such as surgery and postoperative recovery, cardiac catheterization or coronary angioplasty, during drug therapy that may cause bradycardia, and before implantation of a permanent pacemaker

As Prophylaxis after open heart surgery

Acute anterior MI with second-degree or third-degree AV block or bundle branch block

Acute inferior MI with symptomatic bradycardia and/or AV block

Termination of AV nodal reentry or reciprocating tachycardia associated with WPW syndrome, atrial flutter, or ventricular tachycardia

Suppression of ectopic atrial or ventricular rhythm

Electrophysiological studies to evaluate client with brady-dysrhythmias and tachydysrhythmias

Table 30-12 Pacemaker Terminology and Nomenclature*

1974 CRITERIA

I. Chamber Paced	II. Chamber Sensed	III. Mode of Response
V, Ventricle	V, Ventricle	I, Inhibited
A, Atrium	A, Atrium	T, Triggered
D, Atrium and ventricle	D, Atrium and ventricle	D, Atrial triggered and ventricular inhibited
O, None	O, None	O, None (continuous)
		R, Reverse

1981 CRITERIA

I. Chamber Paced	II. Chamber Sensed	III. Mode of Response	IV. Programmability	V. Tachyarrhythmia functions
V, Ventricle	V, Ventricle	I, Inhibited	P, Programmable rate and/or output	B, Burst
A, Atrium	A, Atrium	T, Triggered	M, Multiprogrammability	N, Normal rate competition
D, Atrium and ventricle	D, Atrium and ventricle	D, Atrial triggered and ventricular inhibited	C, Programmable with telemetry	S, Scanning
O, None	O, None	O, None	O, None	E, External

PACEMAKER NOMENCLATURE†

VVI Ventricular demand/ventricular inhibited
AAI Atrial demand/atrial inhibited
DVI AV sequential/ventricular inhibited
VAT Atrial synchronous/P wave triggered
VDD Atrial synchronous/ventricular inhibited
DDD Universal/fully automatic

*Intersociety Commission for Heart Disease code.

†First initial refers to chamber or chambers *paced;* second initial refers to chamber or chambers *sensed;* third initial refers to pacemaker's *response.*

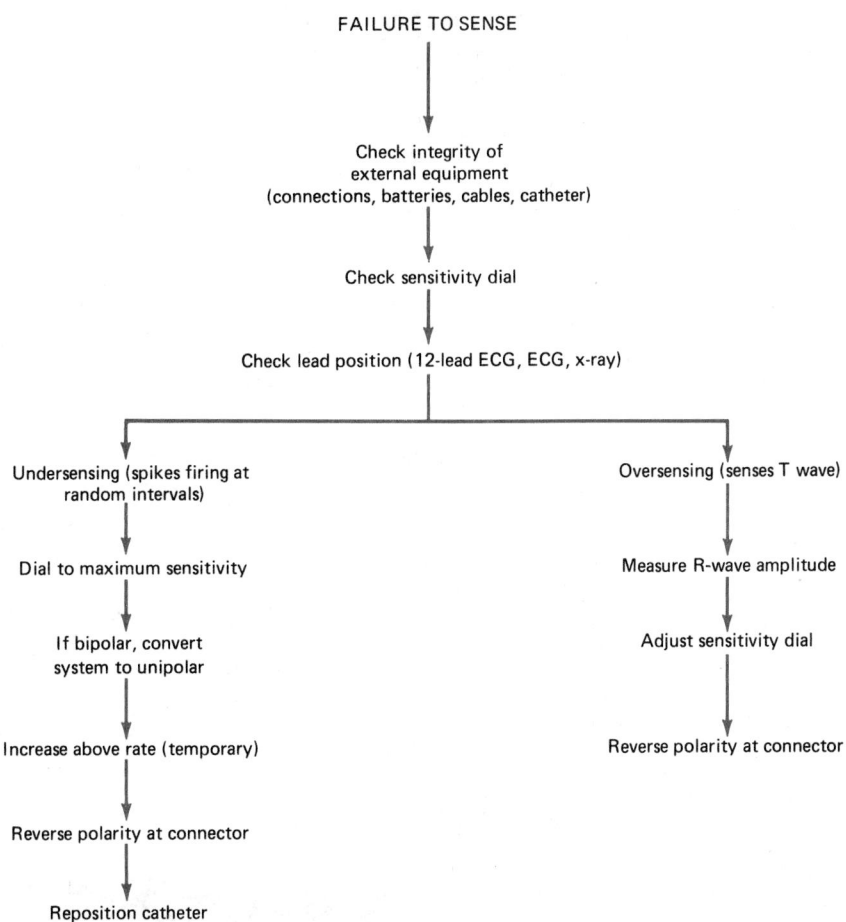

Fig. 30-28   Failure to sense.

the pulse generator can be programmed externally, *P* is in the fourth position of the pacing mode code. If the pacemaker is used to treat tachycardias, the tachydysrhythmia function is indicated in the fifth position of the pacing mode code.

Pacemaker malfunction is manifested by a failure to sense or a failure to capture. *Failure to sense* occurs when the pacemaker fails to recognize spontaneous atrial or ventricular activity and fires inappropriately (Fig. 30-28). Failure to sense may be due to pacer lead fracture, battery failure, or displacement of electrode. *Failure to capture* occurs when the electrical charge to the myocardium is insufficient to produce atrial or ventricular contraction (Fig. 30-29). Failure to capture may be due to pacer lead fracture, battery failure, electrode displacement, or fibrosis at the electrode tip.

Complications of temporary or permanent pacemaker insertion include infection and hematoma formation at the site of insertion of the pacemaker power source, pneumothorax, failure to sense and/or capture with possible bradycardia and significant symptoms, perforation of the atrial or ventricular septum by the pacing wire, and appearance of "end of life" battery parameters on testing the pacemaker. A decrease in CO may also be seen when a ventricular demand/ventricular inhibited mode pacer is inserted because of loss of atrial contractions (atrial "kick").

Measures taken to prevent and assess complications include prophylactic IV antibiotic therapy before and after insertion, assessment of chest x-ray film after insertion to check lead placement and to rule out the presence of a pneumothorax, careful observation of insertion site, and continuous ECG monitoring of client's rhythm. After pacemaker insertion the client is maintained on bed rest for 24 hours, and minimal arm and shoulder activity is allowed to prevent dislodgement of the newly implanted pacemaker leads. The nurse should observe for signs of infection by assessing the incision for redness, swelling, or discharge. Temperature elevation should also be noted. Careful monitoring of the client's rhythm is used to detect problems with sensing or capturing.

The nurse must provide client education in addition to observation for complications after pacemaker insertion. Clients with newly implanted pacemakers have many questions about activity restrictions and fears concerning body image and becoming a "cardiac cripple" after the procedure. The goal of pacemaker therapy should be to enhance physiological functioning and the quality of life.[22] This should be emphasized to the client, and the nurse should give concrete advice on activity restrictions. Basic information for clients with pacemakers is outlined in Table 30-13.

Pacemaker function can be checked by magnet place-

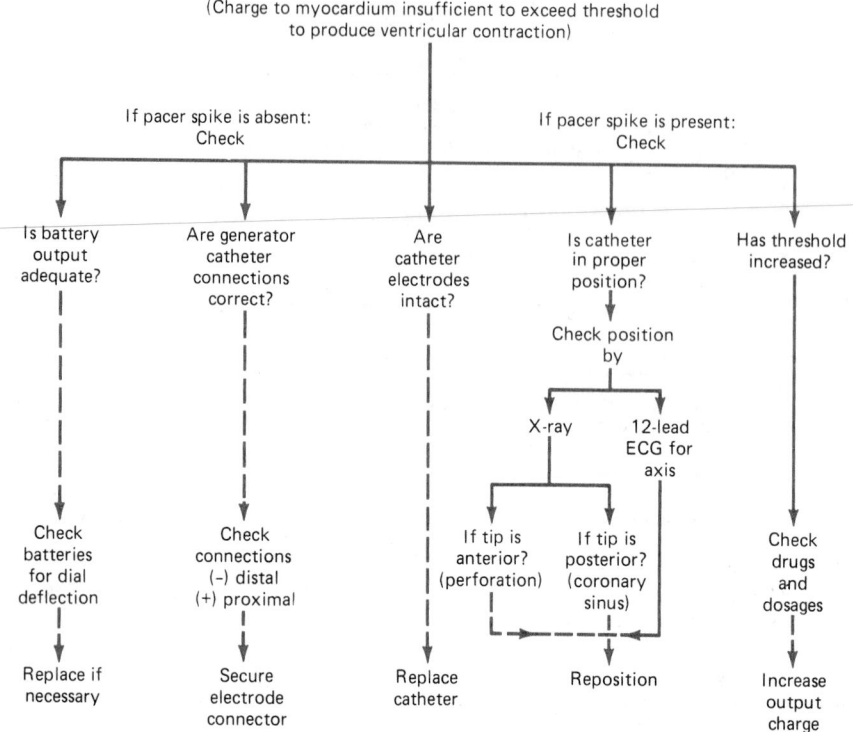

Fig. 30-29 Failure to capture.

Table 30-13 Educational Information for Clients with Pacemakers

Maintain follow-up care with a physician because it is important to check the pacemaker site and to begin regular pacemaker function checks with magnet and ECG evaluation.

Watch for signs of infection at incision site (e.g., redness, swelling, drainage).

Keep incision dry for 1 week after discharge.

For activity restriction, avoid direct blows to generator site. (Avoid contact sports such as football or use of rifle.)

Avoid close proximity to high-output electrical generators or to large magnets such as a magnetic resonance imaging scanner. These devices can reprogram the pacemaker.

Microwave ovens are perfectly safe to use and do not threaten pacemaker function.

Travel without restrictions is allowed. The metal case of a small implanted pacemaker rarely sets off an airport security alarm.

Learn how to take pulse rate.

Carry pacemaker information card at all times, preferably in an easily accessible place such as a wallet or purse.

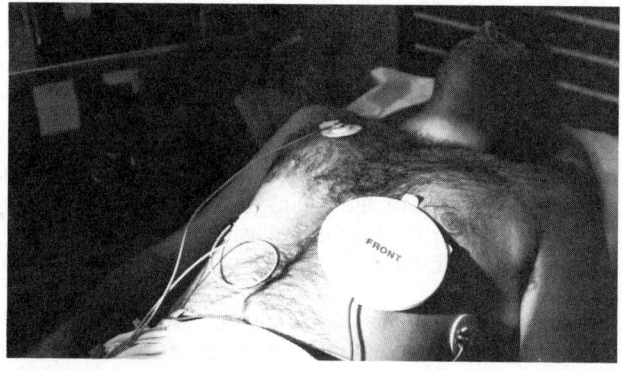

Fig. 30-30 External pacemaker.

External pacemaker. The *external* pacemaker or *transcutaneous* pacemaker has recently been reintroduced as a means of providing adequate HR and rhythm to clients in emergency situations (Fig. 30-30). Placement of the external pacemaker is a noninvasive procedure that should be used only temporarily until a transvenous pacemaker can be inserted or until more definitive therapy is available.

The external pacemaker was used in the 1950s but lost favor in 1959 when internal pacemakers became available. Early external pacemakers were quite painful to use and required high voltage to maintain an acceptable cardiac rhythm. Modern external pacemakers have been modified to allow cardiac stimulation at lower voltage levels. The external pacemaker consists of a power source and a rate- and voltage-control device that is attached to two large electrode pads. One pad is positioned on the anterior part of the chest, usually on the V_2 or V_5 lead position, and the

ment during ECG assessment in the pacemaker clinic, or it can be done from the home using telephone transmitter devices. Clients are sometimes given devices to place on their fingers or directly over the pacemaker battery generator with an attachment to the telephone. In this way the heart rhythm can be transmitted to the pacemaker clinic.

other pad is placed on the back between the spine and the left scapula at the level of the heart.

Before initiating external pacemaker therapy, it is important to tell the client what to expect. The uncomfortable muscle contractions that the pacemaker creates when the current passes through the chest wall should be explained. The client should be reassured that the therapy is temporary and that every effort will be made to adjust the voltage settings of the pacemaker to improve comfort level.[23] Mild analgesia may also be given.

CARDIOPULMONARY RESUSCITATION

Every nurse and physician should be skilled in CPR because *cardiac arrest*, the sudden, unexplained, unexpected cessation of breathing and adequate circulation of blood by the heart, may occur at any time or in any setting. CPR is the process of externally supporting the circulation and respiration of a person who has a cardiac arrest. Resuscitation measures are divided into two components, basic cardiac life support (BCLS) and advanced cardiac life support (ACLS). The American Heart Association establishes the standards for CPR and is actively involved in teaching BCLS and ACLS to health professionals. The American Heart Association recommends that nurses and physicians working with clients be certified in BCLS and ACLS. Certification involves attending formal classes and passing cognitive and motor skill tests.

Basic Cardiac Life Support

BCLS involves the external support of circulation and ventilation for a client with cardiac or respiratory arrest through CPR.[24] Artificial respiration (mouth-to-mouth, mouth-to-mask, mouth-to-nose, mouth-to-stoma) and external chest compression substitute for spontaneous breathing and circulation. The major objective of performing CPR is to provide oxygen to the brain, heart, and other vital organs until appropriate therapeutic management and resuscitation efforts involving advanced life support methods can be initiated or until resuscitation efforts are ordered to be stopped.

Speed is the key to success and is critical to the prevention of biological death or the death of brain cells. CPR must be initiated within 4 to 6 minutes of cardiac or pulmonary arrest. Brain cells begin to die *(brain death)* within 6 minutes of anoxia. It is critical that oxygenated blood be circulated during CPR. Unfortunately, even when CPR is performed with perfect technique, only 25% to 30% of the normal CO is achieved. National standards for knowledge and technique must be met for personnel to be certified to deliver CPR. Assessment of the victim must be stressed in teaching CPR. Each of the broad areas—*A*irway, *B*reathing, and *C*irculation (the ABCs of CPR)—should be reviewed.

Airway and breathing. The first steps in administering BCLS are to confirm absence of breathing and to establish a patent airway. Fig. 30-31 demonstrates opening the airway and performing mouth-to-mouth ventilation. An adult's airway is opened by hyperextending the head. The *head-tilt/chin-lift* manuever is used and involves tilting the head back with one hand and lifting the chin forward with the fingers of the other hand. If no respirations are de-

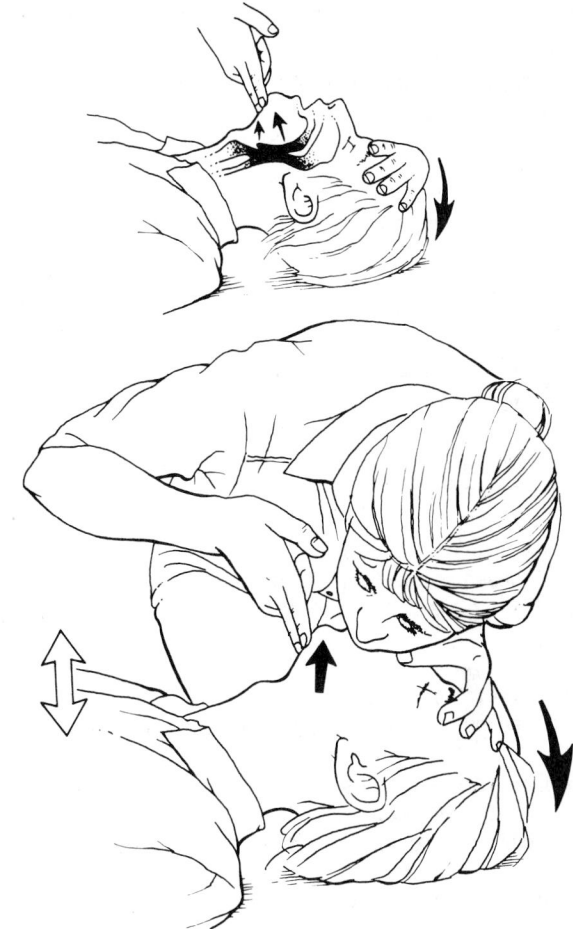

Fig. 30-31 The head-tilt/chin-lift maneuver is used to open the victim's airway to give mouth-to-mouth resuscitation. This procedure is carried out by placing one hand on the victim's forehead and applying firm, backward pressure with the palm to tilt the head back. The chin is lifted and brought forward with the fingers of the other hand.

tected, the rescuer attempts to ventilate the victim with mouth-to-mouth resuscitation. Breaths are given with the victim's nostrils pinched and the rescuer's mouth placed around the victim's mouth to make a tight seal. Two breaths are given by the rescuer, and the rescuer takes a breath between ventilations. The volume of air of each ventilation should be about 800 ml, which can be determined by noting a rise of 1 to 2 inches in the victim's chest. When the victim has a tracheostomy, ventilation should be given through the stoma.

If air flow is obstructed, the rescuer should reposition the head and repeat the attempt to provide ventilation. If the victim cannot be ventilated after repositioning the head, the rescuer should proceed with maneuvers to remove foreign bodies that may be obstructing the airway (Table 30-14).

The subdiaphragmatic abdominal thrust, or *Heimlich maneuver,* is used to move air from the lungs with sufficient force to create an artificial cough intended to move and expel an obstructing foreign body from the airway. With the conscious victim in a standing or sitting position,

Table 30-14 Management of Foreign Body Airway Obstruction

Objectives	Actions
CONSCIOUS VICTIM	
1. Assessment: Determine airway obstruction.	Ask, "Are you choking?" Determine if victim can cough or speak.
2. Act to relieve obstruction.	Perform subdiaphragmatic abdominal thrusts (Heimlich maneuver).*
Be persistent.	Repeat step 2 until obstruction is relieved or victim becomes unconscious.
VICTIM WHO BECOMES UNCONSCIOUS	
3. Position the victim; call for help.	Turn victim on back as a unit, supporting head and neck, face up, arms by sides. Call out, "Help!" If others come, activate emergency medical services.
4. Check for foreign body.	Perform tongue-jaw lift and finger sweep.†
5. Give rescue breaths.	Open the airway with head-tilt/chin-lift. Try to give rescue breaths.
6. Act to relieve obstruction.	Perform subdiaphragmatic abdominal thrusts (Heimlich maneuver 6-10 repetitions).
7. Check again for foreign body.	Perform tongue-jaw lift and finger sweep.
8. Try again to give rescue breaths.	Open the airway with head-tilt/chin-lift. Try to give rescue breaths.
9. Be persistent.	Repeat steps 6 to 8 until obstruction is relieved.
UNCONSCIOUS VICTIM	
1. Assessment: Determine unresponsiveness.	Tap or gently shake shoulder. Shout, "Are you okay?"
2. Position the victim; call for help.	Turn on back as a unit, supporting head and neck, face up, arms by sides. Call out, "Help!" If others come, activate emergency medical services.
3. Open the airway.	Use head-tilt/chin-lift maneuver.
4. Assessment: Determine breathlessness.	Maintain an open airway. With ear over victim's mouth, observe chest. Look, listen, feel for breathing (3-5 seconds).
5. Give rescue breaths.	Make mouth-to-mouth seal. Try to give rescue breaths.
6. Try again to give rescue breaths.	Reposition head. Try rescue breaths again.
7. Activate the emergency medical services system.	If someone responded to the call for help, that person should activate the emergency medical services system.
8. Act to relieve obstruction.	Perform subdiaphragmatic abdominal thrusts (Heimlich maneuver 6-10 repetitions).
9. Check for foreign body.	Perform tongue-jaw lift and finger sweep.
10. Give rescue breaths again.	Open the airway with head-tilt/chin-lift. Try again to give rescue breaths.
11. Be persistent.	Repeat steps 8 to 10 until obstruction is relieved.

Modified from Healthcare provider's manual for basic life support, Dallas, 1988, American Heart Association.
*See Fig. 30-32.
†See Fig. 30-33.

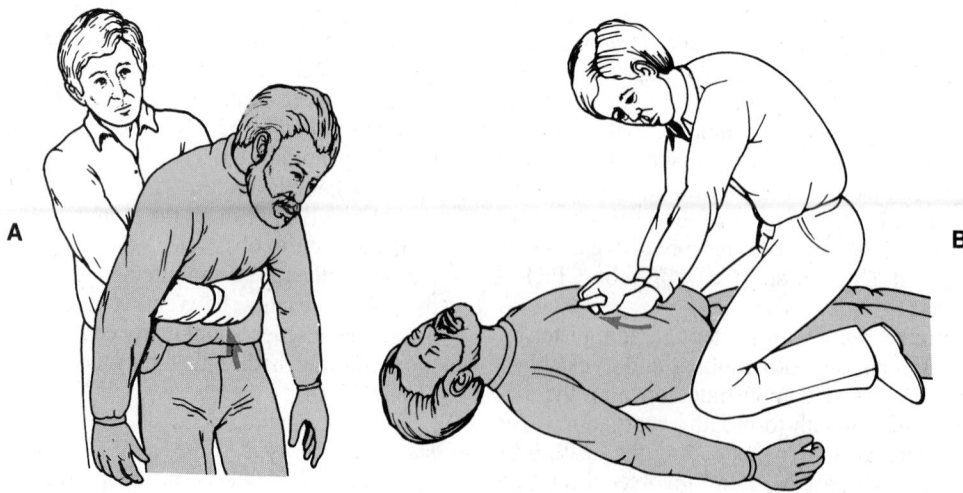

Fig. 30-32 **A,** Heimlich maneuver administered to a conscious (standing) victim of foreign body airway obstruction. **B,** Heimlich maneuver administered to an unconscious (lying) victim of foreign body airway obstruction—astride position.

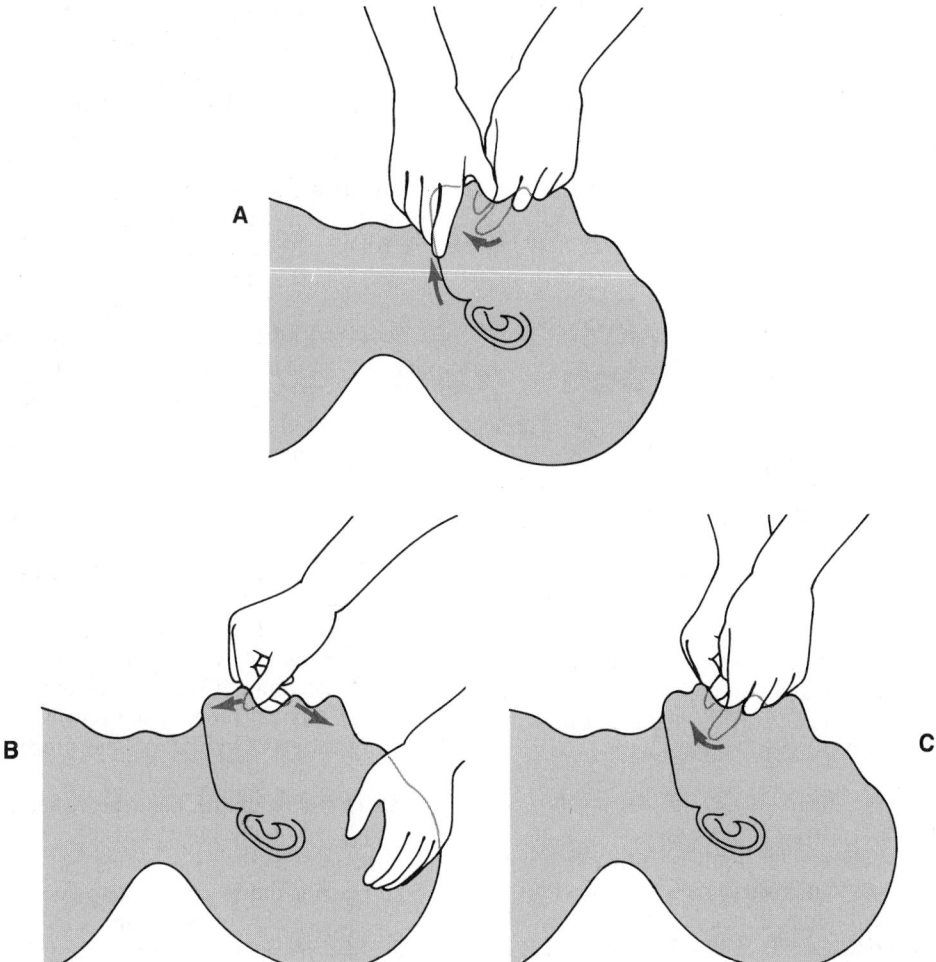

Fig. 30-33 **A,** Finger sweep maneuver administered to an unconscious victim of foreign body airway obstruction. With the victim's head up, the rescuer opens the victim's mouth by grasping both the tongue and the lower jaw between the thumb and fingers and lifting (tongue-jaw lift). This action draws the tongue from the back of the throat and away from the foreign body. The obstruction may be partially relieved by this maneuver. **B,** Crossed-finger technique for opening the airway. If the rescuer is unable to open the mouth with tongue-jaw lift, the crossed-finger technique may be used. The rescuer opens the mouth by crossing the index finger and thumb and pushing the teeth apart. **C,** The index finger of the rescuer's available hand is inserted along the inside of the cheek and deeply into the throat to the base of the tongue. A hooking motion is used to dislodge the foreign body and maneuver it into the mouth for removal.

the rescuer should stand behind the victim, wrap the arms around the victim's waist (Fig. 30-32), and proceed as follows:

1. Make a fist with one hand.
2. Place the thumb side of the fist against the victim's abdomen in the midline, slightly above the navel and well below the tip of the xiphoid process.
3. Grasp the fist with the other hand.
4. Press the fist into the victim's abdomen with a quick, upward thrust.
5. Repeat thrusts until the foreign body is expelled or until the victim becomes unconscious.

With an unconscious victim in a supine position, the rescuer places the heel of one hand against the victim's ab-domen, in the midline slightly above the navel and well below the tip of the xiphoid process; the rescuer places the other hand directly on top of the first (Fig. 30-32). The rescuer presses into the abdomen with 6 to 10 quick, up-ward thrusts, using body weight to perform the maneuver. The rescuer then examines the victim's mouth to see if an obstructing object can be reached by the fingers. A finger sweep maneuver may be employed at this point (Fig. 30-33). If an object is not removed, the rescuer again attempts to ventilate the victim. If the obstruction remains, the pro-cedure is repeated until the obstruction is expelled and the victim can be ventilated. Even if the victim's heart has stopped, cardiac compressions are not started until the vic-tim can be ventilated (i.e. until the airway is cleared).

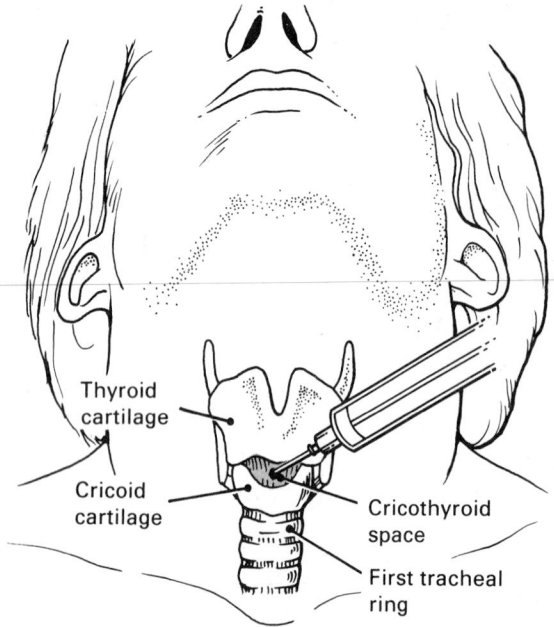

Fig. 30-34 Cricothyroid puncture is performed by inserting a large-gauge needle into the cricothyroid space. This procedure provides a temporary airway in acute airway obstruction.

In cases of advanced stages of pregnancy or marked obesity when the rescuer cannot apply abdominal thrusts effectively, chest thrusts can be employed. The hand position for the application of chest thrusts is the same as that for external cardiac compression. The heel of one hand is placed on the lower half of the sternum. The other hand is placed on top of it with the fingers straight or interlaced. Quick, downward thrusts are then administered.

Cricothyroidotomy.* If attempts at ventilation and removal of the foreign body are not successful and equipment is not available for endotracheal intubation or tracheostomy, a cricothyroidotomy (cricothyroid puncture) may be performed. This procedure provides a temporary airway by puncturing the cricothyroid membrane with a large (12- to 14-gauge) polyethylene needle or scalpel (Fig. 30-34). This method maintains an airway until more definitive therapy can be instituted. Cricothyroidotomy may also be used in other conditions that cause acute airway obstruction (e.g., laryngeal edema from anaphylactic shock).

External cardiac compressions. Cardiac arrest is characterized by the absence of a pulse in the large arteries of an unconscious victim who is not breathing. The carotid artery is used to determine the absence of a pulse. After an airway has been established and two ventilations have been delivered, the rescuer checks the pulse. While maintaining the head-tilt position with one hand on the forehead, the rescuer locates the victim's trachea with two or three fingers of the other hand. The rescuer then slides these fingers into the groove between the trachea and the muscles of the side of the neck where the carotid pulse can

be felt. The technique is more easily performed on the side nearest the rescuer. If no pulse is palpated, chest compressions should be initiated.

The proper technique for administering chest compressions is shown in Fig. 30-35. External chest compression technique consists of serial, rhythmic applications of pressure over the lower half of the sternum. The victim must be in the horizontal supine position when the compressions are performed. The victim must be lying on a flat, hard surface, such as a CPR board (especially manufactured for use in CPR), a head board from a cardiac care unit bed, or if necessary, the floor. The rescuer should be positioned close to the side of the victim's chest.

The following guidelines have been established for proper hand placement (Fig. 30-35, *A*):
1. With the middle index fingers of the hand nearest the victim's legs, the rescuer locates the lower margin of the victim's rib cage on the side next to the rescuer.
2. The fingers are moved up the rib cage to the notch where the ribs meet the sternum.
3. The middle finger is placed on this notch, and the index finger is placed next to it on the lower end of the sternum. (This allows proper placement above the xiphoid process and prevents possible laceration of the liver by the xiphoid process during compressions.)
4. The heel of the hand nearest the victim's head is placed on the lower half of the sternum, close to the index finger of the other hand. The long axis of the heel of the rescuer's hand should be placed on the long axis of the sternum.
5. The first hand is removed from the notch and placed on top of the hand on the sternum so that both hands are parallel to each other.
6. The fingers are extended or interlaced and must be kept off the chest.

The following guidelines have been established for proper compression technique (Fig. 30-35):
1. The elbows are locked into position, the arms are straightened, and the shoulders are positioned directly over the hands so that the thrust for each chest compression is straight down on the sternum.
2. The sternum must be depressed 1.5 to 2 inches (3.8 to 5.0 cm) for the normal-sized adult. The heart is compressed between the sternum and spine.
3. The external chest compression pressure is released to allow blood to flow into the heart. The time allowed for release of compression should be equal to the time required for compression.
4. The hands should not be lifted from the chest or the position changed in any way so that correct hand position is maintained.

Rescue breathing and chest compressions are combined for an effective resuscitation effort of the victim of cardiopulmonary arrest. When there is one rescuer, the rate of compression should be 80 to 100 compressions per minute with a compression/ventilation ratio of 15 compressions to 2 ventilations (Table 30-15). The compression rate for two-rescuer CPR is 80 to 100 per minute, with a compression/ventilation ratio of 5:1 (Table 30-16).

---

*Cricothyroidotomy is considered part of the ACLS.

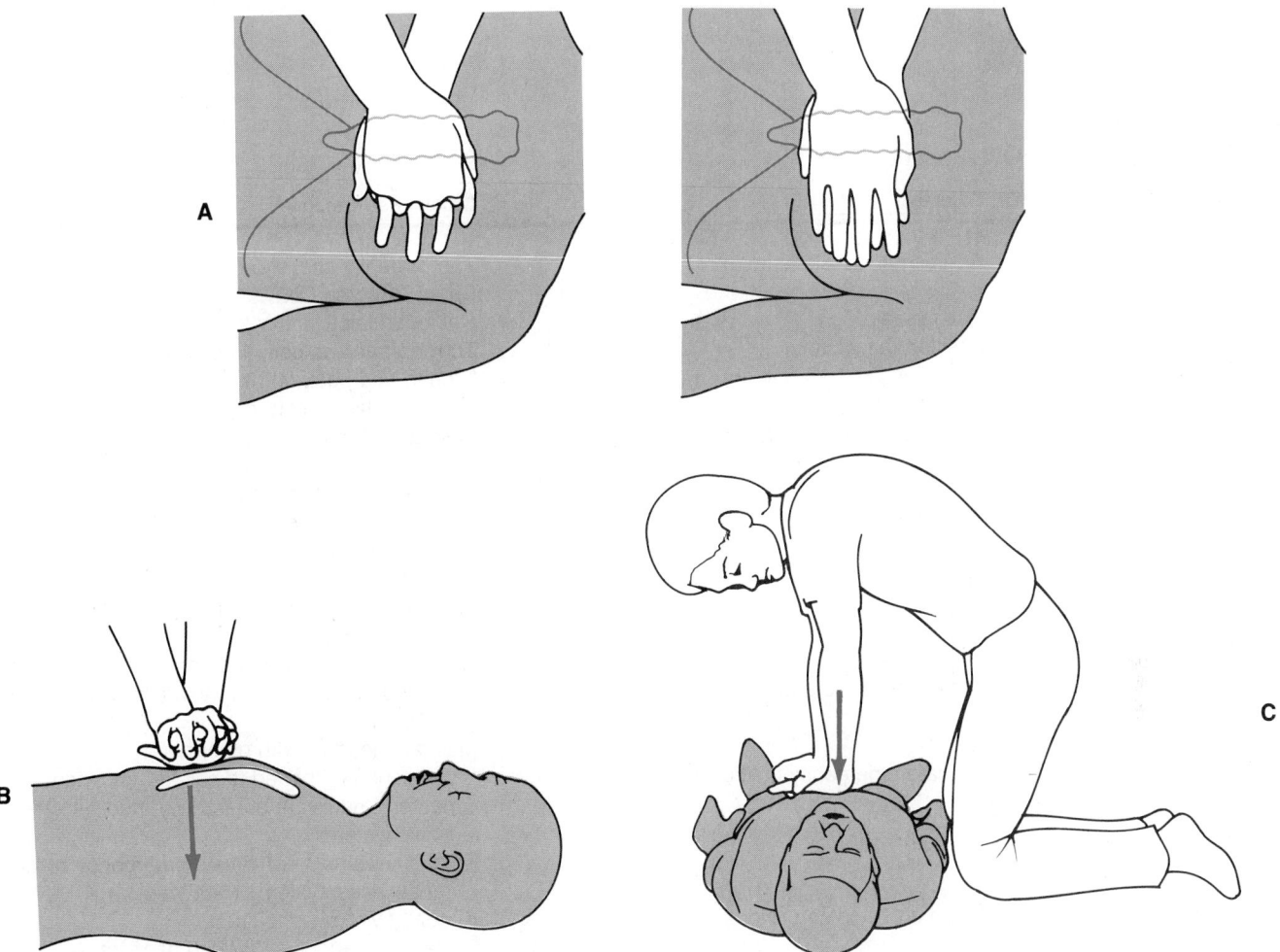

Fig. 30-35 CPR. **A,** Position of the hands during application of external cardiac massage. **B,** When pressure is applied, the lower portion of the sternum is displaced posteriorly with the palm of the hand. **C,** To apply maximum downward pressure, the resuscitator leans forward so that both arms are at right angles to the client's sternum and the elbows are locked.

The victim's condition must be assessed during CPR to determine the effectiveness of compressions and to determine whether the victim has resumed spontaneous circulation and breathing. The pulse should be checked by the ventilating rescuer during the compressions to assess the effectiveness of compressions in two-rescuer CPR. Chest compressions are stopped for 5 seconds at the end of the first minute and every few minutes thereafter to determine whether the victim has resumed spontaneous breathing and circulation. The goal of CPR is the return of spontaneous breathing and circulation, but it is rarely achieved without more definitive therapy with ACLS.

Advanced Cardiac Life Support

ACLS involves a systems approach for effective treatment of cardiac emergencies. It includes BCLS with the addition of more definitive therapy that can be delivered outside the hospital as well as in the hospital.[25,26] Survival rates of victims who have cardiac arrests have been improved by the delivery of BCLS-CPR by lay persons,

along with a well-organized, rapidly responding emergency medical system that provides ACLS (predominantly defibrillation) in the out-of-hospital setting.

Nurses and physicians are certified in the formal ACLS program, which was developed by the American Heart Association in 1974. Table 30-17 lists the ACLS course content that is used to train medical personnel for in-hospital cardiac emergencies. Table 30-18 reviews objectives of drug therapy in cardiac emergencies. An ACLS nurse is required to be skilled in the delivery of emergency cardiac drugs. Establishment and maintenance of a reliable IV line is a primary objective during ACLS. BCLS must be continued during ACLS until breathing and circulation are restored.

Table 30-19 describes drugs and other agents that are commonly used for ACLS. Table 30-20 describes drugs that are frequently used in cardiac emergencies. They are primarily used to treat CHF hypotension, hypertension, and cardiogenic shock associated with acute ischemic heart disease, including acute MI.

Text continued on p. 886

Table 30-15   Adult One-Rescuer CPR

Step	Objective	Critical Performance
1. *Airway*	Assessment: Determine unresponsiveness.	Tap or gently shake shoulder. Shout "Are you OK?"
	Call for help.	Call out "Help!"
	Position the victim.	Turn on back as unit, if necessary, supporting head and neck (4-10 sec).
	Open the airway.	Use head-tilt/chin-lift maneuver.
2. *Breathing*	Assessment: Determine cessation of breathing.	Maintain open airway. With ear over mouth, observe chest: look, listen, feel for breathing (3-5 sec).
	Ventilate twice.	Maintain open airway. Seal mouth and nose properly. Ventilate two times at 1-1.5 sec/inflation. Observe chest rise (adequate ventilation volume). Allow deflation between breaths.
3. *Circulation*	Assessment: Determine absence of pulse.	Feel for carotid pulse on near side of victim (5-10 sec). Maintain head-tilt with other hand.
	Activate emergency medical services system.	If someone responded to call for help, send person to activate emergency medical services system. Total time, step 1—Activate emergency medical services system: 15-35 sec.
	Begin chest compressions.	Kneel by victim's shoulders. Make landmark check before hands are placed. Maintain proper hand position throughout. Keep shoulders over victim's sternum. Maintain equal compression and relaxation. Compress 1.5 to 2 inches. Keep hands on sternum during upstroke. Wait for complete chest relaxation on upstroke. Say any helpful mnemonic (e.g., one-and-two-and-three-and . . .). Remember that compression rate is 80-100/min (15/9–11 sec).
4. Compression/ ventilation cycles	Do four cycles of 15 compressions and 2 ventilations.	Maintain proper compression/ventilation ratio of 15 compressions to 2 ventilations per cycle. Observe chest rise: 1-1.5 sec/inflation; four cycles/52-73 sec.
5. Reassessment	Determine absence of pulse.	Feel for carotid pulse (5 sec). If there is no pulse, go to step 6.
6. Continuation of CPR	Ventilate twice.	Ventilate two times. Observe chest rise: 1-1.5 sec/inflation.
	Resume compression/ventilation cycles.	Feel for carotid pulse every few minutes.

Modified from Healthcare provider's manual for basic life support, Dallas, 1988, American Heart Association.

Table 30-16 Adult Two-Rescuer CPR

Step	Objective	Critical Performance
1. Airway	*One rescuer (ventilator):* Assessment: Determine unresponsiveness.	Tap or gently shake shoulder. Shout "Are you OK?"
	Position the victim.	Turn on back if necessary (4-10 sec).
	Open the airway.	Use a proper technique to open airway.
2. Breathing	Assessment: Determine cessation of breathing.	Look, listen, and feel for breath (3-5 sec).
	Ventilate twice.	Observe chest rise: 1-1.5 sec/inflation.
3. Circulation	Assessment: Determine absence of pulse.	Feel for carotid pulse (5-10 sec).
	State assessment results.	Say "No pulse."
	Other rescuer (compressor): Get into position for compressions.	Put hands, shoulders in correct position.
	Locate landmark notch.	Check landmark.
4. Compression/ ventilation cycles	*Compressor:* Begin chest compressions.	Correct ratio compressions/ventilations is 5/1.
		Compression rate is 80-100/min (5 compressions/3-4 sec).
		Say any helpful mnemonic.
		Stop compressing for each ventilation.
	Ventilator: Ventilate after every fifth compression and check compression effectiveness.	Ventilate 1 time (1-1.5 sec/inflation). Check pulse occasionally to assess compressions.
	(Minimum of 10 cycles)	(Time for 10 cycles: 40-53 sec)
5. Calling for switch	*Compressor:* Call for switch when tired.	Give clear signal to change roles. Compressor completes fifth compression. Ventilator completes ventilation after fifth compression.
6. Switching	Simultaneously switch: *Ventilator:* Move to chest.	Become compressor. Get into position for compressions. Locate landmark notch.
	Compressor: Move to head.	Become ventilator. Check carotid pulse (5 sec). Say "No pulse." Ventilate once (1-1.5 sec/inflation).
7. Continuation of CPR	Resume compression/ventilation cycles.	Repeat step 4.

Modified from Healthcare provider's manual for basic life support, Dallas, 1988, American Heart Association.

Table 30-17 ACLS Course Content

MI
Adjuncts for airway control, ventilation, and supplemental oxygen
Adjuncts for artificial circulation
Dysrhythmias
Electrical therapy in the malignant dysrhythmias
Cardiovascular pharmacology I
Cardiovascular pharmacology II
Acid-base balance
Catheter and infusion-related sepsis
IV techniques
Invasive monitoring techniques
Invasive therapeutic techniques
Postresuscitation management
Special resuscitation situations
Neonatal resuscitation
Resuscitation of infants and children
Medicolegal aspects of CPR and ACLS

Modified from the American Heart Association: Textbook of advanced cardiac life support, Dallas, 1987, American Heart Association, pp v-xiv.

Table 30-18 Objectives of Drug Therapy in Cardiac Emergencies

Correct hypoxemia
Reestablish spontaneous circulation
Optimize cardiac function
Suppress sustained ventricular dysrhythmia
Correct acidosis
Relieve pain
Treat CHF

Modified from American Heart Association: Textbook of advanced cardiac life support, Dallas, 1987, American Heart Association, p 97.

Table 30-19   Drugs and Other Agents Commonly Used in ACLS

Drug	Indications	Route of Administration	Major Pharmacological Effect
Oxygen	Hypoxia, acute MI, cardiopulmonary arrest	Nasal cannula, face mask, mask device, ventilators	Used by all body cells for aerobic metabolism; improves tissue oxygenation
Sodium bicarbonate	Metabolic and respiratory acidosis	IV bolus	Corrects metabolic acidosis by the following formula: $HCO_3^- + H^+ \rightleftharpoons H_2CO_3 \rightleftharpoons CO_2 + H_2O \rightleftharpoons H_2CO_3$
Epinephrine (Adrenalin)	Asystole, electromechanical dissociation, bronchospasm, anaphylaxis	IV bolus or drip, nebulization, endotracheal tube	Stimulates α- and β-receptor sites, resulting in ↑ HR, ↑ myocardial contractile force, ↑ systemic vascular resistance, ↑ arterial blood pressure, ↑ myocardial oxygen consumption, ↑ coronary and cerebral blood flow, ↓ blood flow to kidneys and skin
Atropine	Symptomatic sinus bradycardia, asystole	IV, endotracheal tube	↑ Discharge rate of the SA node (vagolytic action), ↓ refractory period and ↑ speed of conduction through AV node
Lidocaine (Xylocaine)	PVCs, VT, VF	IV, endotracheal tube	↓ Automaticity of Purkinje fibers, ↑ threshold for VF, ↓ conduction velocity and refractory period of Purkinje fibers, prolonged conduction and refractoriness in ischemic tissue
Morphine	Pain with acute MI or acute pulmonary edema	IV	Causes analgesic and sedative effects, ↑ venous pooling, ↓ left ventricular end diastolic pressure, ↓ myocardial oxygen consumption, ↓ left ventricular afterload, ↑ myocardial contractility, ↑ ventricular excitability
Calcium chloride	Lack of clear data demonstrating a beneficial effect of calcium salt administration during CPR	IV	↑ Myocardial contractility, ↑ ventricular excitability
Procainamide (Pronestyl)	PVCs, VT, supraventricular tachycardia	IV	↑ Refractory period in atrium, ↓ excitability in atria and ventricles, ↓ automaticity of pacemaker cells, ↑ threshold to fibrillation, ↑ conduction time
Bretylium (Bretylol)	Resistant VT or VF not responsive to lidocaine, procainamide, defibrillation	IV	Transiently increases blood pressure and dysrhythmias followed by a decrease in blood pressure and dysrhythmias as a result of sympatholytic action, ↑ myocardial contractility, ↑ VF threshold, ↑ refractory period of Purkinje fibers and ventricular muscle
Verapamil	Supraventricular tachycardia	IV	Blocks slow inward current caused by changes in calcium and sodium, causes slow conduction and prolonged refractoriness in AV node

↑, Increases; ↓, decreases; *VT*, ventricular tachycardia; *VF*, ventricular fibrillation; *GI*, gastrointestinal; *CNS*, central nervous system.

Adverse Effects	Nursing Considerations
Oxygen toxicity	In emergency situations, administer oxygen.
Metabolic alkalosis, hypernatremia, water overload, possible worsening of intracellular acidosis	Be aware that drug is used only after more definitive maneuvers have proved unsuccessful. Do not mix it with any other agent.
Transient anxiety, palpitations, headache, tissue necrosis from local injections, increased blood glucose, increased oxygen consumption of heart, hypertension	Correct acidosis before IV administration of epinephrine. Do not mix with alkaline solutions.
Blurred vision, dry mouth, pupil dilatation, difficulty in voiding, increased bronchial secretions, PVCs, VT, or VF (especially in acute MI client)	Give with morphine to counteract vagomimetic effect. Use with extreme caution in clients with myocardial ischemia because it may exacerbate ischemia.
Lethargy, confusion, slurred speech, tingling lips and tongue, disorientation, hypotension convulsions, SA arrest, heart block, bradycardia	Use with caution in clients with slow HRs or heart block. Continuously monitor ECG of clients receiving this drug. Be aware that drug has slower detoxification in clients with liver dysfunction or reduced CO and in clients over the age of 70.
Respiratory depression, hypotension, confusion	Administer with caution. Be aware that morphine is a respiratory depressant. Reverse excessive narcosis with IV naloxone.
Moderate decrease in blood pressure, hypercalcemia, local necrosis if extravasation occurs, bradycardia after rapid administration	Do not mix with sodium bicarbonate. Give slowly if heart is beating (can cause severe bradycardia or sinus arrest). Use cautiously with digitalized client (can enhance toxicity).
GI distress, anorexia, nausea, vomiting, diarrhea; CNS depression and hallucinations; systemic lupuslike syndrome (arthralgia, fever, skin rash); hypotension, convulsions, AV block, PVCs, VF, agranulocytosis	Do not give to client with complete heart block. When giving IV, monitor ECG and blood pressure of client. Stop drug if QRS complex widens or if PR or ST intervals become prolonged.
Postural hypotension, nausea and vomiting, increased sensitivity to catecholamines, aggravation of existing angina pectoris, parotid pain	Watch clients closely for hypersensitivity reaction if they are receiving catecholamine drugs concurrently. In clients with renal failure, watch closely for toxicity.
Hypotension in clients with reduced ventricular function, possible hypotension and/or AV block in those receiving concomitant IV β blocker	Use with extreme caution in clients with sick sinus syndrome or AV block in absence of pacemaker.

Table 30-20 Drugs Commonly Used in Cardiac Emergencies

Drug	Indications	Route of Administration	Major Pharmacological Effect
INOTROPIC VASOACTIVE AGENTS			
Dopamine (Intropin)	Cardiac decompensation, as with CHF or cardiogenic shock; open heart surgery; hypotension	IV	Stimulates dopaminergic, β_2-adrenergic, and α-adrenergic receptors in a dose-dependent fashion: low doses (1-2 μg/kg/min) produce vasodilatation of renal, mesenteric, and cerebral arteries; medium doses (2-10 μg/kg/min) increase CO and modestly increase SVR and preload; high doses (>10 μg/kg/min) cause marked vasoconstriction
Dobutamine (Dobutrex)	Cardiac decompensation, especially with CHF and cardiogenic shock	IV	Stimulates β_1-receptor sites, ↑ myocardial contractility but not HR, slightly stimulates α- and β_2-vascular receptors (does not dilate renal and mesenteric arteries and does not have vasoconstrictive activity at higher doses)
Isoproterenol (Isuprel)	Temporary control of atropine-resistant bradycardia	IV	Stimulates β-receptor sites (β_1 and β_2), ↑ myocardial contractility, ↑ HR, ↑ myocardial oxygen consumption, ↓ SVR, ↓ diastolic pressure (may reduce mean arterial pressure), relaxes smooth muscle in bronchioles and GI tract
Digitalis (Ouabain, digoxin, digitoxin)	Atrial flutter, atrial fibrillation, paroxysmal supraventricular tachycardia, CHF	IV	↑ Myocardial contractility, ↑ rate at which force is developed, ↑ refractory period of AV node, ↑ left ventricular end diastolic volume and pressure, ↑ ventricular automaticity, ↓ atrial automaticity
Amrinone (Inocor)	Severe CHF refractory to diuretics, vasodilators, and conventional inotropic agents	IV	Inhibits phosphodiesterase, has inotropic and vasodilator effects, ↑ CO, ↓ SVR
Norepinephrine (Levophed)	Hypotension when total SVR is low	IV	Acts as α- and β-adrenergic receptor agonist, ↑ myocardial contractility and ↑ peripheral vasoconstriction
VASODILATORS-ANTIHYPERTENSIVES			
Nitroprusside (Nipride)	Hypertensive emergency, acute left ventricular failure	IV	Vasodilates arterioles and venules; causes increased CO in clients with elevated left ventricular filling pressure (increased CO due more to decreased afterload than decreased preload); causes decreased ventricular filling pressure, mean PAP, SVR, and mean arterial pressure

SVR, Systemic vascular resistance; GI, gastrointestinal; ↑, increases; ↓, decreases; VT, ventricular tachycardia; VF, ventricular fibrillation; PAP, pulmonary artery pressure; PCWP, pulmonary capillary wedge pressure.

Adverse Effects	Nursing Considerations
Tachycardia, ectopic dysrhythmias, nausea and vomiting, angina, dyspnea, headache, hypotension, palpitations, vasoconstriction, PVCs	Prevent extravasation by infusing into large vein. Do not mix with alkaline substance. Titrate dose to desired hemodynamic or renal response. Slow rate if an increased diastolic pressure results in a decreased pulse pressure. Continuously monitor ECG and blood pressure.
Marked elevation in HR (30 bpm or more), marked elevation in blood pressure (50 mm Hg), ventricular ectopy, nausea, headache, chest pain, palpitations, shortness of breath	Continuously monitor EGG, blood pressure, PCWP, and CO. Do not mix dobutamine with alkaline substance.
Sinus tachycardia; PVCs; VT; VF; hypotension in presence of hypovolemia, headache, flushing of skin, angina, nausea, tremor, dizziness, weakness, and sweating	Be aware that isoproterenol is contraindicated in the presence of digitalis-induced tachycardias. Use very cautiously in presence of hypokalemia (↑ dysrhythmias). If ventricular irritability occurs, decrease IV infusion rate. Titrate IV dose to achieve HR of 60 bpm.
Cardiac effects of PVCs, junctional rhythms, AV block, VT, VF, PACs	Always assess pulse before giving the drug because many dysrhythmias are caused by digitalis. Monitor ECG when using IV administration. Be aware that reduced renal function, hypercalcemia, and hypokalemia predispose client to digitalis toxicity. When giving drug with quinidine, decrease dose because quinidine reduces renal clearance of digoxin.
Myocardial ischemia, thrombocytopenia, nausea and vomiting, myalgia, fever, hepatic dysfunction	Continuously monitor central hemodynamics. Be aware that drug contains metabisulfite, which is contraindicated in clients allergic to bisulfites.
Increased myocardial oxygen consumption, dysrhythmias	Continuously monitor hemodynamics and ECG. Be aware that ischemic necrosis and sloughing of tissues can occur with extravasations and that drug is contraindicated when hypotension is due to hypovolemia.
Acute effects, including hypotension, tachycardia, increased intracranial pressure; long-term effects, including fatigue, nausea and anorexia, disorientation, psychotic behavior, muscle spasm	Continuously infuse drug because its effect takes 3-5 min. Slow infusion rate if there is excessive increase in HR or lowering of blood pressure. When used for low-output states, monitor ECG, intraarterial pressure, PCWP, and CO. Be aware that the solution must be protected from light to prevent deterioration.

Continued.

Table 30-20   Drugs Commonly Used in Cardiac Emergencies—cont'd

Drug	Indications	Route of Administration	Major Pharmacological Effect
VASODILATORS-ANTIHYPERTENSIVES—cont'd			
Nitroglycerin	Angina pectoris, acute MI, left ventricular failure	IV Sublingual	Relaxes vascular smooth muscle; dilates venous smooth muscle in angina pectoris and MI, inhibiting venous return with reduced ventricular volume, ventricular pressure, and wall stress; dilates large coronary arteries, antagonizes vasospasm, and increases coronary collateral blood flow to ischemic myocardium, reduces left ventricular filling pressure and SVR in CHF
β Blockers Propranolol (Inderal), metoprolol (Lopresser)	Acute MI, angina pectoris, hypertension, atrial fibrillation, atrial flutter, PSVT, refractory VT or VF	IV	Acts as β-adrenergic receptor blocking agent, ↓ HR and myocardial contractility, ↓ myocardial oxygen consumption, depresses automaticity of pacemakers and suppresses ectopic beats, prolongs AV conduction time and refractory period
DIURETICS			
Furosemide (Lasix)	Emergency treatment of pulmonary congestion associated with left ventricular dysfunction, chronic heart failure	IV	Inhibits reabsorption of sodium and chloride in the ascending loop of Henle; has direct venodilating effect that reduces venous return and central venous pressure

R eview Questions

1. All of the following dysrhythmias are considered to be unstable *except*
   a. ventricular tachycardia with ventricular rate of 150 bpm
   b. atrial fibrillation with ventricular rate of 150 bpm
   c. second-degree AV block, Mobitz type II, blood pressure of 70/40
   d. sinus bradycardia, blood pressure of 110/70

2. Recommended treatment for second-degree AV block (Mobitz type I, Wenckebach phenomenon) with stable blood pressure and no symptoms includes
   a. immediate insertion of temporary pacemaker
   b. epinephrine 1 mg IV push
   c. isuprel IV continuous drip
   d. careful observation for symptoms of hypotension

3. Defibrillation is indicated for
   a. third-degree AV block
   b. ventricular fibrillation
   c. ventricular tachycardia
   d. atrial flutter

4. Indications for permanent pacemaker therapy include all of the following *except*
   a. third-degree AV block
   b. chronic atrial fibrillation with slow ventricular response
   c. sick sinus syndrome
   d. asymptomatic sinus bradycardia

5. The compression/ventilation rate for two-person CPR is
   a. 5 compressions to 2 ventilations
   b. 5 compressions to 1 ventilation
   c. 15 compressions to 2 ventilations
   d. 15 compressions to 1 ventilation

6. The primary purpose of the Heimlich maneuver is to
   a. force air from lungs to create a cough
   b. "sweep away" obstructing foreign bodies
   c. deliver manual blows to the back
   d. provide a temporary airway by puncturing the trachea

REFERENCES

1. Andreoli KG and others: Comprehensive cardiac care, ed 6, St Louis, 1987, The CV Mosby Co, p 84.
2. Conover MB: Understanding electrocardiography, arrhythmia and the 12-lead ECG, ed 5, St Louis, 1988, The CV Mosby Co.
3. Moses HW and others: A practical guide to cardiac pacing, Boston, 1983, Little, Brown & Co.
4. Rosen M: The links between basic and clinical cardiac electrophysiology, Circulation 77:251, 1988.

Adverse Effects	Nursing Considerations
Headache, hypotension, bradycardia	Monitor hemodynamics if drug is given IV for CHF. Administer sublingual nitroglycerin while client is sitting or lying down. Treat hypotension with fluid administration.
Bradycardia, hypotension, heart block, fatigue, dizziness, blood sugar disturbances, insomnia, GI distress	Do not use in presence of bradycardia, heart block, and bronchospasm.
Dehydration; hypotension; sodium, potassium, and magnesium depletion; hyperosmolality; metabolic alkalosis; loss of hearing	Inject drug IV slowly over 1 to 2 min.

5. Prystowsky EN: Electrophysiologic-electropharmacologic testing in patients with ventricular arrhythmias, PACE 11:225, 1988.
6. Sergeant LL: Tracking your outpatient's EKG with a Holter monitor, Nursing 10:47, 1986.
7. Kennedy HL and Wiens RD: Ambulatory (Holter) electrocardiography and myocardial ischemia, Am Heart J 117:164, 1989.
8. Rinkenberger RL and others: Invasive and noninvasive evaluation of arrhythmias, Hosp Pract 23:115, 1988.
9. Marriott HJL and Conover MB: Advanced concepts in arrhythmias, St Louis, 1989, The CV Mosby Co.
10. Bigger JT: Definition of benign versus malignant ventricular arrhythmias: targets for treatment, Am J Cardiol 61:501, 1983.
11. Skluth H, Grauer K, and Gums J: Ventricular arrhythmias, an assessment of newer therapeutic agents, Postgrad Med 85:137, 1987.
12. Cardiac Arrhythmia Suppression Trial Study: Preliminary report: effect of encainide and flecainide on mortality in a randomized trial of arrhythmia suppression after myocardial infarction, New Engl J Med 321:406, 1989.
13. Horowitz LN: Drugs and proarrhythmia, Prog Cardiol 1:109, 1989.
14. Robinson KC, McKenna WJ, and Krikler DM: Amiodarone: current perspectives from Europe, Heart Lung 16:636, 1987.
15. Rosen MR and Spinelli W: Some recent concepts concerning the mechanisms of action of antiarrhythmic drugs, PACE 11:1485, 1988.
16. Rotmensch HH and Belhassen B: Amiodarone in the management of cardiac arrhythmias, Med Clin North Am 72:275, 1988.
17. Stanton MS and others: Arrhythmogenic effects of antiarrhythmic drugs: a study of 506 patients treated for ventricular tachycardia or fibrillation, J Am Coll Cardiol 14:209, 1989.
18. Aylward PE and Kerber RE: The technique of electrical countershock, J Crit Illness 8:47, 1986.
19. Kuiper RA: The automatic implantable cardioverter defibrillator as a therapeutic modality for recurrent ventricular tachycardia: a case study, Prog Cardiovasc Nurs 5:6-12, 1990.
20. Cooper DK, Valladares BK, and Futterman LG: Care of the patient with the automatic implantable cardioverter defibrillator: a guide for nurses, Heart Lung 16:640, 1987.
21. Winkle RA and others: Long-term outcome with the automatic implantable cardioverter-defibrillator, J Am Coll Cardiol 13:1353, 1989.
22. Tamarisk NK: Enhancing activity levels of patients with permanent cardiac pacemakers, Heart Lung 17:698, 1988.
23. Persons CB: Transcutaneous pacing: meeting the challenge, Focus Crit Care 14:12, 1987.
24. Albarren-Sotelo R and others: Healthcare provider's manual for basic life support, Dallas, 1988, American Heart Association.
25. Albarren-Sotelo R and others: Textbook of advanced cardiac life support, Dallas, 1987, American Heart Association.
26. Ellstrom K and Bella LD: Understanding your role during a CODE, Nursing 20:37-44, 1990.

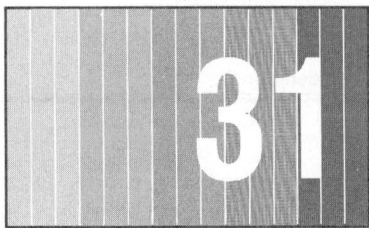

CHAPTER

31

Nursing Role in Management
Inflammatory and Valvular Heart Disease

Nancy Stoetzner Kupper
Ellen Stoetzner Duke

L earning Objectives

1. Describe the etiology, pathogenesis, and clinical manifestations of infective endocarditis and pericarditis.
2. Discuss the therapeutic, pharmacological, and nursing management of infective endocarditis and pericarditis.
3. Explain the importance of prophylactic antibiotic therapy in infective endocarditis.
4. Explain the etiology, clinical manifestations, and management of myocarditis.
5. Describe the etiology, pathogenesis, and clinical manifestations of rheumatic fever and rheumatic heart disease.

6. Discuss the therapeutic and nursing management of clients with rheumatic fever and rheumatic heart disease.
7. Identify the etiologies of congenital and acquired valvular heart diseases.
8. Discuss the pathophysiology and clinical manifestations of the various types of valvular heart problems.
9. Describe the therapeutic and nursing management of valvular heart disease.
10. Describe surgical interventions used in the management of clients with valvular heart problems.

INFLAMMATORY DISORDERS OF THE HEART
Infective Endocarditis

Infective endocarditis is an infection of the endocardial surface with microorganisms present in the lesion.[1] The endocardium, the inner layer of the heart (Fig. 31-1), is contiguous with the heart's valves. Therefore inflammation from infective endocarditis frequently affects the heart's valves.

Infective endocarditis occurs when turbulence within the heart allows certain organisms to infect previously damaged valves or other endothelial surfaces.[2] The damage may occur in individuals with underlying cardiac conditions (Table 31-1). Increased frequency of endocarditis is currently seen in older adults, in clients after prosthetic valve placement, and in intravenous drug abusers. Infective endocarditis may also occur in individuals with no preexisting valvular disorders (Table 31-1).

Before the era of antibiotics, infective endocarditis was almost always fatal. With the advent of penicillin therapy, the prognosis has changed dramatically, and mortality rates are now 20% to 40%.[3] Further appreciable decreases in mortality rates have not occurred, and infective endocarditis continues to pose a significant clinical challenge.

Classification. Two forms of infective endocarditis, *subacute* and *acute*, have been described. The subacute form has a longer clinical course of more insidious onset with less toxicity, and the causative organism is usually of low virulence (most often *Streptococcus viridans*).[1] In contrast, the acute form has a shorter clinical course with a more rapid onset, increased toxicity, and a more pathogenic causative organism (usually *Staphylococcus aureus*).[1]

Etiology and pathophysiology. The term *bacterial endocarditis* has been replaced by *infective endocarditis* because causative organisms may now include fungi, chlamydiae, or rickettsiae as well as bacteria (Table 31-2). In addition to the anatomical changes, a variety of invasive

Reviewed by Marsha Halfman-Franey, R.N., M.S.N., Director, Cardiovascular Nursing Education Program, Arizona Heart Institute, Phoenix, Arizona.

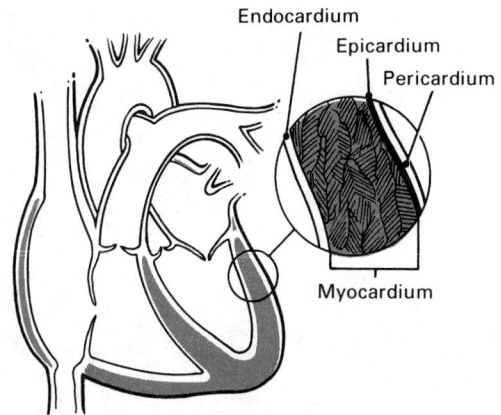

Fig. 31-1 Layers of the heart.

Table 31-1 Predisposing Conditions for the Development of Infective Endocarditis

Cardiac conditions
  Prosthetic heart valves
  Congenital heart disease
  Rheumatic heart disease
  Degenerative heart disease
  Mitral valve prolapse
  Valvular lesions
  Heart murmurs
  Cardiac and prosthetic valve surgery
  Idiopathic hypertrophic subaortic stenosis
  Degenerative heart disease
Immunosuppressive conditions
  Cancer
  Severe burns
  Immunosuppressive therapy
  Radiation therapy
Invasive procedures
  Peripheral arteriovenous fistulas (as used in chronic hemodialysis)
  Indwelling intravenous or intraarterial catheters
  Intravenous drug abuse
  Invasive diagnostic procedures
Alcoholism

Table 31-2 Organisms and Situations Associated with Infective Endocarditis

Organism	Situation
Streptococcus viridans	Dental procedure
S. bovis	GI malignant disorder, older adults
Enterococcus species	GI and GU procedures
Staphylococcus aureus	
Coagulase positive	IV drug use, cardiac surgery, nosocomial infection, parenteral therapy
Coagulase negative	Prosthetic valve
Pseudomonas aeruginosa	IV drug use, cardiac surgery
Serratia marcescens	IV drug use, cardiac surgery
Candida, Aspergillus organisms	Immunocompromised persons

Modified from Scrima DA: Infective endocarditis: nursing considerations, Crit Care Nur 7:48, 1987.

procedures (e.g., surgical interventions, intravenous [IV] injection, and invasive diagnostic procedures) can allow large numbers of organisms to enter the blood stream and trigger the infectious process (see Table 31-1).

Vegetations, the primary lesions of infective endocarditis, consist of fibrin, leukocytes, platelets, and microbes that adhere to the valve surface or endocardium[4] (Fig. 31-2). The loss of portions of these friable vegetations into the circulation results in embolization. In left-sided heart vegetations, systemic embolization occurs progressing to organ (particularly the kidney, spleen, and brain) and limb infarction. Right-sided heart lesions embolize to the lungs.

The infection may spread locally to cause damage to the valves or to their supporting structures. The resulting valvular incompetence and eventual invasion of the myocardium in the ongoing disease results in congestive heart failure (CHF), generalized myocardial dysfunction, and continued sepsis (Fig. 31-3).

Clinical manifestations. The findings in infective endocarditis are nonspecific and can involve multiple organ systems, but fever occurs in more than 90% of clients with endocarditis. Other nonspecific manifestations that may accompany the fever of infective endocarditis include chills, weakness, malaise, fatigue, and anorexia. Arthralgias, myalgias, back pain, abdominal discomfort, weight loss, headache, and clubbing of fingers may occur in subacute forms of endocarditis.

The onset of a new murmur is also frequently noted with infective endocarditis. The aortic and mitral valves are most commonly affected.[5] The murmurs of endocarditis are generally mid-to-late systolic regurgitant types, although they can occur in early diastole or are often absent in tricuspid endocarditis. CHF occurs in up to 80% of clients with aortic valve endocarditis and in approximately 50% of clients with mitral valve endocarditis.[6]

Vascular manifestations of infective endocarditis include *splinter hemorrhages* (black longitudinal streaks) that may occur in the nailbeds. Petechiae may occur as a result of fragmentation and microembolization of vegetative lesions and are common in the conjunctivae, lips, buccal mucosa, and palate and over the ankles, feet and antecubital and popliteal areas. *Osler nodes* (painful, tender, red or purple, pea-size lesions) may be found on the fingertips or toes. *Janeway lesions* (flat, painless, small, red spots) may be found on the palms and soles. Funduscopic examination may reveal hemorrhagic retinal lesions called *Roth's spots.*

Clinical manifestations secondary to embolization in various body organs may also be present. Embolization to the spleen may result in sharp left upper quadrant pain and

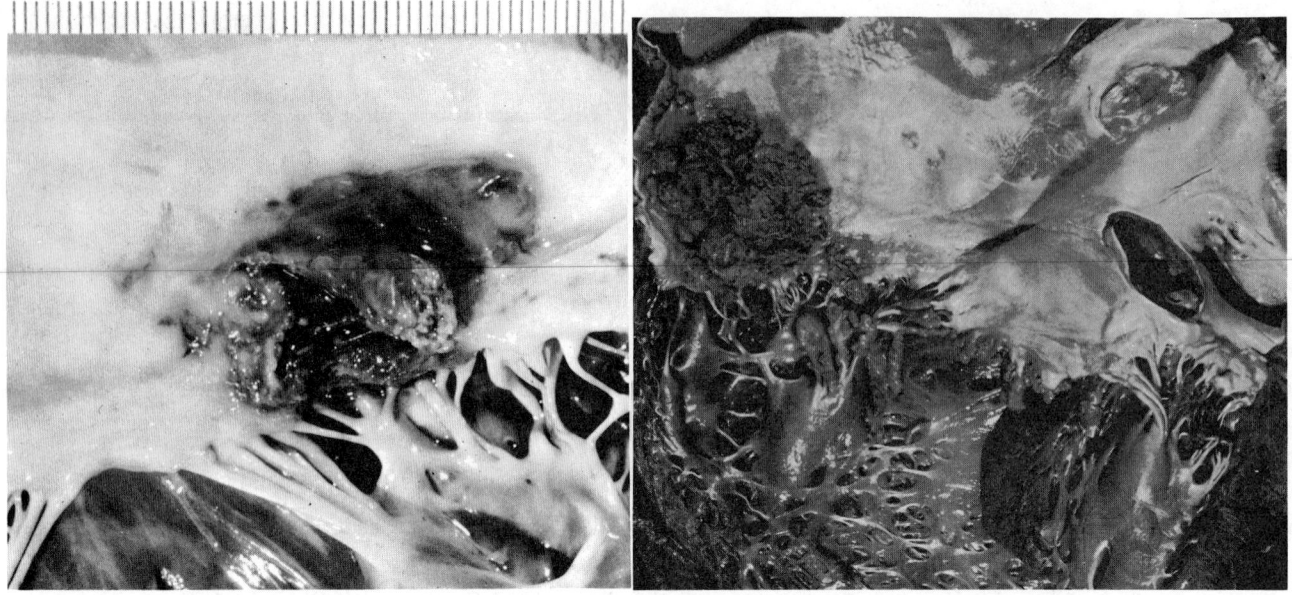

Fig. 31-2 Bacterial endocarditis of the mitral valve (caused by *Streptococcus viridans*). **A,** Ulcerating lesion of a valve also showing evidence of old rheumatic valvulitis (thickening, shortening, and fusing of chordae tendineae). **B,** Different lesion. There is a large vegetation involving the posterior leaflet of the mitral valve and wall of left atrium. (From Kissane JM: Anderson's pathology, ed 9, St Louis, 1990, Mosby—Year Book, Inc, pp 655-656.)

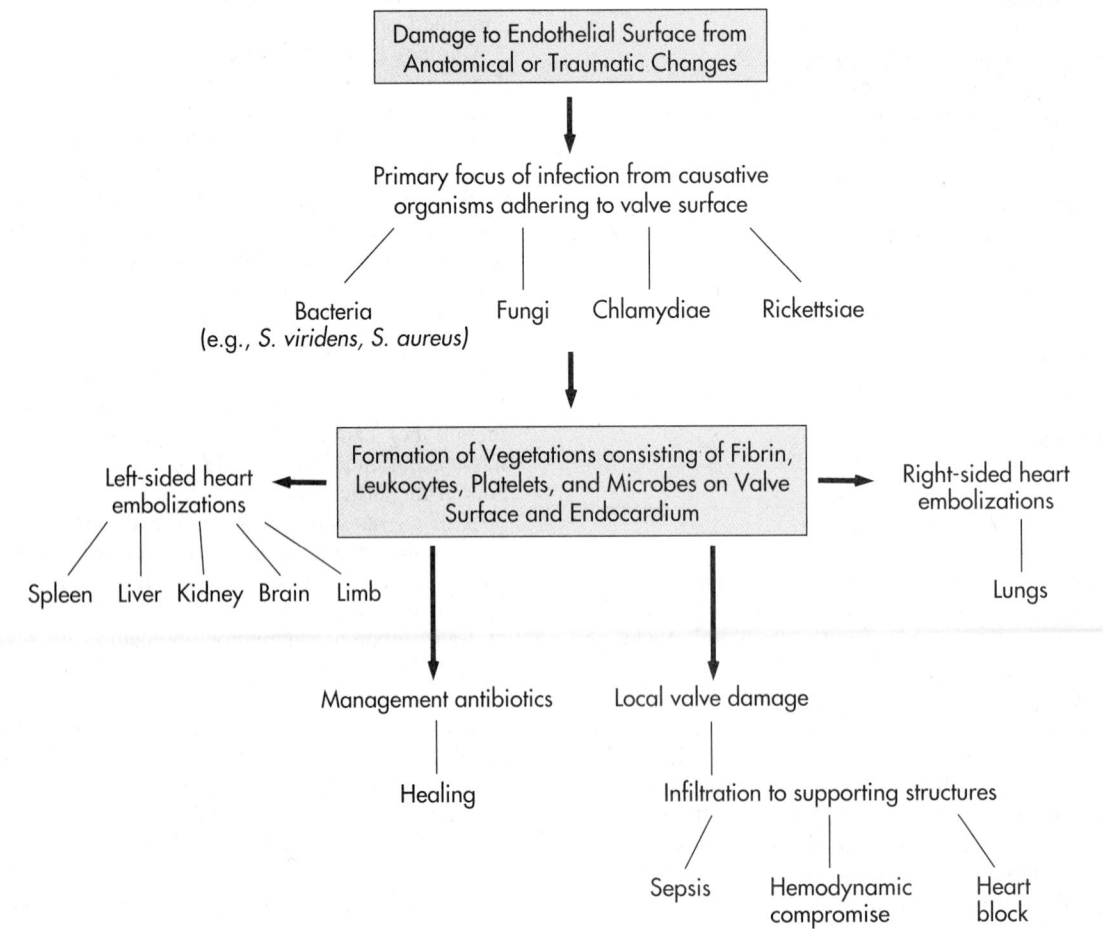

Fig. 31-3 Sequence of events in infective endocarditis.

Table 31-3

Diagnostic and Therapeutic Management: Infective Endocarditis

DIAGNOSTIC

History and physical examination
Blood culture and sensitivity
Chest x-ray film
Electrocardiogram
Echocardiography
Cardiac catheterization

THERAPEUTIC

Appropriate antibiotic therapy
Antipyretics
Rest
Repetition of blood cultures and sensitivity tests
Surgical valve replacement (for severe valvular damage)

Table 31-4 Antibiotic Prophylaxis to Prevent Endocarditis in Cardiac Conditions*

PROPHYLAXIS RECOMMENDED

Prosthetic cardiac valves (including biosynthetic valves)
Most congenital cardiac malformations
Surgically constructed systemic-pulmonary shunts
Rheumatic and other acquired valvular dysfunction
Idiopathic hypertrophic subaortic stenosis
Previous history of bacterial endocarditis
Mitral valve prolapse with insufficiency†

PROPHYLAXIS NOT RECOMMENDED

Isolated secundum atrial septal defect
Secundum atrial septal defect repaired without a patch more than 6 months earlier
Patent ductus arteriosus ligated and divided more than 6 months earlier
Postoperative coronary artery bypass graft surgery

Modified from Shulman ST and others: Prevention of bacterial endocarditis, Circulation 70:1224A, 1984.
*This table lists common conditions but is not all inclusive.
†Definitive data to provide guidance in management of clients with mitral valve prolapse are particularly limited. Generally such clients are at low risk of development of endocarditis, but the risk-benefit ratio of prophylaxis in mitral valve prolapse is uncertain.

splenomegaly. Local tenderness and abdominal rigidity may be present. Embolization to the kidneys may cause pain in the flank, hematuria, azotemia, and glomerulonephritis. Emboli may lodge in small peripheral blood vessels and cause gangrene. Embolization to the brain may cause neurological problems such as hemiplegia, ataxia, aphasia, and change in level of consciousness. Pulmonary emboli may occur in right-sided endocarditis.

Diagnostic studies. Obtaining the client's recent health history is important in assessing infective endocarditis (Table 31-3). Queries should be made regarding any recent dental, urological, surgical, or gynecological procedures including normal or abnormal obstetrical delivery. Previous history of heart disease, recent cardiac catheterization, and skin, respiratory, or urinary tract infections should be documented.

Laboratory data, especially blood cultures, should also be assessed. Positive blood cultures are found in 90% to 95% of clients with infective endocarditis. Three sets (a set consists of one aerobic and one anaerobic culture from one site) should be obtained over a 24-hour period. Negative cultures should be kept for 3 weeks when the clinical diagnosis remains endocarditis because of the possibility of a slow-growing, fastidious, causative organism. The three sets of blood cultures may be obtained at 10-minute intervals if immediate antibiotic therapy is deemed necessary. Blood-culture bottles containing a resin to bind the antibiotic should be used if the client is already receiving antibiotics.[7] Culture-negative endocarditis may occur in those clients who had previous antibiotic therapy, in clients with causative organisms that cannot be grown from blood using routine media (e.g., *Mycobacterium tuberculosis*), or in clients with right-sided infection of the heart.

A mild leukocytosis with average white blood cell (WBC) counts ranging from 10,000 to 11,000/μl and erythrocyte sedimentation rates (ESR) greater than 30 mm/hr are often detectable. Microscopic hematuria and a positive rheumatoid factor may also be present in some clients with endocarditis.

A chest x-ray film is performed to detect the presence of CHF. An echocardiogram may be ordered to detect the presence of valvular vegetations and/or abnormal valve leaflet movement resulting from the growth of vegetations, although this test is insensitive in the detection of prosthetic heart valve vegetations. Two-dimensional echocardiography may be a useful diagnostic tool to identify valvular vegetations, the extent of valvular involvement, and chamber size.

Cardiac valves lie in close proximity to cardiac conductive tissue, especially the atrioventral (AV) node. Because of this, the electrocardiogram (ECG) may reveal varying degrees of heart block (first-degree, Mobitz I and II, complete and bundle branch blocks) and atrial fibrillation.

Cardiac catheterization may be used as a diagnostic tool and is not associated with increased risk for clients with infective endocarditis. The catheterization can supply data about the degree of valvular insufficiency and determine the involvement of more than one valve but should only be performed in the clients who are immediate surgical candidates.[1]

Prophylactic treatment. Clients with various anatomical abnormalities of the heart or great vessels are at an increased risk of contracting infective endocarditis. In approximately 20% of all clients, infective endocarditis occurs after invasive dental or surgical procedures.[8] Antibiotic prophylaxis is recommended for clients with some common cardiac conditions before they undergo certain dental or surgical procedures (Table 31-4). Procedures that require endocarditis prophylaxis are summarized in Table 31-5. Specific antibiotic regimens are recommended for dental, respiratory tract, gastrointestinal (GI), and genitourinary (GU) procedures (Table 31-6). Antibiotic pro-

Table 31-5 Procedures that Require Endocarditis Antibiotic Prophylaxis

OROPHARYNGEAL

All dental procedures likely to produce gingival bleeding (not simple adjustment of orthodontic appliances or shedding of deciduous teeth)
Tonsillectomy and/or adenoidectomy

RESPIRATORY

Surgical procedures or biopsy involving respiratory mucosa
Bronchoscopy, especially with a rigid bronchoscope*

GASTROINTESTINAL

Gallbladder surgery
Colonic surgery
Esophogeal dilatation
Sclerotherapy of esphogeal varices
Colonoscopy
Upper GI endoscopy with biopsy
Proctosigmoidoscopic biopsy

GENITOURINARY

Cystoscopy
Prostatic surgery
Urethral catheterization (especially in presence of infection)
Urinary tract surgery
Vaginal hysterectomy

CARDIAC

Placement of prosthetic heart valves
Surgically constructed systemic pulmonary shunts

OTHER

Incision and drainage of infected tissue

Modified from Shulman ST and others: Prevention of bacterial endocarditis, Circulation 70:1224A, 1984.
*The risk for flexible bronchoscopy is low, but the necessity for prophylaxis is not yet defined.

Table 31-6 Recommended Antibiotic Regimens for Endocarditis Prophylaxis

Use	Agent
DENTAL AND RESPIRATORY TRACT PROCEDURES	
Standard regimen	
Dental procedures that cause gingival bleeding and oral/respiratory tract surgery	Penicillin V 2.0 g orally 1 hr before, then 1.0 g 6 hr later; 2 million units of aqueous penicillin G IV or IM 30-60 min before procedure, 1 million units 6 hr later (for clients unable to take oral medications)
Special regimens	
Parenteral regimen for use when maximum protection desired (e.g., for clients with prosthetic valves)	Ampicillin 1.0-2.0 g IM or IV and gentamicin 1.5 mg/kg IM or IV ½ hr before procedure, followed by 1.0 g oral penicillin V 6 hr later; repeat of parenteral regimen once 8 hr later
Oral regimen for clients allergic to penicillin	Erythromycin 1.0 g orally 1 hr before, then 500 mg 6 hr later
Parenteral regimen for clients allergic to penicillin	Vancomycin 1.0 g IV *slowly* over 1 hr, starting 1 hr before; repeat dose unnecessary
GASTROINTESTINAL AND GENITOURINARY PROCEDURES	
Standard regimen	
For genitourinary/gastrointestinal tract procedures listed in Table 31-5	Ampicillin 2.0 g IM or IV and gentamicin 1.5 mg/kg IM or IV, given ½-1 hr before procedure; one follow-up dose 8 hr later (if appropriate)
Special regimens	
Oral regimen for minor or repetitive procedures in low-risk clients	Amoxicillin 3.0 g orally 1 hr before procedure and 1.5 g 6 hr later
Clients allergic to penicillin	Vancomycin 1.0 g IV *slowly* over 1 hr and gentamicin 1.5 mg/kg IM or IV given 1 hr before procedure; repeat regimen once 8-12 hr later (if appropriate)

Modified from ST Shulman and others: Prevention of bacterial endocarditis, *Circulation* 70:1125A, 1984.

phylaxis should also be instituted in high-risk clients who (1) are to undergo removal or drainage of infected tissue, (2) have indwelling cardiac pacemakers, (3) undergo renal dialysis, and (4) have ventriculoatrial shunts for management of hydrocephalus.

Therapeutic management. Accurate identification of the infecting organism is the key to successful treatment. The appropriate antibiotic is chosen on the basis of sensitivity studies. Treatment of infective endocarditis usually requires 4 to 6 weeks of parenteral single or combination antibiotic therapy (Table 31-7). For clients allergic to penicillin, vancomycin and tobramycin may be used. Some clients require changes in antibiotics because of allergic or other drug-related side effects.

Periodic monitoring of the client's antibiotic serum levels should be performed. Subsequent blood cultures may be done to evaluate the effectiveness of antibiotic therapy. Persistently positive blood cultures indicate improper antibiotic administration, aortic root or myocardial abscess, or the wrong diagnosis (e.g., an infection elsewhere). Fever may persist for several days after treatment has been started and is treated with aspirin, fluids, and rest. Complete bed rest is usually not indicated unless the temperature remains elevated or there are signs of heart damage.

The results of therapeutic management alone are generally poor in clients with fungal endocarditis and prosthetic valve endocarditis.[1] Early valve replacement followed by prolonged therapeutic management is recommended in these situations (see p. 910).

▪ Nursing Management of Infective Endocarditis

Nursing assessment

Subjective and objective data should be obtained from a client with infective endocarditis and are in Table 31-8.[9,10]

Table 31-7 Treatment of Infective Endocarditis

Clinical Situation	Antibiotic Regimen
EMPIRICAL SITUATION	
Acute	Nafcillin, ampicillin, and gentamicin
Subacute	Ampicillin and gentamicin
SPECIFIC PATHOGENS	
Viridans streptococci and nonenterococcal group D streptococci	Penicillin G alone or procaine penicillin and streptomycin or penicillin G and streptomycin
Group D streptococci (enterococcus)	Penicillin G, gentamicin
S. aureus	Nafcillin with or without gentamicin
S. epidermidis	Nafcillin or vancomycin
S. pneumoniae	Penicillin G
Gram-negative bacilli	Antipseudomonal penicillin and aminoglycoside
Fungi	Amphotericin B

Modified from Civetta JM, Taylor RW, and Kirby RR: Critical care, Philadelphia, 1988, JB Lippincott Co, p 997.
*Vancomycin is recommended for the client allergic to penicillin.

Nursing diagnoses

Nursing diagnoses are determined when the problem and etiological factors are supported by clinical data. Nursing diagnoses related to infective endocarditis may include, but are not limited to, those presented in Table 31-9.[11]

Table 31-8

Nursing Assessment of the Client with Infective Endocarditis

SUBJECTIVE DATA

History
Existing: Valvular, congenital, or syphilitic cardiac disease (including valve replacement); previous endocarditis
Recent: Childbirth, obstetrical, or gynecological procedures; invasive techniques including catheterization, cystoscopy, IV therapy, dental or operative procedures; staphylococcal or streptococcal infections
Medications
IV drug abuse, alcohol abuse, immunosuppressive therapy
General
Chills, fatigue, malaise, weakness, exercise intolerance, anorexia, weight loss
Pain
Headache; painful lesions on fingers, toes, skin; chest pain
Integumentary
Diaphoresis, night sweats
Respiratory
Cough, dyspnea on exertion, orthopnea
Cardiovascular
Palpitations
Musculoskeletal
Arthralgias and myalgias
Genitourinary
Back pain, bloody urine

OBJECTIVE DATA

General
Fever
Integumentary
Osler's nodes on extremities; splinter hemorrhages under nailbeds; Janeway's lesions on palms and soles; petechiae of skin, mucous membranes, or conjunctivae; purpura
Respiratory
Tachypnea, rales
Hematological
Anemia
Cardiovascular
Dysrhythmias, tachycardia, new or enhanced murmurs, S_3, S_4, retinal hemorrhages, peripheral edema
Possible findings
Leukocytosis, elevated ESR and cardiac enzymes; positive blood cultures; echocardiogram showing chamber enlargement, valvular dysfunction, and vegetations; chest x-ray film showing cardiomegaly, pulmonary infiltrates; ECG demonstrating ischemia and strain and conduction defects

Table 31-9

 ## NURSING CARE PLAN FOR THE CLIENT WITH INFECTIVE ENDOCARDITIS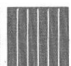

Defining Characteristics	Nursing Interventions	Evaluation Criteria
NURSING DIAGNOSIS: Hyperthermia related to infectious process		
Temperature elevation, diaphoresis, chills, headache, malaise, tachycardia, tachypnea	Monitor vial signs q 4 hr. Report temperature spikes. Administer antipyretics and/or sedatives as ordered. Reduce physical activity. Administer fluids (oral or parenteral) as ordered and tolerated. Administer antibiotics. Monitor blood cultures, WBC count. Wash client with cool water. Cover client with light blankets to prevent shivering.	Normal temperature 97.7° F-99.7° F (36.5° C-37.5° C); normal pulse (60-100 bpm); normal respirations (12-20 breaths/min); absence of chills, diaphoresis, headache
NURSING DIAGNOSIS: Decreased cardiac output related to valvular insufficiency and fluid overload		
Heart murmur, S₃ tachycardia, capillary refill time greater than 3 sec, diminished peripheral pulses, adventitious breath sounds, decrease in urine output, restlessness, confusion	Auscultate heart sounds/rate and rhythm q 4 hr. Monitor for new onset systolic murmur. Assess capillary refill, skin color, and temperature. Assess for jugular venous distension. Assess peripheral, sacral edema. Assess breath sounds q 4 hr. Provide oxygen therapy. Administer diuretics, inotropics, and other medications as ordered. Plan rest periods. Assess hourly urine output. Assess for changes in level of consciousness. Assess BP q 4 hr.	Sufficient cardiac output to maintain systolic BP at 90 mm Hg and urine output greater than 30 ml/hr
NURSING DIAGNOSIS: Potential complication: emboli related to dislodging of vegetations		
Cardiopulmonary effects of chest pain, tachypnea, dyspnea (sudden onset), diminished breath sounds; *renal effects* of decrease in urine output, back pain, hematuria; *splenic effects* of upper left quadrant pain or tenderness, splenomegaly; *Cerebral effects* of anxiety, focal defects, hemiplegia, slurred speech, sensory motor deficits; *GI effects* of abdominal pain, diminished or absent bowel sounds; *peripheral and vascular effects* of splinter hemorrhages, Osler's nodes, Janeway's lesions, diminished peripheral pulses	Assess breath sounds q 4 hr. Assess respiratory rate, rhythm, volume, and use of accessory muscles q 4 hr. Measure intake and output q 1 hr. Monitor color of urine and specific gravity. Assess for abdominal pain. Palpate for enlarged spleen. Assess neurological vital signs as needed. Assess for abdominal pain. Auscultate bowel sounds q 4 hr and as needed. Check temperature and pulses in extremities q 4 hr. Observe skin, eyes, mucous membranes for petechiae. Check fingernails for splinter hemorrhages. Inspect fingers, toes, palms, and soles of feet for nodes. Observe skin surface for lesions. Check peripheral pulses q 4 hr and as needed. Observe for swelling, redness, calf tenderness. Check for Homans' sign. Apply antiembolism stockings. Teach client leg exercises.	Demonstration of adequate circulation to all tissues, absence of complications of embolic episodes

bpm, Beats per minute; *BP,* blood pressure.

Table 31-9

 NURSING CARE PLAN FOR THE CLIENT WITH INFECTIVE ENDOCARDITIS—cont'd

Defining Characteristics	Nursing Interventions	Evaluation Criteria

NURSING DIAGNOSIS: Activity intolerance related to alteration in oxygen transport system secondary to valvular dysfunction

Defining Characteristics	Nursing Interventions	Evaluation Criteria
Fatigue, malaise, weakness, dyspnea, shortness of breath, pallor, cyanosis, confusion, vertigo, increased pulse, increase or decrease in respiratory rate and BP	Assess range of motion (passive) to joints twice a day. Assess active range of motion as tolerated. Plan rest periods between activities. Use footboard and/or overhead trapeze. Monitor vital signs during activity. Monitor for signs of intolerance: tachycardia, hypertension, diaphoresis, shortness of breath. Reduce activity if BP goes down 10 mm Hg. Teach client to check pulse rate. Instruct client to reduce activity if pulse increases > 20 bpm and to not increase activity if resting pulse >100 bpm. Assist with activities as needed.	Completion of activities of daily living with minimal fatigue or physiological distress, maintenance of activity as tolerated

NURSING DIAGNOSIS: Anxiety related to critical illness and prolonged hospitalization

Defining Characteristics	Nursing Interventions	Evaluation Criteria
Insomnia; restlessness; apprehension; withdrawal; helplessness; irritability; elevated pulse rate, BP, respiratory rate	Observe for verbal and physiological signs of anxiety. Allow time for verbalization of fears related to illness. Encourage client to discuss feelings and concerns about illness and hospitalization. Explain how all procedures and activities relate to client's treatment plan. Avoid unnecessary procedures during normal sleep hours. Assess and provide normal sleep aids as possible. Teach client relaxation techniques such as imagery, muscle relaxation.	Recognition and expression of reduction in anxiety, increase in psychological and physiological comfort, demonstration of usual sleep cycles

NURSING DIAGNOSIS: Altered health maintenance related to lack of knowledge about disease and treatment process

Defining Characteristics	Nursing Interventions	Evaluation Criteria
Nonperformance of desired prescribed health behaviors, verbalization of misconceptions about desired or prescribed health behaviors, requests for information	Assess client's knowledge about disease and treatment process. Establish what further information the client needs. Allow time for questions. Discuss symptoms of recurrent infection: fatigue, malaise, chills, elevated temperature, anorexia. Explain need to avoid persons with infections. Encourage early treatment of common infections such as cold and flu. Explain need to report to the physician invasive procedures such as dental or gingival therapy, diagnostic tests, medical and surgical procedures, trauma. Explain significance of prophylactic antibiotic therapy before invasive procedures. Explain the need for good oral hygiene. Discuss names of prescribed medications, dosages, times of administration, purpose, and side effects.	Verbalization of increased understanding of disease process and self-care management

Continued.

Table 31-9

 NURSING CARE PLAN FOR THE CLIENT WITH INFECTIVE ENDOCARDITIS—cont'd

Defining Characteristics	Nursing Interventions	Evaluation Criteria
NURSING DIAGNOSIS: Diversional activity deficit related to restricted mobility and long-term hospitalization (4-6 wk)		
Restlessness and fidgeting; immobile, flat facial expression; unpleasant thoughts or feelings	Discuss the need for diversional activities with client. Explore with client potential diversional activities such as reading, puzzles, watching television, doing handicrafts. Encourage visitors; if not possible, suggest family and friends send cards, letters. Encourage family members to supply materials for the client.	Engagement in identified client diversional activities within prescribed limitation, verbalization of relief of boredom
NURSING DIAGNOSIS: Altered nutrition: less than body requirements related to anorexia		
Reported or recorded inadequate food intake, metabolic need greater than intake, muscle weakness, mental irritability, confusion	Assess food preferences. Weigh client daily, use same scales and at the same time of day. Assess for negative nitrogen balance. Provide caloric intake as ordered to meet body requirements.	Increase in amount and type of nutrient ingested; maintenance of height, weight balance

Nursing interventions

Health maintenance and promotion. The reduction of the incidence of infective endocarditis can be done by identifying individuals who are at risk for the development of endocarditis. Assessment of the client's history and an understanding of the disease process are crucial for planning and implementing appropriate health maintenance strategies (see Table 31-9).

Educating the client is crucial in providing an increased understanding of and adherence to the planned medical regimen. The client should understand the need to avoid persons with infection, especially upper respiratory, and to report cold, flu, and cough symptoms. The importance of avoiding excessive fatigue and the need to plan rest periods before and after activity should be carefully explained to the client. Good oral hygiene, including daily care and regular dental visits, is also important for the client. The client must report to the physician any dental, medical, or surgical procedures that may predispose to bacteremia. The client should understand the significance of the prescribed prophylactic antibiotic therapy before any invasive procedure. Education of the client who is at risk or has had infective endocarditis helps reduce the incidence and reoccurrence of the disease process.

Acute intervention. A client with infective endocarditis has many actual and potential problems that require astute nursing management. Infective endocarditis generally requires treatment with antibiotics for 4 to 6 weeks or a combination of antibiotics. The client may be hospitalized from 2 to 4 weeks.

Physical assessment findings are nonspecific (see Table 31-8) but can help confirm the diagnosis and aid the treatment plans. Fever, chronic or intermittent, is a common early sign. Frequent assessment of body temperature is important because persistent, prolonged temperature elevations may mean that the drug therapy is ineffective. A cooling blanket can be used to control fever.

The client needs adequate periods of physical and emotional rest. Bed rest may be necessary when fever is present or there are complications (e.g., heart damage). Otherwise the client may ambulate and perform moderate activity.

Heart sounds should be assessed with vital signs to detect a change in the character of the cardiac murmur and the presence of extradiastolic sounds. Arthralgia is common and may involve multiple joints and be accompanied by myalgias. The client should be assessed for joint tenderness, range of motion (ROM), and muscle tenderness. The oral mucosa, conjunctivae, upper chest, and lower extremities should be examined for petechiae. A general systems assessment should be completed to facilitate recognition of hemodynamic and embolic complications.

Laboratory data should be monitored to determine the effectiveness of the long-term, high-dose antibiotic therapy received by the client. IV lines should be monitored for patency and antibiotics should be given when scheduled. The client should be monitored continuously for undesirable reactions to drugs. To prevent consequences from immobility, clients should wear antiembolism stockings; perform ROM exercises; and turn, cough, and deep breathe every 2 hours.

Clients may experience anxiety and fear associated with the illness. The nurse must recognize this problem and implement strategies to help reduce the client's fears and anxieties (see Table 31-9).

Chronic management. Management focuses on educa-

Table 31-10 Etiologies of Pericarditis

INFECTIOUS

Viral causes, including coxsackievirus B, coxsackievirus A, echovirus, adenovirus, mumps virus, infectious mononucleosis, varicella, hepatitis B
Bacterial causes, including pneumococci, staphylococci, streptococci, gram-negative septicemia
Tuberculosis
Fungal causes, including histoplasmosis, *Candida* species
Infections, such as toxoplasmosis, Lyme disease

NONINFECTIOUS

Uremia
Acute MI
Neoplasms, such as lung cancer, breast cancer, leukemia, Hodgkin's disease, lymphoma
Trauma after thoracic surgery, pacemaker insertion, cardiac diagnostic procedures
Radiation
Dissecting aortic aneurysm
Myxedema

HYPERSENSITIVE OR AUTOIMMUNE

Delayed postmyocardial-pericardial injury
Postmyocardial infarction (Dressler) syndrome
Postpericardiotomy syndrome
Rheumatic fever
Drug reactions (e.g., from procainamide, hydralazine)
Rheumatological diseases, including rheumatoid arthritis, systemic lupus erythematosus, scleroderma, ankylosing spondylitis

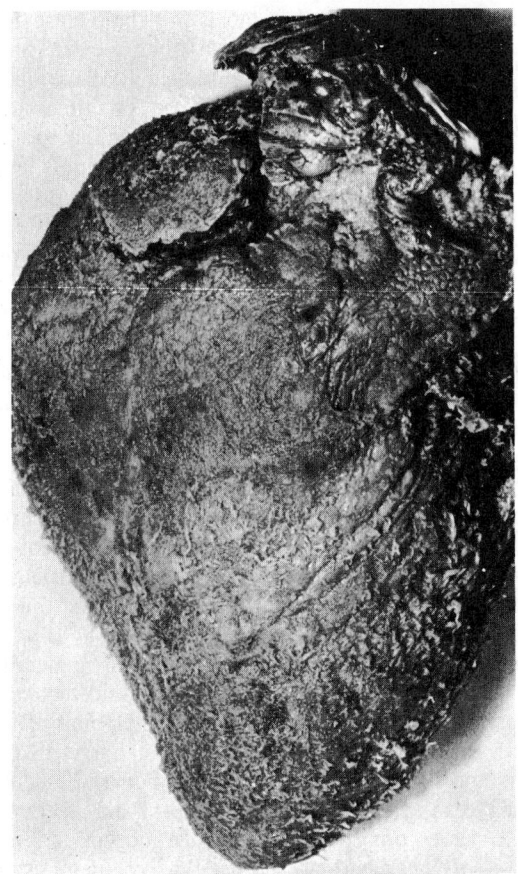

Fig. 31-4 Acute fibrinous pericarditis. There is a shaggy coat of fibrin covering the surface of the heart. (From Anderson WAD and Scotti TM: Synopsis of pathology, ed 10, St Louis, 1980, The CV Mosby Co.)

tion of the client regarding the nature of the disease and on the reduction of the risk of reinfection (see Table 31-9). The client should be instructed about symptoms that may indicate recurrent infection such as fever, fatigue, malaise, and chills and should be aware of the importance of notifying the physician if any of these symptoms occur. The client needs to be instructed about the need for prophylactic antibiotic therapy before any invasive procedure is performed to prevent a reoccurrence (see Table 31-5). The nurse must explain to the client the relationship of follow-up care, good nutrition, and early treatment of common infections (e.g., colds) to maintain good health.

PERICARDITIS
Acute Pericarditis

Pericarditis is a syndrome caused by inflammation of the pericardial sac (the pericardium), which may occur on an acute basis.[12] The pericardium is composed of the inner serous membrane *(visceral pericardium)* that closely adheres to the epicardial surface of the heart and the outer fibrous *(parietal)* layer (Fig. 31-1). The *pericardial space* is the cavity between these two layers and in normal states contains less than 50 ml of serous fluid. Although the pericardium may be congenitally absent or surgically re-

moved, the structure serves a useful anchoring function, provides lubrication from the serous pericardial fluid to decrease friction during systole and diastole, and assists in preventing excessive dilatation of the heart during diastole.

Etiology and pathophysiology. Common causes of acute pericarditis are listed in Table 31-10. Acute pericarditis in the adult client is most often idiopathic with a variety of suspected viral causes, but a proven etiological agent is rarely demonstrated. When a viral agent is identified, the Coxsackievirus B group is the most commonly demonstrated virus and tends to elicit pleuropericarditis in adults (Bornholm disease) and myopericarditis in children. In addition to idiopathic or viral pericarditis, other causes of this syndrome include uremia, bacterial infection, acute myocardial infarction (MI), tuberculosis, neoplasm, and trauma.[13]

The pathological change related to acute pericarditis is acute inflammation. Findings include the presence of polymorphonuclear leukocytes, increased pericardial vascularity, and fibrin deposition on the visceral pericardium, which often reacts to the acute injury by exudation of fluid (Fig. 31-4).

Clinical manifestations. Characteristic clinical manifestations found in acute pericarditis include chest pain, dyspnea, and a pericardial friction rub. The intense, pleuritic chest pain is generally sharpest over the left precordium or retrosternally but may radiate to the trapezius ridge and neck (mimicking angina), or sometimes to the epigastrium or abdomen (mimicking abdominal or other noncardiac pathological conditions). The pain is aggravated by lying supine, deep breathing, coughing, swallowing, and moving the trunk and is eased by sitting up and leaning forward. The dyspnea accompanying acute pericarditis is related to the client's need to breathe in rapid, shallow breaths to avoid chest pain and may be aggravated by fever.

The hallmark finding in acute pericarditis is the *pericardial friction rub*. The rub is a scratching, grating, high-pitched sound believed to arise from friction between the roughened pericardial and epicardial surfaces.[13] It is best heard with the stethoscope diaphragm firmly placed at the lower left sternal border of the chest. The rub does not radiate widely or vary in timing, but it must be frequently auscultated because rubs may be elusive and transient.

Complications. Two major complications that may result from acute pericarditis are *pericardial effusion* and *cardiac tamponade*. Pericardial effusion is generally a rapid accumulation of excess pericardial fluid that occurs in chest trauma. However, a slowly developing effusion may result as in tuberculous pericarditis. Large effusions may compress adjoining structures. Pulmonary tissue compression can cause cough, dyspnea, and tachypnea. Phrenic nerve compression can induce hiccups, and compression of the recurrent laryngeal nerve may result in hoarseness. Heart sounds are generally distant and muffled, although the blood pressure (BP) is usually maintained by compensatory changes.

Cardiac tamponade develops as the pericardial effusion increases in size with failure of compensatory mechanisms to adjust to the continuing altered cardiac compliance. The client with pericardial tamponade is often confused, agitated, and restless and has tachycardia and tachypnea with a low-output state (Table 31-11). The neck veins are usually markedly distended because of jugular venous pressure elevation, and a significant *pulsus paradoxus* is present. Pulsus paradoxus, an inspiratory drop in systolic BP greater than 10 mm Hg, results because the normal inspiratory decline in systolic BP of less than 10 mm Hg is exaggerated in cardiac tamponade. The technique for measurement of pulsus paradoxus is outlined in Table 31-12.

Diagnostic studies. ECG changes in acute pericarditis are key diagnostic clues and evolve over a period of hours to days and weeks (see Table 31-13). Four stages of ECG changes have been described: (1) initial diffuse ST segment elevations that concave upward and are present in all

---

Table 31-11 Clinical Manifestations of Cardiac Tamponade

Decrease in systolic BP
Narrowing pulse pressure
Pulsus paradoxus (>10 mm Hg)
Increase in venous pressure, distension of neck veins
Tachycardia
Tachypnea
Possible friction rub
Muffled heart sounds
Low-voltage ECG
Rapid enlargement of cardiac silhouette on x-ray film
Peripheral cyanosis
Anxiety
Chest pain

Table 31-12 Measurement of Pulsus Paradoxus

1. Make determination during quiet breathing with stable rhythm.
2. Establish systolic pressure.
3. Inflate BP cuff until no sounds are heard with stethoscope.
4. Deflate cuff slowly until sounds are heard on expiration and note the pressure.
5. Deflate cuff until sounds are heard throughout the respiratory cycle and note the pressure.
6. Determine difference that will equal the amount of paradox:

Sounds heard in expiration at	110 mm Hg
Sounds heard throughout cycle	82 mm Hg
Amount of paradox	28 mm Hg

The difference is usually less than 10 mm Hg. If the difference is greater than 10 mm Hg, cardiac tamponade may be present.

Table 31-13

Diagnostic and Therapeutic Management: Acute Pericarditis

DIAGNOSTIC

History and physical examination
Auscultation of chest
ECG
Chest x-ray film
Echocardiography
Pericardiocentesis
Pericardial biopsy
CT scan
Nuclear scan of heart

THERAPEUTIC

Treatment of underlying disease
Bed rest
Aspirin
Nonsteroidal antiinflammatory agents
Corticosteroids
Pericardiocentesis (for large pericardial effusion and/or tamponade)

leads except aV_R and V_1; (2) return of ST segments to baseline with T wave flattening several days later; (3) T wave inversion without the appearance of significant Q waves seen in acute MI; and (4) reversion of T wave changes to normal that may occur weeks or months later.[13] PR segment depression may also be present in the early stages of ST segment changes. These changes are believed to occur because of an injury caused by superficial myocardial inflammation or epicardial injury. Dysrhythmias can accompany these ECG changes but are generally rare occurrences that, when encountered, are usually atrial dysrhythmias in clients with myocardial or valvular pathological conditions in addition to the acute pericarditis.

The chest x-ray film is generally normal or nonspecific in acute pericarditis unless the client has a large pericardial effusion (Fig. 31-5). Echocardiographic findings are much more useful in determining the presence of a pericardial effusion or cardiac tamponade. Additional diagnostic studies such as gallium radionuclide heart scans may be performed, although their sensitivity has not yet been determined.

Laboratory testing, apart from routine studies, focuses on the possible etiology of the pericarditis. For example, elevated blood urea nitrogen (BUN) levels and serum creatinine levels may indicate uremic pericarditis, and a positive tuberculin skin test may suggest tuberculous pericarditis. The fluid obtained during pericardiocentesis (see Fig. 31-6) or the tissue from a pericardial biopsy may also be studied to determine the cause of the pericarditis.

Therapeutic management. Management of acute pericarditis is directed toward identification and treatment of the underlying problem (see Table 31-13). Antibiotics should be used to treat purulent pericarditis. Corticosteroids are generally reserved for pericarditis secondary to systemic lupus erythematosus, for when the client already takes steroids for a rheumatological or other immune system condition, and for those clients who do not respond to nonsteroidal preparations.

The pain and inflammation of acute pericarditis are usually treated with nonsteroidal antiinflammatory agents. High-dose salicylates (300 to 900 mg orally four times a day) or indomethacin (25 to 50 mg orally four times a day) are commonly used. Discriminate and careful administration of corticosteroids is advised because of their numerous side effects such as peptic ulcer disease, sodium retention, hyperglycemia, hypokalemia, and Cushing's syndrome (see Chapter 44). When necessary, prednisone is usually given in a tapering dosage schedule (see Chapter 44).

Pericardiocentesis (Fig. 31-6) should be performed in the presence of acute cardiac tamponade with a reduction of the client's systolic BP of more than 30 mm Hg from the baseline level. Hemodynamic support as the client is prepared for the pericardiocentesis should include administration of volume expanders and inotropic agents.

The procedure is performed in the critical care unit or cardiac catheterization laboratory under sterile conditions and in conjunction with ECG, echocardiogram, and hemo-

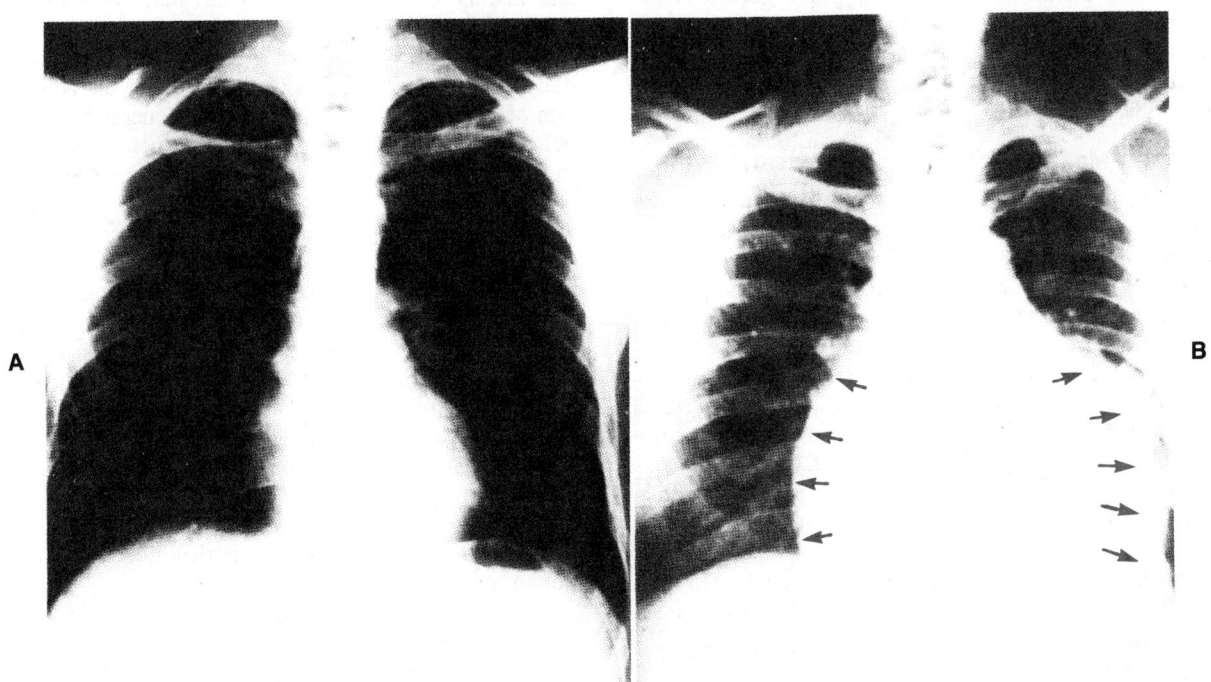

Fig. 31-5 **A,** A normal chest x-ray film. **B,** With pericardial effusion the cardiac silhouette is enlarged with a globular shape *(arrows).* (From Guzzetta CE and Dossey BM: Cardiovascular nursing: bodymind tapestry, St Louis, 1984, The CV Mosby Co, p 772.)

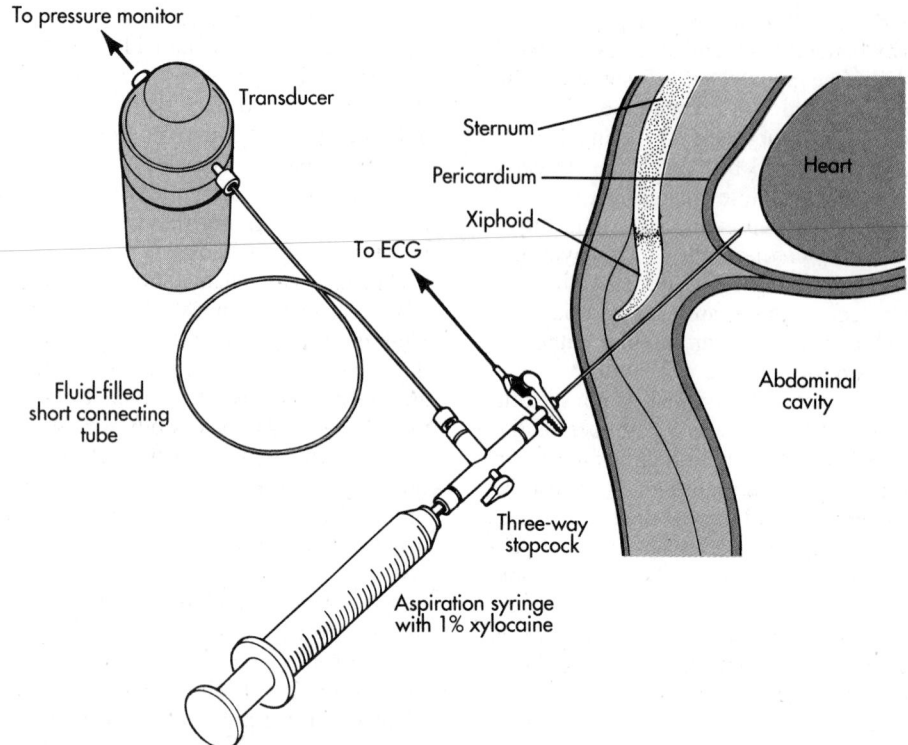

Fig. 31-6 Pericardiocentesis performed under sterile conditions in conjunction with ECG and hemodynamic measurements. (From Lorell BH and Braunwald E: Pericardial disease in heart disease: a textbook of cardiovascular medicine, ed 3, Philadelphia, 1988, WB Saunders Co, p 1500.)

dynamic measurements. A 16 to 18 gauge needle is inserted into the pericardial space to remove fluid for analysis and to relieve cardiac pressure. Complications from pericardiocentesis include pneumothorax, myocardial laceration, and coronary artery laceration.

■ Nursing Management of Acute Pericarditis

The management for the client's pain and anxiety during acute pericarditis are primary nursing considerations. Assessment of the amount, quality, and location of the pain is important, particularly in distinguishing the pain of acute MI (or reinfarction) versus the pain of pericarditis. Careful nursing observations should thus be made regarding ischemic chest pain, which is generally located retrosternal in the left shoulder and arm with a pressurelike, burning quality and is unaffected by posture, and pericarditic chest pain, which is usually located in the precordium, left trapezius ridge with a sharp, pleuritic quality and is often relieved by leaning forward and worsened by recumbency. The ECG should also be assessed to aid in distinguishing these types of pain because acute MI usually involves localized ST segment changes versus the ST segment changes present in all leads except aV_R and V_1 during acute pericarditis.

Pain relief measures include maintaining the client on bed rest with the head of the bed elevated to 45 degrees and providing a padded overbed table for the client. Anti-inflammatory medications prescribed for the client help to alleviate the client's pain. However, because of the potential for GI problems with high-dose use, nursing interventions should be directed toward management of this potential problem. Specific interventions include the administration of these drugs with food or milk generally 30 minutes before or 2 hours after meals and instruction of the client to avoid any alcoholic beverages while taking the medications.

Anxiety-reducing measures for the client with acute pericarditis include providing simple, complete explanations of all procedures performed. These explanations are particularly important for the client during the time the diagnosis of acute pericarditis is being established and for the client who has already experienced an acute MI and has pericarditis (Dressler syndrome).

The real potential for decreased cardiac output (CO) also exists for the client with acute pericarditis because of the possibility of cardiac tamponade. Monitoring for the signs and symptoms of tamponade (see Table 31-11) along with preparations for possible pericardiocentesis are important nursing responsibilities.

Chronic Constrictive Pericarditis

Etiology and pathophysiology. Constrictive pericarditis commonly begins with an initial episode of acute pericarditis (often secondary to neoplasia, radiation, previous surgery, or idiopathic causes) and is characterized by fibrin deposition with a clinically undetected pericardial effusion. Organization and resorption of the effusion slowly follows with progression towards the chronic stage of development consisting of fibrous scarring, thickening of the pericardium from calcium deposition, and eventual obliteration of the pericardial space. The fibrotic, thickened, and adherent pericardium encases the heart, thereby impairing the ability of the atria and ventricles to fill adequately during diastole.

Clinical manifestations. Manifestations of chronic constrictive pericarditis occur over an extended time and mimic those of CHF and cor pulmonale. These include dyspnea on exertion, lower extremity edema, ascites, fatigue, anorexia, and weight loss. The most prominent physical examination finding is elevated jugular venous pressure. Unlike cardiac tamponade, the presence of significant pulsus paradoxus is uncommon. Auscultatory findings include a *pericardial knock,* which is a loud early diastolic sound often heard along the left sternal border.

Diagnostic studies. ECG changes may be nonspecific in chronic constrictive pericarditis but usually consist of low QRS voltage, generalized T wave inversion or flattening, and either P mitrale or atrial fibrillation.[1] The cardiac silhouette on the chest x-ray film may be normal or enlarged depending on the degree of pericardial thickening and the presence of a coexisting pericardial effusion. Echocardiographic findings may reveal a thickened pericardium, but without the presence of a large pericardial effusion, distinctions between the myocardium and epicardium are difficult to ascertain.

Cardiac catheterization pressure tracings are more specific diagnostic tools in constrictive pericarditis. Abnormalities include elevation of the right and left heart pressures with equilibration of these pressures in diastole. Other valuable diagnostic tools used to evaluate this condition are computed tomography (CT) and magnetic resonance imaging (MRI).

▪ Therapeutic and Nursing Management of Chronic Constrictive Pericarditis

Unless the client is free of symptoms or the condition is inoperable, the treatment of choice for chronic constrictive pericarditis is a *pericardiectomy.* The pericardiectomy usually involves complete resection of the pericardium through a median sternotomy with the use of cardiopulmonary bypass. The postoperative prognosis is improved when the surgery is performed earlier in the disease course before development of severe clinical disability. The postoperative nursing care after a pericardiectomy is similar to that of other open heart surgical procedures (see Chapter 29).

Myocarditis

Etiology and pathophysiology. Myocarditis, a focal or diffuse inflammation of the myocardium, has been associated with a variety of etiological agents, including viral, bacterial, rickettsial, mycotic, parasitic, radiation, pharmacological, and chemical factors.[14] Certain medical conditions such as metabolic disorders and collagen-vascular diseases (e.g., systemic lupus erythematosus) may also precipitate myocarditis. Viruses are the most common eti-

ological agent in the United States, with a predominance of RNA viruses (coxsackievirus A and B), echovirus, influenza A and B, and mumps. Myocarditis may also occur when no causative agent or factor can be identified. Myocarditis is frequently associated with acute pericarditis, particularly when it is caused by coxsackievirus B strains or echoviruses.

The pathophysiological mechanisms of myocarditis are poorly understood because there is usually a period of several weeks after the initial infection before the development of manifestations of myocarditis. Immunological mechanisms may play a role in the development of myocarditis. The majority of infections are benign, self-limiting, and subclinical, although viral myocarditis in infants and pregnant women may be virulent.

Clinical manifestations. The clinical features for clients with myocarditis are variable, ranging from a benign course without any overt manifestations to severe heart involvement or sudden death. Fever, fatigue, malaise, myalgias, pharyngitis, dyspnea, lymphadenopathy, and GI complaints are early systemic manifestations of the viral illness.

Early cardiac manifestations appear 7 to 10 days after viral infection and include pericardial chest pain with an associated friction rub because pericarditis often accompanies myocarditis (see p. 897). Cardiac symptoms may progress to CHF (e.g., S_3, rales, jugular venous distention, and peripheral edema), pericardial effusion, syncope, and possibly ischemic pain.

Diagnostic studies. The ECG changes for a client with myocarditis are often nonspecific and reflect associated pericardial involvement including diffuse ST segment abnormalities. Dysrhythmias and conduction disturbances may be present. Laboratory findings are also often inconclusive, with the presence of mild to moderate leukocytosis and atypical lymphocytes, elevated viral titers (virus generally only present in tissue and fluid samples during the initial 8 to 10 days of illness), increased ESR, and elevated levels of enzymes such as the transaminases, creatine phosphokinase, and lactic dehydrogenase.

Histological confirmation of myocarditis is possible through endomyocardial biopsy (EMB), a technique in which several small pieces of myocardial tissue are percutaneously removed from the right ventricle with a special instrument called a *bioptome* and microscopically examined. The biopsy has to be done during the initial 6 weeks of acute illness because this is the period in which lymphocytic infiltration and myocyte damage indicative of myocarditis are present. Special myocardial imaging techniques may also be used in the diagnostic evaluation of myocarditis.

Therapeutic management. The specific treatment for myocarditis has yet to be established and usually consists of managing associated cardiac decompensation. Digoxin, which is often used to treat ventricular failure because it improves myocardial contractility and reduces ventricular rate, should be used cautiously in clients with myocarditis because they are more sensitive to the adverse effects of digoxin and digitalis toxicity may develop with minimum doses. Oxygen therapy, bed rest, restricted activity, and maintenance of standby emergency equipment are general supportive measures used for management of myocarditis.

Immunosuppression therapy with agents such as prednisone, azathioprine, and cyclosporine have been used in a limited number of clients with myocarditis to reduce myocardial inflammation and to prevent irreversible myocardial damage.[15] Administration of immunosuppressive agents is recommended only during the postinfectious stage of the disease, approximately 10 days after onset of initial symptoms, because actual increased tissue necrosis has been demonstrated when these agents are used early in the course of viral myocarditis.[14] The use of steroids for the treatment of myocarditis remains controversial because of the associated serious side effects and lack of clear documentation for their efficacy.

■ Nursing Management of Myocarditis

The potential for decreased CO is an ongoing nursing diagnosis in the care of the client with myocarditis. Interventions should focus on assessment for the signs and symptoms of CHF, instituting measures to decrease cardiac work load (e.g., use of semi-Fowler's position, properly spaced activity and rest periods, and provisions for a quiet environment) with administration, monitoring, and evaluation of ordered medications that increase contractility and decrease preload, afterload, or both.

Clients may be anxious about the establishment of the diagnosis of myocarditis, recovery from myocarditis, and therapy. Measures to facilitate decreased anxiety include monitoring anxiety levels and keeping the client informed about procedures and the diagnosis of myocarditis.

Clients who receive immunosuppressive therapy have additional problems of alteration in immune regulation with the potential for infection and complications related to the therapy. Guidelines for care include monitoring these complications and providing the client with a clean, safe environment according to proper infection control standards. The majority of individuals with myocarditis recover spontaneously. Occasionally, acute myocarditis progresses to chronic dilated cardiomyopathy (see Chapter 29).

Rheumatic Fever and Heart Disease

Rheumatic fever is an inflammatory disease of the heart potentially involving all layers (endocardium, myocardium, and pericardium). The resulting damage to the heart from rheumatic fever is called *rheumatic heart disease,* a chronic condition characterized by scarring and deformity of the heart valves.

Significance. Acute rheumatic fever (ARF) is a complication of up to 3% of sporadic upper respiratory infections caused by group A β-hemolytic streptococci species.[16] Initial and recurrent episodes of ARF are most common from ages 6 through 15. Most recurrences occur within 2 years of the initial episode.[16] Recurrent attacks of rheumatic fever are twice as common between the ages of 11 and 22 as after the age of 22. The frequency of rheumatic recurrences after streptococcal infection is greater in those with rheumatic heart disease than in those who have not had cardiac injury during previous attacks.[17] Attacks do occur

in adulthood. Studies indicate that they are probably more common than previously believed. However, the sequelae of rheumatic heart disease are seen primarily in young adults.

A spectacular decline in the incidence of rheumatic fever was observed in the 1960s and 1970s. By the 1980s, rheumatic fever had virtually disappeared in developed countries such as the United States. However, it does remain common and severe in most of the Third World countries. Antibiotics, notably penicillin, are responsible for the decline in rheumatic fever. Antibiotics given within 9 days of the appearance of streptococcal sore throat, before the immune system fully reacts, can prevent rheumatic complications.[18] A decrease in the prevalence of bacterial strains with the natural ability to trigger rheumatic complications has also contributed to the decline.

Since 1985 a startling reappearance of ARF in the United States has occurred. Outbreaks of the disease have appeared without warning in widely separated, relatively well-to-do communities in the United States and, most dramatically, among military recruits in California and Missouri.[19] In searching for an answer to determine the cause of the reappearance, researchers have focused their efforts on isolating strains of group A streptococci. Researchers have found that the isolated microbes are mucoid strains of the M protein serotypes that were prevalent with epidemic rheumatic fever more than 20 years ago.[19] In the majority of new clients, a sore throat was never noted or reported. The infection that set off the immune system was so mild that the client did not seek care. These reemergent strains are capable of causing rheumatic fever while producing such mild sore throats that no treatment is sought until it is too late to prevent complications.[18]

Etiology. Rheumatic fever almost always occurs as a delayed sequela (usually 2 to 3 weeks) to a group A β-hemolytic streptococcal infection of the upper respiratory system, usually a pharyngeal infection. Streptococcal infections of the skin are not associated with ARF, and some strains of group A β-hemolytic streptococci do not cause rheumatic fever.

In addition to the infecting organisms, other factors play a predisposing role in the development of rheumatic fever. They include socioeconomic factors, familial factors, and the presence of an altered immune response. The incidence of rheumatic fever is higher in low socioeconomic groups and remains a major public health problem in the poorer countries of the Third World.[20] Crowded living conditions may be the major factor contributing to this finding. Neglect, inadequate treatment, poor nutrition, and a lowered state of health may be other reasons why lower socioeconomic groups in the United States and persons in Third World countries are more commonly affected. Rheumatic fever is more likely to develop in people living in urban areas than in rural communities. There also seems to be a familial tendency toward rheumatic fever, which may be genetically related, possibly due to an altered immune response.

Pathophysiology. The correlation of streptococcal pharyngitis with rheumatic fever is conclusive, but the pathogenic mechanisms by which streptococcal infection causes inflammation of the heart and other tissues are not well defined. The organism is not demonstrable in the lesions when rheumatic fever appears several days or weeks after the acute streptococcal infection. Normally, antibodies are produced in response to infections with streptococcal organisms. Episodes of primary and recurrent ARF have been associated with a greater antibody response than those found with uncomplicated streptococcal sore throats.

Manifestations of ARF appear to be related (in susceptible individuals) to an abnormal immunological response to an upper respiratory infection with group A β-hemolytic streptococci. ARF probably affects the heart, joints, central nervous system (CNS), and skin because of an abnormal humoral and cell-mediated immune response to group A streptococcal cell membrane antigens. It is possible that these antigens cross-react with other tissues and bind to receptors on heart, muscle, joint, and brain cells triggering immune and inflammatory responses.[17] However, the direct relationship of this cross-reactive phenomenon to pathology is unproven, and streptococcal-induced autoimmunity as a mechanism to explain the rheumatic process remains a popular but unestablished pathogenetic concept.

Cardiac lesions and valvular deformities. About 40% of ARF episodes are marked by carditis, and all layers of the heart—endocardium, myocardium, and pericardium—may be involved. This generalized involvement gives rise to the term *rheumatic pancarditis*.[16]

Rheumatic endocarditis is found primarily in the valves with swelling and erosion of the valve leaflets. Vegetations form in areas of erosion from deposits of fibrin and blood cells. These lesions initially create fibrous thickening of the valve commissures and chordae tendineae and fibrosis of the papillary muscle (Fig. 31-7). The valves may become stenotic and insufficient. The mitral and aortic valves are most commonly affected; less commonly involved are the tricuspid valve and, rarely, pulmonic valves. Valve leaflets may fuse and become thickened or even calcified, resulting in stenosis. Reduction in the mobility of valve leaflets may occur with failure of the leaflets to appose, resulting in regurgitation.

Myocardial involvement is characterized by Aschoff's bodies, which are nodules formed by a reaction to inflammation, and accompanying swelling and fragmentation of collagen fibers. As Aschoff's bodies age, they become more fibrous and scar tissue is formed in the myocardium. In addition to the Aschoff bodies, a diffuse cellular infiltrate is present in interstitial tissues. This interstitial myocarditis may be more important than the nodular Aschoff bodies in producing heart failure.[21]

Rheumatic pericarditis affects both layers of the pericardium, which become thickened and covered with a fibrinous exudate, and a serosanguineous pericardial fluid may be present. When healing occurs, fibrosis and adhesions develop that partially or completely obliterate the pericardial sac, but constrictive pericarditis does not occur.

These pathophysiological changes in the heart may occur as a result of an initial attack of rheumatic fever; however, recurrent infections may cause further structural damage.

Extracardiac lesions. The lesions of rheumatic fever are systemic, involving especially the connective tissue. The joints (polyarthritis), skin (subcutaneous nodules), CNS (chorea), and lungs (fibrinous pleurisy and rheumatic pneumonitis) can be involved in rheumatic fever.

Clinical manifestations. The diagnosis of ARF is suggested by a clustering of signs and symptoms as well as laboratory findings. When not observed in its most severe form, the disease may be difficult to differentiate from many illnesses with common clinical manifestations. Criteria were established by T.D. Jones in 1944 and revised by the American Heart Association in 1965 to provide a logical basis for diagnosis (Table 31-14). The presence of two major criteria or one major and two minor criteria indicates a high probability of ARF. Either combination must have evidence of an existing streptococcal infection.

Major criteria. Carditis is the most important manifestation of ARF (Table 31-14), with four signs including (1)

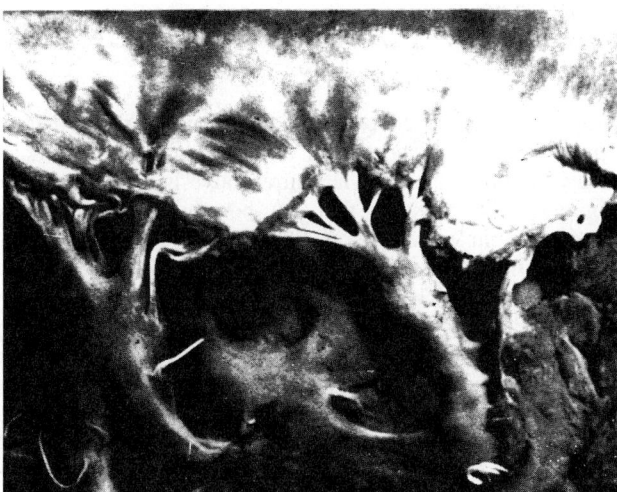

Fig. 31-7 Acute recurrent rheumatic endocarditis involving the tricuspid valve. Verrucae are present along the line of closure of the valve leaflets. Notice thickened chordae tendineae. (From Kissane JM: *Anderson's pathology*, ed 9, St Louis, 1990, Mosby–Year Book, Inc.)

Table 31-14 Modified Jones Criteria for Acute Rheumatic Fever

Major Criteria	Minor Criteria
Carditis	Fever
Polyarthritis	Previous occurrence of rheumatic fever or rheumatic heart disease
Chorea	
Erythema marginatum	
Subcutaneous nodules	Arthralgia
	Prolonged PR interval
	Laboratory findings*

From American Heart Association: Jones criteria (revised) for guidance in the diagnosis of rheumatic fever, Dallas, 1982, American Heart Association.
*See Table 31-15.

an organic heart murmur or murmurs not usually present, usually from mitral or aortic regurgitation, or mitral stenosis; (2) cardiac enlargement and CHF; (3) pericarditis manifested as pericardial friction rubs or signs of effusion; and (4) dysrhythmias.

Polyarthritis, which is not a cause of permanent disability, is the most common finding in rheumatic fever. The inflammatory process affects the synovial membranes of the joint causing swelling, heat, redness, tenderness, and limitation of motion. The arthritis is migratory, affecting one joint and then moving to another. The larger joints are most frequently affected, particularly the knees, ankles, elbows, and wrists. The pain may prevent the person from being able to walk.

Chorea (Syndenham's chorea) is the major CNS manifestation. It is characterized by weakness, ataxia, and choreic movement that is spontaneous, rapid, and purposeless, which tends to intensify with voluntary activity. Females under 18 years of age are primarily affected.

Erythema marginatum lesions are a less common feature of ARF. The bright-pink maplike macular lesions occur mainly on the trunk or inner aspects of the upper arm and thigh but never on the face. The rash is nonpruritic and nonpainful and is neither indurated or raised. It is usually transitory (lasting for a few hours), may recur intermittently for months, and is exacerbated by heat (e.g., a warm bath).

Subcutaneous nodules are firm, small, hard, painless swellings found most commonly over bony prominences (e.g., knees, elbows, spine, scapulae). They frequently are not noticed by the person because the skin overlying the nodules moves freely and is not inflamed.

The presence of the major criteria of ARF vary among children and adults. In contrast to children, polyarthritis is the dominant clinical feature in adults, whereas carditis and the severity of subsequent valvular lesions are less prominent.[22] Two other major criteria, chorea and subcutaneous nodules, are not usually seen in adults, and the occurrence of erythema marginatum is uncommon.

Minor criteria. Minor clinical manifestations (see Table 31-14) are frequently present and are helpful in recognizing the disease. These criteria are too nonspecific to make a definitive diagnosis because they frequently occur in other diseases and are used as supplemental data to confirm the presence of rheumatic fever. Laboratory test abnormalities in rheumatic fever are presented in Table 31-15.

Complications. The course of rheumatic fever cannot be predicted at the onset of the disease, but generalizations can be made on a statistical basis. Within 6 weeks, 75% of ARF attacks abate, and 90% abate within 3 months. Less than 5% last for more than 6 months.[23] Once all evidence of rheumatic inflammation has abated, rheumatic fever does not recur in the absence of a new streptococcal infection. If the initial episode is not associated with carditis, there is little likelihood of subsequent damage if repeated attacks do occur.

A complication that can result from ARF is chronic rheumatic carditis. It results from changes in valvular structure that may occur months to years after an attack of

Table 31-15 Laboratory Test Abnormalities in Acute Rheumatic Fever

ASO titer	>250 IU/ml
ESR	>15 mm/hr in males, >20 mm/hr in females
C-reactive protein	Positive
Throat culture	Positive for streptococci (usually negative)
WBC count	Elevated
Red blood cell parameters (Hct, Hb, RBC)	Mild-to-moderate degree of normocytic, normochromic anemia

Table 31-16

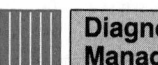
Diagnostic and Therapeutic Management: Rheumatic Fever

DIAGNOSTIC

History and physical examination
ASO titer
Throat culture
ESR
C-reactive protein
WBC count
Chest x-ray film
Echocardiography
ECG

THERAPEUTIC

Bed rest (modified)
Benzathine penicillin 1.2 million units IM or procaine penicillin 600,000 units IM qd for 10 days
Acetylsalicylic acid
Corticosteroids

ARF. Rheumatic endocarditis can result in fibrous tissue growth to valve leaflets and chordae tendineae with scarring and contractures. The mitral valve is most frequently involved. Other valves that may be affected are the aortic and tricuspid valves (see p. 909).

Diagnostic studies. No single diagnostic test exists for rheumatic fever, but the results of combinations of laboratory studies suggest the presence of the disease (Table 31-16). Throat cultures are usually negative at the onset of the disease because of the relatively long latent period of 10 days to several weeks after the precipitating infection. The most specific diagnostic test to confirm a recent group A streptococcal infection is the antistreptolysin (ASO) titer. The ESR and C-reactive protein (CRP) are nonspecific tests indicative of a systemic inflammatory response.

An echocardiogram may show valvular insufficiency and pericardial fluid or thickening. A chest x-ray film may show an enlarged heart if CHF is present. The most consistent electrocardiographic change is delayed AV conduction as evidenced in prolongation of the P-R interval. Other ECG changes are common but nondiagnostic.

Therapeutic management. No specific treatment will cure rheumatic fever. Treatment consists of drug therapy and supportive measures (see Table 31-16). Antibiotic therapy does not modify the course of the acute disease or the development of carditis. Penicillin eliminates residual group A β-hemolytic streptococci remaining in the tonsils and pharnyx and prevents the spread of organisms to close contacts. Salicylates and steroids are the two antiinflammatory agents most widely used in the management of ARF. Both are effective in controlling the fever and joint manifestations. Salicylates are used when arthritis is the main manifestation and steroids if severe carditis is present. Prolonged periods of bed rest have previously been recommended, but now the client without carditis may be ambulatory as soon as acute symptoms have subsided and may return to normal activity when the antiinflammatory therapy has been discontinued. When carditis is present, ambulation is postponed until CHF has been controlled with treatment. Full activities should not be resumed until antiinflammatory therapy has been discontinued.

■ **Nursing Management of Rheumatic Fever**

Nursing assessment

The client should be assessed for risk and etiological factors such as a previous infection by β-hemolytic streptococci, socioeconomic status, and living conditions. Rheumatic fever is five times more likely to occur in a person with a prior history of rheumatic fever than in the general population. A higher incidence of ARF occurs in lower socioeconomic groups and in crowded living conditions. This may be related to poor treatment of streptococcal infections.

Objective assessment should focus on several body systems. The musculoskeletal system should be assessed for signs of polyarthritis: swelling, heat, redness, pain, tenderness, and limitation of motion (particularly the knees, ankles, elbows, and wrists). The skin of the client should be assessed for subcutaneous nodules and erythema marginatum. The procedure involves palpation for subcutaneous nodules over all bony surfaces and along extensor tendons of the hands and feet. The nodules range in size from 1 to 4 cm and are hard, painless, and freely movable. Inspect for erythema marginatum on the trunk and inner aspects of the upper arm and thigh. The erythematous maplike macules do not itch and are not raised. The possible presence of these bright pink macules should be assessed in good light because the rash is difficult to observe.

Auscultatory assessment of the heart should be performed to determine tachycardia, pericardial friction rub, gallop rhythm, diastolic and possibly systolic murmurs, and mitral and aortic murmurs associated with chronic rheumatic fever. The nurse should also assess for signs of CHF effusion and cardiac enlargement, which are related to rheumatic carditis. Chorea is the last major clinical manifestation to assess. Symptoms include involuntary, purposeless, rapid motions; fretfulness; and facial grimaces. Body temperature should be taken for other objective assessment data. The client will usually have a low-grade fever (38° C [100° F]). The client may report subjective symptoms of malaise and abdominal pain.

Nursing diagnoses

Nursing diagnoses of rheumatic fever include, but are not limited to, the following:

1. Activity intolerance related to arthralgia, CHF, and malaise
2. Decreased cardiac output related to dyspnea, tachycardia, and orthopnea secondary to rheumatic carditis or CHF
3. Impaired physical mobility related to polyarthritis, malaise, fatigue, and arthralgia
4. High risk for injury related to involuntary movements secondary to chorea
5. Pain related to polyarthritis
6. High risk for infection transmission related to group A β-hemolytic streptococcal infection
7. High risk for altered health maintenance related to lack of knowledge concerning the need for long-term prophylactic antibiotic therapy and possible disease process sequelae

Nursing interventions

Health promotion and maintenance. Rheumatic fever is one of the few cardiovascular diseases that is preventable. Prevention is frequently classified as primary and secondary. *Primary prevention* involves early detection and immediate treatment of group A β-hemolytic streptococcal pharyngitis. Adequate treatment of streptococcal pharyngitis prevents initial attacks of rheumatic fever. Treatment consists of a single intramuscular (IM) injection of 0.6 to 1.2 million units of benzathine penicillin G or 10 days of oral penicillin G. Erythromycin is substituted for clients who are allergic to penicillin. Oral therapy requires faithful adherence to the full 10-day course of treatment. The nurse's role is educating the community to seek medical attention for symptoms of streptococcal pharyngitis and emphasizing the need for adequate treatment of a streptococcal sore throat.

Secondary prevention focuses on the use of prophylactic antibiotics to prevent recurrent rheumatic fever. A person who has had rheumatic fever is more susceptible to a second attack after a streptococcal infection. The best prevention is monthly injections of benzathine penicillin G.[17] Alternative treatments are daily or twice a day administration of oral penicillin, sulfadiazine, or erythromycin. Prophylactic treatment should continue for life in individuals who had rheumatic carditis as children. Rheumatic fever without carditis after the age of 18 may need only 5 years of prophylactic antibiotic therapy.

Acute intervention. Primary goals of managing a client with ARF are to (1) control and alleviate the infecting organism; (2) prevent cardiac complications; (3) relieve joint pain, fever, and other symptoms; and (4) support the client psychologically and emotionally.

The nurse should administer antibiotics as ordered to treat the streptococcal infection and teach the client that oral antibiotic therapy requires faithful adherence to the full 10-day course of therapy. Respiratory secretion precautions should be maintained for 24 hours after initiation of antibiotic therapy. Tepid sponge baths should be given to relieve fever and antipyretics should be administered as prescribed. Oral fluids should be encouraged if the client is able to swallow, or IV fluids should be administered as prescribed.

Promotion of optimal rest is essential to reduce cardiac work load and diminish the metabolic need of the body. After acute symptoms have subsided, the client without carditis should ambulate. The client may resume normal activity after the antiinflammatory therapy is discontinued. If the client has carditis with CHF, bed rest restrictions should be applied. Again full activity should not be allowed until antiinflammatory therapy is discontinued. Nonstrenuous activities should be encouraged once recovery has begun.

Relief of joint pain is an important nursing goal. Painful joints should be positioned for comfort and proper alignment. Removal of covers from painful joints can be done with a bed cradle. Heat may be applied and salicylates may be administered to relieve joint pain.

Psychological and emotional care can be more important than physical care, especially because children and young adults are the primary clients, and the heart is often viewed as the center of life. Any alteration in cardiac function may be perceived as a threat to the person's body image.

Chronic management. Secondary prevention aims at preventing the recurrence of rheumatic fever. The client with a previous history of rheumatic fever should be taught about the disease process, the possible sequelae, and the continual need for prophylactic antibiotics. The client must be made aware of the high risk of recurrence if a streptococcal infection develops. The client should be informed about the risk of exposure to streptococcal infections from contact with school-age children, individuals in military service, and people in allied health positions. Ongoing client education and reinforcement encourage good health practices and the continuation of prophylactic antibiotic therapy.

The dosage of antibiotics used in prophylaxis of rheumatic fever is not adequate to prevent infective endocarditis. Prophylaxis is necessary if a client with known rheumatic heart disease has dental or surgical procedures involving the upper respiratory, GI, or GU tract. The nurse must explain the difference between these two prophylactic programs.

The client should also be cautioned about the possibility of development of valvular heart disease. The nurse should teach the client to seek medical attention if symptoms such as excessive fatigue, dizziness, palpitations, or dyspnea on exertion develop.

VALVULAR HEART DISEASE

The heart contains two atrioventricular valves, the mitral and tricuspid, and two semilunar valves, the aortic and pulmonic, which are located in four strategic locations to control proper blood flow (Fig. 31-8). Types of valvular heart disease are defined according to the valve or valves affected and the two types of functional alterations, *stenosis* and *regurgitation,* produced by diseased heart valves (Fig. 31-9).

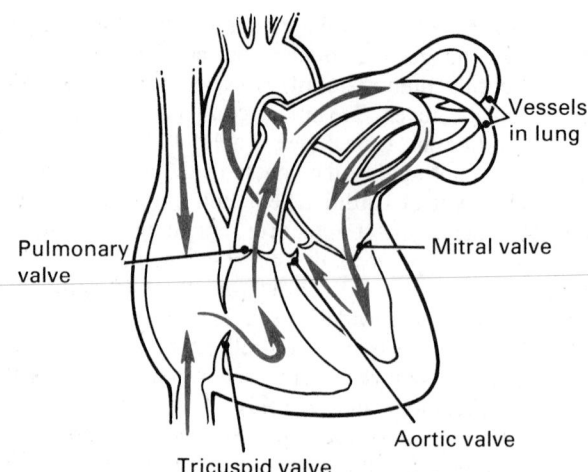

Fig. 31-8   Cross section of valves of the heart.

The pressure on either side of an open valve is normally equal. However, in a stenotic valve the valve orifice is restricted, impeding the forward flow of blood and creating a pressure gradient difference across an open valve.[24] The degree of stenosis is reflected in the pressure gradient differences (i.e., the higher the gradient, the greater the stenosis). In regurgitation (also called *valvular incompetence* or *insufficiency*) the incomplete closure of disease-damaged valve leaflets results in the backward flow of blood.

Valvular disorders occur in children and adolescents primarily from congenital conditions such as tricuspid atresia, pulmonary stenosis, and aortic stenosis (Table 31-17). The incidence of congenital heart disease in the United States is 1 out of every 100 newborns of which 15% to 20% have some type of congenital valvular heart defect.[25] Rheumatic fever is a common cause of adult valvular disease.

Mitral Stenosis

Etiology and pathophysiology. The majority of adult cases of mitral stenosis result from rheumatic fever. Less common causes include congenital mitral stenosis, rheumatoid arthritis, and systemic lupus erythematosus. Because mitral stenosis is primarily the result of recurrent rheumatic endocarditis, the valve leaflets and the chordae tendineae become scarred and develop contractures with adhesions between the two major leaflets at the level of the commissures (the two junctional areas between the two leaflets).[26] The stenotic mitral valve assumes a funnel shape because of the thickening and shortening of the structures composing the mitral valve apparatus (Fig. 31-10). Obstruction to flow across the mitral valve results from these structural deformities and creates a pressure gradient difference between the left atrial and left ventricular chambers during the diastolic filling period of the left ventricle. The flow obstruction increases left atrial pressure and volume with resultant increased pulmonary vasculature pressures and hypertrophy of the pulmonary vessels in cases of chronic left atrial pressure elevations. Pressure overload on the left atrium, the pulmonary vascula-

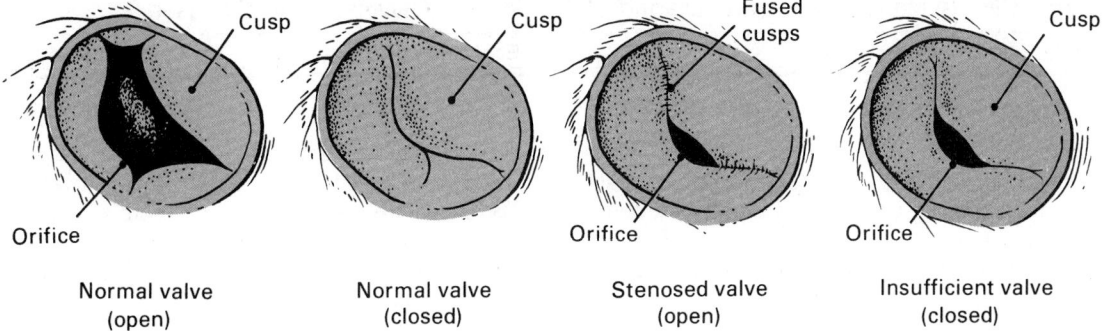

Normal valve (open) Normal valve (closed) Stenosed valve (open) Insufficient valve (closed)

Fig. 31-9 A stenosed valve leads to decreased blood flow through the valve and gradual hypertrophy of the preceding chamber (e.g., a stenosed mitral valve leads to a hypertrophied left atrium). An insufficient valve leads to backward flow through the valve and dilatation of the preceding chamber (e.g., aortic insufficiency leads to a dilated left ventricle).

Table 31-17 Congenital Heart Lesions

Lesion	Description
Ventricular septal defect	Hole in septum between two ventricles
Atrial septal defect	Hole in septum between two atria
Patent ductus arteriosus	Persistence of opening between aorta and pulmonary artery, which normally closes shortly before birth
Pulmonic stenosis	Narrowing of pulmonic valve
Coarctation of aorta	Stricture and narrowing of aorta caused by infolding of wall of aorta
Aortic stenosis	Narrowing of aortic valve
Tetralogy of Fallot	Ventricular septal defect, pulmonic stenosis, aorta overriding two ventricles, and right ventricular hypertrophy
Transposition of great vessels	Reversal of position of aorta and pulmonary artery; origination of aorta from right ventricle, origination of pulmonary artery from left ventricle
Persistent truncus arteriosus	Single vessel exiting the heart to supply blood to pulmonary and systemic circulations
Tricuspid atresia	Absence of communication between right atrium and right ventricle

ture tree, and the right ventricle occurs in chronic mitral stenosis.

Clinical manifestations. Dyspnea, sometimes accompanied by hemoptysis, is the primary symptom of mitral stenosis because of reduced lung compliance.[27] Fatigue and palpitations from atrial fibrillation may also be present. Auscultatory findings generally include a loud or accentuated first heart sound, an opening snap (best heard at the apex with the stethoscope diaphragm), and a low-pitched, rumbling diastolic murmur (best heard at the apex with the stethoscope bell). Clients with mitral stenosis may less frequently have hoarseness, chest pain, seizures, or a cerebrovascular accident from an embolus (Table 31-18).

Mitral Regurgitation

Etiology and pathophysiology. The patency of the mitral valve apparatus depends on the integrity of the mitral leaflets, the mitral annulus, the chordae tendineae, the papillary muscles, the left atrium, and the left ventricle. An anatomical or functional abnormality of any of these

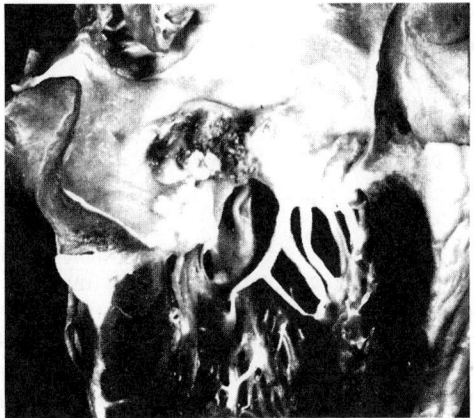

Fig. 31-10 Mitral stenosis. The mitral leaflets are thickened, fused, and ulcerated. The chordae tendineae are also greatly thickened. (From Kissane JM: Anderson's pathology, ed 9, St Louis, 1990, Mosby–Year Book, Inc, p 673.)

Table 31-18 Clinical Manifestations and Diagnostic Findings for Valvular Heart Diseases

Clinical Manifestations	ECG	Echocardiogram	Cardiac Catheterization
MITRAL STENOSIS			
Dyspnea, hemoptysis; fatigue; palpitations; loud, accentuated S_1; opening snap; low-pitched, rumbling diastolic murmur	Right axis deviation, left atrial enlargement, right ventricular hypertrophy, P "mitrale" (wide, M-shaped P wave), atrial flutter or fibrillation	Restricted movement of mitral valve leaflets, decreased size of orifice	Left atrial pressure greater than left ventricular pressure at end of diastole, reduction in CO
MITRAL REGURGITATION			
Weakness; fatigue; dyspnea; peripheral edema, soft S_1; widely split S_2, S_3; pansystolic murmur	P mitrale, left ventricular hypertrophy, atrial flutter or fibrillation	Left atrial enlargement	Dye injection in left ventricle showing regurgitation of blood into left atrium
AORTIC STENOSIS			
Angina pectoris, syncope, heart failure, normal or soft S_1, prominent S_4, crescendo-decrescendo murmur	Left ventricular hypertrophy, left bundle branch block, complete atrioventricular heart block	Restricted movement of aortic valve, diminished orifice	Systolic pressure gradient with left ventricular pressure exceeding left atrial pressure, reduction in CO
AORTIC REGURGITATION			
Exertional dyspnea; orthopnea; nocturnal angina; Corrigan's pulse; soft or absent S_2; S_3 or S_4; soft decrescendo high-pitched diastolic murmur; low-frequency diastolic murmur (Austin-Flint murmur), especially in acute cases	Left ventricular strain or hypertrophy	Left ventricular dilatation	Increase in left ventricular diastolic pressure, aortic root dye injection demonstrating regurgitation of blood into left ventricle
TRICUSPID STENOSIS AND REGURGITATION			
Peripheral edema, ascites, hepatomegaly, presystolic or midsystolic murmur with increased intensity at inspiration (stenosis), pansystolic murmur with increased intensity at inspiration (regurgitation)	Tall, peaked P waves; atrial fibrillation	Right ventricular dilatation and paradoxical septal motion, usually no good visualization of tricuspid valve itself	Pressure gradient across tricuspid valve and increased right atrial pressure (stenosis), reflux of contrast medium into right atrium (regurgitation)

structures can result in regurgitation. Causes of chronic and acute mitral regurgitation are numerous and may be inflammatory, degenerative, infective, structural, or congenital in nature. The majority of cases may be attributed to chronic rheumatic heart disease, isolated rupture of chordae tendineae, mitral valve prolapse, ischemic papillary muscle dysfunction, and infectious endocarditis.[1]

Mitral valve prolapse syndrome, one important cause of mitral regurgitation, involves an abnormal prolapse of the mitral valve into the atria during systole.[28] The syndrome has been described by various names including *Barlow*

syndrome, the *systolic click-murmur syndrome, ballooning mitral cusp syndrome, floppy valve syndrome,* and the *effort syndrome.* Mitral valve prolapse exists in about 4% to 5% of the population, with a 2:1 female-to-male ratio in young adults and a more equal distribution between men and women in middle and older age groups. Causes of mitral valve prolapse have been suggested to be primary or idiopathic (including congenital malformation), secondary (e.g., Marfan's syndrome, rheumatic endocarditis), or an alteration in the CNS or autonomic nervous system. Clients with this syndrome generally have a benign, manageable course unless some severe problems associated with mitral regurgitation develop.

The regurgitant mitral orifice is parallel with the aortic valve, so the burden imposed on the left ventricle and left atrium are determined by the etiology, severity, and duration of the mitral regurgitation. In chronic mitral regurgitation, volume overload on the left ventricle, left atrium, and pulmonary bed is created by the backward flow of blood from the left ventricle into the left atrium during ventricular systole, resulting in varying degrees of left atrial enlargement and left ventricular dilatation. Acute mitral regurgitant states do not result in immediate dilatation of the left atrium or left ventricle. Without these acute changes in compliance to accommodate the regurgitant volume, acute pulmonary edema is produced from the severe pressure overload on the pulmonary vascular bed.

Clinical manifestations. Clients with chronic mitral regurgitation may remain asymptomatic for many years until development of some degree of left ventricular failure. Initial symptoms include weakness, fatigue, and dyspnea that gradually progress to orthopnea, paroxysmal nocturnal dyspnea, and peripheral edema. Palpitations, chest discomfort, fatigue, and anxiety are frequently described by clients with mitral valve prolapse. Auscultatory findings in mitral regurgitation may include an intermittent irregular rhythm, a soft first heart sound, a widely split second heart sound, a third heart sound, and a pansystolic murmur radiating toward the left axilla.

Aortic Stenosis

Etiology and pathophysiology. Congenitally abnormal stenotic aortic valves are generally discovered in childhood, adolescence, or young adulthood. Clients seen later in life acquired the stenosis from traumatic heart disease, calcific degeneration of a bicuspid valve, or senile calcific degeneration of a normal valve. In contrast to mitral stenosis, isolated aortic valve stenosis is almost always nonrheumatic in origin. If it does occur secondary to rheumatic fever, mitral valve disease accompanies the aortic stenosis.

Aortic stenosis results in obstruction to flow from the left ventricle to the aorta during systole. The effect is concentric left-ventricular hypertrophy and increased myocardial oxygen consumption because of the increased myocardial mass. As the disease course progresses and compensatory mechanisms fail, pulmonary hypertension and reduced CO occur.

Clinical manifestations. Symptoms of aortic stenosis (Table 31-18) generally develop when the valve orifice becomes one-third its normal size and classically include angina pectoris, syncope, and heart failure. The prognosis is poor for clients with symptoms and unrelieved obstruction. Survival times from onset of symptoms to time of death are 2 years in clients with heart failure, 3 years in those with syncope, and 5 years in those with angina.[27] Auscultatory findings of aortic stenosis typically reveal a normal or soft first heart sound, a prominent fourth heart sound, and a systolic, crescendo-decrescendo murmur that ends before the second heart sound.

Aortic Regurgitation

Etiology and pathophysiology. Aortic regurgitation may be the result of a primary disease of the aortic valve leaflets, the aortic root, or both. Valve leaflet damage is generally caused by rheumatic fever, infective endocarditis, trauma, degeneration of a biscuspid valve, or rheumatoid disease. Marfan's syndrome, syphilitic aortitis, ankylosing spondylitis, and aortic dissection are diseases that cause aortic regurgitation because of dilatation of the ascending aorta.

The basic physiological consequence of aortic regurgitation is retrograde blood flow from the ascending aorta into the left ventricle resulting in volume overload. The left ventricle initially compensates by dilatation and hypertrophy until myocardial contractility eventually declines and pulmonary hypertension and right ventricular failure develop.

Clinical manifestations. The client with chronic aortic regurgitation generally remains asymptomatic for years and is seen with exertional dyspnea, orthopnea, and paroxysmal nocturnal dyspnea only after considerable myocardial dysfunction has occurred (see Table 31-18). Angina pectoris occurs less frequently in aortic regurgitation than in aortic stenosis. However, a nocturnal angina accompanied by diaphoresis and abdominal discomfort may be present. Clients with acute aortic regurgitation have development of sudden clinical manifestations of cardiovascular collapse with weakness, severe dyspnea, and hypotension that generally constitutes a major medical emergency.

Clients with chronic, severe aortic regurgitation have pulses that are water-hammer or collapsing type with abrupt distention during systole and quick collapse during diastole *(Corrigan's pulse)*. Auscultatory findings may include a soft or absent first heart sound, presence of a third or fourth heart sound, and a soft, decrescendo high-pitched diastolic murmur. A systolic ejection murmur may also be heard, and the *Austin-Flint* murmur, a low frequency diastolic murmur similar to that of mitral stenosis, may be auscultated, particularly in clients with acute aortic regurgitation.

Tricuspid Valve Disease

Etiology and pathophysiology. Tricuspid stenosis is extremely uncommon and occurs almost exclusively in clients with rheumatic mitral stenosis. It is also seen in IV drug users. Tricuspid regurgitation is usually the result of pulmonary hypertension or right ventricular dysfunction.

In tricuspid stenosis, right atrial outflow is obstructed, resulting in right atrial enlargement and elevated systemic venous pressures. Volume overload of the right atrium and ventricle occurs in tricuspid regurgitation.

Clinical manifestations. Since both tricuspid stenosis and tricuspid regurgitation result in the backward flow of blood into the systemic circulation, common manifestations are peripheral edema, ascites, and hepatomegaly. The murmur of stenosis is presystolic (sinus rhythm) or midsystolic (atrial fibrillation), and a pansystolic murmur may be heard in regurgitation. Both types of murmurs dramatically increase in intensity with inspiration.

Pulmonic Valve Disease

Pulmonic valve disease is an uncommon entity and, in the case of pulmonary stenosis, is almost always congenital. Pulmonary regurgitation as an isolated abnormality has a benign course but is generally associated with disease of other valves.

Diagnostic Studies

Diagnosis of valvular heart disease is generally based on the results of an echocardiogram and a cardiac catheterization (see Table 31-18). Chest x-ray results, ECG findings, and the clinical manifestations exhibited by the client also aid in establishing the correct diagnosis.

An echocardiogram provides information on the structure and function of the valves and on enlargement of the chambers. Cardiac catheterization detects pressure changes in the cardiac chambers as well as pressure gradients across the valves. It also quantifies the size of the valve area. An ECG shows variation in the heart rate and rhythm and provides information about possible ischemia or chamber enlargement. A chest x-ray film reveals the heart size and alterations in pulmonary circulation.

Therapeutic Management

Conservative management. An important aspect of conservative management of valvular heart disease (Table 31-19) is prevention of recurrent rheumatic fever and infective endocarditis. Treatment of valvular heart disease depends on the valve involved and the severity of the disease. It focuses on preventing exacerbations of heart failure, acute pulmonary edema, thromboembolism, and recurrent endocarditis. If manifestations of CHF develop, digitalis, diuretics, and a low-sodium diet are recommended. Anticoagulant therapy is used to prevent and treat systemic or pulmonary embolization, and it is also used as a prophylactic measure in clients with atrial fibrillation. Dysrhythmias, especially atrial dysrhythmias, are common with valvular heart disease and are treated with digitalis, antidysrhythmic drugs, or electrical cardioversion. β-Adrenergic blocking drugs may be used to slow the ventricular rate in clients with atrial fibrillation.

Oral nitrates may be prescribed for clients with aortic valvular disease because the resulting peripheral vasodilatation reduces the blood volume returning to the heart and subsequently decreases the pressure gradient between the aorta and the left ventricle, allowing the ventricle to pump more effectively. In addition, nitrates improve coronary artery perfusion and reduce myocardial oxygen consumption.

Percutaneous transluminal balloon valvuloplasty. An alternative treatment for some clients with valvular heart disease is the percutaneous transluminal balloon valvuloplasty (PTBV) procedure (Fig. 31-11). Balloon valvuloplasty has been used for pulmonic, aortic, and mitral stenosis.[29] The procedure, performed in the cardiac catheterization laboratory, involves threading a balloon-tipped catheter from the femoral artery to the stenotic valve so that the balloon may be inflated in an attempt to separate the valve leaflets.[30] A single or double-balloon technique may be used for the PTBV procedure. A typical single balloon (the largest balloons available have a maximum infla-

Table 31-19

Diagnostic and Therapeutic Management: Valvular Heart Disease

DIAGNOSTIC

History and physical examination
Chest x-ray film
ECG
Echocardiography
Cardiac catheterization

THERAPEUTIC

Nonsurgical

Prophylactic antibiotic therapy
   Rheumatic fever
   Infective endocarditis*
Digitalis
Diuretics†
Sodium restriction
Anticoagulant agents
   Warfarin (Coumadin)
   Dipyramidole (Persantine)
   Aspirin
Antidysrhythmic drugs
Oral nitrates
β-Adrenergic blockers
Percutaneous transluminal balloon valvuloplasty

Surgical

Valvuloplasty
Closed commissurotomy
Open commissurotomy
Annuloplasty
Valve replacement

*See Table 31-6.
†See Table 29-6.

tion diameter of 25 mm) is shown inserted through the aortic valve orifice in Fig. 31-12. The double-balloon technique uses combinations of 10, 12, or 15 mm balloons inserted via each femoral artery to allow two balloons to be placed side by side into the valvular orifice, thus permitting a smaller arterial puncture and laceration.[31]

The PTBV procedure is generally indicated for older adult clients and clients who are poor surgical candidates. Complications and postprocedural care requirements are obviously lessened for those undergoing PTBV versus valve replacement, but the long-term results of PTBV have not been determined.

Surgical Interventions

The decision for surgical intervention is based on the client's clinical state as generally appraised through use of the New York Heart Association classification system for functional disability (see Table 29-4). The type of surgery used for a particular client depends on the valves involved, valvular pathology, severity of the disease, and the client's clinical condition.

Reconstructive or reparative procedures are often used

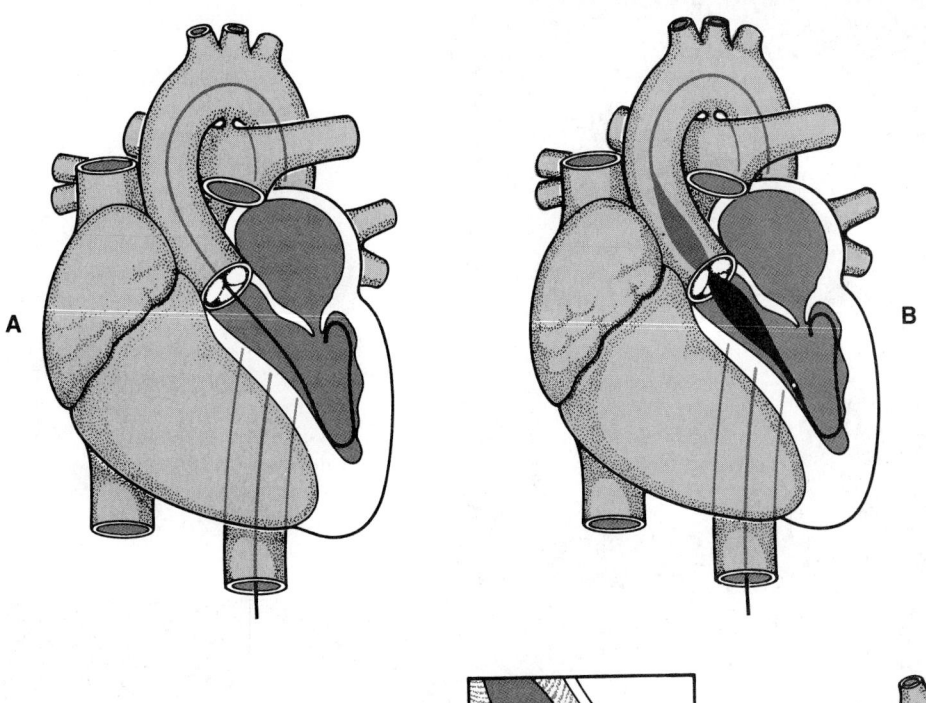

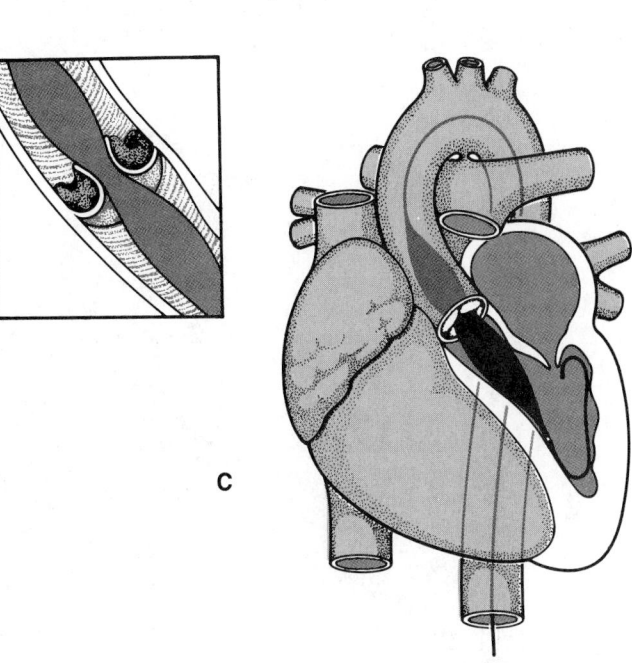

Fig. 31-11 PTBV procedure in a stenotic, calcific aortic valve. **A,** The loop of a wire guide, passed from the right femoral artery retrograde across the aortic valve, is seen nestling at the apex of the left ventricle. This positioning helps prevent perforation of the *C* ventricular wall and minimizes ventricular ectopy. **B,** A 20 mm dilating balloon catheter, having been passed antegrade over the guide wire, is partially inflated; the indentation is caused by the stenosed valve. **C,** Full inflation of the balloon *(inset)* opens the aortic valve orifice. (From Block PC: Balloon valvuloplasty, Cardiol Consult 9:4, 1988.)

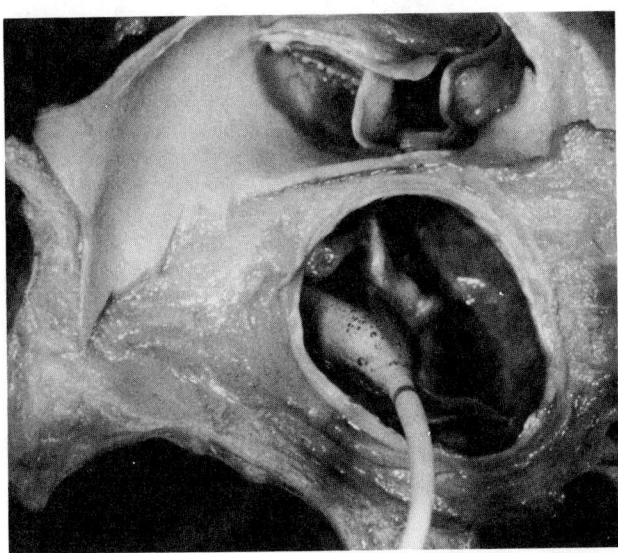

Fig. 31-12 Single balloon inflated through aortic valve orifice in the heart of a 73-year-old man with severe calcific aortic stenosis. Note that balloon does not occupy entire aortic valve opening, thereby allowing the client to maintain perfusion throughout balloon inflation. (From Nichols L and others: Percutaneous aortic valvuloplasty procedure and implications for nursing, Heart Lung 18:357, 1989.)

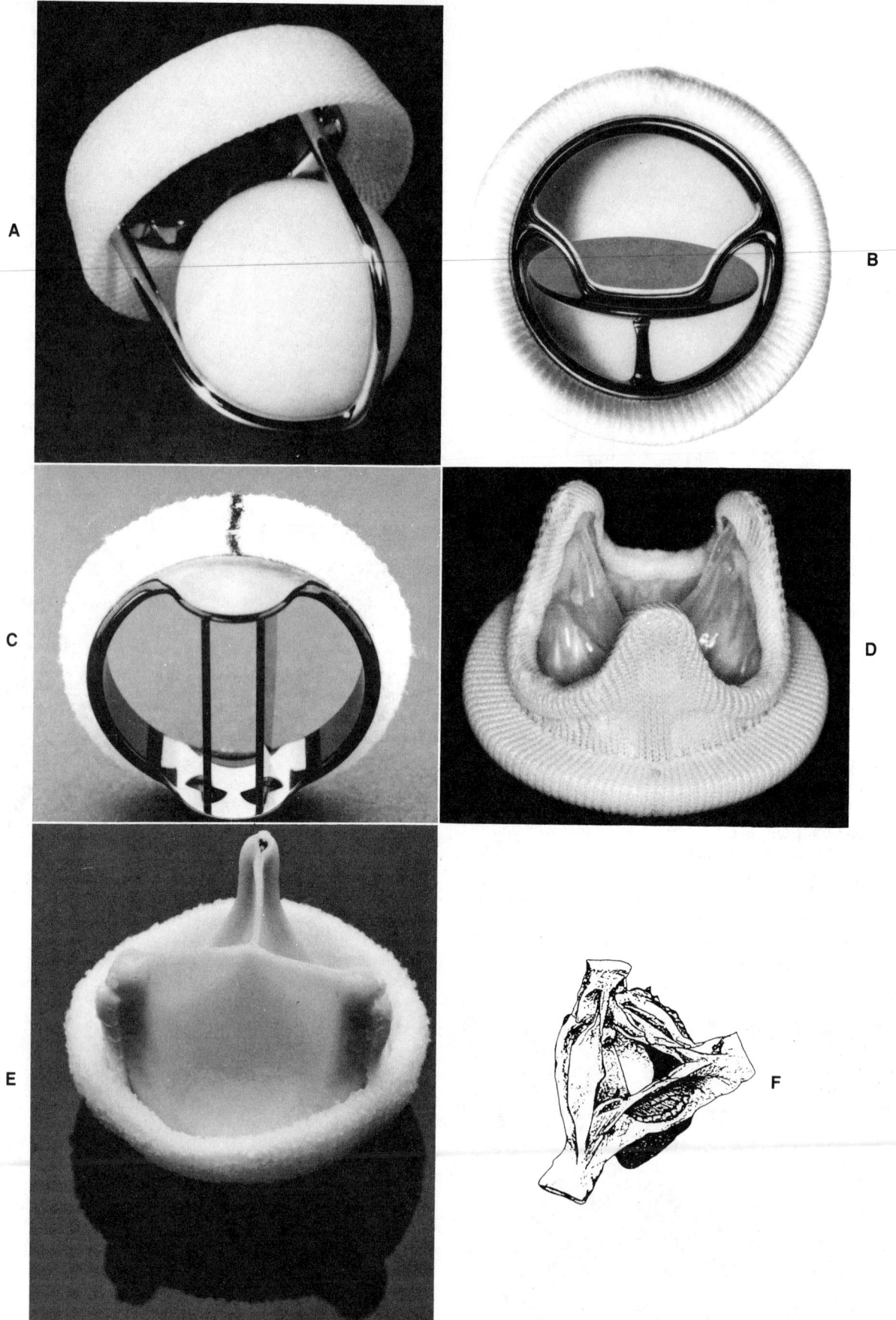

Fig. 31-13 Types of prosthetic and tissue valves. **A,** Caged-ball valve. (Courtesy American Edwards Laboratories, Santa Ana, Calif.) **B,** Tilting-disc valve. **C,** Bi-leaflet valve. **D,** Porcine xenograft. **E,** Pericardial xenograft. (**B, C, E,** Courtesy St. Jude Medical Inc, St. Paul, Minn. **D,** Courtesy Medtronic Inc, Irvine, Calif.) **F,** Homograft. (From Emery RW and Arom KV: The aortic valve, Philadelphia, 1991, Hanley & Belfus, Inc.)

Table 31-20 Types of Prosthetic and Tissue Valves

Type	Description	Advantages	Disadvantages
Caged-ball valve (Starr-Edwards)	Metal cage with several struts mounted on a circular ring, hollow metal or plastic ball (*poppet*) inside of cage	High durability (up to 20 years)	Possibility of blood clots forming on or around valve (thrombogenic) with risk of embolism Need for long-term anticoagulation therapy Very large size
Tilting-disc valve (Bjork-Shiley, Lillehei-Kaster)	Mobile, lens-shaped disc attached to a circular sewing ring by two offset transverse struts, pyrolytic carbon composition	Hemodynamic efficiency High durability	Tendency toward thrombogenicity and embolism Need for long-term anticoagulation therapy
Bi-leaflet valve (St. Jude Medical [SJM] Duromedics)	Two pivoting semicircular discs that open centrally mounted directly onto a sewing ring	Compact size—successful use in children and clients with small aortic roots	Possibility of thrombogenicity and embolism Need for long-term anticoagulation therapy
Porcine xenograft (Hancock, Carpentier-Edwards, Angell-Shiley [no longer manufactured])*	Harvested aortic-valve of pig that is preserved in glutaraldehyde and mounted on a specially designed sewing ring	Low thrombogenicity Need for anticoagulation therapy for only 3 mo after placement	Limited durability (failure rate up sharply after 5-7 yr) Cumbersome structural design
Pericardial xenograft (Ionescu-Shiley)*	Three leaflets composed of pericardium from 16- to 18-month-old calves that are preserved in glutaraldehyde and mounted on a Dacron-covered frame	Low thrombogenicity Need for only short-term anticoagulation therapy Less resistance to blood flow—useful in clients with small aortic roots	Limited durability
Homograft	Harvested aortic valve from human cadaver that is initially frozen until needed for valve replacement, then thawed, trimmed, and sewn into place with special mounting material	Excellent hemodynamics No hemolysis/low risk for embolism Only rare need for anticoagulation therapy	Limited durability No use for mitral or tricuspid valve replacement

*Heterograft.

in mitral or tricuspid valvular heart disease. *Mitral commissurotomy* (valvulotomy) is the procedure of choice for clients with pure mitral stenosis. The less precise *closed* (without cardiopulmonary bypass) method of commissurotomy has generally been replaced by the *open* method in the United States, Canada, and Western Europe.[26] The closed mitral commissurotomy is generally performed in developing nations in which there is a higher number of younger clients with juvenile or third-decade mitral stenosis. Cost considerations are a significant factor.[26] The closed procedure is usually performed with the aid of a transventricular dilator inserted through the apex of the left ventricle into the ostium of the mitral valve (versus previous use of a simple transatrial finger fracture). In contrast, the direct vision or open procedure entails the establishment of cardiopulmonary bypass, removal of thrombi from the atrium and its appendage, commissure incision, and as indicated, separation of fused chordae, splitting of underlying papillary muscle, and debriding of the valve of calcium.

Further reconstruction of the valve may be necessary and can be achieved by *annuloplasty*, a procedure also used in cases of mitral or tricuspid regurgitation. Annuloplasty entails reconstruction of the valve leaflets and the annulus, with or without the aid of prosthetic rings (e.g., a Carpentier ring).

Open surgical *valvuloplasty* involves repair of the valve and/or suturing of torn leaflets. It is primarily performed to treat mitral regurgitation or tricuspid regurgitation. The main advantage of a reparative procedure is that it avoids the risks associated with valve replacement. The disadvantage is that it may not be possible to establish total valve competence.

Prosthetic valves. Although these reparative procedures negate the need for long-term anticoagulation therapy required after prosthetic valve replacement, valvular replacement may still be required for mitral, tricuspid, and occasionally, pulmonic disease. The surgical treatment of choice for combined aortic stenosis and aortic regurgitation is valvular replacement (Fig. 31-13, Table 31-20).

Prosthetic valves have improved since the first caged-ball valve was introduced in 1952. Early valves disintegrated, stuck, became incompetent, changed the structure of chambers, caused emboli, and traumatized blood cells. Newer valves and improved surgical techniques have made valve replacement safer and long-term valvular functioning more effective. A wide variety of valves have been introduced in an attempt to find the most sound, nonthrombogenic, and durable valve.

The two categories of prosthetic valves are *mechanical* and *biological* (tissue) valves. Mechanical valves are made of combinations of metal alloys, pyrolite carbon, and Dacron. Biological valves are usually constructed from animal cardiac tissue. Mechanical prosthetic valves are more durable than biological tissue valves but have an increased risk of thromboembolism, which necessitates the use of long-term anticoagulant therapy. Biological valves offer the client freedom from anticoagulant therapy as a result of their low thrombogenicity. However, their durability is limited by the tendency for early calcification, tissue degeneration, and stiffening of the leaflets. Other problems associated with prosthetic valves include paravalvular leaks and endocarditis.

The choice of a valvular prosthesis depends on many factors. For example, if a client cannot take anticoagulant therapy (e.g., women of childbearing age), a biological valve may be considered. A mechanical valve may be considered for a younger client because it is more durable and lasts longer. In clients over the age of 65 the importance of durability is less of an issue, but the risks of hemorrhage from anticoagulants or noncompliance may be greater. (The care of the client requiring cardiac surgery is discussed in Chapter 29.)

■ Nursing Management of Valvular Disorders

Nursing assessment
Subjective and objective data should be obtained from an individual with valvular disease and are presented in Table 31-21.

Nursing diagnoses
Nursing diagnoses are determined when the problem and etiological factors are supported by clinical data. Nursing diagnoses related to valvular insufficiency may include, but are not limited to, those presented in Table 31-22.

Nursing interventions
Health maintenance and promotion. Prevention of acquired rheumatic valvular disease is achieved by (1) diagnosing and treating the streptococcal infection and (2) providing prophylactic antibiotics for clients with a history of rheumatic fever. Clients at risk for endocarditis must also be treated with prophylactic antibiotics.

Clients must adhere to recommended therapies. People with a history of rheumatic fever, endocarditis, and congenital heart disease should know the symptoms suggestive of valvular heart disease so that they may obtain early medical treatment.

Acute intervention and chronic management. A client with progressive valvular heart disease may require hospitalization or outpatient care for management of CHF, en-

---

Table 31-21

Nursing Assessment of the Client with Valvular Heart Disease

SUBJECTIVE DATA

History
Rheumatic fever, endocarditis, congenital defects, myocardial infarction, chest trauma, cardiomyopathy, syphilis, Marfan's syndrome, pregnancy, staphylococcal and streptococcal infections
Medications
IV drug use
General
Fatigue, weakness, dizziness, syncope
Pain
Anginal or atypical chest pain, neck pain
Respiratory
Dyspnea on exertion, paroxysmal nocturnal dyspnea, cough, hemoptysis, orthopnea
Cardiovascular
Palpitations

OBJECTIVE DATA

General
Fever
Integumentary
Diaphoresis, flushing, cyanosis
Respiratory
Rales, wheezes
Cardiovascular
Abnormal heart sounds, including opening snaps, clicks, thrills, systolic and diastolic murmurs, S_3, and S_4; dysrhythmias, including premature atrial contraction, atrial fibrillation; increase or decrease in pulse pressure; water-hammer pulse; peripheral edema
Neurological
Visual field deficits
Possible findings
Cardiomegaly, valve calcification, pulmonary congestion on chest x-ray film; decrease in excursion, calcification or vegetation of leaflets or prolapse, and chamber enlargement on echocardiogram; atrial and ventricular hypertrophy, dysrhythmias, conduction defects on ECG

---

docarditis, embolic disease, or dysrhythmias. CHF is the most common reason for ongoing medical care.

The nurse's role is implementing and evaluating the effectiveness of therapeutic management. Activity should be designed to consider the client's limitations. An appropriate exercise plan can increase cardiac tolerance. However, restricting activity that regularly produces fatigue and dyspnea should be explained to the client. Smoking should be discouraged. Strenuous physical exercise should be avoided because damaged valves may not be able to handle the required increase in CO. The client should be assisted in planning activities of daily living, with an emphasis on conserving energy, setting priorities, and taking

Table 31-22

NURSING CARE PLAN FOR THE CLIENT WITH VALVULAR HEART DISEASE

Defining Characteristics	Nursing Interventions	Evaluation Criteria

NURSING DIAGNOSIS: Potential complication: decreased cardiac output

Fatigue, malaise, shortness of breath, dyspnea on exertion, paroxysmal nocturnal dyspnea, palpitations, angina, vertigo, cardiac murmur, widened pulse pressure (aortic insufficiency)	Maintain bed rest as ordered. Elevate head of bed 30 to 40 degrees. Monitor BP, apical pulse, respirations q 4 hr and as needed. Auscultate breath sounds q 4 hr and as needed. Administer oxygen as ordered. Auscultate heart sounds q 4 hr and as needed. Monitor cardiac rhythm for changes from baseline. Document and determine dysrhythmia. Administer parenteral therapy as ordered; measure intake and output. Administer inotropic medication as ordered. Assess hemodynamic parameters (e.g., pulmonary artery pressure, pulmonary capillary wedge pressure, CO, central venous pressure) as ordered.	Demonstration of adequate CO

NURSING DIAGNOSIS: Activity intolerance related to insufficient oxygenation secondary to decreased cardiac output

Weakness, fatigue, altered response to activity such as shortness of breath, dyspnea, weak pulse with increase or decrease in rate, BP changes	Assess and monitor client responses to activity (e.g., pulse rate, respirations, BP). Plan rest periods between activities. Organize care to minimize unnecessary disturbance. Assist client with personal care as necessary. Increase activity as tolerated.	Demonstration of cardiac tolerance to increased activity (e.g., stable pulse, respirations, and BP)

NURSING DIAGNOSIS: Potential complication: hypervolemia related to cardiac failure

Peripheral edema; taut, shiny skin; adventitious breath sounds	Assess vital signs q 4 hr. Ausculate breath sounds q 4 hr. Assess for increased or decreased jugular distention. Measure intake and output. Palpate for edema. Assess for weight gain. Restrict sodium as ordered. Monitor laboratory findings, including electrolytes, hemoglobin and hematocrit, BUN and creatinine levels, urinalysis.	Decrease in peripheral edema; clear breath sounds

NURSING DIAGNOSIS: Altered health maintenance related to lack of knowledge about disease process, signs and symptoms of congestive heart failure and infective endocarditis, and prevention strategies

Verbalization of deficiency in knowledge regarding signs and symptoms of heart failure, infective endocarditis, procedures that predispose to bacteremia	Explain nature and cause of disease process. Teach signs and symptoms of heart failure and infective endocarditis and need to report all invasive surgical or diagnostic procedures that may predispose to bacteremia. Explain the importance of notifying the dentist, urologist, and gynecologist of valvular disease. Explain need for good oral hygiene and avoidance of fatigue. Discourage smoking. Explain the need for prophylactic antibiotic therapy.* Discuss the name of prescribed medication, dosage, purpose, and side effects. Instruct client to wear a Medic-Alert bracelet.	Verbalization of knowledge of disease process, complications, and preventive precautions

NURSING DIAGNOSIS: Sleep pattern disturbance related to nighttime awakening secondary to dyspnea and shortness of breath

Awakening during night, daytime fatigue	Elevate head of bed 30 to 40 degrees. Administer oxygen as ordered. Reassure client and remain with client until respirations stabilize. Eliminate environmental noise.	Verbalization of satisfaction with sleep, feeling of being rested on awakening

*See Tables 31-5 and 31-6.

Continued.

Table 31-22

NURSING CARE PLAN FOR THE CLIENT WITH VALVULAR HEART DISEASE—cont'd

Defining Characteristics	Nursing Interventions	Evaluation Criteria
NURSING DIAGNOSIS: Potential complication: systemic and pulmonary emboli		
Dyspnea, pain, diminished or absent peripheral pulses, changes in skin color and temperature	Monitor vital signs and neurological status q 4 hr and as needed. Auscultate breath sounds q 4 hr and as needed. Administer anticoagulants and oxygen as ordered. Assess peripheral pulses. Assess lower extremities for color, warmth, and edema. Reposition q 2 hr. Perform range of motion (active or passive) to extremities q 4 hr. Apply antiembolism stockings.	Absence of signs and symptoms indicative of embolization
NURSING DIAGNOSIS: Pain related to decreased coronary blood flow and increased myocardial oxygen demand secondary to decreased cardiac output		
Complaints of chest pain, nonverbal indicators of pain such as guarding and massaging painful area	Monitor vital signs q 4 hr and as needed. Observe for verbal and nonverbal expressions of pain and discomfort. Decrease activity as ordered. Administer analgesics and nitrates as ordered.	Minimization or control of angina

planned rest periods. Referral to a vocational counselor may be necessary if the client has a physically or emotionally demanding job.

Auscultatory assessment of the heart should be performed to monitor the effectiveness of digitalis, β-adrenergic blocking agents, and antidysrhythmic drugs. When prophylactic anticoagulants are used, the client should be instructed about possible side effects such as bleeding. The client's prothrombin values should be monitored frequently and be maintained at one and one-half to two times the control level. Clients should be instructed to wear a Medic-Alert bracelet.

Urinary output and daily weights should be monitored when diuretics are prescribed. The client's diet should be well-balanced nutritionally with sodium restriction to prevent fluid retention.

The client must understand the importance of prophylactic antibiotic therapy to prevent endocarditis (see Tables 31-4 and 31-5). If the valve disease was caused by rheumatic fever, prophylaxis to prevent recurrence is necessary.

Nurses should help clients achieve and maintain their optimal level of health despite the valvular disorder. Extensive teaching regarding drugs, actions, and side effects is important to achieve compliance. When valvular heart disease can no longer be managed conservatively, surgical intervention is necessary (see Chapter 29).

C ase Study

VALVULAR HEART DISEASE

Mrs. S. is a 54-year-old woman who has received medical care for 10 years. She was told that she had had strep throat as a child. Her rheumatic valve disease was diagnosed 10 years ago when she complained of a persistent cold, palpitations, and

ankle edema. A chest x-ray film and ECG revealed an enlarged left atrium. Auscultation revealed murmurs of mitral stenosis, mitral insufficiency, and aortic insufficiency.

She has an irregular pulse, increasing shortness of breath, and edema. She cannot make the bed without becoming dyspneic. Her physical examination is unchanged, although she has a few rales in the lung bases. She takes digoxin 0.25 mg twice a day.

Discussion Questions

1. Explain the cause of her valvular heart disease. What valves are most likely to become involved with rheumatic heart disease?
2. Differentiate between the pathogenetic characteristics and the clinical manifestations of mitral stenosis and mitral regurgitation.
3. Which other diagnostic procedures are recommended and what may they indicate?
4. In addition to digoxin, what other conservative treatment measures are usually indicated for valvular heart disease?
5. What are the types of valve surgery? Which ones are indicated for Mrs. S.?

R eview Questions

The number of the question corresponds to the same-numbered objective at the beginning of the chapter.

1. The microorganism most often responsible for acute endocarditis is
   a. *Streptococcus viridans*
   b. *Staphylococcus aureus*
   c. *Escherichia coli*
   d. *Pseudomonas* species
2. In the client with infective endocarditis the most common early clinical manifestation is
   a. a new heart murmur
   b. an old, more pronounced heart murmur

c. dyspnea on exertion

d. continuous or intermittent fever

3. The signs of possible embolization in the client with infective endocarditis include all the following *except*

a. rigid, painful abdomen

b. flank pain and hematuria

c. warm, moist extremities

d. confusion and diminished concentration

4. Prophylactic antibiotics are indicated to prevent infective endocarditis for high-risk individuals who

a. are undergoing any dental procedure

b. have acquired a viral respiratory tract infection

c. are entering the third trimester of pregnancy

d. are exposed to acquired immunodeficiency syndrome

5. Which of the following laboratory tests should be ordered for the client with infective endocarditis?

a. sedimentation rate

b. complete blood count

c. serum creatinine

d. blood culture

6. The drug of choice for treating clients with infective endocarditis is

a. penicillin

b. streptomycin

c. tobramycin

d. amphotericin B

7. The pain of pericarditis is

a. dull, aching, and generalized

b. sharp, stabbing, and worsened with inspiration

c. severe, gnawing, and worsened by sitting up

d. acute, piercing, and aggravated by leaning forward

8. The physician is notified immediately whenever the client with pericarditis develops which of the following?

a. a pericardial friction rub heard on auscultation

b. a drop of more than 10 mm Hg in arterial BP pressure during inspiration

c. the development of ST segment changes on the ECG that represent ischemia

d. an x-ray report stating that the cardiac silhouette is slightly increased

9. The most common complications of mitral stenosis include all the following *except*

a. ventricular dysrhythmias

b. pulmonary emboli

c. CHF

d. infective endocarditis

10. The surgical splitting of valve leaflets is identified as a

a. curettage

b. leaflet dilatation

c. valvuloplasty

d. commissurotomy

REFERENCES

1. Civetta JM, Taylor RW, and Kirby RR, eds: Critical care, Philadelphia, 1988, JB Lippincott Co, p 993.

2. von Reyn CF: Infective endocarditis, Hosp Med 23:105, 1987.

3. Lien EA, Solberg CO, and Kalager T: Infective endocarditis 1973-1984 at the Bergen University Hospital: clinical features treatment and prognosis, Scand J Infect Dis 20:239, 1988.

4. Robbins MJ, Eisenberg ES, and Frishman WH: Infective endocarditis: a pathophysiologic approach to therapy, Cardiol Clin 5:545, 1987.

5. Scrima DA: Infective endocarditis: nursing considerations, Crit Care Nurse 7:47, 1987.

6. Chambers HF and Sande MA: Infective endocarditis: basic scheme of pathogenesis, Hosp Med 23:175, 1987.

7. Marrie TJ: Infective endocarditis: a serious and changing disease, Crit Care Nurse 7:31, 1987.

8. Bisno AL: Antimicrobial prophylaxis for infective endocarditis, Hosp Pract 24:209, 1989.

9. Burden LL and Rodgers JC: Endocarditis—when bacteria invade the heart, RN 51:38, 1988.

10. Tucker SM and others: Patient care standards, St Louis, 1988, The CV Mosby Co, p 93.

11. Carpenito LJ: Nursing diagnosis—application and clinical process, Philadelphia, 1989, JB Lippincott Co, p 5.

12. Khan AH: Pericarditis: diagnosis and treatment, Hosp Med 23:43,46,48,52, 1987.

13. Lorell BH and Braunwald E: Pericardial disease. In Braunwald E, ed: Heart disease, ed 3, Philadelphia, 1988, WB Saunders Co, p 1487.

14. Owens-Jones S and Hopp L: Viral myocarditis, Focus Crit Care 15:25, 1988.

15. Grady KL and Constanzo-Nordin MR: Myocarditis: review of a clinical enigma, Heart Lung 18:347, 1989.

16. Smith ND and Abrams J: Valvular heart disease of rheumatic origin, Hosp Med 20:77, 88, 1984.

17. Stollerman GH: Rheumatic fever. In Braunwald E, ed: Harrison's principles of internal medicine, ed 11, New York, 1987, McGraw-Hill Book Co, p 952.

18. Rheumatic fever: making a comeback, Harvard Medical School Health Letter 23:105, 1988.

19. Stollerman GH: Return of rheumatic fever, Hosp Pract 23:100, 1988.

20. Conn HF and others: Conn's current therapy, Philadelphia, 1988, WB Saunders Co, p 92.

21. Stollerman GH: Rheumatic and heritable connective tissue diseases of the cardiovascular. In Braunwald E, ed: Heart disease, a textbook of cardiovascular medicine, ed 3, Philadelphia, 1988, WB Saunders Co, p 1710.

22. Amento EP: Rheumatic fever in children and adults. In Kelley W, ed: Textbook of internal medicine, ed 1, Philadelphia, 1989, JB Lippincott Co, p 1017.

23. Stollerman GH: Acute rheumatic fever and its management. In Hurst JW, ed: The heart, ed 6, New York, 1986, McGraw-Hill Book Co, p 1310.

24. Baas L and Kretton C: Valvular heart disease—its causes, symptoms and consequences, RN 50:30, 1987.

25. Lawrence PS and Wieczorek BH: Congenital valvular heart disease, J Cardiovasc Nurs 1:18, 1987.

26. Rackley CE, Edwards JE, and Karp RB: Mitral valve disease. In Hurst JW, ed: The heart, ed 6, New York, 1986, McGraw-Hill Book Co, p 754.

27. Braunwald E: Valvular heart disease. In Braunwald E, ed: Heart disease—a textbook of cardiovascular medicine, ed 3, Philadelphia, 1988, WB Saunders Co, p 1026.

28. Grass S and Utz SW: Mitral valve prolapse: a review of scientific and medical literature, Heart Lung 15:507, 1986.

29. Babic VV and others: Percutaneous mitral valvuloplasty retrograde, transarterial double-balloon technique utilizing the transseptal approach, Cathet Cardiovasc Diagn 14:229, 1988.

30. Cullen L and Laxson C: Ballooning open a stenotic valve, Am J Nurs 88:987, 1988.

31. Nichols L and others: Percutaneous aortic valvuloplasty procedure and implications for nursing, Heart Lung 18:356, 1989.

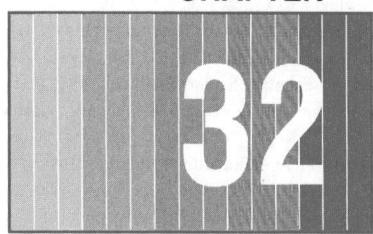

Nursing Role in Management
Vascular Disorders

Jeanne E. Doyle

1. Describe the pathophysiology, clinical manifestations, and surgical management of aortic aneurysms.
2. Outline the perioperative nursing care of a client after aortic aneurysm repair.
3. Describe the pathophysiology, clinical manifestations, and management of aortic dissection.
4. Identify the three risk factors most closely associated with atherosclerosis.
5. Describe the pathophysiology, clinical manifestations, and therapeutic and surgical management of peripheral arterial occlusive disease.
6. Outline the nursing management of the client with acute and chronic arterial insufficiency affecting the lower extremities.

7. Identify three risk factors predisposing to the development of thrombophlebitis.
8. Differentiate between the clinical characteristics of superficial and deep vein thrombophlebitis.
9. Describe the nursing management of the client with deep vein thrombophlebitis.
10. Explain the purpose and actions of commonly used anticoagulants and the nursing role for clients receiving them.
11. Describe the pathophysiology, clinical manifestations, and therapeutic and nursing management of pulmonary emboli.
12. Describe the pathophysiology and nursing management of venous stasis ulcers.

Problems of the vascular system include disorders of the aorta, arteries, veins, and lymphatic vessels. *Peripheral vascular disease* is a term used to describe a wide variety of conditions affecting these vessels in the neck, abdomen, and extremities.

DISORDERS OF THE AORTA
Aneurysms

Aneurysms are outpouchings or dilatations of the arterial wall and are a common problem involving the aorta. Aneurysms of peripheral arteries can also occur but are far less common. Aneurysms occur in men more often than in women, and their incidence increases with age.[1] They are seen most often in clients who are 70 to 80 years old and are considered uncommon before 50 years of age. Significantly, half of all aneurysms greater than 6 cm in diameter rupture within 1 year.[1,2]

Reviewed by Victora A. Fahey, R.N., M.S.N., Vascular Clinical Nurse Specialist, Northwestern Memorial Hospital, Chicago, Illinois.

Pathophysiology. The most common cause of aortic aneurysms is atherosclerosis. Plaques composed of lipids, cholesterol, fibrin, and other debris adhere along and beneath the intima or lining of the artery. Plaque formation causes degenerative changes in the media (middle layer of the arterial wall), leading to loss of elasticity, weakening, and eventual dilatation of the aorta. As these conditions occur, the pulsatile flow of the blood places added stress on the already weakened vessel and causes it to increase in size. The growth rate of aneurysms is unpredictable, but the larger the aneurysm, the greater the risk of rupture.

Atherosclerosis can affect the entire length of the aorta. However, most aneurysms related to atherosclerosis are found in the abdominal aorta, below the level of the renal arteries (see Chapter 28).

Other less common causes of aneurysm formation include syphilis, infections such as tuberculosis and bacterial endocarditis, congenital disorders such as coarctation of the aorta, and trauma.

Classification. Aneurysms are generally divided into two basic classifications, *true* and *false* (Fig. 32-1). A true

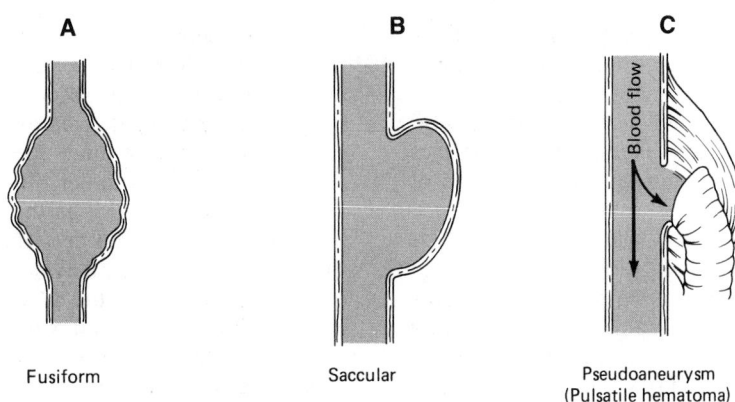

Fig. 32-1   **A,** True fusiform abdominal aortic aneurysm. **B,** True saccular aortic aneurysm. **C,** False or pseudoaneurysm (pulsatile hematoma).

aneurysm is one in which the wall of the artery forms the aneurysm, with at least one vessel layer still intact. Most commonly caused by atherosclerosis, three fourths of true aneurysms occur in the abdomen (Fig. 32-2) and one fourth in the thoracic aorta. Popliteal artery aneurysms rank third in frequency.

True aneurysms can be further subdivided into *fusiform* and *saccular* dilatations. A fusiform aneurysm is circumferential and relatively uniform in shape. A saccular aneurysm is pouchlike and has a narrow neck connecting the bulge to one side of the arterial wall.

A false or pseudoaneurysm is not an aneurysm but a disruption of all layers of the arterial wall resulting in a leak of blood that is contained or tamponaded by surrounding structures. False aneurysms may result from trauma, infection, or disruption of an arterial suture line after bypass surgery. They may also result from arterial leakage after removal of arterial cannulae such as upper extremity arterial catheters and intraaortic balloon pump devices.

Clinical manifestations. Thoracic aneurysms are usually asymptomatic. When manifestations are present, they are varied. The most common manifestation is deep, diffuse chest pain. Aneurysms located in the ascending aorta and the arch can produce hoarseness in the client as a result of pressure on the recurrent laryngeal nerve. Pressure on the esophagus can cause dysphagia. If the aneurysm presses on the superior vena cava, it can cause distended neck veins and edema of the head and arms. Pressure of the aneurysm on pulmonary structures can lead to coughing, dyspnea, and airway obstruction.

Abdominal aneurysms are most often asymptomatic and are often detected on routine physical examination or coincidentally when the client is being examined for an unrelated problem (e.g., abdominal x-ray film, intravenous pyelogram, or abdominal surgery). On physical examination a pulsatile mass in the periumbilical area slightly to the left of the midline may be detected. Bruits (murmurlike sounds resulting from turbulent blood flow) may be audible with a stethoscope placed over the aneurysm.

Symptoms of an abdominal aortic aneurysm may result from compression of nearby anatomic structures, for example, back pain caused by lumbar nerve compression or

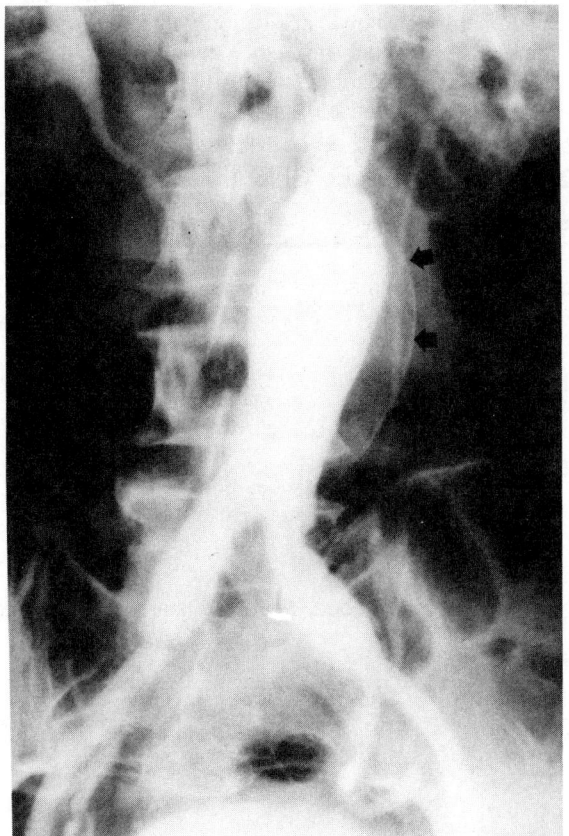

Fig. 32-2   Arteriogram demonstrating fusiform abdominal aortic aneurysm. Note calcification of the aortic wall *(arrows)* and extension of the aneurysm into the common iliac arteries. (Courtesy Jo Menzoian, Boston, Mass.)

epigastric discomfort with or without alteration in bowel elimination resulting from compression on the bowel.

Complications. Complications related to aneurysms can be catastrophic, the most common being rupture. If rupture occurs posteriorly into the retroperitoneal space, bleeding may be tamponaded by surrounding structures, preventing exsanguination. In this case the client has severe back pain and may or may not have back and/or flank ecchymosis as a result of the retroperitoneal bleeding (Turner's sign).

If rupture occurs anteriorly into the abdominal cavity, death from massive hemorrhage is likely. If the client does reach the hospital, presenting signs are manifestations of shock such as tachycardia, hypotension, pale clammy skin, decreased urine output, and altered sensorium, as well as abdominal tenderness on palpation.

Paraplegia is a rare but devastating possible complication. If the blood supply to the spinal cord is severely compromised as a result of rupture, prolonged hypotension, or prolonged clamp time during surgery, permanent paralysis may develop.

Diagnostic studies. Most aneurysms are found on routine physical or x-ray examination. Chest x-ray films are useful in demonstrating the mediastinal silhouette and any abnormal widening of the thoracic aorta. A plain film of the abdomen may show calcification within the wall of an abdominal aortic aneurysm.

When an electrocardiogram (ECG) is performed, it is used to rule out evidence of myocardial infarction (MI) be-

cause some persons may have symptoms suggestive of angina. Echocardiography assists in the diagnosis of aortic insufficiency related to ascending aortic dilatation. Ultrasonography or computerized axial tomography is the most accurate test to determine the anterior to posterior and cross-sectional diameter of the aneurysm and to identify the presence of thrombus in the aneurysm.

Aortography is often performed to locate the exact position of the aneurysm. Any structures receiving their arterial blood supply from the affected part of the aorta can be carefully studied with aortography.

Aortography is done with the use of a local anesthetic. A large needle with a stylet is inserted into the femoral artery, although a subclavian, axillary, brachial, or translumbar approach (through the back directly into the aorta) may also be used. A catheter is inserted and threaded into the artery through the needle. Contrast medium is then injected, and x-ray films are taken with fluoroscopy. When all films have been taken, the catheter is removed. Pressure is applied on the puncture site for 20 minutes or until the bleeding has stopped.

After the procedure the client should be kept in bed and

Table 32-1 Types of Aortic Aneurysm Resection

Location of Aneurysm	Incision Site	Use of Bypass or Hypothermia	Nursing Considerations
Ascending aorta with aortic valve insufficiency	Median sternotomy	Cardiopulmonary bypass and hypothermia are used.	Be aware that if aortic valvular insufficiency is severe, prosthetic valve replacement is performed.
Aortic arch	Median sternotomy	Cardiopulmonary bypass and hypothermia are used. If transverse aorta containing brachiocephalic vessels is involved, extracorporeal perfusion of brain is necessary.	Be aware that cold predisposes client to dysrhythmias. Watch neurological signs.
Descending thoracic aorta	Posterolateral at fourth intercostal space	Hypothermia is used. Cardiopulmonary bypass may be used.	Be aware that Carlen's tube (double-cuffed endotracheal tube) deflates either lung and causes pulmonary stress and atelectasis, that good pulmonary care is important, and that ischemia to spinal cord is common.
Abdominal aortic aneurysm	Xiphoid process to pubis	Bypass and hypothermia are not used. Arterial blood flow to lower extremities can be interrupted for time needed for surgical procedure.	Be aware that graft is placed within artery walls and that this technique prevents graft from eroding into surrounding structures such as bowel.
	Retroperitoneal (left flank, similar to nephrectomy incision)	Bypass and hypothermia are not used.	Be aware that because abdominal cavity is not entered, clients often have fewer problems with gastrointestinal and pulmonary dysfunction and less pain.

remain flat if the femoral site is used for injection. If the translumbar approach is used, the client's hematocrit level should be monitored carefully. Frequent observation of the arterial puncture site is essential to detect any bleeding. The peripheral pulses should be checked at the same time; embolism or vasospasm may occur, blocking arterial flow to the involved arm or leg.

Accurate intake and output should be recorded for at least 24 hours or up until surgery (if scheduled). Monitoring urine output is important for two reasons: (1) the injected contrast material is nephrotoxic and may impair renal function (especially in the client with diabetes) and (2) the contrast material is hyperosmolar and causes marked diuresis. It is important to prevent dehydration, especially in the preoperative client. Additionally, the serum blood urea nitrogen (BUN) and creatinine levels should be compared with pretest values as an indicator of acute renal failure.

Therapeutic management and surgical interventions. The goal of therapeutic management is to prevent rupture of the aneurysm. Therefore early detection and prompt treatment of the client are imperative. Once an aneurysm is suspected, studies are performed to determine its exact size and location. A careful review of all body systems is necessary to identify any coexisting disorders. The carotid and coronary arteries should be assessed for indications of atherosclerotic disease. If obstructions in these vessels are present, they may need to be corrected before the aneurysm repair. Generally, if coexisting problems are not severe, surgery is the treatment of choice. The type of surgery depends on the location of the aneurysm (Table 32-1).

The only effective treatment of an aortic aneurysm is surgery. Surgery to repair a fusiform aneurysm is known as *endoaneurysmorrhaphy*. The technique involves incising the diseased segment of the aorta; removing any intraluminal plaque; inserting a synthetic arterial graft (Dacron or polytetrafluoroethylene), which is sutured to the normal aorta proximal and distal to the aneurysm; and suturing the native aortic wall around the graft (Fig. 32-3). If the iliac arteries are also aneurysmal, the entire diseased segment is replaced with a bifurcation graft (Fig. 32-4).

Before surgery, every effort is made to bring the client to the best possible state of hydration and electrolyte balance. Any abnormalities in coagulation and blood cell count are corrected. Clients may receive antibiotics, enemas, and baths with antiseptics before surgery. However, if the aneurysm has ruptured, the treatment of choice is immediate surgical intervention. Even with prompt care, the mortality rate is high (about 50%) after rupture.

All aneurysm resections require cross-clamping of the aorta proximal and distal to the aneurysm. Because this obstructs blood flow to the lower extremities, the blood is systemically anticoagulated with IV heparin before cross-clamping the aorta. This prevents clotting of pooled blood distal to the aneurysm. Most resections can be completed in 30 to 45 minutes, after which time the clamps are removed and blood flow to the lower extremities is restored.

Fortunately, most abdominal aortic aneurysms originate below the origin of the renal arteries. However, if the an-

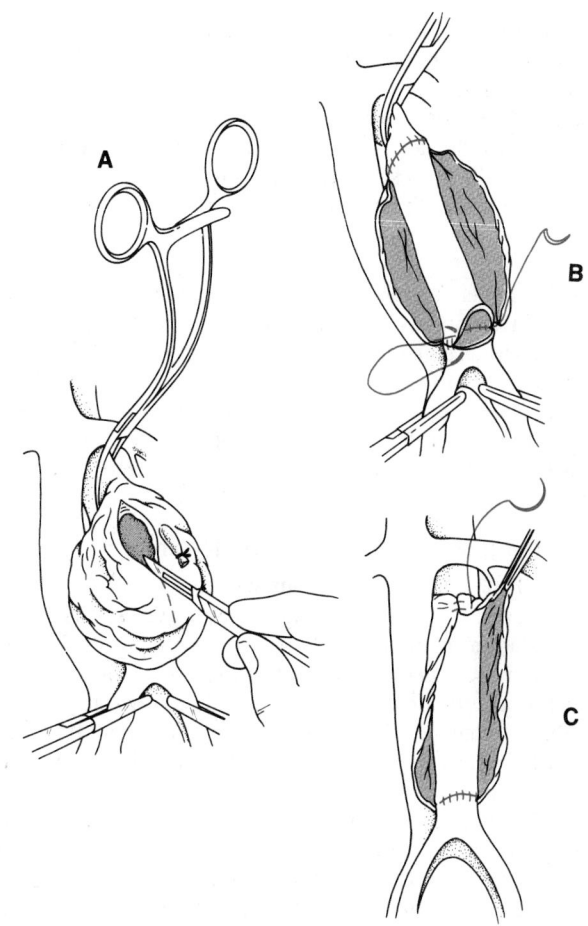

Fig. 32-3 Surgical repair of an abdominal aortic aneurysm. **A,** Incising the aneurysmal sac. **B,** Insertion of synthetic graft. **C,** Suturing native aortic wall over synthetic graft.

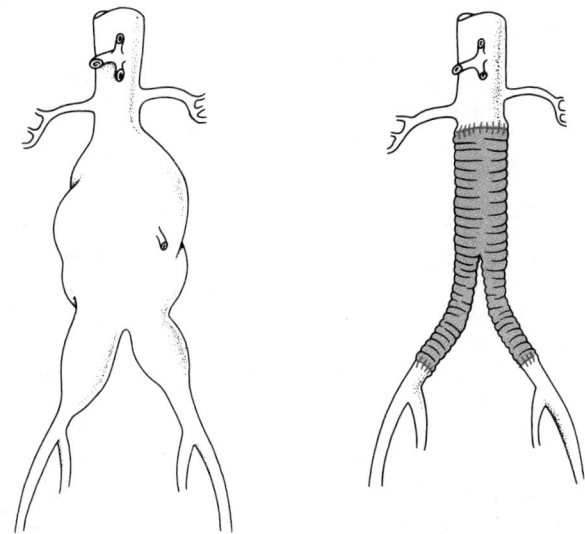

Fig. 32-4 Replacement of aortoiliac aneurysm with a bifurcated synthetic graft.

eurysm extends above the renal arteries or if the cross clamp must be applied above the renal arteries, adequate renal perfusion after removal of the clamp should be ascertained before closure of the abdominal incision.

With saccular aneurysms, it may be possible to excise only the bulbous lesion, repairing the artery by primary closure (suturing the artery together) or by application of an autogenous or synthetic patch graft over the arterial defect.

All clients undergoing aneurysmectomy should be placed in an intensive care unit (ICU) with appropriate support services and equipment postoperatively. When the client arrives in the ICU, an endotracheal tube, an arterial line, a central venous pressure or pulmonary artery catheter, peripheral IV lines, an indwelling catheter, and a nasogastric tube will likely be in place. If the thorax is entered during surgery, chest tubes will also be in place.

■ Nursing Management of Aneurysms

Health promotion and maintenance

The client with an aneurysm may have a variety of manifestations or may be totally free of symptoms. Therefore the nurse must use assessment skills to focus on early detection and treatment. Clients should be urged to receive regular routine physical examinations and should be reminded that any symptom, no matter how minor, must be investigated if it persists.

The incidence of syphilitic aneurysms has declined primarily because people are generally more aware of the manifestations of venereal disease and seek treatment earlier. Nurses need to encourage persons with venereal disease and their contacts to obtain appropriate therapeutic intervention in the course of the disease process. (Sexually transmitted diseases are discussed in Chapter 47.)

Nurses must be aware of cardiovascular disease risk factors and be alert for opportunities to teach health measures to clients in the hospital and the community (see Chapter 28). Trauma victims should be urged to seek medical attention even in the absence of symptoms.

Preoperative care

The nursing role during the preoperative period should include teaching, providing support for clients and their families, and carefully assessing all body systems. It is imperative that problems be identified early and proper intervention instituted (see Chapter 11).

A thorough nursing history and assessment should be performed. Because most aneurysms are atherosclerotic and atherosclerosis is a systemic disease process, it is likely that the disease process is present throughout the body. Therefore it is important for the nurse to watch for signs of cardiac, pulmonary, cerebral, and peripheral vascular problems. Clients should be monitored for signs of rupture of the aneurysm.

Establishing a data baseline is important for later postoperative assessment and intervention. In addition to gathering data, the nurse should observe the client closely for subtle abnormalities. Special attention should be paid to the character and quality of the peripheral pulses, the voice, and the neurological status. Arterial pulse sites in the lower extremities should be marked before surgery.

Postoperative care

In addition to maintaining adequate respiratory function, fluid and electrolyte balance, and pain control (see Chapter 13), the nurse needs to monitor graft patency, renal perfusion, and circulation. The nurse can also assist in preventing ventricular dysrhythmias, infections, and neurological complications (Table 32-2).

Graft patency. Patency of an aortic graft can be assured with maintenance of an adequate systemic blood pressure (BP). Prolonged hypotension may result in thrombosis of the graft as a result of decreased blood flow. Hypovolemia can be avoided by administration of IV fluids and blood components as indicated. Central venous pressure readings should be monitored hourly to help assess the client's state of hydration.

Marked hypertension may cause undue stress on the proximal and distal arterial anastomoses, resulting in leakage of blood or rupture at the suture line. Pharmacological intervention with diuretics or antihypertensive agents may be indicated if severe hypertension persists.

Ventricular dysrhythmias. Ventricular dysrhythmias are usually caused by hypoxia, hypothermia, or unrecognized electrolyte imbalances. Clients with coexisting coronary artery atherosclerosis are prone to dysrhythmias. Nursing interventions include cardiac monitoring and monitoring the results of electrolyte studies and arterial blood gas (ABG) determinations. Persons who return from surgery with hypothermia should be placed on hyperthermia blankets. Urinary output also needs to be monitored carefully.

Infection. The development of a prosthetic vascular graft infection can be a life-threatening complication. Nursing intervention to prevent infection should include ensuring that the client receives a broad-spectrum antibiotic as prescribed to maintain adequate blood levels of the drug. It is important to assess body temperature regularly and to report any elevations. Laboratory data should be monitored because a rising white blood cell (WBC) count may be the first indication of an infection. In addition, the nurse should ensure adequate nutrition, monitor serum albumin levels to ensure proper wound healing, and observe the wound for evidence of poor healing, signs of infection, or any unusual drainage.

All IV, arterial, and central venous catheter insertion sites should be assessed carefully with the use of sterile technique because they are frequently a portal of entry for bacteria. Meticulous perineal care for clients with indwelling urinary catheters is also essential to minimize the risk of urinary tract infection. Incisions should be kept clean and dry.

Gastrointestinal status. After abdominal aneurysm resection, paralytic ileus may develop as a result of the manual manipulation and displacement of the bowel for long periods during surgery. The intestines may become swollen and bruised, and peristalsis ceases for variable intervals.

A nasogastric tube is inserted and connected to low, intermittent suction. This decompresses the stomach and duodenum, prevents aspiration of stomach contents, and decreases pressure on suture lines. The nasogastric tube should be irrigated with normal saline solution as needed,

Table 32-2

 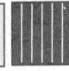

NURSING CARE PLAN FOR THE CLIENT AFTER AORTIC ANEURYSM REPAIR

Defining Characteristics	Nursing Interventions	Evaluation Criteria

NURSING DIAGNOSIS: Potential complication: altered renal perfusion related to renal artery embolism, prolonged hypotension, or prolonged aortic cross-clamping intraoperatively

Urine output <30 ml/hr, history of prolonged hypotension or aortic cross-clamping	Administer IV fluids as ordered. Check and record hourly urinary outputs and CVP. Monitor daily BUN and serum creatinine.	Urine output >30 ml/hr

NURSING DIAGNOSIS: Potential complication: paralytic ileus secondary to bowel manipulation, pain medication, and immobility

Absence of bowel sounds and flatus, abdominal distention, nausea and vomiting	Attach nasogastric tube to low suction. Irrigate with normal saline solution as needed and record drainage. Give frequent oral care while client is receiving nothing orally. Auscultate for bowel sounds q 4-8 hr. Palpate abdomen for distention. Encourage early ambulation when possible. Encourage turning q 2 hr while client is awake.	Normal bowel sounds, return of bowel function

NURSING DIAGNOSIS: High risk for infection related to presence of a prosthetic vascular graft and invasive lines

Elevated body temperature; elevated WBC count, pulse, and RR; purulent drainage from site of invasive line	Administer broad-spectrum antibiotics as ordered. Monitor temperature at least q 4 hr. Monitor WBC count. Use aseptic technique in caring for any indwelling IV line, tubing, or catheter.	Normal body temperature, no signs of infection

NURSING DIAGNOSIS: Potential complication: hypovolemia secondary to hemorrhage, extravascular fluid displacement, or prolonged osmotic diuresis

Decreased BP, increased pulse and RR, bright red bleeding in chest drainage bottle, decreasing mental status	Keep 4 units of packed RBCs available at all times. Observe drainage of chest tube (if inserted) for excessive bleeding. Monitor CVP, BP, and HR q hr and then with decreasing frequency. Check hemoglobin and Hct q 4-6 hr and as needed. Observe abdomen and record girth if abdominal distention appears to be developing.	Hct, BP, and HR within normal range

NURSING DIAGNOSIS: High risk for altered peripheral tissue perfusion related to bypass graft occlusion

Absence of peripheral pulses in lower extremities; cool, pale extremities; sensory changes in extremities; decreased CVP	Assess BP and all peripheral pulses hourly initially and then with decreasing frequency (e.g., q 2 hr, then q 4 hr). Compare extremities for warmth and color. Administer IV fluids at prescribed rates. Check CVP readings hourly.	Patent arterial graft with adequate distal perfusion

NURSING DIAGNOSIS: Potential complication: cardiac dysrhythmia related to hypothermia, electrolyte imbalance, or coexisting coronary artery disease

ECG evidence of dysrhythmias, anxiety, shortness of breath, syncope	Maintain temperature at about 37° C. Administer oxygen as ordered by ventilator or mask. Monitor the results of ABGs and serum electrolytes. Keep lidocaine 100 mg IV bolus at bedside for PVCs and administer as needed.	Baseline preoperative ECG rhythm

CVP, Central venous pressure; *Hct,* hematocrit; *HR,* heart rate; *WBC,* white blood cell, *RR,* respiratory rate.

Continued.

Table 32-2

NURSING CARE PLAN FOR THE CLIENT AFTER AORTIC ANEURYSM REPAIR—cont'd

Defining Characteristics	Nursing Interventions	Evaluation Criteria
NURSING DIAGNOSIS: High risk for sensory/perceptual alteration related to electrolyte imbalance, cerebral hypoxia, altered sensory input, and unfamiliar environment		
Decreased neurological status, confusion	Check chart for preoperative neurological status. Assess neurological status including level of consciousness, pupil size and response to light, movement of extremities, and hand grasp. Orient client frequently to person, time, and place. Provide uninterrupted rest periods, especially while in ICU. Monitor levels of serum electrolytes and ABG.	Return to baseline neurological status

and the amount and character of the drainage should be recorded. The nurse should auscultate for the return of bowel sounds. The passing of flatus can also be a sign of returning bowel function and should be reported.

If the arterial blood supply to the bowel is disrupted during surgery, ischemia or death of intestinal tissue may result. This is evidenced by lack of bowel sounds, fever, abdominal distention, and diarrheal stools. Fortunately, this serious complication is uncommon.

It is unusual for paralytic ileus to persist beyond the fourth postoperative day. While the client is receiving nothing orally (NPO), thorough mouth care should be given every few hours.

Neurological status. Neurological complications can occur after surgical procedures on the aorta, especially when the ascending aorta and arch are involved. Nursing intervention should include assessment of neurological signs (hourly initially after surgery and frequently thereafter) including level of consciousness, pupil size and response to light, ability to move all extremities, and quality of hand grasps (see Chapter 50). These should be recorded in detail with a careful description of the client's response. Any function decreased from the baseline assessment should be reported to the physician immediately.

Circulatory status. The anatomical location of the aneurysm indicates the areas of major concern related to circulatory status. All peripheral pulses should be checked regularly and recorded. This should be done every hour for the first 24 hours and routinely thereafter at frequent intervals. Pulses to be assessed include the dorsalis pedis, posterior tibial, popliteal, and femoral as well as the brachial, radial, carotid, and temporal pulses (see Fig. 26-8).

When checking the pulses, the nurse should mark the location lightly with a ballpoint or felt-tip pen so that others can find them easily. It is also important to note the temperature, color, and movement of the extremities.

It is not unusual for pulses in the lower extremities to be absent briefly after surgery. This is usually due to vasospasm and hypothermia. A decreased or absent pulse in conjunction with a cool, pale, mottled, or painful extremity may indicate embolization of debris from the aneurysm or occlusion of the graft. These findings should be reported to the surgeon immediately.

Renal perfusion. One of the causes of decreased renal perfusion is the possible dislodgement of a fragment of debris from the aorta that subsequently lodges in one or more renal arteries. This can cause obstruction and ischemia of one or both kidneys. Hypotension, poor hydration, prolonged aortic clamping, or blood loss can also lead to decreased renal perfusion.

The client returns from surgery with an indwelling urinary catheter in place. An accurate record of fluid intake and urinary output should be kept until the client resumes the preoperative diet. If hourly urine output drops below 30 ml/hr for 2 consecutive hours, the physician should be notified. Central venous pressure readings also give important information regarding hydration. Daily BUN and serum creatinine studies are performed to evaluate renal function.

Chronic management

Clients may be apprehensive about returning home after major surgery involving the aorta. They should be encouraged to express their concerns and should be reassured that they can return to activities of normal living. Sexual dysfunction in male clients is not uncommon after aneurysm repair surgery. Clients should be taught to observe for changes in color or warmth of the extremities. They can also be taught to take peripheral pulses and to assess changes in their quality.

Aortic Dissection

Aortic dissection, occurring most commonly in the thoracic aorta, is a longitudinal splitting of the medial layer of the artery by a column of blood. Aortic dissection affects men more often than women and occurs most frequently between the fourth and seventh decades of life. If not treated, acute aortic dissection has a 90% mortality rate.[3]

Pathophysiology. Aortic dissection, often misnamed "dissecting aneurysm," results from a small tear in the intimal lining of the artery, allowing blood to "track" between the intima and media; thereby creating a false lumen of blood flow. As the heart contracts, each systolic pulsation causes increased pressure on the damaged area, which further increases the dissection. As it extends proximally or distally, it may occlude major branches of the aorta, cutting off blood supply to the areas such as the brain, abdominal organs, spinal cord, and extremities. Occasionally a small tear develops distally and the blood flow reenters the true vessel lumen.

Arterial dissection differs from an aneurysm in that a false lumen is formed by separation of the intima from the media in dissection. In contrast, a true aneurysm is characterized by an outpouching from a weakened medial layer.

The exact cause of dissection is uncertain. Many authorities believe cystic medial necrosis (destruction of the medial layer elastic fibers) to be the leading cause of the problem. Most people with dissection problems have hypertension. Persons with Marfan's syndrome (a disease of the connective tissue) have a high incidence of dissection. Pregnancy also promotes vascular stress as a result of increased blood volume. Areas that seem to undergo the greatest amount of stress and are thus most prone to dissection are the ascending aorta, the aortic arch, and the descending aorta beyond the origin of the left subclavian artery.

Classification. Aortic dissections are usually identified by the DeBakey classification. *Type I* refers to dissections involving the ascending aorta and the aortic arch and extending into the abdominal aorta. *Type II* refers to dissections involving only the ascending aorta. *Type III* dissections are located in the portion of the aorta distal to the left subclavian artery and extending distally into the thoracic or abdominal aorta.

Clinical manifestations. The client with aortic dissection usually has sudden, severe pain in the back, chest, or abdomen. The pain is described as "tearing" or "ripping." The severe pain may mimic that of MI. As the dissection progresses, pain may be located both above and below the diaphragm. Dyspnea may also be present.

If the arch of the aorta is involved, the client may exhibit neurological deficiencies, including an altered level of consciousness, dizziness, and weakened or absent carotid and temporal pulses. An ascending aortic dissection usually produces some degree of aortic valvular insufficiency, and a murmur is audible on auscultation.[2] Severe insufficiency may produce left ventricular failure with the development of dyspnea and orthopnea caused by pulmonary edema. When either subclavian artery is involved, pulse quality and BP readings may vary between the left and right arms. As the dissection progresses down the aorta, the abdominal organs and lower extremities may begin to demonstrate evidence of altered tissue perfusion.

Complications. A severe complication of dissection of the ascending aortic arch is *cardiac tamponade*, which occurs when blood escapes from the dissection into the pericardial sac. Clinical manifestations include narrowed pulse pressure, distended neck veins, muffled heart sounds, and pulsus paradoxus (see Chapter 31).

Because the aorta is weakened by the medial dissection, it may rupture. Hemorrhage may occur into the mediastinal, pleural, or abdominal cavities.

Dissection can lead to occlusion of the arterial supply to many vital organs. The spinal cord, kidneys, and abdominal structures are the organs most commonly affected. Ischemia of the spinal cord produces symptoms varying from weakness to paralysis in the lower extremities and decreased pain sensation. Renal ischemia is usually mani-

Table 32-3

Diagnostic and Therapeutic Management: Aortic Dissection

DIAGNOSTIC

History and physical examination
ECG
Chest x-ray film
Echocardiography
Aortography

THERAPEUTIC

Bed rest
Pain relief with narcotics
Control of BP
   Trimethaphan (Arfonad)
   Sodium nitroprusside (Nipride)
   Methyldopa (Aldomet)
   Guanethidine (Ismelin)
Propranolol (Inderal)
Aortic resection and repair

fested by low urinary output. The abdomen will show signs of ischemia by decreased bowel sounds and altered bowel elimination.

Diagnostic studies. The diagnostic studies used to assess dissection of the aorta are similar to those performed for aneurysms (Table 32-3). An ECG is done to rule out the possibility of an MI. Left ventricular hypertrophy is a common finding and is possibly related to changes caused by systemic hypertension. A chest x-ray film may show a widening of the mediastinal silhouette, and left pleural effusion is not uncommon. After the client's condition has stabilized, aortography is necessary to assess the extent of the dissection.

Therapeutic management. The goal of therapy for aortic dissection without complications is to lower the BP and myocardial contractility to diminish the pulsatile forces within the aorta (see Table 32-3). The use of trimethaphan (Arfonad) and nitroprusside (Nipride) IV rapidly reduces the BP. Guanethidine (Ismelin) or methyldopa (Aldomet) is administered to provide long-term control. Propranolol (Inderal) is also used to decrease the force of myocardial contractility.

Clients with dissection without complications can safely be treated for a long time. Supportive treatment is directed toward pain relief, blood transfusion (if required), and management of heart failure (if indicated). If the dissection is limited to the descending aorta, conservative therapeutic management is usually adequate to treat the problem. If the dissection involves the ascending aorta, surgery is usually indicated.

Surgery is also indicated when drug therapy is ineffective or when complications of aortic dissection (e.g., heart failure, leaking dissection, occlusion of an artery) are present. The aorta is fragile during the acute phase. Therefore surgery is delayed for as long as possible to allow time for edema in the area of dissection to clear, to permit clotting of the blood in the false lumen, and to allow the healing process to begin.

Surgery for aortic dissection involves resection of the aortic segment containing the intimal tear and replacement with a synthetic graft material. The extent of aortic replacement varies depending on the extent of the dissection.

■ Nursing Management of Aortic Dissection

Nursing management related to an aortic dissection includes keeping the client in bed in a semi-Fowler's position and maintaining a quiet environment. These measures assist in keeping the systolic BP at the lowest possible level. Narcotics and tranquilizers should be administered as ordered. Anxiety and pain must be alleviated because they increase the BP.

Continuous IV administration of antihypertensive agents requires close nursing supervision. A cardiac monitoring device is used, and an intraarterial pressure line is usually inserted (see Chapter 28). The nurse should observe for changes in the quality of peripheral pulses and for signs of increasing pain, restlessness, and anxiety. Vital signs are taken frequently, sometimes as often as every 2 to 3 minutes. A widening pulse pressure may indicate increasing aortic valvular insufficiency. If the blood vessels branching off the aortic arch are involved, decreased cerebral blood flow may alter the sensorium and level of consciousness.

Postoperative care after surgery to correct the dissection is similar to that after aneurysmectomy (see p. 922). The exception is that most clients require continuation of their IV antihypertensive drug therapy.

In preparation for discharge, the nurse needs to focus on client and family teaching. The therapeutic regimen includes antihypertensive drugs, which are usually taken orally. The client needs to understand that these drugs must be taken to control BP. Propranolol can be taken orally to continue to decrease myocardial contractility. It is vitally important that the client understand the drug regimen. The nurse should instruct the client that if the pain returns or other symptoms progress, the client must immediately return to the health care facility.

Aortitis

Aortitis (aortic arch syndrome, Takayasu's disease, pulseless disease) is a rare inflammatory disorder with occlusion of the aorta and one or more of the large arteries that branch off from the thoracic aorta. The terms *aortic arch syndrome* and *pulseless disease* are used to describe this clinical problem.

Occlusion of the carotid and subclavian arteries secondary to aortitis most commonly affects Orientals, particularly young women less than 40 years of age. This disease syndrome is frequently called *Takayasu's disease*. Aortitis of the lower thoracic and abdominal aorta occurring in young women and children in the tropics is similar to Takayasu's disease.

Aortitis is not common in the United States. The most common infectious form is due to syphilis. Noninfectious aortitis has been associated with Hodgkin's disease, scleroderma, rheumatoid arthritis, and ankylosing spondylitis.

Clinical manifestations. Clinical manifestations vary with the extent and location of the occlusion, the degree of collateral circulation, and the number of vessels involved. Initial manifestations of an acute disorder are fever, joint pain, weight loss, malaise, and headache.

After several years, symptoms of peripheral vascular insufficiency appear in the form of a nonspecific inflammatory process. The vessel intima is markedly proliferated, scarred, and fibrotic, and the media is thickened. Pulse deficits can be detected. Vascular bruits and hypertension are also present. Retinal changes and left ventricular failure may result from the hypertension. The mortality rate is about 18%, with the leading causes of death being congestive heart failure (CHF) and cerebrovascular accidents.[4]

Therapeutic management. Management is symptomatic for hypertension and CHF. In general, treatment has not been satisfactory. The role of steroids is not proved. Antibiotics and immunosuppression have not been effective. Surgery may be necessary if vascular insufficiency is severe.

ACUTE ARTERIAL OCCLUSIVE DISORDERS
Pathophysiology

Acute arterial occlusion occurs suddenly without warning signs. It can be caused by embolism, thrombosis of an already narrowed artery, or trauma. Embolization of a thrombus from the heart or an atherosclerotic aneurysm is the most frequent cause of acute arterial occlusion. Heart conditions in which thrombi are prone to develop include infective endocarditis, MI, mitral valve disease, chronic atrial fibrillation, cardiomyopathies (see Chapter 29), and prosthetic heart valves. The thrombi become dislodged and may travel to the lungs if they originate in the right side of the heart or to anywhere in the systemic circulation if they originate in the left side of the heart.

Arterial emboli tend to lodge at sites of arterial branching or in areas of atherosclerotic narrowing. After an acute arterial occlusion the blood supply distal to the embolus decreases. The degree and extent of manifestations produced depend on the size and location of the obstruction, the occurrence of clot fragmentation with embolism to smaller vessels, and the degree of peripheral vascular disease already present.

Sudden local thrombosis may occur at the location of an atherosclerotic plaque. Traumatic injury to the extremity itself may produce partial or total occlusion of a vessel from compression, shearing, or laceration. Acute arterial occlusion may also develop as a result of arterial dissection in the carotid artery or aorta or as a result of iatrogenic arterial injury (e.g., after arteriography) (see p. 925).

Clinical Manifestations

Symptoms usually have an abrupt onset. The exception is when a sudden occlusion is superimposed on preexisting chronic arterial insufficiency. In this case the symptoms may be insidious because collateral circulation is well developed.

Clinical manifestations of acute arterial occlusion include the "five *P*'s": *p*ain, *p*allor, *p*ulselessness, *p*aresthesia, and *poikilothermia* (adaptation of the ischemic limb to its environmental temperature, most often cool). Without immediate intervention, ischemia may progress to tissue necrosis and gangrene. Because nerve tissue is extremely sensitive to lack of oxygen, ischemic neuropathy may persist after revascularization, and it may not be permanent.

Therapeutic Management

With true acute arterial occlusion in the absence of adequate collateral circulation to keep the limb viable, early treatment is essential to save the affected limb. Anticoagulant therapy is initiated immediately to prevent further enlargement of the occluding clot and inhibit embolization. Continuous IV heparin is the agent of choice. The occlusion should be removed as soon as possible. Balloon catheters can sometimes be used and are passed distal and proximal to the site to remove extensions of the clot material. This procedure can be done with the use of local anesthetics. Direct arteriotomy to perform an embolectomy or thromboendarterectomy may be necessary.

If the client remains at risk for further embolization from a persistent source such as chronic atrial fibrillation, long-term treatment includes oral anticoagulation to prevent further acute episodes.

Recently formed emboli may be effectively treated with intraarterial or systemic infusion of a thrombolytic agent such as urokinase or streptokinase. These drugs work by directly dissolving the clot. Although sometimes effective, they are also associated with a fairly high incidence of bleeding complications. Therefore clients should be carefully selected and drug administration should be prescribed and monitored by experienced critical care providers.

Acute Occlusion of the Aortic Bifurcation

Acute occlusion of the aortic bifurcation is an uncommon but catastrophic event. It may occur as a result of a large embolus (saddle embolus), aortic dissection, or sudden thrombosis. A saddle embolus often originates in the heart of a client with chronic atrial fibrillation, mitral valve disease, or following MI. Each of these conditions can result in formation of blood clots on the inside wall of the heart, which can then embolize into systemic circulation when the heart contracts. Acute thrombosis may result from abdominal trauma or chronic atherosclerotic disease.

Clinical manifestations include moderate to severe leg pain. The legs are cold, pale, and pulseless. Total paralysis of both legs may occur.

Treatment is immediate surgical intervention. A saddle embolus can sometimes be removed from the aorta by inserting an embolectomy catheter into the left femoral artery and pulling out the clot. This treatment approach is most effective in the acute stage of occlusion. An aortofemoral bypass may be necessary for aortic thrombosis. Postoperative care is similar to that for abdominal aortic aneurysm surgery.

CHRONIC ARTERIAL OCCLUSIVE DISEASE
Aortoiliac Disease

Slowly progressive atherosclerotic occlusion of the terminal aorta and iliac vessels results in a symptom complex known as *aortoiliac disease* or *Leriche's syndrome*. It predominantly affects men between the ages of 40 to 60 years.

Symptoms depend on the degree of arterial narrowing. A characteristic clinical manifestation is pain in the hip, buttocks, or thighs caused by exercise and relieved by rest. *Intermittent claudication* (development of pain in working muscles while walking but subsiding with rest) in the calf may also be present with superficial femoral or popliteal artery disease. If atherosclerosis has been continuous for a long time, collateral circulation may prevent gangrene of the extremity. Peripheral pulses in the lower extremities are diminished or absent. Impotence is a common problem with aortoiliac disease. The genitalia are supplied with blood through the internal iliac arteries, which may be stenotic or occluded.

In clients with incapacitating symptoms the treatment of choice is surgery, consisting of an aortofemoral bifurcation graft. In certain high-risk clients an extraanatomical bypass (e.g., axillofemoral, femoral-femoral) may be chosen.

Lower Extremity Disease

Peripheral chronic arterial occlusive disease involves progressive narrowing and eventual obstruction of the arteries to the extremities, occurring predominantly in the legs. It may affect the aortoiliac, femoral, popliteal, tibial, or peroneal vessels or any combination of these areas (Fig. 32-5). Chronic arterial occlusion is a slowly progressive, insidious disease primarily attributed to the atherosclerotic process; hence the term *arteriosclerosis obliterans* is used. It usually occurs in the sixth through eighth decades of life, affects primarily men, and has a familial tendency (see Chapter 54).

Etiology and pathophysiology. The leading cause of chronic arterial occlusion is atherosclerosis, which leads to narrowing of the vessel lumen. Atherosclerosis primarily affects larger arteries. The involvement is generally segmental with normal segments interspersed between involved ones. By the time symptoms occur, the vessel is 75% narrowed.[5] The femoral-popliteal area is the site most commonly affected.

The three most significant risk factors for peripheral arterial disease are cigarette smoking, hyperlipidemia, and hypertension. Others are diabetes mellitus, a positive family history, obesity, and a sedentary lifestyle.

Chronic arterial obstruction leads to progressively inadequate oxygenation of the tissues supplied by the obstructed arteries. The pain attributable to ischemia is produced by end products of anaerobic cellular metabolism such as lactic acid. This usually occurs in the larger muscle groups of the legs during exercise. Once the client stops exercising, the metabolites are cleared and the pain subsides. As the disease process becomes advanced, pain develops at rest. This finding indicates insufficient blood flow to the skin and subcutaneous tissues. The client may notice resting foot pain more often at night and achieve partial relief by lowering the limb below heart level (e.g., dangling the leg over the side of the bed).

Clinical manifestations. The severity of the clinical

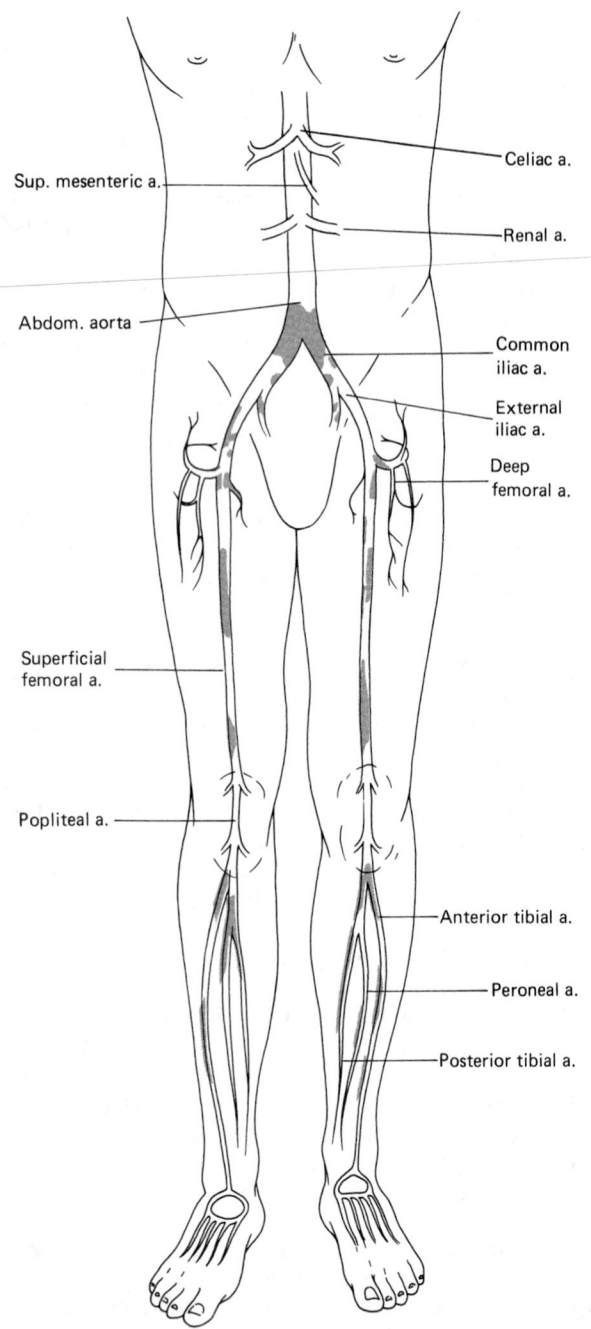

Fig. 32-5 Common anatomical locations of atherosclerotic lesions of the abdominal aorta and lower extremities.

Table 32-4 Chronic Arterial and Venous Insufficiency of the Lower Extremities

Arterial	Venous
No edema	Edema around ankles, sometimes feet
Loss of hair on legs, feet, toes; thickening of nail beds; thinning of skin, overall coolness; dependent rubor	Cyanosis, dermatitis characterized by brown pigmentation; scaling eczema
Ulceration over bony prominences and pressure points on toes and feet	Ulceration around ankle, above or below medial malleoli
Claudication (muscular leg or buttock pain with exercise)	Dull ache or heaviness in calf or thigh
Decreased or absent peripheral pulses	Presence of peripheral pulses

occurs in as many as 30% of clients with aortoiliac occlusion.[6,7]

Ischemic pain at rest occurs as the disease becomes more severe. This is an ominous symptom. Without revascularization the limb will progress to ulceration and gangrenous necrosis. Every attempt is made to save the limb, and surgery is always indicated unless the client is at exceedingly high risk.

Paresthesia, manifested as numbness or tingling occurring in the toes or feet, may result from nerve tissue ischemia. True peripheral neuropathy occurs more commonly in clients with diabetes and in those with progressive longstanding arterial obstruction. It produces excruciating shooting or burning pain in the extremity. It does not follow any particular nerve roots but may be present near ulcerated areas. Gradually diminishing perfusion to nerve tissue cells produces loss of both sensation and deep pain. Therefore injuries to the extremity often go unnoticed.

The physical appearance of the limb as a result of postural changes provides important information about the adequacy of blood flow. Pallor or blanching on elevation indicates significant arterial occlusion. Hyperemia (redness) and a bluish or dusky appearance are observed when the limb is allowed to hang in a dependent position (dependent rubor). The skin becomes shiny and taut and there is a loss of hair on the lower legs. Diminished or absent pedal, popliteal, or femoral pulses may be noted.

Complications. Chronic peripheral arterial disease progresses slowly. Prolonged ischemia leads to atrophy of the skin and underlying structures. Because of the decreased ability to heal, infection and necrosis may result from trauma to the feet. Ischemic ulcers caused by arterial insufficiency most commonly occur over bony prominences on the toes and feet. (This contrasts to ulcers of venous insufficiency, which occur around the malleoli and lower parts of the leg [Table 32-4].) If severe ischemia persists, gangrene can develop. Ischemic ulcers and gan-

manifestations depends on the site and extent of the occlusion as well as the adequacy of collateral circulation (Table 32-4). The classic symptom of peripheral arterial disease is intermittent claudication, defined as ischemic muscle pain that is precipitated by a predictable amount of exercise and relieved by resting. Disease involving the femoral or popliteal arteries may cause claudication in the calf. Occlusive disease of the aortoiliac arteries may produce claudication in the buttocks and upper part of the thighs. If disease extends into the internal iliac (hypogastric) arteries, impotence may result. Sexual dysfunction

Table 32-5

Diagnostic and Therapeutic Management: Chronic Arterial Occlusive Disease

DIAGNOSTIC

History and physical examination including palpation of peripheral pulses
Doppler ultrasound studies
Angiography

THERAPEUTIC

Conservative

Mild analgesic (e.g., codeine)
Reverse Trendelenburg position 10 degrees while in bed
Walking exercises 30 min twice daily as tolerated
Foot care*
Avoidance of extreme temperatures

Surgical

Endarterectomy (done rarely, with localized stenosis)
Bypass graft
Patch graft angioplasty, often in conjunction with bypass
Percutaneous transluminal angioplasty

---

*See Table 43-10.

grene are the most serious complications of chronic arterial disease.

Diagnostic studies. Various tests have been developed to assess blood flow and to outline the vascular system (Table 32-5). A noninvasive test used to determine pulse volume is oscillometry. A pneumatic cuff inflated over the artery measures the amplitude of the pulsations.

Doppler ultrasound consists of a transducer containing a crystal that emits sound waves through a probe. It measures the velocity of blood flow through a vessel. Directional flow can be measured antegrade or retrograde. The Doppler is extremely sensitive to movement of blood. When arterial palpation is difficult, it can sense a weak pulsation even when arterial narrowing or obstruction is severe. Angiography (aortography and femoral arteriography) is used to delineate the location and extent of the disease process.

Duplex imaging, a newer noninvasive test, uses a Doppler system that can systematically map the entire region of an artery in which blood is flowing. It provides a picture similar to that of a conventional arteriogram.

Therapeutic management. Conservative management objectives include (1) protecting the extremity from trauma, (2) slowing the progression of atherosclerosis, (3) decreasing vasospasm, (4) preventing and controlling infection, and (5) improving collateral circulation (see Table 32-5). The client's risk factors should be assessed, and proper intervention should be begun regarding cessation of smoking, weight reduction (if indicated), and control of lipid disorders. Hypertension also needs to be properly managed (see Chapter 27).

Slow, progressive physical activity should be encour-

aged to help develop collateral circulation. For example, the client should be out of bed at least four times per day, walk for 30 minutes twice a day as tolerated and stop if pain occurs (after a rest break the client should continue walking), and keep the foot of the bed in the reverse Trendelenburg position at 10 degrees.

Soaking of the affected part and application of a topical antibiotic may be advised to treat or prevent infection. If ulceration is present, the affected foot should be kept clean and dry. Covering the foot with a dry, sterile dressing helps to maintain cleanliness and protects the limb.

Surgical interventions. Surgical management is indicated (1) when the symptoms of intermittent claudication become incapacitating or (2) when ulceration or gangrene is severe enough to threaten the viability of the limb. The latter problem will likely progress unless arterial circulation can be restored.

Various surgical approaches can be used to improve arterial blood flow beyond a stenotic or occluded artery. The most common is a bypass operation with autogenous vein or synthetic graft material to bypass or carry blood around the lesion (Fig. 32-6).

Other surgical options include *endarterectomy* (opening the artery and removing the obstructing plaque) and *patch graft angioplasty* (opening the artery, removing plaque, and sewing a patch to the opening to widen the lumen).

For clients who are not suitable candidates for more extensive surgery or in whom the surgical options are impossible, blood flow to the periphery may be increased through surgical interruption of sympathetic nerves supplying the blood vessels of the affected limb (sympathectomy). Stimulation of the sympathetic nervous system results in constriction of blood vessels. Sympathectomy prevents this vasoconstriction (i.e., causes permanent dilatation). Upper extremity sympathectomy involves removal of one or more cervical sympathetic ganglia. Lower extremity sympathectomy involves removal of the first, second, and/or third lumbar ganglia. The indications warranting sympathectomy are specific, and it is rarely performed for lower extremity ischemia.

A technique known as *percutaneous transluminal angioplasty,* or angiodilatation involves the use of a special catheter with a cylindrical balloon. When inflated, the balloon dilates the vessel (Fig. 32-7). This procedure is used in certain clients who have localized, accessible lesions. Iliac artery lesions have responded most successfully to percutaneous transluminal angioplasty.

Laser technology, currently being researched, uses laser energy (most commonly from an argon source) to heat the tip of an intravascular catheter. The procedure basically "bores" a hole through an occluded artery.[8-10] Newer devices, called *atherectomy catheters,* are also used inside the artery to "shave" or pulverize plaque lining the arterial wall.[11-13]

Amputation is the least desired surgical option, but it may be required if gangrene is extensive, infection is present in bone (osteomyelitis), and/or all major arteries in the limb are occluded, precluding the possibility of bypass surgery. Every effort is made to preserve as much of the limb as possible so that the potential for rehabilitation with

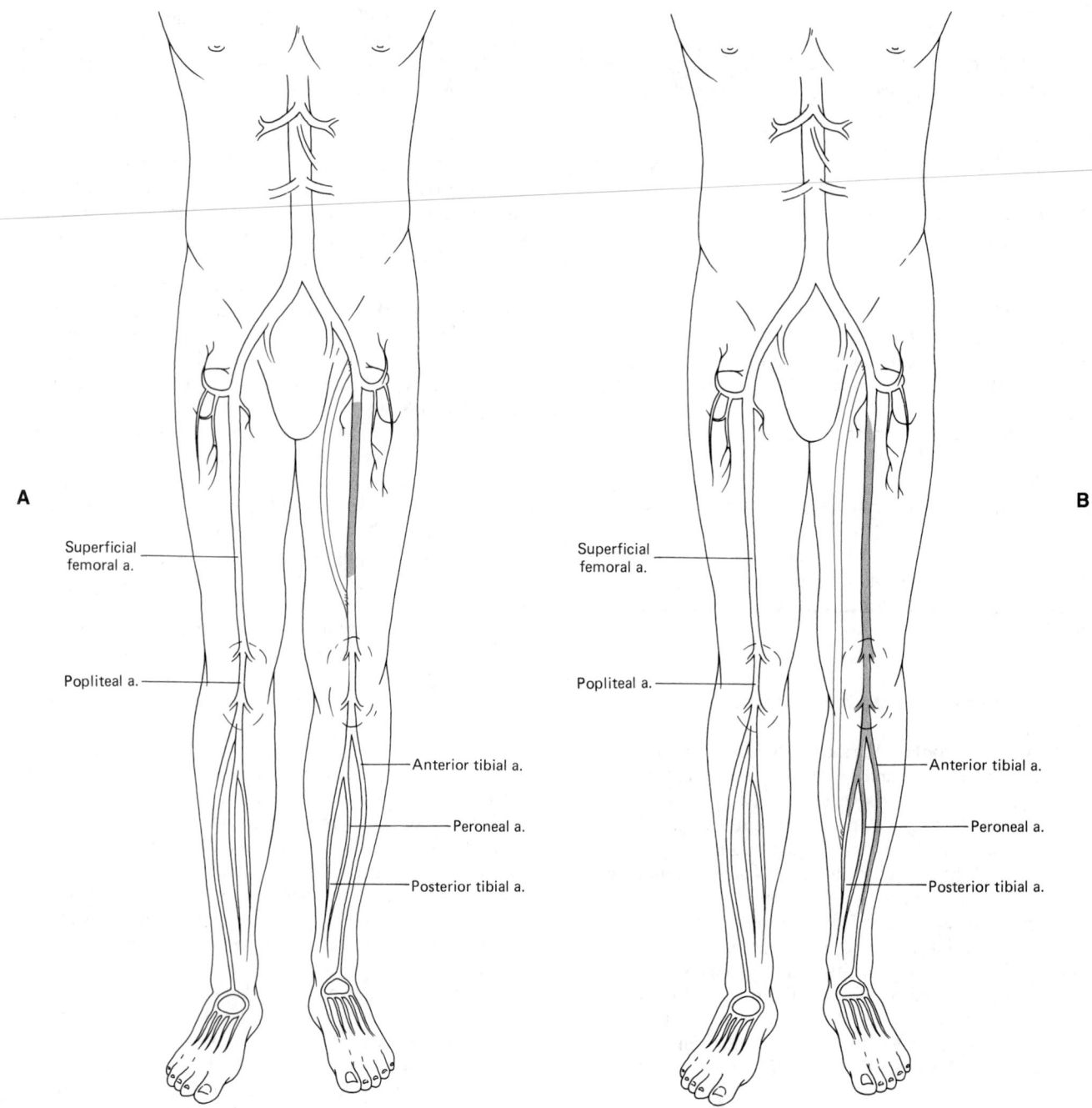

Fig. 32-6 **A,** Femoral-popliteal bypass graft around an occluded superficial femoral artery. **B,** Femoral-posterior tibial bypass graft around occluded superficial femoral, popliteal, and proximal tibial arteries.

an orthotic shoe or prosthesis is optimized (see Chapter 57).

Pharmacological management. Although various drugs are commonly prescribed to treat peripheral arterial occlusive disease, no specific agent is known to be effective except pentoxifylline (Trental), which increases erythrocyte flexibility and reduces blood viscosity, thus improving the supply of oxygenated blood to ischemic muscle.[14] Although it is not conclusive that anticoagulants and antiplatelet aggregating agents such as aspirin and dipyrida-

mole (Persantine) improve circulation through diseased arteries, they are sometimes used after arterial bypass surgery to promote graft patency. Their effectiveness continues to be studied.

Nutritional considerations. If the client has evidence of atherosclerosis, the following should be encouraged:
1. Caloric adjustment so that optimum weight can be achieved
2. Decrease in dietary cholesterol to less than 300 mg/ day

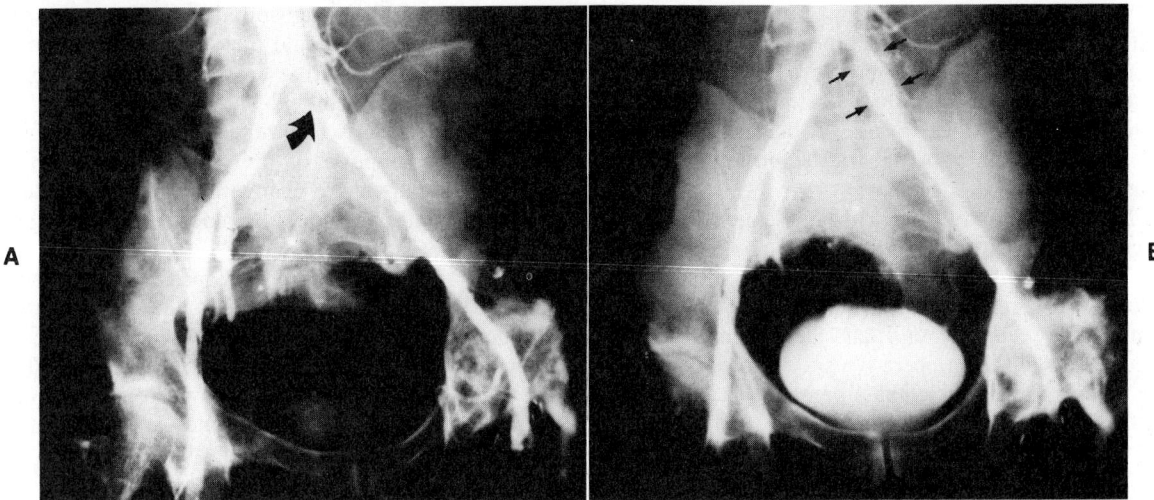

Fig. 32-7 **A,** Tight stenosis of the left common iliac artery *(arrow).* **B,** Dilatation of the left common iliac artery lumen following percutaneous transluminal angioplasty *(arrows).* (Courtesy FW LoGerfo, Boston, Mass.)

3. Substantial reduction in saturated dietary fat (see Table 28-5)
4. Restriction of sodium to 2 g/day if edema is present (see Table 29-7)

▪ Nursing Management of Chronic Arterial Occlusive Disease

Nursing assessment

Subjective and objective data that should be obtained from a client with chronic arterial occlusive disease are presented in Table 32-6.

Nursing diagnoses

Nursing diagnoses are determined when the problems and etiological factors are supported by clinical data. Nursing diagnoses related to chronic arterial occlusive disease may include, but are not limited to, the following:

1. Altered tissue perfusion related to decreased arterial blood flow
2. Impaired skin integrity related to decreased peripheral circulation, altered sensation, and increased susceptibility to infection
3. Pain related to ischemia and exercise
4. Activity intolerance related to imbalance between oxygen supply and demand
5. High risk for injury related to decreased sensation and tissue hypoxia
6. Anticipatory grieving related to potential loss of body part

Nursing interventions

Health promotion and maintenance. The client should be assessed for risk factors and should be taught how to control them (see Table 28-4). The nursing role in client education in the inpatient care facility is important in identifying high-risk clients. The nurse should also be involved at the community level, such as in screening clinics for hypertension. Young people and adults need to be educated

---

Table 32-6

 Nursing Assessment of the Client with Chronic Arterial Occlusive Disease

SUBJECTIVE DATA

History
Positive family history, hypertension, obesity, diabetes, smoking, activity level, high fat intake, stress
Medications
Use of any medications
Pain
Low back, buttock, and leg pain that is precipitated by exercise and that subsides with rest (intermittent claudication); excruciating, burning pain in extremities that may not subside with rest (severe disease)
Reproductive
Impotence

OBJECTIVE DATA

Integumentary
Loss of hair on legs and feet; thick toenails; pallor with elevation; dependent rubor; thin, cool, glossy skin with muscle atrophy; ulcerations over bony areas; gangrene
Cardiovascular
Decreased or absent peripheral pulses, bruits
Neurological
Numbness, tingling in legs or feet
Possible findings
Positive plethysmography, Doppler ultrasonography and/or angiography indicative of occlusive disease

about the hazards of cigarette smoking. The nurse should also assist in teaching diet modification to reduce the intake of animal fat and refined sugars, proper care of the feet, and the avoidance of injury to the extremities. Clients with positive family histories of cardiac, diabetic, or vascular disease need to be encouraged to obtain regular follow-up care.

Acute intervention. After surgical intervention the client is placed in an ICU or recovery area for close observation (see Chapter 13). The operative extremity should be checked every 15 minutes initially and then hourly for color, temperature, capillary refill, and the presence of peripheral pulses distal to the operative site. These findings should be compared with the client's preoperative baseline and with findings in the opposite limb.

When the client is transferred from the recovery room or ICU, nursing care should focus on continued circulatory assessment and monitoring for the development of potential complications (Table 32-7).

Symptoms such as recurrence of severe ischemic pain, loss of palpable pulse or pulses, numbness or tingling, and/or cold temperature change may indicate occlusion of the bypass graft and should be reported to the surgeon immediately.

On the second or third postoperative day, the client should be out of bed three to four times daily. Sitting for prolonged periods of time may be discouraged because leg dependency promotes edema and, depending on the location of the bypass, may impede flow through the graft. Sitting is usually limited to mealtimes and bathroom privi-

Table 32-7

 NURSING CARE PLAN AFTER LOWER EXTREMITY ARTERIAL BYPASS SURGERY

Defining Characteristics	Nursing Interventions	Evaluation Criteria
NURSING DIAGNOSIS: **Potential complication: altered peripheral tissue perfusion related to bypass graft thrombosis**		
Pain below incision site, absent distal pulse, numb or cold extremity	Assess peripheral pulses, color, motion, and sensation of operative limb or limbs every 15 minutes initially, then every hour. Assess client's degree of pain, differentiating incisional pain from ischemic pain. Elevate client's legs slightly. Teach client to keep affected leg straight. Report any significant change in circulatory status to surgeon.	Patent arterial bypass graft
NURSING DIAGNOSIS: **Potential complication: hemorrhage related to vascular surgical procedure and anticoagulation**		
Bleeding, increased HR, decreased BP, restlessness	Monitor Hct every day and as needed. Monitor BP and pulse q 2-4 hr. Observe for overt evidence of excessive incisional bleeding, increased edema, change in color, decreased HR.	Hct, BP, and HR within normal limits; absence of incisional bleeding
NURSING DIAGNOSIS: **Pain related to ineffective pain and comfort measures and surgical procedure**		
Complaints of pain, moaning, facial grimaces, restlessness	Monitor pain medication requirements and effectiveness. Administer analgesics as needed.	Little or no ischemic or incisional pain
NURSING DIAGNOSIS: **High risk for infection related to environmental pathogens and interruption of skin integrity secondary to surgical procedure**		
Elevated body temperature; elevated WBC count, HR, and respiratory rate; purulent drainage from incision; redness, warmth, and swelling around incision	Monitor systemic temperature q 4 hr. Assess incision site for evidence of erythema, warmth, or purulent drainage. Monitor WBC count. Report any suspicion of infection to surgeon.	No wound or graft infection

Hct, Hematocrit; *HR,* heart rate.

leges. If significant swelling develops, a reclining position is preferred with the edematous leg elevated above heart level.

If no complications are present, discharge from the hospital can be anticipated 7 to 10 days postoperatively.

Chronic management. Atherosclerosis is not localized to the lower extremities but is a systemic disease process. The overall approach to the control of atherosclerotic chronic occlusive disease involves management of risk factors. Tobacco in any form is totally contraindicated, not only because of the vasoconstrictive effects of nicotine but also because tobacco smoke impairs transport and cellular utilization of oxygen and increases blood viscosity.[15] Bypass surgery is a symptomatic treatment and does not cure the underlying cause. Continuance of cigarette smoking adversely affects the long-term function of the bypass graft[16] and also results in the development of symptomatic disease in other major arterial beds (e.g., carotid artery disease, coronary artery disease). The health care team must consistently agree to inform clients that they must abstain from smoking. The nurse needs to tell clients about various community agencies and support groups, such as behavior modification and antismoking clinics, if they are unable to stop smoking on their own.

If the client is not a surgical candidate or decides not to have surgery, a plan of care can be implemented to optimize the client's arterial circulation. A progressive exercise program often promotes the development of collateral circulation and enhances venous return. Collateral vessels, usually small insignificant branches of major arteries, often enlarge and carry more blood "around" an occlusive lesion as a compensatory mechanism. The demand for blood and oxygen beyond an arterial blockage is thought to enhance collateral vessel development.

Walking is effective exercise. The client should be instructed to walk only to the point of distress, to rest and allow the discomfort to subside, and then resume walking until distress recurs. This exercise should be done for a prescribed time, usually 30 to 40 min/day, in addition to normal activity.

Both nonoperative and postoperative clients should be taught the importance of meticulous foot care to prevent injury. They should learn to inspect the extremities daily for skin color, mottling, scabs, alterations in the texture of the skin and subcutaneous fat, and reduction or absence of hair growth. Any ulceration or inflammation needs to be reported to the health care provider. Skin temperature should be noted, and capillary refill of the fingers and toes should be tested.

Emphasis on foot care is especially important in the client with both arterial occlusive disease and diabetes, because diabetic neuropathy (i.e., diminished peripheral sensation) increases the susceptibility to traumatic injury (see Table 43-10). These measures also apply to people with vascular disease who do not have diabetes.

The client with chronic arterial disease should avoid long periods of standing or sitting. If prolonged sitting or standing is necessary, the client should plan periodically to walk a few feet, flex the knees, and rotate the ankles. Measures to avoid compromising circulation should be implemented, including avoidance of tight nylon hose and garters, tight bands on socks, and tight waistbands. Shoes should not be laced tightly, and new shoes should be broken in gradually.

Thromboangiitis Obliterans

Thromboangiitis obliterans (Buerger's disease) is a focal, inflammatory, thrombotic disorder of the medium-sized arteries and veins of the lower extremities. Occlusion of the vessel occurs with development of collateral circulation around areas of obstruction. The basic cause is not known. There is a direct relationship to cigarette smoking, since the disease occurs only in smokers. Unlike atherosclerosis, usually no lipid accumulation occurs in the vessel media. The disorder, generally asymmetrical, occurs predominantly in men between 25 and 40 years of age who smoke. A familial tendency has also been observed.

The symptom complex of Buerger's disease is often confused with that of atherosclerotic occlusive disease. The client may have intermittent claudication. The development of rest pain is a premonitory sign of gangrene and may develop in advanced stages of the disease process. Other signs and symptoms may include color and temperature changes in the affected limb or limbs, paresthesia, thrombophlebitis, and cold sensitivity.

Treatment includes avoidance of trauma to the extremity and complete cessation of smoking. Clients are often told that they have a choice between their cigarettes and their legs; they cannot have both. The disorder is difficult to treat. Anticoagulants and vasodilator therapy have met with little success. Amputation, generally below the knee, may be necessary in advanced cases.

Arteriospastic Disease

Arteriospastic disease (Raynaud's phenomenon) is an episodic vasospastic disorder of small cutaneous arteries, most frequently involving the fingers and toes. The exact etiology is not known. The disease occurs primarily in young women. It is seen frequently in association with collagen diseases such as rheumatoid arthritis, scleroderma, and lupus erythematosus. Other contributing factors include occupationally related trauma and pressure to the fingertips as noted in typists, pianists, and those who use hand-held vibrating equipment. Exposure to heavy metals may also be a contributing etiological factor.

The symptoms are usually precipitated by exposure to cold, emotional upsets, and tobacco use. The disorder is characterized by three color changes. Initially, the vasoconstrictive effect produces pallor, which is followed by cyanosis. These changes are subsequently followed by rubor or hyperemia. Because Raynaud's phenomenon is a vasospastic disorder, the pulses are never lost. The client usually describes cold and numbness in the vasoconstrictive phase and throbbing, aching pain; tingling; and swelling in the hyperemic phase. This type of episode usually lasts only minutes but in severe cases may persist for several hours.[5]

If the symptoms persist for several years in the absence of an associated underlying disorder, the diagnosis of primary Raynaud's disease may be made. Complications may include punctate (small hole) lesions of the fingertips and superficial gangrenous ulcers occurring in advanced stages. It is of diagnostic importance to search for an underlying disease. Treatment is generally not required because the symptoms are self-limiting. However, treatment with certain catecholamine-depleting antihypertensive drugs has been encouraging. Oral vasodilators have been used with variable success. Sympathectomy is considered only in advanced cases.

Client education should be directed toward reassurance that no serious underlying disorder is present and that prevention of recurrent episodes is possible. Warm clothing should be worn as protection from the cold, including gloves when the refrigerator-freezer is used or when cold objects are being handled. Moving to a warmer climate is not necessarily beneficial because symptoms may still occur during cooler weather. The client should stop smoking and avoid or learn to cope with anxiety-producing stressful situations.

DISORDERS OF THE VEINS
Thrombophlebitis

The most common disorder of the veins is thrombophlebitis, the formation of a thrombus (clot) in association with inflammation of the vein. The terms *phlebothrombosis* and *phlebitis* have been used to indicate whether the predominant process is thrombus formation or inflammation. In general, the preferred term is *thrombophlebitis* because both clots and inflammation are usually present. The initiating event is usually thrombus formation. Thrombophlebitis is classified as either *superficial* or *deep* (Table 32-8).

In about 65% of all clients receiving IV therapy, superficial thrombophlebitis develops, and in at least 5% of all surgical clients, deep vein thrombophlebitis develops. Of greater significance is that embolization of thrombi from deep veins to the lungs may be fatal and, at the least, results in prolonged hospitalization.

Etiology. Three important factors in the etiology of thrombophlebitis are (1) stasis of venous flow, (2) damage of the endothelium, or inner lining of the vein, and (3) hypercoagulability of the blood. Clients who are at high risk for the development of thrombophlebitis are those who have conditions predisposing them to any of these three disorders (Table 32-9).

Venous stasis. Normal blood flow in the venous system depends on the action of muscles in the extremities and on the functional adequacy of venous valves, allowing flow in one direction only. Venous stasis occurs if these valves are

Table 32-8 Clinical Manifestations of Thrombophlebitis

Clinical Classification	Usual Causes	Usual Location	Clinical Findings	Edema of Extremities	Embolization	Chronic Venous Insufficiency
Superficial	Varicose veins; direct trauma; IV catheters; thromboangiitis obliterans; caustic IV medications such as chemotherapy, radiopaque contrast material; IV drug use	Saphenous veins and their tributaries, forearm	Tender, red, inflamed induration along course of subcutaneous vein (visible and palpable)	Almost never	Almost never	Almost never
Deep Small veins	Postoperatively, before and after childbirth, direct or distant trauma, congestive heart failure, prolonged bed rest, acute febrile disease, sepsis, debilitating disease, malignant disease, blood dyscrasias	Soleal; posterior tibial, other deep calf veins; popliteal; pelvic	Possible tenderness to deep pressure, induration of overlying muscle, minimal or no venous distention	Occasionally	Always a threat	Usually not
Major venous trunks	Systemic lupus erythematosus, pressure of tumors on veins, estrogen therapy, malignant disease, blood dyscrasias, idiopathic cause	Femoral, iliac, inferior or superior vena cava, axillary, subclavian	Swelling, cyanosis, venous distention, mild to moderate pain, tenderness over involved vein (groin or axilla)	Frequently	Always a threat	Frequently

dysfunctional and/or if the muscles of the extremities are inactive. Venous stasis occurs in people who are obese, have CHF, have been on long trips without regular exercise, or are immobile for long periods (e.g., with spinal cord injuries or fractured hips). Also at risk are pregnant women and women in the postpartum period.[17]

Clients with atrial fibrillation are also at high risk because of stagnation of blood and the eddying in blood flow caused by irregular ventricular contractions in response to the fibrillation. Steroid and quinine therapy also predispose clients to stasis and clot formation.

Endothelial damage. Damage to the lining of the vein is caused by trauma or external pressure and occurs any time a venipuncture is performed. Damaged endothelium has decreased fibrinolytic properties, predisposing to the development of thrombus. Increased endothelial damage is sustained when clients receiving IV therapy are receiving high-dose antibiotics, potassium, chemotherapeutic agents, or hypertonic solutions such as contrast media.

Other factors predisposing to endothelial inflammation and damage include the presence of an IV catheter in the same site for longer than 48 hours, the use of contaminated IV equipment, a fracture that causes damage to the blood vessels, diabetes, blood pooling, burns, and any unusual physical exertion that results in muscular strain.

Table 32-9 Risk Factors for Deep Vein Thrombophlebitis and Thromboembolism

---

History of thrombophlebitis
Abdominal and pelvic surgery
Suprapubic prostatectomy
Obesity
Neoplasms, especially hepatic and pancreatic
CHF
Advanced age
Atrial fibrillation
Prolonged immobility
   Bed rest
   Long trip without adequate exercise
   Spinal cord injury
   Fractured hip
MI
Pregnancy
Postpartum period
Estrogen therapy including oral contraceptives
IV therapy
Trauma
Sepsis
Venous cannulation or catheterization
Drug abuse
Cigarette smoking
Excessive vitamin E intake
Hypercoagulable states
   Polycythemia vera
   Severe anemias
   Dehydration or malnutrition
Antithrombin III deficiency

Hypercoagulability of blood. Hypercoagulability of blood occurs in many hematological disorders, particularly polycythemia, severe anemias, and antithrombin III deficiency. Clients with systemic infections in which endotoxins are released also have hypercoagulability. Hypercoagulability also seems to be the contributing factor in idiopathic thrombophlebitis.

Clients who take oral contraceptives (especially those containing estrogen) are at increased risk for thromboembolic disease. Recent studies show that women who take contraceptives and smoke double their risk because of the constricting effect of nicotine on the blood vessel wall. Smoking may also cause hypercoagulability. Hypercoagulability also seems to be the common factor in various malignancies and the associated higher incidence of thromboembolic disease.[18]

Pathophysiology. Red blood cells (RBCs), WBCs, platelets, and fibrin adhere to form a thrombus. A frequent site of thrombus formation is the valve cusps of veins, where venous stasis allows accumulation of blood products. As the thrombus enlarges, increased amounts of blood cells and fibrin collect behind it, producing a larger clot with a "tail" that eventually occludes the lumen of the vein.

If a thrombus only partially occludes the vein and blood flow continues, the thrombus becomes covered by endothelial cells and the thrombotic process stops. If the thrombus does not become detached, it undergoes lysis or becomes firmly organized and adherent within 24 to 48 hours. The organized thrombi may detach and give rise to emboli. The turbulence of blood flow past the thrombus is a major factor contributing to its detachment from the vein wall. These emboli generally flow through the venous circulation, back to the heart, and into the pulmonary circulation, where they may result in pulmonary embolism.

Clinical manifestations. Clinical manifestations of thrombophlebitis vary according to the size and location of the thrombus, and the adequacy of collateral circulation around the obstructive process. Clients with superficial thrombophlebitis may have a palpable, firm subcutaneous cordlike vein. The area surrounding the vein may be tender to the touch, reddened, and warm. A mild systemic temperature elevation and leukocytosis may be present. Edema of the extremity may or may not occur. The most common cause of superficial thrombophlebitis in the arms is IV therapy. The most common cause of superficial thrombophlebitis in the legs is related to varicose veins.

Clients with deep thrombophlebitis may have no symptoms or have unilateral leg edema, pain, warm skin, and a temperature greater than 38° C (100.4° F). If the calf is involved, tenderness may be present on palpation. *Homans' sign,* pain on dorsiflexion of the foot, is a classic but unreliable sign. If the inferior vena cava is involved, both lower extremities may be edematous and cyanotic. If the superior vena cava is involved, both upper extremities as well as the neck and back become edematous and cyanotic.

Complications. The most serious complications of thrombophlebitis are *pulmonary embolism, chronic venous insufficiency,* and *phlegmasia cerulea dolens.* Pulmonary

Table 32-10 Diagnostic Studies in Deep Vein Thrombophlebitis and Pulmonary Embolism

Study	Description and Abnormal Findings
Coagulation studies	
Platelet count, bleeding time, PT, PTT	Elevation if client has underlying blood dyscrasia; decrease possible if client has polycythemia; alteration possible because of previous medications
Noninvasive venous studies	
Venous Doppler evaluation	Determination of venous flow in deep femoral, popliteal, and posterior tibial veins; normal finding of spontaneous flow with variation transmitted by respiration cycle; abnormal finding of absence of flow augmentation with distal compression and proximal release
Impedance plethysmography	Measurement of increase in leg volume induced by obstruction of venous outflow by inflation of thigh cuff: (maximum venous capitance), measurement of speed at which volume decreases on thigh cuff release (venous outflow), abnormal finding of slow outflow
Phleborheography	Recording of small changes in volume through pneumatic cuffs, abnormal findings of noncyclic changes in volume with respiration, diminished or absent venous wave recording, and no elicitation of baseline rise on intermittent cuff compression of foot and calf
^{125}I-labeled fibrinogen scanning	Definition of location of clot and any emboli that may have moved from thrombus site by radionuclide tag of fibrinogen (primarily used in research)
Venogram (phlebogram)	Radiographic definition of location and site of clot, filling defect in vein lumen, and development of collateral circulation
Lung scan (ventilation and perfusion)	Means of determining presence of pulmonary embolism and extent of resulting lung damage, abnormal finding of mismatch between ventilation and perfusion components
Pulmonary arteriogram	Radiographic definition of location and size of pulmonary embolism

PT, Prothrombin time; *PTT,* partial thromboplastin time.

embolism is the most feared complication of thrombophlebitis because of its lethal potential (see p. 943).

Another common complication is chronic venous insufficiency resulting from recurrent thrombophlebitis, with resultant valvular destruction allowing retrograde flow of blood. Persistent edema, increased pigmentation, secondary varicosities, ulceration, and cyanosis of the limb when it is placed in a dependent position may develop in persons with this complication.[19] Signs and symptoms of chronic venous insufficiency often do not develop for many years following deep thrombophlebitis.

Phlegmasia cerulea dolens may develop in clients with severe thrombophlebitis of the lower extremities. It presents as sudden, massive swelling and intense bluish discoloration of the extremity. Gangrene may occur as a result of arterial occlusion resulting from obstruction of venous outflow.

Diagnostic studies. Various diagnostic studies are used to determine the site and extent of the thrombus (Table 32-10).

Therapeutic management

Conservative therapy. The client is usually kept in bed with elevation of the affected extremity until the tenderness has subsided, usually for 5 to 7 days. Warm, moist heat may be used to relieve the pain and treat the inflammation. Mild oral analgesics such as aspirin and codeine are used to relieve pain. For more severe pain, nonsteroidal antiinflammatory agents such as ibuprofen have been used to treat the inflammatory process and accompanying pain (Table 32-11).

Anticoagulant therapy is usually not indicated for superficial thrombophlebitis but is routinely used for deep vein thrombophlebitis. Heparin, administered by continuous IV infusion after an initial bolus dose, is given for up to 10 days and is followed by oral anticoagulants for 3 to 6 months.

If edema is present when the client becomes ambulatory, elastic stockings are recommended. Ideally they should be measured to fit the client once some of the edema has resolved. If edema persists, the use of elastic stockings should be continued after discharge.

Surgical interventions. Most clients are treated conservatively, but a small percentage require surgical intervention (Table 32-11). The primary indication for surgery is to prevent pulmonary emboli. Surgical procedures include venous thrombectomy (rarely performed) and inferior vena cava interruption.

Venous thrombectomy involves the removal of an occluding clot through an incision in the vein. This procedure is done to prevent pulmonary embolism and/or to decrease the risk of the development of chronic venous insufficiency.

Extravascular interruption of the inferior vena cava to prevent pulmonary emboli involves abdominal surgery and application of a partitioning Teflon clip (Fig. 32-8, *A*). Although suture partitioning was once popular, it is rarely done currently.

If clients are too ill for surgical intervention, a caval filter device can be threaded into the right internal jugular vein and into the inferior vena cava below the level of the

Table 32-11

Diagnostic and Therapeutic Management: Deep Vein Thrombophlebitis

DIAGNOSTIC

History and physical examination
Chest x-ray film
CBC count with differential
PT, PTT, platelet count, bleeding time
ECG
Noninvasive venous studies
Venogram of affected limb

THERAPEUTIC
Conservative

Continuous IV heparin
Bed rest with bathroom privileges for bowel movement only
Oral anticoagulants
Full-length elastic hose
Measurement and charting of size of both thighs and calves every morning
Guaiac test on all stools while client is anticoagulated

Surgical

Inferior vena cava interruption
  Clipping
  Plication
Intracaval filter insertion

CBC, Complete blood cell; *PT,* prothrombin time; *PTT,* partial thromboplastin time.

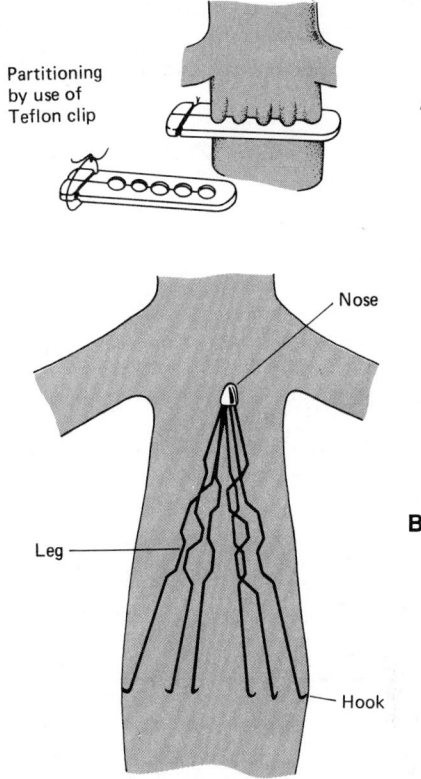

Fig. 32-8 Inferior vena caval interruption techniques to prevent pulmonary embolism. **A,** Partitioning extravascular Teflon clip. **B,** Intravascular Kimray-Greenfield stainless steel filter.

renal veins (Fig. 32-8, *B*) using local anesthesia. The filter device is opened and the spokes penetrate the vessel walls. These devices result in "sieve-type" occlusion, permitting filtration of clots without interruption of blood flow.

Complications after the insertion of the intravascular filter device are rare. They include air embolism, improper placement, and migration of the filter more distally into the venous system. Venous congestion is common and is caused by accumulation of trapped clots at the filter site. At some point, these clots may clog the filter and completely occlude the vena cava. This process is usually so gradual that collateral vessels have a chance to develop and venous flow is maintained. However, development of large collateral venous pathways may provide an alternate route for pulmonary emboli.

Pharmacological management. The goals of anticoagulation therapy in the treatment of thrombophlebitis are to prevent (1) propagation of the clot, (2) development of a new thrombus, and (3) embolization. Anticoagulant therapy does not dissolve the clot. Lysis of the clot begins spontaneously through the body's intrinsic fibrinolytic system (see Chapter 24).

The most commonly used anticoagulants are heparin and coumarin compounds (Table 32-12). Heparin acts directly on the intrinsic and common pathways of blood coagulation (see also Fig. 24-3). Heparin inhibits thrombin-mediated conversion of fibrinogen to fibrin. It also poten-

tiates the actions of antithrombin III, inhibits the activation of factor IX, and neutralizes activated factor X by activating factor X inhibitor.

Coumarin compounds, of which warfarin (Coumadin) is the most commonly used, exert their action indirectly on the coagulation pathway. Warfarin inhibits the hepatic synthesis of the vitamin K-dependent coagulation factors II, VII, IX, and X by competitively interfering with vitamin K. Vitamin K is normally required for the synthesis of these factors.

Oral anticoagulants are begun while heparin is still being administered. An overlap of 3 to 5 days is usually required to maintain therapeutic control of clotting. The clotting status is usually monitored by partial thromboplastin time (PTT) for heparin therapy and prothrombin time (PT) for coumarin derivatives. However, other tests can be used (Table 32-13).

Intramuscular (IM) injection of any drug is contraindicated for the client receiving anticoagulant therapy because of the risk of hematoma formation. Another important precaution involves the concurrent use of other drugs. IV heparin should not be administered with most antibiotics, hydrocortisone, or levarterenol (Levophed). Drug interactions can occur with oral anticoagulants (Table 32-14). A careful drug history should be taken from the client before anticoagulant therapy administration. In addition, the client receiving anticoagulant therapy should be told to seek

Table 32-12 Anticoagulant Therapy

Drug	Route of Administration	Comments
HEPARIN		
Panheprin	Continuous IV infusion by infusion pump	Initial bolus dose of heparin is required. Protamine sulfate should be available as an antidote.
Lipo-Hepin	Intermittent IV infusion q 4 hr	Clotting status is monitored by whole blood clotting time (Lee-White clotting time), PTT, activated clotting time, and activated PTT.
Liquaemin sodium	Intermittent subcutaneous infusion q 6 hr	Aspirin should not be administered to a client taking heparin. Low-dose prophylactic drugs do not alter clotting studies.
COUMARIN DERIVATIVES		
Warfarin (Coumadin, Panwarfin), dicumarol, acenocoumarol (Sintrom)	Oral	Vitamin K should be available as an antidote. Plasma levels may be maintained for up to 5 days. Clotting status is monitored by PT.

Table 32-13 Tests of Blood Coagulation

Test	Drug Monitored	Normal Value	Therapeutic Value
Lee-White whole blood clotting time	Heparin	9-14 min	20-30 min
PT	Warfarin	11-12 sec	20-25 sec
PTT	Heparin	60-90 sec	90-180 sec
APTT	Heparin	24-36 sec	48-60 sec
ACT	Heparin	80-135 sec	3 min

ACT, Activated clotting time; *APTT,* activated partial thromboplastin time.

Table 32-14 Drugs Interacting with Oral Anticoagulants

Drugs Potentiating Response	Drugs Diminishing Response
Anabolic steroids (e.g., Dianabol)	Barbiturates (e.g., secobarbital, phenobarbital)
Clofibrate (Atromid-S)	Cholestyramine (Cuemid, Questran)
Dextrothyroxine (Choloxin)	Ethchlorvynol (Placidyl)
Disulfiram (Antabuse)	Glutethimide (Doriden)
Metronidazole (Flagyl)	Griseofulvin (Grifulvin)
Neomycin	Rifampin (Rifadin, Rimactane)
Oxyphenbutazone (Tandearil)	
Phenylbutazone (Butazolidin)	
Phenyramidol (Analexin)	
Salicylates	
Sulfonamides (Gantrisin)	

medical advice before starting to take any other medications.

Drugs altering platelet function have also shown potential for use in preventing thromboembolic disease. They include acetylsalicylic acid (aspirin), indomethacin (Indo-cin), phenylbutazone (Butazolidin), and dipyridamole (Persantine). The clinical use is undergoing investigation.

■ **Nursing Management of Thrombophlebitis**

Nursing assessment

Subjective and objective data that should be obtained from a client with thrombophlebitis are presented in Table 32-15.

Nursing diagnoses

Nursing diagnoses are determined when the problems and etiological factors are supported by clinical data. Nursing diagnoses related to thrombophlebitis may include, but are not limited to, those presented in Table 32-16.

Nursing interventions

Health promotion and maintenance. Thrombus formation can be prevented in many situations. Prophylactic measures include early ambulation and leg exercises postoperatively, use of elastic stockings (hose), avoidance of dehydration, and low-dose anticoagulant therapy. Heparin (5000 units subcutaneously every 8 to 12 hours) or oral anticoagulants are often recommended for high-risk clients who are predisposed to thrombus formation.

Mechanical methods of prophylaxis, such as the use of intermittent pneumatic compression stockings or boots, help promote venous return, and may also stimulate fibrin-

Table 32-15

Nursing Assessment of the Client with Thrombophlebitis

SUBJECTIVE DATA

History
Previous: Thrombophlebitis, extremity trauma, varicosities.
Recent: Surgery, childbirth, IV therapy, blood infection, smoking, obesity, prolonged bed rest, irregular heartbeat (e.g., atrial fibrillation), COPD, CHF, malignancies, systemic lupus erythematosus, MI, spinal cord injury

Medications
Use of estrogens (including oral contraceptives), steroids, quinine, excessive amounts of vitamin E, IV drug use, IV phenytoin, diazepam, antibiotics, chemotherapy, potassium, contrast dyes

Pain
Pain in area surrounding vein or on palpation or ambulation, positive Homans' sign

OBJECTIVE DATA

General
Fever, anxiety
Integumentary
Red, warm skin around involved vein; increased size of extremity when compared with other side; taut, shiny skin
Cardiovascular
Firm, palpable vein; edema and cyanosis of area
Possible findings
Leukocytosis, abnormal coagulation, anemia or elevated hematocrit and RBC count, positive venous plethysmographic and/or Doppler studies, positive venogram

COPD, Chronic obstructive pulmonary disease.

olytic activity within the vein.[18] These devices are commonly used on high-risk clients while they are hospitalized.

Another important preventive measure is to avoid prolonged standing or sitting in a motionless, dependent position. Frequent knee flexion, ankle rotation, and active walking should be done during long periods of sitting or standing.

Clients should be taught the importance of not smoking and the way to perform deep breathing and range-of-motion exercises. In addition, the nurse should recognize the clients at highest risk for deep vein thrombophlebitis.

Acute intervention. Nursing care for thrombophlebitis is directed toward the reduction of inflammation and the prevention of emboli formation (Table 32-16). Acute intervention in superficial thrombophlebitis involves the use of warm moist packs or soaks, elevation of the affected extremity, removal of an IV catheter if present, and provision of analgesia to minimize pain and inflammation. Some experts advocate surgical intervention if the greater saphenous system of the lower extremity is involved. The greater saphenous vein may be ligated to prevent extension of thrombus into the deep venous system.

Acute intervention in deep vein thrombophlebitis involves IV and oral anticoagulation, 5 to 7 days of bed rest with elevation of the affected extremity, and the use of elastic support (elastic bandages or compression gradient stockings) to promote venous return in the unaffected extemity.

While the client is receiving anticoagulation therapy, the nurse should closely observe for any indication of bleeding, including epistaxis and bleeding gingivae. Urine should be assessed for gross or microscopic hematuria. A smoky appearance to the urine is sometimes noted, and a specimen should be checked daily. Particular attention should be paid to the protection of skin areas that may be traumatized. Surgical incisions should be closely observed for evidence of bleeding. Stools should be tested to determine the presence of occult blood from the gastrointestinal (GI) tract.

The nurse should monitor the hemoglobin and hematocrit levels when a client is receiving anticoagulant drugs (see p. 937). Medication doses are titrated according to the results of clotting studies. The nurse should be cautious about administering either heparin or coumarin without first checking the results of the clotting studies. The antidote for heparin is protamine sulfate and is vitamin K for coumarin. These drugs must be immediately available if hemorrhage occurs.

Chronic management. Elastic stockings, properly measured, fitted, and evenly applied, should be worn when the client becomes ambulatory. These stockings compress superficial veins and prevent venous stasis. The nurse should take care to prevent any pressure under the knee, such as by using pillows or bed gatches. Clients also should be taught to avoid crossing their legs at the knees. These measures will place pressure on the popliteal space, and they will also decrease venous return to the heart.

During all phases of care the nurse should evaluate the client's psychological response. Many clients are apprehensive that their clots will move to the heart or lungs and cause sudden death. All clients should be allowed to verbalize their concerns, and an attempt should be made to clarify misconceptions. Clients hospitalized for long periods of time should be provided with diversion.

Discharge teaching should stress the avoidance of contraceptives for clients with recurrent thrombophlebitis, the hazards of smoking, and the need to avoid constrictive girdles or garters. Exercise programs should be developed with an emphasis on swimming and wading, which are particularly beneficial due to the gentle, even pressure of the water. A balanced program of rest and exercise, along with proper posture, improves arterial filling and venous return.

Dietary considerations for the overweight client are aimed at limiting caloric intake so that the desired weight can be attained. Fat intake may be reduced if lipid or triglyceride levels are above normal for the client's age. Occasionally, sodium limitation is necessary if edema is present. Proper fluid balance is required to prevent additional hypercoagulability of the blood, which may occur in the presence of deficient fluid intake. A well-balanced diet

Table 32-16

 NURSING CARE PLAN FOR THE CLIENT WITH THROMBOPHLEBITIS

Defining Characteristics	Nursing Interventions	Evaluation Criteria
NURSING DIAGNOSIS: Pain related to edema secondary to impaired circulation in extremities		
Complaints of pain in extremity; presence of edema in extremity; redness, tenderness, and warmth around affected vein	Administer analgesics as ordered. Apply continuous warm, moist heat (e.g., K-pad at low heat) if ordered. Keep affected leg elevated. Instruct client not to cross leg at knees. Measure thighs and calves daily.	Relief of pain and reduction of edema
NURSING DIAGNOSIS: Potential complication: pulmonary embolism related to dehydration, immobility, and embolization of thrombus		
Sudden onset of dyspnea, tachypnea, tachycardia, hemoptysis; chest pain; change in mental status	Take vital signs q 4 hr. Report incidence of chest pain or shortness of breath. Use laxative to reduce straining. Maintain adequate hydration. Maintain bed rest to minimize risk of embolism. Administer anticoagulants as ordered. Use elastic stockings when ambulation is started.	No evidence of pulmonary embolism
NURSING DIAGNOSIS: Potential complication: hemorrhage related to anticoagulant medications		
Bright-red bleeding from any body orifice; decreased BP, increased pulse and respiration; restlessness	Administer anticoagulant medications as ordered. Do not give any IM medication. Check PT before giving warfarin and PTT or APTT before giving heparin. Give anticoagulant therapy only if clotting studies are within prescribed limits. Observe client closely for signs of bleeding such as epistaxis, bleeding gingivae, petechiae, ecchymoses, painful joints, incisional bleeding, or melena. Monitor for hemoglobin and/or Hct levels.	Therapy without signs of bleeding
NURSING DIAGNOSIS: High risk for impaired skin integrity related to alteration in peripheral tissue perfusion and possible valvular destruction		
Altered skin pigmentation in lower extremity, pain, open ulcer and edema of lower extremity	Teach client to wear elastic stockings at all times except when sleeping and to change positions when sitting or standing for prolonged periods. Have client elevate legs when sitting.	No evidence of ulcer formation in legs
NURSING DIAGNOSIS: Altered health maintenance related to lack of knowledge about disorder and its treatment		
Many questions or no questions from client	Instruct client on need for routine monitoring of clotting studies. Teach client signs and symptoms of thrombophlebitis and of abnormal bleeding to report to physician. Encourage client to take anticoagulants according to prescribed schedule. Assist client with obtaining Medic-Alert identification to alert others to anticoagulant ingestion. Teach client not to wear garters, girdles, or any constrictive clothing. Encourage dieting to lose weight if indicated. Teach client to avoid rubbing or massaging extremity and to avoid sitting with legs crossed.	Understanding of disease process and treatment, including anticoagulation management, diet and activity, and clothing to be avoided

APTT, Activated partial thromboplastin time; *Hct,* hematocrit.

Table 32-17 Client Education Related to Anticoagulant Therapy

1. Reasons for and basic mechanism of action of anticoagulant therapy and how long anticipated therapy will last
2. Need to take medication at same time each day (preferably in afternoon or evening)
3. Close follow-up with blood tests to assess blood clotting and whether change in drug dosages required
4. Side effects and adverse effects of drug therapy requiring medical attention:
   Any bleeding that does not stop after a reasonable amount of time
   Blood in urine or stool
   Unusual bleeding from gingivae, throat, skin, or nose
   Severe headaches or stomach pains
5. Avoidance of any trauma or injury that might cause bleeding (e.g., vigorous brushing of teeth, contact sports, improperly fitted shoes)
6. Avoidance of aspirin-containing drugs and more than moderate intake of alcohol,
7. Wearing of Medic-Alert bracelet or necklace indicating what anticoagulant is being taken
8. Use of electric razor when shaving
9. Avoidance of marked changes in eating habits such as food fads and crash diets
10. Need to consult with physician before beginning or discontinuing any medication

is important because calcium, vitamin E, and vitamin K all play active roles in the clotting mechanism.

If the client is to be discharged while receiving anticoagulant medication, both the client and the involved family need careful explanations of its dosage, actions, and side effects (Table 32-17).

Varicose Veins

Varicose veins, or varicosities, are dilated, tortuous subcutaneous veins most frequently found in the saphenous system. They may be small and innocuous or large and bulging. *Primary* varicosities are those in which the superficial veins are dilated and the valves may or may not be rendered incompetent. The condition tends to be familial, is characteristically found bilaterally, and is probably caused by congenital weakness of the veins. *Secondary* varicosities result from previous thrombophlebitis of the deep femoral veins with subsequent valvular incompetence. Secondary varicose veins may also occur in the esophagus as varices, in the anorectal area as hemorrhoids, and as abnormal arteriovenous connections (also known as *fistulas* and *malformations*).

Pathophysiology. The basic cause of varicosities is unknown. Superficial veins in the lower extremities become dilated and tortuous with increased venous pressure. The increased venous pressure may be due to congenital weakness of the vein structure, obesity, pregnancy, venous obstruction resulting from thrombosis or extrinsic pressure by tumors, or occupations that require prolonged standing. As the veins enlarge, the valves are stretched and become incompetent, allowing blood flow to be reversed. As back pressure increases and the venous pump (muscle movement that squeezes venous blood back toward the heart) fails, further venous distention results. The increased venous pressure is transmitted to the capillary bed, and edema develops.

Clinical manifestations. Discomfort from varicose veins varies dramatically among people and tends to be worsened by superficial thrombophlebitis. Additionally, many clients voice concern about cosmetic disfigurement. (Fig. 32-9). The most common symptom of varicose veins is an ache or pain after prolonged standing, which is relieved by walking or by elevating the limb. Some clients feel pressure or a cramplike sensation. Swelling may accompany the discomfort. Nocturnal leg cramps, especially in the calf area, may occur.

Complications. Superficial thrombophlebitis is a serious consequence of varicose veins and may occur either spontaneously or after trauma, surgical procedures, or pregnancy. Rupture of varicose veins (although not common) occurs because of weakening of the vessel wall. Ulceration as a result of skin infections or trauma may also develop.

Areas of *chronic venous stasis ulceration* (damaged dermis as a result of decreased tissue perfusion) are usually located near the inner aspect of the ankle, above and behind the medial malleolus.

Diagnostic studies. The Trendelenburg test is a diagnostic procedure that can be performed for the client with varicose veins, although it is rarely used today. The Trendelenburg test is used to assess valvular competence. The client's leg is elevated to 90 degrees and a tourniquet is placed around the thigh with sufficient pressure to occlude the great saphenous vein. The client is then asked to stand and the pattern of filling is observed. No more than 35 seconds should be required for the great saphenous vein to fill with blood from below. If no great rush of venous blood occurs at 60 seconds when the tourniquet is removed, the venous valves are competent and the test result is considered normal.

A Doppler venous examination can detect obstruction and reflux in the venous system with considerable accuracy. Impedance plethysmography provides objective information on deep venous patency.

Therapeutic management. Treatment is usually not indicated if varicose veins are only a cosmetic problem. If incompetency of the venous system develops, therapeutic management involves rest with the feet elevated, elastic support hose, and walking exercise.

Injection sclerotherapy is used more commonly in the treatment of unsightly superficial varicosities.[20] Direct IV injection of a sclerosing agent such as Sotradecol induces inflammation and results in eventual thrombosis of the vein. This procedure can be performed safely in an office setting and causes minimal discomfort. After injection the leg is wrapped with an elastic bandage for 24 to 72 hours to maintain pressure over the vein. Local tenderness subsides within 2 to 3 weeks, and eventually the thrombosed

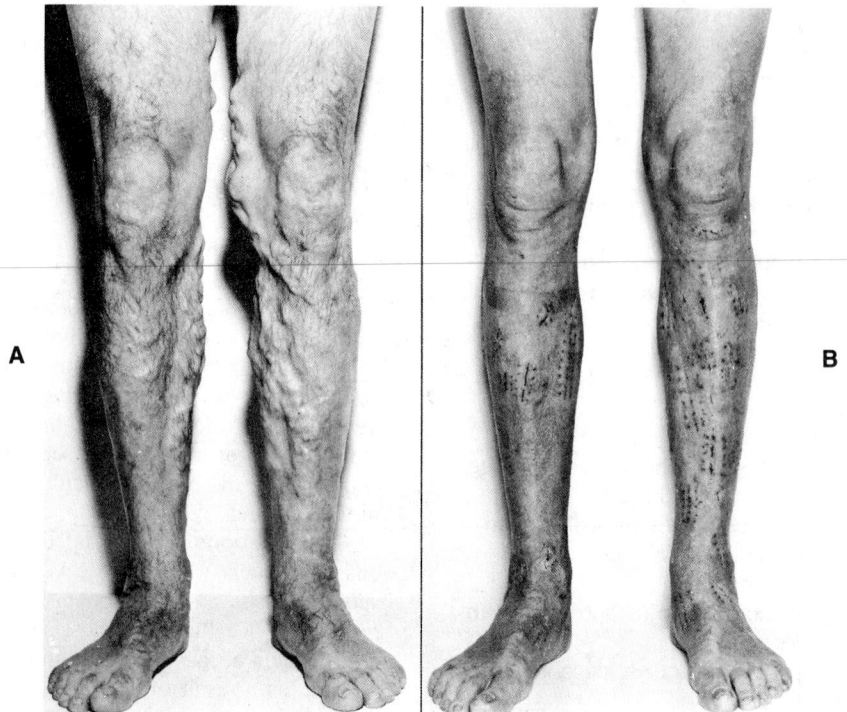

Fig. 32-9   Extensive varicosities (incompetency of the greater saphenous systems). **A,** Appearance preoperatively. **B,** Appearance 2 weeks postoperatively. (From Lofgren KA: Varicose veins. In Haimovici H, ed: Vascular surgery: principles and techniques, New York, 1976, McGraw-Hill, Inc.)

vein disappears. After injection sclerotherapy the client should be advised to wear compression stockings to help prevent the development of further varicosities.

Surgical interventions of varicose veins involve ligation of the entire vein (usually saphenous) and dissection and removal of its incompetent tributaries. Surgical interventions are indicated when chronic venous insufficiency cannot be prevented or controlled with therapy. Recurrent thrombophlebitis in varicose veins is another indication for surgery.

■ Nursing Management of Varicose Veins

Prevention is a key factor related to varicose veins. The nurse should instruct clients to avoid sitting or standing for long periods of time, to maintain ideal body weight, to take precautions against injury to the extremities, and to avoid wearing constrictive clothing.

After vein ligation surgery, the nurse should encourage deep breathing, which helps to promote venous return to the right side of the heart. The extremities should initially be checked hourly for color, movement, sensation, temperature, the presence of edema, and pedal pulses. Bruising and discoloration are considered normal.

Postoperatively, elevation of the extremities at a 15-degree angle is encouraged (except for periods of ambulation) to prevent the development of venous stasis and edema. Elastic stockings or bandages are also used and should be removed once every 8 hours for short periods and reapplied.

Long-term management of varicose veins is directed to-

ward improving circulation, relieving discomfort, improving cosmetic appearance, and avoiding complications such as superficial thrombophlebitis and ulceration. Varicose veins can recur in other veins after the surgical procedure. The client should be taught proper care of the lower extremities, including cleanliness and the use of individually measured elastic hose. The client should be taught to put on the hose while still lying down just before arising in the morning. The importance of periodic positioning of the legs above the heart should be stressed. Overweight clients need assistance with weight reduction. Those whose employment requires prolonged periods of standing or sitting should be encouraged to change their posture as frequently as possible. Pregnant clients with varicosities need appropriate teaching as prescribed by their obstetricians.

Venous Stasis Ulcers

Chronic venous insufficiency can lead to venous stasis ulceration. This condition usually arises as a result of deep venous thrombosis. The basic dysfunction is incompetent valves of the veins. The ulcers usually develop around the ankles, especially in the area of the medial malleoli (Fig. 32-10). Loss of epidermis occurs, and portions of the dermal layer may also be involved depending on the degree of venous stasis. A characteristic brownish coloration of the skin develops because of deposition of melanin and hemosiderin. When capillaries rupture, RBCs are released and disintegrate with subsequent release of hemosiderin.

Clinical manifestations and complications. The skin texture of the lower leg is leathery with a characteristic

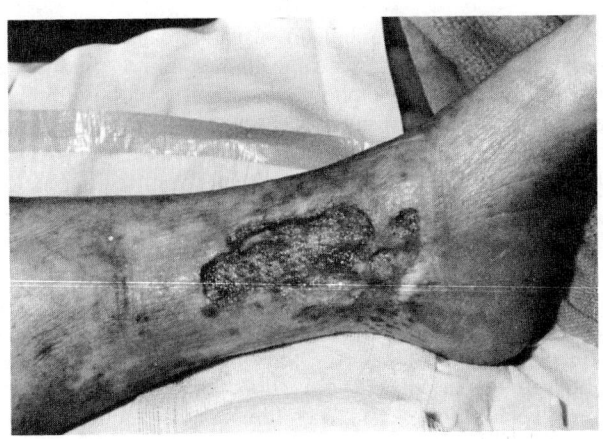

Fig. 32-10 Stasis ulcer associated with postthrombotic venous insufficiency. (From Davis JH: Clinical surgery, St Louis, 1987, The CV Mosby Co.)

red-brown "brawny" appearance. Edema has usually been present for a long time. The ulcer is a concave lesion below the margin of the skin surface and may become extensive. Pain may occur when the limb is in a dependent position or during ambulation. Pain is usually relieved by elevation of the foot.

If the ulcer is untreated, the lesion becomes more extensive, eroding wider and deeper. The likelihood of infection is increased. Scar tissue formation around the rim of the ulcer is found. Poor hygiene, debilitation, and inadequate nutritional status contribute to the severity of the ulcerative lesion.

Therapeutic management. The client is kept in bed with elevation of the extremity. The wound is cleansed with a bacteriostatic solution several times per day followed by the application of a topical dressing. The key to facilitating healing is extrinsic compression to minimize venous stasis, venous hypertension, and edema. Extrinsic compression methods used are elastic bandages, elastic stockings, Unna's boot, and custom-made boots constructed with Velcro straps (Circaid). The affected limb should be wrapped with an elastic bandage to provide compression. A dome paste (Unna's) boot, which hardens into a semirigid cast, is effective at promoting healing and works especially well as an outpatient therapy. It effectively controls edema and requires changes only once or twice weekly.[21]

Newer therapies, focused on promoting healing in a moist environment, are showing increasing promise.[22] Several adhesive hydrocolloid dressings are currently available and, when used in conjunction with extrinsic compression, have proved to be effective in hastening the healing of venous leg ulcers. (Hydrocolloid dressings are discussed in Chapter 7.)

Routine prophylactic antibiotic therapy is not indicated. If infection is evident as manifested by temperature elevation, leukocytosis, or drainage from the site, cultures of the lesion are indicated and appropriate antibiotic therapy is then instituted.

If the ulcer fails to respond to several months of conservative therapy, skin grafting may be indicated. The ulcer is debrided and tissue from a donor site is used (see Chapter 18). Any varicosities in the area of the lesion are removed.

■ Nursing Management of Venous Stasis Ulcers

The client with venous stasis ulcers should elevate the ulcerated leg as much as possible. The nurse should change the dressings as ordered and perform prescribed wound care measures including observation for signs of infection. A balanced diet is encouraged with protein and vitamin supplementation to promote wound healing.

Long-term management of venous stasis ulcers should focus on educating the client in self-care measures because the incidence of recurrence is high. Discharge teaching should include avoidance of trauma to the limbs, proper skin care measures, and application of prescribed elastic support stockings (after complete healing has occurred and swelling is minimized by elevation). Rest periods with elevation of the extremities should also be encouraged. A balanced nutritional program incorporating protein-vitamin supplementation needs to be instituted. Caloric limitation for weight reduction and diabetic diet management are taught when indicated. Once scar formation has occurred, the client should return to a regimen of regular exercise (walking) and periods of leg elevation above the level of the heart.

PULMONARY EMBOLISM
Pathophysiology

Pulmonary embolism is the most common pulmonary complication in hospitalized clients. Although the actual incidence of mortality and morbidity from pulmonary embolism is unknown, it is estimated that nearly 50,000 people die of pulmonary embolism each year in the United States and another 650,000 have nonfatal pulmonary embolisms.[23]

Most pulmonary emboli arise from thrombi in the deep veins of the legs. Other sites of origin include the right side of the heart (especially with atrial fibrillation), upper extremities (rare), and the pelvic veins (especially after surgery or childbirth). Lethal pulmonary emboli originate most commonly in the femoral or iliac veins. Emboli are mobile clots that generally do not stop moving until they lodge at a narrowed part of the circulatory system. The lungs are an ideal location for emboli to lodge due to its extensive arterial and capillary network. The lower lobes are most frequently affected because they have a higher blood flow than the other lobes. Occasionally, the presence of deep vein thrombosis is unsuspected until pulmonary embolism occurs.

Thrombus in the deep veins can dislodge spontaneously. However, a more common mechanism is jarring of the thrombus by mechanical forces, such as sudden standing, and changes in the rate of blood flow, such as those that occur with the Valsalva maneuver.

In addition to dislodged thrombi, rarer causes of pulmonary occlusion include fat emboli (from fractured long bones), air emboli (from improperly administered IV therapy), amniotic fluid, and tumors. Tumor emboli may originate from primary or metastatic malignancies.

Clinical Manifestations

The severity of clinical manifestations depends on the size of the emboli and the size and number of blood vessels occluded. The most common manifestation of pulmonary embolism is sudden onset of unexplained dyspnea, tachypnea, and/or tachycardia. Other manifestations are cough, chest pain, hemoptysis, rales, fever, accentuation of the pulmonic heart sound, and sudden change in mental status as a result of hypoxemia.

Massive emboli may produce sudden collapse of the client with shock, pallor, severe dyspnea, and crushing chest pain. However, some people with massive emboli do not have pain. The pulse is rapid and weak, the BP is low, and an ECG indicates right ventricular strain. When rapid obstruction of 50% or more of the pulmonary vascular bed occurs, acute cor pulmonale may result because the right ventricle can no longer pump blood into the lungs. Death occurs in more than 60% of people with massive emboli.

Medium-sized emboli often cause pleuritic chest pain accompanied by dyspnea, slight fever, and a productive cough with blood-streaked sputum. A physical examination may indicate tachycardia and a pleural friction rub.

Small emboli frequently are undetected or produce vague, transient symptoms. The exception to this is the client with underlying cardiopulmonary disease, in whom even small or medium-sized emboli may result in severe cardiopulmonary compromise. However, repeated small emboli gradually cause a reduction in the capillary bed and eventual pulmonary hypertension. An ECG and chest x-ray film may indicate right ventricular hypertrophy secondary to pulmonary hypertension.

Complications

Pulmonary infarction. Pulmonary infarction (death of lung tissue) occurs in less than 10% of clients with emboli. Infarction is more likely when (1) occlusion of a large or medium-sized pulmonary vessel (greater than 2 mm in diameter), (2) insufficient collateral blood flow from the bronchial circulation, or (3) preexisting lung disease is present. Infarction results in alveolar necrosis and hemorrhage. Occasionally the infarct becomes infected and an abscess may develop. Concomitant pleural effusion is frequently found.

Pulmonary hypertension. Pulmonary hypertension occurs when more than 50% of the cross-sectional area of the normal pulmonary bed is compromised. Pulmonary hypertension also results from hypoxemia. As a single event an embolus does not cause pulmonary hypertension unless it is massive. However, recurrent small to medium-sized emboli may result in chronic pulmonary hypertension. Pulmonary hypertension eventually results in dilatation and hypertrophy of the right ventricle. Depending on the degree of pulmonary hypertension and its rate of development, death may result rapidly or only mild or transient alterations may be produced (see Chapter 21).

Diagnostic Studies

An ECG is not a very sensitive or specific diagnostic measure to detect pulmonary embolism. With small to medium-sized pulmonary emboli it may remain normal or show a combination of changes transiently. As an isolated event, pulmonary embolism usually causes no ECG changes. Dysrhythmias are the most common finding related to pulmonary emboli. Recurrent small pulmonary emboli may eventually produce chronic pulmonary hypertension and ECG changes of right axis deviation with enlargement of the right atrium and right ventricle.

A chest x-ray film is usually not diagnostic unless an infarction has occurred. Even with pulmonary infarction, the chest x-ray film is nondiagnostic in about 50% of clients. Positive findings are best visualized 12 to 24 hours after embolism because variably shaped (round, linear, or occasionally wedge) areas of consolidation are sometimes found in the periphery or lower lobes. Pleural effusions are often noted. The chest x-ray film can be valuable in assessing other pulmonary pathology such as chronic obstructive pulmonary disease and tuberculosis.

A lung scan may be of value in screening for initial (or recurrent) pulmonary embolism, assessing the natural history of the lesion, and evaluating the effectiveness of therapeutic or surgical management. The lung scan has two components and is most accurate when both are performed:

1. *Perfusion scanning* involves IV injection of a radioisotope. A scanning device reflects the adequacy of the pulmonary circulation.
2. *Ventilation scanning* involves inhalation of a radioactive gas such as xenon. Scanning reflects the distribution of gas through the lung. The ventilation component requires the cooperation of the client and may be difficult or impossible to perform in the critically ill, particularly if the client is intubated.

Noninvasive studies and venography are helpful in diagnosing deep vein thrombosis as the likely source of a pulmonary embolism. Additionally, vena cava venography is routinely performed before vena cava interruption.

Pulmonary angiography is an invasive procedure that involves the insertion of a catheter through the antecubital or femoral vein and advancement to the pulmonary artery. Contrast medium is injected to visualize the pulmonary vascular system. This procedure remains the definitive diagnostic test for pulmonary embolism.[24]

ABG analysis is important. The arterial oxygen pressure (Pao_2) is always below normal because of inadequate oxygenation secondary to an occluded pulmonary vasculature. The arterial carbon dioxide pressure ($Paco_2$) is usually below normal due to tachypnea and hyperventilation that occurs with pulmonary emboli. The pH remains normal unless respiratory alkalosis develops as a result of prolonged hyperventilation or to compensate for lactic acidosis caused by shock. ABGs may be greatly influenced by the presence of underlying cardiac and pulmonary disease.

Therapeutic and Pharmacological Management

When the diagnosis of thromboembolic disease has been made, treatment should be instituted immediately (Table 32-18). The objectives of therapeutic treatment are to (1) prevent further growth or multiplication of thrombi in the lower extremities, (2) prevent embolization from the lower extremities to the pulmonary arteries, and (3) provide cardiopulmonary support if indicated.

Conservative therapy. Supportive therapy for the cli-

Table 32-18

**Diagnostic and Therapeutic
Management: Acute Pulmonary Embolism**

DIAGNOSTIC

History and physical examination
Lung scan (perfusion and ventilation)
Chest x-ray film
Continuous ECG monitoring
ABGs
CBC count with differential
Pulmonary angiography
Venogram

THERAPEUTIC

Oxygen by mask or cannula
Establishment of IV route for drugs and fluids
Continuous IV heparin
Bed rest
Narcotics for pain relief
Thrombolytic agents in certain clients
Pulmonary embolectomy in life-threatening situations

CBC, Complete blood cell.

ent's cardiopulmonary status varies according to the severity of the pulmonary embolism. The administration of oxygen by mask or cannula may be adequate for some clients. Oxygen is given in a concentration determined by ABG analysis. In some situations, endotracheal intubation and mechanical ventilation may be needed to maintain adequate oxygenation. Respiratory measures such as turning, coughing, and deep breathing are necessary to prevent or treat atelectasis. If shock is present, vasopressor agents may be necessary to support systemic circulation. If heart failure is present, digitalis and diuretics are used. Pain resulting from pleural irritation or reduced coronary blood flow is treated with narcotics, usually morphine.

Properly managed anticoagulant therapy is effective in the treatment of many clients with pulmonary emboli. Heparin and warfarin (Coumadin) are the anticoagulant drugs of choice. Heparin should be started immediately and is continued as oral anticoagulants are initiated. The dosage of heparin is adjusted according to its effect on the PTT, and that of warfarin is regulated by the PT. Difficulties may be encountered in occasional clients in whom thrombosis or bleeding develops despite an apparently correct dosage.

Anticoagulant therapy for thromboembolic conditions may not be indicated in the presence of blood dyscrasias, hepatic dysfunction causing alteration in the clotting mechanism, injury to the viscera, overt bleeding, a history of cerebrovascular accident, or neurological conditions.

Surgical Interventions

If the degree of pulmonary arterial obstruction is severe (usually greater than 50%) and the client does not respond to conservative therapy, an immediate embolectomy may be indicated. Pulmonary embolectomy is possible with the use of temporary cardiopulmonary bypass. Preoperative pulmonary angiography is necessary to identify and locate the site of the embolus. Fortunately, the need for pulmonary embolectomy is rare.

To prevent further pulmonary embolization, the surgical procedures appropriate for thrombophlebitis may be used (see pp. 936-937). These include insertion of intracaval filter devices and extravascular vena cava interruption (see Fig. 32-8).

Thrombolytic agents. Thrombolytic agents such as urokinase and streptokinase have been shown to dissolve pulmonary emboli within 24 to 48 hours. Streptokinase, obtained from hemolytic streptococci, is thought to activate plasminogen, which is a fibrinolytic enzyme precursor. Urokinase, found in urine, also activates plasminogen. Both agents have been suggested for use in clients with massive emboli or in whom surgery is contraindicated (see Chapter 28). Their use in the treatment of pulmonary emboli is undergoing investigation.

■ Nursing Management of Pulmonary Embolism

Nursing interventions

Health promotion and maintenance. Nursing measures aimed at prevention of pulmonary embolism parallel those for prophylaxis of deep vein thrombophlebitis (see p. 938).

Acute intervention. The prognosis of a client with pulmonary emboli is good if therapy is promptly instituted. The client should be kept in bed in a semi-Fowler's position to facilitate breathing. A patent IV line should be maintained for medications and fluid therapy. The nurse should know the side effects of medications and observe for them. Oxygen therapy should be administered as ordered (see Table 21-13). Careful monitoring of vital signs, ECG, blood gases, and lung sounds is critical to assess the client's status.

The client is usually anxious because of pain, inability to breathe, and fear of death. The nurse should carefully explain the situation and provide emotional support and reassurance to help relieve the client's anxiety. During the acute phase, someone should be with the client as much as possible.

Many clients with pulmonary emboli have been hospitalized for a primary problem such as sepsis, acute respiratory failure, or surgical intervention. The nurse needs to focus on management of the problems caused by the primary disorder and those related to pulmonary emboli.

Chronic management. Clients affected by thromboembolic processes require much psychological and emotional support. In addition to the thromboembolic problems, they may have an underlying chronic illness requiring long-term treatment. To provide supportive therapy, the nurse must understand and differentiate between the various problems caused by the underlying disease and those related to thromboembolic disease.

Long-term management is similar to that for the client with thrombophlebitis (see Tables 32-11, 32-12, and 32-16). Discharge planning is aimed at limiting progression of the condition and preventing complications. The nurse must reinforce the need for the client to return to the health care facility for regular follow-up examination.

C ase Study

THROMBOPHLEBITIS

Shirley J., a 34-year-old woman, was admitted to the hospital with the diagnosis of thrombophlebitis of the left leg. She is on a regular diet at home, smokes two packs of cigarettes per day, and is obese at 185 pounds for her 5-foot 3-inch frame. She knows that she has a bad mitral valve and has previously been treated for "fluttering of the upper portion" of her heart. The only medication she takes is contraceptive pills. She has had a gradual increase in pain and swelling of the left leg. It appears glossy and warm to the touch. She states that it is very tender from midthigh to toe. She has an elevated WBC count and an elevated erythrocyte sedimentation rate. Her temperature is 38° C, and her pulse is irregular at 106 bpm.

Discussion Questions

1. Explain the pathogenesis of thrombophlebitis. What risk factors does Shirley have?
2. Compare superficial thrombophlebitis with deep vein thrombophlebitis in terms of the affected veins and clinical manifestations. Which disorder does Shirley have?
3. What complications may result from thrombophlebitis?
4. What are the main features differentiating arterial vascular and venous vascular problems?
5. What diagnostic tests can be used for thrombophlebitis?
6. Explain the physiological bases for each of the following treatment measures: leg elevation, hot packs, IV heparin, deep-breathing and coughing exercises, and elastic hose.
7. What important things should Shirley be taught to prevent recurrent episodes of thrombophlebitis?

R eview Questions

The number of the question corresponds to the same-numbered objective at the beginning of the chapter.

1. Which of the following statements accurately characterizes aortic aneurysms?
   a. They are most frequently caused by arteriosclerosis.
   b. They occur exclusively in the descending and abdominal aortas.
   c. They are most frequently caused by syphilis.
   d. They most commonly occur in young women after pregnancy.
2. An important nursing measure after an aneurysm repair is to
   a. administer anticoagulant therapy
   b. position the legs in the Trendelenburg position
   c. apply elastic stockings to both feet
   d. palpate the peripheral pulses frequently
3. Aortic dissection
   a. may be asymptomatic
   b. may cause severe chest and back pain
   c. is usually related to hypertension
   d. all the above
4. Which of the following is the most significant atherosclerotic risk factor?
   a. high-roughage diet
   b. sedentary lifestyle
   c. cigarette smoking
   d. elevated high-density lipoprotein
5. Intermittent claudication is a manifestation that occurs as a result of
   a. inadequate blood flow to the muscles during exercise
   b. inadequate blood flow to the skin after application of heat
   c. the beginning of gangrene in the toes
   d. dorsiflexion of the foot when thrombophlebitis is present
6. Which of the following instructions is inappropriate for a client with chronic arterial insufficiency?
   a. Avoid traumatizing or chilling the lower extremity.
   b. Wear an elastic bandage or stocking.
   c. Walk for about 30 to 60 minutes daily or until pain develops.
   d. Check the peripheral pulses daily in both feet.
7. All the following predispose to the development of deep vein thrombophlebitis *except*
   a. elevated WBC count
   b. endothelial damage
   c. stasis
   d. hypercoagulability
8. Deep vein thrombophlebitis is characterized by
   a. redness, heat, and tenderness of the affected area
   b. generalized edema of the involved extremity
   c. pallor and cyanosis of the involved extremity
   d. paresthesia and coolness of the leg
9. Which of the following nursing actions is included in the plan of care for the client with acute lower extremity deep vein thrombophlebitis?
   a. Encourage walking and leg exercises to promote venous return.
   b. Apply topical antibiotics.
   c. Administer anticoagulants as ordered.
   d. Keep client's legs in a dependent position.
10. Which of the following describes the rationale for anticoagulant therapy?
    a. dissolves thromboemboli
    b. prevents platelet aggregation
    c. inhibits the clotting mechanism
    d. activates the clotting mechanism
11. Which of the following best describes the etiology of venous stasis ulceration?
    a. chronic lack of oxygen to the skin
    b. loss of subcutaneous tissue and protective fat
    c. chronic edema, altered skin, pigmentation, and fragility of skin
    d. generalized infection
12. The most common site of origin of pulmonary emboli is the
    a. right side of the heart
    b. peripheral arterial system
    c. pelvic veins
    d. deep veins of the legs

REFERENCES

1. Dalsing MC and Sawchuk AP: Surgery of the aorta. In Fahey VA, ed: Vascular nursing, Philadelphia, 1988, WB Saunders Co, p 190.
2. Doyle JE, Johantgen M, and Vitello-Cicciu J: Vascular disease. In Kinney MR and others, eds: AACN's clinical reference for critical-care nursing, New York, 1988, The CV Mosby Co, p 729.
3. Wheat M: Acute dissection of the aorta. In McCauley K and others, eds: McGoon's cardiac surgery: an interprofessional approach to patient care, Philadelphia, 1985, FA Davis Co.
4. Joyce JW and Hollier LH: The giant cell arteritides: temporal and Takayasu's arteritis. In Bergan JJ and Yao JST, eds: Evaluation and treatment of upper and lower extremity arterial disorders, Orlando, Fla, 1984, Grune & Stratton, pp 465-481.
5. Graham LM and O'Keefe MF: Arterial disease. In Fahey VA, ed: Vascular nursing, Philadelphia, 1988, WB Saunders Co, p 15.
6. Kempczinski R and Birinyi L: Impotence following aortic surgery. In Bernhard V and Towne J, eds: Complications in vascular surgery, Orlando, 1985, Grune & Stratton, pp 311-324.
7. DePalma R: Modern management of impotence associated with aortic surgery. In Bergan JJ and Yao JST, eds: Arterial surgery: new diagnostic and operative techniques, Orlando, 1988, Grune & Stratton.
8. Eagan J: Lasers: applications in cardiovascular atherosclerotic disease in critical care, Nurse Clin North Am 1:311-326, 1989.
9. Eagan J and Vitello-Cicciu J: Laser thermal and balloon angioplasty, J Cardiovasc Nurs 1:74-78, 1987.
10. Gardner R: Lasers in cardiovascular disease, J Cardiovasc Nurs 1:77-79, 1986.
11. Ahn S and Auth D: Removal of focal atheromatous lesions by angioscopically guided high-speed rotary atherectomy, J Vasc Surg 7:292-300, 1988.
12. Kensey K: Recanalization of obstructed arteries with a flexible, rotating tip catheter, Radiology 165:387-389, 1987.
13. Simpson J: Transluminal atherectomy for occlusive PVD, Am J Cardiol 61:96-101, 1988.
14. Nunnelee JD: Medications used in vascular patients. In Fahey VA, ed: Vascular nursing, Philadelphia, 1988, WB Saunders Co, pp 169-183.
15. Kannel WB: Cigarette smoking and peripheral arterial disease, Prim Cardiol 4:13-18, 1986.
16. Provan JL: The effect of cigarette smoking on the long-term success rates of aortofemoral and femoropopliteal reconstructions, Surg Gynecol Obstet 165:49-52, 1987.
17. Bachman JA: Pregnancy and thromboembolic disease, J Soc Peripheral Vasc Nurs 8:11-14, 1990.
18. Fahey VA: Venous thromboembolism. In Fahey VA, ed: Vascular nursing, Philadelphia, 1988, WB Saunders Co, pp 339-365.
19. Doyle JE: Treatment modalities in peripheral vascular disease, Nurs Clin North Am 21:241-253, 1986.
20. Menzoian JO and Doyle JE: Venous insufficiency of the leg, Hosp Pract 24:109-116, 1989.
21. Doyle JE: All leg ulcers are not alike: managing and preventing arterial and venous ulcers, Nursing 13:58-63, 1983.
22. Swanick R: The treatment of venous ulceration, Nursing 18:40-43, 1988.
23. Consensus conference: prevention of venous thrombosis and pulmonary emboli, JAMA 256:744-749, 1986.
24. Alexander J and Zarins C: The diagnosis of pulmonary embolism. In Bergan JJ and Yao JST, eds: Surgery of the veins, Orlando, 1985, Grune & Stratton, pp 447-459.

SECTION V REFERENCES
BOOKS

Abel L: Critical care nursing: a physiologic approach, St Louis, 1986, The CV Mosby Co.

Andreoli KG and others: Comprehensive cardiac care, ed 7, St Louis, 1991, Mosby–Year Book, Inc.

Baumgartner WA, Reitz BA, and Achuff SC: Heart and heart-lung transplantation, Philadelphia, 1990, WB Saunders Co.

Berkey KM, Hanson HI, and Hanson S: Pocket guide to family assessment and intervention, St Louis, 1990, Mosby–Year Book, Inc.

Bowers AC and Thompson JM: Clinical manual of health assessment, ed 3, St Louis, 1988, The CV Mosby Co.

Bullough B and Bullough V: Nursing in the community, St Louis, 1990, Mosby–Year Book, Inc.

Canobbio MM: Volume I: cardiovascular disorders, St Louis, 1990, Mosby–Year Book, Inc.

Christensen PJ and Kenney JW: The nursing process: application of theories, frameworks, and models, ed 3, St Louis, 1990, Mosby–Year Book, Inc.

Clemen-Stone S, Eigsti DG, and McGuire SL: Comprehensive family and community health nursing, ed 2, St Louis, 1987, The CV Mosby Co.

Conover MB: Understanding electrocardiography: arrhythmias and the 12-lead ECG, ed 5, St Louis, 1988, The CV Mosby Co.

Conover MB: Pocket guide to electrocardiography, ed 2, St Louis, 1990, Mosby–Year Book, Inc.

Cookfair J: Nursing process and practice in the community, St Louis, 1990, Mosby–Year Book, Inc.

Daily EK and Schroeder JS: Techniques in bedside hemodynamic monitoring, ed 4, St Louis, 1989, The CV Mosby Co.

DeJardin TR: Clinical manifestations of respiratory disease, ed 2, Chicago, 1990, Year Book Medical Publishers.

Dutcher JP: Modern transfusion therapy, Boca Raton, Fla, 1990, CRC Press.

Edelman CL and Mandle CL: Health promotion throughout the lifespan, ed 2, St Louis, 1990, Mosby–Year Book, Inc.

Francis GS and Alpert JS: Modern coronary care, Boston, 1990, Little, Brown & Co, Inc.

Gazes PC: Clinical cardiology, ed 3, Philadelphia, 1990, Lea & Febiger.

Goodfellow P, ed: Cystic fibrosis, New York, 1989, Oxford University Press.

Gordon M: Manual of nursing diagnosis 1991-1992, St Louis, 1991, Mosby–Year Book, Inc.

Grauer K and Cavallero D: ACLS: certification preparation and a comprehensive review, ed 2, St Louis, 1988, The CV Mosby Co.

Grauer K and Cavallero D: ACLS teaching kit: an instructor's resource, St Louis, 1989, The CV Mosby Co.

Heath M: Workbook to accompany the homemaker/home health aide, St Louis, 1989, The CV Mosby Co.

Hickey PW: Nursing process handbook, St Louis, 1990, Mosby–Year Book, Inc.

Hoeman S: Rehabilitation/restorative care in the community, St Louis, 1990, Mosby–Year Book, Inc.

Hoover KG: Study guide to accompany fundamentals of nursing: concepts, process, and practice, ed 2, St Louis, 1989, The CV Mosby Co.

Jaffe MS and Skidmore-Roth L: Home health nursing care plans, St Louis, 1988, The CV Mosby Co.

Johanson BC and others: Standards for critical care, ed 3, St Louis, 1988, The CV Mosby Co.

Joiner J and others: Management of the patient-ventilator system: a team approach, ed 3, St Louis, 1984, The CV Mosby Co.

Kersten LD: Comprehensive respiratory nursing: a decision-making approach, Philadelphia, 1989, WB Saunders Co.

Kim M, McFarland GK, and McLane AM: Pocket guide to nursing diagnoses, ed 3, St Louis, 1989, The CV Mosby Co.

Lacher M and Redman JR: Hodgkin's disease: the consequences of survival, Philadelphia, 1990, Lea & Febiger.

Levitzky MG, Cairo JM, and Hall SM: Introduction to respiratory care, Philadelphia, 1990, WB Saunders Co.

Magrath I, ed: The non-Hodgkin's lymphomas, Baltimore, 1990, Williams & Wilkins.

Malley WJ: Clinical blood gases: application and noninvasive alternatives, Philadelphia, 1990, WB Saunders Co.

Martin L: Pulmonary physiology in clinical practice: the essentials for patient care and evaluation, St Louis, 1987, The CV Mosby Co.

McFarland GK and McFarlane EA: Nursing diagnosis and intervention: planning for patient care, St Louis, 1989, The CV Mosby Co.

Potter PA: Pocket guide to physical assessment, ed 2, St Louis, 1990, Mosby–Year Book, Inc.

Rau JL: Respiratory care pharmacology, ed 3, Chicago, 1989, Year Book Medical Publishers.

Redman BK: The process of patient education, ed 6, St Louis, 1988, The CV Mosby Co.

Ruppel G: Manuel of pulmonary function testing, ed 5, St Louis, 1991, Mosby–Year Book, Inc.

Sexton DL, ed: Nursing care of the respiratory patient, Norwalk, Conn, 1990, Appleton & Lange.

Stillwell S and Randall E: Pocket guide to cardiovascular care, St Louis, 1990, Mosby–Year Book, Inc.

Sundeen SJ and others: Nurse-client interaction: implementing the nursing process, ed 4, St Louis, 1989, The CV Mosby Co.

Talbot L and Meyers-Marquardt M: Pocket guide to critical care assessment, St Louis, 1989, The CV Mosby Co.

Thompson JM and Bowers AC: Health assessment: an illustrated pocket guide, ed 2, St Louis, 1988, The CV Mosby Co.

Vinsant MO and Spence MI: Common sense approach to coronary care: a program, ed 5, St Louis, 1988, The CV Mosby Co.

Wilkins RL, Sheldon FL, and Krider SJ: Clinical assessment in respiratory care, ed 2, St Louis, 1990, Mosby–Year Book, Inc.

Wilson SF and Thompson JM: Volume II: respiratory disorders, St Louis, 1990, Mosby–Year Book, Inc.

JOURNALS

Ahrens T: Blood gas assessment of intrapulmonary shunting and deadspace, Crit Care Nurs Clin North Am 1:641, 1989.

American Thoracic Society: Standards for the diagnosis and care of patients with COPD and asthma, Am Rev Respir Dis 136:225, 1987.

Ashby D: The patient with peripheral vascular disease, J Post Anesth Nurs 5:112, 1990.

Bauer LE: Discharge of a patient with chronic respiratory failure: part I, Home Healthc Nurse 7:17, 1989.

Bauer LE: Discharge of a patient with chronic respiratory failure: part II, Home Healthc Nurse 7:10, 1989.

Bell TN: Disseminated intravascular coagulation and shock: multisystem crisis in the critically ill, Crit Care Nurs Clin North Am 2:255, 1990.

Black PA: A preventable tragedy: the nurse's role in preventing coronary heart disease, Prof Nurse 5:404, 1990.

Blaisdell MW, Good L, and Gentzler RD: Percutaneous transluminal valvuloplasty, Crit Care Nurse 9:62, 1989.

Bousquet GL: Congestive heart failure: a review of nonpharmacologic therapies, J Cardiovasc Nurs 4:35, 1990.

Bramwell L: Social support in cardiac rehabilitation, Can J Cardiovasc Nurs 1:7, 1990.

Brandt B: Nursing protocol for the patient with neutropenia, Oncol Nurs Forum 17(suppl 1)9, 1990.

Braun LT and Holm K: Preservation of ischemic myocardium through activity management, J Cardiovas Nurs 3:39, 1989.

Brewer-Senerchia C: Thrombolytic therapy: a review of the literature on streptokinase and tissue plasminogen activator with implications for practice, Crit Care Nurs Clin North Am 1:359, 1989.

Brown S and Mann R: Breaking the cycle—control of breathlessness in chronic lung disease, Prof Nurse 5:325, 1990.

Caruthers DD: Infectious pneumonia in the elderly, Am J Nurs 90:56, 1990.

Cholesterol Adult Treatment Panel Report of the National Cholesterol Education Program Expert Panel on Detection, Evaluation, and Treatment of High Blood Cholesterol in Adults, Arch Intern Med 148:36, 1988.

Crowe M and Ultrino C: Psychosocial implications of lung cancer, J Pract Nurs 40:36, 1990.

Derenowski J: Coronary artery disease in Hispanics, J Cardiovasc Nurs 4:13, 1990.

DiLucente LJ: Mimics of coronary artery disease on the electrodiogram, Crit Care Nurse 10:31, 1990.

Dix-Sheldon DK: Pharmacologic management of myocardial ischemia, J Cardiovasc Nurs 3:17, 1989.

Domenico JM: Cardiac arrest following myocardial infarction, J Cardiovasc Nurs 4:56, 1990.

Erickson JM: Blood support for the myelosuppressed patient, Semin Oncol Nurs 6:61, 1990.

Fedorovich C and Littleton MT: Chest physiotherapy: evaluating the effectiveness, Dimens Crit Care Nurs 9:68, 1990.

France-Dawson M: Sickle cell conditions and health knowledge, Nurs Stand 4:30, 1990.

Fukuda N: Outcome standards for the client with chronic congestive heart failure, J Cardiovasc Nurs 4:59, 1990.

Fuller AK: Platelet transfusion therapy for thrombocytopenia, Semin Oncol Nurs 6:123, 1990.

Gavigan M, Kline-O'Sullivan C, and Klumpp-Lybrand B: The effect of regular turning on CABG patients, Crit Care Nurs Q 12:69, 1990.

Gerber RM: Coronary artery disease in the elderly, J Cardiovasc Nurs 4:23, 1990.

Gillette MK and Caruso CC: Intraoperative tissue injury: major causes and preventive measures, AORN J 50:66, 1989.

Goran SF: Vascular complications of the patient undergoing intra-aortic balloon pumping, Crit Care Nurs Clin North Am 1:459, 1989.

Hardy GR: SvO_2 continuous monitory techniques, Dimens Crit Care Nurs 7:8, 1988.

Hickey M: Controlling cor pulmonale, Nursing 20:32E, 1990.

Hoffman L and Wesmiller S: Home oxygen: transtracheal and other options, Am J Nurs 88:464, 1988.

Janson-Bjerklie S: Status asthmaticus, Am J Nurs 90:52, 1990.

Kelleher RM: Cardiac drugs: new inotropes, Crit Care Nurs Clin North Am 1:391, 1989.

Keller C: Coronary artery disease in blacks, J Cardiovasc Nurs 4:1, 1990.

Kennedy GT: Captopril in the treatment of chronic CHF, Crit Care Nurse 10:39, 1990.

Kuhn MM: Nutritional support for the shock patient, Crit Care Nurs Clin North Am 2:201, 1990.

Lee TH and others: Impact of initial triage decisions on nursing intensity for patients with acute chest pain, Med Care 28:737, 1990.

Lindell KO and Wesmiller SW: Using arterial blood gases to interpret acid-base balance, Orthop Nurs 8:31, 1989.

London F: Nursing diagnoses and caring for patients with sickle cell disease, Adv Clin Care 5:12, 1990.

Lynn-McHale D and Shaffer R: Action stat! Ventricular tachycardia: how to control this potentially fatal arrhythmia and prevent cardiac arrest, Nursing 20:33, 1990.

Madsen LA: Tuberculosis today, RN 53:44, 1990.

Martin JS and others: Early triage and treatment of the acute myocardial infarction patient: how fast is fast?, J Emerg Nurs 16:195, 1990.

Menzies A and Stearn R: The future of asthma management, Nurs Stand 4:24, 1990.

Messner RL and Mufson MA: Pneumoccal vaccine: a focus for nursing, Adv Clin Care 5:11, 1990.

Miers LJ and Arnold R: The cardiovascular response to exercise in the patient with congestive heart failure, J Cardiovasc Nurs 4:47, 1990.

Murdaugh C: Coronary artery disease in women, J Cardiovasc Nurs 4:35, 1990.

Nardell EA: Tuberculosis in homeless, residential care facilities, prisons, nursing homes, and other close communities, Semin Respir Infect 4:206, 1989.

Nunnelee JD: Nursing: hope for the vascular patient, J Vasc Nurs 8:19, 1990.

Oniboni AC: Infection in the neutropenic patient, Semin Oncol Nurs 6:50, 1990.

Openbrier DR, Hoffman LH, and Wesmiller SW: Home oxygen therapy: evaluation and prescription, Am J Nurs 88:192, 1988.

Parchert MA and Creason N: The role of nursing in the rehabilitation of women with cardiac disease, J Cardiovasc Nurs 3:57, 1989.

Pavel JN: Red blood cell transfusions for anemia, Semin Oncol Nurs 6:117, 1990.

Petty TL: Drug strategies for airflow obstruction, Am J Nurs 87:180, 1987.

Pierce CD: Transcutaneous cardiac pacing: expanding clinical applications, Crit Care Nurs Clin North Am 1:423, 1989.

Poulton R: Home care program for hemophiliacs, Md Nurs 9:5, 1990.

Rahr VA and Tucker R: Non-Hodgkin's lymphoma: understanding the disease, Cancer Nurs 13:56, 1990.

Rayfield S and Theriot BL: Maximizing safe blood transfusions, Adv Clin Care 5:17, 1990.

Rostad M: Advances in nursing management of patients with lung cancer, Nurs Clin North Am 25:393, 1990.

Schroeder CH: Pulse oximetry: a nursing care plan, Crit Care Nurse 8:50, 1988.

Sipperly ME: Expanding role of coronary angioplasty: current implications, limitations, and nursing considerations, Heart Lung 18:507, 1989.

Stead WW and Dutt AK: Tuberculosis in the elderly, Semin Respir Infect 4:189, 1989.

Suchak BA and Barbon CB: Disseminated intravascular coagulation: a nursing challenge, Orthop Nurs 8:61, 1989.

Traver GA and Leidy NK: Asthma and stress, J Adv Med Surg Nurs 1:25, 1989.

Vaughan P and Brooks C Jr: Adult respiratory distress syndrome: a complication of shock, Crit Care Nurs Clin North Am 2:235, 1990.

Weiner B: Second generation antidysrhythmic agents, Crit Care Nurs Clin North Am 1:417, 1989.

Woodman J and Robinson C: Asthma education—a different approach, Community Outlook May 1990, p 7.

Yoemans AC and Harle MT: Myelodysplastic syndromes, Semin Oncol Nurs 6:9, 1990.

ORGANIZATIONS

American Academy of Facial, Plastic and Reconstructive Surgery, Inc.
1110 Vermont Avenue NW
Washington, DC 20005

American Association of Critical-Care Nurses
One Civic Plaza
Newport Beach, CA 92660

American College of Cardiology
9111 Old Georgetown Road
Bethesda, MD 20814

American Heart Association
7320 Greenville Avenue
Dallas, TX 75231

American Lung Association
1740 Broadway
New York, NY 10019

American Speech-Language-Hearing Association
10801 Rockville Pike
Rockville, MD 20852

Asthma and Allergy Foundation of America
1717 Massachusett Avenue
Suite 305
Washington, DC 20036

Cystic Fibrosis Foundation
6931 Arlington Road, #200
Bethesda MD 20814

International Association of Laryngectomees
c/o American Cancer Society
1599 Clifton Road, NE
Atlanta, GA 30329

Leukemia Society of America, Inc.
733 Third Avenue
New York, NY 10017

National Heart, Lung, and Blood Institute
National Institutes of Health
9000 Rockville Pike
Bethesda, MD 20892

National Hemophilia Foundation
110 Green Street, Room 406
New York, NY 10012

Sickle Cell Disease Foundation of Greater New York
1 West 125th Street, Room 206
New York, NY 10027

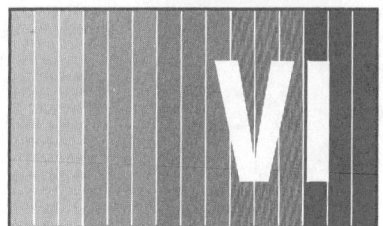

SECTION

VI

PROBLEMS WITH INGESTION, DIGESTION, ABSORPTION, AND ELIMINATION

33

Nursing Assessment

Gastrointestinal System

Rachel Elrod

---

1. Describe the structures and functions of the organs of the gastrointestinal tract.
2. Describe the structures and functions of the liver, gallbladder, biliary tract, and pancreas.
3. Explain the processes of ingestion, digestion, absorption, and elimination.
4. Explain the processes of biliary metabolism, bile production, and bile excretion.
5. Identify the significant subjective and objective data related to the gastrointestinal system that should be obtained from a client.
6. Describe the appropriate techniques used in the physical assessment of the gastrointestinal system.
7. Differentiate normal from common abnormal findings of a physical assessment of the gastrointestinal system.
8. Describe the purpose, significance of results, and nursing responsibilities related to diagnostic studies of the gastrointestinal system.

The main function of the gastrointestinal (GI) system is to supply nutrients to body cells. This is accomplished through the processes of *ingestion* (taking in food), *digestion* (breakdown of food), and *absorption* (transfer of food products into circulation). *Elimination* is the process of excreting waste products of digestion.

The GI system (also called the *digestive system*) consists of the GI tract and its associated organs. Included in the GI tract are the mouth, esophagus, stomach, small intestine, and large intestine. The associated organs are the liver, pancreas, and gallbladder with the duct system (Fig. 33-1).

Psychological or emotional factors such as stress and anxiety influence GI functioning in many people. Stress may be manifested as anorexia, epigastric pain, or diarrhea. However, GI problems should not be solely attributed to psychological factors. Organic and psychologically based problems can exist independently or concurrently. Physical factors such as dietary intake, ingestion of alcohol and caffeine-containing products, cigarette smoking, and fatigue may also affect GI functioning. Some organic

diseases of the GI system such as peptic ulcer disease and ulcerative colitis seem to be related to stress. However, the causal relationship is not completely understood. Both physical and emotional factors affect GI functioning.

STRUCTURES AND FUNCTIONS OF THE GASTROINTESTINAL SYSTEM

The GI tract is a tube about 9 m long extending from the mouth to the anus. The entire tract is composed of four common layers. From the inside to the outside, these layers are (1) mucosa, (2) submucosa, (3) muscle, and (4) serosa. In the esophagus the outer coat is fibrous tissue rather than serosa. The muscular coat consists of two layers: the circular (inner) and the longitudinal (outer).

The GI tract is innervated by the parasympathetic and the sympathetic branches of the autonomic nervous system. The parasympathetic system is mainly excitatory, and the sympathetic system is mainly inhibitory. For example, peristalsis is increased by parasympathetic stimulation and decreased by sympathetic stimulation.

The two types of movement of the GI tract are *mixing* and *propulsion*. These movements are accomplished by peristalsis and rhythmical movements. The secretions of the GI system consist mainly of enzymes and hormones

Reviewed by Sally Brozenec, R.N., Ph.D., Assistant Professor, Rush University College of Nursing, Chicago, Illinois.

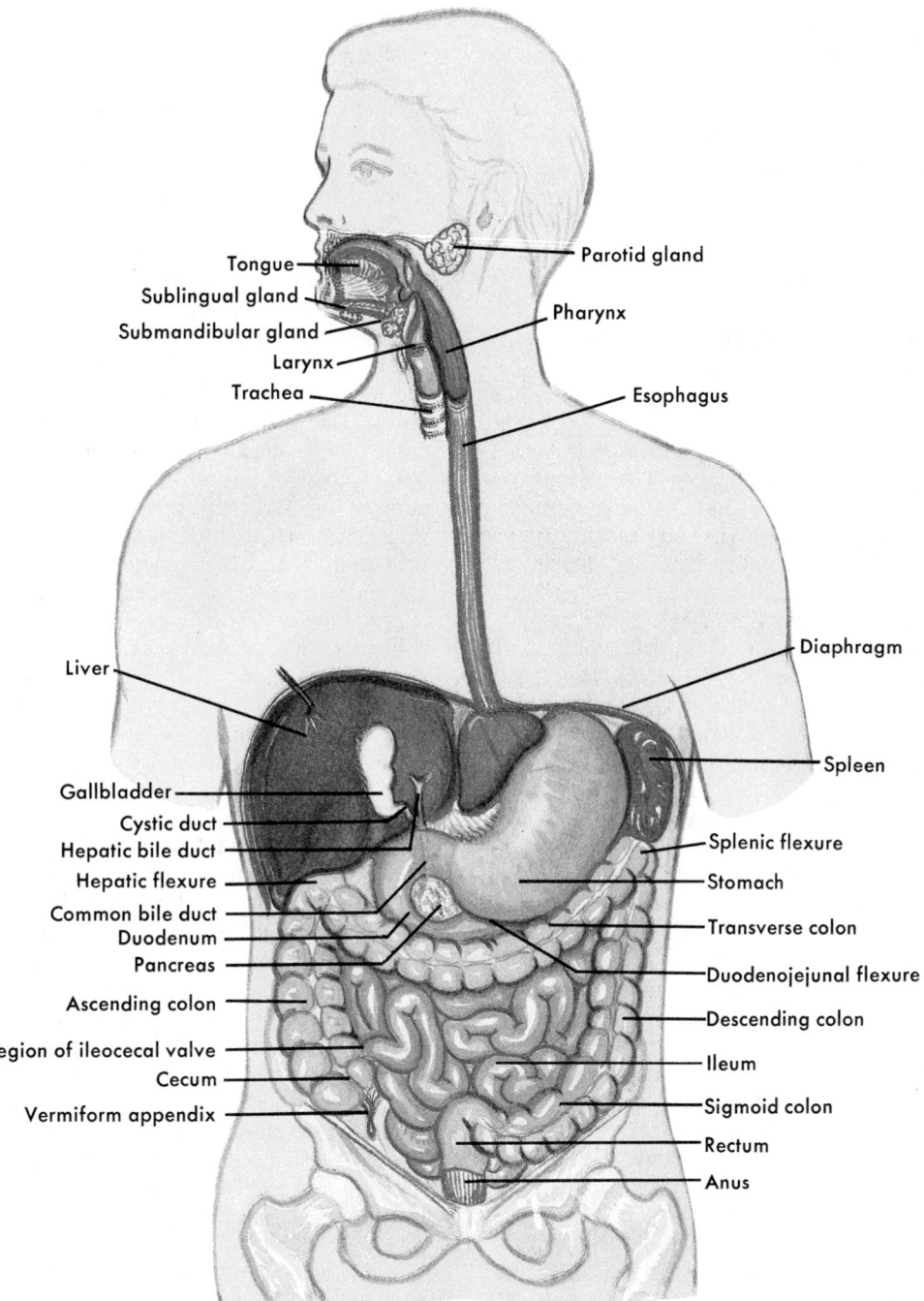

Fig. 33-1 Organs of the GI system. (From Anthony C and Thibodeau G: Textbook of anatomy and physiology, St Louis, 1987, The CV Mosby Co.)

for digestion and mucus to provide protection and lubrication.

The abdominal viscera are almost completely covered by the peritoneum. The two layers of the peritoneum are the parietal, which lines the abdominal cavity wall, and the visceral, which covers the abdominal organs. The peritoneal cavity is the potential space between the parietal and visceral layers. The two folds of the peritoneum are the mesentery and omentum. The mesentery attaches the

small intestine and part of the large intestine to the posterior abdominal wall and contains blood and lymph vessels. The lesser omentum goes from the lesser curvature of the stomach and upper duodenum to the liver, and the greater omentum hangs from the stomach over the intestines like an apron. The omentum contains fat and lymph nodes.

The primary functions of the GI system are (1) ingestion and propulsion (movement) of food; (2) digestion; (3) absorption; (4) delivery to the body of a continual supply of nutrients, electrolytes, and water; and (5) elimination. Each part of the GI system performs different activities to accomplish these functions.

Ingestion and Propulsion of Food

Ingestion is the intake of food. *Deglutition* (swallowing) completes the process of ingestion. A person's appetite or desire to ingest food is a significant factor in how much food is eaten. An appetite center is located in the hypothalamus. It is directly or indirectly stimulated by an empty stomach; decrease in body temperature; hypoglycemia; habit; and the sight, smell, and taste of food. Appetite may be inhibited by stomach distention, illness (especially accompanied by fever), hyperglycemia, nausea and vomiting, and certain drugs (e.g., amphetamines). The economic inability to purchase food supplies may be another factor affecting adequate ingestion, especially in older adults. The organs involved in ingestion and propulsion of food are the mouth, pharynx, and esophagus. Ingestion changes in the older adult include loss of teeth, atrophy and loss of taste buds, and decreased sense of smell, all of which lead to difficulty with ingesting nutrients.

Mouth. The mouth consists of the lips and oral (buccal) cavity. The lips surround the orifice of the mouth and function in speech. The roof of the oral cavity is formed by the hard and soft palate. The oral cavity contains the teeth, used in mastication (chewing), and the tongue. The tongue assists in mastication and deglutition by moving the food backward and keeping it between the teeth. Mucus is secreted by glands on the tongue and helps lubricate the food. The tongue is also important in speech and taste sensation.

Within the oral cavity are three pairs of salivary glands: the *parotid*, *submaxillary*, and *sublingual*. These glands, together with the mucous glands in the mouth, produce saliva. Saliva consists of water, protein, mucin, inorganic salts, and salivary amylase.

Pharynx. The pharynx is a musculomembranous tube that may be divided into the *nasopharynx*, the *oropharynx*, and the *laryngeal pharynx*. The mucous membrane of the pharynx is continuous with the nasal cavity, mouth, auditory tubes, and larynx. The pharynx functions in the act of swallowing and secretes mucus. The *epiglottis* is a lid of fibrocartilage that closes over the larynx during swallowing. The function of the pharynx in ingestion is to provide a route for the food from the mouth to the esophagus.

Esophagus. The esophagus is a hollow, muscular tube that receives food from the pharynx and moves it to the stomach by peristaltic contractions. It is 23 to 25 cm long and 2 cm in diameter. The esophagus is located in the thoracic cavity and starts behind the trachea at the lower end of the pharynx and extends to the stomach. With swallowing, the upper esophageal sphincter (cricopharyngeal muscle) relaxes and a peristaltic wave moves the bolus into the esophagus. The muscular layers contract (peristalsis) and propel the food to the stomach. The gastroesophageal sphincter at the lower end of the esophagus remains constricted except during swallowing, belching, or vomiting. This sphincter prevents gastric reflux.

Digestion and Absorption

Mouth. Digestion begins in the mouth. It involves both mechanical (chewing) and chemical digestion. Saliva is the first secretion involved in digestion, and its main function is to lubricate and soften the food mass, thus facilitating swallowing. The saliva contains ptyalin (amylase), which hydrolyzes starches to maltose.

Stomach. The functions of the stomach are to store food, mix the food with gastric juice and mucin, produce chemical changes, and mechanically change the bolus of food. The stomach also absorbs small amounts of water, glucose, alcohol, and electrolytes.

The stomach lies obliquely in the epigastric, umbilical, and left hypochondriac regions of the abdomen (see Fig. 33-7). The shape and position of the stomach change based on its contents, digestion, and the muscular walls. It always contains gastric fluid and mucus. The three main parts of the stomach are the *fundus, body,* and *antrum* (Fig. 33-2). The pylorus is a small portion of the antrum that lies right before the pyloric sphincter. Sphincter muscles guard the entrance to and exit from the stomach. The *cardiac sphincter* is the opening between the esophagus and stomach; the *pyloric sphincter* is between the stomach and the duodenum.

The serous (outer) layer of the stomach is formed by the peritoneum. The muscular layer, which is smooth muscle, consists of the longitudinal (outer) layer, circular (middle) layer, and the oblique (inner) layer. The mucosal layer forms folds called *rugae,* which contain many small glands. These folds allow the stomach to quadruple in size during digestion. In the fundus are the chief cells, which secrete pepsinogen, and the parietal cells, which secrete hydrochloric acid, water, and the intrinsic factor. The intrinsic factor promotes vitamin B_{12} absorption in the small intestine. Mucus is secreted by glands in the cardiac and pyloric areas. The stomach also secretes an alkaline substance that is protective and prevents autodigestion.

Branches of the vagus nerve of the parasympathetic nervous system innervate the stomach. Parasympathetic stimulation of the stomach increases both peristalsis and secretions. The stomach is also innervated by the sympathetic nervous system. Sympathetic stimulation inhibits gastric secretion and motility.

Small intestine. The two primary functions of the small intestine are digestion and absorption of the end products of digestion. The small intestine is a coiled tube about 7 m in length and from 2.5 cm to 2.8 cm in diameter, diminishing in diameter at the lower end. It extends from the pylorus to the ileocecal valve. The small intestine is composed of the *duodenum,* the *jejunum,* and the *ileum.* The ileocecal valve controls the exit into the large intestine and prevents reflux into the small intestine.

The serous coat of the small intestine is formed by the peritoneum. The mucosa is thick, vascular, and glandular. The circular folds in the mucous and submucous layers provide a greater surface area for secretion of digestive juices and absorption.

The functional units of the small intestine are *villi.* They are present in the entire small intestine. Villi are

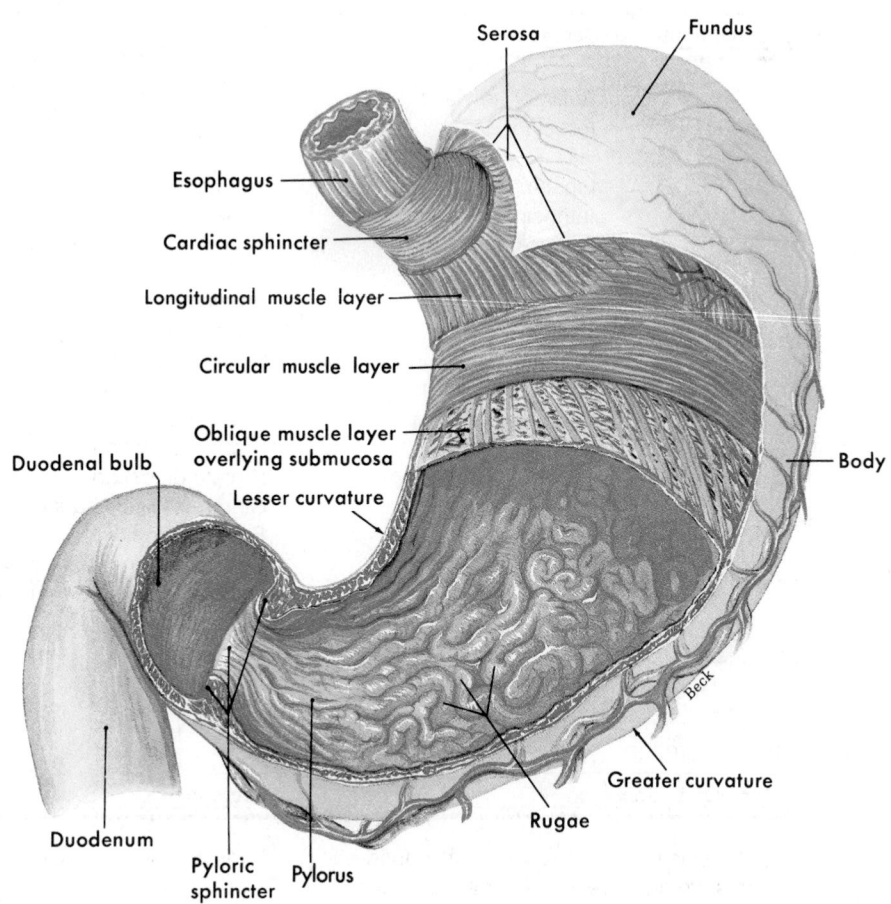

Fig. 33-2 Parts of the stomach. (From Anthony C and Thibodeau G: Textbook of anatomy and physiology, St Louis, 1987, The CV Mosby Co.)

minute, fingerlike projections in the mucous membrane. They contain goblet cells that secrete mucus and absorptive cells that absorb digested foodstuffs. The villi greatly increase the surface area for absorption. Many enzymes on the brush border of the villi digest food substances as they are being absorbed. The *crypts of Lieberkühn* or intestinal glands produce secretions that contain digestive enzymes. *Brunner's glands* in the submucosa of the duodenum secrete mucus.

Both branches of the autonomic nervous system innervate the small intestine. The vagus nerve stimulates motility and secretions, and the sympathetic branch inhibits motility. Pain is relayed through sensory fibers of the sympathetic system. The small intestine receives its blood supply from branches of the hepatic and superior mesenteric artery.

Physiology. Digestion is the physical and chemical breakdown of food into absorbable substances. The GI system functions in digestion by moving food through the GI tract and by secreting substances to break food into smaller particles (Table 33-1).

The process of digestion begins in the mouth where the food is chewed, mechanically broken down, and mixed with saliva. The saliva lubricates the food and starts starch digestion. Salivation is stimulated by chewing movements and the sight, smell, thought, and taste of food. The food is swallowed and passes into the esophagus where peristaltic waves propel it to the stomach.

In the stomach the digestion of proteins begins with minimal digestion of starches and fats. The food is mixed with gastric secretions, which are under nervous system and hormonal control (Tables 33-2 and 33-3). The stomach also serves as a reservoir for food, which is slowly passed into the small intestine. The time food remains in the stomach depends on the nature of the food, but average meals remain from 3 to 4 hours. There is some individual variation in stomach emptying time.

Digestion is completed in the small intestine, where carbohydrates are hydrolyzed to monosaccharides, fats to glycerol and fatty acids, and proteins to amino acids. Chyme (food mixed with gastric secretions) in the small intestine causes mechanical or chemical stimulation, and mixing and peristalsis occur. Secretions responsible for digestion are succus entericus (intestinal juice) from glands in the small intestine, enzymes from the pancreas, and bile from the liver (Table 33-1). Secretions are mainly under nervous system and hormonal control.

When food enters the small intestine, hormones are re-

Table 33-1 Gastrointestinal Secretions

Location	Daily Amount (ml)	Secretion	Action
Salivary glands	1500	Salivary amylase (ptyalin)	Initiation of starch digestion
Stomach	2500	Pepsinogen	Protein digestion
		HCl	Protein digestion
		Lipase	Fat digestion
		Intrinsic factor	Essential for vitamin B_{12} absorption in ileum
Small intestine	3000	Enterokinase	Activation of trypsinogen to trypsin
		Amylase	Carbohydrate digestion
		Peptidases	Protein digestion
		Maltase	Maltose to glucose
		Sucrase	Sucrose to glucose and fructose
		Lactase	Lactose to glucose and galactose
		Lipase	Fat digestion
Pancreas	700	Trypsinogen	Protein digestion
		Chymotrypsin	Protein digestion
		Amylase	Starch to disaccharides
		Lipase	Fat digestion
Liver and gallbladder	1000	Bile	Emulsification of fats and aid in absorption of fatty acids and fat-soluble vitamins (A, D, E, K)

Table 33-2 Phases of Gastric Secretion

Phase	Stimulus to Secretion	Secretion
Cephalic (nervous)	Sight, smell, taste of food—before food enters stomach, result of vagal nerve innervation	Hydrochloric acid, pepsinogen, mucus
Gastric (hormonal and nervous)	Food in antrum of stomach, vagal stimulation	Release of gastrin hormone from antrum into circulation to stimulate increased gastric secretions and motility
Intestinal (hormonal)	Bulk in duodenum and fats in small intestine	Release of intestinal gastrin into circulation to stimulate gastric secretion of pepsin and mucus Release of enterogastrone by intestinal mucosa to cause decreased gastric secretion and motility

Table 33-3 Major Hormones Controlling Gastrointestinal Secretion and Motility

Hormone	Source	Activating Stimuli	Function
Gastrin	Gastric mucosa of pylorus	Stomach distention, partially digested proteins in pylorus	Gastric acid secretion, increased gastric motility, maintenance of lower esophageal sphincter tone
Secretin	Duodenal mucosa	Acid entering small intestine	Inhibition of gastric motility and acid secretion, pancreatic bicarbonate secretion
Cholecystokinin-pancreozymin(CCK-PZ)	Duodenal mucosa	Fatty acids and amino acids in small intestine	Contraction of gallbladder and relaxation of sphincter of Oddi, allowing increased flow of bile into duodenum; release of pancreatic digestive enzymes
Enterogastrone	Duodenal mucosa	Partially digested proteins, fats, and acids in duodenum	Inhibition of gastric secretion and motility, relaxation of sphincter of Oddi, contraction of gallbladder

leased into the bloodstream (Table 33-3). The hormone secretin stimulates the pancreas to secrete fluid with a high concentration of bicarbonate, which neutralizes acid in the chyme. The duodenum also secretes mucus to neutralize hydrochloric acid. The hormone cholecystokinin-pancreozymin (CCK-PZ), produced by the duodenal mucosa, enters the bloodstream and stimulates contraction of the gallbladder and relaxation of the sphincter of Oddi. These actions permit bile to flow from the common bile duct into the duodenum. CCK-PZ also stimulates the pancreas to release pancreatic juices that contain enzymes for hydrolysis of carbohydrates, fats, and proteins.

Absorption is the transfer of the end products of digestion across the intestinal wall to circulation for use by cells. Most absorption occurs in the small intestine. The surface area of the small intestine is greatly increased by its circular folds, villi, and microvilli. The movement of the villi keeps the end products of digestion in contact with the absorbing membrane. Simple sugars (from carbohydrates), fatty acids (from fats), amino acids (from proteins), water, electrolytes, and vitamins are absorbed.

The digestive system seems to adjust well to aging changes. Motor activity and almost all digestive enzyme levels are decreased. Absorption seems to be minimally affected. Fat absorption is moderately decreased, and vitamin B_{12} malabsorption may occur as a result of decreased secretion of intrinsic factor.

Elimination

Large intestine. The large intestine is a hollow muscular tube about 1.5 to 2 m long and 5 cm in diameter. The four parts of the large intestine are (1) the *cecum* and *appendix*, a narrow tube at the end of the cecum; (2) the *colon*: ascending colon on the right side, transverse colon across the abdomen, descending colon on the left side, and the sigmoid colon; (3) the *rectum*; and (4) the *anus*, the terminal portion of the large intestine (Fig. 33-3).

The large intestine is innervated by the parasympathetic nervous system, which stimulates secretions and contraction. The sympathetic nervous system inhibits secretions and motility. The large intestine receives its blood supply mainly from the superior and inferior mesenteric arteries.

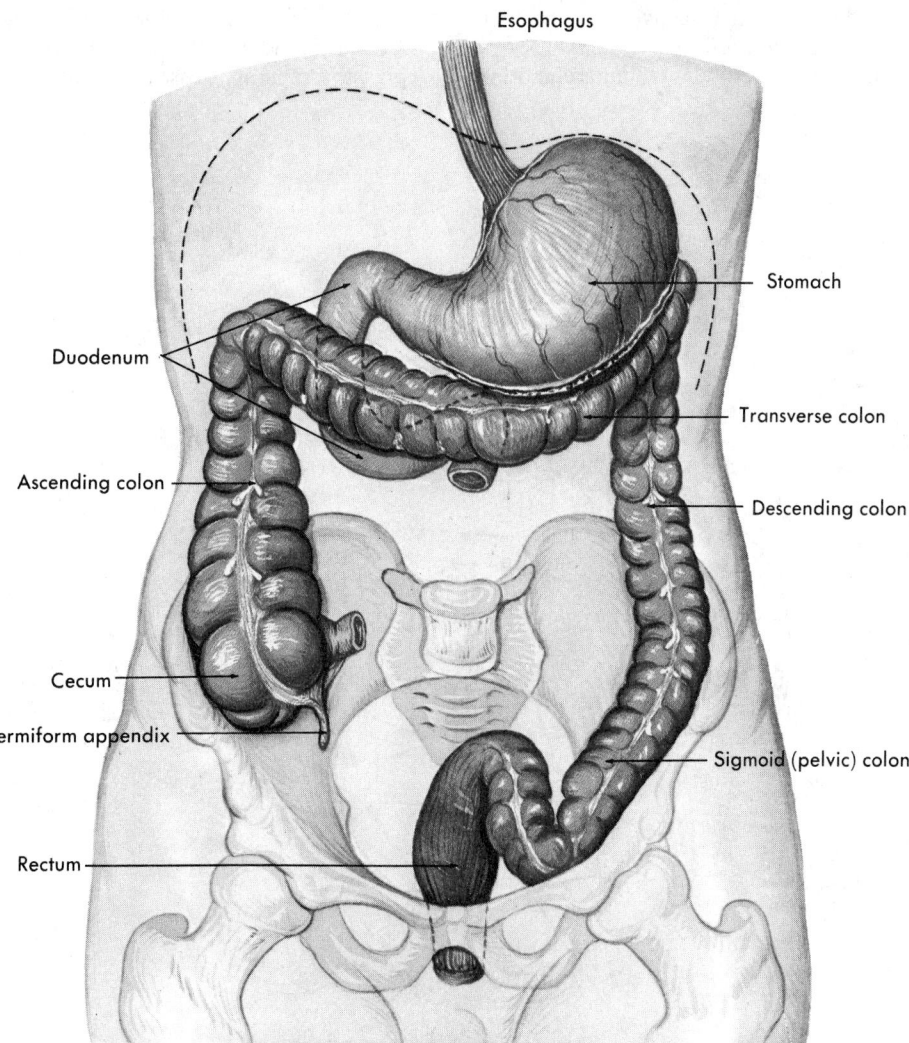

Fig. 33-3   Anatomical locations of the large intestine. (From Anthony C and Thibodeau G: Textbook of anatomy and physiology, St Louis, 1987, The CV Mosby Co.)

The most important function of the large intestine is the absorption of water and electrolytes. It also forms feces and serves as a reservoir for the fecal mass until defecation occurs. Feces are composed of water (75%), bacteria, unabsorbed minerals, undigested foodstuffs, bile pigments, and desquamated epithelial cells. The large intestine secretes mucus, which acts as a lubricant and protects the mucosa.

Microorganisms in the colon are responsible for the putrefaction of proteins not digested or absorbed in the small intestine. These amino acids are deaminated by the bacteria, leaving ammonia, which is carried to the liver and converted to urea. Bacteria in the colon also synthesize vitamin K and some of the B vitamins. Bacteria also play a part in the production of flatus.

The movements of the large intestine are usually slow. When the circular muscles contract, they produce an empty, kneading action called *haustral churning*. Propulsive (mass movements) peristalsis also occurs. When food enters the stomach and duodenum, the gastrocolic and duodenocolic reflexes are initiated, resulting in peristalsis in the colon. These reflexes are more active after the first daily meal and initiate defecation reflexes.

Defecation is a reflex action involving voluntary and involuntary control. Feces in the rectum stimulate sensory nerve endings that produce the desire to defecate. The reflex center for defecation is in the sacral portion of the spinal cord (parasympathetic nerve fibers). These fibers produce contraction of the rectum and relaxation of the internal anal sphincter. When the desire to defecate is felt, the external anal sphincter relaxes voluntarily. Defecation is controlled voluntarily by keeping the external anal sphincter closed.

Defecation can be facilitated by the Valsalva maneuver. This maneuver involves contraction of the chest muscles on a closed glottis with simultaneous contraction of the abdominal muscles. These actions result in an increased intraabdominal pressure. The Valsalva maneuver is contraindicated in people with head injuries, eye surgery, cardiac problems, and liver cirrhosis with portal hypertension. Constipation is common in the older adult and is due to many factors, including inactivity, decreased dietary fiber, depression, drugs, and laxative abuse (see Chapter 37).[1]

Liver, Biliary Tract, and Pancreas

Liver. The liver is the largest internal organ in the body (3 lb in the adult). It lies in the right hypochondriac and epigastric regions. Most of the liver is enclosed in perito-

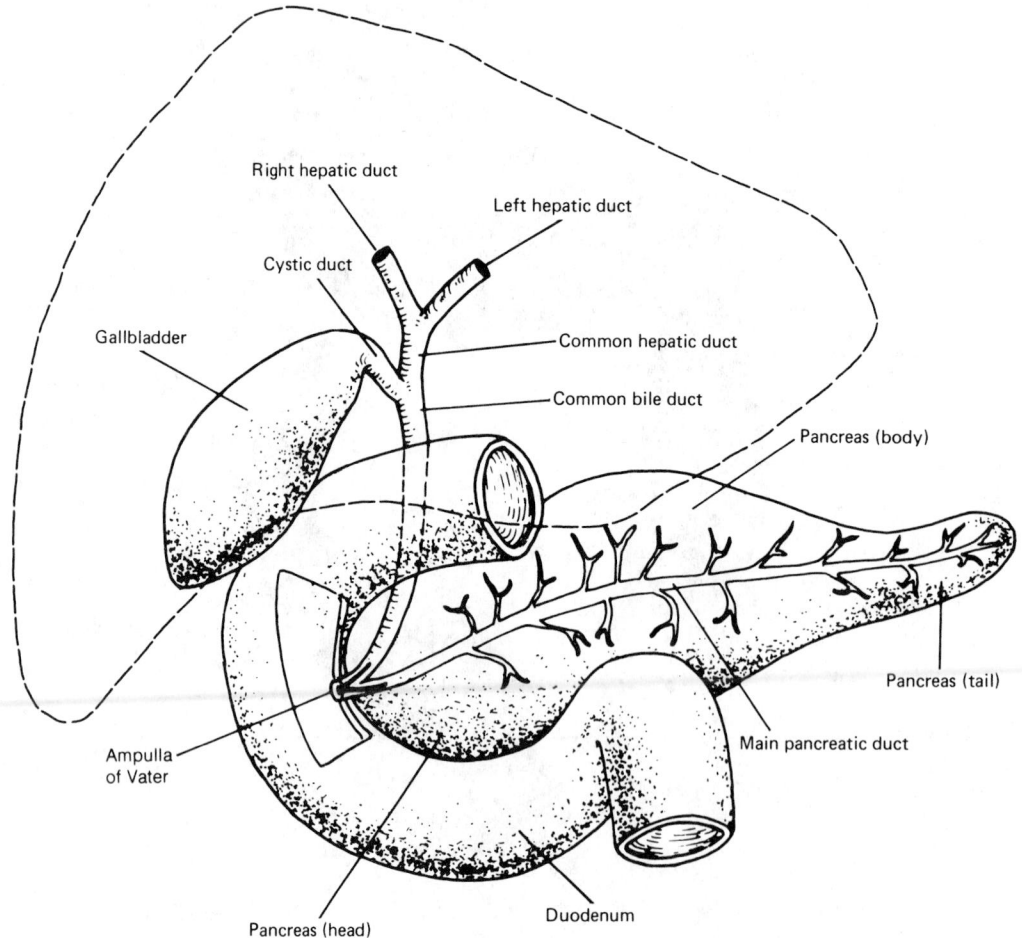

Fig. 33-4 Gross structure of the liver, gallbladder, pancreas, and the duct system. (From Kinney M, Packa D, and Dunbar S: AACN'S clinical reference for critical care nursing, St Louis, 1988, The CV Mosby Co.)

neum. It has a fibrous capsule that divides it into the right and left lobes (Fig. 33-4).

The functional units of the liver are lobules (Fig. 33-5). The lobule consists of rows of hepatic cells arranged around a central vein. The capillaries *(sinusoids)* are located between the rows of hepatic cells and are lined with *Kupffer* cells, which carry out phagocytic activity (removal of bacteria and toxins from the blood). Interlobular bile ducts form from bile capillaries *(canaliculi).* The hepatic cells secrete bile into the canaliculi.

The nerve supply to the liver is from the left vagus and sympathetic celiac plexus. About one third of the blood supply comes from the hepatic artery (branch of the celiac artery), and two thirds comes from the portal vein.

The portal circulatory system brings blood to the liver from the stomach, intestines, spleen, and pancreas. This blood enters the liver through the portal vein. In the liver the portal vein branches and comes in contact with each lobule. The blood in the sinusoids is a mixture of arterial and venous blood.

The liver is essential for life. It functions in the manufacture, storage, transformation, and excretion of a number of substances involved in metabolism. The functions of the liver are numerous but can be classified into four main areas as identified in Table 33-4.

Biliary tract. The biliary tract consists of the gallbladder and the duct system. The gallbladder is a pear-shaped sac on the undersurface of the liver. The function of the gall-

bladder is to concentrate and store bile. It can hold about 45 ml of bile.

Bile is produced by the hepatic cells and secreted into the biliary canaliculi of the lobules. Bile then drains into the interlobular bile ducts, which unite into the two main left and right hepatic ducts. The hepatic ducts merge with the cystic duct from the gallbladder to form the common bile duct (see Fig. 33-4). This duct enters the duodenum at the ampulla of Vater. The sphincter of Oddi keeps the ampulla closed except during digestion.

Bilirubin Metabolism

Bilirubin, a pigment derived from the breakdown of hemoglobin, is constantly being formed (Fig. 33-6). It is bound to albumin because it is insoluble, and this unconjugated bilirubin is transported to the liver. The liver conjugates bilirubin with glucuronic acid. Conjugated bilirubin is soluble and is excreted in bile. Bile also consists of water, cholesterol, bile salts, electrolytes, and phospholipids. Bile salts are needed for fat emulsification.

Bile initially enters the duct system in the canaliculi and flows through the interlobular ducts to the hepatic ducts. From the hepatic duct it can move to the cystic duct or down the common bile duct. Most bile is stored and concentrated in the gallbladder. It is then released into the cystic duct and moves down the common bile duct to enter the duodenum at the ampulla of Vater. In the intestines, most of the bilirubin is reduced to stercobilinogen and uro-

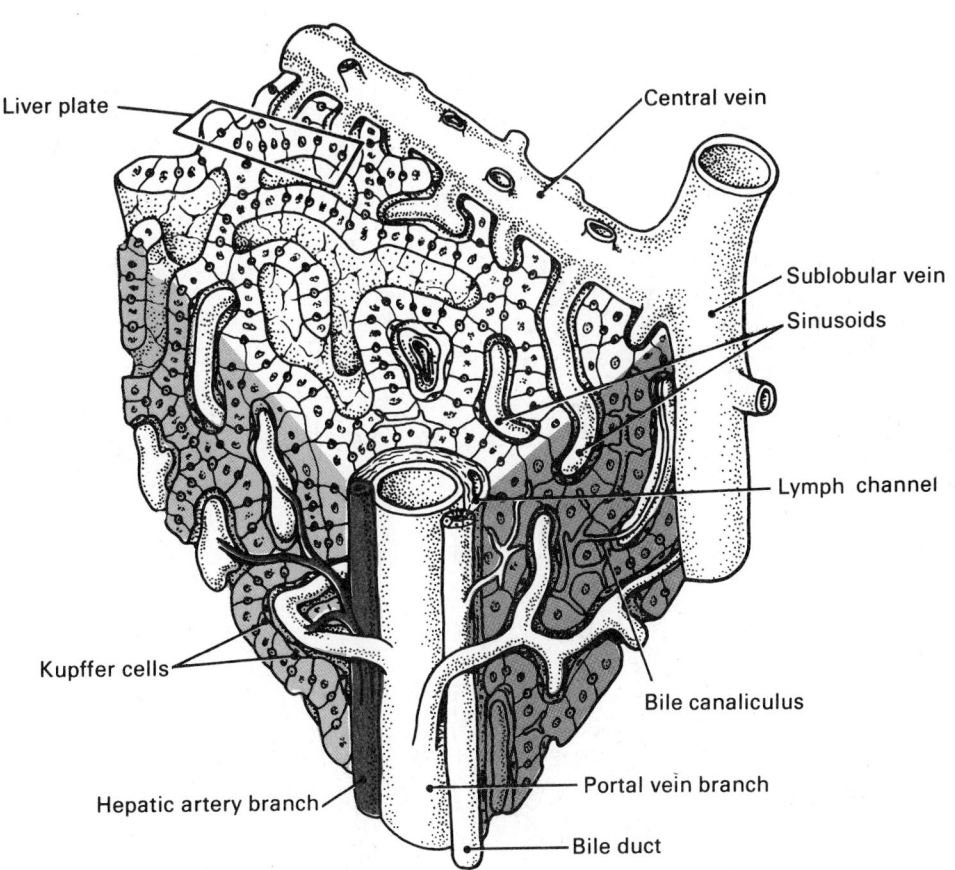

Fig. 33-5 Microscopic structure of liver lobule.

Table 33-4　Major Functions of the Liver

Function	Description
Metabolic functions	
Carbohydrate metabolism	Glycogenesis (conversion of glucose to glycogen), glycogenolysis (process of breaking down glycogen to glucose), gluconeogenesis (formation of glucose from amino acids and fatty acids)
Protein metabolism	Synthesis of nonessential amino acids, synthesis of plasma proteins (except γ-globulin), synthesis of clotting factors, urea formation from NH_3 (NH_3 formed from deamination of amino acids and by action of bacteria on proteins in colon)
Fat metabolism	Synthesis of lipoproteins, breakdown of triglycerides into fatty acids and glycerol, formation of ketone bodies, synthesis of fatty acids from amino acids and glucose, synthesis and breakdown of cholesterol
Detoxification	Inactivation of drugs and harmful substances and excretion of their breakdown products
Steroid metabolism	Conjugation and excretion of gonadal and adrenal steroids
Bile synthesis	
Bile production	Formation of bile, containing bile salts, bile pigments (mainly bilirubin), and cholesterol
Bile excretion	Bile excretion by liver of about 1 L/day
Storage	Glucose in form of glycogen; vitamins, including fat-soluble (A, D, E, K) and water-soluble (B_1, B_2, B_{12}, and folic acid); fatty acids; minerals (iron and copper); amino acids in form of albumin and β globulins
Mononuclear phagocyte system	
Kupffer cells	Ingestion of RBCs, bacteria, and other particles, breakdown of hemoglobin from old RBCs to bilirubin and biliverdin

RBC, Red blood cell.

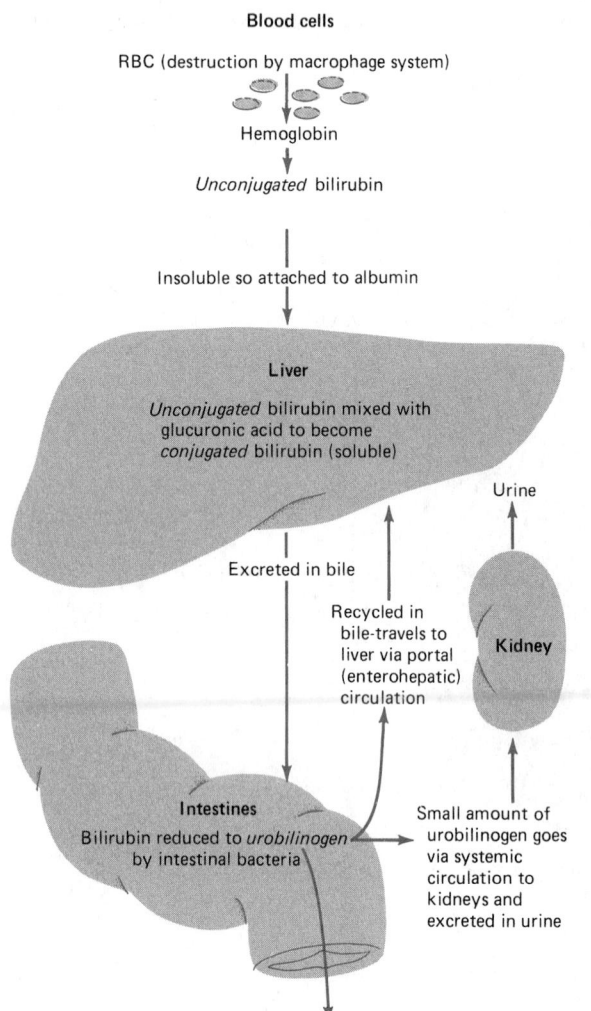

Fig. 33-6　Bilirubin metabolism and conjugation.

bilinogen by bacterial action. These substances account for the brown color of stool. A small amount of conjugated bilirubin is reabsorbed by the blood. Some urobilinogen is reabsorbed by the blood and returned to the liver through the portal circulation (enterohepatic) and excreted in the bile. An insignificant amount of urobilinogen is excreted in the urine.

Pancreas. The pancreas is a long, slender gland lying behind the stomach and in front of the first and second lumbar vertebrae. It consists of the head, body, and tail. The anterior surface is covered by peritoneum. The pancreas contains lobes and lobules. The pancreatic duct extends along the gland and enters the duodenum through the common bile duct (Fig. 33-4). The pancreas has both *exocrine* and *endocrine* functions. Its function as part of the GI system is the exocrine function. Exocrine cells in the pancreas secrete pancreatic enzymes (Table 33-1). The endocrine function is related to the islets of Langerhans, whose β cells secrete insulin and α cells secrete glucagon (see Chapter 42).

Effects of Aging

The process of aging causes changes in the functional ability of the GI system (see Table 33-9). Tooth enamel and dentin wear down and make the teeth susceptible to cavities. Periodontal disease can lead to the loss of teeth. Taste buds decrease, the sense of smell diminishes, and salivary secretions diminish, all of which can lead to a decrease in appetite and make eating less pleasurable.

Motility of the GI system definitely decreases with age, and secretion and absorption are affected to a lesser extent. These changes can lead to hypochlorhydria, delayed gastric emptying, and constipation. The aging process also causes atrophy of the gastric mucosa and villi of the intestine, resulting in decreased secretion of digestive enzymes and protective mucus. The liver size decreases after 50 years of age, but results of liver function tests remain within normal ranges. The liver also loses some ability to metabolize certain drugs. The size of the pancreas is unaffected by aging but does undergo structural changes such as fibrosis, fatty acid deposits, and atrophy. Aging does not cause changes in the structure and function of the gallbladder and bile ducts.

ASSESSMENT OF THE GASTROINTESTINAL SYSTEM

Terminology related to surgery of the GI system is presented in Table 33-5.

Subjective Data

Health history

Past health history. Information should be gathered from the client about the history or existence of the following diseases or problems related to GI functioning: abdominal pain, gastritis, nausea and vomiting, diarrhea and/or constipation, hepatitis, colitis, peptic ulcer, abdominal distention, jaundice, anemia, hiatal hernia, gallbladder disease, dysphagia, and heartburn and/or dyspepsia.

The client should be questioned about previous hospitalizations related to these diseases or problems of the GI

Table 33-5 Surgeries of the Gastrointestinal System

Antrectomy: Removal of antrum portion of stomach
Cecostomy: Opening into cecum
Cholecystectomy: Removal of gallbladder
Cholecystostomy: Opening into gallbladder
Choledochojejunostomy: Opening between common bile duct and jejunum
Choledocholithotomy: Opening into common bile duct for removal of stones
Colostomy: Opening into colon
Esophagoenterostomy: Removal of portion of esophagus with segment of colon attached to remaining portion
Esophagogastrostomy: Removal of esophagus and anastomosis of remaining portion to stomach
Gastrectomy: Removal of stomach
Gastrostomy: Opening into stomach
Glossectomy: Removal of tongue
Hemiglossectomy: Removal of half of tongue
Ileostomy: Opening into ileum
Mandibulectomy: Removal of mandible
Pyloroplasty: Enlargement and repair of pyloric sphincter area
Vagotomy: Resection of branch of vagus nerve

Table 33-6 Hepatotoxic Chemicals and Drugs

Alcohol	Halothane
Arsenic	Isoniazid
Carbon tetrachloride	Propylthiouracil
Chloroform	Sulfonamides
Gold compounds	Thiazide diuretics
Mercury	6-Mercaptopurine
Phosphorus	Methotrexate
Anabolic steroids	Acetaminophen

system. Data should also be obtained related to any abdominal or rectal surgery, including year, cause, postoperative course, and possible blood transfusions.

The health history should include an assessment of the client's past and current use of medications. This is an important part of the assessment, particularly in relation to liver problems. It should include over-the-counter and prescription drugs. Many chemicals and drugs are potentially hepatotoxic (Table 33-6). The nurse should ask the client if antacids are taken, including the kind and frequency. Many people take baking soda (sodium bicarbonate) for an upset stomach. This can be dangerous because it is a systemic antacid that is readily absorbed and can cause metabolic alkalosis. Sodium bicarbonate is also in many over-the-counter effervescent drugs such as Alka-Seltzer.

Data collection should include a dietary history with questions regarding fiber intake, recent weight loss, anorexia, and caffeine use. The nurse should assess the client for allergies to any food and determine what GI symptoms such allergic responses cause. It is also important to assess for over-the-counter laxative abuse.

Family history. It is helpful to determine whether the client has a family history of certain GI diseases and problems. The presence of certain problems may increase the likelihood of similar problems in other family members. The nurse should ask the client about the occurrence of such problems as alcoholism, jaundice, cancer of the GI tract (especially colon), hepatitis, intestinal polyps, peptic ulcers, gallbladder disease, obesity, and diabetes.

Social and personal history

BACKGROUND INFORMATION. The client should be asked about previous occupations involving possible exposure to hepatotoxic chemicals such as carbon tetrachloride, arsenic, phosphorus, and mercury. The nurse should also ask about foreign travel with possible exposure to hepatitis or parasitic infestation.

LIFESTYLE. The client should be assessed in relation to certain habits that have a direct effect on GI functioning. The consumption of alcohol in large quantities has detrimental effects on the mucosa of the stomach and also increases the secretion of acid-pepsin. Alcohol causes fatty infiltration of the liver. The nurse should obtain a history of cigarette smoking. Nicotine is irritating to the entire GI tract mucosa. Cigarette smoking can cause various GI cancers (especially mouth and esophageal cancers), esophagitis, and ulcers.

The nurse should try to determine what is a stressor for the client and what coping mechanisms the client uses to function with these stressors. GI symptoms such as epigastric pain, nausea, and diarrhea develop in many people in response to stressful or emotional situations. Some organic GI problems such as peptic ulcers are related to stress.

The nurse should ask clients about their elimination patterns. What are their regular bowel evacuation habits—frequency, time of day, and normal consistency of stool? What activities or emotions change their regular pattern? The development of the "laxative habit" should be determined. How often does the client take a laxative? What kind is it? A similar inquiry should be made related to enemas. The older adult tends to be constipated and should be questioned about the habitual use of laxatives and what seems to affect personal bowel habits.

A thorough nutritional assessment is essential. A dietary history should be taken and compared with the basic four food groups. The nurse should ask open-ended questions that will allow the client to express beliefs and feelings about the diet. The nurse may need to ask the client to do a 24-hour dietary recall to analyze the adequacy of the diet. The nurse should assist the client in recalling the preceding day's food intake, including early-morning and nighttime intake. The nurse should find out about the intake of snacks, liquids, and vitamin supplements. The nurse must then evaluate the diet in terms of the basic four food groups and try to determine whether the 24-hour recall is typical of the client's usual eating habits. If weekend eating habits vary greatly, the nurse should obtain a separate weekend diet history and assess the client's intake for both quality and quantity of food.

The nurse should ask the client about the use of sugar and salt substitutes and determine fluid and fiber intake.

Inadequate intake of fiber can be associated with constipation and irritable bowel syndrome. The client should be questioned about any changes in appetite, food tolerance, and weight. Anorexia and weight loss may indicate carcinoma.

Food has many social and emotional values as well as physical ones. What is the emotional atmosphere during mealtime? Does the client eat alone? The client's spiritual and cultural beliefs regarding food should be assessed. The nurse should try to determine the economic situation of the client in relation to diet. What percentage of income is spent on food, and how much of this amount is related to culture and how much to economic ability? Are older adults able to prepare their own food? How many hot meals do they have a day? The nurse must remember that although food has different values for each person, it is essential that all nutrients be included.

Review of systems. The client should be questioned in the following areas:

1. Mouth
   a. Dental hygiene—caries, condition of teeth and gingivae, dentures
   b. Bleeding or swelling of gingivae
   c. Dryness or excessive salivation
   d. Lesions
   e. Odors
   f. Sore tongue
   g. Difficulty chewing
2. Ingestion of food and fluids
   a. Painful swallowing (odynophagia)
   b. Difficulty swallowing (dysphagia)
   c. Appetite (increase or anorexia)
   d. Weight change
   e. Intolerance to certain foods
   f. Nausea and vomiting
   g. Indigestion, belching (eructation)
   h. Vomiting of blood (hematemesis)
   i. Location and type of pain
3. Digestion and absorption
   a. Relationship of pain to eating or specific food
   b. Heartburn (pyrosis)
   c. Burning, indigestion (dyspepsia)
4. Elimination
   a. Constipation, diarrhea
   b. Changes in bowel habits
   c. Gas (flatulence)
   d. Blood in stools (melena)
   e. Anal pruritus, burning, pain
   f. Spasms when attempting to defecate (tenesmus)
   g. Frothy stool (steatorrhea)
   h. Distention
   i. Hemorrhoids
5. Hepatic and biliary systems
   a. Jaundice (yellow skin, sclera, or mucous membranes)
   b. Itching (pruritus)
   c. Abdominal edema (ascites)
   d. Dark urine
   e. Clay-colored stools
   f. Hemorrhagic problems (easily produced bruising, purpura, bleeding)

g. Spider angiomas (telangiectasia or spider nevi)

h. Palmar erythema

Objective Data

Physical examination

Mouth

INSPECTION. The lips should be inspected for symmetry, color, and size. They should be observed for abnormalities such as pallor or cyanosis, cracking, ulcers, or fissures. The dorsum (top) of the tongue should have a thin white coating; the undersurface should be smooth. The nurse should observe for any lesions. Using a tongue blade, the nurse should inspect the buccal mucosa and note the color, any areas of pigmentation, and any lesions. Dark-skinned people normally have patchy areas of pigmentation. In assessing the teeth and gums, the nurse should look for caries, loose teeth, abnormal shape and position of teeth, and swelling, bleeding, discoloration, or inflammation of the gingivae. Any distinctive breath odor should be noted.

The pharynx is inspected by tilting the client's head back and depressing the tongue with a tongue blade. The tonsils, uvula, soft palate, and anterior and posterior pillars should be observed. The nurse should have the client say "ah." The uvula and soft palate should rise and remain in the midline.

PALPATION. The nurse should palpate any suspicious areas anywhere in the mouth. Ulcers, nodules, indurations, and areas of tenderness should be palpated. The mouth of the older adult needs careful assessment. Particular attention should be given to dentures (e.g., fit, condition), ability to swallow, and lesions.

Abdomen. Two systems are used to describe anatomically the surface of the abdomen. One system divides the abdomen into four quadrants by a perpendicular line from the sternum to the pubic bone and a horizontal line across the abdomen at the umbilicus (Fig. 33-7 and Table 33-7). The other system divides the abdomen into nine regions (Fig. 33-7), but only the epigastrium, umbilical, and suprapubic or hypogastric regions are commonly addressed. For the abdominal examination, good lighting should shine across the abdomen. The client should be in the supine position and as relaxed as possible. To help relax the abdom-

Table 33-7 Abdominal Structures in Regions of the Abdomen

Right Upper Quadrant	Left Upper Quadrant	Right Lower Quadrant	Left Lower Quadrant
Liver and gallbladder	Left lobe of liver	Lower pole of right kidney	Lower pole of left kidney
Pylorus	Spleen	Cecum and appendix	Sigmoid flexure
Duodenum	Stomach	Portion of ascending colon	Portion of descending colon
Head of pancreas	Body of pancreas	Bladder (if distended)	Bladder (if distended)
Right adrenal gland	Left adrenal gland	Ovary and salpinx	Ovary and salpinx
Portion of right kidney	Portion of left kidney	Uterus (if enlarged)	Uterus (if enlarged)
Hepatic flexure of colon	Splenic flexure of colon	Right spermatic cord	Left spermatic cord
Portion of ascending and transverse colon	Portion of transverse and descending colon	Right ureter	Left ureter

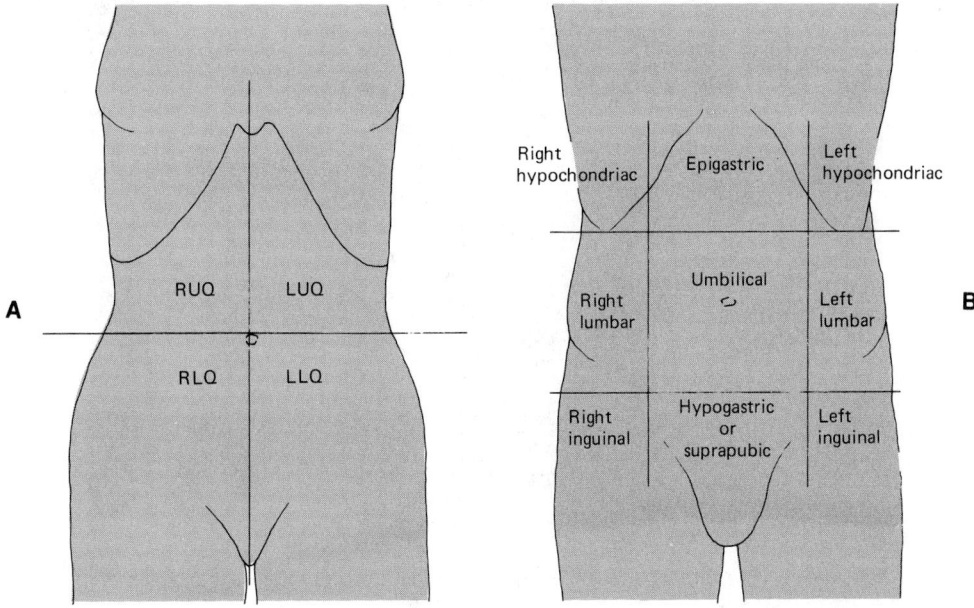

Fig. 33-7 **A,** Abdominal quadrants. **B,** Abdominal regions.

inal muscles, the client should slightly flex the knees and the head of the bed should be raised slightly.

INSPECTION. The nurse should assess the abdomen for skin changes (color, texture, scars, striae, dilated veins, rashes, and lesions), umbilicus (location and contour), symmetry, contour (flat, rounded [convex], concave, protuberant, distention), observable masses (hernias or other masses), and movement (pulsations and peristalsis). A normal aortic pulsation may be seen in the epigastric area. The nurse should look across the abdomen tangentially for peristalsis. Peristalsis is not normally visible in adults but may be visible in thin people.

AUSCULTATION. During examination of the abdomen, auscultation is done before percussion and palpation because these latter procedures may alter the bowel sounds. Auscultation of the abdomen includes listening for increased or decreased bowel sounds and vascular sounds. The diaphragm of the stethoscope is used to auscultate bowel sounds because they are relatively high pitched. The bell of the stethoscope is used to detect lower-pitched sounds. Normal bowel sounds occur 5 to 30 times per minute and sound like high-pitched clicks or gurgles. Before auscultation, warming the stethoscope in the hands helps prevent

abdominal muscle contraction. The nurse should listen in the epigastrium and in all four quadrants. The nurse should listen for bowel sounds for 2 to 5 minutes. Bowel sounds cannot be described as absent until no sound is heard for 5 minutes (in each quadrant). The frequency and intensity of bowel sounds will vary, depending on the phase of digestion. Normally they will sound relatively high pitched and gurgling. Loud gurgles indicate hyperperistalsis and are called *borborygmi*. The bowel sounds will be more high pitched (rushes and tinkling) when the intestines are under tension such as in intestinal obstruction. The nurse should listen for decreased or absent bowel sounds. Terms used to describe bowel sounds include *present, absent, increased, decreased, high pitched, tinkling, gurgling,* and *rushing.* Normally no aortic bruits should be heard. A bruit is a swishing or buzzing sound and represents turbulent blood flow.

PERCUSSION. The purpose of percussion of the abdomen is to determine the presence of fluid, distention, and masses. Sound waves vary according to the density of underlying tissues; the presence of air produces a higher-pitched, hollow sound called *tympany;* the presence of fluid or masses produces a high-pitched sound called *dullness.* The nurse

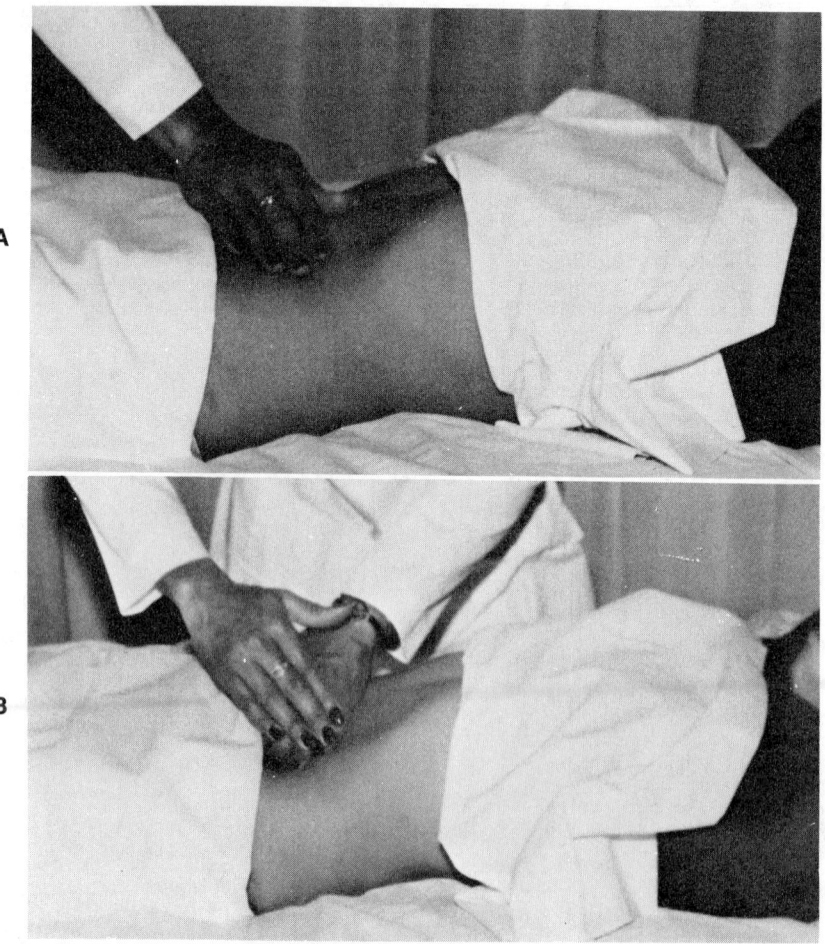

Fig. 33-8 **A,** Light palpation of the abdomen. **B,** Deep palpation of the abdomen (two-hand method).

should lightly percuss all four quadrants of the abdomen and assess the distribution of tympany and dullness. Usually more tympany is present.

To percuss the liver, the nurse should start below the umbilicus in the right midclavicular line and percuss lightly upward until dullness is heard, thus determining the lower border of liver dullness. After the lower border of the liver has been determined, the nurse should start at the nipple line in the right midclavicular line and percuss downward to the area of dullness indicating the upper border of the liver. The height or vertical space between the two areas should be measured to determine the size of the liver. The normal range of liver height in the right midclavicular line is 6 to 12 cm.

PALPATION. *Light palpation* is used to detect tenderness or cutaneous hypersensitivity, muscular resistance, masses, and swelling. It also helps in relaxation for deeper palpation. The nurse should keep fingers together and press gently with the pads of the fingertips, depressing the abdominal wall about 1 cm. Smooth movements should be used and all quadrants palpated (Fig. 33-8).

Deep palpation is used to delineate abdominal organs and masses. The palmar surfaces of the fingers should be used to press more deeply. Again, all quadrants should be palpated. When palpating masses, the nurse should note the location, size, shape, and presence of tenderness. The client's facial expression should be observed during these maneuvers because it will provide nonverbal cues of discomfort or pain.

An alternate method for light and deep abdominal palpation is the two-hand method (Fig. 33-8). One hand is placed on top of the other. The fingers of the top hand apply pressure to the bottom hand. The fingers of the bottom hand feel for organs and masses. The nurse should practice both methods of palpation to determine which one is most effective.

A problem area on the abdomen can be checked for re-

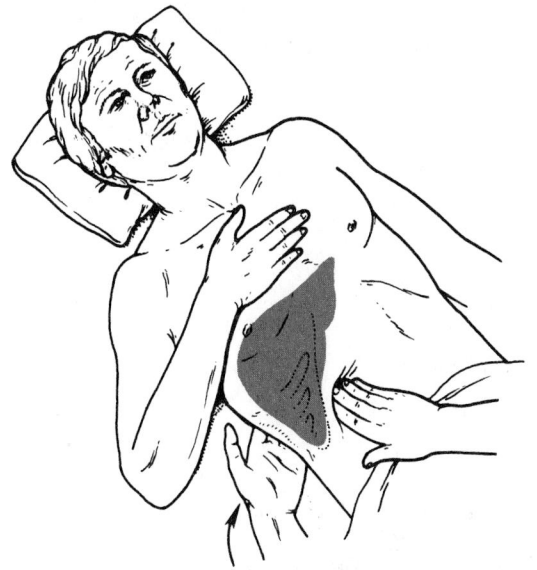

Fig. 33-9 Bimanual technique for palpation of the liver.

bound tenderness by pressing in slowly and firmly over the painful site. The palpating fingers are withdrawn quickly. Pain on withdrawal of the fingers indicates peritoneal inflammation. Because assessing for rebound tenderness may produce pain and severe muscle spasm, it should be done at the end of the examination and only by an experienced practitioner.

To palpate the liver, the nurse's left hand is placed behind the client to support the right eleventh and twelfth ribs (Fig. 33-9). The client may relax on the nurse's hand. The nurse should press the left hand forward and place the right hand on the client's right abdomen lateral to the rectus muscle. The fingertips should be below the lower border of liver dullness and pointed toward the right costal margin. The nurse should gently press in and up. The client should take a deep breath with the abdomen so that the liver drops and is in a better position to palpate. The nurse should try to feel the liver edge as it comes down to the fingertips. The liver edge should feel firm, sharp, and smooth. The surface and contour and any tenderness should be described.[2]

To palpate the spleen, the nurse's left hand reaches over and under the client and supports and presses the client's left lower rib cage forward. The right hand is placed below the left costal margin and presses it in toward the spleen. The nurse should ask the client to breathe deeply. The tip or edge of an enlarged spleen will be felt by the fingertips. The spleen is normally not palpable.[3] If it is palpable, the nurse should not continue because manual compression of the enlarged spleen may cause it to rupture. The standard approach for examining the abdomen can be used on the older adult. Palpation is important because it may reveal a tumor. The abdomen may be thinner and more lax unless the client is obese.[4] If the client has chronic obstructive pulmonary disease, large lungs, or a low diaphragm, the liver may be palpated 1 to 2 cm below the right costal margin.

Rectum. The perianal and anal area should be inspected for color, texture, lumps, rashes, scars, excoriations, fissures, and external hemorrhoids. Any lumps or unusual areas should be palpated with a gloved hand.

For the digital examination of the rectum the gloved, lubricated index finger is placed against the anus while the client strains (Valsalva maneuver). Then, as the sphincter relaxes, the finger is inserted. The finger is pointed toward the umbilicus. The nurse should try to get the client to relax. The finger is inserted into the rectum as far as possible, and all surfaces are palpated. Nodules, tenderness, or any irregularities should be assessed. Particularly in the older adult, a check for occult blood should be included.

Recording of the normal physical assessment of the GI system is found in Table 33-8. Age-related changes in the GI system and differences in assessment findings are recorded in Table 33-9. Common abnormal assessment findings are presented in Table 33-10.

DIAGNOSTIC STUDIES

Many of the diagnostic procedures of the GI system require measures to cleanse the GI tract as well as ingestion or injection of a contrast medium or a radiopaque dye (Ta-

Table 33-8 Normal Physical Assessment of the
Gastrointestinal System

MOUTH

Moist and pink lips; pink and moist buccal mucosa and gingivae without plaques or lesions; teeth in good repair; protusion of tongue in midline without deviation or fasciculations; pink uvula, soft palate, tonsils, and posterior pharynx

ABDOMEN

Flat without masses or scars, bowel sounds in all quadrants, no palpation of liver and spleen, liver 10 cm in right midclavicular line, generalized tympany

ANUS

Absence of lesions, fissures, hemorrhoids

ble 33-11). Often the client has a series of GI diagnostic tests done. A certain sequence is usually followed; for example, a proctoscopy, then a barium enema, and then an upper GI series. The nurse must observe the client closely to ensure adequate hydration and nutrition during the tests. Some diagnostic studies of the GI system are difficult and uncomfortable for the older adult. It may be necessary to individualize and make adjustments. It is particularly important to prevent diarrhea from bowel cleansing procedures and dehydration from prolonged fluid restriction.[5]

Many radiological studies use either barium sulfate or meglumine diatrizoate (Gastrografin) as a contrast medium. Barium sulfate is more effective for visualizing mucosal detail. Gastrografin is water soluble and rapidly absorbed, so it is preferred when a perforation is suspected. Under other circumstances such as suspected aspiration, water-soluble media are contraindicated and barium is preferred because it is inert in the lung.

Table 33-9

 Age-Related Changes of the Gastrointestinal System and Differences in Assessment Findings

Changes	Differences in Assessment Findings
MOUTH	
Loss of teeth	Presence of dentures, difficulty chewing
Decreased taste buds, decreased sense of smell	Diminished sense of taste (especially salt and sweet)
Decreased volume of saliva	Dry oral mucosa
Atrophy of gingival tissue	Poor-fitting dentures
ESOPHAGUS	
Decreased tone and motility	Complaints of pyrosis (heartburn), dysphagia, eructation
ABDOMINAL WALL	
Thinner and less taut	More visible peristalsis, easier palpation of organs
Decrease in number and sensitivity of sensory receptors	Less sensitivity to surface pain
STOMACH	
Decreased acid secretion, atrophy of gastric mucosa, achlorhydria	Food intolerances, signs of anemia as result of vitamin B_{12} malabsorption
SMALL INTESTINES	
Decreased secretion of most digestive enzymes, decreased motility	Complaints of indigestion
LIVER	
Increased size and lowered in position	Easier palpation
LARGE INTESTINE/ANUS/RECTUM	
Decreased anal sphincter tone and nerve supply to rectal area	Fecal incontinence
Decreased muscular tone, decreased motility	Flatulence, abdominal distention, relaxed perineal musculature
Increase in transit time	Constipation, fecal impaction

Radiological Studies

Upper gastrointestinal series. The purpose of an upper GI series (barium swallow) is to observe the movement of a contrast medium through the esophagus and into the stomach by means of fluoroscopy and x-ray examination. It is used to identify esophageal and stomach disorders such as esophageal strictures, varices, polyps, tumors, hiatal hernia, and peptic ulcers in the stomach or duodenum (Fig. 33-10).

The procedure consists of the client swallowing contrast medium and then assuming different positions on the x-ray table. The movement of the contrast medium is observed with fluoroscopy, and several x-ray films are taken (Table 33-11).

Lower gastrointestinal series. The purpose of a lower GI series (barium enema) x-ray film is to observe by means of fluoroscopy the filling of the colon with contrast medium and to observe by x-ray films the filled colon.

This procedure identifies polyps, tumors, and other lesions in the colon.[6] It consists of administering an enema of contrast medium to the client. The air-contrast barium enema provides better visualization of an inflammatory bowel disease, polyps, and tumors but is not tolerated as well in older and immobile clients (Fig. 33-11).

Oral cholecystogram. The purpose of an oral cholecystogram (gallbladder series) is to visualize the gallbladder. It is used to determine the gallbladder's ability to concentrate and store dye and to observe the patency of the biliary duct system. It is a common gallbladder test and may be used to detect gallstones, obstructions of the biliary tract, and other gallbladder disorders.

The procedure consists of an x-ray examination after the oral ingestion of a radiopaque dye. The radiopaque dye used is an organic insoluble iodide such as iopanoic acid (Telepaque, Priodax, or Oragrafin) (Table 33-11).

Text continued on p. 974.

Table 33-10

 Common Assessment Abnormalities of the Gastrointestinal System

Finding	Description	Possible Etiology and Significance
MOUTH		
Ulcer, plaque on lips or in mouth	Sore or lesion	Carcinoma, viral infections
Cheilosis	Softening, fissuring, and cracking of lips at angles of mouth	Riboflavin deficiency
Cheilitis	Inflammation of lips (usually lower) with fissuring, scaling, crusting	Often unknown
Geographic tongue	Scattered red, smooth (loss of papillae) areas on dorsum of tongue	Unknown
Smooth tongue	Red, slick appearance	Vitamin B_{12} deficiency
Leukoplakia	Thickened white patches	Premalignant lesion
Pyorrhea	Recessed gums, purulent pockets	Periodontitis
Herpes simplex	Benign vesicular lesion	Herpesvirus
Candidiasis	White, curdlike lesions surrounded by erythematous mucosa	Exposure to *Candida albicans*
Glossitis	Reddened, ulcerated, swollen tongue	Exposure to streptococci, irritation, injury, vitamin B deficiency, anemia
Acute marginal gingivitis	Friable, edematous, painful, bleeding gingivae	Irritation from ill-fitting dentures, calcium deposits on teeth, food impaction
ESOPHAGUS AND STOMACH		
Dysphagia	Difficulty in swallowing, sensation of food sticking in esophagus	Esophageal problems, cancer of esophagus
Hematemesis	Vomiting of blood	Esophageal varices, bleeding peptic ulcer
Pyrosis	Heartburn, burning in epigastric or substernal area	Hiatal hernia, esophagitis
Dyspepsia	Burning or indigestion	Peptic ulcer, gallbladder disease
Odynophagia	Painful swallowing	Cancer of esophagus, esophagitis
Eructation	Belching	Gallbladder disease
Nausea and vomiting	Feeling of impending vomiting, expulsion of gastric contents through mouth	GI infections, common manifestation of many GI diseases; stress, fear, and pathological conditions

Continued.

Table 33-10

 Common Assessment Abnormalities of the Gastrointestinal System—cont'd

Finding	Description	Possible Etiology and Significance
ABDOMEN		
Distention	Excessive gas accumulation, enlarged abdomen; generalized tympany	Obstruction, paralytic ileus
Ascites	Accumulated fluid within abdominal cavity, eversion of umbilicus (usually)	Peritoneal inflammation, congestive heart failure, metastatic carcinoma, cirrhosis
Bruit	Humming or swishing sound heard through stethoscope over vessel	Partial arterial obstruction (narrowing of vessel), turbulent flow (aneurysm)
Hyperresonance	Loud, tinkling rushes	Intestinal obstruction
Borborygmi	Waves of loud, gurgling sounds	Hyperactive bowel as result of eating
Absent bowel sounds	No auscultation of bowel sounds	Peritonitis, paralytic ileus, obstruction
Absence of liver dullness	Tympany on percussion	Air from viscus (e.g., perforated ulcer)
Masses	Lump on palpation	Tumors, cysts
Rebound tenderness	Sudden pain when fingers withdrawn quickly	Peritoneal inflammation, appendicitis
Nodular liver	Enlarged, hard liver with irregular edge or surface	Cirrhosis, carcinoma
Hepatomegaly	Enlargement of liver, liver edge >1-2 cm below costal margin	Metastatic carcinoma, hepatitis, venous congestion
Splenomegaly	Enlargement of spleen	Chronic leukemia, hemolytic states, portal hypertension, and some infections
Hernia	Bulge or nodule in abdomen, usually appearing on straining	Inguinal (in inguinal canal), femoral (in femoral canal), umbilical (herniation of umbilicus), or incisional (defect in muscles after surgery)
RECTUM		
Hemorrhoids	Thrombosed veins in rectum and anus (internal or external)	Portal hypertension, chronic constipation, prolonged sitting or standing, pregnancy
Mass	Firm, nodular edge	Tumor, carcinoma
Pilonidal cyst	Opening of sinus tract, cyst in midline just above coccyx	Probably congenital
Fissure	Ulceration in anal canal	Straining, irritation
Melena	Abnormal, black, tarry stool containing digested blood	Cancer, bleeding in upper GI tract from ulcers, varices
Tenesmus	Painful and ineffective straining at stool	Ulcerative colitis, diarrhea secondary to GI infection such as food poisoning
Steatorrhea	Fatty, frothy, foul-smelling stool	Chronic pancreatitis, biliary obstruction, malabsorption problems

Table 33-11

Diagnostic Studies of the Gastrointestinal System

Study	Description and Purpose	Nursing Responsibility
RADIOLOGICAL		
Upper GI or barium swallow	Stomach is examined by x-ray with fluoroscopy with contrast medium. Study is used to diagnose structural abnormalities of the esophagus, stomach, and duodenal bulb.	Explain procedure to client and that client will need to drink contrast medium and assume various positions on x-ray table. Keep client NPO for 8-12 hr before procedure. Tell client to avoid smoking after midnight the night before the study. After x-ray test, take measures to prevent contrast medium impaction (fluids, cathartics). Be aware that stool may be white up to 72 hr after test.
Small bowel series	Contrast medium is ingested and flat film taken every 20 min until medium reaches terminal ileum.	Same as for upper GI.
Lower GI or barium enema	Fluoroscopic x-ray examination of colon uses contrast medium, which is administered rectally (enema). Double contrast or air contrast barium enema is test of choice. Air is infused after barium is evacuated.	Before the procedure, administer laxatives and enemas until colon is clear of stool evening before. Administer clear liquid diet evening before. Keep client NPO for 8 hr before test. Instruct client about being given barium by enema. Explain that cramping and urge to defecate may occur during procedure and that client may be placed in various positions on tilt table. After the procedure, give fluids, laxatives, and/or suppositories to assist in expelling barium. Observe stool for passage of contrast medium.
Oral cholecystogram (GB series)	X-ray examination visualizes GB after radiopaque dye such as iopanoic acid (Telepaque) has been ingested orally. Study determines GB's ability to concentrate and store dye and patency of biliary duct system.	Assess client for sensitivity to iodine. Administer radiopaque dye evening before test. Give six tablets (3 g), one q 5 min. Explain that client may need 2 consecutive days of dye ingestion. Keep client NPO after ingestion of dye. Observe for side effects of dye such as nausea, vomiting, diarrhea. May give fatty test meal after x-ray test to check for GB emptying.
Cholangiography IV cholangiogram	X-rays films are used to visualize biliary duct system after IV injection of radiopaque dye.	Keep client NPO for 8 hr. Assess sensitivity to iodine dye. During injection of dye, assess for urticaria, extreme flushing, respiratory distress.
Percutaneous transhepatic cholangiogram	After local anesthesia, liver is entered with long needle (under fluoroscopy), bile duct is entered, bile withdrawn, and radiopaque dye injected. Fluoroscopy is used to determine filling of hepatic and biliary ducts.	Observe client for signs of hemorrhage or bile leakage.
Surgical cholangiogram	Study is performed during surgery on biliary structures, such as GB. Contrast medium is injected into common bile duct.	Explain to client that anesthetic will be used.

CBD, Common bile duct; *GB,* gallbladder; *NG,* nasogastric; *NPO,* nothing taken orally; *Tc-99m,* technetium-99m; *IV,* intravenous.

Continued.

Table 33-11

Diagnostic Studies of the Gastrointestinal System—cont'd

Study	Description and Purpose	Nursing Responsibility
RADIOLOGICAL—cont'd		
Ultrasound	This noninvasive procedure uses high-frequency sound waves (ultrasound waves), which are passed into body structures and recorded as they are reflected (bounced). A conductive gel (lubricant jelly) is applied to the skin and a transducer is placed on the area.	Be aware that bowel must be cleansed because presence of solid material in GI tract causes changes in reflected sounds and that ultrasound is not transmitted well through gas or air. Schedule test before upper GI or barium enema.
Abdominal ultrasound	Study detects abdominal masses (tumors and cysts) and is also used to assess ascites.	Same as above.
Hepatobiliary ultrasound	Study detects subphrenic abscesses, cysts, tumors, cirrhosis and is used to visualize biliary ducts.	Be aware that bowel must be cleansed. Explain procedure to client.
GB ultrasound	Study detects gallstones (high degree of accuracy) and can be used for clients with jaundice or allergic reaction to GB contrast media.	Administer clear liquids for 24 hr before examination. Give laxative evening before and cleansing enema morning of examination. Keep client NPO 8 hr before procedure.
Nuclear imaging scans	Purpose is to show size, shape, and position of organ. Functional disorders and structural defects may be identified. Radionuclide (radioactive isotope) is injected IV and counter (scanning) device picks up radioactive emission, which is recorded on paper. Only tracer doses of radioactive isotopes are used.	Tell client that substances contain only traces of radioactivity and pose little to no danger. Schedule no more than one radionuclide test on the same day. Explain to client need to lie flat during scanning.
Gastric emptying studies	Radionuclide study is used to assess ability of stomach to empty solids or liquids. In solid-emptying study, cooked egg white containing Tc-99m is eaten. In liquid-emptying study, orange juice with Tc-99m is drunk. Sequential images from gamma camera are recorded every 2 min for up to 60 min. Study is used in clients with emptying disorders from peptic ulcer, ulcer surgery, diabetes, or gastric malignancies.	Same as above.
Liver and spleen scans	Client is given IV injection of Tc-99m and positioned under camera to record distribution of radioactivity in liver and spleen. In normal person, intensity of liver and spleen images is equal. Test is useful in detecting hepatomegaly, hepatocellular diseases, hepatic malignancies, and splenomegaly.	Same as above.
Computerized tomography	Noninvasive radiological examination combines special x-ray machine used for tomography (exposures at different depths) with computer. Study detects mainly biliary tract, liver, and pancreatic disorders. Use of contrast medium accentuates density differences and helps detect biliary problems.	Explain procedure to client.

CBD, Common bile duct; *GB*, gallbladder; *NG*, nasogastric; *NPO*, nothing taken orally; *Tc-99m*, technetium-99m; *IV*, intravenous.

Table 33-11

Study	Description and Purpose	Nursing Responsibility
ENDOSCOPIC		

Upper GI endoscopy
  Esophagoscopy
  Gastroscopy
  Gastroduodenoscopy
	Technique directly visualizes mucosal lining of esophagus, stomach, and duodenum with flexible, fiberoptic endoscope. Test may use video imaging to visualize stomach motility. Inflammations, ulcerations, tumors, varices, or Mallory-Weiss tear may be detected.	Before the procedure, keep client NPO for 8 hr. Make sure signed consent is on chart. Give preoperative medication (diazepam or meperidine). Explain to client that local anesthetic may be sprayed on throat before insertion of scope.
		After the procedure, keep client NPO until gag reflex returns. Gently tickle back of throat to determine reflex. Use warm saline gargles for relief of sore throat. Check temperature q 15-30 min for 1-2 hr (sudden temperature spike is sign of perforation).

Proctosigmoidoscopy	Study directly visualizes rectum and sigmoid colon with lighted endoscope. It is usually done with rigid metal scope but may be done with flexible fiberscope. Sometimes special table is used to tilt client into knee-chest position. Test may detect tumors, polyps, inflammatory and infectious diseases, fissures, hemorrhoids.	Administer enemas evening before and morning of procedure. Be aware that client may have clear liquids day before or that no dietary restrictions may be allowed. Explain to client knee-chest position (unless client is older or very ill), need to take deep breaths during insertion of scope, and possible urge to defecate as scope is passed. Encourage client to relax—let abdomen go limp. Observe for rectal bleeding after polypectomy and/or biopsy.
Fiberoptic colonoscopy	Study directly visualizes entire colon up to ileocecal valve with flexible fiberoptic scope. Client's position is changed frequently during procedure to assist with advancement of scope to cecum. Test is used to diagnose inflammatory bowel disease, identify bleeding sites, and dilate strictures. Procedure allows for removal of colonic polyps without laparotomy.	Before the procedure, keep client on clear liquid 1-3 days and NPO for 8 hr. Administer laxatives 1-3 days before and enemas night before. Explain to client same information regarding insertion of scope as for sigmoidoscopy. Explain to client that sedation will be given. Administer alternate preparation of 1 gal of Go-lytely or Colyte evening before (8 oz glass every 10 min). On morning of procedure, allow clear liquids. After the procedure, be aware that client may experience abdominal cramps caused by stimulation of peristalsis because the client's bowel is constantly insufflated with air during procedure. Observe for rectal bleeding and signs of perforation (e.g. malaise, abdominal distention, tenesmus). Check vital signs.
Endoscopic retrograde cholangiopancreatography (ERCP)	Fiberoptic endoscope is inserted through the oral cavity into descending duodenum, then common bile and pancreatic ducts are cannulated. Contrast medium is injected into ducts and allows for direct visualization of structures. Technique can also be used to retrieve a gallstone from distal CBD, dilate strictures, biopsy tumors, diagnose pseudocysts.	Before the procedure, explain procedure to client, including client's role. Keep client NPO 8 hr before procedure. Ensure consent form signed. Administer sedation immediately before and during procedure. Administer antibiotics if needed. After the procedure, check vital signs. Check for signs of perforation or infection. Be aware that pancreatitis is most common complication. Check for return of gag reflex.

Continued.

Table 33-11

Diagnostic Studies of the Gastrointestinal System—cont'd

Study	Description and Purpose	Nursing Responsibility
ENDOSCOPIC—cont'd		
Peritoneoscopy (laparoscopy)	Peritoneal cavity and contents are visualized with laparoscope. Biopsy specimen may also be taken. Double-puncture peritoneoscopy permits better visualization of abdominal cavity, especially liver. Technique can eliminate need for exploratory laparotomy in many clients.	Make sure signed permit is on chart. Keep client NPO 8 hr before study. Administer preoperative sedative medication. Ensure that bladder and bowel are emptied. Instruct client that local anesthetic is used before scope insertion. Observe for possible complications of bleeding and bowel perforation after the procedure.
BLOOD CHEMISTRIES		
Serum amylase	Study measures secretion of amylase by pancreas and is important in diagnosing acute pancreatitis. Level of amylase peaks in 24 hr and then drops to normal in 48-72 hr. Depending on method, *normal finding* is 25-125 U/L.	Obtain blood sample in acute attack of pancreatitis. Explain procedure to client.
Serum lipase	Study measures secretion of lipase by pancreas. Level stays elevated longer than serum amylase. *Normal finding* is 0.2-1.5 U/ml.	Explain procedure to client.
INVASIVE PROCEDURES		
Liver biopsy	Invasive procedure uses needle inserted through small incision between sixth and seventh or eighth and ninth intercostal spaces on the right side to obtain specimen of hepatic tissue.	Before the procedure, check client's coagulation status (PT, clotting or bleeding time). Ensure that client is typed and cross-matched. Take vital signs as baseline data. Explain holding of breath after expiration when needle is inserted. Ensure that informed consent has been signed. After the procedure, check vital signs to detect internal bleeding q 15 min × 2, q 30 min × 4, q 1 hr × 4. Keep client lying on right side for minimum of 2 hr to splint puncture site. Keep client in bed in flat position for 12-14 hr. Assess client for complications such as bile peritonitis, shock, pneumothorax.
MISCELLANEOUS TESTS		
Gastric analysis	Purpose is to analyze gastric contents for acidity and volume. NG tube is inserted and gastric contents are aspirated. Contents are analyzed mainly for hydrochloric acid, but pH, pepsin, and electrolytes may be determined. Histalog and pentagastrin may be used to stimulate hydrochloric acid secretion. Exfoliative cytology may be done to determine whether malignant cells are present. With fasting, *normal acidity* is 2.5 mEq/L and *normal volume* is 62 ml/hr; 30 min after Histalog or pentagastrin administration, *normal acidity* is 1.5 mEq/L and *normal volume* is 110 ml/hr.	Keep client NPO for 8-12 hr. Explain insertion of NG tube. Withhold drugs affecting gastric secretions 24-48 hr before test. Ensure no smoking morning of test (nicotine increases gastric secretion).

CBD, Common bile duct; *GB,* gallbladder; *NG,* nasogastric; *NPO,* nothing taken orally; *Tc-99m,* technetium-99m; *IV,* intravenous.

Table 33-11

Diagnostic Studies of the Gastrointestinal System—cont'd

Study	Description and Purpose	Nursing Responsibility
MISCELLANEOUS TESTS—cont'd		
Fecal analysis	Form, consistency, color are noted. Specimen examined for mucus, blood, pus, parasites, and fat content. Tests for occult blood (guaiac test, Hemoccult, Hematest) are done.	Observe client's stools. Collect stool specimens. Check stools for blood with Hemoccult or Hematest. Keep diet free of red meat for 24-48 hr before guaiac test.
D-Xylose tolerance	Absorption test involves xylose, a monosaccharine, given orally in water. All urine is collected for 5 hr and amount of D-Xylose excreted is measured. *Normal finding* is 20% of xylose excreted in 5 hr.	Keep client NPO for 10-12 hr before test. Ensure that client empties bladder before xylose given orally.
Duodenal drainage	Duodenal contents are aspirated by double-lumen NG tube—one lumen in stomach, the other in duodenum. Stimulant IV drug is given (usually CCK-PZ). Duodenal contents are analyzed for enzymes, blood, bile, malignant cells, cholesterol crystals, and volume.	Explain procedure to client. Insert NG tube. Keep client on NPO status.

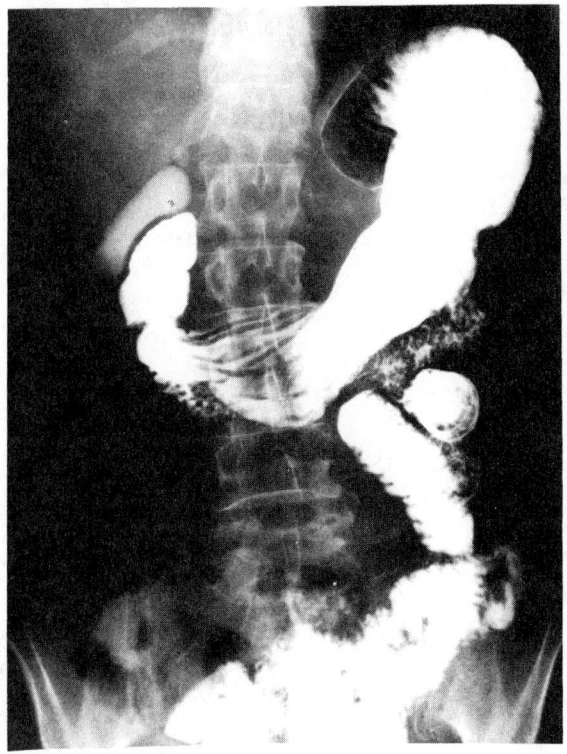

Fig. 33-10   Upper GI tract x-ray film.

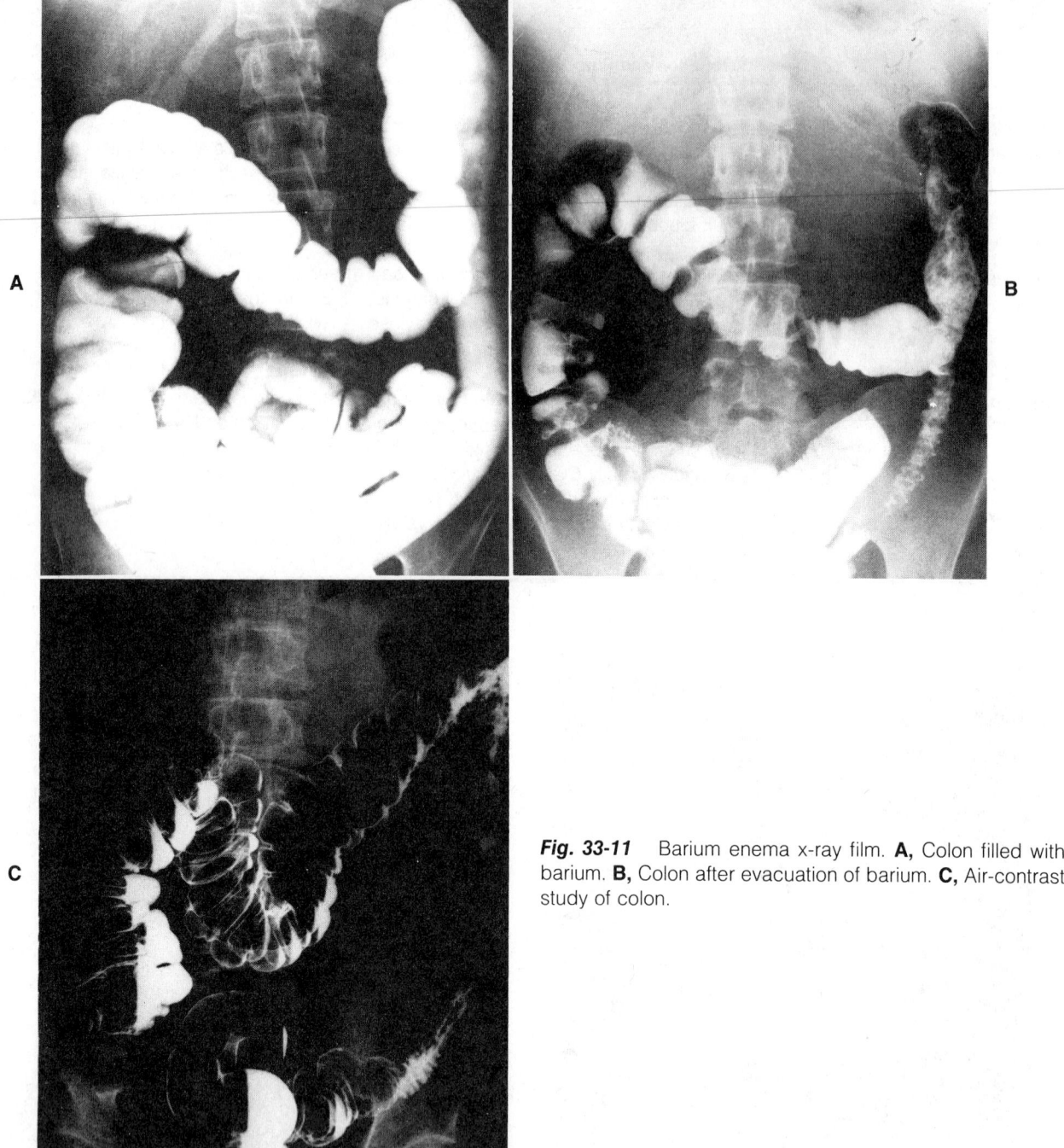

Fig. 33-11 Barium enema x-ray film. **A,** Colon filled with barium. **B,** Colon after evacuation of barium. **C,** Air-contrast study of colon.

Endoscopy

Endoscopy refers to the direct visualization of a body structure through a lighted instrument (scope). Most of the GI tract can be visualized by endoscopy, especially with the flexible fiberoptic scopes.[7] The GI structures that can be examined by fiberoptic endoscopy include the esophagus, stomach, duodenum, colon, and, with the aid of fluoroscopy and x-ray films, the pancreas and biliary tree.

The fiberscope is an instrument channel through which biopsy forceps and cytology brushes may be passed. Cameras may be attached and pictures taken. Endoscopy of the GI tract is frequently done in combination with biopsy and cytological studies. The major complication of GI endoscopy is perforation through the structure being scoped. This complication is decreased with the use of the flexible fiberoptic scopes. All endoscopic procedures require informed, written consent. The specific endoscopy procedures are discussed in Table 33-11.

Table 33-12 Liver Function Tests

Test	Description and Purpose
BILE FORMATION AND EXCRETION	
Serum bilirubin	Measurement of ability of liver to conjugate and excrete bilirubin, allowing differentiation between unconjugated (indirect) and conjugated (direct) bilirubin in plasma
Total	Measurement of direct and indirect total bilirubin *Normal finding* of 0.3-1.3 mg/dl
Direct	Measurement of conjugated bilirubin, elevation in obstructive jaundice *Normal finding* of 0.1-0.3 mg/dl
Indirect	Measurement of unconjugated bilirubin, elevation in hepatocellular and hemolytic conditions *Normal finding* of 0.1-1.0 mg/dl
Urinary bilirubin	Measurement of urinary excretion of conjugated bilirubin *Normal finding* of 0
Urinary urobilinogen	Measurement of urinary excretion of urobilinogen; maximum excretion midafternoon to early evening, collection of total urinary output for 2 hr in afternoon, sent to laboratory in dark container immediately because of oxidization of urobilinogen to urobilin on exposure to air *Normal finding* of 0-4 mg/day
Fecal urobilinogen	Measurement of fecal urobilinogen in stool specimen *Normal finding* of 30-220 mg/100 g stool
DYE EXCRETION TESTS (DETOXIFICATION)	
Indocyanine green	Determination of liver's ability to take up and excrete dye given IV, drawing of blood samples every 5 min for 20-30 min, client on NPO status *Normal finding* of 500-800 ml/m^2 of body surface/min
PROTEIN METABOLISM	
Serum protein levels	Measurement of serum proteins that are manufactured by the liver; measurement of albumin, *normal finding* of 3.5-5.5 g/dl; measurement of globulin, *normal finding* of 2.0-3.5 g/dl Normal total protein of 6-8 g/dl *Normal A/G ratio* of 1.5:1-2.5:1
α-Fetoprotein	Indication of hepatic cancer *Normal finding* of <25 ng/ml
Blood ammonia levels	Conversion of ammonia to urea normally occurring in the liver, elevation in hepatic encephalopathy secondary to liver cirrhosis *Normal finding* of 30-70 μg/dl

Continued.

In addition to diagnostic procedures, many invasive and therapeutic procedures may be done with endoscopes. These include procedures such as polypectomy, sclerosis of varices, laser treatment, cauterization of bleeding sites, papillotomy, common bile duct stone removal, and balloon dilatations. A new and valuable diagnostic procedure is video endoscopy. In this procedure an electronic video endoscope converts electronic signals that can be seen on a television screen.

Liver Biopsy

The purpose of a liver biopsy is to obtain hepatic tissue to be used in establishing a diagnosis such as cirrhosis, hepatitis, and neoplasms. It may also be useful for following the progress of a liver disease.

The two types of liver biopsy are *open* and *closed*. The open method involves making an incision and removing a wedge of tissue. It is done in the operating room with the client under general anesthesia, often concurrently with another surgical procedure. The closed or needle biopsy is an invasive procedure in which the site is infiltrated with a local anesthetic and a needle inserted through a small incision between the sixth and seventh or eighth and ninth intercostal spaces on the right side. The client lies supine with the right arm over the head. The client should be instructed to expire fully and not breathe while the needle is inserted. Nursing assessment before and after a liver biopsy is important (see Table 33-11).

Liver Function Studies

Liver function tests are usually described separately from other GI diagnostic studies. Liver function tests are basically biochemical determinations that reflect hepatic disease. Table 33-12 describes some common liver function tests.

Table 33-12 Liver Function Tests—cont'd

Test	Description and Purpose
HEMOSTATIC FUNCTIONS	
Prothrombin	Determination of prothrombin activity *Normal finding* of 12-15 sec
Vitamin K production	Determination of response of liver to vitamin K, checking of PT necessary 24 hr after injection of vitamin K
SERUM ENZYME TESTS*	
Alkaline phosphatase	Normal presence of high concentrations, excretion in bile, elevation in obstructive jaundice *Normal finding* of 25-90 U/L, *(depending on method and age)*
Serum glutamic-oxaloacetic transaminase (SGOT) or aspartate aminotransferase (AST)	Elevation in liver damage *Normal finding* of 7-40 U/L
Serum glutamic-pyruvic transaminase (SGPT) or alanine aminotransferase (ALT)	Elevation in liver damage *Normal finding* of 5-36 U/L
Lactic dehydrogenase (LDH)	Infrequent use in assessment of liver disease *Normal finding* of 95-200 U/L
γ-Glutamyl transpeptidase	Present in biliary tract (not in skeletal muscle or cardiac), increase in hepatitis and alcoholic liver disease
LIPID METABOLISM	
Serum cholesterol	Synthesis and excretion by liver, increase in biliary obstruction, decrease in extensive liver disease and malnutrition *Normal finding* of 140-220 mg/dl, varying with age
SEROLOGY FOR VIRAL HEPATITIS†	
Hepatitis B surface antigen (HB_sAg) HB_eAg, anti-HB_s, anti-HB_e, anti-HB_c)	Present in blood in early stages of hepatitis B *Normal finding* of negative
Hepatitis A virus	Present in serum and stool early in course of hepatitis A

*Other enzymes that may be assessed are 5'-nucleotidase, aminopeptidase, and cholinesterase.
†See Table 38-3.

R eview Questions

The number of the question corresponds to the same-numbered objective at the beginning of the chapter.

1. The parietal cells in the stomach secrete the intrinsic factor, which
   a. protects and prevents autodigestion
   b. promotes the absorption of vitamin B_{12}
   c. blocks the absorption of the extrinsic factor
   d. inhibits gastric secretion

2. In relation to carbohydrate metabolism the liver forms glucose from amino acids and fatty acids. This process is called
   a. deamination
   b. glycogenesis
   c. gluconeogenesis
   d. glycogenolysis

3. Which of the following statements about the hormone CCK-PZ is true?

a. It is secreted when acid enters the small intestine.
b. It causes relaxation of the gallbladder.
c. It is secreted when the stomach is distended and inhibits gastric acid secretion.
d. It is secreted when fatty acids and amino acids enter the small intestine and causes contraction of the gallbladder.

4. In bilirubin metabolism in the intestines most of the bilirubin is
   a. reduced to urobilinogen by bacterial action
   b. reabsorbed by the blood
   c. conjugated with glucuronic acid
   d. broken down so that it is in an unconjugated form

5. In the review of systems the client should be questioned about ingestion of food and fluids. A significant area to include is

a. melena
b. the relationship of pain to eating or to a specific food
c. dark urine and clay-colored stools
d. steatorrhea
6. On percussion of the abdomen, tympany indicates
a. presence of a mass
b. ascites
c. a bruit
d. presence of air
7. Which of the following findings of an abdominal examination is abnormal?
a. loud, tinkling rushes on auscultation
b. liver dullness
c. inability to palpate spleen
d. no tenderness on palpation
8. The client who has had a liver biopsy should lie on the right side because this position will
a. apply pressure at puncture site
b. prevent shift of ascitic fluid
c. facilitate blood flow to the liver
d. decrease blood flow to the liver

REFERENCES

1. Rowe JW and Besdine RW: Geriatric medicine, ed 2, Boston, 1988, Little, Brown & Co, pp 498-499, 500-501.
2. Bates B: A guide to physical examination and history taking, ed 4, Philadelphia, 1987, JB Lippincott Co, pp 340-343.
3. Swartz MH: Textbook of physical diagnosis, Philadelphia, 1989, WB Saunders Co, pp 344-346.
4. Seidel HM and others: Mosby's guide to physical examination, St Louis, 1987, The CV Mosby Co, pp 401-402.
5. Reichel W, ed: Clinical aspects of aging, ed 3, Baltimore, 1989, Williams & Wilkins, p 188.
6. Fischbach FT: A manual of laboratory diagnostic tests, ed 3, Philadelphia, 1988, JB Lippincott Co, p 604.
7. Dent TL and others, eds: Surgical endoscopy, Chicago, 1985, Year Book Medical Publishers, pp 3-7, 505-507.

Nursing Role in Management
Problems of Ingestion

Rachel Elrod

Ingestion is the process of taking food and fluids into the body via the gastrointestinal (GI) tract. It begins in the mouth with mastication of food by the teeth. Food then passes down the esophagus and into the stomach. It is important that sufficient nutrients be ingested to meet bodily needs. This chapter discusses problems of ingestion that involve the mouth and the esophagus. Oral problems, such as poor dental health, infections and inflammations, and cancer, interfere with ingestion. Esophageal problems may also interfere with swallowing of food and fluids and with passage of the food to the stomach.

Many problems of ingestion make it necessary for the client to use alternative methods of taking in nutrients, either temporarily or permanently. This involves physical and emotional adaptations. The mouth is associated with food, love, and pleasurable sensations. The social implications of not being able to eat are great. Older adults are

Reviewed by Nancy Munn Short, R.N., B.S.N., C.C.R.N., Emergency Department, Duke University Medical Center, Durham, North Carolina.

particularly susceptible to many psychological and physiological problems related to alterations in digestion.

DENTAL PROBLEMS
Dental Caries

Dental caries (decay of teeth) is a general term applied to the decalcification of the mineral components and dissolution of the organic matrix of the teeth. Cavity formation is the clinical evidence of the progression of this process.

Caries development starts when *plaque* builds up and adheres to the teeth. Plaque is a gelatinous substance consisting of bacteria, saliva, and epithelial cells. The tight adherence of plaque to the teeth provides protection for the bacteria (usually lactobacilli and streptococci). Within 30 minutes after eating, these bacteria produce acids from the breakdown of sugars contained in food deposits on the teeth. The acids destroy the outer enamel and later the underlying dentin of the tooth (Fig. 34-1). The decay proceeds and can progress to the pulp of the tooth.

If the decay is not treated, a *pulpitis* develops and ex-

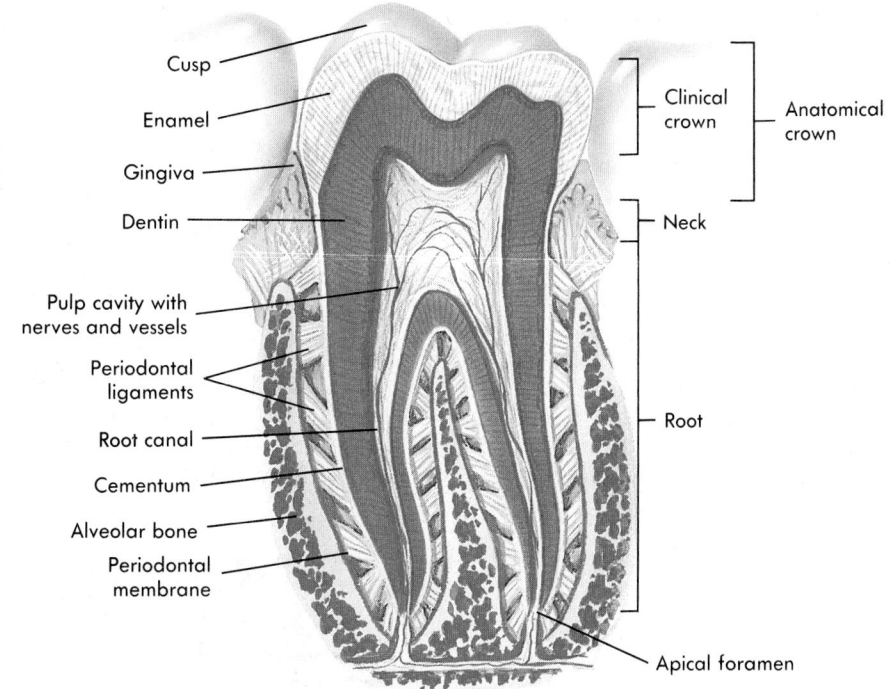

Fig. 34-1 Normal tooth structure. (From Seeley RR, Stephens TD, and Tate P: Anatomy and physiology, St Louis, 1989, The CV Mosby Co, p 735.)

tends to the alveolar bone, forming an abscess. This results in pain, edema of facial structures, and sometimes malaise and fever. During the early stages of pulpitis, pain may be induced by thermal changes, especially cold drinks. In the later stages of pulpitis, heat or reclining may stimulate the onset of more severe pain. At this stage, damage to the pulp is irreversible. Treatment consists of tooth removal or root canal therapy (removal of the pulp and filling of the pulp canal with inert material).

Periodontal Disease

The *periodontium* is the tissue surrounding and supporting the teeth. It is composed of the gingivae (gums), cementum, alveolar bone, and periodontal ligament, which helps to fix the tooth firmly in its bony socket. Periodontal disease is the major cause of tooth loss in adults.[1] Approximately one in four persons has some stage of periodontal disease.[2] Periodontal disease begins with gingivitis and eventually involves the periodontal ligament and the alveolar bone.

Dental plaque is the most important etiological factor in periodontal disease. When plaque calcifies, it forms *calculus,* which is a hard, tenacious mass on the crowns of teeth. *Malocclusion* (faulty relationships between the teeth when the jaws are closed), margins of overextended fillings, and impacted food are other etiological factors that can cause local irritation to the gingivae. Systemic conditions such as diabetes mellitus, thyroid diseases, pregnancy, and vitamin and nutritional deficiencies may modify the person's response to the local etiological factors and make them more susceptible to periodontal disease. The exact role of systemic conditions is unknown.

Certain drugs cause changes, such as inflammation and hyperplasia of the gingiva, which may be related to periodontal disease. Two such drugs are phenytoin (Dilantin) and oral contraceptives.

When the gingivae are irritated from any of the local etiological factors, they become inflamed (Fig. 34-2). The inflammation causes the gingiva to separate from the surface of the tooth. Pockets created between the teeth and the gingivae can collect pus and bacteria (periodontitis). At this stage, bleeding occurs readily, and pus may ooze from the gingiva. Gradually, the bone supporting the teeth is destroyed, and the teeth become very loose. As the periodontal pockets deepen and seal themselves off, periodontal abscesses may occur (Fig. 34-3). At this stage the usual treatment is extraction of the involved tooth or teeth.

■ Nursing Management of Dental Problems
Nursing assessment

The client's teeth should be assessed for caries, missing teeth, displaced teeth, and dental appliances such as dentures, bridges, and crowns. The gingivae (gums) should be assessed for redness, pallor, bleeding, recession, and ulcers. The client should be asked questions regarding dental care and frequency of dental examinations.

Nursing diagnoses

Nursing diagnoses specific to the client with dental problems include, but are not limited to, the following:

1. Altered oral mucous membrane related to ill-fitting dentures, caries, ineffective oral hygiene, or periodontal disease
2. Altered nutrition: less than body requirements related to inability to ingest adequate nutrients because

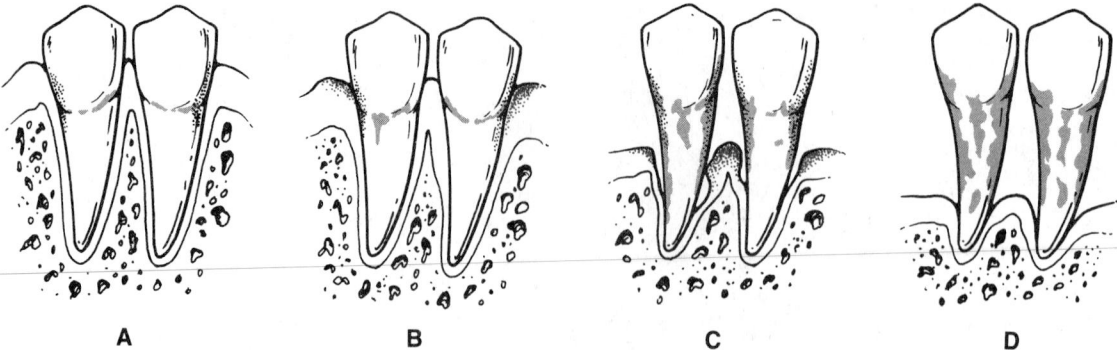

A   **B**   **C**   **D**

Fig. 34-2 Progression of periodontal disease. **A,** Calculus deposits on teeth at gingival line, causing gingivitis. **B,** Gingivae become swollen and tender with spread of inflammation. **C,** Inflammation spreads and pockets develop between teeth and gingivae, which are receding. **D,** The alveolar bone is destroyed and teeth become loose.

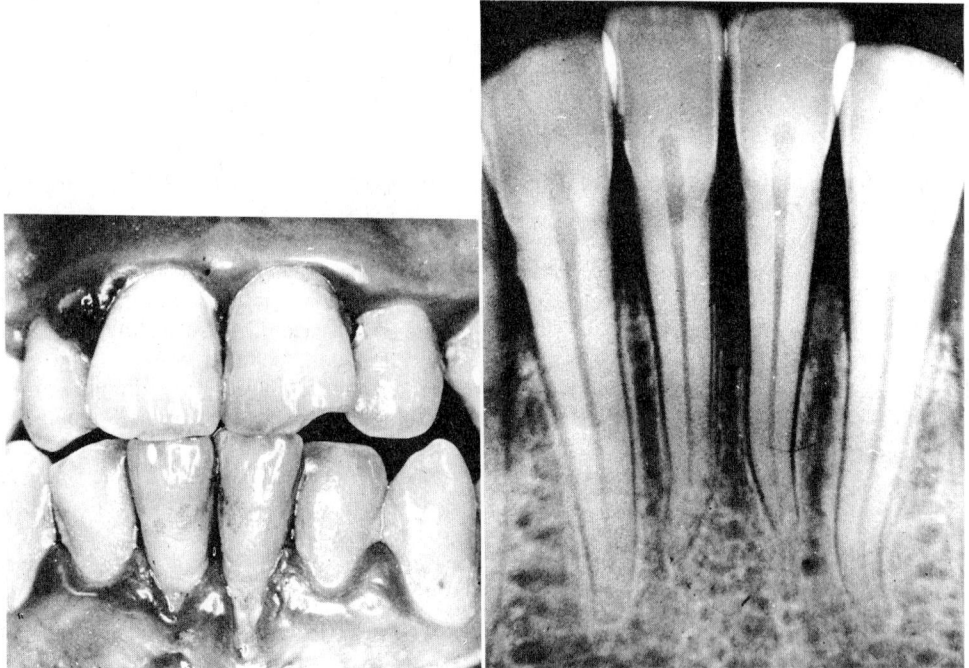

Fig. 34-3 Periodontitis. Signs include edema, periodontal abscess, hemorrhage on slight pressure, tissue recession with retraction of gingival margin, color change from light pink to deep red, loss of tissue in interdental area, horizontal bone loss, and widening of periodontal space. (From Kissane JM, ed: Anderson's pathology, ed 9, St Louis, 1990, Mosby–Year Book, Inc, p 1100.)

of ill-fitting dentures, displaced teeth, gingival disease, dental caries, sensitive teeth, edentulous condition, or oral pain

3. Body image disturbance related to change in appearance of or unattractive teeth, difficulty with eating, or halitosis

4. High risk for noncompliance with regular, periodic dental examinations related to altered perception, lack of motivation, inadequate finances, or lack of knowledge of consequences of noncompliance

Nursing interventions
Health promotion and maintenance

ORAL HYGIENE. Proper oral hygiene is essential to prevent caries and periodontal disease. This involves frequent complete cleaning of the teeth and gingivae with toothbrushing and flossing. The teeth should be brushed after each meal with a soft, rounded-bristle toothbrush. Brushing the teeth should remove food debris and plaque and stimulate the gingivae. The teeth should be brushed by first placing the bristles of the toothbrush next to the gum line and then brushing with a motion away from the gum line.

Flossing should be done at least once a day. It is a useful and important measure for removing plaque between teeth, an area that is not easily accessible to brushing. Flossing is done by gently forcing the floss between the teeth and moving the floss up and down the tooth surface a few times, until it reaches the gum line.

During illness the client may not salivate as usual, which reduces the natural cleaning process of the teeth and mouth. The nurse may need to assume responsibility for dental care and oral hygiene. Swabbing the client's mouth and rinsing it with mouthwash are inadequate measures. Mechanical cleansing is essential to remove the plaque. Either a regular or an electric toothbrush should be used on all surfaces to remove plaque and mechanically stimulate the gingivae to increase blood supply. The client's mouth should be assessed each time oral care is given.

DENTAL EXAMINATIONS. Regular, periodic dental examinations are important to maintain a healthy mouth and teeth. At the time of a dental examination a thorough cleaning with removal of plaque and calculus is done. Caries and early signs of periodontal disease can be detected and treated. The mouth is examined for any signs of oral cancer. For most adults, an examination every 6 to 12 months is adequate. Some persons may require more frequent visits. Persons at risk of infective endocarditis may require prophylactic antibiotics (see Chapter 31).

NUTRITION. Caries develops with increasing frequency in persons who ingest diets high in refined carbohydrates. Because of this finding, a prevention program includes reduction in sugar intake. If sugars are eaten, the teeth should be brushed within 30 minutes of eating. Another aspect of diet therapy that seems to reduce plaque formation is increased vitamin C intake.

FLUORIDE. Fluoridation makes tooth enamel more resistant to the acids produced from the action of bacteria on sugars in the mouth. In drinking water, one part of fluoride per million results in a significant decrease in the decay rate.[1] Many communities consider the fluoridation of drinking water a municipal responsibility and have enacted the necessary legislation. A fluoride solution can be applied topically on the teeth during a dental office visit. In addition, many toothpastes have fluoride added to them and they are recommended by the American Dental Association. Fluoride rinses and tablets are also available for at-home use.

NEW TECHNIQUES. Some chemical methods to inhibit plaque formation and accumulation offer promise. Antimicrobial agents added to mouthwashes, toothpaste, foams, and gels have been tested. They decrease or eliminate bacteria action for a few hours after use. Bonding the teeth with application of a coating solution may protect against decay.

Acute intervention. The nurse may need to refer the client for intervention and care of an acute dental problem. Local manifestations of dental problems include pain that is intermittent and caused by sensitivity to heat or cold stimulation or that is dull and continuous, facial swelling, halitosis, and bleeding or drainage of pus from the mouth. Systemic manifestations include fever, nausea, vomiting, and malaise.

If pulpitis and abscess develop, immediate dental care is needed to prevent further spread of infection to the bone. An opening may be drilled into the pulp chamber, or the gingivae may have to be incised to provide drainage for the abscess. Sometimes a root canal procedure or extraction of a tooth is necessary. After treatment of an abscess, the client can use warm saline rinses. Analgesics may also be required to alleviate the pain.

Extraction of a damaged or defective tooth or one that has a severe abscess may be required. After the extraction the client should apply cold applications (e.g., ice bag, cold washcloth) to the side of the face to reduce swelling and relieve discomfort. Some oozing of blood is expected the first 1 to 2 days. If there is loss of large amounts of bright-red blood, direct pressure should be applied to the bleeding site by the client biting on a gauze pad and the dentist should be notified.

Sometimes the client is hospitalized for the extraction of several teeth, such as when impacted molars are excised or when dentures are required. Postoperatively the client will experience pain and soreness. Ice packs and analgesics are used to relieve the discomfort. Nutrients are liquid to semisoft for a few days. The dentist may order mouthwashes for cleansing and relief of soreness.

Chronic management

DENTURES. The decision to obtain dentures is not easy for most people. They are concerned about changes in cosmetic appearance and the ability to chew food. They need to be assured that dentures will usually decrease the spread of infection, improve nutritional intake, and improve appearance, especially if they have had multiple dental problems preceding the decision to obtain dentures.

Patience must be stressed in the adjustment phase to dentures. It does take time to get used to a different feel and way of chewing. The gingivae should be checked for proper fit and for any signs of gingival irritation. Dentures should be cleaned at least twice a day with salt and sodium bicarbonate or a dentifrice. When the dentures are removed, the client should massage the gums for a few minutes. Some clients prefer to wear their dentures at all times, and there are generally no contraindications to this. In fact, facial contour is better maintained by this practice. If dentures are removed at night, they should be covered with water (especially if they are made of vulcanite) and stored in a safe place.

Clients who wear dentures should be encouraged to obtain regular dental care. Dentures may need to be modified as tissue changes occur from aging, weight changes, or disease processes.

Dental implants are being used in some instances in which the client requires tooth extractions. An implant involves insertion of a titanium post into the bone. The bone fuses with the post and then techniques of restorative dentistry are used to create a crown that is attached to the post.

PERIODONTAL DISEASE. Early treatment of periodontal disease consists of *scaling* and *root planing*. Scaling is the removal of calculus, and root planing is the smoothing of root surfaces. Curettage may be combined with these procedures. This removes the soft tissue lining the pocket and

Table 34-1   Infections and Inflammations of the Mouth

Condition	Etiology	Clinical Manifestations	Treatment
Gingivitis	Neglected oral hygiene, malocclusion, missing or irregular teeth, faulty dentistry, eating of soft rather than fibrous foods	Inflamed gingivae and interdental papillae; bleeding during toothbrushing; development of pus, abscess formation with loosening of teeth (periodontitis)	Prevention through health teaching, dental care, gingival massage, professional cleaning of teeth, fibrous foods, conscientious brushing habits with flossing
Vincent's infection (acute necrotizing ulcerative gingivitis, trench mouth)	Fusiform bacteria; Vincent spirochetes; predisposing factors of worry, excessive fatigue, poor oral hygiene, nutritional deficiencies (vitamins B and C)	Painful, bleeding gingivae; eroding necrotic lesions of interdental papillae; ulcerations that bleed; increased saliva with metallic taste; fetid mouth odor; anorexia, fever, and general malaise	Rest (physical and mental); avoidance of smoking and alcoholic beverages; soft, nutritious diet; correct oral hygiene habits; topical applications of antibiotics; mouth irrigations with hydrogen peroxide and saline solutions
Oral candidiasis (moniliasis or thrush)	*Candida albicans* (a yeast-like fungus), debilitation, prolonged high-dose antibiotic or corticosteroid therapy	Pearly, bluish white "milk-curd" membranous lesions on mucosa of mouth and larynx; sore mouth; yeasty halitosis	Nystatin or amphotericin B as oral suspension or buccal tablets, good oral hygiene
Herpes simplex (cold sore, fever blister)	Herpes simplex virus, type I or II; predisposing factors of upper respiratory infections, excessive exposure to sunlight, food allergies, emotional tension, onset of menstruation	Lip lesions, mouth lesions, vesicle formation (single or clustered), shallow, painful ulcers	Spirits of camphor, corticosteroid cream, mild antiseptic mouthwash, viscous lidocaine, removal or control of predisposing factors, antiviral agents (e.g., acyclovir)
Aphthous stomatitis (canker sore)	Recurrent and chronic form of infection secondary to systemic disease, trauma, stress, or unknown causes	Ulcers of mouth and lips, causing extreme pain; ulcers surrounded by erythematous base	Steroids (topical or systemic), tetracycline oral suspension
Parotitis (inflammation of parotid gland, surgical mumps)	Usually *Staphylococcus* species, *Streptococcus* species occasionally, debilitation and dehydration with poor oral hygiene, NPO status for an extended time	Pain in area of gland and ear, absence of salivation, purulent exudate from duct of gland	Antibiotics; mouthwashes; warm compresses; preventive measures such as chewing gum, sucking on hard candy (lemon drops), adequate fluid intake
Stomatitis (inflammation of mouth)	Trauma; pathogens; irritants (tobacco, alcohol); renal, liver, and hematological diseases; side effect of many cancer chemotherapy drugs	Excessive salivation, halitosis, sore mouth	Removal or treatment of cause, oral hygiene with soothing solutions, topical medications, soft, bland diet

Table 34-2 Oral Tumors

Location	Predisposing Factors	Clinical Manifestations	Treatment
Lip	Constant overexposure to sun and wind, fair complexion, irritation from pipe stem	Indurated, painless ulcer	Surgical excision, radiation
Tongue	Tobacco, irritation, syphilis	Ulcer or area of thickening; soreness or pain; increased salivation, slurred speech, dysphagia, toothache, earache (later signs)	Surgery (hemiglossectomy or glossectomy), radiation
Oral cavity	Poor oral hygiene, tobacco (pipe and cigar smoking, snuff, chewing tobacco), chronic alcoholic intake, chronic irritation (jagged tooth, ill-fitting prostheses, excessive dental calculi, chemical or mechanical irritants)	Leukoplakia; erythroplakia; ulcerations; sore spot; rough area; pain, dysphagia, difficulty in chewing and speaking (later signs)	Surgery (mandibulectomy, radical neck dissection, resections of buccal musoca), radiation, chemotherapy

helps the gums to heal. A *gingivectomy* and *gingivoplasty* may be necessary. In a gingivectomy, tissue and deep pockets are removed. A gingivoplasty involves reshaping of gingival tissue.

In the later stages of periodontal disease, the bone supporting the teeth is often destroyed. At this stage, treatment entails extraction of the teeth and the wearing of dentures.

ORAL INFLAMMATIONS AND INFECTIONS

Oral infections and inflammations that are specific mouth diseases may occur. They may also occur in the presence of some systemic diseases such as leukemia or vitamin deficiency. When oral inflammations and infections are present, they can severely impair the ingestion of food and fluids. Common inflammations and infections of the oral cavity are presented in Table 34-1.

CARCINOMA OF THE ORAL CAVITY

Carcinoma of the oral cavity may occur on the lips or anywhere within the mouth (e.g., tongue, floor of the mouth, buccal mucosa, hard palate, soft palate, pharyngeal walls, and tonsils). Oral carcinoma accounts for about 4% of all cancers. It is more common after the age of 45, with 60 as the average age at onset. Carcinoma of the oral cavity occurs in all ethnic groups. It is more common in men (2:1). Squamous cell carcinoma is the most common oral malignant tumor (more than 90%).[3] The 5-year survival rate of oral cancer is 30%.[4]

Most of the malignant lesions occur on the lower lip in men. Other common sites are the lateral border and undersurface of the tongue, labial commissure, and buccal mucosa. Carcinoma of the lip has the most favorable prognosis of any of the oral tumors. This is probably because lip lesions are more apparent to the client than other oral lesions and are usually diagnosed earlier.

Etiology

Although the cause of carcinoma of the oral cavity is not definitive, there are a number of predisposing factors (Table 34-2). Constant overexposure to the sun and wind is definitely a factor in the development of cancer of the lip. Irritation from the pipe stem resting on the lip is a factor in pipe smokers. Factors that influence intraoral cancer include tobacco (cigar, cigarette, pipe, snuff), excessive alcohol intake, and chronic irritation such as from a jagged tooth or poor dental care. A positive history of use of tobacco and alcohol, past or current, is the most significant etiological factor.[5]

Clinical Manifestations

Leukoplakia, called "white patch" or "smoker's patch," is frequently considered a precancerous lesion. It is a whitish patch on the mucosa of the mouth or tongue. The patch becomes keratinized (hard and leathery) and is sometimes described as hyperkeratosis. Leukoplakia is the result of chronic irritation, especially smoking. *Erythroplasia* (erythroplakia), which is seen as a red velvety patch on the mouth or tongue, is also considered a precancerous lesion.[5]

Cancer of the lip usually appears as an indurated, painless ulcer on the lip. The first sign of carcinoma of the tongue is an ulcer or area of thickening. Soreness or pain of the tongue may occur, especially on eating hot or highly seasoned foods. Some clients experience limitation of movement of the tongue. Later symptoms of cancer of the tongue include increased salivation, slurred speech, dysphagia, toothache, and earache.

Common manifestations of carcinoma of the oral cavity are leukoplakia, erythroplakia, ulcerations, a sore spot, and a rough area (felt with the tongue). Later symptoms are pain, dysphagia, and difficulty in chewing and speaking.

Diagnostic Studies

Biopsy of the suspected lesion with cytological examination is the best definitive diagnostic measure for oral cancer. Oral exfoliative cytology involves scraping of a suspicious lesion and spreading this scraping on a slide. This procedure can help confirm the presence of a cancer. Unlike biopsy, a negative cytological smear cannot be relied on to rule out the possibility of a malignant condition but may be used as a screening test. The toluidine blue test may also be used as a screening test for oral cancer. Toluidine blue is applied topically and stains an area of carcinoma.[6]

Therapeutic Management

Management of oral carcinoma usually consists of surgery, radiation, chemotherapy, or a combination of these (Table 34-3).

Surgical interventions. Surgery remains the most effective treatment, especially for removing the central core of the tumor. Many of the operations are radical procedures involving extensive resections. Various surgical procedures may be performed, depending on the location and extent of the tumor. Some examples are *partial mandibulectomy* (removal of the mandible), *hemiglossectomy* (removal of half of the tongue), *glossectomy* (removal of the tongue), resections of the buccal mucosa and floor of the mouth, and *radical neck dissection*. Composite resections, which are combinations of the various surgical procedures, may be done.

Since cancers of the oral cavity metastasize early to the cervical lymph nodes, a radical neck dissection is commonly performed. It includes wide excision of the involved primary lesion with removal of the regional lymph nodes and deep cervical lymph nodes and their lymphatic channels. In addition, the following structures may also be removed or transected (depending on the primary lesion and its extensiveness): sternocleidomastoid muscle and other closely associated muscles, internal jugular vein, mandible, submaxillary gland, part of thyroid and parathyroid glands, and spinal accessory nerve. A tracheostomy is

commonly performed along with the radical neck dissection. Drainage tubes are inserted into the surgical area and connected to suction to remove fluid and blood (Fig. 34-4). Portable wound suction, as with a Hemovac, is usually used. The radical neck dissection usually involves one side of the neck. If the lesion is in the midline of the oral cavity, simultaneous bilateral neck dissection is done.

Functional neck dissection may be performed as an alternative to radical neck dissection. It involves dissection of the major cervical lymphatic vessels and lateral cervical space but preserves several nerves and vessels, including the sympathetic and vagus nerves and the internal jugular vein.

Life-threatening complications, such as airway obstruction, hemorrhage, and tracheal aspiration, may occur. Airway obstruction must be prevented. Depending on the degree of surgery, a prophylactic tracheostomy is often performed. Hemorrhage can occur because of the vascularity of the head and neck area. Another complication is tracheal aspiration, which may occur up to 1 week after surgery. It occurs because the client is unable to swallow saliva or fluids and aspirates fluid. Other complications include infection, pneumothorax, subcutaneous emphysema or air leak under the skin flaps, and necrosis of the skin flaps. Neural complications can occur as a result of nerve severance during the surgical procedure. The nerves most commonly severed are the spinal accessory nerves and cervical plexus. The facial nerve (cranial nerve), which

Table 34-3

Diagnostic and Therapeutic Management: Oral Carcinoma

DIAGNOSTIC

Oral exfoliative cytology
Biopsy

THERAPEUTIC*

Surgical excision of the tumor
Radical neck dissection
Radiation (internal or external)
Combined surgical excision with radiation
Chemotherapy

---

*Any of the following approaches may be used, depending on the primary lesion and the extent of metastasis.

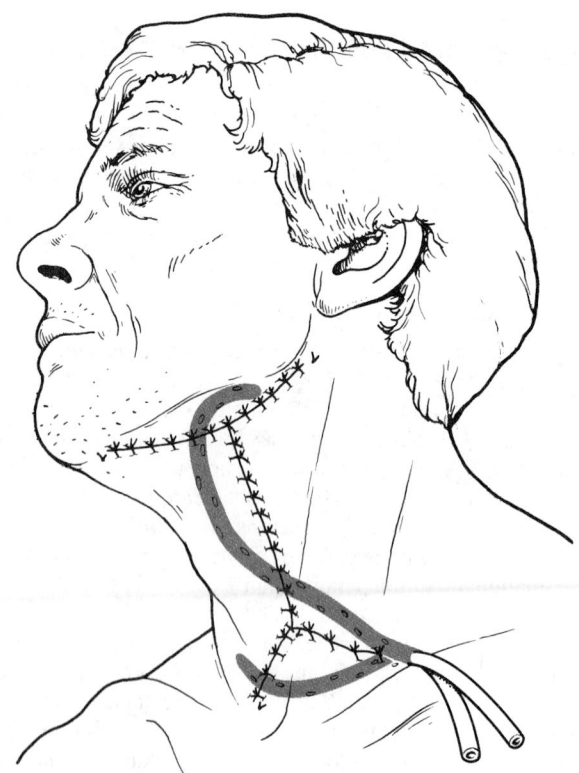

Fig. 34-4 Radical neck incision with suction tubing in place.

passes through the parotid gland, may be affected if this gland is removed.

Radiation and chemotherapy. Radiation is sometimes used before surgery to decrease the size of the tumor. Radiation may also be used postoperatively or palliatively. The type of radiation used may be internal or external. Common forms of internal radiation are the implantation of seeds, such as radon seeds, in gold tubes or molds. External radiation may also be used (see Chapter 9).

Chemotherapy and radiation are used together when the lesions are more advanced or involve several structures of the oral cavity. Chemotherapy may also be used when surgery and radiation fail or as the initial therapy for smaller tumors. Methotrexate (MTX) is the most effective chemotherapeutic agent. Another agent, 5-fluorouracil (5-FU), may be used for small skin lesions. Other chemotherapeutic agents used are cyclophosphamide, bleomycin, vinblastine, hydroxyurea, and cisplatin (see Chapter 9).

Palliative treatment may be the best management when the prognosis is poor, the cancer is inoperable, or the client decides against mutilating surgery. Palliation aims to treat the symptoms and make the client more comfortable. If it becomes difficult to swallow, a gastrostomy may be performed to allow for adequate nutritional intake. Analgesic medication should be given freely to these clients. Frequent suctioning of the oral cavity becomes necessary when swallowing becomes difficult. (Other nursing measures for the terminally ill client are discussed in Chapter 9.)

Nutritional Considerations

After radical neck surgery the client may be unable to take in nutrients through the normal route of ingestion because of swelling, the location of sutures, or difficulty with swallowing. Parenteral fluids will be given for the first 24 to 48 hours. After this time, tube feedings are usually given via a nasogastric or nasointestinal tube that was placed during surgery. Sometimes a temporary feeding gastrostomy may be used. Cervical esophagostomy and pharyngostomy have also been used (see Chapter 35). The nurse must observe for tolerance of the feedings and adjust the amount, time, and formula if nausea, vomiting, diarrhea, or distention occurs. The client is usually taught to do the tube feedings. When the client can swallow, small amounts of water are given. Close observation for choking is essential. Suctioning may be necessary to prevent aspiration.

▪ Nursing Management of Carcinoma of the Mouth

Nursing assessment

Subjective and objective data that should be obtained from a client with carcinoma of the mouth are presented in Table 34-4.

Nursing diagnoses

Nursing diagnoses are determined when the problem and the etiological factors are supported by clinical data. Nursing diagnoses related to carcinoma of the mouth may include, but are not limited, to those presented in Table 34-5.

Nursing interventions

Health promotion and maintenance. The nurse has a significant role in early detection and treatment of carcinoma of the oral cavity. The nurse needs to provide clients with information regarding predisposing factors, such as constant overexposure to the sun and tobacco and other irritants. The nurse should also teach correct oral hygiene and dental care and encourage clients to seek preventive dental care. Risk factors need to be identified. Smoking and the long-term use of smokeless tobacco are the major risk factors for oral cancer.[7] Because early detection of oral carcinoma is very important, clients should be taught to examine their mouths and to recognize danger signals of oral cancer. If any of them are present, the client should be instructed to visit a doctor. Danger signals are as follows:

1. Unexplained pain or soreness in the mouth
2. Unusual bleeding from the oral cavity
3. Dysphagia
4. Swelling or lump in the neck
5. Any ulcerative lesion that does not heal within 1 to 2 weeks

The last signal is very significant; a biopsy of the lesion should probably be performed. The nurse should inspect the client's oral cavity to detect suspicious lesions. Early detection is very important.

Acute intervention. Preoperative care for the client who is to have a radical neck dissection involves consideration of physical and psychosocial needs (Table 34-5). Physical preparation is the same as for any major surgery, with spe-

Table 34-4

Nursing Assessment of the Client with Cancer of the Mouth

SUBJECTIVE DATA

History
Use of alcohol and tobacco, stress, oral and dental hygiene, exposure to wind and sun
Pain
Mouth pain, neck stiffness, dysphagia, difficulty in chewing or speaking
Gastrointestinal
Intolerance to certain foods or temperature of foods, recent weight loss, increased salivation

OBJECTIVE DATA

Lips
Symmetry, color, size, cracking, ulcers, fissures
Tongue
Lesions, soreness, limitation of movement, leukoplakia, erythroplakia
Buccal mucosa
Color, pigmentation, lesions, areas of tenderness, leukoplakia, erythroplakia
Other
Breath odor, increased salivation, slurred speech

Table 34-5

NURSING CARE PLAN FOR THE CLIENT AFTER A RADICAL NECK DISSECTION

Defining Characteristics	Nursing Interventions	Evaluation Criteria

NURSING DIAGNOSIS: Ineffective airway clearance related to viscous secretions secondary to tracheostomy and inability to maintain proper position

Viscous secretions, abnormal breath sounds, respiratory distress, tachypnea, ineffective cough	Position client on side or supine with head turned to one side immediately after surgery. Position in a sitting position as soon as client can tolerate. Suction frequently and carefully. Assess for early signs of respiratory distress. Provide a basin and wipes for saliva and secretions.*	Patent airway, no aspiration of saliva

NURSING DIAGNOSIS: Ineffective breathing pattern related to immobility and pain secondary to surgical incision

Dyspnea, tachypnea, shortness of breath, cyanosis, cough, use of accessory muscles, abnormal breath sounds	Assist client to cough effectively. Support client's neck and head when deep breathing and coughing. Auscultate lungs q 2 hr.	Clear lungs on auscultation, no respiratory distress

NURSING DIAGNOSIS: Acute pain related to surgical procedure and ineffective pain and comfort measures

Communication of pain descriptors; guarding behavior; narrowed self-focus; behaviors indicative of pain, such as restlessness, crying, moaning; facial mask of pain; sympathetic nervous system responses such as diaphoresis and changes in blood pressure, pulse, and respiration rate	Administer mild analgesics. Do not use narcotic analgesics that depress respirations. Support neck and head when moving client. Use gentle suctioning and oral hygiene.	Satisfaction with pain relief

NURSING DIAGNOSIS: Altered nutrition: less than body requirements related to chewing and swallowing difficulties

Inadequate food intake (less than recommended daily allowances), body weight 20% or more under ideal for height and frame, inability to ingest food	Administer tube feedings or total parenteral nutrition as ordered. Observe for tolerance of feedings. Provide privacy when eating. When client starts taking fluids, observe for choking and have suction available. Offer small, frequent, attractively served meals with adequate fluid intake. Monitor caloric intake and weight.	Adequate intake of nutrients, maintenance of body weight

NURSING DIAGNOSIS: Altered oral mucous membranes related to excessive secretions and inability to perform oral hygiene

Oral pain or discomfort, edema, increased secretions, halitosis, weakness, inability or unwillingness to perform oral hygiene	Provide frequent, gentle oral hygiene. Use mouth irrigations with sterile water, normal saline solution, or diluted peroxide. Suction and provide tissues for drooling of saliva. Use Water-Pik or power spray to clean hard-to-reach areas. Apply lubricant to dry lips. Reassure client of your willingness to perform this task.	Clean oral cavity with no infection

*For care of tracheostomy, see Chapter 20.

Table 34-5

 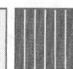

NURSING CARE PLAN FOR THE CLIENT AFTER A RADICAL NECK DISSECTION—cont'd

Defining Characteristics	Nursing Interventions	Evaluation Criteria
NURSING DIAGNOSIS: Impaired verbal communication related to inability to speak secondary to tracheostomy		
Inability to speak	Plan for and provide alternate means of communication (pad and pencil, small chalkboard, "Magic Slate"). Place call button within reach. Visit frequently and assure client that help is available to meet requests.	Use of alternate means of communication
NURSING DIAGNOSIS: Body-image disturbance related to disfiguring surgery, loss of oral communication, and drooling		
Withdrawal, depression, isolation, unwillingness to look at self or assist with care, refusal to see visitors	Assess client's body image concept. Provide privacy. If client drools, instruct to tilt head to side. Encourage attention to personal hygiene and socialization with family and friends. Answer questions honestly about changes in body image. Involve client in self-care. Assure client of self-worth.	Acceptance of altered body image
NURSING DIAGNOSIS: High risk for sexual dysfunction related to altered appearance, altered body image, and self-esteem disturbance		
Verbalization of problem, alterations in achievement of perceived sex role, alteration in relationship with significant other, change of interest in self and others	Encourage discussion regarding sexuality. Encourage client to discuss this problem with sexual partner. Help client realize that sexuality involves more than appearance. Offer support and guidance to sexual partner. Refer to counseling services if needed.	Freedom to discuss and analyze these feelings
NURSING DIAGNOSIS: Anxiety related to lack of knowledge regarding possibilities of reconstructive surgery and prognosis		
Request for information, verbalization of problem, inappropriate or exaggerated behaviors	Provide information about prosthetic devices, speech therapy, and reconstructive surgery. Cooperate with other members of the health care team. Provide opportunities for client to discuss fears about diagnosis and prognosis.	Knowledge of possibilities of reconstructive surgery, realistic plans to resume lifestyle

cial emphasis on oral hygiene. Explanations and emotional support are of special significance and should include postoperative measures relating to communication and feeding. The surgical procedure should be explained to the client and the nurse should make sure that the information is understood.

AIRWAY. Postoperatively, a patent airway is the priority nursing responsibility. The inflammation in the surgical area may press on and compress the trachea. A tracheostomy is commonly done in conjunction with radical neck surgery to ensure an adequate airway. In addition, the client has difficulty swallowing saliva and is at risk of aspiration. A gauze wick placed to direct saliva into an emesis basin or a dental suction tip may be used to remove secretions. If the client has a tracheostomy, frequent suctioning is essential (see Chapter 20). For the client without a tracheostomy, oral or nasopharyngeal suctioning should be done when audible signs of fluid occur or when the client indicates a need for suctioning. The client should be observed for signs of respiratory distress.

POSITIONING. To facilitate drainage from the mouth and to prevent aspiration, positioning is essential. In the immediate and early postoperative period, the client should be lying on the side or supine with the head turned to one side to prevent aspiration. As soon as the client is awake, the head of the bed is usually elevated to promote venous and lymphatic drainage and to facilitate breathing and swallowing. The nurse should provide a basin and mouth wipes to help the client manage the secretions. The basin should be emptied frequently because of the odor of the secretions.

ORAL HYGIENE. Measures must be taken to prevent infection of the oral cavity. Accumulated mucus and old blood provides an excellent medium for microorganisms. Oral hygiene decreases the possibility of infection and also decreases the mouth odor and unpleasant taste for the client. The oral care must be done carefully to prevent trauma. The mouth may be gently irrigated with sterile water, normal saline solution, or diluted hydrogen peroxide. A Water-Pik may be effective for oral irrigations. An applicator soaked with peroxide and saline solution may be used to cleanse the difficult-to-reach areas. The lips should be kept moist with lanolin or lubricant.

WOUND CARE. It is important to observe the dressing for any signs of hemorrhage or constriction. When portable wound suction is used, the nurse should ensure it is functioning properly. The drainage is serosanguineous and gradually diminishes from the initial 80 to 120 ml in 24 hours.

COMMUNICATION. One of the client's postoperative fears is of not being able to talk and to tell the nurse about pain and the need for help. Speech difficulties arise if the client has a tracheostomy or if part of the tongue or palate has been resected. Speech difficulties may occur only temporarily or for a longer time, depending on the amount of tissue removed. Alternate means of communication should have been decided on preoperatively. Suggestions include pad and pencil, small chalkboard, and a Magic Slate. Having the call button within reach is essential. The nurse can provide added assurance and relieve anxiety by frequent visits.

SELF-IMAGE. The nurse should be aware of how the client feels about body alterations. Many clients are sensitive about their appearance. Privacy is important to most clients, especially during eating. The client may have Aeroplast protecting the wound with no dressing and therefore may be reluctant to go outside the room. The nurse should instruct the client to tilt the head to the side to prevent drooling. Assistance with personal hygiene may lessen the client's feelings of a poor body image. The nurse should convey acceptance through both verbal and nonverbal communication and not show repulsion when caring for the client.

The client may go through the grieving process. Support of family, significant others, and friends is important. The nurse should allow the client to verbalize personal feelings about the surgery.

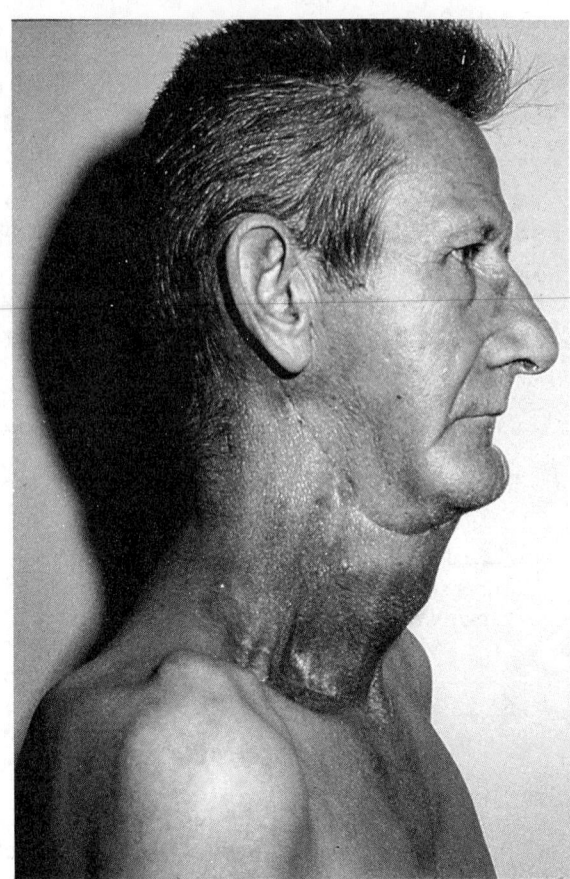

Fig. 34-5 Appearance of the neck following healing after a radical neck dissection. This client also had postoperative external radiation therapy. (Courtesy R. Doberneck, Albuquerque.)

DEPRESSION. Depression is common in clients after radical neck dissections. They may not be able to speak because of the tracheostomy and cannot control their own saliva. The neck and shoulders are numb because of the transected nerves. The facial appearance is significantly altered with swelling, edema, and deformities. Clients need to understand that many of the physical changes are reversible as the edema subsides and the tracheostomy tube is removed (Fig. 34-5). Depression may also be related to the concern about the prognosis. The nurse can help the client through the depression by allowing verbalization of feelings, conveying acceptance, and helping the client regain an acceptable self-concept. Sometimes it is appropriate to obtain a psychiatric referral for clients who are experiencing prolonged or severe depression.

SEXUALITY. The client may feel less desirable sexually and may also feel inadequate. The nurse can assist the client by allowing discussions regarding sexuality and encouraging the client to discuss this problem with the sexual partner. It may be difficult for the client to orally discuss sexual problems because of the alteration in communications. The nurse can allow the client to plan how to communicate with the sexual partner and offer support and guidance to the sexual partner. Helping the client to see that sexuality involves much more than appearance may relieve some anxiety.

Rehabilitative management. Facial disfigurement and other mutilating aspects of radical head and neck surgery may have a major long-term impact on the client's body image and life-style. Many of these surgical procedures leave a deformity, both functionally and cosmetically. It may be difficult for the client to eat and speak, and the altered physical appearance may be embarrassing and depressing. The client may be taught to do various exercises aimed at regaining maximum shoulder function and neck motion. Some clients may have to learn to swallow again. The client may need information about prosthetic devices, speech therapy, and further reconstructive surgery.

Reconstructive surgery should be performed soon after the tumor is removed. Various types of skin grafting are used. It may be necessary to rebuild the nose or the mandible or to close oral cutaneous openings. Prosthetic materials, such as Silastic and Plastigel (which is very soft), are often used to reconstruct various deformities.

MANDIBULAR FRACTURE

Fracture of the mandible may result from trauma to the face or jaws. Maxillary fractures may also occur but are less common than mandibular fractures. The fracture may be simple, with no bone displacement, or it may involve loss of tissue and bone. The fracture may require immediate and sometimes long-term treatment to ensure survival and restore satisfactory appearance and function.

Surgical Interventions

Surgery consists of immobilization, usually by wiring the jaws (intermaxillary fixation). Internal fixation may be accomplished with screws and plates. In a simple fracture with no loss of teeth, the lower jaw is wired to the upper jaw. First, wires are placed around the teeth; then crosswires or rubber bands are used to hold the lower jaw tight against the upper jaw (Fig. 34-6). Arch bars may be used and placed on the maxillary and mandibular arches of the teeth. Vertical wires are placed between the arch bars holding the jaws together. When teeth are missing or if there is bone displacement, other forms of fixation such as

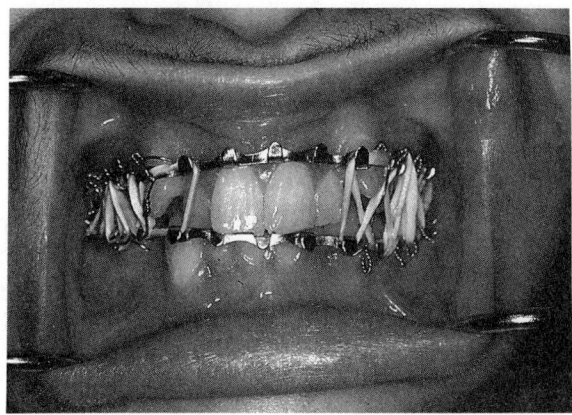

Fig. 34-6 Intermaxillary fixation. (Courtesy RA Weinstein, Denver.)

metal arch bars in the mouth or insertion of a pin in the bone may be used. Usually the immobilization is necessary for only 4 to 5 weeks, since the fractures heal rapidly.

Nutritional Considerations

Ingestion of sufficient nutrients poses a real problem, since the diet must be liquid. The client easily tires of sucking through a straw or laboriously using a spoon. The diet must be planned to include adequate calories and protein. Liquid protein supplements may be helpful to improve the nutritional status. Adequate fluid intake must be included. The nurse needs to work with the dietitian and the client to ensure adequate nutrition. The low-bulk, high-carbohydrate diet and the intake of air through the straw create a problem with flatus and constipation. Ambulation, prune juice, and bulk-forming laxatives may help relieve these problems.

▪ Nursing Management of Mandibular Fracture

Preoperative care

The client should be told preoperatively about the surgical procedure: what it involves, how the face will look, and alterations the surgery will cause. The client needs to be reassured about the ability to breathe normally, speak, and swallow liquids. Usually hospitalization is necessary for only a few days unless there are other bodily injuries or problems.

Postoperative care

Postoperative care should focus on a patent airway, oral hygiene, communication, and adequate nutrition. Two major potential problems in the immediate postoperative period are airway obstruction and aspiration of vomitus. Because the client cannot open the jaws, measures to ensure an airway are essential. The nurse must observe for signs of respiratory distress. The client should be placed on the side with the head slightly elevated immediately after surgery. A wire cutter or scissors (for rubber bands) must be taped to the head of the bed. These may be used to cut the wires or elastic bands in case of an emergency. The wires should be cut only as a last resort—once the client is awake the wires should be cut only in case of cardiac or respiratory arrest. One study demonstrated that it took considerable time to complete the release of fixation and involved increased risk of aspiration of wire fragments.[8]

The physician should explain by means of a picture the appropriate wire or wires to cut, and this should be included in the care plan. In some cases, cutting the wires may allow the entire facial and upper jaw structure to collapse and worsen the problem. A tracheostomy or an endotracheal tray should always be available.

If the client begins to vomit or choke, the nurse should try to clear the mouth and airway. Suctioning may be necessary and may be done by the nasopharyngeal or oral route, depending on the extent of injury and the type of repair. A nasogastric tube may be used for decompression to remove fluids and gas from the stomach to help prevent aspiration. It will also help prevent vomiting. Antiemetics may also be used. The nasogastric tube can later be used as a feeding tube. The nurse should teach the client to clear secretions and vomitus.

Oral hygiene is a very important part of the nursing

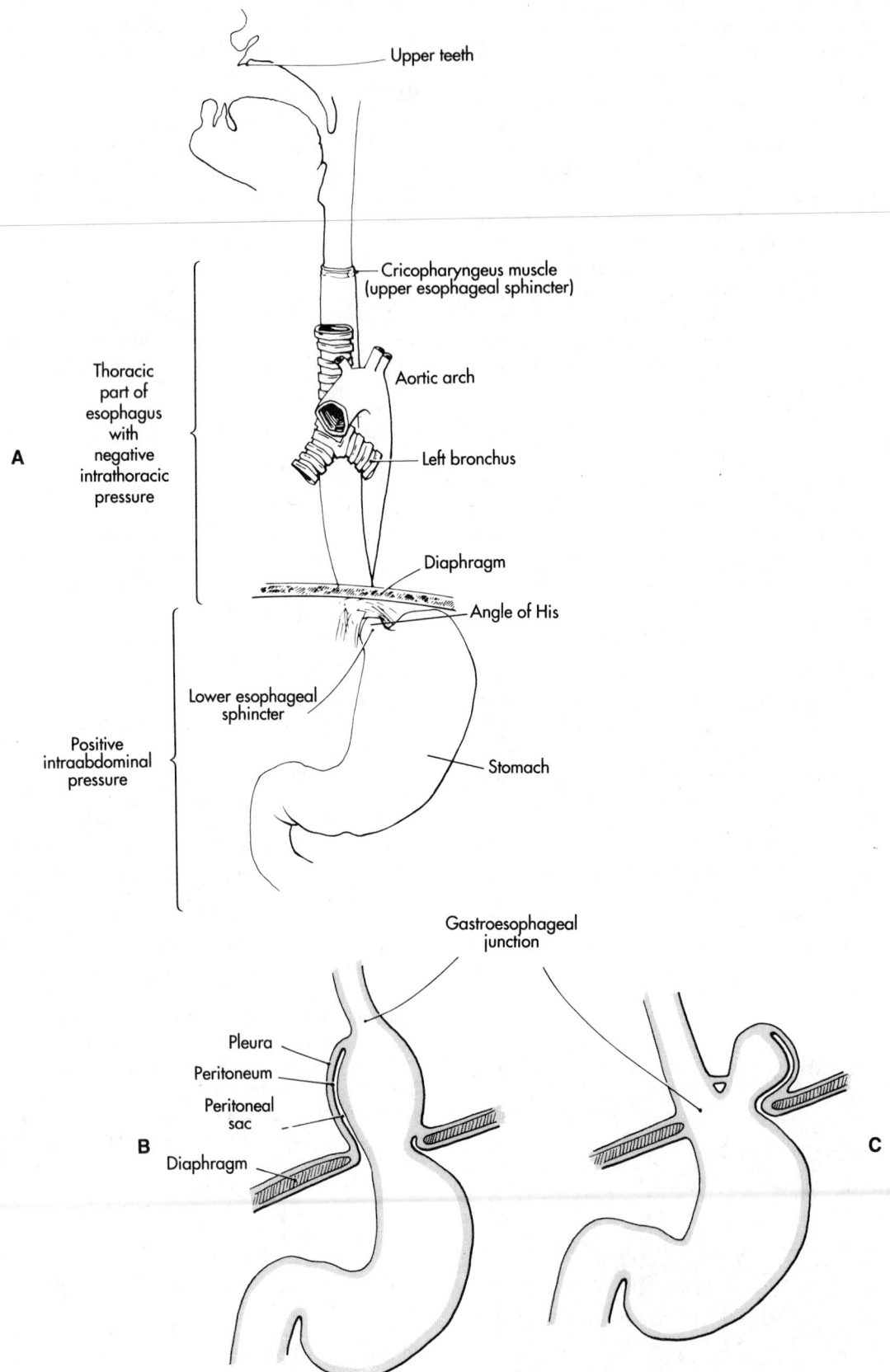

Fig. 34-7 **A,** Normal esophagus. **B,** Sliding hiatal hernia. **C,** Rolling or paraesophageal hernia. (Modified from Price S and Wilson L: Pathophysiology: clinical concepts of disease process, ed 4, St Louis, 1991, Mosby–Year Book, Inc.)

care. The mouth should be rinsed frequently, particularly after meals and snacks, to remove food debris. Warm normal saline solution, water, or alkaline mouthwashes may be used. A soft rubber catheter or a Water-Pik is effective for a thorough oral cleansing. The nurse should inspect the mouth several times a day to see that it is clean. A flashlight is necessary, and a tongue depressor is used to retract the cheeks. The lips and corners of the mouth should be kept moist.

Communication may be a problem, particularly in the early postoperative period. An effective way of communication must be established preoperatively. Some suggestions include a Magic Slate, a pad and pencil, or a small chalkboard. Usually the client can speak well enough to be understood, especially after the first few postoperative days.

The client is usually discharged with the wires in place. The nurse needs to allow the client to verbalize feelings about the altered appearance. Discharge teaching should include oral care, techniques of handling secretions, diet, and how and when to use wire cutters.

HIATAL HERNIA

Hiatal hernia is herniation of a portion of the stomach into the esophagus through an opening, or hiatus, in the diaphragm. It is also referred to as *diaphragmatic hernia* and *esophageal hernia*. Hiatal hernias are classified into two types (Fig. 34-7):

1. *Sliding:* The junction of the stomach and esophagus is above the hiatus of the diaphragm and a part of the stomach slides through the hiatal opening in the diaphragm. It "slides" into the thoracic cavity when the client is supine and usually goes back into the abdominal cavity when the client is standing upright. This is the most common type.
2. *Paraesophageal or rolling:* The esophagogastric junction remains in the normal position, but the fundus and the greater curvature of the stomach roll up through the diaphragm, forming a pocket alongside the esophagus.

Significance

The incidence of hiatal hernia is difficult to determine. Although it is said to be the most common abnormality found on x-ray examination of the upper GI tract, the hernia is often asymptomatic. Hiatal hernias are very common in older adults and occur more frequently in women than in men.[9]

Pathophysiology

Many factors contribute to the development of hiatal hernia. Structural changes, such as weakening of the muscles in the diaphragm around the esophagogastric opening, are usually contributing factors. Factors that increase intraabdominal pressure, including obesity, pregnancy, ascites, tumors, tight corsets, intense physical exertion, and heavy lifting on a continual basis, may also predispose to development of a hiatal hernia. Other predisposing factors are increased age, trauma, poor nutrition, and a forced recumbent position, as when a prolonged illness confines the

Table 34-6 Factors Affecting Lower Esophageal Sphincter Pressure and Reflux in Hiatal Hernia

SUBSTANCES AFFECTING PRESSURE AND TONE

Increase pressure

Antacids	Metoclopramide (Reglan)
Bethanechol (Urecholine)	

Decrease pressure

Fatty foods	Theophylline
Chocolate (theobromine, caffeine)	Diazepam (Valium)
	Morphine sulfate
Peppermint, spearmint	β-Adrenergic blocking drugs
Alcohol	Calcium blockers
Nicotine	Nitrates
Anticholinergics	Prostaglandins
Progesterone	

MEASURES TO PREVENT GASTROESOPHAGEAL REFLUX

Do eat high-protein, low-fat diet; eat small, frequent meals to prevent gastric distention; sleep with head of bed elevated on 4- to 6-inch blocks (gravity fosters esophageal acid clearance); lose weight if overweight.

Do not lie down for 2 to 3 hr after eating, wear tight clothing around the waist, bend over (especially after eating).

Avoid alcohol; smoking (causes an almost immediate, marked decrease in LES pressure) coffee, chocolate, and colas or other soft drinks with caffeine.

person to bed. In some cases, congenital weakness is a contributing factor.

There are no symptoms until the lower esophageal sphincter (LES) becomes incompetent. The LES is the muscle at the point of the junction of the esophagus and the stomach. It encircles the esophagus and has a higher resting tension because of its usual contracted state. This contraction prevents gastric reflux. When the LES pressure is decreased, reflux occurs. Various substances and activities affect LES pressure and tone (Table 34-6). The esophageal mucosa is very sensitive to the acidic gastric secretions, and reflux may cause esophagitis.

Clinical Manifestations

Heartburn (pyrosis) from gastroesophageal reflux is the most common clinical manifestation of hiatal hernia. It is due to irritation of the esophagus by the gastric acids. Heartburn is described as a burning, tight sensation that appears intermittently beneath the lower sternum and spreads upward to the throat or jaw. Heartburn occurs following ingestion of substances that lower the LES pressure (Table 34-6). It is also associated with position, occurring soon or several hours after lying down. Bending over may cause a severe burning pain, which is usually relieved with sitting or standing.

Other common precipitating factors of pain include large meals, alcohol, and smoking. Nocturnal attacks are common, especially if the person has eaten before going to sleep. Heartburn is relieved with milk, alkali substances, or water.

Regurgitation (effortless return of material from stomach into esophagus or mouth) is a fairly common manifestation of hiatal hernia. It is often described as hot, bitter, or sour liquid coming into the throat or mouth. Other symptoms of hiatal hernia include feelings of a lump in the throat or of food stopping, *dysphagia* (difficulty in swallowing), painful swallowing, and bleeding. Frequently the symptoms of hiatal hernia mimic gallbladder disease, peptic ulcer, and angina. Some clients with hiatal hernia have no symptoms.

Complications

Several complications that may occur with hiatal hernia include problems such as hemorrhage from erosion, stenosis, ulcerations of the herniated portion of the stomach, strangulation of the hernia, and regurgitation with tracheal aspiration. Severe chronic esophagitis may follow reflux problems.

Diagnostic Studies

A barium swallow is an important diagnostic measure that may show the protrusion of gastric mucosa through the esophageal hiatus. Esophagoscopy is useful in determining the incompetence of the LES and whether gastric reflux is present. Biopsy and cytological specimens can be taken to differentiate hiatal hernia from carcinoma of the stomach or esophagus and Barrett's esophagus. Esophageal motility studies are sometimes done to determine pressure gradients (Table 34-7).

Therapeutic Management

Conservative therapy. Conservative management consists mainly of various measures to prevent reflux (Table 34-6) and medications that relieve symptoms. Administration of antacids, elimination of constricting garments, avoidance of lifting and straining, elimination of alcohol and smoking, and elevation of the head of the bed are used to meet these goals. If obese, the client is encouraged to lose weight.

Pharmacological Management

Antacids are used to relieve heartburn by their neutralizing effect on hydrochloric acid. They also increase the LES pressure and thus decrease gastroesophageal reflux. They should be taken 1 to 3 hours after meals and at bedtime. Oxaine M, which is an antacid and local anesthetic, may be used for severe pain and pyrosis. Alginic acid and an antacid are sometimes given together (Gaviscon). The alginic acid reacts with sodium bicarbonate and forms a viscous solution that floats to the surface of gastric contents and coats the esophagus, acting as a mechanical barrier to reflux.

Cholinergic drugs, such as bethanechol (Urecholine), may be used to increase LES pressure. Metoclopramide (Reglan), a dopamine antagonist, increases LES pressure and gastric emptying. Histamine H_2-receptor blockers (e.g., ranitidine, cimetidine) have no effect on LES pressure but do decrease gastric acid production. They are particularly helpful for clients with high acid outputs. Sucral-

---

Table 34-7

Diagnostic and Therapeutic Management: Hiatal Hernia

DIAGNOSTIC

Barium swallow
Esophagoscopy

THERAPEUTIC
Conservative

Elevation of head of bed on 4- to 6-inch blocks
High-protein, low-fat diet with avoidance of foods that decrease LES pressure and/or irritate acid-sensitive esophagus
Antacids/Gaviscon
Cholinergic drugs (e.g., bethanechol)
Other drug therapy*

Postoperative surgical

Nasogastric tube to suction
IV fluids with electrolyte replacement
Intake and output
Vital signs every 2 to 4 hr
Pulmonary physiotherapy (turning, coughing, deep breathing, spirometry)
Administration of antiemetic as needed
Administration of analgesic as needed

*See Table 34-8.

Table 34-8 Drug Therapy for Management of Gastroesophageal Reflux

Mechanism of Action	Examples
INCREASED LES PRESSURE	
Cholinergic	Bethanechol (Urecholine)
Dopamine antagonist	Metoclopramide (Reglan)
Antacids	Gelusil, Maalox, Mylanta
ANTISECRETORY	
H_2-receptor antagonists	Cimetidine (Tagamet), ranitidine (Zantac), famotidine (Pepcid)
Acid-suppressing agent	Omeprazole (Losec)
CYTOPROTECTIVE	
Alginic acid-antacid	Gaviscon
Antacids	Gelusil, Maalox, Mylanta
Acid-protective agent	Sucralfate (Carafate)

fate (Carafate), an antiulcer drug, may be used for its cytoprotective properties.

A new drug that may be helpful in controlling reflux, particularily for healing of erosive reflux esophagitis, is omeprazole (Losec). It is a new class of acid-suppressing drug. Omeprazole controls intragastric acidity regardless of the stimulus.[10] (A summary of the pharmacological management is shown in Table 34-8.)

The nurse should observe for and instruct the client about side effects of the medications being taken. Antacids have minimal side effects. Antacids that contain aluminum tend to cause constipation, whereas those that contain magnesium tend to cause diarrhea. Several of the antacids are combinations of aluminum and magnesium designed to minimize these side effects. If the client is taking bethanechol, side effects to observe for include urinary urgency, increased salivation, abdominal cramping with diarrhea, nausea, vomiting, and hypotension. Side effects of metoclopramide include restlessness, anxiety, and insomnia.

If the client is taking cimetidine, the nurse should assess for side effects that include confusion, headache, depression, dizziness, diarrhea, urticaria, rash, and increases in blood urea nitrogen (BUN) and creatinine levels. Side effects of sucralfate include drowsiness, dizziness, nausea, vomiting, constipation, urticaria, and rash.

Nutritional Considerations

A diet high in protein and low in fats is recommended. Fatty foods stimulate the release of cholecystokinin, which decreases LES pressure. Foods that decrease LES pressure such as chocolate, peppermint, and coffee (Table 34-6) should be avoided because they cause reflux. Milk products should be avoided, especially at bedtime, because milk increases gastric acid secretion. Small, frequent meals are advised to prevent overdistention of the stomach. Certain foods (e.g., spicy tomato juice and orange juice) may irritate the acid-sensitive esophagus and thus may have to be avoided. No specific diet is necessary, but foods that cause reflux should be avoided.

■ Nursing Management Related to Conservative Therapy

Clients with hiatal hernia who are being managed need to avoid factors that cause gastroesophageal reflux and thus bring on symptoms. (Measures to prevent reflux are outlined in Table 34-6.) The client who is a smoker should definitely try to stop smoking. Smoking causes an almost immediate marked decrease in LES pressure. The client may need to be referred to other members of the health care team or to community resources for assistance in stopping smoking. The substances that decrease LES pressure and tone should be avoided (see Table 34-6). If stress seems to bring on symptoms, measures to handle stress should be discussed.

Nursing care for the client who is having acute symptoms consists mainly of teaching and encouraging the client to follow the necessary regimen. The nurse should ensure that the head of the bed is elevated correctly (usually on 4- to 6-inch blocks) and that the client does not lie down during the first 2 to 3 hours after eating. This position assists gravity in maintaining the stomach in the abdominal cavity and also helps prevent reflux and tracheal aspiration. Teaching the client to avoid food and activities that cause reflux is important (e.g., late-night eating should be avoided). The client may be taking medications to relieve heartburn, so the nurse will need to observe for side effects and determine whether the medications are relieving symptoms. The client should also be taught possible side effects of medications.

Surgical Interventions

Surgical intervention for hiatal hernia is indicated when conservative therapy fails or when there are complications such as stenosis, strangulation, chronic esophagitis, and bleeding. Very large hiatal hernias and those of the paraesophageal type (because it is a constant problem) are usually repaired surgically.

The objective of surgery is to restore gastroesophageal integrity and prevent gastric reflux. The sphincter must be reinforced. These surgical procedures are termed *valvuloplasties* or *antireflux* procedures. There are basically three slightly varied procedures: the Nissen fundoplication, the Hill gastroplexy, and the Belsey fundoplication (Belsey's Mark IV). The Nissen and the Belsey are the first and second most commonly used operations, respectively.[11]

These three surgical procedures are all variations of fundoplication, which involves "wrapping" the fundus of the stomach around the lower portion of the esophagus in varying degrees. These procedures reduce the hernia, provide an acceptable LES pressure, and prevent movement of the gastroesophageal junction. The Nissen fundoplication is shown in Fig. 34-8. A thoracic or abdominal approach may be used, but the abdominal approach is more common. Postoperative management is summarized in Table 34-7.

Fundoplication prevents reflux in 90% of clients. The success of fundoplication depends on achieving correct tightness of the fundal wrap. If it is too loose, reflux is not

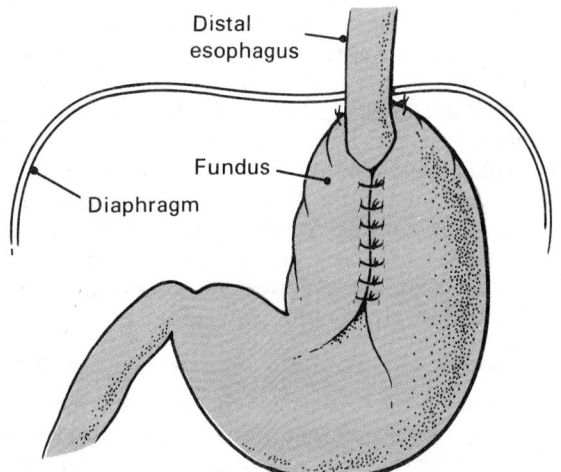

Fig. 34-8 Nissen fundoplication for repair of hiatal hernia. Fundus of stomach is wrapped around distal esophagus and sutured to itself.

prevented. If it is too tight, dysphagia and the gas-bloat syndrome are problems.[12]

An antireflux prosthesis is also available. Called the Angelchik antireflux prosthesis, it is a ring-shaped silicone gel with a tie strap attached. It is tied around the esophagus to prevent the stomach from sliding into the esophagus. Complications of the Angelchik prosthesis include dysphagia, gas-bloat syndrome, and slippage or migration of the prosthesis.[12]

■ Nursing Management Related to Surgical Interventions

Postoperative care focuses on concerns related to prevention of respiratory complications, maintenance of fluid and electrolyte balance, and prevention of infection. If a thoracic approach is used, a chest tube is inserted. Assessment and management related to closed chest drainage are important (see Chapter 21).

Respiratory complications can occur in clients treated with an abdominal approach because of the high abdominal incision. Respiratory assessment should include respiratory rate and rhythm, chest reexpansion, pulse rate and rhythm, and signs of pneumothorax (e.g., dyspnea, chest pain, cyanosis). Coughing and deep breathing are essential to fully expand the lungs. Pulmonary physiotherapy is necessary. The client should not be oversedated with drugs that depress respirations, such as morphine.

The client receives only intravenous (IV) fluids and electrolytes until the return of peristalsis. Extra care should be taken to maintain patency of the nasogastric tube to prevent the need to reinsert the tube. It is dangerous to attempt to replace the tube because of the possibility of perforation of the surgical repair. When peristalsis returns, only fluids are given for 2 to 3 days. Food is added gradually so that the stomach is not overloaded. The nurse must maintain an accurate recording of intake and output and observe for fluid and electrolyte imbalances (see Chapter 10).

After surgical intervention, there should be no symptoms of gastric reflux. The client should be instructed to report such symptoms as heartburn and regurgitation. In the early postoperative period there is usually mild dysphagia due to edema, but it should resolve. The client should report persistent dysphagia, epigastric fullness, and bloating. Immediately after the surgical procedure the client cannot voluntarily vomit or belch, and this may cause the gas-bloat syndrome. If this syndrome persists, medical advice should be sought. A normal diet can be resumed within 6 weeks. The client should avoid foods that are gas forming and should try to prevent gastric distention. Food should be thoroughly chewed.

MALIGNANT NEOPLASMS OF THE ESOPHAGUS

Carcinoma of the esophagus occurs with more frequency now than in previous years, but the incidence is still low. The incidence of squamous cell carcinoma of the esophagus increases with age. There is a higher incidence in blacks and in men. The prognosis is poor.[13]

More than 90% of esophageal cancers are squamous cell carcinomas. A condition called *Barrett's esophagus* or *epithelium* is considered a metaplastic change and may progress to adenocarcinoma of the esophagus. This syndrome is characterized by replacement of areas of the normal squamous epithelium of the esophagus with columnar epithelium. It may result from severe reflux esophagitis.[13]

Pathophysiology

The basic cause of cancer of the esophagus is unknown. Possible predisposing factors are cigarette smoking, excessive alcohol intake, chronic trauma, poor oral hygiene, and spicy foods. The two most important risk factors are smoking and excessive alcohol intake. Certain conditions of the esophagus, such as achalasia, diverticula, and lye burns, are considered premalignant lesions.

The malignant tumor usually appears as an ulcerated lesion. It may have advanced to this stage before symptoms appeared. The majority of tumors are located in the middle and lower portions of the esophagus. The tumor may penetrate the muscular layer and even extend outside the wall of the esophagus. Obstruction of the esophagus occurs in the later stages.

Clinical Manifestations

The onset of symptoms is usually late in relation to the extent of the tumor. Progressive dysphagia is the most common symptom and may be expressed as a substernal feeling as if food is not passing. Initially the dysphagia occurs only with meat, then with soft foods, and eventually with liquids.

Pain develops later and is described as occurring in the substernal, epigastric, or back areas and usually increases with swallowing. The pain may radiate to the neck, jaw, ears, and shoulders. If the tumor is in the upper third of the esophagus, such symptoms as sore throat, choking, and hoarseness may occur. Weight loss is fairly common. When esophageal stenosis is severe, regurgitation of blood-flecked esophageal contents is common.

Complications

Hemorrhage may occur if the cancer erodes into the aorta. Esophageal perforation with fistula formation into the lung or trachea sometimes develops. The tumor may enlarge enough to cause esophageal obstruction. Esophageal carcinoma has a very poor prognosis because of early lymphatic spread and late development of symptoms. The liver and lung are common metastatic sites.

Diagnostic Studies

Barium swallow with fluoroscopy may demonstrate a narrowing of the esophagus at the site of the tumor. Sometimes a crater is visible. Esophagoscopy with biopsy is necessary to make a definitive diagnosis of carcinoma by identification of malignant cells. Endoscopic ultrasonography is a new technique used to detect tumor invasion into the muscularis. Endoscopic ultrasound funnels sound through a series of parts on a probe that fits through a special scope.[14] A bronchoscopic examination may be performed to detect malignant involvement of the trachea. Computerized tomography scanning may be used to more accurately assess the extent of the disease.

Table 34-9

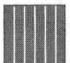

Diagnostic and Therapeutic Management: Carcinoma of the Esophagus

DIAGNOSTIC

Barium swallow
Esophagoscopy with biopsy
Bronchoscopy

THERAPEUTIC

Surgical resection
   Esophagectomy
   Esophagogastrostomy
   Esophagoenterostomy
Radiation
Palliative
   Dilatation
   Stent or prosthesis
   Gastrostomy
   Laser therapy

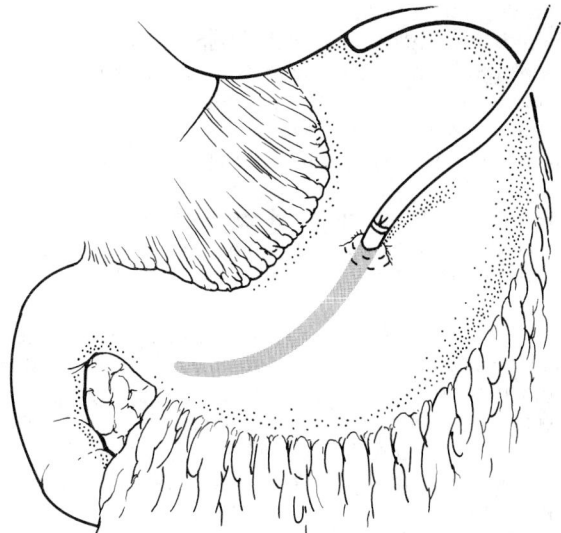

Fig. 34-9 Placement of a gastrostomy tube.

Therapeutic Management

The treatment of carcinoma of the esophagus depends on the location of the tumor and whether invasion or metastasis has occurred (Table 34-9). Surgical removal and radiation are the two methods used. Cancer of the esophagus has a poor prognosis, mainly because in most cases it is not diagnosed until the disease is advanced. Relatively few people are cured. The best results have been obtained with a combination of surgery and radiation.

If the tumor is in the cervical part (upper third) of the esophagus, radiation is usually indicated. A tumor in the lower third of the esophagus is usually resected surgically. In addition, radiation may be used either before or after surgery.

Several types of surgical procedures that can be performed are (1) removal of part or all of the esophagus *(esophagectomy)* with use of a Dacron graft to replace the resected part; (2) resection of a portion of the esophagus and anastomosis of the remaining portion to the stomach *(esophagogastrostomy);* and (3) resection of a portion of the esophagus and anastomosis of a segment of colon to the remaining portion *(esophagoenterostomy)*. The surgical approaches may be thoracic or both abdominal and thoracic.

A gastrostomy may be performed for the purpose of feeding the client (see p. 996). It involves the insertion of a retention or mushroom catheter into the stomach. The catheter is sutured to the abdominal wall (Fig. 34-9).

Surgery may not be done when the client is an older adult or in poor physical health. Palliative therapy consists of restoration of swallowing and maintenance of nutrition and hydration. Palliation can be achieved by dilatation, stent placement, or both. Laser therapy or vaporization of the tumor by means of endoscopy may be used in combination with dilatation. Obstruction recurs as the tumor grows, but laser therapy can be repeated.[14] Sometimes these procedures are combined with radiation therapy.

Other measures for palliation include gastrostomy and esophagostomy.

Dilatation is done with various types of dilators, such as the Celestin tube. Dilatation often relieves dysphagia and allows for improved nutrition. Placement of a stent or prosthesis may help when dilatation is no longer effective. The prostheses are composed of silicone rubber or nylon-reinforced latex tubes with distal and proximal collars.[9] The prosthesis is placed in the esophagus so that food and fluids can pass through the stenotic segment of the esophagus. The prosthesis can be placed endoscopically.

▪ Nursing Management of Esophageal Cancer

Nursing assessment

The client should be assessed for progressive dysphagia and odynophagia (burning, squeezing pain while swallowing). The nurse should question the client regarding the type of substances ingested that cause dysphagia, such as meat, soft foods, and liquids. The client should also be assessed for pain (substernal, epigastric, or back areas), choking, hoarseness, cough, anorexia, weight loss, and regurgitation (sometimes bloody). The client should also be questioned regarding tobacco and alcohol use.

Nursing diagnoses

Nursing diagnoses specific to the client with esophageal cancer include, but are not limited to, the following:

1. Altered nutrition: less than body requirements related to dysphagia, odynophagia, weakness, and radiation therapy
2. Pain related to tumor
3. Anxiety related to diagnosis of cancer, uncertain future, and poor prognosis
4. Anticipatory grieving related to diagnosis of life-threatening malignancy
5. Impaired home maintenance management related to lack of knowledge of disease process and therapeutic regimen, unavailability of a support system, and chronic debilitating disease

Nursing interventions

Health promotion and maintenance. Since the cause of esophageal cancer is not definitive, it is difficult to identify preventive measures. Health counseling needs to focus on elimination of smoking and of excessive alcohol intake. Maintenance of good oral hygiene and dietary habits may also be helpful.

Having the client obtain treatment of esophageal problems, such as achalasia and diverticula, may be helpful, since these are considered premalignant problems. Early diagnosis of esophageal tumors is important but difficult because the onset of symptoms is usually late. Clients should be encouraged to have regular physical examinations and to seek medical attention for any esophageal problems, especially dysphagia. Clients who are at risk of esophageal adenocarcinoma, such as those with Barrett's epithelium, may need regular (yearly) endoscopic screening with biopsy and cytological study.

Acute intervention

PREOPERATIVE CARE. In addition to general preoperative teaching and preparation, particular attention to the client's nutritional needs and oral care is important. Many clients are poorly nourished because of the inability to ingest adequate amounts of food and fluids before surgery. A high-caloric, high-protein diet should be provided. It may have to be in liquid form. Some clients may need IV fluid replacement or total parenteral nutrition. The nurse must keep an accurate intake and output record and assess the client for signs of fluid and electrolyte imbalance.

Meticulous oral care is essential. A thorough cleaning of the mouth, including tongue, gingivae, and teeth or dentures, is necessary. It may be necessary to use swabs or a gauze pad and to really scrub the mouth, including the tongue. Milk of magnesia with mineral oil may be used to remove crust formation. A mixture of mouthwash, ice, and water makes a very refreshing rinse.

Teaching should include information about chest tubes (if a thoracic approach is used), IVs, nasogastric tube, gastrostomy feeding, turning, coughing, and deep breathing (see Chapter 11).

POSTOPERATIVE CARE. The client usually has a nasogastric tube in place, and there may be bloody drainage for 8 to 12 hours. The drainage gradually changes to greenish yellow. Assessment of the drainage, maintenance of the tube, and oral and nasal care are nursing responsibilities.

Because of the location of the incision and the general condition of the client, special emphasis must be placed on prevention of respiratory complications. Turning, coughing, and deep breathing should be done every 2 hours. Use of an incentive spirometer helps in preventing respiratory complications.

The client should be positioned in a semi-Fowler's or Fowler's position to prevent reflux of gastric secretions. When the client can drink fluids or eat, the upright position should be maintained for at least 2 hours after eating to assist the movement of food through the GI tract. Radiation therapy may be given as an adjunct to surgery or as primary therapy (see Chapter 9).

Chronic management. Many clients require long-term follow-up care after surgery or radiation for esophageal cancer. The client needs encouragement and assistance in maintaining adequate nutrition. The client may need a permanent feeding gastrostomy. The client usually has fears and anxieties about a diagnosis of cancer. The nurse should know what the doctor has told the client regarding the prognosis and then provide appropriate counseling. Some communities have resource groups composed of persons with cancer who can serve as support systems. These groups can usually be contacted through the local American Cancer Society.

Referral to a community health nurse may be necessary for continued care of the client (e.g., gastrostomy teaching and follow-up wound care). (Management of the terminally ill client is discussed in Chapter 9.)

Nutritional Considerations

After esophageal surgery, parenteral fluids are given for several days. When fluids are allowed after bowel sounds have returned, 30 to 60 ml of water is given hourly, with gradual progression to small, frequent bland meals. The client should be in an upright position to prevent regurgitation of the fluid. The client is observed for signs of intolerance to or leakage of the feeding into the mediastinum. Symptoms to report that indicate leakage are pain, increased temperature, and dyspnea. Symptoms of food intolerance include vomiting and abdominal distention.

Gastrostomy. A gastrostomy bypasses the esophagus and allows feedings to maintain or restore the client's nutrition. A catheter is placed in the stomach and sutured in place. The connecting end is brought to the surface and sutured to the skin (Fig. 34-9).

A permanent gastrostomy, such as a Janeway, may be used for a client who requires tube feedings over an extended time. These allow for removal of the feeding tube between feedings. A "tube" of gastric tissue is formed and brought out to form a stoma at the skin surface (Fig. 34-10). A small catheter (5 to 10F) is inserted at the skin surface. The stoma forms a seal when the catheter is removed. Problems of leakage and skin irritation are decreased or eliminated.[15]

A gastrostomy tube may be placed by means of *percutaneous endoscopic gastrostomy* (PEG) (Fig. 34-11). The client must have an intact, unobstructed GI tract, and the esophageal lumen must be wide enough to pass the endoscope.[16]

A PEG has several advantages. The procedure itself has fewer risks (no general anesthesia or laporatomy), it can be done at a lower cost, and it requires minimum or no sedation in clients who are severely compromised by their condition. The most frequent complications include aspiration pneumonia, accidental tube removal, wound cellulitis, and clogged tubes.[17]

Feedings can usually be started when bowel sounds are present, usually within 24 hours after catheter placement. The catheter is frequently connected to a pump for continuous feeding. Tap water may be infused within 2 hours after placement. Some important nursing implications for care and feeding of clients with PEGs are listed in Table 34-10.

Feeding. The first gastrostomy feeding consists of either water or glucose in water, 30 to 60 ml at a time with a gradual progression to food. The feeding may consist of

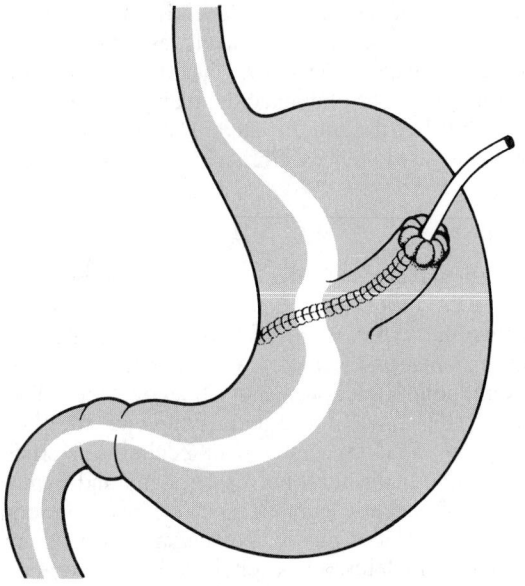

Fig. 34-10 Janeway gastrostomy.

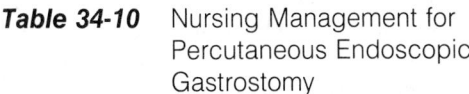

Table 34-10 Nursing Management for Percutaneous Endoscopic Gastrostomy

Assess for bowel sounds before each feeding.
Use liquid diets, not blenderized foods (which may clog tube) for small-bore tubes.
Use liquid medications rather than pills.
Follow other general principles of tube feedings such as elevating head of bed and flushing tube with water.
Assess regularly for complications, such as aspiration, diarrhea, abdominal distention, hyperglycemia, and fecal impaction.

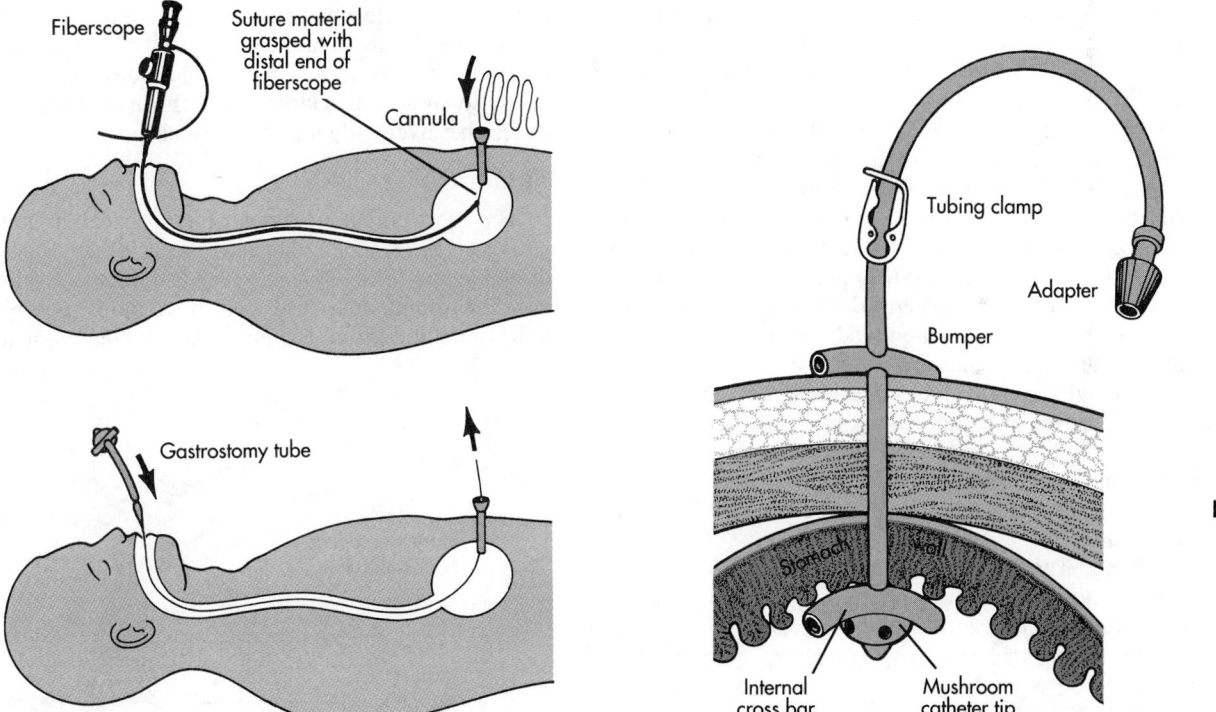

Fig. 34-11 Percutaneous endoscopic gastrostomy. **A,** Gastrostomy tube placement via percutaneous endoscopy. Using endoscopy a gastrostomy tube is inserted through the esophagus into the stomach and then pulled through a stab wound made in the abdominal wall. **B,** A retention disk and bumper secure the tube.

blended foods or a special formula. In the past, tube-feeding formulas have created a problem with diarrhea, but recently lactose-free formulas have decreased this problem. Blenderized feedings promote better bowel function and may be more acceptable psychologically. The feeding should be given at room or body temperature to decrease the likelihood of diarrhea and other GI complaints. Privacy

should be provided. The head should be elevated in a normal eating position and should remain elevated for 30 minutes to 1 hour after the feeding.

Before introducing the feeding, the nurse should aspirate gastric contents and then reinstill and count as part of the feeding. A syringe or funnel is used to introduce the liquid into the tube. A small amount of water is first inserted to make sure the tube is patent. The catheter should be clamped at all times that feedings are not being given to prevent air from entering the tube. It should not be unclamped until the feeding is placed in the syringe or funnel. The feeding is usually 200 to 500 ml (depending on total caloric need) and should be allowed to flow in by gravity over 15 to 20 minutes. After the feeding is finished, the tube should be cleared with water. The client should have an adequate intake of water of up to 2500 ml/24 hr. The catheter is sometimes removed after about 2 weeks and reinserted for each feeding. It should be inserted about 4 to 6 inches.

Continuous feedings by means of an infusion pump are frequently used rather than intermittent feedings. Clients are able to be at home with the infusion pumps.

The pleasurable aspects of eating, such as smelling, seeing, tasting, and chewing the food, are denied the client with a gastrostomy. The client should be allowed to smell, taste, and even chew small amounts of food before the feeding, then the chewed food must be spit out. The client may hesitate to do this because it is not esthetic, but it stimulates salivary and gastric secretions and provides the pleasurable sensations associated with oral intake. The client may become depressed and need frequent encouragement. The nurse should allow expression of feelings about being fed through a tube. Greater satisfaction may be experienced with self-feedings, and the client should be taught self-feeding if possible. The client should be encouraged to sit with the family during meals.

Skin care. Skin care around the gastrostomy is very important because the action of the gastric juice is irritating to the skin. The nurse should try to prevent two possible problems: (1) skin irritation and (2) pulling out of the tube. The skin around the gastrostomy should be assessed daily for signs of redness, excoriation, and maceration. The skin should be kept clean and dry. It should be washed with mild soap and water. A protective ointment (zinc oxide, petrolatum gauze) or a skin barrier (karaya, Stomahesive) may be used on the skin around the gastrostomy. A small dressing may be placed around the tube. Other types of drain/tube pouches may be used if there is a problem with skin irritation.

Teaching. The client or significant others should be taught how to care for the gastrostomy. Teaching should include skin care, care of the tube, and complete information about feedings.

OTHER ESOPHAGEAL DISORDERS
Esophagitis

Esophagitis (inflammation of the esophagus) is common and may occur as a result of chemical irritation from lye or dust and physical irritants such as smoking, very cold or hot liquids, and excessive alcoholic intake. Trauma to the esophagus may also produce inflammation. Achalasia (cardiospasm) and carcinoma may lead to esophagitis.

Reflux esophagitis is very common. It is due to the reflux of gastric contents into the esophagus. A sliding hiatal hernia is a common cause of reflux esophagitis, although it occurs in many clients without hiatal hernia. It is due to an incompetent LES.

Treatment of esophagitis depends on the cause. If strong alkalis or acids cause acute esophagitis, prompt, vigorous treatment is necessary. The treatment of chronic esophagitis includes oral antacids, bland diet, and sleeping with the head of the bed elevated. The goal of treatment is to prevent gastric juices from damaging the esophageal mucosa.

Diverticula

Diverticula are saclike outpouchings of one or more layers of the esophagus. They occur in three main areas: (1) above the upper esophageal sphincter (Zenker's diverticulum), which is the most common; (2) near the esophageal midpoint (traction); and (3) above the LES (epiphrenic)[9] (Fig. 34-12). The main symptoms are dysphagia and regurgitation, especially with Zenker's diverticulum. Traction diverticula may not cause signs and symptoms. The client frequently complains of tasting sour food and smelling a foul odor due to the stagnant food. Complications include malnutrition, aspiration, and perforation.

There is no specific treatment for diverticula. Some clients find they can empty the pocket of food that collects by applying pressure at a point on the neck. The diet may have to be limited to foods that pass more readily (e.g., blenderized foods). Surgical removal of the diverticulum may be necessary if nutrition becomes disrupted. An alternative to surgery is endoscopic division of the septum between the diverticulum and the esophagus.

Strictures

The most common causes of esophageal strictures are strong acids or alkalis that have been ingested and reflux or peptic strictures. Traumas such as throat lacerations and gunshot wounds may also lead to strictures as a result of scar formation from healing. The strictures usually de-

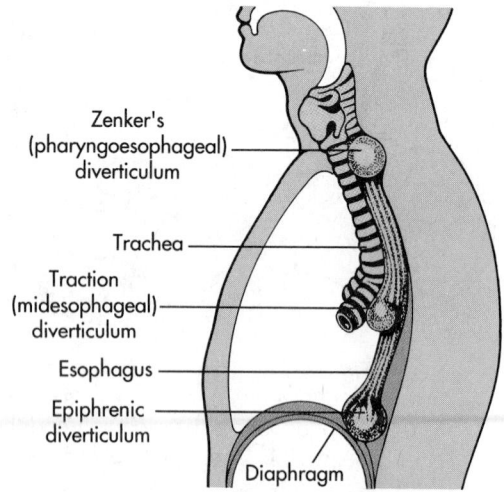

Fig. 34-12 Possible sites for the occurrence of esophageal diverticula. These hollow outpouchings may occur just above the upper esophageal sphincter (Zenker's, the most common type of pulsion diverticulum), near the midpoint of the esophagus (traction), and just above the lower esophageal sphincter (epiphrenic).

velop over a long time. Strictures can be dilated endoscopically using bougies (dilating instruments) or balloon dilators. The newer technique is balloon dilatation, which is done under endoscopy and does not require fluoroscopy.[18] Surgical excision with anastomosis is sometimes necessary. The client may have a temporary or permanent gastrostomy.

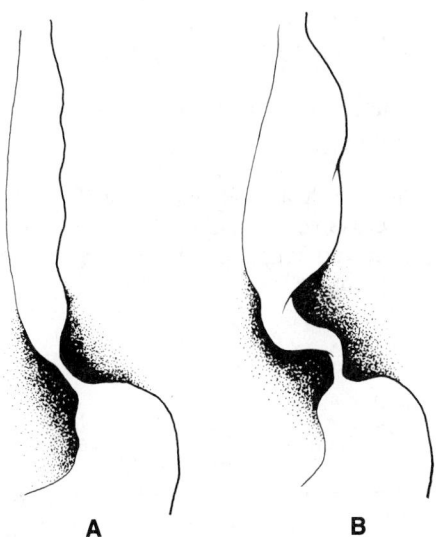

Fig. 34-13 Esophageal achalasia. **A,** Early stage, showing tapering of lower esophagus. **B,** Advanced stage, showing dilated, tortuous esophagus. (From Price S and Wilson L: Pathophysiology: clinical concepts of disease processes, ed 3, St Louis, 1986, The CV Mosby Co, p 236.)

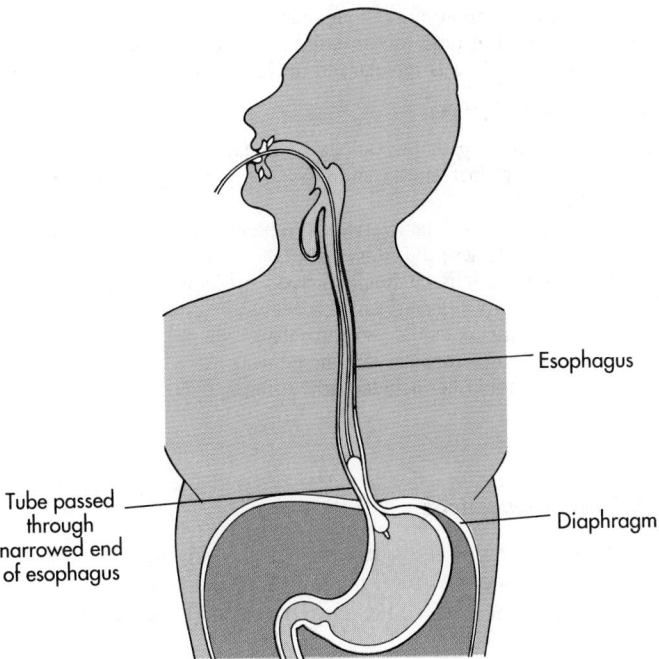

Fig. 34-14 Pneumatic dilatation attempts to treat achalasia by maintaining an adequate lumen and decreasing LES tone.

Achalasia

In achalasia *(cardiospasm),* peristalsis of the lower two thirds (smooth muscle) of the esophagus is absent. LES pressure is increased, along with incomplete relaxation of the lower esophageal sphincter. The result of this condition is dilatation of the lower esophagus (Fig. 34-13). Obstruction of the esophagus at or near the diaphragm also occurs. Food and fluid accumulate in the lower esophagus. The altered peristalsis is due to impairment of the autonomic nervous system innervating the esophagus. Achalasia affects all ages and both genders. The course of the disease is chronic.

Dysphagia is the most common symptom and occurs more frequently with liquids. Substernal chest pain (similar to the pain of angina) occurs during or immediately after a meal. Halitosis and the inability to eructate are other symptoms. Another common symptom is regurgitation of sour-tasting food and liquids, especially when the client is in a horizontal position. Weight loss is typical.

Treatment consists of dilatation, surgery, and drugs. All are directed at relieving the stasis caused by the increased LES pressure, nonrelaxing LES, and aperistaltic esophagus.[19] The aim of therapeutic management is to relieve symptoms. Symptomatic treatment consists of a semisoft bland diet, eating slowly and drinking fluid with meals, and sleeping with the head elevated.

Esophageal dilatation *(bougienage)* is an effective treatment measure for many clients. Pneumatic dilatation of the LES with a balloon-tipped dilator passed orally is usually used. Commonly used dilators for pneumatic dilatation are the Mosher bag, the Tucker mercury dilator, and the Browne-McHardy dilator. They all depend on forcible expansion of a balloon in the lower esophageal sphincter (Fig. 34-14).[9] The forceful dilatation does not restore normal esophageal motility but does provide for emptying of the esophagus into the stomach.

Surgical intervention may become necessary. An *esophagomyotomy* may be performed. In this procedure the muscle fibers that enclose the narrowed area of the esophagus are divided. This allows the mucosa to pouch out through the division in the muscle layer to allow food to be swallowed without obstruction.

A similar procedure is Heller's myotomy (cardiomyotomy), which disrupts the LES in a similar manner and reduces LES pressure. An antireflux procedure is frequently done with the myotomy.[19]

Classes of drugs used in treatment of achalasia include anticholinergics, calcium channel antagonists (nifedipine is one of the best), and long-acting nitrates.

Esophageal Varices

Esophageal varices are dilated, tortuous veins occurring in the lower portion of the esophagus as a result of portal hypertension (see Chapter 38).

FOOD POISONING

Food poisoning is a nonspecific term that describes acute GI symptoms, such as nausea, vomiting, diarrhea, and colicky abdominal pain caused by the intake of contaminated food. Food most commonly causes illness if it is

Table 34-11   Bacterial Food Poisoning

Type	Causative Agent	Sources
Staphylococcal	Toxin from *Staphylococcus aureus*	Meat, bakery products, milk; skin and respiratory tract of food handlers
Clostridial	*Clostridium perfringens*	Meat or poultry dishes cooked at lower temperature (stew or pot pie), rewarmed meat dishes, improperly canned vegetables
Salmonellae	*Salmonella typhimurium* (grows in gut)	Improperly cooked poultry, pork, beef, lamb, and eggs
Botulism	Toxin from *Clostridium botulinum,* ingested toxin absorbed from gut blocking acetylcholine at neuromuscular junction	Improperly canned or preserved food, home-preserved vegetables (most common), preserved fruits and fish, canned commercial products

contaminated with microorganisms or their products. The GI tract is frequently the portal of entry for the microorgansms. The two main types of food poisoning are (1) acute gastroenteritis from bacteria and (2) neurological symptoms from botulism. The most common bacterial food poisonings are presented in Table 34-11.

Foods may be contaminated by poisonous chemicals, such as mercury, arsenic, zinc, and potassium chlorate. Poisoning can also occur from ingestion of poisonous plants (e.g., certain species of mushroom).

The nursing role in relation to food poisoning is mainly health teaching to prevent its occurrence. Teaching should include correct food preparation and cleanliness, adequate cooking, and refrigeration. If the client is hospitalized, nursing care focuses on correction of fluid and electrolyte imbalance from diarrhea and vomiting. With botulism, additional assessment and care relative to neurological symptoms are indicated (see Chapter 55).

C ase Study

HIATAL HERNIA

Mary, 63 years old, has had a sliding hiatal hernia for 10 years. She is 5 feet 2 inches tall and weighs 195 pounds. She used to wear tight corsets but stopped wearing them 2 years ago. In the last year she has had increasing heartburn, especially at night. Mary has currently been on a bland diet and has been taking antacids. She does not like the bland diet.

Mary is admitted to the hospital for a hiatal hernia repair. She is not in acute distress but does complain of the substantial pain and heartburn. She has had some regurgitation. Her vital signs are within normal limits. A barium swallow and an esophagoscopy revealed a large sliding hiatal hernia. It was determined from the esophagoscopy that she has gastric reflux. Mary had a Nissen fundoplication through an abdominal approach. After surgery a nasogastric tube was inserted for suctioning and she was given IV fluids. She is reluctant to move or cough.

Discussion Questions

1. Explain the pathophysiology of a hiatal hernia. What is the difference between a sliding and a paraesophageal hiatal hernia?
2. What are the characteristic symptoms of a hiatal hernia? Which of these did Mary have?
3. Describe a Nissen fundoplication procedure. What is the objective of this surgical procedure?
4. What are potential postoperative complications? What nursing measures prevent them?
5. What should be included in a teaching plan for Mary?

R eview Questions

The number of the question corresponds to the same-numbered objective at the beginning of the chapter.

1. The most effective current method for removing plaque is
   a. physical removal by brushing and flossing
   b. application of a fluoride solution
   c. addition of antimicrobial agents to toothpaste
   d. large doses of vitamin C

Onset of Symptoms (hr)	Symptoms	Treatment	Prevention
1-6	Vomiting, abdominal cramping, diarrhea	Symptomatic, fluid and electrolyte replacement, antiemetics	Immediate refrigeration of foods, monitoring of food handlers
6-12	Diarrhea, abdominal cramps, vomiting (rare)	Symptomatic, antidiarrheal medications	Correct preparation of meat dishes, serving of food immediately after cooking or rapid cooling of food
8-48	Nausea and vomiting, diarrhea, abdominal cramps, fever and chills	Symptomatic, fluid and electrolyte replacement	Correct preparation of food
12-36	GI symptoms of nausea, vomiting, abdominal pain, constipation, distention. Central nervous system symptoms of headache, dizziness, muscular incoordination, weakness, inability to talk or swallow, diplopia, respiratory embarrassment, paralysis, delirium, coma	Maintenance of ventilation, polyvalent antitoxin, guanidine hydrochloric acid (enhances acetylcholine release)	Correct processing of canned foods, boiling of suspected canned foods for 15 min before serving

2. Treatment of Vincent's infection includes
   a. topical application of antibiotics
   b. smallpox vaccinations
   c. viscous lidocaine rinses
   d. amphotericin B suspension
3. Which of the following is *not* considered a predisposing factor for carcinoma of the oral cavity?
   a. pipe smoking
   b. overexposure to the sun
   c. poor dental care
   d. herpesvirus
4. After a radical neck dissection the immediate postoperative goal is
   a. communication
   b. patent airway
   c. prevention of infection
   d. nutritional intake
5. If the client begins to vomit after fixation of mandibular fracture, the nurse should first
   a. cut the wires or elastic bands
   b. place client in lateral position and suction
   c. provide oral hygiene
   d. give an antiemetic
6. The most characteristic symptom of a hiatal hernia is
   a. dysphagia
   b. regurgitation
   c. pyrosis
   d. coughing
7. All the following statements about the management of a client with a hiatal hernia are true *except*

   a. the client should be taught to avoid tight clothing and bending
   b. the overweight client should reduce
   c. the head of the bed may be elevated on blocks
   d. the drug of choice is an anticholinergic
8. The most common symptom of esophageal carcinoma is
   a. sore throat
   b. dysphagia
   c. weight loss
   d. hemorrhage
9. All of the following statements about gastrostomy feedings are true *except*
   a. the feeding may be blended foods or a special formula
   b. the feeding should be warmed to 38° C
   c. the feeding should flow in by gravity
   d. water should be given before and after
10. Which of the following is most likely to cause reflux esophagitis?
    a. outpouching of the muscular layer
    b. impairment of the autonomic nerve plexus
    c. incompetent LES
    d. stricture of the esophagus
11. The food poisoning in which vomiting is the prominent symptom and food sources are meat, bakery products, and milk is
    a. staphylococcal
    b. salmonellae
    c. botulism
    d. clostridial

REFERENCES

1. Goldhaber P and others: Oral manifestations of disease. In Braunwald E and others, eds: Harrison's principles of internal medicine, ed 11, New York, 1987, McGraw-Hill Book Co, p 164.

2. Brunner LS and Suddarth DS: Textbook of medical-surgical nursing, ed 6, Philadelphia, 1988, JB Lippincott Co, p 709.

3. Wyngaarden JB and Smith LH, eds: Cecil's textbook of medicine, ed 18, Philadelphia, 1988, WB Saunders Co, p 687.

4. Schulmeister L: Join the fight against oral cancer, Nursing 17:66, 1987.

5. Prout MN: Early detection of head and neck cancer, Hosp Pract 22:111, 1987.

6. Wyngaarden JB and Smith LH, eds: Cecil's textbook of medicine, ed 18, Philadelphia, 1988, WB Saunders Co, p 679.

7. Stofferman RA: Head and neck. In Davis JH and others, eds: Clinical surgery, St Louis, 1990, Mosby–Year Book, Inc, p 1081.

8. Frost CM and Frost DE: Nursing care of patients with intermaxillary fixation, Heart Lung 12:524, 1983.

9. Croce J: Gastrointestinal problems, Nurse Review, Springhouse, Pa, 1986, Springhouse Corp, pp 29-35.

10. Colin-Jones DG: Histamine-2 receptor antagonists in gastro-esophageal reflux, Gut 30:1305, 1989.

11. Welch CE and Malt RA: Surgery of the stomach, duodenum, gallbladder and bile ducts, N Engl J Med 316:999, 1987.

12. McGouran TCM and others: Is yield pressure at the cardia increased by effective fundoplication? Gut 30:1309, 1989.

13. Goyal RK: Diseases of the esophagus. In Braunwald E and others, eds: Harrison's principles of internal medicine, ed 11, New York, 1987, McGraw-Hill Book Co, p 1237.

14. Waye JD: Expanding uses of therapeutic endoscopy, Hosp Pract 22:143, 1987.

15. Irwin M: Managing leaking gastrostomy sites, Am J Nurs 88:359, 1988.

16. Beck ML: Percutaneous endoscopic gastrostomy, Am J Nurs 89:76, 1989.

17. Starkey JF, Jefferson PA, and Kirby DF: Taking care of percutaneous endoscopic gastrostomy, Am J Nurs 86:42, 1988.

18. Little AG: Esophageal investigation techniques. In Cameron JL, ed: Current surgical therapy, Philadelphia, 1989, BC Decker, p 1.

19. McCallum RW: The management of esophageal motility disorders, Hosp Pract 23:239, 1988.

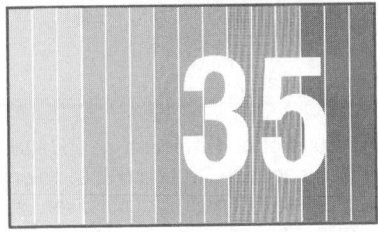

Nursing Role in Management

Problems of Nutrition

Gladys Elizabeth Deters

Learning Objectives

1. Describe the essential components of a nutritionally sound diet and why they are necessary to good health.
2. Describe the common etiological factors, clinical manifestations, and management of vitamin imbalances and malnutrition.
3. Compare the etiological factors, clinical manifestations, and therapeutic and nursing management of bulimia and anorexia nervosa.
4. Differentiate between central and peripheral total parenteral nutrition administration and supplemental tube feedings, including the indications for use, complications, and therapeutic and nursing management.
5. Explain the pathogenesis, complications, and therapeutic and surgical management of obesity.
6. Describe the nursing care related to conservative and surgical management of obesity.

The focus of this chapter is on problems with nutrition. The primary nutritional problems discussed are malnutrition and obesity.

NUTRITIONAL PROBLEMS

Nutritional problems can be found in all age groups, cultures, ethnic groups, and socioeconomic classes and in all parts of the world. Intelligence and wealth do not necessarily preclude the development of poor nutritional habits. The nurse in the roles of care giver, teacher, and resource person can have a profound influence on the health practices of the clients and their families. A strong foundation in the principles of sound nutrition is essential. Together with the physician and the dietitian, the nurse is in a strategic position to assess the dietary practices of clients and provide important information.

The nutritional state of a person or a family may be influenced by many factors. Attitudes toward the importance of food and eating habits are established early in infancy and childhood as a result of parental behavior. Cultural or religious preferences and requirements are frequently reflected in dietary intake. The financial state of a family or an individual often determines the type and amount of nu-

Reviewed by Sally Brozenec, R.N., Ph.D., Assistant Professor, Rush University College of Nursing, Chicago, Illinois.

tritionally sound food that can be purchased. Generally, the lower the socioeconomic status, the poorer the nutritional state. The availability of food sources also contributes to the nutritional state of people. This is usually not a problem in developed countries in which agriculture is well established and productive, but it may be a problem in underdeveloped countries.

Normal Nutrition

Nutrition is the process by which the body uses food for energy, growth, and maintenance and repair of body tissues. Good nutrition in the absence of any underlying disease process results from the ingestion of a balanced diet containing foods from the basic four food groups. The United States Department of Agriculture (USDA) has prescribed the basic four foods comprising milk, meat, fruits and vegetables, and grain. Table 35-1 lists the basic four food groups with daily requirements and examples of common sources.

The essential components of the basic four food groups are carbohydrates, fats, proteins, vitamins, and minerals. *Carbohydrates,* the body's primary source of energy, yield 3.7 calories per gram. Carbohydrates are obtained from the ingestion of starches and sugars, with a small percentage derived from milk and dairy products. Carbohydrates are the chief protein-sparing ingredient in a nutritionally

Table 35-1   Food Groups and Recommended Number of Servings

Group	Nutrients Provided	Number of Servings Daily	Serving Size
Vegetable and fruit	Vitamins A and C, folic acid	4 or more	1-2 cups of or 1 medium-sized lettuce, cucumber, cabbage,* mushrooms, celery, peppers,† greens (all types),* cauliflower,* bean sprouts, green beans, spinach, lemons,* plums, broccoli,† tomato,* carrots,‡ Brussels sprouts,† papayas,* strawberries,† avocado,* beets, grapes, pumpkin, pineapple, peaches,‡ honeydew melon,* apricots,‡ orange juice,† sweet corn, orange, winter squash, apples, pears, bananas, prunes, potato,* raisins, sweet potato‡
Meat	Protein, niacin, thiamine, iron, zinc, vitamin B$_{12}$	2 or more	2 oz of chicken, lean beef, fish, turkey, lean pork chop, ham, pork, refried beans; 2 eggs; 1 cup of dry beans or peas; 2 hot dogs; 4 tbs of peanut butter; ½ cup of nuts
Milk	Calcium, protein, riboflavin, vitamins B$_6$ and B$_{12}$	Children 2-9 yr: 2-3 Children 9-12 yr: 3 or more Teenager: 4 or more Adult: 2 or more Pregnant or lactating women: 4 or more	1 cup of nonfat milk, buttermilk, low-fat milk, plain yogurt, whole milk, flavored (fruit) yogurt, custard, milkshake, or pudding; 1½ oz cheddar cheese or processed cheese; 1½ cups of low-fat cottage cheese or plain cottage cheese; 1¾ cups of ice cream
Bread and cereal	Thiamine, niacin, iron, protein	4 or more	1 slice whole wheat, rye, or white bread; ½ hamburger or hot dog bun; ½ cup of grits, cooked cereals, rice, brown rice, macaroni, or spaghetti; 1 tortilla, pancake, biscuit, muffin, or piece of cornbread; 5 crackers; ½ bagel; 1 cup of presweetened cereal

Modified from Burtis G and others: *Applied nutrition and diet therapy*, Philadelphia, 1988, WB Saunders Co.
*Good source of vitamin C.
†Excellent source of vitamin C.
‡Vitamin A.

sound diet and compose about 45% of the daily caloric needs of the body. In more affluent countries, a carbohydrate-rich diet may provide as much as 70% of total calories.

Fats make up about 35% to 40% of daily caloric needs. One gram of fat yields 9 calories. When stored, fats are found as adipose tissue (primarily triglycerides) in the subcutaneous tissues and in the abdominal cavity. Besides being a major source of body energy, fats act as insulation, which reduces loss of body heat in cold weather and provides padding and protection for vital organs. Fats also help to facilitate the body's absorption of fat-soluble vitamins, and they add satiety to the diet.

Proteins, the third essential component of a well-balanced diet, are obtained from meat, fish, eggs, dairy products, and other vegetarian-type substances. They provide 15% to 20% of daily caloric needs of the body. One gram of protein yields 4 calories. Proteins are very complex nitrogenous organic compounds, of which amino acids are the fundamental units of structure. Amino acids are further divided into *essential* and *nonessential* components. The body is capable of synthesizing nonessential amino acids. However, essential amino acids cannot be synthesized and their availability totally depends on di-

etary sources. An adequate intake of protein is necessary because of the vital role played by the amino acids in biochemical processes in the body. Proteins are essential for tissue growth, repair, and maintenance; body regulatory functions; and energy production.

Vitamins are organic compounds required in small amounts by the body for normal metabolism. Vitamins function primarily in enzyme reactions that facilitate the metabolism of amino acids, fats, and carbohydrates. The body is capable of synthesizing some vitamins in adequate amounts but must rely on a dietary source to meet requirements for others, such as vitamin B$_{12}$. Vitamins are divided into two categories: water-soluble vitamins (C and B complex) and fat-soluble vitamins (A, D, E, and K).

Minerals are inorganic ions (e.g., magnesium, iron) that make up about 4% of the total body weight. When minerals are present in minute amounts, they are referred to as *trace elements* or *micronutrients*. Minerals have a variety of functions in the body, including taking part in enzyme reactions, constituting skeletal structures (calcium, phosphorus, magnesium), and being components of compounds such as hemoglobin (iron), thyroxine (iodine), and vitamin B$_{12}$ (cobalt). Some minerals are stored like the fat-soluble vitamins and can be toxic if taken in excess

Table 35-2 Recommended Daily Caloric Intake

Category	Age (Yr)	Weight (kg)	Weight (lb)	Height (cm)	Height (in)	Energy Needs (kcal)	Energy Needs (Range)
Infants	0.0-0.5	6	13	60	24	kg × 115	(95-145)
	0.5-1.0	9	20	71	28	kg × 105	(80-135)
Children	1-3	13	29	90	35	1300	(900-1800)
	4-6	20	44	112	44	1700	(1300-2300)
	7-10	28	62	132	52	2400	(1650-3300)
Males	11-14	45	99	157	62	2700	(2000-3700)
	15-18	66	145	176	69	2800	(2100-3900)
	19-22	70	154	177	70	2900	(2500-3300)
	23-50	70	154	178	70	2700	(2300-3100)
	51-75	70	154	178	70	2400	(2000-2800)
	76+	70	154	178	70	2050	(1650-2450)
Females	11-14	46	101	157	62	2200	(1500-3000)
	15-18	55	120	163	64	2100	(1200-3000)
	19-22	55	120	163	64	2100	(1700-2500)
	23-50	55	120	163	64	2000	(1600-2400)
	51-75	55	120	163	64	1800	(1400-2200)
	76+	55	120	163	64	1600	(1200-2000)
Pregnant women						+300	
Lactating women						+500	

Table 35-3 Caloric and Protein Needs of a 150 lb (68 kg) Man

Activity	Calories	Protein (g)
Basal	1400	49
Moderate activity (activities of daily living)	2500	70
Postoperative (no complications)	3150	105
Stress response (e.g., to chemotherapy, radiation therapy)	3500	140
Infection	4500+	175+

amounts. The amount needed in the daily diet varies greatly from a few micrograms of trace minerals to a gram or more of the major minerals, such as calcium, phosphorus, and sodium. A well-balanced diet can usually meet the daily requirements of needed minerals. However, deficiency states can occur.

Osteoporosis, a disabling disease in which calcium is lost from the bone, is now recognized as a condition that is prevalent in postmenopausal women. Present data seem to indicate a link to inadequate daily intake of calcium, especially in persons who do not drink milk (see Chapter 58).

The daily caloric requirements of a person are influenced by body build, age, sex, and physical activity. Adjustments are necessary, depending on changes in health status and daily activity level. Table 35-2 summarizes recommended daily calorie intake. Table 35-3 gives an example of calorie and protein needs, depending on activity level.

Nutritional Needs

Children and adolescents. Parents are responsible for setting an example of good nutrition for their children. It has been well documented that obese parents often have obese children. Parental attitudes toward food and eating habits are readily passed on to their children. Parents who have little understanding of what constitutes a well-balanced diet or who cannot or will not learn good nutrition inevitably influence their children to follow the same poor dietary practices. The nurse must help parents to understand the unique food requirements of their children from infancy through adolescence.

Infants and children differ from the adult in several ways. In the first months of life, the infant's gastrointestinal (GI) tract and kidneys are not functionally mature and are therefore limited in the kinds and quantities of nutrients that should be given. In addition, the infant and the child operate at a high basal metabolic rate that consequently leaves little in the way of nutritional reserves.

Adolescence is a particularly vulnerable time for the development of nutritional deficiencies, since this is a time of rapid growth and bodily changes. It is a period during which there is extreme concern with body appearance and social acceptability. Teenage girls are often attracted to fad diets as a means of weight control. Unfortunately, fad diets usually do not follow the basic four food group guidelines and are therefore often nutritionally unsound. Unless good nutritional habits are encouraged and supervised by parents during this developmental period, poor nutritional habits may become established as a way of life. A state of chronic inadequate nutrition may result.

Lower socioeconomic class. Because individuals and families from the lower socioeconomic class must spend a greater percentage of their limited income on food, as the cost of food increases, the tendency is to seek out cheaper foods that may not provide adequate nutrition. Conversely, such persons may prefer to select foods that are more expensive and only marginally nutritious because of their prestige value. The nurse and the dietitian can assist the poor in making food choices that meet nutritional requirements yet stay within their limited resources. Table 35-4 presents low-cost protein supplements.

Older adults. The nutritional requirements of older adults are often overlooked. It is more common to find an undernourished older person than an obese one. As a person grows older there is a concomitant decrease in the basal metabolic rate and in physical activity which lowers the caloric needs for energy. The older person frequently reduces consumption of needed protein, vitamins, and minerals and ingests "empty calories." The reasons given for this alteration in established eating habits can be attributed to living alone, boredom, death of a spouse, disability, and the need to rely on relatives or neighbors for food purchases.

As a group, older adults are less well informed about what constitutes a well-balanced diet. They may be induced to purchase more costly "health foods" at specialty stores under the mistaken assumption that these foods offer more nutrients than foods bought at their local market.

When these factors are added to already existing medical problems, it is easy to see why poor dietary patterns develop. Medical conditions involving the GI tract, such as ulcers, poor dentition, and ill-fitting dentures, contribute to the type and amount of foods that can be eaten. The nurse, working with the nutritionist, must be aware of these common medical and psychosocial factors in older adults and should suggest interventions for overcoming these problems in the teaching or plan of care.

Clients with physical illnesses. Regardless of the cause of the illness, the sick person has increased nutritional needs. Pathological conditions are frequently aggravated by undernutrition, and an existing deficiency state is likely to become more severe during illness. Malnutrition is not an uncommon complication of illness, surgery, or injury. Diseases of the GI tract are accompanied by anorexia, nausea, vomiting, diarrhea, distention, and abdominal cramping. Any combination of these symptoms interferes with normal food consumption. Many clients restrict their dietary intake to a few foods or fluids that are not nutritionally sound out of fear of aggravating the already disturbed GI function.

The malabsorption syndrome, which may result from decreased amounts of necessary enzymes and/or a reduced bowel surface area, can quickly lead to a deficiency state. Treatment of GI disorders with pharmacological agents may result in undesirable side effects and thus alter the normal digestive process. A specific example is seen following the administration of antibiotics. Antibiotics change the normal flora of the intestines, decreasing the body's ability to synthesize some of the B complex vitamins.

Fever accompanies many illnesses, injuries, and infections, with a concomitant increase in the body's basal metabolic rate. Unless there is an increase in the amount of carbohydrates and fats ingested in the diet, protein is used to supply calories, and protein depletion can become a problem.

Hospitalized clients, especially older adults, are at risk of becoming malnourished. Prolonged illness, major surgery, sepsis, draining wounds, burns, hemorrhage, fractures, and immobilization can all contribute to malnutrition. The nurse must assume responsibility, along with the physician and the dietitian, for meeting the client's nutritional needs. The nurse must also be mindful of the requirements of clients who are not overtly ill but who are undergoing diagnostic studies. These clients are usually nutritionally fit on entering the hospital but can develop nutritional problems because of the dietary restrictions imposed by multiple diagnostic studies.

The role of nutrition in the development of disease has long been studied. Investigation of personal dietary habits and the development of cancer has been widely published in recent years. There now appears to be a direct correlation between some types of cancer and dietary intake. A high ingestion of fatty foods appears to be linked with breast and endometrial cancer, and low fiber intake may be associated with some intestinal cancers (see Chapter 9). Further research in this area is needed for a better understanding of diet and disease and especially cancer causation.

Vitamin Imbalances

Vitamin deficiencies are rare in most of the developed countries of the world. When vitamin deficiencies are found, usually several vitamins are involved rather than a single vitamin deficiency. In the United States the recommended dietary allowances (RDA) for essential vitamins and minerals can be obtained by eating a diet consisting of foods from the basic four food groups. When vitamin imbalances do occur, they are usually found among persons such as alcoholics, drug addicts, and the very poor, who follow poor dietary practices. Followers of fad diets or poorly planned vegetarian diets are also subject to a potential deficiency state. Clinical manifestations of vitamin imbalances are most commonly exhibited as neurological manifestations (Table 35-5). The central nervous system

Table 35-4 Low-Cost Protein Supplements*

Brewer's yeast	2⅓ tbs
Cheese	1-in cube
Cottage cheese	¼ cup
Egg	1
Milk, whole, low-fat, skim	⅞ cup
Peanut butter	2 tbs
Pinto beans	¼ cup
Poultry	1 oz
Soybeans (cooked)	1 cup and 2 tsp
Split peas, lentils (cooked)	7 tsp (½ cup)

*Each supplies approximately 7 g of protein, equal to 1 oz of meat.

Table 35-5   Normal Vitamin Requirements and Signs of Imbalance

Vitamin	Normal Daily Requirements		Deficiency Symptoms	Deficiency Signs and Anatomical Changes
A (retinol)	Infants	1400 IU	Dry skin, night blindness, anorexia, eye irritation	Dry, scaly skin; increased susceptibility to infection; xerosis; keratinization of respiratory and GI mucosas; bladder stones; anemia; retarded growth
	Children	2000-3300 IU		
	Men	5000 IU		
	Women	4000 IU		
B₁ (thiamine)	Infants	0.3-0.5 mg	Anorexia and weight loss, insomnia, malaise, irritability, fatigue, paresthesia, muscle cramps, burning feet	Peripheral neuropathy, decreased reflexes, muscle weakness on squatting test, calf muscle tenderness, wrist or foot drop, cardiomyopathy (tachycardia, tachypnea, systemic AV shunt, high-output failure, edema, chest pain), Wernicke's encephalopathy (apathy, lethargy, global confusion, disorientation, nystagmus, ataxia, ocular palsies), Korsakoff's psychosis (retrograde amnesia, lability of emotions, confabulation)
	Children	0.7-1.2 mg		
	Adolescents	1-1.5 mg		
	Adults	1-1.5 mg		
B₆ (pyridoxine)	Infants	0.3-0.6 mg	Irritability, depression, lassitude, anorexia, tingling paresthesia, muscle cramps, painful elbows and shoulders, disequilibrium	Seborrhea involving face, neck, and intertriginous areas; hyperpigmentation of perianal region and legs; acneiform rash on forehead; peripheral neuropathy with motor weakness; tendency to genitourinary tract infections; infantile seizure; glucose intolerance; sideroblastic anemia
	Children	1.3-1.8 mg		
	Adults	1.8-2.2 mg		
C (ascorbic acid)	Infants	35 mg	Lassitude; weakness; irritability; dry, itchy skin; dry mouth; leg and arm pain; tissue swelling	Perifollicular petechiae, follicular hyperkeratosis, ecchymoses, gingivitis, swollen interdental papillae that bleed easily, painful subperiosteal hemorrhage, arthropathy with joint swelling, arterial vascular lesions
	Children	45-50 mg		
	Adults	60 mg		
Folic acid	Infants	30-40 μg	Anorexia, irritability, fatigue, sore tongue, diarrhea, forgetfulness, hostility, paranoid behavior	Glossitis, atrophic enteritis, gastric achlorhydria, malabsorption, megaloblastic anemia, leukopenia, thrombocytopenia, hypersegmented polymorphonuclear cells
	Children	0.1-0.3 mg		
	Adults	0.4 mg		
B₁₂	Infants	0.5-1.5 g	Anorexia, nausea, constipation, fatigue, sore tongue, paresthesias of hands and feet, moodiness, mental slowness, poor memory, agitation, depression, paranoid delusions	Glossitis, atrophic enteropathy, malabsorption, amblyopia, megaloblastic anemia, leukopenia, thrombocytopenia, incoordination, ataxia, organic brain syndrome
	Children	2-3 g		
	Adults	3 g		
D (calciferol)	Infants and children	400 IU	Muscular weakness, excessive sweating, diarrhea and other GI disturbances, bone pain	Active rickets, healed rickets, osteomalacia (generalized skeletal deformities, tender bones)
	Adults	200 IU		
E (tocopherol)	Infants	3-4 mg	Hemolytic anemia (only in newborns)	
	Children	5-7 mg		
	Adolescents	8-10 mg		
	Adults	8-10 mg		

Modified from Willard M: Nutrition for the practicing physician, Menlo Park, Calif, 1982, Addison-Wesley, pp 66-83.
AV, Atrioventricular.

Table 35-6 Vegetarian Protein Sources*

¼ cup beans and ⅔ cup rice
1½ tbs soybeans and ¾ cup rice
⅓ cup sesame seeds and 1 cup rice
¾ cup rice and 1 cup skim milk *or* 5 tbs dry nonfat milk
¾ cup rice and 1¼ oz cheese
2½ tbs beans and ¾ cup bulgur
⅔ cup whole wheat flour and 2½ tbs soy flour
¼ cup beans and 1 cup cornmeal *or* 6 corn tortillas
2½ tbs whole wheat flour and ⅔ cup dry milk and 1 cup cornmeal
⅓ cup beans and 1 oz cheese
¼ cup peanuts and ⅓ cup sunflower seeds

*Each combination provides the same amount of protein available in a 3 oz steak.

(CNS) of the growing child is primarily involved, and the peripheral nervous system is most affected in the adult.

Vegetarian diets. Vegetarian diets can result in a potential vitamin deficiency state. The two large classes of vegetarians are *vegans*, who are pure or total vegetarians and use only plant food, and *lacto-ovo-vegetarians*, who use plant foods and sometimes dairy products and eggs. There are several other types, including the *fruitarians*, but they constitute only a small percentage of the total group. The commonality among all vegetarians is the exclusion of red meat from the diet.

Vegetarianism cannot be considered a nutritional fad, since it is found in all age groups, occupations, and lifestyles. A variety of reasons have been given for following this type of dietary practice, including religious or cultural beliefs, belief that it is a better way of attaining total health, respect for all living beings, ethical-ecological ideals, and economics.

In well-planned vegetarian diets the essential vitamins and minerals are easily obtained. Plant protein, although of a lesser quality than that of animal origin, fulfills most of the protein requirements. Table 35-6 provides an example of vegetable sources of proteins. Lacto-ovo-vegetarians obtain additional protein sources from dairy products and eggs. Milk made from soybeans is an excellent protein source, especially for the true vegan. The one primary deficiency of a strict vegan is lack of vitamin B_{12}. This vitamin can be obtained only from animal protein, special supplements, or foods that have been fortified with the vitamin. Vegans not using vitamin B_{12} supplements are susceptible to the development of megaloblastic anemia and the neurological signs of vitamin B_{12} deficiency. Strict vegetarians and lacto-ovo-vegetarians are also at risk of iron deficiency. Iron-enriched foods or iron supplements (20 mg daily) are recommended and are mandatory during pregnancy, early childhood, adolescence, and after major blood loss.[1]

Megavitamin therapy. Megavitamin therapy refers to the administration of high doses of one or more vitamins, usually 10 to 20 times the RDA. Unless there are serious vitamin deficiencies, megavitamin therapy has no place in maintaining nutrition. The beneficial effects derived from the ingestion of commercially prepared daily vitamins are negligible if a balanced diet is eaten.

The *water-soluble vitamins* (C and B complex) are absorbed only as needed by the body, and the excess is excreted rapidly in the urine. Toxicity from overdoses is rare. However, because the excess is excreted through the kidney and urinary tract, detrimental effects may occur. Vitamin C is uricosuric and may cause the formation of renal stones in susceptible persons when taken in amounts in excess of 10 g/day. When taken in large doses, vitamins function as drugs rather than as nutrients and can cause toxic manifestations.[1]

The *fat-soluble vitamins* (A, D, E, and K) are readily stored and can accumulate to toxic levels. Because most vitamins can be purchased without a prescription, high doses of vitamins A and D can result in serious health hazards, since the excess is not eliminated. Overdose of vitamin A produces headache, blurred vision, nausea, and vomiting. Overdose of vitamin D produces symptoms associated with hypercalcemia. Toxic levels of the fat-soluble vitamins can be reached within a matter of weeks, especially in infants and children.

Eating Disorders

Anorexia nervosa. Anorexia nervosa is a psychiatric condition that results in a severely malnourished state characterized by the vigorous pursuit of thinness and a morbid fear of becoming fat. This condition is found predominantly in adolescent girls. The disorder was first recorded in England in 1684 and was misnamed *anorexia nervosa* because it was thought to be secondary to severe sadness and anxiety. The name has persisted to the present day, even though current research indicates a different causation. Anorexia usually begins during adolescence or early adulthood. It is rare for the illness to occur for the first time in a woman who is over the age of 25; if it does, the eating disorder is usually associated with a severe mental or physical illness.[2]

Anorexia nervosa is now recognized as occurring more often among persons whose sisters and mothers have the disorder than among the general population. It has been reported that there is a higher than expected rate of major depression and bipolar disorder among first-degree relatives of persons who have the condition.[3] In some persons the disorder is associated with stressful life situations with which they are not able to cope adequately. In addition, many were somewhat overweight at the onset of their illness. Common physical signs and symptoms of anorexia nervosa include amenorrhea, bradycardia, hypotension, cold intolerance, dry skin, severe constipation, and edema with altered fluid regulation. Fig. 35-1 presents a schematic drawing of electrolyte problems associated with anorexia.

Once anorexia nervosa has developed, the person will go to almost any extreme to hide eating behaviors from parents or peers. Although eating habits are severely disturbed, the appetite is not suppressed. Frequently there is a history of eating binges followed by self-induced vomiting, use of cathartics, or enemas.

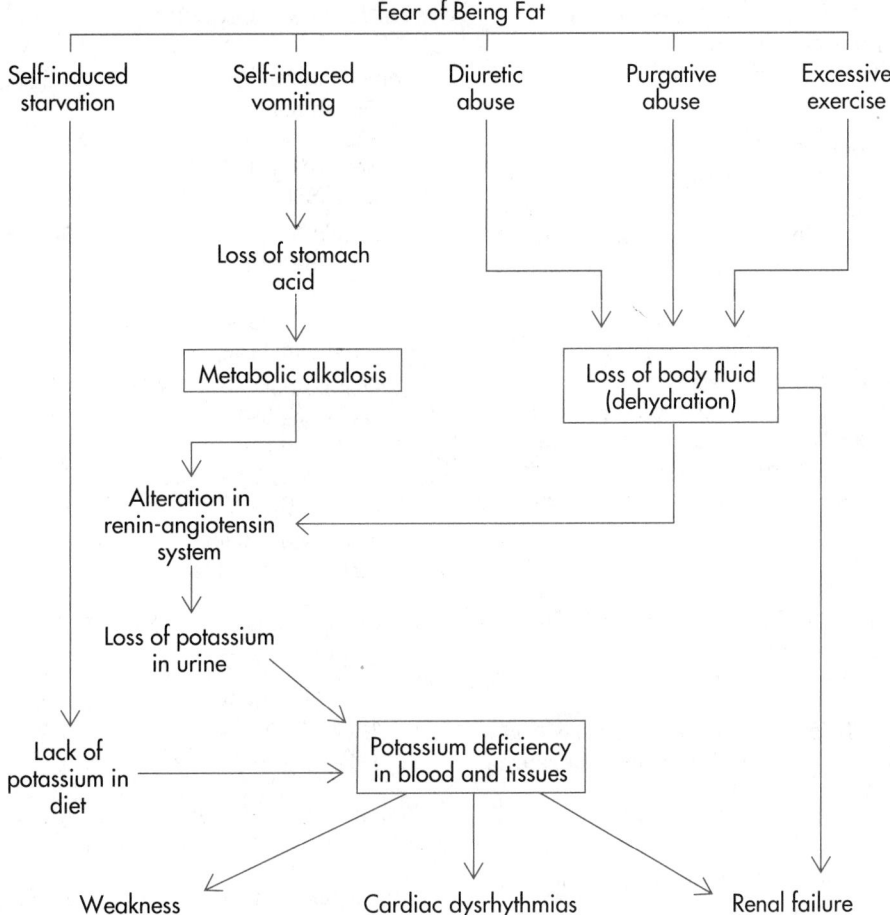

Fig. 35-1 Electrolyte problems in anorexia nervosa. (From Abraham S and Llewellyn-Jones D: Eating disorders: the facts, ed 2, Oxford, England, 1987, Oxford University Press, p 60.)

If the eating pattern is permitted to continue over a prolonged time, body wasting and signs of severe malnutrition are evident. Treatment must involve a combination of improved nutrition and psychiatric care. Hospitalization may be necessary if there are severe physical complications that cannot be managed in an outpatient therapy program. Nutritional replenishment must be closely supervised, not merely for the few pounds the person can rapidly gain but for consistent and ongoing gains.[4] The use of tube or parenteral feedings may be necessary. Improved nutrition, however, is not a cure for anorexia nervosa. The underlying psychological problem must be resolved by identification of the disturbed patterns of family interactions, followed by individual and family counseling.

Bulimia. Bulimia is a disorder that is often confused with anorexia nervosa because bulimia itself is a manifestation of anorexia in some persons. However, the syndrome of bulimia is quite different from anorexia. Bulimia is characterized by compulsive binge eating and purging (through self-induced vomiting, laxative and exercise abuse, and diuretics). Food becomes an obsession and an addiction—an escape from the pressures of life. Unlike persons with anorexia, those caught up in the syndrome of bulimia usually maintain a normal or near-normal body weight (some are even overweight), and the primary symptom is gorging rather than starvation.

Bulimia is increasing in incidence and may be even more prevalent than anorexia nervosa. College-age female students are a population group that seems to be very susceptible to this syndrome. The cause remains unclear but is thought to be similar to that of anorexia nervosa. Drug and alcohol abuse has been reported among persons with bulimia, many of whom are children or siblings of alcoholics. In addition to the psychological considerations, bulimia may cause some physical effects in those persons who binge and purge on a daily basis. Dental problems may develop as a result of constant vomiting. Swollen glands, sore throats, facial puffiness, chronic indigestion, irregular menstrual periods, bloodshot eyes, electrolyte imbalances, and dehydration can also occur. Sudden death due to cardiac arrest or fatal dysrhythmias is not uncommon. Although rare, esophageal tears and gastric rupture secondary to overdistention have been reported.[3]

Persons with bulimia, like those with anorexia, go to great lengths to conceal their abnormal eating habits. As the behavior persists, many problems associated with the

Table 35-7 Diagnostic Criteria for Anorexia Nervosa and Bulimia

ANOREXIA NERVOSA

Refusal to maintain body weight over a minimum normal weight for age and height (e.g., weight loss leading to maintenance of body weight 15% below that expected) or failure to make expected weight gain during period of growth, leading to body weight 15% below that expected

Intense fear of gaining weight or of becoming fat, even though underweight

Disturbance in the way in which body weight, size, or shape is experienced (e.g., the person claims to "feel fat" even when emaciated or believes that one area of the body is "too fat" even when obviously underweight)

Absence of at least three consecutive menstrual cycles when otherwise expected to occur (primary or secondary amenorrhea*)

BULIMIA

Recurrent episodes of binge eating (rapid consumption of a large amount of food in a discrete time)

A feeling of lack of control over eating behavior during the eating binge

Regular practice of self-induced vomiting, use of laxatives or diuretics, strict dieting or fasting, or vigorous exercise to prevent weight gain

A minimum average of two binge-eating episodes a week for at least 3 months

Persistent overconcern with body shape and weight

Modified from American Psychiatric Association: Diagnostic and statistical manual of mental disorders, ed 3, rev, Washington, DC, 1987, American Psychiatric Association.

*A woman is considered to have amenorrhea if her periods occur only following hormone (e.g., estrogen) administration.

Table 35-8 Organizations for Eating Disorders

American Anorexia/Bulimia Association
Department P
133 Cedar Lane
Teaneck, NJ 07666
(201) 836-1800

Anorexia Nervosa and Related Eating Disorders, Inc.
Department P
PO Box 5102
Eugene, Ore 97405
(503) 344-1144

National Anorexic Aid Society
Department P
5796 Karl Road
Columbus, Oh 43229
(614) 436-1112

National Association of Anorexia Nervosa and Associated Disorders, Inc. (ANAD)
PO Box 7
Highland Park, Ill 60035
(312) 831-3438

Overeaters Anonymous*
4025 Spencer St #203
Torrance, Conn 90503

*Consult the Yellow Pages for local chapters.

condition become increasingly hard to deal with effectively. Treatment of bulimia is similar to that described for anorexia nervosa. It consists of individual psychotherapy, nutritional counseling (including discussion of the dangers involved in binge eating and purging), and drug therapy. The use of tricyclic antidepressants (e.g., amitriptyline [Elavil]) is useful for the depression associated with both anorexia nervosa and bulimia. Vitamin, mineral, and iron supplements may be prescribed. However, iron supplementation is not generally required if amenorrhea is present. The return to normal eating habits may take many months to years to accomplish because relapses are frequent. Recovery is difficult; the abnormal eating behavior is very hard to change because binge eating and purging provide the person with a degree of satisfaction and a feeling of control over the body. Table 35-7 compares the current criteria used in the diagnosis of anorexia and bulimia. Table 35-8 lists associations that offer professional help for eating disorders.

Malnutrition

Malnutrition may be defined as an excess, deficit, or imbalance in the essential components of a balanced diet.

Terms such as *undernutrition* and *overnutrition* are also used to describe malnutrition. Undernutrition describes a state of poor nourishment as a result of inadequate diet or diseases that interfere with normal appetite and assimilation of ingested food. Overnutrition refers to the ingestion of more food than is required for body needs as in obesity.

Malnutrition is most prevalent in developing countries in which adequate food sources do not exist, the inhabitants are not well educated about their nutritional needs, and economic and ethnic conditions often preclude the purchase of a balanced diet. As a result of federal nutritional studies, it is now known that undernutrition does exist in scattered parts of the United States. It is usually found in individuals or groups from the lower socioeconomic class.

Types. Protein-calorie malnutrition (PCM) is the most common form of undernutrition and can result from either primary or secondary factors. Primary malnutrition exists when nutritional needs are not met as a result of poor eating habits. Secondary malnutrition is the result of an alteration or defect in ingestion, digestion, absorption, or metabolism. In this type of malnutrition, tissue needs are not met even though the dietary intake would be satisfactory under normal conditions. Secondary malnutrition may occur as a result of GI obstruction, surgical treatment (e.g., after peptic ulcer surgery), cancer, malabsorption syndromes, medications, and infectious diseases.

PCM is due to the ingestion of foods containing deficient amounts of protein (see Table 35-2). In addition to decreased amounts of protein, the diet is generally low in necessary vitamins and minerals. PCM is a serious nutritional problem common throughout the world, affecting every socioeconomic population and every age group. In the United States, where protein intake is high and of good quality, severe malnutrition is less of a problem, but it can occur in high-risk groups.

PCM has long been recognized in infants and children throughout the world by the terms *marasmus* and *kwashiorkor*. Adults with PCM may also be classified by this terminology. Marasmus is the result of a concomitant deficiency of both caloric and protein intake leading to generalized loss of body fat and muscle. Kwashiorkor is caused by a deficiency of protein intake that is superimposed on a catabolic stress event, such as a GI obstruction or surgical procedures, cancer, malabsorption syndromes, and infectious diseases.

Etiology. The following factors increase the potential for the development of malnutrition:

1. Weight loss of one third to one half of the initial body weight from any cause
2. Major surgery, radiation therapy, or chemotherapy
3. Severe burns with exudate high in protein
4. Draining wounds
5. Chronic renal and liver diseases
6. Hemorrhage
7. Bone fractures with prolonged immobilization
8. Malabsorption syndrome
9. Draining pressure sores

Nitrogen loss after severe injury or major surgery may be as much as 20 g/day, excreted as urea, creatinine, and creatine.

Pathophysiology. To better understand the physiological changes that occur in PCM, knowledge of the early phases of the starvation process is essential. Initially, the body selectively uses carbohydrates rather than fat and protein to maintain metabolic function. These carbohydrate stores, found in the liver and muscles, are minimal and may be totally used up within 24 hours. During this early phase of starvation, the only use of protein is in its obligatory participation in cellular metabolism. Once carbohydrate stores are depleted, however, body fat is used for energy to carry on metabolic processes. In prolonged starvation, 90% of calories are provided by fat and protein is conserved. Fat stores are generally depleted in 4 to 6 weeks. At this phase of the starvation process, body proteins can no longer be spared and rapidly decrease, since they are the only remaining body source of energy available.

If the malnourished client has surgery, experiences bodily trauma, or has an infection, the stress response is superimposed on the starvation response. These body insults cause an increase in the metabolic rate, with subsequent increase in energy requirements. Protein stores are no longer spared and are used with increasing frequency for body energy because of the accelerated metabolic energy needs.

As the protein depletion continues, the person enters a state of negative nitrogen balance. Liver function is impaired, and synthesis of new plasma proteins is diminished. The plasma oncotic pressure is decreased because of decreased protein synthesis. The main function of plasma proteins, primarily albumin, is the maintenance of the os-

motic pressure of the blood. Because of this decreased pressure, a shift in body fluids occurs from the vascular space into the interstitial compartment. As protein ingestion decreases and body stores are depleted, albumin eventually leaks into the interstitial space along with the fluid. Edema becomes clinically observable. Often the edema present in the face and legs of the person will mask the muscle wasting that has occurred. Ascites is a classic manifestation of kwashiokor.

As the total blood volume is reduced, the skin appears dry and wrinkled. Along with the shift of fluids to the interstitial space, ions also move. Sodium (normally an extracellular ion) is found in increased amounts in the cell, and potassium (normally an intracellular ion) and magnesium are shifted to the extracellular space. The sodium-potassium exchange pump, which is dependent on adenosine triphosphatase (ATPase), has high energy needs estimated to use 20% to 50% of all calories ingested. When the diet is extremely deficient in calories and essential proteins, the pump will fail, leaving sodium within the cell (along with water), and the cell will expand.

The liver is the body organ that loses the most mass during protein deprivation. It gradually becomes infiltrated with fat secondary to decreased synthesis of lipoproteins. Immediate restoration to the diet of protein and other necessary constituents must be instituted or death will rapidly ensue. The most serious problem associated with PCM in the very young is the probability of mental retardation. In severe malnutrition the development of brain cells is greatly reduced. Brain cells increase most rapidly during fetal life and in the first 5 to 6 months after birth. Once this critical time has passed for brain development, improvement in the nutritional state of the infant will not correct any mental deficiency already incurred.

Clinical manifestations. The adult who is deprived of sufficient protein and calories will have many of the clinical manifestations presented in Table 35-9. The most obvious clinical signs on physical examination are apparent in the skin, eyes, mouth, muscles, and CNS. The speed at which the protein deficiency develops depends on the quantity and quality of the protein intake, caloric value, and the age of the person.

The clinical manifestations are the result of numerous interactions occurring at the cellular level. A change in one area almost automatically effects a change in another. As protein intake is severely reduced, the muscles, which make up the largest reservoir of protein in the body, become wasted and flabby.

Anorexia and diarrhea are common with PCM. Hair lacks its normal luster and falls out easily, and the color ranges from dull red-brown to gray as a result of pigment changes. Most malnourished persons are anemic and are prone to infection. Anemia resulting from PCM is usually due to nutritional deficiencies such as of iron and folic acid.

Infection generally occurs because of the decrease in leukocytes in the peripheral blood. Phagocytosis is altered as a result of the lack of ATP energy necessary to drive the process. The person is more susceptible to all types of infectious processes. Both humoral and cell-mediated immunity are deficient in PCM.

Table 35-9   Signs of Protein-Calorie Malnutrition

Body System	Subclinical Signs	Clinical Signs
Integumentary	Slowed tissue turnover rate, surface temperature 1° F–2° F cooler, diminished febrile response to infection, delayed immune response	Brittle nails, decreased tone and elasticity of skin, xeroderma (dry skin), pigment changes (brown-gray), erythematous seborrheic dermatitis, scrotal dermatitis
Hair		Easy loss of hair, color changes, lack of luster
Eye	Night blindness	Blood vessel growth in cornea, Bitot's spots (gray keratinized epithelium on conjunctiva), dryness of conjunctiva and cornea, pale to red conjunctiva
Gastrointestinal		
Mouth and lips	Reduction in saliva production	Cheilosis (redness and swelling), crusting and ulceration at angle of mouth
Tongue	Mucosa more permeable to bacteria	Raw and red—beefy red, edematous and smooth, atrophy
Teeth	Improper development, delayed eruption	Caries, loose teeth, discolored enamel
Gingivae		Periodontal disease; tendency to bleed easily; receding, pale, and soft
Stomach	Decreased gastric acidity, delayed gastric emptying	Constant hunger, increased incidence of ulcers
Intestines	Decreased motility and absorption, normal flora causing infection from increased permeability of mucosa	Diarrhea and flatulence, protruding abdomen, increased incidence of parasitic diseases
Liver-biliary	Fatty liver, decreased absorption of fat-soluble vitamins	Hepatomegaly
Cardiovascular	Decreased cardiac output, decreased circulation time, decreased hemoglobin, shift in heart position, increased risk of thrombophlebitis	Decreased blood pressure and pulse, slight cyanosis, anemia, body edema
Endocrine	Decreased insulin production	Parotid and thyroid enlargement, polydipsia, polyuria, increased sensitivity to cold
Immunological	Decreased lymphocyte proliferation, decreased albumin levels, decreased antibody production, decreased total protein,	Increased infections, decreased response to skin tests
Musculoskeletal	Decreased growth rate, decreased body stature with chronic PCM, decreased muscle mass	Prominence of bony structures—face, clavicle, scapula, ribs, iliac crests, spinal vertebrae; weak and spindly arms and legs; flat buttocks; weak and flabby muscles; decreased physical activity and ability to work; severe weight loss
Neurological	Loss of ambition, feeling of being old	Depression, confusion, decreased reflexes in legs and ankles, decreased position sense, decreased vibratory sense, paresthesias of hands and feet, syncope
Renal	Negative nitrogen balance, decreased BUN and urine creatinine levels	Nocturia, decreased urinary output
Reproductive	Decreased gonadotropin levels	Amenorrhea, impotence, atrophied breasts
Respiratory	Pulmonary edema, decreased strength of respiratory muscles	Proneness to respiratory infection, decreased respiratory rate, decreased vital capacity

BUN, Blood urea nitrogen.

Table 35-10   Serum Albumin Depletion

Normal value	3.8-4.5 g/dl
Mild depletion	3.0-3.7 g/dl
Moderate depletion	2.5-2.9 g/dl
Severe depletion	<2.5 g/dl

Diagnostic studies. The diagnosis of PCM can be determined by a variety of laboratory studies used in conjunction with physical examination. Serum albumin is useful in the diagnosis of malnutrition. The degree of protein depletion can be identified with the use of the scale in Table 35-10. Serum transferrin levels are an excellent indicator of the loss of proteins. Transferrin, a protein synthe-

Table 35-11   High-Caloric, High-Protein Diet

GENERAL PRINCIPLES

1. A normal diet is supplemented with larger portions to increase the protein and caloric content. It is used for clients with hypermetabolism, burns, excessive stress, and cancer.
2. It is important to eat regularly and to not skip meals or snacks.

Meal	Protein Content (g)	Sample Menu Plans		
Breakfast				
Fruit		Large orange juice	Large apple juice	½ grapefruit
Starch, fat	2	1 toast with butter or jelly	Flour tortilla with butter	Biscuits and gravy
Starch, protein supplement	4	Cream of Wheat with 2 tbs skim milk powder	Atole with 2 tbs skim milk powder	Grits with 2 tbs margarine
		2 poached eggs	2 fried eggs	Omelet with 2 eggs
2 meat	14			
Milk, protein supplement	10	High-protein milk (2 tbs skim milk powder added)	High-protein milk	High-protein milk
Lunch				
4 meat	28	Cheeseburger on bun with double meat patty, lettuce, tomato	2 burritos with extra cheese, meat	Split pea soup with ham hocks
4 starches	8			Grilled cheese sandwich
Vegetable	2		Lettuce and tomato salad with dressing	Watermelon wedge
4 fats		French fried potatoes	Biscochitos	Sugar cookies
Milk, protein supplement	10	High-protein milk shake	High-protein milk	High-protein milk
Dinner				
4 meat	28	Spaghetti with 4 oz meat sauce, parmesan cheese	2 tamales with red chili sauce	4 oz fried chicken
3 starches	6		Spanish rice	Sweet potato
Vegetable	2	Green beans with 2 tbs margarine	Peas with 2 tbs butter	Mustard greens with 2 tbs butter
7 fat			Custard	Biscuit
		Bread with butter		Vanilla ice cream
		Tapioca pudding		
Milk, protein supplement	10	High-protein milk	High-protein milk	High-protein milk
Snack				
Milk	8	Fruit yogurt	Cottage cheese with fruit	½ sandwich with peanut butter
Fruit				Banana
	TOTAL 132			

sized by the liver and used as an iron-transport protein, decreases with the severity of protein deficiency. Serum electrolyte levels demonstrate changes taking place between the intracellular and extracellular spaces. The serum potassium level is often elevated and the serum sodium level decreased. The red blood cell (RBC) count and the hemoglobin level will indicate the presence and degree of anemia. The total lymphocyte count will show a decreased level of lymphocytes. The total lymphocyte count is obtained from the differential white blood cell (WBC) count.

Liver enzyme studies reflect hepatic dysfunction and damage. The serum bilirubin level is usually elevated and is related to the fatty liver infiltrate. Serum vitamin levels are usually diminished in malnutrition. The lowered levels of the fat-soluble vitamins correlate with the elevated se-

rum bilirubin and the clinical signs of steatorrhea. Water-soluble vitamin levels may also be low.

Therapeutic management. PCM, even in its earliest phase, is an easily recognized condition. The affected person is obviously well below ideal on weight-for-height scales according to age and sex. Inspection of the unclothed body reveals loss of muscle mass, muscle wasting, and little evidence of body fat. Diagnosis is not recognized, however, partly because of the body edema masking the deterioration of body muscle and a less than adequate nutritional history. The management of early uncomplicated PCM can be achieved without hospitalization by means of a diet high in calories and protein and close supervision. Table 35-11 gives an example of a high-calorie, high-protein diet.

In severe PCM the client may be hospitalized for correction of fluid and electrolyte imbalances and treatment of infections secondary to compromised status of the immune system. Enteral feeding, both oral and tube feedings, can be used to supplement the diet. In cases of severe PCM, total parenteral nutrition may be initiated.

■ Nursing Management of Malnutrition

Nursing assessment

Regardless of the setting, nurses must become more aware of the nutritional status of their clients. Nursing assessment of the client's nutritional status is presented in Table 35-12. The routine of recording the height and weight often becomes secondary to the client's chief complaint. When PCM is suspected, however, it is of utmost importance for the nurse to record both height and weight as well as to determine the client's position on the height-for-weight chart. If the assessment reveals that the client is well below the average for age and sex, the nurse should record a thorough diet history from the client or the family. The client's nutritional state may not be the reason medical assistance was sought. However, it may well have a bearing on the chief complaint and perhaps may be the underlying reason for the client's being ill. A dietitian should ultimately become involved in the plan of care but the nurse, as the first health professional dealing with the client, should take the initiative in determining the seriousness of the nutritional problems.

The nurse should be aware that psychosocial problems have a direct effect on appetite. This is often overlooked as a cause of undernourishment. A diet history of foods eaten over the past week will reveal a great deal about the client's dietary habits and knowledge of good nutrition. The client's physical state should be thoroughly assessed and documented (see Table 35-12). Each body system should be assessed, in addition to the height and weight

Table 35-12

 Nursing Assessment of the Client with Malnutrition

SUBJECTIVE DATA

History
Recent weight changes; weight problems; appetite changes; number of meals and snacks a day; food preferences and aversions; any dietary problems; history of diseases or surgical procedures that may affect nutritional status; level of physical activity; food allergies or foods that cause indigestion, diarrhea, or gas; change in financial status or family (e.g., loss of spouse)

Medications
Steroids, chemotherapeutic agents, diet pills, alcohol
Gastrointestinal
Use of dentures, difficulty in chewing or swallowing, pain in mouth, anorexia, indigestion, constipation, or diarrhea
Neurological
Paresthesias, loss of position and vibratory sense

OBJECTIVE DATA

General
Height, weight, appearance (e.g., alert, listless, cachectic, posture)
Mouth
Teeth: Dentures, caries, teeth missing, or loose teeth malpositioned
Buccal mucosa: Ulcerations, white patches or plaques, redness, swelling
Gingivae: Spongy, tendency to bleed easily, inflammation, recession, redness
Lips: Dryness, scaliness, swelling, redness and swelling (cheilosis), fever blisters, angular lesions at corners of mouth, fissures or scars (stomatitis)
Tongue: Swelling, scarlet and raw, beefy (glossitis), hyperemic, hypertrophic or atrophic papillae
Eyes
Pale or red conjunctivae, dryness, redness and fissuring of eyelid corners, dryness of eye membrane, soft cornea, dull appearance of cornea
Gastrointestinal
Liver or spleen enlargement
Cardiovascular
Tachycardia, increased blood pressure, dysrhythmias

Musculoskeletal
Flaccidity, poor tone, underdeveloped "wasted" appearance, bowlegs, knock-knees, beaded ribs, chest deformity, prominent scapulas
Neurological
Decrease or loss of reflexes, inattention, irritability, tremor
Integumentary
Hair: Dry, brittle, dull, stringy, thin, sparse, easily plucked, alopecia, color changes
Skin: Rough, dry, scaly, pale, irritated, discolored, petechiae, bruises, edema, darkness under eyes or over cheeks, greasy, scaly areas (nasolabial seborrhea)
Nails: Brittle, ridged, spoon shape
Possible findings
Decreased hemoglobin and hematocrit values; decreased mean corpuscular volume or mean corpuscular hemoglobin (reflective of iron deficiency); increased mean corpuscular volume or mean corpuscular hemoglobin (reflective of folic acid or vitamin B_{12} deficiency); decreased mean corpuscular hemoglobin concentration (reflective of iron deficiency); altered serum electrolyte levels; decreased BUN; decreased serum albumin, transferrin, and prealbumin; decreased peripheral lymphocytes

BUN, Blood urea nitrogen.

and vital signs. Table 35-13 summarizes factors that predispose persons to malnutrition.

Anthropometric measurements that include skinfold thickness at various sites and midarm muscle circumference may be ordered. These measurements are compared to standards for healthy persons of the same age and sex. Nurses often perform these measurements and should know what the results indicate and be able to interpret the outcomes for the client. Skinfold thickness is an indicator of subcutaneous fat stores. The midarm circumference is an indicator of muscle mass or protein stores. Both measurements are decreased in PCM.

Nursing diagnoses

Nursing diagnoses specific to the client with malnutrition include, but are not limited to, the following:

1. Altered nutrition: less than body requirements related to decreased ingestion, digestion, or absorption of food or anorexia
2. Feeding self-care deficit related to decreased strength and endurance, fatigue, and apathy
3. Altered bowel elimination: constipation, diarrhea, or impaction related to poor eating patterns
4. High risk for fluid volume deficit related to deviations affecting access to or absorption of fluids
5. Impaired skin integrity related to poor nutritional state
6. High risk for noncompliance with treatment regimen related to alteration in perception or lack of motivation
7. Activity intolerance related to weakness, fatigue, and inadequate diet

Nursing interventions

Acute intervention. Nurses must avoid the temptation to focus their attention on the other physical problems of the client to the exclusion of the nutritional state. The incidence of nutritional deficiency, especially PCM, is high in hospitalized clients. A number of nutritional studies have indicated that PCM may develop in 25% to 50% of medical and surgical clients hospitalized for 2 weeks or more.[5] Another recent survey on malnutrition revealed an incidence of 44% in general medicine clients and 50% in general surgery clients in a municipal hospital.[6] As a direct

Table 35-13 Persons at Risk for Malnutrition

Those who are grossly underweight or overweight and in whom recent weight loss exceeds 10% of usual body weight or 10 lb per month over several months

Alcoholics

Those without oral intake given ordinary IV solutions for 10 days; older adults for 5 days

Those with nutrient losses from malabsorption, dialysis, fistulas, or wounds or with excessive needs because of hypermetabolism, infection, burns, trauma, or fever

Those given drugs with antinutrient or catabolic properties, such as corticosteroids and oral antibiotics

Modified from Feldman EB: Essentials of clinical nutrition, Philadelphia, 1988, FA Davis Co, p 329.

consequence of these findings, the nurse must become more aware of who is at risk, why, and how to intervene appropriately. Increased calories and protein are required when surgery is performed and when severe trauma, sepsis, or chemotherapy is involved. Wound healing requires increased protein synthesis, increased WBC production, and, in cases of a malignant tumor, increased demands to meet tumor growth. Nitrogen loss is accelerated when fever is present. Despite the return of body temperature to normal, the rate of protein breakdown and resynthesis may be accelerated for several weeks. Major surgery is known to result in many weeks of increased catabolism.[5]

The nurse must have a thorough understanding of nutritional support and the rationale behind orders for such common tasks as daily weights and accurate intake and output records. All too often the busy nurse or the client and family question the need to weigh a person who is in considerable pain and discomfort. Providing the client and family with reasonable explanations can be helpful in gaining their cooperation. Daily weights give an accurate record of body weight gain or loss. These data, in conjunction with accurate recording of foods and fluid intake, produce a clearer picture of the client's nutritional state. To obtain an accurate weight, the nurse should follow a few simple rules, including weighing the client at the same time each day, on the same scale, with the same type or amount of clothing, and preferably with the bladder recently emptied.

The protein and caloric intake required in the malnourished client depends on the cause of the malnutrition, the treatment being employed, and other stressors affecting the client. Table 35-3 gives the requirements of an average 150-pound man in common hospital situations.

If the client is able to take food by mouth, a daily caloric count and diet diary should be maintained to give an accurate record of intake. The nurse and the dietitian working with the client and family can assist in the selection of high-caloric and high-protein foods from a selection list. A knowledge of foods preferred by the client enhances the daily intake and permits more involvement in recovery. Discussion with the client and family about foods that should be eaten to provide high-protein, high-calorie content is important. While the client is still hospitalized, the family can be encouraged to bring the client's favorite foods from home.

It is essential that the client be encouraged to ingest the meats and vegetables served at mealtimes. The drinking of several cups of tea or coffee with the meal may suppress the appetite for the more nutritious foods necessary for complete recovery. Visitors should be discouraged from bringing carbonated beverages or other types of drinks unless they have high caloric value.

The undernourished client usually receives between-meal supplements. These may consist of items prepared in the dietary department or commercially prepared products. Eating these items between meals increases the total daily intake and provides extra calories, proteins, fluids, and nutrients. In addition, multiple small feedings improve the tolerance for food intake by distributing the amount throughout the day.

Table 35-14 Commonly Used Polymeric Formulas

Product	Protein (g/C)	Carbohydrates (% total C)	Lipids (% total C)	Protein (% total C)	Osmolarity (full-strength)	C/ml
Ensure	35.1	54.5	30.5	14	470	1.06
Ensure Plus HN	41.7	53.3	30	16.7	650	1.5
Isocal	32.26	50	37	13	300	1.06
Isocal HCN	37.4	40	45	15	690	2.0
Isotein HN	56.5	52	25	23	300	1.2
Magnacal	35	50	36	14	590	2.0
Meritene liquid	60	46	30	24	505	0.96
Osmolite	35.1	54.6	31.4	14	300	1.06
Osmolite HN	41.8	53.3	30	16.7	490	1.06
Pulmocare	41.7	28.1	55.2	16.7	300	1.5
Sustacal	61.3	55	21	24	620	1.0
Trauma-cal	54.9	38	40	22	490	1.5
Two Cal HN	41.85	43.2	40.1	16.7	690	2.0
Amin-Aid	9.8	64.8	31.5	<1	1125	2.0
Hepatic Aid	26.5	70	19.7	10.2	900	1.6

C, I Calorie; 1 Calorie is equivalent to 1000 calories or 1 kilocalorie (kcal). Modified from Schlichtig R and Ayres S: Nutritional support of the critically ill, Chicago, 1988, Year Book Medical Publishers, Inc, p 153.

Table 35-15 Chemically Defined and Elemental Formulas

Product	Protein (g/C)	Carbohydrates (% total C)	Lipids (% total C)	Protein (% total C)	Osmolarity (full-strength)	C/ml
Criticare HN	35.8	83	3	14	650	1.06
High Nitrogen Vivonex	44.3	81.5	0.8	17.7	810	1.0
Stresstein	58.3	57	20	23	910	1.2
Vivonex	20.6	90.5	1.3	8.2	550	1.0
Vital High Nitrogen	41.7	73.9	9.4	16.7	500	1.0
Reabilan	31.6	52.5	35	12.5	350	1.0
Reabilan HN	42.5	47.5	35	17.5	490	1.33

C, I Calorie; 1 Calorie is equivalent to 1000 calories or 1 kilocalorie (kcal). Modified from Schlichtig R and Ayres S: Nutritional support of the critically ill, Chicago, 1988, Year Book Medical Publishers, Inc, p 153.

Commonly used premixed enteral formulas are listed in Table 35-14. A list of selected commercial elemental diets is found in Table 35-15. Elemental diets are chemically defined, nutritionally sound diets that contain glucose, glucose derivatives, dextrins, amino acids, essential fatty acids, vitamins, and minerals. They are lactose free and leave little residue in the lower bowel. The nurse should be familiar with the commercial products being used in the particular setting, their ingredients, and whether the products can be used as complete meal replacements or only as dietary supplements.

Chronic management. Discharge preparation for both the client and the family is important. They must be carefully instructed on the cause of the undernourished state and ways to avoid the problem in the future. The client must be made aware that undernourishment, whatever the cause, can recur and that adhering to a diet high in protein and calories for a few short weeks cannot restore a normal nutritional state. Many months are needed to reach this goal. Diet instruction is usually carried out by the dietitian, but it is important for the nurse to assess understanding and reinforce the information whenever possible. The client's ability to comply with the dietary instructions must be examined in light of past eating habits, religious and ethnic preferences, age, income, and state of health.

Unless the client and family can be convinced of the necessity for dietary change and have the resources to effect change, it is likely that no long-term benefits will be achieved. Ways should be found in which the client can become involved in the recovery. Keeping a diet diary or a calorie count for a week at a time is one way to analyze eating patterns. These records are also helpful to the health care team in the follow-up care. Self-assessment of progress can be encouraged by having the client get weighed once or twice a week and keep a weight record. The need for continuous follow-up care must be strongly emphasized if rehabilitation is to be accomplished and maintained.

TYPES OF SUPPLEMENTAL NUTRITION
Tube Feeding

Tube feedings may be ordered for the client who is unable to take oral nourishment. Indications for tube feeding, besides PCM, may include those persons who have anorexia, orofacial fractures, head and neck cancer, neurological or psychiatric conditions that prevent oral intake, extensive burns, and those who are receiving chemotherapy or radiation therapy. Tube feedings are easily administered, safer, more physiologically efficient, and less expensive than parenteral nutrition. They are used to provide hyperalimentation by way of the GI tract (alone or as a supplement to oral or parenteral nutrition) or as a treatment for malnutrition.

A nasogastric (NG) tube is most commonly used for short-term feeding problems. If the feedings are necessary over an extended time, other means of feeding may be used, such as an esophagostomy tube, a gastrostomy tube (placed surgically, endoscopically, or percutaneously), or a jejunostomy tube that gives direct access into the jejunum when physiological conditions warrant feeding the client below the stomach pyloric sphincter (see Chapter 34). Jejunostomy is used only when the esophagus and stomach must be bypassed. Procedures that require surgical placement may not be appropriate for a nutritionally depleted person.

Recent advances in the manufacture of feeding tubes made of polyurethane or silicone materials (e.g., Dobbhoff, Duo-Tube, Entriflex, Keofeed, Vivonex tungsten tip) have added to the comfort level of the client in tolerating extended periods of feeding. The older tubes were made of rubber or polyvinyl chloride, which tended to stiffen over time. The new tubes are longer, smaller in diameter, softer, and more flexible, thereby decreasing the possibility of mucosal damage from prolonged placement. In addition, these newer tubes are generally radiopaque, so position can be readily identified by x-ray film. Many of these tubes also have weighted tips, allowing spontaneous passage of the tube through the pylorus into the duodenum. Placement into the intestine helps prevent regurgitation of fluid into the esophagus and subsequent aspiration. These tubes are also more easily placed in the uncooperative or comatose client, since the ability to swallow is not essential during insertion.

The newer, smaller feeding tubes have many advantages over older tubes, such as the Levine tube, yet there are some disadvantages that the nurse must keep in mind. These tubes are more easily blocked when feedings are thick and make irrigation more difficult. They are also susceptible to blockage when oral medications have not been thoroughly crushed and dissolved in water before administration. They can become dislodged by vomiting or coughing and can also become knotted in the GI tract.

The procedure for the administration of tube feeding through a NG tube is standard. The following principles apply:

1. *Client position*: The client should be sitting or lying with head of bed elevated 30 to 45 degrees to prevent aspiration.
2. *Patency of tube*: If feedings are intermittent, the tube should be irrigated with water after each feeding to prevent blockage of the tube. If the feedings are continuous, they should be administered by using an electric or battery-operated feeding pump with a built-in alarm that will sound if the tubing becomes blocked in any way. If no pump is available, the feedings require frequent monitoring of the drip rate so that blockage does not occur from the client's inadvertently lying on the tubing or from too slow a drip rate.
3. *Tube position*: Proper placement of the tube in the stomach should be checked before each feeding or every 4 hours with continuous feedings. Methods used to confirm correct tube placement can include aspiration of stomach contents or injection of 10 ml of air and auscultation over the gastric area for the sound of air entering the stomach. Frequent checking is necessary because the stomach may become atonic, and gastric residual volume may increase with any deterioration of the client's condition. This is especially important when feedings are administered at high infusion rates. For example, when the infusion rate is 25 ml/hr, the total volume that may accumulate in 4 hours in an atonic stomach is 100 ml. At an infusion rate of 100 ml/hr, however, as much as 400 ml may accumulate in 4 hours.[7] The danger of aspiration is then a major care focus. The newer feeding tubes may be passed directly into the bronchus on insertion or may become dislodged and slip into the bronchus without any obvious respiratory symptoms being manifested. Therefore, injection of air to check tube position may be safe and appropriate only when the older, larger, and less flexible tubing is being used. The most accurate assessment for correct tube placement is still by x-ray film.
4. *Administration of feeding*: The principle of gravity is used with the drip method or with a bulb or plunger type of syringe. Applying pressure to force the feeding can damage the gastric mucosa. Pumps may be used. The feeding should be warmed to room temperature before administration. Both the amount and the concentration of the feeding are increased gradually over a few days so that the client will not experience undue side effects, such as nausea or diarrhea. It is important that either the rate or the concentration be increased, and not both at once. It is important to remember that clients still need water replacement, and at least 100 ml should be given every 4 to 6 hours (unless contraindicated).
5. *General nursing considerations*: The client should be weighed daily or several times a week and maintained on accurate intake and output. This permits monitoring of weight gain or loss and tolerance of the feedings. If the client is prone to development of nonketotic-hyperosmolar hyperglycemia, a serious condition that can arise as a result of high glucose intake from feeding formulas, the urine should be checked every 4 hours for sugar and acetone. Feedings that have been opened and not refrigerated or

feedings that have been infusing longer than 8 hours should be discarded. Therefore, feedings should be labeled with the date and time they are initially used. If a pump is used, new pump tubing should be changed every 24 hours.

Problems encountered in clients receiving tube feedings and corrective measures are found in Table 35-16. The use of blenderized foods from a normal diet may be used as tube feedings. The client may psychologically accept these feedings better than commercial products. Normal bowel function is promoted as a result of the fiber and residue content, which is similar to that of a normal diet.

When commercial products are used, it is necessary for the nurse to be aware that concentration, taste, lactose content, osmolarity, and amount of protein, sodium, and fat vary according to manufacturer. The standard concen-

tration is generally 1 kcal/ml. A limited number of flavors are available, and the overuse of one or two flavors, even in tube feedings, can lead over time to dislike and less tolerance.

Osmolarity higher than normal (280 mOsm/L) may be poorly tolerated and result in symptoms of the dumping syndrome (cold sweat, dizziness, distention, weakness, tachycardia, nausea, and diarrhea) (see Chapter 36). Protein content greater than 16% can lead to dehydration unless the client is sufficiently alert to request additional fluids or is given supplemental fluid intake. The nurse must be aware of this potential problem and provide extra fluids through the feeding tube or by mouth. Tube feedings with high sodium content are contraindicated in clients with cardiovascular problems, such as congestive heart failure. High fat content is not advocated for clients suffering from

Table 35-16 Common Problems of Clients Receiving Tube Feedings

Possible Causes	Intervention
VOMITING	
Improper placement of tube	Replace tube in proper position. Check tube position before beginning feeding and q 4 hr if continuous feedings.
Initiation of feeding too soon after placement	Give client time to get adjusted to tube before feeding.
Too fast of feeding	Give feeding by slow drip or via pump slowly. Avoid use of force.
Client in wrong position	Keep head of bed elevated to 30- to 45-degree angle. Have client lie on right side for ½ hr after feeding. Have client sit up on side of bed or in chair. Encourage ambulation unless contraindicated.
Too much of feeding	Check order for amount and number of feedings.
Contamination of formula	Refrigerate unused formula and record date opened. Discard outdated formula q 24 hr. Discard formula left standing for long time.
Air in stomach	Clear tubing of air before feeding. Keep tube feeding container full.
DIARRHEA	
Too fast of feeding, high concentration of formula	Decrease rate of feeding. Check on drugs that may cause diarrhea. Introduce formula gradually from quarter- to half-full strength as tolerated.
Lactose intolerance	Consult physician for change in formula.
Contamination of formula or tubing	Discard old formula. Change tubing q 24 hr.
CONSTIPATION	
No fiber in diet	Consult physician to obtain laxative order. Change formula.
Poor fluid intake	Increase fluid intake.
Drugs	Check on drugs that may be constipating.
DEHYDRATION	
Excessive diarrhea, vomiting	Slow rate or change formula.
Poor fluid intake	Increase intake and check amount and number of feedings. Increase amount if appropriate.
High protein and electrolyte content	Change formula.
Hyperglycemia due to rapid infusion, leading to osmotic diuresis and dehydration	Consult physician. Administer insulin if appropriate. Check urine for sugar and acetone.
SORE NOSE AND THROAT	
Irritation by tube	Provide mouth care q 4 hr. Cleanse nostrils of crusting. Have client gargle with saline or Xylocaine solution if ordered. Change to smaller polyurethane/silicone tube.

GI dysfunction. Some elemental diets use predigested (hydrolyzed) protein and have the advantage of requiring little digestion time and are rapidly absorbed. Disadvantages of predigested protein are the chemical taste and the added expense.

The dietitian can be of considerable assistance to the nursing staff. When close consultation with the nursing staff occurs, existing problems with tube feedings can be quickly and efficiently avoided or resolved.

Total Parenteral Nutrition

When the GI tract cannot be used for the ingestion, digestion, and absorption of essential nutrients, total parenteral nutrition (TPN) may be substituted. Parenteral nutrition (also called *hyperalimentation*) has become a relatively safe and practical method of delivering total nutritional needs by an intravenous (IV) route.

The goal of using TPN is to keep the client in positive nitrogen balance and allow for growth of new body tissue, which can be drastically depleted by prolonged inability to eat normally. Regular IV solutions of 5% dextrose (50 g of dextrose) in water (D₅W) or 5% dextrose in lactated Ringer's solution (D₅LR) contain no protein and have approximately 185 calories per liter. The normal adult requires a minimum of between 1200 and 1500 calories per day to carry out normal physiological function. Clients immediately after severe injury, surgery, or burns and those who are malnourished as a result of medical treatment or disease processes have greatly increased nutritional needs. Some clients may require as many as 10,000 Calories/day. The administration of dextrose solutions sufficient to meet these high caloric requirements would have extreme detrimental effects on the circulatory system, which could result in congestive heart failure or pulmonary edema. Table 35-17 lists the possible indications for the use of TPN.

Table 35-17 Indications for Total Parenteral Nutrition

Acute and chronic renal failure*
Alimentary tract anomalies and fistula
Burns
Chronic diarrhea and vomiting
Complicated surgery or trauma
Diverticulitis
Failure to thrive
GI obstruction
Granulomatous enterocolitis
Hepatic failure (reversible)*
Hypermetabolic states (sepsis, fractures)
Inflammatory bowel disease (Crohn's and ulcerative colitis)
Malabsorption
Malnutrition
Pancreatitis
Severe anorexia nervosa
Severe peptic ulcer disease
Short bowel syndrome

*TPN should be used with extreme caution in this situation.

Composition. Commercially prepared TPN base solutions are available for both central and peripheral use. These base solutions contain dextrose and nitrogen in the form of amino acids or protein hydrolysates. They may also contain minimal amounts of electrolytes or vitamins. However, because the amounts of each are limited, they may not meet the requirements of each individual client. The hospital pharmacy adds the necessary electrolytes (e.g., sodium, potassium, chloride, calcium, magnesium, and phosphate), vitamins, and trace elements (e.g., zinc, copper, chromium, and manganese).

Calories. Calories in TPN are supplied primarily by carbohydrates in the form of dextrose (20% to 50%). The administration of between 100 and 150 g of dextrose (1 g equaling 3.7 cal) daily has a protein-sparing effect. Since most clients receiving TPN are nutritionally depleted, their daily caloric needs are well above the average. These clients must receive 2000 calories or more each day. The administration of 1000 ml of a 50% dextrose (500 g of dextrose) solution or 2000 ml of 25% dextrose provides about 1850 calories.

Nitrogen. The normal healthy man needs about 56 g of protein daily. In a nutritionally depleted client under the stress of illness or surgery, requirements can exceed 150 g per day to ensure a positive nitrogen balance. Standard base solutions of TPN provide approximately 5 to 6 g of nitrogen (32 to 37 g of protein equivalent) or about 128 to 140 calories per bottle (1 g equals 4 cal).

Electrolytes. Assessment of individual requirements should take place daily at the beginning of therapy and then several times a week as the treatment progresses. The following are normal daily electrolyte requirements:

Sodium: 60 to 200 mEq
Potassium: 50 to 160 mEq
Chloride: 100 to 200 mEq
Magnesium: 20 to 30 mEq
Phosphate: 30 to 100 mEq

The base solutions used by many hospitals already contain electrolytes. If the client requires more or less than this amount, the solutions must be ordered daily by the physician.

Trace elements. Zinc, copper, manganese, cobalt, and iodine must be ordered according to the client's condition and needs. Because zinc stores may become depleted within a week or two of starting TPN, the physician needs to monitor these levels closely and add amounts according to the client's requirements.

Vitamins. The daily addition of a multivitamin preparation to 1 L of TPN generally meets the vitamin requirements. If multivitamin infusion is used, the vitamin B₁₂ requirement may be met without the need for supplemental injections. It is necessary for the physician to order vitamin K and folic acid separately. Folic acid, 500 μg, is given daily. Intramuscular (IM) vitamin K may be ordered depending on the results of the prothrombin time.

Methods of administration. TPN may be administered by two routes, *central* and *peripheral*. Central parenteral nutrition is given through a catheter inserted into the subclavian vein and subsequently threaded into the superior vena cava. Central hyperalimentation is indicated when

Table 35-18 Complications of Total Parenteral Nutrition

SEPSIS

Fungus
  Candida species (accounts for 50% to 70% of infections)
Gram-positive bacteria
  Staphylococcus aureus
  Staphylococcus epidermidis
  Streptococcus, α or nonhemolytic, species
  Enterococcus species
Gram-negative bacteria
  Klebsiella species
  Pseudomonas species
  Escherichia coli
  Enterobacter species
  Proteus species

METABOLIC PROBLEMS

Glucose metabolism
  Hyperglycemia and hypoglycemia
  Glycosuria
  Hyperosmolar nonketotic coma
  Osmotic diuresis
  Ketoacidosis
Amino acid metabolism
  Serum amino acid imbalances
  Elevated serum ammonia
  Prerenal azotemia
Calcium and phosphorus metabolism
  Hypophosphatemia
  Hypercalcemia and hypocalcemia
  Hypervitaminosis and hypovitaminosis (vitamin D)
Essential fatty acid deficiency

CENTRAL CATHETER

Insertion
  Air embolus
  Pneumothorax
  Hydrothorax
  Hemorrhage
Dislodgement
Thrombosis of great vein

long-term nutritional support is necessary, when the client has high protein and caloric requirements, and when suitable peripheral veins are not available. Peripheral hyperalimentation is administered through a large peripheral vein when nutritional support is needed for only a short time, protein and caloric requirements are not excessively high, the risk of a central catheter is too great, or nutritional support is used to supplement inadequate oral intake.

Central and peripheral parenteral nutrition differ in tonicity, which is measured in milliosmoles (mOsm, the concentration of particles in a fluid). Blood, which is isotonic, measures about 280 mOsm/L. The standard IV solutions of D_5W and normal saline are isotonic. Central hyperalimentation solutions measure 1600 mOsm/L and are very hypertonic due to the high glucose content, which ranges from 20% to 50%. Central hyperalimentation must be infused in a large central vein so that rapid dilution can occur. The use of a peripheral vein causes irritation and thrombophlebitis. Peripheral hyperalimentation is less hypertonic (using only 20% glucose) and can be safely administered through a large peripheral vein, although phlebitis can occur. Standard base solutions are now manufactured for parenteral use.

All TPN solutions should be prepared by a pharmacist or a trained technician using strict aseptic techniques under a hooded laminar flow unit. Nothing should be added to hyperalimentation solutions after they are prepared in the pharmacy. The danger of drug incompatibilities and contamination is very high. The fewer personnel involved in the preparation and administration of TPN, the less danger of infection for the client. In most hospitals the physician must order the TPN solution daily. In this way the solution and additives can be adjusted to the client's current needs. Each bottle of solution indicates the glucose and protein content, all additives, the time mixed, and the date and time of expiration. In general, solutions are good for 24 to 36 hours and must be refrigerated until ½ hour before being used.

Complications. Complications of TPN can be divided into three special categories: sepsis, metabolic problems, and problems with the central catheter line. The major complications of each category are presented in Table 35-18.

■ Nursing Management of Total Parenteral Nutrition

Peripheral hyperalimentation is a source of IV nutrition that may be given concurrently with oral nourishment. A large peripheral vein can be used because the solution is less hypertonic and therefore less irritating. The peripheral injection site should be observed for signs of phlebitis. The site is changed at least every 48 hours, depending on established hospital policy. The preparation and administration of peripheral nutrition follow the same criteria as outlined for central hyperalimentation (Table 35-19).

Catheter placement. The placement of the catheter into a large central vein for TPN is performed by the physician. The vein most commonly used is the subclavian, although the innominate or jugular veins may be used. The procedure is the same as for the insertion of a central venous pressure line and should be done under strict aseptic conditions. The use of sterile gowns, gloves, drapes, and masks is mandatory. The nurse must be ready to clarify or reinforce information already given the client regarding the need for initiating TPN by vein.

During the catheter insertion, the client is placed supine in the Trendelenburg position with a rolled towel between the scapulae. This position increases venous pressure in the subclavian vein, thus distending it, and provides the best access route for catheter insertion. Chest and neck hair may be shaved to eliminate a source of contamination. The skin is prepared by cleansing with an iodine antiseptic solution over the shoulder, neck, and chest area on the side where the catheter is to be inserted. The iodine must

Table 35-19

NURSING CARE PLAN FOR CLIENTS RECEIVING TOTAL PARENTERAL NUTRITION

Defining Characteristics	Nursing Interventions	Evaluation Criteria

NURSING DIAGNOSIS: High risk for infection related to placement of a central venous access catheter, inadequate aseptic practices, and decreased resistance

Inadequate body defenses due to open wound for TPN line, use of bacteriogenic solution, inadequate nutrition	Refrigerate solution until ½ hour before using. Use aseptic technique when connecting IV tubing and filter to central catheter. Label tubing and filter with time and date. Change filter q 24 hr and tubing with each bottle or according to institutional policy. Check expiration date. Change occlusive dressing over catheter site according to institutional policy, using aseptic technique (e.g., sterile gloves, mask). Observe for signs of inflammation and infection. Monitor vital signs q 4 hr.	No manifestation of infection, normal body temperature, negative blood cultures

NURSING DIAGNOSIS: Potential complication: hyperglycemia and electrolyte imbalances

Elevated fasting blood sugar, polyuria, polydipsia, polyphagia, blurred vision, dizziness, nausea and vomiting, dehydration, fatigue, deep labored breathing, loss of consciousness; glycosuria; severe stress (surgical, trauma, emotional upset); electrolyte imbalance	Monitor blood glucose level daily. Check urine sugar and acetone q 4 hr. Notify physician of 3+ or 4+ readings. Administer regular insulin if ordered. Initial TPN therapy must be gradually increased over 24 to 48 hr. Maintain accurate infusion rate. Check every ½ hour or use an infusion pump (e.g., IVAC). Watch for kinks and obstruction or disconnected tubing. Never increase or decrease flow rate by more than 10%. Observe for signs of hyperglycemia (e.g., thirst, polyuria, confusion). Observe for hypoglycemia (e.g., sweating, hunger, weakness, tremors). Never stop TPN abruptly unless it is replaced by another glucose source. Taper TPN gradually. Monitor serum electrolyte levels daily. Check for symptoms of hyperkalemia (muscle weakness, flaccid paralysis, cardiac dysrhythmias, abdominal cramps, diarrhea) and hypokalemia (general weakness, decreased muscle tone, weak or irregular pulse, low blood pressure, shallow respirations, abdominal distention, and ileus).*	Blood sugar within normal range, serum electrolytes within normal range

NURSING DIAGNOSIS: Potential complication: air embolus secondary to incorrect insertion position

Abnormal blood gases, cough, cyanosis, pain, anxiety, fatigue, respiratory rate and depth changes, altered chest excursion, shortness of breath	On catheter insertion, place client in Trendelenburg position with rolled towel between scapulae. Instruct client to take a deep breath and hold while needle is inserted into subclavian vein (Valsalva maneuver). Use same position and Valsalva maneuver when changing tubing to prevent air from being sucked into vein. Reconnect catheter to IV tubing immediately. If air embolism is suspected, observe for sudden onset of dyspnea, decreased blood pressure, chest pain, and hemoptysis. Place client in Trendelenburg position with left side down to "trap" air in right atria. Continue to observe for shock, cough, and shortness of breath. Notify physician immediately.	No signs of impaired breathing

*Other manifestations of electrolyte imbalances are discussed in Chapter 10.   *Continued.*

Table 35-19

NURSING CARE PLAN FOR CLIENTS RECEIVING TOTAL PARENTERAL NUTRITION—cont'd

Defining Characteristics	Nursing Interventions	Evaluation Criteria

NURSING DIAGNOSIS: Impaired physical mobility: arm, shoulder, and chest related to muscle or nerve trauma secondary to catheter insertion and position restrictions and pain

Inability to move upper body at will, decreased muscle strength and control, neuromuscular impairment (brachial plexus injury), pain on movement	Observe client for pain in shoulder and sensory change. Assist with range of motion within position restrictions. Assist with activities of daily living. Administer pain medication as ordered.	Satisfactory movement of upper body, achievement of activities of daily living, satisfactory pain control

NURSING DIAGNOSIS: Anxiety related to inability to ingest food and fluids; uncertain outcome; lack of knowledge regarding catheter position and rationale, benefits, and management of TPN

Restlessness and apprehension, expression of concern regarding changes in life events, frequent questioning regarding care of catheter and TPN line	Instruct client on rationale and benefits of TPN and care of line. Give approximate length of time TPN will be used. Illustrate catheter position by drawings and pictures. Reassure client the catheter will not move into the heart. Describe the advantages of physical activity. Provide range-of-motion exercise that client can perform while in bed. Encourage ambulation.	Knowledge of rationale for and care of TPN line

be removed by scrubbing the skin with 70% alcohol, which prevents an iodine skin burn, reduces any allergic reactions, and helps destroy the cell walls of bacteria found on the skin surface.

In some institutions the skin is first scrubbed with soap and water, followed by defatting of the skin with acetone or ether. The use of a defatting agent is questionable because surface lipids have an antimicrobial property and are known to significantly reduce the number of organisms such as *Staphylococcus aureus* and *Candida albicans*. Use of acetone in the skin preparation is known to remove these antimicrobial substances.

After draping of the area and application of a local anesthetic, a Silastic catheter is inserted through a large-bore needle into the right or left subclavian vein. The client is instructed to take a deep breath and to stop breathing (Valsalva maneuver) when the needle is inserted. This will temporarily stop the positive pressure associated with normal ventilation and prevent air from being sucked into the subclavian vein, which could cause an air embolus or pneumothorax. If the client is unconscious or intubated, a Valsalva maneuver can be performed by means of a manual resuscitation bag. The catheter is then threaded into the superior vena cava. A skin suture may be used to stabilize the catheter; there is not total agreement on its necessity, as it is often a source of infection.

A standard isotonic IV solution is infused through the central line until x-ray film confirms proper placement of the catheter tip in the superior vena cava and not in the jugular vein or heart. The catheter insertion site is covered with an iodine ointment, and an occlusive dressing is placed over it. The date is marked on the dressing.

Complications frequently associated with catheter placement are hemorrhage, hydrothorax and pneumothorax, air embolus, and catheter and venous thrombosis. It is important that the tip of the catheter not lie within the right atrium. TPN solution is hyperosmolar, and the catheter tip can cause erosions of the atrial tissue with subsequent infection.[7]

Proper placement of a catheter for central hyperalimentation is illustrated in Fig. 35-2. Once established, the central catheter should not be used for the administration of blood or antibiotics, for the drawing of blood samples, or for central venous pressure monitoring.

Administration of solution. Sepsis is one of the major concerns with TPN solutions. It is essential that proper aseptic techniques be followed. The use of a millipore filter to trap bacteria and precipitate is controversial. The nurse should adhere to institutional protocol. When the filter is used, it should be placed proximal to the catheter hub. Filters are changed every 24 hours, and new IV tubing is changed with each new bottle of TPN. Tubing and filter should be clearly labeled with the date and the time they are put into use. When a new tubing or filter is attached to the central catheter, the client should be asked to perform the Valsalva maneuver so that the chance of an air embolus is reduced while the catheter is open and not connected to an infusion source. Luer-Lok connections should be used and taped as an added safeguard to prevent an accidental break in the continuity of the line.

At the beginning of TPN therapy, the solution is infused at a gradually increasing rate over a 24- to 48-hour period. In this way the pancreas can adapt to the increased amount of glucose in the circulation by producing more in-

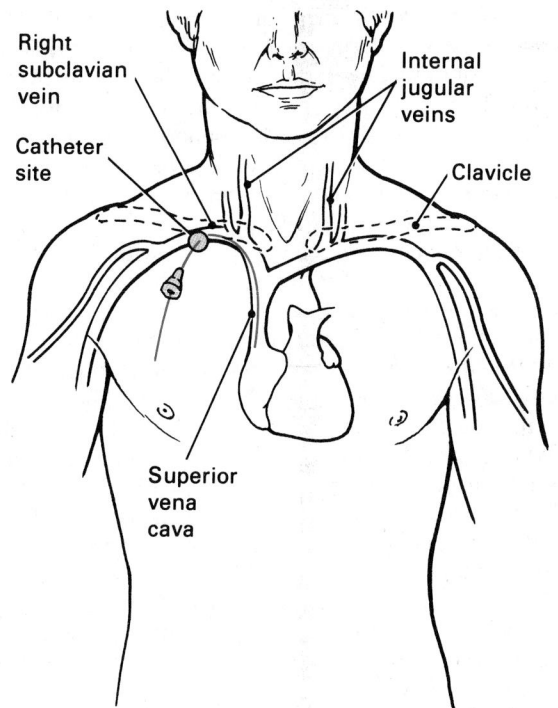

Fig. 35-2 Placement of a catheter for total parenteral nutrition.

sulin. The urine should be tested for sugar and acetone every 4 to 6 hours while the client is receiving hyperalimentation. Glycosuria of 1+ or 2+ is expected during the first few days of therapy. However, readings of 3+ or 4+ require either the addition of regular insulin to the solution or the administration of insulin on a sliding-scale schedule. (Sliding scale is explained in Chapter 43.) Blood glucose levels can be checked with a glucose-testing meter (see Chapter 43). If these are available, they are more accurate indicators of the client's blood glucose level than urinary determinations.

Nurses must be aware that speeding or slowing the infusion rate is contraindicated. Speeding up the rate results in a large amount of glucose entering the circulation. Endogenous insulin levels are not adequate to handle this increase in glucose, and a hyperosmolar state results. The renal tubules are unable to reabsorb the glucose and it spills into the urine. Conversely, slowing the rate results in a hypoglycemic state, since it takes time for the pancreatic islet cells to adjust to a reduced glucose level. Checking the amount infused and the rate every ½ hour is recommended. An infusion pump should be used during administration of TPN so that the infusion rate can be maintained and an alarm will sound if the tubing becomes obstructed. Before setting up and administering TPN, the nurse must check the label and ingredients in the solution to see that they are what the physician ordered. Solutions must also be examined for signs of contamination, such as a cloudy appearance. If contamination is suspected, the solution should be promptly returned to the pharmacy for replacement. It is the nurse's responsibility to ensure that the TPN solution is discontinued and replaced with a new solution

if it is still infusing at the end of 24 hours. This is necessary because of the high glucose concentration of the solution. At room temperature, the solution is a perfect setting for the rapid growth of microorganisms.

Vital signs should be monitored every 4 hours. Daily weights give an indication of the client's nutritional status as therapy progresses. Body weight is considered the sum of the changes in protein, fat, and water. Body water fluctuates more from day to day than does protein or fat. Analysis must be made of whether gains or losses in weight are due to fluid gained from edema, fluid lost through diuresis, or actual increase or decrease in true body weight. Blood levels of glucose, electrolytes, protein, a complete blood count, and enzyme studies are followed daily or every other day. Correlation of these important values assists the nurse in assessing the client's progress toward a more nutritionally balanced state.

Dressings covering the catheter site are changed according to institutional protocol, from every other day to once a week. Frequently, specially trained nurses from the IV team or the nutritional support team are responsible for the dressing changes. Some institutions allow the staff nurses to carry out dressing changes after special instruction. The procedure for changing the dressing is similar to that followed during the catheter insertion. The institutional routine should be followed with respect to appropriate use of acetone, betadine, and alcohol for the dressing change. The site is carefully observed for signs of inflammation and infection. Phlebitis can readily occur in the vein as a result of the hypertonic infusion and can become infected. Many clients receiving central TPN are immunosuppressed and are more susceptible to opportunistic infections. Many are receiving chemotherapy or corticosteroids and antibiotics, which will mask signs of infection.

If sutures are used to anchor the catheter, they may become infected. If an infection is suspected during dressing change, a culture specimen of the site and drainage should be sent for analysis and the physician should be notified immediately. The use of an occlusive dressing protects the wound from contamination.

If the client exhibits signs and symptoms of a systemic infection, the catheter tip is usually suspect unless another cause can be found. Cultures of blood, sputum, urine, draining wound, and the catheter tip, if it has been removed, are done at once. A chest x-ray film is taken to detect any pulmonary infection. The current bottle of TPN solution with tubing and filter should also be cultured and replaced with an entire new setup. When the catheter tip is the source of infection, antibiotic therapy is generally not necessary, since removal of the catheter will eliminate the problem. A new central line may be immediately established or replaced by a peripheral route. It is important that a glucose source be provided to prevent rebound hypoglycemia.

Weaning. The same precautions should be followed in weaning from TPN as when therapy is being initiated, except in inverse order. The flow rate must be gradually decreased over a period of 4 to 6 hours while oral intake is increased. If an emergency situation precludes a slow weaning process, other dextrose-containing fluids should be administered without interruption. For clients who are going to surgery the TPN should be discontinued ahead of the scheduled operation time. At the time the catheter is removed by the physician, the site is immediately covered with iodine ointment and an occlusive dressing is applied. The dressing should be changed daily until the wound heals. Oral nourishment should be encouraged, and a careful record of intake should be maintained. Daily weights and laboratory analysis of serum levels continue.

Home parenteral nutrition. Home parenteral nutrition is now an accepted mode of nutritional therapy for persons who do not require hospitalization but who benefit from continued nutritional support. With proper instruction in catheter care, aseptic technique in mixing and handling of the IV solutions and tubing, and side effects to watch for, some clients have been successfully treated at home for many months. The client with cancer is a prime candidate for this therapy.

Intravenous Fat Emulsion

The first infusion of fat emulsions occurred during the 1920s in Japan. Further research was delayed until after World War II. Recently the FDA approved the use of 10% and 20% intralipid fat emulsion solutions. These lipid emulsions provide approximately 1.1 kcal/ml (10% solutions) and 2 kcal/ml (20% solutions).

The contents of intralipid fat emulsion are listed in Table 35-20. The use of IV fat is indicated for the following clients:

1. Those receiving peripheral hyperalimentation who require an additional caloric source
2. Those receiving long-term (more than 5 days) hyperalimentation who require a source of essential fatty acids
3. Those receiving central hyperalimentation who have excessive caloric needs

The administration of fat emulsion is contraindicated in clients with a disturbance in fat metabolism and should be used with caution in clients who are in danger of fat embolism and those with pancreatitis, liver damage, pulmonary disease, anemia, blood coagulation disorders, and allergy to eggs.

Intralipid solution is isotonic and is used as the primary caloric substrate in complete peripheral TPN solutions. The FDA now allows up to 60% of calories to be provided as lipid administered IV. It can be infused separately, or when it is used with TPN, the fat emulsion is given as a supplemental source of calories because essential fatty ac-

Table 35-20 Standard Contents of Intralipid Fat Emulsion (500 ml)

Soybean triglycerides	10%
Egg yolk phospholipids	1.2%
Glycerin	2.25%
Water	500 ml
Osmolarity	280 mOsm/L
Electrolytes	None
Total calories	550

ids are not included in the standard preparations of TPN. Prolonged use of TPN can lead to a fatty acid deficiency, which is manifested by dermatitis and loss of hair. Recent pharmacological advances now permit the direct mixing of lipid emulsion with dextrose and amino acids in a single 3-liter bag suitable for peripheral infusion.[7]

Intralipid solutions should be refrigerated until 1 hour before administration. Special tubing is provided by the manufacturer, and new tubing is used with each bottle. Nothing is to be added to the solution before administration. Intralipid should not be filtered. When peripheral hyperalimentation is being run at the same time (unless with the use of the premixed TPN and intralipid solution), the fat emulsion should be connected below the filter through a Y injection site as close as possible to the injection site. As with TPN solutions, fat emulsion should begin at a slow rate, usually 1 ml/min for the first 15 minutes. If no reaction is observed, the rate may be increased to 125 ml/hr. Adverse reactions that can occur are allergic manifestations, dyspnea, cyanosis, fever, flushing, phlebitis, chest and back pain, and pain at the IV site. IV fat may be ordered daily or at least two to three times per week, depending on the caloric needs or fatty acid requirements of the client. A major benefit derived from IV fat administration is that a large number of calories can be provided in a relatively small amount of fluid. This is especially beneficial when the client is at risk of fluid overload.

OBESITY
Significance

Obesity is one of the major health problems found in our society. In the United States, obesity is the most common nutritional problem. The term *obesity* is generally used when the body's fat composition is above normal, with normal being 15% to 20% for men and 20% to 25% for women. It can be classified as mild, moderate, severe, or morbid when weight exceeds ideal body weight by 15% to 30%, 30% to 50%, 50% to 100%, or more than 100%, respectively.[8] The term *overweight* has often been used to define obesity; yet the terms are not identical. Overweight refers to excess in body weight in relation to a standard for height. Obesity refers to excess body fat.

In obese persons a variety of diseases occur in excess of the expected rate. These include hypertension, hyperlipidemia, diabetes, gout, cardiovascular disease, gallbladder disease, and menstrual and ovarian irregularities. Most agree that obesity is hazardous to health and detrimental to well-being and, because of its multiple biological concomitants and its promotion of atherogenic traits, obesity constitutes a major health problem. It is pure fallacy to attribute obesity only to the prosperous middle-aged man or woman or to those of lower socioeconomic status. Obesity can occur in anyone and at any time during the life cycle.

Formation of Adipose Tissue

The formation of adipose tissue, unless determined to be secondary to an organic etiological factor, can occur only when a person consumes more food than is required to carry out normal physiological function and growth. The excess is stored as adipose tissue in layers beneath the skin surface, the omentum, the mesentery, and in fat pads that normally surround the kidneys and the heart. The process of reaching an obese state is usually insidious. The person may be completely unaware of changes in eating habits or body size until looking in a mirror or discovering the need for a larger clothing size.

Adipose tissue present in obesity is of the same composition as fat tissue normally found in smaller amounts in the same areas. It consists of clumps of fat cells together with supporting tissue, such as blood vessels, lymphatic vessels, and fibrous tissue. Although adipose tissue is very high in neutral fat, it also contains water, protein, and a small amount of glycogen. The size of the adipose tissue mass is the sum of the number of adipose cells and the adipose cell size, which is determined by the amount of triglyceride found within the cell.

Obesity research has demonstrated that expansion of the tissue mass occurs as a result of an increase in cell size *(hypertrophic obesity)* or an increase in cell size and cell number *(hypertrophic-hyperplastic obesity)*. Until recently it was believed that fat cells increased in number only until puberty. After puberty, if a person absorbed more energy from food than was expended by metabolic processes or by exercise, the excess energy was converted into fat and was stored in the existing fat cells, which increased in size. Research shows that the fat cell is capable of expanding to a 1000-fold increase in volume.[9] It is now known that when faced with fat storage at any age, the fat cell first increases in size and, when a critical size is achieved, divides to form new fat cells.[10] Additional research indicates that weight loss achieved by dietary means ceases when the size of the fat cell reaches its normal size. This suggests that the size of the fat cell may be the determinant of the amount of weight lost, whereas the number of fat cells may determine the body weight at which this limit is reached.[9]

The adipose tissue mass in early-onset obesity is distributed universally over the entire body; the adipose tissue mass in adult-onset obesity is centrally distributed. Fig. 35-3 shows a client with extreme juvenile-onset obesity; Fig. 35-4 shows a client with extreme adult-onset obesity.

An understanding of how adipose tissue is formed has considerable impact on methods of weight loss and of reduction of the adipose tissue mass in the adult. Severe dietary restrictions do not decrease the number of fat cells present but do result in a decrease in the size of the cells. The saying "once a fat cell, always a fat cell" is unfortunately true and is based on scientific fact.

Pathophysiology

Many factors have been investigated in an effort to identify their relationship and influence on the occurrence of obesity. The following questions should be considered in assessment of the client with obesity:

1. What is the psychological importance of food?
2. Is intake influenced by hunger?
3. Do the taste and appearance of food and physical factors in the environment make some persons more sensitive and propel them to excess eating habits?
4. Is there an emotional problem that creates a need for oral gratification?
5. Are there any stressors influencing the person's eating patterns?

The children of obese parents tend to be obese. Obesity tends to affect several persons within a family, but whether this tendency is genetically controlled or influenced by a shared environment has not been determined.

An aspect of obesity that is currently a major area of research is the metabolic adaptive response of the hypothalamus and energy balance. The lateral and ventral parts of the hypothalamus control appetite and, as a result, influence eating behavior. Hypothalamic adaptation apparently develops in any person who starves and reduces weight below the established "set point." The concept is that in every person the hypothalamus has a set point for energy balance, above which energy conservation becomes increasingly less efficient and below which energy conser-

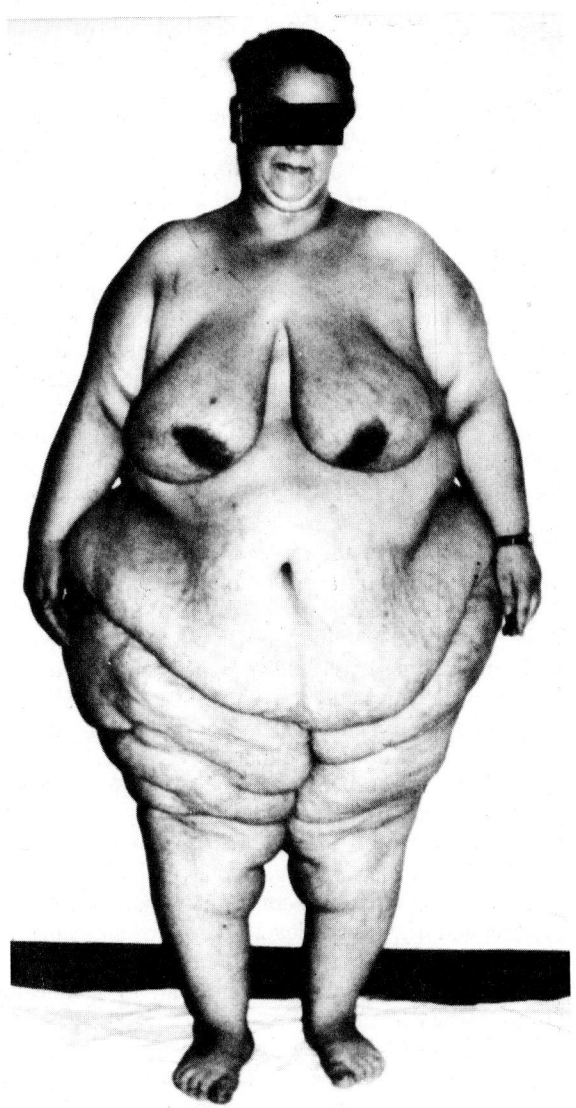

Fig. 35-3 Extreme juvenile-onset obesity. (From Mancini R and others: Medical complications of obesity, London, 1979, Academic Press, Inc.)

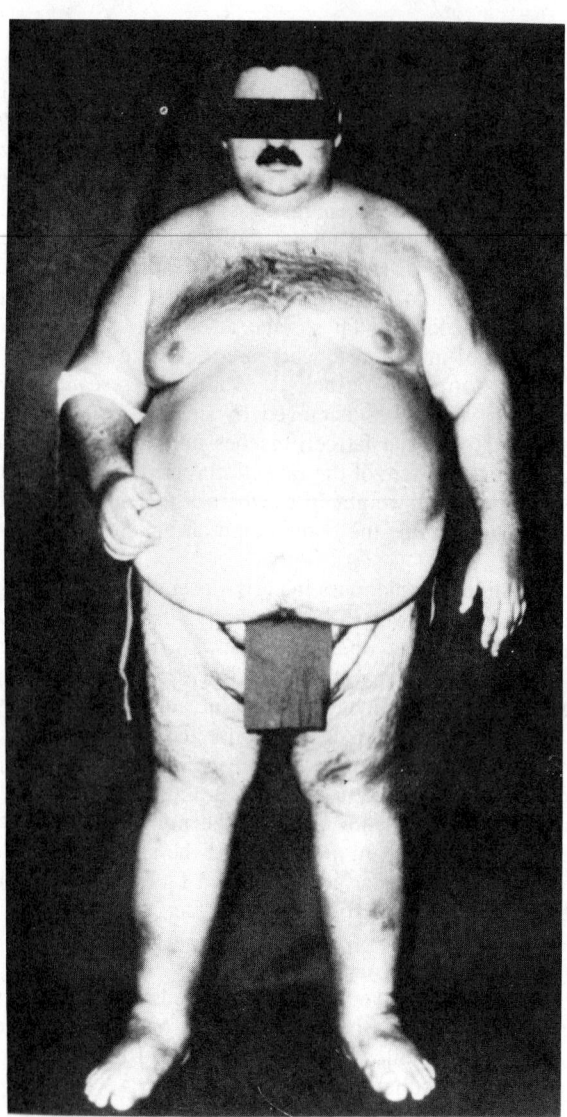

Fig. 35-4 Extreme adult-onset obesity. (From Mancini R and others: Medical complications of obesity, London, 1979, Academic Press, Inc.)

vation becomes increasingly more efficient. This homeostatic mechanism accounts for the fact that most adults keep their weight remarkably constant, despite large swings in energy input and expenditure.

This ability of the body to conserve energy as dieting continues may account for the failure of sustained weight loss to occur even though caloric intake is drastically curtailed. It could also account for why the obese person, no matter what dietary regimen is followed, tends to remain extremely overweight.

Most obese persons have a sedentary lifestyle; they usually have a nonstrenuous indoor occupation and engage in few, if any, spirited recreational activities. Their energy needs are considerably less than are the requirements of a construction worker who also plays tennis several times a week. Thus an obese person with sedentary habits only adds to an already positive energy balance by not engaging in activities that burn off some excess fatty tissue through energy-consuming exercises.

Complications

The medical and social problems associated with obesity are numerous. The medical problem may be a direct result of too much fat, or the medical problem may have an adverse effect on obesity. Cardiovascular and respiratory problems are very common in obese persons. Many clients experience dyspnea on exertion, orthopnea, paroxysmal nocturnal dyspnea, drowsiness, and somnolence. In addition, these clients are prone to the development of polycythemia secondary to low oxygenation of arterial blood. Polycythemia results in an increased viscosity of the circulating blood volume and sluggish flow throughout all vessels and capillaries. As a result, obese clients may have occlusion of vessels and clotting abnormalities. Heart size increases as body weight increases, since the heart must work harder to maintain adequate circulation. Hypertension is the most common cardiovascular disease associated with obesity. The presence of polycythemia creates considerable strain on the heart because of the increased RBC count and plasma volume. Therefore obesity can precipitate hypertrophy of the heart, especially of the left ventricle.

The Pickwickian syndrome, which is known as *obesity hypoventilation,* has long been recognized as a result of extreme obesity. The bellows action of the chest wall is compromised, and there is dysfunction of the central respiratory control center. The movement of the muscles of the chest wall and the diaphragm is reduced because of the weight of the fatty tissue mass. Hypoventilation results in a state of chronic hypercapnia. The increased carbon dioxide level affects the respiratory control center, causing an abnormal body response to the high carbon dioxide level. The manifestations are cyanosis, dyspnea, edema, and somnolence. In addition, most clients have a reduced vital capacity and polycythemia. Blood gas exchange is also directly affected. Although the Pickwickian syndrome is rare, caution should always be used when sedatives are used for the morbidly obese person, since these drugs can precipitate severe respiratory complications.

The incidence of diabetes mellitus is quite high in obese persons. Excessive food intake stimulates hyperinsulinemia. Through a negative-feedback mechanism, excessive insulin levels decrease the number of insulin-receptor sites on adipose cells. The loss of insulin-receptor sites decreases the amount of glucose that can enter the cells. This promotes high levels of blood glucose. Weight reduction reverses this process.

Gallstone formation in the obese client is also quite common. The incidence of gallstones rises as the body weight increases. There is a concomitant rise in the serum cholesterol and triglyceride levels as well as an increase in body weight. These levels tend to fall as obesity is corrected. The high levels can also contribute to the development of coronary heart disease.

Excessive weight on the weight-bearing joints (hips and knees) and the lower spine can cause much pain and discomfort. Although obesity has not been implicated as a cause of degenerative joint disease, it is a predisposing factor. Obesity may contribute to the pathogenesis of osteoarthritis in multiple joints in which the disease process has already started.

Other complications associated with obesity are menstrual irregularities, infertility, endometrial cancer, and fatty liver infiltration. Understandably, the life expectancy of an obese person can be shortened as a result of the problems encountered.

In addition to the many physical complications associated with obesity, the client may suffer from long-standing emotional and social problems. Society puts great emphasis on attaining and maintaining the healthy and vigorous look. Those who deviate from this prescribed standard often meet with discrimination and disdain. The very fat person may find it difficult to obtain a desired job, social acceptance at school, or membership in organizations. Choice of clothing is often limited in style, color, size, and quantity. These socioemotional problems may be manifested in poor self-esteem and body image.

Diagnostic Studies

The management of obesity must be well planned and have the total commitment of the physician and the client. Although less than 5% of all cases of obesity are of organic origin, diagnostic evaluation for such conditions must be a first step in the treatment process. A thorough history and physical examination are necessary and will reveal the extent and duration of the obese state.

There is no definite agreement on a technique for determining who is obese. Several methods are currently in use. One widely used method is to compare the client's weight to a standardized weight-for-height chart and then designate the client to be a percentage overweight. Table 35-21 provides a standardized weight-for-height chart. Normal weight depends largely on body build. A limitation of this method of assessing obesity can be seen from the following example: A person who inherits a medium frame and bulky muscle mass may be considered 20% overweight according to the standardized chart and yet not be obese.

A more scientific method of determining the amount of body fat is by measuring skin fold thickness with special calipers at one of four body sites: biceps, triceps, subscapular, or suprailiac. Accurate estimates of body fat are then derived as a result of correlations established with body density from anthropometric charts. Although considered a more exact technique, this method also has limitations. As a person ages, total body fat increases, as does the skin fold thickness for the fatty tissue at each site. The disadvantage of this method of calculating the degree of obesity is that the standards for the skin fold thickness are generally obtained from healthy young men and women, 20 to 30 years of age, and do not consider age-related changes.

The least reliable technique and yet perhaps the most frequently used is direct observation of the client. A subjective assessment of total body fat is made. The ideal body is one that has only a thin layer of adipose tissue covering the skeletal frame. When a roll of excess subcutaneous adipose tissue is seen, the client is considered obese.

Diagnostic studies may include a chest film and barium contrast studies of the upper and lower GI tracts. An oral cholecystogram may be performed, since the incidence of gallstones is high in obese clients. Arterial blood gases

Table 35-21 Desirable Weights for Men and Women (According to Weight in Pounds According to Frame, Ages 25 and Over)

Height	Small	Medium	Large
MEN			
5′ 2″	128-134	131-141	138-150
5′ 3″	130-136	133-143	140-153
5′ 4″	132-138	135-145	142-156
5′ 5″	134-140	137-148	144-160
5′ 6″	136-142	139-151	146-164
5′ 7″	138-145	142-154	149-168
5′ 8″	140-148	145-157	152-172
5′ 9″	142-151	148-160	155-176
5′10″	144-154	151-163	158-180
5′11″	146-157	154-166	161-184
6′	149-160	157-170	164-188
6′ 1″	152-164	160-174	168-192
6′ 2″	155-168	164-178	172-197
6′ 3″	158-172	167-182	176-202
6′ 4″	162-176	171-187	181-207
WOMEN			
4′10″	102-111	109-121	118-131
4′11″	103-113	111-123	120-134
5′	104-115	113-126	122-137
5′ 1″	106-118	115-129	125-140
5′ 2″	108-121	118-132	128-143
5′ 3″	111-124	121-135	131-147
5′ 4″	114-127	124-138	134-151
5′ 5″	117-130	127-141	137-155
5′ 6″	120-133	130-144	140-159
5′ 7″	123-136	133-147	143-163
5′ 8″	126-139	136-150	146-167
5′ 9″	129-142	139-153	149-170
5′10″	132-145	142-156	152-173
5′11″	135-148	145-159	155-176
6′	138-151	148-162	158-179

From 1983 Metropolitan Life Insurance Company weight tables by height and size of frame for people aged 25 to 59, in 1-inch shoes and wearing 5 pounds of indoor clothing for men or 3 pounds for women.

(ABGs) and pulmonary function tests may be performed to assess respiratory status.

The physician explores genetic and endocrine factors in the workup. Etiological factors such as hypothyroidism, hypothalamic tumors, Cushing's syndrome, hypogonadism in men, or polycystic ovarian disease in women are studied. Laboratory tests of liver function, fasting glucose level, triglyceride level, and low- and high-density lipoprotein cholesterol levels assist in evaluating the cause of obesity.

Therapeutic Management

Conservative therapy. When no organic cause can be found for obesity, a supervised plan of care should be devised that will lead to successful weight reduction. The

Table 35-22 1200-Calorie-Restricted Weight-Reduction Diet*

GENERAL PRINCIPLES

1. Eat regularly. Do not skip meals.
2. Measure foods to determine the correct portion size.
3. Avoid concentrated sweets, such as sugar, candy, honey, pies, cakes, cookies, and regular sodas.
4. Reduce fat intake by baking, broiling, or steaming foods.
5. Maintain a regular exercise program for successful weight loss.

Meal	Exchanges			
Breakfast	1 meat	1 scrambled egg	1 hard-boiled egg	1 oz ham
	2 bread	1 slice toast ¾ cup dry cereal (unsweetened)	1 flour tortilla ½ cup Cream of Wheat	2 griddle cakes with diet syrup
	1 fruit	½ small banana	⅓ cup orange juice	⅓ cup pineapple juice
	1 fat	1 tsp margarine 1 sausage link†	1 slice bacon	1 tsp margarine
	1 dairy	1 cup low-fat milk	1 cup low-fat milk	1 cup low-fat milk
	Beverage	Coffee	Coffee	Coffee
Lunch	2 meat	1 slice bologna 1 slice cheese	Cheese enchiladas (made with 2 oz cheese, 2 corn tortillas, chili sauce)	2 oz baked breaded pork chop
	2 bread	2 slices bread		1 corn muffin
	Vegetable	Lettuce, pickles	Tomato wedges	Spinach
	1 fruit	Fresh grapes (12)	2 canned peach halves (packed in water)	Fresh orange
	Beverage	Diet soda	Artificially sweetened lemonade	Unsweetened iced tea
Dinner	2 meat	2 oz roast beef	Chili con carne (made with ½ cup ground beef, ½ cup pinto beans, and chili powder)	2 oz baked chicken
	1 bread	Baked potato (with 1 tsp margarine†)		Corn on the cob with 1 tsp margarine
	Vegetable	Cooked carrots	Tossed salad and 1 tbs salad dressing†	Okra
	1 fruit	¾ cup strawberries	Fresh apple	Fruit cocktail (packed in water)
	1 milk	1 cup low-fat milk	1 cup low-fat milk	1 cup low-fat milk

*For 1000 calories, omit 1 fruit exchange and change low-fat milk to skim milk. For 1500 calories, add 1 meat, 1 fruit, and 2 fat exchanges. Change low-fat milk to whole milk. For 1800 calories, add 2 bread, 3 meat, 3 fat, and 1 fruit exchanges. Change low-fat milk to whole milk.
†1 extra fat exchange allowed for each cup of 2% low-fat milk; 2 extra fat exchanges allowed for each cup of skim milk.

plan should focus primarily on dietary reduction and a sensible exercise program.

A good reducing diet should contain foods from the basic four food groups and should be as similar to the client's usual eating pattern as is permissible. A diet that includes adequate amounts of fruits and vegetables provides enough bulk to prevent constipation and meet daily vitamin A and C requirements. Lean meat, fish, and eggs provide sufficient protein and the B complex vitamins. The amount of caloric intake may need to be restricted to 800 to 1500 calories per day, depending on the client's age, weight, nutritional status, and length of time estimated for ideal weight to be achieved. Table 35-22 contains a sample 1200-calorie reducing diet.

Because most obese persons are sedentary, a planned exercise program should be implemented in conjunction with caloric reduction. There is no evidence that exercise promotes an increase in appetite or leads to dietary excess. In fact, exercise frequently has just the opposite effect. Walking is considered the best type of exercise for the obese person, since it is the easiest form of physical activity that can be performed safely.

Medications have been used in the treatment of obesity but only as adjuncts to a good diet and exercise program. These drugs are used to suppress appetite. Although a variety of drugs have been used, diuretics, laxatives, antispasmodics, thyroid hormone, amphetamines, and amphetaminelike adrenergic drugs are the most commonly prescribed. Amphetamines do suppress the appetite and facilitate weight loss. However, when the pharmacological effects of the drug wear off or the drug is discontinued, the appetite generally returns and weight gain is resumed unless food reduction and the exercise program are maintained. Amphetamines should never be prescribed for extended periods or under conditions in which supervised control may not be possible. There is always a potential for drug abuse and dependence. These drugs should be used with caution in clients with hypertension, cardiovascular disease, or hyperthyroidism because of the drugs' sympathomimetic effects, which can aggravate these conditions. Some states have banned the use of amphetamines in the treatment of obesity.

Surgical Interventions

Surgical interventions are never the primary method of weight reduction and should be used only after the more conventional treatments have failed.

For a client to be selected for any of the operations for morbid obesity, the following criteria are considered:

1. Massive obesity for 5 years
2. Failure to reduce weight with other forms of therapy
3. Body weight 100 pounds above the ideal for age, sex, and height
4. No serious endocrine problem causing the obesity
5. Absence of other medical conditions (liver disease, alcoholism, cardiovascular or pulmonary disease, inflammatory bowel disease, cancer)
6. Psychiatric and social stability
7. Availability of a team of physicians to provide immediate and long-term care
8. Presence of a high-risk condition that weight loss would ameliorate

Some physicians believe that low intelligence, possible pregnancy, and age are limiting factors to the consideration of surgical intervention. Clients below the age of 20 or over the age of 50 are frequently discouraged from seeking surgical treatment. Weight reduction is more difficult to achieve with increasing age, and the complications that accompany these procedures are more devastating with age. The surgical procedures used in the treatment of obesity are presented in Table 35-23.

Lipectomy. Lipectomy (adipectomy) is performed to remove unsightly flabby folds of adipose tissue. Clients who choose adipectomies do so for cosmetic reasons. In some clients, up to 15% of the total fat cells are removed from the breasts, abdomen, and lumbar and femoral areas. There is no evidence that a regeneration of adipose tissue occurs at the surgical sites. However, it must be emphasized to the client that surgical removal does not prevent obesity from recurring, since lifetime eating habits often

Table 35-23 Surgical Procedures Used in the Treatment of Obesity

Purpose	Procedure
Reduction of adipose tissue	Lipectomy
	Liposuction
Reduction in food intake	Jaw wiring
	Gastroplasty
	Gastric bypass
	Intragastric balloon
Reduction in food absorption	Intestinal bypass

remain the same. Although body image and self-esteem may be enhanced by such procedures, these operations are not without complications. The dangerous effects of general anesthesia and the potential for poor wound healing in the obese client cannot be overemphasized. It is more useful for the majority of clients contemplating adipectomy to be instructed in preventive health measures, such as slow weight reduction to maintain and preserve tissue integrity, the value of exercise, and behavior-modification techniques.

Liposuction. A surgical procedure recently introduced is called *liposuction* or *suction-assisted lipectomy*. The current use is for cosmetic purposes and not for weight reduction. This surgical intervention helps to improve facial appearance or body contours. A candidate for this type of surgery is one who has achieved weight reduction but who has excess fat under the chin, along the jawline, in the nasolabial folds, over the abdomen, or around the waist and upper thighs. The procedure is relatively easy to perform and free of complications. A long, hollow, stainless steel cannula is inserted through a small incision over the fatty tissue to be suctioned. The purpose of this type of surgery is to improve body appearance, thereby enhancing body image and self-concept.

Jaw wiring. During the past few years many obese clients have had their jaws wired in an attempt to achieve weight reduction. The client is able to speak after the procedure but is able to ingest only fluids. This type of obesity treatment does achieve weight loss but does not change the basic eating patterns of the person when the wires are removed. Weight is usually regained. While the jaw is wired, the client must carry wire cutters at all times. Both the client and the family need to be instructed in the use of wire cutters in times of emergency such as vomiting, choking, and cardiac arrest. Compliance with a meticulous oral hygiene regimen is essential while the wires are in place. Frequent dental checkups are advisable during this period because irritation to the cheeks and gingivae may occur from the wires. Routine brushing and gingival stimulation are encouraged. (The nursing care of clients with wired jaws is discussed in Chapter 34.) At present, jaw wiring is more acceptable when performed before gastric bypass surgery or gastroplasty, when immediate weight loss is advantageous to the outcome of this more hazardous surgical intervention.

Table 35-24   Surgical Interventions for Morbid Obesity

Jejunoileal Bypass	Gastric Bypass	Gastroplasty	
		Gastric Partitioning	Gastric Vertical Banding
METHOD OF WEIGHT LOSS			
Controlled malabsorption	Reduced gastric capacity	Reduced gastric capacity	Reduced gastric capacity
ANATOMICAL CHANGE			
End-to-end jejunileal by-pass	Roux-en-Y procedure	Small gastric pouch	Small gastric pouch

ADVANTAGES			
None—complications outweigh any advantages.	A great and sustained weight loss is obtained. A better state of health results than with jejunileal bypass.	Procedure is easy to perform. No anastomosis is necessary. A more normal anatomy and physiology are maintained.	Procedure is easy to perform. No anastomosis is necessary. A more normal anatomy and physiology are maintained.

Intragastric balloon. A recent innovation used to control oral intake is the cylindrical plastic balloon called the *gastric bubble*. Following introduction into the stomach by endoscopy, the balloon is inflated, thus reducing the size of the stomach to a size similar to that achieved by gastroplasty. Initially the gastric bubble was acclaimed as the new nonsurgical means to weight loss. With further use, significant side effects such as stomach ulcers and the potential for perforation are now recognized. The bubble has been known to collapse spontaneously in the stomach, requiring surgical removal, and it has caused intestinal obstruction. The chief advantage of this weight-control measure is its ease of insertion. Prolonged use of the gastric bubble will determine its proper place as a weight-control strategy.

Surgical bypass procedures and gastroplasty. The obese client may be considered a candidate for an intestinal bypass (jejunoileal), a gastric bypass, or gastroplasty (gastric partitioning and vertical banding) (Table 35-24). Generally these surgical procedures are indicated only for clients who are morbidly obese (body weight two times or more above normal) and who have failed to lose weight with all other prescribed weight-loss regimens.

The *jejunoileal bypass* procedure results in weight loss by producing malabsorption. In this procedure, the proximal jejunum is anastomosed to the last 4 inches of ileum.

The remainder of the small intestine is left undisturbed. As a result, almost 90% of the small intestine is bypassed and malabsorption is achieved.

The jejunoileal bypass is no longer performed by many surgeons because of the many complications associated with it. Most of the long-term complications are related to malabsorption from the short functioning intestine, the toxic effects from overgrowth of coliform bacteria in the excluded bowel, or combinations of these factors.

The *gastric bypass* operation induces weight loss by reducing food intake and producing only minimal malabsorption. With the Roux-en-Y surgical procedure, the stomach size is reduced. The procedure consists of stapling the stomach without transection to create a 30 to 45 ml pouch and a gastrojejunostomy. The Roux-en-Y gastric bypass is now considered the "gold standard" for gastric restrictive procedures.[11] The chief contraindications to this surgical procedure are history of peptic ulcer disease, coronary artery disease, malignant lesions, drug dependence, alcohol abuse, and psychiatric problems.

Gastroplasty (gastric partitioning or vertical banding) is a third type of surgical procedure that is used to induce weight loss in the morbidly obese person. When the *partitioning procedure* is used, the stomach is partitioned into a small upper portion and a large distal portion by dividing the stomach, either by surgical transection or by the placement of two rows of staples. A small channel is left open in both operations so that ingested food and fluid can slowly pass through from the small upper portion into the larger distal end. The new upper gastric pouch holds approximately 2 to 3 ounces of food or fluid at any one time.

The other form of gastroplasty is *vertical banding*. This procedure consists of the placement of vertical staples to create a pouch and channel for food flow. The channel is reinforced with prosthetic material. This procedure has achieved considerable success in the management of weight loss.

Gastroplasty has several advantages over the gastric bypass operation. It is technically easier to perform, especially when stapling is used. If reversal of the procedure is required, removal of the staples is easier than the difficult procedure of converting the gastric bypass. In addition, symptoms of the dumping syndrome and malabsorption are eliminated.

■ Nursing Management of the Obese Client

Nursing assessment

The nurse, working closely with the physician and dietitian, plays a major role in the planning and management of the obese client. By asking specific and leading questions, the nurse can often obtain information that the client may withhold out of embarrassment or shyness or because of being a poor historian. Information that can assist the nurse in understanding obese clients and provide a basis for intervention is presented in Table 35-25. The nurse must provide acceptable reasons for such personally intrusive questions, respond to the client's concerns about diagnostic tests, and interpret test outcomes. The client's answers to questions must be treated with respect, understanding, and a nonjudgmental attitude, regardless of neg-

Table 35-25 Nursing Assessment of the Obese Client

Client's perception of cause of obesity

Frequency of eating

Factors that contribute to overeating, such as boredom, time of day, stress

Physical problems associated with obesity, such as cardiac problems, chronic joint pain, respiratory problems, diabetes mellitus

Psychosocial problems related to obesity, such as feelings of rejection, isolation, guilt, or shame

Detailed family history of possible genetic or endocrine cause of obesity

Reproductive history, including menstrual and menopausal history

Adult- or juvenile-onset obesity

Dietary patterns and history from the past week, including types and amount of food ingested

Attitude related to a long-term commitment to a weight-loss program

History of compliance with prescribed reducing diets in the past

Factors that influenced success or failure of past reducing plans

Resources to support a reducing diet, both personal and financial

ative personal feelings the nurse may have about obesity and working with "fat" people.

Anthropomorphic measurements are an integral part of the assessment of obese persons. The nurse may perform these measurements and explain their significance to the client. Measurements used with the obese person include skin fold thickness as well as height, weight, waist and hip size, and calculation of the waist to hip ratio. This ratio provides supplementary data about the adverse metabolic impact of the person's obesity. Accumulation of fat cells in the gluteal-femoral area may be metabolically inert except during the latter part of pregnancy and during lactation. Fat distributed over the abdomen and upper body (neck, arms, and shoulders) and known as *android obesity* is associated with a greater cardiovascular risk of hypertension, diabetes mellitus, dyslipidemia, ischemic heart disease, stroke, and death. The nurse should emphasize that this type of obesity be treated vigorously. When the fat distribution is peripheral (gluteal-femoral), it is called *gynecoid obesity*. The client should be informed that this type of obesity carries a better prognosis but may be more difficult to reduce.[5,12]

As part of the initial nursing physical assessment, each body system needs to be examined with particular attention to the organ system in which the client has expressed a problem or concern. Providing specific documentation on these areas assists the physician with a more in-depth history and physical examination.

Nursing diagnoses

Nursing diagnoses specific to the client with obesity include, but are not limited to, the following:

1. Altered nutrition: more than body requirements related to excessive intake in relation to metabolic need and decreased activity
2. Impaired physical mobility related to excessive body weight
3. Social isolation related to alterations in physical appearance and perceived unattractiveness
4. High risk for impaired skin integrity related to alterations in nutritional state (obesity), immobility, excess moisture, and multiple skin folds
5. Ineffective breathing pattern related to decreased lung expansion from obesity
6. High risk for noncompliance with treatment regimen related to alteration in perception and/or lack of motivation
7. Body-image disturbance related to deviation from usual or expected body size and inability to lose or retain weight loss

Nursing interventions

Diet teaching. The only effective method of treating obesity is to restrict dietary intake so that it is below energy requirements. It is rare to find an overweight person who has not at some time attempted to lose weight. Some have met with limited and temporary success, and others have met only with failure. It is likely that the great majority of these persons attempted weight loss by trying out one of the many fad diets that offer the enticement to eat and get slim. Fad diets in general claim weight loss quickly and inexpensively. Although it is true that body weight is lost initially, it is not fat but body water that is lost. The normal fat cell is composed of about 80% fat, 18% water, and 2% protein. It is also a storage area for glycogen. Glycogen is known to bind with water. Because most reducing diets severely restrict carbohydrate, the body's glycogen stores become depleted within a few days. It is only when the glycogen-water pool is almost depleted of energy that adipose tissue is burned up to release energy for bodily functions.

Obese clients need to understand that following a well-balanced, low-caloric diet is the most sensible approach to weight loss and will have a more satisfying and long-lasting result than fad diets. Table 35-22 presents an example of a weight-reduction diet.

The degree of success of any reducing diet depends on the amount of weight to be lost. A moderately obese person will obviously attain the goal more easily than will a massively obese person. Adult-onset obesity is much more amenable to successful treatment than the obesity of juvenile onset. In juvenile-onset obesity, the eating patterns have been present for many years and the number of fat cells is usually much higher. As a result, more drastic dieting efforts and perseverance are necessary to achieve weight reduction.

Motivation is the essential ingredient for achievement of success. The obese client must see the need for weight loss and the advantages that will accrue. The nurse can assist by helping the client to look at eating patterns through a diet diary. A frank discussion of eating habits helps the client to realize that often eating is done not because of hunger but because of bad habits picked up over time. The bad habits must be changed or weight loss will be only temporary.

Setting a realistic goal, such as losing 1 to 2 pounds per week, must be agreed on at the outset. Trying to lose too much too fast usually results in a sense of frustration and failure for the client. The nurse can help the client understand that losing large amounts of weight in a short period of time causes the adipose tissue to lose elasticity and tone and become unsightly folds of flabby tissue. Slower weight loss offers better cosmetic results. Inevitably, the client reaches plateau periods during which no weight is lost. These plateaus may last from several days to several weeks. It is especially important that the client know that these are normal occurrences encountered during weight reduction to prevent discouragment or frustration and giving up of the prescribed dietary plan. A weekly check of body weight is a good method of monitoring progress. Daily weighing is not recommended because of the frequent fluctuations resulting from retained urine and feces. The client should be instructed to weigh at the same time of day, wearing the same type of clothing.

There is no firm agreement on the number of meals to be eaten when a person is on a diet. Some nutritionists advocate several small meals a day because the body's metabolic rate is temporarily increased immediately after eating. When several small meals a day are ingested, more calories are burned. There seems to be general agreement that consumption of most of the daily caloric intake at a large evening meal results in less weight loss than when the calories are evenly distributed throughout the day.

When a person is first starting on a dietary program, food portions should be weighed in order to stay within the dietary guidelines. After a time, weighing may not be necessary because the client can make accurate judgments of size and weight. A list of permitted foods serves as a good reference and permits an occasional meal to be eaten at a restaurant. The client who carefully follows the prescribed diet will not need to take vitamin supplements. Appropriate fluid intake should be encouraged. Alcoholic beverages are usually not permitted on a reducing diet because they increase the caloric intake and are low in nutritional value.

Exercise teaching. Once an exercise program has been outlined for the client, the nurse can reinforce instruction and help individualize it to the client's time schedule and physical limitations. The nurse should point out that engaging in weekend exercise only or in spurts of strenuous activity is not advantageous and can actually be dangerous. Joining a health spa can be one mechanism of getting exercise. However, sitting in a sauna and trying to spot-reduce a specific part of the body do not constitute an appropriate daily program. Walking, swimming, and cycling are more sensible forms of exercise and have more long-range benefits. The combination of a good reducing diet and an exercise program can have profound effects on the client's achievement of weight loss. A major benefit derived from exercise involving the long muscles is cardiovascular conditioning.

Many psychological benefits can be derived from an exercise program. Reduction in tension and stress, better-quality sleep and rest, decreased desire to eat excessively, increased stamina and energy, improved self-concept and self-confidence, better attitudes toward work and play, and increased optimism about the future can be achieved.

Drug therapy teaching. The role of the nurse in relation to drug therapy should center around teaching about proper administration and side effects. Emphasis should be on the dangers of drug dependence and tolerance. The modification of dosage without consultation with the physician or the nurse can have detrimental effects. The nurse should reemphasize that the diet and exercise regimens are the cornerstone of permanent weight loss. Medications are only psychological aids that do not help the client change eating behavior. The purchase of over-the-counter diet aids should be discouraged.

Behavior-modification training. The person who is on any type of restrictive dietary program is often encouraged to join a group of other obese persons who are receiving professional counseling to help them modify their eating habits. The assumption behind behavior modification is that obesity is a learned disorder caused by overeating and that the critical difference between an obese person and a nonobese person is in the way they eat. Therefore most behavior-modification programs deemphasize the diet and focus on how the person eats. Participants are taught to restrict their eating to designated meals and to increase the amount of physical activity in their lives. Persons who have undergone behavior therapy are more successful in maintaining their losses over an extended time than those who followed a diet alone.

Many self-help groups are available to the person who wants to learn more about successful dieting and who likes the support of others having the same problems and experiences. TOPS (Take Off Pounds Sensibly) is the oldest nonprofit organization of this type. Behavioral modification is an integral part of the program, along with nutrition education. Weight Watchers International, Inc. is probably the most successful commercial weight-reduction enterprise. Weight Watchers offers a food plan that is nutritionally balanced and practical to follow, and it has used behavior-modification techniques since 1974. Other self-help groups and organizations are Overeaters Anonymous, Weight Losers, Trim Clubs, Inc., and the Diet Workshop, Inc. These groups offer diet education, exercise plans, and behavior modification.

There has been a proliferation of commercial weight-reduction centers across the nation. Many of these programs are staffed by nurses and require an initial physical examination by a physician before a client is accepted for weight reduction. These weight-reduction centers are costly and are therefore prohibitive to those in the lower socioeconomic class. Many of these programs also offer special prepackaged foods and supplements that must be purchased as part of the weight-reduction plan. Only these prescribed foods and drinks are to be consumed until an agreed-on amount of weight is lost. The client is encouraged to buy the same type of foods for the maintenance phase of the program, lasting from 6 months to a year. Behavior-modification training is incorporated within these programs as well. Although persons who follow this type of program are likely to lose weight, once they leave the program the weight is usually regained because they tend to resume prior eating behaviors and return to the foods previously eaten.

A new concept of influencing health behavior and better employee health has occurred recently. Programs on health teaching and maintenance have been started at the place of employment. The rationale for such programs is that better health repays the cost of the programs through improved work performance, decreased absenteeism, and, eventually, less hospitalization. Weight-reduction and hypertension programs have been instituted and are very popular with employees.

Preoperative care. Special considerations are necessary in the care of clients who are admitted to the hospital for surgical treatment of obesity, especially the morbidly obese. Most nursing units are not prepared to meet the needs of a client who is often too large for a typical hospital or recovery room bed or who has arms or legs that even a large-size blood pressure cuff will not fit. To eliminate embarrassment for the client and frustration for the staff, plans for these special needs must be made before the client's admission. Oversized blood pressure cuffs should be ready for use when the client arrives. A private room may be necessary for privacy of the client and to accommodate the bed and sitting arrangements. A strongly reinforced trapeze bar should be placed over the bed to facilitate movement and positioning. In some cases a specially constructed chair may have to be built and beds joined together to allow the client to sit and sleep in comfort.

A care-planning conference should be a priority so that even simple nursing care measures do not become impossible tasks. Consideration should be given to such things as how the client will be weighed, how the client will be transported throughout the hospital, and how simple physical assessment strategies may have to be adjusted to accommodate the morbidly obese client. Anticipating ahead of time the need to use the hospital's meat or freight scales saves time and energy later for both the staff and the client. Another need is a wheelchair with removable arms that is large enough to accommodate the client and that will easily pass through doorways. Strategies for bathing, turning, and ambulating the client, including the number of extra hands needed to carry out these measures, are invaluable when the actual need arises. Special gowns are also needed. Routine physical assessment strategies do not work well with a morbidly obese female client who has numerous layers of skin folds covering the chest and abdomen in addition to huge, pendulous breasts obscuring the area to be assessed. Without identifying alternatives or unique methods of dealing with this problem, assessment of respiratory status and bowel sounds or even wound inspection will be unpleasant.

Wound infection is one of the most common complications after surgery. Because of the many layers of flabby skin folds, especially in the abdominal area, preoperative skin preparation is very important. Frequently, the client is instructed to take several showers a day for several days before admission to the hospital. Careful cleansing with soap and warm water of the abdominal area from the breasts to below the waist is emphasized.

The client must be instructed in the proper coughing technique, deep breathing, and methods of turning and positioning to prevent pulmonary complications after surgery. The use of a spirometer may be introduced before surgery. Because most obese clients breathe shallowly, use of the spirometer helps prevent and alleviate postoperative lung congestion.

All clients admitted for major bypass surgery, gastroplasty, or partitioning procedures have an NG tube inserted during surgery and attached to suction after surgery. Allowing the client to see a typical tube and explaining why it is necessary is a good method of involving the client in the plan of care. The client should know that oral nourishment will be impossible for a few days after the surgery and that IV fluids will be the main source of intake. Hyperalimentation nutritional support may be necessary for some clients.

Early ambulation is mandatory for these clients. It is essential the client know that it is usually necessary to get out of bed very soon after surgery and with increasing frequency thereafter—generally three to four times each day. The dangers of thrombophlebitis and measures to counteract its development are a routine part of preoperative teaching. The client should know that elastic stockings or elastic wraps will be applied to the legs and that active and passive range-of-motion exercises will be a frequent part of daily care. Low-dose heparin will also be ordered. (General preoperative nursing care is discussed in Chapter 11.)

Postoperative care. The client experiences considerable abdominal pain after the operation. Administration of pain medications should be given as frequently as necessary during the immediate postoperative period. The nurse must remember that IM medications must be given with an extra long needle, such as a spinal needle, so that the medication is administered into the muscle and not into the subcutaneous tissue, which will delay absorption. Because prevention of pulmonary complications is a major nursing goal, it must be anticipated that the client will not fully cooperate when having a great deal of discomfort. In addition, the large amount of truncal adipose tissue, especially on the abdomen and chest, compromises respiratory ability. Keeping the head of the bed elevated at a 30-degree angle at all times facilitates ventilatory efforts. Encouraging and assisting the client to turn, cough, and deep breathe at least every 1 to 2 hours prevents atelectasis and pneumonia. Frequent mouth and nose care also helps breathing efforts, since the NG tube is inserted through one nostril.

Position changes and range-of-motion exercises are instituted immediately after surgery and carried out every 1 to 2 hours. Ambulatory efforts are begun on the evening of surgery. The nurse should enlist the assistance of other staff members during these initial efforts while encouraging the client to help.

The abdominal wound requires frequent observation for amount and type of drainage, condition of the sutures, and signs of infection. The incision must be protected against undue straining that accompanies turning and coughing. Wound dehiscence and wound healing are potential problems with all obese clients. Monitoring the vital signs assists in identifying problems such as infection.

It is important that the NG tube be kept patent and in the correct position. Vomiting is a common occurrence following gastric bypass and gastric partitioning procedures. If patency is blocked or the tube requires repositioning, the physician should be notified at once. The upper gastric pouch is very small, and irrigating the tube with too much solution or manipulating tube position can lead to disruption of the anastomosis or staple line. In most cases the NG tube can be removed in about 48 hours or when bowel sounds have resumed.

Skin care should be carried out several times each shift. Perspiration may be excessive at times. The many layers of flabby skin should be kept clean and dry so that this source of irritation is eliminated. Clients who have jejunoileal bypass experience severe diarrhea early in their postoperative period. This is due to malabsorption created by surgical shortening of the small intestine. Meticulous care of the skin around the anal area and administration of antidiarrheal medications must be initiated immediately. For the client who has an indwelling catheter perineal care is important so that a urinary tract infection can be avoided.

Clear liquids are given orally when tolerance is established. The amount offered at first is necessarily limited to about 1 ounce, which is to be sipped slowly. More solid types of food are given to the client who has had bypass surgery as progress is made through the postoperative recovery period. Clients who have had gastroplasty surgery are kept on a fluid diet for a longer time. The need for a liquid diet only is based on the rationale that the ingestion of too much fluid or foods can cause disruption of the staple or suture line, leading to leakage and possible peritonitis.

Discharge teaching. Clients who have undergone major surgical treatment for their obesity have not been successful in following a prescribed diet. Now they are forced to reduce their oral intake as a result of the anatomical changes brought about by the operative procedure. These clients find they must adhere to a reduced intake because of their concern for abdominal distention, cramping abdominal pain, increased and foul-smelling flatus, and frequent diarrhea.

Weight loss is considerable during the first 6 to 12 months. Most weight is lost by those who have bypass surgery. It is during this time that the client must learn to adjust intake sufficiently to maintain a stable weight. Although behavior modification was not an intended outcome when these surgical procedures were devised, it becomes an unexpected secondary gain. The diet generally prescribed should be high in protein and low in carbohydrates, fat, and roughage and consist of six small feedings daily. Fluids should not be ingested with the meal, and in some cases, fluids should be restricted to less than 1000 ml/day. Fluids and foods high in carbohydrate tend to promote diarrhea and symptoms of the dumping syndrome.

Vitamin deficiencies are a long-term concern after bypass surgery due to the induced malabsorption and the body's inability to absorb important vitamins such as A, C, and D. B_{12} supplements are usually prescribed on a permanent basis because absorption of this vitamin takes place in the ileum. Ileal absorption capacity is drastically reduced by the surgical intestinal bypass. The client should be aware of the signs and symptoms of vitamin deficiencies as well as electrolyte imbalances (Table 35-5). It is often necessary to replace iron, calcium, and potassium to maintain required physiological levels.

Diarrhea may continue for several years after intestinal bypass. Some clients still pass as many as six to eight stools a day at the end of a year. Proper diet and use of antidiarrheal medications must be clearly understood by the client. Other troublesome problems frequently encountered after intestinal bypass are urinary and biliary stones, polyarthritis, and polymyalgia. Late complications can also be anticipated after gastric bypass or gastroplasty. Some of the complications seen with intestinal bypass surgery occur, including anemia, vitamin deficiencies, diarrhea, and psychiatric problems. Failure to lose weight or loss of too much weight may be caused by the surgical formation of too large a stomach pouch or of an outlet that is much too small, respectively. Peptic ulcer formation, the dumping syndrome, and small bowel obstruction may be seen late in the recovery and rehabilitative stage.

Long-term follow-up care must be stressed because of the many complications found late in the recovery period. The client must be encouraged to strictly adhere to the prescribed diet and to keep the physician informed of any changes in physical or emotional condition. Some clients have been known to overeat when they return home and to gain rather than lose weight.

Reversal of the surgical procedures may be required for some clients. Reversal of the gastric bypass is extremely difficult due to the technical nature of the procedure. The jejunoileal bypass can be reversed or restored more easily. Rationales for revisional surgery include hepatic failure, weight loss below ideal weight, debilitating weakness, severe psychiatric problems, intractable electrolyte deficiencies, pulmonary tuberculosis, and renal failure.

The nurse must anticipate and recognize several potential psychological problems after surgery. Some clients express guilt feelings over the fact that the only way they could lose weight was by surgical means rather than by the "sheer willpower" of reduced dietary intake. The nurse should be ready to provide support so that these clients do not dwell on negative feelings.

Many morbidly obese clients who blamed their feelings of social inferiority or inadequacies on their appearance before bypass surgery may suffer from episodes of depression. A possible hypothesis for the depression is the result of their altered body image and therefore the loss of a major coping strategy. By 6 to 8 months after surgery, considerable weight loss has occurred, and they are able to clearly see how much their appearance has changed. Massive weight loss often leaves the client with large quantities of flabby skin that result in body image as well as hygienic problems. Reconstructive surgery at least 1 full year after the initial surgery may alleviate this unsightly situation. Reduction of the breasts, upper arms, thighs, and excess abdominal skin folds are possible solutions.

Discussion of this possible outcome with the client before surgery and again during the rehabilitation phase of recovery helps facilitate the client's adjustment to a new body image and social reintegration.

C ase Study

OBESITY

Helen, a 42-year-old woman, came to the Obesity Clinic asking to be placed on a weight-reduction program. She is 5 feet 3 inches tall and weighs 232 pounds. The normal weight for Helen's medium body frame is 121 to 135 pounds. She stated that she has been overweight since her first pregnancy at the age of 22. She explained that she gained additional weight with each subsequent pregnancy (four in all). She has never been able to maintain any weight loss, even though she has tried many popular reducing plans throughout the years.

Helen's gallbladder was removed 3 years ago because of gallstones. Before the surgery her physician put her on a 1200-calorie reducing diet. She was able to lose 30 pounds in 4 months but admits she eventually went off the diet because she was not losing weight fast enough and was discouraged. She has since regained all the weight lost plus an additional 15 pounds.

During the past year, Helen has noticed that she becomes short of breath with minimal exertion. She also complains of a chronic low backache and sore knees after being on her feet for even a short time. As a result, she is unable to engage in social activities outside her home or to perform household chores as in the past.

Physical examination reveals Helen to be morbidly obese. Auscultation of breath sounds reveals "wheezes" throughout the lung fields with a respiratory rate of 28 per minute. Pulmonary function tests show a greatly reduced vital capacity. Blood gas determinations show a $Paco_2$ of 45 mm Hg. All endocrine evaluations are within normal limits, with the exception of a fasting blood sugar of 135 mg/dl.

Discussion Questions

1. How does adipose tissue form within the body?
2. What is the difference between juvenile-onset obesity and adult-onset obesity? Which type does Helen have?
3. What are the dangers inherent in following fad diets for quick weight loss?
4. What are the possible complications of obesity from a medical and social standpoint?
5. What is the pathophysiology of Helen's pulmonary and joint discomfort?
6. What are the merits of a good weight-reduction program and how should the nurse counsel the obese client?
7. What are the surgical interventions available to the obese person for the purpose of weight reduction?

R eview Questions

The number of the question corresponds to the same-numbered objective at the beginning of the chapter.

1. Vegans who use only plant food may be at risk of a deficiency in
   a. essential amino acids
   b. fat-soluble vitamins
   c. vitamin B_{12}
   d. water-soluble vitamins

2. The clinical manifestations commonly exhibited by the person with PCM include all the following *except*
   a. weak, flabby muscles
   b. severe weight loss
   c. hepatomegaly
   d. normal blood pressure and pulse

3. Common characteristics of both bulimia and anorexia nervosa include all the following *except*
   a. concealment of abnormal eating habits
   b. menstrual irregularities
   c. distorted body image
   d. intense fear and dislike of being or becoming obese

4. The nurse working with a client receiving total parenteral nutrition should know that
   a. central hyperalimentation may be administered through the femoral vein
   b. *Pseudomonas* organisms are a frequent cause of sepsis
   c. the rate of administration must never be increased or decreased abruptly
   d. the central catheter can be used for monitoring central venous pressure

5. The term *morbid obesity* is applied when a person's weight exceeds ideal body weight by
   a. 20%
   b. 100%
   c. 50%
   d. 30%

6. The most serious and difficult long-term complication following jejunoileal bypass surgery for morbid obesity is
   a. hepatic failure
   b. gallstones
   c. anemia
   d. dumping syndrome

REFERENCES

1. Burtis G, Davis J, and Martin S: Applied nutrition and diet therapy, Philadelphia, 1988, WB Saunders Co, p 87.
2. Sholevar G: Anorexia nervosa and bulimia. In Field H and Domangue B, eds: Eating disorders throughout the life span, New York, 1987, Praeger Publishers, p 31.
3. American Psychiatric Association: Diagnostic and statistical manual of mental disorders, ed 3, Washington, DC, 1987, American Psychiatric Association, pp 66-68.
4. Mickley D: Eating disorders, Hosp Pract 23:77, 1988.
5. Feldman E: Essentials of clinical nutrition, Philadelphia, 1988, FA Davis Co, p 329.
6. Lerman R: Malnutrition in hospitalized patients, Hosp Pract 21:22, 1986.
7. Schlichtig R and Ayres S: Nutritional support of the critically ill, Chicago, 1988, Year Book Medical Publishers, Inc, pp 147-164.
8. Conn H: Health and obesity: an overview in health and obesity, New York, 1982, Haven Press, p 1.
9. Field H and Domangue B, eds: Eating disorders throughout the life span, New York, 1987, Praeger Publishers, p 77.
10. Abraham S and Lewellyn-Jones D: Eating disorders: the facts, New York, 1987, Oxford University Press, p 113.
11. Bivins B and others: Surgery for morbid obesity: a continuing challenge, Henry Ford Hosp Med J 36:105, 1988.
12. Fachnine JD: Morbidity and treatment of clinically important obesity: an internal medicine perspective, Henry Ford Hosp Med J 36:109, 1988.

CHAPTER

36

Nursing Role in Management

Problems of Digestion

Gladys Elizabeth Deters

L earning Objectives

1. *Describe the pathogenesis, complications, and therapeutic and nursing management of a client with nausea and vomiting.*
2. *Differentiate between acute and chronic gastritis, including the causes, pathophysiology, and therapeutic and nursing management.*
3. *Explain the common causes, clinical manifestations, and therapeutic and nursing management of a client with upper gastrointestinal bleeding.*
4. *Compare and contrast gastric and duodenal ulcers, including pathogenesis, clinical manifestations, complications, and therapeutic and nursing management.*
5. *Explain the anatomical and physiological changes and the common complications that result from surgical procedures for gastric ulcer.*
6. *Describe the clinical manifestations and the therapeutic, surgical, and nursing management of a client with cancer of the stomach.*

NAUSEA AND VOMITING

Nausea and vomiting are the most common manifestations of gastrointestinal (GI) diseases. Although each manifestation can occur independently, they are usually closely related and treated as one problem. They are also found in a wide variety of conditions that are unrelated to GI disease. Nausea and vomiting are frequent accompaniments of pregnancy, infectious diseases, central nervous system (CNS) disorders (e.g., meningitis, CNS lesion), circulatory problems (e.g., congestive heart failure), side effects of drugs (e.g., digitalis, antibiotics), metabolic disorders (e.g., uremia), and psychological stimulation (e.g., stress, fear).

A single episode of nausea accompanied by vomiting in an adult may have no significant relationship to GI disease. If vomiting occurs several times, however, it is extremely important that the cause be identified.

Nausea is a feeling of discomfort in the epigastrium with a conscious desire to vomit. Anorexia usually accompanies nausea and is brought on by unpleasant stimulation involving any of the five senses. Generally, nausea occurs

before vomiting and is characterized by contraction of the duodenum and by slowing of gastric tone and motility.

Vomiting is the forceful ejection of partially digested food from the upper GI tract. It occurs when the gut becomes overly irritated, excited, or distended. Immediately before the act of vomiting, the person becomes aware of the need to vomit. Most of the physiological changes occur in the stomach and duodenum. The autonomic nervous system is activated and results in sympathetic stimulation, causing tachycardia, tachypnea, and diaphoresis. In addition, parasympathetic stimulation causes relaxation of the esophageal sphincter, an increase in gastric motility, and a pronounced increase in salivation. These manifestations are experienced immediately preceding the vomiting episode.

Vomiting is a complex phenomenon that requires the coordinated activities of several structures, including closure of the glottis, deep inspiration with contraction of the diaphragm in the inspiratory position, closure of the pylorus, relaxation of the stomach and cardiac sphincter, and contraction of the abdominal muscles with increasing intraabdominal pressure. These simultaneous activities force the stomach contents up through the esophagus, into the pharynx, and out the mouth. The stomach has a passive role in these activities.

Reviewed by Sally Brozenec, R.N., Ph.D., Assistant Professor, Rush University College of Nursing, Chicago, Illinois.

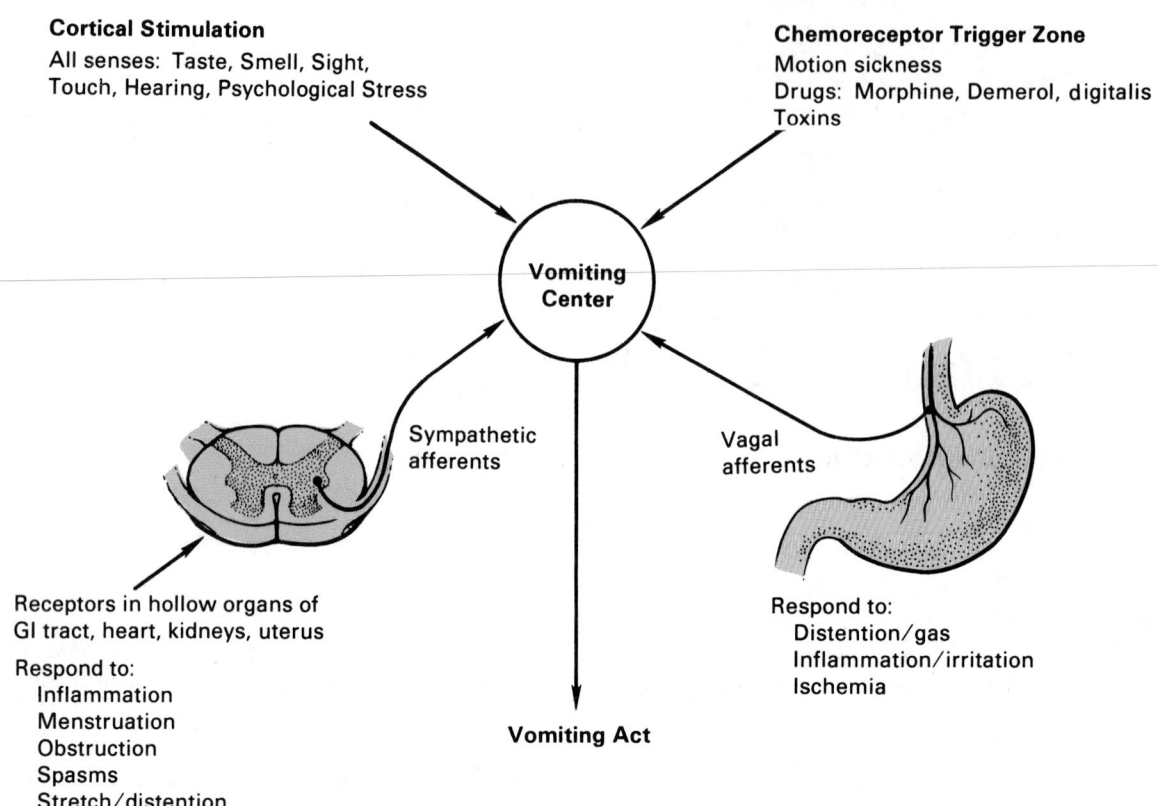

Cortical Stimulation
All senses: Taste, Smell, Sight, Touch, Hearing, Psychological Stress

Chemoreceptor Trigger Zone
Motion sickness
Drugs: Morphine, Demerol, digitalis
Toxins

Vomiting Center

Sympathetic afferents

Vagal afferents

Receptors in hollow organs of GI tract, heart, kidneys, uterus

Respond to:
Inflammation
Menstruation
Obstruction
Spasms
Stretch/distention

Respond to:
Distention/gas
Inflammation/irritation
Ischemia

Vomiting Act

Fig. 36-1 Stimuli involved in the act of vomiting.

Pathophysiology

Emetic impulses are transmitted to the vomiting center located in the medulla by afferent stimulation of the vagus and sympathetic nervous system. Visceral receptors are located in the GI tract, kidneys, heart, and uterus. When irritated, these receptors can stimulate the vomiting center and the vomiting reflex (Fig. 36-1).

In addition, the chemoreceptor trigger zone (CTZ) located on the floor of the fourth ventricle in the brain responds to vestibular impulses associated with motion sickness and chemical stimuli of drugs and toxins. The CTZ then transmits these impulses directly to the vomiting center. Emotions, stress, unpleasant sights and odors, and pain are all capable of triggering vomiting. When nausea and vomiting are prolonged and severe, dehydration can rapidly occur. In addition to water, essential electrolytes dissolved in body fluids are also lost. As vomiting persists, there may be severe electrolyte imbalances, loss of extracellular fluid volume, decreased plasma volume, and eventually circulatory failure.

Severe nausea and vomiting may precipitate a metabolic problem or be the direct result of a metabolic crisis. It is not uncommon to find nausea and vomiting associated with such conditions as uremia, hyperthyroidism, hyperparathyroidism and hypoparathyroidism, diabetic acidosis, Addison's disease, and hypertensive crisis. When vomiting is severe, metabolic alkalosis results from loss of hydrochloric acid and acids from the extracellular fluids. Metabolic acidosis as a result of severe vomiting is less common than metabolic alkalosis. Acidosis can occur when contents from the small intestines are vomited because of the loss of bicarbonate. Weight loss is evident within a short time when vomiting is severe.

The threat of aspiration is a constant concern when vomiting is severe. This is especially dangerous in older adults and in the client who is weak and debilitated. The client who cannot adequately manage self-care should be put in a semi-Fowler's or side-lying position.

Therapeutic Management

The goals of therapeutic management are to (1) determine and treat the underlying cause of the nausea and vomiting and (2) provide symptomatic relief of nausea and vomiting. Determining the cause is often difficult because nausea and vomiting are presenting manifestations of many conditions of the GI tract and disorders of other body systems.

A careful history elicits important information regarding times when the vomiting occurs, precipitating factors, and a description of the contents of the vomitus. Differentiation must be made between vomiting, regurgitation, and projectile vomiting. *Regurgitation* is a process in which partially digested food is slowly brought up from the stomach. It is seldom preceded by retching or vomiting. *Projectile vomiting* is a very forceful projection of stomach contents without nausea and is characteristic of CNS lesions.

The presence of a fecal odor and bile after prolonged

Table 36-1 Medications for Relief of Nausea and Vomiting

Classification	Generic Name	Trade Name
Antiemetic/ antipsychotic	Chlorpromazine	Thorazine
	Haloperidol	Haldol
	Perphenazine	Trilafon
	Prochlorperazine	Compazine
	Promazine	Sparine
	Metoclopramide	Reglan
	Trifluoperazine	Stelazine
	Triflupromazine	Vesprin
Antihistamine	Buclizine	Bucladin-S
	Cyclizine	Marezine, meclizine
	Dimenhydrinate	Dramamine
	Diphenhydramine	Benadryl
	Promethazine	Phenergan
Others	Benzquinamide	Emete-Con
	Diphenidol	Vontrol
	Thiethylperazine maleate	Torecan
	Trimethobenzamide HCl	Tigan

vomiting is indicative of intestinal obstruction beyond the pylorus. A functioning ileocecal valve ordinarily prevents the backflow of fecal contents from the colon into the small intestines. The presence of bile may suggest obstruction below the ampulla of Vater or bile reflux gastritis. The presence of partially digested food several hours after a meal is indicative of gastric outlet obstruction or delay in gastric emptying.

The color of the emesis has value in determining the presence of blood and the location of the blood source. Vomitus with a "coffee ground" appearance is associated with blood that has remained in the stomach and changed to a dark brown as a result of its interaction with gastric acid. Bright red blood indicates active bleeding suggestive of a Mallory-Weiss tear (in the mucosal lining of the lower esophagus or cardia of stomach), bleeding gastric or duodenal ulcer or neoplasm, or bleeding esophageal varices.

The time of day at which the vomiting occurs is often helpful in ascertaining causation. Early-morning vomiting is a frequent occurrence in pregnancy and in uremia associated with renal disease. Emotional stressors with no evident functional disorder may elicit vomiting during or immediately after the ingestion of a meal.

The indications for using drugs in the treatment of nausea and vomiting depend on the cause of the problem (Table 36-1). Because the cause cannot always be readily determined, medications must be used with caution. The use of antiemetics before the cause of the vomiting is established can lead to masking of the underlying disease process and delay of diagnosis and treatment. Drugs that inhibit nausea and vomiting act on the vomiting center, the CTZ, and peripheral nerves. Many drugs, including antiemetics, antipsychotics, and antihistamines, can control

nausea and vomiting. Because many of these drugs have anticholinergic actions, they are contraindicated for clients with glaucoma, prostatic hypertrophy, pyloric or bladder neck obstruction, and biliary obstruction. They share many common side effects, which include dry mouth, hypotension, sedative effects, rashes, and GI disturbances such as constipation.

Nutritional Considerations

Clients with severe vomiting require intravenous (IV) fluid therapy with electrolyte replacement until they are able to tolerate oral intake. In some cases a nasogastric (NG) tube and suction may have to be used to decompress the stomach. Once the symptoms have subsided, oral nourishment beginning with clear liquids may be started. Extremely hot or cold liquids are not usually well tolerated. Carbonated beverages at room temperature and with the carbonation gone and warm tea are more easily tolerated. Broth is usually an excellent liquid choice because of its electrolyte content. Gatorade is also high in electrolyte content and is often used to treat dehydration. The addition of dry toast or crackers seems to alleviate the feeling of nausea and helps prevent vomiting.

As the client's condition improves, a diet high in carbohydrate and low in fatty foods should be provided. Such items as a baked potato, plain gelatin, cereal with milk and sugar, and hard candy may be added. Foods that are known to be poorly tolerated include coffee, spicy foods, and highly acidic foods. Food should be eaten slowly and in small amounts so that overdistention of the stomach is avoided. When solid foods have been reintroduced fluids should be taken between meals rather than with meals. It is advised that the client remain quietly relaxed for approximately 1 hour after meals.

■ Nursing Management of the Client with Nausea and Vomiting

Nursing assessment

Each client with a history of prolonged and persistent nausea or vomiting requires a thorough nursing assessment before the generation of a specific plan of care. Although the conditions that may be associated with nausea and vomiting are numerous, the nurse should have a basic understanding of some of the more common conditions and should be able to identify clients who are at high risk. A knowledge of the physiological mechanisms involved in nausea and vomiting and the demonstration of a genuine regard for the client's suffering are essential. Subjective and objective data that should be obtained from those experiencing these symptoms, regardless of underlying cause, are presented in Table 36-2.

Nursing diagnoses

Nursing diagnoses specific to the client experiencing nausea and vomiting include those found in Table 36-3 and the following:

1. Anxiety related to fear of stimulating recurrence of nausea and vomiting and lack of knowledge related to etiology and consequences of prolonged nausea and vomiting
2. Self-care deficit related to fatigue and discomfort of prolonged nausea and vomiting

Table 36-2

Nursing Assessment of the Client with Nausea and Vomiting

SUBJECTIVE DATA

History
GI disorders, chronic indigestion, food allergies, pregnancy, stress, fear, infection, CNS disorders, recent travel, bulimia, metabolic disorders, cancer, cardiovascular disease

Medications
Use of antiemetics, digitalis, opiates, ferrous sulfate, aspirin, aminophylline, alcohol, antibiotics; general anesthesia; chemotherapy

General
Weakness, anorexia, weight loss

Gastrointestinal
Amount, frequency, character, and color of vomitus; dry heaves; onset and duration; abdominal tenderness

OBJECTIVE DATA

General
Lethargy, sunken eyeballs

Integumentary
Pallor, dry mucous membranes, poor skin turgor

Gastrointestinal
Amount, frequency, character (projectile), content (undigested food, blood, bile, feces), and color of vomitus (red, "coffee ground," green-yellow)

Urinary
Decreased output, concentrated urine

Possible findings
Altered serum electrolytes (especially hypokalemia), metabolic alkalosis, abnormal upper GI findings or abdominal x-ray films

---

3. Altered oral mucous membranes related to prolonged and persistent vomiting and inadequate oral hygiene
4. Altered health maintenance related to lack of knowledge of appropriate food and fluid intake and of management of recurrent episodes of nausea and vomiting

Nursing interventions

The majority of persons who experience nausea and vomiting can be managed at home. The client and the family will be grateful to the nurse who can provide simple instructions on how to deal successfully with the unpleasant sensations of nausea, discuss methods of prevention, and provide strategies to manage and resolve vomiting episodes.

A number of sensations accompany nausea just before the episode of vomiting, including retching, increased salivation, and diaphoresis. Although these sensations cannot be entirely eliminated, they can be diminished to a degree. The occurrence of nausea or vomiting may be minimized if measures are taken to keep the immediate environment quiet, free of noxious odors, and well ventilated. The avoidance of sudden changes of position and unnecessary activity is also helpful in this regard. Use of relaxation techniques, frequent rest periods, and diversional tactics help prevent nausea and vomiting or facilitate a more rapid recovery from their effects. Cleansing the face and hands with a cool washcloth and mouth care between episodes increase the person's comfort level. When the symptoms occur, all foods and medications should be stopped until the acute phase is past. If a medication is suspected as the cause, the physician should be notified immediately so that either the dosage can be altered or a new medication can be prescribed. The client should be reminded that stopping the drug without consulting the physician may eliminate the immediate cause of the nausea and vomiting but that omission of the prescribed medication may have detrimental effects on health or the disease state.

When food is identified as the precipitating cause of nausea and vomiting, the nurse should help the client solve the problem. What food was it? When was it eaten? Has this food caused problems in the past? Is anyone else in the family sick?

When the client believes some foods and fluids can be tolerated, the nurse might suggest that it would be helpful to begin with clear liquids such as warm cola beverages, Gatorade, tea or broth, dry crackers or toast, and then plain gelatin. Bland foods are generally well tolerated in small amounts. Rest and a relaxed environment free of noxious odors add to the client's general comfort. An antiemetic drug may be taken only if recommended by the physician. Taking over-the-counter drugs for relief of symptoms may make the condition worse. When nausea and vomiting persist regardless of home treatment strategies, hospitalization may be necessary for diagnosis of the underlying problem. Hospitalization is always a stressful event, and when it is associated with nausea and vomiting of unknown etiology, the client's condition may worsen as a consequence.

Until a diagnosis is confirmed, the client is kept on NPO status and given IV fluids. Antiemetic medications may be withheld or administered with caution because they may mask the underlying condition. An NG tube connected to low suction may be necessary for those with persistent vomiting. Keeping the stomach empty helps eliminate the stimulus to vomit.

With prolonged vomiting, there is a possibility of dehydration and electrolyte imbalances. The nurse must plan care that includes an accurate record of intake and output, monitoring of vital signs, assessment for signs of dehydration, proper positioning to prevent possible aspiration in the susceptible client, and observation for changes in the client's general physical comfort and mentation.

The measures for home care maintenance are also appropriate in the hospital setting. Because the client is more acutely ill and less able to perform these strategies alone, the nurse must take responsibility for providing physical and emotional support, maintaining a quiet, odor-free environment, and giving explanations regarding the laboratory and diagnostic tests ordered.

Table 36-3

 NURSING CARE PLAN FOR THE CLIENT WITH NAUSEA AND VOMITING

Defining Characteristics	Nursing Interventions	Evaluation Criteria
NURSING DIAGNOSIS: Nausea and vomiting		
Nausea and vomiting	Offer reassurance and explanations. Remove visual stimuli and source of odors immediately. Provide mouth care. Change soiled gown and linens. Keep clean emesis basin and tissues within easy reach. Use diversional activities, if appropriate. Maintain quiet environment, restrict visitors, and avoid unnecessary procedures or activities. Administer antiemetics and pain medications as ordered. Instruct client to take several deep breaths and swallow to prevent nausea. Prevent sudden changes in position. Keep head of bed elevated. Instruct client to avoid foods and beverages that stimulate nausea and vomiting.	Cessation of nausea and vomiting, verbalization of satisfaction with care
NURSING DIAGNOSIS: Fluid volume deficit related to prolonged vomiting and inability to ingest, digest, or absorb food and fluids		
Decreased urine output and increased concentration, increased pulse rate, hypotension (postural), decreased intake, nausea, decreased skin turgor, dry skin and mucous membranes, increased serum sodium, decreased potassium	Keep client on NPO status until able to tolerate foods and fluids by mouth. Administer and monitor amount and type of IV fluid. Administer antiemetic or pain medications as prescribed. Record amount and frequency of vomitus. Maintain accurate intake and output records. Weigh daily in acute phase. If ordered, maintain NG tube to low suction. Check patency, type, and amount of drainage. Provide frequent mouth care. Assess skin tone and turgor for degree of dehydration. Monitor laboratory results of sodium, potassium, and chloride. Routinely test vomitus for pH, bile, blood. Document amount, frequency, odor, and consistency of emesis. Notify physician of results and changes in vomiting pattern.	No signs of dehydration
NURSING DIAGNOSIS: Anxiety related to lack of knowledge of treatment plan and follow-up care		
Verbalization of lack of knowledge, threat to health status, apprehension, tension; fear of unspecific outcomes and recurrence of symptoms	Explain rationale for plan of care and diagnostic tests ordered. Teach about relationship between nausea and vomiting and foods, medications, treatment regimens, and psychosocial factors. Outline instructions or steps to take if nausea and vomiting recur after discharge.	Early diagnosis of underlying disease process, development of trusting and helpful relationship, verbalization of understanding of causative factors and purpose of therapeutic interventions
NURSING DIAGNOSIS: High risk for altered nutrition: less than body requirements related to nausea and vomiting		
Lack of interest in or aversion to food, perceived or actual inability to ingest food, weight loss	Assure client appetite will return when nausea and vomiting are controlled. Maintain IV feedings or total parenteral nutrition until oral intake is possible. Instruct client to resume eating cautiously with bland, nonirritating foods.	Gradual return to usual weight and eating habits

Those who are already hospitalized for other health problems are also prone to episodes of nausea and vomiting. These include the postoperative client who is recovering from the effects of the surgical procedure and anesthesia, pain, and adverse reactions to medications and treatment. Nausea and vomiting are common side effects in cancer clients being given chemotherapy drugs or radiation therapy. (A comprehensive review of nursing care for the client who is receiving chemotherapy and radiation therapy is found in Chapter 9.)

GASTRITIS

Gastritis, inflammation of the gastric mucosa, is one of the most common problems affecting the stomach. Approximately 50% of adults have mild gastritis during their lifetime.

Types

Gastritis may be acute or chronic and may be diffuse or localized. Table 36-4 lists the types of gastritis.

Acute gastritis is an inflammatory condition that may be the result of drugs (e.g., aspirin, digitalis, butazolidin, indomethacin), large amounts of alcohol, coffee, cigarette smoking, some contaminated foods (*Staphylococcus* and *Salmonella* organisms), food allergies, and CNS lesions. Steroidal and nonsteroidal antiinflammatory drugs are known to inhibit the synthesis of prostaglandins, which results in increased acid secretion in the stomach.

Excesses of spicy, irritating foods and metabolic conditions such as uremia have also been implicated as causing acute gastritis. The symptoms of acute gastritis include anorexia, nausea and vomiting, epigastric tenderness, and a feeling of fullness. Hemorrhage is commonly associated with alcohol abuse and at times may be the only presenting symptom. Acute gastritis is self-limiting, lasting from a few hours to a few days, with complete healing of the mucosa expected.

Chronic gastritis has an increasing incidence with age, with most cases occurring after the age of 50. Chronic gastritis is frequently the result of repeated insults by the causative agents of acute gastritis, or it may be idiopathic in origin. The presence of chronic gastritis is often related to symptoms associated with other diseases, such as gastric cancer.

Chronic irritation and inflammation to the mucosa from repeated alcohol abuse, drugs, stress, and caustic substances can eventually lead to atrophic gastritis and gastric atrophy. Pernicious anemia is known to develop with progressive atrophic gastritis. Symptoms of chronic atrophic gastritis range from absence of symptoms to distention, pain, and nausea and vomiting after eating. Misdiagnosis is common, since the symptoms are similar to those of mild indigestion and often go untreated.

Pathophysiology

There is considerable evidence that gastritis is the result of a breakdown in the normal gastric barrier. Consequently, there is back diffusion of hydrogen and sodium ions from the gastric lumen. The mucosal barrier normally protects the stomach tissue from autodigestion by acid. When the barrier is broken, acid can diffuse back into the mucosa. This allows hydrochloric acid to enter and thereby increase the secretion of pepsinogen and the release of histamine from mast cells. The combined result of these occurrences is tissue edema, loss of plasma into the gastric lumen with disruption of capillary walls, and possible hemorrhage.

Factors that are known to alter the diffusion barrier are chronic alcohol abuse, excess ingestion of aspirin, reflux of duodenal contents after gastric surgery, ischemia, and uremia. The ingestion of even small amounts of aspirin in susceptible persons is known to result in asymptomatic GI bleeding manifested by positive stool tests for occult blood. After a severe drinking episode, acute damage to the gastric mucosa can range from local degeneration of superficial epithelial cells to desquamation and destruction of the mucosa, with mucosal congestion, edema, and hemorrhage.[1] Gastritis is known to occur after reflux of bile salts from the duodenum into the stomach as a result of anatomical changes after surgical procedures such as gastroduodenostomy and gastrojejunostomy. Progressive gastric atrophy from chronic breakage in the protective mucosal barrier causes the chief and parietal cells to eventually malfunction. As the mass of the acid-secreting parietal cells decreases, hypochlorhydria (partial atrophy) or achlorhydria exists. In some clients, gastric cancer develops. When the acid-secreting cells do not function, the source of intrinsic factor is also lost. Intrinsic factor, which normally combines with vitamin B_{12}, is unavailable, and thus vitamin B_{12} cannot be absorbed in the ileum.

The intrinsic factor protects vitamin B_{12} from digestion by the GI enzymes. Eventually the body's stores of vitamin B_{12} in the liver are depleted and a deficiency state exists. Lack of this important vitamin, which is essential for the growth and maturation of red blood cells (RBCs), results in the development of pernicious anemia. Because there is a high frequency of circulating antibodies in clients with pernicious anemia, it is suggested that atrophic gastritis may be an autoimmune disease.[2]

Diagnostic Studies

Proper diagnosis of gastritis is frequently delayed or completely missed because the symptoms are nonspecific. Endoscopic examination with biopsy must be performed to obtain a definitive diagnosis, especially when the history indicates chronic gastritis. Radiographic studies are not helpful, since the superficial mucosa is generally involved

Table 36-4 Types of Gastritis

Acute	Chronic
Acute corrosive gastritis	Atrophic gastritis
Acute erosive gastritis	Bile reflux gastritis
Acute hemorrhagic gastritis	Chronic corrosive gastritis
Acute superficial gastritis	Chronic superficial gastritis
Stress ulcers	Giant hypertrophic gastritis (Zollinger-Ellison type)

and changes will not show clearly on x-ray film. A complete blood count (CBC) may demonstrate the presence of anemia from blood loss. Stools are tested for the presence of occult blood. A gastric analysis, although currently not used as much, demonstrates the amount of hydrochloric acid present, with achlorhydria being a common sign of severe atrophic gastritis. Cytological examination is done to rule out gastric carcinoma.

Therapeutic Management

Elimination of the cause and its avoidance in the future are generally all that is needed to treat acute gastritis. The plan of care is supportive and similar to that described for nausea and vomiting. During the acute phase, bed rest, nothing by mouth, and IV fluids are prescribed. Fluids and electrolytes lost through vomiting and occasionally diarrhea are replaced. In severe cases an NG tube may be used, either for lavage of the precipitating agent from the stomach or in conjunction with suction to keep the stomach empty and free of noxious stimuli. Antiemetics are given for nausea and vomiting. Antacids have proved beneficial in the relief of abdominal discomfort by reducing the amount of gastric acid secreted or by raising intragastric pH to above 6. The addition of H_2 antagonists, such as ranitidine or cimetidine, to the medical regimen also inhibits gastric acid secretion. Clear liquids are resumed when the acute symptoms have subsided, with gradual reintroduction of solid, bland foods. Acute gastritis with hemorrhage is treated with transfusion and fluid replacement. Surgical intervention with partial gastrectomy, vagotomy, or pyloroplasty may be necessary if treatment fails.

The treatment of chronic gastritis focuses on evaluating and eliminating the specific cause (e.g., cessation of alcoholic intake, abstinence from drugs). Pernicious anemia must be treated by regular injections of vitamin B_{12} (see discussed in Chapter 25). An individualized bland diet and use of antacids is recommended. The use of cigarettes is contraindicated in all forms of gastritis.

▪ Nursing Management of Acute Gastritis

Nursing interventions during acute gastritis are similar to those described in Table 36-3 for the client with nausea and vomiting. Dehydration can occur rapidly in severe gastritis accompanied by vomiting. Keeping the client on NPO status and quiet and monitoring of IV fluids is essential. If hemorrhage is considered likely, frequent checking of vital signs and testing the vomitus for blood are indicated. Elimination of the cause of the gastritis results in rapid improvement in the client's condition. Identification of the causative agent is important to prevent future gastric irritation. A bland diet consisting of six small feedings a day and the use of an antacid after meals helps the client maintain normal gastric function. It is essential that the nurse have knowledge of the action and therapeutic effects of H_2 antagonists to teach the client and monitor drug effects.

The care of the client with chronic atrophic gastritis and gastric atrophy is also supportive. There is no known cure, although corticosteroids have been somewhat successful in regeneration of parietal cells. With advanced gastric atrophy, vitamin B_{12} injections are necessary for the lifetime of the client. Discussion of the continued need for this essential vitamin must be included in the plan of care. The client should also be encouraged to avoid causative factors and to follow the prescribed diet and medication regimen. Because the incidence of gastric cancer is higher in clients who have a history of chronic gastritis, especially atrophic gastritis, close medical follow-up should be stressed.

UPPER GASTROINTESTINAL BLEEDING
Etiology and Pathophysiology

Although the most serious loss of blood from the upper GI tract is characterized by a sudden onset, insidious occult bleeding can also be a major problem. The severity of bleeding depends on whether the origin is venous, capillary, or arterial. Suspicion of bleeding from an arterial source may be aroused when the bleeding is profuse and the blood is bright red. The bright red color indicates that the blood has not been in contact with the stomach's acid secretions. In contrast, "coffee ground" vomitus reveals that the blood and other contents have been in the stomach for some time and have been changed by contact with gastric secretions. This type of bleeding may have come from the slower flow of a venous or capillary origin. Melena (tarry stools) indicates slow bleeding from an upper GI source. The darker the color of the stool, the longer the passage of blood through the intestines, resulting in further degradation of hemoglobin. A massive upper GI hemorrhage is generally defined as a loss of more than 1500 ml of blood or loss of 25% of intravascular blood volume.

Discovering the cause of the bleeding is not always an easy task. A variety of areas in the GI tract may be involved, and there may be many different reasons for the blood loss. Table 36-5 lists the common causes of bleeding.

Medication induced. The overuse of some medications, either prescribed by the physician or self-administered, has been definitely implicated as a cause of upper GI bleeding. Clients who take aspirin or aspirin-containing compounds regularly may be at risk of bleeding episodes. Aspirin and other antiinflammatory drugs, such as phenylbutazone, indomethacin, and corticosteroids, can cause irritation and erosion of the gastric mucosa. Erosion into the blood ves-

Table 36-5 Common Causes of Upper Gastrointestinal Bleeding

DRUG INDUCED	STOMACH-DUODENUM
Salicylates	Peptic ulcer disease
Corticosteroids	Stress ulcer
Phenylbutazone	Hemorrhagic gastritis
Indomethacin	Carcinoma
	Polyps
ESOPHAGUS	
	SYSTEMATIC DISEASES
Esophageal varices	
Esophagitis	Blood dyscrasias
Mallory-Weiss syndrome	Leukemia
	Uremia

sels is always a potential danger and a frequent cause of bleeding.

Aspirin-containing products are currently being sold without prescriptions as over-the-counter drugs. It is not unusual for clients to deny the use of aspirin yet be self-medicating with aspirin-containing drugs, such as Alka-Seltzer, Bufferin, and Excedrin. A careful history of all commonly used medications is therefore necessary whenever upper GI bleeding is suspected.

Esophageal origin. Bleeding from an esophageal source is most likely the result of chronic esophagitis, esophageal varices, or bleeding from a tear in the mucosa near the esophageal-gastric junction. Chronic esophagitis can be caused by the ingestion of chemicals irritating to the mucosa (e.g., lye) or hot, spicy, irritating foods. Alcohol and cigarettes are known irritants to the esophageal mucosa. An incompetent cardiac sphincter, which permits reflux of the acidic stomach contents back into the esophagus, can lead to chronic irritation and erosion. Severe retching and vomiting can cause a tear in the esophageal mucosa and cause severe bleeding (Mallory-Weiss syndrome). Esophageal varices usually occur secondary to cirrhosis of the liver.

Branches of the vena cava and the azygos vein from the systemic circulation converge with the smaller vessels of the lower esophagus. These vessels are inelastic and become engorged and tortuous because of increased pressure exerted upon them secondary to portal hypertension. Anything that may increase the pressure (e.g., coughing, sneezing, trauma) or result in mechanical irritation (e.g., vomiting, irritation, or erosion) may result in sudden, massive bleeding. (Esophageal varices are discussed in Chapter 38.)

Stomach and duodenal origin. Erosion of a blood vessel by a peptic ulcer located in the stomach or duodenum must always be considered as a possible cause of upper GI bleeding. Ulcers frequently penetrate blood vessels. The left gastric artery may be penetrated by a gastric ulcer and the superior pancreaticoduodenal artery by a duodenal ulcer.

Stress ulcers, which may occur after severe burns, trauma, or major surgery, erode more superficial blood vessels than does a peptic ulcer. They may also cause bleeding from erosion of a larger blood vessel. Gastritis produced by ingestion of drugs, alcohol, or the reflux of bile contents commonly results in bleeding. Gastric carcinoma can be the cause of a steady blood loss as it grows and ulcerates through the mucosa and blood vessels located within its path. Hematemesis and melena are commonly associated with cancer of the stomach.

Systemic diseases. Systemic diseases (e.g., leukemia, blood dyscrasias) that interfere with normal blood clotting must be considered whenever upper GI bleeding occurs.

Emergency Assessment and Management

Although approximately 75% of clients who have massive hemorrhage will spontaneously stop bleeding, the cause must be identified and treatment initiated immediately. In spite of advances in intensive care, intravascular monitoring, and fiberoptic endoscopy, there has been little change in the mortality rate for upper GI bleeding, which has remained approximately 10% for the past 40 years.[3]

Although a complete history of events leading to the bleeding episode is important in discovering the cause of the blood loss, it should be deferred until emergency care has been initiated. The immediate physical examination must include a systemic evaluation of the client's condition with emphasis on blood pressure, rate and character of pulse, peripheral perfusion with capillary refill, and observation for the presence or absence of neck vein distention. Vital signs should be monitored every 15 to 30 minutes. Signs and symptoms of shock must be evaluated, and treatment should be started as soon as possible (see Chapter 27). The client's respiratory status is carefully assessed, along with a thorough abdominal examination. The presence or absence of bowel sounds should be assessed and noted. A tense, rigid, boardlike abdomen may indicate a perforation and peritonitis.

Once the immediate interventions have begun, the client or family should answer the following questions: Is there a history of previous bleeding episodes? Has weight loss been a recent problem? Has the client received blood transfusions in the past and were there any transfusion reactions? Is there a religious preference that prohibits the use of blood or blood products? Are there any other illnesses that may contribute to bleeding or interfere with treatment (e.g., congestive heart failure, diabetes mellitus)?

Laboratory studies are ordered and include a CBC, blood urea nitrogen (BUN), serum electrolytes, blood glucose, prothrombin time, liver enzymes, arterial blood gases (ABGs), and a type and cross-match for possible blood transfusions. All vomitus and stools should be tested for the presence of gross and occult blood. A urinalysis provides information on the presence of blood in the urine, and the specific gravity gives an immediate indication of the client's hydration status.

Therapeutic Management

An open IV line with a large-gauge needle (Nos. 16 to 18) should be established for fluid and blood replacement. The type and amount of fluids infused are dictated by physical and laboratory findings. It is generally best to begin with an isotonic crystalloid solution (e.g., Ringer's lactate). Unless contraindicated by cardiac or renal insufficiency, whole blood or fresh frozen plasma is preferred over packed red cells for replacement of lost volume in massive bleeding. Packed red cells do not contain clotting factors that are depleted during major hemorrhagic events. (The use of blood transfusions and volume expanders is discussed in Chapters 25 and 27, respectively.) The hemoglobin and hematocrit values are not of immediate assistance in estimating the degree of blood loss but provide a baseline for guiding further treatment. The initial hematocrit may be normal and not reflect the loss until about 4 to 6 hours after fluid replacement has taken place, since initially the loss of plasma and RBCs is equal. When upper GI bleeding is less profuse, infusion of isotonic saline solution followed by packed red cells permits restoration of the hematocrit more quickly and does not create complications of fluid volume overload.

For most clients who are bleeding profusely an indwelling catheter will be inserted so that urine volume can be accurately assessed hourly. A central venous pressure line may be inserted so that the client's hydration can be monitored more easily. When a history of valvular heart disease, coronary artery disease, or congestive heart failure is elicited or when pulmonary edema is a factor, a pulmonary artery catheter may be necessary (see Chapter 28). A central venous pressure line is capable of monitoring right-sided heart pressure and function but does not reflect accurate left ventricular function. When the client is vomiting blood, an NG tube is indicated. A large tube passed through the mouth may be more beneficial than a small one passed through the nose. Passage through the mouth is easier, but no tube should ever be advanced against resistance because of the likelihood of damaging the gastric mucosa or causing perforation. Aspiration of stomach contents through the tube facilitates the removal of clots from the stomach and alleviates the client's need to vomit.

In most cases, bleeding ceases spontaneously without any intervention. However, for many years it has been common practice to lavage the stomach with cool or ice water or saline solution through an NG tube to induce local vasoconstriction of the bleeding vessel. The value of lavage is now in question. Recent studies indicate that ice water lavage has no effect on the rate of bleeding from gastric ulcers and may actually impede the body's normal coagulation mechanism.[4] Advocates of gastric lavage claim that when emergency endoscopy is necessary, lavage ensures that blood will not interfere with endoscopic visualization of the gastric mucosa.

If used, the amount of iced solution instilled should be no more than 2000 ml/hr. The usual procedure is to instill 50 to 100 ml each time, leave it in place for several minutes, and then aspirate it or allow drainage by gravity. The majority of clients who are bleeding from the stomach show diminished blood flow in about 30 to 45 minutes with this method. The addition of a vasoconstrictor to lavage solutions may also be used in some institutions. Such drugs as levarterenol (diluted in saline solution) have demonstrated the ability to help control hemorrhage from erosive gastritis.

Diagnostic Studies

As soon as the bleeding is under control and the client's condition is more stable (usually within 12 to 24 hours), the exact cause and location of the bleeding should be determined. The most useful diagnostic tools are fiberoptic panendoscopy, angiography, and barium contrast studies.

Fiberoptic panendoscopy. Fiberoptic panendoscopy should be used before either angiography or barium studies. This diagnostic tool is very accurate in identifying the specific source of the bleeding. When the procedure is performed by a skilled practitioner, bleeding from severe gastritis can be easily distinguished from that of a gastric or duodenal ulcer.

Angiography. Angiography has been used effectively in diagnosing upper GI bleeding. It is effective when the bleeding is profuse (more than 1 ml/min) and obscures the bleeding site from the endoscope. Opponents of angiography state that its diagnostic ability is not definitive in many cases. In addition, the procedure requires preparation and setup time and may not be appropriate for a high-risk, unstable client. In this procedure a catheter is placed into the left gastric or superior mesenteric artery and advanced until the site of bleeding is discovered. Angiography is an invasive procedure and should be undertaken only if the client has no allergies to the contrast medium, has adequate hydration and urinary output, and has no cardiovascular contraindications.

Barium contrast studies. Barium contrast studies have less immediate value in the identification of major bleeding sites during the acute phase of treatment. They are of little value if the bleeding is due to gastritis or a shallow superficial ulcer. Barium studies can document an actual lesion but cannot verify that it is the bleeding source. If barium is used initially as a diagnostic tool and the bleeding intensifies, the barium will obscure and delay endoscopy and angiography until it has been cleared from the stomach.

Surgical Interventions

Surgical interventions are indicated when bleeding continues regardless of the therapy provided. A high percentage of clients are known to have another massive hemorrhage within 5 years after the first bleeding episode. Some physicians regard surgical therapy as necessary when the client continues to bleed after rapid transfusion of up to 2000 ml of whole blood or remains in shock after 24 hours. The choice of operation is determined by the site of the hemorrhage. In addition, the surgeon must consider the age of the client, since mortality rates increase considerably over the age of 60. It is essential that the operation be performed as soon as the need has been established.

Pharmacological Management

Drug therapy can be started after the bleeding site has been identified and bleeding has slowed or ceased. The drugs most commonly used in the management of upper GI bleeding are antacids, histamine H_2-receptor antagonists, and vasopressin. Table 36-6 reviews their mechanism of action in relation to upper GI bleeding.

Antacids have long been known to neutralize hydrochloric acid secreted by the parietal cells of the stomach and therefore are the drugs of choice in the treatment of peptic ulcer. It has only recently been confirmed that antacids help in the healing process as well. Antacids have the ability to neutralize hydrochloric acid, increase the pH of gastric contents to above 5, and therefore inhibit the activation of pepsinogen to pepsin. The most frequently used antacid preparations are magnesium hydroxide, magnesium trisilicate, aluminum hydroxide, calcium carbonate, and sodium bicarbonate (see Table 36-11). Aluminum hydroxide and magnesium trisilicates are the most useful because they are nonabsorbable. Calcium carbonate and sodium bicarbonate are absorbable, and prolonged use can lead to systemic alkalosis.

The neutralizing effects of antacids taken on an empty stomach last only 20 to 30 minutes. When antacids are taken after meals, the effects may last as long as 3 to 4

Table 36-6 Drug Therapy for Gastrointestinal Bleeding

Drug	Source of GI Bleeding	Mechanism of Action
Antacids*	Duodenal ulcer, gastric ulcer, acute gastritis (corrosive, erosive, and hemorrhagic)	Neutralizes acid and maintains gastric pH above 5.5, elevated pH inhibits activation of pepsinogen
Histamine H_2-receptor antagonists Cimetidine (Tagamet), ranitidine (Zantac), famotidine (Pepcid), nizatidine (Axid)	Duodenal ulcer, gastric ulcer, esophagitis, acute gastritis (especially hemorrhagic)	Inhibits action of histamine at H_2 receptors of parietal cells and decreases acid secretion
Vasopressin	Acute gastritis (corrosive, erosive, and hemorrhagic)	Causes vasoconstriction and increases smooth muscle activity of the GI tract, reduces pressure in the portal circulation and arrests bleeding

*See Table 36-11.

hours. After the acute phase of bleeding, from whatever the cause, has diminished, antacids are generally administered hourly, either orally or through the NG tube. If the tube is in place, the stomach contents should be aspirated and tested periodically for pH. If pH is less than 5, intermittent suction may be used, or the frequency or dosage of the antacid may be increased.

Some physicians order instillation of from 60 to 180 ml of an antacid via the NG tube, clamp the tube 15 minutes, and then test gastric contents for pH. If pH is below 7, a comparable amount of antacid is again instilled, and the process is repeated until a neutral pH is attained. Antacids are then added regulary or intermittently to maintain a neutral pH. This regimen has demonstrated control of bleeding from a variety of causes (see Table 36-6).

Histamine H_2-receptor antagonists cimetidine (Tagamet), ranitidine (Zantac), and famotidine (Pepcid) are well established in the treatment of peptic ulcer disease and in the prophylactic treatment of clients at risk of stress-related upper GI hemorrhage. Although these drugs have no proven ability to control active bleeding, they have become part of standard treatment protocols. These drugs inhibit the action of histamine at the H_2 receptors of parietal cells and thereby decrease acid secretion. The neutralizing effects of each of these medications are much longer than those of regular antacid therapy (lasting up to about 5 hours for cimetidine and 13 hours for ranitidine).

Vasopressin (Pitressin), which is posterior pituitary extract, can produce vasoconstriction and is used to treat upper GI bleeding. It may be administered systemically through a vein or intraarterially at the local site of actual bleeding. It should be given with caution to clients with a known history of vascular diseases or hypersensitivity to vasopressin.

In clients who do not respond to vasopressin therapy, selective embolization of the bleeding vessel may be performed. The procedure is carried out while the catheter is still within the artery. Fragments of Gelfoam (gelatin foam) 2.5 mm in size are placed within the artery, or a mixture of Gelfoam powder and Renografin-76 (contrast medium) can be injected into the bleeding artery. The anticipated result in both cases is occlusion of the vessel.

These procedures offer a promising method of controlling upper GI hemorrhage.

The use of the endoscopic examination has expanded recently because of the ability to perform transendoscopic electrocoagulation. Bleeding sites can be cauterized locally, which obviates the necessity of a surgical procedure. This procedure has proved useful in stopping the bleeding of gastritis, Mallory-Weiss syndrome, bleeding peptic ulcers and polyps, and gastric ulcer. Endoscopic thermal techniques now available to treat upper GI hemorrhage include (1) electrocoagulation, (2) heat probe, (3) argon laser, and (4) neodymium: yttrium-aluminum-garnet (ND:YAG) laser. These new thermal techniques are expensive and cumbersome, especially the laser. The heat probe is considered faster, safer, and more effective than the laser. It coagulates tissue by the direct application of a heating element to the bleeding site.[4]

The injection of a sclerosing agent into the bleeding site holds promise in controlling upper GI bleeding. It is a simple procedure that requires little client preparation. An agent such as epinephrine (a vasoconstrictor) is diluted and injected through the biopsy portal of the endoscope, causing the formation of submucosal deposits around the bleeding site. The resultant vasoconstriction and local inflammation compress the site, and bleeding is controlled.[4] Although further investigation is necessary, the use of thermal endoscopic techniques does hold hope for clients who are considered poor surgical risks. The need for transfusions and the length of hospital stay are reduced, thus making these techniques attractive alternatives.

Sedatives to control agitation and restlessness should be administered cautiously. They make accurate assessment of the client's condition more difficult. Anticholinergic drugs are contraindicated in acute upper GI bleeding episodes.

■ Nursing Management of Upper Gastrointestinal Bleeding

Nursing assessment

As the nurse begins care of the client admitted with upper GI bleeding, a thorough and accurate nursing assessment is an essential first step. Subjective and objective

Table 36-7

Nursing Assessment of the Client with Upper Gastrointestinal Bleeding

SUBJECTIVE DATA

History
Precipitating events before bleeding episode, peptic ulcer disease, previous bleeding episodes and treatment, family history of bleeding disorders, smoking or alcohol use, stress-related situations

Medications
Use of aspirin, nonsteroidal antiinflammatory drugs, corticosteroids, anticoagulants

General
Fever, bleeding from other sites

Pain
Epigastric pain

Gastrointestinal
Vomiting, diarrhea, cramps

OBJECTIVE DATA

General
Vital signs, intake and output

Integumentary
Clammy, cool, pale skin; pale mucous membranes, nailbeds, and conjunctivae; spider angiomas; jaundice; ascites; edema

Possible findings
Decreased hematocrit and hemoglobin; hematuria; guaiac-positive stools, emesis, or gastric aspirate; decreased levels of clotting factors; elevated liver function studies; abnormal upper GI studies or endoscopy results

---

data that should be obtained from the client or significant others are presented in Table 36-7.

Nursing diagnoses

Nursing diagnoses specific to the client with upper GI bleeding include, but are not limited to, the following:

1. Anxiety related to upper GI bleeding; hospitalization; pain and discomfort; and lack of knowledge of the outcome, disease process, and management
2. Fluid volume deficit related to loss of blood
3. Altered renal and cerebral tissue perfusion
4. Decreased cardiac output related to loss of circulatory volume
5. Pain and discomfort
6. Potential complication: hypovolemic shock

Nursing interventions

Health promotion and maintenance. Although not all cases of upper GI bleeding can be anticipated and prevented, the nurse shares responsibility with the physician in trying to identify clients who are at high risk and in carrying out anticipatory guidance. Clients with a history of chronic gastritis or peptic ulcer disease should always be considered in the high-risk category because of the increasing incidence of bleeding associated with chronic irritation or chronic ulcers. Clients who have had one major bleeding episode are very likely to have another within a few years. These clients must be instructed to avoid irritat-

ing foods, prevent or decrease stress-inducing situations at home or at work, and take only prescribed medications. Over-the-counter medications can be harmful, since their contents may include drugs that are contraindicated because of their potential irritating effects on the mucosa. These clients should be instructed in the methods of testing their vomitus or stools for the presence of occult blood. Positive results should be promptly reported to the physician or the nurse. Close and frequent follow-up care is very important for all clients with ulcers because recurrence rates are high.

The client who requires regular administration of ulcerogenic drugs, such as aspirin, corticosteroids, or nonsteroidal antiinflammatory drugs (e.g., indomethacin), should receive instructions regarding the potential adverse effects these agents may have on the GI mucosa. These drugs should be avoided if at all possible. However, if aspirin must be prescribed, enteric-coated tablets can be substituted for regular tablets. Taking the medications at mealtimes or with snacks will lessen the potential irritating effects. The use of an antacid along with the prescribed medication is usually beneficial. These clients should also be instructed in testing for occult blood in vomitus and stool and the follow-up measures necessary if positive results are obtained.

When the nurse is working with the client who has a history of cirrhosis of the liver with esophageal varices, the instructions must be specific regarding the importance of avoiding known irritants, such as alcohol and hot, spicy, irritating foods. The prompt treatment of an upper respiratory tract infection should be stressed. Severe coughing or sneezing can create increased pressure on the already fragile varices and may result in massive hemorrhage.

Clients who are known to have blood dyscrasias or liver dysfunction or who are taking cancer chemotherapy drugs have a potential bleeding problem because of the alteration in their normal clotting mechanism. When these clients also have a history of ulcer disease, gastritis, varices, or drug and alcohol abuse, they should be carefully instructed regarding their disease process and medications, and they should be closely observed for bleeding.

Acute intervention. The care of the client who is bleeding from an unknown upper GI source requires continuous and diligent nursing care and assessment. The client cannot provide specific information about the cause of the bleeding until the immediate physical needs are met. An immediate nursing assessment should be performed while getting the client ready for initial treatment. The assessment should include the client's level of consciousness, vital signs, appearance of neck veins, skin color, and capillary refill. The abdomen should be checked for distention, guarding, and peristalsis. Immediate determination of vital signs indicates whether the client is in shock from blood loss and also provides a baseline blood pressure and pulse by which to monitor the progress of treatment. Signs and symptoms of shock include low blood pressure; rapid, weak pulse; increased thirst; cold, clammy skin; and restlessness. Vital signs should be monitored every 15 to 30 minutes, and the physician should be informed of any significant changes.

When obtaining vital signs, the nurse should consider the client's age and physical condition. Taking the blood pressure and pulse with the client lying down and then sitting will indicate postural changes that occur after acute blood loss. If the pulse rate increases more than 20 beats per minute (bpm) and the systolic blood pressure decreases 10 mm Hg, the blood loss is generally estimated to exceed 1 L. The older the client, the more changes in vital signs should be expected.[5]

The client should be approached in a calm and assured manner to help decrease the level of anxiety. Caution should be used before administering sedatives for restlessness because it is one of the warning signs of shock and may be masked by the medication.

Once an infusion has been started, the IV line must be maintained as a vehicle for fluid or blood replacement. An accurate intake and output record is essential so that the client's hydration status can be assessed. Urine output should be measured hourly. A rate of at least 30 ml/hr indicates adequate renal perfusion. Lesser amounts may indicate renal ischemia secondary to loss of blood volume. Urine specific gravity should be measured because it will give additional information regarding the client's hydration status. Consistent readings greater than 1.025 (normal is 1.005 to 1.025) indicate that the urine is very concentrated and that there is probably a low blood volume. The physician needs to be kept informed of these important parameters so that the IV solutions can be increased or decreased accordingly. If the client has a central venous pressure line in place, readings must be recorded every 1 to 2 hours. These readings indicate more accurately the circulating blood volume as it returns to the right side of the heart. Readings below 6 cm H_2O may indicate hypovolemia. Readings of about 15 cm H_2O may indicate that fluid replacement has been administered too quickly or in excess amounts. Older adults and clients with a history of cardiovascular problems should be observed closely for signs of fluid overload. This can be accomplished easily with the placement of a pulmonary artery catheter. However, the threat of volume overload and pulmonary edema must be a constant concern in all clients who are receiving large amounts of IV fluids within a short time. Therefore, auscultation of breath sounds and close observation of respiratory effort are important. Many institutions require an electrocardiogram (ECG) of each client over 40 years of age as standard procedure. It is well to keep in mind that foods such as beets or even swallowed mouthwash can give vomitus a bloody appearance. Unless the contents of the vomitus are checked for occult blood, false information may be recorded. Swallowed blood from a nosebleed must also be accurately noted to avoid misdiagnosis of an upper GI bleeding episode. When an NG tube is inserted, the nurse must pay special attention to keeping it in proper position and observing the aspirate for blood.

The majority of upper GI bleeding episodes cease spontaneously, even without intervention. Although the use of cool or iced gastric lavage has become standard treatment in many institutions, its effectiveness is of questionable value. Therefore the nurse must understand the rationale for this therapy and the results that are anticipated. Either cool or iced tap water or saline solution may be used. Water has the advantage of being able to break up large clots more easily than saline solution, is less expensive, and is always available. A disadvantage of tap water is that it may create more electrolyte imbalance than would an isotonic saline solution.

Instillation of approximately 50 to 100 ml at a time into the stomach generally results in decreased bleeding if the blood is gastric in origin. Instilling too much can increase the client's discomfort, especially if distention is already present. Instillation of too small an amount and aspirating too soon does not allow enough time for the cold fluid to cause vasoconstriction in the bleeding area.

The lavage fluid may be aspirated from the stomach or drained by gravity. When aspiration is the method used, it is important not to aspirate if resistance is felt. The tip of the NG tube may be up against the gastric mucosal lining. The constant pressure from attempts to aspirate the lavage fluid may cause erosion of the mucosa. When resistance is a factor, the nurse should use gravity as the alternative method of gastric drainage.

Close monitoring of vital signs, especially in clients with heart problems, is important because dysrhythmias may occur as a result of the close proximity of the cold, fluid-filled stomach to the heart. Keeping the client warm and the head of the bed elevated provides more comfort and prevents possible aspiration problems. The head of the bed should always be elevated when antacids are being instilled through an NG tube. Serious pulmonary complications can result if aspiration occurs. The nurse must chart the results of the lavages promptly and accurately.

The nurse caring for a client with upper GI bleeding should be well informed as to what constitutes blood in the stools. Black, tarry stools are not usually associated with a brisk hemorrhage but do indicate the presence of bleeding of prolonged duration. Bright red blood in the stool is usually from a source in the lower bowel. When vomitus contains blood but the stool contains no gross or occult blood on Hematest, the hemorrhage is considered to have been of short duration.[5] Menses and bleeding hemorrhoids should be ruled out as possible sources of blood in the stools.

Monitoring the client's laboratory studies enables the nurse to estimate the effectiveness of therapy. The hemoglobin and hematocrit are usually evaluated every 4 to 6 hours or more often and provide an accurate estimation of volume lost after rehydration has taken place. At first the hematocrit may not accurately reflect the amount of blood lost or the amount of blood replaced and will appear falsely high or low. Assessing the client's BUN level also provides data on the degree of blood lost, but not for about 24 to 48 hours. The BUN level is generally elevated with a significant hemorrhage, since blood proteins are subjected to bacterial breakdown in the GI tract. Renal disease as a cause of an elevated BUN level should be ruled out. Many clients receive oxygen by mask or by nasal prongs so that the circulating blood is ensured of an adequate oxygen content. Clients with emphysema should be observed very closely for signs of carbon dioxide narcosis when receiving oxygen (see Chapter 21).

When oral nourishment is begun, the client is observed for symptoms of nausea and vomiting and a recurrence of bleeding. Feedings initially consist of clear fluids or milk and are given hourly until tolerance is determined. These feedings help neutralize the gastric secretions and assist in the mucosal repair. Gradual introduction of bland foods follows if the client exhibits no signs of discomfort.

Antacids are one of the primary medications administered after upper GI bleeding. Anticipating the effects of the prescribed preparations can be helpful in providing better care. The nurse should know that preparations containing calcium or aluminum can result in constipation, while those with magnesium cause diarrhea. Although these preparations are nonabsorbable and result in fewer systemic problems, magnesium products must be used with care in clients with renal insufficiency. Administering the antacid preparation accurately and on schedule is important if the stomach pH is to be maintained at a level no lower than 5.

Clients in whom hemorrhage was the result of chronic alcohol abuse require close observation for the beginning of delirium tremens as withdrawal from alcohol takes place. Symptoms indicating the beginning of delirium tremens are agitation, uncontrolled shaking, sweating, and vivid hallucinations. (Cirrhosis of the liver is discussed in Chapter 38.)

The client and the family need to be taught how to avoid future bleeding episodes. Ulcer disease, drug or alcohol abuse, and liver and respiratory diseases can all result in upper GI bleeding. The client and the family must be made aware of the consequences of noncompliance with diet and drug therapy. It must be emphasized that no medications (especially aspirin) other than those prescribed by the physician should be taken. Smoking and alcohol should be eliminated because they are sources of irritation and interfere with tissue repair. The need for long-term follow-up care may be necessary due to the possibility of another bleeding episode. The client and the family should be instructed on what to do if an acute hemorrhage occurs in the future.

PEPTIC ULCER

Peptic ulcer is an erosion of the GI mucosa resulting from the digestive action of hydrochloric acid and pepsin. Any portion of the GI tract that comes into contact with gastric secretions is susceptible to ulcer development; this includes the lower esophagus, the stomach, the duodenum, and the margin of gastrojejunal anastomosis after surgical procedures. It is estimated that approximately 10% of men in the United States and 4% of women will have duodenal ulcers during their lifetime.[6]

Types

Peptic ulcers can be classified as *acute* or *chronic,* depending on the degree of mucosal involvement (Fig. 36-2), and *gastric* or *duodenal,* according to location. Acute ulcers are associated with superficial erosion and minimal inflammation. They are of short duration and resolve quickly when the cause is identified and removed. A chronic ulcer is one of long duration, eroding through the muscular wall with the formation of fibrous tissue. It is present continuously for many months or intermittently throughout the person's lifetime. A chronic ulcer is at least four times as common as an acute erosion.[7] Gastric and duodenal ulcers, although defined as peptic ulcers, are distinctly different in their etiology and incidence (Table 36-8). Generally, the treatment of ulcers is quite similar.

Gastric ulcers. Although gastric ulcers can occur in any portion of the stomach, they are most commonly found on the lesser curvature in close proximity to the antral junction. Before the beginning of the twentieth century, gastric ulcers were more common than duodenal ulcers, and they were found predominantly in young women. Since the turn of the century, the incidence of gastric ulcers has decreased, and these are now surpassed in incidence by duodenal ulcers by a ratio of 4:1. Gastric ulcers remain more prevalent in women and in older adults.

The mortality rate from gastric ulcers is greater than that from duodenal ulcers and is attributed to the fact that the peak incidence occurs in persons over 50 years of age.

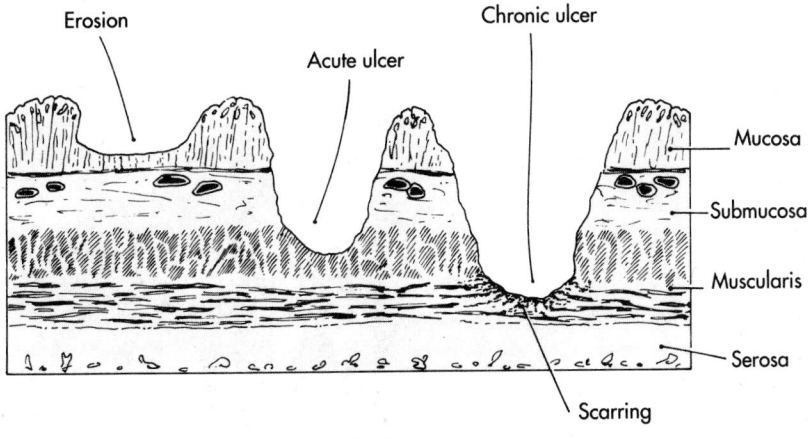

Fig. 36-2 Peptic ulcers, including an erosion, acute ulcer, and chronic ulcer. Both the acute and chronic ulcer may penetrate the entire wall of the stomach. (From Price S and Wilson L: Pathophysiology: clinical concepts of disease processes, ed 4, St Louis, 1991, Mosby–Year Book, Inc.)

Table 36-8 Gastric and Duodenal Ulcers

Lesion	Location of Lesion	Gastric Secretion	Incidence	Clinical Manifestations	Recurrence Rate	Complications
GASTRIC ULCER						
Superficial; smooth margins; round, oval, or cone-shaped	Predominantly antrum, also in body and fundus	Normal to decreased	Greater in women; peak age, fifth to sixth decade; decreasing number of cases; more common in lower socioeconomic class and in unskilled laborers; increased with smoking, drug and alcohol abuse, incompetent pyloric sphincter; increased in stress ulcers, after severe burns, head trauma, and major surgery	Burning or gaseous pressure in high left epigastrium and back and upper abdomen, occasional nausea and vomiting, weight loss, pain 1-2 hr after meals, relief of pain with food or liquids (if penetrating ulcer, aggravation of discomfort with food)	High	Hemorrhage, perforation, and obstruction
DUODENAL ULCER						
Penetrating (associated with deformity of duodenal bulb from recurrent healing of ulcers)	First 1-2 cm of duodenum	Increased	Decreasing incidence, especially in men; equal incidence in women after menopause and men; increased incidence in close relatives; peak age, 35-45 yr; all occupations, increased association with psychological pressures; increased with smoking and alcohol ingestion; increased in blood group O; increased association with chronic obstructive pulmonary disease, cirrhosis, pancreatic disease, hyperparathyroidism, Zollinger-Ellison syndrome, chronic renal failure	Burning, cramping, pressurelike pain across midepigastrium and upper abdomen; back pain with posterior ulcers; pain 2-4 hr after meals and midmorning, midafternoon, middle of night; periodic and episodic; pain relief with antacids and sometimes food; occasional nausea and vomiting	High	Hemorrhage, perforation, and obstruction

Duodenal ulcer may occur at any age, but the incidence is especially high between the ages of 35 and 45 years. Contrary to common belief, gastric ulcers are not more prevalent among those in executive or managerial positions. Persons from the lower socioeconomic class and manual or unskilled workers are more prone to gastric ulcers.

Gastric ulcers have been attributed to various factors that lead to acute episodes or to chronic involvement. Acute gastric lesions can be precipitated by stressful situations and drugs. The development of stress ulcers has been known since the late eighteenth century, when they were first described in association with severe body trauma. Later, Curling established the relationship between gastroduodenal ulcers and severe burns.

The stress ulcer is a form of erosive gastritis. It is believed that the body of the stomach undergoes a period of transient ischemia to the gastric mucosa in association with hypotension, severe injury, extensive burns, and complicated surgery. Multiple superficial erosions result, and these may bleed. The ischemia is due to decreased capillary blood flow or the opening of arteriovenous shunts secondary to hypotension so that blood flow bypasses the gastric mucosa. This results in an imbalance between the destructive properties of gastric acid and destruction of the stomach's mucosal barrier, especially in the fundic portion, which results in ulceration.[8]

Drugs that are unwisely prescribed or taken indiscriminately can cause acute gastric ulcers and in some cases can lead to development of chronic ulcers. Drugs most often implicated include aspirin, corticosteroids, indomethacin, phenylbutazone, and reserpine. Other known causative factors of gastric ulcer formation are chronic alcohol abuse, gastritis, bile reflux gastritis from an incompetent pyloric sphincter, and coffee. Caffeine is known to stimulate gastric acid secretion. Cigarette smoking is positively linked with gastric ulcer. One proposed theory is that smoking causes a reduction of pancreatic bicarbonate secretion, thus creating an increased pH in the duodenum. In addition, nicotine seems to enhance reflux of duodenal contents into the antrum of the stomach. The ingestion of hot, rough, or spicy foods has been suggested as a causative factor, but there is no concrete evidence to substantiate this claim.

Research into a genetic cause for ulcers has shown that some members of the same family are more prone to develop gastric or duodenal ulcers. Evidence is not complete, however, and the ulcer development could just as well be due to the sharing of the same environment. Gastric ulcer personality has not been demonstrated, yet ulcer-prone persons do appear to react to stress with more frustration, fear, anxiety, and guilt than those who are less predisposed to ulcer formation.

The pain associated with gastric ulcer is located high in the epigastrium and occurs spontaneously about 1 to 2 hours after meals. The pain is described as "burning" or "gaseous." The pain can occur when the stomach is empty or when food has been ingested. If the ulcer has eroded through the gastric mucosa, food tends to aggravate rather than alleviate the pain. Some persons do not experience any pain until the presence of the ulcer is demonstrated

through a serious complication, such as hemorrhage or perforation.

It is rare for gastric ulcers to become malignant, but transformation may occur in about 1% of all cases.[9] When there is any doubt, a biopsy of the gastric mucosa should be performed to differentiate between a benign ulcer and a malignant neoplasm.

Duodenal ulcers. Duodenal ulcers account for about 80% of all peptic ulcers. Although duodenal ulcers often occur in persons susceptible to psychological pressures and anxieties, this theory of causation requires more study. It is known that duodenal ulcer can develop in anyone, regardless of occupation or socioeconomic group. Although duodenal ulcers still affect more men than women, the incidence of duodenal ulcer has followed a downward trend in men and a steady increase in women. The explanation for this change has not been clearly identified. However, some believe that the overuse of aspirin and increased consumption of alcohol by women may partially account for this increased incidence.[10]

Pregnancy appears to protect women from having ulcers. Estrogen and progesterone have demonstrated positive effects on ulcer healing. Progesterone has also been noted to lower acid secretion to a small degree. There is evidence that in women past menopause, who no longer have this endocrine protection, ulcers develop at the same rate as in men.

As with gastric ulcers, some persons within certain families are more prone to duodenal ulcer formation. Supporting a genetic etiology is the fact that persons with blood group O have an increased incidence of duodenal ulcers.

The development of duodenal ulcers is associated with a high acid secretion by gastric parietal cells. Several diseases have been identified with a high risk of duodenal ulcer development; these include chronic obstructive pulmonary disease, cirrhosis of the liver, chronic pancreatitis, hyperparathyroidism, chronic renal failure, and the Zollinger-Ellison syndrome. A high gastric acid concentration is believed to be the factor common to all these conditions. Some argue that medications prescribed in the treatment of these conditions may also have detrimental effects on the gastric mucosa. Alcohol ingestion and heavy smoking habits are also associated with duodenal ulcer formation since both are known irritants to the GI mucosa.

It is common for persons with ulcers to have no pain or other symptoms. The gastric and duodenal mucosae do not have pain sensory fibers, which may account for this phenomenon. When pain does occur with duodenal ulcer, it is described as "burning" or "cramplike." It is most often located in the midepigastrium region beneath the xyphoid process. Ulcers located on the posterior aspect of the duodenum can be manifested by back pain. The pain usually occurs 2 to 4 hours after meals and is relieved by antacids and sometimes foods that neutralize and dilute the gastric acid. A characteristic of duodenal ulcer is its tendency to occur continuously for a few weeks or months and then disappear for a time, only to recur some months later. Some clients claim their symptoms worsen in the spring and fall of the year, thus strengthening the concept of a seasonal trend in occurrence. This course of events usually lasts throughout the entire life span of the ulcer.

Pathophysiology

Protein digestion can occur only in an acid environment. Hydrochloric acid is secreted by the parietal cells at a pH of 0.8. After mixing with the stomach contents, the pH reaches 2 to 3, a highly favorable range of acidity for pepsin activity. Pepsinogen, the precursor of pepsin, is activated to pepsin in the presence of hydrochloric acid and a pH of 2 to 3. When the stomach acid level is neutralized by the presence of food or antacids, the pH of hydrochloric acid is increased to 3.5 or more. At a pH of 3.5 or more, pepsin has little or no proteolytic activity and soon becomes inactive.

Peptic ulcers develop only in the presence of an acid environment. Hydrochloric acid and pepsin must be present for normal digestion to take place in the stomach. The typical person with a gastric ulcer has normal to less than normal gastric acidity compared with the person with a duodenal ulcer. However, intraluminal acid does seem to be essential for a gastric ulcer to occur, since it has been well established that clients with pernicious anemia and achlorhydria rarely have gastric ulcers. In addition, inhibition of gastric acid secretion by histamine H_2-receptor blockers does accelerate the healing of benign gastric ulcers.

The stomach is normally protected from autodigestion by the gastric mucosal barrier. The GI tract has a very high cell turnover rate, and the surface mucosa of the stomach is renewed about every 3 days. As a result of this high turnover rate, the mucosa can continually repair itself except in extreme instances when the cell breakdown surpasses the cell renewal rate. Normally, water, electrolytes, and water-soluble substances (e.g., glucose) can easily pass through the barrier. However, the mucosal barrier prevents the back diffusion of acid from the gastric lumen through the mucosal layers to the underlying tissue.

Under specific circumstances the mucosal barrier can be impaired and back-diffusion of acid can occur. When the barrier is broken, hydrochloric acid freely enters the mucosa and injury to the tissues occurs. This results in cellular destruction and inflammation. Histamine is released from the damaged mucosa, resulting in vasodilatation and increased capillary permeability. The released histamine is then capable of stimulating further secretion of acid and pepsin.

A variety of agents are known to destroy the mucosal barrier. It is estimated that 5% to 10% of all gastric ulcers are drug induced. Ulcerogenic drugs, such as aspirin and aspirinlike agents, inhibit synthesis of mucus and prostaglandins and cause abnormal permeability. Corticosteroids have the ability to decrease the rate of mucous cell renewal and thereby decrease its protective effects. Lipid-soluble cytotoxic drugs can pass through the barrier and destroy it.

When the mucosal barrier is disrupted, there is a compensatory increase in blood flow. This phenomenon can occur in several ways. Prostaglandinlike substances and histamine act as vasodilators, thus increasing capillary blood flow. As blood flow increases within the affected mucosa, hydrogen ions are rapidly removed from the area, buffers are delivered to help neutralize the hydrogen ions present, nutrients necessary for cell function arrive, and the rate of mucosal cell replication increases.[11] When blood flow is not sufficient to carry out these events, tissue injury results. When the increase is sufficient to dilute, buffer, and remove the excess, tissue damage may be minimal or may result in no injury at all. Fig. 36-3 shows a representation of the interrelationship between the mucosal blood flow and disruption of the gastric mucosal barrier.

Although gastric ulcers are characterized by a normal to low secretion of gastric acid, the back-diffusion of acid is greater with chronic gastric ulcers than with duodenal ulcers or in the normal person. Therefore, the critical pathological process in gastric ulcer formation may not be the amount of acid that is secreted but the amount that is able to penetrate the mucosal barrier.

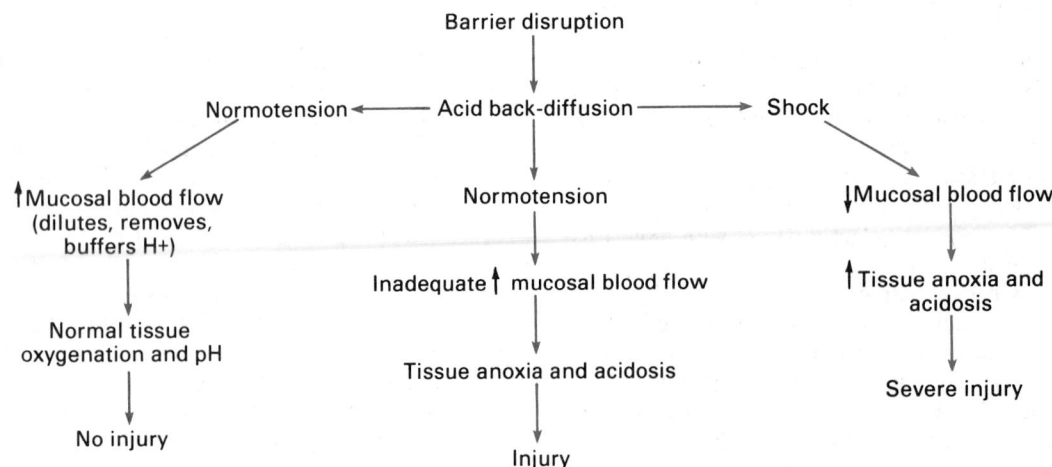

Fig. 36-3 The relationship between mucosal blood flow and disruption of the gastric mucosal barrier.

The gastric mucosa is also protected from the damage of ulceration by two other mechanisms. First, mucus is secreted by superficial mucous cells and forms a layer that can entrap or slow the diffusion of hydrogen ions across the mucosal barrier. Second, bicarbonate is secreted by the gastric and duodenal mucosa, and this helps neutralize hydrogen in the lumen of the GI tract.

Increased vagal nerve stimulation from a variety of causes, including emotions, causes hypersecretion of hydrochloric acid and pepsin. Increased concentrations of acid can alter the mucosal barrier. Duodenal ulcers are associated with high acid content. The fact that persons with duodenal ulcers are prone to be vulnerable to the effects of emotional stressors may be one reason acid levels are above normal. It has been suggested that the continual response of the parietal cells to maximal stimulation results in hyperplasia of the cell mass. There is also an increase in gastrin levels in most persons with duodenal ulcer.

There has been some controversy concerning the role of the gram-negative organism, *Campylobacter pylori,* in peptic ulcer disease. Evidence seems to indicate a strong association between a *C. pylori* infection and type B gastritis. In addition, *C. pylori* is one of the few organisms able to survive in the normally acid gastric environment. Recent reports show that the organism actually proliferates and may have a direct link with hydrogen ion, pepsin, and increased mucosal susceptibility to ulcer formation.[12] Further study will determine whether this organism does play a role in the development of peptic ulcer.

Complications

The three major complications of chronic peptic ulcer disease are hemorrhage, perforation, and gastric outlet obstruction. All are considered emergency situations and are initially treated conservatively. However, surgery may become necessary at any time during the course of the therapy.

Hemorrhage. Hemorrhage is the most common complication of peptic ulcer disease. It develops from erosion of the granulation tissue found at the base of the ulcer during healing or from erosion of the ulcer through a major blood vessel. Duodenal ulcers account for a greater percentage of upper GI bleeding than gastric ulcers.

Perforation. Perforation is considered the most lethal complication of peptic ulcer. Perforation is commonly seen in large penetrating duodenal ulcers that have not healed and are located on the posterior mucosal wall (Fig. 36-4). Perforated gastric ulcers are most frequently located on the lesser curvature of the stomach. Even though duodenal ulcers are more prevalent and perforate more frequently, mortality rates associated with perforation of gastric ulcers are higher. The older age of the client with gastric ulcers, who often has other concurrent medical problems, is thought to be the crucial factor.

Perforation of a peptic ulcer occurs when the ulcer penetrates the serosal surface, with spillage of either gastric or duodenal contents into the peritoneal cavity. The size of the perforation is directly proportional to the length of time the client has had the ulcer. The larger the perforation, the longer the history of the ulcer. Small perforations seal themselves and result in a cessation of symptoms; larger perforations require immediate surgical closure. Spontaneous sealing occurs as a result of large amounts of fibrin being produced in response to the perforation. This leads to fibrinous fusion of the duodenum or gastric curvature to adjacent tissue, mainly the liver.

The clinical manifestations of perforation are characterized by their sudden and dramatic onset. The client experiences sudden, severe upper abdominal pain that quickly spreads throughout the abdomen. The visceral and parietal layers of the peritoneum have an abundance of pain receptors, and this contributes to the abrupt, intense pain experienced. There may be shoulder pain if the spillage causes irritation to the phrenic nerve. The abdominal muscles are contracted so that they appear rigid and boardlike as they attempt to protect the abdomen from further injury. The client's respirations become shallow and rapid. Bowel sounds are usually absent. Nausea and vomiting may occur but are generally absent. Most clients have a history of ulcer disease or recent symptoms of indigestion.

The contents entering the peritoneal cavity from the stomach or duodenum contain a variety of ingredients, including air, saliva, food particles, hydrochloric acid, pepsin, bacteria, bile, and pancreatic juices. A bacterial peritonitis may occur within 6 to 12 hours, followed by paralytic ileus. The intensity of the peritonitis is proportional to the amount and duration of the spillage through the perforation. It is difficult to determine from the sudden onset of symptoms whether gastric or duodenal ulcer is the cause, since the clinical characteristics of perforation are the same (see Chapter 37).

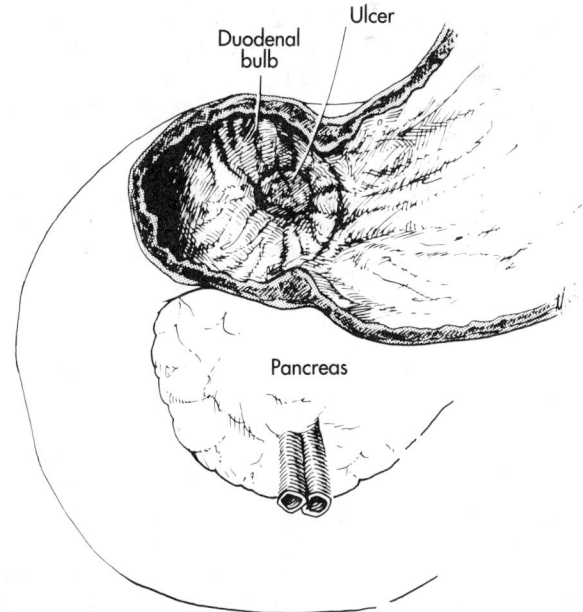

Fig. 36-4 Duodenal ulcer of the posterior wall penetrating into the head of the pancreas, resulting in a walled-off perforation. (From Price S and Wilson L: Pathophysiology: clinical concepts of disease processes, ed 4, St Louis, 1991, Mosby–Year Book, Inc.)

Gastric outlet obstruction. The most common cause of gastric outlet obstruction is duodenal ulceration. At times ulcers located in the antrum and the prepyloric and pyloric regions may also cause obstruction. In the early phase of obstruction (often referred to as the *compensated phase*), gastric emptying is normal to near normal. This phase may be associated with large peristaltic waves. Over time, excessive peristalsis creates hypertrophy of the stomach wall. After long-standing obstruction the stomach enters the *decompensated phase,* which results in dilatation and atony. The obstruction is not totally due to fibrous scar tissue because active ulcer formation is associated with edema, inflammation, and pylorospasm, all of which contribute to the narrowing of the pylorus.

The client with gastric outlet obstruction generally has a long history of ulcer pain. Ulcerlike pain of short duration or complete absence of pain is more indicative of a malignant obstruction. The pain progresses to a more generalized upper abdominal discomfort that becomes worse toward the end of the day as the stomach fills and dilates. Relief may be obtained by belching or by self-induced vomiting. Vomiting is very common and often projectile. The vomitus contains food particles that were ingested many hours or even a day or two before the vomiting episode. There is often an offensive odor if the contents have been dormant in the stomach for a time. The client who vomits frequently will be anorectic, with evident weight loss, and thirsty and will have an unpleasant taste in the mouth. Constipation is a common complaint that usually results from dehydration and lack of roughage in the diet.

The client with gastric outlet obstruction may show a swelling in the upper abdomen indicating dilatation of the stomach. Loud peristalsis can be heard, and visible peristaltic waves are often observed passing across the abdomen from left to right. If the stomach is grossly dilated, it is possible to palpate it as well.

An upper GI examination with barium as contrast medium is helpful in making a diagnosis and demonstrates the presence of an active ulcer crater or scarring from previously healed ulcers. Barium normally should pass from the stomach within 2 hours, but with gastric outlet obstruction, 50% of the barium remains on follow-up films up to 6 hours later.

Diagnostic Studies

The diagnostic measures used to determine the presence and location of a peptic ulcer are similar to those with acute upper GI bleeding. *Fiberoptic endoscopy* is the procedure most often used. It is more reliable than barium contrast studies because of the maneuverability of fiberoptic scopes for viewing the entire gastric and duodenal mucosa. These procedures can also be used to determine the degree of ulcer healing after treatment. When gastric malignancy is a possibility, the endoscope can be used in obtaining tissue specimens for biopsy.

Barium contrast studies, although widely used, are not accurate in identifying shallow, superficial ulcers because of failure of the barium to properly fill the ulcer crater. X-ray studies are also ineffective in differentiating a peptic ulcer from a malignant ulcer. In addition, x-ray films do not readily demonstrate the degree of healing that can be visually determined with the endoscope. Barium studies are of benefit in the diagnosis of pyloric obstruction due to recurrent ulcers.

Exfoliative cytology is valuable when there is a need to distinguish between a benign and a malignant ulcer. The test consists of examining exfoliated cells that are found in various body secretions or scraped from mucous membranes. A sample of these cells can be obtained during gastroscopic examination. Although the accuracy of this examination for determining the presence of a gastric tumor has proven value, it should not stand alone as a diagnostic tool because of the danger of false results.

Gastric analysis has questionable value in the diagnosis of peptic ulcer disease because in many clients gastric secretions are normal in amount and composition. However, it can provide important data in (1) identifying a possible gastrinoma (Zollinger-Ellison syndrome), (2) determining the amount of gastric hyperacidity, and (3) evaluating the results of therapy such as vagotomy and histamine H_2-antagonist drug therapy. Several methods may be used to determine the amount of gastric secretions. An NG tube can be placed into the antrum with the use of fluoroscopy and the secretions collected overnight for a 12-hour period. The hydrochloric acid concentration is calculated and compared with equivalents already established for persons who do not have ulcers, those with gastric and duodenal ulcers, and those with Zollinger-Ellison syndrome. The accuracy of this method is not good because the NG tube may become plugged or aspiration methods may be inconsistent. Augmented histamine or pentagastrin stimulation may be more accurate in estimating the degree of acid secretion. In these tests the stomach's ability to secrete gastric juice is studied after stimulation with either betazole HCl (Histalog) or pentagastrin.

Laboratory analysis, including a CBC, urinalysis, liver enzyme studies, serum amylase determination, and stool examination, should be performed. The CBC may indicate the presence of anemia secondary to bleeding from the ulcer. The liver enzyme studies help to determine any liver problems, such as cirrhosis, that may complicate the treatment of the ulcer. The urine and stool are routinely tested for the presence of blood. The serum amylase determination is frequently ordered if posterior penetration of the pancreas is suspected. It provides data on pancreatic function.

Therapeutic Management

Conservative management. When the client's clinical manifestations and health history suggest the diagnosis of a peptic ulcer and diagnostic studies confirm its presence, a medical regimen is instituted (see Table 36-9). The regimen consists of adequate rest, dietary interventions, medications, elimination of smoking, and long-term follow-up care. The aim of the treatment program is to decrease the amount of gastric acidity, enhance mucosal defense mechanisms, and minimize the harmful effects on the mucosa. Hospitalization of the client is not always necessary during the initial treatment phase.

Adequate rest, both physical and emotional, is important in the treatment process. A quiet, calm environment at home or on the job is not easy to achieve and may require some modifications in the client's daily routine. The benefits derived from the elimination of stressors help to decrease the stimulus for overproduction of gastric secretions. Moderation in daily activity is essential. Excessive physical activity can result in increased gastric secretions through increased motor activity.

Dietary changes are necessary so that foods and beverages irritating to the client can be avoided or eliminated. An individualized bland diet consisting of six small meals a day is usually prescribed in the regimen. However, there is considerable controversy over the actual therapeutic benefits derived from this type of diet, since the rationale for a bland diet is not supported by scientific evidence. Therefore no specific diet seems totally appropriate in the treatment of ulcer disease. Each client should be instructed to eat and drink foods and fluids that do not cause any distressing and harmful side effects. Alcohol and caffeine-containing products should be eliminated because of their irritating effects (see p. 1051).

Medications are a vital part of therapy. The client must be well informed about each drug prescribed, why it is ordered, and the expected benefits. Strict adherence to the prescribed regimen of drugs is mandatory. Drug therapy that includes the use of antacids, histamine H_2-receptor antagonists, and anticholinergics is shown in Table 36-10. Aspirin and nonsteroidal anti-inflammatory drugs should be discontinued. When these medications must be continued, enteric coated or highly buffered preparations are more suitable.[6]

Smoking, although not a primary cause of peptic ulcer, has an irritating effect on the mucosa, increases gastric motility, and delays mucosal healing. It should be eliminated completely or severely reduced. The combination of adequate rest and abstinence from smoking accelerates ulcer healing.

The healing of a peptic ulcer requires many weeks of therapy. Pain disappears after 3 to 6 days, but ulcer healing is much slower. Complete healing may take 3 to 9 weeks, depending on ulcer size and treatment regimen employed. Healing of the ulcer should be assessed by means of x-ray studies or endoscopic examination. Barium contrast films can be used to measure adequately the healing of a gastric ulcer. However, it should be noted that endoscopic examination is the only accurate measure of duodenal ulcer healing.

Because recurrence of peptic ulcer is frequent, interruption or discontinuation of therapy can have detrimental results. The client must be encouraged to comply with therapy and continue with follow-up care for at least 1 year. If changes in lifestyle were part of the prescribed therapy, they should be maintained. Antacids and H_2-receptor antagonists are usually stopped after the ulcer has healed or are prescribed in the form of low-dose maintenance therapy. No other medications, unless prescribed by the physician, should be taken because they may have an ulcerogenic effect. Finally, the client and the family should be told what to do in the event pain and discomfort recur or blood is noted in the vomitus or stools.

Table 36-9

Diagnostic and Therapeutic Management: Peptic Ulcer

DIAGNOSTIC

Complete blood count
Urinalysis
Liver enzymes
Serum electrolytes
Fiberoptic endoscopy
Upper GI barium-contrast study
Gastric analysis
Exfoliative cytology

THERAPEUTIC
Conservative management

Adequate rest
Bland diet (six small meals a day)
Cessation of smoking
Medications
    Antacids
    H_2-receptor blocking agents
    Anticholinergics
    Sucralfate
    H^+, K^+-ATPase inhibitors
    Prostaglandins
Stress reduction

Acute exacerbation without complications

NPO
NG suction
Bed rest to moderate light activity
Cessation of smoking
IV fluid replacement
Medications
    Antacids
    H_2-receptor blocking agents
    Anticholinergics
    Sedatives

Acute exacerbation with complications (hemorrhage, perforation, obstruction)

NPO
NG suction
Bed rest
IV fluid replacement (whole blood, packed RBCs, Ringer's lactate)
Stomach lavage

Surgical intervention

Perforation—simple closure with omentum graft
Gastric outlet obstruction—pyloroplasty and vagotomy
Ulcer cure
    Billroth I and II
    Vagotomy and pyloroplasty

Table 36-10 Drug Therapy for Peptic Ulcer Disease

ACID SUPPRESSION

Neutralization
  Antacids*
Decreased secretion
Acetylcholine antagonist
  Anticholinergics
H_2-receptor antagonists
  Cimetidine (Tagamet)
  Ranitidine HCl (Zantac)
  Famotidine (Pepcid)
  Nizatidine (Axid)
Gastrin-receptor antagonist
  Proglumide†
H^+, K^+-ATPase inhibitor
  Omeprazole†

CYTOPROTECTION

Sucralfate (Carafate)
Colloidal bismuth
Bismuth subsalicylate (Pepto-Bismol)

ANTISECRETORY AND CYTOPROTECTION

Prostaglandin analogs
Misoprostol (Cytotec)

OTHERS

Tricyclic antidepressants (e.g., amitriptyline [Elavil])
Carbenoxolone

Modified from Achkar E: Medical treatment of peptic ulcer disease, Hosp Formulary 24:80, 1989.
*See Table 36-11.
†Currently under investigation in the United States.

Acute exacerbation. The recurrence rate for both gastric and duodenal ulcers is high after therapeutic treatment. The client with an acute exacerbation of peptic ulcer can usually be treated with the same regimen used for conservative management. However, the situation is considered more serious because of the chronicity of the ulcer and the possible complications of perforation, hemorrhage, and obstruction.

An acute exacerbation is frequently accompanied by bleeding, increased pain and discomfort, and nausea and vomiting. One method of symptom relief involves the placement of an NG tube into the stomach, with intermittent suction for about 24 to 48 hours. The rationale is to keep the stomach empty and to remove any stimulus for hydrochloric acid and pepsin secretion. Major disadvantages of this intervention are esophageal and gastric mucosal irritation and erosion from the NG tube itself. When an NG tube is used, close observation is required so that symptoms are not made worse.

If there is a history of an incompetent pyloric sphincter allowing reflux of duodenal contents into the stomach, maintenance of an empty stomach decreases the stimulus

for pancreatic enzyme secretion as well. This period of stomach rest eliminates any causative factors that may have precipitated the acute exacerbation and permits the resolution of edema and inflammation of the mucosa. Fluids and electrolytes are replaced by IV infusion until the client is able to tolerate oral feedings without distress.

Blood or blood products may be administered if bleeding has occurred. Careful monitoring of the vital signs, intake and output, laboratory studies, and signs of impending shock are important during this acute episode.

Endoscopic examination is usually performed on each client sometime during the acute period. The guidelines for using endoscopy include (1) severe systemic disease, (2) lack of improvement within 7 to 10 days of treatment, and (3) persistent symptoms at the end of the treatment regimen. Other clients who benefit from endoscopic examination are those who have recurrent ulcer disease, who suffer complications or are at high risk of complications, who are over 50 years of age with a personal or family history of gastric cancer, or who have symptoms suggestive of gastric cancer.[6]

Inspection reveals the degree of inflammation or bleeding as well as the ulcer location. It is important to ascertain the presence of a prepyloric or pyloric ulcer that can cause gastric outlet obstruction.

When endoscopic examination reveals no major problems and the client's physical condition stabilizes, the plan of care for the client should follow the same regimen of diet, activity, and medications as used in conservative management. A 5-year follow-up program is recommended after acute exacerbation. An increase in the healing rate is achieved after conservative treatment, but the treatment plan cannot prevent the scar formation that can result in gastric outlet obstruction. Approximately 42% to 88% of ulcers recur.

Perforation. The immediate focus of therapeutic management of a client with a perforation is to stop the spillage of gastric contents into the peritoneal cavity and restore blood volume. An NG tube is inserted into the stomach to provide continuous aspiration and gastric decompression to halt spillage through the perforation. Although duodenal aspiration is not achieved as promptly, placement of the tube as near to the perforation site as possible facilitates decompression.

Circulating blood volume must be replaced with lactated Ringer's and albumin solutions. These solutions substitute for the fluids lost from the vascular and interstitial space as the peritonitis develops. Blood replacement in the form of packed RBCs may be necessary. Unless contraindicated, a central venous pressure line and an indwelling catheter should be inserted and monitored hourly. Clients with a history of cardiac disease require ECG monitoring or placement of a pulmonary artery catheter for more accurate assessment of left ventricular function. Broad-spectrum antibiotic therapy should be started immediately to treat the bacterial peritonitis. Administration of pain medications provides comfort.

This regimen may be all that is required for some clients whose perforations seal spontaneously. When the perforation cannot be corrected by conservative management, surgical closure must be carried out as soon as blood volume is restored. It is generally believed that clients with uncorrected hypovolemia should not be subjected to any surgical procedure for approximately 12 hours. This length of time is viewed as sufficient to adequately initiate decompression measures, restore lost blood volume, and stabilize the client's condition.

The operative procedure involving the least risk to the client is simple oversewing of the perforation and reinforcement of the area with a graft of omentum. The excess gastric contents are suctioned from the peritoneal cavity during the surgical procedure. Before surgical closure some surgeons irrigate with warm Ringer's lactate solution or instill an antibiotic solution into the abdominal cavity to help counteract the peritonitis.

There is controversy regarding the need for more definitive surgical treatment of a perforated ulcer than can be achieved with simple closure. Other types of surgical procedures used depend on the location of the peptic ulcer and the surgeon's preference. If cure of the ulcer is the ultimate goal, the surgical procedures may include gastric resection or vagotomy and pyloroplasty.

Gastric outlet obstruction. The aim of therapy for gastric outlet obstruction is to decompress the stomach, correct any existing fluid and electrolyte imbalances, and improve the client's general state of health. An NG tube is inserted into the stomach and attached to continuous suction to remove excess fluids and undigested food particles. With continuous decompression for several days the stomach has the opportunity to regain its normal muscle tone, the ulcer can begin healing, and the inflammation and edema will subside.

The tube is clamped after several days of suction, and gastric residue is measured periodically. The frequency and amount of time the tube remains clamped are proportional to the amount of aspirate obtained and the comfort level of the client. A method commonly followed is to clamp the tube overnight for approximately 8 to 12 hours and to measure the gastric residue in the morning. When the aspirate falls below 200 ml, it is considered to be within a normal range and the client can begin oral intake of clear liquids. Initially, oral fluids are begun at 30 ml/hr and then gradually increased in amount. The client must be watched carefully for signs of distress or vomiting. As the amount of gastric residue decreases, solid foods are added and the tube is removed.

IV fluids and electrolytes are administered according to the degree of dehydration, vomiting, and electrolyte imbalance indicated by laboratory studies. Pain relief results from the decompression measures, and analgesics are usually not necessary. Such drugs as anticholinergics are not recommended for clients with gastric outlet obstruction because they reduce gastric motility and gastric emptying. Antacid and histamine H_2-receptor antagonist therapy is an integral part of treatment if the obstruction has been determined on endoscopic examination to be the result of an active ulcer. Pyloric obstruction may be removed nonsurgically by balloon dilatations performed through the endoscope. Surgical intervention may be necessary to remove scar tissue (see p. 1064). Drug therapy in the management of peptic ulcer disease has made significant advances in recent years (see Table 36-10).

Pharmacological Management

Antacids. Antacids are the initial drugs of choice in the treatment of peptic ulcers. They decrease gastric acidity and the acid content reaching the duodenum. By raising the pH level to above 3.5, antacids effectively inactivate pepsin's proteolytic activity. In addition to their neutralizing effects, some antacids, such as aluminum hydroxide, can bind to bile salts, thus decreasing their detrimental effects on the gastric mucosa.

Antacids consist of systemic and nonsystemic types. Systemic antacids, such as sodium bicarbonate, are very soluble and are absorbed into the circulation. Their long-term use can lead to systemic alkalosis; therefore they are rarely used in ulcer treatment. The nonsystemic antacids are insoluble and poorly absorbed. The common commercial nonsystemic antacids consist of calcium carbonate, magnesium hydroxide, or aluminum hydroxide as single preparations or in various combinations (Table 36-11).

Table 36-11 Composition of Antacid Preparations

Ingredient	Trade Name
Single substance	
Aluminum carbonate	Basaljel
Aluminum hydroxide gel tablets	Amphojel/Alu-Cap
Aluminum phosphate	Phosphaljel
Calcium carbonate	Alka-2, Tums
Dihydroxyaluminum aminoacetate	Robalate
Dihydroxyaluminum sodium carbonate	Rolaids
Magaldrate	Riopan
Magnesium carbonate	
Magnesium hydroxide	Mag-Ox, Maox
Mixtures of aluminum hydroxide and magnesium salts	
	Aludrox
	A-M-T
	Cremalin
	Delcid
	Gaviscon
	Gelusil and Gelusil M
	Maalox
	Mylanta
	WinGel
Mixtures of calcium carbonate and aluminum and magnesium hydroxides	
	Camalox
	Ducon
Mixtures of calcium carbonate, magnesium carbonate, and magnesium oxide	
	Alkets

Table 36-12 Side Effects of Antacid Therapy

Antacid	Reactions
Aluminum hydroxide gels	Constipation, phosphorus depletion with chronic use
Calcium carbonate	Constipation or diarrhea, hypercalcemia, milk-alkali syndrome, renal calculi
Magnesium preparations	Diarrhea, hypermagnesemia, phosphorus-depletion syndrome
Sodium preparations	Milk-alkali syndrome if used with large amounts of calcium, sodium toxicity if on sodium restrictions

The preparation may be in liquid or tablet form. A large number of tablets may be required to equal the same dose of a liquid preparation. Since the tablets are chewable, much of the medication is left coating the teeth and gingivae instead of the stomach.

It has long been recognized that antacids ingested on an empty stomach are quickly evacuated and only partially used. Because the duration of action is only about 30 minutes, best results are obtained when they are prescribed 1 and 3 hours after meals and at bedtime. More frequent administration has resulted in poor tolerance and reduced long-term compliance. Acid secretion is also known to occur with higher doses and frequency by maintaining a high antral pH, which in turn stimulates release of gastrin.

The physician must consider the type and dosage of antacid prescribed because of the adverse effects some of these preparations have on the health status or on other medications the client may be taking (Table 36-12). Preparations high in sodium, such as Titralac, Di-Gel, and Amphojel, should be used with caution in older adults and in clients with cirrhosis of the liver, hypertension, congestive heart failure, and renal disease. Magnesium preparations should not be prescribed for clients in renal failure because of the risk of magnesium toxicity. The most frequent side effect experienced with magnesium antacids is diarrhea. Aluminum hydroxide causes constipation. The combination of aluminum and magnesium salts seems to lessen the side effects of both.

Antacids have the capacity to interact unfavorably with some medications. They can enhance the absorption of drugs such as dicumarol and amphetamines. The action of digitalis preparations can be potentiated when taken in combination with calcium or magnesium antacids. In some instances, antacids may decrease the absorption rates of prescribed drugs, such as tetracycline. Therefore it is important to inform the physician of any drugs that are being taken before antacid therapy is begun.

The dosage of antacid must often be adjusted by the physician so that the amount prescribed has the capacity of neutralizing the acid present. It is generally recommended that each dose of an antacid be capable of neutralizing 100 mEq of hydrochloric acid. Any alteration in dosage should be carefully communicated to the client and the family, along with the rationale for the change so that compliance is more likely. The adjustment of antacids by the client must be avoided. Taking too much or too little of an antacid can compromise its effectiveness and may lead to unpleasant side effects or an increase in ulcer discomfort.

For active gastric and duodenal ulcers, the prescribed treatment period varies from 4 to 8 weeks or until healing is demonstrated through endoscopic or barium contrast studies. Many physicians recommend daily maintenance doses of an antacid to minimize ulcer recurrence.

Compliance with long-term antacid therapy seems to diminish with time. The client fails to take the correct dose or stops taking the drug altogether. Many persons stop therapy because they find it inconvenient to keep the necessary daily supply at work, when traveling, or at home. For some clients it is embarrassing to be seen taking medications generally known to be prescribed for people with ulcers.

Histamine H$_2$-receptor antagonist. The use of the histamine H$_2$-receptor antagonists cimetidine (Tagamet), ranitidine (Zantac), famotidine (Pepcid), and nizatidine (Axid) is now a standard component of most ulcer treatment regimens. Histamine is believed to be the final intracellular activator of hydrochloric acid secretion. These drugs block the action of histamine on the H$_2$ receptors and thus reduce hydrochloric acid secretion and accelerate ulcer healing. Commonly used antihistamine drugs have no effect on gastric acid secretion.

Histamine H$_2$-blocker drugs may be administered orally or IV. Their therapeutic effects are considerably longer than those of antacids, some lasting for up to 12 hours. In addition, the drugs have demonstrated capabilities in the healing of gastric and duodenal ulcers. When the oldest of the H$_2$ blockers, cimetidine and ranitidine, are compared, the latter clearly has several advantages: (1) it is 5 to 12 times more potent and therefore has a longer duration of action; (2) optimal dosage can be achieved on a bid (twice a day) schedule versus qid (four times a day) for cimetidine; (3) it inhibits nocturnal acid secretion for a longer time period; (4) it has fewer side effects (headache, dizziness, malaise, neutropenia, thrombocytopenia, and elevated liver enzyme levels) than cimetidine (granulocytopenia, gynecomastia, diarrhea, fatigue, dizziness, rash, and mental confusion in older adults); (5) it is capable of healing ulcers that were resistant to cimetidine therapy.

Famotidine (Pepcid) and nizatidine (Axid) are the newest of these drugs now available. They are considered more potent at reduced dosage levels. Side effects appear to be minimal. Muscle cramps, headache, and constipation have been associated with the use of famotidine. Somnolence, sweating, and urticaria have occurred with nizatidine. Both drugs can be administered with antacids. Although side effects are minimal, additional adverse reactions may become apparent with continued use.

Anticholinergic drugs. Anticholinergic drugs are often ordered in the treatment of peptic ulcer disease. These drugs decrease cholinergic stimulation of gastric secretions. There is divided opinion concerning their efficacy in

Table 36-13 Anticholinergic Drugs Used in the Treatment of Peptic Ulcer

Trade Name	Generic Name
Antrenyl Bromide	Oxyphenonium bromide, atropine sulfate
Banthine	Methantheline bromide
Bentyl	Dicyclomine
Cantil	Mepenzolate bromide
Darbid	Isopropamide iodide
Daricon	Oxyphencyclimine
Donnatol	Belladonna and phenobarbital
Pamine	Methscopolamine bromide
Pro-Banthine	Propantheline bromide
Robinul	Glycopyrrolate

preventing recurrences and their therapeutic effectiveness in alleviating symptoms and preventing complications. Because of their tendency to decrease gastric motility, they should be avoided in gastric ulcer in which stasis of secretions increases the client's pain and discomfort. Their use is associated with a high incidence of side effects, such as dry mouth and skin, flushing, thirst, tachycardia, dilated pupils, blurred vision, and urine retention. Anticholinergics must be prescribed with caution in clients with narrow-angle glaucoma, prostatic hypertrophy, and gastric outlet obstruction. It has been predicted that the use of anticholinergics may decline as a result of the acceptance of histamine H_2-receptor antagonists. Anticholinergics, however, are able to potentiate the benefits of antacids and cimetidine. Therefore their use in ulcer therapy is likely to continue for the present. Commonly prescribed anticholinergic medications are listed in Table 36-13.

Other drug therapy. In addition to the standard drug therapy for ulcers, several new medications are available. Sucralfate (Carafate) is used for the short-term treatment of duodenal ulcers. Its ability to accelerate ulcer healing is thought to be a result of the formation of an ulcer-adherent complex covering the ulcer and thereby protecting it from erosion from pepsin, acid, and bile salts. Sucralfate does not have acid-neutralizing capabilities. It has proven to be cytoprotective of the stomach and possibly the duodenum. Its action is most effective at a low pH, and it should be given at least 30 minutes before or after an antacid. Adverse side effects are minimal. However, it does bind with cimetidine, digoxin, warfarin (Coumadin), phenytoin, and tetracycline, causing reduced bioavailability of these drugs.[13]

Colloidal bismuth or bismuth subsalicylate (Pepto-Bismol) has demonstrated ability to facilitate healing of peptic ulcer. It is effective against *Campylobacter pylori*, which has recently been identified as the organism present in large numbers of clients with gastritis or gastric and duodenal ulcers. This drug is nonabsorbable and causes black stool.

Misoprostol (Cytotec) is a new prostaglandin synthetic analogue. It has both protective and antisecretory effects on gastric mucosa. Misoprostol is the only drug approved in the United States for the prevention of gastric ulcers induced by nonsteroidal antiinflammatory drugs and aspirin. A major advantage of misoprostol is that it does not interfere with the therapeutic effects of aspirin and nonsteroidal antiinflammatory drugs. It is believed that persons who require chronic nonsteroidal antiinflammatory drug therapy, such as those with osteoarthritis and who are over 60 years of age, benefit from the use of misoprostol because it causes fewer complications of gastric ulcer and less frequent need for hospitalization.[14] Chronic users of aspirin and nonsteroidal antiinflammatory drugs have been at risk of complications of gastric ulcer.

H^+, K^+-ATPase inhibitors, such as the investigational drug omeprazole, have shown ability to suppress gastric acid secretion. Studies indicate that it heals duodenal ulcer in 88% to 100% of the cases after 6 weeks' treatment.[4] Omeprazole is not yet approved for use in the United States.

Tricyclic antidepressants (e.g., imipramine, doxepin) have duodenal ulcer healing rates close to those obtained with cimetidine. The mode of action is not fully understood but appears similar to that of anticholinergic agents.

Metoclopramide (Reglan) is a procainamide derivative that is sometimes prescribed in ulcer disease. It appears to enhance gastric motility and emptying but has no effect on acid or gastrin secretion. Metoclopramide is used in the treatment of gastric ulcers. Through its ability to stimulate motility and gastric emptying, the stasis or prolonged retention of acid-stimulating food or drugs in the stomach is prevented. Metoclopramide should never be used in clients with upper GI hemorrhage or mechanical obstruction or in whom perforation is suspected. The drug therapy selected for the client is often determined by the cost and drug availability.

Nutritional Considerations

There are no specific diets or foods that are totally useful in treating peptic ulcer disease. The client is encouraged to eat as normally as possible. If certain foods result in pain or discomfort, they should be avoided. The critical aspect is individualization of the dietary plan.

Food acts as a buffer for gastric secretions. The buffering action of food lasts about 60 minutes and is then followed by an increase in the concentration of acid in the secretions. Dietary orders vary according to the preference of the physician, but there is general agreement that foods eaten should be those that are well tolerated by the client and eaten on a regular schedule of six meals a day. The rationale for ingesting many meals a day instead of three large ones is that the stomach should never be totally empty. In this way, gastric motility is decreased, gastric acid is neutralized, and the digestive action on the mucosa is minimal. Gastric contractions increase in intensity when the stomach is empty or distended with large amounts of food.

Dietary instructions should include a sample diet with a list of foods that usually cause distress and should therefore be eliminated from the diet. Foods known to irritate the gastric mucosa include hot, spicy foods and pepper; alcohol; carbonated beverages; tea; coffee; and broth (meat extract). They are contraindicated because they have no known buffering capacity yet are able to stimulate gastric acid secretion. Foods high in roughage, such as raw fruit, salads, and vegetables, may irritate an inflamed mucosa. If these foods are well chewed, this seems to be less of a problem.

Protein is considered the best neutralizing food, but it also stimulates gastric secretions. Carbohydrates and fats are the least stimulating to acid secretion, but they do not neutralize well. The client must determine a suitable combination of these essential nutrients without causing undue distress to the ulcer disease.

Historically, milk was an essential part of ulcer therapy until it was learned that milk proteins and calcium are stimulants to gastric acid production. For this reason, milk as part of diet therapy for ulcers was out of favor for a time. Recent investigations have demonstrated that milk not only can neutralize gastric acidity but also contains prostaglandins and growth factors, both of which are known to protect the GI mucosa from injury.

■ Nursing Management of Peptic Ulcer

Nursing assessment

Subjective and objective data that should be obtained from a client with peptic ulcer disease are presented in Table 36-14.

Nursing diagnoses

Nursing diagnoses are determined when the problem and the etiological factors are supported by clinical data. Nursing diagnoses related to peptic ulcer may include, but are not limited to, those presented in Table 36-15.

Nursing interventions

Health promotion and maintenance. Clients in whom peptic ulcer disease has been diagnosed have specific teaching needs that must be met to prevent and avoid recurrence or complications. General instructions should cover aspects of the disease process itself, nutritional therapy, medication, possible changes in lifestyle, and regular follow-up care.

Knowing the cause of the ulcer and understanding the disease process may motivate the client to become more involved in care and increase compliance with therapy. The client needs to understand the diet plan and why it is essential for recovery and health maintenance. The nurse and the dietitian should elicit a dietary history from the client and plan for ways in which the ulcer diet can be easily incorporated into the client's home and work setting. The client who is following a diet prescribed for another illness needs to know how to balance the two so that the two conditions are not harmed by dietary interventions.

The client does not always provide the physician with accurate information regarding habitual use of alcohol or cigarettes. The nurse may be looked upon as less threatening and more understanding of these habits than the physician. The nurse should use these interactions as opportunities to provide useful information about the detrimental effects of alcohol and cigarettes on ulcer disease.

The nurse should instruct the client about prescribed medications, including their actions, side effects, and in-

Table 36-14

Nursing Assessment of the Client with Peptic Ulcer

SUBJECTIVE DATA

History
Positive family history, stress, alcohol abuse, cigarette smoking, gastrinoma, chronic renal failure, chronic obstructive pulmonary disease, serious illness or trauma
Medications
Use of aspirin, corticosteroids, indomethacin, phenylbutazone
General
Weight loss, anorexia
Pain
Duodenal ulcers: Burning, epigastric pain occurring 2 to 4 hours after meals and relieved by food
Gastric ulcers: Pain occurring 1 to 2 hours after meals and made worse by food; worse at night
Gastrointestinal
Pyrosis, belching, nausea and vomiting, dyspepsia, abdominal tenderness, dark stools

OBJECTIVE DATA

General
Anxiety, irritability
Gastrointestinal
Epigastric tenderness
Possible findings
Anemia; guaiac-positive stools; abnormal upper GI, endoscopic, and barium studies

herent dangers if omitted for any reason. The client should know why over-the-counter medications (e.g., aspirin) should not be taken unless approved by the physician. Because antacids are a large part of therapy and may be bought without prescription, the client must be informed that interchanging brands without checking with the physician or nurse can lead to harmful side effects.

Efforts should be made to obtain more information about the client's psychosocial status. Knowledge of lifestyle, occupation, and coping behaviors can be helpful to the plan of care. The client may be reluctant to talk about personal subjects, the stress experienced at home or on the job, the ordinary method of coping, or dependence on drugs or alcohol. Unfortunately, the client does not often see the relationship between lifestyle or occupation and ulcer disease. It is important to listen for subtle clues from the client's statements and to observe for behavior that broadens this data base.

When the occupation, related work habits, home, or environment have been implicated as factors in peptic ulcer development, the client must be made aware of these stressors, how to avoid them in the future, or how to cope with them successfully if they cannot be altered. Vocational or psychological counseling may be necessary so that fatigue and repeated emotional upsets can be avoided.

Table 36-15

 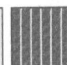

NURSING CARE PLAN FOR THE CLIENT WITH PEPTIC ULCER

Defining Characteristics	Nursing Interventions	Evaluation Criteria

Conservative Management

NURSING DIAGNOSIS: **Pain related to increased gastric secretions, decreased mucosal protection, and ingestion of gastric irritants**

Defining Characteristics	Nursing Interventions	Evaluation Criteria
Burning cramplike pain in epigastrium and abdomen; pain onset 1 to 2 hr after meals with gastric ulcer; pain onset 2 to 4 hr after meals (midmorning, midafternoon) and middle of night with duodenal ulcer; pain relieved by food, liquids, or antacids; occasional nausea and vomiting	Determine pain characteristics from verbal description and physical assessment data. Reinforce need to comply with peptic ulcer disease management plan.	Verbalization of satisfaction with pain control

NURSING DIAGNOSIS: **Impaired home maintenance management related to lack of knowledge of long-term management of peptic ulcer disease**

Defining Characteristics	Nursing Interventions	Evaluation Criteria
Frequent questions about home care, incorrect responses to questions about peptic ulcer disease	Explain ulcer disease process at client's level of understanding. Help client identify stressors and initiate modifications in daily routine. Discuss diet plan and assist with implementation at home and in work setting. Provide rationale for the elimination of alcohol, spicy foods, coffee, tea, and carbonated beverages from diet. Explain the harmful effects of smoking. Provide information on medication actions and side effects. Caution against strenuous exercise and activity.	Verbalization of plan to modify lifestyle and incorporate therapeutic regimen into lifestyle

NURSING DIAGNOSIS: **Noncompliance with medical regimen related to unwillingness to modify lifestyle and lack of understanding of consequences of not following treatment plan**

Defining Characteristics	Nursing Interventions	Evaluation Criteria
Missed appointments, persistence of symptoms, disease progression with evidence of complications, partially used or unused medications, evidence of dietary indiscretions, failure to set and achieve health-enhancing goals	Emphasize that disease process requires commitment to therapeutic regimen and long-term follow-up care. Discuss dangers of dietary indiscretions, alcohol ingestion, and smoking. Discuss why over-the-counter drugs must not be taken without physician's approval. Offer encouragement and helpful ways client can incorporate plan of care into pattern of living. Inform client what to do if symptoms of ulcers occur.	Willingness to adhere to and knowledge of plan of care

Acute Exacerbation Management

NURSING DIAGNOSIS: **Acute pain related to acute exacerbation of disease process and inadequate comfort measures**

Defining Characteristics	Nursing Interventions	Evaluation Criteria
Verbalization of increase in pain, nonverbal indicators of pain, such as moaning, crying, doubling up	Encourage bed rest or light activity. Provide quiet, relaxed environment and limit visitors. Administer medications as ordered.	Satisfaction with pain management

Continued.

Table 36-15

 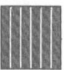

NURSING CARE PLAN FOR THE CLIENT WITH PEPTIC ULCER—cont'd

Defining Characteristics	Nursing Interventions	Evaluation Criteria

NURSING DIAGNOSIS: Nausea and vomiting related to acute exacerbation of disease process and inadequate comfort measures

Verbalization of increase in nausea and/or vomiting	Maintain NPO status. Maintain NG tube to suction; explain rationale. Check patency frequently. Provide mouth and nose care q 4 hr. Check vomitus or aspirate for occult blood.	Decrease or absence of nausea and vomiting, increase in client comfort

NURSING DIAGNOSIS: Ineffective individual coping: depression and frustration related to exacerbation and possible complications of disease process

Perception of powerlessness, anxiety and fear of unknown, inability to effectively self-manage symptoms, perception of loss of control	Assess coping skills. Suggest more effective ways to deal with health status. Assist client and family to understand why the ulcer may have recurred. Reeducate client about diet and drugs. Offer reassurance and faith in plan. Suggest vocational or psychological counseling if indicated.	Expression of satisfaction with coping strategies, active role in personal health care

NURSING DIAGNOSIS: Potential complication: hemorrhage secondary to eroded mucosal tissue

Evidence of hematemesis, bright red or melena stool; abdominal pain or discomfort; symptoms of shock (lower blood pressure, cool, clammy skin, cyanosis, dyspnea, tachycardia, decreased urine output); history of peptic ulcer and chronic gastritis; history of previous treatment of peptic ulcers; recent ingestion of nonsteroidal antiinflammatory drugs and aspirin	If ordered, maintain NG tube for suction and ensure its patency by lavaging. If ulcer is actively bleeding, observe aspirate for amount and color, suggesting brisk or slow bleed. Take vital signs every 15 to 30 min. Maintain IV infusion line. If blood is replaced, observe for transfusion reaction. Record intake and output. Watch for signs of impending shock. Reassure client and family. Remain calm and confident in plan of care. Monitor laboratory studies of hematocrit and hemoglobin. Administer medications as ordered.	No evidence of bleeding, hemoglobin and hematocrit within normal ranges, stable vital signs

NURSING DIAGNOSIS: Potential complication: perforation of GI mucosa secondary to impaired mucosal tissue integrity

Report of sudden, severe onset of abdominal pain; client in fetal position; rigid, boardlike abdomen; change in vital signs (hypovolemic shock); change in bowel sounds from normal to hypoactive to absent; anxious and fearful appearance	Observe for manifestations of perforation, such as sudden, severe abdominal pain; rigid, boardlike abdomen; pain to shoulders; increasing distention; decreasing bowel sounds. Monitor vital signs every 15 to 30 min. Maintain NG tube to suction. Administer pain medication. Monitor IV fluids. Observe for signs of hypovolemic shock. Prepare client for emergency diagnostic tests and possible surgical intervention. Assess for allergies to antibiotics.	Satisfactory level of pain control, identification of and management for perforation

The need for long-term follow-up care must be stressed. Because therapeutic management is frequently followed by a recurrence of the ulcer disease, the client should be encouraged to seek immediate intervention if symptoms of the disease recur.

Acute intervention. During the acute exacerbation of an ulcer, the client generally complains of increased pain and nausea and vomiting, and some may have evidence of bleeding. Initially, many clients attempt to cope with the symptoms at home before receiving medical assistance.

Very often during this acute phase all that is necessary for the client's immediate recovery is to maintain NPO status for a few days, with an NG tube to intermittently suction and replace fluids. The rationale for this therapy must be conveyed to the anxious client and the family. They must be made to understand that the advantages far outweigh any temporary discomfort imposed by the presence of the tube. Regular mouth care alleviates the dry mouth. Cleansing and lubrication of the nares facilitates breathing and decreases soreness. Gastric contents should be analyzed for acid level, blood, bile, or other irritating substances. When the stomach is kept empty of gastric secretions, the ulcer pain diminishes and ulcer healing begins. Usually this form of intervention is effective, and the client reacts with gratitude and cooperation.

Because the client is receiving nothing by mouth, IV fluids are ordered. The type and amount administered are directly related to the fluid lost, the manifestations exhibited by the client, and the results of the hemoglobin, hematocrit, and electrolyte determinations. The nurse should be aware of any other current health problem that could be adversely affected by the type of fluid used or the rate of the infusion. Constant monitoring of these parameters provides information on the hydration status and the effectiveness of treatment. Vital signs are initially taken at least hourly so that shock can be detected and treated. This is especially important if the client had a bleeding episode or if blood is present in the gastric aspirate or stool.

Physical and emotional rest are conducive to ulcer healing. The client's immediate environment should be quiet and restful, and visitors should be restricted. The use of a mild sedative or tranquilizer has beneficial effects when the client is anxious and apprehensive. The nurse must use good judgment before sedating a person who is becoming increasingly restless. There is danger that the medication will mask the signs of shock secondary to upper GI bleeding.

If the client's condition improves without progression of symptoms (e.g., increased pain, vomiting, hemorrhage), the regimen outlined for conservative medical management is followed. All too frequently, an acute exacerbation is accompanied by one or more complications, especially hemorrhage and perforation and, to a lesser extent, obstruction.

HEMORRHAGE. Changes in the vital signs and an increase in the amount and redness of the aspirate often signal massive upper GI bleeding. It is important to maintain the patency of the NG tube so that blood clots do not obstruct the tube. If the tube becomes blocked, the client can develop abdominal distention. When there is an increased amount of blood in the gastric contents, the client's pain is often decreased because the blood helps to neutralize the acidic gastric contents. This is an important point to recognize whenever the pain previous to this episode has been constant or unrelieved by suction or drugs.

The nurse needs to monitor the results of the hemoglobin and hematocrit determinations. Awareness of the significance of the report and ability to correlate the data to the client's signs and symptoms can be lifesaving. (The nursing intervention for upper GI bleeding is discussed in more detail on p. 1056.)

PERFORATION. When there is sudden, severe abdominal pain unrelated in intensity and location to the pain that brought the client to the hospital, the nurse must recognize the possibility of ulcer perforation. When any person with an ulcer, particularly a chronic duodenal ulcer, demonstrates these manifestations, perforation should be suspected and the physician notified immediately.

Perforation is indicated by a rigid, boardlike abdomen, severe generalized abdominal and shoulder pain, drawing up of the knees, and shallow, grunting respirations. The bowel sounds that may have been normal or hyperactive previously may diminish and become absent.

Vital signs are important parameters and should be promptly recorded and taken every 15 to 30 minutes. The nurse should temporarily stop all oral or NG medications and feedings until the physician can be reached and a definitive diagnosis made. If perforation does exist, anything taken internally can add to the spillage into the peritoneal cavity and increase discomfort. If IV fluids are being administered at the time of the perforation, the rate should be maintained or increased as the plasma volume becomes depleted.

The symptoms experienced by the client are very frightening. The reaction of the nursing staff must be one of calm reassurance in spite of the seriousness of the situation. Simple explanations of the need for chest and abdominal x-ray films help diminish the client's anxiety and give some insight into the diagnostic plan. Indicating why frequent samples of blood are necessary lessens confusion and resistance.

When perforation is confirmed, the nurse should ensure that any known allergies the client has have been recorded on the chart. This is important because antibiotic therapy is usually started and careful observation for allergic reactions must be made. When the perforation fails to seal spontaneously, surgical closure is necessary and is performed as soon as possible. There is often little time to prepare the client and the family thoroughly for the surgical intervention, yet some instructions can be carried out while the immediate therapy is begun. If major reconstructive surgery is anticipated, the client and the family may question the need when the problem is only a small hole. To answer this type of question, the nurse must first have an understanding of the usual operative procedures being used and, in addition, must know that unless the surgery can cure the ulcer that caused the perforation, the client may need more surgery in the future. (Nursing management of peritonitis is discussed in Chapter 37.)

GASTRIC OUTLET OBSTRUCTION. Gastric outlet obstruction is a complication of peptic ulcer disease that can occur at any time. Because the onset of symptoms is usually gradual, the condition is not generally as serious an emergency as hemorrhage or perforation. Obstruction is a possible complication when the client has a history of an ulcer that is located close to the pylorus. Relief of symptoms is easily achieved by constant NG aspiration of stomach contents. This allows edema and inflammation to subside and then permits normal flow of gastric contents through the pylorus.

Obstruction can also occur during the treatment of an acute episode of peptic ulcer exacerbation. If these symptoms are experienced while the client is still on NPO status, the patency of the NG tube should be suspected. Regular irrigation of the tube with a saline solution facilitates proper functioning. It may be helpful to reposition the client from side to side so that the tube tip is not constantly lying against the mucosal surface.

When oral feedings have been resumed and symptoms of obstruction are observed, the physician should be promptly informed. Generally, all that is necessary is to resume gastric aspiration so that the edema and inflammation resulting from the acute episode have more time to resolve. IV fluids with electrolyte replacement keep the client hydrated during this period. Clamping the NG tube and checking for gastric retention have to be done. It is important to maintain accurate intake and output records, especially of the gastric aspirate. The client should be kept aware of why these symptoms are being experienced and should be assured that the condition will improve shortly. In some instances in which treatment is not successful, surgery may be performed after the acute phase has passed.

Chronic management. The client who has recurrence of ulcer disease following initial healing must learn to live with a disease that is chronic. The client may be angry and frustrated, especially if the prescribed mode of therapy has been faithfully followed and failed to halt the extension of the disease process.

Unfortunately, many clients do not comply with the plan of care originally designed, and they experience repeated exacerbations. Clients quickly learn that they experience no discomfort when they omit prescribed medications or indulge in occasional dietary indiscretions. Often they make no or little alteration in lifestyle. After an acute exacerbation the client is often more amenable to following the plan of care and open to suggestions for changes in lifestyle. Changes are difficult for most people and may be met with resistance. This reaction itself can result in hypersecretion and hypermotility and cause a delay in ulcer healing.

If the client has been instructed to stop smoking or to avoid the use of alcohol, the benefits of such a request must be measured against the detrimental physical and emotional outcomes. The client may fare better from a reduction in their use rather than from total elimination. Although alcohol and smoking are known to interfere with ulcer healing, they frequently serve as coping mechanisms. From the client's point of view, the anguish caused by their total elimination may outweigh the benefits to be gained from abstention. The goal, however, should always be total cessation. A client with chronic ulcers needs to be aware of the complications that may result from the disease, the clinical manifestations indicating their presence, and what to do until the physician can be seen.

Surgical Interventions

The indications for surgical treatment of ulcers are decided on an individual basis. About 20% of clients with ulcers need surgical intervention. Because there is a high recurrence rate for both duodenal and gastric ulcers and complications increase with the duration of the ulcer, many physicians believe that surgery is necessary after therapy has been tried and proved unsuccessful. The following criteria are used as general indications for surgical intervention:

1. Intractability: Failure of the ulcer to heal or recurrence of the ulcer after therapy
2. Previous history of hemorrhage or increased risk of bleeding during treatment
3. Prepyloric or pyloric ulcers (both have high recurrence rates)
4. Concurrent condition, such as severe burns, trauma, or sepsis
5. Multiple ulcer sites
6. Drug-induced ulcers, especially when withdrawal from the drug may put the person at risk
7. Possible existence of a malignant ulcer

A variety of surgical procedures are used to treat ulcer disease. They usually involve a partial gastrectomy, vagotomy, and/or pyloroplasty. Partial gastrectomy with removal of the distal two thirds of the stomach and anastomosis of the gastric stump to the duodenum is called a *gastroduodenostomy* or *Billroth I* operation. Partial gastrectomy with removal of the distal two thirds of the stomach and anastomosis of the gastric stump to the jejenum is called a *gastrojejunostomy* or *Billroth II* operation. In both procedures the antrum and the pylorus are removed. Because the duodenum is bypassed, Billroth II operation is the preferred surgical procedure for the repair of duodenal ulcers and prevention of their recurrence. Figure 36-5 is a schematic drawing of the Billroth I and II procedures.

Vagotomy is the severing of the vagus nerve, either totally (truncal) or selectively at some point in its innervation to the stomach. In a truncal vagotomy the nerve is severed bilaterally in both the anterior and the posterior trunk. Selective vagotomy consists of cutting the nerve at a particular branch of the vagus nerve, which results in denervation of only a portion of the stomach, such as the antrum or the parietal cell mass.

Pyloroplasty consists of surgical enlargement of the pyloric sphincter to facilitate the easy passage of contents from the stomach. It is most commonly done after vagotomy or to enlarge an opening that has been constricted from scar tissue. A vagotomy causes decreased gastric motility. A pyloroplasty accompanying vagotomy increases gastric emptying.

The combination of a Billroth I or II procedure with vagotomy has the advantage of eliminating the ulcer and the stimulus for ulcer development. Surgical intervention results in removal of most of the parietal cell mass of the stomach and thus decreases the secretion of hydrochloric

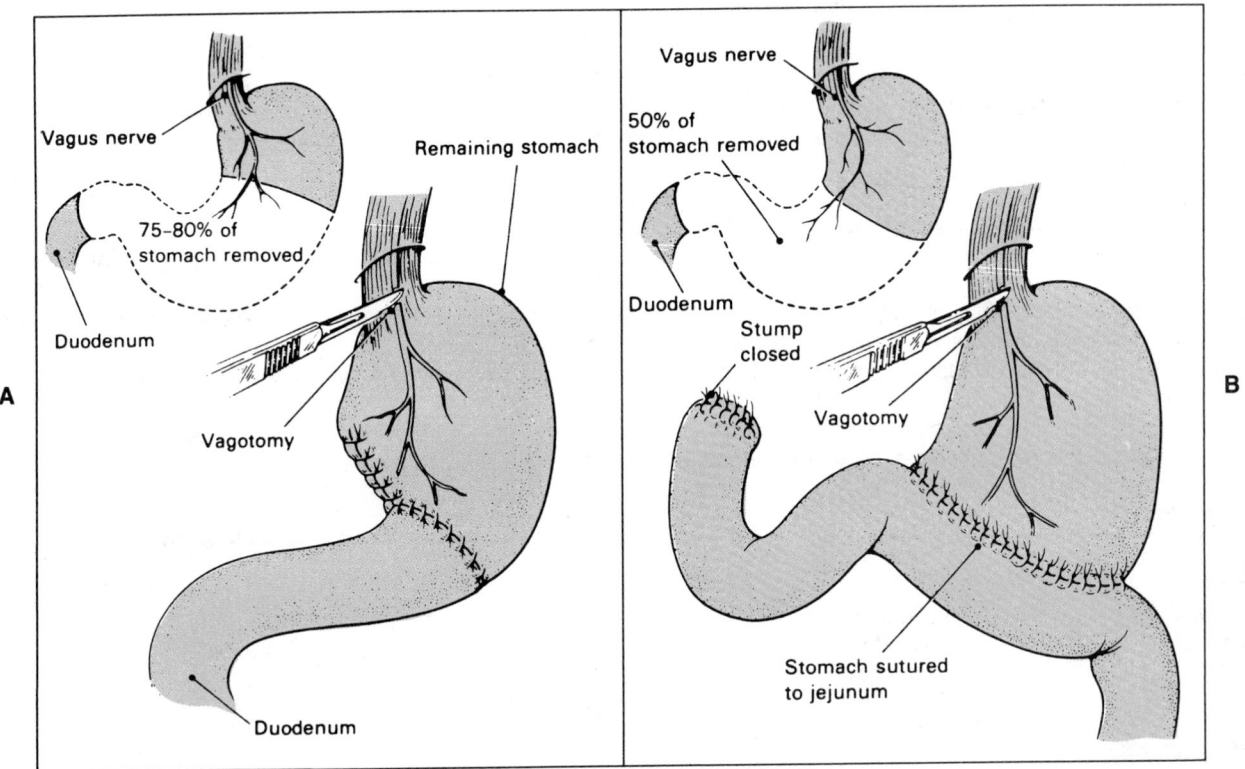

Fig. 36-5 **A,** Billroth I. **B,** Billroth II.

acid and pepsin. Surgical removal of the antrum results in removal of the source of gastrin secretion. (Gastrin normally stimulates parietal and chief cells.) Vagotomy eliminates the stimulus of hydrochloric acid and gastrin hormone secretion because of vagal stimulation.

Postoperative complications. The most common postoperative complications from peptic ulcer surgery are (1) the dumping syndrome, (2) postprandial hypoglycemia, and (3) bile reflux gastritis.

Dumping syndrome. The dumping syndrome is the direct result of surgical removal of a large portion of the stomach and the pyloric sphincter. These changes drastically reduce the reservoir capacity of the stomach. Although the dumping syndrome is more commonly experienced after a Billroth II gastrectomy, it can occur after any gastric reconstruction and vagotomy.

The dumping syndrome is associated with meals containing hyperosmolar chyme. Normally, gastric chyme enters the small intestine in small amounts, and shifts in fluid from the extracellular space are minimal. After surgery, however, the stomach no longer has control over the amount of gastric chyme entering the small intestine. Consequently a large bolus of hypertonic fluid enters the intestine and results in fluid being drawn into the bowel. This creates a decrease in plasma volume. A secondary consequence of this fluid shift is distention of the bowel lumen, which stimulates increased intestinal motility and the urge to defecate.

The dumping syndrome is experienced by approximately one third to one half of clients after peptic ulcer surgery. The onset of symptoms occurs at the end of a meal or within 15 to 30 minutes after eating. The client usually describes feelings of generalized weakness, sweating, palpitations, and dizziness. These symptoms are attributed to the sudden decrease in plasma volume. The client complains of abdominal cramps, borborygmi, and the urge to defecate. These manifestations occur when the bolus of hypertonic fluid causes extracellular fluid to shift into the small intestine. These manifestations usually last for no longer than an hour after meals.

Treatment consists of several simple measures. In most cases the symptoms are self-limiting and disappear completely within several months to a year after surgery. Interventions prescribed for the client are diet instruction, rest, and reassurance. The diet should consist of six small dry feedings daily that are low in carbohydrate, restricted in refined sugars, and contain moderate amounts of protein and fat. Sample menu plans are presented in Table 36-16. Fluids may be taken between meals but not with the meal. The client should plan short rest periods of at least 30 minutes after each meal. The recumbent position is the most beneficial if the client can arrange for it. Reassuring the client that the unpleasant symptoms are usually of short duration is helpful in gaining cooperation. A small percentage of clients experience long-term problems and may require further reconstructive surgery.

Postprandial hypoglycemia. This condition is considered a variant of the dumping syndrome, since it is the result of uncontrolled gastric emptying of a bolus of fluid high in carbohydrate into the small intestine. The bolus of

Table 36-16   Dietary Interventions for Postgastrectomy Dumping Syndrome

PURPOSE

To slow the rapid passage of food into the intestine; to control symptoms of the dumping syndrome (dizziness, sense of fullness, diarrhea, tachycardia), which sometimes occur following a partial or total gastrectomy

DIET PRINCIPLES

1. Meals are divided into six small feedings to avoid overloading intestines at mealtimes.
2. Fluids should not be taken with meals, but at least 30 to 45 minutes before or after meals. This helps prevent distention or a feeling of fullness.
3. Concentrated sweets (e.g., honey, sugar, jelly, jam, candies, sweet pastries, sweetened fruit) are avoided because they sometimes cause dizziness, diarrhea, and a sense of fullness.
4. Protein and fats are increased to promote rebuilding of body tissues and meet energy needs. Meat, cheese, eggs, and milk products are specific foods to increase in the diet.
5. Amount of time these restrictions should be followed varies. The health care provider decides the proper amount of time to remain on this prescribed diet according to the client's clinical condition and progress.

Exchanges	Sample Menu Plans		
Breakfast			
1 meat	1 poached egg	1 fried egg	1 oz ham
1 starch	1 slice toast	1 corn tortilla	2 biscuits with 2 tsp
Fat	2 sausage	2 slices bacon	gravy
	Margarine	Margarine	
10 AM snack			
1 starch	¾ cup dry cereal	½ cup atole	½ cup grits with 2 tbs
½ cup milk	½ cup milk	½ cup milk	margarine added
1 fruit	½ fresh banana	2 unsweetened canned	⅓ cantaloupe
	Sugar substitute	peach halves	½ cup buttermilk
		Sugar substitute	
Lunch			
2 meat	Grilled cheese sand-	1 burrito with 1 oz	2 oz fried fish
2 starch	wich with 2 oz	meat, 1 oz cheese,	½ cup buttered rice
1 vegetable	cheese, lettuce	½ cup pinto beans, 1	½ cup mustard greens
1 fruit	2 unsweetened pear	flour tortilla	1 fresh apple
Fat	halves	½ diet gelatin dessert	1 slice bread
		with fruit cocktail	
		added	
2 PM snack			
1 meat or substitute	½ cup plain yogurt	½ cup cottage cheese	2 tsp peanut butter
1 starch	2 graham crackers	5 soda crackers	1 slice bread
Dinner			
2 meat	2 oz tomato meatloaf	2 tamales	2 oz fried pork chop
1 starch	½ cup mashed pota-	½ cup buttered corn	½ cup black-eyed peas
Vegetable	toes with gravy	1 fresh orange	½ cup buttered carrots
1 fruit	½ cup buttered green		1 fresh plum
Fat	beans		
	½ cup unsweetened		
	applesauce		
8 PM snack			
1 meat	½ sandwich with 1	1 corn tortilla with 1 oz	½ sandwich with 1
1 starch	slice bread, 1 oz	melted cheese and	slice bread, 1 slice
Vegetable	roast beef, lettuce,	green chili	salami, lettuce, may-
Fat	mayonnaise		onnaise

concentrated carbohydrate results in hyperglycemia and the release of excessive amounts of insulin into the circulation. A secondary hypoglycemia then occurs, with symptoms appearing about 2 hours after meals. The symptoms experienced are the ones observed in any hypoglycemic reaction and include sweating, weakness, mental confusion, palpitations, tachycardia, and anxiety.

The immediate ingestion of sugared fluids or candy relieves the hypoglycemic symptoms. The treatment of this type of hypoglycemia is similar to that of the dumping syndrome. To avoid similar occurrences, the client should be instructed to limit the amount of sugar consumed with each meal and to eat small, frequent meals with moderate amounts of protein and fat.

Bile reflux gastritis. Gastric surgery that involves the pylorus, either reconstruction or removal, can result in reflux alkaline gastritis. It is recognized that prolonged contact of bile, especially bile salts, causes damage to the gastric mucosa. Chronic gastritis of this form may result in the back-diffusion of hydrogen ions through the gastric mucosa. Paradoxically, peptic ulcer may recur after surgical treatment that was intended as a cure.

The symptoms associated with reflux alkaline gastritis are continuous epigastric distress that increases after meals. Vomiting relieves the distress but only temporarily. The administration of cholestyramine resin (Questran), either before or with meals, has met with considerable success. Cholestyramine binds with the bile salts that are the source of irritation in this condition. Aluminum hydroxide antacids have also been used in the treatment of this condition.

Preoperative care. Surgical intervention is the treatment of choice for peptic ulcer when conservative therapeutic management has been unsuccessful. Surgery also may be performed after an acute exacerbation, when the ulcer is complicated by sudden perforation or increased bleeding, or to relieve gastric outlet obstruction. The wishes of the client for surgical intervention must also be considered, especially when repeated hospitalizations have been required. The client may openly request surgery as the only hope for a cure.

When surgery is planned with the goal of curing the ulcer disease, the surgeon should provide necessary information about the procedure and the expected outcome so that the client can make an informed decision. The nurse can help the client and the family by clarifying and interpreting their questions. A discussion of the surgical procedure accompanied by a diagram or picture showing the anatomical changes that will result should be incorporated into the preoperative care. Instructions should be clear on what to expect after surgery including comfort measures, pain relief, coughing and breathing exercises, use of the NG tube, and IV fluid administration (see Chapter 11).

Postoperative care. Care of the client after major abdominal surgery is similar to the postoperative care after abdominal laparotomy (Table 37-16). An NG tube is used to decompress the remaining portion of the stomach so that the suture line can be rested and there is time for the resolution of edema and inflammation resulting from surgical trauma.

The gastric aspirate must be carefully observed for color, amount, and odor during the immediate postoperative period. The color of the aspirate is expected to be bright red at first, with a gradual darkening within the first 24 hours after surgery. Normally the color changes to yellow-green within 36 to 48 hours. If the tube becomes clogged during this period, the physician may order periodic gentle irrigations with normal saline solution. If the tube needs to be replaced or repositioned, the physician must be called on to perform this task because of the danger of perforating the gastric mucosa or disrupting the suture line.

It is essential that the NG suction be working and that the tube remain patent so that increased gastric secretions do not put a strain on the anastomosis. This can lead to distention of the remaining portion of the stomach and result in (1) rupture of the sutures, (2) leakage of gastric contents into the peritoneal cavity, (3) hemorrhage, and (4) possible abscess formation. A fecal odor from the aspirate is abnormal and may indicate reflux of large intestinal contents into the operative area. The nurse should observe the client for signs of decreased peristalsis and lower abdominal discomfort that may indicate impending intestinal obstruction. Accurate intake and output records must be kept. Vital signs are monitored and recorded every 4 hours.

The client should be kept comfortable and free of pain by the administration of the prescribed medications and by frequent changes in position. The incision is relatively high in the epigastrium and may interfere with deep-breathing and coughing measures. Splinting the area with a pillow while gently and persistently encouraging the client to put forth the best efforts possible helps prevent pulmonary complications. Splinting also protects the abdominal suture line from rupture during coughing. The dressing must be observed for signs of bleeding or odor and drainage indicative of an infection. Ambulation is encouraged and is increased daily after the first postoperative day.

While the NG tube is connected to suction, IV therapy is maintained. Potassium and vitamin supplements are added to the infusion until oral feedings are resumed. Sometimes before the NG tube is removed, the client is started on oral feedings of clear liquids to determine the tolerance level. The stomach is aspirated within an hour or two to assess the amount remaining and its color and consistency. When fluids are well tolerated, the tube is removed and fluids are increased in frequency with a slow progression to regular foods. The regimen of six small meals a day is begun.

Discharge planning and instruction should be started as soon as the immediate postoperative period is successfully passed. Dietary instructions may be given by the dietitian and reinforced by the nursing staff. Because the stomach's reservoir has been greatly diminished after gastric resection, the meal size must be reduced accordingly. The client must be advised to eliminate drinking fluids with meals as had been done in the past. Dry foods with a low carbohydrate content and moderate protein and fat content are better tolerated until the client has had time to adjust. These dietary changes, with the incorporation of a short rest period after each meal, facilitate digestion and eliminate most of the problems of the dumping syndrome. The client should be informed that feelings of weakness, palpitations, and dizziness may occur unless there is complete adherence to the diet instructions. Reassurance that following these simple dietary measures will result in freedom from symptoms within a few months is essential to long-term compliance.

Postprandial hypoglycemic reaction can be avoided if these dietary instructions are followed with special emphasis on eating foods low in sugar content. Although only a very small percentage of clients experience alkaline reflux gastritis, the client must be cautioned to notify the physician of any continuous epigastric distress after meals that is similar to that felt before surgery.

Pernicious anemia is a long-term complication that may occur after partial gastrectomy. However, it is seen more often when the entire stomach is surgically removed. Pernicious anemia is caused by the loss of intrinsic factor, which is produced by the parietal cells. Depending on the amount of parietal cell mass removed in surgery, the client may eventually require ongoing regular injections of vitamin B_{12}. Vitamin B_{12} is normally stored in the liver. Total depletion of vitamin B_{12} stores usually takes several years.

Because the client is generally returning to the same home and work environment and because the basic personality has not changed, there is always the danger of ulcer redevelopment, especially at the site of the anastomosis. Adequate rest, nutrition, and avoidance of known stressors are keys to complete recovery. Avoiding the use of medications not prescribed by the physician should be reemphasized, along with restrictions on smoking and alcohol use. If the client is willing to make these kinds of adjustment in lifestyle, a successful rehabilitation is more likely.

CANCER OF THE STOMACH

Although the rate of stomach cancer has been steadily declining in the United States since the 1930s, an estimated 23,000 new cases, with 13,700 deaths, were projected for the year 1990.[15] Of the GI cancers, gastric cancer ranks fourth behind colorectal cancer in incidence. Costa Rica and Japan have the highest incidence rates in the world. Cancer of the stomach is more prevalent in males of the lower socioeconomic class, primarily those living in urban areas. Stomach cancer is typically at an advanced stage when diagnosed and is not amenable to surgical resection.

Etiology

Many factors have been implicated in the development of gastric cancer, yet no single causative agent has been identified. It is believed that a diet of smoked, highly salted or spiced foods may have a carcinogenic effect. A genetic etiology has been postulated because of the greater than normal occurrence of stomach cancer in immediate family members. Some research studies lend support to a genetic cause. For example, persons with blood group A have a greater incidence of gastric cancer than is found in the general population. However, other studies dispute this claim. At the present time there is no universally accepted genetic connection.

Other predisposing factors associated with a high incidence of gastric cancer are atrophic gastritis, pernicious anemia, benign gastric polyps, and achlorhydria. The relationship between chronic peptic ulcers of the stomach and the development of gastric cancer is still controversial. Malignant transformation of a benign chronic ulcer does occur but accounts for less than 5% of all gastric cancers. It is known that persons with achlorhydria or pernicious anemia are more likely to develop gastric cancer than those with normal gastric acid production. When lymph nodes are involved at the time of diagnosis, the 5-year survival is approximately 16%.[7]

Pathophysiology

Malignant tumors of the stomach may be present for a long time and may have spread to adjacent organs before any distressing symptoms occur. The tumor may grow to large dimensions without obstructing the lumen of the stomach simply because the lumen itself is so large. The mean interval from onset of symptoms to consultation with a physician may be as long as 6 months. This long delay is largely attributed to the vague, intermittent abdominal distress experienced by the client. Unfortunately, this type of early symptom is experienced by most healthy persons at one time or another as a result of dietary indiscretions, nervous tension, and anxiety.

Gastric cancer can occur in any portion of the stomach, with the majority located near the pylorus and the antrum along the lesser curvature. Tumors located at the cardia and fundus are associated with a poor prognosis. These tumors typically infiltrate rapidly to the surrounding tissue, the regional lymph nodes, and the liver. Clients with tumors located along the lesser curvature have a better survival rate.[16] Adenocarcinomas account for more than 90% of the cancers, and sarcomas (comprising lymphomas and leiomyomas) make up the rest.

The tumor growth is insidious and follows a pattern of continuous infiltration. Cancer of the stomach may spread by direct extension along the mucosal surface and infiltrate through the gastric wall. Once the stomach wall has been penetrated by tumor growth, adjacent organs and structures that may become involved are the esophagus, duodenum, omentum, liver, and pancreas. Distant metastasis is facilitated by the rich lymphatic plexuses in the stomach wall. Seeding of tumor cells into the peritoneal cavity may occur late in the course of the disease. Evidence of spread to the peritoneal cavity is manifested by ascites and by spread to the ovaries.

Clinical Manifestations

The clinical manifestations exhibited by persons with gastric cancer can be categorized by signs and symptoms of anemia, peptic ulcer disease, or indigestion. Anemia is a common occurrence with stomach cancer. It is caused by chronic blood loss as the lesion erodes through the mucosa or as a direct result of pernicious anemia, which develops when intrinsic factor is lost. The person appears pale and weak and complains of fatigue, weakness, dizziness, and, in extreme cases, shortness of breath. The stool is positive for occult blood.

The symptoms of gastric malignancy are sometimes

identical to those of peptic ulcer. The pain and discomfort can actually be alleviated by belching and the use of antacids and diet restrictions.

Manifestations related to indigestion include vague epigastric fullness with feelings of early satiety after meals. Weight loss, dysphagia, and constipation frequently accompany epigastric distress. When nausea, vomiting, and hematemesis occur, they may indicate obstruction at the gastric outlet or may be a warning of impending hemorrhage.

The early detection of gastric cancer is difficult because of the diversity of symptoms. On physical examination, the client may be pale and lethargic if anemia is present. When the appetite has been poor and weight loss has been considerable, the client may appear cachectic. A mass can often be detected beneath the abdominal wall and is seen to move with each inspiration. On palpation, the mass may be felt in the epigastrium. Masses that are predominantly in the antrum of the stomach are generally found to the left of the midline. Masses located to the right of midline usually tend to be metastases to the liver or indicate involvement of the perigastric lymph nodes. Supraclavicular lymph nodes that are hard and enlarged and located on the left side are suggestive of metastasis via the thoracic duct from the stomach lesion. The presence of ascites is an obviously unfavorable sign.

Diagnostic Studies

The diagnostic studies for gastric malignancy include laboratory analysis of blood, stool, and gastric secretions. Blood chemistry studies assist in the determination of anemia and its severity. Liver enzymes and serum amylase may indicate liver and pancreatic involvement or other abnormalities related to their dysfunction. Stool examination provides evidence of occult or gross bleeding. A gastric analysis indicates the level of hydrochloric acid present in the fasting stomach. Washings obtained during the gastric analysis can be used for the exfoliative cytological examination. The test demonstrates the histological changes indicative of malignancy. However, this test should never be used as the sole diagnostic criterion because false readings are sometimes obtained.

The carcinoembryonic antigen (CEA) radioimmunoassay test is used as an adjunctive diagnostic tool for cancer of the GI tract. CEA is a glycoprotein that is found in significant amounts in embryonic life, especially in the large intestine. It is also found in some adult clients with GI carcinomas. Elevated levels of CEA may indicate malignancy, yet CEA may be elevated in persons who smoke and also in those with benign lesions. Therefore, while the CEA test may be of some use in the preoperative workup of a client with suspected cancer of the stomach, it should never be used as the only diagnostic tool. (CEA is also discussed in Chapters 9 and 37.)

Barium x-ray films may demonstrate defects in peristalsis, tone, secretion, motility, and spasm of the stomach. On x-ray examination the malignant ulcer crater is more irregular around the edges and more elevated than the craters found with benign peptic ulcers. Barium studies do not always detect small lesions of the cardia and fundus.

Endoscopic examination of the stomach should be per-

formed along with barium x-ray studies. Lesions that go undetected on x-ray film can be more easily viewed and biopsied when the fiberoptic scope is used. The stomach can be distended with air during the procedure so that the mucosal folds can be stretched. Fixation of the mucosa is indicative of malignancy.

Therapeutic Management

When the diagnosis of gastric malignancy has been confirmed, the treatment of choice is surgical removal of the tumor. The preoperative management of clients with gastric cancer focuses on the correction of nutritional deficits, transfusions for the treatment of anemia, and replacement of blood volume (Table 36-17).

Transfusions of whole blood or packed RBCs correct the anemia and increase the blood volume. If a gastric lesion has been located at or near the pylorus and is causing gastric outlet obstruction, gastric decompression may be necessary before surgery. When the tumor has extended into the transverse colon and partial colon resection is also required, special preparation of the bowel is necessary. This preparation may include a low-residue diet, enemas to cleanse the bowel, and the use of antibiotics to reduce the intestinal bacteria. Clients with achlorhydria who do not have gastric acid available to destroy the bacteria may also need antibiotic bowel preparation. Recent studies indicate that the use of prophylactic antibiotics reduces postoperative complications by 10%.

Correction of malnutrition is vital if surgery is planned. Malnutrition is associated with increased postoperative complications and mortality rates. The possible explana-

---

Table 36-17

Diagnostic and Therapeutic Management: Gastric Cancer

DIAGNOSTIC

History and physical examination
CBC
Urinalysis
Stool examination
Liver enzymes
Serum amylase
Upper GI barium study
CEA
Exfoliative cytology
Fiberoptic endoscopy and biopsy
Gastric analysis

THERAPEUTIC

Surgery
    Subtotal gastrectomy—Billroth I or II
    Total gastrectomy with esophagojejunostomy
Adjuvant therapy
    Radiation therapy
    Chemotherapy
    Combination radiation therapy and chemotherapy

tion for this is the advanced disease found in most clients, making surgical resection unsuitable.[17]

Surgical Interventions

The surgical intervention used in the treatment of stomach cancer may consist of the procedure used for surgery for peptic ulcer disease. The specific surgery employed is determined by the location and extent of the lesion, the client's physical condition, and preference of the surgeon. When metastasis is widespread at the time of diagnosis, surgical intervention may be only palliative.

The surgical aim is to remove as much of the stomach as necessary to remove the tumor and a margin of normal tissue. When the lesion is located in the cardia or high in the fundus, a total gastrectomy with esophagojejunostomy is performed. This procedure involves anastomosis of the lower end of the esophagus to the jejunum (Fig. 36-6). Lesions located in the antrum or the pyloric region are generally treated by either a Billroth I or a Billroth II procedure. When metastasis has occurred in adjacent organs, such as the spleen, ovaries, or bowel, the surgical procedures must be modified and extended as necessary.

The chance of a complete cure by surgical means is decreased considerably when the lymph nodes are involved. Survival rates are considerably shortened when organs adjacent to the stomach show evidence of invasion at the time of surgical intervention.

Adjuvant therapy. Surgery is the only definitive means of achieving a cure. However, when the client cannot physically withstand a surgical procedure or when surgical cure is not feasible, radiation or chemotherapy alone or in combination may be used. Neither radiation therapy nor chemotherapeutic agents have been very successful when used as the primary mode of treatment. Radiation therapy has proved to be of little value except in certain instances of obstruction of the cardia. The radiosensitivity of gastric cancers is quite low, and it has been estimated that only 10% will respond to radiotherapy.

Preoperative radiation is usually not done because of the risk of poor wound healing of the anastomosis of the gastric stump to the bowel. When radiation is used as a palliative measure, the tumor mass can be decreased, with temporary relief of the cardia or pyloric obstruction. Postoperative radiation has not been widely used, nor has it increased survival rates. The combination of chemotherapy and radiation is now being used for clients who are not candidates for surgical excision. The success rate with combination chemotherapy has met with only temporary relief of symptoms, and long-term survival rates have not shown significant improvement.

Until recently, single-agent chemotherapy for gastric cancer has proved of little value. Agents that have been identified as having some effect on gastric cancer are 5-FU, BCNU, methyl CCNU, doxorubicin (Adriamycin), and triazinate. A better response rate in clients with advanced gastric cancer is now found when chemotherapeutic agents are used in combination, such as FAT (5-FU, doxorubicin, and triazinate). The hope for better outcomes with the use of chemotherapy depends on finding new ways of administering old drugs, finding new drugs, and determining new drug combinations. The hope for the ultimate cure of clients with gastric cancer now seems to lie in the combined efforts of surgery, radiation, and chemotherapy. The role of biological response modifiers is still under investigation for use in gastric cancer. (These therapies are discussed in Chapter 9.)

■ Nursing Management of Gastric Cancer

Nursing assessment

The assessment of a person with possible gastric cancer is similar to that for one with peptic ulcer disease (see Table 36-14). Important data to be obtained from the client and the family should include a nutritional assessment, a psychosocial history, the client's perceptions of the health problem and the need for hospitalization, and the physical examination of the client.

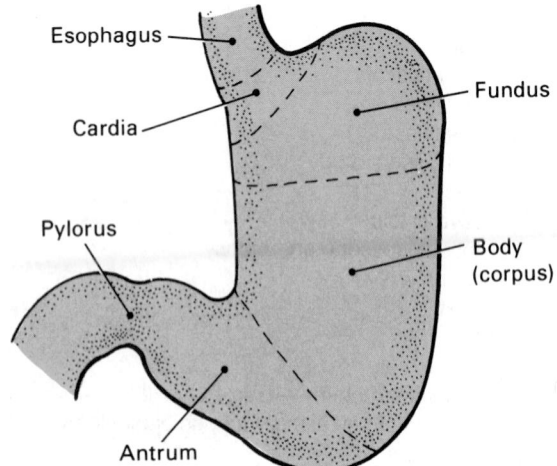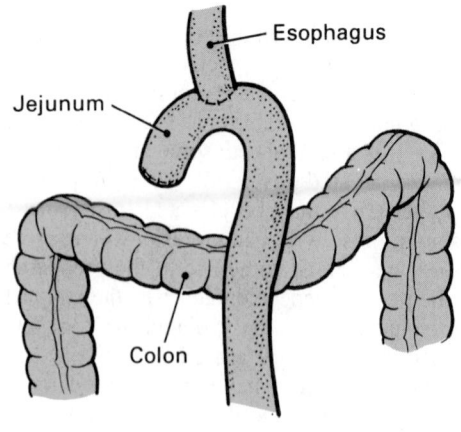

Fig. 36-6 A total gastrectomy for gastric cancer (total gastrectomy with esophagojejunostomy).

The nutritional assessment must elicit information regarding appetite, changes in eating patterns over the previous 6 months, and the role of highly seasoned or salty foods as a regular part of the diet. It is necessary to ascertain the client's normal weight and any changes that may have occurred in the past few months. Unexplained weight loss is common in many types of cancer before diagnosis. A history of vague symptoms of dyspepsia, early satiety, feeling full after consuming even a small amount of food, or reporting symptoms of gas pain should help the nurse differentiate these typical gastric cancer symptoms from those of peptic ulcer. As with peptic ulcer clients, the nurse should determine whether pain is present, where and when it occurs, and how it is relieved. When the pain has been controlled with ingestion of foods, fluids, or antacids for a period of time but now continues or worsens regardless of interventions, gastric cancer may be the underlying cause.

Psychosocial and demographic data include age, present or previous occupation, and financial status. Gastric cancer can occur at any age, but the risk is more prevalent in men in the fifth to the sixth decade of life. A family history of cancer, especially if it is gastric cancer, puts a person at greater than normal risk.

It is important to determine the client's personal perception of the health problem and method of coping with hospitalization, diagnostic tests, and procedures and the way personal crisis was managed in the past. The possibility of a diagnosis of cancer and a treatment regimen that may include surgery, chemotherapy, or radiation treatment forecasts a prolonged stressful period and a possibly fatal outcome. Therefore it is essential that the nurse learn as much as possible about what the client and the family understand and how well they will be able to handle and support the client if tests result in an unfavorable diagnosis and complex treatment interventions are planned. If surgery is probable, the nurse should assess what the client expects from surgery (cure or palliation) and how that client has responded to any previous surgical procedures.

A complete physical examination reveals the client's current functional abilities, the presence of other health problems, and an estimate on how well the client may respond to therapy. A state of cachexia may be evident if the nutritional state has been compromised for an extended time. Malnourished clients do not respond well to chemotherapy or radiation therapy and are poor surgical risks.

Nursing diagnoses

Nursing diagnoses specific to the client with gastric cancer include, but are not limited to, the following:

1. Altered nutrition: less than body requirements, related to inability to ingest, digest, or absorb nutrients
2. Activity intolerance related to generalized weakness, abdominal discomfort, and nutritional deficits
3. Anxiety related to lack of knowledge of diagnostic tests, unknown diagnostic outcome, disease process, and therapeutic regimen
4. Pain related to underlying disease process and side effects of surgery, chemotherapy, or radiation therapy

5. Anticipatory grieving related to perceived unfavorable diagnosis and impending death

Nursing interventions

Health promotion and maintenance. The nursing role in the early detection of cancer of the stomach is focused primarily on identification of clients who are at high risk. The nurse should be aware of symptoms associated with gastric cancer, method of spread, and the significant findings on physical examination. The nurse should understand that the cure rate is often quite dismal because symptoms arise late in the course of the disease process, are vague, and often mimic other conditions, such as peptic ulcer.

The nurse must be alert to problems suggesting gastric cancer, such as poor appetite, weight loss, fatigue, and persistent gastric distress. If any of these manifestations are present, medical attention should be obtained and the necessary diagnostic tests performed. The role of diet in the causation of gastric cancer should be well understood by the nurse so that the client at risk can be taught acceptable dietary alternatives. Some researchers suggest that 15% to 20% of all stomach cancers can be prevented by changing dietary patterns.[18]

In addition, any client with a positive family history of gastric cancer should be encouraged to undergo diagnostic evaluation if manifestations of anemia, peptic ulcer, or vague epigastric distress are present. It is imperative that the nurse recognize the possible existence of stomach cancer in a client who is treated for peptic ulcer and who fails to gain relief after 3 weeks of diet and prescribed medications. The ulcer, if it is benign, should show signs of healing on x-ray study.

Acute intervention

PREOPERATIVE CARE. When the diagnostic tests confirm the presence of a malignancy, the client and the family generally react with shock, disbelief, and depression, regardless of how thoroughly they may have been prepared for this possible outcome. The psychological impact of the diagnosis, added to the physical distress already being experienced, can be quite devastating. Throughout this period the nurse must give emotional and physical support, provide information, clarify test results, and maintain a positive attitude with respect to the client's immediate recovery and long-term survival.

On admission to the hospital, the client may be in poor physical condition. Surgery may have to be delayed while the client is made more physically sound to withstand the strain of major surgery. A positive nutritional state enhances wound healing as well as the ability to withstand infection and other possible postoperative complications. The nursing staff should recognize the necessity for surgical delay and the advantages to be gained for the client. Many clients have been anorectic for a long time and have lost considerable body weight. The nutritional state is improved by a well-balanced diet, along with the administration of supplemental vitamins. Most clients are able to tolerate several small meals a day rather than three regular meals. The diet may be supplemented by a variety of commercial liquid supplements (see Tables 35-14 and 35-15) and vitamins. The nurse is challenged to find innovative ways of persuading the client to eat when lack of appetite and state of mind make eating difficult and unrewarding. Getting the client's family to assist with meals and encourage intake may be beneficial. If the client is unable to ingest oral feedings, it may be necessary to provide for nutritional needs with tube feedings or parenteral hyperalimentation.

If needed, blood replacement and fluid volume restoration may be carried out in the preoperative period. Because anemia is usually present, whole blood may be administered. If the client has cardiovascular problems, the use of packed RBCs may be substituted so that circulatory overload does not complicate the course of treatment. Close observation for reactions to the transfusions is important. Monitoring the hemoglobin and hematocrit levels provides information on the progress of therapy.

The preoperative teaching plan before gastric surgery for cancer is much the same as that for peptic ulcer surgery. When the anticipated surgery involves the resectioning of a portion of the colon, the nurse should explain the need for enemas and antibiotic therapy in bowel preparation.

POSTOPERATIVE CARE. Postoperative care of the client with gastric carcinoma is similar to that following a Billroth I or II procedure. When the surgical intervention has involved a total gastrectomy, the plan of care is somewhat different. The operation performed usually requires some resectioning of the lower esophagus along with the removal of the entire stomach and anastomosis of the esophagus to the jejunum. The chest cavity must be entered, and drainage is accomplished by the insertion of chest tubes. (Chest surgery and drainage tubes are discussed in Chapter 21.) After total gastrectomy, the NG tube does not drain a large quantity of secretions because removal of the stomach has eliminated the reservoir capacity. The NG tube is removed after several days, when peristalsis has resumed. Small amounts of clear fluid may then be started. The client requires close observation for signs of leakage of the fluids at the anastomosis as evidenced by an elevation in the temperature and increasing dyspnea. When fluids are well tolerated without distress, the amount may be increased along with the addition of some solid foods. Meals consist of six to eight small feedings a day, and this pattern will be necessary for the lifetime of the client.

As a consequence of a total gastrectomy, clients experience the symptoms of the dumping syndrome. Unfortunately, weight loss is very common, and these clients never do well nutritionally the rest of their lives. Postoperative wound healing may be impaired because of avitaminosis. This necessitates the IV or oral replacement of vitamins B_{12}, C, D, and K and the B complex vitamins. Because these vitamins are absorbed primarily in the upper part of the small intestine, they must be replaced, since the duodenum has been bypassed in the surgical procedure.

Clients who have a Billroth I or II operative procedure should receive the same postoperative care as those who have had peptic ulcer surgery. These clients are also subject to the same type of postoperative complications as the dumping syndrome and postprandial hypoglycemia.

Clients with advanced malignant disease can be offered only palliative treatment. The chemotherapy agent found most useful for controlling symptoms of gastric cancer is 5-FU. When this medication or any of the combination drugs is prescribed, the nurse must have current information regarding the action and side effects of the drugs. The client should be made aware of the potential benefits and hazards that can result from the chemotherapy. (The care of the client receiving chemotherapy is discussed in detail in Chapter 9.)

Radiation therapy can be used as an adjuvant to surgery or for palliation. Clients are generally quite fearful of radiation and may develop many misconceptions regarding its value and dangers. To reassure the client and ensure completion of the designated number of treatments, the nurse must provide detailed instruction. Because most therapy is completed on an outpatient basis, the nurse should assess the client's knowledge of radiation, care of the skin, the need for good nutrition and fluid intake during therapy, and the appropriate use of antiemetic drugs. (Specific care of the client receiving radiation therapy is discussed in Chapter 9.)

Chronic management. Before the client is discharged, the need for teaching should be reviewed. Most dietary measures useful after peptic ulcer surgery are applicable after surgery for gastric carcinoma. Plans should be made for the relief of pain, including comfort measures and the judicious use of analgesics. Wound care, if needed, must be taught to the primary caregiver in the home situation. Dressings, special equipment, or special services may be required for the client's continued care at home. A list of community agencies that are available for assistance can be provided before the client goes home. The services of the American Cancer Society are especially helpful.

When treatment in the form of chemotherapy or radiation therapy is to be continued after discharge, a referral to the public health nurse may be beneficial. The public health nurse can assist with recovery, determine the degree of client compliance, and be a sympathetic health care provider with whom the client can consult.

Long-term follow-up must be stressed. The client must be encouraged to comply with the prescribed dietary and medication regimens, keep appointments for chemotherapy administration or radiation treatments, and keep the physician informed of changes in physical condition. (Dealing with the long-term management of the cancer client is discussed in Chapter 9.)

C **ase Study**

PEPTIC ULCER

Bill, a 40-year-old bus driver, is admitted to the hospital for the first time since a duodenal ulcer was diagnosed 11 months ago. He states that he followed the prescribed bland diet and took Maalox and ranitidine as his physician ordered for approximately 3 months. At that time, an endoscopic examination revealed complete healing of the ulcer. Bill, fortified by this good news, reverted to his previous eating habits and began enjoying several beers each evening. He also did not comply with the maintenance medications prescribed by his physician.

Several weeks before admission, Bill was under unusual job pressure when it became necessary for him to drive his bus overtime for several hours each day because several drivers were on vacation. He began experiencing epigastric pain about 2 hours after meals and sometimes at night—pain only briefly relieved by taking an antacid. On several occasions he noted that his stools were darker than their usual brown color.

On the evening before admission, Bill had a disagreement with his wife and drank a six-pack of beer. He soon began experiencing severe epigastric distress that was unrelieved by antacids or by a ranitidine tablet he had left over from his initial prescription. He vomited once and noted that the vomitus was streaked with blood. At that time he decided to call his physician.

On physical examination, Bill was found to have epigastric tenderness on palpation. He appeared pale and extremely anxious. Blood studies done on admission indicated the presence of anemia with a hemoglobin value of 10 g/dl. A stool examination was positive for occult blood.

Discussion Questions

1. Discuss the pathophysiological changes that occur in duodenal ulcer.
2. Differentiate between duodenal and gastric ulcers.
3. Explain the reason for Bill's anemia and guaiac-positive stool.
4. Which diagnostic examinations would be most appropriate during his acute episode?
5. What is the role of the nurse during an acute exacerbation of peptic ulcer?
6. Discuss the plan of nursing care necessary in the prevention of further acute episodes.
7. List the possible complications of peptic ulcer and the nurse's role in the care of each.

R eview Questions

The number of the question corresponds to the same-numbered objective at the beginning of the chapter.

1. The least useful measure in the treatment of a client with severe nausea and vomiting is
   a. maintenance of a clean and odor-free environment
   b. high-carbohydrate and low-fat diet
   c. high-protein diet and antispasmodics
   d. elevation of head of bed to prevent aspiration
2. Which of the following is not a cause of acute gastritis?
   a. absence of vitamin B_{12} in food intake
   b. ingestion of drugs such as aspirin
   c. foods contaminated with *Staphylococcus* or *Salmonella* organisms
   d. ingestion of large amounts of alcohol
3. In the care of the client who has a sudden, severe upper GI bleeding episode, the nursing management includes all the following *except*
   a. administration of anticholinergics and stool softeners
   b. gastric lavages
   c. central venous pressure monitoring
   d. fluid replacement with volume expanders or blood transfusions

4. Which of the following statements describes the differences between a gastric and duodenal ulcer?
   a. Duodenal ulcer pain occurs 2 to 4 hours after meals and in the middle of the night.
   b. Duodenal ulcers have increased in incidence in men and women over the past 20 years.
   c. Gastric ulcer pain is periodic and episodic.
   d. Duodenal ulcers have a malignant potential.
5. Which of the following statements does not accurately describe the dumping syndrome?
   a. Symptoms arise from a bolus of hyperosmolar fluid entering the intestines.
   b. Symptoms are experienced 2 to 3 hours after meals.
   c. Complaints of weakness, sweating, dizziness, and abdominal cramps are common.
   d. Symptoms are self-limiting and disappear in about 6 to 12 months.
6. Which of the following diagnostic tests is least helpful in accurately diagnosing stomach cancer?
   a. gastroscopy
   b. gastric analysis
   c. CEA
   d. exfoliative cytology

REFERENCES

1. Domschke S and Domschke W: Gastroduodenal damage due to drugs, alcohol and smoking, Clin Gastroenterol 3:419, 1984.
2. Garrity T and Jeffries G: Gastritis: is it a distinct clinical entity? In Barkin J and Rogers A, eds: Difficult decisions in digestive diseases, Chicago, 1989, Year Book Medical Publishers, Inc, p 80.
3. Hahn S and Goldberg R: Bleeding in the upper gastrointestinal tract: what is the rationale for endoscopic intervention? In Barkin J and Rogers A, eds: Difficult decisions in digestive diseases, Chicago, 1989, Year Book Medical Publishers, Inc, p 487.
4. Kandel G: Management of nonvariceal upper GI hemorrhage, Hosp Pract 25:167-184, 1990.
5. Eastwood G: Upper GI bleeding: differential diagnosis and management (part 1), Hosp Med 23:57-85, 1987.
6. Katz K and Hollander D: Outpatient management of duodenal ulcer disease, Hosp Med 24:95-103, 1988.
7. Dancygier H and Classen M: Endoscopy of peptic ulcer. In Brooks F, Cohen S, and Soloway R, eds: Peptic ulcer disease, New York, 1985, Churchill Livingstone, pp 18-26.
8. Levinson M: Gastric stress ulcer, Hosp Pract 24:59-67, 1989.
9. Lechago J: Histology of peptic ulcer. In Brooks F, Cohen S, and Soloway R, eds: Peptic ulcer disease, New York, 1985, Churchill Livingstone, p 38.
10. Spiro H: Duodenal ulcer, Hosp Pract 20:70D-E, 1985.
11. Meeroff JC: Ulcer disease in the upper gastrointestinal tract, Hosp Pract 19:204, 1984.
12. Caldwell H and Marshall B: *Campylobacter pylori* and peptic disease: therapeutic implications, Drug Therapy 19:92-105, 1989.
13. Karb V: GI drugs: histamine antagonists, sucralfate and metoclopramine, J Neurosci Nurs 20:202, 1988.
14. Marble D and Ward J: Managing NSAID-induced peptic ulcer, Drug Therapy 19:34-45, 1989.
15. Silverberg E, Boring C, and Squires T: CA 40:9-26, 1990.
16. Wang J: Stomach cancer, Semin Oncol Nurs 4:258, 1988.
17. Viste A and others: Postoperative complications and mortality after surgery for gastric cancer, Ann Surg 207:12, 1988.
18. Frank-Stromborg M: The epidemiology and primary prevention of gastric and esophageal cancer, Cancer Nurs 12:57, 1989.

Nursing Role in Management
Problems of Absorption and Elimination

Barbara Henzel

---

1. Explain the common etiologies and therapeutic and nursing management of diarrhea, fecal incontinence, and constipation.
2. Describe common causes of an acute abdomen and nursing care of the client following an exploratory laparotomy.
3. Describe the nursing management for a client with acute appendicitis.
4. Identify the therapeutic and nursing management of peritonitis.
5. Describe the common etiologies, clinical manifestations, and management of gastroenteritis.
6. Compare and contrast ulcerative colitis and Crohn's disease, including pathophysiology, clinical manifestations, complications, and therapeutic and nursing management.
7. Differentiate among mechanical, neurogenic, and vascular bowel obstructions, including causes and therapeutic and nursing management.
8. Describe the clinical manifestations and surgical and nursing management of cancer of the colon and rectum.

9. Explain the anatomical and physiological changes that result from a sigmoid colostomy, a transverse colostomy, and an ileostomy.
10. Describe the preoperative and postoperative therapeutic and nursing management of a client having bowel surgery.
11. Compare and contrast a colostomy and an ileostomy in relation to nursing care and client teaching.
12. Differentiate between diverticulosis and diverticulitis, including clinical manifestations and therapeutic and nursing management.
13. Compare and contrast the types of hernias, including etiology and surgical and nursing management.
14. Describe the types of malabsorption syndrome and appropriate management of sprue syndrome and lactase deficiency.
15. Describe the types, clinical manifestations, and therapeutic and nursing management of anorectal conditions.

DIARRHEA, BOWEL INCONTINENCE, AND CONSTIPATION
Diarrhea

Etiology. Diarrhea is not a disease but a symptom. The term *diarrhea* may mean different things to different clients. It is commonly referred to as an increase in frequency of stools, stool volume, or looseness of stool. The multiple causes of diarrhea include increased intestinal se-

cretion, decreased intestinal absorption, increased intestinal motility, and a combination of these (Table 37-1).

Clinical manifestations and complications. Diarrhea may be acute or chronic. Acute diarrhea most commonly results from infection. Symptoms of the infection may include explosive watery diarrhea, abdominal cramping, fever, nausea, vomiting, malaise, and tenesmus. Leukocytes, blood, and mucus may be present in the stool, depending on the causative agent (Table 37-2). Diarrhea is usually considered chronic when it persists for at least 2 weeks or when it subsides and returns more than 2 to 4 weeks after the initial episode.

Reviewed by Debra Broadwell-Jackson, R.N., Ph.D., C.E.T.N., Associate Professor, Nell Hodgson Woodruff School of Nursing, Emory University, Atlanta, Georgia.

Severe diarrhea may be debilitating and life threatening. Clients may have severe dehydration, electrolyte disturbances, and hypovolemia. Diarrhea is one of the major causes of death in the world, especially in infants. Malabsorption and malnutrition are sequelae of chronic diarrhea. Perianal skin excoriation may develop in any type of diarrhea.

Therapeutic management. Accurate diagnosis and management require a thorough history, physical examination, and when indicated, laboratory tests. A history of travel, medication, diet, previous surgery, and interpersonal contacts, as well as family history, should be obtained. Blood tests may identify anemia, elevated white blood cell (WBC) count, iron and folate deficiencies, and electrolyte disturbances. Stools may be examined for the presence of blood, mucus, leukocytes, and parasites. Stool cultures help in identifying infectious agents. Measurement of stool electrolytes and osmolarity may help determine whether the diarrhea is secretory or caused by decreased absorption and is usually performed in clients with chronic diarrhea. Measurement of fat in the stool is helpful in differentiating between steatorrhea and secretory diarrhea. Upper and lower barium studies may be helpful in detecting mucosal disease. Endoscopy may also be used to visualize the mucosa and to obtain specimens for diagnosis.

The treatment of diarrhea is based on the cause and is aimed at replacement of fluid and electrolytes and decreasing the number, volume, and frequency of stools. Oral solutions containing glucose and electrolytes (e.g., Gatorade, Pedialyte) are often sufficient to replace losses due to mild diarrhea. Antidiarrheal agents may be given to coat and protect mucous membranes, inhibit gastric motility,

Table 37-1 Causes of Diarrhea

SECRETORY

Excess accumulation of fluid in the intestinal lumen due to increased intestinal secretion and increased intestinal motility

Infectious: Cholera, *Escherichia coli, Shigella, Salmonella, Staphylococcus, Clostridium difficile,* viral agents (rotavirus), and parasitic agents *(e.g., Giardia lamblia)*

Hormonal: Carcinoid (increased serotonin), Zollinger-Ellison syndrome (increased gastrin), vasoactive intestinal peptide–secreting adenoma of pancreas and medullary, carcinoma of the thyroid (increased calcitonin)

Exudate producing: Inflammatory bowel disease, pseudomembranous colitis, amebiasis, shigellosis

Other: Partial colonic obstruction, villous adenoma, increased bile salts, alcohol, caffeine

Drugs: Laxatives, antibiotics

DECREASED ABSORPTION

Excess accumulation of fluid due to mucosal disease, increased intestinal motility, or ingestion of poorly absorbable material (osmotic)

Mucosal disease: Tropical sprue, Crohn's disease, Whipple's disease, radiation injury, ulcerative colitis

Osmotic: Lactase deficiency, laxatives

Other: Decreased surface area due to surgical resection or mucosal disease

INCREASED MOTILITY

Irritable bowel syndrome, vagotomy, diabetic autonomic neuropathy

Table 37-2 Causes of Acute Infectious Diarrhea

	Onset	Duration	Symptoms
VIRAL			
Rotavirus, Norwalk	18-24 hr	24-48 hr	Explosive watery diarrhea, nausea, vomiting, abdominal cramps
BACTERIAL			
Escherichia coli	4-24 hr	3-4 days	4 or 5 loose stools per day, nausea, malaise, low-grade fever
Shigella	24 hr	7 days	Watery stools containing blood and mucus, fever tenesmus, urgency
Salmonellae	6-48 hr	2-5 days	Watery diarrhea, fever, nausea
Campylobacter species	24 hr	<7 days	Profuse, watery diarrhea; malaise; nausea; abdominal cramps; low-grade fever
Clostridium perfringens	8-12 hr	24 hr	Watery diarrhea, abdominal cramps, vomiting
PARASITIC			
Giardia lamblia	1-3 wk	Few days to 3 mo	Sudden onset; foul, explosive, watery diarrhea; flatulence; epigastric pain and cramping; nausea
Entamoeba histolytica	4 days	Weeks to months	Frequent soft stools with blood and mucus (in severe cases, watery stools), flatulence, distention, cramping, fever, leukocytes in stool

Table 37-3 Antidiarrheal Drugs

Type	Mechanism of Action	Examples
Demulcent	Soothes, coats, and protects membrane	Bismuth subsalicylate (Pepto-Bismol); calcium polycarbophil (Mitrolan-OTC); activated charcoal; kaolin, pectin, hyoscyamine sulfate, atropine sulfate, and hyoscine hydrobromide (Donnagel)*; donnagel and opium (Donnagel-PG)*
Anticholinergic	Inhibits gastric motility	Donnagel,* Donnagel-PG,* diphenoxylate HCl with atropine sulfate (Lomotil, Colonaid), loperamide HCl (Imodium)†
Narcotic	Quiets CNS	Camphorated tincture of opium (paregoric); Donnagel-PG; paregoric, pectin, and kaolin (Parepectolin); tincture of opium, homatropine methylbromide, and pectin (Dia-Quel liquid OTC)‡

*Also absorbent, which contributes to the adhesiveness of the stool.
†Has cholinergic and noncholinergic actions.
‡Also an anticholinergic.

Table 37-4

Nursing Assessment of the Client With Diarrhea

SUBJECTIVE DATA

History
Usual bowel habits, ingestion of coarse and spicy foods, recent travel, infections, stress, diverticulitis or malabsorption, metabolic disorders, inflammatory bowel disease or irritable bowel syndrome
Medications
Use of laxatives, magnesium-containing antacids, antibiotics, methyldopa, digitalis, colchicine; over-the-counter antidiarrheal medications
General
Weight loss, weakness, anorexia, thirst
Pain
Tenesmus, abdominal pain and cramping
Gastrointestinal
Amount, frequency, color and character of stools; borborygmi; bloating; abdominal tenderness

OBJECTIVE DATA

General
Lethargy, sunken eyeballs, fever, malnutrition
Integumentary
Pallor, dry mucous membranes, poor skin turgor, perianal excoriation
Gastrointestinal
Amount, frequency, character (sudden onset, alternating diarrhea and constipation); color and consistency of stool; hyperactive bowel sounds; abdominal distention; presence of pus, blood, mucus, or fat in stools; fecal impaction
Urinary
Decreased output, concentrated urine
Possible findings
Abnormal serum electrolyte levels; anemia; leukocytosis; eosinophilia; positive stool cultures; presence of ova, parasites, leukocytes, blood, or fat in stools; abnormal sigmoidoscopic or colonoscopic findings; abnormal lower gastrointestinal series

and quiet the central nervous system (CNS) (Table 37-3). They should not be given over a prolonged time. Antibiotics are usually not indicated in treatment of diarrhea and in some cases may alter bowel flora sufficiently to increase diarrhea.

Acute diarrhea is often self-limiting in the adult. The mucous membrane lining is usually not destroyed from the inflammatory process. Symptoms continue until the irritant or causative agent is excreted.

Chronic or excessive diarrhea can result in serious problems. If there is excessive loss of fluids containing sodium and potassium, parenteral hyperalimentation with vitamin supplements may be required.

■ Nursing Management of Acute Infectious Diarrhea

Nursing assessment

Nursing assessment should begin with a thorough history and physical examination (Table 37-4). The client should be asked to describe the symptoms. Questions should focus on the duration, frequency, character and consistency of stool, and associated symptoms. A medication history should include use of antibiotics, laxatives, and other drugs known to cause diarrhea. Recent travel, excessive stress, and health and family history should be discussed. Dietary history should include questions about eating habits, appetite, and food intolerances, especially milk and dairy products.

Physical examination begins with obtaining orthostatic vital signs and height and weight. The client's skin should be inspected for poor turgor, dryness, and areas of breakdown. The abdomen should be inspected for distention, palpated for tenderness, and auscultated for bowel sounds.

Nursing diagnoses

Nursing diagnoses are determined when the problem and etiological factors are supported by clinical data. Nursing diagnoses related to acute infectious diarrhea may include, but are not limited to, those presented in Table 37-5.

Nursing interventions

Strict medical asepsis is important because acute diarrhea is potentially infectious. Enteric isolation precautions are usually instituted if an infection is suspected. All cases

Table 37-5

 NURSING CARE PLAN FOR THE CLIENT WITH ACUTE INFECTIOUS DIARRHEA

Defining Characteristics	Nursing Interventions	Evaluation Criteria
NURSING DIAGNOSIS: Diarrhea related to acute infectious process		
Frequent loose, watery stools	Monitor frequency, amount, color, consistency of stools. Record intake and output. Administer antidiarrheal agents as ordered. Follow hospital procedure for enteric precautions. Use strict medical asepsis when handling bedpan, linens, or client. Monitor vital signs q 4 hr. Administer antiinfective medications as ordered.	Normal bowel elimination, afebrile
NURSING DIAGNOSIS: Fluid volume deficit related to excessive fluid loss and decreased fluid intake secondary to vomiting and/or diarrhea		
Dry skin and mucous membranes; poor skin turgor; hypovolemia; hypotension; tachycardia; decreased urine output; electrolyte imbalance—decreased sodium, decreased potassium; decreased level of consciousness	Assess for skin turgor changes, sunken eyes, rapid pulse, and anorexia. Monitor intake and output. Monitor sodium and potassium levels and report abnormalities to physician. Monitor vital signs q 4 hr. Weigh client daily. Administer IV fluids as ordered. Increase intake of fluids as tolerated to at least 3000 ml/day. Assess mouth for dryness. Note client's complaints of thirst. If client is not vomiting, administer fluids, such as Gatorade or Pedialyte. Medicate with antidiarrheals as ordered.	Normal vital signs; normal skin turgor; pink, moist mucous membranes; urine output >30 ml/hr; normal serum electrolytes; return to baseline mental status
NURSING DIAGNOSIS: Impaired skin integrity of perianal area related to contact with diarrheal stools and inadequate perianal hygiene		
Redness, swelling, possible ulceration of skin, pain during elimination	Initiate care measures for skin and mucous membranes of perianal area. Cleanse area with warm water after each bowel movement, rinsing well and patting dry with a soft towel. Apply ointment to promote healing. Use an anesthetic ointment or spray foam.	No evidence of skin breakdown in perianal area
NURSING DIAGNOSIS: Acute pain and abdominal cramping related to increased GI motility		
Guarding, doubling over, change in affect, verbal complaints, tachycardia, diaphoresis	Provide restful, stress-free environment. Provide comfort measures. Administer antidiarrheals and anticholinergics as ordered.	Verbalization of satisfactory comfort level
NURSING DIAGNOSIS: High risk for infection transmission related to lack of knowledge in prevention of reinfection or transmission of infectious disease		
Recurrence of diarrhea, fever, and other presenting symptoms; evidence of same symptoms in family members	Explain importance of reporting changes in stools. Assist client in identifying factors that precipitated diarrhea. Stress importance of good hand-washing techniques. Explain importance of seeking medical care when diarrhea and other symptoms begin.	No recurrence of symptoms, knowledge of disease process and preventive measures

of acute diarrhea should be considered infectious until the cause is determined.

Hand washing is the most important measure in prevention of the transfer of microorganisms. Hands should be washed before and after contact with each client and when excretions of any kind are handled. Clients should be taught the principles of hygiene, medical asepsis, and the potential dangers of an illness that is infectious to themselves and others. Proper handling as well as cooking and storage of food should be discussed with clients suspected of having infectious diarrhea.

Bowel Incontinence

Etiology and pathophysiology. Knowledge of the mechanisms involved in fecal continence is helpful in understanding the condition. Normally the contents of the bowel pass into the rectum, causing rectal distention. Sensory receptors in the surrounding pelvic muscles provide the sensation of rectal filling. This causes a reflex relaxation of the internal anal sphincter and contraction of the external anal sphincter. Sensory receptors located in the anal canal can distinguish between solid stool, liquid stool, and gas. The combination of contraction of the abdominal muscles, relaxation of the pelvic muscles, squatting (which straightens the anorectal angle), and voluntary relaxation of the external anal sphincter allows for elimination of feces. Fecal incontinence may be due to multiple causes (Table 37-6).

Therapeutic management. Diagnosis and effective management require a thorough history and physical examination with appropriate diagnostic studies.[1] In all cases a rectal examination should be performed, followed by examination with a flexible sigmoidoscope. Internal prolapse, increased perineal descent, and rectocele may be identified by rectal examination. Flexible sigmoidoscopy may identify inflammation, tumors, fissures, and other rec-

*tal-sigmoid pathology. Other studies often ordered are barium enema, colonoscopy, and anorectal manometry.

Treatment of incontinence depends on the underlying cause. Medications may be given for diarrhea or fecal impaction. Loperamide may be useful in reducing diarrhea and increasing sphincter tone.[2] A high-fiber diet (see Table 37-10), along with increased fluid intake, should be given unless contraindicated, as in clients with colonic inertia. Bowel training programs are usually effective, even with clients who lack total sphincter function.[3]

Biofeedback therapy is 70% effective in treating incontinence in clients with intact sphincter function, preserved mental status, and motivation to learn.[4,5] Biofeedback requires education, reinforcement, and concentration. It is a safe, painless, and inexpensive treatment for fecal incontinence. Surgery should be considered only when therapeutic treatment fails, in cases of full-thickness prolapse, and when the sphincter needs repair.

Fecal incontinence due to fecal impaction can be a common problem in the older adult. A rectal examination may help to identify the presence of an impaction. If the impaction is higher in the bowel, an abdominal x-ray examination is indicated. Fecal impaction usually resolves after enemas and manual disimpaction.

■ Nursing Management of Fecal Incontinence
Nursing assessment

Fecal incontinence is not only an embarrassment to the client but also a potential hazard to normal skin integrity. It is necessary to make an assessment of the client's general condition to identify the best alternative for managing the client with fecal incontinence. The nurse should identify normal bowel habits and current symptoms, including frequency and nature of the stools.

A neurological assessment that includes evaluation of mental status can be helpful in identifying the most effective treatment for the client. Assessment should also include history of multiple or traumatic childbirths, previous anorectal surgery, and injury.

Nursing diagnoses

Nursing diagnoses are determined when the problem and the etiological factors are supported by clinical data. Nursing diagnoses specific to the client with fecal incontinence include, but are not limited to, the following:

1. Potential for impaired skin integrity of the perianal area due to incontinence of stool
2. Bowel incontinence due to trauma, inflammation, neurological disorder, relaxation of pelvic muscles, or fecal impaction
3. Social isolation related to embarrassment and odor
4. Self-esteem disturbance related to inability to control bowel functions

Nursing interventions

Prevention and treatment of fecal incontinence may be alleviated by implementing a bowel training program. The client should be put on a bedpan, assisted to a bedside commode, or walked to the bathroom at a regular time daily to assist with reestablishment of bowel regularity. A good time to establish this pattern is within 30 minutes after breakfast each day if there is no conflict with the hos-

---

Table 37-6 Causes of Fecal Incontinence

TRAUMATIC	NEUROLOGICAL
Obstetric	Stroke
Postsurgical	Tumor
Hemorrhoidectomy	Degenerative disease
Anterior resection	Iatrogenic drug intoxication
Fistulectomy	Multiple sclerosis
Anorectal surgery	Diabetes mellitus
Spinal cord injuries	Dementia
INFLAMMATION	**OTHER**
Infection	Pelvic floor relaxation
Trauma	Perineal descent
Radiation	Loss of elasticity of rectum (age related)
	Fecal impaction
	Diarrhea
	Medications

pital routine. If the usual bowel habits differ from this pattern, efforts should be made to adhere to the client's individual timing.

If these techniques are ineffective in reestablishing bowel regularity, a bisacodyl (Dulcolax) or glycerin suppository may be inserted 15 to 30 minutes before the usual evacuation time. This stimulates the anorectal reflex and often can be discontinued when a regular pattern is reestablished.

Maintenance of skin integrity is of upmost importance, especially in the bedridden and older adult client. Nursing management may necessitate drainage tubes, use of incontinence briefs, and meticulous skin care. Tubes and catheters are usually not recommended because their use over an extended period may decrease responsiveness of the rectal sphincter and cause ulceration of the rectal mucosa. Use of incontinence briefs may be helpful in maintaining skin integrity if changed frequently, but this can be demeaning and humiliating to the client. Meticulous cleaning after each stool is required. Washing, rinsing, thorough drying, and application of a protective barrier are essential to the maintenance of skin integrity. Because the client may have several stools each day, maintaining skin integrity is a time-consuming task for the nurse and the family.

Perianal pouching is an alternative in the management of fecal incontinence. Pouching provides skin protection and fecal containment as well as comfort and dignity.

Because odor is often a problem, deodorant sprays and room deodorizers may be used. For the client who is confined to bed for an extended time, a mattress with a round opening may be obtained. For the client who is ambulatory, a chair (regular or special commode wheelchair) may be used. Regardless of the mobility of the client, the nurse must make sure the skin is clean, odorless, and intact.

Constipation

Etiology. Millions of persons suffer from constipation. Despite its prevalence, little is known about its pathophysiology.[6] *Constipation* may be defined as a decrease in frequency of bowel movements from what is "normal" for the individual; hard, difficult-to-pass stool; a decrease in stool volume; and retention of feces in the rectum. Normal bowel elimination may vary from three times a day to once every 3 days.[7] Because of such a wide variation, it is important to determine the severity of constipation on the basis of the client's normal pattern of elimination.

Frequently constipation may result from lack of dietary fiber, inadequate fluid intake, and lack of exercise. If proper preventive measures are subsequently taken, this type of constipation should not recur. Constipation may also be due to sociocultural beliefs, environmental constraints, ignoring the urge to defecate, chronic laxative abuse, and multiple organic causes (Table 37-7).

Clients may imagine they are constipated. They may believe they should have a daily bowel movement or expect passage of stool the same time every day. This can result in chronic laxative abuse and possibly cathartic colon syndrome, whereby the colon becomes dilated and atonic. Change in diet, in mealtime, or in the client's daily routine are a few environmental factors that may cause constipation. Depression, stress, and ignoring of the urge to defecate can also result in constipation.

Ignoring the urge to defecate causes the muscles and membranes in the rectal area to become insensitive to the presence of feces. The prolonged retention of feces in the rectum results in drying of stool because of the reabsorption of water from the feces. The harder and drier the feces, the worse the constipation.

Clinical manifestations and complications. The clinical presentation of constipation may vary from a chronic discomfort to an acute event mimicking an "acute abdomen." Other clinical manifestations are presented in Table 37-8.

Hemorrhoids are the most common complication of chronic constipation.[7] They result from venous engorgement due to repeated Valsalva maneuvers (straining) and venous compression from hard impacted stool. In the presence of obstipation or fecal impaction, colonic perforation

Table 37-7　Organic Causes of Constipation

COLONIC DISORDERS	SYSTEMIC DISORDERS
Luminal or extraluminal obstructing lesions	**Metabolic/endocrine**
Inflammatory strictures	Diabetes mellitus
Volvulus	Hypothyroidism
Intussusception	Pregnancy
Irritable bowel syndrome	Hypercalcemia
Diverticular disease	Pheochromocytoma
Rectocele	
	Collagen vascular disease
DRUG INDUCED	Scleroderma
Antacids (calcium and aluminum)	Amyloidosis
Antidepressants	
Anticholinergics	**Neurogenic disorders**
Antipsychotics	Hirschsprung's disease
Antihypertensives	Neurofibromatosis
Barium sulfate	Autonomic neuropathy (pseudoobstruction)
Iron supplements	Multiple sclerosis
Bismuth	Parkinson's disease
Calcium supplements	Spinal cord lesions or injury

Table 37-8　Clinical Manifestations of Constipation

Hard, dry stool	Increased flatulence
Abdominal distention	Nausea
Abdominal pain	Anorexia
Decreased frequency of bowel movements	Headache
	Palpable mass
Straining	Stool with blood
Rectal pressure	Dizziness
Tenesmus	

may occur. This may be life threatening and cause abdominal pain, nausea, vomiting, fever, and an elevated WBC count. An abdominal x-ray study showing the presence of free air can diagnose perforation.

Fecal impaction may also cause stercoral ulcers (ulcers of the colonic mucosa that result from pressure necrosis). These are most commonly seen in older adults. Solitary rectal ulcers may also occur and may result from straining.

Valsalva's maneuver, which occurs during straining to pass a hardened stool, may cause serious problems in clients with congestive heart failure, cerebral edema, hypertension, and coronary artery disease. During straining, the client takes a deep inspiration, the breath is held, and the glottis closes and traps the air. The abdominal muscles contract and try to push against the colon. Increases in intraabdominal pressure and intrathoracic pressure occur. The heart slows temporarily (bradycardia), and the cardiac output is decreased with a transient drop in arterial pressure.

When the client relaxes, there is decreased thoracic pressure and a sudden flow of blood into the heart, causing tachycardia. Immediately the arterial pressure rises momentarily. These changes may be fatal for the client who cannot compensate for sudden overload of blood flow to the heart after straining.

Therapeutic management. A thorough history and physical examination should be performed so that the underlying cause of constipation can be identified and treatment be started. Abdominal series, barium enema, colonoscopy or sigmoidoscopy, and anorectal manometry may be helpful in determining an organic cause. Most cases of constipation can be managed with diet therapy, an exercise program, and cathartic agents (laxatives) (Table 37-9). Laxatives should always be used with caution because they may become a cause of constipation with chronic overuse.

Clients with severe constipation due to a motility disorder may require more intensive treatment. Studies such as

Table 37-9 Cathartic Agents

Category	Mechanisms of Action	Example	Onset of Action	Comments
Bulk forming	Absorbs water; increases bulk, thereby stimulating peristalsis	Metamucil, Perdiem, Konsyl, Hydrocil	Usually within 24 hr	Contraindicated in clients with abdominal pain, nausea, and vomiting and in clients suspected of having appendicitis, biliary tract obstruction, or acute hepatitis; needs to be taken with fluids
Stimulants	Increase peristalsis by irritating colon wall and stimulating nerves that innervate it	Anthraquinone drugs Cascara sagrada, senna Phenolphthalein drugs Ex-Lax, Correctol, Feen-a-Mint, Bisacodyl, Dulcolax	Usually within 12 hr	Cause melanosis coli (brown or black pigmentation of colon), are most widely abused laxatives, should not be used in clients with impaction or obstipation
Stool softeners and lubricants	Lubricate intestinal tract and soften feces, making hard stools easier to pass; do not affect peristalsis	Mineral oil, dioctyl sodium, sulfosuccinate, Colace, Peri-Colace, Doxidan	Softeners up to 72 hr, lubricants up to 8 hr	Can block absorption of fat-soluble vitamins such as vitamin K, which may increase risk of bleeding among clients on anticoagulants
Saline and osmotic solutions	Cause retention of fluid in intestinal lumen due to osmotic effect	Magnesium salts Magnesium citrate, MOM Sodium phosphates Fleets enema, Phospho-soda Lactulose Polyethylene glycolsaline solutions Go-Lytely, Colyte	15 min to 3 hr	Magnesium-containing products may cause hypermagnesemia in clients with renal insufficiency

anorectal manometry, radioactive transit studies, and sigmoidoscopic rectal biopsies should be performed before treatment. The use of metoclopramide (Reglan) and second- and third-generation prokinetic agents, domperidone and cisapride, are effective in clients who are unresponsive to conventional therapy. In clients with unrelenting constipation a subtotal colectomy with ileorectal anastomosis is the procedure of choice.[7]

Enemas should be limited in their use to treat constipation. They are fast acting and are beneficial in the immediate treatment of constipation. Soapsuds enemas should be avoided because they may lead to colitis. Oil-retention enemas may be used to soften fecal impactions.

Nutritional considerations. An important role of the nurse is teaching the client the importance of dietary measures to prevent constipation. Many clients experience an improvement in their symptoms when they simply increase their intake of dietary fiber and fluids. Dietary fiber is found in two forms: insoluble and soluble in water. Both are contained in most foods, but some foods are higher in soluble fiber (Table 37-10).

Insoluble fiber remains essentially unchanged by the time it reaches the colon, and it is found in higher concentrations in whole wheat and bran. Soluble fibers form gel-like substances that add viscosity to the digested contents, causing decreased gastric emptying and decreased transit time in the small intestine. This affects glucose absorption and cholesterol metabolism, which may be beneficial in the management of diabetes, atherosclerosis, and cholesterol gallstones. Soluble fiber is found in oat bran, fruits, vegetables, and psyllium.

The diet should also include a fluid intake of at least 3000 ml/day. The nurse should encourage the selection of foods the client likes and is able to prepare and foods that are affordable. The client's understanding of the diet and the importance of dietary fiber is important to ensure compliance.

■ Nursing Management of Constipation
Nursing assessment

Subjective and objective data that should be obtained from a person with constipation are presented in Table 37-11.

Nursing diagnoses

Nursing diagnoses are determined when the problem and the etiological factors are supported by clinical data. Nursing diagnoses related to constipation may include, but are not limited to, those presented in Table 37-12.

Nursing interventions

Nursing management should be based on the client's symptoms (see Table 37-12). Emphasis should be placed on maintenance of a high-fiber diet, increasing fluid intake, and a regular exercise program. Clients should be taught to establish a regular time to defecate and not to suppress the urge to defecate. In many persons the urge to defecate occurs after breakfast because of the stimulation of the gastrocolic reflex. The client should be discouraged from using laxatives and enemas to achieve fecal elimination.

Proper position is important when defecating. For a cli-

Table 37-10 High-Fiber Diet*

	Fiber per Serving (g)	Size of Serving	Calories per Serving
VEGETABLES			
Asparagus	3.5	½ cup	18
Beans			
Navy	8.4	½ cup	80
Kidney	9.7	½ cup	94
Lima	8.3	½ cup	63
Pinto	8.9	½ cup	78
String	2.1	½ cup	18
Broccoli	3.5	½ cup	18
Carrots, raw	1.8	½ cup	15
Corn	2.6	½ medium ear	72
Peas, canned	6.7	½ cup	63
Potatoes			
Baked	1.9	½ medium	72
Sweet	2.1	½ medium	79
Squash			
Acorn	7.0	1 cup	82
Tomato, raw	1.5	1 small	18
FRUITS			
Apple	2.0	½ large	42
Banana	1.5	½ medium	48
Blackberries	6.7	¾ cup	40
Orange	1.6	1 small	35
Peach	2.3	1 medium	38
Pear	2.0	½ medium	44
Raspberries	9.2	1 cup	42
Strawberries	3.1	1 cup	45
GRAIN PRODUCTS			
Bread			
Rye	0.8	1 slice	62
White	0.7	1 slice	64
Whole wheat	1.3	1 slice	59
Cereal			
All Bran (100%)	8.4	⅓ cup	70
Corn Flakes	2.6	¾ cup	70
Shredded Wheat	2.8	1 biscuit	70
Crackers			
Graham	1.4	2 squares	53
Popcorn	3.0	3 cups	62
Rice			
Brown	1.6	⅓ cup	72
White	0.5	⅓ cup	76

Modified from Dietary fiber: an overview for physicians, Chicago, 1985, Searle Consumer Products, Inc.
*Recommended for clients with diverticulosis, irritable bowel syndrome, constipation, hemorrhoids, colon cancer, atherosclerosis, hyperlipidemia, and diabetes.

Table 37-11

Nursing Assessment of the Client With Constipation

SUBJECTIVE DATA

History
Usual elimination patterns, exercise, fluid and food intake, colorectal disease, neurological dysfunction, anorectal pain, bowel obstruction, environmental changes, cancer, stress

Medications
Use of aluminum antacids, anticholinergics, antidepressants, antihistamines, antipsychotics, diuretics, narcotics, iron, laxatives, enemas

General
Anorexia, malaise, weakness, headache, dizziness

Pain
Abdominal pain on defecation and tenesmus

Gastrointestinal
Frequency, amount, and consistency of stools; defecation difficulty; bloating; flatus; diarrhea (if impacted); nausea; rectal pressure

OBJECTIVE DATA

General
Lethargy

Integumentary
Anorectal fissures, hemorrhoids, abscesses

Gastrointestinal
Abdominal distention, fecal impaction, hypoactive or absent bowel sounds, stool consistency and amount

Possible findings
Guaiac-positive stools, abdominal x-ray study demonstrating stool in colon

ent in bed, the bedpan should be placed and the head of the bed should be elevated as high as the client can tolerate. For the person who can sit on a toilet, a footstool may be placed in front of the toilet. Placing the feet on the footstool promotes flexion of the thighs, which assists in defecation.

The client with poor muscle tone should be encouraged to exercise the abdominal muscles and can be taught to contract the abdominal muscles several times a day. Situps and straight leg raises can also be used to improve abdominal muscle tone.

Some clients may have to be encouraged to increase their social activities as well as their physical activity; this is especially true of older adults, who may become depressed and socially isolated because of multiple factors. Inactivity can lead to constipation. These clients should be encouraged and assisted in establishing social contacts and activities outside their homes.

INFLAMMATORY DISEASE
Acute Abdomen

Etiology. The client with an acute abdomen has acute onset of abdominal pain requiring prompt decision making and surgical intervention.[8] Causes of an acute abdomen are varied (Table 37-13). Therefore many disorders must be ruled out before a diagnosis is confirmed.

Clinical manifestations. Pain is the most important presenting symptom. The client may also complain of abdominal tenderness, vomiting, diarrhea, constipation, flatulence, fatigue, bleeding, and an increase in abdominal girth.

Therapeutic management. Diagnosis begins with a complete history and physical examination. Physical examination should include a rectal and pelvic examination. A complete blood cell (CBC) count, urinalysis, abdominal x-ray films, and an electrocardiogram (ECG) are done ini-

Table 37-12

 NURSING CARE PLAN FOR THE CLIENT WITH CONSTIPATION

Defining Characteristics	Nursing Interventions	Evaluation Criteria
NURSING DIAGNOSIS: Constipation related to inadequate dietary intake of fiber, inadequate fluid intake, and decreased physical activity		
Hard, dry stools; straining; painful defecation; abdominal distention; decreased frequency of defecation; headache; increased flatulence	Provide client with a list of high-fiber foods. Encourage a minimum of 20 g of fiber intake daily. Teach role of fiber and fluids in prevention of constipation. Encourage fluid intake of at least 3000 ml/day. Discuss benefits of exercise. Assist in establishing a regular exercise program. Discuss importance of responding to urge to defecate. Teach and assist in establishing regular elimination pattern. Provide privacy. Monitor and document bowel activity. Administer and document results of prescribed agents. Teach correct use of laxatives.	High-fiber diet consisting of 20 to 30 g of fiber per day; fluid intake of 3000 ml/day; increased physical activity; establishment of regular pattern of elimination

tially. Pregnancy tests should be performed in women of childbearing age who have acute abdominal pain. The findings of these studies may provide some information as to the cause of the acute abdomen. Prehospital care of the client with an acute abdomen or abdominal trauma is presented in Tables 37-14 and 37-15.

The goal of management is to identify and treat the cause. The physician attempts to make a differential diagnosis when the client is seen with an acute abdomen, since there are many causes of abdominal pain that do not require surgery (see Table 37-13).

In addition to being a therapeutic measure, surgery can also be diagnostic. Operative exploration is usually done after a careful examination of the client and is justified when "look and see" is better than "wait and see." The surgical procedure is an exploratory laparotomy, in which an opening is made through the abdominal wall into the peritoneal cavity to determine the cause of an acute abdomen.

■ Nursing Management of Acute Abdomen
Nursing assessment

Vital signs should be taken immediately. Orthostatic blood pressure and pulse rate should be obtained to determine hypovolemic changes. An elevated temperature may indicate an inflammatory or infectious process. The abdomen should be inspected for distention, masses, abnormal

---

Table 37-13 Causes of Acute Abdomen

Abdominal penetrating trauma	Pancreatitis
Acute ischemic bowel	Pelvic inflammatory disease
Appendicitis	Peptic ulcer
Bowel obstruction with perforation or necrosis	Perforated GI malignancy
Cholecystitis	Peritonitis
Diverticulitis with peritonitis	Ruptured abdominal aneurysm
Foreign body perforation	Ruptured ectopic pregnancy
Gastritis	Ruptured ovarian cyst
Gastroenteritis	Ulcerative colitis
Mesenteric adenitis	Uterine rupture
	Volvulus

Table 37-14

 Prehospital Emergency Care of the Client with an Acute Abdomen*

Possible etiologies: Inflammation (e.g., appendicitis, cholecystitis, pancreatitis, ulcerative colitis, gastritis, pelvic inflammatory disease), obstruction or perforation of an abdominal organ, gastrointestinal bleeding, or vascular problems (e.g., ruptured aortic aneurysm, mesenteric vascular occlusion)

CLINICAL MANIFESTATIONS

Abdominal pain or tenderness—diffuse or localized
Abdominal distention
Abdominal rigidity
Nausea and vomiting
Bleeding from GI tract (e.g., hematemesis, melena)
Manifestations of shock (e.g., decreased blood pressure, rapid pulse rate) if associated with bleeding

MANAGEMENT

Monitor airway and be prepared to support respiration.
Be on alert for vomiting. Have suction equipment ready.
Administer high-flow oxygen via nasal cannula.
Monitor vital signs.
Start IV line with large-gauge needle.
Position client in a comfortable position.
Try to determine any precipitating causes and history of underlying conditions.

*See Chapter 59 for a general discussion on measures related to prehospital emergency care.

Table 37-15

 Prehospital Emergency Care of the Client with Abdominal Trauma*

Etiology: Blunt or penetrating abdominal trauma due to automobile accidents, knife or gunshot wounds, falls, and fights

CLINICAL MANIFESTATIONS

Evidence of bruising on abdominal wall or penetration of skin
Rigid, distended abdomen with tender, rebound pain
Radiation of pain to shoulder and back
Preferred position lying still with legs up in fetal position
Nausea and vomiting
Rapid, shallow breathing
Increased pulse rate
Decreased blood pressure
Bloody urine

MANAGEMENT

Remove all clothing to carefully assess for injury.
Control all bleeding and cover all open wounds with sterile dressing.
Monitor for any respiratory distress, especially if client vomits.
Start IV line with large-gauge needle.
Monitor vital signs.
Be alert for vomiting. Have suction equipment available.
If there is a penetrating impaled object in abdomen, *do not remove.* Stabilize with bulky dressing and tape securely in place.
Cover any protruding organs or tissue with sterile moist dressing and apply occlusive tape to secure.
Apply oxygen via nasal cannula, especially if client is in shock.
Immobilize client if pelvic fracture is suspected.

*See Chapter 59 for a general discussion on measures related to prehospital emergency care.

Table 37-16

NURSING CARE PLAN FOR THE CLIENT FOLLOWING LAPAROTOMY

Defining Characteristics	Nursing Interventions	Evaluation Criteria
NURSING DIAGNOSIS: Pain related to surgical incision and inadequate pain control measures		
Complaints of pain, body posturing and sounds indicative of pain, unwillingness to move in bed or to ambulate	Assess for pain and give pain medication every 3 to 4 hr as ordered for first 72 hr. Splint incision with pillows during coughing, deep breathing, and moving. Position client comfortably.	Verbalization of satisfactory level of pain control
NURSING DIAGNOSIS: Nausea and vomiting related to decreased motility, GI distention, and narcotics		
Complaints of nausea, vomiting of gastric contents, lack of or diminished bowel sounds, abdominal distention	Administer antiemetic medications as ordered. Assess sensitivity to pain narcotics. Maintain patency of NG tube, if present. Assess for bowel sounds and abdominal distention. Keep client on NPO status until bowel sounds return. Limit unpleasant sights, smells, and stimuli.	Relief of nausea and vomiting
NURSING DIAGNOSIS: Ineffective airway clearance related to sedation, pain, immobility, and location of incision		
Shallow, labored respiratory pattern; decreased breath sounds; rhonchi; productive cough; fever	Monitor vital signs q 4 hr. Report temperature elevation, labored respirations. Have client cough and deep breathe 10 times q 2 hr for 72 hr. Splint operative site with pillows during coughing and deep breathing. Turn client q 2 hr. Auscultate lungs q 4 hr. Assess breathing pattern and rate. Ambulate client at least three times a day, beginning the first postoperative day. Have client assume semi-Fowler's position while in bed.	Lungs clear to auscultation; nonlabored, deep respirations; absence of fever
NURSING DIAGNOSIS: Constipation related to immobility, pain, medication, and decreased motility		
Decreased or absent bowel sounds, abdominal pain, abdominal distention, inability to pass flatus or stool	Assess abdomen for distention and bowel sounds every shift. Check for passage of flatus and bowel movement and record. Administer laxative as ordered if client has not had bowel movement in 4 days. Encourage frequent position changes and ambulation as tolerated. Encourage increased fluid intake as tolerated.	Normal bowel sounds within 72 hr; soft, formed bowel movement within 4 days; abdomen soft to palpation

pulsation, scars, and discolorations. Bowel sounds should be auscultated. Bowel sounds are diminished or absent in acute peritonitis. Palpation should be gentle.

A thorough assessment of the client's symptoms should be made to determine the onset, location, intensity, duration, frequency, and character of pain. Assessment of vomiting should include the amount, color, consistency, and odor of the vomitus. Bowel habits should also be carefully assessed.

Nursing interventions

Preoperative care. Emergency preparation of the client with an acute abdomen is usually limited to a CBC count and typing and cross-matching of blood. Catheterization, preparation of the abdominal skin, and the passage of a na-

sogastric (NG) tube may be done in the emergency room or operating room. (Preoperative care is discussed in Chapter 11.)

Postoperative care. The nurse prepares the room with equipment for gastric suctioning. When the client returns from surgery, the NG tube is connected to suction as ordered (Table 37-16).

The purpose of the NG tube is to empty the stomach of secretions and gas and thus prevent gastric dilatation. (Gastrointestinal [GI] peristaltic activity is impaired because of the manipulative procedures of the surgery and anesthesia.) Low intermittent suctioning is ordered to prevent trauma to the gastric mucosa.

Drainage from the tube may be dark brown to dark red

for the first 12 hours. Later it should be light yellowish brown, or it may have a greenish tinge because of the presence of bile. If a dark red color continues or if bright red blood is observed, the physician should be notified at once of the possibility of hemorrhage. "Coffee ground"–like granules in the drainage are due to the presence of small amounts of blood that have been chemically acted on by gastric secretions.

The NG tube is checked frequently for patency. The tube may become obstructed with mucus, sediment, or old blood. An order is usually written to irrigate the tube with 20 to 30 ml of normal saline solution if needed. Repositioning the tube may facilitate drainage.

An accurate record of intake and output, including emesis and gastric drainage, is essential. The nurse should assess serum electrolyte values, since prolonged gastric suctioning will result in deficiencies of sodium, chloride, potassium, and bicarbonate.

The NG tube is removed when peristalsis returns, usually 24 to 72 hours after surgery. Motility of the stomach normally returns within 24 to 48 hours. Motility of the small intestine usually resumes within 24 hours, whereas return of large intestine motility may take as long as 3 to 5 days. Peristaltic activity is assessed by auscultation for bowel sounds.

Mouth care and nasal care are essential. The client tends to breathe through the mouth while the NG tube is in place. In addition, increased nasal secretions and crusting result from mechanical stimulation of the NG tube.

Parenteral fluids are administered to provide the client with fluids and electrolytes until bowel sounds return. Occasionally, ice chips may be ordered because they aid in the flow of saliva and prevent drying. When bowel sounds return, fluids and food are increased gradually. The diet may be supplemented with multivitamins and iron.

Nausea and vomiting are not uncommon after abdominal surgery. These problems are often self-limiting. Observation is important in determining the cause. Antiemetics such as promethazine (Phenergan), hydroxyzine (Vistaril), prochlorperazine (Compazine), or trimethobenzamide (Tigan) may be ordered.

Abdominal distention and gas pains are also common after surgery; these are due to swallowed air and impaired peristalsis resulting from immobility, manipulation of abdominal contents during surgery, and side effects of anesthesia. The pain can be so uncomfortable that medications to stimulate peristalsis, such as bethanechol (Urecholine) or neostigmine methylsulfate (Prostigmin), may be given. A rectal tube or moist heat on the abdomen may be effective in relieving distention. The physician should be informed of abdominal distention and rigidity. Gradually, as intestinal activity increases, distention and gas pains decrease.

Emotional support from the nursing staff is important. Honest, clear, concise explanations of all procedures in language the client and the family can understand help to allay anxiety.

Rehabilitative management. Preparation for discharge begins when the client returns from the operating room. Instructions to the client and the family should include any modifications in activity, care of the incision, diet, and drug therapy. Small, frequent meals high in calories should be taken initially, with a gradual increase in intake of food as tolerated.

Normal activities should be resumed gradually, with planned rest periods. The client should be aware of possible complications after surgery and should notify the physician immediately if vomiting, pain, weight loss, incisional drainage, or changes in bowel functions occur.

Chronic Abdominal Pain

Chronic abdominal pain may originate from abdominal structures or may be referred from a site with the same or a similar nerve supply. Some common causes are irritable bowel syndrome, peptic ulcer disease, diverticulitis, chronic pancreatitis, hepatitis, cholecystitis, pelvic inflammatory disease, and vascular insufficiency. Psychogenic pain should also be considered (see Chapter 51).

Diagnosis of chronic abdominal pain presents a challenge. Assessment should begin with a thorough history and identification of the specific pain pattern. Character and severity of pain, location, duration, and onset should be determined. The assessment should also include the relationship of pain to meals, defecation, activity, and factors that increase or decrease the pain. Deep pain, usually of visceral or somatic origin, is more characteristic of chronic abdominal pain. It is usually described as dull, aching, or diffuse. (Specific causes of abdominal pain are discussed on p. 1083 and in Chapter 38.)

New technologies, such as endoscopy, computed tomography (CT) scans, magnetic resonance imaging (MRI), laparoscopy, and radiographic barium studies, have lessened the need for exploratory laparotomy but have not lessened the frustrations experienced by the clinician attempting to make a diagnosis.

Appendicitis

Appendicitis is an inflammation of the appendix, a narrow blind tube that extends from the inferior part of the cecum. It occurs in 6% of the general population. Peak incidence is between the ages of 11 and 30 years, and the condition occurs equally in both sexes.[8]

Etiology. The most common causes of appendicitis are obstruction of the lumen by a *fecalith* (accumulated feces) (Fig. 37-1), foreign bodies, intramural thickening due to lymphoid hyperplasia, or tumor of the cecum or appendix. Obstruction results in distention, venous engorgement, and the accumulation of mucus and bacteria that can lead to gangrene and perforation.

Clinical manifestations. Appendicitis typically begins with periumbilical pain, followed by anorexia, nausea, and vomiting. The pain is persistent and continuous, eventually shifting to the right lower quadrant and localizing at McBurney's point (located halfway between the umbilicus and the right iliac crest). Further assessment of the client reveals localized tenderness, rebound tenderness, and muscle guarding. The client usually prefers to lie still, often with the right leg flexed. Low-grade fever may or may not be present, and coughing aggravates pain. Rovsing's sign may be elicited by palpation of the left lower quadrant, causing pain to be felt in the right lower quadrant. Complications of acute appendicitis are perforation, peritonitis,

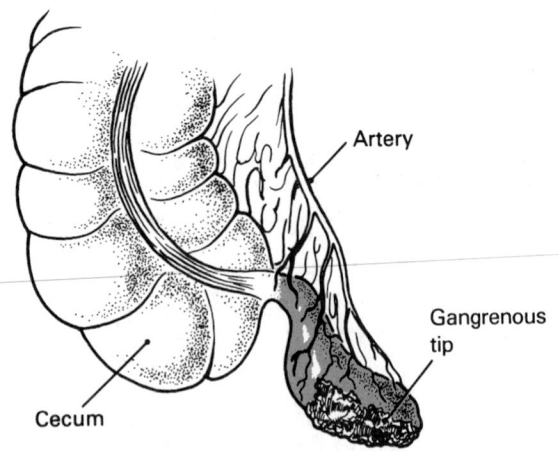

Fig. 37-1 In appendicitis the blood supply of the appendix is impaired by bacterial infection in the wall of the appendix, which may result in gangrene.

and abscesses. Early diagnosis and treatment are important to prevent these serious complications.

Therapeutic management. Examination of the client includes a complete history and physical examination (particularly palpation of the abdomen) and a differential leukocyte count. A urinalysis may be done to rule out genitourinary (GU) conditions that mimic the manifestations of appendicitis.

The treatment of appendicitis is immediate surgical removal if the inflammation is localized. If the appendix has ruptured and there is evidence of peritonitis or an abscess, conservative treatment, consisting of antibiotic therapy and parenteral fluids, may be used to prevent sepsis and dehydration for 6 to 8 hours before an appendectomy is performed.

■ Nursing Management of Appendicitis

The client with abdominal pain is encouraged to see a physician and to avoid self-treatment, particularly the use of laxatives and enemas. The increased peristalsis from these procedures may cause perforation of the appendix. Until the client is seen by a physician, nothing should be taken by mouth (NPO) to ensure that the stomach will be empty in the event surgery is needed. An ice bag may be applied to the right lower quadrant to decrease the flow of blood to the area and impede the inflammatory process. Heat is never used because it may cause the appendix to rupture. Surgery is usually performed as soon as a diagnosis is made. Postoperative recovery is usually short and rapid (4 to 7 days).

Postoperative nursing management is similar to postoperative care of the client after laparotomy (see Table 37-16). In addition, the client should be observed for evidence of peritonitis. Ambulation begins the day of surgery or the first postoperative day. The diet is advanced to general as tolerated. The client is usually discharged on the second or third postoperative day, and normal activities are resumed 2 to 3 weeks after surgery.

Table 37-17 Causes of Peritonitis

GENERALIZED	LOCALIZED*
Perforated ulcer, gallbladder, or colonic diverticulum	Appendicitis
	Diverticulitis
Spontaneous bacterial peritonitis	Inflammatory bowel disease (e.g., Crohn's disease, ulcerative colitis)
Ruptured ovarian cyst	Pelvic inflammatory disease
	Pancreatitis
	Cholecystitis
	Hepatitis

*Conditions may result in generalized peritonitis by rupture into the peritoneal cavity.

Peritonitis

Peritonitis results from a localized or generalized inflammatory process of the peritoneum. It may appear in acute and chronic forms, and it may be caused by trauma or rupture of an organ containing chemical irritants or bacteria, which are released into the peritoneal cavity. Examples of a chemical peritonitis include gastric ulcer perforation and ruptured ectopic pregnancy. A chemical peritonitis is commonly followed by bacterial invasion. Bacterial peritonitis can be caused by a traumatic injury (e.g., gunshot wound, ruptured appendix), or it can be secondary to other diseases or conditions (e.g., pancreatitis, peritoneal dialysis) (Table 37-17).

Pathophysiology. The response of the peritoneum to the leakage of contents is localization of the offending agent by attempting to "wall" it off. If the attempt fails, peritonitis worsens. The tissue begins to swell, and fibrinous exudate develops. Adhesions may be formed. These adhesions may shrink and disappear when the infection is eliminated. Normally, peritoneal injuries heal without formation of adhesions unless other factors, such as infection, ischemia, or foreign substances, are present.

Clinical manifestations. Pain is the most constant symptom of peritonitis, followed by ascites.[9] A universal sign is tenderness over the involved area. Rebound tenderness, muscular rigidity, and spasm are other major signs of irritation of the peritoneum. Abdominal distention, fever, tachycardia, tachypnea, nausea, vomiting, and altered bowel habits may also be present. These manifestations vary, depending on severity and acuteness of the underlying cause. Complications of peritonitis include hypovolemic shock, septicemia, ileus, and organ failure.

Diagnostic studies. A CBC is done to determine leukocytosis and hemoconcentration (Table 37-18). An abdominal paracentesis may be performed to determine blood, bile, pus, bacteria, and amylase content. Paracentesis should always be done when ascites is present. An x-ray examination of the abdomen shows dilatation of the large and small bowels with edema of the wall of the small bowel. Air may be seen under the diaphragm.

Ultrasound and CT scans may be useful in identifying

Table 37-18

Diagnostic and Therapeutic Management: Peritonitis

DIAGNOSTIC

CBC
Serum electrolytes
Abdominal x-ray film
Abdominal paracentesis and culture of fluid
CT scan or ultrasound
Peritoneoscopy

THERAPEUTIC

Preoperative or nonoperative

NPO status
Fluid replacement
Antibiotic therapy
NG suction
Analgesics
Preparation for surgery to include the above and total parenteral nutrition

Postoperative

NPO status
NG tube to low-intermittent suction
Semi-Fowler's position
IV fluids with electrolyte replacement
Total parenteral nutrition as needed
Antibiotic therapy
Blood transfusions as needed
Sedatives and narcotics

---

the presence of ascites and localized lesions. Peritoneoscopy may be helpful in clients without ascites. Direct visualization of the peritoneum can be obtained along with biopsy specimens for diagnosis.

Therapeutic management. The goals of management of peritonitis are to identify and eliminate the cause, combat infection, and prevent complications. Clients with milder cases of peritonitis or those who are poor surgical risks may be managed nonsurgically. Treatment consists of antibiotics, NG suction, analgesics, and intravenous (IV) fluid administration. Clients who require surgery need preoperative preparation consisting of the aforementioned treatment. These clients are usually placed on total parenteral nutrition (TPN) because of increased nutritional requirements.

■ Nursing Management of Peritonitis

Nursing assessment

It is important to determine whether the client has had a traumatic injury or has been exposed to chemical irritants or bacteria. The assessment of pain is very important. Identifying the location of pain may help the physician determine the cause of peritonitis. The client should be assessed for the presence and quality of bowel sounds, in-

creasing abdominal distention, fever, and manifestations of hypovolemic shock.

Nursing diagnoses

Nursing diagnoses specific to the client with peritonitis include, but are not limited to, the following:

1. Abdominal pain related to inflammation of the peritoneum and abdominal distention
2. High risk for fluid volume deficit related to collection of fluid in peritoneal cavity as a result of trauma, infection, or ischemia
3. Potential complication: hypovolemic shock
4. Altered nutrition: less than body requirements due to nausea and vomiting
5. Anxiety related to uncertainty of cause or outcome of condition and pain

Nursing interventions

The client with peritonitis is very ill and needs skilled supportive care. Accurate monitoring of fluid intake and output and electrolyte status is necessary to determine replacement therapy.

The nurse should provide rest and a quiet environment; keep the client on NPO status; monitor vital signs frequently; and assess cardiac, renal, and pulmonary function. Analgesics should be given for pain, and sedatives should be given to allay anxiety. If the client has surgery, drains are inserted to remove purulent drainage and excessive fluid. Postoperative care of the client is similar to the care of the client with an exploratory laparotomy (see Table 37-16).

Gastroenteritis

Gastroenteritis is an inflammation of the mucosa of the stomach and small intestine. Clinical manifestations include nausea, vomiting, diarrhea, abdominal cramping, and distention. Fever, leukocytosis, and blood or mucus in the stool may be present. Causative agents are varied (see Table 37-2). Most cases are self-limiting. Until vomiting has ceased, the client should be on NPO status. If severe dehydration has occurred, IV replacement of fluids may be necessary. Fluids containing glucose and electrolytes (e.g., Gatorade) should be given as soon as tolerated. If the causative agent is identified, appropriate antibiotic, antimicrobial, or antiinfective medication is given.

■ Nursing Management of Gastroenteritis

Accurate monitoring of intake and output is important for successful replacement of lost fluid. Strict medical asepsis and enteric precaution should be instituted when indicated. The client should be instructed in the importance of proper food handling and preparation of food to prevent infections, such as salmonellosis and trichinosis. The importance of rest and increased fluid intake as symptomatic treatment measures for gastroenteritis should be stressed.

Symptomatic nursing care is given for nausea, vomiting, and diarrhea (see Tables 36-3 and 37-5). The nurse should assess complaints of pain, vomiting, and diarrhea because gastroenteritis is often confused with appendicitis. To allay the client's apprehension, the nurse should explain that gastroenteritis usually runs an acute course with no sequelae. Chronically malnourished, older adult, and debilitated clients are at greater risk of complications and often need to be hospitalized for severe gastroenteritis.

IRRITABLE COLON

Irritable colon, which is also called *irritable bowel syndrome* (IBS) and *spastic colon,* is a motility disorder and symptom complex that involves intermittent and recurrent abdominal symptoms. The most common presenting symptom is abdominal pain associated with a change in bowel habits. The client may experience constipation, diarrhea, or alternating diarrhea and constipation. Other symptoms commonly found include pain relieved by defecation, abdominal distention, excessive flatulence, urge to defecate, and sensation of incomplete evacuation. Symptoms usually occur in the same way in each person. Stress or psychological factors, as well as ingestion of food, have been identified as major factors that precipitate IBS symptoms. In addition, IBS has been referred to as a disorder of the "waking state."[10] It is unusual for symptoms to awaken a person from sleep. In Western societies, twice as many women as men have IBS. In approximately 50% of the clients, the disorder is diagnosed before the age of 35 years.[10]

The key to accurate diagnosis is a thorough history and physical examination. Emphasis should be on presenting symptoms, past health history (including psychosocial aspects), family history, and drug and dietary history. Diagnostic tests should be selectively used to rule out more serious life-threatening disorders with symptoms similar to those of IBS, such as colon cancer, peptic ulcer disease, and malabsorption disorders.

The physician should establish a strong relationship with the client at the onset of treatment. The client needs reassurance that the symptoms are functional. The client should be encouraged to verbalize concerns and anxiety. A diet containing at least 20 g/day of dietary fiber should be initiated (see Table 37-10). This may also include the addition of psyllium-containing products (e.g., Metamucil).

Clients whose primary symptoms are abdominal distention and increased flatulence should be advised to eliminate common gas-producing foods such as broccoli and cabbage from the diet, and to substitute yogurt for milk products if there is lactose intolerance. Anticholinergic agents, such as dicyclomine (Bentyl), may be helpful if taken before meals to alleviate the pain associated with ingestion of food. For clients with high levels of anxiety a mild sedative or tranquilizer may be ordered but should be prescribed for only a short time.

INFLAMMATORY BOWEL DISEASE

Crohn's disease and ulcerative colitis are immunologically related disorders that are referred to as inflammatory bowel disease (IBD). These disorders are characterized by chronic, recurrent inflammation of the intestinal tract. Clinical manifestations are varied and may be debilitating.

Although there has been extensive research on the etiology of IBD, the cause remains unknown. Possible causes include (1) an infectious agent (e.g., virus, bacteria) because IBD produces mucosal changes in the colon similar to those of infectious diarrhea, although no consistent pathogen has been identified; (2) an autoimmune reaction

due to the presence of immunologically mediated conditions and immune-related disorders, such as systemic lupus erythematosus, ankylosing spondylitis, and erythema nodosum; (3) food allergies (although this has not been substantiated); and (4) heredity, inasmuch as multiple familial recurrences have been documented. In one study, 84% of identical twins of clients were affected with Crohn's disease.[11] Another study showed that ulcerative colitis occurred 10 to 20 times more often in first-degree relatives of clients with Crohn's disease than in the general population.[12] For years IBD (especially ulcerative colitis) was thought to be due to psychosomatic factors, such as severe emotional stress. It is now believed that these emotional changes result from and are not the cause of the disease.

Ulcerative Colitis

Ulcerative colitis is characterized by inflammation and ulceration of the colon and rectum. It may occur at any age but peaks between the ages of 15 and 40 years. Ulcerative colitis affects both sexes but has a higher incidence in women. It is more common in Jewish and upper middle-class urban populations.

Pathophysiology. The inflammation of ulcerative colitis is diffuse and involves the mucosa and submucosa with alternate periods of exacerbations and remissions (Table 37-19). The disease usually begins in the rectum and sigmoid colon and spreads up the colon in a continuous pattern (Fig. 37-2).

The mucosa of the colon is hyperemic and edematous in the affected area. Multiple abscesses develop in the crypts of Lieberkühn (intestinal glands). As the disease advances, the abscesses break through the crypts into the submucosa, leaving ulcerations. These ulcerations also destroy the mucosal epithelium, causing bleeding and diarrhea. Losses of fluid, protein, and electrolytes occur because of the decreased mucosal surface area for absorption. Areas of inflamed, undermined mucosa form pseudopolyps. Granulation tissue develops, and the mucosa musculature becomes thickened, shortening the colon.

Clinical manifestations. Ulcerative colitis may appear as an acute fulminating crisis or, more commonly, as a chronic disorder with mild to severe acute exacerbations that occur at unpredictable intervals over many years. The major symptoms of ulcerative colitis are bloody diarrhea and abdominal pain. Pain may vary from the mild lower abdominal cramping associated with diarrhea to the severe, constant abdominal pain associated with acute perforations. With mild disease, diarrhea may consist of one or two semiformed stools containing little blood. The client may have no other systemic manifestations. In severe fulminating cases, diarrhea is bloody, contains mucus, and occurs 10 to 20 times a day. In addition, fever, weight loss greater than 10% of total body weight, anemia, tachycardia, and dehydration are present. Toxic megacolon and perforation may ensue. Acute fulminant colitis is present in only 6% to 10% of clients with severe ulcerative colitis.[13]

Complications. Complications of ulcerative colitis may be classified into those that are *intestinal* and those that are *extraintestinal.* Intestinal complications of ulcerative coli-

Table 37-19 Ulcerative Colitis and Crohn's Disease

Characteristic	Ulcerative Colitis	Crohn's Disease
Age	Young to middle aged	Young
Location	Starts distally and spreads in a continuous pattern up the colon	Occurs anywhere along GI tract in characteristic skip lesions; most frequent site is terminal ileum
Distribution	Continuous	Segmental
Depth of involvement	Mucosa and submucosa	Entire thickness of bowel wall (transmural)
Small-bowel involvement	Minimal	Common
Fistulas	Rare	Common
Strictures	Rare	Common
Anal abscesses	Rare	Common
Granulomas	Absent	Common
Perforation	Common	Rare
Toxic megacolon	Common	Rare
Malabsorption	Minimal incidence	Common
Diarrhea	Common	Common
Abdominal crampy pain	Possible	Common
Fever (intermittent)	During acute attacks	Common
Weight loss	Common	Severe
Rectal bleeding	Common	Rare
Tenesmus	Severe	Rare
Pseudopolyps	Common	Rare
Cobblestoning of mucosa	Rare	Common
Carcinoma	Increased incidence after 10 years of disease	Minimal risk
Recurrence after surgery	Cure with colectomy	60% or more recurrence after segmental resections of small or large intestine

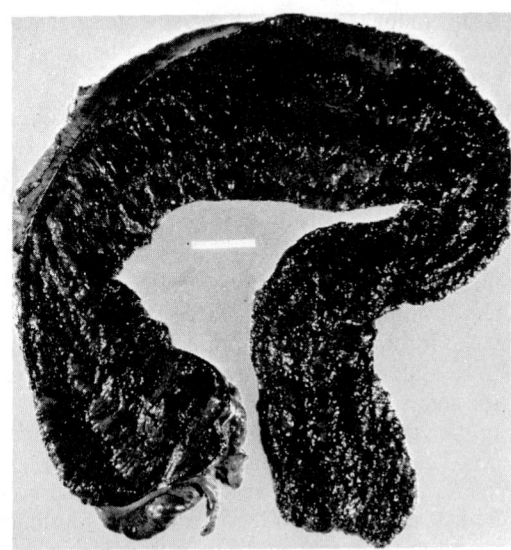

Fig. 37-2 Chronic ulcerative colitis. (From Kissane JM: Anderson's pathology, ed 9, St Louis, 1990, Mosby–Year Book, Inc, p 1162.)

tis include hemorrhage, strictures, perforation, toxic megacolon, and colonic dilatation. Hemorrhage is a result of inflamed, ulcerated mucosa and is usually controlled with conservative therapy. Massive hemorrhage is unusual and requires emergency surgery. Strictures are less common in ulcerative colitis than in Crohn's disease and are seen most often in clients with severe, long-standing disease. Perforation is most often associated with toxic megacolon but may occur alone. Most cases of perforation occur in the left side of the colon. Toxic megacolon occurs in approximately 3% of persons with ulcerative colitis.[13,14] Colonic dilatation, most often in the transverse colon, occurs as a result of severe acute inflammation of the entire colonic wall.

Extraintestinal complications can be divided into three groups: (1) colitis-related, (2) related to small-bowel pathology, and (3) nonspecific complications[15] (see Table 37-20). Colitis-related manifestations are associated with active inflammation and often respond to treatment of the underlying bowel disease. These manifestations can involve the joints, skin, mouth, and eyes. Skin lesions such as erythema nodosum and pyoderma gangrenosum are among the most frequently seen extraintestinal manifestations. Complications related to small-bowel pathology depend on severity and extent of small-bowel involvement, and they tend to persist in the absence of active inflammation. These are more often seen with Crohn's disease. Nonspecific complications occur in a small percentage of clients and have no correlation with the activity of the underlying disease.

Clients who have had ulcerative colitis for more than 10 years are at greater risk of colon cancer. The risk of cancer depends on age at onset, duration, and extent of disease.

Table 37-20 Extraintestinal Manifestations of Ulcerative Colitis

COLITIS RELATED

Joints
    Peripheral arthritis (colitic)
    Ankylosing spondylitis
    Sacroiliitis
    Finger clubbing
Skin
    Erythema nodosum
    Pyoderma gangrenosum
Mouth
    Aphthous ulcers
Eye
    Conjunctivitis
    Uveitis
    Episcleritis

RELATED TO SMALL-BOWEL PATHOLOGY

Malabsorption
Gallstones
Kidney stones

NONSPECIFIC

Liver disease—primary sclerosing cholangitis
Osteoporosis
Amyloidosis
Peptic ulcer disease

Table 37-21

 Diagnostic and Therapeutic Management: Ulcerative Colitis

DIAGNOSTIC

Fiberoptic colonoscopy
Sigmoidoscopy
Barium enema
CBC, sedimentation rate
Stool for blood, culture and sensitivity, and indirect hemagglutination
Complement fixation test

THERAPEUTIC
Mild and moderate disease

Low-roughage diet and no milk or milk products
Antimicrobial therapy
Corticosteroids
Anticholinergic therapy
Antidiarrheal agents

Severe (fulminant) disease

IV fluids with electrolytes
Blood transfusions
NPO status
NG tube to low suction
Antimicrobial therapy
Corticosteroids
Surgery if no improvement (colon resection with ileostomy)

Clients should be periodically screened with surveillance colonoscopy. Biopsy specimens should be taken every 10 cm throughout the entire colon.

Diagnostic studies. Several studies are appropriate for diagnosis of bowel abnormalities (Table 37-21). Blood studies should include a CBC, serum electrolyte level, and serum protein electrophoresis. A CBC typically shows iron deficiency anemia due to blood loss. An elevated WBC count may indicate toxic megacolon or perforation. Decreases in serum electrolytes, such as sodium, potassium, and magnesium, are due to fluid and electrolyte losses from diarrhea and vomiting. Hypoalbuminemia is a result of protein loss in the bowel. The stool should be examined for blood, pus, and mucus. Stool cultures should be obtained to rule out infectious causes of inflammation.

A double-contrast barium enema may show areas of granular inflammation with ulcerations. The colon may appear narrow and shortened and pseudopolyps may be present. A double-contrast study (in which air is introduced into the bowel after the expulsion of barium) is more effective in detecting mucosal abnormalities in ulcerative colitis.

Examinations with a flexible sigmoidoscope and a colonoscope allow direct visualization of the mucosa of the large intestine. Sigmoidoscopy visualizes the rectum, the sigmoid colon, and the descending colon; colonoscopy visualizes the entire large intestine. The extent of inflammation, ulcerations, pseudopolyps, strictures, and lesions may be identified. Biopsy specimens may be taken for definitive diagnosis.

Therapeutic management. The goals of treatment are to (1) rest the bowel, (2) control the inflammation, (3) combat infection, (4) correct malnutrition, (5) alleviate stress, and (6) provide symptomatic relief (see Table 37-21). The mainstays of therapy are sulfasalazine (Azulfidine) and corticosteroids. Most clients can eventually be maintained on sulfasalazine alone. Corticosteroids are usually indicated for flare-ups of the disease. Hospitalization is indicated if the client fails to respond to steroid therapy, if fever or abdominal pain develops, or if complications are suspected.

Drug therapy is the most important aspect of treatment (Table 37-22).[16] Sulfasalazine, a combination of sulfapyridine and 5-aminosalicylic acid (5-ASA), is the principal drug used. It is effective in the maintenance of clinical remission and in the treatment of mild to moderately severe attacks. After remission is obtained, therapy is continued with a gradual reduction over several months. The maintenance dose is usually continued for at least 1 year. Further reduction of the dosage increases the number of relapses.[17]

Corticosteroids are of proven benefit in the management of active ulcerative colitis. Oral prednisone or prednisolone is effective in treatment of mild to moderate disease without systemic manifestations. If remission is not

Table 37-22 Drugs Used to Treat Ulcerative Colitis

Category	Action	Examples
Anticholinergic	Decrease in GI motility and secretions and relief of smooth muscle spasms	Methantheline bromide (Banthine) Propantheline (Pro-Banthine) Oxyphencyclimine (Daricon)
Sedatives	Quieting of CNS without inducing sleep or analgesia	Diazepam (Valium) Flurazepam (Dalmane)
Antidiarrheal	Decrease in GI motility	Diphenoxylate (Lomotil)
Antimicrobial	Prevention or treatment of secondary infection	Cephalothin sodium (Keflin) Sulfasalazine (Azulfidine)
Steroids	Antiinflammatory	Corticosteroids (cortisone, prednisone)
Immunosuppressives	Suppression of immune response	Azathioprine (Imuran)
Hematinics and vitamins	Correction of iron deficiency anemia and promotion of healing	Iron dextran injection (Imferon) Iron sorbitex (Jectofer) Vitamin B_{12}

achieved, the client requires hospitalization and IV therapy. Clients with severe attacks and systemic manifestations require hospitalization and IV corticosteroid therapy. Clients are placed on a regimen of bowel rest and fluids, and electrolytes are administered IV. Hydrocortisone enemas and foams are effective in treatment of colitis limited to the rectosigmoid area. Rectal foams are usually administered in 5 ml volumes, and clients generally prefer them over enemas because of the ease of administration. Enemas are the preferred choice if the disease spreads beyond the sigmoid colon. Retention enemas have been shown to deliver medication into the descending colon and beyond in clients with active disease. Although steroids are reported to bring remission in 60% to 85% of cases, studies have also shown they do not necessarily prolong remission. Clients should be monitored for signs of Cushing's syndrome, hypertension, hirsutism, and mood swings. In some cases, psychosis may develop.

5-ASA (the active form of sulfasalazine) and 4-ASA, given as retention enemas, are effective in the treatment of left-sided ulcerative colitis and proctitis. Topical salicylate therapy is the treatment of choice in clients with localized disease. 5-ASA (mesalamine [Rowasa]) is also being given orally. The acrylic-coated tablets provide delivery of the drug more distally in the intestine.

Immunosuppressive drugs (e.g., 6-mercaptopurine [6-MP], azathioprine[Imuran]) have been used in some cases in the treatment of ulcerative colitis when a client has failed to respond to any of the usual medications and before surgery is considered. More recently methotrexate and cyclosporine have been evaluated for their effectiveness in the treatment of ulcerative colitis.

Surgical interventions. Approximately 85% of clients with ulcerative colitis go into remission with conservative therapy and nursing care, but 15% to 20% require surgery. Surgery is indicated if the client fails to respond to treatment; if exacerbations are frequent and debilitating; or if there is massive bleeding, perforation, strictures, obstruction, or changes that suggest carcinoma has developed.

Four surgical procedures used to treat ulcerative colitis are (1) total proctocolectomy with permanent ileostomy; (2) total proctocolectomy with continent ileostomy (Kock pouch); (3) total colectomy with ileorectal anastomosis; and (4) total colectomy with rectal mucosa stripping, ileal reservoir, and ileoanal anastomosis. Total proctocolectomy with ileostomy is the standard surgical procedure. It is a one-stage operation and is considered curative. Complications are minimal. Disadvantages relate to the need for a permanent ileostomy. (For care of the client with an ileostomy, see pp. 1109-1110.)

A variation from the traditional ileostomy is the continent ileostomy or Kock pouch (Fig. 37-3). This method eliminates the need for the client to wear an external appliance or bag over the stoma. The stoma is usually covered with a cap or dressing in case of mucus leakage. The pouch is not used for clients with Crohn's disease because the pouch itself may become diseased. This procedure is considered curative for ulcerative colitis but has a higher complication rate than the traditional ileostomy.

An internal pouch in the distal segment of the ileum is made surgically (see Fig. 37-3). The intestine is split, a fold is made, and a one-way nipple valve is created and sutured into place on the abdomen (see Fig. 37-3). The pouch acts as a reservoir and is drained at regular intervals on insertion of a catheter. During surgery a catheter is inserted into the pouch to allow suture lines to heal and to allow fixation of scar tissue around the valve to prevent slippage. The catheter may stay in place for up to 3 weeks. Once the catheter is initially removed, insertions to remove contents are begun every 3 to 4 hours and are gradually decreased until the capacity of the reservoir increases. Eventually catheter insertions are needed only three to four times a day. The client eventually determines the frequency by the changes in sensation of pressure in the pouch.

A continuous leakage of fluid is prevented by the one-way valve created at the internal end of the ileum from the stoma to the ileal pouch. Pressure created when the pouch fills with feces forces the valve to close. The majority of complications that arise are a result of valve failure. Valve failure has been reported as high as 40%. "Pouchitis" is another complication seen after this surgery, and manifes-

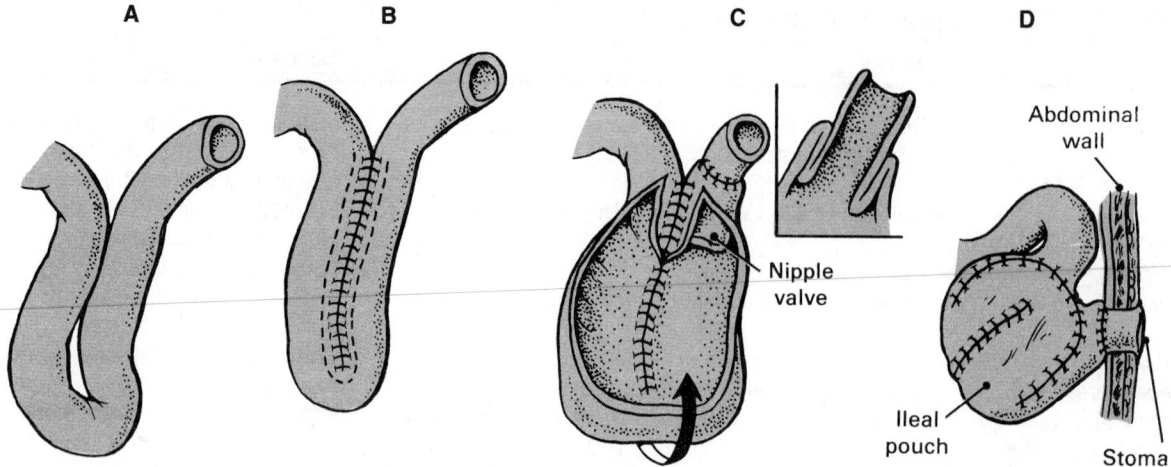

Fig. 37-3 Surgical formation of continent ileostomy (Kock pouch). **A,** Loop of terminal ileum. **B,** Both limbs sutured together and incised in a U shape. **C,** Pouch created with nipple valve. **D,** Pouch sutured to abdominal wall.

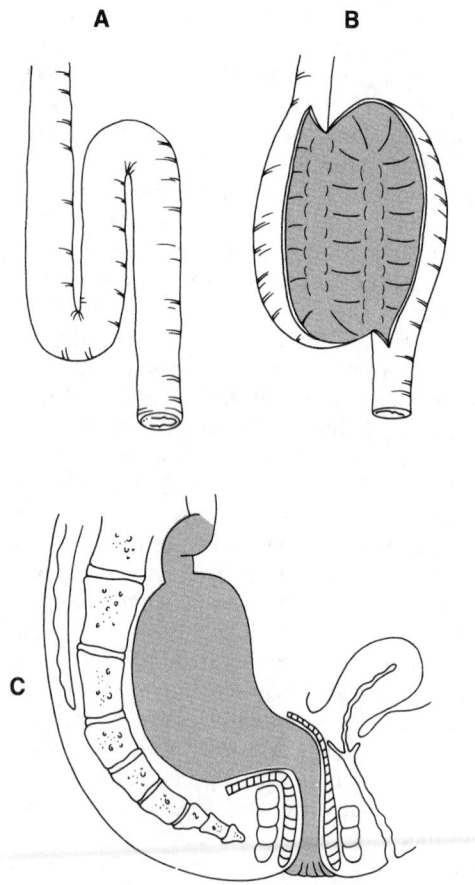

Fig. 37-4 Endorectal ileoanal anastomosis. **A,** Formation of a reservoir. **B,** Posterior suture lines completed. **C,** Terminal ileum anastomosed to anus within rectal stump.

tations are fever, malaise, and watery diarrhea. The lining appears red and inflamed, and biopsies show nonspecific inflammation. Clients usually respond to treatment with metronidazole.

Total colectomy with ileorectal anastomosis is not often performed. It is used primarily to avoid or delay a permanent ileostomy. This procedure is contraindicated in clients with rectal disease, sphincter incompetence, or Crohn's disease. A more widely performed procedure involves total colectomy and ileoanal anastomosis with the formation of an ileal reservoir (Fig. 37-4). Rectal mucosa is removed, and the internal and external anal sphincters remain intact. This is considered curative surgery, and clients remain continent. This is technically a more difficult procedure to perform, and it is always done in two stages. Clients with Crohn's disease, sphincter incompetence, or severe rectal disease are not candidates for this procedure.

Nutritional considerations. An important and major factor in the treatment of ulcerative colitis is diet. Therefore the dietitian is an important member of the team and should be consulted early in the course of the disease. The goals of diet management are to provide adequate nutrition without exacerbating symptoms, to correct and prevent malnutrition, to replace fluid and electrolyte losses, and to alleviate weight loss. The diet for each client must be individualized.

Traditionally during the acute phase the client may be on NPO status. When food is permitted, a high-calorie, high-protein, low-residue diet (Table 37-23) with vitamin and iron supplements is frequently prescribed. Special dietary restrictions are not usually necessary. Some physicians allow the client to eat anything that does not cause symptoms. Cold foods, high-residue foods (whole-wheat bread, cereal with bran, nuts, raw fruit), and smoking increase intestinal motility and should be avoided.

Often enteral supplements and parenteral nutrition are necessary. Clients with systemic manifestations, significant fluid and electrolyte losses, or malabsorption may

Table 37-23 Low-Residue Diet

PURPOSE

The low-residue diet provides foods low in fiber, which will result in a reduced amount of fecal material in the lower intestinal tract.

GENERAL PRINCIPLES

1. This diet eliminates foods that are indigestible or stimulating to the intestinal tract to reduce the amount of residue in the colon. Foods should be included or excluded according to the following list.
2. Hot and cold foods should be eaten slowly.
3. Milk products are limited to 2 cups daily. For a more restricted-residue diet, milk should be eliminated.

Food	Foods Included	Foods Excluded
Beverages	Carbonated drinks, coffee, tea, cocoa, strained fruit juices	Alcohol, fruit juices with pulp
Bread	White bread, rolls, rusk, melba toast, crackers	Bread and crackers containing whole grain flour or bran; any hot breads such as biscuits, muffins, waffles, or pancakes
Cereals	Cooked refined or strained cereals: Cream of Wheat, Cream of Rice, farina, grits, dry cereals without bran, noodles, spaghetti, and macaroni	Whole grain cereals; cereals containing bran, nuts, and raisins; Shredded Wheat
Meat	Lean, tender ground beef, lamb, pork, veal or fish, broiled, stewed, or baked; canned tuna or salmon; shellfish; crisp bacon, chicken or turkey without skin, liver; creamy peanut butter	Fried, smoked, pickled, or cured meats, highly seasoned ham, fried fish, luncheon meats
Egg	All but fried	Fried or uncooked eggs
Cheese	Milk, cheese (American, cheddar), cottage cheese	All other cheese
Milk	Limit to 1-2 cups (if tolerated), including that used in cooking; plain yogurt	Fruit yogurt
Fats	Butter, margarine, cream, oil, crisp bacon, mayonnaise, plain gravy	Any other; rich or spiced gravies
Soup	Cream and vegetable soups made from foods allowed and with milk allowed, bouillon, broth; strained vegetable juices	Cream and vegetable soups from foods not allowed (peas and dried beans)
Vegetables	Tender carrots, beets, or asparagus; strained vegetables; potatoes without skins; vegetable juices	Raw vegetables, all vegetables not strained, dried beans, peas, and legumes
Fruit	Strained fruit juices, ripe bananas, applesauce, pears, peaches, peeled apricots, Napoleon cherries, baked apple (no skin)	Raw fruits, fruits with skins, seeds
Desserts	Plain desserts (custards and puddings, plain ice cream from milk allowance), sherbet, plain gelatin desserts, angel food cake, sponge cake, plain butter cake, plain cookies	Nuts, coconut, raisins, rich desserts (pies, rich cakes, cobblers)
Condiments	Allspice, cinnamon, mace, paprika, salt, ground thyme, sugar, vinegar, lemon juice	All others

SAMPLE MENU PLAN

Breakfast	**Lunch**	**Dinner**
½ cup applesauce	Roast beef sandwich on 2 slices white bread (no lettuce or tomato)	Baked chicken
½ cup Cream of Wheat	1 tbs mayonnaise	Mashed potato
Scrambled egg	2 sugar cookies	Cooked carrots
White toast	Canned peach halves	White bread
Butter or jelly	Coffee	Butter
1 cup milk		Angel food cake
Coffee		1 cup milk
		Coffee

need parenteral hyperalimentation or enteral feedings, such as elemental diets. Elemental diets (see Table 35-15) are high in calories and nutrients, are lactose-free, and are absorbed in the proximal small intestine, which allows the more distal bowel to rest. (Elemental diets are discussed in Chapter 35.)

Parenteral hyperalimentation allows for a positive nitrogen balance while resting the bowel. Vitamins, minerals, electrolytes, and other important nutrients can be administered to promote healing and correct nutritional deficiencies.

Iron dextran (Imferon) intramuscularly (IM) by Z-track or IV may be necessary if anemia is severe. In clients receiving long-term sulfasalazine therapy, folic acid deficiency may develop and supplementation may be necessary. Clients with small-bowel disease, ileal resection, or malabsorption may need monthly injections of vitamin B$_{12}$. Potassium supplements may be necessary if corticosteroid therapy is used, since hypokalemia can result in toxic megacolon.

■ Nursing Management of Ulcerative Colitis
Nursing assessment
Subjective and objective data that should be obtained from a person with ulcerative colitis are presented in Table 37-24.

Nursing diagnoses
Nursing diagnoses are determined when the problem and etiological factors are supported by clinical data. Nursing diagnoses related to ulcerative colitis may include, but are not limited to, those presented in Table 37-25.

Nursing interventions
Nursing care of the client with ulcerative colitis is directed toward an intensive therapeutic and supportive program (see Table 37-25). Emotional support is important, since clients with ulcerative colitis often have a tendency to be insecure, dependent, and sensitive. It is important that the nurse establish a good working relationship and encourage the client to talk about self and daily activities. Honesty, patience, and understanding are crucial in the relationship with the client. An explanation of all procedures and treatment is necessary and may allay some apprehension. Appropriate diversional activity should be used to move the client's attention away from the intestinal tract. Psychotherapy may be indicated if the client is experiencing emotional problems, but the nurse needs to recognize that the client's behavior may result from factors other than emotional ones. Any person who has 10 to 20 bowel movements a day and has rectal discomfort may be anxious, frustrated, discouraged, and depressed. This experience may invoke fears, insecurities, and stress in the client. Along with other team members, the nurse can assist the client to accept the chronic condition and have an optimistic view with the possibility of cure after surgery. The nurse may find that inadequate coping mechanisms in the client with ulcerative colitis are due to early onset of the disease (at 10 to 15 years of age), which may have interfered with usual, expected growth, development, and maturation.

Table 37-24

Nursing Assessment of the Client With Ulcerative Colitis

SUBJECTIVE DATA

History
Positive family history, ethnicity, infection, food intolerance
Medications
Use of antidiarrheal medications
General
Fatigue, anorexia, weight loss, malaise
Pain
Lower abdominal pain (worse before defecation), cramping, tenesmus
Gastrointestinal
Frequent bloody stools containing mucus and pus, nausea and vomiting

OBJECTIVE DATA

General
Pallor, dry mucous membranes and poor skin turgor, emaciated appearance, intermittent fever
Integumentary
Anorectal excoriation
Gastrointestinal
Abdominal distention, hyperactive bowel sounds
Possible findings
Anemia; leukocytosis; electrolyte imbalance; guaiac-positive stool; abnormal proctosigmoidoscopic, colonoscopic, and barium enema findings

---

Bed rest may be ordered if the client is critically ill. An alternating-pressure mattress, foam pads, or sheepskin may be used to prevent skin breakdown. A sedative or tranquilizer may be prescribed to ensure rest.

The nurse should allow the client extra time to eat. Some uninterrupted planned time allows the nurse to get to know the client and allows the client to build trust. In addition to teaching related to treatment, medications, diet, tests, and the disease and its management, discussion of everyday topics should also be a part of diversional therapy.

Rest is important in the management of ulcerative colitis. Clients may lose much sleep because of frequent episodes of diarrhea and abdominal pain. Nutritional deficiencies and anemia leave the client feeling weak and listless. Activities should be scheduled around the rest periods. The nurse should also set limits and follow through because the client can be demanding. A positive attitude when giving care is most helpful in the management of ulcerative colitis. The client needs to know and understand that the nurse wants to help and does not consider the care repugnant.

Until diarrhea is controlled, the client must be kept clean, dry, and free of odor. A bedpan and wipes should be kept within reach of the client. The bedpan should be emptied as soon as possible. A deodorizer should be

Table 37-25

NURSING CARE PLAN FOR THE CLIENT WITH ULCERATIVE COLITIS

Defining Characteristics	Nursing Interventions	Evaluation Criteria

NURSING DIAGNOSIS: Altered health maintenance related to lack of knowledge of course of disease, appropriate lifestyle adjustments, and nutritional and pharmacological interventions

Questioning about disease and treatment, poor decisions about activities of daily living	Provide information about the disease. Refer to dietitian to teach about specific dietary needs. Teach about the relationships of stress to the disease. Teach stress-reduction techniques.	Correct information about disease and treatment

NURSING DIAGNOSIS: Sleep pattern disturbance related to frequent stools

Numerous interruptions of sleep, fatigue during waking hours with resultant frequent naps	Provide measures to reduce bowel irritability, such as medications ordered. Instruct client to refrain from nicotine and caffeine. Encourage client in use of usual sleeping routines.	Verbalization of feeling of being rested with improved sleep pattern

NURSING DIAGNOSIS: Diarrhea related to irritated bowel and intestinal hyperactivity

Frequent diarrheal stools (>10 per day)	Monitor frequency and character of stools. Maintain food and fluid restrictions. Teach client to avoid nicotine, caffeine, and foods or fluids irritating to bowel. Administer antidiarrheal medications as prescribed.	Fewer stools, firmer stools

NURSING DIAGNOSIS: Anxiety related to possible social embarrassment, unfamilar environment, diagnostic tests, and treatment

Expression of concerns about effect of disease on social relationships, questions about hospitalization, withdrawal	Monitor signs of anxiety. Encourage open discussion of feelings about diagnosis. Explain all treatments, diagnostic tests, and medications. Provide privacy.	Verbalization of less anxious feeling, relaxed facial expression

NURSING DIAGNOSIS: Potential complication: hypovolemia and electrolyte imbalances

Tachycardia, hypotension, weakness, dizziness, poor skin turgor, pallor, sunken eyes, rectal bleeding, abnormal serum electrolytes, urine output <30 ml/hr	Assess and document skin turgor, color, and temperature q 4 hr. Maintain accurate intake and output records; include stool volumes. Monitor hourly urine outputs in severely ill clients and notify physician of output <30 ml/hr. Monitor vital signs q 4 hr or more frequently if client unstable. Monitor serum electrolyte values. Notify physician of hypokalemia, hyponatremia. Administer IV fluids, blood products as ordered. Encourage oral intake (at least 3000 ml/day) when tolerated.	Maintenance of fluid balance as evidenced by normal vital signs, good skin turgor, urine output >30 ml/hr, normal serum electrolytes

NURSING DIAGNOSIS: Altered nutrition: less than body requirements related to decreased nutrient intake, increased nutrient loss through diarrhea, and decreased absorption of intestine

Anorexia, nausea, and vomiting; weight loss; weakness, lethargy; anemia; change in hair, skin, and mucous membranes due to nutrient and vitamin deficiencies	Assess and document signs of malnutrition: hair loss; dry skin; bleeding, cracked gingivae; muscle weakness. Record daily weights. Monitor intake and output. Perform ongoing calorie counts. Administer IV fluids and TPN as ordered. Give and instruct client on well-balanced, low-residue diet with small, frequent feedings. Administer nutritional supplements, as ordered. Assess client's food likes and dislikes. Assist in determining what foods are tolerated by client. Teach client to take small bites, eat slowly, chew well.	Maintenance of body weight within normal range, adequate nutritional intake, increased strength and activity tolerance

Continued.

Table 37-25

NURSING CARE PLAN FOR THE CLIENT WITH ULCERATIVE COLITIS—cont'd

Defining Characteristics	Nursing Interventions	Evaluation Criteria
NURSING DIAGNOSIS: Impaired skin integrity of perianal area related to diarrhea, immobility, and altered nutritional status		
Frequent loose, watery stools; erythema, redness of perianal area; discomfort around perianal area during and after evacuation; poor nutritional intake; prolonged bed rest	Assess skin for signs of breakdown. Cleanse perianal area after each bowel movement with mild soap and warm water and dry thoroughly. Provide sitz baths for comfort and hygiene. Apply protective ointment. If client is on bed rest, change position frequently, at least q 2 hr. Monitor fluid and nutrient intake. Encourage increased intake of proteins to promote healing. Instruct client and family on proper skin care techniques.	Maintenance of skin integrity, prevention of skin breakdown
NURSING DIAGNOSIS: Ineffective individual coping related to chronic disease, lifestyle changes, stress, and chronic pain		
Inability to express feelings and concerns; display of dependent, attention-getting behavior	Identify ineffective behaviors in client and institute plan of care. Include other staff members and family to set limits. Encourage client's expression of feelings. Discuss reasons for limitations. Offer reassurance and psychological support. Know limitations and refer to counseling when appropriate.	Development of healthy coping behaviors

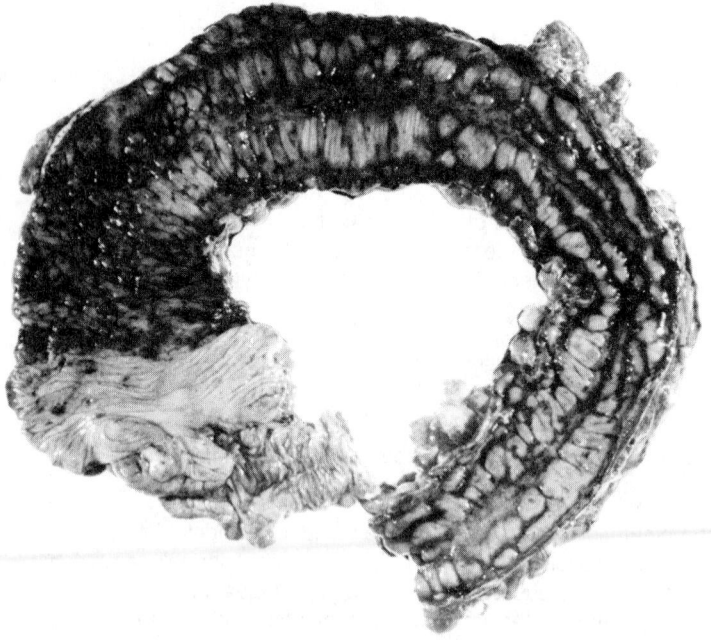

Fig. 37-5 Granulomatous colitis (Crohn's disease of colon) involving almost entire large bowel. (From Kissane JM: Anderson's pathology, ed 9, St Louis, 1990, Mosby–Year Book, Inc, p 1163.)

placed in the room. Antidiarrheal agents should be administered as ordered. If the client has continuous diarrhea, the enterostomal therapy nurse or therapist may give helpful suggestions. Meticulous perianal skin care using plain water (no harsh soap) is necessary to treat and prevent skin breakdown. Dibucaine (Nupercaine), witch hazel, or other soothing compresses and/or prescribed ointment and sitz baths may reduce irritation and relieve discomfort of the anus.

Crohn's Disease

Crohn's disease is a chronic, nonspecific inflammatory disorder of unknown origin that can affect any part of the GI tract. It was once thought to be a disease specific to the small intestine and was called *regional enteritis*. Later it was described in the large intestine and referred to as *granulomatous colitis*. In 1968, the International Congress of Gastroenterology decided to call the disease that affected the entire gut *Crohn's disease*.[18]

Crohn's disease may occur at any age but occurs most often between the ages of 15 and 30 years. Both sexes are affected, with a slightly higher incidence in women. Similar to ulcerative colitis, it occurs more often in Jewish and upper middle-class urban populations. The incidence of Crohn's disease is slightly lower than that of ulcerative colitis.

Pathophysiology. Crohn's disease is characterized by inflammation of segments of the GI tract (Fig. 37-5). It can affect any part of the GI tract but is most often seen in the terminal ileum, jejunum, and colon. Involvement of the esophagus, stomach, and duodenum is rare. The inflammation involves all layers of the bowel wall (i.e., transmural). Areas of involvement are usually discontinuous, with segments of normal bowel occurring between diseased portions. This pattern of involvement is referred to as *skip lesions*. Typically ulcerations are deep and longitudinal and penetrate between islands of inflamed edematous mucosa, causing the classic cobblestone appearance. Thickening of the bowel wall occurs, as well as narrowing of the lumen with stricture development. Abscesses or fistula tracts that communicate with other loops of bowel, skin, bladder, rectum, or vagina may develop. Histologically, granulomas are present in 50% to 70% of all clients.

Clinical manifestations. The manifestations depend largely on the anatomical site of involvement, extent of the disease process, and presence or absence of complications. The onset of Crohn's disease is usually insidious, with nonspecific complaints such as diarrhea, fatigue, abdominal pain, weight loss, and fever. Early diagnosis may be more difficult than for ulcerative colitis. The principal symptoms of Crohn's disease are diarrhea and abdominal pain. Diarrhea is usually nonbloody and is a result of the inflammatory process or malabsorption. Pain may be severe and intermittent or constant, depending on the cause. Other manifestations include abdominal cramping and tenderness, abdominal distention, fever, and fatigue. Extraintestinal manifestations, such as arthritis and finger clubbing, may precede the onset of bowel disease. As the disease progresses, there is weight loss, malnutrition, dehydration, electrolyte imbalances, anemia, increased peristalsis, and pain around the umbilicus and right lower quadrant.

Crohn's disease is a chronic disorder with unpredictable periods of recurrence and remission. Attacks are intermittent, usually recurring over a period of several weeks to months, with diarrhea and abdominal pain subsiding spontaneously.

Complications. Complications are common in Crohn's disease. Scar tissue from the inflammation narrows the lumen of the intestine and may cause strictures and obstruction, a frequent complication. Fistulas are a cardinal feature and may develop between segments of bowel. Cutaneous fistulas, common in the perianal area, and rectovaginal fistulas also occur. Fistulas communicating with the urinary tract may cause serious urinary tract infections. Inflammation of the intestines may involve all layers, predisposing the client to perforation and the formation of intraabdominal abscesses and peritonitis.

Impaired absorption may occur from damaged areas of the intestinal mucosa causing various nutritional abnormalities. Fat malabsorption causes a deficiency in the fat-soluble vitamins (A, D, E, and K). The client may have an intolerance to gluten (a protein found in barley, rye, and wheat).

Systemic complications are similar to those of ulcerative colitis and include arthritis, liver disease, cholelithiasis (especially with ileal involvement), ankylosing spondylitis, pyoderma gangrenosum, erythema nodosum,

Table 37-26

Diagnostic and Therapeutic Management: Crohn's Disease

DIAGNOSTIC

CBC
Stool for occult blood
X-ray film of small bowel
Barium enema
Proctosigmoidoscopic examination
Flexible sigmoidoscopy

THERAPEUTIC

High-calorie, high-vitamin, high-protein, low-residue, milk-free diet
Antimicrobial agents
Corticosteroid drugs
Supplementary parenteral nutrition
Elemental diet
Physical and emotional rest
Surgery to treat complications*

*See Table 37-27.

and uveitis. Renal disorders are common, especially nephrolithiasis secondary to increased oxalate absorption.

Diagnostic studies. Diagnosis of Crohn's disease can be made by means of a thorough history and physical examination to establish clinical signs and symptoms, barium studies, and endoscopy (Table 37-26). Laboratory studies may determine electrolyte disturbances and the presence of anemia. Barium studies are useful in determining location and extent of the disease and may reveal classic findings, such as stricturing of the ileum (string sign), cobblestoning of the mucosa, fistulas, and skip areas of abnormal and normal mucosa. A small-bowel barium enema is preferred over an upper GI x-ray series with small-bowel follow-through for defining mucosal abnormalities. Endoscopic studies, such as colonoscopy and sigmoidoscopy, are useful in detecting such early mucosal changes as patchy inflammation, small ulcerations, and skip areas that may not be seen radiographically. Biopsies may be performed to determine the presence of granulomas.

Therapeutic management. The goal of therapeutic management is to control the inflammatory process, relieve symptoms, correct metabolic and nutritional problems, and promote healing. Drug therapy and nutritional support are the mainstays of treatment.

Sulfasalazine is effective when the disease involves the large intestine but is much less effective when only the small intestine is involved. Corticosteroid therapy is effective in reducing inflammation and suppressing disease. The dosage and the route of administration depend on the severity of the illness and the area involved. Once clinical symptoms subside, the dosage should be tapered. Immunosuppressive agents (6-MP, azathioprine) may be tried if repeated trials with corticosteroids fail. Clients require close monitoring because of the serious side effects of these drugs. Metronidazole is useful in treating Crohn's disease of the perianal area. Marked exacerbations have been reported when the drug is stopped.

A major advance in nutrient therapy has been the elemental diet and TPN (see Chapter 35). Parenteral hyperalimentation may be given to clients with severe disease, small-bowel fistulas, or short-bowel syndrome. It is given before and after surgery to promote wound healing, reduce complications, and hasten recovery. The elemental diet provides a high-calorie, high-nitrogen, fat-free, no-residue substrate that is absorbed in the proximal small bowel. This diet can be given to most clients with Crohn's disease, even during acute exacerbations.

The diet should otherwise be low in residue, roughage, and fat but high in calories and protein. It may be difficult to maintain adequate absorption during periods of disease exacerbation and even during periods of remission. The client usually responds favorably when milk and milk products are excluded from the diet. Lactose, a disaccharide produced from milk digestion, may not be adequately absorbed because of the inability of the damaged mucosa of the intestine to produce adequate amounts of lactase. High-fat diets are poorly tolerated because of the malabsorptive deficit caused by loss of absorbing mucosa and altered bile salt metabolism. Adequate absorption may be difficult to maintain during periods of disease exacerbation and even during periods of remission.

Vitamin deficiencies may develop as a result of malabsorption. Vitamin B_{12} injections every month may be needed because of the inability of the terminal ileum to absorb this vitamin.

Balloon dilatation of strictures may be effective in relieving symptoms in some clients. This is usually performed through a colonoscope or under fluoroscopic guidance. Strictures most often dilated are those in the colon or small bowel.

Surgical interventions. Surgery is used in clients with severe symptoms that are unresponsive to therapy and in those with life-threatening complications. The majority of clients with Crohn's disease eventually require surgery at least once in the course of their disease. Indications for surgery are outlined in Table 37-27. Unlike ulcerative colitis, which can be cured by total proctocolectomy, Crohn's disease is not cured by surgery. The recurrence rate after surgery is high. The surgical procedure depends on the affected area and the condition of the client. Conservative intestinal resection with anastomosis of healthy bowel is the procedure of choice.

■ Nursing Management of Crohn's Disease

Acute care of the client is very similar to that of the client with ulcerative colitis (see Table 37-25). As the client's condition improves, the nurse should allow for more self-care, provide frequent rest periods, and advise the client of the importance of rest and avoidance or control of emotional stress. Initially this may be difficult for the client when told the nature of the disease and the limitations of the treatment. Special skin care may be needed by clients who have perianal fistulas or abscesses. Postoperative care should be the same as for exploratory laparotomy (see p. 1084 and Table 37-16).

In the majority of clients with Crohn's disease the course is chronic and intermittent, regardless of the site of involvement. The client and significant others may need help in setting realistic short- and long-term goals. Teaching is important and should include (1) the importance of rest and diet management, (2) perianal care, (3) action and side effects of medications, (4) symptoms of recurrence of disease, (5) the time to seek medical care, and (6) use of diversional activities to reduce stress.

INTESTINAL OBSTRUCTION

Intestinal obstruction occurs when intestinal contents cannot pass through the GI tract, and it requires prompt treatment. The obstruction may be partial or complete. The causes of intestinal obstruction can be classified as *mechanical* or *nonmechanical*.

Mechanical

Mechanical obstruction may be caused by an occlusion of the lumen of the intestinal tract. Most intestinal obstructions occur in the small intestine, most often in the ileum.[19] Mechanical obstruction is the most common cause of intestinal obstruction (Fig. 37-6). Adhesions account for 50%, hernias for 15%, and neoplasms for 15% of obstructions of the small intestine.[20] Adhesions normally develop after abdominal surgery. Obstruction can occur within days of surgery or years later. Carcinoma is the most common cause of large-bowel obstruction, followed by volvulus and diverticular disease.

Nonmechanical

A nonmechanical obstruction may result from a neuromuscular or vascular disorder. Paralytic (adynamic) ileus is the most common form of nonmechanical obstruction. It occurs to some degree after any abdominal surgery. Other causes of paralytic ileus include inflammatory reactions, such as acute pancreatitis, acute appendicitis, electrolyte abnormalities, and thoracic or lumbar spinal fractures.

Pseudoobstruction is an apparent mechanical obstruction of the intestine without demonstration of obstruction by radiographic methods. Pseudoobstruction may be caused by collagen vascular diseases and neurological and endocrine disorders, but mostly it is found to be idiopathic.

Vascular obstructions are rare and are due to an inter-

Table 37-27 Indications for Surgical Management of Crohn's Disease

Drainage of abdominal abscess	Intestinal obstruction
	Massive hemorrhage
Failure to respond to conservative therapy	Perforation
	Secondary hydronephrosis
Fistulas	
Growth retardation	Severe anorectal disease
Inability to decrease steroids	Suspicion of carcinoma

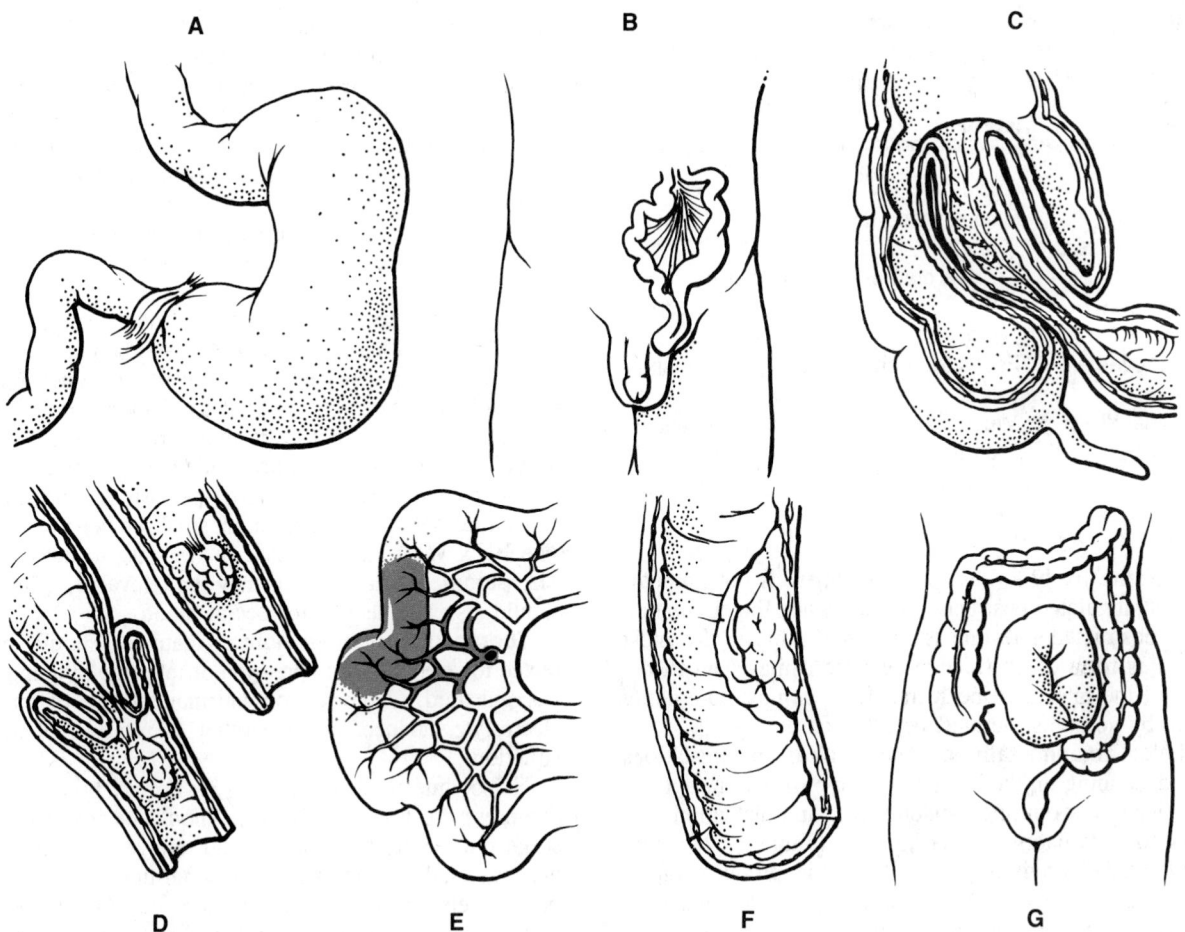

Fig. 37-6   Bowel obstructions. **A,** Adhesions. **B,** Strangulated inguinal hernia. **C,** Ileocecal intussusception. **D,** Intussusception due to polyps. **E,** Mesenteric occlusion. **F,** Neoplasm. **G,** Volvulus of the sigmoid colon.

ference with the blood supply to a portion of the intestines. The most common causes are emboli and atherosclerosis of the mesenteric arteries. The celiac, inferior, and superior mesenteric arteries supply blood to the bowel. Emboli may originate from thrombi in clients with chronic atrial fibrillation, diseased heart valves, and prosthetic valves. Venous thrombosis may be seen in low-blood-flow states, such as heart failure and shock.

Pathophysiology. Normally 6 to 8 L of fluid enters the small bowel daily. Most of the fluid is absorbed before it reaches the colon. About 75% of intestinal gas is swallowed air.[19] Bacterial metabolism produces methane and hydrogen gases. Fluid, gas, and intestinal contents accumulate proximal to the intestinal obstruction. This causes distention, and the distal bowel may collapse. The distention reduces the absorption of fluids and stimulates intestinal secretions. As the fluid increases, so does the pressure in the lumen of the bowel. The increased pressure leads to an increase in capillary permeability and extravasation of fluids and electrolytes into the peritoneal cavity. Edema, congestion, necrosis from impaired blood supply, and possible rupture of the bowel may occur. The retention of fluid in the intestine and peritoneal cavity can lead to a se-

vere reduction in circulating blood volume and result in hypotension and hypovolemic shock.

The electrolyte-rich fluids, which are normally reabsorbed in the bowel, are retained in the bowel and subsequently lost into the peritoneal cavity. The location of the obstruction determines the extent of fluid, electrolyte, and acid-base imbalances. If the obstruction is high, as in the pylorus, metabolic alkalosis may result from the loss of hydrochloric acid from the stomach through vomiting or NG intubation.

When the obstruction is located in the small bowel, dehydration occurs rapidly. Dehydration and electrolyte imbalance do not occur early in large-bowel obstruction. If the obstruction is below the proximal colon, most GI fluids have been absorbed before reaching the point of the obstruction. Solid fecal material accumulates until symptoms of discomfort appear. Reverse peristalsis may cause vomiting of fecal material very late in the bowel obstruction.

Simple obstructions of the intestine involve blockage of the lumen in one spot. A closed-loop obstruction occurs when the lumen is blocked in two different spots (e.g., volvulus). This results in an isolated segment of bowel and obstruction proximal to that segment. Strangulation and

Table 37-28 Clinical Manifestations of Small and Large Intestinal Obstructions

Clinical Manifestation	Small Intestine	Large Intestine
Onset	Rapid	Gradual
Vomiting	Frequent and copious	Rare
Pain	Colicky, cramp-like, intermittent	Low-grade crampy abdominal pain
Bowel movement	Feces for a short time	Absolute constipation
Abdominal distention	Minimally increased	Greatly increased

gangrene are likely to develop if treatment is not immediate. A strangulated obstruction occurs when the circulation to the obstructed intestine is impaired. This is the most dangerous form of obstruction because it may lead to necrosis of the intestine (incarcerated). It is most commonly caused by volvulus, hernias, or adhesions.

Clinical manifestations. The clinical manifestations vary, depending on the location of the obstruction, and include nausea, vomiting, abdominal pain, distention, inability to pass flatus, and obstipation (Table 37-28). Obstruction located high in the small intestine produces rapid-onset, sometimes projectile vomiting with bile-containing vomitus. Vomiting from more distal obstructions of the small intestine is more gradual in onset. The vomitus may be orange-brown and foul smelling because of bacterial overgrowth. In some cases it may be feculent. Vomiting may be entirely absent in large-bowel obstruction if the ileocecal valve is competent; otherwise, the client may eventually vomit feculent material.

Abdominal pain in high intestinal obstructions is usually relieved by vomiting. Persistent, colicky abdominal pain is seen with lower intestinal obstruction. A characteristic sign of mechanical obstruction is pain that comes and goes in waves. This is due to intestinal peristalsis trying to move bowel contents past the obstructed area. In contrast, paralytic ileus produces a more constant generalized discomfort. Strangulation causes severe, constant pain that is rapid in onset.

Abdominal distention is a common manifestation of all intestinal obstructions. It is usually absent or minimally noticeable in high obstructions of the small intestine and markedly increased in lower intestinal obstructions. Abdominal tenderness and rigidity are usually absent unless strangulation or peritonitis has occurred.

Auscultation of bowel sounds reveals high-pitched sounds above the area of obstruction. Audible borborygmi are often noted by the client. The client's temperature rarely rises above 37.8° C (100° F) unless strangulation or peritonitis has occurred.

Diagnostic studies. A thorough history and physical examination should be performed. Abdominal x-rays are the most useful diagnostic aids. Upright and lateral abdominal x-ray films show the presence of gas and fluid in the intestines. The presence of intraperitoneal air indicates perforation. Barium enemas are helpful in locating large intestinal obstructions. Sigmoidoscopy or colonoscopy may provide direct visualization of an obstruction in the colon.

Laboratory tests are important and provide essential information. A CBC and serum electrolyte, amylase, and blood urea nitrogen (BUN) determinations should be made. An elevated WBC count may indicate strangulation or perforation; elevated hemoglobin and hematocrit values may reflect hemoconcentration. Lowered values indicate bleeding from a neoplasm or strangulation with necrosis. Serum electrolytes should be monitored frequently. They provide essential information on the client's fluid and electrolyte balance. Serum sodium, potassium, and chloride concentrations are decreased in small-bowel obstruction. The BUN value may increase in response to dehydration. The serum amylase level may be elevated. The stool should also be checked for occult blood.

Therapeutic management. Treatment should be directed toward (1) decompression of intestine by removal of gas and fluid, (2) correction and maintenance of fluid and electrolyte balance, and (3) relief or removal of the obstruction.

NG or intestinal tubes (Fig. 37-7) may be used to decompress the bowel. NG tubes should be inserted before surgery to empty the stomach and relieve distention. They are also used instead of nasointestinal tubes to treat partial or complete small-bowel obstruction. Intestinal tubes, such as the Cantor or Miller-Abbott tubes, are passed into the small intestine. They are 10 feet (300 cm) long and mercury weighted. Insertion of an intestinal tube is controversial. Use of a long intestinal tube is difficult and time consuming. Some physicians believe there is inadequate gastric decompression once the tube is in the small intestine. A higher incidence of postoperative complications and longer hospitalizations were noted in a group of clients treated with intestinal tubes as compared with those treated with NG tubes.[21] NG or intestinal tubes are effective in the treatment of clients with neurogenic obstruction who do not require surgery.

Decompression of the large intestine should be attempted unless necrosis or perforation is present. Enemas, rectal tubes, sigmoidoscopy, and colonoscopy may be used. Sigmoidoscopy may successfully reduce a sigmoid volvulus. Colon-decompression catheters may be passed through partially obstructed areas via a colonoscope to decompress the bowel before surgery.

IV infusions that contain normal saline solution and potassium should be given to maintain fluid and electrolyte balance. Total parenteral hyperalimentation may be necessary in some cases to correct nutritional deficiencies, improve the client's nutritional status before surgery, and promote postoperative healing.

Most mechanical obstructions are treated surgically. They may involve simply resecting the obstructed segment of bowel and anastomosing the remaining healthy bowel. Partial or total colectomy, colostomy, or ileostomy may be

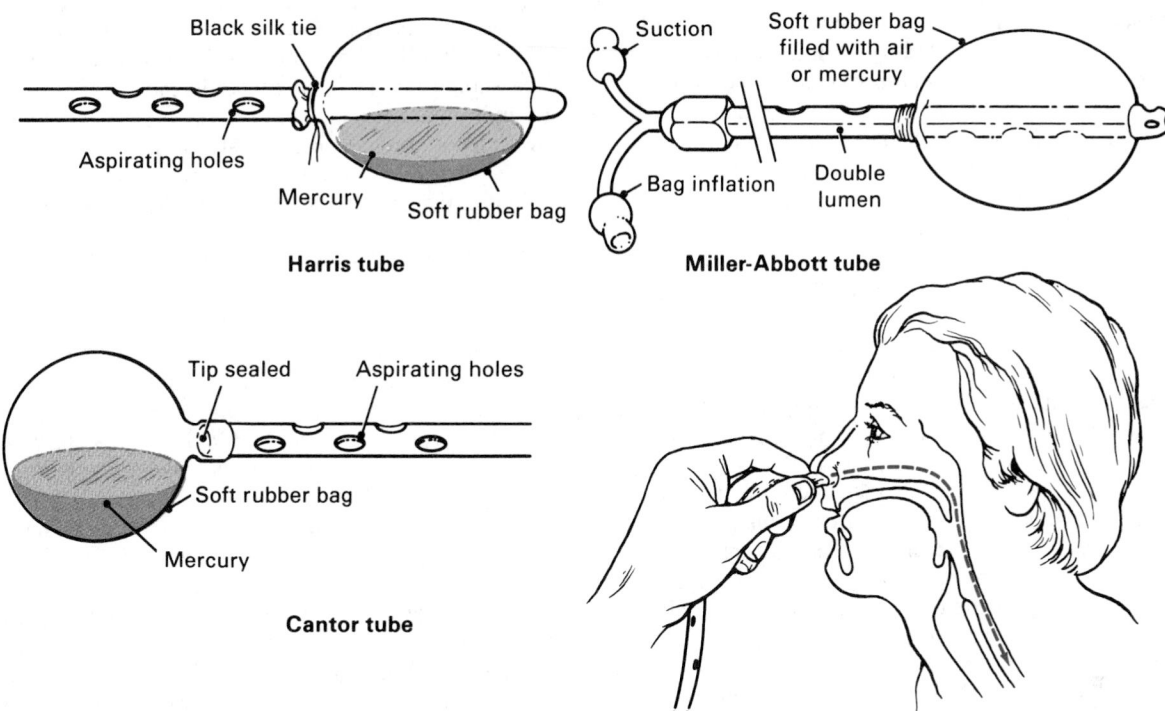

Fig. 37-7 Intestinal tubes used for decompression.

required when extensive obstruction or necrosis is present. Occasionally obstructions can be removed nonsurgically. A colonoscope can be used to remove polyps, to dilate strictures, and to remove and necrose tumors with a laser.

■ Nursing Management of Intestinal Obstruction

Nursing assessment

Intestinal obstruction is a potential life-threatening condition. Signs and symptoms are varied. Nursing assessment must begin with a detailed client history and physical examination. The type and location of obstruction usually cause characteristic symptoms. The nurse should determine the location, duration, intensity, and frequency of abdominal pain and whether abdominal tenderness or rigidity is present. Onset, frequency, color, odor, and amount of vomitus should be recorded. Bowel function, including passage of flatus, needs to be determined. The nurse should auscultate for bowel sounds and document character and location; inspect the abdomen for scars, palpable masses, and distention; and observe for muscle guarding and tenderness.

Nursing interventions

The client should be monitored closely for signs of dehydration and electrolyte imbalance. A strict intake and output record should be maintained. All vomitus and tube drainage should be included. IV fluids should be administered as ordered. Serum electrolyte levels should be monitored closely. Clients with a high obstruction are more likely to have metabolic alkalosis; clients with a low obstruction are at greater risk of metabolic acidosis. Clients are often restless and constantly change their position to relieve the pain. Analgesics may often be withheld until

the obstruction is diagnosed because they may mask other signs and symptoms and decrease intestinal motility. The nurse should provide comfort measures, promote a restful environment, and keep distractions and visitors to a minimum. Nursing care of the client after surgery for an intestinal obstruction is similar to care of the client after a laparotomy (see Table 37-16).

Care of nasogastric and intestinal tubes

Although the physician usually inserts intestinal tubes, the nurse assists with the procedure. Insertion is easier if the client relaxes, takes deep breaths, and swallows when instructed. Mouth care is extremely important. Vomiting leaves a terrible taste in the client's mouth, and fecal odor may be present. The client breathes through the mouth, drying the mouth and lips, when an NG tube is in place. The nurse should encourage and assist the client to brush the teeth frequently. Mouthwash and water for the client to use in rinsing the mouth and petroleum jelly or water-soluble lubricant for the lips should be provided at the bedside.

The client's nose should be checked for signs of irritation from the NG tube. This area should be cleaned and dried daily with application of a water-soluble lubricant and retaping of the tube. NG and intestinal tubes should be checked every 4 hours for patency. The client may be placed on a schedule to clamp the tube every 2 hours for 1 hour, or for 3 out of every 4 hours before removal of the tube.

POLYPS OF THE LARGE INTESTINE

Colonic polyps arise from the mucosal surface of the colon and project into the lumen. They may be *sessile* (flat, broad-based and attached directly to the intestinal wall) or *pedunculated* (attached to the intestinal wall by a thin stalk). They may be found anywhere in the large intestine but are most commonly found in the rectosigmoid area. Rectal bleeding or occult blood in the stool are the most common symptoms, although most polyps are asymptomatic.

Types

The most common types of polyp are hyperplastic and adenomatous. Hyperplastic polyps originate from the epithelium and are nonneoplastic growths. They rarely grow larger than 5 mm in size and never cause clinical symptoms. Other benign (nonneoplastic) polyps include inflammatory polyps, lipomas, and juvenile polyps (Table 37-29).

Adenomatous polyps are characterized by neoplastic changes in the epithelium. They are closely linked to colorectal adenocarcinoma. Structurally, there are three types, with tubular adenomas being the most prevalent. The risk of cancer in the polyp increases with polyp size and villous structure. Villous adenomas have a higher risk of containing cancer than tubular adenomas.

Hereditary polyposis syndromes are rare and may be neoplastic or nonneoplastic in nature. They are characterized by multiple polyps that at times number in the thousands and that are located in the large intestine and sometimes in other areas of the GI tract. Clients with familial adenomatous polyposis have a 100% chance of having colon cancer by the age of 40. Total colectomy with ileostomy is the treatment of choice.

■ Therapeutic and Nursing Management of Polyps

Diagnosis of polyps is made by barium enema, sigmoidoscopy, and colonoscopy. All polyps are considered abnormal and should be removed. In clients whose polyps are identified through barium enema, removal (polypec-tomy) should be done through a colonoscope or a sigmoidoscope.[22,23] If the polyp is not removable, a biopsy specimen should be taken for tissue diagnosis.[24,25] Surgery is not indicated unless carcinoma is present or in certain cases of polyposis. The client should be observed for rectal bleeding, fever, severe abdominal pain, and abdominal distention that may indicate hemorrhage or perforation.

CANCER OF THE COLON AND RECTUM
Significance

Colorectal cancer is the second most common cause of cancer death in the United States.[26] It accounts for about 20% of all deaths due to cancer in the United States. Cancer of the colon and rectum may occur at any age but is most prevalent over the age of 50. The 5-year survival rate remains under 50% and has not changed in several decades.

The incidence of cancer at specific sites in the colon varies (Fig. 37-8). In both sexes, the incidence of right colon cancers has increased and cancers in the rectum have decreased. The highest percentage of colorectal cancers in the United States are currently located in the cecum, ascending colon, and sigmoid colon.[27] Approximately 20% of colorectal cancers are within reach of the examining finger, and 50% are within reach of the sigmoidoscope.[25]

Pathophysiology

The causes of colorectal cancer remain unclear. Groups at high risk of colorectal cancer have been identified (Table 37-30). Age is a risk factor in both men and women. The risk for development in the general population increases slightly after the age of 40, and then rises rapidly in the following decades.

Diet is the most important environmental factor that has been associated with colorectal cancer. The high-caloric, high-fat Western diet has been closely associated with development of colon cancer.

Adenocarcinoma is the most common type of colon

Table 37-29 Types of Polyps of the Large Intestine

NEOPLASTIC	NONNEOPLASTIC
Epithelial polyps (adenomatous)	Epithelial polyps (hyperplastic)
Tubular adenoma	Hereditary polyposis syndromes (hamartomatous polyposis syndrome)
Tubular villous adenoma	
Villous adenoma	Familial juvenile polyposis
Hereditary polyposis syndromes (adenomatous polyposis syndrome)	Peutz-Jeghers syndrome
Familial adenomatous polyposis	Inflammatory polyps
Gardner syndrome	Pseudopolyps
	Benign lymphoid polyp
	Submucosal polyps
	Lipomas
	Leiomyomas
	Fibromas

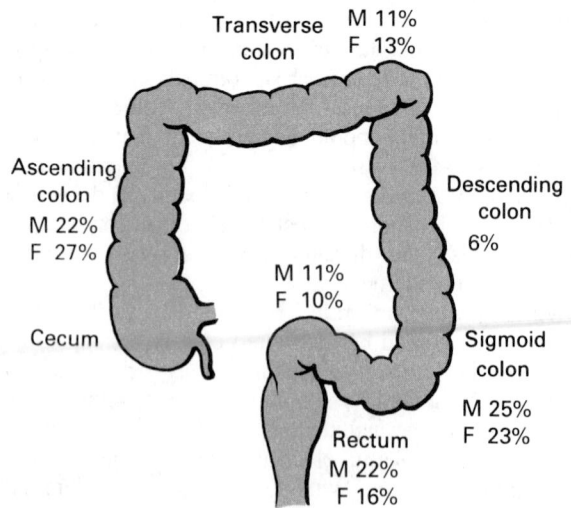

Fig. 37-8 Incidence of cancer. Two thirds of all colon cancers occur in the rectosigmoid and rectum. Percentages listed for men and women.

Table 37-30 Predisposing Factors for Colorectal Cancer

Age	Family history of colorectal cancer
Familial polyposis	
Colorectal polyps	Previous history of colorectal cancer
Chronic inflammatory bowel disease	History of genital or breast cancer (women)

Table 37-31

Diagnostic and Therapeutic Management: Cancer of the Colon

DIAGNOSTIC

Sigmoidoscopy
Barium enema
Colonoscopy
Rectal examination
CBC
Testing of stools for occult blood
CEA test
Liver function studies
CT scan of abdomen

THERAPEUTIC

Surgery
Radiation therapy
Chemotherapy

cancer. Most colorectal cancers appear to arise from adenomatous polyps.[26] All tumors tend to spread through the walls of the intestine and into the lymphatic system. Tumors commonly spread to the liver because the venous blood flow from the colorectal tumors is through the portal vein.

Clinical Manifestations

Clinical manifestations of colon cancer are usually nonspecific or do not appear until the disease is far advanced. Cancer on the right side of the colon gives rise to clinical manifestations that are different from those on the left side of the colon. Rectal bleeding, the most common presenting symptom of colorectal cancer, is most often seen with left-sided lesions. Other commonly seen manifestations of left-sided lesions include alternating constipation and diarrhea, change in stool caliber (narrow, ribbonlike), and sensation of incomplete evacuation. Obstruction symptoms appear earlier with left-sided lesions because of the smaller lumen size.

Cancers of the right side of the colon are usually asymptomatic. Vague abdominal discomfort or crampy, colicky abdominal pain may be present. Iron deficiency anemia and occult bleeding dictate further investigation. Weakness and fatigue result from anemia.

Diagnostic Studies

A thorough history with close attention to family history should be obtained, and a physical examination should be performed initially (Table 37-31). The digital rectal examination is the most important aspect of the physical examination, since many rectal cancers are within reach of the finger. If colorectal cancer is suspected, examination with the flexible sigmoidoscope and an air-contrast barium enema (in combination) are often performed. Colonoscopy is the procedure of choice if a questionable lesion is seen on barium enema or sigmoidoscopy. Synchronous lesions may be present at other sites in the colon, and tissue diagnosis may be made by brushing or biopsy during the procedure. Before surgery, a colonoscopy should be performed.

Laboratory studies should include a CBC, clotting studies, and liver function tests. A CT scan of the abdomen may be helpful in detecting liver metastases, retroperitoneal and pelvic disease, and depth of penetration of tumor into the bowel wall. A CT scan should be done before surgery. Transanal intraluminal ultrasound is being used to determine the extent of rectal wall involvement.

Table 37-32 Dukes' Staging System for Colorectal Carcinoma

Classification	Description
A	Negative nodes, limitation of lesion to mucosa
B_1	Negative nodes, extension of lesion through mucosa but still within bowel wall
B_2	Negative nodes, extension through entire bowel wall
C_1	Positive nodes, limitation of lesion to bowel wall
C_2	Positive nodes, extension of lesion through entire bowel wall
D	Presence of distant, unresectable metastases

A carcinoembryonic antigen (CEA) test is often performed, although it is not specific for colon cancer. A normal level of CEA does not exclude the possibility of a malignant condition. This test is used most effectively in following the progress of a client after surgery. Return to normal of a previously elevated CEA indicates successful removal of tumor. In contrast, persistent postoperative elevated or increasing CEA levels suggest residual tumor or tumor spread.

Therapeutic Management

Prognosis and treatment correlate with pathological staging of the disease. Several methods of staging are currently being used. The most widely known is Dukes' classification (Table 37-32). Surgical removal of the primary lesion is the treatment for Dukes' stages A, B, and C.

Prognosis for Dukes' stage A is 90% to 100% 5-year survival compared to less than 15% with Dukes' stage D.

The most recent classification of colorectal cancer is the TNM system, which is based on pathological assessment and includes data from the history and physical examination and presurgical endoscopic and laboratory evaluations. *T* describes the extent of the primary tumor; *N* represents the location and number of lymph nodes involved; and *M* indicates the presence of distant metastasis. Cancer of the colon can also be divided into stages, with *stage O* representing cancer in situ, *stage 1* corresponding to Dukes' A and B_1, *stage II* corresponding to B_2, *Stage III* corresponding to C_1 and C_2, and *Stage IV* to Dukes' D.

Several noninvasive procedures may be performed through a colonoscope to treat certain types of colorectal cancer effectively. Endoscopic polypectomy is a highly effective and safe procedure.[22,26] Adequate treatment is thought to be obtained if the resected margin of the polyp is free of cancer, the cancer is not poorly differentiated, and there is no apparent lymphatic or blood vessel involvement. Laser therapy may be used to ablate nonresectable tumors. This is usually used only as palliative therapy in clients with obstructive symptoms.

Surgical Interventions

Surgery is the only curative treatment of colorectal cancer. The type of surgery performed is determined by the location and extent of the cancer. Success of surgery depends on resection of the tumor with an adequate margin of healthy bowel and resection of the regional lymph nodes.

Right hemicolectomy is performed when the cancer is located in the cecum, ascending colon, hepatic flexure, or transverse colon to the right of the middle colic artery. A portion of the terminal ileum, the ileocecal valve, and the appendix are removed and an ileotransverse anastomosis is performed. A *left hemicolectomy* involves resection of the left transverse colon, the splenic flexure, the descending colon, the sigmoid colon, and the upper portion of the rectum.

Clear margins are most difficult to obtain with rectal carcinoma. Location of the rectal lesion determines the surgical procedure to be performed. There must be enough rectum left to ensure a secure anastomosis, or an abdominal-perineal resection is indicated. *Abdominal-perineal resection* is most often performed when the cancer is located within 5 cm of the anus.

In the abdominal-perineal resection, an abdominal incision is made and the proximal sigmoid is brought through the abdominal wall in a permanent colostomy. The distal sigmoid, rectum, and anus are removed through a perineal incision. The perineal wound may be closed around a drain or left open with packing to allow healing by granulation. Complications that can occur are delayed wound healing, hemorrhage, persistent perineal sinus tracts, infections, and urinary tract and sexual dysfunction.

Low anterior resection may be indicated for tumors of the rectosigmoid and the mid to upper rectum. The use of EEA staplers has allowed lower and more secure anastomoses. The stapler is passed through the anus, where the colon is stapled to the rectum. This technique has made it possible to resect lesions as low as 5 cm from the anus.

Sphincter-sparing procedures are being performed on clients who are poor operative risks and for clients with early disease. The number of these procedures may increase with continued early detection and surveillance. In these procedures a local resection is performed and the anal sphincters are left intact.

Radiation Therapy and Chemotherapy

Radiation may be used preoperatively or as a palliative measure for clients with advanced lesions. As a palliative measure, its primary objective is to reduce the tumor size and provide symptomatic relief. (For discussion on radiation therapy, see Chapter 9.) Chemotherapy is used as a palliative treatment. No drug is available that can cure malignant colon or rectal tumors. The most commonly used drugs are 5-fluorouracil (5-FU) and methotrexate. Nitrosoureas, BCNU, and MeCCNU are sometimes used in combination with 5-FU.

■ Nursing Management of Colon and Rectal Cancer

Nursing assessment

Subjective and objective data that should be obtained from a client with cancer of the colon or rectum are presented in Table 37-33.

Nursing diagnoses

Nursing diagnoses specific to the client with cancer of the colon or rectum include, but are not limited to, the following:

1. Altered bowel elimination: change in bowel habits, alternating constipation and diarrhea, and rectal bleeding
2. Abdominal pain and cramping related to difficulty in passing stools due to partial or complete obstruction from tumor
3. Fear related to diagnosis of colon cancer, surgical or therapeutic interventions, and life expectancy

Nursing interventions

Health promotion and maintenance. The current recommendations from the American Cancer Society for colorectal cancer screening in clients who are not at high risk include annual digital rectal examination and fecal testing for occult blood beginning at the age of 40. Starting at the age of 50, flexible sigmoidoscopy should be done every 3 to 5 years, after 2 negative examinations 1 year apart. Positive findings should be followed with colonoscopy or air-contrast barium enema.[24,25]

High-risk clients should be screened differently. Screening usually begins with colonoscopy and fecal occult blood testing, and continued follow-up varies according to risk factors.

Acute intervention. Acute nursing care for clients with colon resections is similar to care of the client having a laparotomy (see Table 37-16). For example, the client may undergo an abdominal-perineal resection. In addition to general preoperative teaching and ostomy care instructions, the client should be informed of the extent of the surgical procedure and the amount of care necessary to fa-

Table 37-33

Nursing Assessment of the Client With Colorectal Cancer

SUBJECTIVE DATA

History
Family history of cancer; previous breast or gynecological cancer; familial polyposis; villous adenoma; adenomatous polyps; Gardner syndrome; chronic ulcerative colitis or Crohn's disease; dietary intake of fat, fiber, and highly refined carbohydrates; asbestosis

Medications
Use of any medications affecting bowel function

General
Weight loss, weakness, fatigue, anorexia

Pain
Abdominal and low back pain, tenesmus (late symptoms)

Gastrointestinal
Change in bowel habits, alternating diarrhea and constipation, bleeding, nausea and vomiting, mucoid stools, decrease in stool caliber, feelings of incomplete evacuation, increased flatus, urgency, black and tarry stools

OBJECTIVE DATA

General
Pallor, cachexia, lymphadenopathy (later signs)

Gastrointestinal
Palpable abdominal mass, distention, ascites and hepatomegaly (liver metastasis)

Possible findings
Anemia; guaiac-positive stools; palpable mass on digital rectal exam; positive proctosigmoidoscopy, colonoscopy, or barium enema; positive biopsy

---

cilitate complete wound healing. The client should be taught side-to-side positioning and made to understand that short walks are better than sitting. The nurse should teach and assist the client in proper positioning for taking a sitz bath. The client may not know that the sitz bath and positioning are sources of comfort. The client may experience phantom rectal sensation because the sympathetic nerves responsible for rectal control are not severed during the surgery. The nurse must be astute in distinguishing phantom sensations from perineal abscess pain. An explanation to the client may allay anxieties.

A well-developed, consistent nursing plan of care should be coordinated early. The implementation of this plan will facilitate the healing process and hasten the client's rehabilitation.

After an abdominal-perineal resection there are three wounds: (1) an abdominal incision through which the colon is severed, (2) a left abdominal incision or stab wound that forms the colostomy, and (3) an incision in the perineum.

The management of the perineal incision differs among physicians. Three techniques are used: (1) packing of the entire open wound, (2) partial closure with Penrose drains for open drainage, and (3) primary closure of the perineal wound with closed-suction drainage of the pelvic cavity. The type of management of the perineal wound is individualized. The open and packed method is used in clients with extensive perirectal and perianal infections, contamination during surgery, or uncontrollable bleeding in the pelvic wound. When infection or contamination is minimal, a partial closure with drains is used. Primary closure is the preferred method in all other clients. An indwelling catheter is placed in the perineal wound and connected to low continuous suction. This usually remains until drainage is less than 50 ml/24 hr (approximately 3 to 5 days).

Clients who have open and packed wounds require meticulous postoperative care. The packing is usually left in place for 2 to 5 days. Packing the pelvic cavity for prolonged periods may result in sepsis and rigidity of the cavity wall and impede the healing process. The nurse should examine the wound regularly and record bleeding, excessive drainage, and unusual odor. The packing is usually removed in stages. When all packing is removed, the perineal wound is usually irrigated daily with normal saline solution, Betadine, or hydrogen peroxide solution to remove tissue debris and to facilitate healing. Irrigations are done several times a day, and an aseptic technique is always used.

If the wound is partially closed and drains are in place, the nurse must continue assessment. The incision is observed for suture integrity, signs and symptoms of wound inflammation, and infection. The drainage is examined and observations are recorded.

When the primary closure technique is used, the catheters are left in place for approximately 3 to 5 days; during this time, drainage is examined and observations are recorded. The area around the catheters is observed for signs of inflammation and is kept clean and dry. The nurse should observe for signs of edema, erythema, drainage around the suture line, fever, and an elevated WBC count.

Warm sitz baths (38° C to 41° C) for 10 to 20 minutes are usually given three to four times a day to assist in tissue debridement, provide comfort, and increase circulation to the area. Moist heat causes vasodilatation, which allows more oxygen to flow to the affected area. Sitz baths of more than 20 minutes may result in too much vasodilatation, causing congestion and discomfort.

The client may complain of pain and itching in and around the wound. There is no physiological explanation for the sensations that are felt, but a careful examination should be made to rule out delayed wound healing. Antipruritic agents and sitz baths are usually ordered.

The perineal dressing is reinforced and changed frequently because the drainage is profuse for several hours after surgery. All drainage is carefully assessed for amount, color, and consistency. The drainage is usually serosanguineous. The rectal area is kept as clean as possible to prevent odor and skin irritation. The client's position should be changed frequently from side to side. There is usually considerable pain from the perineal area. Because the dressing is changed often, a T binder or Fuller shield is used to hold the dressing in place without causing excoriation of the skin and discomfort to the client from frequent removal of tape.

The perineal wound may not be completely healed before discharge. After discharge the client is usually seen by the physician, the home health nurse, and the enterostomal therapist in an outpatient clinic. The wound is usually irrigated and debrided; if necessary, the infected area may be cauterized with silver nitrate. The skin around the wound should be assessed for loose hair. Shaving may be necessary to prevent the development of a chronic draining sinus. The nurse should report the drainage because it may also indicate the presence of a foreign body, fistula, osteomyelitis, or rectal tissue not removed during surgery. The client and significant others are taught management of the wound and the procedure to take a sitz bath at home. The client and the family should be aware of all community services available for assistance.

Sexual dysfunction is a possible complication of an abdominal-perineal resection and should be included in the plan of care. Although the effect of the procedure depends on the technique used, the subject should be discussed intelligently and tactfully by the surgeon, with follow-up as necessary by other members of the health care team. The nurse should understand that erection, ejaculation, and orgasm involve different nerve pathways and that a dysfunction of one does not mean total sexual dysfunction. The enterostomal therapy nurse is an important member of the team and can often provide correct and factual information concerning sexual dysfunction resulting from an abdominal-perineal resection.

Chronic management. Psychological support for the client as well as for the family is important. The recovery period is long and the possibility of recurrence of cancer is ever present. The overall 5-year survival rate for all clients undergoing resection for colon cancer is less than 50%.[14] This presents a problem for the client and health care providers because of the often painful, debilitating, and demoralizing manifestations produced by the recurrent disease and the lack of any effective palliative therapy. Chemotherapy may be used as an adjuvant measure for the client with evidence of local or distant metastasis. (The special needs of the cancer client are discussed in Chapter 9.)

OSTOMY SURGERY
Types

An *ostomy* is created when the proximal end of the intestine is brought through the abdominal wall and sutured to the skin (Table 37-34). It may be permanent or temporary. The opening is called a *stoma*. Fecal matter is diverted through the stoma to the outside of the abdominal wall.

An *ileostomy* is an opening from the ileum through the abdominal wall and is also referred to as a *conventional* or *Brooke ileostomy*. It is most commonly used in surgical treatment of ulcerative colitis and familial polyposis.

A *cecostomy* is an opening between the cecum and the abdominal wall. Both cecostomies and ascending colostomies are uncommon. They are usually temporary and most often are used for fecal diversion before surgery or for palliation.

A *colostomy* is an opening between the colon and the abdominal wall. The proximal end of the colon is sutured to the skin (Fig. 37-9). A *temporary colostomy* is usually performed to rest the bowel, to protect an end-to-end anastomosis after bowel resection, or as an emergency measure following abdominal trauma (e.g., gunshot wound). Diverticulitis is the most common reason for a temporary colostomy. Temporary colostomies are usually located in the transverse colon. Loop colostomy and double-barrel colostomy are most commonly performed as temporary colostomies, but they may be permanent.

A *double-barrel colostomy* is performed on clients with diverticular disease or obstruction from tumor in the descending and sigmoid colon. The colon is resected, and both ends are brought through the abdominal wall, creating two stomas. The proximal stoma is where stool is eliminated. The distal stoma is nonfunctional and is often called a *mucous fistula*.

A *loop colostomy* is made when a loop of bowel is brought out above the skin surface and held in place by a plastic rod (Fig. 37-10). This prevents the colon from slipping back into the abdominal cavity. The loop of colon may be opened during surgery, but most often it is opened 3 to 5 days after surgery by means of electrocautery. This

Table 37-34 Colostomy and Ileostomy

	Colostomy			
	Ascending	**Transverse**	**Sigmoid**	**Ileostomy**
Stool consistency	Semiliquid	Semiformed	Formed	Liquid to semiliquid
Fluid requirement	Increased	Possibly increased	No change	Increased
Bowel regulation	No	Uncommon	Yes	No
Appliance and skin barriers	Yes	Yes	Dependent on regulation	Yes
Irrigation	No	Possible	Possible every 24-48 hr	No
Indications for surgery	Perforating diverticulitis in lower colon; trauma; inoperable tumors of colon, rectum, or pelvis; rectovaginal fistula	Same as for ascending	Cancer of the rectum or rectosigmoidal area	Ulcerative colitis, diseased or injured colon, birth defect, familial polyposis, trauma, cancer

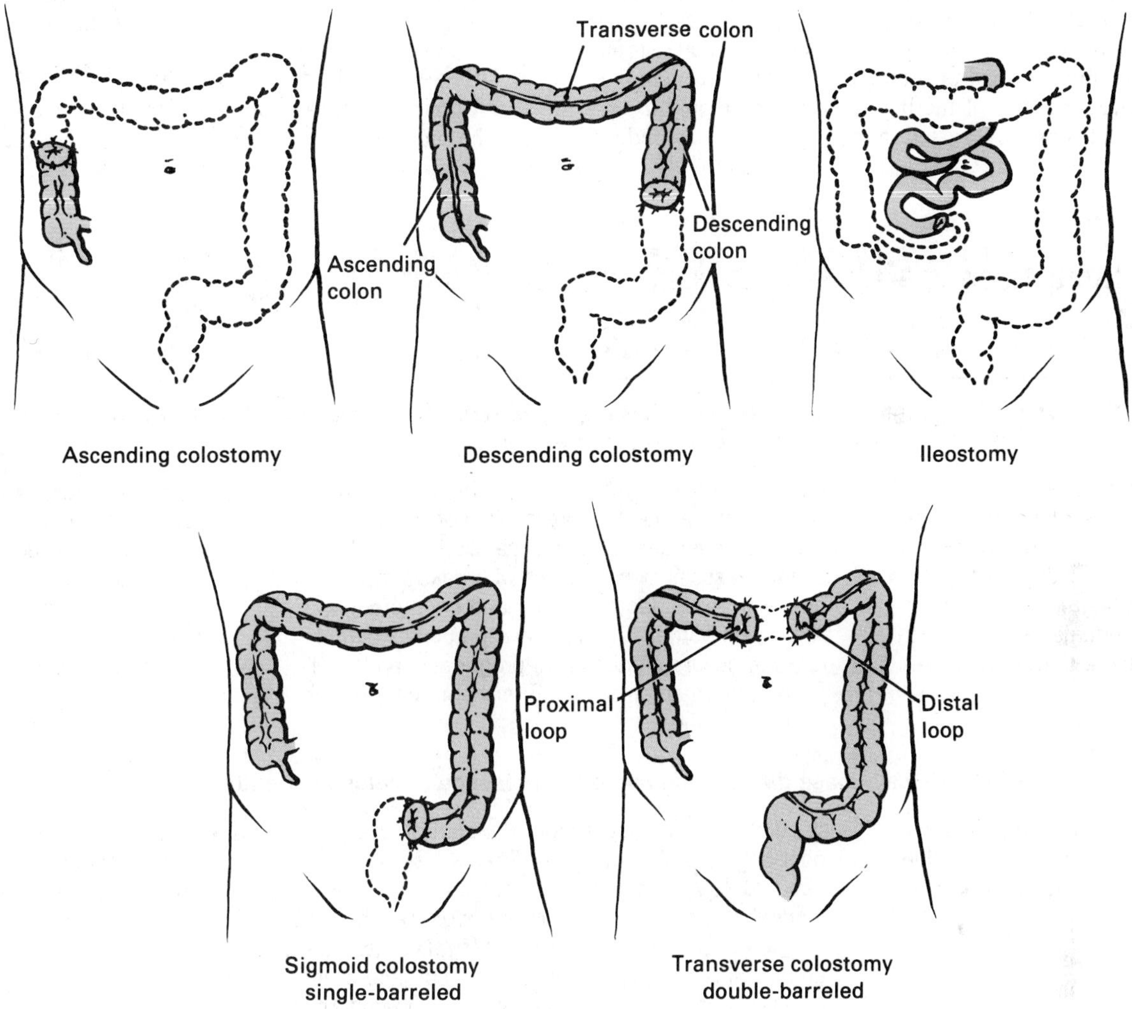

Transverse colon

Ascending colon

Descending colon

Ascending colostomy

Descending colostomy

Ileostomy

Proximal loop

Distal loop

Sigmoid colostomy
single-barreled

Transverse colostomy
double-barreled

Fig. 37-9 Types of ostomies.

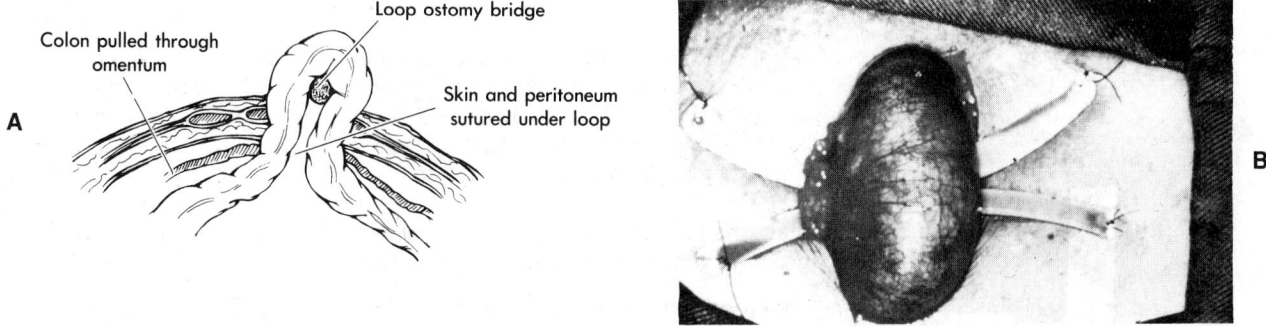

Loop ostomy bridge

Colon pulled through omentum

Skin and peritoneum sutured under loop

A

B

Fig. 37-10 **A,** Loop colostomy. (From Gruendemann BJ and Meeker MH: Alexander's care of the patient in surgery, ed 9, St Louis, 1991, Mosby–Year Book, Inc.) **B,** Loop colostomy. (Courtesy Hollister Incorporated.)

is not a painful procedure, since the bowel has no sensory nerve endings, and it usually is done at the client's bedside. Loop colostomies are performed more often than double-barrel colostomies as temporary procedures.

A *permanent-end colostomy* consists of a single stoma from the proximal end of the severed colon, with removal of the distal portion of the bowel. Most commonly a permanent colostomy is located in the sigmoid or descending colon. Permanent colostomies are performed when an abdominal-perineal resection is done. They may also be created after traumatic abdominal injuries and surgical resection of a bowel perforated from diverticulitis.

■ Nursing Management of Ostomy Surgery

Preoperative care. The physician should explain in detail the procedure to be done. Psychological preparation is

Table 37-35

 NURSING CARE PLAN FOR THE CLIENT WITH A COLOSTOMY

Defining Characteristics	Nursing Interventions	Evaluation Criteria
NURSING DIAGNOSIS: High risk for impaired skin integrity of peristomal area related to irritation from fecal drainage and lack of knowledge of skin care		
Erythematous, inflamed skin around stoma with burning and itching, poorly fitting appliance with leakage, lack of adequate skin care and failure to use skin barrier	Have enterostomal nurse see client before the operation to mark stoma site in area free of creases and folds for better seal of appliance. During pouch change, assess skin for signs of breakdown. Clean area with mild soap and water and dry thoroughly. Apply skin barrier. Change pouch routinely before leakage occurs. Teach client proper skin and appliance care. Plan for outpatient or home visit for continued teaching.	Normal skin integrity, intact pouch seal, client knowledgeable about proper technique of skin care and application of appliance
NURSING DIAGNOSIS: Body-image disturbance related to presence of colostomy and malodor		
Verbalization of embarrassment or shame due to malodor or presence of stoma	Instruct client on measures for odor control, use of odor-proof pouch, pouch deodorants, use of room deodorants when pouch is emptied, and avoidance of foods that are known to increase odor. Teach client how to conceal pouch under clothing. Discuss normal emotional response to stoma and encourage client to express feelings. Encourage family members to participate. Provide client with information on local United Ostomy Association.	Adjustment to altered body image, control of odor
NURSING DIAGNOSIS: Altered health maintenance related to lack of knowledge of long-term management of colostomy		
Frequent questioning about colostomy care	Assess and instruct client in irrigation procedure. If client is not candidate for irrigation, teach care of permanent appliance. Instruct client to avoid foods that cause diarrhea and increase flatus. Plan follow-up care. Provide contact person if questions arise.	Ability to manage care of colostomy by client or identification of home-support system
NURSING DIAGNOSIS: Altered sexuality patterns related to perceived loss of sexual appeal and possibility of accidental seepage of fecal material during sexual activity		
Verbalization of concern about activating intimate relations with spouse or significant other	Encourage discussion of meaning of sexuality to client and significant other. Discuss ways to avoid seepage and conceal colostomy stoma and/or appliance during intimate relations. If appropriate, arrange visit with person of same sex with colostomy to discuss sexual concerns and share potential solutions. Encourage use of perfumes or fragrant body oils during sexual activity.	Confidence in ability to resume previous sexual activity

very important. The family and the client usually have many questions concerning the procedure. If available, an enterostomal therapy nurse or therapist should visit with the client and the family. The client and the family should understand the extent of surgery as well as the type of ostomy and its care.

If the physician agrees, a trained ostomy visitor from the United Ostomy Association can provide meaningful psychological support. The client has the opportunity to see a person who has adjusted well and who has experienced some of the same feelings and concerns. The family will also benefit from the visit.

Bowel preparation before surgery decreases the chance of a postoperative infection by cleansing the bowel of feces and bacteria. Orally administered osmotic lavages (e.g., Go-Lytely, Colyte) have shortened the classic 72-hour preparation with clear liquids, cathartics, and enemas. IV and oral antibiotics are given. Nonabsorbable neomycin and erythromycin are given orally to decrease intracolonic bacterial counts.

Colostomy care. Postoperative nursing care should focus on assessing the stoma, protecting the skin, selecting the appliance, and assisting the client to adapt psychologically to a changed body (Table 37-35).

The stoma should be pink. A dusky blue stoma indicates ischemia, and a brown-black stoma indicates necrosis. The nurse should assess and document stoma color every 8 hours until the stoma remains pink for 3 days. There is mild to moderate swelling of the stoma the first 2 to 3 weeks after surgery. A skin barrier should next be applied to protect the peristomal suture line and skin surrounding the stoma. Solid skin barriers include stomahesive (Convatec), karaya, and Comfeel (Coloplast). Liquids that dry to a thin-film skin barrier include Skin-Gel (Hollister) and Skin-Prep (United). The skin should be washed with warm water and dried thoroughly before the barrier is applied.

With an open-ended, transparent, plastic, odor-proof pouch it is easy to protect the skin and to observe and collect the drainage. The pouch must fit snugly to prevent leakage around the stoma. The size of the stoma is determined with a stoma-measuring card. Although the pouch is usually applied after surgery, the colostomy does not function until 2 to 4 days postoperatively when peristalsis has been adequately restored. An exception to this is when a temporary colostomy is performed and the stoma is opened in the operating room with no bowel preparation being done previously.

The volume, color, and consistency of the drainage are recorded. Each time the appliance is changed, the condition of the skin is observed for irritation or excoriation. An appliance should *never* be placed directly on irritated skin.

The diet for the client with a colostomy is individualized. Usually a low-residue diet is ordered to decrease the amount of bulk and undigested food, to allow the stoma and bowel to heal, and to decrease the swelling from surgery. The client should be taught to avoid foods that cause gas, diarrhea, or constipation or that are odor-forming (Table 37-36). If the client introduces one food at a time, foods that cause problems can be easily identified. The goal is to return to a normal preoperative diet.

A colostomy in the ascending and transverse colon has semiliquid stools and is more difficult to regulate than a colostomy on the left side of the colon. The client needs to be instructed to use a drainable pouch. A colostomy in the sigmoid or descending colon has semiformed or formed stools and can be regulated by the irrigation method. The client may or may not wear a drainage pouch. A nondrainable pouch should have a gas filter.

Colostomy irrigations. Colostomy irrigations are intended to regulate bowel function. The irrigations stimulate the bowel to function at a specific time every day or every other day. If control is achieved, there should be little or no spillage between irrigations. The client who establishes regularity may need to wear only a pad or cover over the stoma. The client who cannot or chooses not to establish regularity by irrigations must wear an appliance at all times.

All equipment should be assembled before the irrigation. A commercially obtained irrigation set usually has all the equipment needed. The nurse should encourage the client to watch the procedure and explain each step (Table 37-37). The cone tip on the tubing controls the depth of insertion and dilates the stoma. If resistance is met, force should not be used because perforation of the intestine can result. The procedure should not be rushed and time should be given so that the client will feel relaxed.

Discharge to the home should not occur until the client or a family member is comfortable with and knows the procedure and has returned the demonstration. The client should be able to identify all necessary equipment and supplies, perform skin care, control odor, care for the stoma, identify signs and symptoms of complications, know the importance of fluids and food in the diet, have names and addresses of the United Ostomy Association, and know when to seek medical care.

Ileostomy care. Care of the ileostomy is presented in Table 37-38. The client should be seen preoperatively by

Table 37-36 Guide to Food Selection for the Client with an Ostomy

ODOR PRODUCING	DIARRHEA CAUSING
Eggs	Alcohol
Garlic	Beer
Onions	Cabbage family
Fish	Spinach
Asparagus	Green beans
Cabbage	Coffee
Broccoli	Spicy foods
Alcohol	Fruits (raw)
GAS FORMING	**CONSTIPATING**
Beans	Nuts
Cabbage family	Raisins
Onions	Popcorn
Beer	Seeds
Carbonated beverages	Chocolate
Cheeses, strong	Vegetables (raw)
Sprouts	Celery
	Corn

Table 37-37   Equipment and Procedure for Colostomy Irrigation

EQUIPMENT

Lubricant

Irrigation set (1000 to 2000 ml container, tubing with irrigating tip, clamp)

Irrigating sheath or sleeve with belt

Toilet tissue to clean around the colostomy

Bag for soiled dressing

PROCEDURE

1. Place 500 to 1000 ml of warm water (not to exceed 40.5° C, 105° F) in container. At first give only 500 ml or less. Gradually increase amount to 1000 ml.
2. Ensure comfortable position. Client may sit in chair in front of toilet.
3. Clear tubing of all air by flushing it with fluid.
4. Attach tubing to irrigating cone.
5. Hang container on hook or IV pole 40 to 53 cm (18 to 24 inches) above stoma (about shoulder height).
6. Apply irrigating sheath and place bottom end in bedpan or toilet bowl.
7. Lubricate catheter.
8. Insert catheter 7 to 10 cm (3 to 4 inches). If resistance is met, perform digital examination to remove feces or check for muscle spasms. *Never* use force—the bowel can perforate.
9. Release clamp or squeeze bulb to begin flow. Give only 500 ml at first. Gradually increase amount each day to 1000 ml maximum.
10. Allow the solution to flow slowly over 15 minutes.
11. If cramping occurs, stop the flow of solution for a few seconds. Lower the level of the container to lessen the force of flow of solution.
12. Clamp the tubing and remove irrigating tip when the desired amount has entered.
13. Allow 20-30 minutes for the solution and feces to be expelled. Close off the irrigating sheath at the bottom to allow ambulation.
14. Cleanse, rinse, and dry peristomal skin well.
15. Replace the colostomy drainage pouch.
16. Wash and rinse all equipment and hang to dry.

an enterostomal therapy nurse or therapist. A site for the stoma located in the right lower quadrant of the abdomen should be determined. Skin folds, scars, bony prominences, and creases need to be avoided. Proper placement of the stoma is important for adherence of the pouch without leakage. An ileostomy stoma protrusion of at least 1 to 1.5 cm makes care easier. When the stoma is flat, seepage occurs and the skin becomes denuded. Drainage is constant and extremely irritating to the skin. Regularity cannot be established. An appliance needs to be worn at all times. An open-ended drainable pouch is worn by the client so that the drainage can be emptied as needed. The drainable pouch is usually worn for several days before being changed, as long as leakage does not occur around the stoma. If pouch leakage occurs, the pouch should be promptly removed, the skin should be cleansed, and a new appliance should be placed. A solid skin barrier should always be used, and a two-piece pouching system is recommended after the operation. The system contains a skin barrier that adheres to the skin and a snap-on pouch. The pouch can be removed for observation of the stoma without disturbing the skin barrier.

Immediately after surgery, intake and output must be accurately monitored. The client should be observed for signs and symptoms of fluid and electrolyte imbalance, particularly potassium, sodium, and fluid deficits. In the first 24 to 48 hours after surgery the amount of drainage from the stoma may be negligible. After this period, there will be an increase in flatus and liquid (approximately 1000 to 2000 ml a day), which decreases as the stool becomes pasty with the prescribed diet. If the small bowel has been shortened as a result of resections in Crohn's or other disease, the drainage from the ileostomy may not decrease. The ileal stoma often bleeds easily when it is touched because it is a mucous membrane. The client should be told that minimal oozing of blood is normal.

The importance of fluid and electrolyte balance must be understood by the client. The client should be instructed to drink at least 1 to 2 L of fluid daily, and more may be necessary when diarrhea occurs and in the summer when perspiration is increased. Diarrhea from an ileostomy produces acidosis from the loss of bicarbonate. The physician may instruct the client to take an electrolyte solution at home (1 teaspoon of salt and 1 teaspoon of baking soda in 1 quart of water). Fluids rich in electrolytes should be encouraged. A commercial drink such as Gatorade is helpful in maintaining electrolyte balance.

Usually a low-roughage diet is ordered initially. Foods that produce diarrhea, increased flatus, and malodor should be avoided. Later there are no dietary restrictions except for foods that are troublesome for the client. Return to a normal presurgical diet is the goal.

Adaptation to an ostomy. Acceptance of the ostomy is the first step toward total recovery. The client experiences a grief reaction to loss of a body part as well as an alteration in body image. Each person uses different coping mechanisms. The adjustment period for the ostomy client depends on the individual lifestyle.

Psychological support during the grieving process may be needed. There are usually concerns about body image, sexual activity, family responsibilities, and changes in lifestyle. The client may become resentful and have fears of odor or soiling. Support from the nursing staff, allowing the client to verbalize freely, and talking to another person with an ostomy may help the ostomate work through personal feelings.

The client should not be forced to learn to care for the ostomy. The nurse should watch for clues that the client is ready. Teaching at the appropriate time is an important part of the care and can contribute to a smooth adjustment process.

Activities of daily living are resumed within 6 to 8 weeks. Very heavy lifting should be avoided. The client's physical condition determines when sports may be re-

Table 37-38

NURSING CARE PLAN FOR THE CLIENT WITH AN ILEOSTOMY

Defining Characteristics	Nursing Interventions	Evaluation Criteria

NURSING DIAGNOSIS: High risk for impaired skin integrity related to irritation from fecal drainage secondary to improper location of appliance, inadequate skin care, or sensitivity to appliance material

Inflamed, erythematous skin; leaking ileal contents from around pouch	Assess skin around stoma for signs of irritation. Inspect pouch to make sure seal is tight and no leakage is present. When pouch is changed, clean skin with warm water. Dry thoroughly. Always apply solid skin barrier before applying pouch. Empty pouch when it is one-third to one-half full to prevent seal from leaking. Instruct client in skin care and pouch-changing techniques.	Dry, clean, and intact skin around stoma

NURSING DIAGNOSIS: High risk for fluid volume deficit related to excess fluid loss and inadequate oral intake

Weakness, poor skin turgor, sunken eyes, hypotension, tachycardia, hypokalemia, hyponatremia, oliguria	Record intake and output and include ileostomy drainage. Monitor ileostomy drainage and notify physician of watery drainage. Monitor vital signs q 4 hr. Report urine output <30 ml/hr. Ensure fluid intake of at least 3000 ml/day in the initial postoperative period. Instruct client that fluid intake should be at least 1000 ml/day and will need to increase during very hot weather, when client is perspiring excessively, and during episodes of diarrhea. Monitor serum electrolytes. Instruct client on signs and symptoms of sodium, potassium, and fluid deficits.*	Normal serum electrolytes, normal vital signs, good skin turgor, urine output >30 ml/hr

NURSING DIAGNOSIS: Altered nutrition: less than body requirements related to lack of knowledge of appropriate foods and decreased appetite

Weight loss, vitamin and mineral deficiencies, inability to tolerate certain foods	Reassure client that a normal diet can be tolerated but that certain foods may need to be avoided. Gradually introduce foods and begin with low-residue diet. Introduce one food at a time. Teach client to chew food slowly and thoroughly. Give list of foods to avoid.† Arrange visit with dietitian if indicated.	Selection and planning of dietary intake to maintain weight at optimum level

NURSING DIAGNOSIS: Body-image disturbance related to change in body structure and possible perceived sexual dysfunction

Withdrawn behavior, depression, inability to verbalize fears and concerns, reluctance to learn about or participate in ileostomy care	Encourage verbalization of feelings. Reassure client and be supportive. Be sensitive to clues of grief and denial. Involve client in self-care but do not abandon. Encourage family members to participate in care. Provide thorough instructions on skin care, appliance application, complications, United Ostomy Association, and places to buy equipment. Assure client that a change in lifestyle is not necessary. Assess concern over sexual functioning. Counsel and refer if indicated. Plan follow-up postoperative discharge.	Verbalization of positive feelings about resuming role responsibilities and self-care

NURSING DIAGNOSIS: Impaired home management related to lack of knowledge of long-term ileostomy management

Frequent questions regarding immediate and long-term issues related to ileostomy care	Teach client or family ileostomy care related to appliance care, nutrition, personal hygiene, and emotional factors. Assure client of ability to manage long-term care. Advise client of problems, such as fever or diarrhea, that should be referred to health care provider.	Verbalization of confidence in ability to manage ileostomy care after discharge by client and/or family

*See Chapter 10.
†See Table 37-36.

sumed. Bathing and swimming are not prohibited. Water does not harm the stoma.

Ostomy clients are often confronted with sexual concerns. They fear sexual failure and offending a sexual partner. The capacity to enjoy sexual intercourse is not decreased.

The male client has varying sexual responses, ranging from full potency to complete loss of orgasm. Those who are orgasmic may have retrograde ejaculation, in which the seminal fluid is propelled backward into the bladder. This retrograde ejaculation causes the urine to have a milky color. Other problems frequently encountered are impotence, sterility, and ejaculatory incompetence. The nurse must pay particular attention to the client's response to the surgery as well as to the responses of significant others. Temporary or permanent impotence may be brought about through fear of failure, fear of offending the sexual partner, or depression from the losses experienced.

The female client usually does much better than the male in relation to sexual functioning. She is generally able to have intercourse, be orgasmic, and remain fertile. In many clients, sexual responses may be enhanced because the ostomy took care of a diseased organ or physical problem. Other female clients may fear that they are unlovable and untouchable and that their sexual relationships will be lost.

Pregnancy is possible; however, a limit to the number of pregnancies may be recommended by the physician on the basis of the client's physical condition and the philosophy of the physician. The person with an ostomy who becomes pregnant should have regular medical care.

Sexual concerns should be discussed with the client and the partner. If the nurse feels uncomfortable doing this, appropriate counseling should be obtained. Additional information is available from enterostomal therapy nurses and therapists and from the United Ostomy Association.

MECKEL'S DIVERTICULUM

Meckel's diverticulum of the ileum is a result of incomplete obliteration of the vitelline duct (narrow channel connecting the yolk sac with the intestine). It is the most frequent congenital anomaly of the intestinal tract and is usually located within 100 cm of the ileocecal valve. It most often remains asymptomatic, but 60% of clients with symptoms are under 2 years of age and one third are less than 1 year of age.[27] The diverticulum may contain all types of intestinal mucosa but most often contains gastric mucosa.

Bleeding or hemorrhage is the most common complication from ulceration of the ileal mucosa. Clients may have classic "currant jelly" stools. Other complications include intestinal obstruction, diverticulitis, umbilical discharge, and perforation with peritonitis. The treatment is surgical resection of the diverticulum.

DIVERTICULOSIS AND DIVERTICULITIS

A diverticulum is a saccular dilatation or outpouching of the mucosa through the circular smooth muscle of the intestinal wall. Clinically, diverticular disease occurs in two forms—diverticulosis and diverticulitis. Multiple non-

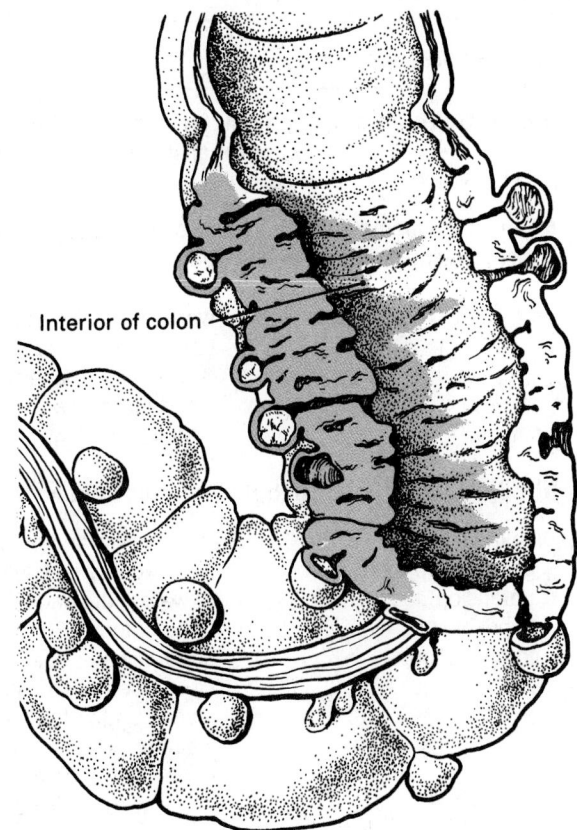

Interior of colon

Fig. 37-11 Diverticula are outpouchings of the colon. When they become inflamed, the condition is diverticulitis. The inflammatory process can spread to the surrounding area in the intestine.

inflamed diverticula are present with diverticulosis. The client is most often free of symptoms but may have some abdominal discomfort. In diverticulitis, inflammation of the diverticula occurs (Fig. 37-11). Diverticula may occur at any point within the GI tract but are most commonly found in the sigmoid colon.

Pathophysiology

Diverticular disease is a very common GI disorder that affects 10% of the population by the age of 40, and 50% are affected by the age of 80.[28] It affects men and women equally, but men seem to have a higher complication rate.

There is no known cause of diverticular disease, but deficiency in dietary fiber has been associated with it. The disease is more prevalent in Western populations that consume diets that are low in fiber and high in refined carbohydrates, and it is virtually unknown in areas of the world, such as rural Africa, where high-fiber diets are consumed.

When diverticula form, the smooth muscle of the colon wall becomes thickened. Lack of dietary fiber slows transit time and more water is absorbed from the stool, making it more difficult to pass through the lumen. Decreased bulk of the stool, combined with a more narrowed lumen in the sigmoid colon, causes high intraluminal pressures. These factors are believed to contribute to the formation of diverticula.

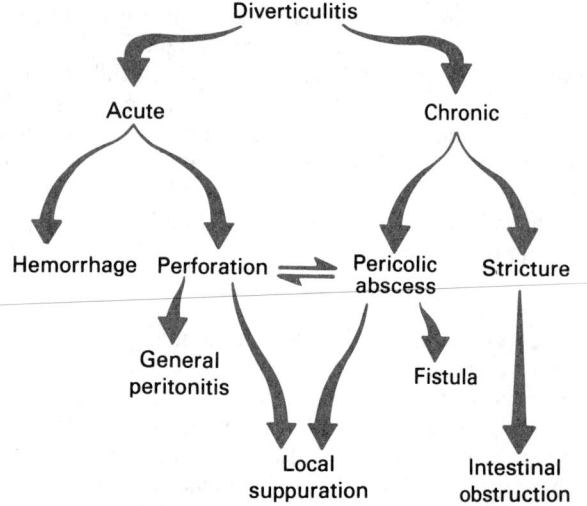

Fig. 37-12 Complications of diverticulitis.

The cause of diverticulitis is related to the retention of stool and bacteria in the diverticulum, which form a hardened mass called a *fecalith*. This causes inflammation and usually small perforations. Inflammation of the diverticulum spreads to the surrounding area in the intestines (Fig. 37-12), causing the tissue to become edematous. Abscesses may form, or complete perforation with peritonitis may occur.

Clinical Manifestations

The majority of clients with diverticulosis have no symptoms. Those with symptoms typically have crampy, abdominal pain located in the left lower quadrant that is usually relieved by passage of flatus or bowel movement. Alternating constipation and diarrhea may be present.

In clients with diverticulitis, abdominal pain is localized over the involved area of the colon. A tender, left lower quadrant mass may be felt on palpation of the abdomen. Fever, chills, and leukocytosis may be present.

Complications of diverticulitis include perforation with peritonitis, abscess and fistula formation, bowel obstruction, ureteral obstruction, and bleeding. Bleeding is a common complication of diverticulitis and is manifested by maroon stools or hematochezia. Bleeding usually stops spontaneously.

Diagnostic Studies

A barium enema is typically used to diagnose diverticular disease. A CBC, urinalysis, and fecal occult blood test should be performed (Table 37-39). A colonoscopy should be performed on clients with symptoms to rule out possible hidden polyps or lesions. Clients with acute diverticulitis should not have barium enema or colonoscopy because of the possibility of perforation.

Therapeutic Management

Uncomplicated diverticular disease is treated with a high-fiber diet and bulk laxatives, such as psyllium hydrophilic mucilloid (Metamucil). Anticholinergic drugs such

---

Table 37-39

Diagnostic and Therapeutic Management: Diverticulosis and Diverticulitis

DIAGNOSTIC

Stool for occult blood
Barium enema
Sigmoidoscopy
Colonoscopy
CBC
Urinalysis
Blood culture

THERAPEUTIC

Uncomplicated diverticular disease

High-residue diet
Bulk laxatives
Stool softeners
Anticholinergics
Mineral oil
Bed rest
Clear liquid diet
Oral antibiotics

Acute diverticulitis

Antibiotics
NPO status
IV fluids
Possible colon resection for obstruction or hemorrhage
Bed rest
NG suction

---

as dicyclomine (Bentyl) and Donnatol may be used to relieve discomfort due to spasm of the bowel.

In acute diverticulitis, antibiotic therapy is required. The client is also maintained on bed rest to decrease intestinal motility, is kept on NPO status, and the WBC count is monitored. An NG tube may be necessary.

Surgical intervention is necessary to drain abscesses or to resect an obstructing inflammatory mass. The usual surgical procedures involve resection of the involved colon with a temporary diverting colostomy. The colostomy is reanastomosed after the colon is healed.

▪ Nursing Management of Diverticulosis and Diverticulitis

Clients should be provided with a full explanation of their condition. The better they understand the disease process and adhere to the prescribed regimen, the less likely the exacerbation of the disease and the onset of complications.

Uncomplicated diverticular disease is primarily treated by a high-fiber diet (see Table 37-10). Fluids should be increased because fibers retain water, thus decreasing the amount absorbed by the body. If the client is obese, a reduction in weight is needed.

Increased intraabdominal pressure should be avoided

because it may precipitate an attack. Factors that increase intraabdominal pressure are straining at stool, vomiting, bending, lifting, and tight, restrictive clothing.

In acute diverticulitis, the goal of treatment is to allow the colon to rest and the inflammation to subside. The client is kept on NPO status and bed rest and given parenteral fluids. The client needs to be observed for signs of possible peritonitis.

When the acute attack subsides, oral fluids progressing to a semisolid diet are allowed. Ambulation is also permitted. At this stage the client needs to be observed for a recurrent attack. If the client has a bowel resection or colostomy, the nursing care is the same as for these procedures.

HERNIAS

A hernia is a protrusion of a viscus through an abnormal opening or a weakened area in the wall of the cavity in which it is normally contained. A hernia may occur in any part of the body, but it usually occurs within the abdominal cavity. If the hernia can be placed back into the abdominal cavity, it is known as *reducible*. The hernia can be reduced by manipulation, or it can occur without manipulation when the person lies down. If the hernia cannot be placed back into the abdominal cavity, it is known as *irreducible* or *incarcerated*. In this situation the intestinal flow may be obstructed. When the hernia is irreducible and the intestinal flow and blood supply are obstructed, the hernia is *strangulated*. The result is an acute intestinal obstruction.

Types

The *inguinal* hernia is the most common type of hernia and occurs at the point of weakness in the abdominal wall where the spermatic cord in men and the round ligament in women emerge (Fig. 37-13). When the protrusion escapes through the inguinal ring and follows the spermatic cord or the round ligament, it is termed an *indirect* hernia. When it escapes through the posterior inguinal wall it is a *direct* hernia. An inguinal hernia is more frequent in men.

A *femoral* hernia occurs when there is a protrusion through the femoral ring into the femoral canal. It occurs below the inguinal (Poupart's) ligament as a bulge. It becomes strangulated easily and occurs more frequently in women. The *umbilical* hernia occurs when the rectus muscle is weak or the umbilical opening fails to close after birth. This type is found most commonly in children.

Ventral or *incisional* hernias are due to weakness of the abdominal wall at the site of a previous incision. It is found most commonly in clients who are obese, who have had multiple surgical procedures in the same area, and who have had inadequate wound healing because of poor nutrition or infection.

Clinical Manifestations

A hernia commonly occurs over the involved area when the client stands or strains. There may be some discomfort as a result of tension. Severe pain is caused if the hernia becomes strangulated. In this situation the clinical manifestations of a bowel obstruction, such as vomiting, crampy abdominal pain, and distention, are found.

Therapeutic Management

Diagnosis is based on history and physical examination findings. Surgery is the treatment of choice for hernias to prevent the possible complication of strangulation. Umbilical hernia is not usually repaired surgically because it may reduce itself if left alone until the child gets older. The surgical repair of a hernia is known as a *herniorrhaphy*. The reinforcement of the weakened area with wire, fascia, or mesh is known as a *hernioplasty*. When there is strangulation, necrosis and gangrene may develop if immediate care is not given. A bowel resection of the involved area or a temporary colostomy may be needed to treat a strangulated hernia.

■ Nursing Management of Hernias

Some clients with hernias may wear a truss, which is a pad placed over the hernia and held in place with a belt. The truss is worn to keep the hernia from protruding. If a client wears a truss, the nurse should check for skin irritation caused by the continual rubbing of the truss.

After a hernia repair, the client may have difficulty voiding. Therefore the nurse should observe for a distended bladder. An accurate intake and output record is important. Scrotal edema is a painful complication after an inguinal hernia repair. A scrotal support with application

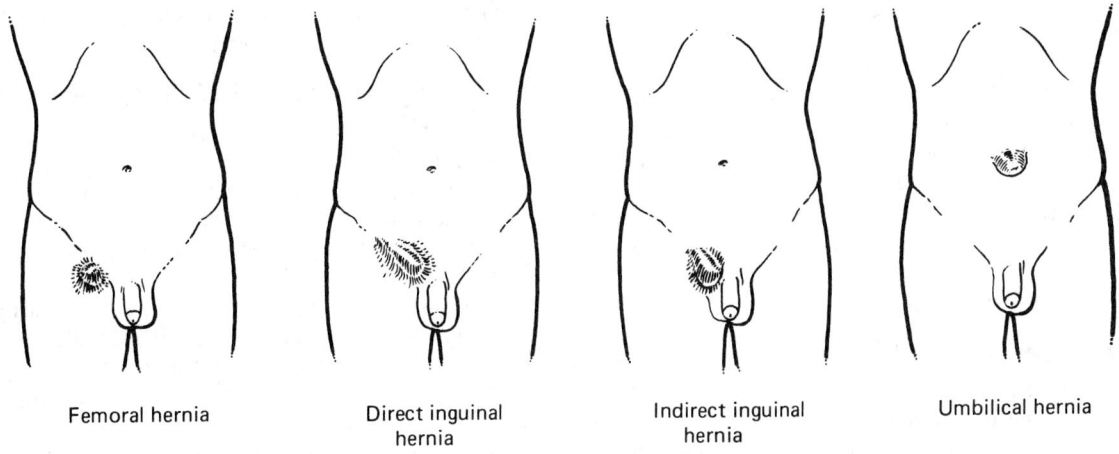

Femoral hernia   Direct inguinal   Indirect inguinal   Umbilical hernia
                        hernia   hernia

Fig. 37-13   Types of hernias.

of an ice bag may help relieve pain and edema. Coughing is not encouraged, but deep breathing and turning should be done. If the client needs to cough or sneeze, the incision should be splinted during coughing, and sneezing should be done with the mouth open.

After discharge the client may be restricted from heavy lifting for 6 to 8 weeks. Some surgeons do not put any limitations on physical activities.

MALABSORPTION SYNDROME

Malabsorption results from impaired absorption of fats, carbohydrates, proteins, minerals, and vitamins. The stomach, small intestine, liver, and pancreas regulate normal digestion and absorption. Nutrients are ordinarily broken down through the digestive process so that absorption can take place through the intestinal mucosa into the bloodstream. If there is an interruption in this process at any point, malabsorption may occur. Several problems can cause malabsorption (Table 37-40). They can be classified into malabsorptions caused by (1) biochemical or enzyme deficiencies, (2) bacterial proliferation, (3) disruption of small-intestine mucosa, (4) disturbed lymphatic and vascular circulation, and (5) surface area loss.[29] Lactose intolerance is the most common malabsorption disorder, followed by inflammatory bowel disease, nontropical (celiac) and tropical sprue, and cystic fibrosis.

The most common clinical manifestation of malabsorption is *steatorrhea* (fatty stools). Bulky, foul-smelling stools that float in water and are difficult to flush are characteristic of steatorrhea (Table 37-41).

Table 37-40 Common Causes of Malabsorption

BIOCHEMICAL OR ENZYME DEFICIENCIES

Lactase deficiency
Biliary tract obstruction
Pancreatic insufficiency
  Cystic fibrosis
  Chronic pancreatitis
  Zollinger-Ellison syndrome

BACTERIAL PROLIFERATION

Tropical sprue
Parasitic infection

SMALL INTESTINAL MUCOSAL DISRUPTION

Celiac disease
Whipple's disease
Crohn's disease

DISTURBED LYMPHATIC AND VASCULAR CIRCULATION

Lymphoma
Ischemia
Lymphangiectasia
Congestive heart failure

SURFACE AREA LOSS

Billroth II gastrectomy
Short-bowel syndrome
Distal ileal resection, disease, or bypass

Table 37-41 Clinical Manifestations of Malabsorption

Manifestations	Pathophysiology
GASTROINTESTINAL	
Weight loss	Malabsorption of fat, carbohydrates, and protein leading to loss of calories; marked reduction in caloric intake or increased use of calories
Diarrhea	Impaired absorption of water, sodium, fatty acids, bile, or carbohydrates
Flatulence	Bacterial fermentation of unabsorbed carbohydrates
Steatorrhea	Undigested and unabsorbed fat
Glossitis, cheilosis, stomatitis	Deficiency of iron, riboflavin, vitamin B_{12}, folic acid, and other vitamins
HEMATOLOGICAL	
Anemia	Impaired absorption of iron, vitamin B_{12}, and folic acid
Hemorrhagic tendency	Vitamin C deficiency
	Vitamin K deficiency inhibiting production of clotting factors II, VII, IX, and X
MUSCULOSKELETAL	
Bone pain	Osteoporosis from impaired bone formation
	Osteomalacia secondary to hypocalcemia, hypophosphatemia
Tetany	Hypocalcemia, hypomagnesemia
Weakness, muscle cramps	Anemia, electrolyte depletion (especially potassium)
Muscle wasting	Protein malabsorption
NEUROLOGICAL	
Altered mental status	Dehydration
Paresthesias	Vitamin B_{12} deficiency
Peripheral neuropathy	Vitamin B_{12} deficiency
Night blindness	Thiamine deficiency
	Vitamin A deficiency
INTEGUMENTARY	
Bruising	Vitamin K deficiency
Dermatitis	Fatty acid deficiency, zinc deficiency, niacin and other vitamin deficiencies
Brittle nails	Iron deficiency
Hair thinning and loss	Protein deficiency
CARDIOVASCULAR	
Hypotension	Dehydration
Tachycardia	Hypovolemia, anemia
Peripheral edema	Protein malabsorption, protein loss in diarrhea

Screening tests available for malabsorption include qualitative examination of stool for fat (Sudan stain), a 72-hour stool collection for quantitative measurement of fecal fat, and the D-xylose absorption-excretion test, which is a good screening test for carbohydrate absorption (see Table 33-11). Other diagnostic studies include three different kinds of breath test: (1) the bile acid breath test, which is used to evaluate bile-salt malabsorption or malabsorption from bacterial overgrowth; (2) the triolein breath test, which measures carbon dioxide excretion after ingestion of a radioactive triglyceride; and (3) the excretion of breath hydrogen after ingestion of lactose, which is a sensitive, specific, and noninvasive test for detection of lactase deficiency. The rationale for the hydrogen breath test is that bacterial metabolism is the only source of hydrogen production in human beings and most of this occurs in the colon.

A pancreatic secretin test may be performed to rule out pancreatic insufficiency. Endoscopy may be used to obtain a small bowel biopsy specimen for diagnosis. Radiographic studies of the esophagus, stomach, and small intestine may be indicated. A small-bowel enema is frequently performed to identify abnormal mucosal patterns.

Laboratory studies that are frequently ordered include a CBC, determinations of prothrombin time, serum vitamin A and carotene levels, serum electrolytes, cholesterol, and calcium. Two causes of malabsorption are sprue and lactase deficiency.

Sprue

Two closely related malabsorption conditions are *nontropical sprue* and *tropical sprue*. Tropical and nontropical sprue are found in adults. Nontropical sprue is most commonly referred to as *celiac sprue* (especially in children) but is also called *adult celiac disease* and *gluten-induced enteropathy*.

Etiology. In celiac disease there is marked atrophy and flattening of the villi. As a result, absorption within the small intestine is reduced. The proposed reason for the injury to the villi is a hypersensitivity response initiated by gluten and gliadin (a breakdown product of gluten). Gluten is a protein found in wheat, rye, barley, and oats. The hypersensitivity leads to an inflammatory response of the mucosa.

Tropical sprue is a chronic disorder acquired in endemic tropical areas. The exact cause is unknown, but the disorder has been linked to an infectious agent. Folate deficiency is also believed to play a role in the development of this disease. Clinically, it resembles nontropical sprue.

Clinical manifestations. Generalized symptoms include steatorrhea (bulky, foul-smelling, yellow-gray, greasy stools), diarrhea, weight loss, signs of multiple vitamin deficiencies, abdominal distention, and excessive flatulence.

Therapeutic management. Treatment of sprue syndrome is based on the underlying cause. In nontropical sprue, a gluten-free diet usually leads to clinical recovery. Wheat, barley, oats, and rye products should be avoided. Soybean flours may be used. Corticosteroids are also used to treat nontropical sprue, but only in severely ill clients who have not responded to a gluten-free diet. The basis for this treatment is that the inflammatory response is mediated by an immunological response.

Tropical sprue is treated with broad-spectrum antibiotics (e.g., tetracycline) in conjunction with folic acid therapy. The client who responds to this therapy and achieves a remission is usually maintained on folic acid.

Lactase Deficiency

Lactase deficiency is a condition in which the lactase enzyme is deficient or absent. Lactase is the enzyme that breaks down lactose into two simple sugars—glucose and galactose. Although primary lactase deficiency seems to be hereditary, milk intolerance may not become clinically evident until late adolescence or early adulthood. About 5% of the adult population has primary lactase deficiency. The highest incidence is found in African and North American blacks, American Indians, Mexican-Americans, and Jews. Acquired lactase deficiency is often seen in other GI diseases in which the mucosa has been damaged, including ulcerative colitis, Crohn's disease, gastroenteritis, and sprue syndrome.

Clinical manifestations. The symptoms of lactose intolerance include bloating, flatulence, crampy abdominal pain, and diarrhea. They may occur within ½ hour to several hours after drinking a glass of milk or ingesting a milk product. The diarrhea of lactose intolerance results from fluid secretion into the small intestines, responding to the osmotic action of undigested lactose.

■ Therapeutic and Nursing Management of Lactase Deficiency

Many lactose-intolerant persons are aware of their milk intolerance and avoid milk. A lactose intolerance test can be performed to rule out milk allergies. The client is given 50 to 100 mg of lactose orally. Blood samples are drawn before the consumption of lactose and at 15-, 30-, 60-, and 90-minute intervals. Failure of the blood sugar to increase more than 20 mg/dl is suggestive of lactase deficiency. Results of the hydrogen breath test after ingestion of lactose are abnormal.

Treatment consists of eliminating lactose from the diet by avoiding milk and milk products. A lactose-free diet is given initially and is gradually advanced to a low-lactose diet as tolerated by the client. The objective of care is to teach the importance of adherence to the diet. Many lactose-intolerant persons may not exhibit symptoms if lactose is taken in small amounts. In some persons, lactose may be tolerated better if taken with meals.

The client needs to be aware that milk, ice cream, cottage cheese, and cheese have a high lactose content. If the milk has been fermented (e.g., cultured buttermilk, yogurt, sour cream), the client with low lactase levels may tolerate it better.

Lactase enzyme (Lactaid) is available commercially as an over-the-counter product. It is mixed with milk and breaks down the lactose before the milk is ingested.

ANORECTAL PROBLEMS
Hemorrhoids

Hemorrhoids are dilated varicose veins of the anus and rectum. They may be internal (occurring above the internal

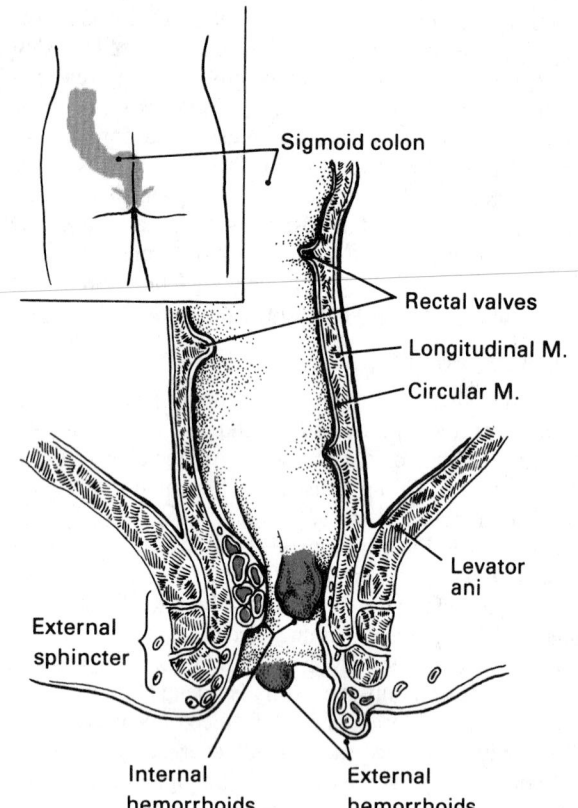

Fig. 37-14   Anatomical structures of the rectum and anus with external and internal hemorrhoids.

sphincter) or external (occurring outside the external sphincter) (Fig. 37-14). Hemorrhoids occur most frequently in persons between the ages of 20 to 50. In affected persons, hemorrhoids appear periodically, depending on amount of anorectal pressure.

Pathophysiology. Hemorrhoids develop when the flow of blood through the veins of the hemorrhoidal plexus is impaired. Internal hemorrhoids may become constricted and painful. They are the most common cause of bleeding with defecation. The amount of blood lost at one time may be small but may lead to iron deficiency anemia over time. External hemorrhoids are reddish blue and seldom bleed or cause pain unless a vein ruptures. If the blood clots in external hemorrhoids, they become inflamed, painful, and are said to be *thrombosed.*

Hemorrhoids may be caused by many factors, including pregnancy, prolonged constipation, straining in an effort to defecate, heavy lifting, prolonged standing and sitting, and portal hypertension as found in cirrhosis.

Therapeutic management. Hemorrhoids are diagnosed by inspection, digital examination, proctoscopy, or examination with the flexible sigmoidoscope. Therapy should be directed toward the causes and the client's symptoms. A high-fiber diet and increased fluid intake will prevent constipation and reduce straining, which allows engorgement of the veins to subside. Ointments such as Nupercaine, creams, suppositories, and witch hazel compresses are used to shrink the mucous membranes and relieve discom-

fort. Stool softeners may be ordered to keep the stools soft, and sitz baths may be ordered to relieve pain.

Application of ice packs for a few hours, followed by warm packs, may be used for thrombosed hemorrhoids. Another conservative treatment involves use of a sclerosing solution, such as 5% phenol in oil, or a combined solution of quinine and urea may be injected into the submucous tissue surrounding the hemorrhoids, causing a fibrosing and shrinking of the supporting tissues.

Internal hemorrhoids may be ligated with a rubber band. The constrictive effect impairs circulation, and the tissue becomes necrotic, separates, and sloughs off. There is some local discomfort with this procedure, but no anesthetic is required. Aspirin or propoxyphene (Darvon) is usually given for discomfort. Anal dilatation and lateral sphincterotomy may be performed to reduce vascular engorgement by reducing sphincter pressure. Other methods, such as infrared photocoagulation, bipolar diathermy, and cryotherapy, are used to treat the mucosa.

A *hemorrhoidectomy* is the surgical excision of hemorrhoids. Surgery is indicated when there is prolapse, excessive pain or bleeding, or large hemorrhoids. In general, hemorrhoidectomy is reserved for clients with severe symptoms related to multiple thrombosed hemorrhoids or marked protrusion. Surgical removal may be done by cautery, clamp, or excision. One surgical approach is to leave the area open so that healing takes place by secondary intention. In another approach the hemorrhoids are removed, the tissue is sutured, and healing takes place by primary-intention wound healing.

▪ Nursing Management of Hemorrhoids

Conservative nursing management for the client with hemorrhoids includes teaching measures to (1) prevent constipation, (2) avoid prolonged standing or sitting, (3) properly use over-the-counter medications available for hemorrhoidal symptoms, and (4) seek medical care for severe symptoms of hemorrhoids (e.g., excessive pain and bleeding, prolapsed hemorrhoids) when necessary.

Pain is a common problem after a hemorrhoidectomy. The nurse must be aware that although the procedure is minor, the pain is severe and narcotics are usually given initially.

Sitz baths are started 1 to 2 days after surgery. A warm sitz bath provides comfort and keeps the anal area clean. A sponge ring in the sitz bath helps relieve pressure on the area. Initially the client should not be left alone because of the possibility of weakness or fainting.

Packing may be inserted into the rectum to absorb drainage. A T binder may hold the dressing in place. If packing is inserted, it usually is removed the first or second postoperative day. The nurse should assess for rectal bleeding. The client may be embarrassed when the dressing is changed, and privacy should be provided. The client usually dreads the first bowel movement and often resists the urge to defecate. Pain medication may be given before the bowel movement to reduce discomfort.

A stool softener such as dioctyl sodium sulfosuccinate (Colace) is usually ordered the first few postoperative days. If the client does not have a bowel movement within 2 to 3 days, an oil retention enema is given.

Discharge teaching includes the importance of the diet, care of the anal area, symptoms of complications (especially bleeding), and avoidance of constipation and straining. Sitz baths are recommended for 1 to 2 weeks. The physician may order a stool softener to be taken for a time. Hemorrhoids may recur. Occasionally anal strictures develop and dilatation is necessary. Regular checkups are important in the prevention of any further problems.

Anal Fissure

An anal fissure (fissura in ano) is a skin ulcer or a crack in the lining of the anal wall that is caused by trauma or local infection. It is frequently associated with constipation and subsequent stretching of the anus from hard feces. The most common clinical manifestations are painful spasms of the anal sphincter and severe, burning pain during defecation. Some bleeding may occur, and constipation results because of fear of pain associated with bowel movements.

Conservative treatment consists of bowel regulation with mineral oil and stool softeners. Sitz baths and anal anesthetic suppositories (Anusol) are also ordered. Surgical treatment usually consists of excision of the fissure. Postoperative nursing care is the same as the care for the client who has had a hemorrhoidectomy.

Anorectal Abscess

An anorectal abscess is a localized infection with pus in the fatty tissue of the anorectal area (Fig. 37-15). It is usually caused by an infection. The most common causative organisms are *Escherichia coli*, staphylococci, and streptococci. Clinical manifestations include pain, foul-smelling pus, tenderness and swelling near the anus, and elevated temperature.

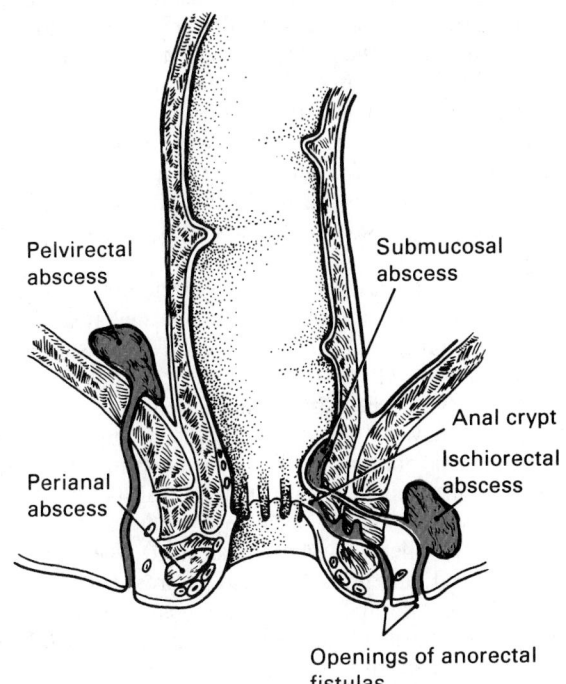

Fig. 37-15 Common sites of anorectal abscesses and fistula formation.

Surgical treatment consists of making an opening into the abscess to drain the pus. If packing is used, it should be impregnated with petroleum jelly and the area should be allowed to heal by granulation. The packing is changed every day, and moist, hot compresses are applied to the area. Care must be taken to avoid soiling the dressing during urination or defecation. A low-residue diet is given. The client may leave the hospital with the area open. Discharge teaching should include wound care, the importance of sitz baths, thorough cleaning after bowel movements, and follow-up visits to the physician.

Anorectal Fistula

An anal fistula is an abnormal tunnel leading out from the anus or rectum. It may extend to the outside of the skin, the vagina, or the buttocks. Anorectal fistulas are a complication of Crohn's disease. This condition often precedes an anorectal abscess.

Feces may enter the fistula and cause an infection. There may be persistent blood-stained, purulent discharge or stool leakage from the fistula. The client may have to wear a pad to prevent staining of clothes.

Surgical treatment involves a fistulotomy or a fistulectomy. In a fistulotomy the fistula is opened and healthy tissue is allowed to granulate. A fistulectomy is an excision of the entire fistulous tract. Gauze packing is inserted and the wound is allowed to heal by granulation. Care is the same as after a hemorrhoidectomy.

Pilonidal Sinus

A pilonidal sinus is a small tract under the skin between the buttocks in the sacrococcygeal area. It is thought to be of congenital origin. It may have several openings and is lined with epithelium and hair, thus the name *pilonidal* ("a nest of hair").

The skin is moist, and movement of the buttocks causes the short, wiry hair to penetrate the skin. The irritated skin becomes infected and forms a pilonidal cyst or abscess. There are no symptoms unless there is an infection. If it becomes infected, the client complains of pain and swelling at the base of the spine.

The formed abscess requires incision and drainage. The wound may be closed or left open to heal by secondary intention. The wound is packed and sitz baths are ordered.

Nursing care includes hot, moist heat applications when an abscess is present. The client is usually more comfortable lying on the abdomen or side. The client should be instructed to avoid contaminating the dressing when urinating or defecating and to avoid straining whenever possible.

C | ase Study

ULCERATIVE COLITIS

Marie, a 37-year-old woman, is admitted for the fifth time in an 11-month period with acute ulcerative colitis. She complains of severe diarrhea (10 to 15 stools a day with blood and mucus), intestinal cramping, anorexia, nausea, and vomiting. She is dehydrated, has a temperature of 38° C (100.4° F), and is crying.

Marie stated she takes Azulfidine and prednisone. During the past 72 hours she has not taken any medication because of the nausea and vomiting.

On physical examination, palpation over the colon revealed abdominal tenderness and an enlarged liver. Blood studies done on admission revealed iron deficiency anemia and a low serum albumin value.

Discussion Questions

1. Explain the pathophysiological changes that occur in ulcerative colitis.
2. How does ulcerative colitis differ from Crohn's disease?
3. Explain the reason for Marie's anemia and low serum albumin.
4. What would a proctosigmoidoscopic examination reveal during the acute phase?
5. List three nursing goals for Marie and a plan for implementation of care to meet these goals.
6. What are the complications of ulcerative colitis and the role of the nurse in preventing their occurrence?

Review Questions

The number of the question corresponds to the same-numbered objective at the beginning of the chapter.

1. Common treatment measures for the client with constipation are
   a. low-residue diet and anticholinergic drugs
   b. stool softeners and high-residue diet
   c. antiemetics and low-fiber diet
   d. enemas and high fluid intake
2. Nursing care of a client after an exploratory laparotomy includes
   a. antacids through NG tube every 2 hours
   b. irrigation of NG tube with sterile water every 2 to 3 hours
   c. assessment of bowel sounds in all four quadrants
   d. assessment of the number and character of stools the first 2 postoperative days
3. Which of the following is not a common clinical manifestation of acute appendicitis?
   a. prolonged diarrhea
   b. WBC of 18,000/μl
   c. nausea and vomiting
   d. constipation
4. The physician asks to be notified if any signs of rupture of the appendix occur. For which of the following should notification occur?
   a. nausea and vomiting
   b. tenderness in the right lower quadrant
   c. sudden, sharp pain in the right lower quadrant
   d. elevated temperature of 37.8° C (100° F)
5. Common clinical manifestations of gastroenteritis are
   a. abdominal cramps, nausea, and vomiting
   b. fever, diarrhea, and leukopenia
   c. anorexia, pain, and constipation
   d. vomiting, fever, and constipation

6. Which of the following statements regarding the difference between ulcerative colitis and Crohn's disease is accurate?
   a. Crohn's disease is more likely to be treated with a colectomy.
   b. Ulcerative colitis is characterized by skip lesions.
   c. Crohn's disease is more likely than ulcerative colitis to result in cancer.
   d. Both diseases are characterized by remissions and exacerbations.
7. Intestinal obstruction can occur due to
   a. adhesions and paralytic ileus
   b. intussusception and dehydration
   c. volvulus and varices
   d. atresias and telangiectasia
8. In carcinoma of the large intestine there is a higher incidence of bowel obstruction in the
   a. ascending colon because of its narrow lumen
   b. transverse colon because of its semisolid content
   c. ileocecal valve because of the semiliquid content
   d. sigmoid region because of the narrow lumen and fecal consistency
9. Physiological changes occurring after an ileostomy necessitate
   a. stoma irrigations
   b. skin care around the stoma
   c. avoidance of low-residue diets
   d. the need to wear a belted appliance
10. Bowel preparation for a colostomy with nonabsorbable antibiotics is done primarily to
    a. reduce the bacterial flora in the colon
    b. prevent diarrhea
    c. prevent constipation
    d. prevent additional formation of ammonia
11. During a colostomy irrigation the client may experience cramping. If this occurs, the nurse should
    a. slow the flow by lowering the container
    b. discontinue the irrigation at once
    c. reduce the temperature of the irrigation solution
    d. insert the catheter about 1 inch farther
12. In contrast to diverticulitis, the client with diverticulosis
    a. often has no symptoms
    b. has rectal bleeding
    c. has localized crampy pain
    d. has abscesses
13. Hernias are commonly found in any of the following sites *except*
    a. epigastrium
    b. inguinal ring
    c. umbilicus
    d. femoral ring
14. In nontropical sprue the client's diet must be
    a. gluten-free, high-protein, high-caloric
    b. gluten-free, low-fat, low-protein
    c. milk-free, high-protein, high-caloric
    d. low-caloric, low-protein, high-fat

15. Hemorrhoids are characterized by all of the following *except*
    a. tendency toward constipation
    b. internal or external
    c. bleeding after bowel movement
    d. dilatation of the rectal arteries

REFERENCES

1. Shiau Y: Clinical and laboratory approaches to evaluate diarrheal disorders, Crit Rev Clin Lab Sci 25:43-63, 1987.
2. Thorne GM: Gastrointestinal infections—dietary interactions, J Am Coll Nutr 5:487-499, 1986.
3. Drossman D: What can be done to control incontinence associated with the irritable bowel syndrome? Am J Gastroenterol 84:355-357, 1989.
4. Hanauer S: Fecal incontinence in the elderly, Hosp Pract 23:105-112, 1988.
5. MacLeod J: Management of anal incontinence by biofeedback, Gastroenterology 93:291-294, 1987.
6. Krevsky B, Maurer A, and Fisher R: Patterns of colonic transit in chronic idiopathic constipation, Am J Gastroenterol 84:127-132, 1989.
7. Ogorek CP and Reynolds J: Chronic constipation, diagnosis and treatment, Endosc Rev 4:47-53, 1987.
8. Chobanian S and VanNess M: Manual of clinical problems in gastroenterology, Boston, 1988, Little, Brown & Co, pp 111-113.
9. Sleisenger MH and Fordtran JS: Gastrointestinal disease, pathophysiology, diagnosis and management, ed 4, Philadelphia, 1989, WB Saunders Co, p 1934.
10. Friedman G: Irritable bowel syndrome: a practical approach, Am J Gastroenterol 84:863-867, 1989.
11. Field LL and Boyd N: Genetic markers and inflammatory bowel disease: immunoglobulin allotypes (GM, KM) and protease inhibitor, Am J Gastroenterol 84:753-755, 1989.
12. Lashner BA and others: Prevalence and incidence of IBD in family members, Gastroenterology 91:396-400, 1986.
13. Ginsburg AL: Management of inflammatory bowel disease, Gastroenterol Clin North Am 18:73, 1989.
14. LaMont JT and Kandel GP: Toxic megacolon in ulcerative colitis, early diagnosis and management, Hosp Pract 21:102A-102Z, 1986.
15. Swartz ML: Beyond the scope: a nursing view of the extraintestinal manifestations of IBD, Gastroenterol Nurs 12:3-9, 1989.
16. Goldstein F: Some effects of drug laws and regulations on the practice of medicine, with particular emphasis on inflammatory bowel disease, Am J Gastroenterol 83:1091-1097, 1988.
17. Das KM: Sulfasalazine therapy in inflammatory bowel disease, Gastroenterol Clin North Am 18:1-20, 1989.
18. Black M: Crohn's disease, pathophysiology, diagnosis and management, Gastroenterol Nurs 11:259-262, 1989.
19. McConnell E: Meeting the challenge of intestinal obstruction, Nursing 87 17:34-41, 1987.
20. Holder WD: Intestinal obstruction: gastroenterologic emergencies, Gastroenterol Clin North Am 17:317-340, 1988.
21. Brolin R and Crosna M: Mast B: use of tubes and radiographs in the management of small bowel obstruction, Ann Surg 206:126-133, 1987.
22. Cranley JP and others: When is endoscopic polypectomy adequate therapy for colonic polyps containing invasive carcinoma? Gastroenterology 91:419, 1986.
23. Christie JP: Malignant colon polyps—cure by colonoscopy or colectomy, Am J Gastroenterol 79:543, 1984.
24. Gryska P, VonRyll R, and Cohen AM: Screening asymptomatic patients at high risk for colon cancer with full colonoscopy, Dis Colon Rectum 30:18-20, 1987.
25. Warden MJ and others: Role of colonoscopy and flexible sigmoidoscopy in screening for colorectal cancer, Dis Colon Rectum 30:52-54, 1987.
26. Luk GD: Colorectal cancer, Gastroenterol Clin North Am 17:654-656, 1988.
27. Sleisenger MH and Fortran JS: Gastrointestinal disease, pathophysiology, diagnosis, and management, ed 4, Philadelphia, 1989, WB Saunders Co, pp 1519-1553.
28. Nemec R: Diverticular disease of the colon; manual of clinical problems in gastroenterology, Boston, 1988, Little, Brown & Co, pp 122-124.
29. Fineman V and Henzel B: Malnutrition: primary and secondary problems: nutritional disorders, metabolic problems, Springhouse, Pa, 1988, Springhouse, pp 38-57.

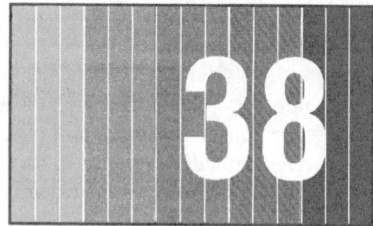

38

Nursing Role in Management

Problems of the Liver, Biliary Tract, and Pancreas

Rachel Elrod

L earning Objectives

1. Differentiate between the three types of jaundice, including common causes and diagnostic findings.
2. Differentiate between the types of viral hepatitis, including etiology, pathophysiology, clinical manifestations, complications, and therapeutic management.
3. Describe the nursing management of the client with viral hepatitis.
4. Explain the etiology, pathogenesis, clinical manifestations, complications, and therapeutic and surgical management of cirrhosis of the liver.
5. Describe the nursing management of the client with cirrhosis.
6. Describe the types, clinical manifestations, and management of carcinoma of the liver.

7. Describe the pathophysiology, clinical manifestations, complications, and therapeutic and surgical management of acute and chronic pancreatitis.
8. Describe the nursing management of the client with pancreatitis.
9. Explain the clinical manifestations and management of carcinoma of the pancreas.
10. Explain the pathophysiology, clinical manifestations, complications, and therapeutic and surgical management of gallbladder disorders.
11. Describe the nursing management of the client undergoing therapeutic or surgical treatment of cholecystitis and cholelithiasis.

JAUNDICE

Jaundice, a yellowish discoloration of body tissues, results from an alteration in normal bilirubin metabolism or flow of bile into the hepatic or biliary duct systems. It is a symptom rather than a disease. Jaundice results when the concentration of bilirubin in the blood becomes abnormally increased. The bilirubin level has to be about three times normal (total serum bilirubin is 2 to 3 mg/dl) for jaundice to occur. Jaundice can usually first be detected in the sclera and skin.

Most of the body's bilirubin is formed from the breakdown of hemoglobin (from erythrocytes) by macrophages (see Fig. 33-6). This unconjugated (indirect) bilirubin is

released into the circulation and is not water soluble, so it is bound to albumin. Because unconjugated bilirubin is not water soluble and cannot be filtered in the kidneys, it is not excreted in the urine. In the liver the unconjugated bilirubin is conjugated with glucuronic acid to form conjugated (direct) bilirubin, which is water soluble. Conjugated bilirubin is secreted into bile, which flows through the hepatic and biliary duct system into the small intestine. In the large intestine, bilirubin is converted to urobilinogen, which is further catabolized to stercobilinogen. Urobilinogen and stercobilinogen give the characteristic brown color to feces. Some urobilinogen is reabsorbed into the portal circulation and returned to the liver. Normally a very small amount of urobilinogen is excreted in urine.

The three types of jaundice are classified as hemolytic, hepatocellular, and obstructive.

Reviewed by Nancy Munn Short, R.N., B.S.N., C.C.R.N., Emergency Department, Duke University Medical Center, Durham, North Carolina.

Table 38-1 Diagnostic Findings in Jaundice

	Hemolytic	Hepatocellular	Obstructive
Serum bilirubin			
Unconjugated (indirect)	↑	↑	Somewhat ↑
Conjugated (direct)	Normal	↑	Moderately ↑
Urine bilirubin	Negative	↑	↑
Urobilinogen			
Stool	↑	Normal to ↓	Negative
Urine	↑	Normal to ↑	Negative

Hemolytic Jaundice

Hemolytic (prehepatic) *jaundice* is due to an increased breakdown of red blood cells (RBCs), which produces an increased amount of unconjugated bilirubin in the blood. The liver is unable to handle this increased load. Consequently, the level of unconjugated bilirubin in the blood rises (Table 38-1). Because unconjugated bilirubin is not water soluble, it is not excreted in the urine. However, increased urobilinogen is produced because of the liver's increased conjugation and excretion of bilirubin. This may result in darker urine and stool. Causes of hemolytic jaundice include blood transfusion reactions, sickle cell crisis, and hemolytic anemia.

Hepatocellular Jaundice

Hepatocellular (hepatic) *jaundice* results from the liver's altered ability to take up bilirubin from the blood or to conjugate or excrete it. Both unconjugated and conjugated bilirubin serum levels increase (see Table 38-1). Because conjugated bilirubin is water soluble, it is excreted in the urine. The urinary urobilinogen may be normal or increased, depending on the diseased liver's ability to take up urobilinogen from the portal circulation. Fecal urobilinogen is normal or decreased, depending on the degree of intrahepatic blockage from fibrosis or inflammation. The most common causes of hepatocellular jaundice are hepatitis, cirrhosis, and hepatic carcinoma.

Obstructive Jaundice

Obstructive (posthepatic) *jaundice* is due to impeded or obstructed flow of bile through the liver or biliary duct system. The obstruction may be intrahepatic or extrahepatic. Intrahepatic obstructions are due to swelling or fibrosis of the liver's canaliculi and bile ducts. This can be caused by damage from liver tumors, hepatitis, or cirrhosis. Causes of extrahepatic obstruction include common bile duct obstruction from a stone, sclerosing cholangitis, and carcinoma of the head of the pancreas.

Laboratory findings show an elevation of both unconjugated and conjugated bilirubin and urine bilirubin (see Table 38-1). There is more of an increase of conjugated bilirubin than of unconjugated bilirubin. Because bilirubin does not enter the intestines, there is decreased to no fecal or urinary urobilinogen. With complete obstruction, the stools are clay-colored.

VIRAL HEPATITIS

Hepatitis is an inflammation of the liver. Acute viral hepatitis is the most common type. The types of viral hepatitis are A, B, non-A, non-B, and delta (hepatitis D). Hepatitis may also be caused by drugs and other chemicals (see Table 33-6). Occasionally hepatitis is caused by bacteria, such as streptococci, *Salmonella* organisms and *Escherichia coli*.

Each year there are 50,000 to 60,000 clinically recognized cases of viral hepatitis in the United States. Because of incomplete reporting, the actual number is thought to be several times higher. Most cases of each type of hepatitis occur among young adults. The incidence of hepatitis A in the United States increased 26% between 1983 and 1988, accounting for 50% of reported cases of hepatitis in 1988. It is most common in children and young adults. The incidence of hepatitis B decreased 18% by 1988, but it is still higher than a decade ago.[1]

Almost 80% of adults over the age of 50 who live in cities have hepatitis A antibodies in their blood, indicating previous infection. By middle age approximately 40% of the population in North America and Western Europe have acquired immunity to hepatitis A.[2]

Etiology

Increasing knowledge in the past decade regarding the viruses that cause hepatitis has been due to the discovery of immunological markers for the viral antigens and antibodies. Hepatitis viruses A, B, and non-A, non-B have been identified. Non-A, non-B includes two types of hepatitis—parenterally transmitted (PT) and enterically transmitted (ET).[1] PT non-A, non-B hepatitis is probably caused by two different agents, one of which has been identified. This agent is an RNA virus and is proposed as hepatitis C virus.[3] Other viruses known to damage the liver include cytomegalovirus, Epstein-Barr virus, herpesvirus, coxsackievirus, and rubella virus.[4] Current terminology regarding viral hepatitis is presented in Table 38-2.

The only way to distinguish the various forms of viral hepatitis is by the presence of the antigens and antigenic subtypes and the subsequent development of antibodies to them. Epidemics of hepatitis are consistently due to hepatitis A virus; 20% to 60% of episodic or sporadic hepatitis is caused by hepatitis B virus or non-A, non-B virus. Infection with each virus provides immunity to that virus (homologous immunity). The client can still develop another type of viral hepatitis. Characteristics of the hepatitis viruses A, B, and non-A, non-B are summarized in Table 38-3.

Hepatitis A virus. The hepatitis A virus (HAV) is an RNA virus. It is found in feces 2 or more weeks before the onset of symptoms, 3 to 4 weeks before jaundice, and before there is an elevation in serum glutamic-oxaloacetic transaminase (SGOT) or aspartate aminotransferase (AST) level. The virus persists in the stool for 1 week after the onset of jaundice. It is present in the blood only briefly. Anti-HAV (antibody to hepatitis A virus) appears in the serum as the stool becomes negative for the virus. It stays in serum indefinitely. The finding of anti-HAV in the serum indicates that the client has had a prior sensitization to hepatitis A virus.

Table 38-2 Terminology Related to Viral Hepatitis

Term	Description
Hepatitis A virus (HAV)	Agent formerly known as infectious hepatitis virus, responsible for hepatitis A infection, present in stool early in course of hepatitis A, RNA virus
IgG anti-HAV	Antibody to HAV, detection during acute illness and present indefinitely
IgM anti-HAV	Specific class antibody to HAV, indication of recent infection with hepatitis A
Hepatitis B virus (HBV)	Agent formerly known as serum hepatitis virus, responsible for hepatitis B infection, present in serum, DNA virus
Hepatitis B surface antigen (HB$_s$Ag)	Group of proteins forming outer coat of HBV; formerly known as Australian antigen and hepatitis-associated antigen; present in serum, body fluids, and hepatocytes in >80% of clients with hepatitis B
Anti-HB$_s$	Antibody to HB$_s$Ag, usually first detectable in convalescence, probably protective antibody, indication of past infection and immunity to HBV
Hepatitis B core antigen (HB$_c$Ag)	Antigenic determinant of core of HBV
Anti-HB$_c$	Antibody to HB$_c$Ag, detectable during and after acute phase of illness
Hepatitis B e-antigen (HB$_e$Ag)	Circulating in serum only, correlation with infectivity of virus
Anti-Hb$_e$	Antibody to HB$_e$Ag, may not be detectable until late in convalescence, presence in serum of HB$_s$Ag carrier suggesting lower titer of HBV
Non-A, non-B hepatitis (NANB)	Forms of viral hepatitis caused by agents other than HAV and HBV, RNA retrovirus
Parenterally transmitted non-A, non-B virus (PT-NANB)	At least two viruses, one known as hepatitis C virus; epidemiologically similar to hepatitis B
Enterically transmitted non-A, non-B virus (ET-NANB)	Cause of epidemics in Africa, Asia, and Mexico
Hepatitis D virus (HDV)	Agent responsible for hepatitis D or delta infection, infection only in the presence of HBV
Anti-HDV	Antibody to delta antigen, indication of present or past infection with delta virus

Table 38-3 Hepatitis A, B, and C Viruses

Characteristic	Hepatitis A	Hepatitis B	Hepatitis C
Incubation period	15-50 days (average 28)	45-160 days (average 120)	14-180 days
Mode of transmission	Fecal-oral (fecal contamination and oral ingestion)	Percutaneous and permucosal; infective blood or body fluids at birth, from sexual contact, from contaminated needles	Parenteral (percutaneous)
Sources of infection and spread of disease	Crowded conditions; poor personal hygiene; poor sanitation; contaminated food, milk, water, and shellfish; persons with subclinical infections	Contaminated needles, syringes, and blood products; sexual activity (heterosexual with multiple partners or with infected persons, homosexual activity); asymptomatic carriers	Blood and blood products, needles and syringes
Virus in feces	3-4 weeks before jaundice	Possible but degraded	No
Virus in serum	Briefly	HB$_s$Ag in serum throughout clinical course	Yes
Carrier state	No	Yes	Yes
γ Globulin (prophylaxis)	Immune serum globulin	Hepatitis B immune globulin or immune serum globulin	Some trials with immune globulin
Diagnostic tests	Anit-HAV IgM, anti-HAV IgG	HB$_s$Ag, HB$_e$Ag, anti-HB$_s$, anti-HB$_c$, anti-HB$_e$	Anti-HCV
Vaccine	Being developed	Manufacture from serum containing HB$_s$Ag or from recombinant vaccine by yeast, provision of immunity to HDV by vaccine	No

HB$_s$Ag, Hepatitis B surface antigen; *HA Ag,* hepatitis A antigen; *HB$_e$AG,* hepatitis B e-antigen; *anti-HB$_s$,* antibody to HB$_s$AG; *anti-HB$_c$,* antibody to hepatitis B core; *anti-HB$_e$,* antibody to HB$_e$Ag; *anti-HCV,* antibody to hepatitis C virus.

Hepatitis B virus. Hepatitis B virus (HBV), which is a DNA virus, is a complex structure with three distinct antigenic particles:

1. Hepatitis B surface antigen (HB_sAg) is a group of proteins that form the outer coat of the hepatitis B virus. It is produced in large amounts by the host liver cells in response to the virus. It is easily detectable in the serum, is present in serum several weeks before jaundice, and persists throughout the clinical course of the disease.

2. Hepatitis B core antigen (HB_cAg) is the antigenic material in the core of the virus. It is probably infectious but it cannot be detected in the blood. The antibody (anti-HB_c) can be detected.

3. Hepatitis B e-antigen (HB_eAg) is found in circulating blood. It is present only in HB_sAg-positive persons. It seems to be associated with the development of chronic liver disease after acute hepatitis B. The e antigen is also present in clients with chronic liver disease who are HB_sAg carriers. The presence of HB_sAg correlates with the time of highest infectivity.[4]

Each antigen has a corresponding antibody that is elicited during an attack of acute viral hepatitis (see Table 38-2). These antibodies can be detected in the serum of persons with prior exposure to the antigenic virus. The presence of anti-HB_s indicates immunity to hepatitis B.

Non-A, non-B hepatitis. Researchers have recently identified an agent responsible for non-A, non-B (NANB) PT hepatitis. It has been named hepatitis C virus (HCV). HCV is one agent responsible for PT hepatitis. There is at least one agent for ET hepatitis. ET-NANB hepatitis is transmitted via the fecal-oral route. It occurs in Africa, Asia, and Mexico.[1] It is a retrovirus (RNA virus). Hepatitis C virus exhibits characteristics of chronic self-perpetuation in the host and stubborn survival in blood. Both epidemiologically and clinically, is more similar to HBV than to HAV. It appears to be the cause of 80% to 90% of cases of transfusion-associated hepatitis. It also occurs in drug abusers, clients in chronic care institutions, health care workers, hemodialysis clients, and renal transplant recipients. There is a carrier state associated with HCV hepatitis.

Pathophysiology

Liver. The pathophysiological changes in the types of viral hepatitis are similar. Hepatitis involves widespread inflammation of liver tissue. Liver cell damage consists of hepatic cell degeneration and necrosis. There is proliferation and enlargement of the Kupffer cells. Inflammation of the periportal areas may interrupt bile flow. Cholestasis may occur. The liver cells regenerate in an orderly manner, and if no complications occur, they should resume their normal appearance and function during convalescence.

Systemic effects. The antigen-antibody complexes between the virus and its corresponding antibody form a circulating immune complex in the early phases of hepatitis. The presence of circulating immune complexes activates the complement system (see Chapter 8). The clinical manifestations of this activation are rash, angioedema, arthritis, fever, and malaise. Glomerulonephritis and vasculitis have also been found secondary to immune complex disease.

Clinical Manifestations

A large number of clients, especially the younger ones, have no symptoms. The clinical manifestations of viral hepatitis may be classified into three phases: (1) the preicteric or prodromal phase, (2) the icteric phase, and (3) the posticteric or convalescent phase (Table 38-4).

Preicteric phase. The *preicteric phase* precedes jaundice and lasts from 1 to 21 days. This is the period of maximal infectivity. Gastrointestinal (GI) symptoms may include anorexia; nausea; abdominal (right upper quadrant) discomfort; and sometimes vomiting, constipation, or diarrhea. The anorexia is frequently severe and is thought to be due to a toxin produced by the diseased liver. The client may find food repugnant and, if a smoker, have a distaste for cigarettes. There is also a decreased sense of smell. Weight loss occurs during the preicteric phase. Other symptoms during this phase are malaise, headache, fever (low-grade), arthralgias, and skin rashes. Physical examination reveals hepatomegaly, lymphadenopathy, and sometimes splenomegaly.

Icteric phase. The *icteric phase* lasts 2 to 4 weeks and is characterized by jaundice. Jaundice results when bilirubin diffuses into the tissues. The urine may darken because of excess bilirubin being excreted by the kidneys. If conjugated bilirubin cannot flow out of the liver because of obstruction or inflammation of the bile ducts, the stools will be light or clay-colored. Pruritus sometimes accompanies the jaundice, especially if cholestasis is present. The pruritus occurs as a result of the accumulation of bile salts beneath the skin.

Table 38-4 Clinical Manifestations of the Phases of Hepatitis

Preicteric	Icteric	Posticteric
Anorexia	Jaundice	Malaise
Nausea, vomiting	Pruritus	Easy fatigability
Right upper quadrant discomfort	Dark urine	Hepatomegaly
Constipation or diarrhea	Bilirubinuria	
Decreased sense of taste and smell	Light stools	
	Fatigue	
Malaise	Continued hepatomegaly with tenderness	
Headache	Feeling of well-being	
Fever	Weight loss	
Arthralgias		
Urticaria		
Hepatomegaly		
Splenomegaly		
Weight loss		

When jaundice occurs, the fever usually subsides. The GI symptoms usually remain, and some fatigue may continue. The liver is usually enlarged and tender. Toward the end of this phase, when the jaundice is receding, the client may experience a feeling of well-being.

Posticteric phase. The convalescent stage of the *posticteric phase* begins as jaundice is disappearing and lasts weeks to months, with an average of 2 to 4 months. During this period the client's major complaint is malaise and easy fatigability. Hepatomegaly remains for several weeks, but splenomegaly subsides during this period. Relapses may occur, and the disappearance of jaundice does not mean the client has totally recovered.

General considerations. Not all clients with viral hepatitis have jaundice. This is referred to as *anicteric hepatitis* and occurs more frequently in children. A high percentage of persons with HAV are anicteric and do not have symptoms.

There is some slight variation in manifestations between the types of hepatitis. In hepatitis A the onset is more acute and the symptoms are usually mild, flulike manifestations. In hepatitis B the onset is more insidious and the symptoms are usually more severe. There may be fewer GI symptoms. Extrahepatic manifestations of HBV include glomerulonephritis and polyarteritis nodosa. These manifestations are thought to be due to the deposition of circulating HB_sAg and its antibody in tissue and subsequent complement activation.

Complications

Most clients with viral hepatitis recover completely with no complications. The mortality rate is very low, with about 1% in HBV and even lower in HBA.[2] The mortality rate is higher in older adults and those with underlying debilitating diseases. Complications that can occur include chronic persistent hepatitis, chronic active hepatitis, fulminant viral hepatitis, and cirrhosis of the liver.

Chronic persistent hepatitis. The most common complication of viral hepatitis is chronic persistent hepatitis in which there is a delayed convalescent period. It is usually benign and is characterized by fatigue and hepatomegaly. Liver function tests may remain abnormal for several years.

Chronic active hepatitis. Chronic active hepatitis is characterized by the persistence of signs and symptoms of hepatitis and abnormal liver function tests for more than 6 months. It is distinguished from chronic persistent hepatitis by liver biopsy. The ongoing process of liver necrosis is likely to progress to cirrhosis. Steroid therapy may be used, especially in clients with severe symptoms. However, there is some controversy regarding its usefulness. Antiviral agents are being evaluated in the treatment of chronic hepatitis. Interferon and adenine arabinoside are two that are being studied extensively.[5]

HB_sAg-positive clients whose serum remains positive for HB_eAg are more likely to have chronic active hepatitis. In addition, alteration in the client's cellular immune response may be important in the development of the chronic HB_sAg carrier state and consequent progression from acute hepatitis B to chronic active hepatitis. This finding may explain why clients with chronic renal failure who are undergoing hemodialysis when hepatitis B develops are more at risk of chronic active hepatitis. (Persons with chronic renal failure are known to have a depressed cellular immune response.)

The HB_sAg persists longer than 6 months in approximately 10% of the clients. These clients also have elevated aminotransferase levels and are considered to have chronic hepatitis.

Fulminant hepatitis. Fulminant viral hepatitis is a clinical syndrome that results in severe impairment or necrosis of liver cells and potential liver failure.[4] Fulminant viral hepatitis develops in a very small percentage of clients. The disorder may occur as a complication of NANB hepatitis or HBV, particularly HBV accompanied by infection with delta virus. Toxic reactions to drugs and congenital metabolic disorders may also cause fulminant hepatitis. Hepatocellular failure with death usually occurs.

Delta hepatitis. The hepatitis delta virus can infect only those persons who have active hepatitis B or who are carriers. The virus is a defective RNA virus that cannot survive on its own and requires the helper function of a DNA virus such as hepatitis B. The importance of hepatitis delta virus relates to its clinical virulence. It can transform asymptomatic or mild chronic hepatitis B infection to severe, progressive chronic active hepatitis and cirrhosis and can accelerate the course of chronic active hepatitis B. Delta virus is also a contributing factor in a substantial proportion of cases of fulminant hepatitis B.[6] Delta hepatitis can occur as a primary infection along with HBV (coinfection) or in a carrier of hepatitis B (superinfection).[7]

Diagnostic Studies

In viral hepatitis many of the liver function tests show significant abnormalities. These findings assist in determining decreased liver function. The common abnormalities are identified in Table 38-5.

Physical assessment reveals hepatic tenderness, hepatomegaly, and splenomegaly. The liver is palpable. A liver biopsy is not indicated unless the diagnosis is in doubt or a more severe form of hepatitis is suspected.

Simple, widely available serological tests for the detection of HAV and anti-HAV are now available. These are radioimmunoassays (RIAs) and enzyme-linked immunosorbent assays (ELISAs).

A diagnostic test available for recent hepatitis A is the IgM antibody test. The IgM anti-HAV appears early and peaks within a few weeks of the onset of symptoms and then declines when the HAV disappears from the stool. The IgG anti-HAV also appears early in the disease but remains in the blood indefinitely. The presence of IgG anti-HAV indicates previous HAV infection and immunity to reinfection.[2] The client who has no IgM antibody but does have IgG does not have acute hepatitis A but has had it in the past and is now immune to it.

Hepatitis B is confirmed by the finding of HB_sAg in the serum. The presence of HB_sAg and anti-HB_s aids in the establishment of a definitive diagnosis. In the early stages hepatitis B can be diagnosed by the presence of HB_sAg, and during the convalescent stage, it can be diagnosed by

Table 38-5   Diagnostic Findings in Hepatitis

Test	Abnormal Finding	Etiology
Transaminase (aminotransferase)		
SGOT (AST)	Elevation	Liver cell injury
SGPT (ALT)	Elevation in preicteric phase; decrease as jaundice disappears	Liver cell injury
Alkaline phosphatase	Some elevation	Impaired excretory function of the liver
Serum proteins		
γ Globulin	Normal or increase	Liver damage
Albumin	Normal or decrease	Liver damage
Serum bilirubin (total)	Elevation to about 8-15 mg/dl	Hepatocellular damage
Urinary bilirubin	Elevation	Conjugated hyperbilirubinemia
Urinary urobilinogen	Elevation 2-5 days before jaundice	Diminished reabsorption of urobilinogen
Prothrombin time	Prolonged	Decreased absorption of vitamin K in intestine with decreased production of prothrombin by liver
HAV—fecal	Presence in hepatitis A until jaundice disappears	Antigen in feces
HAV—serum	Presence in hepatitis A (brief)	Antigen in serum
HB$_s$Ag—serum	Positive in hepatitis B	Surface antigen in serum
IgG anti-HAV	Positive in hepatitis A	Development early in disease
IgM anti-HAV	Early appearance in hepatitis A	Indication of recent hepatitis A infection
Anti-HB$_s$	Presence during convalescent stage of hepatitis B	Indication of immunity to hepatitis B

Table 38-6

Diagnostic and Therapeutic Management: Viral Hepatitis

DIAGNOSTIC

Liver function studies
Hepatitis serology
   HB$_s$Ag (HB$_e$Ag in some cases)
   Anti-HB$_s$
   Anti-HB$_c$
   Anti-HAV

THERAPEUTIC

High-calorie, moderate- to high-protein, high-carbohydrate, low-fat diet
Vitamin supplements
Rest—degree of strictness varying

the presence of the anti-HB$_s$. Currently tests for NANB hepatitis consist of tests to exclude HAV, HBV, cytomegalovirus, and Epstein-Barr virus.[8] It is hoped that with the recent identification of the HCV, there will be a more definitive test for the identification of NANB hepatitis.

Therapeutic Management

There is no specific treatment or therapy for viral hepatitis. Emphasis is on measures to rest the body and assist the liver in regenerating (Table 38-6). Adequate nutrients and rest seem to be most beneficial for healing and liver cell regeneration. Dietary emphasis is on a well-balanced diet that the client can tolerate (see p. 1127).

Rest reduces the metabolic demands on the liver, increases the blood supply to the liver, and thus promotes cell regeneration. Strict bed rest may be considered during the icteric phase. Many physicians believe that strict bed rest is not essential and that alternating periods of activity and rest are adequate. The type of rest ordered may depend on the severity of symptoms, the client's degree of fatigue, and the degree of changes in the liver function tests, particularly the enzymes.

Pharmacological Management

There are no specific drug therapies for the treatment of viral hepatitis. Steroid therapy is usually reserved for the client who is extremely ill, has chronic active hepatitis, or seems in danger of having fulminating hepatitis. Dosage may be as high as 80 mg per day in cases of acute illness. Corticosteroids increase the appetite and improve the sense of well-being. They also improve the metabolism of cholesterol and in this way decrease bilirubin levels and cholestasis. Therefore jaundice and pruritus are decreased.

Supportive drug therapy may include antiemetics, such as dimenhydrinate (Dramamine) or trimethobenzamide (Tigan). Phenothiazines should not be used because of their possible cholestatic and hepatotoxic effects. If the client requires a sedative or hypnotic drug, diphenhydramine (Benadryl) or chloral hydrate may be used.

Immune globulin is used in the prevention and modification of viral hepatitis. Immune serum globulin (ISG) is effective for hepatitis A and offers some protection against hepatitis B because it contains varying amounts of the hepatitis B antibody. ISG is adequate except in a definite contact exposure. Hepatitis B immune globulin (HBIG) is prepared from plasma of donors with a high titer of anti-HB$_s$. HBIG is very expensive. ISG provides temporary passive immunity and is recommended in cases of exposure to hepatitis A from close (household) contact in persons who are not positive for anti-HAV and for travelers to foreign countries. HBIG provides temporary passive immunity and is recommended for exposure when the source of exposure has a positive test for HB$_s$Ag. Examples include accidental needle sticks, mucosal contact, sexual exposure, and transmission to a neonate.[5] There are two vaccines available for hepatitis B (Heptavax-B and Recombivax-HB).

Nutritional Considerations

No special diet is required in the treatment of viral hepatitis. However, a diet high in carbohydrates with moderate to high protein and low fat content is usually recommended. Adequate calories are important because the client usually loses weight. If fat content is poorly tolerated because of lack of bile in the intestines, it should be reduced. Basically the specific foods on the diet are dictated by the client. Vitamin supplements, particularly B complex and vitamin K, are frequently used.

If anorexia, nausea, and vomiting are severe, intravenous (IV) solutions of glucose or supplemental tube feedings may be used. Fluid and electrolyte balance must be maintained.

■ Nursing Management of Hepatitis

Nursing assessment
Subjective and objective data that should be obtained from a person with hepatitis are presented in Table 38-7.

Nursing diagnoses
Nursing diagnoses are determined when the problem and the etiological factors are supported by clinical data. Nursing diagnoses related to hepatitis may include, but are not limited to, those presented in Table 38-8.

Nursing interventions
Health maintenance and promotion. Viral hepatitis is a community health problem. The nurse must assume a significant role in the control and prevention of this disease. It is helpful to first understand the epidemiology of the different types of viral hepatitis before considering appropriate control measures.

HEPATITIS A. Epidemics of viral hepatitis are almost always due to HAV. The mode of transmission of HAV is predominantly fecal-oral (mainly by ingestion of food or liquid infected with the virus) and rarely parenteral. Poor hygiene, crowded situations, and poor sanitary conditions are all factors related to hepatitis A. The disease occurs more frequently in underdeveloped countries. Infected food handlers may be a source of infection. Certain foods, such as contaminated milk, water, and shellfish, are other sources of infection. The eating of raw shellfish from contaminated waters is a current source of infection.

Table 38-7

 Nursing Assessment of the Client with Hepatitis

SUBJECTIVE DATA

History
IV drug and alcohol abuse; hemophilia, blood transfusions, or hemodialysis; exposure to infected persons; ingestion of contaminated food or water; sexual promiscuity; exposure to benzene or carbon tetrachloride; ingestion of poison mushrooms; crowded, unsanitary living conditions; exposure to contaminated needles; recent travel

Medications
Use and misuse of acetaminophen, phenytoin, halothane, methyldopa

General
Malaise, headache, weight loss, fatigue, anorexia, distaste for cigarettes (in smokers)

Pain
Right upper quadrant pain and tenderness

Integumentary
Pruritus, urticaria

Gastrointestinal
Nausea and vomiting, light-colored stools, diarrhea, feeling of fullness in right upper quadrant

Urinary
Dark urine

Musculoskeletal
Arthralgias, myalgias

OBJECTIVE DATA

General
Low-grade fever, lethargy, lymphadenopathy

Integumentary
Rash, angioedema, jaundice, icteric sclera, injection sites

Gastrointestinal
Hepatomegaly, splenomegaly

Possible findings
Abnormal liver function tests; anemia; serological tests positive for hepatitis, including HB$_s$Ag, anti-HB$_s$, anti-HB$_c$, anti-HAV, elevated serum bilirubin; abnormal liver scan; positive liver biopsy

There does not seem to be a chronic carrier state for HAV. The virus is present in feces during the incubation period, so it can be carried by persons who have undetectable, subclinical infections. It can also be transmitted by clients with anicteric hepatitis A.

Preventive measures include personal and environmental hygiene and health education to promote good sanitation. Hand washing is essential and is probably the most important precaution. Health teaching should include careful hand washing after bowel movements and before eating.

According to the Centers for Disease Control (CDC) guidelines, enteric or disease-specific precautions should be followed for the client with hepatitis A. Hospitals deter-

Table 38-8

NURSING CARE PLAN FOR THE CLIENT WITH VIRAL HEPATITIS

Defining Characteristics	Nursing Interventions	Evaluation Criteria
NURSING DIAGNOSIS: Altered nutrition: less than body requirements related to anorexia, nausea, and reduced metabolism of nutrients by liver		
Inadequate food intake; perceived inability to ingest food; lack of interest in food; aversion to eating; actual or potential metabolic needs in excess of intake, with or without weight loss	Offer frequent small feedings, provide oral care before meals. Allow client to choose food items. Serve highest-calorie and protein nutrients at time of day client feels most like eating. Provide attractively served meals in pleasant surroundings. Assess nutritional status.	Adequate nutritional intake; maintenance of normal body weight
NURSING DIAGNOSIS: Activity intolerance related to fatigue, weakness, increased energy utilization associated with increased basal metabolic rate due to viral infection, and inadequate nutritional status		
Verbal report of fatigue or weakness, altered response to activity (blood pressure, pulse, respirations)	Plan rest periods. Increase client's activity gradually as allowed and tolerated. Conserve client's strength. Teach client to monitor and control activities that provoke fatigue.	Increased tolerance for activity
NURSING DIAGNOSIS: Anxiety related to lack of understanding of diagnosis, anticipated changes in lifestyle, and fear of prognosis and complications		
Increased tension, apprehension, fright, distress, restlessness, insomnia, trembling, expression of concern regarding changes in health status	Assess level of anxiety. Provide reassurance and comfort. Convey sense of empathic understanding (e.g., touch, quiet presence). Ascertain and support current coping skills. Encourage verbalization of fear and anxiety. Explain tests, procedures, and health maintenance behaviors.	Description of own anxiety and coping patterns, verbalization of increase in psychological and physiological comfort
NURSING DIAGNOSIS: Upper abdominal pain related to inflammation of the liver		
Communication of pain descriptors, guarding behavior, narrowed self-focus, behaviors indicative of pain (e.g., moaning)	Administer mild analgesic as ordered. Use nursing care measures to help relieve the discomfort or pain (e.g., position changes, back rub, relaxation, diversion, guided imagery).	Verbalization of decreased discomfort, absence of objective signs of discomfort or pain, relaxed demeanor
NURSING DIAGNOSIS: Body-image disturbance related to stigma of having a communicable disease, change in appearance (jaundice), and possible alterations in lifestyle and roles (alcohol consumption, drug use, restriction of sexual activity)		
Verbal and/or nonverbal response to actual or perceived change in structure or function	Clarify misconceptions regarding limitations. Encourage participation in self-care. Instruct client in ways to prevent spread of hepatitis. Assist client in expressing feelings. Allow client to ask questions, and encourage client.	Adaptation to changes in appearance, verbalization of understanding of body changes, seeking of information

Table 38-8

NURSING CARE PLAN FOR THE CLIENT WITH VIRAL HEPATITIS—cont'd

Defining Characteristics	Nursing Interventions	Evaluation Criteria

NURSING DIAGNOSIS: Altered health maintenance related to lack of knowledge of follow-up care

Frequent questions about transmission of disease, activities allowed, and general follow-up care	Teach client basic facts about illness, modes of transmission, diet, activities allowed, avoidance of alcohol, and need for follow-up care.	Verbalization of understanding of follow-up care, planning of follow-up visit with health-care provider

NURSING DIAGNOSIS: Fatigue related to flulike symptoms secondary to viral infection

Malaise, nausea, vomiting, diarrhea, fever	Apply heat to aching muscles and joints as ordered. Monitor intake and output. Provide small feedings as tolerated. Medicate as needed for fever. Provide periods of uninterrupted rest.	Verbalization of increased comfort

Table 38-9   Isolation Precautions for Hepatitis

	Hepatitis A	Hepatitis B	Hepatitis Non-A, Non-B
Mask	No	No	No
Gloves	Yes, for touching infective material	Yes, for touching infective material when handling feces if GI bleeding	Yes, for touching infective material
Gowns	If soiling likely (feces)	If soiling likely (blood or body fluids)	If soiling likely (blood or body fluids)
Private room	Only if client hygiene poor	No	No
Infective material	Feces (possible)	Blood and body fluids	Blood and body fluids
Length of precautions	7 days after onset of jaundice	Until negative for HB_sAg	Duration of illness

mine which precautions (enteric or disease-specific) they wish to use. Table 38-9 outlines the isolation precautions for hepatitis A, B, and non-A, non-B. (For enteric precautions, see Table 7-15.)

Because the peak excretion of HAV occurs about the time of the onset of symptoms and is not detectable by the time the enzymes such as the SGOT (AST) reach their peak, it is not necessary to enforce precautions for the entire icteric period. Isolation precautions should be maintained for about 1 week from the onset of jaundice. Family and significant others should be given clear, concise instructions and explanations regarding the isolation procedures. However, if the client goes home after the communicable time period, no further isolation precautions are necessary.

A major preventive measure for hepatitis A is administration of ISG. Because clients with hepatitis A are most infectious just before the onset of symptoms, those exposed (through household contact) should be given ISG within 1 to 2 weeks of exposure. If the contact has anti-

HAV antibodies, the ISG is not necessary. ISG may not prevent infection, but it will modify the illness to a subclinical infection. ISG provides 6 to 8 weeks of passive protection. It may also be used as a prophylactic measure for travelers to foreign countries that have a high incidence of hepatitis. A vaccine for active immunization against hepatitis A is being developed but is not yet available.[5]

HEPATITIS B. It was previously thought that HBV was transmitted only by percutaneous inoculation with contaminated needles, instruments, blood, and blood products. Now it is known there are other modes of transmission. HB_sAg has been detected in almost every body fluid: (1) vaginal secretions, (2) menstrual fluids, (3) semen, (4) saliva, (5) respiratory secretions, (6) tears, (7) gastric juice, (8) synovial fluid, and (9) cerebrospinal fluid. When the HB_sAg is found in these secretions, it is in even higher concentrations in the blood.

Nonpercutaneous transmission is not as common as percutaneous transmission, but it does occur, particularly among sexual partners of HB_sAg carriers, both with and

without symptoms. HBV is definitely transmitted by sexual intercourse. The venereal route is probably the most predominant means of nonpercutaneous spread, where transmission occurs via permucosal routes. In some areas the incidence among male homosexuals has surpassed IV drug abuse as a source of infection. Kissing and sharing of food items may spread the virus via saliva. There is very little, if any, likelihood of enteric transmission because the HBV is degraded by intestinal mucosal enzymes and enzymes from the bacterial flora. If GI bleeding occurs, the feces can be contaminated with the virus from the blood.

There are symptom-free carriers of HBV (0.1% to 0.5% of the general population in the United States), with an even higher incidence of carriers among medical and other health care workers. The HB_sAg level remains elevated in carriers (HB_sAg-positive on at least two occasions at least 6 months apart). Liver enzyme values may be normal.[8] The carriers of hepatitis B may have low-grade disease, a normal liver, or a severe chronic liver disease. A positive test for anti-HB_s in adults indicates that they have had hepatitis B or the vaccine.

Control and prevention of hepatitis B focuses on identification of possible exposure via percutaneous and sexual transmission. Good hygienic practices, including handwashing, are important. A condom is advised for sexual intercourse and the partner should be vaccinated. Razors, toothbrushes, and other personal items should not be shared. Close contacts of the client with hepatitis B who are HB_sAg negative and antibody negative should be vaccinated.[5] Other measures include the use of washed RBCs and the screening of blood donors for HB_sAg. Clients who have anti-HB_s in their blood and receive transfusions seem to be protected from hepatitis B. An added control measure then is to administer blood containing anti-HB_s.

The nurse must be aware of the groups at high risk of contracting hepatitis B. These include hemodialysis clients, other clients receiving frequent transfusions, workers in hemodialysis units and blood chemistry laboratories, IV drug abusers, persons with a homosexual lifestyle, prison inmates, and household and sexual partners of HBV carriers.

According to CDC guidelines, universal precautions should be followed for the client with hepatitis B. This includes use of disposable needles and syringes, which should be disposed of in puncture-resistant disposal units without bending or breaking. With the use of universal precautions, many agencies have no specific isolation procedures for hepatitis A or B. (See Table 38-9 for the necessary precautions for hepatitis B. Table 8-28 outlines universal precautions.) Because HBV remains in the blood for a much longer time than HAV remains in the stool, isolation is usually carried out during the client's entire hospitalization.

Antiviral chemotherapy (e.g., interferons) is being attempted to try to eliminate the chronic HBV carrier state. Passive immunization for postexposure prophylaxis may be provided with either ISG or HBIG. The ISG seems to offer some protection against hepatitis B. There is a formalin-treated hepatitis B vaccine made from purified HB_sAg-containing particles (Heptavax-B). The vaccine is made from the plasma of chronic HB_sAg carriers. The vaccine is given in a series of three intramuscular (in the deltoid) injections. The second one is administered within 1 month of the first one, and the third one within 6 months after the first. The cost is about $150 for the series. The vaccine is 90% to 95% effective. Only minor adverse reactions have been reported—transient fever and soreness at the injection site. Some persons do not want to take Heptavax-B vaccine because of fear of contracting acquired immunodeficiency syndrome. There is no evidence of contamination of the vaccine with the human immunodeficiency virus.[9] The vaccine is recommended to provide active immunity to hepatitis B in high-risk clients and health care providers.

The CDC recommends vaccination for health care providers who are frequently exposed to blood and other body fluids. Included among high-risk clients are users of illicit drugs, homosexual men, persons with hemophilia, sexual contacts, household members of carriers, and dialysis clients. Because passive immunization with HBIG does not interfere with the response to the vaccine, both may be administered after needle-stick exposure and sexual contact exposure.

An alternative vaccine (Recombivax HB) is now also available. This vaccine is genetically engineered, being produced by a recombinant strain of yeast. The two vaccines—Heptavax-B and Recombivax HB—are similar in effectiveness, safety, route of administration, and immunization schedule.[9] Preventive and control measures for hepatitis A and B are summarized in Table 38-10.

HEPATITIS NON-A, NON-B. The majority of cases of transfusion-associated hepatitis involve NANB hepatitis. This also occurs in drug abusers, clients in chronic care institutions, health care workers, and dialysis clients. At this time less is known about hepatitis NANB. Because it resembles HBV epidemiologically, similar precautions are used for NANB and HBV. Excluding blood donors with elevated SGPT (ALT) levels reduces the incidence of NANB hepatitis. Also, paid donors and donors with a history of hepatitis should be excluded.[5]

Control of hepatitis in hospital personnel

HEPATITIS A. Hepatitis A is rarely transmitted from clients to personnel. When this does occur, it is associated with clients with undiagnosed hepatitis who are hospitalized for other problems. Usually these clients are incontinent of feces.

HEPATITIS B. Transmission of HBV occurs when there is parenteral or mucosal exposure to HB_sAg-positive blood from clients who have acute hepatitis B or who are carriers. These two groups of persons have high concentrations of HBV in the blood and serous fluids. The risk of contracting hepatitis B from clients is definitely related to contact with blood or body fluids. Client contact without contact with blood is not considered a risk factor. The greatest risk to health care workers is from contact with symptom-free carriers. About 1% of clients admitted to large metropolitan hospitals are HB_sAg-positive. Most of these (90%) are not routinely identified. Because of this, it has been suggested that certain groups with a high carrier rate have routine HB_sAg determinations. Included are persons with

Table 38-10   Preventive Measures for Viral Hepatitis

Hepatitis A	Hepatitis B
Hand washing	*Percutaneous transmission*
Good personal hygiene	Screening of blood donors for HB$_s$Ag
Environmental sanitation	Administration of washed RBCs
Control and screening of food handlers (especially while carrying virus)	Administration of blood containing anti-HB$_s$ when possible
Enteric precautions (before jaundice)	Use of disposable needles and syringes
ISG	*Sexual transmission*
Early administration to those exposed (during incubation period)	Administration of HBIG to sexual partners of HB$_s$Ag-positive persons
Use as prophylaxis for travelers to tropical and developing countries	Testing of sexual partners for susceptibility (test for anti-HB$_c$)
	Administration of hepatitis B vaccine series for sexual partners
	Use of condom for sexual intercourse
	Avoidance of sharing of toothbrushes and razors (treated as sexual exposure)
	General measures
	Hand washing
	Registration of carriers
	Passive immunization
	ISG (for exposure)
	HBIG (one-time exposure [needle stick, contact with material from mucous membrane])
	Active immunization
	Vaccine (high-risk persons, household and sexual contacts of HBV carriers, health care providers)

Table 38-11   Measures to Prevent Transmission of Hepatitis Viruses from Clients to Personnel*

Hepatitis A	Hepatitis B	Hepatitis Non-A, Non-B
Always maintain good personal hygiene.	Use blood precautions	Use blood precautions.
Wash hands.	Wash hands.	Wash hands.
Follow isolation precautions when caring for client with hepatitis A.	Have minimal contact with blood or blood-contaminated excretions.	Have minimal contact with blood or blood-contaminated excretions.
	Handle the blood of clients as potentially infective.	Handle the blood of clients as potentially infective.
	Dispose of needles properly.	Dispose of needles properly.
	Administer ISG after exposure by needle sticks or mucosal contact.	
	Administer HBV vaccine to high-risk hospital personnel, such as those who have more physical exposure to blood; some hospitals use serology screening to determine vaccine use.	

*A suggested guideline for general practice to prevent the nurse from contracting viral hepatitis from undiagnosed clients and carriers is for the nurse to wear disposable gloves when handling (1) soiled bedpans, urinals, and catheters and (2) client's bed linens soiled by body excreta or secretions. Universal precautions should be followed during the care of all clients (see Table 8-28).

drug abuse problems, chronic liver disease, chronic renal failure, Hodgkin's disease, leukemia, Down syndrome, and polyarteritis nodosa.[1]

The principal mode of transmission of HBV in the hospital is parenteral. Examples of parenteral transmission include accidental needle sticks and transfusion of contaminated blood or blood products. Other forms of transmission may include contamination of fresh cutaneous scratches or abrasions, burns, and contamination of mucosal surfaces with infective serum, saliva, or semen.

NON-A, NON-B HEPATITIS. Transmission is usually due to percutaneous needle exposure or other blood exposure and undetected parenteral transmission. Measures to prevent transmission of the viruses from clients to personnel are presented in Table 38-11. Very rarely do health care workers infect client contacts.

Acute intervention

JAUNDICE. The nurse should assess for the degree of jaundice. In light-skinned persons the jaundice is usually observed first in the sclera of the eyes and later in the skin.

In dark-skinned persons, jaundice is observed in the hard palate of the mouth and inner canthus of the eyes. Ictotest reagent tablets may be used to detect urinary bilirubin. Comfort measures to relieve pruritus (if present), headache, and arthralgias are helpful (see Table 38-8).

ISOLATION. When the client with suspected viral hepatitis is admitted to the hospital, universal precautions should be instituted by health care personnel until the type of hepatitis can be determined.

NUTRITION. An important measure in assisting liver cells to regenerate is adequate nutrition (see p. 1127). Ensuring that the client receives adequate nutrients is not always easy. The anorexia and extreme distaste for food cause nutritional problems. Dietary assessment must be considered. The nurse should try to determine whether there is something that appeals to the client in spite of the anorexia. Small, frequent meals may be preferable to three large ones and may also help to prevent nausea. Frequently, clients with hepatitis find that anorexia is not as severe in the morning, so it is easier to eat a good breakfast than a large dinner. Measures to stimulate the appetite, such as mouth care, antiemetics, and attractively served meals in pleasant surroundings, should be included in the nursing care plan. Other measures that may be tried to counteract the anorexia are carbonated beverages and avoidance of very hot or very cold foods.

REST. Rest is essential and is another factor in promoting liver cell regeneration. The nurse must assess the client's response to the rest and activity plan and modify it accordingly. The care plan should include appropriate time schedules for rest and activity, with scheduled rest periods uninterrupted by visitors or nursing staff. If the client is on strict bed rest, measures to prevent respiratory and circulatory complications should be initiated. Assessment of the liver function tests and other symptoms should continue as a guide to activity.

Psychological and emotional rest are as essential as physical rest. Strict bed rest may produce anxiety and extreme restlessness in some clients and may be more damaging than reasonable ambulation. Diversional activities, such as reading and hobbies (for example, knitting, stamp collecting), may help the client. The client should be assisted to understand the temporary nature of symptoms, especially sexual abstinence, during the period of communicability.

Chronic management. To assist the client to complete recovery, the nurse must assess the client's knowledge of nutrition and provide the necessary dietary teaching. Rest and adequate nutrition are especially important until studies show that liver function has returned to normal. The client must be cautioned about overexertion and the need to follow the physician's advice about when it is safe to return to work.

The client should be assessed for any manifestations indicative of complications. Bleeding tendencies with increasing prothrombin time, symptoms of encephalopathy, or markedly abnormal liver function tests indicate problems, and the client should be assessed and treated promptly.

The client should be instructed to have regular follow-up for at least 1 year after the diagnosis of hepatitis. Because relapses are fairly common, the client should be instructed about symptoms of recurrence. Alcohol should be avoided for 1 year because it is detoxified in the liver and may interfere with recovery.

Clients who remain positive for HB_sAg are carriers and should never be blood donors. The client with hepatitis B should also be instructed to use condoms when engaging in sexual intercourse until the enzyme levels are near normal or tests for HB_sAg are negative.

TOXIC AND DRUG-INDUCED HEPATITIS
Etiology

Liver injury and death may occur after the inhalation, parenteral injection, or ingestion of certain chemical substances (see Table 33-6). The two major types of chemical hepatotoxicity are toxic and drug induced. Agents producing *toxic hepatitis* (carbon tetrachloride, gold compounds, acetaminophen) are generally systemic poisons or are converted in the liver to toxic metabolites. Liver necrosis generally occurs within 2 to 3 days of acute exposure to a toxic substance.

Idiosyncratic drug reactions produce *drug-induced hepatitis*. Such agents as halothane, isoniazid, chlorothiazides, methotrexate, and α-methyldopa may produce idiosyncratic reactions because of (1) client susceptibility (metabolic reactivity) to these agents or (2) immunologically mediated hypersensitivity responses. Liver injury may occur at any time during or shortly after exposure. Some responses occur 2 to 5 weeks after exposure.

Clinical Manifestations and Therapeutic Management

Toxic and drug-induced hepatitis are similar to viral hepatitis in the pathophysiological changes in the liver and the clinical manifestations. The usual presenting clinical findings are anorexia, nausea, vomiting, hepatomegaly, splenomegaly, and abnormal liver function studies. Treatment is largely supportive, as in acute viral hepatitis. Recovery may be rapid if the hepatotoxin is identified and removed. Liver transplantation may be necessary.

CIRRHOSIS OF THE LIVER

Cirrhosis is a chronic progressive disease of the liver characterized by extensive degeneration and destruction of the liver parenchymal cells. The liver cells attempt to regenerate, but the regenerative process is disorganized, resulting in abnormal blood vessel and bile duct relationships from the fibrosis. The overgrowth of new and fibrous connective tissue distorts the liver's normal lobular structure, resulting in lobules of irregular size and shape with impeded vascular flow. Cirrhosis may have a very insidious, prolonged course.

Cirrhosis is ranked as the fourth leading cause of death in persons after the age of 40. The highest incidence occurs between the ages of 40 and 60, and it is twice as common in men as in women. Excessive alcohol ingestion is the single most common cause of cirrhosis.[10]

Etiology

The four types of cirrhosis, in order of incidence, are as follows:

1. *Laennec's cirrhosis* (also called *portal, nutritional,* or *alcoholic cirrhosis*) is usually associated with alcohol abuse. Alcoholism is the most important etiological factor in cirrhosis. The first change in the liver from excessive alcohol intake is an accumulation of fat in the liver cells. Uncomplicated fatty changes in the liver are potentially reversible if the person stops drinking alcohol. If the alcohol abuse continues, widespread scar formation occurs throughout the liver.

2. *Postnecrotic cirrhosis* is a complication of toxic or viral hepatitis. Broad bands of scar tissue form within the liver.

3. *Biliary cirrhosis* is associated with chronic biliary obstruction and infection. There is diffuse fibrosis of the liver, with jaundice as the main feature.

4. *Cardiac cirrhosis* results from long-standing severe right-sided heart failure in clients with cor pulmonale, constrictive pericarditis, and tricuspid insufficiency.

Pathophysiology

In cirrhosis, cell necrosis occurs, and the destroyed liver cells are replaced by scar tissue. The normal lobular architecture becomes nodular. Eventually irregular, disorganized regeneration, poor cellular nutrition, and hypoxia due to an inadequate blood flow and scar tissue result in less functioning liver tissue.

The specific cause of cirrhosis remains a mystery and cannot be determined in many clients. It is known that cirrhosis occurs with greatest frequency among alcoholics. There continues to be some controversy as to whether the cause is the alcohol or the malnutrition that frequently coexists with chronic ingestion of alcohol. There have been cases of nutritional cirrhosis resulting from extreme dieting or malnutrition. It is believed that the combined impact of malnutrition and alcohol is especially damaging to liver cells. Alcohol is known to produce necrosis of cells and fatty infiltration with formation of fibrous septa. There is evidence that alcohol alone can cause liver damage.[4] Some persons seem to have a predisposition to cirrhosis, regardless of their dietary or alcoholic intake.

Clinical Manifestations

Early manifestations. The onset of cirrhosis is usually insidious but may be sudden. GI disturbances are common early symptoms and include anorexia, dyspepsia, flatulence, nausea and vomiting, and change in bowel habits (diarrhea or constipation). These symptoms occur as a result of the liver's altered metabolism of carbohydrates, fats, and proteins. The client may complain of abdominal pain described as a dull, heavy feeling in the right upper quadrant or epigastrium. The pain is due to swelling and stretching of the liver capsule, spasm of the biliary ducts, and intermittent vascular spasm. Other early manifestations are fever, lassitude, slight weight loss, and enlargement of the liver and spleen. The liver is palpable in many clients with cirrhosis.

Later manifestations. Later symptoms may be severe and result from liver failure and portal hypertension. Jaundice, peripheral edema, and ascites develop gradually. Other late symptoms include skin lesions, hematological disorders, endocrine disturbances, and peripheral neuropathies (Fig. 38-1). In the advanced stages the liver becomes small and nodular.

Jaundice. Jaundice results from the functional derangement of liver cells and compression of bile ducts by connective tissue overgrowth. Jaundice occurs as a result of the decreased ability to conjugate and excrete the bilirubin. The jaundice may be minimal or severe, depending on the degree of liver damage. It is usually hepatocellular jaundice. If obstruction of the biliary tract occurs, obstructive jaundice also results and is usually accompanied by pruritus. The pruritus is due to an accumulation of bile salts underneath the skin.

Skin lesions. Various skin manifestations are commonly seen in cirrhosis. *Spider angiomas* (telangiectasia or spider nevi) are small, dilated blood vessels with a bright red center point and spiderlike branches. They occur on the nose, cheeks, upper trunk, neck, and shoulders. *Palmar erythema* (red areas that blanch with pressure) is located on the palms of the hands. Both of these lesions are attributed to an increase in circulating estrogen as a result of the liver's inability to inactivate it.

Hematological problems. Hematological problems include thrombocytopenia, leukopenia, anemia, and coagulation disorders. Thrombocytopenia, leukopenia, and anemia are probably due to the splenomegaly. Splenomegaly results from backup of blood from the portal vein into the spleen. Overactivity of the enlarged spleen results in increased removal of blood cells from circulation. The anemia is also due to inadequate RBC production and survival. Other factors involved in the anemia relate to poor diet, poor absorption of folic acid, and bleeding from varices.

The coagulation problems result from the liver's inability to produce prothrombin and other factors essential for blood clotting. Coagulation problems are manifested by hemorrhagic phenomena or bleeding tendencies, such as epistaxis, purpura, petechiae, easy bruising, gingival bleeding, and heavy menstrual bleeding.

Endocrine disturbances. Several symptoms relating to the metabolism and inactivation of adrenocortical hormones, estrogen, and testosterone occur in cirrhosis. Normally the liver inactivates these hormones. When the damaged liver is unable to do this, various manifestations occur. In the male, gynecomastia, loss of axillary and pubic hair, testicular atrophy, and impotence with loss of libido may occur as a result of estrogen accumulation. In younger females amenorrhea may occur, and in older females there may be vaginal bleeding. The liver fails to metabolize aldosterone adequately, and this results in hyperaldosteronism with sodium and fluid retention.

Peripheral neuropathy. Peripheral neuropathy is a common finding in alcohol-associated cirrhosis. It is prob-

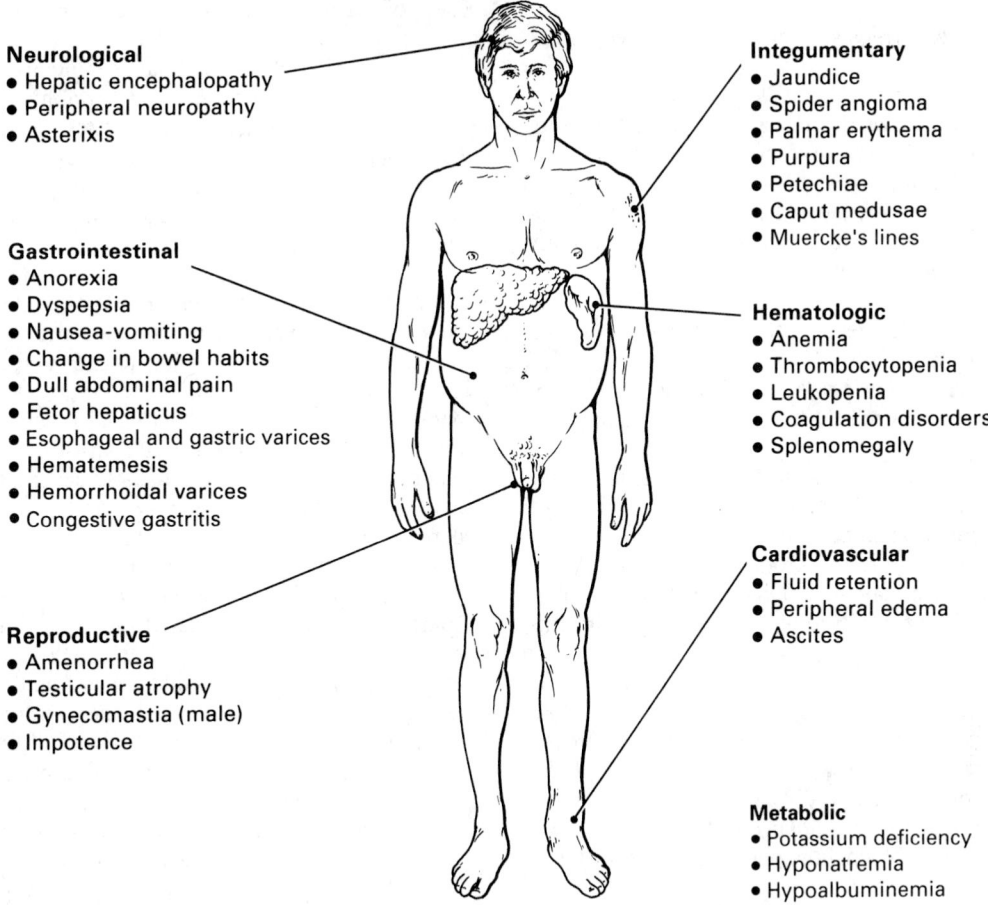

Neurological
• Hepatic encephalopathy
• Peripheral neuropathy
• Asterixis

Gastrointestinal
• Anorexia
• Dyspepsia
• Nausea-vomiting
• Change in bowel habits
• Dull abdominal pain
• Fetor hepaticus
• Esophageal and gastric varices
• Hematemesis
• Hemorrhoidal varices
• Congestive gastritis

Reproductive
• Amenorrhea
• Testicular atrophy
• Gynecomastia (male)
• Impotence

Integumentary
• Jaundice
• Spider angioma
• Palmar erythema
• Purpura
• Petechiae
• Caput medusae
• Muercke's lines

Hematologic
• Anemia
• Thrombocytopenia
• Leukopenia
• Coagulation disorders
• Splenomegaly

Cardiovascular
• Fluid retention
• Peripheral edema
• Ascites

Metabolic
• Potassium deficiency
• Hyponatremia
• Hypoalbuminemia

Fig. 38-1   Systemic clinical manifestations of liver cirrhosis.

ably due to a dietary deficiency of thiamine, folic acid, and vitamin B_{12}. The neuropathy usually results in mixed nervous system symptoms, but sensory symptoms may predominate. Clinical manifestations of cirrhosis of the liver are numerous and may eventually involve the total body (see Fig. 38-1).

Complications

Major complications of cirrhosis are portal hypertension with resultant esophageal varices, peripheral edema and ascites, hepatic encephalopathy (coma), and hepatorenal syndrome.

Portal hypertension and esophageal varices. Because of the structural changes in the liver from the cirrhotic process, there is compression and destruction of the portal and hepatic veins and sinusoids. These changes result in obstruction to the normal flow of blood through the portal system, resulting in portal hypertension. There are many pathophysiological changes that result from portal hypertension. Collateral circulation develops in an attempt to reduce this high portal pressure and also to reduce the increased plasma volume and lymphatic flow. The common areas where the collateral channels form are in the lower esophagus (the anastomosis of the left gastric vein and the azygos veins), the anterior abdominal wall, the parietal peritoneum, and the rectum. Varicosites may develop in

areas where the collateral and systemic circulations communicate, resulting in *esophageal and gastric varices, caput medusae* (ring of varices around the umbilicus), and *hemorrhoids*.

Esophageal varices (graded I to IV) are a common complication, occurring in anywhere from two thirds to three fourths of clients with cirrhosis. These collateral vessels contain little elastic tissue and are quite fragile. They tolerate the high pressure poorly, and the result is distended, tortuous veins that bleed easily. Large varices are more likely to bleed.

Clients with bleeding esophageal varices have a high mortality rate. These varices are the most life-threatening complication of cirrhosis. The mortality rate is 67% to 75% in clients with severe liver dysfunction.[11] Recurrence of bleeding is very high.

The varices rupture and bleed in response to ulceration and irritation. Factors producing ulceration and irritation include alcohol ingestion; swallowing of poorly masticated food; ingestion of coarse food; acid regurgitation from the stomach; and increased intraabdominal pressure caused by nausea, vomiting, straining at stool, coughing, sneezing, or lifting heavy objects. The client may have melena or hematemesis. There may be slow oozing or massive hemorrhage. Massive hemorrhage is a medical emergency.

Table 38-12   Factors Involved in the Development of Ascites

Factor	Mechanism
Portal hypertension	Increase in resistance of blood flow through liver
Increased flow of hepatic lymph	Weeping of protein-rich lymph from surface of cirrhotic liver, intrahepatic blockage of lymph channels
Decreased serum colloidal oncotic pressure	Impairment of liver synthesis of albumin, loss of albumin into peritoneal cavity
Hyperaldosteronism	Increase in aldosterone secretion stimulated by decreased renal blood flow, impairment of liver metabolism of aldosterone
Impaired water excretion	Reduction in renal vascular flow and excessive serum levels of ADH

Peripheral edema and ascites. Peripheral edema sometimes precedes ascites, but in some clients its development coincides with or occurs after ascites. Edema results from (1) decreased colloidal osmotic pressure from impaired liver synthesis of albumin and (2) increased portocaval pressure from portal hypertension. Peripheral edema occurs as ankle and presacral edema.

Ascites is the accumulation of serous fluid in the peritoneal or abdominal cavity. It is a common manifestation of cirrhosis. When the blood pressure is elevated in the liver, as occurs in portal cirrhosis, proteins can be transported from the blood vessels via the larger pores of the sinusoids (capillaries) into the lymph space. When the lymphatic system is unable to carry off the excess proteins and water, they will leak through the liver capsule into the peritoneal cavity. The osmotic pressure of the proteins pulls additional fluid into the peritoneal cavity (Table 38-12).

A second mechanism of ascites is hypoalbuminemia resulting from the inability of the liver to synthesize albumin. The hypoalbuminemia results in decreased colloidal osmotic pressure. A third mechanism of ascites, hyperaldosteronism, results when aldosterone is not metabolized by damaged liver cells. The increased level of aldosterone causes increased amounts of sodium to be reabsorbed by the renal tubules. This retention of sodium by cirrhotic clients as well as an increase in the antidiuretic hormone (ADH) causes additional water retention in these clients. There is also a reduction in renal blood flow and glomerular filtration. The fact that the diseased liver does not metabolize estrogen as effectively may also contribute to the edema and ascites.

Hypokalemia is common and is due to an excessive loss of potassium ions because of the effects of aldosterone. Low potassium levels can also result from diuretic therapy used to treat the ascites.

Ascites is manifested by abdominal distention with weight gain (Fig. 38-2). If the ascites is severe, the umbilicus may be everted. Abdominal striae with distended ab-

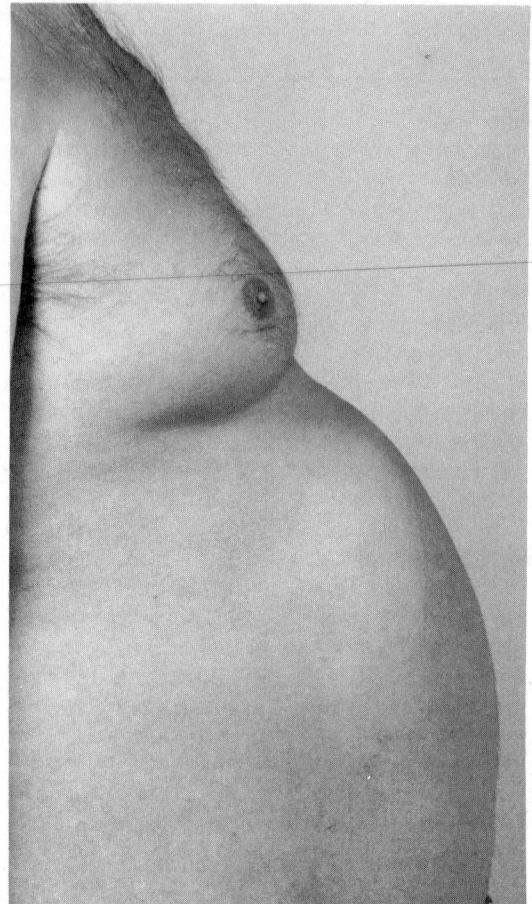

Fig. 38-2   Ascites and gynecomastia associated with cirrhosis of the liver. Photograph was taken after a paracentesis was performed.

dominal wall veins may be present. The client has a dehydrated appearance—dry tongue and skin, sunken eyeballs, and muscle weakness. There is also a decrease in urinary output.

Hepatic encephalopathy. Hepatic encephalopathy or coma is a frequent terminal complication in liver disease. *Encephalopathy* is a more descriptive term than *coma*. Hepatic encephalopathy can occur in any condition in which liver damage causes blood to enter the systemic circulation without liver detoxification. There is a high mortality rate associated with hepatic encephalopathy.

A number of etiological factors are involved in hepatic encephalopathy. The main pathogenic agent is nitrogenous ammonia, which is a cerebral toxin. A major source of ammonia is the bacterial and enzymatic deamination of amino acids in the intestines. The ammonia that results from this deamination process normally goes to the liver via the portal circulation and is converted to urea, which is excreted by the kidneys. When the blood is shunted past the liver via the collateral anastomoses or the liver is unable to convert ammonia to urea, large quantities of ammonia remain in the systemic circulation. The ammonia crosses the blood-brain barrier and produces neurological toxic manifestations.

Table 38-13 Factors Precipitating Hepatic Encephalopathy

Factor	Mechanism
GI hemorrhage	Increase in ammonia in GI tract
Constipation	Increase in ammonia from bacterial action on feces
Hypokalemia	Increase in renal production of ammonia, which enters systemic circulation; potassium ions needed by brain to metabolize ammonia
Hypovolemia	Increase in blood ammonia by causing hepatic hypoxia; impairment of cerebral, hepatic, and renal function due to decreased blood flow
Infection	Increase in catabolism, increase in cerebral sensitivity to toxins
Cerebral depressants (e.g., narcotics)	No detoxification by liver, causing increase in cerebral depression
Metabolic alkalosis	Facilitation of transport of ammonia across blood-brain barrier, increase in renal production of ammonia
Paracentesis	Loss of sodium and potassium ions, decrease in blood volume
Dehydration	Potentiation of ammonia toxicity
Increased metabolism	Increase in work load of liver
Diuretics	Increase in renal formation of ammonia, possibly resulting in azotemia, which increases endogenous ammonia production; hypokalemia also possible
Uremia (renal failure)	Retention of nitrogenous metabolites

Other toxic substances that may contribute to hepatic encephalopathy are false neurotransmitter substances, methionine, and short-chain fatty acids. It is currently believed that the liver may produce substances necessary for normal brain functioning. When the diseased liver can no longer produce these substances, encephalopathy may result. A number of factors may precipitate hepatic encephalopathy, mostly because they increase the amount of circulating ammonia (Table 38-13).

Clinical manifestations of encephalopathy are changes in neurological and mental responsiveness, ranging from lethargy to deep coma. In the early stages, manifestations include euphoria, depression, apathy, irritability, memory loss, confusion, yawning, drowsiness, insomnia, agitation, slow and slurred speech, emotional lability, impaired judgment, hiccups, slow and deep respirations, hyperactive reflexes, and a positive Babinski reflex.

Clinical manifestations of impending coma include disorientation as to time, place, or person. A characteristic symptom is *asterixis* or flapping tremors (liver flap). This may take several forms, the most common involving the arms and hands. When asked to hold the arms and hands stretched out, the client is unable to hold this position and there will be a series of rapid flexion and extension movements of the hands. Other signs of asterixis are rhythmic movements of the legs with dorsiflexion of the foot and rhythmic movements in the face with strong closure of the eyelids.

Fetor hepaticus occurs in some clients with encephalopathy. It is a musty, sweet odor of the client's breath. This odor is from the accumulation of methionine (an amino acid containing sulfur) resulting from the liver's inability to metabolize it.

Impairments in writing involve difficulty in moving the pen or pencil from left to right and apraxia (the inability to construct simple figures). Other signs include hyperventilation, hypothermia, and grimacing and grasping reflexes.

Table 38-14 Bilirubin Metabolism Abnormalities in Cirrhosis*

Type	Finding
Serum bilirubin	
Unconjucated	↑
Conjugated	↑
Urine bilirubin	↑
Urobilinogen	
Stool	Normal, ↓
Urine	Normal, ↑

*These are bilirubin metabolism abnormalities occurring with *hepatocellular jaundice,* the most frequent type of jaundice with cirrhosis.

Hepatorenal syndrome. Hepatorenal syndrome is a serious complication of cirrhosis. It is characterized by functional renal failure with advancing azotemia, oliguria, and intractable ascites. There is no structural abnormality of the kidneys. The exact cause of the renal failure is unknown, but it is thought to be associated with altered renal hemodynamics and possible cortical vessel constriction, which is caused by either a prostaglandin deficiency or increased serum angiotensin. The syndrome frequently follows diuretic therapy, GI hemorrhage, or paracentesis. Hepatic encephalopathy is also associated with the deterioration in renal function. Treatment measures include salt-poor albumin, salt and water restrictions, and diuretic therapy. Treatment is usually unsuccessful.

Diagnostic Studies

A liver profile in cirrhosis demonstrates abnormalities in most of the liver function studies (see Table 33-12). Enzyme levels—alkaline phosphatase, SGOT (AST), SGPT (ALT), and lactic acid dehydrogenase—are elevated because of the release of these enzymes from damaged liver

cells. Protein metabolism tests show decreased total protein, decreased albumin, and increased globulin levels. The liver does not synthesize γ globulins but does synthesize albumin. The globulin level often increases in cirrhosis and indicates increased synthesis or decreased removal. γ Globulins (antibodies) are produced in the lymphatic system, spleen, and bone marrow. Fat-metabolism abnormalities are reflected by decreased cholesterol levels. Dye excretory tests, such as the indiocyanine green (ICG) test, show retention of the dye. The prothrombin time is prolonged and bilirubin metabolism is altered (Table 38-14). Liver biopsy may be performed to identify liver cell changes and alterations in the lobular structure. Differential analysis of ascitic fluid is helpful in establishing a diagnosis.

Therapeutic Management

Rest. Although there is no specific therapy for cirrhosis, certain measures can be taken to promote liver cell regeneration and prevent or treat complications (Table 38-15). Rest is significant in reducing metabolic demands of the liver, reducing the hepatic blood flow, and allowing for recovery of liver cells. At various times during the progress of cirrhosis the rest may have to take the form of complete bed rest.

Ascites. The focus of management of the client with ascites is sodium restriction and diuretics. Rest is very important, since bed rest decreases sodium retention. However, complete bed rest may not be necessary unless the client has massive ascites. Bed rest initially frequently mobilizes some of the fluid. There should also be accurate assessment and control of fluid and electrolyte balance. Salt-poor albumin may be used to help maintain intravascular volume and adequate urinary output by increasing plasma colloid osmotic pressure. A low-sodium diet is prescribed. The client is usually not on restricted fluids unless severe ascites develops.

Diuretic therapy is an important part of management. Frequently a combination of drugs that work at more than one kidney tubular site is more effective. Spironolactone (Aldactone) is very effective, even in clients with severe sodium retention. Spironolactone is an antagonist of aldosterone and is potassium sparing. Other potassium-sparing diuretics are amiloride (Midamor) and triamterene (Dyrenium). A high-potency loop diuretic, such as furosemide (Lasix), is frequently used in combination with a potassium-sparing drug. Chlorothiazide (Diuril) or hydrochlorothiazide may also be used, but the thiazide diuretics are not as potent as the loop diuretics.

A paracentesis (needle puncture of the abdominal cavity) is usually safe. However, it is reserved for the client with impaired respiration or abdominal pain due to severe ascites. It is not a suitable form of chronic therapy.

Peritoneovenous shunt. A surgical procedure provides for the continuous reinfusion of ascitic fluid into the venous system. Called the *LaVeen peritoneovenous shunt*, it consists of a tube and a one-way valve. The tube runs from the abdominal cavity through the peritoneum, under the subcutaneous tissue, and into the jugular vein or superior vena cava (Fig. 38-3). The valve opens when the pres-

Table 38-15

Diagnostic and Therapeutic Management: Cirrhosis of the Liver

DIAGNOSTIC

Liver function studies
Liver biopsy
Esophagoscopy
Serum electrolytes
Prothrombin time
CBC
Stool for occult blood
Upper GI
24-hour urine for NaCl

THERAPEUTIC

Administration of 3000-calorie, high-carbohydrate, low- to moderate-protein, low-fat diet (depending on stage); low sodium for ascites
Administration of B-complex vitamins
Complete bed rest with bathroom privileges
No alcohol
Administration of diuretics
Management of complications

CBC, Complete blood count.

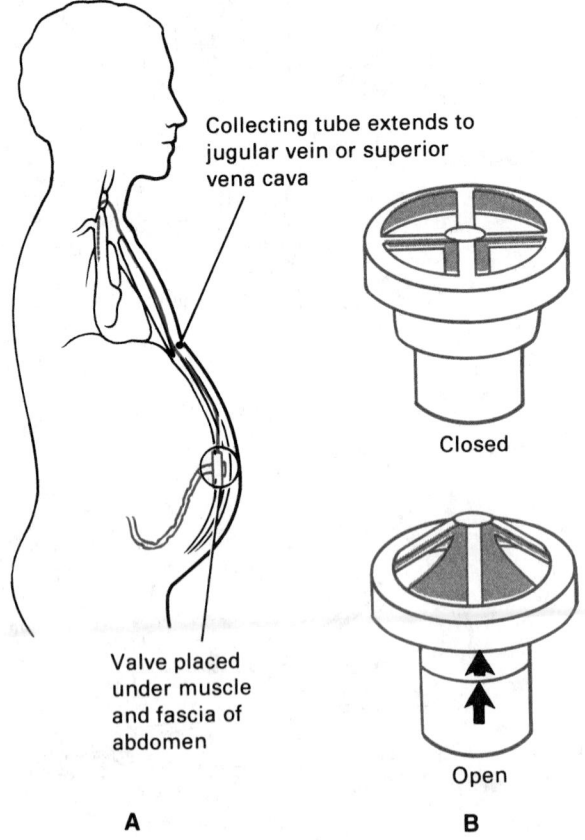

Fig. 38-3 LeVeen continuous peritoneal-venous shunt. **A,** Collecting tube. **B,** Valve in closed and open position.

sure in the peritoneal cavity is 3 to 5 cm H_2O higher than that in the superior vena cava. This allows the ascitic fluid to flow into the venous system. The client's inspiration increases the intraperitoneal pressure, causing the valve to open. Another shunt, the Denver shunt, has a subcutaneous pump that irrigates the tubing when manually compressed. This shunting of the ascitic fluid causes an improvement in hemodynamic factors and increases sodium and fluid excretion. Urine output is also increased.

Esophageal varices. The main therapeutic goal related to esophageal varices is avoidance of bleeding and hemorrhage. Persons who have esophageal varices should avoid ingesting alcohol, aspirin, and irritating foods. Upper respiratory infections should be treated promptly, and coughing should be controlled.

Management related to bleeding esophageal varices includes emergency, therapeutic, and prophylactic interventions. Management measures used are vasopressin and somatostatin, β blockers, balloon tamponade, sclerotherapy, ligation of varices, and shunt therapy. Much controversy surrounds which is the best method to use and under what circumstances.

When bleeding occurs, the first step is to make a definitive diagnosis. This is very important because clients with cirrhosis can also bleed from erosive gastritis, peptic ulcers, and Mallory-Weiss tears. The diagnosis is made by endoscopic examination as soon as possible. Lavage with a wide-bore nasogastric (NG) tube (e.g., Ewald) may be done to remove blood and clots to prepare the client for endoscopy. Measures to control bleeding are then initiated. Vasopressin (Pitressin) administration and balloon tamponade are considered effective "stopgap" measures for this. Vasopressin produces vasoconstriction of the splanchnic arterial bed, decreased portal blood flow, and decreased portal hypertension. It can be given either IV or by intraarterial infusion into the superior mesenteric artery. However, IV use is just as effective as intraarterial. Nitroglycerin and sodium nitroprusside (Nipride) are sometimes used together with vasopressin. This seems to decrease some of the side effects of vasopressin while maintaining results. Somatostatin may be used instead of vasopressin to decrease splanchnic blood flow.

Balloon tamponade controls the hemorrhage by mechanical compression of the varices. The Sengstaken-Blakemore tube is used for this purpose (Fig. 38-4). It has two balloons: gastric and esophageal. It has three lumens: one for the gastric balloon, one for the esophageal balloon, and one for gastric aspiration. When inflated, the gastric

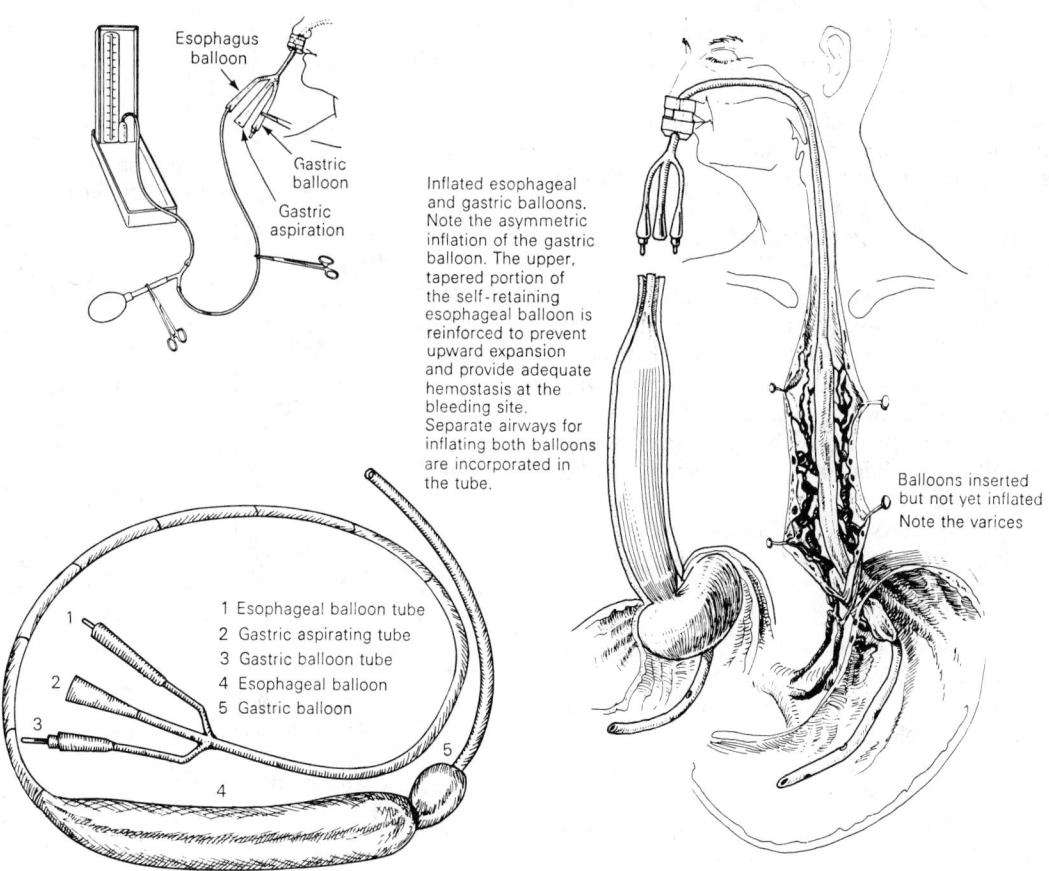

Fig. 38-4 Esophageal tamponade accomplished with Sengstaken-Blakemore tube. (Courtesy Davol Rubber Company, Providence, RI.)

and esophageal balloons put mechanical compression on the varices. The gastric balloon anchors the tube in position and also applies pressure to any bleeding gastric varices. The Minnesota tube, a variation of the Blakemore tube, also has an esophageal aspiration port.

Propranolol (Inderal), a β blocker, can be given orally to prevent recurrent GI bleeding. It reduces portal venous pressure. This effect is due to reduced cardiac output and possibly constriction of splanchnic vessels. Because it reduces hepatic blood flow, it can enhance the possibility of hepatic encephalopathy.

Sclerotherapy is the injection of a sclerosing solution into the varices. It is usually done endoscopically, but percutaneous transhepatic obliteration may be used. This procedure obliterates the short gastric veins supplying the esophageal varices. A catheter is passed through the skin and liver to the portal vein and to the gastric veins to obliterate the varices. Endoscopic sclerotherapy requires repeat treatments. Sclerotherapy may be used therapeutically, prophylactically, and as an emergency measure. It is more

difficult during an active bleeding episode, and there are more complications. Sclerotherapy does not work on gastric varices. In several studies, sclerotherapy was successful in controlling bleeding in 90% of acute hemorrhages.[4] Currently, endoscopic ligation of esophageal varices is also being done.

Various surgical shunting procedures may be used to decrease portal hypertension by diverting some of the portal blood flow, at the same time still allowing adequate liver perfusion. Currently, the shunts most commonly used are the portacaval shunt and the distal splenorenal shunt (Fig. 38-5). Shunts are indicated more after a second major bleeding episode. Although a prophylactic portacaval shunt lessens bleeding, it does not prolong life. Clients die of hepatic encephalopathy caused by the diversion of the ammonia past the liver and into the systemic circulation. The distal splenorenal shunt (Warren shunt) leaves portal venous flow intact (Fig. 38-4), and because of this, it has a lower incidence of hepatic encephalopathy. With time, however, the flow of blood through the liver decreases.

Supportive measures during an acute variceal bleed include administration of fresh frozen plasma and packed RBCs, vitamin K (Aquamephyton), and H_2 blockers such as cimetidine (Tagamet). Neomycin administration may be started to prevent hepatic encephalopathy from the extra load of protein on the liver.

Hepatic encephalopathy. The goal of management of hepatic encephalopathy is the reduction of ammonia formation. This consists mainly of protein restriction and reduction of ammonia formation in the intestines. The degree of protein restriction is determined by the client's state of responsiveness. The protein restriction may range from 0 to 40 g a day.

Several measures to reduce ammonia formation in the intestines are used. Sterilization of the intestines with antibiotics such as neomycin sulfate, which are poorly absorbed from the GI tract, is one method. Neomycin is given orally or rectally. This reduces the bacterial flora of the colon. Bacterial action on protein in the feces results in ammonia production. Cathartics and enemas are also used to decrease bacterial action. Constipation should be prevented.

Lactulose (Cephulac) may also be used to treat hepatic encephalopathy. This is a synthetic ketoanalog of lactose. In the colon, it is split into lactic acid and acetic acid, which decrease the pH from 7.0 to 5.0. The acidic environment discourages bacterial growth. The increased availability of hydrogen ions encourages the conversion of ammonia to ammonium ion (NH_4^+), which is excreted in the stool. Lactulose also has a cathartic effect. It is usually given orally but may be given as a retention enema.

Levodopa is a recently used drug in the treatment of encephalopathy. It is a precursor of dopamine and norepinephrine. Use of levodopa is based on the theory that there is a deficiency of dopamine and norepinephrine in encephalopathy because they are replaced by false transmitters (amines from breakdown of dietary proteins). Normally these are destroyed by liver enzymes, which the diseased liver can no longer do.

Control of hepatic encephalopathy also involves treat-

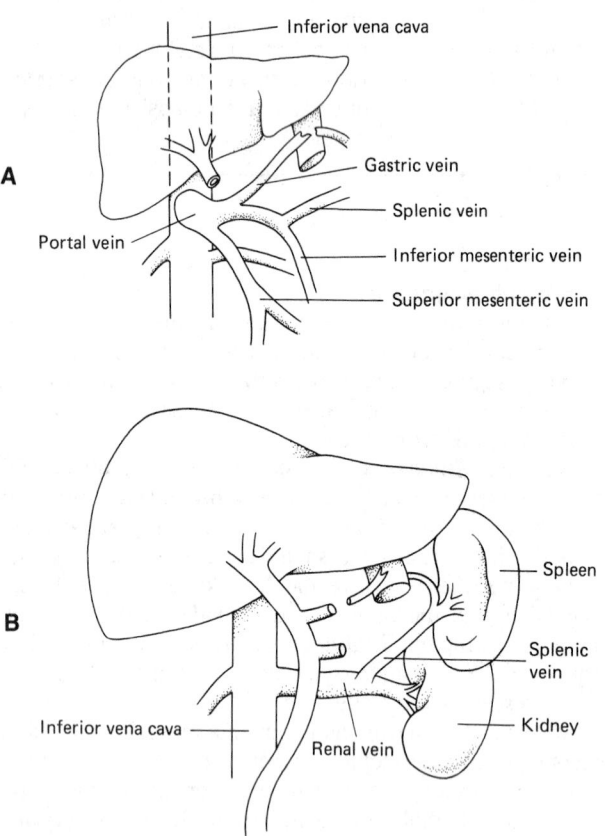

Fig. 38-5 Portosystemic shunts. **A,** Portacaval shunt. The portal vein is anastomosed to the inferior vena cava diverting blood from the portal vein to the systemic circulation. **B,** Distal splenorenal shunt. The splenic vein is anastomosed to the renal vein. The portal venous flow remains intact while esophageal varices are selectively decompressed. (The short gastric veins are decompressed.) The spleen conducts blood from the high pressure of the esophageal and gastric varices to the low pressure renal vein.

ment of precipitating causes (Table 38-13). This involves controlling GI hemorrhage and removing the blood from the GI tract to decrease the protein in the intestine. Electrolyte and acid-base imbalances and infections should also be treated.

Pharmacological Management

There is no specific drug therapy for cirrhosis. However, a number of medications are used to treat symptoms and complications of advanced liver disease (Table 38-16).

Nutritional Considerations

The diet for the client with cirrhosis without complications is high in calories (3000 per day) with high carbohydrate content, moderate to high protein, and moderate to low fat. The amount of protein varies depending on the degree of liver damage and the danger of encephalopathy. Some physicians order 1.5 g of protein per kilogram of body weight to maintain plasma osmotic balance and promote liver cell regeneration. In some situations the client may be given a reduced quantity of protein to reduce the risk of encephalopathy. Vitamin supplements are usually given. Foods high in protein include meat, fish, poultry, eggs, and dairy products. High-protein nourishment in the form of eggnogs, milkshakes, or protein supplements may be used, particularly for the client who is malnourished.

The client with edema formation is on a low-sodium diet. The degree of sodium restriction varies depending on the client's condition. The client needs instruction regarding the degree of restriction. Table salt is the most common source of sodium. Sodium is also present in baking soda, baking powder, and some over-the-counter medications. Foods that are high in sodium content include canned soups and vegetables, salted snacks such as potato chips, nuts, smoked meats and fish, crackers, breads, olives, pickles, catsup, and beer.

The nurse must remember that some medications (e.g., antacids) contain sodium. The antacid Riopan is low in sodium. Carbonated beverages tend to be high in sodium, and low-sodium and sodium-free carbonated drinks are available. Clients should be advised to read labels. Foods high in protein usually have large amounts of sodium. Alternative protein supplements that are low in sodium may have to be used. The client and the family need assistance to make the diet more palatable by the use of seasonings such as garlic, parsley, onion, lemon juice, and spices.

The client with hepatic encephalopathy is on a very-low-protein to no-protein diet (Table 38-17). Foods allowed include toast, cereal, rice, tea, fruit juices, and hard candies. Sufficient carbohydrate intake must be provided to maintain an intake of 1500 to 2000 calories to prevent hypoglycemia and catabolism. IV or tube feedings may be required.

■ Nursing Management of Cirrhosis

Nursing assessment
Subjective and objective data that should be obtained from an individual with cirrhosis are presented in Table 38-18.

Table 38-16 Medications Used in Cirrhosis

Medication	Mechanism of Action
Vasopressin (Pitressin)	Hemostasis and control of bleeding in esophageal varices, constriction of splanchnic arterial bed
Propranolol	Reduction of portal venous pressure, prevention of GI bleeding
Neomycin sulfate	Decrease in bacterial flora, decreasing formation of ammonia
Lactulose (Cephulac)	Acidification of feces in bowel and trapping of ammonia, causing its elimination in feces
Levodopa	Conversion to dopamine, which has been displaced with amines from protein breakdown
Diuretics	
Spironolactone (Aldactone)	Blocking of action of aldosterone, potassium sparing
Chlorothiazide (Diuril)	Thiazide that acts on proximal tubule to decrease reabsorption of sodium and potassium ions and water
Furosemide (Lasix)	Rapid action on distal tubule and Henle's loop to prevent reabsorption of sodium and potassium ions and water

Nursing diagnoses
Nursing diagnoses are determined when the problem and the etiological factors are supported by clinical data. Nursing diagnoses related to cirrhosis may include, but are not limited to, those presented in Table 38-19.

Nursing interventions
Health maintenance and promotion. The client with cirrhosis may be faced with a very prolonged course and the possibility of serious, life-threatening problems and complications. The nurse should be a resource person in helping the client achieve the highest level of wellness. The client and the family need to understand the importance of continuous health care and medical supervision. They should be taught symptoms of complications and when to seek medical attention.

Measures to achieve and maintain a remission should be encouraged. These include proper diet, rest, avoidance of potentially hepatotoxic over-the-counter drugs, and abstinence from alcohol. Abstinence from alcohol is very important and results in improvement in most clients. The nurse must realize the difficulty this poses for some clients. The nurse's own attitude regarding the client whose cirrhosis is attributed to alcohol abuse should be explored. Care should be given without rejection and moralizing. The alcoholic client should be treated with a caring attitude. The nurse also has the responsibility of public education regarding the effects of alcohol and other substances that are toxic to the liver.

Table 38-17 Low-Protein Diet for Hepatic Failure

GENERAL PRINCIPLES

Limit protein to 20 g per day at onset of severe hepatic failure.
Protein must be from protein sources with high biological value.
Diet must be high in calories.
Fat is limited only to prevent early satiety.
Protein is increased in diet by 10 g increments as tolerated without causing signs and symptoms of hepatic encephalopathy.
Sodium is also usually restricted as well as fluid when edema and ascites are present.

Meal	Sample Menu Plans*		
Breakfast			
1 fruit, calorie supplement 1 low-protein bread 1 egg (protein) Fat, calorie supplement ¼ cup milk (2 g protein)	½ cup grape juice with 2 tbs Polycose powder† French toast made with low-protein bread, 1 egg, 3 tsp salt-free butter and syrup ¼ cup milk	¼ cup cranberry juice with 2 tbs Polycose powder Low-protein toast with 3 tsp salt-free butter and 2 tsp jelly 1-egg omelet with 3 tsp salt-free butter ¼ cup milk	¼ cup prune juice with 2 tbs Polycose powder Low-protein toast with 3 tsp salt-free butter 1 egg fried in 3 tsp salt-free butter ¼ cup milk
Snack			
Calorie supplement	Jelly beans	Hard candy	Sugar mints
Lunch			
2 starch (4 g protein) 1 vegetable (2 g protein) 1 fruit, calorie supplement Fat, calorie supplement	¼ cup half and half ½ cup Cream of Wheat with 3 tsp salt-free butter Applesauce with whipped topping or Lipomul‡ Small tossed salad with 3 tbs oil and vinegar§ Peas with 3 tsp salt-free butter	¼ cup half and half ½ cup cornmeal (atole) with 3 tsp salt-free butter Small guacamole salad Gelatin with whipped topping or Lipomul Corn with 3 tsp salt-free butter	¼ cup half and half ½ cup grits with 3 tsp salt-free butter Cucumbers in sour cream Peaches with whipped topping or Lipomul Sweet potatoes with brown sugar and 3 tsp salt-free butter
Snack			
Calorie supplement	Low-protein cookies	Low-protein bread cubes with whipped cream and strawberries	Popsicles made with Polycose
Dinner			
1 starch (2 g protein) 1 vegetable (2 g protein) 1 low-protein bread ¼ cup milk (2 g protein) Fat, calorie supplement	½ baked potato 3 tsp salt-free butter Low-protein bread ¼ cup sour cream ½ cup green beans with 3 tsp salt-free butter and 2 tsp jelly ¼ cup milk	½ cup fried potatoes with 1 tsp melted salt-free butter ½ cup zucchini with 3 tsp salt-free butter Low-protein toast with 3 tsp salt-free butter and 2 tsp marmalade ¼ cup milk	½ cup mashed potatoes ½ cup fried okra Low-protein toast with 3 tsp salt-free butter and 2 tsp jam ¼ cup milk

*The diet plan contains approximately 20 g protein.
†Polycose is a brand-name product made by Ross Laboratories.
‡Lipomul is a fat emulsion made by Upjohn.
§Crisp food should be avoided because of the possibility of esophageal varices.

Table 38-18

Nursing Assessment of the Client with Cirrhosis

SUBJECTIVE DATA

History
Alcohol abuse; previous hepatitis; chronic biliary obstruction and infection; severe right-sided heart failure; exposure to carbon tetrachloride, benzene derivatives, or other hepatotoxic agents

Medications
Adverse reaction to any medication; use of anticoagulants, aspirin

General
Anorexia, weakness, fatigue, weight loss

Pain
Dull, right upper quadrant or epigastric pain

Integumentary
Pruritus, dry skin

Hematological
Bleeding and bruising tendencies

Gastrointestinal
Dyspepsia, nausea and vomiting, pale stools, change in bowel habits

Urinary
Dark urine

Reproductive
Impotence, amenorrhea

Neurological
Numbness, tingling of extremities

OBJECTIVE DATA

General
Cachexia, wasting of extremities

Integumentary
Icteric sclera, jaundice, petechiae, ecchymoses, spider angiomas, alopecia, edema, palmar erythema, loss of axillary and pubic hair

Cardiovascular
Peripheral edema, ascites

Gastrointestinal
Abdominal distention, palpable liver and spleen, foul breath, GI bleeding, red tongue, hemorrhoids

Reproductive
Gynecomastia and testicular atrophy (men), impotence, loss of libido, amenorrhea, and heavy menstrual bleeding (women)

Neurological
Altered mentation, asterixis

Possible findings
Anemia, thrombocytopenia; leukopenia; abnormal liver function studies; elevated coagulation studies, ammonia, and bilirubin levels; abnormal abdominal ultrasound and liver scan; positive liver biopsy

Acute intervention. The focus of nursing care for the client with cirrhosis is on conserving the client's strength (see Table 38-19). Rest assists the liver to restore itself. Complete bed rest may not always be necessary. When the client requires complete bed rest, measures to prevent pneumonia, thromboembolic problems, and decubitus ulcers should be taken. The activity and rest schedule may be modified according to signs of clinical improvement (e.g., decreasing jaundice, improvement in liver function studies). Major concerns of the nurse in determining appropriate nursing care measures to meet the need for rest involve regulation of the physical, emotional, and social climate.

Anorexia, nausea and vomiting, pressure from ascites, and poor eating habits all create problems in maintenance of an adequate intake of nutrients. The nursing measures relating to nutrition for clients with hepatitis also apply here. Oral hygiene before meals may improve the client's taste sensation. Between-meal nourishments should be available so that they can be provided at times when the client can best tolerate them. Food preferences should be provided whenever possible. Explanations to the client and the family of the reason for any dietary restrictions should be provided.

Nursing assessment and care should include the client's physiological response to cirrhosis. Is jaundice present? Where is it observed—sclera, skin, hard palate? What is the progression of jaundice? If the jaundice is accompanied by pruritus, measures to relieve itching should be carried out. Cholestyramine (Questran) may be ordered to help relieve the pruritus. The color of the urine and stools should be noted.

Edema and ascites are frequent manifestations of cirrhosis and require nursing assessments and interventions. Accurate calculation and recordings of intake and output, daily weights, and measurements of extremities and abdominal girth help in the ongoing assessment of the location and extent of the edema. If the client can assume a kneeling position when abdominal girth measurement is taken, the abdominal fluid will go to the most dependent part of the abdomen. This gives the best measurement of abdominal girth. For many clients, girth must be measured in the standing or lying position. Where the measurements are taken should be recorded and should be a part of the nursing care plan.

Dyspnea is a frequent problem for the client with ascites. A semi-Fowler's or Fowler's position allows for maximal respiratory efficiency. Pillows can be used to support the arms and chest and may increase the client's comfort and ability to breathe.

Meticulous skin care is essential because the edematous tissues are subject to breakdown. An alternating–air pressure mattress or other special mattress should be used. A turning schedule (minimum of every 2 hours) must be adhered to rigidly. The abdomen may be supported with pillows. If the abdomen is taut, cleansing must be done very gently. This client tends to move very little because of the abdominal discomfort and dyspnea. Therefore range-of-motion exercises are helpful, and measures such as coughing and deep breathing to prevent respiratory problems

Table 38-19

NURSING CARE PLAN FOR THE CLIENT WITH CIRRHOSIS

Defining Characteristics	Nursing Interventions	Evaluation Criteria

NURSING DIAGNOSIS: **Altered nutrition: less than body requirements related to anorexia, impaired utilization and storage of nutrients, nausea, and loss of nutrients from vomiting**

Lack of interest in food, aversion to eating, reported inadequate food intake, perceived inability to ingest food	Provide oral care before meals. Administer antiemetics as ordered. Provide small, frequent meals with nourishments at times the client can best tolerate them. Determine food preferences and allow these whenever possible. Provide attractively served meals in pleasant surroundings.	Adequate intake of nutrients, maintenance of normal body weight

NURSING DIAGNOSIS: **Impaired skin integrity related to edema, ascites, and pruritus**

Complaints of pruritus; areas of excoriation due to scratching; taut, shiny skin over edematous areas; areas of skin breakdown	Restrict sodium intake as ordered. Restrict fluids if ordered. Administer prescribed diuretics. Observe for side effects and hypokalemia. Monitor intake and output. Assess location and extent of edema by weighing client at the same time each day, taking daily measurements of extremities and of abdominal girth (same location each time). Provide meticulous skin care. Reposition client at least q 2 hr. Do range-of-motion exercises. Elevate edematous areas. Have client use special mattress, such as alternating-air pressure or egg crate mattress. Clip client's nails short and keep clean. Administer antipruritic medication as ordered. Provide diversions and distractions.	Maintenance of skin integrity, relief of pruritus

NURSING DIAGNOSIS: **Ineffective breathing pattern related to pressure on diaphragm and reduced lung volume secondary to ascites**

Dyspnea, shortness of breath, tachypnea, cyanosis, cough, changes in respiratory rate, depth, or pattern, changes in pulse	Place client in semi-Fowler's or Fowler's position. Support the arms and chest with pillows. Auscultate chest for rales. Assess respiratory rate and rhythm.	Ability to breathe with minimal difficulty, effective breathing pattern, absence of cyanosis and other signs and symptoms of hypoxia

NURSING DIAGNOSIS: **High risk for injury related to diminished sensory perception secondary to peripheral neuropathy**

Numbness and tingling of lower extremities, decreased sensation in lower extremities	Prevent excess stimulation or trauma to extremities. Do not use restrictive bed linens. Instruct client to avoid tight clothing. Use care with heat and cold applications. Assist with ambulation.	No injury due to decreased sensory perception

NURSING DIAGNOSIS: **Potential complication: bleeding related to bleeding tendency secondary to altered clotting factors**

Epistaxis, purpura, petechiae, easy bruising, gingival bleeding, heavy menstrual bleeding, hematuria, melena	Provide gentle nursing care. Provide assistance with ambulation. Observe for bleeding from body orifices, urine, and stool. Use smallest-gauge needle possible when giving injection and apply gentle but prolonged pressure after injection. Advise use of soft-bristle toothbrush. Teach client to avoid straining at stool, vigorous blowing of nose, and coughing. Observe for signs of thrombocytopenia such as purpura on the forearms, axillae, and skin. Monitor laboratory results (hematocrit, hemoglobin, and prothrombin time).	Minimal bleeding, no hemorrhage

Continued.

Table 38-19

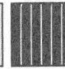

NURSING CARE PLAN FOR THE CLIENT WITH CIRRHOSIS—cont'd

Defining Characteristics	Nursing Interventions	Evaluation Criteria
NURSING DIAGNOSIS: Activity intolerance related to fatigue, anemia, ascites, dyspnea, treatment schedule, and cardiac deconditioning		
Fatigue or weakness, abnormal heart rate or blood pressure, altered response to activity and weakness	Conserve client's strength. Provide activity and rest as required by regulating physical, emotional, and social climate. Monitor hemoglobin and hematocrit readings. Plan scheduled rest periods for client.	Feeling of being rested, increase in tolerance for activity
NURSING DIAGNOSIS: High risk for infection related to leukopenia and increased susceptibility to environmental pathogens		
Evidence of risk factors, including leukopenia, altered immune response, and altered circulation	Monitor client's temperature every 2 to 4 hr. Observe for any local and systemic manifestations of infection. Protect from others with infections. Monitor white blood cell count.	Absence of infections, normal body temperature
NURSING DIAGNOSIS: Body-image disturbance related to change in appearance and body function		
Verbalization of dissatisfaction with appearance, avoidance of contact with others, disparaging remarks about self and body, preoccupation with body	Assess client's response. Present an accepting attitude. Be a supportive listener. Care for the client with concern and warmth. Explain the changes. Assure client and family jaundice is not permanent. Encourage actions to promote appearance, such as use of makeup.	Acceptance of altered body image
NURSING DIAGNOSIS: Altered health maintenance related to lack of knowledge regarding importance of consistent follow-up care, signs and symptoms of complications, proper diet, and alcohol restrictions		
Reports or demonstrations of an unhealthy practice or lifestyle (e.g., substance abuse, alcohol), expressions of inaccurate perception of health status, verbalization of deficiency in knowledge or skill	Explain to client and family importance of continuous health care. Teach client and family symptoms of complications and when to seek medical attention. Teach proper diet. Teach client to avoid potentially hepatotoxic over-the-counter drugs. Encourage abstinence from alcohol. If client has esophageal varices, instruct to avoid aspirin and control cough. Have client avoid spicy and rough foods and activities that increase portal pressure, such as straining at stool, coughing, sneezing, and retching and vomiting.	Maintenance of state of wellness at highest level possible for client

should be implemented. The lower extremities may be elevated. If scrotal edema is present, a scrotal support provides some comfort.

When the client is taking diuretics, the serum levels of sodium, potassium, chloride, and bicarbonate should be monitored. The client should be observed for signs of fluid and electrolyte imbalance, especially hypokalemia. Hypokalemia may be manifested by cardiac dysrhythmias, hypotension, tachycardia, and generalized muscle weakness. Hyponatremia is manifested by muscle cramping, weakness, lethargy, and confusion.

Observations and nursing care in relation to hematolog-

Table 38-19

	NURSING CARE PLAN FOR THE CLIENT WITH CIRRHOSIS—cont'd	
Defining Characteristics	**Nursing Interventions**	**Evaluation Criteria**

NURSING DIAGNOSIS: Total self-care deficit related to weakness, fatigue, balance and gait disturbance, and dyspnea

Inability to initiate or complete self-care activities	Assess client's ability to care for self. Perform activities of care client cannot do. Maintain positive caring attitude while giving care. Encourage client to resume self-care activities when able.	Achievement of client's care needs

NURSING DIAGNOSIS: Sleep pattern disturbance related to frequent assessments and treatments, discomfort, and inability to assume usual sleep position due to orthopnea

Interruption in sleep cycles, complaints of tiredness, frequent napping	Plan care to allow uninterrupted period for sleep. Assist client to assume comfortable position for sleep.	Verbalization of feeling of being rested, longer periods of uninterrupted sleep

NURSING DIAGNOSIS: Ineffective airway clearance related to inability to remove and swallow secretions and bleeding from esophageal varices

Ineffective cough; inability to remove airway secretions; abnormal breath sounds; abnormal respiratory rate, rhythm, depth	Suction client (oral and pharyngeal areas) frequently. Place in semi-Fowler's position. Have scissors near bed to cut tube, if necessary. (Indications include increased respiratory rate, cyanosis, dyspnea). Encourage client to expectorate. Provide emesis basin and tissues. Provide frequent oral and nasal care to provide relief from taste of blood and irritation from mouth breathing.	Patent airway; expectoration of saliva as necessary

NURSING DIAGNOSIS: Altered peripheral tissue perfusion related to bleeding esophageal varices

Pallor; cool, clammy skin; decrease in blood pressure; tachycardia; rapid, shallow respirations	Monitor vital signs every hour. Administer IV fluids and blood products as ordered.	Blood pressure and pulse within normal limits

NURSING DIAGNOSIS: Sensory/perceptual alterations related to increased formation of ammonia secondary to hepatic encephalopathy and mobility restrictions

Inappropriate responses to environmental stimuli	Assess and record client's neurological status at least q 2 hr. Include an exact description of client's behavior. Encourage fluids (if not restricted) and give laxatives and enemas as ordered to decrease production of ammonia. Provide low-protein or no-protein diet as ordered. Limit physical activity. Control factors known to precipitate coma.*	No reduction in sensory/perceptual status

*See Table 38-13.

ical disorders (bleeding tendencies, anemia, increased susceptibility to infection) are the same as for the client with advanced liver disease (see Table 38-19).

The nurse must assess the client's response to the altered body image resulting from the jaundice, spider angiomas, palmar erythema, ascites, and gynecomastia. The client may experience a great deal of anxiety regarding these changes. The nurse should explain these phenomena and should be a supportive listener. Nursing care with concern and warmth regardless of physical changes helps the client maintain self-esteem.

When the client experiences manifestations of advanced

liver disease, other problems such as bleeding esophageal varices and hepatic encephalopathy must be considered.

BLEEDING ESOPHAGEAL VARICES. If the client has esophageal varices in addition to cirrhosis, the nurse must be observant of any signs of bleeding from the varices, such as hematemesis and melena. If hematemesis occurs, the nurse should assess the client for hemorrhage, call the physician, and be ready to assist with whatever treatment is used to control the bleeding. If mechanical compression is used, the nurse should obtain the esophageal-gastric balloon.

The initial nursing task related to insertion of the Sengstaken-Blakemore tube is to explain the use of the tube and how it will be inserted. The balloons should be checked for patency. Sometimes the stomach is lavaged with saline solution before insertion of the tube. It is usually the physician's responsibility to insert the tube. The deflated tube is inserted through the nose into the stomach (see Fig. 38-3). The gastric balloon is inflated with 150 to 250 ml of air and the tube is retracted until resistance is felt. Traction may be applied (¾ to 1¼ pounds) to hold the tube securely in place and prevent downward movement. The tube is secured by placement of a piece of sponge or foam rubber at the nostrils (nasal cuff). This protects the mucosal surfaces from irritation and injury. The esophageal balloon is then inflated with air. A sphygmomanometer is used to maintain and measure the desired pressure at 20 to 40 mm Hg. The position of the balloons is verified by x-ray film. Sometimes it is helpful to have the client wear a football helmet with the tube secured to the mouth guard. This stabilizes the tube and applies traction. Traction causes ulceration of the nasal mucosa and can be used for only short intervals (2 to 3 hours) at a time.

Sometimes iced saline lavage is used to help control the bleeding. (Nursing care of upper GI bleeding is discussed in Chapter 36.) The nurse must assure that the right amount of pressure is maintained for the correct time. Constant tension and an upward pull on the stomach initiate contraction of the stomach that may lead to retching and increased portal pressures. Sometimes the esophageal balloon is deflated every 8 to 12 hours to avoid necrosis. Each lumen must be labeled to avoid confusion. The NG lumen may be connected to suction to remove blood and keep the stomach empty.

Nursing care includes monitoring for complications of rupture or erosion of the esophagus, regurgitation and aspiration of gastric contents, and occlusion of the airway by the balloon. If the gastric balloon breaks or is deflated, the esophageal balloon will slip upward, obstructing the airway and causing asphyxiation. If this happens, the nurse must cut the tube or deflate the esophageal balloon. Scissors should be kept at the bedside. Regurgitation can be minimized by oral and pharyngeal suctioning and by keeping the client in a semi-Fowler's position.

The client is unable to swallow saliva because of the inflated esophageal balloon occluding the esophagus. With the Minnesota tube, which has an esophageal aspiration lumen, this problem can be alleviated. The nurse should encourage the client to expectorate and should provide an emesis basin and tissues. Frequent oral and nasal care provides relief from the taste of blood and irritation from mouth breathing.

The client is extremely ill at this stage. The crises of the bleeding and the ordeal of the Sengstaken-Blakemore tube create a great deal of psychological trauma. Emotional support and gentle caring must be provided.

HEPATIC ENCEPHALOPATHY. The focus of nursing care of the client with hepatic encephalopathy is on sustaining life and assisting with measures to reduce the formation of ammonia. The nurse should assess (1) the client's level of responsiveness (e.g., reflexes, pupillary reactions, orientation), (2) sensory and motor abnormalities (e.g., hyperreflexia, asterixis, motor coordination), (3) fluid and electrolyte imbalances, (4) acid-base imbalances, and (5) the effect of treatment measures.

The neurological status, including an exact description of the client's behavior, should be assessed and recorded at least every 2 hours. Care of the client with neurological problems should be based on the severity of the encephalopathy.

Nursing measures to prevent constipation should be instituted to decrease the production of ammonia. Drugs, laxatives, and enemas should be given as ordered. Encouragement of fluids may also help, if not contraindicated. The client should not strain at stool because this may cause bleeding of the hemorrhoidal varices. Any GI bleeding may worsen the coma. The client who is taking lactulose should be assessed for diarrhea. The correct dosage of lactulose produces two to four semiformed stools a day.

Factors that are known to precipitate coma should be controlled as much as possible (see Table 38-13). Because exercise produces ammonia as a by-product of metabolism, the physical activity of the client must be limited. Hypokalemia should be controlled.

The client is on either a very-low-protein or a no-protein diet, neither of which is very palatable. Foods and fluids high in carbohydrate should be given because the liver is not synthesizing and storing glucose. The client may require tube feedings or parenteral hyperalimentation if an adequate diet cannot be ingested.

Chronic management. Cirrhosis is a chronic disease. The client is affected not only physically but also psychologically, socially, and economically. Major adjustments may be required to make lifestyle changes, especially if alcohol abuse is the primary etiological factor. The nurse should provide information regarding community support programs such as Alcoholics Anonymous, for help with alcohol abuse.

Adequate explanations, along with written instructions, related to fluid or dietary restrictions should be given to the client and the family. Other health teaching should include instruction about adequate rest periods, how to detect early signs of complications, skin care, drug therapy precautions, observation for bleeding, and protection from infection. Counseling information regarding sexual problems may be needed. Referral to a community health nurse may be helpful to ensure adequate client compliance with prescribed therapy.

CARCINOMA OF THE LIVER

Primary carcinoma (originating in the liver) is quite rare. Metastatic carcinoma of the liver is more common.

Hepatocellular carcinoma is the most common malignant tumor of the liver. The remaining primary tumors are cholangiomas or bile duct carcinomas. A high percentage of clients with primary cell carcinoma have cirrhosis of the liver. Hepatitis B is also commonly associated with hepatocellular carcinoma. Men have a higher incidence of primary liver cancer.[4]

The liver is a common site of metastatic growth due to its high rate of blood flow and extensive capillary network. Cancer cells in other parts of the body are commonly carried to the liver via the portal circulation.

The malignant cells cause the liver to be enlarged and misshapen. Hemorrhage and necrosis in the liver are common. Lesions may be singular or numerous and nodular or diffusely spread over the entire liver. Some tumors infiltrate into other organs such as the gallbladder or into the peritoneum or diaphragm. Primary liver tumors commonly metastasize to the lung.

Clinical Manifestations

It is difficult to diagnose carcinoma of the liver. It is particularly difficult to differentiate it from cirrhosis in its early stages, since many of the clinical manifestations (e.g., hepatomegaly, weight loss, peripheral edema, ascites, and portal hypertension) are similar. Other common manifestations include dull abdominal pain in the epigastric or right upper quadrant region, jaundice, anorexia, nausea and vomiting, and extreme weakness. Clients frequently have pulmonary emboli. Tests used to assist in the diagnosis are a liver scan, hepatic arteriography, endoscopic retrograde cholangiopancreatography, and a liver biopsy. The test for α-fetoprotein (AFP) may be positive. AFP helps to distinguish primary cancer from metastatic cancer.

Therapeutic Management

Treatment of cancer of the liver is largely palliative. Surgical excision (lobectomy) is sometimes performed if the tumor is localized to one portion of the liver. Usually surgery is not feasible because the cancer is too far advanced when it is detected. Surgical excision offers the only chance for cure of liver cancer. Management is very similar to that for cirrhosis (see pp. 1137-1140). Chemotherapy may be used, but there is usually a poor response. Hepatic artery perfusion with 5-fluorouracil may be attempted.

Nursing intervention for the client with liver carcinoma focuses on keeping the client as comfortable as possible. Because this client manifests the same problems as any client with advanced liver disease, the nursing interventions discussed for cirrhosis of the liver apply. (See Chapter 9 for care of the client with cancer.)

The prognosis for cancer of the liver is very poor. The cancer grows rapidly, and death may occur within 4 to 7 months as a result of hepatic encephalopathy or massive blood loss from GI bleeding.

LIVER TRANSPLANTATION

The first human liver transplant was performed in 1963 at the University of Colorado by Dr. Thomas Starzl.[12] In the last decade, liver transplantation has become a practical therapeutic option for many adults and children with irreversible liver disease. It improves the quality of life for end-stage liver clients. Indications for liver transplantation include congenital biliary abnormalities, inborn errors of metabolism, hepatic malignancy (confined to the liver), sclerosing cholangitis, and chronic end-stage liver disease. Cirrhosis of the liver is a major indication in adults. Liver transplants are not recommended for the client with widespread malignant disease.

The major postoperative complications are rejection and infection. Other problems associated with liver transplantation include vascular anomalies, coagulation problems such as hemorrhage and thrombosis, and biliary reconstruction. Rejection is not as major a problem as in kidney transplants. The liver seems to be less susceptible to severe rejection than the kidney. Cyclosporine is an effective immunosuppressant drug and its use, as well as improvements in surgical technique and postoperative care, has reduced morbidity and mortality. Cyclosporine depresses T-helper cell function and preserves T-suppressor cell function (see Chapter 41). It does not cause bone marrow suppression and does not impede wound healing. Other immunosuppressants used include azathioprine (Imuran), corticosteroids, and the monoclonal antibody OKT3.[13]

The preferred anastomosis for biliary tract reconstruction is a *choledochocholedochostomy* (direct anastomosis between the common bile ducts of the recipient and the donor). This procedure retains the sphincter of Oddi and therefore prevents ascending cholangitis. An alternative procedure is a *choledochojejunostomy* (anastomosis between the donor's common bile duct and the recipient's jejunum). This procedure is used if the recipient's duct is diseased, absent, or too small.

The client who has had a liver transplant requires competent and highly skilled nursing care, either in an intensive care unit (ICU) or in some other specialized unit. Liver function tests, cholangiograms, and coagulation studies are used to assess functioning of the new liver and to identify complications or problems.

ACUTE PANCREATITIS
Significance

Acute pancreatitis is an acute inflammatory process of the pancreas. The degree of inflammation varies from mild edema to severe hemorrhagic necrosis.

In the United States the overall prevalence of acute pancreatitis is about 0.5%. It is most common in middle-aged men and women, but affects more men than women. The severity of the disease varies according to the extent of pancreatic destruction. Some clients recover completely, others have recurring attacks, and chronic pancreatitis develops in others.

Etiology and Pathophysiology

Many factors can cause injury to the pancreas. The primary etiological factors are biliary tract disease and alcoholism. In the United States the most common cause is alcoholism, followed by gallbladder disease. Other less common causes of acute pancreatitis include trauma; viral infections; penetrating duodenal ulcer; cysts; abscesses;

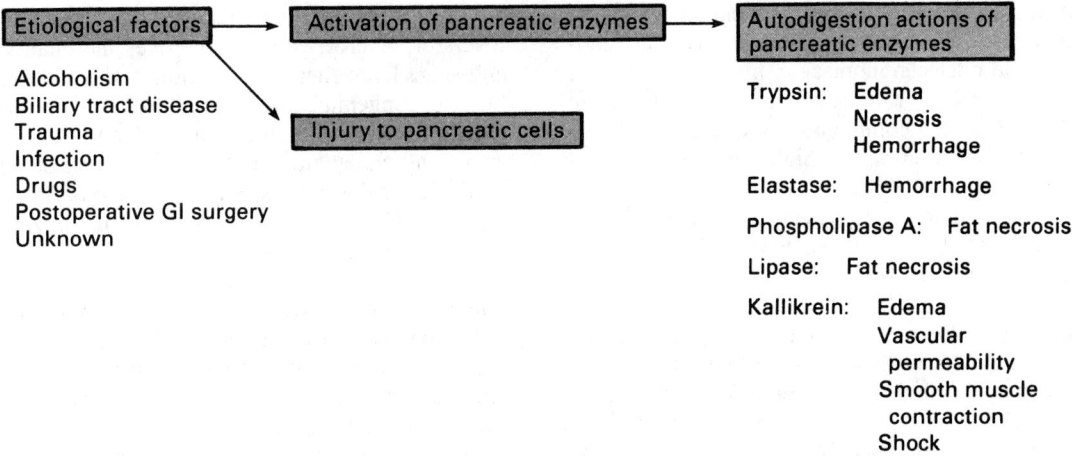

Fig. 38-6 Pathogenic process of acute pancreatitis.

certain drugs (corticosteroids, thiazide diuretics, oral contraceptives); and metabolic disorders such as hyperparathyroidism, hyperlipidemia, and renal failure. Pancreatitis may occur after surgical procedures on the pancreas, stomach, duodenum, or biliary tract. Pancreatitis can also occur after endoscopic retrograde cholangiopancreatography (ERCP) (see Table 33-11). In some cases the cause is not known (idiopathic).

The most common pathogenic mechanism is believed to be autodigestion of the pancreas (Fig. 38-6). The etiological factors cause injury to pancreatic cells or activation of the pancreatic enzymes in the pancreas rather than in the intestine. It is not clear how the activation of pancreatic enzymes occurs. One possible cause is believed to be the reflux of bile acids into the pancreatic ducts through an open or distended sphincter of Oddi. This reflux may occur because of gallstones impacted at the ampulla of Vater, atony and edema of the sphincter, or obstruction of pancreatic ducts and pancreatic ischemia.

Trypsinogen is an inactive proteolytic enzyme produced by the pancreas. Normally it is released into the small intestine via the pancreatic duct. In the intestine it is activated to trypsin by enterokinase. Normally trypsin inhibitors in the pancreas and plasma bind and inactivate any trypsin that is inadvertently produced. In pancreatitis, activated trypsin is present in the pancreas. This enzyme can digest the pancreas and also activate other proteolytic enzymes such as elastase and phospholipase.

Elastase and phospholipase A play a major role in autodigestion of the pancreas. Elastase is activated by trypsin and causes hemorrhage by producing dissolution of the elastic fibers of blood vessels. The phospholipase A is probably activated by trypsin and bile acids and causes fat necrosis.

It is not entirely clear how alcohol causes acute pancreatitis. One theory is that it stimulates secretion and production of hydrochloric acid, which stimulates pancreatic secretions. Alcohol may also cause regurgitation of duodenal contents into the pancreatic duct, resulting in inflammation.[10]

The pathophysiological involvement of acute pancreatitis ranges from edematous pancreatitis (which is mild and self-limiting) to necrotizing pancreatitis (in which the degree of necrosis correlates with the severity of manifestations).

Clinical Manifestations

Abdominal pain is the predominant symptom of acute pancreatitis. The pain is usually located in the left upper quadrant but may be in the midepigastrium. It commonly radiates to the back because of the retroperitoneal location of the pancreas. The pain has a sudden onset and is described as severe, deep, and continuous. It is aggravated by eating and frequently has its onset when the client is recumbent; it is not relieved by vomiting. The pain may be accompanied by flushing, cyanosis, and dyspnea. The client may assume various positions involving flexion of the spine in an attempt to relieve the severe pain. The pain is due to distention of the pancreas, peritoneal irritation, and obstruction of the biliary tract.

Other manifestations of acute pancreatitis include nausea and vomiting, low-grade fever, leukocytosis, hypotension, tachycardia, and jaundice. Abdominal tenderness with muscle guarding is common. Bowel sounds may be decreased or absent. Ileus may occur and causes marked abdominal distention. The lungs are frequently involved, with rales present. Intravascular damage from circulating trypsin may cause areas of cyanosis or greenish to yellow-brown discoloration of the abdominal wall. Other areas of ecchymoses are the flanks (Grey Turner's spots or sign, a bluish flank discoloration) and the periumbilical area (Cullen's sign, a bluish periumbilical discoloration). These result from seepage of blood-stained exudate from the pancreas.

Shock may occur because of hemorrhage into the pancreas or toxemia from the activated pancreatic enzymes. The increased formation of kinin peptides (activated by trypsin), such as kallikrein and bradykinin, causes vasodilatation, increased capillary permeability, and altered vasomotor tone. Hypovolemia also occurs as a result of exudation of blood and plasma proteins into the retroperitoneal space.

Table 38-20   Diagnostic Studies in Acute Pancreatitis

Laboratory Test	Abnormal Finding	Etiology
PRIMARY TESTS		
Serum amylase	Increased (>200 Somogyi units/dl)	Pancreatic cell injury
Serum lipase	Elevated	Pancreatic cell injury
Urinary amylase	Elevated	Pancreatic cell injury
SECONDARY TESTS		
Blood glucose	Hyperglycemia	Impairment of carbohydrate metabolism due to β-cell damage and release of glucagon
Serum calcium	Hypocalcemia	Saponification of calcium by fatty acids in areas of fat necrosis
Serum triglycerides	Hyperlipidemia	Unknown

Complications

Two significant local complications of acute pancreatitis are *pseudocyst* and *abscess*. A pancreatic pseudocyst is a cavity continuous with or surrounding the outside of the pancreas. The pseudocyst is filled with necrotic products and liquid secretions, such as plasma, pancreatic enzymes, and inflammatory exudates. As pancreatic enzymes escape from the pseudocyst, the serosal surfaces next to the pancreas become inflamed with subsequent formation of granulation tissue leading to encapsulation of the exudate. Symptoms of pseudocyst are abdominal pain, palpable epigastric mass, nausea, vomiting, and anorexia. The serum amylase level frequently remains elevated. These cysts sometimes resolve spontaneously but may perforate, causing peritonitis, or rupture into the stomach or duodenum. Treatment consists of an internal drainage procedure with a Roux-en-Y anastomosis between the pancreatic duct and the jejunum.

A pancreatic abscess is a large fluid-containing cavity within the pancreas. It results from extensive necrosis in the pancreas. It may become infected or perforate into adjacent organs. Manifestations of an abscess include upper abdominal pain, abdominal mass, high fever, and leukocytosis. Pancreatic abscesses require prompt surgical drainage.

The main systemic complications of acute pancreatitis are pulmonary complications (pleural effusion, atelectasis, and pneumonia) and tetany due to hypocalcemia. The pulmonary complications are probably due to the passage of the exudate containing pancreatic enzymes from the peritoneal cavity through transdiaphragmatic lymph channels. Hypocalcemia results from fixation of calcium by fatty acids in areas of fat necrosis and increased levels of circulating glucagon. The glucagon causes an increase in excretion of calcium in the urine.

Diagnostic Studies

The primary diagnostic tests for acute pancreatitis are serum amylase and lipase and urinary amylase levels. The serum amylase level is the criterion most commonly used. It may elevate to levels greater than 200 Somogyi units per deciliter. The serum amylase is usually elevated early and remains elevated for 24 to 72 hours.

The serum lipase is also elevated in acute pancreatitis and is a helpful complementary test because other disorders (e.g., mumps, cerebral trauma, renal transplantation) may also cause an increase in serum amylase.

There is an increase in urinary amylase, which may persist several days beyond the elevation of serum amylase. Urinary amylase may be increased to more than 3600 U per day. Normally a timed collection (e.g., a 2-hour collection) is a more dependable measure than a randomly collected urinary specimen.

The renal amylase-creatinine clearance test estimates the amount of blood cleared of amylase by the kidney per minute. The finding that the renal clearance of amylase is higher than the creatinine clearance in acute pancreatitis has led to the suggestion that the amylase-creatinine clearance ratio is a more specific test than urinary amylase clearance. It is a significant finding for assessment of acute pancreatitis if the renal clearance of amylase is greater than the clearance of creatinine.

Other laboratory abnormalities include hyperglycemia, hyperlipidemia, and hypocalcemia (Table 38-20). There is a high incidence of hyperlipidemia with recurrent pancreatitis.

ERCP is diagnostic for gallstones, pancreatic cysts, and abscesses. A combination of laboratory studies and ERCP is usually used to help make the diagnosis. An ultrasound scan of the pancreas may also be used.

Therapeutic Management

Objectives of therapeutic management of acute pancreatitis include (1) relief of pain, (2) prevention or alleviation of shock, (3) reduction of pancreatic secretions, (4) control of fluid and electrolyte imbalance, (5) prevention or treatment of infections, and (6) removal of the precipitating cause, if possible (Table 38-21).

A primary consideration is the relief and control of pain. Meperidine (Demerol) is preferred because it causes less spasm of the smooth muscles of the ducts than opiate drugs. It may be combined with an antispasmodic. How-

Table 38-21

 Diagnostic and Therapeutic Management: Acute Pancreatitis

DIAGNOSTIC

Serum amylase
Serum lipase
Two-hour urinary amylase and renal amylase clearance
Blood sugar
Serum calcium
Triglycerides
Flat plate of the abdomen
Pancreatic ultrasound scan
CT scan of the pancreas
ERCP

THERAPEUTIC

Meperidine IM
NPO with NG tube to suction
Cimetidine or ranitidine IV
Albumin (if shock present)
IV calcium gluconate (10%) (if tetany present)
Lactated Ringer's solution

CT, Computerized tomography.

ever, atropinelike drugs should be avoided when paralytic ileus is present because they may contribute to the problem. Other medications that relax smooth muscles (spasmolytics), such as nitroglycerin or papaverine, may be used.

If shock is present, blood volume replacements are used. Plasma or plasma volume expanders such as dextran or albumin may be given. Fluid and electrolyte imbalances are corrected with lactated Ringer's solution or other electrolyte solutions. Central venous pressure readings may be used to assist in determination of fluid-replacement requirements.

It is important to reduce or suppress pancreatic enzymes to decrease stimulation of the pancreas and allow it to rest. This is accomplished in several ways. First, the client is allowed to take nothing by mouth (NPO). Second, NG suction may be used to reduce vomiting and gastric distention and to prevent gastric digestive juices from entering the duodenum. These measures suppress pancreatic secretion. Certain drugs may also be used for this purpose (see Table 38-22).

The inflamed and necrotic pancreatic tissue is a good source for bacterial growth. Therefore infections should be prevented. There is some controversy about the prophylactic use of antibiotics. It is important to monitor the client closely so that antibiotic therapy can be instituted early if infection occurs.

Peritoneal lavage or dialysis has been used to remove the kinin and phospholipase A–containing exudate from the peritoneal cavity. This has proved beneficial in some cases of severe acute pancreatitis. It prevents early death but has little effect on overall mortality. Endoscopic papil-lotomy may be used to remove an impacted gallstone from the common bile duct when the pancreatitis is due to the stone.

Surgical intervention may be indicated when the diagnosis is uncertain and in clients who do not respond to conservative therapy. Surgery is necessary for an abscess, acute pseudocyst, and severe peritonitis. Percutaneous drainage of a pseudocyst can be performed, and a drainage tube is left in place. Surgical treatment of associated biliary tract disease may be necessary.

Pharmacological Management

Several different drugs may be used in the treatment of both acute and chronic pancreatitis (Table 38-22). A number of drugs are used in an effort to suppress pancreatic secretion, but these drugs have not proved very effective in the management of pancreatitis.

Nutritional Considerations

Initially the client with acute pancreatitis is on NPO status to reduce pancreatic secretion. When food is allowed, small, frequent feedings are given. The diet is usually high in carbohydrate content because that is the least stimulating to the pancreas. The diet combines high carbohydrate intake with low fat and high protein intake. It is bland with no stimulants (e.g., caffeine) and no alcohol. Supplemental fat-soluble vitamins may be given. The client may require supplemental commercial liquid preparations. If severe nutritional deficiencies exist, total parenteral nutrition (hyperalimentation) may be used (see Chapter 35).

■ Nursing Management of Acute Pancreatitis

Nursing assessment
Subjective and objective data that should be obtained from a person with acute pancreatitis are presented in Table 38-23.

Nursing diagnoses
Nursing diagnoses are determined when the problem and the etiological factors are supported by clinical data. Nursing diagnoses related to acute pancreatitis may include, but are not limited to, those presented in Table 38-24.

Nursing interventions
Health maintenance and promotion. The major factors involved in health promotion are (1) assessment of clients for predisposing and etiological factors of pancreatitis and (2) encouragement of early treatment of these factors to prevent occurrence of acute pancreatitis. The nurse should encourage the early diagnosis and treatment of biliary tract disease such as cholelithiasis. The client should be encouraged to eliminate alcohol intake, especially if there have been any previous episodes of pancreatitis. Attacks of pancreatitis become milder or disappear with the discontinuance of alcohol use.

Acute intervention. Because abdominal pain is a prominent symptom of pancreatitis, a major focus of nursing care is the relief of pain (Table 38-24). Giving the prescribed medications before the pain becomes too severe makes the medication more effective. The nurse should ascertain how long the pain medication provides relief. Mea-

Table 38-22 Drugs Used in Treatment of Acute and Chronic Pancreatitis

Drug	Mechanisms of Action
ACUTE PANCREATITIS	
Meperidine (Demerol)	Relief of pain
Nitroglycerin or papaverine	Relaxation of smooth muscles and relief of pain
Antispasmodics (e.g., dicyclomine [Bentyl], propantheline bromide [Pro-Banthine])	Decrease of vagal stimulation, motility, pancreatic outflow (inhibition of volume and concentration of bicarbonate and enzymatic secretion); contraindicated in paralytic ileus
Acetazolamide (Diamox) (carbonic anhydrase inhibitor)	Reduction in volume and bicarbonate concentration of pancreatic secretion
Antacids	Neutralization of gastric secretions; decrease in hydrochloric acid stimulation of secretin and pancreozymin, which stimulates production of pancreatic secretions
Cimetidine (Tagamet), ranitidine (Zantac)	Decrease in hydrochloric acid by inhibiting histamine
Calcium gluconate	Treatment of hypocalcemia to prevent or treat tetany
Adrenocortical steroids	Use only for seriously ill clients with hypotension or shock
Aprotinin (Trasylol)	Antitryptic and antikallikreinic actions
Glucagon	Reduction in pancreatic inflammation and decrease in serum amylase, suppression of pancreatic secretion
Somatostatin	Inhibition of pancreatic secretions
CHRONIC PANCREATITIS	
Pancreatin (Viokase)	Replacement therapy for pancreatic enzymes
Insulin	Treatment for diabetes if it occurs or for hyperglycemia

Table 38-23

 Nursing Assessment of the Client with Acute Pancreatitis

SUBJECTIVE DATA

History
Alcohol abuse, biliary tract disease, abdominal trauma or surgery, duodenal ulers, infection, metabolic disorders
Medications
Use of thiazides, estrogens, corticosteroids, azathioprine, sulfonamides, opiates, and furosemide
General
Weakness, anorexia
Pain
Severe midepigastric or left upper quadrant pain that may radiate to the back, aggravation with food and alcohol intake
Respiratory
Dyspnea
Gastrointestinal
Nausea and vomiting

OBJECTIVE DATA

General
Restlessness, anxiety, flushing, low-grade fever, diaphoresis
Integumentary
Discoloration of abdomen and flanks, jaundice
Respiratory
Tachypnea, basilar rales
Cardiovascular
Tachycardia, hypotension
Abdominal distention and tenderness, diminished bowel sounds
Gastrointestinal
Possible findings
Elevated serum amylase and lipase, leukocytosis, hyperglycemia, elevated urine amylase, abnormal ultrasound and CT scans of pancreas

CT, Computerized tomography.

Table 38-24

 NURSING CARE PLAN FOR THE CLIENT WITH ACUTE PANCREATITIS

Defining Characteristics	Nursing Interventions	Evaluation Criteria
NURSING DIAGNOSIS: Acute pain related to distention of pancreas, peritoneal irritation, obstruction of bilary tract, and ineffective pain and comfort measures		
Communication of pain descriptors, guarding behavior, narrowed self-focus, behaviors indicative of pain (e.g., moaning), diaphoresis, blood pressure, pulse, and respiratory rate changes	Give ordered analgesic and antispasmodic medications before pain gets too severe. Ascertain how long the medication provides relief. Make assessments regarding the pain, its severity, location, other accompanying symptoms, and precipitating factors. Provide comfort measures, such as positioning client comfortably with frequent changes in position and diversional activities.	Reports of satisfaction with pain control
NURSING DIAGNOSIS: Fluid volume deficit related to nausea, vomiting, NG suction, and restricted oral intake		
Thirst, increased fluid output, altered intake, dry skin and mucous membranes, decreased skin turgor, decreased oral intake	Give antiemetics as ordered. Measure and describe emesis. Provide oral hygiene after emesis. Observe for manifestations of metabolic alkalosis in severe vomiting.	Maintenance of adequate intake of fluids and electrolytes as evidenced by normal skin turgor, moist mucous membranes, stable weight
NURSING DIAGNOSIS: Potential complication: fluid and electrolyte imbalance related to loss of fluids into peritoneal cavity		
Excessive loss of fluids and electrolytes resulting in confusion, anorexia, diarrhea, seizures, muscle weakness, paralytic ileus, dysrhythmias, metabolic alkalosis, muscle cramps, mental changes, tetany	Observe for manifestations of hypokalemia, hyponatremia, hypocalcemia, and hypochloremia. Monitor serum laboratory results. Observe for jerking, irritability, and muscular twitching. Monitor serum calcium laboratory reports. Give calcium gluconate as ordered.	Normal serum electrolytes, absence or control of tetany
NURSING DIAGNOSIS: Potential complication: hemorrhagic shock related to elastase dissolving blood vessel walls		
Pallor; cool, clammy skin; hypotension; tachycardia; increased respirations	Monitor vital signs every 1-2 hr. Assess for continuing or increasing signs of shock. Assess hourly output for decreased urinary output.	Blood pressure within normal limits, no signs of shock
NURSING DIAGNOSIS: Impaired gas exchange related to pain, irritation near diaphragm, and ineffective cough		
Shortness of breath, dyspnea, cyanosis, tachypnea, cough, respiratory depth changes	Observe for fever or respiratory symptoms such as dyspnea, tachypnea. Have client turn, cough, and deep breathe every 1-2 hr. Place client in semi-Fowler's position to promote deeper respirations. Auscultate lungs q 2 hr.	Absence of respiratory infections, normal breath sounds, absence of signs and symptoms of hypoxia

Table 38-24

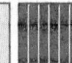

NURSING CARE PLAN FOR THE CLIENT WITH ACUTE PANCREATITIS—cont'd

Defining Characteristics	Nursing Interventions	Evaluation Criteria
NURSING DIAGNOSIS: Altered oral mucous membranes related to NG tube and NPO status		
Dry mouth, oral pain or discomfort, coated tongue, stomatitis, halitosis, oral lesions or ulcers, lack of or decreased salivation	Give oral and nasal care every 1-2 hr. Moisten client's nostrils and lips with water-soluble lubricant. Assess oral mucosa.	Moist lips and nares, absence of parotitis and stomatitis
NURSING DIAGNOSIS: Altered health maintenance related to lack of knowledge of preventive measures, diet restrictions, restriction of alcohol intake, and follow-up care		
Verbalization of the problem, request for information, inaccurate follow-through of instruction	Teach client (1) to abstain from alcohol; (2) to restrict fats and use more carbohydrates in diet; (3) to avoid rich, rough, and stimulating foods; and (4) to correctly measure blood glucose levels and to observe for steatorrhea. Assess client's understanding of prescribed regimen. Provide details on follow-up care. Suggest follow-up if alcohol use problematic.	Verbalization of understanding of condition or disease process and treatment, initiation of lifestyle changes and participation in treatment regimen, planning for follow-up care
NURSING DIAGNOSIS: Altered nutrition: less than body requirements related to anorexia, dietary restrictions, nausea, loss of nutrients from vomiting, and impaired digestion resulting in decreased use of nutrients		
Weight loss, weakness, fatigue, weight below normal for height and age	Monitor weight and laboratory values. Observe stools for steatorrhea. Administer total parenteral nutrition if ordered. Implement measures to reduce pain and nausea. Provide oral care before and after meals. If oral intake is allowed, provide small portions of appealing foods. Obtain dietary consult if indicated.	Weight appropriate for height, no further weight loss, adequate energy to perform activities of daily living

sures such as comfortable positioning, frequent changes in position, and relief of nausea and vomiting assist in reducing the restlessness that usually accompanies the pain. Some clients experience lessened pain by assuming positions that flex the trunk and draw the knees up to the abdomen. It is important to control the pain and restlessness because they increase body metabolism and subsequent stimulation of pancreatic secretions.

Nursing measures for the client who is on NPO status or has an NG tube should be employed. Frequent oral and nasal care to relieve the dryness of the mouth and nose is comforting to the client. Oral care is essential to prevent parotitis. If the client is taking anticholinergics to decrease GI secretions, there will be additional dryness of the mouth caused by the side effects of the drug. If the client is taking antacids to suppress secretions, they should be sipped slowly or inserted in the NG tube. The nurse must regularly assess the functioning of the suction.

A vital part of the nursing care plan for this client is ob-

servation for electrolyte imbalances. Frequent vomiting, along with gastric suction, may result in decreased chloride, sodium, and potassium levels. Because hypocalcemia can also occur, the nurse must observe for symptoms of tetany, such as jerking, irritability, and muscular twitching. The client should be assessed for a positive Chvostek's or Trousseau's sign. Calcium gluconate as ordered should be given to treat symptomatic hypocalcemia.

The client with acute pancreatitis is susceptible to infections. The nurse should observe for fever and other manifestations of infection. Respiratory infections are common due to the retroperitoneal fluid raising the diaphragm, which causes the client to take shallow, guarded abdominal breaths. Measures to prevent respiratory infections include turning, coughing, deep breathing, and assuming a semi-Fowler's position.

Other important assessments are observation for signs of paralytic ileus, renal failure, and mental changes. Glucometer determination of the blood glucose level should be

done to assess damage to the β cells of the islets of Langerhans in the pancreas.

After pancreatic surgery the client may require special wound care for an anastomotic leak or a fistula. Measures to prevent skin irritation should be used. These include skin barriers such as Stomahesive, karaya paste or Colley-Seel, pouching, and drains. In addition to protecting the skin, pouching also provides a more accurate determination of fluid and electrolyte losses and increases client comfort. Sterile pouching systems are available. The nurse may want to consult with a clinical specialist or an enterostomal therapist, if available.

Chronic management. Because frequent doses of narcotics may be required for this client during the acute stage, follow-up for assessment of possible narcotic addiction may be indicated. This is a more likely problem with chronic pancreatitis than in the client with acute pancreatitis. Counseling regarding abstinence from alcohol is very important to prevent the client from experiencing future attacks of acute pancreatitis and development of chronic pancreatitis.

Dietary teaching should include restriction of fats because they stimulate the secretion of pancreozymin, which then stimulates the pancreas. Carbohydrates are less stimulating to the pancreas, so they should be encouraged (see p. 1150).

Early detection makes it possible to correct mental changes by treating the cause before overt psychotic behavior is manifested. Possible causes of mental changes include sepsis, anorexia, toxicity from cellular breakdown products, and withdrawal from alcohol.

The client and the family should be given instructions regarding the recognition and reporting of symptoms of diabetes mellitus or steatorrhea (foul-smelling, frothy stools). These changes indicate possible destruction of pancreatic tissue. The nurse should make sure the client fully understands the prescribed regimen. Each aspect must be explained. The importance of taking the required medications and following the recommended diet should be stressed.

CHRONIC PANCREATITIS
Pathophysiology

Chronic pancreatitis is progressive destruction of the pancreas with fibrotic replacement of pancreatic tissue. Strictures and calcifications may also occur in the pancreas. There are actually several types of chronic pancreatitis, but they all have a common underlying pathophysiological disorder. The two major types are *chronic obstructive pancreatitis* and *chronic calcifying pancreatitis.* Chronic pancreatitis may follow acute pancreatitis, but it may also occur in the absence of any history of an acute condition.

Chronic obstructive pancreatitis is associated with biliary disease. The most common cause is inflammation of the sphincter of Oddi associated with cholelithiasis. Cancer of the ampulla of Vater, duodenum, or pancreas can also cause this type of chronic pancreatitis.

In chronic calcifying pancreatitis there is inflammation and sclerosis, mainly in the head of the pancreas and around the pancreatic duct. This type of chronic pancreatitis is the most common form. It is also called *alcohol-induced pancreatitis.* Increases in heavy social drinking have produced a higher incidence in countries in which the disease was previously considered rare. In the United States, chronic pancreatitis is found almost exclusively in alcoholics. As with cirrhosis, there seems to be a metabolic abnormality that predisposes a person who drinks to the direct toxic effect of the alcohol on the pancreas.

In chronic calcifying pancreatitis the ducts are obstructed with protein precipitates. These precipitates block the pancreatic duct and eventually calcify. This is followed by fibrosis and glandular atrophy. Pseudocysts and abscesses commonly develop.

Clinical Manifestations

As with acute pancreatitis, a major manifestation of chronic pancreatitis is abdominal pain. The client may have episodes of acute pain, but it usually is chronic (recurrent attacks at intervals of months or years). The attacks may become more and more frequent until they are almost constant, or they may diminish as the pancreatic fibrosis develops. The pain is located in the same areas as in acute pancreatitis but is usually described as a heavy, gnawing feeling or sometimes as burning and cramplike. The pain is not relieved with food or antacids.

Other clinical manifestations include symptoms of pancreatic insufficiency, including malabsorption with weight loss, constipation, mild jaundice with dark urine, steatorrhea, and diabetes mellitus. The steatorrhea may become quite severe with voluminous, foul, fatty stools. Some abdominal tenderness may be found.

Diagnostic Studies

Laboratory findings in chronic pancreatitis include increased serum amylase (200 to 600 Somogyi U/dl), increased serum bilirubin, and increased alkaline phosphatase levels. There is usually mild leukocytosis and an elevated sedimentation rate.

The secretin stimulation test is probably the most useful test in diagnosing chronic pancreatitis. Secretin is given IV, and gastric-duodenal secretions are collected with a double-lumen tube for separate gastric and duodenal aspiration. In chronic pancreatitis there is reduced volume of secretions and reduced bicarbonate concentration (less than 90 mEq/L). Normally, secretin stimulates the production of pancreatic fluid high in bicarbonate content.

Other abnormal diagnostic findings are hyperglycemia and fatty stools (steatorrhea) found in fecal fat determination. Neutral fat is indicative of maldigestion. Arteriography and x-ray films may demonstrate fibrosis and calcification.

ERCP involves cannulation and visualization of the pancreatic and common bile ducts through a fiberoptic endoscope that is inserted into the esophagus and then into the duodenum. The common bile duct and the pancreatic duct are then cannulated. Contrast dye can be injected into the ducts for visualization. Changes in the pancreatic ductal system, such as gross dilatation and microcysts, can be visualized through the use of ERCP.

Therapeutic and Pharmacological Management

When the client with chronic pancreatitis is experiencing an acute attack, the therapeutic management is identical to that for acute pancreatitis. At other times the focus is on prevention of further attacks, relief of pain, and control of pancreatic exocrine and endocrine insufficiency. It sometimes takes large, frequent doses of analgesics to relieve the pain, and narcotic addiction may become a problem.

Diet, pancreatic enzyme replacement, and control of the diabetes are measures used to control the pancreatic insufficiency. The diet is bland, low-fat, high-carbohydrate, and high-protein. The client does not tolerate fatty, rich, and stimulating foods, and these should be avoided to decrease pancreatic secretions and demands on the pancreas. Alcohol must be totally eliminated.

Antacids and anticholinergic drugs may be given to decrease hydrochloric acid, which stimulates pancreatic activity. Cimetidine (Tagamet) and ranitidine (Zantac), which inhibit histamine and thus decrease hydrochloric acid secretion, may be used for the same purpose. Pancreatic enzymes such as pancreatin (Viokase) and pancrelipase (Cotazym) contain amylase, lipase, and trypsin and are used to replace the deficient pancreatic enzymes. They are usually enteric coated to prevent their digestion by gastric acid activity. Bile salts are sometimes given to facilitate the absorption of the fat-soluble vitamins (A, D, E, and K) and prevent further fat loss. If diabetes develops, it is controlled with insulin or oral hypoglycemic drugs.

Treatment of chronic pancreatitis sometimes requires surgery. When biliary disease is present or if obstruction or pseudocyst develops, surgery may be indicated. Other operations performed are procedures to divert bile flow or relieve ductal obstruction. A choledochojejunostomy diverts bile around the ampulla of Vater where there may be spasm or hypertrophy of the sphincter. In this procedure the common bile duct is anastomosed into the jejunum. If the pancreatic sphincter is fibrotic, a sphincterotomy enlarges it. Pancreatic drainage procedures relieve ductal obstruction. One type is the Roux-en-Y pancreatojejunostomy in which the pancreatic duct is opened and an anastomosis is made with the jejunum. Total pancreas transplantation and islet cell transplantation are experimental techniques currently being studied in clinical trials to provide long-term replacement of endocrine function.

▪ Nursing Management of Chronic Pancreatitis

Except during an acute episode, the focus of nursing management is on chronic care and health promotion. The client should be instructed to take measures to prevent further attacks. Dietary control, along with consistency of other treatment measures such as taking pancreatic enzymes, is essential. The pancreatic extracts are usually given with meals or can be given with a snack. The nurse should observe the client's stools for steatorrhea to help determine the effectiveness of the enzymes. The client and the family need instructions regarding observation of stools.

If diabetes has developed, blood sugars or urinary glucose and acetone levels have to be monitored, and the cli-

ent will need diabetic teaching (see Chapter 43). The client who is taking antacids should be instructed to sip the medication slowly, and the nurse should make certain it is taken as ordered to help control gastric acidity. Antacids should be taken after meals. Both the antacid and the pancreatic enzymes may be left at the bedside to prepare the client for self-management at home.

Alcohol must be avoided, and the client may need assistance with this problem. If the client has developed a dependence on alcohol or narcotics, referral to other agencies or resources may be necessary.

CARCINOMA OF THE PANCREAS

The incidence of carcinoma of the pancreas is increasing. There were 28,100 new cases in the United States in 1990. It is the fourth leading cause of death from cancer. It is 30% more common in men and 50% more common in blacks. The risk increases with age.[14]

Most of the tumors are adenocarcinomas originating from the epithelium of the ductal system. More than half the tumors occur in the head of the pancreas. As the tumor grows, the common bile duct becomes obstructed and jaundice develops. Tumors starting in the body or tail often remain silent until their growth is quite advanced.

It may be difficult to differentiate cancer of the pancreas from chronic pancreatitis. The prognosis of a client with cancer of the pancreas is very poor. Most clients die within 5 to 12 months, and the 5-year survival rate is very low.

Etiology

The cause of cancer of the pancreas remains unknown. There seems to be some relationship between pancreatic cancer, diabetes mellitus, and chronic pancreatitis. However, it is not clear whether the cancer follows these diseases or whether these diseases occur as a result of pancreatic cancer. Recently, investigators believe a potential etiological factor may be a chemical carcinogen, but organ-specific carcinogens have not been identified. It is known that pancreatic cancer can be induced with chemicals such as nitrosoureas. Cigarette smoking is now firmly established as a significant risk factor in the development of cancer of the pancreas. Pancreatic cancer develops twice as frequently in persons with a history of heavy cigarette use (more than two packs a day) as in nonsmokers. The carcinogens from the tobacco probably reach the pancreatic ducts by bile reflux or via the bloodstream. Another risk factor is the Western diet, particularly the high fat content. Increased consumption of meat has also been implicated. Methods of processing foodstuffs may also be involved as a possible risk factor for cancer of the pancreas. The role of coffee as a contributing factor is still being investigated, but according to one study, coffee consumption increased the risk.[15]

Clinical Manifestations

Common clinical manifestations of pancreatic cancer include abdominal pain (dull, aching), anorexia, nausea, rapid and progressive weight loss, and jaundice. Pain is very common and is probably caused by perineural inva-

sion by the tumor. The pain is located in the upper abdomen or left hypochondrium and frequently radiates to the back. It is frequently related to eating, and it also occurs at night. The weight loss is due to poor digestion and absorption caused by lack of digestive juices from the pancreas.

Diagnostic Studies

Better diagnostic measures are needed for detection of pancreatic cancer, since most of the current methods detect only advanced stages. Cytological examination of the pancreatic juice may reveal malignant cells. The secretin test frequently results in decreased volume of pancreatic juice with normal bicarbonate and enzyme production. There are currently no specific blood tests diagnostic of pancreatic cancer. Carcinoembryonic antigen (CEA) is elevated in a high percentage of clients with advanced disease, but it is also increased with other types of cancers and even some benign conditions. The CEA plasma level is therefore probably more useful in assessing the client's response to treatment than in diagnosis. The pancreatic oncofetal antigen (POA), as well as other tumor markers, have been studied, but the results are too nonspecific to be of much value. Currently, monoclonal antibodies are also being studied.

Ultrasonography detects abnormalities of the pancreas but cannot distinguish cancer from other pancreatic disorders such as pancreatitis. Since this is a noninvasive procedure, it may be used in some situations. Computerized tomography (CT) scans are very effective in identifying a solid tumor mass and other changes such as lymph node spread. Pancreatic arteriography demonstrates occlusion of the celiac axis and the superior mesenteric artery.

With ERCP it is possible to get excellent x-ray visualization of the pancreatic ducts. In pancreatic cancer, findings include obstruction or narrowing of a major duct and frequently saccular dilatations of smaller peripheral ducts. Material for cytology and biopsy may show malignant cells. ERCP is usually considered to be the best diagnostic test.

Therapeutic Management

Surgery provides the most effective treatment of cancer of the pancreas. The classic surgery is a *radical pancreaticoduodenectomy* or *Whipple's procedure* (Fig. 38-7). This entails resection of the proximal pancreas (proximal pancreatectomy), the adjoining duodenum (duodenectomy), the distal portion of the stomach (partial gastrectomy), and the distal segment of the common bile duct. An anastomosis of the pancreatic duct, common bile duct, and stomach to the jejunum is done. A total pancreatectomy is currently a popular therapeutic measure. Sometimes a simple bypass procedure, such as a cholecystojejunostomy to relieve biliary obstruction, may be used as a palliative measure. Some surgeons suggest a more radical resection, such as a total pancreaticoduodenectomy with splenectomy. Biliary stents (e.g., Cotton-Leung stent) can be used as a palliative measure when tumors compress the bile duct.

Radiation therapy alters survival rates very little but is effective for pain relief. External radiation is usually used, but implantation of internal radiation seeds into the tumor

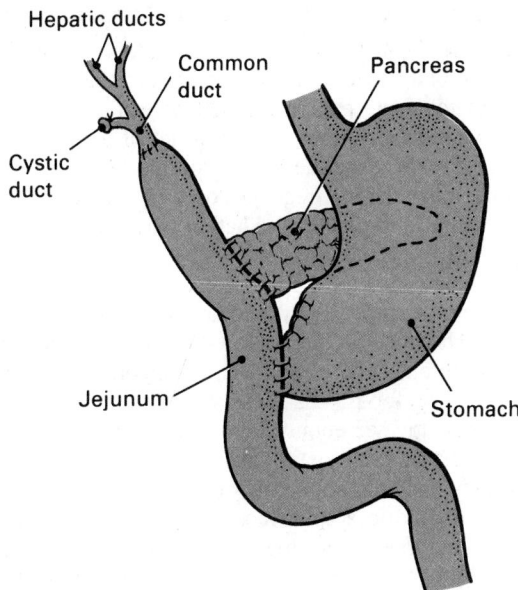

Fig. 38-7 Whipple procedure or radical pancreaticoduodenectomy. This surgical procedure involves resection of the proximal pancreas, adjoining duodenum, distal portion of the stomach, and distal portion of the common bile duct. An anastomosis of the pancreatic duct, common bile duct, and stomach to the jejunum is done.

has been used. Chemotherapy has limited success. Combinations of drugs such as 5-FU and BCNU produce a better response than single chemotherapeutic agents. Immunotherapy is sometimes attempted (see Chapter 9). Adjuvant therapy, which uses surgical resection, radiation, and chemotherapy, is believed by some to be the most effective way to manage the almost always fatal cancer of the pancreas.

■ Nursing Management of Carcinoma of the Pancreas

Because the client with carcinoma of the pancreas has many of the same problems as the client with pancreatitis, nursing care includes the same measures (see pp. 1151-1155). The nurse should provide symptomatic and supportive nursing care. Medications and comfort measures to relieve pain should be provided before the client reaches the peak of pain. Psychological support is essential, especially during times of anxiety or depression, which seem to occur frequently in these clients.

Adequate nutrition is an important part of the nursing care plan. Frequent and supplemental feedings may be necessary. Measures to stimulate the appetite as much as possible and to overcome anorexia, nausea, and vomiting should be included in the nursing care. Because bleeding can result from impaired vitamin K production, the nurse should assess for bleeding from body orifices and mucous membranes. If the client is undergoing radiation therapy, the nurse must observe for adverse reactions, such as anorexia, nausea, vomiting, and skin irritation.

This client will not live long and this will probably be

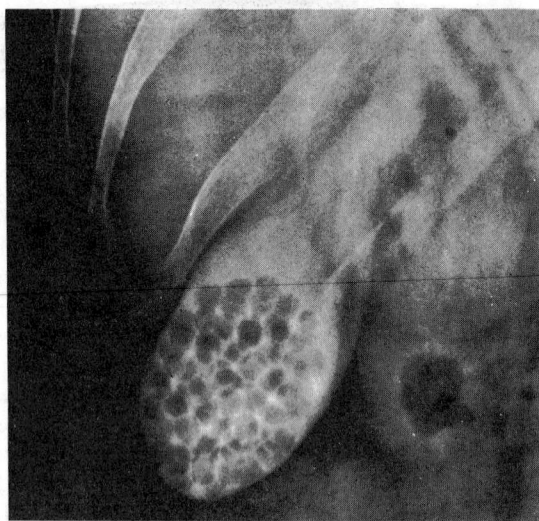

Fig. 38-8   X-ray film of a gallbladder with gallstones.

communicated by the physician. A significant component of the nursing care is helping the client and the family or significant others through the grieving process.

DISORDERS OF THE BILIARY TRACT

The most common disorder of the biliary system is *cholelithiasis* (stones in the gallbladder) (Fig. 38-8). *Cholecystitis* (inflammation of the gallbladder) is usually associated with cholelithiasis. The stones may be lodged in the neck of the gallbladder or in the cystic duct. Cholecystitis may be acute or chronic. These conditions usually occur together.

Significance

Gallbladder disease is a common health problem in the United States. It is estimated that 10% of the adults in the United States have cholelithiasis.[16] *Cholecystectomy* (removal of the gallbladder) ranks among the most common surgical procedures performed in the United States.[17] The incidence of cholelithiasis is higher in women, in multiparous women, and in persons over the age of 40. Postmenopausal women on estrogen therapy are at somewhat greater risk of having gallbladder disease than are women who are taking birth control pills. Oral contraceptives alter the character of bile, resulting in increased cholesterol saturation. Other factors that seem to increase the occurrence of gallbladder disease are a sedentary lifestyle, a familial tendency, and obesity. Obesity causes increased secretion of cholesterol in bile. Gallbladder disease is more common in white people than in Asians and blacks. There is an especially high incidence in the Native American population, particularly in the Navajo and Pima tribes.

Pathophysiology

Cholecystitis. Cholecystitis is most commonly associated with stones. When it occurs in the absence of stones, it is thought to be due to bacteria reaching the gallbladder via the vascular or lymphatic route or chemical irritants in the bile. *E. coli* is the most common bacterium involved.

Streptococci and salmonellae are also common causative bacteria. Other etiological factors include adhesions, neoplasms, extensive fasting, anesthesia, and narcotics.

Inflammation is the major pathophysiological condition and may be confined to the mucous lining or involve the entire wall of the gallbladder. During an acute attack of cholecystitis the gallbladder is edematous and hyperemic. It may be distended with bile or pus. The cystic duct is also involved and may become occluded. The wall of the gallbladder becomes scarred after an acute attack. Decreased functioning occurs if large amounts of tissue are fibrosed.

Cholelithiasis. The actual cause of gallstones is unknown. Basically, cholelithiasis develops when the balance that keeps cholesterol, bile salts, and calcium in solution is altered so that precipitation of these substances occurs. Conditions that upset this balance include infection and disturbances in the metabolism of cholesterol.

It is known that in clients with cholelithiasis the bile secreted by the liver is supersaturated with cholesterol (lithogenic bile). The bile in the gallbladder also becomes supersaturated with cholesterol. Whenever bile is supersaturated with cholesterol, precipitation of cholesterol will occur.

A high percentage of gallstones are precipitates of cholesterol. Other components of bile that precipitate into stones are bile salts, bilirubin, calcium, and protein. The stones sometimes have a mixed consistency. Mixed cholesterol stones, which are predominantly cholesterol, are the most common gallstones.

These changes in the composition of bile are probably very significant in the formation of gallstones. Stasis of bile leads to progression of the supersaturation and changes in the chemical composition of the bile. Immobility, pregnancy, and inflammatory or obstructive lesions of the biliary system decrease bile flow. Hormonal factors during pregnancy may cause delayed emptying of the gallbladder.

The stones may remain in the gallbladder or migrate to the cystic duct or to the common bile duct. They cause pain as they pass through the ducts and may lodge in the ducts and produce an obstruction. Small stones are more likely to move into a duct and cause obstruction. Table 38-25 depicts the changes and manifestations that occur when the stones obstruct the common bile duct. If the blockage occurs in the cystic duct, the bile can continue to flow into the duodenum directly from the liver. When the bile in the gallbladder cannot escape, however, this stasis of bile may lead to cholecystitis.

Clinical Manifestations

Manifestations of cholecystitis vary from indigestion to moderate to severe pain, fever, and jaundice. Initial symptoms of acute cholecystitis include indigestion and pain and tenderness in the right upper quadrant, which may be referred to the right shoulder and scapula. Manifestations of inflammation, such as leukocytosis and fever, occur. Acute cholecystitis may be present, with sudden onset of midepigastric or right upper quadrant pain radiating to the back and right shoulder. The pain is accompanied by rest-

Table 38-25 Clinical Manifestations Caused by Obstructed Bile Flow

Clinical Manifestation	Etiology
Obstructive jaundice	No bile flow into duodenum
Dark amber urine, which foams when shaken	Soluble bilirubin in urine
No urobilinogen in urine	No bilirubin reaching small intestine to be converted to urobilinogen
Clay-colored stools	Same as above
Pruritus	Deposition of bile salts in skin tissues
Faulty absorption or lack of absorption of fat-soluble vitamins (A, D, E, and K)	No bile in small intestine to emulsify fat; without bile, excretion of fatty acids in stool with loss of fat-soluble vitamins
Intolerance for fatty foods (nausea, sensation of fullness, anorexia)	No bile in small intestine for fat digestion
Bleeding tendencies	Lack of or decreased absorption of vitamin K resulting in decreased production of prothrombin
Steatorrhea	No bile salts in duodenum, preventing fat emulsion and digestion

lessness, diaphoresis, and nausea and vomiting. Physical findings include right upper quadrant tenderness and abdominal rigidity. Symptoms of chronic cholecystitis include a history of fat intolerance, dyspepsia, heartburn, and flatulence.

Cholelithiasis may produce severe symptoms or none at all. Many clients have "silent cholelithiasis." The severity of symptoms depends on whether the stones are stationary or mobile and whether obstruction is present. When a stone is lodged in the ducts or when stones are moving through the ducts, spasms may result. The spasms are the tissues' responses to the stone in an attempt to move it forward. This sometimes produces very severe pain, which is termed *biliary colic* even though the pain is rarely colicky. It is more often steady. The pain can be excruciating and accompanied by tachycardia, diaphoresis, and prostration. The severe pain may last up to an hour, and when it subsides there is residual tenderness in the right upper quadrant. The attacks of pain frequently occur 3 to 6 hours after a heavy meal or when the client assumes a recumbent position. When total obstruction occurs, symptoms related to bile blockage are manifested (see Table 38-25).

Complications

Complications of cholecystitis include subphrenic abscess, pancreatitis, cholangitis (inflammation of biliary ducts), biliary cirrhosis, fistulas, and rupture of the gallbladder, which can produce bile peritonitis.

Many of the same complications can occur from cholelithiasis, including cholangitis, biliary cirrhosis, carcinoma, and peritonitis. Choledocholithiasis (stone in the common bile duct) may occur, producing symptoms of obstruction.

Diagnostic Studies

Ultrasonography is probably the best means of diagnosing gallstones (Table 33-11). It is especially useful for clients with jaundice, since it does not depend on liver function, and for clients who are allergic to contrast medium. It is very accurate in detecting stones (90% to 95%).

An oral cholecystogram allows for the visualization of stones when they are radiopaque. An IV cholangiogram outlines both the gallbladder and the ducts, so gallstones that have moved into the ductal system can be visualized. Percutaneous transhepatic cholangiography may be used to diagnose obstructive jaundice and to locate stones within the bile ducts. Bile taken during ERCP is sent for culture to identify any possible infecting organism.

Laboratory tests may demonstrate abnormalities in some of the liver function tests and an increased white blood cell (WBC) count as a result of inflammation. Both the direct and indirect bilirubin levels are elevated, as is the urinary bilirubin level if there is an obstructive process present. If the common bile duct is obstructed, no bilirubin will reach the small intestine to be converted to urobilinogen. Serum enzymes, such as alkaline phosphatase, SGOT (AST), and LDH, may be elevated. The serum amylase is increased if there is pancreatic involvement.

Therapeutic Management

Cholecystitis. During an acute episode of cholecystitis the focus of treatment is on (1) control of pain, (2) control of possible infection with antibiotics, and (3) maintenance of fluid and electrolyte balance (Table 38-26). Treatment is mainly supportive and symptomatic. If nausea and vomiting are severe, gastric decompression may be used to prevent further gallbladder stimulation. Anticholinergics to decrease secretions (which prevent biliary contraction) and counteract smooth muscle spasms may be administered. Analgesics are given to decrease the pain.

Cholelithiasis. There are currently several options for therapeutic management of cholelithiasis. These include extracorporeal shock-wave lithotripsy (ESWL), cholesterol solvents such as methyl tertiary terbutyl ether (MTBE), oral drugs that dissolve stones, endoscopic sphincterotomy, and surgery. Supportive treatment, similar to that given for cholecystitis, may also be necessary. If the stones cause an obstruction, additional treatment consists of replacement of fat-soluble vitamins, administration of bile salts to facilitate digestion and vitamin absorption, and a low-fat diet.

In ESWL a biliary lithotriptor uses high-energy shock waves to disintegrate gallstones. The client must have a functioning gallbladder. An ultrasound scan is first done to locate the stones and to determine where to direct the shock waves. The shock waves are directed through the abdomen as a water-filled cushion is pressed against the area. It usually takes 1 to 2 hours to disintegrate the

stones. After they are broken up, the fragments pass through the common bile duct and into the small intestine.[18]

Endoscopic sphincterotomy (papillotomy) is especially effective in removing common bile duct stones (Fig. 38-9). The endoscope is passed to the duodenum. With an electrodiathermy knife attached to the endoscope, the sphincter of Oddi is widened by incision of the sphincter muscle. The stones are removed with a balloon or basket.[19]

Still in the investigational stage is the instillation of MTBE into the gallbladder via a percutaneous catheter. MTBE dissolves cholesterol stones within hours. Its safety has not been established.[20] Oral bile acids are also used to dissolve stones (see p. 1160).

The procedure of choice for most clients is still a cholecystectomy. This is a safe procedure with minimal morbidity, and it requires only a brief hospitalization.

Surgical interventions. Surgical intervention for cholelithiasis is frequently indicated and may consist of any one of several procedures (Table 38-27). The most common surgical approach is through a right subcostal incision. A T tube is inserted into the common bile duct during surgery when a common bile duct exploration is part of the surgical procedure (Fig. 38-10). This ensures patency of the duct until the edema produced by the trauma of exploring and probing the duct has subsided. It also allows the excess bile to drain while the small intestine is adjusting to receiving a continuous flow of bile.

Table 38-26

Diagnostic and Therapeutic Management: Cholelithiasis

DIAGNOSTIC

Ultrasound
Cholecystogram or IV cholangiogram
Liver function studies
WBC count

THERAPEUTIC
Conservative treatment

IV fluids
NPO with NG tube—later progressing to low-fat diet
Antiemetics
Analgesics (e.g., meperidine)
Fat-soluble vitamins (A, D, E, and K)
Anticholinergics
Bile salts
Antibiotics
ERCP with sphincterotomy

Postsurgical treatment

Analgesics
Low Fowler's position
Progressive surgical diet
Change of dressing as needed
T tube (if common bile duct exploration performed)

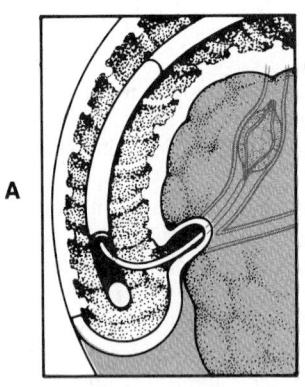

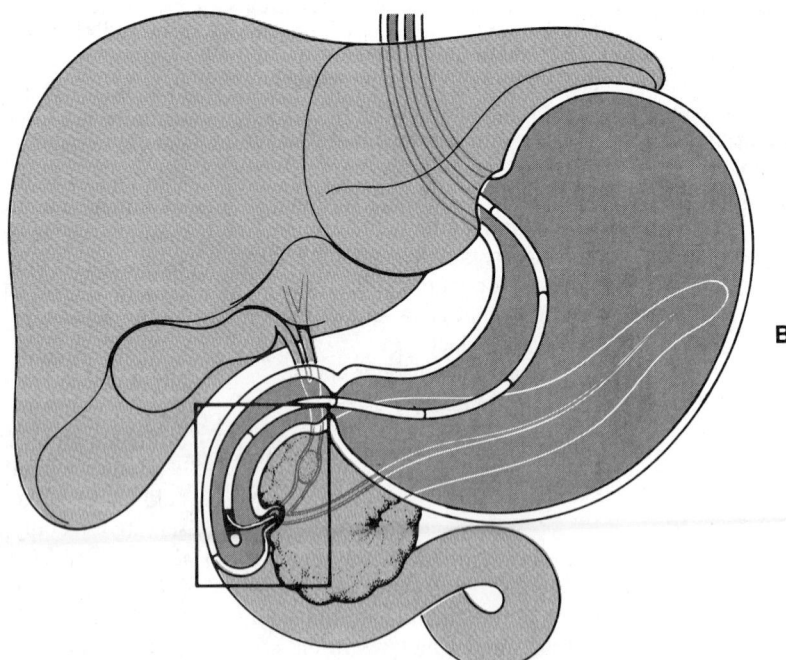

Fig. 38-9 **A,** During endoscopic sphincterotomy, flexible endoscope is advanced through the mouth and stomach until its tip sits in the duodenum opposite the common bile duct. **B,** After widening the duct mouth by incising the sphincter muscle, the physician advances a basket attachment into the duct and snags the stone.

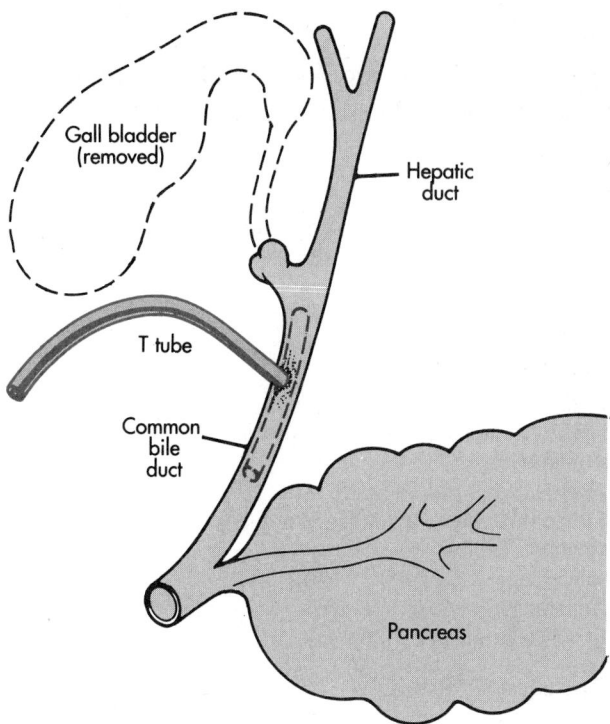

Fig. 38-10 Placement of T tube. *Dotted lines* indicate parts removed.

Table 38-27 Gallbladder Surgery Procedures

Name	Description
Cholecystectomy	Removal of gallbladder
Cholecystostomy (usually an emergency)	Incision into gallbladder (usually for removal of stones)
Choledocholithotomy	Incision into common bile duct for removal of stones
Cholecystogastrostomy	Anastomosis between stomach and gallbladder
Cholecystoduodenostomy	Anastomosis between gallbladder and duodenum to relieve obstruction at distal end of common bile duct
Endoscopic cholecystectomy	Removal of gallbladder via laparoscopy using a dissecting laser

Another type of surgical procedure that has recently been introduced is the *endoscopic cholecystectomy (laparoscopic laser cholecystectomy)*, in which the gallbladder is removed through one of four small punctures in the abdomen. A 1 cm puncture is made slightly above the umbilicus, and the surgeon inflates the abdominal cavity with 3 to 4 L of carbon dioxide to improve visibility. A laparoscope, which has a camera attached, is then inserted into the abdomen. Two additional punctures are made just below the ribs, one on the right anterior axillary line and the other on the right midclavicular line. These punctures are used for insertion of grasping forceps. A dissection laser is inserted into the fourth puncture, which is made just right of the midsection. (The incision sites may vary.)

Using closed-circuit monitors to visualize the abdominal cavity, the surgeon retracts and dissects the gallbladder and removes it with grasping forceps.

This procedure is relatively minor, with few complications. Most clients experience minimal postoperative pain and are discharged the day of surgery or the day after. In most cases they are able to resume normal activities and return to work after 2 or 3 days.

Transhepatic biliary catheter. The transhepatic biliary catheter can be used preoperatively in biliary obstruction and in hepatic dysfunction secondary to obstructive jaundice. It can also be inserted when inoperable liver, pancreatic, or bile duct carcinoma obstructs bile flow. The catheter is inserted under fluoroscopy and involves percutaneous insertion across the liver parenchyma into the common bile duct and duodenum. It decompresses obstructed extrahepatic bile ducts so that bile can flow freely. After insertion, the catheter is connected to a drainage bag. The skin around the catheter insertion site has to be cleansed daily with an antiseptic. It is important to observe for bile leakage at the insertion site. Depending on the reason the catheter was inserted, the client may be discharged with it in place.

Pharmacological Management

The most common drugs used in the treatment of gallbladder disease are analgesics, anticholinergics (antispasmodics), fat-soluble vitamins, and bile salts.

Meperidine (Demerol) is used if a narcotic analgesic is required. This causes less spasm in the ducts than opiates such as morphine sulfate. Amyl nitrite and nitroglycerin may be used to relax the smooth muscle of the biliary tract. If nitroglycerin is given, the nurse should observe for side effects of nausea, vomiting, flushing of the skin, and hypotension.

Anticholinergics such as atropine and other antispasmodics may be used to relax the smooth muscle and decrease ductal tone. Papaverine also has a relaxing effect on smooth muscle. Nursing observations for side effects of drugs and relief of the pain should be made.

If the client has chronic gallbladder disease or any biliary tract obstruction, fat-soluble vitamins (A, D, E, and K) will probably be given. Bile salts may be administered to facilitate digestion and vitamin absorption.

Hydrocholeretic drugs may be administered following gallbladder surgery when a T tube is in place or with conservative therapy as long as there is no obstruction. These drugs stimulate the production of bile of a low specific gravity. Examples are bile salts such as dehydrocholic acid (Decholin) and florantyrone (Zanchol).

For treatment of pruritus, cholestyramine (Questran) may provide relief. This is a resin that binds bile salts in the intestine, increasing their excretion in the feces. Cholestyramine is administered in powder form and should be mixed with milk or juice. The nurse should observe for side effects of nausea, vomiting, diarrhea or constipation, and skin reactions.

Modest success is being demonstrated with the use of chenodeoxycholic acid (CDCA, chenodiol, Chenix) to dissolve or prevent the formation of cholesterol gallstones. Chenodiol reduces the cholesterol secretion in bile, converting bile supersaturated with cholesterol to bile unsaturated with cholesterol. It also dissolves stones by solubilizing cholesterol. Therapy may take anywhere from 6 months to 2 years for dissolution of the stones, and low-dose therapy is recommended to prevent recurrence. Chenodiol is recommended for clients with small radiolucent stones who are poor surgical risks. The main side effects are cramps and diarrhea, but these are usually not severe. Ursodeoxycholic acid (UDCA)-ursodiol (Actigall) is very similar to CDCA but causes less diarrhea. It is very expensive. These drugs may be used after ESWL to prevent formation of other stones.[20]

Nutritional Considerations

The major dietary modification for a client with cholelithiasis and cholecystitis is a low-fat diet (see Table 28-5). If obesity is a problem, a reduced-caloric diet is indicated. The low-fat diet prevents excess stimulation of the gallbladder. Foods that are avoided include dairy products such as whole milk, cream, butter, whole milk cheese, and ice cream; fried foods; rich pastries; gravies; and nuts. Many clients have fewer problems if they eat smaller, more frequent meals.

After gallbladder surgery the client is given nothing by mouth for 24 to 48 hours. The diet is advanced according to the client's tolerance. The amount of fat in the postoperative diet depends on the client's tolerance of fat. A low-fat diet may be helpful if the flow of bile is reduced (usually only in the early postoperative period) or if the client is overweight. Sometimes the client is instructed to restrict fats for 4 to 6 weeks. Otherwise no special dietary instructions are needed other than to eat nutritious meals and avoid excessive fat intake.

▪ Nursing Management of Gallbladder Disease
Nursing assessment

Subjective and objective data that should be obtained from a person with gallbladder disease are presented in Table 38-28.

Nursing diagnoses

Nursing diagnoses are determined when the problem and the etiological factors are supported by clinical data. Nursing diagnoses related to gallbladder disease may include, but are not limited to, those presented in Table 38-29.

Nursing interventions

Health maintenance and promotion. The nurse should assume responsibility for recognition of predisposing factors of gallbladder disease in general health screening. Ethnic groups in which the disease is more common, such as Native Americans, should be taught initial manifestations and instructed to seek medical care if these manifestations occur. The client with chronic cholecystitis does not have acute symptoms and may not seek help until jaundice and biliary obstruction occur. Earlier detection in these clients is beneficial so that they can be treated with a low-fat diet and monitored more closely.

Table 38-28

Nursing Assessment of the Client with Cholecystitis or Cholelithiasis

SUBJECTIVE DATA

History
Positive family history, activity level, obesity, ethnicity, multiparity, infection, previous abdominal surgery, cancer, extensive fasting, pregnancy, diabetes, cirrhosis
Medications
Use of estrogen or oral contraceptives
General
Weight loss, chills, anorexia
Pain
Moderate to severe pain in right upper quadrant that may radiate to the back or scapula (biliary colic)
Integumentary
Dry, itchy skin
Gastrointestinal
Indigestion, fat intolerance, nausea and vomiting, dyspepsia, pyrosis, flatulence, clay-colored stools
Urinary
Dark urine

OBJECTIVE DATA

General
Fever, restlessness
Integumentary
Jaundice, icteric sclera
Respiratory
Tachypnea, splinting during respirations
Cardiovascular
Tachycardia
Gastrointestinal
Palpable gallbladder, abdominal guarding and distention
Possible findings
Elevated liver function tests and bilirubin, leukocytosis, abnormal gallbladder ultrasound, positive oral cholecystogram or IV cholangiogram

Acute intervention. Nursing objectives for the client undergoing conservative therapy include (1) relieving pain, (2) relieving nausea and vomiting, (3) providing comfort and emotional support, (4) maintaining fluid and electrolyte balance and nutrition, (5) making accurate assessments for effectiveness of treatment, and (6) observing for complications.

This client is frequently experiencing severe pain. The medications ordered to relieve the pain should be given as required by the client and before the pain becomes more severe. The nurse should assess what medications relieve the pain and how much medication is required. Observations for side effects of the medications must be part of the continued assessment. Nursing comfort measures, such as a clean bed, comfortable positioning, and oral care, are appropriate.

Some clients have more severe nausea and vomiting than others. For these clients it may be necessary to use

Table 38-29

NURSING CARE PLAN FOR THE CLIENT FOLLOWING A CHOLECYSTECTOMY

Defining Characteristics	Nursing Interventions	Evaluation Criteria
NURSING DIAGNOSIS: Acute pain related to surgical incision and ineffective pain and comfort measures		
Communication of pain descriptors, guarding behavior, narrowed self-focus, behaviors indicative of pain (e.g., moaning), diaphoresis, blood pressure, pulse, and respiratory rate changes	Administer ordered analgesic frequently enough to ensure that the client will move about. Provide comfort measures. Reposition client as needed. Help client support incision when coughing and deep breathing and getting out of bed.	Reports of satisfaction with pain control
NURSING DIAGNOSIS: Ineffective breathing pattern related to splinted or guarded respirations secondary to pain		
Dyspnea, shortness of breath, tachypnea, cyanosis, cough, respiratory depth changes, changes in respiratory rate or pattern, changes in pulse	Assist client to cough and deep breathe every hour. Auscultate lung sounds q 2-4 hr. Plan a schedule with client and ensure that analgesia is given as needed to make it easier to cough, deep breathe, and move about. Support incision with pillow or hands. Encourage early ambulation. When client is in bed, place in low Fowler's position.	Normal breath sounds, respiratory rate of 12-16/min
NURSING DIAGNOSIS: Potential complication: paralytic ileus related to decreased peristalsis secondary to surgery and immobility		
Failure to pass gas or feces, abdominal distention and tenderness, absence of bowel sounds	Keep client on NPO status until bowel sounds are present. Maintain IV fluid administration at prescribed rate. Provide oral care q 1-2 hr. Auscultate for bowel sounds q 4 hr. Encourage ambulation 3 or 4 times a day if not contraindicated.	Normal bowel sounds, normal nutritional intake
NURSING DIAGNOSIS: High risk for impaired skin integrity related to heavy, irritating drainage from surgical area		
Disruption of epidermal and dermal tissue, erythema, denuded skin, lesions, pruritus, drainage from surgical area	Keep dressing dry and clean. Use Montgomery straps to reduce skin irritation from frequent removal of tape. Observe and record type of drainage. Cleanse skin carefully with warm water and pat dry.	Surgical area free from redness and signs of irritation
NURSING DIAGNOSIS: Altered health maintenance related to lack of knowledge of postoperative management, diet, and activity restrictions		
Verbalization of problem, request for information, inaccurate follow-through of instruction	Instruct client to avoid heavy lifting for 4 to 6 wk. Provide dietary teaching plan if client is required to remain on low-fat diet or if put on a weight-reduction program. Assist client to arrange necessary follow-up care.	Knowledge of activity level and dietary restrictions, planning for follow-up care, return to usual lifestyle

gastric decompression. The elimination of intake of food and fluids also prevents further stimulation of the gallbladder. Oral hygiene, care of nares, accurate intake and output measurements, and maintenance of suction should be a part of the nursing care plan for this client. For clients with less severe nausea and vomiting, antiemetics are usually adequate. When the client is vomiting, comfort measures such as frequent mouth rinses should be provided. Any vomitus should be immediately removed from the client's view.

If pruritus occurs with jaundice, measures to relieve itching are necessary. Such measures include baking soda or Alpha Keri baths, lotions such as those containing calamine, antihistamines, soft old linen, and control of the temperature (not too hot and not too cold). The client's nails should be kept short and clean. Clients should be taught to rub with their knuckles rather than scratch with their nails when they cannot control the scratching.

A significant portion of the nursing care plan for this client centers on accurate assessment of progression of the symptoms and development of complications. The nurse must be knowledgeable of and observe for signs of obstruction of the ducts by stones. These include jaundice; clay-colored stools; dark, foamy urine; steatorrhea; fever; and increased WBC count.

When symptoms of obstruction are present (see Table 38-25), the nurse must be aware of the possibility of bleeding as a result of decreased prothrombin production. Common sites to observe for bleeding are the mucous membranes of the mouth, nose, gingivae, and injection sites. If injections are given, a small-gauge needle should be used and gentle pressure applied after the injection. The nurse should know what the client's prothrombin time is and use this as a guide in the assessment process.

Assessment for infections includes monitoring of vital signs. A temperature elevation with chills and jaundice may indicate choledocholithiasis.

Nursing care of the client after endoscopic papillotomy includes assessment to detect complications such as pancreatitis, perforation, infection, and bleeding. The client's vital signs should be monitored. Abdominal pain and fever may indicate pancreatitis. The client should be on bed rest for several hours and should have nothing by mouth until the gag reflex returns.

CARE AFTER SURGICAL INTERVENTION. Preoperative care is essentially the same as for any abdominal surgical procedure (see Chapter 37). The nurse should be aware of such details as whether the client will have an NG tube, since these are frequently not used for gallbladder surgery. Client teaching should include information regarding the types of drainage tubes that will be used postoperatively.

Postoperative nursing care is discussed in Table 38-29. Adequate ventilation and prevention of respiratory complications are important objectives for this client. The high incision in the right subcostal region is near the diaphragm, and the client is reluctant to take deep breaths because of the pain this causes.

If the client has an NG tube, it will probably be in for 24 to 48 hours. When bowel sounds are heard, the client is given clear liquids, with progression to a surgical soft diet and then to a low-fat or regular diet. The nurse should observe tolerance to the diet and assist in any required dietary instruction.

The client may have a Penrose drain or a Jackson-Pratt drain inserted into a stab wound near the incision. This allows for drainage and prevents accumulation of fluid and serous drainage in the area from which the gallbladder was removed. If there is serosanguineous bile-tinged drainage, the dressing should be changed frequently. The wound should be kept dry and clean because bile is irritating to the skin. When changing the dressing, the nurse should use sterile technique, clean around the drain (if indicated), and take special care not to dislodge the drain. Currently many clients have no drains and may have a dressing for only 24 to 48 hours.

If the client has a T tube, part of the nursing care plan is related to maintaining bile drainage and observation of the T-tube functioning and drainage. The T tube is connected to a closed gravity drainage system. Nursing care in relation to the T tube is summarized in Table 38-30. If the Penrose or Jackson-Pratt drain or the T tube is draining large amounts, it is helpful to use a sterile pouching system to protect the skin.

Chronic management. When the client is on a conservative therapy, long-term nursing management depends on symptoms and on whether surgical intervention is being planned. Dietary teaching is usually necessary. The diet is usually low in fat, and sometimes a weight-reduction diet is also recommended. The client may need to take fat-soluble vitamin supplements. The nurse should provide instructions regarding observations the client should make indicating obstruction (stool and urine changes, jaundice, and pruritus). Continued health care is important, and its significance should be explained and stressed.

The client may be discharged as soon as 3 to 5 days after a cholecystectomy. If a T tube has been inserted, hospitalization may be extended or the client may go home with the T tube in place. The T tube is usually left in place for 7 to 10 days. In that case the client must be taught how to care for the tube and to report symptoms such as excessive drainage, jaundice, and light-colored stools. The client should be instructed to avoid heavy lifting for 4 to 6 weeks. Usual sexual activities, including intercourse, should be resumed as soon as the client feels ready unless given other instructions by the physician.

Sometimes the client is required to remain on a low-fat diet for 4 to 6 weeks. If so, a dietary teaching plan is necessary. A weight-reduction program may be helpful if the client is overweight. Most clients tolerate a regular diet with no difficulties but should avoid excessive fats.

Approximately 20% of all clients who have cholecystectomies for gallstones have postoperative GI complaints. The most common is upper abdominal pain and is called *postcholecystectomy syndrome*.[21] It may be caused by residual calculi, recurring calculi, stricture of the duct, or infection around the common bile duct. Surgical intervention may be necessary to correct the cause of the problem. Fiberoptic endoscopy is effective in the management of many of these clients (see p. 1159).

Table 38-30 Nursing Care of a Client with T Tube

Nursing Care	Rationale
Observe amount and color of drainage: Initially bloody and then greenish brown after several hours	To determine excess bleeding and whether bile is flowing and not blocking up in liver or leaking into peritoneal cavity; increased bile flow after it has started to decrease possible indication of ductal obstruction below tube
Approximately 400 ml/day after first few days; decrease in amount as bile begins to follow normal route; drainage of more than 1000 ml/day should be reported to physician	
Observe for drainage around tube; may need to use sterile pouching system	To prevent irritating effects of bile on skin
Do not irrigate, aspirate, or clamp tube without an order	To promote free-flowing bile
Maintain client in low Fowler's position	To promote bile drainage
Maintain correct level of drainage bag as ordered	To allow for gravity drainage of bile
Follow orders for raising level of bag and/or clamping; observe for pain, chills, fullness, and nausea	To check patency of common bile duct
Assist client to turn and ambulate without dislodging or kinking tube	To prevent dislodgment and maintain patency
If tube is clamped for 1-2 hr before and after meals, assess client's response	To determine whether bile is aiding digestion
Observe for indications that bile is flowing through normal channels: Brown stools Decreased amount of drainage from tube No signs of jaundice	To determine when bile is flowing through normal channels and when T-tube removal is possible (usually 7-10 days)

CANCER OF THE GALLBLADDER

Primary cancer of the gallbladder is rare. The majority of gallbladder carcinomas are adenocarcinomas. There seems to be a definite relationship between cancer of the gallbladder and chronic cholecystitis and cholelithiasis. Approximately 80% of clients with gallbladder malignancy also have gallstones.

The early symptoms of carcinoma of the gallbladder are insidious and are similar to those of chronic cholecystitis and cholelithiasis, which makes diagnosis difficult. Later symptoms are usually those of biliary obstruction. Cancer of the gallbladder has a very poor prognosis.

Treatment is mainly symptomatic and supportive. Sometimes the tumor is resected. Chemotherapy and radiotherapy are seldom used because they are neither curative nor palliative.

Nursing management involves supportive care with special attention to nutrition, hydration, skin care, and pain relief. Many of the nursing care measures used for clients with cholecystitis and cholelithiasis (see pp. 1161-1163) are frequently applied, as well as nursing care measures for the client with cancer (see Chapter 9).

C ase Study

CIRRHOSIS OF THE LIVER

Ronald is a 42-year-old man admitted in a hepatic coma. He has had cirrhosis of the liver for 10 years. He is an admitted alcoholic and has been drinking heavily for 15 years. He says he has been "sober" for the past 2 years. Review of old records reveals progressive weakness, anorexia, weight loss, jaundice, pedal edema, ascites, and mental disorientation.

On admission, Ronald is stuporous and has twitching, asterixis, and fetor hepaticus. He appears thin, malnourished, and very ill. Assessment reveals 4+ pitting edema of the lower extremities, ascites, jaundice, spider angiomas, and purpura. Both the liver and the spleen are palpable.

Previous liver biopsy findings
Fatty liver (at 36 years of age)
Cirrhosis with some necrosis (at 40 years of age)

Present laboratory values		*Medications and diet*
Total bilirubin	11 mg/dl	Lactulose 20 ml qid
Serum enzymes	SGOT 180 U/L	Neomycin 1 g qid
	SGPT 525 U/L	Aldactone 100 mg bid
	LDH 450 U/L	Thiamine 100 mg q d
Serum ammonia	220 μg/dl	IM
Hematocrit	24%	
Prothrombin time	30 sec	40 g protein, 2 g sodium diet

Discussion Questions

1. What are possible causes of cirrhosis? What type of cirrhosis does Ronald have?
2. Describe the pathophysiological changes that occur in the liver as cirrhosis develops. Explain the results of Ronald's two liver biopsies.
3. List Ronald's clinical manifestations of liver failure. For each manifestation, explain the pathophysiological bases.
4. Explain the significance of the results of his laboratory values.
5. What is the cause of hepatic coma? What measures should be instituted to control or decrease the ammonia level?

6. Ronald was being closely observed for the possibility of GI bleeding. Why is this considered a possible complication?
7. In the early stages of cirrhosis, what can be done to control the disease?
8. Identify the purpose of each medication Ronald is taking.
9. What is the reason for the special diet therapy for him?

Review Questions

The number of the question corresponds to the same-numbered objective at the beginning of the chapter.

1. A major problem in hepatocellular jaundice is with the
   a. production of unconjugated bilirubin
   b. conjugation and excretion of bilirubin
   c. flow of bile through the bile ducts
   d. excessive breakdown of erythrocytes
2. With hepatitis in the prodromal (preicteric) phase, which of the following is expected?
   a. sudden onset of jaundice
   b. weight loss
   c. acute yellow atrophy
   d. flulike symptoms
3. When caring for the client with viral hepatitis the *most* important precaution is probably
   a. gowning and gloving
   b. hand washing
   c. using disposable dishes
   d. getting an injection of ISG
4. A client with cirrhosis of the liver
   a. has a tendency to bleed and hyperventilate
   b. is prone to infection and metabolic alkalosis
   c. shows signs of jaundice and ascites
   d. develops decreased body temperature and pruritus
5. When caring for a client with hepatic encephalopathy the nurse may give enemas, provide a low-protein diet, and limit physical activity. These measures are done to
   a. eliminate potassium ions
   b. decrease the production of ammonia
   c. increase the production of ammonia
   d. decrease portal pressure
6. Which of the following statements about carcinoma of the liver is false?
   a. Surgical excision of the tumor is highly successful.
   b. Nursing intervention focuses on symptomatic and comfort measures.
   c. The prognosis is very poor.
   d. It is difficult to distinguish primary from metastatic tumors.
7. The most common pathogenic mechanism in acute pancreatitis is
   a. cellular disorganization
   b. lack of secretion of enzymes
   c. autodigestion
   d. overproduction of enzymes
8. Teaching measures for the client with chronic pancreatitis should include all the following *except*
   a. consistency of taking pancreatic enzymes with meals
   b. observation of stools for signs of steatorrhea
   c. monitoring of urinary glucose and acetone levels
   d. high-protein, moderate-fat, low-carbohydrate diet
9. Identify the false statement about carcinoma of the pancreas.
   a. Cigarette smoking is a significant risk factor.
   b. Most of the tumors are adenocarcinomas.
   c. The most effective treatment is external radiation.
   d. An important nursing measure is assisting the client with the grieving process.
10. A significant factor in the formation of gallstones seems to be
    a. chemical irritants in the bile
    b. supersaturation of bile with cholesterol
    c. bacteria reaching the gallbladder via the vascular route
    d. an increase in the bile acid pool size
11. To which of the following complications should the nurse give highest priority on the nursing care plan of the client following a cholecystectomy?
    a. respiratory problems
    b. thrombophlebitis
    c. abdominal distention
    d. wound infection

REFERENCES

1. Centers for Disease Control: Protection against viral hepatitis: recommendations of the Immunization Practices Advisory Committee, MMWR 39:RR-2, 1, 3, 8-9, 1990.
2. Schiff L and Schiff ER, eds: Diseases of the liver, ed 3, Philadelphia, 1987, JB Lippincott Co, pp 163, 461-465.
3. Stollerman GH, ed: Capsule and comment, Hosp Pract 24:49, 1989.
4. Gitnick G, ed: Principles and practice of gastroenterology and hepatology, New York, 1988, Elsevier.
5. Rakel RE, ed: Conn's current therapy 1990, Philadelphia, 1990, WB Saunders Co, p 460.
6. Nishioka NS and Dienstag JL: Delta hepatitis: a new scourge? N Engl J Med 312:1515, 1985.
7. Lettau LA and others: Outbreak of severe hepatitis due to delta and hepatitis B viruses in parenteral drug abusers and their contacts, N Engl J Med 317:1256, 1987.
8. Hollinger FB: Serologic evaluation of viral hepatitis, Hosp Pract 22:101-114, 1987.
9. Pachter A: Should nurses receive the hepatitis B vaccine? Nursing 18:51, 1988.
10. Ruppert S: Gastrointestinal problems, Nurse Review, Springhouse, Pa, 1986, Springhouse Corp, p 99.
11. Quinless FW: Severe liver dysfunction, Focus Crit Care 12:24-32, 1985.
12. Whiteman K and others: Liver transplantation, Am J Nurs 90:69-72, 1990.
13. Sabesin SM and Williams JW: Current status of liver transplantation, Hosp Pract 22:75-86, 1987.
14. American Cancer Society: Cancer facts and figures 1990, Atlanta, 1990, pp 12, 14.
15. Patel PH and Thomas E: Carcinoma of the pancreas, Hosp Pract 22:131, 1987.

16. Rakel RE, ed: Conn's current therapy 1990, Philadelphia, 1990, WB Saunders Co, p 422.
17. Ruppert S: Gastrointestinal problems, Nurse Review, Springhouse, Pa, 1986, Springhouse Corp, p 116.
18. Petersen BT: Biliary lithotripsy, Hosp Pract 25:23-30, 1990.
19. Lancaster SL: Clinical news, gallstone lithotripsy, Am J Nurs 12:1629-1630, 1988.
20. Willis DA, Harbit MD, and Julius LM: Gallstone alternatives to surgery, RN 53:44-50, 1990.
21. Gitnick G, ed: Principles and practice of gastroenterology and hepatology, New York, 1988, Elsevier, p 961.

SECTION VI REFERENCES

BOOKS

Bayless TM: Current management of inflammatory bowel disease, St Louis, 1989, The CV Mosby Co.

Bayless TM: Current therapy in gastroenterology and liver disease, vol 3, ed 3, St Louis, 1989, The CV Mosby Co.

Corman ML: Colon and rectal surgery, ed 2, Philadelphia, 1989, JB Lippincott Co.

Eastwood GL, ed: Premalignant conditions of the gastrointestinal tract, New York, 1991, Elsevier Science Publishing Co, Inc.

Fisher Rl: Malabsorption and nutritional status and support, gastroenterology clinics of North America, Philadelphia, 1989, WB Saunders Co.

Funk SG and others, eds: Key aspects of comfort: management of pain, fatigue and nausea, New York, 1989, Springer Publishing Co.

Gibson RS: Principles of nutritional assessment, New York, 1990, Oxford University Press.

Guthrie HA and Bagby RS: Introductory nutrition, St Louis, 1989, The CV Mosby Co.

Prinsley DM and Sandstead HH, eds: Nutrition and aging, New York, 1990, Alan R Liss, Inc.

Rombeau JL and Caldwell MD, eds: Enteral and tube feeding, ed 2, Philadelphia, 1990, WB Saunders Co.

Sleisenger MH and Fordtran JS: Gastrointestinal disease, pathophysiology, diagnosis, and management, ed 4, Philadelphia, 1989, WB Saunders Co.

Tolonen M: Vitamins and minerals in health and nutrition, New York, 1990, E Horwood.

US National Research Council Committee on Diet and Health: Diet and health: implications for reducing chronic disease risk, Washington, DC, 1989, National Academy Press.

US National Research Council Subcommittee on the Tenth Edition of RDA's, Food and Nutrition Board: Recommended dietary allowances, ed 10, Washington, DC, 1989, National Academy Press.

Weinsier RL, Heimburger DC, and Butterworth CE: Handbook of clinical nutrition: clinician's manual for the prevention, diagnosis, and management of nutritional problems, ed 2, St Louis, 1989, The CV Mosby Co.

Williams JW, ed: Hepatic transplantation, Philadelphia, 1990, WB Saunders Co.

Williams SR: Essentials of nutrition and diet therapy, ed 5, St Louis, 1989, The CV Mosby Co.

Zakim D and Bayer TD, eds: Hepatology: a textbook of liver disease, ed 2, Philadelphia, 1990, WB Saunders Co.

JOURNALS

Abernathy GB and others: Efficacy of tub feeding in supplying energy requirements of hospitalized patients, JPEN 13:387, 1989.

Basilisco G and others: Risk factors for first operation in Crohn's disease, J Gastroenterol 84:749, 1989.

Beckermann S and Galloway S: Elective resection of the liver: nursing care, Crit Care Nurse 9:40, 1989.

Cerrato PL: Is America really constipated? RN 52:81, 1989.

Choi M and others: *Salmonella* outbreak in a nursing home, J Am Geriatr Soc 38:531, 1990.

Collins AS: Gastrointestinal complications in shock, Crit Care Nurs Clin North Am 2:269, 1990.

Crocker KS: Gastrointestinal manifestations of the acquired immunodeficiency syndrome, Nurs Clin North Am 24:395, 1989.

Dennison AR and others: The management of hemorrhoids, J Gastroenterol 84:475, 1989.

Eisenberg P: Enteral nutrition: indications, formulas, and delivery techniques, Nurs Clin North Am 24:315, 1989.

Fernandez-Banares F and others: Vitamin status in patients with inflammatory bowel disease, J Gastroenterol 84:744, 1989.

Front ME, Wise SR, and Carey LC: Common bile duct strictures: diagnosis, management, follow-up, AORN J 52:57, 1990.

Haderstorfer B, Whitehead W, and Schuster M: Intestinal gas production from bacterial fermentation of undigested carbohydrate in irritable bowel syndrome, Am J Gastroenterol 84:375, 1989.

Hallak A: Spontaneous bacterial peritonitis, J Gastroenterol 84:345, 1989.

Hennessy K: Nutritional support and gastrointestinal disease, Nurs Clin North Am 24:373, 1989.

Jeffres C: Complications of acute pancreatitis, Crit Care Nurse 9:38, 1989.

Kohn CL and Keithley JK: Enteral nutrition: potential complications and patient monitoring, Nurs Clin North Am 24:339, 1989.

Loos FD: Acute pancreatitis: a critical nursing challenge, Can Crit Care Nurs J 6:5, 1989.

Naccarato M and Kresevic D: Caring for adults who have cystic fibrosis, Am J Nurs 89:1462, 1989.

O'Reilly M and Mulry K: Postanesthesia care of renal and biliary lithotripsy patients, J Post Anesth Nurs 4:382, 1989.

Ragan JA: Lasers in gastroenterology, Nurs Clin North Am 25:685, 1990.

Rice PS and Phaosawasdi K: Understanding idiopathic chronic constipation: an understated problem, Gastroenterol Nurs 12:90, 1989.

Rowland GA, Marks DA, and Torres WE: The new gallstone destroyers and dissolvers, Am J Nurs 89:1473, 1989.

Shapiro M: The gastroenterologist and the treatment of hemorrhoids: is it about time? J Gastroenterol 84:493, 1989.

Willis DA, Harbit MD, and Julius LM: Gallstones: alternatives to surgery, RN 53:44, 1990.

ORGANIZATIONS

American Dental Association
211 East Chicago Avenue
Chicago, IL 60611

American Digestive Disease Society
60 East 42nd Street, Room 411
New York, NY 10165

Canadian Foundation of Ileitis and Colitis
21 Saint Claire Avenue, East, Suite 301
Toronto, Ontario, Canada M4T 1L9

Hollister, Inc.
2000 Hollister Drive
P.O. Box 250
Libertyville, IL 60048

International Association for Enterostomal Therapy, Inc.
2081 Business Center Drive, Suite 290
Irvine, CA 92715

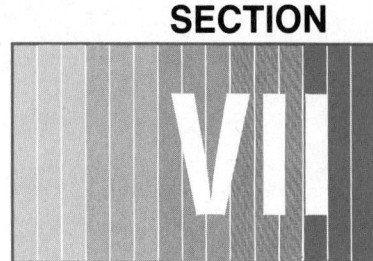

SECTION VII

PROBLEMS WITH URINARY FUNCTION

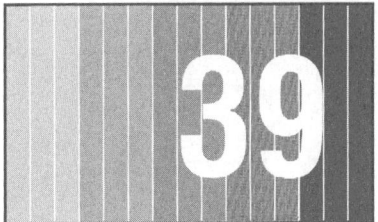

39

Nursing Assessment
Urinary System

Sharon Mantik Lewis

"Bones can break, muscles can atrophy, glands can loaf, even the brain can go to sleep without immediate danger to survival. But should the kidneys fail . . . neither bone, muscle, gland, nor brain could carry on."[1] This statement underlines the importance of kidneys to our lives. Adequate functioning of the kidneys is essential to maintenance of a healthy body. If the kidneys fail to function and care is not given, death is inevitable within 2 to 3 weeks.

The kidney is the principal organ of the urinary system. Besides the two kidneys, there are two ureters, a urinary bladder, and a urethra in the urinary system (Fig. 39-1). The other organs can be thought of as storage and drainage channels for the urine after it is formed in the kidneys.

The primary function of the kidney is to regulate the volume and composition of extracellular fluid. Its excretory function is secondary to this regulatory function. The

Reviewed by Evelyn Butera, R.N., M.S., C.N.N., Manager, Education Services, Northwest Kidney Center, Seattle, Washington.

secretory functions of the kidney include renin secretion, erythropoietin production, vitamin D activation, and acid-base balance regulation.

STRUCTURES AND FUNCTIONS OF THE URINARY SYSTEM
Kidneys

Macrostructure. The two kidneys are bean-shaped organs that are retroperitoneal (behind the peritoneum) on either side of the vertebral column. Each kidney weighs 120 to 170 g (4 to 6 ounces) and is usually about 12 cm (5 inches) long. The right kidney, with the liver above it, is lower than the left. The right kidney is at the level of the twelfth rib. An adrenal gland lies on top of each kidney.

Each kidney is surrounded by a considerable amount of fat and connective tissue that serve to support and maintain it in position. The surface of the kidney is covered by a thin, smooth layer of fibrous membrane called the *capsule*. The *hilus* serves as the entry site for the renal artery and nerves and the exit site for the vein and ureter.

On a longitudinal section of the kidney (Fig. 39-2), the internal structure can be visualized. The outer layer is referred to as the *cortex,* and the inner layer is called the *medulla*. The medulla consists of a number of *pyramids*. The apices of these pyramids are called *papillae*. They enter *calyces*. Minor calyces merge to form major calyces. These form a funnel-shaped sac called the *renal pelvis*. The lumen of the pelvis decreases to form the ureter.

Microstructure. The functional unit of the kidney is the *nephron*. Each kidney has more than 1 million nephrons. A nephron is composed of a glomerulus, Bowman's capsule, and a tubular system. The tubular system consists of the proximal convoluted tubule, the loop of Henle, and the distal convoluted tubule (Fig. 39-3). Several nephrons converge into a collecting duct, which eventually merges into a minor calyx.

Blood supply. A blood supply of about 1200 ml/min, which is 20% to 25% of the cardiac output, flows to the two kidneys. It reaches them via the renal artery, which arises from the aorta and enters the kidney through the hilus (Fig. 39-4). The renal artery divides into secondary

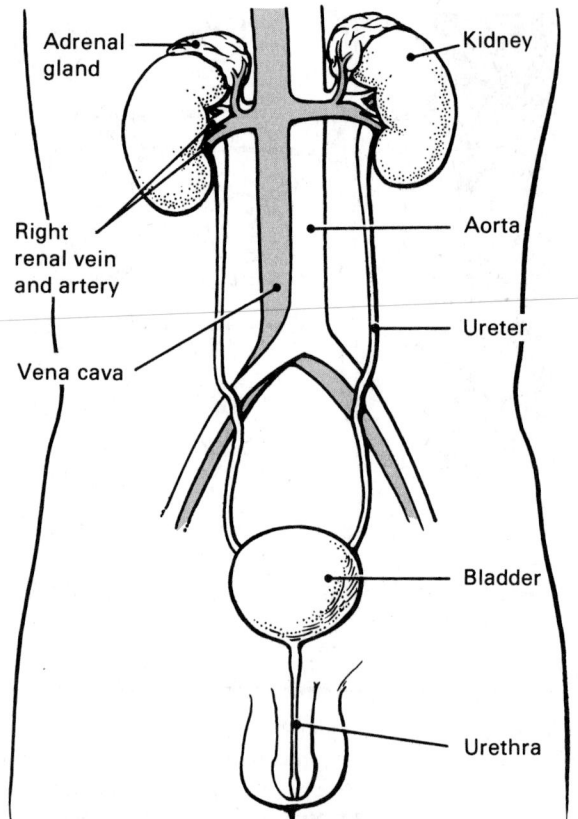

Fig. 39-1 Organs of the male urinary system.

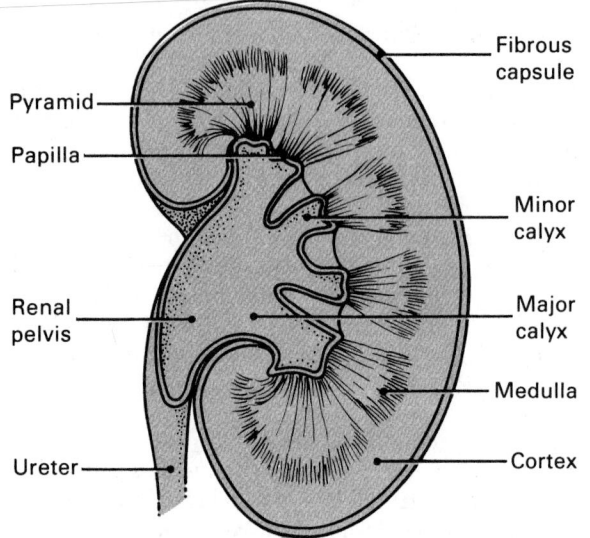

Fig. 39-2 Longitudinal section of the kidney.

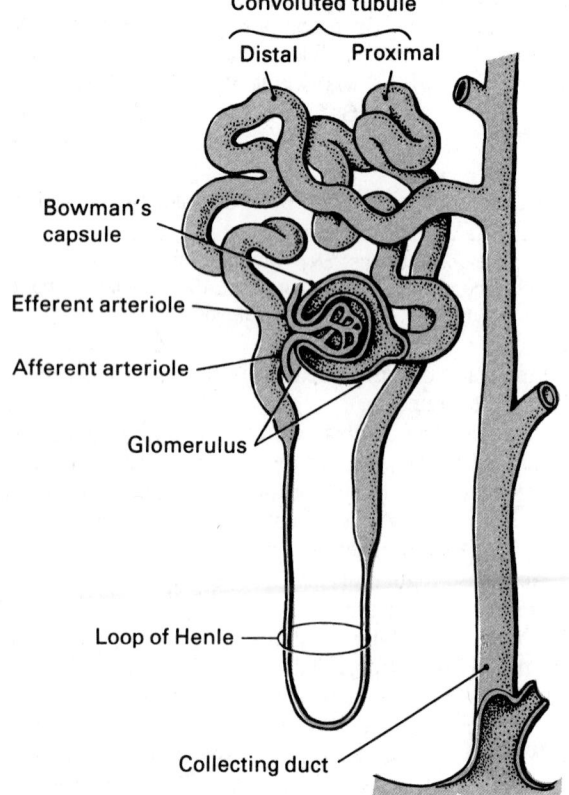

Fig. 39-3 Nephron of the kidney.

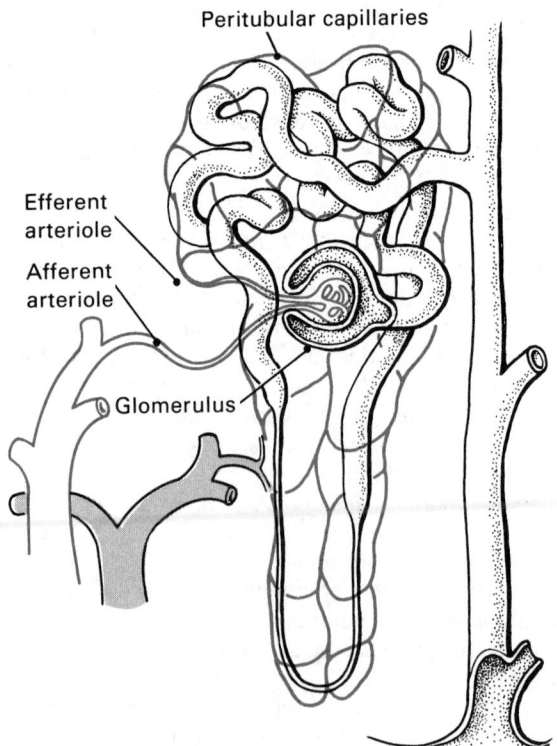

Fig. 39-4 Blood supply of the nephron.

branches and then into still smaller branches, each of which eventually forms an *afferent arteriole*. The afferent arteriole divides into a capillary network called a *glomerulus*, which is a tuft of up to 50 capillaries. The capillaries of the glomerulus eventually unite in the *efferent arteriole*. This again splits up to form a capillary network called the *peritubular capillaries*, which, as the name suggests, surround the tubular system.

Physiology of Urine Formation

Glomerulus. Urine formation starts at the glomerulus where blood is filtered. The blood flow to the glomeruli of both kidneys is about 1200 ml/min. A semipermeable membrane surrounding the outer surface of the glomerulus allows for filtration (Fig. 39-3). The pressure of the blood within the glomerular capillaries causes blood to be filtered into Bowman's capsule, where it begins to pass down to the tubule. Filtration is more rapid in the glomerulus than in ordinary tissue capillaries because of the porosity of the glomerular membrane. The ultrafiltrate is similar in composition to blood except that it lacks blood cells, platelets, and large plasma proteins. Capillary permeability is increased in many renal diseases, permitting plasma proteins to pass into the urine.

The amount of blood filtered by the glomeruli in a given time is referred to as the *glomerular filtration rate* (GFR). The normal GFR is about 125 ml/min. However, on the average only 1 ml/min leaves as urine.

Tubular function. Because the glomerular membrane functions to filter substances chiefly by size, provision is made for the reabsorption of essential materials and the excretion of nonessential ones (Table 39-1). The tubules and collecting ducts carry out these functions by means of reabsorption and secretion (Fig. 39-5). *Reabsorption* refers to the passage of a substance from the lumen of the tubules through the tubule cells and into the capillaries. It involves both active and passive transport. *Tubular secretion* refers to the passage of a substance from the capillaries through the tubular cells into the lumen of the tubule.

In the proximal convoluted tubule about 80% of the electrolytes are reabsorbed. Normally, all the glucose, amino acids, and protein are reabsorbed. Hydrogen ions (H^+) and creatinine are secreted into the filtrate.[2]

In the loop of Henle, reabsorption continues. In the ascending limb, chloride ions (Cl^-) are actively reabsorbed, followed passively by sodium ions (Na^+). About 25% of the filtered sodium is reabsorbed here. The loop of Henle is also very important in conserving water and thus concentrating the filtrate.

Two important functions of the distal convoluted tubules are final regulation of water balance and acid-base balance. In the distal tubule the role of certain hormones becomes important. Antidiuretic hormone (ADH), released by the posterior pituitary, is required for water reabsorption. In the presence of ADH the tubules become more permeable to water, allowing it to return to circulation. In the absence of ADH the tubules are practically impermeable to water and any water in them leaves the body as urine.

In the presence of aldosterone (released from the adrenal cortex) acting on the distal tubule, reabsorption of Na^+

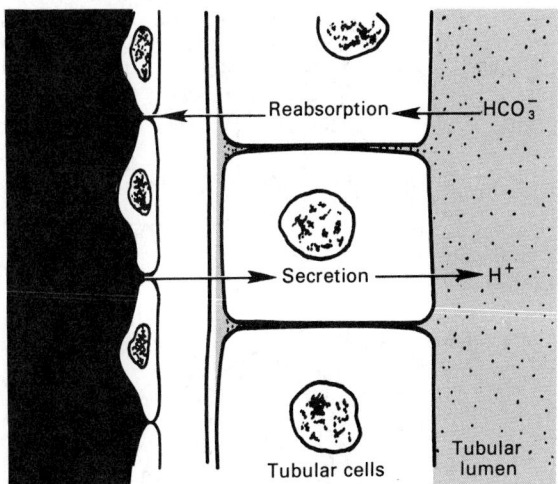

Fig. 39-5 Reabsorption and secretion in the tubules.

Table 39-1 Functions of the Components of the Nephron

Component	Function
Glomerulus	Filtration
Proximal tubule	Reabsorption of 80% of electrolytes and water, reabsorption of all glucose and amino acids, reabsorption of HCO_3^-, secretion of H^+ and creatinine
Loop of Henle	Reabsorption of Na^+ and Cl^- in ascending limb, concentration of filtrate
Distal tubule	Secretion of K^+, H^+, ammonia; reabsorption of water (regulated by ADH); reabsorption of HCO_3^-; regulation of Ca^{2+} and PO_4^{2-} by parathormone; regulation of Na^+ and K^+ by aldosterone
Collecting duct	Reabsorption of water (ADH required)

HCO_3^-, Bicarbonate ions; H^+, hydrogen ions; Na^+, sodium ions; Cl^-, chloride ions; K^+, potassium ions; *ADH*, antidiuretic hormone; Ca^{2+}, calcium ions; PO_4^{2-}, phosphate ions.

and the water occurs. In exchange for Na^+, potassium ions (K^+) are excreted.

Parathormone is released from the parathyroid gland. It is secreted in the presence of low serum calcium levels. It causes increased tubular reabsorption of calcium ions (Ca^{2+}) and decreased tubular reabsorption of phosphate ions (PO_4^{2-}). Therefore, serum Ca^{2+} levels are increased.

Acid-base regulation involves reabsorbing and conserving most of the bicarbonate (HCO_3^-) and secreting excess H^+. The distal tubule functions in different ways to maintain the pH of extracellular fluid (ECF) within a range of 7.35 to 7.45 (see Chapter 10). In the distal tubule, K^+ ions are also secreted into the filtrate.

When the filtrate leaves the distal tubule and enters the collecting duct, it is called *urine*. Final concentration of water may occur in the collecting duct.[3]

The basic function of nephrons is to clean or clear blood plasma of unnecessary substances. After the glomer-

ulus has filtered the blood, the tubules separate the unwanted from the wanted portions of tubular fluid. The wanted portions are returned to the blood and the unwanted portions pass into urine. Of every 125 ml filtered, about 1 ml becomes urine; 124 ml is returned to the blood.

Ureters

The ureters are tubes 25 to 35 cm (10 to 12 inches) long and 2 to 8 mm (0.08 to 0.3 inch) in diameter that convey urine to the bladder from the kidneys. One to five peristaltic contractions per minute assist in the transportation of urine from the kidneys to the bladder. The ureters are profusely innervated with sympathetic and parasympathetic nerve fibers. The afferent nerve fibers from the ureters play an important role in stimulating the acute severe pain (renal colic) associated with the lodging and passing of ureteral calculi.

Where the ureters enter the bladder, a fold of mucous membrane serves as a ureterovesical valve, which prevents the backflow of urine into the ureters when the bladder contracts. Because the renal pelvis holds only 3 to 5 ml of urine, damage to the kidneys can result from a backflow of urine.

Bladder

The urinary bladder is a collapsible storage bag composed of muscular elastic tissue that is capable of considerable distention. Its primary function is to serve as a reservoir for urine.

On the average, 200 to 250 ml of urine in the bladder causes moderate distention and the urge to urinate. When the quantity of urine reaches 400 ml, the person feels uncomfortable. The process of emptying the bladder is known as *micturition;* the terms *voiding* and *urination* are also used. The capacity of the bladder varies with the individual, ranging from 1000 to 1800 ml.

The desire to urinate depends on the integrity of the stretch receptors in the bladder wall. The distention of the bladder stimulates stretch receptors, causing reflex contraction of the bladder and simultaneous relaxation of the internal sphincter. This is followed by relaxation of the external sphincter, which is under voluntary control, and emptying of the bladder. Parasympathetic nerve fibers in the bladder are actively involved in micturition, coordinating bladder contraction, and relaxation of the sphincters.

Voluntary contraction of the external sphincter, which is composed of skeletal muscle, is a learned response. It depends on proper neurological function. Injury to the nerves supplying the bladder, urethra, spinal cord, or motor area of the cortex may lead to incontinence. Any pain or difficulty in urinating is abnormal and requires immediate medical attention.

The mucous membrane of the bladder wall has phagocytic ability. The unidirectional flow of urine from the kidney to the bladder also guards against ascending infection.

Normal urine output is approximately 1500 ml/day, which varies with food and fluid intake. The volume of urine produced at night is less than one half of that formed during the day as a result of hormonal influences. This diurnal pattern of urination is normal. Most persons urinate five to six times a day and occasionally at night.

Urethra

The urethra is a small tube that leads from the bladder to the exterior of the body. Its primary function is to discharge urine. In the female it is 3 to 5 cm (1 to 2 inches) long and lies behind the symphysis pubis and anterior to the vagina. The male urethra, which is about 20 cm (8 inches) long, originates at the bladder and extends the length of the penis. It serves as the passageway for urine as well as semen.

Normally, the urethra contains some bacteria. The turbulent flow of urine through the urethra flushes it free of debris and bacteria. The mucous membrane lining the urethra secretes mucus that is bacteriostatic.

Other Renal Functions

In addition to its function in regulating the volume and composition of ECF, the kidney also has a function in production of erythropoietin, production and secretion of renin, and activation of vitamin D.

Erythropoietin is produced and released in response to decreased oxygen tension in the renal blood supply. Erythropoietin stimulates the production of red blood cells (RBCs) by the bone marrow. A deficiency of erythropoietin leads to anemia in renal failure.

Vitamin D is metabolized by the kidney from an inactive form to an active metabolite. Interference with this function contributes to renal osteodystrophy (see Chapter 41).

Renin is important in the regulation of blood pressure (Fig. 39-6). It is released from the granular cells of the afferent arteriole. These cells, together with the macula densa cells of the distal convoluted tubule and the mesangial cells, form the *juxtaglomerular apparatus.* Renin is

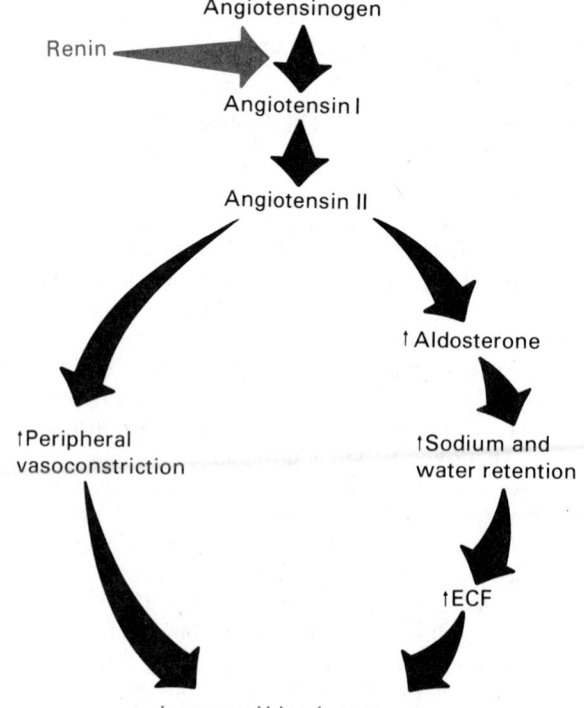

Fig. 39-6 Renin-angiotensin mechanism.

released in response to decreased arterial blood pressure, renal ischemia, ECF depletion, norepinephrine, and increased urinary Na^+ concentration. Renin catalyzes the splitting of the plasma protein angiotensinogen into angiotensin I, which is subsequently converted to angiotensin II. Angiotensin II stimulates the release of aldosterone from the adrenal cortex, and this causes Na^+ and water retention, leading to an increased ECF volume. Angiotensin II also causes increased peripheral vasoconstriction. The increase in ECF and vasoconstriction causes an elevation in blood pressure, which normally acts to inhibit renin release. Excessive renin production may be a contributing factor in the etiology of renal hypertension (see Chapter 27).

Prostaglandins. Prostaglandins (PGs) are a structurally related group of 20-carbon fatty acids with a 5-carbon ring. They are synthesized by most body tissues from the precursor, arachidonic acid, in response to appropriate stimuli. PGs, which are involved in the regulation of cell function and host defenses, exert their influence primarily on cells or tissues that are close to the site where they are synthesized. (See Chapter 7 for a more detailed discussion of prostaglandins.)

In the kidney, PG synthesis occurs primarily in the medulla. The kidneys secrete a variety of PGs. These PGs have a vasodilating action in addition to increasing renal blood flow and promoting Na^+ excretion. They counteract the vasoconstrictor effect of angiotensin and norepinephrine. Renal PGs may have a systemic effect in lowering blood pressure by decreasing systemic vascular resistance.[4]

The significance of these PGs is related to the role of the kidney in causing hypertension. In renal failure with a loss of functioning parenchymal tissue, these renal vasodilator factors are also lost. This may be one factor that contributes to the common finding of hypertension in renal failure (see Chapter 41).

ASSESSMENT OF THE URINARY SYSTEM
Subjective Data

Health history
Past health history. The client should be questioned about the existence or history of diseases that are known to be related to renal problems. These include (1) hypertension, (2) diabetes mellitus, (3) gout, (4) connective tissue disorders (e.g., systemic lupus erythematosus, scleroderma), (5) skin or upper respiratory infections of streptococcal origin, (6) urinary tract infections, (7) urinary calculi, and (8) infectious disease. The client should also be questioned about any previous hospitalizations related to these diseases as well as any urinary tract problems during past pregnancies. The duration, severity, and client's perception of any problems should be elicited. If the client has ever been catheterized or has had diagnostic studies involving instrumentation of the urinary tract or use of contrast media, this information should be noted.

An assessment of the client's current and past use of medication is important. This should include over-the-counter drugs as well as prescription drugs. Many prescription drugs are known to be nephrotoxic agents (Table

Table 39-2 Nephrotoxic Agents	
ANTIBIOTICS	**OTHER AGENTS**
Amikacin	Captopril
Amphotericin B	Carbon tetrachloride
Bacitracin	Cisplatin
Cephalosporins	Cyclosporine
Colistin	Ethylene glycol
Gentamicin	Gold
Kanamycin	Heavy metals
Neomycin	Methotrexate
Polymyxin B	Nitrosoureas (e.g., carmustine)
Streptomycin	Nonsteroidal antiinflammatory agents (e.g., ibuprofen, indomethacin)
Sulfonamides	
Tobramycin	Phenacetin
	Quinine
	Rifampin
	Salicylate (large quantities)

39-2). Certain drugs may alter the quantity and character of urine output. Anticoagulants may cause hematuria, diuretics change the volume of urine output, and drugs such as phenazopyridine hydrochloride (Pyridium) and nitrofurantoin (Macrodantin) change its color.

Family history. The presence of certain renal or urological problems in a family history increases the likelihood of similar problems occurring in a family member. The nurse should ask about family members who have had any of the diseases referred to in the past health history as well as polycystic renal disease, congenital urinary tract abnormalities, and Alport's syndrome (hereditary nephritis).

Social and personal history
BACKGROUND INFORMATION. The client should be asked about past employment in an occupation that involved exposure to chemicals. Carbon tetrachloride, phenol, and ethylene glycol are examples of nephrotoxic chemicals. The combination of carbon tetrachloride and alcohol is known to cause tubular necrosis.

LIFESTYLE. It has been shown that persons living in certain areas of the United States (Great Lakes, Southwest, Southeast) have a higher than normal incidence of urinary calculi. This may be due to the higher mineral content of the soil and water.

The client's diet may be important in identifying factors contributing to calculi formation. Some persons who drink large quantities of milk or ingest other products high in Ca^{2+} have high concentrations of Ca^{2+} in their urine. Fluid intake should also be assessed. Dehydration may contribute to formation of calculi, urinary infections, and renal failure.

The level of activity should also be assessed. A sedentary person is more likely than an active one to have stasis of urine, which can predispose to infection and calculus

Table 39-3 Clinical Manifestations of Disorders of
the Urinary System

GENERAL MANIFESTATIONS

Fatigue	Itching
Headaches	Excess thirst
Blurred vision	Chills
Elevated blood pressure	Changes in body weight
Anorexia	Changes in mentation
Nausea and vomiting	

RELATED TO URINARY SYSTEM

Pain

Dysuria
Flank or costovertebral angle
Groin
Suprapubic

Changes in urine output

Polyuria
Oliguria
Anuria

Changes in patterns of urination

Frequency
Nocturia
Dysuria
Hesitancy of stream
Change in stream
Urgency
Retention
Incontinence
Stress incontinence
Enuresis

Changes in urine consistency

Hematuria
Pyuria
Concentrated
Dilute
Color (red, brown, yellowish green)

Edema

Facial (periorbital)
Ankle
Ascites
Anasarca
Sacral

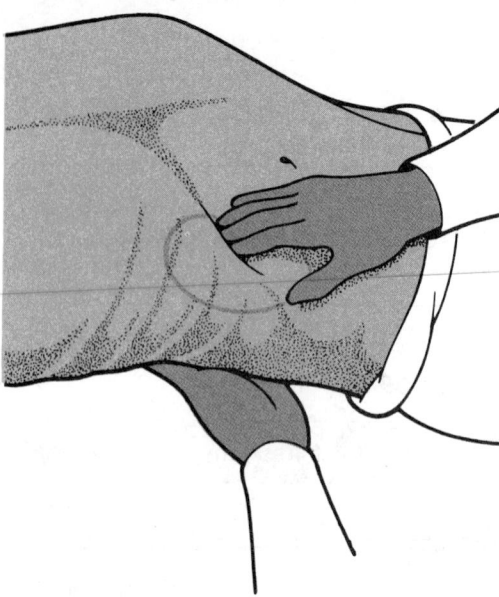

Fig. 39-7   Palpating the right kidney.

Skin: Pallor, yellowish-gray cast, excoriations, changes in turgor, bruises, texture (e.g., rough, dry skin)
Mouth: Stomatitis and urinous breath odor
Face, abdomen, and extremities: Generalized edema, abdominal mass from bladder distention or malignant tumor
Weight gain: Secondary to edema
General state of health: Fatigue, lethargy, and diminished alertness

Palpation. The kidneys are posterior organs protected by the abdominal organs, the ribs, and the heavy back muscles. A landmark useful in locating the kidneys is the costovertebral angle (CVA) formed by the rib cage and the vertebral column. The normal-sized left kidney is rarely palpable because it is overlain by the spleen. Occasionally, the lower pole of the right kidney is palpable.

To palpate the right kidney, the examiner's left hand is placed behind and supporting the client's right side between the rib cage and the iliac crest (Fig. 39-7). The right flank is elevated with the left hand and the right hand is used to palpate deeply for the right kidney. The lower pole of the right kidney may be felt as a smooth, rounded mass that descends on inspiration. If the kidney is palpable, its size, contour, and tenderness should be noted. Kidney enlargement is suggestive of hydronephrosis, neoplasm, polycystic disease, or a renal abscess.[5]

The urinary bladder is normally not palpable unless it is distended with urine. If the bladder is full, it may be felt as a smooth, round, firm organ and is sensitive to palpation.

Percussion. Tenderness in the flank area may be detected by means of fist percussion. This is performed by striking the fist (kidney punch) of one hand against the dorsal surface of the other hand, which is placed flat along the posterior CVA margin. Normally, a firm blow in the flank area should not elicit pain. If CVA tenderness and pain are found, a kidney infection may be present.

formation. Demineralization of the bones may also occur in a person with limited physical activity.

A history of past and present drug intake is very important. There are many potentially nephrotoxic agents that a client may be taking, as either prescription or nonprescription drugs. The client should be asked about cigarette smoking, which is associated with many diseases (including bladder cancer), especially in women.

Review of systems. A person with a marked decrease in renal function may manifest dysfunctions of multiple body systems. Therefore it is necessary to discuss the functioning of the total body as well as to ask questions related specifically to the urinary system. The questions related to the general assessment are important because they can reveal common clinical manifestations of renal disease. The occurrence of a combination of these findings increases the likelihood of an underlying renal disorder. Clinical manifestations of disorders of the urinary system that should be investigated are shown in Table 39-3.

Objective Data

Physical examination

Inspection. The nurse should assess for changes in the following:

Table 39-4 Normal Physical Assessment of the Urinary System

No CVA tenderness
Nonpalpable kidney and bladder
No palpable masses

Normally, a bladder is not percussible until it contains 150 ml of urine. If the bladder is full,[6] dullness is heard above the pubic symphysis. A distended bladder may be percussed as high as the umbilicus.

Auscultation. The diaphragm of the stethoscope may be used to auscultate over both CVAs and in the upper abdominal quadrants. With this technique, the abdominal aorta and renal arteries are auscultated for bruits (an abnormal murmur), which indicate interference with the blood supply to the kidneys.

Table 39-5

Common Assessment Abnormalities of the Urinary System

Finding	Description	Possible Etiology and Significance
Dysuria	Painful or difficult urination	Sign of urinary tract infection and wide variety of pathological conditions
Frequency	Increased incidence of urinating	Acutely inflamed bladder, retention with overflow, excess fluid intake
Enuresis	Involuntary nocturnal urinating	Symptomatic of lower urinary tract disorder
Hesitancy	Delay or difficulty in initiating urinating	Partial urethral obstruction
Urgency	Strong desire to urinate	Inflammatory lesions in bladder or urethra, acute bacterial infections
Hematuria	Blood in the urine	Cancer of genitourinary tract, blood dyscrasias, renal disease, urinary tract infection, stones in kidney or ureter
Burning on urination	Stinging pain	Urethral irritation
Pneumaturia	Passage of urine containing gas	Fistula connections between bowel and bladder, gas-forming urinary tract infections
Retention	Inability to urinate, even though bladder contains excessive amount of urine	Finding after pelvic surgery, childbirth, catheter removal; urethral stricture or obstruction; neurogenic bladder
Pain	Presence over suprapubic area (related to bladder), urethral pain (irritation of bladder neck), flank (CVA) pain	Infection, urinary retention, foreign body in canal, urethritis, pyelonephritis, renal colic or stones
Incontinence	Inability to voluntarily control discharge of urine	Neurogenic bladder, bladder infection, injury to external sphincter
Stress incontinence	Involuntary urination with pressure such as sneezing or coughing	Weakness of sphincter control
Nocturia	Frequency of urination at night	Renal disease with impaired concentrating ability, bladder obstruction, congestive heart failure, diabetes mellitus, finding after renal transplant
Polyuria	Large volume of urine in a given time	Diabetes mellitus, diabetes insipidus, chronic renal failure, diuretics, excess fluid intake
Anuria	Technically no urination (classification of anuria when 24-hr urine output < 100 ml)	Acute renal disease, end-stage renal disease, bilateral ureteral obstruction
Oliguria	Diminished amount of urine in a given time (24-hr urine output of 100 to 400 ml)	Severe dehydration, shock, transfusion reaction, kidney disease

Table 39-4 shows how to record the normal physical assessment findings of the urinary system. Table 39-5 presents common assessment abnormalities of the urinary system.

Renal Function in the Older Adult

Anatomical changes in the aging kidney include a 20% to 30% decrease in size and weight between the ages of 30 and 90 years.[7] This loss in renal mass is predominantly in the cortex. The aging nephron fails as a unit because glomerular and tubular function appear to decrease at the same rate. By the seventh decade of life, 30% to 50% of glomeruli have lost their function because of sclerosis or other abnormalities.[8] Blood flow to and within the kidney also decreases. There is no evidence that atherosclerotic vascular disease is primarily responsible for the age-related changes in the kidney.[9]

Physiological changes in the aging kidney include a decreased renal blood flow, decreased GFR, and decreased ability to conserve Na^+, dilute or concentrate urine, and excrete an acid load.[9] Under normal conditions, the aging kidney is able to maintain homeostasis, but after abrupt changes in blood volume, acid load, or other insults, the kidney may not be able to function effectively. Table 39-6 shows the assessment changes in the urinary system that are associated with aging.

DIAGNOSTIC STUDIES

Diagnostic studies are important in locating and understanding problems of the urinary system. The accuracy of the findings of these studies is influenced by (1) adherence to the proper procedures related to the study and (2) cooperation of the client in restricting fluids, collecting urine specimens, and lying quietly on the x-ray table.

Many radiological studies require the use of a bowel preparation the evening before the study. Commonly used bowel preparations include enemas, castor oil, magnesium citrate, and bisacodyl (Dulcolax) tablets or suppositories. Sometimes a further bowel preparation is required the morning of the study. The purpose of bowel preparations is to clear the lower gastrointestinal (GI) tract of feces and gas. Because the kidneys lie in a retroperitoneal location, the contents of the colon may obstruct visualization of the urinary tract. If a bowel preparation is not properly done, the study may be unsuccessful and have to be rescheduled.

When a client has repeated diagnostic studies on consecutive days, it is important to prevent dehydration. It is not uncommon to have a client take nothing by mouth (NPO) after midnight, spend all morning in the x-ray department, return too late for lunch or too tired to eat, sleep all afternoon, and be on NPO status after midnight again because of studies the next day. Severe dehydration, especially in a diabetic, debilitated, or older client, may lead to acute renal failure. The nurse is responsible for ensuring that a client undergoing diagnostic studies is properly hydrated and given correct nourishment between studies.

Another important nursing responsibility related to diagnostic studies is providing the client with an adequate explanation of the procedure. The period during a diagnostic workup is typically a very anxious one for most clients. The fear inherent in not knowing what is wrong is often worse than the diagnosis itself. Additional anxiety is caused by the unknown nature of the procedure. Clients need to know what the procedure involves and its basic

Table 39-6

 Age-Related Changes of the Urinary System and Differences in Assessment Findings

Changes	Differences in Assessment Findings
KIDNEY	
Decrease in amount of renal tissue	Less palpable
Decrease in number of nephrons and renal vascular bed, thickened basement membrane of Bowman's capsule and glomeruli	Decrease in creatinine clearance, increase in BUN level
Decrease in function of loop of Henle and tubules	Alterations in drug excretion, nocturia; loss of normal diurnal excretory pattern due to decreased ability to concentrate urine, less concentrated urine
URETER, BLADDER, AND URETHRA	
Decrease in elasticity and muscle tone	Palpable bladder after urination due to retention
Weakening of urinary sphincter	Stress incontinence (especially during Valsalva maneuver), dribbling of urine after urination
Decrease in bladder capacity and sensory receptors	Frequency, urgency, nocturia, overflow incontinence
Estrogen deficiency leading to relaxed pelvic floor; prostatic enlargement; uninhibited bladder contractions	Stress incontinence, dribbling

BUN, Blood urea nitrogen.

purpose, where it will be done, how long it takes, and whether it will hurt. These things should be explained at a level appropriate to their understanding. Clients should also be instructed on their responsibility during a particular study (e.g., to lie flat on the table or to keep the legs straight).

Diagnostic studies of the urinary system often cause embarrassment and emotional stress to the client. Examination of the urinary system may be perceived as an intrusion on a very personal body area. The nurse should alleviate anxiety by providing privacy and protecting the modesty of the client.

Urine Studies

Urinalysis. In evaluating disorders of the urinary tract, one of the first studies done is a urinalysis (Tables 39-7 and 39-8). This test may provide information about possible abnormalities, indicate what further studies need to be done, and supply information on the progression of a diagnosed disorder (e.g., diabetes mellitus).

For a routine urinalysis, a specimen may be collected at any time of the day. However, it is best to obtain the first specimen urinated in the morning. This concentrated specimen is most likely to contain abnormal constituents if they are present in the urine. The specimen should be examined within 1 hour of urinating. If it is not, bacteria multiply rapidly, RBCs hemolyze, casts disintegrate, and the urine becomes alkaline as a result of urea-splitting bacteria. If it is not possible to send the specimen to the laboratory, it should be refrigerated. However, to obtain the best results, the nurse should try to coordinate specimen collection with routine laboratory hours.

The results of a urinalysis usually include a description of the appearance, specific gravity (mass and density), osmolality (total solute concentration), pH, glucose, ketones, and protein in the urine and a microscopic examination of urine sediment for white blood cells (WBCs), RBCs, and casts (see Table 39-8).

Composite urine collections. Composite urine specimens are collected over a period that may range from 2 to 24 hours. The purpose of a composite specimen is to examine or measure specific components, such as electrolytes, sugar, protein, 17-ketosteroids, catecholamines, and creatinine. These specimens may have to be refrigerated, or preservatives may have to be added to the container used for collecting urine.

For collection of a composite urine specimen, the client is instructed to urinate and discard the urine. This time is noted as the start of the test. All urine from subsequent urinations is saved in a container for the designated period. Finally, at the end of the period, the client is asked to urinate and this urine is added to the container.

Creatinine clearance. One of the most common composite indicators used to analyze urinary system disorders is creatinine clearance. Creatinine is a waste product produced by muscle breakdown. Urinary excretion of creatinine is a measure of the amount of active muscle tissue in the body, not of body weight. Therefore, persons with larger muscle mass have higher values. Because almost all

creatinine in the blood is normally excreted by the kidneys, creatinine clearance is the most accurate indicator of renal function. The result of a creatinine clearance closely approximates that of the GFR. A blood specimen for serum creatinine determination should be obtained during the period of urine collection. Creatinine clearance is calculated as follows:

Creatinine clearance (ml/min) =
$$\frac{\text{Urine creatinine (mg/ml)} \times \text{Urine volume (ml/min)}}{\text{Serum creatinine (mg/ml)}}$$

Creatinine levels remain remarkably constant for each person because they are not significantly affected by protein ingestion, muscular exercise, water intake, or rate of urine production. Normal creatinine clearance values range from 85 to 135 ml/min. After the age of 40, the creatinine clearance rate decreases at a rate of about 1 ml/min per year.

Radiological Studies

Intravenous pyelogram. The purpose of an intravenous pyelogram (IVP) or excretory urogram is to visualize the urinary tract. The presence, position, size, and shape of the kidneys, ureters, and bladder can be evaluated. Cysts, tumors, lesions, and obstructions cause a distortion in the normal appearance of these structures.

The procedure consists of injecting an intravenous (IV) dose of radiopaque dye, which circulates in the blood and is excreted by the kidneys into the urine. During injection of the dye, the client may experience warmth, a flushed face, and a salty taste. After injection, films are taken sequentially. (A *rapid-sequence IVP* has x-ray films taken every minute for the first 5 minutes.) The sequencing of films is planned so that dye excretion can be followed from the cortex of the kidney to the bladder. A film taken at 45 minutes allows for visualization of the bladder. The presence of bladder atony or outlet obstruction also can be detected by a posturination film, which shows the residual volume of urine in the bladder.

Preparation of the client the evening before the test consists of giving a cathartic or an enema to eliminate feces and air from the colon. Fluids are withheld for 8 hours before testing to produce slight dehydration so that the dye will concentrate. Clients with significantly decreased renal function should not have an IVP because the dye will not be properly excreted by the kidneys.

The client should also be assessed for a possible allergic reaction to the dye. The contrast medium is typically an iodine derivative. A person with iodine sensitivity may have an anaphylactic reaction after dye injection. A person with a known allergy to iodine or seafood should not have an IVP. During dye injection, the client should be observed for signs of respiratory distress, urticaria, decrease in blood pressure, and other signs of anaphylaxis. Emergency drugs such as epinephrine (Adrenalin) and diphenhydramine (Benadryl) and cardiopulmonary resuscitation equipment should be available in the room. After the procedure, the nurse should encourage the client to force fluids to assist in flushing out the dye.

Text continued on p. 1182.

Table 39-7

Diagnostic Studies of the Urinary System

Study	Description and Purpose	Nursing Responsibility
URINE STUDIES		
Urinalysis	Study is a general examination of urine to establish baseline information or provide data in establishing a tentative diagnosis and determining further studies to be ordered.*	Try to obtain first urinated morning specimen. Ensure that specimen is examined within 1 hr of urinating. Wash perineal area if soiled with menses, fecal material.
Creatinine clearance	Creatinine is a waste product of protein breakdown (primarily body muscle mass). Clearance of creatinine by the kidney approximates the GFR. *Normal finding* is 85-135 ml/min.	Collect 24-hour urine specimen. Discard first urination when test is started. Save urine from all subsequent urinations for 24 hr. Instruct client to urinate at end of 24 hr, and add specimen to collection. Ensure that serum creatinine clearance is determined during the 24-hr period.
Urine culture ("clean catch")	Study is done to confirm suspected urinary tract infection and identify causative organisms. Normally, bladder is sterile, but urethra contains bacteria and a few WBCs. If properly collected, stored, and handled: < 10,000 organisms per milliliter indicates no infection, 10,000-100,000/ml is usually not diagnostic and test may have to be repeated, > 100,000/ml indicates infection.	Use sterile container for collection of urine. Touch only outside of container. For females, separate labia with one hand and clean meatus with other hand, using at least three sponges (saturated with cleansing solution) in a front-to-back motion. For males, retract foreskin (if present) and cleanse glans with at least three cleansing sponges. After cleansing, instruct client to start urinating, stop, and then continue voiding in sterile container. (The initial voided urine flushes out most contaminants in the urethra and perineal area.) Inform physician of need for catheterization if client is unable to cooperate with this procedure.
Concentration test	Study evaluates renal concentration ability. Concentration is measured by specific gravity readings. *Normal finding* is 1.020-1.035.	Instruct client to fast after given time in evening (in usual procedure). Collect three urine specimens at hourly intervals in morning.
Residual urine	Study determines amount of urine left in bladder after urinating. Finding may be abnormal in problems with bladder innervation, sphincter impairment, or urethral strictures. *Normal finding* is ≤ 50 ml urine (increases with age).	If residual urine test is ordered, catheterize client immediately after urinating. If a large amount of residual urine is obtained, be aware that physician may want catheter left in bladder.
Protein determination Dipstick (Albustix, Combistix)	Test detects protein (primarily albumin) in urine. *Normal finding* is 0-trace.	Dip end of stick in urine and read result by comparison with color chart on label. Grading is from 0 to 4+. Use with caution. A positive result may not indicate significant proteinuria. Be aware that some medications may give false-positive reading.
Quantitative test	A 12- or 24-hr collection gives a more accurate result of the amount of protein in urine. Persistent proteinuria usually indicates renal disease. *Normal finding* is 0-150 mg/24 hr, consisting mainly of albumin.	Perform 24-hour urine collection.

*See Table 39-8.

Continued.

Table 39-7

	Diagnostic Studies of the Urinary System—cont'd	
Study	**Description and Purpose**	**Nursing Responsibility**
BLOOD CHEMISTRIES		
BUN	Study is most commonly used to identify presence of renal problems. Concentration of urea in blood is regulated by rate at which kidney excretes urea. *Normal finding* is 10-30 mg/dl.	Be aware that in interpretation of BUN, nonrenal factors may cause increase (e.g., rapid cell destruction from infections and GI bleeding, trauma, athletic activity with excessive muscle breakdown, steroid therapy).
Creatinine	Study is more reliable than BUN as a determinant of renal function. Creatinine is end product of muscle and protein metabolism and is liberated at constant rate. *Normal finding* is 0.5-1.5 mg/dl. Results are higher in males.	Explain test and watch for postpuncture bleeding.
BUN/creatinine ratio	*Normal finding* is 10:1.	
Uric acid	Study is used as a screening test for kidney disease as well as indication of disorders of purine metabolism such as gout. Values depend on renal function as well as rate of purine metabolism and dietary intake of food rich in purines. *Normal finding* is 2.5-5.5 mg/dl (female) and 4.5-6.5 mg/dl (male).	Explain test and watch for postpuncture bleeding.
Sodium	Sodium is main extracellular electrolyte determining blood volume. Usually values stay within normal range until late stages of renal failure. *Normal finding* is 135-145 mEq/L.	Explain test and watch for postpuncture bleeding.
Potassium	Kidneys are responsible for excreting majority of body's potassium. In renal disease, K^+ determinations are critical because K^+ is one of the first electrolytes to become abnormal. Elevations of > 6 mEq/L can lead to muscle weakness and cardiac dysrhythmias. *Normal finding* is 3.5-5.5 mEq/L.	Explain test and watch for postpuncture bleeding.
Calcium	Calcium is main mineral in bone and aids in muscular contraction, neurotransmission, and clotting. In renal disease, decreased absorption of Ca^{2+} leads to renal osteodystrophy.* *Normal finding* is 9-11 mg/dl (4.5-5.5 mEq/L).	Explain test and watch for postpuncture bleeding.
Phosphorus	Phosphorus balance is inversely related to Ca^{2+} balance. In renal disease, phosphorus levels are elevated. Soft tissue calcification may occur if both Ca^{2+} and phosphorus are elevated.† *Normal finding* is 2.8-4.5 mg/dl.	Explain test and watch for postpuncture bleeding.
Bicarbonate	Most clients in renal failure have metabolic acidosis and low serum HCO_3^- levels. *Normal finding* is 20-30 mEq/L.	Explain test and watch for postpuncture bleeding.
RADIOLOGICAL		
Kidneys, ureters, bladder	Study involves flat-plate x-ray examination of abdomen and pelvis and delineates size, shape, and position of kidneys.	Perform bowel preparation (if ordered).

BUN, Blood urea nitrogen; *IVP*, intravenous pyelogram; *IV*, intravenous; *CT*, computerized tomography; *CBC*, complete blood count.
*See Table 39-8.
†See Chapter 41.

Table 39-7

Diagnostic Studies of the Urinary System—cont'd

Study	Description and Purpose	Nursing Responsibility
RADIOLOGICAL—cont'd		
IVP or excretory urogram	X-ray examination visualizes urinary tract after IV injection of radiopaque dye.	Evening before procedure, give cathartic or enema to empty colon of feces and gas. Keep client on NPO status 8 hr before procedure. Before procedure, assess client for iodine sensitivity to avoid anaphylactic reaction. Inform client that procedure involves lying on table and having serial x-rays taken. After procedure, force fluids (if permitted) to flush out dye.
Nephrotomogram	X-ray film is taken with rotating tubes. Test delineates segments of the kidney at different levels. Multiple exposures are taken to visualize specific sections of the kidney after IV injection of radiopaque dye.	Explain procedure to client. Prepare client as for IVP.
Retrograde pyelogram	X-ray film of urinary tract is taken after injection of radiopaque dye into kidneys. Cystoscope is inserted and ureteral catheters are inserted through it into renal pelvis. Dye is injected through catheters.	Prepare client as for IVP. Inform client that pain may be experienced from distention of pelvis and discomfort from cystoscope. Inform client that general anesthesia may be given for procedure.
Renal arteriogram (angiogram)	Study is performed by injecting radiopaque dye into renal artery via catheter inserted into femoral artery. Purpose is to visualize renal blood vessels.	Prepare client evening before procedure by giving cathartic or enema. The morning of the procedure, give preoperative medication to sedate and relax client. Before injection of dye, test client for iodine sensitivity. After procedure, check insertion site for bleeding and take peripheral pulses in involved leg every 30 to 60 min to detect occluded blood flow.
Ultrasound	Small external ultrasound probe is attached to client. Conductive gel is applied to the skin. Noninvasive procedure involves passing sound waves into body structures and recording images as they are reflected back. Computer interprets tissue density based on sound waves and displays it in picture form. Study is most valuable in detection of renal or perirenal masses, differential diagnosis of renal cysts, solid masses, and identification of obstructions. It can safely be used in clients with renal failure.	Explain procedure to client.
CT scan	Study provides excellent visualization of kidneys. Kidney size can be evaluated; tumors, abscesses, suprarenal masses (e.g., adrenal tumors, pheochromocytomas), and obstructions can be detected. Advantage of CT over ultrasound is its ability to distinguish subtle differences in density. Use of IV-administered contrast medium during CT accentuates density of renal tissue and helps differentiate masses.	Explain procedure to client.

Continued.

Table 39-7

Diagnostic Studies of the Urinary System—cont'd

Study	Description and Purpose	Nursing Responsibility
RENAL RADIONUCLIDE IMAGING		
Renal scan	Radioactive isotopes are injected IV. Radiation detector probes are placed over kidney and scintillation counter monitors radioactive material in kidney. Purpose is to show blood flow, glomerular filtration, tubular function, and excretion. Radioisotope distribution in kidney is scanned and mapped. Test is useful in showing location, size, and shape of kidney and in generally assessing blood perfusion and ability to secrete urine. Abscesses, cysts, and tumors may appear as *cold spots* because of presence of nonfunctioning tissue.	Perform no dietary or activity restriction. Inform client that no pain or discomfort should be felt while test is carried out.
ENDOSCOPY		
Cystoscopy	Study involves use of tubular lighted scope to inspect bladder. Lithotomy position is used. It may be done using local or general anesthesia.	Before procedure, force fluids or give IV fluids if general anesthesia is to be used. Ensure consent form is signed. Explain procedure to client. Give preoperative medication. After procedure, explain to client that burning on urination, pink-tinged urine, and urinary frequency are expected effects after cystoscopy. Do not let client walk alone immediately after procedure because orthostatic hypotension may occur. Offer warm sitz baths, heat, mild analgesics to relieve discomfort.
Cystogram	Radiopaque dye is instilled into bladder via cystoscope or catheter. Purpose is to visualize bladder and evaluate vesiculoureteral reflux.	Explain procedure to client. If done via cystoscope, follow nursing care related to cystoscopy.
Cystometrogram	Study involves insertion of catheter and instillation of water or saline solution into bladder. Measurements of pressure exerted against bladder wall are recorded. Purpose is to evaluate bladder tone.	Explain procedure to client. Observe client for manifestations of urinary infection after procedure.
INVASIVE PROCEDURE		
Renal biopsy	Technique is usually done as a skin (percutaneous) biopsy through needle insertion into lower lobe of kidney. Purpose is to obtain renal tissue for examination to determine type of renal disease or to follow progress of renal disease.	Before procedure, ascertain coagulation status through client history, CBC, hematocrit, prothrombin time, bleeding/clotting time. Type and cross match client for 2 units of blood. Ensure consent form is signed. Be aware that IVP or ultrasound study is done before biopsy. After procedure, apply pressure dressing to biopsy site and check frequently for bleeding. Keep client on bed rest for up to 24 hr. Take vital signs frequently. Observe urine for gross bleeding. Determine microscopic bleeding by use of dipstick. Assess client for flank pain.

Table 39-8 Urinalysis Findings

Test	Normal	Abnormal Finding and Significance
Color	Amber-yellow	Dark-smoky color suggests hematuria. Yellowish brown to olive green indicates excessive bilirubin. Orange red or orange brown caused by phenazopyridine (Pyridium) or urobilin in excess. Cloudiness of freshly voided urine indicates infection.
Smell	Aromatic	On standing, urine becomes more ammonialike in smell. In urinary tract infections, urine smells unpleasant.
Protein	0-150 mg/24 hr 0-18 mg/dl	Persistent proteinuria is characteristic of acute and chronic renal disease, especially involving glomeruli. In absence of disease, positive reading may be caused by high-protein diet, strenuous exercise, dehydration, fever, or emotional stress. Vaginal secretions may contaminate urine specimen and give positive reading.
Glucose	None	Glycosuria indicates diabetes mellitus or low renal threshold for glucose reabsorption (if blood glucose level is normal). Small amounts may be found after glucose loading (e.g., glucose tolerance test).
Ketones	None	Altered carbohydrate and fat metabolisms indicate diabetes mellitus and starvation. Findings can also be seen in dehydration, starvation, vomiting, and severe diarrhea.
Bilirubin	None	Presence of bilirubinuria is as significant as jaundice in detection of liver disorders. Bilirubin may appear in urine before jaundice becomes visible or may be present in persons with hepatic disorders who do not have recognizable jaundice.*
Specific gravity	1.003-1.030	Specific gravity of morning urine specimen reflects maximum concentrating ability of kidney and is 1.025 to 1.030. Low specific gravity indicates dilute urine and possibly excessive diuresis. High specific gravity indicates dehydration. If it becomes fixed at about 1.010, this indicates renal inability to concentrate urine, suggesting that kidney is progressing to end-stage renal disease.
Osmolality	300-1300 mOsm/kg	Measurement is more accurate method than specific gravity for determining diluting and concentrating ability of kidneys. Deviations from normal indicate tubular dysfunction. Findings indicate if kidney has lost ability to concentrate or dilute urine.
pH	4.0-8.0 (average, 6.0)	If more than 8.0, finding may be due to standing of urine or urinary tract infections because bacteria decompose urea to form ammonia. If less than 4.0, may indicate respiratory and metabolic acidosis.
RBC	0-4/hpf	Bleeding in urinary tract is caused by calculi, cystitis, neoplasm, glomerulonephritis, tuberculosis, kidney biopsy, or trauma.
WBC	0-5/hpf	Increased number of WBCs in urine (pyuria) indicates urinary tract infection or inflammation.
Casts	None-occasional hyaline	Casts are molds of the renal tubules and may contain protein, WBCs, RBCs, or bacteria. Noncellular casts are hyaline in appearance, and a few may be found in normal urine. Casts indicate renal dysfunction or urinary tract infections.
Culture for organisms	No organisms in bladder, $< 10^4$ organisms/ml result of normal urethral flora	Bacteria counts $>10^5$/ml indicate urinary tract infection. Organisms most commonly found in urinary tract infections are *Escherichia coli, Proteus vulgaris,* staphylococci, and streptococci.

hpf, High powered field.

*See Chapter 38 for further discussion.

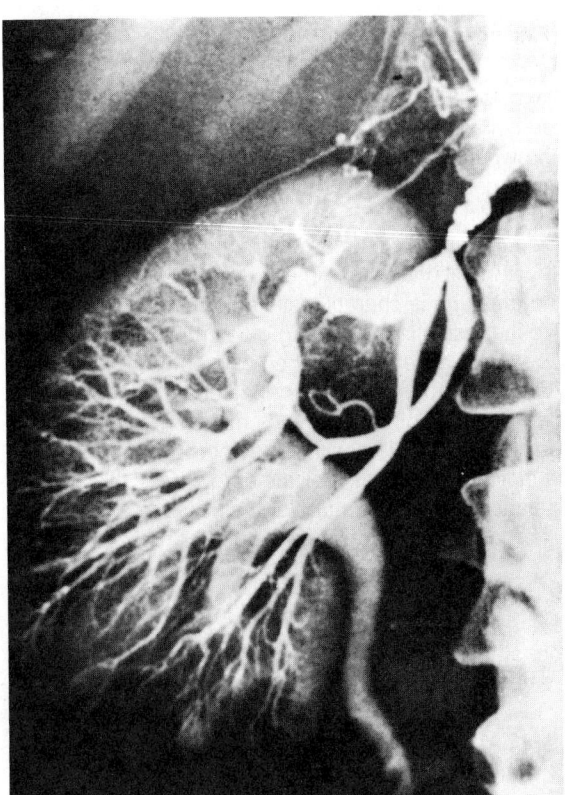

Fig. 39-8 Renal arteriogram showing stenosis of the right renal artery. (From Price SA and Wilson LM: Pathophysiology: clinical concepts of disease processes, ed 4, St Louis, 1991, Mosby–Year Book, Inc.)

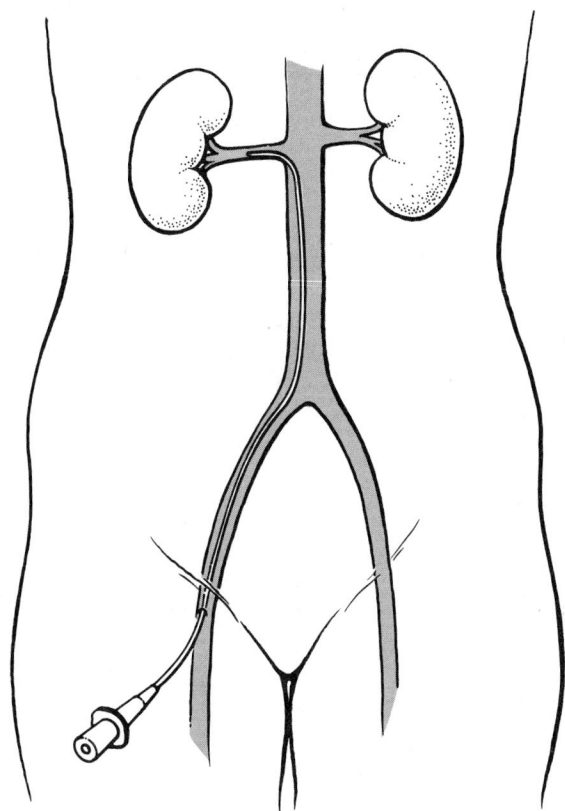

Fig. 39-9 Catheter insertion for a renal arteriogram.

Retrograde pyelogram. A retrograde pyelogram evaluates the same structures as an IVP. This is an x-ray visualization of the kidneys, ureters, and bladder after direct injection of a dye into the kidney via a ureteral catheter introduced through a cystoscope. It may be done if an IVP does not visualize the urinary tract or if the client is allergic to the dye or has decreased renal function.

The dangers associated with a retrograde pyelogram are similar to those related to cystoscopy, including the risk of infection and the use of anesthesia (see pp. 1183-1184).

Renal arteriogram. The purpose of a renal arteriogram (angiogram) is to visualize the renal blood vessels. The findings of an arteriogram can assist in diagnosing renal artery stenosis, additional or missing renal blood vessels, and renovascular hypertension and in differentiating between a renal cyst and a renal tumor (Fig. 39-8). Renal arteriograms are also included in the workup of a potential renal transplant donor.

The evening before the procedure, the client is given a cathartic to eliminate fecal material from the colon. The morning of the procedure, a preoperative medication is given to relax and sedate the client.

Most arteriograms are done in the x-ray department by a specially trained physician. The client is given a local anesthetic at the site of catheter insertion. A catheter is usually inserted into the femoral artery and passed up the aorta to the level of the renal arteries (Fig. 39-9). A contrast medium (dye) is then injected to outline the renal blood supply, and x-ray films are taken. The client may experience a transient warm feeling along the course of the blood vessel when the dye is injected.

After the catheter is removed, a pressure dressing is placed over the femoral injection site. It is important to observe for bleeding at the site. The client is usually kept on bed rest for 12 to 24 hours. Peripheral pulses in the involved leg should be taken at least every 30 to 60 minutes to detect occlusion of blood flow due to a thrombus. Complications that may result from a renal arteriogram include thrombus, embolus, local inflammation, and hematoma.

Digital subtraction angiography. Because of potential complications, the renal arteriogram is being replaced by digital subtraction angiography (DSA) in many hospitals that have the facilities to perform this procedure. Utilizing computer technology, this procedure permits visualization of the arteries after an IV injection of contrast medium.

A primary advantage of DSA is that it requires small peripheral venous injections of contrast medium compared with the relatively large doses that must be injected via arterial cannulation for a renal arteriogram. (See Table 26-6 for a further description of DSA.)

Renal radionuclide imaging. Renal scans involving the use of radionuclides are useful in evaluating the anatomical structures, perfusion, and function of the kidneys. Different institutions use different imaging techniques. In

general, the following radionuclides are used for these purposes:

Anatomical structures: Technetium 99m(^{99m}Tc)-labeled compounds such as dimercaptosuccinic acid (DMSA) or glucoheptonate

Perfusion and function: Iodine 131-labeled *o*-iodohippurate (Hippuran) and ^{99m}Tc-labeled diethylenetriaminepentaacetic acid (DTPA)

Infection or abscesses: Gallium 67 citrate

For this procedure a radioactive isotope is injected IV. Radiation detector probes are placed over the kidney, and a scintillation counter monitors the appearance and disappearance of the radioactive material in the kidney.

The results reveal the difference between the two kidneys with respect to blood flow, tubular function, and excretion. A normal scan shows symmetrical functioning of both kidneys. Normally, the distribution of activity is recorded throughout the kidneys. A lesion (e.g., a tumor) is indicated by the absence of radioactivity in an involved area and appearance of the resultant defect on the scan. In renovascular disease, an area with decreased blood flow can readily be visualized. This study is particularly useful in detecting renal vascular disease, acute renal failure, and upper urinary tract obstruction and in monitoring the function of a transplanted kidney.

Usually, there are no dietary or activity restrictions related to preparation of the client. During the test the client should feel no pain or discomfort. No special precautions are needed in the use of radioactive material, since only tracer doses are used.

Renal biopsy. The purpose of a renal biopsy is to determine the nature and extent of renal disease. This information can be used in establishing a diagnosis and following the progress of a disease as well as in determining the treatment. Biopsy material can be obtained through an open biopsy or a closed percutaneous needle biopsy. An open biopsy is rarely performed because it requires a surgical procedure with anesthesia. A percutaneous needle biopsy is more common. It is usually done in the x-ray department or in the client's room, although it may be done in the operating room.

Absolute contraindications to a percutaneous renal biopsy are bleeding disorders, the presence of a single kidney, and uncontrolled hypertension. Relative contraindications include suspected renal infection, hydronephrosis, and possible vascular lesions.

Because one danger of a biopsy is hemorrhage, the client's coagulation status should be assessed before the procedure. This includes a health history, complete blood count (CBC), hematocrit, prothrombin time, and bleeding or clotting time determinations. The client may also be typed and cross-matched for two units of blood.

An IVP or ultrasound examination is done to determine the position and location of the kidneys as a guide to needle insertion. Preparation also includes explaining the procedure to the client and discussing any concerns. A signed consent form is required before a biopsy is performed.

The procedure consists of having the client lie prone, with a pillow or sandbag used to elevate the abdomen and expose the kidneys. With the IVP or ultrasound findings used as a guide, the position of the kidney is marked on

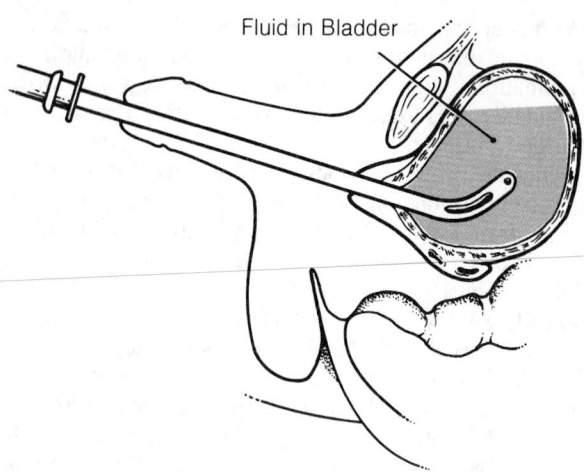

Fig. 39-10 Cystoscopic examination of a bladder in a male.

the body. Local anesthesia is used and a biopsy needle is inserted into the kidney just below the twelfth rib. The client is instructed to hold a breath while the biopsy specimen is being taken.

After the procedure, a pressure dressing is applied and the client is kept prone for 30 to 60 minutes. Usually the client should remain on bed rest for 24 hours. Vital signs should be taken every 5 to 10 minutes the first hour and then with decreasing frequency. The biopsy site should be inspected frequently for bleeding. Serial urine specimens should be assessed for gross and microscopic hematuria. A dipstick can be used to test for bleeding, even when hematuria is not obvious. The physician may order all urine sent for laboratory analysis to detect possible hematuria. The client should also be assessed for flank pain.

Complications of a renal biopsy include renal hemorrhage, hematoma, and infection. Even if no complications occur, the client should be instructed to avoid lifting heavy objects for 5 to 7 days.

Endoscopy

Cystoscopy. The main purpose of cystoscopy is to inspect the interior of the bladder with a tubular lighted scope called a cystoscope (Fig. 39-10). Cystoscopes can be used to insert ureteral catheters, remove calculi, obtain biopsy specimens of bladder lesions, and treat bleeding lesions. In most cases, bladder disorders can be determined by cystoscopic examination.

The client is given a preoperative medication for sedation about 1 hour before the procedure. Cystoscopy is usually done in a cystoscope room in the x-ray department or in the operating room. A signed consent form is required. Fluids may be forced before the procedure to ensure a continuous flow of urine. If general anesthesia is given, IV fluids may be used to maintain adequate fluid intake.

The cystoscopic examination may be performed with local or general anesthesia, depending on the needs and condition of the client. The client is put in a lithotomy position. Most of the pain associated with cystoscopy results from spasms and contractions of bladder sphincters. Relaxation and deep breathing by the client alleviate some of

the bladder and sphincter spasms. A local anesthetic is instilled into the urethra before scope insertion. During the examination, saline solution is inserted slowly to distend the bladder; this allows better visualization but will cause an urge to urinate.

After the procedure, the client can expect to have burning on urination, blood-tinged urine, and urinary frequency from the irritation of scope insertion and manipulation. The nurse should observe for bright red bleeding, which is not a normal reaction. The client should not be allowed to walk without assistance immediately after the procedure because postural hypotension may result from blood flow back to the legs after the client has been in a lithotomy position. After the procedure, the nurse is responsible for forcing fluids and administering mild analgesics, sitz baths, and heat to decrease the client's discomfort. Complications that may result from cystoscopy include urinary retention, urinary tract hemorrhage, bladder infection, and perforation of the bladder.

Cystogram. The purpose of a cystogram is to outline and visualize the bladder and evaluate the ureterovesical valves for reflux. In addition to suspected vesicoureteral reflux, indications for a cystogram include a neurogenic bladder and recurrent urinary tract infections. A cystogram can also delineate abnormalities of the bladder, such as diverticula, calculi, and tumors. The procedure involves instillation of a radiopaque dye into the bladder, which may be done via a cystoscope or a catheter.

A voiding cystourethrogram is a voiding study of the bladder opening and urethra. The bladder is filled with radiopaque dye. During urination, films are taken to visualize the bladder and urethra. After urination, another film is taken to assess for residual urine. A voiding cystourethrogram can detect abnormalities of the lower urinary tract, urethral stenosis, bladder neck obstruction, and prostatic enlargement.

Cystometrogram. The purpose of a cystometrogram is to evaluate bladder tone. It is usually ordered if a client has incontinence or neurogenic dysfunction of the bladder.

The procedure consists of insertion of a retention catheter while the client is in a supine position. A liter bottle of saline solution or water and a cystometer are connected to the catheter. Fluid is instilled at a constant rate, and the pressure exerted against the bladder wall is measured. The client is asked to indicate when the urge to void is first experienced (usually after 100 to 200 ml has been instilled). Fluids are instilled until urgency occurs (350 to 450 ml) or until it is determined that this sensation is absent. After the catheter is withdrawn the client is asked to empty the bladder, and the amount of residual urine is determined. During the study a cholinergic drug such as bethanechol (Urecholine) may be given to determine whether it will enhance the tone of a flaccid bladder. However, an anticholinergic drug may be given to promote relaxation of a hyperactive bladder.

R **eview Questions**

The number of the question corresponds to the same-numbered objective at the beginning of the chapter.

1. The main function of the pelvis of the kidney is to
   a. give structural support to the kidney
   b. serve as a collecting chamber for urine
   c. regulate the concentration of the filtrate
   d. serve as the entry and exit site for blood vessels
2. The action of ADH causes
   a. increased sodium reabsorption
   b. decreased sodium reabsorption
   c. increased water reabsorption
   d. decreased water reabsorption
3. A client related a history of the following diseases. Which is known to be related to renal problems?
   a. measles
   b. diabetes mellitus
   c. gastric ulcer
   d. jaundice
4. Which of the following statements regarding the physical assessment of the urinary system is accurate?
   a. An empty bladder is palpable as a small nodule.
   b. Auscultation is used to listen to urine in the bladder.
   c. The client lies prone when the kidneys are palpated.
   d. The flank area is percussed with a firm blow.
5. Which of the following findings of a physical assessment of the urinary system is considered normal?
   a. easily palpable left kidney
   b. CVA tenderness elicited by a kidney punch
   c. nonpalpable left kidney
   d. palpable bladder to the level of the pubic symphysis
6. An important nursing responsibility after a renal arteriogram is to
   a. encourage ambulation 2 to 3 hours after the study
   b. apply warm, wet sponges to the insertion site
   c. palpate peripheral pulses in the leg
   d. keep the client on NPO status for 4 hours after the study
7. Which of the following is considered a normal constituent of urine?
   a. ketones
   b. creatinine
   c. amino acids
   d. bacteria

REFERENCES

1. Smith HW: Fish to philosopher, Boston, 1953, Little, Brown & Co, p 4.
2. Vander AJ: Renal physiology, ed 3, New York, 1985, McGraw-Hill Book Co.
3. Groer MW and Shekleton ME: Basic pathophysiology: a holistic approach, ed 3, St Louis, 1989, The CV Mosby Co, pp 893-894.
4. Dunn MJ: Clinical effects of prostaglandins in renal disease, Hosp Pract 19:99-113, 1984.
5. Stark JL: A quick guide to urinary tract assessment, Nursing 18:57-58, 1988.
6. McConnell EA: Assessing the bladder, Nursing 15:44-46, 1985.
7. Brown WW: Geriatric nephrology and urology—1989, Peritoneal Dialysis International 9:27-28, 1989.
8. Beck LH: Kidney function and disease in the elderly, Hosp Pract 26:75-90, 1990.
9. Roy AT and others: Renal failure in older people: UCLA grand rounds, J Am Geriatr Soc 38:239-253, 1990.

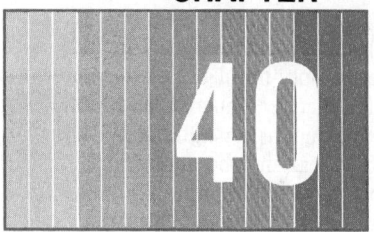

CHAPTER

40

Nursing Role in Management
Renal and Urological Problems

Sharon Mantik Lewis

Learning Objectives

1. Describe the pathophysiology, clinical manifestations, and therapeutic and pharmacological management of cystitis, urethritis, and pyelonephritis.
2. Explain the nursing management of urinary tract infections.
3. Describe the immunological mechanisms involved in glomerulonephritis.
4. Explain the clinical manifestations and therapeutic and nursing management of acute poststreptococcal glomerulonephritis, Goodpasture's syndrome, and chronic glomerulonephritis.
5. Describe the common causes, clinical manifestations, and therapeutic and nursing management of nephrotic syndrome.
6. Compare and contrast the etiology, clinical manifestations, and therapeutic and nursing management of various types of urinary calculi.
7. Explain the common causes and management of renal trauma, renal vascular problems, congenital abnormalities, and hereditary renal problems.
8. Describe the mechanisms of renal involvement in metabolic and connective tissue disorders.
9. Describe the clinical manifestations and management of renal and bladder cancer.
10. Describe the common causes and management of bladder dysfunctions.
11. Differentiate among ureteral, suprapubic, nephrostomy, and urethral catheters with respect to indications for use and nursing responsibilities.
12. Explain the nursing management of the client undergoing nephrectomy or urinary diversion surgery.

Renal and urological disorders encompass a spectrum of clinical problems. The diverse causes of these disorders may involve infectious, immunological, obstructive, metabolic, collagen-vascular, traumatic, congenital, neoplastic, and neurological mechanisms. This chapter discusses the therapeutic and nursing management of clients with specific disorders of the kidneys, ureters, bladder, and urethra. An effective management plan must deal with the significant psychosocial problems that may arise for these clients. These issues include anxiety about discussing problems related to the genitalia, embarrassment related to exposure during examination and treatment, and fear of changes in body image or body function. (Acute and chronic renal failure is discussed in Chapter 41.)

INFECTIOUS DISORDERS OF THE URINARY SYSTEM
Significance

Urinary tract infections (UTIs) are the second most common bacterial disease; at least 8000 persons die each year of infections of the kidney. In addition, more than 100,000 persons are hospitalized annually for an average of 6 to 7 days because of renal infections.[1] Infections of the urinary tract may appear as a variety of disorders. The common factor is a microbial invasion of the tissues of the urinary tract, most often by *Escherichia coli* (Table 40-1). Bacterial counts of 10^5 organisms or more generally indicate a UTI. However, bacterial counts as low as 10^2 to 10^3 in clients with symptoms are indicative of UTI.

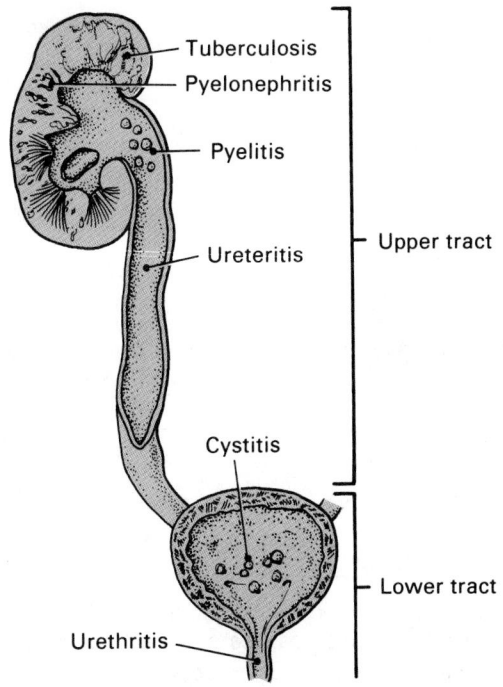

Fig. 40-1 Sites of infectious processes in the urinary tract.

Table 40-1 Bacteria Most Commonly Causing Urinary Tract Infections

*Escherichia coli**	*Pseudomonas aeruginosa*
Klebsiella aerobacter	*Staphylococcus saprophyticus*
Proteus mirabilis	*Streptococcus* species
Enterobacter	

*Causes about 80% of cases in persons who do not have urinary tract structural abnormalities or calculi.

The infections may be broadly classified as upper and lower UTIs (Fig. 40-1). Infections may be localized in a specific site, such as the kidney (pyelonephritis) or bladder (cystitis), but there is always the possibility that the bacteria will invade the remainder of the urinary tract. Infections that are resistant to treatment are often associated with structural abnormalities of the urinary tract.

It is often difficult to determine the location of the infection on the basis of clinical manifestations and diagnostic findings. The client may have both an upper and a lower UTI. Some clients may be free of symptoms. The frequency of UTIs varies with age and sex (more frequent in women), and the condition may be acute or chronic.

Recurrent UTIs can be classified as *relapses* (recurrence with the same strain of bacteria that occurs within 1 to 2 weeks of stopping antibiotic therapy) or *reinfections* (recurrence with a new strain). Most relapses result from unresolved renal infections.

Etiology

Defense mechanisms. The urinary tract above the urethra is normally sterile. Several physiological and mechan-

ical defense mechanisms assist in maintaining sterility and preventing UTIs. These defenses include normal voiding with complete emptying of the bladder, normal phagocytic ability of the bladder mucosa and urine, ureterovesical junction competence, peristaltic activity that propels urine toward the bladder, and the antibacterial effect of the zinc concentration in prostatic fluid. An alteration in any of these defense mechanisms increases the risk of contracting a UTI.

The following factors may predispose a client to infection:

1. Renal scarring from previous infections
2. Diminished ureteral peristalsis during pregnancy
3. Urinary retention for any reason
4. Presence of a foreign body such as a urinary catheter
5. Vesicoureteral reflux of urine in a retrograde direction from the bladder toward the kidney
6. Humoral or cellular immune deficiency in an otherwise normal urinary tract
7. Female gender
8. Presence of calculi
9. Clinical disorder such as neurogenic bladder

Source of urinary tract infections. The organisms that usually cause UTIs are introduced via the ascending route from the urethra. Most infections are due to gram-negative aerobic bacilli normally found in the gastrointestinal (GI) tract. A common factor contributing to ascending infection is urological instrumentation (e.g., catheterization and cystoscopic examinations). Instrumentation allows bacteria that are normally present at the opening of the urethra to enter the urethra or bladder. Sexual intercourse may result in bacteriuria, which is usually asymptomatic. Currently there is controversy about the relation between sexual intercourse and UTIs.

Rarely do UTIs result from a hematogenous route, where blood-borne bacteria secondarily invade the kidneys, ureters, or bladder from elsewhere in the body. For a kidney infection to occur from hematogenous transmission, there must be prior injury to the urinary tract, such as obstruction of the ureter, damage caused by stones, or renal scars.

An important source of UTIs is hospital-acquired, or *nosocomial,* infection. The cause of nosocomial infection is often *E. coli* and, less frequently, *Pseudomonas* organisms. Urological instrumentation, particularly with an indwelling urinary catheter, is the most common predisposing factor. UTIs account for about 40% of all nosocomial infections, and about 80% of these infections result from catheterization.[1]

The occurrence of UTIs is often related to the presence of abnormalities of the urinary tract, such as strictures and obstructions. An untreated UTI can lead to chronic pyelonephritis and a progressive decrease in renal function. If no abnormality exists, uncomplicated pyelonephritis rarely leads to progressive renal damage and renal failure.

Cystitis

Pathophysiology. Although the majority of clients with cystitis are women, other groups with a high incidence are older men and young children (especially girls). These age and sex variations in the frequency of cystitis are related to

anatomical differences or pathological changes in the groups at risk. The adult female urethra is short, and its proximity to the rectum and vagina predisposes the client to the risk of bladder contamination. Bacterial contamination of the bladder can result from poor personal hygiene practices and sexual intercourse.

In children and older men, UTIs are often associated with other preexisting problems. In children, vesicoureteral reflux is usually the preexisting abnormality. In men, the longer urethra (of which the proximal two thirds is normally sterile) and the antibacterial property of prostatic secretions provide protection from bacterial infections unless there are predisposing causes. In older men, the infection is usually related to obstruction caused by benign prostatic hypertrophy (see Chapter 49).

Not all bacterial invasions of the bladder result in UTI or cause spread to the upper urinary tract (pyelonephritis). Once cystitis has occurred, it may remain localized in the urinary bladder for years without ascension to the kidney. Although the bacterial infection may be self-limiting, suspected UTI should be evaluated even in clients who have no symptoms.

Clinical manifestations. The manifestations of cystitis are frequency and urgency of urination, suprapubic pain, dysuria, and foul-smelling urine. In some persons, hematuria and pyuria may be present. The presence of fever, nausea and vomiting, and flank tenderness usually indicates pyelonephritis. About one half of all persons with significant bacteriuria have no symptoms. The incidence of asymptomatic bacteriuria increases greatly with age.[2]

Diagnostic studies. Examining the urine for the presence of white blood cells (WBCs) by means of either a microscope or a urine dipstick is important in evaluating a person who complains of dysuria. The definitive diagnosis of cystitis is made on examination of a urine Gram stain or by urine culture. The best method for obtaining the urine culture is a midstream technique, also called *clean-catch urine.* (See Table 39-7 for the technique.) If a satisfactory specimen cannot be obtained with this method, catheterization may be used. This procedure carries a 1% to 2% risk of introducing microorganisms into the bladder and causing a UTI.

As an alternative to standard overnight culture methods, rapid methods to detect bacteriuria have been developed to provide results in 1 to 2 hours. These include photometry and bioluminescence.[3] A test used to differentiate upper and lower UTIs involves analysis of bacteria found in urine for the presence of antibody coating. In this test, bacteria from clients with pyelonephritis demonstrate antibody coating on their surfaces. In contrast, no surface antibodies can be found on bacteria from clients with cystitis.

Therapeutic management. Once cystitis has been diagnosed, appropriate antimicrobial therapy is initiated. The therapeutic management of cystitis is summarized in Table 40-2.

Pharmacological management. Many drugs are effective against organisms that cause UTIs. The most effective and least expensive drugs are the sulfonamides, including sulfisoxazole (Gantrisin) and sulfamethoxazole (Gantanol). Other drugs that are used are nalidixic acid (NegGram),

Table 40-2

Diagnostic and Therapeutic Management: Cystitis

First Infection—Symptomatic

DIAGNOSTIC

Urinalysis
Urine for culture and sensitivity
Antibody-coated bacteria test

THERAPEUTIC*

Administration of antimicrobials for 7 days
Administration of single dose of oral antibiotic (amoxicillin, ampicillin, sulfisoxazole, trimethoprim-sulfamethoxazole, ciprofloxacin)
Administration of 3-day course of oral antibiotics (trimethoprim-sulfamethoxazole or norfloxacin)
Encouragement of fluid intake of 3000 ml/day
Repeat of urine culture

Recurrent Infection

DIAGNOSTIC

Urinalysis
Urine for culture and sensitivity
Evaluation of urinary tract (e.g., IVP, voiding cystourethrogram, cystoscopy, pelvic examination)

THERAPEUTIC

Administration of antimicrobials for 10-14 days based on sensitivity testing
Administration of prophylactic drug (e.g., trimethoprim-sulfamethoxazole) for repeated recurrent infections
Encouragement of fluid intake of 3000 ml/day
Repeat of urine culture

IVP, Intravenous pyelogram.
*See text for description of different treatment protocols.

nitrofurantoin (Furadantin, Macrodantin), and methenamine mandelate (Mandelamine). Methenamine achieves its desired effect by decomposing to formaldehyde and ammonia. The urinary pH should be less than 6 for methenamine to be effective. The urinary pH should be tested to ensure the activity of the drug.

Systemic antibiotics such as ampicillin, amoxicillin, cephalosporins, and aminoglycosides (gentamicin, tobramycin) are used. Phenazopyridine hydrochloride (Pyridium) may be used in cystitis to provide an analgesic effect on the urinary mucosa. This drug should relieve the burning sensation. The azo dye in the drug stains the urine reddish orange. It is important to tell clients about the color change so that they do not think it is related to the infection.

Sulfamethaxazole and trimethoprim (Bactrim, Septra) have proved to be an effective drug combination in the treatment of UTIs, especially recurrent ones. When these drugs are used together, resistance to them seems to develop less rapidly.

Single-dose therapy has been effective in clients when the infection is localized to the bladder and the organism is sensitive to antibiotics. Single-dose therapy results in lowered cost, increased compliance, and decreased potential for resistant organisms. If there is involvement of the kidney or if the client is an older adult or has diabetes, single-dose therapy is not appropriate. All clients treated with a single course of antibiotics should have follow-up cultures. Clients who have positive cultures after single-dose therapy should be assumed to have upper UTIs and should be treated for them. The antibody-coated bacteria test can distinguish between infections involving only the bladder and those affecting the kidney. Many clinicians are now treating uncomplicated infections with a 3-day course of antibiotics. As with single-dose therapy, candidates for 3-day therapy must be chosen to exclude those with upper UTIs.[4] Antibiotic therapy is not usually recommended for asymptomatic bacteriuria unless symptoms develop or there is evidence of obstructive uropathy in the symptom-free client.

■ Nursing Management of Cystitis

Nursing interventions

Health promotion and maintenance. Health promotion and maintenance measures include recognizing the groups with a higher than normal incidence of UTIs. Health promotion activities can help decrease the frequency of infections and promote early detection of infection. These activities include teaching preventive measures, such as emptying the bladder when the urge to urinate is first felt, drinking at least eight glasses of water a day, and wiping the perineal area from front to back after urination and defecation. In addition, it is important to teach the client to identify symptoms such as difficulty or pain on urinating, foul-smelling urine, and frequency and urgency of urination.

The nurse can play a major role in the prevention of nosocomial infections. Debilitated persons, older adults, clients with severe underlying disease (such as cancer, cirrhosis, or diabetes), and clients being treated with immunosuppressive drugs, long-term corticosteroid therapy, or radiation are at high risk of UTIs. Clients undergoing instrumentation of the urinary tract are also at risk of the development of nosocomial infections.

For clients at risk of nosocomial urinary infections, it is important to provide good perineal hygiene, especially after a bedpan is used. Incontinence should be avoided by answering the call light quickly or offering the bedpan or urinal at frequent intervals to the bedridden client. If a catheter has been inserted, special catheter care measures must be employed (see p. 1210).

Acute intervention. Acute intervention for a client with cystitis includes forcing fluids if this is not contraindicated. It is sometimes difficult to get clients to maintain an adequate fluid intake because they think it will increase their feelings of urgency. Treatment of cystitis does not usually require hospitalization.

The client needs to be instructed about the prescribed drug therapy. Common side effects of the drugs should be explained, and the client should be told to notify the physician if they occur.

The urine should be examined for gross or microscopic hematuria, malodor, and sediment. The client should be instructed to observe for any changes in the color or consistency of the urine as a sign of the effectiveness of therapy.

Chronic management. Chronic management of a client with UTI emphasizes the need for the client's compliance with the medication regimen. It is the nurse's responsibility to educate the client about the need for ongoing care. This includes taking antimicrobial medication as ordered until all the pills are gone, not just until symptoms subside; maintaining adequate fluid intake of 2000 to 3000 mL/day; emptying the bladder when the urge to urinate occurs or at least every 2 to 3 hours; urinating after intercourse; and discontinuing use of a diaphragm (if used).

The client must understand the need for follow-up care with urine culture to determine that the infection has been adequately treated. Relapse with bacteria of the same species usually occurs within 1 to 2 weeks after completion of therapy. If the client has been compliant, relapse suggests possible renal involvement in the infectious process. For clients who have more than two infections every 6 months, the use of long-term prophylactic therapy may be appropriate. Low-dose antibiotics after sexual intercourse may also be of benefit in preventing episodes of infection.

Urethritis

The clinical manifestations of inflammation of the urethra (urethritis) are the same as those of cystitis. A definitive diagnosis is made by obtaining a sterile urine specimen when the bladder is catheterized, indicating that the site of infection is the urethra rather than the bladder. Causes of urethritis include a bacterial or viral infection, *Trichomonas* and monilial infection (especially in women), gonorrhea (especially in men), and chlamydia. (Gonococcal urethritis is discussed in Chapter 47.)

Treatment is based on identifying and treating the cause and providing symptomatic relief. In chlamydial infections, doxycycline should be used. Women with negative urine cultures and no pyuria do not usually respond to antibiotics. Hot sitz baths without perfumed bath oil or bath salts may relieve the symptoms. The client should be instructed to avoid the use of vaginal deodorant sprays, to properly cleanse the perineal area after bowel movements and urination, and to avoid intercourse until symptoms subside.

Urethral Syndrome

Symptoms of dysuria, urgency, and frequency unaccompanied by significant bacteriuria (i.e., less than 10^2 to 10^3 per milliliter of urine) have been called the acute *urethral syndrome*. Clinically, these clients cannot be readily distinguished from those with cystitis. When present, bacteria are usually *E. coli* or staphylococci. If few or no bacteria are detected, *Chlamydia trachomatis* or *Neisseria gonorrhoeae* (both sexually transmitted pathogens) may be the cause. (Detection of *Chlamydia* organisms requires tissue culture or immunological testing for chlamydial antigen in urethral or cervical specimens.) Chlamydial infection is less likely to cause hematuria and suprapubic pain than bacterial infection.

Treatment depends on the causative agent. If bacteria are involved, the treatment is similar to that for cystitis. These clients respond well to single-dose therapy. In women with chlamydial infection, doxycycline should be used. Simultaneous treatment of the client's sexual partner may be recommended.

Acute Pyelonephritis

Etiology. Pyelonephritis is an acute or chronic inflammatory process of the renal pelvis and parenchyma of the kidney. Generally, the inflammatory process is caused by bacterial invasion. Most infections are caused by the normal inhabitants of the intestinal tract (e.g., *E. coli*).

Pyelonephritis can develop via the ascending route following cystitis. Another preexisting factor often is present. In children, it is usually associated with vesicoureteral reflux or other urinary tract abnormalities. In adults, common preexisting factors are bladder tumors, prostatic hypertrophy, strictures, and urinary stones. Repeated attacks of acute pyelonephritis, especially in the presence of these abnormalities, can result in chronic pyelonephritis. The infection commonly starts in the renal medulla and then spreads to the adjacent cortex. The infected portion of the kidney heals, resulting in fibrosis and scarring.

Clinical manifestations. The clinical manifestations of acute pyelonephritis vary from mild lassitude to the sudden onset of chills, fever, vomiting, malaise, flank pain, dysuria, and frequent urination. Symptoms of cystitis may or may not be present. The clinical manifestations usually subside within a few days, even without specific therapy. However, bacteriuria and/or pyuria may persist.

On the basis of symptoms and clinical findings, it is often difficult to differentiate between clients with infections confined to the bladder and those with renal involvement. Clients with kidney infections may have symptoms related to cystitis or may have no symptoms. The most promising and practical approach to this problem appears to be the determination of whether antibody-coated bacteria are present in the urine.

Therapeutic management. The therapeutic management of acute pyelonephritis is summarized in Table 40-3, and the diagnostic findings are given in Table 40-4. Urine cultures should always be obtained when pyelonephritis is suspected. Intravenous pyelograms (IVP) or excretory urograms are usually not obtained in the early stages of pyelonephritis to prevent the possible spread of infection.

An essential principle of therapeutic management is to consider factors that may be contributing to the infection, such as an obstruction or urinary tract anomaly. In addition to an IVP, this involves the use of other diagnostic procedures such as a cystourethrogram and cystoscopy. It is essential to obtain follow-up urine cultures to determine the effectiveness of therapy.

Pharmacological management. Clients with mild symptoms may be treated for 14 days (see Table 40-3). Intravenous (IV) antibiotics are often given initially. If they appear to be successful, the client may be discharged on an oral form of the antibiotic. Relapses may be treated with a 6-week course of antibiotics. Reinfections may be treated as individual episodes of disease or managed with long-term antibiotic therapy. Antibiotic prophylaxis may

Table 40-3

Diagnostic and Therapeutic Management: Acute Pyelonephritis

DIAGNOSTIC

Urinalysis
Urine for culture and sensitivity, Gram stain
IVP, ultrasound, CT scan
WBC count
Blood culture (if bacteremia suspected)
Antibody-coated bacteria test

THERAPEUTIC

Mild symptoms
  Outpatient management or short hospitalization for IV antibiotics
  Administration of oral antibiotics (e.g., trimethoprim-sulfamethoxazole, ciprofloxacin) for 14 days
  Fluid intake of 3000 ml/day
  Follow-up urine cultures
Severe symptoms
  Hospitalization
  Parenteral antibiotics (e.g., aminoglycoside [amikacin, gentamicin], cephalosporin [cefoxitin, cefoperazone])
  Fluid intake of 3000 ml/day
  Follow-up urine cultures

Table 40-4   Diagnostic Findings in Acute Pyelonephritis

Test	Findings
Urinalysis	Cloudy, foul-smelling urine; pyuria; large quantities of bacteria, pus, RBCs, WBCs, casts on microscopic examination; antibody-coated bacteria; increase in urinary pH
Blood	Elevation in WBC count, possible positive blood cultures
IVP, ultrasound, CT scan	Enlargement of involved kidney or kidneys, abscesses in renal tissue, structural abnormalities

also be used for recurrent infections. The effectiveness of therapy is evaluated in accordance with the presence or absence of bacterial growth on urine culture.

■ Nursing Management of Urinary Tract Infection

Nursing assessment

Subjective and objective data that should be obtained from a client with a UTI are presented in Table 40-5.

Nursing diagnoses

Nursing diagnoses specific to the client with a UTI include, but are not limited to, those presented in Table 40-6.

Nursing interventions

Health promotion and maintenance. Health promotion and maintenance measures are similar to those for cystitis.

Table 40-5

 Nursing Assessment of the Client with a Urinary Tract Infection

SUBJECTIVE DATA

History
Previous urinary tract infections; urinary calculi, stasis, reflux, strictures, or retention; recent urological instrumentation (catheterization, cystoscopy, surgery); neurogenic bladder; pregnancy; prostatic hypertrophy; sexually transmitted disease; renal failure; bladder cancer; polycystic kidney disease

Medications
Use of antibiotics, anticholinergics, antispasmodics

General
Upper UTI: Chills, fever, lassitude, malaise, anorexia
Lower UTI: Suprapubic or low back pain, bladder spasms, dysuria

Gastrointestinal
Nausea and vomiting with upper UTI

Urinary
Frequency, urgency, hesitancy, nocturia, burning on urination

OBJECTIVE DATA

Gastrointestinal
Abdominal rigidity with upper UTI

Urinary
Hematuria, foul-smelling urine
Upper UTI: Tender, enlarged kidney; decreased urinary output

Possible findings
Leukocytosis; urinalysis positive for bacteria, pyuria, RBCs, and WBCs; positive urine culture; antibody-coated bacteria test (positive in pyelonephritis, negative in cystitis); IVP, voiding cystourethrogram and cystoscopy demonstrating abnormalities of urinary tract

---

In addition, it is important that the client receive early treatment for cystitis to prevent ascending infections. Because clients with structural abnormalities of the urinary tract are at high risk of infection, the need for regular medical care should be stressed.

Acute and chronic intervention. Nursing interventions vary, depending on the severity of symptoms (see Table 40-6). These interventions include teaching the client about the disease process with emphasis on (1) the need to continue medications as prescribed, (2) the need for a follow-up urine culture to ensure proper management, and (3) identification of recurrence or relapse of infection. In addition to antibiotic therapy, the client should be encouraged to drink at least eight glasses of fluid every day. Increased fluid intake should be continued, even after the infection has been treated. Additional comfort measures include administration of phenazopyridine hydrochloride (Pyridium), a urinary analgesic. Inform the client that this drug causes reddish-orange urine. Antispasmodics may also be ordered to relieve acute distress. Clients with frequent relapses or reinfections may be treated with long-term low-dose antibiotics. Understanding the rationale for therapy is important to enhance client compliance.

Chronic Pyelonephritis

Chronic pyelonephritis (also called *chronic interstitial nephritis*) is not the result of an isolated episode of acute pyelonephritis unless there are predisposing factors, such as obstruction, neurogenic bladder, or vesicoureteral reflux. Chronic pyelonephritis is usually the end result of long-standing UTIs with recurrences, relapses, and reinfections.

The pathological changes indicate that there have been repeated episodes of chronic inflammation and scarring. Grossly, both kidneys are irregularly and asymmetrically scarred. The renal pelvis and calyces are deformed, blunted, and dilated.

Clinical features of chronic pyelonephritis include a history of recurrent acute infections leading to progressive destruction of functioning nephrons resulting in chronic renal insufficiency. During active infection, urine cultures are positive and leukocyte casts are found on urinalysis. End-stage chronic pyelonephritis is not easily distinguished from other causes of chronic renal failure. IVP, renal biopsy, renal ultrasound, or CT scan may be useful in delineating the severity of renal involvement after the infection has been resolved.

The level of renal function can vary in chronic pyelonephritis. Clients may have improvement in function after an acute exacerbation. Chronic pyelonephritis may progress to chronic renal failure. (Therapeutic and nursing care of the client with chronic renal failure are discussed in Chapter 41.)

Renal Tuberculosis

Renal tuberculosis is rarely a primary lesion. It is usually secondary to tuberculosis of the lung. In 4% to 8% of clients with pulmonary tuberculosis, the tubercle bacilli reach the kidneys via the bloodstream. Onset occurs 5 to 8 years after the primary infection. The most common manifestations include frequent urination, burning on voiding, and epididymitis (in men). Infrequently, renal colic, lumbar and iliac pain, and hematuria may be present. A diagnosis is based on localization of tubercle bacilli in the urine and on IVP findings.

Long-term complications of renal tuberculosis depend on the duration of the disease before treatment. Scarring of the renal parenchyma and the development of ureteral strictures occur. The earlier treatment is initiated, the less likely is the development of renal failure. (Nursing and therapeutic management for the client with tuberculosis are discussed in Chapter 21.)

IMMUNOLOGICAL DISORDERS OF THE KIDNEY
Significance

Immunological processes involving the urinary tract predominantly affect the renal glomerulus. Glomerular disease is found in about one half of all clients with severe renal disease. The disease process results in inflammation

Table 40-6

NURSING CARE PLAN FOR THE CLIENT WITH A URINARY TRACT INFECTION

Defining Characteristics	Nursing Interventions	Evaluation Criteria

NURSING DIAGNOSIS: Ineffective thermoregulation related to infection

Defining Characteristics	Nursing Interventions	Evaluation Criteria
Elevation in temperature, tachycardia, tachypnea, chills	Monitor vital signs q 2-4 hr. Administer antipyretics and antibiotics as ordered. Ensure adequate hydration via oral or IV route. Monitor intake and output. Cover client lightly and keep client dry. Prevent chilling.	Normal temperature, no chills

NURSING DIAGNOSIS: Pain related to dysuria, urgency, frequency, and bladder spasms secondary to inflammation and tissue trauma

Defining Characteristics	Nursing Interventions	Evaluation Criteria
Pain on urination, flank pain, suprapubic pain, lower back pain, bladder spasms; statement that pain is present	Palpate abdomen and percuss flank to identify painful area. Position client for comfort. Administer analgesics, antispasmodics, and azo dyes as ordered and note their effectiveness. Apply heating pad to painful area. Alert client that azo dyes will color urine. Encourage fluid intake. Encourage bed rest during acute phase.	Satisfactory pain control or absence of pain

NURSING DIAGNOSIS: Altered patterns of urinary elimination: frequency, urgency, incontinence, or nocturia related to UTI

Defining Characteristics	Nursing Interventions	Evaluation Criteria
Urgency, frequency, nocturia, incontinence, hematuria; verbalization of concern over altered elimination pattern	Instruct client regarding reason for symptoms. Force fluids up to 3000 ml/day (e.g., daytime, 1500 ml; evening, 1000 ml; nighttime, 500 ml). Administer IV fluids as ordered. Obtain urine for culture and sensitivity. Administer antimicrobial medication as ordered. Instruct client about good perineal care and cleansing after each bowel movement. Observe urine for color, odor, amount, and frequency.	No evidence of infected urine, normal urination pattern

NURSING DIAGNOSIS: High risk for reinfection related to lack of knowledge regarding prevention of recurrence and signs and symptoms of recurrence

Defining Characteristics	Nursing Interventions	Evaluation Criteria
Recurrent UTI, lack of knowledge of measures to prevent reinfection	Instruct client about the need to force fluids to 3000 ml/day unless contraindicated. Explain rationale for use of medications, times, and method of administration. Explain need for follow-up care. Instruct client on appropriate hygiene, including careful cleansing of perineal region, wiping from front to back after urinating, cleansing with soap and water after each bowel movement. Explain the importance of emptying the bladder before and after intercourse. Instruct client to urinate when the urge occurs or at least q 2-3 hr. Instruct client to avoid bath salts, oils, and vaginal sprays, which can irritate the urethral meatus, and to observe for symptoms of recurrence to be reported, such as changes in urinating habits, character of urine, flank pain, or incontinence.	Negative urine culture, no symptoms of UTI

of all glomeruli (glomerulonephritis). It affects both kidneys equally. Although the glomerulus is the primary site of inflammation, tubular, interstitial, and vascular changes also occur.

Glomerulonephritis is divided into a number of classifications, which may describe (1) the extent of damage (diffuse or focal), (2) the initial cause of the disorder (e.g., lupus erythematosus, scleroderma, streptococcal infection), or (3) the extent of changes (minimal or widespread). Minimal-change glomerulonephritis is responsible for more than 50% of all cases of nephrotic syndrome in children and about 20% of all cases in adults.

Etiology and Pathophysiology

Two types of antibody-induced injury can initiate glomerular damage. In the first type, the antibodies have specificity for antigens within the glomerular basement membrane (GBM). These are called *anti-GBM antibodies.* Immunoglobulins and complement are deposited along the basement membrane. The mechanism that causes a person to develop antibodies against its GBM is not known. Production of *autoantibodies* (antibodies to one's own tissue) may be stimulated by a structural alteration in the GBM or by a reaction of the basement membrane with an exogenous agent (e.g., hydrocarbon, viruses).

In the second type of immune process, the antibodies react with circulating nonglomerular antigens and are randomly deposited as immune complexes along the GBM. On electron microscopy of renal tissue sections, they appear as "lumpy-bumpy" deposits. In this immune complex process, the antigens do not come from the glomeruli but from either endogenous circulating native DNA or exogenous sources (e.g., bacteria, viruses, chemicals, and drugs). Bacterial products appear to be important in poststreptococcal glomerulonephritis as well as in endocarditis. Viral agents have been recognized in certain cases of glomerulonephritis that develop after hepatitis and measles.

All forms of immune complex disease are characterized by an accumulation of antigen, antibody, and complement in the glomeruli, which can result in tissue injury. The immune complexes activate complement (see Chapter 7). Complement activation results in the release of chemotactic factors that attract polymorphonuclear leukocytes and cause the release of histamine and other vasoactive amines. The intrinsic clotting pathway may also be activated. The end result of these processes is glomerular injury as a result of inflammation.

Clinical Manifestations

There are many clinical manifestations of glomerulonephritis. They may include varying degrees of hematuria (ranging from microscopic to gross) and urinary excretion of various formed elements, including RBCs, WBCs, and some granular casts. Proteinuria and elevated blood urea nitrogen (BUN) and serum creatinine levels are other manifestations. In most cases, recovery from the acute illness is complete. When progressive involvement occurs, however, the result is destruction of renal tissue and marked renal insufficiency.

The client's history provides important information related to glomerulonephritis. It is necessary to assess exposure to drugs, immunizations, microbial infections, and viral infections such as hepatitis. It is also important to evaluate the client for more generalized conditions involving immune disorders, such as lupus erythematosus and systemic progressive sclerosis (scleroderma).

Acute Poststreptococcal Glomerulonephritis

Acute poststreptococcal glomerulonephritis (APSGN) is most common in children and young adults, but all age groups can be affected.[5] APSGN develops 5 to 21 days after an infection of the pharynx or skin by certain nephro-toxic strains of group A β-hemolytic streptococci (e.g., streptococcal sore throat, tonsillitis, impetigo). The person produces antibodies to the streptococcal antigen. Although the specific mechanism is not known with certainty, the antigen-antibody complexes are deposited in the glomeruli and activate complement. Complement activation causes an inflammatory reaction to the injury. The response to the injury is also a decrease in the filtration of metabolic waste products from the blood and an increase in the permeability of the glomerulus to larger protein molecules.

Clinical manifestations and complications. The clinical manifestations of APSGN appear as a variety of signs and symptoms, which may include generalized body edema, hypertension, oliguria, hematuria with a smoky or rusty appearance, and proteinuria. Fluid retention occurs as a result of decreased glomerular filtration. The edema appears initially in low-pressure tissue, such as that around the eyes (periorbital edema), but later progresses to involve the total body as ascites or peripheral edema in the legs. Smoky urine is indicative of bleeding in the upper urinary tract. The degree of proteinuria varies with the severity of the glomerulonephropathy. Hypertension primarily results from increased extracellular fluid volume.

Clients with APSGN may have abdominal or flank pain. Sometimes the client may have no symptoms, with the problem being found on routine urinalysis.

More than 95% of clients with APSGN recover completely or improve rapidly with conservative management. The prognosis for adults is less favorable than for children. Chronic glomerulonephritis develops in 5% to 15% of the affected persons, and irreversible renal failure occurs in less than 1% of clients.[6]

Diagnostic studies. The diagnosis of APSGN is based on a complete history and physical examination and laboratory studies (Table 40-7) to determine the presence or history of a group A β-hemolytic streptococcus in a throat

---

Table 40-7

| **Diagnostic and Therapeutic Management: Acute Glomerulonephritis** |

DIAGNOSTIC

History and physical examination
Urinalysis
CBC
Serum levels, including BUN, creatinine, albumin
Complement studies and ASO titer
Renal biopsy (if indicated)

THERAPEUTIC

Bed rest
Sodium and fluid restriction
Administration of loop diuretics (furosemide, ethacrynic acid)
Antihypertensive therapy
Adjustment of dietary protein intake to level of uremia and proteinuria

or skin lesion. An immune response to the streptococcus is often demonstrated by assessment of antistreptolysin O (ASO) titers. The finding of decreased complement components (especially C1q, C3, and C4) is indicative of an immune-mediated response. A renal biopsy may be performed to confirm the presence of the disease.

Therapeutic management. The therapeutic management of ASPGN focuses on symptomatic relief (Table 40-7). Bed rest is recommended until the signs of glomerular inflammation (proteinuria, hematuria) and hypertension subside. Edema is treated by restriction of sodium and fluid intake and by administration of loop diuretics such as furosemide and ethacrynic acid. Severe hypertension is treated with antihypertensive drugs. Dietary protein intake may be restricted if there is evidence of an increase in nitrogenous wastes (e.g., elevated BUN value). The restriction varies with the degree of proteinuria.

Penicillin or erythromycin should be given only if the streptococcal infection is still present. Steroids and cytotoxic drugs have not been shown to be of value.

■ Nursing Management of Acute Poststreptococcal Glomerulonephritis

Nursing interventions

Health promotion and maintenance. One of the most important ways to prevent the development of APSGN is to encourage early diagnosis and treatment of sore throats and skin lesions. If streptococci are found in the culture, treatment with appropriate antibiotic therapy (usually penicillin) is essential. The client needs to be encouraged to take the full course of antibiotics to ensure that the bacteria have been eradicated. Good personal hygiene is an important factor in preventing the spread of cutaneous streptococcal infections.

Acute intervention. The nursing management of acute glomerulonephritis is specific to the client's symptoms. An important nursing measure is helping the client plan adequate rest to allow the kidneys to heal. The client may need assistance in the management of fluid and dietary restrictions. (Low-protein, low-sodium, fluid-restricted diets are discussed in Chapter 41.) Other nursing measures are described in Table 40-8.

Goodpasture's Syndrome

Goodpasture's syndrome, an example of cytotoxic (type II) autoimmune disease, is characterized by the presence of circulating antibodies against GBM and alveolar basement membrane.[7] Although the primary target organ is the kidney, the lungs are involved by way of cross-reactivity. The pathological nature of the syndrome results when binding of the antibody causes an inflammatory reaction mediated by complement fixation and activation (see Chapter 7). Type A_2 influenza viruses, hydrocarbons, penicillamine, and unknown genetic factors stimulate autoantibody production.

Goodpasture's syndrome is a rare disease that is seen mostly in young men. The clinical manifestations include hemoptysis, pulmonary insufficiency, rales, rhonchi, renal involvement with hematuria and renal failure, weakness, pallor, and anemia. Pulmonary hemorrhage usually occurs and may precede glomerular abnormalities by weeks. Abnormal diagnostic findings include low hematocrit and hemoglobin readings, elevated BUN and serum creatinine levels, hematuria, and proteinuria.

■ Therapeutic and Nursing Management of Goodpasture's Syndrome

Until recently, the prognosis for clients with Goodpasture's syndrome was poor. Therapeutic management consists of corticosteroids, immunosuppressive drugs (e.g., azathioprine), plasmapheresis (see Chapter 8), and dialysis. Renal transplantation can be attempted, once the circulating anti-GBM antibody titer decreases. In selected clients with severe pulmonary hemorrhage, bilateral nephrectomy has been helpful. The exact mechanism for improvement has not been proved.

Nursing management appropriate for a critically ill client who is experiencing symptoms of acute renal failure and respiratory distress is instituted. Death is often secondary to respiratory hemorrhage. (Nursing interventions for a client in acute renal failure are discussed in Chapter 41, and nursing interventions for a client with respiratory failure are discussed in Chapter 23.) Because this syndrome is rare and primarily affects previously healthy young men, support and understanding of the client and the family are of major importance. The client and the family need instruction concerning current therapy, medications, and complications of the disease process.

Rapidly Progressive Glomerulonephritis

Rapidly progressive glomerulonephritis (RPGN) is characterized by sudden onset and rapid deterioration of renal function. Renal failure may occur within weeks to months in contrast to chronic glomerulonephritis, which develops insidiously and progresses over many years.

RPGN can occur in a variety of situations: (1) as a complication of inflammatory or infectious disease (e.g., APSGN), (2) as a complication of a multisystemic disease (e.g., systemic lupus erythematosus, Goodpasture's syndrome), (3) as an idiopathic disease, or (4) in association with the use of certain drugs (e.g., penicillamine).

Treatment of RPGN has included corticosteroids, cytotoxic agents, anticoagulants, and antithrombotic agents. Plasmapheresis has recently been used.[8] More than one half of clients with RPGN progress to end-stage renal disease within 6 months after the diagnosis of the illness. Dialysis therapy and transplantation are used to maintain clients with RPGN. RPGN may recur after a renal transplant.

Chronic Glomerulonephritis

Chronic glomerulonephritis is a syndrome that reflects the end stage of glomerular inflammatory disease. Most types of glomerulonephritis and nephrotic syndrome can eventually lead to chronic glomerulonephritis.

The syndrome is characterized by proteinuria, hematuria, and the slow development of uremic syndrome (see Chapter 41) as a result of decreasing renal function. Chronic glomerulonephritis does not usually follow an acute course. It progresses insidiously toward renal failure and uremia over a few to as many as 30 years.

Table 40-8

NURSING CARE PLAN FOR THE CLIENT WITH ACUTE GLOMERULONEPHRITIS

Defining Characteristics	Nursing Interventions	Evaluation Criteria

NURSING DIAGNOSIS: Fluid volume excess related to sodium and water retention and renal dysfunction

Edematous extremities; taut, shiny skin; tachypnea, crackles, elevated blood pressure	Maintain diet and fluid restrictions as ordered (e.g., low sodium, limiting of fluid intake to 1200 ml). Monitor intake and output. Administer diuretics as ordered. Assess skin turgor. Help client turn q 2 hr. Elevate edematous extremities. Give skin care q 4 hr. Ensure that active or passive range-of-motion exercises are done q 2-4 hr. Assess respiratory status q 4 hr and observe for pulmonary edema. Weigh client daily. Monitor blood pressure q 2-4 hr. Instruct client to report symptoms related to elevated blood pressure (headaches, blurred vision, loss of balance, nosebleeds). Limit activity as ordered. Administer antihypertensives as ordered. Instruct client about antihypertensives, including rationale for use, method of administration, and side effects.	Absence of edema, blood pressure within normal range

NURSING DIAGNOSIS: Ineffective individual coping: depression related to chronicity of disease, lack of social support, lack of knowledge regarding disease process and treatment, and perceived helplessness

Verbalization of concern about disease process, lack of support system, sad affect	Encourage client to verbalize fears. Instruct client about disease process. Explain treatment before implementation. Involve family and client in planning care.	Verbal indication that explanations are understood, verbal and behavioral indication of reduction of anxiety

NURSING DIAGNOSIS: Activity intolerance related to fatigue, weakness, protein depletion, elevated vital signs, depression, interrupted sleep, and treatment regimen

Verbalization of inability to move about freely or meet personal needs, increase in vital signs with activity, dyspnea on exertion	Monitor vital signs as ordered. Check laboratory values for electrolyte imbalances, protein balance, and anemia. Plan care with client to provide for rest periods. Provide quiet environment. Assist in positioning client for comfort. Provide supportive care.	Increase in ability to tolerate activity

NURSING DIAGNOSIS: High risk for altered health maintenance related to chronicity of illness, complex medical regimen, and lack of knowledge regarding fluid intake, signs and symptoms of recurrence, medications, and prevention of recurrence

Questions or incorrect answers about disease management	Instruct client during hospital stay to prepare for home self-care, including diet and fluid restrictions (individualized according to degree of renal dysfunction); monitoring of daily weight; measurement of urine output and awareness of character of urine; reporting of any pyuria, dysuria, or hematuria; rationale, dose, and side effects of medications; need for rest and relaxation; need to avoid crowds in cold weather and people with respiratory infections; and preventive measures for UTIs.	Compliance with medication and health care regimen, ability to identify symptoms to be reported to physician

Chronic glomerulonephritis is often found coincidentally when an abnormality on a urinalysis or elevated blood pressure is detected. It is quite common to find that the client has no recollection or history of acute nephritis or any renal problems. A renal biopsy may be performed to determine the exact cause and nature of the glomerulonephritis. However, many institutions now prefer to use ultrasound and CT scanning as diagnostic measures. (Management of chronic renal failure is discussed in Chapter 41.)

NEPHROTIC SYNDROME
Clinical Manifestations

The term *nephrotic syndrome* describes a clinical course that can be associated with a number of disease conditions. Some of the more common causes of nephrotic syndrome are listed in Table 40-9. The characteristic manifestations include edema, massive proteinuria, hyperlipidemia, and hypoalbuminemia.[9] The increased glomerular membrane permeability found in nephrotic syndrome is responsible for the massive excretion of protein in the urine. This results in decreased serum protein and subsequent edema formation.

The diminished plasma oncotic pressure from the decreased serum proteins stimulates hepatic lipoprotein synthesis, which results in hyperlipidemia. Initially, cholesterol and low-density lipoproteins are elevated. Later the triglyceride level is also increased. Fat bodies (fatty casts) commonly appear in the urine.

Table 40-9 Causes of Nephrotic Syndrome

PRIMARY GLOMERULAR DISEASE

Membranous proliferative glomerulonephritis
Primary nephrotic syndrome
Focal glomerulonephritis
Inherited nephrotic disease

EXTRARENAL CAUSES

Multisystem disease
  Systemic lupus erythematosus
  Diabetes mellitus
  Amyloidosis
Infections
  Bacterial (streptococcal, syphilis)
  Viral (hepatitis, human immunodeficiency virus infection)
  Protozoal (malaria)
Neoplasms
  Hodgkin's disease
  Solid tumors of lungs, colon, stomach, breast
  Leukemias
Allergens (e.g., bee sting, pollen)
Drugs
  Penicillamine
  Nonsteroidal antiinflammatory drugs
  Captopril
  Heroin

Immune responses, both humoral and cellular, are deficient in nephrotic syndrome. As a result, infection is an important cause of morbidity and mortality. Skeletal abnormalities, including hypocalcemia, blunted calcemic response to parathyroid hormone, hyperparathyroidism, and osteomalacia, may occur.

Hypercoagulability with thromboembolism is potentially the most serious complication of nephrotic syndrome. The renal vein is the site most commonly involved. Pulmonary emboli occur in about 40% of nephrotic clients with thrombosis.

Therapeutic Management

Treatment of nephrotic syndrome is symptomatic. The goals are to (1) relieve edema and (2) cure or control the primary disease. Therapeutic management of the edema includes the cautious use of loop diuretics and a low-salt, high-protein diet. IV albumin has not been beneficial as replacement therapy because it is rapidly lost in the urine. Albumin is used only in severe *anasarca* (generalized edema) or severe orthostatic hypotension and hypovolemia.

Corticosteroids and cyclophosphamide (Cytoxan) are used for the treatment of severe cases of nephrotic syndrome. Prednisone has been effective to varying degrees in persons with lipoid nephrosis, membranous glomerulonephritis, proliferative glomerulonephritis, and lupus nephritis. Management of diabetes and treatment of edema are the only measures used for diabetic nephrosis.

▪ Nursing Management of Nephrotic Syndrome

A major nursing intervention for a client with nephrotic syndrome is related to edema. It is important to assess the edema by weighing the client daily, accurately recording intake and output, and measuring abdominal girth or extremity size. Comparing this information daily provides the nurse with a tool for assessing the effectiveness of treatment. The edematous skin needs careful cleaning. Trauma should be avoided, and the effectiveness of diuretic therapy must be monitored.

The client has the potential to become malnourished from the excessive loss of protein in the urine. Maintaining a high-protein diet that is also low in sodium is not always easy. The protein intake should be 1.0 to 1.5 g/kg of body weight. The client is usually anorexic. Serving small, frequent meals in a pleasant setting may encourage better dietary intake.

Because the client is susceptible to infection, measures should be taken to avoid exposure to persons with known infections. Persons with nephrotic syndrome are often ashamed of their edematous appearance and need support in dealing with an altered body image.

RENAL DISEASE AND ACQUIRED IMMUNODEFICIENCY SYNDROME

Clients with acquired immunodeficiency syndrome (AIDS) can have a variety of renal manifestations, ranging from mild fluid and electrolyte abnormalities to progressive renal impairment resulting in end-stage renal disease.[10] The incidence of renal disease associated with hu-

man immunodeficiency virus (HIV) is about 10% and is highest among IV drug users.[11]

HIV-associated renal syndromes include the following:

1. *Proteinuria and nephrotic syndrome,* which occurs in about 10% of clients with HIV infection.[10] It may be the presenting sign of HIV infection in some persons.

2. *HIV-associated nephropathy* (HIVAN), which is characterized by proteinuria, progressive azotemia, absence of hypertension, large kidney size on renal imaging studies, and unusually rapid progression to end-stage renal disease.

3. *Acute renal failure,* which is most commonly seen in clients with AIDS who are critically ill with HIV-related infection or malignancy. Both oliguric and nonoliguric forms of renal failure can occur. The natural cause of acute renal failure secondary to AIDS is similar to acute renal failure associated with other acute illnesses (see Chapter 41). Survival and recovery usually depend on the treatment of the primary cause of renal failure and support of renal function by dialysis.

OBSTRUCTIVE UROPATHIES

The outflow of urine from the kidney may be obstructed anywhere along the urinary tract from the ureteropelvic junction to the terminal urethra. Obstruction is a predisposing factor in the development of UTIs and chronic pyelonephritis.

Two general classifications of urinary tract obstructions are *congenital* and *acquired.* Congenital obstructions most commonly involve a stricture, or narrowing, of the ureter.

Acquired obstructions include tumors (prostatic or bladder), scar tissue or fibrosis, and foreign bodies such as urinary calculi. Common causes of urinary obstruction are shown in Fig. 40-2. Functional obstruction can occur from neurological lesions that result in a neurogenic bladder. Pelvic or abdominal neoplasms may also result in urinary tract obstruction. The symptoms and pathological features associated with urinary obstruction depend on the site and on whether the obstruction is partial or complete.

The distention of the renal pelvis and calyces from an obstruction to normal urine flow is termed *hydronephrosis* (Fig. 40-3). *Hydroureter,* or dilatation of the ureter, may also result from obstructed urinary flow. In an obstructive process, urine production continues; eventually, sustained

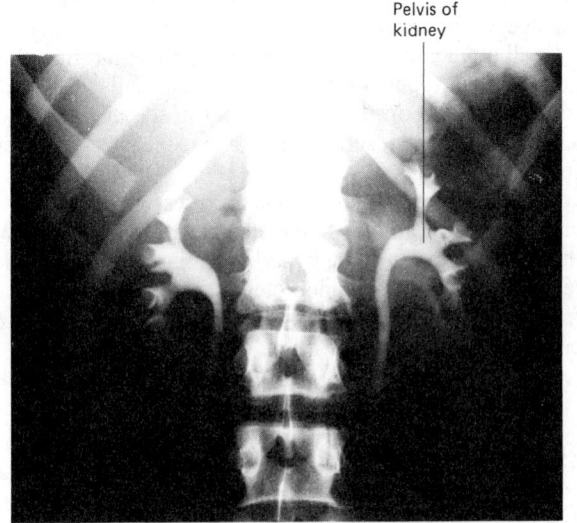

Fig. 40-3 **A,** Normal IVP. **B,** IVP showing hydronephrosis and hydroureter. (Courtesy Harborview Medical Center, University of Washington, Seattle.)

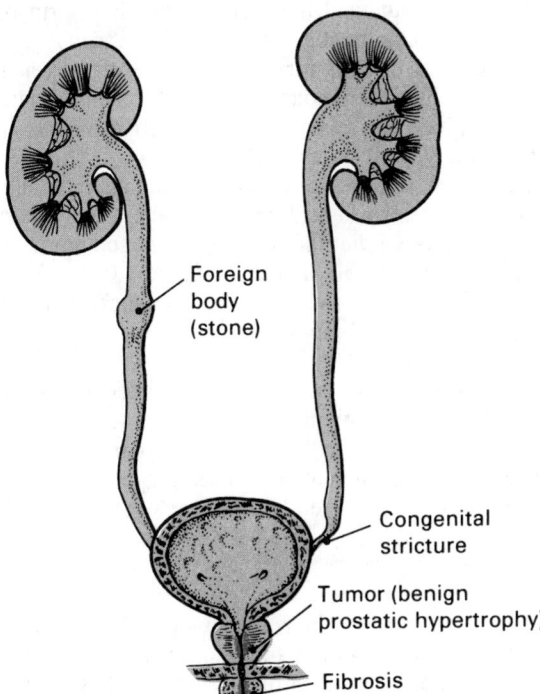

Fig. 40-2 Common causes of urinary tract obstruction.

or intermittent high pressure may develop, resulting in destruction of renal tissue. If the pressure remains low or moderate, the kidney may continue to dilate, with no noticeable loss of function. There is an increased risk of pyelonephritis because of urinary stasis and reflux. If only one kidney is involved and the other kidney is functioning, the client may be free of symptoms. If both kidneys or only one functioning kidney is involved (e.g., if the client has only one kidney), disturbances in renal function (e.g., increased BUN or serum creatinine levels) are found. If the obstruction progresses, oliguria or anuria develops. Often episodes of oliguria are followed by polyuria if the obstruction is a stone that becomes dislodged. Treatment requires location and relief of the blockage. This can include insertion of a tube (e.g., urethral or ureteral), surgical correction of the disease process, or diversion of the urinary stream above the level of blockage.

Renal Calculi

Significance. Kidney stones (nephrolithiasis) are common, with 1 in 1000 persons in the United States hospitalized annually because of urinary stones. In the United States, the incidence of urinary stone disease is highest in the Southeast and Southwest, followed by the Midwest. Except for struvite (an infected stone), which is more common in women, stone disorders are more common in men. The majority of clients are between 20 and 55 years of age. Stone formation is more frequent in whites than in blacks. The incidence is also higher in persons with a family history of stone formation. Recurrence of stones can occur in up to 80% of clients. There is seasonal variation, with stone formation occurring more often in the summer months, thus raising the question of the role of dehydration in this process. Stone formation in the kidney also seems to increase in incidence as countries become more industrialized, whereas the incidence of bladder stones decreases.[12]

Table 40-10 Factors in the Development of Urinary Tract Calculi

CLIMATE

High atmospheric temperature resulting in increased fluid loss, low urine volume, and increased solute concentration in urine

DIET

Large intake of dietary proteins increasing uric acid excretion, excessive amounts of tea or fruit juices elevating urinary oxalate level, large intake of calcium and oxalate

GENETIC FACTORS

Family history of stone formation, cystinuria, gout, or renal acidosis

LIFESTYLE

Sedentary occupation, immobility

Etiology. Many factors are involved in the incidence and type of stone formation, including dietary, genetic, climatic, lifestyle, and occupational influences (Table 40-10). Many theories have been proposed to explain the formation of stones in the urinary tract. No single theory can account for stone formation in each case. It is known that in the kidneys of stone formers, a mucoprotein is formed, which is the matrix for the stone. Urinary pH, solute load, and inhibitors in the urine affect the formation of stones. The higher the pH, the less soluble are calcium and phosphate. The lower the pH, the less soluble are uric acid and cystine. Other important factors in the development of stones include obstruction with urine stasis and urinary infection with urea-splitting bacteria (e.g., *Proteus* organisms). These bacteria cause the urine to become alkaline and contribute to the formation of calcium phosphate stones. Stones in the lower urinary tract (bladder or urethra) are found primarily in older men with prostatic enlargement and UTI.

Types. The term *calculus* refers to the stone and *lithiasis* refers to stone formation. There are five major categories of stones: (1) calcium phosphate, (2) calcium oxalate, (3) uric acid, (4) cystine, and (5) struvite (magnesium ammonium phosphate) (Table 40-11).

Clinical manifestations. Clinical manifestations of calculi include hematuria, abdominal or flank pain, and renal colic. The type of pain is determined by the location of the stone (Fig. 40-4). If the stone is trapped in a calyx or in the renal pelvis, pain may be absent. If it produces obstruction in a calyx or at the ureteropelvic junction, the client may experience dull pain or even colic. Pain resulting from the passage of a calculus down the ureter is intense and colicky. The client may be in mild shock with cold, moist skin. Costovertebral tenderness may be present. Other clinical manifestations include the presence of urinary infection accompanied by fever, vomiting, nausea, and chills.

Diagnostic studies. Diagnostic studies useful in the evaluation and management of renal lithiasis include urinalysis, urine culture, cystoscopy, IVP, retrograde pyelogram, CT scan, ultrasound, stone analysis for metabolic contents, and measurement of the urine and serum levels of various substances involved in stone formation (e.g., calcium, phosphate, oxalate, uric acid). A careful history, including previous stone formation and familial stone formation, is useful. Measurement of urine pH is useful in the diagnosis of struvite stones and renal tubular acidosis (alkaline pH) and uric acid stones (tendency to acidic pH). X-ray examination of kidneys, ureters, and bladder (KUB) may be done to pinpoint the location, number, and size of radiopaque stones (see Fig. 40-5). An IVP or retrograde pyelogram can further localize the degree and site of obstruction and confirm the presence of nonradiopaque stones (uric acid, cystine). Retrieval and analysis of kidney stones are very important in the diagnosis of the underlying problem contributing to stone formation. Chemical and crystallographic analysis can be done.

Therapeutic management. Evaluation and management of a client with renal lithiasis consist of two concurrent approaches. The first approach is directed toward

Table 40-11 Types of Urinary Calculi

Urinary Stone	Incidence (%)	Characteristics	Predisposing Factors	Therapeutic Measures
Calcium oxalate*	35-40	Small, often possible to get trapped in ureter, more frequent in men than in women	Idiopathic hypercalciuria, hyperoxaluria, independent of urinary pH	Increase hydration. Reduce dietary oxalate.‡ Give thiazide diuretics, phosphate therapy. Give cholestyramine to bind oxalate. Give calcium lactate to precipitate oxalate in GI tract.
Calcium phosphate	8-10	Mixed stones (typically), with struvite or oxalate stones	Alkaline urine, primary hyperparathyroidism	Treat other stones.
Struvite	10-15	Three to four times as common in women as in men, always an association with UTIs, large staghorn type (usually)†	UTIs (usually *Proteus* organisms)	Administer antimicrobial agents, acetohydroxamic acid. Surgical intervention used to remove stone. Take measures to acidify urine.
Uric acid	5-8	Predominant in men, high incidence in Jewish men	Gout, acid urine, inherited condition	Reduce urinary concentration of uric acid. Alkalinize urine. Administer allopurinol.
Cystine	1-2	Genetic autosomal recessive defect, defective absorption of cystine in GI tract and kidney, excess concentrations causing stone formation	Acid urine	Increase hydration. Give D-penicillamine to prevent cystine crystallization. Give sodium bicarbonate to maintain alkaline urine.

*Calcium stones can exist as calcium oxalate, calcium phosphate, or a mixture of both (accounts for about 30% of all stones). Calcium stones account for 70% to 85% of all stones.
†See Fig. 40-4.
‡See Table 40-12.

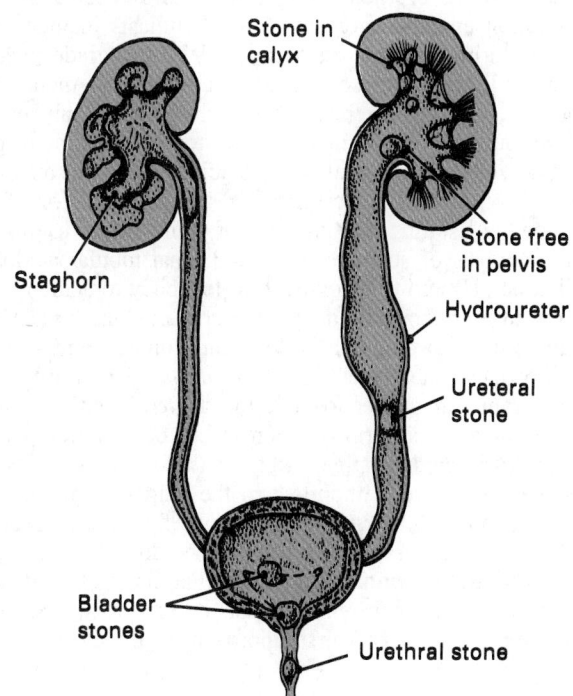

Fig. 40-4 Location of calculi in the urinary tract.

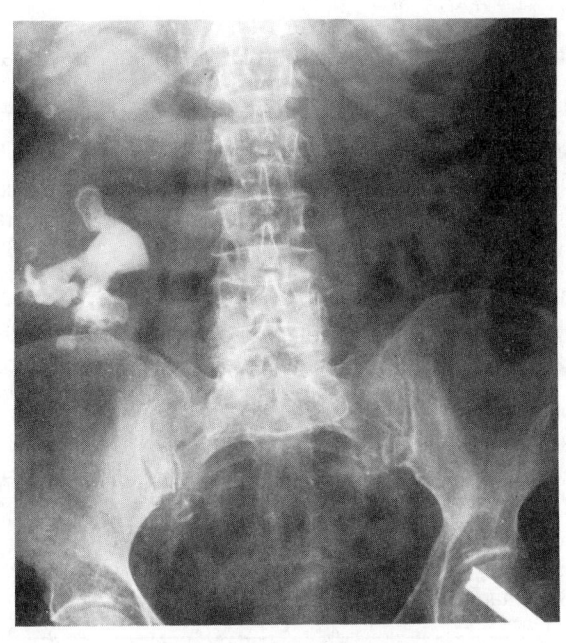

Fig. 40-5 X-ray film of a staghorn calculus. (Courtesy Harborview Medical Center, University of Washington, Seattle.)

management of the acute attack. This involves treating the symptoms of pain, infection, or obstruction as indicated for the individual client. An adequate fluid intake of 3000 to 4000 ml/day to produce a minimum urine output of 2 L/day is recommended. About 90% of stones pass spontaneously.

The second approach is directed toward evaluation of the etiology of the stone formation to prevent further development of stones. Information to be obtained from the client includes family history, geographical residence, nutritional assessment including the intake of vitamins A and D, whether lifestyle is sedentary, history of periods of prolonged illness with immobilization or dehydration, and any history of disease or surgery involving the GI or genitourinary (GU) tract.

Proper therapy for metabolically active stone formers requires a concerted therapeutic and nursing management approach, with primary emphasis on teaching and on developing a therapeutic regimen with which the client can reasonably comply (see Table 40-11). Adequate hydration, reduction of dietary oxalate, and reduction in the use of soda and coffee can decrease the incidence of calcium stones. When calcium urolithiasis is associated with hyperuricosuria (even in the absence of hypercalciuria), the use of allopurinol may be helpful. Excessive dietary intake of calcium and vitamin A or D should be evaluated and corrected. A thiazide diuretic such as hydrochlorothiazide reduces urinary calcium excretion and is used to treat stone formers who have idiopathic hypercalciuria. Phosphate compounds may be given to reduce hypercalciuria, decrease the intestinal absorption of calcium, and enhance the urinary excretion of crystal inhibitors such as pyrophosphate.

The treatment of uric acid stones is aimed at increasing the urinary pH to make the uric acid more soluble (e.g., alkalinizing the urine by increasing the intake of bicarbonate) and reducing the urinary concentration of uric acid. Maintenance of adequate hydration (3 L/day) is helpful in reducing the uric acid concentration of the urine. A low-purine diet (Table 40-12) may be prescribed. If the urate output is high as a result of endogenous production, allopurinol is given.

Treatment of struvite stones requires control of infection. This may be difficult if the stone remains in place. In addition to antibiotics, acetohydroxamic acid may be used in the treatment of kidney infections that result in the continual formation of struvite stones. Acetohydroxamic acid, an inhibitor of the chemical action caused by the persistent bacteria, can be used effectively to retard struvite stone formation. If the infection cannot be controlled, the stone may have to be removed surgically.

Surgical interventions. Indications for surgical stone removal include the following:

1. Stones too large for spontaneous passage
2. Stones associated with bacteriuria or symptomatic infection
3. Stones causing impaired renal function
4. Stones causing persistent pain, nausea, or ileus
5. Inability of client to be treated medically

If the stone is located in the bladder, a *transurethral lithol-*

Table 40-12 Foods High in Purine, Calcium, and Oxalate

PURINE

High: Sardines, herring, mussels, sweetbreads, liver, kidney, goose, venison, meat soups

Moderate: Chicken, salmon, crab, veal, mutton, bacon, pork, beef, ham

CALCIUM

Milk, cheese, ice cream, yogurt, foods containing flour, all beans (except green beans), lentils, fish with fine bones (e.g., sardines, kippers, herring, salmon), dried fruits, nuts, chocolate, cocoa, Ovaltine, sauces containing milk

OXALATE

Spinach, rhubarb, asparagus, cabbage, tomatoes, beets, nuts, celery, parsley, runner beans, chocolate, cocoa, instant coffee, Ovaltine, tea

apaxy may be performed. In this operation an instrument is inserted into the bladder via the urethra, and the stone is crushed and then washed out with irrigating solution. Small stones in the distal ureter may be removed transurethrally with instruments that snare the stone. These are referred to as *baskets* and consist of a special catheter with filaments attached so that when the catheter is passed beyond the stone and gradually withdrawn, the stone becomes entangled in the filaments. If this procedure is not successful, one or two ureteral catheters may be left in place to dilate the ureter and extraction can be attempted again in a few days. If extraction is not successful or if the stone is above manipulation range in the ureter, *lithotripsy* (stone crushing) or open surgery is indicated.

Lithotripsy techniques include *percutaneous ultrasonic lithotripsy* and *extracorporeal shock-wave lithotripsy*. In percutaneous ultrasonic lithotripsy an ultrasonic probe is placed in the renal pelvis via a percutaneous nephroscope and is positioned against the stone. (The client is given general or spinal anesthesia for this procedure.) The probe produces ultrasonic waves, which break up the stone. A continuous saline irrigation flushes out the stone particles, and all outflow drainage is strained so that the particles can be analyzed. Without ultrasound the calculi can also be removed by forceps or basket extraction. Complications are rare but include hemorrhage, sepsis, and abscess. Postoperatively, clients usually complain of severe colic type pain. The first few voidings are bright red, and as the bleeding subsides, the urine becomes dark red or turns a smoky color. Antibiotics are usually given for 2 weeks to reduce the risk of infection.

In extracorporeal shock-wave lithotripsy, a noninvasive procedure, the client is anesthetized (spinal or general) and placed in a water bath.[13] The affected kidney is positioned under water over a high-voltage spark generator, which produces high-energy acoustic shock waves that shatter the stone without damaging the surrounding tissues. The stone is broken down into fine gravel, which is excreted into the

client's urine within a few days after the procedure. A primary advantage of these techniques compared with open surgery is the decrease in the length of hospitalization and the client's earlier return to normal activities.[14]

The type of open surgery needed depends on the location of the stone. A *nephrolithotomy* is an incision into the kidney to remove a stone. A *pyelolithotomy* is an incision into the renal pelvis to remove a stone. If the stone is located in the ureter, a *ureterolithotomy* is performed. A *cystotomy* may be indicated for bladder calculi. For open surgery on the kidney or ureter, a flank incision directly below the diaphragm and across the side is usually the preferred surgical approach.

Nutritional considerations. A high fluid intake (at least 3000 to 4000 ml/day) to produce a urine output of at least 2 L/day is recommended during or after an episode of urolithiasis. (For specific dietary intervention, see Table 40-12.) Increasing the fluid intake is especially important for clients who are active in sports, live in dry climates, perform physical exercise, or work in occupations that require outdoor work or a great deal of physical activity that can lead to dehydration.

Another preventive measure concerns the client who is on bed rest or is relatively immobile for a prolonged time. It is important to maintain a high fluid intake as well as prevent urinary stasis by turning the client every 2 hours and helping the client to sit or stand if possible.

■ Nursing Management of Renal Calculi

Nursing assessment

Subjective and objective data that should be obtained from a client with renal lithiasis are presented in Table 40-13.

Nursing diagnoses

Nursing diagnoses specific to a client with renal lithiasis include, but are not limited to, those presented in Table 40-14.

Nursing interventions

Acute intervention. In the acute phase, it is important to determine whether the stone has passed. All urine voided by the client should be strained through gauze in an effort to detect the stone. Forcing fluids and encouraging ambulation help the stone pass down the urinary tract. The client should not walk if pain is present during an attack of renal colic. Narcotics may be required for renal colic because the pain is excruciating. (For other nursing measures see Table 40-14.)

If the cause of the stone formation is determined, it is important for the nurse to teach the client ways to prevent its recurrence. Dietary restrictions are related to the type of stone. For example, restricting milk and milk products may help persons who are at risk of developing calcium phosphate stones. Diets that restrict purines may be helpful to clients at risk of developing uric acid stones.

Stones that do not pass spontaneously must be removed. The nursing care of a client with a transurethral litholapaxy is discussed in Table 40-15. (Nursing care for a client with an open surgical approach is discussed on p. 1212.)

Chronic management. Stone formation can be prevented and the recurrence rate can be greatly reduced. Fol-

---

Table 40-13

Nursing Assessment of the Client with Renal Lithiasis

SUBJECTIVE DATA

History
Positive family history; recent or chronic UTI; bed rest; immobilization; previous obstruction or kidney disease with urinary stasis; dietary intake of purines, calcium, oxalate, phosphates; fluid intake; gout; prostatic hypertrophy, hypertension
Medications
Use of antibiotics, phosphates, thiazides, antihypertensives, sodium bicarbonate, allopurinol, analgesics
General
Fever, chills
Pain
Acute, severe, colicky pain in flank, back, abdomen, groin, or genitalia; dysuria
Gastrointestinal
Diarrhea, nausea and vomiting
Urinary
Decreased urinary output, feeling of bladder fullness, burning with urination, urgency, frequency

OBJECTIVE DATA

General
Anxiety, guarding
Integumentary
Warm, flushed skin or pallor with cool, moist skin (mild shock)
Gastrointestinal
Abdominal distention, absence of bowel sounds
Urinary
Oliguria, hematuria, tenderness on palpation of renal areas, passage of stone or stones
Possible findings
Elevated BUN and serum creatinine levels; RBCs, WBCs, pyuria, crystals, casts, minerals, bacteria on urinalysis; elevated creatinine, uric acid, calcium, phosphorus, oxalate, or cystine values on 24-hour urine sample; calculi or anatomical changes on IVP of KUB; direct visualization of obstruction on cystoureteroscopy

---

low-up care includes monitoring the client's compliance with fluid and dietary recommendations. Periodic urine cultures may be indicated. Testing the pH of the urine is important, especially to assess the effectiveness of acidifying or alkalinizing agents. It is important to emphasize the need to avoid inadvertent dehydration from excessive exercise and to increase fluid needs during illness.

Strictures

Strictures may occur in the bladder neck, urethra, or ureters. A *stricture* is a narrowing of the lumen and is sometimes congenital but is usually acquired. Strictures of the neck of the bladder may be congenital or may result from chronic prostatitis in men or cystitis in women.

Table 40-14

NURSING CARE PLAN FOR THE CLIENT WITH ACUTE RENAL LITHIASIS

Defining Characteristics	Nursing Interventions	Outcome
NURSING DIAGNOSIS: Pain related to irritation of stone and inadequate pain control or comfort measures		
Complaints of pain, facial grimacing, restlessness	Monitor fluid intake up to 3000-4000 ml/day unless contraindicated. Assess pain and administer pain medication as ordered. Apply moist heat to flank area as needed. Schedule activity as tolerated between attacks of renal colic.	Minimal or no pain, verbalization of decrease in pain
NURSING DIAGNOSIS: Anxiety related to uncertain outcome and lack of knowledge regarding possible surgery		
Expressions of concern about future treatments, withdrawn demeanor, emotional lability	Explain surgical or nonsurgical procedure (include insertion of urethral catheters). Allow client to express feelings of anxiety, fear of surgery.	Expression of relief of anxiety
NURSING DIAGNOSIS: Altered health maintenance related to lack of knowledge about prevention of recurrence, diet, fluid requirements, and symptoms of recurrence		
Questions that indicate inadequate knowledge of disorder	Instruct client during initial hospital stay to prepare for home self-care, including forcing fluids to 3000 ml/day unless contraindicated and diet restrictions and rationale.* Inform client about rationale, dose, frequency, and side effects of medication. Tell client to strain all urine through a piece of gauze (if necessary) and to bring stone to physician for analysis. Educate client about symptoms of recurrence to be reported (e.g., hematuria, flank pain).	Verbalization of correct self-care measures
NURSING DIAGNOSIS: Potential complication: urinary obstruction related to presence of stone in path of urine flow		
Complaints of urgency along with inability to void	Monitor urine output and fluid intake. Monitor for bladder distention. Notify physician of oliguria. Strain all urine. Save stone and send for analysis as ordered.	Urine output satisfactory in relation to fluid intake

*See Table 40-12.

Causes of urethral strictures include trauma from accidents (e.g., those resulting in fractured pelvis), gonorrheal infections, and urethral instrumentation. Ureteral strictures may be caused by severe or chronic infection, radiation therapy, and retroperitoneal abscess formation from inflammatory bowel disease and perforation.

Strictures can sometimes be avoided by the proper management of inflammatory processes or traumatic injuries. Treatment of existing strictures includes dilatation, use of a catheter for temporary or permanent drainage for ureteral or urethral strictures, and surgery. Nursing interventions include preparing and informing the client about the procedure and assessing the client's need for management, education, and follow-up.

RENAL TRAUMA

A continued increase in the incidence of traumatic renal injuries is related to an increase in the mechanization and speed of transportation and to the increase in violent crimes and injuries.[15] The majority of incidents occur in men less than 30 years of age. Blunt trauma is the most frequent cause. Injury to the kidney should be considered in multiple injuries, traffic accidents, and falls. It is especially likely when the client strikes the abdomen, flank, or back and when fractures of the spine or ribs or penetrating injuries have occurred. The determining factor in the mortality rate is the severity of the associated injuries.

Clinical findings include a history of trauma to the area of the kidneys. Gross or microscopic hematuria may be present. Diagnostic studies include urinalysis, IVP with cystography, ultrasound, and CT GU evaluation. Renal arteriography may also be used. Both the injured kidney and the noninvolved kidney should be evaluated to provide information for further management. In cases of blunt trauma, surgical intervention is often not required, although it is needed for penetrating renal injuries.

Table 40-15

NURSING CARE PLAN FOR THE CLIENT WITH TRANSURETHRAL EXTRACTION OF RENAL LITHIASIS

Defining Characteristics	Nursing Interventions	Evaluation Criteria
NURSING DIAGNOSIS: Altered patterns of urinary elimination: decreased output and hematuria related to trauma or blockage of urinary catheters		
Decrease in urinary output, bloody urine	Monitor urine output q hr. Assess patency of catheters hourly. Prevent blockage of catheter. Document amount and character of urine. Be aware that urine may be slightly bloody initially because of irritation from the stone and surgical manipulation.	Patent catheters
NURSING DIAGNOSIS: High risk for infection related to introduction of bacteria from lower urethra into bladder		
Elevation in temperature; chills; cloudy, foul-smelling urine	Monitor vital signs. Observe for fever. Report any fever or chills to physician. Administer antipyretics if indicated. Force fluids unless contraindicated. Note character and color of urine. Observe for cloudy, foul-smelling urine. Administer antibiotics as ordered. If irrigation of ureteral catheter is ordered, use strict aseptic technique with 3 ml of sterile saline solution.	Absence of infection
NURSING DIAGNOSIS: Pain related to inflammation and inadequate pain control or comfort measures		
Complaints of bladder spasms, flank pain	Maintain patency of catheters. Observe for kinks in catheter or lack of urine output. Administer medications for pain as ordered. Explain cause of pain or spasms to client. Assess pain. Be aware that persistent pain may be due to perforation of bladder or obstruction of ureteral catheter.	Absence of or relief from pain

Nursing interventions vary with the type and extent of associated injuries. Specific interventions related to renal trauma include monitoring intake and output, observing for hematuria, determining the presence of myoglobinuria, assessing the cardiovascular status, and monitoring potentially nephrotoxic antibiotics.

RENAL VASCULAR PROBLEMS

Vascular problems involving the kidney include (1) nephrosclerosis, (2) renal artery stenosis, and (3) renal vein thrombosis.

Nephrosclerosis

Nephrosclerosis consists of sclerosis of the small arteries and arterioles of the kidney. There is decreased blood flow, which results in patchy necrosis of the renal parenchyma. Ischemic necrosis and destruction of glomeruli with subsequent fibrosis also occur.

Benign nephrosclerosis usually occurs in adults 30 to 50 years of age. It is caused by vascular changes resulting from hypertension as well as from the arteriosclerotic process. The arteriosclerotic vascular changes account for most of the loss of renal function associated with aging.

There is a direct relation between the degree of nephrosclerosis and the severity of hypertension. The client with benign nephrosclerosis may have normal renal function in the early stages. The only detectable abnormality may be hypertension.

Accelerated nephrosclerosis, or *malignant nephrosclerosis,* is associated with malignant hypertension, a complication of hypertension characterized by a sharp increase in blood pressure with a diastolic pressure greater than 130 mm Hg. Clients are usually young adults, with a male predominance of 2:1. Renal insufficiency progresses rapidly, with death occurring secondary to uremia in half of the clients.

Treatment of benign nephrosclerosis is the same as that of essential hypertension (see Chapter 27). Malignant nephrosclerosis is treated with aggressive antihypertensive therapy (see Chapter 27). The availability and use of antihypertensives have improved the prognosis for clients with benign nephrosclerosis. Renal dysfunction and renal failure (in some persons) constitute one of the major complications of hypertension. The prognosis for clients with malignant hypertension is poor, with the major cause of death related to renal failure.

Renal Artery Stenosis

Renal artery stenosis is a partial occlusion of one or both renal arteries and their major branches. It can be due to atherosclerotic narrowing or fibromuscular dysplasia. Renal artery stenosis accounts for 2% to 5% of all cases of hypertension.

Renal artery stenosis is considered a major cause of hypertension when it develops abruptly, especially in clients under 20 or over 50 years of age and in clients with no familial history of hypertension. This contrasts with the age distribution for essential hypertension, which is 30 to 50 years of age. A renal arteriogram is the best diagnostic tool for identifying renal artery stenosis.

Surgical revascularization of the kidney is indicated when blood flow is decreased enough to cause renal ischemia or when evidence indicates that renovascular hypertension is present and surgical intervention may cause the client to become normotensive. The surgical procedure usually involves anastomoses between the kidney and another major artery, usually the splenic artery or aorta. Percutaneous transluminal angioplasty may be an alternative for clients who are not good candidates for surgery (see Chapter 32). In selected cases of unilateral renal involvement with high renin production, unilateral nephrectomy may be indicated.

Renal Vein Thrombosis

Renal vein thrombosis may occur unilaterally or bilaterally. Glomerulonephritis, amyloidosis, diabetic glomerulosclerosis, thrombophlebitis of the pelvic and femoral veins, and dehydration resulting from excessive use of diuretics predispose the client to bilateral vein thrombosis. Unilateral thrombosis may result from external trauma, perinephric abscess, retroperitoneal tumors, renal biopsy, renal tumors, surgery near or on the renal hilus, and nephrotic syndrome as a result of membranous glomerulonephritis.

The client has symptoms of flank pain, hematuria, or fever or has nephrotic syndrome. Anticoagulation is important in treatment because there is a high incidence of pulmonary emboli. Steroids may be used in clients with nephrosis. Surgical thrombectomy may be performed instead of or along with anticoagulation.

HEREDITARY RENAL DISEASES

Hereditary renal diseases involve developmental abnormalities of the renal parenchyma. These abnormalities either are isolated or are part of more complex malformation syndromes. The majority of inherited structural abnormalities are cystic. However, cysts may also develop as a result of obstructive uropathies, metabolic derangements, or neurological diseases.

Polycystic Renal Disease

There are two forms of hereditary polycystic renal disease. It may be manifested in childhood or adulthood. The childhood form of polycystic disease is a rare autosomal recessive disorder that is often rapidly progressive.

The adult form of polycystic disease is an autosomal dominant disorder. It is latent for many years and is usu-

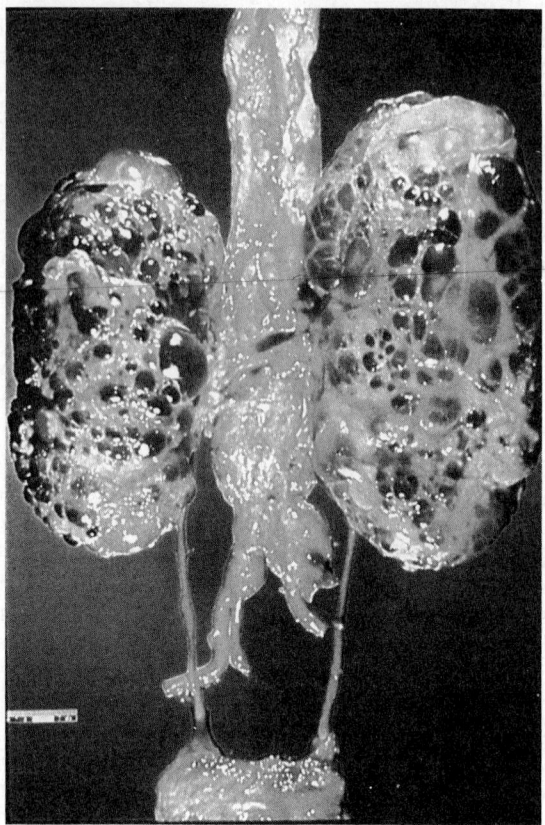

Fig. 40-6 Polycystic kidneys. (From Schreiner G and Heptinstall R: Chronic renal failure, famous teachings in modern medicine, New York, MEDCOM, Inc.)

ally manifested at about 40 years of age. It involves both kidneys and occurs in both men and women. The cortex and the medulla are filled with thin-walled cysts that are several millimeters to several centimeters in diameter (Fig. 40-6). The cysts enlarge and destroy surrounding tissue by compression. They are filled with fluid and may contain blood or pus.

Clinical manifestations. In the client with polycystic disease, symptoms appear when the cysts begin to enlarge. A common early symptom of adult cystic disease is flank pain, which is either steady and dull or abrupt in onset as well as episodic and colicky. On physical examination, palpable bilateral enlarged kidneys are often found. Other clinical manifestations include hematuria, UTI, and hypertension. Diagnosis is based on clinical manifestations, family history, IVP, ultrasound, or CT scan.

Therapeutic management. There is no specific treatment for polycystic kidney disease. A major aim of treatment is to prevent infections of the urinary tract or to treat them with appropriate antibiotics if they occur. Nephrectomy may be necessary if pain, bleeding, or infection becomes a chronic, serious problem.

When the client begins to experience progressive renal failure, the therapeutic and nursing interventions are determined by the remaining renal function. Nursing measures are those used for management of end-stage renal disease

(see Chapter 41). They include diet modification, fluid restriction, medications, assisting the client to accept the chronic disease process, and assisting the client and the family to deal with the altered body image, financial concerns, and other issues related to the hereditary nature of the disease.

Clients who have adult polycystic disease often have had children by the time their disease is diagnosed. Each child of a parent with the gene has a 50% chance of having the disease. The client will need appropriate counseling regarding plans for having more children. In addition, genetic counseling resources should be provided for the children.

Medullary Cystic Disease

Medullary cystic disease is a hereditary disorder that occurs in two forms. The *recessive* form is associated with renal failure before the age of 20; the *dominant* form is associated with renal failure after the age of 20. Most cysts are located in the medulla. The kidneys are asymmetrical in shape and are significantly scarred. (Treatment of infection, anemia, hypertension, and other aspects of end-stage renal disease are discussed in Chapter 41.)

Alport's Syndrome

Alport's syndrome is also known as *chronic hereditary nephritis*. It is inherited as an autosomal dominant disorder. Males are affected earlier and more severely than females. Frequently there is an associated sensorineural hearing deficit. The disease is frequently diagnosed in the first decade of life. The basic defect is altered synthesis of the GBM. Clients most commonly have hematuria and progressive uremia. Treatment is supportive. Steroids and cytotoxic drugs are not effective. The disease does not recur after kidney transplantation.

CONGENITAL ABNORMALITIES OF THE URINARY SYSTEM

Congenital malformations of the urinary system are of concern for several reasons. An estimated 10% of persons have malformations of the excretory system that are potentially significant. These malformations may be the preexisting causes of infection, hypertension, or the development of calculi. Congenital disorders involve abnormalities in the amount, position, form, and differentiation of renal tissue. Congenital disorders include (1) exstrophy of the bladder, (2) horseshoe kidney, (3) solitary kidney, (4) anomalies of origin and termination of the renal blood vessels, and (5) an abnormal number or structure of the ureters.

Exstrophy of the bladder is a rare condition that can include anomalies of the bladder (everted on the abdominal wall), pubic bones, and GU system. Initially, the upper urinary tract is not involved. However, if the condition is not corrected, obstruction with resulting hydronephrosis and hydroureter develops. Surgical closure should be performed within the first 48 hours of life. Depending on the anomalies involved, some type of urinary diversion surgery may be required.

Horseshoe kidney involves fusion of both kidneys. The condition can result in a number of problems. Clients may have episodes of abdominal pain. The horseshoe kidney is more susceptible in abdominal trauma. The areas of the kidneys that are fused have poor drainage of urine, and this can predispose to stasis of urine, infection, and formation of calculi. Nursing interventions include teaching related to health care follow-up, symptoms to be reported, and proper treatment and prevention of UTIs and the development of calculi.

RENAL INVOLVEMENT IN METABOLIC AND CONNECTIVE TISSUE DISEASES

Various metabolic and connective tissue disease processes may have an effect on renal function. The pathophysiological effects on the renal parenchyma are not always specific to each process. The clinical course of renal involvement is that of chronic progressive nephropathy, which can result in uremia and death. Therapeutic management includes treatment of the primary disorder along with symptomatic relief of the renal involvement. If renal involvement progresses to chronic renal failure, management includes dialysis or transplantation (see Chapter 41). Nursing interventions include teaching the client about the primary disease process, the renal involvement, and the resulting need to comply with dietary and fluid restrictions and medication.

Diabetes mellitus may affect the kidney in several ways. Microangiopathic changes in diabetes consist of diffuse glomerulosclerosis, involving thickening of the GBM and nodular glomerulosclerosis (Kimmelstiel-Wilson syndrome), which is characterized by nodular lesions. Nodular glomerulosclerosis is reasonably specific for type I diabetes mellitus. Diabetic clients prone to glomerulonephropathy (e.g., the presence of trace proteinuria or retinopathy) require careful monitoring of insulin requirements. Diabetic glomerulopathy can result in chronic renal failure. Clients with diabetes are especially susceptible to UTIs. Primary nursing interventions include teaching the client about the increased risk of UTIs, the appropriate preventive measures, and when to seek additional medical care (see Chapter 43).

Gout is a syndrome of acute attacks of arthritis due to hyperuricemia (see Chapter 58). Monosodium urate crystals deposited within joints are responsible for the syndrome. Renal disease may develop as a result of damage caused by deposition of uric acid crystals in the renal interstitium and tubules.

Amyloidosis is a disease manifested by altered structure and function caused by deposition of a hyaline substance (amyloid) in a variety of organs. The hyaline consists largely of protein. Kidney involvement is very common in amyloidosis. Proteinuria is often the first clinical manifestation.

Systemic lupus erythematosus (SLE) is a connective tissue disorder characterized by the involvement of several tissues and organs, particularly the joints, skin, and kidneys (see Chapter 58). Clinical manifestations of lupus nephritis are similar to those of other forms of glomerulonephritis. Most frequently found are microscopic hematuria and significant proteinuria. Renal failure frequently occurs

in SLE and has a poor prognosis. The long-term course of SLE is extremely variable. Steroids are effective for clients with severe renal disease. Recently, plasma exchange therapy has been used.

Scleroderma (progressive systemic sclerosis) is a disease of unknown etiology characterized by widespread alterations of connective tissue and by vascular lesions in many organs (see Chapter 58). In the kidney, vascular lesions are associated with fibrosis. An immune complex mechanism has been postulated as a possible etiological factor. The severity of renal involvement varies. Clients who develop severe renal lesions have a poor prognosis. Once uremia develops, about 70% die within 3 years.

NEOPLASTIC DISORDERS OF THE URINARY TRACT
Renal Tumors

Tumors of the kidney are responsible for approximately 8000 deaths per year. They arise from the cortex or pelvis (and calyces). Tumors arising from both areas may be benign or malignant. However, malignant tumors are more frequent. *Renal cell carcinoma* (adenocarcinoma) is the most common type. Adenocarcinoma is twice as frequent in men as in women and is typically discovered when the person is 50 to 70 years old. Risk factors include cigarette smoking, gender, and family history. There are no characteristic early symptoms. Generalized symptoms of weight loss, weakness, and anemia are the earliest manifestations. The classic manifestations of gross hematuria, flank pain, and a palpable mass are those of advanced disease. The most common sites of metastases include the lungs, liver, and long bones. Renal cystic disease and associated renal carcinomas may develop in persons undergoing renal dialysis (see Chapter 41).

Several studies are used to diagnose adenocarcinoma of the kidney. The excretory urogram and the retrograde pyelogram can identify changes in the renal outline (e.g., elongated calyces, invasion of the renal pelvis, calcification). Studies done to differentiate between a tumor and a cyst include nephrotomography, arteriography, ultrasound, percutaneous needle aspiration, CT, and magnetic resonance imaging (MRI). Small renal tumors are found earlier because of the increased use of CT scans and MRI.

The staging of the tumor is presented in Table 40-16. The treatment of choice is a radical nephrectomy. Radiation therapy is indicated in inoperable cases, with incomplete tumor removal, and when there are metastases to bone or lungs. At present, chemotherapy is not effective.

Table 40-16 Staging for Renal Carcinoma

Stage	Description
I	Limitation to renal capsule
II	Spreading to perirenal fat
III	Regional lymph node involvement, tumor thrombus in renal vein or vena cava, involvement of lymph nodes and renal vein or vena cava
IV	Presence of distant metastases

Biological response modifiers, including α interferon, tumor necrosis factor, and interleukin 2, are under investigation in the treatment of metastatic disease.[16] α Interferon is the most beneficial agent currently available.

The course is variable. Survival of clients at 5 years without lymph node involvement is about 70%. In the presence of distant metastases, survival at 5 years is less than 10%. (For a discussion of nursing care after nephrectomy, see p. 1212.)

Wilms' Tumor

Wilms' tumor is a common renal tumor of infants and children. Of these tumors, 40% are hereditary, with an autosomal dominant mode of transmission. The most common clinical manifestation is abdominal swelling or distention. This distention is often noticed by the parents or is found on a routine examination. Other symptoms include pain, fever, hematuria, and hypertension. Diagnostic studies for Wilms' tumor include ultrasound and renal arteriography.

Therapeutic treatment includes surgical removal of the involved kidney and radiation therapy. Radiation therapy is used postoperatively as well as for inoperable tumors, bilateral tumors, and metastases. Chemotherapy with actinomycin D and vincristine is also frequently used. Survival is greater than 85% if there are no distant metastases.

Cancer of the Bladder

The most frequent malignant tumor of the urinary tract is carcinoma of the bladder. Most bladder tumors are papillomatous growths within the bladder. Cancer of the bladder is most common between the ages of 50 and 70 years and is at least twice as common in men as in women. The etiology of the tumor can involve cigarette smoking, exposure to dyes used in the rubber and cable industries, and chronic abuse of phenacetin-containing analgesics. Chronic bladder infections and calculous disease are involved in the etiology of carcinoma of the squamous cell type.

Gross hematuria is the most common clinical finding and the first in 75% of clients. Bladder irritability with dysuria, frequent urination, and intermittent bleeding may also be noted.

Bladder cancer can be classified as superficial, invasive, or metastatic. Superficial carcinomas are seen in clients with carcinoma in situ, mucosal involvement, and submucosal involvement. Clients with invasive disease have cancers that have progressed into the muscle, surrounding fat, or both.

Therapeutic management. Therapeutic management is outlined in Table 40-17. Surgical interventions include five possible procedures. *Cystoscopic resection and fulguration* (electrosurgery) is used for the diagnosis and treatment of superficial lesions with a low recurrence rate. This procedure is also used to control bleeding in clients who are poor operative risks or who have advanced tumors. With this technique the tumor mass is excised by means of a blade inserted through the cystoscope. The remaining portions of the tumor are cauterized.

A second technique, *laser photocoagulation,* is also

Table 40-17

 Diagnostic and Therapeutic Management: Carcinoma of the Bladder

DIAGNOSTIC

Urinalysis
IVP
Cystoscopy with biopsy
Cytology studies
CT scan

THERAPEUTIC

Surgical treatment
    Cystoscopic resection and fulguration
    Laser photocoagulation
    Open loop resection or fulguration
    Segmental cystectomy
    Total cystectomy
Radiation
Chemotherapy

---

used to treat superficial bladder cancers. This procedure can be repeated any number of times for recurrence. The advantages of laser include bloodless destruction of the lesion, minimal risk of perforation, and lack of need for a urinary catheter.

A third technique used is *open loop resection* (snaring of polyp-type lesions) or fulguration. It is used for the control of bleeding, for large superficial tumors, and for multiple lesions. Treatment for large lesions entails a *segmental resection* of the bladder.

Postoperative management of clients who have had one of these three surgical procedures includes instructions to drink 2500 to 3000 ml of fluid per day, measurement of intake and output, avoidance of alcoholic beverages, use of analgesics and stool softeners (if necessary), and sitz baths to promote muscle relaxation and reduce urinary retention. The nurse should also help the client and the family cope with fears about cancer, surgery, and sexuality and should emphasize the importance of regular follow-up care.

When the tumor is invasive or involves the trigone (the area where ureters insert into the bladder) and the client otherwise has a good life expectancy and no demonstrated metastases beyond the pelvic area, a *total cystectomy* with urinary diversion is the treatment of choice (see p. 1215).

Radiation therapy is used with cystectomy or as the primary therapy when the cancer is inoperable or when surgery is refused. Chemotherapy with local instillation of thiotepa is of some use in the treatment of superficial recurring lesions. Thiotepa is an alkylating agent that is pharmacologically related to nitrogen mustard. It is directly instilled into the client's bladder and retained for about 2 hours. The position of the client is changed every 15 minutes for maximum contact in all areas of the bladder. The usual protocol is one treatment a week for 4 weeks.

Other intravesical chemotherapeutic agents include doxorubicin and mitomycin. Intravesical therapeutic agents that are under investigation include bacillus-Calmette-Guerin (BCG) and α interferon. Cyclophosphamide, vinblastine, doxorubicin (Adriamycin), methotrexate, and cisplatin are systemic chemotherapeutic agents used in treating bladder cancer.

URINARY INCONTINENCE AND RETENTION

An estimated 8 to 10 million people in the United States suffer from urinary incontinence or the inability to control the passage of urine from the bladder.[17] Incontinence exacts physical (infection, pressure sores, perineal rashes), psychosocial (embarrassment, isolation, depression), and economic costs. However minor the problem, incontinence can cause severe psychological distress. Incontinence is not an inevitable consequence of aging; in most cases among older adults, it can be significantly improved or corrected.[18] Retention is the inability to urinate in spite of the presence of urine in the bladder. Both incontinence and retention may occur in the same person.

Normal Bladder Function

Storage of urine in the bladder is mediated by relaxation of the detrusor muscle (which provides the propulsive force for emptying the bladder) and closure of the sphincters. The detrusor muscle is controlled by the parasympathetic autonomic nervous system through the pelvic nerves from sacral spinal cord segments S2, S3, or S4. The smooth muscle of the trigonal portion of the bladder between the ureteral orifices and the posterior area of the bladder outlet is innervated by the sympathetic nervous system, in which α receptors predominate. This layer of muscle acts as an involuntary internal sphincter. The external urethral sphincter and perineal muscles are under voluntary control.

The sensation of bladder fullness is transmitted via sensory nerves to the sacral cord. If not suppressed by cortical control, the sacral cord discharges motor impulses by reflex that cause powerful sustained detrusor contraction. Urination can be prevented by means of cortical suppression of the reflex arc or voluntary contraction of the external sphincter and perineal muscles. Urination occurs when detrusor contraction is coordinated with sphincter relaxation.

Causes of Urinary Incontinence

Anything that interferes with bladder or urethral sphincter control can result in urinary incontinence. Congenital disorders that produce incontinence include exstrophy of the bladder, epispadias, spina bifida with myelomeningocele, and ectopic ureteral orifice. Acquired disorders are described in Table 40-18. *Neurogenic bladder* is a general term referring to any bladder dysfunction resulting from a central nervous system (CNS) neurological disorder. There are numerous causes of this condition, including such problems as CNS tumors, cerebrovascular accidents, multiple sclerosis, diabetic neuropathy, and spinal cord injury. A person with a neurogenic bladder may have problems with urgency, frequency, incontinence, inability to uri-

Table 40-18 Acquired Disorders Causing Urinary Incontinence

Type	Description	Causes	Treatment
Stress incontinence	Sudden increase in intraabdominal pressure causes involuntary passage of urine. It can occur during coughing, heavy lifting, straining, or laughing.	Condition is found most commonly in women with relaxed pelvic musculature (frequently from obstetrical complications or multiple pregnancies). Structures of the female urethra atrophy when deprived of estrogen. Condition is found in men after prostrate surgery for benign prostatic hypertrophy or prostatic carcinoma.	Perineal muscle exercises (e.g., Kegel exercises), weight loss if client is obese, insertion of vaginal pessary, estrogen vaginal creams, condom catheters or penile clamp
Urge incontinence	Condition occurs randomly when involuntary urination is preceded by warning of few seconds to few minutes. Leakage is periodic but frequent. Nocturnal frequency and incontinence are common. Condition may appear with varying severity during psychological stress.	Condition is caused by uncontrolled contraction or overactivity of detrusor muscle. Bladder escapes central inhibition and contracts reflexly. Conditions include CNS disorders (e.g., cerebrovascular disease, Alzheimer's disease, brain tumor, Parkinson's disease), bladder disorders (e.g., carcinoma in situ, radiation effects, interstitial cystitis), interference with spinal inhibitory pathways (e.g., malignant growth in spinal cord, spondylosis), and bladder outlet obstruction as well as conditions of unknown etiology.	Treatment of underlying cause, instruction to have client urinate more frequently, anticholinergic drugs (e.g., propantheline), imipramine at bedtime, calcium channel blockers, condom catheters
Overflow (paradoxical) incontinence	Conditioin occurs when the pressure of urine in overfull bladder overcomes sphincter control. Leakage of small amounts of urine is frequent throughout the day and night. Urination may also occur frequently in small amounts. Bladder remains distended and is usually palpable.	Disorder is caused by outlet obstruction (prostatic hypertrophy, bladder neck obstruction, urethral stricture) or by underactive detrusor muscle due to myogenic or neurogenic factors (e.g., herniated disk, diabetic neuropathy). It may also occur after anesthesia and surgery (especially procedures such as hemorrhoidectomy, herniorrhaphy, cystoscopy). Neurogenic bladder (flaccid type) is another cause.	Urinary catheterization to decompress bladder, implementation of Credé's or Valsalva maneuver, prazosin (α-adrenergic blocker) to decrease outlet resistance, bethanechol to enhance bladder contractions, intermittent catheterization, surgery to correct underlying problem

Continued.

Table 40-18 Acquired Disorders Causing Urinary Incontinence—cont'd

Type	Description	Causes	Treatment
Reflex incontinence	Condition occurs when no warning or stress precedes periodic involuntary urination. Urination is frequent, is moderate in volume, and occurs equally during the day and night.	Spinal cord lesion above S2 interferes with CNS inhibition. Disorder results in detrusor hyperreflexia and interferes with pathways coordinating detrusor contraction and sphincter relaxation.	Treatment of underlying cause, bladder decompression to prevent ureteral reflux and hydronephrosis, intermittent self-catheterization, α-adrenergic blocker (e.g., prazosin) to relax internal sphincter, diazepam or baclofen to relax external sphincter, prophylactic antibiotics, surgical sphincterotomy
Incontinence after trauma or surgery	Vesicovaginal fistula (connection between bladder and vagina) may occur in females. Alteration in continence control in male involves proximal urethral sphincter (bladder neck and prostatic urethra) and distal urethral sphincter (external striated muscle).	Vesicovaginal fistulas may occur during pregnancy, after delivery of baby, as result of hysterectomy or invasive cancer of cervix, or after radiation therapy. It is found as postoperative complication after transurethral, perineal, or retropubic prostatectomy.	Surgery to correct fistula, urinary diversion surgery to bypass urethra and bladder, external condom catheter, penile clamp, placement of artificial implantable sphincter

Table 40-19 Neurogenic Bladder

Type	Spinal Cord Lesion	Characteristics
Upper motor neuron (spastic, automatic, hyperreflexive, uninhibited)	Damage above S2, S3, or S4 segments (e.g., from cerebrovascular accident, Parkinson's disease, spinal cord injuries)	Intact but involuntary micturition reflex, hypertrophied detrusor muscle with reduced bladder capacity, frequent uncontrollable urgency incontinence
Lower motor neuron (flaccid, nonreflexive, atopic, hypotonic)	Damage at S2, S3, or S4 segments (e.g., from tumors of sacral part of spinal cord, diabetes)	No control of micturition; large capacity for urine in bladder because of no sensation or desire to void, resulting in urinary retention; bladder muscle damage, cystitis, and renal infections from overdistention; incontinence only when bladder becomes so full that small amounts of urine are forced out (overflow incontinence)
Mixed motor neuron	Cortical damage (e.g., from brain tumor, trauma)	Diminished perception of bladder fullness and decreased ability to empty the bladder, urgency to void but inability to control urgency

nate, and obstruction-like symptoms. Long-term problems include formation of calculi, infection, and progressive deterioration in renal function. A simplified classification of neurogenic bladder is listed in Table 40-19. (A more detailed description of neurogenic bladder is found in Chapter 55.)

Retention can be found in association with incontinence but can also be independent of incontinence. Drugs that may cause retention include (1) antihypertensives (e.g., methyldopa [Aldomet], hydralazine [Apresoline]), (2) antiparkinsonian drugs (e.g., levodopa), (3) antihistamines, (4) anticholinergics (e.g., atropine, belladonna), (5) antispasmodics (e.g., belladonna), (6) sedatives, and (7) anesthesia (especially spinal anesthesia).

Postoperative urinary retention is not uncommon and is related to preoperative medication (atropine and sedatives

are frequently used), anesthesia, supine position after surgery, and low fluid intake. Postoperative retention may also be related to the effects of surgical manipulation of the bladder nerves.

Another cause of retention is urethral obstruction, which may be caused by congenital urethral stenosis, benign prostatic hypertrophy, fecal impaction, or tumors (involving bladder outlet or large, displaced uterine myomas). Psychological problems may also contribute to urinary retention. Psychogenic urinary retention is found more commonly in women than in men.

Diagnostic Studies

A complete history and physical examination (with particular attention to the GU system) are essential to obtain information on the client's past and current urination patterns, current physical health, and underlying reasons for incontinence. A drug history, including both prescription and over-the-counter drugs, may provide information on possible reasons for retention.

Diagnostic tests of urological dysfunction are essential in evaluation of the function and structure of the urinary tract, especially the bladder. These tests may include IVP, cystoscopy (including urethroscopy), cystometrography, electromyography (to assess sphincter, perineal, and muscle activity), and catheterization for residual urine.

Therapeutic Management

Treatment should correct the factors responsible for incontinence or retention if possible (see Table 40-18). (Bladder training programs are described in Chapter 55.)

Surgical intervention may be indicated to correct the incontinence. The surgical approach varies, depending on the underlying problem. For example, a transurethral resection of the prostate is used to treat benign prostatic hypertrophy. Urethral strictures are dilated or sounded. A common surgical intervention for stress incontinence is the Marshall-Marchetti procedure, which involves suspending the urethra and bladder neck by suturing the anterior vaginal wall on each side to the periosteum of the pubic bones and lower rectum.

Pharmacological Management

Anticholinergic agents such as methantheline (Banthine), propantheline (Pro-Banthine), and oxybutynin (Ditropan) are used to treat spastic bladders by suppressing the unwanted contractions that occur when the bladder has only a small volume of urine. Parasympathomimetics (cholinergics) such as bethanechol (Urecholine) and neostigmine (Prostigmin) are used to treat flaccid bladders by stimulating bladder contractions. α-Adrenergic blockers such as prazosin (Minipress) and phenoxybenzamine (Dibenzylene) can be used to relax spastic bladder necks. Sympathomimetics such as ephedrine and phenylephrine may be used to increase bladder neck and urethral tone (which may decrease in stress incontinence). Diazepam (Valium) and dantrolene (Dantrium) can be used to relax spastic external sphincters. Imipramine (Tofranil) and calcium channel blockers (e.g., nifedipine) reduce detrusor contractions and improve continence.

■ Nursing Management of Urinary Incontinence

The nurse must recognize both the physical and the emotional problems that accompany incontinence. The client's dignity, privacy, and feelings of self-worth must be maintained or enhanced. Most persons suffering from incontinence can be helped with proper diagnosis and modern therapeutic approaches.

A client with stress incontinence should be taught to do pelvic floor (perineal) muscle exercises (Kegel exercises).[19] The client should be sitting in a chair with legs slightly apart and feet flat on the floor and then should be told to contract the pelvic muscles, pressing the buttocks together as though trying to stop the urge to urinate. These exercises should be repeated 10 to 20 times four times a day. To see how effective these exercises are, the client can try to start and stop the urine flow while urinating.

Nursing measures aimed at maintaining urinary continence include frequent palpation to assess for bladder distention and offering the urinal or bedpan or helping the client to the bathroom every 2 hours or at scheduled times. Assuming the usual position for urination (standing for the man and sitting for the woman) and applying pressure over the bladder area often aid in urination. The nurse should be sure the client has privacy and is not rushed when trying to urinate. Techniques to stimulate urination include running water in the sink, placing hands in water, and pouring warm water over the perineum. In addition, the nurse should ensure that the client maintains a high fluid intake during the day.

Fluid restriction, diapers, and keeping a urinal in place at all times are only temporary measures to reduce the occurrence or effects of incontinence. Long-term use of these measures discourages continence and can lead to dehydration and skin problems.

If bladder retraining cannot be achieved, external appliances or intermittent self-catheterization may be indicated. Several external appliances that prevent soiling, decrease odor, and improve body image are available for men. External appliances for women are not useful in most situations. Intermittent self-catheterization using a clean technique can be taught to selected clients. Keeping the skin clean and dry is essential to prevent skin irritation and breakdown.

INSTRUMENTATION

A catheter is a tubular instrument made of rubber, plastic, metal, or other material and is used to drain or inject gases or fluids through a body passage. The process of inserting the catheter into a body cavity or passage is termed *catheterization*. The nursing responsibility includes understanding the reason for catheterization, the scientific principles involved, and the appropriate care of the client after catheterization.

The reasons for urinary catheterization are listed in Table 40-20. Two reasons that are *not* indications for catheterization are (1) routine acquisition of a sterile specimen for laboratory analysis and (2) convenience of the nursing staff or the client's family. The risks of nosocomial infection are too high to allow catheterization of a client for the convenience of hospital personnel or family members.

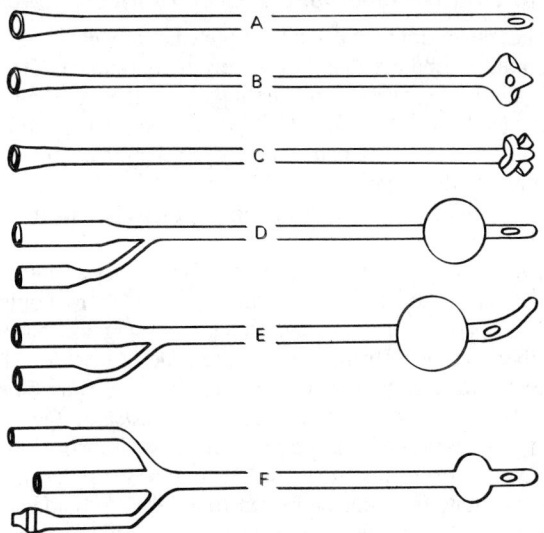

Fig. 40-7 Different types of commonly used catheters. Simple urethral catheter (*A*), mushroom or dePezzar (can be used for suprapubic catheterization) (*B*), winged-tip or Malecot (*C*), indwelling with inflated bag (*D*), indwelling with Coude tip (*E*), and three-way indwelling (the third lumen is used for irrigation of the bladder) (*F*). (From Moidel HC and others: Nursing care of the patient with medical-surgical disorders, ed 2, New York, 1976, McGraw-Hill Book Co, p 1081.)

Table 40-20 Indications for Urinary Catheterization

1. Relief of urinary retention caused by lower urinary tract obstruction, paralysis, or inability to void
2. Bladder decompression preoperatively and operatively for lower abdominal or pelvic surgery
3. Facilitation of surgical repair of urethra and surrounding structures
4. Splinting of ureters or urethra to facilitate healing after surgery or other trauma in area
5. Instillation of medications into bladder
6. Accurate measurement of urinary output in critically ill client
7. Measurement of residual urine after urination
8. Study of anatomical structures of urinary system

Catheters should be the final means of providing the client with a dry environment for prevention of skin breakdown and protection of dressings or skin lesions.

Urinary catheterization is commonly used in the management of the hospitalized client. However, it is not without serious risks. The urinary tract is the most common site of nosocomial infections. Urinary catheterization is a major cause of UTIs. Scrupulous aseptic technique is mandatory when a urinary catheter is inserted. After insertion, maintenance and protection of the closed drainage system are major nursing responsibilities. Irrigation of the catheter should *not* be routinely performed.

Nursing management should include assessment of the client's capacity for bladder training or use of external de-

vices and for fluid management. While the client has a catheter in place, nursing actions should include maintaining patency of the catheter, providing for the comfort and safety of the client, restoring bladder tone in anticipation of catheter removal, and preventing infection. Attention should be given to the psychological implications of urinary drainage. Concerns of the client can include embarrassment related to exposure of the body, an altered body image, and fear concerning the care of the catheter that results in increased dependency of the client.

Catheters vary in construction materials, tip shape (Fig. 40-7), and size of the lumen. Catheters are sized according to the French scale. Each French unit equals 0.33 mm of diameter. The diameter measured is the internal diameter of the catheter. The size used varies with the size of the individual. In women, urethral catheter sizes 14 to 16 F are the most common; in men, sizes 16 to 18 F are used. Problems resulting from too small a catheter include possible obstruction of the urinary flow by blood clots or mucus plugs and difficulty in passing the catheter if resistance is met in the urethra. The primary problem resulting from too large a catheter is tissue erosion secondary to excessive pressure on the meatus or urethra. Four routes are used for urinary tract catheterization: urethral, ureteral, suprapubic, and via a nephrostomy tube.

Urethral Catheterization

The most common route of catheterization is insertion of the catheter through the external meatus into the urethra, past the internal sphincter, and into the bladder. Specific procedures for insertion of the urethral catheter are found in fundamental nursing textbooks. Several principles that should be considered in the management of clients with urethral catheters include the following:

1. Indwelling urinary catheters should be used *only* when absolutely necessary and never solely for the convenience of the care givers. Their use should be discontinued as early as possible.
2. Catheterized clients, particularly those who are ambulatory, should receive appropriate instruction regarding catheter care.
3. A sterile, closed drainage system should always be used. The distal urinary catheter and the proximal drainage tube should not be disconnected except for catheter irrigation. Unobstructed downhill flow must be maintained. The collecting bag should be emptied regularly and kept below the level of the bladder. Poorly functioning catheters should be replaced. Leg bags should not be used for short-term clients because the risk of bacterial infection is too great.
4. Perineal care (one to two times per day and when necessary) should include cleaning of the meatus-catheter junction with antiseptic soap. Following this, an antimicrobial ointment may be applied. Lotion or powder should not be used near the catheter. The catheter should be properly secured to the leg to prevent movement and urethral traction.
5. Sterile technique must be used whenever the collecting system is opened. Catheter irrigation is performed only when obstruction is suspected. If fre-

quent irrigations are necessary for catheter patency, a triple-lumen catheter, permitting continuous irrigations within a closed system, is preferable. Small volumes of urine for culture can be aspirated from the distal catheter by means of a sterile syringe and a 21-gauge needle. The puncture site must first be prepared with a tincture of iodine and/or alcohol solution. Many drainage systems are now equipped with a sampling port. Silicone or plastic catheters do not self-seal. Urine for chemical analysis (e.g., glucose, electrolytes) can be obtained from the drainage bag.

6. When the client is catheterized for less than 2 weeks, routine catheter change is not necessary. For chronic indwelling catheters, replacement is necessary when concretions can be palpated in the catheter or when malformations of the catheter occur. With long-term use of catheters, leg bags may be used. If the collection bag is reused, it should be washed in soap and water and rinsed thoroughly. When not reused immediately, it should be filled with ½ cup of vinegar. The vinegar, discarded before reuse, is effective against *Pseudomonas* organisms and eliminates odors.

Ureteral Catheters

Ureteral catheters are placed through the ureters into the renal pelvis (Fig. 40-8). The catheters are inserted either (1) by being threaded up the urethra and bladder to the ureters under cystoscopic observation or (2) by surgical insertion through the abdominal wall into the ureters. Ureteral catheters are used after surgery to splint the ureters and prevent them from being obstructed by edema or other trauma. The urine volume from the ureteral catheters should be recorded separately from that of other urinary catheters. Clients are usually kept on bed rest while ureteral catheters are in place until specific orders indicate that ambulation is permissible.

The placement of ureteral catheters should be checked frequently, and tension of the catheter should be avoided. These catheters drain urine from the renal pelvis, which has a capacity of 3 to 5 ml. If the volume of urine in the renal pelvis increases, tissue damage to the pelvis will result from pressure. Therefore ureteral catheters should not be clamped. If the physician orders irrigation of the ureteral catheter, strict aseptic technique is required. If output is decreased, the physician should be notified immediately. Drainage should be checked often (at least every 1 to 2 hours). It is normal for some urine to drain around the ureteral catheter into the bladder. Accurate recording of urine output from both the ureteral and the urethral catheters is essential.

Suprapubic Catheters

Suprapubic catheterization is the simplest and oldest method of urinary diversion (Fig. 40-9). The two methods of insertion of a suprapubic catheter into the bladder are (1) through a small incision in the abdominal wall and (2)

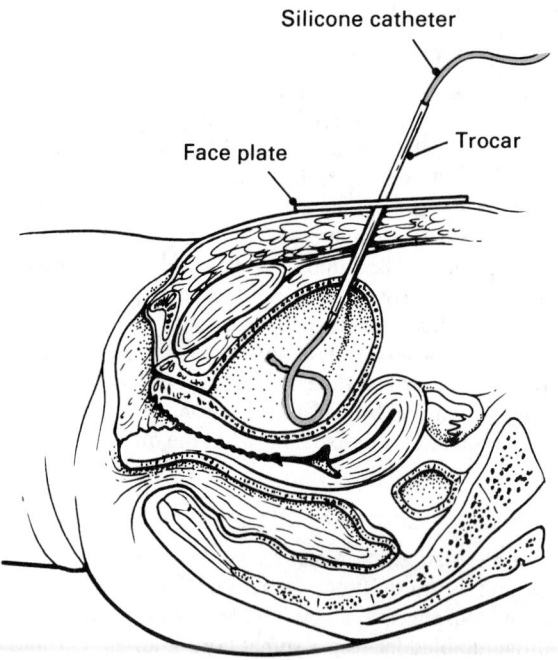

Silicone catheter

Face plate

Trocar

Fig. 40-9 Silicone suprapubic catheter in place within the bladder. The catheter is inserted through a small incision or by puncture with a trocar. It is threaded through the trocar into the bladder. When the catheter is in place, the trocar is removed. The catheter is secured to the abdominal wall with a faceplate, which is sutured to the abdominal wall. The catheter is attached to a drainage system. For permanent use, the catheter should be changed at least every 6 months.

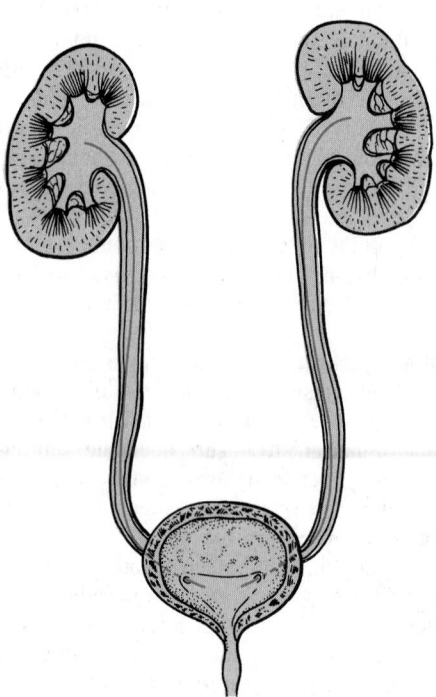

Fig. 40-8 Ureteral catheters.

by the use of a trocar. Suprapubic catheters are placed while the client is under general anesthesia when another surgical procedure is being performed or at the bedside with a local anesthetic. The catheters are usually sutured into place. The nursing responsibility includes taping the catheter to prevent dislodgment. The care of the tube and catheter is similar to that of the urethral catheter. Stomahesive is effective around the insertion site in protecting the skin from breakdown.

Suprapubic catheters are used in temporary situations such as bladder, vesical neck, prostate, and urethral surgery. Advantages include a reduced incidence of UTI and increased comfort and convenience for the client. Suprapubic catheterization may be used instead of urethral catheterization, especially in the young or infant male and when a urethral catheter cannot be inserted.

Suprapubic catheters are prone to poor drainage because of mechanical obstruction of the catheter tip by the bladder wall, sediment, and clots. Nursing interventions to ensure patency of the tube include (1) preventing tube kinking by coiling the excess tubing, (2) having the client turn from side to side, and (3) milking the tube. If these measures are not effective, the catheter is irrigated with sterile technique after a physician's order has been obtained.

If the client experiences bladder spasms that are difficult to control, urinary leakage may result. Urecholine or belladonna and opium (B + O) suppositories may be prescribed to decrease bladder spasms.

Nephrostomy Tubes

Nephrostomy tubes (catheters) are inserted on a temporary basis to preserve renal function when a complete obstruction of the ureter is present. They are inserted directly into the pelvis of the kidney and attached to connecting tubing for closed drainage. The principles are the same as those of ureteral catheters. That is, the catheter should never be kinked, laid upon, or clamped. If the client complains of excessive pain in the area or if there is excessive drainage around the tube, the catheter should be checked for patency. If irrigation is ordered, strict aseptic technique is required. Sterile saline solution (3 ml) may be ordered for the irrigation. Infection and secondary stone formation are complications associated with the insertion of nephrostomy tubes.

Intermittent Catheterization

An alternative approach to long-term indwelling catheterization is intermittent catheterization. It is being used with increasing frequency in conditions characterized by neurogenic bladder (e.g., spinal cord injuries, chronic neurological diseases). This type of catheterization may also be used in the oliguric and anuric phases of acute renal failure to reduce the possibility of infection from an indwelling catheter. The main goal of intermittent catheterization is to prevent urinary retention and stasis.

The technique consists of inserting a urethral catheter into the bladder every 3 to 5 hours. The bladder is emptied and the catheter is removed. Lubricant is only necessary for men. The catheter may be inserted by the client or the care provider.

In the hospital, sterile technique is used. For home care, a clean technique that includes good hand washing with soap and water is used. There has been no significant increase in infection with the use of an appropriate clean technique. The client is taught to observe for signs of UTI so that treatment can be instituted early. If indicated, some clients are placed on a regimen of prophylactic antibiotics.

RENAL AND UROLOGICAL SURGERY
Renal and Ureteral Surgery

The most common indications for nephrectomy are a renal tumor, polycystic kidneys that are bleeding or severely infected, massive traumatic injury to the kidney, and the elective removal of a kidney from a donor. As mentioned previously (see p. 1199), surgery involving the ureters and kidneys is most commonly performed to remove calculi that become obstructive.

The basic needs of the client undergoing renal and ureteral surgery are similar to those of any client who experiences surgery (see Chapters 11 to 13). In addition, it is especially important preoperatively to ensure adequate fluid intake and a normal electrolyte balance. The client should be told that there will probably be a flank incision on the affected side and that surgery will require a hyperextended, side-lying position. This position frequently causes the client to experience muscle aches after surgery. If a nephrectomy is planned, the client needs to be assured that one working kidney is sufficient to maintain normal renal function. Specific postoperative needs of a client are related to urine output, respiratory status, and abdominal distention.

Urine output. In the immediate postoperative period, urine output should be determined at least every 1 to 2 hours. Drainage from various catheters should be recorded separately. Catheters or tubes should not be clamped or irrigated without a specific order. The total urine output should be at least 30 to 50 ml/hr. It is also important to assess for urine drainage on the dressing and to estimate the amount. Daily weighing of the client is important. The same scale should be used, properly balanced, and the client should have on similar clothing and dressings each time.

It is important to observe and monitor the color and consistency of urine. Urine with increased amounts of mucus, blood, or sediment may occlude the drainage tubing or catheter.

Respiratory status. Renal surgery is usually performed through a flank incision just below the diaphragm and frequently involves removal of the twelfth rib. Postoperatively, it is important to ensure adequate ventilation. The client is often reluctant to turn, cough, and deep breathe because of the incisional pain. Adequate pain medication should be given to ensure the client's comfort and ability to perform coughing and deep-breathing exercises. Frequently, additional respiratory devices such as an incentive spirometer are used every 2 hours while the client is awake. In addition, early and frequent ambulation assists in maintaining adequate respiratory function.

Abdominal distention. Abdominal distention is present to some degree in most clients who have had surgery on

Table 40-21 Types of Urinary Diversion Surgery

Type	Description	Advantages	Disadvantages	Special Considerations
Ureterosigmoidostomy	Ureters are excised from bladder and anastomosed into sigmoid colon. Urine flows into colon and empties via rectum.	No need for external drainage appliances, urinary control via rectum	Urination via rectum necessary every 2-3 hr, absorption of fluid and electrolytes via bowel mucosa, possibility of hypochloremic acidosis, possibility of reflux from colon to kidney, high risk of ascending UTI	Frequent elimination is needed to prevent fluid and electrolyte problems and reflux. Enemas are usually contraindicated. Flatus causes stress incontinence. Flatus needs to be expelled in toilet. Rectal catheter may have to be inserted for drainage while client is sleeping.
Ileal conduit	Ureters are implanted into part of ileum or colon that has been resected from intestinal tract. Abdominal stoma is created.	Relatively good urine flow with few physiological alterations	External appliance necessary to continually drain urine	Surgical procedure is more complex. Postoperative complications may be increased. Reabsorption of urea by ileum occurs. Meticulous attention is necessary to care for stoma and collecting device.
Cutaneous ureterostomy	Ureters are excised from bladder and brought through abdominal wall, and stoma is created. Ureteral stomas may be created from both ureters, or ureters may be brought together and one stoma created.	No need for major surgery as ileal conduit	External appliance necessary because of continuous urine drainage, possibility of stricture or stenosis of small stoma	Periodic catheterizations may be required to maintain patency of stomas.
Nephrostomy	Insertion of catheter into pelvis or kidney. Procedure may be done to one or both kidneys and may be temporary or permanent. It is most frequently done in advanced disease as palliative procedure.	No need for major surgery	High risk of renal infection, predisposition to calculus formation from catheter	Nephrostomy tube may have to be changed every month. Catheter must never be clamped.

their kidneys or ureters. It is most commonly due to paralytic ileus from reflex paralysis caused by manipulation and compression of the bowel during surgery. Oral intake is restricted until bowel sounds are present (usually 24 to 48 hours after surgery). IV fluids of at least 3000 ml/day should be given until the client can ingest an equivalent amount of oral fluids. Clients can usually eat a regular diet by the fourth postoperative day.

Urinary Diversion

Removal of the urinary bladder (cystectomy) with diversion of the urine to an external device may be performed in several conditions, including cancer of the bladder, neurogenic bladder, congenital anomalies, strictures, trauma to the bladder, and chronic infections with deterioration of renal function.[20] Several types of surgical procedures are performed (Table 40-21 and Fig. 40-10). The

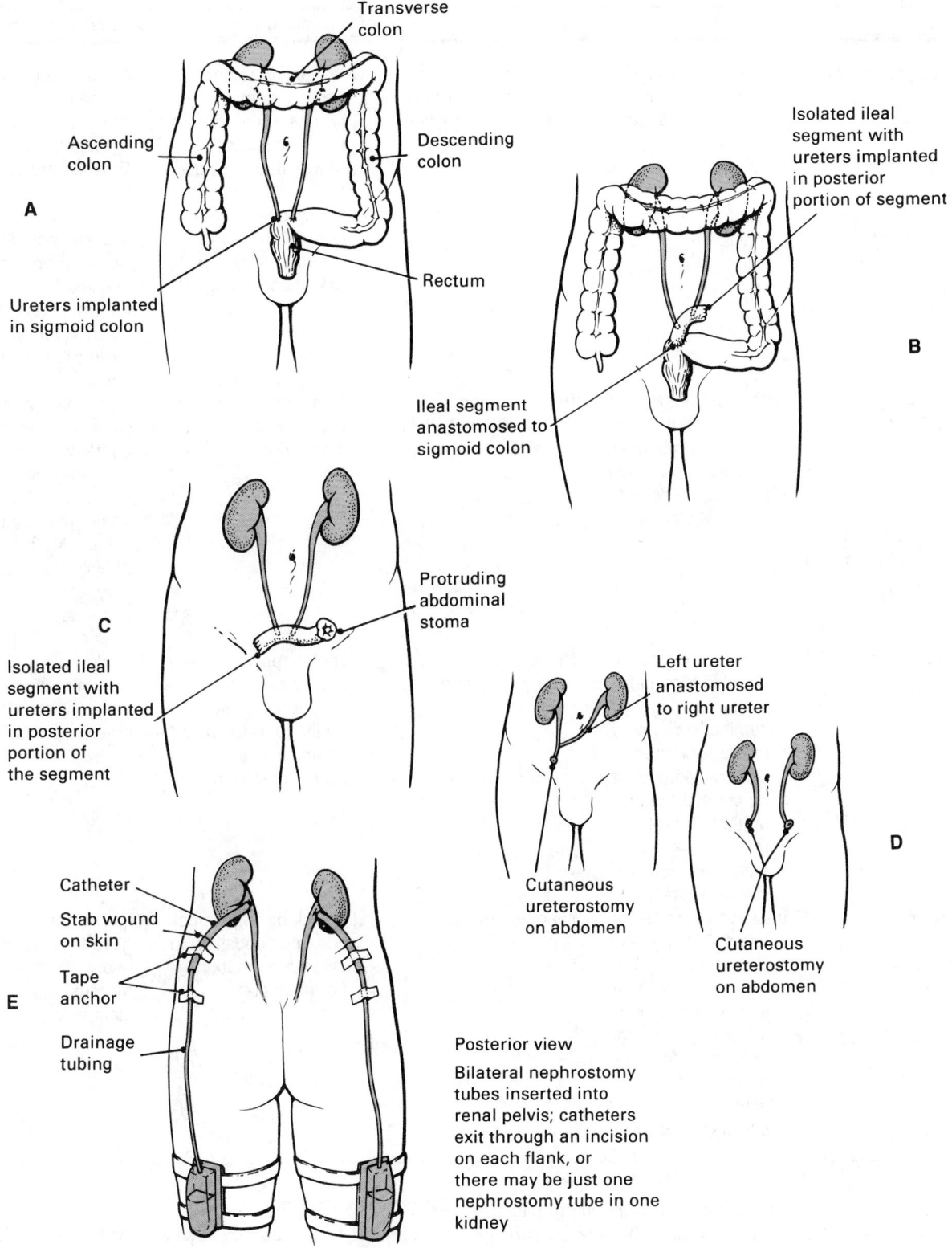

Fig. 40-10 Methods of urinary diversion. **A,** Ureterosigmoidostomy. **B,** Ureteroileosigmoidostomy. **C,** Ileal loop (or ileal conduit). **D,** Ureterostomy (transcutaneous ureterostomy and bilateral cutaneous ureterostomies). **E,** Nephrostomy. (From Jones D and others, eds: Medical-surgical nursing: a conceptual approach, ed 2, New York, 1982, McGraw-Hill Book Co, p 235.)

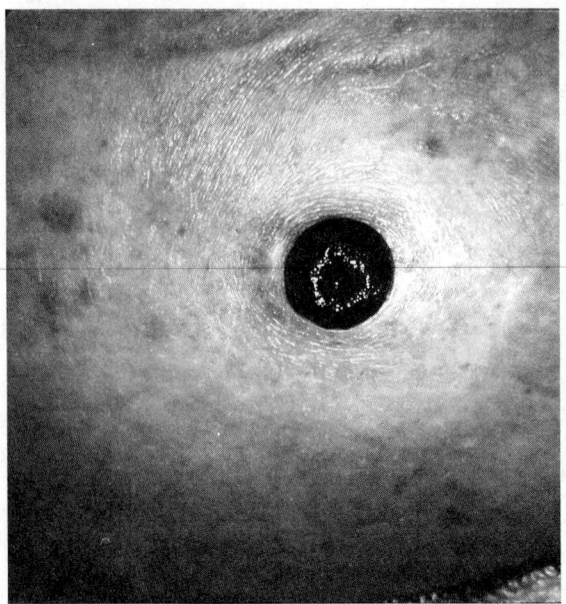

Fig. 40-11 Ideal urinary stoma. It is symmetrical, has no skin breakdown, and protrudes about 1.5 cm; the mucosa is a healthy red and the configuration is flat when the client is upright and supine. (Courtesy Lynda Brubacher, Virginia Mason Hospital, Seattle.)

most common type of surgery is the *ileal conduit (ileal loop)*. In this procedure a 15.2 to 20.3 cm (6 to 8 inch) segment of the ileum is converted into a conduit for urinary drainage. The colon is used (colon conduit) instead of the ileum with increasing frequency. The ureters are anastomosed into one end of the conduit and the other end of the bowel is brought out through the abdominal wall to form a stoma (Fig. 40-11). While the segment of bowel remains supported by the mesentery, it is completely isolated from the intestinal tract. The bowel is anastomosed and continues to function normally. Because there is no valve and no voluntary control over the stoma, drops of urine flow from the stoma every few seconds, requiring the use of a permanent external collecting device.

The disadvantages of this procedure compared with cutaneous ureterostomy and the use of permanent nephrostomy tubes are the extent of the surgical procedure, increased postoperative complications, reabsorption of urea by the ileum, and the attention required to care for the stoma and the collecting device. Disadvantages of cutaneous ureterostomy include stricture of the stoma, whereas those of permanent nephrostomy tubes include maintenance of patency of the tubes and a higher incidence of pyelonephritis.

Preoperative management. The client awaiting cystectomy and ileal conduit is given a great deal of information. The nurse must assess ability and readiness to learn before initiating a teaching program. If the client is not ready to learn, the teaching plan should be adjusted. The client's anxiety and fear may be decreased by the information. However, the anxiety and fear may also interfere with learning. The client's family should be involved in the

teaching process. A discussion of the social aspects of living with a stoma (including clothing, changes in body image and sexuality, exercise, and odor) provides the client with facts that may allay some fears. Concerns about the effect on sexual activities should be discussed. A visit from an ostomate may be very helpful at this time. Additional interventions are presented in Table 40-22.

Postoperative management. Nursing interventions during the postoperative period (see Table 40-22) should be planned to prevent surgical complications such as postoperative atelectasis and shock (see Chapter 13). After pelvic surgery, there is an increased incidence of thrombophlebitis. With removal of part of the bowel, there is an increased incidence of paralytic ileus and small-bowel obstruction. A nasogastric tube is necessary for 3 to 5 days.

Specific attention should be given to preventing injury to the stoma and maintaining urine output. Mucus is present in the urine because it is secreted by the intestines as a result of the irritating effect of the urine. The client should be told that this is a normal occurrence. A high fluid intake is encouraged to "flush" the ileal conduit.

The skin around the stoma requires meticulous care. Alkaline encrustations with dermatitis may occur when alkaline urine comes in contact with exposed skin (Fig. 40-12). Changing of appliances is discussed in Table 40-23. A properly fitting appliance is essential to prevent skin problems. The appliance should be about 0.2 cm (0.1 inch) larger than the stoma. It is normal for the stoma to shrink within the first few weeks after surgery. The urine is kept acidic to prevent alkaline encrustations.

Acceptance of the surgery and of alterations in body image is needed to ensure the client's best adjustment. Concerns of the client include fear that the stoma will be offensive to others and will interfere with sexual, personal, professional, and recreational activities. The client should know that very few if any activities will be restricted as a result of the urinary diversion.

Discharge planning includes teaching the client symptoms of obstruction or infection and care of the ostomy. The client is fitted for a permanent appliance 7 to 10 days after surgery and may need to be refitted at a later time, depending on the degree of stoma shrinkage. Appliances are made of a variety of products, including natural and synthetic rubbers, plastics, and metals. Regardless of the type, all appliances have a faceplate that adheres to the skin, a collecting pouch, and an opening to drain the pouch. The faceplate may be secured to the skin with glues, adhesives, or adhering synthetic wafers. If improperly fitted or applied, the faceplate may cause skin problems (Fig. 40-13). The client needs information on where to purchase supplies, emergency telephone numbers, location of ostomy clubs, and follow-up visits with an enterostomal therapist as indicated.

Continent Urinary Diversions

Recently, continent cutaneous urinary diversions requiring intermittent catheterization rather than bag drainage have become popular. A variety of surgical procedures are available that preserve the upper urinary tracts; avoid reflux and obstruction of the ureters; and create a reservoir

Table 40-22

NURSING CARE PLAN FOR THE CLIENT WITH AN ILEAL CONDUIT

Defining Characteristics	Nursing Interventions	Evaluation Criteria

NURSING DIAGNOSIS: Anxiety related to effects of procedure on lifestyle and relationships; lack of knowledge regarding surgical procedure, appliance, and its use; and postoperative pain management

Defining Characteristics	Nursing Interventions	Evaluation Criteria
Frequent questions about surgical procedure; drawn facies; pallor, sweating, restlessness, inability to sleep, talkativeness; increase in vital signs; feeling of apprehension, tension, nervousness	Instruct client in preoperative, operative, and postoperative procedures including diet, medications, nasogastric tubes, IVs, NPO status, enemas, pain management, turning, coughing and deep breathing, and leg exercises. Mark stoma site before surgery with consideration of skin folds, old scars, abdominal muscles, clothing lines, and client's predominant use of right or left hand. Demonstrate how to apply appliance and use equipment. Allow client to wear appliance filled with water under clothing to determine how it will feel. Answer questions honestly and provide emotional support. Assess understanding and emotional response of client and significant others. Arrange for visit with person with an ostomy or with enterostomal therapist.	Demonstration of knowledge about surgical preoperative, operative, and postoperative procedures, including both stoma and appliance

NURSING DIAGNOSIS: High risk for ascending UTI related to surgical procedure, ureteral obstruction, chronic use of external appliance, and incorrect or inadequate stoma care

Defining Characteristics	Nursing Interventions	Evaluation Criteria
Elevation in body temperature, pain in back or abdomen, bloody or cloudy urine, decrease in urinary output	Empty appliance q 2-3 hr or when one-third full of urine. Use bedside drainage bag at night to prevent reflux of urine into conduit. Instruct client about symptoms to be reported, including absence of urine, blood in urine, pain in back or abdomen, elevated temperature, malaise, increase in abdominal girth, nausea and vomiting. Encourage high fluid intake of 2000-3000 ml/day. Inform client that no specific diet is required but that cranberry juice may help decrease odor. Give vitamin C to keep urine acidic. (Alkaline urine irritates the skin.)	No UTI

NURSING DIAGNOSIS: Body-image disturbance related to effects of loss of body parts and change in body function on lifestyle or relationships

Defining Characteristics	Nursing Interventions	Evaluation Criteria
Negative feelings about self, refusal to look at or touch stoma or participate in self-care, expression of concern about effect on family and lifestyle	Encourage client to share feelings. Demonstrate willingness to listen and answer questions. Provide information about surgery and expected effects. Determine the need for additional support (e.g., psychiatric support, visit by an ostomate). Encourage gradual involvement in self-care.	Verbal and/or behavioral indication of acceptance of changes in image and function

NURSING DIAGNOSIS: Altered health maintenance related to lack of knowledge regarding stoma and appliance care

Defining Characteristics	Nursing Interventions	Evaluation Criteria
Expression of concern about how to manage ileal conduit, frequent questions or inaccurate responses regarding stoma care	Demonstrate proper method of changing stoma bag and have client give return demonstration. Change temporary bag.* Demonstrate care and procedure to use in changing permanent appliance.* Have client give return demonstration with explanation.	Demonstration of ability to change stoma bag and cleanse stoma, demonstration of ability to maintain permanent appliance

*See Table 40-23.

Table 40-22

NURSING CARE PLAN FOR THE CLIENT WITH AN ILEAL CONDUIT—cont'd

Defining Characteristics	Nursing Interventions	Evaluation Criteria
NURSING DIAGNOSIS: High risk for impaired skin integrity related to ill-fitting appliance, inadequate hygiene, and lack of knowledge regarding stoma care		
Improperly fitted appliance, reddened and irritated skin around stoma	Check appliance position. Observe stoma for any bleeding or eroded areas. Cleanse stoma as ordered. Allow no tight clothing or binders over stoma.	Intact, viable stoma; clean and intact skin surrounding stoma
NURSING DIAGNOSIS: Potential complication: paralytic ileus related to surgical manipulation of bowel		
Absence of bowel sounds, abdominal distention, cramping pain, nausea and vomiting	Maintain patency of nasogastric tube. Encourage early ambulation. Administer IV fluids as ordered. Monitor fluid and electrolyte levels. Assess for presence or absence of bowel sounds, flatus, and bowel movements.	Normal bowel sounds, absence of nausea and vomiting
NURSING DIAGNOSIS: Potential complication: thrombophlebitis related to surgery involving pelvic manipulation		
Diminished or absent lower extremity pulses; positive Homans' sign; swelling, warmth, and pain in legs	Teach client method to do range-of-motion exercises for legs while in bed and instruct client to keep legs uncrossed. Turn or help client turn q 2 hr while in bed. Increase activity level gradually and have client ambulate as soon as possible. Provide elastic wraps or support hose for legs as ordered. Administer anticoagulants if ordered.	Absence of Homans' sign and swelling, warmth, or pain in legs
NURSING DIAGNOSIS: High risk for altered sexuality patterns related to perceived or actual effects of surgery on sexual activity		
Verbalization of concern over future sexual function, lack of understanding by significant other	Provide accurate information related to sexual activity. Provide information about penile implant when appropriate. Provide information and support for spouse or significant other.	Verbalization of feelings about changes in sexuality and sexual function

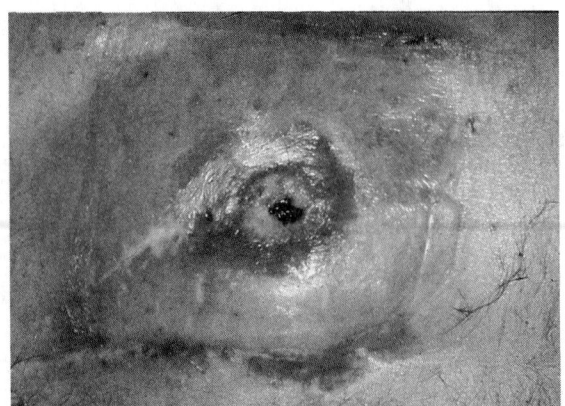

Fig. 40-12 Ammonia salt encrustation secondary to alkaline urine. (Courtesy Lynda Brubacher, Virginia Mason Hospital, Seattle.)

Table 40-23 Guidelines for Changing Ileal Conduit Appliances

TEMPORARY APPLIANCE

1. Cut hole in bag to fit over stoma (pouch 3.2 mm [⅛ inch] larger than stoma).
2. Remove old bag.
3. Clean area gently and remove old adhesive.
4. Wash area with warm water.
5. Place wick (rolled-up 4 × 4 inch pad) over stoma to keep area dry during rest of procedure.
6. Dry skin around stoma.
7. Apply tincture of benzoin or other skin protectant around stoma to area where bag will be placed.
8. Apply bag by first smoothing its edges toward side and lower portion of body.
9. Remove wick and complete application of bag.
10. If client is usually in bed, apply bag so that it lies toward side of body.
11. If client is ambulatory, apply bag so that it lies toward center of body.
12. Connect drainage tubing to bag.
13. Keep drainage bag on same side of bed as stoma.

PERMANENT APPLIANCE

1. Keep appliance in place for 2 to 14 days.
2. Change appliance when fluid intake has been restricted for several hours.
3. Have client sit or stand in front of mirror.
4. Moisten edge of faceplate with adhesive solvent and gently remove.
5. Clean skin with adhesive solvent.
6. Wash skin with warm water. (Client may shower.)
7. Dry skin and inspect.
8. Place wick (rolled up 4 × 4 inch pad) over stoma to keep skin free of urine.
9. Apply skin cement to faceplate and skin.
10. Place appliance over stoma.
11. Wash removed appliance with soap and lukewarm water; soak in distilled vinegar; rinse with lukewarm water and air-dry.

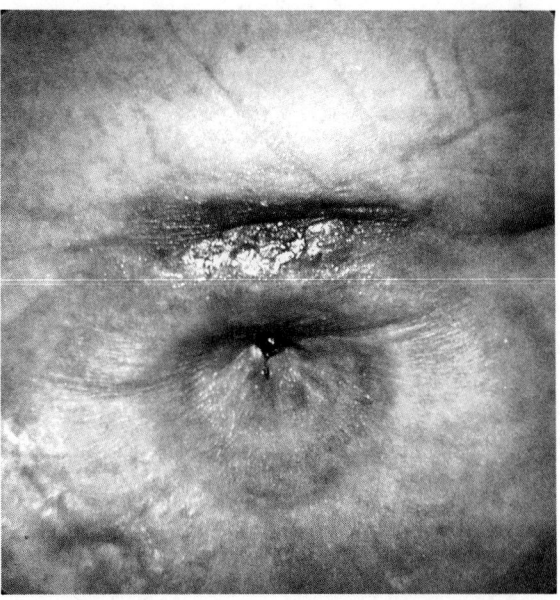

Fig. 40-13 Retracted urinary stoma with pressure sore from faceplate above stoma. (Courtesy Lynda Brubacher, Virginia Mason Hospital, Seattle.)

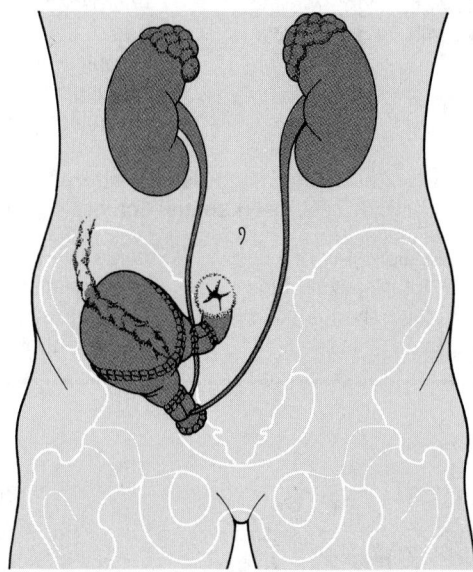

Fig. 40-14 Creation of a Kock pouch with implantation of ureters into one intussuscepted portion of the pouch and creation of a stoma with the other intussuscepted portion.

with a high capacity, low pressure, and the ability to be emptied.

The Kock pouch, the Mainz pouch, and the Indiana continent urinary reservoir are three types of continent urinary reservoirs. The Kock pouch for urinary diversion is a variation of the one used for creation of a continent ileostomy to treat ulcerative colitis (see Chapter 37 and Fig. 37-4). In this procedure a segment of the ileum is used to create a pouch, and two different portions of the ileum are intussuscepted. The ureters are anastomosed to one of the intussuscepted portions, and the other intussuscepted limb is used to create an external stoma (see Fig. 40-14).

A Mainz pouch, a variation of the Kock pouch, is created from the ileum and cecum. The ureters are tunneled through the wall of the colon and into the pouch. The stoma can be placed in a suprapubic position or directly in the umbilicus.

The Indiana continent urinary reservoir uses a portion of the terminal ileum, ascending colon, and cecum to create the reservoir. The ureters are implanted in the reservoir. The stoma can be placed on the abdomen, attached to a portion of the urethral stump, or attached to the anterior vaginal wall. Long-term follow-up is needed to compare the results of these and other urinary reservoirs.

With continent urinary diversion procedures, an external drainage collection pouch is not necessary because

urine is not draining continuously through the stoma. The client needs to learn to perform intermittent self-catheterization to drain the urine. Catheterization is usually done every 4 to 5 hours. The client is taught a clean technique for inserting and caring for the catheter. Although continent urinary diversion requires a stoma, it can be reassuring to the client to know that no external appliance is needed.

C ase Study

URINARY TRACT INFECTION

Janet, a 28-year-old woman, has had a history of painful urination for 5 months. Intermittently, she has had fever, chills, and back pain. Recently, she has had frequent urination with the passage of small volumes of urine.

On physical examination, she was in no acute distress. Vital signs included a temperature of 38° C (100.4° F), a pulse rate of 80, and a blood pressure of 100/70. She had bilateral flank pain and upper abdominal tenderness to palpation. A urine specimen for culture and sensitivity was obtained.

Discussion Questions

1. What are the most common organisms that cause UTIs?
2. What factors predispose a client to a UTI?
3. What are the clinical manifestations of UTIs? Which symptoms did Janet have?
4. What is the difference between upper and lower UTIs?
5. What can the nurse do to help Janet prevent another UTI?

R eview Questions

The number of the question corresponds to the same-numbered objective at the beginning of the chapter.

1. The organisms that cause pyelonephritis most commonly reach the kidneys by which of the following means?
   a. descending infection
   b. ascending infection
   c. bloodstream
   d. lymphatic system
2. Women who are especially susceptible to UTIs should
   a. take prophylactic sulfonamides for the rest of their lives
   b. drink at least 2 to 3 L of fluid per day
   c. take tub baths with bubble bath
   d. cleanse themselves from the rectum to the urethra after toileting
3. The immunological mechanisms involved in glomerulonephritis include all of the following *except*
   a. activation of complement resulting in release of chemotactic factors
   b. deposition of immune complexes along the GBM
   c. destruction of glomeruli by proteolytic enzymes contained in the GBM
   d. release of kinins and vasoactive amines
4. Clinical manifestations of acute pyelonephritis include

   a. elevated blood pressure
   b. albuminuria and edema
   c. bacteria and WBCs in the urine
   d. hematuria and hemoptysis
5. The edema that occurs in nephrotic syndrome is due to
   a. increased hydrostatic pressure caused by sodium retention
   b. decreased colloidal osmotic pressure caused by loss of serum albumin
   c. decreased aldosterone secretion from adrenal insufficiency
   d. increased colloidal osmotic pressure caused by increased serum albumin
6. Clinical manifestations of renal calculi include
   a. dribbling at the end of urination and pyuria
   b. severe flank pain and hematuria
   c. frequency of urination and polyuria
   d. urgent, uncontrollable urination
7. Which of the following is inherited as an autosomal dominant disorder?
   a. adult-onset polycystic renal disease
   b. horseshoe kidney
   c. malignant nephrosclerosis
   d. exstrophy of the bladder
8. Renal tissue changes that may occur in diabetes mellitus include
   a. glomerulosclerosis and pyelonephritis
   b. renal sugar-crystal calculi and cysts
   c. lipid deposits in the glomerulus and nephrons
   d. uric acid calculi and nephrolithiasis
9. The classic manifestations of advanced renal adenocarcinoma include all the following *except*
   a. palpable mass
   b. gross hematuria
   c. flank pain
   d. renal colic
10. Which of the following measures is not appropriate for a bladder-training program for incontinence?
    a. limiting fluid intake at bedtime
    b. muscle-strengthening exercises
    c. scheduled voiding times
    d. use of retention catheters during the night
11. A client with a ureterolithotomy returns from surgery with a nephrostomy tube in place. Which of the following should be included in nursing care?
    a. Notify the physician of a nephrostomy tube drainage of more than 30 ml/hr.
    b. Irrigate the nephrostomy tube with 10 ml of normal saline solution as needed.
    c. After nausea has subsided, force fluids of at least 2 to 3 L/day.
    d. Encourage client to drink fruit juices and milk.
12. A client has had a cystectomy and ileal conduit diversion performed. Four days postoperatively, mucus shreds are seen in the drainage bag. The nurse should
    a. notify the physician
    b. notify the charge nurse
    c. chart it as a normal observation
    d. irrigate the drainage tube

REFERENCES

1. National Institute of Arthritis, Diabetes, and Digestive and Kidney Disease: Urinary tract infections, Washington, DC, 1985, National Institute of Health.
2. Stamm W and Turck M: Urinary tract infection and pyelonephritis. In Wilson JD and others: Harrison's principles of internal medicine, ed 12, New York, 1990, McGraw-Hill Book Co, Inc, pp 538-543.
3. Johnson JR and Stamm WE: Urinary tract infections in women: diagnosis and treatment, Ann Intern Med 111:906-917, 1989.
4. Johnson MA: Urinary tract infections in women, Am Fam Physician 41:565-571, 1990.
5. Tejani A and Inguilli E: Poststreptococcal glomerulonephritis: current clinical and pathologic changes, Nephron 55:1-5, 1990.
6. Earle DP: Poststreptococcal acute glomerulonephritis, Hosp Pract 20:84E-84BB, 1985.
7. Jones DA and others: Goodpasture's syndrome revisited, NC Med J 51:411-415, 1990.
8. Cole E: Plasma exchange in rapidly progressive glomerulonephritis, Apheresis 1:257-262, 1990.
9. Bernard DB: Nephrotic syndrome: a clinical approach, Hosp Pract 25:114-130, 1990.
10. Seney FD and others: Acquired immunodeficiency syndrome and the kidney, Am J Kidney Dis 16:1-13, 1990.
11. Schoenfeld P and Feduska NJ: Acquired immunodeficiency syndrome and renal disease: report of the National Kidney Foundation–National Institutes of Health Task Force on AIDS and Kidney Disease, Am J Kidney Dis 16:14-25, 1990.
12. Coe FL and Favus MJ: Nephrolithiasis. In Wilson JD and others: Harrison's principles of internal medicine, ed 12, New York, 1990, McGraw-Hill Book Co, Inc, pp 1202-1206.
13. Mackety CJ: Lasers in urology, Nurs Clin North Am 25:697-709, 1990.
14. Jones DJ and others: The changing practice of percutaneous stone surgery, Br J Urol 66:1-5, 1990.
15. Sox MA and Fabian TC: The pelvis. In Moore EE and others: Early care of the injured patient, ed 4, Philadelphia, 1990, BC Decker, pp 176-181.
16. Debruyne FMJ and others: New prospects in the management of metastatic renal cell carcinoma: experimental and clinical data, Uro-oncology: current status and future trends, 1990, Willey-Liss, pp 243-255.
17. Diokno AC and others: Prevalence of urinary incontinence and other urological symptoms in the noninstitutionalized elderly, J Urol 135:1022-1025, 1986.
18. Resnick NM: Diagnosis and treatment in the institutionalized elderly, Semin Urol 7:117-123, 1989.
19. Burns PA and others: Treatment of stress incontinence with pelvic floor exercises and biofeedback, J Am Geriatr Soc 38:341-344, 1990.
20. Gleeson MJ and Griffith DP: Urinary diversion, Br J Urol 66:113-122, 1990.

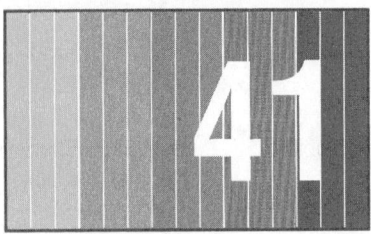

CHAPTER

41

Nursing Role in Management
Acute and Chronic Renal Failure

Sharon Mantik Lewis
Barbara Wood
JoAnn Seppelt

Learning Objectives

1. Differentiate between acute and chronic renal failure.
2. Differentiate among the causes of prerenal, intrarenal, and postrenal acute renal failure.
3. Describe the clinical course of reversible acute renal failure.
4. Explain the therapeutic and nursing management for a client in the oliguric and diuretic phases of acute renal failure.
5. Describe the systemic effects of chronic renal failure.
6. Explain the conservative management of and the related nursing care for clients with chronic renal failure.
7. Differentiate between peritoneal dialysis and hemodialysis in terms of purpose, indications for use, advantages and disadvantages, and nursing responsibilities.
8. Compare common vascular access sites used for hemodialysis.
9. Compare dialysis and renal transplantation as methods of treatment for end-stage renal disease.
10. Describe the nursing role for clients in the preoperative, intraoperative, and postoperative stages of kidney transplantation.
11. Explain the long-term problems of the client with a kidney transplant.

Renal failure is severe impairment or total lack of kidney function. In renal failure there is an inability to excrete metabolic waste products and functional disturbances of all body systems as well. Renal failure is classified as *acute* or *chronic*. Acute renal failure most commonly has a rapid onset. In contrast, chronic renal failure usually develops insidiously over time.

Although acute renal failure is potentially reversible, the mortality rates remain distressingly high in spite of advances in treatment. The focus in chronic renal failure has changed from treating a terminally ill client to dealing with a person who has a manageable chronic disease that requires long-term care. The change in focus is due to the life support system of dialysis and to improved techniques in renal transplantation.

Reviewed by Evelyn Butera, R.N., M.S.N., C.N.N., Manager, Education Services, Northwest Kidney Center, Seattle, Washington.

ACUTE RENAL FAILURE

Acute renal failure is a clinical syndrome characterized by a rapid decline in renal function with progressive *azotemia*, an accumulation of nitrogenous waste products such as blood urea nitrogen (BUN) and serum creatinine. *Uremia* is the clinical situation in which azotemia progresses to a symptomatic state. Acute renal failure is usually associated with a decrease in urinary output to less than 400 ml/day (oliguria), although it is possible to have normal or increased urinary output. There is no correlation between the amount of urine produced and the severity of the renal failure.

Acute renal failure may develop insidiously with progressive elevations of BUN, creatinine, and potassium without oliguria. Most commonly, acute renal failure occurs in previously healthy individuals and generally follows an identifiable trauma or contact with a nephrotoxic agent. The most common cause of acute renal failure is related to surgical procedures.

Table 41-1 Common Causes of Acute Renal Failure

PRERENAL	INTRARENAL	POSTRENAL

Decrease in vascular volume from the following:
    Hemorrhage
    Burns
    Prolonged diarrhea or vomiting
Decrease in cardiac output from the following:
    Myocardial infarction
    Cardiac dysrhythmias
    Congestive heart failure
    Surgery (e.g., open-heart)
Intravascular pooling of blood from the following:
    Septic shock
    Anaphylaxis
Renal vascular obstruction from the following:
    Thrombosis of renal arteries
    Bilateral renal vein thrombosis
	Nephrotoxic injury from the following:
	    Hemolytic blood transfusion reaction (hemoglobin blocks tubules)
	    Severe crushing injury (myoglobin released from muscles blocks tubules)
	    Chemicals (ethylene glycol, mercuric chloride, carbon tetrachloride, lead, arsenic)
	    Drugs (aminoglycosides [gentamicin, tobramycin, amikacin], amphotericin B, phenacetin, cisplatin)
	    Radiographic contrast agents
	Acute glomerulonephritis
	Acute pyelonephritis
	Toxemia of pregnancy
	Malignant hypertension
	Systemic lupus erythematosus
	Drug-induced acute interstitial nephritis (penicillins, cephalosporins, nonsteroidal antiinflammatory agents, sulfonamides, rifampicin)
	Hepatorenal syndrome
		Calculi formation
		Benign prostatic hypertrophy
		Neoplasms (bladder and pelvic organs)
		Renal papillary necrosis
		Obstruction in collecting ducts (sulfonamides, uric acid crystals)
		Trauma (to back, pelvis, or perineum)
		Strictures
		Spinal cord disease

Other terms used synonymously with acute renal failure are *renal shutdown, acute tubular necrosis,* (ATN), and *acute tubular insufficiency.* Even though ATN is often used interchangeably with acute renal failure, the former term actually describes a *type* of acute renal failure.

Etiology and Pathophysiology

The etiologies of acute renal failure are multiple and complex. They are categorized according to similar pathogenesis into prerenal, intrarenal (or renal parenchymal), and postrenal causes (Table 41-1).

Prerenal causes consist of factors outside the kidneys that impair renal blood flow and lead to decreased glomerular perfusion. Prerenal disease can lead to intrarenal disease because prolonged renal ischemia can lead to tubular necrosis.

Intrarenal causes include conditions of actual damage to the renal tissue (parenchyma) leading to malfunctioning of nephrons. Primary renal diseases such as acute glomerulonephritis and acute pyelonephritis may lead to acute renal failure. More commonly, ATN is the predisposing insult. ATN may be caused by hemoglobin released from hemolyzed red blood cells (RBCs) or myoglobin released from necrotic muscle cells. Hemoglobin and myoglobin block the tubules and cause renal vasoconstriction. Nephrotoxic chemicals and drugs can cause obstruction of intrarenal structures by crystallization or actual damage to the epithelial cells of tubules.

Postrenal causes involve mechanical obstruction of urinary outflow. As the flow of urine is blocked, urine backs up into the renal pelvis. Usually anuria (no urine output), rather than oliguria, occurs in obstructive disorders. The most common causes are calculi, trauma, and tumors.

The two major mechanisms that lead to acute renal destruction are renal ischemia and nephrotoxic injury (Fig. 41-1). Acute renal failure that results from these types of damage is usually referred to as acute tubular necrosis (ATN). Severe renal ischemia causes a disruption in the basement membrane and patchy destruction of the tubular epithelium. Nephrotoxic agents cause necrosis of tubular epithelial cells, which slough off and plug the tubules. Nephrotoxic injury usually leaves the basement membrane intact. ATN is potentially reversible if the basement membrane is not destroyed and if the necrotic tubular epithelium regenerates.

Possible pathological processes involved in acute renal failure include the following[1,2]:

1. *Renal vasoconstriction:* Ischemia stimulates renin release, which activates the angiotensin-aldosterone system and results in constriction of peripheral and renal afferent arterioles. With decreased blood flow there is decreased glomerular capillary pressure and glomerular filtration rate (GFR) as well as tubular dysfunction and, ultimately, oliguria.

2. *Cellular edema*: Ischemia causes anoxia, which leads to endothelial cell edema. Cellular edema raises tissue pressures above capillary flow pressure, so blood flow through the arterioles may still be altered after treatment of the underlying condition. Inadequate renal blood flow further depresses the GFR.

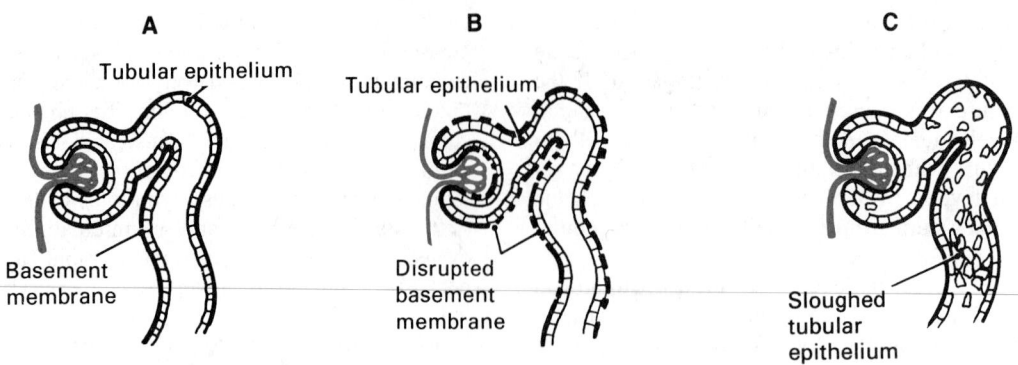

Fig. 41-1   Nephron destruction in acute renal failure. **A,** Normal nephron. **B,** Damage from renal ischemia results in patchy necrosis of the tubule. The lumen may also be blocked by casts. **C,** Damage from nephrotoxic agents.

3. *Decreased glomerular capillary permeability*: Ischemia alters glomerular epithelial cells and thus decreases glomerular capillary permeability. This in turn reduces the GFR, which significantly reduces tubular blood flow and leads to tubular dysfunction.
4. *Intratubular obstruction*: When tubules are damaged, interstitial edema occurs and necrotic epithelial cells accumulate in the tubules. This accumulated debris also lowers the GFR by obstructing the tubules and increasing intratubular pressure.
5. *Leakage of glomerular filtrate*: Glomerular filtrate leaks back into plasma through holes in the damaged tubular membranes, which decreases intratubular fluid flow.

Clinical Course

Clinically, acute renal failure may progress through the phases of oliguria, diuresis, and recovery. In some situations the client does not recover from acute renal failure, and chronic renal failure results.

Oliguric phase. The most common initial manifestation of acute renal failure is oliguria caused by a reduction in the GFR. The oliguria usually occurs within 1 to 7 days of the causative event. If the cause is ischemia, oliguria may occur within 24 hours, but when nephrotoxic drugs are involved, it may be delayed for as long as a week. Initially, the presence of anuria is rare unless the precipitating cause is a urinary obstructive disorder. (*Acute nonoliguric renal failure* may also occur. In this situation, the onset may be relatively insidious with hypervolemia or an elevated BUN as the first presenting abnormality.) The duration of the oliguric phase may range from a few days to several weeks. Some cases have lasted for several months. The average duration is about 10 to 14 days, but it rarely exceeds 4 weeks. The longer the oliguric phase lasts, the poorer is the prognosis.

It is important to distinguish prerenal oliguria from oliguria of acute renal failure. In prerenal oliguria there is no damage to the renal tissue. The oliguria is caused by a decrease in circulating blood volume (e.g., as a result of shock, burns, severe dehydration) and is potentially reversible. (Some causes of acute renal failure are also potentially reversible.) Prerenal oliguria is characterized by urine with a high specific gravity and a low sodium concentration. In contrast, oliguria of acute renal failure is characterized by urine with a low specific gravity and a high sodium concentration. Prerenal oliguria can be corrected by means of fluid, blood, or plasma replacement to increase renal perfusion.

The manifestations of the oliguric phase of acute renal failure are changes in urinary output, fluid and electrolyte abnormalities, and uremia. The nurse must be alert for the presenting signs and symptoms of these changes.

Urinary changes. Urinary output may decrease to less than 20 ml/hr. The urine may be bloody. A urinalysis may show casts, RBCs, white blood cells (WBCs), a specific gravity fixed at around 1.010, and urine osmolality at about 300 mOsm/L. This is the same specific gravity and osmolality as for plasma, reflecting tubular damage with a loss of concentrating ability by the kidney. Proteinuria may be present if the renal failure is related to glomerular membrane dysfunction.

Fluid volume excess. When urinary output decreases, fluid retention occurs. The neck veins enlarge, the pulse becomes more bounding, and edema and hypertension may develop. Fluid overload can eventually lead to congestive heart failure and pulmonary edema.

Metabolic acidosis. In renal failure the kidneys cannot synthesize ammonia or excrete acid metabolites. The bicarbonate level decreases because bicarbonate is used up in buffering hydrogen ions. In addition, defective reabsorption and regeneration of bicarbonate occur. The client may develop Kussmaul's (rapid, deep) respiration to increase the excretion of carbon dioxide. Kussmaul's respiration is a compensatory mechanism for acidosis.

Sodium balance. Damaged tubules cannot conserve sodium. Consequently, the urinary excretion of sodium may increase, resulting in normal or below normal levels of serum sodium. However, excessive intake of sodium can lead to volume expansion, hypertension, and congestive heart failure.

Potassium excess. The serum potassium levels increase, since the normal ability of the kidneys to excrete 80% to 90% of the body's potassium is impaired. If the acute renal failure was caused by massive tissue trauma, the damaged cells release potassium to the extracellular fluid. Thus clients with tissue injury may have higher serum potassium levels. In addition, acidosis enhances the movement of potassium from intracellular to extracellular fluid.

When potassium levels exceed 6 mEq/L, treatment must be initiated immediately to prevent cardiac dysrhythmias. Before clinical signs of hyperkalemia are apparent, the electrocardiogram (ECG) will show tall, peaked T waves, widening of the QRS complex, and ST depression. Progressive changes in the ECG, which are related to increasing potassium levels, are depicted in Fig. 10-12.

Calcium deficit. A low serum calcium level results from decreased gastrointestinal (GI) absorption of calcium

Table 41-2 Clinical Manifestations of Acute Uremia

Body System	Clinical Manifestations
Urinary	↓ Urinary output
	Proteinuria
	Casts
	↓ Specific gravity
	↓ Osmolality
	↑ Urinary sodium
Cardiovascular	Volume overload
	Congestive heart failure
	Hypotension (early)
	Hypertension (after development of fluid overload)
	Pericarditis
	Pericardial effusion
	Dysrhythmias
Respiratory	Pulmonary edema
	Kussmaul's respiration
Gastrointestinal	Nausea and vomiting
	Anorexia
	Stomatitis
	Bleeding
	Diarrhea
	Constipation
Hematological	Anemia (development within 48 hr)
	Leukocytosis
	Defect in platelet functioning
Neurological	Lethargy
	Convulsions
	Asterixis
	Memory impairment
Others	↑ Susceptibility to infection
	↑ BUN
	↑ Creatinine
	↑ Potassium
	↓ pH
	↓ Bicarbonate

↓, Decreased ↑, increased.

and elevated serum phosphate levels that are due to its decreased excretion by the kidneys. Normally, most plasma calcium is found ionized (physiologically active form) or bound to protein. In renal failure it is unusual for hypocalcemia to be symptomatic because acidosis keeps more calcium in an ionized form. Sometimes a low serum level of ionized calcium may cause symptoms of tetany.

Azotemia. The BUN and serum creatinine levels are elevated. If the client is experiencing rapid catabolism (e.g., because of infections, fever, severe injury, or GI bleeding), the BUN will be further elevated.

Eventually, all body systems become involved in the acute uremic syndrome (Table 41-2). The extrarenal manifestations are generally similar to those found in clients with chronic uremia (see Fig. 41-3).

Diuretic phase. The diuretic phase begins with a gradual increase in daily urine output of 1 to 3 L/day but may reach 3 to 5 L/day. Although urine output is increasing, the kidneys are still not completely healed.[3] The high urine volume is due to osmotic diuresis from the high urea concentration and the inadequate concentrating ability of the tubules.

At this stage, the uremia may still be very severe, as reflected by low creatinine clearances and elevated serum creatinine and BUN levels. The client must be monitored for deficits in sodium, potassium, and water caused by excessive losses in the urine. The diuretic phase may last 1 to 3 weeks.

Recovery phase. The recovery phase begins when the GFR increases so that BUN and serum creatinine levels start to stabilize and then decrease. Although the major improvements occur within the first 1 to 2 weeks of this phase, renal function continues to improve for up to 12 months after acute renal failure.

The mortality rate from acute renal failure varies from 30% to 60%, depending on the cause. Many deaths are related to the underlying disease. However, the most common cause of death is secondary infection. The incidence of infection is highest in individuals in whom surgery or traumatic injury contributed to renal failure. The presence of infection may go unrecognized, since clients with renal failure do not necessarily have a temperature elevation in response to an infection.

Some individuals do not recover and progress to chronic renal failure. Older adult clients recover normal renal function less frequently than younger clients. Among the individuals who recover, the vast majority achieve clinically normal renal function with no evidence of later decline in renal function or complications such as hypertension.

Therapeutic Management

The therapy for prerenal oliguria is aimed at restoring blood volume and causing diuresis. Diuretic therapy consisting of loop-acting diuretics (furosemide and ethacrynic acid) or an osmotic diuretic (mannitol) can be used to increase the renal blood flow and the GFR. These diuretics are used selectively in attempts to prevent acute renal failure. If acute renal failure is already established, forcing fluids and diuresis is not effective and may in fact be harmful.

There is no specific therapeutic management for acute renal failure. Because the renal lesions are potentially reversible, the primary goal of treatment is to maintain the client in as normal a state as possible while the kidneys are repairing themselves (Table 41-3). The precipitating cause is determined and corrected if possible. Management is focused on controlling the client's symptoms and preventing complications. Conservative therapy may be all that is necessary until renal function resumes. However, the general trend now is to initiate early and frequent dialysis to keep the client as free of symptoms as possible and to prevent complications.

Fluid intake must be closely monitored during the oliguric phase. The common rule for calculating fluid replacement is to consider all losses (e.g., urine, diarrhea, vomitus, blood) plus 500 ml for insensible losses in a 24-hour period. For the next 24-hour period, the client's fluid intake is restricted to the previous day's losses. For example, if a client excreted 300 ml of urine on Tuesday with no other losses, fluid replacement on Wednesday would be 800 ml.

Hyperkalemia is the most important sudden hazard in acute renal failure because it can cause life-threatening cardiac dysrhythmias. The various therapies used to decrease potassium levels are listed in Table 41-4. The first measures described in the table constitute only temporary treatment and do not result in a decrease in total body potassium.

The most common indications for the use of dialysis in acute renal failure include (1) volume overload, (2) potassium level greater than 6 mEq/L, (3) metabolic acidosis (serum bicarbonate level less than 15 mEq/L), (4) BUN level greater than 120 mg/dl, and (5) any other signs of uremic intoxication (e.g., encephalopathy, pericarditis, bleeding).

Hemodialysis has the advantage of efficiency and shorter duration compared with peritoneal dialysis. However, it is technically more complicated and requires anticoagulation therapy. Rapid biochemical changes may induce side effects such as hypotension and disequilibrium syndrome. Peritoneal dialysis is simpler but carries the risk of peritonitis, is less efficient in the catabolic client, and takes a longer time. Peritoneal dialysis may be preferred for individuals with intracranial bleeding or cardiovascular instability. Hemodialysis is preferred for hypercatabolic clients and for clients who have had abdominal or thoracic trauma and/or surgery. Continuous arteriovenous hemofiltration may also be used in the treatment of acute renal failure.

Nutritional Considerations

In the past, the regimen of fluid restriction and nutritional therapy was designed so that body weight would decrease by 0.25 to 0.5 kg/day from the loss of body tissue catabolized on the low-protein diet. Today these severe restrictions are usually not necessary except during the interval between the diagnosis of oliguria and the establishment of dialysis and a nutritional regimen. However, a steady weight or weight gain during this interval usually indicates hypervolemia.

If the client does not receive adequate nutrition, catabolism of body protein will occur. This causes increased urea, phosphate, and potassium levels. The major goal of nutritional management is to decrease catabolism of the body's protein. Carbohydrate intake should be 100 g/day to prevent ketosis from fat breakdown and gluconeogenesis from protein breakdown. Protein intake is generally 1.0

Table 41-3

 Diagnostic and Therapeutic Management: Acute Renal Failure

DIAGNOSTIC

History and physical examination
Identification of precipitating cause
Serum creatinine and BUN levels
Serum electrolytes
Urinalysis

THERAPEUTIC

Treatment of precipitating cause
Fluid restriction (500 ml plus fluid loss)
Dietary management
Measures to lower potassium*
Total parenteral nutrition (if indicated)
Intralipid infusions (if indicated)
Initiation of dialysis (if necessary)

*See Table 41-4.

Table 41-4 Therapies to Lower Serum Potassium Levels

HYPERTONIC GLUCOSE AND INSULIN (IV ADMINISTRATION)

Potassium moves into cells with glucose in the presence of insulin.

SODIUM BICARBONATE (IV ADMINISTRATION)

Therapy can correct acidosis and causes shift of potassium into cells.

CALCIUM GLUCONATE (IV ADMINISTRATION)

Therapy is generally used in advanced cardiac toxicity. Calcium antagonizes the cardiac effects of potassium.

DIALYSIS

Hemodialysis can bring potassium levels to normal within 1-2 hr. Peritoneal dialysis may take 4-8 hr to achieve the same effect.

SODIUM POLYSTYRENE SULFONATE (KAYEXALATE)

Cation-exchange resin (sodium for potassium) is administered by mouth or retention enema. Therapy removes 1 mEq of potassium per gram of drug and is mixed in water with sorbitol to produce osmotic diarrhea.

DIETARY RESTRICTIONS

Daily potassium intake is limited to 2 g (50 mEq).

IV, Intravenous.

to 1.5 g/kg. Essential amino acid supplements (e.g., Amin-Aid) may be given for amino acid and caloric supplementation, either orally or through tube feedings. Potassium and sodium are regulated in accordance with plasma levels. Dietary fat intake is increased so that the client gets at least 35 to 45 calories/kg body weight per day. Intralipid (fat emulsions) infusions can also be given as a nutritional supplement, and they provide a good source of nonprotein calories (see Chapter 35). If a client cannot obtain an adequate oral intake, total parenteral nutrition (TPN) can be used (see Chapter 35). TPN is most commonly used in clients who have had extensive surgical procedures, trauma, burns, or altered GI function. Clients treated with TPN may need daily hemodialysis or continuous arteriovenous hemofiltration to remove the accumulation of excess fluid.

■ Nursing Management of Acute Renal Failure
Nursing interventions

Health maintenance and promotion. Prevention of acute renal failure is primarily directed toward (1) identifying and monitoring high-risk populations and (2) controlling industrial chemicals and nephrotoxic drugs. In the hospital the clients at greatest risk for developing acute renal failure are those who have experienced massive trauma, major surgical procedures, extensive burns, cardiac failure, sepsis, or obstetrical complications. These clients must be monitored carefully for intake and output, fluid and electrolyte balance, and possible blood transfusion reactions. Extrarenal losses of fluid from vomitus, diarrhea, hemorrhage, and increased insensible losses must be assessed and recorded. Intake and output records and each client's weight provide valuable indicators of fluid volume status. Aggressive diuretic therapy for a client with cardiac failure can lead to inadequate renal vascular perfusion.

Streptococcal infections must be identified and treated with antibiotics. Compliance with the antibiotic regimen is critical to eliminate the source of infection. Complications of streptococcal infection include acute poststreptococcal glomerulonephritis and rheumatic heart disease.

Older adult clients or those with diabetes who are undergoing multiple diagnostic studies need special attention to prevent them from becoming dehydrated. Individuals with urinary tract infections need prompt treatment and careful follow-up care. Other persons who are considered at risk are those with hypertension or connective tissue disorders (e.g., systemic lupus erythematosus) and those taking oncolytic drugs that cause hyperuricemia.

Industrial and agricultural chemicals and products (organic solvents, insecticides, cleaning agents) need to be monitored regularly regarding their safety for both the employee and the general population. Individuals who are taking drugs that are potentially nephrotoxic need to have their renal function monitored with serum creatinine and BUN determinations (Table 39-2). Clients should be cautioned about the abuse of over-the-counter analgesics, since some of these are also potentially nephrotoxic drugs.

Acute intervention. The client with acute renal failure is critically ill and suffers not only from the effects of a renal disease but often from those of the nonrenal disease or condition (e.g., surgery, cardiac disease) that contributed to the renal failure. The nursing staff may become overly concerned with the client's urinary output and forget to focus on the client as a total person with many physical and emotional needs. Usually the changes caused by renal failure come on suddenly. Both the client and the family need assistance in understanding that the functioning of the whole body can be disrupted by renal failure. These changes are potentially reversible, since the kidneys can repair themselves.

The nursing role in managing fluid and electrolyte balance is important during the oliguric and diuretic phases. Observing and recording the accurate intake and output of fluids cannot be overemphasized. Daily weights measured with the same scale at the same time each day are essential in evaluating and detecting excessive gains or losses of body fluid (one pound is equivalent to about 500 ml of fluid). The nurse must be knowledgeable about the common signs and symptoms that result from hypervolemia (in the oliguric phase) or hypovolemia (in the diuretic phase), hypernatremia or hyponatremia, hyperkalemia or hypokalemia, and other electrolyte imbalances that may occur in acute renal failure (see Chapter 10). Hyperkalemia is a leading biochemical cause of death in acute renal failure. Most typically, hyperkalemia is manifested with impairment in neuromuscular status and cardiac conduction. Muscle weakness, abdominal cramps, flaccid paralysis, and absence of deep tendon reflexes are signs of neuromuscular impairment. Cardiac conduction abnormalities to watch for include a prolonged PR interval, prolonged QRS interval, peaked T wave, and depressed ST segment.

Because infection is the leading cause of death in acute renal failure, meticulous aseptic technique is critical. The use of an indwelling catheter should be avoided. If acute renal failure is diagnosed in a client, the catheter may be removed. The client should be protected from other individuals with infectious diseases. The nurse should be alert for local manifestations of infection (e.g., swelling, redness, pain) as well as systemic manifestations (e.g., anorexia, malaise, leukocytosis) because an elevated temperature may not be present. If antibiotics are used to treat an infection, the type and dosage must be considered because the kidney is the route of excretion for many antibiotics.

Respiratory complications, especially pneumonitis, can be prevented: humidified oxygen, intermittent positive-pressure breathing, turning, coughing, and deep breathing are measures the nurse can use to help the client maintain adequate respiratory ventilation.

Skin care and measures to prevent decubiti should be performed, since the client usually develops edema as well as muscle loss. Mouth care is important to prevent stomatitis, which develops when urea irritates the mucous membranes.

Chronic management. Recovery from acute renal failure is highly variable and depends on the underlying illness, the general condition and age of the client, the length of the oliguric phase, and the management of the client. The rest of the body as well as the kidneys has experienced a major insult. Good nutrition, rest, and limited ac-

tivity are necessary to restore the client to a functioning state. The diet should be high in calories, and protein intake should be regulated in accordance with renal function. Follow-up care and regular evaluation of renal function are necessary. The client should be taught the signs and symptoms of recurrent renal disease, especially manifestations of fluid and electrolyte imbalances. Measures to prevent the recurrence of acute renal failure must be emphasized.

The long-term convalescence of 3 to 12 months may cause social and financial hardships for the family, and appropriate counseling and referrals should be performed. Occasionally, renal function deteriorates and manifestations of chronic renal failure develop. If the kidneys do not recover, the client progresses to chronic renal failure.

Acute Renal Failure in Older Adults

Older adults are more susceptible than younger adults to acute renal failure. Although decreased renal reserve function is the primary risk factor, age itself and impaired function of other organ systems are independent risk factors. The aging kidney is less able to withstand changes in hydration, solute load, and cardiac output. Common causes of acute renal failure in older adults include dehydration, hypotension, diuretic therapy, aminoglycoside therapy, obstructive disorders (e.g., prostatic hypertrophy), surgery, infection, and radiocontrast agents. The prognosis after acute renal failure is generally worse in older adults than in younger persons. The mortality rate after acute renal failure is 5% to 25% higher in older adults than in younger persons, and death is usually due to infection, GI hemorrhage, or myocardial infarction.[4]

CHRONIC RENAL FAILURE

Chronic renal failure involves progressive, irreversible destruction of both kidneys. The disease process progresses until many nephrons are destroyed and replaced by scar tissue. Although there are many different causes of chronic renal failure (Fig. 41-2), the end result is a systemic disease involving every body organ. (The specific disease processes are discussed in Chapter 40.)

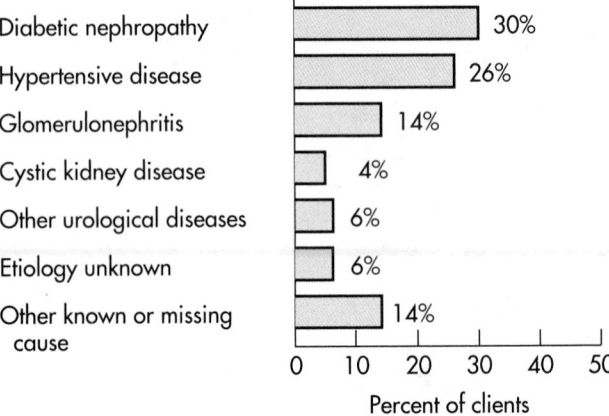

Diabetic nephropathy	30%
Hypertensive disease	26%
Glomerulonephritis	14%
Cystic kidney disease	4%
Other urological diseases	6%
Etiology unknown	6%
Other known or missing cause	14%

0 10 20 30 40 50
Percent of clients

Fig. 41-2 Primary renal disease leading to end-stage renal failure. (From United States Renal Data System, Washington, DC, 1989, Department of Health and Human Services.)

The kidneys have a remarkable functional reserve. Up to 80% of the GFR may be lost with few overt changes in the functioning of the body. Humans are born with 2 million nephrons and can survive (albeit with difficulty) with as few as 20,000.[5] In the vast majority of cases the individual passes through the early stages without recognizing the disease state because the functioning nephrons can compensate. The prognosis and course of chronic renal failure are highly variable. Some individuals live normal, active lives with compensated renal failure, whereas others may rapidly progress to end-stage renal failure.

Although there are no distinct stages in chronic renal failure, the disease progression may be divided into three stages:

1. *Diminished renal reserve*: This stage is characterized by normal BUN and serum creatinine levels and an absence of symptoms.
2. *Renal insufficiency*: This stage occurs when the GFR is about 25% of normal. BUN and serum creatinine levels are slightly increased. Easy fatigue and weakness are common symptoms. As the renal failure progresses, headaches may occur. Nocturia and polyuria occur as a result of the kidneys' loss of ability to concentrate urine.
3. *End-stage renal failure or uremia*: The last stage occurs when the GFR is less than 5% to 10% of normal or when creatinine clearances are less than 5 to 10 ml/min. It is at this stage that most clients begin to have symptoms.

Significance

In the United States over 160,000 individuals have end-stage renal disease (ESRD).[6] Each year over 55,000 people die from various diseases of the kidneys.[6] During the 1970s, dramatic changes in the focus of treatment of chronic renal disease occurred. In July 1973 the federal government enacted a law that provided financial assistance for all persons who had ESRD and required treatment.* Before 1973, treatment was available only to those who could afford the cost of chronic dialysis or renal transplantation.

Since 1973, many deaths have been prevented through the use of maintenance dialysis and renal transplantation. The majority of clients (more than 130,000) are treated with dialysis because of a lack of donated organs, because many clients do not want transplants, or because clients are medically unsuitable for the transplantation procedure.[6] With the expansion of dialysis programs each year, an increasing percentage of older individuals and clients with systemic disease (diabetics and clients with stable cancer) are being maintained on dialysis.

Because of the End-Stage Renal Disease Medicare Program in the United States, almost every client, regardless of age, is offered dialysis. Clients between 55 and 64 years old are now the fastest growing group entering the Medicare Renal Disease Program.[7] In general, transplantation is not an option for older adults unless they are con-

---

*Currently, Medicare pays 80% of the cost of dialysis when the client has been on chronic dialysis for 3 months or has begun home training.

sidered "young older adults" with few, if any, associated diseases.

The increasing number of older adults with ESRD has changed the data relating various diseases to the development of renal failure. Before the mid 1970s, glomerulonephritis and interstitial nephritis were the most common causes. Currently, hypertension and diabetes are the leading causes of renal failure.

Clinical Manifestations

As renal function progressively deteriorates, every organ system becomes involved. The clinical manifestations are due to retained uremic toxins including urea, creatinine, phenols, hormones, abnormal electrolyte concentrations, and many other substances.[8] Uremic syndrome is a total body disease that causes disturbances in the various organ systems (Fig. 41-3). It is important to recognize that the manifestations of uremia vary among clients.

Urinary system. In the stage of renal insufficiency, the most noticeable sign is polyuria that is due to the inability of the kidneys to concentrate urine. Clients notice this most frequently at night when they must arise several times to urinate (nocturia). Because of the decrease in renal concentrating ability, the specific gravity of urine gradually becomes fixed at around 1.010 (the osmolar concentration of plasma). As renal failure progresses, oliguria, and later, anuria occur. If the client is still producing urine, common findings are proteinuria with casts, pyuria, and hematuria.

Metabolic disturbances

Azotemia. As creatinine clearance decreases, the BUN and serum creatinine levels increase. The BUN levels are influenced by protein intake, fever, and catabolic rate. Serum creatinine and creatinine clearance are better indicators of renal function than BUN. As BUN increases, nausea, lethargy, fatigue, vomiting, diarrhea, and headaches become common complaints.

The serum creatinine level in an older adult client with ESRD is lower than the level that is expected in a younger person with the same degree of renal dysfunction. Decreased muscle mass, decreased muscle activity, and decreased meat consumption account for this phenomenon.

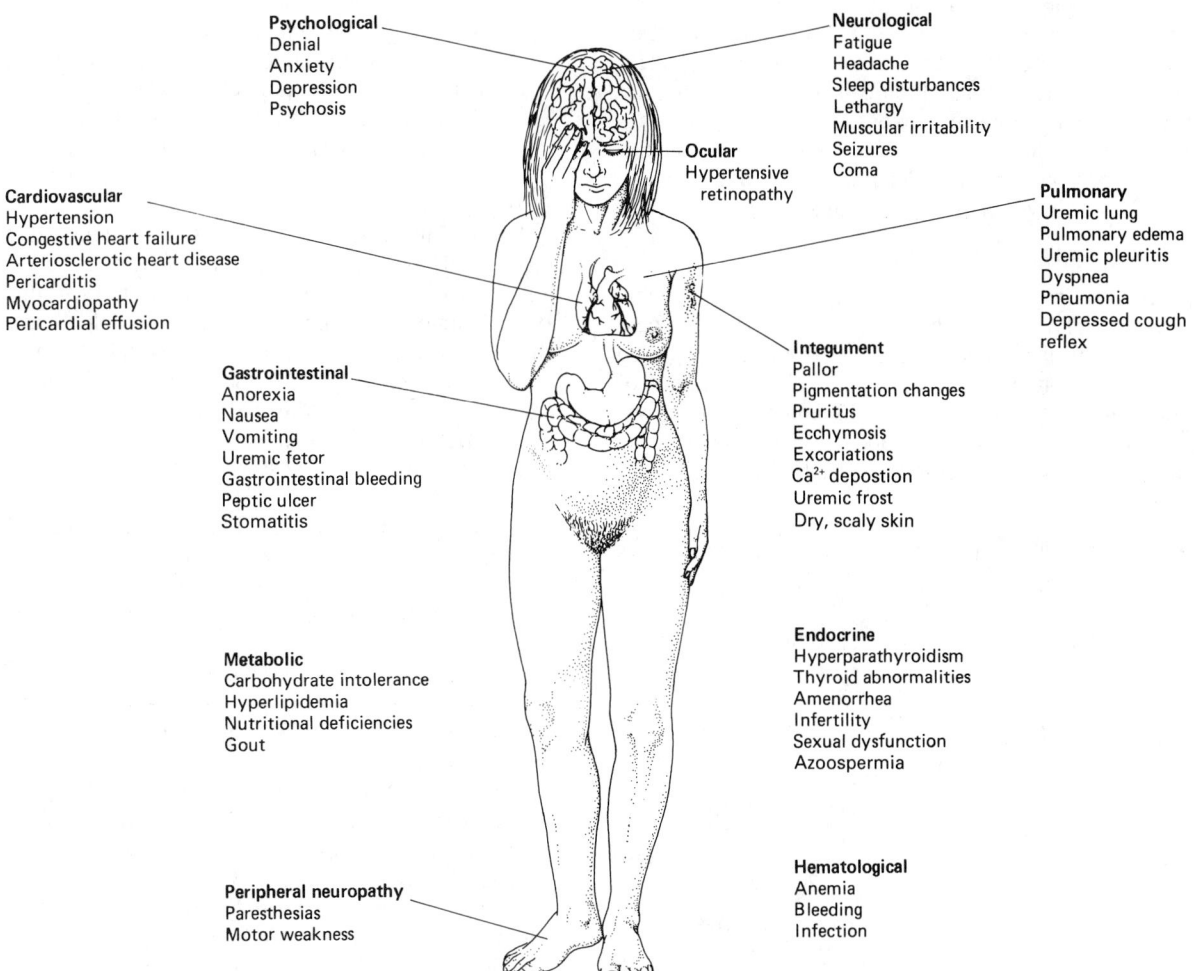

Psychological
Denial
Anxiety
Depression
Psychosis

Neurological
Fatigue
Headache
Sleep disturbances
Lethargy
Muscular irritability
Seizures
Coma

Ocular
Hypertensive
retinopathy

Cardiovascular
Hypertension
Congestive heart failure
Arteriosclerotic heart disease
Pericarditis
Myocardiopathy
Pericardial effusion

Pulmonary
Uremic lung
Pulmonary edema
Uremic pleuritis
Dyspnea
Pneumonia
Depressed cough reflex

Gastrointestinal
Anorexia
Nausea
Vomiting
Uremic fetor
Gastrointestinal bleeding
Peptic ulcer
Stomatitis

Integument
Pallor
Pigmentation changes
Pruritus
Ecchymosis
Excoriations
Ca^{2+} depostion
Uremic frost
Dry, scaly skin

Metabolic
Carbohydrate intolerance
Hyperlipidemia
Nutritional deficiencies
Gout

Endocrine
Hyperparathyroidism
Thyroid abnormalities
Amenorrhea
Infertility
Sexual dysfunction
Azoospermia

Peripheral neuropathy
Paresthesias
Motor weakness

Hematological
Anemia
Bleeding
Infection

Fig. 41-3 *Clinical manifestations of chronic uremia. (Modified from Hekelman F and Ostendarp C: Nephrology nursing, New York, 1979, McGraw-Hill Book Co, Inc.)*

The uric acid level also increases and can lead to precipitation of uric acid crystals, causing gouty arthritis. The actual incidence of gout is low.

The initial treatment for azotemia is protein restriction. As BUN decreases, the nausea, vomiting, and fatigue usually become less noticeable.

Carbohydrate intolerance. Defective carbohydrate metabolism is due to impaired glucose utilization resulting from cellular insensitivity to the normal action of insulin. The exact nature of this insulin resistance is unclear but may be related to circulating insulin antagonists, alterations in hormone receptors, or abnormalities of transport mechanisms. Moderate hyperglycemia, hyperinsulinemia, and abnormal glucose tolerance tests are common findings. Insulin and glucose metabolism may improve (but not to normal values) after the initiation of dialysis. Individuals who have diabetes mellitus and then become uremic may require less insulin than they did before the onset of chronic renal failure. The insulin doses of insulin-dependent diabetics must be individualized and monitored carefully.

Elevated triglycerides. The hyperinsulinemia stimulates hepatic production of triglycerides, and the assimilation of triglycerides by peripheral tissues is diminished. Almost all clients with uremia develop hyperlipidemia, which is usually a type IV profile with elevated very low-density lipoproteins (VLDLs), normal low-density lipoproteins (LDLs), and lowered high-density lipoproteins (HDLs). The reason for the altered lipid metabolism is related to decreased levels of the enzyme lipoprotein lipase, which is important in the breakdown of lipoproteins. Type IV hyperlipidemia is a definite risk factor for accelerated atherosclerosis (see Chapter 28). This dysfunction compounds the problem in diabetics with renal disease who already have increased atherosclerotic changes.

The serum level of triglycerides does not usually decrease after dialysis is started. In clients who are on chronic peritoneal dialysis, it frequently becomes higher as a result of the increased amounts of glucose absorbed from the peritoneal dialysate fluid.

Electrolyte imbalances

Potassium. Hyperkalemia is the most serious electrolyte problem associated with renal failure. Fatal dysrhythmias can occur when the serum potassium level reaches 7 to 8 mEq/L. Hyperkalemia results from the failure of the excretory ability of the kidneys, the breakdown of cellular protein with the subsequent release of potassium, and acidosis, which contributes to the shift of potassium from intracellular to extracellular spaces.

Metabolic acidosis. Metabolic acidosis results from the impaired ability of the kidneys to excrete the acid load (primarily ammonia) and from defective reabsorption and regeneration of bicarbonate. Plasma bicarbonate usually stabilizes at a new steady state at around 16 to 20 mEq/L. It usually does not progress below this level because hydrogen ion production is usually balanced by buffering from demineralization of the bone (the phosphate buffering system). Kussmaul's respiration is less prominent in chronic than in acute renal failure and reduces the severity of acidosis by increasing carbon dioxide excretion.

Magnesium. Magnesium is primarily excreted by the kidneys. Hypermagnesemia is generally not a problem unless the client experiences a sudden intake of magnesium (e.g., from milk of magnesia, magnesium citrate, antacids containing magnesium).

Sodium. Sodium levels can range from low to high. Hypernatremia does not usually develop until the later stages of renal failure. Sodium retention can contribute to edema, hypertension, and congestive heart failure. Sodium intake needs to be individually determined.

Hematological system

Anemia. The anemia associated with chronic renal failure is classified as normocytic, normochromic, reflecting hypoproliferative activity of the bone marrow. Anemia remains relatively stable at hematocrit levels varying from 15% to 35%. Clients on chronic peritoneal dialysis may have higher hematocrits than those on long-term hemodialysis. The main cause of anemia is decreased production of erythropoietin by the kidney, resulting in decreased erythropoiesis by the bone marrow. Other factors contributing to anemia are nutritional deficiencies, decreased RBC life span, increased hemolysis of RBCs, the need for frequent blood samples, and bleeding from the GI tract.[9] For clients on maintenance hemodialysis, blood loss in the dialyzer may also contribute to the anemic state. Folic acid is dialyzable, and if it is not adequately replaced in the diet or by drugs, megaloblastic anemia may develop in a client on chronic hemodialysis. In addition, elevated levels of parathyroid hormone (produced in these clients to compensate for low serum calcium levels) may constitute a uremic toxin, inhibiting erythropoiesis and shortening survival of RBCs as well as stimulating bone marrow fibrosis, which can result in decreased numbers of hematopoietic cells.

Bleeding tendencies. The most common cause of bleeding in uremia is a qualitative defect in platelet function. This dysfunction is due to impaired platelet aggregation and impaired release of platelet factor 3. The altered platelet function, hemorrhagic tendencies, and GI bleeding are usually reversible by means of hemodialysis or peritoneal dialysis. In addition, there are alterations in the coagulation system with increased concentrations of both factor VIII and fibrinogen found in the serum of these clients.

Infection. Infectious complications are due to changes in leukocyte function and altered immunological response and function. A diminished inflammatory response occurs as a result of an altered chemotactic response by both neutrophils and monocytes. This impairment significantly decreases the accumulation of WBCs at the site of injury or infection. Both cellular and humoral immune responses are also suppressed. Characteristic clinical findings include lymphopenia, lymphoid atrophy (especially of the thymus), decreased antibody production, and suppression of the delayed hypersensitivity response. Other factors contributing to the increased risk of infection include protein malnutrition, the uremic effect on mucous membranes, hyperglycemia, and the presence of external trauma (e.g., from catheters, needle insertions into vascular access sites).

Cardiovascular system. The most common cardiovascular abnormality is hypertension, which is usually due to

sodium retention and increased extracellular fluid volume. In some individuals, increased renin production contributes to the problem (Fig. 39-6). Hypertension accelerates atherosclerotic vascular disease, produces intrarenal arterial spasm, and eventually leads to left ventricular hypertrophy and congestive heart failure. Hypertension also causes retinopathy and encephalopathy.

Congestive heart failure from left ventricular hypertrophy can lead to pulmonary edema. Peripheral edema is also commonly present. Cardiac dysrhythmias may result from hyperkalemia, hypocalcemia, and decreased coronary artery perfusion.

Uremic pericarditis develops and occasionally progresses to a pericardial effusion and cardiac tamponade. Pericarditis is manifested by a friction rub, chest pain, hypotension, pulsus paradoxus, and low-grade fever.

The vascular changes from long-standing hypertension and the accelerated atherosclerosis from elevated triglyceride levels account for cardiovascular complications (e.g., myocardial infarction, cerebrovascular accident) being the leading cause of death for clients on maintenance dialysis.

Respiratory system. Respiratory changes include Kussmaul's respiration, dyspnea from congestive heart failure, pulmonary edema, uremic pleuritis (pleurisy), pleural effusion, and a predisposition to respiratory infections, which may be related to decreased pulmonary macrophage activity. The sputum is thick and tenacious. The cough reflex is depressed. "Uremic lung," or uremic pneumonitis, is typically found in chronic renal failure and shows up as an interstitial edema on chest x-ray examination. This condition usually responds to vigorous dialysis treatments.

Gastrointestinal system. Every part of the GI system becomes affected as a result of inflammation of the mucosa by excessive urea. Mucosal ulcerations, found throughout the GI tract, are caused by the increased ammonia produced by bacterial breakdown of urea. Stomatitis with exudations and ulcerations, a metallic taste in the mouth, and a urinous odor of the breath are commonly found. Anorexia, nausea, and vomiting contribute to weight loss. Peptic ulcer disease can also be found in clients with chronic renal failure. Diarrhea may occur because of hyperkalemia and altered calcium metabolism. Constipation is a frequent complication of aluminum hydroxide medications (antacids), which are taken to lower phosphate levels.

Neurological system. Neurological changes are expected as renal failure progresses. The exact cause of these changes is unknown, but they may be partially attributed to increased nitrogenous waste products, electrolyte imbalances, and axonal atrophy and demyelination of nerve fibers. High levels of uremic toxins have been implicated in axonal damage.

A general depression of the central nervous system (CNS) results in lethargy, apathy, decreased ability to concentrate, fatigue, and altered mental ability. Convulsions and coma may result from hypertensive encephalopathy and an extremely elevated BUN. Dialysis encephalopathy (dialysis dementia) has also been associated with aluminum toxicity.

Peripheral neuropathy is initially manifested by a slowing of nerve conduction to the extremities. The client complains of a restless leg syndrome and may describe it as "bugs crawling inside the leg." Paresthesia, especially of both feet and legs, may be described by the client as a burning sensation. Eventually, motor involvement may lead to bilateral footdrop, various degrees of paralysis, muscular weakness and atrophy, and loss of deep tendon reflexes. Muscle twitching, jerking, asterixis, and nocturnal leg cramps also occur.

No treatment for neurological problems, except dialysis and transplantation, is available. Sensory impairment is often a signal to start dialysis. Dialysis may reduce the symptoms and halt the progress of neuropathies, but not necessarily. Motor neuropathy may not be reversible. The problem of neuropathy is compounded in the diabetic who has not only diabetic neuropathy but also the neuropathies of renal failure.

Musculoskeletal system. Renal osteodystrophy is a syndrome of skeletal changes found in chronic renal failure. It is due to alterations in calcium phosphate metabolism (Fig. 41-4). Normally, the calcium phosphate ratio maintains the electrolytes in an insoluble state. As the GFR decreases, phosphate is not excreted by the kidney. Calcium phosphate complexes form and are deposited in various parts of the body (metastatic calcification). Low serum calcium stimulates a rise in parathyroid hormone, which causes bone resorption of calcium. This eventually leads to demineralization of the bones and an elevated alkaline phosphatase level.

Normally, the kidney metabolizes vitamin D (formed in the skin or ingested) to its active form. The active form of vitamin D is needed for adequate calcium absorption from the GI tract. In renal failure the kidney fails to activate vitamin D, and calcium absorption is thus impaired.

The changes resulting from increased phosphate retention, bone resorption of calcium, inadequate calcium absorption, and elevated parathyroid hormone levels lead to the following conditions:

1. *Osteomalacia*: This condition results from lack of mineralization of newly formed bone secondary to hypocalcemia. Most commonly this is due to aluminum accumulation, since the primary route for excretion is through the kidneys.
2. *Osteitis fibrosa*: This condition results from calcium resorption from the bone and replacement with fibrous tissue. This is primarily caused by elevated parathyroid hormone levels.
3. *Metastatic calcification* (soft-tissue calcification): This condition results from calcium phosphate deposits in soft tissues of the body. Common sites are the blood vessels, joints, lungs, muscles, myocardium, and eyes. "Uremic red eye" is due to the irritation of the deposits. Arterial calcification in the fingers and toes may cause gangrene.

Integumentary system. The most noticeable change in the integumentary system is a yellowish discoloration of the skin. This change is due to the absorption and retention of urinary chromogens that normally give the characteristic color to urine. The skin also appears pale as a result of

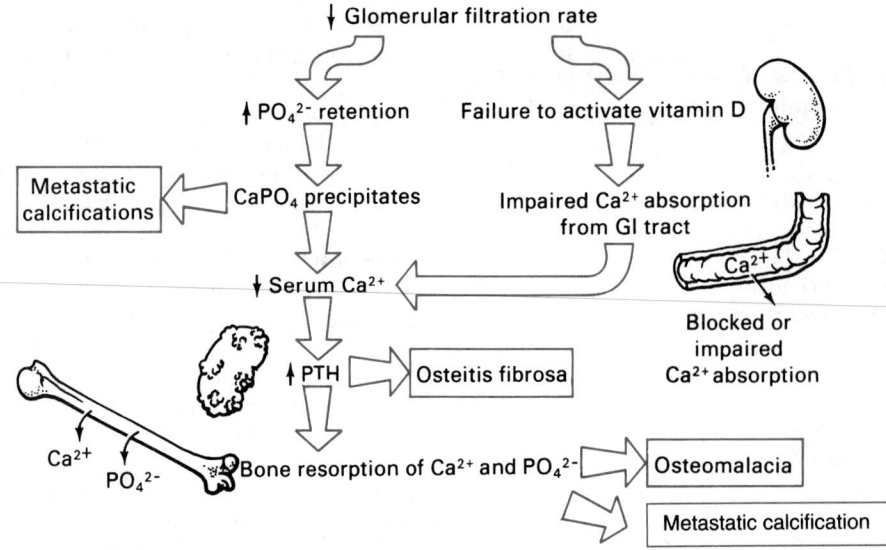

Fig. 41-4 Mechanisms of renal osteodystrophy.

anemia and is dry and scaly because of a decrease in oil-gland activity. Decreased perspiration results from a decrease in size of the sweat glands.

Pruritus most commonly results from a combination of the dry skin, calcium phosphate precipitations in the skin, and sensory neuropathy. The itching may be so intense that it can lead to bleeding or infection. Pruritus also may be due to uremic frost, which results from urea crystallization on the skin. Uremic frost is usually seen only when BUN levels are extremely high.

The hair is dry and brittle and may fall out. The nails are thin, brittle, and ridged. Petechiae and ecchymoses may be present and are due to clotting abnormalities.

Reproductive system. Both sexes characteristically experience infertility and a decrease in libido. Women usually have decreased levels of estrogen, progesterone, and luteinizing hormone, causing anovulation and menstrual changes (usually amenorrhea). Menses and ovulation may return after dialysis is started. Men experience loss of testicular consistency, decreased testosterone levels, and low sperm counts. Sexual dysfunction may also be due to anemia, which causes fatigue and decreased libido. In addition, peripheral neuropathy can cause impotence in men and anorgasmy in women. Additional factors for changes in sexual function are psychological problems (e.g., anxiety, depression), physical stress, and side effects of medication.

Sexual function may improve with maintenance dialysis and may return to normal with successful transplantation. Some dialysis clients and many kidney transplant recipients have parented children.

Endocrine system. All clients with chronic renal failure exhibit some clinical manifestations of hypothyroidism. Tests of thyroid function yield low to low-normal levels for serum triiodothyronine (T_3) and thyroxine (T_4) levels. Neither the clinical significance nor the exact reason for these findings is known.

Psychological changes. Personality and behavior changes, emotional lability, withdrawal, and depression are commonly observed. Fatigue and lethargy contribute to the client's feeling of sickness. The changes in body image caused by edema and integumentary disturbances lead to further anxiety and depression. Decreased ability to concentrate and lessened mental activity make the client appear dull and uninterested in the environment. The client is faced with significant changes in lifestyle, occupation, family responsibilities, and financial status. The client's future depends on drugs, dietary restrictions, dialysis, and possibly another person's kidney.

Conservative Management

When a client is diagnosed as having chronic renal insufficiency, conservative management is attempted before maintenance dialysis begins (Table 41-5). Every effort is made to detect and treat potentially reversible causes of renal failure (e.g., cardiac failure, dehydration, pyelonephritis, nephrotoxins, lower urinary tract obstruction). Conservative management is directed toward (1) preserving existing renal function, (2) treating the symptoms, (3) preventing complications, and (4) providing for the client's comfort. Conservative management primarily consists of pharmacological and nutritional intervention.

Pharmacological management

Hyperkalemia. Acute hyperkalemia is usually treated with intravenous (IV) glucose and insulin or IV 10% calcium gluconate (Table 41-4). Dietary restrictions of protein and foods high in potassium are needed. Sodium polystyrene sulfonate (Kayexalate), a cation-exchange resin, is used to lower potassium levels. The exchange resin, administered orally or rectally, exchanges 1 mEq of sodium for 1 mEq of potassium. The potassium is bound to the resin, which is excreted in the stool. Since Kayexalate is constipating, a bulk laxative (usually sorbitol) is given. The client should be told to expect some diarrhea.

Table 41-5

Diagnostic and Therapeutic Management: Chronic Renal Failure

DIAGNOSTIC

Identification of reversible renal disease
   Renal biopsy
   Radiographic studies
Hematocrit and hemoglobin level
BUN, serum creatinine, and creatinine clearance levels
Serum electrolytes
Urinalysis and urine culture

THERAPEUTIC

Correction of extracellular fluid volume overload or deficit
Dietary restrictions
Multivitamins
Maintenance of hematinic and androgen levels
Administration of phosphate-binding antacids
Antihypertensive therapy
Measures to lower potassium*
Adjustment of drug dosages to degree of renal function

---

*See Table 41-4.

Hypertension. Treatment of hypertension initially consists of sodium and fluid restriction and the administration of furosemide (Lasix). The antihypertensive drugs used are methyldopa (Aldomet), hydralazine (Apresoline), captopril (Capoten), propranolol (Inderal), minoxidil (Loniten), and clonidine (Catapres) (see Chapter 27). β-Adrenergic antagonists such as propranolol may decrease renin release. The blood pressure should be measured in supine, sitting, and standing positions to effectively monitor the antihypertensive drugs. The blood pressure should be maintained below 150/100 mm Hg. However, too vigorous treatment can cause a hypotensive reaction in a client who has compensated for long-standing hypertension.

Renal osteodystrophy. Initially, dietary restriction of protein also decreases phosphate intake. Aluminum hydroxide gels and antacids (e.g., Amphojel, Basaljel, and Alternagel) are used to bind the phosphate, which is then excreted in the stool. Magnesium-containing antacids should not be given because magnesium is not eliminated by the malfunctioning kidneys, and the kidneys do not bind phosphate as effectively as aluminum-containing antacids. Phosphate binders should be administered with each meal to be effective. Aluminum hydroxide is available in liquid, tablet, capsule (Alu-Caps), and cookie form (Phos-Lo cookies); if the client finds one form unpalatable, another form may be substituted. Because aluminum hydroxide contributes to constipation, stool softeners are usually prescribed. Excessive absorption of aluminum may occur, and this can lead to aluminum bone disease (osteomalacia) and in some instances, dialysis encephalopathy. Calcium carbonate and calcium acetate are currently being used more frequently as substitutes for aluminum phosphates.[10,11] When administered with meals, calcium carbonate forms relatively insoluble complexes with dietary phosphates and is excreted in the feces.

If hypocalcemia persists in spite of controlled serum phosphate levels, supplemental calcium may be given. The active form of vitamin D is commercially available in oral preparations such as calcitriol (Rocaltrol) and calcifediol (Calderol) and in injection form as calcitriol (Calcijex). It is important to lower the phosphate level before administering calcium or vitamin D because these drugs may contribute to soft-tissue calcification if both calcium and phosphate levels are elevated. If renal osteodystrophy remains severe, a subtotal parathyroidectomy may be performed to decrease the synthesis and secretion of parathyroid hormone.

The most common methods for evaluating the status of the bone disease are skeletal x-ray examination, bone scans, bone biopsy, and bone densitometry.

Anemia. The most important cause of renal anemia is a decreased production of erythropoietin. With the introduction of recombinant DNA technology, human erythropoietin can now be made in large amounts and is now available for the treatment of anemia.[12,13] It can be administered IV during dialysis or subcutaneously. Erythropoietin has been very effective in treating anemia. Clinically, a significant increase is usually not seen for 2 to 3 weeks. Clients who are receiving erythropoietin have an improved cardiac performance as well as an enhanced quality of life.

A common adverse effect of human erythropoietin is the development or aggravation of hypertension. The underlying mechanism is unclear but may be related to the hemodynamic changes (e.g., increased whole blood viscosity) that occur as the client's anemia is corrected. Another side effect of erythropoietin is the development of functional iron deficiency as a result of the increased demand for iron in newly synthesized hemoglobin.

Regular maintenance dialysis marginally increases erythropoiesis. Supplemental folic acid (1 mg or more daily) is usually given. Most clients receive oral iron supplements. Parenteral iron is used if iron deficiencies persist in spite of oral iron intake. Orally administered iron should not be taken at the same time as aluminum hydroxide antacids because the aluminum binds the iron.

Androgen therapy (nandrolone decanoate, fluoxymesterone, and testosterone propionate) stimulates RBC production in some but not all clients. Side effects reported with long-term androgen treatment in men include increased muscular bulk, improved sexual function, and priapism. Side effects in women include hirsutism, voice changes, and acne.

Blood transfusions should be avoided in treating anemia unless the client experiences an acute blood loss or has symptomatic anemia (i.e., dyspnea, excess fatigue, tachycardia, palpitations). Undesirable effects of transfusions are the suppression of erythropoiesis as a result of a decrease in the hypoxic stimulus, the transmission of hepatitis, and the possibility of an iron overload.

Complications of drug therapy. Most drugs are excreted partially or totally by the kidneys. Drug dosages must be adapted to the degree of renal failure. Drug toxicity is a serious problem in clients with uremia. Delayed and decreased elimination leads to an accumulation of drugs in the body. Increased sensitivity to the drug may result as drug levels increase in the blood and tissues.

Table 41-6   Daily Nutritional Requirements for Clients with Chronic Renal Failure*

	Conservative Management	Hemodialysis	Peritoneal Dialysis
Fluid allowance	Urine output plus 500 ml	Urine output plus 1000 ml	No restriction
Protein†	0.5 g/kg body weight	1.0-1.5 g/kg IBW	1.5-2.0 g/kg IBW
Calories	35-40 kcal/kg EDW	35-40 kcal/kg EDW	35-40 kcal/kg IBW
Fat	Determined by caloric requirement	Determined by caloric requirement	Determined by caloric requirement
Carbohydrate	Unlimited intake of sugars and starches, bread and cereal products limited because of protein limit	Same as for conservative management	30% of calories to unlimited intake
Iron	No supplementation	900 mg supplement	500-900 mg supplement
Potassium	40-70 mEq	40-70 mEq	No restriction
Sodium	1-3 g	2-4 g	No restriction
Phosphorus	700-1200 mg	700-1200 mg	700-1200 mg
Calcium	1000-2000 mg	1000-1500 mg	1000-1500 mg
Folic acid	1.0 mg supplement	1.0 mg supplement	1.0 mg supplement

IBW, Ideal body weight; *EDW,* estimated dry weight.
*Contributed by Beverly J. Spears, R.D., New Mexico Artificial Kidney Center, Albuquerque, NM.
†At least 70% of protein intake should be of high biological value (e.g., coming from eggs, milk, and meat).

Digitalis preparations are excreted largely by the kidneys. Digitalization and maintenance drug dosages may have to be adjusted. Dialysis does not affect body levels of digoxin, but it does affect potassium levels, which can potentiate the action of digitalis.

Aminoglycosides (gentamicin, kanamycin, tobramycin), cephaloridines, penicillin in high doses, and tetracyclines are potentially nephrotoxic. Aspirin, which inhibits platelet aggregation, can produce significant bleeding in a uremic client.

Nutritional considerations

Protein restriction. Before the use of maintenance dialysis, Giovannetti and Giordano designed a 20 g, high-quality protein diet to prevent the accumulation of nitrogenous waste products. This diet provided the essential amino acids from eggs and milk. No meat was allowed. In addition to eggs and milk, low-protein vegetables, noodles, butter balls, and high-carbohydrate foods were included. Client acceptance of this dietary regimen was poor, and clients were malnourished as well as vitamin deficient.

The current diet is designed to be as normal as possible to maintain good nutrition (Table 41-6). For the client who is not undergoing dialysis, one guide is to restrict protein intake to 0.5 g/kg of ideal body weight (IBW) when the creatinine clearance is less than 20 ml/min. Some treatment centers use a routine 40 g protein diet (Table 41-7). Because this diet is deficient in vitamins, multivitamins are prescribed. Once the client is started on dialysis, protein intake can be increased to 1.0 to 1.5 g/kg of IBW. Dietary protein guidelines for clients on peritoneal dialysis differ from those for clients on hemodialysis. Because excessive amounts of protein are lost in the dialysate during peritoneal dialysis, the protein intake must be high enough to compensate for the losses so that the nitrogen balance is maintained. The recommended protein intake is 1.5 to 2.0 g/kg of IBW. For all clients with renal failure, at least 70% of protein intake should come from eggs, milk, poultry, and meat; these foods are considered to have high biological value because they contain the essential amino acids.

Sufficient calories from carbohydrates and fat are needed to minimize catabolism of body protein and maintain body weight. Therefore 100 g of carbohydrates and an appropriate amount of fat are prescribed to maintain an intake of 2000 to 2500 calories per day (see Table 41-6 for specific guidelines).

Lowering the protein intake decreases the metabolic end products of urea, potassium, phosphate, and hydrogen. As the BUN level decreases, the symptoms of nausea, vomiting, fatigue, and headache become less troublesome.

Commercially prepared products that are high in calories and low in protein, sodium, and potassium are available. Liquid and powder preparations include Cal-Power, HY-Cal, Controlyte, and Polycose. Products containing only the essential amino acids (Amin-Aid) can also be used as dietary supplements.

Water restriction. Water intake depends on the daily urine output. Generally, 500 ml (from insensible loss) plus an amount equal to the urine output is allowed for a client with chronic renal failure who is not on dialysis. This amount of fluid is in addition to the fluid found in food. Foods that are liquid at room temperature (e.g., Jell-O and ice cream) should be counted as fluid intake. The fluid allotment should be spaced throughout the day so that the client does not become uncomfortable from thirst. During chronic hemodialysis, fluid intake is adjusted so that ideally the client gains no more than 1.0 to 1.5 kg between dialyses.

Sodium and potassium restriction. The amount of sodium and potassium restriction depends on the ability of the kidneys to excrete these electrolytes. Sodium-restricted diets may vary from 500 to 2300 mg (1 mEq = 23 mg of sodium), depending on the degree of edema and hyperten-

Table 41-7 Diet Plan for Clients with Renal Failure

GENERAL PRINCIPLES

1. Protein, sodium, potassium, phosphorus, and fluids are controlled to meet each client's needs.
2. Protein sources should be of high biological value.
3. High-sodium foods and high-potassium foods should be avoided.
4. Sufficient calories and nutrients are provided to meet daily requirements.

Meal	Exchanges	Sample Menu Plans*		
Breakfast	1 fruit	60 ml grape juice	60 ml apple juice	Applesauce
	1 bread	Toast or corn flakes	Tortilla	Grits
	1 meat	Scrambled egg	Fried egg	Poached egg
	3 fats	2 tsp margarine or butter	2 tsp butter	2 tsp butter
		30 ml cream	30 ml cream	30 ml cream
		Jelly	Jam	Jam
	Beverage	250 ml decaf coffee	250 ml decaf coffee	250 ml decaf coffee
	Dairy	120 ml milk	120 ml milk	120 ml milk
Lunch	1 meat	Salt-free tuna, ¼ cup	2 enchiladas (using ¼ cup ground beef, 2 corn tortillas, and shredded lettuce)	Fried chicken leg
	2 breads	2 slices bread		Cornbread
				½ cup rice
	Vegetable	Lettuce and cucumber	Chili sauce	Zucchini
	Fruit	Canned plums	Canned pears	Canned peaches
	2 fats	2 tbs salt-free mayonnaise	2 tbs oil for cooking	1 tsp butter
		Hard candy	Jelly beans	1 tbs oil for cooking
				Hard candy
	Beverage	250 ml carbonated beverage	250 ml carbonated beverage	250 ml carbonated beverage
Dinner	1 meat	1 oz fried fresh fish	1 oz chicken	1 oz pork
	1 bread	½ cup mashed potatoes (using presoaked potatoes)	1 salt-free corn or flour tortilla to make chicken taco	Salt-free corn on the cob
	Vegetable	Salt-free green peas	Tossed salad	Salt-free green beans
	Fruit	Fruit cocktail	Canned pineapple	Grapes
	3 fats	30 ml cream	30 ml cream	2 tsp butter
		1 tbs fat for cooking	2 tbs salt-free dressing	
		1 tsp butter		
	Beverage	250 ml fruit punch	250 ml fruit punch	250 ml fruit punch
		250 ml decaf coffee	250 ml decaf coffee	250 ml decaf coffee
Snack		120 ml gelatin dessert with whipped topping	180 ml Popsicle	Butter balls
		140 ml carbonated beverage†	80 ml carbonated beverage	320 ml carbonated beverage

*Each diet plan contains 40 g protein, 40 mEq potassium, 2 g sodium, and 1500 ml fluid. To increase the protein to 60 g, the dietitian can add 3 oz meat; 1 egg and 2 oz meat; 120 ml milk, 1 egg, and 1½ oz meat; or 120 ml milk and 2½ oz meat. With the increase in protein, the potassium level also increases to 60 mEq.
†Coke is an acceptable beverage.

sion. (The average daily intake of sodium is 8 to 15 g.) Sodium and salt should not be equated because the sodium content in 1 g of sodium chloride is equivalent to 400 mg of sodium. The client should be instructed to avoid foods known to be high in sodium such as cured meats, pickled foods, canned soups and stews, frankfurters, cold cuts, soy sauce, and salad dressings. Some salt substitutes should not be used because they contain potassium chloride.

Controlled dietary restrictions of potassium range from 1500 to 2500 mg (1 mEq = 39 mg of potassium). For every 20 g increase in dietary protein, the potassium intake is increased by 500 mg. This makes it virtually impossible to restrict potassium to 40 mEq (1.6 g) in an 80 g protein diet because most foods that are high in protein are also high in potassium. Foods with high potassium levels that should be avoided are dried fruits, legumes, oranges, bananas, melons, deep green and deep yellow vegetables, beans, and peas (see Table 41-8).

Low-protein diets. Recent research indicates that a low-protein (0.4 to 0.6 g/kg), low-phosphorus diet supplemented with amino acids and their ketoanalogues can actu-

Table 41-8 High-Potassium Foods*

FRUITS

1 medium tangerine, 108 mg	1 fresh pear, 230 mg	1/10 wedge honeydew melon, 351 mg
1/2 cup fresh pineapple, 113 mg	1/2 cup prune juice, 300 mg	1 nectarine, 406 mg
1/2 cup pineapple juice, 188 mg	3 apricots, 301 mg	1 medium banana, 440 mg
1 dried fig, 126 mg	1/2 cup apricot nectar, 188 mg	10 dried prunes, 448 mg
1/2 grapefruit, 170 mg	1 fresh peach, 308 mg	10 dates, 518 mg
1/2 cup grapefruit juice, 200 mg	1/2 fresh papaya, 337 mg	1/2 cup raisins, 553 mg
1 medium orange, 194 mg	1/4 cantaloupe	1/2 avocado, 680 mg
1/2 cup orange juice, 241 mg		

COOKED VEGETABLES

1/2 cup broccoli, 200 mg	2½-in diameter tomato, 222 mg	1/2 cup rhubarb, 274 mg
1/2 cup rutabagas, 200 mg	1/2 cup tomato juice, 276 mg	1/2 cup pumpkin, 294 mg
1/2 cup pared and boiled potatoes, 221 mg	1/2 cup Brussels sprouts, 228 mg	1/2 cup winter squash, 316 mg
1 baked potato, 782 mg	1/2 cup pinto beans, 234 mg	1/2 cup mashed parsnips, 398 mg
1/2 cup yams, 215 mg	1/2 cup vegetable juice cocktail, 268 mg	Artichokes, 458 mg

MISCELLANEOUS

1 tbs wheat germ, 57 mg	1 cup bran cereal, 137 mg	1 tbs light molasses, 183 mg
1 slice whole grain bread, 72 mg	10 pecans, 54 mg	1 tbs dark molasses, 585 mg
1 slice white bread, 25 mg	10 peanuts, 127 mg	1 oz chocolate, 235 mg
1 oz meat, 85 mg	10 walnuts, 223 mg	1 cup milk, 351 mg
1 tbs cocoa, 106 mg		

*39 mg potassium = 1 mEq potassium.

ally slow the progression of renal failure.[14] Keto acids of essential amino acids have been used as a dietary supplement in Europe and are now being used on a limited basis in the United States. The rationale for using this treatment is that in the body, nonessential amino acids transfer amine groups to the essential keto acids synthesizing essential amino acids. Thus the nitrogen present in nonessential amino acids is used and the total nitrogen intake is kept to an absolute minimum. Keto acid supplements are available in liquid preparations.

■ Nursing Management of Chronic Renal Failure

Nursing interventions

Acute intervention. The specific nursing management related to various problems is included in the nursing care plan for clients with chronic renal failure (Table 41-9). In addition, it is very important to educate clients because they are responsible for their own diets, medications, and follow-up care for their disease. They should weigh themselves daily, learn to take daily blood pressures (if possible), and identify signs and symptoms of edema, hyperkalemia, and other electrolyte imbalances. Clients and their families need to understand the importance of strict dietary adherence. The dietitian and the nurse need to meet with clients and families on a continuing basis to assist them in diet planning. A diet history and consideration of cultural variations make diet planning and adherence more easily achieved goals.

Clients need a complete understanding of their drugs, the dosages, and the common side effects. It may be help-

ful to make a list of the medications and the times of administration that can be posted in their homes in convenient locations. Clients need to be instructed to avoid certain over-the-counter drugs such as aspirin, laxatives, and antacids that contain magnesium.

It is important that clients be motivated to assume the primary role in the management of their disease. The period of conservative management provides a good opportunity to evaluate each client's ability to manage the disease. This is a critical factor in considering each client as a candidate for home dialysis or transplantation.

Chronic management. The length of time a client can be maintained on conservative management is highly variable and depends on the progression of renal failure. When conservative therapy is no longer effective, dialysis and transplantation are the only measures that can be used to prolong life.

While the client is being maintained on conservative management, the decision regarding future therapies, if any, should be made. This must be done before complications such as bleeding, progressive neuropathies, and persistent congestive heart failure occur. Dialysis is more effective in preventing complications than in treating them.

Clients and their families need a clear explanation of what is involved in dialysis and transplantation. If alternative treatments are presented early enough in the course of therapy, clients will have an opportunity to carefully consider their choices. They need to be informed that if they choose dialysis, the option of transplantation still remains.

Table 41-9

 NURSING CARE PLAN FOR THE CLIENT WITH CHRONIC RENAL FAILURE

Defining Characteristics	Nursing Interventions	Evaluation Criteria

NURSING DIAGNOSIS: Fluid volume excess related to inability of kidney to excrete fluid, inadequate dialysis, excessive fluid intake, and elevated plasma sodium levels

Edema, hypertension, bounding pulse, peripheral venous distention, weight gain, shortness of breath, pulmonary edema	Restrict fluid and sodium intake as ordered. Maintain a low-sodium diet. Administer prescribed diuretics. Weigh client daily. Monitor fluid intake and output. Observe and record amount of periorbital, sacral, and peripheral edema. Provide skin care with special emphasis on edematous areas. Evaluate edematous areas. Reposition client q 2 hr. Auscultate chest for rales. Observe for dyspnea.	Absence or control of edema, no evidence of dyspnea, dry weight remaining within 2 pounds of client's established dry weight, blood pressure within limits defined for client

NURSING DIAGNOSIS: Potential complication: hypertension related to sodium and water retention and alterations of renin-angiotensin system

Elevated blood pressure, headache, dizziness, shortness of breath, chest pain, edema	Take vital signs q 4 hr (with client lying, sitting, standing). Administer antihypertensive medications as ordered. Observe for orthostatic hypotension and other side effects of medication. Instruct client to change positions slowly. Explain to client the actions and side effects of drugs.	Maintenance of blood pressure within acceptable range of client

NURSING DIAGNOSIS: Potential complication: hyperkalemia related to decreased renal excretion, increased tissue catabolism, and shift of potassium into extracellular fluid related to metabolic acidosis

Serum potassium > 5.5 mEq/L, muscle weakness, dysrhythmias, paresthesias, intestinal colic and diarrhea, tall T waves on ECG	Discuss with client importance of following prescribed diet and avoiding foods high in potassium. Monitor serum potassium and notify physician of elevated levels. Be prepared to administer treatment for hyperkalemia.*	Maintenance of serum potassium at <6 mEq/L, no signs of hyperkalemia on ECG

NURSING DIAGNOSIS: High risk for injury: fracture related to altered calcium and phosphate absorption, metabolism, and excretion; decreased vitamin D metabolism; and metastatic calcifications

Hypocalcemia, elevated serum phosphate levels, muscle pain, limited mobility of joints, deposition of calcium phosphate in joints and other places, demineralization of bone	Monitor serum calcium and phosphate levels. Observe for manifestations of bone pain. Provide range-of-motion exercises and encourage ambulation. Administer aluminum hydroxide, calcium supplements, and vitamin D as ordered. (Give aluminum hydroxide with meals.) Observe for and prevent constipation when aluminum hydroxide is used. Observe for hypercalcemia when using calcium supplement. Explain to client the potential for fracture. Assist with ambulation. Provide safe environment.	Slowing of bone disease, serum calcium and phosphorus levels within normal range for client, no bone fractures

NURSING DIAGNOSIS: Impaired skin integrity related to decrease in oil and sweat gland activity, deposition of calcium phosphate precipitants, capillary fragility, and neuropathy

Itching, bruising, dry skin; yellow-gray skin; edema; skin inflammation or infection; excoriation	Assess skin for changes in color, texture, turgor, and vascularity. Inspect client for bruises, purpura, and signs of infection. Provide skin care q 4-8 hr with tepid water, xipamide (Aquaphor), or bath oils. Apply ointments or creams (lanolin, Aquaphor) for comfort and to relieve itching. Administer antihistamines and antipruritics as prescribed. Trim client's nails short and keep them clean. Monitor serum calcium and phosphate levels.	Freedom from itching and skin dryness; intact, clean skin that is free from infection

*See Table 41-4.

Table 41-9

 NURSING CARE PLAN FOR THE CLIENT WITH CHRONIC RENAL FAILURE—cont'd

Defining Characteristics	Nursing Interventions	Evaluation Criteria

NURSING DIAGNOSIS: Potential complication: peripheral neuropathy related to effects of uremia on peripheral nerves

Decreased sensation in feet, numbness and burning of feet, muscle cramps, restlessness of legs, loss of muscle strength, foot-drop	Explain to client reason for neuropathy. Prevent trauma and excess stimulation to extremities. Instruct client to avoid tight clothing and restricting bed linens. In collaboration with physical therapy department, develop exercise regimen to maintain prescribed level of activity. Assess adequacy of dialysis therapy.	No paresthesia or pain, safe and comfortable ambulation and activities of daily living

NURSING DIAGNOSIS: Activity intolerance related to anemia secondary to uremia, bleeding, and blood loss during dialysis

Fatigability, poor tolerance for activity, decreased hematocrit and RBC count, pallor, dyspnea, tachycardia	Administer hematinics as ordered (at different times than aluminum hydroxide antacids). Do not administer folic acid before or during hemodialysis. Assess client's response to activity. Provide adequate periods of rest. Teach client to plan activities to avoid fatigue. Watch for any bleeding sites. Instruct client to use soft toothbrush for oral care. Monitor hematocrit readings.	Maintenance of hematocrit in stable range, performance of activities of daily living without undue fatigue

NURSING DIAGNOSIS: High risk for infection related to suppressed immune system, malnutrition, and skin breakdown secondary to dialysis, access sites, and uremic changes in skin

Chills, fever, tachycardia; redness, swelling, and/or drainage in area of break in skin	Provide frequent oral and personal hygiene. Instruct client to avoid exposure to people with infections. Turn, cough, and deep breathe client q 2 hr. Watch for local and systemic manifestations of infection. Maintain aseptic technique when performing dialysis.	Absence of infections, WBC count within normal range

NURSING DIAGNOSIS: Altered nutrition: less than body requirements related to restricted intake of nutrients, nausea, vomiting, anorexia, stomatitis, and altered metabolism of nutrients

Loss of appetite, loss of weight, alterations in electrolyte balance, unpleasant taste in mouth, elevated BUN level	Measure and describe vomitus. Administer antiemetics as ordered. Provide frequent mouth care. Provide small, frequent meals. Allow client freedom in choosing food and fluid intake within limitations. Provide at least 2000-2500 cal/day and restrict protein. Provide hard candy, gum, and lollipops to improve taste. Monitor weight, BUN, serum creatinine, albumin, total protein, and serum electrolytes.	Maintenance of ideal body weight, no blood in vomitus and stool, maintenance of albumin and total protein within acceptable limits, maintenance of BUN and serum creatinine within acceptable limits

NURSING DIAGNOSIS: Constipation related to decreased mobility, antacid intake, fluid restrictions, dietary modification, or electrolyte imbalances

Lack of usual bowel elimination	Administer stool softeners as prescribed. Teach client to avoid over-the-counter laxatives that contain magnesium.	Resumption of usual bowel elimination pattern

NURSING DIAGNOSIS: Diarrhea related to GI inflammation secondary to urea or hyperkalemia or as side effect of sorbital-Kayexalate treatment

Frequent, loose-to-watery stools	Record and measure stool. Monitor electrolytes (especially potassium and calcium levels) when client has persistent diarrhea.	Resumption of usual bowel elimination pattern

Continued.

Table 41-9

NURSING CARE PLAN FOR THE CLIENT WITH CHRONIC RENAL FAILURE—cont'd		
Defining Characteristics	**Nursing Interventions**	**Evaluation Criteria**

NURSING DIAGNOSIS: Sensory/perceptual alterations related to CNS changes induced by uremic toxins

Confusion, slowing of thought processes, decreased attention and memory span, disorientation, changes in sensorium (e.g., somnolence, stupor), changes in mood (e.g., irritability, depression), changes in behavior (e.g., withdrawal)	Provide explanation of effects of uremia on nervous system. Assess client's level of consciousness and mental status at regular intervals. Discuss significant material for brief rather than long time periods. Allow client time to respond. Validate client's understanding of what is discussed. Provide for orientation (e.g., calendar, radio). Teach family how to evaluate mental changes and when to refer to physician.	Mental alertness and appropriate interaction with environment

NURSING DIAGNOSIS: High risk for sexual dysfunction related to effects of uremia on endocrine system and the psychosocial impact of renal failure and its treatment

Amenorrhea, failure to ovulate, and decreased libido in women Impotence, atrophy of testicles, gynecomastia, azoospermia in men	Discuss meaning of sexuality with client and significant other. Encourage client and partner to discuss feelings openly and to use other means of sexual expression besides intercourse. Explore new patterns of sexual activity if previous patterns lead to anxiety. Emphasize importance of giving and receiving love and affection as opposed to performing.	Expression of satisfaction with sexual relationship by client and significant other

NURSING DIAGNOSIS: Anticipatory grieving related to loss of kidney function

Expression of feelings of sadness, anger, inadequacy, hopelessness	Listen to concerns of client. Allow client time to mourn loss of body function. Include family members in discussions of client's concerns.	Progression toward acceptance of chronic disease

NURSING DIAGNOSIS: Self-esteem disturbance related to enforced lifestyle changes, dependency on dialysis, chronic fatigue, cost of treatment, occupational problems, and role maintenance

Expression of feelings of inadequacy and unworthiness, concerns about family finances and functioning	Provide opportunity for client to discuss concerns. Refer client to social worker and for counseling if indicated. Assure client of self-worth. Encourage client and significant others to share feelings.	Expression of positive feelings about self, participation in treatment regimen, adaptation of lifestyle to changing health status

If transplantation does not work, they can return to dialysis. Many persons with chronic renal failure have received more than one kidney transplant.

DIALYSIS*

Dialysis refers to the movement of fluid and molecules across a semipermeable membrane from one compartment to another. Clinically, dialysis is a technique in which substances move from the blood through a semipermeable membrane and into a dialysis solution (dialysate). Dialysis

is used to correct fluid and electrolyte imbalances, to remove waste products and drugs, and to take the place of renal function in acute and chronic renal failure. The two methods of dialysis are *peritoneal dialysis* and *hemodialysis* (Table 41-10). In peritoneal dialysis the peritoneal membrane is used as the dialyzing surface. In hemodialysis an artificial membrane (usually made of cellulose-based materials) is used as the dialyzing surface that is in contact with the client's blood.

Dialysis is begun when the client's uremic state can no longer be adequately managed conservatively. A general guideline is to start dialysis when the GFR is less than 5 to 10 ml/min. However, this criterion varies widely in differ-

---
*Portions of the section on dialysis were contributed by Barbara Wood, R.N., New Mexico Artificial Kidney Center, Albuquerque, New Mexico.

Table 41-10 Peritoneal Dialysis and Hemodialysis

Peritoneal Dialysis		Hemodialysis	
Advantages	**Disadvantages**	**Advantages**	**Disadvantages**
Immediate initiation in almost any hospital	Bacterial or chemical peritonitis	Rapid fluid removal	Vascular access problems
Less complicated than hemodialysis	Protein loss into dialysate	Rapid removal of urea and creatinine	Dietary and fluid restrictions
Portable system with CAPD	Exit-site and tunnel infections	Effective potassium removal	Heparinization necessary
Fewer dietary restrictions	Self-image problems with catheter placement	Less protein loss	Extensive equipment necessary
Relatively short training time	Hyperglycemia	Lowering of serum triglycerides	Disequilibrium and hypotension during dialysis
Usable in clients with vascular access problems	Aggravated hyperlipidemia	Home dialysis possible	Added blood loss that contributes to anemia
Less cardiovascular stress	Surgery for catheter placement		Specially trained personnel necessary
Better blood pressure control	Contraindication in clients with multiple abdominal surgery or trauma		
Home dialysis possible			
Preferable for diabetics			

ent clinical situations, and the physician determines when to start dialysis on an individual basis. Certain uremic complications, including encephalopathy, neuropathies, uncontrollable hyperkalemia, pericarditis, and accelerated hypertension, indicate a need for immediate dialysis.

General Principles

Solutes and water move across the membrane from the blood to the dialysate or from the dialysate to the blood in accordance with concentration gradients. The principles of diffusion, osmosis, and ultrafiltration are involved in dialysis (Fig. 41-5). *Diffusion* is the movement of solutes from an area of greater concentration to an area of lesser concentration. In renal failure, urea, creatinine, uric acid, and electrolytes (potassium, phosphate) move from the blood to the dialysate with the net effect of lowering their concentration in the blood. RBCs, WBCs, and large plasma proteins are too large to diffuse through the membrane.

Osmosis is the movement of fluid from an area of lesser to an area of greater concentration of solutes. Glucose is added to the peritoneal dialysate bath and creates a greater osmotic gradient across the membrane to remove excess fluid from the blood.

Ultrafiltration results when a pressure gradient across the dialyzer membrane is created by an increased pressure in the blood compartment (positive pressure) or a decreased pressure in the dialysate compartment (negative pressure). Extracellular fluid moves to the dialysate because of the pressure gradient. In peritoneal dialysis, excess fluid is removed by increasing the osmolality of the dialysate with the addition of glucose. In hemodialysis, excess fluid is removed by creating a pressure differential between the blood and the dialysate solution with a combination of positive pressure in the blood compartment and/or negative pressure in the dialysate compartment.

The dialysate solution usually contains an electrolyte composition similar to that of normal plasma. The concen-

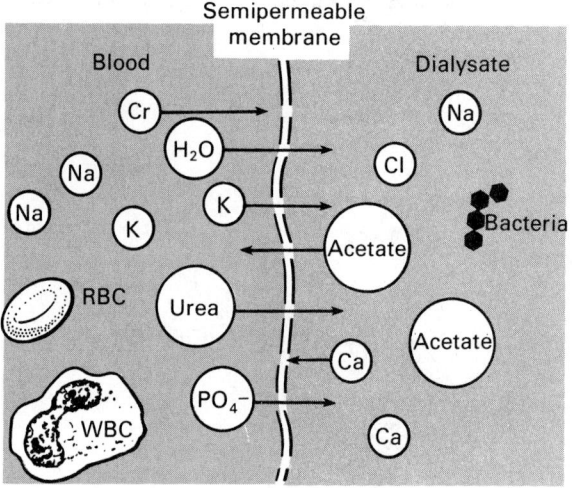

Fig. 41-5 Osmosis and diffusion across a semipermeable membrane.

tration of the dialysis solution may be individually determined on the basis of the client's needs.

Peritoneal Dialysis

Although peritoneal dialysis was first used in 1923, it did not come into widespread use for chronic treatment until the 1970s with the development of a soft, pliable peritoneal catheter and the introduction of the concept of continuous peritoneal dialysis. In recent years the use of peritoneal dialysis to treat both acute and chronic renal failure has increased considerably. The large area of the peritoneum makes it a very good semipermeable membrane for performing clinical dialysis.

Catheter placement. Peritoneal access is obtained by inserting a catheter through the anterior abdominal wall (Fig. 41-6). The prototype of the catheter that is used was

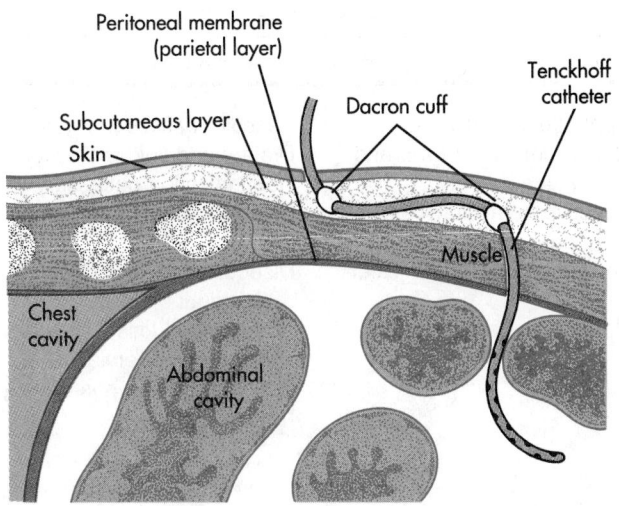

Peritoneal membrane (parietal layer)

Subcutaneous layer

Skin

Dacron cuff

Tenckhoff catheter

Muscle

Chest cavity

Abdominal cavity

Fig. 41-6 Tenckhoff catheter used in peritoneal dialysis.

developed by Tenckhoff in 1968 and is made of silicone rubber tubing (Fig. 41-6). The current version of this catheter is about 25 cm long and has one or two Dacron cuffs at the subcutaneous and peritoneal ends of the percutaneous tunnel to anchor the catheter securely and to seal out organisms and prevent their migration down the shaft from the skin. Within a few weeks, fibrous tissue grows into the Dacron cuff, anchors the catheter in place, and prevents bacterial penetration into the peritoneal cavity. The tip of the catheter rests in the peritoneal cavity and has many perforations spaced throughout the tubing to allow fluid to flow in and out of the catheter. Other types of catheters for chronic peritoneal dialysis are variations of the Tenckhoff catheter, including the Toronto-Western, Purdue-Column Disc, and Gore-Tex catheters (Fig. 41-7).[15]

The technique for catheter placement varies. Although it is possible to place a permanent catheter in the peritoneal cavity with a trocar, it is usually done via surgery so that its placement can be directly visualized. Preparation of the client for catheter insertion includes emptying the

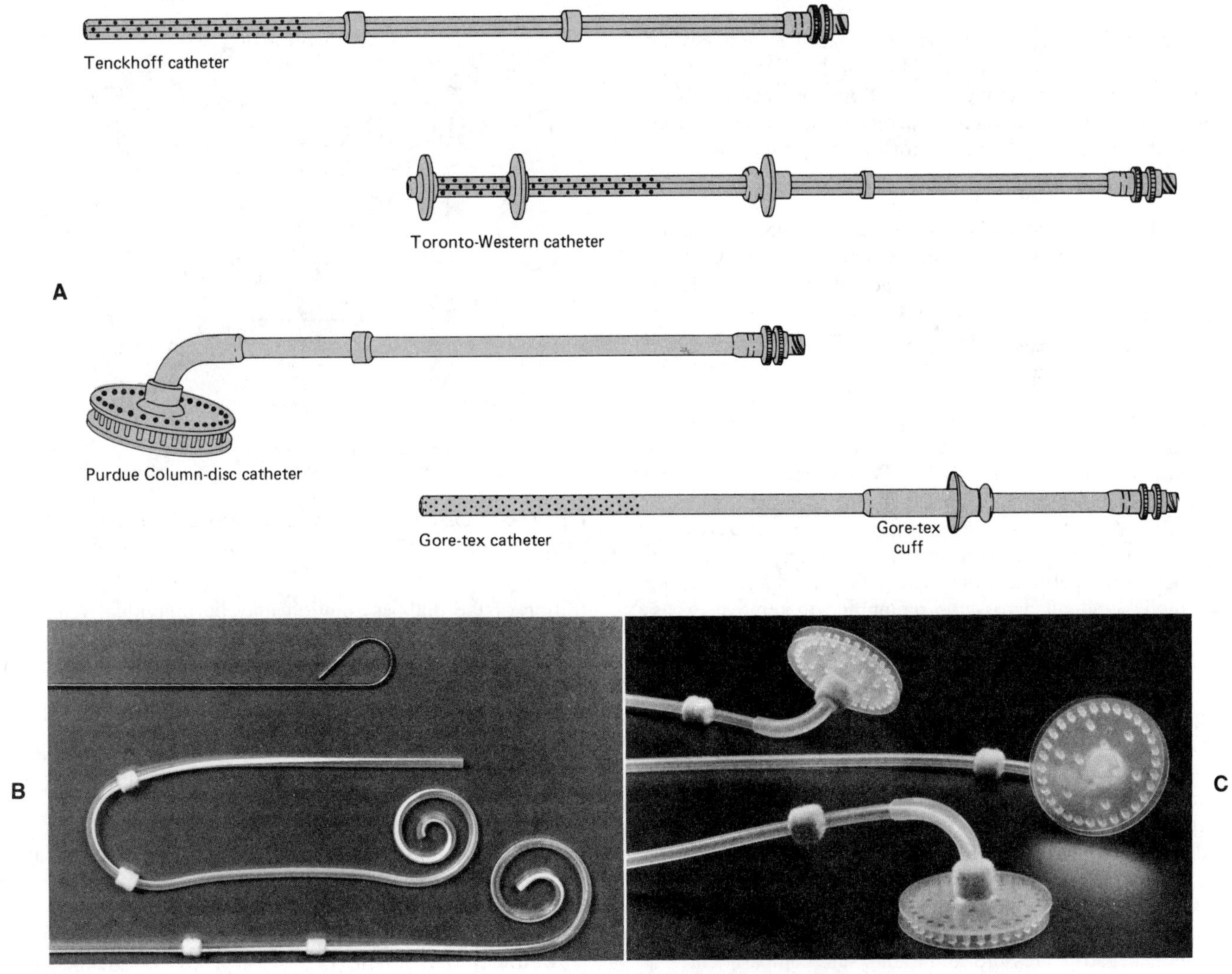

Tenckhoff catheter

Toronto-Western catheter

A

Purdue Column-disc catheter

Gore-tex catheter

Gore-tex cuff

B

C

Fig. 41-7   **A,** Peritoneal catheters used for peritoneal dialysis. **B,** Bent neck curl catheter. **C,** Disc catheter. (**B** and **C** courtesy Quinton Instruments, Seattle, Wash.)

bladder, weighing the client, and obtaining a signed consent form. In the nonsurgical approach an area approximately 2 cm below the umbilicus is anesthetized with a local anesthetic and the abdomen is distended with dialysis solution. A trocar, with the catheter threaded through or over it, is inserted into the peritoneal cavity. When the client feels pressure in the rectal area and has the urge to defecate, the trocar is withdrawn and the catheter is in place. In the surgical approach a midline umbilical incision is made and the catheter is implanted under direct manipulation and visualization. After the catheter is inserted, the skin is cleaned with an antiseptic solution, and a sterile dressing is applied. Complications of catheter insertion include perforation of the bladder, bowel, or a blood vessel and the introduction of bacteria.

The catheter is connected to a sterile tubing system and anchored to the abdomen with tape. The catheter is irrigated immediately with heparinized dialysate (usually 500 ml) to clear blood and fibrin from it. This procedure helps prevent the catheter from clogging and causing poor drainage and inflow. Before the start of peritoneal dialysis, it is preferable to allow a waiting period of 7 to 14 days for proper sealing of the catheter and for tissue ingrowth into the cuffs.

Some centers start dialysis 5 to 7 days after catheter insertion. About 2 to 4 weeks after catheter implantation, the exit site should be clean, dry, and free of redness and tenderness. Once the catheter incision site is healed, the client may shower and then pat the catheter and exit site dry. Daily catheter care includes the application of an antiseptic solution and a sterile dressing as well as examination of the catheter site for signs of infection (Fig. 41-8). If cared for properly, a catheter should last at least 18 months.

Dialysis solutions and cycle. Dialysis solutions are available commercially in 1- or 2-liter (and sometimes smaller or larger volumes) plastic bags (Dianeal, Inpersol) with glucose concentrations of 1.5%, 2.5%, and 4.25%. The electrolyte composition is similar to that of plasma except that potassium is usually in low concentrations in the dialysate. The dialysis solution is warmed to body temperature to increase peritoneal clearance, prevent hypothermia, and make the client more comfortable.

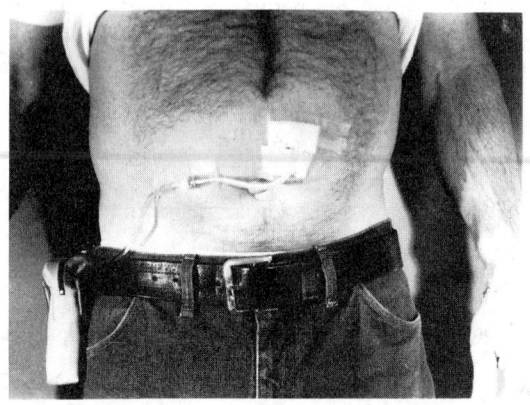

Fig. 41-8 Placement of peritoneal catheter.

Fluid removal during peritoneal dialysis depends on osmotic forces, and glucose is the most effective osmotic agent. However, the problems arising from high rates of peritoneal glucose absorption such as obesity, hypertriglyceridemia, and control of blood glucose levels in diabetics have led to a search for alternative osmotic agents. Many of these agents are currently under investigation.

The three phases of the peritoneal dialysis cycle are *inflow, dwell time* (equilibration), and *drain time*. During inflow, 2 L of solution is infused over about 10 minutes. The flow rate may be decreased if the client becomes uncomfortable. After the solution has been infused, the inflow clamp is closed before air enters the tubing.

The next part of the cycle is dwell time or equilibration, which allows for diffusion and osmosis between the client's blood and the peritoneal cavity. The amount of dwell time depends on the method of peritoneal dialysis. Drain time takes 10 to 20 minutes and may be facilitated by gently massaging the abdomen or changing the client's position. The cycle starts again with the infusion of another 2 L of solution. For manual peritoneal dialysis, a period of about 20 to 30 minutes is required to complete an exchange.

Peritoneal dialysis systems. Three types of peritoneal dialysis currently being used are intermittent peritoneal dialysis (IPD), continuous ambulatory peritoneal dialysis (CAPD), and continuous cyclic peritoneal dialysis (CCPD).[16]

Intermittent peritoneal dialysis. For IPD, automated cycler equipment is used to deliver the dialysate (Fig. 41-9). The client dialyzes three to five times per week (usually overnight) for about 8 hours per treatment. The automated cycler times and controls the inflow and outflow of the peritoneal dialysate. Alarms and monitors are built into the system to make it safe for clients to dialyze while they sleep. Between the dialyses the abdomen is empty. It may be easier to teach clients and their families to use the peritoneal dialysis machines at home compared with the hemodialysis equipment. In addition to its use in chronic dialysis, IPD is usually the preferred peritoneal dialysis method for treating acute renal failure. An advantage of IPD is that the system remains closed for the duration of dialysis, thus reducing the risk of infection.

Continuous ambulatory peritoneal dialysis. CAPD is carried out manually by exchanging 1.5 to 3 L (usually 2 L) of peritoneal dialysate four to five times daily with dwell times of 4 to 8 hours. One schedule, for example, starts the three exchanges at 7 AM, 12 noon, and 5 PM, and the fourth exchange at 10 PM. In this procedure the person instills 2 L of dialysate from a collapsible plastic bag into the peritoneal cavity through a disposable plastic tube (called the *line* or *transfer set*). The tube is secured to the permanent catheter on one end and attaches to the bag on the other end by means of a device (commonly called a *spike*). After instillation, the client closes the tubing with a clamp and the bag is folded and concealed in the client's clothing. Some of the newer devices allow the bag to be disconnected between exchanges. After the equilibration period the dialysate (effluent) is drained from the peritoneal cavity by unwrapping the bag, lowering it to the

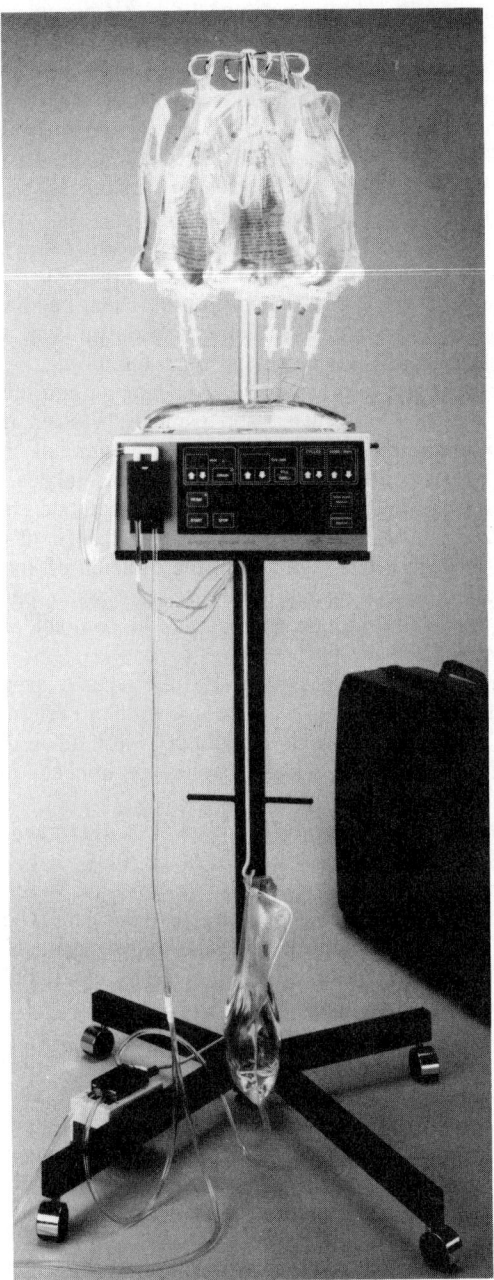

Fig. 41-9 Automated peritoneal dialysis cycler. (Courtesy Abbott Laboratories, Abbott Park, Ill.)

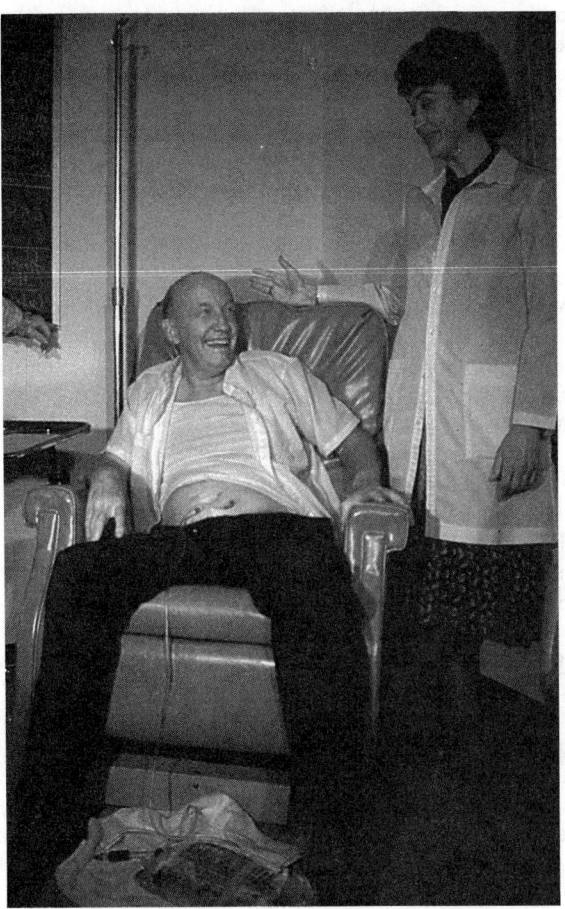

Fig. 41-10 Drain period for a CAPD client.

floor, and releasing a clamp on the tubing; the solution drains out in 10 to 20 minutes (Fig. 41-10). The bag is then disconnected and discarded. A new 2 L bag of dialysate solution is attached to the tube and the cycle is started again. It is critical in peritoneal dialysis to maintain sterile technique. Several tubing connections and devices are commercially available to help maintain a sterile system.

Continuous cyclic peritoneal dialysis. CCPD is a combination of IPD at night and CAPD during the day.[17] In CCPD the client is connected to an automated cycler for a time—usually at bedtime. The machine cycles four to six exchanges and up to 2 hours per exchange. The client dis-

connects from the machine after the cycles are complete, and the abdomen is filled with dialysate until the client reconnects to the machine. CCPD is usually done 6 to 7 days a week. For CCPD, the system is opened only twice a day, once to connect at night and once to disconnect in the morning. Thus the threat and actual incidence of peritonitis are greatly reduced. The main disadvantages of CCPD are the need to use mechanical equipment and the need to remain connected to the cycler throughout the night.

Contraindications for peritoneal dialysis include the following:

1. History of multiple abdominal surgical procedures or severe pathology (e.g., severe pancreatitis, diverticulitis)
2. Recurrent abdominal wall hernias
3. Advanced peripheral vascular disease
4. Excessive obesity with large abdominal wall and fat deposits
5. Preexisting vertebral disease (e.g., chronic back problems)
6. Severe obstructive pulmonary disease

Complications

Infection. Infection of the peritoneal catheter exit site is most commonly caused by *Staphylococcus aureus* or *S. epidermidis*. Superficial exit-site infection caused by these

organisms is frequently resolved with antibiotic therapy. Clinical manifestations of an exit-site infection include redness at site, tenderness, and drainage. If not treated immediately, subcutaneous tunnel infections usually result in abscess formation and may cause peritonitis and thus necessitate catheter removal.[18]

Peritonitis. Peritonitis results from contamination of the solution or tubing or from progression of exit-site or tunnel infections. The primary clinical manifestation of peritonitis is a cloudy peritoneal effluent that has a WBC count of over 100 cells per microliter (particularly neutrophils). Antibiotics are started by mouth, IV, or intraperitoneally. Repeated infections may necessitate the removal of the peritoneal catheter and termination of dialysis. Gastrointestinal manifestations may also be present, including diffuse abdominal pain, diarrhea, vomiting, abdominal distention, and hyperactive bowel sounds. Fever may or may not be present. Peritonitis is usually due to *S. aureus* or *S. epidermidis* (from skin flora). The formation of adhesions in the peritoneum can result from repeated infections, and this decreases the peritoneal membrane's ability as a dialyzing membrane. Cultures, Gram stains, and a cell count and a differential of peritoneal effluent are used to confirm the diagnosis of peritonitis.

Abdominal pain. Although it is not severe, a common complication is pain caused by the low pH of the dialysate solution, peritonitis, intraperitoneal irritation (which usually subsides in 1 to 2 weeks), and placement of the catheter. Pain occurs when the tip of the catheter touches the bladder, bowel, or peritoneum. A change in the placement of the catheter should correct this problem. An infusion of dialysate that is too rapid may cause referred pain in the shoulder. If the infusion rate is decreased, the pain usually subsides.

Outflow problems. When outflow fails shortly after catheter placement, it may be due to a kink in the tunnel segment of the catheter, omentum wrapped around the catheter, or migration of the catheter out of the pelvic region. Outflow problems after the catheter has settled into place are often due to a full colon; bowel evacuation frequently relieves the problem.

Hernias. Because of continuous increases in intraabdominal pressures, hernias develop in predisposed individuals such as multiparous women and older adult men. However, after hernia repair, peritoneal dialysis can be continued.

Lower back problems. Increased intraabdominal pressure can cause or aggravate lower back pain. The lumbosacral curvature is increased by intraperitoneal infusion of dialysate. Orthopedic binders and a regular exercise program for the back muscles have been beneficial for some clients.

Bleeding. Dialysis fluid on the first exchange may be pink or slightly bloody because of the trauma of catheter insertion. Gross bleeding indicates injury to the abdominal wall.

Pulmonary complications. Atelectasis, pneumonia, and bronchitis may occur from repeated upward displacement of the diaphragm, resulting in decreased lung expansion. The longer the dialysis period, the greater is the likelihood of pulmonary complications. Frequent repositioning and deep-breathing exercises help alleviate pulmonary complications.

Protein loss. Plasma proteins, amino acids, and polypeptides are lost in the dialysate fluid because of the permeability of the peritoneal membrane. The amount of loss may be as much as 9 to 12 g/day. This protein loss may be increased up to 40 g/day during episodes of peritonitis. The client can maintain a positive nitrogen balance with satisfactory protein intake.

Encapsulating sclerosing peritonitis. *Encapsulating sclerosing peritonitis* is a term applied to the development of a thick fibrous membrane that surrounds and compresses the bowel. Intestinal obstruction and strangulation are common complications.

Loss of ultrafiltration. Loss of ultrafiltration is associated with encapsulating sclerosing peritonitis. It can also occur as a result of unknown reasons and is associated with rapid glucose absorption.

Effectiveness of and adaptation to chronic peritoneal dialysis. The use and popularity of chronic peritoneal dialysis is increasing. The technique offers a short training program, independence, and ease of traveling. Clinically, clients on CAPD do at least as well as clients on hemodialysis, and sometimes better. There are few or no dietary restrictions, and greater mobility is possible than with conventional hemodialysis. The major disadvantage is the possibility of developing peritonitis. As further improvements in techniques (e.g., improved connecting and sterilizing devices, in-line filters, improved catheters) are made, the incidence of peritonitis should decrease.

Peritoneal dialysis is indicated especially for individuals who have vascular access problems and respond poorly to the hemodynamic stresses of hemodialysis (e.g., the older adult client with diabetes and cardiovascular disease). Diabetics with end-stage renal failure do better on peritoneal dialysis than on hemodialysis. The advantages of peritoneal dialysis for diabetics include better blood pressure control, stable cardiovascular status without rapid fluid shifts, better control of blood sugars by intraperitoneal insulin (which can often eliminate the need for subcutaneous insulin), and avoidance of the risk of retinal hemorrhage from heparin use during hemodialysis.

■ Nursing Management of the Client on Peritoneal Dialysis

Nursing care of the client on peritoneal dialysis is usually done on an outpatient basis except for the emergency hospitalization of a client with chronic renal failure. The peritoneal dialysis nurse is responsible for assessing the client regarding dialysis exchanges or for assisting the hospital staff in performing the peritoneal dialysis procedure.

The hospital staff assist the client by warming the peritoneal dialysis solution and adding medication and by performing the exchange if the client is unable to do so. Clients must be weighed daily (with the peritoneum empty) to properly assess volume status. Guidelines for weight gain or loss are set by the physician or peritoneal dialysis nurse.

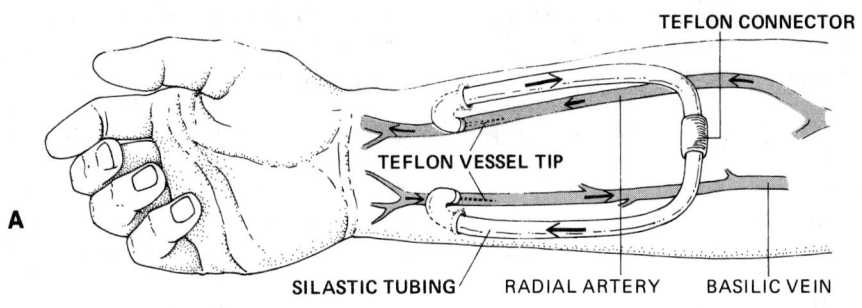

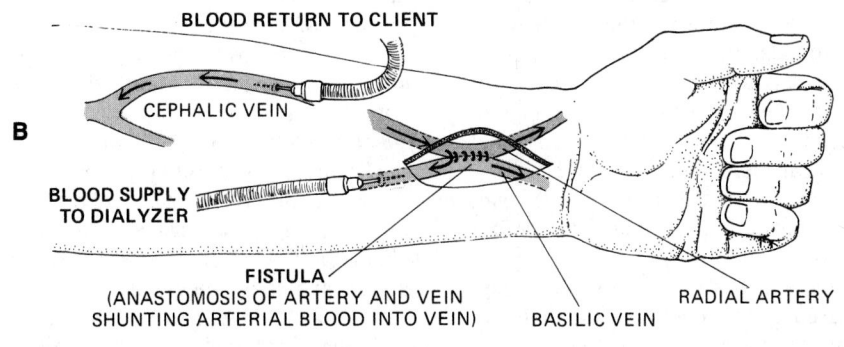

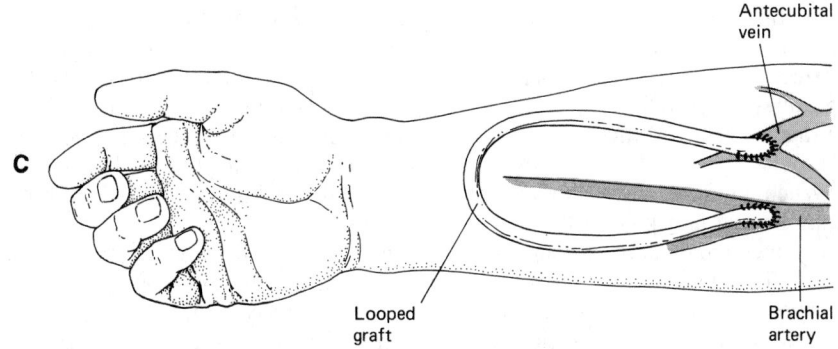

Fig. 41-11 Methods of vascular access for hemodialysis. **A,** External cannula or shunt. **B,** Internal AV fistula. (From Kagan L: Renal disease: a manual of patient care, New York, 1979, McGraw-Hill Book Co, Inc.) **C,** Looped graft in forearm.

Hemodialysis

In 1943, Willem Kolff in the Netherlands performed the first dialysis on a human being with the use of a rotating-drum dialyzer. After coming to the United States during World War II, he established dialysis treatment in the 1950s.

Vascular access sites. Vascular access is one of the major problems with hemodialysis. Before 1960, hemodialysis required the insertion of needles into arterial and venous vessels for each dialysis. Chronic dialysis was not possible with this technique. In 1960, Scribner developed a Teflon silicone rubber cannula that could be inserted into the radial artery and into an adjacent forearm vein (Fig. 41-11, *A*). The cannula is implanted subcutaneously and connected by silicone rubber tubing that exits from the skin. The two ends are connected by a U-shaped shunt. The external access cannula is commonly referred to as an *external shunt*. The shunt can be disconnected for dialysis to allow arterial blood to flow through the artificial kidney and return to the venous side. Another external cannula, the Thomas femoral shunt, consists of silicone rubber tubing implanted in the thigh using the femoral artery and vein. A Dacron faceplate appliqué is sutured to the femoral vessel walls. The external shunt caused many complications. Therefore it has been phased out for chronic dialysis. Its primary use today is as a temporary access device while an internal fistula is developing or while a graft is healing.

Internal arteriovenous fistulas and grafts. In 1966 the use of the subcutaneous internal arteriovenous fistula (Fig.

41-11, *B*) was introduced by Cimino and Brescia. An arteriovenous (AV) fistula is created in the forearm or thigh by a side-to-side, end-to-side, or end-to-end anastomosis between an artery (usually radial or ulnar) and a vein (usually cephalic). The fistula provides for arterial blood flow through the vein. The increased pressure of the arterial blood flow through the vein makes the vein accessible for venipuncture and allows it to handle the high blood flows required for hemodialysis.

Modifications of the internal AV fistula have incorporated saphenous or umbilical vein grafts, bovine grafts, and synthetic materials (Dacron, Teflon) to form a "bridge" between the arterial and venous blood supplies.[19] These devices and grafts are surgically anastomosed between an artery (usually brachial) and a vein (usually antecubital) (Fig. 41-11, *C*). The synthetic materials are relatively resistant to infectious organisms, which makes them very valuable because of the multiple needle sticks required in hemodialysis.

The fistula requires 1 to 6 weeks to mature sufficiently for use. Similarly, when a fistula is created with grafting material, an interval of 2 to 6 weeks is usually necessary to allow for healing and decreases in edema, although some institutions use it earlier than this. Two 14- to 16-gauge needles are inserted into the engorged vein or graft with the use of local anesthesia to obtain vascular access, and they are attached via tubing to dialysis lines. Normally, a thrill can be felt by palpating the area of anastomosis and a bruit can be heard with a stethoscope. Blood pressures and venipuncture should not be performed on the affected extremity.

The subcutaneous AV fistula is much less likely to clot and become infected than the external cannula. Good fistulas seem to get better as the years go by, although grafted devices are not as good as simple AV fistulas. The main problem of AV fistulas is thrombosis that results from several years of use. Some people develop distal ischemia (steal syndrome) because of the bypass of arterial blood. Another complication is the development of an aneurysm at the fistula site. Although infections are not common, when the site surrounding a grafted device becomes infected, it results in a serious problem that is frequently associated with bacteremia.

Temporary vascular access. In some situations when temporary vascular access is required, percutaneous cannulation of the subclavian, internal jugular, or femoral vein is used. A flexible Teflon, silicone rubber, or polyurethane catheter is inserted into these large veins and provides easy access to circulation without the need for the client to have surgery or to sacrifice a peripheral artery or vein. The procedure for percutaneous cannulation is similar to the method of insertion of a central venous pressure line (see Chapter 26). Catheters can have either a single or a double lumen. If a single-lumen catheter is used, a special device is also used during dialysis to alternate the flow of blood into and out of the dialysis machine (Fig. 41-12). Percutaneous cannulas in subclavian or jugular veins can be left in place for 3 to 12 weeks. Femoral-vein cannulas can remain in place for only 2 to 3 days.

A disadvantage of femoral-vessel cannulization is the

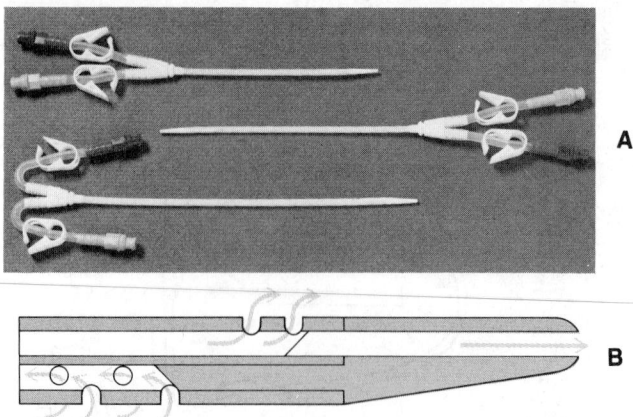

Fig. 41-12 Temporary double-lumen-single-needle vascular access catheter for acute hemodialysis. **A,** The soft, flexible dual-lumen polyurethane tube is attached to a Y hub. (Courtesy Quinton Instrument Company, Seattle, Wash.) **B,** Blood is withdrawn continuously through the outer lumen upstream and returned through the inner lumen downstream, thus reducing recirculation.

short time the catheter can remain in place. If these vessels are used for vascular access, repeated venipunctures are needed for the course of acute dialysis. Complications of femoral catheterization consist of femoral-vein thrombosis with pulmonary emboli (especially if the treatment is prolonged), infections, immobility (while catheter is in use), and inadvertent blood-vessel punctures with hematoma formation. Technical complications of subclavian-vein catheterization include brachial plexus lesions, hemothorax, and pneumothorax; a moderate risk of infection also exists. The patency of the subclavian catheter is usually maintained with intermittent injections of heparin. While the catheter is in place, the client is usually comfortable and can be ambulatory. No medications should be administered or blood withdrawn from this catheter. Trained dialysis staff may inject heparin into the lumen of the catheter at the end of dialysis and remove the heparin before starting dialysis.

Combined internal-external atraumatic vessel devices that can be implanted in the upper arm or the thigh have been developed. One type, called *Hemasite,* consists of a titanium T-shaped body surrounded by Dacron velour with Gore-Tex grafts attached to both ends of the T. The neck of the device exits through the skin, and the external part is fitted with a special device that can be interfaced with the blood tubing sets. The main problems with this device are infection and clotting. The primary advantage is that it spares the client the pain of repeated needle punctures.

When dialysis is indicated, there are several possible ways to approach treatment. The first procedure consists of simultaneously creating an external shunt and an internal AV fistula. The external shunt can be used until the AV fistula is ready. When the internal fistula is ready, the external fistula is removed. The second procedure consists of creating a subcutaneous AV fistula or hemodialyzing via a subclavian catheter until the AV fistula is ready. The third

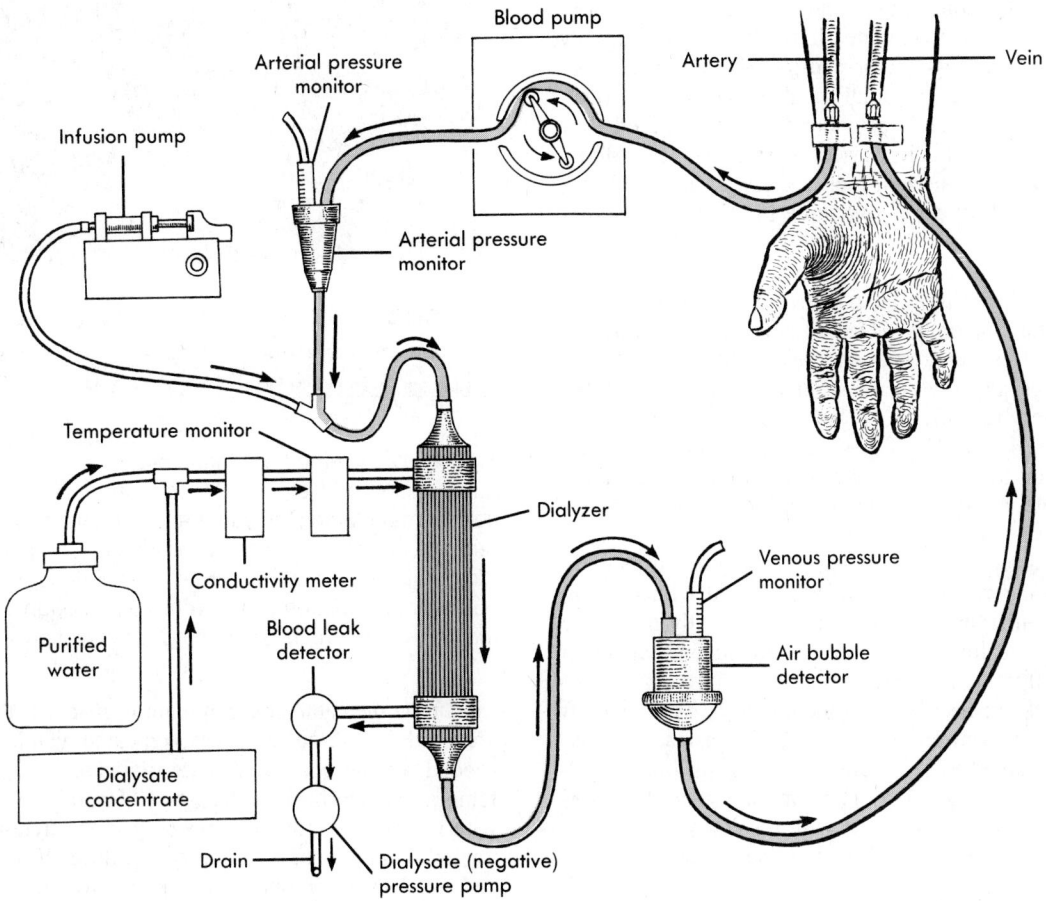

Fig. 41-13 Components of a hemodialysis system. (From Thelan LA, Davie JK, and Urden LD: Textbook of critical care nursing: diagnosis and management, St Louis, 1990, Mosby–Year Book, Inc, p 651.)

procedure involves surgically creating the AV fistula while the client is being maintained on conservative therapy, well in advance of ESRD.

Dialyzers. Although rarely used today, the coil dialyzer was the first type of dialyzer used in which blood flowed through a series of cellophane tubes. Historically, this was later replaced by a flat plate dialyzer (Kiil), in which blood flowed between sheets of membrane outside of which the dialysate passed.

In hemodialysis a semipermeable membrane made of cellulose-based materials is primarily used in the form of a hollow fiber kidney, which contains thousands of fibers packed in a cylinder (Fig. 41-13). The blood circulates through the fibers, and dialysis fluid flows between them with dialysis occurring across the membrane. Various dialyzers differ in regard to surface area, membrane composition and thickness, clearance of waste products, and removal of fluid.

Most dialysis units now reprocess and reuse the dialyzers for the same client after cleaning and subsequent disinfection. The advantages of reprocessing and reusing are considerable, and economic reasons represent the primary advantage. With reuse, the dialyzers become more biocompatible so that there are fewer side effects from blood/membrane interactions during the dialysis procedure. A major concern with reprocessing and reuse is potential residual contamination from disinfectant in the dialyzer.

Procedure. After the venipunctures the needle closest to the fistula delivers "arterial" blood to the dialyzer. The dialyzer is usually primed with saline solution. Heparin is added to the blood as it flows into the dialyzer. Once the blood enters the extracorporeal circuit, it is propelled through the dialyzer by a blood pump at a flow rate of 100 to 300 ml/min, while the dialysate (warmed to body temperature) circulates in the opposite direction at a rate of 300 to 900 ml/min. Anticoagulation therapy is required to prevent clotting of blood in the dialyzer and blood lines. Most units use routine heparinization, which consists of a loading dose given at the initiation of dialysis and smaller doses given throughout the treatment. The last dose is usually given in the last hour before the end of dialysis treatment to prevent excessive site bleeding after dialysis. Blood is returned from the dialyzer via the "venous" lines to the client.

In addition to the dialyzer, the other piece of equipment is a dialysate delivery and monitoring system (Fig. 41-14). It pumps the dialysate fluid as well as the blood through the dialyzer. Adjustments can be made for ultrafiltration

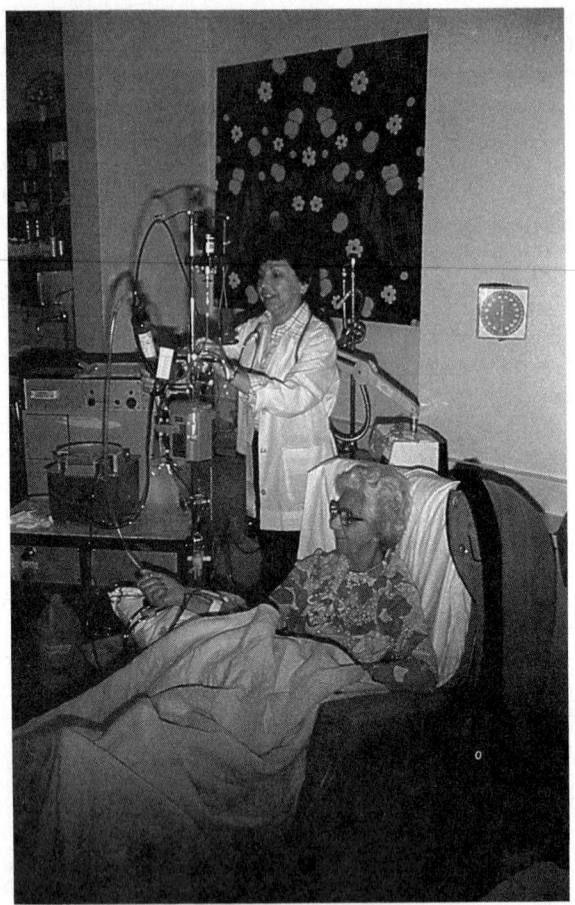

Fig. 41-14 Hemodialysis delivery system.

by creating a positive pressure in the blood side or a negative pressure (transmembrane pressure) on the dialysate side or by a combination of both. The dialysis system has an alarm system to warn of blood or air leaks; alterations in dialysate temperature, concentration, or pressure; and extremes in blood pressure readings.

Dialysis is terminated by turning off the blood flow pump, clamping the arterial inflow line, and flushing the dialyzer with saline solution to return all blood to the client. The needles are then removed from the client, and firm pressure is applied to the venipuncture sites.

Before beginning treatment, the nurse must complete an assessment that includes fluid status (weight, blood pressure, lung and heart sounds), condition of vascular access, temperature, and general condition of the skin. The difference between the last postdialysis weight and the present predialysis weight determines the ultrafiltration. Ideally, no more than 1.0 to 1.5 kg should be gained between treatments. While the client is on dialysis, vital signs should be taken at least every 30 to 60 minutes, since rapid changes may occur in the vascular system.

Most maintenance dialysis units use reclining chairs in an attempt to create a nonhospital environment. Most people sleep, read, talk, or watch television during dialysis. Hemodialysis usually lasts 2 to 4 hours and occurs three times per week. While clients are attached to dialysis ma-

chines, they can engage in meaningful interaction with the staff.

Settings. Hemodialysis can be done in an inpatient (hospital) or an outpatient (clinic or hospital) setting. Inpatient dialysis is used for treating seriously ill clients. In outpatient dialysis the client comes to the hospital or a satellite unit for treatment. The client may choose self-care in either setting with backup support from trained personnel if needed.

Another choice of setting for hemodialysis is the home. In 1963, home hemodialysis training was started. Today, about 15% of clients on hemodialysis use it. One of the main advantages of home dialysis is that it allows greater freedom in choosing dialysis times. The main reasons that more people do not use home dialysis are (1) lack of a trained partner, (2) inadequate space or facilities at home, (3) fear of unexpected problems outside the hospital setting, and (4) medical problems that warrant close supervision while the client is on hemodialysis.

Complications

Disequilibrium syndrome. Disequilibrium syndrome develops as a result of rapid changes in the composition of the extracellular fluid. Urea, sodium, and other solutes are removed more rapidly from the blood than from the cerebrospinal fluid and the brain. The higher osmotic gradient in the brain cells allows fluid to pass into these cells, causing cerebral edema. Manifestations include nausea, vomiting, confusion, restlessness, headaches, twitching and jerking, and occasionally seizures. In addition, the rapid changes in osmolality may cause muscle cramps and contribute to hypotension. Treatment consists of slowing the rate of dialysis and infusing hypertonic saline solution, albumin, or mannitol to draw fluid from the brain cells back into circulation.

Hypotension. Hypotension that occurs during hemodialysis primarily results from rapid removal of vascular volume (hypovolemia), decreased cardiac output, and decreased systemic vascular resistance. The drop in blood pressure during dialysis may precipitate lightheadedness, nausea, vomiting, seizures, and coronary ischemia. The usual treatment for hypotension includes a decrease in pressure gradient, infusion of 0.9% saline solution (100 to 200 ml), placement of the client in Trendelenburg's position to improve cerebral blood flow, and decreasing of the rate of fluid removal. If a client experiences recurrent hypotensive episodes, a reassessment of dry weight, dialyzer size, and blood pressure medications may have to be done.

Muscle cramps. Muscle cramps are a common problem in clients on dialysis and are associated with significant discomfort and pain. They can result from too rapid removal of sodium and water or from neuromuscular hypersensitivity.

Loss of blood. Blood loss may result from residual blood in the dialyzer, from accidental separation of cannula tubing or dialysis membrane rupture, as a side effect of heparinization, or from bleeding after the removal of needles at the end of dialysis. In a client who has received too much heparin, postdialysis bleeding can be considerable.

Hepatitis. The cause of hepatitis in clients on dialysis is related to blood transfusions. In addition, clients are frequently free of symptoms because of their immunocompromised state, but they do become carriers of hepatitis B. In the past, hepatitis was usually associated with the hepatitis B virus. However, the incidence of hepatitis B has decreased with frequent testing for hepatitis B surface antigen (HB_sAg), separation of infected dialysis clients, the use of disposable equipment, and the use of disposable gloves when needles are inserted and removed. In addition, hepatitis B vaccine has been given to clients and personnel in dialysis units. Currently, non-A, non-B hepatitis is responsible for the majority of cases of hepatitis in dialysis populations. (Hepatitis is discussed in more detail in Chapter 37.)

Sepsis. Sepsis is often related to infections of vascular access sites. Bacterial endocarditis can occur because of the frequent and prolonged access to the vascular system that is required for dialysis.

Intractable ascites. Intractable ascites is being reported with increasing frequency during the course of chronic dialysis. Although the exact cause is unknown, most cases seem to be related to repeated fluid overload, poor nutrition, and cardiomyopathy. Although some clients overcome ascites, the prognosis is generally poor.[20]

Dialysis encephalopathy. Dialysis encephalopathy, a progressive neurological impairment, is characterized by speech disturbances, dementia, lack of muscle coordination, and myoclonic seizures. A frequent cause of this problem is aluminum toxicity. Aluminum toxicity may result from aluminum in water sources used in the dialysate solution, ingestion of aluminum-containing antacids, and a decreased ability of the kidneys to excrete aluminum. Aluminum can be removed from dialysis fluid by water purification systems, and new phosphate-binding antacids that are not aluminum based are being investigated. Chelation therapy with deferoxamine infusion has been used to promote a rapid release of aluminum from bone and tissue stores.

Acquired cystic kidney disease. Acquired cystic kidney disease is the development of multiple cysts in the kidneys of clients on chronic dialysis. Possible causes for the development of renal cysts include (1) occlusion of renal tubules by epithelial hyperplasia or fibrosis, (2) accumulation of uremic metabolites, and (3) toxic substances from dialysis equipment and dialysate fluid. The cysts are very susceptible to hemorrhage, and bleeding into the cystic kidney may cause hematuria or hemorrhage into the retroperitoneal space.

Increased incidence of cancer. There is a significant increase in the incidence of neoplasms in clients with renal failure who have not had transplants as compared with the general population.[21,22] The increased incidence is most commonly found for tumors such as those of the lung, breast, uterus, colon, and prostate.

Effectiveness of and adaptation to hemodialysis. Hemodialysis is still an imperfect technique in treating ESRD. It cannot replace the metabolic and hormonal functions of the kidneys. Hemodialysis can relieve most of the symptoms of chronic renal failure and, if started early

enough, can prevent certain complications. However, it does not alter the accelerated atherosclerosis and may only partially correct anemia.

The yearly death rate of clients on maintenance dialysis has increased from about 10% to close to 20%. The major reason for this is the increased proportion of older adult clients (older than 65 years of age) who are now receiving dialysis as maintenance therapy. The majority of deaths are due to cardiovascular-related disease (cerebrovascular accident or myocardial infarction); infectious complications are the second leading cause of death. Many of the complications associated with chronic renal failure continue into the transplantation period and can affect the success of a kidney transplant.

Individual adaptation to maintenance hemodialysis varies considerably. Initially, many clients feel very positive about the machine because it makes them feel better. Some people come to hospitals or satellite units for dialysis because they know that if they are not treated, they will get very sick and die. Dependence on a machine is a reality. Many clients have dreams about being tied to the machine. Depression and suicidal tendencies may be manifested in noncompliance with a diet or drug therapy or in a large weight gain. A primary nursing goal is to help clients regain or maintain positive self-esteem and continue to be productive in society.

Hemofiltration

Continuous arteriovenous hemofiltration (CAVH) is an alternative or adjunctive method of treating acute and chronic renal failure (Fig. 41-15). CAVH provides a

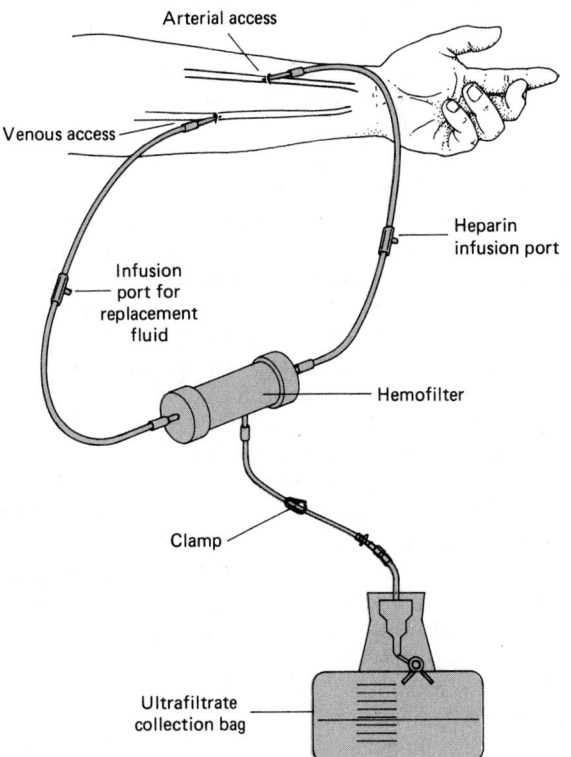

Fig. 41-15 Continuous AV hemofiltration.

means by which solutes and fluids can be removed slowly and continuously.[23,24] CAVH is especially useful in individuals with fluid overload regardless of the cause of the overload (e.g., acute renal failure with or without hemodynamic instability, pulmonary edema). If a client with acute renal failure has severe manifestations of uremia (e.g., hyperkalemia, pericarditis), hemodialysis is indicated for therapy rather than hemofiltration. However, hemofiltration can be used in conjunction with hemodialysis for continuous fluid removal.

The device is a highly permeable hollow fiber hemofilter. This filter removes plasma water and nonprotein solutes, which are collectively called *ultrafiltrate*. Vascular access is achieved by means of an AV Scribner external shunt, cannulation of the femoral artery and vein, or a double-lumen subclavian catheter. The systemic blood pressure provides the force to achieve sufficient blood flow through the hemofilter. When the hydrostatic pressure exceeds the oncotic pressure, water and nonprotein solutes pass out of the filter into the extracapillary space and drain through the ultrafiltrate port into a collection device. The remaining fluid continues through the filter and returns to the client through the venous access site. While the ultrafiltrate pours out of the hemofilter, fluid and electrolyte replacements can be infused into the venous port. This fluid is designed to replace volume and solutes such as sodium, chloride, bicarbonate, and glucose and is free of unwanted solutes such as creatinine, urea, potassium, and phosphates. Total parenteral nutrition can also be infused to provide for the intake of essential nutrients. The infusion rate of replacement fluids is determined in accordance with the ultrafiltration rate to control weight reduction and fluid and electrolyte elimination. Replacement fluid may also be infused into the arterial port and is called *predilutional fluid replacement*. This method of fluid replacement allows for greater clearance of urea.

Like hemodialysis, CAVH provides for the removal of fluid, electrolytes, and solutes. However, several of its features differ from hemodialysis, including the following:

1. It is continuous rather than intermittent.
2. It functions by means of convection rather than by osmosis and diffusion.
3. It relies on a client's blood pressure rather than a pump to propel blood.
4. It has few or no effects on cardiovascular stability (e.g., disequilibrium syndrome).
5. It does not require the specialized skills of a hemodialysis nurse.

CAVH also makes it possible to administer parenteral nutrition and drug therapy in clients who are on fluid restrictions. However, hemodialysis and peritoneal dialysis remain the best maintenance therapies for clients with chronic renal failure.

CAVH can be continued as long as 30 to 40 days, but the hemofilter may have to be changed every 12 to 48 hours because of loss of filtration efficiency or clotting. The ultrafiltrate is clear yellow, and specimens are obtained every 4 to 6 hours for evaluation of serum chemistries. If the ultrafiltrate becomes bloody or blood tinged, a possible rupture in the filter membrane should be suspected. Capillary leakage necessitates changing the hemofilter.

During CAVH the nurse must monitor fluid and electrolyte balance. Hourly intake and output measurements as well as daily weights must be recorded. Vital signs and hemodynamic pressures should be monitored hourly. Although reductions in central venous pressure and pulmonary artery pressure are expected, there should be little change in mean arterial pressure or cardiac output. Assessment and care of the vascular access sites are important.

An alternative to CAVH is *continuous arterial venous hemodialysis* (CAVHD). During CAVHD a bag of dialysis solution is connected to the end of the hemofilter opposite the ultrafiltration port, creating a diffusion gradient. The advantage of CAVHD is that urea and creatinine clearances are greater than those during CAVH. The increased rate of solute removal can reduce the incidence of uremia, acidosis, and electrolyte imbalances. High ultrafiltration rates can be achieved by changing the glucose concentration of the dialysis solution to create a greater osmotic gradient.

TRANSPLANTATION*

The first kidney transplant in the United States was performed in 1954 in Boston between identical twins. After 7 years the recipient died of a myocardial infarction at age 29. Advances in immunosuppressive drug therapy and tissue typing in the 1960s made transplantation available to a broader range of people.

Today in the United States, over 100,000 individuals have received kidney transplants. Although a successful transplant restores all aspects of renal function, its availability depends on a suitable donor and appropriate tissue matching.

Preoperative Period

Living related donor selection and preparation. Living related donors (LRDs) provide 15% to 20% and cadaveric donors provide 80% to 85% of all donated kidneys. LRDs are usually parents, siblings, or children. Physiological and psychological assessments of a potential donor are done. Histocompatibility studies and blood typing are done first. If the results match those of the recipient, the prospective donor's complete history is taken, and a complete physical examination, including chest x-ray examination, urinalysis, urine culture, intravenous pyelogram, ECG, complete blood count (CBC), electrolyte studies, glucose tolerance tests, BUN, serum creatinine, creatinine clearance, aortogram, and renal arteriogram, is performed.

Cadaveric donors. Cadaveric donors are most commonly trauma victims. The kidneys are suitable only if they have not been subjected to ischemia or trauma. The generally accepted age for cadaveric donors is 5 to 55 years, although suitable kidneys have been obtained from younger and older donors. Donors must be free of systemic disease (e.g., diabetes mellitus, malignancies) and

---

*Portions of the section on transplantation were contributed by JoAnn Seppelt, R.N., Director of Transplant Services, University of New Mexico Hospital, Albuquerque, New Mexico.

infection and must have normal kidney function. Permission from the donor's immediate family is required after determination of brain death. Even if the donor carries a signed donor card, consent from the closest relative is required.

A nationwide computerized service is available for persons with ESRD who are on an active transplant list. When a kidney is procured in one area of the county but there is no suitable recipient, the computer service is used to find the most suitable recipient in another area.

After the kidneys are removed from the cadaveric donor, they are flushed with an electrolyte solution and can then be transported in a sterile environment in a compact watertight container filled with ice. This method is called *cold preservation* or *hypothermic storage*. With this method, kidneys can be preserved for up to 48 hours.

The development of kidney preservation machines has increased the viability of kidneys. These machines pump a cold perfusate (albumin or commercially prepared albumin perfusates containing electrolytes) through the renal artery. The perfusate is cold (5° C to 10° C), which allows for a decreased metabolic rate. Kidneys have been adequately perfused for up to 72 hours, providing additional time for transportation, tissue typing, and preparation of the recipient. Although it does increase the viability of the kidney, the perfusion pump is technically difficult to operate and is not used in many areas of the country.

The limited availability of LRDs has turned the focus to cadaveric donors. Although there are over 130,000 people on maintenance dialysis, only about 9000 transplants are performed each year. Currently, more than 16,000 people are waiting for kidney transplants.[25]

Recipient selection and preparation. A successful transplant can now be achieved in circumstances previously thought to carry too high a risk of failure or death (e.g., in a client with diabetes mellitus). The age range within which transplants are performed continues to widen. At the lower end it now extends into the first year of life, and at the higher end there is no well-defined or widely agreed on cutoff point. Contraindications to transplantation include disseminated malignancies, refractory cardiac failure, chronic respiratory failure, extensive vascular disease, chronic infection, and psychosocial disorders (e.g., alcoholism, drug addiction). A hepatitis B carrier state is an adverse factor but not a contraindication to transplantation.

In addition to a determination of ABO blood types and human leukocyte antigens (HLAs) as baseline screening data, the potential recipient's serum should be screened regularly for HLA antibodies. These antibodies often appear transiently or permanently after blood transfusion or rejection of a transplanted kidney.

In clients on hemodialysis, preoperative dialysis is usually required unless the last routine dialysis was completed within the previous 24 hours. The main purpose of dialysis in this situation is to correct hyperkalemia and hypervolemia. Possible sites of infection, including the lungs, urinary tract, and vascular access sites, should be carefully assessed and treated with appropriate antibiotics.

Histocompatibility studies. Histocompatibility testing is performed to determine the degree of similarity between

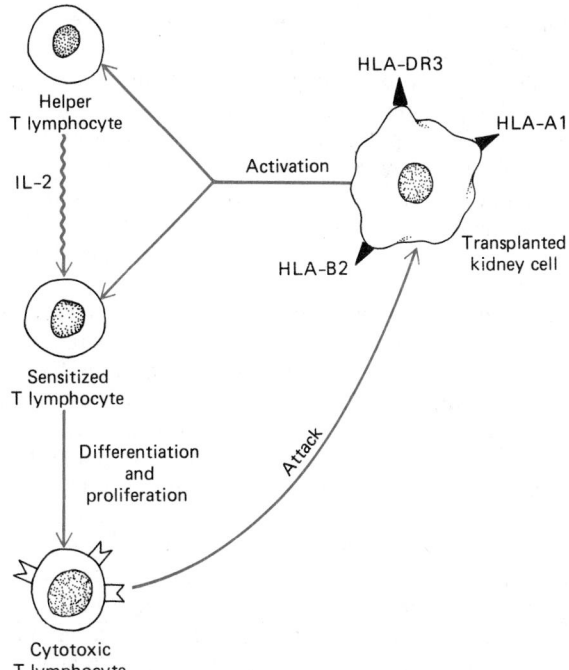

Fig. 41-16 The mechanism of action of T-cytotoxic lymphocyte activation and attack of renal transplanted tissue.

donor and recipient antigens. ABO blood group antigens are important in determining histocompatibility and are matched. In addition, the HLA antigens, which determine the acceptance or rejection of transplanted tissue, are determined (see Chapter 8). All recipients and donors express HLA antigens on all nucleated cells. The HLA antigens initiate the process of rejection and serve as targets of the immunological attack against the grafted organ (Fig. 41-16).

The HLA complex is located on chromosome 6 in humans. Major HLA loci that have been identified in this region include A, B, C, D, and D-related (DR) (see Fig. 8-9). Each locus may have multiple alleles and more alleles are being discovered. Each person has two antigens for each locus, one inherited from each parent. Because the genes that code for HLA are closely linked, they are inherited as a group or haplotype. One haplotype is inherited from each parent (see Fig. 8-9). After HLA testing, the potential kidney to be transplanted is considered an *HLA-one haplotype match*, *HLA-identical (two-haplotype match)*, or *non-HLA-identical (HLA mismatch)*.

The purpose of histocompatibility testing is to identify the antigens at each locus. A serological test is used to type for the antigens at HLA-A, HLA-B, and HLA-C loci with lymphocytes taken from peripheral blood or lymph nodes. For kidney transplantation the antigens at the A and B loci are the ones usually considered. The total time required for HLA typing is about 4 hours for HLA-A and HLA-B.

A mixed lymphocyte culture assesses the antigen match at the D locus. In this test, lymphocytes from the recipient are incubated for 5 to 7 days with lymphocytes from the donor. The degree of proliferation of lymphocytes corre-

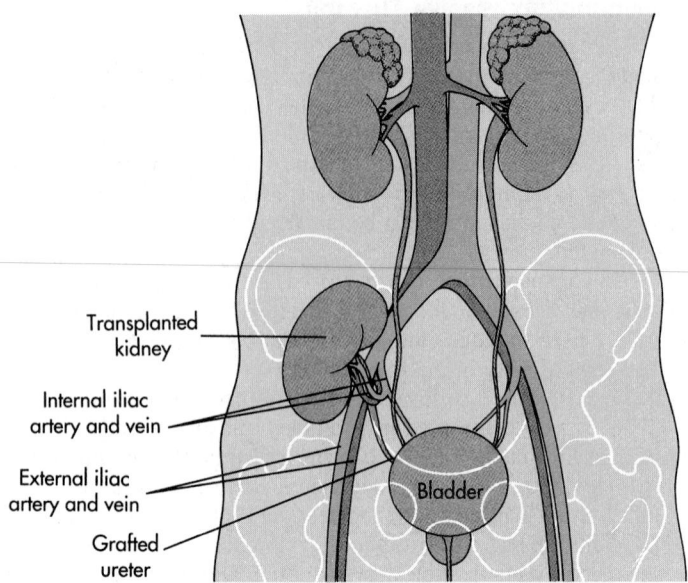

Transplanted kidney

Internal iliac artery and vein

External iliac artery and vein

Bladder

Grafted ureter

Fig. 41-17 Surgical placement of transplanted kidney.

lates with the degree to which the donor cells are recognized as foreign. This is the in vitro equivalent of the response expected in vivo. Because this test takes so long, it is not used for cadaveric donors. HLA-DR typing is done by means of a serological test similar to HLA-A and HLA-B typing to assess for D-antigen compatibility in cadaveric transplant situations. Since D and DR loci are so closely linked on the chromosome, the products of these two loci are probably inherited together. Typing for DR takes about 6 hours.

A tissue typing crossmatch uses serum from the recipient mixed with donor lymphocytes to test for any preformed cytotoxic (anti-HLA) antibodies to the donated kidney. The recipient may have been exposed to antigens similar to those of the donor by means of previous blood transfusions, pregnancy, a previous kidney transplant, or bacteremia. This procedure takes about 3 to 5 hours and is used in both LRDs and cadaveric donors. A positive crossmatch indicates cytotoxic antibodies and is a contraindication to transplantation. If transplanted, this type of kidney will immediately undergo hyperacute rejection.

In cadaveric transplantation an attempt is made to match as many antigens as possible between the HLA-A, HLA-B, and HLA-DR loci. The effect of a good match is less important in the era of new immunosuppressive medication. However, this is a matter of controversy.

Pretransplant blood transfusions. In the past, clients were purposefully transfused with blood before transplantation because of a demonstrated improvement in graft survival. This applied to donor-specific transfusions in the LRD situation as well as random transfusions in cadaveric transplantation. With the advent of cyclosporine, the immunological advantage of purposeful pretransplantation transfusions is no longer clear. In addition, the risk of complications such as hepatitis and preformed antibodies has made many clients unwilling to accept transfusions.

Surgical Procedure

For an LRD kidney transplant, two surgical teams are used. One team carefully removes the donor kidney attached to artery, vein, and ureter. After the kidney is removed, it is core-cooled by flushing with an electrolyte solution at approximately 10° C. Frequently, mannitol is added to this solution to increase osmolality. The kidney is then carried to the operating room with the recipient.

The donated kidney is surgically implanted in the iliac fossa because the iliac blood vessels are easy to expose (Fig. 41-17). When either kidney from the donor is equally satisfactory, the left is usually chosen because it has a longer renal vein. The renal artery is anastomosed to the internal iliac (hypogastric) artery or the external iliac artery. The renal vein is attached to the external iliac vein. The donor's ureter is implanted into the recipient's bladder.

Bilateral nephrectomies of the recipient's kidneys are not performed unless the client has uncontrollable hypertension, infection, bleeding in the kidneys, or ureteral reflux.

Postoperative Care

Recipient. The nursing care for a recipient is similar to that for any client who has had major surgery. The immediate postoperative care consists of careful monitoring of fluid and electrolyte balances and intake and output. A massive diuresis may occur in response to renal ischemia. IV fluids are adjusted hourly according to the urine output and the state of hydration. A common order for replacement is 30 ml/hr plus an amount that equals urine output. An indwelling catheter is inserted and urine output is monitored hourly. The catheter is removed as soon as possible but may be left in place up to 3 days to allow the suture line in the bladder to become more stable. While the catheter is in place, observing for patency of the tubing and providing catheter care are very important.

The abdominal dressing should be checked for both blood and urine drainage. Urinary leakage may be present if the ureteral anastomosis is not securely implanted in the bladder. It may also result from ureteral obstruction of the newly implanted ureter. Careful, frequent monitoring of vital signs is also critical. A low-grade fever may be a sign of rejection or infection.

Vigorous pulmonary exercises are needed to increase ventilation and drainage of secretions. Coughing and deep breathing can be combined with the use of incentive spirometry. The client can be turned to the surgical side. Usually, frequent and early ambulation is encouraged.

Mouth care is very important because of ulcerations that occur as a result of renal failure and steroid therapy. Mycostatin mouthwashes are usually prescribed.

Most clients feel very good as their renal function returns. Occasionally, the new kidney does not produce urine immediately. If this occurs, the client must be dialyzed until adequate renal function begins. This is often a time of great discouragement for the hopeful client. The client should be reassured that this is not uncommon, especially in recipients of cadaveric donated kidneys.

Donor. The usual postoperative care is similar to that after a nephrectomy (see Chapter 40). Often the donor re-

mains the forgotten person as all of the attention is focused on the transplanted kidney in the recipient. The pain of a nephrectomy is greater than that of the iliac fossa incision experienced by the recipient. Nephrectomy often requires partial rib resection and entry into the pleural space. In contrast to the recipient, who feels better as renal function is restored, the donor feels very sick for 2 to 3 days. Urine culture, renal function, and a complete blood count are reassessed before discharge, and the donor is followed up at regular intervals. Most donors are ready to be discharged from the hospital in 6 or 7 days and can usually return to work in a month.

The majority of related kidney donors have positive psychological reactions because the donation provides a boost in self-image and elation because of the improved health of a close family member. If the kidney does not function immediately or is rejected, the donor may feel disappointed and guilty. The donor is a healthy individual who sacrificed a kidney and took a leave from work and family. Each donor must always face the unanswered question of what will happen if the remaining kidney is injured or becomes diseased.

Immunosuppressive Therapy

Immunosuppressive therapy is used to suppress the body's immune response to the foreign kidney (Table 41-11). Azathioprine (Imuran), corticosteroids, and cyclosporine are the standard drugs ordered. These drugs are usually started on the day of transplantation. However, the method of administration can vary from center to center. All three medications must be taken daily while the graft is still functioning.

Cyclophosphamide (Cytoxan) has been found to be an adequate substitute for azathioprine. However, it is primarily used to reduce the dose of azathioprine if the client develops toxicity in the liver.

Cyclosporine (cyclosporin A), first used in Europe in 1978, is now being used in all kidney transplant centers in the United States. The mechanism of action of this fungus extract is to prevent the production and release of interleukin 2 from T-helper lymphocytes (Fig. 41-16). Since the proliferation and maturation of T-cytotoxic lymphocytes is mediated by interleukin 2, cyclosporine alters the cell-mediated immune attack against the transplanted kidney. This drug does not cause bone marrow depression or alter the

Table 41-11 Immunosuppressive Therapy for Renal Transplant Recipients

Agent	Route of Administration	Mechanism of Action	Adverse Side Effects
Azathioprine (Imuran)	IV, PO	Is derivative of 6-mercaptopurine, interferes with purine synthesis and inhibits DNA and RNA synthesis, inhibits proliferation of T lymphocytes	Bone marrow suppression (leukopenia, anemia, thrombocytopenia), drug-induced hepatitis, oral lesions, increased susceptibility to infection
Corticosteroids Prednisone Methylprednisolone (Solu-Medrol)	PO IV	Suppress inflammatory response, prevent proliferation of T-cytotoxic lymphocytes	Cushingoid syndrome (peptic ulcer, GI bleeding, aseptic necrosis, sodium and water retention, acne, muscle weakness, fat dystrophy, capillary fragility, delayed healing, hyperglycemia, mood alterations); bacterial, fungal, and viral infections
Cyclophosphamide (Cytoxan)	PO	Is alkylating agent; interferes with DNA, RNA, and protein synthesis	Alopecia, leukopenia, hemorrhagic cystitis
ALG, ATG	IV, IM	Has unknown mechanism, is directed against lymphocytes, reduces circulating lymphocytes, decreases lymphocyte proliferation	Serum sickness, fever and chills, anaphylactic shock, rash, local phlebitis, thrombocytopenia
Cyclosporine (Cyclosporin A, Sandimmune)	PO, IV	Prevents production and release of interleukin 2, inhibits maturation of T-cytotoxic lymphocyte precursors	Hepatotoxicity, nephrotoxicity, lymphomas, infections, skin rashes, hirsutism, hypertension, tremors, gingival hyperplasia, breast fibroadenoma, nausea, and anorexia
OKT3 (Orthoclone OKT3)	IV push	Masks T-cell receptor for foreign antigens that recognize HLA mismatch between donor and recipient	Fever, headache, vomiting, chills, diarrhea, hypotension, bronchospasm, infection, aseptic meningitis

PO, Orally; *IM,* intramuscular; *ALG,* antilymphocytic globulin; *ATG,* antithymocytic globulin.

normal inflammatory response. Cyclosporine is used in conjunction with steroids or a combination of steroids and azathioprine. Many of the side effects of cyclosporine, which are listed in Table 41-11, are dose related.

Antilymphocyte globulin (ALG) and antithymocyte globulin (ATG) are also used as immunosuppressive therapy in many transplant centers. These agents are prepared by immunizing horses, rabbits, or goats with lymphoblasts (for ALG) or thymocytes (for ATG). Human thymocytes are obtained from the thymic tissue of cadavers or from clients who are undergoing cardiac surgery. The ALG or ATG is then purified and given to humans. The actual mechanism of action of ALG and ATG is not known. These polyclonal antibody preparations, which are directed against lymphocytes, induce lymphopenia and decrease the proliferative response of T lymphocytes, possibly as a result of the generation of T-suppressor lymphocytes. Current experience suggests that ALG and ATG should be used at the onset of an acute rejection rather than as maintenance immunosuppressive therapy.

In contrast to the polyclonal antibody preparations of ALG and ATG, monoclonal antibodies are used for treating acute rejection episodes (see Chapter 8). OKT3 was the first of these monoclonal antibodies to be used in clinical transplantation.[26] OKT3 is a mouse monoclonal antibody that reacts with the T3 antigen found on the surface of human thymocytes and mature T cells. Thus OKT3 is an antiantigen-receptor antibody that interferes with the immunological function of the T lymphocyte, the pivotal cell in the response to graft rejection. This agent reverses 95% of acute rejection episodes. OKT3 is administered IV push daily for 10 to 14 days.

Within minutes after the initial infusion of OKT3, circulating T cells become essentially undetectable. Adverse reactions are usually experienced with the first, second, and third injections and include a febrile response beginning 30 to 60 minutes after infusion. The most exciting aspect of monoclonal antibody therapy is the possibility of developing immunosuppressive protocols with highly uniform activity directed toward only selected T-cell subsets rather than toward the entire lymphocyte population.

Immunosuppressives affect the entire body, not just the transplanted kidney. This puts the client at great risk for infection. More specific immunosuppressive therapy aimed only at the foreign kidney, not the total body, is needed.

Complications

Rejection

Hyperacute rejection. Hyperacute (humoral-mediated) rejection occurs minutes to hours after transplantation. Renal vessels thrombose and the kidney dies. Preformed antibodies from pregnancy, blood transfusions, or previous transplants react with recipient antigens in the donor kidney. There is no treatment and the transplanted kidney is removed. Hyperacute rejection can be prevented by avoiding the transplantation of a kidney to the HLA-antigens of which the recipient has been sensitized.

Acute rejection. Acute rejection most commonly occurs 4 days to 4 months after transplantation. This type of rejection is mediated by the recipient's T-cytotoxic cells, which attack the foreign kidney. It is not uncommon to have at least one rejection episode, especially with cadaveric-donated kidneys. These episodes are usually reversible with immunosuppressive therapy, which usually consists of increased doses of steroids, ALG, ATG, and OKT3.

Signs of rejection include decreasing creatinine clearance, increasing serum creatinine, elevated BUN levels, fever, weight gain, decreased urine output, increasing blood pressure, and a swollen and painful transplant site. Most of these features are uncommon in a client receiving cyclosporine, which makes it difficult to distinguish between acute rejection and nephrotoxicity as a side effect of the drug.

Chronic rejection. Chronic rejection is a process that occurs over months or years. It is associated with a gradual occlusion of the renal blood vessels. Signs include proteinuria, hypertension, steady weight gain, and increasing serum creatinine levels. There is no definitive therapy for this type of rejection. Treatment is mainly supportive (physiological and psychosocial). This type of rejection is difficult to manage and is not associated with the optimistic prognosis of acute rejection.

Infections. Infections are common and serious complications of immunosuppressive therapy. Respiratory infections are the most frequent cause of death from infection. The client is at greatest risk during the early months when maximum dosages of immunosuppressives are administered. The client with a compromised immune system is very susceptible to infection from opportunistic organisms. Bacterial infections (pneumonia, urinary tract, and wound) are usually caused by endogenous organisms. *Pneumocystis carinii* (a parasitic protozoan), *Legionella* organisms (gram-negative bacteria), and *Mycobacterium tuberculosis* are also common causes of respiratory infections. Viral infections (cytomegalovirus) occur frequently after prolonged steroid therapy. Fungal infections (e.g., *Candida, Cryptococcus* organisms) can occur anywhere and are difficult to treat.

Malignancies. The incidence of malignancies (5% to 6% of clients) in kidney transplant recipients is 100 times greater than that in the general population. In general, the primary reason for this increased incidence is related to an altered immune system, which is due to the effect of immunosuppressive therapy. The malignancies include cancer of the skin and lips, lymphomas, and Kaposi's sarcoma.

Recurrence of renal disease. Recurrence of the same type of renal disease that destroyed the original kidney takes place in 15% of kidney transplant recipients. It is most common with certain types of glomerulonephritis and can result in the loss of a functioning kidney transplant.

Vascular disease. Clients who receive transplants as well as those who remain on hemodialysis have an increased incidence of atherosclerotic vascular disease. The exact reasons for this are not known. It may be due to an inability to alter the process that started with renal failure or to hypertension and hyperlipidemia that are present and enhanced by steroid therapy.[27] Table 41-12 covers dietary instruction after transplantation.

Table 41-12 Dietary Instructions to the Client After a Kidney Transplant

Rationale for diet
  After you have had a kidney transplant, most of the dietary restrictions you followed before the surgery are no longer needed. However, you will need to follow a salt-restricted, high-protein diet with special attention to weight control.
Salt
  A low-salt diet (2 g of sodium) helps prevent fluid retention and controls blood pressure.
Protein
  Your body needs increased dietary protein for two reasons:
    1. To repair body tissue damaged during the transplant
    2. To replace protein broken down by steroid medications
Calories
  Because some of your new medications can cause high blood sugar levels, increased appetite, and excessive weight gain, you should try to avoid high-caloric foods (sweets, sugar, fried foods, soda, potato chips) as much as possible. Snack on low-caloric foods (vegetables, fruits, plain yogurt) to help satisfy your hunger.

From Dietary Department, University of New Mexico Hospitals, Albuquerque, NM.

Aseptic bone necrosis. Aseptic necrosis of the hips, knees, or both can occur in kidney transplant recipients. This problem is primarily due to the side effects of chronic steroid therapy and may be potentiated by altered calcium metabolism. Currently, there is no intervention to prevent this complication.

Adaptation to and Effectiveness of Transplantation

If a transplant is successful, the client has the potential to return to nearly normal functioning. Most clients feel so improved that euphoria predominates for a while. Some of the euphoria is due to the effect of the steroids. The question of rejection (if and when) is a continual fear. The longer a person goes without rejection, the better the prognosis. Even if a kidney is rejected, the alternatives of dialysis and another transplant are available.

Most people who have successful transplants believe that it was worth all the risks to feel so good. These individuals suffer the greatest depression when the kidney is rejected after many months or years. They need to be reassured that they have done nothing (other than possibly failing to comply with drug therapy) to cause the rejection to occur.

The prolongation of life in chronic renal failure puts clients in an unusual situation. First they wonder whether they can learn to accept death, and then there is hope for life with dialysis. Next they ask a healthy relative to donate a kidney or they receive a cadaveric kidney transplant. Then they live through months wondering how long this new kidney will last.

The leading causes of death after transplantation are infection and cardiovascular disease. If the transplant is successful, the quality of life is much better than that offered by maintenance dialysis.

The use of cyclosporine and OKT3 has dramatically improved graft survival in the past 5 years. The 3-year client and graft survival rates for LRD transplant recipients are now 95% and 85%, respectively; for cadaveric transplant recipients, 3-year client and graft survival rates are 80% and 70%, respectively.

When the transplant fails, the client usually returns to dialysis and can continue on dialysis or wait for another transplant. Because immunosuppressive therapy is still inadequate, a major research goal is to develop more specific and less toxic drugs.

C ase Study

CHRONIC RENAL FAILURE

Curt had been treated for acute glomerulonephritis at the age of 5. At that time, his urine showed proteinuria and hematuria. At the age of 11 he was diagnosed as having recurring acute glomerulonephritis. He had no follow-up care during the next 10 years. At the age of 21 he began noticing weakness on walking, paresthesia, dyspnea on exertion, headaches, diplopia, and swollen hands and feet. His skin was yellowish and sallow. He complained of some itching. A diagnostic workup showed the following:

Serum creatinine	15.4 mg/dl
Creatinine clearance	4.0 ml/min
BUN	156 mg/dl
Potassium	6.8 mEq/L
Bicarbonate	12.0 mEq/L
Hematocrit	20%
Blood pressure	146/100
Chest x-ray examination	Cardiomegaly and pulmonary edema

He was diagnosed as having chronic glomerulonephritis, and an internal AV fistula was surgically created. He was started on hemodialysis 3 times weekly.

His therapeutic management consisted of the following:
  Alu-Caps
  Methyldopa (Aldomet)
  Multivitamins
  Ferrous gluconate
  Folic acid
  Diet consisting of 60 g protein, 2 g sodium, 1500 ml fluid per day

Discussion Questions

1. Explain the basic pathological changes that resulted in the development of chronic glomerulonephritis.
2. Identify the abnormal diagnostic study results and explain why each would occur. What is their significance for nursing observation and care?
3. Explain why Curt developed each of his clinical manifestations. What is the appropriate nursing intervention for each one?
4. What is the purpose of Curt's therapeutic management?
5. Explain the principles of hemodialysis and how it works to treat renal failure.

R eview Questions

The number of the question corresponds to the same-numbered objective at the beginning of the chapter.

1. Which of the following best describes acute renal failure?
   a. complete absence of renal blood flow
   b. sudden reduction in renal function
   c. rapid increase in urine output with azotemia
   d. gradual increase in the GFR

2. Common causes of ATN include
   a. septic abortion and acute glomerulonephritis
   b. blood transfusion reaction and carbon tetrachloride inhalation
   c. acute pyelonephritis and ureteral calculi
   d. congestive heart failure and hepatorenal syndrome

3. During the diuretic phase of acute renal failure, which of the following serum electrolyte imbalances is most likely to develop?
   a. increased potassium and decreased sodium
   b. increased potassium and increased sodium
   c. decreased potassium and increased sodium
   d. decreased potassium and decreased sodium

4. If a client in the oliguric phase of acute renal failure has urinated 300 ml during the previous 24 hours, how much fluid should the client have during the next 24 hours?
   a. 300 ml
   b. 500 ml
   c. 800 ml
   d. 1000 ml

5. Demineralization of the bones can occur in uremic syndrome because
   a. uremic toxins prevent calcium from combining with bone matrix
   b. secondary hyperparathyroidism causes mobilization of calcium out of the bones
   c. dietary restrictions to combat uremia prevent calcium intake
   d. metabolic acidosis prevents normal bone formation

6. The following measures are used in the management of chronic renal failure. For which one is the correct rationale given?
   a. Kayexalate to reduce peripheral edema
   b. aluminum hydroxide to decrease serum phosphate
   c. calcitriol to decrease serum calcium
   d. methyldopa to increase urine output

7. Nursing care for a client on chronic peritoneal dialysis includes all of the following *except*
   a. encouraging protein intake of high biological value
   b. decreasing the inflow rate if referred shoulder pain is experienced
   c. changing the peritoneal catheter every 2 to 3 weeks
   d. instructing the client that fluid intake is unrestricted

8. A common complication associated with internal AV fistulas is
   a. infection
   b. palpable thrill
   c. thrombosis
   d. bleeding

9. Complications of renal transplantation include
   a. hepatitis and hypertension
   b. malignancies and vascular disease
   c. steal syndrome and infection
   d. bleeding and osteodystrophy

10. Which of the following factors have to be compatible in the donor and recipient before a renal transplant can be considered?
    a. gender and HLA
    b. familial relationship and Rh factor
    c. ABO blood groups and tissue crossmatch
    d. age and ABO blood groups

11. The most common problem associated with immunosuppressive therapy is
    a. anemia
    b. thrombocytopenia
    c. predisposition to infection
    d. hypercoagulation

REFERENCES

1. Baer CL: Acute renal failure: recognizing and reversing its deadly course, Nursing 20:34-39, 1990.
2. Epstein FH and Brown RS: Acute renal failure: a collection of paradoxes, Hosp Pract 23:171-194, 1988.
3. Norns MKG: About acute renal failure, Nursing 19:21, 1989.
4. Beck LH: Kidney function and disease in the elderly, Hosp Pract 23:75-90, 1988.
5. Maher JF: Replacement of renal function by dialysis, ed 3, Boston, 1989, Kluwer Academic Publishers.
6. United States Renal Data System, 1987.
7. United States Congress, Office of Technology Assessment: Life-sustaining technologies and the elderly, Pub No OTA-BA-306, Washington, DC, 1987, US Government Printing Office.
8. Fine LG: The uremic syndrome: adaptive mechanisms and therapy, Hosp Pract 22:63-73, 1987.
9. Paganini EP: A review of anemia associated with chronic renal disease: primary and secondary mechanisms, Semin Nephrol 9:3-8, 1989.
10. Williams B and others: The use of calcium carbonate to treat the hyperphosphatemia of chronic renal failure, Nephrol Dial Transplant 4:725-729, 1989.
11. Martis L, Serkes KD, and Nolph KD: Calcium carbonate as a phosphate binder: is there a need to adjust peritoneal dialysate calcium concentrations for patients using $CaCO_3$? Peritoneal Dial Int 9:325-328, 1989.
12. Hatch FE: Reversing the anemia of renal failure, Hosp Pract 25:25-34, 1990.
13. Eschbach JW and Adamson JW: Recombinant human erythropoietin: implications for nephrology, Am J Kid Dis 11:203-209, 1988.
14. Ihle BU and others: The effect of protein restriction on the progression of renal insufficiency, N Engl J Med 321:1773, 1989.
15. Hickman RO and Watkins S: Peritoneal dialysis access: an introduction, Dial Transplant 17:10-12, 1988.
16. Twardowski ZJ: Peritoneal dialysis: current technology and techniques, Postgrad Med 85:161-182, 1989.
17. Diaz-Buxo JA: Current status of continuous cyclic peritoneal dialysis (CCPD), Peritoneal Dialysis International 9:9-14, 1989.
18. Strangio L: Peritoneal dialysis made easy, Nursing 18:43-46, 1988.

19. Hickman RO and Watkins S: A review of hemodialysis catheters and access devices, Dial Transplant 16:481, 1987.

20. Gluck Z and Nolph KD: Ascites associated with end-stage renal disease, Am J Kid Dis 10:9-18, 1987.

21. Boileau M and others: Renal adenocarcinoma and end-stage kidney disease, J Urol 138:603-606, 1987.

22. Port FK and others: Neoplasms in dialysis patients: a population-based study, Am J Kid Dis 14:119-123, 1989.

23. Dirkes SM: Making a critical difference with CAVH, Nursing 19:57-60, 1989.

24. Paradiso C: Hemofiltration: an alternative to dialysis, Heart Lung 18:282-290, 1989.

25. Hull A: UNOS, HCFA data confirms dismal year for organ procurement, Nephrol News Issues 4:14-17, 1990.

26. Trusler LA: OKT3: nursing considerations for use in acute renal transplant rejection, ANNA J 17:299-303, 1990.

27. Gammarino M: Renal transplant diet: recommendations for the acute phase, Dial Transplant 16:497-502, 1987.

SECTION VII REFERENCES

BOOKS

Brumfitt W and Hamilton-Miller JMC: Urinary tract infections, vol 1, St Louis, 1990, Mosby–Year Book, Inc.

Carlton CE, ed: Controversies in urology, Chicago, 1989, Year Book Medical Publishers.

Chan JCM and Gill JR Jr, eds: Kidney electrolyte disorders, New York, 1990, Churchill Livingstone, Inc.

Gardner KD and Bernstein J, eds: The ceptic kidney, Boston, 1990, Kluwer Academic Publishers.

Gatto GRD, ed: Urinary tract infections, Boston, 1989, Kluwer Academic Publishers.

Glassock RJ: Current therapy in nephrology and hypertension, vol 3, ed 3, St Louis, 1990, Mosby–Year Book, Inc.

Jacobson HR, Striker GE, and Klahr S: Nephrology, St Louis, 1990, Mosby–Year Book, Inc.

Nissenson AR, Fine RN, and Gentile EC: Clinical dialysis, ed 2, Norwalk, Conn, 1990, Appleton & Lange.

Resnick MI, Caldamone AA, and Spirnak JP: Decision making in urology, vol 2, ed 2, St Louis, 1990, Mosby–Year Book, Inc.

Resnick MI and Pak CYC: Urolithiasis: a medical and surgical reference, Philadelphia, 1990, WB Saunders Co.

Teter CF, Faller N, and North C, eds: Nursing for continence, Philadelphia, 1990, WB Saunders Co.

Wein AJ: Voiding function and dysfunction: a logical and practical approach, Chicago, 1988, Year Book Medical Publishers.

JOURNALS

Ader K, Pierce LL, and Salter JP: Urinary tract infections: a quality assurance rehabilitation nursing perspective, Rehabil Nurs 15:193, 1990.

Ashby D: Hyponatremia after transurethral resection of the prostate, J Post Anesth Nurs 3:121, 1988.

Baer CL: Assessing flank pain, Nursing 19:75, 1989.

Bavendam TG: Stress urinary incontinence in women, J Enterostomal Ther 17:57, 1990.

Brennan C: Lithotripter treatment of kidney stones in outpatient surgery, J Post Anesth Nurs 4:170, 1989.

Danziger CH: Uremic neuropathy and treatment with renal transplantation, ANNA J 16:67, 1989.

Finocchiaro DN and Herzfeld ST: Understanding autonomic dysreflexia, Am J Nurs 90:56, 1990.

Gharbieh PA: Renal transplant: surgical and psychologic hazards, Crit Care Nurs 8:58, 1988.

Gilbert V and Gobbi M: Making sense of . . . bladder irrigation, Nurs Times 85:40, 1989.

Lancaster LE: Renal response to shock, Crit Care Nurs Clin North Am 2:221, 1990.

Mackety CJ: Lasers in urology, Nurs Clin North Am 25:697, 1990.

Manion BA: Lyme disease in chronic renal failure: CAPD therapy, ANNA J 17:320, 1990.

McLean MH: Implanting an artificial urinary sphincter, Can Oper Room Nurs J 7:5, 1989.

Miles B: Elderly people: incontinence, Nursing (London) 3:26, 1989.

Newman DK and Smith DA: Incontinence: the problem patients won't talk about, RN 52:42, 1989.

Plawecki HM, Freiberg G, and Plawecki JA: Increasing organ donation in the black community, AANA J 16:321, 1989.

Roe BH: Use of bladder washouts: a study of nurses' recommendations, J Adv Nurs 14:494, 1989.

Rudolphi DM: Renovascular hypertension diagnosis to discharge: a case study, J Vasc Nurs 8:6, 1990.

Smith MF: Renal trauma: adult and pediatric considerations, Crit Care Nurs Clin North Am 2:67, 1990.

Stark JL: A quick guide to urinary tract assessment, Nursing 18:56, 1988.

Storrar ML: Urinary diversion and bladder reconstruction, NATNEWS 27:11, 1990.

Switters DM: Assessing leakage from around the urethral catheter, Urol Nurs 9:8, 1989.

Systems of life no 171: senior systems—36: urinary incontinence—2: promoting continence, Nurs Times 85:61, 1989.

Taylor T: Preventing complications from hemodialysis, Dimens Crit Care Nurs 9:210, 1990.

Walpert N: An orderly look at calcium metabolism disorders, Nursing 20:60, 1990.

Watson R: An improved urinary sheath, Nurs Elder 2:12, 1990.

Webster D: Comparing patients' and nurses' views of interstitial cystitis: a pilot study, Urol Nurs 10:10, 1990.

Weiskittel P and Sommers MS: The patient with lower urinary tract trauma, Crit Care Nurs 9:53, 1989.

Wheeler V: A new kind of loving? The effect of continence problems on sexuality, Prof Nurs 5:492, 1990.

Wilson M: Securing indwelling ureteral catheters during lithotripsy, Urol Nurs 9:20, 1989.

ORGANIZATIONS

American Nephrology Nurses Association
North Woodbury Rd, Box 56
Pitman, NJ 08071

American Urological Association Allied
11512 Allecingie Parkway
Richmond, VA 23235

National Kidney Foundation
30 East 33rd Street
New York, NY 10016

United Ostomy Association
36 Executive Park, Suite 120
Irvine, CA 92714

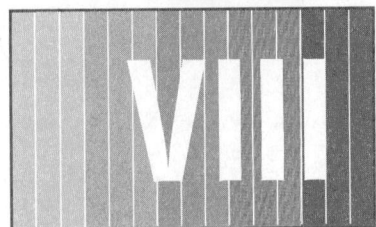
PROBLEMS RELATED TO REGULATORY MECHANISMS

CHAPTER

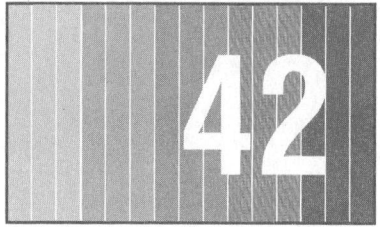

Nursing Assessment
Endocrine System

Linda B. Haas

L earning Objectives

1. Identify the common characteristics and functions of hormones.
2. Identify the locations of the endocrine glands.
3. Describe the functions of hormones secreted by the pituitary, thyroid, parathyroid, and adrenal glands and the pancreas.
4. Describe the locations and roles of hormone receptors.
5. Identify significant subjective and objective data related to the endocrine system that a nurse should obtain from a client.
6. Describe the technique used in physical assessment of the thyroid gland.
7. Differentiate normal from abnormal findings in assessment of the endocrine system.
8. Describe age-related changes in the endocrine system and differences in assessment findings.
9. Describe the purpose and significance of results of and nursing responsibilities for diagnostic studies of the endocrine system.

The endocrine system is an integrated chemical communication and coordination system that enables reproduction, growth and development, and regulation of energy. With the nervous system, it maintains the internal homeostasis of the body and coordinates responses to environmental changes and stress. The endocrine system is composed of glands or glandular tissues that synthesize, store, and secrete chemical messengers (hormones) that affect specific target organs and body tissues through the bloodstream. The specificity of this system is determined by the affinity of receptors on the target organs and tissues for a particular hormone. The endocrine glands include the hypothalamus, pituitary, thyroid, parathyroids, adrenals, kidneys, pancreatic islets, ovaries, and testes (Fig. 42-1) (see Chapters 39 and 45).

STRUCTURES AND FUNCTIONS OF THE ENDOCRINE SYSTEM
Glands

Exocrine glands. Exocrine glands pass along their secretions through ducts that empty outside the body or into

Reviewed by Florencetta Hayes Gibson, R.N., M.S.N., C.N.S., Assistant Professor, School of Nursing, Northeast Louisiana University, Monroe, Louisiana.

the lumen of the organ lined with the same embryonic epithelium as the gland. For example, the exocrine secretions of the sweat glands are discharged directly onto the surface of the skin. Exocrine secretions of the pancreas, called *enzymes,* are secreted into the pancreatic duct and transported to the intestine.

Endocrine glands. Endocrine organs (glands and cells) are ductless but highly vascularized. They synthesize hormones and secrete them into the bloodstream, where they influence specific target tissues.

Hormones

Characteristics. A hormone is a chemical substance synthesized and secreted by a specific organ or tissue and carried by the blood to other sites in the body where its actions are exerted. Most hormones have common characteristics, including (1) circulation through the blood, (2) secretion in minute but effective amounts at predictable but variable rates, (3) binding to specific cellular receptors to change intracellular metabolism, and (4) variable alteration of the rates of physiological responses of target tissues. A newly discovered chemical messenger believed to be a hormone is called a *factor* until its chemical structure has been determined.

Some hormones (e.g., somatostatin, vasoactive intesti-

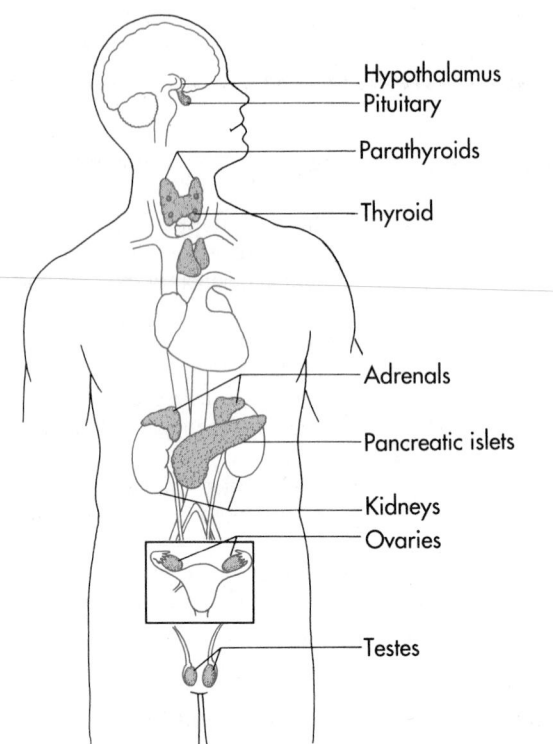

Fig. 42-1 Location of the major endocrine glands. The parathyroid glands actually lie on the posterior surface of the thyroid.

- Hypothalamus
- Pituitary
- Parathyroids
- Thyroid
- Adrenals
- Pancreatic islets
- Kidneys
- Ovaries
- Testes

nal peptide) are synthesized and secreted by several tissues and stimulate different physiological responses depending on the source and target tissue. For example, somatostatin is found in several areas of the brain, including the part of the hypothalmus that contols the anterior pituitary. In this instance, somatostatin inhibits growth hormone and thyroid-stimulating hormone (TSH) release. Somatostatin is also synthesized and secreted by the δ cells of the endocrinepancreas where it inhibits insulin and glucagon release, probably in a paracrine manner.

Structure. Structurally the major hormones are amines, peptides (proteins), or steroids. Amine hormones, derived from the amino acid tyrosine, include the catecholamines and dopamine, which bind to cell membrane receptors, and thyroid hormones, which bind to receptors in the cell nucleus. Peptide hormones, because of their large size and lipid insolubility, are unable to penetrate cell membranes and bind to receptors on the cell membranes. The hormone-receptor complex then activates intracellular processes and ultimately the activity of genes. Steroid hormones, secreted by the adrenal cortices and gonads, are synthesized from cholesterol, are lipid soluble, and are able to diffuse into cells and bind to specific receptors in the nucleus.

Hormones may also be classified in terms of their solubility in aqueous solutions. Hormones transported in blood bound to plasma proteins such as steroids and thyroid hormones have limited water solubility. Water-soluble, non-protein-bound hormones such as peptides and catecholamines circulate freely.

Functions. Hormones alter the rate of many physiological activities. Important hormonal functions are related to reproduction, responses to stress and injury, ionic and energy metabolism, and growth and development. Table 42-1 summarizes the major hormones, their synthesizing glands, target organs or systems, and functions.

Hormone-Receptor Interaction

Hormone receptors. The specificity of hormone–target cell interaction is determined by receptors.[1] Receptors or binding sites are glycoprotein macromolecules of the target cell that interact with a hormone in the first step of the action of a hormone.[2] The receptor actually allows the substance to recognize the cell. Steroid and thyroid hormone receptors are in the nucleus of the target cell, whereas receptors for other hormones span the cell membrane.

Intracellular hormone-receptor complexes, such as those seen in steroid hormone action, occur in the cell nucleus, where they stimulate or inhibit the synthesis of messenger ribonucleic acid (mRNA). This mRNA migrates to the cytoplasm, where it stimulates the synthesis of new protein (Fig. 42-2). Peptide hormone and catecholamine receptors are located on the cell membrane. The hormone-receptor complex stimulates or inhibits intracellular cyclic adenosine monophosphate (cAMP), a secondary messenger. cAMP exerts its action by activating kinases to regulate intracellular enzyme activity (Fig. 42-3).

Thyroid hormones act at several cellular sites. Specific receptors exist on the cell membranes and within the mitochondria and nucleus. At the cell membrane, the hormone-receptor complex stimulates nutrient transport; in the mitochondria, the complex increases metabolic energy; and at the nuclear level, it promotes synthesis of structural and functional cellular components.

Regulation of Hormonal Secretion

The regulation of endocrine activity is controlled by specific mechanisms of varying levels of complexity. These mechanisms stimulate or inhibit hormone synthesis and secretion. One such mechanism, *simple feedback,* which may be negative or positive, is based on the blood level of a particular substance. This substance may be a hormone or other chemical compound regulated by or responsive to a hormone.

In *negative feedback,* high levels of the substance inhibit hormone synthesis and secretion, and low levels stimulate hormone synthesis and secretion. Negative feedback is similar to the functioning of a thermostat in which cold air in a room activates the thermostat to release heat, and hot air turns off the thermostat to prevent more warm air from entering the room. A physiological example of this is the relation between calcium and parathyroid hormone (PTH). Low blood calcium levels stimulate the parathyroid glands to release PTH, which acts on bone, the intestine, and the kidneys to increase blood calcium levels. The increased blood calcium levels then inhibit further PTH release (Fig. 42-4).

In *positive feedback,* high levels of a substance stimulate hormone synthesis and secretion, and low levels inhibit hormone synthesis and secretion. An example of pos-

Table 42-1 Major Hormones

Hormones	Target Organ or System	Functions
ANTERIOR PITUITARY		
Growth hormone or somatotropin*	Multiple sites (e.g., skeletal system, glands)	Growth of all tissue, organic metabolism
Thyroid-stimulating hormone or thyrotropin	Thyroid gland	Synthesis and release of thyroid hormone, growth and function of thyroid (stimulation of thyroidal iodine uptake)
Adrenocorticotropic hormone or corticotropin	Adrenal cortex	Growth of adrenal cortex, secretion of corticosteroids
Prolactin or lactogen	Breasts	Stimulation of milk production, protein synthesis, mammary gland development
Gonadotropic hormones* (e.g., follicle-stimulating and luteinizing hormones)	Reproductive organs	Sex cell production, sex hormone secretion, reproductive organ growth
β-lipotropin		Stimulation of target organs for the release of hormones, growth and development of target organs
POSTERIOR PITUITARY		
Oxytocin†	Reproductive system, breasts	Milk secretion, uterine motility
Antidiuretic hormone or vasopressin†	Renal system, vascular smooth muscle	Resorption of water, peristalsis
THYROID		
Thyroxine	All body tissues	Energy metabolism
Triiodothyronine		Growth and development, metabolism, control of body temperature
Calcitonin	Plasma	Regulation of calcium and phosphate blood levels, stimulation of bone demineralization
PARATHYROIDS		
Parathyroid hormone or parathormone	Bone, intestine, kidneys	Regulation of calcium blood levels (bone demineralization)
ADRENAL MEDULLA		
Epinephrine or adrenalin	Fuel for metabolic system, cardiovascular system	Response to stress, organic metabolism, increase of cardiac output
ADRENAL CORTEX		
Cortisol or hydrocortisone	Cardiovascular system, fuel for metabolic system	Organic metabolism, response to stress
Androgens (e.g., testosterone and androsterone)	Reproductive system	Masculinization, growth and sexual activity in women

Modified from Vander AJ and others: Human physiology: the mechanisms of body function, New York, 1985, McGraw-Hill Book Co, Inc, p 232.
*These hormones are synthesized in the hypothalamus; the anterior pituitary stores and secretes them.
†These hormones are synthesized in the hypothalamus; the posterior pituitary stores and secretes them.
‡GI hormones are also called *GI regulatory peptides* because they function in paracrine and neurotransmitter manners as well as hormones.

Table 42-1   Major Hormones—cont'd

Hormones	Target Organ or System	Functions
ADRENAL CORTEX—cont'd		
Aldosterone	Kidney	Regulation of sodium and potassium balance and thus electrolyte and water balance
Norepinephrine	Cardiovascular system	Response to stress
PANCREAS		
Insulin	All body systems	Regulation of energy metabolism
Glucagon	Liver	Same as above
Somatostatin or growth hormone–release inhibiting hormone	Pancreas	Inhibition of insulin and glucagon
GONADS		
Women: ovaries		
Estrogen	Reproductive system, breasts	Development of secondary sex characteristics, preparation of uterus for fertilization and fetal development
Progesterone	Reproductive system	Preparation of uterus for fertilization and fetal development
Men: testes		
Testosterone	Reproductive system	Development of secondary sex characteristics, production of sperm
KIDNEYS		
Erythropoietin	Bone marrow	Stimulation of red blood cell production
LIVER		
Somatomedin C	Skeletal system	Bone growth
HEART		
Atrial natriuretic factor	Kidneys	Water excretion
GASTROINTESTINAL TRACT‡		
Gastrin	Stomach	Stimulation of acid, enzyme, water, electrolyte secretion
	Pancreas	Stimulation of enzyme, water, electrolyte secretion
Cholecystokinen	Gallbladder	Stimulation of contraction
	Pancreas	Stimulation of enzyme secretion
Secretin	Pancreas	Stimulation of water and bicarbonate secretion, enhancement of insulin release
Vasoactive intestinal peptide (VIP)	Pancreas	Stimulation of pancreatic secretions
	Liver	Stimulation of glycogenolysis and gluconeogenesis
	Intestine	Regulation of motility and ion and water transport

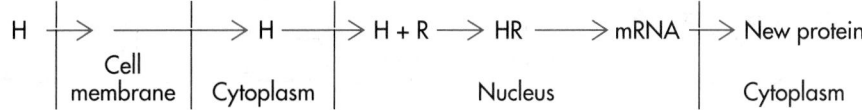

Fig. 42-2 Hormone-receptor action: steroid hormones. Hormone *(H)* diffuses through the cell membrane and cytoplasm and combines with its receptor *(R)* in the nucleus to form a hormone-receptor complex *(HR)*, which affects formation of new mRNA. New mRNA then diffuses to the cytoplasm where it makes new protein.

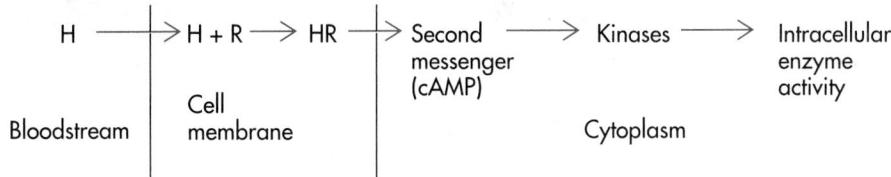

Fig. 42-3 Hormone-receptor action: peptide hormones and catecholamines. Hormone *(H)* binds to receptor *(R)* in the cell membrane to form hormone-receptor complex *(HR)*. The HR activates second messengers (e.g., cAMP) at the membrane's inner surface. The second messenger activates kinases in the cytoplasm. The kinases regulate intracellular activity.

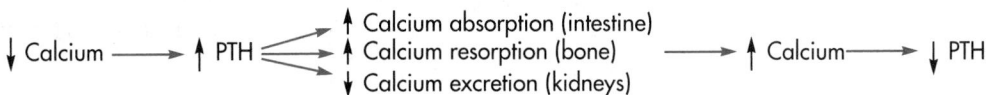

Fig. 42-4 Simple negative feedback: calcium and PTH.

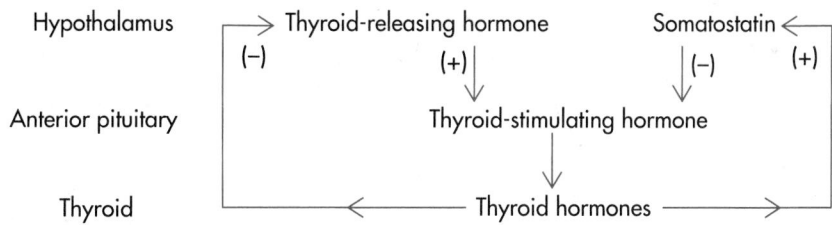

Fig. 42-5 Hypothalamic-pituitary–target gland feedback loop (TRH, TSH, thyroid hormones). Stimulatory (+) and inhibitory (−) feedback effects are shown.

itive feedback is the stimulatory effect of increased luteinizing hormone (LH) levels on ovarian estradiol secretion during the menstrual cycle.

Another level of complexity exists in feedback systems. An example of this is regulation of thyroid hormones (Fig. 42-5). TSH, or thyrotropin, from the anterior pituitary is activated by thyrotropin-releasing hormone (TRH) and is inhibited by somatostatin, both of which are secreted by the hypothalamus. In addition, low levels of thyroxine (T_4) and triiodothyronine (T_3) stimulate TSH release. Conversely, high circulating levels of a thyroid hormone inhibit TSH secretion.

An example of a complex feedback system is insulin regulation (Table 42-2). High levels of circulating glucose, amino acids, and fats (as seen after a meal) stimulate insu-

lin secretion. In addition, gastrointestinal (GI), or enteric, hormones such as gastrin and secretin enhance insulin release after a meal, as does vagal stimulation. After pure protein ingestion, glucagon stimulates insulin secretion. Insulin secretion is inhibited by low circulating levels of glucose and amino acids, high circulating levels of steroids and catecholamines (as seen in stress), hypokalemia, and other pancreatic hormones such as glucagon and somatostatin.

In addition to chemical regulation, some endocrine glands are directly affected by the activity of the nervous system. Nervous system involvement can result from stress; it is initiated by the central nervous system (CNS) and implemented by the autonomic nervous system.[3]

Another regulatory mechanism affecting many hor-

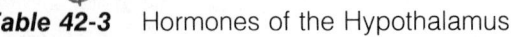

Cortisol related to energy related Hormones

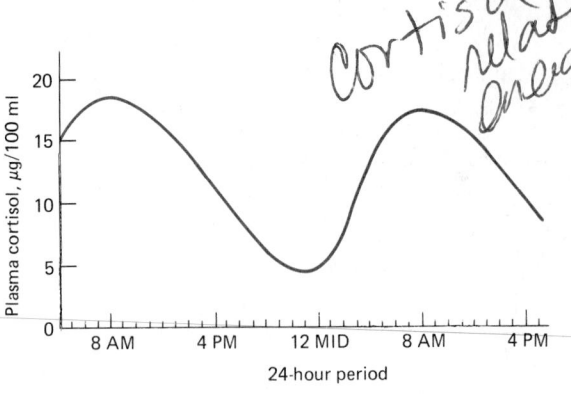

Fig. 42-6 Circadian rhythm of cortisol secretion.

Table 42-2 Factors Influencing Insulin Secretion

STIMULATE SECRETION	INHIBIT SECRETION
↑ Glucose levels	↓ Glucose levels
↑ Amino acid levels	↓ Amino acid levels
↑ Gastrointestinal hormone levels	↓ Potassium levels
↑ Vagal stimulation	↑ Steroid hormone levels
	↑ Catecholamine levels
	↑ Somatostatin levels
	↑ Glucagon levels (usually)
	↑ Insulin levels

monal secretions involves the *rhythms* of secretions. These rhythms originate in brain structures. A common physiological rhythm is the *diurnal (circadian) rhythm*, in which a hormone level fluctuates predictably during a 24 hours. These rhythms may be related to sleep-wake or dark-light cycles. For example, cortisol rises early in the day, declines toward evening, and rises again toward the end of sleep to peak by morning (Fig. 42-6). Growth hormone (GH) and prolactin secretion peak during sleep. TSH secretion is also maximum during sleep and ebbs 3 hours after a person wakens in the morning. The menstrual cycle is an example of a body rhythm that is longer than 24 hours (*ultradian*). These rhythms must be considered when interpreting laboratory data results related to hormone levels.

Neuroendocrine System

The nervous and endocrine systems are interrelated and interdependent. Autonomic nerves control endocrine gland blood flow and hormone secretion, and hormones have a regulatory effect on nervous tissue. For example, testosterone and estrogen affect the hypothalamic neuronal synthesis and release of follicle-stimulating hormone (FSH) and LH. Hormones can also influence behavior. In addition, substances can be hormones in one instance and neurotransmitters or modulators in another. For example, catecholamines are hormones when they are secreted by the adrenal medulla and neurotransmitters when they are secreted by nerve cells in the brain.[4] The differentiating factor is the mode of transport. When epinephrine travels through the bloodstream, it is a hormone. When it travels across synaptic junctions, it is a neurotransmitter.

Table 42-3 Hormones of the Hypothalamus

RELEASING HORMONES

CRH
TRH
Growth hormone–releasing hormone or somatotropin-releasing hormone
Gonadotropin-releasing hormone
Prolactin-releasing factor (e.g., vasoactive intestinal peptide)

INHIBITING HORMONES

Prolactin-inhibiting hormone
Somatostatin (inhibits TRH, GH, and TSH)
Dopamine (inhibits TSH and prolactin)

Hypothalamus

The hypothalamus and the pituitary gland integrate communication from the nervous and endocrine systems. CNS input is mediated by hypothalamic hormones and neurotransmitters (norepinephrine, dopamine, serotonin, and acetylcholine), which helps to regulate pituitary hormone secretion and has extrapituitary effects (e.g., influences secretion, metabolism, and transport of protein in the target organ).[5] Hypothalamic hormones can stimulate or inhibit the synthesis and release of anterior pituitary hormones (Table 42-3). Several hypothalamic hormones (e.g., somatostatin, TRH, and corticotropin-releasing hormone [CRH]) are synthesized and secreted in other areas of the body.

The hypothalamus and pituitary gland communicate via veins called the median eminence portal system (Fig. 42-7). The hypothalamus secretes releasing and inhibiting hormones that travel through the portal system to the anterior pituitary, where they interact with specific receptors and rapidly stimulate the synthesis and release of anterior pituitary hormones (Table 42-3).

Pituitary Gland

The pituitary gland (*hypophysis*) weighs about 0.6 g and is located in the sella turcica at the base of the brain above the sphenoid bone. It is connected to the hypothalamus by the infundibular (hypophyseal) stalk. The pituitary consists of two parts, the anterior (*adenohypophysis*) and the posterior (*neurohypophysis*) lobes.

Anterior pituitary. The anterior lobe accounts for 80% of the gland by weight. Anterior pituitary function is regulated by the integrated effects of hypothalamic releasing and inhibiting hormones and feedback effects from circulating hormones. Hormones secreted by the anterior pituitary include GH, TSH, adrenocorticotropic hormone (ACTH), prolactin, gonadotropic hormones (e.g., FSH and LH), and β-lipotropin (see Table 42-1).

Posterior pituitary. The posterior pituitary is an extension of the hypothalamus. The cell bodies of neurons that carry posterior pituitary hormones are in the hypothalamus, and the axons terminate in the posterior pituitary. The posterior pituitary lies ■ behind the anterior pituitary

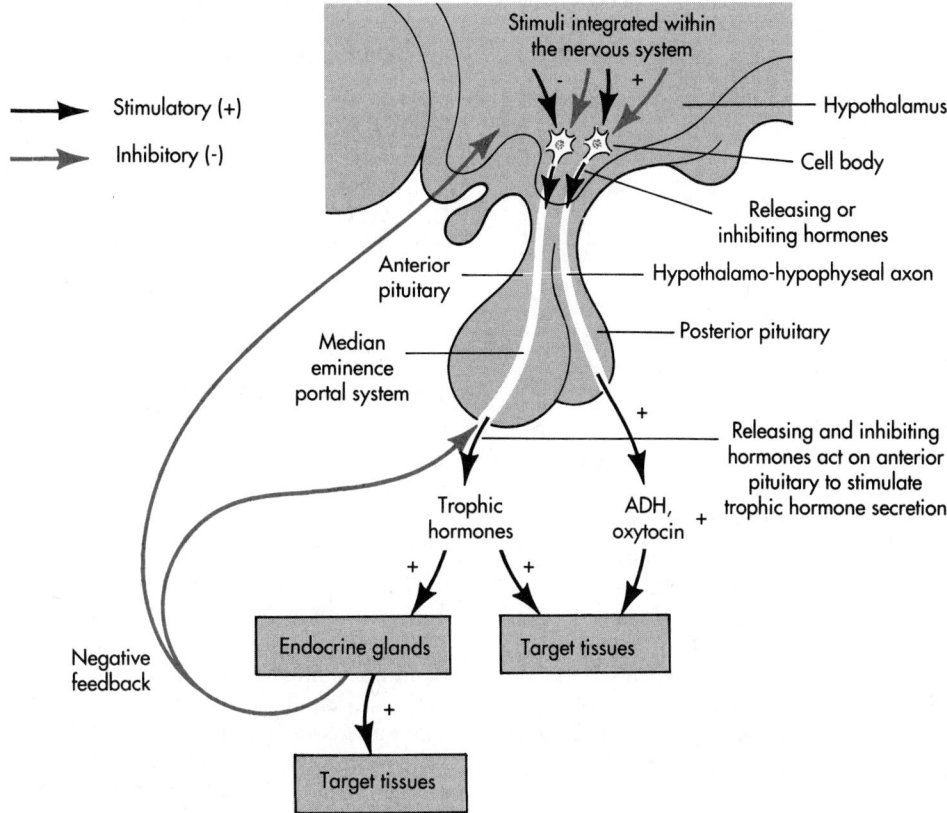

Fig. 42-7   Relationship among the hypothalamus, pituitary, and target tissues. Stimuli cause hypothalamic neurons to secrete releasing (+) or inhibitory (−) hormones. (Modified from Seeley RR, Stephens TD, and Tate P, eds: Anatomy and physiology, St Louis, 1989, Times Mirror/Mosby College Publishing, p 523.)

and consists of pituicytes, unmyelinated nerve fibers, and the terminals of axons. The hormones of the posterior pituitary, antidiuretic hormone (ADH) or vasopressin and oxytocin, are produced in the hypothalamus as prohormones, travel down the nerve fibers, and are stored in the posterior pituitary near capillaries. The hormones are released into the general circulation after appropriate stimulation.

The major physiological role of ADH is regulation of water volume by controlling renal water excretion. ADH is also a potent vasoconstrictor and potentiates the effects of CRH. The most important stimulus to ADH secretion is increased osmotic pressure of body water as reflected by increased plasma osmolality (a measure of solute concentration of circulating blood). Plasma osmolality is increased by decreased extracellular fluid or increased sodium concentration. The increased plasma osmolality activates hypothalamic osmoreceptors, which are extremely sensitive, specialized neurons. These activated osmoreceptors then stimulate ADH release. Therefore when body fluids become highly concentrated, osmoreceptors cause ADH release; thus a major effect of ADH is to enhance fluid retention by increasing cell permeability in the collecting tubules of the kidney and to enhance reabsorption of water. In the absence of ADH, dilute urine is excreted.

Nonosmotic stimuli to ADH secretion include decreased blood volume, hypotension, angiotensin, nausea, vomiting, hypoglycemia, and many pharmacological agents. ADH release is inhibited by hypothermia, β-adrenergic agents, and alcohol.[6]

Oxytocin stimulates milk ejection from the mammary gland, contraction of uterine smooth muscle, and possibly prolactin release. Secretion of oxytocin is increased by vaginal stimulation and stimulation of touch receptors in nipples as well as by hemorrhage and psychological stress. Oxytocin secretion is inhibited by loud noises, severe pain, and increased temperature.[7]

Thyroid Gland

The thyroid gland is located in the anterior portion of the neck in front of the trachea. It consists of two encapsulated lateral lobes connected by a narrow isthmus. It is a highly vascular organ.

The major function of the thyroid gland is the production, storage, and release of the thyroid hormones, T_4 and T_3. T_4 is the precursor for T_3, which is the more active hormone. About 10% of circulating T_3 is secreted directly by the thyroid gland, and the remainder is obtained by peripheral conversion of T_4.

Iodine is necessary for the synthesis of thyroid hormone. T_4 and T_3 affect the metabolic rate, caloric requirements, oxygen consumption, carbohydrate and lipid metabolism, growth and development, brain functions, and

nervous system activity. More than 99% of thyroid hormones circulate bound to plasma proteins, the majority to thyroid-binding globulin and the remainder to prealbumin and albumin. Only the unbound, "free" hormones and those bound to albumin are biologically active.

Thyroid hormone production and release is stimulated by TSH. Low circulating levels of thyroid hormone stimulate the release of TRH by the hypothalamus and anterior pituitary. High circulating thyroid hormone levels downregulate the number of TRH receptors of the TSH-producing cells of the pituitary and also decrease TSH secretion.

Calcitonin is a hormone produced by thyroid C cells (neuroendocrine cells). It is secreted in response to high circulating calcium levels and GI hormones. Secretion is inhibited by somatostatin. In pharmacological doses, calcitonin inhibits bone resorption and increases renal excretion of calcium and phosphate, thereby lowering calcium levels. The physiological significance of calcitonin is not known.[8]

Parathyroid Glands

The parathyroid glands are small, oval structures arranged in pairs behind each thyroid lobe. Occasionally they are found in the chest. There are usually four glands. The major cell type of the glands are epithelial, and the gland is richly supplied with blood by fenestrated capillaries from the inferior and superior thyroid arteries. The parathyroids secrete PTH or parathormone. Its major role is to regulate the blood level of calcium. PTH acts on bone, the kidneys, and indirectly, the GI tract. In bone, PTH stimulates bone resorption and inhibits bone formation to release calcium and phosphate into the blood. The renal effect of PTH is to increase calcium reabsorption and phosphate excretion by the tubules. In addition, PTH stimulates the renal conversion of vitamin D to its most active form (1,25-dihydroxyvitamin D_3). This active vitamin D then enhances the intestinal absorption of calcium.

PTH is free of pituitary and hypothalamic control. The secretion of this hormone is directly regulated by a feedback system. When the serum calcium level is low, PTH secretion increases; when the serum calcium level rises, PTH secretion falls (Fig. 42-4).

Adrenal Glands

The adrenal glands, whose major function is to protect a person from acute and chronic stress, are small, paired, highly vascularized glands located near the upper poles of each kidney and lateral to the lower thoracic and upper lumbar vertebrae. Each gland weighs about 4 g and consists of two parts, the inner medulla and the outer cortex; each has distinct functions.

Adrenal medulla. The adrenal medulla constitutes 10% of the gland and consists of sympathetic postganglionic neurons with axons. The medullae secrete the catecholamines, epinephrine (the major hormone), and norepinephrine. Catecholamines, usually considered neurotransmitters, are hormones when secreted from the adrenal medullae; they are hormones as they are released into the circulation and transported to their target organs. They exert their effects after binding to adrenergic receptors. Cate-

cholamines have widespread effects on all body systems (see Chapters 5 and 50).

Adrenal cortex. The adrenal cortex, the outer part of the adrenal gland, constitutes 90% of the gland. It secretes more than 50 steroid hormones, which are classified as glucocorticoids, mineralocorticoids, and androgens. Glucocorticoids (e.g., cortisol) are named for their effects on glucose metabolism. Mineralocorticoids are essential for the maintenance of fluid and ion balance. Adrenal androgens (sex steroids) are produced and secreted in small but significant amounts with small amounts of estrogen.

Glucocorticoids. Cortisol is the most abundant and potent glucocorticoid. It is necessary to maintain life. About 92% of circulating cortisol is bound to transcortin (corticosteroid-binding globulin). The free cortisol (8%) binds with receptors in the cytoplasm and nucleus of a target cell. The hormone-receptor complex exerts cortisol's effects within the nucleus of the target tissue. Cortisol is episodically secreted in a diurnal pattern (Fig. 42-6). A major function of cortisol is to increase hepatic gluconeogenesis and decrease peripheral glucose use in the fasting state. In addition, cortisol contributes to differentiation and development; lipid, protein, and nucleic acid metabolism; and physiological responses to many hormones. It is also critical in the body's response to stress.[10] In the liver, cortisol stimulates the synthesis of protein and nucleic acids (anabolism), whereas in the periphery, it stimulates protein breakdown (catabolism). In addition, glucocorticoids stimulate lipolysis in adipose tissue, thereby mobilizing glycerol and free fatty acids.

Other effects of glucocorticoids include their antiinflammatory action and supportive actions in stressful situations. Cortisol combats inflammation by stabilizing the membranes of cellular lysosomes and preventing increased capillary permeability. The lysosomal stabilization reduces the release of proteolytic enzymes and thereby their destructive effects on surrounding tissue. Cortisol helps maintain vascular integrity and responsiveness and fluid volume and has mineralocorticoid effects because it can bind to mineralocortoid receptors.[11] A marked increase in the rate of cortisol secretion by the adrenal cortex can aid the body in coping more effectively with stressful situations (see Chapter 5). The secretion of cortisol is under the control of ACTH from the anterior pituitary and is maintained by a self-regulating feedback mechanism.

Mineralocorticoids. Aldosterone, a potent mineralocorticoid, functions at the renal collecting tubule to promote renal reabsorption of sodium and excretion of potassium and hydrogen ions and, to a lesser extent, calcium and magnesium ions. Aldosterone synthesis and secretion are stimulated by angiotensin II, hyponatremia, and hyperkalemia.

Adrogens and other sex hormones. Adrenal androgens are the third class of steroids synthesized and secreted by the adrenal cortex. They cause masculization.

The adrenal cortex also secretes estrogen and progesterone. In men, estrogen contributes little to reproductive activity. In women, adrenal androgens may function in sexuality and libido. In postmenopausal women, the adrenal cortex is the major source of endogenous estrogen (see Chapters 48 and 49).

Pancreas

The pancreas, a long, tapered, lobular, soft gland that weighs between 60 and 90 g, lies behind the stomach, anterior to the first and second lumbar vertebrae. The pancreas performs exocrine and endocrine functions. The islets are the areas of endocrine activity; they release their secretions into the portal circulation. The secretions are also paracrine. (Paracrine secretions diffuse to neighboring cells to exert their action, rather than traveling to their target tissues through the bloodstream like endocrine secretions.) The islets account for less than 2% of the gland and consist of α, β, and δ cells. Glucagon is synthesized by the α cells, insulin by the β cells, and gastrin and somatostatin by the δ cells.

Glucagon. Glucagon is synthesized and released from pancreatic α cells in response to low levels of blood sugar, protein ingestion, and exercise. It stimulates hepatic glycogenolysis and gluconeogenesis and enhances adipose tissue lipolysis. Usually, glucagon and insulin function in a reciprocal manner to maintain normal blood glucose levels (euglycemia). The exception is after ingestion of a high-protein carbohydrate-free meal, in which case both hormones are secreted. In this instance, glucagon counteracts the inhibitory effect of insulin on gluconeogenesis, and euglycemia is maintained.

Insulin. Insulin is the principal regulator of the metabolism and storage of ingested carbohydrates, fats, and amino acids. It facilitates glucose diffusion across cell membranes in most tissues, although the brain, the lens of the eye, hepatocytes, erythrocytes, and cells in the intestinal mucosa and kidney tubules are not dependent on insulin for glucose use. An increased blood glucose level is the major stimulus for insulin synthesis and secretion. Other stimuli to insulin secretion are increased amino acid levels; GI hormones, which enhance the response to glucose; and vagal stimulation. Insulin secretion is usually inhibited by low blood glucose levels, glucagon, somatostatin, hypokalemia, and catecholamines (see Table 42-2).

A major effect of insulin on glucose metabolism occurs in the liver, where the hormone enhances glucose incorporation into glycogen and triglyceride by altering enzymatic activity and inhibiting gluconeogenesis. In peripheral tissues, insulin facilitates glucose transport into cells, transport of amino acids across muscle membranes and their synthesis into protein, and transport of triglyceride into adipose tissue. Thus insulin is a storage, or anabolic, hormone.

The endocrine system is concerned with the regulation of body processes and the maintenance of internal homeostasis despite vastly changing substrates, as is seen in glucose homeostasis after food ingestion. After a meal, insulin is responsible for the storage of nutrients (anabolism). In the fasting state (during which ingested glucose is not readily available), hormones such as cortisol and glucagon break down stored complex fuels (catabolism) to provide simple glucose as fuel for energy.

Heart

Atrial natriuretic factor (ANF) is a peptide hormone produced by atrial myocytes; it helps maintain fluid homeostasis. Its release is stimulated by stretch receptors associated with venous return to the right atrium. These receptors are in turn stimulated by fluid excess, cold water immersion, increased plasma osmolality, and sodium intake. ANF stimulates diuresis by increasing the glomerular filtration rate, which increases sodium and chloride excretion. ANF also inhibits renin and the action of angiotensin II at the adrenal glands.[12]

Prostaglandins

The prostaglandins(PGs) are not hormones in the classic sense but are a group of closely related lipid compounds that because of their short half-lives, act in an autocrine manner; that is, they exert their effects on the cells that synthesize and secrete them. PGs are types of eicosanoids, a class of compounds that are oxidation products of long-chain polyunsaturated fatty acids found in the cell membrane. PGs are formed in all body tissues except red blood cells (RBCs). They are synthesized and released in response to appropriate stimuli, often trauma. PGs are involved in hormone responses at the cellular level and are thought to modulate hormone action. Several classes of PGs have been identified, including PGE, PGF, PGD and PGI.[13]

Pharmacological effects of PGs include the release of anterior pituitary peptides, bronchodilatation and constriction, GI motility, inhibition of lymphocyte proliferation, platelet inhibition, enhanced renin release, uterine contraction, cervical ripening, and vasoconstriction and dilatation.[13] PGs are used therapeutically to initiate labor and to induce abortion. Blockage of the effects of PGs with nonsteroidal antiinflammatory agents has therapeutic effects. For example, because primary dysmenorrhea is believed to be caused by excess $PGF_{2\alpha}$ and PGE_2 during menstruation, these painful cramps can often be successfully treated with such agents.

Effects of Aging

Normal aging has many effects on the endocrine system (Table 42-4). This can be manifested by events such as changes in a hormone's basal level, response to stimuli, transport of the hormone, target organ responsiveness, and catabolism. Often one change such as decreased response to stimuli is offset by another such as decreased metabolic clearance rate so that the net effect is normal hormone levels. Because radioimmunoassays of hormone levels have become widely available (see p. 1272), problems previously attributed to age-related endocrine changes have been found to be the effects of other illnesses on the endocrine system.

Assessment of the effects of aging on the endocrine system is difficult because the subtle changes of aging often occur with symptoms of endocrine disorders.[14] However, there are endocrine changes with clinical significance. Aging is associated with decreased hypothalamic neurotransmitters, and the hypothalamus is less sensitive to feedback inhibition. In addition, alterations in PTH secretion are often seen and may be related to the bone changes seen in older adults. Besides endocrine changes related to aging, the nurse must be aware that endocrine problems may oc-

Table 42-4   Endocrine System in Normal Aging

Hormone	Basal Level	Secretion	MCR	Target Organ Response	Clinical Significance
POSTERIOR PITUITARY					
Oxytocin					
ADH	↑	↑	—	↓ (renal)	Hyponatremia, syndrome of inappropriate ADH
ANTERIOR PITUITARY					
GH	↓	↓	—	—	
TSH	↑	↑	—	?	
ACTH	—	—	—	—	—
Prolactin	↑	↑	?	?	Decreased response to surgical stress
LH and FSH	↑	↑	?	↓	
THYROID					
T₄	—	↓	↓		—
T₃	↓	—			Increased hypothyroidism
PARATHYROIDS					
PTH	↑	↑	?	?	Hypercalcemia, hypercalciuria
ADRENAL CORTEX					
Cortisol	—	↓	↓	↓	Decreased response to stress
Androgens	↓	↓	?	?	
Aldosterone	↓	↓	↓	?	Decreased response to sodium restriction and upright posture
ADRENAL MEDULLA					
Epinephrine	—		—	↓	Decreased response to β-blockers (e.g., less decreased heart rate and cardiac output)
Norepinephrine	↑	↑	↑	↓	Increased peripheral and α-adrenergic sympathetic nerve activity
PANCREAS					
Insulin	↑	↓	—	↓	Impaired glucose tolerance
GONADS					
Estrogen	↓	↓	?	?	Increased hot flashes, osteoporosis, decreased vaginal secretions
Testosterone	↓	↓	?	?	Decreased ejaculatory force
KIDNEYS					
Renin	↓	↓	?	?	Decreased response to sodium restriction, upright posture
Vitamin D	↓	N/A	?	?	Decreased intestinal absorption of calcium

MCR, Metabolic clearance rate; ↑, increased; ↓, decreased; —, no change; ?, no data or conflicting data; *N/A,* not applicable.

cur differently in older adults than in younger persons. Altered PTH secretion (see p. 1338) usually manifests as hyperparathyroidism. However, the older adult often has altered mental status, fatigue, and generalized weakness rather than the kidney stones and peptic ulcers seen in younger persons. In addition, thyroid disorders often exhibit different symptoms in the older client.[14] The symptoms of hypothyroidism in the older adult are usually similar to those in younger persons but are more likely to be overlooked because the symptoms—fatigue, mental impairment, sluggishness, and constipation—can be attributed solely to aging. In addition, older persons with hypothyroidism have more disturbances of the CNS, such as syncope, convulsions, dementia, and coma. They often have pitting edema and deafness. Older clients with hyperthyroidism frequently have manifestations related only to

the cardiovascular system, such as palpitations, angina, atrial fibrillation, and breathlessness. They may also have depression, anorexia, constipation, and weight loss (apathetic hyperthyroidism). Thus signs and symptoms often attributed to 'old age' may constitute indications of endocrine problems.

ASSESSMENT OF THE ENDOCRINE SYSTEM

Hormones affect every body tissue and system, causing great diversity in the signs and symptoms of endocrine dysfunction. Therefore assessment of the endocrine system is often difficult and requires keen clinical skills to detect manifestations of disorders. Endocrine dysfunction may result from deficient or excessive hormone secretion, transport abnormalities, an inability of the target tissue to respond to a hormone (resistance), or inappropriate stimulation of the target-tissue receptor.

Endocrine disorders may have nonspecific or very specific manifestations. For example, weight loss may be a sign of panhypopituitarism, hyperthyroidism, occasionally hypothyroidism, Addison's disease, pheochromocytoma, relative or absolute insulin lack, or hyperparathyroidism. Alternatively, it may be due to malignancy, GI or emotional problems, or a well-planned weight reduction program. A careful health history will yield data to help sort out possible causes. Some signs of endocrine dysfunction are specific, such as the classic "polys" (polyuria, polydipsia, and polyphagia) in diabetes mellitus and exophthalmos in hyperthyroidism. Specific signs do not cause the assessment problems that the more common nonspecific signs and symptoms do.

Certain guidelines (see Chapter 3) should be used in the assessment of endocrine dysfunction. Nonspecific changes should alert the clinician to the possibility of endocrine changes. The most common nonspecific symptoms are fatigue and depression, often accompanied by other manifestations. The latter includes changes in energy level, alertness, sleep patterns, mood, affect, weight, skin, hair, personal appearance, and sexual function (Table 42-5).

Assessment of the endocrine system includes growth and development patterns, weight distribution and changes, and comparisons of these factors with normal findings. Height should be measured in all clients.* The charts used should be race specific because significant racial differences exist in normal children. For example, white children as a rule are smaller than black children but are larger than those from Asian races. Familial patterns

*The reader is referred to a pediatric text for normal height and weight charts for infants and children.

Table 42-5 Nonspecific Manifestations of Hormone Dysfunction

Manifestations	Panhypopituitary Hormone	ADH	Thyroid Hormone	Cortisol	Mineralocorticoids	Insulin	PTH
	↓	↑ ↓	↑ ↓	↑ ↓	↑ ↓	↑ ↓	↑ ↓
Nutrition and elimination							
Weight	↓		↓ ↑	↑ ↓		↓ ↓	↓
Appetite	↓		↑ ↓	↑ ↓		↑ ↓	↓
Growth abnormality (children)	+		+	+ +		+	+
Abdominal pain			+ +	+		+	+
Stool output	↓		↑ ↓				↓
Urine output		↓ ↑			↑	↑	↑
Cardiovascular system							
Blood pressure		↑ ↓		↑	↑	↑	
Pulse			↑ ↓	↑		↑	
Anemia	+		+ +	+			+
Neurological system							
Temperature			↑ ↓	↑		↓ ↑	
Sleep disturbances	+	+	+	+ +		+	+
Convulsions	+	+	+	+		+	+
Mood							
Depression or apathy	+	+ +	+	+ +		+	+ +
Skin							
Body hair	↓		↓ ↓	↑			↓
Pigmentation	↓		↓	↑ ↓			↓
Reproductive or sexual system							
Male dysfunction	+		+ +	+ +	+	+	+
Female dysfunction	+		+ +	+ +		+	

↑, Increased; +, present; ↓, decreased.

should always be assessed. A helpful guide in growth assessment is that approximate normal growth rates are 3 in/yr from ages 1 to 7 and 2 in/yr from ages 8 to 15. Heights more than three standard deviations below the mean should be investigated.[15] Approximate average heights for children and young teenagers can be estimated on the basis of age using the following formula:

$$\text{Height (inches)} = 2.5 \times \text{Age (years)} + 30$$

In adults, weight may indicate endocrine dysfunction (see Table 35-21). A client's percentage of ideal body weight (IBW) may be obtained by dividing the actual weight by the ideal or optimal weight for height and multiplying by 100. A client who is 120% greater than optimal body weight is considered obese.[16] Ideal weight may also be estimated by the following formulas:

$$\text{Men: IBW} = (\text{height in inches} - 60) \times 4 + 120$$

$$\text{Women: IBW} = (\text{height in inches} - 60) \times 4 + 110$$

The nurse should note the percentage above or below IBW. A weight increase of more than 1 kg/day usually indicates fluid retention.

Subjective Data

Health history

Past health history. During an assessment the client or a significant other should be specifically questioned about previous endocrine abnormalities or the presence of the following manifestations or events:

1. Delay or acceleration in growth and development
2. History of a major blow to the head
3. Increases in the size of the head, hands, or feet in the adult (e.g., change in ring, glove, or shoe size)
4. Abnormal secondary sex characteristics (e.g., facial hair in women, decreased need for shaving in men, changes in the amount and distribution of axillary and pubic hair in both genders)
5. Problems with menstruation and pregnancies in women
6. Increased or decreased thirst and urination
7. Visual changes
8. Difficulty in swallowing, change in neck size
9. Hypertension
10. Nephrolithiasis (kidney stones)
11. Changes in hair distribution, skin and hair color and texture
12. Changes in appetite and weight
13. Changes in memory, ability to concentrate, energy level
14. Sleep disturbances
15. Increased sympathetic nervous system activity (e.g., nervousness, palpitations, sweating, tremors)

The client should be questioned about the general state of health and whether there have been any changes. The nurse also asks whether any problem has affected the client's ability to function at work, at home, or in society. The nurse further inquires about previous hospitalizations, surgeries, chemotherapies, radiation treatments (especially of the neck), and medications (specifically hormones or steroids) for any of these problems.

Family history. Hereditary and constitutional factors can play a major role in the cause of endocrine problems. The client should be questioned about the following conditions in family members:

1. Diabetes mellitus or insipidus
2. Hyperthyroidism or hypothyroidism, goiter
3. Hypertension or hypotension
4. Obesity
5. Infertility
6. Growth problems
7. Pheochromocytoma (neoplastic tumor of the adrenal medulla or sympathetic ganglia)
8. Autoimmune diseases (e.g., Addison's disease)
9. Adrenal hyperplasia

Further information may be elicited by asking additional questions such as the following: Are there any other members of your family who have or have had a similar problem? This frequently uncovers evidence of a familial factor that cannot be found in any other way.

Social and personal history

BACKGROUND INFORMATION. Stressors of all kinds affect the endocrine system. Areas that can cause a great deal of stress should be investigated. Clients should be asked about their place of employment, kind of work, ability to meet job requirements, and the amount of stress involved. The nurse asks whether the job provides an adequate income. Marital status and usual coping patterns are also discussed. The nurse then determines whether previous coping patterns are still successful. It is often useful to ask family members or a significant other about behavior changes.

LIFESTYLE. If the client has a specific problem, an appropriate history should be taken and the system involved should be assessed. For instance, a chief complaint of tachycardia indicates the need for a cardiovascular assessment and for information related to stress, diet, exercise, and sleep. The clinician must also remember the possibility of endocrine dysfunction and must assess for hyperthyroidism. The lack of clear-cut endocrine symptoms requires a conscientious and detailed health history.

Review of systems. If an endocrine problem is suspected, the nurse must investigate many systems because of the systemic effects of hormones. If the information is not gathered under the review of a specific system, the client should be asked about the following information:

1. *General data:* Weight changes, energy level, sleep patterns, diaphoresis, weakness, heat intolerance
2. *Growth and development patterns:* Growth pattern, occurrence of growth spurts, size of parents and siblings
3. *Hair:* Changes in amount, texture, distribution, color, breakage
4. *Head:* Changes in size, shape, symmetry, movement; headache
5. *Eyes and vision:* Changes in shape, symmetry, appearance, size, acuity; swelling on awakening; pain; blurred vision, diplopia; burning, "gritty" feeling
6. *Nose:* Symptoms of nasal obstruction, (e.g., snoring, noisy nasal breathing), change in sense of smell

7. *Voice:* Changes; hoarseness
8. *Integumentary system:* Generalized and local changes in skin color or pigmentation, especially over joints; scars, striae, creases; ability to tan; bruising; moisture and texture, dryness, oiliness, scaling; rate of healing
9. *Nails:* Changes in growth, texture, ridges, separation from nail bed, brittleness
10. *Respiratory system:* Dyspnea, history of tuberculosis, date and results of last tuberculosis test
11. *Cardiovascular system:* Palpitations, dyspnea on mild exertion, hypertension, evidence of lightheadedness or dizziness, especially when assuming sitting or upright positions
12. *Gastrointestinal system:* Changes in appetite, thirst, bowel habits; dysphagia; abdominal pain or discomfort; nausea, vomiting; character and color of stool; usual eating pattern, food preferences; alcohol consumption
13. *Urinary system:* Changes in amount, color, odor of urine; nocturia; evidence of kidney stones (e.g., hematuria, pain)
14. *Reproductive and sexual system:* Libido, changes in size or shape of genitalia, breast discharge.
    a. Female: Menarche, menstrual abnormalities or changes, menopause, infertility, pregnancies, births, birth weights of children, lactation (particularly after last pregnancy)
    b. Male: Erectile function (e.g., difficulty achieving or maintaining erection), ability to have a morning erection, infertility
15. *Neurological system:* Headache, nervousness, neuromuscular excitability, dizziness, syncope, convulsions, hallucinations, sensory or motor changes, paresthesias (especially around the mouth [perioral] or in the hands or feet), memory loss, irritability, depression, altered thought and speech patterns
16. *Musculoskeletal system:*
    a. Muscles: Weakness, wasting, twitching, aching (especially when reaching above head), climbing stairs, or rising from a chair, spasms
    b. Joints: Pain, stiffness
    c. Bones: Pain, fractures, increase in size (adult), decrease in height, increase in width of hands or feet

Objective Data

Physical examination
Mental-emotional status. Throughout the examination the client's orientation, alertness, memory, affect, personality, anxiety, and speech pattern should be objectively assessed.

Inspection. The nurse should observe the client's general appearance, including physical growth and development, level of consciousness and orientation, and appearance and appropriateness of dress. Endocrine dysfunction can subtly or markedly affect the size, shape, color, and maturation of the body. Assessment should include the following:

1. *Body size:* Height and weight compared with a table of standards or estimation of normality; size of head and extremities, proportionality and posture; facial features
2. *Integumentary system:* Skin color, pigmentation, texture, coarseness, leather texture, excessive thinness, size of sweat glands, diaphoresis, acne, striae, ecchymosis, vitiligo (patchy loss of pigmentation)
3. *Hair:* Texture, distribution, brittleness, alopecia (patchy baldness)
4. *Face:* Color; erythema, especially on cheeks (plethora); pained, anxious expression
5. *Eyes:* Eyebrows, hair distribution; visual acuity, lens opacity; shape, position, movement of eyelids; lid lag; visual fields; extraocular movements; edema
6. *Nose:* Mucosa, noisy breathing
7. *Mouth:* Buccal mucosa, condition of teeth, malocclusion and mottling, tongue size and fasciculations, size and shape of jaw
8. *Voice:* Huskiness or hoarseness, volume, pitch, slurring
9. *Neck:* Symmetry, alignment; forceful carotid pulsations; unusual bulging of the thyroid lobes behind the sternocleidomastoid muscles; trachea in midline; dullness, thickening, flabbiness of vocal cords; polyps; gray-brown hyperpigmentation on posterior neck and axillae (acanthosis nigricans). (Observation should be made first in the normal position, preferably with side lighting, then in slight extension, and then as the client swallows some water.)
10. *Extremities:* Size, shape, symmetry, proportionality (distance from symphysis pubis to foot: approximately half of total height), edema
    a. Hands: Tremors (a piece of paper is placed on outstretched fingers, palm down, to assess fine tremors); muscle strength, grip, thenar wasting, Dupuytren's contracture, clubbing
    b. Legs: Muscle weakness (assessed by having the seated client extend one leg to a horizontal position; ability to hold this position for 2 minutes usually indicates normal muscle strength), bowing, color and amount of hair, size of feet, corns, calluses, pedal pulses
    c. Toes: Maceration, fissures, deformities
11. *Reflexes:* Particularly deep tendon reflexes, relaxation time
12. *Pulses:* Rate and force
13. *Thorax:* Gynecomastia in men
14. *Abdomen:* Increased pigmentation of scars, purplish striae, pain on light palpation
15. *Genitalia:* Decreased hair distribution (diamond pattern in women may indicate virilizing tumor), size of testes, clitoral enlargement

Palpation. The thyroid is the only palpable endocrine gland. Thyroid palpation requires considerable practice, as well as validation by an experienced examiner. Palpation

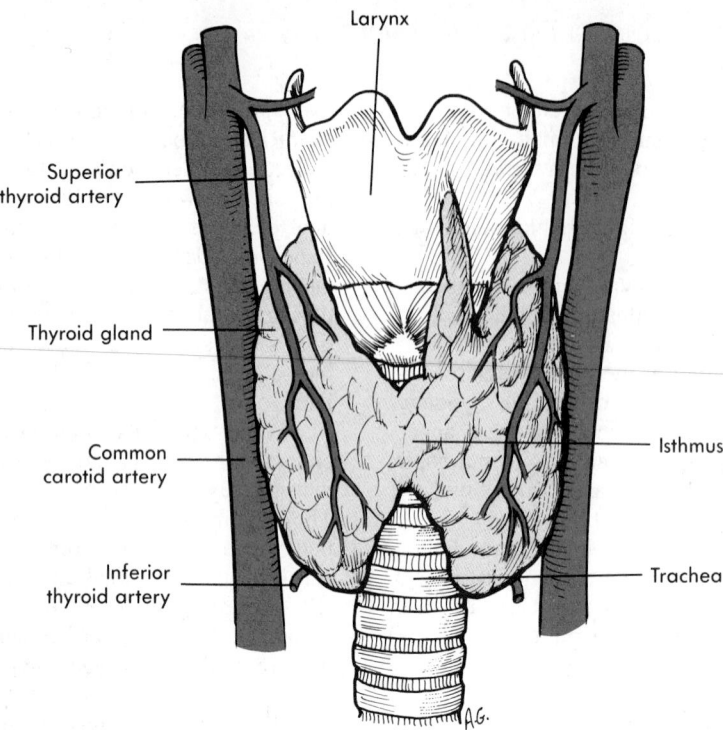

Fig. 42-8 Frontal view of thyroid gland. (From Seeley RR, Stephens TD, and Tate P: Anatomy and physiology, St Louis, 1989, Times Mirror/Mosby College Publishing, p 528.)

can cause the release of thyroid hormone into the circulation, increasing the client's symptoms and potentially causing a thyroid storm (see Chapter 44). In clients with visibly enlarged thyroids, palpation of the thyroid should be deferred if a more experienced clinician will be examining the client.

To palpate the thyroid, the nurse identifies other midline neck structures (Fig. 42-8). The thyroid can be palpated anteriorly and posteriorly, although posterior palpation is easier and more common. Water should always be available for the client to swallow as part of this examination.

ANTERIOR PALPATION. Standing in front of the client, the nurse, using the pads of the index and middle fingers, palpates below the cricoid cartilage for the thyroid isthmus. The client swallows water while the nurse feels for the isthmus rising up under the fingers. The fingers are then moved laterally to the anterior border of the sternocleidomastoid muscle, and each lateral lobe is palpated before and while the client swallows water.

POSTERIOR PALPATION. The examiner stands behind the client. With the thumbs of both hands resting on the nape of the client's neck, the nurse, with the index and middle fingers of both hands, feels for the thyroid isthmus and for the anterior surfaces of the lateral lobes. To facilitate the examination of each lobe and to relax the neck muscles, the nurse asks the client to flex the neck slightly forward and to the right. The thyroid cartilage is displaced to the right by the left hand and fingers. The nurse palpates with the right hand after placing the thumb deep and behind the sternocleidomastoid muscle with the index and middle fin-

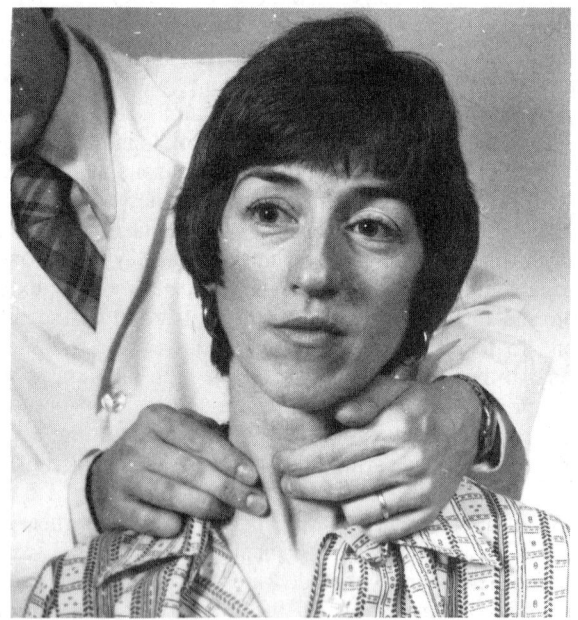

Fig. 42-9 Posterior palpation of the thyroid gland.

gers in front of it; the area is palpated with the right hand (Fig. 42-9). While this is done, the client is asked to swallow water. This procedure is then repeated on the left side. The thyroid is palpated for its size, shape, symmetry, and tenderness and for any nodules. In the average person the thyroid is often not palpable. If palpable, it usually feels

smooth with a firm consistency and is not tender with gentle pressure. Nodules, enlargement, asymmetry, or hardness is abnormal, and the client should be referred for further evaluation.

Vital signs. Assessment of vital signs should include the following:

1. Temperature: Elevation or hypothermia (a special thermometer is needed to evaluate hypothermia)
2. Respirations: Change in rate or rhythm
3. Blood pressure: Widening of the pulse pressure, hypotension, or hypertension or orthostatic hypotension (see Chapter 27); orthostatic and pulse changes
4. Heart sounds: Systolic murmur at apex or pulmonic area (possible indication of increased blood flow as a result of hyperthyroidism)

Other assessment skills. Percussion and auscultation are not normally part of an endocrine assessment, except with an enlarged thyroid, where bruits may be heard over the lateral lobes with the stethoscope diaphragm.

DIAGNOSTIC STUDIES

Accurately performed laboratory tests aid and confirm diagnoses of problems of the endocrine system. These tests can measure absolute hormone levels and estimate the production, transport, and catabolism of hormones. Hormones with fairly constant basal levels (e.g., T_4 and insulin) require only a single measurement. Hormones with pulsatile secretion (e.g., LH and testosterone) may require multiple samples with a measurement taken from pooled aliquots. Notation of sample time on the laboratory slip and sample is important for hormones with circadian or sleep-related secretion (e.g., cortisol and GH).

On occasion, multiple blood sampling is indicated, such as in suppression tests (e.g., dexamethasone suppression) and stimulation tests (e.g., glucose tolerance). To decrease client discomfort and minimize the effects of stress hormones, the nurse initiates an intravenous (IV) infusion of normal saline solution with a stopcock between the extension and the infusion tubing. After insertion of the infusion, 15 to 30 minutes should be allowed for stress hormones to normalize. Baseline samples are then drawn, the appropriate medication is given through the stopcock, and samples are withdrawn through the stopcock at the appropriate times. A heparin lock may be used in place of the saline infusion. It is necessary to draw and discard 1.5 to 3 ml from the client before drawing the sample for measurement. This prevents saline or heparin dilution.

In general, tests of endocrine function require client fasting and elimination of most environmental stimuli. This requires inactivity throughout the test; such inactivity can be achieved with bed rest with the head of the bed elevated or through the use of a recliner chair. Clients should refrain from smoking or taking food or fluids by mouth. A thorough explanation of the test and the reasons for reducing environmental stimuli reassures clients and helps them cooperate. Clients should be monitored frequently during the test, not just when samples are being taken.

During endocrine testing there are instances in which simultaneous blood and urine samples or special preservatives are needed for samples. The nurse ensures thorough client instruction, as well as correct and complete sample collection. When a client is having multiple endocrine testing, such as with suspected pituitary disease, a fluid volume deficit may occur. Nursing interventions in this instance include recording the amount of blood and urine taken per test, assessing for dehydration, and promptly notifying the physician if blood loss through sample collection is excessive or the client becomes dehydrated. Using the saline infusion method helps offset fluid volume deficit.

Several types of laboratory tests are used to determine endocrine status, including radioimmunoassay, immunometric assay, radioreceptor assay, and in vitro bioassays.[17] The radioimmunoassay, a displacement assay, uses antibodies specific for a hormone or parts of a hormone and can measure very small amounts of circulating hormones. It is used for peptide, steroid, and thyroid hormones. Immunometric assays can measure minute hormone levels and are used for TSH measurements. Radioreceptor assays measure the ability of a hormone to bind to its receptor. Highly sensitive in vitro bioassays, used for peptide and steroid hormones, incubate plasma with tissue extracts or cultured cells to measure the effects of hormone-receptor interaction. In addition to hormone levels, hormone receptors can be measured. Receptor measurements are useful in states of hormone resistance such as those seen with insulin, PTH, and vitamin D.

Specific diagnostic studies related to the endocrine system are summarized in Table 42-6. Because of the interrelatedness of the endocrine system, nursing intervention is focused on reducing the stress and anxiety often associated with diagnostic testing. Unless nursing measures related to client instruction and expectations are initiated, the effect of stress hormones can produce inaccurate and misleading results.

Normal values and collection procedures vary among laboratories. It is therefore important to check with the laboratory doing the testing to determine the correct procedure and normal values.

SUMMARY

The endocrine system is responsible for maintaining the body's internal homeostasis, despite an ever-changing internal and external environment. The endocrine system is complicated and characterized by signals, signal transport, and responses to those signals. The signals let the body know that environmental alterations such as fuel intake, lack of fuel, or stress have occurred. The endocrine system then uses the added fuel, produces more fuel when needed, or fights the stress. The classic endocrine tissues involved in maintaining homeostasis are the hypothalamus; the pituitary, thyroid, parathyroid, and adrenal glands; the pancreas; and the gonads. However, research is showing that other tissues, such as those in the heart, kidneys, and intestine, also have endocrine functions. In addition, the interrelationship between the nervous system and the endocrine system is an area of intense research. This neuroendocrine system seems to stimulate and integrate the functions of both systems.

Text continued on p. 1280.

Table 42-6

Diagnostic Studies of the Endocrine System		
Study	**Description and Purpose***	**Nursing Responsibility**
PITUITARY STUDIES		
Serum studies		
GH	This test evaluates GH hypersecretion. After an overnight fast, GH should be less than 5 nanograms (ng)/ml in men and less than 10 ng/ml in women. Values greater than 50 ng/ml suggest acromegaly.	Inform client that blood sample will be drawn. Make sure that client takes nothing by mouth after midnight and that there is no smoking. Ensure that bed rest was prescribed and maintained because if samples are drawn from client who walked to the laboratory or who is stressed from venipuncture, abnormally high levels may result. Send samples to laboratory immediately. Observe venipuncture site for bleeding or hematoma formation.
Somatomedin C (sulfation factor)	This screening test evaluates GH; it is less variable than GH because it is not subject to circadian rhythm and fluctuations. It cannot be used to diagnose GH deficiency in children under 4 years of age. *Normal values* are 135-250 ng/ml; low levels indicate GH deficiency, and high levels indicate GH excess. Values elevate during puberty and pregnancy.	Observe venipuncture site for bleeding or hematoma formation.
Oral glucose tolerance test	This test can confirm GH excess. GH level tests are done with glucose level tests. GH levels should be less than 2 ng/ml at some time during test; GH values of greater than 2 ng/ml indicate GH excess.	Ensure that client has been fasting. (Same as pancreatic studies.)
Test to determine GH release after exercise	This screening test evaluates GH reserve in suspected hypopituitarism. After client runs up 2 flights of stairs or exercises to raise pulse rate to 180 bpm, single sample is drawn. Values are affected by many drugs. With children with GH level greater than 20 ng/ml and with adults with GH level greater than 6 ng/ml, no further testing is required.	Have client fast. Explain procedure. Monitor pulse rate before and after exercise. Send sample to laboratory immediately.

*See Chapter 44.

Continued.

Table 42-6

Diagnostic Studies of the Endocrine System—cont'd

Study	Description and Purpose*	Nursing Responsibility
PITUITARY STUDIES—cont'd **Serum studies—cont'd**		
Study to evaluate insulin-induced hypoglycemia	This test is used in examination of clients with suspected hypopituitarism. IV injection of regular insulin is given, based on body weight (usually 0.1 units [U]/kg). Basal samples of GH, cortisol, and glucose are drawn. Blood samples are drawn at 30, 45, 60, and 90 minutes after injection. If test is terminated because of hypoglycemia (glucose level less than 60 mg/dl), samples are drawn for GH and cortisol levels 30 minutes after IV dextrose. GH level should rise twofold to threefold over baseline levels. Response is subnormal or absent in GH deficiency.	Ensure that client fasted overnight (water is allowed) and that bed rest was prescribed. Have 5% cortisone, 20 ml of 50% dextrose, and IV solution of 5% glucose at bedside for use if severe hypoglycemia occurs and test will continue. Continually assess client's mental status because seizures, cardiac dysrhythmias, and coma can result from hypoglycemia. (Test is contraindicated in clients with seizure disorders, cardiac disease, hypocortisolism, and hypothyroidism.) Assess capillary glucose levels immediately with glucose reagent strips or meters. Note on laboratory slips times that blood is drawn. Provide 25 g glucose after last sample.
Prolactin level	This test evaluates prolactin levels. Decreased levels in postpartum woman attempting to nurse may be associated with Sheehan's syndrome.* *Normal values* are up to 23 ng/ml (nonlactating); levels greater than 200 ng/ml indicate pituitary tumors.	Have client fast. Inform client that blood sample will be drawn. Draw blood at least 2 hours after client awakens. Observe venipuncture site for bleeding or hematoma formation.
Gonadotropin levels: FSH, LH	These studies are useful in distinguishing primary gonadal problems from pituitary insufficiency. Normal levels vary according to age and sex. In women, there are marked differences during menstrual cycle and in postmenopausal period. Levels are low in pituitary insufficiency and high in primary gonadal failure. In women, values for FSH are: basal rate—5-20 milli-International Units (mIU)/ml; ovulatory surge—12-30 mIU/ml; and postmenopausal level—greater than 50 mIU/ml. In women, values for LH are: basal rate—5-25 mIU/ml; ovulatory surge—25-100 mIU/ml; and postmenopausal level—greater than 50 mIU/ml. In men, values for FSH and LH are 5-20 mIU/ml.	Ensure that client has fasted. Inform client that 3 blood samples may be drawn 30 minutes apart. For women, note on laboratory slip time of menstrual cycle or whether she is postmenopausal.

*See Chapter 44.

Table 42-6

Diagnostic Studies of the Endocrine System—cont'd

Study	Description and Purpose*	Nursing Responsibility
PITUITARY STUDIES—cont'd		
Serum studies—cont'd		
Water deprivation test	This test is used to differentiate causes of polyuria, including pituitary diabetes insipidus (DI), nephrogenic DI, syndrome of inappropriate ADH, and psychogenic polydipsia. Two units of ADH or vasopressin diluted in saline solution is administered intravenously for 2 hours. With normal clients and clients with psychogenic DI, urine osmolality is greater than 600 mOsm/kg and plasma osmolality is less than 300 milliosmoles (mOsm)/kg after ADH administration. With clients with pituitary DI, plasma osmolality is greater than 300 mOsm/kg; with dilute urine, it is less than 270 mOsm/kg. With clients with nephrogenic DI, there is little or no response to ADH.	Have client discontinue tea, coffee, alcohol, and smoking after midnight. Obtain baseline weight and urine and plasma osmolality. Ensure that fluid is withheld. Weigh client and take three postural blood pressure (BP) measurements (lying and standing BP measurements separated by 2 minutes) hourly. Assess urine hourly for volume and specific gravity. Send hourly samples for urine osmolality. Draw sample for plasma osmolality when (1) urine samples are collected and (2) orthostatic hypotension and postural tachycardia appear. Assess weight at 4, 6, 7, and 8 hours.
Radiological studies		
Skull x-ray films, computed tomography (CT) scan, nuclear magnetic resonance (NMR) scan	These tests are useful in evaluating sella turcica for volume, enlargement, or erosion when disease of hypothalamic pituitary axis is suspected. Compare with normal measurement of sella turcica in relation to client's height.	Ask client to lie as still as possible; explain that tests are painless and noninvasive. Explain procedure.
THYROID STUDIES		
Serum studies		
T_4 RIA	This test measures total serum level of T_4. It is useful in evaluating thyroid function and monitoring thyroid therapy. *Normal values* are 5-12 µg/dl.	Inform client that fasting is not necessary. Inform client that blood samples will be drawn. Observe venipuncture site for bleeding or hematoma formation.
T_3 RIA	This test measures serum levels of T_3. It is helpful in diagnosing hyperthyroidism if T_4 levels are normal. *Normal values* are 65-195 ng/dl	Inform client that fasting is not necessary. Inform client that blood samples will be drawn. Observe venipuncture site for bleeding or hematoma formation.
T_3 resin uptake	This study indirectly measures binding capacity of thyroid-binding globulin. *Normal values* are 25%-35%.	Inform client that fasting is not necessary. Inform client that blood samples will be drawn. Observe venipuncture site for bleeding or hematoma formation.

Continued.

Table 42-6

Diagnostic Studies of the Endocrine System—cont'd

Study	Description and Purpose*	Nursing Responsibility
THYROID STUDIES—cont'd		
Serum studies—cont'd		
Free T_4 test	This study measures active component of total T_4. *Normal values* are 1.0-3.5 ng/dl.	Inform client that fasting is not necessary. Inform client that blood samples will be drawn. Observe venipuncture site for bleeding or hematoma formation.
Free T_3 test	This test measures active component of total T_3. *Normal values* are 0.25-0.65 ng/dl.	Inform client that fasting is not necessary. Inform client that blood samples will be drawn. Observe venipuncture site for bleeding or hematoma formation.
Thyroid ^{131}I uptake (radioactive iodine uptake)	This study provides direct measure of thyroid activity. It is useful for evaluation of functional activity of solitary thyroid nodules. Small tracer dose of ^{131}I is given orally or intravenously. Serum uptake measurements are drawn at 2 to 4 and at 24 hours. *Normal serum values* for 2-4 hours are 3%-10% and for 24 hours, they are 5%-30%. Values are affected by drugs, seafood, certain radiographic contrast media, and antiseptics containing iodine.	Instruct client to discontinue thyroid medication and to start T_3 (Cytomel) 25 mg 2-3 times/day for 4 weeks. Tell client to report for further testing in 10-14 days. Collect 24-hour urine specimen.
TSH (S-TSH, immunoradiometric) level	This test measures level of TSH, which is markedly elevated in primary hypothyroidism. *Normal values* are 0.3-5.4 microunits (μU)/ml	Inform client that fasting is not necessary. Inform client that blood sample will be drawn. Observe venipuncture site for bleeding or hematoma formation.
Calcitonin level	High calcitonin level with normal serum calcium level is associated with medullary thyroid carcinoma. *Normal values* are less than or equal to 0.155 ng/ml for men and 0.105 ng/ml for women.	Ensure that client has fasted. Inform client that blood sample will be drawn. Observe venipuncture site for bleeding or hematoma formation.
Radiological studies		
Thyroid scan	This study is used to evaluate nodules of the thyroid. Tracer dose of technetium is given intravenously. Scanner passes over thyroid and makes graphic record of radiation emitted. Normal thyroid scan reveals homogeneous pattern with symmetrical lobes.	Determine whether other tests requiring iodine preparation (IV pyelogram, saturated solution of potassium iodine, or barium enema) have been done within 30 days (can invalidate test). Explain procedure to client.
PARATHYROID STUDIES		
Serum studies		
PTH RIA	This test measures PTH level in serum. Normal range depends on assay used; check with laboratory. This study must be interpreted in terms of concomitantly drawn serum calcium level.	Ensure that client has fasted overnight. Inform client that blood sample will be drawn. Observe venipuncture site for bleeding or hematoma formation.

*See Chapter 44.
†See Chapter 39.

Table 42-6

Diagnostic Studies of the Endocrine System—cont'd

Study	Description and Purpose*	Nursing Responsibility
PARATHYROID STUDIES—cont'd **Serum studies—cont'd**		
Total calcium level	This study measures total serum calcium to help detect bone and parathyroid disorders. Hypercalcemia can indicate primary hyperparathyroidism, and hypocalcemia can indicate hypoparathyroidism. *Normal values* are 9.0-11.0 mg/dl or 4.5-5.5 milliequivalents (mEq)/L.	Ensure that client has fasted overnight. Inform client that blood sample will be drawn. Observe venipuncture site for bleeding or hematoma formation. Ensure that prolonged tourniquet application does not cause falsely elevated values. Adjust total calcium for albumin levels. Use following formula: Total serum calcium (mg/dl) − albumin (g/dl) + 4.0 = adjusted total serum calcium.
Phosphorus level	This study measures inorganic phosphorus. Hyperphosphatemia indicates hypoparathyroidism or renal failure; hypophosphatemia indicates hyperparathyroidism. Phosphorus and calcium levels are inversely related. *Normal values* are 2.8-4.5 mg/dl.	Ensure that client has fasted overnight. Inform client that blood sample will be drawn. Observe venipuncture site for bleeding or hematoma formation.
1,25-Dihydroxyvitamin D$_3$ level	This test is used to evaluate calcium and phosphorus levels and bone disease. *Normal values* are 15-60 picograms (pg)/ml.	Ensure that client has fasted. Inform client that blood sample will be drawn. Observe venipuncture site for bleeding or hematoma formation.
Urine studies		
Calcium levels	This test is used for evaluating parathyroid activity if client's diet is stable (10-20 mg/kg calcium/day). *Normal values* for men are less than 275 mg/24 hours, and for women, they are less than 250 mg/24 hours.	Collect 24-hour urine specimen. Instruct client regarding 24-hour urine collection.†
Phosphorus levels	This study is used for evaluating parathyroid activity. It measures phosphorus content in urine. Phosphorus level depends on calcium and phosphorus intake. Phosphorus and PTH levels are inversely related. If diet is relatively stable (0.9-1.3 g phosphorus/day), normal excretion for adult is less than 1000 mg.	Instruct client regarding 24-hour urine collection.†
Radiological studies		
Skeletal x-ray films, CT scans	These tests are used to determine bone disease and osteoporosis. Fractures or deformities can be caused by the demineralization produced by excessive PTH.	Monitor client's exposure to x rays. Inform client that tests are painless and noninvasive and that no special preparation is required for x-ray studies. For CT scan, give client radiolabeled bone-seeking agent 4 hours before scan.

Continued.

Table 42-6

Diagnostic Studies of the Endocrine System—cont'd

Study	Description and Purpose*	Nursing Responsibility
ADRENAL STUDIES **Serum studies**		
Cortisol levels	This test measures amount of cortisol in serum and evaluates status of adrenocortical function. *Normal values* are 5-25 μg/dl at 8 AM, 3-10 μg/dl at 4 PM. (This level is usually half the 8 AM level.)	Ensure that client has fasted. Inform client that blood sample will be taken. Observe venipuncture site for bleeding and hematoma formation. Ensure collection of properly timed blood sample. Draw specimen early in morning when cortisol levels are highest. Mark time on laboratory slip. Minimize stress to avoid raising level.
Aldosterone levels	This study assesses mineralocorticoid production. *Normal values* are 5 to 20 ng/dl (upright posture) and 8.5 ng/dl (supine posture).	Ensure that client has been on high-salt diet (greater than 120 mEq/24 hours for 4 days). Maintain client in recumbent position for 8 hours before test. Ensure that test is performed before 9 AM.
ACTH stimulation test	This study is used to evaluate adrenal function. After baseline samples are drawn, 250 μg synthetic ACTH is given as IV or IM bolus; samples are drawn 30 and 60 minutes after bolus. Baseline ACTH sample is often drawn in case results are abnormal. Plasma cortisol at 60 minutes should be (1) greater than baseline and (2) greater than 20 μg/dl.	Inject ACTH with a plastic syringe and collect samples for ACTH in plastic, heparinized tubes. Administer test with continuous-infusion method. Monitor site and rate of IV infusion. Ensure sample collection at appropriate times.
Dexamethasone suppression tests (most common overnight dexamethasone suppression test)	This test assesses adrenal function and is especially helpful if hyperactivity is suspected. It is useful in evaluation of Cushing's syndrome. Dexamethasone (Decadron), 2 mg, is given between 11 PM and midnight to suppress secretion of corticotropin-releasing factor. Plasma cortisol sample is drawn 8 hours later. Cortisol level less than 5 μg/dl indicates normal adrenal response (50% decrease in cortisol production).	Ensure that client has fasted. Inform client that blood sample will be taken. Observe venipuncture site for bleeding and hematoma formation. Make sure that acutely ill clients or those under stress are not tested. ACTH may override suppression. Screen client for drugs such as estrogen and glucocorticoids, which may give false-positive results. Ensure accurate timing of medication and sample collection.
Metyrapone suppression test	This study is used to evaluate feedback response of hypothalamus and pituitary and adrenal glands and to differentiate causes of endogenous glucocorticoid overproduction. Metyrapone (30 mg/kg) is given at midnight. Sample is drawn at 8 AM for plasma 11-deoxycortisol (Compound S), cortisol, and ACTH. Normal response is 11-deoxycortisol: 7-22 μg/dl and ACTH greater than 250 pg/dl. To validate blockage by metyrapone, cortisone must be (1) less than 8 μg/dl and (2) less than 45% of Compound S level.	Weigh client. Administer metyrapone with milk and snack at midnight. (Note that metyrapone can cause gastrointestinal distress and confusion.) Draw ACTH into heparinized plastic tube with plastic syringe. Ensure that client has not ingested estrogens, phenytoin, and phenobarbital because these substances invalidate test.

*See Chapter 44.
†See Chapter 39.

Table 42-6

Diagnostic Studies of the Endocrine System—cont'd

Study	Description and Purpose*	Nursing Responsibility
ADRENAL STUDIES—cont'd **Urine studies**		
17-Ketosteroid levels	This test measures androgen metabolites in urine and evaluates adrenal cortical and gonadal function. *Normal values* are 10-22 mg/day for men and 6-16 mg/day for women.	Instruct client regarding 24-hour urine collection.† Tell client that specimen must be kept refrigerated or iced during collection. Determine whether preservative is required for method used.
Aldosterone levels	This test measures urinary aldosterone level to evaluate adrenal function. It is useful in determining therapy for hypertension. *Normal values* are 5-250 µg/24 hours.	Ensure that client is on unrestricted diet with normal salt intake and no medication for 3 weeks before collection. Instruct client regarding 24-hour urine collection.†
Free cortisol levels	This is preferred test to evaluate hypercortisolism. It can also be used to screen for endogenous glucocorticoids. *Normal values* are less than 100 mg/24 hours.	Instruct client regarding 24-hour urine collection and avoidance of stressful situations and excessive physical exercise. Tell client that some drugs (e.g., reserpine, diuretics, phenothiazines, and amphetamines) may elevate levels. Ensure that client is on low-sodium diet.
Vanillylmandelic acid levels	This study measures urinary excretion of catecholamine metabolite and is helpful in diagnosing pheochromocytoma. *Normal values* are less than 8 mg/24 hours; pheochromocytoma is indicated with values of 10-250 mg/24 hours.	Keep 24-hour urine collection at pH of less than 3.0 with hydrochloric acid as preservative. Know that newer methods are not affected by dietary intake. Consult with laboratory or physician about client discontinuing any drugs 3 days before urine collection.
PANCREATIC STUDIES **Serum studies**		
Fasting blood sugar (FBS) levels	This study measures circulating glucose level. *Normal serum values* for adults are 70-110 mg/dl and for pregnant women, they are 60-90 mg/dl.	Ensure that client has fasted 12 hours overnight. Inform client that blood sample will be drawn. Observe venipuncture site for bleeding or hematoma formation.
Oral glucose tolerance tests	A. This 2-hour test is used to diagnose diabetes mellitus if FBS is equivocal. Client drinks 75 g of glucose; samples for glucose are drawn immediately and at 30, 60, and 120 minutes. *Normal values* are less than 200 mg/dl at 30, 60, and 90 minutes and less than 140 mg/dl at 120 minutes. B. This 5-hour test is used to evaluate hypoglycemia. Client drinks 100 g of glucose; samples for glucose are drawn immediately and at 30, 60, 90, 120, 180, 240, and 300 minutes. Baseline cortisol level test is done if client becomes symptomatic. Clients with reactive hypoglycemia have adrenergic symptoms and glucose less than 60 mg/dl between 30 minutes and 5 hr after glucose ingestion.	Ensure that tests are not done in clients who are malnourished, confined to bed for over 3 days, or severely stressed. Instruct client to refrain from smoking and caffeine and to fast for 12 hours before test. Ensure that client's diet 3 days before test included 150-300 g of carbohydrate with intake of at least 1500 calories/day. Screen for estrogens, phenytoin, and corticosteroids, and check for hypokalemia, which may impair glucose tolerance. Simultaneously monitor glucoses with capillary glucose reagent strips or reflectance meters.

Table 42-6

 Diagnostic Studies of the Endocrine System—cont'd

Study	Description and Purpose*	Nursing Responsibility
PANCREATIC STUDIES—cont'd **Serum studies—cont'd**		
Capillary glucose monitoring	This test is used to give instant glucose values with glucose oxidase method. Capillary values (whole blood) are usually 10%-15% less than serum values.	Obtain large drop of blood from clean finger, touch strip to drop of blood (not finger), time accurately, and compare colors in good lighting, if using visual method. Use automatic finger-puncture device if available. Be sure to change section of device that touches clients' fingers between clients.
Glycosylated hemoglobin levels	This test measures degree of glucose control during previous 3 months (life span of hemoglobin molecule). *Normal values* are less than 7% (values vary widely, check with laboratory).	Inform client that fasting is not necessary and that blood sample will be drawn. Observe venipuncture site for bleeding or hematoma formation.
Urine studies		
Glucose level (Clinistix, Labstix, Multistix, Clinitest)	This test estimates amount of glucose in urine by using reducing substance. Results have wide range from negative (no glucose) to 2% (large amount of glucose).	Use freshly voided urine specimen collected at appropriate time. Know that many different drugs alter glucose readings and that errors are great if directions for timing are not followed exactly. Follow package directions.
Ketone level (Acetest, Ketostix, Labstix, Multistix)	This test measures amount of acetone excreted in urine as result of incomplete fat metabolism. Positive result can indicate lack of insulin and diabetic acidosis.	Use freshly voided urine specimen. Test is often done with glucose test. Directions must be followed exactly. Certain drugs can produce false-positive and false-negative results.
Glucose and acetone level (Keto-diastix)	This study measures glucose and acetone levels.	Know that large amounts of urinary acetone may depress glucose measurement.

*See Chapter 44.

Because the endocrine system affects the entire body, dysfunction can effect many physical, psychological, and social body responses. The changes caused by dysfunction can be obvious but are more often subtle, particularly in the early stages. Therefore assessment of the endocrine system requires many assessment and diagnostic skills. Changes are often attributed to many other causes, including normal aging. Laboratory diagnoses are therefore important in the assessment of the endocrine system. A major role of nursing in laboratory assessments is ensuring that the client understands the tests and preparations for them and that samples are collected and labeled correctly.

R *eview Questions*

The number of the question corresponds to the same-numbered objective at the beginning of the chapter.

1. Which of the following is considered a major characteristic of all endocrine hormones?
   a. They exert their effects on neighboring cells.
   b. They are regulated by negative feedback.
   c. They require binding to receptors to initiate cellular effects.
   d. They are composed of amino acids.
2. Tissues that secrete hormones are almost always
   a. contained within encapsulated, discrete glands
   b. highly vascularized
   c. associated with ducts
   d. located in the cranial or abdominal areas
3. Glucocorticoids, secreted by the adrenal glands, are involved in
   a. oxygen use
   b. aldosterone stimulation
   c. TSH inhibition
   d. the stress response

4. A characteristic of all hormone receptors in the endocrine system is that they
   a. determine the specificity of the cellular response
   b. are protein macromolecules
   c. are located on the cell membrane
   d. stimulate second messengers

5. Which information would the nurse elicit if endocrine dysfunction is suspected?
   a. breathing difficulties
   b. varicosities
   c. energy level
   d. blistering

6. When a normal thyroid gland is palpable, it should feel
   a. nodular
   b. hard
   c. asymmetrical
   d. smooth

7. Which of the following is an abnormal finding in an endocrine assessment?
   a. weight of 130 pounds in a woman who is 57 inches tall
   b. height of 50 inches in a 7-year-old child
   c. drop in systolic blood pressure from 150 to 128 mm Hg 2 minutes after moving from a sitting to a standing position
   d. drop in diastolic blood pressure from 88 to 82 mm Hg 2 minutes after moving from a lying to a sitting position

8. There is a relationship between bone changes seen in aging and
   a. insulin
   b. PTH
   c. T_4
   d. ADH

9. Which of the following tests is most likely to be ordered to evaluate the activity of a solitary thyroid nodule?
   a. TSH
   b. T_3
   c. magnetic resonance imaging
   d. thyroid uptake

REFERENCES

1. Vander AJ, Sherman JH, and Luciano DS: Human physiology: the mechanisms of body function, ed 4, New York, 1985, McGraw-Hill Book Co, Inc, p 233.
2. Baxter JD and others: Introduction to the endocrine system. In Felig P and others: Endocrinology and metabolism, ed 2, New York, 1987, McGraw-Hill Book Co, Inc, p 3.
3. Tepperman J and Tepperman HM: Metabolic and endocrine physiology, ed 5, Chicago, 1987, Year Book Medical Publishers, pp 35-41.
4. Ojeda SR and Griffin JE: Organization of the endocrine system. In Griffin JE and Ojeda RO: Textbook of endocrine physiology, New York, 1988, Oxford University Press, p 4.
5. McCann SM: The anterior pituitary and hypothalamus. In Griffin JE and Ojeda RO: Textbook of endocrine physiology, New York, 1988, Oxford University Press, p 71.
6. Baylis PH: Vasopressin and its neurophysin. In Degroot LJ, ed: Endocrinology, ed 2, Philadelphia, 1989, WB Saunders Co, p 216.
7. Samson WK: The posterior pituitary and water metabolism. In Griffin JE and Ojeda RO, eds: Textbook of endocrine physiology, New York, 1988, Oxford University Press, p 106.
8. Breslau NA: Calcium homeostasis. In Griffin JE and Ojeda RO, eds: Textbook of endocrine physiology, New York, 1988, Oxford University Press, p 286.
9. Kaplan NM: The adrenal glands. In Griffin JE and Ojeda RO, eds: Textbook of endocrine physiology, New York, 1988, Oxford University Press, p 245.
10. Feldman D: Mechanism of action of cortisol. In DeGroot LJ, ed: Endocrinology, ed 2, Philadelphia, 1989, WB Saunders Co, p 1557.
11. Baxter JD and Tyrell JB: The adrenal cortex. In Felig P and others: Endocrinology and metabolism, ed 2, New York, 1987, McGraw-Hill Book Co, Inc, p 552.
12. Ehrlich EN: Electrolyte metabolism. In DeGroot LJ, ed: Endocrinology, ed 2, Philadelphia, 1989, WB Saunders Co, p 1588.
13. Myers A and others: The eicosanotides: prostaglandins, thromboxane, and leukotrines. In DeGroot LJ, ed: Endocrinology, ed 2, Philadelphia, 1989, WB Saunders Co, p 2480.
14. Luskv KL: Growth and development. In Griffin JE and Ojeda RO, eds: Textbook of endocrine physiology, New York, 1988, Oxford University Press, p 215.
15. Bray GA: Obesity: an endocrine perspective. In DeGroot LJ, ed: Endocrinology, ed 2, Philadelphia, 1989, WB Saunders Co, p 2305.
16. MacLennan WJ and Peden NR: Metabolic and endocrine problems in the elderly, London, 1989, Springer-Verlag, p 17.
17. Griffin JE: Assessment of endocrine function. In Griffin JE and Ojeda RO, eds: New York, 1988, Oxford University Press, p 56.

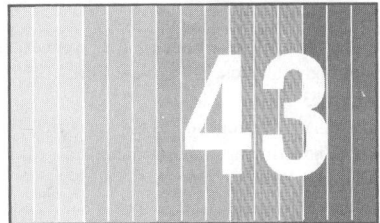

CHAPTER

43

Nursing Role in Management
The Client with Diabetes

Virginia Valentine

SIGNIFICANCE

Diabetes mellitus is a serious health problem throughout the world. An estimated 12 million people have diabetes in the United States alone. It is estimated that 1 in 20 people in the United States may have diabetes mellitus. It is the fifth leading cause of death by disease in this country and the leading cause of new cases of blindness. It increases the risk of coronary artery disease fourfold or more.[1] The staggering cost in human suffering and diabetes-related expenses (estimated at $4.8 billion annually) warrants a sound knowledge base to provide nursing care for clients with diabetes.[2]

PATHOPHYSIOLOGY

Diabetes mellitus is not a single disease but a chronic systemic syndrome characterized by hyperglycemia caused by a decrease in the secretion or activity of insulin. These insulin alterations result in disordered metabolism of car-

bohydrate, fat, and protein and, in time, structural abnormalities in a variety of organs and organ systems, especially the heart, kidneys, and eyes. The complications arise primarily from microangiopathy, macroangiopathy, and neuropathy. In addition, diabetes mellitus is associated with complications of pregnancy.[3]*

Normal Insulin Metabolism

Insulin is a hormone produced by the β cells in the islets of Langerhans in the pancreas. In normal conditions, insulin is continuously released into the bloodstream in small amounts (a basal rate), with increased release (bolus) when food is ingested (Fig. 43-1). The activity of released insulin lowers blood glucose and facilitates a stable, normal glucose range of approximately 70 to 120 mg/dl. The average amount of insulin secreted daily by an adult is approximately 40 to 50 units or 0.6 U/kg of body weight. Other hormones (glucagon, epinephrine, growth hormone, cortisol, and somatostatin) work to counter the effects of insulin and are often referred to as *counterregulatory hormones* because they stimulate glycogen release and thereby increase blood glucose levels. Insulin and these counterregulatory substances provide a sustained but regulated release of glucose for energy during food intake and periods of fasting and normally maintain blood glucose levels within the normal range. Some researchers believe that an abnormal production of any or all these hormones may be present in diabetes.[4]

Once insulin is released into the bloodstream from the β cells, it is routed through the liver. Within the liver, approximately 50% to 70% of received insulin is extracted from the blood. Insulin is formed from proinsulin after cleavage of the C-peptide chain (Fig. 43-2).[5] The presence of C peptide in serum and urine is a useful indicator of β-cell function.[5] The remaining insulin (now active A- and B-peptide chains) functions to promote glucose transport

<hr>

Reviewed by Joan Colgin, R.N., B.S.N., C.D.E., Endocrine Associates of Dallas P.A., Program Director and Research Coordinator, Dallas, Texas.

<hr>

*Gestational diabetes mellitus and management of the pregnant client with diabetes is a specialized area not covered in this chapter. The reader is advised to consult an obstetrical text for information about this area.

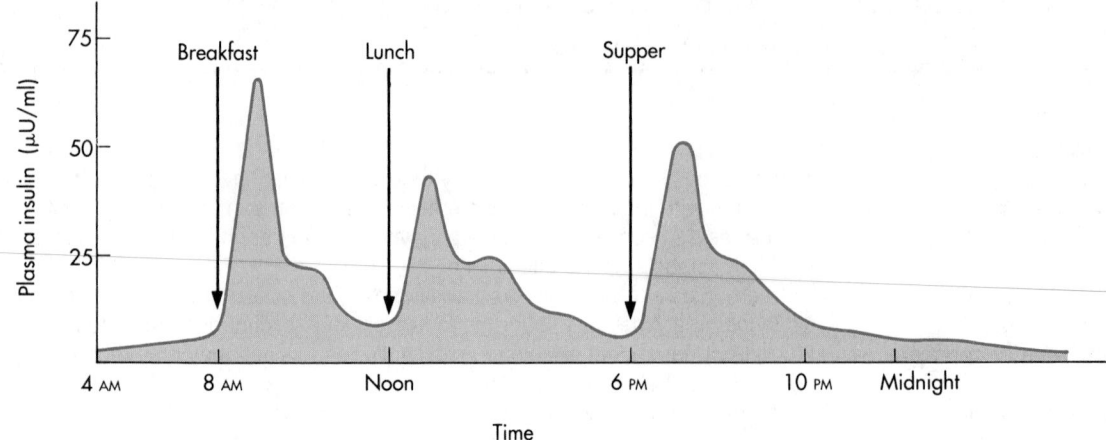

Fig. 43-1 In the first hour or two after meals, insulin concentrations rise rapidly in blood and peak at about 1 hour. After meals, insulin concentrations promptly decline toward preprandial values as carbohydrate absorption from the gut declines. After carbohydrate absorption from the gut is complete and during the night, insulin concentrations are low and fairly constant with a slight increase at dawn. (From Diabetes mellitus, Indianapolis, 1988, Eli Lilly, Inc, p 195.)

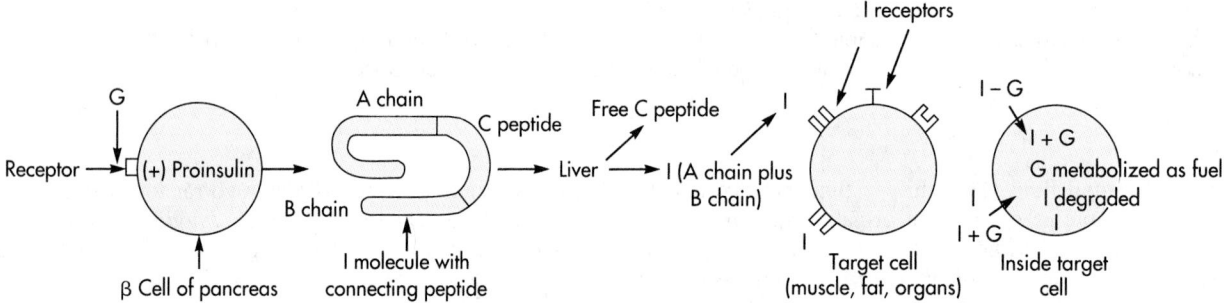

Fig. 43-2 Insulin formation-function pathway. *I*, Insulin; *G*, glucose. (From Price M: Insulin and oral hypoglycemic agents, Nurs Clin North Am 18:688, 1983.)

from the bloodstream across the cell membrane to the cytoplasm of the cell. The rise in plasma insulin after a meal stimulates storage of glucose as glycogen in liver and muscle, enhances fat deposition in adipose tissue, inhibits protein degradation, and accelerates the processes of amino acid transport into cells and protein synthesis. The fall in insulin level during normal overnight fasting facilitates the release of stored glucose from the liver, protein from muscle, and fat from adipose tissue.[6] For this reason insulin is known as the *storage hormone.*

Skeletal muscle and adipose tissue have specific receptors for insulin and are considered to be insulin-dependent tissues. Other tissues (e.g., brain, liver, and blood cells) do not directly depend on insulin for glucose transport but on an adequate glucose supply.

As shown in Fig. 43-2, the absolute lack or decreased insulin activity may occur at several points along the insulin formation-function pathway from many different causes. *Prereceptor defects* include destruction of β cells from β-cell antibodies; circulating insulin antagonists such as cortisol, growth hormone, glucagon, and catechola-

mines; and circulating insulin antibodies. *Receptor defects* include decreased binding of insulin to insulin-specific receptors and a decreased number of insulin-specific receptors. Examples of conditions with receptor defects are obesity, glucocorticoid and oral contraceptive treatment, acromegaly, and circulating insulin-receptor antibodies. Postreceptor defects include abnormal coupling between insulin and the glucose transport system, enzymatic defects in glucose metabolism, and a defect in intracellular use. Because of these possibilities for malfunctioning, diabetes mellitus must be considered a heterogeneous disease not amenable to only one treatment regimen.

Clinical Manifestations

Normally, insulin and its counterregulatory hormones maintain blood glucose within a range of 70 to 120 mg/dl. Elevated blood glucose levels produce symptoms related to the degree of actual or relative insulin deficiency. When an absolute insulin deficiency or decreased insulin activity occurs, glucose is not used properly. Glucose remains in the bloodstream and produces an osmotic effect on intracellu-

Table 43-1 Types of Diabetes Mellitus and Other Categories of Glucose Intolerance

Classes	Distinguishing Characteristics
CLINICAL	
Diabetes mellitus	
Insulin-dependent diabetes mellitus, type I	Clients may be of any age, are usually thin, and usually have abrupt onset of signs and symptoms with insulinopenia before age 30. They often have strongly positive urine ketone tests in conjunction with hyperglycemia and depend on insulin therapy to prevent ketoacidosis and to sustain life.
Non-insulin-dependent diabetes mellitus, type II (obese or nonobese)	Clients are usually older than 30 yr at diagnosis, are obese, and have relatively few classic symptoms. They are not prone to ketoacidosis except during periods of stress. Although not dependent on exogenous insulin for survival, they may require it for adequate control of hyperglycemia.
Other types of diabetes mellitus	Clients have certain associated conditions or syndromes.
Impaired glucose tolerance (obese or nonobese)	Clients have plasma glucose levels that are higher than normal but not diagnostic for diabetes mellitus.
Other types of impaired glucose tolerance	Clients have certain associated conditions or syndromes.
Gestational diabetes mellitus	Clients have onset or discovery of glucose intolerance during pregnancy.
STATISTICAL RISK	
Previous abnormality of glucose tolerance	Clients have normal glucose tolerance and history of transient diabetes mellitus or impaired glucose tolerance.
Potential abnormality of glucose tolerance	Clients have never had abnormal glucose tolerance but have a greater than normal risk of diabetes mellitus or impaired glucose tolerance developing.

lar and interstitial fluid. This shift in fluid balance results in clinical symptoms of frequent urination *(polyuria)* and thirst *(polydipsia)*. Without sufficient insulin the client may experience hunger *(polyphagia)* as the body turns to other energy sources besides glucose: first fat and then protein. Varying degrees of polyuria, polydipsia, and polyphagia are the hallmark symptoms of diabetes mellitus.

Acute and chronic complications from hyperglycemia are closely associated with the type of diabetes mellitus and the circumstances in which it occurs (see p. 1299).

Classification

The diagnostic label of *diabetes mellitus* carries many psychological and socioeconomic ramifications and therapeutic requirements. Therefore accurate classification of the degree and type of glucose intolerance and diabetes is important. Based on knowledge about diabetes, a system for the diagnosis and classification of degree and type was developed by the National Diabetes Data Group of the National Institutes of Health in 1979.[7] The classification system is based on not only the presence and degree of hyperglycemia but also the presenting history and symptoms (see Table 43-1). The classification scheme also includes persons who have had or who are having glucose intolerance without overt signs of diabetes mellitus. Recognition of this difference allows persons at higher risk for diabetes to be followed without being misclassified or mismanaged.

The diagnosis of diabetes mellitus is made when the fasting plasma glucose level exceeds 140 mg/dl on at least two occasions or when at least two random blood glucose measurements exceed 200 mg/dl. *Impaired glucose tolerance* is classified as a fasting plasma glucose higher than normal but lower than those considered diagnostic for diabetes mellitus.

ETIOLOGY

Diabetes mellitus is not a single disease. It is a heterogeneous syndrome for which several theories of etiology have been proposed. Current theories link the causes of diabetes, singly or in combination, to genetic, autoimmune, viral, and environmental factors such as obesity and stress. As reflected in Table 43-1, there are primarily two types of diabetes mellitus: *type I,* in which insulin production by the β cells is reduced or completely absent and for which the management requires insulin replacement, and *type II,* which is the more prevalent type of diabetes mellitus (approximately 80% of clients). Table 43-2 depicts the distinguishing manifestations of types I and II diabetes mellitus.

Type I: Insulin-Dependent Diabetes Mellitus

In type I diabetes, β-cell destruction is attributed to a genetic predisposition coupled with one or more viral agents and/or a possible autoimmune reaction. This autoimmune reaction may or may not be triggered by a virus. Three viruses that have been implicated are mumps, rubella, and coxsackievirus B. It is not known conclusively that these are the only factors involved.

The complexity may be better appreciated in light of current information about histocompatibility locus antigens

Table 43-2 Characteristics of Type I and Type II Diabetes Mellitus

Factor	Type I	Type II
Age at onset	Usually in young persons but possible at any age	Usually >age 35 yr but possible at any age
Type of onset	Usually abrupt	Insidious
Genetic susceptibility	HLA-related DR3, DR4, and others	Frequent genetic background, no relation to HLA
Environmental factors	Virus, toxins, autoimmune stimulation	Obesity, nutrition
Islet cell antibody	Present at outset	Absent
Endogenous insulin	Minimal or absent	Possibly excessive, adequate but delayed secretion or reduced but not absent secretion
Nutritional status	Thin, catabolic state	Obese or possibly normal
Symptoms	Thirst, polyuria, polyphagia, fatigue	Frequently none, or mild
Ketosis	Prone, at onset or during insulin deficiency	Resistant except during infection or stress
Control of diabetes	Often difficult with wide glucose fluctuation	Variable, control with diet and exercise
Dietary management	Essential	Essential, possibly sufficing for glycemic control
Insulin	Required for all	Required for 20%-30%
Sulfonylurea	Not efficacious	Efficacious
Vascular and neurological complications	In majority of clients after ≥5 yr diabetes	Frequent

Modified from Diabetes mellitus, Indianapolis, 1988, Eli Lilly, Inc, p 4.

(HLAs), which are proteins on the cell surface controlled by genes on chromosome 6. (See Chapter 8 for a discussion of HLA antigens and disease associations.) Five groups of these antigens—A, B, C, D, and DR—have been recognized, and these groups can appear in many variations. Results of family studies confirm that susceptibility to type I diabetes is strongly linked to the HLA DR3/DR4 locus.[8] The variations most often associated with type I diabetes are those that are positive for one or more of the following HLA types: B8, DR3, B15, and DR4.[9] Theoretically, when these genetic defects are exposed to viral infections, the β cells are destroyed directly or an autoimmune process is triggered, which in turn destroys the β cells. A combination of both processes may occur. Current research continues to seek genetic markers to identify persons at risk for type I diabetes who are free of symptoms and to study immunological sequences that may be manipulated to prevent or cure type I diabetes.

Genetic counseling for parents is based on statistical risk. If one child has type I diabetes, other siblings have a 5% to 10% chance of type I diabetes developing (up to 45% if the sibling is an identical twin). If a parent has type I diabetes, the risk to the offspring is 25% to 40%.

The onset and progression of hyperglycemic symptoms are usually more rapid and acute in type I diabetes, and successful treatment depends on insulin replacement. If the disease process is allowed to progress without treatment, diabetic ketoacidosis with nausea and vomiting, electrolyte imbalance, weight loss, and muscle wasting may develop. Without treatment (i.e., insulin) ketoacidosis can progress to coma and death.

Once treatment is initiated, clients with type I diabetes may go into a remission (often called the *honeymoon phase*). This phase is not known to last much beyond a year (although recent immunosuppression research studies have demonstrated a remission of 2 years or more for clients with type I diabetes treated within 6 weeks of diagnosis), and diabetes management must be resumed again.[9]

Type II: Non-Insulin-Dependent Diabetes Mellitus

Approximately 80% of diabetes mellitus is type II non-insulin-dependent diabetes mellitus. There are two recognized subtypes of type II: obese and nonobese (see Table 43-1). Type II diabetes has a strong genetic influence, but no correlation with HLA type has been found. This type of diabetes is most often associated with a population more than 40 years of age, particularly among those who are overweight, but type II has also been identified in younger age groups. It was formerly termed *maturity-onset diabetes in the young.*

Another distinguishing feature of this type of diabetes mellitus is an endogenous insulin supply sufficient to inhibit the development of diabetic ketoacidosis (DKA), which occurs when endogenous insulin is markedly reduced or absent. The pathophysiological factors that have been identified in type II diabetes include (1) reduced production or overproduction of insulin secretion, (2) decreased tissue (fat, muscle) responsiveness to insulin as a result of receptor and/or postreceptor defects, and (3) abnormal hepatic glucose regulation. Obesity appears to play a major role in type II obese diabetes by downregulating insulin receptors in skeletal muscle and fat cells; that is, the number of available insulin receptors is decreased. The development of these events is often referred to as *periph-*

eral insulin resistance. A reduced-caloric diet for the obese type II client tends to reverse this phenomenon.[10] Type II clients may benefit from oral hypoglycemic agents, which have been found to be physiologically effective in several ways, including increasing insulin production, improving cell receptor binding, and regulating hepatic glucose production.

In type II diabetes mellitus the onset of hyperglycemic symptoms may occur over a long period and the person may "adjust" to the persistent feelings of fatigue, thirst, polyuria, and blurred vision without realizing that the diabetes disease process is producing the symptoms. If the client with type II diabetes has marked hyperglycemia (e.g., 500 to $\geq$1000 mg/dl), a sufficient endogenous insulin supply may prevent DKA from occurring, but fluid and electrolyte loss may become severe and lead to hyperosmolar coma. (See p. 1302 for the sequence of events associated with hyperosmolar hyperglycemia.) During precipitating and acute situations (such as acute illness), clients with type II diabetes may briefly require insulin administration. It is also possible for the type II client to have DKA if a precipitating stress event is severe and strains the available endogenous insulin supply. The fact that some persons with type II diabetes may require insulin during times of stress or for treatment of hyperosmolar hyperglycemia does not mean that these persons are insulin dependent or will require long-term insulin treatment.[11]

Genetic counseling for the type II group is based on a known higher familial risk. The siblings of a person with type II diabetes are at a 25% risk for type II diabetes developing, whereas the offspring of parents with type II diabetes have a 10% chance of the disease developing. Children and young adults with type II diabetes have a 50% chance of transmitting the disease to their children.[12]

DIAGNOSTIC STUDIES

The classification system in Table 43-1 depends on appropriate and accurate diagnostic techniques. Urine tests are not sufficient for diagnosing diabetes mellitus because variables such as age, medications, and a normally low renal threshold for glucose may show glycosuria without the presence of diabetes or glucose intolerance.

When overt symptoms of hyperglycemia—polyuria, polydipsia, and polyphagia—together with fasting blood glucose levels of 200 mg/dl or greater are present, further glucose tolerance tests are usually not warranted. However, when oral glucose tolerance tests are used, the accuracy of test results depends on adequate client preparation and attention to the many factors that may influence the outcome of such tests. For example, factors that can induce falsely elevated values include recent sharp restrictions of dietary carbohydrate, acute illness, medications such as contraceptives and glucocorticosteroids, and restricted activity such as bed rest. Clients with impaired gastrointestinal (GI) absorption may also have false-negative test results. Table 43-3 outlines the initial assessment and management when diabetes mellitus is the suspected diagnosis.

Because diabetes is a multisystem, multiproblem disease, all laboratory studies must be correlated with clinical

Table 43-3

 Diagnostic and Therapeutic Management: Diabetes Mellitus

DIAGNOSTIC

Complete history and physical examination
Blood tests, including fasting blood glucose, postprandial blood sugar, glycosylated hemoglobin, cholesterol and triglyceride levels, blood urea nitrogen and creatinine, electrolytes
Urine for complete urinalysis, culture and sensitivity, glucose and acetone
Funduscopic examination
Neurological examination
Blood pressure
Monitoring of weight

THERAPEUTIC

Calculated food plan
Exercise plan
Insulin or oral hypoglycemia agent (if indicated)
Dental examination
Podiatric examination
Specific teaching and follow-up programs

findings. The most common finding in overt diabetes mellitus is an elevated blood glucose level (>140 mg/dl). Glucose values differ depending on the source of the sample and the site from which it is taken, the timing in relation to meals, and the time of day. Arterial and capillary plasma values tend to be higher than whole blood and venous blood samplings. Postprandial (after meals) and late afternoon values also tend to be higher. Age also makes a difference. The American Diabetes Association (ADA) recommends adding 10 mg/dl to the normal value for each decade more than age 50 years.

In the presence of abnormal insulin utilization, fat metabolism is altered. This results in elevations of lipid, cholesterol, and triglyceride levels that are associated with the vascular disorders of diabetes.

The results of urine tests for glucose and acetone depend on age, severity of diabetes, and renal function. Blood glucose is a better measurement of glycemic status because glycosuria may not be evident when hyperglycemia is present (see p. 1279). The presence of ketonuria and elevated serum ketones accompanied by marked hyperglycemia is the heralding sign of DKA. In persons without diabetes who fast, ketonuria also develops as a result of fat breakdown but without accompanying hyperglycemia.

Glycosylated hemoglobin is a measurement that is useful in determining glycemic levels over time. The hemoglobin of red blood cells (RBCs) attracts a certain amount of glucose (approximately 5% to 7% in the nondiabetic person). When blood glucose is elevated over time or when the person has frequent wide fluctuations in glycemic levels, the amount of glucose attached to the hemoglo-

bin molecule increases. The glucose remains attached to the RBC for the life of the cell. Therefore a glycosylated hemoglobin test indicates the overall glucose control for the past 120 days. Laboratory methods may differ in this assay because some methods measure the entire glycosylated hemoglobin molecule whereas other methods measure only a specific glycosylated hemoglobin, hemoglobin A_1, or hemoglobin A_{1c}. Depending on the method used, levels more than 7% or 9% are considered to be abnormally elevated. Diseases affecting RBCs (e.g., sickle cell anemia) also affect the glycosylated hemoglobin results and should be taken into consideration in the interpretation of this test result.[13]

Proteinuria is a sign of early nephropathy. Analysis for microalbuminuria may show early nephropathy long before routine urinalysis displays proteinuria. Microalbuminuria tests are now the recommended method for early detection of nephropathy. The presence of protein in the urine as detected by microalbuminuria urinalysis should be followed with a 24-hour urine correction for determination of creatinine clearance and serum creatinine. Diagnostic tests requiring the use of fluorescein dyes should be approached with extreme caution in clients with proteinuria. Clients with serum creatinine levels of 4 to 6 mg/dl or greater may have irreversible deterioration of renal function and oliguria after an intravenous (IV) pyelogram or angiogram. Also, clients with diabetes in the later stages of renal disease may require a reduction in insulin dose as a result of both a decrease in caloric intake and an alteration in insulin function and metabolism in chronic renal failure.[14]

The Doppler instrument is used to diagnose the presence or degree of peripheral vascular disease. It is a device similar to an electronic stethoscope that amplifies sound. The procedure is noninvasive and can measure blood pressure in the lower extremities and blood flow velocity. It can indicate areas of stenosis or occlusion and can be used as one of the indicators for additional diagnostic testing with angiopathy.

THERAPEUTIC MANAGEMENT

Management of diabetes mellitus is primarily aimed at achieving a balance of diet, activity, and medications together with appropriate monitoring and client and family education (Fig. 43-3). These components are equally necessary for good control of diabetes.

NUTRITIONAL CONSIDERATIONS

Dietary management is the cornerstone of therapy for diabetes. In both type I and type II diabetes, an individually calculated, balanced diet is of primary importance. In type I diabetes, insulin replacement is also necessary, but it must be prescribed in conjunction with an appropriate diet.

Dietary Adherence

A potentially difficult adjustment for the client with diabetes is the need to comply with an individually prescribed diet. Diet and eating patterns have special meanings for each client in regard to emotions, culture, and re-

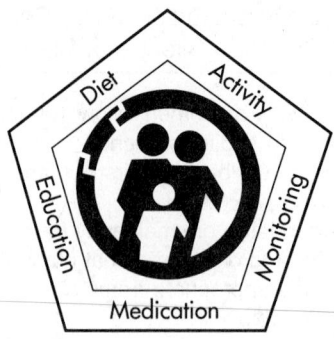

Fig. 43-3 The five aspects of diabetes management make up the complete program for good control. (From Diabetes mellitus, Indianapolis, 1988, Eli Lilly, Inc.)

ligion. Many people are aware that a well-balanced diet is healthy, but most people find it difficult to adhere to a special diet all the time. Reinforcement and encouragement are essential if a successful dietary program is to be followed.

The attainment or maintenance of desirable or reasonable body weight is a dietary goal for the client with diabetes. The emotional impact of diabetes on a client who uses food to relieve stress presents a strong challenge to the nurse. Frequently a contract between nurse and client with inherent reinforcement for adherence may be helpful. Behavior modification techniques may be successful for long-term weight control. Crash or fad diets should be avoided.

Calculating a Diabetic Diet

A diabetic diet is calculated individually according to the client's ideal body weight, occupation, age, and activities. For the adult, calories are based on desirable body weight and activity needs (Table 43-4). For persons with type I diabetes, who are usually lean at diagnosis, it is important that adequate calories be prescribed. Calorie levels for meal plans should be based on the client's nutrition history and usual food intake. Additional calories can be added to promote weight gain or subtracted to promote weight loss. This is usually based on the baseline number of calories plus or minus 10%. Weight loss diets should contain between 1000 and 1200 calories for the adult to avoid protein breakdown. Although fasting has been used with success in short-term treatment of obese type II diabetic clients, it must be done under strict medical supervision.

Once caloric needs are determined in relation to the need to lose, maintain, or gain weight, the proportions of carbohydrates, protein, and fat are calculated. The distribution of daily calories averages 50% to 60% from carbohydrates (of which 90% to 95% should be complex carbohydrates), 20% from protein, and 30% from fat (of which 20% should be polyunsaturated). The diet should also include 10 to 15 g of fiber.[15]

Many different systems are available to achieve these dietary goals, such as "points" (a simplified method of tracking calories), and menu plans and exchange lists for

Table 43-4   General Guidelines for Calculating a Diet for a Client with Diabetes

1. Determine DBW. For women, allow 100 lb for first 5 ft and 5 lb for each additional inch: _____DBW
   For men, allow 106 lb for the first 5 ft and 6 lb for each additional inch: _____DBW
2. For adjusting to large or small body frame, multiply DBW by 10%. Add or subtract that number for DBW according to the appropriate frame size. If client does not feel comfortable with calculated DBW, client's idea of desired weight should be the initial goal, with renegotiation of DBW later.
3. Multiply DBW by 10. This is the baseline number of calories.
4. Adjust calories for activity needs with the following guidelines:

Sedentary:	DBW × 3
Moderate:	DBW × 5
Strenuous:	DBW × 10

   (Most people belong to the sedentary group. Strenuous activity includes skilled athletes and heavy laborers such as jackhammer users.)
5. Take the number from step 4 and add it to the answer in step 3. This will be the total number of daily calories required to maintain the person's DBW. To have client lose weight, subtract 500 cal from this total. To have client gain weight, add 500 cal to this total.

Example: 40-year-old woman, 5 ft 8 in tall, small frame, sedentary:

   100 + (8 × 5) = 140 DBW
   Minus 10% for small body = 126 lb
      (adjusted) DBW
   10 × 126 = 1260 cal for baseline
   126 × 3 = 378 cal for activity
   1260 + 378 = 1638 total daily cal for
      weight maintenance

The next step is to divide the total daily calories into meal apportionments with prescribed amounts of carbohydrates, proteins, and fat.

DBW, Desirable body weight.

Table 43-5   Meal Plan and Exchange Lists

1800-CAL MEAL PLAN

	Breakfast	Lunch	Dinner	HS
Milk	1	1	1	
Bread/starch	2	2	2	1
Fruit	1	1	1	
Vegetable		1	1	
Meat	2	2	2	1
Fat	2	2	1	1

EXCHANGE LIST EXAMPLES

Milk exchange	**Amount/serving**
Milk (skim)	1 cup
Milk (2%)	1 cup
Yogurt (plain, low fat)	1 cup

Fruit/juice exchange	**Amount/serving**
Orange juice	½ cup
Banana	½
Cherries	10 large

Meat/protein exchange	**Amount/serving**
Egg	1
Poultry	1 oz
Frankfurter	1

Vegetable exchange	**Amount/serving**
Green beans (plain)	1 cup
Mushrooms (plain)	1 cup
Tomato juice	½ cup

Bread/starch exchange	**Amount/serving**
Hamburger bun (large)	½
Cooked cereal	½ cup
Corn	⅓

Fat exchange	**Amount/serving**
Mayonnaise	1 tsp
Bacon	1 strip
Butter	1 tsp

The exchange lists are based on material in the *Exchange Lists for Meal Planning* prepared by committees of the American Diabetes Association, Inc, and the American Dietetic Association in cooperation with the National Institute of Arthritis, Metabolism, and Digestive Diseases and the National Heart and Lung Institute, National Institutes of Health, Public Health Service, U.S. Department of Health, Education and Welfare. Used with permission.
HS, Hour of sleep.

meal planning from the American Diabetes Association and the American Dietetic Association. All methods reflect the seven dietary guidelines published by the U.S. Food and Drug Administration.

Exchange Lists

Individual dietary prescriptions may be converted into a meal plan based on the exchange list system of the American Diabetes Association. An exchange list divides all foods except concentrated carbohydrates into one of six categories or food groups: milk, meats, vegetables, fats, breads, and fruits. Each food group is calculated to include the specific quantity of food allowed according to standard household measurements. Each food quantity is equal to one food exchange. Calories are not listed for each food, but the overall meal plan is set to provide the daily number of calories prescribed by the physician. The meal plan explains how many food exchanges are allowed for each food group per meal. All the foods within the specific food groups are allowed for variety as long as the quantity is taken into account. Table 43-5 shows a sample 1800-calorie meal plan and an excerpt from the exchange lists. Diet strategies differ between type I and type II diabetes and

Table 43-6 Dietary Strategies for Type I and Type II Diabetes Mellitus

Factor	Type I	Type II
Total calories	Increase in caloric intake possibly necessary to achieve desirable body weight and restore body tissues	Reduction in caloric intake necessary for obese clients
Effect of diet	Diet and insulin necessary for glucose control	Diet alone possibly sufficient for glucose control
Distribution of calories	Equal distribution of carbohydrate through meals or adjustment of carbohydrate for insulin activity	Equal distribution not essential
Consistency in daily intake	Necessary for glucose control	Desirable for weight reduction
Uniform timing of meals	Crucial for NPH/Lente insulin programs, flexibility with multidose regular insulin	Desirable but not essential
Intermeal and bedtime snacks	Frequently necessary	Not recommended
Supplement for exercise programs	Carbohydrate 20 g/hr for moderate physical activities	Necessary if client controlled on sulfonylurea or insulin

Modified from Diabetes mellitus, Indianapolis, 1988, Eli Lilly, Inc, p 87.

should be considered when planning dietary management (Table 43-6). Complete exchange lists and calculated diets for different caloric requirements are available from the American Diabetes Association.

An area receiving increased attention and research is "glycemic indices," which refer to the status of foods as simple (quick acting) or complex carbohydrate. For example, raw potatoes release glucose more slowly during digestion; however, the same starches are altered by heat when cooked and are more quickly available for absorption. This type of information is useful in considering ways to select and prepare foods for more predictable glycemic control.[16]

Diet Education

Most often the dietitian initially teaches the principles of the diabetic diet. However, the nurse should be knowledgeable about diabetes dietary principles to answer questions and to help the client make appropriate selections and decisions. The nurse should include the family of the client when teaching the diet plan. Particular attention and teaching efforts should be directed to the person who will be cooking. It is important, however, that the responsibility for maintaining a diabetic diet not fall to someone other than the client with diabetes. Reliance on another person to make health decisions fosters dependence and should be avoided except in special situations.

Principles that both the nurse and dietitian should teach and reinforce include the following:

1. Eat according to the prescribed meal plan: No two meal plans are alike. A meal plan is individualized to reflect the dietary needs related to a specific client's desirable body weight (DBW), occupation, age, activities, and type of diabetes. Individual responses to a dietary prescription should be monitored, and appropriate adjustments should be made when necessary.

2. Never skip meals: This is particularly critical for clients taking insulin or oral hypoglycemic agents (OHAs). The body requires food at regularly spaced intervals throughout the day. Insulin and OHAs are prescribed to fit this schedule. Omission or delay of meals may result in hypoglycemia.

3. Learn to recognize appropriate food portions: Practice can result in accurate portion allotments.

Areas of Concern

Alcohol. Alcohol is high in calories, has no nutritive value, and promotes hypertriglyceridemia. In addition, it has detrimental effects on the liver (see Chapter 38). The inhibitory effect of alcohol on gluconeogenesis can cause severe hypoglycemia. A client can reduce this risk by eating carbohydrates when drinking alcohol. Alcohol may produce a disulfiram (Antabuse) effect (nausea and vomiting, flushing, respiratory distress, chest pain) proportional to the amount ingested with certain OHAs.

However, if the client chooses, a drink can be calculated into the diabetic diet by substituting 45 calories of alcohol for one fat exchange. One drink has approximately 135 calories and equals three fat exchanges. When possible, clients with diabetes should drink on a full stomach, use sugar-free mixes, and drink dry, light wines.

Dietetic foods. The word *dietetic* is confusing because it does not always refer to a lack of calories. The caloric value of dietetic foods should be determined by reading the label. If no caloric value is listed, calories must be counted in the meal plan from the appropriate exchange group.

Dietetic foods are expensive and, although convenient, are not necessary. The client can be taught to make intelligent decisions regarding the use of nondietetic foods by reading labels. For example, foods with sugar, mannitol, or sorbitol listed as the first two ingredients should be avoided. The increasing availability of foods prepared with

artificial sweeteners allows greater freedom in the diet. Recipes that use artificial sweeteners are available.

PHARMACOLOGICAL MANAGEMENT

The two types of glucose-lowering agents used in the treatment of diabetes are insulin and OHAs.

Insulin

Indications for use. Exogenous insulin is needed when a client has inadequate insulin to meet specific metabolic needs and the combination of dietary management, exercise, and oral agents cannot maintain a satisfactory blood glucose level. Exogenous insulin is required for the management of type I diabetes. Exogenous insulin may be prescribed for clients with type II diabetes during periods of severe stress, such as illness or surgery, or when attempts at glycemic control by means of diet, exercise, and/or OHAs fail.

Exogenous insulin has commonly been obtained from the pancreases of pigs and cows. These two forms of insulin are similar to human insulin protein chains, with pork insulin being more similar to human insulin. However, these sources have become expensive to obtain, and although the purification process for extracting the insulin islets has improved to where only minuscule amounts of foreign protein are present, these substances can initiate insulin allergies. Insulins marked "purified" have had nearly all extraneous pancreatic proteins removed. Recently human insulin has been made commercially available.

Human insulin is produced by genetically altering common bacteria by recombinant DNA technology. This insulin exhibits chemical and biological properties identical to human insulin produced by human β cells. The advantage of these new insulins is a reduced allergic response and a more predictable insulin activity. The purified and human insulins are preferred for clients with newly diagnosed type I diabetes, clients who demonstrate insulin allergies, clients with gestational diabetes, and clients who are pregnant.

Types. In addition to origin and purity, insulins differ in regard to onset, peak action, and duration (Fig. 43-4). The specific properties of each type of insulin are matched with the client's diet and activity. Not all clients respond to insulin exactly as shown in Table 43-7. The action times are listed as anticipated guidelines. Human insulin may have slightly less activity time.

All insulin preparations start with regular insulin as a base; zinc is added (to make Lente insulin), and zinc and protamine are added to make NPH and PZI to prolong the action of insulin. These binding agents can cause an allergic reaction at the injection site. Regular insulin is prescribed when a rapid onset of glucose-lowering action is needed, such as before meals and during periods of acute illness, surgery, or stress. Only regular insulin can be administered IV; thus it is used in emergencies.

Insulins are commonly used in combination to mimic the normal endogenous insulin secretion (see Fig. 43-1). The timing of insulin administration in relation to meals is important. Regular insulin should be taken 20 to 30 minutes before meals to ensure the onset of action in conjunction with meal absorption. Examples of insulin combination regimens, onset, peak, and descriptions of the advan-

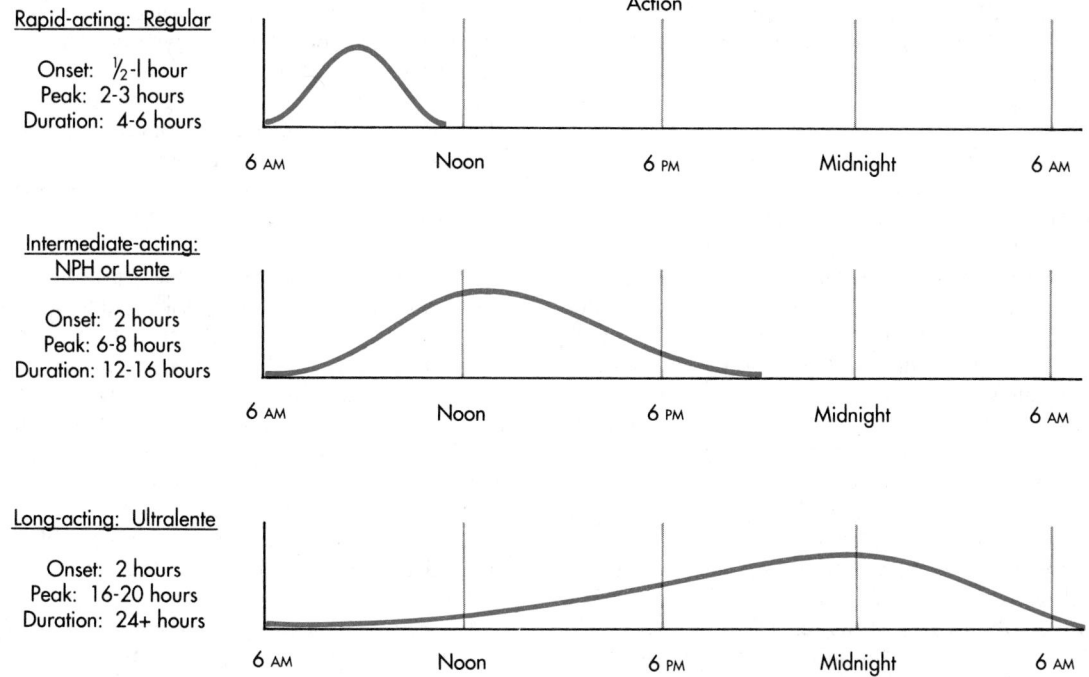

Fig. 43-4   Commercially available insulin preparations. Insulin is available in beef, beef and pork, and purified pork preparations and as human insulin. Premixed insulins of regular and NPH are also available.

Table 43-7 Insulin Regimens

Regimen	Type of Insulin Used	Time Administered and Expected Time-Action Curve*	Advantages	Disadvantages
Single dose	Intermediate insulin (I)	7 AM (I) — Noon — 6 PM — Midnight — 7 AM	One injection should cover noon and PM meal. Hypoglycemia during sleep is not problem.	No fasting, breakfast, or nighttime coverage of hyperglycemia is necessary.
Split-mixed dose (20/30 premix)	Intermediate and regular insulin (I + R)	7 AM (I + R) — Noon — 6 PM — Midnight — 7 AM	Two injections provide coverage for 24 hr.	Two injections are required. Client is "locked" into set meal pattern.
Split-mixed dose	Intermediate and regular insulin (I + R)	7 AM (I + R) — Noon — 7 PM (R) — 9 PM (I) — Midnight — 7 AM	Three injections provide coverage for 24 hr, particularly during early AM hours. Potential is reduced for 2-3 AM hypoglycemia.	Three injections are required.
Multiple dose	Intermediate and regular insulin (I + R)	7 AM (R) — Noon (R) — 7 PM (R) — 9 PM (I) — 7 AM	More flexibility is allowed at mealtimes and for amount of food intake.	Four injections are required. Premeal blood glucose checks, establishing and following individualized algorithm as necessary.
Multiple dose† (split dose long-acting insulin [Ultra Lente])	Regular insulin and longest-acting insulin (R + LA)	7 AM (R+LA) — Noon (R) — 7 PM (R) — Midnight — 7 AM	Insulin delivery pattern more closely simulates normal endogenous insulin pattern. Some flexibility is allowed in food intake pattern. Regimen gives a basal insulin coverage and regular insulin covers meal blood sugar excursions.	Requires three or four injections and blood glucose check premeal and on retiring. Establishing and following individualized algorithm are necessary.

*Short-acting insulin ⎯⎯⎯; intermediate and long-acting insulin - - - - - - - -
†Insulin delivery through the pump is similar to this regimen.

tages and disadvantages of each regimen are presented in Table 43-14. Ideally, regimens should be mutually selected by the client and the health care provider. The criteria for selection are based on the type of diabetes and the required, desired, and feasible levels of glycemic control.

Because a single injection of a modified insulin rarely provides adequate glycemic control for most insulin-dependent clients, supplementation with regular insulin is mixed with the modified insulin in the same syringe to avoid unnecessary injections. On the basis of current insulin formulations and use, the effect of NPH and regular insulin mixed in any proportion is the same as if the two were injected separately. The commercially available 70:30 mixtures of NPH and regular insulin appear to have the same activity as their component insulins given at separate injection sites.

Mixing human regular and Lente insulins results in blunting of the usual peak action of the regular insulin, presumably because the excess zinc in the Lente insulin binds regular insulin. Although this blunting effect occurs, the client may be instructed to mix Lente and regular insulins with the regular insulin dose adjusted to compensate for the effect.

As a protein, insulin requires special storage considerations. Heat and freezing alter the insulin molecule. Insulin in use may be left at room temperature for up to 4 weeks unless the room temperature is higher than 30° C (85° F) or below freezing. Extra insulin may be stored in the refrigerator. The same principles apply for a client with diabetes who is traveling. Insulin can be stored in a thermos or cooler to keep it cool (not frozen) if the client is traveling in hot climates.

Administration. Because insulin is inactivated by gastric juices, it must be administered by injection. Daily administration of insulin is most commonly done by means of subcutaneous (SC) injection, although intramuscular (IM) or IV administration of regular insulin can be done when immediate onset of action is desired. The half-life of regular insulin in the circulation is 4 minutes, necessitating a continuous IV infusion for administration rather than a bolus IV injection. The steps in SC insulin injection are outlined in Table 43-8. The technique should be taught to new insulin users and reviewed periodically with long-term users. It should never be assumed that because insulin is being used, the client knows and practices the correct insulin injection technique. Inaccurate preparation is often caused by poor eyesight. Air bubbles in the syringe may not be seen, or the scale on the syringe may be read improperly. Administration systems, such as the insulin "pen," are available for visually impaired persons.

The client receiving mixed insulins (e.g., regular and an intermediate-acting insulin) needs to learn the proper technique for combining both in the same syringe if commercially prepared premixed insulins cannot be used (Fig. 43-5). Insulins should not be mixed if they differ in purity or species origin.

Recommended sites for insulin injection are noted in Fig. 43-6. The speed with which peak serum concentrations are reached varies with the anatomical site for injection. The fastest absorption is from the abdomen, then the deltoid area, thigh, and buttock. Because of the variability

Table 43-8   Preparing for Insulin Injection

1. Wash hands thoroughly.
2. Roll intermediate insulin bottle between palms of hands to mix insulin. *Note:* Always inspect insulin bottle before using it for first time. Make sure that it is of proper type and concentration, expiration date has not passed, and top of bottle is in perfect condition.
3. Prepare insulin injection in same manner as for any injection.
4. Select proper injection site and inject following procedure for any SC injection.* In sites where SC tissue is adequate, inject commercial insulin needles at 90-degree angle. For sites with minimal SC tissue, pinch up skin and insert needle at 45-degree angle.
5. If blood appears in syringe after needle is inserted, select new site for injection. Aspiration of syringe is not necessary.
6. After injecting insulin, apply some pressure with alcohol swab or cotton ball at site when withdrawing needle.
7. Hold swab in place for few seconds but do not massage.
8. Destroy and dispose of single-use syringe safely. *Note:* When instructing clients to self-inject insulin, use the following guidelines (if appropriate): (1) syringe does not need to be aspirated after injection and (2) disposable syringes can be reused for several injections.

*See Fig. 43-6.

in absorption and the decreased frequency of lipoatrophy in clients treated with human or purified pork insulins, rotation of injection sites is no longer the recommended injection technique when these types of insulin are used. The client should rotate the injection sites within a particular area, such as the abdomen, for a period and then, if rotation to the thigh is desired, the client can adjust the regimen to the new peak and action times for the new site.

The client should also be cautioned about injecting into a site that is to be exercised. For example, the client should not inject insulin into the thigh and then go jogging. Exercise of the area containing the injection site together with the application of heat may increase the rate of absorption and speed the onset of insulin action.

Insulin administration also requires the appropriate syringe. Most commercial insulin is available as U100, indicating that each milliliter contains 100 U of insulin. U100 insulin must be used with a U100-marked syringe. For users taking smaller doses of insulin, insulin syringes with larger black lines are marked for 25, 30, or 50 U and are available for use with U100 insulin. Before the development of U100 insulin, insulin was available in concentrations of U40 and U80. Limited supplies of U40 are still available. If clients use this form of insulin, the syringe should be appropriately matched.

Innovations. Continuous SC insulin infusion is currently being accomplished through insulin pumps. The pump devices are able to deliver insulin continuously in titrated amounts through tubing attached to a small pump device on one end and to a needle on the other end, which

1. Wash hands.
2. Gently rotate intermediate insulin bottle.
3. Wipe off tops of insulin vials with alcohol sponge.
4. Draw back amount of air into the syringe that equals total dose.

5. Inject air equal to NPH dose into NPH vial. Remove syringe from vial.

6. Inject air equal to regular dose into regular vial.

7. Invert regular insulin bottle and withdraw regular insulin dose.

8. Without adding more air to NPH vial, carefully withdraw NPH dose.

Fig. 43-5   Mixing insulins. This step-order process avoids the problem of contaminating regular insulin with intermediate-acting insulin. As a general rule, the two insulins being mixed should be of the same brand. (From Price M: Insulin and oral hypoglycemic agents, Nurs Clin North Am 18:692, 1983.)

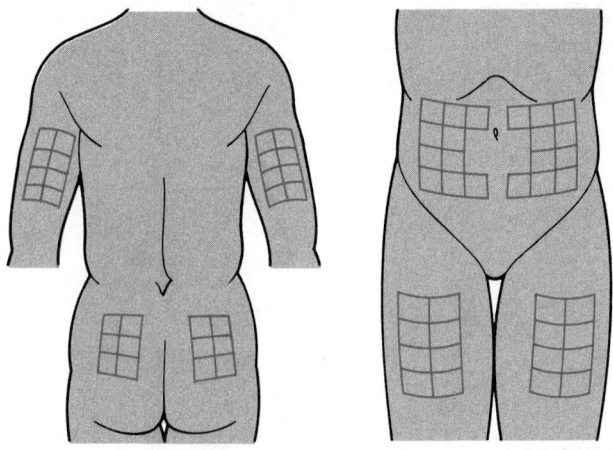

Fig. 43-6   Injection sites for insulin.

is placed subcutaneously in the skin. The wearer can inject a premeal bolus through the apparatus and achieve a nearly normal insulin delivery for 24 hours. Although they offer the advantage of tight glycemic control and only one needle change every 48 to 72 hours, these devices are expensive and require vigorous client participation in glucose monitoring and decision making about the regimen.

An alternative to the insulin pump is intensive therapy, which consists of several daily insulin injections together with frequent self-monitoring of blood glucose and dietary adherence. Studies have shown comparable control outcomes in clients receiving intensive therapy. Because the required client participation is similar, intensive therapy may be instituted before the initiation of pump use.[17] Because of the specialized nature of these insulin delivery devices, expert guidance from a physician and a nurse educator is essential.

Problems. Hypoglycemia, insulin allergies, lipodystrophy, and Somogyi effect are the problems associated with insulin therapy.

Allergic reactions. There are three types of allergic reactions to insulin. Local reactions may occur as itching, erythema, and burning around the injection site. Local reactions may be self-limiting within 1 to 3 months or may improve with a low dose of antihistamine.

A "true" insulin allergy is a systemic response with urticaria and possibly anaphylactic shock generally resulting from the use of animal insulins. Fortunately, this type of allergy is rare, particularly since human insulin has become available. A more common type of allergy is insulin resistance, in which antibodies are formed against the insulin and actually bind to the insulin molecules and render them inactive. The insulin molecule may be released at a later, unpredictable time to trigger unanticipated peaks in insulin action. An insulin allergy may be the suspected problem when insulin requirements approach 100 U/day.

This type of allergy is seen more often in clients who start insulin therapy, enter a brief remission in diabetes, and then resume insulin when the remission is over. For this reason the client may receive a low dose of insulin (<10 U) during the honeymoon period. Most of these reactions can be avoided through the use of insulin with greater purity.

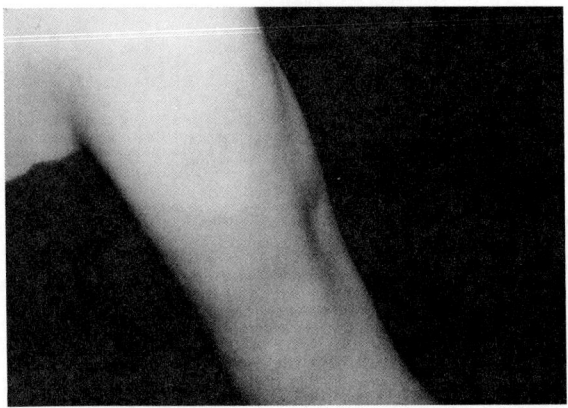

Fig. 43-7 Lipodystrophy of the arm.

Lipodystrophy. Lipodystrophies (hypertrophy or atrophy of SC tissue) may occur if the same injection sites are used frequently without a daily or weekly rotation (Fig. 43-7). The use of hypertrophied sites may result in erratic insulin absorption. Purified pork or human insulin may be used to treat the lipoatrophy by injecting at the edge of the lipoatrophic area. This stimulates fat cells to regenerate tissue. Lipoatrophies have been most commonly associated with beef or beef and pork insulin and rarely with human insulin. Hypertrophy, a thickening of the SC tissue, eventually regresses if the client does not use the site for at least 6 months.

Somogyi effect and dawn phenomenon. The Somogyi effect is characterized by wide differences in early morning (low) and postprandial (high) glucose levels (Fig. 43-8). The blood glucose level drops below normal in response to too much insulin (see p. 1303 for the causes of hypoglycemia). Counterregulatory hormones are released, stimulating lipolysis, gluconeogenesis, and glycogenolysis, which in turn produce rebound hyperglycemia and ketosis. The danger of this effect is that when blood glucose is measured, the client (or even the health care professional) may assess the situation as hyperglycemia and increase the insulin dose. The Somogyi effect is associated with the occurrence of undetected hypoglycemia during

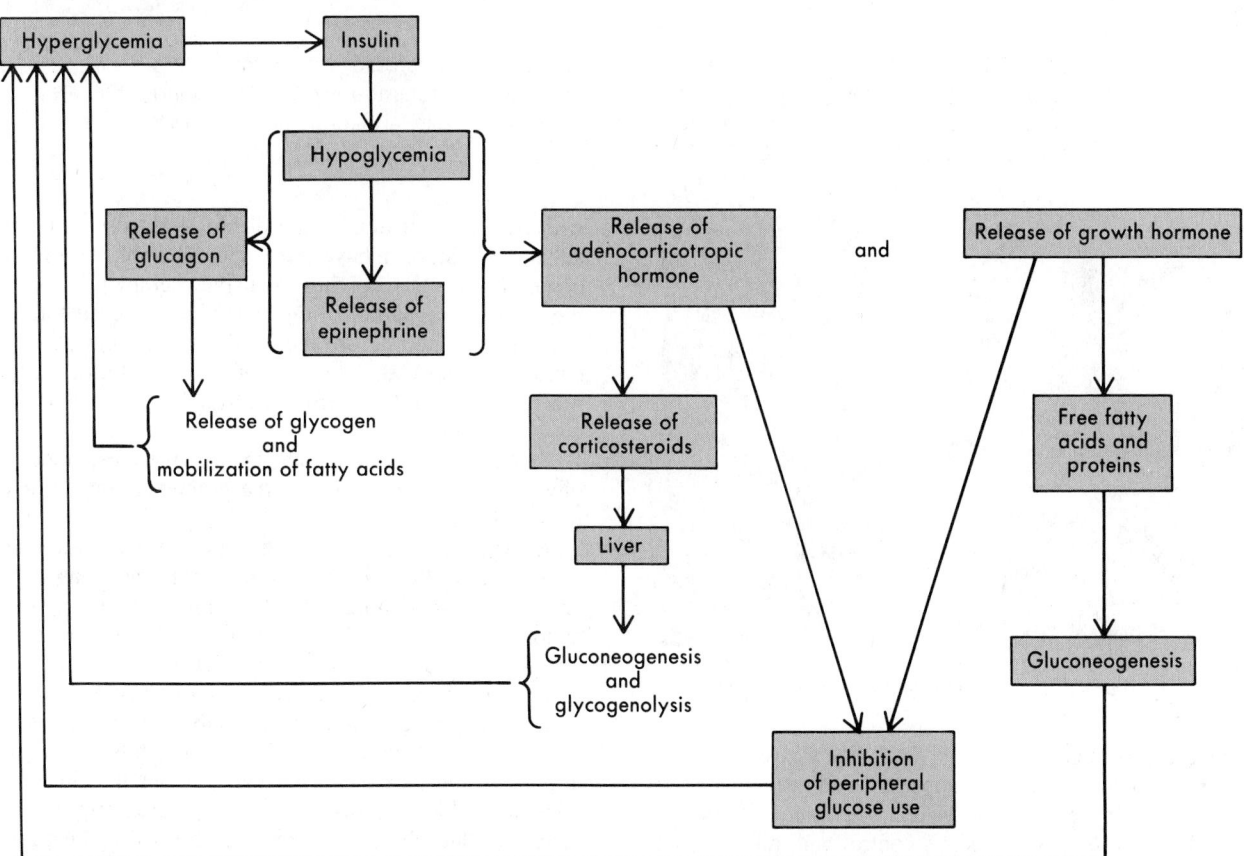

Fig. 43-8 The Somogyi effect. (From McCance KL and Huether SE: Pathophysiology: the biological basis for disease in adults and children, St Louis, 1990, Mosby–Year Book, Inc, p 623.)

sleep, although it can happen at any time. The client may report headaches on awakening and may recall night sweats or nightmares. When the Somogyi effect occurs at night, the client's blood glucose is elevated on awakening in the morning.

With dawn phenomenon, hyperglycemia is also found on awakening in the morning and ketonuria may be present. The cause is theorized to be a dawn release of endogenous growth hormone and/or cortisol. Both are counterregulatory hormones to insulin and raise the blood glucose level. The dawn phenomenon affects the majority of diabetics and tends to be most severe when growth hormone is at its peak in adolescence and young adulthood.

Careful assessment is required to document each phenomenon because the treatment for each differs.[18] The treatment for Somogyi effect is less insulin. The treatment for dawn phenomenon is an adjustment in the timing of insulin administration and/or an increase in insulin. The assessment must include insulin dose, injection sites, and variability in the time of meals or insulin administration. In addition, the client is asked to measure and document bedtime, 3 AM, and morning fasting blood glucose levels on several occasions.

■ Nursing Management Related to Insulin

Nursing responsibilities for clients receiving insulin include proper administration, assessment of the client's use of and response to insulin therapy, and education of the client regarding administration, adjustment to, and side effects of insulin. Table 43-9 lists guidelines for the nurse

assessing a client using glucose-lowering agents, including insulin and OHAs.

The client with newly diagnosed diabetes should be assessed for the ability to understand the purpose of insulin therapy; the interaction of insulin, diet, and activity; and the ways side effects may be manifested. The client or significant other also has to be able to prepare and inject the insulin. If the client or family lacks the psychomotor skills to prepare insulin, the nurse may have to find additional resources to assist the client.

Some clients find it difficult to inject themselves. This may be due to fear of the needle or anger and lack of acceptance of the disease. The nurse needs to determine the emotions and attitude of the client and family regarding insulin therapy.

Follow-up assessment of clients who have been using insulin therapy also includes an inspection of insulin sites for allergic reactions, a review of insulin preparation and injection technique, a history pertaining to the occurrence of hypoglycemic episodes, and the client's method for handling hypoglycemic episodes. A review of the client's record of urine and/or blood glucose tests is also important in assessing overall glycemic control.

Oral Hypoglycemic Agents

Sulfonylureas were found to have blood glucose–lowering effects during research on their antibiotic properties in the 1940s. The first generation of these drugs to be used in the treatment of diabetes mellitus included tolbutamide (Orinase), acetohexamide (Dymelor), tolazamide (Toli-

Table 43-9 Assessing the Client Treated with Glucose-Lowering Agents

For client with newly diagnosed diabetes or for reevaluation of GLA regimen

Cognitive	Is client or responsible other able to understand why insulin or OHAs are being used as a part of diabetes management? Is client or responsible other able to understand concepts of asepsis, combining insulins, insulin-OHA actions, and side effects? Is client able to remember to take >1 dose/day? Does client take medications at right times in relation to meals?
Psychomotor	Is client or responsible other able to prepare and administer accurate doses of GLA?
Affective	What emotions and attitudes are client and responsible others displaying in regard to diagnosis of diabetes and insulin or OHA treatment?

For follow-up of GLA-treated client

Effectiveness of therapy	Is client having symptoms of hyperglycemia? Does blood glucose and urine record show good or poor control? Is glycosylated hemoglobin consistent with glucose records?
Side effects of GLA therapy	Is atrophy or hypertrophy present at injection sites? Has client had hypoglycemic episodes? If so, how often? What time of day? Are there complaints of nightmares, night sweats, or early morning headaches? Has client had skin rash or GI upset since taking OHA?
Self-management behaviors	If client is having hypoglycemic episodes, how are those episodes managed? How much insulin or OHA is client taking and at what times of day? Is client adjusting insulin or OHA dose? Under what circumstances and by how much? Has exercise pattern changed? Is client adhering to number of prescribed calories? Are meals taken at times corresponding to peak insulin action?

GLA, Glucose-lowering agent.

Table 43-10 First-Generation and Second-Generation Oral Hypoglycemic Agents

Name	Dosage	Duration of Action	Metabolism and Excretion
FIRST-GENERATION SULFONYLUREAS			
Tolbutamide (Orinase)	500-3000 mg 2-3 times/day	6-12 hr (half-life of 4-5 hr)	Rapidly metabolized in liver, 100% excreted in urine
Acetohexamide (Dymelor)	250-1500 mg 2 times/day	12-24 hr (half-life of 1-2 hr)	Rapidly metabolized in liver, 60% excreted in urine
Tolazamide (Tolinase)	100-1000 mg 1-2 times/day	12-24 hr (half-life of 7 hr)	Metabolized in liver, 85% excreted in urine
Chlorpropamide (Diabinese)	100-500 mg/day	36-60 hr (half-life of 36 hr)	99% excreted by urine, virtually nonmetabolized by liver
SECOND-GENERATION SULFONYLUREAS			
Glipizide (Glucotrol)	2.5-40 mg/day	10-24 hr (half-life of 2-4 hr)	Metabolized in liver, excreted in urine (60%-90%) and bile (5%-20%)
Glyburide (Micronase, Diabeta)	1.25-20 mg/day	24 hr (half-life of 10 hr)	Metabolized in liver, excreted in urine (50%) and bile (50%)

Modified from Price M: Insulin and oral hypoglycemic agents, Nurs Clin North Am 18:702, 1983.
*Side effects can be minimized if OHA choice is matched appropriately to client needs. OHAs are not appropriate for ketosis-prone clients and pregnant clients and should be used cautiously if at all in clients with renal or hepatic dysfunction. There is <5% incidence of side effects.

nase), and chlorpropamide (Diabinese). A second generation of sulfonylureas, approved for use in the United States in 1984, includes glipizide (Glucotrol) and glyburide (Micronase, Diabeta).

Indication for use. OHAs are not oral insulin or a substitute for insulin. The client must have some functioning endogenous insulin for OHAs to be effective. They are thought to act by stimulating the β cells to release insulin and by increasing insulin sensitivity to receptors on insulin-sensitive tissue. They may also reduce hepatic glucose production.

The ideal client for OHAs is a type II nonobese person more than 40 years of age who has had diabetes for less than 5 years. In the client with newly diagnosed diabetes, therapy with OHAs may not be started until the client has been given an opportunity to try dietary control. Even if OHA therapy is initially successful, the client may eventually fail to maintain control and insulin therapy may have to be initiated.

A study in 1970 indicated that cardiovascular deaths were more frequent in clients treated with OHAs (e.g., tolbutamide) than in those treated with insulin or diet therapy alone.[19] Although the results of this study have been disputed, many physicians are still reluctant to prescribe oral agents and prefer to use methods of treatment such as diet, exercise, and/or insulin.

Types. As with insulin, the sulfonylureas differ in terms of dosage, absorption time, peak action, and duration. Second-generation sulfonylureas offer the advantages of lower doses, fewer side effects, and partial biliary excretion. The action, dosage, and side effects of first- and second-generation OHAs are listed in Table 43-10.

Disadvantages. OHAs, which are broken down by the kidney, should be used cautiously if at all in clients with renal disease. Sulfonylureas, which are metabolized by the liver, should also be avoided in cases of impaired liver function. Clients with allergies to sulfonamides should use OHAs cautiously if at all. The sulfonylureas can cause side effects such as nausea and vomiting, diarrhea, skin allergies, and hematological disorders, although these effects are less common in second-generation OHAs. A small percentage of clients taking alcohol while receiving an OHA may have an Antabuselike effect (i.e., nausea, vomiting, flushing, respiratory distress, and chest pain). Symptoms are usually proportional to the amount of alcohol ingested.

The hypoglycemic action of OHA can be enhanced and prolonged by means of the concurrent administration of drugs such as anticoagulants, salicylates, alcohol, and propranolol. Drugs that can oppose OHA action include thyroid preparations, corticosteroids, and thiazide diuretics.[20]

■ Nursing Management Related to Oral Hypoglycemic Agents

Nursing responsibilities for clients taking OHAs are similar to those for clients taking insulin. Proper administration, assessment of the client's use of and response to the OHA, and education of the client and the family about OHA are all part of the nurse's function. Table 43-8 lists guidelines for the nurse assessing a client starting therapy with OHAs and the follow-up assessment.

The assessment done by the nurse can be invaluable in determining the most appropriate oral agent for a client. The assessment includes the client's mental status, eating

Metabolites	Side Effects*
None	GI upset, skin rash, photosensitivity reactions, diasulframlike reactions with alcohol, hypoglycemia
One metabolite with two and one-half times hypoglycemic potency of parent compound	GI upset, skin rash, photosensitivity reactions, diasulframlike reactions with alcohol, hypoglycemia
Six metabolites, three with weak hypoglycemic properties	GI upset, skin rash, photosensitivity reactions, diasulframlike reactions with alcohol, hypoglycemia
None	GI upset, skin rash, photosensitivity reactions, diasulframlike reactions with alcohol, hypoglycemia
Two inactive metabolites	Fewer side effects than first generation, decrease in drug interaction with other compounds, hypoglycemia
Two inactive metabolites	

habits, home environment, attitude toward diabetes, and use of oral agents. For example, if the client is older, lives alone, or has difficulty remembering to follow a medication and diet schedule, a shorter-acting OHA may be preferable. Some clients may assume that their diabetes is not a serious condition if they are taking only a pill for glycemic control. Clients need to understand the importance of diet and not skipping meals. Clients should not take extra pills if they have overeaten and should not take a dose any later than the evening meal. The client also needs to know that hypoglycemic reactions may be severe and prolonged and that physician supervision may be necessary, particularly for older clients.

Clients should also be instructed to contact a physician if periods of illness or extreme stress occur. During such a period, insulin therapy may be required to prevent or treat hyperglycemic symptoms and hyperglycemic hyperosmolar nonketosis (HHNK).

Other Drugs Affecting Blood Glucose Levels

The client with diabetes may be concurrently taking other medications. Both the client and the health care provider must be aware of drug interactions that can potentiate hypoglycemic and hyperglycemic effects. For example, β-adrenergic drugs block the hepatic glycogenolytic response that occurs in response to hypoglycemia. Thiazide diuretics can also potentiate hyperglycemia by inducing potassium loss. A list of medications that may influence glycemic control is presented in Table 43-11. Medications may have to be changed or dosages adjusted if the client is also taking glucose-lowering agents (GLAs).

Table 43-11 Medications with Effects on Blood Glucose

GLUCOSE-LOWERING EFFECT

Acetaminophen	Fenfluramine	Probenecid
Alcohol	Insulin	Salicylates in large
β Blockers	Monoamine oxidase	doses
Biguanides	inhibitors	Sulfonylureas
Dicumarol		

OCCASIONAL GLUCOSE-RAISING EFFECT

Acetazolamide	Calcitonin	Nicotine
Asparaginase	Ethacrynic acid	Nifedipine
Caffeine in large doses	Morphine	

COMMON GLUCOSE-RAISING EFFECT

Arginine hydrochloride	Furosemide	Lithium
Barbiturates	Glucagon	Marijuana
Corticosteroids	Glucose	Phenothiazines
Diazoxide	Glycerin/glycerol	Phenytoin
Epinephrine	Levodopa	Thiazide diuretics

EXERCISE

Regular, consistent exercise is considered an essential part of diabetic management. Exercise contributes to weight loss, reduction of triglycerides and cholesterol, increased muscle tone, and improved circulation. In type I diabetes, exercise may increase insulin sensitivity, thereby necessitating a lowering of the insulin dose. In type II diabetes, exercise contributes to weight loss and improves insulin binding on cell receptors. However, the client should be aware that exercise is perceived by the body as a stress and that counterregulatory hormones are increased to ensure that adequate glucose is readily available. As a result, hyperglycemia may occur in situations of poorly controlled diabetes or in insulin-dependent clients who exercise at a time of day when insufficient insulin is available. Additional information about exercise and diabetes that is important for both the client and the health care provider to know includes the following:

1. Exercise does not have to be vigorous to be effective. The blood glucose–reducing effects of exercise can be attained with mild exercise such as brisk walking. The exercises selected should be enjoyable to foster regularity.
2. Exercise is best done after meals, when the blood glucose level is rising.
3. Exercise plans should be individualized for each client and monitored by the health care provider.
4. Clients should be encouraged to monitor their own blood glucose before, during, and after exercise to determine the effect exercise has on their blood glucose level at particular times of the day.
5. The client should be alerted to the possibility of delayed exercise-induced hypoglycemia, which may occur several hours after the completion of exercise.
6. The client taking a GLA should not have to forgo the enjoyment of planned or spontaneous exercise. The client can be taught to compensate for extensive planned and spontaneous activity by monitoring blood glucose level to make adjustments in the insulin dose (if taken) and food intake.

Hypoglycemia is likely to occur if the insulin-dependent client exercises at a time when the GLA action is peaking or if exercise is strenuous and prolonged and carbohydrate is not replaced. This can also occur if a normally sedentary client with diabetes has an unusually active day. Exercise can be scheduled about 1½ hours after a meal or a 10 to 15 g carbohydrate snack can be eaten before exercising to avoid hypoglycemia. For every 45 minutes to 1 hour of strenuous exercise such as tennis, the client should repeat the 10 to 15 g carbohydrate snack. (See Table 43-12 for guidelines on calories burned per hour for different activities.)

Hyperglycemia may occur if exercise is scheduled at a time when insulin action is waning. When the insulin dose is insufficient to cover the amount of exercise, the increase in blood glucose created by the counterregulatory hormones may not be curtailed. Again, the client can guard against this situation by scheduling exercise when sufficient insulin is available. Some clients may have to inject a small bolus of regular insulin if the blood glucose level

Table 43-12 Activities Affecting Energy

Light Activity (100-200 cal/hr)	Moderate Activity (200-350 cal/hr)	Vigorous Activity (400-900 cal/hr)
Driving a car	Active housework	Aerobic exercise
Fishing	Bicycling	Bicycling
Light housework	Bowling	Hard labor
Secretarial work	Brisk walking	Ice skating
Teaching	Dancing	Outdoor sports
Walking casually	Gardening	Running
	Golf	Soccer
	Roller skating	Tennis
		Wood chopping

is elevated before exercising to prevent progressive hyperglycemia.[21]

MONITORING BLOOD GLUCOSE

Glucose levels must be determined daily to monitor the interactions and effect of diet, exercise, and medication on an individual diabetic regimen. Detection of extreme or episodic hyperglycemia is necessary to avoid DKA and HHNK. Traditionally, monitoring has been accomplished by checking for the presence and degree of glycosuria. This technique provides only gross, semiquantitative information. Many factors affect urine test results, such as age, medications, disease, and the individual renal threshold. Urine testing also cannot measure the presence or degree of hypoglycemia. Urine testing for ketonuria, however, is a valuable aid in determining the advent of DKA and is recommended for all clients with type I diabetes when they are having hyperglycemia or illness. Second voided specimens, which were previously recommended for clients using urine testing, have been shown to constitute an unnecessary step.

Self-Monitoring

Self-monitoring of blood glucose (SMBG) is the more reliable technique for measuring blood glucose. Commercially available glucose-testing products, including disposable lancets and lancet holders, are widely available. A small drop of capillary blood (usually from a finger stick) is dropped onto a reagent strip. After a specified time, the strip is read either visually or by a machine. The machines are either reflectance meters or sensors. Reflectance meters work by measuring the amount of light reflected onto a strip that has reacted with a color change in response to the reaction of glucose with the reagent strip. Sensors use the measurement of conductivity of electricity as it is affected by the glucose in the blood. The technology of SMBG is a rapidly changing field with newer and more convenient systems being introduced every year. A diabetes educator should be consulted to learn the latest in monitoring technology.

Many meters are computerized and are becoming increasingly sophisticated. Some models are capable of storing "memory" of previous blood glucose tests. These tests

can be retrieved to provide a more complete picture of blood glucose fluctuations over time and to guide adjustment to the regimen.

The technique for using a blood glucose–monitoring product accompanies each product. However, the following steps can be taught to all self-monitoring clients:

1. Hands are washed in warm water. Cleaning the site with alcohol is not necessary and may even interfere with test results.
2. If it is difficult to obtain an adequate drop of blood for testing, the client should warm the hands in warm water or let the arms hang dependently for a few minutes before the finger puncture is made.
3. The puncture is made on the side of the finger pad rather than near the center. Fewer nerve endings are along the side of the finger pad.
4. The puncture should be only deep enough to obtain a sufficiently large drop of blood. Unnecessarily deep punctures may cause pain and bruising.

The advantages of SMBG are that it ensures immediate information about blood glucose levels and produces accurate records with daily glucose fluctuations and trends. SMBG is the preferred glucose-monitoring method for clients with type I diabetes. Type II clients may also benefit from SMBG by seeing the correlation between dietary choices and blood glucose levels. As weight is lost and blood glucose levels are lowered, the obese type II client may also gain reinforcement from SMBG.[22]

The frequency of monitoring depends on the glycemic goals the client and physician set and the intensity of the treatment regimen. Clients receiving two or more injections per day may want to test before meals every day. If the glycemic control is relatively stable, the client may elect to test two or more times a day on certain days of the week. Testing is most often done before meals but can be done any time the client needs to know the way a factor, such as exercise or stress, is affecting the blood glucose level. The frequency of recording SMBG results to guide therapy decisions should be mutually determined by the health care provider and the client.

Ideally, clients should be motivated to learn not only SMBG technique but also how to interpret the results. Most clients find that SMBG brings about physiological and emotional benefits as well as a willingness to be an active partner in the treatment. Achieving the desired level of client participation also requires time and effort from the health care professional. The nurse involved in this aspect of management should anticipate a close working relationship with the client for a period of 3 to 6 months as the client learns refinements of the technique and appropriate decision making regarding changes in diet, medication, and exercise. A client who is visually impaired, color blind, or limited in manual dexterity needs careful evaluation of the glucose-monitoring method most appropriate for that client's needs. Reflectance meters are now commercially available for the visually impaired.

COMPLICATIONS

With the discovery and initial administration of insulin, it was believed that a cure for diabetes had been found.

However, 70 years of insulin therapy has proved that insulin is not the total answer in regard to the treatment of diabetes. Hyperglycemia-related problems do not cause death as often as they did before insulin was discovered. Other chronic complications of long-term therapy are responsible for more than 75% of all diabetic deaths.

The acute problems of diabetes are associated with severe, untreated hyperglycemia (e.g., DKA and HHNK) or the hypoglycemic side effects of treatment with GLAs.

Chronic problems are primarily those of end organ disease from microangiopathy, macroangiopathy, and neuropathy. Hyperglycemia also plays a role in these complications, but the extent of this role has not yet been determined. Hyperglycemia may damage cells and tissue in at least two ways:

1. Metabolic dysfunction in the breakdown of glucose may lead to accumulation of damaging by-products (e.g., sorbitol).
2. Glucose becomes abnormally bound to protein structures of the body and produces deleterious effects in nerves and blood vessels over time.

Animal experiments and many clinical observations suggest that normalization of blood glucose may protect against the development of complications. More conclusive evidence in human beings should come from controlled clinical trials currently under way, including the Diabetes Control and Complications Trial sponsored by the National Institutes of Health. This comparative trial of conventional and intensive insulin therapy is evaluating the effect of glycemic control on already established early retinopathy and on the genesis of changes in clients without retinopathy soon after diagnosis.[23]

Acute Metabolic Complications

The acute problems of DKA and HHNK coma arise from events associated with hyperglycemia and insufficient insulin. Another problem that may arise from too much insulin or an excessive dose of an OHA is hypoglycemia (also referred to as *insulin reaction* or *low blood glucose*), which occurs when the level of available blood glucose falls. It is important for the health care provider to be able to distinguish between hyperglycemia and hypoglycemia because hypoglycemia can constitute a serious threat and requires *immediate* attention. Table 43-13 compares the manifestations, causes, management, and prevention of hyperglycemia and hypoglycemia (see also p. 1303).

Diabetic ketoacidosis. DKA, also referred to as *diabetic acidosis* and *diabetic coma,* may develop quickly or during several days or weeks. It can be caused by too little insulin accompanied by increased caloric intake, physical or emotional stress, or undiagnosed diabetes. DKA is most likely to occur in type I diabetes but may be seen in type II in conditions of severe illness or stress when extra demand is placed on the pancreas to produce insulin.

When the insulin supply is insufficient, glucose cannot be properly used for cellular energy. In response to cellular starvation, the body releases and breaks down stored fats and protein to provide the needed energy. Free fatty acids from stored triglycerides are released and metabolized in the liver in such large quantities that ketones are

Table 43-13 Hyperglycemia and Hypoglycemia

Hyperglycemia	Hypoglycemia	Hyperglycemia	Hypoglycemia
MANIFESTATIONS*		**TREATMENT**	
Blood glucose >500 mg/dl	Blood glucose <50 mg/dl	Physician's attention	Immediate ingestion of 5-20 g of simple carbohydrates
Increase in urination	Cold, clammy skin	Continuance of diabetic medication as ordered	Ingestion of another 5-20 g of simple carbohydrates in 15 min if no relief obtained
Increase in appetite followed by lack of appetite	Numbness of fingers, toes, mouth	Frequent checking of blood and urine specimens and recording of results	Contacting of physician if no relief obtained
Weakness, fatigue	Rapid heartbeat	Hourly drinking of fluids	Discussion with physician about medication dosage
Blurred vision	Emotional changes		
Headache	Headache		
Glycosuria	Nervousness, tremors		
Nausea and vomiting	Faintness, dizziness	**PREVENTIVE MEASURES**	
Abdominal cramps	Unsteady gait, slurred speech	Taking of prescribed dose of medication at proper time	Taking of prescribed dose of medication at proper time
Progression to DKA or HHNK	Hunger	Accurate administration of insulin	Accurate administration of insulin
	Changes in vision	Maintenance of diet	Ingestion of all ordered diet foods at proper time
	Negative, double-voided urine specimen	Maintenance of good personal hygiene	Provision of compensation for exercise
	Seizures, coma	Adherence to sick-day rules when ill	Ability to recognize and know symptoms and treat them immediately
CAUSES		Checking of blood for glucose as ordered	Carrying of simple carbohydrates
Too much food	Alcohol intake without food	Contacting of physician regarding ketonuria	Education of friends, family, fellow employees about symptoms and treatment
Too little or no diabetic medication	Too little food—delayed, omitted, inadequate intake		Checking of blood for glucose as ordered
Inactivity	Too much diabetic medication		Wearing of diabetic identification
Emotional, physical stress	Too much exercise without compensation		
Poor absorption of insulin	Diabetic medication or food taken at wrong time		
	Loss of weight without change in medication		
	Use of β blockers blocking recognition of symptoms		

*There is usually a gradual onset of symptoms in hyperglycemia and a rapid onset in hypoglycemia.

formed (ketonemia). Excess ketones upset the pH balance, and acidosis develops. More water is lost as ketones are excreted (ketonuria) in an attempt to balance the pH (Fig. 43-9).

Gluconeogenesis from protein is the last resource used by the body as a compensatory response to provide a cellular energy source. The result is an increase in blood glucose and nitrogen. However, because of the prevailing insulin deficiency, this glucose resource cannot be used and the blood glucose level rises further, adding to the osmotic diuresis. Dehydration and loss of electrolytes, particularly potassium, ensue. The client's skin becomes dry and loose, and the eyeballs become soft and sunken. Hypotension with a weak, rapid pulse may develop.

Vomiting caused by the acidosis results in more fluid and electrolyte losses. The continual bicarbonate loss adds to the acidosis. Finally, Kussmaul's respirations (rapid, deep breathing associated with dyspnea) begin to remove carbonic acid through the exhalation of carbon dioxide. Acetone is noted on the breath as a sweet, fruity odor.

Renal failure may eventually occur from hypovolemic shock. This failure causes the retention of ketones and glucose, and the acidosis progresses. The client becomes comatose as a result of the neurological stressors of dehydration, electrolyte imbalance, and acidosis. If the condition is not treated, death is inevitable.

Therapeutic management. Before the advent of self-monitoring of blood glucose, clients with DKA required hospitalization for treatment. Today, hospitalization may not be required. In instances where fluid and electrolyte imbalance is not severe and self-monitoring of blood glucose can be done by the client or someone in the household, less severe forms of DKA may be managed on an outpatient basis. However, other factors, such as presence of fever, nausea and vomiting, or diarrhea; altered mental status; nature of the cause of the ketoacidosis; and availability of frequent communication with the physician (every few hours), must also be considered in this decision.

Regardless of the setting in which it occurs, DKA is a serious condition that proceeds rapidly and must be treated

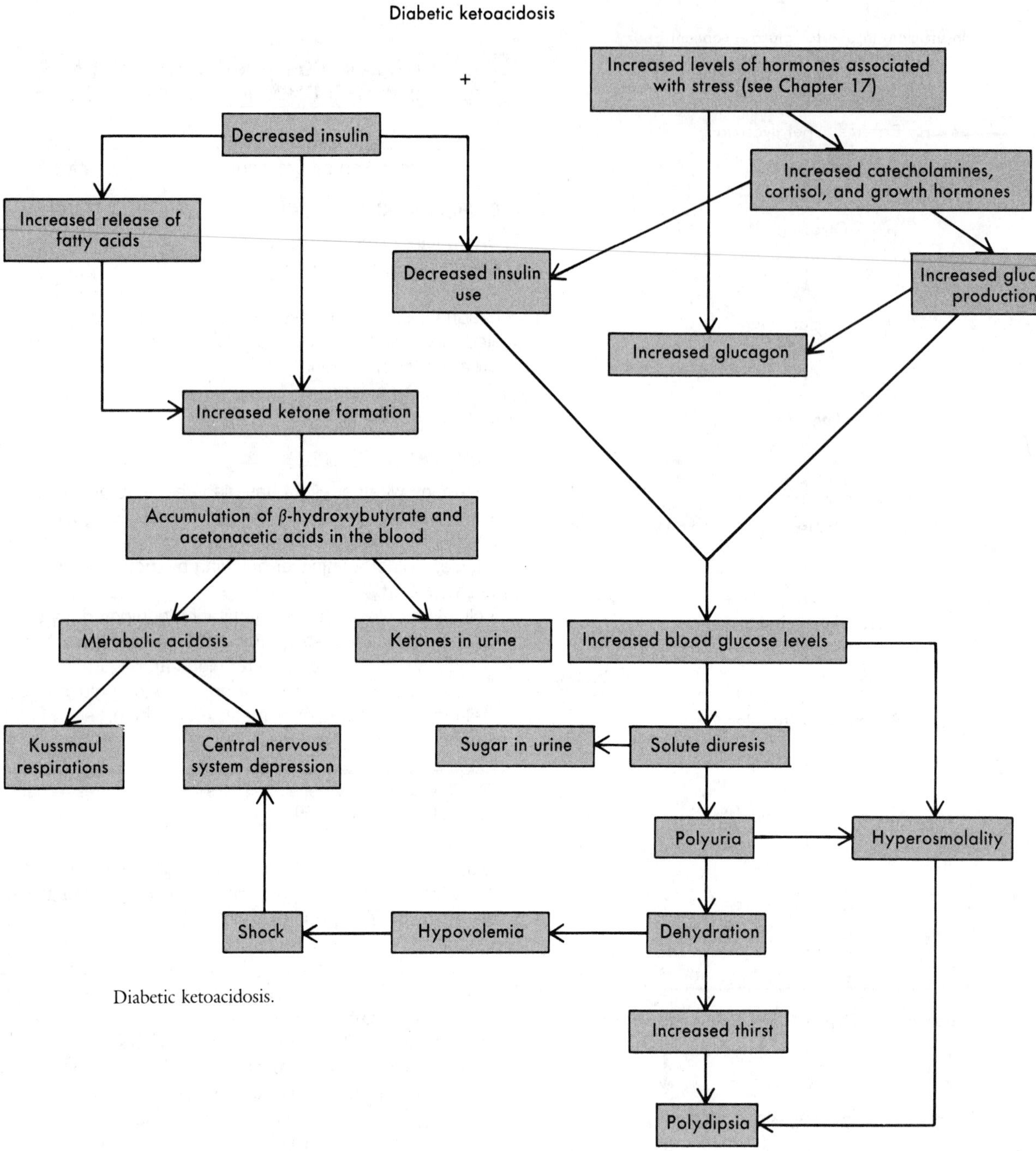

Diabetic ketoacidosis

Fig. 43-9 Diabetic ketoacidosis. (From McCance KL and Huether SE: Pathophysiology: the biological basis for disease in adults and children, St Louis, 1990, Mosby−Year Book, Inc, p 621.)

promptly. See Table 43-14 for the prehospital care of a client with DKA. Treatment is aimed at (1) immediate administration of insulin, (2) replacement of fluid to correct hypovolemia, and (3) replacement of electrolytes to correct imbalances.

The preferred treatment for DKA is the low-dose insulin IV infusion method. In this method a loading dose (0.15 U/kg) of insulin is administered, then 0.1 U/kg of insulin in normal saline solution are administered hourly by carefully titrated IV infusion. This insulin therapy is continued until a blood glucose level of 250 mg/dl is reached. The risk of hypoglycemia and hypokalemia may be reduced with this method.[24] When the blood glucose level reaches 250 mg/dl, a solution containing 5% to 10% glucose (e.g., 5% dextrose in saline solution) is given to prevent hypoglycemia along with IV or SC insulin as needed to maintain blood glucose control.

Fluid and electrolyte therapy is aimed at replacing ex-

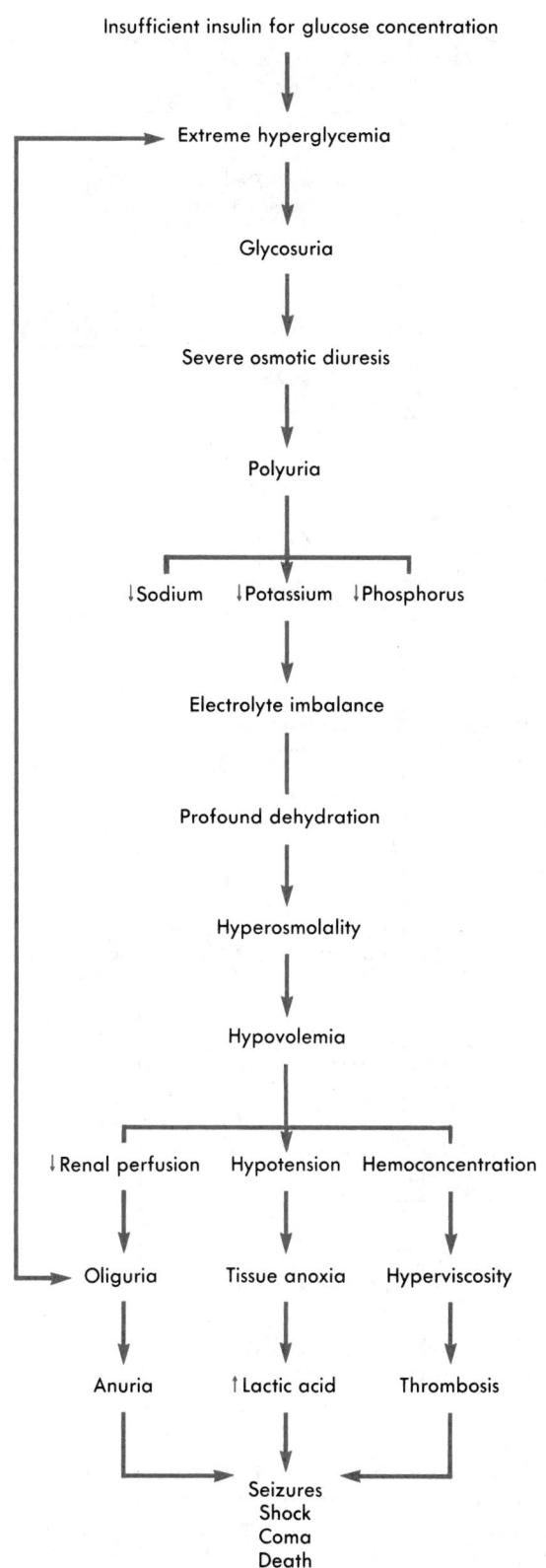

Fig. 43-10 Pathophysiology of HHNK. (From Thelan LA, Davie JK, and Urden LD: Textbook of critical care nursing: diagnosis and management, St Louis, 1990, Mosby–Year Book, Inc, p 751.)

Table 43-14

 Prehospital Emergency Care of the Client with Diabetic Ketoacidosis*

Etiology: Undiagnosed and/or untreated diabetic condition, insulin not taken as prescribed, presence of infection

CLINICAL MANIFESTATIONS

Dry mouth, thirst
Abdominal pain
Vomiting
Gradually increasing restlessness, confusion, stupor
Red, dry, warm skin; eyes that appear sunken
Breath odor of acetone
Rapid, weak pulse
Labored breathing

MANAGEMENT

Determine whether client has diabetes, time of last food intake, and time and amount of last insulin injection.
Give high-carbohydrate snack such as sugar or orange juice. Do not administer anything by mouth unless client is fully alert.
If client has blood glucose monitoring equipment available, check blood glucose level. If glucose level is <70 mg/dl and client is alert, administer high-carbohydrate treatment such as juice or sugar drink. If blood glucose is elevated >400 mg/dl or meter reads "high," seek emergency medical assistance.

*See Chapter 59 for a general discussion on measures related to prehospital emergency care.

tracellular and intracellular water and deficits of sodium, chloride, bicarbonate, potassium, phosphate, magnesium, and nitrogen. The principal goal of potassium therapy is to prevent hypokalemia. Regardless of the initial plasma potassium value, the total body potassium deficit is large. Early potassium replacement is essential because hypokalemia remains a significant cause of unnecessary and avoidable mortality during treatment of DKA.[25]

Assessment of blood pressure, pulse, and tissue turgor; cardiac monitoring; and determination of central venous pressure give some indications of the degree of hypovolemia. Bicarbonate is usually not given to correct acidosis unless the condition is severe (pH < 7.0). Indiscriminate use of bicarbonate may reverse acidosis too quickly and result in severe hypokalemia, which can produce potentially fatally cardiac dysrhythmias.

Hyperglycemic hyperosmolar nonketosis. HHNK occurs in the client with diabetes who is able to produce enough insulin to prevent DKA but not enough to prevent severe hyperglycemia, osmotic diuresis, and extracellular fluid depletion (Fig. 43-10). The increasing hyperglycemia causes intracellular dehydration because of a shift of fluid from the intracellular to the extracellular space. This causes neurological abnormalities such as somnolence, coma, seizures, hemiparesis, and aphasia. HHNK often occurs in the older adult client with type II diabetes. There

Table 43-15

Diagnostic and Therapeutic Management: Diabetic Ketoacidosis and Hyperglycemic Hyperosmolar Nonketosis

DIAGNOSTIC

Blood work, including immediate blood glucose, complete blood cell count, ketones, pH, electrolytes, blood urea nitrogen, blood gases
Urinalysis, including specific gravity, pH, sugar, acetone

THERAPEUTIC

Administration of regular insulin
Administration of IV fluids
Electrolyte replacement
Recording of intake and output
Central venous pressure monitoring (if indicated)
Assessment of blood glucose level
Assessment of blood and urine for ketones
Cardiac monitoring

---

is usually a history of inadequate fluid intake, increasing mental depression, and polyuria.

Therapeutic management. HHNK constitutes a medical emergency. This acute complication has a mortality rate of 5% to 40%.[26] The immediate therapy to reverse this hyperosmolar state consists of the rapid administration of IV solutions. From 6 to 20 L of fluid may have to be given during the first 24 to 48 hours. Depending on the degree of dehydration, either 0.9% or 0.45% sodium chloride is used. Regular insulin is given intravenously to aid in reducing the hyperglycemia. When blood glucose levels fall to 250 mg/dl, IV fluids containing glucose should be administered. Electrolytes are monitored and replaced as needed. Vital signs, intake and output, tissue turgor, and cardiac monitoring are assessed to monitor fluid and electrolyte loss.

The management for both DKA and HHNK is similar except that HHNK requires greater fluid replacement (Table 43-15). Once the client is stabilized, attempts to detect and correct the underlying precipitating cause should be initiated.

▪ Nursing Management of Diabetic Ketoacidosis and Hyperglycemic Hyperosmolar Nonketosis

The nurse's role in the acute management of the client with DKA or HHNK closely parallels the role in therapeutic management. As an inpatient, the client is closely monitored with appropriate blood and urine tests. The nurse is responsible for monitoring blood glucose and urine for output and ketones as well as using laboratory data to direct care.

Areas that need monitoring are (1) administration of IV fluids to correct dehydration, (2) administration of insulin therapy to reduce blood glucose and serum acetone, (3) administration of electrolytes to correct electrolyte imbalance, (4) assessment of renal status, (5) assessment of the

cardiopulmonary status related to hydration and electrolyte levels, and (6) monitoring of the level of consciousness.

The nurse must also monitor the signs of potassium imbalance resulting from hypoinsulinemia and osmotic diuresis (see Chapter 10). When treatment for hyperglycemia is begun with insulin, potassium loss may initially be increased. As insulin is replaced, potassium moves back into the cell. This movement of potassium into and out of extracellular fluid influences cardiac functioning. For this reason, cardiac monitoring is a useful aid in detecting hyperkalemia and hypokalemia because characteristic changes indicating potassium excess or deficit are observable on electrocardiographic readings.

Vital signs should be assessed often to determine the presence of fever, hypovolemic shock, tachycardia, and Kussmaul's breathing.

Hypoglycemia. Hypoglycemia, or low blood glucose, occurs when proportionately too much insulin is in the blood for the available glucose. This causes the blood glucose level to drop to less than 50 mg/dl. This type of hypoglycemia is different from the condition commonly termed *reactive* hypoglycemia (see p. 1316).

Hypoglycemic symptoms may also occur when a very high blood glucose level falls too rapidly (e.g., a blood glucose level of 300 mg/dl falling quickly to 180 mg/dl). Although the blood glucose level is above normal by definition and measurement, the sudden metabolic shift can evoke hypoglycemic symptoms. This type of situation can be induced by too vigorous treatment of hyperglycemia with insulin.

The balance between blood glucose and insulin can be disrupted by the administration of too much insulin, the ingestion of too little food, unusual amounts of exercise, and delayed eating. Insulin reactions can occur at any time, but most reactions occur when the GLA is at its peak of action or when the client's daily routine is disrupted without adequate adjustments in diet, medications, and/or activity. Although hypoglycemia is more common with insulin therapy, it can occur with OHAs and may be severe and persist for an extended time as a result of the longer half-lives of active metabolites of some OHAs.

A decrease in available blood glucose can result in a sympathetic nervous system response with the release of epinephrine. This results in manifestations of cold sweats, weakness, trembling, nervousness, irritability, pallor, and increased heart rate. The clinical manifestations of hypoglycemia vary with each client. The brain depends on a constant supply of glucose because it is unable to store glucose or glycogen. If that supply is inadequate, the client will experience confusion, fatigue, and abnormal behavior that can resemble alcoholic intoxication.

In recent years the physiology of glucose recovery has been shown to depend on glucagon and epinephrine. In type I diabetes, secretion and utilization of one or both of these substances may be impaired. As a result, some type I clients do not have the early warning symptoms produced by epinephrine. Rather, they have neuroglycopenia, that is, the more advanced symptoms of cerebral glucose deficit. The symptoms of this condition are irritability, irrational behavior, dizziness, tremors, and loss of conscious-

ness. This may result from the development of autonomic neuropathy or from treatment with β-adrenergic blocking agents.[17] These clients must be managed with intensive education and instruction in the prevention of hypoglycemia.

■ Therapeutic and Nursing Management of Hypoglycemia

The preferred treatment of hypoglycemia is prevention. However, if hypoglycemia occurs, the client should be able to reverse the situation before medical assistance is required. The client's ability to do this depends on the state of alertness and ability to swallow and the availability of a quick-acting carbohydrate source.

At the first sign of hypoglycemia the client should ingest 5 to 20 g of a simple (fast-acting) carbohydrate, such as 120 ml of orange juice, 120 ml of regular soft drink, two packets of sugar, or five or six hard candies. Overtreatment with large quantities of quick-acting carbohydrates such as a whole candy bar should be avoided.

If the symptoms are still present after 10 to 15 minutes, ingestion of 5 to 20 g of carbohydrate should be repeated.[27] Once the symptoms have improved, the client should eat a longer-lasting carbohydrate such as bread or milk to prevent symptoms from recurring. Commercial products such as gels or tablets containing specific amounts of quick-acting carbohydrate are convenient for carrying in a purse

---

Table 43-16

Diagnostic and Therapeutic Management: Hypoglycemia

DIAGNOSTIC

Stat blood glucose
History (if possible)

THERAPEUTIC

Determination of cause of hypoglycemia (after correction of condition)

Conscious client

Administration of 5-20 g of quick-acting CHO (e.g., 6-8 oz regular soda pop, 1 tbs syrup or honey, 4 tsp jelly, 6-8 oz orange juice, 2½ tsp sugar, commercial dextrose products [per label instructions])
Repetition of treatment in 15 min (if no improvement)
Administration of additional food of longer-acting CHO (e.g., slice of bread, 4 oz milk) (after subsiding of symptoms)
Immediate notification of physician or emergency service (if client outside hospital) (if symptoms not subsiding after two to three administrations of quick-acting CHO)

Worsening symptoms or unconscious client

SC or IM injection of 1 mg of glucagon
Administration of 50 ml 50% IV glucose

CHO, Carbohydrate.

---

or pocket to be used in such situations. High-fat foods and high-protein foods are not to be used initially to correct hypoglycemia. These food sources are metabolized too slowly to be effective as immediate treatment.

If there is little discernible improvement in the client's condition after two to three doses of 5 to 20 g of simple carbohydrate within 30 minutes or if the client is not alert enough to swallow, 1 mg of glucagon may be administered with the same technique used for an insulin injection. Glucagon stimulates a strong hepatic response to convert glycogen to glucose. Once the client is receiving medical care, a concentrated glucose solution may also be administered slowly intravenously until the client regains consciousness. Blood glucose level must be carefully monitored during the treatment. (See Table 43-16 for a summary of therapeutic and nursing management.)

With effective treatment, hypoglycemia can be quickly reversed. Once the acute hypoglycemia has been reversed, the nurse should explore with the client the reasons why the situation developed. This assessment may indicate the need for additional education of the client and the family to avoid future episodes of hypoglycemia. The danger of hypoglycemic reactions must be stressed because memory and learning impairment can result from repeated episodes of severe hypoglycemia.

DKA, HHNK, and hypoglycemia constitute potentially life-threatening situations and may be frightening to the client and the family. The nurse should attempt to keep the family members informed about the client's progress to relieve their anxiety. The nurse's calm, competent manner in caring for the client can provide assurance to the acutely ill client and the family.

Chronic Complications

Angiopathy. *Angiopathy,* or blood vessel disease, is estimated to account for the majority of deaths among clients with diabetes. Many factors are being investigated in the development of angiopathy. These chronic blood vessel dysfunctions are divided into two categories: macroangiopathy and microangiopathy.

Macroangiopathy. *Macroangiopathy,* or disease of large and medium-sized blood vessels, is essentially atherosclerosis and arteriosclerotic vascular disease characterized by a higher frequency and earlier onset than in the nondiabetic population.

The degree of vascular damage appears to be related to the duration of the diabetes, not to its severity. Although atherosclerotic plaque formation is believed to have a genetic origin, its development seems to be promoted by the altered lipid metabolism common to diabetes (Table 43-17). Tight glucose control may help delay the atherosclerotic process.

The complications resulting from macroangiopathy are cerebrovascular, cardiovascular, and peripheral vascular disease. Although genetic makeup cannot be altered, a client with diabetes can diminish the risk factors that aggravate macroangiopathy, such as obesity, smoking, hypertension, high fat intake, and low activity level.

Microangiopathy. *Microangiopathy,* or disease of the small blood vessels, is different from macroangiopathy in

Table 43-17 Mechanisms of Macrovascular Disease in Diabetes

CELLULAR MECHANISMS

Arterial endothelial cell injury (sorbitol accumulation, hypoxia, hypertension, immune complexes)
Foam cell activation (smooth muscle cell migration, monocyte/macrophage activation)

HEMOSTATIC MECHANISMS

Platelet dysfunction (aggregation, thromboxane production, growth factor release)
Clotting factor abnormalities (raised fibrinogen, factor VII, factor VIII, reduced fibrinolysis)
Cell-cell forces (RBC rigidity)

LIPOPROTEIN ABNORMALITIES

Hypertriglyceridemia (increased VLDL, remnant particles, reduced lipoprotein lipase activity, reduced HDL in type II diabetes mellitus)
Hypercholesterolemia (increased LDL in type II diabetes mellitus)
Apolipoprotein abnormalities (e.g., glycosylation)

OTHER MECHANISMS

Chronic renal disease secondary to diabetes (raised VLDL, LDL; lowered HDL; hypertension)
Increased arterial wall proteoglycans (charge trapping of lipoproteins, local cell activation)
Abnormalities of collagen, fibronectin (synthesis, glycosylization)
Insulin-induced lipogenesis, esterification
Intramural coronary vascular (meso and micro) disease

Modified from Diabetes mellitus, Indianapolis, 1988, Eli Lilly, Inc, p 299.
HDL, High-density lipoprotein; *LDL,* low–density lipoprotein; *VLDL,* very low–density lipoproteins.

Table 43-18 Pathophysiological Factors in Diabetic Angiopathy

Endothelial function	Decreased prostacyclin production, decreased plasminogen activity, decreased lipoprotein lipase activity, increased von Willebrand factor, endothelial leakage
Platelet function	Increased adhesiveness, increased thromboxane production, increased aggregation
Smooth muscle	Proliferation of tissue
Lipid and lipoprotein metabolism	Increased VLDL, increased LDL, increased cholesterol, decreased HDL
Coagulation	Increased clot size, increased clotting factors, increased fibrinogen and fibrin production, decreased plasminogen activity
Venous system	Venous dilatation
RBC function	Increased erythrocyte aggregation, decreased erythrocyte deformability
Oxygen transport	Increased glycosylated hemoglobin, decreased response to 2,3-DPG
Capillary basement membrane	Thickening of basement membrane
WBC function	Decreased adherence, decreased random migration, decreased chemotaxis, decreased phagocytosis, decreased effectiveness

Modified from Spies E: Vascular complications associated with diabetes mellitus, Nurs Clin North Am 18:722, 1983.
VLDL, Very–low density lipoprotein; *LDL,* low-density lipoprotein; *HDL,* high-density lipoprotein; *DPG,* diphosphoglycerate.

that it is specific to diabetes (Table 43-18). Microangiopathy is the result of thickening of the basement membranes in the capillaries and arterioles. Although microangiopathy can be found throughout the body, the areas most noticeably affected are the eyes (retinopathy), the kidneys (nephropathy), and the skin (dermopathy). Thickening of the basement membrane has been found in some persons with diabetes before or at the time of diagnosis or before the onset of symptoms of diabetes mellitus. However, clinical manifestations usually do not appear until 15 to 20 years after the onset of diabetes.[28]

Peripheral vascular disease. *Peripheral vascular disease* (PVD) is a combination of microangiopathy and macroangiopathy as well as clotting abnormalities. The legs and feet are most often affected in diabetes mellitus, and associated problems account for 20% of hospitalizations of clients with diabetes. The sequelae of PVD can lead to infection, gangrene, and amputation. Signs of PVD include intermittent claudication, pain at rest, cold feet, loss of hair, delayed capillary filling, and dependent rubor. The disease is diagnosed by means of history, Doppler findings, and angiography (see p. 731). Management centers

on control or reduction of risk factors, particularly smoking, high cholesterol intake, and hypertension. Antibiotics are necessary when infection is present. If the infection cannot be reversed with antibiotic therapy, amputation may be necessary. Proper care of the feet is crucial for the client with PVD; guidelines for foot care are listed in Table 43-19.

Diabetic retinopathy. The term *retinopathy* literally means disease of the retina; however, *diabetic retinopathy* refers to the microangiopathic process seen in clients with diabetes. After 10 years with diabetes mellitus, 50% of clients demonstrate diabetic retinopathy; after 15 years, approximately 80% of clients have some retinal disease.

Retinopathy is classified as (1) background retinopathy, (2) preproliferative retinopathy, and (3) proliferative retinopathy. The types are outlined in Table 43-20. In background retinopathy, the more common form, partial occlusion of the small blood vessels in the retina causes the development of microaneurysms in the capillary walls. These microaneurysms are so weak that capillary fluid leaks out, causing retinal edema and eventually hard exudates or intraretinal hemorrhages. Vision may be affected if the macula is involved.

Preproliferative retinopathy is distinct from background retinopathy and indicates further destruction of retinal capillaries.

Proliferative retinopathy, the more severe form, involves the retina and the vitreous. When retinal capillaries become occluded, new blood vessels are formed (neovascularization) to supply the retina with blood. These new vessels hemorrhage easily and may produce vitreous contraction. The vessels are torn and bleed into the vitreous cavity, preventing light from reaching the retina. The client sees black or red spots or lines. If these new blood vessels pull the retina while the vitreous contracts, causing a tear, partial or complete retinal detachment will occur. If the macula is involved, vision is lost.

The two most common forms of treatment of diabetic retinopathy are photocoagulation and vitrectomy. Photocoagulation by laser converts light energy into heat and coagulates the tissue in the area where the light is directed. It is particularly useful with neovascularization because the laser obliterates new vessels, stopping the hemorrhage. It can be done on an outpatient basis in a short time.

Vitrectomy is the aspiration of blood, membrane, and fibers from the inside of the eye through a small incision just behind the cornea. This form of surgery is particularly useful for the treatment of organized vitreous hemorrhage and traction retinal detachments.

Persons with diabetes are also prone to other visual problems. Glaucoma occurs as a result of the occlusion of the outflow channels as a result of neovascularization. This type of glaucoma is difficult to treat and often results in blindness. Cataracts occur with increasing frequency in the client with diabetes. Although the process is similar to that of senile cataracts, it occurs at an earlier age in the client with diabetes. Diabetic retinopathy may occur concurrently with nephropathy and parallel its progression.[8]

Table 43-19 Guidelines for Foot Care

1. Wash feet daily with a mild soap and *warm* water. Test water temperature with hands first.
2. Pat feet dry gently, especially between toes.
3. Examine feet daily for cuts, blisters, swelling, and red, tender areas. Do not depend on feeling sores. If eyesight is poor, have others inspect feet.
4. Use lanolin on feet to prevent skin from drying and cracking. Do not apply between toes.
5. Use mild foot powder on sweaty feet. Powder feet only, not shoes.
6. Do not use commercial remedies to remove calluses or corns.
7. Cleanse cuts with warm water and mild soap, covering with clean dressing. Do not use iodine, rubbing alcohol, or strong adhesives.
8. Report skin infections or nonhealing sores to health care provider immediately.
9. Cut toenails straight across, even at ends of toes. Do not cut down corners. Soak nails before cutting.
10. Separate overlapping toes with cotton.
11. Break in new shoes slowly. Avoid open-toe, open-heel, and high-heel shoes. Leather shoes are preferred to plastic ones. Wear slippers with soles. Do not go barefoot. Shake out shoes before use.
12. Wear clean, absorbent (cotton or wool) socks or stockings that have not been mended. Colored socks must be colorfast.
13. Do not wear clothing that leaves impressions, hindering circulation.
14. Do not use hot water bottles or heating pads to warm feet. Wear socks for warmth.
15. Guard against frostbite.
16. Exercise feet daily either by walking or by flexing and extending feet in suspended position. Avoid prolonged sitting, standing, and crossing of legs.

Table 43-20 Types of Diabetic Retinopathy

Type	Pathological Alteration
Background	Microvasculature of retina of eye is damaged. Capillaries become damaged, resulting in development of microaneurysms (seen as tiny red dots on retina).
Preproliferative	Possible progression from background retinopathy represents further destruction of retinal capillaries and development of capillary dropout.
Proliferative	Abnormal blood vessels grow on surface of retina. Vessels can grow into chamber of vitreous surface and can hemorrhage, filling vitreous chamber with blood.

Modified from Guthrie D: Diabetes education: a core curriculum for health professionals, Chicago, 1988, American Association of Diabetes Educators.

Nephropathy. *Diabetic nephropathy* is now the leading cause of clients' receiving end-stage renal disease (ESRD) therapy in the United States. Mild proteinuria develops in 70% of persons with diabetes mellitus and may progress to more serious involvement and ESRD. This occurs as a result of microvascular abnormalities associated with diabetes mellitus, but these processes are not clearly understood.

Microangiopathy in the kidneys causes diffuse and nodular glomerulosclerosis. Diffuse glomerulosclerosis affects the basement membranes of all glomerular capillaries, usually in both kidneys. The basement membranes become thickened and leaky. Sclerosis of glomerular vascular tufts leads to progressive renal failure. In nodular glomerulosclerosis (Kimmelstiel-Wilson lesions), nodules develop in the glomeruli. In advanced cases most glomeruli are involved. In more than 70% of clients, the course of diabetes nephropathy is complicated by the presence of hypertension. The monitoring and treatment of hypertension is the most important part of diabetes management and is believed to be a significant factor in controlling the progression of nephropathy.[24] (See Chapter 27 for a discussion of hypertension and Chapter 41 for a discussion of acute and chronic renal failure.)

ESRD requires treatment by either dialysis or kidney transplantation. Clients in the later stages of nephropathy may require an adjustment in insulin and OHAs because of a loss of the insulin-degradative function of the kidneys and an abnormal peripheral insulin response.[29]

Neuropathy. *Neuropathy* is probably one of the most common complications of diabetes in adults. However, its cause is unclear. Mononeuropathic conditions (i.e., single nerve branch involvement) are theorized to develop from microangiopathy, whereas the more diffuse neuropathic conditions are attributed to metabolic defects and the accumulation of by-products in the nerve tissue. The result is reduced nerve conduction and demyelinization. Neuropathy can precede, accompany, or follow the diagnosis of diabetes.

The two major categories of diabetic neuropathy are (1) neuropathic conditions of the peripheral nervous system, including symmetrical peripheral polyneuropathy, mononeuropathic disorders, and diabetic amyotrophy, and (2) autonomic neuropathic conditions, including cardiovascular abnormalities, GI abnormalities, urinary bladder abnormalities, and sexual dysfunction.

Symmetrical peripheral polyneuropathy affects all the extremities but most often affects the legs. Symmetrical peripheral polyneuropathy is usually bilateral and symmetrical and is thought to be due to both metabolic and vascular mechanisms. Clients have pain and paresthesias. The pain, described as burning, cramping, crushing, or tearing, is usually worse at night and may occur only at that time. It may be relieved by walking.

The paresthesias are associated with tingling, burning, and itching sensations. Complete or partial loss of sensitivity to touch and temperature is common. Foot injury and ulcerations can occur without the client ever having pain (Fig. 43-11). Clients report that they feel as if they were walking on pillows or that their feet were numb. At times the skin becomes so sensitive (hyperesthesia) that even light pressure from bed sheets cannot be tolerated. Neuropathy in the hands causes atrophy of the small muscles, limiting fine movement (Fig. 43-12).

Mononeuropathic conditions tend to occur unilaterally and are characterized by a sudden onset of pain with weakness or paralysis. Although the extremities are most often affected, cranial nerves III, IV, and VI may be involved.

No direct treatment for neuropathy is known. Treatment is aimed at relief of symptoms, particularly pain. Medications commonly used include tricyclic antidepressants and topical creams (e.g., capsaicin [Axsain, Zostrix]). Better glucose control may also aid in the reduction of symptoms. As nerve conduction improves, the pain may initially increase before relief is noted. A class of drugs referred to as *aldose-reductase inhibitors* is currently under investigation for treatment of complications of diabetes such as neuropathic disorders and retinopathy. These drugs reverse some of the biochemical and physiological changes believed to underlie these complications.[30] It is hoped that they will block the development of complications as well as relieve symptoms.[31]

Neuropathy affecting the autonomic nervous system may produce nocturnal diarrhea, postural hypotension, im-

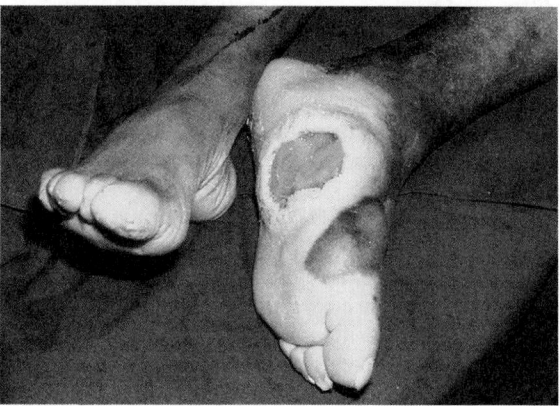

Fig. 43-11 Neuropathy: neurotrophic ulceration.

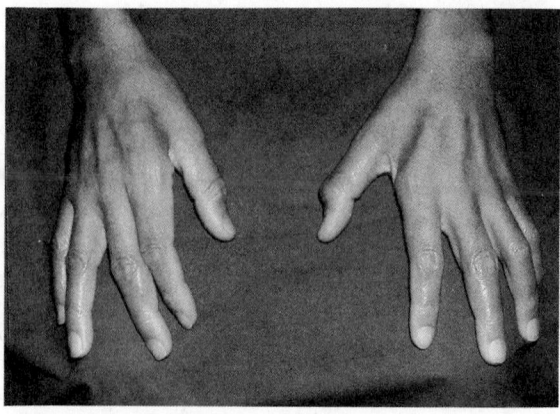

Fig. 43-12 Diabetic neuropathy: muscle atrophy.

potence, and neurogenic bladder. Nocturnal diarrhea is not associated with abdominal cramping. It affects few persons with diabetes and does not disturb diabetic control. Gastroparesis diabeticorum is delayed gastric emptying that can produce anorexia, nausea, vomiting, and persistent feelings of fullness. Gastroparesis can trigger hypoglycemia by delaying food absorption. Metoclopramide, a dopamine depleter, stimulates esophageal and gastric emptying and has been used in the treatment of gastroparesis.

The cardiovascular abnormalities associated with autonomic neuropathy are postural hypotension, resting tachycardia, and painless myocardial infarction. Clients with postural hypotension should be instructed to change from a lying or sitting position slowly. If postural hypotension is severe, medication may have to be prescribed.

Reports of the prevalence of impotence among men with diabetes vary from 30% to 60%. Impotence associated with diabetes mellitus is believed to result from damage to the sacral parasympathetic nerves. Determining whether impotence is of organic or psychological origin is an important part of the assessment. Organic impotence usually develops insidiously, whereas psychological impotence is often acute in onset. Measuring nocturnal penile tumescence (extent and duration of penile erection) during rapid eye movement phases of sleep is one assessment method to establish the presence of organic disease. Nonsurgical devices and surgical prosthetic implantations have been developed that make vaginal penetration possible. Decreased libido is a problem with some women with diabetes, as is monilial and nonspecific vaginitis. Organic impotence or sexual dysfunctioning in either the male or the female client requires sensitive therapeutic counseling for both the client and the client's partner.[32]

A neurogenic bladder develops as sensation in the inner wall decreases, causing urinary retention. Clients with retention have infrequent voiding, difficulty in voiding, and a weak stream of urine. Emptying the bladder every 3 hours in a sitting position helps prevent stasis and subsequent infection. Tightening the abdominal muscles during voiding and using Credé's maneuver (mild massage downward over the lower abdomen and bladder) may also help with complete bladder emptying. Cholinergic drugs such as bethanechol chloride (Urecholine) may be used. The client may also have to learn self-catheterization (see Chapters 40 and 55).

Neuropathic arthropathy, or Charcot's joints, results in ankle and foot changes that ultimately lead to joint dysfunction and foot-drop. These changes occur gradually and promote an abnormal distribution of weight over the foot. New pressure points emerge, and neuropathic ulcers often develop. The ulcers resemble a "BB shot" or "punched out" wound and are initially painless when peripheral polyneuropathy is present. Infection is a danger and may penetrate to underlying bone tissue, necessitating the long-term use of antibiotics and weeks of avoidance of weight bearing on the affected limb. The ideal treatment is prevention. Table 43-19 outlines rules for foot care that can reduce the client's risk for infection and possible amputation.

The treatment of neuropathic disorders involves good diabetic control and supportive care. There is no known cure. Clients under relatively good glycemic control appear to have a lower incidence of neuropathy than those with poorly controlled disease. However, neuropathy can occur despite good control.

Skin changes. *Skin disorders* such as diabetic dermopathy and necrobiosis lipoidica diabeticorum are attributed to microangiopathy. *Shin spots* are brown spots located on the anterior surfaces of the lower extremities. They are harmless and painless and initially measure less than 1 cm in diameter. *Necrobiosis lipoidica diabeticorum,* which is believed to be the result of trauma, consists of lesions similar to those of diabetic dermopathy but is more likely to be associated with ulcerations and necrosis. The lesions are reddish yellow and atrophic. Skin grafts are sometimes required because of the slow healing of the lesions. Necrobiosis lipoidica diabeticorum is present most often in insulin-dependent women and may precede the onset of overt diabetes.

Infection. Clients with diabetes are more susceptible to *infections* than other clients. The mechanisms for this phenomenon include a defect in the mobilization of inflammatory cells and an impairment of white blood cells (WBCs) in the process of phagocytosis. Recurring or persistent infections such as *Candida albicans* as well as boils and furuncles in the undiagnosed client often lead the health care provider to suspect diabetes. Loss of sensation (neuropathy) may delay the detection of an infection.

Persistent glycosuria may encourage bladder infections, especially in a neurogenic bladder. Decreased circulation as a result of angiopathy can prevent or delay the healing process. Protein waste during hyperglycemia and DKA is also responsible for poor healing. Antibiotic therapy has prevented infection from being a major cause of death in diabetics. The treatment of infections must be prompt and vigorous.

■ Nursing Management of Diabetes Mellitus

Nursing assessment

Initial subjective and objective data that should be obtained from a person with diabetes mellitus are presented in Table 43-21. After the initial assessment, periodic client assessments should be done on a schedule as outlined in Table 43-22.

Nursing diagnoses

Nursing diagnoses are determined when the problem and etiological factors are supported by clinical data. Nursing diagnoses related to diabetes mellitus may include, but are not limited to, those found in Table 43-23.

Nursing interventions

Health promotion and maintenance. Nurses may be involved in any or all aspects of management, but the focus of nursing care has two aims: (1) to care for the client during acute episodes and (2) to assist the client in learning to live with diabetes everyday. Both foci require the nurse to be thoroughly familiar with diabetes and its management and to educate the client with diabetes about all aspects of the disease.

Table 43-21

Nursing Assessment of the Client with Diabetes Mellitus

SUBJECTIVE DATA

History

Positive family history, mumps, rubella, coxsackievirus or other viral infections, chronic pancreatitis, Cushing's syndrome, acromegaly

Recent: Infection, surgery, trauma or stress, obesity, compliance with diet, activity level, pregnancy, size of babies

Medications

Use of and compliance with insulin or OHAs; use of glucocorticosteroids, diuretics, phenytoin (Dilantin)

General

Weakness, fatigue, thirst, hunger, malaise, irritability, weight loss (in type I), weight gain (in type II)

Pain

Abdominal pain, headache

Integumentary

Itching, skin infections, poor healing (especially involving the feet)

Gastrointestinal

Nausea and vomiting, constipation or diarrhea

Urinary

Frequent urination, nocturia, incontinence

Reproductive

Impotence, frequent vaginal infections

Neurological

Blurred vision, numbness or tingling in extremities

Musculoskeletal

Muscle weakness

OBJECTIVE DATA

General

Fruity breath, dehydration

Integumentary

Dry, inelastic skin; pigmented lesions (on legs); ulcers (especially on feet)

Cardiovascular

Cool extremities, loss of hair on toes

Neurological

Cataracts, vitreal hemorrhages, altered reflexes

Musculoskeletal

Muscle wasting

Possible findings

Serum electrolyte abnormalities; fasting blood glucose level >140 mg/dl; glucose tolerance test >200 mg/dl; leukocytosis; elevated blood urea nitrogen, creatinine, triglycerides, glycosylated hemoglobin; glycosuria; ketonuria; albuminuria

---

The nurse may request consultation with a diabetes educator who is certified by the American Association of Diabetes Educators. Certified diabetes educators have met stringent preparation and experience criteria and have demonstrated expertise in the field of diabetes education.

Table 43-22 Periodic Assessment for a Client with Diabetes

Item	Initial Visit	Every 3 Mo	Every 12 Mo
Assessment of glycemic control			
Symptoms of hypoglycemia	X	X	
Symptoms of hyperglycemia	X	X	
Record of blood tests	X	X	
Glycosylated hemoglobin	X	X	
Assessment for complications			
Postural blood pressure and pulse	X	X	
Weight	X	X	
Funduscopic	X	X	
Primary provider	X		
Ophthalmologist			X
Cardiac examination	X		X
Neurological examination			
Sensory: pinprick vibration sense	X		X
Motor: ankle reflexes, muscle bulk and tone	X		X
Pelvic exam as indicated for vaginal discharge		prn	
Extremities			
Feet: calluses, toenails, ulcers	X	X	
Peripheral pulses			
Dorsalis pedis	X		X
Posterior tibial	X		X
Popliteal	X		X
Femoral	X		X
Assessment for education			
Diet	X	X	
Medication management	X	X	
Monitoring skills	X	X	
Laboratory			
Blood glucose level	X	X	
Blood urea nitrogen/creatinine	X		X
Urinalysis for proteinuria	X		X
Electrocardiogram	X*		X
Fasting cholesterol level	X		
Fasting triglycerides level	X		

*If appropriate to age and history.

The certified diabetes educator is designated with the initials CDE after the name.*

The effect of the diagnosis of diabetes cannot be overestimated, and an assessment of the client's perception of what it means to have diabetes must be carefully assessed before client education is designed and implemented. The nurse should foster a positive attitude about the prescribed regimen and assist the client in developing an individual-

---

*For information regarding certified diabetes educators in your area or regarding the certification process, contact The American Association of Diabetes Educators, 500 N. Michigan Ave, Suite 1400, Chicago, Ill 60611.

Table 43-23*

NURSING CARE PLAN FOR THE CLIENT WITH DIABETES

Defining Characteristics	Nursing Interventions	Evaluation Criteria

Acute management

NURSING DIAGNOSIS: Potential complication: DKA and HHNK related to excess blood glucose

DKA: Increase in urination; vomiting; somnolence; dehydration; dry, loose skin; hypotension with weak, rapid pulse; coma; hyperglycemia >250 mg/dl, presence of urine ketones, pH <7.3; HHNK: hyperglycemia >500 mg/dl, serum osmolality >300 mOsm/kg, absence of ketonuria	Administer insulin per physician order. Monitor plasma glucose and ketone levels. Administer fluid and electrolyte replacement as ordered. Monitor input and output and vital signs for signs and symptoms of inadequate tissue perfusion. Assess for precipitating factors. Monitor cardiac activity.	Blood glucose within normal limits, restoration of circulatory volume and electrolyte balance, understanding of precipitating factors and prevention behaviors

NURSING DIAGNOSIS: Potential complication: hypoglycemia related to low blood glucose

History of too much insulin, too little food, unusual amounts of exercise, or delayed eating; cold sweats; weakness; trembling; nervousness; irritability; pallor; increase in heart rate; confusion; fatigue; abnormal behavior	Check blood glucose if time permits (e.g., when symptoms are mild). Provide quick-acting carbohydrate source; give orally if client is alert enough to swallow. Repeat oral dose in 10-15 min if no improvement. If no improvement or client is comatose, administer 1 mg glucagon subcutaneously or 30-50 ml of 50% IV dextrose per physician order. When client improves and is alert, provide long-acting carbohydrate or next scheduled meal. Assess for precipitating factors.	Blood glucose within normal limits, understanding of precipitating factors and steps to prevent or treat future episodes

Chronic management

NURSING DIAGNOSIS: Noncompliance related to complexity of treatment regimen, anger and grief about diagnosis, or insufficient financial resources

Verbalization of frustration over complexity of treatment regimen, avoidance of opportunities to participate in self-care, lack of attention at education classes	Complete diabetes assessment. Develop education plan on basis of assessment. Include family and/or significant other. Make referrals as necessary to social worker, counselor, or certified diabetes educator. Reassure client of ability to learn required information to care for self.	Positive statements about ability to manage self-care, participation as partner with health care provider

*This care plan is intended to be used for persons with newly diagnosed diabetes.

ized management plan. Learning goals should be mutually determined by the client and the nurse on the basis of individual needs as well as therapeutic requirements. The nurse needs to assess the client's feelings and facilitate acceptance of diabetes mellitus and its treatment over time.

Acute intervention. Nurses are involved with the care of clients with diabetes in many acute situations, such as DKA, hypoglycemia, and HHNK. Other areas of acute intervention relate to management during stress, such as during acute illness and surgery.

STRESS OF ACUTE ILLNESS AND SURGERY. Both emotional and physical stress can increase the blood glucose level and result in hyperglycemia. However, it is impossible to avoid stress totally in life situations such as deaths in the family, job interviews, and final examinations. These situations may require extra insulin to avoid hyperglycemia.

Common stress-evoking situations include acute illness and the controlled stress of surgery. The client with diabetes who has a minor illness such as a cold or the flu should continue drug therapy and food intake. A carbohydrate li-

Table 43-23*

NURSING CARE PLAN FOR THE CLIENT WITH DIABETES—cont'd

Defining Characteristics	Nursing Interventions	Evaluation Criteria

Chronic management—cont'd

NURSING DIAGNOSIS: Altered health maintenance related to lack of knowledge of adequate exercise program, diet and weight control, administration and potential side effects and complications of GLA, glucose monitoring, and care during acute minor illness

Defining Characteristics	Nursing Interventions	Evaluation Criteria
Frequent questioning regarding all aspects of diabetic management, inaccurate responses to direct questions about diabetic management	Complete diabetes assessment with special attention to exercise behaviors. Plan individualized exercise program with client. Review steps to prevent hyperglycemia and hypoglycemia.	Participation in exercise program to meet therapeutic goals (e.g., weight loss, improved insulin sensitivity, improved muscle tone, endurance)
	Complete diabetes assessment with specific attention to diet. Review diet and problem areas with client. Counsel on weight loss if appropriate. Refer to dietitian.	Dietary preparation and intake appropriate for GLA and client
	Complete diabetes assessment with special attention to GLA administration. Review administration; have client give return demonstration of insulin injection. Assess injection sites. Review symptoms and treatment of hypoglycemia.	Safe, effective administration of GLA with minimal or no side effects
	Complete diabetes assessment and review client glucose record. Demonstrate glucose testing. Have client give return demonstration. Review glucose records with client and explain how to identify trends. Remind client to call physician if blood glucose is >250 mg and ketonuria present.	Demonstration of proper blood glucose testing, recording of measurements, appropriate use of records to alter regimen
	Review effect of stress on glycemic control. Review sick-day care. Assist client in devising a sick-day plan, including foods to have on hand, and family member or friend who can be with client during illness episode. Review symptoms needing attention of physician, including blood glucose level >250 mg/dl, ketonuria, fever, nausea and vomiting.	Verbalization of steps for sick-day care; verbalization plan of action for self in event of illness; verbalization of symptoms lasting >24 hr that require immediate physician attention, including fever, nausea, and vomiting

Continued.

quid substitution such as regular soft drinks, gelatin dessert, or beverages such as Gatorade may be necessary. The client should understand that food intake is important during this time because the body requires extra energy to deal with the stress of the illness. Extra insulin may be necessary to meet this demand without DKA concurrently developing.

Blood glucose monitoring should be done every 1 to 2 hours by either the client or a person who can assume responsibility for care during the illness. Urine output and the presence and degree of ketonuria should be monitored, particularly when fever is present. Fluid intake should be increased to prevent dehydration, with a minimum of 4 oz/hr for an adult.

The client should be instructed to contact the health care provider when a blood glucose level more than 250 mg/dl, fever, ketonuria, and nausea and vomiting occur. The health care provider should supervise the necessary adjustments in the treatment regimen during times of stress. Eventually, the well-informed client will be able to

Table 43-23*

NURSING CARE PLAN FOR THE CLIENT WITH DIABETES—cont'd

Defining Characteristics	Nursing Interventions	Evaluation Criteria

Chronic management—cont'd

NURSING DIAGNOSIS: **High risk for infection related to depressed immune system, inadequate circulation, and environmental pathogens**

Redness, swelling, and/or pus at trauma or pressure site; fever	Complete diabetes assessment. Assess oral cavity, skin, pulses, particularly lower extremities and pedal pulses. Review skin and foot care. Have client give return demonstration of foot care. Review signs of infection, including redness, swelling, pus.	Verbalization of steps of prevention (skin care, foot care, regular dental care), verbalization and demonstration of care for minor cuts and burns, verbalization of signs of infection and need for intervention

NURSING DIAGNOSIS: **Self-esteem disturbance related to lifestyle changes imposed by diabetes and its treatment, stigma of having a chronic illness, and frustration at progression of disease despite careful management**

Negative feelings about self, resistance to incorporating treatment regimen into lifestyle, refusal to acknowledge diagnosis	Encourage client to discuss diagnosis and its implications. Suggest attending diabetes education classes. Suggest creative approaches to problems with clients. Assure client of continued value and self-worth.	Verbalization of positive attitude about self and ability to manage disease, planning for continued contact with health care provider for health monitoring

*This care plan is intended to be used for persons with newly diagnosed diabetes.

Name			Phone		
Address					
Physician			Phone		
Address					
INSULIN	DOSAGE	TIME	ORAL MEDICATION	DOSAGE	TIME
Regular			Orinase		
PZI			Diabinese		
Globin			Dymelor		
NPH			Tolinase		
Lente			DBI		
Semilente			DBI TD		
Ultralente					
			Date		

I am a DIABETIC

If unconscious or behaving abnormally, I may be having a reaction associated with diabetes or its treatment.

If I can swallow give me sugar, candy or a sweet drink. If I do not recover promptly, call a physician or send me to the hospital.

If I am unconscious or cannot swallow, do not attempt to give me anything by mouth, but call a physician or send me to the hospital immediately.

Fig. 43-13 Diabetic alerts: Clients with diabetes should carry a card and wear a bracelet or necklace that states they have diabetes. If the client with diabetes is unconscious, these measures will ensure prompt and appropriate attention.

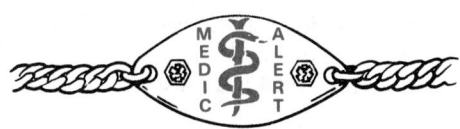

make most adjustments independently on the basis of past successful experiences.

Surgery is controlled stress, and adjustments in the diabetes regimen can be planned to ensure glycemic control. Clients are given IV fluids and insulin immediately before, during, and after surgery when there is no oral intake. Type II clients receiving OHAs usually have the OHAs discontinued 48 hours before surgery and are treated with insulin during the surgical period. The client should understand that this is a temporary measure and is not to be interpreted as a worsening of diabetes.

Nurses caring for an unconscious surgical client receiving insulin must be alert for hypoglycemic signs such as sweating, tachycardia, and tremors. Nurses should be aware that blood glucose monitoring must also be done frequently.

Chronic management

PERSONAL HYGIENE. The potential chronic complications of infections, neuropathy, and microangiopathy require the client with diabetes to participate in good hygiene practices related to skin and dental care. Because of susceptibility to periodontal disease and pyorrhea, daily brushing and flossing should be encouraged. When dental work must be done, the dentist should be informed that the client has diabetes.

Daily baths should be part of routine care, with particular emphasis given to foot care (see Table 43-19). If cuts, scrapes, or burns occur, they should be treated promptly. The area should be washed, and a nonabrasive or nonirritating antiseptic ointment must be applied. The area should be covered with a dry, sterile pad. If the injury does not begin to heal within 24 hours or if signs of infection develop, the health care provider should be notified immediately.

DIABETIC IDENTIFICATION AND TRAVEL. Clients should be instructed to carry identification at all times indicating that they have diabetes. An identification card (Fig. 43-13) can supply valuable information, such as the name of the health care provider and the type and dose of insulin or OHA. A Medic-Alert bracelet or necklace should be worn by all persons with diabetes. Police, paramedics, and many private citizens are aware of the need to look for this identification when working with sick or unconscious people.

Travel for clients with diabetes requires planning in advance. They should have all supplies in carry-on luggage and with them at all times. This includes insulin, syringes, quick-acting carbohydrate, and glucagon. Extra insulin should be available in case a bottle breaks or gets lost. If the client is planning a trip out of the country, it is wise to have a letter from the physician explaining that the client has diabetes and requires all the materials, particularly syringes, for ongoing health care.

Some travel involves time changes such as traveling coast to coast or across the international date line. The client should contact the health care provider to plan an appropriate insulin schedule. Many clients find it easier and more predictable to take only regular insulin every 4 to 6 hours to cover their insulin needs while on long airplane trips instead of trying to anticipate the peak of intermediate

insulin and the availability of meals. During travel, most clients find it helpful to keep their watches set to the time of the city of origin until they reach their destination. The key to travel when taking insulin is to know the type of insulin being taken, its onset of action, and the anticipated peak time. Meals or carry-along food can then be planned around this schedule.

Diabetes education

The major educational objective is a level of self-management appropriate to the individual client. Ideally, the client should be taught about the disease and encouraged to achieve self-management with guidance only from the health care provider. The more in control the client with diabetes can feel, the more likely the client is to accept and adhere to the management program. The basis of self-management is a sound educational program related to diabetes. A knowledgeable client should be able to make minor adjustments in insulin dosage and diet prescription to compensate for special circumstances, such as illness or increased exercise.

Not all clients with diabetes are capable of self-management. If the client is not able to manage the disease, a family member may be able to assume this role. If the client or the family cannot make decisions related to diabetes management, the nurse may identify appropriate resources outside the family. These resources can assist the client and the family in outlining a feasible treatment program that meets their capabilities. Client and health care provider resources are listed at the end of the chapter.

The American Diabetes Association offers pamphlets, booklets, and a bimonthly magazine called *Diabetes Forecast* for clients of all ages. Affiliates of the American Diabetes Association are located in all states. The American Diabetes Association also publishes materials and sponsors conferences for health care professionals concerned with diabetes research and management. It bestows recognition on education programs that meet the national standards of diabetes education and can provide a list of these programs. Drug companies manufacturing diabetes-related products also have free educational material for clients and health care providers.

Treatment programs take time to learn. The theory and textbook information are only the beginning. Clients must then incorporate the information into their own lifestyles. The health care provider who educates clients and their families understands that the education process initially takes weeks to months and provides periodic reassessment after the basics have been learned and integrated.

Another useful strategy is to divide the teaching content into the level that must be learned right away and the level that can be scheduled for another time. Levels of diabetes education include (1) survival, (2) home management, and (3) improvement of lifestyle. These levels are outlined in Table 43-24. The levels provide the diabetes educator with some structure for client education and relieve the expectation that the client will have to be taught everything in a short time.[33]

In 1984 the National Diabetes Advisory Board established a set of standards to be used for ensuring the quality of diabetes client education programs. The American Dia-

Table 43-24 Levels of Diabetes Education

LEVEL 1

Educational guidelines for initial management of diabetes

Provides content required at time of diagnosis and represents basic or survival needs. Level is based on limitations of client and family to accept and/or assimilate all there is to know about diabetes at time of diagnosis and limitations of some settings to provide additional education.

Aims

Educational activities provide client and family with initial knowledge and skills to enable person to get along (survive) at time of initial diagnosis of diabetes.

LEVEL 2

Educational guidelines for home management of diabetes

Places emphasis on increasing knowledge and flexibility as some experience is gained in living with diabetes. This is perceived as essential for every client but must be tailored to individual needs and capacity. This type of educational experience is preferably offered in a nonhospital environment as close to home as possible.

Aims

Educational activities provide client and family with diabetes skills and knowledge to participate in home management of duties. Goal is to enable client and family to become self-sufficient in daily management of diabetes. Client and family members play an integral role in diabetes care and should be regarded as equal members of the health care team.

LEVEL 3

Educational guidelines for improvement of lifestyle

Presents form of advanced learning viewed as enriching client's life with flexibility, insight, and self-determination. Most clients are forced to discover this information by trial and error through experience. Although no educational program can or should entirely replace personal experience, process need not be experienced by each person.

Aims

Educational offerings are aimed at increasing client's and family's understanding of diabetes and focus on individual needs. Improved lifestyle suggests intelligent participation by client in management of needs. Flexibility in management enables client to participate in activities and ultimately leads to greater self-determination.

Modified from American Diabetes Association and American Association of Diabetes Educators: Guidelines for diabetes care, New York, 1981, American Diabetes Association.

betes Association then developed a set of review criteria that specify the conditions under which each standard is to be met for a diabetes education program to be "recognized." It is believed that meeting the national standards and obtaining recognition will result in improvement in the overall quality of diabetes client education programs. In addition, recognition is seen as a prerequisite to obtaining third-party reimbursement for client education services nationally.[34]

Assessment of learning needs. After the initial diagnosis of diabetes has been made, the lifelong process of client education begins. The nurse's understanding of diabetes mellitus is central to a successful teaching program. An assessment of the client's knowledge of diabetes and lifestyle preferences is useful in planning the teaching program. Table 43-25 is an example of a diabetes client education record that can provide the nurse with a framework related to the client's learning needs. Based on the information obtained from the record, an educational plan can be developed to meet the client's individual needs. Table 43-26 is a summary of educational needs that can be used to track the progress of the client's educational program. The nurse should assess the client's knowledge base fre-

quently so that gaps in knowledge or incorrect or inaccurate ideas can be quickly corrected. The record can be reviewed with the client to outline and contract for additional educational information. The record can also provide an efficient way for other health care providers to be aware of what the client knows or needs to learn.

Clients are often treated in outpatient diabetes clinics. Frequently these clinics are staffed by diabetes nurse specialists. These specialists have preparation beyond the baccalaureate degree in diabetes and work collaboratively with physicians to manage clients with diabetes. The diabetes nurse specialist is also often available to the nursing staff for consultation in the acute-care setting. The diabetes outpatient clinic can provide specialized instruction, group interaction, and contact with other persons with diabetes. Often such clinics are run in accordance with the team concept. Consequently, an endocrinologist, a diabetes nurse specialist, dietitian, podiatrist, counselor, and social worker may be available to the client at one visit.

Follow-up nursing management

Although the educational emphasis is on self-care, clients should be encouraged to also see themselves as partners in care with the health care provider. In addition to

Table 43-25 Diabetes Client Education Record

___

1. Demographic information   Date:_____
Name:_____   Age:_____
Race:_____Sex (circle): M F   Participant status (circle): Inpatient Outpatient
Level of education:_____   Occupation:_____
Physician's name:_____   Marital status (circle): Single Married Widowed Divorced
2. General medical condition
Height:_____ Weight:_____ % Ideal weight:_____ Blood pressure:_____
Hb$_{A1c}$:_____ Total cholesterol level:_____ HDL:_____ Triglycerides level:_____
Allergies:_____
Other medications:_____
Other medical problems:_____
Present health status:_____
_____

3. Diabetes history
Type of diabetes:_____   Duration of diabetes:_____
Treatment plan (check): _____Insulin _____OHAs _____Diet alone
Monitoring system: Type_____ Test times_____ Product_____ Usual AM value_____
Attach monitoring log, if appropriate.
Name/type of insulin or OHA: Dose   Times taken
_____   _____   _____
_____   _____   _____
Describe any side effects to OHAs/insulin:_____
Complications (check):
_____Retinopathy_____ Neuropathy _____Renal_____ Foot_____ Macrovascular _____Other (specify)_____
Describe:_____
Incidences of DKA, hypoglycemia, hyperglycemia (date, etc.):_____
4. Dietary habits
If prescribed, daily caloric intake:_____ Food or foods to avoid:_____
Indicate times of Breakfast_____ Lunch_____ Dinner_____
Attach dietary recall data or nutrition workup, if appropriate.
5. Physical activity habits
Does client have regular exercise program (20 min, 3 days/wk)?_____ Yes _____No
     If yes, indicate:
        Type   Duration   Intensity (Circle)
     _____   _____   Light   Medium   Heavy
     _____   _____   Light   Medium   Heavy
     _____   _____   Light   Medium   Heavy
6. Diabetes education history
Prior diabetes education? Client ___Yes ___No   Significant Other___ Yes ___No
Prior education:_____
Special educational needs:_____
Will significant other participate in program? Yes___ No___   Relationship:_____
7. Source of referral (check one)
___Physician ___Self-referred ___Facility staff ___Community agency ___Other (specify):_____
8. Social history
Cigarettes/day:_____ Alcoholic drinks/wk:_____
No. in household:_____ Relationship:_____
Types of health/medical insurance:_____

___

Modified from Meeting the standards: a manual for completing the ADA application for recognition, Alexandria, Va, 1989, American Diabetes Association, Inc.

Table 43-26 Summary of Educational Needs Assessment/Progress Form

Content Area	Preprogram*		Taught†	Postprogram‡	
Client			Date/initial/method		
1. Understands general facts of diabetes	Y	N		Y	N
2. Is well adjusted psychologically in relation to diabetes	Y	N		Y	N
3. Adequately or appropriately involves family in diabetes care	Y	N		Y	N
4. Understands and practices effective nutritional management	Y	N		Y	N
5. Understands benefits of and engages in appropriate exercise	Y	N		Y	N
6. Monitors blood or urine glucose levels appropriately	Y	N		Y	N
7. Properly uses insulin or OHAs	Y	N		Y	N
8. Knows relationship among nutrition, exercise, and medication	Y	N		Y	N
9. Recognizes and responds appropriately to symptoms of hypoglycemia and hyperglycemia	Y	N		Y	N
10. Understands effects of illness on diabetes management and responds appropriately	Y	N		Y	N
11. Practices proper hygiene (skin care, foot care, dental care) to prevent complications of diabetes	Y	N		Y	N
12. Cooperates in therapeutic management and rehabilitation of diabetes complications	Y	N		Y	N
13. Understands benefits and responsibilities of self-management in diabetes	Y	N		Y	N
14. Effectively uses available health care systems	Y	N		Y	N
15. Makes appropriate use of community resources	Y	N		Y	N

Modified from Meeting the standards: a manual for completing the American Diabetes Association application for recognition, Alexandria, Va, 1989, American Diabetes Association, Inc.
N, No; *Y,* yes.
*Preprogram: Did client know content before education?
†Taught: Was content taught? Put date, initials (instructor's name must accompany initials at least once); method of instruction (L, lecture; D, demonstration; R, return demonstration; V, video; X, other); and format (1/1, one to one; CL, classroom; G, group; SI, self-instruction module).
‡Postprogram: Did client know content after education?

carrying out the daily management routines, maintaining a schedule of regular follow-up to assess the progress of the disease and additional education are necessary. Table 43-22 outlines a suggested follow-up schedule to aid in the long-term care of a client with diabetes.

REACTIVE HYPOGLYCEMIA

Many people claim to have reactive hypoglycemia. However, reactive hypoglycemia occurs infrequently in persons other than those with diabetes treated with insulin or sulfonylureas. It results from an uncompensated reduction in blood glucose level. The symptoms are similar to those of the hypoglycemia of diabetes: sudden onset of hunger, diaphoresis, tremulousness, weakness, nervousness (adrenergic) and headache, confusion, slurred speech, behavioral aberrations, focal neurological signs, and coma (neuroglycopenic). These symptoms mimic the effects of anxiety and stress and are often misinterpreted.[35]

Idiopathic hypoglycemia (i.e., hypoglycemia of no known cause) is particularly difficult to document. Various physiological disturbances have been suggested, but subtle abnormalities of insulin response to food (particularly excessive or delayed secretion) seem the most likely possibilities.[35] A definite diagnosis can be made only if the plasma glucose concentration is less than 50 mg/dl accompanied

by symptoms of hypoglycemia and relieved by eating. The usual treatment is a diet balanced in protein and carbohydrate with frequent small meals.

If a client claims to have reactive hypoglycemia, it should be determined whether this has been medically diagnosed or self-diagnosed. Because of the similarity to symptoms of anxiety reaction, careful assessment of the symptoms and the treatment is important.

C *ase Study*

DIABETIC KETOACIDOSIS

John, a 34-year-old man, was admitted to the emergency room after he was found comatose in his apartment by his landlord. Diabetes had been diagnosed within the last year, and he was taking a total of 48 U of insulin: 12 U of regular insulin plus 20 U of NPH before breakfast, 8 U of regular insulin before dinner, and 8 U of NPH at bedtime. His landlord, who is also a friend and is familiar with John's treatment regimen, stated that John had stomach flu for the past week and stopped taking insulin a few days ago when he was unable to eat. The landlord did a quick finger stick to check John's blood glucose and reported the results as >600 mg/dl.

On physical examination the client was found to have DKA. His breathing was deep and rapid, and his breath smelled of

acetone. His face was flushed and his skin was dry. His serum acetone was 3+ with Acetest tablets, and a stat blood glucose revealed a glucose level of 730 mg/dl. Blood pH was 7.26.

Discussion Questions

1. Briefly explain the pathophysiology of the development of DKA in this client.
2. What clinical manifestations of DKA did the client manifest?
3. What were the precipitating factors in this case?
4. What distinguished this case history from one of HHNK and hypoglycemia?
5. What educational needs must be met before the client's discharge?

Review Questions

The number of the question corresponds to the same-numbered objective at the beginning of the chapter.

1. Which of the following describes diabetes mellitus?
   a. curable
   b. systemic
   c. communicable
   d. idiopathic
2. Insulin-dependent diabetes is the result of
   a. β-cell destruction
   b. high consumption of sugar
   c. insulin resistance at the cell membrane
   d. too much insulin
3. A clinical manifestation indicative of DKA is
   a. cold sweats
   b. Kussmaul's breathing
   c. hyperreflexia
   d. edema
4. The only type of insulin suitable for IV administration is
   a. NPH
   b. regular
   c. Lente
   d. PZI
5. For the client with diagnosed diabetes, a diabetic diet must be followed
   a. until the blood glucose level returns to normal
   b. only for type I diabetes
   c. only during periods of additional stress
   d. as long as the client lives
6. The first topic the diabetic client should be taught is
   a. an exercise program
   b. diet control
   c. survival skills
   d. weight loss measures
7. The appropriate instruction for the client with diabetes related to skin care is
   a. use of heat to increase the blood supply
   b. avoidance of softening lotions and creams
   c. daily inspection of all skin surfaces
   d. use of iodine on cuts and abrasions

REFERENCES

1. National Diabetes Data Group: Diabetes in America, Washington, DC, 1984 US Government Printing Office, pp 11-13.
2. Sinnock P and Bauer DW: Reimbursement issues in diabetes, Diabetes Care 7:291-296, 1984.
3. Shuman CR: Diabetes mellitus: definition, classification, and diagnosis. In Galloway JA, Potvin JH, and Shuman CR, eds: Diabetes mellitus, Indianapolis, 1988, Eli Lilly, Inc, p 2.
4. Blackard WG: Insulin deficiency. In Davidson JK, ed: Clinical diabetes mellitus, New York, 1986, Thieme, p 54.
5. Davidson MB: Diabetes mellitus: diagnosis and treatment, New York, 1986, John Wiley & Sons, p 400.
6. Feldman JM: Pathophysiology of diabetes mellitus. In Galloway JA, Potvin JH, and Shuman CR, eds: Diabetes mellitus, Indianapolis, 1988, Eli Lilly, Inc, p 29.
7. National Diabetes Data Group classification and diagnosis of diabetes mellitus and other categories of glucose intolerance, Diabetes 28:1039, 1979.
8. Rotter JI and Remoen DL: The genetics of diabetes, Hosp Pract 15:79, 1987.
9. Elsenbarth GS: Type I diabetes mellitus: a chronic autoimmune disorder, N Engl J Med 314:1360-1368, 1986.
10. Olson OC: Diagnosis and management of diabetes mellitus, New York, 1988, Raven Press, p 135.
11. Lebovitz H, ed: Physician's guide to noninsulin-dependent (type II) diabetes: diagnosis and treatment, ed 2, Alexandria, Va, 1988, American Diabetes Association.
12. Pyke DA: Diabetes and heredity. In Galloway JA, Potvin JH, and Shuman CR, eds: Diabetes mellitus, Indianapolis, 1988, Eli Lilly, Inc, p 21.
13. Davidson MB: Diabetes mellitus: diagnosis and treatment, vol 1, New York, 1986, John Wiley & Sons, Inc.
14. Sperling M, ed: Physician's guide to insulin-dependent (type I) diabetes, ed 1, Alexandria, Va, 1988, American Diabetes Association.
15. Kohn H and Goddard K: A comparison of the American Diabetes Association's 1984 diabetic dietary recommendations with the food intake of individuals with type II diabetes mellitus, Diabetes Educator 11:25-29, 1985.
16. Nestel PJ and others: Effects of a high-starch diet with lower high fiber content on post-absorptive glucose utilization and glucose production in normal subjects, Diabetes Care 7:207, 1984.
17. Hughes B: Diabetes management: the time is right for tight glucose control, Nursing 5:63, 1987.
18. Stephenson JM and Schernthaner G: Dawn phenomenon and Somogyi effect in IDDM, Diabetes Care 12:245-251, 1989.
19. University Group Diabetes Program: A study of the effects of hypoglycemic agents on vascular complications in patients with adult onset diabetes: mortality results, Diabetes 19(suppl 2):747-830, 1970.
20. Berger M: Oral agents in the treatment of diabetes mellitus. In Davidson JK, ed: Clinical diabetes mellitus, New York, 1986, Thieme.
21. Brown SP and Thompson WR: The therapeutic role of exercise in diabetes mellitus, Diabetes Educator 14:202-206, 1988.
22. Consensus statement of the American Diabetes Association: Self-monitoring of blood glucose, Diabetes Care 13(suppl):41, 1990.
23. Ahern J and others: The diabetes control and complications trial (DCCT): the trial coordinator perspective, report by the DCCT research group, Diabetes Educator 15:236-241, 1989.
24. Neuman G and Cohen MP: Testing for microalbuminuria, Diabetes Prof Winter:1-7, 1989.
25. Sabo CE and Michael SR: Diabetic ketoacidosis: pathophysiology, nursing diagnosis, and nursing interventions, Focus Crit Care 16:21-28, 1989.
26. Kitabchi AE and Rumbak M: The management of diabetic emergencies, Hosp Pract 6:129-160, 1989.
27. Lumley WA: Recognizing and reversing insulin shock, Nursing 9:34-41, 1989.

28. Singer A: Peripheral vascular disease and the diabetic foot: clinical evaluation, Practical Diabetol 6:12, 1989.

29. Amerlin R: Early diabetic nephropathy: diagnosis and treatment, Practical Diabetol 8:21, 1989.

30. Benfield P: Aldose reductase inhibitors and late complications of diabetes, Drugs 2:43, 1986.

31. Broadstone VL and others: Diabetic peripheral neuropathy, part I: sensorimotor neuropathy, Diabetes Educator 13:30-35, 1987.

32. Zasler N: Managing erectile dysfunction with external devices, Practical Diabetol 8:1-9, 1989.

33. Guthrie DW, Hinnen D, and DeShetler E: Diabetes education: a core curriculum for health professionals, Chicago, 1988, American Association of Diabetes Educators, p 314.

34. Meeting the standards: a manual for completing the American Diabetes Association Application for Recognition of Diabetes Patient Education Programs, Alexandria, Va, 1989, American Diabetes Association.

35. Kitabcki AE and Goodman RC: Hypoglycemia pathophysiology and diagnosis, Hosp Pract 30:45, 1987.

DIABETES INFORMATION RESOURCES

American Diabetes Association
   National Service Center
   1660 Duke St.
   Alexandria, VA 22314
American Association of Diabetes Educators
   500 N. Michigan Ave.
   Suite 1400
   Chicago, IL 60611
Juvenile Diabetes Foundation
   23 E. 26th St.
   New York, NY 10010

CHAPTER

44

Nursing Role in Management

Endocrine Problems

Linda B. Haas

Learning Objectives

1. Describe the pathophysiology, clinical manifestations, and therapeutic and nursing management of clients with imbalances of hormones produced by the anterior pituitary.
2. Describe the pathophysiology, clinical manifestations, and therapeutic and nursing management of clients with imbalances of hormones produced by the posterior pituitary.
3. Describe the pathophysiology, clinical manifestations, and nursing management of clients with thyroid enlargement or dysfunction.
4. Describe the pathophysiology, clinical manifestations, and therapeutic and nursing management of clients with imbalances of hormones produced by the parathyroids.
5. Describe the pathophysiology, clinical manifestations, and therapeutic and nursing management of clients with imbalances of hormones produced by the adrenal cortices.
6. Describe the pathophysiology, clinical manifestations, and therapeutic and nursing management of clients with imbalances of hormones produced by the adrenal medullae.
7. Name the endocrine disorders characterized by excesses and deficits in fluid volume and define the appropriate nursing interventions.
8. Describe the systemic effects of short- and long-term use of corticosteroid therapy.
9. List the nursing assessments, interventions, rationale, and expected outcomes related to client education for chronic management of endocrine problems.

This chapter deals with problems related to hormones produced by the anterior and posterior pituitary, thyroid, parathyroid, and adrenal glands. (Diabetes mellitus is discussed in Chapter 43; problems related to the reproductive system in Chapters 48 and 49; and the concept of stress, in Chapters 1 and 5.)

HEALTH MAINTENANCE AND PROMOTION

The goal of health maintenance activities is to maintain or restore the highest level of health for the individual. For the client with an endocrine problem, the nursing process should be directed toward (1) careful assessment to detect the early and subtle changes that indicate dysfunction, particularly in caring for clients with conditions that may predispose them to endocrine dysfunction; (2) prevention of

hormone imbalance; (3) support when irreversible dysfunction or its manifestations occur or when lifestyle changes are indicated; and (4) reduction of future risks or complications. Nurses perform the meticulous assessment of the usual and potential stressors that interact with the endocrine system, note subtle changes in biopsychosocial parameters, and plan interventions focusing on the maintenance of homeostasis and client education. Significant others should be included in the plan of care whenever possible.

The nurse's role in the management of the client with endocrine dysfunction includes the following actions:

1. Assessment
   a. Physical, psychological, and social parameters related to endocrine function
   b. Usual coping patterns and support systems
   c. Emotional, physical, and environmental stressors (past, current, and potential)
   d. Familial patterns

Reviewed by Florencetta Gibson, R.N., M.Ed., M.S.N., Assistant Professor, School of Nursing, Northeast Louisiana University, Monroe, Louisiana.

Table 44-1 Information Related to Drug Therapy

Correct dosage and time schedule
Correct route and technique for administration
Side effects
Extraneous influences that may interfere with response to medication (e.g., stress)
Signs and symptoms that indicate need to increase, decrease, or discontinue prescribed medication
Signs and symptoms that indicate need to contact primary care provider
Knowledge that lifetime replacement is usually necessary
Plan for regular follow-up care
Necessity of wearing an identification or medical alert device at all times

2. Development of nursing diagnoses on the basis of nursing assessment
3. Establishment of expected outcomes related to each diagnosis within the realm of the client's psychobiological and social limitations
4. Interventions
   a. Preparation, support, and encouragement in the management of diagnostic and acute phases to promote effective coping
   b. Education for long-term health maintenance, including verbal and written instructions with demonstrations and return demonstrations, if applicable (Table 44-1)
   c. Information about when to seek help and the availability of community resources for optimal health maintenance
   d. Education, referral, and support in diet modification (if applicable)
   e. Education in the most appropriate methods of dealing with present and potential stressors (building on the client's past and current positive coping mechanisms)

Education and strategies for coping with a chronic disease and the alterations involved in a client's self-image and lifestyle are a major focus of the nursing care for a client with an endocrine dysfunction.

Often, the signs and symptoms of endocrine dysfunctions are vague (see Table 42-5) and attributable to a myriad of physical and psychological disorders, including hypochondriasis. They are often overlooked by clients, families, and clinicians until very prominent symptoms occur, sometimes with irreversible pathology. A nurse with a sound knowledge base related to endocrine problems and good assessment skills can often detect endocrine problems early. (See Chapter 42 for a discussion of the assessment of the endocrine system.)

Promotion of endocrine health maintenance requires that adequate nutrients be provided for hormone production. The importance of adequate nutrition is illustrated by the thyroid enlargement and marginal hypothyroidism that can develop in individuals with iodine deficiencies. However, iodine is only one of a number of elements required for normal hormone production. Protein and thyroid hormones incorporate amino acids in their molecules. To maintain adequate endocrine function, the diet must contain adequate protein, minerals, and vitamins.

Although steroid hormones are synthesized from cholesterol, the nutritional (exogenous) cholesterol requirements are uncertain. Cholesterol is produced endogenously in the liver, and high cholesterol levels have been associated with cardiovascular disease. Research has shown a strong positive correlation between serum cholesterol levels and atherosclerosis, which contributes to the leading cause of death in Western societies.[1] Clients on a typical American diet are apt to consume excess cholesterol (greater than 300 mg/day). Only cachectic individuals and those suffering from malabsorption and debilitating diseases such as cancer and anorexia nervosa should not monitor their dietary cholesterol intake to avoid excess.

Disruptions in rhythmic patterns produce asynchronism between body requirements and hormone production. The distress experienced by jet travelers and shift workers is characteristic of this asynchronism. Changes in the routine of living should be minimized. If sudden marked alterations are unavoidable, the individual should attempt to minimize other stressors as much as possible to lessen the total stress level.

Stress markedly alters the rate and patterns of hormone production and disrupts natural rhythms. Strategies should be developed to keep stress within manageable limits. Stress is also a potent stimulus to the endocrine system. Many acute endocrine conditions first appear after a major stressor, such as the death of a close family member, has been experienced. Unusual stress is also a factor in exacerbations of chronic conditions. (See Chapter 5 for a discussion of techniques for stress management.)

Most endocrine problems are chronic, with signs and symptoms that may subside with proper treatment, care, education, and self-management by the client or family. Consistent adherence to daily self-management regimens and follow-up care can frequently prevent acute episodes. Some individuals require only continuing treatment with medications and periodic evaluation. Others have exacerbations or concurrent illness and require hospitalization. Careful assessment, management, and education of the client and family can have a positive effect on the course and outcome of problems associated with the endocrine system.

In general, endocrine problems are caused by overproduction or underproduction of hormones, transport abnormalities, inability of target tissues to respond to hormones, or problems with feedback mechanisms. Endocrine disorders are often described as primary or secondary. In *primary disorders* the defect is in the gland producing the hormone. Examples are tumors that cause abnormal hormone secretion, autoimmune disease in which antibodies attack the gland, and inborn errors of metabolism. *Secondary disorders* are related to increased or decreased stimulation of the glands, usually by a tropic hormone. This is illustrated by hypothyroidism, which is due to lack of thyroid-stimulating hormone (TSH) stimulation, and Cushing's disease, which is due to excess ACTH caused by a pituitary adenoma.

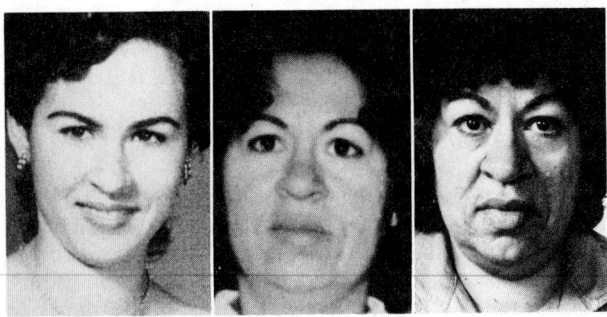

Fig. 44-1 Progressive development of acromegalic features. (Courtesy Linda Haas, Seattle.)

PITUITARY GLAND
Disorders of the Anterior Pituitary

Growth hormone excess. Growth hormone (GH), an anabolic hormone, promotes protein synthesis and mobilizes glucose and free fatty acids. Overproduction of GH, which is usually due to a benign pituitary adenoma, causes gigantism or acromegaly characterized by bone overgrowth. *Gigantism* results when the onset occurs before closure of the epiphyses and while the long bones are still capable of longitudinal growth. The onset usually occurs in early childhood but may occur at puberty. The excessive growth is usually proportional. These children may grow as tall as 8 feet and weigh over 300 lb. Although rare, these tumors constitute 20% of pituitary tumors diagnosed in childhood.[2] The children are not healthy and usually die in early adulthood.

Acromegaly, although also rare, is the more common abnormality that is caused by GH excess. Symptoms begin insidiously in the third and fourth decades of life, and both genders are affected equally. When the problem develops after epiphyseal closure, bones increase in thickness and width. Physical features include enlargement of the hands, feet, and paranasal and frontal sinuses; and deformities of the spine and mandible (Fig. 44-1). In addition, enlargement of soft tissue (e.g., tongue, skin, abdominal organs) causes manifestations such as speech difficulties, coarsening of facial features, and abdominal distention. Persons with acromegaly may exhibit diaphoresis, oily skin, peripheral neuropathy, and proximal muscle weakness.

The enlarged pituitary can exert pressure on surrounding structures, leading to visual disturbances and headaches. Because GH mobilizes stored fat for energy, it increases levels of free fatty acids in the blood and predisposes clients to atherosclerosis. The hormone also antagonizes the action of insulin and can cause hyperglycemia. Prolonged stimulation by GH is diabetogenic (see Chapter 43).

Diagnostic studies. In addition to the history and physical examination, diagnosis of growth hormone excess requires evaluation of plasma GH and somatomedin C levels. Skull x-ray films may show a large sella turcica and increased bone density. Computerized tomography (CT) scanning with contrast media and magnetic resonance imaging (MRI) are used for further evaluation and tumor localization.

Therapeutic management. The therapeutic goal in gigantism and acromegaly is to return GH levels to normal. This may be accomplished by means of surgery, irradiation, pharmacological intervention, or a combination of these three. Surgery, the usual treatment of choice, is most commonly accomplished with the transsphenoidal approach, in which an incision is made in the inner aspect of the upper lip and gingiva. The sella turcica is entered through the floor of the nose and sphenoid sinuses. The goal of transsphenoidal microsurgery is to remove only the GH-secreting adenoma. However, the pituitary is destroyed or removed in some instances. Removal of the entire pituitary results in permanent deficiencies of hormones of the anterior pituitary. Rather than replacing the tropic hormones, which requires parenteral administration, the essential hormones produced by target organs (glucocorticoids, thyroid hormone, and certain sex hormones) can be given orally. Testosterone needs to be self-administered intramuscularly (IM) every 2 weeks. Hormone replacement must be continued throughout life.

External irradiation normalizes GH levels in 30% to 60% of clients treated in this manner. If a tumor is large or has a great deal of supersellar extension, surgery may be followed by irradiation. Pharmacological treatment is accomplished with bromocriptine, a dopamine agonist that reduces GH levels to within the normal range. The GH-lowering effect of this drug is seldom complete or permanent.

The prognosis depends on age at onset, age when treatment is initiated, and tumor size. Usually, bone growth can be arrested and soft-tissue hypertrophy can be reversed. However, diabetic and cardiac complications may continue in spite of treatment.

■ Nursing Management of Excess Growth

Nurses should assess the signs and symptoms of abnormal tissue growth and physical size in all clients. Assessment of children includes evaluation of growth and development with the use of growth charts (see Chapter 42).

Markedly accelerated growth, especially if greater than 12 to 15 cm (5 to 6 inches) per year and if inconsistent with familial patterns, constitutes cause for medical referral. Adults should be questioned about increases in hat, ring, glove, and shoe size. Clients can be questioned about changes in appearance seen in serial photographs.

When first seen, clients usually have experienced undesirable changes in appearance and may have marked alterations in self-image. They also commonly exhibit symptoms of diabetes mellitus such as polydipsia, polyuria, and blurred vision. Cardiovascular disease may be present. Clients need unconditional acceptance by health care workers and considerable emotional support during the periods of diagnosis and treatment. They should be carefully monitored for hyperglycemia and cardiovascular symptoms such as angina pectoris, hypertension, and congestive heart failure.

Individuals treated surgically need skilled neurosurgical nursing and must be prepared before surgery for postoperative care. Nursing interventions include discussion of ambulation, pain control, activity, and hormone replacement. Clients should be instructed to avoid vigorous coughing,

sneezing, and straining at stool to prevent cerebrospinal fluid leakage from the point at which the sella turcica was entered.[3]

After surgery in which a transsphenoidal approach has been used, the head of the client's bed should be elevated at a 30-degree angle at all times. This avoids pressure on the sella turcica and decreases headaches, a frequent postoperative problem. Mild analgesia is given for headaches.

Any clear nasal drainage should be tested for glucose. The use of glucose oxidase reagent strips is adequate for this purpose. The presence of glucose indicates that the drainage consists of cerebrospinal fluid. Complaints of persistent and severe generalized or supraorbital headache may indicate cerebrospinal fluid leakage into the sinuses. A cerebrospinal fluid leak usually resolves within 72 hours when treated with head elevation and bed rest. If the leak persists, daily spinal taps may be done to reduce pressure and allow the fossa to heal. Intravenous (IV) antibiotics are usually administered when there is a cerebrospinal fluid leak to prevent meningitis. Clients must avoid bending for any reason for 2 months after a transsphenoidal hypophysectomy to avoid disrupting the surgical site. It is important that clients' families be aware of the need for clients to avoid straining and bending so that they can assist them whenever necessary. Constipation should be prevented by the use of stool softeners and laxatives.

If the pituitary is removed *(hypophysectomy)*, hormone replacement is necessary. Immediately after surgery, the client may exhibit signs of diabetes insipidus because of the loss of antidiuretic hormone, which is stored in the posterior lobe of the pituitary. Vasopressin (Pitressin) is given IM as needed on the basis of an output that exceeds 800 to 900 ml over 2 hours or if the specific gravity is below 1.004. If the entire pituitary gland was removed, the need to replace antidiuretic hormone is permanent.

Because the source of ACTH may have been removed, cortisone replacement may be necessary. Careful client education is necessary when cortisone must be taken regularly. Target gland hormone insufficiency results from lack of tropic hormone from the pituitary. Lifelong replacement therapy is necessary.

Hypopituitarism causes infertility because of deficient sex hormones. In addition, gamete (ova and sperm) production ceases because of lack of stimulation from the gonadotropins. However, if an individual with deficient gonadotropins wishes to have children, these hormones may be replaced with intermittent subcutaneous infusions.

Because surgery may involve the possible destruction of the pituitary with permanent hormone deficiencies and possible altered fertility, clients need assistance in working through the grieving process associated with these losses. It is important that clients be aware of the consequences if surgery is not done so that an informed decision can be made. The need for continued drug therapy reduces the client's perception of independence and requires considerable emotional adjustment. The nurse must consider the emotional impact of a hypophysectomy when counseling the client and planning the educational program related to hormone replacement.

Excesses of other tropic hormones. Excesses of other tropic hormones and overproduction of a single anterior pi-

tuitary hormone usually produce syndromes related to hormone excess from the target organ. If ACTH is involved, Cushing's disease (ACTH excess) results. If TSH levels are excessive, hyperthyroidism develops.

In some instances, excess secretion of a pituitary hormone may be appropriate, such as when there are alterations in the negative feedback system. (See Chapter 42 for a discussion of negative feedback.) In adults, hypersecretion of the pituitary gonadotropins, follicle-stimulating hormone, and luteinizing hormone (LH) occurs in primary gonadal failure. The resultant low levels of sex hormones cause oversecretion of gonadotropins by the pituitary and are not indicative of intracranial disease. Thus excess FSH and LH may indicate a pathological gonadal process such as orchitis or may be a normal consequence of aging. Sex hormone replacement therapy normalizes gonadotropin activity but does have side effects (see Chapters 48 and 49).

In some situations, symptoms of excess gonadotropins signify pituitary disease and are indications for prompt referral for definitive diagnosis. This is true of inappropriate lactation in either gender and precocious puberty in children.

Prolactin-secreting adenomas (prolactinomas) are the most frequently occurring pituitary tumor. Women may have galactorrhea, menstrual abnormalities, or infertility. In men, impotence and decreased libido and sperm density may result. Treatment is achieved with surgery, radiation, or pharmacological intervention.

Hypofunction. *Hypopituitarism* is a rare disorder and involves a decrease in one or more of the anterior pituitary hormones. Primary hypofunction may be due to infections, autoimmune disorders, tumors, or destruction of the gland. Failure to secrete GH is the most common abnormality, followed by deficiencies of the gonadotropins, TSH, corticotropin, and prolactin.[4] Thus infertility may be caused by primary gonadal failure or may be the first indication of pituitary hypofunction. In the latter case, the gonads lack tropic hormone stimulation. The most common cause of pituitary hypofunction is a tumor, but destruction of the pituitary can also result from trauma, irradiation, and surgical procedures. Cranial irradiation used in the treatment of leukemia may cause hypothalamic dysfunction, which often results in pituitary dysfunction.

In women, hypofunction can follow a postpartum hemorrhage. This is called *postpartum pituitary necrosis*, or *Sheehan's syndrome*. Sheehan's syndrome should be suspected when failure to lactate and amenorrhea occur in a client with a history of postpartum hemorrhage. Panhypopituitarism may develop over a span of 10 to 15 years. The hypoxia of the pituitary during hemorrhagic shock at parturition produces slow degeneration and necrosis of the gland.[5] The client does not lactate after childbirth and is subsequently infertile because of a lack of prolactin and gonadotropins. Later, hypothyroidism develops and is followed by glucocorticoid deficiency. Because of the lethargy and apathy that are characteristic of these two hormone deficiencies, affected women rarely seek treatment. They are at high risk for alienation from husbands and significant others, who may misinterpret their lack of energy and motivation as signs of laziness or mental illness. Inability to fulfill the requirements for employment and ca-

reer advancement opportunities can lead to downward social mobility. Many women with Sheehan's syndrome are diagnosed only after an acute addisonian crisis. Some are never diagnosed or treated because they succumb to this life-threatening condition.

Decreased pituitary hormone secretion is associated with anorexia nervosa (see Chapter 35). This condition usually affects young women with distorted body images. They decrease caloric intake and increase exercise levels to the point at which body weight and body fat percentage fall below a critical level for normal hypothalamic-pituitary gonadotropin function, leading to amenorrhea. Decreased circulating thyroid hormone with inadequate TSH response and cortisol and androgen abnormalities occur.

Clinical manifestations. Clinical findings vary with the degree and speed of onset of pituitary dysfunction and are related to hyposecretion of the target glands. The symptoms are often nonspecific and commonly include weakness, fatigue, headache, sexual dysfunction, fasting hypoglycemia, dry and sallow skin, diminished tolerance for stress, and poor resistance to infection. Premature, fine wrinkling around the eyes and mouth is common. Psychiatric symptoms include apathy, mental slowness, and delusions. Orthostatic hypotension may also occur. If a pituitary tumor exerts pressure on the optic chiasma, there may be asymmetrical visual field changes. If the tumor is large, blindness in one or both eyes may occur.

Hyposecretion of GH during childhood results in growth retardation. Growth may be normal for the first year or two but then slows progressively. Intelligence is usually normal. When pituitary hypofunction affects gonadotropins, sexual development is impaired and features remain childlike. Replacement therapy with GH is limited to prepubertal children to allow normal growth to occur.[6] There are no obvious manifestations of GH deficiency in adults.

In adult women, menstrual irregularities, diminished libido, and changes in secondary sex characteristics (e.g., decreased breast size) are the first signs of pituitary insufficiency and related gonadotropin deficiencies. If the cause is Sheehan's syndrome, lactation fails and subsequent infertility occurs. Men experience testicular atrophy, diminished spermatogenesis, loss of libido along with impotence, and decreased facial hair and muscular mass.

If hypopituitarism is not detected and treated, the client eventually develops deficiencies of thyroid hormone and the adrenal corticosteroids. The latter deficiency causes a tendency toward shock and may result in an episode of acute adrenal insufficiency (refractory and life-threatening shock stemming from sodium and water depletion).

Therapeutic management. Treatment of hypopituitarism consists of surgery, or irradiation for the removal of a tumor, permanent hormone replacement, and a nutritious diet. Replacement therapy is carried out with corticosteroids, thyroid hormone, and sex hormones. Gonadotropins can sometimes restore fertility.

■ Nursing Management of Anterior Pituitary Insufficiency

A primary role of the nurse in relation to anterior pituitary insufficiency is assessment and recognition of subtle

signs and symptoms. Clients with hypopituitarism may first exhibit symptoms in stressful situations such as trauma or surgery. In addition, hypopituitarism may be detected in clients with complaints of failure to grow, infertility, or amenorrhea. Failure to grow is indicative of pituitary dwarfism, and infertility and amenorrhea can be signs of Sheehan's syndrome.

Children affected by pituitary dwarfism exhibit slow but proportional growth. Except for their small size, they may appear completely normal. When the age of puberty is reached, however, sexual maturation may not occur. If it does proceed, the epiphyses close, ending all possibility of further growth despite hormone replacement. For this reason and because normal stature and psychosocial development are more likely to be achieved with early initiation of treatment, these children must be identified and treated early. (See a pediatric text for a complete discussions of pituitary dwarfism.)

The nurse should be alert for the possibility of Sheehan's syndrome and refer for diagnosis and treatment any woman with the following characteristics:

1. A history of hemorrhage or other hypoxic episode during the birth of her youngest child
2. Failure to lactate after this birth
3. Failure of pubic hair, shaved during delivery, to regrow
4. Scanty, irregular, or absent menses
5. A decrease in secondary sex characteristics (or complaints of being "less womanly" than formerly)
6. Signs and symptoms of hypothyroidism
7. Signs and symptoms of glucocorticoid insufficiency without the bronzing of the skin associated with that condition

Although Sheehan's syndrome has been considered a relatively rare condition, there is evidence that it has been seriously underdiagnosed. The disease is devastating to affected women, but it is reversible, in large part, with hormone replacement.

If the disease is not detected and treated early, the woman is likely to need considerable help in rebuilding her life. Marital, vocational, or psychological counseling may be needed, and appropriate referrals should be made. The nature of the physiological problem should be explained to significant others, and their help should be enlisted in the rehabilitative process.

Disorders of the Posterior Pituitary

The hormones secreted by the posterior pituitary are antidiuretic hormone (ADH) (also called *vasopressin*) and oxytocin. ADH contributes to fluid balance by controlling renal reabsorption of free water (Fig. 44-2). It also has potent vasoconstrictive properties. Oxytocin controls lactation and uterine contractions. Oxytocin excess is not recognized as a clinical problem. This hormone is administered pharmacologically in the management of labor.

Syndrome of inappropriate antidiuretic hormone. The syndrome of inappropriate antidiuretic hormone (SIADH) occurs when ADH is released in amounts far in excess of those indicated by the plasma osmotic pressure (Fig. 44-3). SIADH is characterized by fluid retention, dilutional hyponatremia, hypochloremia, concentrated urine (greater

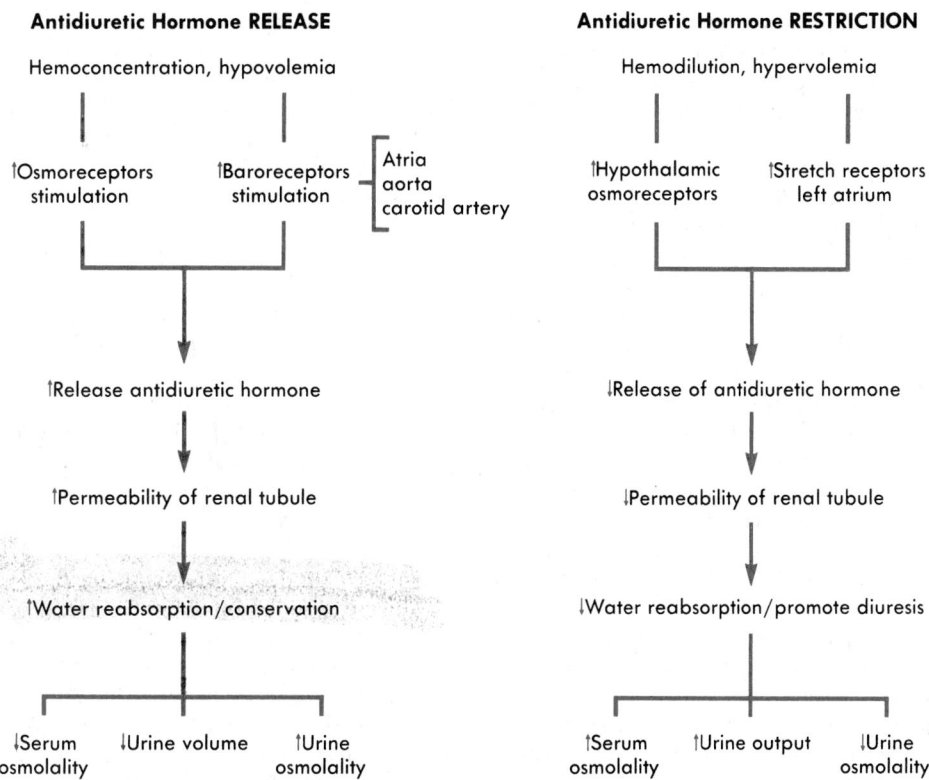

Fig. 44-2 Physiology of the release and restriction of antidiuretic hormone. (From Thelan LA, Davie JK, and Urden LD: Textbook of critical care nursing: diagnosis and management, St Louis, 1990, Mosby–Year Book, Inc, p 734.)

than 50 to 100 mOsm/kg), lack of intravascular volume depletion, and normal renal function.

Causes and clinical manifestations. SIADH has various causes (Table 44-2). When no cause for SIADH is apparent, the diagnosis of idiopathic SIADH is made. This disorder is especially prevalent in older adult clients.[7] Ectopic production by carcinomas is not a primary pituitary disorder but has similar manifestations and nursing care. Bronchogenic carcinoma is the most common ADH-secreting tumor. Other pulmonary conditions, such as pneumonia, lung abscess, and positive-pressure breathing, have been associated with SIADH. The syndrome is also associated with such diverse conditions as trauma (all types but most frequently head trauma), meningitis, subarachnoid hemorrhage, peripheral neuropathy, delirium tremens, Addison's disease, psychoses, vomiting, stress, and many medications.[8]

The excess ADH increases renal tubular permeability and reabsorption of water into the circulation. Consequently, extracellular fluid volume expands, plasma osmolality declines, the glomerular filtration rate rises, and sodium levels decline.

The problems related to volume excess include low urinary output and weight gain without edema. As plasma osmolality and serum sodium levels decline, cerebral edema may occur, leading to lethargy, anorexia, confusion, headache, convulsions, and coma. Other effects of hyponatremia include muscle cramps and weakness.

Therapeutic management. The diagnosis of SIADH is made by means of simultaneous measurement of urine and serum osmolality. The serum osmolality is much lower than the urine osmolality, indicating the inappropriate excretion of a concentrated urine in the presence of very dilute serum. There are low levels of blood urea nitrogen (BUN), serum creatinine, and albumin and an ADH level that is inappropriate for the serum osmolality.

Treatment is aimed at restoring normal fluid balance and osmolality. Fluids are restricted to 800 to 1000 ml per day. If fluid restriction alone does not improve the symptoms, IV 4.5% saline solution may be administered. A diuretic such as furosemide may be used to promote diuresis if cardiac symptoms develop. Because of the increased potassium excretion this medication causes, potassium supplements may be needed. SIADH tends to be self-limiting when caused by head trauma or drugs but chronic in nature when associated with tumors or metabolic diseases. Treatment of the underlying cause is indicated to improve the clinical course. In chronic symptomatic SIADH, demeclocycline (Declomycin, 900 to 1200 mg/day), a tetracycline that causes nephrogenic diabetes insipidus, is useful. This drug blocks the action of ADH at the level of the distal and collecting tubules, regardless of where ADH is secreted.

■ Nursing Management of Syndrome of Inappropriate Antidiuretic Hormone

Careful nursing assessment of clients who have had surgery or those susceptible to the syndrome (Table 44-2) can help in the early detection of SIADH. Nurses should be alert for low urinary output with a high specific gravity, a

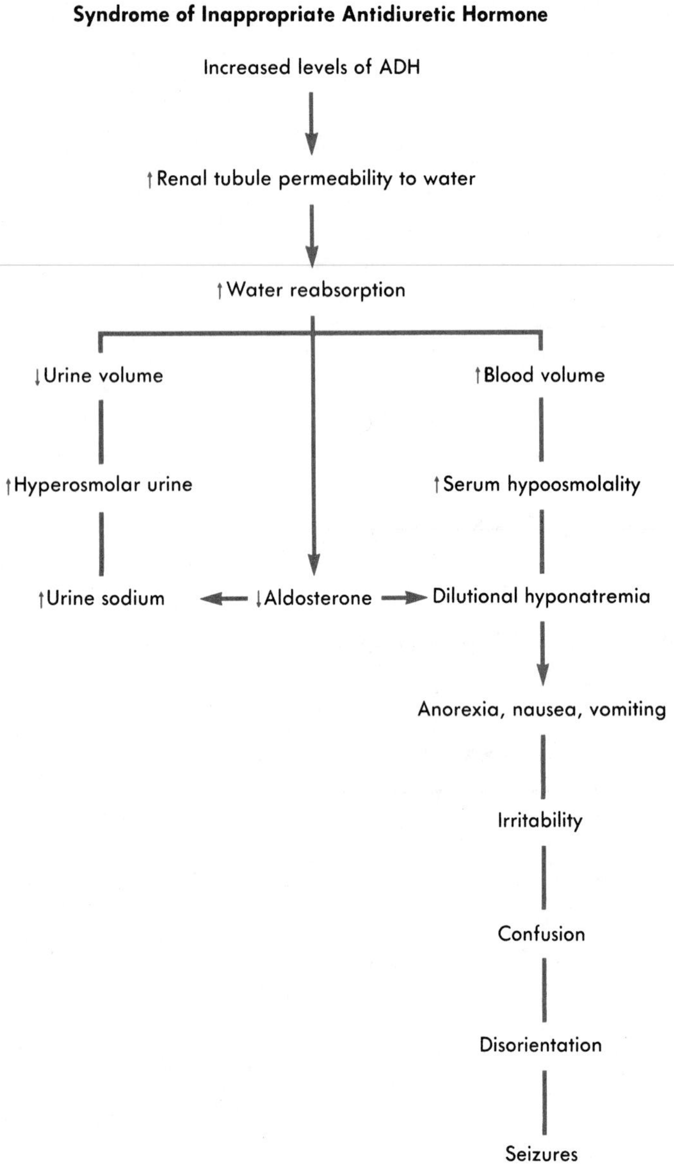

Syndrome of Inappropriate Antidiuretic Hormone

Increased levels of ADH

↓

↑Renal tubule permeability to water

↓

↑Water reabsorption

↓Urine volume   ↑Blood volume

↑Hyperosmolar urine   ↑Serum hypoosmolality

↑Urine sodium ← ↓Aldosterone → Dilutional hyponatremia

Anorexia, nausea, vomiting

Irritability

Confusion

Disorientation

Seizures

Fig. 44-3 Pathophysiology of SIADH. (From Thelan LA, Davie JK, and Urden LD: Textbook of critical care nursing: diagnosis and management, St Louis, 1990, Mosby–Year Book, Inc, p 763.)

sudden weight gain, or a serum sodium decline. If a client has SIADH, nursing measures include the assessments and interventions presented in Table 44-3.[9]

When SIADH is chronic, clients must learn to manage their treatment regimens. Fluids are restricted to 800 to 1000 ml/day. If the drinking of liquids is an aspect of socialization, the client should be assisted in planning fluid intake to save liquid allowances for social occasions. Clients may be treated with a diuretic to remove excess fluid volume. The diet should be supplemented with sodium and potassium, especially if diuretics are prescribed. Salts of these electrolytes must be well diluted to prevent gastrointestinal (GI) irritation or damage. They are best taken at mealtime to allow mixing with and dilution by food. Clients should be taught the symptoms of fluid and electro-

Table 44-2 Causes of the Syndrome of Inappropriate Antidiuretic Hormone

Ectopic production of tumors
   Bronchogenic carcinoma
   Carcinoma of duodenum
   Carcinoma of pancreas
Nonneoplastic diseases
   Trauma
   Pulmonary disease
   Central nervous system disorders
   Other endocrine disease
Drugs
   Oxytocin
   Vincristine
   Chlorpropamide
   Thiazide diuretics
   Clofibrate
   Carbamazepine
   Nicotine
   Anesthetics

Modified from Felig P and others, eds: Endocrinology and metabolism, New York, 1987, McGraw-Hill Book Co, Inc, p 369.

Table 44-3 Nursing Management of the Client with SIADH

ASSESSMENT*

Accurate hourly intake (oral and parenteral) and output
Hourly measurement of urine specific gravity
Daily weights
Level of consciousness
Observation for hyponatremia every 2 hr (decreased neurological function, convulsions, nausea and vomiting, muscle cramping)
Monitoring of heart and lung sounds, blood pressure

INTERVENTIONS

Restriction of total fluid intake to no more than 1000 ml/day (including that taken with medications); restriction of oral intake to 700 ml < urine output until normalization of serum sodium (if appropriate)
Positioning head of bed flat or with no more than 10 degrees of elevation to enhance venous return to heart and increase left atrial filling pressure, reducing ADH release
Positioning side rails up because of potential alterations in mental status
Turning of client every 2 hours, proper positioning, range-of-motion exercise, massage (if client bedridden)
Use of seizure precautions such as padded side rails, accessible padded tongue blade, and dim lighting
Assistance with ambulation
Provision of frequent oral hygiene

*Use a flow sheet for assessment documentation.

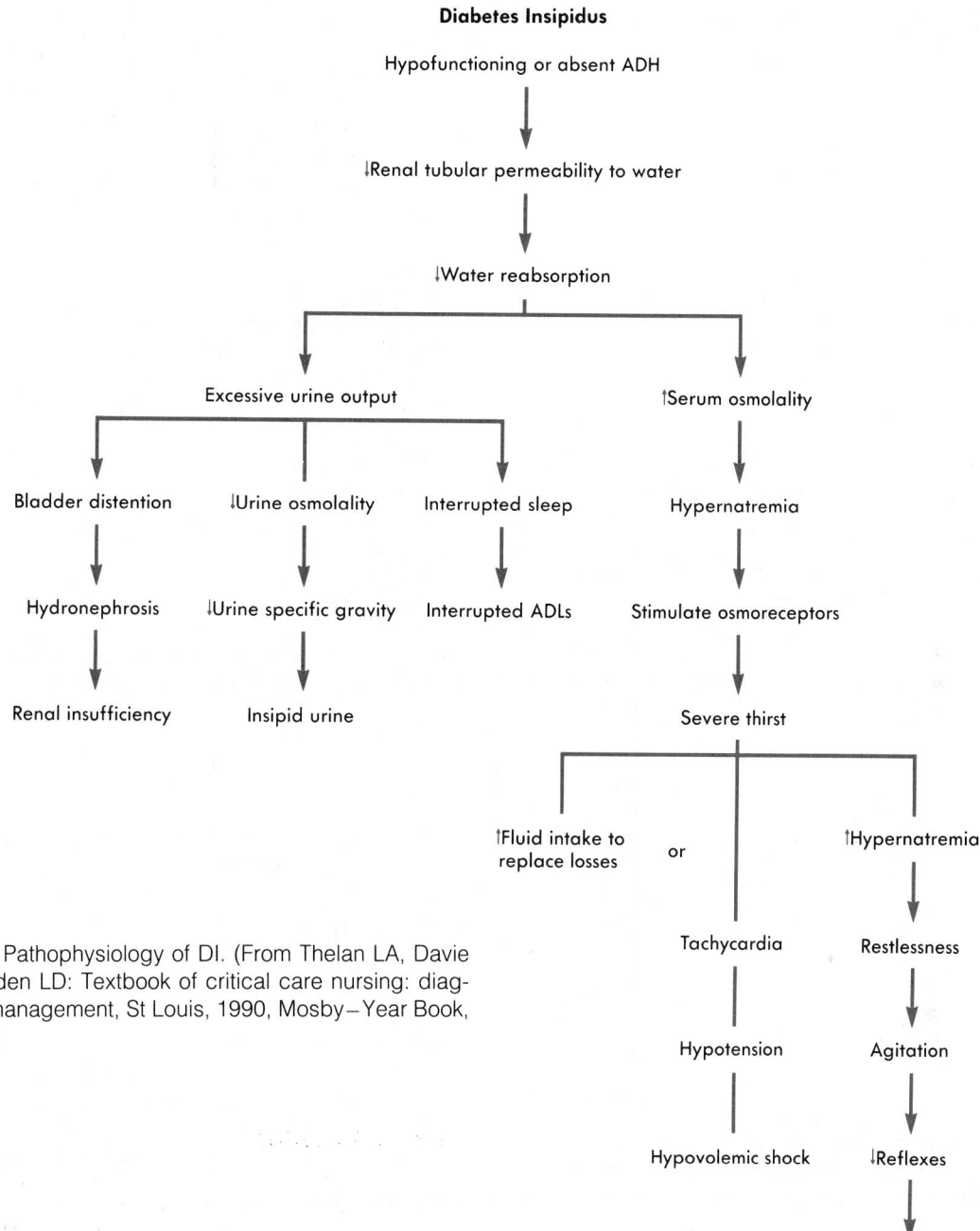

Fig. 44-4 Pathophysiology of DI. (From Thelan LA, Davie JK, and Urden LD: Textbook of critical care nursing: diagnosis and management, St Louis, 1990, Mosby–Year Book, Inc, p 755.)

lyte imbalances, especially those involving sodium and potassium, so that they can monitor their responses to treatment (see Chapter 10). If a client is to be treated with demeclocycline, the need for close follow-up care should be stressed because of the nephrotoxic side effects and the potential for increased susceptibility to fungal infection that is associated with this drug.

Diabetes insipidus. Central diabetes insipidus (DI) is an uncommon syndrome of posterior pituitary hypofunction characterized by increased thirst (polydipsia) and increased urination (polyuria) (Fig. 44-4). It results from ADH deficiency, which prevents the kidneys from reabsorbing water. An estimated 30% of cases have no appar-

ent cause (i.e., are idiopathic).[10] The remainder are due to brain tumors, pituitary surgery, head trauma, granulomatous disease, central nervous system (CNS) infections, and vascular disorders. Central DI may also be caused by osmoreceptor destruction.

Clinical manifestations. The outstanding characteristic of DI is the excretion of large quantities of urine (up to 5 to 20 L/day) with a very low specific gravity. In the milder form, urinary output may be lower (2 to 4 L/day). The majority of clients compensate for the water loss by drinking huge quantities of water so that serum osmolality is normal or only moderately elevated. Clients are usually fatigued from nocturia. If compensation is not possible, severe fluid

volume deficit results. This is manifested by weight loss, poor tissue turgor, hypotension, tachycardia, constipation, and shock. These symptoms are related to rising serum osmolality and hypernatremia.

Therapeutic management. Since polydipsia and polyuria (usually defined as output of greater than 250 ml of urine/hr) may be pituitary (central), renal (nephrogenic), or psychological (psychogenic) in origin, identification of the cause is the initial step in therapeutic management. A complete history is taken, and a complete physical is done; the possibility of an emotional disturbance leading to psychogenic polydipsia is ruled out. This condition is associated with overhydration and hypervolemia rather than with the dehydration and hypovolemia observed in DI. A water deprivation test is usually done to confirm the diagnosis of central DI (see Table 42-8).

DI that is a result of head trauma or surgery is usually self-limiting and improves with treatment of the underlying problem. The goal of treatment is maintenance of fluid and electrolyte balance. This may be accomplished by the administration of increased amounts of fluid and/or by hormone replacement with ADH administered by injection or inhalation. Chlorpropamide, clofibrate, and thiazide diuretics may be prescribed. For long-term therapy, desmopressin acetate, an analogue of ADH that is administered as a nasal preparation and does not have the vasoconstrictive effect, or pitressin tannate in oil (a slowly absorbed IM preparation of ADH) is prescribed.

■ Nursing Management of Diabetes Insipidus

Nursing care of the client with DI is based on the clinical symptoms. Because of the polyuria, severe dehydration and hypovolemic shock may occur. Fluids must be replaced. This can be done with oral or IV replacement, depending on the client's condition and ability to drink copious amounts of fluids. Adequate fluids should be kept at the bedside. Accurate records of intake and output, urine specific gravity, and daily weights are mandatory in the assessment of fluid volume status. Fluid volume deficit manifested by hypotension, tachycardia, and rapid, shallow respirations can be detected early by frequent assessment. Polyuria and nocturia can cause disturbances in rest and sleep patterns. Clients are often listless, tired, and discouraged. Support and reassurance that the sleep disturbances are temporary are helpful. Perineal care should be done at least twice daily in bedridden female clients to cleanse urine from the perineum.

If a water deprivation test is done, the client's baseline weight, pulse, urine and plasma osmolarities, specific gravity of urine, and blood pressure are obtained. All fluids are withheld for 8 to 16 hours. The client may be anxious. Reassurance that the test will be stopped if fluid volume deficit becomes severe helps allay anxiety. The client should be observed throughout the test because of the craving to drink. During the test, the client's blood pressure is assessed hourly and urine osmolality is measured. Weight is assessed every 2 hours. The test continues until urine osmolalities stabilize (hourly increase less than 30 mOsm/kg in 2 consecutive hours) or body weight declines by 3%.[10]

Clients affected by transient DI are usually hospitalized. In this situation, the nurse administers the prescribed form of ADH. Pitressin tannate in oil should be warmed to body temperature before use and rolled to thoroughly mix the oil and drug. Solutions of protein hormones such as ADH should be protected from excessive heat, freezing, and vigorous agitation to prevent denaturation of the protein molecule. Desmopressin acetate is administered as a nasal preparation. It is the preferred treatment for clients with hypertension or cardiovascular disease. Overmedication with either preparation can precipitate volume excess. Clients should be assessed for weight gain, headache, restlessness, and chest pain. The adequacy of treatment is assessed by monitoring fluid intake and output and specific gravity of urine. Increased urine volume with lower specific gravity is related to an inadequate pharmacological effect and the physician should be notified immediately.

Clients who require long-term ADH replacement need instruction in self-management. Desmopressin acetate is usually taken intranasally twice daily. Nasal irritation, headache, and nausea may indicate overdosage, whereas failure to improve may indicate underdosage. If Pitressin tannate in oil is used, client instruction in IM injection should include verbal and written directions and more than one return demonstration before discharge. If hospitalized, clients should give their own injections. If in an ambulatory care setting, they can practice with normal saline solution. Discussions and handouts should include the following instructions about the use of the medication:

1. Store in a cool, dry place (at temperatures between 4.4° C [40° F] and 26.7° C [80° F]) that is protected from light.
2. Warm to body temperature before use and roll to mix drug and oil thoroughly.
3. Inject IM every 1 to 3 days, depending on the response.
4. Report angina or signs of volume excess (weight gain, headache, restlessness) to clinician immediately.
5. Wear a medical identification bracelet at all times.

THYROID GLAND

Thyroid hormones—thyroxine (T_4) and triiodothyronine (T_3), which is the more active form—regulate energy metabolism and growth and development. Thyroid disorders are manifested as hyperfunction, hypofunction, inflammation of the thyroid, or enlargement (goiter). A goiter may interfere with surrounding structures and can be associated with increased, normal, or decreased hormone production.

Hyperthyroidism

Hyperthyroidism (hyperfunction of the thyroid) results from excessive circulating levels of T_4, T_3, or both. It is second only to diabetes mellitus among noniatrogenic-occurring endocrine diseases. The incidence is six times greater in women than in men, and the highest frequency is in the 30- to 50-year-old age group. Iodine deficiency is believed to predispose clients to this and other thyroid diseases; a greater incidence occurs in iodine-poor geographic

locations (goiter belt). The most common form of hyperthyroidism is Graves' disease, followed by multinodular goiter.

Types

Graves' disease. Graves' disease is a multisystem autoimmune syndrome marked by increased production of thyroid hormone. Clients with a genetically determined abnormality of immune regulation become sensitized to and develop antibodies against various antigens within their thyroid gland and often to other tissues as well. Most clients with Graves' disease have hyperthyroidism and diffuse thyroid hyperplasia. Exophthalmos may be present.

Antibodies that stimulate thyroid tissue are found in the serum of individuals with Graves' disease. These antibodies, known collectively as *thyroid-stimulating antibodies* (TSAbs) stimulate the TSH receptor and activate the production of thyroid hormones inappropriately.

Graves' disease occurs more frequently in young women. A concordance rate of 50% in identical twins indicates genetic and environmental components in the expression of the disease. The disease is characterized by remissions and exacerbations, with or without treatment. It may progress to destruction of thyroid tissue, causing hypothyroidism. Precipitating factors such as insufficient io-

---

Table 44-4   Clinical Manifestations of Thyroid Hormone Dysfunction

Hypofunction	Hyperfunction	Hypofunction	Hyperfunction
CARDIOVASCULAR		**MUSCULOSKELETAL**	
Increased capillary fragility	Systolic hypertension	Fatigue	Fatigue
Decreased pulse rate	Increased rate and force of	Weakness	Muscle weakness
Varied changes in blood	cardiac contractions	Muscular aches and pains	Proximal muscle wasting
pressure	Bounding, rapid pulse	Slow movements	Pretibial myxedema
Cardiac hypertrophy, weak	Increased cardiac output		Dependent edema
contractility	Cardiac hypertrophy		
Distant heart sounds	Systolic murmurs	**NERVOUS**	
Anemia	Dysrhythmias	Apathy	Difficulty in focusing eyes
Tendency to develop con-	Palpitations	Lethargy	Nervousness
gestive heart failure, an-	Atrial fibrillation (more com-	Forgetfulness	Fine tremor (of fingers and
gina, myocardial	mon in older adults)	Slowed mental process	tongue)
infarction	Angina	Hoarseness	Insomnia
		Slow, slurred speech	Lability of mood
RESPIRATORY		Prolonged relaxation of	Restlessness
Dyspnea	Increased respiratory rate	deep tendon muscles	Personality changes of irri-
Decreased breathing capac-	Dyspnea on mild exertion	Stupor	tability, agitation
ity		Paresthesias	Exhaustion
		Anxiety, depression	Hyperreflexia of tendon re-
GASTROINTESTINAL		Polyneuropathy	flexes
Decreased appetite	Increased appetite		Depression, fatigue, apathy
Nausea and vomiting	Weight loss		(in older adults)
Weight gain	Increased peristalsis		Lack of ability to concen-
Constipation	Diarrhea		trate
Distended abdomen	Increased bowel sounds		
Enlarged, scaly tongue	Splenomegaly	**REPRODUCTIVE**	
		Prolonged menstrual peri-	Menstrual irregularities
INTEGUMENTARY		ods or amenorrhea	Amenorrhea
Dry, thick, inelastic, cold	Warm, smooth, moist skin	Decreased libido	Decreased libido
skin	Thin, brittle nails detached	Infertility	Impotence in men
Thick, brittle nails	from nail bed (onycholy-		Gynecomastia
Dry, sparse, coarse hair	sis)		
Poor turgor of mucosa	Hair loss	**OTHER**	
Generalized interstitial	Palmar erythema	Increased susceptibility to	Intolerance to heat
edema	Fine silky hair	infection	Increased sensitivity to
Puffy face	Premature graying (in men)	Increased sensitivity to nar-	stimulant drugs
Decreased sweating	Diaphoresis	cotics, barbiturates, anes-	Exophthalmos
Pallor	Vitiligo	thesia	Elevated basal temperature
		Intolerance to cold	Lid lag, stare
		Decreased hearing	Goiter
			Rapid speech

dine supply, infections, and emotions may interact with genetic factors that control immunological and metabolic abnormalities to cause Graves' disease.[11]

Multinodular goiter. This condition is characterized by small, discrete, autonomously functioning nodules that secrete thyroid hormone. If associated with signs of hyperthyroidism, a nodule is termed *toxic adenoma.* The frequency of toxic multinodular goiter is highest in women in the sixth and seventh decades of life. There is usually a history of preexisting goiter for years before the onset of demonstrable hyperthyroidism. The manifestations are slower to develop and usually less severe than in Graves' disease. It is usually not associated with exophthalmos. These thyroid nodules may be benign or malignant.

Clinical manifestations. The clinical manifestations of hyperthyroidism are related to the effects of excess thyroid hormones in two ways. The first is their direct effect of increasing metabolism, and the second is their effect on the sympathetic nervous system. Thyroid hormones increase the number of β-adrenergic receptors, thereby increasing sensitivity to the activity of catecholamines, even though the absolute levels of epinephrine and norepinephrine are not elevated.[11] (The manifestations of hyperthyroidism are summarized in Table 44-4.) A client with advanced disease may exhibit many of the symptoms, whereas in a client in the early stages of the disease process, the only signs may be weight loss and increased nervousness.

Exophthalmos. Exophthalmos (proptosis), in which the eyeballs protrude from the orbits, is due to increased deposits of fat and fluid in the retroorbital tissues (Fig. 44-5). This sign, which is seen in 20% to 40% of clients with Graves' disease, is most likely autoimmune in nature. In exophthalmos the upper lids are usually retracted and elevated, and the eyeballs are forced outward with the sclera above the iris visible. This produces the characteristic stare and protrusion. Exophthalmos is usually bilateral but can be unilateral or asymmetrical. When the eyelids do not close completely, the epithelial surfaces become dry and irritated. Serious complications such as corneal ulcers and eventual loss of vision can occur.

Complications. Hyperthyroid crisis (thyroid storm, thyrotoxicosis) is an acute manifestation of all hyperthyroid symptoms. It is potentially a fatal situation, but death is rare when treatment is vigorous and initiated early. Treatment is aimed at reducing the circulating thyroid hormone level by appropriate drug therapy and extracorporeal removal of thyroid hormone. Support therapy such as fever reduction and fluid replacement is also initiated. The cause is presumed to be stressors such as infection, trauma, or surgery in a client with preexisting hyperthyroidism, either diagnosed or undiagnosed. Manifestations include severe tachycardia, heart failure, shock, hyperthermia (up to 40.7° C [105.3° F]), restlessness, agitation, abdominal pain, delirium, and coma. Measures must be taken to prevent death.

Diagnostic studies. Serum levels of T_4 can be measured with radioimmunoassay techniques (see Table 42-8) and will be elevated. T_3 resin uptake (T_3RU) is also elevated. T_3RU varies inversely with the amount of thyroid hormone that is protein bound and therefore inactive; that is, a high T_3RU indicates that more hormone than normal is biologically active. Free T_4 and T_3 is usually elevated in hyperthyroidism. A subnormal TSH level, as determined by the sensitive TSH (S-TSH) immunoradiometric assay, indicates hyperthyroidism. These tests are accurate measures of circulating thyroid hormone and its efficacy.

Further diagnostic evaluation may include a thyroid-releasing hormone (TRH) stimulation test. The failure of TSH to respond to TRH indicates an autonomously functioning thyroid that has led to pituitary suppression of TSH.[12] Most clients with Graves' disease do not respond to this test. In addition, the electrocardiogram (ECG) may show tachycardia, atrial fibrillation, and alterations in P and T waves.

Therapeutic management. The goal of management is to block the adverse effects of thyroid hormones and stop their oversecretion. This is accomplished by means of (1) pharmacotherapy with antithyroid drugs and β-adrenergic receptor blockers, (2) thyroid ablation with radioactive iodine, and (3) subtotal thyroidectomy after adequate preparation (Table 44-5). The choice of treatment is influenced by the client's age, the severity of the disorder, complicating features (including pregnancy), and the client's preferences. If surgery is to be performed, the client is usually given antithyroid drugs to produce a euthyroid state. Any other associated disorders, such as cardiac disease or diabetes mellitus, must also be controlled before surgery.

For thyroidectomy to be effective, approximately 90% of thyroid tissue must be removed. If too much tissue is taken, the gland will not regenerate after surgery and hypothyroidism will develop. During the surgical procedure, extreme care must be taken to avoid injuring the recurrent laryngeal nerves and the parathyroid glands.

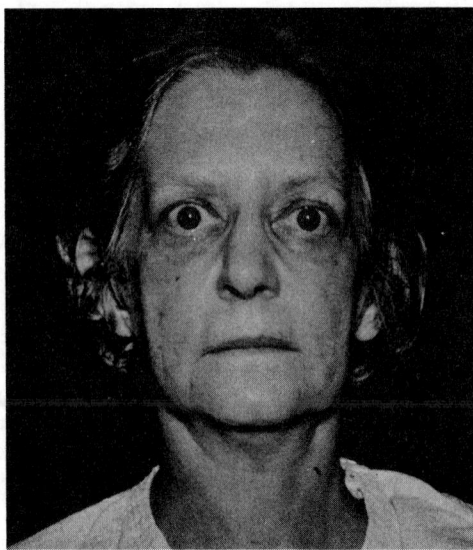

Fig. 44-5 Exophthalmos secondary to Graves' disease. (From Prior JA, Silberstein JS, and Slang JM: Physical diagnosis: the history and examination of the patient, ed 6, St Louis, 1981, The CV Mosby Co.)

Table 44-5

Diagnostic and Therapeutic Management: Hyperthyroidism

DIAGNOSTIC

Complete history and physical examination
Ophthalmologic examination
ECG
Laboratory tests
  Serum T_3RU, T_4, free T_3, TSH levels
  TRH stimulation test
Nuclear medicine-thyroid scan

THERAPEUTIC

Graves' disease

Antithyroid drugs
  Propylthiouracil
  Methimazole
β-Adrenergic blockers such as propranolol (Inderal)
Ablation of thyroid tissue
  Radioactive iodine (^{131}iodine)
  Subtotal thyroidectomy
High-caloric diet

Multinodular goiter

Antithyroid drugs
  Propylthiouracil
  Methimazole
Ablation of thyroid tissue by radioactive iodine

Pharmacological management

Antithyroid drugs. The most commonly used antithyroid drugs are classified as *thioamides*. Propylthiouracil and methimazole (Tapazole) are the most commonly used drugs clinically. These drugs block the synthesis of thyroid hormones. Propylthiouracil also blocks peripheral conversion of T_4 and T_3. Although there is considerable individual variation, improvement usually begins 1 to 2 weeks after the initiation of therapy and good results are seen within 4 to 8 weeks. Therapy is usually continued for 6 months to 2 years to allow for spontaneous remission. The two major disadvantages of antithyroid drugs are client noncompliance and a high incidence of recurrence of the disease once the drugs are discontinued. Indications for use include Graves' disease in young clients, thyrotoxicosis during pregnancy, and the need to render a client euthyroid before surgery.

Iodine. Iodine in large doses blocks the release of thyroid hormone. Its maximal effect is usually seen within 1 to 2 weeks. After that time a reduction in the therapeutic effect may be seen, and long-term iodine therapy is not effective in controlling hyperthyroidism. Usually one drop of a saturated solution of potassium iodide is administered twice daily before surgery. Iodine decreases the size and vascularity of the thyroid, making resection safer and easier. Administration of propylthiouracil, with iodine therapy added 7 to 10 days before surgery, is a common method for surgical preparation of a client with hyperthyroidism.

β-Adrenergic blockers. Propranolol is the most frequently used β-adrenergic blocker. It relieves the symptoms of hyperthyroidism that result from increased β-adrenergic receptors caused by excess thyroid hormones. These symptoms include heat intolerance, palpitations, nervousness, tremor, and muscle weakness. Propranolol is used in conjunction with other antithyroid treatment and rapidly relieves symptoms that cause discomfort to the client with hyperthyroidism. Propranolol is not used in clients with asthma or heart disease. Atenolol may be used instead.

Radioactive iodine. Radioactive iodine (radioiodine or RAI) limits thyroid hormone secretion by damaging or destroying thyroid tissue. It is administered orally, with the dose determined by estimated thyroid weight. This treatment is effective but is associated with a high incidence of hypothyroidism.[13] RAI has a delayed response, and maximum effects may not be evident for 2 to 3 months. However, it is effective and inexpensive and can be administered on an outpatient basis. The client is treated with propylthiouracil or propranolol before and for the first 3 months after therapy for relief of hyperthyroid symptoms until the effects of irradiation become apparent. Thyroid ablation with ^{131}I is not indicated in children or in pregnant women because RAI crosses the placenta and destroys the fetal thyroid.

■ Nursing Management of Hyperthyroidism

Nursing assessment

Subjective and objective data that should be obtained from an individual with hyperthyroidism are presented in Table 44-6.

Nursing diagnoses

Nursing diagnoses are determined when the problem and etiological factors are supported by clinical data. Nursing diagnoses related to hyperthyroidism may include, but are not limited to, those presented in Table 44-7.

Nursing interventions

Acute intervention

ENVIRONMENT. A restful, calm, quiet room should be provided because increased metabolism causes sleep disturbances. Provision of adequate rest may be a challenge due to the client's irritability and restlessness. Interventions may include (1) placing the client in a cool room, away from very ill clients and noisy, high-traffic areas; (2) using light bed coverings and changing the linen frequently if the client is diaphoretic; (3) encouraging and assisting with exercise involving large muscle groups (tremors can interfere with small-muscle coordination) to allow the release of nervous tension and restlessness; and (4) establishing a supportive, trusting relationship to help the client cope with aggravating events and lessen anxiety. A primary nurse or consistent nursing staff may be particularly beneficial to the client with hyperthyroidism.

Nursing interventions with the client's significant others include assisting them to perform the nursing interventions as well as (1) instructing them in the nature of the client's

illness to enable them to understand the physical and emotional manifestations the client experiences, (2) exploring or suggesting ways they can help reduce stressful situations, (3) providing a nonjudgmental atmosphere for them to express difficulties in accepting and dealing with the client's demands and behavior, and (4) restricting visitors who upset the client.

EYE CARE. If exophthalmos is present, there is a potential for corneal injury related to irritation and dryness. Some clients may also have orbital pain. Nursing interventions to relieve eye discomfort and prevent corneal ulceration include application of methylcellulose drops to soothe and moisten conjunctival membranes. Salt restriction may help reduce periorbital edema. Elevation of the client's head promotes fluid drainage from the periorbital area. (Clients should sit upright as much as possible.) Dark glasses reduce glare and prevent irritation from dust and dirt. If the eyelids cannot be closed, they should be lightly taped shut for sleep. To maintain flexibility, the client should be taught to exercise the intraocular muscles several times a day, by turning the eyes in the complete range of motion. Good grooming can be helpful in reducing the loss of self-esteem that results from an altered body image. If the exophthalmos is severe, treatment may involve suturing the eyelids together, administration of corticosteroids, irradiation of retroorbital tissues, orbital decompression, or corrective lid or muscle surgery.

Nutritional considerations. The potential for nutritional deficits usually exists with an increased metabolic rate. A high-calorie diet (4000 to 5000 kcal/day) may be ordered to satisfy hunger and prevent tissue breakdown. This is accomplished with six full meals a day and snacks high in protein, carbohydrates, minerals, and vitamins, particularly B-complex vitamins and ascorbic acid. (Ascorbic acid is required for collagen synthesis.) The protein allowance should be 1 to 2 g/kg of ideal body weight. Increased carbohydrates should compensate for disturbed metabolism, provide energy, and spare protein. Recommended foods should be kept readily available. The nurse should weigh the client daily to monitor adequacy of diet, since weight increases are usually desirable. Offering fluids frequently prevents volume deficit related to diaphoresis and insensible loss. Highly seasoned and high-fiber foods should be avoided, since they stimulate the already hypermotile GI tract. Substitutes should be provided for caffeine-containing liquids such as coffee, tea, and cola, the stimulating effects of which augment increased restlessness and disturbances of the sleep pattern. Milk is an excellent food source that provides both calcium and protein. A dietitian should be consulted for guidance in meeting the nutritional needs of a client with hyperthyroidism.

▪ Nursing Management of the Client Receiving Radioactive Iodine Therapy

RAI therapy is usually done on an outpatient basis and is the therapy of choice for older adults. Because the usual therapeutic dose of iodine is only 7 to 10 mCi, no radiation safety precautions are necessary. Clients should be instructed that radiation thyroiditis and parotiditis are possible and may cause dryness and irritation of the mouth and

---

Table 44-6

 Nursing Assessment of the Client with Hyperthyroidism

SUBJECTIVE DATA

History
Positive family history of thyroid disorders or pernicious anemia, preexisting goiter, increased iodine intake, exposure to head and neck radiation
Recent: Infection, trauma, surgery
Medications
Use of thyroid hormones
General
Weight loss, nervousness, emotional lability, irritability, increased appetite, fatigue, insomnia, heat sensitivity
Pain
Headache, chest pain, abdominal pain
Integumentary
Itching, sweating
Respiratory
Dyspnea on exertion
Cardiovascular
Palpitations
Gastrointestinal
Diarrhea, nausea
Urinary
Polyuria
Reproductive
Decreased libido, impotence, gynecomastia (in men); amenorrhea (in women)
Musculoskeletal
Muscle weakness

OBJECTIVE DATA

General
Exophthalmos, infrequent blinking, restlessness, agitation, rapid speech and body movements, hyperthermia, enlarged thyroid
Integumentary
Warm, diaphoretic, velvety skin; thin, loose nails; hair loss; palmar erythema; diffuse increased pigmentation
Respiratory
Tachypnea
Cardiovascular
Tachycardia, bounding pulse, systolic murmurs, hypertension, diffuse and brawny edema of legs and feet, dysrhythmias
Neurological
Hyperreflexia, diplopia, tremors (of hands, tongue, eyelids)
Musculoskeletal
Muscle wasting
Possible findings
Elevated serum T_3, T_4, and T_3 resin uptake and iodine levels; negative serum TRH stimulation test; chest x-ray film showing cardiac hypertrophy

Table 44-7

NURSING CARE PLAN FOR THE CLIENT WITH HYPERTHYROIDISM

Defining Characteristics	Nursing Interventions	Evaluation Criteria
NURSING DIAGNOSIS: Sleep pattern disturbance related to anxiety, environmental stimulation, disruption of normal sleep pattern, and caffeine intake		
Complaints of restlessness, irritability, insomnia, fatigue; awakening during the night	Promote continuation of usual practices related to rest and sleep unless contraindicated. Decrease environmental stimuli. Administer frequent back rubs with effleurage. Approach client with calm, unhurried demeanor. Work efficiently when with client. Encourage quiet diversions. Encourage frequent short walks during the day. Encourage maintenance of usual bedtime ritual. Administer antithyroid drugs as ordered. Administer sedatives as needed. Eliminate caffeine (e.g., coffee, tea, cola, chocolate) from diet.	Decrease in purposeless movements, verbalization of feeling of being rested on awakening
NURSING DIAGNOSIS: Activity intolerance related to fatigue, exhaustion, and heat intolerance secondary to hypermetabolism		
Complaints of weakness, inability to perform usual activities, short attention span, memory lapses, dyspnea, tachycardia, irritability	Assist client with self-care as needed. Limit ambulation to short walks. Schedule activities of daily living and treatments to promote adequate rest periods.	Decrease in perception of weakness and fatigue
NURSING DIAGNOSIS: Ineffective thermoregulation related to impaired temperature adaptation and altered perception of ambient temperature		
Verbalization of feelings of excess warmth; wearing of inappropriately scant amount of clothing; elevated temperature; warm, moist skin; diaphoresis	Maintain cool environmental temperature. Provide light, loose clothing. Bathe client frequently. Change linen frequently.	Decrease in perspiration, increase in comfort
NURSING DIAGNOSIS: High risk for injury: corneal ulceration related to decreased blinking or inability to close eyelids secondary to exophthalmos		
Complaints of eye pain, feeling of grittiness or "sand" in eyes; proptosis; inability to close eyelids completely; lid lag; lid retraction; visible sclera above iris; "stare"	Instruct client to wear dark glasses. Restrict client's salt intake. Raise head of bed at night. Teach client to exercise extraocular muscles daily. Cover client's eyes with mask or tape shut if eyes will not close.	No evidence of corneal damage
NURSING DIAGNOSIS: High risk for trauma related to fine muscle tremors, fatigue, inattentiveness, incoordination		
Complaints of inability to perform tasks requiring small muscles; restlessness, fatigue; fine-muscle tremors; uncoordinated movements; pretibial myxedema	Assist client as necessary with tasks requiring fine motor skills. Reduce environmental hazards. Assist client with ambulation. Teach client safety practices.	No accidental injury.

Table 44-7

NURSING CARE PLAN FOR THE CLIENT WITH HYPERTHYROIDISM—cont'd

Defining Characteristics	Nursing Interventions	Evaluation Criteria

NURSING DIAGNOSIS: Altered nutrition: less than body requirements related to hypermetabolism and inadequate diet

Complaints of weight loss, hunger, clothing too large; less than optimal body weight	Teach and provide high-calorie, high-vitamin, high-mineral diet that includes between-meal and bedtime snacks. Weigh client daily. Monitor BUN and albumin levels. Arrange dietary consultation if indicated.	Maintenance of weight (or gain in weight), alleviation (or prevention) of nutritional deficiency; verbalization of satisfaction with diet

NURSING DIAGNOSIS: Anxiety related to lack of knowledge about management and course of disease, hypermetabolism, and presence of hypertension

Inability to verbalize information regarding medication and low-sodium foods, verbalization of inability to cope with stresses and increased metabolic activities	Teach client about disease management, including medication regimen, potential for hypertension, chronic nature of disease, and dietary implications. Promote rest and relaxation. Teach client strategies for coping with stress. Administer medications as ordered.	Verbalization of knowledge of management and course of disease, verbalization of decrease in anxiety

NURSING DIAGNOSIS: Potential complication: congestive heart failure

Complaints of dyspnea, fatigue, chest pain; edema; cardiac enlargement; atrial fibrillation; diaphoresis	Reduce environmental stressors. Promote rest and relaxation. Assess tolerance to activity. Discourage physical activity that is not well tolerated. Administer cardiotonics as ordered. Monitor vital signs and cardiac status frequently.	No indicators of congestive heart failure

throat. Relief may be obtained with frequent sips of water, ice chips, or the use of a salt and soda gargle three to four times per day. This gargle is made by dissolving 1 teaspoon of salt and 1 teaspoon of baking soda in 2 cups of warm water. The discomfort should subside in 3 to 4 days. If it persists, the client should contact a clinician. Because of the high frequency of hypothyroidism after RAI, clients and significant others should be instructed about the symptoms of hypothyroidism and the need to seek medical help if these symptoms occur.

■ Nursing Management of the Client Experiencing Thyroid Surgery

Preoperative care

When subtotal thyroidectomy is the treatment of choice, the client must be adequately prepared to avoid postoperative complications. The signs and symptoms of hyperthyroidism are alleviated as much as possible, and cardiac problems must be controlled before surgery. If iodine is used, the client must be assessed for signs of iodine toxicity such as swelling of buccal mucosa and other mucous membranes, excessive salivation, nausea and vomiting, and skin reactions. If these reactions occur, iodine administration should be discontinued and the physician should be notified. Iodine should be mixed with water or juice, sipped through a straw, and administered after meals.

Preoperative teaching should include comfort and safety measures in which the client can participate. Coughing, deep breathing, and leg exercises should be practiced, and their importance should be explained. The client should be taught how to support the head manually while turning in bed, since this maneuver minimizes stress on the suture line after surgery. Range-of-motion exercises of the neck should be practiced. The nurse should explain routine postoperative care such as IV infusions. The client should be told that talking is likely to be difficult for a short time after surgery.

Postoperative care

The hospital room must be prepared for the client. Oxygen, suction equipment, and a tracheostomy tray should be readily available. A tracheostomy tray is required in the event that airway obstruction occurs. Although this happens rarely, it constitutes an emergency situation. Recurrent laryngeal nerve damage leads to vocal cord paralysis. If there is paralysis of both cords, spastic airway obstruction will occur, requiring an immediate tracheostomy.

Respiration may also become difficult because of excess swelling of the neck tissues, hemorrhage, and hematoma formation. Laryngeal stridor (harsh, vibratory sound) may occur during respiration as a result of tetany, which occurs when the parathyroid glands are removed or damaged during surgery. Calcium salts such as calcium gluconate and calcium chloride should be readily available for IV administration to treat tetany.

After a thyroidectomy the nurse should do the following:

1. Assess every 2 hours for 24 hours for any signs of hemorrhage or tracheal compression such as irregular breathing, neck swelling, frequent swallowing, sensations of fullness at the incision site, choking, and blood on the anterior or posterior dressings. Bleeding is assessed by feeling behind the neck for moisture.
2. Place the client in a semi-Fowler's position; support the head with pillows, avoiding flexion of the neck and any tension on the suture lines.
3. Monitor vital signs. Complete the initial assessment by checking for signs of tetany (e.g., tingling in toes, fingers, or around the mouth; muscular twitching; apprehension) and by evaluating difficulty in speaking and hoarseness. (Some hoarseness is to be expected for 3 to 4 days after surgery because of edema.)
4. Control postoperative pain by giving medication. Meperidine and morphine are commonly prescribed.

If postoperative recovery is uneventful, the client is ambulated the first day, takes fluid as soon as tolerated, and eats a soft diet by the second day after surgery.

Nursing interventions

Chronic management. Follow-up care is very important to clients who have undergone thyroid surgery. Hyperthyroidism may recur after a period of time, requiring further treatment. Hormone balance should be monitored periodically to ensure that normal function has returned. Most clients experience a period of relative hypothyroidism after surgery because of the marked reduction in the size of the thyroid. The remaining tissue usually hypertrophies, recovering the capacity to produce the hormone needed by the body. The administration of thyroid hormone is avoided because exogenous hormone inhibits pituitary production of TSH and delays or prevents the restoration of normal gland function and thyroid tissue regeneration.

The client can do a great deal to prevent complications and promote a return to normal function during the hypothyroid period after surgery. Caloric intake must be reduced markedly below the amount that was required before surgery to prevent weight gain. Some surgeons may suggest avoiding foods that contain thyroid-inhibiting substances (goitrogens) (Table 44-8). Adequate iodine is necessary to promote thyroid function, but excesses inhibit the thyroid. Seafood once or twice a week or normal use of iodized salt should provide sufficient intake. Regular exercise helps stimulate the thyroid and should be encouraged. Exposure to alternating extremes of temperature, such as hot and cold showers, also promotes thyroid hyperplasia

Table 44-8 Common Exogenous Goitrogens

FOODS

Potent goitrogens
  Turnips
  Rutabagas
  Soybeans (especially when fed to infants in formula)
  Skins of peanuts
  Milk from kale-fed cattle
Less potent goitrogens
  Seafood
  Green leafy vegetables
  Peanuts
  Peaches
  Peas
  Strawberries
  Carrots
  Cabbage
  Mustard seed
  Radishes

DRUGS

Thyroid inhibitors
  Propylthiouracil
  Methimazole
  Carbimazole
  Iodine in large doses
Others
  Sulfonamides
  Salicylates
  p-Aminosalicylic acid
  Phenylbutazone
  Lithium

but is not acceptable to many individuals because of cold intolerance. High environmental temperature should be avoided because it inhibits thyroid regeneration.

The neck incision should be lubricated and range-of-motion exercises should be carried out three or four times daily to promote comfort and return of full range of motion. The client should be taught movements that cause flexion, extension, rotation, and lateral bending of the neck. The appearance of the incision may be quite distressing to the client. The client should be reassured that the scar will fade in color and eventually assume the appearance of a normal neck wrinkle. Scarves, jewelry, high collars, or other coverings can effectively camouflage a fresh scar.

Regular follow-up care is necessary. Clients should be seen biweekly for a month and then at least semiannually to assess for the development of hypothyroidism. If a complete thyroidectomy has been performed, the client needs instruction in lifelong thyroid replacement (with medication). Failure of thyroid function is considered by some authorities to be the normal end stage of Graves' disease. Clients should be taught the signs and symptoms of progressive thyroid failure and should be instructed to seek medical care if these develop. Hypothyroidism is relatively

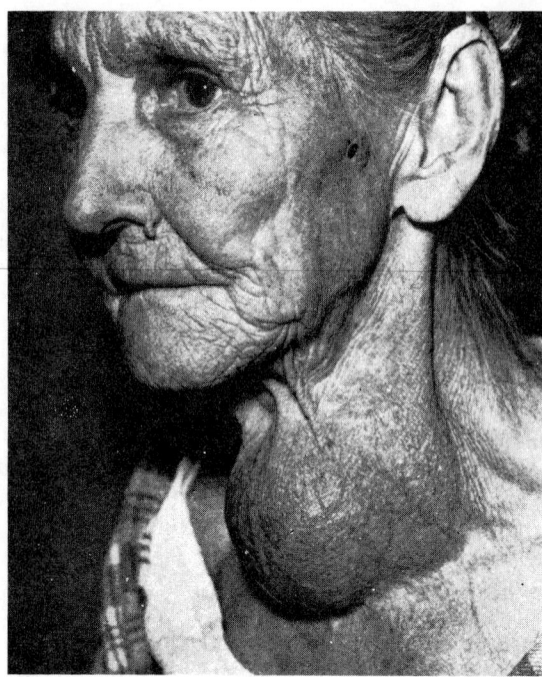

Fig. 44-6 Simple goiter. (From Anthony CA and Thibodeau GA: Textbook of anatomy and physiology, St Louis, 1987, The CV Mosby Co, p 370.)

easy to control with oral administration of thyroid preparations.

Thyroid Enlargement

Enlargement of the thyroid gland is called *goiter* (Fig. 44-6). Goiter may result from hypertrophy caused by excess TSH stimulation, which can be caused by inadequate circulating thyroid hormones. Goiter may also be caused by growth-stimulating immunoglobulins and other growth factors. Goitrogens (see Table 44-8), which inhibit synthesis of thyroid hormone, can cause goiter but usually only in individuals who live in iodine-deficient areas.

T_4 and T_3RU are measured to determine whether a goiter is associated with hyperthyroidism or hypothyroidism. Thyroid antibodies are measured to assess for thyroiditis. Goiters are usually treated with thyroid hormone to suppress TSH. Surgery to remove excess thyroid tissue may also be performed.

Thyroid nodules. A thyroid nodule—a palpable deformity of the thyroid gland—may be benign or malignant. Malignant tumors of the thyroid gland are rare. The major sign of thyroid cancer is the appearance of a hard, painless nodule in an enlarged thyroid. A thyroid scan shows whether nodules on the thyroid are "hot" or "cold." When a person is given tracer doses of ^{131}I, tumors on the thyroid may take up the radioactive iodine. These are called *hot* nodules and are nearly always benign. Ultrasonography and MRI may also be used to aid in diagnosis. Benign nodules are usually not dangerous, but they can cause tracheal compression if they become too large. Because few malignancies use iodine and many are cystic in nature, they usually show up as cold spots in the thyroid scan.

Measurement of serum calcitonin is also helpful in diagnosis, since increased levels are associated with medullary thyroid carcinoma.

Neoplasms are treated by means of surgical removal. Surgical procedures may range from simple removal of the tumor to total thyroidectomy with bilateral neck dissection. Many thyroid cancers are TSH-dependent, and thyroid hormone in hyperphysiological doses is often prescribed to inhibit pituitary secretion of TSH. Nursing care for the client with thyroid tumors is similar to care for the client who has undergone thyroidectomy and also includes general nursing measures for the client with cancer (see Chapter 9).

Thyroiditis. Thyroiditis is an inflammatory process in the thyroid and can have several causes. Subacute granulomatous thyroiditis (de Quervain's thyroiditis), which presents with hyperthyroidism, is thought to be due to a viral infection, whereas acute thyroiditis is due to bacterial infection. Both have an abrupt onset. Autoimmune thyroiditis (Hashimoto's thyroiditis), leading to hypothyroidism, is insidious in onset. Hashimoto's thyroiditis is a chronic autoimmune disease in which thyroid tissue is replaced by lymphocytes and fibrous tissue. It is the most common cause of goiterous hypothyroidism in the United States.

T_4 and T_3 are initially elevated in subacute and acute thyroiditis but may become depressed with time. Thyroid hormone levels are usually low in chronic Hashimoto's thyroiditis. Suppression of radioactive iodine uptake indicates a low thyroid reserve and subacute thyroiditis. Thyroid antibodies are present in Hashimoto's thyroiditis.

Recovery from thyroiditis may be complete in weeks or months without treatment. If the condition is bacterial in origin, treatment may include specific antibiotics or surgical drainage. In subacute and acute forms, salicylates are used, followed by corticosteroids if there is no response to the salicylates within 72 hours. Thyroid hormone may be used if the client shows signs and symptoms of hypothyroidism. Propranolol or atenolol may be used for the cardiovascular symptoms of a hyperthyroid condition.

Nursing care of clients with thyroiditis includes education regarding normal thyroid function and what is happening in the client's specific instance. Other nursing interventions depend, in part, on the therapeutic management. Nursing orders include reassurance, support, and assistance during the recovery period. Acetaminophen may be used to alleviate thyroid discomfort. Clients should be instructed to remain under close health supervision and report any change in symptoms so that progress can be monitored.

Clients with thyroiditis of autoimmune origin may be susceptible to other autoimmune diseases such as Addison's disease, pernicious anemia, and premature gonadal failure. They should be taught the signs and symptoms of these disorders, particularly Addison's disease. Since stress may aggravate these autoimmune diseases, stress management is an important part of client education (see Chapter 5). These clients should also be given a list of common goitrogens (see Table 44-8) and encouraged to avoid them as much as possible.

Clients receiving thyroid hormone replacement or corticosteroids must be taught the expected side effects of these drugs and measures to manage them. They should also be instructed in unexpected side effects and told when and to whom these should be reported. Toxic symptoms should be clearly defined, and the client should be instructed to report them. Table 44-3 lists signs of hyperthyroidism that are the same as toxic symptoms of thyroid hormone replacement. Table 44-11 lists signs of hypercortisolism that are similar to drug toxicity. Client handouts written in understandable language should accompany instruction. The handouts should be reviewed with the client to assess understanding, and information should be clarified when necessary. Clients treated surgically need care similar to that for those undergoing thyroidectomy.

Hypothyroidism

Hypothyroidism usually results from insufficient circulating thyroid hormone as a result of a variety of abnormalities. All hypothyroid states have certain features in common, regardless of the cause. Some differences depend on the client's age at onset of the deficiency.

Causes. Hypothyroidism may occur in infancy *(cretinism)*, childhood, or adulthood. Cretinism is caused by thyroid hormone deficiencies during fetal or early neonatal life. It can be caused by maternal iodine deprivation or congenital thyroid abnormalities. Juvenile hypothyroidism has causes similar to those seen in adults and requires prompt diagnosis and treatment to prevent developmental retardation.

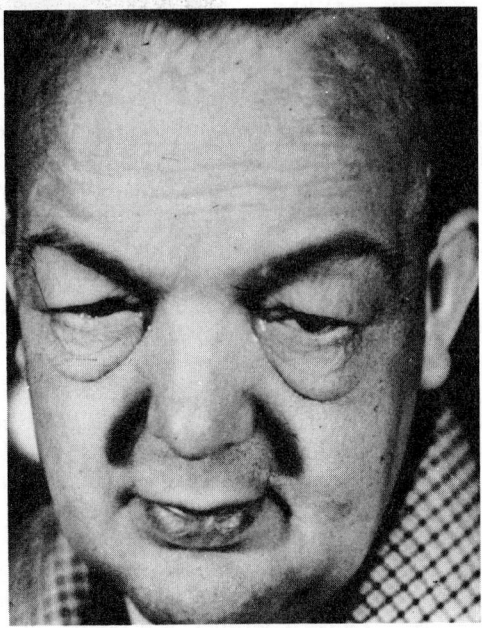

Fig. 44-7 Myxedema, a condition produced by hyposecretion of the thyroid gland during the adult years. Note the edema around the eyes and facial puffiness. (From Prior JA, Silberstein JS, and Slang JM: Physical diagnosis: the history and examination of the patient, ed 6, St Louis, 1981, The CV Mosby Co.)

In the adult the most common cause of primary hypothyroidism is atrophy of the thyroid gland, considered to be the end result of both Hashimoto's thyroiditis and Graves' disease. These conditions involve autoimmune processes in which the thyroid gland is gradually destroyed by endogenous antibodies. Thyroid deficiency also occurs when pituitary TSH production is inadequate. Iatrogenic causes of hypothyroidism include surgical removal of the thyroid, destruction of the thyroid gland by radiation, and surgical removal of the pituitary. Occasionally, hypothyroidism develops as a result of the ingestion of goitrogens (Table 44-8). Persons with underlying autoimmune disease are particularly susceptible to goitrogens.

Although the typical client with hypothyroidism is a woman over 50, the disease can occur at any age and in either gender. An increased incidence has been correlated with the use of radioactive iodine. Hypothyroidism is more common in iodine-deficient areas of the world, such as Zaire and Nepal.

Clinical manifestations. The major manifestations of cretinism are defective physical development and mental retardation. Although affected infants appear normal at birth, cretinism should be suspected when there is a long gestational period and failure to thrive. Affected infants may exhibit squinting, excessive sleeping, thickened skin and lips, enlarged tongue, a hoarse cry, dull facial expression, respiratory difficulty, supraclavicular and periorbital edema, umbilical hernia, and hypothermia.

Cretinism occurs in 1 of 4500 births in the United States. Early recognition is essential for normal physical and mental development. All states require neonatal screening for cretinism with a simple heel capillary blood test. Cretinism causes irreversible mental retardation and dwarfism. When treatment with hormone replacement is begun soon after birth, normal physical and intellectual development will ensue.[14]

Hypothyroidism in childhood is usually due to autoimmune thyroiditis. A prevalence of 1.3% to 6% has been reported in schoolchildren. Intellectual development is normal, but physical and sexual development is altered. The face remains childlike, and eruption of permanent teeth and sexual maturation are delayed. In addition, there is a high frequency of other autoimmune diseases.[15]

Hypothyroidism in adults is characterized by an insidious and nonspecific slowing of body processes; personality changes; fatigue and lethargy; and generalized, interstitial nonpitting edema. The mucinous edema *(myxedema)* occurs in severe, long-standing hypothyroidism. The term *myxedema* is often used synonymously with hypothyroidism. The mucinous edema causes characteristic facies with puffiness, periorbital edema, and masklike affect (Fig. 44-7). Mental changes observed in hypothyroidism include impaired memory, slowed speech, decreased initiative, and somnolence. In addition, cold intolerance, dry and coarse skin, muscle weakness and swelling, overall weakness, constipation, weight gain, hair loss, brittle nails, hoarseness, and menorrhagia are common.

Unless hypothyroidism occurs after thyroidectomy or during treatment with antithyroid drugs, the onset of

symptoms may occur over months to years. The symptoms are so insidious that medical attention is seldom sought. The client's family and friends are often unaware of the changes. The severity of the symptoms depends on the degree of thyroid hormone deficiency.

The clinical manifestations of hypothyroidism result from the long-term physiological effects of thyroid hormone deficiency. They may involve any body system but are more pronounced in those systems with high protein turnover: the cardiovascular, GI, reproductive, and hematopoietic systems.

Hypothyroid heart disease includes cardiomyopathy, pericardial effusion, and coronary atherosclerosis. Bradycardia and weakened cardiac contractility lead to decreased cardiac output. (Pericardial effusion, however, seldom results in hemodynamic compromise.) Increased cholesterol and triglyceride levels and the accumulation of mucopolysaccharides in the intima of small blood vessels can result in coronary atherosclerosis. It is seldom symptomatic because of the decreased myocardial oxygen consumption that has been observed in this disease.

GI motility is decreased in clients with hypothyroidism, and achlorhydria (absence of hydrochloric acid) is common. Constipation, which is a common complaint, may progress to obstipation and, rarely, to intestinal obstruction. The underlying metabolic disease makes the individual a very high-risk candidate for surgery.

Women with hypothyroidism frequently complain of menorrhagia. Some affected individuals have been treated for this condition for long periods and may have undergone hysterectomy before the underlying endocrine disorder was diagnosed. In addition, anovulatory cycles with infertility may occur.

Anemia is a common feature of hypothyroidism. Erythropoietin levels may be low or normal. Oxygen demand is decreased in the periphery, and there is hypocellular bone marrow. The result is a low hematocrit. Other hematopoietic effects are vitamin B_{12}, iron, and folate deficiencies and a predisposition to bruising.

The brain is affected by diminished cerebral blood flow related to decreased cardiac output. This is manifested by mental sluggishness, inattentiveness, memory loss, lethargy, and changes in affect. Although some individuals

with hypothyroidism exhibit a jocular air regarding their condition, others appear depressed. They express distress and describe an impaired self-image in regard to their disabilities and altered appearance. Although clients with hypothyroidism sleep long hours, decreases in stage 3 and stage 4 sleep occur.

Complications

Myxedema coma. The mental sluggishness, drowsiness, and lethargy of hypothyroidism may progress gradually or suddenly to marked impairment of consciousness or coma. This situation constitutes a medical emergency. Myxedema coma can be precipitated by infection, drugs (especially narcotics, tranquilizers, and barbiturates), exposure to cold, and trauma. It is characterized by subnormal temperature, hypotension, and hypoventilation. For the client to live, vital functions must be supported, and IV thyroid hormone must be administered.

Diagnostic studies. T_4, T_3, and T_3RU levels are usually low in hypothyroidism. These values, correlated with symptoms gathered from the history and physical examination, confirm the diagnosis. Serum TSH levels help determine the cause of hypothyroidism. Serum TSH is high when the defect is in the thyroid and low when it is in the pituitary or hypothalamus. An increase in TSH after TRH injection suggests hypothalamic dysfunction, whereas no change is compatible with anterior pituitary dysfunction (Table 44-9).

Therapeutic management. The primary objective in treating hypothyroidism is restoration of a euthyroid state as safely, rapidly, and inexpensively as possible by means of replacement therapy. Therapeutic management of adults includes gradual replacement of thyroid hormones and a low-calorie diet to promote weight loss. Lifelong therapy is usually required for both adults and children.

Pharmacological management. Synthetic oral thyroxine (Synthroid, Levothroid, Noroxine) is the drug of choice to treat hypothyroidism. In young, otherwise healthy clients, the maintenance replacement dose can be started at once. In older adult clients and those with compromised cardiac status, a small initial dose is recommended because the usual dose may overstimulate metabolic activity of the heart and circulatory system. The resultant oxygen demand may cause angina and cardiac dysrhythmias. Any chest pain experienced by a client starting thyroid replacement should be reported, and ECG and serum cardiac enzyme tests must be performed. The dose is increased at 3- to 4-week intervals. It is important that clients take their replacement medication regularly.

■ Nursing Management of Hypothyroidism

Nursing assessment

It is important to question the client who is suspected of having hypothyroidism about weight gain, mental changes, fatigue, slowed and slurred speech, cold intolerance, skin changes such as increased dryness or thickening, constipation, and dyspnea. The client should be assessed for bradycardia; distended abdomen; dry, thick, cold skin; thick, brittle nails; paresthesias; and muscular aches and pains.

Table 44-9 Diagnostic Studies in Hypothyroidism

Study	Finding
Serum T_3RU	Low
Serum T_3	Low
Serum T_4	Low
Serum cholesterol	Increased
ECG	Bradycardia, low voltage
Serum TSH	High (if thyroid diseased), low (if pituitary diseased)
TRH stimulation test	Increase in TSH if hypothalamus decreased, no change in TSH if pituitary diseased

Nursing diagnoses

Nursing diagnoses specific to the client with hypothyroidism include, but are not limited to, the following:

1. Pain related to cold intolerance
2. High risk for impaired skin integrity related to decreased tissue perfusion and oxygenation
3. Altered nutrition: more than body requirements related to hypometabolism
4. Constipation related to GI hypomotility
5. Activity intolerance related to fatigue, hypometabolism, slowed mental processes, and decreased cardiac output and breathing capacity

Nursing interventions

Acute intervention. The following nursing interventions contribute to the recovery of a client with hypothyroidism:

1. Provide a comfortable, warm environment because of the client's intolerance to cold.
2. Take measures to prevent skin breakdown. Use soap sparingly and apply an emollient or lotion. An alternating-pressure mattress may be helpful.
3. Avoid using sedatives. If they must be given, give the lowest possible dose and closely monitor mental status, level of consciousness, and respirations.
4. Prevent constipation by gradually increasing exercise, administering stool softeners, increasing bulk in the diet, and promoting regular bowel habits. Avoid enemas because they produce vagal stimulation, which can be hazardous to clients with cardiac disease.
5. Teach the client the nature of the thyroid hormone deficiency, self-care practices necessary to recovery, and signs and symptoms to monitor.

For assessment of the client's progress, vital signs, body weight, fluid intake and output, and visible edema should be monitored. Cardiac assessment is especially important because the cardiovascular response to the hormone determines the medication regimen. Energy level and mental alertness should be noted. These should increase within 2 to 14 days and continue to rise steadily to normal levels.

Chronic management. Repeated client education is imperative. Often the hypothyroid client needs more time than usual to comprehend all of the necessary information. It is important to provide written instructions, to repeat the information often, and to assess the client's comprehension level regularly. The need for lifelong drug therapy must be stressed. The signs of hypothyroidism or hyperthyroidism that indicate hormone imbalance should be included in the teaching plan. It is sometimes difficult for the client to recognize signs of overdosage or underdosage; therefore, a family member or friend should be included in the instruction process. Forgetfulness is an early indication of thyroid deficiency.

The client must be taught to contact a clinician immediately if signs of overdose such as orthopnea, dyspnea, rapid pulse, palpitations, nervousness, or insomnia appear. Clients with diabetes mellitus should test their capillary blood sugar at least daily, since the euthyroid state frequently increases insulin requirements. In addition, thyroid preparations potentiate the effects of other common drug groups, such as anticoagulants, antidepressants, and digitalis compounds.

With treatment, striking transformations occur in both appearance and mental function. Most adults return to a normal state. Cardiovascular conditions and (occasionally) psychosis may persist despite corrections of the hormone imbalance. Relapses occur if treatment is interrupted.

PARATHYROIDS
Hyperparathyroidism

Hyperparathyroidism is a condition involving increased secretion of parathyroid hormone (PTH). PTH helps regulate calcium and phosphate levels by stimulating bone resorption, renal tubular reabsorption of calcium, and activation of vitamin D. Until recently, this dysfunction was considered rare. With the advent of routine evaluation of serum calcium levels, however, the true prevalence in the general population is estimated to be 0.5%, and the annual incidence in women over 60 years of age is estimated to be 1.8%.[16]

Hyperparathyroidism is classified as primary, secondary, or tertiary. *Primary disease* may be caused by tumors in or hyperplasia of the parathyroid glands, leading to a derangement of calcium, phosphate, and bone metabolism. The most common cause is a single adenoma (in 84% of cases). *Secondary hyperparathyroidism* appears to be a compensatory response to abnormal states that induce or cause hypocalcemia, the main stimulus of parathyroid activity. Disease conditions associated with secondary hyperparathyroidism include vitamin D deficiencies, malabsorption, chronic renal failure, and hyperphosphatemia. *Tertiary hyperparathyroidism* is observed in clients who have had kidney transplants after a long period of dialysis treatment for chronic renal failure (see Chapter 41).

Primary hyperparathyroidism is twice as common in women and usually occurs between the ages of 30 and 70. The peak incidence is in postmenopausal women. Previous head and neck irradiation may predispose a client to the development of parathyroid adenoma.[17] Increased PTH has a multisystem effect (Table 44-10). In the bones, subperiosteal bone resorption, decreased bone density, cyst formation, and general weakness can occur as a result of the effect of PTH on osteoclastic and osteoblastic activity.

In the kidneys the excess calcium cannot be reabsorbed, leading to hypercalciuria. The calcium in the urine, along with the large amount of phosphate excreted in the urine, can lead to calculi formation. In addition, the glomerular filtration rate decreases, and proximal renal tubular acidosis may occur. The effect of increased PTH on the intestines leads to an increase in the absorption of calcium in the presence of increased vitamin D production by the kidneys. The hypercalcemia can lead to increased secretion of gastrin and pepsin, resulting in peptic ulcer disease. An increase in pancreatitis is also observed.

Clinical manifestations and complications. Hyperparathyroidism presents with varying symptoms, which may include weakness, loss of appetite, constipation, increased need for sleep, and shortened attention span. Major signs include loss of calcium from bones (osteoporo-

Table 44-10 Clinical Manifestations of Parathyroid Dysfunction

System	Hypofunction	Hyperfunction
Cardiovascular	Decreased contractility of heart muscle Decreased cardiac output Prolongation of QT and ST intervals on ECG Dysrhythmias	Dysrhythmias Shortened QT interval on ECG Hypertension
Gastrointestinal	Abdominal cramps Urinary and fecal incontinence (in older adults)	Vague abdominal pain Anorexia Nausea and vomiting Constipation Pancreatitis Peptic ulcer disease Cholelithiasis Weight loss
Integumentary	Dry, scaly skin Hair loss on scalp and body Brittle nails, transverse ridging Changes in developing teeth, lack of tooth enamel	Skin necrosis Moist skin
Musculoskeletal	Fatigue Weakness Painful muscle cramps Skeletal x-ray changes, osteosclerosis Soft-tissue calcification Difficulty in walking	Skeletal pain Backache Weakness, fatigue Pain on weight bearing Pathological fractures of long bones Compression fractures of spine Decreased muscle tone
Nervous	Personality changes Psychiatric manifestations of depression, anxiety Irritability Memory impairment Headache Convulsions Positive Chvostek's sign and/or Trousseau's phenomenon Tremor Paresthesias of perioral area, hands, feet Hyperactive deep-tendon reflexes Disorientation, confusion (in older adults)	Personality disturbances Emotional irritability Memory impairment Psychosis Delirium, confusion, coma Incoordination Hyperactive deep-tendon reflexes Abnormalities of gait Psychomotor retardation
Renal	Urinary frequency	Hypercalciuria Kidney stones (nephrolithiasis) Urinary tract infections Polyuria
Other	Eye changes, including lenticular opacities, cataracts, papilledema Hyperventilation	Corneal calcification on slit-lamp examination

sis), broken bones, kidney stones (nephrolithiasis), and peptic ulcer. Asymptomatic cases are being identified with increasing frequency with routine calcium screening. Serum calcium is usually elevated, and serum phosphate is decreased. Neuromuscular abnormalities are characterized by muscle weakness, particularly in the proximal muscles of the lower extremities. The serious complications of hyperparathyroidism are renal failure, collapse of vertebral bodies, and long bone and rib fractures.

Diagnostic studies. Serum calcium levels usually exceed 10 mg/dl. Because of its inverse relation with calcium, the serum phosphorus level is usually below 3 mg/

dl. Other elevations include PTH, urine calcium, serum chloride, uric acid, creatinine, amylase (if pancreatitis is present), and alkaline phosphatase (if bone disease has already begun). If bone changes are present, radiological studies may reveal subperiosteal resorption, bone cysts, demineralization of bones, loss of the lamina dura of the teeth, and tumors of the long bones. ECG studies may reveal shortened QT intervals, prolonged QR intervals, and abnormal QRS complexes.

Therapeutic management. The objective of treatment is to relieve symptoms and prevent complications caused by excess PTH. The choice of therapy depends on the ur-

gency of the clinical situation, the degree of hypercalcemia, the underlying disorder, the status of renal and hepatic function, the clinical presentation of the client, and the particular advantages and disadvantages of the different therapeutic modalities.

Parathyroid tumors should be removed surgically. The parathyroids occasionally lie in ectopic sites such as the mediastinum. This situation requires a highly skilled surgeon to open the chest and explore the area behind the sternum. Generally, a single gland is removed if an adenoma is the cause of the hyperparathyroidism. When cancer is the cause, all of the parathyroids are removed.

If the symptoms are mild and in older adult clients or those at increased surgical risk from other health problems, a conservative management approach is followed. This includes an annual examination that includes tests for serum calcium, phosphorus and alkaline phosphatase levels and renal function, x-ray films to assess for metabolic bone disease, and measurement of urinary calcium excretion.

Specific management measures include maintenance of a high fluid intake, limitations of calcium intake, sodium intake of 8 to 10 g/day to replace losses, and phosphorus replacement unless contraindicated by a high risk for urinary calculi formation. Continued ambulation and the avoidance of immobility are also critical aspects of management. The client is monitored regularly with serum calcium and creatinine clearance tests. Annual x-ray examinations of the hand will indicate subperiosteal bone resorption.

Pharmacological management. Mithramycin, an antihypercalcemic agent, has been shown to effectively lower serum calcium within 48 hours; however, because of toxic side effects, its use is limited to clients with metastatic parathyroid carcinoma and severe bone disease. Postmenopausal women show improvement of primary hyperparathyroidism with estrogen therapy.

In severe hyperparathyroidism, normal saline solution is administered IV to correct fluid volume deficit and promote calcium excretion. Furosemide is also given orally or IV to decrease renal tubular resorption of calcium. Propranolol (Inderal) may be used to inhibit the action of catecholamines, which stimulate PTH secretion.

■ Nursing Management of Hyperparathyroidism

Nursing assessment
Subjective and objective data that should be collected from an individual with hyperparathyroidism are presented in Table 44-11.

Nursing diagnoses
Nursing diagnoses are determined when the problem and etiological factors are supported by clinical data. Nursing diagnoses related to hyperparathyroidism may include, but are not limited to, those presented in Table 44-12.

Nursing interventions
If surgery is performed, close monitoring of the client's vital signs is required. Other aspects of care are similar to that after thyroidectomy. The major postoperative complications are tetany and fluid and electrolyte disturbances.

Table 44-11

 Nursing Assessment of the Client with Hyperparathyroidism

SUBJECTIVE DATA

History
Family history of multiple endocrine neoplasias, familial hyperparathyroidism, previous head or neck x-ray examinations, vitamin D deficiency, malabsorption, malnutrition, chronic renal failure

Medications
Compliance with renal failure medications (e.g., phosphate binders, calcium supplements)

General
Weakness, irritability, anorexia, increase in sleeping, depression, malaise, fatigue, weight loss

Pain
General skeletal pain, backaches, bone pain on weight bearing, renal colic, dysuria, abdominal pain

Gastrointestinal
Constipation, nausea and vomiting

Urinary
Polyuria

Musculoskeletal
Muscle weakness, arthralgias

OBJECTIVE DATA

General
Apathy

Cardiovascular
Hypertension, dysrhythmias (especially bradycardias)

Neurological
Drowsiness, slow mentation, confusion, delirium, poor coordination

Musculoskeletal
Osteoporosis, fractures, decreased muscle tone

Possible findings
Elevated serum calcium (>10 mg/dl), PTH, chloride, alkaline phosphatase, uric acid, creatinine; decreased serum phosphate (<3 mg/dl), bicarbonate; guaiac positive stool and emesis (peptic ulcer); subperiosteal bone resorption on x-ray examinations; enlarged parathyroids on ultrasonography

Tetany is usually apparent early in the postoperative period but may develop over several days. Mild tetany, characterized by unpleasant tingling of the hands and around the mouth, may be present but should abate without problems. If tetany becomes more severe (e.g., muscular spasms or laryngospasms develop), IV calcium may be given. Strict monitoring of intake and output is necessary to evaluate volume and electrolyte status. Calcium, potassium, phosphate, and magnesium levels are assessed frequently. Mobility is encouraged because it promotes calcification of the bones. If surgery is not performed, treatment to relieve symptoms and prevent complications is carried out.

Table 44-12

NURSING CARE PLAN FOR THE CLIENT WITH HYPERPARATHYROIDISM

Defining Characteristics	Nursing Interventions	Evaluation Criteria
NURSING DIAGNOSIS: Activity intolerance related to muscle weakness and fatigue secondary to low calcium levels		
Complaints of weakness and fatigue; inability to use stairs, arise from chairs; pain on weight bearing	Assist with ambulation and limit ambulation to short walks. Assist client with self-care as needed. Plan activities of daily living and treatment to allow for adequate rest periods. Provide client with walker or cane, as necessary.	Decrease in perception of fatigue and weakness, no accidental injury
NURSING DIAGNOSIS: Altered health maintenance related to lack of knowledge of need for low-calcium, acid-ash diet and high fluid intake		
Inability to verbalize knowledge of or to make selection of foods low in calcium and acid-ash, need for increased fluid intake or plan to increase fluid intake, hypercalciuria, urinary tract infection	Consult dietitian. Reinforce dietary teaching. Ensure that client has visual aids or written handouts. Include family in dietary instructions. Instruct client about symptoms of renal stones. Strain urine for stones. Keep fluids within easy reach and offer frequently. Provide low-calcium, acid-ash diet. (Omit milk and milk products; include additional cranberries, prunes, and plums.) Encourage fluid intake to point of moderate overhydration (4000 ml plus fluid output per day). Instruct client regarding proper diet and fluid intake. Consult with physician concerning possible prescription of ascorbic acid to acidify urine. Assess client for flank pain and hematuria and report immediately.	No renal stones, prompt detection and early treatment of renal stones, verbalization of plan by client and family to adhere to dietary instructions
NURSING DIAGNOSIS: Altered nutrition: less than body requirements related to loss of appetite, nausea, vomiting, and personality disturbances		
Complaints of loss of appetite, nausea; refusal to socialize; inability to recall instructions; vomiting, guarding of abdominal area; irritability; self-isolation	Administer mouth care frequently with use of flavored mouthwash or toothpaste. Eliminate noxious odors from environment. Encourage eating with others in sitting or dining room. Serve small amounts of food frequently.	Maintenance of adequate food and fluid intake, maintenance of stable weight
NURSING DIAGNOSIS: Constipation related to dehydration and inactivity		
Complaints of less than usual number of stools, rectal fullness and pressure, pain on defecation; hard stools, <3 stools per week; diminished bowel sounds	Encourage fluid intake to point of moderate overhydration. Administer prune juice daily. Maintain diet high in bulk. Request order for stool softener from physician. Encourage frequent, short walks. Promote maintenance of regular habit of defecation consistent with preadmission pattern.	Regular evacuation (preferably daily) of soft or formed stools, prompt detection of constipation or impaction
NURSING DIAGNOSIS: High risk for injury: fractures and joint contractures related to decreased bone density, weakness, improper body alignment, and immobility		
Complaints of bone and joint pain, weakness, backache; impaired mobility, unsteady gait, uncoordinated movements; decrease in mental status	Maintain client in good body alignment. Assist client with ambulation. Reduce safety hazards in environment. Maintain bed in low position. Warn transportation aides and other hospital departments such as radiology department about handling and positioning client during tests.	No occurrence of deformity or accidental injury

Continued.

Table 44-12

 NURSING CARE PLAN FOR THE CLIENT WITH HYPERPARATHYROIDISM—cont'd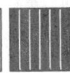

Defining Characteristics	Nursing Interventions	Evaluation Criteria
NURSING DIAGNOSIS: Body-image disturbance related to weight loss, weakness, fatigue, and mental status changes		
Verbalization of negative feelings about self; weakness, fatigue; inability to cope with usual activities; expression of feelings of hopelessness; hostile, angry behavior; self-isolation; weight loss	Encourage client to ventilate feelings about physical and emotional changes. Compliment client when appropriate. Reassure client that fatigability and depression will improve when hormone imbalance is corrected. Encourage short walks to sitting room or solarium. Ascertain which activities the client has enjoyed in past; encourage continued involvement in those activities that are appropriate to setting and client's condition. Reduce amount of gray and blue colors in environment; increase red, orange, and pure tones of yellow.	Statements and actions indicative of improved self-image, more positive mental outlook
NURSING DIAGNOSIS: Sensory/perceptual alterations related to slowed mentation, depression, and drowsiness		
Disorientation, inappropriate behavior or response, difficulty in concentrating	Orient client as indicated. Provide calm, restful environment. Explain actions in simple language. Avoid confusion and overstimulation. Monitor and record level of consciousness and orientation every shift.	Maintenance of reality-based orientation, appropriate actions and reactions

Hypoparathyroidism

Hypoparathyroidism, or inadequate circulating PTH, is not a common endocrine problem. It is characterized by hypocalcemia resulting from a lack of PTH to maintain serum calcium levels. PTH resistance at the cellular level may also occur (pseudohypoparathyroidism). This is a genetic defect resulting in hypocalcemia in spite of normal or high PTH levels and is often associated with hypothyroidism and hypogonadism.

Causes. The most common cause of hypoparathyroidism is accidental removal of or damage to the vascular supply of the glands during neck surgery (e.g., thyroidectomy, radical neck surgery).[18] Idiopathic hypoparathyroidism resulting from absence, fatty replacement, or atrophy of the glands is a rare disease that usually presents early in life and may be associated with other endocrine disorders. Affected clients may have parathyroid antibodies. Hypomagnesemia is increasingly being recognized as a cause of hypoparathyroidism. Hypomagnesemia, as seen in alcoholism or malabsorption, impairs PTH secretion and its action on bone and kidneys.

Clinical manifestations. The clinical features of hypoparathyroidism are due to a low serum calcium level (see Table 44-9). Sudden decreases in calcium ion concentration give rise to a syndrome called *tetany*. This state is characterized by tingling of the lips, hands, and occasionally feet, leading to increased muscle tension, paresthesias, and stiffness. Dysphagia, painful tonic spasms of smooth and skeletal musculature, a constricted feeling in the throat, and laryngospasms are also present. Chvostek's

sign (facial muscle spasm when the face is tapped below the temple) and Trousseau's phenomenon (carpopedal spasm when arterial circulation is interrupted by applying a blood pressure cuff for 3 minutes [see Fig. 10-13]) are usually positive. Respiratory function may be severely compromised by accessory muscle spasm and airway obstruction that are due to laryngospasms. Clients are usually markedly anxious and apprehensive. Abnormal laboratory findings include decreased serum calcium and PTH levels and increased serum phosphate levels.

Therapeutic management. The main objectives of treatment are (1) to treat tetany when present and (2) to prevent long-term complications by maintaining eucalcemia. Tetany is treated with IV infusion or slow push of calcium salts. Long-term therapy consists of the administration of vitamin D and possibly supplemental calcium and oral phosphate binders.

Pharmacological management. Emergency treatment of tetany requires the administration of IV calcium. Generally, 5 to 20 ml of a 10% solution is infused at a rate not to exceed 0.5 ml/min. Calcium salts can cause hypotension and cardiac arrest; thus, a slow IV push is required.[19] In addition, these salts can cause venous irritation and inflammation if leakage occurs into extravascular tissues. For long-term management, oral calcium supplements may be prescribed. Calcium carbonate, an antacid, is readily available but may alter acid-base balance. Calcium gluconate is available in tablet form and should be chewed into fine particles. It should be ingested when there is acid in the stomach and therefore should be taken at the end of

a meal. Oral calcium supplements are administered in four divided doses daily.

Hormone replacement is not used to treat hypoparathyroidism because of antibody formation, expense, and the need for parenteral administration. Vitamin D is used in chronic and resistant hypocalcemia to enhance intestinal calcium absorption and bone resorption. The preferred preparations are 1,25(OH)$_2$ vitamin D and 1,α25 dihydroxycholecalciferol (calcitriol, Rocaltrol). These drugs are more potent, raise calcium levels more rapidly, and are more quickly metabolized than previously used vitamin D preparations. The last factor is important, since vitamin D is a fat-soluble vitamin and can be toxic.

■ Nursing Management of Hypoparathyroidism

Nursing interventions

Acute intervention. Nursing care of a client with hypoparathyroidism requires close assessment for signs of tetany. The client should be observed closely for carpopedal spasm (Trousseau's phenomenon) while blood pressures are being taken because it is an early sign of tetany. Periodic assessment for Chvostek's sign is advisable. Tingling in the finger tips and around the mouth, irritability, anxiety, apprehension, muscular hypertonicity, and cramps may precede acute tetany.

If tetany or generalized muscle cramps develop, rebreathing may partially alleviate the symptoms. If clients can cooperate, they should be instructed to breathe in and out of a paper bag. This reduces carbon dioxide excretion from the lungs, increases carbonic acid levels in the blood, and lowers body pH. Because both solubility and the degree of ionization of calcium are enhanced in acidic environments, the proportion of total body calcium available in physiologically active form is increased, temporarily relieving the functional hypocalcemia. A client who is incapacitated by muscle spasms may be rebreathed by the nurse. The nurse places the open end of a plastic or rubber glove over the client's mouth and nose at the end of exhalation. The glove inflates with exhaled air, which is subsequently rebreathed. The glove should be removed every three to four respirations to allow one inhalation of fresh air to maintain adequate oxygenation.

IV calcium salts should be available at the bedside for treatment of acute tetany. Calcium salts must be infused slowly because high blood levels can cause serious cardiac dysrhythmias or cardiac arrest. Clients who have been digitalized are particularly vulnerable. Because ventricular standstill occurs in systole, this type of arrest is less likely than others to respond to resuscitation. ECG monitoring is appropriate. Side rails should be padded as a seizure precaution. Clients should be kept in a nonstimulating environment, assisted with hygienic needs, and given support and encouragement until they are free of symptoms.

Chronic management. Clients with hypoparathyroidism need instruction in the management of long-term diet and drug therapy. A high-calcium diet includes foods such as dark green vegetables, soy beans, and tofu. Calcium supplements are best administered 2 to 3 hours after meals. The client should be told that foods containing oxalic acid (e.g., spinach and rhubarb), phytic acid (e.g.,

bran and whole grains), and phosphorus reduce calcium absorption. Although calcium carbonate often leads to constipation and flatulence, bran and whole grain foods should not be used for treatment. Alternative nursing interventions may include providing stool softeners, adequate fluids, and fresh fruits.

The client should be instructed with written handouts about the signs and symptoms of hypocalcemia and hypercalcemia. The client should also be instructed to report these signs and symptoms to a clinician as soon as possible if they do occur. If manifestations of hypocalcemia occur, calcium supplementation should be increased. The need for lifelong treatment and health supervision should be stressed. The client's calcium levels should be monitored three to four times a year. Treatment modification is often necessary because hypercalcemia can develop without apparent cause. Thorough client instruction and frequent serum calcium assessment should allow a normal life expectancy. Clients need support and encouragement to continue cooperating with the regimen. They often dislike taking so many pills.

ADRENAL CORTEX
Cushing's Syndrome

Cushing's syndrome is a spectrum of clinical abnormalities caused by an excess of corticosteroids, particularly glucocorticoids. There are three main classifications of corticosteroids. *Glucocorticoids* regulate organic metabolism and are critical in the physiological stress response. *Mineralocorticoids* regulate sodium and potassium excretion. *Androgens* contribute to growth and development in both genders and to sexual activity in adult women. Several conditions can cause Cushing's syndrome (Table 44-13). Other causes include primary adrenal tumors and ectopic corticotropin production by extrapituitary-adrenal tumors (usually of the lung or pancreas). Cushing's disease and primary adrenal tumors are more common in females, whereas ectopic corticotropin production is more common in males. Spontaneously occurring Cushing's syndrome is most common in young to middle-aged adults.[20] Iatrogenic Cushing's syndrome can result from prolonged use of glucocorticoids.

Clinical manifestations. The clinical manifestations of Cushing's syndrome affect most body systems and are related to excess levels of corticosteroids (Table 44-14). Although manifestations of glucocorticoid excess usually predominate, symptoms of mineralocorticoid and androgen excess may also be apparent.

Table 44-13 Causes of Cushing's Syndrome

Corticotropin-secreting pituitary tumor (Cushing's disease)
Cortisol-secreting neoplasm within the adrenal cortex that can be either carcinoma or adenoma
Excess secretion of corticotropin by carcinoma of lung or other malignant growth outside either adenohypophysis or adrenals
Prolonged administration of high doses of corticosteroids

Table 44-14   Clinical Manifestations of Adrenal Cortical Hormone Dysfunction

System	Hypofunction	Hyperfunction
GLUCOCORTICOIDS		
General appearance	Weight loss, fever	Truncal (centripedal) obesity, thin extremities, rounding of face (moon face), fat deposits on back of neck and on shoulders ("buffalo hump")
Integumentary	Bronzed or smoky hyperpigmentation of face, neck, hands (especially creases), buccal membranes, nipples, genitalia, and scars (if pituitary function normal); vitiligo	Thin, fragile skin; purplish-red striae; petechial hemorrhages; bruises; florid cheeks (plethora); acne; poor wound healing
Cardiovascular	Hypotension, tendency to develop refractory shock, vasodilatation	Hypervolemia, hypertension, edema of lower extremities
Gastrointestinal	Anorexia, nausea and vomiting, cramping abdominal pain, diarrhea	Increase in secretion of pepsin and hydrochloric acid, anorexia
Urinary		Glycosuria, hypercalcinuria, kidney stones
Musculoskeletal	Fatigability	Muscle wasting in extremities, fatigue, osteoporosis, awkward gait, back and joint pain, weakness, growth retardation (in children)
Immune	Propensity toward autoimmune diseases	Inhibition of immune response, suppression of allergic response, inhibition of inflammation
Hematological	Anemia, lymphocytosis	Leukocytosis, lymphopenia, polycythemia, increased coagulability
Fluids and electrolytes	Hyponatremia, dehydration, hyperkalemia	Sodium and water retention, edema, hypokalemia
Metabolic	Hypoglycemia, insulin sensitivity	Glucose intolerance, negative nitrogen balance, hyperlipidemia
Emotional	Neurasthenia, depression, exhaustion or irritability, confusion, delusions	Psychic stimulation, euphoria, irritability, hypomania to depression, emotional lability
MINERALOCORTICOIDS		
Fluid and electrolytes	Sodium loss, decreased volume of extracellular fluid, hyperkalemia	Marked sodium and water retention, tendency toward edema, marked hypokalemia
Cardiovascular	Hypovolemia, tendency toward shock, decreased cardiac output, decreased heart size	Hypertension
ANDROGENS		
Integumentary	Decreased axillary and pubic hair (in women)	Hirsutism, acne
Reproductive	No effect in men, decreased libido in women	Menstrual irregularities in women, enlargement of clitoris, gynecomastia (in males)
Musculoskeletal	Decrease in muscle size and tone	Increase in muscle development

Glucocorticoid excess produces marked changes in personal appearance (Figs. 44-8 and 44-9). Obesity, facial plethora (redness), hirsutism, menstrual disorders, hypertension, and muscle weakness may be present. Catabolic processes are predominant, and wound healing is delayed. Mood disturbances (irritability, anxiety, euphoria), insomnia, irrationality, and occasionally, psychoses may occur.

The clinical presentation, as revealed by the history and physical examination, is the first indication of Cushing's syndrome. Of particular importance are (1) a combination of centripetal obesity and protein wasting as indicated by slender extremities and thin, friable skin; (2) "moon facies" (fullness of the face); (3) purplish-red striae on the abdomen, breast, or buttocks, which are usually depressed below the skin surface; (4) premenopausal osteoporosis; and (5) unexplained hypokalemia. Adrenal androgen excess may cause pronounced acne. In women, menstrual disorders and hirsutism are common.

Diagnostic studies. Abnormal findings may include polycythemia, hypokalemia, hyperglycemia, glycosuria, and osteoporosis as observed on x-rays. Plasma cortisol levels may be elevated, with loss of diurnal variation. Plasma corticotropin may be low, normal, or elevated depending on the underlying problem. When Cushing's syndrome is suspected, a 24-hour urine collection for free cortisol and a low-dose dexamethasone suppression test (see Chapter 42) are done. If these results are abnormal, a high-dose suppression test is done. False-positive results can occur in depressed clients, those under acute stress, and those who are practicing alcoholics. CT scanning and MRI may be used for tumor localization.

Therapeutic management. The treatment of choice for Cushing's disease is transsphenoidal surgical removal of the pituitary adenoma. Adrenalectomy is indicated for adrenal tumors or hyperplasia. Clients with ectopic corticotropin-secreting tumors are managed with treatment of the neoplasm. In inoperable cases or in cases in which residual disease remains, treatment with *o,p'* DDD (mitotane) may be used. This drug suppresses cortisol production, alters peripheral metabolism of steroids, and decreases plasma and urine steroid levels by actually killing adrenocortical cells. The action of this drug results in a "medical adrenalectomy." Metyrapone and aminoglutethimide may be used to inhibit cortisol synthesis. Occasionally, bilateral adrenalectomy is necessary (Table 44-15).

When surgical treatment of Cushing's syndrome is contraindicated, irradiation and pharmacological therapy may be used. Irradiation is most effective in children with Cushing's disease. Drug therapy includes mitotane, metyrapone, and aminoglutethimide. The relatively common side effects of these agents include anorexia, nausea and vomiting, depression, vertigo, skin rashes, and diplopia. Ketoconazole, which inhibits synthesis of gonadal and adrenal steroids, may also be used. The side effects from this medication are fewer than those of other adrenal suppressants. Radiation and drug therapy may be combined.

If Cushing's syndrome has developed during the course of prolonged administration of steroids, one or more of the following alternatives may be tried: (1) gradual discontinuance of steroid therapy, (2) reduction of the steroid dose,

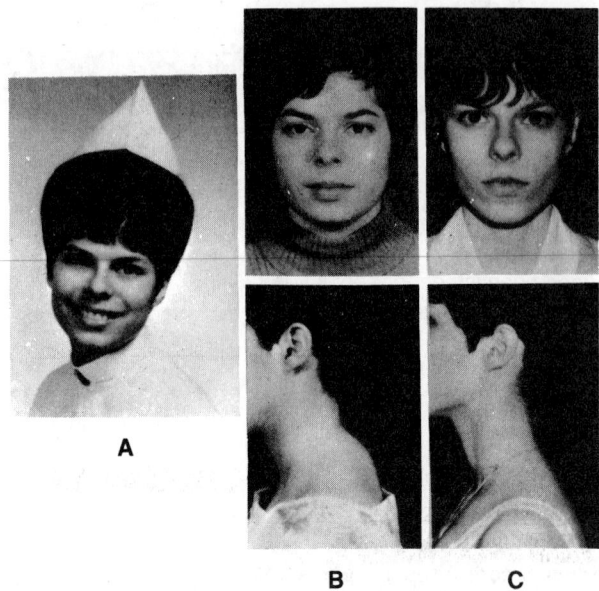

Fig. 44-8 A woman with Cushing's syndrome due to right adrenal cortical adenoma. **A,** Client at age 18, 2 years before surgery. **B,** Client at age 20, 1 month before surgery. **C,** Client at age 21, 1 year after surgery. (From Petersdorf RG and others, eds: Harrison's principles of internal medicine, vol 2, ed 12, New York, 1991, McGraw-Hill Book Co, Inc, p 1721.)

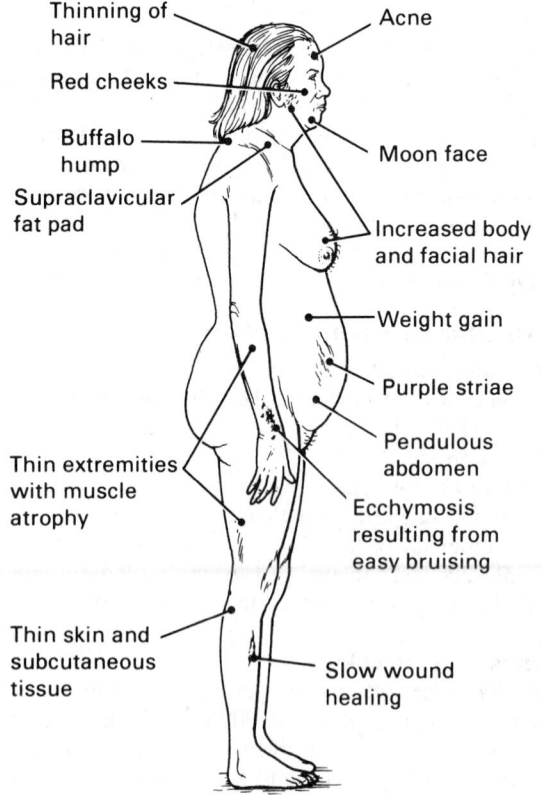

Fig. 44-9 Common characteristics of Cushing's syndrome.

Table 44-15

Diagnostic and Therapeutic Management: Cushing's Syndrome

DIAGNOSTIC

Complete history and physical examination
Plasma cortisol levels for diurnal variations
Complete blood count
Blood chemistries for sodium, potassium, glucose
Dexamethasone suppression test
24-hour urine for free cortisol
Examination of visual fields
CT scan, MRI

THERAPEUTIC

Adrenal cortical adenoma, carcinoma, or hyperplasia
  Surgical adrenalectomy
  Medical adrenalectomy
Pituitary corticotropin hypersecretion
  Transsphenoidal resection of microadenoma
  Radiation
  Treatment with hypothalamic serotonin antagonist
   (cyproheptadine)
Surgical removal of nonendocrine corticotropin-producing
  tumors, adrenalectomy (if tumors inoperable)
Discontinuance of or alteration in administration of exoge-
  nous corticosteroids

---

and/or (3) conversion to an alternate-day regimen. Gradual discontinuance is necessary to avoid potentially life-threatening adrenal insufficiency. An alternate-day regimen is a dosing regimen in which twice the daily dosage of a shorter-acting corticosteroid is given every other morning to minimize hypothalamic-pituitary-adrenal suppression, growth suppression, and altered habitus. This regimen is not used when the corticosteroids are given as physiological replacements.

■ Nursing Management of Cushing's Syndrome

Nursing assessment

Subjective and objective data that should be obtained from a client with Cushing's syndrome are presented in Table 44-16.

Nursing diagnoses

Nursing diagnoses are determined when the problem and etiological factors are supported by clinical data. Nursing diagnoses related to Cushing's syndrome may include, but are not limited to, those presented in Table 44-17.

Nursing interventions

Acute intervention. The client with Cushing's syndrome is seriously ill and debilitated. Because the therapeutic interventions have many side effects, the focus of daily assessment is on signs and symptoms of hormone and drug toxicity and complicating conditions such as cardiovascular disease, diabetes mellitus, infection, nephroli-

Table 44-16

Nursing Assessment of the Client with Cushing's Syndrome

SUBJECTIVE DATA

History
Pituitary tumor (Cushing's disease); adrenal, pancreatic, or pulmonary neoplasms; weight gain; frequent infections; GI bleeding; alcoholism
Medications
Use of corticosteroids
General
Weakness, emotional lability, anxiety, increased appetite, insomnia, fatigue
Pain
Headache; back, joint, and rib pain
Integumentary
Prolonged wound healing, easy bruising
Urinary
Polyuria
Reproductive
Amenorrhea, impotence, decreased libido
Neurological
Poor concentration and memory
Musculoskeletal
Muscle weakness

OBJECTIVE DATA

General
Truncal obesity, supraclavicular fat pads, buffalo hump, moon facies
Integumentary
Plethora; hirsutism; thin, friable skin; acne; petechiae; purpura; hyperpigmentation; purplish-red striae on breasts, buttocks, and abdomen
Cardiovascular
Hypertension, edema
Reproductive
Gynecomastia (in males), enlarged clitoris
Neurological
Poor coordination
Musculoskeletal
Muscle wasting, thin extremities
Possible findings
Hypokalemia, hyperglycemia, leukocytosis, polycythemia, elevated plasma cortisol and corticotropin levels; abnormal dexamethasone suppression test; elevated free cortisol, 17 ketosteroids on urine testing; osteoporosis on chest x-ray examination

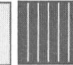

Table 44-17

NURSING CARE PLAN FOR THE CLIENT WITH CUSHING'S SYNDROME

Defining Characteristics	Nursing Interventions	Evaluation Criteria

NURSING DIAGNOSIS: High risk for infection related to exposure to environmental pathogens and suppression of immune system secondary to hypercortisolism

Immunosuppressive therapy, inadequate protein stores, proteinuria, muscle wasting, poor wound healing	Assess potential infection sites such as urinary and respiratory tracts, skin, and IV lines. Monitor temperature and white blood cell count. Provide private room, if possible. Maintain meticulous asepsis and prevent contact with contagious individuals. Instruct client in self-care practices to avoid infection (e.g., hand washing). Refer client to dietitian for high-protein diet instruction. Instruct client and family in signs and symptoms of infection and to report these to clinician immediately.	Infection not developed; detection and treatment of any infectious process, verbalization of signs and symptoms of infection by client and family, planning to provide high-protein diet by client and family

NURSING DIAGNOSIS: High risk for injury: fracture related to decreased muscle strength, fatigue, osteoporosis, and increased protein catabolism

Complaints of weakness, fatigue, back and rib pain; difficulty in ambulating, impairment in mobility; impairment in judgment; drowsiness; hypocalcemia	Assist client as necessary with ambulation and self-care. Provide cane or walker as necessary. Keep side rails up if client's judgment is impaired. Provide quiet environment and rest periods as indicated. Refer to dietitian for instruction in high-calcium diet. Reinforce dietary instructions. Instruct client and family in provision of a safe environment (e.g., non-skid surfaces in wet areas, use of railings, good lighting). Orient client to new surroundings.	No accidental injury, ability of client and family to list high-calcium foods

NURSING DIAGNOSIS: Altered nutrition: more than body requirements related to increased appetite, high caloric content of foods, and inactivity

Statement of increased appetite; preference for fatty, sweet foods; weight 10% or more than optimum for height; inappropriate menu choices	Obtain dietary consult for instruction in low-caloric, high-nutrition diet (including protein and calcium). Reinforce dietary instructions. Assist with appropriate menu choices. Provide low-calorie, high-vitamin snacks. Instruct in or refer to psychologist for instruction in behavior modification techniques related to eating.	Maintenance of body weight or loss of no more than 1 to 2 lb per week

NURSING DIAGNOSIS: Sensory/perceptual alterations related to hormone imbalance

Complaints of "feeling blue," sadness, helplessness, worthlessness, insomnia; euphoric statements; self-isolation; distressed, tearful, sad appearance; inability to concentrate; poor grooming and personal hygiene; hypomanic behavior	Explain to client and family that feelings are related to hormone imbalance. Provide quiet diversionary activities. Ensure adequate rest periods, short periods of socialization. Provide resources for adequate grooming. Assist client and family in problem solving. Instruct client in relaxation techniques.	Verbalization of feelings about client's emotional state by client and family, identification and verbalization of personal strengths and coping mechanisms, exhibition of good grooming and personal hygiene

Continued.

Table 44-17

NURSING CARE PLAN FOR THE CLIENT WITH CUSHING'S SYNDROME—cont'd

Defining Characteristics	Nursing Interventions	Evaluation Criteria
NURSING DIAGNOSIS: Self-esteem disturbance related to altered body image, emotional lability, and diminished physical capabilities secondary to hormone imbalance		
Verbalization of negative feelings regarding personal appearance, inability to perform usual activities, poor grooming and hygiene, truncal obesity, moon face, acne, plethora, buffalo hump, excess body hair, bruises, edema	Explain to client and family that physical and emotional changes are related to hormone imbalance. Accept and respect client as a person. Encourage good grooming and use of attractive attire. Compliment client when appropriate. Reassure client that most manifestations of disease will disappear when hormone imbalance is corrected.	Verbalization of acceptance of appearance by client and family, use of self-care methods to improve appearance
NURSING DIAGNOSIS: Impaired skin integrity related to excess steroids, immobility, and altered skin fragility		
Edema; thin, fragile skin; impaired healing	Protect client from bumping and bruising. Change client's position frequently. Provide good skin care, particularly to edematous areas and areas over bony prominences. Assist client with ambulation as tolerated.	Intact skin

thiasis, and pathological fractures. Daily nursing assessment includes the following:

1. Vital signs every 4 hours, particularly blood pressure
2. Daily weights (gain possibly indicating volume excess)
3. Signs and symptoms of infection, especially pain, loss of function, and purulent drainage, since other signs and symptoms of inflammation may be minimal or absent
4. Location, time, and duration of abdominal pain
5. Signs of abnormal thromboembolic phenomena, such as sudden chest pain, dyspnea, or tachypnea
6. Capillary or urine glucose
7. Bone pain or limitations of range of motion, especially in the lower back
8. Changes in mental status, particularly depression

Clients need a great deal of emotional support. Changes in appearance such as centripedal obesity, multiple bruises, hirsutism in females, and gynecomastia in males can be very distressing. Clients may feel unattractive, repulsive, or unwanted. The nurse can help by remaining sensitive to those feelings and offering respect and unconditional acceptance. Clients can be reassured that the physical changes and much of the emotional lability stem from the hormone toxicity and will resolve with normal hormone levels. If the cortisol hypersecretion is caused by pituitary hypersecretion of corticotropin, a transsphenoidal tumor resection may be done.

Interventions related to surgery. If treatment involves surgical removal of the adenoma, the primary tumor, or one or both of the adrenal glands, nursing care will have an additional focus on preoperative and postoperative care. Surgery on glandular structures poses risks beyond those of other types of operations. Because glands are highly vascular, the risk of hemorrhage is increased. Manipulation of glandular tissue during surgery may release large amounts of hormone into the circulation, producing marked fluctuations in the metabolic processes affected by these hormones.

PREOPERATIVE MANAGEMENT. Before surgery the client should be brought to optimal physical condition. Hypertension and hyperglycemia are controlled and hypokalemia is corrected with diet and potassium supplements. A high-protein diet helps correct the protein depletion caused by excess glucocorticoids.

Although adrenalectomy is uncommon, clients experiencing this procedure should be aware that IV infusions and nasogastric suctioning are likely after surgery. Information and instruction about exercises, coughing, and deep breathing are particularly important, since clients are prone to thrombosis and infection. If the surgical approach is abdominal, the incision will be high in the abdomen, increasing the difficulty in coughing and deep breathing.

POSTOPERATIVE MANAGEMENT. Because of hormone fluctuations, blood pressure, fluid balance, and electrolyte levels tend to be unstable after surgery. High doses of cortisone are administered IV during surgery and for several days af-

terward to ensure adequate responses to the stress of the procedure. If large amounts of endogenous hormone have been released into the systemic circulation during surgery, the client is likely to develop hypertension, increasing the risk of hemorrhage. High levels of cortisone also increase susceptibility to infection and delay healing.

Any rapid or significant changes in blood pressure, respirations, or heart rate should be reported. Fluid intake and output should be monitored carefully and assessed for potential imbalance. The critical period for circulatory instability ranges from 24 to 48 hours after surgery. IV corticosteroids are given, and the dose and rate of flow are adjusted to the client's clinical manifestations and fluid and electrolyte balance. Oral doses are given as tolerated. The IV line may be kept in place after IV corticosteroids are withdrawn to keep a line open for quick administration of corticosteroids or vasopressors.

If cortisone dosage is tapered too rapidly after surgery, acute adrenal insufficiency may develop. Vomiting after the nasogastric tube is removed, increased weakness, dehydration, and hypotension may indicate hypocortisolism. In addition, clients may complain of painful joints, pruritus, or peeling skin, and they may experience severe emotional disturbances. These signs and symptoms should be reported so that drug doses can be adjusted. The nurse must constantly be alert for signs of glucocorticoid imbalance. After surgery the client is usually maintained on bed rest until the blood pressure stabilizes. The nurse must be alert for subtle signs of postoperative infections, since the usual immune and inflammatory responses are suppressed. Meticulous care must be used when changing the dressing and during any other procedures that necessitate access to body cavities, to circulation, or to areas under the skin so that infection is prevented.

CHRONIC INTERVENTION. The discharge instructions are based on the client's lack of endogenous cortisol and resulting inability to react to stressors physiologically. Clients should wear Medic-Alert bracelets at all times and carry medical identification and instructions in a wallet or purse. Exposure to extremes of temperature, infections, and emotional disturbances should be avoided as much as possible. Stress may produce or precipitate acute adrenal insufficiency because any remaining adrenal tissue cannot meet the increased hormonal demands. Many clients can be taught to adjust their corticosteroid replacement therapy in accordance with their stress levels. The nurse should consult with each client's physician to determine the parameters for dosage changes if this plan is feasible. If clients cannot adjust their own medication or if weakness, fainting, fever, or nausea and vomiting occur, clients should contact their physicians for a possible adjustment in corticosteroid dosage. Lifetime replacement therapy is required by many clients, but it may take several months to adjust the hormonal dose satisfactorily.

Adrenocortical Insufficiency

Adrenocortical insufficiency (hypofunction of the adrenal cortex) may be primary (Addison's disease) or secondary due to a lack of corticotropin. In Addison's disease, all three classes of adrenal steroids (glucocorticoids, mineral-ocorticoids, and androgens) are reduced. In secondary adrenocortical insufficiency, corticosteroids and androgens are deficient but mineralocorticoids rarely are. Corticotropin deficiency may be caused by pituitary disease or suppression of the hypothalamic-pituitary axis as a result of the administration of exogenous glucocorticoids.[21]

Addison's disease. The most common cause of Addison's disease (which is a rare condition) is idiopathic atrophy, an autoimmune disease in which adrenal tissue is destroyed by antibodies formed against the client's own adrenal tissue. Often, other endocrine conditions are present, such as polyglandular endocrine failure. In the past, tuberculosis was a common cause of Addison's disease, but this is now rare in areas in which tuberculosis is controlled. Less common causes include hemorrhage, infarction, fungal infections (e.g., histoplasmosis, coccidioidomycosis), acquired immunodeficiency syndrome (AIDS), and metastatic cancer.[20] Iatrogenic Addison's disease may be due to anticoagulant therapy (causing adrenal hemorrhage), antineoplastic chemotherapy, bilateral adrenalectomy, or abrupt withdrawal of exogenous steroids.

Clinical manifestations. Progressive weakness, weight loss, and anorexia are primary features at diagnosis. Skin hyperpigmentation, a striking feature, is seen primarily in sun-exposed areas of the body, at pressure points, over joints, and in creases, especially palmar creases. It is most likely due to increased secretion of β-lipotropin or corticotropin, caused by hypocortisolism and the resultant lack of negative feedback on these tropic hormones. Other frequent manifestations are hypotension, hyponatremia, hyperkalemia, nausea and vomiting, and diarrhea. The most dangerous feature of Addison's disease is hypotension, which may cause shock, especially during stress. Circulatory collapse from this cause is unresponsive to the usual treatment (vasopressors and fluid replacement) and requires glucocorticoid administration to stabilize the hypotension.

Acute adrenal insufficiency. Adrenocortical insufficiency may be primary as a result of destruction of the adrenal cortex or secondary because of a lack of corticotropin stimulation. Clients with primary adrenal disease are cachectic, darkly pigmented, and hypotensive, whereas those with secondary adrenal insufficiency have pale skin and complain of weakness, lethargy, fatigability, loss of appetite, and nausea. Clients with either primary or secondary adrenocortical insufficiency are at risk for acute adrenal insufficiency (addisonian crisis), which is a life-threatening emergency caused by insufficient adrenocortical hormones or a sudden marked decrease in these hormones. It may occur during (1) stress (e.g., from infection, surgery, trauma, hemorrhage, or psychological distress), (2) sudden withdrawal of adrenocortical hormone replacement therapy (which is often done by a client who lacks knowledge of the importance of replacement therapy), (3) adrenal surgery, or (4) sudden pituitary gland destruction (pituitary apoplexy).

Severe manifestations of cortisol and aldosterone deficiencies are exhibited, including hypotension (particularly postural), tachycardia, dehydration, confusion, hyponatremia, hypoglycemia, and hyperkalemia. GI manifesta-

tions include nausea, vomiting, diarrhea, and vague abdominal pain.

Diagnostic studies. The diagnosis of Addison's disease is made in conjunction with the presence of clinical features, along with low cortisol levels. Other abnormal laboratory findings include hyperkalemia, hypochloremia, hyponatremia, hypoglycemia, and increased BUN level. Urine-free cortisol is low. A failure of cortisol levels to rise in response to ACTH stimulation indicates primary adrenal disease. A positive response to corticotropin points to probable pituitary disease (see Table 42-8).

Therapeutic and pharmacological management. Tuberculosis is treated if present. The mainstay of treatment is replacement therapy with glucocorticoids and mineralocorticoids (Table 44-18). Glucocorticoids are divided into doses: two thirds in the morning and one third in the afternoon. Mineralocorticoids are given once daily, preferably in the evening. This dosage schedule reflects normal circadian rhythm in endogenous hormone secretion and decreases the side effects associated with steroid replacement therapy. When any illness or stress associated with daily living occurs—mild or acute—glucocorticoid dosage must be increased to prevent adrenal crisis. Examples of situations requiring steroid adjustment are the flu, extraction of teeth, and rigorous physical activity such as playing tennis on a hot day or running a marathon. The client should take two to three times the usual dose and notify the clinician. When in doubt, it is better to err on the side of overreplacement. If vomiting or diarrhea occurs, as may happen with the flu, the clinician must be notified immediately because electrolyte replacement may be necessary. In addition, these symptoms may be early indicators of crisis. Overall, however, clients who take their medications consistently can anticipate a normal life.

Management of acute adrenocortical insufficiency (addisonian crisis) requires immediate glucocorticoid replacement therapy. Treatment must be vigorous and directed toward shock management. IV hydrocortisone 100 mg every 6 hours, sodium, fluids, and dextrose (for hypoglycemia) are necessary for 24 hours or until blood pressure returns to normal.[20]

■ Nursing Management of Addison's Disease

Nursing assessment

Nursing assessment related to the client with Addison's disease includes assessment of subjective data such as weight loss, increased paleness, loss of body hair, anorexia, salt craving, nausea and vomiting, cramping abdominal pain, and diarrhea. Clients may also complain of exhaustion, profound weakness, inability to perform usual activities, muscle aches, lightheadedness, lack of interest in usual activities and relationships, confusion, inability to tolerate any stress, decreased libido, and amenorrhea.

Objective data found in the nursing assessment may include emaciation, pale skin (but bronzed in sun-exposed areas, scars, buccal mucosa, and genitalia), and sparse body hair (particularly axillary and genital). Skin tenting (delayed return of skin to flat position after pinching) may be observed with poor skin turgor. Hypotension (particularly postural), decreased cardiac output and heart size, muscle wasting, and weakness may also be present. Laboratory values may indicate hyponatremia, hyperkalemia, hypoglycemia, low serum cortisol, increased serum corticotropin, decreased 24-hour urine-free cortisol, and lack of response to corticotropin stimulation test (see Table 42-8). Irritability, confusion, disorientation, or depression may also be noted.

Nursing diagnoses

Nursing diagnoses related to the client with Addison's disease may include, but are not limited to, the following:

1. Activity intolerance related to weakness and hypotension
2. Self-care deficit related to weakness, lack of interest, and depression
3. Potential complication: hypotension related to volume depletion
4. Altered nutrition: less than body requirements related to weakness, anorexia, and nausea and vomiting
5. Self-esteem disturbance related to inability to perform usual activities, loss of hair, skin hyperpigmentation, and diagnosis of chronic illness
6. Altered health maintenance related to lack of knowledge of management of lifelong hormonal replacement therapy
7. Decreased cardiac output related to low blood pressure and volume depletion
8. Altered sexuality patterns related to weakness, malaise, depression, and changing self-concept

Nursing interventions

Acute intervention. Because the client is physiologically unstable, frequent nursing assessment is necessary. Vital signs and signs of fluid volume deficit and electrolyte imbalance should be assessed every 30 minutes to 4 hours for the first 24 hours depending on the client's instability. In addition, the following nursing assessments and orders should be included: daily weighing, diligent steroid administration, protection against exposure to infection (reverse isolation), and complete assistance with daily hygiene.

Table 44-18

Diagnostic and Therapeutic Management: Addison's Disease

DIAGNOSTIC

Complete history and physical examination
Plasma cortisol levels
Serum electrolytes
ACTH-stimulation test
Tuberculin test
CT scan

THERAPEUTIC

Daily cortisone replacement (two thirds on awakening in morning, one third in late afternoon)*
Daily fluorocortisone in afternoon*
Salt additives for excess heat or humidity

---

*For conditions of normal daily stress in individuals with usual daytime activity.

Clients should be protected from noise, light, and environmental temperature extremes. They cannot cope with these stresses, since they cannot produce corticosteroids.

Clients usually respond by the second day and can start oral corticosteroid replacement. Because discharge frequently occurs before the usual maintenance dose of 30 to 40 mg of corticosteroids is reached, clients should be instructed on the importance of keeping scheduled follow-up appointments.

Chronic management. The nurse has an important role in the long-term management of Addison's disease. Because of the serious nature of the disease and the need for lifelong replacement therapy, a well-organized and carefully presented teaching plan is vital to the health of the client. Table 44-19 outlines the major areas that must be included in the teaching plan. The nurse should consult with the client's physician to determine whether any special problems or topics must be included in the plan.

Because clients with Addison's disease are unable to tolerate physical or emotional stress, long-term care revolves around recognizing the need for additional replacement medication and techniques for stress management. Clients who can control or manage the degree of stress they experience maintain better hormone balance than those who cannot. The nurse should help clients develop good coping skills and techniques for handling stress.

A hormone-deficient client receiving glucocorticoid replacement is less apt to exhibit toxic symptoms from the medication than a client receiving pharmacological doses of these drugs. Because the aim of replacement therapy is to return to normal hormone levels, nursing care is designed to help the client maintain hormone balance and manage the medication regimen.

Dosage schedules are designed to mimic the diurnal rhythm of endogenous glucocorticoid production. Two thirds of the daily dose should be taken on arising at the beginning of the day; the remaining one third should be taken about 8 hours later. Because glucocorticoids are stimulating to the CNS, they may cause insomnia if taken late in the evening. The need for glucocorticoid hormone is proportional to stress levels. A client who cannot produce endogenous hormone must adjust the dose of exogenous hormone to the stress level. Doses are usually doubled when minor stress occurs (e.g., a respiratory infection or a visit to the dentist) and tripled when major stress occurs.

Clients must be taught the signs and symptoms of glucocorticoid deficiency and excess. These should be reported to their physicians so that dosages may be adjusted to each client's need. It is also important that clients wear identification bands stating that they have Addison's disease so that appropriate therapy can be initiated in case of an unexpected trauma, accident, or crisis.

Clients should have an emergency kit with them at all times. The kit should consist of 100 mg of IM hydrocortisone, syringes, and instructions for use. Clients and significant others should be instructed in how to give an injection in case the replacement therapy cannot be taken orally.

GLUCOCORTICOID THERAPY

Cortisone and related glucocorticoids are used to relieve the signs and symptoms associated with many disease processes (Table 44-20). The long-term administration of glucocorticoids in therapeutic doses often leads to serious complications and side effects; therefore, glucocorticoid

---

Table 44-19 Client Education Related to Addison's Disease

Names and dosages of drugs
Actions of drugs
Symptoms of overdosage and underdosage
Conditions requiring increased medication (e.g., trauma, infection, surgery, emotional crisis)
Course of action to take relative to changes in need for medication
    Increase in dose of glucocorticoid
    Administration of large dose of glucocorticoid IM
    Consultation with clinician
Prevention of infection and need for prompt and vigorous treatment of existing infections
Need for lifelong replacement therapy
Need for lifelong medical supervision
Need for medical identification device

Table 44-20 Pharmacological Uses of Glucocorticoids

HORMONE REPLACEMENT

Adrenal insufficiency	Congenital adrenal hyperplasia

THERAPEUTIC EFFECT

Arthritis	Eye disease
Rheumatoid carditis	Inflammation
Nephrotic syndrome	Skin diseases
Collagen diseases	GI diseases
Giant cell arteritis	Chronic ulcerative colitis
Mixed connective tissue disorders	Inflammatory bowel disease
Polymyositis	Nontropical sprue
Polyarteritis nodosa	Regional enteritis
Systemic lupus erythematosus	Neurological disease
Allergic reactions	Prevention of cerebral edema and increased intracranial pressure
Anaphylaxis	
Bee stings	Malignancies, some tumors
Contact dermatitis	
Drug reactions	Head trauma
Serum sickness	Liver diseases
Urticaria	Alcoholic hepatitis
Pulmonary diseases	Chronic active hepatitis
Aspiration pneumonia	Subacute necrotic necrosis
Bronchial asthma	
Chronic obstructive pulmonary disease	Immunosuppression (after organ transplantation)

therapy is not recommended for minor chronic conditions. Rather, therapy should be reserved for diseases in which there is a risk of death or permanent loss of function and conditions in which short-term therapy is likely to produce remission or recovery. The potential benefits of treatment must always be weighed against the risks.

Effects

The therapeutic actions of glucocorticoids include the following:

1. Antiinflammatory action: Glucocorticoids stabilize lysosomal membranes, thus inhibiting release of proteolytic enzymes during inflammation; inhibit phagocytosis; and prevent or suppress redness, swelling, tenderness, heat, and local edema.
2. Immunosuppression: Glucocorticoids cause atrophy of lymphoid tissue, suppress cell-mediated hypersensitivity, and decrease production of lymphocytes and antibodies.
3. Maintenance of normal blood pressure: Glucocorticoids potentiate the vasoconstrictor effect of norepinephrine and act on the renal tubules to increase sodium resorption and enhance potassium and hydrogen excretion. Retention of sodium (and subsequently water) increases blood volume and helps maintain blood pressure.
4. Carbohydrate and protein metabolic effect: Glucocorticoids have an antiinsulin effect and can induce glucose intolerance by increasing glycogenolysis and insulin resistance. They also stimulate the breakdown of protein for gluconeogenesis, which can lead to muscle wasting. Although corticosteroids mobilize free fatty acids and redistribute fat in cushingoid patterns, the mechanism for this process is unknown. Corticosteroids also decrease the conversion of T_4 to T_3.

Complications

Beneficial and toxic effects of the glucocorticoids stem from their physiological actions. A beneficial effect in one situation may be a harmful one in another. Thus the vasopressive effect of the hormone is critical in enabling the organism to function in stressful situations but can produce hypertension when the substance is used for drug therapy. Inhibition of cell division is therapeutic and sometimes curative in the treatment of malignancies, but it slows healing after trauma or surgery. Suppression of inflammation and the immune response may help save the lives of the victim of anaphylaxis and the transplant recipient, but it causes reactivation of latent tuberculosis and greatly reduces resistance to other infections. Specific side effects related to glucocorticoid therapy are listed in Table 44-21.

■ Nursing Management of the Client Receiving Glucocorticoid Therapy

Many clients receive glucocorticoid therapy for nonendocrine reasons (see Table 44-20), and thorough instruction is necessary to ensure client cooperation. Steroids are taken once daily or once every other day. They should be taken early in the morning with food to decrease gastric irritation. These medications are usually administered for

Table 44-21 Side Effects of Glucocorticoid Therapy

Susceptibility to infection is increased. Infection develops more rapidly and spreads more widely in the cushingoid individual.

Blood pressure is increased due to excess blood volume and potentiation of vasoconstrictor effects. Hypertension in turn predisposes client to cardiac failure.

Glucose intolerance affects more than 90% of individuals with cushingoid patterns.

Protein depletion decreases bone formation, density, and strength and predisposes client to pathological fractures, especially compression fractures of the vertebrae (osteoporosis).

Decreased mucus production predisposes client to stomach and duodenal ulceration (peptic ulcer).

Clients undergoing surgery are at increased risk for dehiscence and evisceration. Healing is delayed.

Hypokalemia may develop, and potassium supplements may be indicated.

Skeletal muscle atrophy occurs, and muscle weakness predisposes client to accidental injury.

Suppression of pituitary corticotropin synthesis occurs. Glucocorticoid deficiency is likely if hormones are withdrawn abruptly.

Hypocalcemia related to anti–vitamin D effect may occur.

Mood and behavior changes (feelings of invulnerability and depression) may be observed.

Fat from extremities is redistributed to trunk and face.

---

chronic conditions, and client education is a major nursing intervention. Because exogenous corticosteroid administration may suppress endogenous corticotropin and therefore endogenous cortisol (suppression is time- and dose-dependent), the danger of abrupt cessation of glucocorticoid therapy must be emphasized to clients and significant others. Further instruction and interventions to minimize the side effects and complications of glucocorticoid therapy include the following:

1. A diet high in protein, calcium (at least 1500 mg/day), and potassium but low in fat and concentrated simple carbohydrates such as sugar, honey, syrups, and candy
2. Assistance in identifying measures to ensure adequate rest and sleep, such as daily naps and avoidance of caffeine late in the day
3. Instruction about how to recognize edema and ways to restrict sodium intake to less that 2000 mg/day if it occurs
4. Instruction in weekly home monitoring of blood pressure or location of places near home, such as fire stations, where blood pressure may be monitored regularly if home monitoring is not possible
5. Instruction in urine or capillary glucose monitoring, symptoms of hyperglycemia (e.g., polydipsia, polyuria, blurred vision), and glycosuria (glucose in the urine) and the need to report hyperglycemic symptoms and glycosuria

6. Instruction to notify a clinician if the client experiences postprandial heartburn or epigastric pain that is not relieved by antacids
7. Instruction in safety measures, such as getting up slowly and using good lighting to avoid accidental injury
8. Instruction about maintaining good hygiene practices and avoiding contact with persons with colds or other contagious illnesses so that infection is avoided

Disorders of Aldosterone Secretion

Primary hyperaldosteronism. Primary hyperaldosteronism (aldosteronism) is characterized by excessive aldosterone secretion caused by adrenal adenoma (65%) or bilateral adrenal hyperplasia (34%). This disorder is seen in 0.05% to 2% of clients with essential hypertension. It is more common in women, and the usual age of diagnosis is between 20 and 50 years. The main effects of aldosterone are sodium retention and potassium excretion. Thus the hallmark of this disease is hypertension with hypokalemia.

The most common features are sodium retention and excessive urinary potassium loss. The hypernatremia leads to hypertension and headache. The hypokalemia causes generalized muscle weakness, tiredness, cardiac dysrhythmias, glucose intolerance, nocturia, and metabolic alkalosis that may lead to tetany.[22] Edema is not evident because the excess sodium is not retained in the intravascular space.

The diagnosis should be suspected in all clients with hypokalemia and hypertension who are not being treated with diuretics. It is confirmed by increased plasma aldosterone, serum sodium, and potassium levels; 24-hour urine collection for sodium and potassium levels; an IV saline infusion test; and decreased plasma renin activity. Adenomas are localized by means of a CT scan.

The treatment for adenoma is unilateral adrenalectomy. Before surgery, clients should be treated with a low-sodium diet, potassium-sparing diuretics, and antihypertensive agents to control serum potassium levels and blood pressure. Hypertension and hypokalemia are treated with potassium-sparing diuretics or angiotensin-converting enzyme inhibitors. Spironolactone (Aldactone) is a competitive antagonist for the mineralocorticoid receptor in the terminal distal tubule and collecting duct and increases excretion of sodium and water and retention of potassium. Potassium supplements and sodium restrictions are also necessary. Potassium supplementation and a potassium-sparing diuretic should not be started simultaneously because of the danger of hyperkalemia. Clients with bilateral hyperplasia are treated therapeutically with spironolactone (Aldactone); amiloride (Midamor), which is a potassium-sparing diuretic; or aminoglutethimide, which blocks aldosterone synthesis.[23]

Nursing care includes careful assessment for signs of hypokalemia, tetany, fluid and electrolyte imbalance, and cardiovascular status. Blood pressure should be monitored frequently before and after surgery because unilateral adrenalectomy is successful in controlling hypertension in only 50% of clients with adenoma.

Clients receiving maintenance therapy with spironolactone (Aldactone) or amiloride (Midanor) need instruction regarding the possible side effects of gynecomastia, impotence, and menstrual disorders as well as knowledge about the signs and symptoms of hypokalemia and hyperkalemia. Clients should be taught how to monitor their own blood pressure and the need for frequent monitoring. The need for continued health supervision should be stressed.

Secondary hyperaldosteronism. Secondary hyperaldosteronism is a pathological condition that occurs in response to an extraadrenal stimulus, often angiotensin, renal artery stenosis, or juxtaglomerular cell tumors. If treatment of the primary disorder is not possible, angiotensin-converting enzyme inhibitors are useful in inhibiting the powerful vasoconstrictive property of this substance.

Adrenogenital syndrome. The adrenal glands normally produce small amounts of androgen. Overproduction of these hormones leads to adrenogenital syndromes such as congenital adrenal hyperplasia.[24] Causes of congenital adrenal hyperplasia syndromes are tumors and congenital enzymatic deficiencies leading to hypocortisolism. The hypocortisolism causes increased corticotropin, which overstimulates the adrenals and causes hypertrophy and excess androgen production.[25] The onset of symptoms may occur from birth to early adult life. Males show precocious sexual development, and females show signs of masculinization and menstrual irregularities.

Adrenal Medulla

Pheochromocytoma. Disorders of the adrenal medulla are rare. There are no specific diseases caused by insufficiency of catecholamines (epinephrine and norepinephrine). The most common disorder of the adrenal medulla is pheochromocytoma, a neoplasm that produces excessive catecholamines. Most of these tumors (95%) are benign and encapsulated.[26] Pheochromocytoma can occur at any age and in either gender, but it is found most commonly in clients between the ages of 40 and 60.

The most striking clinical features are episodic hypertension, hypermetabolism, and hyperglycemia. Attacks of paroxysmal hypertension are due to sympathetic nervous system stimulation and are often accompanied by anxiety, palpitations, and profuse sweating. Attacks may be provoked by exercise, sexual activity, hyperventilation, compression or palpation of the tumor, postural change, emotional distress, surgery, and major trauma.[27] Additional symptoms may include throbbing and severe headaches, vasomotor changes (e.g., pallor, facial flushing, pupil dilatation), orthostatic hypotension, and visual blurring. The duration of the attacks may vary from a few minutes to several hours.

■ Therapeutic and Nursing Management of Pheochromocytoma

Measurement of urinary metanephrines is the simplest and most reliable test. Values are elevated in at least 90% of persons with pheochromocytoma. CT scans and MRI are used for tumor localization.

Treatment consists of surgical removal of the tumor. Although rare, this is one of the few conditions in which dangerously high blood pressure can be corrected surgically.

Case finding is an important nursing function. Any client with hypertension accompanied by symptoms of sympathoadrenal discharge should be referred to a physician for definitive diagnosis.

Before surgery the client is hospitalized for treatment to correct symptoms such as hypovolemia and cardiovascular complications to decrease the risk of surgery. Sympathetic blocking agents are administered to reduce the blood pressure and alleviate other symptoms of catecholamine excess. Because this management may result in orthostatic hypotension, the client must be advised to make postural changes cautiously. Clients need rest, nourishing food, and emotional support during this period. Preoperative and postoperative care is similar to the interventions for any client undergoing adrenalectomy except that blood pressure fluctuations from catecholamine imbalances tend to be severe and need to be carefully monitored.

C ase Study

GRAVES' DISEASE

Sally C., a 43-year-old woman, was admitted to a large county hospital with a fever of 40.6° C (105° F). Her history included recent job loss because of inability to cope with job stress, fatigue, unintentional weight loss, insomnia, palpitations, and heat intolerance. Her evaluation included an endocrine workup, and she was diagnosed as having Graves' disease. A subtotal thyroidectomy was planned for 2 months later, and she was started on propylthiouracil and propranolol.

Discussion Questions

1. What caused the client's symptoms and what prompted the endocrine workup? Why would an endocrine workup not have been done?
2. What laboratory tests were done to diagnose Graves' disease? What were the probable results?
3. Why was surgery delayed and what was the purpose of the pharmacological intervention?
4. What are the client's immediate learning needs and her learning needs before and after surgery?
5. What are the nursing interventions for successful long-term management of this client after the subtotal thyroidectomy?

R eview Questions

The number of the question corresponds to the same-numbered objective at the beginning of the chapter.

1. The client with GH excess exhibits all of the following *except*
   a. hypoglycemia
   b. abnormal bone growth
   c. abdominal distention
   d. visual changes
2. Clients who have experienced intracranial surgery or head trauma are more likely than clients who have experienced other types of surgery or trauma to develop
   a. diabetes mellitus
   b. hyperthyroidism
   c. Cushing's syndrome
   d. SIADH
3. A client with an enlarged thyroid usually exhibits all of the following *except*
   a. history of goiter
   b. exophthalmos
   c. hyperthyroidism
   d. female gender
4. If the parathyroid glands are removed accidentally during neck surgery, the client may develop
   a. kidney stones
   b. difficulty in swallowing
   c. thyroid crisis
   d. tetany
5. An important nursing intervention when caring for a client with Cushing's syndrome is to
   a. administer steroids in equal doses
   b. protect the client from exposure to infection
   c. restrict protein intake
   d. observe for signs of hypotension
6. After an adrenalectomy for pheochromocytoma, the client is most apt to experience
   a. hyperglycemia
   b. marked sodium and water retention
   c. hypokalemia
   d. marked fluctuations in blood pressure
7. Nursing assessment for fluid volume imbalance includes all of the following *except*
   a. urine acetone
   b. intake and output
   c. urine specific gravity
   d. daily weighings
8. The side effects of steroid therapy include all of the following *except*
   a. cushingoid appearance
   b. peptic ulcers
   c. insomnia
   d. hypoglycemia
9. The client needs to know that the best time to take cortisone for replacement purposes is
   a. every other day on awakening
   b. regularly by the clock, at 6- or 8-hour intervals
   c. on arising and in the late afternoon
   d. once a day at bedtime

REFERENCES

1. Lipid Research Clinics Program: The Lipid Research Clinics coronary primary prevention trial results: I. reduction in incidents of coronary heart disease, J Am Med Assoc 25:1351, 1984.
2. Frohman LA: Diseases of the anterior pituitary. In Felig P and others, eds: Endocrinology and metabolism, ed 2, New York, 1987, McGraw-Hill Book Co, Inc, p 301.
3. Resio MJ: Nursing diagnosis: alteration in oral/nasal mucous membranes related to trauma of transsphenoidal surgery, J Neurosci Nurs 16:112, 1986.
4. Carlson HE: Pituitary disease. In Hershman JM, ed: Endocrine pathophysiology: a patient oriented approach, ed 3, Philadelphia, 1988, Lea & Febiger, p 21.
5. Christy NP and Warren MP: Other clinical syndromes of the hypothalamus and anterior pituitary including tumor mass effects. In DeGroot L, ed: Endocrinology, ed 2, Philadelphia, 1989, WB Saunders Co, p 431.

6. Rogol A: Anabolic steroid therapies for growth disorders, Hosp Pract 24:89, 1989.

7. Kannan CR: Essential endocrinology, New York, 1986, Plenum Medical Book Co.

8. German K: Fluid and electrolyte problems associated with diabetes insipidus and syndrome of inappropriate ADH, Nurs Clin North Am 22:785, 1987.

9. Patterson LM and Norojan EL: Diabetes insipidus versus syndrome of inappropriate antidiuretic hormone, Dimens Crit Care Nurs 8:226, 1989.

10. Culpepper RM, Hebert SC, and Andreoli TE: The posterior pituitary and water metabolism. In Wilson JD and Foster DM, eds: Williams textbook of endocrinology, ed 7, Philadelphia, 1985, WB Saunders Co, p 637.

11. McKenzie JM and Fakarija M: Hyperthyroidism. In DeGroot L, ed: Endocrinology, ed 2, Philadelphia, 1989, WB Saunders Co, p 654.

12. Hay ID and Klee GG: Thyroid dysfunction, Endocrinol Metab Clin North Am 17:494, 1988.

13. Mathewson MK: Thyroid disorder, Crit Care Nurse 7:74, 1987.

14. Tiwary CM: Neonatal screening for metabolic and endocrine diseases, Nurse Pract 12:28, 1987.

15. Fisher DA: Thyroid disease in the neonate and in childhood. In DeGroot L, ed: Endocrinology, ed 2, Philadelphia, 1989, WB Saunders Co, p 74.

16. Habener JF and Potts JT Jr: Primary hyperparathyroidism—clinical features. In DeGroot L, ed: Endocrinology, ed 2, Philadelphia, 1989, WB Saunders Co, p 954.

17. Stewart AF and Broadus AE: Mineral metabolism. In Felig P and others, ed: Endocrinology and metabolism, ed 2, New York, 1987, McGraw-Hill Book Co, Inc, p 1379.

18. Parfitt AM: Surgical, idiopathic, and other varieties of parathyroid hormone-deficient hypoparathyroidism. In DeGroot L, ed: Endocrinology, ed 2, Philadelphia, 1989, WB Saunders Co, p 1056.

19. Govoni LE and Hayes JE: Drugs and nursing implication, Norwalk, Conn, 1988, Appleton & Lange, p 183.

20. Baxter JD and Tyrrell JB: The adrenal cortex. In Felig P and others, eds: Endocrinology and metabolism, ed 2, New York, 1987, McGraw-Hill Book Co, Inc, p 600.

21. Schira MG: Steroid-dependent states and adrenal insufficiency. In Chambers JK, ed: Common fluid and electrolyte disorders, Nurs Clin North Am 22:837, 1987.

22. Bardin CW: Current therapy in endocrinology and metabolism—3, Toronto, 1988, BC Decker.

23. Melby JC: Diagnosis and treatment of primary aldosteronism and isolated hypoaldosteronism. In DeGroot L, ed: Endocrinology, ed 2, Philadelphia, 1989, WB Saunders Co, p 1706.

24. Young WF and Klee GG: Primary aldosteronism. In Young WF and Klee GG, eds: Diagnostic evaluation of endocrine disorders II, Endocrinol Metab Clin North Am 17:367, 1988.

25. Ehrlich EN: Electrolyte metabolism: secondary aldosteronism and compensatory increases in aldosterone secretion. In DeGroot L, ed: Endocrinology, ed 2, Philadelphia, 1989, WB Saunders Co, p 1602.

26. Benowitz NL: Diagnosis and management of pheochromocytoma, Hosp Pract 25:163, 1990.

27. Feldman JM: Diagnosis and management of pheochromocytoma, Hosp Pract 24:175, 1989.

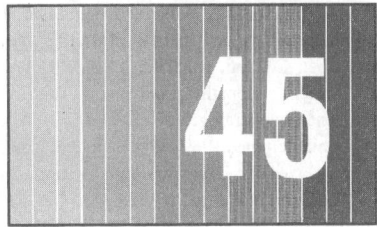

Nursing Assessment

Reproductive Systems

Ellen Frances Olshansky

L earning Objectives

1. Describe the structures and functions of the male and female reproductive systems.
2. Explain the functions of the major hormones essential to the structure and function of the reproductive systems.
3. Describe the physiological and psychological changes of a man and a woman during the stages of sexual response.
4. Describe age-related changes in the reproductive systems and differences in assessment findings.
5. Identify significant subjective and objective data related to the reproductive systems and information about sexual function that should be obtained from a client.
6. Describe noninvasive techniques used in physical assessment of the reproductive systems.
7. Differentiate normal from common abnormal findings of a physical assessment of reproductive systems.
8. Describe the purpose, significance of results, and nursing responsibilities related to diagnostic studies of the reproductive systems.

To accurately assess the male and female reproductive systems, the nurse must understand (1) the structure and function of the reproductive organs, (2) the interrelationship of the hypothalamus, pituitary gland, and gonads, and (3) the biopsychosocial aspects of sex and sexuality.

STRUCTURES AND FUNCTIONS OF THE MALE AND FEMALE REPRODUCTIVE SYSTEMS

The reproductive system is interrelated with other systems, including the neurological, endocrine, and urinary systems. It is responsible for the continuation of the species through fertilization, implantation, maintenance of pregnancy, and birth of a baby. The reproductive system is also directly related to sexuality and thus is intricately interwoven into the complex, highly sensitive, and frequently stress-laden psychosocial mores and values about sex.

Reviewed by Steve R. Toussaint, R.N., M.S.N., Assistant Professor of Nursing, Linfield College, Good Samaritan School of Nursing, Portland, Oregon.

Male Reproductive System

The male reproductive system consists of the external structures—the penis and scrotum—and the internal structures, including the prostate gland, seminal vesicles, and several ducts (Fig. 45-1). The *scrotum* lies within the scrotal sac, which is a thin, loose outer layer of skin over a more muscular internal layer. The scrotum consists of two halves divided by a septum; each half contains a testis, epididymis, and spermatic cord. The testis is an ovoid, smooth, firm organ measuring 2 to 2.5 cm in depth and 2 to 3 cm in width. Within the testes are the *seminiferous tubules,* where spermatozoa (sperm) are formed at a rate of 10 to 30 billion per month. The tubules lead into a system of small ducts that conduct sperm to the *epididymis*.

The epididymis is a soft, cordlike structure that measures almost 530 cm in length if stretched out. It lies in the anterior plane and along the posterolateral surface of each testis. This organ may be considered to be a large duct. It stores the sperm as they mature and until they are released by ejaculation or until they disintegrate and are reabsorbed by the body (Fig. 45-2). The *ductus deferens* extends from the epididymis to a point close to the prostate gland, where

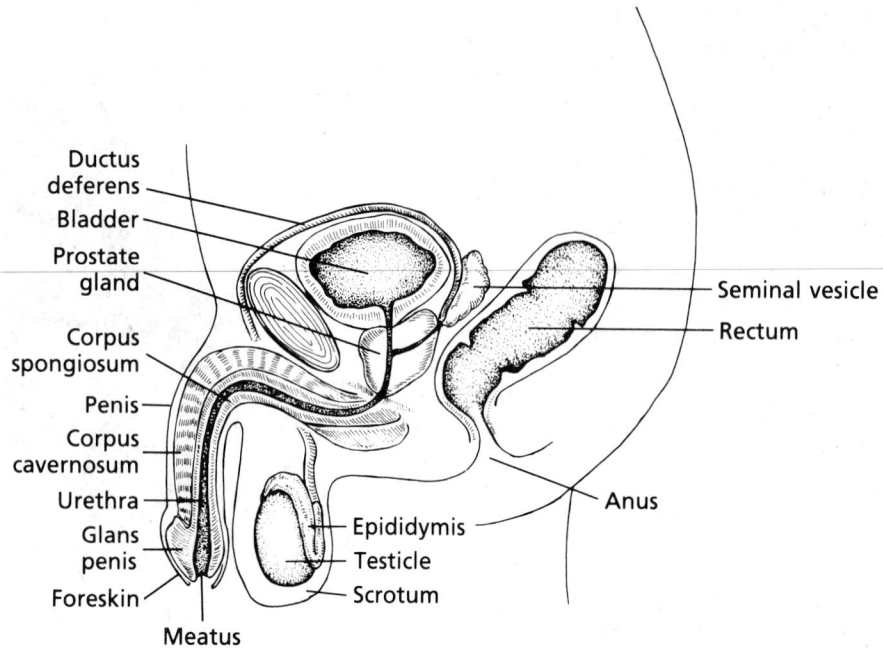

Fig. 45-1 External and internal male sex organs. (From Potter PA and Perry AG: Fundamentals of nursing: concepts, process and practice, ed 2, St Louis, 1989, The CV Mosby Co, p 1326.)

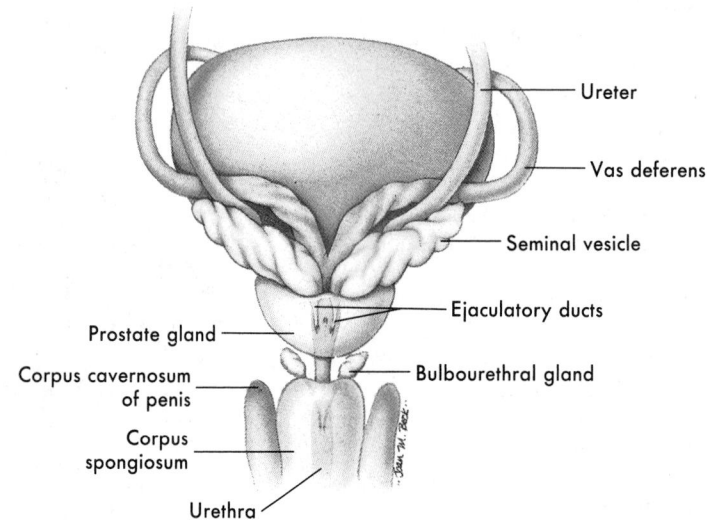

Fig. 45-2 Formation of the ejaculatory ducts by union of the seminal vesicles with the ductus deferens just before entrance into the prostate gland. The ejaculatory ducts open into the prostatic portion of the urethra. (From Anthony CP and Thibodeau GA: Textbook of anatomy and physiology, ed 12, St Louis, 1987, Times Mirror/Mosby College Publishing, p 724.)

it becomes the *ejaculatory duct* and enters the urethra. The duct system emerging from each testis conveys sperm into the urethra.

The spermatic cord contains not only the ductus deferens but also the arteries, veins, and lymph vessels that supply the testis and epididymis. All of these structures are enclosed by the cremaster muscle and by layers of fascia. The cord enters into the inguinal canal through the external inguinal ring. There the cord ends, and its components, primarily the ductus deferens, continue the backward course toward the scrotum.

The prostate, seminal vesicles, and Cowper's (bulbourethral) glands are the accessory glands of the male reproductive system. These glands produce and secrete seminal fluid, which contains sperm. The *prostate gland* is below the bladder. Its posterior surface approximates the rec-

tal wall. The normal prostate measures 2 cm in width and 3 cm in length and is divided into right and left lateral lobes and an anteroposterior median lobe. The *seminal vesicles* lie just behind the bladder and between the rectum and bladder. The ducts of the seminal vesicles fuse with the ductus deferens to form the ejaculatory ducts that enter the prostate gland. *Cowper's glands* lie on each side of the urethra and slightly posterior to it just below the prostate. The ducts of these glands enter directly into the urethra. The secretion from the prostate accounts for the largest amount of ejaculate fluid. In comparison, the seminal vesicles and Cowper's glands contribute a minimum amount of fluid to the ejaculate. Fig. 45-2 follows the route of sperm from production to ejaculation.

The urethra extends from the bladder through the prostate and ends in a slitlike opening (meatus) on the ventral side of the *glans,* the end of the penis. The glans is covered by a fold of skin, the prepuce (or foreskin), which forms at the junction of the glans and the shaft of the penis. There is no prepuce in the circumcised male. The broadened segment of the glans at the junction is the *corona.* The shaft of the penis consists of (1) erectile tissue, the corpus cavernosum and corpus spongiosum; (2) the fibrous sheath that encases the erectile tissue; and (3) the urethra. The skin covering the penis is thin, loose, and essentially hairless.

Female Reproductive System

The female reproductive system consists of the breasts, uterus, ovaries, fallopian tubes, vagina, and external genitalia (the vulva), as well as ligaments and pelvic bones.

Breasts. The breasts are a secondary sex characteristic that develops during puberty in response to estrogen. Cyclical hormonal changes lead to regular changes in breast tissue to prepare them for lactation when fertilization and pregnancy occur. The breasts are also considered a major organ of sexual stimulation and response.

The breasts extend from the second to the sixth ribs, with the tail reaching the axilla (Fig. 45-3). The fully mature breast is dome shaped and contains a pigmented center called the *areola.* The areolar region contains *Montgomery's tubercles,* which are sebaceouslike glands that assist in moistening the nipple. The nipple itself contains 15 to 20 minute openings that lead into ducts forming the *lactiferous sinuses,* where milk is stored during lactation. Ducts (secondary tubules) extend and branch from the lactiferous sinuses outward, eventually ending in lobules called *alveoli* or *acini* of the breasts. The alveoli secrete milk during lactation.* The breast's rich lymphatic network drains primarily into the axillary, infraclavicular, and supraclavicular channels. This system is often responsible for the metastasis of a malignancy from the breast to other parts of the body (Fig. 45-4). The fibrous and fatty tissue that supports and separates the channels of the mammary duct system is primarily responsible for the varying sizes and shapes of the breasts in individuals.

Pelvic organs. The *ovaries* are usually located on either side of the uterus, just behind and below the fallopian

---

*Refer to maternity texts for a discussion of breast changes during pregnancy.

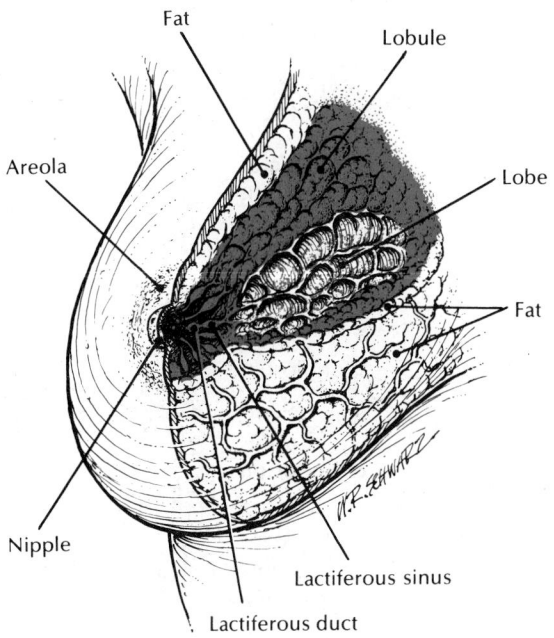

Fig. 45-3 The female breast. (From Malasanos L, Barkauskas V, and Stoltenberg-Allen K: Health assessment, ed 4, St Louis, 1990, Mosby–Year Book, Inc, p 282.)

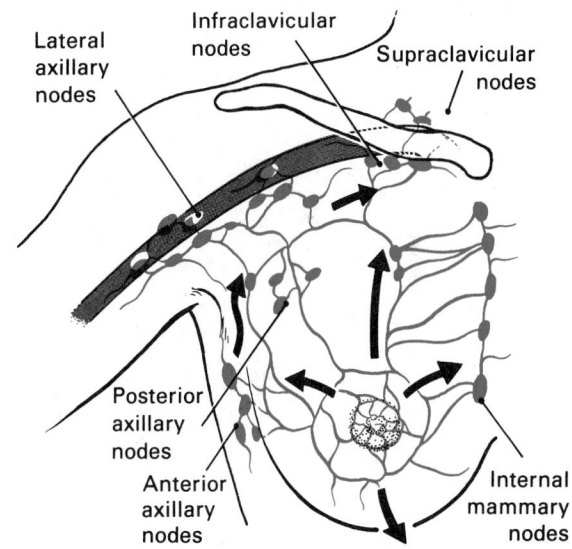

Fig. 45-4 Lymphatic drainage of the breast. *Arrows* indicate direction of drainage.

(uterine) tubes (Fig. 45-5). The ovaries are firm and solid, averaging 1.5 cm in width, 3 cm in length, and 2 cm in depth. They function in ovulation and secretion of the two major reproductive hormones, estrogen and progesterone. The outer zone of the ovary contains follicles with germ cells, or oocytes. Each follicle contains a primordial (immature) oocyte surrounded by granulosa and theca cells. These two layers protect and nourish the oocyte until the follicle reaches maturity and ovulation occurs. Not all fol-

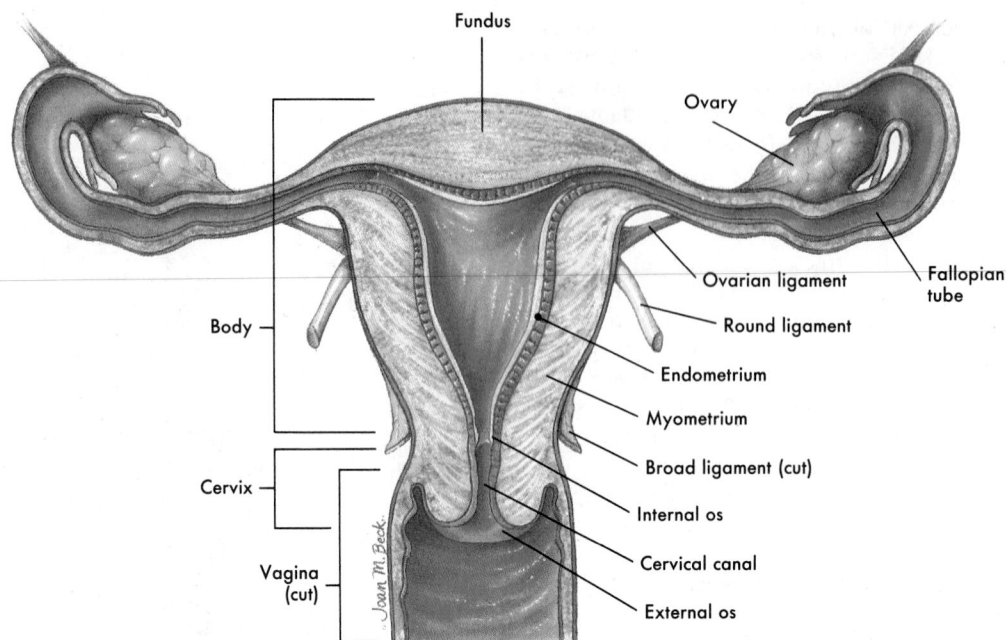

Fig. 45-5 Anatomy of the female reproductive tract. (From Seeley RR, Stephens TD, and Tate P: Anatomy and physiology, St Louis, 1989, Times Mirror/Mosby College Publishing, p 857.)

licles reach maturity, however. In a process called *atresia,* the primordial follicles degenerate and are reabsorbed by the body; thus the number of follicles declines from 2 to 4 million at birth to approximately 400,000 at menarche. This number continues to decrease throughout a woman's reproductive years. [1]

Normally, each month during a woman's reproductive years, one follicle reaches maturity, and the oocyte is ovulated, or expelled, from the ovary through the stimulus of the gonadotropic hormones, follicle-stimulating hormone (FSH), and luteinizing hormone (LH). The oocyte then travels up the fallopian tubes for fertilization by a sperm.

The distal ends of the fallopian tubes consist of fingerlike projections called *fimbriae* that "massage" the ovaries at ovulation to help extract the mature ovum. The tubes, which average 12 cm in length, extend from the fimbriae to the superior lateral borders of the uterus. Fertilization usually takes place within the outer one third of the tubes.

The *uterus* is a pear-shaped, hollow, muscular organ (Fig. 45-4). It is located between the bladder and the rectum. In the mature nulliparous (never pregnant) female the uterus is approximately 6 cm in length and 4 cm in width. The uterine walls are composed of an outer or serosal layer; a middle muscular layer, the *myometrium;* and an inner mucosal layer, the *endometrium.*

The uterus consists of the fundus, body (or corpus), and cervix. The body forms about 80% of the uterus and connects with the cervix at the isthmus, or neck.

The *cervix* is the lower portion that invaginates (projects into) into the anterior wall of the vaginal canal. It constitutes about 15% to 20% of the uterus in the nulliparous female. The cervix consists of the *ectocervix,* or the outer portion that protrudes into the vagina, and the *endo-*

cervix, or the canal in the opening of the cervix. The ectocervix is covered with squamous epithelial cells, giving it a smooth, pinkish appearance. The endocervix contains a lining of columnar epithelial cells, giving it a rough, reddened appearance. The junction at which the two kinds of epithelial cells meet is called the *squamocolumnar junction* and contains the cells that must be examined in a Papanicolaou (Pap) smear for accurate screening for malignancies. Endocervical cells must be present in the sample taken for a Pap smear to ensure that the squamocolumnar junction, or transformation zone, has been tested. Samples should also be routinely taken from the vaginal posterior fundus, as well as from all areas on the cervix, vagina, and vulva that look abnormal. [2] The columnar epithelium under hormonal influence provides enough elasticity at labor for the cervix to stretch so that a fetus can exit. Otherwise, the cervical canal is 2 to 4 cm long and is relatively tightly closed. The cervix allows sperm to enter the uterus and allows menses or products of conception to be expelled.

The entrance of sperm into the uterus is facilitated by mucus produced by the cervix under the influence of estrogen. Under normal conditions at ovulation, cervical mucus becomes watery and more abundant; it can stretch several inches (*spinnbarkhert*) and looks like egg whites. This mucus allows easy entrance of sperm into the uterus. Postovulatory cervical mucus, resulting from the influence of progesterone, is thick and inhibits sperm passage. Knowledge of these physiological changes is used in natural approaches to family planning.

The anterior and posterior peritoneal covering of the uterus is called the *broad ligament.* It separates the uterus from the bladder and rectum but does not provide support

for the uterus or adnexa (ovaries and tubes). The cardinal ligaments, which extend from the isthmus of the uterus to the pelvic wall, also offer only minimal support. The round ligament, which extends anteriorly to the labia majora, provides some support but is easily weakened by pregnancy. The firmest support for the uterus is provided by the uterine sacral ligaments, which pull the uterus back and away from the vaginal orifice.

The *vagina* is a tubular structure 8 to 10 cm in length that is lined with squamous epithelium. The secretions of the vagina consist of cervical mucus, desquamated epithelium, and, during sexual stimulation, a direct transudate. These fluids protect against vaginal infection. The muscular and erectile tissue of the vaginal walls allow enough dilatation and contraction to accommodate the passage of the fetus during labor as well as penetration of the penis during intercourse. The anterior vaginal wall lies along the urethra and bladder. The posterior vaginal wall is adjacent to the rectum.

The female *pelvis* consists of four bones: two hipbones (also called the *innominate bones:* the *ilium,* the *ischium,* and the *os pubis*), the sacrum, and the coccyx. These bones are very important during birth and are often a determining factor of the ability of a woman to deliver a child vaginally. Knowledge of these bones and the landmarks that they form in the pelvis allows the practitioner to determine pelvic measurements and the potential for a woman's pelvis to accommodate the birth of a full-term fetus.

The pelvis is also divided into the true pelvis and the false pelvis. The true pelvis encompasses the brim, cavity, and outlet and is the bony passageway through which the fetus passes during birth. The false pelvis consists of the superior portion of the iliac bones, above the brim.[3]

External genitalia. The external portion of the female reproductive system (Fig. 45-6), commonly called the *vulva,* consists of the mons pubis, labia majora, labia minora, clitoris, urethral meatus, ducts of Skene's glands, vaginal orifice, and Bartholin's glands.

The mons pubis is a fatty layer lying over the pubic bone. It contains coarse hair that lies in an upside-down triangular pattern. (The male hair pattern is diamond shaped.) The labia majora are folds of adipose tissue that form the outer borders of the vulva. These hair-covered folds contain sweat glands and sebaceous glands. The hairless labia minora form the borders of the vaginal orifice and extend anteriorly to enclose the clitoris.

In a virgin the vaginal orifice usually contains a thin membrane called the *hymen,* which varies the size of the vaginal orifice between individuals from pinhole size to an opening large enough to allow two fingers to enter. Frequently, the hymen is torn during first sexual intercourse, and only tags remain. In many societies the bleeding that occurs with this tearing has been used to validate virginity. However, not all hymens are torn by the first intercourse. Some are already well stretched or were torn through childhood activity or accidents.

The *clitoris* is homologous (similar) to the male penis; it is the erectile tissue that becomes engorged during sexual excitation. It lies anterior to the urethral meatus and

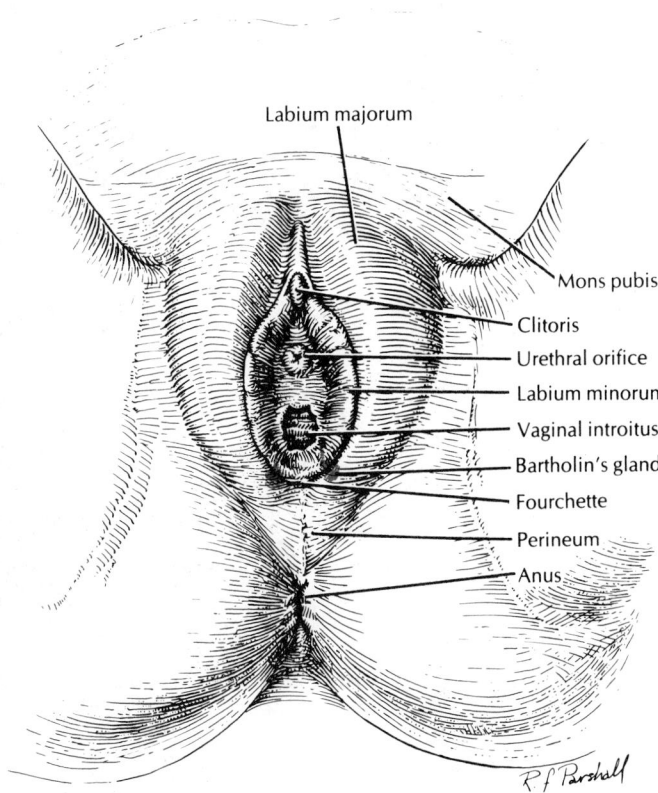

Fig. 45-6   External female genitalia. (From Malasanos L, Barkauskas V, and Stoltenberg-Allen K: Health assessment, ed 4, St Louis, 1990, Mosby–Year Book, Inc, p 1330.)

vaginal orifice and is usually covered by the prepuce or hood.

Skene's glands and ducts lie alongside the urethral meatus and have no known function. They are homologous to the male prostate. Bartholin's glands, which are at the posterior and lateral aspects of the vaginal orifice, secrete a thin, mucoid material believed to contribute slightly to lubrication during sexual intercourse. These glands are not usually palpable unless sebaceous-like cysts form or an infection arises.

Neuroendocrine Regulation

The hypothalamus and pituitary gland (see Chapter 42) and the gonads (organs of reproduction) secrete hormones on which the processes of ovulation, spermatogenesis (formation of sperm), and fertilization, as well as the formation and function of the secondary sex characteristics, depend (Fig. 45-7). The hypothalamus secretes gonadotropic-releasing hormones (GnRHs), which stimulate the pituitary gland to secrete its hormones: FSH, LH, interstitial cell stimulating hormone (ICSH), and luteotropic hormone (LTH), or prolactin. The gonadal hormones are estrogen, progesterone, and testosterone.

In women, FSH production by the pituitary stimulates the growth and maturity of follicles to cause ovulation. The mature follicle produces estrogen, which in turn suppresses the release of FSH. In men, FSH stimulates the seminiferous tubules to produce sperm.

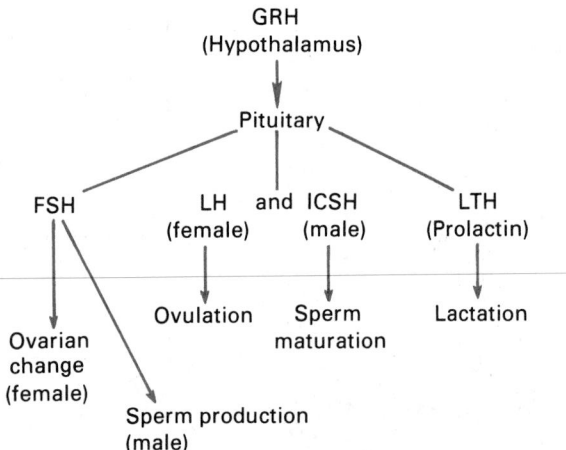

Fig. 45-7 The hypothalamic-pituitary-gonadal axis. Only the major pituitary hormone actions are depicted.

Table 45-1 Gonadal Feedback Mechanisms

TONIC CENTER (NEGATIVE FEEDBACK)

↓ Estrogen → ↑ GnRH → ↑ FSH → ↑ estrogen
        (hypo-   (pituitary) (ovaries)
        thalamus)

CYCLIC CENTER (POSITIVE FEEDBACK)

↑ Estrogen → ↑ GnRH → ↑ LH
        (hypo-   (pituitary)
        thalamus)

TESTES (NEGATIVE FEEDBACK)

↓ Testosterone → ↑ GnRH →
              (hypothalamus)
↑ FSH and ICSH → ↑ testoster-
(pituitary)   one (testes)

LH contributes to the ovulatory process because it stimulates an estrogen surge thought to be responsible for this process. It also causes the development of the ruptured follicle into a corpus luteum (see p. 1362), which secretes progesterone. This hormone maintains the richly vascular state of the uterus (secretory phase) in preparation for fertilization and implantation. In men, LH induces the secretion of testosterone by the testes.

ICSH is responsible for the production of testosterone by the interstitial cells of the testes and thus is essential for the full maturation of sperm. Prolactin has no known function in men but, with other hormones, stimulates the development and growth of the mammary glands in women. During lactation, it initiates and maintains milk production.

The gonadal hormones in women, estrogen and progesterone, are produced by the ovaries. Estrogen is essential to the development and maintenance of (1) the secondary sex characteristics, (2) the phase of the menstrual cycle immediately after menstruation (proliferative phase), and (3) uterine changes essential to pregnancy. Estrogen has also been found in the urine of men, although its role and importance are not well understood. In men, this hormone is produced in the adenal cortex.

Progesterone plays a major role in the menstrual cycle but most specifically in the secretory phase. Like estrogen, progesterone is involved in the bodily changes associated with pregnancy. Adequate progesterone is necessary to maintain the viability of an implanted embryo.

The major gonadal hormone of men, testosterone, is produced by the testes. Testosterone is responsible for the development and maintenance of secondary sex characteristics, as well as for adequate spermatogenesis.

The circulating levels of gonadal hormones are controlled primarily by a negative feedback process. Receptors within the hypothalamus are sensitive to the circulating blood levels of the hormones (Table 45-1). Increased levels of hormones stimulate a hypothalamic response to decrease the high circulating levels. Likewise, low circulating levels provoke a hypothalamic response that increases the low circulating levels. For example, if the circulating level of testosterone is low, the hypothalamus is stimulated to secrete GnRH. This stimulates the pituitary to secrete greater amounts of FSH and ICSH, which in turn causes an increase in the production of testosterone. The high levels of testosterone then stimulate a decrease in the production of GRH and thus of FSH and ICSH.

In women, however, there is a slight variation. The circulating levels are controlled through a combination of a negative and a positive feedback system. The tonic center operates as a negative feedback control mechanism, as in men. When circulating estrogen levels are low, the tonic center of the hypothalamus is stimulated to increase its production of GnRH. GnRH stimulates the pituitary to secrete greater amounts of FSH, resulting in higher levels of estrogen production by the ovaries. Reciprocally, higher levels of circulating estrogen result in a decreasing secretion of GnRH and thus a decrease in the secretion of FSH by the pituitary.

In contrast, the cyclic center of the hypothalamus represents a positive feedback control mechanism. Thus with high levels of circulating estrogen, a greater level of GnRH is produced, resulting in an increased level of LH from the pituitary. Likewise, lowered levels of estrogen result in a lowered level of LH.

Menstrual Cycle

The major functions of the ovaries are the secretion of hormones and ovulation. These functions are accomplished during the normal menstrual cycle, a monthly process mediated by the hormonal activity of the hypothalamus, pituitary, and ovaries. Menstruation occurs each month during which an egg is not fertilized (Fig. 45-8). The menstrual cycle is divided into three phases labeled in relation to uterine and ovarian changes: (1) the proliferative or follicular phase, (2) the secretory or luteal phase, and (3) the menstrual phase. The length of an average menstrual cycle ranges from 20 to 40 days.

The menstrual cycle begins with the first day of menstruation, which lasts 3 to 5 days. During this time, estro-

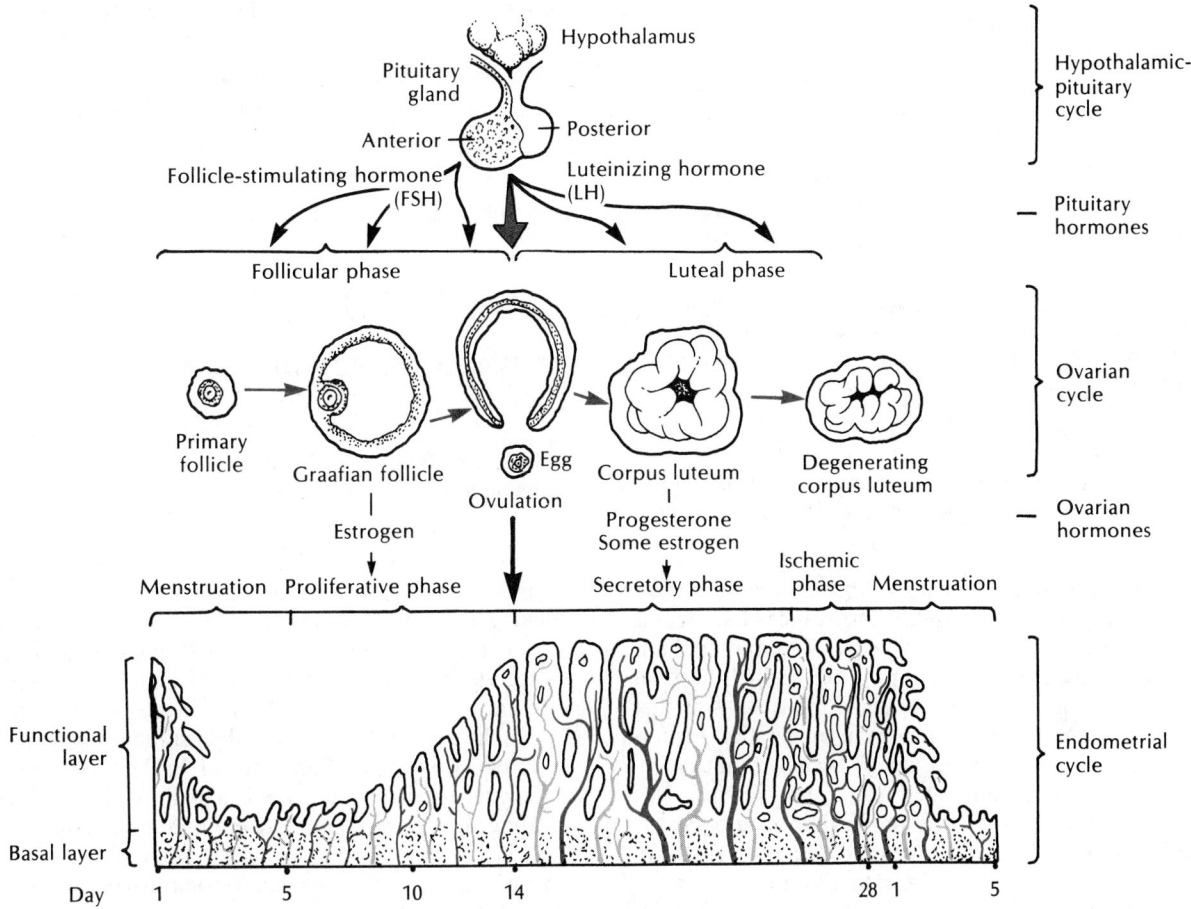

Fig. 45-8 Changes associated with a normal menstrual cycle. (From Bobak IM, Jensen MD, and Zalar MK: Maternity and gynecologic care: the nurse and the family, ed 4, St Louis, 1989, The CV Mosby Co, p 1332.)

gen and progesterone levels are low, but FSH levels are elevated. Under the stimulation of FSH, one follicle fully matures. (The mechanism that usually ensures only one follicle reaching maturity is not known.) The mature follicle stimulates estrogen production, causing a negative feedback with resulting decreased FSH secretion.

Although initial follicular maturity is stimulated by FSH, complete maturity and ovulation occur only with the presence of LH. With increasing estrogen secretion, there is a surge of LH, which facilitates ovulation. After ovulation, LH promotes the development of the corpus luteum.

The fully developed corpus luteum continues to secrete estrogen and initiates progesterone secretion. If fertilization occurs, high levels of estrogen and progesterone continue to be secreted as a result of the continued activity of the corpus luteum from stimulation by human choriotropic hormone (HCG). If fertilization does not occur, menstruation results because of a decrease in estrogen and progesterone production.

During the follicular changes in the ovary, the endometrial lining of the uterus also undergoes change. As larger amounts of estrogen are produced, the endometrial lining proliferates; that is, there is increased cellular growth, including an increase in the length of blood vessels and glandular tissue.

With ovulation and increased levels of progesterone, the luteal, or secretory, phase begins. In this phase the blood vessels begin to coil, which increases the surface area of the vascular supply. The glandular tissues mature and secrete a glycogen-rich substance, and the glandular ducts dilate. If the corpus luteum regresses (fertilization does not occur) and estrogen and progesterone levels fall, the endometrial lining can no longer be supported. As a result, the blood vessels contract, and tissue begins to slough (fall away). This sloughing is menses.

Menopause

Menopause is the cessation of menses for the remainder of a woman's lifetime. It is usually diagnosed if 1 year of _amenorrhea_ (absence of menstruation) has occurred without signs of other problems. The average age at which menopause occurs is 48 to 52 years, but this can vary.[5] The climacteric is the period during which symptoms of approaching menopause begin, menopause actually occurs, and equilibrium after menopause is established (Table 45-2). Ovulation decreases over a period of years.[6] In a sense the stage for menopause is set during fetal life. Approximately 2 to 4 million eggs are present during week 20 of fetal life, although the number begins to decline at

Table 45-2 Common Manifestations During the Climacteric

PREMENOPAUSAL

Irregular menses
Vasomotor instability (hot flashes)
Nervousness

MENOPAUSAL

Cessation of menses
Frequent vasomotor symptoms
Atrophy of genitourinary tissue (e.g., vaginal epithelium)

POSTMENOPAUSAL

Atrophic vaginitis
Occasional vasomotor symptoms
Atrophy of genitourinary tissue with decreased support
Osteoporosis

Table 45-3 Structural Homologues of the Male and Female Reproductive Systems

Male	Female
Penis	Clitoris
Scrotal ridge	Labia minora
Scrotum	Labia majora
Testes	Ovaries
Cowper's glands	Bartholin's glands
Prostate	Skene's ducts
Prostatic utricle (blind pouch of urethra)	Vagina

this time. The average female ovulates only 400 to 500 times during a lifetime. Many follicles undergo *atresia* and then are called atretic follicles.[7] About 40 to 50 years after birth the full store of oocytes becomes exhausted. As this decline reaches lower levels during the climacteric, the amount of estrogen produced also begins to decline.

This reduced level of estrogen leads to a reduced frequency of ovulation. The atrophy of secondary sex characteristics partially results from these lowered estrogen levels. Sources of estrogen other than the ovary, such as the adrenal glands, become very important in maintaining estrogen-dependent tissues. The blood levels of FSH increase as much as tenfold to twentyfold in response to lower estrogen. These elevated FSH levels may take several years to subside to postmenopausal levels.

The reason for "hot flashes" or vasomotor instability is not clearly understood. However, lowered estrogen levels result in hot flashes, and the more sudden the withdrawal of estrogen, as with removal of the ovaries, the more likely that the symptoms will be severe (if no replacement is provided). These symptoms subside over time, with or without replacement therapy. Autonomic nervous system instability may also be related to emotional irritability during the climacteric, but this "symptom" has been greatly exaggerated in literature and myth. Atrophy of the vaginal epithelium often causes vaginal dryness responsible for mild to moderate dyspareunia (painful intercourse). This can lead to unnecessary and premature cessation of sexual activity. Dryness is a problem that can be easily corrected with hormonal creams. In general, the extent and severity of the symptoms of the climacteric vary and are not easily predicted, even with a detailed history of family patterns.

Osteoporosis, a condition in which the amount of bone mass is deficient because of increased bone resorption, is quite prevalent in menopausal women. This condition puts women at a much greater risk for sustaining fractures of the spine, vertebrae, wrist, and hips. Such fractures can be life-threatening in older women.

The symptoms of menopause and particularly the risk of osteoporosis create a dilemma in the care of menopausal women. The use of estrogen replacement therapy often reduces the risk of such symptoms but can create other potentially serious side effects, such as cancer of the uterus and hypertension. Adequate calcium intake and exercise are also important factors in the prevention of osteoporosis (see Chapter 57).

Phases of Sexual Response

It is helpful to look at the structural homologues in the male and female reproductive systems to understand sexual response (Table 45-3). Masters and Johnson describe sexual response in terms of the excitement, plateau, orgasmic, and resolution phases.[7]

Orgasm does not occur in every sexual encounter. In addition, orgasm does not depend on anatomical features such as size of the penis or vaginal canal. Sexual response is a complex interplay of psychological and physiological phenomena and thus is subject to the effects of everyday stress, as well as illness or crisis.

Male sexual response. The penis and urethra are essential to the transport of sperm into the vagina and cervix during intercourse. This transport is facilitated by erection of the penis in response to sexual stimulation during the excitement phase. Erection results from the filling of the large venous sinuses within the erectile tissue of the penis. In the flaccid state the sinuses hold only a small amount of blood, but during the erected state they are congested with blood. Because the penis is richly endowed with neurons from the sympathetic, parasympathetic, and pudendal nerve endings, it is readily stimulated to erection. The loose skin of the penis becomes taut as a result of the intense venous congestion. This erectile tautness allows for easy insertion into the vagina.

As the man reaches the plateau phase, the erection is maintained, and a small increase in diameter occurs as a result of a slight increase in vasocongestion. There is also an increase in testicular size. Sometimes a change in color occurs in the glans penis, which becomes more reddish-purple.

The subsequent contraction of the penile and urethral musculature during the orgasmic phase propels the sperm outward through the meatus. In this process, termed *ejaculation,* sperm are released into the ductus deferens during contractions. They advance through the prostate, where

Table 45-4

Age-Related Changes of the Reproductive System and Differences in Assessment Findings

Changes	Differences in Assessment Findings
MALE	
Penis	
Decreased subcutaneous fat, decreased skin turgor	Easily retractable foreskin (if uncircumcised), decrease in size, fewer sustained erections
Testes	
Decreased testosterone production	Decrease in size, change in position (lower), increase in firmness
Prostate	
Benign hypertrophy of unknown cause	Enlargement
Breasts	
Enlargement	Gynecomastia (abnormal enlargement)
FEMALE	
Breasts	
Decreased subcutaneous fat, increased fibrous tissue, decreased skin turgor	Less resilient, looser, more pendular tissue
Vulva	
Decreased skin turgor	Atrophy, decreased amount of pubic hair, decreased size of clitoris
Vagina	
Atrophy of tissue, decreased muscle tone	Pale mucosa, dryness of mucosa, less intense sexual response, relaxation of outlets
Urethra	
Decreased muscle tone	Cystocele (protrusion of bladder through vaginal wall)
Uterus	
Decreased thickness of myometrium	Decrease in size
Ovaries	
Decreased estrogen and progesterone production	Nonpalpable ovaries

they are bathed in fluid from the prostate and seminal vesicles. The sperm continue their path through the urethra, receiving a small amount of fluid from the Cowper's glands, and are finally ejaculated through the urinary meatus. Orgasm is marked by the rapid release of the vasocongestion and myotonia that have developed. In other words, the rapid release of muscular tension (through rhythmic contractions) occurs primarily in the penis, prostate, and seminal vesicles.

After ejaculation, a man enters the resolution phase. During this phase the penis undergoes involution, gradually returning to its unstimulated, flaccid state.

Female sexual response. The changes that occur in a woman during sexual excitation are similar to those in a man. In response to stimulation the clitoris swells (becomes congested, as does the penis in a man) and vaginal

lubrication increases from secretions from the cervix and Bartholin's glands and sweating of the vaginal walls. This initial response is the excitation phase.

As excitation is maintained in the plateau phase, the vagina expands and the uterus is elevated (in the male, an increase in testicular size). In the orgasmic phase, contractions occur in the uterus from the fundus to the lower uterine segment. There is a slight relaxation of the cervical os, which helps the entrance of sperm, and rhythmic contractions of the vagina. Muscular tension is rapidly released through rhythmic contractions in the clitoris, vagina, and uterus. This phase is followed by a resolution phase in which these organs return to their pre-excitation state.

Effects of aging on sexual responses. With advancing age, changes occur in the male and female reproductive systems. In women, many of these changes are related to

Table 45-5 Age-Related Changes of Sexual
Function

MALE

Increased stimulation necessary for erection
Decreased need to ejaculate
Decreased ability to attain erection
Negative attitude by society toward sexual relations among
  older adults
Possible decreased response to sexual stimuli

FEMALE

Decreased vaginal lubrication
Possible decreased response to sexual stimuli
Negative attitude by society toward sexual relations among
  older adults

---

decreased estrogen production associated with menopause. Table 45-4 lists age-related changes that should be considered when caring for an older adult.

Gradual changes resulting from advancing age occur in the sexual responses of men and women (Table 45-5). These changes occur at different rates and to varying degrees. The cumulative effects of these changes, as well as the negative social attitude toward sexuality in older adults, can affect the sexual practices of people in this age group. Nurses have an important role in working with such clients who are concerned about their sexuality. Nurses should emphasize the normalcy of sexual activity in older adults. Counseling may be necessary to help older clients accommodate to these physiological changes.[8]

ASSESSMENT OF THE MALE AND FEMALE REPRODUCTIVE SYSTEMS
Subjective Data

Health history. As in other systems, a thorough review of data is not confined only to the reproductive systems. Because problems in other systems are often interrelated with problems and stresses within the reproductive system, the nurse must elicit general information, as well as information specifically relating to the reproductive system.

Past health history

PEDIATRIC AND ADULT ILLNESSES. Common pediatric illnesses that affect reproductive functioning are mumps and rubella. The occurrence of mumps in young men has been associated with an increase in sterility. In the health history the nurse should elicit whether male clients have had mumps, been immunized, or had indications of sterility.

Rubella is of primary concern to women of childbearing age. If rubella occurs during the first 3 months of pregnancy, the possibility of congenital anomalies is increased. For this reason, nurses should encourage immunization for all women of childbearing age who have not been immunized for rubella or have not already had the disease; however, women should not be immunized if they are already pregnant. Women are also advised not to conceive for at least 3 months after immunization.

Chronic diseases that affect the functioning of the re-

productive system must be assessed. The nurse must ascertain whether the client has had diabetes. Men frequently experience impotency problems that are due in part to the chemical imbalances of diabetes. In women with diabetes, pregnancy and the use of oral contraceptives constitute risks to health. The morbidity and mortality rates of women with diabetes are increased with pregnancy or oral contraceptive use. Likewise, a history of cardiovascular disease in women, including hypertension, thrombophlebitis, and angina, causes a higher incidence of morbidity and mortality with pregnancy or oral contraceptive use. Anemia is also relevant to women's reproductive health. Anemia can result from or be aggravated by menstrual flow. Fear of painful intercourse can occur in women because of physiological changes of vaginal atrophy and decreased vaginal lubrication.

In men, strokes may cause physiological or psychological impotence. Men who have suffered heart attacks frequently experience impotence. Often, this impotence is due to fear of causing another heart attack. The interviewer must be sensitive to this concern. Questions asked about the illness may show such a fear and thus indicate a need for counseling and support regarding sexual and cardiac needs.

Oral contraceptive use is often contraindicated in clients with neurological dysfunction such as seizures or migraine headaches; these conditions can be aggravated by such contraceptives. Cholecystitis and hepatitis may also be contraindications for oral contraceptives; cholecystitis is often aggravated by oral contraceptives, and liver disease generally precludes the use of estrogen products because they are metabolized by the liver. Other contraindications to oral contraceptive use may be asthma or other chronic obstructive respiratory problems because progesterone thickens respiratory secretions.

Questions relating to endocrine disorders, particularly hypothyroidism and hyperthyroidism, must also be raised because these disorders directly interfere with women's menstrual cycles and with sexual performance in men. Finally, men and women should be assessed for kidney and urinary tract disorders because sexual functioning and reproductive capacity can be impeded with genitourinary problems.

HOSPITALIZATIONS AND SURGERIES. Any hospitalizations or surgeries should be noted in the health history. However, particular note of certain surgeries should be taken (Table 45-6). Therapeutic or spontaneous pregnancy interruptions are also determined at this time.

MEDICATIONS. A pharmacological profile of prescribed and over-the-counter drugs is necessary for all clients. Particularly relevant in assessment of the reproductive system is the use of diuretics (sometimes prescribed for premenstrual edema), tranquilizers (which may interfere with sexual performance), and antihypertensives (which have been implicated in impotence). Thus clients who use drugs such as methyldopa (Aldomet), clonidine, guanethidine, and hydralazine must be closely assessed for these problems. Diuretics are least often associated with impotence.

In women, the use of oral contraceptives or other hormones should be noted. The nurse must also note the use

Table 45-6 Surgeries for the Reproductive Systems

Surgery	Definition
MEN	
Herniorrhaphy	Repair of hernia
Prostatectomy	Removal of prostate gland
Vasectomy	Removal of part of ductus deferens
Repair of testicular torsion	Correction of axial rotation of spermatic cord, which cuts off blood supply to the testicle, epididymis, and other structures
Varicocelectomy	Repair of varicose vein of scrotum
WOMEN	
Dilatation and curettage (D & C)	Dilatation of uterus and scraping of endometrium, performed to diagnose disease of uterus, correct heavy or prolonged vaginal bleeding, or empty uterus of products of conception
Cryosurgery	Use of subfreezing temperature to destroy tissue, especially in treatment of malignancy
Tubal ligation	Tying off of fallopian tubes
Repair of cystocele	Correction of protrusion of urinary bladder through vaginal wall
Repair of rectocele	Correction of protrusion of rectum and posterior vaginal wall into vagina
Hysterectomy	Removal of uterus
Oophorectomy	Removal of one or both ovaries
Salpingectomy	Removal of one or both fallopian tubes

of drugs such as marijuana, barbiturates, amphetamines, and phencyclidine hydrochloride (PCP) or "angel dust," which can have serious behavioral or physiological impacts on the functioning of the reproductive system.

ALLERGIES. The nurse must ensure that clients are not allergic to sulfonamides, penicillin, and rubber or latex. Sulfonamides and penicillin are used frequently in the treatment of genitourinary symptoms, including vaginitis (inflammation of the vaginal tissues). Rubber or latex is an essential ingredient in diaphragms and some condoms. An allergy to these substances precludes their use as contraceptive methods.

OCCUPATIONAL HISTORY AND ENVIRONMENTAL EXPOSURES. A thorough health history includes information about the client's occupation and potential hazards associated with it. Exposure to toxic chemicals, for example, can affect sexual functioning and reproductive capacity.

FAMILY HISTORY. A family history of cancer, particularly cancer of the reproductive organs, is essential to an adequate reproductive health history. Determination of a familial tendency for diabetes mellitus, hypothyroidism, hyperthyroidism, hypertension, stroke, angina, myocardial infarction, endocrine disorders, or anemia is also important.

In addition, the nurse should obtain data related to in utero exposure to diethylstilbestrol (DES). DES was frequently administered to women to prevent spontaneous abortions during the 1940s and 1950s, with some decline in use during the 1960s. It is associated with cervical adenosis and cervical and vaginal adenocarcinoma in women exposed to it in utero. Male offspring of DES mothers experience congenital anomalies such as structural defects of the genitourinary tract and decreased semen levels.

SOCIAL AND SEXUAL HISTORY. Assessment of the reproductive system is incomplete without a knowledge of the client's social history. The nurse should know whether a woman uses cigarettes, alcohol, caffeine, or other drugs because these substances can be detrimental to a fetus and cigarette smoking can increase the risk of morbidity in women using contraceptives. These substances may also adversely affect sperm count in men. Men may also suffer from impotence or decreased libido.

Patterns of sexual relationships also provide important information. A history of multiple sexual partners increases the risk of contracting a sexually transmitted disease (STD). For a woman, this can increase the risk of pelvic inflammatory disease (PID), which can compromise her ability to have a baby. A history of homosexual or bisexual relationships may also place a person at increased risk for developing the human immunodeficiency virus (HIV), although HIV infections also occur in the heterosexual population.

The extent and depth of the interview regarding sexuality depend primarily on the expertise of interviewers and the needs and willingness of the client. Before taking a sexual history, interviewers should assess their own comfort with their own sexuality because discomfort in questioning is obvious to the client. Interviews must be done in an environment that provides reassurance, confidentiality, and a nonjudgmental attitude. It is best to begin with the least sensitive areas and then move to more sensitive areas. For this reason, sexual histories are frequently initiated during the review of the genitourinary and gynecological systems. Early questioning can thus relate to menstruation, the onset of puberty, and the presence or absence of symptoms of genitourinary problems. The use of

Table 45-7 Sexual History Format

How long have you been sexually active?
How frequently do you have penile-vaginal intercourse?
How frequently do you masturbate?
How many sexual partners do you have?
What is your sexual preference?
How frequently do you have oral sex?
How frequently do you have rectal intercourse?
What STDs have you had (e.g., gonorrhea, syphilis, herpes)?
What contraceptive method are you using?
How often do you use a contraceptive method?
Do you consider your contraceptive method satisfactory?
Do you consider your sex life satisfactory?
How often have you experienced impotence or difficulty with vaginal lubrication or pain with intercourse?
How has your sex life changed?
How would you like to see your sex life change?
How would your partner rate your sex life?

these questions thus provides an introductory period for care providers and client before they move into more sensitive areas.

Questions about sexuality should always be asked in a straightforward manner. Questions that ask "Why?" are not conducive to objective interviewing. Questions should be asked in a manner that assumes that clients have done everything. This prevents individuals from feeling guilty or unique. For example, nurses should not ask, "Do you masturbate?" Rather, they should ask, "How often do you masturbate?" If clients do not masturbate, they can simply state that they do not. If clients masturbate, they are more likely to indicate this because the question has been worded without judgment. Table 45-7 outlines questions appropriate for an initial assessment or annual examination.

The nurse should routinely ask questions related to sexual health because such information is an integral component of overall general health. Men should be questioned about their ability to achieve and maintain erections. This may be approached by questioning the frequency with which they find it difficult to do so. Women should be questioned about pain with intercourse or difficulty with penetration. Indications of sexual dysfunction may require referral or consultation with a sexual counselor.

A thorough genitourinary history must also be collected for the assessment of the reproductive system to be complete.

GYNECOLOGICAL AND OBSTETRICAL HISTORY. Every woman who enters the health care system should have a complete obstetrical and gynecological history taken (Table 45-8). The history provides 80% to 90% of the data essential to accurate assessment, planning, and intervention for clients with reproductive problems.

The first review questions usually refer to the breast.

The nurse asks the client whether she performs a monthly breast self-examination (BSE) (see Chapter 46). The nurse inquires about previous or present breast lumps or masses to screen for breast cancer, one of the leading causes of death in women. A breast lump is the most common sign of cancer. If a lump is present, its onset, size, and consistency should be noted. The nurse also asks whether there has been an increase or a decrease in the size and shape of the lump since its onset or discovery. The client is also questioned about breast pain or tenderness. She should describe the degree and severity of pain; breast pain or tenderness is not usually present with a malignant mass, particularly in the early stages.

Nipple discharge in a woman who is not pregnant or lactating is another important symptom of problems. The nurse asks about the color, consistency, amount, and odor of the discharge. Discharge not related to lactation or pregnancy must be further investigated.

The presence of a breast mass must also be evaluated in relation to a woman's menstrual cycle because the breasts often become more cystic during the luteal phase of the cycle. The ideal time to assess a woman's breasts is about day 10 of her menstrual cycle. The nurse also inquires about a history of breast cancer in a woman's mother, maternal aunt, and sister because such a history increases the client's risk as well.

Menstrual history data are used in the detection of pregnancy, infertility, and numerous other gynecological concerns. An accurate gynecological assessment requires an accurate menstrual history. A menstrual history should contain the following data: age at onset of menstruation, average length of cycle, usual duration of menstruation (number of days), and usual amount. The amount is usually best determined by ascertaining the number of pads or tampons used per day and the amount of saturation (small, medium, or large). Other important information includes dysmenorrhea and premenstrual symptoms such as headache, tension, and fluid retention.

Changes in the usual menstrual pattern must be explicitly described to determine whether the change is transient and unimportant or connected with a more serious gynecological problem. Spotting or bleeding between menstruations, excessive menstrual bleeding (menorrhagia), lack of menstruation (amenorrhea), and postcoital bleeding are examples of such problems. Changes in menstrual patterns created by the use of contraceptive pills or intrauterine devices (IUDs) must be identified. Contraceptive pills usually decrease the amount and duration of flow, whereas IUDs may cause an increase in the amount and duration. IUDs also frequently increase the severity of dysmenorrhea.

A general gynecological history should rule out pelvic pain, exposure to STDs, vaginal infections, and the presence of symptoms such as vaginal discharge and dyspareunia. Finally, the nurse should obtain a clear obstetrical history, including therapeutic and spontaneous abortions (pregnancy interruptions). These data provide the basis for family planning and fertility counseling most relevant to the individual.

Table 45-8 Gynecological and Obstetrical History Format

GENERAL GYNECOLOGICAL INFORMATION

External genitalia
___Pain
___Rashes
___Other
___Vaginal discharge
Amount_____
Color_____
Consistency_____
Odor_____
___Pain during intercourse
___Bleeding after intercourse
___STDs
   ___*Trichomonas vaginalis* ___Gonorrhea
   ___Chlamydiae   ___Syphilis
   ___*Haemophilus ducreyi* ___Herpes
   ___Other (nonspecific)
___Yeast infection *(Candida albicans)*
Last Pap smear_____ Abnormal_____
             (yes or no)
___Uterine fibroids   Treatment if any_____
___Endometriosis_____
___Ovarian cyst_____
Did your mother take hormones when she was
  pregnant with you?_____
  (yes or no or not sure)
Any difficulties in getting pregnant?_____
  (yes, no, or has not tried yet)

OBSTETRICAL INFORMATION

___Number of pregnancies
___Number of deliveries
___Number of live births
___Number of spontaneous abortions (miscarriages)
___Number of therapeutic abortions
___Number of ectopic pregnancies (tubal)
___Number of cesarean sections
Problems during pregnancy, if any_____
_____
_____

MENSTRUAL INFORMATION

Age at onset_____
Last menstrual period_____
Cycle (frequency)_____Irregular periods_____
                Length_____
Duration of each menses_____
Number of pads or tampons used on heaviest days
Clots_____Spotting (other than during menses)___
Dysmenorrhea (describe)_____
Treatment_____
Change in flow or amount_____
Menopause_____Menopausal symptoms_____
Estrogen replacement_____(yes or no)
If menopausal, have you noticed any vaginal bleeding?
_____
Birth control method (if applicable)_____
Length_____Previous methods_____

BREAST INFORMATION

___Breast lumps (location)_____
_____
_____
___Treatment, if any_____
_____
___Mammogram (date)_____
_____
___Breast pain
  Onset_____
  Severity_____
  Previous occurrence_____
___Breast discharge
  Onset_____
  Amount_____
  Color_____
  Odor and consistency_____
  Breast-feeding_____(yes or no)
Where are you in your menstrual cycle (if any breast
  abnormality is found)?_____
___Breast self-examination
  Frequency_____

Objective Data

Physical examination. The examination of the external genitalia uses inspection and palpation.

Male genitalia. An examination may be performed with the client lying or standing. The standing position is preferred. The examiner should be seated in front of the standing client. The use of a glove is recommended.

PUBES. The nurse observes the diamond-shaped pattern of hair distribution. The absence of hair is not normal. The skin is also evaluated.

PENIS. The nurse notes the size and skin texture of the penis and any lesions, scars, and swelling. The location of the urethral meatus, as well as the presence or absence of a foreskin, should be noted. The foreskin is retracted to note cleanliness and is replaced over the glans after observa-

tion. The glans are compressed to note any discharge and its amount, color, and odor if present. The nurse also palpates the penile shaft for tenderness or masses and observes the ventral and dorsal aspects.

SCROTUM AND TESTES. The nurse performs a complete skin examination by lifting each testis to inspect all sides of the scrotal sac. Palpation of the scrotum is done to note changes in consistency or the presence of masses. The client should also be taught self-testicular examination (see Chapter 49).

INGUINAL REGION AND SPERMATIC CORD. The examiner inspects the inguinal regions for rashes, lesions, or lymphadenopathy, which may suggest pelvic organ infection. The nurse has the client cough or bear down and notes any conspicuous bulging in the inguinal canals. The nurse also palpates

Table 45-9 Recording the Normal Physical Assessment of the Reproductive Systems

MALE
Penis and scrotum
Normal hair distribution

Skin

No lesions or inflammation
Circumcised penis
Meatus patent, no discharge
Testes smooth, firm, 2 cm in width and 3 cm in length
No masses, slight tenderness

Epididymis

Nontender
No masses
No inguinal hernias

FEMALE
Breasts

Symmetrical
Nipples everted, no dimpling
No nipple discharge
No masses, lesions, or tenderness
No axillary nodes
Appropriate for age and parity

Vulva

Normal hair distribution
No lesions, redness, swelling, or masses
Patent vaginal orifice, no discharge
Nonpalpable Skene's ducts and Bartholin's glands, no tenderness
Intact clitoris and urethral meatus

---

the area for any bulging as the client again coughs or bears down.

The spermatic cord is located posteriorly in the scrotal sac. The nurse follows the cord on each side. The inguinal region is gently palpated using the forefinger or small finger and pushing up through the loose scrotal skin to the abdominal wall along the inguinal region. The internal inguinal ring meets and impedes the finger. At this point, the client again bears down and coughs. The nurse determines whether the strain produces bulging of the intestines through the ring (a hernia), requiring medical care.

ANUS AND PROSTATE. The sphincter and perineal regions are inspected for lesions, masses, and hemorrhoids. A digital examination is required for all clients who have symptoms of prostate trouble, such as difficulty in voiding and the urge to void frequently; this examination is performed annually for men over 40.

Female breasts and external genitalia. Physical examination of women often begins with inspection and palpation of the breasts and then proceeds to the abdomen. Examination of the abdomen provides an opportunity to de-

tect pain or masses that may involve the genitourinary system.

BREASTS. The nurse compares the size, shape, and position of both breasts and notes any nipple discharge and the amount, color, and consistency if present. The size, shape, location, and consistency of lumps or masses in either breast, the axilla, and supraclavicular area are described. The nurse also determines whether the lump is movable or stationary. The client should be taught the techniques of BSE (see Chapter 46).

EXTERNAL GENITALIA. The mons pubis, labia majora, labia minora, perineum, and anal region are inspected for characteristics of skin, hair distribution, and contour. Lesions, swelling, and discharge are noted.

The nurse separates the labia to fully inspect the clitoris, urethral meatus, vaginal orifice, hymen, perineum, and anal region. Any inflammation or cysts on Bartholin's glands or Skene's glands are noted.

INTERNAL PELVIC EXAMINATION. During the speculum examination, the nurse observes the walls of the vagina and cervix for inflammation, discharge, polyps, and suspicious growths. During this examination, it is possible to take a Pap smear and collect secretions for culture and study under the microscope (i.e., wet smears).

After the speculum examination, a bimanual examination is performed to allow assessment of the size, shape, and consistency of the uterus, ovaries, and tubes.* (The tubes are not normally palpable.) Table 45-9 illustrates a recording format for the physical assessment findings of the male and female reproductive systems. Tables 45-10 through 45-12 summarize common assessment abnormalities of the breasts, the female reproductive system, and the male reproductive system.

DIAGNOSTIC STUDIES

Many diagnostic tests used to assess problems of other body systems also provide valuable data in the assessment of the reproductive systems. Table 45-13 summarizes the most commonly used diagnostic studies in the assessment of the reproductive systems and the nurse's responsibility regarding these diagnostic tests. It is also the nurse's responsibility to ensure that the client understands the purpose of any test being performed.

Urine Studies

Pregnancy testing. Detection of pregnancy is generally validated by measuring the output of HCG in the urine by means of an immunological assay test. The three most commonly used methods are latex inhibition, hemagglutination inhibition, and latex agglutination from an antigen-antibody response. The hemagglutination test is the most sensitive but takes 2 hours to perform. The latex methods can be performed in 2 minutes and are considered adequate for screening purposes. They are most accurate if performed 6 weeks after the last normal menstrual period.

Home pregnancy test kits are also sold over the counter. Positive results are based on the presence of HCG. These

---

*Refer to a physical examination text for details of the pelvic and bimanual examination.

Text continued on p. 1377.

Table 45-10

Common Assessment Abnormalities of the Breast

Finding	Description	Possible Etiology and Significance
Nipple inversion or retraction	Recent onset, reddening, pain, unilateral	Abscess, inflammatory cancer
	Recent onset (usually within past year), unilateral presentation, lack of tenderness	Neoplasm
Nipple secretions		
Galactorrhea (female)	Milkiness, no relationship to lactation, unilateral or bilateral or intermittent or consistent presentation	Drug therapy, particularly phenothiazines, tricyclic tranquilizers, methyldopa; hypofunction or hyperfunction of thyroid or adrenal glands; tumors of hypothalamus or pituitary gland; excessive estrogen; prolonged suckling or breast foreplay
Galactorrhea (male)	Milkiness, bilateral presentation	Chorioepithelioma of testes
Purulent	Gray-green or yellow color; frequent unilateral presentation; association with pain, erythema, induration, nipple inversion	Puerperal (after birth) mastitis (inflammatory condition of breast) or abscess
	Same as above but usually without nipple inversion	Infected sebaceous cyst
Serous discharge	Clear appearance, unilateral or bilateral or intermittent or consistent presentation	Intraductal papilloma
Dark green or multicolored discharge	Thickness, stickiness, and frequent bilateral presentation	Mammary duct ectasia (dilatation of mammary ducts)
Serosanguineous or bloody drainage	Unilateral presentation	Papillomatosis (widespread development of nipplelike growths), intraductal papilloma, carcinoma (male and female)
Scaling or excoriation of nipple	Unilateral or bilateral presentation, crusting, possible ulceration	Paget disease, eczema, infection
Nodules, lumps, or masses	Multiple bilateral, well-delineated, soft or firm, mobile cysts; pain; premenstrual occurrence	Fibrocystic disease
	Rubbery consistency, fluid-filled interior, pain	Mammary duct ectasia
	Soft, mobile, well-delineated cyst, absence of pain	Lipoma, fibroadenoma
	Erythema, tenderness, induration	Infected sebaceous cysts, abscesses
	Usually singular, hard irregularly shaped, poorly delineated, nonmobile	Neoplasm

Table 45-11

Common Assessment Abnormalities of the Female Reproductive System

Finding	Description	Possible Etiology and Significance
Vulvar discharge	Cottage-cheese consistency, frequent itching and inflammation, lack of odor	Candidiasis (*Candida* or yeast infection), vaginitis
	Grayish color, copious flow, frothy appearance, vulvar irritation	*Gardnerella vaginalis*
	Purulent odor, grayish-green or yellow color	*Trichomonas vaginalis*
	Bloody color	*Chlamydia trachomatis, Neisseria gonorrhoeae,* menstruation, trauma, cancer
Vulvar erythema	Bright or beefy red color, itching	*Candida albicans*
	Reddened base, painful vesicles or ulcerations	Genital herpes
	Macules or papules, itching	Chancroid (STD), contact dermatitis, scabies, pediculosis
Vulvar growths	Soft, fleshy growth; lack of tenderness	Condyloma acuminatum
	Flat and warty appearance, lack of tenderness	Condyloma latum
	Same as either of above, possible pain	Neoplasm
	Reddened base, vesicles, and small erosions; pain	Lymphogranuloma venereum, genital herpes, chancroid
	Indurated, firm ulcers; lack of pain	Chancre (syphilis), granuloma inguinale
Abdominal pain or tenderness	Intermittent or consistent tenderness in right or left lower quadrant	Salpingitis (infection of fallopian tubes), ectopic pregnancy, ruptured ovarian cyst, PID, tubal or ovarian abscess
	Periumbilical location, consistent occurrence	Cystitis, endometritis (inflammation of endometrium)

Table 45-12

Common Assessment Abnormalities of the Male Reproductive System

Finding	Description	Possible Etiology and Significance
Penile growths or masses	Indurated, smooth, disklike appearance; absence of pain; singular presentation	Chancre
	Papular to irregularly shaped ulceration with pus, lack of induration	Chancroid
	Ulceration with induration and nodularity	Cancer
	Flat, wartlike nodule	Condyloma latum
	Elevated, fleshy, moist, elongated projections with single or multiple projections	Condyloma acuminatum
	Localized swelling with retracted, tight foreskin	Paraphimosis (inability to replace foreskin in its normal position after retraction), trauma
Vesicles, erosions or ulcers	Painful, erythematous base; vesicular or small erosions	Genital herpes, balanitis (inflammation of glans penis), chancroid
	Painless, singular, small erosion with eventual lymphadenopathy	Lymphogranuloma venereum, cancer
Scrotal masses	Localized swelling with tenderness, unilateral or bilateral presentation	Epididymitis (inflammation of epididymis), testicular torsion, orchitis (mumps)
	Swelling, tenderness	Incarcerated hernia
	Unilateral or bilateral presentation; swelling without pain; translucent, cordlike or wormlike appearance	Hydrocele (accumulation of fluid in outer covering of testes), spermatocele (swelling of epididymis or sperm ducts), varicocele (varicose condition of veins of portion of spermatic cord), hematocele (accumulation of blood within scrotum)
	Firm, nodular testes or epididymis; frequent unilateral presentation	Tuberculosis, cancer
Penile discharge	Clear to purulent color, minimal to copious flow	Urethritis or gonorrhea, *Chlamydia trachomatis,* trauma
Penile or scrotal erythema	Macules and papules	Scabies, pediculosis
Inguinal masses	Bulging, unilateral presentation during straining	Inguinal hernia
	Shotty, 1 to 3 cm nodules	Lymphadenopathy

Table 45-13

Diagnostic Studies of the Male and Female Reproductive Systems

Study	Description and Purpose	Nursing Responsibility
URINE STUDIES		
Pregnancy testing (Pregnosticon Dri Dot [latex inhibition test], Gravindex, Pregnosticon Accuspheres [hemagglutination-inhibition])	HCG is detected in urine to ascertain whether woman is pregnant. Hydatidiform mole and chorioepithelioma (in men and women) may also be detected. Positive result is a cloudy solution. Negative result is a clear solution.	Instruct client to obtain first morning specimen. Tell her that accuracy of test is greatest 6 weeks after last menstrual period. Obtain thorough menstrual history from client, including birth control methods. Determine presence or absence of presumptive signs of pregnancy (e.g., breast changes or increased whitish vaginal discharge).
Hormone testing		
Total estrogen levels	Urine estrogen levels are used to detect ovarian pathology, hyperadrenalism, interstitial cell tumor of the testes, liver disease, and ectopic pregnancy. A 24-hour urine collection is required. Normal levels vary, depending on menstrual cycle.	Instruct client to save all urine for 24 hours and to keep it refrigerated.
Pregnanediol levels	Progesterone levels are assessed. It is most commonly used to detect corpus luteum cysts and sometimes threatened abortions. It may also be used to determine adrenal cortical function and causes of amenorrhea. Normal levels vary according to menstrual cycle or length of gestation.	Instruct client to collect all urine for 24 hours and to keep it refrigerated.
Testosterone levels	Tumors and developmental anomalies of the testes can be detected.	Instruct client to collect 24-hour urine specimen. Keep it refrigerated. Collect genitourinary and reproductive system history.
BLOOD STUDIES		
Prolactin assay	This test detects pituitary dysfunction and causes of amenorrhea.	Ensure that client has fasted. Inform client that blood sample will be drawn in morning. Observe venipuncture site for bleeding or hematoma formation.
Serum HCG radioimmunoassay (RIA)	Same as pregnancy testing.	Instruct client to have blood drawn in laboratory. (Elicit where she is in her menstrual cycle, whether she has missed menses, and if so, how late she is.)
Serum androstenedione and testosterone levels	These tests ascertain whether elevated androgens are due to adrenal or ovarian dysfunction. Serum testosterone is also drawn to assess cause of amenorrhea.	Collect health history to eliminate potential sources of interference with accuracy of results (i.e., use of steroids or barbiturates or presence of hypothyroidism or hyperthyroidism).
Serum progesterone RIA	This study is frequently used to detect functioning corpus luteum cyst. It may also be used in determining adrenal pathology.	Ensure that client has fasted. Inform client that blood sample will be drawn in morning. Observe venipuncture site for bleeding or hematoma formation. Instruct client that serum must be drawn around day 24 or 25 of cycle for greatest accuracy.

Continued.

Table 45-13

Diagnostic Studies of the Male and Female Reproductive Systems—cont'd

Study	Description and Purpose	Nursing Responsibility
BLOOD STUDIES—cont'd		
Serum estradiol RIA	This test measures ovarian function. It is particularly useful in assessing estrogen-secreting tumors and status of precocious female puberty. Normal values depend on laboratory that performs test and should be obtained from that laboratory.	Ensure that client has fasted. Inform client that blood sample will be drawn in morning. Observe venipuncture site for bleeding or hematoma formation.
Human placental lactogen (HPL)	This hormone is detected in maternal serum as early as 6 weeks gestation. It plays a role in the metabolic processes of pregnancy.	Tell the client that fasting is unnecessary. Inform client that blood sample will be drawn in morning. Observe venipuncture site for bleeding or hematoma formation.
SYPHILIS STUDIES		

Nontreponemal serological tests
  Wassermann (complement fixation)
  Venereal Disease Research Laboratory (VDRL) (flocculation)
  Rapid plasma reagin (RPR) (agglutination)
	These tests are nonspecific antibody tests used to detect syphilis. Positive readings can be made within 1 to 2 weeks after appearance of primary lesion (chancre) or 4 to 15 weeks after initial infection.	Tell the client that fasting is unnecessary. Inform client that blood sample will be drawn in morning. Observe venipuncture site for bleeding or hematoma formation. Obtain data to determine presence or absence of problems such as hepatitis and autoimmune diseases that may interfere with accuracy of results.

Treponemal test Fluorescent treponemal antibody absorption (FTA-ABS)	This test detects syphilis antibodies. It also detects early syphilis with great accuracy. It is usually performed if results of nontreponemal testing are questionable.	Tell the client that fasting is unnecessary. Inform client that blood sample will be drawn in morning. Observe venipuncture site for bleeding or hematoma formation.
MISCELLANEOUS STUDIES		
Dark-field microscopy	Direct examination of specimen obtained from potential syphilitic lesion (chancre) is performed to detect treponema.	Avoid direct skin contact with open lesion.
Wet mounts	Direct microscopic examination of specimen of vaginal discharge is performed immediately after collection. This determines presence or absence and number of *Trichomonas* organisms, bacteria, white and red blood cells, and candidal buds or hyphae. Other clues or causes of inflammation or infection may be determined.	Explain procedure and purpose to client. Instruct client not to douche before examination. Prepare for collection of specimens (glass slide, 10% to 20% potassium hydroxide [KOH] solution, sodium chloride [NaCl] solution, and cotton-tipped applicators).
Cultures	Culture of specimens of vaginal, urethral, or cervical discharge is taken and used to assess presence of gonorrhea, chlamydia, or yeast. Rectal and throat cultures may also be taken, depending on data obtained from sexual history.	Obtain specific contact and sexual history inclusive of oral and rectal intercourse. Instruct against douching before examination. Obtain urethral specimen from men before they void. Instruct women who are sexually active with multiple partners to have at least a yearly culture. Instruct sexually active men to have any discharge evaluated immediately to rule out gonorrhea strains that do not cause classic symptoms of dysuria.
Gram stain	This presumptive test is used for rapid detection of gonorrhea. Presence of gram-negative intracellular diplococci generally warrants initiation of treatment.	Same as above.

Table 45-13

Diagnostic Studies of the Male and Female Reproductive Systems—cont'd

Study	Description and Purpose	Nursing Responsibility
CYTOLOGICAL STUDIES		
Pap smear	Microscopic study of exfoliated cells via special staining and fixation technique detects malignancy. Cells most commonly studied are those obtained directly from endocervix, cervix, vaginal pool, and endometrial lining of the uterine cavity.	Instruct women who are sexually active and who are over 18 to have yearly Pap smears. Arrange for smear at midcycle time. Instruct clients not to douche for at least 24 hours before examination. Collect careful menstrual and gynecological history.
Nipple discharge test	Cytological study of nipple discharge is performed.	Indicate whether hormonal preparations are being taken by client. Instruct client during demonstration of breast self-examination or examination of breasts that nipple discharge should always be evaluated.
RADIOLOGICAL STUDIES		
Soft tissue mammography	X-ray image of breast tissue on photographic film is used to assess breast masses, recent breast enlargement, and nipple discharge to detect malignancy. It is usually outpatient procedure.	Instruct client about risks (radiation) and advantages of the examination.
Contrast mammography	This test is used to evaluate abnormal nipple discharge. It is particularly effective in detecting nonpalpable intraductal papillomas. Test consists of injection of radiopaque dye in breast duct.	Determine actual or possible allergy to contrast medium.
Xeroradiography	It is similar to mammogram, except recordings are made on photocopy paper rather than x-ray film.	Same as mammography.
Ultrasonography (ultrasound)	This test measures and records high-frequency sound waves as they pass through tissues of variable density. It is very useful in detecting masses greater than 3 cm such as ectopic pregnancies, IUDs, ovarian cysts, and hydatidiform moles.	Instruct client that test is accurately performed only with a full bladder. Tell client to not empty bladder for at least 1½ to 2 hours before examination.
OPERATIVE PROCEDURES		
Breast biopsy	Histological examination of excised breast tissue is performed.	Before surgery, instruct client about operative procedures and sedation. After surgery, perform wound care and instruct client about breast self-examination.
Hysterosalpingogram	This test involves instillation of radioscopic dye through cervix into uterine cavity and subsequently through and out fallopian tubes. Spot x-ray images are taken to detect abnormalities of uterus and its adnexa (ovaries and tubes) as dye progresses through them. Test may be most useful in diagnostic assessment of fertility (i.e., to detect adhesions near ovary, an abnormal uterine shape, or blockage of tubal pathways).	Inform client about procedure and that it may be fairly uncomfortable. Determine possibility of dye allergy.

Continued.

Table 45-13

Diagnostic Studies of the Male and Female Reproductive Systems—cont'd

Study	Description and Purpose	Nursing Responsibility
OPERATIVE PROCEDURES—cont'd		
Colposcopy	Direct visualization of cervix with binocular microscope allows study of cellular dysplasia and vascular and tissue abnormalities of cervix. This test is used as a follow-up study for abnormal Pap smears and for examination of women exposed to DES in utero. Biopsy of cervix may be taken during colposcopic examination. This test is valuable in decreasing number of false-negative cervical biopsies.	Instruct client about this outpatient procedure. Inform client that this examination is similar to speculum examination. Explain purpose of procedure and prepare client for it.
Conization	Cone-shaped sample of squamocolumnar tissue of cervix is removed for direct study.	Explain purpose and method of procedure and that it requires use of surgical facilities and anesthesia. Instruct client to rest for at least 3 days after procedure. Also discuss necessity for 3-week follow-up check.
Culdotomy, culdoscopy, and culdocentesis	Culdotomy is incision made through posterior fornix of cul-de-sac and allows visualization of peritoneal cavity (specifically, uterus, tubes, and ovaries). Culdoscope can then be used to study these structures closely. This is valuable technique in fertility evaluations. Withdrawal of fluid (culdocentesis) allows examination of fluid type.	Explain purpose and method of procedure. Prepare client for vaginal operation with preoperative instruction and sedation. Perform assessment of bleeding and discomfort after surgery.
Peritoneoscopy (laparoscopy)	This test allows visualization of pelvic structures via special fiberoptic scopes inserted through small abdominal incisions. Instillation of carbon dioxide into cavity improves visualization. This technique is used in diagnostic assessment of uterus, tubes, and ovaries.	Explain purpose and method of procedure. Before surgery, instruct client about procedure, prepare abdomen, and reassure client about sedation. Tell client to rest for 1 to 3 days after surgery.
D & C	This operative procedure dilates cervix and allows curetting of endometrial lining. Curetted material is studied histologically. This test is used in assessment of abnormal bleeding patterns and cytological evaluation of lining.	Before surgery, instruct client about procedure and sedation. Tell client that overnight hospitalization may be required. Perform postoperative assessment of degree of bleeding (frequent pad check during first 24 hours).
FERTILITY STUDIES		
Semen analysis	Semen is assessed for volume (2 to 5 ml), viscosity, sperm count (greater than 20 million/ml), sperm motility (60% motile), and percent of abnormal sperm (60% with normal structure).	Instruct client to bring in fresh specimen within 2 hours after ejaculation.
Basal body temperature assessment	This measurement indicates indirectly whether ovulation has occurred. (Temperature rises at ovulation and remains elevated during secretory phase of normal menstrual cycle.)	Instruct client to take her temperature using special basal temperature thermometer (calibrated in tenths of degrees) every morning before getting out of bed. Tell client to record temperature on graph.

Table 45-13

	Diagnostic Studies of the Male and Female Reproductive Systems—cont'd	
Study	**Description and Purpose**	**Nursing Responsibility**
FERTILITY STUDIES—cont'd		
Huhner test	Mucus sample from cervix is examined within 2 to 8 hours after intercourse. Total number of sperm is assessed in relation to number of live sperm. This test is performed to determine whether cervical mucus is "hostile" to passage of sperm from vagina into uterus.	Instruct couples to have intercourse at estimated time of ovulation and be present for test within 2 to 8 hours after intercourse.
Endometrial biopsy	In this outpatient procedure, small curette is used to obtain piece of endometrial lining to assess endometrial changes common to progesterone secretion after ovulation.	Tell client that test must be performed in postovulation portion of cycle and that local anesthesia is used. Explain that procedure should cause only short period of uterine cramping. Instruct client to rest after procedure.
Hysterosalpingogram	Same as operative procedures.	Same as operative procedures.
Serum progesterone	Same as blood studies.	Same as blood studies.

tests are 97% accurate, but a negative test should be repeated in 2 weeks to achieve the greatest accuracy.[12] Serum pregnancy tests have also been developed. They are almost 100% accurate.

Hormone studies. Although estrogen studies are performed, the results are frequently inaccurate because of the complex metabolic pathways by which estrogen is broken down. Testosterone is a major precursor to estrogen formation, and its presence in urine can be measured in men and women.

Blood Studies

Recently, serum pregnancy tests using radioimmunoassays have been developed. One radioimmunoassay is the β subunit of HCG, which is so sensitive that a pregnancy can be detected before a woman misses her menstrual period.[9]

Prolactin assay is used primarily in the workup of a client with amenorrhea. High levels of prolactin are normally associated with low levels of estrogen such as those that occur during lactation. However, the same finding can occur with pituitary adenomas.

Serum progesterone and estradiol are commonly tested in ovarian function assessment, particularly for amenorrhea. In addition, hormonal blood studies are essential components of a thorough fertility workup.

Syphilis Studies

The types of tests performed to diagnose syphilis are nontreponemal and treponemal. Nontreponemal tests such as the VDRL test and the RPR card test are inexpensive and reliable. These tests detect the presence of antibodies in the serum of infected clients. Nonspecific antibodies can be produced during many pathological processes, especially some types of autoimmune diseases, and can yield false-positive test results.

Treponemal tests such as the FTA-ABS are highly reliable and should be used after a weakly positive or questionable VDRL. This test measures specific antibodies to *Treponema pallidum*. The FTA-ABS does not assess the adequacy of treatment of syphilis; the FTA-ABS remains reactive even after treatment.

Miscellaneous Studies

The most specific and direct examination for syphilis is dark-field microscopy. Unfortunately, the chancre is frequently gone by the time that symptoms occur, so the test cannot be performed. Other miscellaneous tests of secretions involve wet mounts, cultures, and stains to detect specific reproductive problems (see Table 45-13).

Cytological Studies

The Pap smear is a screening test to detect cervical cancer. It is performed by obtaining cells from the cervical canal, preferably the endocervix, as well as from the vagina and placing these cells in a fixative to be examined by a cytologist for cellular abnormalities. Pap smears are more accurate if performed at midcycle or during the secretory phase of the menstrual cycle because there is a greater likelihood that abnormal cells will be detected during these times. A Pap smear should be performed annually or more frequently in women with a history of dysplasia or exposure to DES. Pap smears are necessary in women who have had a hysterectomy because abnormal vaginal cells can sometimes be detected.

A negative Pap test does not rule out endometrial cancer. Specific tests are available to obtain a smear directly from the endometrium. Uterine aspiration and cannulation

into the uterine cavity make it possible to obtain endometrial tissue. Cytological study of any nipple discharge is also done.

Radiological Examinations

Mammography has become one of the most frequently used diagnostic tools in reproductive system assessment (see Chapter 46). Unfortunately, its frequent use has been highly criticized because of the potential risks of radiation. However, increased awareness of the risks from radiographic studies has resulted in valuable improvements in the technique of mammography, particularly in lowering the exposure per examination. The American Cancer Society recommends that a mammogram be performed on all women who are free of symptoms at 35 to 40 years of age. This baseline mammogram should be done earlier in a woman with a history of breast cancer in her family. Mammograms every 1 to 2 years are recommended for women between ages 40 and 49 and yearly after age 50.[10]

R | eview Questions

The number of the question corresponds to the same-numbered objective at the beginning of the chapter.

1. Which of the following structures make up the accessory organs of the male reproductive system?
   a. scrotum, ductus deferens, seminal vesicles, and urethra
   b. penis, testes, epididymis, and spermatic cord
   c. prostate, Cowper's glands, seminal vesicles
   d. testes, spermatic cord, prostate, and seminal vesicles
   e. penis, prostate, seminal vesicles, and Cowper's glands
2. Which of the following hormones are produced by the gonadal organs?
   a. LTH, progesterone, testosterone, and FSH
   b. GnRH, estrogen, and testosterone
   c. FSH, LH, and ICSH
   d. estrogen, progesterone, and testosterone
   e. estrogen, testosterone, and FSH
3. Female orgasm is the result of which of the following events?
   a. clitoral swelling and increased vaginal lubrication
   b. rapid release of vasocongestion and myotonia in the external and internal reproductive structures
   c. clitoral swelling, vaginal lubrication, and uterine elevation
   d. vaginal enlargement and secretion with penile insertion
   e. fallopian tube and uterine contractions
4. Decreased muscle tone in the aging female reproductive system can result in
   a. nonpalpable ovaries
   b. gynecomastia
   c. cystocele
   d. pendulous breasts
5. Which of the following are not significant to data collection regarding past health history for the assessment of male and female reproductive systems?

a. client's stature, physical strength, and appearance
b. presence or absence of measles, mumps, and rubella immunizations
c. hypertension, prostate surgery, and dilatation and curettage
d. allergies to rubber, breast surgery, and vasectomy
e. anemia, mother's use of DES, and dysmenorrhea

6. Which of the following is not a part of the physical examination of a man?
   a. palpation of testes and epididymis
   b. palpating for Bartholin's glands and Skene's ducts
   c. palpation for inguinal hernia
   d. inspection for penile discharge
   e. palpation of spermatic cord
7. Vaginal discharge and penile discharge may indicate which of the following diseases?
   a. syphilis
   b. gonorrhea
   c. balanitis
   d. epididymitis
   e. endometriosis
8. Because mammography requires the judicious use of radiography, which of the following criteria should be followed for breast mammography?
   a. Only women under 35 years of age should have a mammogram.
   b. Women over the age of 35 with a high risk for breast cancer should not have a yearly mammogram.
   c. Women over the age of 50 should have a yearly mammogram.
   d. Mammography should be performed only when a discernible mass of 3 months' duration is found.
   e. A mammography should be performed only in conjunction with breast biopsy.

REFERENCES

1. Griff RT and Schreiber JR: The ovary. In Yen SSC and Jaffe RB, eds: Reproductive endocrinology, Philadelphia, 1986, WB Saunders Co.
2. Morris JM: The abnormal Pap smear. In Glass RH, ed: Office gynecology, ed 3, Baltimore, 1988, Williams & Wilkins.
3. Bennett VR and Brown LK: Myles textbook for midwives, ed 11, Edinburgh, 1989, Churchill Livingstone.
4. Speroff L, Glass RH, and Kase NG: Clinical gynecologic endocrinology and infertility, ed 4, Baltimore, 1989, Williams & Wilkins.
5. Green S: Menopause, naturally: preparing for the second half of life, San Francisco, 1984, Volcano Press.
6. Neeson JD: Normal reproductive anatomy and physiology. In May KA and Mahlmeister LR, eds: Comprehensive maternity nursing, ed 2, Philadelphia, 1990, JB Lippincott Co.
7. Masters WH and Johnson E: Human sexual response, Boston, 1966, Little, Brown & Co.
8. Stoklosa J: Counseling men about disability, illness, and aging. In Swanson JM and Forrest KA, eds: Men's reproductive health, New York, 1984, Springer Publishing.
9. May KA and Mahlmeister LR: Comprehensive maternity nursing, ed 2, Philadelphia, 1990, JB Lippincott Co.
10. Marchant DJ: Benign diseases of the breast. In Glass RH, ed: Office gynecology, ed 3, Baltimore, 1988, Williams & Wilkins.

CHAPTER

46

Nursing Role in Management
Breast Disorders

Idolia Cox Collier

L *earning Objectives*

1. *Perform breast examination using the proper techniques on the client.*
2. *Teach breast self-examination, including rationale, technique, and reasons for referral.*
3. *Describe the causes, clinical manifestations, and therapeutic and nursing management of common benign breast disorders.*
4. *Describe the risk factors, pathophysiology, clinical manifestations, and therapeutic management of breast cancer.*
5. *Identify the types, indications, and complications of surgical interventions for breast cancer.*
6. *Explain the physical and psychological preoperative and postoperative aspects of nursing management for the client undergoing a mastectomy.*
7. *Describe the indications, types, and management related to reconstructive breast surgery.*

Breast disorders represent a significant health concern to women. Nearly every woman experiences some type of fibrocystic changes in her breasts. For one in nine American women, a breast disorder is diagnosed as a malignancy. Whether benign or malignant, intense feelings of shock, fear, and denial often accompany the initial discovery of a breast problem. These feelings are associated as much with the possible loss of a breast as with the fear of cancer itself.

Throughout history, the female breast has been regarded as a symbol of beauty, sexuality, and motherhood. For many women, identity and femininity are closely related to the breast. The threat of mutilation or loss of a breast may be devastating for the woman because of the significant psychological, social, sexual, and body-image implications associated with it.

Reviewed by Michelle Goodman, R.N., M.S., Oncology Clinical Nurse Specialist, Section of Medical Oncology, Rush Presbyterian St. Luke's Medical Center, Assistant Professor of Nursing, Rush University College of Nursing, Chicago, Illinois.

HEALTH PROMOTION AND MAINTENANCE
Early Detection

Health promotion and maintenance practices apply to all women, regardless of the presence of benign or malignant conditions. The most important practices related to breast problems are the regular performance of proper breast self-examination (BSE) and routine mammography. It is critical that breast lesions be detected early, diagnosed accurately, and treated promptly. A variety of factors influence disease-free states and overall survival after the diagnosis of breast cancer. However, many studies have demonstrated a better prognosis when the malignancy is small and the axillary lymph nodes are not involved.[1] Early diagnosis through mammography, BSE, and regular clinical examination is therefore a significant factor affecting mortality. Although there is increasing debate about the benefit of BSE, the practice is still encouraged because it has been demonstrated that between 85% and 90% of all breast cancers are discovered by women themselves.[2] Mammography will detect a breast tumor at an earlier stage than that which is achievable with BSE.[3] The frequency of these examinations is determined by the client's

Table 46-1 Risk Factors for Breast Cancer

Risk Factors	Increased	Decreased	Comments
Age	Older	Younger	Nearly two thirds found in postmenopausal women
Age at menarche	12 years of age or younger	13 years of age or older	Active menstruation for 40 years or more resulting in twice the breast cancer risk of menstrual activity for less than 30 years
Age at menopause	55 years of age or older	Before age 45	
Age at first full-term pregnancy	First full-term birth at age 30 or older or nulliparity	First full-term birth before age 30	
Atypical (precancerous) changes on breast biopsy	Present	Absent	Five times the risk of breast cancer when present
Family history of breast cancer	Present	Absent	Maternal first-degree relatives, particularly when premenopausal and/or bilateral

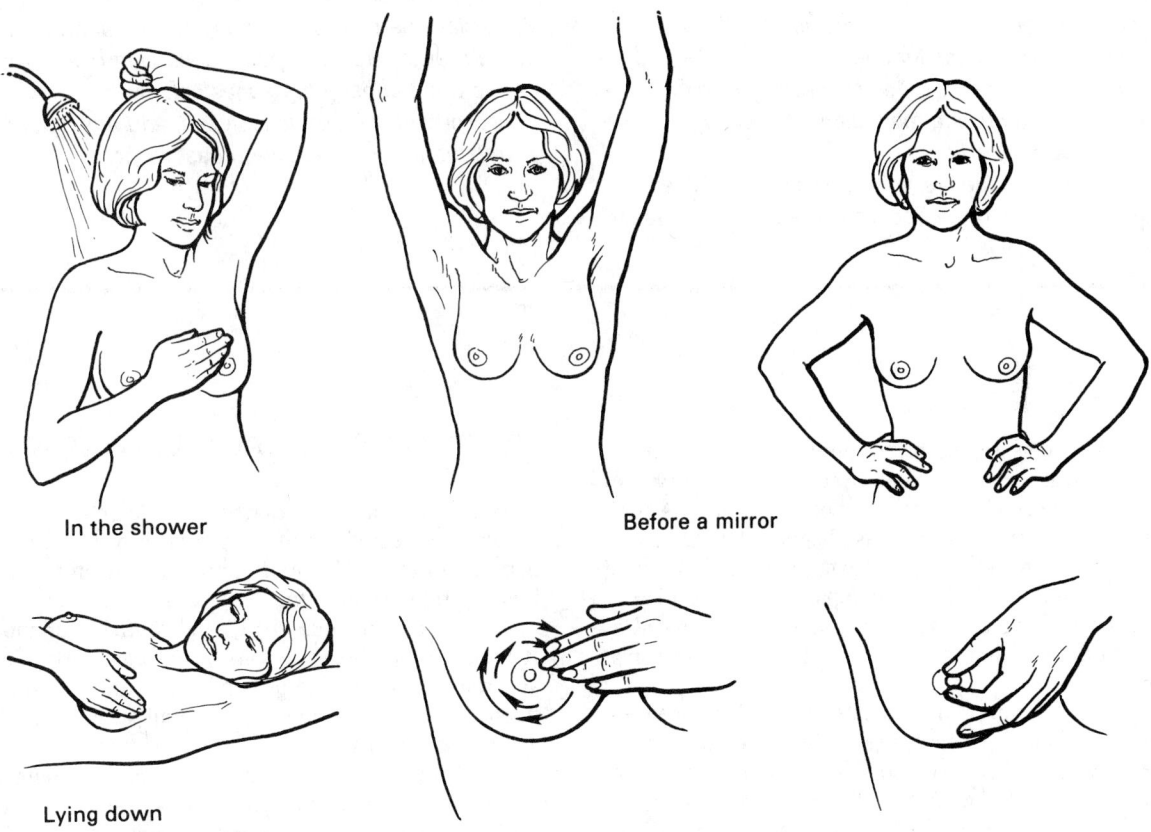

In the shower

Before a mirror

Lying down

Fig. 46-1 Breast self-examination. (Modified from 'How to examine your breast,' Atlanta, American Cancer Society.)

age and the presence of risk factors in her history (Table 46-1). Current guidelines accepted by the American Cancer Society, the National Cancer Institute, and the American College of Radiology regarding breast surveillance practices include the following:

1. Monthly BSE starting at age 20
2. Physical examination of the breasts performed by a physician every 3 years between ages 20 and 35 and every year thereafter
3. Baseline mammographic examination for clients be-

tween the ages of 35 and 39, an annual or biennial mammogram for clients between the ages of 40 and 49, and an annual mammogram for clients 50 years of age or older[4]

Although the reasons that women report for failing to practice regular BSE have changed somewhat over the years, the vast majority of women still do not regularly examine their breasts. A national survey on breast cancer conducted by the National Cancer Institute in 1979 showed that 90% of women were aware of BSE technique and that 75% practiced it at least once a year.[5]

More recent studies have found that 15% to 27% of participants perform monthly BSE. Approximately 43% to 54% reported less than monthly performance, whereas 30% did not practice BSE at all.[6,7] Factors that increase BSE compliance include a reminder system, confidence in BSE skill, encouragement from physicians and significant others, and BSE instruction that involves the client's active participation.

Nurses teaching BSE must emphasize that early detection and treatment enhance survival rates. Efforts must be directed toward teaching women the importance of BSE, how to perform it, what to do if a problem is detected, and the importance of clinical examination and mammography.

The technique for BSE has been established by the American Cancer Society (Fig. 46-1). BSE should be done monthly at a regular time. In premenopausal women, this is best done 7 days after the start of menstruation. At this time, hormonal stimulation of the breasts is at its lowest point. In most women, nodularity and tenderness will be minimal. Postmenopausal women and women who have had hysterectomies should set a regular date for monthly BSE. The monthly date of a birthday or the first day of the month are common choices for many women.

The examination should be done in good light and should include inspection before a mirror and careful, systematic palpation. The entire breast should be examined. The woman should be taught the BSE procedure by a nurse or doctor using the woman's own hand on her breast. A gentle circular motion over wet, soapy skin is particularly useful. The client should be told what to look for, such as a lump, nipple discharge, nipple retraction, redness, pain or tenderness, dimpling of the skin, and edema. Some teaching techniques involve using silicone breast models that simulate normal and abnormal breast tissue to help women learn to identify problems. The client should be shown the normal variations in her own breasts so that she will be able to detect changes. Finally, she should be reminded that most breast problems are not related to malignancy.

Follow-Up Care

If a problem is suspected, the woman should see her primary care provider or contact a comprehensive breast center as soon as possible so that additional diagnostic studies can be promptly initiated. If the problem is not serious, the woman's anxiety can be quickly relieved. Even when the client faithfully practices BSE, she should have an annual breast examination by a nurse or physician. The care evidenced by the clinician in performing BSE reinforces the practice of BSE by the client.

ASSESSMENT OF BREAST DISORDERS

The most frequently encountered breast disorders in women are fibrocystic disease, carcinoma, fibroadenoma, intraductal papilloma, and ductal ectasia including dilated ducts. In men, gynecomastia is overwhelmingly the most frequently observed disorder.

Many factors must be considered when the nurse is assessing a breast problem. Gender and age are important variables. Only 1% of breast carcinoma occurs in males. Benign lesions occur more frequently in premenopausal women. Breast cancer is predominantly found in postmenopausal women, and the incidence increases with age and family history.

Risk factors in the client's history must be evaluated. The history of the breast disorder assists in establishing the diagnosis. The presence of nipple discharge, pain, rate of growth, and correlation with the menstrual cycle should all be investigated.

The size and location of the lump or lumps should be carefully documented. Additionally, the physical characteristics of the lesion, such as consistency, mobility, and shape, should be assessed. If nipple discharge is present, the color and consistency should be noted, as well as whether it occurs from single or multiple ducts or from one or both breasts.

Diagnostic Studies

Several techniques can be used to screen for breast disease or provide diagnosis for a suspicious physical finding. Mammography is an x-ray technique used to visualize the internal structure of the breast (Fig. 46-2). Approximately 2 million women have mammography annually. Mammography can detect nonpalpable tumors. The minimum size

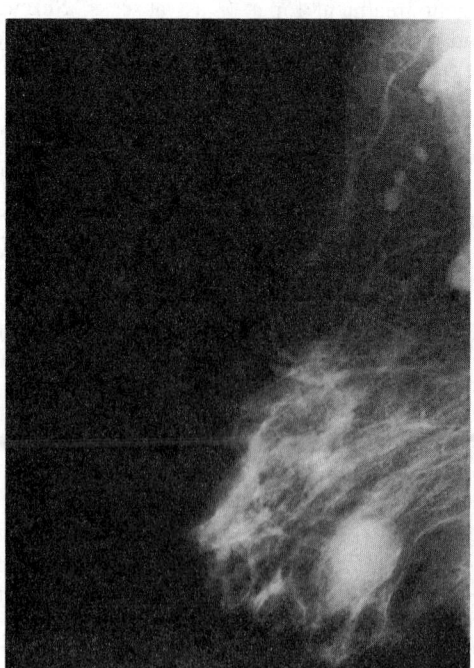

Fig. 46-2 Mammogram indicating the presence of carcinoma. Note enlarged axillary lymph nodes due to tumor involvement.

detectable by physical examination is 1 cm. Comparative mammography may show early cancer tissue changes. The diagnostic accuracy of mammography in combination with physical examination is thought to be greater than 90%.[8] Improved imaging techniques have reduced the radiation exposure that accompanies mammography to insignificant levels. Therefore the benefits of mammography outweigh the risks from radiation exposure. Other breast imaging procedures that are used to evaluate benign and malignant breast problems are listed in Table 45-12.

BENIGN BREAST PROBLEMS
Breast Infections

Mastitis. *Mastitis* is an inflammatory condition that occurs most frequently in lactating women. *Lactational mastitis* presents as a localized area that is erythematous, painful, and tender to palpation. Fever is usually present. The infection develops when organisms, usually staphylococci, gain access to the breast through a cracked nipple. Preparation of the breast for nursing by nipple rolling and toughening can decrease the incidence of lactational mastitis. In its early stages, mastitis can be cured with antibiotics. It is not necessary that nursing cease unless an abscess is forming and/or a purulent drainage is noted. The mother may wish to use a nipple shield or to hand-express milk from the involved breast until the pain subsides. The client should see her physician promptly to begin a course of antibiotic therapy.

Lactational breast abscess. If mastitis persists after several days of antibiotic therapy, a *lactational breast abscess* may have developed. In this condition the skin may become red and edematous over the involved breast, often with a corresponding palpable mass, and the client may have an elevated temperature. Antibiotics alone constitute insufficient treatment for a breast abscess. Surgical incision and drainage is necessary. The drainage is cultured, and therapy with an appropriate antibiotic is begun.

Fibrocystic Disease

Fibrocystic disease (FCD) is a benign breast condition characterized by changes in breast tissue. The changes include the development of excess fibrous tissue, hyperplasia of the epithelial lining of the mammary ducts, proliferation of mammary ducts, and cyst formation.[9] The use of the term *disease* is incorrect, since the cluster of problems is actually an exaggerated response to hormonal influence. However, FCD is used because it is the generally accepted name for the problem. Lumps can appear in both breasts and are often found in the upper, outer quadrants. It is the most frequently occurring breast disorder.

Fibrocystic changes occur most frequently in women between the ages of 35 and 50 but often begin in women as young as 20 years old. Changes tend to subside after menopause. The cause of FCD is thought to be hormonally influenced because of the relation of this condition to active ovarian function. Other factors that may play a role include nulliparity, stress, and nutrition. FCD is often exacerbated in the premenstrual phase and relieved after menstruation.

Symptoms of FCD include one or more palpable lumps that are usually round, well delineated, and freely movable within the breast. The consistency of the lump is related to the amount of fluid within it. There may be accompanying discomfort ranging from tenderness to pain. The lump is usually observed to increase in size and perhaps in tenderness before menstruation. Cysts may enlarge or shrink rapidly. Nipple discharge associated with FCD is often milky, watery-milky, yellow, or green.

Therapeutic management. With the initial discovery of a discrete mass in the breast by a woman or her physician, aspiration or surgical biopsy may be indicated. With large or frequent cysts, surgical removal may be favored over repeated aspiration. If no fluid is found on aspiration, if the fluid that is found is hemorrhagic, or if a residual mass remains, an excisional biopsy should be done.

Clients with cystic changes should be encouraged to return regularly for follow-up examinations throughout life. They should also be taught BSE so that they can detect any problems. Severe FCD may make palpation of a malignant lesion more difficult. Any new lumps should be evaluated, and changes in symptoms should be reported and investigated. Cancer does not develop from cysts.

Many types of treatment have been suggested for fibrocystic breasts. These include dietary, therapeutic, and surgical approaches such as a low-salt diet, analgesics, diuretics, restrictions of methylxanthines such as caffeine, vitamin therapy, hormone therapy, antihormone therapy, and subcutaneous mastectomy. In Europe, bromocriptine (Parlodel) and antiestrogens [e.g., tamoxifen (Nolvadex)] have been effective in relieving nodularity; however, they have not yet been approved by the Food and Drug Administration for use in the United States. Danazol has been approved as a treatment for FCD.

Danazol decreases follicle-stimulating hormone (FSH) and luteinizing hormone (LH) leading to amenorrhea and anovulation. The ensuing reduction of estrogen stimulation by this drug results in decreased pain and nodularity.[9] It may take 3 to 6 months for the effects of danazol to be noted. Side effects can be severe, including masculinization, hypoestrogenic effects, and hepatic dysfunction, but they do not usually occur with the dosage used to treat FCD.

Abstention from all forms of methylxanthines (e.g., caffeine, theophylline, and theobromide) is a promising therapy. Clients can actively participate by conscientiously eliminating caffeine from their diets. Because caffeine is mildly addicting, some clients may experience headaches as they withdraw it from their diets. Because stress is a contributing factor in breast discomfort, efforts should be directed toward the reduction of stress. Many of these approaches are considered experimental. Their large numbers indicate the uncertainty surrounding the cause of FCD.

The role of the nurse in the care of the client with FCD is primarily one of teaching. Clients should be told that they may expect recurrence of the cysts in one or both breasts until menopause and that cysts may enlarge or become painful just before menstruation. Clients should be reassured that cysts do not "turn into" cancer. They should be instructed to have any new lump examined promptly. Clients should be carefully instructed in BSE, using their own breasts. Teaching breast models can also be used if available.

Fibroadenoma

Fibroadenoma is a common tumor of the breast in American women. It generally occurs in women between 15 and 25 years of age and is the most frequent cause of breast tumors in women under 25 years of age. Fibroadenomas tend to develop more frequently in black women. They are usually small, painless, round, well delineated, and very mobile. They may be soft but are usually solid, firm, and rubbery in consistency. There is no accompanying retraction or nipple discharge. The lump is usually painless. In cases of fibroadenoma the tumor may appear as a single unilateral mass, although multiple bilateral fibroadenomas have been reported. The tumor grows slowly and often stops growing when it reaches a size of 2 to 3 cm. Tumor size is not affected by menstruation. However, pregnancy can stimulate dramatic growth. Fibroadenomas are rarely associated with cancer, although a very small number (less than 1%) of these tumors may be cystosarcoma phylloides, which are cancerous.[10]

Therapeutic management. Fibroadenomas are detected easily by physical exam and are often visible on mammography. Definitive diagnosis, however, requires biopsy and tissue examination by a pathologist. Treatment is by excision, which is not urgent in women under 25 years of age. In women over 35 years of age, all new lesions should be examined by means of excisional biopsy. Fibroadenomas are not reduced by radiation and are not affected by hormone therapy.

The nurse frequently has the opportunity to counsel young women with fibroadenoma. During this contact the benign nature of the lesion should be stressed, follow-up examinations should be encouraged, and BSE should be carefully taught.

Nipple Discharge

Nipple discharge may occur spontaneously or as a result of nipple manipulation. A milky secretion is due to inappropriate lactation as a result of such problems as drug therapy, endocrine problems, and neural disorders. It may also be idiopathic.

Secretions can also be serous, grossly bloody, or brown to green. These may be caused by either benign or malignant disease. A slide can be made of the secretion to detect specific disease. Diseases associated with nipple discharge include malignancies, cystic disease, intraductal papilloma, and ductal ectasia. Treatment depends on identification of the cause. In most cases, nipple discharge is not related to malignancy.

Intraductal papilloma. Intraductal papillomas are benign, wartlike growths found in the mammary ducts, usually near the nipple. Typically, there is an associated bloody discharge. A lump is rarely present. Intraductal papillomas usually affect women 45 to 50 years of age. A single duct or several ducts may be involved. Treatment includes excision of the papilloma and the involved duct or duct system.

Ductal ectasia. Ductal ectasia is a benign breast disease of perimenopausal and postmenopausal women involving the ducts in the subareolar area. It usually involves several bilateral ducts. Nipple discharge is the primary symptom. This discharge is multicolored and sticky. Ductal ectasia is initially painless but may progress to burning, itching, and pain around the nipple as well as swelling in the areolar area. Inflammatory signs are often found, the nipple may retract, and the discharge may become bloody in more advanced disease. Ductal ectasia is not associated with malignancy. If an abscess develops, warm compresses and antibiotics are usually effective treatments. Therapy consists of close follow-up examinations and/or surgical excision of the involved ducts.

Age-Related Breast Changes

Loss of subcutaneous fat and structural support and atrophy of mammary glands often result in pendulous breasts in the postmenopausal woman. The nurse should encourage older women to wear a well-fitting bra. Adequate support can improve physical appearance and reduce pain in the back, shoulders, and neck. It can also prevent *intertrigo* (dermatitis caused by friction between opposing surfaces of skin). Surgical lifting of sagging breasts is possible and may be desirable when reconstruction after a mastectomy is performed (see p. 1393).

The decrease in glandular tissue makes breast masses easier to palpate. Rib margins may be palpable in the older adult woman and may cause concern. The nurse should encourage older clients to continue BSE and to have annual mammograms and clinical examinations, since the incidence of breast cancer increases with age.

Male Breast Problems

Although the vast majority of breast problems occur in women, it is also important that men know how to examine their breasts. A thorough examination of the male breast should be a routine part of a physical examination. Gynecomastia, a transient enlargement of one or both breasts, is the most common breast problem in men.

Pubertal gynecomastia. Pubertal hypertrophy caused by increased estrogen production is seen most often in boys between the ages of 13 and 17. It is usually limited, although occasionally the localized hypertrophy may measure 2 to 3 cm in size. Pubertal hypertrophy is almost always self-limiting, and disappears within 4 to 6 months of onset. Parents and the affected boy should be reassured that in almost all cases this is a normal physiological phenomenon that will disappear spontaneously and will require no treatment. Rarely, unilateral gynecomastia in the young male may be marked and fail to regress. This is the only indication for surgical intervention.

Senescent gynecomastia. Senescent hypertrophy of the breast occurs between the ages of 50 and 70 years. A probable cause is the elevation in plasma estrogen in older adult men as the result of an increase in the peripheral conversion of androgens to estrogens with age. Though initially unilateral, the tender, firm, centrally located enlargement may become bilateral. When gynecomastia is characterized by a discrete, circumscribed mass, it must be diagnosed to differentiate it from the rarer breast cancer in males. Senescent hypertrophy requires no treatment and generally regresses within 6 to 12 months.

Gynecomastia may also be a symptom of other problems. It is seen accompanying developmental abnormalities of the male reproductive organs. It may also accom-

pany organic diseases, including testicular tumors, cancer of the adrenal cortex, pituitary adenomas, hyperthyroidism, and liver disease. Gynecomastia may occur as a side effect of drug therapy, particularly with administration of estrogens and androgens, digitalis, isoniazid, ranitidine, and spironolactone. Use of heroin and marijuana can also cause gynecomastia.

BREAST CANCER

Breast cancer poses a threat to life. In addition, the treatment can involve such a degree of disfigurement that it is a potential threat to a woman's self-image.

Significance

Breast cancer is the most common malignancy in American women. This disease develops in one in nine women. It is second only to lung cancer as the leading cause of death from cancer in women. The mortality rate of 27 per 100,000 women has changed little in 45 years. Each year in the United States, approximately 130,000 cases of breast cancer occur and about 41,000 women die of the disease.[11]

Etiology and Risk Factors

Although the etiology is not completely understood, a number of factors are thought to relate to the cause of breast cancer. Heredity or genetically transmitted susceptibility is considered to play a role. Hormonal influences are considered important. A number of external factors have been considered as contributory, including diet, obesity, viruses, and use of alcohol. Environmental factors such as chemicals and radiation may play a role.

Factors that place a client at higher risk for breast cancer have been identified (Table 46-1). Women are at greater risk than men, since 99% of breast cancer occurs in women. Increasing age also increases the risk of developing breast cancer. Breast cancer is rare in women under 25 years of age and predominates in women over the age of 60.[12] Positive family history is an important risk factor, especially if the involved member with breast cancer was premenopausal, had bilateral disease, and was a first-degree relative (i.e., mother, sister, daughter). The role of family history, however, is often overestimated. Risk factors appear to be cumulative; therefore, the presence of other risk factors may greatly increase the overall risk, especially for those with a positive family history.[12] Identification of risk factors indicates an increased need for careful surveillance of the client and careful instruction in BSE.

Clinical Manifestations

Breast cancer is usually first detected as a single lump in the breast. It occurs most often in the upper, outer quadrant of the breast (Fig. 46-3). The rate at which the lesion grows varies considerably. Slow-growing lesions are often associated with a lower mortality rate. On palpation, breast cancer is characteristically hard, irregularly shaped, poorly delineated, and nonmobile. It is painless and nontender in 90% of cases.

Only 5% to 10% of breast cancers present as nipple dis-

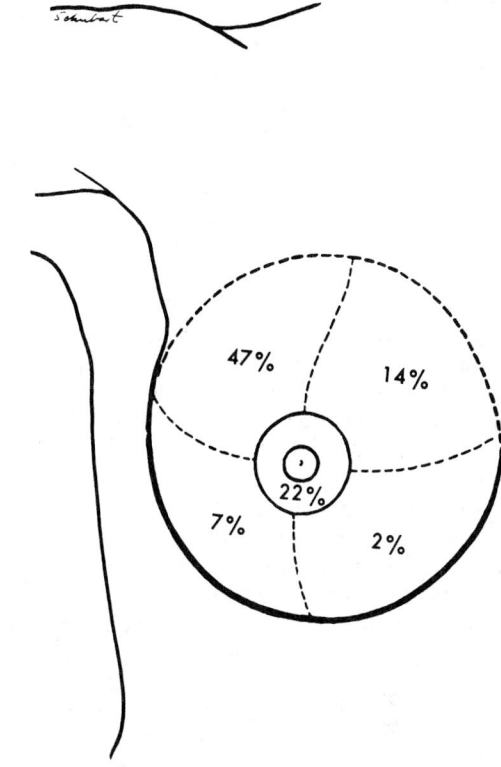

Fig. 46-3 Distribution of carcinomas in different areas of the breast. (From del Regato JA, Spjut HN, and Cox JD: Cancer: diagnosis, treatment and prognosis, St Louis, 1985, The CV Mosby Co, p 717.)

charge. The discharge is usually unilateral and may be clear or bloody. Nipple retraction may occur. Often, there is edema of the skin over the breast, giving it a characteristic appearance like that of an orange peel *(peau d'orange)*. In late stages, infiltration, induration, and dimpling of the overlying skin may occur (Fig. 46-4).

Definitive diagnosis of malignancy can be made only by means of histological examination of biopsied tissue. Biopsy technique may be either needle aspiration and cytological examination or open surgical biopsy.

Complications

The main complication of breast cancer is systemic disease. Long-term follow-up studies have shown that metastasis may occur early in the disease with or without lymph node involvement. Advanced disease usually involves a recurrence months or years after primary treatment, but it may exist at the time of initial diagnosis.

Locally advanced disease involves a tumor that is large and has invaded adjacent structures. Local recurrence is defined as a new tumor appearing at or near the site of an original tumor. The majority of recurrences appear within 3 years of the diagnosis of breast cancer and may locally involve skin, breast tissue, chest wall, and lymph nodes.

Widely disseminated or metastatic disease involves the growth of colonies of cancerous breast cells in parts of the

Table 46-2   Common Sites of Breast Cancer Recurrence and Metastasis

Site	Clinical Presentation
Local recurrence	
Skin	Firm, discrete nodules; occasionally pruritic, usually painless
Regional recurrence	
Lymph nodes	Enlarged nodes in axilla or supraclavicular area, usually nontender, superior vena caval obstruction due to enlarged supraclavicular nodes (oncological emergency), pain in shoulder and arm of affected side
Distant metastases	
Skeletal metastasis	Localized pain of gradually increasing intensity, percussion tenderness at involved sites, pathological fracture due to involvement of bone cortex, hypercalcemia due to skeletal metastasis or endocrine therapy
Spinal cord metastasis	Progressive back pain, localized and radicular; muscular weakness, usually in lower extremities; paresthesias in one or more extremities; bowel and/or bladder sphincter dysfunction; paralysis due to epidural spinal cord compression
Brain metastasis	Headache, unilateral sensory loss, focal muscular weakness, hemiparesis, incoordination (ataxia), visual defects, speech disorder (dysphasia), impaired cognition, behavioral and/or mental changes, loss of sphincter control, papilledema, persistent nausea and vomiting, seizure activity, progressive loss of consciousness
Pulmonary metastasis (including lung nodules and pleural effusions)	Dependent on sites and extent of pulmonary metastases; chest pain, dyspnea on exertion, shortness of breath, tachypnea, nonproductive cough (not present in all clients); adventitious breath sounds, dullness to percussion, restricted chest-wall expansion on affected side with pleural effusion
Liver metastasis	Abdominal distension; right lower-quadrant abdominal pain sometimes with radiation to scapular area; nausea and vomiting, anorexia, weight loss; weakness and fatigue; hepatomegaly, ascites, jaundice; peripheral edema; elevated liver function tests
Bone marrow metastasis	Anemia; infection; increased bleeding, bruising, petechiae; weakness and fatigue; mild confusion, lightheadedness; dyspnea

Modified from Engelking C: Recurrent breast cancer: physical and psychological sequelae, Innov Oncol Nurs 5:2, 1989.

body distant from the breast. Metastases primarily occur through the lymphatic chains, principally those of the axilla (see Fig. 45-4). Prognosis is directly related to the number of nodes involved. Distant metastasis occurs through the bloodstream when either the end of the lymphatic chain is reached or the tumor directly invades a vessel. The organs most frequently invaded by metastasis are bone, lung, brain, liver, and bone marrow. However, metastatic disease can be found in any distant site (Table 46-2).

Therapeutic Management

There are wide variations in the therapeutic management of breast cancer (Table 46-3). The most important factor in prognosis is the extent of the disease at the time of diagnosis, which is referred to as the *stage*. The therapeutic regimen is often dictated by the clinical stage classification of the cancer (Table 46-4). Although surgical removal of the involved breast has historically been the mainstay of treatment, this is not always the case today. (Side effects and appropriate nursing management of specific treatment modalities for cancer are discussed in Chapter 9.)

Surgical Interventions

Halsted radical mastectomy was once the preferred surgical method. Currently, the modified radical mastectomy involving total removal of the breast and axillary lymph

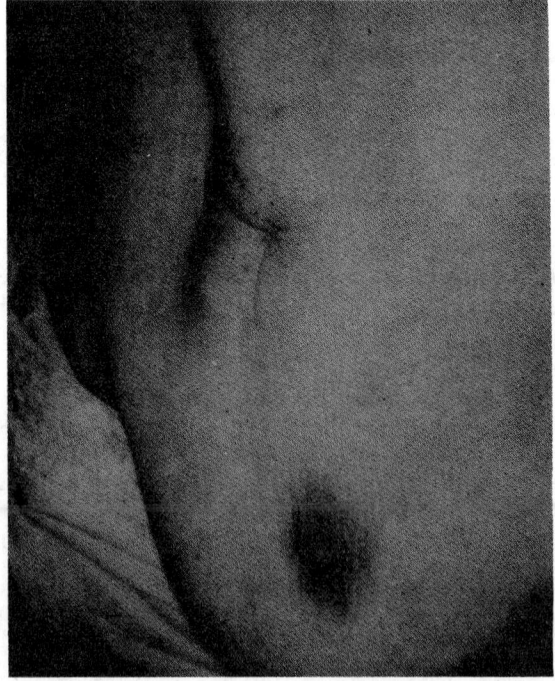

Fig. 46-4   Dimpling of skin over primary carcinoma of breast in upper, outer quadrant. (From Schwartz A and others: Principles of surgery, ed 5, New York, 1989, McGraw-Hill Book Co, Inc, p 558.)

Table 46-3

 Diagnostic and Therapeutic Management: Breast Cancer

DIAGNOSTIC

History of risk factors
Physical examination of breast and lymphatics
Mammography
Biopsy
Estrogen receptor assay

Staging

Complete blood count, platelet count
Calcium, phosphorus, liver function tests
Chest x-ray examination
Liver scan
Bone scan

THERAPEUTIC

Surgery
  Lumpectomy*
  Simple mastectomy*
  Modified radical mastectomy
  Radical mastectomy
  Extended radical mastectomy
Radiation therapy
  Primary radiotherapy
  Adjuvant radiotherapy
  Palliative radiotherapy
Chemotherapy
  Adjuvant chemotherapy
  Chemotherapy of recurrent disease
Hormonal therapy†
  Hormones (e.g., tamoxifen, aminoglutethimide)
  Surgical hormonal therapy

*With or without axillary node sampling or dissection.
†If estrogen receptor positive.

nodes is the most common surgical intervention. Breast-sparing approaches, such as lumpectomy with and without radiation therapy, are currently being performed. Surgical options for breast cancer are summarized in Table 46-5.

Recently it has been recommended that a biopsy and breast removal be performed in two stages. This allows the pathologist to make a definitive diagnosis. The client also does not enter the operating room uncertain of her diagnosis and then return to the recovery room with her breast amputated. The two-step approach has positive psychological benefits for the client in that she may participate in decision making and benefit from anticipatory support.[13] No adverse effects have been reported from this two-stage management.

Lymphedema of the arm on the affected side is a distressing complication after a Halsted radical mastectomy in about 50% of clients. Approximately 10% are severely affected. The client may experience heaviness, pain, impaired motor function in the arm, and numbness and par-esthesias of the fingers as a result of lymphedema. Lymphedema can occur as a result of the excision or irradiation of lymph nodes.[14] When the axillary nodes cannot return lymph fluid to the central circulation, the fluid accumulates in the arm, causing obstructive pressure on the veins and venous return. Cellulitis and progressive fibrosis can result from lymphedema.

Although lymphedema is not always preventable, it can be controlled somewhat after surgery by means of frequent and sustained elevation of the arm, regular use of a custom-fitted sleeve, and treatment with an inflatable sleeve (pneumomassage).

An additional problem that clients may encounter is stiffness in the shoulder joint on the affected side. An extreme case may be referred to as *frozen shoulder*. Gentle exercise, started as soon as possible after surgery, helps relax muscles and promote joint movement. Clients should not exercise beyond the point of pain.

In addition to potential physical complications, women may experience emotional problems after mastectomy, including anxiety, insomnia, depression, passive thoughts of suicide, and feelings of worthlessness and shame. These feelings are more common in younger women. Older women tend to focus more on the cancer itself.[13]

After surgery, the client must be followed up for the rest of her life at regular intervals. Most clients have professional examinations every 2 to 4 months for 2 years and every 6 months thereafter in addition to monthly BSE. The client must have yearly mammography of the remaining breast or breast tissue.

The decision to recommend adjuvant therapy after surgery depends on the number of diseased nodes, menstrual status, age, cell type, size and extent of the cancer, presence or absence of estrogen receptors, and other preexisting health problems that can complicate treatment.

Recently, analysis of malignant breast cells by flow cytometry has provided additional information that may be useful in predicting the risk of recurrent or metastatic breast disease. The technique requires a laser-powered flow cytometer to measure certain characteristics of malignant cells, which are difficult to evaluate by microscopy. Factors most commonly evaluated by flow cytometry are DNA content (ploidy) and proliferative capacity (S-phase fraction). These measurements correlate strongly with current predictors of recurrence and may even be superior indicators of prognosis. Now, however, this diagnostic procedure is still under investigation and is not used as a single determining factor in treatment planning.[15,16]

Radiation therapy. The three situations in which radiation therapy may be used for breast cancer are (1) as the primary treatment to destroy the tumor or as a companion to surgery to prevent local recurrence, (2) to shrink a large tumor to operable size, and (3) as the palliative treatment for pain caused by local recurrence and metastases.

Primary radiation therapy. When radiation therapy is the primary treatment, it is usually performed after local excision of the breast mass. It is considered to be an acceptable alternative to mastectomy when the cancer is detected at a very early stage. The breast and the regional lymph nodes (in some cases) are irradiated daily over the

Table 46-4 Staging and Grouping of Breast Cancer

PRIMARY TUMOR (T)
Clinical/diagnostic classification

T_X No detection of tumor possible
T_0 No evidence of primary tumor
T_{is}* Carcinoma in situ (e.g., intraductal carcinoma, lobular carcinoma in situ, Paget's disease of the nipple with no tumor)
T_1 Tumor 2 cm or less in greatest dimension
    T_{1a} Tumor 0.5 cm or less in greatest dimension
    T_{1b} Tumor more than 0.5 cm but not more than 1 cm in greatest dimension
    T_{1c} Tumor more than 1 cm but not more than 2 cm in greatest dimension
T_2† Tumor more than 2 cm but not more than 5 cm in greatest dimension
T_3† Tumor more than 5 cm in greatest dimension
T_4 Tumor of any size with direct extension to chest wall or skin
    T_{4a} Fixation to chest wall
    T_{4b} Edema (including *peau d'orange*), ulceration of skin of breast, or satellite skin; confinement of nodules to same breast
    T_{4c} Fixation to chest wall and edema, ulceration of skin, and confinement of nodules to same breast
    T_{4d} Inflammatory carcinoma

NODAL INVOLVEMENT (N)
Clinical/diagnostic classification

N_X No lymph node involvement
N_0 No evidence of regional lymph node metastasis
N_1 Metastasis to movable ipsilateral axillary lymph nodes
N_2 Metastasis to ipsilateral axillary lymph nodes fixed to one another or other structures
N_3 Metastasis to ipsilateral internal mammary lymph nodes

DISTANT METASTASIS (M)

M_X No distant metastasis
M_0 No evidence of distant metastasis
M_1 Distant metastasis (including metastasis to ipsilateral supraclavicular lymph nodes)

STAGE GROUPING

Stage 0	T_{is}	N_0	M_0
Stage I	T_1	N_0	M_0
Stage IIA	T_0	N_1	M_0
	T_1	N_1	M_0
	T_2	N_0	M_0
Stage IIB	T_2	N_1	M_0
	T_3	N_0	M_0
Stage IIIA	T_0	N_2	M_0
	T_1	N_2	M_0
	T_2	N_2	M_0
	T_3	N_1, N_2	M_0
Stage IIIB	T_4	Any N	M_0
	Any T	N_3	M_0
Stage IV	Any T	Any N	M_1

Modified from American Joint Committee on Cancer: Staging: manual for staging of cancer, ed 3, Philadelphia, 1988, JB Lippincott Co.
*Paget's disease associated with a tumor is classified according to the size of the tumor.
†Chest wall includes ribs, intercostal muscles, and serrated anterior muscle but not pectoral muscles.

Table 46-5   Surgical Approaches to Breast Cancer

Procedure	Definition
Local excision, lumpectomy, or tylectomy	Removal of tumor and small margin of normal tissue, overlying skin left in place, axillary nodes (if removed) taken through separate incision
Partial mastectomy, segmental mastectomy, or wedge resection	Removal of tumor and 2 to 3 cm wedge of normal tissue surrounding it and portion of overlying skin
Quadrantectomy	Removal of quarter of breast containing tumor, including skin and most axillary lymph nodes
Total mastectomy or simple mastectomy	Removal of entire breast, most or all axillary lymph nodes and chest wall muscles remaining
Modified radical mastectomy	Removal of entire breast and some, but not all, axillary lymph nodes, major chest-wall muscles remaining
Halsted radical mastectomy	Removal of entire breast, skin, chest-wall muscles, and axillary lymph nodes
Extended radical mastectomy	Halsted radical mastectomy and removal of internal mammary lymph nodes

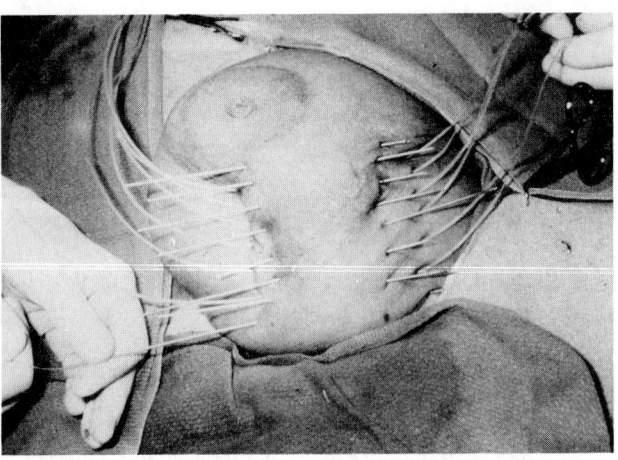

Fig. 46-5   Placement of seed holders for an iridium seed implant. (Courtesy John Breneman, Cincinnati.)

course of approximately 4 to 5 weeks. An external beam of radiation is used to deliver an approximate total dose of 4500 to 5000 cGy (4500 to 5000 rads; 1 rad = 1 cGy). A "boost" treatment to the full breast may also be given, either before or after therapy has been completed. The boost is a dose of radiation delivered to the area in which the original tumor was located. It can be given by external beam and usually adds ten treatments to the total number given. Alternatively, the boost can be given internally through the use of an interstitial radioactive implant (Fig. 46-5).

The radioactive substance, usually iridium-192, is in the form of "seeds" that resemble short pieces of pencil lead on a nylon thread. The seeds are inserted into "seed holders," hollow plastic tubes that are inserted through the breast during surgery. "Dummy seeds," which resemble the real ones but are not radioactive, are used in the operating room to prevent unnecessary radiation exposure to hospital staff. The dummy seeds are removed when the woman returns to her room and radioactive seeds are then substituted. The implant remains in place for about 2 days to deliver an approximate dose of 20 cGy (2000 rads). Once the implant is removed, radiation precautions are no longer required, and routine visiting procedures can be resumed.

Esophagitis, tracheitis, fatigue, skin changes, and breast edema may be temporary side effects of external beam radiation therapy. Chemotherapy may be used systemically to enhance the local effects of irradiation. (Nurs-

ing management of the client receiving radiation therapy is discussed in Chapter 9.)

Radiation therapy as adjunct to surgery. Although an uncommon treatment mode, preoperative radiation therapy can reduce the size of a large tumor mass to operable proportions by destroying the cancer cells. Additionally, because the malignant cells are partially or completely destroyed, the rate of local recurrence decreases. The disadvantages of potential delayed wound healing and increased lymphedema do not seem to outweigh the advantages of preoperative radiation in cases in which the cancer is locally advanced.

The decision to use radiation therapy after mastectomy is based on the probability of the presence of local residual cancer cells. Irradiating the area will not prevent the appearance of distant metastasis at a later date. The site of radiation therapy (lymph nodes, chest wall, or both) depends on the degree of possible spread of the cancer. Although radiation therapy can reduce the local recurrence rate, it has not altered the long-term survival rate of clients.[17]

Palliative radiation therapy. In addition to reducing the primary tumor mass with a resultant decrease in pain, radiation therapy is also used to stabilize symptomatic metastatic lesions in such sites as bone, soft-tissue organs, the brain, and the chest. Radiation therapy relieves pain and is often successful in controlling recurrent or metastatic disease for long periods.

Systemic therapy. The goal of systemic therapy is to destroy or control tumor cells that have spread to distant sites. The vast majority of women with breast cancer have no evidence of metastatic disease at the time of diagnosis. However, the 5-year relapse rate is approximately 50% when one to three nodes are malignant. When more than four nodes are involved, the rate increases to nearly 80%.[1] Because of the high risk for recurrent disease, nearly all women with evidence of node involvement should be offered some type of systemic therapy. Certain women, particularly those who are premenopausal, are known to be at higher risk for recurrent or metastatic disease. These

women are often recommended for systemic therapy even when no evidence of node involvement is found.

Current types of systemic therapy available for breast cancer treatment include chemotherapy, hormonal manipulation, and biological response modifiers.

Chemotherapy refers to the use of cytotoxic drugs to destroy cancer cells. The greatest benefits from chemotherapy have been achieved among premenopausal women with node findings that are positive for malignancy. Some studies indicate improved outcomes for postmenopausal women as well.[18,19]

Breast cancer is one of the solid tumors that is most responsive to drug therapy. More than a dozen agents that have a positive effect have been identified. The use of combinations of drugs is clearly superior to the use of single drugs. A common combination-therapy protocol includes cyclophosphamide, doxorubicin, methotrexate, and 5-fluorouracil (CAMF).

Combinations of different types of chemotherapeutic agents have been shown to have a greater antitumor effect than single-agent therapy. The benefit of combination treatment probably results from the use of drugs that have different actions on cell growth and division.

Because healthy cells are also affected by chemotherapy, a variety of side effects accompany their use. Usually systems and organs with rapidly growing cells are the most strongly affected. The most common side effects involve the gastrointestinal (GI) tract, bone marrow, and hair follicles, resulting in nausea, anorexia, weight loss, fatigue, irritability, and alopecia.[20]

Hormonal therapy. Estrogen can promote growth of breast cancer cells if the cells are estrogen dependent. If the source of estrogen is removed, the events that cause cellular transformation do not occur and tumor regression may occur. The source of estrogen can be removed by surgical ablation (e.g., oophorectomy, adrenalectomy, and hypophysectomy) or with additive hormonal therapy. Hormonal therapy is widely used to treat recurrent or metastatic cancer but may occasionally be used as an adjuvant to primary treatment.[21]

Two advances have increased the use of hormone therapy. First, reliable tests (hormone receptor assays) have been developed to identify women who are likely to respond to hormone therapy. Both estrogen and progesterone receptor status of the tumor can be determined. The importance of the assay is its ability to predict whether hormone manipulation is a treatment of choice for clients with breast cancer, either at the time of initial therapy or if the cancer recurs. Second, drugs that can inactivate the hormone-secreting glands as effectively as surgery or radiation, without the side effects of these therapies or the need to supplement other hormones no longer secreted by the ablated gland, have been developed.

Not all breast malignancies are estrogen dependent. Although normal breast tissue contains receptor sites for hormones, malignant cell transformation alters these receptor sites in some cells. If a malignant cell retains hormone receptor sites, it continues to be dependent on estrogen for cell division. The receptor sites that are altered as a result of malignant transformation are no longer controlled by hormones. Premenopausal and perimenopausal women are more likely to have tumors that are not hormone dependent, whereas women who are past menopause are likely to have hormone-dependent tumors.[22] Chances of tumor regression observed with hormone manipulation are minimal in women whose tumors are lacking estrogen and progesterone receptors. Receptor status probably has no relation to response to chemotherapy. Receptor states may change following hormonal therapy, radiotherapy, or chemotherapy.

Tamoxifen is the usual first choice of treatment in postmenopausal, estrogen-receptor-positive women with or without nodal involvement. It is also the first choice of treatment for premenopausal women with estrogen-receptor-positive tumors without nodal involvement. Tamoxifen, an anti-estrogen, blocks the estrogen-receptor sites of malignant cells and is commonly used to prevent or treat recurrent breast cancer. In premenopausal, nodal-positive, estrogen-receptor-positive women, combination chemotherapy is the usual treatment choice.

Additional drugs that may be used to suppress hormone-dependent breast tumors include megestrol acetate (Megace), diethylstilbestrol (DES), fluoxymesterone (Halotestin), and aminoglutethimide (Cytadren). Less common hormone-deprivation strategies include bilateral oopherectomy, adrenalectomy, and hypophysectomy.

Biological response modifiers. The use of biological response modifiers represents an attempt to stimulate the body's natural defenses to recognize and attack cancer cells (see Chapter 9).

■ Nursing Management of Breast Cancer

Throughout interactions with a client with breast cancer, the nurse must keep in mind the extensive psychological impact of the disease. All aspects of care must include sensitivity to the client's altered body image. An open relationship in which the client can express her fears and feelings is essential. The nurse can help meet the client's psychological needs by doing the following:

1. Assisting her to develop a positive but realistic attitude
2. Reinforcing that she is living, not dying, in spite of the diagnosis of breast cancer
3. Encouraging her to verbalize her anger and fears of cancer, disfigurement, and potential sexual rejection by her partner
4. Promoting open communication of thoughts and feelings between the client and her family
5. Providing accurate and complete answers to questions about her disease and treatment options
6. Offering information about community resources, such as Reach to Recovery, Encore, and local support groups

Nursing assessment

Subjective and objective data that should be obtained from an individual suspected of having or diagnosed as having breast cancer are presented in Table 46-6.

Nursing diagnoses

Nursing diagnoses related to the care of a client after a modified radical mastectomy may include, but are not limited to, those presented in Table 46-7.

Table 46-6

 Nursing Assessment of the Client with Breast Cancer

SUBJECTIVE DATA

History

Positive family history (especially mother or sister); previous unilateral breast cancer; exposure to excessive radiation; menstrual history (early menarche with late menopause); parity; age when first child born; FCD; previous endometrial, ovarian, or colon cancer; dietary fat and alcohol intake; obesity; chronic psychological stress (in women); Klinefelter's syndrome, testicular atrophy (in men)

Medications

Use of estrogens, especially as postmenopausal hormone replacement therapy and in oral contraceptives

General

Anorexia (possible indicator of metastasis)

Pain

No pain in 90% of clients; headache, bone or brain pain (possible indicators of metastasis)

Reproductive

Palpable lump found on BSE; unilateral nipple discharge (clear, milky, or bloody); change in breast contour, size, or symmetry

OBJECTIVE DATA

General

Anxiety, axillary and supraclavicular lymphadenopathy

Respiratory

Pleural effusions (possible indicator of metastasis)

Gastrointestinal

Hepatomegaly, jaundice; ascites, edema (possible indicators of liver metastasis)

Reproductive

Hard, irregular, nonmobile breast lump most often in upper, outer sector, possibly fixated to fascia or chest wall; nipple retraction, erosion; edema ("orange peel"), erythema, induration, infiltration, or dimpling (in later stages)

Possible findings

Finding of lump on breast examination; positive results of mammography, thermography, or ultrasonography; positive results of biopsy

---

Nursing interventions
Acute intervention

PREOPERATIVE. The client needs to be provided with sufficient information to ensure informed consent. Some clients need extensive, detailed information. For others, this only increases anxiety. Sensitivity to individual needs is essential.

Preoperative diagnostic studies must be completed. Teaching in the preoperative phase includes instruction in turning, coughing and deep breathing, a review of postoperative exercises, and explanation of the recovery period from the time of surgery until discharge.

POSTOPERATIVE. In addition to the usual postoperative nursing measures, the client who has had a modified radical mastectomy needs specific nursing interventions.

Restoring arm function on the affected side after mastectomy is one of the most important goals of nursing activities. The client should be placed in a semi-Fowler's position with the arm on the affected side elevated on a pillow. Flexing and extending the fingers should begin in the recovery room with daily increase in activity. (Information pertaining to arm exercises and care also apply to women who have had an axillary node dissection after lumpectomy or simple mastectomy.) Postoperative mastectomy exercises are instituted gradually at the surgeon's direction (Fig. 46-6). These exercises are designed to prevent contractures and muscle shortening, maintain muscle tone, and improve lymph and blood circulation. The difficulty and pain encountered by the client in performing the previously simple tasks included in the exercise program may cause frustration and depression.

Postoperative discomfort can be minimized by administering analgesics about 30 minutes before initiating exercises. If showering is permitted, the flow of warm water over the involved shoulder often has a soothing effect and reduces joint stiffness. Whenever possible, the same nurse should work with the client so that progress can be commended and problems can be identified.

Measures to prevent or reduce lymphedema must be used by the nurse and taught to the client. The affected arm should never be dependent, even while the person is sleeping. Blood pressure readings, venipunctures, and injections should not be done on the affected arm. Elastic bandages should not be used in the early postoperative period because they inhibit collateral lymph drainage. The client must be instructed to protect the arm on the operative side from even minor trauma such as a pin prick or sunburn. If trauma occurs, the area should be washed thoroughly with soap and water. A topical antibiotic ointment and a bandage or other sterile dressing should be applied. The physician must be advised, and the site of injury must be observed closely for evidence of inflammation. The client must know and understand that she is at risk of developing lymphedema for the rest of her life.

When lymphedema is acute, an intermittent pneumatic compression sleeve can be used. This device applies mechanical massage to the arm. Manual massage is also effective in mobilizing subcutaneous accumulations of fluid. Elevation of the arm so that it is level with the heart, diuretics, and isometric exercises may be recommended to reduce the fluid volume in the arm. The client may need to wear an elastic pressure-gradient sleeve during waking hours to maintain maximum volume reduction.

Psychological care.

The nurse can promote the client's recovery by arranging a visit from a Reach to Recovery volunteer if the service is available. Medical approval for this visit is usually necessary, although the client can request a visit herself after discharge from the hospital. The "Reach to Recovery Program" of the American Cancer Society is a rehabilitation program for women who have had breast surgery. It is designed to help them meet their psychological, physical, and cosmetic needs.[23] The volun-

Table 46-7

NURSING CARE PLAN FOR THE CLIENT AFTER A MODIFIED RADICAL MASTECTOMY

Defining Characteristics	Nursing Interventions	Evaluation Criteria
NURSING DIAGNOSIS: Pain related to surgical incision and manipulation of tissue		
Verbalization regarding presence and degree of pain at operative area	Administer analgesics as prescribed. Position arm to prevent tension and provide support. Encourage use of noninvasive pain management strategies such as distraction and relaxation.	Absence of or tolerable level of pain
NURSING DIAGNOSIS: Self-care deficit related to decreased arm and shoulder mobility		
Limitation in self-care participation	Flex and extend fingers in postoperative care area and continue throughout postoperative period. Carry out postmastectomy exercises. Assist client to resume activities of daily living as tolerated or as directed by physician. Emphasize bilateral activity of upper extremities.	Return to usual arm and shoulder function
NURSING DIAGNOSIS: Self-esteem disturbance related to altered body image and loss of body part		
Verbalization of concern about appearance and feelings of loss of femininity, depression, refusal to view incision, fear of intimacy	Arrange for Reach to Recovery visitor, if available. Provide information regarding prosthesis fitting and breast reconstruction (if client is interested). Assist client to verbalize feelings and encourage open communication with significant others. Share information regarding community resources (e.g., support groups, information services) and breast reconstruction.	Verbalization of feelings about surgery and change in body image
NURSING DIAGNOSIS: Fear related to diagnosis of cancer		
Questioning, insomnia, lack of attention, crying	Encourage client to talk about diagnosis of cancer. Provide accurate information. Encourage verbalization of feelings. Provide opportunity for significant others to discuss situation.	Verbalization of fear, evidence of support of significant others
NURSING DIAGNOSIS: Altered sexuality patterns related to loss of body part, fatigue, and anxiety regarding diagnosis		
Decrease in sexual desire and responsiveness, perception of sexual activities as undesirable	Assess cause, adaptation to loss, and personal ability to intervene. If appropriate, refer client and partner for therapy, counseling, or support.	Adaptation to altered body image, satisfying sexual relationships
NURSING DIAGNOSIS: Altered health maintenance related to lack of knowledge regarding BSE and signs and symptoms to report to physician		
Acknowledgment of lack of information about and/or confidence in performing BSE; lack of information about plans for follow-up care, signs and symptoms of recurrent or metastatic disease	Teach or evaluate BSE performance. Reinforce importance of annual mammogram. Provide information about signs and symptoms to report to physician (e.g., new and persistent bone pain, weakness, constipation, visual disturbances, confusion, new lump in breast or chest wall).	Early recognition of recurrent or metastatic disease

Continued.

Table 46-7

 NURSING CARE PLAN—cont'd

Defining Characteristics	Nursing Interventions	Evaluation Criteria

NURSING DIAGNOSIS: Potential complication: lymphedema related to edema on operative side and lack of knowledge of preventive measures

Edema in hand and/or arm on operative side, which increases with dependent positioning; heaviness; localized pain; lack of knowledge of preventive measures	Instruct client about self-care strategies and precautions to reduce risk of lymphedema. Do not perform venipunctures or take blood pressure measurements in affected arm. Avoid dependent arm position. Elevate arm and hand on pillow. Restrict abducting arm for first week. Perform hand and wrist movements, elbow flexion, and extension hourly or as indicated. Encourage participation in activities of daily living and self-care as much as possible. Use elastic sleeve if ordered.	Maintenance of usual size and shape of hand and arm

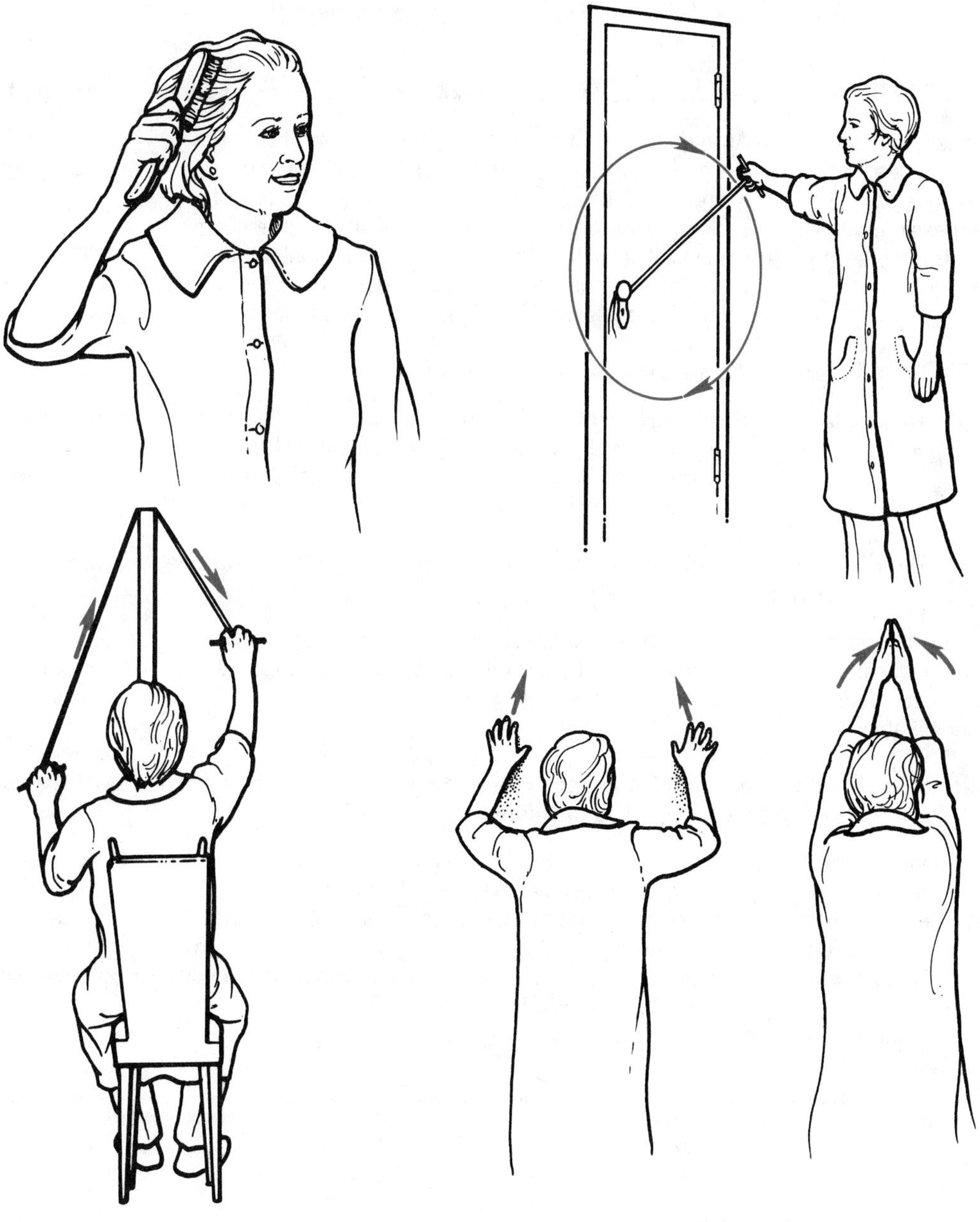

Fig. 46-6 Postoperative mastectomy exercises.

teers, who are all women who have had mastectomies, can answer questions about what to expect at home, how to tell people about the surgery, and what prosthetic devices are available. If a Reach to Recovery volunteer is not available, it is the nurse's responsibility to be knowledgeable about the needs of the client after a mastectomy. The American Cancer Society and the National Cancer Institute can provide excellent material to assist the nurse in meeting the special needs of women with breast cancer.

The professional staff must never underestimate the tremendous psychological impact that a radical mastectomy can have on the client. Emotional complications are common. The nurse's accepting, concerned attitude can do a great deal to relieve the feelings of anger and depression experienced by many clients.

Chronic management. The nurse should explain the follow-up routine to the client and emphasize the importance of beginning and continuing BSE and annual mammography. Symptoms that should be reported to the clinician include new back pain, weakness, constipation, and confusion. If adjuvant therapy is to be used, the client should have specific instructions about appointment times and treatment locations.

The nurse should stress the importance of wearing a well-fitting prosthesis. A variety of products are available to meet the specific needs of individual clients. Well-trained salespersons can help the client select a suitable prosthesis. There are both physical and psychological advantages to the use of a prosthesis; the return of a normal external appearance is an especially important one.

The implications of a mastectomy on the sexual identity and relationships of the client vary.[24] A preoperative sexual assessment provides helpful baseline data that the nurse can use to plan postoperative interventions. Often, the husband, sexual partner, and/or family members may need assistance in dealing with their emotional reactions to the diagnosis and surgery for them to act as effective means of support for the client.[25] There are no physical reasons for a mastectomy to prevent sexual satisfaction. If difficulty in adjustment or another problem develops, counseling may be necessary to deal with the emotional component of a mastectomy and the diagnosis of cancer.

Usually, initial coping mechanisms begin to lose effectiveness at about 3 months, and a peak period of psychological disturbance occurs for the client. Special nursing interventions are necessary, in terms of both psychological support and self-care education, if a recurrence of cancer is found.

Paget's Disease

Paget's disease is a breast malignancy characterized by a persistent eczematoid lesion of the nipple and areola with or without a palpable mass. Itching, bloody nipple discharge, erosion, and ulceration may be present. Diagnosis of Paget's disease is confirmed by pathological examination of the surgical specimen.

The treatment of Paget's disease is a simple or modified radical mastectomy. The nursing care for the client with Paget's disease is the same as the care for a client with any breast carcinoma.

MAMMOPLASTY

Mammoplasty is the surgical change in the size and/or shape of the breast. It may be done electively for cosmetic purposes to either enlarge or reduce the size of the breasts. It may also be done to reconstruct the breast after a mastectomy.

Health care providers should remain nonjudgmental toward women who desire mammoplasty. The desire to alter the appearance of the breasts has special significance for each client as she attempts to alter or recreate her body image. The client's motives should not be questioned. It is important, however, that the client have a realistic idea about what mammoplasty can accomplish and about possible complications such as hematoma formation, hemorrhage, and infection. If an implant is involved, capsular contracture and loss of the implant are possible.

Breast Augmentation

In augmentation mammoplasty (the procedure to enlarge the breasts) an implant is placed in a surgically created pocket between the capsule of the breast and the pectoral fascia. Most implants are silicone envelopes filled with a fluid such as dextran, saline, or silicone. Because of their resemblance to the human breast, implants filled with silicone are the most widely used.

Breast Reduction

For some women, large breasts can be a source of great embarrassment. They can interfere with normal daily activities such as walking, typing, and driving a car. Overly large breasts can also lead to back, shoulder, and neck problems. They may make stylish dressing more difficult. Reduction in the size of the breasts can have positive effects on both the psychological and the physical health of the client. Reduction mammoplasty is performed by resecting wedges of tissue from the upper and lower quadrants of the breast. The excess skin is removed, and the areola and nipple are relocated on the breast.

Breast Reconstruction

Breast reconstruction can be done after mastectomy. Recent strides in techniques have made this surgery a satisfactory alternative for many women.[26] The possibility of breast reconstruction may encourage women to seek professional help if a breast lump is detected. As women are demanding more information about and participation in treatment decisions, breast reconstruction is becoming more common and accepted.

Indications. The main indication for breast reconstruction is to improve the woman's self-image and to overcome feelings of loss. Present techniques cannot restore lactation, nipple sensation, or erectility. Therefore the erotic functions of the breast are not present. Although the breast will never return to its premastectomy appearance, the reconstructed appearance usually represents an improvement over the mastectomy scar (Fig. 46-7). The contour of the breast is restored without the use of an external prosthesis.

Timing of reconstruction. Controversy exists over the appropriate time lapse from mastectomy to reconstructive

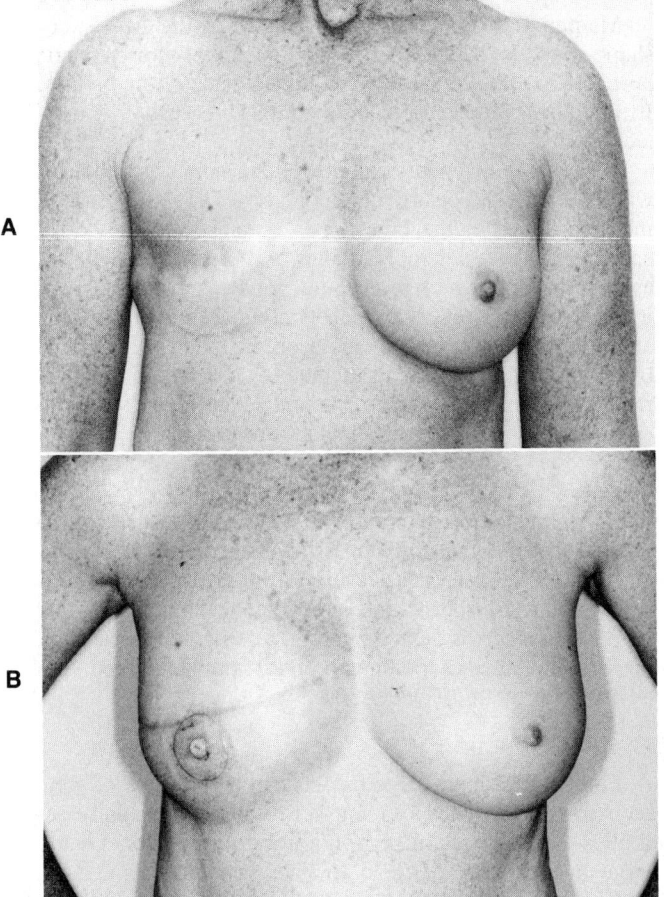

Fig. 46-7 A, Appearance of chest following right modified radical mastectomy. **B,** Appearance of chest following breast reconstruction using a tissue expander. (Courtesy Michael Leadbetter, Cincinnati.)

surgery. Some surgeons believe that reconstruction should not be attempted until there has been a lapse of 6 to 12 months from the time of surgery. Others believe that the timing of reconstruction surgery should be individualized, based on the need for postoperative chemotherapy or radiation and the psychological needs of the client.[27] The timing of reconstruction ranges from 5 days to 5 years after surgery.[27] Early reconstruction does not retard or influence further treatment or adversely affect predicted survival.

Techniques of reconstruction. The extent of the reconstruction depends on the type of mastectomy done. If extensive chest-wall defects are not present, a tissue expander can be used to stretch the skin and muscle at the mastectomy site.[28] Placement of the expander can be performed at the time of mastectomy or at a later date. The tissue expander, which is deflated at the time of surgery, is gradually filled by weekly injections of sterile water or saline solution, which stretch the skin and muscle. Once the tissue is adequately stretched, the expander is surgically removed, and the permanent implant is inserted. Some expanders are designed to remain in place and become the implant, eliminating the need for a second surgical procedure.

If insufficient muscle is left after mastectomy or if the chest wall has been irradiated, myocutaneous flaps may be

used to repair the soft-tissue defects. Flaps are most often taken from the back (latissimus dorsi muscle) or the abdomen (transverse rectus abdominis muscle). An implant may be used in addition to the flap, if the flap does not provide the desired cosmetic result alone. Reconstruction of the nipple-areolar complex is optional.

The natural response to the presence of a foreign substance is the formation of a fibrous capsule around the implant. If excessive capsular formation occurs as a result of infection, hematoma, trauma, or reaction to a foreign body, a contracture can develop, resulting in a deformed breast. Surgeons differ in their approaches to the prevention of contracture formation, although gentle manual massage around the implant is routine. Prevention of the problems that cause excessive capsule formation is critical. Other postoperative complications include skin ulceration, hypertrophic scar formation, intercostal neuralgia, and wound infection.

■ Nursing Management of Mammoplasty

Mammoplasty may be done in the outpatient surgical area, or it may involve overnight hospitalization. General anesthesia is used. Drains are generally placed in the surgical site to prevent hematoma formation and then removed 2 to 3 days after surgery. The drainage must be examined for color and odor to detect postoperative infection. The client's temperature should also be monitored. Dressings should be changed as necessary with the use of sterile technique. In cases in which a nipple graft has been performed, the dressings should not be disturbed for 7 to 10 days. After surgery the client needs to be assured that the appearance of the breast will improve when sutures are removed and healing is completed. Blackening of the reimplanted nipple immediately after the operation is expected. The client should be instructed to wear a bra that provides good support continuously for 2 to 3 days after mammoplasty. Depending on the extent of the operation, most women can resume normal activities within 2 to 3 weeks. Strenuous exercise may not be appropriate until several weeks later.

C ase Study

BREAST CANCER

Irene J., a 40-year-old woman, discovered a lump in her breast while doing her monthly BSE. The following day, she saw her physician, who confirmed the presence of the lump and ordered a mammogram. The mammogram showed a solid mass with associated microcalcifications. Mrs. J. was hospitalized for a biopsy procedure, which confirmed the presence of a malignancy. A right modified radical mastectomy was scheduled in 2 days.

Discussion Questions

1. What risk factors related to breast cancer should be asked about when taking the client's health history?
2. What are the characteristics of the malignant growth determined by palpation?
3. What is the preoperative and postoperative nursing management for this client?
4. What methods should be used to help this client and her family adjust to the impending change in her body image?

5. What are the possible complications the client may face after a modified radical mastectomy?

6. What are common postoperative exercises that this client will need to practice?

Review Questions

The number of the question corresponds to the same-numbered objective at the beginning of the chapter.

1. In the BSE procedure recommended by the American Cancer Society, palpation of the breast while lying down involves
   a. a top-to-bottom motion
   b. a left-to-right motion
   c. a right-to-left motion
   d. a circular motion

2. In addition to monthly BSE, all women over the age of 50 should
   a. have their breasts examined yearly by a professional
   b. have their breasts examined and mammography done yearly
   c. have mammography yearly
   d. have no additional examination

3. A round, well-delineated, palpable lump that may increase in size premenstrually each month and disappear at menopause is characteristic of
   a. FCD
   b. fibroadenoma
   c. intraductal papilloma
   d. ductal ectasia

4. Breast cancer occurs
   a. with equal frequency in men and women
   b. with equal frequency throughout the life span
   c. more frequently in women who have borne children and lactated
   d. more frequently in postmenopausal women

5. Removal of the breast, pectoralis major fascia, and axillary tail of the breast is called
   a. modified radical mastectomy
   b. lumpectomy
   c. simple mastectomy
   d. standard radical mastectomy (Halsted procedure)

6. Measures to prevent or reduce lymphedema include all of the following *except*
   a. positioning of the affected arm in a dependent position
   b. protection of the affected arm from trauma
   c. early institution of postmastectomy exercises
   d. early postoperative use of elastic bandages

7. The primary indication for breast reconstruction is to
   a. restore sensation and erectility
   b. restore lactation
   c. improve the client's self-image
   d. return the breast to its premastectomy appearance

REFERENCES

1. Henderson IC and others: Cancer of the breast. In Davita VT, Hellman S, and Rosenberg SA, eds: Cancer: principles and practice, Philadelphia, 1989, JB Lippincott Co, p 1197.

2. Baird S, McCorkle R, and Grant M, eds: Cancer nursing, Philadelphia, 1991, WB Saunders Co, pp 202-203.

3. Owen P and Long P: Facilitating adherence to ACS and NCI guidelines for breast cancer screening, AAOHN J 37:153, 1989.

4. Kase NG, Weingold AB, and Gershenson DM: Principles and practice of clinical gynecology, ed 2, New York, 1990, Churchill Livingstone, p 688.

5. National Cancer Institute: National survey on breast cancer: a measure of progress in public understanding, NIH Pub No 81-2306, Nov, 1980, US Department of Health and Human Services.

6. Rutledge DN and Davis GT: Breast self-examination compliance and the health belief model, Oncol Nurs Forum 15:175, 1988.

7. Chanpion VL: Attitudinal variables related to intention, frequency, and proficiency of breast self-examination in women 35 and over, Res Nurs Health 11:238, 1988.

8. Frankl G: Screening and detection of breast cancer. In Lippman ME, Lichter AS, and Danforth DN, eds: Diagnosis and management of breast cancer, Philadelphia, 1988, WB Saunders Co, p 10.

9. Ellerhorst-Ryan JM, Turba E, and Stahl DL: Evaluating benign breast disease, Nurs Pract J 13:13, 1988.

10. McDaniel MD and Chrichlow RW: Cystosarcoma phylloides. In Strombeck J and Rosato FE, eds: Surgery of the breast, New York, 1986, Thieme, Inc, p 151.

11. Silverberg E and Lubera JA: Cancer statistics, 1989, Ca 39:3, 1989.

12. Danforth DN, Lichter AS, and Lippman ME: Diagnosis of breast cancer. In Lippman ME, Lichter AS, and Danforth DN, eds: Diagnosis and management of breast cancer, Philadelphia, 1988, WB Saunders Co, p 50.

13. Valanis BG and Rumpler CH: Helping women to choose breast cancer treatment alternatives, Cancer Nurs 8:168, 1985.

14. Kissin MW and others: Risk of lymphoedema following treatment of breast cancer, Br J Surg 73:580, 1986.

15. Dressler LG and others: DNA flow cytometry and prognostic factors in 1331 frozen breast cancer specimens, Cancer 61:420, 1988.

16. Clark GM and others: Prediction of relapse or survival in patients with node-negative breast cancer by DNA flow cytometry, N Engl J Med 320:627, 1989.

17. Lichter AS and Findlay PA: Radiation therapy as an adjuvant to surgery in the treatment of operable breast cancer. In Lippman ME, Lichter AS, and Danforth DN, eds: Diagnosis and management of breast cancer, Philadelphia, 1988, WB Saunders Co, p 228.

18. Davidson NE and Lippman ME: Adjuvant therapy for breast cancer. In Lippman ME, Lichter AS, and Danforth DN, eds: Diagnosis and management of breast cancer, Philadelphia, 1988, WB Saunders Co, p 348.

19. Abeloff MD and Beveridge RA: Adjuvant chemotherapy of breast cancer—the consensus conference revisited, Oncology 2:21, 1988.

20. Knobf MK: Physical and psychological distress associated with adjuvant chemotherapy in women with breast cancer, J Clin Oncol 4:678, 1986.

21. Goodman M: Concepts of hormonal manipulation in the treatment of cancer, Oncol Nurs Forum 15:639, 1988.

22. Dunne CF: Hormonal therapy for breast cancer, Cancer Nurs 11:288, 1988.

23. Cohen RJ: Diagnosis: breast cancer, Hosp Med 20:92, 1984.

24. Schwarz A and others: Nursing care plans: sexuality and treatment of breast cancer, Oncol Nurs Forum 11:16, 1984.

25. Northouse L: Longitudinal study of the adjustment of patients and husbands to breast cancer, Oncol Nurs Forum 16:511, 1989.

26. Muller C: Postmastectomy reconstruction . . . a new life, Can OR Nurs J 5:28, 1987.

27. Schain WS and others: The sooner, the better: a study of psychological factors in women undergoing immediate versus delayed breast reconstruction, Am J Psychiatry 142:40, 1985.

28. D'Angelo T and Gorrell C: Breast reconstruction using tissue expanders, Oncol Nurs Forum 16:23, 1989.

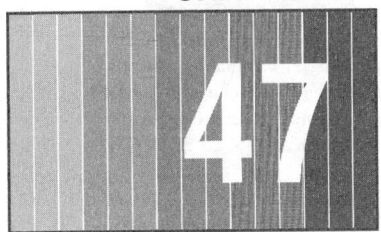

CHAPTER

47

Nursing Role in Management
Sexually Transmitted Diseases

Linda C. Carnago

L *earning Objectives*

1. *Identify the contributory factors to the high incidence of sexually transmitted diseases.*
2. *Explain the etiology, clinical manifestations, complications, and diagnostic abnormalities of gonorrhea, syphilis, genital herpes, Chlamydia trachomatis, infections, acquired immunodeficiency syndrome, and condylomata acuminata.*
3. *Explain the therapeutic and pharmacological management of gonorrhea and syphilis.*
4. *Compare primary genital herpes with recurrent genital herpes.*
5. *Identify individuals at risk for acquiring acquired immunodeficiency syndrome and the usual means of transmission of the disease.*
6. *Identify nursing assessment and nursing diagnoses for clients who are suspected of having a sexually transmitted disease.*
7. *Describe the nursing role in the prevention and control of sexually transmitted diseases.*
8. *Describe the physiological and psychological nursing interventions for the client with a sexually transmitted disease.*

SEXUALLY TRANSMITTED DISEASES

Sexually transmitted diseases (STDs) are infectious diseases usually associated with intimate sexual contact. They are often referred to as *venereal diseases*. The existence of syphilis and gonorrhea is generally known, but there are over 20 diseases that can be sexually transmitted (Table 47-1). Several STDs are more common in tropical and semitropical areas, such as chancroid and granuloma inguinale. However, the mobility of modern society is increasing their occurrence in other areas of the world. Diseases that are associated with sexual transmission can also be contracted by routes other than sexual means, such as through blood, blood products, and accidental inoculation.

Significance

In the United States, all cases of gonorrhea and syphilis must be reported to the state or local health officer. In spite of this requirement, there are many unreported and undiagnosed cases. Gonorrhea ranks first and syphilis ranks third among the reported communicable diseases in the United States. The incidence of gonorrhea steadily in-

creased after 1966 but began to decline in 1975. This trend continued in 1987, with a decline of 9.9% in reported cases, possibly influenced by more focused control activities, changes in surveillance and reporting, and changes in host factors. Teenagers and young adults accounted for 25% to 40% of all gonorrhea cases reported. Most states have enacted laws that permit examination and treatment services for minors without parental consent.

The incidence of primary and secondary syphilis has changed since 1941 (Fig. 47-1), presumably as a result of factors such as availability of penicillin. In 1987, a 25% increase in infectious syphilis was reported. This is the largest single year increase since 1960.[1] Possible reasons for the increase include the following:

1. Prostitutes, among others, may transmit the disease by offering sexual favors for nonintravenous drugs such as crack cocaine.
2. Spectinomycin, which does not appear to cure coincubating syphilis, was routinely used to treat resistant strains of gonorrhea.
3. Resources available for syphilis control were decreased. The fact that there was an increase in the number of women (32.9%) with syphilis will probably affect the incidence of congenital syphilis.[2] In the last 40 years, treat-

Reviewed by Lynn Hanson, N.P., M.S., University of California, San Francisco, Faculty Gynecology Practice, San Francisco, California.

Table 47-1 Sexually Transmitted Diseases and Diseases Associated with Sexual Transmission

Bacterial infection
  Syphilis*
  Gonorrhea*
  Chancroid*
  Granuloma inguinale*
  Gardnerella vaginalis vaginitis
  Neisseria meningitidis
  Group B β-hemolytic streptococcal infections
Viral infections
  Genital herpes
  Condyloma acuminatum
  Molluscum contagiosum
  Cytomegalovirus infection
  Viral hepatitis type B*
Chlamydia trachomatis infections
  Lymphogranuloma venereum*
  Chlamydial cervicitis/urethritis
Mycoplasma infections
Trichomoniasis
Candidiasis
Pubic lice
Scabies
Reiter's disease
Acquired immunodeficiency syndrome†

---

*Reportable diseases.
†A total of 38 states requires or has legislation pending that requires reporting of persons infected with human immunodeficiency virus.

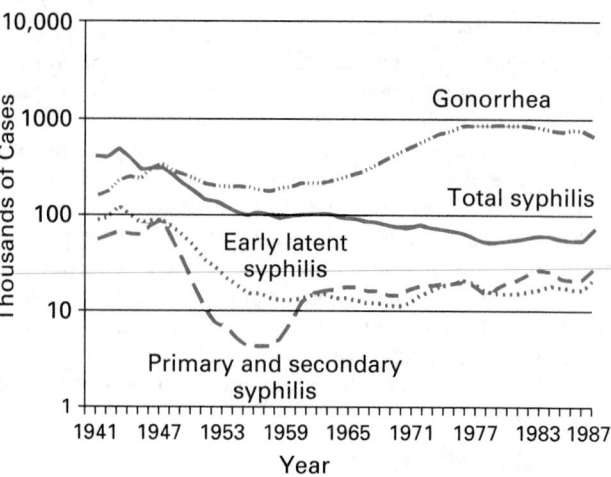

Fig. 47-1 Reported cases of syphilis and gonorrhea in the United States from 1941 to 1987. (From HEW PHS Center for Disease Control: Sexually transmitted disease statistics, Atlanta, Oct 1988.)

ment of large numbers of clients with syphilis has produced a 98% reduction in the complications of this disease.

Because genital herpes, *Chlamydia trachomatis* infections, and condylomata acuminata (genital warts) are not reportable diseases, their true incidence is difficult to determine. Researchers have estimated that approximately 400,000 to 600,000 new cases of genital herpes occur each year and that recurrent episodes exceed several million annually.[3] The disease has gained attention because of its association with neonatal infection and cervical cancer. Infections caused by *C. trachomatis* are the most prevalent STDs in the United States today.[4] Nongonococcal urethritis is at least twice as common as gonococcal urethritis among sexually active men.[5] Chlamydial infections are a common cause (25% to 30%) of pelvic inflammatory disease (PID).[6] Genital warts have become increasingly common, with an estimated annual incidence of one-half to 1 million cases. There is concern over the strong association between specific types of warts and genital cancer.[7]

As of June 1991, over 175,000 cases of acquired immunodeficiency syndrome (AIDS) and more than 110,000 AIDS-related deaths had been reported to the Centers of Disease Control (CDC). Groups at highest risk of acquiring AIDS continue to be homosexual or bisexual men and nonintravenous drug users (56%). Others at high risk in-

clude female or heterosexual male intravenous drug users (IVDU), sex partners or children IVDUs, and individuals with other or unknown risk factors (e.g., homosexual IVDUs, transfusion recipients, hemophiliacs) (see Fig. 8-10).[8]

Factors Affecting Incidence

There are contributing factors to the increased incidence of STDs. Earlier reproductive maturity and expanded longevity have resulted in a longer sexual life span. The increase in the total population has resulted in an increase in the number of susceptible hosts. Greater sexual freedom, changing roles of women, changes in the institution of marriage and the family, decreased social control by religious institutions, and increased emphasis on sexuality by the media are also factors. In addition, increased leisure time, inexpensive travel, and urbanization have brought together people of varying cultural backgrounds and value systems. Codes of behavior from the new environment are usually adopted and may result in the exploration of new forms of sexual conduct.

Changes in methods of contraception are also reflected in the incidence of venereal disease. The condom is considered to be the only contraceptive device that is prophylactic in regard to venereal disease. Recent studies suggest that condom use is increasing in selected populations but is still infrequent.[9] Commonly used oral contraceptives cause the secretions of the cervix and vagina to become more alkaline. This change produces a more favorable environment for the growth of venereal disease organisms at those sites. It has been demonstrated that women who take oral contraceptives have a lower risk of PID as a result of the ability of the cervical mucus to act as a barrier against bacteria. However, *Chlamydia* species, the leading cause of nongonococcal PID, may be enhanced by oral contraceptive use.[10,11] Intrauterine device users are also at risk of PID.[12]

GONORRHEA

The causative organism of gonorrhea is *Neisseria gonorrhoeae,* a gram-negative diplococcus. It may invade any mucosal surface of the body but is most likely to invade the moist linings of the urinary and genital organs of both sexes. The disease is spread by direct physical contact with an infected host, usually during sexual activity. Neonates can develop a gonococcal infection after passage through an infected birth canal. The delicate gonococcus is easily killed through drying, heating, or washing with an antiseptic solution. Consequently, indirect transmission by instruments or linens is rare. The incubation period is 3 to 4 days. The disease confers no immunity to subsequent reinfection.

Clinical Manifestations

Men. The initial site of infection in heterosexual men is usually the anterior urethra. Symptoms of urethritis consisting of dysuria and profuse, purulent urethral discharge develop within 3 to 5 days after infection. Men generally seek medical assistance early in the disease because their symptoms are usually obvious and distressing. In less than 5% of cases, men with urethral gonorrhea have no symptoms.[13]

Women. Most women who contract gonorrhea are free of symptoms or have minor symptoms that are often overlooked, making it possible for them to remain a source of infection. A small number of women may complain of vaginal discharge, dysuria, or frequency of urination. Changes in menstruation may be a symptom, but they are often disregarded by the woman. After the incubation period, redness and swelling occur at the site of contact, which is usually the cervix or urethra. A purulent exudate often develops, with a potential for abscess formation. The disease may remain local or can spread by direct tissue extension to the uterus, fallopian tubes, and ovaries. Although the vulva and vagina are uncommon sites for a gonorrheal infection, they may become involved when little or no estrogen is present, such as in prepubertal girls and postmenopausal women.

General. Anorectal gonorrhea may be present, particularly in homosexual men, and is usually caused by anal intercourse. Gonococcal proctitis in women probably results from rectal coitus as well as contamination from infected vaginal secretions. Most clients with rectal infections have no significant symptoms. A small percentage of individuals develop gonococcal pharyngitis resulting from orogenital sexual contact. When the gonococcus can be demonstrated by culture, individuals of either gender are infectious to their sexual partners.

Complications

Because men often seek treatment early in the course of the disease, they are less likely to develop complications. The complications that do occur in men are prostatitis, urethral strictures, and sterility from orchitis or epididymitis. Because women who are free of symptoms seldom seek treatment, complications are more common and usually constitute the reason for seeking medical attention. PID, bartholinian abscess, ectopic pregnancy, and infertility are the main complications of gonorrhea in women. A small percentage of infected persons, mainly women, may develop a disseminated gonococcal infection (DGI). The appearance of skin lesions, fever, arthralgia, or arthritis usually causes the client to seek medical help.

Newborn prophylaxis. Almost all states have a health department regulation or law requiring the instillation of a prophylactic drug such as erythromycin (0.5%) or silver nitrate into the eyes of all newborns.[14] Therefore the incidence of gonorrheal eye infections in newborns (ophthalmia neonatorum) is relatively uncommon today. Untreated infected infants develop permanent blindness.

Diagnostic Studies

The most reliable way to confirm gonococcal infection is to demonstrate the organism by means of smear or culture. The immediate identification of *N. gonorrhoeae* is usually made with Gram-stained smears made from the discharge of secretions. The slides should be interpreted by a clinician or technician with experience so that a correct diagnosis is made initially, since some clients fail to return for follow-up care. Cultures of the discharge or secretion can provide definitive diagnosis after incubation for 24 to 48 hours. No effective blood test is available for the diagnosis of gonorrhea.

For men a presumptive diagnosis of gonorrhea is made if there is a history of sexual contact with an infected individual followed by a urethral discharge within a few days. Typical clinical manifestations combined with a positive Gram-stained smear of purulent discharge from the penis gives an almost certain diagnosis. Culture of discharge is indicated for men whose smears are negative in the presence of strong clinical evidence.

Making a diagnosis of gonorrhea in women on the basis of symptoms is difficult because most women are symptom free or have complaints that may be confused with other conditions. Smears and purulent discharge do not establish a diagnosis of gonorrhea because the female genitourinary (GU) tract normally harbors a large number of organisms that resemble *N. gonorrhoeae*. A culture must be done to confirm the diagnosis. Although the cervix is the most common site, specimens may also be taken from the urethra, anus, or oropharynx to confirm the diagnosis. The CDC recommends that all women treated for gonorrhea have a rectal culture done. A specific culture medium (Thayer-Martin), which encourages the growth of the gonococcus, is used. If laboratory facilities are not readily accessible, special holding media are available.

Therapeutic and Pharmacological Management

A history of sexual contact with a partner known to have gonorrhea is considered good evidence for the presence of gonorrhea. Because of a short incubation period and high infectivity, treatment is instituted without awaiting culture results, even in the absence of any sign or symptom. The treatment of gonorrhea in the early stage is curative. Traditionally, the drug of choice for gonorrheal therapy was penicillin, but changes have been made because of resistant strains of *N. gonorrhoeae* and the incidence of coexisting chlamydial infection (Table 47-2).

Recently, a rapid increase of cases of gonorrhea caused by resistant strains of *N. gonorrhoeae* has been identified (Fig. 47-2). The three most important strains from a public health standpoint are penicillinase-producing resistance to penicillin (first appearing in 1976), chromosomally mediated resistance to penicillin (first appearing in 1983), and plasmid-mediated high-level tetracycline resistance (first appearing in 1985).[15]

Table 47-2

Diagnostic and Therapeutic Management: Gonorrhea

DIAGNOSTIC

History and physical examination
Smear and culture
Serological testing for syphilis

THERAPEUTIC

Initial therapy*
  Ceftriaxone 250 mg IM once or spectinomycin 2 g IM once plus doxycycline 100 mg orally twice a day for 7 days; possible substitution of erythromycin base of stearate 500 mg four times a day for 7 days (when tetracyclines are contraindicated, as in pregnant women and prepubertal children)
  Test for syphilis
  Confidential counseling and testing for human immunodeficiency virus infections
  Follow-up cultures 3 to 7 days after completion of treatment
Case finding
Treatment of contacts
Instruction on abstinence from sexual intercourse and alcohol
Reexamination and reculture (at least once)
Repeat of serological test for syphilis at 1 month

IM, Intramuscular.
*Adapted from Center for Disease Control: STD treatment guidelines, MMWR 38:8, 1989.

No clinical distinction occurs between infections caused by resistant or sensitive strains of *N. gonorrhoeae*. Therefore it was anticipated that there would be (1) increased numbers of disease-related complications (e.g., PID, DGI), (2) extended periods of infectiveness resulting in increased numbers of sex partners becoming infected, and (3) increased cost of treatment.[16] As a result, ceftriaxone, an effective cephalosporin, became part of the treatment plan. The high frequency (45%) of coexisting chlamydial and gonococcal infections has led to the addition of doxycycline to the treatment regimen. Clients with coincubating syphilis are likely to be cured by the same drugs.

All sexual contacts of clients with gonorrhea must be treated to prevent reinfection after resumption of sexual relations. The "ping-pong" effect of reexposure, treatment, and reinfection can cease only when infected partners are treated simultaneously. Additionally, the client should be advised to abstain from sexual intercourse and alcohol for 2 to 4 weeks. Sexual intercourse allows the infection to spread and can retard complete healing as a result of vascular congestion. Alcohol has an irritant effect on the healing urethral walls. Men should be cautioned against squeezing the penis to look for further discharge. Follow-up examination and reculture should be done at least once after treatment, usually in 4 to 7 days. Relapse, reinfection, and complications should be treated appropriately.

SYPHILIS
Etiology and Pathophysiology

Not all people who are exposed to syphilis acquire the disease; some appear resistant to infection. The causative organism for syphilis is *Treponema pallidum,* a spirochete. It is extremely fragile and easily destroyed by drying, heating, or washing. The organism is thought to enter the body through very small breaks in the skin or mucous membrane. Its entrance is facilitated by the minute tissue damage that often occurs during intercourse. In addition to sexual contact, syphilis may be spread through contact with infectious lesions, blood transfusions, and sharing of needles among drug addicts. Congenital syphilis is transmitted from an infected mother to the fetus in utero. The incubation period ranges from 10 to 90 days but is usually

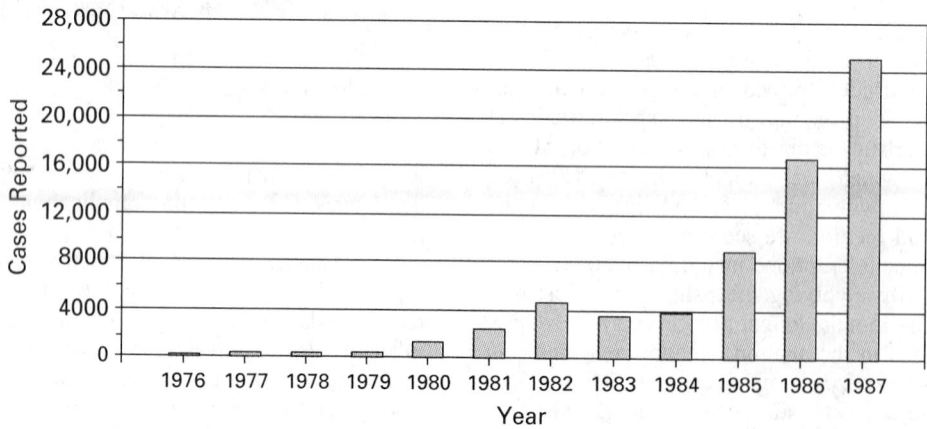

Fig. 47-2 Total antibiotic resistant gonorrhea in the United States from 1976 to 1987. (From HEW PHS Center for Disease Control: Sexually transmitted disease statistics, Oct 1988.)

Table 47-3 Stages of Syphilis

Clinical Stage	Characteristic Findings	Communicability	Duration of Stage
Primary	Chancre	Exudate from chancre highly infectious	3-8 wk
Secondary	Widespread (cutaneous eruptions) and systemic symptoms (6-12 wk after chancre, malaise, arthralgia, headache, occasionally liver and kidney dysfunction)	Exudate from skin and mucous membrane lesions highly infectious	1-2 yr
Latent	Absence of signs or symptoms	Noninfectious after 4 years, possible placental transmission	Throughout life or progression to late stage
Late*	Appearance 3 to 20 years after initial infection	Noninfectious	Chronic (without treatment), possibly fatal
Benign	Gummas (chronic, destructive lesions affecting any organ of body, especially skin, bone, liver, mucous membranes)	Spinal fluid possibly containing organism	
Cardiovascular	Aortic valve insufficiency or saccular aneurysm of thoracic aorta, aortitis		
Neurosyphilis	General paresis (personality changes from minor to psychotic, tremors, physical and mental deterioration)		
	Tabes dorsalis (ataxia, areflexia, paresthesias, lightning pains, damaged joints [Charcot's joints])		

*Several forms such as cardiac and CNS occur in approximately 25% of untreated cases.

considered to be 3 weeks. Immunity to reinfection may develop if the disease persists.

Syphilis is a disease of the blood vessels. The host tissues react to the presence of *T. pallidum* multiplying in the lymphatics and perivascular spaces by (1) capillary dilatation and swelling and proliferation of the endothelium and (2) a perivascular infiltration of lymphocytes, plasma, giant cells, and fibroblasts, with the formation of new blood vessels. Scar tissue formation is the method of healing of syphilis. The severity and extent of the damage vary according to the state of immunity of the host tissue.

Clinical Manifestations

Syphilis presents a variety of signs and symptoms that can mimic a number of less serious diseases. Consequently, it is more difficult to recognize syphilis than other venereal diseases. If it is not treated, specific clinical stages are characteristic of the disease progression (Table 47-3). Chancres, which are painless indurated lesions found on the penis, vulva, nipples, and lips and in the mouth, vagina, and rectum, are seen in the primary stage (Fig. 47-3). Cutaneous eruptions include a bilateral, symmetrical rash usually involving the palms and soles; mucous patches in the mouth, tongue, or cervix; *condyloma-lata* (moist papules) in the anal and genital area; *alopecia* (hair loss); and generalized lymphadenopathy (Fig. 47-4). These findings are characteristic of the secondary stage.

Complications

Complications of the disease occur chiefly in late syphilis. This stage is rare today and should never occur, since

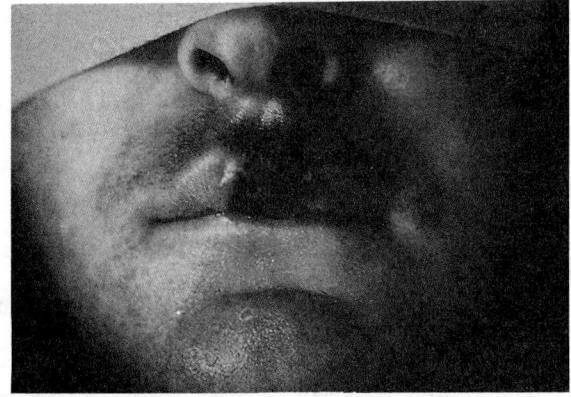

Fig. 47-3 Primary syphilis chancre on upper lip. (Courtesy USPHS, Washington, DC.)

it can be prevented by treatment with antibiotics in the earlier stages. Therapy for complications treats the symptoms.

The *gummas* (chronic, destructive lesions affecting any organ of the body) of benign late syphilis may produce irreparable damage to bone, liver, or skin but seldom result in death. In cardiovascular syphilis, formation of aneurysms and scarring of the aortic valve may occur. The resulting aneurysm may press on structures such as intercostal nerves, resulting in pain. The possibility of rupture exists as the aneurysm increases in size. Scarring of the aortic valve results in aortic valve insufficiency and, eventually, heart failure.

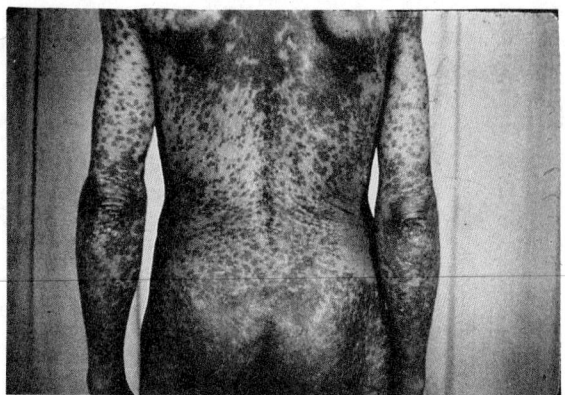

Fig. 47-4 Generalized posterior cutaneous eruptions in secondary syphilis. Distribution of lesions is bilateral and symmetrical. (Courtesy USPHS, Washington, DC.)

Neurosyphilis (general paresis) is responsible for degeneration of the brain with mental deterioration. Evidence of other neurological deficits may be present. Problems related to sensory nerve involvement are a result of *tabes dorsalis* (progressive locomotor ataxia). There may be sudden attacks of pain anywhere in the body, which can confuse the diagnosis of conditions such as peptic ulcer. Loss of vision and position sense in the feet and legs can also occur. Walking may become even more difficult as joint stability is lost. (Late syphilis is also discussed in Chapter 54.)

Diagnostic Studies

The first step in diagnosis is obtaining a detailed history relevant to sexual behavior. A physical examination should be done to identify any suspicious lesions as well as other significant signs and symptoms.

The presence of spirochetes on dark-field microscopy of tissue scrapings from primary or secondary lesions can confirm a clinical diagnosis of syphilis. Nonspecific antitreponemal antibodies can be detected by tests such as VDRL and rapid plasma reagin. These nontreponemal tests are suitable for screening purposes and usually become positive 10 to 14 days after the appearance of a chancre. Fluorescent treponemal antibody absorption and *T. pallidum* hemagglutination detect specific antitreponemal antibodies and are suitable for confirming the diagnosis.

False negatives and false positives do occur with nontreponemal tests. False negatives may occur during primary syphilis before the body has had time to produce reagin antibody. False positives may occur with other diseases or conditions such as hepatitis, infectious mononucleosis, smallpox vaccination, collagen diseases, narcotic addiction, and aging. Positive nontreponemal test results should be followed by more specific treponemal tests to rule out other causes. Specific changes related to cell count, estimation of total protein, cerebrospinal fluid, and one or more tests for antibody are diagnostic of asymptomatic neurosyphilis.

If a client is treated early in the course of the disease on the basis of history and symptoms, the serological testing

Table 47-4

 Diagnostic and Therapeutic Management: Primary Syphilis

DIAGNOSTIC

History and physical examination
Dark-field microscopy
Nontreponemal or treponemal serological testing
Testing for human immunodefiency virus antibody

THERAPEUTIC

Appropriate drug therapy*
Case finding
Treatment of contacts
Surveillance
    Repeat of quantitative nontreponemal tests at 3, 6, and 12 mo
    Examination of cerebrospinal fluid at 1 yr if treatment involving alternative antibiotics

*See Table 47-5.

may not indicate the presence of syphilis. Once a person has positive serological findings for syphilis, indicating the presence of antibodies, these findings may remain positive for an indefinite period in spite of successful treatment.

Therapeutic and Pharmacological Management

Therapeutic management of syphilis is aimed at eradication of all syphilitic organisms (Table 47-4). However, treatment cannot reverse damage that is already present in the late stage of the disease. Parenteral penicillin remains the treatment of choice for all stages of syphilis. To date, there is no evidence to suggest a decrease in the effectiveness of penicillin against *T. pallidum*. Table 47-5 describes therapy for the various stages of syphilis and is in accordance with United States Public Health Service recommendations. All stages of syphilis should be treated.

Appropriate antibiotic treatment of maternal syphilis before the eighteenth week of pregnancy prevents infection of the fetus. Appropriate treatment after 18 weeks of pregnancy cures both mother and fetus because the antibiotics can cross the placental barrier. All clients with neurosyphilis must be carefully followed with periodic serological testing, clinical evaluation at 6-month intervals, and repeat cerebrospinal fluid examinations for at least 3 years. Specific therapeutic management is based on the presenting symptoms.

GENITAL HERPES

There are two types of infection caused by herpes simplex virus (HSV)—type 1 and type 2. In general, type 1 strain (HSV-1) causes infection above the waist, involving infections of the gingivae, dermis, upper respiratory tract, and central nervous system (CNS). Type 2 strain (HSV-2) most frequently involves the genital tract and perineum (i.e., below the waist). However, either strain can cause disease on the mouth or the genitals. HSV-1 can be transmitted from mouth to genitals, and HSV-2 can be trans-

Table 47-5 Drug Therapy for Syphilis

Stage	Benzathine Penicillin G (IM)	Aqueous Crystalline Penicillin G (IV)	Other Antibiotics*
Early syphilis (primary, secondary, and early latent)†	2.4 megaunits divided in two doses at single visit		Tetracycline hydrochloride or erythromycin, 500 mg orally four times a day for 14 days‡
Syphilis lasting more than 1 yr†	2.4 megaunits weekly for three doses, totaling 7.2 megaunits		Tetracycline hydrochloride or erythromycin, 500 mg orally four times a day for 30 days‡
Symptomatic neurosyphilis		12-24 megaunits daily for 10 days, totaling 120-240 megaunits, followed by benzathine penicillin G 2.4 megaunits IM weekly for three doses	

Modified from Centers of Disease Control: STD treatment guidelines of USPHS, Atlanta, 1989, Centers for Disease Control.
IM, Intramuscular; *IV*, intravenous.
*Given when penicillin is contraindicated.
†Includes pregnant women.
‡Erythromycin estolate and tetracycline are not recommended for syphilitic infection in pregnant women because of potential adverse effects on both mother and child.

mitted from genitals to mouth through oral-genital contact.

Because HSV is readily inactivated at room temperature and by drying, airborne and fomitic spread have not been documented as a significant means of transmission. The virus enters through the mucous membrane or breaks in skin during contact with an infected person. When a person is infected with HSV, the virus may persist within the individual for life.

The initial infection is usually an HSV-1 infection, commonly occurring in childhood. The primary HSV-2 infection usually occurs when sexual activity begins. In contrast to other venereal diseases, the infection can recur completely unrelated to additional venereal contact and produce a syndrome similar to the primary infection. The incubation period is 3 to 7 days.

Clinical Manifestations

Clients with primary HSV-2 infections initially complain of burning or tingling at the site of inoculation. Vesicular lesions, which may occur bilaterally on the penis, scrotum, vulva, perineum, perianal region, vagina, or cervix, contain large quantities of infectious viral particles (Fig. 47-5). The lesions rupture and form shallow, moist ulcerations. Finally, crusting and epithelialization of the erosions occur. Primary infections tend to be associated with local inflammation and pain accompanied by systemic manifestations of fever, headache, malaise, myalgia, and inguinal lymphadenopathy.

Urination may be painful, and retention may occur as a result of HSV urethritis and/or cystitis, as well as from urine touching active lesions. A purulent vaginal discharge may develop with HSV cervicitis. The duration of symptoms and the frequency of complications are greater in women. Many HSV-2 infections are asymptomatic; the exact percentage is unknown. Transmission of genital herpes therefore can occur by means of sexual contact with an excretor of virus who is free of symptoms. Primary lesions are generally present for 17 to 20 days, but new lesions sometimes continue to develop for 6 weeks. Clients are thought to be infectious until the lesions are completely healed.

After the first infection, HSV-2 establishes latency in the sacral ganglia and may be reactivated periodically. Recurrent attacks occur in about 50% to 80% of all cases during the year following the primary episode. Stress, sexual activity, sunburn, and fever tend to trigger recurrence. Many clients can predict a recurrence by noticing early symptoms of tingling, burning, and itching at the site where lesions eventually arise. The symptoms of recurrent episodes are less severe, and the unilateral lesions heal within 10 to 12 days with recurrent episodes. With time the recurrent lesions generally occur less frequently.

Complications

Complications of genital herpes frequently involve the CNS, causing aseptic meningitis and lower motor neuron damage. Neuron damage may result in atonic bladder, impotence, and constipation. The most common complication is autoinoculation of the virus to extragenital sites such as fingers (whitlow), lips, and breasts.

Pregnancy. Lesions in pregnant women persist longer than in nonpregnant women, and the symptoms seem to be more severe. The incidence of abortion is higher if an HSV-2 infection is contracted during the first 20 weeks of pregnancy. The development of disseminated neonatal herpesvirus infections carries a high incidence of infant

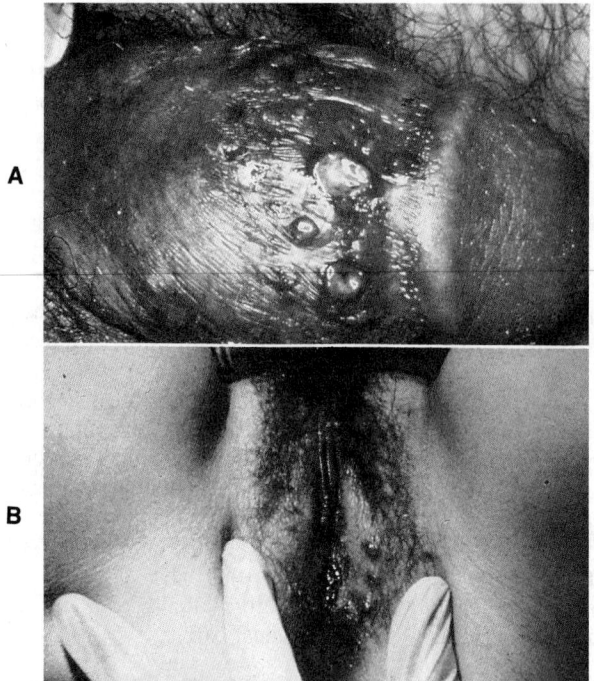

Fig. 47-5 HSV-2 in a male and a female client. Vesicular lesions on **A,** penis and **B,** perineum. (Courtesy USPHS, Washington, DC.)

Table 47-6

 Diagnostic and Therapeutic Management: Genital Herpes

DIAGNOSTIC

History and physical examination
Viral isolation by tissue culture
Cytological examination of vesicular exudate for multinucleated giant cells

THERAPEUTIC

Primary infection
    Acyclovir 200 mg orally five times daily for 7-10 days or until clinical resolution
Recurrent infection
    Acyclovir 200 mg orally five times daily for 5 days or acyclovir 800 mg orally two times daily for 5 days
    Acyclovir (5%) ointment
Attempt to identify trigger mechanisms
Yearly Pap smear
Abstinence from sexual contact while lesions present
Provision of symptomatic interventions

Modified from Center for Disease Control: STD treatment guidelines, Atlanta, 1989.

mortality. A positive cervical viral culture usually indicates the need for cesarean section, since most infections to neonates occur during passage through the birth canal.

Cervical cancer. Epidemiological evidence has linked genital herpes infections in women with carcinoma of the cervix. Both diseases have similar predisposing factors, such as intercourse at an early age and multiple sex partners.

Although data do not show with certainty that herpesvirus initiates a process resulting in cervical cancer, the association appears to be valid.[17] Therefore women who have had genital herpesvirus infections should be particularly conscientious about having a regular Papanicolaou (Pap) smear taken. Recently, attention has been focused on human papillomavirus as another possible link in cervical cancer.

Diagnostic Studies

Diagnosis of genital herpes is usually based on the client's symptoms and history. The diagnosis can be confirmed through viral isolation from active lesions by means of tissue culture. Tzanck or Pap-stained smears from lesions show the cellular characteristics of viruses. Recently a new, easy to perform sensitive antibody test—HerpCheck—was approved for use.[18] This test can detect HSV within 4 hours. It can provide for early treatment of infected newborns and reduce the need for cesarean section.

Therapeutic and Pharmacological Management

The skin lesions of genital herpes heal spontaneously unless secondary infection occurs. Symptomatic treatment

such as good genital hygiene and the wearing of loose-fitting cotton undergarments should be encouraged (Table 47-6). The lesions should be kept clean and dry. To ensure complete drying of the perineal area, women may use a hair dryer set on a cool setting. Frequent sitz baths may soothe the area and reduce inflammation. Pain may require a local anesthetic such as lidocaine (Xylocaine) or systemic analgesics such as codeine and aspirin. Clients are advised to abstain from sexual contact while lesions are present and for 10 days after lesions heal.[19]

Currently, acyclovir (Zovirax), a purine analogue that inhibits herpetic viral replication, is being prescribed. Although not a cure, acyclovir shortens the duration of viral shedding and healing time of genital lesions in primary and recurrent outbreaks and suppresses recurrences with daily use. Continued use of oral acyclovir for 1 to 2 years is safe and effective. Once the drug is discontinued, however, recurrences return to their pretreatment frequency.[20,21] Adverse reactions to acyclovir are mild and include headache, occasional nausea and vomiting, and diarrhea. The safety of systemic acyclovir for treatment of pregnant women has not been established. Acyclovir ointment (5%) can be applied to lesions of genital herpes or mucocutaneous herpes infections. IV acyclovir is reserved for severe or life-threatening infections. Hospitalization is required, and nephrotoxicity has been observed with its use.

CHLAMYDIAL INFECTIONS

C. trachomatis is recognized as a genital pathogen responsible for an increasing variety of clinical illnesses (e.g., nongonococcal urethritis [NGU] and cervicitis). Be-

cause chlamydial infections closely parallel gonococcal infections, clinical differentiation may be difficult. The incubation period of 1 to 3 weeks is longer than that of gonorrhea, and the symptoms are often milder. The high incidence of recurrences may be due to failure to treat the sexual partners of infected persons.

Clinical Manifestations and Complications

As with gonorrhea, chlamydial infections result in a superficial mucosal infection that can become more invasive. Men with NGU generally complain of dysuria, frequency of urination, and a mucoid or watery urethral discharge that may be noted only on arising in the morning. Women with cervicitis are generally free of symptoms, although some have a mucopurulent vaginal discharge. A large number of women with chlamydial cervicitis have been found to have a male partner with NGU.

Complications often develop from poorly managed, inaccurately diagnosed, or undiagnosed chlamydial infections. Infection in men may result in epididymitis with possible infertility and Reiter's disease. (Reiter's disease is an arthritis disorder of men, usually associated with conjunctivitis or urethritis.) Women may develop hypertrophic erosion of the cervix, salpingitis leading to PID, and infertility. Preliminary studies have shown an association of *C. trachomatis* with cervical dysplasia. Proctitis is associated with rectal intercourse. *Chlamydia* infection may be transmitted from a mother to the newborn, causing inclusion conjunctivitis or pneumonia.

Diagnostic Studies and Therapeutic Management

Chlamydial infections are diagnosed by excluding gonorrhea. If no gram-negative intracellular diplococci are found on the Gram-stained smear of male urethral discharge or the sediment of first-catch urine specimen, a culture is done. If both are negative and signs of inflammation are present (e.g., polymorphonuclear leukocytes [PMNs] on the Gram-stained smear), a diagnosis of NGU-*Chlamydia* infection or cervicitis may be made. Endocervical smears and monoclonal antibody tests are done to diagnose the infection in women. Culturing for chlamydial organisms should be done if the laboratory facilities are available. Antigen-detection methods have been developed that offer a low-cost alternative to culture, but these tests are not ideal.

Chlamydial infections respond to treatment with tetracycline or doxycycline. For tetracycline the dosage is 500 mg orally four times a day for at least 7 days. For doxycycline the dosage is 100 mg two times a day for at least 10 days. Doxycycline is more expensive than tetracycline. Follow-up care should include advising the client to return if symptoms persist or recur.

CONDYLOMATA ACUMINATA

Condylomata acuminata (genital warts), which are caused by human papillomavirus (HPV), are seen frequently in young, sexually active adults. The genitalia and anorectal region as well as urethral, bladder, and oral mucosa may be affected. The incubation period of the warts is 1 to 6 months.

Clinical Manifestations and Complications

Condylomata acuminata lesions are discrete single or multiple papillary growths that are white to gray. The warts may grow and coalesce to form large, cauliflower-like masses. In men the warts may occur on the penis and scrotum, around the anus, or in the urethra. In women the warts may be located on the vulva, vagina, and cervix and in the perianal area.

During pregnancy, genital warts tend to grow rapidly. Cesarean section may be indicated if the birth canal becomes blocked by massive warts. An infected mother may transmit the condition to her newborn. Bleeding on defecation may occur with anal warts.

Recent research has linked HPV to squamous cell carcinoma of the genital organs in women.[22] A percentage of women who have confirmed HPV cervical infections can be expected to progress to cervical intraepithelial neoplasia within a year if untreated. A high proportion of clients with carcinoma of the vulva, vagina, and cervix or squamous cell carcinoma of the penis have a history of preexisting condylomata.[23] Therefore clients with genital warts should receive regular medical care.

Diagnostic Studies and Therapeutic Management

Diagnosis may be made on the basis of the gross appearance of the lesions. However, the warts may be confused with condylomata lata of secondary syphilis, carcinoma, or benign neoplasms. Serological testing and biopsy should be done to rule out these conditions. Cytological testing (e.g., Pap smear), colposcopy, anoscopy, and histological examination of tissues are used in the detection of HPV. Virapap, a test that uses DNA hybridization techniques, determines the presence and type of HPV. Currently, HPV virus cannot be confirmed by culture.

Genital warts are difficult to treat and often require multiple office visits using a variety of treatment modalities. One common treatment is the use of 50% to 85% trichloroacetic acid applied directly to the wart surface. Petroleum jelly is applied to the surrounding normal skin to minimize irritation before a small amount of trichloroacetic acid is applied to the wart with a cotton swab. A sharp stinging pain if often felt with initial acid contact but this quickly subsides. Trichloroacetic acid is not washed off after treatment and can be used in pregnant women.

Podophyllin (10% to 25%) is recommended therapy for small external genital warts. When podophyllin (a cytotoxic agent) is used, it is applied carefully to each wart, avoiding normal tissue, and it should be thoroughly washed off in 1 to 4 hours. This substance encourages the sloughing of skin containing viral particles. Podophyllin has local (e.g., pain, burning) and systemic (e.g., nausea, dizziness, leukopenia, respiratory distress) toxic symptoms. It is contraindicated in pregnant women. If the warts do not regress, treatments such as cryotherapy with liquid nitrogen, electrocautery, laser therapy, 5-fluorouracil 5% cream, and surgical excision may be indicated.

ACQUIRED IMMUNODEFICIENCY SYNDROME

AIDS is caused by human immunodeficiency virus (HIV). Monoclonal antibody analysis has demonstrated

that clients with AIDS have a depressed ratio of T-helper cells to T-suppressor cells. Consequently, too few cells turn on the body's immune response and too many cells turn off the process. With the body's disease-fighting immune system weakened, the client becomes vulnerable to opportunistic diseases such as *Pneumocystis carinii* pneumonia (PCP) and *Kaposi's sarcoma* (a type of skin cancer) as well as other opportunistic infections. (HIV infection and AIDS are discussed in Chapter 8.)

■ Nursing Management of Sexually Transmitted Diseases

Nursing assessment

Subjective and objective data that should be obtained from a person with a sexually transmitted disease are presented in Table 47-7.

Nursing diagnoses

Nursing diagnoses specific to the client with a sexually transmitted disease include, but are not limited to, the following:

1. High risk for infection transmission related to inadequate personal and genital hygiene and lack of knowledge about mode of transmission
2. High risk for anxiety related to impact of condition on relationships, disease outcome, and lack of knowledge of disease
3. Pain related to genital lesions and dysuria
4. Self-esteem disturbance related to change in body image
5. High risk for noncompliance due to lack of knowledge of possible complications and confusion about therapy

Nursing interventions

Health promotion and maintenance. Many approaches to curtailing the spread of venereal diseases have been advocated and have met with varying degrees of success. Sexual abstinence is a certain method of avoiding all venereal diseases, but few adults consider this a feasible alternative to sexual expression. Limiting sexual intimacies outside of a well-established monogamous relationship can reduce the risk of contracting venereal disease. There are also specific procedures that if followed consistently, can aid in preventing a venereal infection. Certain STD agents (HSV-2, *C. trachomatis*, HPV) have been linked with cervical intraepithelial neoplasia (CIN), a precancerous lesion that appears to be an STD itself. It is now commonly believed that carcinomas of the cervix originate from CIN. Therefore, an annual Pap smear should be mandatory for clients at risk for STDs. The nurse should counsel clients in regard to these measures.

MEASURES TO PREVENT INFECTION. An inspection of the sexual partner's genitals before coitus is recommended. The presence of discharge, sores, blisters, or rash should be viewed with concern. A client who is aware of specific signs and symptoms of infection can intelligently make the decision to continue the sexual interaction with modifications or elect not to have sexual relations. Clients should remember that when they have sex, they expose themselves to the infections of everyone with whom the partner has ever had sex. Men should be told that some protection is provided if

Table 47-7

 Nursing Assessment of the Client with a Sexually Transmitted Disease

SUBJECTIVE DATA

History
Exposure to individuals with STDs, multiple partners, pregnancy

Medications
Use of oral contraceptives; allergy to any antibiotic, especially penicillin

General
Malaise, chills, fever

Pain
Tenesmus; painful, burning lesions; headache; dysuria; dyspareunia

Integumentary
Itching at infected site, alopecia

Gastrointestinal
Pharyngitis, oral lesions

Urinary
Frequency, urinary retention, urethral discharge

Reproductive
Vaginal discharge, presence of genital or perianal lesions

Musculoskeletal
Arthralgias

OBJECTIVE DATA

General
Lymphadenopathy (generalized or inguinal)

Integumentary
Syphilis: Primary: painless, indurated genital or perianal lesions; secondary: bilateral, symmetrical rash on palms, soles, or entire body
Genital herpes: Painful genital or anal vesicular lesions
Condylomata: Single or multiple gray or white genital or anal warts (possibly becoming massive)
Chlamydial: Painless vesicle or papule

Gastrointestinal
Purulent rectal discharge (indicator of gonorrhea), rectal lesions

Urinary
Urethral discharge, erythema, proctitis

Reproductive
Cervical discharge, lesions, inflamed Bartholin's glands

Possible findings:
Gonorrhea: Positive Gram stain, smears, and cultures for gram-negative diplococci within PMNs
Syphilis: Positive findings on VDRL and RPR, spirochetes on dark-field microscopy
Genital herpes: Positive tissue culture for HSV-2
Chlamydia: Positive culture for *Chlamydia* organism

they void immediately following intercourse and wash their genitalia and the adjacent areas with soap and water. Women may also benefit from postcoital voiding, washing, and douching. Spermicidal jellies and creams have a mild detergent effect that may reduce the risk of contracting STDs. These same barriers can serve as supplementary lubrication, thereby decreasing irritation and chances for development of an entry for the organism.

Proper use of a condom provides a highly effective mechanical barrier to infection. The condom should be undamaged and correctly in place throughout all phases of sexual activity. The use of a spermicidal foam in the vagina such as nonoxynol-9 (which inactivates most STD agents) and concurrent use of a condom can further reduce risk of disease.[24] Clients should be given specific verbal and written instructions on the proper use of condoms (Table 8-27). The objections to condom usage, such as interference with spontaneity and the presence of a barrier, should be discussed by the partners. Many men find the use of condoms objectionable, although it need not interfere with sexual satisfaction. Most women cannot tell the difference when a condom is used.

Sexual contact with persons known or suspected to have AIDS should be avoided (see Chapter 8). Sexually active homosexual men can reduce their risk by minimizing the number of their sexual contacts. Anal intercourse should be eliminated, and condoms should be used if sexual contacts continue.

SCREENING PROGRAMS. Screening programs that are used to find infected clients can also help prevent certain STDs. For many years, there have been various screening programs to find cases of syphilis. Concern over cost effectiveness of these programs while the disease prevalence was low has resulted in only 16 states requiring premarital blood tests for syphilis.[25] A total of 49 states require prenatal testing for syphilis.[26] Other screening programs such as those carried out as part of hospital admission physicals have also been discontinued. At the same time, several states are proposing premarital HIV screening. The cost and the concern over the possibility of destroying current working relationships with high-risk populations are deterrents to the adoption of these programs. Some states prefer the educational approach, requiring that couples receive AIDS-related literature or undergo counseling.[26]

Screening programs have been developed and implemented for gonorrhea. These programs involve women because women are more likely to have asymptomatic gonorrhea and thereby serve as sources of infection. Routine gonorrheal cultures during women's pelvic examinations are being performed as a major part of these programs. Their effectiveness is well documented. Mass application of screening programs for genital chlamydial infections, genital herpes, and HPV will be possible when rapid, cost-effective tests are developed.

CASE FINDING. Interviewing and case finding are other processes used to control venereal disease. These activities are directed toward locating and examining all contacts of each known client with venereal disease as soon as possible after sexual exposure so that effective treatment can be initiated. Trained interviewers may often find cases even if they are supplied with only limited information. The caseworkers, who are often nurses, are aware of the social implications of these diseases and the need for discretion. Sexual contacts are often not informed about the origin of the information naming them as a contact so that greater cooperation and privacy is ensured.

EDUCATIONAL AND RESEARCH PROGRAMS. Nurses can actively encourage their communities to provide better education about STDs for their citizens. Teenagers, who are known to have a high incidence of infection, should be a prime audience for such educational programs. Hot-line services, physician extenders, and outreach programs sponsored by the CDC are effective. The National Gay Task Force and the Herpes Resource Center were established to provide education and support where needed. Knowledge and understanding of the disease can decrease the venereal disease epidemic. Currently, efforts are being made to develop a serological test for gonorrhea and effective immunizing agents for syphilis, gonorrhea, genital herpes, HPV, and AIDS. The development of venereal disease vaccines is viewed by many clinicians as a prerequisite for eradication of venereal diseases.

Acute intervention

PSYCHOLOGICAL SUPPORT. The diagnosis of venereal disease may be met with a variety of emotions such as shame, guilt, anger, and a desire for vengeance. The nurse should try to help clients verbalize their feelings and provide counseling. Couples in marital or committed relationships are confronted with an added problem when venereal disease is diagnosed. The realization of sexual activity by one of the partners with a person outside the relationship must be faced. Other concerns relative to their relationship are present, and the acute problem may serve as an incentive to do other problem solving. Support and counseling for the couple are needed. A referral for professional counseling to explore the implications of venereal disease in their relationship may be indicated.

Clients who have contracted genital herpes are faced with the fact that repeated infections can occur and that no cure is available. This can be frustrating and disruptive to their physical, emotional, and social lives. The fear of spontaneous abortion and neonatal infection and the potential for cervical cancer are also serious concerns. Helping the client identify and avoid any factors that may precipitate the condition is indicated. Informing the client that the incidence and severity of recurrences will decrease over time can provide a degree of support.

HPV infections involve a prolonged course of treatment. Clients can become frustrated and distressed because of frequent office visits, associated costs, the potential for unpleasant side effects as a result of treatment, and the effect of the infection on their future health and sexual relationships. Tremendous support and a willingness to listen to the client's concerns are needed.

The psychological burden of clients with AIDS can be devastating. The clients are often young or early middle-aged men who may face discrimination, social isolation, gradual loss of independence, and eventually the prospect of a fatal disease. Many may dwell on the relation between their illness and their lifestyle, especially if they have not

come to grips with their homosexuality. Opportunities for the client and significant others to explore their feelings and deal with their anxieties should be provided.

COMPLIANCE AND FOLLOW-UP. Nurses working in public health facilities, clinics, or other outpatient settings are more likely to care for clients with STDs than nurses in hospitals. These nurses are in a position to explain and interpret treatment measures such as the purpose and possible side effects of prescribed drugs and the need for follow-up care. Nursing care plans for clients with primary syphilis and gonorrhea are presented in Tables 47-8 and 47-9.

Fortunately, single-dose treatment for gonorrhea and syphilis helps prevent the problems associated with noncompliance with drug therapy. Clients requiring multiple-dose therapy should be given special instructions in completing the prescribed regimen and should be informed about problems of noncompliance. Clients with herpes virus should be instructed to use a rubber glove when applying acyclovir to prevent autoinoculation to other body sites. All clients should return to the treatment center for a repeat culture from the infected sites or serological testing at designated times to determine the effectiveness of the treatment. Informing the client that cures are not always obtained on the first treatment can reinforce the need for a follow-up visit. Clients should also be advised to inform their sexual partners of the need for treatment, regardless of whether they are free of symptoms or experiencing symptoms.

HYGIENE MEASURES. The client with venereal disease should have certain hygiene measures emphasized. An important measure is frequent hand washing and bathing; this results in the destruction of many of the causative organisms of venereal disease. Bathing and cleaning of the involved areas can provide local comfort and prevent secondary infection. Douching may spread the infection and is therefore generally contraindicated. The synthetic materials used in most undergarments frequently increase or exacerbate local irritations by trapping moisture. Cotton undergarments provide better absorption and are cooler and more comfortable for the client with venereal disease.

Table 47-8

 NURSING CARE PLAN FOR THE CLIENT WITH PRIMARY SYPHILIS

Defining Characteristics	Nursing Interventions	Evaluation Criteria
NURSING DIAGNOSIS: High risk for infection transmission related to inadequate personal and genital hygiene and lack of knowledge about mode of transmission		
Unawareness of hygienic precautions, infectious discharge from lesion, questioning about mode of transmission	Instruct client in hygienic measures, including good hand washing and wearing of cotton undergarments. Use precautions regarding linen and hand washing for initial 24 hr of treatment. Investigate need for treatment of sexual partners with antibiotics. Instruct client regarding abstinence or use of condoms and mode of transmission.	Description of appropriate hygienic measures and mode of transmission, absence of discharge, no spread of infection to others
NURSING DIAGNOSIS: High risk for altered health maintenance related to lack of knowledge of acute and follow-up measures and possibility of reinfection		
Noncompliance with follow-up care, belief that medication is curative	Explain reasons for return visits to clinic at specified intervals. Inform client that blood samples will be taken at each visit. Assist with case finding. Explain precautions necessary to prevent reinfection, such as use of condoms, inspection of partner's genitalia, voiding, and washing of genitalia after intercourse. Inform client that there is no development of immunity to disease.	Compliance with appropriate follow-up protocol, statement of reasons for follow-up care, knowledge of precautionary measures, absence of reinfection
NURSING DIAGNOSIS: Anxiety related to effect of condition on relationships and lack of knowledge of further stages of disease and management		
Emotional reaction to diagnosis of syphilis	Encourage verbalization. Counsel client and sexual partner, if indicated. Describe signs of secondary syphilis. Reaffirm need for compliance with follow-up care.	Acceptance of diagnosis, knowledge of symptoms of secondary syphilis or late disease, statement of need to comply

Table 47-9

NURSING CARE PLAN FOR THE CLIENT WITH GONORRHEA

Defining Characteristics	Nursing Interventions	Evaluation Criteria
NURSING DIAGNOSIS: High risk for infection transmission related to lack of knowledge of precautionary measures		
Infectious genital discharge, initial infection	Administer medications as ordered after checking for any allergies. Instruct client in hygienic measures of hand washing, bathing, and wearing of cotton undergarments.	Absence of discharge, no further spread of infection
NURSING DIAGNOSIS: Pain related to dysuria		
Complaints of burning on urination, urgency, frequency	Encourage fluids. Monitor intake and output. Administer analgesia as ordered. Use sitz baths.	Absence of dysuria
NURSING DIAGNOSIS: High risk for anxiety related to impact of condition on relationships, disease outcome, and lack of knowledge of disease		
Emotional response of anger and restlessness to diagnosis, requesting of information about signs and symptoms of complications	Allow client and sexual partner to verbalize concerns. Investigate need for counseling. Instruct client about symptoms of complications and need to report problems such as difficulty in voiding, chills, fever, dysuria, and urethral discharge.	Decrease or absence of anxiety related to diagnosis, knowledge of signs and symptoms
NURSING DIAGNOSIS: High risk for altered health maintenance related to lack of knowledge of appropriate follow-up measures and possibility of reinfection		
Unawareness of disease process, hygienic precautions, and follow-up procedure; noncompliance with follow-up care	Explain precautions to take, such as being selective about sexual partners, using condoms, voiding and washing genitalia after coitus. Inform client regarding absence of immunity. Instruct client regarding return to clinic within 4-7 days after completion of treatment for cultures. Assist with case finding.	No reinfection, compliance with follow-up protocol

SEXUAL ACTIVITY. Sexual abstinence is indicated during the communicable phase of the disease. If sexual activity occurs before treatment of the client has been completed, the use of condoms can prevent the spread of infection and reinfection. The client can also choose to relate to a partner in an intimate way that avoids both coitus and oral-genital contact.

Chronic management. Because many venereal diseases are cured with a single dose or short course of antibiotic therapy, many persons are casual about the outcome of these diseases. The consequences of this attitude can include delays in treatment, noncompliance with instructions, and subsequent development of complications. The complications are serious and costly; they can result in disfigurement and destruction of important tissues and organs.

Surgery and prolonged therapy are indicated for many clients with disease-related deformity. Major surgical procedures such as resection of an aneurysm or aortic valve replacement may be necessary to treat cardiovascular problems. Pelvic surgery and procedures may include lysis of adhesions, dilatation of strictures, reconstructive tuboplasty, and in vitro fertilization. Secondary infections may occur because of the location of the lesions. These infections may be severe, requiring more therapy than the original problem.

C *ase Study*

SYPHILIS

Bob J., a 48-year-old man, was admitted to the hospital after a minor traffic accident. During his physical examination a painless indurated lesion that appeared to be a chancre was discovered on his penis. His sexual history revealed that his only sexual partner other than his wife was a woman he had met 3 weeks earlier while on a business trip. A tentative diagnosis of syphilis was made.

Discussion Questions

1. How can the diagnosis of syphilis be established?
2. How could Bob have prevented the infection?
3. What are the possible complications if Bob is not treated?
4. What are the implications of this diagnosis for Bob's relationship with his wife?
5. What measures should Bob have his wife take?
6. What instructions should be given to Bob regarding follow-up care?

R eview Questions

The number of the question corresponds to the same-numbered objective at the beginning of the chapter.

1. Factors that have led to an increase in STDs include
   a. longer sexual life span
   b. increased social controls
   c. better reporting of venereal diseases
   d. improved antibiotic therapy
2. If a men goes without treatment for gonorrhea, he may develop
   a. reinfection with the microorganisms
   b. an immunity to the microorganisms
   c. ureteritis, pyelonephritis, and nephritis
   d. prostatitis, epididymitis, and orchitis
3. Ceftriaxone is prescribed for gonorrhea to
   a. decrease side effects of treatment
   b. treat all strains of organism
   c. provide single-dose therapy
   d. defray the cost of therapy
4. Recurrent genital herpes
   a. can be cured with the use of acyclovir
   b. is generally milder than the initial infection
   c. lasts for 7 to 21 days
   d. does not interfere with sexual activity
5. AIDS can be transmitted by all of the following *except*
   a. air currents
   b. contaminated needles
   c. blood transfusion
   d. sexual contact
6. Nursing assessment findings of clients suspected of having a sexually transmitted disease include all of the following *except*
   a. paresthesias of extremities
   b. lesion of the skin or genitalia
   c. complaints of rectal and urinary discomfort
   d. presence or absence of unusual discharges
7. The prime audience for the nurse to reach in regard to venereal disease control is
   a. primary grade students
   b. teenagers
   c. unmarried adults
   d. homosexuals
8. Emotional support is best given to the client with a venereal disease through
   a. offering of many alternatives
   b. concerned listening
   c. isolation from others
   d. emphasis on duration of disease

REFERENCES

1. US Department of Health and Human Services, Public Health Services: Division of sexually transmitted diseases and STD laboratory program annual report, Atlanta, 1987-1988, Centers for Disease Control.
2. Centers for Disease Control: Continuing increase in infectious syphilis—United States, MMWR 37:38, 1988.
3. Centers for Disease Control: Genital herpes infection—United States—1966-1984, MMWR 35:402, 1986.
4. Centers for Disease Control: STD treatment guidelines, MMWR 38:29, 1989.
5. Cates W: Epidemiology and control of sexually transmitted diseases: strategic evaluation, Infect Dis Clin North Am 1:11, 1987.
6. Whelan M: Nursing management of the patient with *Chlamydia trachomatis* infection, Nurs Clin North Am 23:880, 1988.
7. Stone K: Epidemiologic aspects of genital HPV infection, Clin Obstet Gynecol 32:114, 1989.
8. Centers for Disease Control: First 100,000 cases of acquired immunodeficiency syndrome—United States, MMWR 38:561, 1989.
9. Centers for Disease Control: Condoms for prevention of sexually transmitted diseases, MMWR 37:135, 1988.
10. Washington J and others: Oral contraceptives, *Chlamydia trachomatis* infections and pelvic inflammatory disease, JAMA 253:2249, 1985.
11. Peterson H and Lee N: The health effects of oral contraceptives: misperceptions, controversies and continuing good news, Clin Obstet Gynecol 32:350, 1989.
12. Lee NC and others: The intrauterine device and pelvic inflammatory disease revisited: new results from the women's health study, Obstet Gynecol 32:6, 1988.
13. Parish L and Gschnaet F: Sexually transmitted diseases: a guide to clinicians, New York, 1989, Springer-Verlag, p 63.
14. US Department of Health Education and Welfare, Public Health Services: Venereal disease control laws—summary, Atlanta, 1972, Centers for Disease Control.
15. Zenilman J, Cates W, and Morse T: *Neisseria gonorrhoeae:* an old enemy rearms, Infect Dis Med Letol Obstet Gynecol 7:5s, 1986.
16. Centers for Disease Control: Antibiotic resistant strains of *Neisseria gonorrhoeae:* policy guidelines, MMWR 36:2s, 1987.
17. Robertson S and others: Clinical practice in sexually transmissible diseases, ed 2, New York, 1989, Churchill Livingstone, p 319.
18. Baker D and others: Clinical evaluation of new herpes simplex virus ELISA: a rapid diagnostic test for herpes simplex virus, Obstet Gynecol 73:322, 1989.
19. Kellum M and Loucks A: Genital herpes infections: diagnosis and management, Nurs Pract 7:322, 1989.
20. Baker D and others: One year suppression of frequent recurrences of genital herpes with acyclovir, Obstet Gynecol 73:86, 1989.
21. Mastow S and others: Suppression of recurrent genital herpes by single daily dosages of acyclovir, Am J Med 85:33, 1988.
22. Selvaggi S: Cytologic detection of condylomas and cervical intraepithelial neoplasia of the uterine cervix with histologic correlation, Ca 58:2076, 1986.
23. Enterline J and Leonardo J: Condylomata acuminata, Nurs Pract 14:10, 1989.
24. Centers for Disease Control: Condoms for prevention of sexually transmitted diseases, MMWR 37:135, 1988.
25. Centers for Disease Control: Survey of states mandatory premarital serology testing, Atlanta, Feb 3, 1987, p 1-4.
26. Centers for Disease Control: Prenatal examination laws, Atlanta, Aug 1979.

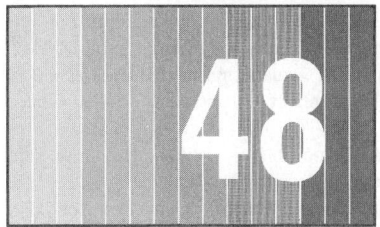

Nursing Role in Management
Female Reproductive Problems

Linda C. Carnago

Although problems related to female reproductive organs are discussed and written about more openly today, misconceptions, fears, and embarrassment about gynecological problems are still common. The nurse plays an important role in (1) disseminating knowledge about health-promoting measures, (2) providing clarification and reassurance when indicated, and (3) assisting the client in seeking help to obtain early recognition and treatment of potentially serious problems.

Reviewed by Kathryn A. Patterson, C.N.M., Ph.D., Assistant Professor, Maternity Nursing, Women's Health Nurse Practitioner Program, University of Hawaii, School of Nursing, Honolulu, Hawaii.

DISORDERS OF MENSTRUATION

Menstruation is a periodic discharge of blood and disintegrating endometrium after a normal ovulatory cycle.[1] This process remains an essentially normal event, occurring approximately every 28 days. However, there may be considerable variation in the days between cycles and in the duration, amount, and character of bleeding, which can be associated with reproductive problems.

Health Maintenance and Promotion

Before the nurse can begin to do health teaching, the client's knowledge of the characteristics of the menstrual cycle should be assessed. Table 48-1 includes these char-

Table 48-1 Characteristics of Menstrual Cycle and Related Client Education

Characteristic	Client Education
MENARCHE	
Occurs between ages of 9 and 18 yr, average age at onset is 12 or 13 yr	See physician regarding possible endocrine or developmental abnormality when delayed.
INTERVAL	
Usually is 27-31 days, but regular cycles as short as 17 or as long as 45 days are considered normal if pattern is consistent for individual	Keep written record to identify own pattern of menstrual cycle. Expect some irregularity in premenopausal period. Be aware that drugs (phenothiazines, narcotics, contraceptives) and stressful life events can result in missed periods.
DURATION	
Menstrual flow generally lasts 2-8 days	Realize that pattern is fairly constant but that wide variations do exist.
AMOUNT	
Average menstrual flow is 30-100 ml per period; amount varies among women and in the same woman at different times; it is usually heaviest first 2 days	Count pads or tampons used per day. The average tampon or pad completely saturated absorbs 20-30 ml. Very heavy flow is indicated by complete soaking of 2 pads in 1-2 hr. Know that flow increases then gradually decreases in premenopausal period. IUD or drugs such as anticoagulants and thiazides can produce heavy menses.
COMPOSITION	
Menstrual discharge is mixture of endometrium, blood, mucus, and vaginal cells; it is dark red and less viscous than blood and usually does not clot	Realize that clots indicate heavy flow or vaginal pooling.

IUD, Intrauterine device.

acteristics and related client education. When this information is discussed and explained, the client becomes aware that variations do exist for the "normal" menses and that knowledge can help dispel apprehension and fear. If the client's menstrual cycle pattern does not fall within the range of normal, the nurse should urge her to seek prompt medical attention.

Many old wives' tales are told concerning activities allowed during menstruation. The nurse should be prepared to clarify the facts. The client should be assured that bathing and hair washing are safe. A daily warm tub bath can actually relieve some of the associated pelvic discomfort. Women can swim, exercise, have intercourse, and basically, behave like healthy persons.

Frequent changing of tampons or pads meets comfort and hygiene needs during menstruation. The selection of internal or external sanitary protection is a matter of personal preference. Tampons are convenient and make menstrual hygiene easier, whereas pads may provide better protection.

Premenstrual Syndrome

Premenstrual syndrome (PMS) is the name given to a group of physical and psychological symptoms that occur cyclically, usually 7 to 14 days before the onset of menstruation, and that subside with the menstrual flow. A symptom-free week usually occurs before ovulation. Included among the physical symptoms are breast discomfort, peripheral edema, weight gain, abdominal bloating, episodes of binge eating, and headache. Anxiety, depression, irritability, and mood swings are some of the psychological symptoms. PMS may actually consist of several subgroups categorized as anxiety and irritability, hyperhydration, appetite changes, and depression.[2] Episodes of antisocial behavior and incidents of suicide and child abuse have been described coinciding with PMS. The syndrome can occur at any time between menarche and menopause, but the majority of women seeking treatment for PMS are 30 to 40 years of age.[3] Although the precise incidence has not been determined, it is estimated that 30% to 40% of menstruating women are affected.

Etiology. Proposed etiological factors are as diverse as the symptoms of PMS. Imbalances of ovarian hormones, prolactin, and aldosterone, prostaglandin excess, hypoglycemia, deficiencies of vitamin B and magnesium, changes in endorphin activity and in the hypothalamic-pituitary axis, and psychological dysfunction have been implicated. There is support for each of the potential causes, but none seems to explain PMS completely.

Clinical manifestations. PMS is diagnosed by exclusion. A complete health, gynecological, obstetrical, and psychological history as well as a thorough physical exam-

ination are necessary to rule out any underlying conditions, such as thyroid dysfunction, uterine fibroids, or psychopathology that may account for the premenstrual symptoms. In addition, no helpful biomedical or laboratory markers are available in establishing the diagnosis.

The number and severity of symptoms that should be present to confirm the diagnosis have not been established. The client's symptoms and her menstrual cycle can be correlated through the use of a prospective daily diary in which menstrual experiences and basal body temperature are recorded. The menstrual diary must show identical symptoms in at least two consecutive cycles to support the diagnosis of PMS.[4] A slight rise in the basal body temperature identifies the timing of ovulation. Comparison of the two records shows an absence of symptoms in the follicular phase and the presence of complaints in the luteal phase, which resolve with the onset of menstruation.[5]

Therapeutic management. Nonpharmacological and pharmacological strategies are used in treating the client with PMS (Fig. 48-1). The nonpharmacological approach emphasizes diet manipulation, exercise, stress management, and education and counseling. Clients who eat a nutritious, well-balanced diet and limit their salt, refined sugar, and caffeine intake note that symptoms of edema, increased appetite, and irritability lessen. Vitamin supplementation, especially vitamin B_6 (pyridoxine), is recommended. A dosage of 100 mg of vitamin B_6 daily partially relieves symptoms of dizziness, nausea, and withdrawal behavior. Because excess vitamin B_6 increases the risk of peripheral neuropathy (characterized by ataxia and profound changes in vibratory and position sensation), regular evaluation to assess symptoms of neuropathy is needed.[6] Most of the symptoms of peripheral neuropathy are reversible when vitamin B_6 is discontinued. Naturally occurring vitamin B_6 may be found in such foods as pork, milk, egg yolk, and legumes. Oral contraceptives can cause deficiencies in both vitamin B_6 and magnesium.

Exercise results in a release of endorphins, leading to mood elevation. Aerobic exercises have a tranquilizing effect on muscular tension. The client's lifestyle and interests need to be considered when an exercise program is being planned. Because fatigue tends to exaggerate the symptoms, adequate rest in the premenstrual period is a priority. Explanation, reassurance, and exploration of any psychological aspects should also be done. The use of recognized techniques for stress reduction, including yoga,

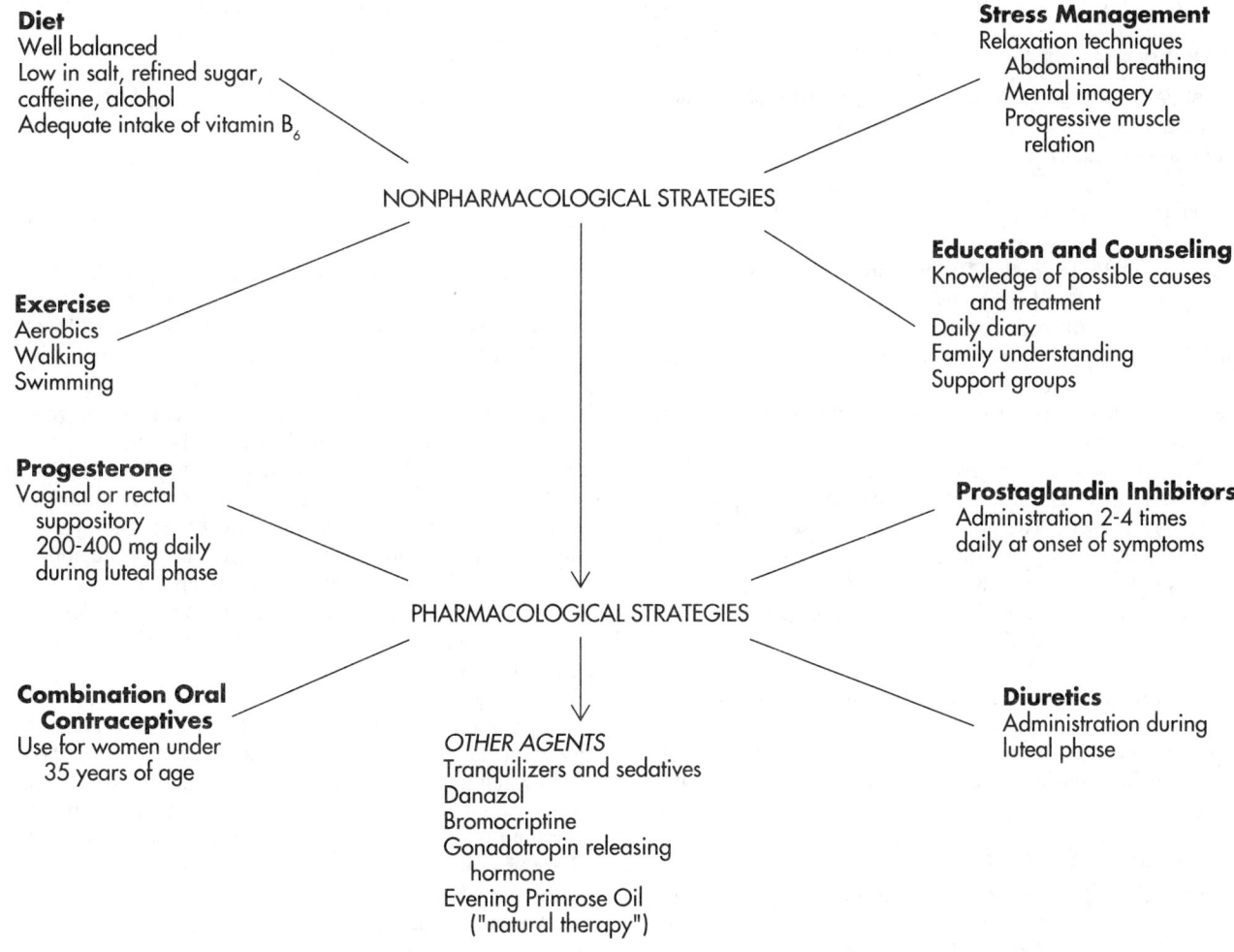

Fig. 48-1 Treatment strategies for PMS.

meditation, imaging, and biofeedback training, should be encouraged.

Clients should be educated and counseled regarding PMS and the current theories on its etiology and treatment. Counseling should involve listening and reassurance as well as provision of factual information. Spouses or significant others need to be informed about the nature of PMS because their understanding and support will be important in the client's daily life. Joining a PMS support group can also be beneficial for some clients.

Pharmacological management. Pharmacological treatment strategies should be considered when symptoms persist. Presently, no single drug is being prescribed for the treatment of PMS symptoms. One therapy is used for a time, and if no improvement is observed, another approach is tried. Progesterone has been widely advocated, but its use remains controversial because results have not been as beneficial as originally thought. The precise role of ovarian hormones in PMS is still unclear. Excessive synthesis of prostaglandins is thought to trigger PMS symptoms, and antiprostaglandin inhibitors such as mefenamic acid (Ponstel) have been prescribed. These medications are effective in reducing depression, pain, headache, and tension. Diuretics such as spironolactone (Aldactone) have improved the symptoms of abdominal bloating and weight gain. Other agents used include combined oral contraceptives, tranquilizers or sedatives, bromocriptine (Parlodel), danazol, gonadotropin-releasing hormone analogues, and Evening Primrose Oil ("natural therapy").

An increasingly aware public is demanding assistance with the distress PMS causes women and their families. As a result, many clinics now offer counseling and treatment for clients with PMS. However, women should be counseled to be cautious in seeking care for PMS because the cause is not completely understood, the treatment is not definitive, and the potential for quackery is high.

Dysmenorrhea

Dysmenorrhea is defined as pain or discomfort associated with menstrual flow. The degree of pain and discomfort varies with the individual. The two types of dysmenorrhea are *primary,* in which pelvic organs are normal, and *secondary,* in which a diagnosed pelvic disease or condition is the underlying cause of the condition. Approximately 50% of all women experience dysmenorrhea, making it one of the most common gynecological problems.[7]

Etiology. Current evidence suggests that prostaglandin $F_{2\alpha}$ ($PGF_{2\alpha}$) and prostaglandin E_2 (PGE_2) released from the endometrium at the time of menstruation cause primary dysmenorrhea.[8] The sequential stimulation of the endometrium by estrogen, followed by progesterone, results in a dramatic increase in prostaglandin production by the endometrium. Prostaglandins increase myometrial contractions and cause constriction of small endometrial blood vessels, with consequent tissue ischemia, endometrial disintegration, bleeding, and pain. Dysmenorrhea may be caused by excessive tissue ischemia resulting from increased intrauterine pressure, vessel constriction, and decreased uterine

blood flow. Women who do not ovulate do not experience dysmenorrhea because progesterone or its withdrawal is a prerequisite for prostaglandin release within the uterus.

Secondary dysmenorrhea often occurs well before the onset of menses and may persist for a longer time during the flow than primary dysmenorrhea. Secondary dysmenorrhea is due to pelvic diseases such as endometriosis, chronic pelvic inflammatory disease, uterine leiomyomas, and adenomyosis. Various diagnostic and therapeutic measures are used when secondary dysmenorrhea is suspected.

Clinical manifestations. Primary dysmenorrhea usually occurs within 3 years of menarche. Characteristic manifestations include lower midabdominal pain that is colicky in nature, with radiation to the lower back and upper thighs. The abdominal pain is often accompanied by nausea, diarrhea, fatigue, headache, and a general sense of malaise. The pain usually begins at the onset of menstruation and lasts for 12 to 72 hours, with the most severe pain occurring on the first day.

Secondary dysmenorrhea usually occurs after the woman has experienced problem-free periods for some time. The pain, which may be unilateral, is generally more constant in nature and may continue throughout the period.

Therapeutic management. A major management goal is to distinguish primary from secondary dysmenorrhea.[9] Taking of a complete health history and performing a physical examination should be the first procedure. If the history is suggestive and pelvic examination findings are normal, the problem is usually treated as primary dysmenorrhea.

Treatment of dysmenorrhea varies depending on the severity of the disability and the individual client's response. Many clients with dysmenorrhea respond well to symptomatic therapy, including rest, reassurance, local heat, and mild analgesics. Since dysmenorrhea is a recurring problem, the use of narcotics is discouraged because addiction is a possibility.

Pharmacological management. Two groups of drugs considered highly effective for primary dysmenorrhea are prostaglandin synthetase inhibitors (PGSIs) and oral contraceptives. PGSIs inhibit production or action of prostaglandins in the menstrual fluid and subsequent uterine activity.

The PGSIs used are nonsteroidal antiinflammatory agents such as ibuprofen (Motrin, Advil, Nuprin), naproxen (Naprosyn), and mefenamic acid (Ponstel). Ibuprofen, naproxen, and mefenamic acid significantly decrease the frequency and severity of symptoms.[10] One of these drugs is prescribed to be taken just before menses (for women who can accurately predict the onset of menses) or at the time of onset of menses. Therapy usually continues four times daily for the first 3 to 4 days of the period. If there is a possibility of pregnancy, the use of PGSIs is precluded.

The most common side effects of PGSIs include dizziness and gastrointestinal (GI) distress. The taking of food with the drug may relieve the latter problem. A history of asthma or peptic ulcers should be reported to the physician because PGSIs are contraindicated in this situation.

Oral contraceptives may be the first line of treatment if

they are also the woman's contraceptive choice. With the suppression of ovulation by oral contraceptives, the production of prostaglandins is also suppressed. Because dysmenorrhea occurs most frequently in young women, there are few contraindications to the use of oral contraceptives.

Surgical treatment is usually reserved for women who have undergone every form of therapy and psychiatric evaluation. In these clients a laparoscopy is performed to evaluate chronic pelvic pain.

■ Nursing Management of Dysmenorrhea

Clients often ask nurses what can be done when minor discomforts associated with some cycles occur. The client should be aware that relief may be obtained by lying down for short periods, drinking hot beverages, applying heat to the abdomen, and taking a mild analgesic. When medications are prescribed, the nurse may be the person who teaches the client about their use. The nurse can also suggest noninvasive pain-relieving practices such as distraction and guided imagery (see Chapter 51). These practices may increase the client's feeling of control and self-reliance.

Other long-term health care measures that can decrease the discomfort of dysmenorrhea are available and should be used. These include (1) regular exercise, (2) maintenance of proper nutritional habits, (3) avoidance of constipation, (4) maintenance of good body mechanics, and (5) avoidance of worry, mental strain, and overfatigue, particularly during the time preceding menstrual periods. Staying active and interested in activities may also help. The nurse's approach to the problem of dysmenorrhea must be thoughtful and sensitive. The counsel and supportive therapy given can provide a foundation for coping with this common problem.

Menstrual Irregularities

The ovarian cycle is more unstable and vulnerable to disruptive influences in its early (adolescence) and late phases (premenopausal). Therefore abnormal bleeding is more common at the beginning and end of the active menstrual life.

Types

Amenorrhea. The absence of menses refers to the failure to menstruate before the age of 17 (primary amenorrhea) and cessation of menses for 6 months or more after they have become established (secondary amenorrhea). Amenorrhea probably occurs in less than 5% of clients. The common causes of amenorrhea are listed in Table 48-2.

Menorrhagia. Menorrhagia is an increased duration or amount of menstrual bleeding at the time of a normal period. In the early reproductive years, it may be associated with an endocrine problem or blood dyscrasia. A single episode of excessive bleeding may indicate a spontaneous abortion or ectopic pregnancy. Uterine tumors, including carcinoma, are common causes of menorrhagia. Pelvic inflammatory disease, endometriosis, the use of an intrauterine device (IUD), and drugs such as anticoagulants and thiazides can also produce heavy menses.

Metrorrhagia. Metrorrhagia is bleeding or spotting between menstrual periods. Slight midcycle (mittelschmerz)

Table 48-2 Causes of Amenorrhea

HYPOTHALAMIC-PITUITARY AXIS

Reversible CNS-mediated insults (e.g., emotional stress, anorexia nervosa or severe dieting, strenuous exercise, post-pill syndrome, chronic or acute illness)
Prolactinoma and other causes of hyperprolactinemia (e.g., drugs)
Craniopharyngioma and other brainstem or parasellar tumors
Congenital conditions (e.g., isolated gonadotropin deficiency)*
Trauma (e.g., head injury with hypothalamic contusion)
Infiltrative processes (e.g., sarcoidosis)
Vascular disease (e.g., hypothalamic vasculitis)

OVARIES

Autoimmune disease (often involving thyroid, adrenal, and islet cells)
Premature menopause (idiopathic) or resistant-ovary syndrome
Polycystic ovary disease
Tumors
Congenital or genetic conditions (e.g., Turner's syndrome)*
Infection (e.g., mumps oophoritis)
Toxins (especially alkylating chemotherapeutic agents)
Irradiation
Trauma, torsion (rare)

UTEROVAGINAL OUTFLOW TRACT

Asherman's syndrome (postcurettage loss of endometrium)
Müllerian dysgenesis*

HORMONAL SYNTHESIS AND ACTION

Male pseudohermaphroditism (e.g., testicular feminization)*
17-Hydroxylase deficiency*

Modified from Veldhuis JD: Management of amenorrhea, Hosp Pract 23:43, 1988.
CNS, Central nervous system.
*Usually presents as primary amenorrhea.

spotting, associated with the decrease of estrogen levels before ovulation, is a common occurrence and is not considered metrorrhagia. *Intramenstrual bleeding* refers to uterine blood loss at a time other than menstruation and may be caused by (1) uterine lesions such as fibroids, polyps, hyperplasia, and carcinoma; (2) cervical erosion and carcinoma; and (3) pelvic inflammatory disease. Clients who are taking contraceptives may have metrorrhagia, which is referred to as *breakthrough bleeding.*

Reasons for changes in the usual pattern of menstruation vary, as does the associated degree of concern. One explanation involves a change in lifestyle. Changes in marital status, recent moves, undue excitement, financial stresses, and other emotional crises can cause amenorrhea or unusual bleeding. These effects demonstrate the strong influences that psychological factors have on endocrine function and should be considered when the client comes for evaluation. When menorrhagia or metrorrhagia occurs,

the possibility of pelvic neoplasm must always be considered.

Therapeutic management. Because the causes of menstrual irregularities are multiple and varied, diagnostic and therapeutic measures vary as well. Initially, a detailed health history is obtained and a careful physical examination, including a pelvic examination, is performed. An assessment of the actual loss of blood is attempted. Pregnancy, chronic disease, recent physical or psychic stress, and a possible drug-induced menstrual disturbance are ruled out. A wide range of tests and procedures relative to a tentative diagnosis are then performed. The client may be referred to a gynecological endocrinologist for further investigation of the problem.

Treatment of menstrual irregularities is determined by the specific disorder and the age of the client. Conservative treatment consists of hormonal therapy. Progesterone given in a single course for a problem of short duration or for three to four menstrual cycles may result in the return of normal ovarian function and control of excessive bleeding. When estrogen as well as progesterone problems exist, a trial of 3 to 4 months of oral contraceptives is given, often resulting in normal cycling. The dosage of oral contraceptives is adjusted if breakthrough bleeding occurs.

Treatment of any psychogenic cause of menstrual irregularities involves giving ample amounts of reassurance and understanding. Psychotherapy may be indicated for the underlying emotional problem.

Surgical interventions. Surgical interventions include a variety of procedures such as dilatation and curettage (D & C), polypectomy, cauterization (destruction of tissue by a chemical or by heat), myomectomy (removal of uterine tumor without removal of the uterus), and hysterectomy.

D & C is the most frequently performed gynecological procedure. *Dilatation* is the widening of the cervical canal with a dilator, and *curettage* is the scraping of the lining of the uterus with a curet. A D & C is considered both a diagnostic and a therapeutic measure. A diagnostic D & C is performed to identify a lesion in the endocervix or endometrium. A therapeutic D & C is done for an incomplete abortion and to correct excessive or prolonged bleeding. Dilatation of the cervix may be done to treat dysmenorrhea or sterility due to cervical stenosis. A D & C is most often done as an outpatient procedure, but overnight hospitalization may be indicated.

■ Nursing Management of Menstrual Irregularities

Nursing interventions

Acute intervention. The amount of vaginal bleeding the client experiences should be accurately assessed. The number of pads used as well as the degree of saturation should be reported and recorded. The client's fatigue level, along with variations in blood pressure and blood count, should be noted, since anemia and hypovolemia may be present.

When a client is scheduled for a D & C, food intake is restricted after midnight the evening before the procedure. The procedure may be done in the operating room, in a free-standing surgery center, or in the physician's office, with the client under local or general anesthesia. Even if the choice is local anesthesia, the client should be prepared to receive general anesthesia if this becomes necessary.

Postoperatively, the client's vital signs should be checked every 15 minutes until stable. The amount of vaginal bleeding should be noted, and a pad count should be kept. Some abdominal cramping, pelvic discomfort, or back pain is usual. These problems should be relieved with mild analgesics (e.g., aspirin, acetaminophen). Persistent pain should be reported to the physician, since the uterus is occasionally perforated during the procedure.

Because the client is discharged within 1 to 6 hours after the operation, teaching is an especially important aspect of nursing care. Specific instructions for self-care must be provided, including the following:

1. Avoid the use of tampons or douching and refrain from intercourse until examination the second week after the operation.
2. Expect a vaginal discharge during the healing process. It should be lighter in amount than the usual menses and from dark red to dark brown, and it should last no longer than 1 week.
3. Avoid strenuous activity for 1 week, but a return to usual activities 2 days after recovery from anesthesia is usually appropriate.
4. Report any signs of infection, such as fever, chills, foul-smelling discharge, heavy bleeding, and pelvic pain.

The client should also be told that the subsequent menstrual period is not usually affected.

Chronic management. Treatment of menstrual problems is not always adequate. For example, a D & C for metrorrhagia may be helpful for a time, but then the problem may recur. Continued use of contraceptives may become undesirable because of the client's age or state of health. If abnormal bleeding persists, the client generally becomes frustrated and worried and wants something done to correct the condition. If abdominal bleeding persists, hysterectomy may be the treatment of choice. The nurse may play an important role in addressing the concerns some women express about physical, sexual, and emotional changes after a hysterectomy. Other women, who do not wish to become pregnant, may be relieved to have an end to persistent bleeding. Assessment of the individual woman provides the direction for the counseling.

Menopause

The *climacteric* is the transitional period in the life of a woman during which reproductive function gradually diminishes and then ceases. It lasts approximately 15 to 20 years, from about the ages of 40 to 60. During this period, monthly menses occur less frequently and are irregular, and the flow decreases in amount. The *menopause* is the physiological cessation of menses associated with decreased ovarian function occurring during the climacteric. (The terms *climacteric* and *menopause* are often erroneously used to mean the same thing.) It is diagnosed when a year has passed without menstruation. Natural menopause usually occurs between the ages of 47 and 52 years. Artificially induced menopause occurs after irradiation of the ovaries, surgical removal of both ovaries, or hysterectomy. Regardless of the cause, menopause results in defi-

Table 48-3 Signs and Symptoms of Estrogen Deficiency

Vasomotor
  Hot flashes
Genitourinary
  Atrophic vaginitis
  Dyspareunia secondary to poor lubrication
  Dysuria
Psychological
  Emotional lability
  Change in sleep pattern
  Decreased REM sleep
Skeletal
  Increased fracture rate, particularly of vertebral bodies
    but also of humerus, distal radius, and upper femur
Cardiovascular
  Decreased high-density lipoproteins
Dermatological
  Diminished collagen content of skin

REM, Rapid eye movement.

ciency or absence of estrogen. The signs and symptoms of estrogen deficiency are listed in Table 48-3.

Clinical manifestations

Physical. The most common physical symptoms directly related to menopause are hot flashes and atrophic vaginal changes. These changes are physiological responses to decreasing estrogen levels. The hot flashes are described as a sensation of warmth, beginning in the upper part of the chest and spreading to the neck, face, and upper extremities, followed by profuse perspiration and sometimes chilling. These sensations last from several seconds to 5 minutes and occur most often at night, thereby disturbing sleep. A hot flash can be triggered by situations that affect body temperature, such as eating of a hot meal, hot weather, drinking of an alcoholic beverage, stress, and warm clothing. Hot flashes are not well understood, but apparently they are the result of instability between the hypothalamus and the autonomic nervous system brought about by a decline in estrogen.[11]

Atrophic vaginal changes secondary to decreased estrogen include thinning of the mucosa and disappearance of rugae. Vaginal secretions also decrease and become more alkaline. Because of these changes, the vaginal canal is easily traumatized and susceptible to infection.

Many physical changes in menopausal women are frequently associated with the process of aging rather than just decreased ovarian functioning. These changes include a redistribution of fat, a tendency to gain weight more easily, muscle and joint pain, loss of elasticity of skin, and atrophy of the external genitalia and breast tissue.

Psychological. During the time of menopause, women also begin to reevaluate and redefine their roles. Frustration over lost dreams, guilt feelings about previous failures, boredom with lack of challenge, and discouragement over diminishing horizons can develop into a variety of symptoms. These symptoms include emotional lability, anxiety, depression, insomnia, fatigue, palpitations, and headache. Menopause is often more difficult for a woman who perceives her ability to reproduce as her main reason for living and a way to prove her self-worth.

Therapeutic management. Significant beneficial effects as well as potential risks are associated with the use of hormonal replacement therapy (HRT) in postmenopausal women. The decision as to whether, when, and how to use HRT and the duration of its use are controversial. The lowest effective dose of estrogen for the shortest possible time is prescribed by some physicians, whereas others advocate long-term therapy to the age of 70 or beyond.[12,13] Low-dose estrogen effectively controls disabling vasomotor symptoms. Approximately 80% of women can accept and tolerate hot flashes without treatment if they are assured that the hot flashes will stop within 1 to 5 years.

When atrophic vaginal changes occur, estrogen vaginal creams or suppositories (e.g., Premarin) provide effective and rapid relief. These are administered daily for about a week and thereafter once or twice a week, depending on the client's response. Because substantial systemic absorption of estrogen occurs with vaginal use, the risks related to systemic estrogen therapy should be considered.

HRT may be prophylactic against osteoporosis and perhaps against cardiovascular disease. Prevention of osteoporosis results in arresting or slowing the process of demineralization from the bone. The loss of minerals, especially calcium, from bone begins with the onset of the climacteric around the age of 40. Effective therapy should begin before demineralization occurs and should continue throughout the menopausal and postmenopausal periods. Adequate calcium supplementation and regular weight-bearing exercise are needed to maintain bone regeneration and prevent bone loss, regardless of whether HRT is used. (See Chapter 57 for a discussion of osteoporosis.) Estrogen is capable of reducing low-density lipoproteins and increasing high-density lipoproteins. However, a cause-and-effect relationship between decreased levels of estrogen and the increased incidence of cardiovascular disease in postmenopausal women is not well established.[14]

Endometrial cancer is a high-risk potential for women taking only estrogen replacement because unopposed estrogen may induce endometrial hyperplasia and ultimately adenocarcinoma. The addition of a progestin for the last 7 to 10 days of the cycle reduces this risk. However, the cycling of estrogen and progesterone mimics the normal menstrual cycle, resulting in the reestablishment of menses. An increase in the incidence of gallstones and hypertension has also been noted in women taking HRT. Because HRT involves lower doses of estrogen, the risk of thrombophlebitis and stroke is not observed as it may be in women who use oral contraceptives.

Postmenopausal estrogen replacement does not appear to substantially increase the risk of the development of breast cancer, although estrogen may play a permissive or supportive role in the disease process, especially in higher doses and for a longer duration.[15,16] There is also no good evidence that progestins reduce the risk of breast cancer. Because progestins may adversely affect lipoproteins and

thus increase cardiovascular mortality, the use of progestins in a woman who has no uterus is unnecessary and possibly detrimental.

A distinction between the menstrual irregularities that are basically physiological features of menopause and the development of pathological conditions such as polyps or cancer must be made. This entails a careful physical as well as pelvic examination, cervical cytological study, and curettage of the cervix and endometrium. Once pathological conditions are ruled out, several months of hormonal therapy may be considered.

Symptoms attributed to aging and psychological factors should be treated. Tranquilizers and sedatives may be prescribed for symptoms of insomnia and emotional manifestations, but *not* at the expense of ignoring the need to resolve the grieving problems that often accompany menopause. Women must be listened to in a nonjudgmental fashion. Efforts should be made to help the client reevaluate her life and make realistic plans for the future.

Pharmacological management. Before HRT is begun, a careful health history should be obtained to document whether a family tendency for cancer, hypertension, cardiovascular disease, or osteoporosis exists. A complete physical examination, including breast and pelvic examinations, a Papanicolaou (Pap) smear, endometrial biopsy, and a baseline blood pressure, is also performed. Conjugated estrogen (a mixture of natural estrogens) is given cyclically in a dosage ranging from 0.3 to 1.25 mg per day, with the medication omitted 5 to 7 days per month. The addition of progestins in a dosage of 2.5 to 10 mg per day during the last 7 to 10 days of estrogen administration initiates shedding of the endometrium and thus prevents endometrial hyperplasia. Other cycling schedules, such as dosages of both estrogen and a progestin given daily through the entire month, may also be prescribed. Women on this regimen should be prepared for some regular withdrawal menstrual bleeding. This withdrawal bleeding often subsides when the client has been on this drug combination for some time.[16]

A new method of administering estrogen, transdermal estradiol (Estraderm), is now available. Patches are applied to a clear, dry area on the trunk of the body and are worn either continuously or for the first 21 days of the cycle. Each patch delivers a lower dose of estrogen and has to be changed only twice a week. Progestin should be given if the uterus is still present.

A woman's decision to initiate HRT must be an informed one. The therapeutic limits of the replacement therapy and its benefit-risk ratio must be explained. The woman will have to be seen by her health care provider every 6 months to 1 year, at which time she will be reexamined. An endometrial biopsy should be performed after 2 years of treatment. Estrogen should not be used by clients with unexplained vaginal bleeding, known or suspected estrogen-dependent neoplasia, acute liver disease or chronic impaired liver function, renal insufficiency, acute vascular thrombosis, or neuroophthalmological vascular diseases.[17]

Estrogens, such as Premarin, Estinyl, and Ogen, and progestins, such as Norlutin and Provera, are also administered cyclically. The original dose may be tapered and then discontinued after a few years of therapy. By this time the acute symptoms have usually subsided. The nurse should be alert to the possible side effects of the drugs and should be able to interpret them for the client. Hormonal replacement may be continued as part of a plan to prevent the development or worsening of osteoporosis. The side effects include weight gain, breast and pelvic discomfort due to engorgement, headache, GI disturbances, vaginal discharge, and skin pigmentation. These symptoms usually result from an excessive estrogen dosage or are an initial response to therapy. They can be reduced by decreasing the dosage, or they may resolve spontaneously with continued use of the drugs. The most potentially significant side effect of estrogen is vaginal bleeding, which often occurs as a withdrawal effect when estrogen is used cyclically. Because postmenopausal bleeding may also be a sign of cancer, any unexpected bleeding should be reported promptly to the physician for investigation.

■ Nursing Management of Menopause

When menopause occurs, women have almost as many years of their adult lives ahead of them as behind them. During this period a woman can choose to foster good health, vitality, and attractiveness, or she can perceive that menopause is the beginning of a prolonged degenerative process. Nurses can help women work through changes that occur by providing health teaching as well as reassurance.

The client's understanding of the physiology of menopause needs to be assessed, since this may affect reactions to the changes and compliance with the therapeutic approach. The client should be made aware that the symptoms she is experiencing are normal and will pass after a time. Many misconceptions about menopause have been perpetuated and should be clarified by the nurse to reduce unnecessary anxiety.

Diet and exercise are important areas of health education for the menopausal woman. A daily intake of about 30 cal/kg with maintenance of sound nutrition is recommended for the menopausal woman. A decrease in metabolic rate and careless eating habits and not menopause result in weight gain and related fatigue. An adequate intake of calcium and vitamin D can maintain healthy bones and thereby counteract the effect of decreased estrogen that tends to make bones grow lighter and more fragile. The recommended daily allowance (RDA) of calcium for the average woman is 800 to 1000 mg per day. The RDA for osteoporosis prevention is 1200 to 1400 mg per day. The RDA for vitamin D is 400 IU; no increase is recommended for osteoporosis prevention.[18] Dairy products should be ingested in moderate amounts, whereas intake of junk foods, soft drinks, and protein should be decreased because these foods raise phosphate levels and therefore lower calcium levels.

A regular program of exercise and physical activity can improve circulation, maintain good muscle tone, and delay some aspects of aging for women in menopause. Exercise stimulates osteoblastic activity, thereby delaying osteoporosis. Activities such as brisk walks, bicycling, and

gardening are healthy and enjoyable. Development of new interests can help ease tension and anxiety.

Sexual function can continue with little change in the vast majority of postmenopausal women. Cessation of menstruation and ability to bear children should not be equated with cessation of sexual capability. Femininity and libido do not disappear with menopause. An older woman is often capable of greater warmth, sensitivity, and humanity in her sexual relationships than she was as a very young woman.[13] Atrophic changes in vaginal epithelium associated with inadequate lubrication may lead to *dyspareunia* (painful coitus). Petrolatum or K-Y jelly is often effective in dealing with this problem. An active sex life helps increase lubrication and maintain the pliability of vaginal tissues. The client should be given an opportunity to discuss concerns candidly.

Some of the symptoms of menopause, such as hot flashes, are self-limiting, and the concern for them decreases with time. The burden of birth control and the fear of pregnancy no longer exist. A few women may need extended counseling to assist them in resolving their psychological problems. Psychiatric help may also be indicated. The use of appropriate printed material for client education to supplement discussion is often effective.

CONTRACEPTION AND BIRTH CONTROL

The role of women in society is changing. Many of these changes have been brought about and encouraged by the women's liberation movement. Many women wish to pursue careers in addition to family and childbearing roles. Recently, many more avenues have opened up to women, and women are eager and willing to explore them. With the advent of effective methods of contraception and abortion, pregnancy is seen as a voluntary experience. Women can now make choices about family size and spacing in keeping with their newer lifestyles. Poor health or genetic problems of either partner and the mutual desire for fewer children may be motivators for the use of current methods of family planning. Each individual can therefore make a personal choice regarding reproduction based on conscience or desire. These practices can result in planned pregnancies at desired intervals.

Significance

The rapid growth of population has been identified as a threat to natural resources and to the quality of life for all. Consequently, the issue of population control is influenced by political and economic factors balanced against sociocultural constraints for each social group. Because of this situation, women may expect a high priority to be placed on the development of a contraceptive with a high degree of safety, effectiveness, and availability. However, sociocultural constraints often inhibit actions that appear to be logical and practical approaches to the problem of population growth. For example, despite increasing pregnancies among adolescents, adequate and accurate contraceptive information is rarely provided to teenagers. Despite growing concern over the number of children born into an adverse socioeconomic environment, there are efforts to restrict the option of abortion for poor women. Women are often left to consider the health consequences and economic risk-benefit ratio between pregnancy and contraception. These factors often leave women in a moral dilemma in their decision making about contraceptives.

Contraceptive Methods

An ideal contraceptive is one that is safe, simple to use, inexpensive, and reversible and does not interfere with the act of intercourse. No single method that meets all these criteria is yet available. *Temporary* contraceptives provide protection for individuals who wish to avoid or delay pregnancy. To be effective, they must be used correctly and consistently. *Permanent* methods of birth control such as sterilization are becoming increasingly acceptable to men and women. Sterilization is often chosen by persons who have completed their families or who wish to remain childless. Table 48-4 summarizes the common contraceptive methods, their use, side effects, and related client education. (Male sterilization is discussed in Chapter 49.)

Medroxyprogesterone acetate (Depo-Provera), a less common contraceptive that prevents ovulation, is given as an injection once every 3 months. It allows spontaneity of sex, but its side effects of irregular bleeding and prolonged amenorrhea after being discontinued (resulting in infertility) have limited its use in the United States. A female condom that is basically a combination of a diaphragm and a condom has recently been developed.[19] Additional methods of contraception that are being investigated include progestogen implants inserted under the skin, vaginal rings, male contraceptives, prostaglandins for induction of menses, and an antipregnancy vaccine.[20]

Male contraception includes a device and steroidal and nonsteroidal agents. The only device is the condom (a barrier). This form of contraception has attracted renewed interest for the protection it provides against sexually transmitted diseases and acquired immunodeficiency syndrome (AIDS). Research on steroidal contraceptives continues. The latest study is investigating a combined use of GnRH with testosterone and reports that when given intramuscularly daily for 10 days, this combination suppressed gonadotropins and inhibin. It is not known whether this suppression will persist during a longer treatment period, or whether it will reliably induce azoospermia. There have been no reported side effects.[21]

Research continues on the cottonseed derivative, gossypol. This drug alters sperm structure and motility and decreases sperm production. However, because of complications, slow onset of action, slow return of fertility, and difficulties in the mode of administration (currently available only in injection form), most researchers agree that the product will not be ready for marketing for at least 5 years.[22]

■ Nursing Management of Contraception and Birth Control

Persons desire to prevent conception for a number of reasons related to personal convenience, economics, social values, and lifestyle. The nurse is in a position to counsel individuals and couples about birth control. The nurse can assist them by presenting concise, factual, unbiased infor-

Table 48-4 Methods of Birth Control

Description	Side Effects and Complications	Client Education

TEMPORARY

Oral contraceptives

Description	Side Effects and Complications	Client Education
Combination pill containing mixture of estrogen and progesterone (standard and low-dose) taken usually on 5th through 25th day of each cycle, prevention of ovulation, changes in endometrium, alterations in cervical mucus and tubal transport, simple and unobtrusive in use, 99% effective, failure due to irregular or incorrect use; minipill containing progestin only, inhibition of ovulation not always occurring, prevention of implantation 96%-98% effective	Side effects of weight gain, nausea and vomiting, spotting and breakthrough bleeding, postpill amenorrhea, breast tenderness, headache, chloasma, irritability, nervousness, depression, and decreased libido; complications of benign liver tumors, gallstones, myocardial infarction, thromboembolism, stroke(smokers over age of 35 yr at higher risk); contraindications of history of cardiovascular or liver disease, hypertension, breast or pelvic cancer and caution with diabetes mellitus, sickle cell anemia	Instruct client in correct use of pills. Tell client to take pill same time each day; when pill is forgotten one day, take two next day. Review side effects, contraindications. Explain that client should report cramps or swelling of legs, chest pain. Discuss need for periodic (every 6-12 months) checkup that involves weight, BP, Pap smear, hematocrit. Review danger signs of drug. Take drug history, asking about use of phenytoin, phenobarbital, antibiotic (ampicillin), which affect contraceptive action. Inform client that method is usually not recommended for persons over age 35. Discourage smoking.

IUD

Description	Side Effects and Complications	Client Education
Insertion into uterus of flexible objects made of plastic or copper wire (nonmedicated or medicated with substance altering uterine environment), usually with attached string that protrudes into vagina; contraception probably prevented by inflammatory response in endometrium, preventing implantation; after insertion, no additional equipment necessary; 97%-99% effective; failure mainly due to undetected expulsion	Increased menstrual flow, intramenstrual bleeding and cramping, especially during early months of use; possible complications of ectopic pregnancy, pelvic infection, perforation of uterus, infertility	Discuss techniques and experience of insertion and removal. Inform client that insertion may be more difficult and expulsion and complications greater in nulliparous clients. Instruct client to check for string in vagina after each period; report to physician if unable to locate. Discuss need for annual pelvic examination and Pap smear.

Diaphragm

Description	Side Effects and Complications	Client Education
Dome-shaped latex cup with circular metal spring (varies in size) covering cervix, coating of inner surface with spermicide before insertion, provision of mechanical barrier to sperm, prescription method, fitting by professional, recurrent motivation to use necessary, 87% effective, failure due to improper fitting or placement of device	Allergy to latex, spermicide	Demonstrate how to hold, insert, and remove device, using model. Allow for insertion and removal practice sessions. Advise client that insertion may be any time before coitus, but removal should be 6-8 hr after coitus. Tell client that bowel and bladder should be emptied before insertion. Give instructions for cleansing and storing, checking for holes or deterioration. Advise client that diaphragm must be refitted following pregnancy, weight loss, or weight gain. Advise client that it is not suitable if severe pelvic relaxation is present.

BP, Blood pressure.

Continued.

Table 48-4 Methods of Birth Control—cont'd

Description	Side Effects and Complications	Client Education
TEMPORARY—cont'd		
Vaginal sponge		
Cup-shaped disposable polyruethane sponge that is impregnated with spermicide, removal loop located on bottom; provision of 24 hr mechanical and chemical barrier that traps and absorbs sperm,; one size; available without prescription; 89%-90% effective; failure due to improper placement	Allergy or irritation to sponge and/or spermicide; risk of toxic shock syndrome uncertain, but with no greater incidence than for tampon use	Ascertain client's ability to palpate cervix, properly place moistened sponge over cervix, and remove (gently to avoid tearing). Inform client that removal is aided by bearing down and that sponge remains in place 6 hr after coitus. Advise client that it is not suitable if severe pelvic relaxation is present or during menses.
Cervical cap		
Rubber thimble-shaped shield covering cervix held in place only by suction, spermicide in inner surface providing mechanical barrier to sperm, fitting by professional, effectiveness similar to diaphragm, failure due to dislodgement and improper fit	Allergy to rubber and/or spermicide, possible cervical irritation or erosion from suction	Provide sufficient time for practice with insertion and removal (more time than for diaphragm). Give instruction for cleaning, storing, and inspecting for damage. Inform client that it can be used with abnormalities of vaginal canal but not with cervical inconsistencies or pelvic inflammatory disease.
Condom		
Thin rubber sheath fitting over erect penis and providing mechanical barrier to sperm, simple method to use, no prescription necessary, 85% effective, failure due to tearing or slipping during coitus	Possible allergy to rubber, possible decrease in sensation and interference with foreplay	Advise client to roll sheath along entire penis, leaving slack at end to receive semen. Inform client that sharp object (e.g., fingernails) may tear condom. Tell client to hold sheath in place when penis is withdrawn to prevent emptying of sperm in or near vagina.
Spermicide		
Insertion into vagina by means of applicator or aerosol spray, provision of chemical barrier to cervical os, simple method to use, no prescription necessary, 80% effective, failure due to uncertain dispersion and retention of agent within vagina	Possible allergies in either partner	Instruct client on proper insertion of spermicide. Advise on application just before *each* act of coitus. Inform client that use is chiefly for women with infrequent coitus.
Rhythm method		
Periodic abstinence during fertile portion of menstrual cycle; strong motivation, self-control necessary; compliance with all religious doctrines; 60%-65% effective; failure due to difficulty in determining precise day of ovulation, irregularity of menses		Discuss methods to establish baseline menstrual patterns and identify ovulation. Give instructions in use of calendar or basal body temperature method to determine ovulation and fertile period.

Table 48-4   Methods of Birth Control—cont'd

Description	Side Effects and Complications	Client Education
PERMANENT		
Tubal		
Variety of abdominal and vaginal surgical procedures (laparotomy, laparoscopy, culdoscopy) that permanently bar sperm and ovum from meeting; crushing, ligating, clipping, or plugging of fallopian tubes (potentially reversible procedure); 99.96% effective; failure due to recanalization of fallopian tubes, erroneous ligation	Bowel injury, hemorrhage, or infection	Determine whether temporary contraceptives were used and reason for client's dissatisfaction. Counsel regarding effects of procedure on physiology and sexual performance. Assist in obtaining written informed consent for procedure. Inform client that procedure requires short-term hospitalization or can be done on outpatient basis.
Hysterectomy		
Surgical removal of uterus, 100% effective	Bladder infection, vascular disorders, infection, hemorrhage, pain, psychological adjustment	Assess or counsel regarding understanding of extent of surgery, altered physiology, complications, and sexual performance. Inform client of increased cost and recuperation time.
Vasectomy		
Bilateral surgical ligation and resection of ductus deferens, 100% effective	Hematoma, swelling, psychological adjustment	Inform client that procedure is usually done as outpatient procedure and takes 15-30 min. Tell client that alternative form of contraception is needed until no sperm is seen on examination. Explain that procedure does not affect masculinity.

mation about methods available, including their benefits and risks. The couple should choose a method that is most compatible with their personal circumstances. This should be a method that they will use and feel comfortable using (Fig. 48-2).

Women who are considering sterilization as a contraceptive method have common concerns about pain associated with the procedure, the effects of sterilization, and possible complications. Counseling should provide accurate information about these concerns and allow the individuals to explore their feelings about ending reproductive functioning. When motives are healthy and the woman is well-adjusted, sterilization will not adversely affect sexual functioning, physiology, or self-concept.

With the increased interest in family planning, nurses should know the available resources for contraceptive referral within their communities. *Planned Parenthood* is a resource that is available in most areas. Literature dealing with contraception should also be provided for persons who demonstrate an interest in it.

When the person has made a decision on the method of contraception, counseling in the proper use of the method must be given. The nurse should evaluate the client's real understanding of the method chosen and provide explanations and interpretation if necessary. The client should also be aware of an alternative method of contraception if emergencies such as misplacing of a diaphragm occur at an inopportune time.

Women who use contraceptives but wish to eventually have a family should understand the risks of deferring pregnancy. Fertility increases to a peak at 24 years of age and then declines, with a rapid fall after age 30. Fetal and maternal risks also increase with age. Women with progressive conditions such as heart disease should be advised to have their families as early as possible.

INFERTILITY

Infertility is the failure to conceive after a year or more of unprotected, adequately timed intercourse. Approximately 15% of couples in the United States are involuntarily infertile. Professional intervention can help about 40% of these couples achieve a pregnant state.

In determining the cause of infertility and in treating it, both man and woman must be evaluated. A factor relating to the woman is found in no more than one half of barren marriages. Proper study and the subsequent therapeutic measures require time (often a year or more) and patience for results to be obtained. A trusting relationship between the health professionals and the infertile couple should be established early in the investigative process.

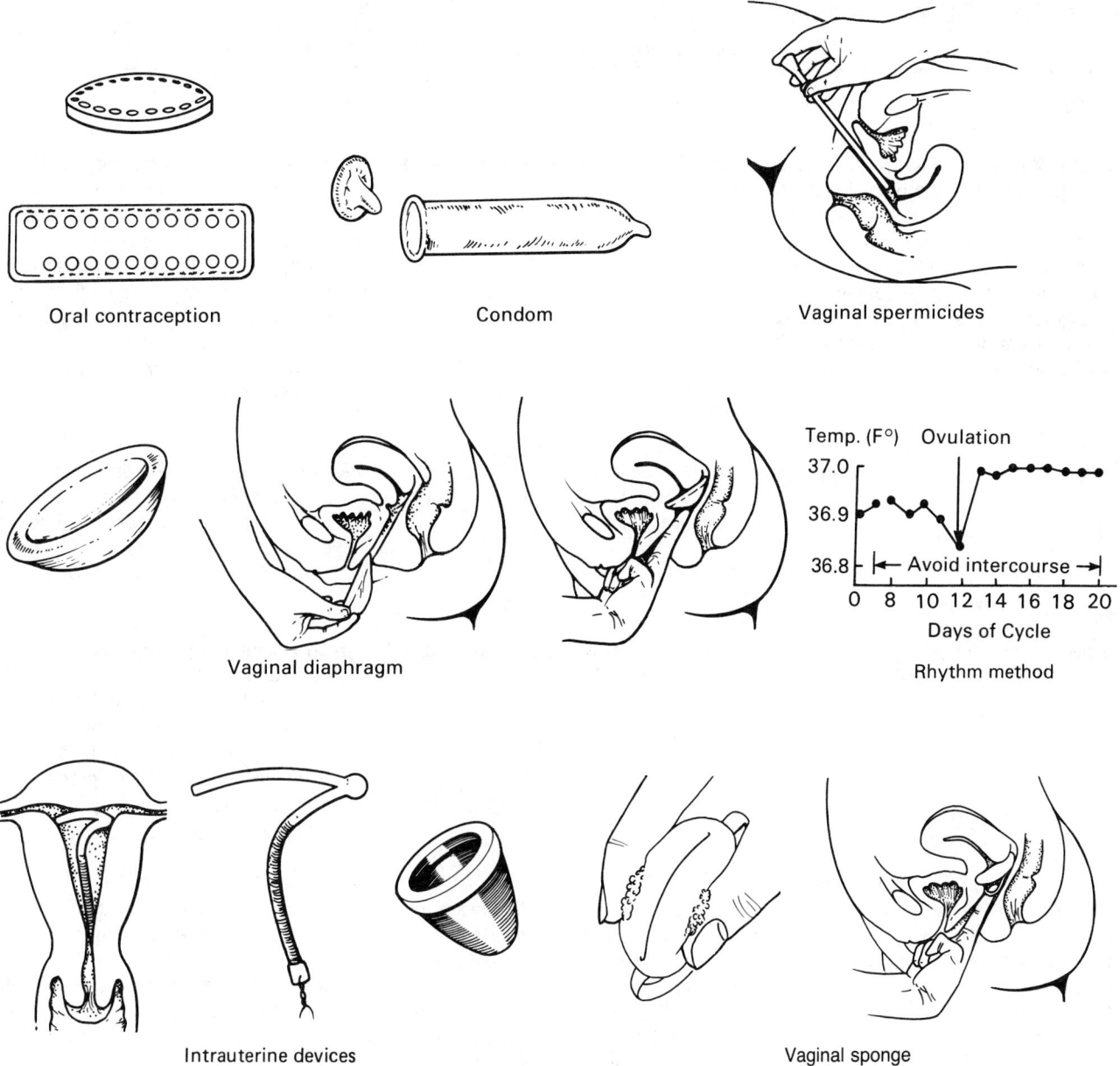

Oral contraception

Condom

Vaginal spermicides

Vaginal diaphragm

Rhythm method

Intrauterine devices

Vaginal sponge

Fig. 48-2 Temporary contraceptive methods and devices. (From Govan ADT, Hodge C, and Callander R: Gynecology illustrated, ed 3, New York, 1985, Churchill Livingstone.)

Etiology

A complete list of the causes of female infertility is extensive. The following are found most frequently: anovulation, tubal disease, and abnormalities of the cervical mucus or uterus. Other possible causes include systemic debility, psychological stress, marital and sexual maladjustment, and lack of knowledge about reproductive functioning. (Male infertility is discussed in Chapter 49.) In some instances the fertility problem is attributed to the couple rather than to one of the partners. Immune factors (antisperm agglutinating and immobilizing antibodies found in either partner), infrequent intercourse, and nonoptimal sexual techniques may be implicated.

Diagnostic Studies

After a detailed history is obtained and a general physical examination of the woman is performed to rule out any related medical or gynecological disease, several basic tests are performed to evaluate whether the cause is female infertility. These tests include ovulatory studies, tubal patency studies, and postcoital studies.

Ovulatory studies. A *basal body temperature record* is kept to determine whether there is regular ovulation. The woman is instructed to take and record her temperature on awakening and before any activity. The same site (e.g., oral) should be used each time. Any cause for variation, such as sleeplessness or illness, should be noted. As ovu-

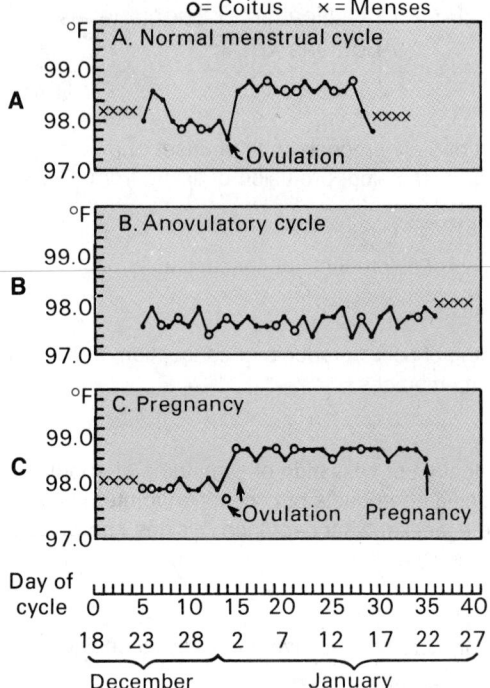

Fig. 48-3 Basal body temperature chart. **A,** Typical biphasic temperature curve indicative of ovulation and normal progesterone effect. **B,** Irregular monophasic curve characteristic of anovulatory cycles. **C,** Ovulatory curve with sustained temperature elevation following conception and the first missed period.

lation approaches, the production of estrogen increases and may cause a drop in temperature. When ovulation occurs, progesterone is produced, causing a 0.3° C to 0.4° C (0.5° F to 0.7° F) rise in temperature. The temperature graph and the readings (Fig. 48-3) therefore detect ovulation and suggest the timing of intercourse if pregnancy is desired. Rigid adherence to a schedule can produce psychological stress sufficient to inhibit sexual relations.

Simple rapid ovulation production kits are now available for use by clients at home. These kits are generally used daily to measure luteinizing hormone (LH) levels in urine samples. Ovulation occurs about 28 to 36 hours after the first rise of LH, so intercourse can be properly timed to ovulation.[23] Other tests for ovulation include cervical and vaginal smears, endometrial biopsy, and plasma progesterone determinations.

Tubal patency studies. Tubal disease (occlusion or lack of peristalsis) is assessed most commonly by means of *hysterosalpingography*. This procedure consists of the radiological visualization of the uterus and tubes by injection through the cervix of a radiopaque dye. Tubal patency and any distortions of the endometrial cavity can be determined. A laxative or an enema is given to the client before the test so that distention or gas shadows will be prevented, thereby making the x-ray film easier to read. The client may experience moderate cramping and should be observed for signs of a possible allergic reaction to the dye. Culdoscopy or laparoscopy, in which the tubes may be visualized directly while a dye is injected into the cervix, is also used to detect tubal disease. Tubal insufflation (Rubin's test), which involves the introduction of carbon dioxide through the cervix via a cannula, is rarely used today to determine tubal patency.

Postcoital studies. Examination of the cervical mucus can reveal whether it undergoes favorable changes at ovulation, enabling penetration, survival, and normal progression of the sperm. A *postcoital examination* can determine whether the cervical environment is favorable for the sperm. The woman is asked to have intercourse about the time ovulation is expected and 2 to 12 hours before being seen by the physician. Douching or bathing should be avoided before the test. The cervical and vaginal secretions are aspirated and examined for the number and motility of sperm present.

Therapeutic Management

The management of infertility problems depends on the cause. If infertility is secondary to an ovarian disturbance, supplemental hormone therapy to restore and maintain ovulation may be attempted. Drugs used to induce ovulation include clomiphene citrate (Clomid), human menopausal gonadotropin (Pergonal), and bromocriptine (Parlodel).

When an actual mechanical tubal block exists, a reparative surgical procedure can be attempted. However, only a small percentage of normal intrauterine term pregnancies have followed tuboplasty.

Poor cervical mucus may be a result of chronic cervicitis or inadequate estrogenic stimulation. Careful cauterization of the cervix may eradicate the chronic cervicitis, and the administration of estrogens can improve the quantity and quality of the cervical mucus.

Improving the client's general health may help, especially when a debilitating or chronic illness is present. Removing or reducing psychological stress can improve the emotional climate, making it more conducive to achievement of pregnancy. Education of the client (couple) regarding the probable time of ovulation and appropriate coital technique may also be indicated.

In selected cases, *artificial* (donor) *insemination,* or the introduction of semen into the female genital tract, can be an effective treatment. The selection of the donor is carried out with great care, with attention to his general state of health, genetic background, and blood type. Male sterility is the usual reason for the use of insemination.

In vitro fertilization (IVF), another technique used, is the removal of mature oocytes from the woman's ovarian follicle via laparoscopy, followed by fertilization of the ova with the partner's sperm in a petri dish. When fertilization and cleavage have occurred, the resulting embryos are transferred into the woman's uterus. The procedure requires 2 to 3 days to complete and is used in cases of fallopian tube obstruction, oligospermia, and unexplained infertility. IVF still has a relatively low rate of success; it is costly and emotionally stressful, but it has become a recognized and accepted method of therapy for infertile couples.

Two other approaches are used for infertile couples. *Gamete intrafallopian transfer* (GIFT) involves the placement of gametes, sperm and oocytes, into the woman's fallopian tubes through laparoscopy. *Nonsurgical ovum transfer* (surrogacy) is performed when a woman signs a contract or volunteers to be artificially inseminated and gives the baby that was conceived to the semen donor. Noncoital reproduction poses many medical, ethical, legal, and social concerns.

If an incurable barrier to conception exists or if the program of therapy has failed to achieve pregnancy after a period of 1 year, the possibility of adoption should be seriously considered.

■ Nursing Management of Infertility

The nurse has a major responsibility for teaching and providing emotional support throughout the infertility-testing period. Feelings of anger and frustration between the partners may heighten as so many tests are performed. The problem of infertility can generate great tension in a marriage. Shame and guilt may be precipitated when other persons become involved in this intimate area of a relationship. Recognizing and taking steps to deal with the psychological and emotional factors that surface can assist the couple to better cope with the situation.

Provisions for giving information and emotional support by the nurse continue as therapeutic measures are attempted. Once the cause of fertility is determined, the client with the problem may need help with gender identity related to the inability to conceive. Clients should be given ample opportunities to talk over their concerns.

ABORTION

An abortion is the termination of a pregnancy before the fetus is legally viable. As defined legally, *viability* varies between 20 and 28 weeks of gestation and between 300 and 1000 g of weight. Abortions are classified as *spontaneous*, occurring naturally with no artificial means, or *induced*, occurring as a result of mechanical or medicinal interruption. *Miscarriage* is the lay term indicating the unintended termination of a pregnancy.

Spontaneous Abortion

Spontaneous abortion occurs in about 30% to 40% of all conceptions. Fetal or maternal abnormalities are the chief causes of these abortions. Spontaneous abortions are subdivided into the categories outlined in Table 48-5 so that they can be differentiated clinically.

Therapeutic management. The presence of uterine cramping serves as an aid to diagnosis of vaginal bleeding as a spontaneous abortion. This symptom is usually absent in vaginal bleeding caused by other conditions, such as polyps. Laboratory findings provide little information on which to base a diagnosis. Pregnancy tests may remain positive for about 2 weeks after fetal death. Sonographic examination of the pelvis can have diagnostic and prognostic value for clients who are threatening to abort.

Treatment for a spontaneous abortion is limited. Bed rest, sedation, and abstention from sexual activity are recommended when a diagnosis of threatened abortion is

Table 48-5 Classification of Spontaneous Abortions

INEVITABLE

History of early pregnancy, then onset of moderate bleeding and cramping; protusion of tissue from dilated cervix

COMPLETE

Expelling of all products of conception

INCOMPLETE

Retaining of some products of conception, mainly placenta and membranes

MISSED

Fetal death, but cessation of symptoms of abortion and retaining of products of conception in uterus for more than 4 weeks; disappearance of signs and symptoms of pregnancy

HABITUAL

Three or more consecutive pregnancies ending in abortion

made. The client is advised to report any bleeding to the physician. An estimated 80% of clients proceed to abortion regardless of management. A D & C is generally performed after spontaneous abortion to minimize blood loss, reduce the chance of secondary infection, and shorten convalescence. For the habitual aborter who is found to have an incompetent cervical os, the cervix may be tightened surgically by placement of a purse-string suture through it (Shirodkar's operation). At delivery the suture is removed by the physician to allow a vaginal delivery, or the suture is retained and delivery is by cesarean section.

■ Nursing Management of Spontaneous Abortion

It may be necessary for the client who is threatening to abort to be admitted to the hospital. Vital signs are monitored, and an estimation of blood loss is made. Measures are taken to restrict activity and reduce stress to provide the needed physical and mental rest. Any tissue or suspicious clots that are passed are saved to be examined for traces of fetus and placenta. The possibility of losing the pregnancy may be very distressing to the client. Sympathy, support, reassurance, and someone to talk to are particularly appreciated.

Induced Abortion

Indications for induced abortion include (1) preservation of life or health of the mother; (2) avoidance of birth of an offspring with a serious developmental or hereditary disorder; and (3) inability of parents to support or care for the child, conception after rape, and parents with mental incompetence or severe emotional problems. Therapeutic abortions are performed in the hospital or in a clinic on an outpatient basis. Abortion for medical and social reasons is now available to more than half the world's population, making it one of the most commonly performed surgical procedures.

In 1973 the United States Supreme Court *(Roe v. Wade)* reached a decision establishing that abortion is a matter between the woman and her physician within certain limits. In 1989 the Supreme Court turned control of abortion back to the states (the Webster decision). As a result there is confusion and uncertainty about the restrictions and accessibility of abortion within each state. Viability testing, public funding for abortions, parental role in a teenager's decision for an abortion, standards for abortion clinics, and informed consent are issues that the states are addressing.

Techniques. The decision about which technique to use depends on the length of the pregnancy and the woman's condition. Early abortion methods include menstrual extraction, suction curettage, and D & C. Late or second-trimester abortions include intrauterine instillation of drugs and hysterotomy. Table 48-6 summarizes the methods of abortion in current use, including the advantages and disadvantages of each.

Early pregnancies can also be terminated by a recently developed pill, RU 486 (mifepristone). RU 486 is a progesterone antagonist that prevents implantation of a fertilized ovum. Approximately 48 hours after 600 mg of RU 486 is taken orally, an injection or vaginal suppository of prostaglandin is given, causing the uterus to contract and expel its contents, usually within 24 hours. A period of heavy bleeding usually ensues and side effects of cramps, nausea, and fatigue may occur. RU 486 appears to be a reasonable alternative to surgical abortion, but it is not available for use in the United States.[24]

■ Nursing Management of Induced Abortions

Because physical and psychological complications can arise after abortion procedures, the decision to have an abortion warrants careful consideration. The woman and her significant others need support and acceptance. Some clients benefit from counseling before the procedure, especially when the decision to have an abortion involves conflict. The specific procedure planned must be explained to each client. At times the overriding need to have the pregnancy terminated does not allow detailed explanations or teaching to be absorbed. Anxiety, loneliness, and fear are emotions often experienced before and during the procedure. Friends or family may not be present to support the client. The nurse can be an important factor in the client's experience of the event.

Follow-up care includes instructions on signs and symptoms of possible complications and the importance of avoiding sex, tampons, and douching until reexamination. The client is instructed to return for reexamination in 2 weeks. Some depression is common, and the client should be prepared for this before discharge. Contraception can be initiated during the client's return visit in accordance with her needs and desires.

ECTOPIC PREGNANCY

An ectopic pregnancy is the implantation of the fertilized ovum anywhere outside the uterine cavity. The most frequent site is the fallopian tube, but the location may be ovarian, abdominal, or cervical (Fig. 48-4). Any blockage of the tube or reduction of tubal peristalsis impedes or delays the passage of the zygote to the uterine cavity and can result in tubal fertilization. Salpingitis, adhesions, tumors, tubal surgery, and hormonal imbalances as well as the presence of an IUD can predispose a woman to ectopic pregnancy. The number of ectopic pregnancies per live births has been steadily increasing for the past 15 years.[25] The most commonly cited reason is the increased number of cases of sexually transmitted diseases (STDs) with their sequelae of distorted and scarred fallopian tubes. Although implantation occurs, the tubal environment is not favorable. The thin tubal wall can expand only minimally with growth of the gestational sac before it ruptures, accompanied by tearing into its blood supply and intraabdominal bleeding. The profuse bleeding that occurs with ruptured ectopic pregnancy is the reason it is one of the leading causes of maternal death. The fetus usually dies. Tubal pregnancy has been known to interfere with the future reproductive ability of many women.

Clinical Manifestations

The majority of women with tubal pregnancy exhibit subacute and atypical symptoms. The chief complaints are menstrual irregularity, vaginal spotting (which occurs after fetal death and estrogen withdrawal), and crampy pain in the lower abdomen (due to tubal distention). Significant pelvic or abdominal tenderness may not be present on physical examination. Generally, there is a gradual drop in the hemoglobin level.

Some women experience vaginal bleeding, followed by the sudden development of acute abdominal pain, indicating rupture of the tube. The pain, often accompanied by vomiting and fainting, is associated with referred shoulder pain caused by diaphragmatic irritation. The abdomen becomes distended with blood and may be tight and tender to touch. Hypovolemic shock may result, as manifested by its classic signs and symptoms. An obvious emergency situation exists.

Therapeutic Management

Ectopic pregnancy generally represents a diagnostic challenge, not only because of its vague manifestations but also because of its similarity to a wide variety of other pelvic and abdominal disorders such as salpingitis, spontaneous abortion, rupture of a cyst, appendicitis, and peritonitis. Ultrasonography, which determines the presence or absence of an intrauterine gestational sac, and serum radioimmunoassay, which identifies the human chorionic gonadotropin (HCG) level as an indication of pregnancy, are the first diagnostic tests performed. When the signs and symptoms are more pronounced, culdocentesis (aspiration of the cul-de-sac) for unclotted blood or a laparoscopy is used to confirm the diagnosis.

Once the diagnosis of ectopic pregnancy is made, surgery should proceed immediately. The client may be given a transfusion to relieve shock and restore a satisfactory blood volume for safe anesthesia and surgery. A salpingostomy or salpingotomy may be done to remove the products of conception from an unruptured tubal pregnancy. Salpingectomy is more commonly performed, es-

Table 48-6 Induced Abortion

Method	Length of Pregnancy	Procedure	Advantages	Disadvantages
EARLY ABORTION				
Menstrual extraction or regulation	Usually up to 2 wk after first missed period	Catheter is inserted through cervix into uterus, and suction is applied. Endometrium and contents of uterus are aspirated.	Low cost, simple, performance at outpatient facility without anesthesia or cervical dilatation, minimally traumatic	Continuation of pregnancy possible, potential for uterine injury and bleeding
Suction curettage	10-12 wk	Cervix is usually dilated, uterine aspirator is introduced, and suction is applied, removing endometrial tissue and implanted pregnancy.	Outpatient procedure, most often involving local anesthesia, 1- to 2-day recovery period	Infection, uterine perforation possible
D & C	10-16 wk (approximate)	Cervix is dilated, and products of conception are removed by scraping uterine walls with a curet.	Safe and effective procedure for more advanced pregnancy, outpatient procedure with general anesthesia, 2-day recovery period	More psychological trauma, more expensive, greater risk with general anesthesia and more invasive procedure
LATE ABORTION				
Instillation of drugs Hypertonic saline solution	After 16 wk	About 200 ml of amniotic fluid is withdrawn, and a similar amount of 20% normal saline solution is injected. Uterus is apparently irritated and begins to contract within 12-36 hr. Contractions may be assisted with IV oxytocin.	Inexpensive, readily available, feticidal	Hypernatremia, infection, hemorrhage, disseminated intravascular coagulation, more emotional trauma because of time required
Prostaglandins		Amniocentesis is done, and 8 ml of prostaglandin is inserted into amniotic sac, resulting in stimulation of smooth muscle of uterus. Expulsion of uterine contents occurs within 24 hr.	Fast induction, no need for surgery	Nausea and vomiting, abdominal cramps, cervical laceration, delivery of live fetus, high cost
Hysterotomy	16-20 wk	Miniature cesarean section is performed. Incision is made into uterus and contents are removed.	Concurrent sterilization procedure possible	More difficult and expensive in time and money, surgical incision with possible complications

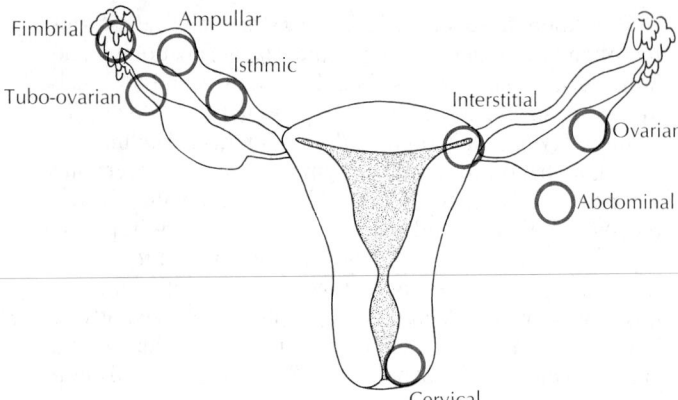

Fig. 48-4 Sites of implantation of ectopic pregnancies. Order of frequency of occurrence is ampulla, isthmus, interstitium, fimbria, tuboovarian ligament, ovary, abdominal cavity, and cervix (external os). (From Bobak I, Jensen M, and Zalar M: Maternity and gynecologic care, ed 4, St Louis, 1989, The CV Mosby Co, p 1401.)

pecially if the contralateral tube appears normal. All gross abdominal blood and clots are removed to prevent intraperitoneal adhesions.

▪ Nursing Management of Ectopic Pregnancy

Nursing care depends on the condition of the client. Before diagnosis has been confirmed, the nurse should be alert to signs of increasing pain and vaginal bleeding that may indicate rupture of the tube has occurred. Vital signs are monitored closely, along with signs of shock. Explanations and preparation for diagnostic procedures are given when appropriate. Preparation of the client for abdominal surgery may follow rapidly. The client's emotional status should be assessed. Reassurance and support for the surgery should be given to both the client and her family.

RAPE
Significance

Rape is defined legally as unlawful carnal knowledge of a person by force and without the person's consent. Carnal knowledge can entail completed coitus or even the slightest penetration of the male penis into the female genitalia. The desire for control and contempt or hostility toward women in general are often associated with rape.

The number of rapes, particularly against women, is increasing at an alarming rate. The Uniform Crime Reports for the United States published by the Federal Bureau of Investigation show that there were 94,504 reported cases of rape in 1989, representing 6% of all crimes of violence. This number in 1989 is a 2.2% increase over 1988 (92,486 cases) and a 14% increase of the number for 1980.[26] At the same time, many cases of rape are unreported because of the fear and embarrassment of the victims. There is no legal requirement that the rape of an adult be reported. Some women feel that they would not be able to withstand the stresses of prosecution or that they would be met with disbelief and humiliation from the police, the medical staff, or their peers.

Table 48-7

Prehospital Emergency Care of the Client Who Has Been Sexually Assaulted*

Etiology: Carnal knowledge of a person (male or female) without consent, by compulsion through force, threat, fraud

CLINICAL MANIFESTATIONS

Emotional or physical manifestations of shock
Hysteria, crying, anger
Decreased level of consciousness
Hyperventilation
Pain in genital area or from extragenital injuries
Bleeding from inflicted wounds
Contusions over face and body

MANAGEMENT

Assess client's emotional state.
Get a complete account of the incident.
Assess for any obvious bodily injuries.
Treat any *urgent* medical problems (e.g., bleeding wounds, fractures).
Monitor vital signs.
Prepare to treat for shock.
Do not cleanse the client; keep the client from cleansing, douching, or urinating.
Save any evidence found (e.g., fragments of clothing, tissue, blood, hair); bag each piece of evidence separately; label outside with client's name, date, time, and place where evidence was found and transport it with client to hospital (ensure that this follows local protocol).
Protect the client's privacy, support the client as much as possible.

---

*See Chapter 59 for a general discussion of measures related to prehospital emergency care.

Clinical Manifestations

Physical injuries. Rape may result in genital and extragenital injuries, pregnancy, and venereal disease. Genital injuries appear less frequently and are generally of a minor nature, such as bruises and lacerations to the perineum, hymen, vulva, vagina, cervix, and anus. Some women have sustained lacerations of the ligaments supporting the uterus, resulting in uterine displacement, and severe lacerations of the vagina, requiring extensive surgical reconstruction and repair. Dyspareunia and vaginismus (painful spasms of the vagina) have developed as a consequence. Approximately 9% percent of all homicides are related to rape and sex offenses.[27]

In general, the more serious injuries involve extragenital areas, such as the face, neck, and extremities, and often occur after the rape. Fractures, subdural hematomas, cerebral concussions, and intraabdominal injuries have resulted in the need for hospitalization. Rape is an act of violence with sex as the weapon rather than a sexual act. Table 48-7 outlines the prehospital care of the client who has been sexually assaulted.

Table 48-8 Checklist for Evaluation of Alleged Rape

1. Medicolegal
   Valid written consent for examination, photographs, laboratory tests, release of information, and laboratory samples
   Appropriate "chain of evidence" documentation
2. History
   Current health status and past history
   Age, parity, and gravidity
   Menstrual and contraceptive history
   Time of last coitus before assault
   Activities performed after assault (e.g., changed clothes, bathed, douched, urinated, brushed teeth)
   History of assault (who, what, when, where, why)
   Penetration, ejaculation, condom, extragenital acts
3. General physical examination
   Vital signs and general appearance
   Extragenital trauma—mouth, breasts, neck
   Cuts, bruises, scratches (photograph taken)
4. Pelvic examination
   Vulvar trauma, erythema, hymen, anal and rectal status
   Matted hairs or free hairs
   Vaginal examination with unlubricated speculum for foreign body, discharge, blood, lacerations
   Uterine size
   Adnexa, especially hematomas
5. Laboratory samples
   Saline irrigation of vagina with 2 ml solution and swab; acid phosphatase, blood groups
   Vaginal smears—Pap and Gram stain
   Oral or rectal swabs and smears, if indicated
   Blood samples—VDRL serology, blood group and type, pregnancy test, alcohol; serological testing for HIV and hepatitis B infection, if appropriate, with repetition 8-12 wk later
   Cultures—cervix and other areas if indicated (gonococcal and chlamydial)
   Combing and clipping of scalp hairs
   Fingernail scrapings
   Combing of pubic hairs
   Clipping of matted pubic hairs
   Clipping of pubic hair
6. Treatment
   Care of injuries and emotional trauma
   Antibiotic prophylaxis for venereal disease, if appropriate; ceftriaxone 250 mg IM followed by doxycycline 100 mg orally bid for 7 days
   Protection against pregnancy if any risk with diethylstilbestrol (DES), 25 mg bid for 5 days or ethinyl estradiol, 0.5 mg daily for 5 days
   Protection of legal rights
   Recommendation of continued follow-up and services of rape crisis center
   Repetition of gonorrhea and chlamydial culture 14 to 21 days later
   Repetition of serological testing 8 to 12 wk later
   Pregnancy test if appropriate

Emotional trauma. The emotional trauma of a rape victim often affects the victim's future sexual functioning and intimate relationships. The initial reaction of most women to rape is shock, disbelief, and emotional breakdown, including crying, agitation, and incoherence. Feelings of fear, humiliation, degradation, embarrassment, anger, and the need for revenge and self-blame are commonly expressed. Within several days to weeks after the rape the woman displays controlled behavior and a return to normal life patterns. It is believed that the victim's real feelings at this time may be hidden under her calm, composed affect. The long-term results of the rape include the integration and resolution of the experience. This progressive pattern of behavior has been described as the *rape trauma syndrome*.[28] Rape trauma syndrome is an accepted NANDA nursing diagnosis. Some time is needed for the woman to complete this process; not all women are able to achieve full resolution of the rape experience. Many victims develop phobias, such as fear of crowds. Others are unable to resume their usual sexual patterns or have frightening dreams that persist for long periods. Counseling may be helpful.

Social effects. The support and acceptance offered rape victims by their significant others are important in reducing the sociological crisis of rape. The men in the victim's life take on a greater significance. How they respond to the situation will affect her future relations with them and with all men. They may have serious problems resolving the incident and may need as much help as the victim.

Changes in residency and place of employment may occur as a consequence of the experience because of fear or inability to maintain previous relationships. Rape trauma dramatically disrupts the homemaking and parenting roles normally performed by the adult woman. The victim's husband and family have a tremendous potential for both negative and positive influence. They can revictimize the victim and increase her burden in resolving the rape, or they can provide the victim with support and find support themselves in resolving a shared crisis. In one survey, 50% of sexual assault victims were separated from their husbands or lovers within 2 to 3 years after the attack.[29]

Therapeutic Management

When the victim of a rape is admitted to the emergency room or clinic, a specific chain of events occurs (Table 48-8). A signed informed consent is obtained from the victim before rape data are collected. All materials gathered are well documented, labeled, and given to the appropriate person, such as the pathologist or a police officer. The materials are handled by as few people as possible, and signatures of all responsible for keeping and handling the data are obtained. Many items can be used as evidence if the victim chooses to file a complaint. Consequently, the integrity of the material must be maintained. The nurse's involvement in the medicolegal process depends on the policies of the individual institution.

A gynecological and sexual history and an account of the assault (who, what, when, where, why), as well as a general physical and pelvic examination, add further information about the rape incident. Laboratory tests are done

primarily to determine the presence of sperm in the vagina and to rule out the possibility of venereal disease and pregnancy.

During the treatment period the client's physical injuries are attended to and prophylaxis for venereal disease and pregnancy is administered. The client's immediate and long-term need for emotional support is given special consideration.

The physician cannot legally (see definition, p. 1427) state that rape occurred. The physician can swear findings show that sexual intercourse took place and that injury was inflicted. These findings, along with others such as the police report and examination of the rape scene, can form the foundation for the rapist's conviction.

■ Nursing Management of Rape

All women should be aware of rape-prevention tactics (Table 48-9). They should also be encouraged to learn some basic techniques of self-defense. Local high schools and the YWCA usually have self-defense classes in which formal instruction is given. Practicing the various techniques with a friend builds up a woman's confidence in her ability to fight back. Learning self-defense can make the woman less vulnerable and more self-reliant.

When a rape victim is brought to the clinic or emergency room, she should be given the highest priority for care and treatment. A quiet, private area should be used for the initial assessment and the examinations that follow. The client should not be left alone. Whenever possible, the same nurse should remain with her throughout her stay and provide needed emotional support. The client's actions and words as she describes the rape incident may be inconsistent, confused, and inappropriate. The nurse should maintain a nonjudgmental attitude, leaving moral and legal judgment to others.

Table 48-9   Rape Prevention Tactics

See that there are lights at all entrances to your home.

Keep your doors locked and do not open them to a stranger; ask for identification if a service person comes to the door.

Do not advertise that you live alone; list only your initials with your last name in the telephone directory or on the mailbox; never reveal to a caller that you are home alone.

Avoid walking alone in deserted areas; walk to the parking lot with a friend; be sure you see each other leave.

Have your keys ready as you approach your car or home.

Keep all doors locked and windows up when driving.

Never get on an elevator with a suspicious person; pretend you have forgotten something and get off.

Say what you mean in social situations; be sure your voice and body language reflect your response.

Carry a loud whistle and use it when you think you are in danger.

Yell "fire" if you are attacked and run toward a lighted area.

The client usually has many feelings and thoughts about the rape and generally wants to talk about them to an interested listener. Talking may help the client feel better and gain understanding of her reactions to the incident. When the nurse listens carefully, the client feels she is not alone and is better able to gain control over the situation.

The nurse should assess the client's stress level before preparing her for the various procedures that will follow. The client's coping mechanisms are supported when she knows what to expect and what is expected of her, as well as why the particular procedure must be done. Because the pelvic examination may trigger a flashback of the rape, the nurse should answer all related questions before the examination and urge the client to relax as much as possible.

Following the examinations, the client's physical comfort needs should be considered. She may need safety pins or needle and thread for her torn clothing or a cool drink to relieve her thirst. Most women who have been raped feel dirty and will appreciate a place to wash as well as use a mouthwash, especially if oral sex was involved.

The nurse can also further emphasize and elaborate on any prescribed treatment. The client's understanding of the possible side effects of the medications given should be assessed. The client is urged to see her own physician or to return for a follow-up examination and venereal disease testing. Many rape victims are unaware of the availability of compensation (a law in most states) and appreciate information about the application process. This compensation is to assist them in paying for emergency services and for emotional injuries that may temporarily interfere with their ability to work.[30]

When the client is discharged, the nurse should make certain she has transportation home. If friends or family members are not available, the hospital or clinic should attempt to work out an arrangement with an appropriate community resource. The client should not be sent home alone.

Many communities today have rape crisis centers. These public service organizations have trained professional and nonprofessional volunteers who provide an emotional support system for rape victims on request. Their programs provide advocacy to ensure dignified treatment of the victim throughout the medical and police procedures, short-term counseling for the victim and her family, and court assistance and public education on rape-related issues. The nurse should be able to give the client the names and local telephone numbers of such organizations.

The rape victim generally has many concerns about her sexuality. Long-term counseling may be necessary to permit the crisis to stabilize. The nurse can assist the client in obtaining the needed counseling while providing continued reassurance and emotional support.

INFLAMMATION AND INFECTIONS OF THE VAGINA, CERVIX, AND VULVA

Infection and inflammation of the vagina, cervix, and vulva tend to occur when the natural defenses of the acid vaginal secretions (maintained by sufficient estrogen levels) and the presence of Döderlein's bacilli (*Lactobacillus* organisms) are disrupted. The woman's resistance may

Table 48-10 Inflammations and Infections of the Vagina, Cervix, and Vulva

Etiology	Clinical Manifestations and Diagnostic Methods	Management
SIMPLE VAGINITIS		
Variety of organisms, including *Escherichia coli* and staphylococci	Vulvar irritation, profuse yellowish mucoid discharge, diagnosis by cultures to identify infecting organism	Appropriate antibiotic, local or systemic approach, vinegar douche, β-lactose vaginal suppository (to restore normal vaginal flora), sitz baths
CANDIDIASIS		
Candida albicans (fungus); normal resident of mouth, GI tract, and vagina; predisposing factors of pregnancy, oral contraceptive use, antibiotics, steroid therapy, diabetes, obesity, douching	Pruritus; thick, white curdy odorous discharge; bright red and swollen vagina and vulva; difficult to cure; recurrence likely; diagnosis by microscopic examination of discharge under 10% potassium hydroxide solution	Miconazole nitrate (Monistat) or clotrimazole (Gyne-Lotrimin) suppositories, each 200 mg intravaginally hs for 3 days; nystatin (Mycostatin) vaginal suppository bid for 14 days (virtually nontoxic but less effective)
TRICHOMONIASIS		
Trichomonas vaginalis (protozoan); infection of paraurethral glands in both sexes; sexual transmission but possible transmission through shared bathing facilities, washcloths, or douche equipment	Profuse, thin, frothy, yellow-gray malodorous discharge; intense pruritus and excoriation of vulvar tissues; hemorrhagic spots ("strawberry spots") on cervix and vaginal walls; diagnosis by microscopic examination under saline wet mount or by culture	Metronidazole (Flagyl) 2.0 g PO in single dose for client and partner simultaneously (unpleasant metallic taste, vomiting when taken with alcohol, no use in early pregnancy)
NONSPECIFIC VAGINITIS		
Gardnerella vaginalis, Corynebacterium vaginale; gram-negative pleomorphic coccobacillus possibly sexually transmitted or normal vaginal inhabitant in certain conditions	Thin, homogeneous, foul-smelling grayish white discharge; normal vaginal epithelium, absence of pruritus and burning, diagnosis by wet mount or Gram stain of secretions	Metronidazole (Flagyl) 500 mg PO bid for 7 days or clindamycin 300 mg PO bid for 7 days when Flagyl contraindicated
ACUTE AND CHRONIC CERVICITIS		
Chlamydia trachomatis, Neisseria gonorrhoeae, streptococci, staphylococci, *Escherichia coli;* repeated episodes of acute cervicitis leading to abnormal healing process	Yellow mucopurulent discharge; intermenstrual and/or postcoital spotting; inflamed and irritated cervix with varying amounts of ulceration; eversion of mucosa around os; pelvic pain in severe cases; backache; urinary disturbances; diagnosis by positive whiff test (detection of fishy odor with drop of potassium hydroxide on discharge), saline wet mount, Pap smear, visualization of cervical lesions, cultures to identify infecting organism	Appropriate antibiotics, treatment of both partners, cervical cauterization or cryosurgery if chronic condition
BARTHOLINITIS		
Escherichia coli, Trichomonas vaginalis, Neisseria gonorrhoeae, staphylococci, streptococci	Erythema around Bartholin's gland; swelling, edema, and pain of labia and introitus on affected side; development of bartholinian abscess; diagnosis by examination of external genitalia and by cultures to identify infecting organism	Appropriate antibiotics, surgical drainage of abscess, excision of gland in clients with chronic bartholinitis

also be decreased as a result of aging, poor nutrition, and the use of drugs that alter the mucosa. The causative organisms gain entrance to the areas through contaminated hands, clothing, and douche nozzles and during intercourse, surgery, and childbirth. Table 48-10 relates the specific etiological factors, clinical manifestations and diagnostic methods, and therapeutic management of common inflammations and infections.

■ Nursing Management of Inflammation and Infections of the Vagina, Cervix, and Vulva

Normally the endocervical glands secrete a clear exudate, which may become cloudy and take on a slight odor as it passes through the vagina. The amount of discharge may increase (physiological leukorrhea) at ovulation, just before menstruation, during pregnancy and sexual excitement, and during use of oral contraceptives. When changes in the amount, color, character, or odor of the discharge occur, they usually indicate an infection (pathophysiological leukorrhea).

Women need to know what situations increase the risk of vaginal, cervical, and vulvar infections. Excessive douching, for example, can be harmful because it destroys the vagina's natural resistance to disease. Douching more than once every week or two can cause these results.

Drugs such as oral contraceptives, antibiotics, and steroids may produce changes in the vaginal flora, which may trigger an infection. Clients taking these medications need to know of their predisposition to infection. Cleanliness after urinating and defecating should be stressed. It may be necessary to review the importance of using daily health and hygienic practices with some clients. Instructions to seek care when symptoms arise should also be given.

The nurse should assess the client's response to a diagnosis of vaginal or cervical infection. A discharge may affect the client's body image, making her feel unclean. A client's psychosocial concerns may include sexual transmission, the partner's uncertain monogamy, and threats to fertility. Clarifying the nature, spread, and implications of the infection is necessary to decrease anxiety and dispel myths.

A variety of treatment measures are prescribed for vaginal, cervical, and vulvar infections. Because these measures are usually carried out by the client, her understanding of them and her ability to perform the treatment correctly must be assessed. Vaginal suppositories, ointments, and creams are often used when infection occurs. Instructions in their use are best given with the aid of a model of the pelvis. The importance of hand washing before and after their insertion should be stressed. The client should be advised to remain recumbent for 30 minutes after insertion to allow for absorption and to prevent loss of the medication from the vagina. There may be some drainage from the vagina. If the client is concerned about this, she can wear a minipad. During treatment the client should refrain from intercourse or request that her partner use a condom.

Heat in the form of a sitz bath, perineal irrigation, and douche is often prescribed to reduce inflammation, promote healing, and provide comfort. Instructions in their use should be given as indicated. Disposable sitz baths that fit over the toilet bowl are available, although the bathtub serves the same purpose. A text on fundamentals of nursing should be consulted for correct douching technique.

Local measures, such as avoidance of scratching, excessive moisture (including too frequent bathing), tight clothing, and wearing of underpants or pantyhose with a cotton crotch, are also advocated. Chafing, increased heat and moisture, and interference with normal ventilation promote favorable conditions for the growth of fungal, protozoal, and bacterial agents. The nurse can teach the client to recognize signs of successful therapy as well as those indicating the need to contact the physician.

When reinfection occurs readily, the possibility of a symptom-free male carrier or the presence of undiagnosed diabetes mellitus should be investigated. A review of the prescribed treatment measures for possible misunderstandings and a check on compliance with drug therapy may also be indicated.

If the client has cauterization or cryosurgery for chronic cervicitis, specific instructions are necessary. These instructions are similar to those following a D & C. The client should also know that an unpleasant vaginal discharge caused by the sloughing of destroyed cells may persist for 3 weeks. Cryosurgery involves the freezing and removal of abnormal cervical tissue through the use of a probe and liquid nitrogen. The treatment is quick and almost painless. The client will have a watery discharge for 2 weeks. Topical antiseptic creams may be prescribed during the 7- to 8-week healing period.

Toxic Shock Syndrome

Toxic shock syndrome (TSS) is an acute condition caused by the toxin of a local infection of *Staphylococcus aureus,* which can invade through any part of the body. TSS usually occurs in women who are menstruating and using tampons or who have chronic vaginal infections. It has also occurred in nonmenstruating women, men, and children. In these cases, TSS was associated with cellulitis, abscesses, insect bites, infected wounds, and influenza.[31] TSS is characterized by the sudden onset of high fever; vomiting; diarrhea; and a red, macular, palmar or diffuse rash followed by desquamation of the skin of the hands and feet. It may involve multiple organ systems and proceed to hypotension, shock, sepsis, shock lung, disseminated intravascular clotting, and acidosis. Treatment is symptomatic and supportive.

Because TSS has been linked to the use of tampons during menstruation, it is recommended that superabsorbent tampons not be used. They provide a favorable milieu for bacterial growth because they can absorb a large amount of menstrual blood and may be left in place longer than other tampons. The nurse should advise clients to alternate tampons with sanitary napkins, using the latter at night. When tampons are used, they should be changed regularly and inserted carefully to avoid abrasions. Good hand washing techniques should always be used. Organisms gain entrance into the circulatory system through abrasions in the vagina. Women who have had TSS are at risk of recurrence and should be instructed not to use tampons until *S. aureus* is no longer present in the vaginal flora.[32]

PELVIC INFLAMMATORY DISEASE

Pelvic inflammatory disease (PID) is an infectious condition of the pelvic cavity that may involve the fallopian tubes (salpingitis), ovaries (oophoritis), pelvic peritoneum, and pelvic vascular system.

Etiology

The frequent causative organisms of PID are *Neisseria gonorrhoeae,* chlamydiae, mycoplasmata, streptococci, and anaerobes. Any of these organisms may gain entrance during sexual intercourse or after abortion, pelvic surgery, or childbirth. Users of IUDs are also at risk of getting the condition. PID is a common complication of gonorrhea and chlamydial infections. The infection can be acute or chronic.

Clinical Manifestations

The client with acute PID seeks medical attention because of crampy, continuous, bilateral lower abdominal pain. Movement or ambulation increases the pain. Irregu-

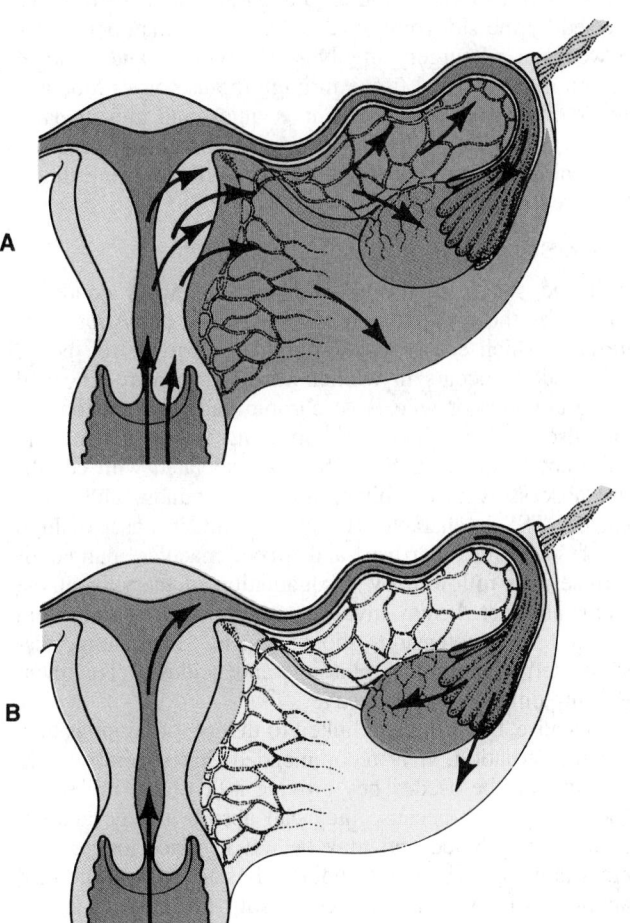

Fig. 48-5 Common routes of the spread of PID. **A,** Direct spread of bacterial infection other than *Neisseria gonorrhoeae.* **B,** Direct spread of *Neisseria gonorrhoeae.* (From Pernell M and Benson R: Current obstetric and gynecologic diagnosis and treatment, ed 6, Norwalk, Conn, 1987, Appleton & Lange.)

lar vaginal bleeding and a vaginal discharge, occasionally greenish or brownish yellow and foul smelling, frequently accompany the pain. Dysuria, dyspareunia, fever, and chills may also be present. Nausea and vomiting are seen in advanced cases.

Once introduced, the infection spreads by two typical routes. One route is along the uterine endometrium to the tubes and into the peritoneum (Fig. 48-5). Salpingitis, pelvic peritonitis, or tuboovarian abscess may result. The second route is primarily through the uterine or cervical lymphatics, across the parametrium, to the tubes or ovaries. Pelvic cellulitis and sometimes thrombophlebitis of the pelvic veins can occur.

Chronic PID can result if the acute phase of the condition does not respond to treatment or if treatment is inadequate. Chronic PID is characterized by persistent dull pelvic aching, secondary dysmenorrhea, dysfunctional uterine bleeding, and periodic bouts of acute symptoms.

Complications

Frequently the client is rendered sterile as a result of adhesions and strictures that may develop in the fallopian tubes. They can result in closure of the fallopian tubes because of scarring and adhesions. Ectopic pregnancy may result when a tube is partially obstructed because the sperm may pass through the stricture but the fertilized ovum cannot reach the uterus. The pelvic and tubal ovarian abscesses may "leak" or rupture, resulting in pelvic or generalized peritonitis. Embolic episodes may occur following thrombophlebitis of the pelvic veins. As the general circulation is flooded with bacterial endotoxins from the infected areas, septic shock may result.

Diagnostic Studies

The first step in the diagnosis of PID is obtaining a careful health history and performance of a physical examination. Often there is a history of a recent acute infection of the lower genital tract. An abdominal examination usually reveals the presence of pain and tenderness in both lower quadrants. Movement of the pelvic organs during vaginal examination increases the pain. Masses that are fixed and poorly defined may be found, indicating enlargement of the fallopian tubes or ovaries or abscess formation. The leukocyte count and the erythrocyte sedimentation rate are assessed and are generally found to be elevated, thereby confirming the presence of an infectious process. Culture and Gram stains are done on material taken from the vagina, cervix, or cul-de-sac of Douglas. Laparoscopy is performed to visualize the reproductive organs and to obtain specimens from the tubal mucosa for culture studies. Ultrasonic examinations can aid in diagnosing abscesses and following the progress of healing with treatment.

Therapeutic Management

Risk factors, such as multiple sexual partners, sexual activity in female teenagers, low socioeconomic status, IUD contraception, previous PID, and contact with untreated male sexual partners, are considered when planning education for clients with PID.[33]

Treatment of PID may be on an outpatient basis or may require hospitalization. The client is given a combination of antibiotics such as cefoxitin and doxycycline to provide broad coverage against the causative organisms.[34] Instructions are given to avoid coitus and douching, restrict general activities, get adequate rest and nutrition, and return to the clinic for reevaluation in 48 to 72 hours if symptoms persist or increase.

If outpatient treatment is not successful or if the client is acutely ill or in severe pain, admission to the hospital is indicated. There, maximum doses of parenteral antibiotics can be given. Some physicians believe the addition of cortisone to the antibiotics serves to reduce the inflammation, allowing for faster recovery and improvement in subsequent fertility. Application of heat to the lower abdomen or sitz baths may be used to improve circulation and decrease pain. Bed rest in the semi-Fowler's position promotes drainage of the pelvic cavity by gravity and may prevent the development of abscesses high in the abdomen. Analgesics to relieve pain and intravenous (IV) fluids to prevent dehydration are also prescribed. Sexual partners of women with PID should also be treated as possible sources of infection.

Indications for surgery include the presence of residual masses (abscesses) with the potential for rupture and peritonitis, failure of the client to respond to conservative management, and a history of frequent exacerbations. The abscess may be drained without laparotomy, or it may be necessary to remove the infected areas along with the uterus, tubes, and ovaries. The extent of the disease, as well as the age and condition of the client determine the extent of the surgery. The childbearing function in young women is preserved whenever possible.

■ Nursing Management of Pelvic Inflammatory Disease

Nursing assessment
Subjective and objective data that should be obtained from a client with PID are presented in Table 48-11.

Nursing diagnoses
Nursing diagnoses are determined when the problem and the etiological factors are supported by clinical data. Nursing diagnoses related to PID may include, but are not limited, to those presented in Table 48-12.

Nursing interventions
Health maintenance and promotion. Prevention, early recognition, and prompt treatment of vulvar, vaginal, and cervical infections can help prevent PID and its serious complications. If the nurse knows the factors that predispose a person to the development of PID, she can identify clients who are at risk and take appropriate measures.

Gynecological surgery, childbearing, and abortion tend to lower the resistance and make the client more susceptible to infection. In these instances, careful medical and surgical asepsis is imperative to prevent the introduction of organisms into the reproductive tract. The nurse should counsel the client to seek medical attention for any unusual vaginal discharge or possible infection of the reproductive organs. The client should be encouraged by the awareness that some discharges are not indicative of infection and

that early diagnosis and treatment of an infection can prevent complications. Routine cultures for *Neisseria gonorrhoae* and chlamydiae should be taken at the time a pelvic examination is being done on every sexually active woman. Women should be informed of the methods of preventing infection as well as the signs of infection in their partners.

Acute intervention. During the acute phase of the condition, frequent perineal cleansing is indicated to prevent the spread of the infection (see Table 48-12). The character, amount, color, and odor of the vaginal discharge are recorded. Excoriation of the vulva may occur from the vaginal discharge. Frequent checks of the vital signs and the degree of abdominal pain can give clues about the effectiveness of therapy. An explanation of the limited activity (bed rest in a semi-Fowler's position) increases client cooperation.

Table 48-11

Nursing Assessment of the Client with Pelvic Inflammatory Disease

SUBJECTIVE DATA

History
Use of IUD; previous PID; multiple sexual partners; exposure to partner with urethritis; previous STD; infertility; recent childbirth, abortion, or pelvic surgery

Medications
Use of and allergy to any antibiotics

General
Malaise, fever, chills

Pain
Lower abdominal and pelvic pain; low back pain; pain on fundal palpation and cervical motion; onset of pain just after a menstrual period; dysmenorrhea, dyspareunia, dysuria

Gastrointestinal
Nausea and vomiting, diarrhea or constipation

Urinary
Frequency, urgency

Reproductive
Abnormal vaginal bleeding and menstrual irregularity, vulval pruritus, vaginal discharge

OBJECTIVE DATA

Reproductive
Mucopurulent cervicitis, vulval maceration, vaginal discharge (heavy and purulent to thin and mucoid), tenderness on motion of cervix and uterus

Abdomen
Tenderness, presence of inflammatory masses

Possible findings
Leukocytosis, elevated erythrocyte sedimentation rate, positive culture of secretions or endocervical fluid, pelvic inflammation and positive endometrial biopsy on laparoscopic examination, abscess or inflammation on ultrasonography

Table 48-12

NURSING CARE PLAN FOR THE CLIENT WITH PELVIC INFLAMMATORY DISEASE

Defining Characteristics	Nursing Interventions	Evaluation Criteria
NURSING DIAGNOSIS: Acute pain related to infectious process		
Crampy lower abdominal pain, guarding behavior, altered muscle tone	Assess degree of pain. Provide comfort measures (e.g., backrub, nonstimulating environment, heat to lower abdomen). Administer analgesics as ordered.	Verbalization of satisfactory level of pain control
NURSING DIAGNOSIS: High risk for infection transmission related to vaginal discharge and lack of knowledge of proper hygiene and appropriate sexual practices regarding precautionary measures		
Purulent vaginal discharge, inadequate hand washing, improper disposal of perineal pads	Observe, report, and record color, amount, character, and odor of discharge. Use and teach strict medical asepsis when in contact with discharge (e.g., proper hand washing, careful handling and disposal of perineal pads). Explain need for precautions related to vaginal discharge and encourage client's participation in them. Provide frequent perineal care. Advise client against sexual contact while infected.	Decrease in or no vaginal discharge, knowledge and use of medical asepsis
NURSING DIAGNOSIS: Anxiety related to imposed activity restrictions, perceived loss of control, and lack of knowledge of outcome on reproductive status and course of disease		
Restlessness, frequent questioning about restricted activity and outcome, few visitors, irritability, impatience, crying spells	Maintain bed rest in semi-Fowler's position. Explain need for limited activity. Provide diversional activities. Provide stimulation and orientation (e.g., radio, clock). Allow client to help in planning care. Place in room with clients who are oriented to and interested in surroundings. Discuss possible outcomes of disease process. Provide time for client to ventilate feelings. Listen and interact therapeutically. Provide counsel for client and significant others. Clarify course of disease.	Accurate discussion of possible outcomes of disease process on reproductive status and course of disease, acceptance of possible outcome and restrictions
NURSING DIAGNOSIS: Impaired skin integrity related to vaginal drainage		
Excoriated, painful, reddened perineal area	Provide and teach gentle perineal cleansing technique q 3-4 hr. Avoid excessive warmth from covers or clothing. Teach front-to-back wiping technique.	Satisfactory perineal care, no excoriation in perineal area

Efforts must be made to prevent spread of the infection to others. Proper hand washing with a germicidal soap and use of universal precautions when handling and disposing of soiled perineal pads are required. Disinfection of utensils, bedpans, and all items in direct contact with the client is an additional measure that can be used to contain the infection. The need for these precautions should be explained to the client, and her participation in them should be encouraged.

Chronic management. The client with chronic PID experiences chronic pelvic discomfort and requires repeated treatment. Her emotional response to the disease and the therapy should be assessed. The client may feel well one day and develop distressing discomforts the next. She may become discouraged and depressed. The nurse should be aware of these feelings and provide the client with emotional support as well as clarification about the course of the disease.

The client may have guilt feelings about the problem, especially if it was associated with a venereal disease. She may also be concerned about the possibility of becoming sterile. Discussion with the client and significant others re-

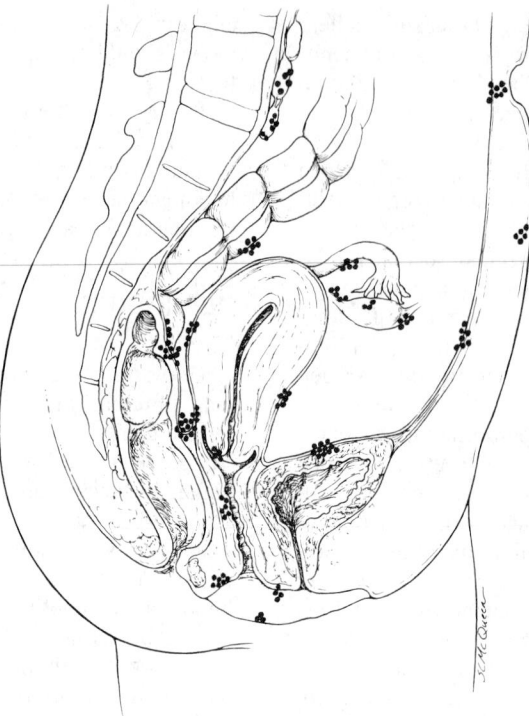

Fig. 48-6   Common sites of endometriosis. (From Droegemueller W and others: Comprehensive gynecology, St Louis, 1987, The CV Mosby Co.)

garding these feelings and concerns can assist her to cope more effectively with them.

ENDOMETRIOSIS

Endometriosis is a condition characterized by the presence and proliferation of endometrial tissue in sites outside the endometrial cavity. The most frequent sites are in or near the ovaries, the uterosacral ligaments, and the uterovesical peritoneum. They can be in many other locations, however, such as the stomach and spleen. The tissue responds to the hormones of the ovarian cycle and undergoes a minimenstruation similar to the uterine endometrium. Active endometriosis is found most commonly in nulliparous women between the ages of 25 and 40. It appears to cause infertility in 10% to 30% of all cases.

Etiology

Although many theories about the cause of endometriosis have been advanced, the more commonly held theory concludes that small bits of endometrial tissue are "regurgitated" back up the uterine tube and escape into the abdomen during menstruation. As the ectopic endometrium menstruates, the blood collects in cystlike nodules that have a characteristic bluish black look. Nodules in the ovaries are sometimes called *chocolate cysts* because of the thick, chocolate-colored material they contain.

Clinical Manifestations

The symptoms may be vague and diffuse because of the multiple sites affected. Some clients have no symptoms, and the disease is discovered incidental to abdominal surgery. More commonly, the client complains of pelvic pain that takes the form of secondary dysmenorrhea. The pain is described as dull, aching, or cramping in the lower abdominal region, occurring 1 to 2 days before menses and diminishing after the onset of flow. It may be related to hemorrhagic distention of the cystlike nodules or to escape of bloody discharge into the peritoneal cavity. Other symptoms include backache, abnormal uterine bleeding, dyspareunia, and painful defecation.

When a cyst ruptures, the pain may be acute and the resulting irritation promotes the formation of adhesions, which fix the affected area to another pelvic structure. The adhesions may become severe enough to cause a bowel obstruction or painful micturition. Adhesions involving the uterus, tubes, or ovaries may result in infertility.

Therapeutic Management

Diagnosis is frequently confirmed by a history of the characteristic symptoms of the condition and the palpation of firm nodular lumps in the adnexa on bimanual examination. Visualization of the typical bluish nodes with culdoscopy, laparoscopy, or during a laparotomy establishes a definite diagnosis (Fig. 48-6). The treatment of endometri-

osis is influenced by the client's age, her desire to bear children, and the severity of the symptoms. With menopause, ovarian atrophy begins and hormonal stimulation declines, usually leading to the disappearance of the symptoms.

Observation and mild analgesia are used initially when symptoms are not severe or incapacitating. Regular follow-up examinations at least once yearly to check on further progression of the disease are needed so that necessary changes in the plan of management can be made. Pregnancy and lactation often result in the relief of symptoms, since menstruation ceases during this time. Continuous use (for 9 months) of combined progestin and estrogen softens and regresses endometrial tissue. Ovulation is suppressed and pseudopregnancy (hyperhormonal amenorrhea) is produced. However, because of troublesome side effects, this treatment modality is used less frequently today. The hormonal treatment of choice is danazol (Danocrine), a synthetic androgen that inhibits the anterior pituitary. When given in dosages of up to 800 mg/day for 6 to 9 months, the drug produces a pseudomenopause (ovarian suppression), with consequent atrophy of ectopic endometrial tissue. Subjective relief of symptoms is noted within 6 weeks of danazol use. Side effects include weight gain, acne, hot flashes, and hirsutism. The associated cost is a major drawback.

Endometriosis is controlled but not cured by hormonal therapy. Persistent lesions give rise to subsequent recurrences once the menstrual cycle is reestablished.

Surgical Interventions

Surgical treatment may be conservative or radical. Conservative surgery is usually used in the management of young women. It involves removal or destruction of endometrial implants and lysing or excision of adhesions by means of laparoscopic laser surgery and laparotomy. Efforts are made to conserve all tissues necessary to maintain fertility.[35] Radical surgery is generally performed in women approaching menopause. It involves removal of the uterus, tubes, ovaries, and as many endometrial implants as possible. Hysterectomy with removal of as many implants as possible but with preservation of all or part of the ovarian tissue is recommended for the young woman who does not want children but wishes to have cyclical ovarian function.

■ Nursing Management of Endometriosis

Nurses should encourage women to have regular physical examinations in an effort to identify early symptoms of endometriosis. Client education about the disease process can clarify and dispel false ideas and fears. Dysmenorrhea after years of relatively pain-free menses and infertility after a period of trying to achieve pregnancy may serve as clues to the presence of this disease and should be reported and investigated.

When the symptoms are less severe, a "wait-and-see" approach may be used. Education of the client and reassurance that a health-threatening situation does not exist may permit her to accept the treatment and live with the minor discomfort. The nurse is often the person who counsels the

client in the use of drugs. The action of the prescribed hormones should be explained, as well as the possible side effects.

If surgery is the treatment selected, the nursing care is similar to the general preoperative and postoperative care of a client undergoing abdominal surgery. The nurse needs to know the extent of the procedure so that appropriate postoperative teaching can be done.

BENIGN TUMORS OF THE FEMALE REPRODUCTIVE SYSTEM
Leiomyomas

Etiology. Leiomyomas (fibroids, myomas, fibromyomas, fibromas) are the most common benign tumors of the female genital tract. At least 25% of women over 35 years of age have uterine leiomyomas. The incidence appears higher in black women. The cause of leiomyomas is unknown, but they are thought to depend on ovarian hormones, growing slowly during the reproductive years and undergoing atrophy with the advent of menopause. These tumors are composed mainly of smooth muscle and fibrous connective tissue.

Clinical manifestations. About half of the women with leiomyomas develop symptoms, the most common being menorrhagia. Pain is rarely experienced with leiomyomas, but it is associated with infection or twisting of the pedicle from which the tumor is growing. Dysmenorrhea and dyspareunia may occasionally occur. Pressure on surrounding organs may result in rectal, bladder, and lower abdominal discomfort. Large tumors may cause a general enlargement of the lower abdomen. These tumors are sometimes associated with abortion and infertility.

Therapeutic management. Diagnosis is usually based on the characteristic pelvic findings of an enlarged uterus distorted by nodular masses. The presence of a malignant tumor is ruled out before treatment is begun. Treatment depends on the symptoms, the age of the client, her desire to bear children, and the location and size of the tumor or tumors. An intravenous pyelogram should be obtained to detect urethral compression with resulting hydronephrosis. If the symptoms are minor, the physician may elect to follow the client closely for a time. In the young woman who wishes to have children, a myomectomy is performed. In cases of large leiomyomas, the treatment is hysterectomy (see p. 1440).

Cervical Polyps

Cervical polyps are benign pedunculated lesions that generally arise from the endocervical mucosa and are seen protruding through the external os on speculum examination of the cervix and vagina. Polyps are a characteristic bright cherry-red and are soft and fragile in consistency. They are generally small, measuring less than 3 cm in length, and may be single or multiple. Their origin is unknown. Symptoms are usually not present, but metrorrhagia and bleeding after straining and coitus can occur. Polyps are prone to infection. When the polyp is small, it can be excised in an outpatient procedure. If the point of attachment of the polyp cannot be identified and is not accessible to cautery, a polypectomy is performed in an op-

erating room. All tissue removed is sent for pathological review, since polyps occasionally undergo malignant changes.

Ovarian Tumors

Benign tumors of the ovary are many and varied. The cause of most of them is unknown. For purposes of clarity, they are divided into nonneoplasms and neoplasms. *Nonneoplasms* are usually simple cysts surrounded by a thin capsule and are seen mainly during the reproductive years. *Neoplasms* of the ovaries are fluid-filled cysts that are frequently bilateral and may be benign or malignant (see p. 1439).

Ovarian tumors are often asymptomatic until they are large enough to cause pressure in the pelvis. Constipation, urinary frequency, a full feeling in the abdomen, anorexia, and peripheral edema may occur, depending on the size and location of the tumor. There may be an increase in abdominal girth. Pelvic pain may be present if the tumor is growing rapidly. Severe pain results when the cyst twists on its pedicle (twisted ovarian cyst).

Pelvic examination reveals a mass or an enlarged ovary that demands further investigation. Laparoscopy or exploratory laparotomy is often performed to confirm the diagnosis. During surgical treatment, attempts are made to save as much ovarian function as possible. Surgery usually involves removal of one or both ovaries.

MALIGNANT TUMORS OF THE FEMALE REPRODUCTIVE SYSTEM
Cervical Cancer

Carcinoma of the cervix is the sixth most frequent malignancy in women, behind cancer of the breast, colon, rectum, endometrium, lung, and ovary.[36] It occurs predominantly in women between the ages of 30 and 50. The incidence is higher among black and Hispanic women than among white women. An increased risk of cervical cancer is associated with low economic status, early marriage, early sexual activity, several partners (particularly those with poor penile hygiene), multiple pregnancies, a history of untreated chronic cervicitis, venereal disease (e.g., venereal warts), viral infections, papilloma, HSV II, and smoking. Nearly 29% of deaths due to cervical cancer are attributable to cigarette smoking.[37] Sexual contact is the principal risk factor for cervical cancer.

The number of deaths from cervical cancer has fallen steadily over the past 40 years. This is attributable to better early diagnosis with the widespread use of the Pap test. Its high-detection efficiency permits treatment at a time (stage 0) when cure is almost certain.

In the late 1960s, several cases of cervical (and vaginal) carcinoma were reported in adolescent girls. Subsequent studies revealed that diethylstilbestrol (DES) had been administered to their mothers during pregnancy. Enough evidence has accumulated to recommend that DES not be used during pregnancy. Daughters of women who ingested DES are encouraged to have regular gynecological examinations.

Currently, there is a resurgence of cervical carcinoma in young women. Risk varies directly with an increase in number of sexual partners and with early incidence of first intercourse. These circumstances, along with certain serotypes of papillomavirus, have resulted in detection of cervical cancer in women in their early twenties. Preventive education should be directed toward counseling on delaying sexual activity and the use of barrier and spermicidal contraceptives.

Women should be taught and motivated to report any abnormal vaginal bleeding to a physician, particularly during the menopausal period. A thorough yearly gynecological examination, including a Pap test, is urged by most sources. In its recent guidelines, the American Cancer Society recommends annual Pap tests beginning with the onset of sexual activity. Following three negative Pap tests, less frequent tests may be recommended by the physician.[38] The effect of many women having this examination has been a dramatic reduction in the occurrence of invasive cancer of the cervix.

The fears and anxieties that arise in relation to cancer are many and varied. All women have seen and heard accounts of the disfigurement, tissue destruction, and disabilities that seem to follow cancer. Nurses should emphasize the positive fact that early discovery improves the prognosis and hinders the occurrence of more serious outcomes. The important goal of disease prevention is again the major concern.

Persons at high risk, such as those with family histories of cancer or prolonged local tissue irritation, are special cases. They should be sought out and encouraged to have frequent examinations for the appearance of cancer.

Clinical manifestations. Early cervical cancer is generally asymptomatic, but leukorrhea and intermenstrual bleeding eventually occur. The discharge is usually thin and watery but becomes dark and foul smelling as the disease advances, suggesting the presence of an infection. The vaginal bleeding is initially only spotting, but as the tumor enlarges, it becomes heavier and more frequent. Pain is a late symptom and is followed by weight loss, anemia, and cachexia.

Diagnostic studies. A Pap test, the Schiller iodine test (see Chapter 45), colposcopy, and a biopsy may be used to diagnose cancer of the cervix. (Details of the Pap test are given in Chapter 45.) The classification for cytological findings used by many laboratories is given in Table 48-13. The current trend is to use descriptive terms such as *benign, moderate dysplasia,* and *squamous cell carcinoma* to report test results.

The World Health Organization has developed an international classification of cancer of the cervix with stages

Table 48-13 Classification of Cytological Findings of Pap Tests

Class I	No abnormal or atypical cells
Class II	Atypical but no evidence of malignancy
Class III	Suggestive but not conclusive for malignancy
Class IV	Strongly suggestive of malignancy
Class V	Conclusive for malignancy

Table 48-14 International Classification of Clinical Stages of Carcinoma of the Cervix

Stage	Extent	Treatment	5-Year Survival Rate (%)*
Stage 0	In situ, intraepithelial	Cervical conization, total hysterectomy, cryosurgery, laser surgery	95-100
Stage I	Strict confinement to cervix (no consideration of extension to corpus)		75-85
Stage IA	Microinvasive (early stromal invasion)	Radiation or surgery	
Stage IB	All other cases of stage I	Radiation, Wertheim's hysterectomy	
Stage II	Extension beyond cervix but not to pelvic wall, involvement of vagina but not as far as lower third		
Stage IIA	No obvious parametrial involvement	Radiation, Wertheim's hysterectomy	65-75
Stage IIB	Obvious parametrial involvement	Radiation; if this fails, pelvic exenteration may be required	50-65
Stage III	Extension to pelvic wall, no cancer-free space between tumor and pelvic wall on rectal examination, involvement of lower third of vagina, hydronephrosis or nonfunctioning kidney	Radiation	20-30
Stage IIIA	No extension to pelvic wall		
Stage IIIB	Extension to pelvic wall and/or hydronephrosis or nonfunctioning kidney		
Stage IV	Extension beyond true pelvis or clinical involvement of the mucosa of bladder or rectum, no stage IV classification with bullous edema alone	Radiation, surgery (e.g., exenteration)	1-10
Stage IVA	Spread to adjacent organs		
Stage IVB	Spread to distant organs		

*Statistics are compiled from a variety of references. Those most generally agreed on are used here.

from 0 to IV (Table 48-14). Stage 0, the preinvasive stage of carcinoma in situ of the cervix, is limited to the epithelial layer. A period of 5 to 10 years may elapse between the preinvasive stage and a stage I lesion, making the prognosis good for early diagnosis. Stage IV involves cancer that has extended outside the reproductive tract.

The finding of an abnormal Pap smear (with the exception of class V) indicates the need for additional procedures, such as colposcopy and biopsy, before a definitive diagnosis of cancer can be made. Colposcopy involves examination of the cervix with a binocular microscope with low levels of magnification ($10\times$ to $40\times$). The procedure discloses epithelial abnormalities and suggests areas for biopsy. As a result, it improves the rate of detection for cervical cancer and can lead to more focused treatment.

The type and extent of the biopsy vary with the abnormality seen. A punch biopsy may be done on an outpatient basis with special punch biopsy forceps. Because there are few nerve endings in the cervix, little discomfort is experienced by the client. When conization (the excision of a cone-shaped section of the cervix with a scalpel) is used, surgical facilities are required. The client should be observed for excessive bleeding after a cone biopsy.

Therapeutic management. Treatment of cancer of the cervix is guided by the stage of the tumor and the client's age and general state of health (see Table 48-14). Conization may be the only type of therapy needed for carcinoma

in situ if analysis of the removed tissue demonstrates that a wide area of normal tissue surrounds the excised malignancy. Laser treatments, in which a directed infrared beam causes the boiling and vaporization of intracellular water, is very effective in the destruction of dysplastic tissue. Cautery and cryosurgery may also be used (see p. 1431). Fertility is preserved with these four procedures. Invasive cancer of the cervix is treated with surgery, radiation, or a combination of the two to remove or destroy the involved areas and lymphatic drainage. Surgical procedures commonly carried out include radical hysterectomy (Wertheim) and pelvic exenteration (see p. 1442). Radiation may be external (e.g., cobalt) or internal (e.g., radium). The extent of the radiation depends on the stage.

Systemic or regional chemotherapy has been disappointing in most cases of recurrent cervical cancer. Previously irradiated areas are especially difficult to treat because the capillary blood supply is diminished, resulting in poor drug delivery to the tumor bed. However, some clients experience an improved sense of well-being with chemotherapy.

Endometrial Cancer

Cancer of the endometrium (uterus) has become the most common gynecological malignancy, accounting for about 50% of female genital tract neoplasms. Possible factors contributing to the increased incidence include obe-

sity, aging of the general population, better reporting of cases, and more widespread prescribing of estrogens for postmenopausal women.[39] Obesity is the most important risk factor because it increases estrogen production and availability.[40]

Endometrial cancer grows slowly, metastasizes late, and is amenable to therapy if diagnosed early. It is associated with women who are between the ages of 50 and 70, nulliparous, obese, hypertensive, or diabetic or who had a late menopause or prolonged unopposed estrogen-only replacement therapy. The first symptom of endometrial cancer is abnormal uterine bleeding, usually in postmenopausal women. Pain occurs late in the disease process, and other symptoms that may arise are related to metastasis to other organs.

D & C, endometrial biopsy, and smears are used to diagnose endometrial cancer. D & C and endometrial biopsy may require hospitalization, whereas the smears are taken in an office procedure in which endometrial tissue is "aspirated" from the uterus. The Pap test is not a reliable diagnostic tool for endometrial cancer. Treatment is by total hysterectomy and bilateral salpingo-oophorectomy. Surgery may be preceded by irradiation, either externally with cobalt or internally with intracavitary radium.

Chemotherapy is reserved for recurrences or distant metastases. Progesterone therapy (e.g., Megace) is the treatment of choice when the progesterone receptor status is positive and the tumor is well differentiated. Cytoxic chemotherapy is considered when progesterone therapy is unsuccessful.

Ovarian Cancer

Cancer of the ovary seems to be linked to nulliparity, infertility, endometriosis, and celibacy. Multiple pregnancies and early age at first birth actually seem to reduce the risk of ovarian cancer. It occurs more frequently in women between the ages of 40 and 65 and has a high familial incidence. It is the leading cause of death related to gynecological conditions in the United States.

In its early stages, ovarian cancer is asymptomatic. As the malignancy grows, a variety of symptoms, such as an increase in abdominal girth, bowel and bladder dysfunction, pain, and ascites accompanied by dyspnea, occur. An ovarian malignancy should be considered when abnormal uterine bleeding occurs.

There are no specific tests or procedures to aid in the diagnosis of ovarian cancer other than the pelvic examination. When a suspicious mass in the ovarian area is palpated, an exploratory laparotomy is performed to establish the diagnosis. If the mass is malignant, treatment depends on the surgical staging of the disease. The usual treatment for stage I malignancies is a total abdominal hysterectomy and bilateral salpingo-oophorectomy with removal of as much of the tumor as possible (i.e., tumor debulking). The remaining tissues in the abdomen and pelvis are carefully scrutinized. Ascitic fluid is submitted for cytological study and appropriate biopsies are performed to determine the stage of the disease.

The addition of chemotherapy or the instillation of intraperitoneal radioisotopes is usually suggested for stage I disease. Clients with stage II disease may receive external abdominal and pelvic irradiation, intraperitoneal irradiation, or systemic combined chemotherapy after tumor-reducing surgery. After completion of systemic chemotherapy, a "second-look" surgical procedure is often performed to determine whether there is any evidence of disease. If no disease is found, the chemotherapy is stopped and the client is monitored for recurrent disease. Combined chemotherapy or occasionally whole-abdomen irradiation is used in stage III and stage IV diseases.

Unfortunately, many malignancies have metastasized to the peritoneum, omentum, or bowel surface before discovery of the tumors. In these situations the prognosis is poor. Recurrent ascites causing shortness of breath and discomfort may require frequent paracenteses, but the fluid accumulates again in a few days. Irradiation and chemotherapy may be used to shrink the size of the tumor, relieving pressure and pain.

Vulvar Cancer

Cancer of the vulva is relatively rare, occurring mainly among women over 50 years of age. The malignancy is visible, accessible, and relatively slow growing.

Cancer of the vulva may follow leukoplakia (irregular white patches on vulva mucosa that produce intense pruritus) or other conditions causing chronic irritation of the area. The client may initially experience pruritus, soreness of the vulva, discharge, or bleeding but tends to ignore these symptoms. Edema of the vulva and pelvic lymphadenopathy develop as the disease progresses.

Diagnosis of vulvar cancer is done by means of pelvic examination and biopsy. The treatment for vulvar cancer is vulvectomy. The extensiveness of the surgery depends on the size and site of the malignancy. If it is in situ, a simple vulvectomy (surgical excision of the vulva) is done. If the cancer is invasive, a radical vulvectomy with superficial and deep lymph node dissection is indicated. Irradiation is not generally used in this area because the tissues do not tolerate it well.

■ Nursing Management of Malignant Tumors

Nursing assessment

Malignant tumors of the female reproductive system can be found in the cervix, endometrium, ovaries, and vulva. Clients with any of these malignant tumors may experience a variety of clinical manifestations, including leukorrhea (white discharge from the vagina), irregular vaginal bleeding, vaginal discharge, increase in abdominal pain and pressure, bowel and bladder dysfunction, and vulvar itching and burning.

Nursing diagnoses

Nursing diagnoses specific to the female client with malignant tumors of the reproductive system include, but are not limited to, the following:

1. Anxiety related to threat to biological integrity and lack of knowledge related to disease process and prognosis
2. Pain related to pressure secondary to enlarging tumor
3. Body-image disturbance related to loss of body part
4. Altered sexuality patterns related to physiological limitations and fatigue

5. Ineffective breathing pattern related to presence of ascites
6. Anticipatory grieving related to poor prognosis of the disease

Nursing interventions

Health maintenance and promotion. Although early diagnosis and treatment of cancer of the genital tract have improved, a relatively high associated death rate remains. The chief reason may be that women do not sufficiently participate in good preventive care. In their many contacts with women, nurses can play a major role in advocating such care. To carry out this mission successfully, nurses have to be well informed about genital tract malignancies, especially their early signs and symptoms, and the various diagnostic studies and treatment measures available. In spite of the known effectiveness of the Pap test in detecting cervical malignancy, two out of five women do not have routine Pap smears.

SURGICAL PROCEDURES ON THE FEMALE REPRODUCTIVE SYSTEM
Types

A variety of surgical procedures (Table 48-15) are carried out when benign or malignant tumors of the genital tract are found. A hysterectomy may be done either vaginally or abdominally. A vaginal route is used when vagi-

Table 48-15 Surgical Procedures on the Female Reproductive Tract

Type of Surgery	Description
Subtotal hysterectomy	Removal of uterus without cervix (rarely done today)
Total hysterectomy	Removal of uterus and cervix
Panhysterectomy (TAH-BSO)	Removal of uterus, cervix, fallopian tubes, and ovaries*
Simple vulvectomy	Excision of vulva with wide margin of skin
Radical vulvectomy	Excision of tissue from anus to few cm above symphysis pubis (skin, labia majora and minora, and clitoris) with superficial and deep lymph node dissection
Vaginectomy	Removal of vagina
Radical hysterectomy (Wertheim)	Panhysterectomy, partial vaginectomy, and dissection of lymph nodes in pelvis
Pelvic exenteration (total)	Radical hysterectomy, total vaginectomy, removal of bladder with diversion of urinary system and resection of bowel with colostomy
Anterior pelvic exenteration	Above operation without bowel resection
Posterior pelvic exenteration	Above operation without bladder removal

*See Fig. 48-7, *A.*

nal repair is to be done in addition to removal of the uterus. The abdominal route is used when large tumors are present and the pelvic cavity is to be explored or when the tubes and ovaries are to be removed at the same time. The abdominal route can present more postoperative problems because it involves an incision and the opening of the abdominal cavity. In both vaginal and abdominal hysterectomies the ligaments that support the uterus are attached to the vaginal cuff so that normal depth of the vagina is maintained.

Nursing Management of Tumors
Acute surgical intervention

All clients experience a degree of anxiety when surgery is contemplated, but the prospect of major gynecological surgery may heighten these concerns. Some women may fear a loss of femininity and worry about possible changes in their secondary sex characteristics. Others may experience feelings of guilt, anger, or embarrassment. Still others may focus on the effect surgery will have on their reproductive and sexual functions. There are also women who view the whole process as annoying or who are relieved by the thought of no longer having to worry about becoming pregnant. Each client must be understood in light of her fears and concerns and must be approached and evaluated individually. The nurse who exhibits interest and a willingness to listen can provide considerable psychological support.

Hysterectomy. Preoperatively, the client is prepared physically for surgery with the standard perineal or abdominal preparation and shave. A vaginal douche and enemas may be given, according to the preference of the surgeon. The bladder should be emptied before the client is sent to the operating room. An indwelling catheter is often inserted preoperatively.

After surgery the client who has had a hysterectomy will have an abdominal dressing (abdominal hysterectomy) or a sterile perineal pad (vaginal hysterectomy). Table 48-16 presents a nursing care plan for the client after a total abdominal hysterectomy. The dressing should be observed frequently for any sign of bleeding during the first 8 hours after surgery. A moderate amount of serosanguineous drainage on the perineal pad is expected.

The client may experience urinary retention postoperatively because of temporary bladder atony resulting from edema or nerve trauma. This problem is more acute when a radical hysterectomy has been performed. At times an indwelling catheter is used for 1 to 2 days postoperatively to maintain constant drainage of the bladder and prevent strain on the suture line. If an indwelling catheter is not used, catheterization may be necessary if the client has not urinated for 8 hours postoperatively. If residual urine is suspected after the removal of an indwelling catheter, catheterization is done to prevent bladder infection caused by pooling of urine. A serious surgical complication is the accidental ligation of a ureter. Any complaint of backache or decreased urine output should be reported to the surgeon.

Abdominal distention may develop from the sudden release of pressure on the intestines when a large tumor is

Table 48-16

NURSING CARE PLAN FOR THE CLIENT WITH A TOTAL ABDOMINAL HYSTERECTOMY

Defining Characteristics	Nursing Interventions	Evaluation Criteria

NURSING DIAGNOSIS: Altered patterns of urinary elimination: retention related to loss of bladder tone, uncomfortable urinating position, and pain

Distension of bladder, voiding of small amounts, difficulty using bedpan and commode, limited activity	Measure intake and output. Encourage fluids orally within limitations of diet. Palpate bladder for distension. Catheterize as ordered. Provide privacy during client's attempts to urinate. Give perineal care every shift. Report any complaints of backache and decreased output. Provide routine catheter care if indwelling catheter is in place.	Urination without difficulty in sufficient quantities

NURSING DIAGNOSIS: Potential complication: paralytic ileus related to surgical manipulation of bowel and immobility

Distension of abdomen, complaints of gas pains, limited food and fluid intake, decreased bowel sounds	Auscultate, percuss, palpate abdomen for presence of flatus. Encourage ambulation q 4 hr. Insert rectal tube as ordered.	Soft, flat abdomen and expulsion of flatus; soft, formed stool before discharge

NURSING DIAGNOSIS: Potential complication: thromboembolic phenomenon related to immobility and irritation of vessels of pelvis and upper thigh

Recent surgery, limited leg exercises, presence of calf tenderness	Observe lower extremities for warmth, color, blanching, and sensation q 8 hr. Report and record signs and symptoms noted. Help client change position q 2 hr while in bed. Avoid high Fowler's position and pressure under knees. Carry out active-passive exercises q 2 hr. Reapply antiembolism stockings every shift. Ambulate q 4 hr.	Normal circulation with no signs of inflammation of lower extremities

NURSING DIAGNOSIS: Body-image disturbance related to perceived loss of feminity and future inability to conceive

Crying, weeping, depression; verbalization of perceived loss of femininity or ability to conceive	Provide factual information regarding anticipated bodily changes. Provide information on hormone replacement. Encourage discussion with client, significant others, and health professionals.	Accurate statement of effects of hysterectomy, verbalization of confidence in ability to adjust to postsurgical state

NURSING DIAGNOSIS: Altered sexuality patterns related to perceived lack of desirability and fatigue secondary to surgery and lack of knowledge regarding resumption of sexual activity

Frequent questioning about future sexual response, lack of desire to resume presurgical sexual practices	Facilitate discussion of sexuality with significant other. Reassure client that energy and desire will return after a period of convalescence. Explain psychological and physiological implications of hysterectomy related to a woman's sexuality.	Optimism that satisfactory sexual practices can be resumed when indicated by surgeon

NURSING DIAGNOSIS: Altered health maintenance related to lack of knowledge regarding resumption of sexual activity, activity restrictions, and HRT

Questioning about postdischarge plans related to resumption of sexual activity, presurgery occupational and leisure activity, and advisability of HRT	Encourage expression of concerns. Assess knowledge level. Provide information regarding HRT. Initiate discussion of sexual activity with significant other. Provide timetable for gradual resumption of presurgery activity.	Confidence in ability to make appropriate decisions related to sexual activity, occupational and leisure activity, and HRT

removed or from paralytic ileus secondary to anesthesia and pressure on the bowel. Food and fluids may be restricted if the client is nauseated. A rectal tube may be prescribed to relieve abdominal flatus, and ambulation is encouraged. A Fleet enema or suppository is frequently given on the third postoperative day. Ambulation is encouraged to help relieve the problem.

Special care must be taken to prevent the development of thrombophlebitis of the vessels of the pelvis and upper thigh. Frequent changes of position and the avoidance of high Fowler's position and pressure under the knees minimize stasis and pooling of blood. Special attention must be given to clients with varicosities. Leg exercises to promote circulation and the use of antiembolism stockings or elastic bandages can be helpful.

The client often feels depressed for several days. This response may be due to hormonal changes. She may experience periodic crying spells, sometimes called "hysterectomy blues," resulting from wide vacillation in estrogen and progesterone levels. The loss of a body part may bring about grieflike responses that occur when any great loss is sustained. Sympathetic understanding and care are needed during this period. Families, especially partners, must understand and accept these responses.

Before discharge, the nurse should be certain that the client knows what changes will occur in her body because of the surgery (e.g., she will not menstruate if a total hysterectomy was performed). If the ovaries have been removed, she may experience hot flashes within days and other menopausal changes gradually. Her discharge planning should include immediate and long-range limitations. Intercourse should be avoided until the wound is healed (about 4 to 6 weeks). However, intercourse is not contraindicated once healing is complete. Sutures at the top of the vagina can tear and produce considerable bleeding if genital sex is engaged in too early or is too unrestrained. Secondary sex characteristics are not affected unless the ovaries have been removed. If a vaginal hysterectomy is performed, the woman needs to know that there may be a temporary loss of vaginal sensation. She should be reassured that sensation will return in several months.

Physical restrictions are limited for a short time. Heavy lifting should be avoided for 2 months. Activities that may increase pelvic congestion, such as dancing and walking swiftly, should be avoided for several months, whereas activities such as swimming may be both physically and mentally helpful. Wearing a girdle is allowed and may provide comfort. Once the client has been assured that healing is complete, all previous activity can be resumed.

Salpingectomy and oophorectomy. Postoperative care of the woman who has undergone removal of a fallopian tube (salpingectomy) or an ovary (oophorectomy) is similar to that for any client having abdominal surgery. One exception is that if a large ovarian cyst is removed, there may be abdominal distention due to the sudden release of pressure in the intestines. An abdominal binder may provide relief until the distention subsides.

When both ovaries are removed (bilateral oophorectomy), surgical menopause results. The symptoms are similar to those of regular menopause but may be more severe because of the sudden withdrawal of hormones. Attempts are made to leave at least a portion of an ovary. Replacement therapy with estrogen is given to most clients to preserve secondary sex characteristics and to avoid symptoms of menopause unless the surgery has been done because of malignancy.

Vulvectomy. Although cancer of the vulva is relatively uncommon, the extent of the required surgery and the psychological implications for the client demand the best in nursing management. It is important that the nurse recognize the extent of a vulvectomy and the fact that it is a means of diagnosing a cancer. An honest, open attitude with the client and her partner preoperatively can be most helpful in the postoperative period.

After a vulvectomy the client returns to the unit with a wound in the perineal area extending to the groin. The wounds may be covered or left exposed and frequently have drains attached to portable suction (e.g., Hemovac). A heavy pressure dressing is often in place for the first 24 to 48 hours. The wounds are cleaned with normal saline solution or an antiseptic twice daily. Solutions can be applied with an aseptic bulb syringe or a Water Pic machine. A heat lamp or a hair dryer is then used to dry the area. Wound care must be meticulous to prevent infection, which results in delayed healing.

Special attention to bowel and bladder care is needed. A low-residue diet and fecal softeners prevent straining at stool and wound contamination. An indwelling catheter is used to provide urinary drainage. Great care is taken not to dislodge the catheter because the extensive edema in the area would make its reinsertion very difficult. Heavy, taut sutures are often used to close the wounds, resulting in severe discomfort for the client. In other instances the wound may be allowed to heal by granulation. Analgesics may be required frequently to control pain. Careful positioning of the client through the use of strategically placed pillows provides comfort. Ambulation is usually begun on the second postoperative day, but this varies with the preference of the surgeon. Anticoagulant therapy to prevent vascular complications is common.

Because the surgery causes mutilation of the perineal area and the healing process is slow, the client is likely to become discouraged. Opportunities for the client to express her feelings and concerns about the operation should be provided. The client needs specific instructions in self-care before she is discharged. She should be told to report any unusual odor, fresh bleeding, or perineal pain. Home care nursing can benefit the client during her adjustment period. Sexual function is often retained. Whether clitoral sensation is retained may be critical to some women, particularly if it was a primary source of orgasmic satisfaction. A discussion of alternative methods of achieving sexual satisfaction may also be indicated.

Pelvic exenteration. When other forms of therapy are ineffective in checking the spread of cancer and stage IV is identified, pelvic exenteration may be performed. Candidates for this procedure are selected on the basis of their likelihood of surviving the surgery and their ability to adjust to and accept the imposed limitations.

The postoperative care involves that of a client who has had a radical hysterectomy, an abdominal perineal resection, and an ileal conduit (Fig. 48-7). The physical, emo-

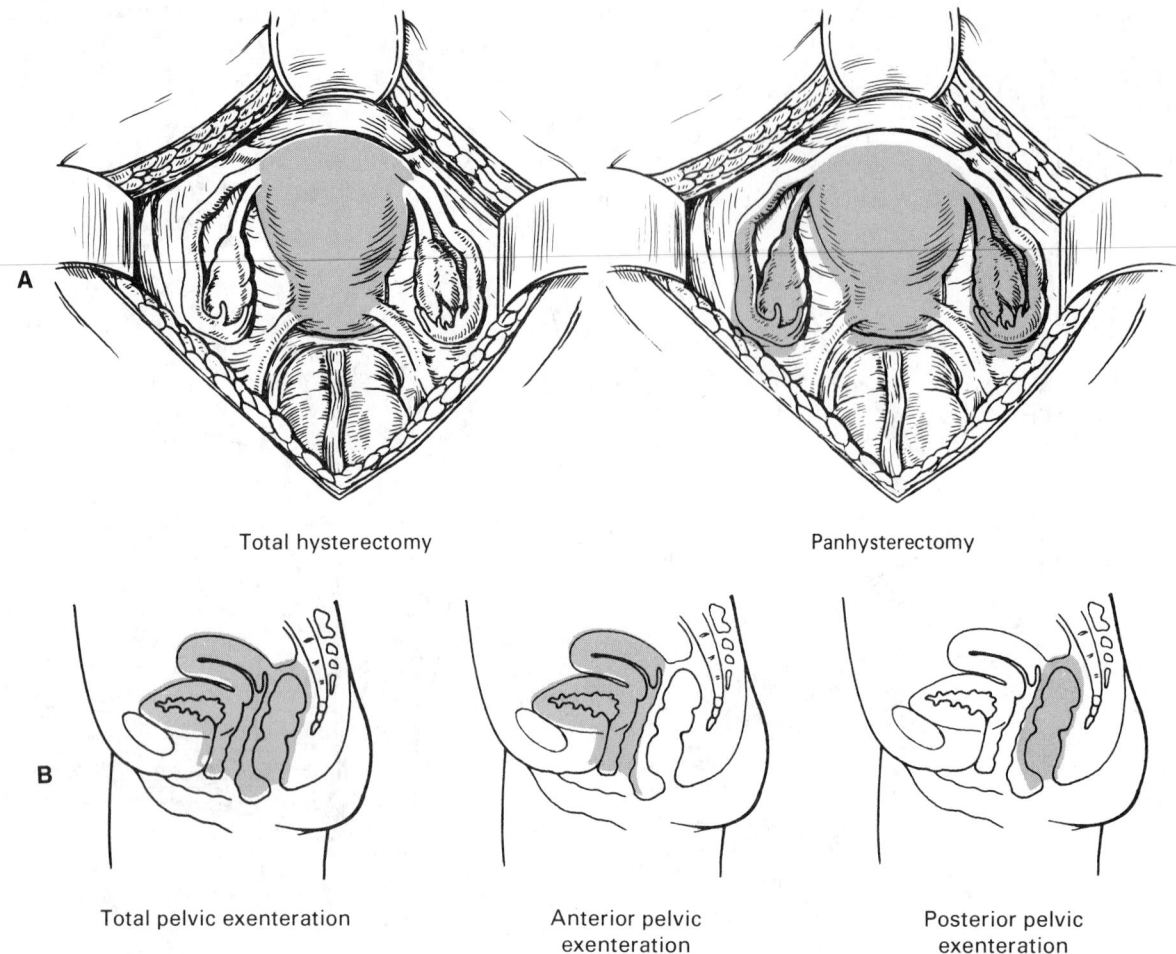

Total hysterectomy

Panhysterectomy

Total pelvic exenteration

Anterior pelvic
exenteration

Posterior pelvic
exenteration

Fig. 48-7 Surgical procedures and related organ removal for tumors of the female reproductive tract. **A,** Hysterectomy. **B,** Pelvic exenteration. (From Govan ADT, Hodge C, and Callander R: Gynecology illustrated, ed 3, New York, 1985, Churchill Livingstone.)

tional, and social adjustments to life on the part of the woman and her family are great. There are urinary or fecal diversions in the abdominal wall, the sexual function of the vagina is lost, and menopause may occur (estrogen therapy is frequently contraindicated).

The client's rehabilitative process should keep pace with her acceptance of the situation. Much understanding and support is needed from the nursing staff. The client should be gently encouraged to regain her independence. She needs to verbalize her feelings about her altered body structure to an interested and concerned listener. The family should be included in the plan of care.

The client is told to return to her physician or clinic at specified intervals. Early recurrence of the cancer may then be identified and treated. At this time the client's physical and emotional adjustment to the changes in body image produced by the surgery and her ability to carry out any treatment measures can also be assessed. Additional teaching and counseling can then be provided.

RADIATION THERAPY FOR UTERINE CANCER
Internal Radiation

Internal radiation is used in the management of cervical and endometrial cancer because of the accessibility of

these body parts and the favorable results obtained. Radium and cesium are two commonly used isotopes. In preparation of the client for the treatment, a cleansing enema is given to prevent displacement of the isotope. An indwelling catheter is inserted to prevent a distended bowel or bladder from coming into contact with the radioactive source.

A variety of applicators have been developed for intracavitary treatment. Some are inserted as multiple small irradiators (e.g., Heyman's capsules, Fig. 48-8, *A*), whereas others consist of a central tube (tandem) with irradiators placed on each side of the cervix (vaginal ovoids).

The applicator may contain the radioactive material when it is inserted into the endometrial cavity and vagina of an anesthetized client in the operating room. This is known as *preloading*. In the *afterloading* technique (Fig. 48-8, *B*) the applicator is implanted in the operating room but is not loaded with the radioactive material until its correct placement is checked by x-ray film and the client has returned to her room. Radiation exposure to the client is precisely controlled. The radiation exposure to the physician and other personnel involved in the implantation is reduced when the afterload technique is used. The applicator is secured with vaginal packing and is left in place from 24

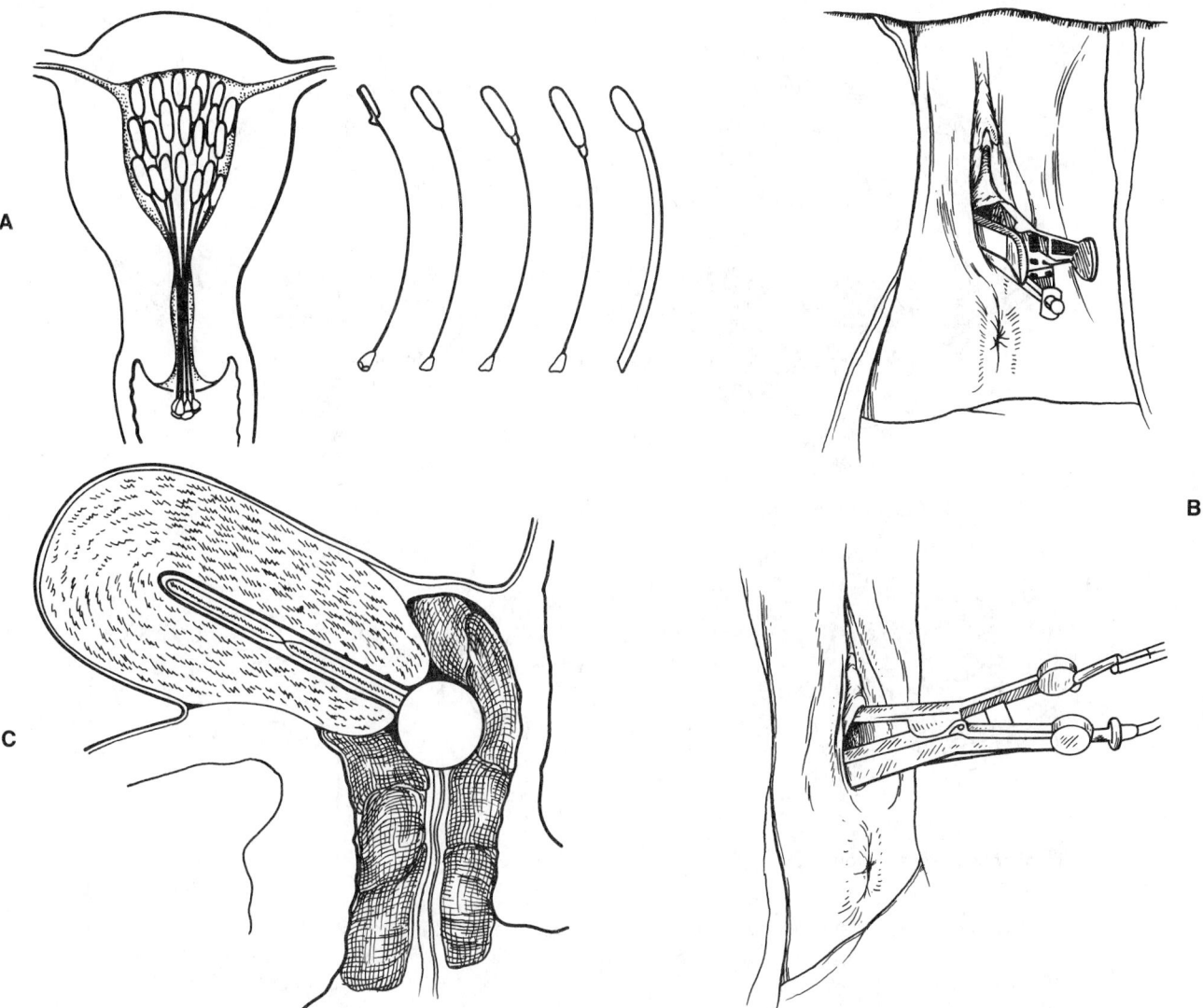

Fig. 48-8 Intracavitary radiation for uterine cancer. **A,** Heyman's capsules: various sizes and capsules in place. (From Green T: Gynecology: essential of clinical practice, ed 3, Boston, 1977, Little, Brown & Co.) **B,** Applicator in position ready to be loaded (afterloading). (From Hikemeyer R: Nursing care in radium therapy, Nurs Clin North Am 2:92, 1967.) **C,** Radiation applicator secured in position with gauze packing. (From Garry M and others: Gynecology illustrated, ed 2, New York, 1979, Churchill Livingstone.)

to 72 hours (Fig. 48-8, *C*). The radiologist determines the exact amount of radioactive substance to be used and the hours it will be left in place so that destruction of cancer cells can occur with minimal damage to normal cells.

During the treatment the client is placed in a private room and is on absolute bed rest. She may be turned from side to side. The presence of an intrauterine applicator produces uterine contractions that may require analgesics. The destruction of cells results in a foul-smelling vaginal discharge, and a deodorizer is helpful. Nausea, vomiting, diarrhea, and malaise may develop as a systemic reaction to the radiation.

Nurses should stay in the immediate area no longer than is necessary to give proper care and attention, and no nurse should attend the client for more than ½ hour a day.

The nurse may stay at the foot of the bed or at the entrance to the room to minimize radiation exposure. Visitors should stay 6 feet away from the bed and limit visits to less than 3 hours a day. The reasons for these precautions should be explained to the client and her visitors. (A more detailed discussion of nursing care of the client with an internal implant is given in Chapter 9.)

At the end of the prescribed period of radiation, the radioactive material and the catheter are removed. A cleansing douche is given. The client is allowed to ambulate and is usually discharged from the hospital the next morning. Complications that may arise after radiation of the uterus include fistulas (vesicovaginal, ureterovaginal), cystitis, phlebitis, hemorrhage, and fibrosis. If fibrosis occurs, the vaginal wall becomes smaller in diameter and shorter. Di-

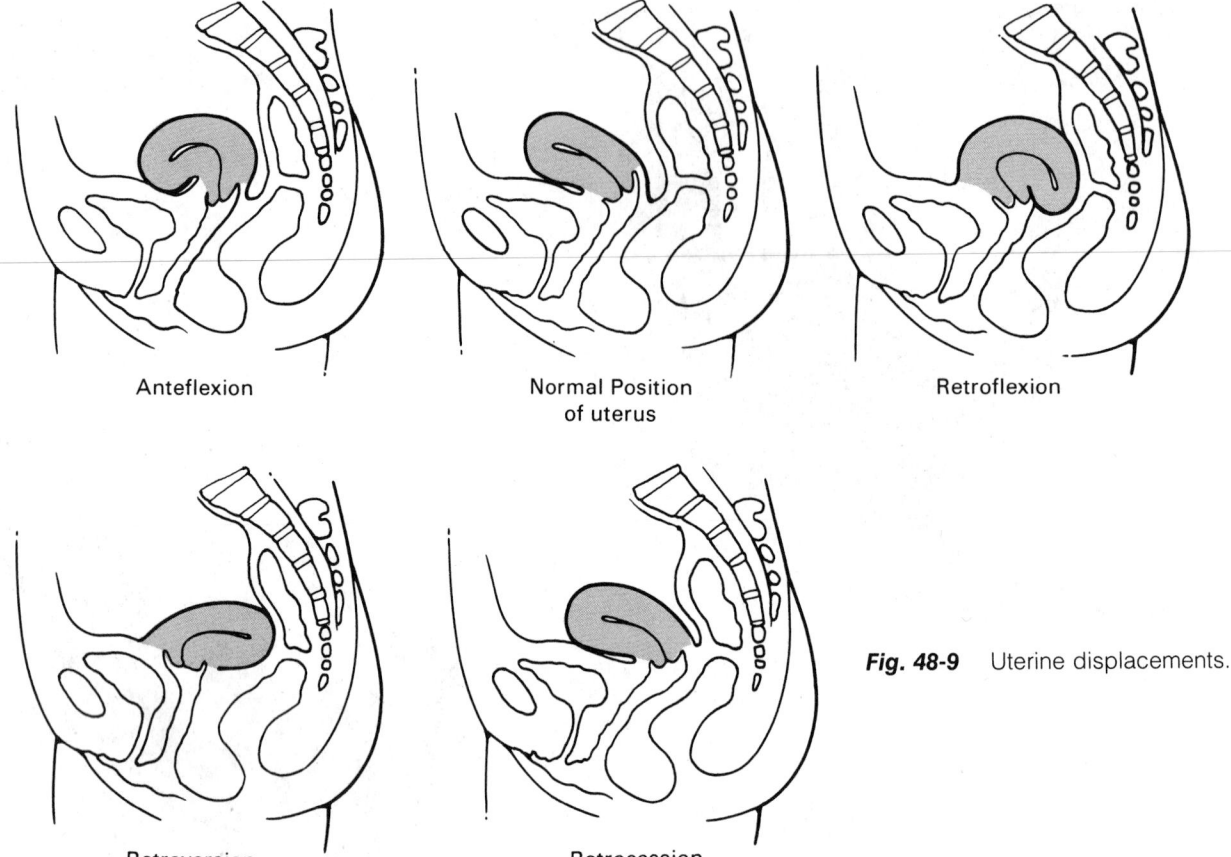

Anteflexion

Normal Position
of uterus

Retroflexion

Retroversion

Retrocession

Fig. 48-9   Uterine displacements.

latation of the vagina through intercourse or the use of an obturator is indicated. The client is urged to report any unusual symptoms or complaints to her physician.

After internal radiation the client may be concerned about resumption of sexual activity. Application of a lubricant and increased foreplay can aid in vaginal lubrication. Reassurance that intercourse is not contraindicated for either party is important.

External Radiation

Pelvic radiation is delivered by supervoltage equipment, such as a linear accelerator and cobalt 60. The treatment period usually extends for 4 to 6 weeks. The care of the client receiving external pelvic radiation is the same as it is for treatment elsewhere in the body (see Chapter 9). The client should be told to urinate immediately before the treatment to avoid trauma to the bladder. Radiation side effects, including enteritis and cystitis, may occur. These are natural reactions to radiotherapy and are not due to an overdose. Informing the client in advance of the possible side effects and what measures to use lessens the impact when side effects do occur.

UTERINE STRUCTURAL ABNORMALITIES

The uterus normally flexes anteriorly about 45 degrees and is movable. The cervix points downward and posteriorly. The filling of the bladder or bowel may cause a change in uterine position. Displacement of the uterus as well as of the bladder and rectum can be either congenital or acquired as a result of stretching and weakness of muscles of the pelvic floor and the ligaments that support the uterus. The acquired displacement of these structures is frequently due to injuries sustained during childbirth or surgery, closely occurring pregnancies, tumors, inflammatory disease, and the loss of tissue elasticity associated with aging.

Uterine Displacement

The uterus may be displaced in several ways. Anterior displacement, or *anteflexion*, occurs when the body of the uterus is flexed forward. Posterior displacements include *retroflexion* (flexed backward) and *retroversion* (tilted backward). These positional differences are most often simple anatomical variations from the most frequent uterine location and axial direction in midpelvis and in moderate anteversion (Fig. 48-9).

Retroversion is encountered in 20% or more of otherwise normal, symptom-free women. As an anatomical variation, retroversion is usually innocent of the variety of pelvic symptoms often ascribed to it, such as backache, infertility, menorrhagia, pregnancy complications, dysmenorrhea, and dyspareunia. Treatment involves the use of exercise therapy to stretch and strengthen the uterine ligaments and pelvic muscles. One exercise has the client assume the knee-chest position (causing the uterus to fall forward) for a few minutes several times a day. Another appropriate exercise is called Kegel's exercise, in which the client tightens the muscles of the perineum as if to stop

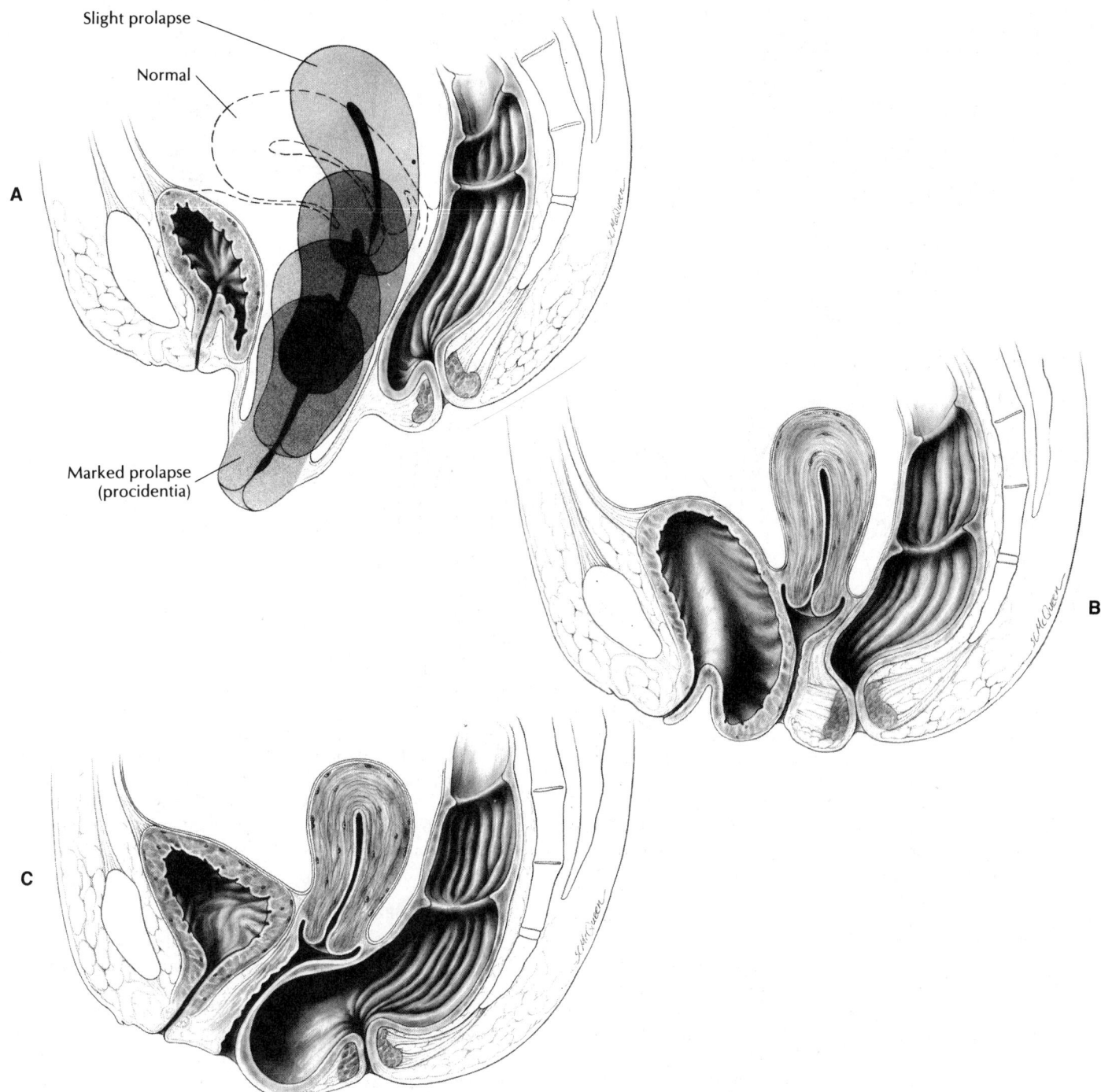

Slight prolapse

Normal

A

Marked prolapse
(procidentia)

B

C

Fig. 48-10 **A,** Uterine prolapse. **B,** Cystocele. **C,** Rectocele. (From Bobak IM and others: Maternity and gynecologic care, ed 4, St Louis, 1989, The CV Mosby Co.)

the flow of urine. The tension should be maintained for 5 seconds at a time, with the exercise repeated in sets of 10 and repeated 10 times during the day.

Another treatment for uterine displacement is the use of a pessary (a rubber or plastic appliance placed in the vagina for uterine support). Before insertion of the vaginal pessary, the uterus is manually replaced in its normal position. Once inserted, the pessary holds the cervix in a posterior position, thus allowing the uterus to fall forward.

When the pessary is properly positioned, the client is unaware of its presence and experiences no difficulty in voiding or during intercourse. Because a pessary irritates the vaginal mucosa, the client should be instructed to douche regularly to remove excess vaginal debris. The client should discuss symptom relief with her physician 6 weeks after insertion of the pessary. The pessary may be changed or removed at this time.

However, if the uterus is retroverted and adherent pos-

teriorly, it is noted as secondary or acquired retroversion and is often associated with PID and endometriosis. The underlying disease is responsible for posterior retraction. Treatment is directed toward resolving the underlying cause if it can be found. A uterine suspension (shortening of the round ligaments) may be the treatment of choice for acquired retroversion.[41] This surgery ensures the maintenance of an anterior position of the uterus.

Uterine Prolapse

Downward displacement or *prolapse* of the uterus through the pelvic floor and vaginal outlet is traditionally rated as first-degree (the cervix comes down to the introitus), second-degree (the cervix protrudes through the introitus), or third-degree (procidentia—the entire uterus protrudes through the introitus) prolapse (Fig. 48-10, *A*). The client complains of a feeling of "something coming down." She may have dyspareunia, a dragging or heavy feeling in the pelvis, backache, and bowel or bladder problems if cystocele or rectocele is also present. Stress incontinence is a common and troubling problem. When second- or third-degree uterine prolapse occurs, the protruding cervix and vaginal walls are subjected to constant irritation, and tissue changes may occur.

Surgery generally involves a vaginal hysterectomy with anterior and posterior repair of the vagina and underlying fascia. In situations in which surgery is contraindicated, pessaries are used to correct the prolapse. A variety of pessaries are available for the different degrees of prolapse. Every 3 to 4 months the pessary is cleaned and replaced by the client, if possible, or by her physician. She is also checked for signs of excessive irritation. Pessaries that are unattended for long periods are associated with erosion, fistulas, and an increased incidence of vaginal carcinoma.

Cystocele and Rectocele

If a prolapse of the uterus occurs, the uterus pulls structures such as the bladder, rectum, and urethra down or out of position. This type of displacement results in disorders such as *cystocele* (a herniation of the bladder into the vagina) and *rectocele* (a herniation of the bowel into the vagina) (Fig. 48-10, *B* and *C*).

A cystocele or a rectocele may cause a dragging pain in the back and in the pelvis. A cystocele often causes urinary symptoms such as incontinence (especially with activities that increase intraabdominal pressure, for example, coughing and lifting), frequency, and urgency. A rectocele may cause bowel symptoms such as constipation and incontinence of gas or liquid feces. Infection, hemorrhoids, and cystitis may occur as complications of these conditions.

In the early stages of cystocele or rectocele, perineal exercises may be used to strengthen the weakened muscles. A pessary may be placed when surgery is contraindicated or refused. Surgery designed to tighten the vaginal wall is generally the method of treatment. A cystocele is corrected with a procedure called an *anterior colporrhaphy*, whereas a *posterior colporrhaphy* is done for a rectocele. If further surgery is needed to relieve stress incontinence, procedures to support the urethra and restore the proper angle between the urethra and the posterior bladder wall are used. In a Marshall-Marchetti procedure, the urethra is supported by a series of sutures placed through the anterior vaginal wall on either side of the urethra and then through the periosteum of the pubic bone. The Stamey procedure, which is less invasive, suspends the bladder by way of sutures passed adjacent to the ureterovesical junction.[42]

■ Nursing Management of Uterine Structural Abnormalities

Nurses can play an active part in preventing the incidence of uterine prolapse. They can encourage pregnant clients to seek qualified obstetrical care early in the pregnancy. Better care during the maternity cycle has helped reduce the occurrence of the problem. Nurses can also teach perineal exercises (e.g., Kegel's) during the postpartum period. As part of the preoperative preparation for vaginal surgery, a cleansing douche may be ordered the morning of surgery. A cathartic and a cleansing enema are usually given when a rectocele repair is scheduled. A perineal shave is done. The nurse can assist the client in understanding any limitations that surgery may impose on sexual and reproductive capacity, since misunderstandings frequently occur.

In the postoperative period, the goals of care are to prevent wound infection and pressure on the vaginal suture line. This necessitates perineal care at least twice a day and after each episode of urination or defecation.

A heat lamp may be used to help dry the area and enhance the healing process. An ice pack applied locally may relieve the initial perineal discomfort and swelling. A disposable glove filled with ice and covered with a cloth works well in these instances. Later, sitz baths are generally used.

After an anterior colporrhaphy, an indwelling catheter is usually left in the bladder for 4 days to allow the local edema to subside. The catheter keeps the bladder empty, thereby preventing strain on the sutures. Catheter care with an antiseptic is generally done twice daily. After posterior colporrhaphy, straining at stool is avoided by means of a low-residue diet and the prevention of constipation. Mineral oil is usually given each night.

Discharge instructions should be reviewed before the client leaves the hospital. They include the use of douches or mild laxatives as needed; restriction of heavy lifting and prolonged standing, walking, or sitting; and avoidance of intercourse until the physician gives permission. There may be a loss of vaginal sensation, which can last for several months. The client needs to be reassured that this situation is temporary.

FISTULAS

A fistula is an abnormal opening between internal organs or between an organ and the exterior of the body. Fistulas can occur as a result of injury during delivery, surgery, radiation therapy, and disease processes, such as carcinoma. They may develop between the vagina and the bladder, urethra, ureter, or rectum. When *vesicovaginal fistulas* (between the bladder and the vagina) develop, some urine leaks into the vagina, whereas with *rectovaginal fistulas* (between the rectum and the vagina), flatus and

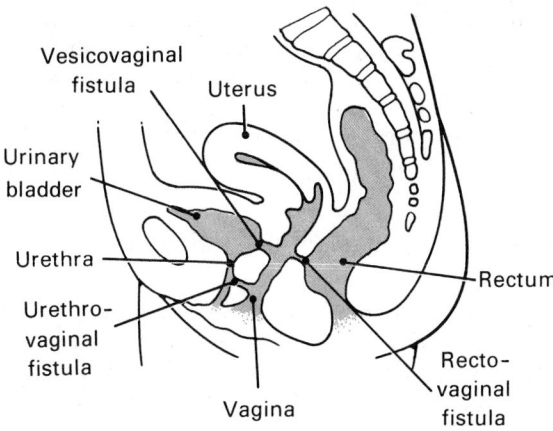

Fig. 48-11 Common fistulas involving the vagina.

feces escape into the vagina (Fig. 48-11). In both instances, excoriation and irritation of the vaginal and vulvar tissues occur and may lead to severe infections. In addition to wetness, offensive odors may develop, causing embarrassment and severely limiting socialization.

■ Therapeutic and Nursing Management of Fistulas

Because small fistulas may heal spontaneously within a matter of months, treatment can be postponed. If the fistula does not heal, surgical excision is required. Inflammation and tissue edema must be eliminated before surgery is attempted. This may involve a wait of up to 6 months for the surgery. The fistulectomy may result in the client's having an ileal conduit or temporary colostomy.

Perineal hygiene is of great importance, both preoperatively and postoperatively. The perineum should be cleansed every 4 hours. Warm sitz baths should be taken 3 times daily if possible. Perineal pads should be changed frequently. Deodorizing and comfort measures such as douches or powders and local heat are used. Douches should be given with low pressure to avoid further damage to the tissues. A low-residue diet and high enemas may be given to reduce the constant flow of feces. The client should be encouraged to maintain an adequate fluid intake. Encouragement and reassurance by the staff are needed in helping the client cope with her problems.

Postoperatively, nursing care emphasis is on avoidance of stress on the repaired areas and prevention of infection. Care should be taken so that the indwelling catheter is draining at all times. Oral fluids should be urged to provide for internal catheter irrigation. Minimal pressure and strict asepsis are used if catheter irrigation becomes necessary. The first stool after bowel surgery may be purposely delayed to prevent contamination of the wound. Later, stool softeners or mild laxatives may be given. (See Chapter 40 for care of a client with an ileal conduit and Chapter 37 for care of a client with a colostomy.) Surgical repair of fistulas is not always effective, even in the best conditions. Supportive nursing care for the client and her significant others therefore is especially important.

C ase Study

TOTAL ABDOMINAL HYSTERECTOMY

Mrs. Marion P., a 40-year-old woman with two children, has been having menorrhagia and occasionally metrorrhagia for the past 5 months. She consulted her physician, who obtained a complete history and performed a physical examination. On pelvic examination, several large, firm masses in the body of the uterus, thought to be leiomyomas, were palpated. On the basis of these findings, the physician advised Mrs. P. to have a hysterectomy. Initially she was reluctant to undergo such an operation, but after deliberating the matter for a week she gave her consent.

Mrs. P. was admitted to the hospital for a total abdominal hysterectomy. After surgery she was returned to her room with an indwelling catheter in place and both legs wrapped in full-length antiembolism stockings.

Discussion Questions

1. What are the common causes of menorrhagia and metrorrhagia?
2. What clinical manifestations may result from leiomyomas?
3. What is the physical and psychological preoperative preparation that should be given to this client?
4. What observation should be made in the client's immediate postoperative period?
5. What possible complications, including their basis for development, can arise after abdominal hysterectomy?

R eview Questions

The number of the question corresponds to the same-numbered objective at the beginning of the chapter.

1. Primary dysmenorrhea is usually
   a. due to overexertion
   b. rare in the teenager
   c. idiopathic
   d. due to uterine pathophysiology
2. Postoperative care following a D & C includes
   a. observing the suture line
   b. checking on bowel activity
   c. doing a pad count
   d. expecting severe cramps
3. The client in climacteric may experience
   a. vasomotor reactions
   b. irregular menstrual periods
   c. dyspareunia
   d. all the above
4. The use of oral contraceptives may result in
   a. perforation of the uterus
   b. thromboembolic disorders
   c. infection of the uterus
   d. few side effects
5. An induced abortion
   a. occurs without apparent cause
   b. occurs with mechanical intervention
   c. is always illegal
   d. produces few psychological effects
6. Genital injuries resulting from rape may include
   a. bruises and lacerations of the perineum and cervix

 b. lacerations of the uterine ligaments
 c. both a and b
 d. neithor a nor b
7. A prominent symptom of cervicitis is
 a. leukorrhea
 b. urinary frequency
 c. severe perineal pain
 d. vaginal hemorrhage
8. Symptoms of PID may include
 a. itching, fever, backache
 b. malaise, menorrhagia, polyps
 c. rectal bleeding, nausea, vomiting
 d. vaginal discharge, fever, abdominal pain
9. A complication of endometriosis is
 a. frequent pregnancies
 b. adhesions
 c. dehydration
 d. hemorrhage
10. A common complaint of women with uterine fibroids is
 a. constant cramping pain
 b. urinary dribbling
 c. menorrhagia
 d. sterility
11. The diagnosis of endometrial cancer is best made by
 a. D & C
 b. Schiller iodine test
 c. Pap smear
 d. culdoscopy
12. Discharge instructions for the client who has had a hysterectomy include
 a. take frequent brisk walks
 b. resume normal activities
 c. do not wear a girdle
 d. avoid sexual activity until the wound is healed
13. Nursing responsibilities related to intracavitary radiation for uterine cancer include
 a. allowing the client bathroom privileges only
 b. maintaining absolute bed rest for the client
 c. remaining at the bedside 1 hour a day for care
 d. limiting visitors to 5 hours a day
14. Management of the client with a retroverted uterus includes
 a. insertion of a pessary
 b. immediate uterine suspension
 c. vaginal hysterectomy
 d. anterior and posterior colporrhaphy
15. A vesicovaginal fistula results in
 a. fecal incontinence
 b. leakage of urine from the bladder
 c. leakage of fecal material into the vagina
 d. leakage of urine from the vagina

REFERENCES

1. Ledger W and others, eds: Obstetrics and gynecology, ed 8, St Louis, 1987, The CV Mosby Co, p 76.
2. Jones H, Wentz A, and Burnett L: Novak's textbook of gynecology, ed 11, Baltimore, 1988, Williams & Wilkins, p 253.
3. Johnson S: The epidemiology and social impact of premenstrual symptoms, Clin Obstet Gynecol 30:371, 1987.
4. Wickes S: Premenstrual syndrome, Prim Care 13:480, 1988.
5. Keye W: General evaluation of premenstrual symptoms, Clin Obstet Gynecol 30:404, 1987.
6. Kendall K and Schurr P: The effects of vitamin B_6 supplementation on premenstrual symptoms, Obstet Gynecol 70:149, 1987.
7. Kase NG, Weingold A, and Gershenson DM: Principles and practice of clinical gynecology, ed 2, New York, 1990, Churchill Livingstone, p 483.
8. Ryan KJ, Berkowitz R, and Barbieri RL: Kistner's gynecology: principles and practice, ed 5, Chicago, 1990, Year Book Medical Publishers, p 56.
9. Dawood MY, McGuire J, and Demers L, eds: Premenstrual syndromes and dysmenorrhea, Baltimore, 1985, Urban & Schwarzenberg, Inc, p 85.
10. Shapiro S: Treatment of dysmenorrhea and premenstrual syndrome with non-steroidal antiinflammatory drugs, Drugs 36:484, 1988.
11. Speroff L, Glass R, and Kase N: Clinical gynecologic endocrinology and fertility, ed 4, Baltimore, 1989, Williams & Wilkins, p 136.
12. Jones H, Wentz A, and Burnett L: Novak's textbook of gynecology, ed 11, Baltimore, 1988, Williams & Wilkins, p 440.
13. Collins J: Menopause, Prim Care 15:605, 1988.
14. Collins J: Menopause, Prim Care 15:602, 1988.
15. Ryan KJ, Berkowitz R, and Barbieri RL: Kistner's gynecology: principles and practice, ed 5, Chicago, 1990, Year Book Medical Publishers, p 470.
16. Kase N, Weingold A, and Gershenson D: Principles and practice of clinical gynecology, ed 2, New York, 1990, Churchill Livingstone, p 351.
17. Kase N, Weingold A, and Gershenson D: Principles and practice of clinical gynecology, ed 2, New York, 1990, Churchill Livingstone, p 350.
18. Barber HR: Perimenopausal and geriatric gynecology, New York, 1988, Macmillan Publishing Co, p 200.
19. Connell E: Barrier contraceptives, Clin Obstet Gynecol 32:380, 1989.
20. Monier M and Laird M: Contraceptives: a look at the future, Am J Nurs 4:499, 1989.
21. Bagatell CJ and others: A comparison of the suppressive effects of testosterone and a potent new gonadotropin-releasing hormone on gonadotropin and inhibin levels in normal men, J Clin Endocrinol Metab 69:43, 1989.
22. Bagatell CJ and others: A comparison of the suppressive effects of testosterone and a potent new gonadotropin-releasing hormone on gonadotropin and inhibin levels in normal men, J Clin Endocrinol Metab 69:48, 1989.
23. Jacobs L: Initial clinical survey of the infertile couple, Prim Care 15:586, 1988.
24. Rodger M and Baird D: Induction of therapeutic abortion in early pregnancy with mifepristone in combination with prostaglandin pessary, Lancet 1:1414, 1987.
25. Centers for Disease Control: Ectopic pregnancy—United States, 1986, MMWR 38:484, 1989.
26. US Department of Justice: Uniform crime reports for the United States, Washington DC, 1989, US Government Printing Office, p 16.
27. US Department of Justice: Uniform crime reports for the United States, Washington DC, 1989, US Government Printing Office, p 14.
28. Burgess A and Holmstrom L: Rape crisis and recovery, Englewood Cliffs, NJ, 1979, Prentice-Hall, Inc, p 35.
29. Hecks D: The patient who's been raped, Emerg Med 20:108, 1988.
30. Foley T and Davies M: Rape: nursing care of victims, St Louis, 1983, The CV Mosby Co, p 157.
31. MacDonald K and others: Toxic shock syndrome: a newly recognized complication of influenza and influenza-like illness, JAMA 257:1053, 1987.

32. Scott J and others: Danforth's obstetrics and gynecology, ed 6, Philadelphia, 1990, JB Lippincott Co, p 740.

33. Labadie L and Rhule R: Management of genital infections, Emerg Med Clin North Am 5:447, 1987.

34. Centers for Disease Control: Sexually transmitted disease treatment guidelines, MMWR 38:32, 1989.

35. Wilson E: Surgical therapy for endometriosis, Clin Obstet Gynecol 31:859, 1988.

36. American Cancer Society: Fact and figures—1990. ACS Pub No 90-4235M-#508-LE, Atlanta, 1990, American Cancer Society, p 8.

37. Centers for Disease Control: Chronic disease reports: deaths from cervical cancer—United States, 1984-1986, MMWR 38:652, 1989.

38. American Cancer Society: Summary of current guidelines for cancer-related checkup: recommendations, ACS Pub No 3347.10-PE, Atlanta, 1988, American Cancer Society.

39. Kaplan A: Endometrial carcinoma, Hosp Med 23:79, 1989.

40. Ryan KJ, Berkowitz R, and Barbieri RL: Kistner's gynecology: principles and practice, ed 5, Chicago, 1990, Year Book Medical Publishers, p 211.

41. Hale R and Krieger J: Gynecology: a concise testbook, New York, 1983, Medical Examination, p 227.

42. Fowler J and Crowley J: Stress urinary incontinence: endoscopic suspension of vesical neck, AORN J 45:924, 1987.

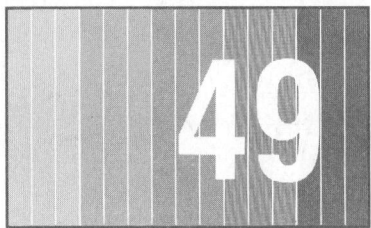

CHAPTER

49

Nursing Role in Management

Male Genitourinary Problems

Cindy Meredith

Learning Objectives

1. *Describe the pathophysiology, clinical features, and therapeutic management of problems affecting the male reproductive system.*
2. *Describe the nursing management of problems affecting the male reproductive system.*
3. *Explain the nursing role in the management of problems related to male sexual functioning.*
4. *Identify the psychological and emotional implications of problems related to the male reproductive organs.*

Table 49-1   Measures to Minimize Embarrassment for the Male Client

1. Ensure privacy.
2. Drape carefully so that only the area examined is exposed.
3. Determine that client understands the terminology used for his body parts.
4. Use an open, nonjudgmental attitude toward the client's sexual practices.
5. Ensure confidentiality.

Problems of the male reproductive system are a source of anxiety for many men. This anxiety is related to manipulation and exposure of the genitalia, discussion of intimate topics, and fear of possible pathological conditions related to the male reproductive organs. Anxiety and fear may cause the client to delay seeking help for a problem or practicing health-promoting behaviors. Specific nursing measures that can minimize embarrassment for the male client should be used when he seeks health care (Table 49-1). The nursing role in the management of problems of the male reproductive system can involve a wide range of problems in any of the various structures (Fig. 49-1).

PROBLEMS OF THE PROSTATE GLAND
Benign Prostatic Hypertrophy or Hyperplasia

Significance. The most common problem of the adult male reproductive system is benign prostatic hypertrophy or hyperplasia (BPH). This problem occurs in about 50% of men more than 50 years of age and 75% of men more than 70 years of age. Benign prostatic hypertrophy is most likely to develop in the median and lateral lobes of the

Reviewed by Steve Toussiant, R.N., M.S.N., Assistant Professor of Nursing, Linfield College, Good Samaritan School of Nursing, Portland, Oregon.

prostate, and cancer is most likely to develop in the posterior lobe (Fig. 49-2).

Pathophysiology. BPH begins with small nodules in the gland. Although the cause of the development of these nodules is not completely understood, it is thought that they are an overgrowth of smooth muscle and connective tissue resulting from endocrine changes associated with aging. Excessive accumulation of dihydroxytestosterone in the prostate, stimulation of estrogen, and local growth hormone action have been proposed as causes. Glandular tissue also increases.

Problems arise when the gland enlarges to where the proximal urethra is partially or completely obstructed, which results in urinary retention. At rectal examination, the benign hypertrophic gland feels firm and enlarged.

Clinical manifestations. The client seeks assistance for relief of the symptoms related to urinary obstruction. Symptoms are usually very gradual in onset and may not be noticed by the client until hypertrophy of the prostate gland is far advanced. The first symptom experienced is often nocturia (awakening at night to void) caused by decreasing bladder capacity from an enlarging prostate. A small urinary stream, hesitancy (difficulty in starting the stream), and dribbling at the end of voiding are also symptoms. A urinary tract infection may be present as a result of the obstructive process.

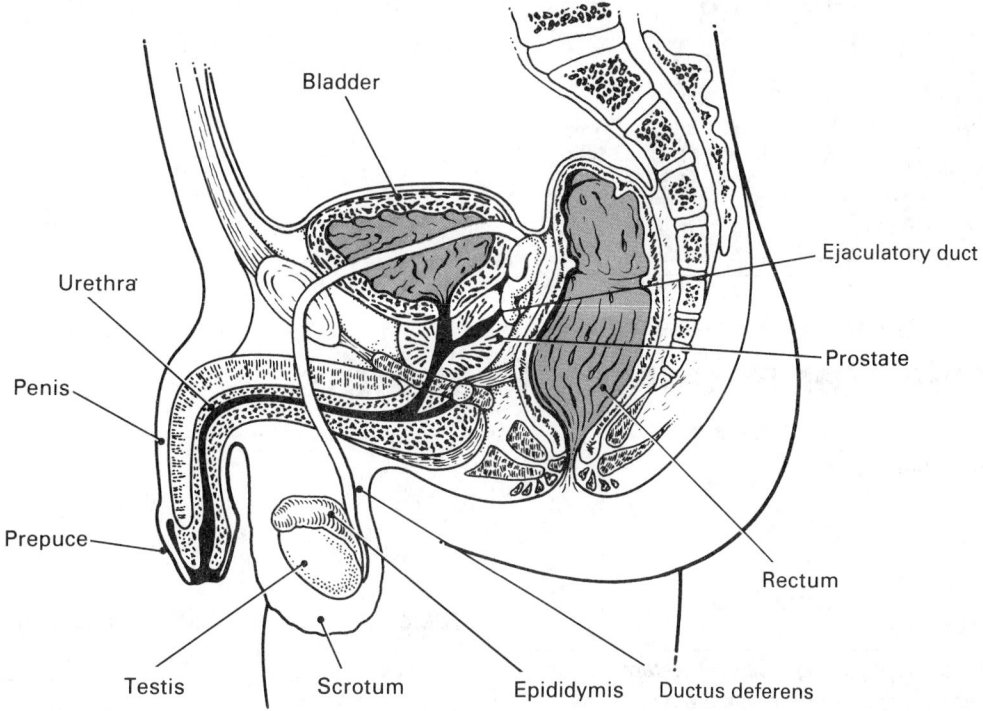

Fig. 49-1 Areas of the male reproductive system in which problems are likely to develop.

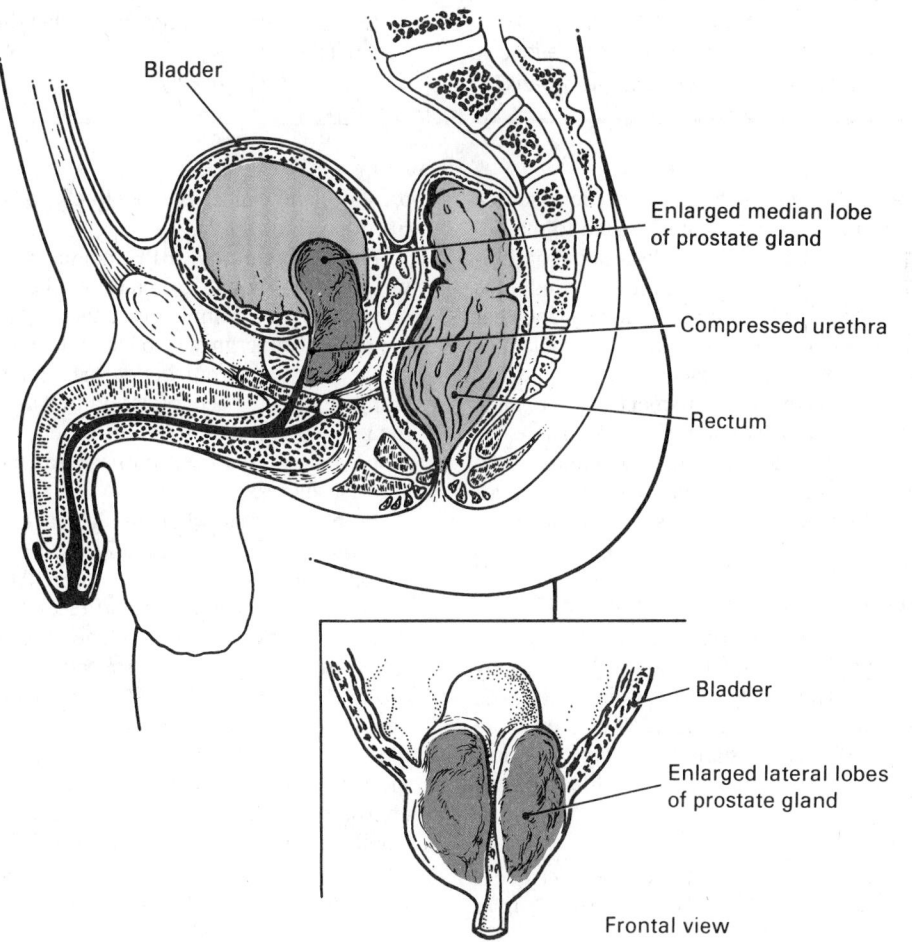

Fig. 49-2 Benign prostatic hypertrophy of the median lobe.

Complications. The client with BPH is at increased risk for urinary tract infection because of failure of the bladder to empty completely. The residual urine provides a favorable environment for bacterial growth. Calculi may develop as a result of the alkalinization of the residual urine. Breakage of tiny overstretched blood vessels of the bladder may produce hematuria.

More serious complications resulting from urinary retention are abnormally distended ureters *(hydroureters)*, destruction of the kidney's parenchyma from the back pressure of the urine *(hydronephrosis)*, and pyelonephritis. These complications can lead to renal failure.

Diagnostic studies. The most common sign of BPH is enlargement of the prostate on rectal palpation. In addition, urinalysis may indicate alkalinity and the presence of infection. In the early stages of BPH, the specific gravity of the urine may be unchanged or elevated because the client may restrict fluid intake to decrease the need to void. If hydronephrosis with renal impairment has occurred, the specific gravity will be low. If BPH has been a long-standing problem, the blood urea nitrogen (BUN) and creatinine levels may be elevated because of renal involvement.

A cystoscopic examination shows the encroachment of the prostate gland into the urethra. Small hemorrhagic areas may be present in the bladder.

Transrectal and suprapubic ultrasonography are valuable in evaluating the size of the prostate. This procedure estimates prostatic volume and weight to facilitate treatment of BPH.

Therapeutic management. The goal of therapeutic management is to restore bladder drainage. This may be temporarily accomplished by catheterization; however, the catheter does not resolve the underlying problem of prostatic enlargement. Several experimental, nonsurgical techniques used for treatment of BPH have the same objective as surgical treatment—to relieve the client's symptoms and to prevent or treat the complication of BPH. One treatment includes medication in an attempt to either alleviate the symptoms or shrink the growth of the prostatic tissue. Treatment with antiandrogens, luteinizing hormone–releasing hormone (LH-RH) agonists, and gonadotropin-releasing hormone (GnRH) analogues is used to improve urodynamics and decrease prostate volume. These approaches require an indefinite period of treatment because urinary function reverts to pretreatment levels when the medication is stopped.[1]

Localized application of heat is used in an attempt to reduce the size of the prostatic tissue.[2] Although experimental, this approach appears to be a promising alternative for clients with mild disease who are poor candidates for surgery. One technique to achieve a desired temperature of 43° C or greater involves the intracavitary placement in the urethra of a radiating microwave antenna that emits heat. This procedure results in highly significant increases in urine flow rate, decreases in postvoid residual urine capacity, and decreases in frequency of nocturia.[1] Mild side effects include occasional problems of bladder spasm, hematuria, and dysuria.

Another alternative treatment is a prostatic balloon device that dilates the urethra to enlarge the passage and allow for free flow of urine.[3,4] The balloon is inflated for ap-

proximately 10 to 20 minutes, and the client may experience mild pain and urinary urgency. After dilatation the balloon is removed, and the urethra is assessed for indication of increased diameter. If the procedure is successful, an indwelling catheter is left in place for the first 24 hours to monitor urinary output and the degree of hematuria. The dilatation procedure may be repeated if the first attempt was unsuccessful. Complications resulting from this procedure have been rare, and the short-term results are encouraging. The procedure is not a permanent solution to the problem of an enlarged prostate but does offer a nonsurgical, cost-saving option to appropriate clients, particularly those at high risk for surgery. The balloon technique is contraindicated in clients with atonic bladder because dilatation alone will not properly empty the bladder.

The primary treatment of BPH is surgery (Table 49-2). The selection of a surgical approach to remove the adenomatous tissue depends on the size and position of the prostatic enlargement (Fig. 49-3).

The type of surgery selected depends on the client's degree of debility and reproductive outlook. The nurse can help the client ask appropriate questions regarding the impact of a particular type of surgery on sexual functioning.

Transurethral resection. The transurethral resection (TUR) approach is the most common route for partial removal of the prostate. TUR accounted for 95% of prostatectomies performed on Medicare recipients in 1985.[5] This approach is useful for removal of the medial lobe surrounding the urethra. No external surgical incision is made because a resectoscope is passed through the urethra to excise and cauterize prostatic tissue. A large (No. 18 to 22) three-way indwelling catheter with a 30 ml balloon con-

Table 49-2

Diagnostic and Therapeutic Management: Benign Prostatic Hypertrophy

DIAGNOSTIC

Rectal examination
Prostatic ultrasound with or without guided needle biopsy
Cystoscopy
Urinalysis with culture
Renal studies
    BUN
    Serum electrolyte and serum creatine levels
    Intravenous pyelogram

THERAPEUTIC

Catheterization
High fluid intake
Antibiotics
Antiandrogen therapy
Prostatic balloon
Surgery
    Transurethral incision or resection
    Suprapubic resection
    Retropubic resection
    Perineal resection

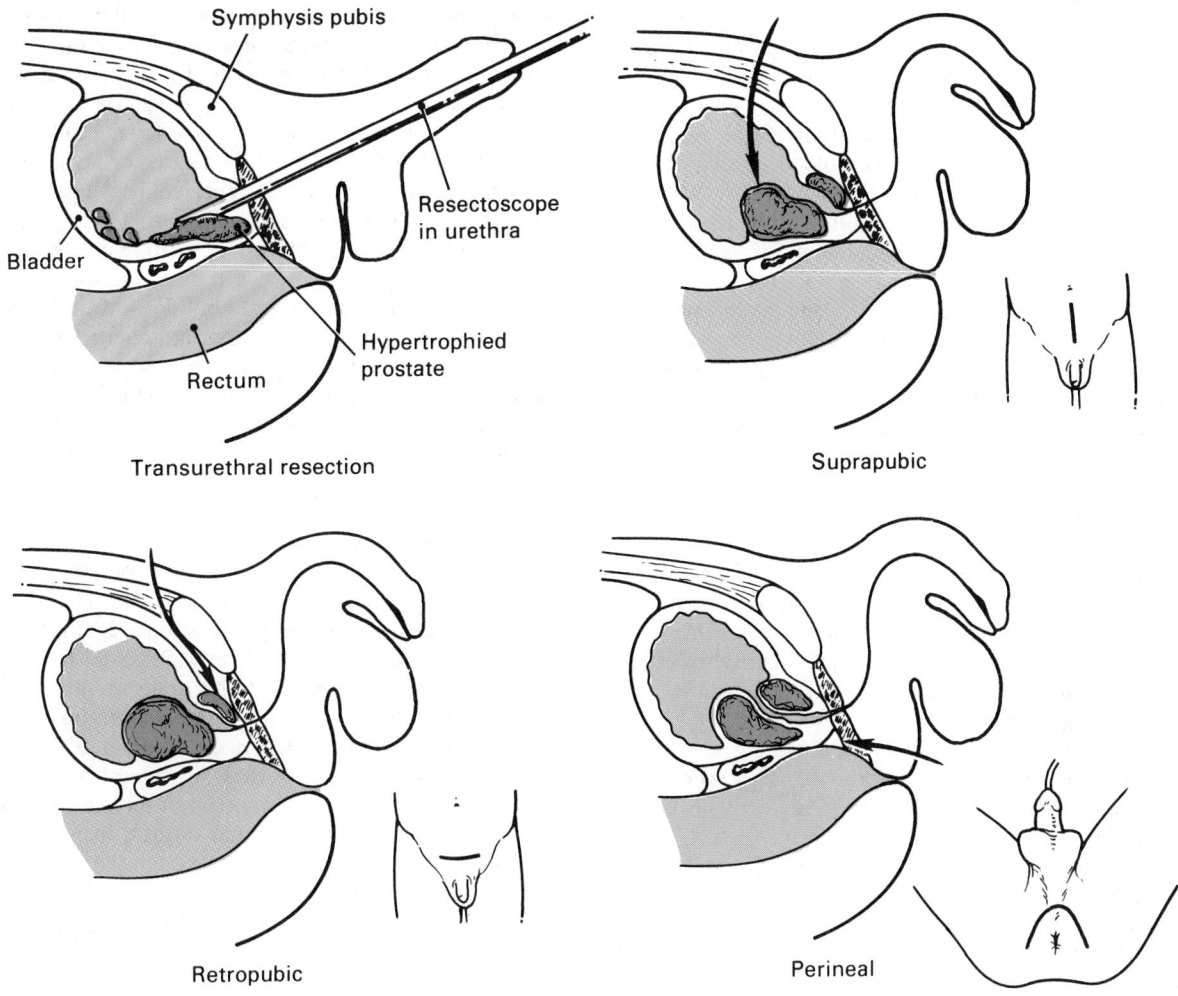

Fig. 49-3   Four types of prostatectomy.

taining 30 to 60 ml of sterile water is usually inserted into the bladder after the procedure to provide hemostasis and facilitate urinary drainage. Bladder irrigation, continuous or intermittent, is usually done for at least 24 hours to prevent obstruction from mucous threads and blood clots. A TUR is often the surgery of choice for the debilitated client or for the client with moderate prostatic enlargement. The advantages of TUR are that it does not involve an external incision and is unlikely to result in erectile dysfunction or long-term incontinence. A disadvantage is that it does not completely remove all prostatic tissue, leaving the potential for recurrence of hyperplasia.

Transurethral incision of the prostate. In high-risk clients or those with mild obstruction, transurethral slits or incisions are made into the prostatic tissue to relieve bladder neck obstruction.[5] The client is discharged with an indwelling catheter for the first 24 hours to monitor output and hematuria. Advantages of transurethral incision of the prostate (TUIP) include maintenance of antegrade ejaculation, short operating time, and minimal complications. The disadvantages are that it is a temporary solution and may not provide adequate relief from obstructive symptoms, it is most effective on a small gland of less than 20 g,

cancer of the prostate may be missed, and rectal injury may occur, depending on the location of the incision.[6]

Suprapubic resection. The suprapubic approach is used when an extremely large mass of tissue obstructs the urethra. The prostate is approached through a low midline abdominal incision through the bladder to the anterior aspect of the prostate. This technique completely removes the gland. After surgery a cystotomy catheter is left in place through the abdominal incision to prevent pressure on the suture line. An indwelling catheter with a 30 ml balloon is placed in the urethra. This approach allows better exploration, but it has an increased risk of urinary tract infections, incontinence, and hemorrhage.

Retropubic resection. The retropubic approach is used to remove a large mass located high in the pelvic area. It is the most common approach for a radical prostatectomy with pelvic lymph node dissection. A low midline abdominal incision is made into the prostate gland. After surgery the client has a large indwelling catheter with a 30 ml balloon placed in the urethra. A Penrose drain may be left in the abdominal incision site to aid in the removal of drainage from the area. Both suprapubic and retropubic resections are difficult in the client who is obese.

The bladder is not incised in this approach, and direct visualization of the prostate is possible. The risk of hemorrhage remains high.

Perineal resection. The perineal approach is used to remove a large mass located low in the pelvic area and is often used with cancer of the prostate. The incision is made between the scrotum and the anus. Because of the possibility of inadvertently entering the rectum, the bowel is prepared with enemas, antibiotics, and a low-residue diet. After surgery an indwelling catheter with a 30-ml balloon is left in the urethra. A Penrose drain may be placed in the incision site to promote drainage of the area. Although all open procedures carry the risk of erectile dysfunction, the perineal approach is most likely to result in impotence. Urinary incontinence may also be a problem.

The Campbell-Walsh procedure is a nerve-sparing surgical technique that greatly reduces the incidence of erectile dysfunction and it is used primarily with the retropubic approach. Clients should be encouraged to discuss this procedure with their physicians before surgery.[7]

A prophylactic vasectomy may be done with an open prostatectomy to decrease the risk of ascending epididymitis. The major postoperative complications of these types of surgery are hemorrhage, infection, and bladder spasm.

■ Nursing Management of Benign Prostatic Hypertrophy

Nursing interventions

Health maintenance and promotion. Since the cause of BPH is poorly understood, the focus of health promotion is on early detection and treatment. Men should have a prostate examination at least yearly after 40 years of age.

Some men find that the ingestion of drugs such as alcohol and caffeine tends to increase prostatic symptoms. If this happens, the client should avoid these drugs.

Clients with obstructive symptoms should be advised to urinate when they first feel the urge to minimize urinary stasis and acute urinary retention. Fluid intake should be maintained at a normal level to avoid dehydration or fluid overload. The client may believe that if he restricts his fluid intake, his symptoms will be less severe, but this only increases the chance of an infection developing. However, if the client rapidly increases his intake of fluids beyond what the urethra can eliminate, hydronephrosis can develop more readily because of the obstruction to urine elimination.

Acute intervention

PREOPERATIVE CARE. The objectives of preoperative care of the client about to undergo prostatectomy are (1) restoration of urinary drainage, (2) treatment of any urinary tract infection, and (3) client education, especially related to sexual functioning.

Urinary drainage must be restored before surgery. Prostatic obstruction may have resulted in retention or inability to void. A urethral catheter such as a coudé catheter may be needed to restore drainage. If a sizable obstruction of the urethra exists, a filiform catheter with sufficient rigidity to pass the obstruction may be inserted by a urologist. Aseptic technique is important at this time to avoid introducing bacteria into the bladder.

Any infection of the urinary tract must be treated before surgery. Restoring drainage, forcing fluids, and providing a diet high in acid ash-producing foods are helpful in clearing the infection. Antibiotics are usually given.

The client is usually concerned about the impending surgery in regard to his sexual functioning. Data gathered during the health history related to the sexual history will identify possible problem areas. The nurse should provide an opportunity for the client to express his concerns. The client needs to know how the surgery will affect sexual functioning and whether a vasectomy is planned. The consequences of this in regard to his ability to father children should be explored. The surgical consent form should indicate whether a vasectomy is to be performed. Except in the perineal approach, a prostatectomy does not usually result in erectile dysfunction. All types of prostatic surgery generally result in some degree of retrograde ejaculation. The client should be informed that the ejaculate may be decreased in amount or totally absent. Retrograde ejaculation is not harmful because the fluid is simply eliminated during the next urination.

POSTOPERATIVE CARE. Nursing responsibilities focus on assessing and preventing complications and restoring urinary control and sexual expression (Table 49-3). The main complications of prostatectomy are hemorrhage, bladder spasms, and infection. The plan of care should be adjusted to the type of surgery, the reasons for surgery, and the client's response to surgery.

After prostatectomy the bladder may be continuously irrigated with sterile normal saline solution or another prescribed solution that removes clotted blood from the bladder and ensures drainage of urine. Some form of irrigation (continuous or intermittent) may be used for 24 hours or until no clots are noted draining from the bladder.

Blood clots are normal after a prostatectomy for the first 24 to 36 hours. However, large amounts of bright red blood in the urine can indicate hemorrhage. Postoperative hemorrhage may occur from displacement of the catheter or increases in abdominal pressure. Release or displacement of the catheter dislodges the 30 ml balloon that provides counterpressure on the operative site. Traction on the catheter may be applied to provide counterpressure on the bleeding site in the prostate, decreasing bleeding. Such traction can result in local necrosis. Pressure should therefore be relieved on a scheduled basis by qualified personnel. Activities that increase abdominal pressure, such as sitting or walking for prolonged periods and straining to have a bowel movement, should be avoided in the postoperative recovery period.

Bladder spasms are a distressing complication for the client after transurethral and suprapubic prostatectomy and occur as a result of irritation of the bladder mucosa from the insertion of the resectoscope, the presence of a catheter, and clots leading to obstruction of the catheter. The client should be instructed not to attempt to urinate around the catheter, because this increases the likelihood of spasm. If bladder spasms develop, the catheter should be checked for clots. If present, the clots should be removed by irrigation so that urine can flow freely. Belladonna and opium suppositories, along with relaxation techniques, are

Table 49-3

NURSING CARE PLAN FOR THE CLIENT UNDERGOING TRANSURETHRAL RESECTION

Defining Characteristics	Nursing Interventions	Evaluation Criteria
Preoperative		
NURSING DIAGNOSIS: Pain: bladder distention related to prostatic obstruction secondary to enlarged prostate		
Complaints of distended bladder and need to void, palpable bladder, no urine output	Insertion of indwelling catheter (usually done by urologist); monitor intake and output. Percuss bladder every shift for distention. Assess comfort status. Ensure patency of catheter.	No complaints of discomfort because of bladder distention
NURSING DIAGNOSIS: High risk for urinary infection related to indwelling catheter, inadequate oral intake, environmental pathogens, and urinary stasis		
Elevated temperature; cloudy, foul-smelling urine	Monitor temperature. Do urinalysis for culture. Give client 8 oz of fluid every waking hour. Observe strict aseptic technique for catheter care. Observe color and characteristics of urine.	No evidence of urinary tract infection
NURSING DIAGNOSIS: Anxiety related to actual or potential sexual dysfunction, diagnosis, and lack of knowledge regarding surgical procedure and postoperative care		
Verbalization of anxiety about impact of surgery on sexuality; questioning or inaccurate comments about surgical course	Perform standard preoperative teaching. Assess client's concerns related to sexual functioning and correct misconceptions and inaccuracies. Provide opportunity for private conversation for client to ask personal questions. Assure client that a TUR does not usually cause problems in sexual functioning. Inform client about retrograde ejaculation.	Decrease in anxiety about effect of surgery and sexuality and surgical course as shown by accurate knowledge base, correct responses to questions, calm demeanor
Postoperative		
NURSING DIAGNOSIS: Potential complication: hemorrhage related to surgical procedure		
Large amounts of bright red blood in urine; symptoms of shock such as rapid pulse and lowering blood pressure	Observe urinary drainage and report bright red bleeding in larger than expected quantities immediately. Monitor blood pressure, pulse, and respirations and report abnormalities. Maintain catheter drainage. Do not perform rectal treatments such as enemas or rectal temperatures (except belladonna and opium suppositories for bladder spasms).	No evidence of hemorrhage
NURSING DIAGNOSIS: Pain: bladder spasms related to irrigations and clots, surgical procedure, and ineffective pain and comfort measures		
Expression of pain from spasms; nonverbal signs of pain such as moaning, crying, legs drawn to abdomen	Maintain patency of catheter. Irrigate catheter if occluded with clots. Instruct client not to urinate around catheter. Give belladonna and opium suppository as needed. Instruct client in relaxation techniques.	No complaints of discomfort because of bladder spasms
NURSING DIAGNOSIS: High risk for infection: urinary related to indwelling catheter, environmental pathogens, and inadequate oral intake		
Febrile, diaphoretic, presence of indwelling catheter, self-restriction of fluid intake, cloudy urine	Monitor temperature q 4 hr first 48 hr postoperatively. Give client 8 oz of water hourly. Observe strict aseptic technique for catheter care.	No evidence of infection

Table 49-3

NURSING CARE PLAN—cont'd

Defining Characteristics	Nursing Interventions	Evaluation Criteria

Postoperative—cont'd

NURSING DIAGNOSIS: Altered health maintenance related to lack of knowledge regarding need for follow-up care and activity restriction postoperatively

| Unawareness of potential for prostatic cancer; questioning or inaccurate comments about postoperative activity | Teach client that some prostatic tissue is present that could become malignant. Reinforce need for annual examination. Instruct client to avoid heavy lifting, straining during defecation, or prolonged periods of travel until surgeon approves such activity. | Annual prostatic examination, no postoperative bleeding because of inappropriate activity |

NURSING DIAGNOSIS: Altered pattern of urinary elimination: dribbling related to poor sphincter control

| Inappropriate leakage of urine | Teach client exercises to control urinary stream (Kegel's exercises). Advise client about devices to control dribbling. | Absence or control of dribbling |

used to relieve the pain and decrease spasm. The catheter is removed 2 to 6 days after surgery. The client should urinate within 6 hours after catheter removal. If he cannot, a catheter must be reinserted for a day or two. If the problem continues, the nurse should instruct the client in the self-catheterization procedure.

Sphincter tone may be poor immediately after surgery, resulting in incontinence or dribbling. This is a common but distressing situation for the client. Sphincter tone can be strengthened by having the client practice Kegel exercises (pelvic floor muscle technique) 10 to 20 times per hour. The client may also practice starting and stopping the stream several times during urination. Usually it takes several weeks to achieve control. In some instances, control of urine may never be fully regained. Continence can improve for up to 12 months. If continence has not been achieved by that time, the client can be instructed to use a penile clamp, condom catheter, or incontinent briefs to avoid embarrassment from dribbling. An occlusive cuff that serves as an artificial sphincter can be surgically implanted to restore continence. The nurse should assist the client in developing practices that will allow him to socialize and interact with relatives and friends.

The client should be observed for signs of *postoperative infection*. If an external wound is present, the area should be observed for redness, heat, swelling, and purulent drainage. Careful aseptic technique should be used when irrigating the bladder, since bacteria can be introduced into the urinary tract. Proper care of the catheter is important. The catheter should be connected to a closed drainage system and should not be disconnected unless it is being removed, changed, or irrigated. The secretions that accumulate around the meatus should be cleansed daily with soap and water. Special care must be taken if a perineal incision is present because of the proximity of the anus. Rectal treatments (except belladonna and opium suppositories) such as rectal temperatures and enemas should be avoided because they may initiate bleeding.

Dietary intervention is important in the postoperative period to prevent the client from straining while moving his bowels. Straining increases the intraabdominal pressure, which can lead to bleeding of the operative site. A diet high in fiber produces a soft and easily passed stool.

Rehabilitative management. After prostatic surgery the client may be concerned about erectile dysfunction. Physiological impotence occurs when the perineal nerves are cut or damaged during a radical prostatectomy. The degree of concern is often related to anxiety over loss of sex role, degree of self-esteem, and quality of sexual interaction between the client and his sexual partner. Sexual counseling may be necessary if erectile dysfunction becomes a chronic problem. Clients may also require counseling regarding treatment options.

If a vasectomy is to be performed, the client should be prepared preoperatively to accept the ensuing sterility. Many men experience retrograde ejaculation after prostatectomy because of trauma to the internal sphincter. Semen is discharged into the bladder at orgasm and may produce cloudy urine when the client urinates after orgasm. The nurse should discuss these problems with the client and his partner and allow them to ask questions and express their concerns.

The bladder may take up to 2 months to return to its normal capacity. The client should be instructed to drink at least 1 L of fluid per day and to urinate every 2 to 3 hours to irrigate the urinary tract. Because the client may be experiencing incontinence or dribbling, he may believe that decreasing fluid intake will relieve this problem.

The client must be advised that he should continue to have yearly rectal examinations, particularly if he has had a TUR. Hyperplasia can recur in the remaining prostatic tissue and again cause obstruction. Because the entire prostate is not resected during the TUR, the client is still at risk for the development of prostatic cancer (Table 49-3).

Table 49-4 Whitmore-Jewett Staging Classification of Prostate Cancer

Stage A: Clinically unrecognized
A1   <5% of prostatic tissue neoplastic
A2   >5% of prostatic tissue neoplastic, all high-grade tumors
Stage B: Clinically intracapsular
B1   Nodule <2 cm and surrounded by palpably normal tissue
B2   Nodule >2 cm or multiple nodules
Stage C: Clinically extracapsular, localized to periprostatic area
C1   Minimal extracapsular extension
C2   Large tumors involving seminal vesicles and/or adjacent structures
Stage D: Metastatic disease
D1   Pelvic lymph node metastases or ureteral obstruction causing hydronephrosis
D2   Distant metastases to bone, viscera, or other soft tissue structures

Modified from Crawford ED, ed: Current genitourinary cancer surgery, Philadelphia, 1990, Lea & Febiger, p 152.

Cancer of the Prostate

Significance. Although rarely found in men less than 60 years of age, cancer of the prostate is the second most common form of cancer in men. Approximately 86,000 new cases are diagnosed each year, and about 25,000 deaths occur each year in the United States from this form of cancer. Screening for prostatic cancer is done by means of palpation of the gland during rectal examination. The nodules that are palpated are examined by means of thin needle biopsy or through a surgical biopsy method. Unfortunately, 80% or more of prostatic cancers are already metastatic when first diagnosed. Stage B lesions treated with traditional radical prostatectomy yield a 10-year survival rate of 50% to 79%, with 10% to 15% of clients experiencing incontinence and 30% to 60% becoming impotent postoperatively. The Walsh nerve-sparing surgical technique has resulted in a dramatic decrease in loss of erectile dysfunction.[8]

Prostatic cancer is staged on the basis of growth of the tumor (Table 49-4). Surgery is the most accurate method of staging because the extent of the growth of the tumor can only be assessed by means of inspection during the operation and the results of pathology reports of lymph nodes.

Pathophysiology. Prostatic cancer is an androgen-dependent adenocarcinoma. Factors such as sexual activity, social or economic class, and alcohol use are not epidemiologically significant. A higher incidence exists related to age (60 years of age or older) and in black men and married men.

The tumor is slow growing and usually begins in the posterior or lateral portions of the prostate and spreads by continuity to the seminal vesicles, urethral mucosa, bladder wall, and external sphincter. The cancer later spreads through the perineural lymphatic system to the regional lymph nodes. The veins from the prostate seem to be the mode of spread to the pelvic bones, head of the femur, lower lumbar spine, liver, and lungs.

Clinical manifestations and complications. Prostate cancer is asymptomatic in the early stages. Eventually the client may have symptoms similar to those of benign prostatic hypertrophy, including urinary obstruction, hesitancy, dribbling, frequency, urgency, hematuria, nocturia, and retention. The prostate feels hard, enlarged, and fixed on rectal examination. The enlargement is usually unilateral. When coupled with urinary symptoms, pain in the lumbosacral area that radiates down to the hips or legs is strongly indicative of metastasis.

Early recognition and treatment of this tumor is required to control growth and prevent metastasis. The tumor can spread to pelvic lymph nodes, bones, bladder, lungs, and liver. Once the tumor has spread to distant sites, the major problem becomes the management of pain. As the cancer spreads to bone, pain can become very severe, especially in the back and legs because of compression of the spinal cord (see Chapter 51).

Diagnostic studies. Improved diagnostic techniques have greatly enhanced the physician's ability to detect cancer of the prostate at an earlier stage. The rectal examination is an effective screening method to detect an enlarged prostate. Ultrasonography of the prostate allows the physician to visualize the outer lobes of the prostate and pinpoint potential cancer sites. When a suspicious area is located, a special biopsy needle can be inserted, and the specimen is then examined. Ultrasonography with guided-needle biopsy provides a method of early detection and treatment of prostatic cancer.[9-12]

Elevated prostatic acid phosphate (PAP) and prostate specific antigen (PSA) levels may also be indicative of cancer of the prostate.[13] However, these tests have many false-positives and false-negatives that limit their usefulness for screening purposes. Prostatic activity before the blood test, such as intercourse, masturbation, rectal examination, or prostatic massage, may account for the lack of specificity of these tests. In stage D, serum acid phosphatase is increased as a result of metastasis. Serum alkaline phosphatase becomes elevated as new bone is formed at the site of bone metastasis. At this stage, osteoblastic changes are seen on x-ray films of the bones of the pelvis, spine, ribs, and skull. Bone scans of metastatic areas show abnormal findings.

Therapeutic management. A unique feature of prostatic cancer is that cell growth initially depends on the presence of androgens. Orchiectomy (removal of the testis) is the usual means of decreasing androgen production in the adult male. This procedure has many emotional overtones for men. Estrogen treatment can be substituted for orchiectomy and can cause regression of the size of the prostate and disappearance of metastatic bone lesions. The minimum dose of estrogens capable of suppressing plasma testosterone to castration levels is used. Estrogen therapy often results in gynecomastia, mood swings, and total loss of erectile functioning. Although more emotionally traumatic to the man, orchiectomy does not have as many

Table 49-5

Diagnostic and Therapeutic Management: Prostatic Cancer

DIAGNOSTIC

Rectal examination

Prostatic ultrasonography with biopsy, needle aspiration, open biopsy

Blood chemistry, including serum acid and alkaline phosphatase, PSA, PAP

Radiological evaluation for bone metastases

THERAPEUTIC
Stage A

Continued medical follow-up, observation, TUR or total prostatectomy, pelvic lymphadenectomy

Stage B

Total prostatectomy or radiation therapy with or without lymphadenectomy

Stage C

Radical resection of prostate, radiation therapy to pelvis, hormonal manipulation (experimental) or orchiectomy

Stage D

Hormone therapy, radiation to metastatic bone areas

Table 49-6

Nursing Assessment of the Client with Cancer of the Prostate

SUBJECTIVE DATA
History

Age, race, positive family history, prostatic hypertrophy, sexually transmitted diseases, fat intake, exposure to cadmium or rubber textiles, urban living environment

Medication

Use of any medications affecting urinary tract (e.g., morphine, anticholinergics, MAO inhibitors, tricyclic antidepressants)

General

Possible indicators of metastasis such as weight loss, anorexia, fatigue, malaise

Pain

Possible indicators of metastasis such as dysuria, bone pain, low back pain radiating to legs or pelvis

Urinary

Hesitancy or straining to start stream, urgency, retention with dribbling, frequency, nocturia, weak stream, hematuria

OBJECTIVE DATA
General

Pelvic lymphadenopathy (late sign)

Urinary

Hard, enlarged, and fixed prostate on rectal examination

Musculoskeletal

Pathological fractures (metastasis)

Possible findings

Elevated serum PAP enzyme assay, elevated serum acid phosphatase (metastasis), positive biopsy results

---

physical side effects as estrogen therapy. Although estrogen therapy does not usually prolong life, it is effective in relieving pain and urinary obstruction. Estrogens and orchiectomy are usually reserved for stage D prostatic cancer.

Estrogen treatment is declining in popularity because of the side effects and reduced effectiveness in decreasing androgens. Luteinizing hormone (LH) antagonists (Lupron) that block androgens at the pituitary level are increasing in use. This medication is expensive and requires subcutaneous injections. Therapeutic management of the four stages of prostatic cancer is summarized in Table 49-5.

■ Nursing Management of Prostatic Cancer

Nursing assessment

Subjective and objective data that should be obtained from an individual with cancer of the prostate are presented in Table 49-6.

Nursing interventions

Health promotion and maintenance. One of the most important roles for nurses in relation to prostatic cancer is to encourage clients to have an annual prostate examination to increase early detection of this malignant tumor. Men more than 40 years of age should begin the practice of having an annual rectal examination.

Acute intervention. Preoperative and postoperative phases of therapy are the same as for benign prostatic hypertrophy. However, an additional consideration is con-

cern for the client's psychological response to a diagnosis of cancer. The nurse needs to provide psychological support for the client and his family to help them cope with the diagnosis of cancer (see Chapter 9). Prostatic cancer, when recognized and treated in the early stage, is a highly curable disease.

Rehabilitative management. Because cure is possible for prostatic cancer stages A, B, and C, treatment is more aggressive, and both surgical intervention and pelvic radiation may be used. The nurse needs to consider the long-term side effects of pelvic radiation such as incontinence, erectile dysfunction, scarring, and bowel necrosis in preparing the client for radiation treatment. Radiation therapy for stage D prostatic cancer is for palliative relief of pain from metastatic bone lesions.

Prostatitis

Pathophysiology. A number of inflammatory conditions can affect the prostate gland. The most common form of prostatitis is *abacterial* or *prostatosis.* Acute prostatitis and chronic prostatitis due to bacterial causes are less common.

Abacterial prostatitis may follow a viral illness or may be secondary to a sudden decrease in sexual activity, particularly in a younger adult. The cause of this problem is not known, but it is probably a noninfectious process.

Bacterial prostatitis is commonly associated with urethritis or an infection of the lower urinary tract. Commonly suspected organisms are *Escherichia coli, Enterobacter* organisms, *Proteus* species, *Chlamydia trachomatis,* and group D streptococci.[14] Organisms are believed to reach the prostate from the bloodstream or the urethra.

Clinical manifestations and complications. Acute bacterial prostatitis most often affects young males resulting in symptoms of fever, chills, dysuria, urethral discharge, and a congested and very tender prostate.

The symptoms of chronic prostatitis are variable and generally milder than those of acute prostatitis; they include backache, perineal pain, mild dysuria, and frequency. Factors that may contribute to chronic prostatitis include urethral obstruction, persistent infections above the urethra, and prostatic pathological conditions such as hyperplasia and prostatic calculi. The prostate feels irregularly enlarged, firm, and slightly tender on palpation.

The complications of prostatitis are epididymitis and cystitis. Chronic prostatitis can predispose the client to recurrent urinary tract infections. Sexual functioning may be affected in regard to postejaculation pain, variable libido problems, and relative impotence. Prostatic abscess is a rare complication.

Diagnostic studies. If a client with prostatitis has a fever, the white blood cell (WBC) count may be elevated. The urine is often cloudy with a foul odor. The client is instructed to void into two or three separate containers for a *split specimen urinalysis*. The first container shows many more WBCs and bacteria than subsequent containers. Palpation of the prostate gland may be normal or may include enlargement, tenderness, and calculi in long-standing cases.

Table 49-7

Diagnostic and Therapeutic Management: Bacterial Prostatitis

DIAGNOSTIC

Rectal examination
Complete blood count
Semen culture
Split specimen urinalysis

THERAPEUTIC

Acute bacterial type
 Double strength sulfamethoxazole and trimethoprim
  (Bactrim DS, Septra DS) for 30 days, tetracycline 500
  mg four times a day for 7 days, or erythromycin 500
  mg four times a day for 7 days
 Analgesics, stool softeners, sitz baths
Chronic type
 Sulfamethoxazole and trimethoprim for 12 weeks
 Sitz baths, prostatic massage, intercourse, masturbation

Therapeutic management. Therapeutic management of acute bacterial prostatitis usually consists of an antibiotic that concentrates in the prostate. Most antibiotics cannot penetrate the prostate because the very low pH of the gland precludes solubility of the drugs. Exceptions are tetracycline and the combination of sulfamethoxazole and trimethoprim.

Therapeutic management of chronic prostatitis is much more controversial (Table 49-7). Long-term antibiotics, vigorous prostatic massage, sitz baths, and stool softeners are sometimes prescribed. The efficacy of these measures other than for comfort has not been shown.

■ Nursing Management of Chronic Prostatitis

The client with chronic prostatitis should be instructed regarding the long-term nature of the problem. Because the prostate can serve as a source of urinary tract infection, fluid intake should be kept at a high level. Antibiotics may have to be taken for a number of months. Activities that drain the prostate—intercourse, masturbation, and prostatic massage—will probably help in the long-term management of this problem. Chronic prostatitis may eventually lead to erectile dysfunction, and the client may need to seek treatment.

PROBLEMS OF THE PENIS

Health problems of the penis are rare if sexually transmitted infectious diseases are excluded (see Chapter 47). The problems may be divided into congenital problems, problems of the prepuce, problems with the erectile mechanism, and cancer.

Congenital Problems

Hypospadias is present when the urethral meatus is located on the ventral surface of the penis anywhere from the corona to the perineum. Therapeutic treatment for hypospadias is usually not necessary unless there is an associated chordee, or bending under of the penis during erection, which may prevent intercourse, or for cosmetic reasons or emotional well-being.

Epispadias, opening of the urethra on the dorsal surface of the penis, is a complex birth defect that is usually associated with other genitourinary (GU) tract defects. Corrective surgery is usually done in early childhood.

Problems of the Prepuce

Problems of the prepuce rarely occur because circumcision has been so widely practiced in the United States for the past 40 to 60 years. *Paraphimosis* is edema of the retracted foreskin, preventing normal return over the glans. If this occurs, circumcision or dorsal slit of the prepuce may be required because the blood supply is cut off and necrosis may result.

Problems of the Erectile Mechanism

Priapism is a painful erection, lasting longer than 6 hours. The client may be unable to urinate. Causes of priapism include thrombosis of the veins of the corpora cavernosa, leukemia, sickle cell anemia, diabetes, degenerative lesions of the spine, neoplasms of the spinal cord, and

cocaine use. Treatment may include sedatives, injection of vasoconstrictors directly into the penis, aspiration of the corpora cavernosa with a large-bore needle, or the surgical creation of a shunt to drain the corpora. After an episode of priapism, the client may be unable to ever achieve an erection.

Cancer

Cancer of the penis is rare and usually is seen only in men who were not circumcised as infants. The tumor begins as a warty lesion that may be mistaken for a venereal wart. The majority of malignancies (95%) are well-differentiated squamous cell carcinomas.[15] Treatment in the early stages is laser removal of the growth or a partial penectomy. A radical resection may be done if the cancer has spread. Clients have a 60% to 90% 5-year survival rate of tumors confined to the penis. The survival rate drops to 10% to 30% with distant metastasis.

PROBLEMS OF THE SCROTUM AND ITS CONTENTS
External Problems

The skin of the scrotum is susceptible to a number of common dermatoses. The most common conditions of the scrotal skin are fungal infections, dermatitis (neurodermatitis, contact, and seborrheic), and parasitic infections (scabies and lice). These conditions involve discomfort for the client but have few if any severe complications (see Chapter 17).

Internal Problems

Problems that develop inside the scrotum usually are first noticed as a mass or scrotal edema. Some problems produce pain, whereas others do not. The conditions affecting scrotal contents that are seen most frequently in the adult are epididymitis, hydrocele, spermatocele, varicocele, orchitis, torsion, and testicular cancer (Fig. 49-4).

Epididymitis. *Epididymitis* is an inflammatory process of the epididymis, usually secondary to an infectious process, trauma, or urinary reflux down the vas. Swelling may progress to the point that the epididymis and testis are indistinguishable. The problem may be associated with prostatitis and is usually painful. The use of antibiotics is controversial in the absence of a specific infection. Treatment consists of bed rest with elevation of the scrotum and use of ice packs. Ambulation places the scrotum in a dependent position and increases pain. Most tenderness subsides within 1 week, although swelling may last for weeks or months.

Hydrocele. A *hydrocele* results from interference with lymphatic drainage of the scrotum with swelling of the tunica vaginalis that surrounds the testis. The mass transillu-

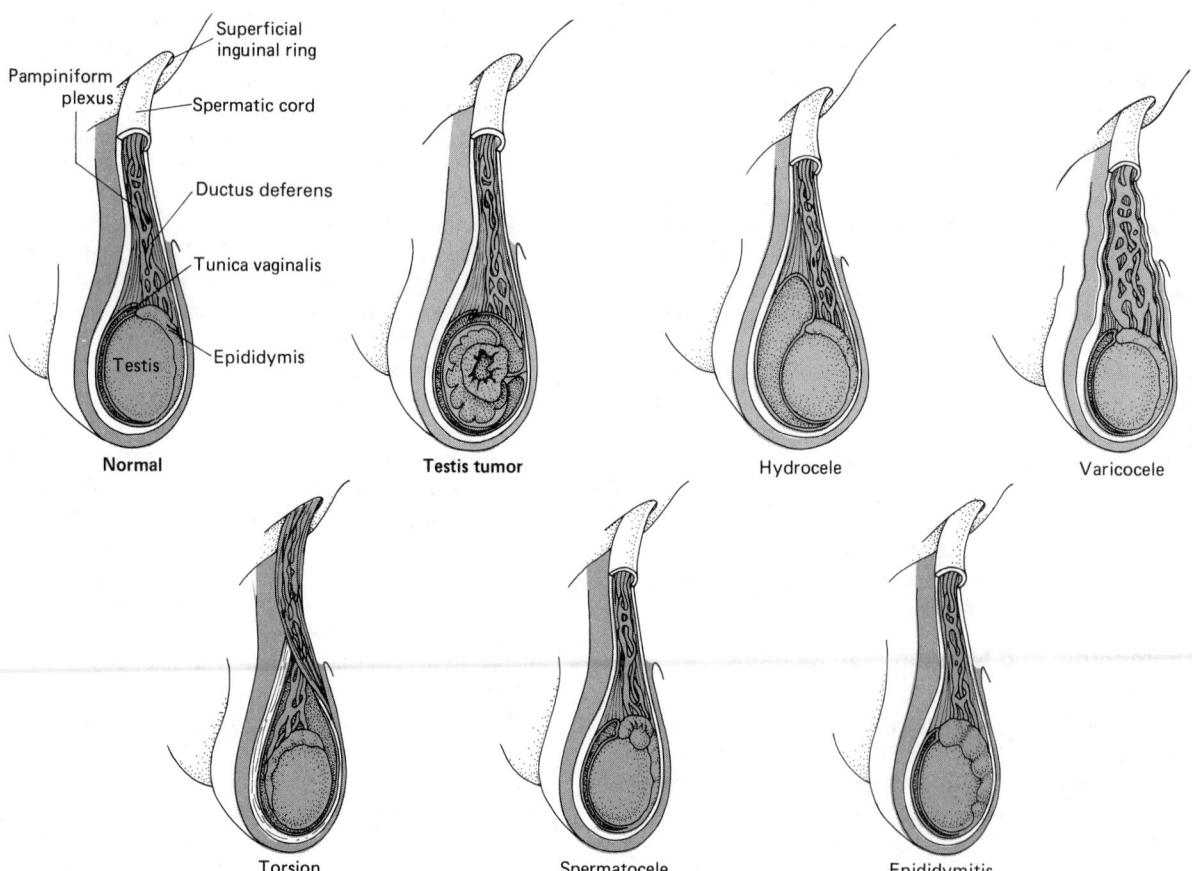

Fig. 49-4   Scrotal masses. (From Babayan RK: Evaluation of scrotal masses, Hosp Pract 20:51-52, 1985.)

minates with a bright light. No treatment is indicated unless the swelling becomes very large and uncomfortable in which case surgical drainage of the mass is done.

Spermatocele. A *spermatocele* is a firm, sperm-containing cyst of the epididymis that is visible with transillumination. The cause is unknown. Surgical removal is the treatment, and it is important for the client to be able to distinguish this cyst from cancer when performing self-examination.

Varicocele. A *varicocele* is a dilatation of the veins that drain the testes. The scrotum feels wormlike when palpated. The cause of the problem is unknown. The varicocele is usually located on the left side of the scrotum as a consequence of retrograde blood flow from the left renal vein. Surgery is indicated if the client is infertile, since persistent varicoceles are associated with 40% to 50% of the causes of infertility.

Torsion. Although rare, *torsion*, which involves a twisting of the testes and epididymis, is seen most commonly at puberty. This problem usually follows some form of strenuous exercise. Torsion constitutes a surgical emergency. The client experiences pain, tenderness, nausea, and vomiting, but urinary complaints, fever, and WBCs or bacteria in the urine are usually not found. The pain does not subside with rest or elevation of the scrotum.

Tumors of the testes

Significance and etiology. Testicular tumors make up about 0.7% of all forms of cancer of the male. They occur in 2 per 100,000 males per year, with the peak age of incidence between 20 and 40 years of age.[16] Testicular tumors are much more common in clients who have had undescended testicles (cryptorchidism).

Testicular tumors may develop from the cellular components of the testis or from the embryonal precursors (germinal tumors). Nongerminal tumors are very rare and usually benign and can occur at any age. Germinal tumors are almost always malignant.

Pathophysiology. Germinal tumors may have a slow or rapid onset depending on the type. The client may notice a lump in his scrotum as well as scrotal swelling. The scrotal mass is usually nontender and very firm and cannot be transilluminated. Back pain or gynecomastia is associated with metastasis. Clients with germinal cell tumors produce increased amounts of human chorionic gonadotropin (HCG), which can be measured in the plasma.

The prognosis for clients with testicular cancer has improved, and 75% obtain complete remission of the disease if it is detected in the early stages.[16]

■ Therapeutic and Nursing Management of Testicular Cancer

As with many forms of cancer, survival of the client is closely associated with early recognition of the tumor. The scrotum is easily examined, and beginning tumors are usually palpable. The nurse should teach the client how to do a self-examination and should particularly focus on clients with a history of an undescended testis or a previous testicular tumor (Fig. 49-5).

The procedure for self-examination is not difficult. The

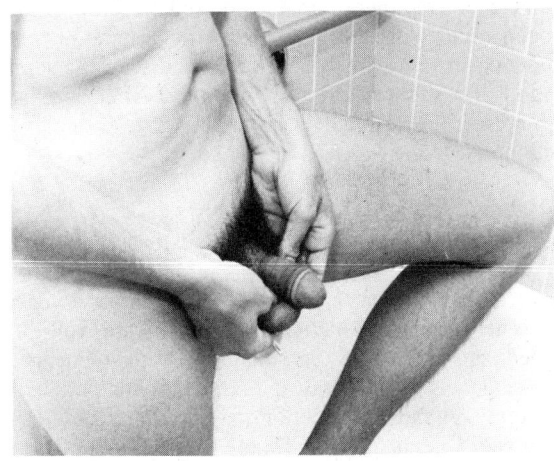

Fig. 49-5 Testicular self-examination.

client may indicate some reluctance to examine his own genitals. With encouragement the client can learn this simple procedure. He should be encouraged to do self-examinations frequently until he is comfortable with the procedure. The scrotum should be examined once a month.

The guidelines for self-examination of the scrotum are as follows:

1. Do the examination while the scrotum is warm because the testes retract toward the perineum when cold. During a shower or bath is a good time for examination.
2. Use both hands to palpate the scrotal contents. Roll each testicle between the thumb and first three fingers until the entire surface has been covered.
3. Identify the structures. The testicles should feel round and smooth, like hard-boiled eggs. Differentiate the testis from the epididymis. The epididymis is not as smooth as the egg-shaped testis. One testis may be larger than the other. Size is not as important as texture. Check for lumps, irregularities, pain in the testicles, and a dragging sensation. Locate the spermatic cord, which is usually firm and smooth.
4. Choose a consistent day of the month that is easy to remember to examine the testicles. The examination can be done more frequently if desired.
5. Notify the doctor at once if any abnormalities are found.

The nurse should make this procedure as simple and uncomplicated for the client as possible. The client needs to practice to develop familiarity with his body. However he wishes to become familiar is correct for him.

Therapeutic management of testicular cancer involves surgical removal of the affected testis and the cord and resection of the regional and paraaortic lymph nodes. Radiation of the remaining lymph nodes and single or multiple chemotherapeutic agent regimens such as bleomycin, vincristine, cisplatin, and vinblastine are also used after surgery depending on the histological conditions and disease stage.

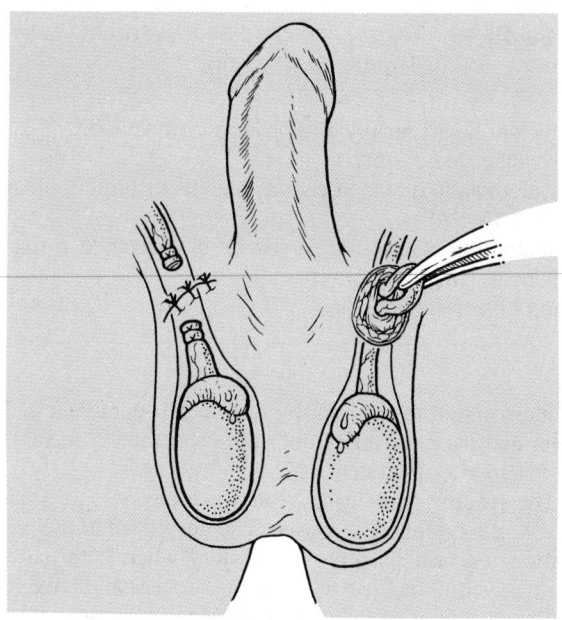

Fig. 49-6 Vasectomy procedure.

SEXUAL FUNCTIONING
Vasectomy

Vasectomy is the bilateral surgical ligation and/or resection of the ductus deferens performed for the purpose of sterilization (Fig. 49-6). The procedure requires only 15 to 30 minutes and is usually performed with the client under local anesthesia on an outpatient basis. Vasectomy is considered a permanent form of sterilization, although some successful reversals *(vasovasotomy)* have been reported.

After vasectomy the client will not notice any difference in the quantity of the ejaculate, since its major component is seminal fluid. The client will need to use an alternative form of contraception until semen examination reveals no sperm. This usually requires at least 10 ejaculations or 6 weeks to evacuate sperm distal to the anastomotic site. Sperm cells continue to be produced by the testes but are absorbed by the body rather than passing through the ductus deferens. In rare instances there may be a spontaneous reanastomosis of the ductus deferens, resulting in restoration of fertility.

Vasectomy does not affect the production of hormones, ejaculation, or the physiological mechanisms related to sexuality. Occasionally postoperative hematoma and swelling of the scrotum occur. Psychological adjustment may be a problem after surgery. It may be very difficult for the client to separate vasectomy from castration at a subconscious level. Some men may develop erectile dysfunction or may feel the need to become much more sexually active than they were in the past to prove their masculinity. Careful discussion of the procedure and its outcome before the surgery can be helpful in detecting clients who may have problems with psychological adjustment. Surgery should be delayed for these clients.

Erectile Dysfunction

Significance. Data show that 1 out of every 10 men in the United States experiences erectile dysfunction.[17] The problem is increasing in all segments of the sexually active male population. In younger men the increase is attributed to an increase in substance abuse, such as recreational drugs and alcohol. Middle-aged men are being affected by modern medical technology such as major organ transplants, bypass surgeries, and chemotherapeutic agents. The older population (men over the age of 70) are living longer, fuller lives and expect to remain sexually active, regardless of any existing medical conditions. Stress factors associated with modern lifestyles are affecting every part of the age continuum and contribute greatly to the psychological causes of erectile failure.[17-20]

Pathophysiology. Erectile dysfunction is the inability to attain or maintain an erect penis that allows satisfactory sexual performance. This problem occurs at some time for almost all sexually active males. The problem can occur at any age, although it is most common among males between the ages of 55 and 65 years. When the problem occurs during more than 25% of sexual encounters, the client needs intervention.

Erection is a vasocongestive engorgement of the corpora cavernosa and the corpus spongiosum of the penis. Problems occur when these spaces fail to fill when desired or when they empty before orgasm. Two classifications of erectile dysfunction are *primary dysfunction,* in which the client has never been able to have an adequate erection with any type of sexual experience, and *secondary dysfunction,* in which the client has lost the ability to perform or is able to have an erection in only a particular way. Some men can only have an erection with a full bladder or masturbation; others have an erection with a particular partner but not with others. A functional erection requires not only desire but also adequate blood supply, nerve innervation, and hormone balance.

Clinical manifestations and complications. The causes for the disorder may be physiological, psychological, or both (Table 49-8). The major complication of this problem is that the client's inability to perform sexually can cause stress in his interpersonal relationships and may preclude sex role functioning. Table 49-9 lists age-related changes in sexual performance. Explanation of these age-related changes may be all that is necessary to reassure an anxious older client in regard to his own sexuality.

Diagnostic studies. Rapid advances have been made in the diagnosis and treatment of erectile dysfunction in the past 5 years. Until 10 years ago, a man's problem was generally labeled as "psychological" unless he had severe diabetes or total paralysis. With the advent of modern technology, 50% to 80% of the causes are being attributed to physiological reasons and can be determined by the diagnostic studies in Table 49-10.

Therapeutic management. The treatment for erectile dysfunction is based on the cause. Treatment of psychological causes of erectile dysfunction is usually done by a qualified therapist. The approach may be behavioral or psychological, or in some clients it may involve therapeu-

Table 49-8   Causes of Erectile Dysfunction

Psychogenic

Excessive stress in family, work, or interpersonal relationships
Depression
Fatigue
Fear of failure to perform

Vascular

Aortic aneurysm
Arteriosclerosis of pelvic blood vessels
Aortofemoral bypass

Neurological and nerve conduction

Electroshock therapy
Multiple sclerosis
Parkinson's disease
Peripheral neuropathic conditions
Sympathectomy
Tumors or transection of spinal cord
Trauma to spinal cord
Spina bifida
Central nervous system disorders

Genitourinary

Perineal or suprapubic prostatectomy
Postpriapism
Postkidney transplant
Cystectomy
Long-term dialysis
Phimosis
Varicocele
Hydrocele

Endocrine

Addison's disease
Diabetes mellitus
Obesity
Thyrotoxicosis
Myxedema
Pituitary tumor
Testosterone deficiency
High levels of prolactin

Cardiorespiratory

Angina pectoris
Myocardial infarction
Emphysema
Atherosclerosis
Postcardiac surgery

Anatomical

Congenital deformities of the penis (e.g., hypospadias)
Peyronie disease

Drug induced

Caffeine
Nicotine, marijuana, cocaine
Alcohol
Antihypertensives
Diuretics
Antidepressants
Major tranquilizers
Antineoplastic agents
Drugs for Parkinson's disease
Narcotics
Estrogens

Table 49-9   Age-Related Changes in Sexual Performance*

Time lag between perceiving sexual opportunity and full erection
Diminished size and rigidity of the penis at full erection
Increased time interval to ejaculation
Changed nature of ejaculation with less spurting and lessened intensity of feeling
Shortened period between ejaculation and flaccidity
Increase in time to next reaction to sexual stimulation

*For almost all men by the age of 45 to 50 years.

Table 49-10   Diagnostic Studies Related to Erectile Dysfunction

Complete health history and physical examination
Psychological evaluation
Blood profile (e.g., blood chemistries, testosterone, prolactin, PSA, PAP)
Vascular flow studies (e.g., injection of vasodilators, duplex Doppler, cavernosogram)
Sleep tumescence studies

tic intervention to temporarily restore self-confidence. The client and partner usually develop a satisfactory sexual relationship after treatment.

The specific problem is treated if a physiological cause of erectile dysfunction exists. The results of these interventions are usually quite satisfactory when both partners are involved in the decision-making process and have realistic expectations of the treatment. Many treatment options are available to the male experiencing erectile dysfunction due to physiological causes.

Pharmacological management. Whenever possible, collaboration should occur between the primary physician providing the medical care and the urologist treating the erectile dysfunction. Elimination of or substitution for a medication that causes erectile dysfunction (e.g., methyldopa, propranolol) is sometimes all that is necessary to alleviate the problem.

Yohimbine (Yocan), an oral medication, is a mild vasodilator and reported aphrodisiac. It is often used in conjunction with other forms of therapy and may serve to provide a placebo effect or boost the confidence of the client.

Testosterone therapy is administered as a pill, sublingual tablet, transdermal patch, or intramuscular (IM) injection. Careful evaluation of the man's serum testosterone level and prostate condition must precede introduction of this therapy. Administration of testosterone to a man with normal levels of hormone production may actually suppress the body's natural ability to produce testosterone. Testosterone is contraindicated in men with cancer of the prostate due to its ability to cause proliferation of the prostatic cancer cells.

Intracorporeal injection therapy is an innovative treatment option that is still considered experimental. A vasoactive medication (e.g., papaverine or prostaglandin E_1) is injected directly into the corporeal body by a 25 to 27 gauge syringe. Within 15 to 30 minutes an erection is obtained, which may last for up to 2 hours. The dose is regulated on a individual basis to prevent the side effect of priapism. Home injection therapy instruction is given to those men that are suitable candidates for the therapy.[20] The treatment is ineffective in men with severe vascular problems.

Aids or devices. Suction devices applied to the penis produce a vacuum within a cylinder, thereby pulling blood up into the corporeal bodies. A penile ring or other device placed around the base of the penis causes vasoconstriction and prevents detumescence (subsidence of swelling).[21]

Table 49-11 Types of Penile Prostheses

Type	Action
NONINFLATABLE	
Small-Carrion	Simple, nonmechanical de-
Finney	vices that provide firm-
Jonas-Silver	ness for penetration;
Mentor semirigid	surgically simple and eco-
American Medical Sys- tems 600	nomical; use of local an- esthesia; problems of
Duraphase	concealment
INFLATABLE	
Brantley-Scott (AMS-700)	Hydraulic devices that pro-
Mentor GFS	vide most natural erection
Uni-flate 1000	and detumescence and increase girth/diameter, more complex and ex- pensive, skill and dexter- ity necessary to inflate and deflate
SELF-CONTAINED	
Hydroflex	Compact devices that pro-
Omniphase	vide mid-range erection
Flexi-flate	properties, surgically sim- ple, most expensive

Special care must be taken in using these devices to prevent tissue damage. Suction devices are sometimes used in conjunction with intracorporeal injection therapy in those clients with moderate-to-severe venous leaks of the penile veins.

Some clients do not require penetration for satisfactory sexual expression and may use a vibrator or dildo (rubber penis). Clients experiencing temporary loss of erection or who are awaiting surgical interventions use a variety of methods to achieve sexual satisfaction. Sexual counselors or therapists acting as consultants provide support and offer alternative forms of sexual expression.

Electronic stimulators in the form of rectal probes provide direct stimulation to damaged nerve endings that innervate the sympathetic and parasympathetic pathways involved in producing an erection. Their primary use is in clients with spinal cord injuries and multiple sclerosis. Presently, the devices have limited availability.

Surgical interventions. When impotence arises from inadequate blood flow into the penis, revascularization of the corporeal bodies may be beneficial. If a venous leak occurs, ligation of the affected veins may provide a solution. Careful vascular diagnostic studies are completed first to determine whether the problem is insufficient blood flowing into the corporeal bodies or a rapid loss of blood from the area that prevents the maintenance of an erection. Bypass grafts and venous ligation have limited success in older men because of the rapid obstruction of the graft and the natural tendency to form collateral circulation around the ligated vessel.[22]

Penile implants have provided surgical management of erectile dysfunction for more than 20 years.[23] The paired devices are implanted into the corporeal bodies to provide an erection firm enough for penetration. The three basic types of implants are the noninflatable (semirigid), the inflatable (two- and three-piece systems), and the self-contained devices (Table 49-11). All provide a usable erection and should be chosen carefully based on the client's mental and physical capabilities, surgical risk factors, personal lifestyle, and insurance and financial resources. The ability to satisfy both partners should also be considered.

The surgical procedure may be done on an outpatient basis, with clients being monitored at home by home care nurses. Recovery time varies from 6 to 8 weeks. Clients considered to be at high risk for complications include those with uncontrolled diabetes and those with severe circulatory problems. Clients should be advised that a prosthesis will not restore ejaculation or tactile sensations if they were absent before surgery. Sexual counseling is often recommended before and after surgery to deal with unrealistic expectations and restore communication techniques.

■ Nursing Management of Erectile Dysfunction

The client experiencing erectile dysfunction requires a great deal of emotional support for both himself and his partner. Men often do not feel comfortable discussing their problems with other men because of society's expectations of a man's sexual abilities. The man may experience and demonstrate isolation from support systems, and he may also lose self-esteem, which can eventually lead to loss of role functions.

The client needs reassurance that confidentiality will be maintained. In conjunction with therapeutic treatment, it often becomes necessary to provide counseling and therapy for the couple to establish realistic expectations and develop meaningful communication patterns. The majority of men wait an average of 2 years before seeking medical assistance. They are often highly motivated and expect immediate solutions to their problems. The health care team should provide a support system and accurate information as soon as possible.

Pain management of clients experiencing surgical interventions generally consists of administration of prescribed analgesics and elevation and application of ice to the scrotum for the first 48 hours postoperatively. The normal course for healing ranges from 4 to 6 weeks. Resumption of sexual activities before complete healing may result in infection, extrusion, erosion, or rupture. Clients should also be instructed to use a water-soluble lubricant and approach penetration slowly and at a comfortable angle.

Infertility

The male is the cause of infertility in about one third of childless marriages. Infertility can be due to disorders of the hypothalamic-pituitary system, disorders of the testes, and abnormalities of the ejaculatory system. Endocrine causes of male infertility, although rare, are listed in Table 49-12. A careful health history, including sexual practices, and a physical examination are the initial diagnostic mea-

Table 49-12 Endocrine Causes of Male Infertility

Androgen excess	Hyperthyroidism
Diabetes mellitus	Hypothyroidism
Estrogen excess	Hypogonadism
Glucocorticoid excess	Hyperprolactinemia

sures in an infertility study. Examination can disclose a varicocele, a treatable cause of male infertility. The use of drugs with a known effect on testicular function such as chemotherapy drugs, ketoconazole, Azulfidine, and cimetidine should also be documented.

The first test in an infertility study is a semen analysis. Additional tests helpful in determining the etiology include plasma testosterone and serum LH and follicle-stimulating hormone (FSH) measurements. A testicular biopsy may be necessary to differentiate between ductal obstruction and maturation arrest. The specific cause of infertility is often not determined.

The nurse should be concerned and tactful in dealing with the male client undergoing infertility studies. For many men, fertility and masculinity are equated. The nurse must be sensitive to the problem of gender identity with the infertile male. Infertility can seriously strain a marriage, and the couple may require counseling if conception will never be possible. (Female infertility is discussed in Chapter 48.)

C ase Study

TESTICULAR CANCER

Jon is a 20-year-old man. One morning while showering, he noticed a firm, nontender nodule on his left testis. He thought nothing of the nodule, but over the next 3 months he became increasingly worried, because the nodule was becoming larger. After careful examination the nurse practitioner at the college student health office referred Jon to a urologist that afternoon. Jon was hospitalized that evening, and results of surgical biopsy confirmed the diagnosis of embryonal testicular cancer.
The recommended treatment for Jon included surgical removal of the testis and the cord along with resection of the regional and paraaortic lymph nodes. He was told that he should also undergo radiation and chemotherapy after surgery.

Discussion questions

1. What are the key signs and symptoms of testicular cancer?
2. What are the types of testicular cancer?
3. What are Jon's chances for survival?
4. How could Jon's chances for complete recovery have been enhanced?
5. Design a teaching plan to prepare this client to successfully perform genital self-examination.

R eview Questions

The number of the question corresponds to the same-numbered objective at the beginning of the chapter.
1. The major risk factor currently identified for the development of BPH is
   a. multiple sexual partners
   b. smoking
   c. frequent urinary tract infections
   d. age
2. Prevention of bladder spasms immediately after prostatectomy is best done by
   a. forcing fluids
   b. keeping the catheter free of clots
   c. elevating the head of the bed
   d. having the client ambulate
3. The nurse can inform the client that after vasectomy the client will be
   a. immediately sterile
   b. unable to ejaculate in a normal manner
   c. unable to contract venereal diseases
   d. able to resume his usual sexual functioning
4. The nurse can decrease the client's discomfort over care involving his reproductive organs by
   a. assuring privacy for care
   b. making sure that the client understands the terminology being used for his body parts
   c. maintaining a nonjudgmental attitude toward his sexual practices
   d. all the above

REFERENCES

1. Sapozink MD and others: Transurethral hyperthermia for benign prostatic hyperplasia: preliminary clinical results, J Urol 143:944, 1990.
2. Linder A and others: Local hyperthermia of the prostate gland for the treatment of benign prostatic hypertrophy and urinary retention: a preliminary report, Br J Urol 60:567, 1987.
3. Reddy PK and others: Balloon dilation of the prostate for treatment of benign hyperplasia, Urol Clin North Am 13:529-534, 1988.
4. Reddy PK, Wasserman N, and Sidi AA: Balloon dilation of the prostate: can it help the patient with BPH? Contemp Urol, Feb-Mar 1989, pp 44-53.
5. Orandi A: Transurethral incision of prostate compared with transurethral resection of prostate in 132 matching cases, J Urol 138:810-815, 1987.
6. Li MK and Ng ASM: Bladder neck resection and transurethral resection of the prostate: a randomized prospective trial, J Urol 138:807, 1987.
7. Walsh PC: Radical pelvic surgery with preservation of sexual function, Ann Surg 208:391-400, 1987.
8. Walsh PC: Radical prostatectomy, preservation of sexual function, cancer control: the controversy, Urol Clin North Am 14:663-673, 1987.
9. Gluck R, Cohen M, and Warner R: Transrectal ultrasound in early detection of clinical stage A prostate cancer, Urology 31:58-61, 1989.
10. Lee F, Torp-Pederson ST, and McLeary RD: Diagnosis of prostate cancer by transrectal ultrasound, Urol Clin North Am 16:663-673, 1989.
11. Gluck R, Cohen M, and Warner R: Transrectal ultrasound in early detection of clinical stage A prostate cancer, Urology 34:58-61, 1989.

12. Scardino PT and others: Staging of prostate cancer: the value of ultrasonography, Urol Clin North Am 16:713-734, 1989.
13. Hardeman SW, Wake RW, and Soloway MS: Two new techniques for evaluating prostate cancer: the role of prostate-specific antigen and transrectal ultrasound, Postgrad Med 86:197-198, 201, 204, 1989.
14. Weidner W, Schiefer HG, and Krauss H: Role of *Chlamydia trachomatis* and mycoplasms in chronic prostatitis, a review, Urol Int 43:167-173, 1988.
15. Crawford ED and Dawkins CA: Cancer of the penis. In Skinner DG and Tieskovsky G, eds: Diagnosis and management of genitourinary cancer, Philadelphia, 1988, WB Saunders Co, 549-563.
16. Skinner DG and Lieskowsky DG: Management of early stage non-seminomatous germ cell tumors of the testis. In Skinner DG and Tieskovsky DG, eds: Diagnosis and management of genitourinary cancer, Philadelphia, 1988, WB Saunders Co, 516-523.
17. Berger RE and Berger D: Biopotency: a guide to sexual success, Emmaus, Penn, 1987, Rodale Press, pp 1-16.
18. Kaye KW: Impotence: a current understanding and approach, J Enterostom Ther 14:117-124, 1987.
19. Meredith C: ROMP: a self-help group for impotent men, Am Urol Assoc Allied J 6:7-8, 1985.
20. Lue TF and Zorgniotti AW: Patient guide: treatment for impotence, Med Aspects Human Sexuality 21:29-30, 1987.
21. Nadig PW, Ware JC, and Blumoff R: Noninvasive device to produce and maintain an erection-like state, Urology 27:126-131, 1986.
22. Williams G and others: Diagnosis and treatment of venous leakage: a curable cause of impotence, Br J Urol 61:151-155, 1988.
23. Bretan PN: History of the prosthetic treatment of impotence, Urol Clin North Am 16:1-5, 1989.

SECTION VIII REFERENCES

BOOKS

Adler M, ed: Diseases in the homosexual male, New York, 1988, Springer-Verlag.
Bardin CW: Current therapy in endocrinology and metabolism, vol 3, ed 3, St Louis, 1988, The CV Mosby Co.
Becker KL and Bilezikian JP, eds: Principles and practice of endocrinology and metabolism, Philadelphia, 1990, JB Lippincott Co.
Brownlee M and Sherwood LM: Diabetes mellitus and its complications, St Louis, 1990, Mosby–Year Book, Inc.
Dittmar SS: Rehabilitation nursing: process and application, St Louis, 1989, The CV Mosby Co.
Falk SA, ed: Thyroid disease: endocrinology, surgery, nuclear medicine, and radiotherapy, New York, 1990, Raven Press.
Fogel CT and Lauver D: Sexual health promotion, Philadelphia, 1990, WB Saunders Co.
Friessen SR and Thompson NW, eds: Surgical endocrinology: clinical syndromes, ed 2, Philadelphia, 1990, JB Lippincott Co.
Guthrie DW, Hinnen D, and Deshetler E: Diabetes education: a core curriculum for health professionals, Chicago, 1988, American Association for Diabetes Educators.
Kase N, Weingold A, and Gershenson D: Principles and practice of clinical gynecology, ed 2, New York, 1990, Churchill Livingstone, Inc.
Kerstein MD, ed: Diabetes and vascular disease, Philadelphia, 1990, JB Lippincott Co.
Keye WR Jr, ed: Laser surgery in gynecology and obstetrics, ed 2, Chicago, 1990, Year Book Medical Publishers.
Lubinski R: Dementia and communication, St Louis, 1990, Mosby–Year Book, Inc.
MacLennan WJ and Pedea NR: Metabolic and endocrine problems in the elderly, New York, 1989, Springer-Verlag.
McLaughlin DS, ed: Lasers in gynecology, Philadelphia, 1991, JB Lippincott Co.
Meeting the standards: a manual for completing the American Diabetes Association application for recognition of diabetes patient education programs, Alexandria, Va, 1989, American Diabetes Association.
Mitchell GW Jr and Bassett LW, eds: The female breast and its disorders, Baltimore, 1990, Williams & Wilkins.
Montague DK: Disorders of male sexual function, Chicago, 1988, Year Book Medical Publishers.
Noone RB: Plastic and reconstructive surgery of the breast, St Louis, 1990, Mosby–Year Book, Inc.
Parish L and Gschnaet F: Sexually transmitted diseases: a guide for clinicians, New York, 1989, Springer-Verlag.
Rifkin H and Porte D Jr, eds: Ellenberg and Rifkin's diabetes mellitus: theory and practice, ed 4, New York, 1990, Elsevier Science Publishing Co, Inc.
Robertson D and others: Clinical practice in sexually transmissible diseases, ed 2, New York, 1989, Churchill Livingstone, Inc.
Scott J and others: Dansforth's obstetrics and gynecology, ed 6, Philadelphia, 1990, JB Lippincott Co.
Skinner DG and Lieskowsky G: Diagnosis and management of genitourinary cancer, Philadelphia, 1988, WB Saunders Co.
Speroff L, Glass R, and Kase N: Clinical gynecologic endocrinology and fertility, ed 4, Baltimore, 1989, Williams & Wilkins.

JOURNALS

Baker D and others: Clinical evaluation of a new herpes simplex virus ELISA: rapid diagnostic test for herpes simplex virus, Obstet Gynecol 73:322, 1989.
Baker D and others: One year suppression of frequent recurrences of genital herpes with oral acyclovir, Obstet Gynecol 73:84, 1989.
Bertorelli AM: Nutrition counseling: meeting the needs of ethnic clients with diabetes, Diabetes Educ 16:285, 1990.
Booth DE and Morris CL: Hypeparathyroidism: the overlooked disorder, J Gerontol Nurs 16:16, 1990.
Cagno JM: Diabetes insipidus, Crit Care Nurse 9:86, 1989.
Cawley M, Kostic J, and Cappello C: Informational and psychosocial needs of women choosing conservative surgery/primary radiation for early stage breast cancer, Cancer Nurs 13:90, 1990.
Centers for Disease Control: Continuing increase in infectious syphilis—United States, MMWR 37:35, 1988.
Centers for Disease Control: 1989 STD treatment guidelines, MMWR 38:1, 1989.
Connell E: Barrier contraceptives, Clin Obstet Gynecol 32:377, 1989.
Crooks CE and Jones SD: Educating women about the importance of breast screenings: the nurse's role, Cancer Nurs 12:161, 1989.
Dellasega C: Self-care for the elderly diabetic, J Gerontol Nurs 16:16, 1990.
Dunne CF: Hormonal therapy for breast cancer, Cancer Nurs 11:288, 1988.
Edwards J: Lasers in gynecology, Nurs Clin North Am 25:673, 1990.
Eichhorst B: Contraception, Prim Care 15:437, 1988.
Ensign J, Rowe J, and Kowalski K: Premenstrual syndrome: etiology and treatment possibilities, AORN J 47:962, 1988.
Enterline J and Leonardo J: Condylomata acuminata, Nurse Pract 14:9, 1988.
Estey Al, Tan MH, and Mann K: Follow-up intervention: its effect on compliance behavior to a diabetes regimen, Diabetes Educ 16:291, 1990.
Francis B: Hypothyroidism, Adv Clin Care 5:29, 1990.

Galuk D: The nurse (as) diabetes educator, Adv Clin Care 5:27, 1990.

Gray ME: Factors related to practice of breast self-examination in rural women, Cancer Nurs 13:100, 1990.

Hahn R and others: Prevalence of HIV infection among intraveous drug users in the United States, JAMA 261:2677, 1989.

Higgs DJ: The patient with testicular cancer: nursing management of chemotherapy, Oncol Nurs Forum 17:243, 1990.

Hoops S: Renal and retinal complication in insulin-dependent diabetes mellitus: the art of changing the outcome, Diabetes Educ 16:221, 1990.

Kapila R and Kloser P: Women and AIDS: an overview, Med Asp Human Sex 22:92, 1988.

Kaplan A: Endometrial carcinoma, Hosp Med 25:79, 1989.

Kreisberg RA, Rose LI, and Russo GJ: Skin signs in endocrine disease, Patient Care 23:73, 1989.

Ladenson PW and Ragland G: Endocrine emergencies, Patient Care 22:36, 1988.

Lamb MA: Psychosexual issues: the woman with gynecologic cancer, Semin Oncol Nurs 6:237, 1990.

Levin ME: Diabetic foot lesions: pathogenesis and management, J Enterostomal Ther 17:29, 1990.

McKeon V: Cruel myths and clinical facts about menopause, RN 52:52, 1989.

Melman A: Evaluation and management of erectile dysfunction, Surg Clin North Am 68:965, 1989.

Michael SR and Sabo CE: Nursing management of the diabetic patient receiving nutritional support, Focus Crit Care 17:331, 1990.

Mohler JL and others: Fine-needle core and aspiration biopsy: a new method for diagnosis of prostatic carcinoma, Cancer 63:1846, 1989.

Monier M and Laird M: Contraceptives: a look at the future, AJN 4:497, 1989.

Montague DK: Penile prosthesis: an overview, Urol Clin North Am 16:7, 1989.

Nettina S: When patients with genital herpes turn to you for answers, Nurs 19:61, 1989.

Nielsen BB and East D: Advances in breast cancer: implications for nursing care, Nurs Clin North Am 25:365, 1990.

Northouse LL: The impact of breast cancer on patients and husbands, Cancer Nurs 12:276, 1989.

Olson RL and Mitchell ES: Self-confidence as a critical factor in breast self-examination, JOGNN 18:476, 1989.

Reddy PK and Wasserman N: A new technique for outpatient transurethral dilation of the prostate. Paper presented at the eighty-fourth annual meeting of the American Urological Association, Dallas, 1989.

Roberto PL: Diabetic nephropathy: causes, complications, and considerations, Crit Care Nurs Clin North Am 2:55, 1990.

Rosenberg CS: Wound healing in the patient with diabetes mellitus, Nurs Clin North Am 25:247, 1990.

Rosenthal M: Menopausal mood disorders, Hosp Med 25:120, 1989.

Schultz PN: Hypopituitarism in patients with a history of irradiation to the head and neck area: diagnoses and implications for nursing, Oncol Nurs Forum 16:823, 1989.

Tackenberg JN: Cryolumpectomy: another option for breast cancer, Nursing 20:32J, 1990.

Ternulf-Nyhlin K: A contribution of qualitative research to a better understanding of diabetic patients, J Adv Nurs 15:796, 1990.

Treybig M: Primary dysmenorrhea or endometriosis? Nurs Pract 14:8, 1989.

Tulman L and Fawcett J: A framework for studying functional status after diagnosis of breast cancer, Cancer Nurs 13:95, 1990.

Washington A and others: Oral contraceptives, *Chlamydia trachomatis* infection and pelvic inflammatory disease, JAMA 253:2246, 1988.

Woolard DG, Larson JL, and Hudson L: Screening for *Chlamydia trachomatis* at a university health service, JOGNN 18:145, 1989.

Yeates S and Blaufuss J: Managing the patient in diabetic ketoacidosis, Focus Crit Care 17:240, 1990.

Yeatts RP and Clontz DM: Graves' ophthalmopathy, J Ophthalmic Nurs Technol 9:126, 1990.

ORGANIZATIONS

American Association of Diabetes Educators
500 North Michigan Avenue
Suite 1400
Chicago, IL 60611

American College of Nurse-Midwives
1522 K Street, NW, Suite 1000
Washington, DC 20005

American Diabetes Association
505 8th Avenue
New York, NY 10018

Nurse Association of the American College of Obstetricians and Gynecologists
409 12th Street, SW
Washington, DC 20024

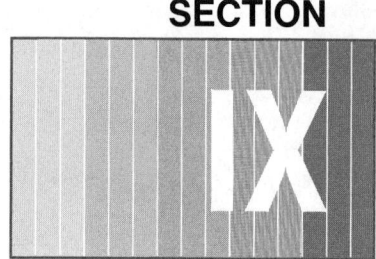
PROBLEMS RELATED TO MOVEMENT AND COORDINATION

CHAPTER

50

Nursing Assessment
Neurological System

Judith M. Ozuna

L earning Objectives

1. Describe the functions of neurons and neuroglia.
2. Explain the electrochemical aspects of nerve impulse transmission.
3. Explain the anatomical location and function of the cerebrum, brainstem, cerebellum, spinal cord, peripheral nerves, and cerebrospinal fluid.
4. Identify the major arteries supplying the brain.
5. Describe the functions of the 12 cranial nerves.
6. Compare the functions of the two divisions of the autonomic nervous system.
7. Describe age-related changes in the neurological system and differences in assessment findings.
8. Identify the significant subjective and objective data related to the nervous system that should be obtained from a client.
9. Describe the techniques used in the physical assessment of the nervous system.
10. Differentiate normal from common abnormal findings of a physical assessment of the nervous system.
11. Describe the purpose, significance of results, and nursing responsibilities related to diagnostic studies of the nervous system.

STRUCTURES AND FUNCTIONS OF THE NERVOUS SYSTEM

The human nervous system is a highly specialized system responsible for the control and integration of the body's many activities. The nervous system can be divided into the central nervous system (CNS) and the peripheral nervous system (PNS). The CNS consists of the brain and spinal cord. The PNS consists of the cranial and spinal nerves and peripheral components of the autonomic nervous system. Before considering higher-order structures and their functions, cellular elements and nerve impulse transmission are discussed.

Cells of the Nervous System

The nervous system is made up of two types of cells, *neurons* and *neuroglia*. Although neuroglial cells are more numerous, they are mainly supportive to the neuron, the primary functional unit of the nervous system. Neurons are nonmitotic; that is, they do not replicate and cannot re-

place themselves if they are irreversibly damaged. Neuroglia, however, are mitotic and can replicate themselves.

Neurons. The neurons of the nervous system come in many different shapes and sizes, but they all share common characteristics: (1) excitability, or the ability to generate a nerve impulse; (2) conductivity, or the ability to transmit the impulse to other portions of the cell; and (3) the ability to influence other neurons, muscle cells, and glandular cells by transmitting nerve impulses to them.

A typical neuron consists of a cell body, an axon, and several dendrites (Fig. 50-1). The *cell body* containing the nucleus and cytoplasm is the metabolic center of the neuron. *Dendrites* are short processes extending from the cell body. They receive nerve impulses from the axons of other neurons and conduct impulses toward the cell body. The nerve *axon* projects varying distances from the cell body, ranging from several micrometers to more than a meter. Its function is to carry nerve impulses to other neurons or to end organs. The end organs are smooth and striated muscles and glands. Axons may be myelinated or unmyelinated. Many axons present in the CNS and the PNS are covered by a segmentally interrupted myelin sheath composed of a white, lipid substance that acts as an insulator

Reviewed by Marylou Muwaswes, R.N., M.S., Assistant Clinical Professor, School of Nursing, University of California, San Francisco, California.

for the conduction of impulses. Generally, the smaller fibers are unmyelinated.

Neuroglia. Neuroglia, or glial cells, provide support, nourishment, and protection to neurons and make up about 85% of the cells of the CNS. Different types of glial cells have specific functions. *Oligodendroglia* produce the myelin sheath of nerve fibers in the CNS (Schwann cells myelinate nerve fibers in the periphery) and are primarily found in the white matter of the CNS. *Astrocytes* are found primarily in gray matter; however, their physiological importance is not well understood. They are thought to provide structural support to neurons and their delicate processes, to form the blood-brain barrier with the endothelium of the blood vessels, and to play an indirect role in synaptic transmission (conduction of impulses between neurons). In damaged brain, they appear to act as phagocytes for neuronal debris, and they proliferate to form scar tissue (gliosis) in the CNS. *Ependymal cells* line the brain ventricles and aid in the secretion of cerebrospinal fluid. *Microglia* are relatively rare in normal CNS tissue. They migrate to areas of CNS damage and act as phagocytes to remove neural debris. Most tumors in the CNS are composed of neuroglia because neurons do not have the capacity to replicate themselves.

Nerve Regeneration

Once a neuron dies, it is not replaced. At birth the human body contains all the nerve cells it will ever have. The body cannot make new nerve cells. If only the axon of the nerve cell is damaged, however, the cell attempts to repair itself. When damaged, all nerve cells attempt to grow back to their original destinations by sprouting many branches from the damaged ends of their axons. Unfortunately, excessive gliosis (scarring) in the CNS prevents the new nerve branches from making their former connections to other neurons.

In the PNS (outside the brain and spinal cord), injured nerve fibers can successfully regenerate by growing within the protective myelin sheath of the supporting Schwann cells if the cell body is intact. Chances for normal regeneration are greatest when the separated ends of the peripheral nerves are close or the nerve sheaths are preserved. Complete functional recovery is likely if the separated nerves are correctly reattached.[1]

Nerve Impulse

The purpose of a neuron is to initiate and receive messages about events both within and outside the body. The initiation of a neuronal message (nerve impulse) involves the generation of an *action potential,* which is an electrical impulse that travels along the axon. When the impulse reaches the end of the nerve fiber, it is transmitted across the junction between nerve cells (synapse) by a chemical interaction involving neurotransmitters. This chemical interaction generates another action potential in the next neuron. These events are repeated until the nerve impulse reaches its destination.

Action potential. When nerve cells are in a resting (nonactive) state, the inside of the cell carries a negative electric charge relative to the outside of the cell. Sodium

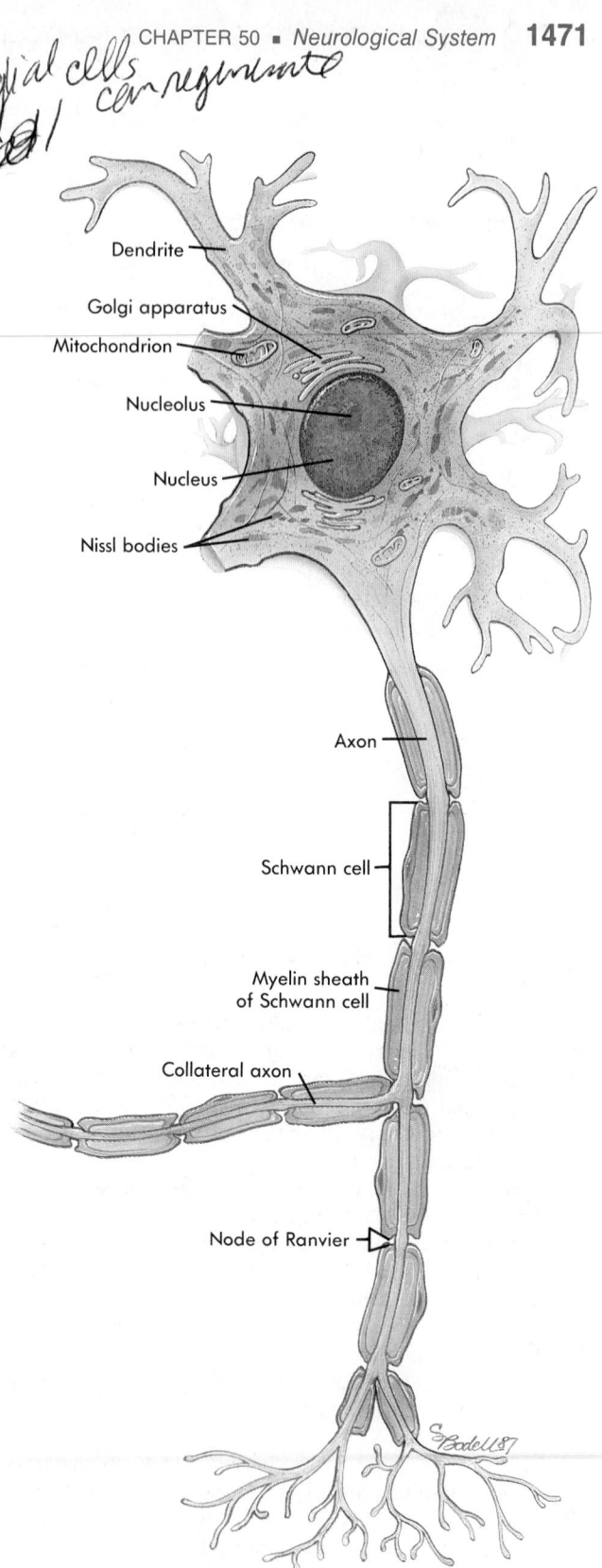

Fig. 50-1 Structural features of neurons: dendrites, cell body, and axons. (From Seeley R, Stephens T, and Tate P: Anatomy and physiology, St Louis, 1989, Times Mirror/ Mosby College Publishing, p 339.)

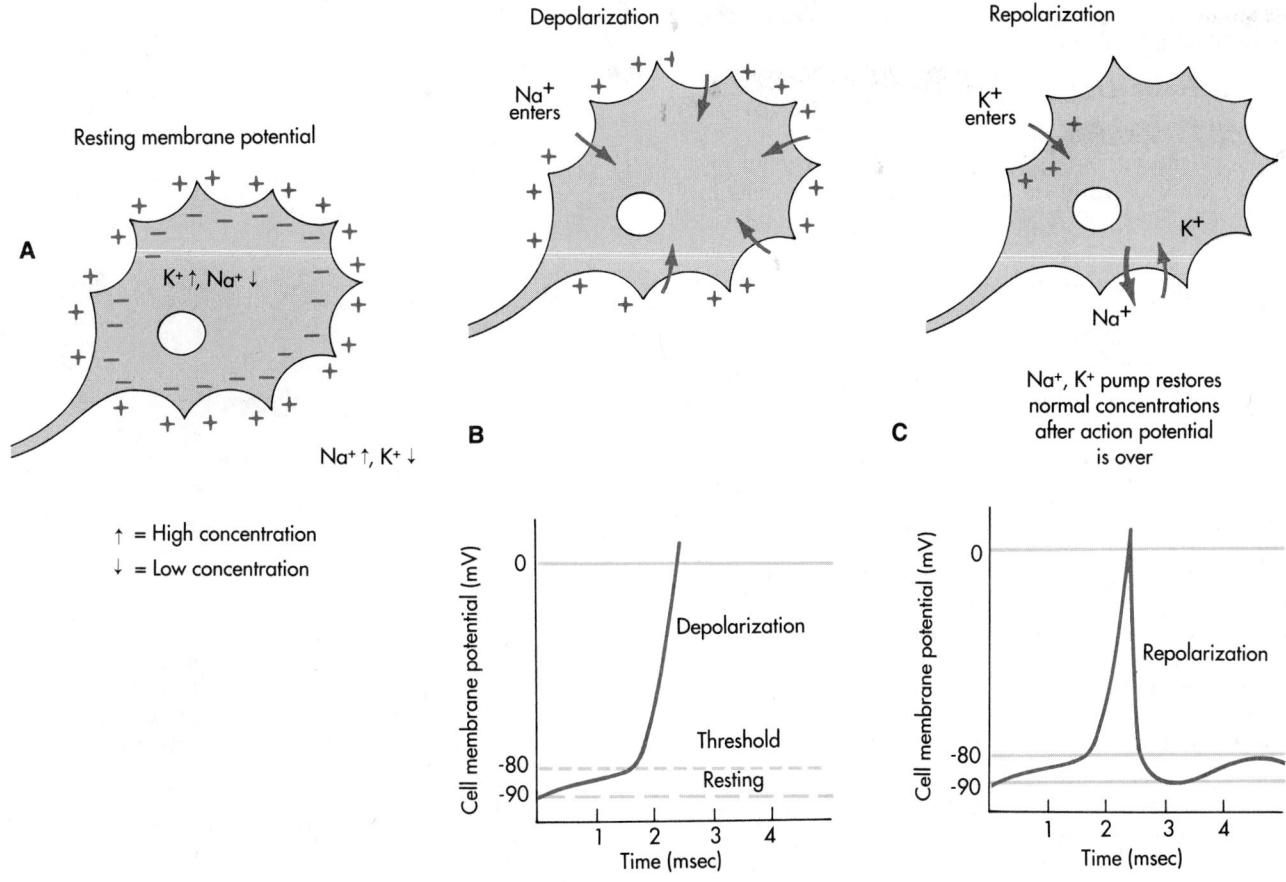

Fig. 50-2 **A,** Resting membrane potential. **B,** Depolarization. **C,** Repolarization.

ions (Na$^+$) are in high concentration outside the cell, and potassium (K$^+$) ions are in high concentration inside the cell. The difference in electric charge across the cell membrane is called the *resting membrane potential*. An action potential occurs when a stimulus is of sufficient magnitude to alter the membrane potential.

During the action potential the cell membrane becomes more permeable to Na$^+$, allowing the ions to move readily into the cell. The resulting change in the voltage across the cell membrane is called *depolarization*. The inside of the cell temporarily becomes positive relative to the outside. After rapid depolarization, *repolarization* (the inside of the cell becoming negative relative to the outside) is facilitated by a slower increase in K$^+$ permeability, which in turn is caused by the depolarization associated with entry of Na$^+$ into the cell (Fig. 50-2). The whole process of depolarization and repolarization of the nerve cell membrane takes only 1 to 2 milliseconds. With repeated action potentials the cells accumulate Na$^+$. An active metabolic process within the cell is required to move Na$^+$ out of and K$^+$ back into the cell. This metabolic process is accomplished by the Na$^+$, K$^+$ pump that acquires energy from the breakdown of adenosine triphosphate (ATP).

The action potential has an all-or-none quality; that is, once the cell depolarizes enough to cause an action potential, the size of the action potential is independent of the strength of the stimulus. When an action potential is initi-

ated at one point of a neuron, it is transmitted along the axon without losing its intensity.

The myelination of nerve axons facilitates the conduction of an action potential. Many peripheral nerve axons have gaps, called *nodes of Ranvier,* at regular intervals in the myelin sheath surrounding them. An action potential traveling down one of these axons hops from node to node without traversing the insulated membrane segment between nodes. making the action potential travel much faster than it would otherwise. This is called *saltatory* (hopping) *conduction.* In an unmyelinated fiber the wave of depolarization traverses the entire length of the axon, each portion of the membrane becoming depolarized in turn. Fig. 50-3 compares nerve impulse transmission of myelinated and unmyelinated fibers.

Synapse. A synapse is the structural and functional junction between two neurons. It is the point at which the nerve impulse is transmitted from one neuron to another. The essential structures of synaptic transmission are a *presynaptic terminal,* a *synaptic cleft,* and a *receptor site* on the postsynaptic cell (Fig. 50-4). When a nerve impulse reaches the end of the axon (presynaptic terminal), it causes release of a chemical substance (neurotransmitter) from tiny vesicles within the terminal. This release depends on influx of calcium (Ca^{2+}), which occurs when the action potential traveling down the axon causes depolarization of the nerve terminal. The neurotransmitter then

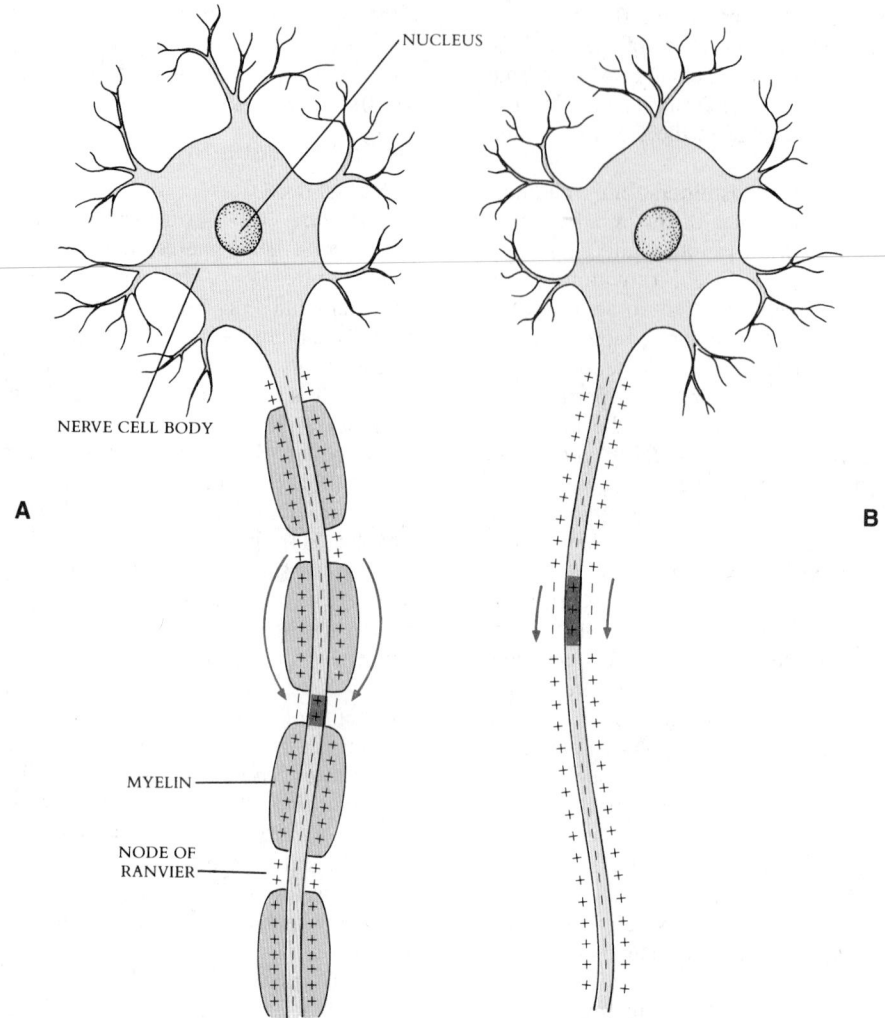

Fig. 50-3 **A,** Saltatory conduction. **B,** Depolarization in an unmyelinated fiber. (From Raven PH and Johnson GB: Biology, ed 2, St Louis, 1989, Times Mirror/Mosby College Publishing.)

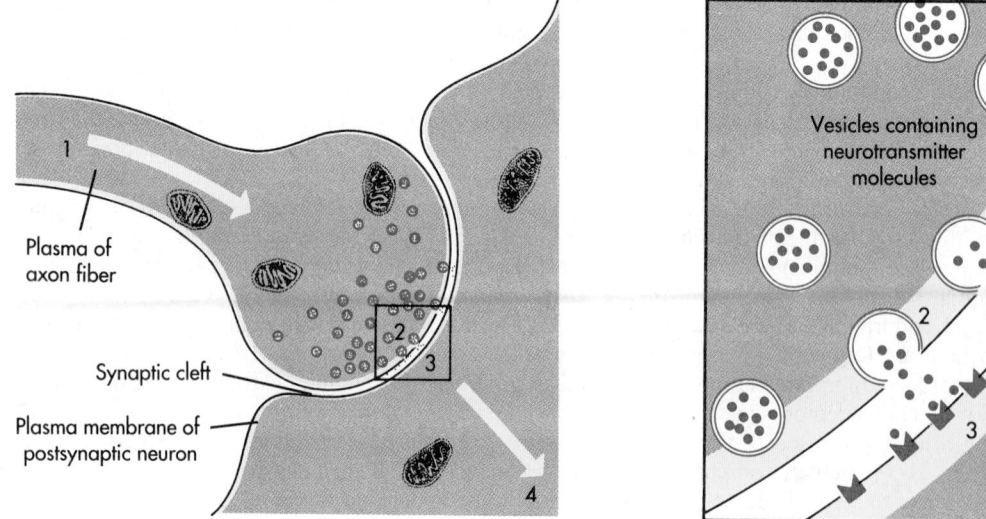

Fig. 50-4 A synapse. *1,* Presynaptic action potential; *2,* vesicles release neurotransmitter molecules; *3,* postsynaptic receptors; *4,* postsynaptic action potential.

crosses the microscopic space (synaptic cleft) between the two neurons and attaches to receptor sites of the receiving (postsynaptic) neuron. This causes a change in the permeability of the postsynaptic cell membrane to specific ions such as Na^+ and K^+ and a change in the electrical potential of the membrane.

Neurotransmitters. Neurotransmitters are chemical agents involved in the transmission of an impulse across the synaptic cleft. Some neurotransmitters are *excitatory:* they cause an increase in Na^+ permeability within the cell membrane, increasing the likelihood that an action potential will be generated. This type of synaptic input results in an excitatory postsynaptic potential. Other neurotransmitters are *inhibitory:* they cause an increase in permeability of K^+ and chloride ions (Cl^-), decreasing the likelihood that an action potential will be generated. This type of synaptic input results in an inhibitory postsynaptic potential.

Each of the hundreds to thousands of synaptic connections of a single neuron has an influence on that neuron. The net effect of the input is sometimes excitatory and sometimes inhibitory. The net effect of the synaptic input depends on the number of presynaptic neurons that are releasing neurotransmitters on the postsynaptic cell and their type of influence (excitatory or inhibitory). A presynaptic cell that releases an excitatory neurotransmitter does not always cause the postsynaptic cell to depolarize enough to generate an action potential. However, when many presynaptic cells release excitatory neurotransmitters on a single neuron, the sum of their input is enough to generate an action potential. The presynaptic input can be summed by the number of presynaptic cells firing *(spatial summation)* and/or by the frequency of firing of a single presynaptic cell *(temporal summation)*. Summation usually occurs by both events.

The effect of a excitatory or inhibitory neurotransmitter depends on which ion channels in the postsynaptic membrane are influenced by that neurotransmitter. In mammals the neurotransmitters that are known to generally have an excitatory influence are acetylcholine, norepinephrine, serotonin, dopamine, and histamine. The ones that generally have an inhibitory influence are γ-aminobutyric acid, glutamate, and glycine.

Neurotransmitters continue to combine with the receptor sites at the postsynaptic membrane until they are inactivated by enzymes, taken up by the presynaptic endings, or diffused away from the synaptic region. In addition, neurotransmitters can be affected by drugs and toxins, which can modify their function or block their attachment to receptor sites on the postsynaptic membrane.

Interesting neurotransmitter substances discovered in 1975 are the enkephalins and endorphins. These are endogenous peptides, all of which are fragments of the hormonal protein β-lipotropin, that have morphinelike properties. After the discovery of opiate receptor sites in the brain and spinal cord during drug abuse research, investigators searched for endogenous opiatelike compounds. These compounds were assumed to exist because there were naturally occurring receptors for them. The compounds were isolated, and their chemical makeup was identified from brain extracts. They were proved to have morphinelike properties by the fact that their analgesic-an-

esthetic effects were reversed by the administration of naloxone, a narcotic antagonist. The pituitary gland contains high levels of β-endorphin. Enkephalins are known to exist in the intestine as well as in the CNS.[2]

Central Nervous System

Spinal cord

Structure. Major structural components of the CNS are the cerebral hemispheres, the cerebellum, the brainstem, and the spinal cord. The spinal cord is continuous with the brainstem and exits from the cranial cavity through the foramen magnum. A cross section of the spinal cord (Fig. 50-5) reveals gray matter that is centrally located in an H shape and is surrounded by white matter. Gray matter contains the cell bodies of voluntary motor neurons and preganglionic autonomic motor neurons, as well as cell bodies of association neurons *(interneurons)*. Certain subdivisions within the gray matter have been identified (see Chapter 51). White matter contains the axons of the ascending sensory and descending (suprasegmental) motor fibers. The myelin surrounding these fibers gives them their white appearance. Specific ascending and descending pathways in the white matter can be identified. The spinal pathways or tracts are named for the point of origin and the point of destination (e.g., spinocerebellar tract [ascending], corticospinal tract [descending]). The major spinal pathways are presented in Fig. 50-5.

Ascending tracts. In general, the ascending tracts carry specific sensory input to higher levels of the CNS. This input comes from special sensory endings (receptors) in the skin, muscles and joints, viscera, and blood vessels, and it enters the spinal cord by way of the dorsal roots of the spinal nerves. The *fasciculus gracilis* and the *fasciculus cuneatus* (commonly called the *dorsal* or *posterior columns*) carry impulses concerned with touch, deep pressure, vibration, position sense, and kinesthesia (appreciation of movement). The *spinocerebellar tracts* carry subconscious information about muscle tension and body position to the cerebellum for coordination of movement. This information is not consciously perceived. The *spinothalamic tracts* carry pain and temperature sensations.

Although the functions of these pathways are generally accepted, other ascending tracts may also carry sensory modalities. The symptoms of various neurological diseases suggest that additional pathways for touch, position sense, and vibration exist.

Descending tracts. Descending tracts carry impulses that are responsible for muscle movement. Among the most important descending tracts are the *corticobulbar* and *corticospinal tracts* collectively, called the *pyramidal tract*. These tracts carry volitional impulses from the cortex to the cranial and peripheral nerves, respectively. Another group of descending motor tracts carries impulses from the *extrapyramidal system,* which includes all motor systems (except the pyramidal system) concerned with voluntary movement. It includes descending pathways originating in the brainstem, the basal ganglia, and the cerebellum. The motor output exits the spinal cord by way of the ventral roots of the spinal nerves.

Lower and upper motor neurons. Lower motor neurons (LMNs) are the final common pathway for higher mo-

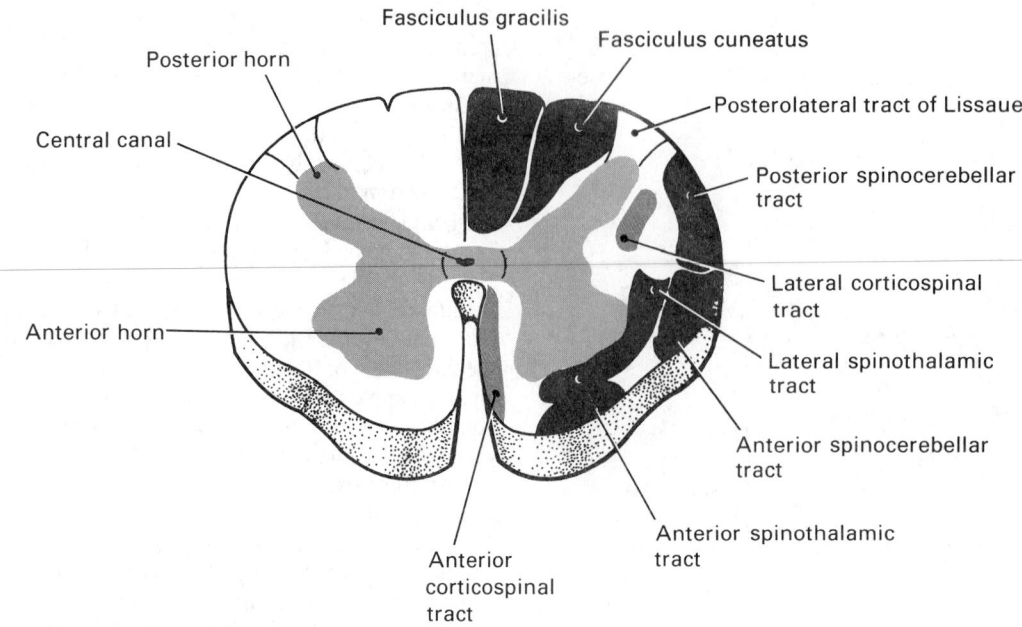

Fig. 50-5 Schematic cross section of spinal cord showing arrangement of gray matter and white matter. Major ascending (sensory) tracts of the white matter are indicated in *black;* major descending (motor) tracts are in *red.*

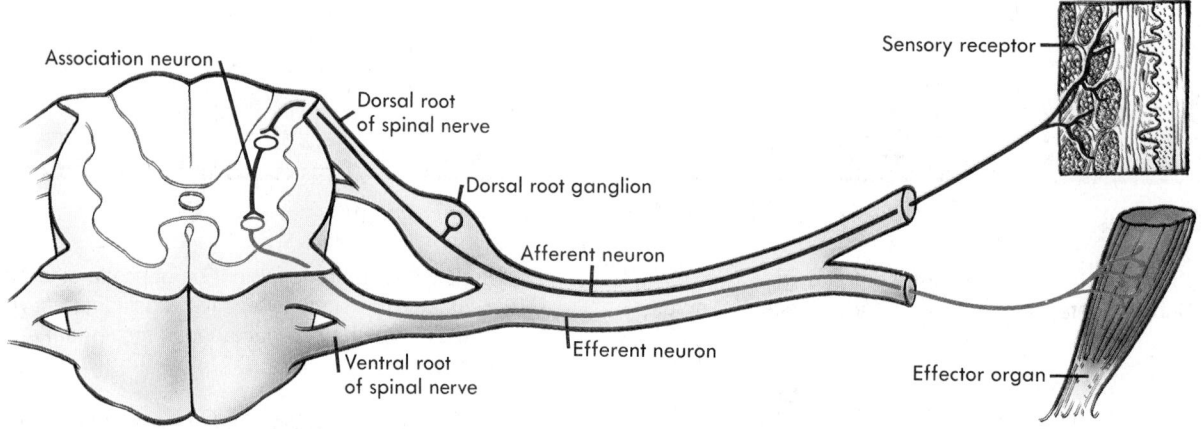

Fig. 50-6 Basic diagram of a reflex arc, including the sensory receptor, afferent neuron, association neuron, efferent neuron, and effector organ. (From Seeley R, Stephens T, and Tate P: Anatomy and physiology, St Louis, 1987, Times Mirror/Mosby College Publishing, p 354.)

tor centers to influence skeletal muscle, the effector organ for movement. The cell bodies of LMNs, which send axons to innervate skeletal muscles of the arms, trunk, and legs, are located in the anterior horn of the corresponding segments of the spinal cord (e.g., cervical segments contain LMNs for the arms). LMNs for skeletal muscles of the eyes, face, mouth, and throat are located in the corresponding segments of the brainstem. These cell bodies and their axons make up the somatic motor components of the cranial nerves. LMN lesions generally cause weakness or paralysis, denervation atrophy, hyporeflexia or areflexia, and decreased (flaccid) muscle tone.

Upper motor neurons (UMNs) include all supraspinal motor neurons that influence skeletal muscle movement. These neurons are located in the brainstem and cerebral cortex. UMN lesions generally cause weakness or paralysis, disuse atrophy, hyperreflexia, and increased (spastic) muscle tone.

Reflex arc. A *reflex* may be defined as an involuntary response to a stimulus. The components of a monosynaptic reflex arc (the simplest kind of reflex arc) are a receptor organ, an afferent neuron, an effector neuron, and an effector organ (e.g., skeletal muscle). The afferent neuron synapses with the efferent neuron in the gray matter of the spinal cord. A reflex arc is shown in Fig. 50-6. More complex reflex arcs have other neurons in addition to the affer-

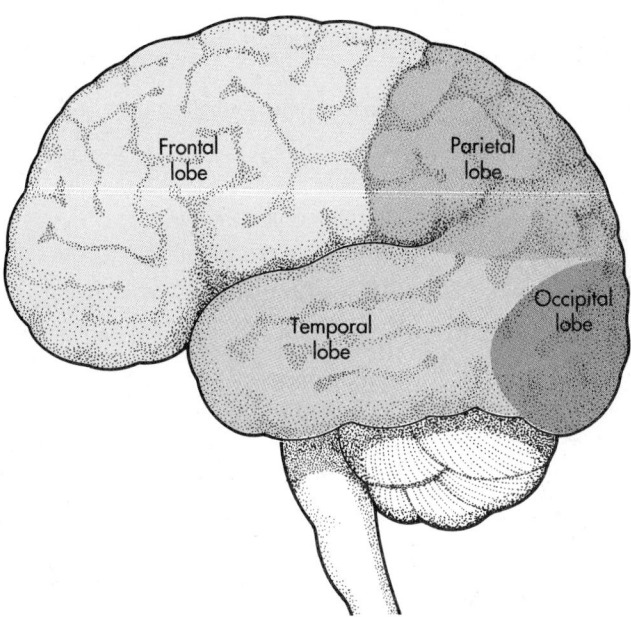

Fig. 50-7 Right hemisphere of cerebrum, lateral surface, showing major lobes of the brain.

ent neuron influencing the effector neuron. In the spinal cord, reflex arcs play an important role in maintaining muscle tone, which is the basis for body posture.[3]

Brain

The brain can be divided into three major components—cerebrum, brainstem, and cerebellum.

Cerebrum. The cerebrum is composed of the right and left hemispheres. Both hemispheres can be further divided into four major lobes: frontal, temporal, parietal, and occipital (Fig. 50-7). These divisions are useful to delineate portions of the neocortex (gray matter), which makes up the outer layer of the cerebral hemispheres. Neurons in specific parts of the neocortex are essential for various highly complex and sophisticated aspects of mental functioning, such as language, memory, and appreciation of visual-spatial relationships.

The functions of the cerebrum are multiple and complex. Specific areas of the cerebral cortex are associated with specific functions. Table 50-1 summarizes the location and function of the parts of the cerebrum.

Brainstem. The brainstem includes the midbrain, the pons, and the medulla (Fig. 50-8). Ascending and descending fibers pass through the brainstem going to and from the cerebrum and cerebellum.

The cell bodies, or nuclei, of cranial nerves III through XII are in the brainstem, as in the *reticular formation*, a

Table 50-1 Location and Function of the Parts of the Cerebrum

Part	Location	Function
Cortical areas		
Motor		
Primary	Precentral gyrus	Controls initiation of movement on opposite side of body
Supplemental	Anterior to precentral gyrus	Facilitates proximal muscle activity, including activity for stance and gait, and spontaneous movement and co-ordination
Sensory		
Somatic	Postcentral gyrus	Registers body sensations (e.g., temperature, touch, pressure, pain) from opposite side of body
Visual	Occipital lobe	Registers visual images
Auditory	Superior temporal gyrus	Registers auditory inputs
Association areas	Parietal lobe	Integrates somatic and special sensory inputs
	Posterior temporal lobe	Integrates visual and auditory inputs for language comprehension
	Anterior temporal lobe	Integrates past experiences
	Anterior frontal lobe	Controls higher-order processes (e.g., judgment, insight, reasoning, problem solving, planning)
Basal ganglia	Near lateral ventricles of both cerebral hemispheres	Controls and facilitates learned and automatic movements
Thalamus	Below basal ganglia	Relays sensory and motor inputs to cortex and other parts of cerebrum
Hypothalamus	Below thalamus	Regulates endocrine and autonomic functions (e.g., feeding, sleeping, emotional and sexual response)
Limbic system	Lateral to hypothalamus	Influences affective (emotional) behavior and basic drives such as feeding and sexual behavior

diffusely arranged group of neurons and their axons that extends from the medulla to the thalamus and hypothalamus. Its functions include relaying sensory information, influencing excitatory and inhibitory control of spinal motor neurons, and controlling vasomotor and respiratory activity. The reticular activating system is part of the reticular formation and is the regulatory system for arousal, a component of consciousness.

The vital centers concerned with respiratory, vasomotor, and cardiac function are located in the medulla. The brainstem also contains the centers for sneezing, coughing, hiccupping, vomiting, sucking, and swallowing.

The basal ganglia, the thalamus, the hypothalamus, and the limbic system are also located in the cerebrum. The basal ganglia are a group of paired structures located centrally in the cerebrum and midbrain; most of them are on both sides of the thalamus. The function of the basal ganglia is to modulate the initiation, execution, and completion of voluntary movements and automatic movements associated with skeletal muscle activity, such as swinging of the arms while walking, swallowing saliva, and blinking.

The thalamus lies directly above the brainstem (Fig. 50-9) and is the major relay center for sensory and other afferent (i.e., cerebellar) inputs to the cerebral cortex. The hypothalamus is located just inferior to the thalamus and

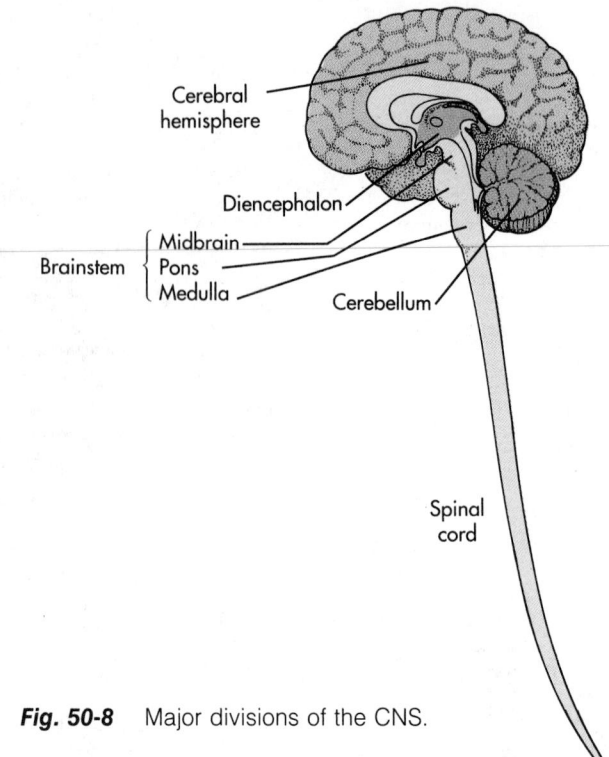

Fig. 50-8   Major divisions of the CNS.

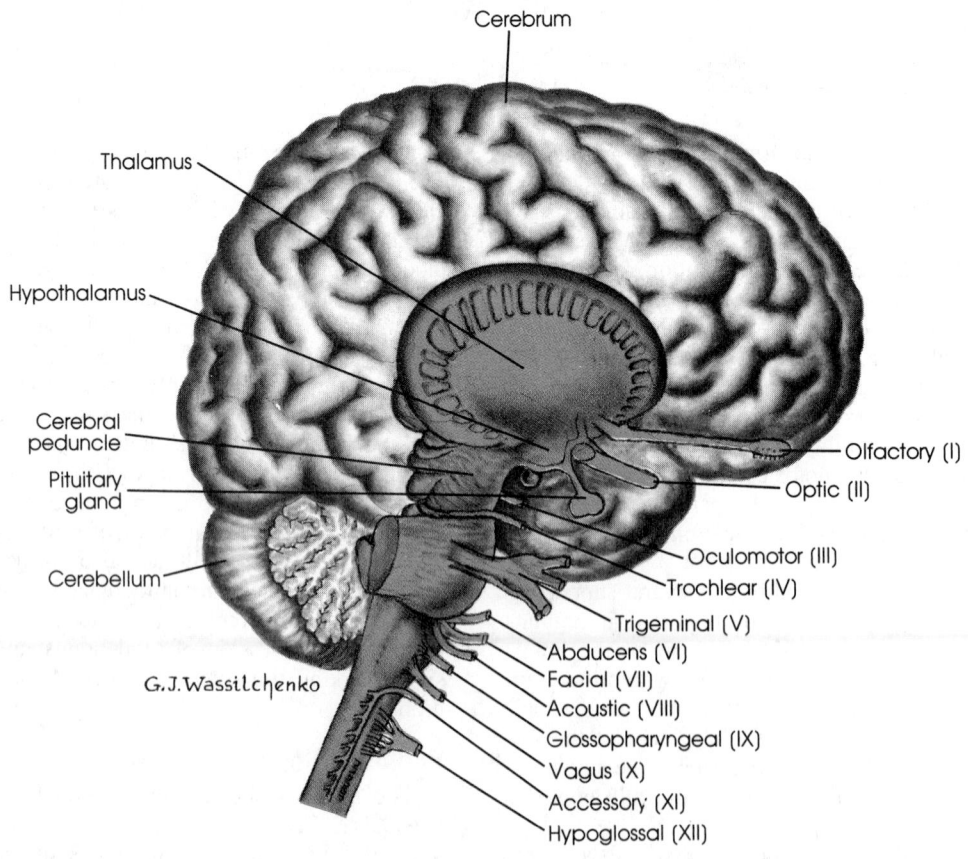

Fig. 50-9   The diencephalon (thalamus and hypothalamus) and cranial nerves. (From Rudy EB: Advanced neurological and neurosurgical nursing, St Louis, 1984, The CV Mosby Co.)

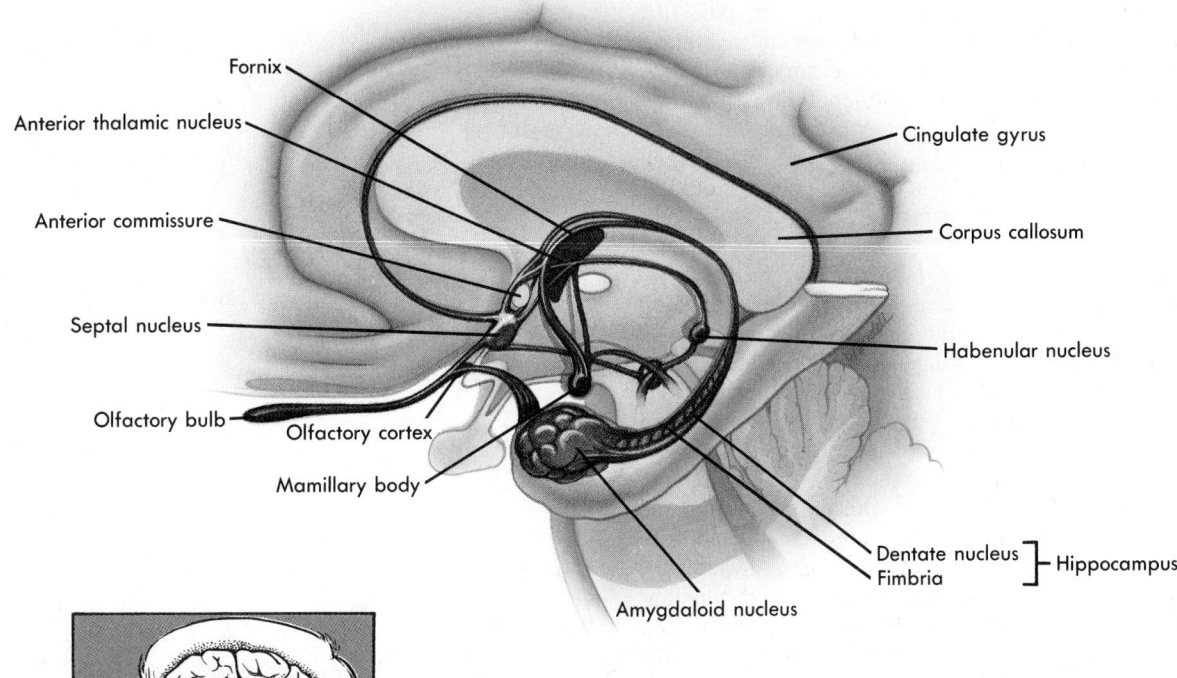

Fig. 50-10 Limbic system. (From Seeley R, Stephens T, and Tate P: Anatomy and physiology, St Louis, 1989, Times Mirror/Mosby College Publishing, p 378.)

slightly in front of the midbrain. It regulates the autonomic and the neuroendocrine systems. The limbic system is a phylogenetically old part of the human cerebrum. It is located near the inner surfaces of the cerebral hemispheres (Fig. 50-10) and is concerned with emotion, aggression, feeding behavior, and sexual response.

Cerebellum. The cerebellum is located in the posterior part of the cranial fossa, along with the brainstem, under the occipital lobe of the cerebrum. The function of the cerebellum is to coordinate voluntary movement and to maintain trunk stability and equilibrium. It influences motor activity by connecting to the motor cortex, brainstem nuclei, and their descending pathways. To perform these functions, the cerebellum receives information from the cerebral cortex, muscles, joints, and inner ear.

Ventricles and cerebrospinal fluid. Several supporting structures located within the CNS are important in regulating neuronal function and physical support of the brain. The *ventricles* are four fluid-filled cavities within the brain that connect with one another and with the spinal canal. The lower portion of the fourth ventricle becomes the spinal canal in the lower part of the brainstem. The spinal canal is located in the center and extends the full length of the spinal cord.

The ventricles and spinal canal are filled with an average of 135 ml of *cerebrospinal fluid* (CSF). CSF circulates within the subarachnoid space that surrounds the brain, brainstem, and spinal cord. This fluid provides cushioning for the brain and spinal cord, allows fluid shifts from the cranial cavity to the spinal cavity, and carries nutrients. The formation of CSF in the choroid plexus in the ventricles seems to involve both passive diffusion and active transport of substances.[4] CSF resembles an ultrafiltrate of blood plasma. Although CSF is continually being formed, many physiological factors influence its rate of formation. The CSF circulates throughout the ventricles and seeps into the subarachnoid space surrounding the brain and spinal cord. It is absorbed primarily through the arachnoid villi—tiny projections into the subarachnoid space—and into the intradural venous sinuses and eventually into the venous system. The analysis of CSF composition provides useful diagnostic information related to certain nervous system diseases. Measurement of CSF pressure is sometimes done in clients with actual or suspected intracranial diseases. Increases in intracranial pressure, indicated by increased CSF pressure, can lead to herniation of the brain and compression of vital brainstem structures. The signs marking this event are part of the herniation syndrome.

Peripheral Nervous System

The PNS includes all the neuronal structures that lie outside the CNS. It consists of cranial and spinal nerves, their associated ganglia (groupings of cell bodies), and portions of the autonomic nervous system.

Spinal nerves. The spinal cord can be seen as a series of spinal segments, one on top of another. In addition to the cell bodies, each segment contains a pair of dorsal (af-

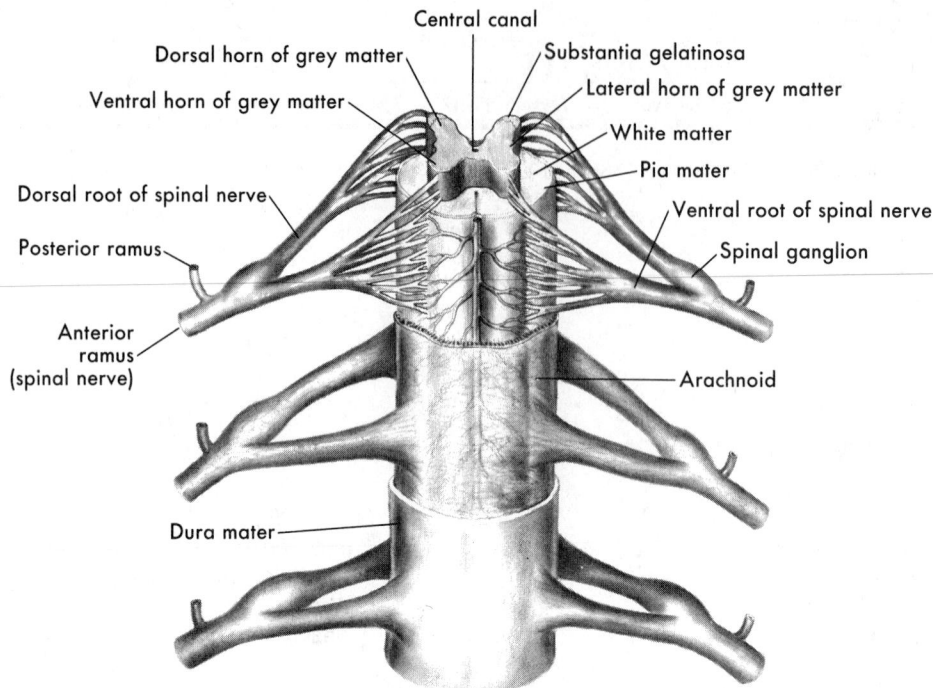

Fig. 50-11 Cross section of spinal cord showing attachments of spinal nerves. (From McCance K and Huether S: Pathophysiology: the biological basis for disease in adults and children, St Louis, 1990, The CV Mosby Co, p 363.)

ferent) sensory nerve fibers or roots and ventral (efferent) motor fibers or roots, which innervate a specific region of the neck, trunk, or limbs. This combined motor-sensory nerve is called a *spinal nerve* (Fig. 50-11). The cell bodies of the voluntary motor system are located in the anterior horn of the spinal cord gray matter. The cell bodies of the autonomic (involuntary) motor system are located in the anterolateral portion of spinal cord gray matter. The cell bodies of sensory fibers are located in the dorsal root ganglia just outside the spinal cord. On exiting the spinal column, each spinal nerve divides into *ventral* and *dorsal rami,* a collection of motor and sensory fibers that eventually go to peripheral structures (e.g., skin, muscle, viscera). The sympathetic ganglia are attached to the ventral rami of the spinal nerves by gray and white *rami communicantes.*

A *dermatome* is the area of skin innervated by the sensory fibers of a single dorsal root of a spinal nerve. A *myotome* is a muscle group innervated by the primary motor neurons of a single ventral root. These are simple components in the embryonic stage of human development. However, the dermatomes and myotomes of a given spinal segment overlap with those of adjacent segments in the adult because of the development of ascending and descending collateral branches of nerve fibers. The dermatomes give a general picture of somatic sensory innervation by spinal segments.

Cranial nerves. The cranial nerves (CNs) are the 12 paired nerves composed of cell bodies with fibers that exit from the cranial cavity. Unlike the spinal nerves, which always have both afferent sensory and efferent motor fibers, some CNs have only afferent and some only efferent fi-

bers; others have both. Table 50-2 summarizes the motor and sensory components of the CNs. Fig. 50-9 shows the position of the CNs in relation to the brain and spinal cord. Just as the cell bodies of spinal nerves are located in specific segments of the spinal cord, the nuclei of the CNs are located in specific regions (segments) of the brainstem. Exceptions are the nuclei of the olfactory nerves and the optic nerves: the primary cell bodies of the olfactory nerve are located in the nasal epithelium and those of the optic nerve are in the retina. CN XI is a spinal nerve, and its efferent fibers migrate upward before exiting the neuroaxis at the level of the medulla.

Autonomic nervous system. The autonomic nervous system (ANS) governs involuntary functions of cardiac muscle, smooth (involuntary) muscle, and glands. Until recently it was thought that these functions could not be consciously controlled. However, research in biofeedback and studies of Asian cultures indicate that many of these "involuntary" functions can be voluntarily affected.

The ANS is divided into two components, *sympathetic* and *parasympathetic,* which are anatomically as well as functionally different. These two systems function together to maintain a relatively balanced internal environment. The ANS is considered an efferent system and consists of a presynaptic neuron, a synapse, and a postsynaptic neuron.

The preganglionic cell bodies of the sympathetic nervous system (SNS) are located in spinal segments T1 to L2. The sympathetic ganglia, which contain the cell bodies of the postganglionic neurons, lie close to the spinal column, along the vertebral bodies in the rami communicantes. These ganglia and the connecting nerves are called

Table 50-2 Cranial Nerves

Nerve	Sensory Fibers			Motor Fibers		Functions
	Receptors	Cell Bodies	Termination	Cell Bodies	Termination	
I Olfactory	Nasal mucosa	Nasal mucosa	Olfactory bulbs (relay of neurons to olfactory cortex)			Sense of smell
II Optic	Retina	Retina	Nucleus in thalamus (lateral geniculate body), termination of some fibers in superior colliculus of midbrain			Vision
III Oculomotor	External eye muscles except superior oblique and lateral rectus	?	?	Midbrain (oculomotor nucleus and Edinger-Westphal nucleus)	External eye muscles except superior oblique and lateral rectus, termination of fibers from Edinger-Westphal nucleus in ciliary ganglion and then ciliary and iris muscles	Eye movements, regulation of size of pupil, accommodation, proprioception (muscle sense)
IV Trochlear	Superior oblique	?	?	Midbrain	Superior oblique muscle of eye	Eye movements, proprioception
V Trigeminal	Skin and mucosa of head, teeth	Gasserian ganglion	Pons (sensory nucleus)	Pons (motor nucleus)	Muscles of mastication	Sensations of head and face, chewing movements, muscle sense
VI Abducens	Lateral rectus	?	?	Pons	Lateral rectus muscle of eye	Abduction of eye, proprioception
VII Facial	Taste buds of anterior two thirds of tongue	Geniculate ganglion	Medulla (nucleus solitarius)	Pons	Superficial muscles of face and scalp	Facial expressions, secretion of saliva, taste
VIII Acoustic Vestibular branch	Semicircular canals and vestibule (utricle and saccule)	Vestibular ganglion	Pons and medula (vestibular nuclei)			Balance or equilibrium sense
Cochlear or auditory branch	Organ of Corti in cochlear duct	Spiral ganglion	Pons and medulla (cochlear nuclei)			Hearing

Modified from Anthony CP and Thibodeau GA: Textbook of anatomy and physiology, ed 12, St Louis, 1987, Times Mirror/Mosby College Publishing, pp 266-267.
?, Unknown.
*Not confirmed.

Table 50-2 Cranial Nerves—cont'd

Nerve	Sensory Fibers			Motor Fibers		Functions
	Receptors	Cell Bodies	Termination	Cell Bodies	Termination	
IX Glosso-pharyngeal	Pharynx; taste buds and other receptors of posterior one third of tongue	Jugular and pe-trous ganglia	Medulla (nucleus solitarius)	Medulla (nucleus ambiguus)	Muscles of phar-ynx	Taste and other sensations of tongue, swal-lowing move-ments, secretion of saliva, aid in reflex control of blood pressure and respiration
	Carotid sinus, carotid body	Jugular and pe-trous ganglia	Medulla (respira-tory and vaso-motor centers)	Medulla at junc-tion of pons (nucleus saliva-torius)	Otic ganglion and then parotid gland	
X Vagus	Pharynx, larynx, carotid body, thoracic and abdominal vis-cera	Jugular and no-dose ganglia	Medulla (nucleus, solitarius), pons (nucleus of cranial nerve V)	Medulla (dorsal motor nucleus)	Ganglia of vagal plexus and then muscles of pharynx, lar-ynx, thoracic and abdominal viscera	Sensations and movements of organs sup-plied (e.g., slowing of heart, increase in peristalsis, contraction of muscles for voice produc-tion)
XI Spinal accessory	?	?	?	Medulla (dorsal motor nucleus of vagus and nucleus ambig-uus)	Muscles of tho-racic and ab-dominal viscera and pharynx and larynx	Shoulder move-ments, turning movements of head, move-ments of vis-cera, voice production, proprioception*
				Anterior gray col-umn of first five or six cervical segments of spinal cord	Trapezius and sternocleido-mastoid muscle	
XII Hypo-glossal	?	?	?	Medulla (hypo-glossal nu-cleus)	Muscles of tongue	Tongue move-ments, proprio-ception*

the *paravertebral chain*. The major neurotransmitter re-leased by the postganglionic fibers of the SNS is norepi-nephrine, whereas the neurotransmitter released by the preganglionic fibers is acetylcholine.

In contrast, the preganglionic cell bodies of the para-sympathetic nervous system are located in the brainstem and the sacral spinal segments (S2 to S4). The parasympa-thetic ganglia are located in or near the structures that they innervate. Acetylcholine is the neurotransmitter released at both preganglionic and postganglionic nerve endings.

The ANS provides dual and often reciprocal innervation

to many structures. For example, the SNS increases the rate and force of the heartbeat and the parasympathetic nervous system decreases the rate and force. The SNS di-lates bronchi and bronchioles of the lungs, and the para-sympathetic nervous system constricts them. Some struc-tures are innervated by only one system (e.g., the hair fol-licles and the sweat glands, which are innervated only by the SNS). Table 50-3 compares the SNS and parasympa-thetic nervous system.

The result of SNS stimulation is activation of mecha-nisms required for "fight or flight," a mass response

Table 50-3 Sympathetic and Parasympathetic Nervous Systems

Visceral Effector	Effect of Sympathetic Nervous System*	Effect of Parasympathetic Nervous System†
Heart	Increase in rate and strength of heartbeat (β receptors)	Decrease in rate and strength of heartbeat
Smooth muscle of blood vessels		
Skin blood vessels	Constriction (α receptors)	No parasympathetic fibers
Skeletal muscle blood vessels	Dilatation (β receptors)	No parasympathetic fibers
Coronary blood vessels	Dilatation (β receptors)	No parasympathetic fibers
Abdominal blood vessels	Constriction (α receptors)	No parasympathetic fibers
Blood vessels of external genitals	Ejaculation (contraction of smooth muscle in male ducts (e.g., epididymis, ductus deferens)	Dilatation of blood vessels causing erection in male
Smooth muscle of hollow organs and sphincters		
Bronchi	Dilatation (β receptors)	Constriction
Digestive tract, except sphincters	Decrease in peristalsis (β receptors)	Increase in peristalsis
Sphincters of digestive tract	Contraction (α receptors)	Relaxation
Urinary bladder	Relaxation (β receptors)	Contraction
Urinary sphincters	Contraction (α receptors)	Relaxation
Eye		
Iris	Contraction of radial muscle, dilatation of pupil	Contraction of circular muscle, constriction of pupil
Ciliary	Relaxation, accommodation for far vision	Contraction, accommodation for near vision
Hairs (pilomotor muscles)	Contraction producing goose pimples or piloerection (α receptors)	No parasympathetic fibers
Glands		
Sweat	Increase in sweat (neurotransmitter, acetylcholine)	No parasympathetic fibers
Digestive (e.g., salivary, gastric)	Decrease in secretion of saliva; not known for others	Increase in secretion of saliva
Pancreas, including islets	Decrease in secretion	Increase in secretion of pancreatic juice and insulin
Liver	Increase in glycogenolysis (β receptors), increase in blood glucose level	No parasympathetic fibers
Adrenal medulla‡	Increase in epinephrine secretion	No parasympathetic fibers

Modified from Anthony CP and Thibodeau GA: Textbook of anatomy and physiology, St Louis, 1987, Times Mirror/Mosby College Publishing, p 313.
*Neurotransmitter is norepinephrine unless otherwise stated.
†Neurotransmitter is acetylcholine unless otherwise stated.
‡Sympathetic preganglionic axons terminate in contact with secreting cells of the adrenal medulla. Thus the adrenal medulla functions as a "giant sympathetic postganglionic neuron."

throughout the body. In contrast, the parasympathetic nervous system is geared to act in localized and discrete regions. It serves to conserve and restore the energy stores of the body.

Cerebral Circulation

The blood supply of the brain arises from the *internal carotid arteries* (anterior circulation) and the *vertebral arteries* (posterior circulation). Knowledge of the distribution of the major arteries of the brain and the area supplied is essential for understanding and diagnosing the signs and symptoms of cerebral vascular disease and trauma.

Each internal carotid artery supplies the ipsilateral hemisphere, whereas the basilar artery, formed by the junction of the two vertebral arteries, supplies structures within the posterior fossa (cerebellum and brainstem). The circle of Willis arises from the basilar artery and the two internal carotid arteries (Fig. 50-12). This vascular circle may act as a safety valve when differential pressures are present in these arteries. It also may function as an anastomotic pathway when occlusion of a major artery occurs. In general, the two *anterior cerebral arteries* supply the medial portion of the frontal lobes. The two *middle cerebral arteries* supply the outer portions of the frontal, parietal,

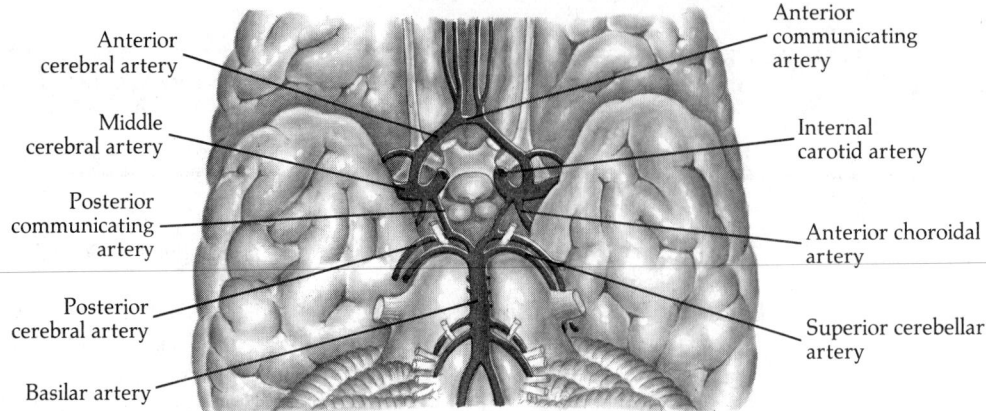

Fig. 50-12 Circle of Willis. (From Thompson JM and others: Mosby's manual of clinical nursing, ed 2, St Louis, 1989, The CV Mosby Co, p 263.)

and superior temporal lobes. The two *posterior cerebral arteries* supply the medial portions of the occipital and inferior temporal lobes. Venous blood drains from the brain through the dural sinuses, which form channels that drain into the two jugular veins.

Blood-brain barrier. The blood-brain barrier is a physiological barrier between blood capillaries and brain tissue. The structure of brain capillaries differs from that of other capillaries in certain ways. Some substances that normally pass readily into most tissues are prevented from entering brain tissue. This barrier protects the brain from certain potentially harmful agents while allowing nutrients and gases to enter. Because the blood-brain barrier affects the penetration of pharmaceutical agents, only certain drugs can enter the CNS from the bloodstream. Lipid-soluble compounds enter the brain easily, whereas water-soluble and ionized drugs enter the brain and spinal cord slowly.

Protective Structures

Meninges. The meninges are three layers of protective membranes that surround the brain and spinal cord. The thick *dura* forms the outermost layer, followed by the *arachnoid* and *pia*. The falx cerebri is a fold of the dura that separates the two cerebral hemispheres and prevents expansion of brain tissue in cases such as rapidly growing tumors and acute hemorrhage. The expanding brain must squeeze under this structure, causing displacement toward the side opposite the lesion. The tentorium cerebelli is a fold of dura that separates the cerebral hemispheres from the posterior fossa (which contains the brainstem and cerebellum). Expansion of mass lesions in the cerebrum force the brain to herniate through the opening created by the brainstem. This is referred to as *tentorial herniation*.

The arachnoid mater is a delicate, impermeable membrane that lies between the thick dura mater and the pia mater and directly covers the brain and spinal cord. The subarachnoid space lies between the arachnoid and pia mater. This space is filled with CSF. Structures passing to and from the brain and the skull or its foramina (holes through which blood vessels and nerves enter and exit the intracranial compartment) must pass through the subarach-

noid space. Therefore all cerebral arteries and veins lie in this space, as do the cranial nerves. A large subarachnoid space is in the region of the third and fourth lumbar vertebrae, which is the area penetrated to obtain CSF during a lumbar puncture. (The spinal cord itself ends between the first and second lumbar vertebrae.)

Skull. The bony skull protects the brain from external trauma. It is composed of 8 cranial bones and 14 facial bones.

The structure of the skull cavity explains the physiology of head injuries (see Chapter 53). Although the top and sides of the inside of the skull are relatively smooth, the bottom surface is uneven. It has many ridges, prominences, and foramina. The largest hole is the *foramen magnum*, through which the brainstem extends to the spinal cord. This foramen offers the only major space for the expansion of brain contents during increased intracranial pressure.

Vertebral column. The vertebral column protects the spinal cord, supports the head, and provides for flexibility. The vertebral column is made up of 33 individual vertebrae: 7 cervical, 12 thoracic, 5 lumbar, 5 sacral (fused into one), and 4 coccygeal (fused into one). Each vertebra has a central opening through which the spinal cord passes. The vertebrae are held together by a series of ligaments. Intervertebral disks occupy the spaces between vertebrae.

Effects of Aging on the Neurological System

The high rate of metabolic activity of neurons and their lack of replication make them particularly vulnerable to wear with age. One associated age-related change involves the decline in brain concentration of neurotransmitter substances. Age-related changes in the biosynthetic capabilities of neurons affect neuronal activity, changes in neurotransmitters, and changes in the neuronal membranes with which these neurotransmitters interact at synapses.[5]

Many changes in assessment result from age-related changes in the various components of the neurological system. Table 50-4 lists these changes and associated assessment differences.

Table 50-4

Age-Related Changes of the Neurological System and Differences in Assessment Findings

Component	Changes	Differences in Assessment Findings
CENTRAL NERVOUS SYSTEM		
Brain*	Reduction in cerebral blood flow and metabolism	Alterations in selected mental functioning
	Decrease in efficiency of temperature-regulating mechanism	Decrease in body temperature, impairment of ability to adapt to environmental temperature
	Decrease in number of neurotransmitters, disruption in integration as result of loss of neurons	Repetitive movements, tremors
PERIPHERAL NERVOUS SYSTEM		
Cranial and spinal nerves	Decrease in conduction time in some nerves	Decrease in reaction time in specific nerves
	Cellular degeneration, death of neurons	Decrease in speed and intensity of neuronal reflexes
	Decrease in oxygen supply, changes in basal ganglia caused by vascular changes	Changes in gait and ambulation (e.g., extrapyramidal, Parkinson-like gait); diminished kinesthetic sense
FUNCTIONAL DIVISIONS		
Motor	Decrease in muscle bulk	Diminished strength and agility
	Decrease in electrical activity	Decrease in reactions and movement time
Sensory†	Decrease in sensory receptors caused by degenerative changes and involution of fine corpuscles of nerve endings	Diminished sense of touch; inability to localize stimuli; decrease in appreciation of pain, touch, temperature, and peripheral vibrations
	Decrease in electrical activity	Slowing of or alteration in sensory reception
	Atrophy of taste buds	Signs of malnutrition, weight loss
	Degeneration and loss of fibers in olfactory bulb	Diminished sense of smell
	Degenerative changes in nerve cells in vestibular system of inner ear, cerebellum, and proprioceptive pathways in nervous system	Poor ability to maintain balance, widened gait
Reflexes	Possible decrease in deep tendon reflexes	Below-average reflex score
	Decrease in sensory conduction velocity as result of myelin sheath degeneration	Sluggish reflexes, slowing of reaction time
RETICULAR FORMATION		
Reticular activating system	Modification of hypothalamic function, reduction in stage IV sleep	Increase in frequency of spontaneous awakening together with tiredness, interrupted sleep, insomnia
AUTONOMIC NERVOUS SYSTEM		
SNS and ANS	Morphological features of ganglia, slowing of ANS response	Orthostatic hypotension, systolic hypertension

*See Table 4-2 for the effects of aging on adult mental functioning.
†Specific changes related to the eye are in Table 14-3, and specific changes related to the ear are in Table 14-7.

ASSESSMENT OF THE NEUROLOGICAL SYSTEM
Subjective Data

Health history. Three points should be considered in taking the history of clients with neurological problems.[6] One is to avoid suggesting symptoms to the client. Caution must be used to not suggest certain symptoms to the client or ask leading questions such as "Is your headache throbbing?" or "Are you weak on the right side?" It is better to ask open-ended questions such as "What is your headache like?" or "What is it about your right side that bothers you?" A second point is that the mode of onset and the course of the illness are especially important aspects of the history. Often the nature of a neurological disease process can be described by these facts alone, and the nurse should elicit all pertinent data in the history of the present illness, especially data related to characteristics and progression of the symptoms. The third point is that because many neurological diseases affect a client's mental functioning, mental status must be accurately assessed before assuming that the history is factual. If the client cannot be considered a reliable source, the health history should be obtained from a person who has firsthand knowledge of the client's problems and complaints. In many instances a health history cannot be obtained, and the clinician must proceed with objective data only.

The health history helps guide the approach of the neurological examination; that is, it can direct the clinician toward the parts of the neurological system that need to be assessed closely. If the client's primary complaint is dizziness, the examination may be closely focused on visual, vestibular, and cerebellar functions rather than on somatic motor and sensory functions.

Many chief complaints, including behavioral changes, alteration in level of consciousness, developmental problems, paroxysmal disorders, infectious processes, pain, motor or sensory aberrations, and trauma, should alert the clinician to the need for a detailed neurological examination. In addition to being a primary complaint, neurological problems often result from other problems such as alcoholism and metastatic lesions.

Past health history. When eliciting data about health history, the nurse should ask the client specific questions about diabetes, pernicious anemia, cancer, infections, and hypertension because these conditions can affect the nervous system. Any hospitalizations, injuries, or surgeries related to the neurological system should be noted. Particular attention should be given to eliciting a careful medication history related especially to the use of sedatives, narcotics, tranquilizers, and mood-elevating drugs, including over-the-counter drugs of these categories.

The perinatal history may reveal exposure to toxic agents such as viruses, alcohol, tobacco, drugs, and irradiation, which are known to adversely influence the development of the nervous system. It may reveal a difficult labor and delivery, which can cause brain damage resulting from such events as hypoxia, forceps delivery, and Rh incompatibility.

Growth and developmental history can be important in ascertaining whether nervous system dysfunction was present at an early age. The nurse should specifically inquire about major developmental tasks such as walking and talking. Success at school or identified problems in an educational setting are other important pieces of developmental data to gather. Often this information is not available when the older client is interviewed. If the client cannot provide a detailed developmental history, the nurse should proceed with the history gathering and avoid distressing the client by further probing.

Family history. The purpose of gathering a careful family history is to determine whether the neurological problem has a hereditary or congenital background. Specifically, the client should be questioned about familial history of such disorders as epilepsy, amyotrophic lateral sclerosis, Huntington's disease, muscular dystrophy, mental retardation, dementia, stroke, and psychiatric problems.[7]

Personal and social history. The standard information gathered in the client profile can provide a great deal of information related to actual or potential neurological problems. A major area to assess is the presence of change in any previously established routine of daily living. Changes related to sleep, exercise, recreation, occupation, stressors, and sexual practices can have specific neurological implications and need to be carefully investigated.

Review of systems. Specific problems to inquire about related to review of systems include the following: (1) general behavior change; (2) mood change; (3) loss of consciousness; (4) anxiety or nervousness; (5) seizures; (6) speech problems; (7) memory deficits; (8) motor problems such as imbalance, paralysis, tic, or tremor; and (9) sensory problems such as pain or paresthesia (tingling sensation). After a careful review of system information, the nurse should ask someone who knows the client well whether any mental or physical changes have been noticed in the client. The client with a neurological problem is often not aware of it or is unable to provide enough specific data to aid in the diagnosis. (For a list of age-related changes in nervous system function see Table 4-8.)

The ability to participate in sexual activity should also be assessed because many nervous system diseases can affect sexual response. Cerebral lesions may inhibit the desire phase or reflex responses of the excitement phase. Brainstem and spinal cord lesions may partially or completely interrupt the connections between the brain and effector systems necessary to achieve intercourse. Neuropathies and spinal cord lesions that affect sensation, especially in the erotic zones, may decrease desire. Finally, autonomic neuropathies and lesions of the sacral cord and cauda equina may prevent reflex activity of the sexual response. Despite these possible problems, persons with dysfunction of physical sexual response do not lose their sexuality and can achieve intimacy and affection without physical intercourse.

General survey. The general survey statement can provide important data related to the neurological status of a client such as grooming habits, behavioral observations, facies, gait, posture, and communication patterns. In addition to providing currently useful data, a well-written general survey provides the nurse with baseline data for future comparison.

Objective Data

Neurological examination. The standard neurological examination was developed over many years by physicians to help them determine the presence, location, and nature of disease of the nervous system. The examination is divided into six categories: mental status, cranial nerves, motor, cerebellar, sensory, and reflex areas. The choice of particular items of the examination depends on the purpose for which it is done. If a comprehensive baseline assessment of neurological functioning is desired, all components of the examination are done. However, if a specific problem is to be evaluated, only certain components may be assessed. For example, if a client's primary complaint is lack of feeling in the feet, the examination may be focused only on movement and sensation of the lower limbs. Similarly, if a client comes into the emergency room after a head injury and is unconscious, a specific examination is conducted because the client is not able to respond to verbal instructions.

A different approach to the neurological examination has been proposed for nursing purposes. The primary purposes of the nursing neurological examination are to determine the effects of neurological dysfunction on daily living in light of the client's and the family's ability to cope with the neurological deficits. Although the method of gathering data may be the same, the interpretation of the data is different from the medical model. The standard medical model of the neurological examination can also be used for nursing purposes. Nurses and physicians share the responsibility for assessing life-threatening neurological dysfunction.

Mental status. Assessment of mental status (cerebral functioning) gives an indication of how the client is functioning as a whole and how the client is adapting to the environment. It involves assessment of complex and high-level cerebral functions that are governed by many areas of the cerebral cortex. Much of the area covered in this part of the examination is assessed during the history and therefore does not need to be assessed further. For example, language and memory can be assessed when the client is asked for details of the illness and significant past events. The client's cultural and educational background should be taken into account when assessing mental status.

Components of the mental status examination are as follows:

1. *General appearance and behavior:* This component includes motor activity, body posture, dress and hygiene, facial expression, and speech.
2. *Content of consciousness:* The client must be conscious before other functions can be determined. The nurse should note orientation to time, place, person, and situation, as well as memory, fund of information (general knowledge), insight, judgment, problem solving, and calculation. Common questions are "Who were the last three presidents?" "What does 'a stitch in time saves nine' mean?" "Subtract 7 from 100, and keep subtracting 7." The nurse should consider whether the client's plans and goals match the physical and mental capabilities.
3. *Mood and affect:* The nurse should note agitation, anger, depression, or euphoria and appropriateness of these states. Questions should be directed to bring out the feelings of the client.
4. *Thought content:* The nurse should note illusions, hallucination, delusions, or paranoia.
5. *Intellectual capacity:* The nurse should note retardation, dementia, and intelligence.

Cranial nerves. Testing of each CN is essential in the neurological examination (see Table 50-2).

OLFACTORY NERVE. After determination that both nostrils are patent, the olfactory nerve (CN I) is tested by asking the client to close one nostril, close the eyes, and sniff from a bottle containing coffee, spice, soap, or some other readily recognized odor. The same is done for the other nostril. Generally, olfaction is not tested unless the client has some disturbance with smell. Chronic rhinitis, sinusitis, and heavy smoking can often decrease the sense of smell. Disturbance in ability to smell may be associated with a tumor involving the olfactory bulb, or it may be the result of a basilar skull fracture that has damaged the olfactory fibers as they pass through the delicate cribriform plate of the skull.

OPTIC NERVE. Visual fields and visual acuity are assessed to test the function of the optic nerve (CN II). Visual fields are assessed by confrontation. The examiner, positioned directly opposite the client, asks the client to close one eye, look directly at the bridge of the examiner's nose, and indicate when an object (finger, pencil tip, head of pin) presented from the periphery of each of the four visual field quadrants is seen (Fig. 50-13). The same test is repeated for the other eye. The examiner is used as a control because both examiner and client are sharing the same visual field. It is important to remember that the nasal side of the visual field is narrower because of the nasal bridge. Visual field defects may be due to lesions of the optic nerve, optic chiasm, or tracts that extend through the temporal, parietal, or occipital lobes. Visual field changes resulting from brain lesions are usually either a hemianopsia (half of the visual field is affected) or a quadrantanopsia (one fourth of the visual field is affected).

Visual acuity is tested by asking the client to read a Snellen chart from 20 feet away. The number on the lowest line that the client can read with 50% accuracy is recorded. The client should wear glasses if appropriate, unless they are used only for reading. The eyes should be tested individually and together. If a Snellen chart is not

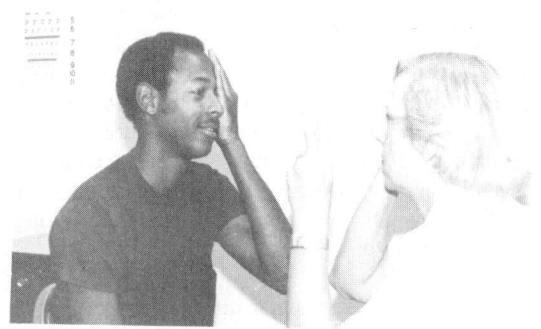

Fig. 50-13 Assessment of visual fields by gross confrontation.

available, the client should be asked to read newsprint for a gross assessment of acuity. The distance required from client to newsprint for accurate reading should be recorded. Acuity may not be testable by these means if the client does not read English, is retarded, or is aphasic.

Funduscopy reveals the physical condition of the optic disk (head of the optic nerve) as well as the retina and blood vessels. It is routinely done when the optic nerve is tested. Optic nerve atrophy and papilledema can be detected by this method.*

OCULOMOTOR, TROCHLEAR, AND ABDUCENS NERVES. Because the oculomotor (CN III), trochlear (CN IV), and abducens (CN VI) nerves help move the eye, they are tested together. The client is asked to follow the examiner's finger as it moves horizontally and vertically (making a cross) and diagonally (making an X). If there is weakness or paralysis of one of the eye muscles, the eyes do not move together and the client has a disconjugate gaze. The presence and direction of *nystagmus* (fine, rapid jerking movements of the eyes) is observed at this time, even though it is most often indicative of vestibulocerebellar problems. Other functions of the oculomotor nerve are tested by checking for pupillary constriction and for convergence (eyes turning inward) and accommodation (pupils constricting with near vision). To test pupillary constriction, the examiner shines a light into the pupil of one eye and looks for ipsilateral constriction of the same pupil and contralateral (consensual) constriction of the opposite eye. The size and shape of the pupils should be noted. The optic nerve must be intact for this reflex to occur. Testing for pupillary constriction is an important component of the neurological assessment of clients at risk for herniation syndrome (see Chapters 52 and 53). Because the oculomotor nerve exits at the top of the brainstem at the tentorial notch, it can be easily compressed by expanding mass lesions in the cerebral hemispheres. The result is a pupil that does not constrict to light; it may become dilated because the sympathetic input to the pupil acts unopposed. Convergence and accommodation are tested by having the client focus on the examiner's finger as it moves toward the client's nose. Another function of the oculomotor nerve is to keep the eyelid open. Damage to the nerve can cause ptosis (drooping eyelid).

TRIGEMINAL NERVE. The sensory component of the trigeminal nerve (CN V) is tested by having the client identify light touch (cotton) and pinprick in each of the three divisions (ophthalmic, maxillary, and mandibular) of the nerve on both sides of the face. The client's eyes should be closed during this part of the examination. The motor component is tested by asking the client to clench the teeth and palpating the masseter muscles just above the mandibular angle. The corneal reflex test evaluates CN V and VII simultaneously. It involves applying a cotton wisp strand to the cornea. The sensory component of this reflex (corneal sensation) is innervated by the ophthalmic division of CN V. The motor component (eye blink) is innervated by CN VII. This reflex is not normally tested in clients who are awake and alert because other tests evaluate these two

nerves. However, for clients with a decreased level of consciousness, the corneal reflex test provides an opportunity to evaluate the integrity of the brainstem at the level of the pons because the fibers of CN V and VII have connections in this area.

FACIAL NERVE. The facial nerve (CN VII) innervates the muscles of facial expression. Its function is tested by asking the client to raise the eyebrows, close the eyes tightly, purse the lips, draw back the corners of the mouth in an exaggerated smile, and frown. The examiner should note any asymmetry in the facial movements because they can indicate damage to the facial nerve. Although taste discrimination of salt and sugar in the anterior two thirds of the tongue is a function of this nerve, it is not routinely tested unless a peripheral nerve lesion is suspected.

ACOUSTIC NERVE. The cochlear portion of the acoustic (vestibulocochlear) nerve (CN VIII) is tested by having the client close the eyes and indicate when a ticking watch or the rustling of the examiner's fingertips is heard as the stimulus is brought closer to the ear. Each ear is tested individually, and the distance from the client's ear to the sound source when first heard is recorded. This test identifies only gross deficits in hearing. For more precise assessment of hearing, an audiometer is used (see Chapter 14). The vestibular portion of this nerve is not routinely tested unless the client complains of dizziness, vertigo, or unsteadiness or has auditory dysfunction. If this is the case, caloric testing, which is beyond the scope of routine testing, may be done.

GLOSSOPHARYNGEAL AND VAGUS NERVES. Because both these nerves innervate the pharynx, they are tested together. The glossopharyngeal nerve (CN IX) is primarily sensory. In the gag reflex (bilateral contraction of the palatal muscles initiated by stroking or touching either side of the posterior pharynx or soft palate with a tongue blade) the sensory component is mediated by CN IX, the major motor component by the vagus nerve (CN X). It is important to assess the gag reflex in clients who have a decreased level of consciousness or a disease involving the throat musculature. If the reflex is weak or absent, the client is in danger of aspirating food or secretions. The strength and efficiency of swallowing is important to test in these clients for the same reason. Another test for the awake, cooperative client is to have the client phonate by saying "ah" and to note the bilateral symmetry of elevation of the soft palate. Any asymmetry can indicate weakness or paralysis. Swallowing is also assessed.

SPINAL ACCESSORY NERVE. The spinal accessory nerve (CN XI) is tested by asking the client to shrug the shoulders against resistance and to turn the head to either side against resistance. There should be smooth contraction of the sternomastoid and trapezius muscles. Symmetry of muscle bulk should also be noted.

HYPOGLOSSAL NERVE. The hypoglossal nerve (CN XII) is tested by asking the client to protrude the tongue. It should protrude in the midline. The client should also be able to push the tongue to either side against the resistance of a tongue blade. Again, any asymmetry can indicate weakness or paralysis.

Motor system. The motor system examination includes assessment of bulk, tone, and power of the major muscle

---

*See an ophthalmoscopic text for specifics of the funduscopic examination.

groups of the body as well as assessment of balance and coordination. The examiner tests strength by asking the client to push or pull against the resistance of the examiner's arm as it opposes flexion and extension of the client's muscle. The client should be asked to offer resistance at the shoulder, elbow, wrist, hips, knees, and ankles. The client's grip strength can also be tested. Mild weakness may be tested by having the client extend both arms forward at shoulder height with palms up while the eyes are closed. Mild weakness of the arm is demonstrated by downward drifting of the arm and/or pronation of the palm (pronator drift). Any weakness or asymmetry of strength between the same muscle groups of the right and left side should be noted.

Tone is tested by passively moving the limbs through their range of motion; there should be a slight resistance to these movements. Abnormal tone is described as *hypotonia* (flaccidity) or *hypertonia* (spasticity). Involuntary movements (e.g., tics, tremor, myoclonus, athetosis, chorea, dystonia) should be noted.

Cerebellar function is tested by assessing balance and coordination. A good screening test for both balance and muscle strength is to observe the client's station (posture while standing) and gait. The examiner should note the pace and rhythm of the gait and observe the arm swing. (The arms should move symmetrically and in the opposite direction of the leg on the same side.) The client's ability to ambulate is a key factor in determining the amount of nursing care that is needed and the risk of injury due to falling. The Romberg test is conducted after observing the client walk. The client should stand with feet together and eyes open. Balance should be easily maintained. The client is asked to close both eyes while maintaining the same position. Balance should continue to be maintained with minimum swaying.

Coordination can be easily tested in several ways. The finger-to-nose test involves having the client alternately touch the nose with the index finger, then touch the examiner's finger. The examiner repositions the finger while the client is touching the nose so that the client must adjust to a new distance each time the examiner's finger is touched. These movements should be performed smoothly and accurately. Other tests include asking the client to pronate and supinate both hands rapidly and to do a shallow knee bend, first on one leg, then on the other. Dysarthria or slurred speech should be noted because it is a sign of discoordination of the speech muscles.

The heel-to-shin test involves having the client place one heel on the opposite shin below the knee and moving the heel down the shin to the ankle. This is repeated for the other leg. These movements should flow smoothly without jerking or hesitation.

Sensory system. Several modalities are tested in the somatic sensory examination. Each modality is carried by a specific ascending pathway in the spinal cord before it reaches the sensory cortex.

There are some general guidelines for performing the sensory examination. The client should always have the eyes closed to avoid visual clues. The examiner should avoid giving verbal cues such as, "Is this sharp?" The sensory stimulus should be applied in such a way that the client does not expect it; that is, the examiner should avoid rhythmical application of the stimulus. In the routine neurological examination, sensory testing of the four extremities is sufficient. However, if a disturbance in sensory function of the skin is identified, the boundaries of that dysfunction should be carefully delineated.

LIGHT TOUCH. Light touch is usually tested first. The examiner gently strokes a cotton wisp over each of the four extremities and asks the client to indicate when the stimulus is felt by saying "touch." (The sensory examination of the trigeminal nerve may be delayed until this time because the same material for testing sensation is used.)

PAIN AND TEMPERATURE. Pain is tested by touching the skin with the sharp end of a pin. This stimulus is irregularly alternated with a simple touch stimulus with the dull end of the pin to determine whether the client can distinguish the two stimuli. Extinction or inhibition is assessed by simultaneously stimulating opposite sides of the body symmetrically with either a pain or a touch stimulus. Normally, the simultaneous stimuli are appreciated; appreciation of only one may indicate a parietal lobe lesion.

The sensation of temperature is tested by applying tubes of warm and cold water to the skin and asking the client to identify the stimuli with the eyes closed. If pain sensation is intact, assessment of temperature sensation may be omitted because both sensations are carried by the same ascending pathways.

VIBRATION SENSE. Vibration sense is assessed by applying a vibrating C-128 tuning fork to the fingernails and/or bony prominences of the hands, legs, and feet. The examiner asks the client if the vibration, or "buzz" is felt. The examiner then asks the client to indicate when the vibration ceases. The examiner stops the vibration with the hand as desired.

POSITION SENSE. Position sense is assessed by placing the thumb and forefinger on either side of the client's forefinger or great toe and gently moving the finger up or down. The client is asked to indicate the direction in which the digit is moved.

CORTICAL SENSORY FUNCTIONS. Several tests evaluate cortical integration of sensory perceptions (which occurs in the parietal lobes). *Two-point discrimination* is assessed by placing the two points of a calibrated compass on the tips of the fingers and toes. The minimum recognizable separation is 4 to 5 mm in the fingertips and much more elsewhere. This test is important in diseases of the sensory cortex and in peripheral nerve disease. *Graphesthesia* is tested by having the client identify numbers traced on the palm of the hands. *Stereognosis* is tested by having the client identify the size and shape of easily recognized objects (e.g., coins, keys, a safety pin) placed in the hands. *Sensory extinction* or *inattention* is evaluated by touching both sides of the body simultaneously. An abnormal response occurs when the client perceives the stimulus only on one side. The other stimulus is "extinguished."

Reflexes. Skeletal muscles contract when their tendons are stretched because of reflexes. A simple muscle stretch reflex is initiated by briskly tapping the tendon of a stretched muscle, usually with a reflex hammer (Fig. 50-

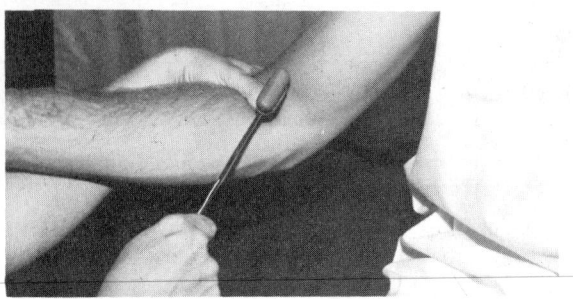

Fig. 50-14 The examiner strikes a swift blow over a stretched tendon to elicit a stretch reflex.

14). The response (muscle contraction of the corresponding muscle) is measured as follows: 0 = absent, 1 = weak response, 2 = normal response, 3 = exaggerated response, 4 = hyperreflexia with clonus. *Clonus*, an abnormal response, is a continued rhythmic contraction of the muscle after the stimulus has been applied.

In general, the biceps, triceps, brachioradialis, and patellar and Achilles tendons are tested. The examiner elicits the biceps reflex by placing the thumb over the biceps tendon in the antecubital space and striking the thumb with a hammer. The client should have the arms partially flexed at the elbow with the palms up. The normal response is flexion of the arm at the elbow or contraction of the biceps muscle that can be felt by the examiner's thumb.

The triceps reflex is elicited by striking the triceps tendon above the elbow while the client's arm is flexed. The normal response is extension of the arm or visible contraction of the triceps.

The brachioradialis reflex is elicited by striking the radius 3 to 5 cm above the wrist while the client's arm is relaxed. The normal response is flexion and supination at the elbow or visible contraction of the brachioradialis muscle.

The patellar reflex is elicited by striking the patellar tendon just below the patella. The client can be sitting or lying as long as the leg being tested hangs freely. The normal response is extension of the leg with contraction of the quadriceps.

The Achilles tendon reflex is elicited by striking the Achilles tendon while the client's leg is flexed at the knee and the foot is dorsiflexed at the ankle. The normal response is plantar flexion at the ankle.

Table 50-5 is an example of how to record a normal neurological assessment. Common abnormal assessment findings of the neurological system are presented in Table 50-6.

Nursing approach. The premise of the nursing approach is that the primary purpose of nursing is to help clients cope effectively with deficits in self-care and in activities of daily living. Consequently, the neurological examination should be viewed in terms of functional disabilities rather than dysfunction of component parts of the nervous system. The effects of the disabilities on the client's ability for self-care, movement, and desired activities of daily living should be the focus. This includes understanding, communicating, remembering, seeing, speaking, feeling,

Table 50-5 Recording the Normal Neurological Examination*

MENTAL STATUS

Alert and oriented status, orderly thought processes, appropriate mood and affect

CRANIAL NERVES†

Smell intact to soap and coffee; visual fields full to confrontation; visual acuity 20/20 in both eyes; intact extraocular movements; no nystagmus; pupils equal, round, reactive to light and accommodation; intact facial sensation to touch and pinprick; facial movements full; intact gag and swallow reflexes; symmetrical elevation of soft palate; full strength with head turning and shrugging of shoulders against resistance; midline protrusion of tongue

MOTOR SYSTEM

Normal gait and station; normal tandem walk; negative Romberg test; normal and symmetrical muscle bulk, tone, strength; smooth performance of finger-nose, heel-shin movements

SENSORY SYSTEM

Intact sensation to light touch, position sense, vibration, pinprick, heat and cold, two-point discrimination; intact stereognosis and graphesthesia

REFLEXES‡

Biceps, triceps, brachioradialis, patellar, and Achilles tendon reflexes 2+ bilaterally; downgoing toes with plantar stimulation

---

*If some portion of the neurological examination was not done, this should be indicated (e.g., "Smell not tested").
†May also be recorded as "CN I to XII intact."
‡May also be recorded as drawing of stick figure indicating reflex strength at appropriate sites.

---

moving, walking, and integrated regulatory functions such as elimination and temperature regulation. In addition, the nursing approach involves inquiry about where the neurological lesion is located on the basis of history and examination to determine what other effects the lesion may have on daily functioning.[8]

All functions of the nervous system can be categorized in six areas: consciousness, mentation, movement, sensation, integrated regulation, and coping with disability. Table 50-7 lists the functions involved in each of these categories and thus forms the basis of nursing neurological assessment.

DIAGNOSTIC STUDIES

The diagnostic studies of the nervous system are presented in Table 50-8.

Laboratory Studies

Cerebrospinal fluid analysis. CSF analysis provides information about a variety of CNS diseases. Normal CSF

Table 50-6

Common Assessment Abnormalities of the Nervous System

Finding	Description	Possible Etiology and Significance
Altered consciousness	Inability to speak, obey commands, open eyes appropriately with verbal or painful stimulus*	Intracranial lesions, metabolic disorder, psychiatric disorders
Anisocoria	Inequality of pupil size	Lesion, injury, or intracranial pressure in area of midbrain
Agnosia	Inability to determine meaning or significance of sensory stimulus	Cerebral cortex lesion
Apraxia	Inability to perform learned movements, defect in motor planning	Cerebral cortex lesion
Aphasia	Loss of language faculty (language comprehension, language expression, or both)	Cerebral cortex lesion
Analgesia	Loss of pain sensation	Lesion in spinothalamic tract or thalamus, lack of or damage to sensory nerve endings

Anesthesia
  Hyperesthesia
  Hypoesthesia
	Absence of sensation
	Increase in sensation
	Decrease in sensation
		Lesions in spinal cord, thalamus, sensory cortex, or peripheral sensory nerve

Anosognosia	Inability to recognize bodily defect or disease	Lesions in right parietal cortex, common in right-sided stroke
Astereognosis	Inability to recognize form of object by touch	Lesions in parietal cortex
Ataxia	Lack of coordination of movement	Lesions of sensory pathways, cerebellum; anticonvulsant, sedative, hypnotic drug toxicity (including alcohol)
Muscle atrophy (disuse or denervation atrophy)	Wasting away or diminution in size of muscle	Suprasegmental (upper motor neuron) lesions, segmental (lower motor neuron) lesions
Bladder dysfunction Atonic (autonomous)	Absence of muscle tone and contractility, enlargement of capacity, no sensation of discomfort, overflow with large residual, inability to voluntarily empty or empty by reflex	Early stage of spinal cord injury
Hypotonic	More ability than atonic bladder but less than normal	Interruption of efferent pathways from bladder
Hypertonic	Increase in muscle tone, diminished capacity, reflex emptying, dribbling, incontinence	Lesions in pyramidal tracts (efferent pathways)
Diplopia	Double vision	Lesions affecting nerves of extraocular muscles, cerebellar toxicity
Dysarthria	Lack of coordination in articulating speech	Lesions in cerebellum or pathway of cranial nerves (including brainstem); anticonvulsant, sedative, or hypnotic drug toxicity (including alcohol)
Dyskinesia	Impairment of power of voluntary movement, resulting in fragmentary or incomplete movements	Disorders of basal ganglia, idiosyncratic reaction to psychotropic drugs
Dysphagia	Difficulty in swallowing	Lesions involving motor pathways of CN IX, X (including lower brainstem)
Extensor plantar response (Babinski sign)	Upgoing toes with plantar stimulation	Suprasegmental or upper motor neuron lesion

*See Table 52-2.

Table 50-6

 Common Assessment Abnormalities of the Nervous System—cont'd

Finding	Description	Possible Etiology and Significance
Homonymous hemianopsia	Loss of vision in one side of visual field	Injury or lesions in area of optic tract or its radiations to occipital cortex
Hemiplegia	Paralysis in one side	Stroke and other lesions involving motor cortex
Nystagmus	Jerking or bobbing of eyes as they track moving object	Lesions in cerebellum, brainstem, vestibular system; anticonvulsant, sedative, hypnotic toxicity (including alcohol)
Ophthalmoplegia	Paralysis of eye muscles	Lesions in brainstem or CN III, IV, VI
Opisthotonus	Extreme arching of back with retraction of head	Meningitis, tonic phase of grand mal seizure
Papilledema	"Choked disk," swelling of optic nerve head	Increase in intracranial pressure
Paraplegia	Paralysis of lower extremities	Spinal cord transection or mass lesion (thoracolumbar region)
Quadriplegia	Paralysis of all extremities	Spinal cord transection or mass lesion (cervical region)

fluid is clear, colorless, and free of red blood cells (RBCs) and contains few proteins. Normal CSF values are listed in Table 50-9.

Lumbar puncture. Lumbar puncture is the most common method of obtaining CSF for analysis. It is contraindicated in the presence of increased intracranial pressure or infection at the site of puncture.

Nurses often assist in this procedure because it is usually done in the client's room. Before the procedure the nurse should have the client empty the bladder. The client should lie in the lateral recumbent position, with the back as near as possible to the edge of the bed. The nurse should assist the client to draw up the knees to the abdomen and flex the head to the chest. This helps separate the vertebrae so that the needle can be inserted more easily.

Using strict sterile technique, the physician inserts a long needle below the third lumbar vertebra. This may cause some local discomfort. There is no danger of injuring the spinal cord, since the cord terminates between the first and second lumbar vertebrae. However, the client may have some pain radiating down the leg or muscle twitching if the spinal root is irritated by the needle. The nurse can assure the client that this is temporary and that the client is not in danger of being paralyzed.

A manometer is attached to the needle, and CSF pressure is determined *after* the client is asked to relax and extend the legs. If this is not done, the pressure appears abnormally high. CSF is withdrawn in a series of tubes and sent for analysis. Some examiners believe that the client should be kept lying flat for a few hours after the procedure to avoid "spinal headache," which is presumably caused by loss of the cushioning effect of CSF as a result of leakage of CSF at the puncture site. The prone position may be effective in preventing CSF leakage. Other clinicians do not believe that the lying position is necessary be-

Table 50-7 Functional Categories in Nursing Neurological Assessment

CONSCIOUSNESS

Arousal	Self-awareness

MENTATION

Thinking	Language
Remembering	Problem solving
Perceiving	

MOVEMENT

Expressing (facial)	Transferring
Speaking	Eating (chewing, swallowing)
Walking	Blinking (combined movement and sensation)

SENSATION

Seeing	Feeling (e.g., touch, temperature, pain, pressure, position, form, shape)
Smelling	
Hearing	

INTEGRATED REGULATORY FUNCTION

Eating (ingesting, digesting)	Circulation
Eliminating	Temperature control
Breathing	Sexual response
	Emotion

COPING WITH DISABILITY

Self-care competence	Coping (e.g., adapting, supporting, growing)
Role competence	

Modified from Mitchell PH and others: Neurological assessment for nursing practice, Reston, Va, 1984, Reston Publishing, p 7.

Table 50-8

Diagnostic Studies of the Nervous System

Study	Description and Purpose	Nursing Responsibility
CEREBROSPINAL FLUID ANALYSIS		
Lumbar puncture	CSF is aspirated by needle insertion in L4-5 interspace to assess many CNS diseases.	Assist client to assume and maintain lateral recumbent position with knees flexed. Ensure maintenance of strict aseptic technique. Ensure labeling of CSF specimens in proper sequence. Keep client flat 6 to 24 hr depending on physician preference. Encourage fluids. Monitor neurological and VS. Administer analgesia as needed.
RADIOLOGICAL		
Skull and spine films	Simple x-ray films of skull and spinal column are done to detect fractures, bone erosion, calcifications, abnormal vascularity.	Explain that procedure is noninvasive. Explain positions to be assumed.
Cerebral angiography	Serial x-ray visualization of intracranial and extracranial blood vessels is performed to detect vascular lesions and tumors of brain. Radiopaque contrast medium is used.	Withhold preceding meal. Explain that client will have hot flush of head and neck when dye is injected. Administer premedication. Explain need to be absolutely still during procedure. Monitor neurological and VS every 15 to 30 min first 2 hr, every hr next 6 hr, then every 2 hr for 24 hr. Maintain pressure dressing and ice to injection site. Maintain bed rest until client is alert and VS are stable. Report any signs of change in neurological status.
Computerized tomography (CT)	Computer-assisted x-ray film of several levels or thin cross-sections of the brain are done to detect problems such as hemorrhage, tumor, cyst, edema, infarction, brain atrophy, hydrocephalus.	Explain that procedure is noninvasive (if no dye used). Observe for allergic reaction and note puncture site (if dye used). Explain appearance of scanner. Instruct client on need to remain absolutely still during procedure.
Myelography	X-ray film of spinal cord and vertebral column after injection of dye into subarachnoid space is used to detect spinal lesions (e.g., ruptured disk, tumor).	Administer preprocedure sedation as ordered. Instruct client to empty bladder. Inform client that test is performed with client on tilting table that is moved during test. Note that specific postprocedural management depends on whether oil- or water-based contrast medium is used. Encourage fluids. Monitor neurological and VS.
Magnetic resonance imaging (MRI)	Internal body parts are visualized by means of magnetic energy. No invasive procedures are required unless dye is used.	Screen client for metal parts in body. Instruct client on need to lie very still for up to 1 hr.
Echoencephalography (EEG)	Ultrasonography is used to detect midline shift of intracranial contents as a result of mass lesions.	Explain that procedure is noninvasive.
Radioisotope brain scan	Specialized scanning of brain after oral, intravenous, or intraarterial administration of radioisotope is performed to detect mass lesions or vascular abnormalities.	Inform client that only tracer dose is used and that there is no radioactive danger. Explain that after administration of radioisotope, scanner will move overhead.

VS, Vital signs.

Table 50-8

 Diagnostic Studies of the Nervous System—cont'd

Study	Description and Purpose	Nursing Responsibility
ELECTROGRAPHIC		
Electroencephalography	Electrical activity of brain is recorded by scalp electrodes to evaluate cerebral disease, CNS effects of systemic diseases, brain death.	Inform client that procedure is painless and without danger of electric shock. Withhold stimulants. Inform that client may be asked to perform various activities such as hyperventilation during test. Determine whether any medications (e.g., tranquilizers, anticonvulsants) should be withheld. Resume medications after test. Assist client to wash electrode paste out of hair.
Electromyography	Electrical activity associated with innervation of skeletal muscle is recorded by insertion of needle electrodes to detect myopathic conditions and peripheral nerve disease.	Inform client of slight discomfort associated with insertion of needles.
Evoked potentials	Electrical activity associated with nerve conduction along sensory pathways is recorded by electrodes placed on skin and scalp. Stimulus generates the impulse. Procedure is used to diagnose disease, locate nerve damage, and monitor function intraoperatively.	Explain procedure to client.
Visual evoked potentials	Electrical activity in visual pathway is recorded with rapidly reversing checkerboard pattern on television screen. One eye is tested at a time.	Explain procedure to client.
Brainstem auditory evoked potentials	Electrical activity in auditory pathway is recorded with earphones that produce clicking sounds. One ear is tested at a time.	Explain procedure to client.
Somatosensory evoked potentials	Electrical activity in certain peripheral nerves is recorded with mild electrical pulse (several per sec).	Inform client that stimulus may cause mild discomfort or muscle twitch.

cause headache seems to develop in some clients despite precautions. Meningeal irritation (nuchal rigidity) or signs and symptoms of local trauma (hematoma, pain) may develop in some clients.

Radiological Studies

Cerebral angiography. Cerebral angiography is indicated when vascular lesions or tumors are suspected. A catheter is inserted into the femoral (sometimes brachial) artery. It is then passed up the artery to the aortic arch and into the base of a carotid or a vertebral artery for injection of radiopaque dye. A series of x-ray films is taken in a timed sequence so that pictures of the arteries, smaller vessels, and veins can be obtained (Fig. 50-15). This study can help localize and determine the presence of abscesses, aneurysms, hematomas, arteriovenous malformations, arterial spasm, and certain tumors.

Because this is an invasive procedure, adverse reactions

Table 50-9   Normal Cerebrospinal Fluid Values

Parameter	Normal Value
Specific gravity	1.007
pH	7.35
Appearance	Clear, colorless
RBCs	None
WBCs	0-8/μL
Protein	
Lumbar	15-45 mg/dl
Cisternal	15-25 mg/dl
Ventricular	5-15 mg/dl
Glucose	45-75 mg/dl
Microorganisms	None
Opening pressure with lumbar puncture	60-150 mm H_2O

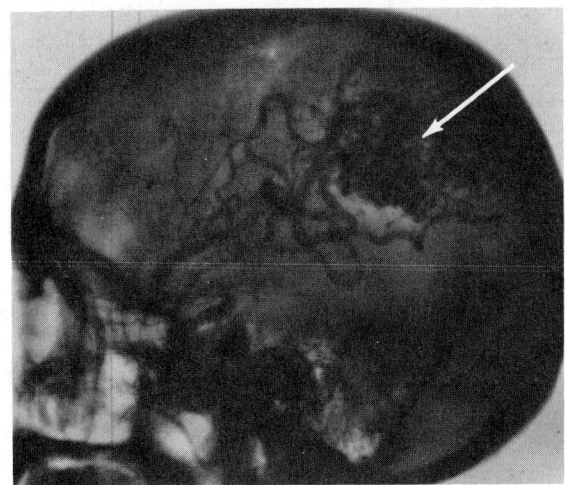

Fig. 50-15 Cerebral angiogram illustrating an arteriovenous malformation (arrow).

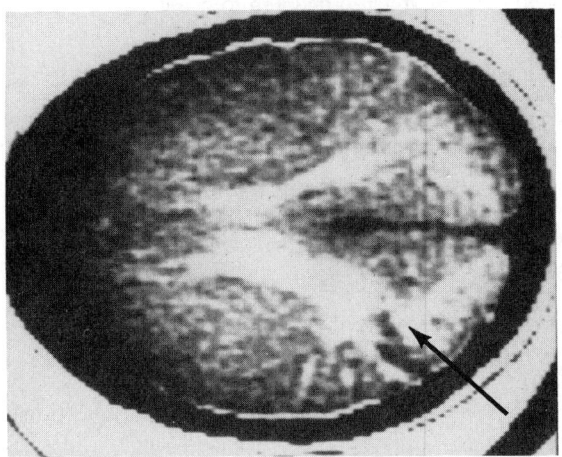

Fig. 50-16 CT scan of a client with an arteriovenous malformation. Dilated right lateral ventricle and enhancement of the AVM just posterior to the right ventricle is observed (arrow).

may occur. The client may have an allergic (anaphylactic) reaction to the contrast medium. This reaction usually occurs immediately after injection and may require emergency resuscitation measures in the procedure room. The most common precaution for nurses to take in caring for the client after the return to the room is observation for bleeding at the catheter puncture site (usually the groin). A pressure dressing and ice are usually placed on the site to aid hemostasis and prevent swelling.

Computerized tomography. Computerized tomography (CT) scan has revolutionized neuroradiology. It has greatly reduced the use of other diagnostic studies such as pneumoencephalography, ventriculography, echoencephalography, and radioisotope brain scan. It is noninvasive, although intravenous (IV) injection of contrast medium may be used to enhance visualization of the blood vessels and

identify disruptions in the blood-brain barrier, and can be done on an outpatient basis. A series of x-ray films scanning different levels of the brain are compiled with computer assistance and presented in a series of black-and-white pictures (Fig. 50-16). These pictures, which illustrate "slices" of the brain, can show hemorrhages of all types, tumors, cysts, edema, infarction, brain atrophy, and hydrocephalus. CT scans do not illustrate structures in the posterior fossa and the base of the brain as well as some other tests such as myelography and magnetic resonance imaging (MRI).

Magnetic resonance imaging. MRI became available in the mid-1980s. Rather than using x-ray films, this method involves two kinds of magnetism. The client is placed within a giant magnetic field that aligns the protons of hydrogen ions in the body's cells. Bursts of radio-frequency magnetism are introduced to flip the protons out of alignment. When the radio-frequency magnetism is turned off, the protons realign. The resulting magnetic field change is picked up by the machine and is processed by a computer. A vivid black-and-white picture of slices of the brain is then produced.

MRI is useful in evaluating brain and spinal cord edema, hemorrhage, infarction, blood vessels, neoplasms, and bone lesions. Because MRI yields greater contrast in the images of soft-tissue structures than the CT scan, it is the diagnostic test of choice in several neurological diseases.

Myelography. Myelography is used to visualize the spinal column and the subarachnoid space when a spinal lesion is suspected. The most common lesion for which this test is used is a herniated or protruding intervertebral disk. Other lesions include spinal tumors, adhesions, syringomyelia, bony deformations, and arteriovenous malformations. The test involves x-ray filming of the spinal column after injection of the contrast medium into the subarachnoid space by catheter. Water-soluble iodine dyes such as iopamidol (Isovue) are used most often because they are absorbed into the bloodstream and excreted by the kidneys. Preparation for this procedure is the same as for lumbar puncture. Before the dye is injected, clients must be asked whether they have any allergies, specifically whether they have had any anaphylactic or hypotensive episodes from other dyes. After myelography the head of the client's bed should be elevated 30 degrees for a few hours so that the dye does not gravitate toward the brain.

Headache is the most common complaint after myelography. It may be accompanied by nausea and occasionally vomiting. The nurse should observe the client for any changes in neurological status and provide a quiet, comfortable environment after the procedure.

Electrographic Studies

Electroencephalography. The technique of Electroencephalography (EEG) is the recording of the electrical activity of the brain by 8 to 16 electrodes placed on specific areas of the scalp. This test is done to evaluate not only cerebral disease but also the CNS effects of many metabolic and systemic diseases and to determine brain death. Among the cerebral diseases assessed by EEG are epi-

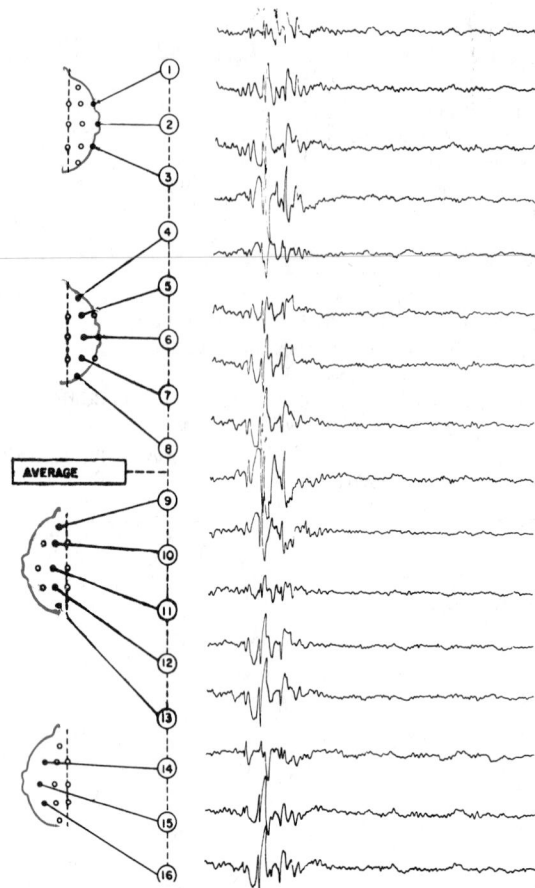

Fig. 50-17 EEG showing a generalized epileptic discharge.

lepsy, mass lesions (e.g., tumor, abscess, hematoma), cerebrovascular lesions, and brain injury (Fig. 50-17). The procedure is noninvasive. Clients sometimes have the misconception that the recording electrodes will give them an electric shock. They should be assured that this is not so and that the procedure is similar to electrocardiography.

Electromyography. Electromyography (EMG) is the recording of electrical activity associated with innervation of skeletal muscle. The recording is displayed on a cathode-ray oscilloscope and may be played on a loudspeaker for simultaneous analysis. Needle electrodes are inserted into the muscle to record specific motor units because recording from the skin is not sufficient. Normal muscle at rest shows no electrical activity. Typical electrical activity occurs when the muscle contracts. This activity may be altered in diseases of muscle itself (e.g., myopathic conditions) or in disorders of muscle innervation (e.g., segmental or lower motor neuron lesions, peripheral neuropathic conditions). Fibrillations are spontaneous, independent contractions of individual muscle fibers that can be detected only by EMG. They appear on EMG 1 to 3 weeks after a muscle has lost its nerve supply.

Evoked potentials. Evoked potentials are recordings of electrical activity associated with nerve conduction along sensory pathways. The activity is generated by a specific sensory stimulus related to the type of study (e.g., checkerboard patterns for visual evoked potentials, clicking sounds for auditory evoked potentials, and mild electrical pulses for somatosensory evoked potentials). Electrodes placed on specific areas of the skin and scalp record electrical activity, which is stored and averaged by a computerized instrument. A wave pattern appears on a screen and is printed on paper. Peaks in the wave pattern correspond to conduction of the stimulus through certain points along the sensory pathway (e.g., peripheral nerve, brainstem, and cortical areas). Increases in the normal time from stimulus onset to a given peak (latency) indicate slowed nerve conduction or nerve damage. Indications for this test include evaluation of disease of the optic nerve such as optic neuritis in multiple sclerosis, acoustic neuroma, and other diseases that may affect the visual or auditory pathways.

R eview Questions

The number of the question corresponds to the same-numbered objective at the beginning of the chapter.

1. The primary function of the neuron is to
   a. regulate extracellular fluid concentrations
   b. supply nutrients to other cells in the CNS
   c. transmit information to, from, and within the CNS
   d. maintain arousal
2. Nerve impulses are transmitted
   a. between neurons by chemical synaptic mechanisms and within a neuron by action potentials
   b. between neurons by action potentials and within a neuron by action neurotransmitters
   c. between neurons and neuroglia to the periphery
   d. between neurons and tiny capillaries
3. Two CNS structures essential for the execution of smooth, coordinated movement are
   a. cerebellum and hypothalamus
   b. hypothalamus and basal ganglia
   c. basal ganglia and occipital cortex
   d. basal ganglia and cerebellum
4. The middle cerebral arteries supply
   a. the medial portion of the frontal lobes
   b. the outer portions of the frontal, parietal, and superior temporal lobes
   c. the posterior fossa
   d. the occipital lobes
5. Unlike spinal nerves, some cranial nerves
   a. have only an efferent motor component
   b. have only an afferent sensory component
   c. carry "special senses"
   d. all the above
6. The net result of activation of the SNS is
   a. hibernation
   b. sensory overload
   c. seizure activity
   d. preparation for fight or flight
7. The decreased sensory receptors associated with aging result in
   a. increased pain perception

b. sluggish reflexes
c. inability to localize stimuli
d. orthostatic hypotension

8. Data regarding the perinatal and growth and development history are important because they may
   a. indicate early damage to the CNS
   b. indicate genetic factors
   c. reveal aspects of mothering
   d. a and b

9. To assess for nystagmus, the nurse asks the client to
   a. follow the finger as it approaches the nose
   b. identify familiar objects placed in the hand with eyes closed
   c. follow the nurse's finger laterally and hold the gaze
   d. bend from the waist with arms hanging freely

10. Disturbances of higher cortical functions include
    a. ataxia, agnosia, paraplegia
    b. analgesia, ataxia, diplopia
    c. apraxia, agnosia, aphasia
    d. paraplegia, analgesia, aphasia

11. A common nursing responsibility for studies involving invasive procedures is
    a. observation of the puncture site
    b. application of pressure bandage to puncture site
    c. a and b
    d. assuring a fasting state

REFERENCES

1. Fitzgerald MJT: Neuroanatomy, London, 1985, Bailliere Tindall, p 17.
2. Snyder S: Opioid peptides in the brain. In Schmidt F and Worden F, eds: The neurosciences, fourth study program, Cambridge, Mass, 1979, MIT Press, pp 1057-1068.
3. Snell RS: Clinical neuroanatomy, Boston, 1987, Little, Brown & Co, p 156.
4. Afifi AK and Bergman RA: Basic neuroscience, ed 2, Baltimore, 1986, Urban and Schwarsenberg, p 441.
5. Yurich AG and others: The aged person and the nursing process, Norwalk, Conn, 1989, Appleton & Lange, p 618.
6. Adams R and Victor M: Principles of neurology, New York, 1985, McGraw-Hill Book Co, Inc, p 4.
7. Bird TD: Medical genetics and clinical neurology. In Bearn AS, Motulsky AG, and Childs B, eds: New York, 1985, Praeger, p 3.
8. Mitchell PH and others: Neurological assessment for nursing practice, Reston, Va, 1984, Reston Publishing.

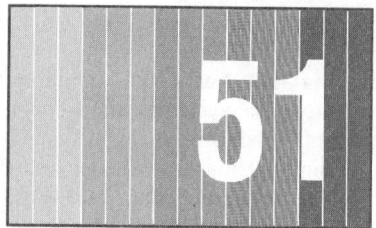

Nursing Assessment and Role in Management

Pain

Barbara J. Boss

Pain is a complex phenomenon. The understanding of this phenomenon has undergone and is still undergoing change. Increased knowledge plus the demonstrated need and demand for an integrated, holistic multidisciplinary approach to pain management has continued to lead to (1) an increase in the number and types of therapeutic modalities used to manage pain by different health care professionals and (2) an emphasis on approaching the client experiencing pain from a whole-person perspective. Pain management is a specialty area of health care practice and requires a multidisciplinary approach. The nurse has an important role on this multidisciplinary team. The nursing assessment and management of pain continue to become more complex.

Reviewed by Kathleen A. Puntillo, R.N., M.S., Doctoral Candidate, Physiological Nursing, University of California, San Francisco; Associate Professor, School of Nursing, Sonoma State University, Rohnert Park, California.

DEFINITION

Pain is a complex biopsychosocial phenomenon. No simple, clear-cut definition exists. A purely physiological definition, such as "pain is a protective mechanism," is not adequate because the behavioral manifestations of pain are socially and culturally determined.

Some pain has a positive value. Pain may serve as a warning signal that the body is experiencing tissue damage, preventing a person from continuing a task that could cause serious injury. Pain may aid in locating and diagnosing the cause of a problem and may serve as a way to measure treatment effectiveness. Fear of pain prevents some persons from pursuing potentially harmful activities and may encourage some persons to take care of themselves.

Because pain is a complex concept and experience, a useful definition to guide nurses in the assessment and management of clients experiencing pain is that *pain is whatever the person experiencing the pain says it is, existing whenever the person says it does.*[1] This definition recognizes pain as a personal, private experience.

COMPONENTS

Pain has three components: a sensory-discriminative component, an affective-motivational component, and a cognitive-evaluative component. The sensory-discriminative component is the recognition of the sensation as painful (perception of pain). The affective-motivational component of pain makes up the emotional and behavioral dimensions of the pain experience. The cognitive component involves the responses to the pain experience that are determined by past experiences, learned behaviors, conditioned responses, and the person's analysis and interpretation of the situation.

Pain can also be viewed as having a perceptive component and a reactive component. The *perceptive component* involves the sensation being experienced (perceived) as one of pain; hence it is equivalent to the sensory-discriminative component. The *reactive component* includes responses elicited by the pain perception and involves phys-

iological, psychological, behavioral, and cognitive responses to pain. The affective-motivational and the cognitive-evaluative components of pain are part of this reactive component.

PHYSIOLOGICAL BASES OF PAIN
Pain Stimuli

Pain is often due to actual or potential tissue damage and is caused by a physical or chemical stimulus. Noxious (painful) stimuli result from a mechanical, heat, or chemical source. The mechanical sources of pain are predominantly sharp objects. A noxious heat stimulus is an excessive degree of radiant heat (greater than 45° C). Chemical mechanisms are the most common stimuli that produce painful sensations and include exogenous substances, such as acids, bases, and other caustic chemical agents, and endogenous pain-inducing substances released from damaged cells. The endogenous pain-inducing substances include potassium, histamine, serotonin, the plasma kinins (e.g., bradykinin), acetylcholine, an acid pH, substance P, and the prostaglandins. Substance P, somatostatin, and other neuropeptides also mediate pain transmission.

Nociceptors

Receptors act as transducers converting mechanical, heat, or chemical stimuli into electric impulses. Free (undifferentiated) nerve endings are receptors for pain (noxious stimulus).[2] Pain receptors are called *nociceptors*.

Some receptors respond to only one type of pain stimuli, such as intense noxious mechanical stimuli or noxious heat stimuli; these are called *unimodal* or *specific nociceptors*. Other receptors respond to noxious stimuli but also serve as receptors for non-pain-producing stimuli such as pressure. These receptors are called *polymodal* or *wide-dynamic-range nociceptors*.[2]

Pain-Impulse Transmission

The typical means of pain receptor excitation is by the release of cellular chemicals such as bradykinin and prostaglandins. Substance P is released from virtually all small, unmyelinated free nerve endings. A burst of action potentials at the nerve ending is stimulated. If the threshold level is reached, transmission of a nerve impulse begins. The nociceptive threshold does not normally differ among individuals, even of different racial or cultural backgrounds.[3] However, the nociceptive threshold can be lowered or raised in a person under certain circumstances (see p. 1500).[4] Lowering the nociceptive threshold means that a stimulus of lower-than-normal intensity can initiate a nerve-impulse transmission. Raising the nociceptive threshold means that a stimulus has to be of greater-than-normal intensity to evoke a nerve impulse.

Pain Pathways

Pain impulses spread along the nerve fiber ascending from receptors toward the spinal cord (or toward the brainstem in the head region) through afferent nerve fibers. A first neuron is either a fine, myelinated A-delta fiber or an unmyelinated C fiber. A-delta fibers mediate sharp, prickling pain. C fibers mediate a burning sensation.[2] Fibers of both types pass through the dorsal root of the spinal nerve and synapse with a second neuron in the dorsal horn.

Direct spinothalamic tract. Pain is predominantly conveyed in the anterolateral system of the spinal cord via one of two spinal cord–brainstem nociceptive pathways—the direct (lateral) spinothalamic tract (neospinothalamic pathway) and the indirect spinoreticular tract (Fig. 51-1). The direct spinothalamic tract is partially composed of nociceptive neurons that originate primarily in laminae I, IV, V, and VI of the dorsal horn, decussate (cross) at about the same level of the cord by passing through the anterior white commissure, and then ascend in the lateral funiculus of the spinal cord. These neurons synapse throughout the brainstem, and only a small portion of the fibers ascend directly to the posterior thalamus. This tract is thought to convey information about the spatial and temporal aspects of pain sensations. Pain sensations conducted by this pathway are experienced as sharp and well localized.

Indirect spinoreticular tract. The indirect spinoreticular tract (paleospinal pathway) is a more complex pathway composed primarily of small C fibers. It is concerned exclusively with transmission of pain impulses.[2] The nociceptive neurons are found primarily in laminae V, VII, and VIII of the dorsal horn. After decussating, the fibers ascend as the ventral spinoreticular tract through the brainstem, where many of the fibers terminate. The remaining fibers that do not synapse in the brainstem continue to ascend upward to terminate in the medial thalamus. This pathway is concerned with unpleasant sensations of a diffuse and burning nature. Visceral sensations are thought to be conveyed in this system as well.

Because these brainstem areas have numerous connections with the hypothalamus and the limbic system, the connections play an important role in the affective-motivational component of pain. It is also believed that the connections to the hypothalamus are at least partly responsible for the response of the autonomic nervous system to pain. Increased hypothalamic activity results in increased sympathetic tone, tachycardia, increased cardiac output, and hypertension.[5]

Release of stress hormones, the activation of the limbic system, and the interpretation the person places on the pain experience trigger the anxiety, apprehension, and suffering experienced. These emotional responses give rise to the behaviors exhibited by persons in pain.

Pain Perception

Pain perception is the threshold for recognition (awareness) of pain, that is, the point at which a person experiences pain. Pain perception probably takes place at the thalamic level. Pain perception does not vary among persons of different racial or cultural backgrounds. Pain perception within an individual, however, can be raised by decreasing the level of consciousness with the use of analgesics and anesthetics and by deep brain stimulation (see p. 1507).

From the posterior thalamic neurons, pain impulses are probably transmitted to the somatic sensory area and the posterior parietal area of the cortex. The medial thalamic neurons have fibers that project to the frontal cortex.[2]

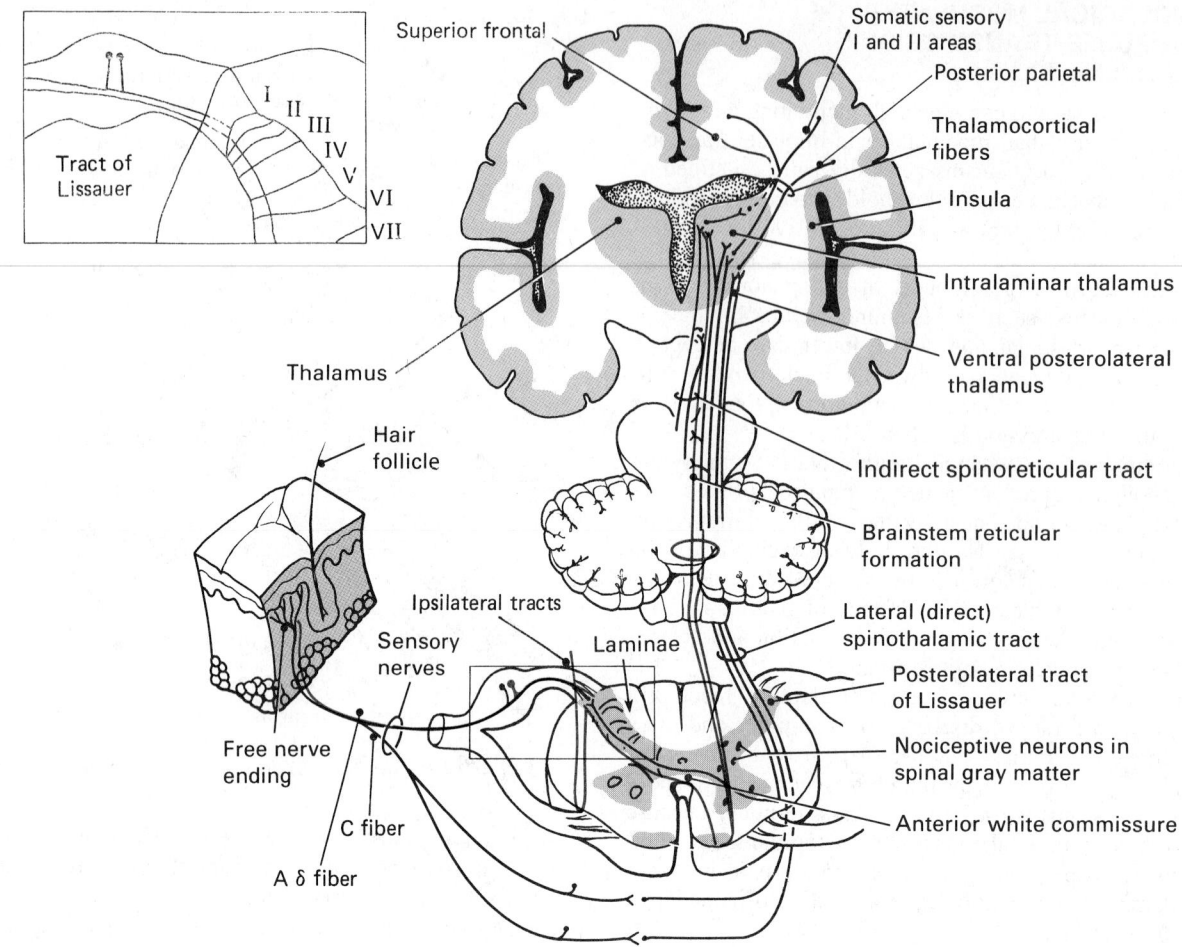

Fig. 51-1   The pain pathways.

The cortex is presumed to provide analysis and interpretation of the pain experience. The interpretation of the type, quality, and meaning of the pain is influenced by such factors as personality, cultural background, experiences, physical and psychological conditioning, and motivation.[5]

Pain Tolerance

Pain tolerance is the point at which a person feels that the pain can no longer be tolerated.[3] Pain tolerance is the amount of pain a person is willing to endure. It varies among individuals and within the same individual. This highly individual dimension has a large component of social and cultural conditioning. Pain tolerance is essentially a learned response.

Descending Systems in Pain Modulation

Besides the pain-impulse transmission upward to higher brain centers, some impulses synapse with motor neurons in the same and adjacent spinal cord segments to produce reflex responses, including skeletal muscle spasm, vasoconstriction, and decreased gastrointestinal (GI) and genitourinary (GU) function. Other automatic reflexes elicited higher in the nervous system by the pain impulse alter the rate and depth of breathing.

In addition, as pain information is transmitted to higher centers, various central nervous system (CNS) structures function to change the ascending information. This is accomplished through a descending (efferent) system that can alter or inhibit the pain impulse transmission. The cerebral cortex, the gray matter of the midbrain surrounding the aqueduct of Sylvius (the periaqueductal gray matter), and certain neurons in the pons and medulla can profoundly change pain-impulse transmission.[2]

Endogenous Pain Control

Endogenous pain control involves a pain-inhibiting system that is composed of three levels. A descending pathway activated by ascending pain impulses inhibits the pain-transmission neurons at the spinal cord level. This system is thought to be mediated in part by endogenous opiates. At the midbrain level, endogenous opiates are released. These endogenous opiates are capable of producing analgesia. They also serve as transmitter substances exciting descending fibers, which in turn activate a system of serotonin-containing cells at the medullary level. This system transmits inhibitory impulses to the cells in the dorsal horn. A major neurotransmitter in this system is serotonin. Normal concentration of this transmitter is necessary for adequate function of the descending pain system.

PHYSIOLOGICAL MODULATION OF PAIN-IMPULSE TRANSMISSION
Facilitating Mechanisms

The nervous system contains both facilitating and inhibiting mechanisms that modulate pain-impulse transmission. Facilitating mechanisms generally can be defined as those factors that lower pain threshold or pain perception.

Progressive sensitization is the progressive lowering of the pain threshold. One cause of progressive sensitization is the presence of large amounts of endogenous pain-inducing substances, such as histamine, serotonin, the kinins, and the prostaglandins, which lower the nociceptive threshold.[6] These agents can lower the nociceptive threshold so that pain receptors fire with normal touch. Thus pain-impulse transmission is enhanced.

Facilitation occurs when a stimulus that is normally not strong enough to produce a nerve impulse "primes" the succeeding neuron so that a second similar stimulus can evoke a nerve impulse. The threshold of excitation of the succeeding neuron is lowered by the preceding neuron's activity. Thus the person's experience of pain can be intensified, even when the degree of stimulation and the extent of tissue damage remain constant.

Pain receptors, however, are nonadapting receptors. They maintain a rate of discharge over minutes and often hours. Since the primary purpose of pain is to protect the person, this failure to adapt (exhibit a decreasing responsiveness to stimuli) is useful in acute tissue injury because it urges the person to take measures to stop the tissue damage. However, in ongoing acute or chronic pain in which tissue damage is not continuing, this feature of nonadaptation is a disadvantage.

Inhibiting Mechanisms

Inhibiting mechanisms generally are those factors that increase the pain threshold and decrease pain perception. Inhibitory mechanisms that influence pain-impulse transmission are at least partly mediated through the release of endogenous opiates.

A group of neuropeptides with morphinelike (opiate) properties, called *endorphins* (from *endogenous* and *morphine*), play a major role in the body's chemical defense against pain. Another major group of endogenous opiates consists of the *enkephalins*, which inhibit the transmission of pain impulses. These substances differ in molecular size, site of origin, and site of action.

Enkephalins. Within the nervous system, enkephalins have been found in high concentration in several areas of the brain and in the dorsal horns of the spinal cord, where synapsing of nociceptive fibers and enkephalin-containing fibers occurs. Concentrations of enkephalins are found in the central gray matter of the brainstem, the substantia gelatinosa, and the thalami at sites of termination of the spinothalamic systems.[5]

The enkephalins are released into the synaptic cleft. The released enkephalins are either rapidly inactivated by specific enzymes or attracted to and bind with opiate receptors found on nociceptive fibers to inhibit the activity of the cell.[2] For example, in the dorsal horn of the spinal cord the presence of enkephalin attached to the opiate-re-

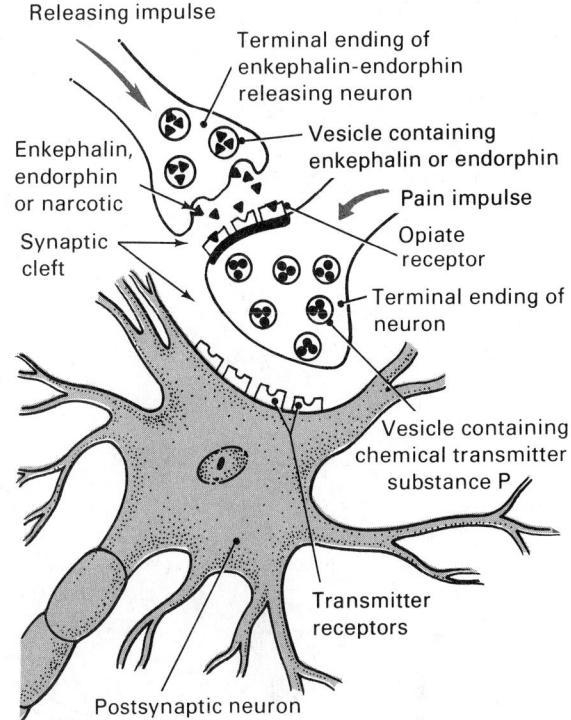

Fig. 51-2   The enkephalin-endorphin receptor sites.

ceptor site partially depolarizes the nociceptive neuron, resulting in a reduction in the amount of pain-inducing transmitter substance released. This results in a decrease in the intensity and firing rate of the impulses transmitted to the next ascending neuron (Fig. 51-2).

The opiate receptors are the receptor sites at which morphine and other narcotic molecules act to block the transmission of nociceptive impulses. The activity of the endogenous opiates can be blocked by opiate antagonists such as naloxone (Narcan).

Endorphins. The endorphins are found in great concentration in the hypothalamus and the pituitary gland. Although several have been isolated, β-endorphin is the most potent and presumed to be the most important.[2] β-Endorphin binds firmly to the opiate receptor, but it is not activated nearly as rapidly as the enkephalins. β-Endorphin has a wide range of effects. Its actions include analgesia, catatonic posturing, and behavioral disturbances. β-Endorphin appears to be released in combination with adrenocortical hormone (ACTH) in response to extreme stress.

Evidence now exists to indicate that the placebo response is caused by the release of endogenous opiates. The placebo somehow causes the individual to mobilize endogenous opiates. It is now thought that persons who have a deficiency of endogenous opiates are far more likely to have chronic pain syndromes. This is supported by the finding that persons with chronic pain syndromes have significantly lower endogenous opiate levels.[7]

PAIN THEORIES

Over the years, three types of pain theories have predominated—the specificity theory, the gate-control the-

ory, and the pattern theories. More recently, the thalamic neuron theory and the endogenous pain-control theory have gained recognition.

Specificity Theory

The specificity theory, the earliest of the pain theories, was proposed first by Descartes in the seventeenth century. It holds that there are distinct pain receptors—the free nerve endings in the tissues. These peripheral pain receptors are stimulated by a specific type of sensory input only and function only as pain receptors. No other type of receptor can generate nerve impulses that can be experienced as pain.

Although some receptors are specialized, it is doubtful that these specific receptors have direct and constant access to the higher brain centers. Each impulse is probably not automatically interpreted only as pain. The theory does not satisfactorily explain pain tolerance, especially the modulation of the pain experience by variables such as social factors, cultural influences, personality, and pain experiences. The theory also does not account for many of the clinical pain syndromes, such as causalgia, phantom-limb pain, and peripheral neuralgia.[8] The theory does provide the rationale for ablative neurosurgical procedures.

Pattern Theories

The pattern theories of pain were proposed because the specificity theory was inadequate to explain all aspects of the pain experience. These theories do not hold that there are specific receptors for pain. Pain is experienced because various sensory receptors are stimulated in a certain pattern. Pain is the result of intense receptor stimulation, producing a certain pattern of nerve impulses that is coded within the CNS to signify pain.

As a further development, the sensory interaction pattern theory states that small-diameter fibers carry pain patterns while large-diameter fibers inhibit pain transmission. In abnormal syndromes such as neuralgias and postinfectious pain, it is theorized that the large inhibitory fibers are lost. The pattern theories have contributed to the understanding of pain, but the alteration of pain perception by psychological factors is not explained by either of the pattern theories.

Thalamic Neuron Theory

The thalamic neuron theory places the source of a chronic pain syndrome in the thalamus. The theory suggests that thalamic neurons normally transmitting sensory impulses become autonomous. A state of prolonged hypersensitivity develops. Normal sensory impulses are experienced as pain when transmitted by these hyperexcitable neurons. The theory states that the thalamic neurons are more prone to develop a hyperexcitable state, especially when repeatedly stimulated.

This theory moves pain generation from the periphery or the spinal cord to the thalamus. It suggests that continuous or repeated stimulation—for example, an acute tissue injury—can generate a hyperexcitable state and implies that it is essential to prevent large numbers of pain impulses from reaching the thalamus after acute injury.

Gate-Control Theory

The gate-control theory of pain was first proposed in 1965 and was expanded in 1967 and 1976. According to this theory, the perception of pain does not depend on specific pain receptors. Pain results from a balance of input to central transmission cells through myelinated (innocuous) and small unmyelinated (noxious) C fibers. This input is under the influence of substantia gelatinosa (SG) cells that inhibit central transmission cells when excited. Myelinated fibers excite SG cells, leading to the inhibition of transmission cells by the SG. Conversely, unmyelinated C fibers inhibit SG cells, allowing for the central transmission of pain impulses.

The gate theorists hold that two other pain-inhibiting mechanisms besides stimulating large-A-fiber inhibitory transmissions exist—the *central biasing mechanism,* thought to be located in the reticular formation of the brainstem, and the *central control mechanism,* located in the thalamus and cerebral cortex. To function, the central biasing mechanism requires visual, auditory, or other sensory stimuli, including that generated by distraction and injury. It is postulated to be capable of sending impulses down the spinal cord to close the pain gate in the dorsal horn, thus inhibiting pain-impulse transmission.

The central control mechanism is thought to be activated by stimulation of the dorsal horn transmission cells. Selective brain processes that regulate or modulate the gate-control system are triggered. At this level, attention, experience, emotions, anxiety, anticipation, culture, expectations, suggestion, and other factors are able to regulate and therefore exert control over the pain input.

Although empirical support for the theory has not been generated, the gate-control theory has clinical significance because it provides insight into previously unexplained aspects of pain, such as how the meaning of a pain-producing situation for the individual, a person's unique history of pain, and the present state of mind can not only influence reaction to pain but greatly affect perception of pain.[2] Since its publication in 1965, the gate-control theory has generated a fruitful search for additional pain-management techniques. The gate-control theory and the inhibiting mechanism of endogenous opiates support such therapies as rubbing, massage, touch, acupuncture, and electrical stimulation.

EFFECT OF AGING ON PAIN PERCEPTION

The effects of aging on factors that affect pain and pain perception are contradictory. However, the general consensus is that the pain threshold increases with age.[9] Recognition of pain by the aging client may be affected by impairments of the peripheral nervous system or CNS, drug therapy, and cognitive impairments. Other factors relative to pain, such as the meaning of the pain, cultural influence, past pain experience, and acceptability of pain behaviors, are the same in older adults and in younger persons.

The aged client may have a decreased number of pain receptors and decreased receptor sensitivity. A stronger nociceptive stimulus may be required under ordinary circumstances to initiate nociceptive impulse transmission.

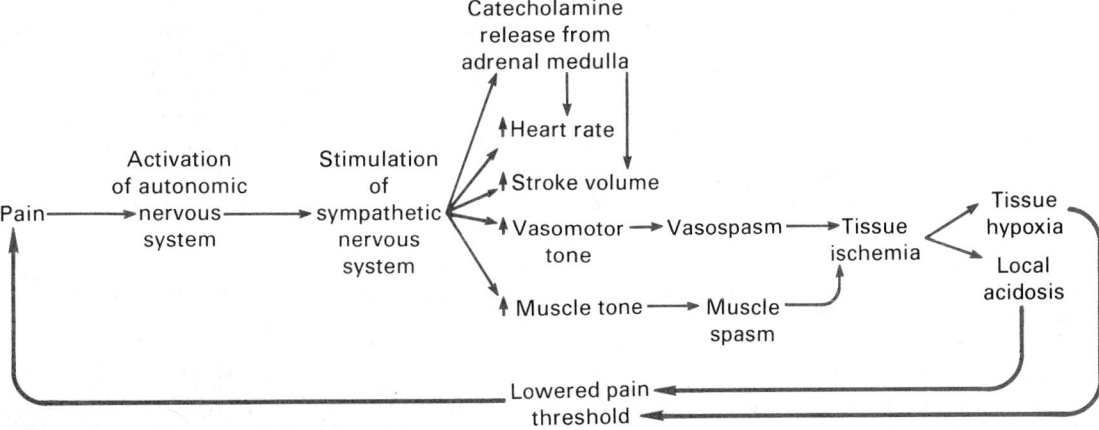

Fig. 51-3   The acute pain cycle.

Because transmission time is slightly increased, reaction time is also increased. Thus the older adult may have sustained greater tissue damage than a younger client before recognizing and reacting to the nociceptive stimulus. For example, it is common for older adults to have very advanced appendicitis, even peritonitis, before they experience the associated abdominal pain.

The age-related reduction in pain incidence is unexplained. However, in addition to alterations in neural pathways, there may be differences in the psychological disposition to report pain. This may lead to pain being underrecognized and inadequately assessed and treated in older adults. Depression manifested by vegetative signs, such as increased sleep and lassitude, may result when the older adult experiences chronic pain.

TYPES OF PAIN SYNDROME
Acute Pain Syndromes

Acute pain can be described as an unpleasant sensory, perceptual, and emotional experience produced by tissue damage that is caused by disease, accidental injury, surgical operation, or certain other therapeutic procedures.[3] Once the cause of the pain is known, acute pain has no useful purpose. This type of pain is only a source of anxiety and suffering, and if the pain is not stopped, it elicits autonomic reflexes that result in physiological dysfunction.[9] The uncontrolled acute pain cycle is shown in Fig. 51-3. Increased sympathetic nervous system activity results in significant increases in cardiac output and blood pressure, thus increasing cardiac work load, metabolism, and oxygen consumption.[10] This cycle must be broken by an effective pain management protocol.

Postoperative pain. A prototype for an acute pain syndrome is postoperative pain. The quality, quantity, and duration of pain are related to the nature of the surgical procedure.[10,11] Any trauma, including surgical trauma, results in tissue damage. Pain-inducing substances released in the traumatized tissue may lower the pain threshold *(progressive sensitization);* thus normally innocuous (nonnoxious) stimuli are experienced as painful *(allodynia).* The length of the incision contributes directly to the amount of pain-inducing substance released. The duration and extent of the surgery also contribute directly to the amount of trauma.[11] A transverse incision generally produces less postoperative pain than a vertical or diagonal incision because fewer nerves and muscles and less fascia are severed.[11,12] Incisions involving the thoracic and upper abdominal areas are frequently associated with greater postoperative pain because of movement with each respiration. Clients with anorectal surgery and surgery involving the back region often experience greater postoperative pain because of muscle spasms.[11]

Because skin and soft tissues are well supplied with free nerve endings, incisional pain is experienced as sharp and well localized. Clients describe incisional pain as sharp, cutting, tearing, or stabbing. With prolonged stimulation, such as that from tension on the sutures, the pain tends to develop a burning quality. Deeper tissues, such as muscles, tendons, ligaments, joints, bones, and arteries, have fewer nerve endings; thus the ability to clearly localize the pain is diminished. Pain is experienced as more diffuse and tends to radiate to adjacent areas. Clients tend to describe somatic pain as dull and aching. Pain from various deep structures differs; for example, pain associated with a punctured artery tends to be diffuse and dull, whereas pain from periosteal damage is sharp.[13] Trauma to visceral structures, pleura, or peritoneum can produce sharp but diffuse tenderness, pain, or intense referred pain. Fear and anxiety are both part of the affective-motivational component of postoperative pain (see Chapter 13).

Referred pain. Acute pain syndromes may arise from ischemia of a viscus due to pressure or impaired blood supply. Visceral pain is often experienced as a vaguely localized but often severe pain on the surface of the skin, and the affected skin surface area may be distant from the damaged viscus. This phenomenon is known as *referred pain.* Several explanations have been offered to account for the misinterpretation of the source of the pain. Currently the most accepted hypothesis states that the afferent pathway from the involved viscus and the afferent pathways from the involved skin areas converge on the same spinal cord neuron. Thus impulses transmitted centrally by this second neuron lead to misinterpretation of the location of the pain (Fig. 51-4).

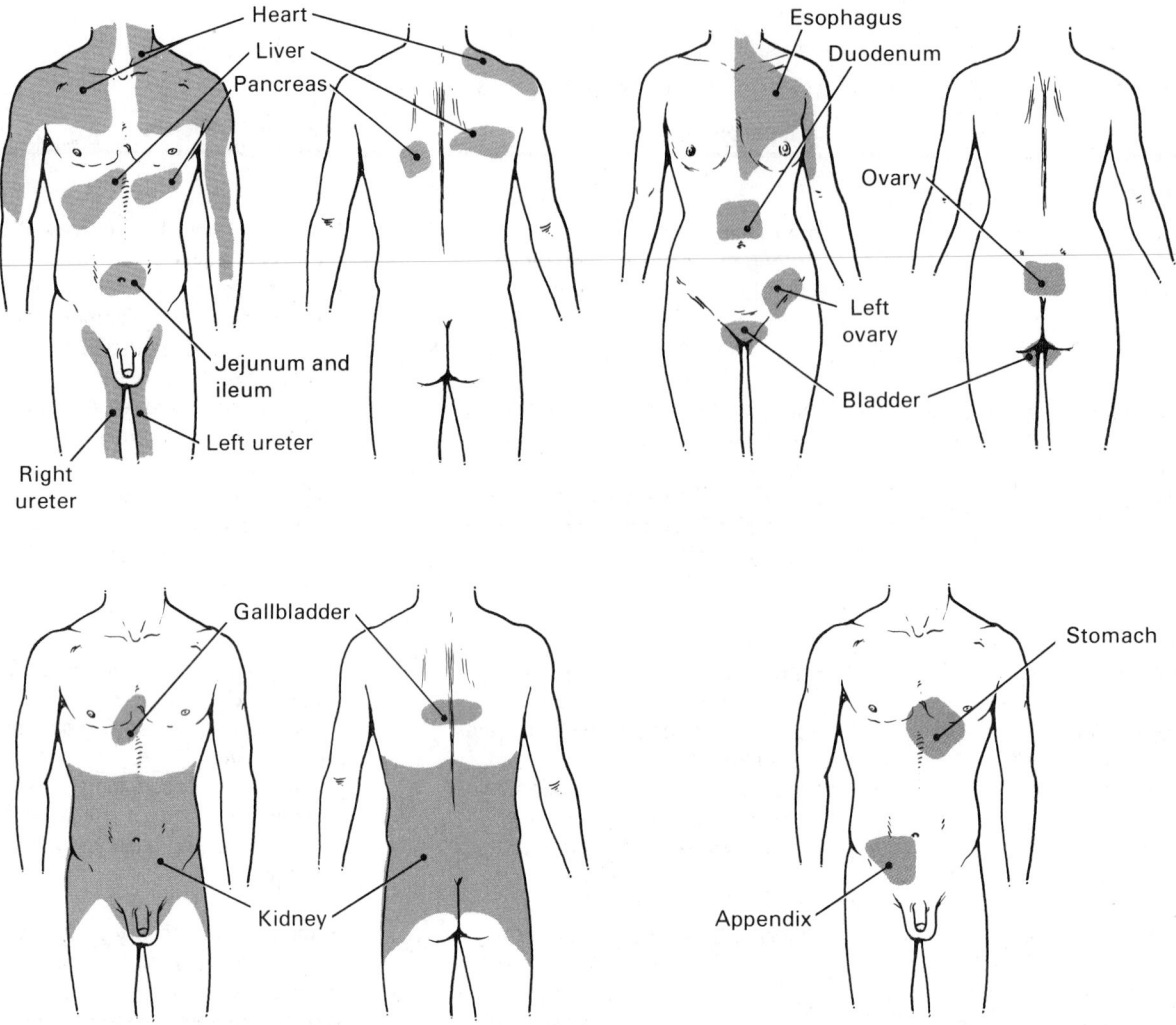

Fig. 51-4　Typical surface locations of pain originating from stimuli in visceral organs.

Chronic Pain Syndromes

Chronic pain is a continuous or regularly recurring pain that extends over a period of 6 months or more. Intractable pain is severe chronic pain that is incapacitating and resistant to the usual therapeutic measures.

Chronic pain is different from acute pain and presents additional problems. In chronic pain syndromes a persistent disease factor or pathological state may be present. In such instances the pain serves as a constant reminder of the threat to function, integrity, and possibly life itself, but chronic pain is also a disease. The client becomes anxious and frustrated. Chronic pain affects the person's entire life. Life begins to revolve around the pain, and the total person may be affected. The client's family is also affected by the chronic pain state.

The causes of chronic pain syndromes can be categorized as posttraumatic, postinfectious, degenerative, vascular, cancer, and idiopathic (cause unknown). These causes may produce any one of three major chronic pain states—central pain, peripheral pain, and peripheral-central pain.[14] Central pain may emerge when the CNS has been injured or involved by the disease process. Pain of

peripheral origin arises when the peripheral nerves are traumatized, compressed, or become dysfunctional in some other way. Peripheral-central pain emerges when peripheral nervous system and CNS tissues are contributing to the pain experience (Table 51-1).

Posttraumatic pain syndromes. A posttraumatic pain syndrome often occurs after accidental injury and is characterized by persistence of the pain long after the damaged tissues have healed. The severity of the posttraumatic pain experience exceeds what would normally be expected after the degree of tissue injury. Posttraumatic pain syndromes include such conditions as chronic low-back pain, herniated disk syndromes, posttraumatic head pain, postsurgical pain syndromes, and causalgias. If the pain is not brought under control, pain trigger zones surrounding the painful areas may extend, involving other body parts.

Pain associated with cancer. The pain associated with cancer may take the form of acute pain at certain times and chronic pain at others. Most persons with cancer do not initially experience pain. Some never suffer physiological pain from the malignant process. However, many experience pain in the later stages of their disease.[6]

Table 51-1   Peripheral, Central, and Peripheral-Central Pain Syndromes

Pain	Description	Precipitating Factors
PERIPHERAL NERVE PAIN		
Nerve-root compression	Intermittent, radicular, stabbing pain along one or more nerve roots	Any activity stretching nerve (intensification of pain)
Neuralgias	Pain along course of nerves	Viral infections; conditions such as diabetes mellitus, vitamin deficiency, ischemia, and ingestion of toxins, in which axons degenerate
Trigeminal neuralgia (tic douloureux)	Brief, paroxysmal, extreme pain, usually along one division of trigeminal nerve	Eating, talking, cold, air currents, or spontaneous occurence
Postherpetic pain	Sudden explosive pain along cutaneous distribution of nerve following herpes zoster	Aggravation with cutaneous stimuli, noise, stress
CENTRAL PAIN		
Spinal cord		
Tabetic pain	Paresthesias, poorly localized pain sensations	Involvement of sensory fibers entering spinal cord
Multiple sclerosis	Paresthesias, poorly localized pain sensations	Involvement of ascending sensory pathways
Trauma	Paresthesias, poorly localized pain sensations	Involvement of ascending sensory pathways
Low-back pain	Highly variable pain syndrome	Trauma involving ascending sensory pathways
Brainstem		
Direct tissue damage	Highly variable pain syndrome	Stimulation of sensory pathways, initiating transmission of impulses interpreted as pain
Thalamic pain syndrome	Deep, paroxysmal, and excruciating pain, often burning and causalgia-like, in contralateral extremities	Damage to ventroposterior lateral nucleus of thalamus
Cerebrum		
Pain of cortical origin	Disturbed sensations on contralateral side of body similar to nerve-root pain	Inadequate understanding at present
Headache	Highly variable pain syndrome	Vasodilatation of cerebral vessels, muscle contraction, traction on pain-sensitive structures, meningeal irritation, pressure
PERIPHERAL-CENTRAL PAIN		
Causalgia	Spontaneous severe burning pain in distal portion of extremities; initial vasodilatation and later vasoconstriction and trophic skin, subcutaneous tissue, bone, and joint changes	Result of acute peripheral nerve injury (often more than 6 mo after injury), aggravation with cold, touch, emotions, visual stimuli, auditory stimuli, or startle response
Phantom limb pain	Paresthesias; feelings of coldness and heaviness; cramping, shooting, burning, or crushing pain	Presence of pain in limb before amputation

The pain associated with a progressive cancerous process may involve several physiological mechanisms that induce pain. The compression of neural tissues produces a continuous, stabbing, or sharp, well-localized pain that follows the neural distribution of the involved nerve. Paresthesias (abnormal sensations such as "pins and needles" or burning sensations) are often experienced. Infiltration of the integument, fascia, or other tissues results in localized pain that is initially dull and aching but becomes more severe as the tumor enlarges. Obstruction of a viscus causes a true visceral pain described as full, diffuse, boring, and poorly localized.

Sudden occlusion of a tube, such as the ureter, may produce a severe, cramping, colicky pain. The pain associated with obstruction of a blood vessel depends on the type of vessel occluded: occlusion of an artery results in ischemic pain, whereas occlusion in the venous system or the lymphatic system results in dull, diffuse, burning, and aching pain. Tissue damage results in inflammation, and the inflammatory process produces tenderness and sensitivity to touch. In the person with late-stage cancer this inflammation is often complicated by infection and necrosis of the involved tissues.

The pain associated with necrosis is severe and often excruciating and tends to be unresponsive to most treatment regimens. The bone destruction often resulting from metastasis is another frequent cause of cancer pain. The pain is sharp and lancinating. Although it is often continuous, the pain is more severe on movement.

The physiological and psychological impact of pain associated with cancer is often greater than that of nonmalignant chronic pain syndromes. Physical deterioration is usually more severe because the person is often anorectic as a result of chemotherapy or radiation therapy.

MULTIDISCIPLINARY PAIN-MANAGEMENT TECHNIQUES

Therapeutic techniques to manage pain syndromes are generally directed at altering either the sensory-discriminative or the affective-motivational and cognitive-evaluative components of pain. Comprehensive, holistic pain-management programs use a multidisciplinary approach using a combination of techniques directed at all components of pain.

Alteration of the Sensory-Discriminative Component

Many techniques to alter the sensory-discriminative pain component induce an analgesic (pain-free) or an anesthetic (sensation-free) state. Analgesia can be achieved through dermal stimulation using techniques such as massage, pressure, vibration, heat, cold, externally applied preparations, and transcutaneous electrical nerve stimulation (TENS) and are supported by the gate-control theory of pain. Deep-structure stimulation by percutaneous electrical nerve stimulation, acupuncture, dorsal cord stimulation, and deep brain stimulation also produce analgesia. Endogenous opiate mobilization has been demonstrated to account for the analgesia produced by TENS, acupuncture, and deep brain stimulation.[15] TENS and dorsal column

stimulation act through presynaptic inhibition. Narcotic analgesics provide exogenous opiates. An anesthetic state can be produced by nerve block or by neurosurgical or radiological interruption of the pain pathway.

Another means to alter the sensory-discriminative pain component is to block release of endogenous pain-inducing substances. Many nonnarcotic analgesics act to inhibit activation or release of these substances.

Dermal stimulation

Types. Dermal (cutaneous) stimulation to produce analgesia is defined as noninjurious stimulation of the client's skin for the purpose of pain relief.[1] Dermal stimulation may be provided by the client or someone else. The dermal stimulation methods differ related to convenience, cost, need for a physician's prescription, precautions, contraindications, and trained health care professionals who may provide the intervention. A major difference from the client's perspective is that the various methods produce different sensations.

Pressure is an instinctual response to pain. An injured part is reflexly clutched and pressure is applied. Dermal stimulation that uses a pressure method harnesses this automatic response in a deliberate fashion. Pressure may be applied with the fingertips, the ball of the thumb, the heel of the hand, the entire hand, or the knuckles. At times both hands are used. Occasionally a hard but smooth object, such as a sandbag, may be used to apply pressure.

Acupressure is a specific pressure technique that involves application of pressure, massage, or both to specified points on the skin. These points are the same as the traditional acupuncture points. Pressure is applied with the thumb, the tip of the index finger, or the palm of the hand.

Massage of an injured body part with rubbing is also an instinctual response. This response can be deliberately tapped to manage pain. Many massage techniques exist. Examples include moving the hands or fingers over the skin slowly or briskly with long strokes or in circles (superficial massage) or applying firm pressure to the skin to maintain contact while massaging the underlying tissues (deep massage). Relaxation is also often induced by massage. Specific massage techniques are involved in some forms of acupressure and in trigger-point massage. Cold massage to trigger points is also used. Other manipulative procedures include passive movement (mobilization) techniques applied locally and regionally and single, high-velocity thrusts to joints and soft tissue.[16]

The application of *cutaneous vibration* and high-frequency energy, such as by ultrasound, short- and longwave diathermy, and microwave, is used to provide pain relief.[17] The pain relief may be immediate, or it may require several minutes to occur. The duration of the pain relief is highly variable. Many different vibration devices exist, varying in size and shape to meet individual needs. A physician's prescription is not necessary for the purchase of a vibratory device.

Heat therapy is the application of either moist or dry heat to the skin. Heat therapy can be either superficial or deep. Superficial dry heat can be applied by means of an electrical device, such as a heating pad, a heat cradle, or a gooseneck or infrared lamp, or by nonelectrical means,

such as hot-water bottles and exposure to the sun. Superficial moist heat can be obtained nonelectrically from hydrocollator (moist heat) packs, soaks, showers, baths, whirlpools, and Hubbard tanks and by wrapping the body part in plastic to trap body heat.[5] Electric heating pads designed to provide moist heat are also available. Physical therapy departments provide deep-heat therapy through such techniques as short-wave diathermy, microwave diathermy, and ultrasound therapy (Fig. 51-5).

Heat therapy generally involves intermittent applications of heat for short periods of time, but some therapy methods, such as trapping of body heat, may be continued for prolonged periods or may be continuous.

Cold therapy involves the application of either moist or dry cold to the skin. Dry cold can be applied by means of an ice bag, moist cold by means of towels soaked in ice water, cold hydrocollator packs, or immersion in a bath or under running cold water. Icing, with ice cubes or blocks of ice made to resemble Popsicles, is another technique used for pain relief. Ice massage is a technique combining cold therapy and massage; the ice is applied evenly over the area of pain with slow up-and-down strokes for about 10 minutes.[1] Physical therapists sometimes use ethyl chloride or "vasocoolant" sprays as part of a cold-therapy regimen.

Cold therapy is used for a variety of painful conditions, including posttraumatic pain and postoperative pain (especially that following orthopedic procedures) and with bursitis, osteomyelitis, and muscle spasms. In addition, contrast baths (alternating hot and cold applications) and hydrotherapy used in conjunction with relaxation, passive movement exercises, and breathing exercises may be used to treat pain.[18]

Externally applied preparations, such as ointments, lotions, gels, liniments, and balms (most of which are over-the-counter products), are sometimes applied to the skin to achieve pain relief. Although these agents contain various substances, two common ingredients are menthol and methyl salicylate (oil of wintergreen). The salicylate component is absorbed from the skin. On application, these agents usually produce a strong hot or cold sensation and should not be used after massage or a heat treatment. Massage also intensifies the sensation. Skin testing is advisable when the client has not used the particular agent before, since the strengths of the agents vary and various intensi-

ties of sensation are produced. Relief of pain is reported for muscle pain, joint pain, headache, and visceral pain associated with gas, distention, and endometriosis.

TENS involves the delivery of an electric current through electrodes applied to the skin surface over the painful region, at trigger points, or over a peripheral nerve. A TENS system consists of two or more electrodes connected by lead wires to a stimulator (Fig. 51-6). The stimulator is usually about the size of a pack of cigarettes and is battery operated. The batteries are usually rechargeable. Most stimulators may be worn and used 24 hours a day. The system can also be disassembled for intermittent use by detaching the stimulator and wires while leaving the electrodes in place. A physician's order is required to initiate this therapy.

Experimentation with different stimulators, different electrode placements, and different frequency settings is often necessary to achieve therapeutic results with TENS. If one stimulator is not effective in providing pain relief, another should be tried. Multiple sites of stimulation may also be tried during successive trials to determine the most effective site for pain modulation.

Conventional (high-frequency) TENS units that use alternating current set at a rate of 40 to 400 Hz (cycles per second) typically produce rapid analgesia (within 20 minutes), but the effectiveness is brief. With low-frequency TENS (1 to 5 Hz) the onset of analgesia is slow, but the effect lasts much longer.[19]

The person receiving high-frequency TENS experiences paresthesias during the treatments. The voltage and the

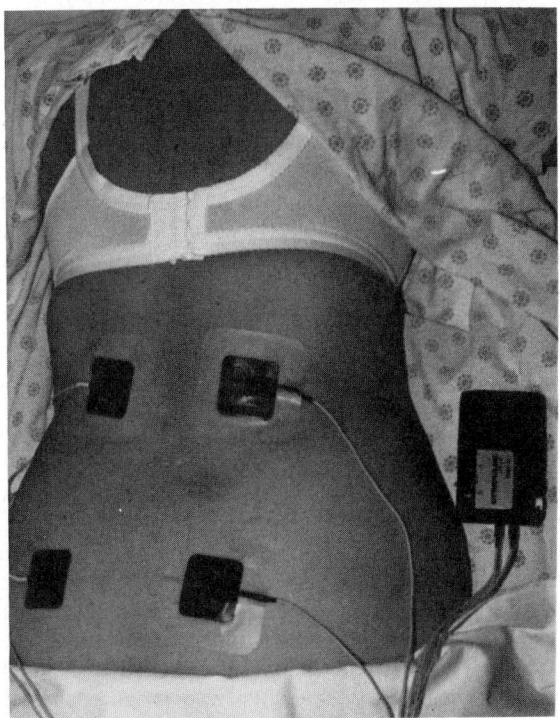

Fig. 51-6 Initial TENS treatment being given by physical therapy department to assess value in pain relief.

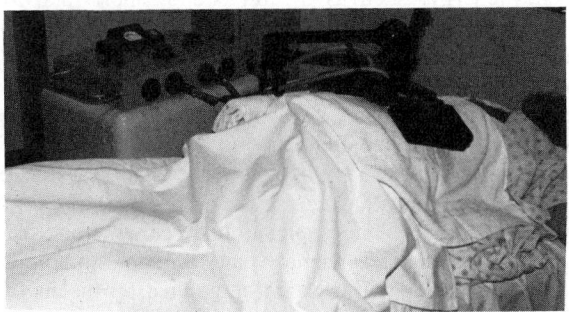

Fig. 51-5 Client receiving heat treatment by diathermy.

rate of stimulation are altered according to the client's response to the paresthesias. Some therapists set low-frequency TENS at an amplitude to produce strong rhythmic muscular contractions, whereas other therapists set amplitude according to client tolerance and relief.[3]

The pain relief produced by low-frequency TENS is believed to be the result of mobilization of endogenous opiates. The relief provided by high-frequency TENS may be mediated by another unidentified mechanism. TENS is used most commonly to treat chronic pain in adults. Pain relief has been reported in low-back pain, cervical (neck) syndrome, arthritis, sciatica, tic douloureux, postherpetic neuralgia, peripheral nerve injuries, brachial plexus injuries, and stump and phantom limb pain.[20] TENS has been used in children with chronic pain syndromes and with acute pain. During the actual application of TENS, acute postoperative pain is reduced. Postoperative pulmonary and GI tract complications can also be minimized with the use of TENS. Pain relief after discontinuance of TENS varies.

Contraindications for the use of TENS are not firmly established. TENS is not currently recommended for clients with cardiac pacemakers or with a history of myocardial ischemia or dysrhythmias. TENS is not applied over broken skin or anesthetic areas; in areas of the carotid sinuses, or laryngeal and pharyngeal muscles; or in the eyes.[20]

Guidelines. Any type of dermal stimulation should initially be of moderate intensity and then increased or decreased to achieve optimal pain relief. The most effective intensity for dermal stimulation is slightly less than the intensity that produces discomfort in persons with normal skin—frequently a stimulation of slightly above moderate intensity.[1,21,22]

Dermal stimulation may be continuous or intermittent. The duration of most cutaneous stimulation is 10 to 30 minutes; however, ice massage rarely lasts longer than 10 minutes. When firm pressure is applied to trigger points or acupuncture points, steady pressure is usually not maintained more than a few seconds.

The frequency of dermal stimulation should be determined by how long pain relief persists following stimulation. When the pain recurs, the dermal stimulation is reapplied. An arbitrary schedule (such as tid or qid) may be established in an institutional setting. On an outpatient basis, dermal stimulation is scheduled by appointment.

Continuous application of most dermal stimulation methods is impractical. If the client needs continuous stimulation to achieve pain relief, TENS or a menthol product may be the most practical solution.[1]

Generally, dermal stimulation is applied directly over the painful area, around the painful site, or just proximal and distal to the painful area. *Trigger-point stimulation* is an effective alternative in some instances. A trigger point is a small hyperirritable area with a taut band in the muscle or connective tissue, often just below the skin, that causes pain when it is stimulated sufficiently.[23] Trigger points may exist in the painful area or at a point distant from the actual pain. There is a strong association between trigger points and acupuncture points for pain.[1] Although pressure on a trigger point may produce a dull, aching discomfort,

continued pressure may relieve the pain. Pressure with massage and ice massage are also used for trigger-point stimulation.

Another possible area of stimulation is over peripheral nerves that innervate the painful area. This type of stimulation is most readily accomplished by TENS. Contralateral stimulation may be necessary when a painful area is too sensitive to be directly stimulated or when the painful area is not accessible because of a covering. The reason for the effectiveness of contralateral stimulation is not known. Contralateral stimulation is also used with phantom limb pain. If the aforementioned alternatives are unacceptable, unrelated areas can be stimulated.

Use of cutaneous stimulation techniques must be individualized to the client and the particular type of pain. The client may have strong preferences regarding the type of dermal stimulation used and the area to be stimulated. Individual needs relate to cost, convenience, intensity of stimulation, and duration of stimulation. Although success rates vary, 50% of the persons using some type of dermal stimulation achieve 50% to 100% reduction of pain.[24]

Deep-structure stimulation

Percutaneous electrical nerve stimulation. Deeper peripheral tissues can be stimulated through percutaneous electrical nerve stimulation or acupuncture. Percutaneous electrical nerve stimulation is a preliminary step designed to evaluate the potential usefulness of a permanently implanted device. It is accomplished by insertion of a needle to which a stimulator is attached near a large peripheral or spinal nerve. The amount of electric current is regulated to provide the maximum pain relief. If the percutaneous stimulation successfully reduces the client's pain, a permanent peripheral nerve stimulator is surgically implanted. A special electrode is placed around the nerve, and an internal receiver is implanted subcutaneously at waist level on the anterior chest wall. The client activates the receiver by means of a special transmitter and antenna as needed for optimum pain relief.

Acupuncture. Acupuncture involves the insertion of needles at specified cutaneous sites. The needles are activated by hand or by low-voltage electric current. Onset of analgesia may not be immediate, but once the endogenous opiates have been mobilized, the technique's pain-relieving capacities extend beyond the period of actual stimulation.

Dorsal cord or deep brain stimulation. CNS stimulation can be achieved through dorsal cord stimulation or deep brain stimulation. Dorsal cord stimulation is an alternative pain-management technique to percutaneous electrical nerve stimulation when the pain involves large areas, such as the lower extremities or the back. During a laminectomy, electrodes are implanted intradurally in the dorsal aspect of the spinal cord. The level of implantation is determined by the pain location. A receiver is implanted subcutaneously on the anterior chest wall at waist level. The antenna and the transmitter system are similar to those used in permanent peripheral nerve stimulation.

Electrical stimulation of certain regions of the brain, including areas of the frontal lobes, thalamus, midbrain, lower brainstem, caudate nucleus of the basal ganglion,

and internal capsule, produces long-lasting analgesia, called *stimulus-produced analgesia*. This analgesia is specific to pain. Motor function, affect, and other behavior responses are unaffected. At least two pain-modulating systems are involved. In the periventricular gray system, the release of enkephalin is hypothesized to activate neurons that exert an inhibitory action on small pain afferents. Pain syndromes responsive to morphine are treated with periaqueductal and periventricular deep brain stimulation. Central pain is best treated with internal capsule and lateral thalamus stimulation, although the mechanism of action is unclear.[25]

Analgesic therapy. Analgesic agents used in pain management interfere with pain transmission at peripheral, spinal cord, or lower brain center sites by blocking release of endogenous pain-transmitter substances. Some drugs also alter perception and response to pain.

Narcotic analgesics. Narcotic analgesics (opiate agonists) include natural, semisynthetic, and synthetic drugs that bind to opiate-receptor sites in the CNS to block pain transmission. For example, in the dorsal spinal cord, binding blocks the release of pain-transmitter substances such as substance P. Most narcotic drugs are capable of relieving severe pain. However, tolerance of the analgesic effects and physical dependence may occur. These drugs tend to alter perception of the pain experience and behavioral response to the pain. In addition, the common side effects of respiratory depression, nausea, vomiting, ileus, and urinary retention encourage the use of alternate pain-relief methods.

Mixed agonist-antagonists. A related group of narcotic agents, the agonist-antagonists, provide relief similar to that produced by other narcotics. These agents have decreased receptor activity, which is associated with analgesia, respiratory depression, dependence, and euphoria. When given alone, they provide satisfactory analgesia. However, when given in combination with other narcotic analgesics, symptoms of acute withdrawal, such as anxiety or hallucinations, or loss of all analgesia may occur. These agents also have a greater tendency to produce undesirable psychiatric effects than do other narcotics. Included in this agonist-antagonist group are butorphanol (Stadol), nalbuphine (Nubain), and pentazocine (Talwin).

Partial agonists. Buprenorphine (Buprenex), a related narcotic agent, has a lower risk of abuse and does not produce the psychiatric effects seen with the agonist-antagonist drugs. The drug precipitates withdrawal if taken with other narcotic analgesics.

Nonsteroidal antiinflammatory drugs. Nonsteroidal antiinflammatory drugs (NSAIDs) are nonnarcotic medications that include aspirin and other salicylates, acetaminophen, and the nonsalicylate NSAIDs such as indomethacin (Indocin), naproxen (Naprosyn), and phenylbutazone (Butazolidin). NSAIDs generally have analgesic properties equal to those of aspirin and have similar antiinflammatory effects. However, the analgesic effectiveness of each agent varies greatly among individuals.

Nonsteroidal analgesics tend to act at peripheral sites to reduce pain, often by inhibiting transmitter-substance mobilization. The peripheral analgesic effects of the NSAIDs are attributed primarily to prostaglandin inhibition. Prostaglandin increases sensitivity of nerves to bradykinin, a pain-inducing substance. With reduction of the amount of prostaglandins, the amount of pain from bradykinin is reduced. These drugs do not bind to opiate-receptor sites. NSAIDs relieve mild to moderate pain and do not cause drug tolerance, physical dependence, or CNS depression.

Because of the differing actions and sites of action for these two categories of analgesic drugs, nonnarcotic drugs and NSAIDs are often used simultaneously. Thus several sites and two components of pain are attacked at one time; there is also an additive effect on the degree of analgesia. Side effects of NSAIDs include fluid retention, gastric ulceration and blood loss, tinnitus, and prothrombinemia. They are particularly useful in the treatment of low-back pain, migraine, cancer, postoperative pain, dysmenorrhea, and the rheumatic diseases.

Serotonin blockers. Drugs that alter serotonin synthesis, release, reuptake, or receptor sites are also used to alter the sensory-discriminative component of pain. Tricyclic antidepressants, such as amitriptyline (Elavil), imipramine (Tofranil), and doxepin (Sinequan), block serotonin reuptake, making more serotonin available at the synaptic level in the descending pain-blockading pathways. Thus analgesia is produced and the effects of other analgesic agents are enhanced.

Adjuvants. Certain drugs are used to elicit complementary effects or counteracting effects to minimize undesirable side effects associated with the analgesic agents. For example, caffeine is used to produce mood elevation, a decreased sense of fatigue, and increased alertness. If a narcotic agent is being used, the caffeine often counters the depressant side effects of the narcotic. Similarly, other stimulants such as amphetamines are used to increase alertness and counter the depressant effects. The enhanced alertness is believed to improve the person's ability to concentrate and thus assist with distraction.

Potentiators. Another group of drugs called *potentiators* is used to intensify the action of narcotic agents, thus increasing the degree and duration of analgesia. Drugs commonly used as potentiators include promethazine (Phenergan), hydroxyzine (Atarax, Vistaril), meprobamate (Equanil, Miltown), and diazepam (Valium). These drugs have an additive effect or are antianxiety agents rather than true potentiators.

Pain cocktails. Brompton's cocktail (Brompton's Mix, Pain Cocktail, or Hospice Mix) is an oral liquid narcotic mixture. The ingredients commonly used in pain cocktails include a narcotic such as morphine or methadone, a stimulant such as amphetamine, an antiemetic such as prochlorperazine (Compazine), and a flavoring agent such as cherry syrup or alcohol. Variation in drugs for the individual client's needs is common. The mixture is taken regularly rather than on an as-needed basis.

Anesthesia. Nerve blocks and neurosurgical or radiological procedures are used to reduce pain. A functional part of the nervous system is temporarily or permanently destroyed to interrupt pain transmission.

Nerve blocks. Nerve blocks are accomplished with the use of local anesthetics or neurolytic agents. Initially, tem-

porary nerve blocks with local anesthetics are used to isolate the involved pain pathway and to determine the possible effectiveness of a permanent blocking procedure for the particular individual. Typically, the local anesthetic effects last for only a few hours. The effects of neurolytic agents such as alcohol, phenol, or saline last for weeks to months; therefore these agents are used for a more long-lasting effect.

Nerve blocks have been a successful pain-management technique for more localized chronic pain states, such as peripheral vascular disease, trigeminal neuralgia, causalgia, and some cancer pain. A nerve block was formerly considered advantageous in managing localized pain caused by malignancy and in debilitated clients who could not withstand a surgical procedure for pain relief. This use is currently being reevaluated in view of the increasing life expectancy of persons being treated for malignancies and the availability of other therapeutic modalities. Consequently, the employment of nerve blocks has been reduced.[26]

Neurosurgical interventions. Neurosurgical interventions are accomplished by surgical resection or thermocoagulation, including radio frequency coagulation. Interventions that destroy the sensory division of a peripheral or spinal nerve are classified as neurectomies, rhizotomies, and sympathectomies. Neurosurgical procedures that ablate the lateral spinothalamic tract are classified as cordotomies if the tract is interrupted in the spinal cord or tractotomies if the interruption is in the medulla or the midbrain of the brainstem. (Fig. 51-7 identifies the sites of neuro-

surgical procedures for pain relief.) Surgical resection of the lateral spinothalamic tract is rare today because a percutaneous approach is available. Both cordotomy and tractotomy can be performed with the aid of local anesthesia by a percutaneous technique in which the pain fibers are isolated by fluoroscopy and a radio-frequency lesion is created.

Neurosurgical interventions involving the thalamus or frontal lobe region of the brain are carried out through a stereotaxic procedure. Long electrodes or other probes are inserted deep into the brain tissue and positioned by the use of external points or landmarks of the skull. The tissue is destroyed by thermocoagulation or other means.

Intractable pain may be controlled by surgery, such as a pituitary resection. This type of procedure is used only for severe, intractable pain that does not respond to other therapeutic measures. Ablative procedures are less frequently used today with the availability of good analgesic methods to control pain.

Alteration of the Affective-Motivational and Cognitive-Evaluative Components

Techniques to alter the affective-motivational and cognitive-evaluative components of pain include a variety of cognitive strategies, behavioral approaches, and hypnosis. Many of the behavioral approaches, such as biofeedback, autogenic training, and relaxation strategies, necessitate biogenic training.

Cognitive strategies

Distraction. Cognitive strategies that are designed to affect the affective-motivational and cognitive-evaluative components of pain include distraction, imagery, and meditation. Distraction involves redirection of attention on something away from the pain.[26] The distraction stimuli may be external events, internal activities, or bodily sensations. Distraction techniques help the client cope with the pain being experienced.

Imagery. Imagery is purposeful or therapeutic use of imagination.[27] For pain relief the individual's own imagination is used to develop sensory images that focus away from the pain sensation and emphasize other sensory experiences and pleasant memories. Guided imagery provides a mental substitute for the pain. Specific images have been developed for use in pain relief to bring about removal of the pain. These include the techniques of breathing out the pain, the ball of healing energy, and the healthy body image.[1]

Another imagery technique is to use images in the course of conversation. For example, the client is helped to "pretend your body is a puppet on a string," "let your body go limp all over," or "try to feel like a limp dishrag." To explain a therapeutic measure, the nurse may tell the client that "this will loosen the knots you describe in the back of your neck," "this is stretching out the back muscles to stop the spasms," "the heat is melting away the pain," or "the heat is driving away the pain." Use of images the client has used to describe the pain may be particularly effective.

A similar imagery technique is brief instruction. The client is told to "think of the sensation as unusual, not

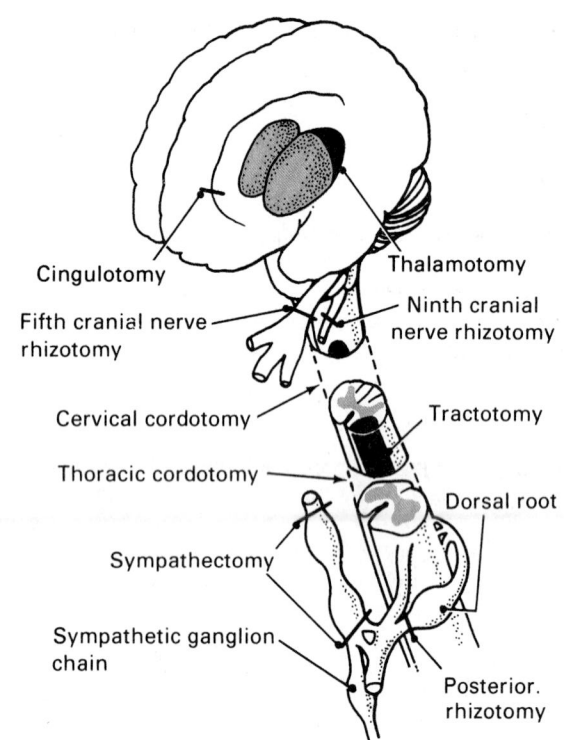

Fig. 51-7 Sites of neurosurgical procedures for pain relief.

Cingulotomy
Fifth cranial nerve rhizotomy
Cervical cordotomy
Thoracic cordotomy
Sympathectomy
Sympathetic ganglion chain
Thalamotomy
Ninth cranial nerve rhizotomy
Tractotomy
Dorsal root
Posterior rhizotomy

Table 51-2 Relaxation Strategies

Rhythmic breathing*

1. Provide a quiet environment.
2. Help the client get comfortable by elevating the legs with the knees bent (relaxing the leg, back, and abdominal muscles) or supporting the neck with a pillow. Check to see that arms and legs are not crossed.
3. Instruct client to close eyes and to breathe in and out slowly, saying, "Breathe in, two, three, four; breathe out, two, three, four."
4. Once rhythmic breathing is established, instruct client to listen to your voice, and with a low and steady voice, instruct client to do the following:
   Breathe in and out slowly and deeply.
   Try to breathe from the abdomen.
   Feel more relaxed with each exhalation.
   Try to identify your own special feeling of relaxation (e.g., light and weightless or very heavy).
   While you are breathing, let your imagination take you to a place you remember as peaceful and pleasant; look around, listen to the sounds, feel the air, notice the smells.
   When you are ready to end this relaxation exercise, count silently from one to three; on one, move your lower body; on two, move your upper body; on three, breathe in deeply, open your eyes, and while breathing out slowly, say silently: "I am relaxed and alert." Stretch as if just waking up.

Progressive relaxation*

1. Follow steps 1, 2, and 3 of rhythmic breathing.
2. Once client is breathing slowly and comfortably, instruct client to focus with each exhalation on a particular area of the body, starting with the feet, tensing and then relaxing them, while *feeling* the part relax.
3. Instruct client to tense and then relax the calves, knees, and so on.

Relaxation by sensory pacing

1. Follow steps 1 and 2 of rhythmic breathing.
2. Instruct client to slowly repeat and finish either in a low voice or to self each of the following sentences:
   Now I am aware of seeing. . .
   Now I am aware of feeling. . .
   Now I am aware of hearing. . .
   Instruct client to repeat and complete each sentence four times, then three times, then twice, and finally once.
3. Instruct client to allow the eyes to close when they feel heavy.

Relaxation by color exchange

1. Follow steps 1, 2, and 3 of rhythmic breathing.
2. Instruct client to notice any tension, tightness, aches, or pains in the body and to give that sensation the first color that comes to mind.
3. Instruct client to breathe in pure white light from the universe and send the light to the tense/painful place in the body, letting the white light surround the color of the discomfort.
4. Instruct client to exhale the color of the discomfort and let the white light take its place.
5. Instruct client to continue breathing in the white light and exhaling the color of the discomfort, allowing the white light to fill the entire body and bring about a sense of peace, well-being, and energy.

Modified autogenic relaxation

1. Follow steps 1, 2, and 3 of rhythmic breathing.
2. Instruct client to repeat each of the following phases to self four times, saying the first part of the phrase while breathing in for 2 to 3 seconds, holding the breath for 2 to 3 seconds, then saying the last part of the phrase while breathing out for 2 to 3 seconds:

Breathing in	*Breathing out*
I am	relaxed
My arms and legs	are heavy and warm
My heartbeat	is calm and regular
My breathing	is free and easy
My abdomen	is loose and warm
My forehead	is cool
My mind	is quiet and still

---

*In conditioning of a relaxation response, a "signal breath" involving deep inhalation through the nose and forceful exhalation through the mouth is the key. This signal breath precedes and follows each run through the exercise.

Table 51-2 Relaxation Strategies—cont'd

Relaxing with music

1. Provide client with a tape recorder and headset.
2. Ask client to select a favorite cassette of slow, quiet music.
3. Instruct client to get into a comfortable position (either sitting or lying down but with arms and legs uncrossed) and to close eyes and listen to the music through the headset.
4. Instruct client to imagine floating or drifting with the music while listening.

Rhythmic massage

1. Massage near the area of pain in a circular, firm manner.
2. Avoid tender, red, or swollen areas.

painful," "concentrate on other things," "think of your hand as dull and insensitive," or "think of your hand as a wax hand or a rubber hand and not really part of your body."[1]

Images that suggest return to health are also helpful. They increase therapeutic physiological functioning. Examples of such images are "the food is supplying nutrients to repair the damaged tissues" or "the heat is bringing increased blood flow to the area to cleanse the tissues and carry away the wastes."

Hypnosis. Hypnosis is a state of altered consciousness characterized by extreme responsiveness to suggestion. Through hypnosis the client is separated from the analytical and judgmental component of the thought processes so that acceptance of suggestion is possible. Hypnosis is induced artificially in a subject by means of verbal suggestion from the hypnotist or by the subject's concentration on some object. Although it requires training, hypnosis can be used successfully for some persons whose pain syndromes involve a tension component or a psychogenically based set of symptoms. This technique decreases tension by reducing fear and anxiety and by enhancing the person's optimism and sense of well-being. Hypnotic suggestion can also be used to induce analgesia, for sensory-imagery conditioning, and to induce a relaxation state.

Behavioral approaches. *Relaxation* strategies elicit the relaxation response. The positive effects of relaxation include reducing the effects of stress, decreasing acute anxiety, acting as a distraction from the pain, alleviating skeletal muscle tension or contraction, producing a state of increased susceptibility to suggestions of comfort, combating fatigue, facilitating sleep, and enhancing the effectiveness of other pain-relief measures.[28] Elicitation of the relaxation response requires a quiet environment, a comfortable position, a mental device as a focus of concentration (e.g., a word, a sound, the heartbeat, or the person's breathing), and a passive attitude.[29] Relaxation strategies include deep-breathing regimens, heartbeat breathing, music, slow and rhythmic breathing, and progressive relaxation exercises with a trainer (Table 51-2).

Relaxation techniques are used in biofeedback, autogenic training, meditation, yoga, Zen practices, imagery, and hypnosis. *Autogenic training* involves learning to self-regulate bodily functions, such as heart rate, breathing rate, blood flow, and muscle tension.

Biofeedback applies operant conditioning principles. Through an attached monitoring device, such as an electrocardiograph (ECG), electroencephalograph (EEG), or electromyelograph, the client is provided with information about a physiological function that is not normally available. The physiological signal itself is transformed, amplified, and then displayed on a monitor or by means of an auditory feedback system. With this increased awareness of the physiological state and with special training, the individual can learn to modify a particular physiological state.

Several principles of pain control seem to be involved in biofeedback, including the principle of distraction, induction of a relaxed state, and development of control over the pain. Biofeedback has been used to treat chronic pain syndromes with a stress-related component. Several types of biofeedback training have been used in pain management: Electromyogram feedback has been used for muscle-contraction (traction) headache. EEG feedback trains the person to produce alpha brain wave activity, which is believed to be incompatible with the experiencing of pain. Finger temperature feedback is used for migraine. When the client learns to increase peripheral circulation, sympathetic nervous system activity in the cranial blood vessels is decreased. Temporal artery pulse amplitude feedback is also used to treat migraine by teaching the person to reduce temporal artery dilatation.

Behavioral programs. The primary goal of behavioral programs is to reduce the number and frequency of pain behaviors by means of medication management, exercise, and family retraining. Baseline data related to medication use, activity level, and client-family interactions are collected. Medication intake is systematically reduced and converted to the oral route. The liquid form is often used. A program of scheduled activity is initiated. The exercise regimen starts at baseline or less and is gradually increased along with recreational activities. Family retraining is directed toward assisting family members to identify ways by which they reinforce pain behaviors and then teaching family members alternate ways of interacting. Other management techniques used in behavioral programs may include hypnosis, biofeedback, vocational counseling, and marital therapy.

Therapeutic touch. Therapeutic touch is a process by which the therapist acts as a channel for environmental and

PAIN CONTROL ASSESSMENT QUESTIONNAIRE

This questionnaire has been developed for you to describe your pain. Answer the questions as best you can. There are no right or wrong answers. A treatment plan will be written with you from your description of pain.

1. Please mark with an "X" on the drawing where you have pain.

   You may mark more than one area. If you do, label them "a," "b," "c," etc.

2. On a scale of 0–10, if 0 was no pain and 10 the worst pain imaginable, mark where your pain is:

   0 1 2 3 4 5 6 7 8 9 10

3. Describe your pain in your own words.

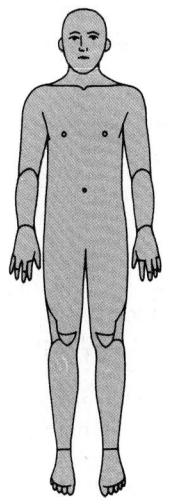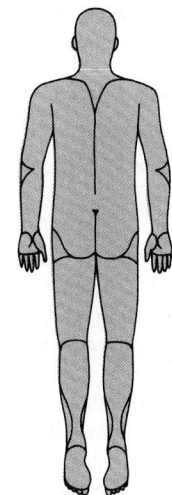

4. Is your pain always present?   YES   NO

5. Does your pain come and go?   YES   NO

6. Does your pain spread?   YES   NO

7. How long have you been having this pain?

8. When is your pain most uncomfortable?

   What activities were you doing at the time?

9. When you experience pain, do you have any of the following?

   □ change in appetite
   □ nausea and vomiting
   □ constipation
   □ difficulty urinating
   □ coughing
   □ change in breathing
   □ dizziness
   □ confusion
   □ insomnia
   □ depression
   □ anger
   □ anxiety
   □ fatigue
   □ change in ability to work
   □ change in sexual function

   What do you find helps to relieve these symptoms?

   _____
   _____
   _____
   _____
   _____
   _____
   _____
   _____
   _____
   _____
   _____
   _____
   _____
   _____

10. Using the pain scale, what level of pain would be acceptable to you at this time? (0 is no pain and 10 is the worst pain imaginable.)

    0 1 2 3 4 5 6 7 8 9 10

Thank you for completing this questionnaire. We will develop a treatment plan from this questionnaire and discuss this plan with you. Periodically you will be asked to evaluate and update your plan as needed.

Fig. 51-8   Example of a pain assessment questionnaire. (From Wheat BZ: Pain management: a cooperative effort between patient and nurse, Stanford Nurse 6:5, 1984.)

universal energy through the therapist's mental concentration and focusing to effect a relief of pain.[30] Therapeutic touch may be used for all types of pain. It may be used as the single mode of treatment or in combination with other techniques according to the client's needs.

Comprehensive pain-management programs. Most comprehensive pain-management programs began in the early 1970s. This approach involves comprehensive assessment and problem identification by an interdisciplinary team. The treatment plan includes elimination of drug dependence, therapeutic measures to reduce the pain, physical rehabilitation, psychological rehabilitation for the client and family, and the return of control over the pain-management program to the client. A comprehensive multidisciplinary pain assessment and pain profile, along with a complete physical and laboratory evaluation, are the first

steps. Whether the client is withdrawn from the medication being used and a new drug regimen is initiated or the current drug regimen is simply titrated downward depends on the individual pain-management center.

For example, 10 mg of intramuscular (IM) morphine may be replaced by the equivalent oral methadone dose of 20 mg; 75 mg of IM meperidine may at first be changed to the equivalent oral dose (300 mg), then changed to 200 mg of oral meperidine with 650 mg of aspirin and 650 mg of acetaminophen. The oral meperidine may be gradually decreased. For 64 mg of oral codeine, a substitution of 32 mg of oral codeine and 650 mg of aspirin may be made and then converted to 650 mg of aspirin and 650 mg of acetaminophen. For dosage reduction of narcotic agents, 20% of the total daily dosage is usually withdrawn every 2 days for morphine and its derivatives and every 3 days for methadone.

Generally, treatment is aimed at achieving maximum mobilization and relief of pain with the use of physical and psychological treatment techniques. Physical reconditioning is initiated slowly. A sound and reasonably vigorous exercise program is gradually established. Physical treatment modalities initiated may include massage, pressure, heat therapy, cold therapy, vibration, TENS, and acupuncture. An equally important component of chronic pain management is psychotherapy and a cognitive-behavioral approach.[27] The client is taught skills to help cope with the pain while cognitive restructuring is addressed. Biofeedback training is often used. Psychological counseling for both the client and the family is a critical component. Persons who have been in pain for a prolonged time may have markedly altered their interpersonal relationships and communication patterns with family, friends, and health care personnel. The chronic stress of the pain may have left their lives in shambles. Most authorities recommend an intensive program of psychological therapy over a short time, dealing with issues in the present, rather than the more traditional prolonged therapy.[8]

In a holistic pain-management program, the client learns to draw on inner resources and to assume responsibility for practicing skills that will help to cope with the pain. The person is helped to use family and significant others effectively. The client learns to manage the pain.

ASSESSMENT OF PAIN

The goals of pain assessment are (1) to attempt to truly understand the client's pain experience, (2) to identify the causative factor or factors, and (3) to identify modulating factors that are influencing the pain experience. Fig. 51-8 presents an example of a pain-assessment questionnaire.

Detection of Physical Sources

When a client is experiencing pain, the cause of the pain should be sought so that it can be removed if possible. The nurse should observe for signs of physical sources of pain, including trauma, inflammation, ischemia, distention (especially of a viscus), perforation of a viscus, and muscle spasm. In many cases there may be a secondary pain source. For example, the postoperative client may have a distended bladder that needs to be decompressed.

Searching for the cause of pain is especially important with the onset of an acute pain episode, but it must be remembered that clients with chronic pain syndromes may also have a related or unrelated acute pain experience.

Data Collection

The following data should be collected from the client who is experiencing pain, whether acute or chronic[1]:
1. Brief but thorough explanation of pain location
2. Mode of onset
3. Precipitating or associated factors
4. Detailed description of how pain evolved
5. Quality and characteristics of pain (e.g., dull, aching, shooting)
6. Duration, intensity, and severity of pain
7. Change in pain since it was first perceived
8. Measures that relieve the pain
9. Associated signs and symptoms, such as autonomic nervous system responses
10. Meaning of pain experience

Clinical observation should be used to expand or clarify data collected from the client. The nurse should also conduct a general survey of the client that includes the following:
1. Client's appearance
2. Client's motor behavior (e.g., facial expression, posture, gait, motor activity)
3. Client's affective behavior (e.g., affect, crying, withdrawal, irritability)
4. Client's verbal behavior (e.g., expressions of anger, frustration, hopelessness or despair, fear, anxiety)

Responses elicited by a pain stimulus should be noted, including (1) brainstem-level automatic responses such as rise in blood pressure, increased heart rate, increased cardiac output, rapid irregular respirations, and dilated pupils and (2) spinal-level reflex responses such as decreased GI motility resulting in nausea, vomiting, and distention; decreased urinary output; bronchospasm; and increased muscle tension. Besides collecting the aforementioned assessment data, the nurse may need to (1) inspect and palpate the painful area, (2) identify trigger points of pain, (3) test the range of motion of involved joints, and (4) test the location, degree, and type of decreased sensation or increased hypersensitivity. Trigger points can be identified by pressing carefully and systematically throughout the painful area and at distances from the area of pain.[8]

In chronic pain situations, the following assessment data should also be collected:
1. A brief but thorough review of history and experiences with pain[1]
2. Past treatments and results of those treatments
3. Current pain-management protocol
4. General effect of pain on activity level and lifestyle
5. Methods used to cope with pain of various intensities

Pain-assessment scales. Different pain-assessment scales exist. There are verbal descriptor scales, visual analogue scales, and multidimensional scales. *Verbal descriptor scales* consist of three to five numerically ranked descriptor words, such as *none, slight, mild, moderate,* or

Visual Analog Scale

No
pain

Worst
pain
possible

McGill Pain Questionnaire

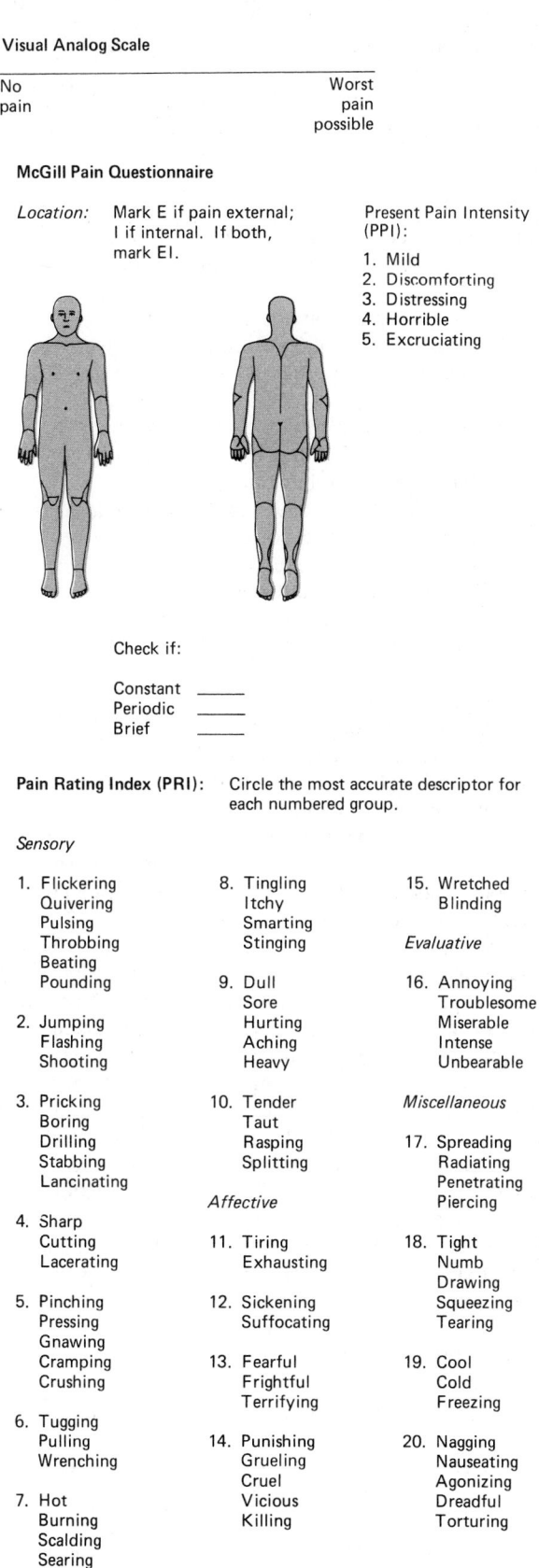

Location: Mark E if pain external; I if internal. If both, mark EI.

Present Pain Intensity (PPI):
1. Mild
2. Discomforting
3. Distressing
4. Horrible
5. Excruciating

Check if:

Constant _____
Periodic _____
Brief _____

Pain Rating Index (PRI): Circle the most accurate descriptor for each numbered group.

Sensory

1. Flickering
   Quivering
   Pulsing
   Throbbing
   Beating
   Pounding

2. Jumping
   Flashing
   Shooting

3. Pricking
   Boring
   Drilling
   Stabbing
   Lancinating

4. Sharp
   Cutting
   Lacerating

5. Pinching
   Pressing
   Gnawing
   Cramping
   Crushing

6. Tugging
   Pulling
   Wrenching

7. Hot
   Burning
   Scalding
   Searing

8. Tingling
   Itchy
   Smarting
   Stinging

9. Dull
   Sore
   Hurting
   Aching
   Heavy

10. Tender
    Taut
    Rasping
    Splitting

Affective

11. Tiring
    Exhausting

12. Sickening
    Suffocating

13. Fearful
    Frightful
    Terrifying

14. Punishing
    Grueling
    Cruel
    Vicious
    Killing

15. Wretched
    Blinding

Evaluative

16. Annoying
    Troublesome
    Miserable
    Intense
    Unbearable

Miscellaneous

17. Spreading
    Radiating
    Penetrating
    Piercing

18. Tight
    Numb
    Drawing
    Squeezing
    Tearing

19. Cool
    Cold
    Freezing

20. Nagging
    Nauseating
    Agonizing
    Dreadful
    Torturing

Fig. 51-9 Examples of pain assessment scales. (Modified from Melzack R: The McGill pain questionnaire, McGill University, Montreal, Canada, 1975.)

severe. The number of the word chosen determines the intensity of the pain experience. *Visual analogue scales* usually consist of a straight line, which represents a continuum of pain intensity. Verbal anchors—no pain to the worst pain possible—are placed at either end of the scale. The length of the line may vary, but it is most commonly 10 cm (Fig. 51-9). The time frame can vary to fit the situation.

Multidimensional measures tap more than intensity dimensions of the pain experience. For example, a two-dimensional scale with a sensory component and a distress component has been developed. The physical sensation of the pain is rated from 0 to 100. On the distress scale the distress caused by the pain is ranked from slight distress, moderate distress, very distressing, to just bearable. The McGill Pain Questionnaire has four parts: location of the pain; sensory, affective, evaluative, and miscellaneous qualities of the pain; and two intensity measurements (see Fig. 51-9). Each word in a group has a score—its order in the group. The number values of the words chosen by the client are added in each category for a category score and totaled for a total pain score.

■ Nursing Management of Pain Syndromes

The nursing goals of pain management are the same as those of other members of the health team: (1) to alter the sensory-discriminative pain component and (2) to alter the affective-motivational and cognitive-evaluative components of pain. The American Nurses' Association's Division of Medical-Surgical Nursing Practice and the American Association of Neuroscience Nurses' *Neuroscience Nursing Practice: Process and Outcome Criteria for Selected Diagnoses* address the nurse's role in pain management in the diagnostic category on sensation. The component of the diagnostic category that focuses on pain is presented in Table 51-3. A critical element in the nursing management of a client with a pain syndrome is the establishment of a trusting relationship and a good rapport with the client and the family. The client and the family need to know that (1) the nurse considers the pain significant and understands that chronic pain may totally disrupt a person's life; (2) the nurse's goal is to help the client cope with the pain by using techniques to help with relaxation, comfort, the sense of aloneness and isolation, and protection from depersonalization; and (3) the nurse will help the client maintain or regain control over the environment. A priority with clients who have chronic pain is to let it be known that the nurse believes the person has pain and to explain some of the physiological mechanisms that operate in chronic pain.

Establishment of a Nurse-Client Relationship

Nursing actions that promote the establishment of an effective relationship with the person who is experiencing pain and with the family should include the following:

1. *Clarify responsibilities in pain relief:* What is the nurse going to do? What are the client and the family expected to do?
2. *Believe the client:* The client needs to be able to trust the nurse to believe in the pain. Nursing activ-

Table 51-3　Standard for Nursing Diagnosis of Chronic Pain

Nursing Diagnosis of Chronic Pain	Process Criteria	Outcome Criteria
Defining characteristics* Communication of pain or discomfort Behaviors 　Restlessness or agitation 　Avoidance of activity 　Altered muscle tone 　Preoccupation with or guarding of 　　painful part 　Irritability 　Fatigue 　Emotional lability 　Withdrawal 　Disruption of cycle of sleeping and 　　waking 　Disruption of eating pattern	Acknowledgment of existence of pain Assistance with identification of situations and factors that precipitate or intensify pain Assistance with adjustment of lifestyle to reduce pain-producing situations and factors Assistance with use of prescribed pain regimens for maximum benefit Collaboration with pain-management specialists to develop appropriate cutaneous, affective, and cognitive treatment modalities Collaboration with other care providers to establish management program Education of client, family, and significant others about nature of pain Provision of guidance regarding anticipated lifestyle changes Provision of opportunities for client to verbalize feelings related to chronicity of pain Provision of positive reinforcement for health-promoting behaviors and encouragement of appropriate use of caregivers and support systems	Client participation in developing, carrying out, and evaluating management plan Client report of improved sense of well-being and increased satisfaction with relationships, lifestyle, and self Client report of engaging in positive social interactions with others Support of family and significant others of management plan

Modified from American Nurses' Association: Neuroscience nursing practice: process and outcome criteria for selected diagnoses, Kansas City, Mo, 1985, American Nurses' Association.
*One or more of the listed characteristics.

ities to relieve pain convey concern and trustworthiness. This message can also be conveyed verbally to the client by saying "I know you are in pain." The nurse needs to help the family to believe the client.

3. *Respect the client's response to pain:* Nurses should accept the right of the client to respond to the pain in the necessary manner. The family also needs help in this area. The client may also need help to accept the response to the pain; the behavior may be less than expected by the client and the family.

4. *Collaborate with the client:* The client should be encouraged to use coping techniques that have been effective in the past. The client and the family should be assisted to use personal resources more effectively. The client's expectations of a nurse must also be met, even if those expectations do not entirely conform to the job description or to the nurse's role perception. The client and the family should be helped to participate actively in setting goals for pain relief.

5. *Explore the pain with the client:* Nurses need to find out the meaning of the pain to the individual enduring the pain and to the family.

6. *Be with the client often:* Nurses should act as buffers for the client and the family during difficult times.[31] The nurse's physical presence may reassure or distract the client, or it may offer variety, thus relieving the pain.

Nursing Measures Related to the Sensory-Discriminative Component

Physical measures. Nursing measures to alter the sensory-discriminative pain component include nursing actions that stimulate large-diameter A fibers, such as (1) applying electrical stimulation, vibration, or counterirritation by means of heat or cold therapy as ordered by the physician and (2) providing cutaneous stimulation through pressure, massage, and bathing (Fig. 51-10). This aspect of nursing management cannot be overemphasized and should be taught to the client and the family.

Anxiety, pain, and immobility increase muscular tension. Nursing management of pain syndromes must include measures to reduce this muscular tension, including frequent position changes, positioning that supports body parts, early ambulation, heat applications, and measures to promote relaxation, such as massage and back rubs. These measures should also be taught to the client and the family.

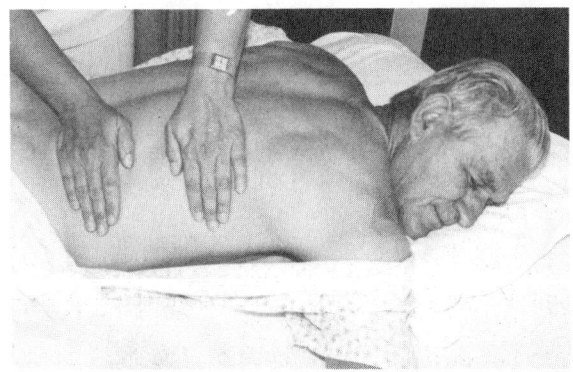

Fig. 51-10 A back rub is a time-honored method of providing cutaneous stimulation.

Analgesia. The nursing management of pain syndromes also involves establishing and maintaining an effective analgesic regimen. The use of a preventive approach to pain is crucial. The client should be medicated before painful procedures and activities that can be expected to produce pain. If these procedures or activities are planned so that they occur when the client's analgesic has reached its peak effectiveness, the pain will be decreased and the client's ability to participate will be increased. Moreover, if the client is medicated before the pain begins to increase rather than when it becomes severe, far less medication is required. This may minimize the drug side effects that often aggravate the pain. The client and the family may need to be taught when to ask for pain medication. Administration may also be time controlled, with the medication given regardless of the presence or absence of pain.

Nurses, family members, and clients need to remember that an IM injection is not necessarily the only or best route of administration for pain medication. The oral route and a subcutaneous injection are alternate routes in almost all pain syndromes, including acute pain experiences. Good pain control can be achieved by these approaches. The oral route prevents the problems inherent in the prolonged use of IM injections. A larger dose must be ordered to achieve effective pain relief when the oral route is used.

Self-medication programs for persons using oral analgesics have been successful. The individual is given a 24-hour supply of medication and keeps a record of the medication taken. Evidence of drug abuse or drug loss by clients has not been reported in the literature. Persons on such programs have shown decreased anxiety, decreased pain, and increased self-esteem and control.

Another route often overlooked but particularly useful when the client cannot take the analgesic by mouth is the rectal route. Rectal suppositories that are effective for pain relief include hydromorphone (Dilaudid), oxymorphone (Numorphan), and morphine.[32]

A preventive approach should be employed when either the oral or the rectal route is used. Absorption of the drug is slower than with IM injections, and therefore more time is needed for the drug to provide effective pain relief. Families should be taught to use this preventive approach.

Currently, creams and lotions containing 10% triethano-lamine salicylate (Aspercreme, Myoflex cream) are available. These agents have been recommended by the manufacturers for joint and muscle pain. Although no sensation is experienced when they are applied at or near the pain source, the aspirinlike substance is absorbed locally. This route of administration avoids gastric irritation, but the other side effects of high-dose salicylate are not necessarily prevented.

Continuous intravenous (IV) infusion of morphine is another method that has been extremely effective in providing pain control. The morphine is most commonly mixed with 5% dextrose in water but any IV solution is compatible with the drug. A microdrip infusion set using an infusion control pump is used. Usually a secondary line is added to the primary IV line after incompatibilities are checked. Morphine is incompatible with solutions containing drugs such as sodium bicarbonate, heparin, and aminophylline.

Another type of IV system is client-controlled analgesia (demand analgesia). In client-controlled analgesia, a dose of narcotic is delivered through an indwelling IV catheter when the person pushes a button. This places the client in control and eliminates waiting for medication to be brought and given. The syringe pump, however, will deliver the drug only as frequently as the preset interval. This delivery system has been used primarily for acute pain, with satisfactory results.

Continuous extravascular infusion provides a means to infuse local anesthetics or analgesics. The sites for catheter placement for this type of infusion include the epidural space, brachial plexus, celiac plexus, and lumbar sympathetic chain and regionally along nerves. Continuous extravascular infusion has been used for both acute and chronic pain. The drug concentration varies with each individual client. The anesthetic or analgesic agent is usually delivered in 300 ml of normal saline solution with an infusion rate adjusted to the degree of pain and to the physiological responses to the medication, such as hypotension, bradycardia, or respiratory depression, during the first 24 hours. After that time, the dosage is gradually titrated downward.

Perispinal narcotic therapy is extremely effective. An epidural catheter is used to deliver a preservative-free narcotic, such as morphine, meperidine (Demerol), or fentanyl (Sublimaze), into the epidural space by bolus injection (intermittent epidural infusion or epidural client-controlled analgesia) or continuous infusion (epidural morphine pump). An intrathecal morphine pump can provide a continuous morphine infusion into the subarachnoid space through an intrathecal catheter. These modalities have become popular. Prompt recognition and treatment of side effects and complications are necessary, and meticulous catheter care is required.

Preventive measures. Institution of preventive measures to minimize joint and muscle stiffness is important to the pain-management regimen. As severe pain subsides, the client tends to become more aware of the pain associated with joint and muscle tenderness. The nurse should establish a passive range-of-motion program and, if not contraindicated by the client's condition, an active exer-

cise regimen for the client. The exercise program reduces the stiffness and helps to release any muscle spasms that may be present. Both client and family should be taught the exercise regimen. The client should be encouraged to move about as much as possible within the medically prescribed activity order.

The nurse must also prevent painful complications that result from immobility, including decubitus ulcers, contractures, and thrombophlebitis. Because pain can be intensified by distention of a viscus, constipation should be prevented by ensuring that the client is mobilized as soon as possible and given laxatives as necessary. Because urinary retention can cause or increase pain, intake and output should be monitored and the bladder percussed to assess the degree of distention. Foley catheters should be checked frequently to ensure patency and free flow of urine.

The client should be helped to identify the precipitating factors that cause pain. Measures to prevent the pain should then be instituted and taught to the client and family.

Pain management must include methods to promote rest and sleep. Research has clearly established that persons deprived of rapid-eye-movement sleep and deep sleep (phases III and IV) become irritable and fatigued and have increased sensitivity to pain. The client must be allowed to sleep undisturbed for at least 2 hours at a time, and comfort measures, analgesics and hypnotics, and relaxation techniques should be used to promote sleep.

A well-balanced diet high in the B complex vitamins and tryptophan is recommended. The B complex vitamins and tryptophan enhance optimal neurological functioning and nervous system repair. Sugars, caffeine, nicotine, and alcohol should be kept to a minimum.

Nursing Measures Related to the Affective-Motivational and Cognitive-Evaluative Components

Behavioral measures. Nursing actions designed to alter the affective-motivational and cognitive-evaluative components of pain (noninvasive or self-control strategies) include anticipatory guidance, effective use of others, and assistance of the client and the family to use behavioral approaches that involve relaxation and conditioning, stress inoculation, and cognitive strategies such as distraction and imagery.

Anticipatory guidance. The client should be prepared as much as possible regarding pain experiences. This is referred to as *anticipatory guidance.* By preparing the client for what to expect, the nurse can help reduce anxiety and clarify misinformation and misinterpretation. Knowing what to expect helps the client cope with the unknown. The following are areas of client teaching:

1. Occurrence, onset, and duration of pain
2. Quality, location, and severity of pain
3. Information on how personal safety is being ensured
4. Underlying cause of pain
5. Methods of pain relief

In the anticipatory phase of the pain experience some anxiety mobilizes the development of coping strategies. This is an important point when nurses are dealing with clients who are to have a painful experience. These clients cannot be reassured that there will be little or no pain, but they must be helped to identify ways to cope with the expected pain.

Family teaching and the family-nurse relationships are extremely important. Assessment of the family and friends and their interaction with the client is essential in the presence of a pain syndrome. Relationships are often inappropriate and stressful. Nursing interventions to teach the family and friends and to provide information on more effective coping techniques for themselves as well as strategies to help the client are essential.

Relaxation technique. In behavioral approaches the client should be encouraged to continue to do whatever has proved relaxing. The client should be taught to use those relaxation techniques that have some appeal. Teaching relaxation techniques to the client and the family is beginning to assume a larger role in the nursing management of pain.

Conditioning. Certain pain-relief measures result in relief frequently enough for *classic conditioning* to take place. Nurses can help the client benefit from this phenomenon by deliberately pairing relief methods. For example, the nurse should teach a relaxation technique to be used each time a pain medication is given. One result of this is the additive effect gained from two measures used simultaneously. A second result is the conditioned response gained over time so that eventually the relaxation technique alone will have the same effect without the use of pain medication.

Behavior modification (*operant conditioning*) is based on the principle that the frequency of a behavior may be increased or decreased by the use of reinforcement. Positive reinforcement results in an increase in the frequency of the behavior. Nurses can use behavior modification by giving praise and attention to the client who is willing to try new pain relief methods or who engages in behaviors unrelated to pain. The client's attempts to progress toward recovery should be praised and noticed. Silence or ignoring nonbeneficial behavior is also important. The family should be taught to provide positive reinforcement, ignore nonbeneficial behavior, and use silence.

Stress inoculation. Stress inoculation training involves a three-stage approach to behavioral change. First, the meaning of the clinical manifestations is taught. The client is then taught coping strategies that are incompatible with the pain experience and pain behavior. Finally, the client is taught how to use this new knowledge and awareness in the pain situation. Nurses participate in all phases of stress inoculation training, assisting the client to progress through the stages.

Behavioral programs. In behavioral programs, nurses assess and document pain behaviors in clients and families. In addition, they work with clients on their medication regimens. Nurses play a major role in reinforcing "well" behaviors and promoting attendance at prescribed therapies, exercise, and other beneficial assignments.

Cognitive strategies. When assisting the client to use cognitive strategies, the nurse must remember that the cli-

ent's ability to use *distraction* effectively to decrease the pain experience does not mean that the pain is not severe. Clients and family members, as well as some health care personnel, need to understand this aspect. Distraction techniques remove pain from the center of attention, thereby increasing pain tolerance and decreasing the response to the pain experience. The pain, however, is real.

Part of the nurse's role is to encourage the client to use the distraction techniques that have been found helpful in the past. The nurse should also assist the client to use these distraction techniques. Family members also need to be taught how to assist the client to use these techniques effectively. Both client and family need support in adopting them.

The nurse should use *imagery* in conversation with the client. Then the nurse should assist the client with imaging by encouraging the client to relive past events and asking for a detailed description of a pleasant event or scene. When the client focuses on only one sensory modality—for example, what the mountain looked like—the nurse should ask about other sensory modalities, such as sound, smell, or temperature. Involving multiple senses helps reinforce the image. The technique can also be taught to family members.

Clients, especially children, are often more accepting of the use of imagery than health care professionals. Nurses are sometimes reluctant to teach clients these techniques for fear of disapproval from physicians or other nurses or because the techniques seem "unscientific." However, research findings support the relationship between imagery and alpha brain wave activity associated with relaxation and sleep.

Conscious suggestion involving the use of voice and carefully chosen words to help the conscious and aware person relax may be effectively used to assist the person in pain. Conscious suggestion, unlike hypnosis, uses suggestion with the conscious alert person. The first step is a disarming statement that seems likely to have come from the client's own mouth. For example, "You want yourself to relax, don't you?" The suggestions are subtle. The first statement is positive, but it always implies a subtle command "you want to." The emphasis is on the "*you want* to, don't you?" This is followed with more suggestions. For example, "You are going to let yourself relax, aren't you?" The nurse is selling relaxation to the client.

Many of these techniques elicit behaviors that are incompatible with pain. For example, relaxation is incompatible with muscle tension. Talking about a scenic view is incompatible with thinking about pain. Rhythmic breathing is incompatible with the breath holding and gasping that are associated with pain. Eliciting of behaviors that are incompatible with pain is part of the nursing management of the client experiencing pain.

Emotional considerations. Depression and anger are often experienced by the person in pain and by the family. These feelings of anger and depression can often be reduced by helping the client and family to gain control over the pain and to feel less isolated. The nurse should encourage the client and family to express feelings. The client needs to be assured that these feelings are common and

may need assistance to maintain a reality orientation about the direction of the anger. The establishment of an activity program such as an exercise, occupational therapy, or recreational therapy regimen can be an effective measure to reduce depression. The client may need antidepressant or mood-elevating drugs as much as or more than pain medication.

Preserving the client's energy for enjoyable activities is also important. The nurse must first identify the activities that are most important or pleasurable for the client. Together they must find ways for the client to carry out these activities by reorganizing priorities and schedules and perhaps changing some rules and regulations. Providing periods of rest and sleep may also be necessary to allow the client to have the energy needed for those activities that are deemed important.

EVALUATION OF THE PAIN-MANAGEMENT PROTOCOL

In acute and chronic pain situations, the nurse should evaluate the effectiveness of the pain-relief measures taken by nursing and other health care personnel. The effectiveness of individual pain-relief measures and of the total pain-management protocol must be judged. These judgments are made by comparing the client's motor, autonomic, affective, and cognitive responses before the intervention with responses after the intervention. Both subjective and objective data enter into the evaluation, but it must be remembered that the client is the final judge.

If the client says that the relief measures are not adequate, the nurse should reassess the pain and also consider the following questions[1]:

1. Are a variety of pain-relief measures being used? (If not, additional measures should be added.)
2. Are the pain-relief measures being used before the pain becomes severe? (If not, an anticipatory analgesia regimen should be implemented.)
3. Is what the client believes will be effective included in the pain-management protocol? (If not, the reasons should be determined.) Can classic conditioning be used if the client cannot keep receiving what is perceived as most effective?
4. Is the client willing and able to be a more active participant in the pain management? (If not, the reasons should be determined.) How can the client be helped to become more active?
5. Can the client be encouraged to try the pain-relief measure one or two more times, especially if some additional measures are implemented?

A revised pain-management protocol should then be formulated and implemented.

NEEDS OF CAREGIVERS

Working with clients who are experiencing pain generates stress in nurses as well as in other health care personnel. Pain, like death, is one of the most universally frightening experiences, not only for those experiencing it but also for those witnessing it. The client's fear of the pain and feelings of powerlessness to control the pain elicit an awareness of the nurse's own vulnerability and limitations.

Fear and a sense of powerlessness may be evoked. These affectual experiences and the stress they engender may elicit defense mechanisms and inappropriate coping behaviors, such as alienation from or avoidance of the client and the family and denial of the severity of the pain experience or of the fact that the client has any pain at all.

Nurses working with clients experiencing pain need self-insight and value clarification. They need peer group involvement, not only to assist with value clarification but to offer support, guidance, and perhaps counseling on an ongoing informal and formal basis. In addition, consultation from experts in the area of pain management may be necessary. Nurses also need ongoing in-service or continuing education to correct the myths and misconceptions that prevail about pain and pain management, such as the exaggerated fears of addicting clients, which often results in the withholding of pain medication. Another educational need of nurses is to keep abreast of the rapidly expanding knowledge in the area of pain and pain management and to acquire additional skills in this area.

C ase Study

ACUTE HEAD PAIN

Mrs. M. is a 26-year-old woman admitted from the emergency room with incapacitating head pain of 3 days' duration. She complains of generalized pounding pain involving her entire head and neck that has become gradually worse over the last 3 days. She is now curled up in bed on her left side and refuses to move. She states that moving "makes the pain unbearable." She has been unable to eat or drink for the past 48 hours because of nausea and vomiting. Her vital signs are as follows: temperature, 37.7° C (99.8° F); blood pressure, 90/50; pulse rate, 125; respiration rate, 24. The muscles of her neck and upper back are tense. She has been crying since admission. Mrs. M. is married to a first-year general surgery resident. She has a 6-month-old daughter and a 2-year-old son. She and her husband are from the Northeast and moved to a southern university town 9 months ago, when her husband started his residency program. Both families live in New York.

Discussion Questions

1. What are the components of pain specifically related to Mrs. M?
2. What physiological factors are contributing to the head pain? What can be done to decrease or eliminate these factors?
3. What are the clinical manifestations of an uncontrolled acute pain cycle? Which of these does Mrs. M. manifest?
4. What can the nurse do to help alleviate Mrs. M.'s pain?
5. What other nursing problems besides pain does this client have? What are the appropriate nursing interventions for each?

R eview Questions

The number of the question corresponds to the same-numbered objective at the beginning of the chapter.

1. Which is the most comprehensive definition of pain?
   a. a harmful stimulus that signals current or impending tissue damage
   b. a pattern of responses that operates to protect the individual from harm
   c. an unpleasant sensation or sense of hurt experienced by the individual
   d. an individualized hurting experience that has a perceptual component and a response component
2. Pain perception occurs at the level of the
   a. spinal cord
   b. reticular activating system
   c. thalamus
   d. cerebral cortex
3. A modulating factor that increases the pain threshold is
   a. sensitization facilitation
   b. enkephalin release
   c. nonadaptation of pain receptors
4. The gate-control theory of pain provides a theoretical basis for all the following therapeutic modalities *except*
   a. ablative neurosurgical procedures
   b. massage
   c. electrical nerve stimulation
   d. exercise regimens
5. Factors that may cause pain perception to vary within the same individual are
   a. presence of fatigue
   b. degree of motivation
   c. level of anxiety
   d. all the above
6. Pathophysiological consequences of an untreated acute pain syndrome include
   a. local alkalosis
   b. increased urinary output
   c. decreased peristalsis
   d. decreased muscle tone
7. What assessment data are *not* critical to planning care for the client who is experiencing a chronic pain syndrome?
   a. cause of the pain
   b. the client's experiences with pain
   c. methods used by the client to cope with the pain
   d. factors precipitating or associated with the pain
8. Mobilization of the endogenous opiates is achieved by which of the following management techniques?
   a. narcotic analgesics
   b. electrical nerve stimulation
   c. acupuncture
   d. deep brain stimulation to the thalamus
9. A method of cutaneous stimulation that is an independent nursing action is
   a. electrical nerve stimulation
   b. acupuncture
   c. pressure, rubbing, and massage
   d. application of external counterirritants

REFERENCES

1. McCaffery M: Nursing management of the patient with pain, Philadelphia, 1979, JB Lippincott Co, p 11.
2. Kelly DD: Representations of pain and analgesia. In Kandel ER and others, eds: Principles of neural science, New York, 1985, Elsevier, p 332.

3. Bowsher D: Acute and chronic pain and assessment. In Wells PE and others, eds: Pain management in physical therapy, Norwalk, Conn, 1988, Appleton & Lange, p 12.

4. Martin JH: Receptor physiology and submodality coding in the somatic sensory system. In Kandel ER and others, eds: Principles of neural science, New York, 1985, Elsevier, p 290.

5. Wells N: Pain: acute and chronic. In Mitchell P and others, eds: AANN's neuroscience nursing phenomena and practice human responses to neurologic health problems, Norwalk, Conn, 1988, Appleton & Lange, p 388.

6. Payne R: Cancer pain anatomy, physiology and pharmacology, Cancer 63:2267, 1989.

7. Meinhart NT and McCaffery M: Pain: a nursing approach to assessment and analysis, Norwalk, Conn, 1983, Appleton-Century-Crofts, p 68.

8. Conway-Rutkowski BL: Carini and Owens' neurological and neurosurgical nursing, St Louis, 1982, The CV Mosby Co, pp 222-223.

9. Matteson MA and McConnell ES: Gerontological nursing: concepts and practice, Philadelphia, 1988, WB Saunders Co, p 349.

10. Henthorn TD and Krejcie TC: Postoperative pain management. In Tollison CD, ed: Handbook of chronic pain management, Baltimore, 1989, Williams and Wilkins, p 551.

11. Sweeney SS: OR observations: key to postop pain, AORN J 32:394-396, 1980.

12. Bonica JJ: Pain, New York, 1980, Raven Press.

13. McCauley K and Polomano RC: Acute pain: a nursing perspective with cardiac surgical patients, Top Clin Nurs 2:46, 1980.

14. Krishnan KRR and others: Systems approach to chronic pain syndromes. In France RD and Krishnan KRR, eds: Chronic pain, Washington, DC, 1988, American Psychiatric Press, pp 17-19.

15. Bowsher D: Modulation of nociceptive input. In Wells PE and others, eds: Pain management in physical therapy, Norwalk, Conn, 1988, Appleton & Lange, p 34.

16. Wells N: Pain, acute and chronic. In Mitchell P and others, eds: AANN's neuroscience nursing phenomena and practice human responses to neurologic health problems, Norwalk, Conn, 1988, Appleton & Lange, p 182.

17. Low JL: Shortwave diathermy, microwave, ultrasound and interferential therapy. In Wells PE and others, eds: Pain management in physical therapy, Norwalk, Conn, 1988, Appleton & Lange, pp 116, 156.

18. Skinner AT and Thomson AM: Hydrotherapy. In Wells PE and others, eds: Pain management in physical therapy, Norwalk, Conn, 1988, Appleton & Lange, pp 239-250.

19. Bengston R and Warfield CA: Physical therapy for pain relief, Hosp Pract 8:840, 1984.

20. Frampton V: Transcutaneous electrical nerve stimulation and chronic pain. In Wells PE and others, eds: Pain management in physical therapy, Norwalk, Conn, 1988, Appleton & Lange, p 107.

21. Gammon GD and Staff I: Studies on the relief of pain by counterirritation, J Clin Invest 20:13-20, 1941.

22. Melzack R: Prolonged relief of pain by brief, intense transcutaneous somatic stimulation, Pain 1:357-373, 1975.

23. Prithui Raj P: Practical management of pain, Chicago, 1986, Year Book Medical Publishers, p 571.

24. Shealy NC: Holistic management of chronic pain, Top Clin Nurs 2:6, 1980.

25. Sundaresan N and others: Neurosurgery in the treatment of cancer pain, Cancer 63:2372, 1989.

26. Ferrer-Brechner T: Anesthetic techniques for the management of cancer pain, Cancer 63:2343, 1989.

27. Breitbart W: Psychiatric management of cancer pain, Cancer 63:2339, 1989.

28. Turk DC and others: Pain and behavioral medicine: a cognitive-behavioral perspective, New York, 1983, Guilford Press, pp 269-270.

29. Benson H: The relaxation response, New York, 1975, William Morrow & Co.

30. Wright SM: The use of therapeutic touch in the management of pain, Nurs Clin North Am 22:707, 709, 1987.

31. McCaffery M: How to relieve your patients' pain fast and effectively with oral analgesics, Nursing 10:63, 1980.

32. Inturrisi CE: Management of cancer pain pharmacology and principles of management, Cancer 63:2315, 1989.

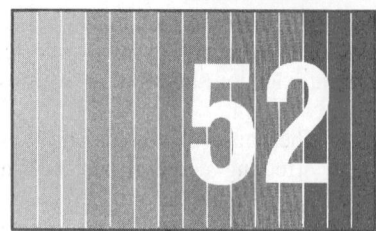

CHAPTER

52

Nursing Role in Management
Intracranial Problems

Connie A. Walleck

UNCONSCIOUSNESS

Unconsciousness is a state caused by many different health problems. Because intracranial problems often result in unconsciousness, they are the focus of this chapter. The same general principles of care of an unconscious client apply, regardless of the cause of the unconscious state.

Unconsciousness is an abnormal state in which the client is unaware of self or environment. Unconsciousness can range from a brief episode, such as fainting, to the prolonged unconsciousness of coma from which the person cannot be roused, even with vigorous external stimuli. Between these two extremes are degrees of unconsciousness varying in length and severity. Unconsciousness itself is not a diagnosis or a disease but rather a manifestation of a large number of pathophysiological processes, including

Reviewed by Marylou Muwaswes, R.N., M.S., Assistant Clinical Professor, University of California, San Francisco, School of Nursing, San Francisco, California.

trauma, metabolic disturbances, mass lesions, and infections. Therapeutic and nursing management is aimed at determining and correcting the cause of the unconsciousness, maintaining the bodily functions of the client, supporting the vital functions, and protecting the client from injury and the hazards of immobility.

Etiology

Consciousness involves two aspects: arousal and content.[1] The *arousal component* of consciousness refers to a state of wakefulness dependent on the activity of the reticular activating system (RAS), a network of nerve fibers and cell bodies that is located in the reticular formation in the central part of the brainstem and has neural connections to many parts of the nervous system. An intact RAS can maintain a state of wakefulness, even in the absence of a functioning cortex. The *content component* of consciousness refers to the ability to reason, think, and feel and to react to stimuli with purpose and awareness. These activi-

Table 52-1 Causes of Unconsciousness

Supratentorial mass lesions	**Subtentorial lesions**
Epidural hematoma	Brainstem infarction
Subdural hematoma	Brainstem tumor
Intracerebral hematoma	Brainstem hemor-
Cerebral infarction	rhage
Brain tumor	Cerebellar hemor-
Brain abscess	rhage
	Cerebellar abscess

Metabolic and diffuse cerebral disorders

Ischemia-anoxia
Postictal states and concussion
Infection (meningitis, encephalitis)
Subarachnoid hemorrhage
Exogenous toxins
Endogenous toxins and deficiencies

ties are mediated by the cerebral hemispheres, commonly called the *higher centers*. Intellect and emotional functions are also controlled by these centers.

Interruption of impulses from the RAS or alteration of the functioning of the cerebral hemispheres can cause unconsciousness. Any condition that widely alters the function of the hemispheres or that depresses or destroys the upper brainstem results in an impaired consciousness. Many specific etiological events can result in unconsciousness. Causes can be grouped according to pathophysiological mechanisms such as supratentorial mass lesions, subtentorial mass lesions or destructive lesions, and metabolic and diffuse cerebral disorders (Table 52-1). Psychiatric disorders such as depression, catatonia, and schizophrenia can also result in failure to respond to the environment.

Supratentorial mass lesions generally interfere with consciousness by compressing and shifting the cerebral contents and causing pressure on the upper brainstem containing the RAS. These lesions, occurring above the tentorium, may include trauma (e.g., lacerations or contusions, subdural or epidural hematomas), subarachnoid hemorrhage, intracerebral hemorrhage or infarction, tumors, and abscesses. The most serious consequence of a supratentorial mass lesion is the possibility of herniation of the cerebral hemisphere through the tentorial notch, causing compression of the brainstem. Another form of herniation can occur if the brain shifts laterally, forcing the cingulate gyrus under the falx and compressing the blood vessels of the opposite hemisphere.

Subtentorial mass or destructive lesions occur below the tentorium and interfere with consciousness by compressing or destroying the RAS above the midpons. Pontine or cerebellar hemorrhage, infarction, tumor, or abscess can affect the subtentorial area of the brain.

Metabolic and diffuse cerebral disorders of either intracranial or extracranial origin can cause alterations in the conscious state. These disorders can cause disturbances in cerebral metabolism that regulates cellular nutrition, electrolyte balance, oxygen and carbon dioxide regulation, and

enzymatic functions. Specific metabolic problems that can cause unconsciousness include uremia, diabetes, hypoglycemia, alcohol intoxication, barbiturate overdose, and lead poisoning.

Regardless of the cause of the unconscious state, two major reactions affecting cerebral metabolism generally occur: cerebral ischemia-anoxia and cerebral edema. The most common physiological problem of metabolic brain disease is a decreased oxygen uptake. Cerebral ischemia-anoxia, both focal and global, is managed by instituting measures to ensure adequate systemic circulation. Cerebral edema and the resulting increased intracranial pressure may be treated by hyperventilation, hyperosmotic drugs, dehydration, and steroids.[2]

Psychiatric or psychogenic disorders can cause unconsciousness. Although the neurological system is intact, the client does not react to the environment. A psychiatric referral is appropriate when the possibility of organic disease has been ruled out.

Unconscious State

The client's state of consciousness is defined by both behavior and the pattern of brain activity recorded by an electroencephalogram (EEG). In the most profound state of unconsciousness the client does not respond to deep pain. Corneal and pupillary reflexes are absent. The client cannot swallow or cough and is incontinent of urine and feces. The EEG pattern demonstrates decreased or absent neuronal activity. This client is in a coma.

Behavior. The nurse may find it helpful to conceptualize states of consciousness as a continuum. This continuum of electrical activity in the brain ranges from the hyperexcitable state of seizure to the hypoexcitable state of coma. The normal level of alertness is between these two states, with abnormalities ranging from slight disorientation to profound coma. A variety of terms have been used to describe points on the continuum, but they tend to be confusing (e.g., the term *lethargy* has a variety of meanings). Rather than relying on these terms, the nurse needs to learn appropriate assessment techniques and to describe the level of consciousness by noting the specific behaviors observed. When a deviation from the normal state of consciousness occurs, a more structured method of observation should be initiated. This type of systematic approach to nursing assessment is illustrated in Fig. 52-1 and consists of assessing the level of consciousness by the Glasgow coma scale and body functions.

Glasgow coma scale. Because of the confusion and ambiguity that surround terms describing altered states of consciousness, the Glasgow coma scale (GCS) was developed in 1974. The three areas assessed in this method correspond to the definition of coma as the inability of a client to speak, obey commands, or open the eyes when a verbal or painful stimulus is applied.[3] Specific assessments evaluate the client's response to varying degrees of stimuli. Three indicators of response are evaluated, including eye opening, best verbal response, and best motor response (Table 52-2). Specific behaviors that are seen as responses to the testing stimulus in each of these three areas are given a numerical value and can be plotted on a graph.

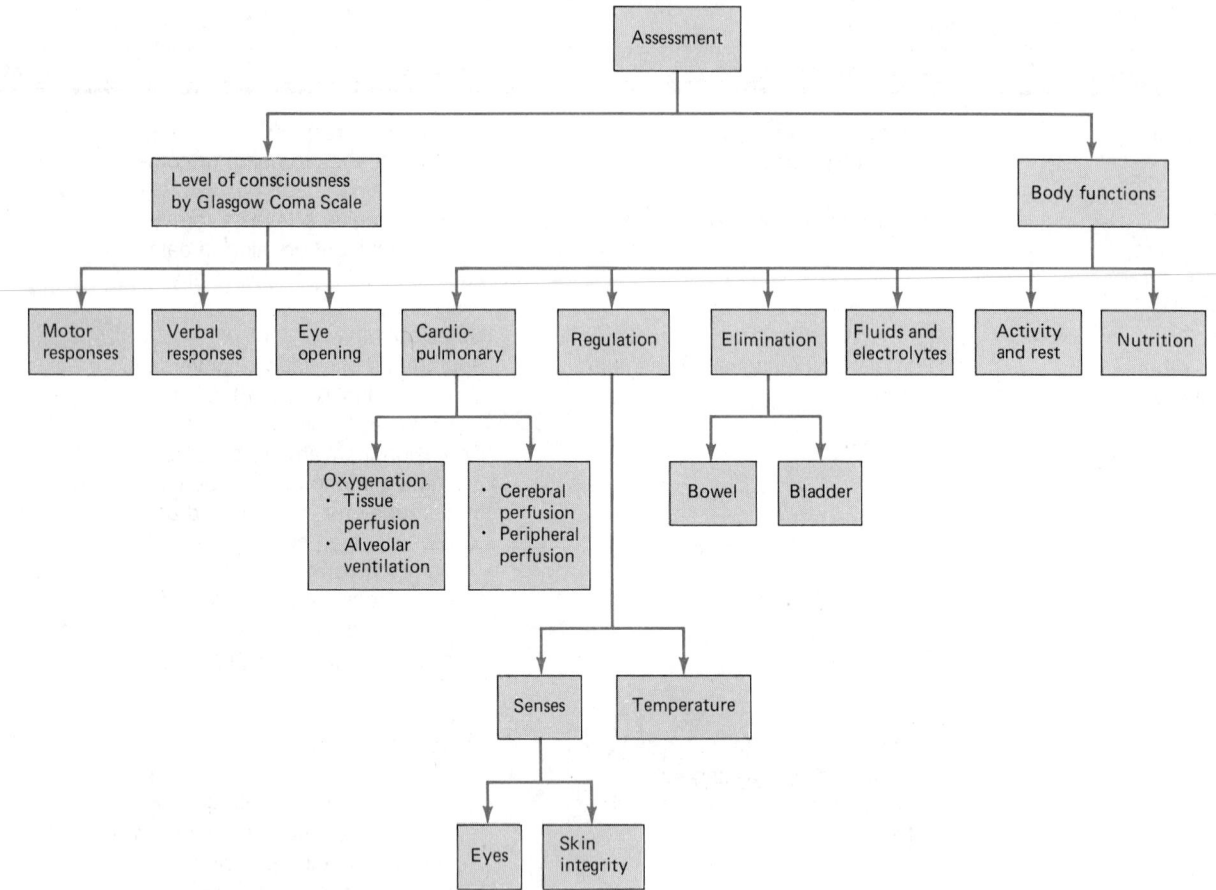

Fig. 52-1   A systematic approach to nursing assessment of the unconscious client. (From Wong J, Wong S, and Dempster JK: Care of the unconscious patient: a problem-oriented approach, Am Assoc Neurosci Nurses 16:145, 1984.)

The clinician's responsibility is to elicit the best response on each of the scales: the higher the scores are, the higher the level of brain functioning. The graph visually plots a place on the consciousness continuum to determine whether the client is stable, improving, or deteriorating. The subscale scores are particularly important if a client is untestable in one area. For example, severe periorbital edema may make eye opening impossible. In addition, the score for each can be added to give a sum. This sum can be interpreted by comparing it to the score of 15 for a fully alert person and the lowest possible score of 3. A score of 7 or less is generally considered coma level.

The GCS offers several advantages in the assessment of the unconscious client. It is specific and structured, allowing different clinicians to arrive at the same conclusion regarding the client's status. It saves time for the assessor because the ratings are done with numbers rather than with lengthy descriptions. The GCS is also specific enough to discriminate between different or changing states.

The GCS is used to assess the level of consciousness only. Other components of the neurological assessment include pupillary checks, extremity strength testing, and, if appropriate, corneal reflex testing.

Monitoring of body functions. In addition to assessing the neurological state of the unconscious client, various body functions, such as respiration and elimination, also need to be monitored. Adequate circulation and respiration are most vital and should always be the first body function evaluated.

INTRACRANIAL PRESSURE

Understanding the mechanisms associated with intracranial pressure (ICP) is important in caring for clients with many different neurological problems. The skull is like a closed box with three essential volume components: brain tissue, blood, and cerebrospinal fluid (CSF) (Fig. 52-2). Under normal conditions in which intracranial volume remains relatively constant, the balance of these components maintains ICP. This relatively constant volume is explained by the Monro-Kellie hypothesis, which states that if the volume added to the cranial vault equals the volume displaced from it, total intracranial volume will not change.

Other factors that influence ICP under normal circumstances are changes in (1) arterial pressure, (2) venous pressure, (3) intraabdominal and intrathoracic pressure, (4) posture, (5) blood gases, and (6) temperature (especially hypothermia).[4] The degree to which these other factors increase or decrease ICP depends on the ability of the brain to accommodate to the changes.

Table 52-2 Glasgow Coma Scale

Category of Response	Appropriate Stimulus	Response	Score
Eyes open	Approach to bedside	Spontaneous response	4
	Verbal command	Opening of eyes to name or command	3
	Pain (pressure on proximal nail bed)*	Lack of opening of eyes to previous stimuli but opening to pain	2
		Lack of opening of eyes to any stimulus	1
		Untestable	U
Best verbal response	Verbal questioning with maximum arousal	Appropriate orientation, conversant, correct identification of self, place, year, and month	5
		Confusion, conversant, but disorientation in one or more spheres	4
		Inappropriate or disorganized use of words (e.g., cursing), lack of sustained conversation	3
		Incomprehensible words, sounds (e.g., moaning)	3
		Lack of sound, even with painful stimuli	1
		Untestable	U
Best motor response	Verbal command (e.g., "raise your arm, hold up two fingers")	Obedience of command	6
	Pain (pressure on proximal nail bed)	Localization of pain, lack of obedience but presence of attempts to remove offending stimulus	5
		Flexion withdrawal,† flexion of arm in response to pain without abnormal flexion posture	4
		Abnormal flexion, flexing of arm at elbow and pronation, making a fist	3
		Abnormal extension, extension of arm at elbow usually with adduction and internal rotation of arm at shoulder	2
		Lack of response	1
		Untestable	U

*Produces least interrater variability.
†Added to the original scale by many centers.

Regulation and Maintenance

Normal intracranial pressure. Normal ICP is the pressure exerted by the brain tissue, blood volume, and CSF volume within the skull. ICP can be measured by means of a water manometer or a pressure transducer. With the client in the lateral recumbent position, the pressure is generally recorded at 80 to 180 cm H_2O with the use of the water manometer. When the client is lying with a 30 degree elevation of the head and the pressure is measured intracranially, it is 0 to 15 mm Hg with the use of the pressure transducer. A sustained pressure above the upper limit is considered abnormal.

Normal compensatory adaptations. Within certain limits, the body can compensate for changes in the volume components of the skull to maintain normal ICP. The body does this by making small changes in any of the three components. Specific changes initially involved in compensation include increased CSF absorption and displacement into the spinal subarachnoid space and collapse of the cerebral veins and dural sinuses. Other mechanisms that assist in compensation are (1) distensibility of the dura, (2) increased venous outflow, (3) decrease in CSF production, (4) changes in intracranial blood volume, and (5) slight compression of brain tissue.[5]

However, these compensatory adaptations to changes in volume are limited. Initially, increased volume produces no increase in ICP. If the volume increase continues, ICP rises dramatically and decompensation occurs.[5]

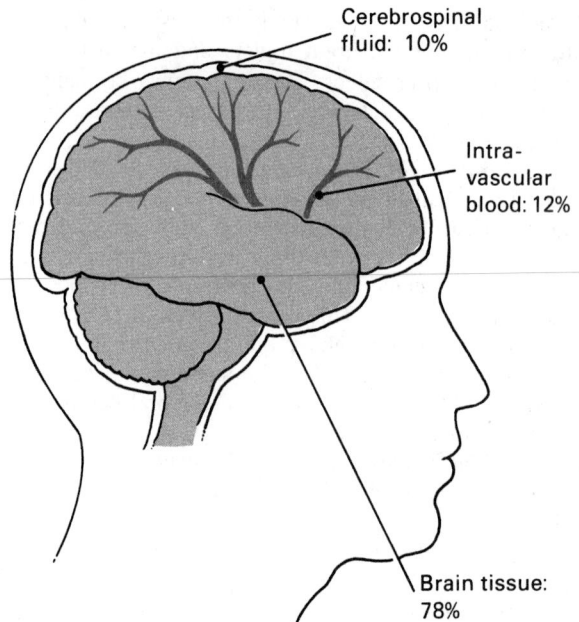

Fig. 52-2 Components of the brain.

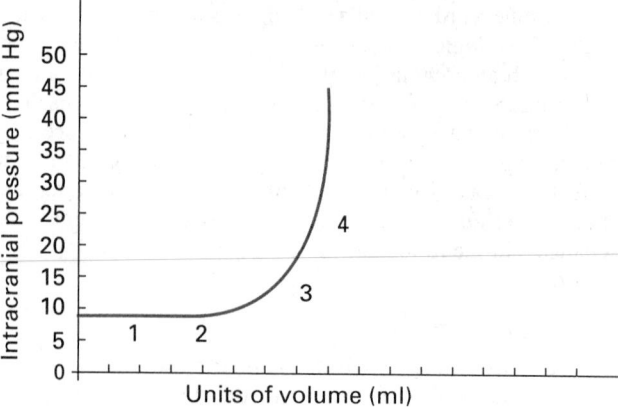

Fig. 52-3 Intracranial volume-pressure curve.

Table 52-3 Calculation of Cerebral Perfusion Pressure

CPP = MAP − ICP
MAP = diastolic pressure + ⅓ pulse pressure
Example: Systemic blood pressure = 122/84
     MAP = 97
     ICP = 12 mm Hg
     CPP = 85 mm Hg

Autoregulation of cerebral blood flow. The brain has the ability to regulate its own blood flow in response to its metabolic needs in spite of wide fluctuations in systemic arterial pressure. *Autoregulation* is defined as the automatic alteration in the diameter of the cerebral blood vessels that maintains a constant blood flow to the brain during changes in systemic arterial pressure. The purpose is to maintain the cerebral perfusion pressure within normal limits. The lower limit at which autoregulation is effective in a normotensive person is a mean arterial pressure (MAP) of 50 mm Hg. Below this, cerebral blood flow decreases and symptoms of cerebral ischemia, such as syncope and blurred vision, occur. The upper limit of autoregulation is 150 mm Hg. When this pressure is exceeded, the constrictor response is lost and the blood-brain barrier is disrupted; the result is an increase in cerebral edema.

The *cerebral perfusion pressure* (CPP) is the pressure needed to ensure blood flow to the brain. Its pressure is equal to the MAP minus the ICP (CPP = MAP − ICP). This formula is clinically useful, although it does not consider the effect of systemic vascular resistance.[2] As the CPP decreases, autoregulation fails and cerebral blood flow decreases. A CPP of 30 mm Hg is incompatible with life. Table 52-3 shows how to calculate the cerebral perfusion pressure.

The maintenance of blood flow to the brain is critical because the brain requires a constant supply of oxygen and glucose. Normal cerebral blood flow is 30 to 50 ml/100 g of tissue per minute (approximately 700 ml/min). The brain also uses 20% of the body's oxygen and 25% of its glucose.[6] Under normal circumstances, autoregulation is maintained by three physiological mechanisms: ICP changes, cerebral vasodilatation, and metabolic factors.

Pressure changes. The concept of the pressure-volume curve can be used to represent the stages of increased ICP (intracranial hypertension) (Fig. 52-3). At stage 1 on the curve, the brain is in total compensation, with accommodation and autoregulation intact and no increase in ICP. At stage 2, there is a reduction in cerebral blood flow, which places the client at risk of increased ICP. At stage 3, any small addition of volume causes a great increase in pressure. There is a loss of autoregulation, and there may be symptoms indicating increased ICP, such as systolic hypertension with an increasing pulse pressure, bradycardia, and respiratory slowing (*Cushing's triad*). With the loss of autoregulation and the rise in the systolic blood pressure as a result of the Cushing response, decompensation occurs. The ICP passively follows the blood pressure. Finally, when the client is in stage 4, the ICP rises to terminal levels with little increase in volume. Herniation occurs as the brain tissue shifts from the compartment of greater pressure to a compartment of lesser pressure.

Cerebral vasodilatation. Cerebral arteries dilate when the cerebral oxygen tension falls below 50 mm Hg. This dilatation decreases cerebral vascular resistance in an effort to raise oxygen tension. If oxygen tension is not raised, anaerobic metabolism begins, resulting in an accumulation of lactic acid. In an acid environment, an increase in vasodilatation and a further increase in blood flow occur.

Metabolic factors. Oxygen tension, carbon dioxide tension, and hydrogen ion concentration affect cerebral vessel tone. An increase in the partial pressure of arterial carbon dioxide ($Paco_2$) is the most potent vasodilator. A severely low Pao_2 and a high hydrogen ion concentration (acidosis) are also potent cerebral vasodilators.[6]

Extreme cardiovascular changes such as asystole and pathophysiological states such as diabetic coma can alter or abolish autoregulation globally. Trauma and tumors can alter autoregulation focally. When autoregulation is lost, the size of the cerebral vessels is directly influenced by any changes in systemic blood pressure, hypoxia, or the effects of catecholamines. Without appropriate intervention, increasing ICP can progress to loss of consciousness, changes in neurological function, brain herniation, and death.

Increased Intracranial Pressure

Increased ICP is a life-threatening situation that results from an increase in any or all of the three components of the skull—brain tissue, blood, and CSF. Cerebral edema is an important factor related to increased ICP.

Cerebral edema. A variety of conditions are associated with cerebral edema (Table 52-4). Regardless of the cause, cerebral edema results in an increase in tissue volume that carries the potential for increased ICP. The extent and severity of the original insult are the factors that determine the degree of cerebral edema.

Three types of cerebral edema—vasogenic, cytotoxic, and interstitial edema—have been distinguished, and more than one type may be present from one insult in the same client.[7] *Vasogenic cerebral edema* is the most common type, occurs mainly in the white matter, and is attributed to changes in the endothelial linings of cerebral capillaries. These changes allow leakage of macromolecules from the capillaries into the surrounding extracellular space, resulting in an osmotic gradient favoring flow of water from the intravascular to the extravascular component. A variety of insults, such as brain tumors, abscesses, and ingested toxins, may cause an increase in the permeability of the blood-brain barrier and produce an increase in the extracellular fluid volume. The speed and extent of the spread of the edema fluid are influenced by the systemic blood pressure, the site of the brain injury, and the extent of the blood-brain barrier defect. This edema may be manifest in focal neurological deficits, disturbances in consciousness, and severe increased ICP.

Cytotoxic cerebral edema results from local disruption of the functional or morphological integrity of cell membranes. Causes of cytotoxic cerebral edema are destructive lesions or trauma to brain tissue resulting in cerebral hypoxia, sodium depletion, and syndrome of inappropriate antidiuretic hormone. This type of cerebral edema results in movement of fluid and protein from the extracellular space directly into the cells, with subsequent swelling and loss of cellular function. Cytotoxic cerebral edema occurs most often in gray matter.

Interstitial cerebral edema is the result of periventricular diffusion of ventricular CSF in a client with uncontrolled hydrocephalus. It can also be caused by enlargement of the extracellular space as a response to systemic hyponatremia. Osmotic particles and fluid move into the cells to equilibrate with the hypoosmotic interstitial fluid. Regardless of the cause of cerebral edema, manifestations of increased ICP result unless compensation is adequate.

Mechanisms. Increased ICP can be caused by several clinical problems, including (1) a mass lesion, such as a hematoma, contusion, or rapidly growing tumor; (2) cerebral edema associated with brain tumors, head injury, or brain inflammation; or (3) metabolic coma. These cerebral insults may result in hypercapnia, cerebral acidosis, impaired autoregulation, and systemic hypertension, which promote the formation and spread of cerebral edema.[8] This edema distorts brain tissue, further increasing ICP, which leads to even more tissue hypoxia and acidosis. Fig. 52-4 illustrates the progression of increased ICP.

Unless there is a reduction in ICP, brainstem compression occurs. As the intracranial mass continues to increase, herniation of the brain from one compartment to another can occur.

Complications. The major complication of uncontrolled increased ICP is cerebral herniation (Fig. 52-5). The three major patterns of supratentorial brain shift are *cingulate* (lateral beneath the falx) herniation, *central* or *transtentorial* (downward) herniation, and *uncal* (lateral and downward) herniation. These patterns are distinguished by the direction of the shift and by the cerebral structures involved. Regardless of the specific intracranial shift, displacement and herniation cause a potentially reversible pathophysiological process to become irreversible. Ischemia and edema are further increased, compounding the preexisting problem. Compression of the brainstem and cranial nerves may be fatal. Fig. 52-6 illustrates symptoms of supratentorial increased ICP from the early phase through herniation.

Subtentorial and infratentorial herniations force the cerebellum and brainstem downward through the foramen magnum. If compression of the brainstem is unrelieved, respiratory arrest may occur.

Clinical manifestations. The clinical manifestations of increased ICP can take many forms, depending on the cause, location, and rate at which the pressure increase oc-

Table 52-4 Conditions Associated with Cerebral Edema

Mass lesions	Vascular insult
Neoplasm (primary and metastatic)	Infarct (thrombolic and embolic)
Abscess	Venous sinus thrombosis
Hemorrhage (intracerebral and extracerebral)	Anoxic and ischemic episodes
Head injuries	Toxic or metabolic encephalopathic conditions
Hemorrhage	Lead or arsenic intoxication
Contusion	Renal failure
Posttraumatic brain swelling	Liver failure
Neurosurgical procedures involving brain manipulation	Reye's syndrome

Modified from Edelman AS and Weiss MG: Cerebral edema: techniques for monitoring and options for management, *Consultant* 25:59, 1985.

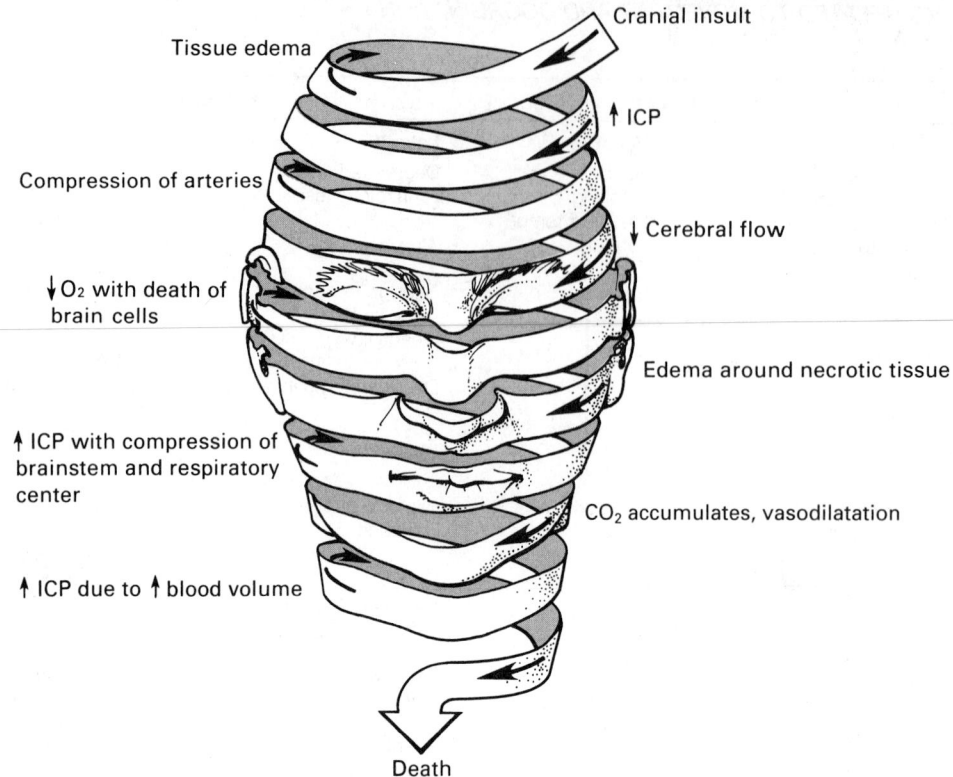

Fig. 52-4 Progression of increased ICP. (From Snyder M and Jackle M: Neurologic problems: a critical care nursing focus, Bowie, Md, 1981, Brady, p 52.)

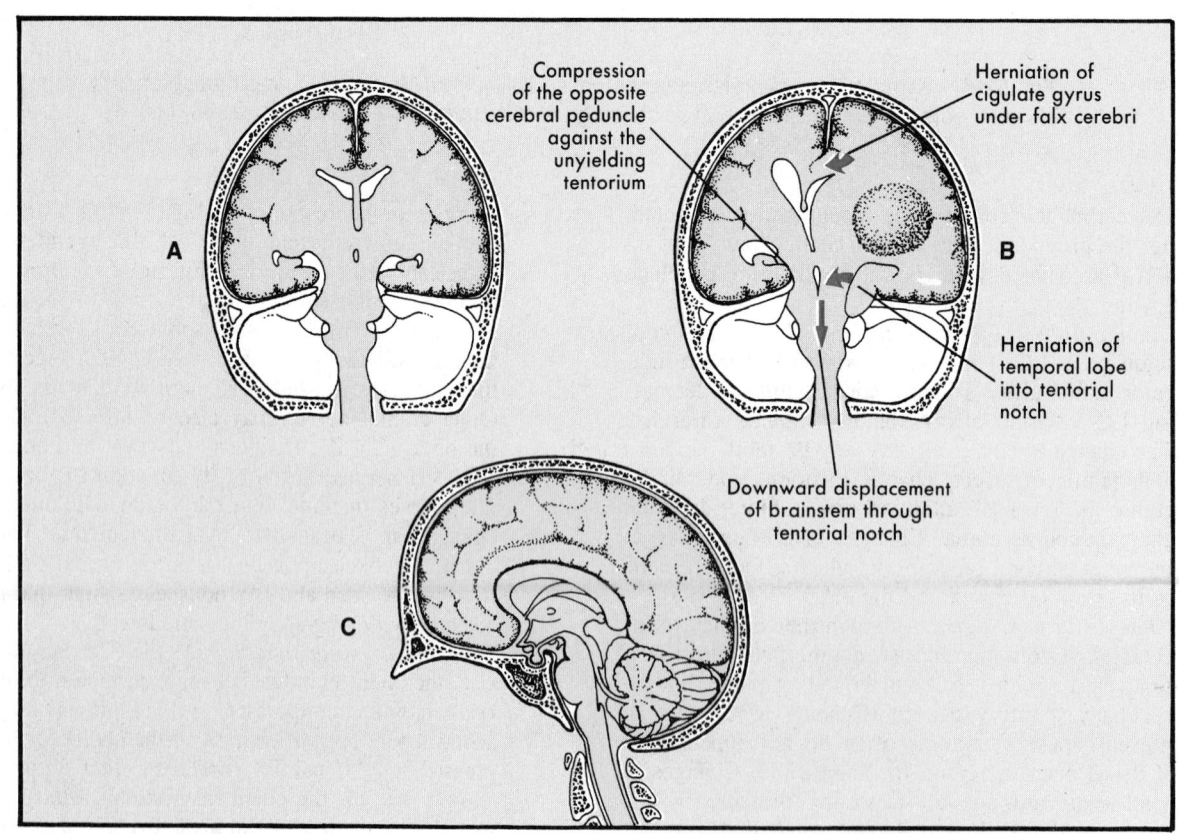

Fig. 52-5 Herniation. **A,** The normal relationship of intracranial structures. **B,** Shift of intracranial structures. **C,** Downward herniation of the cerebellar tonsils into the foramen magnum. (From McCance KL and Huether SE: Pathophysiology: Biological basis for disease in adults and children, St Louis, 1990, The CV Mosby Co, p 469.)

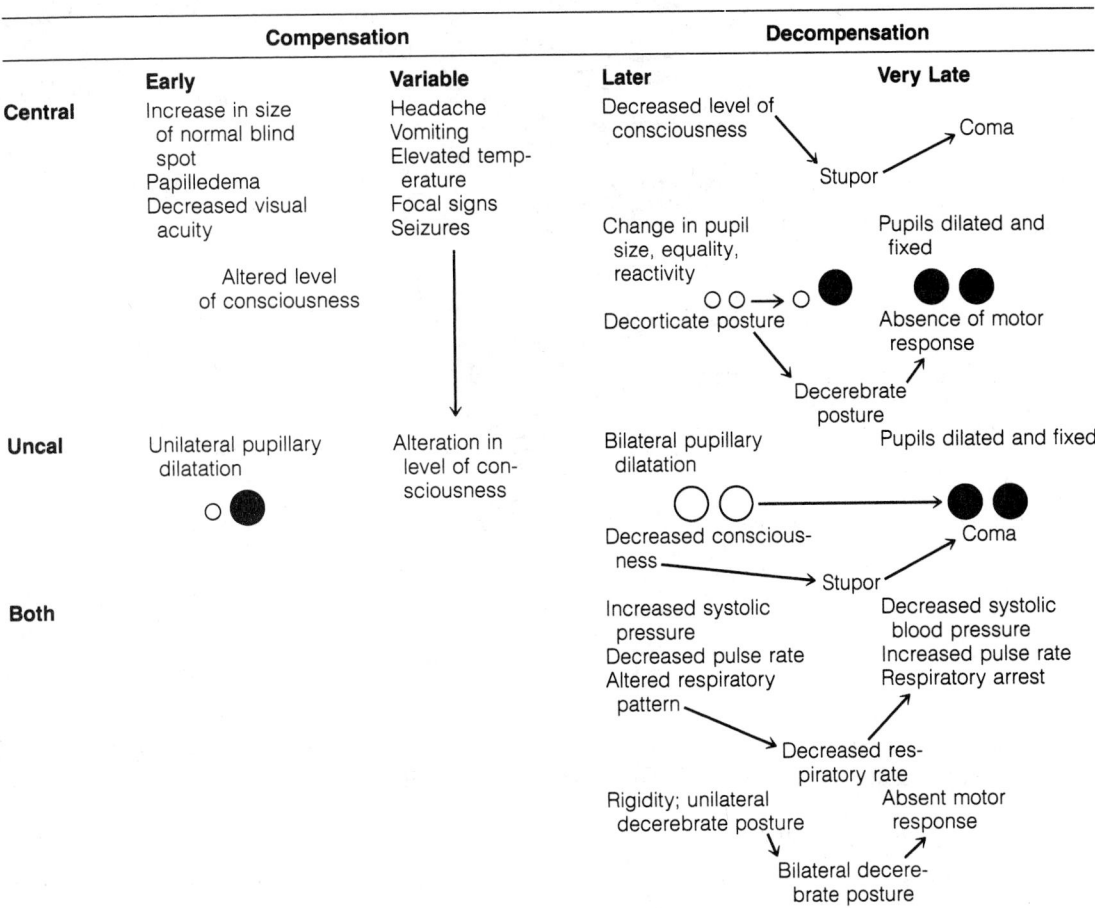

Fig. 52-6 Symptoms of supratentorial increased ICP. (From Moidel HC and others, eds: Nursing care of the patient with medical-surgical disorders, ed 2, New York, 1976, Mc-Graw-Hill Book Co, Inc, p 868.)

curs. The earlier the condition is recognized and treated, the better the prognosis. The clinical manifestations of increased ICP associated with supratentorial lesions include the following:

1. *Change in level of consciousness:* The level of consciousness (LOC) is a sensitive and important indicator of the client's neurological status. A decreasing LOC should always be investigated carefully. The change in consciousness may be subtle, such as a flattening of affect, change in orientation, or decrease in level of attention, or a more dramatic change such as coma. Changes in LOC are due to impaired cerebral blood flow, which affects the cells of the cerebral cortex and the RAS.

2. *Changes in vital signs:* Although the complex of increasing systolic pressure (widening pulse pressure), bradycardia with a full and bounding pulse, and irregular respiratory pattern (Cushing triad) may be present, these symptoms often do not appear until ICP has been increased for some time. Changes in vital signs are due to increasing pressure on the pons, medulla, hypothalamus, and thalamus. A change in body temperature may also be noted.

3. *Ocular signs:* Compression of the oculomotor nerve (CN III) results in dilatation of the ipsilateral pupil, sluggish or no response to light, inability to move the eye upward, and ptosis of the eyelid. These signs can be the result of a shifting of the brain from midline, which compresses the trunk of the cranial nerve, paralyzing the pupil sphincter. A fixed, unilaterally dilated pupil is a neurological emergency that indicates transtentorial herniation of the brain. Other cranial nerves may also be affected, such as the optic (CN II), trochlear (CN IV), and abducens (CN VI) nerves. Signs of dysfunction of these cranial nerves include blurred vision, diplopia, and changes in extraocular eye movements. Papilledema, a choked optic disk seen on retinal examination, is also seen and is a nonspecific sign that is associated with long-standing increased ICP.

4. *Decrease in motor function:* As the ICP continues to rise, the client manifests changes in motor ability. A contralateral hemiparesis or hemiplegia may be seen, depending on location of the source of the increased ICP. If painful stimuli to elicit a motor response is used, the client may exhibit a localization to the stimuli or a withdrawal from it. Decorticate (flexor) and decerebrate (extensor) posturing may also be elicited by noxious stimuli (Fig. 52-7). Decorticate posture consists of internal rotation and

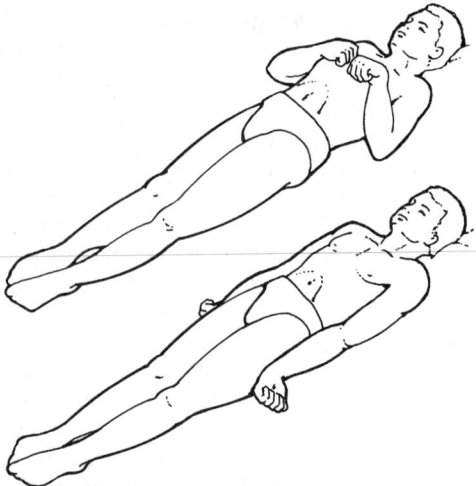

Fig. 52-7   Decorticate and decerebrate posturing. (From Thelan LA, Davie JK, and Urden LD: Textbook of critical care nursing, ed 1, St Louis, 1990, Mosby–Year Book, Inc, p 526.)

adduction of the arms with flexion of the elbows, wrists, and fingers as a result of interruption of voluntary motor tracts. Extension of the legs may also be seen. Decerebrate posture may indicate more serious damage and results from disruption of motor fibers in the midbrain and brainstem. In this position the arms are stiffly extended, adducted, and hyperpronated. There is also hyperextension of the leg with plantar flexion of the foot.

5. *Headache:* Although the brain itself is insensitive to pain, compression of other intracranial structures such as the walls of arteries and veins and the cranial nerves can produce headache. The headache is often continuous but worse in the morning. Straining or movement may accentuate the pain.

6. *Vomiting:* Vomiting, usually not preceded by nausea, is often a nonspecific sign of increased ICP. This is called *unexpected vomiting* and is related to pressure changes in the cranium. Projectile vomiting may also be seen in children and is related to increased ICP.

It is often difficult to identify increased ICP as the cause of coma. Loss of consciousness also confuses the interpretation of clinical signs, making it difficult to follow the progression of the increasing ICP.

Diagnostic studies. Diagnostic studies are aimed at identifying the presence and the underlying cause of increased ICP. Computerized tomography (CT) scanning has revolutionized the diagnosis of increased ICP. It is generally the initial test and can be used to differentiate the many conditions that can cause increased ICP and to evaluate therapeutic options. CT scans are particularly helpful in clients who have experienced trauma or who have tumors. Other tests that may be used include cerebral angiography, EEG testing, cerebral blood flow studies, and evoked potential studies. New diagnostic tests, such as the positron emission transaxial tomography (PETT) scan and magnetic resonance imaging (MRI), may prove to be even

Table 52-5

Diagnostic and Therapeutic Management: Increased Intracranial Pressure

DIAGNOSTIC

Complete history and physical examination
Vital signs, neurological checks, ICP measurements (via intraventricular catheter, subdural bolt, or epidural transducer) every hour
Skull, chest, and spinal x-ray studies
CT scan, EEG, angiography
Cerebral blood flow studies, MRI imaging, PETT scan
Laboratory studies, including CBC, coagulation profile, electrolytes, creatinine, ABGs, ammonia level, general drug and toxicology screen, CSF protein, cells, and glucose
ECG

THERAPEUTIC

Elevation of head of bed to 30 degrees with head in neutral position
Intubation and controlled ventilation to $Paco_2$ of 27 to 33 mm Hg
Good pulmonary toilet
Maintenance of fluid balance with 0.5 normal saline solution, assessment of osmolality
Maintenance of systolic arterial pressure between 100 and 160 mm Hg
Maintenance of CPP >70 mm Hg
Maintenance of normothermia
Adequate sedation
Drug therapy
   Osmotic diuretics (mannitol, urea, glycerol)
   Loop diuretics (furosemide, ethacrynic acid)
   Glucocorticosteroids (methylprednisolone, dexamethasone)
ICP monitoring

CBC, Complete blood count; *ABGs,* arterial blood gases; *ECG,* electrocardiogram.

more helpful in diagnosing the cause of increased ICP. In general, a lumbar puncture is not performed when this condition is suspected because of the possibility of cerebral herniation from the sudden release of the pressure in the skull from the area above the lumbar puncture.

Therapeutic management. The goals of therapeutic management (Table 52-5) are to identify and treat the underlying cause of increased ICP and to support brain function. A careful history is an important diagnostic aid that can direct the search for the underlying cause.

The prehospital management of the client with actual or potential increased ICP is important to prevent secondary injury to the brain. Table 52-6 outlines the prehospital care of the unconscious client. Once the client has been transported to the tertiary care facility, aggressive therapeutic management is needed.

While the cause of increased ICP is being sought, the condition itself must be treated aggressively to interrupt the cycle. Ensuring adequate oxygenation to support brain

Table 52-6

Prehospital Emergency Care of the Unconscious Client*

Possible etiologies: Head and neck trauma, drug overdose, meningitis, encephalitis, metabolic conditions (e.g., diabetic coma, liver failure, uremia, carbon dioxide narcosis), cardiac arrest, exogenous toxins (e.g., ethylene glycol, salicylates), cerebrovascular accident

CLINICAL MANIFESTATIONS

Unarousable state
Altered neurological and vital signs
Pupillary changes
Involuntary movements
Flaccidity of muscles with depressed reflexes
Decerebrate or decorticate posturing
Unresponsiveness to painful stimuli

MANAGEMENT

Assess for patent airway; if no gag reflex is present intubate client.
Assist ventilation if needed.
Administer 100% oxygen.
Assess and monitor vital signs, cardiac rhythm, neurological signs, and LOC.
Start IV line with large-bore needle.
Administer 50% dextrose (50 ml IV); if possible, give thiamine (50 mg slowly IV) first.
If there is possibility of narcotic overdose, administer naloxone (0.4 mg IV).
Try to determine cause of unconsciousness.
Check for peculiar breath odors (e.g., acetone, alcohol).
Assess body surface for trauma.
Examine ears for bleeding or otorrhea.

*See Chapter 59 for a general discussion of measures related to prehospital emergency care.

---

function is the first step in the management of increased ICP. An endotracheal tube or tracheostomy may be necessary to maintain adequate ventilation. Arterial blood gas (ABG) analysis guides the oxygen therapy. The goal is to maintain the arterial oxygen pressure (Pao_2) at 100 mm Hg or greater. It may be necessary to maintain the client on a ventilator to ensure adequate oxygenation.

A mild hyperventilation to maintain a $Paco_2$ of 27 to 30 mm Hg can have an effect on cerebral blood flow. The lowering of the $Paco_2$ leads to a constriction of the cerebral blood vessels, reducing cerebral blood flow and thereby decreasing the ICP.[9] This positive effect assumes that the brain will respond to hypocapnia by vasoconstriction. Lowering the $Paco_2$ below 20 mm Hg can cause ischemia and a worsening of the increased ICP.

If the condition is caused by a mass lesion, such as a tumor or hematoma, surgical removal of the mass is the best management (see p. 1545). Nonsurgical intervention for the reduction of tissue volume related to cerebral tissue swelling and cerebral edema includes the use of diuretics, glucocorticosteroids, and fluid restriction.

Pharmacological management. Drug therapy plays an important part in the management of increased ICP. Osmotic and loop diuretics are used to reduce the volume of brain water, and the glucocorticosteroids are thought to control the cerebral edema.

Osmotically active agents have been used for more than 50 years to treat cerebral tissue swelling. The principle governing the use of hypertonic solutions is the removal of fluid from the cerebral tissues in response to a vascular osmotic gradient established between the brain and the intravascular compartment. To be effective, the agent must remain in the intravascular compartment. In cases of brain injury and damage to the blood-brain barrier, the osmotic withdrawal is from normal tissue, where the vessels and blood-brain barrier are intact, rather than from edematous tissue. The beneficial effects must be attributed to a decrease in the bulk of normal tissue. However, if a major disruption of the blood-brain barrier occurs, this form of therapy may be more harmful than beneficial, since the hypertonic solution can pass into the edematous tissue and lead to a rebound phenomenon.[10]

Agents such as mannitol (Osmitrol), glycerol, and urea are available for use in osmotherapy. Mannitol (25%) is the most widely used agent and is given intravenously in doses ranging from 0.5 to 2 g/kg. For optimal effect, rapid administration with attention to preventing fluid overload is recommended. An advantage of glycerol is that it can be given orally and provides calories for energy. This drug decreases ICP by osmotic effects, decreases CSF production, and increases cerebral blood flow to ischemic areas of the brain.[10] Fluid and electrolyte status must be monitored when these drugs are used. Mannitol and urea may be contraindicated if renal disease is present and if serum osmolality is elevated. The effect of these hypertonic solutions is rapid and short lived.

Recent studies have demonstrated the positive effect on increased ICP of loop diuretics such as furosemide (Lasix) and ethacrynic acid (Edecrin). These diuretics inhibit sodium and chloride reabsorption in the ascending limb of the loop of Henle and cause a reduction in the rate of CSF production by 40% to 70%, thus reducing the ICP.[6] This lowering of pressure enhances the clearance of tissue fluid.

In spite of the controversy over the value of corticosteroid therapy in certain forms of cerebral edema, glucocorticosteroids have been used extensively in the treatment of cerebral edema. Dexamethasone (Decadron), a semisynthetic steroid, is the most commonly used steroid, and studies have demonstrated that it effectively reduces the quantity of vasogenic edema.

The mode of action of steroids is not completely known. It is theorized that they act by their stabilizing effect on the cell membrane. Steroids are also thought to improve neuronal function by improving cerebral blood flow and restoring autoregulation. Steroids are most beneficial in clients who have brain tumors with peritumoral edema. Research indicates that high-dose dexamethasone treatment is not effective in improving the outcome of severe head injuries.[11]

Complications associated with the use of steroids include hyperglycemia, increased incidence of infections, and gastrointestinal (GI) bleeding. Clients receiving ste-

roids should concurrently be given antacids or H$_2$ blockers such as cimetidine (Tagamet) to prevent GI bleeding. Fluid intake should be monitored because of the potential for hyponatremia. Since hyperglycemia has also been associated with steroid use, glucose levels of the blood and urine should be monitored regularly.

Pharmacological control of the cerebral metabolic rate is effective in controlling ICP. High-dose barbiturates (e.g., pentobarbital and thiopental) cause a decrease in increased ICP. A secondary effect is a reduction in cerebral edema and a more uniform blood supply to the brain.[12] Monitoring capabilities should be available when this treatment is used.

Research is ongoing for other agents that may be useful in controlling the metabolic rate. These agents include phenytoin, lidocaine, and calcium channel blockers.[13] Their mechanisms are not well understood, but their effect on preventing the formation of cerebral edema and controlling ICP is promising.

Fluid restrictions. Moderate dehydration to maintain serum osmolality can be effective in reducing cerebral edema. Fluids should be restricted to 65% to 75% of normal requirements. A lowering of serum osmolarity and an increase in cerebral edema occur if 5% dextrose in water is used for the administration of piggyback medications. If an intravenous (IV) drug routine is used, 0.45% or 0.9% sodium chloride is the preferred solution.[9] The use of fluid restriction to reduce tissue volume should be evaluated on the basis of clinical factors such as urine output, insensible fluid loss, serum and urine osmolality, and the client's condition.

Nutritional considerations. All clients must have their nutrition needs met, regardless of their state of consciousness or health. The client with increased ICP is in a hypermetabolic and hypercatabolic state and in need of glucose to provide the necessary fuel for the metabolism of the injured brain. If the client cannot maintain an adequate oral intake, other means of meeting the nutritional requirements such as a nasogastric tube or total parenteral nutrition should be initiated (see Chapter 35). Because certain types of feedings are low in sodium, added salt may be necessary. In addition to added minerals, free water may also be needed to meet the fluid needs of the client. Because malnutrition promotes continued cerebral edema, maintenance of optimal nutrition is imperative.

■ Nursing Management of Increased Intracranial Pressure

Regardless of the cause of unconsciousness, the unconscious client is managed as if there were actual or potential increased ICP. The goals of nursing management are to (1) maintain function, (2) monitor neurological changes, and (3) prevent complications secondary to immobility and the decreased LOC.

Nursing assessment

Subjective data about the unconscious client can be obtained from family members or other persons who are familiar with the client. Events preceding the unconscious state should be investigated. Fig. 52-1 presents a systematic approach to assessment of the unconscious client. This information, coupled with data for the GCS (see Table 52-

2), provides the knowledge base on which a nursing care plan can be formulated.

Ongoing assessment of the client with increased ICP is an important aspect of nursing care. Careful recording of the assessment is equally important. Fig. 52-8 illustrates a typical neurological clinical flow sheet used to display a client's neurological status over time.

The general plan of the neurological assessment is to evaluate the client's mental status, cranial nerve functioning, motor functioning, sensory status, cerebellar functioning, and reflexes. This schema helps the nurse organize the assessment to gather the data needed (see Chapter 50 for a discussion of the neurological assessment). If the client is critically ill, an abbreviated neurological assessment using the GCS, pupillary checks, and certain cranial nerve evaluations is made by the nurse on an ongoing basis.

In addition to the GCS score, other indicators of neurological function should be examined. Pupil size and reaction are essential components of the neurological check. The pupils are compared to one another for size, movement, and response (Fig. 52-9). If the oculomotor nerve is compressed by supratentorial pressure, the pupil on the affected side becomes larger until it fully dilates. If ICP continues to increase, both pupils dilate.

Pupillary reaction is tested with a flashlight. The normal reaction is brisk constriction when the light is shone directly into the eye. A consensual response (a slight constriction in the opposite pupil) should also be noted at the same time. A hyperactive or sluggish reaction can indicate early pressure on the third cranial nerve. A fixed pupil shows no response to light stimulus, which usually indicates increased ICP.

Evaluation of other cranial nerves can be included in the neurological check. Eye movements controlled by cranial nerves III, IV, and VI can be examined in the client who is awake and can be used to assess the function of the brainstem. In the unconscious client, extraocular eye movements are not specifically tested. Testing the corneal reflex gives information on the functioning of cranial nerves V and VII. If this reflex is absent, routine eye care should be initiated to prevent corneal abrasion (see Chapter 15).

Eye movements of the uncooperative or unconscious client can be elicited by reflex with the use of head movements (oculocephalic) and caloric stimulation (oculovestibular) (see Chapter 15).[14] To test the oculocephalic reflex (doll's-head or "doll's eyes" phenomenon), the nurse rotates the client's head briskly while holding the eyelids open. A positive response is movement of the eyes across the midline in the direction opposite the rotation. Next, the nurse quickly flexes and then extends the neck. Eye movement should be opposite the direction of head movement—up when the neck is flexed and down when it is extended. Abnormal responses can aid in locating the intracranial lesion. This test should not be attempted if a cervical spine problem is suspected. (The oculovestibular reflex is discussed in Chapter 15.)

Motor strength is tested by asking the client who is awake to squeeze the nurse's hands to compare strength in the hands. The palmar drift test is an excellent measure of strength in the upper extremities. The client raises the

Neurological Assessment Record

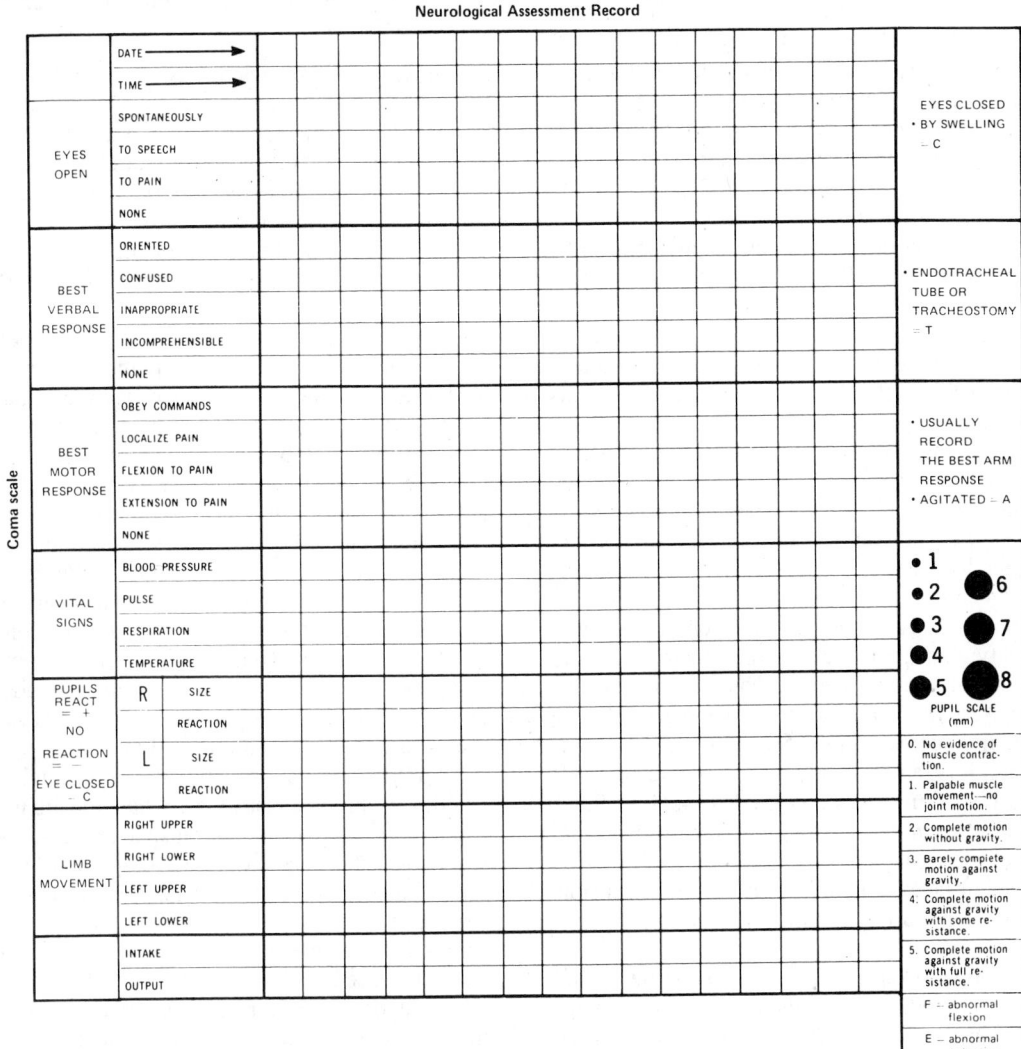

Fig. 52-8 Neurological clinical flow sheet. (From Kinney MR and others, eds: AACN's clinical reference for critical care nursing, St Louis, 1988, The CV Mosby Co.)

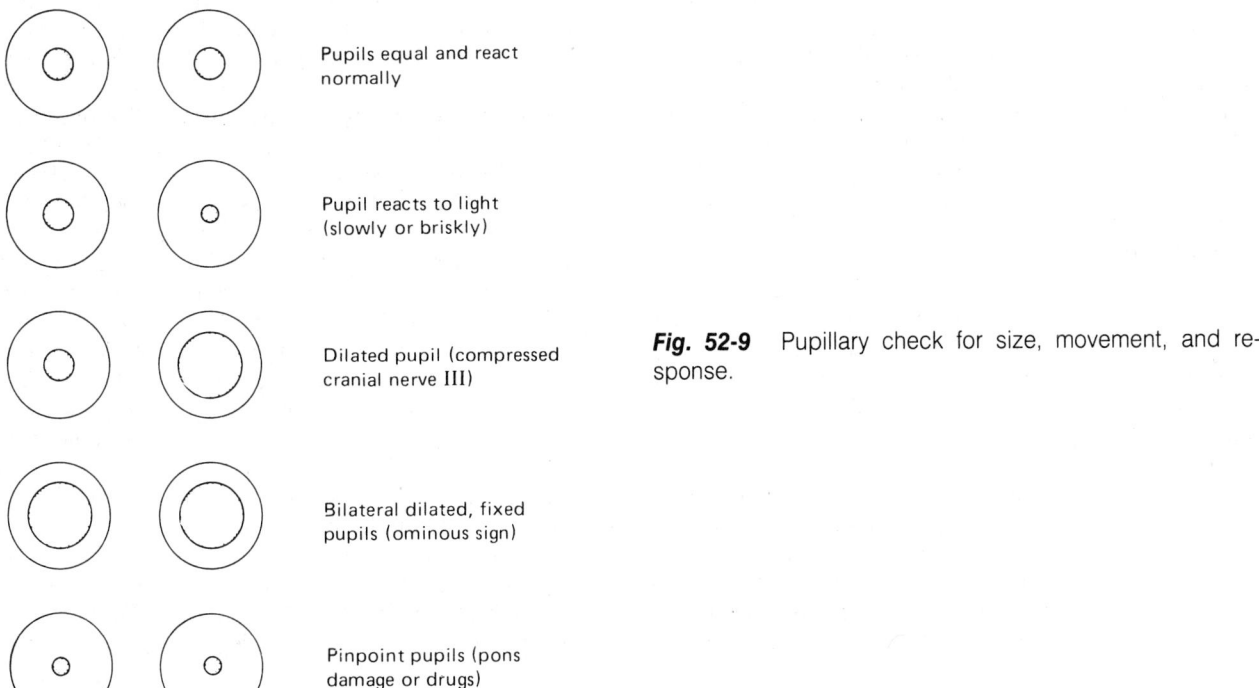

Pupils equal and react normally

Pupil reacts to light (slowly or briskly)

Dilated pupil (compressed cranial nerve III)

Bilateral dilated, fixed pupils (ominous sign)

Pinpoint pupils (pons damage or drugs)

Fig. 52-9 Pupillary check for size, movement, and response.

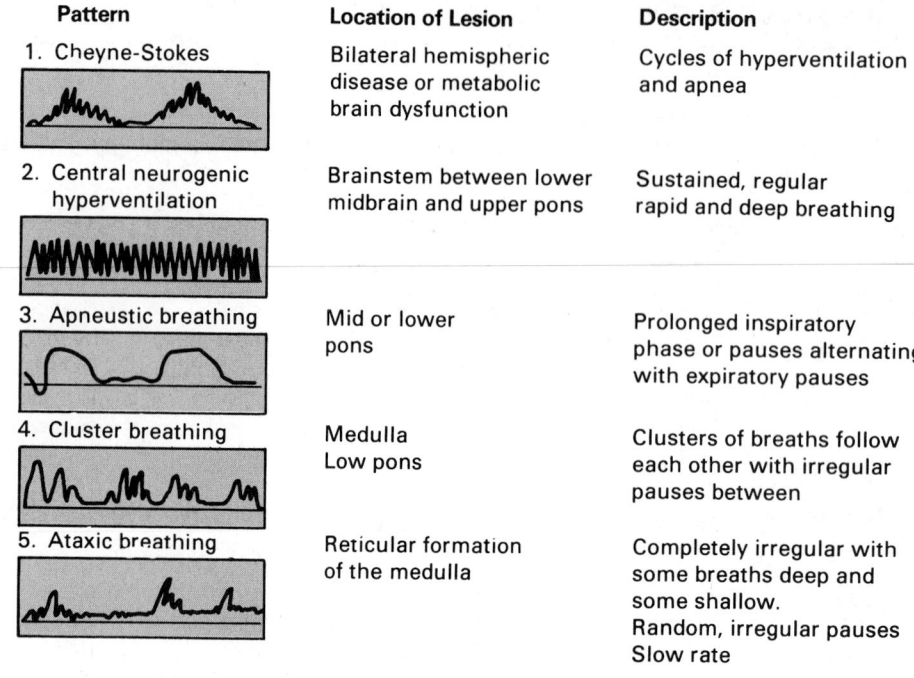

Pattern	Location of Lesion	Description
1. Cheyne-Stokes	Bilateral hemispheric disease or metabolic brain dysfunction	Cycles of hyperventilation and apnea
2. Central neurogenic hyperventilation	Brainstem between lower midbrain and upper pons	Sustained, regular rapid and deep breathing
3. Apneustic breathing	Mid or lower pons	Prolonged inspiratory phase or pauses alternating with expiratory pauses
4. Cluster breathing	Medulla Low pons	Clusters of breaths follow each other with irregular pauses between
5. Ataxic breathing	Reticular formation of the medulla	Completely irregular with some breaths deep and some shallow. Random, irregular pauses Slow rate

Fig. 52-10   Common abnormal respiratory patterns associated with coma.

arms in front of the body with the palmar surface facing upward. If there is any weakness in the upper extremity, the palmar surface turns downward and the arm drifts downward. Bending the knees up in bed is a good assessment of lower extremity strength. All four extremities should be tested for strength.

Motor strength of the unconscious or uncooperative client can be assessed by observation of spontaneous movement. If no spontaneous movement is possible, the client should be stimulated with pain, and the response should be noted. Resistance to movement during passive range-of-motion exercises is another measure of strength.

The vital signs, including blood pressure, pulse, respiratory rate, and temperature, should also be systematically recorded. The nurse needs to be aware of the Cushing triad, since this indicates severe increased ICP. Besides recording respiratory rate, the nurse should also note the respiratory pattern (Fig. 52-10).

Nursing diagnoses

The nursing diagnoses are supported by the data obtained on assessment and include those associated with increased ICP and unconsciousness. Clients with one or both of these serious problems require the highest level of nursing care because they are usually totally dependent on the nurse. Nursing diagnoses related to the unconscious client are presented in Table 52-7.

Nursing interventions

Maintenance of respiratory function. Maintenance of a patent airway is critical in the client with increased ICP and is a primary nursing responsibility. As the LOC decreases, the client is at increased risk of airway obstruction if the tongue drops back and occludes the airway and secretions accumulate. Altered breathing patterns may become evident. Airway patency can be aided by keeping the client lying on one side, with frequent position changes.

Snoring sounds, which may indicate obstruction, should be noted. The client should be suctioned as necessary to remove accumulated secretions. An oral airway facilitates breathing and provides an easier suctioning route in the comatose client.

The nurse must use measures to prevent hypoxia and hypercapnia. Proper positioning of the head is important. Elevation of the head of the bed 30 degrees enhances respiratory exchange and aids in decreasing cerebral edema. Suctioning and coughing can cause transient increases in ICP and decreases in Pa_{O_2}. Suctioning should be kept to a minimum and should be of short duration (less than 15 seconds), with the administration of oxygen and hyperventilation using a manual bag ventilation (e.g., Ambu Bag) before and after to prevent decreases in Pa_{O_2}. *Optimum oxygenation* is defined as a Pa_{O_2} of greater than 100 mm Hg.

Abdominal distention can interfere with respiratory function and should be prevented. Insertion of a nasogastric tube to aspirate the stomach contents can prevent distention, vomiting, and possible aspiration.

ABGs should be measured and evaluated regularly (see Chapter 19). The appropriate ventilatory support can be ordered on the basis of Pa_{O_2} and Pa_{CO_2} values. The nurse should be aware if a mild hyperventilation (Pa_{CO_2} of 27 to 33 mm Hg) is desired.

Unless the client is on ventilatory support, the use of narcotic sedatives and opiates should be avoided. Besides depressing respirations, these agents can also cloud the client's LOC. A narcotic that does not increase ICP, depress respiration, or cloud LOC should be selected to control pain. A nonnarcotic analgesic can be used in the client with increased ICP for an extended period. Agitation and restlessness should be evaluated, and appropriate drugs should be used, if indicated. Narcotics and opiates may be used in a client on a mechanical ventilator who is also un-

Table 52-7

 NURSING CARE PLAN FOR THE UNCONSCIOUS CLIENT

Defining Characteristics	Nursing Interventions	Evaluation Criteria

NURSING DIAGNOSIS: Ineffective airway clearance related to unconsciousness, immobility, and inability to mobilize secretions

Inability to maintain proper position, ineffective cough, inability to clear secretions, rales on auscultation, thick secretions	Maintain client's side-lying position, keeping head of bed elevated. Ensure patent airway. Have oxygen available. Suction frequently. Monitor ABGs or oxygen saturation by pulse oximetry. Perform chest physical therapy at least q 4 hr. Observe client for signs of decreased oxygenation, including changes in LOC and cyanosis.	Decreased risk of aspiration, demonstration of increased air exchange as measured by ABGs within normal limits, clear chest x-ray film, clear breath sounds in all lobes of the lungs

NURSING DIAGNOSIS: Ineffective breathing patterns related to loss of central nervous system integrative function and immobility

Hypoventilation or hyperventilation as measured by ABGs; altered respiratory pattern, such as Cheyne-Stokes, central neurogenic hyperventilation, apneustic; $Pao_2 <$ 60 mm Hg, $Paco_2 >$ 45 mm Hg	Describe and document breathing pattern and breath sounds. Monitor ABGs. Implement ventilatory support as ordered. Suction client as needed. Provide frequent rest periods to prevent respiratory fatigue. Monitor use of respiratory depressant drugs, such as barbiturates and narcotics.	Adequate oxygenation as demonstrated by $Pao_2 >$ 80 mm Hg, clear chest x-ray film, normal breathing pattern

NURSING DIAGNOSIS: Altered cerebral tissue perfusion related to cerebral tissue swelling

GCS $<$ 8; agitation; altered thought process; elevated systolic blood pressure, bradycardia, and widened pulse pressure; intracranial pressure $>$ 15 mm Hg	Monitor client's neurological status at least every hour initially; assess level of consciousness and document. Monitor ICP and calculate CPP.* Limit care activities that increase intracranial pressure (e.g., suctioning, hip flexion). Provide comfort measures. Provide rest periods after care activity. Elevate head of bed 30 to 45 degrees at all times. Hyperventilate client to maintain $Paco_2$ at 27 to 33 mm Hg. Monitor reactions to all medications, especially diuretics and sedatives. Maintain intracranial monitoring device.	No further deterioration in LOC, ICP $<$ 20 mm Hg, CPP $>$ 60 mm Hg; stable vital signs

NURSING DIAGNOSIS: Altered nutrition: less than body requirements related to hypermetabolism and inability to take food and fluids

Decreased LOC, self-care deficit for feeding, hyperthermia ($>$38.3° C [101° F]), metabolic needs in excess of intake, weight loss	Assess fluid status and document intake and output hourly initially. Check skin turgor. Monitor electrolytes. Weigh client daily. Maintain fluid restrictions as ordered. Evaluate swallowing abilities. Advance client to high-protein, high-caloric feedings (enteral or oral as indicated). Auscultate bowel sounds. Elevate head of bed during and after feedings. Provide adequate free water as indicated.	Adequate caloric intake to maintain weight and promote healing, maintenance of weight within 5 pounds of admission weight, normal electrolytes

NURSING DIAGNOSIS: Impaired skin integrity related to nutritional deficit, self-care deficit, and immobility

Inability to move or change position, dry skin, fever, weight loss $>$ 10 lb, abrasions or lacerations	Assess skin frequently, especially over bony prominences and around genitalia and buttocks. Turn client at least q 2 hr as indicated. Provide fluids to prevent dehydration. Use low-air-loss beds as indicated. Cleanse all abrasions and lacerations. Massage skin as indicated.	Absence of skin breakdown

*See Table 52-3.

Table 52-7

 NURSING CARE PLAN FOR THE UNCONSCIOUS CLIENT—cont'd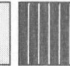

Defining Characteristics	Nursing Interventions	Evaluation Criteria

NURSING DIAGNOSIS: High risk for infection related to immobility, monitoring devices, invasive lines, and compromised immune system

Hyperthermia (temperature > 101° F), exudate around catheter insertion sites (IV, Foley's, intracranial), lethargy, abnormal chest x-ray film with breath sounds, foul-smelling urine	Observe strict sterile technique when assisting with insertion and maintenance of ICP-monitoring devices and all invasive lines. Maintain integrity of all closed systems. Monitor and record any leakage of fluid from nose (rhinorrhea), ears (otorrhea), or around ICP monitoring site and invasive lines. Take temperature rectally at least q 4 hr. Monitor for signs of meningitis (e.g., change in LOC, fever, increased WBC count, nuchal rigidity, photophobia). Obtain cultures as ordered.	Lack of fever, free of wound infection, normal white blood cell count, and chest x-ray film

NURSING DIAGNOSIS: Self-care deficit, total, related to unconscious state

Decreased LOC, inability to follow commands or move purposefully, sedation to control metabolic rate	Assess level of motor and sensory abilities at least q 4 hr. Bathe client daily. Turn client q 2 hr as indicated. Perform range-of-motion exercises at least q 4 hr as tolerated. Begin bowel program as soon as possible. Allow family to participate in care. Allow client to participate in care when able. Monitor nutritional intake. Monitor intake and output. Provide catheter care.	Meeting of all physical and psychosocial needs, absence of skin breakdown, bowel movement at least every other day, adequate urine output

NURSING DIAGNOSIS: High risk for injury related to seizure activity and environmental hazards

Decreased LOC; cranial nerve II, III, IV, V, VI deficits; motor and/or sensory deficits or loss; seizure activity	Assess environment for hazards. Make sure side rails are up at all times. Maintain bed in low position. Monitor for seizure activity. Pad side rails. Place airway at bedside. Document all seizure activity. Assess client's motor and sensory abilities frequently. Orient client to environment when appropriate. Stay with client during any seizure activity.	Absence of injury, control of seizures, safe environment

NURSING DIAGNOSIS: Anxiety of family members related to lack of knowledge concerning nature and prognosis of coma

Frequent questioning by family regarding client's condition, unrealistic expectations for recovery, expressions of anxiety over lack of knowledge	Encourage family members to ask questions of health care team. Spend time with family members, especially when they are at the bedside. Explain all procedures thoroughly to them. Encourage regular family conferences with physicians, nurses, and other health care team members. Provide support to family members.	Increase in knowledge of family members, adequate information base on which family members can make decisions about future care

NURSING DIAGNOSIS: Altered family processes related to comatose family member

Inability to adapt to health crisis of family member, lack of communication or miscommunication among family members	Teach and assist family members to provide care to ill family member. Facilitate family communication and realistic planning for needs of ill family member. Provide accurate information to family regarding client's situation. Initiate referrals as indicated.	Verbalization of feelings by family members and participation in care of ill member, use of appropriate referrals

dergoing ICP monitoring. At times, it may even be necessary to use paralytic agents such as pancuronium (Pavulon) or curare to ensure optimal ventilatory support (see Chapter 23). The client should then be fully monitored.

Fluid and electrolyte balance. Fluid and electrolyte disturbances can have an adverse effect on ICP. Free water needs to be minimized to prevent an increase in cerebral edema. IV fluids should be closely monitored with the use of a limited-volume device or a volume-control apparatus for accuracy. Intake and output, with insensible losses and daily weights taken into account, are important parameters in the assessment of fluid balance.

Electrolyte determinations should be made daily, and any abnormal values should be discussed with the physician. It is especially important to monitor glucose, sodium, potassium, and serum osmolality measurements. Urinary output is monitored to detect problems related to diabetes insipidus (e.g., increased urinary output related to a decrease in antidiuretic hormone secretion) and syndrome of inappropriate secretion of antidiuretic hormone (SIADH), which results in decreased urinary output. Besides urinary output, the serum sodium and osmolality are also used to diagnose diabetes insipidus and SIADH. Diabetes insipidus may result in severe dehydration unless treated. The usual treatment is fluid replacement, aqueous pitressin, pitressin in oil, or desmopressin acetate (see Chapter 44). SIADH results in a dilutional hyponatremia that may produce cerebral edema, changes in LOC, seizures, and coma.

Monitoring of intracranial pressure. In 1960, a technique was refined for the continuous monitoring of ICP by insertion of a catheter into the ventricles. Over the last 25 years, the technology for monitoring ICP has improved greatly and is regularly used in clients with suspected increased ICP who may benefit from treatment and in whom the underlying process is thought to be self-limiting. Clients with irreversible pathological processes or advanced neurological decline caused by primary or metastatic lesions may not be monitored. The measurement of ICP is valuable in detecting the early rise of ICP and client response to treatment and in providing information necessary for clinical decisions.

There are three ways to monitor ICP: epidural sensor, subdural subarachnoid bolt, and intraventricular catheter (Fig. 52-11). The *epidural sensor* is a self-contained fiberoptic transducer introduced into the epidural space. It is the least invasive of the three techniques and is appropriately used to measure trends in ICP.

The *subdural subarachnoid bolt* is the most commonly used of the ICP-monitoring devices. It can be placed with the use of a local anesthetic. It is a relatively accurate device and is less invasive than the intraventricular catheter. The risk of infection is also less with the bolt than with the intraventricular catheter. One disadvantage of the device is that there is decreased accuracy at high pressure.

An *intraventricular catheter*, which is introduced into the frontal horn of the lateral ventricle in the nondominant hemisphere, offers the most accurate way to measure ICP. Although the highest rate of infection is associated with this monitoring system and intracranial hemorrhage can be precipitated, the advantage of having a two-way system allowing instillation of fluid and the drainage of CSF makes it the optimal monitoring system.

The waveform seen when the ICP is normal has a steep upward systolic slope, followed by a downward diastolic slope with a dicrotic notch (Fig. 52-12, *A*). This waveform

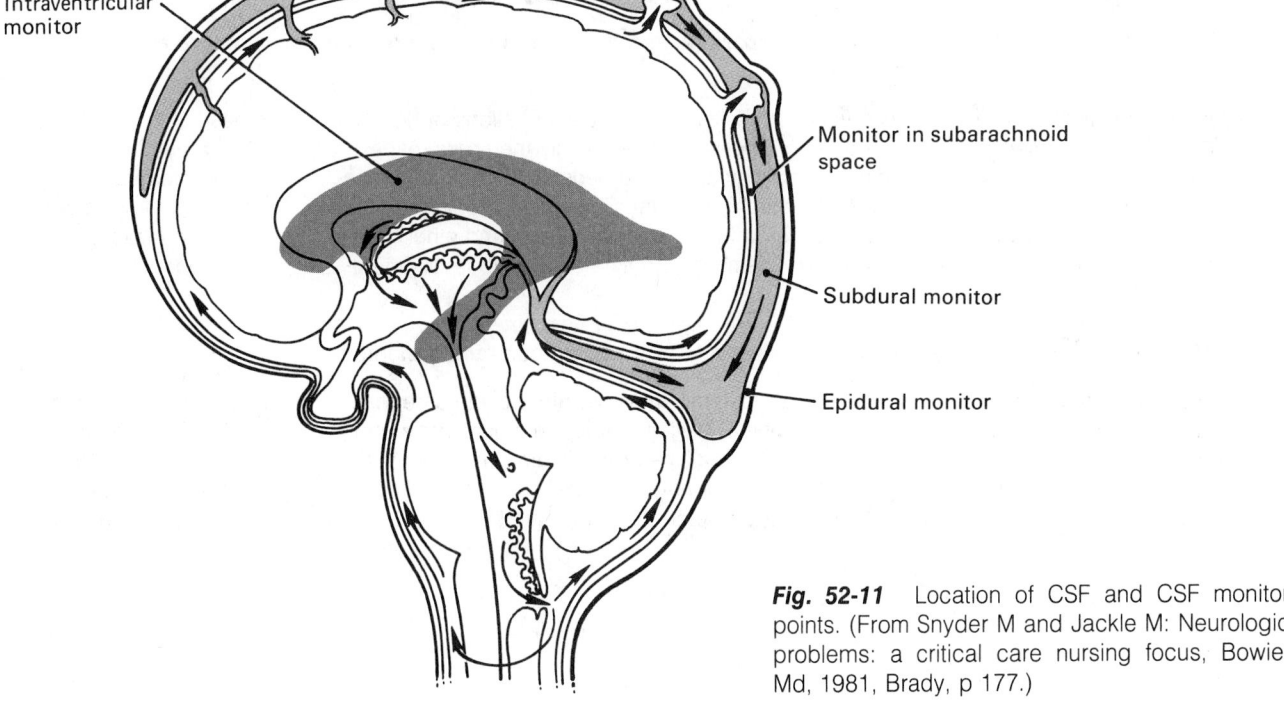

Intraventricular monitor

Monitor in subarachnoid space

Subdural monitor

Epidural monitor

Fig. 52-11 Location of CSF and CSF monitor points. (From Snyder M and Jackle M: Neurologic problems: a critical care nursing focus, Bowie, Md, 1981, Brady, p 177.)

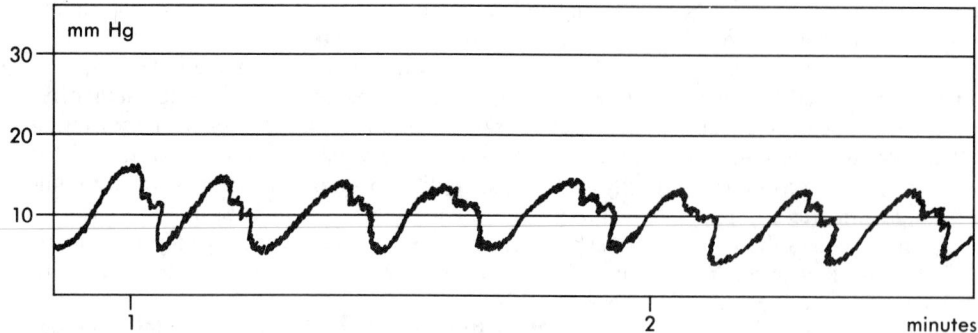

A, Normal ICP waveform—4 to 15 mm Hg.

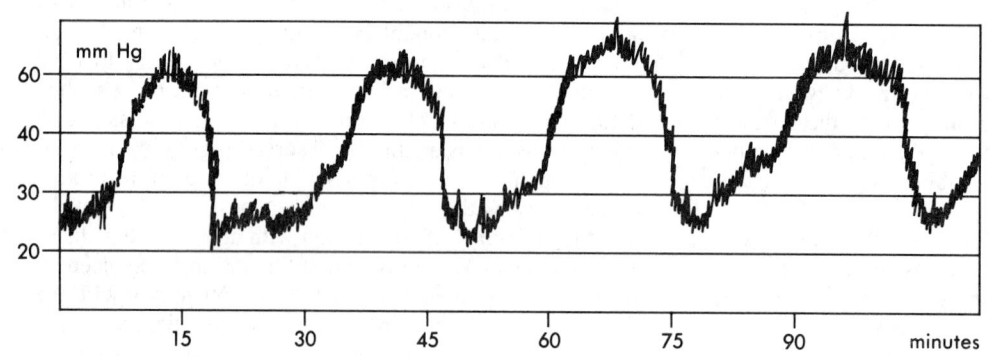

B, A waves (plateau waves)—50 to 100 mm Hg—may occur briefly with changes in intrathoracic pressure; if sustained, may indicate precipitous rise in ICP and compromised compensation; eventually, irreversible brain damage occurs.

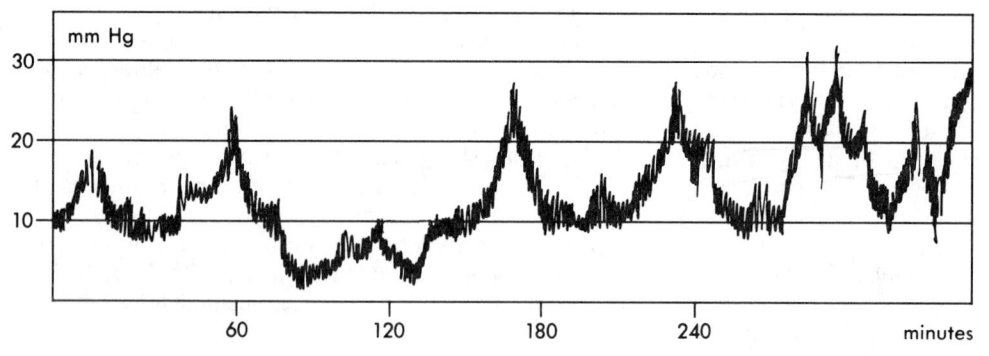

C, B waves—jagged sawtooth pattern with transient elevations to 50 mm Hg occurring every 1 to 2 minutes: may reflect decreasing ability to compensate; and may precede A waves.

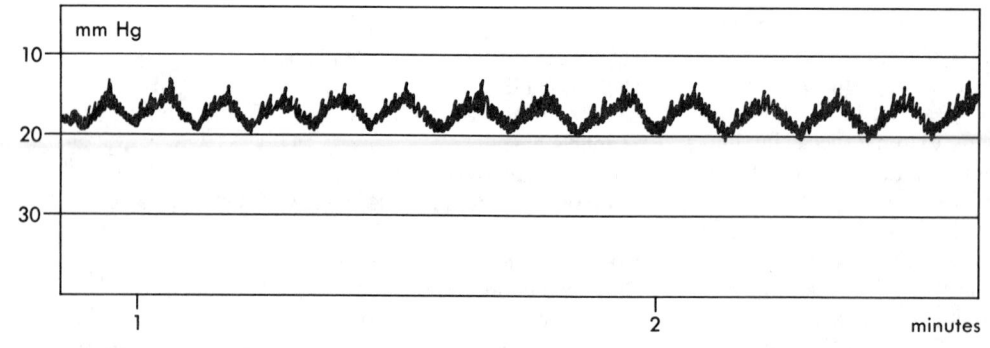

D, C waves—rhythmic oscillations; may vary with respirations or changing blood pressure; not dangerous.

Fig. 52-12   Monitoring ICP. (From Johanson BC and others: Standards for critical care, ed 3, St Louis, 1988, The CV Mosby Co, pp 272-273.)

indicates an ICP measurement between 4 and 15 mm Hg and usually appears continuously.[15]

Three distinct wave patterns seen in association with pathological conditions have been described. These patterns are called *A (or plateau) wave*, *B wave*, and *C wave* (Fig. 52-12). These abnormal waves may not be seen in the clinical monitoring situation. Plateau waves are indicative of severe ICP problems. They are described as elevations in ICP of 50 to 100 mm Hg lasting from 5 to 20 minutes. During these elevations the CPP may be less than 40 mm Hg. These waveforms represent a neurological emergency and must be treated at the onset for irreversible brain damage to be prevented. B waves are smaller increases in ICP (20 to 50 mm Hg) and last only about 2 minutes. These waveforms are seen with changes in the respiratory pattern and are thought to be precursors of A waves. The C waves are slight elevations from baseline, and their significance has not been determined.

Inaccurate ICP readings can be caused by CSF leaks around the monitoring device, obstruction of the intraventricular catheter or bolt, difference in the height of the bolt and the transducer, kinks in the tubing, and the Valsalva maneuver.[10]

Careful monitoring of the amount of CSF drained is essential. A closed system should be used to decrease the chance of infection. The amount of fluid to be drained should be ordered by the physician. A major complication of this type of drainage system occurs when the fluid is removed too rapidly, causing a decompression and potential herniation as a result of the sudden drop in pressure. Another complication of rapid decompression is development of a subdural hematoma.

Nursing care of the client with increased ICP who is being monitored is complex. Prevention of infection by use of strict aseptic technique during dressing changes is imperative. Maintenance of the intactness of the system is also critical to ensure that ICP readings are accurate, since treatment is generally based on the pressures. Recording of the amount and color of the drainage is also important in caring for the client with an intraventricular catheter drainage system.

Body position. Clients with increased ICP should be maintained in the head-up position. The head of the bed should always be elevated to at least 30 degrees unless a concurrent cervical neck injury has been identified. Elevation of the head of the bed promotes venous drainage from the head via the valveless jugular system, directly decreasing vascular congestion, which can produce cerebral edema. Along with elevation of the head of the bed, the nurse must take care to prevent extreme neck flexion, which can cause venous obstruction and contribute to increased ICP.

Care should be taken to turn the client with slow, gentle movements because rapid changes in position may increase ICP. Caution should be used to prevent discomfort in turning and positioning of the client because pain or agitation also increases pressure. Increased intrathoracic pressure also contributes to increased ICP by impeding venous return; thus coughing, straining, and the Valsalva maneuver should be avoided. Extreme hip flexion should be avoided to decrease the risk of raising the intraabdominal pressure, which can restrict movement of the diaphragm and cause respiratory distress. The client should be turned at least every 2 hours.

Decorticate or decerebrate posturing is a reflex response in some clients with increased ICP. Turning, skin care, and even passive range of motion can elicit the posturing reflexes. Attempts should be made to provide needed physical care activities to minimize complications of immobility, such as atelectasis and contractures. In cases of severe posturing reflexes, these activities may have to be done less frequently, because posturing can cause increases in ICP.

Protection from injury and environmental management. The client with increased ICP and a decreased LOC needs protection from self-injury. Confusion, agitation, and the possibility of seizures can put the client at risk of injury. Restraints should be used judiciously in the agitated client. If restraints are absolutely necessary to keep the client from removing tubes or falling out of bed, they should be secure enough to be effective, and the skin area under the restraints should be observed regularly for irritation. Agitation may increase with the use of restraints, which indicates the need for other measures to protect the client from injury. Light sedation with agents such as haloperidol (Haldol) or lorazepam (Ativan) may be needed. Having a family member or significant other stay with the client may have a calming effect. For the client with seizures or at risk of seizure activity, seizure precautions should be instituted. They include padded side rails, an airway at the bedside, accurate and timely administration of anticonvulsants, and close observation.

The client can benefit from a quiet, nonstimulating environment. The nurse should always use a calm, reassuring approach. Touching and talking to the client, even one who is in coma, is always an appropriate care approach. The nurse needs to create a balance between sensory deprivation and sensory overload for the client with increased ICP.

Contributory factors. Relationships exist between nursing care activities and increases in ICP. Table 52-8 lists some of the factors that have been identified as contribu-

Table 52-8 Etiological Factors for Increased Intracranial Pressure

Hypercapnia ($Paco_2 > 42$ mm Hg)
Hypoxemia ($Pao_2 < 50$ mm Hg)
Cerebral vasodilating agents (e.g., halothane anesthesia, antihistamines)
Valsalva maneuver
Body positions (e.g., prone, flexion of neck, extreme hip flexion)
Isometric muscle contractions
Coughing or sneezing
Rapid-eye-movement sleep
Emotional upset
Arousal from sleep

Modified from Hickey J: The clinical practice of neurological and neurosurgical nursing, Philadelphia, 1986, JB Lippincott Co, p 263.

tors to increased ICP. Nurses should be alert to these factors and should attempt to minimize them. Nursing management of the client with increased ICP is one of the most important aspects of the care provided these clients.

Psychological considerations. Besides the carefully planned physical care provided clients with increased ICP, the nurse must also be aware of the psychological well-being of the clients and their families. Anxiety over the diagnosis and the prognosis for the client with neurological problems can be distressing to the client, family, and nursing staff. The nurse's competent and assured manner in performing the care needed by the client is reassuring to everyone involved. Short, simple explanations are appropriate and allow the client and the family to acquire the amount of information they desire. The nurse should assess the family members' desire and need to assist in providing care for the client and allow for their participation as appropriate.[9]

HEAD TRAUMA

Head injury includes any trauma to the scalp, skull, or brain. The term *head trauma* is used primarily to signify craniocerebral trauma, which includes an alteration in consciousness—no matter how brief.

Head trauma has a high potential for poor outcome. Factors that are important in predicting a poor outcome include the presence of an intracranial hematoma, increasing age of the client, abnormal motor responses, impaired or absent eye movements or pupil light reflexes, early sustained hypotension, hypoxemia or hypercapnia, and elevation of ICP over 20 mm Hg in spite of artificial ventilation.[16]

Significance

Statistics regarding the occurrence of head injuries are incomplete because many victims die at the scene of the accident or the condition is considered minor and health care is not sought. An estimated 1 to 3 million persons suffer head injuries each year in the United States.[17] Mortality related to head injury is approximately 24 per 100,000 persons in the United States. Motor vehicle accidents are the most common cause of head injury. Other causes include falls, assaults, sports-related injuries, and recreational accidents.

Types

Scalp lacerations. Scalp lacerations are the most minor of the head traumas. Because the scalp contains many blood vessels with poor constrictive abilities, most scalp lacerations are associated with profuse bleeding. The major complication associated with scalp laceration is infection.

Skull fractures. Skull fractures frequently occur with head trauma. There are four major types of skull fracture (Table 52-9). Fractures may be closed or open, depending on the presence of a scalp laceration or extension of the fracture into the air sinuses or dura. The type and severity of a skull fracture depend on the velocity, momentum, direction of injuring agent, and site of impact. Specific manifestations of a skull fracture are generally associated with the location of the injury (Table 52-10).

Table 52-9 Types of Skull Fractures

Description	Cause
LINEAR	
Break in continuity of bone without alteration of relationship of parts	Low-velocity injuries
COMMINUTED	
Multiple linear fractures with fragmentation of bone into many pieces	Direct, high-momentum impact
DEPRESSED	
Displacement of comminuted fragments	Indentation due to powerful blow
COMPOUND	
Depressed skull fracture and scalp laceration with communicating pathway to intracranial cavity	Severe head injury

Table 52-10 Clinical Manifestations of Skull Fractures by Location

Location	Syndrome or Sequelae
Frontal fracture	Exposure of brain to contaminants through frontal air sinus; possible association with air in forehead tissue, CSF rhinorrhea, or pneumocranium
Orbital fracture	Periorbital ecchymosis (raccoon eyes)
Temporal fracture	Boggy temporal muscle due to extravasation of blood, benign oval-shaped bruise behind ear in mastoid region (Battle's sign), CSF otorrhea
Parietal fracture	Deafness, CSF or brain otorrhea, bulging of tympanic membrane due to blood or CSF facial paralysis, loss of taste, Battle's sign
Posterior fossa fracture	Occipital bruising resulting in cortical blindness, visual field defects; rare appearance of ataxia or other cerebellar signs
Basilar skull fracture	CSF or brain otorrhea, bulging of tympanic membrane by blood or CSF, Battle's sign, tinnitus or hearing difficulty, facial paralysis, conjugate deviation of gaze, vertigo

Modified from Davis JE and Mason B: Neurologic critical care, New York, 1979, Van Nostrand Reinhold, pp 111-112.

A specialized type of linear fracture occurs when the fracture occurs at the base of the skull—a basilar skull fracture. This fracture generally crosses a sinus and tears the dura (e.g., frontal or temporal) and is associated with leakage of CSF. Rhinorrhea (CSF leakage from the nose) or otorrhea (CSF leakage from the ear) generally confirms that the fracture has traversed the dura. Two methods of testing can be used to determine whether the fluid leaking from the nose or ear is CSF. The first method is to test the leaking fluid with a Dextrostik or Testape strip to determine whether glucose is present. CSF gives a positive reading for sugar. If blood is present in the fluid, however, testing for the presence of sugar is unreliable because blood contains glucose. In this event, the nurse should look for the "halo" or "ring" sign. To perform this test, the nurse allows the leaking fluid to drip onto a white pad (4 × 4) or towel and observes the drainage. Within a few minutes the blood coalesces into the center, and a yellowish ring encircles the blood if CSF is present. The color, appearance, and amount of leaking fluid must be noted because both tests can give false-positive results. The major potential complications of this type of fracture are intracranial infections and hematoma as well as meningeal and brain tissue damage.

Minor head trauma. Brain injuries are categorized as being minor or major. *Concussion* (a sudden transient mechanical head injury with disruption of neural activity and a change in the LOC) is considered a minor head injury. The client may not lose total consciousness with this injury.

Signs of concussion include a brief disruption in LOC, amnesia for the event (retrograde amnesia), and headache. The manifestations are generally of short duration. If the client has not lost consciousness or if the loss of consciousness lasts less than 5 minutes, the client is usually discharged from the care facility with instructions to notify the physician if symptoms persist or if behavior changes are noted.

The *postconcussion syndrome* is seen anywhere from 2 weeks to 2 months after the concussion. Symptoms include persistent headache, lethargy, personality and behavior changes, shortened attention span, and changes in intellectual ability. It is believed that this syndrome can significantly affect the client's abilities to perform activities of daily living.

Although concussion is generally considered benign and usually resolves spontaneously, the symptoms may be preliminary to a more serious, progressive problem. At the time of discharge it is important to give the client and family instructions for observation and accurate reporting of symptoms or changes in neurological status.

Major head trauma. Major head trauma includes contusions and lacerations. Both injuries represent severe trauma to the brain. Contusions and lacerations are generally associated with closed injuries.

A *contusion* is a bruising of the brain tissue with a potential for the development of areas of necrosis, pulping infarction, hemorrhage, and edema. Contusion frequently occurs at the site of a fracture. With contusion, the phenomenon of coup-countre coup injury is often noted. Because of movement of the brain inside the skull, damage occurs both at the site of the direct impact of the brain on the skull and at a secondary area of damage on the opposite side away from injury, leading to multiple contused areas. Bleeding around the contusion site is generally minimal, and the blood is reabsorbed slowly. Neurological assessment demonstrates focal findings and a generalized disturbance in the LOC. Seizures are a common complication of brain contusion.

Lacerations involve actual tearing of the brain tissue and occur frequently in association with depressed and compound fractures and penetrating injuries. Tissue damage is severe, and surgical repair of the laceration is impossible because of the texture of the brain tissue. If bleeding is deep into the brain parenchyma, focal and generalized signs are noted.

When major head trauma occurs, many delayed responses are seen, including hemorrhage, hematoma formation, seizures, and cerebral edema. Intracerebral hemorrhage is generally associated with cerebral laceration. This hemorrhage is manifest as a space-occupying lesion accompanied by unconsciousness, hemiplegia on the contralateral side, and a dilated pupil on the ipsilateral side. As the hematoma expands, symptoms of increased ICP become more severe. Prognosis is generally poor for the client with a large intracerebral hemorrhage. Subarachnoid hemorrhage and intraventricular hemorrhage can also occur secondary to head trauma.

Epidural hematoma. An epidural hematoma is a neurological emergency and is usually associated with a linear fracture crossing a major artery in the dura, causing a tear. It can have a venous or arterial origin. Venous epidural hematomas are associated with a tear of the dural venous sinus and develop slowly. With arterial hematomas, the middle meningeal artery lying under the temporal bone is frequently torn. Hemorrhage occurs into the epidural space, which lies between the dura and the inner surface of the skull (Fig. 52-13, *A*). Because this is an arterial hemorrhage, the hematoma occurs rapidly and under high pressure. Symptoms often include unconsciousness at the scene or a brief lucid interval followed by headache, focal findings, and a decreasing LOC. Without rapid intervention, mortality approaches 100%.[18] Death is generally related to herniation.

Subdural hematoma. A subdural hematoma usually results from injury to the brain substance and its parenchymal vessels (Fig. 52-13, *B*). The veins that drain the brain's surface into the sagittal sinus are the source of most subdural hematomas. Because a subdural hematoma is usually venous in origin, the hematoma is much slower to develop a mass large enough to produce symptoms. However, a subdural hematoma may be caused by an arterial hemorrhage, in which case it develops more rapidly. Subdural hematomas may be acute, subacute, or chronic (Table 52-11).

After the initial bleeding of the veins, a subdural hematoma may appear to enlarge over time as the breakdown products of the blood draw fluid into the subdural space to reach isotonicity. An acute subdural hematoma manifests signs within 48 hours of the injury. The signs and symp-

toms are similar to those associated with brain tissue compression in increased ICP and include decreasing LOC and headache. The client appears drowsy and confused. The ipsilateral pupil dilates and becomes fixed. A subacute subdural hematoma usually occurs within 2 to 14 days of the injury. Failure to regain consciousness may point to this possibility.

A chronic subdural hematoma develops over weeks or months after a seemingly minor head injury. The peak incidence of chronic subdural hematoma is in the sixth and seventh decades of life when a potentially larger subdural space is available as a result of brain atrophy. With atrophy, the brain remains attached to the supportive structures, but tension is increased and it is subject to tearing. The larger size of the subdural space also accounts for the focal symptoms rather than the signs of increased ICP as the presenting complaint. Chronic alcoholics are also prone to cerebral atrophy and subsequent development of subdural hematoma.

Delay in diagnosis in the older adult can be attributed to the fact that the symptoms mimic other health problems in persons of this age group, including vascular disease and senile dementia. Somnolence, confusion, lethargy, and memory loss are associated with other health problems in addition to subdural hematoma. The client has a history of head trauma in only 60% to 70% of cases.

Therapeutic Management

In addition to measures to treat cerebral edema and manage increased ICP, the principal treatment of head injuries is timely diagnosis and surgery if necessary. For the client with concussion and contusion, observation and management of increased ICP are the primary management strategies.

The treatment of skull fractures is usually conservative. For depressed fractures and fractures with loose fragments,

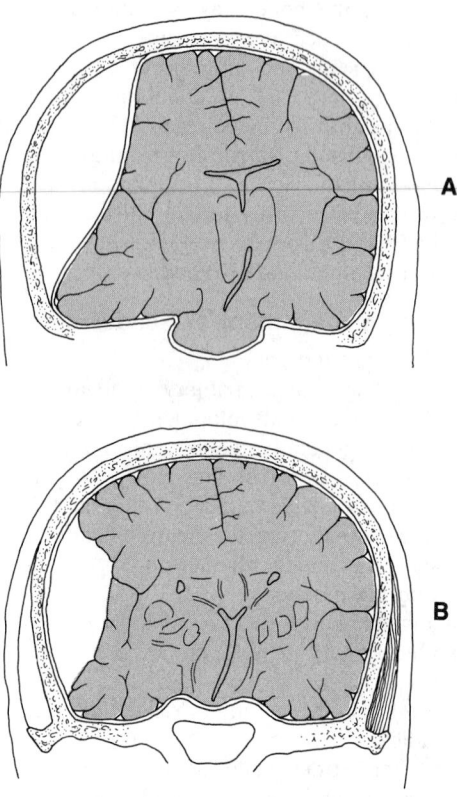

Fig. 52-13 **A,** Epidural hematoma in the temporal fossa, usually a result of laceration of the middle meningeal artery. **B,** Subdural hematoma, usually a result of laceration of the subdural veins. (From Price S and Wilson L, eds: Pathophysiology: clinical concepts of disease processes, ed 4, St Louis, 1991, Mosby–Year Book, Inc.)

Table 52-11 Acute, Subacute, and Chronic Subdural Hematomas

Occurrence After Injury	Progression of Symptoms	Treatment	Type of Trauma
ACUTE			
24-48 hr	Immediate deterioration	Craniotomy, evacuation and decompression	Severe
SUBACUTE			
48 hr-2 wk	Initial unconsciousness, gradual improvement, deterioration over hours, dilatation of pupils, ptosis	Evacuation and decompression	Severe
CHRONIC			
Weeks, months (longer than 20 days)	Nonspecific, nonlocalizing progression; progressive alteration in LOC	Evacuation and decompression, membranectomy	Trivial, nonexistent, or forgotten (recollection of incident by only 60% to 71% of persons)

a craniotomy is necessary to elevate the depressed bone and remove the free fragments. If large amounts of bone are destroyed, the bone may be removed and a cranioplasty will be needed at a later time.

In cases of acute subdural and epidural hematomas the blood must be removed. A craniotomy is generally performed to visualize the bleeding vessels so that they can be properly coagulated. Burr-hole openings may be used in an extreme emergency for a more rapid decompression, followed by a craniotomy to stop all bleeding. A drain is generally placed postoperatively for several days to prevent any reaccumulation of blood.

■ Nursing Management of Head Trauma

Nursing assessment

The client with a head injury is always considered to have the potential for development of increased ICP. The data collected generally include information gathered for the unconscious client (see Fig. 52-1). The most important aspects of the objective data are noting the GCS score (see Table 52-2), monitoring the neurological status (see Fig. 52-8), and determining whether a CSF leak has occurred.

Nursing diagnoses

Nursing diagnoses specific to the client who has sustained a head injury include, but are not limited to, the following:

1. High risk for eye injury related to loss of protective reflexes
2. Hyperthermia related to increased metabolism, infection, and loss of cerebral integrative function secondary to possible hypothalamic injury
3. Impaired physical mobility related to decreased LOC and treatment-imposed bed rest
4. Pain related to headache, nausea, and vomiting
5. Sensory/perceptual alterations related to cerebral injury and intensive care unit environment
6. Potential complication: increased ICP secondary to cerebral edema
7. Anxiety related to abrupt change in health status, hospital environment, and lack of knowledge of seriousness of health problem
8. High risk for infection related to environmental contamination secondary to open wound
9. Altered cerebral tissue perfusion related to interruption of cerebral blood flow associated with cerebral hemorrhage, hematoma, and edema
10. Self-esteem disturbance related to altered appearance of head and face and dependence on others

Nursing interventions

Health maintenance and promotion. One of the best ways to prevent head injuries is to prevent car and motorcycle accidents. The nurse can be active in campaigns that promote driving safety and can speak to driver education classes regarding the dangers of unsafe driving and of driving after drinking alcohol. The wearing of seat belts in cars and the use of helmets for riding on motorcycles are the most effective measures for increasing survival after accidents. States are increasingly active in passing legislation requiring the use of automobile safety devices for both children and adults. The speed limit of 55 mph has dra-

Table 52-12

Prehospital Emergency Care of the Client with Head Injury*

Etiology: Head trauma causing a disruption in normal brain activity, which may occur as a result of a motor vehicle accident, falls, fights, sports-related injuries, and recreational accidents

CLINICAL MANIFESTATIONS

Obvious scalp lacerations
Breaks or depressions in the skull
Bruises, contusions on face
Unequal pupils
Asymmetrical facial movements
Garbled speech
Decreased LOC, irritability, violent behavior
Unconsciousness
Increased blood pressure, decreased pulse rate
Inability to control bowel and bladder activity
Dripping of blood or clear fluid from nose or ears

MANAGEMENT

Establish and maintain airway.
Remove any items (e.g., tissue, teeth) that may have broken off and can block airway.
Determine LOC and monitor neurological and vital signs and cardiac rhythm.
Immobilize and stabilize head and neck for transport.
Assess for scalp wounds and skull fractures.
Observe for rhinorrhea, otorrhea, or other clues of CSF leakage.
Control any bleeding.
Administer oxygen by cannula.
If client exhibits signs of shock, look for other associated injuries.
Start IV line with large-gauge needle.
Do not overheat client but control environment and body covering to prevent shivering.

---

*See Chapter 59 for a general discussion of measures related to prehospital emergency care.

matically reduced fatalities within the United States. The wearing of protective helmets by lumberjacks, construction workers, miners, horseback and bicycle riders, and sky divers is also recommended. The nurse should be familiar with data on outcomes with and without safety devices in working with groups who oppose safety legislation as an infringement of personal freedom. Young parents should be educated in the proper use of car seats and restraints for their children. The nurse should also teach younger children about safety precautions for bicycle riding, skateboarding, and contact sports.

Acute intervention. Action taken at the scene of the accident can have an important impact on the outcome of the head injury. Table 52-12 lists the prehospital care of the client with a head injury.

The general nursing management of the head-injured

client may initially consist only of observation for changes in neurological status. This action is critically important because the client's condition may deteriorate rapidly, necessitating emergency surgery. Appropriate preoperative and postoperative nursing interventions are initiated if surgery is anticipated.

The nurse should explain the need for frequent neurological assessments to both the client and the family. Behavioral manifestations associated with head injury can result in a frightened, disoriented client who is combative and resists help. The nurse's approach should be calm and gentle. Restraints should be avoided if possible because they often produce agitation, which further elevates ICP. A family member may be available to stay with the client and thus prevent increasing anxiety and fear.

The nurse should perform neurological assessments at intervals based on the client's condition. The GCS is useful in assessing the level of arousal (see Table 52-4). Indications of a deteriorating neurological state, such as a decreasing LOC or a lessening of motor strength, should be reported to the physician, and the client's condition should be closely monitored.

Much of the nursing care for the brain-injured client relates to the unconscious state and increased ICP (see p. 1531). However, there may be specific problems that require nursing intervention.

Eye problems may include loss of corneal reflex, periorbital ecchymosis and edema, and diplopia. Loss of the corneal reflex may necessitate taping the eyes shut, suturing the eyelids to prevent abrasion, and administering eye drops to lubricate. Preorbital ecchymosis and edema disappear spontaneously, but warm and cold compresses provide comfort and hasten the process. Diplopia can be relieved by use of an eye patch.

Hyperthermia may occur from infection or injury to the hypothalamus. Increased metabolism secondary to hyperthermia increases metabolic waste, which in turn produces further cerebral vasodilatation.

Nursing measures specific to the care of the immobilized client, such as those related to bladder and bowel function, skin care, and infection, are also indicated. If CSF rhinorrhea or otorrhea occurs, the nurse should inform the physician immediately. The client should lie flat in bed unless contraindicated by increased ICP. A loose collection pad may be placed under the nose or over the ear. No dressing should be placed into the nasal or ear cavities. The client should be cautioned not to sneeze or blow the nose. Nasogastric tubes should not be used, and nasotracheal suctioning should not be performed on these clients.

Nausea and vomiting may be a problem and can be alleviated by antiemetic medication. Headache can usually be controlled with aspirin or small doses of codeine.

If the client's condition deteriorates, intracranial surgery may be necessary (see p. 1545). A burr hole or craniotomy may be indicated, depending on the underlying injury that is causing the symptoms.

The client is often unconscious before surgery, making it necessary for a family member to sign the consent form for surgery. This is a difficult and frightening time for the client's family and requires sensitive nursing management. The suddenness of the situation makes it especially difficult for the family to cope.

The emergency nature of the surgery may prevent the usual careful preoperative preparation. The nurse should consult with the neurosurgeon to determine specific preoperative nursing measures.

Chronic management. Once the condition has stabilized, the client is usually transferred to a general neurological unit for rehabilitation. As with any craniocerebral problem, there may be chronic problems related to motor and sensory deficits, communication, memory, and intellectual functioning. Many of the principles of nursing management of the client with a stroke are appropriate (see Chapter 54). With time and patience, many of the chronic problems subside or disappear. Outward appearance is not a good indicator of how well the client will function in the home or work environment.

Seizure disorders are seen in approximately 5% of clients with a nonpenetrating head injury. In 25% of clients who develop a seizure disorder, the onset is 4 or more years after the initial injury. Anticonvulsants are not used prophylactically but are generally instituted after a witnessed seizure or if an EEG demonstrates subclinical seizure activity. Phenytoin (Dilantin) is the anticonvulsant of choice in posttraumatic seizure activity.

The mental and emotional sequelae of brain trauma are often the most incapacitating problems. It is estimated that more than 60% of clients with head injuries who have been comatose for more than 6 hours undergo some personality change. They may suffer loss of concentration and memory and defective memory processing. Personal drive may decrease; apathy and apparent laziness may increase. Euphoria and lability, along with a seeming lack of awareness of the seriousness of the injury, mark their affect. The client's behavior may indicate a loss of social restraint, judgment, tact, and emotional control.

Progressive recovery may continue for 6 months or more before a plateau is reached and a prognosis for recovery can be made. Specific nursing management in the posttraumatic phase depends on specific residual deficits.

In all cases the family must be given special consideration. They need to understand what is happening, and they must be taught appropriate interaction patterns. The nurse must give guidance and referrals for financial aid, child care, and other personal needs and must assist the family in involving the client in family activities whenever possible.

The family often has unrealistic expectations of the client as the coma begins to recede. The family expects full return to pretrauma status. In reality, the client experiences a reduced awareness and ability to interpret environmental stimuli. The nurse needs to prepare the family for the emergence of the client from coma and must explain that the process of awakening often takes several weeks.

When the time for discharge planning arrives, the family and the client may benefit from very specific posthospital instructions to avoid family-client friction. Special "no's" that may be appropriately suggested by the neurosurgeon, neuropsychologist, and nurse include *no* drinking

Table 52-13 Major Intracranial Tumors

Tumor	Tissue of Origin	% of All Brain Tumors	Usual Locations	Malignant or Benign
Gliomas				
Astrocytoma	Supportive tissue, glial cells and astrocytes	20	White matter of frontal and temporal lobes in adults, lateral cerebellar lobes in children	Moderately malignant, grades I and II
Glioblastoma multiforme	Primitive stem cell (glioblast)	20	Cerebral hemispheres	Highly malignant and invasive, grades III and IV
Oligodendroglioma	Glial cells and dendrites	2	Cerebral hemispheres, most in frontal lobe, some in basal ganglia and cerebellum	Benign (encapsulation and calcification)
Ependymoma	Ependymal epithelium	1	Lateral and fourth ventricles in children and young adults (usual)	Benign to highly malignant, most benign and encapsulated
Medulloblastoma	Supportive tissue	1	Posterior fossa, fourth ventricle, brainstem in children	Highly malignant and invasive, metastatic to spinal cord and remote areas of brain
Meningioma	Endothelial cells, fibrous tissue elements, transitional cells, angioblasts	25	Arachnoid villi, dura, half over convexity of hemisphere and half at base of hemisphere	Benign, encapsulation outside brain substance
Acoustic neuroma (neurofibroma)	Sheath of vestibular portion of CN VIII	5	Site between pons and cerebellum	Benign or low-grade malignancy, encapsulation
Pituitary adenoma	Pituitary glandular tissue	10	Pituitary gland	Usually benign
Vascular tumors Hemangioblastoma Arteriovenous malformation	Overgrowth of arteries and veins enlarging from feeder vessels	3	Parietal cortex near middle cerebral vessels	Benign
Metastatic tumors	Lungs, breast, kidney, thyroid, prostate	8	Cerebral cortex, diencephalon	Malignant

of alcoholic beverages, *no* driving, *no* use of firearms, *no* work with hazardous implements and machinery, and *no* unsupervised smoking.[19]

INTRACRANIAL TUMORS
Significance

Tumors within the cranial cavity cause approximately 2% of all deaths. Approximately 15,000 cases of brain tumor are diagnosed each year, accounting for 10% to 15% of all malignant disease. Brain tumors rank tenth in men and twelfth in women as causes of cancer death.

Types

Tumors of the brain may be primary, arising from tissues within the brain, or secondary, due to metastasis from a malignant neoplasm elsewhere in the body. Brain tumors arise from within the brain and may be found in any location. They are generally classified according to the tissue from which they arise. If malignant, the tumor is graded according to general cancer staging procedures. Brain tumors may be classified as (1) inside the brain substance (e.g., gliomas, vascular tumors) or (2) outside the brain substance (e.g., meningiomas, cranial nerve tumors). Probably more than half of the intracranial tumors are malignant; they infiltrate the brain parenchyma and are not amenable to complete surgical removal. Other tumors may be histologically benign but are so located that complete removal is not possible. Brain tumors are more commonly seen in middle age, but they may occur at any age.

Unless treated, all intracranial tumors eventually cause death from increasing tumor volume leading to increased ICP. Brain tumors rarely metastasize outside the central nervous system (CNS) because of their containment by structural (meninges) and physiological (blood-brain) barriers. Table 52-13 compares the major intracranial tumors.

Clinical Manifestations

The clinical manifestations of intracranial tumors are generally due to the local destructive effects of the tumor, the resulting accumulation of metabolites, the displacement of structures, obstruction of CSF flow, and the effects of edema and increased ICP on the cerebral function.

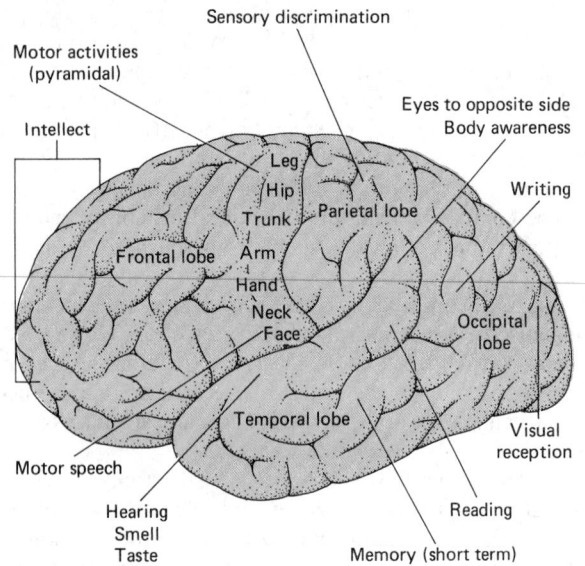

Fig. 52-14 Each area of the brain controls a particular activity.

The rate of growth and the appearance of manifestations depend on the location, size, and rate of growth of the tumor. Fig. 52-14 illustrates the functional areas of the cerebral cortex and can be used as a guide to correlate local manifestations with the location of the tumor.

A wide range of possible clinical manifestations are associated with brain tumors. In some circumstances a slight decrease in mental acuity may be the only symptom. In other cases there may be a dramatic event such as a seizure. In others, the manifestations of increased ICP may be apparent. Finally, manifestations may clearly indicate the location of the tumor by an alteration in the function controlled by the affected area.

Complications

If the tumor mass obstructs the ventricles or occludes the outlet, ventricular enlargement (hydrocephalus) can occur. Surgical treatment is needed to relieve the pressure and involves placement of a ventriculoatrial, a ventriculovagular, a ventriculopleural, or a ventriculoperitoneal shunt. A catheter is placed in the ventricle to provide the drainage, and a distal catheter is tunneled through the skin to drain into the right atrium, the pleural cavity, or the peritoneum. Rapid decompression can cause prostration and headache, so the client is gradually introduced to the upright position. The client should be instructed to avoid contact sports that may result in a blow to the valve or shearing of the catheter. If signs of increased ICP, such as headache, blurred vision, vomiting without nausea, decreasing LOC, or restlessness occur, the physician should be notified. Signs of an infected shunt, such as high fever, persistent headache, and stiff neck, warrant investigation.

Therapeutic Management

Treatment goals are aimed at (1) identifying tumor type and location, (2) removing or decreasing tumor mass, and (3) preventing or managing increased ICP (Table 52-14).

Table 52-14

Diagnostic and Therapeutic Management: Intracranial Tumors

DIAGNOSTIC

History and physical examination
Neurological examination
EEG
CT scan, MRI imaging, PETT scan
Skull x-ray study
Visual field examination
Brain scan
Biopsy

THERAPEUTIC

Dexamethasone (IV)
Anticonvulsant therapy
Surgical excision
Radiation therapy
Chemotherapy
Biological response modifiers
Hyperthermia

The type and location of the tumor are determined by several diagnostic measures. A careful history and physical examination may provide data with respect to location. A CT scan and a brain isotope scan are used to diagnose the location of the lesion. Newer diagnostic tools such as the PETT scan and MRI provide more reliable diagnostic information. The EEG is useful but of less importance. A lumbar puncture is seldom diagnostic and carries with it the risk of cerebral herniation. Angiography can be used to determine blood flow to the tumor and further localize the tumor.

Surgical Interventions

Surgical removal is the preferred treatment for brain tumors. However, the outcome depends on the type and location of the tumor. Meningiomas and oligodendrogliomas can usually be completely removed, whereas the more invasive gliomas and medulloblastomas can be only partially removed. Surgery reduces tumor mass, which decreases ICP and provides relief of symptoms with an extension of survival time. Tumors located in the deep central areas of the dominant hemisphere, the posterior corpus collosum, or the upper brainstem cause extensive neurological damage and are considered inoperable.

Radiation and Chemotherapy

Radiation therapy lengthens survival in clients with malignant gliomas, especially when it is combined with partial surgical removal. Clients with less malignant tumors respond to radiation with longer survival time and decreased tumor recurrence. Edema and rapidly increasing ICP may be a complication of radiation therapy but can be managed with high doses of corticosteroids.

Normally the blood-brain barrier prohibits the entry of most drugs into the brain parenchyma. The most malignant

tumors abolish the blood-brain barrier in the area of the tumor, allowing chemotherapeutic agents to be used to treat the malignancy.[20] An effective group of chemotherapeutic drugs called the *nitrosoureas* (CCNU and BCNU) are particularly effective in treating brain tumors. Other drugs being used include methotrexate (previously called amethopterin) and procarbazine (Matulane). Brain tumors that cannot be totally removed may be treated with a combination of steroids, surgery, radiation, and chemotherapy (see Chapter 9).

Many techniques to control and treat brain tumors are currently under investigation; these include radium implants into the tumor bed, local hyperthermia, and biological response modifiers. Although progress in treatment has increased length and quality of survival of clients with gliomas, death is still inevitable.

■ Nursing Management of Brain Tumor and Craniotomy

Nursing assessment

The subjective and objective data of the client with a brain tumor include the data the nurse collects for the unconscious client. In addition to the assessment data listed in Fig. 52-8, the initial assessment should be structured to provide baseline data of the neurological status and the information needed to design a realistic, individualized care plan. Areas to be assessed include the LOC and content of consciousness, motor abilities, sensory perception, integrated function (including bowel and bladder function), balance and proprioception, and the client's and the family's coping abilities. Watching a client perform activities of daily living and listening to the client's conversation are convenient ways to perform part of the neurological assessment. Having the client or the family explain the problem can be very helpful in determining the client's limitations and can also provide the nurse with information about the client's insight into the problems. All initial data should be accurately recorded to provide a baseline for comparison to determine whether the client's condition is improving or deteriorating.

Interview data are as important as the actual physical assessment. Questions concerning medical history, intellectual abilities and educational level, and history of nervous system infections and trauma should be asked. Determination of the presence of seizures, syncope, pain, and headaches or other pain is important in planning care for the client.

Nursing diagnoses

The client with a brain tumor who has undergone a craniotomy requires complex postoperative care. The nursing diagnoses used for the unconscious client and the client with head injury may be appropriate for the client after craniotomy. Additional nursing diagnoses are presented in Table 52-15.

Nursing interventions

Acute intervention

BEHAVIORAL CHANGES. A primary or metastatic tumor of the frontal lobe can cause behavioral and personality changes. Loss of emotional control, confusion, disorientation, memory loss, and depression may be signs of a frontal lobe lesion. These behavioral changes are often not perceived by the client but can be very disturbing and even frightening to the family. These changes can also cause a distancing to occur between the family and the client. Assisting the family in understanding what is happening to the client and supporting the family through this diagnostic phase are very important roles for the nurse.

The confused client with behavioral instability can be a challenge. Protecting the client from self-harm is an important part of nursing care. At times when the client's behavior is manifested by rage and aggression, the nurse must also be concerned about self-protection. Close supervision of activity, use of side rails, judicious use of restraints, padding of the rails and the area around the bed, and a calm, reassuring approach to care are all essential techniques in the care of these clients.

Perceptual problems associated with frontal lobe and parietal lobe tumors contribute to a client's disorientation and confusion. Minimization of environmental stimuli, creation of a routine schedule, and use of reality orientation can be incorporated into the care plan for the confused client.

PHYSICAL CHANGES. Seizures frequently occur with brain tumors. These are managed with anticonvulsant drugs. Seizure precautions should be instituted for the protection of the client. Some behavioral changes seen in the client with a brain tumor are a result of seizure disorders and can improve with control of the seizures by means of drugs (see Chapter 54).

Motor and sensory dysfunctions are problems that interfere with the activities of daily living. Alterations in mobility must be managed, and the client needs to be encouraged to provide as much self-care as physically possible. Self-image often depends on the client's ability to participate in care within the limitations of the physical deficits.

Language deficits can also occur in clients with brain tumors. Motor (expressive) and/or sensory (receptive) dysphasias may occur. The disturbance in communication can be frustrating for the client and may interfere with the nurse's ability to meet the client's needs. Attempts should be made to establish a communication system that can be used both by the client and the staff.

Nutritional intake may be decreased because of the client's feeding inability, loss of appetite, or loss of desire to eat. Assessing the nutritional status of the client and ensuring adequate nutritional intake are important aspects of care. The client may need encouragement to eat or, in some cases, may have to be fed orally, parenterally, by nasogastric tube, or by total parenteral nutrition.

SURGICAL INTERVENTIONS. The general preoperative and postoperative nursing care for the client undergoing cranial surgery is similar, regardless of the cause. Table 52-16 lists indications for a craniotomy.

The client (if conscious and coherent) and the family will be gravely concerned about the potential physical and emotional problems that can result from surgery. The uncertainty regarding prognosis and outcome requires compassionate nursing care in the preoperative period.

Preoperative teaching is important in allaying the fears of the client and the family and also in preparing them for

Table 52-15

NURSING CARE PLAN FOR THE CLIENT WITH A CRANIOTOMY

Defining Characteristics	Nursing Interventions	Evaluation Criteria

NURSING DIAGNOSIS: Potential complication: increased ICP related to postoperative cerebral edema

Altered LOC, dysphagia, headache, pupil inequality, decreased respirations and pulse rate, elevated systolic blood pressure with widened pulse pressure, swelling around surgical site, elevation of bone flap	Establish baseline of neurological function immediately on client's return from operating room. Perform neurological checks every hour until the client stabilizes; then every 4 hr for at least 72 hr postoperatively. Report significant changes. Measure and record ICP every 1-4 hr. Maintain monitoring equipment in functioning condition. Provide aseptic care of insertion site. Protect equipment from being dislodged. Administer diuretics and corticosteroids as ordered. Position client with head of bed elevated to 30 degrees. Avoid neck and hip flexion. Prevent constipation and straining with defecation. Manage elevated temperature.* Use measures to decrease agitation and hyperactivity. Assess surgical site for signs of elevation of flap during dressing change.	No permanent decrease in neurological functioning

NURSING DIAGNOSIS: Ineffective breathing pattern related to decreased LOC, immobility, positioning, and impaired coughing

Change in pulse and respiratory rates from baseline, adventitious breath sound	Assess all respiratory parameters q 2 hr for 72 hr, then every 4-8 hr. Draw and evaluate ABGs regularly. Give oxygen by prongs or mechanical ventilator until ABGs are stable for at least 24-72 hr. Encourage gentle coughing and turning and position client on side with head slightly hyperextended if LOC is decreased. Suction client gently and for only brief periods if necessary. Hyperventilate and hyperoxygenate before and after each coughing or suctioning session. Observe for gastric distention; insert nasogastric tube if indicated and maintain patency. Report any consistent alterations in breathing patterns such as apnea or central neurogenic hyperventilation. Be aware of possible need for tracheotomy or endotracheal tube with artificial ventilation. Culture any abnormal secretions.	Patent airway, absence of rales or rhonchi, ABGs within normal limits; absence of respiratory distress or infection, normal breath sounds

NURSING DIAGNOSIS: Pain related to craniotomy, position, environmental stimuli, and ineffective pain or comfort measures

Report of headache; behaviors indicative of head pain such as shielding eyes, holding head, pained expression	Assess location, type, duration, degree, and severity of pain. Administer mild analgesics as ordered, and evaluate effects. Position as comfortably as possible, as for increased ICP. Keep environment quiet, darken room, put cool cloth on client's eyes.	Decrease in complaints of pain, ability to rest

NURSING DIAGNOSIS: Altered nutrition: less than body requirements related to inability to feed self, difficulty swallowing, and decreased LOC

Inability to feed self, decreased response to environment, coughing and choking when attempting to swallow, weight loss, poor skin turgor, abnormal electrolyte levels	Evaluate ability to swallow. Advance client to high-protein, high-caloric, small frequent feedings as tolerated. Feed client if necessary. If client is unable to eat, administer tube feedings every 3-4 hr or total parenteral nutrition as ordered.	Normal electrolyte level, absence of negative nitrogen balance or excessive weight loss

*See Table 52-19.

Continued.

Table 52-15

NURSING CARE PLAN FOR THE CLIENT WITH A CRANIOTOMY—cont'd

Defining Characteristics	Nursing Interventions	Evaluation Criteria
NURSING DIAGNOSIS: High risk for infection related to incision, drains, monitoring devices, and presence of environmental pathogens		
Fever, drainage, redness at tube sites and incision, multiple sites for pathogen entry	Use meticulous aseptic technique. Provide catheter and drain care according to institutional policy. Monitor vital signs and laboratory values. Maintain adequate nutritional and fluid intake.	Absence of signs of local or systemic infection
NURSING DIAGNOSIS: Potential complication: CSF leak from nose or ears related to surgical incision		
Clear or slightly yellow drainage from ears or nose	Assess for drainage from ears or nose. Test drainage for glucose, report to physician if positive. Carry out cultures of nose and throat. Do not plug nose or ears with cotton; use loose "snuffer" type of gauze dressing for comfort (change frequently). Watch for temperature elevation, irritability, headache, or nuchal rigidity and report immediately. Administer antibiotics if ordered.	Sealing of leak in 1-2 wk, absence of meningitis
NURSING DIAGNOSIS: Self-esteem disturbance related to physical appearance resulting from surgery		
Refusal to look at self or participate in self-care, crying or anger about appearance, social withdrawal	Encourage client to express feelings about appearance. Explain the rate of hair regrowth. Provide information about wigs or hairpieces if requested. Encourage the use of scarves in women and hats in men. Reassure client about self-worth.	Acceptance of the temporary nature of appearance, maintenance of normal activities
NURSING DIAGNOSIS: Self-care deficit (total) related to decreased LOC, weakness, or postoperative status		
Inability or unwillingness to perform activities of daily living	Provide for total self-care requirements of the client, including hygiene and skin care and tube feeding or total parenteral nutrition. Turn client at least q 2 hr. Maintain indwelling catheter patency, assess need for enema or suppository. Maintain range of motion of all joints. Provide oral hygiene q 2 hr. Keep client's eyes closed to prevent corneal damage.	Provision of all self-care needs
NURSING DIAGNOSIS: Sensory/perceptual alteration related to altered sensory reception, transmission, or integration secondary to neurological surgery		
Possible disorientation; altered sight, hearing, taste, or smell; decreased LOC	Assess client's ability to speak, see, hear, taste, and smell. Orient client to surroundings. Describe surroundings when sight is impaired. Eliminate extraneous noise. Provide stimulation for all senses.	Maintenance of highest possible level of contact with environment

the postoperative period. The client and the family should be given general information concerning the type of operation that will be performed and what can be expected immediately after the operation. Explaining that the client's hair will be shaved to allow for better exposure and prevention of contamination may prevent unnecessary concern over this task. The head is usually shaved in the operating room after induction of anesthesia. The family should also be informed that the client will be taken to an intensive care unit or to a special care unit after the operation.

The primary goal of care after a craniotomy is prevention of increased ICP (see Table 52-15). The turning and positioning of the client sometimes depends on the site of the operation. If the surgical approach is in the posterior fossa, the client is generally kept flat or at a slight eleva-

Table 52-16   Indications for Craniotomy

Indication	Cause	Manifestations	Procedure
Intracranial viral infection	Bacteria	Early findings: stiff neck, headache, fever, weakness, seizures; later findings: seizures, hemiplegia, speech disturbances, ocular disturbances, unconsciousness	Excision or drainage of abscess
Hydrocephalus	Overproduction of CSF, obstruction to flow, defective reabsorption	Early findings: mental changes, disturbances in gait; later findings: memory impairment, urinary incontinence, increased tendon reflexes	Placement of ventriculovenous, ventriculopleural, or ventriculoperitoneal shunt
Intracranial tumors	Benign or malignant cell growth	Change in LOC, pupillary changes, sensory or motor deficit, papilledema, seizures, personality changes	Excision or partial resection of tumor
Intracranial bleeding	Rupture of cerebral vessels due to trauma or cardiovascular accident	Epidural: momentary unconsciousness, lucid period, then rapid deterioration; subdural: headache, seizures; pupillary changes	Surgical evacuation through burr holes or craniotomy
Skull fractures	Trauma to skull	Headache, CSF leakage, cranial nerve deficit	Debridement of fragments and necrotic tissue, elevation and realignment of bone fragments
Arteriovenous malformation	Congenital tangle of arteries and veins (frequently in middle cerebral artery)	Headache, intracranial hemorrhage, seizures, mental deterioration	Excision or embolization of malformation
Aneurysm repair	Dilatation of weak area in arterial wall (usually near anterior portion of circle of Willis)	Before rupture: headache, lethargy, visual disturbance; after rupture: violent headache, decreased LOC, visual disturbances, motor deficit	Dissection and clipping of aneurysm

tion (10 to 15 degrees). Lying on the back will be prevented as much as possible, and flexion of the neck will be avoided to protect the suture line. The maximum swelling in the operative area occurs within 24 to 48 hours after the surgery.

With an incision over the skull in the anterior or middle fossae, the client returns from the operating room with the head elevated at an angle of 30 to 45 degrees. If a bone flap has been removed (craniectomy), care should be taken not to have the client positioned on the operative side.

The dressing should be observed for color, odor, and amount of drainage. The physician should be notified immediately of any excessive bleeding or clear drainage. Checking drains for placement and assessing the area around the dressing are also important.

Frequent assessment of the neurological status of the client is essential during the first 48 hours. Besides the neurological functions, fluids, electrolyte levels, and osmolality are monitored closely to detect changes in sodium regulation, the onset of diabetes insipidus, or severe hypovolemia.

The dressing is usually in place for 3 to 5 days. Scalp care should include meticulous care of the incision to prevent wound infection. The area should be cleansed with povidone-iodine (Betadine) or a similar antiseptic-disinfectant. Cleansing should be followed by application of an antibiotic ointment according to procedure. Once the dressing is removed, use of an antiseptic soap for washing the scalp may also be beneficial. The psychological impact of baldness can be alleviated by the use of a wig, turban, or cap after the incision has completely healed. For the client who is receiving radiation, use of a sunblock and head covering should be advocated if any exposure to the sun is planned.

Chronic management. The rehabilitative potential for a client after intracranial surgery depends on the reason for the surgery, the postoperative course, and the client's general state of health. Nursing interventions must be based on a realistic appraisal of these factors. An overall goal for the nurse is to foster independence for as long as possible and to the highest degree possible.

Specific rehabilitation potential cannot be determined

until cerebral edema and increased ICP subside postoperatively. Care must be taken to maintain as much function as possible through measures such as careful positioning, meticulous skin and mouth care, regular range-of-motion exercises, bowel and bladder care, and adequate nutrition.

Referrals may be made to other specialists on the health care team. For example, the speech therapist may be helpful to the client who has a speech problem. The needs and problems of each client should be addressed individually because many variables affect the plan.

Mental and emotional residual deficits are often more difficult for the client and the family to accept than motor and sensory losses. The nurse can provide much help and support during the adjustment phase and in long-range planning.

The mental and physical deterioration of the client, including seizures, personality disorganization, apathy, and wasting, is difficult for both family and health professionals to endure. Although progress is continuously being made to help the client with a brain tumor by means of chemotherapy, conventional and interstitial radiation, and biological response modifiers, the prognosis remains grim.

INFLAMMATORY CONDITIONS OF THE BRAIN

Meningitis, encephalitis, and brain abscesses are the most common inflammatory conditions of the brain and spinal cord. Inflammation can be caused by bacteria, viruses, fungi, and chemicals (e.g., contrast media used in diagnostic tests or blood in the subarachnoid space). CNS infections may enter from the bloodstream, by extension from a primary site, by extension along cranial and spinal nerves, and in utero. Bacterial infections are the most common, and the organisms usually involved are *Streptococcus pneumoniae, Haemophilus influenzae, Neisseria meningitides, Staphylococcus aureus,* and *Meningococcus* organisms. Bacterial meningitis carries the highest mortality and is considered a medical emergency.[21]

Meningitis

Pathophysiology. Meningitis is an acute inflammation of the pia mater and the arachnoid membrane surrounding the brain and the spinal cord. Therefore meningitis is always a cerebrospinal infection. The organisms usually gain entry to the CNS through the upper respiratory tract or bloodstream, but they may enter by direct extension from penetrating wounds of the skull or through fractured sinuses in basal skull fractures.

Meningitis usually occurs in the fall, winter, or early spring and is often secondary to viral respiratory disease. Children under 6 years of age, older adults, and persons who are debilitated are more often affected than the general population. *S. pneumoniae* causes about 30% of the cases.

The inflammatory response to the infection tends to increase CSF production, with a moderate increase in pressure. The purulent secretion produced quickly spreads to other areas of the brain through the CSF. If this process extends into the brain parenchyma or if a concurrent encephalitis is present, cerebral edema and increased ICP become more of a problem. All clients with meningitis must be observed closely for manifestations of increased ICP,

which are thought to be a result of swelling around the dura, increased CSF volume, and endotoxins produced by the bacteria.

Clinical manifestations. Fever, severe headache, and nuchal rigidity (resistance to flexion of the neck) are key signs of meningitis. Positive Kernig's sign and Brudzinski's sign (see Chapter 50), photophobia, a decreased LOC, and signs of increased ICP may also be present. Seizures occur in some cases. With meningitis the headache becomes progressively worse and may be accompanied by vomiting and irritability. If the infecting organism is *Meningococcus,* a skin rash is common and petechiae may be seen.

Complications. The most common complication of meningitis is residual neurological dysfunction. Cranial nerve dysfunction often occurs with cranial nerves III, IV, VI, VII, or VIII in bacterial meningitis. The dysfunction usually disappears within a few weeks. Hearing loss may be permanent after bacterial meningitis but is not a complication of viral meningitis.

Cranial nerve irritation can have serious sequelae. The optic nerve (CN II) is compressed by increased ICP. Papilledema is often present, and blindness may occur. When the oculomotor (CN III), trochlear (CN IV), and abducens (CN VI) nerves are irritated, ocular movements are affected. Ptosis, unequal pupils, and diplopia are common. Irritation of the trigeminal nerve (CN V) is evidenced by sensory losses and loss of the corneal reflex, and irritation of the facial nerve (CN VII) results in facial paresis. Irritation of the vestibulocochlear nerve (CN VIII) causes tinnitus, vertigo, and deafness.

Hemiparesis, dysphasia, and hemianopsia may also occur. These signs usually resolve over time. If resolution does not occur, it suggests a cerebral abscess, subdural empyema, subdural effusion, or a persistent meningitis. Acute cerebral edema may occur with bacterial meningitis, causing seizures, third nerve palsy, bradycardia, hypertensive coma, and death.

A noncommunicating hydrocephalus may occur if the exudate causes adhesions that prevent the normal flow of the CSF from the ventricles. CSF reabsorption by the arachnoid villi may also be obstructed by the exudate. Surgical implantation of a shunt is the only treatment.

A complication of meningococcal meningitis is the *Friderichsen-Waterhouse syndrome.* The syndrome is manifest by petechiae, disseminated intravascular coagulopathy, and adrenal hemorrhage.

Disseminated intravascular coagulopathy is a serious complication of meningitis (see Chapter 25). It is the cause of death in about 1% of clients with meningitis.

Diagnostic studies. A major diagnostic tool is examination of the CSF. Variations in the CSF depend on the causative organism. Protein levels in the CSF are usually elevated and are higher in bacterial than in viral cases. Decreased CSF glucose concentration is common to bacterial meningitis and may be normal in viral meningitis. The CSF is purulent and turbid in bacterial meningitis; it may be the same or clear in viral meningitis. The most predominant white blood cell (WBC) type in the CSF during inflammatory disorders of the brain is the polymorphonuclear (PMN) leukocyte (Table 52-17). Cultures of blood,

Table 52-17   Cerebral Inflammatory Conditions

Causative Organisms	CSF Pressure (60-150 mm H$_2$O)	CSF WBC Count (0-8/μl)	Protein* (15-45 mg/dl)	Glucose (45-75 mg/dl)	Appearance	Diagnostic Studies	Treatment
MENINGITIS							
Bacteria, yeasts, fungi, viruses, pneumococci, streptococci	Increased	500/μl (mainly PMN)	High	Low or absent	Turbid	Stained smears and cultures	Antibiotics with sensitivity tests
ENCEPHALITIS							
Bacteria, fungi, parasites, herpes simplex virus, other viruses	Normal to slight increase, increase with increased ICP	<500/μl, PMN (early), lymphocytes (later)	Slight increase	Normal	Clear	Viral studies	Supportive, prevention of symptoms of increased ICP, vidarabine (Vira-A)
BRAIN ABSCESS							
Streptococci, staphylococci through bloodstream	Increased	25-300/μl (PMN)	Normal	Low or absent	Clear	CT scan, EEG, skull x-ray film	Antibiotics, incision and drainage

*Lumbar.

sputum, and nasopharyngeal secretions are taken before the start of antibiotic therapy to identify the causative organism.

X-ray films of the skull may demonstrate infected sinuses. CT scans are usually normal in uncomplicated meningitis. In other cases, CT scans may reveal evidence of increased ICP or hydrocephalus.

Therapeutic management. Rapid diagnosis based on history and physical examination is crucial because the client is usually in a crisis state when health care is sought (Table 52-18). When meningitis is suspected, antibiotic therapy is instituted after the collection of specimens for cultures, even before the diagnosis is confirmed. Diagnostic measures include lumbar puncture and analysis of CSF. Eye grounds should be examined for papilledema before lumbar puncture for identification of possible increased ICP.

Penicillin and ampicillin are the drugs of choice. Chloramphenicol is used for persons who are allergic to penicillin. Nafcillin can be used for gram-negative organisms. These drugs are effective because of their ability to penetrate the blood-brain barrier.

▪ Nursing Management of Meningitis

Nursing interventions

Health promotion and maintenance. Prevention of respiratory infections through vaccination programs for pneumococcal pneumonia and influenza should be supported by nurses. In addition, early and vigorous treatment of respi-

Table 52-18

Therapeutic Management: Cerebral Inflammatory Problems

DIAGNOSTIC

History and physical examination
Analysis of CSF
CBC, electrocyte levels, glucose, prothrombin time, platelet count
Routine urinalysis
Blood cultures (twice)
Urine specific gravity (every 4 hr)
CT scan
EEG
Skull x-ray studies
Brain scan

THERAPEUTIC

Strict bed rest
IV fluids
Penicillin IV
Chloramphenicol IV
Codeine for headache
Aspirin for temperature above 38° C (100.4° F)
Hypothermia
Clear liquids as desired/tolerated
Phenytoin IV

Table 52-19

 NURSING CARE PLAN FOR THE FEBRILE CLIENT

Defining Characteristics	Nursing Interventions	Evaluation Criteria

NURSING DIAGNOSIS: Hyperthermia related to infection and abnormal temperature regulation by hypothalamus from increased ICP

Defining Characteristics	Nursing Interventions	Evaluation Criteria
Signs of infections or increased ICP, fever	Take client's temperature every 2-4 hr. Administer antipyretic drugs orally or rectally q 4 hr. Keep environment temperature at 21.1° C (70° F). Avoid heavy layers of clothing or bed covers. Give tepid sponge baths (half alcohol, half water). Use skin lotion to prevent drying. Change linen frequently if client is diaphoretic. Use hypothermia blanket. Reduce temperature gradually. Protect extremities with sheepskin or by wrapping in soft towels. Apply lotion frequently to entire body. Sedate if necessary to prevent chilling. Implement measures to treat causative disorder.	Core body temperature of 37.8° C (100° F), absence of damage to skin as result of antipyretic measures

NURSING DIAGNOSIS: High risk for fluid volume deficit related to increased metabolic rate, diaphoresis, and decreased oral intake

Defining Characteristics	Nursing Interventions	Evaluation Criteria
Rapid respirations; damp skin, clothing, and bed clothes; unwillingness or inability to ingest fluids; signs of dehydration such as dry lips and tongue, poor skin turgor, sunken eyes	Monitor fluid intake to 3-4 L/day if tolerated. Monitor vital signs every 2-4 hr. Administer IV fluids if necessary. Monitor intake and output accurately; give careful estimate of insensible losses. Assess client for dehydration.	Absence of signs of dehydration

NURSING DIAGNOSIS: Altered nutrition: less than body requirements related to increased caloric need secondary to increased metabolic rate and decreased oral intake

Defining Characteristics	Nursing Interventions	Evaluation Criteria
Decreased or absent food intake, weight loss	Weigh client daily. Give high-caloric, high-protein, easily digested food and fluids. Help client balance activity and rest.	Absence of weight loss

NURSING DIAGNOSIS: Sensory/perceptual alteration related to decreased LOC

Defining Characteristics	Nursing Interventions	Evaluation Criteria
Inaccurate interpretation of environment, signs of fear or anxiety, disorientation, restlessness, reports of auditory or visual hallucinations	Administer sedative medication as ordered. Keep room quiet; dim lights. Use calm, reassuring approach. Avoid use of restraints. Assist and support client during uncomfortable or frightening diagnostic procedures.	Minimal disorientation, lack of evidence of agitation

NURSING DIAGNOSIS: Pain related to headache, muscle and joint aches, and malaise secondary to pressure on nerves and presence of infectious exudate

Defining Characteristics	Nursing Interventions	Evaluation Criteria
General discomfort of head, joints, and muscles; apathy; grimacing on movement; reluctance to talk or move; noncompliance with treatment measures	Administer mild analgesia as needed. Assist client to position of comfort in bed. Encourage gentle range of motion and leg exercises. Massage muscles as needed. Control environment to encourage rest.	Expression of satisfaction with pain relief, increase in participation in treatment plan

NURSING DIAGNOSIS: Potential complication: seizure activity secondary to cerebral irritation

Defining Characteristics	Nursing Interventions	Evaluation Criteria
Generalized seizure activity	Protect client by keeping side rails up and padded. Administer sedative and anticonvulsant medications as ordered. Initiate vigorous nursing interventions to reduce fever.	Minimal or absence of seizure activity, lack of evidence of physical injury

ratory and ear infections is important. Persons who have close contact with anyone who has meningitis should be given prophylactic antibiotics.

Acute intervention. The client with meningitis is usually acutely ill. The fever is high and resistant to aspirin. Head pain is severe. Irritation of the cerebral cortex may result in seizures. The changes in mental status and LOC depend on the level of ICP.

Initial assessment should include vital signs, neurological evaluation, fluid intake and output, and evaluation of lung fields and skin. These should be reassessed at intervals based on the client's condition and recorded carefully.

Head pain and neck pain secondary to movement require attention. Codeine provides some pain relief without undue sedation for most clients. The client should be assisted to a position of comfort, often curled up with the head slightly extended. The head of the bed should be slightly elevated when permitted after lumbar puncture. A darkened room and a cool cloth over the eyes relieve the discomfort of photophobia.

For the delirious client, additional low lighting may be necessary to decrease hallucinations. All clients suffer some degree of mental distortion and hypersensitivity and may be frightened and misinterpret the environment. Every attempt should be made to minimize environmental stimuli and the resulting exaggerated perception. Restraints should be avoided. Padded side rails with sheets tied to the four corners to keep the client from getting out of bed may be used to prevent injury. Arm boards secured with multiple layers of stretch gauze (e.g., Kerlix) protects the IV infusion site. A familiar person at the bedside has a calming effect. The nurse needs to be efficient with care but also to project an attitude of caring and of unhurried gentleness. The use of touch and a soothing voice to give simple explanations of activities is helpful. If seizures occur, appropriate observations should be made and protective measures should be taken. Anticonvulsant medications are administered as ordered. Problems associated with increased ICP are also managed (see p. 1531).

Fever must be vigorously managed because of its effect of increasing cerebral edema and seizures (Table 52-19). In addition, neurological damage may result from an extremely high temperature over a prolonged time. Aspirin should be administered because it is useful in reducing fever and its antiinflammatory effects are therapeutic. However, if the fever is resistant to aspirin, more vigorous means are necessary. The automatic cooling blanket is the most efficient. Care should be taken to not reduce the temperature too rapidly because shivering may result, causing a rebound effect and increasing the temperature. The extremities should be wrapped in sheepskin, soft towels, or a blanket covered with a sheet to protect them from "frostbite." Skin care should be given frequently to prevent breakdown. If a cooling blanket is not available or desirable, tepid sponge baths with water may be effective in lowering the temperature. The skin needs to be protected from excessive drying or injury.

Because high fever greatly increases the metabolic rate and thus insensible fluid loss, the client should be assessed for dehydration and adequacy of intake. Diaphoresis fur-

ther increases fluid losses, which should be estimated and included in an intake and output record. Replacement fluids should be calculated as 800 ml for respiratory losses and 100 ml for each degree of temperature above 38° C (100.4° F). The designated antibiotic schedule must be followed to maintain therapeutic blood levels. Observations should be made for side effects of the drugs used.

With the exception of meningococcal meningitis, meningitis usually no longer requires isolation. However, good aseptic technique is essential to protect the client and the nurse.

Chronic management. After the acute period has passed, the client requires several weeks of convalescence before normal activities can be resumed. In this period, good nutrition should be stressed, with an emphasis on a high-protein, high-caloric diet in small, frequent feedings.

Muscle rigidity may persist in the neck and the back of the legs. Progressive range-of-motion exercises and warm baths are useful. Activity should be gradually increased as tolerated, but adequate bed rest and sleep should be encouraged. Quiet activities that are based on an assessment of individual interests should be encouraged to prevent boredom.

Residual effects are uncommon in meningococcal meningitis, but pneumococcal meningitis can result in sequelae such as dementia, epilepsy, deafness, hemiplegia, and hydrocephalus. Vision, hearing, cognitive skills, and motor and sensory abilities should be assessed after recovery, with appropriate referrals as indicated. Meningitis in infancy may have "silent" neurological sequelae, which are manifest as learning and behavior problems when the child reaches school age.

Throughout the acute and convalescent periods the nurse should be aware of the anxiety and stress experienced by the client's significant others. Meningitis is generally considered a serious and usually fatal illness by the general public. The family needs to be supported and involved in care as much as possible.

Encephalitis

Encephalitis is an acute inflammation of the brain and is usually caused by a virus. Many different viruses have been implicated in encephalitis, some of them associated with certain seasons of the year and endemic to certain geographical areas. Epidemic encephalitis is transmitted by ticks and mosquitoes. Nonepidemic encephalitis may occur as a complication of measles, chickenpox, or mumps.

Encephalitis is a serious, sometimes fatal disease. Mortality ranges from 5% to 20%, with the highest fatality in encephalitis caused by herpes simplex and eastern and Venezuelan equine viruses. Manifestations resemble those of meningitis, but they have a more gradual onset. They include headache, high fever, convulsions, and change in LOC. Therapeutic and nursing management is symptomatic and supportive. Cerebral edema is a major problem, and hypertonic solutions and steroids are used to control it. The disease is characterized by diffuse damage to the nerve cells of the brain, perivascular cellular infiltration, proliferation of glia, and increasing cerebral edema. The

sequelae of encephalitis include mental deterioration, amnesia, personality changes, and hemiparesis.

Vidarabine suspension (Vira-A) is used in the treatment of herpes simplex encephalitis. It has been shown to reduce mortality from 70% to 28%, although neurological complications may not be reduced. For maximal benefit, the medication must be started before the onset of coma. The potential toxicity of vidarabine requires that nurses be knowledgeable about the method of administration and the side effects. Acyclovir is also used for the treatment of herpes simplex encephalitis. It has fewer side effects than vidarabine and is often the preferred treatment.

Brain Abscess

Brain abscess is an accumulation of pus within the brain tissue that can result from a local or systemic infection (Fig. 52-15). Direct extension from ear, tooth, mastoid, or sinus infection is the primary cause. Other sites for abscess formation include septic venous thrombosis from pulmonary infection, bacterial endocarditis, skull fracture, and an unsterile neurological procedure. Streptococci and staphylococci are the primary infective organisms.

Manifestations are similar to those of meningitis and encephalitis and include headache and fever. Signs of increased ICP may include drowsiness, confusion, and seizures. Focal symptoms may be present and reflect the local area of the abscess. For example, visual field defects or psychomotor seizures are common with temporal lobe abscess, whereas occipital abscess may be accompanied by visual impairment and hallucinations.

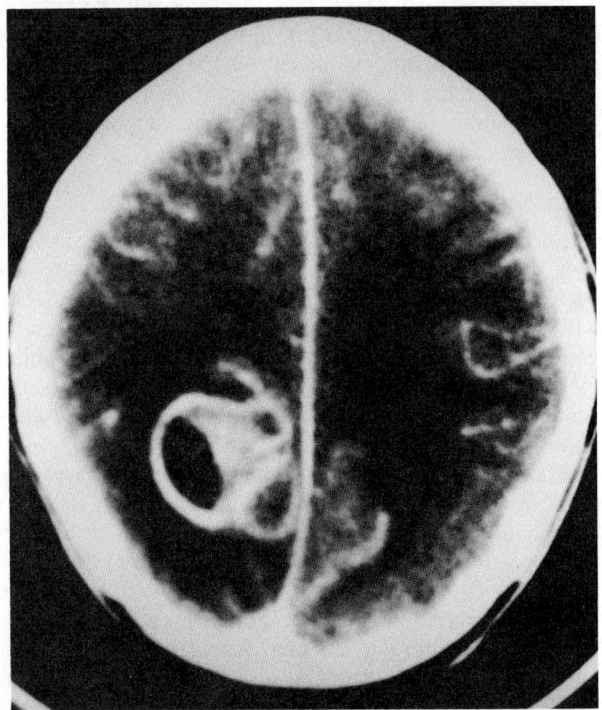

Fig. 52-15 CT scan showing brain abscess. (From Marshal SB and others: Neuroscience critical care, Philadelphia, 1990, WB Saunders Co, p 269.)

Antimicrobial therapy is the primary treatment for brain abscess. Other manifestations are treated symptomatically. If pharmacological management is not effective, the abscess may need to be drained or removed if it is encapsulated. In untreated cases, mortality approaches 100%. Epilepsy occurs in approximately 30% of the cases. Nursing measures parallel those for meningitis or for increased ICP.

Other infections of the brain include subdural empyema, osteomyelitis of the cranial bones, epidural abscess, and venous sinus thrombosis after periorbital cellulitis.

Human Immunodeficiency Virus

The impact of the human immunodeficiency virus (HIV) infection of the brain is just beginning to be identified. An estimated 10% of persons who have acquired immunodeficiency syndrome (AIDS) have neurological complaints as their first symptoms, and another 40% eventually have significant neurological problems.[22] Complications of HIV infection include the AIDS-dementia complex, also known as *subacute HIV encephalopathy*, primary lymphoma, and toxoplasmosis.

The AIDS-dementia complex is characterized by diffuse, progressive changes in personality, memory loss, clumsiness, and incontinence. The major therapeutic interventions include zidovudine (AZT), psychotherapy, and psychotropic drugs.

Primary lymphoma is seen as multiple lesions with a rapid onset of symptoms. Seizures are common in clients with these lesions. The therapeutic management of the lymphoma includes radiation therapy and chemotherapy. Anticonvulsants are used to manage seizures.

Opportunistic infections accompany HIV infection. In the brain, toxoplasmosis is an opportunistic infection. Generally, the client has a rapid onset of symptoms similar to those of a brain abscess. Treatment is symptomatic but may also include drugs such as pyrimethamine (Daraprim), sulfadiazine (Mierosulfan), and clindamycin (Cleocin). Other infections identified in clients with AIDS include cytomegalovirus, papovavirus, and cryptococcal meningitis. (HIV infections are discussed in Chapter 8.)

C ase Study

HEAD INJURY

Thomas M. is a 44-year-old man who was admitted to the intensive care unit yesterday with a diagnosis of possible concussion as a result of a motor vehicle accident. Information from the ambulance attendant suggests that the client may have fallen asleep while driving home, run off the road, and hit a telephone pole. He was unconscious briefly after the accident but was alert on admission, although he did not remember what had happened to him or why he was at the hospital. During morning report, the staff reported that he had become very agitated and verbally and physically abusive and that the staff had to resort to the use of full leather restraints. His wife went home in tears, distressed by his aggressive behavior. As he became increasingly noisy, IV diazepam was ordered. The nurse reported early the next morning that he was "nice and quiet," with vital signs and laboratory test findings within normal

limits. Neurological assessments were not done because the staff did not want to wake him.

Now that the client is being assessed at 8 AM, it is noted that he cannot be aroused except by painful stimuli. Observation shows Cheyne-Stokes respirations, and during the apneic phase, he assumes decorticate posture. His pupils are small (4 mm) but reactive. The Babinski sign is positive. Blood pressure is 150/62; pulse rate is 60 beats per minute.

Discussion Questions

1. What could have been the cause of Mr. M's combative behavior?
2. Analyze the management he received in the first 12 hours. What, if anything, should have been done differently?
3. What were the causative factors in his change of status by the morning?
4. What do the signs and symptoms suggest for Mr. M.'s area of brain involvement?
5. On the basis of the nursing assessment, what are the priority interventions?
6. What could be said to Mrs. M. about her husband's condition? What additional data might be elicited from her?

R eview Questions

The number of the question corresponds to the same-numbered objective at the beginning of the chapter.

1. Unconsciousness always indicates
   a. inability to respond to external stimuli
   b. easy return to the alert state
   c. unawareness of self or environment
   d. a common underlying cause
2. The basic mechanism of unconsciousness is interference between the cerebral hemispheres and the
   a. pons
   b. RAS
   c. medulla
   d. autonomic nervous system
3. Appropriate nursing management for the unconscious client with a problem related to airway obstruction includes all of the following *except*
   a. suction as needed
   b. keep in side-lying position
   c. use oral airway up to 48 hr
   d. hyperextend the neck
4. Clinically significant increased ICP is defined as
   a. any pressure elevation over 15 mm Hg
   b. sustained pressure of 50 mm Hg for at least 2 hours
   c. transient pressure over 100 mm Hg during a sneeze
   d. sustained pressure of 100 mm Hg for more than 15 minutes
5. Which of the following compensatory mechanisms is physiologically useful in alleviating pressure changes within the cranial cavity?
   a. herniation of the temporal lobes through the tentorial notch
   b. displacement of CSF into the spinal subarachnoid space

   c. decreased absorption of CSF by the venous system
   d. expansion of the venous system
6. Which of the following admitting medical orders might be written for a client with proven or suspected increased ICP?
   a. ambulation every 4 hours
   b. IV administration of 5% dextrose in water at 150 ml/hr
   c. use of hyperthermia blanket and temperature at 36° C (96.8° F)
   d. meperidine hydrochloride, 100 mg as needed for pain
7. At the lower pontine–upper medullary level, which of the following abnormal signs is most often noted?
   a. high blood pressure with wide pulse pressure
   b. decorticate posture
   c. pinpoint, reactive pupils
   d. neurogenic hyperventilation
8. The best position for the client with increased ICP is
   a. increase of head-of-bed angle to 30 degrees, with client lying on back or side and without neck or hip flexion
   b. supine position with bed flat, head turned to left
   c. high Fowler's position with knee flexion and elevation of legs
   d. increase of head-of-bed angle to 30 degrees, with client lying on side with hips and knees flexed
9. Shock waves are strongly transmitted to the brain through the skull in which of the following types of direct head injury?
   a. depressed fracture (open)
   b. linear fracture (open)
   c. closed
   d. penetrating
10. The main general focus of treatment for the client with head injury is
    a. prevention or management of increased ICP
    b. prevention of future head injuries
    c. prevention of infection
    d. surgery
11. The combination treatment of choice for brain tumors that cannot be totally removed surgically includes all the following *except*
    a. radiation
    b. chemotherapy
    c. cryosurgery
    d. steroids
12. Effective management of negative behavioral manifestations resulting from an intracranial tumor should focus on
    a. teaching of the client's spouse or significant other assertive behavior
    b. isolation for the safety of the client and of others
    c. explanations to the client how disturbing the behavior is to others

    d. assistance for family members in handling their feelings

13. Nursing care for the client after a craniotomy includes
    a. frequent neurological assessments, maintenance of the client flat in bed for 48 hours, and limited IV fluids progressing to oral feedings
    b. ICP measurements, ambulation as soon as tolerated, and suctioning every 2 hours
    c. neurological checks, change of head dressing every 4 hours, and gentle pulmonary toilet
    d. frequent neurological checks, elevation of head of bed to 30 degrees, and avoidance of neck and hip flexion

14. The three key signs and symptoms that are primary clues to meningitis are
    a. severe headache, fever (39° C, 102° F), nuchal rigidity
    b. general irritability, nausea and vomiting, fever 39° C (102° F)
    c. severe headache, fever (37.2° C to 37.8° C, 99° F to 100° F), anorexia
    d. nuchal rigidity, normal temperature, lassitude

15. The most critical assessments for the nurse to perform for the client with a cerebral inflammatory problem include
    a. pain, neurological checks, GI functions
    b. neurological checks, seizures, breath sounds
    c. pain, seizures, skin check
    d. neurological checks, breath sounds, skin check

REFERENCES

1. Plum F and Posner JB: Diagnosis of stupor and coma, ed 3, Philadelphia, 1980, FH Davis Co.
2. Drummond BL: Preventing increased intracranial pressure: nursing can make a difference, Focus Crit Care 17:116, 1990.
3. Jennett B and Teasdale G: Aspects of coma after severe head injury, Lancet 23:878, 1977.
4. Fishman RA: Cerebrospinal fluid in diseases of the nervous system, Philadelphia, 1980, WB Saunders Co.
5. Mitchell PH: Decreased behavioral arousal. In Mitchell PH and others, eds: AANN's neuroscience nursing, Norwalk, Conn, 1988, Appleton & Lange, p 76.
6. Prough DS and Roger AT: Physiology and pharmacology of cerebral blood flow and metabolism, Crit Care Clin (Neurol Crit Care) 5:713, 1989.
7. Thurel C, Ragguena JL, and Habib AA: Cerebral edema. In Tinker J and Rapin M, eds: Care of the critically ill patient, New York, 1983, Springer-Verlag, pp 741-743.
8. Pfenninger EG and others: Early changes of intracranial pressure, perfusion pressure, and blood flow after acute head injury, J Neurosurg 70:774, 1989.
9. Marshal SB and others: Neuroscience critical care: pathophysiology and patient management, Philadelphia, 1990, WB Saunders Co, p 193.
10. Rogers AT and Stump DA: Cerebral physiologic monitoring, Crit Care Clin (Neurol Crit Care) 4:849, 1989.
11. Dearden NM and others: Effect of high dose dexamethasone on outcome from severe head injury, J Neurosurg 64:81, 1986.
12. Marshal SB and others: Neuroscience critical care: pathophysiology and patient management, Philadelphia, 1990, WB Saunders Co, pp 199-200.
13. Raeburn D and Gonzales RA: CNS disorders and calcium antagonists, Trends Pharmacol Sci 9:117, 1988.
14. Zegeer LS: Oculocephalic and vestibulo-ocular responses: significance for nursing care, J Neurosci Nurs 21:46, 1989.
15. Smith RN: Intervention alternative: nervous system. In Hudak CM and others: Critical care nursing: a holistic approach, Philadelphia, 1990, JB Lippincott Co, p 545.
16. Ward JD: Axioms on head injury, Hosp MD 20:15, 1984.
17. Gennarelli TA and others: Mortality of patients with head injury and extracranial injury treated in trauma centers, J Trauma 29:1193, 1989.
18. McGinnis GS: Central nervous system. I. Head injuries. In Cardona VC and others, eds: Trauma nursing: from resuscitation through rehabilitation, Philadelphia, 1988, WB Saunders Co, p 397.
19. Hickey J: The clinical practice of neurological and neurosurgical nursing, ed 2, Philadelphia, 1986, JB Lippincott Co, p 254.
20. Marshal SB and others: Neuroscience critical care: pathophysiology and patient management, Philadelphia, 1990, WB Saunders Co, pp 477-478.
21. Sapien GM and others: Pediatric nursing care, St Louis, 1990, Mosby–Year Book, Inc, p 417.
22. Scherer P: How AIDS attacks the brain, Am J Nurs 90:46, 1990.

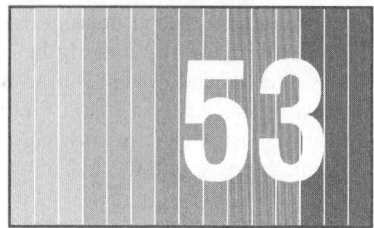

53

Nursing Role in Management
Stroke Client

Christina M. Mumma

---

earning Objectives

1. *Describe the incidence and risk factors of stroke.*
2. *Explain the mechanisms that affect cerebral blood flow.*
3. *Describe the atherosclerotic process.*
4. *Compare and contrast the pathophysiology of strokes caused by thrombosis, embolism, and intracranial hemorrhage.*
5. *Correlate the clinical manifestations of stroke with the underlying pathophysiology.*

6. *Describe diagnostic study abnormalities commonly found in stroke.*
7. *Describe the therapeutic, pharmacological, and dietary management of the stroke client.*
8. *Describe the acute nursing management of the stroke client.*
9. *Describe the rehabilitative nursing management of the stroke client.*
10. *Explain the psychosocial impact of a stroke on clients and their families.*

A *cerebrovascular accident* (CVA or stroke) is the abrupt or rapid onset of a neurological deficit resulting from disease of the blood vessels that supply the brain.[1] The term *stroke* is used to describe an event that can be caused by a number of different pathological processes.[2] For most persons who suffer strokes, the stroke seems to "just happen" without warning. However, a warning sign or symptom may have occurred and gone unrecognized.

Regardless of the cause, the parts of the brain damaged by the loss of blood supply can no longer perform their specific cognitive, sensory, motor, or emotional functions. The resulting impairments can be slight or severe and temporary or permanent.

SIGNIFICANCE

Stroke is ranked third among all causes of death in the United States, exceeded only by heart disease and cancer. A 30% decrease in the incidence of stroke has occurred during the past 20 years. However, stroke continues to be a major public health problem in terms of both mortality

---

Reviewed by Virginia Printz-Fedderson, R.N.C., C.N.R.N., M.S.N., Education Nurse Specialist, Lovelace Medical Center, Albuquerque, New Mexico.

and permanent disability. An estimated 500,000 first strokes occur each year, of which one fourth to one third are fatal. Stroke is often considered a disease of the older adult because approximately 60% to 75% of all strokes occur in persons over 65 years of age. About 40% of those who survive a stroke are left with moderate to severe disability and require assistance with activities of daily living.[3,4]

Stroke has significant economic effects on clients and families and on the total economy. The combined direct and indirect costs of stroke are estimated to be greater than $14 billion per year in the United States.[5] The heavy toll in terms of human suffering and disruption of lives must also be considered, although this figure is not calculable in economic terms. The need for continued improvement in the control of risk factors and the prevention of stroke is critical.

RISK FACTORS

Considerable research has been conducted to determine the risk factors most closely associated with stroke. These factors may be divided into two categories: (1) nonreversible and (2) potentially reversible. Risk of stroke increases for persons with more than one of the risk factors.

The nonreversible risk factors include gender, age,

race, and heredity. The overall incidence of stroke is higher for men than for women. The risk of stroke is markedly increased with advancing age. Blacks are more likely than whites to have a stroke, probably because they have a higher incidence of hypertension. There is sometimes a hereditary pattern to the occurrence of strokes, although the inherited factor or factors are not clear.

The risk factors that are potentially reversible include hypertension, cardiac disease, diabetes mellitus, blood lipid abnormalities, and certain lifestyle habits. The most important risk factor associated with stroke is hypertension. Available evidence suggests that treatment of hypertension is the only significant contributor to the prevention of stroke.[2] The evidence of a link between stroke and the other potentially reversible risk factors has been inconclusive. There is general agreement about the increased risk of stroke associated with cardiac disease and diabetes mellitus. There is, however, little agreement about the effects of the other potentially alterable risk factors on stroke proneness. Most of the lifestyle risk factors associated with coronary artery disease are much less clearly linked to stroke (see Chapter 28). These risk factors include obesity, cigarette smoking, alcohol use, and a diet high in saturated fats and cholesterol.

Excessive intake of alcohol may indirectly increase the risk of stroke because of the association between alcohol use and hypertension. Cigarette smoking may also indirectly affect stroke risk because of the association between cigarette smoking and coronary heart disease. Obesity may contribute to risk of stroke because of the higher blood pressure associated with it. There is no conclusive evidence of higher risk of stroke due to dietary intake of fats, inactivity, salt intake, or stress. Research shows, however, that there may be an increased risk of stroke among women who use oral contraceptives.[2]

PATHOPHYSIOLOGY
Regulation of Cerebral Blood Flow

Because the neurons of the brain do not have regenerative capabilities, the prevention of cerebral damage is important. For adequate cerebral functioning, blood flow must be maintained at 750 to 1000 ml/min, which is one fifth of the cardiac output. If this blood flow is interrupted, as in a stroke, neuronal metabolism is altered in 30 seconds, metabolism ceases in 2 minutes, and cellular death occurs in 5 minutes. Once the neuron is dead, its function is lost unless another part of the brain can be trained to take over the lost function.

The cerebrovascular system is very adaptive. It maintains a constant blood flow to the brain in spite of marked changes in the systemic circulation. The factors that affect cerebral blood flow can be divided into extracranial and intracranial factors.

Extracranial factors. The extracranial factors are primarily related to the circulatory system. They include (1) systemic blood pressure, (2) cardiac output, and (3) viscosity of the blood. During activities of daily living there are marked variations in local oxygen requirements. Alterations in cardiac output, vasomotor tone, and distribution of blood flow are effective in maintaining constant cerebral

perfusion. The mean arterial blood pressure has to fall below 70 mm Hg or rise above 160 mm Hg before the cerebral blood flow is altered, and cardiac output has to be reduced by one third before cerebral blood flow is reduced. Changes in blood viscosity increase or decrease cerebral blood flow. Anemia increases flow, and polycythemia reduces it.

Intracranial factors

Metabolic factors. Metabolic alterations are important intracranial factors involved in the regulation of cerebral blood flow. Metabolic factors that result in vasodilatation with restoration of blood flow toward normal include high carbon dioxide concentration and low oxygen tension. Carbon dioxide, however, is the most potent regulator of cerebral blood flow. An increase in hydrogen ion concentration also increases cerebral blood flow. Alone or in combination, these metabolic factors can maintain adequate cerebral blood flow in normal situations.

Blood vessels. The condition of the blood vessels supplying the brain also influences the cerebral blood flow (see Chapter 50). Many persons have congenital anomalies in the cerebrovascular system. These anomalies include tortuosity, coiling, kinking, and arteriovenous malformations. These congenital anomalies may interfere with cerebral blood flow and are common sites for the development of atherosclerotic diseases. Atherosclerosis from any cause increases resistance in the blood vessels and further reduces blood flow.

Collateral circulation is another factor related to cerebral blood flow. Collateral circulation develops in response to a decrease in normal blood flow. The circle of Willis contains many collateral circulatory connections and is responsible for the greater part of collateral circulation.

Collateral vessels should maintain cerebral blood flow in the event of damage to the main blood supply. However, they cannot always do so. Individual differences in the state of the collateral circulation when a stroke occurs are the factors that determine whether major loss of function results.

Intracranial pressure. Intracranial pressure (ICP) is another factor that influences cerebral blood flow (see Chapter 52). Among the causes of increased ICP are stroke, neoplasms, trauma, and hydrocephalus. Increased ICP compresses the brain and reduces cerebral blood flow. Greatly reduced cerebral blood flow may result in cerebral infarction.

Both extracranial and intracranial factors may be involved in a stroke. The initial insult may be related to one or more of these factors. For example, when an intracranial hemorrhage occurs, the continuity of the vascular system is interrupted. The lost blood and the edema secondary to the inflammatory process cause an increase in ICP. This interferes with cerebral perfusion, and carbon dioxide and hydrogen ion concentration increase, leading to a further increase in ICP.

ATHEROSCLEROSIS

Atherosclerosis, a common pathophysiological process in stroke (see Chapter 28), is usually involved in the development of a thrombosis and is often implicated in

strokes caused by emboli. (The role that atherosclerosis plays in the development of thrombosis and emboli is shown in Fig. 28-4.) Initially, an abnormal infiltration of lipids occurs in the intima of the arteries. This fatty streak may develop into an atherosclerotic plaque. These plaques often develop where there is increased turbulence in the blood, as at the bifurcation of an artery or a tortuous area (Fig. 53-1). Turbulence may later damage the atherosclerotic plaque, resulting in a loss of intimal continuity or ulceration. Platelets and fibrin aggregate on the roughened surface. Parts of the plaque may break off and travel to a narrower distal artery. Cerebral infarction occurs at the point where the blood supply is cut off.

Types

Strokes may be classified as either ischemic or hemorrhagic on the basis of their underlying pathophysiology (Table 53-1). Ischemic strokes result from a decreased blood flow to the brain secondary to partial or complete occlusion of an artery. They occur much more frequently than hemorrhagic strokes. The most common types of ischemic stroke are thrombotic and embolic. Hemorrhagic strokes are generally the result of spontaneous bleeding into the brain tissue itself (intracerebral or intraparenchymal hemorrhage) or into the subarachnoid space and/or the ventricles (subarachnoid hemorrhage).

Thrombosis. Thrombosis is the formation of a blood clot or coagulum that results in the narrowing of the lumen of a blood vessel with eventual occlusion. It is the most common cause of cerebral infarction. Two thirds of the strokes due to thrombosis are associated with hypertension or diabetes, both of which are conditions that accelerate the atherosclerotic process. Thrombosis may be preceded by prodromal warnings, such as paresthesias (abnormal sensations), paresis (decreased strength and motility of an extremity), and aphasia (disturbance of language function). These transient periods of neurological deficit called

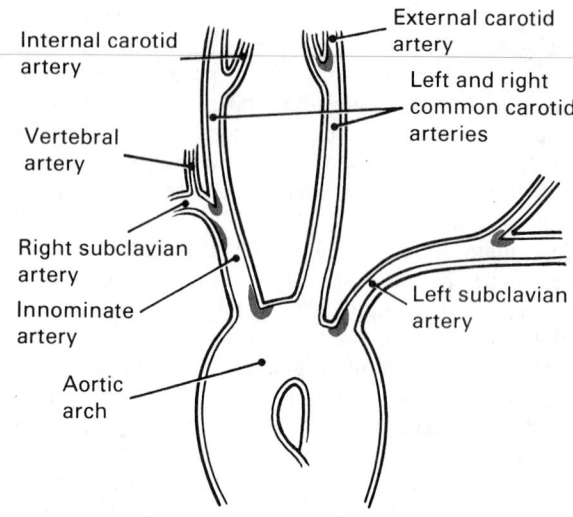

Fig. 53-1 Common sites for the development of atherosclerosis in extracranial and intracranial arteries. The main locations are just above the common carotid bifurcation (most common site) and the start of the branches from the aorta, innominate, and subclavian arteries.

Table 53-1 Types of Stroke

Type	Gender/Age	Warning	Time of Onset	Course/Prognosis
ISCHEMIC				
Thrombotic	Men more than women, oldest median age	TIA (30%-50% of cases)	During or after sleep	Stepwise progression, some improvement (usual), recurrence in 20%-25% of survivors
Embolic	Men more than women	TIA (uncommon)	Lack of relationship to activity, sudden onset	Single event, some improvement (usual), recurrence common without aggressive treatment of underlying disease
HEMORRHAGIC				
Intracerebral	Slightly higher in women	Headache (25% of cases)	Activity (often)	Progression over 24 hr; poor, fatality more likely with presence of coma
Subarachnoid	Slightly higher in women, youngest median age	Headache (common)	Activity (often), very sudden onset	Single sudden event (usual), fatality more likely with presence of coma

(handwritten annotation: Tia - w/sign headache)

transient ischemic attacks (TIAs) can signal a developing lesion.

A stroke caused by thrombosis usually occurs during or after a period of repose or sleep. It is characterized by intermittency or erratic progression of signs and symptoms. The resultant ischemia leads to edema and congestion of the affected area. The manifestations usually peak within 72 hours and are often secondary to the developing edema. The degree of involvement depends on the rapidity of onset, the size of the lesion, and the presence of collateral circulation. As edema subsides, some improvement is usually apparent within 2 weeks. In most cases, maximal improvement is attained in 12 to 24 weeks, although some clients continue to show improvement as long as 2 years after the stroke.

Embolism. Cerebral embolism is the occlusion of a cerebral artery by an embolus, resulting in necrosis and edema of the area supplied by the involved blood vessel. Embolism is the second most common cause of stroke. The majority of emboli originate in the endocardial (inside) layer of the heart, with plaques or tissue breaking off from the endocardium and entering the circulation. The embolus lodges at the point where an artery becomes too narrow for it to pass and causes ischemic infarction. Cardiac diseases or situations that contribute to the development of emboli include chronic atrial fibrillation, myocardial infarction, valvular disease, valve replacements, rheumatic heart disease, and infective bacterial endocarditis. Atherosclerotic plaques in the extracranial arteries are a second source of emboli. The emboli from the heart or extracranial arteries usually travel up through the carotid system and lodge in the middle cerebral artery or in one of its branches. Emboli are increasingly being implicated in TIAs.

The clinical picture of an embolic stroke is more varied than that of a thrombotic stroke. It can affect any age group. An embolic stroke secondary to rheumatic heart disease may involve young to middle-aged adults. An embolus arising from an atherosclerotic plaque is more common in older adults. A prodromal warning is less common than with thrombosis. The onset of the stroke is usually sudden and unrelated to activity. The client usually maintains consciousness, although a headache may develop on the side where the embolus is lodged. Prognosis is related to the amount of brain tissue deprived of its blood supply. For example, if the embolus lodges in the main stem of the middle cerebral artery, most of the lateral cerebral hemisphere suffers ischemic damage and the prognosis is poor. More frequently, however, the embolus breaks apart, sending smaller particles to lodge downstream in smaller branches of the arterial tree. This phenomenon accounts for the marked improvement frequently seen after embolic stroke. However, recurrence of embolic stroke is common unless the underlying cause is aggressively treated.

Intracerebral hemorrhage. Intracerebral hemorrhage, or bleeding into the brain tissue itself, can occur spontaneously in clients with hypertension or atherosclerosis of the intracranial blood vessels. These conditions cause degenerative changes in the walls of the arteries, resulting in rupture and subsequent hemorrhage. As a result of this type of hemorrhage, the escaping blood creates a mass that compresses and displaces the brain. In a large hemorrhage, herniation of the brain tissue may occur, usually resulting in coma and death. The prognosis for survival is worse for hemorrhagic than for ischemic strokes. Mortality rates as high as 50% to 60% have been reported for intracerebral hemorrhage. The outlook has improved with the increased use of computerized tomography (CT) scanning with resultant earlier diagnosis and more definitive treatment. The prognosis for survival and recovery is related to the extent and location of the hemorrhage.

Subarachnoid hemorrhage. A subarachnoid hemorrhage due to the rupture of an intracranial aneurysm may occur after trauma or physical exertion but usually happens during normal daily activities. Approximately one third of subarachnoid hemorrhages occur during sleep. The first symptom is usually a sudden severe headache. Loss of consciousness may occur and is associated with a poor prognosis for recovery. Unlike other types of stroke, a massive subarachnoid hemorrhage may cause sudden death. Signs of meningeal irritation, such as nuchal rigidity and Kernig's and Brudzinski's signs, are usually present. Fever is common. Focal signs, such as hemiparesis or aphasia, may not be seen.

Initially a clot forms at the site of a ruptured aneurysm. As the clot begins to dissolve and vasospasm subsides, the chance of renewed bleeding increases. Reduced activity and the prevention of straining are critical parts of the management of a ruptured aneurysm to decrease the possibility of clot disruption.

Temporal Development

Recent work has been done by the National Institute of Neurological Disorders and Stroke on the classification of cerebrovascular diseases. The classification of the temporal development of CVAs includes TIA, reversible ischemic neurological deficit, stroke in evolution or progressing stroke, and completed stroke (stable stroke).[2] Knowledge of this classification is useful in planning nursing care.

Transient ischemic attack. A TIA is a brief episode of neurological deficit that passes without apparent residual effects. The deficits usually last less than 30 minutes but may last for up to 24 hours. There is no sign of permanent neurological deficit between attacks. Of persons who have one TIA, about one third will have no further TIAs, about one third will have more than one TIA and not have a completed stroke, and about one third will eventually have a completed stroke.[2,6] A widely held hypothesis is that TIAs are caused by microemboli breaking off from atherosclerotic plaques in the extracranial arteries and temporarily interrupting cerebral oxygenation.[7] Although embolic occurrence is most common, a TIA may be caused by decreased cerebral blood flow.[8] A TIA is considered a warning signal and is usually a sign of advanced atherosclerotic disease of cerebral arterial supply. A client with symptoms of TIA needs to seek medical care promptly.

A TIA must be differentiated from other causes of cerebral ischemia, such as a developing subdural hematoma or an increasing tumor mass. Cardiac monitoring and tests of-

ten reveal an underlying cardiac condition that is responsible for the clot formation. Medications that prevent platelet aggregation—aspirin, dipyridamole (Persantine)—as well as anticoagulant medications may be prescribed for long-term therapy after a TIA.

The signs and symptoms vary according to the part of the brain affected. The anatomical location of the neurological deficit can be identified on the basis of clinical manifestations. If the carotid system is involved, the client may report a temporary loss of vision in one eye, a transient hemiparesis, or a sudden inability to speak. Common symptoms of TIA related to vertebral-basilar insufficiency are tinnitus, vertigo, darkened or blurred vision, diplopia, ptosis, dysarthria, dysphagia, and unilateral or bilateral numbness or weakness.

Reversible ischemic neurological deficit. The term *reversible ischemic neurological deficit* is sometimes used if the neurological deficit remains after 24 hours but leaves no residual signs or symptoms after days to weeks. This is considered by some to be a completed stroke with minimal to no residual deficit.

Stroke in evolution. A stroke in evolution, or a progressing stroke, develops over a period of hours or days. This pattern of progression is most characteristic of an enlarging intraarterial thrombus. A stepwise or intermittent progression of deteriorating neurological findings is common. However, any stroke may have a gradual progression of manifestations for up to 72 hours after the infarct. The progression of manifestations correlates with the degree of edema secondary to the inflammatory process.

Completed stroke. When the neurological deficit remains unchanged over a 2- to 3-day period, the stroke is called a *completed stroke* (stable stroke). An embolic stroke may demonstrate this characteristic from the onset. With the exception of stroke secondary to a ruptured aneurysm, a completed stroke signals readiness for more aggressive rehabilitative treatment. If a ruptured aneurysm is the suspected cause, activity may be restricted for as long as 3 to 4 weeks to reduce the possibility of additional hemorrhage.

CLINICAL MANIFESTATIONS

The concept of stroke evokes a common mental picture. However, this picture varies markedly from client to client. The manifestations of stroke depend on (1) the anatomical site of the lesion, (2) the rate of onset, (3) the size of the lesion, and (4) the presence of collateral circulation. Table 53-2 lists symptoms seen when specific cerebral arteries are involved, regardless of whether the CVA is due to thrombosis, embolus, or hemorrhage. The physical disabilities are usually easy to identify. The language and spatial-perceptual problems are more subtle and difficult to recognize; consequently, these problems are often ignored or misunderstood. Figure 53-2 illustrates the manifestations of right-sided and left-sided stroke.

Neuromotor

Motor deficits are the most obvious manifestations of stroke. These symptoms are caused by the destruction of motor neurons in the pyramidal pathway. This destruction

can result in the loss of skilled voluntary movements (akinesia), impairment of integration of movements, and alterations in muscle tone and reflex activity. The hyporeflexia that initially occurs with the stroke progresses to hyperreflexia for most clients.

These losses follow characteristic patterns. Because the pyramidal pathway decussates at the lower end of the medulla, a stroke in the right hemisphere of the brain causes paralysis of the left side. The upper and lower extremities of the involved side may be affected to different degrees, depending on the part of the cerebral circulation that was compromised. The middle cerebral artery distribution is the most common site for cortical strokes, leading to greater weakness in the upper extremity than in the lower extremity. The shoulder tends to rotate internally and the hip rotates externally. The foot is plantar flexed and inverted. A period of flaccidity (hypotonia) may last for a few days to several weeks. Flaccidity is usually followed by spasticity (hypertonia). During the spastic stage the deep tendon reflexes are exaggerated. The Babinski reflex is present.

Problems with motor control may affect nutrition and respiration as well as mobility. In addition to experiencing difficulty with self-feeding, the client may have impairment of swallowing (dysphagia) because of weakness of the mouth and throat muscles. The swallow reflex may also be diminished or absent. This problem is generally more severe with a brainstem stroke (bulbar dysphagia), but it may also be seen with a cortical stroke (pseudobulbar dysphagia). The client may be unable to swallow secretions and consequently is susceptible to aspiration pneumonia.

Problems related to the motor control of elimination are more complex. Fortunately, such problems are usually transient. When the stroke is confined to one hemisphere, the prognosis for return to normal bladder function is excellent. The reflex arc remains intact, a partial sensation of bladder filling remains, and the client maintains partial voluntary control over urination.[2] Initially, the client may experience frequency, urgency, and incontinence. Bladder training is facilitated if started immediately. Since a retention catheter may interfere with this process, it should be used only during the most acute period of the stroke if absolutely necessary. Motor control of the bowel is usually not a problem. However, the client is prone to constipation. This is attributed to immobility, weakened abdominal muscles, decreased oral intake, inability to communicate the need to defecate, and lack of response to the defecation reflex.

Communication

The left hemisphere is dominant for language in all right-handed and in the majority of left-handed persons. When the stroke occurs in the dominant hemisphere, the client may experience communication difficulties, or *aphasia*.[9] Language disorders involve the expression and the comprehension of written or spoken words. When the lesion involves Wernicke's area of the brain, the client experiences *receptive* aphasia; neither the sounds of speech nor its meaning can be distinguished, and comprehension of

Table 53-2   Clinical Manifestations Related to Specific Cerebral Artery Involvement

MIDDLE CEREBRAL ARTERY INVOLVEMENT

Blockage of main stem
  Contralateral paralysis
  Contralateral anesthesia: loss of proprioception, fine touch, localization
  Aphasia of dominant side
  Nondominant side: neglect of opposite side, dysmetria
  Homonymous hemianopsia, conjugate-gaze paralysis

ANTERIOR CEREBRAL ARTERY INVOLVEMENT

Occlusion of stem*
Occlusion distal to anterior communicating artery
  Contralateral sensory and motor deficits of leg and foot
  Contralateral weakness of proximal upper extremity
  Urinary incontinence (possibly unrecognized by client)
  Contralateral grasp and sucking reflexes
  Apraxia
  Possible cognitive impairment
  Distractibility

POSTERIOR CEREBRAL ARTERY INVOLVEMENT†

Anterior and proximal occlusion
  Thalamogeniculate branch occlusion (thalamic syndrome, Dejerine-Roussy syndrome)
    Contralateral sensory loss: deep and cutaneous with varying degrees (e.g., greater pain and temperature loss than touch or position sense, or the reverse, or presence of loss in only part of body)
    Temporary hemiparesis
    Homonymous hemianopsia
    Thalamic pain: later with recovery; unpleasant, diffuse, contralateral; occurrence or response after stimulus; possible depression and distortion of taste
  Paramedian branch occlusion: central midbrain and subthalamus
    Weber's syndrome: oculomotor palsy with contralateral paralysis
    Stupor or coma
    Possible contralateral ataxic tremor
Cortical occlusion
  Branches to temporal and occipital lobes
  Possible incomplete homonymous hemianopsia, usually in upper fields
  Dominant hemisphere
    Dyslexia, dyscalculia (inability to perform mathematical calculations)
    Anomia: most severe for colors
    Moderate recent memory deficit
  Nondominant hemisphere
    Topographical disorientation (surroundings)
    Anomia: faces
Upper basilar artery occlusion (bilateral)
  Eye deficits
    Bilateral homonymous hemianopsia
    Total blindness (cortical)
    Central vision loss
    Paracentral vision loss
    Visual hallucinations
    Apraxia of ocular movement
  Possible severe memory loss
  Inability to count or name objects

---

*There is usually no problem if the stem is occluded near the anterior communicating artery because perfusion from the opposite side is maintained.
†The site of occlusion, the origin of the basilar arteries, and the arrangement of the circle of Willis are involved in the type of deficit seen. This can occur from a thrombus or embolus.
‡If both vessels are of adequate size and there is contralateral blood flow, there may be no visible deficit.

VERTEBRAL ARTERY INVOLVEMENT‡

Blockage of lateral medulla (involvement of one or more arteries—most frequent in occurrence)
   Contralateral decrease in pain, temperature sense
   Ipsilateral Horner's syndrome: miosis, ptosis, decreased sweating
   Hoarseness
   Dysphagia
   Ipsilateral paralysis of palate and vocal cord
   Nystagmus, diplopia, oscillopsia, vertigo, nausea, vomiting
   Ipsilateral ataxia of limbs: falling or toppling to ipsilateral side
   Loss of taste
Posterior medulla block
   Ipsilateral cerebellar ataxia
Posteroinferior cerebellar artery occlusion: sudden vertigo, nausea, vomiting, ataxia, nystagmus

BASILAR ARTERY INVOLVEMENT

General
   Bilateral motor and sensory deficits of all extremities
   Diplopia
   Nystagmus
   Blindness or lesser degree of visual impairment
   Ataxia
   Coma
Branches
   Superior cerebellar
      Severe ipsilateral cerebellar ataxia
      Nausea and vomiting
      Slurred speech
      Contralateral loss of pain and temperature, including face
      Partial deafness
      Ipsilateral Horner's syndrome
   Anterior inferior cerebellar
      Ipsilateral deafness
      Vertigo, nausea, vomiting
      Nystagmus
      Tinnitus
      Cerebellar ataxia
      Ipsilateral Horner's syndrome
      Conjugate lateral-gaze paralysis
      Contralateral pain and temperature loss
      Hemiplegia (dependent on location of infarction)

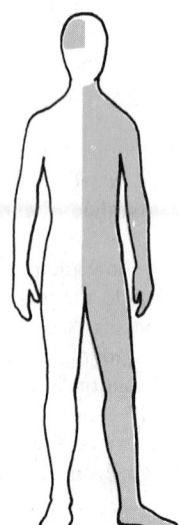

Right brain damage:
- Paralyzed left side
- Spatial-perceptual deficits
- Behavioral style: quick, impulsive
- Memory deficits: performance
- Indifference to the disability

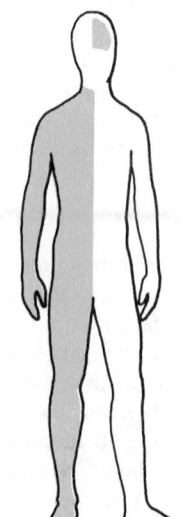

Left brain damage:
- Paralyzed right side
- Speech-language deficits (if left brain dominant)
- Behavioral style: slow, cautious
- Memory deficits: language
- Distress and depression in relation to the disability

Fig. 53-2   Manifestations of right-sided and left-sided stroke.

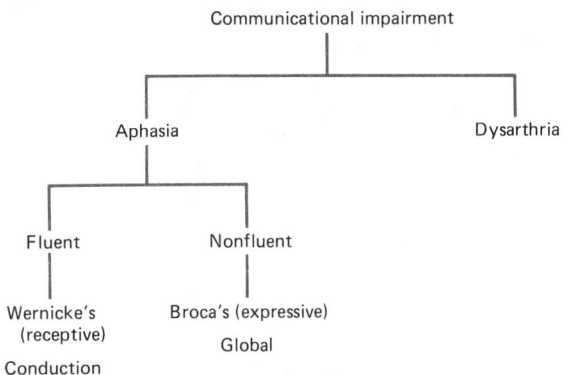

Fig. 53-3 Types of communicational impairment common after stroke.

both written and spoken language is impaired. The lesion causing *expressive* aphasia affects Broca's area, the motor area for speech. This client has difficulty in speaking and writing. Aphasias may be classified as either nonfluent or fluent (Fig. 53-3). In *nonfluent* aphasia the client speaks very little and produces speech slowly and with obvious effort. In *fluent* aphasia the client may speak, but the phrases have little meaning because of impaired comprehension. Conduction aphasia is a type of fluent aphasia in which the lesion is in the pathway between Broca's and Wernicke's areas. Most aphasias are mixed, with some impairment of both expression and understanding. A massive lesion may result in *global* aphasia, in which virtually all language function is lost.

Another communication problem that many stroke clients experience is *dysarthria*, or slurred speech. Dysarthria results from a disturbance in muscular control and produces impairment of pronunciation, articulation, and phonation. Dysarthria does not result in any disturbance of language function itself. However, an occasional stroke client may be unfortunate enough to have both aphasia and dysarthria.

Affective

Clients with a stroke may demonstrate loss of control of their emotions. Their emotional responses may be exaggerated or unpredictable. This is compounded by the depression experienced with the change in body image and the frustration related to communication problems. It may be difficult to tell whether the client is crying because of emotional lability or depression.

Intellectual

Both memory and judgment may be impaired in a client who has had a stroke. These impairments are experienced in right- and left-sided lesions. A left-sided lesion is more likely to result in memory problems related to language; a right-sided lesion usually causes problems related to spatial-perceptual content. The client with a left-sided lesion tends to be overly cautious in matters of judgment. In contrast, the client with a right-sided lesion may be quick and impulsive. Both may experience difficulty in making generalizations, which interferes with the ability to learn.

Spatial-Perceptual

A stroke in the right hemisphere is more likely to cause deficits in spatial-perceptual orientation, although they can occur with damage to the left hemisphere as well. These spatial-perceptual deficits may be divided into four categories. The first relates to the client's erroneous perception of self and illness. This deficit follows lesions of the parietal lobe. Clients may deny their illnesses or their own body parts. The second category concerns the client's erroneous perception of self in space. The client may neglect all input from the affected side. This may be compounded by homonymous hemianopsia, in which blindness occurs in the corresponding halves of the visual fields of both eyes. In addition, the client has difficulty with spatial orientation such as judgment of distances. The third spatial-perceptual deficit is agnosia, the inability to recognize an object by sight, touch, or hearing. The fourth deficit is apraxia, the inability to carry out learned sequential movements on command.

DIAGNOSTIC STUDIES

After a stroke, various diagnostic studies are carried out in an effort to determine the cause of the stroke and as a basis for decisions about therapeutic and/or surgical treatment (Table 53-3). A CT scan is the primary diagnostic test used after a stroke. It can indicate the size and location of the lesion. CT testing is also useful in differentiating between infarction and hemorrhage. Serial CT scans are often used to determine the effectiveness of treatment and to evaluate the course of healing.

Certain neurodiagnostic tests such as skull x-ray studies, brain scan, lumbar puncture, and electroencephalogram (EEG) that were formerly used in the diagnosis of stroke are currently used much less. Although the skull x-ray study is usually normal after a stroke, there may be a pineal shift with a massive infarction. A brain scan shows increased uptake of radioactive media in infarction.

Although not performed routinely, a lumbar puncture may show a transient increase in leukocytes in the cerebrospinal fluid (CSF). The presence of blood in the CSF is indicative but not diagnostic of hemorrhage. A lumbar puncture is usually not done in the presence of increased ICP because of the danger of herniation from a sudden decrease in pressure. An EEG may show low-voltage, slow waves in ischemic infarction. If hemorrhage is the cause of the stroke, the EEG may show high-voltage slow waves. Arteriography can demonstrate areas of cervical and cerebrovascular occlusion, atherosclerotic plaques, and malformation of vessels. If the suspected cause of the stroke includes emboli from the heart, cardiac diagnostic tests should be done (Table 53-3).

Newer diagnostic tests used in some medical centers to aid in the diagnosis of stroke include magnetic resonance imaging (MRI), positron emission transaxial tomography (PETT), and digital subtraction angiography (DSA). MRI uses a magnetic field instead of radiation to produce a picture of the brain that is superficially similar to that of a CT scan. MRI is considered by some to be the best imaging method to differentiate hemorrhagic from nonhemorrhagic infarcts. The use of MRI in the diagnosis of stroke is expected to increase in the future. PETT shows the chemical

Table 53-3 Diagnostic Tests for Suspected Cerebrovascular Accident

Distinction between CVA and nonvascular causes of acute neurological deficit (e.g., tumor, encephalitis, subdural hematoma)
    Radionuclide scan (brain scan)
    CT scan
    EEG
    CSF*
    Angiography
Distinction between cerebral hemorrhage and infarction
    CT scan
    Magnetic resonance imaging
    CSF*
    Angiography
Distinction between superficial and deep cerebral infarction
    CT scan
    EEG
Evaluation of etiology of CVA
    Carotid circulation
    Carotid Doppler
    Carotid ultrasonic scan
    Carotid angiography (evaluation for carotid endarterectomy or extracranial-intracranial bypass)
    Cardiac assessment
    Electrocardiogram
    Cardiac enzymes
    Echocardiography
    Holter monitor (evaluation for dysrhythmias)

*For CSF testing, a lumbar puncture is avoided if elevation of ICP is suspected.

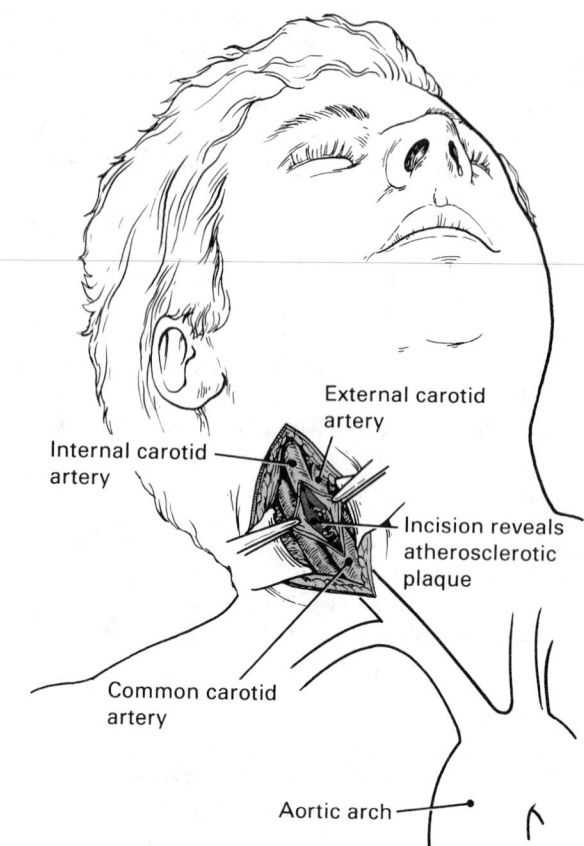

Fig. 53-4 Carotid endarterectomy. The atherosclerotic plaque in the internal carotid artery is removed to prevent impending cerebral infarction.

activity of the brain and provides an excellent depiction of the extent of tissue damage after a stroke. Less active or diseased tissue appears darker than healthy, active cells. Major research efforts are aimed at perfecting this technique to aid in the diagnosis and treatment of brain disease.[2]

DSA involves the intravenous (IV) or arterial injection of a contrast agent to produce good visualization of neck vessels and the large vessels of the circle of Willis. Intraarterial injection of contrast material has almost completely replaced IV DSA because the arterial approach requires a smaller bolus of contrast fluid and produces superior results.[2] It is considered safer than cerebral angiography because less vascular manipulation is required. However, conventional intraarterial angiography is still needed for examination of intracranial arteries. Because angiography is potentially dangerous as a result of the possibility of dislodging an embolus or of causing vasospasm or further hemorrhage, it is used only when no other safer test can provide the needed information.

THERAPEUTIC MANAGEMENT
Prevention

Once a stroke has occurred, the impact of therapeutic management is limited. The priority of therapy is therefore prevention—both the prevention of infarction in the client with a TIA and the prevention of recurrence in the client

who has had a stroke. Clients with known risk factors, such as diabetes, hypertension, or cardiac dysfunction, should be followed closely. Measures designed to prevent the development of a thrombus or embolus are used. For men, the administration of aspirin (ASA) or dipyridamole (Persantine) has decreased the incidence of stroke. However, these antiplatelet aggregants have been of questionable benefit in the treatment of women, although the reason for this is not known. Anticoagulants are also used for clients with TIAs, although the possibility of hemorrhage must be considered.

The most common surgical procedures used to reduce the frequency of TIAs and the danger of impending stroke are endarterectomy and extracranial-intracranial (EC-IC) bypass. Both are designed to maintain cerebral blood flow, and both must be performed before an infarction occurs or the hazards outweigh the benefits. An endarterectomy is used to remove an atherosclerotic plaque that is obstructing an extracranial artery and reducing blood flow to the brain. The most common sites of atherosclerotic plaque development are the regions of the common carotid bifurcation and the arch of the aorta. During the procedure the arteries are clamped above and below the plaque. An incision slightly larger than the plaque is made, and the plaque is removed. During this period the brain receives blood through the vertebral-basilar system and the other internal carotid artery (Fig. 53-4). If these blood vessels also have

a compromised blood flow as a result of atherosclerosis, a temporary shunt may be placed. This decision is based on EEG readings and cerebral blood flow measurements. A patch graft is sewed in to close the artery, or the artery is closed primarily. The blood pressure during surgery is maintained above 170 mm Hg to maintain critical perfusion pressure.

EC-IC bypass is used for intracranial problems when the obstruction cannot be removed directly. Although there are a number of variations, the procedure usually involves anastomosing a branch of an extracranial artery to an intracranial artery just beyond the obstruction. Branches of the middle cerebral artery are most commonly used. A burr hole is drilled in the skull and is used to connect the extracranial artery to the involved intracranial artery. In this way an intracranial occlusion is bypassed.

Acute Management

The focus of therapeutic management of the stroke client is (1) the preservation of life, (2) the prevention of additional brain damage, and (3) the lessening of disability. The diagnostic tests used to determine the cause of the

stroke are the same for all types of stroke; the treatment differs according to type of stroke and whether the aim of treatment is prevention, management during the acute phase, or long-term rehabilitation (Table 53-4).

The first goal of therapeutic management is to maintain a patent airway, which may be compromised because of a decreased consciousness. Interventions to accomplish this goal must be initiated at the scene of the stroke to prevent cerebral anoxia and permanent brain damage. Table 53-5 outlines key aspects of prehospital care of the stroke client. Oxygen, an artificial airway, or possibly intubation and mechanical ventilation may be indicated.

The client is monitored closely for signs of increasing neurological deficit. Therapeutic, surgical, and pharmacological interventions may be appropriate, depending on the reason for the increasing deficit.

Because of cerebral edema, the fluid and electrolyte balance must be carefully controlled. Initially, the client retains fluids because of the stress response (increased antidiuretic hormone and aldosterone). Inappropriate secre-

---

Table 53-4

 Therapeutic Management: Stroke

PREVENTION

Thrombotic stroke
  Control of hypertension
  Control of diabetes mellitus
Embolic stroke of cardiogenic origin
  Anticoagulation therapy for clients with atrial fibrillation
  Treatment of underlying condition
Intracerebral hemorrhage
  Control of hypertension
Surgical intervention for clients with aneurysms at risk of bleeding

TREATMENT IN ACUTE PHASE

Thrombotic TIAs
  Anticoagulation
  Antiplatelet aggregation
  Endarterectomy
  EC-IC bypass
Progressing stroke (strokes in evolution)
  Anticoagulation
Completed stroke with mixed neurological deficit
  Treatment of brain edema
Embolic stroke of cardiogenic origin
  Treatment of underlying cause
Intracerebral hemorrhage
  Treatment of brain edema, surgical decompression, if indicated
Subarachnoid hemorrhage
  Surgical extirpation (dependent on size and location of hemorrhage)

Table 53-5

 Prehospital Emergency Care of the Client with a Stroke*

Etiology: Sudden vascular compromise causing disruption of blood flow to the brain, which can be caused by thrombosis, trauma, aneurysm, embolism, or hemorrhage

CLINICAL MANIFESTATIONS

Alteration in level of consciousness
Weakness, numbness, paralysis of portion of body
Speech or visual disturbances
Severe headaches
Increased pulse rate
Flushed or pale face
Respiratory distress
Unequal pupil activity
Drooping of facial features on affected side, difficulty in swallowing
Seizures
Loss of bowel and bladder control
Nausea and vomiting

MANAGEMENT

Assess for patent airway.
Position client with head elevated to decrease ICP.
Assess and monitor neurological and vital signs; monitor cardiac rhythm.
Remove all dentures and bridges.
Keep client warm and quiet.
Start IV line with large gauge needle.
Administer oxygen.
Take seizure precautions.
Assess for any precipitating events.

---

*See Chapter 59 for a general discussion of measures related to prehospital emergency care.

tion of antidiuretic hormone may occur. This may be partially offset by the client's inability to drink or by highly concentrated tube feedings. All factors must be considered before fluids are ordered.

The physician usually tries to keep the client slightly dehydrated yet provide enough fluids to prevent capillary sludging. Adequate fluid intake during the acute phase is usually 1000 ml/day. When the period of acute stress is over, the fluid requirements increase as diuresis starts. Fluid requirements may be met with an additional 1000 ml of 5% dextrose in water per day. If the client is unable to eat within 5 to 7 days, parenteral hyperalimentation or tube feedings are instituted.

Three therapeutic approaches have been used with varying success to prevent additional brain damage. The first and most effective is the use of measures designed to reduce cerebral edema, which interferes with metabolism of the viable cells. Although a temporary phenomenon, this interference may result in the death of additional cells or even of the person. Dehydrating agents, such as mannitol, glycerol, or urea, may be employed. These hyperosmotic agents tend to draw fluid from the interstitial spaces into the vascular system. Corticosteroids are also used to reduce cerebral edema. The second approach used to prevent additional brain damage involves measures designed to reduce the metabolic needs of the brain. Hypothermia and barbiturate therapy are among the treatments that have been attempted for this purpose, although neither has proved effective. The third therapeutic approach is designed to promote cerebral blood flow. Vasodilators, hypertensive agents (treatment to increase blood pressure), and hyperventilation therapy have all been attempted but have been of little proven value.[7]

When a cerebral hemorrhage is the result of rupture of an aneurysm, surgical intervention may be appropriate. Early surgery to decrease the danger of rebleeding and to facilitate management of vasospasm has become more widely accepted.[10] Clips may be placed on either side of the aneurysm. The aneurysm may be wrapped or reinforced with muscle.

If the client's condition or the location of the aneurysm indicates that internal repair is inadvisable, external repair may be attempted. This involves clamping of the common carotid artery, a procedure that requires perfusion of the affected hemisphere by circulation from the opposite side. The adequacy of this circulation is determined by angiogram and isotope blood flow studies.

Chronic Management

After the stroke has stabilized for 12 to 24 hours, therapeutic management shifts from the preservation of life to the lessening of disability. At this point the client may be evaluated by a physiatrist—a physician who specializes in physical medicine and rehabilitation. Depending on the available resources and the client's estimated rehabilitation potential, the physiatrist may recommend that the client be transferred to a rehabilitation unit. Other possible approaches may be (1) to initiate various rehabilitation treatments in the acute-care setting, (2) to have the client participate in rehabilitation therapy on an outpatient basis, or

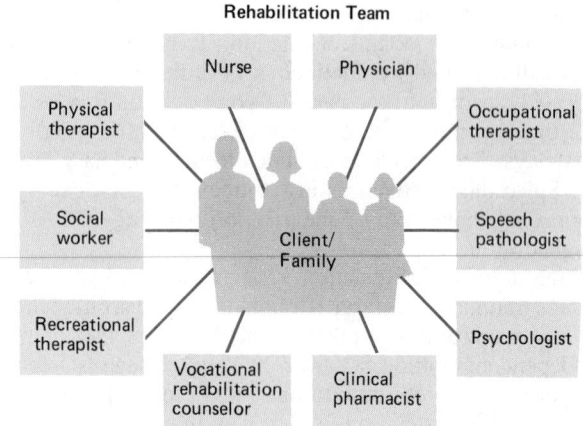

Fig. 53-5 Representative membership of the rehabilitation team.

(3) to set up a home care rehabilitation program in which therapists treat the client in the client's home.

As part of the long-term therapeutic management after a stroke, various members of the health care team may be involved in the effort to return the client to optimal functioning. The exact composition of the team depends on the needs of the client and the resources of the involved institution (Fig. 53-5).

PHARMACOLOGICAL MANAGEMENT
Hyperosmotic Agents

When the cerebral edema accompanying a stroke threatens to cause herniation, a dehydrating agent is used. IV mannitol is the drug of choice. This hyperosmotic agent reduces the ICP caused by edema. It must be used with caution in clients with renal dysfunction because the increased circulatory volume may compromise damaged kidneys. Side effects of mannitol include fever, angina, pulmonary congestion, headache, and blurred vision.

Urea and glycerol may also be used as hyperosmotic agents. However, urea has a rebound effect that may eventually increase the ICP. Glycerol is metabolized into sugar and cannot be used for clients with diabetes. These drugs are not used as often as mannitol. With any of these agents, the nurse must carefully monitor intake and output, body weight, electrolytes, and serum osmolality. The client can become dehydrated.

Corticosteroids

Dexamethasone (Decadron) is also used to treat the client with a stroke. When this drug is used, the initial dose is tapered over a period of 7 to 10 days. Dexamethasone acts as an antiinflammatory agent to break the cycle of increasing ICP by reducing the inflammatory reaction. Although commonly used, its benefit in the treatment of stroke is questionable. Additional research is needed.

Anticoagulants

Heparin is used as an anticoagulant in the treatment of TIAs, thrombotic strokes, and strokes in evolution. It exerts its effect by the activation of plasma antithrombin and

the subsequent inactivation of thrombin. Heparin is used as the first step in anticoagulation. It is most effective when administered by continuous IV infusion at a rate of 1000 U/hour or until the partial thromboplastin time is 1½ to 2 times normal. The duration of treatment is usually 7 to 10 days. Complications include bleeding and easy bruising. Since its effectiveness in the treatment of stroke syndromes is controversial, the risk of bleeding has to be weighed in terms of benefits.

Long-term anticoagulation is accomplished by the oral administration of warfarin (Coumadin, Panwarfin), which inhibits prothrombin synthesis and decreases the vitamin K–dependent clotting factors. The usual dosage is 5 to 10 mg per day. A prothrombin time of 1½ to 2 times normal is desirable. The duration of treatment in stroke syndromes is 3 to 6 months. Excessive bleeding is the primary complication. (Table 32-17 lists the nursing implications related to anticoagulant therapy and client education.)

A client taking warfarin on a long-term basis needs to know the following:

1. Signs of anticoagulant overdosage
2. Drugs with which warfarin interacts
3. Rationale for avoiding modifications in diet
4. Importance of avoiding trauma
5. Importance of a Medic-Alert bracelet
6. Need for routine blood testing

Platelet Aggregation Inhibitors

Platelet aggregation inhibitors, which interfere with platelet function, are used in the management of TIAs and symptoms of progressing stroke. Aspirin and dipyridamole are two such agents.

Acetylsalicylic acid (aspirin, ASA) is used in men to prevent platelet aggregation at the site of an atherosclerotic plaque. The dosage of 320 mg qid or 640 mg bid is administered orally. The complications of gastrointestinal (GI) bleeding may be reduced by administering the aspirin with meals. Aspirin is contraindicated in clients with peptic ulcer disease and must be used with caution when anticoagulants are also being taken. The duration of treatment is indefinite.

Dipyridamole (Persantine) also inhibits platelet aggregation. It is used alone or with aspirin in the treatment of TIAs. It is administered orally in doses of 50 to 75 mg qid (or tid with aspirin). Complications include nausea and vomiting, which can be managed by administration of the drug with meals. Duration of treatment is indefinite.

NUTRITIONAL CONSIDERATIONS

After the acute phase, the dietitian can assist in determining the appropriate daily caloric intake based on the client's overall size, weight, and activity level. Residual physical problems (e.g., paralysis of the dominant arm) and psychosocial problems (e.g., depression) must also be considered in relation to a nutritional plan.

If the client is unable to take in an adequate diet orally, tube feeding may be initiated, usually by the nasogastric route. Most commercially prepared formulas provide about 100 cal/100 ml. Sustagen, Isocal, and Ensure are examples of complete nutritional formulas. The latter two are also low in lactose and residue. Because tube feedings tend to be hyperosmotic, they may dehydrate the client. If a quantity is given at one time, it needs to be preceded and followed by water. Cramping and diarrhea are common side effects of tube feedings. These can usually be controlled by administration of small, frequent, less concentrated feedings at room temperature. It may also be helpful to use a formula that contains fiber (e.g., Enrich). (Tube feedings are discussed in Chapter 35.)

Although the client may experience diarrhea from the tube feedings, more commonly the client who has had a stroke tends to be constipated. The following dietary measures aid in the prevention of constipation:

1. Fluid intake of 2500 to 3000 ml daily unless contraindicated
2. Prune juice, 120 ml, or stewed prunes daily
3. Cooked fruit three times daily
4. Cooked vegetables three times daily
5. Whole-grain cereal or bread three to five times daily

In combination with a regular schedule, privacy, a footstool to increase abdominal pressure, and exercise, these dietary measures are very effective in preventing constipation.

■ Nursing Management of Stroke

Nursing assessment

Subjective and objective data that should be obtained about a person who has had a stroke are presented in Table 53-6. The subjective data include examples of questions asked of the client or persons who are familiar with the client. These questions help the nurse to determine the client's experience of the stroke from the client's personal perspective. The objective data include specific physical assessment findings commonly associated with stroke (e.g., hemiparesis, dysphagia, aphasia).

Nursing diagnoses

Nursing diagnoses are determined when the problem and the etiological factors are supported by clinical data. Nursing diagnoses related to stroke may include, but are not limited to, those presented in Table 53-7.

Nursing interventions

Health promotion and maintenance. To reduce the incidence of stroke, the nurse needs to focus teaching efforts toward stroke prevention for persons with known risk (e.g., clients with TIAs, hypertension, or diabetes mellitus). The significance of other potentially reversible risk factors for the occurrence of stroke is unclear. However, control of risk factors implicated in coronary artery disease may indirectly help to prevent stroke. (For the nurse's role in management of these risk factors see Chapter 28.) In any health care setting and for the population as a whole, nurses can play a major role in the promotion of a healthy lifestyle. An overall program to prevent events such as stroke includes the recognition that people are responsible to some degree for their own health and for the health of future generations.

Acute intervention

RESPIRATORY PROBLEMS. During the acute phase of a stroke the nursing priority is management of respiratory function. Stroke clients are particularly vulnerable to respiratory

problems. Advancing age and immobility make them particularly susceptible to atelectasis. With dysphagia or coma, aspiration pneumonia may develop. In coma the tongue tends to fall back and obstruct the airway. This problem requires that the client be positioned in a side-lying position.

An oropharyngeal airway may be used during the first 24 to 48 hours. This airway holds the tongue in place, preventing airway obstruction and providing access for suctioning. If the client is unable to breathe without an airway after 48 hours, a tracheostomy is performed. A suction machine should be available in the room. Coughing and deep breathing are helpful to the client who has had a stroke. However, because these activities increase ICP, they should not be used in a hemorrhaging client or when the possibility of herniation is imminent. In most clients who have had a stroke, an obstructed airway is more harmful than increased ICP secondary to coughing.

NEUROLOGICAL PROBLEMS. The client's neurological status needs to be monitored closely to detect stroke in evolution or increased ICP. The level of consciousness, mental status, pupillary responses, movement and strength of extremities, and vital signs are checked at regular intervals. The frequency of neurological checks (see Chapter 52) depends on the condition of the client. A decreasing level of consciousness, the earliest and most sensitive sign of increasing ischemia in the brain, should prompt the nurse to check the client more frequently. Such a change should be reported promptly to the attending physician.

CARDIOVASCULAR PROBLEMS. Nursing goals for the cardiovascular system are designed to maintain homeostasis. Because of advancing age or heart problems, many clients have decreased cardiac reserve after a stroke. Fluids are retained because of increased production of antidiuretic hormone and aldosterone secondary to stress. Fluid retention plus overhydration can result in fluid overload. It can also increase cerebral edema. The nurse therefore should closely monitor intake and output. IV therapy is also carefully regulated. In the initial stages, fluids may be limited to 1000 ml/day or approximately 42 ml/hr. Every effort needs to be made to ensure a constant flow rate and to avoid a sudden rush of IV fluid. Manifestations of fluid overload are rales, dyspnea, shortness of breath, and coughing. In addition, the nurse should regularly assess for other cardiovascular problems, such as hypertension and cardiac dysrhythmias.

After a stroke the client is at risk of thrombophlebitis and deep-vein thrombosis in the weak or paralyzed lower extremity. This risk is related to both immobility and decreased muscle pumping activity in the extremity. The most effective prevention is to keep the client moving. Active range-of-motion exercises should be taught if the client has any voluntary movement in the affected extremity. For the client with hemiplegia, passive range-of-motion exercises should be done at least several times a day. Additional measures often used to prevent thrombophlebitis include positioning to minimize the effects of dependent edema and use of elastic or support hose. Intermittent pneumatic compression stockings may be ordered for long-term bedridden clients.

Table 53-6

 Nursing Assessment of the Client with a Stroke

SUBJECTIVE DATA

History
Positive family history, race, hypertension; previous stroke, TIA(s), aneurysm, cardiac disease, including recent myocardial infarction, dysrhythmias, congestive heart failure, valvular disease, infective endocarditis; alcohol abuse, smoking, hyperlipidemia, diabetes, gout (onset, duration, progression, and resolution of symptoms)

Medications
Use of oral contraceptives, use of and compliance with antihypertensive and anticoagulant agents

General
Weakness, easy fatigability, vertigo, anorexia

Pain
Headache, possibly sudden and severe (hemorrhage)

Gastrointestinal
Nausea and vomiting, dysphagia

Neurological
Loss of movement and sensation, visual disturbances, syncope, disturbances in taste and smell; tingling, numbness, weakness on one side

OBJECTIVE DATA

General
Emotional lability, lethargy, apathy or combativeness, fever

Respiratory
Loss of cough reflex, labored or irregular respirations, tachypnea, rhonchi (aspiration), airway occlusion (tongue), apnea

Cardiovascular
Hypertension, tachycardia, carotid bruit

Gastrointestinal
Loss of gag reflex, bowel incontinence, decreased or absent bowel sounds

Urinary
Incontinence

Neurological
Contralateral motor and sensory deficits, including weakness, paresis, paralysis, anesthesia; unequal pupils, hand grasps; akinesia, aphasia (expressive, receptive, global), agnosias, alexia, hemiattention, apraxia, visual deficits, perceptual or spatial disturbances, altered level of consciousness (drowsiness to deep coma) and Babinski sign, decreased followed by increased deep tendon reflexes, flaccidity followed by spasticity, amnesia, ataxia, personality change, nuchal rigidity, seizures

Possible findings
Polycythemia, positive CT and MRI scans showing size and location of lesion, positive Doppler ultrasonography and cerebral angiography

Table 53-7

NURSING CARE PLAN FOR THE CLIENT WITH A STROKE

Defining Characteristics	Nursing Interventions	Evaluation Criteria
NURSING DIAGNOSIS: Impaired physical mobility related to generalized weakness, muscle atrophy, or paralyzed extremities		
Decreased physical activity; limited range of motion; decreased muscle strength, control, or mass; minimal repositioning	Assess and document range of motion, transfer abilities, and positioning ability. Administer passive or active range of motion exercises to affected extremities at least tid. Position correctly with support pillows according to procedures. Encourage as much self-mobility as possible. Teach and assist family and client with positioning techniques; document progress.	Transfer and ambulation at maximal level of ability
NURSING DIAGNOSIS: Impaired verbal communication related to residual aphasia		
Refusal or inability to speak, word-finding problems, use of inappropriate words, inability to follow verbal directions	Assess exact communication deficits and strengths. Intervene as appropriate. Use short, simple questions that elicit "yes" and "no" answers. Use gestures. Speak slowly and allow adequate time for response.	Demonstration of ability to communicate needs effectively
NURSING DIAGNOSIS: Self-care deficit (partial to total) related to motor weakness, paralysis, and loss of ability to effectively perform activities of daily living		
Observation or valid report of inability to eat, bathe, use toilet, dress, or groom independently	Assess and document level of self-care. Encourage independence, providing supervision or assistance as needed. Follow through with techniques for activities of daily living recommended by occupational or physical therapist. Observe and coach family and attendants in performing activities of daily living with client.	Performance of activities of daily living by client or with assistance from family or staff
NURSING DIAGNOSIS: Sensory/perceptual alteration: visual deficit related to visual field cut, diplopia, and ptosis secondary to decreased circulation to brain		
Behavioral evidence or verbal report of inability to see objects in affected area of visual field	Assess and document amount of visual field impairment. Teach client to turn head and scan environment. Early in care, approach client on unaffected side. Provide visual stimulation. Place objects in client's field of vision. Give physical and verbal cues to aid in path finding. Later in care, approach client on affected side and encourage client to turn head. Place objects on involved side and assess ability to compensate. For diplopia, use an eye patch.	Bringing of objects into field of vision, scanning with eyes, expression of satisfaction with vision
NURSING DIAGNOSIS: Altered pattern of urinary elimination: incontinence related to impaired impulse to void or inability to reach toilet or manage tasks of voiding		
Flow of urine at unpredictable times, urination before reaching appropriate receptacle, nocturia	Assess and record client's continent and incontinent voidings to determine patterns. Note color and character of urine daily and as needed. Provide intake of 2000 ml/day unless contraindicated. If indwelling catheter is used, give perineal cleansing and catheter care every shift and as needed. Offer urinal or commode q 2 hr and as needed.	Absence of urinary tract infection; satisfactory control by natural or artificial method

Table 53-7

 NURSING CARE PLAN FOR THE CLIENT WITH A STROKE—cont'd

Defining Characteristics	Nursing Interventions	Evaluation Criteria

NURSING DIAGNOSIS: Constipation related to immobility, inadequate fiber or bulk intake, and impaired defecation impulse

Lower frequency or less amount of stool than usual pattern, sensation of rectal fullness or pressure or abdominal discomfort, decreased bowel sounds, distended abdomen	Discuss previous bowel habits with family and client and establish program. Teach client and family about high-fiber foods to include in diet. Instruct to insert dentures at mealtime so client can eat high-roughage foods. Provide privacy for bowel program. Involve client and family in making appropriate changes. Document on nursing care plan; give suppository, stool softeners, if needed.	Regular formed stool at least every other day with no incontinence

NURSING DIAGNOSIS: High risk for ineffective airway clearance related to inability to raise secretions

Weak, ineffective cough; bronchial congestion; adventitious breath sounds; changes in color, amount, and consistency of sputum	Observe for increase in pulmonary secretions, changes in color of secretions, and temperature elevation. Auscultate lungs for diminished breath sounds daily and as needed. Suction as needed. Instruct client and family in feeding program and emergency measures.	Ability to expectorate secretions

NURSING DIAGNOSIS: Impaired swallowing related to weakness or paralysis of affected muscles

Drooling, difficulty in swallowing, choking	Physical assessment to determine ability to swallow and presence of gag reflex. Have client sit upright for meals and for 30 minutes afterward. Teach client to take small bites and place in unaffected side of mouth, keep chin down, and stroke throat to stimulate swallowing. Give thick shakes, foods with texture, and cold foods. If problem with sputum and saliva production, avoid milk products. After client has eaten, check oral cavity for pocketed food and teach client and family this technique. Give oral care after meals. Notify dietitian of need to change food texture or fluids as needed. Provide quiet environment and supervision as needed. If choking occurs, do not interfere unless difficulty in breathing develops, then use back blows, abdominal thrusts, and suction as needed.	No signs or symptoms of aspiration, ability to tolerate foods and fluids without choking

NURSING DIAGNOSIS: Altered nutrition: less than body requirements related to difficulty or inability to feed self, immobility, and possible depression

Weight loss, inadequate food and fluid intake, altered taste sensation, fatigue, listlessness, thirst, weight loss, dry skin, decreased skin turgor, weakness	Weigh client on admission and every other day as needed. Request nutritious snacks between meals and at bedtime if indicated. Evaluate previous eating patterns and food preferences to enhance appetite. Perform interventions as for choking, aspiration. Assist with eating. Assess for dehydration. Measure intake and output for 3 days or until satisfactory balance is achieved. Monitor adequate fluid intake. Have client sit upright while drinking.	Adequate intake of food and fluids, stable weight or weight change as recommended by dietitian

Continued.

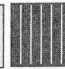

Table 53-7

NURSING CARE PLAN FOR THE CLIENT WITH A STROKE—cont'd		
Defining Characteristics	Nursing Interventions	Evaluation Criteria

NURSING DIAGNOSIS: Self-esteem disturbance related to actual or perceived loss of function

Refusal to touch or look at affected body parts, increasing dependence on others, refusal to participate in self-care	Encourage client to verbalize feelings. Spend time with client, using good listening techniques. Establish achievable goals. Explain all procedures and involve client in planning goals. Offer praise for every success and step of progress. Involve client as soon as possible in rehabilitation program. Refer for counseling or medical-psychiatric evaluation if indicated.	Verbalization of feelings and concerns, appropriate socialization with family and staff, realistic goal setting

MUSCULOSKELETAL PROBLEMS. The nursing goal for the musculoskeletal system is to maintain function. This is accomplished by the prevention of joint contractures and muscular atrophy. In the acute phase, range-of-motion exercises and positioning are important nursing interventions. Passive range-of-motion exercise is begun on the first day of hospitalization. If the stroke is due to a cerebral hemorrhage, the movements are limited to the limbs. The client is taught to actively exercise the affected limbs as soon as possible. (Muscle atrophy secondary to lack of innervation and to inactivity can develop in as little as a month.)

The paralyzed side needs special attention when the client is positioned. Each joint should be positioned higher than the joint proximal to it. Specific deformities on the affected side of the hemiplegic client that nurses must be aware of are shoulder adduction; flexion contractures of the hand, wrist, and elbow; external rotation of the hip; and plantar flexion of the foot. Subluxation of the shoulder on the affected side is common and not preventable. However, careful positioning and moving of the affected arm may prevent the development of a painful shoulder condition. Immobilization of the affected upper extremity may precipitate a painful shoulder-hand syndrome.

Use of a footboard is not recommended for positioning a stroke client in bed. Rather than preventing plantar flexion (foot drop), the sensory stimulation of a footboard against the bottom of the foot increases plantar flexion. A trochanter roll should be used to prevent external rotation of the hip when the client is in the supine position. However, even therapeutic interventions can be detrimental if the client is allowed to remain in any position too long.

INTEGUMENTARY PROBLEMS. The skin of the client who has had a stroke is particularly susceptible to breakdown because of loss of sensation and diminished circulation. These deficits are caused by interference with the nerve supply to the blood vessels of the affected side. The problem is compounded by the age of the client and possible incontinence. Pressure points should be examined and massaged with each turning. If an area of redness develops, the client should be turned more frequently. The client should not be left in any position longer than 2 hours.

Time spent lying on the paralyzed side should be limited to 30 minutes at a time. In addition, the skin needs to be kept clean and dry. An emollient may be beneficial for the older adult or dehydrated client. Special mattresses that are filled with water or air or that provide alternating pressure may help in relieving pressure areas. If an area of redness develops and does not return to normal color when pressure is relieved, the epidermis and dermis are damaged and should not be massaged, since massage will cause greater damage. Control of pressure is the single most important factor in the prevention and treatment of skin breakdown. Vigilance is required for pressure sores to be prevented.

GASTROINTESTINAL PROBLEMS. The stress of illness contributes to a catabolic state that can interfere with recovery. Although neurological and respiratory problems take priority in the acute phase of stroke, nutritional requirements should be addressed as soon as the client is medically stable. The client may be maintained for 5 to 7 days on IV fluids. Facial weakness on the affected side and dysphagia (difficulty swallowing) present special problems. If the client is conscious, oral feeding should be considered.

The first oral feeding should be approached with caution because the gag reflex may be impaired. Before initiation of feeding, the gag reflex may be assessed by gently stimulating the back of the throat with a tongue blade (Fig. 53-6). If a gag reflex is present, the client will gag spontaneously. If it is absent, the feeding should be deferred and exercises to stimulate swallowing should be started. The speech therapist or the occupational therapist is usually responsible for designing this program.[11] However, the nurse may be called on to develop the program in some clinical settings. To assess swallowing ability, the nurse should elevate the head of the bed to an upright position (unless contraindicated) and give the client a small amount of crushed ice or ice water to swallow. If the gag reflex is present and the client is able to swallow safely, the nurse may proceed with the feeding. Mouth care before feeding helps stimulate sensory awareness and salivation and can facilitate swallowing. The client should remain in a high Fowler's position, preferably in a chair with the head

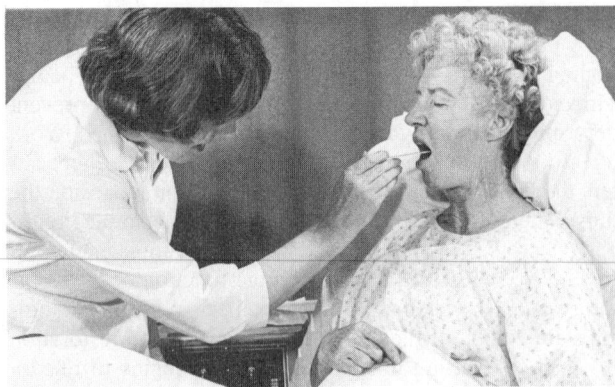

Fig. 53-6 Before initiating oral feeding, the nurse should check for the presence of a gag reflex.

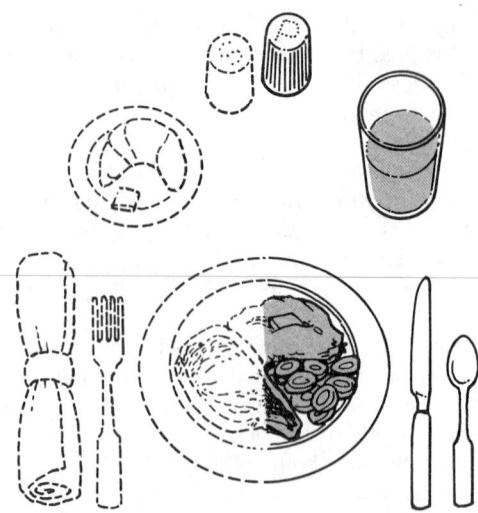

Fig. 53-7 Spatial/perceptual deficits in stroke. Perception of a client with homonymous hemianopsia shows that food on the left side is not seen and thus ignored.

Table 53-8 Communicating with a Client Who Has Aphasia

Treat the client as an adult.

Present one thought or idea at a time.

Keep questions simple or ask questions that can be answered with "yes" or "no."

Organize the client's day by preparing and following a schedule (the more familiar the routine, the easier it will be for the person with aphasia).

Make use of gestures or demonstration as an acceptable alternative form of communication. Encourage this by saying "Show me . . ." or "Point to what you want."

Speak with normal volume and tone.

Allow body contact (e.g., the clasp of a hand or touching) as much as possible. Realize that touching may be the only way the client can express feelings.

Give the client time to process information and generate a response before repeating a question or statement.

Decrease environmental stimuli that may be distracting and disrupt communication efforts.

flexed forward for the feeding and for 30 minutes after the feeding. Foods should be easy to swallow and provide enough texture, temperature (fairly hot or fairly cold), and flavor to stimulate a swallow reflex. Pureed foods are not usually the best choice because they are often bland and too smooth and at room temperature by the time the client is fed. Thin liquids are often difficult to swallow and may promote coughing. Milk products should be avoided because they tend to increase the viscosity of mucus and increase salivation. Food should be placed on the unaffected side of the mouth. The nurse should ensure that the atmosphere is unrushed and nonstressful. Each feeding must be followed by scrupulous oral hygiene, since food tends to collect on the affected side of the mouth.

The most common bowel problem is constipation. The client should be checked every 2 days for impaction. Because diet, fluids, and exercise are limited during the acute phase of stroke, a laxative or a stool softener may have to be used. It is often the responsibility of the nurse to request these medications. Suppositories may be necessary to relieve constipation. Enemas are used only if suppositories and digital stimulation are ineffective, because they cause vagal stimulation and increase ICP.

GENITOURINARY PROBLEMS. In the acute stage of stroke, the primary genitourinary problem is poor bladder control, resulting in incontinence. Efforts should be made to promote normal bladder function and avoid the use of an indwelling catheter. If an indwelling catheter is used initially, it should be removed as soon as the client is medically and neurologically stable. Long-term use of an indwelling catheter promotes the development of a urinary tract infection and prolongs bladder retraining. An intermittent catheterization program may be used for clients with urinary retention. An adequate fluid intake is critical for bladder retraining. A commode, bedpan, or urinal should be offered every 2 hours. A condom catheter may be used for men.

COMMUNICATION PROBLEMS. During the acute stage the nurse's role in meeting the psychological needs of the client is primarily supportive. An alert client is usually very anxious due to lack of understanding of what has happened and inability to communicate. Extensive evaluation and treatment of language and communication deficits are usually done after the client's condition has stabilized. In the acute phase the client's response to one or two simple questions should give the nurse a guideline for structuring explanations and instructions. If the client cannot understand words, gestures may be used to support the verbal cues. It may help to speak slowly and calmly and to use relatively simple words (Table 53-8). The stroke client with aphasia may be easily overwhelmed by verbal stimuli.

SENSORY/PERCEPTUAL PROBLEMS. Homonymous hemianopsia (blindness in the same half of each visual field) is a common problem after a stroke (Fig. 53-7). Persistent disre-

gard of objects in part of the visual field should alert the nurse to this possibility. The client needs to learn to compensate for these deficits. After the initial stress of the illness, the nurse may begin placing items necessary for activities of daily living on the affected side. Initially, the nurse compensates for the perceptual problem by arranging the environment within the client's perceptual field. Later the client is instructed to consciously attend to the neglected side. The position of the affected arm or leg in space must be checked by the client to prevent unfelt trauma.

In the clinical situation it is often difficult to distinguish between a visual field cut and a neglect syndrome. Both problems may occur with strokes affecting either the right side or the left side of the brain. A person may be unfortunate enough to have both homonymous hemianopsia and a neglect syndrome, which increase the inattention to the affected side. A neglect syndrome results in decreased safety awareness and puts the client at considerable risk of injury. Immediately after the stroke the nurse must anticipate potential safety hazards and provide protection from injury. This involves the use of careful observation while the client is awake or the use of side rails and soft vest restraints. The use of restraints is sometimes contraindicated if their use agitates the client.

Other visual problems may include diplopia, loss of the corneal reflex, and ptosis, particularly if the stroke is in the vertebrobasilar distribution (see Table 53-2). Diplopia is often treated with the use of an eye patch. If the corneal reflex is absent, the client is at risk of a corneal abrasion and should be observed closely and protected against eye injuries. There are no definitive nursing interventions to use for ptosis, and the problem is usually not severe after a stroke.

COPING PROBLEMS. A stroke is usually a sudden, extremely stressful event for both the client and close family members. If the client is married, it is often as if the stroke had happened to the couple. An older couple may perceive the stroke as a very real threat to life and to their accustomed lifestyle. Reactions to this threat vary considerably but may involve (1) fear and apprehension, (2) denial of the severity of the stroke, (3) depression, and (4) anger. During the acute phase of caring for the stroke client and the family, nursing intervention designed to facilitate coping involves providing information and emotional support.

Explanations to the client about what has happened and about diagnostic and therapeutic procedures should be clear and understandable. It will be particularly challenging to keep the aphasic client adequately informed. Tone, demeanor, and touch may also be used to convey support.

The client's family should be given a careful, detailed explanation of what has happened to the client. However, if the family is extremely anxious and upset during the acute phase, explanations may have to be repeated at a later time. Because family members usually have not had time to prepare for the illness, they may need assistance in arranging care for family members or pets and for transportation and finances. A social service referral is often helpful.

Rehabilitative management. In the past several years there has been increasing emphasis on rehabilitation after a stroke. Rehabilitation is the process of maximizing the client's capabilities and resources to promote optimal functioning related to physical, mental, and social well-being. Three goals of rehabilitative management are to prevent deformity, maintain function, and restore function.[12] Work toward the first two goals begins at the time the client enters the health care system. For example, on admission the nurse attempts to prevent deformity in the hemiplegic client by proper positioning and range-of-motion exercises. In addition, measures to maintain the function of the respiratory and GI systems are implemented. With physiological stabilization of the client, the focus shifts to restoration of function. During this stage the client begins to relearn and to regain control over bodily actions and functions that are deficient or lost because of the stroke. These activities may focus on speech, walking, bowel and bladder control, and activities of daily living.

Because no member of the health team has all the knowledge and skills necessary for rehabilitation, a team approach is usually used. The rehabilitation team works together to achieve the client's goals. This requires a great deal of communication and coordination. The nurse is in a good position to facilitate this process and is often the key person in successful rehabilitation efforts. The client's participatory decision making during the rehabilitative phase is essential to goal achievement after a stroke. In addition to client and family, nurse, and physiatrist, members of the rehabilitation team may include representatives from the following disciplines: physical therapy, occupational therapy, speech pathology, recreational therapy, social service, psychology, clinical pharmacy, pastoral care, and vocational counseling. Physical therapists focus on mobility, progressive ambulation, transfer techniques, and equipment needed for mobility. The main emphasis of occupational therapy is on retraining for activities of daily living, such as eating, dressing, hygiene, and other activities that involve fine motor skills. Occupational therapists also perform cognitive and perceptual evaluation and retraining.

The long-term management of the stroke client is focused on rehabilitation. The problems the stroke client has are caused by or are a response to a neurological deficit. Table 53-7 provides an example of a nursing care plan for the stroke client. Many of the nursing interventions outlined in the care plan are initiated in the acute phase and continued throughout the rehabilitation phase of care.

MUSCULOSKELETAL SYSTEM. In the rehabilitation of the musculoskeletal system the nurse initially emphasizes the functions the client needs to eat, toilet, and walk around the room. Before the initiation of any intervention the nurse needs to assess the stage of recovery of muscle function. If the muscles are still flaccid after several weeks, the prognosis for regaining function is poor and the focus of care is on preventing additional loss. Most clients begin to show signs of spasticity with exaggerated reflexes within 48 hours. This actually denotes progress. As improvement continues, small voluntary movements of the hip or shoulder may be accompanied by involuntary movements in the rest of the extremity (synergy). In the final stage of recovery the client acquires voluntary control of isolated muscle groups.

Balance training is an initial rehabilitative effort and begins with the client sitting up in bed or on the edge of the bed. The nurse must be alert for dizziness or syncope as a result of vasomotor instability.

Next the client needs to learn to transfer from the bed to an armchair or a wheelchair. The chair is placed next to the bed on the client's unaffected side. The client rises to a standing position facing the chair. When the client is stable in the standing position, the unaffected hand is placed on the far arm of the chair. The client turns and sits down. The nurse may provide minimal assistance by standing at the client's weak side, supporting the affected arm and blocking the affected knee to keep it from buckling. In some rehabilitation settings a Bobath approach (neurodevelopmental treatment) is used in work with stroke clients. The goal of a Bobath approach is to help the client gain control over patterns of spasticity by inhibiting abnormal reflex patterns. Therapists and nurses who use a Bobath approach focus on (1) encouraging normal muscle tone, (2) encouraging normal movement, and (3) promoting bilateral functions.[13,14] If therapists and nurses are using a Bobath approach, transfers are taught to unaffected and affected sides to facilitate more normal, bilateral functioning.

Support or assistive devices, such as canes, walkers, or leg braces, may eventually be needed but are not used unless absolutely necessary. If they are used, the physical therapist usually selects the most appropriate ones for the client. The nurse needs to incorporate physical therapy activities into the daily routine of the client for additional practice and repetition of the rehabilitative efforts.

GASTROINTESTINAL SYSTEM. Inability to self-feed and lack of bowel regularity are two common GI problems after a stroke. The inability to feed oneself is very frustrating and may result in malnutrition. The easiest solution is to have the client switch hands for eating. The unaffected hand may be clumsy at first, but the end result is usually better than can be achieved with assistive devices. However, eating with only one hand is still a challenge. Assistive devices, such as a rocker knife, a plate guard, and a nonslip mat to keep the plate from sliding, are particularly useful eating aids (Fig. 53-8). Removal of unnecessary items from the tray or table can reduce spills and resulting embarrassment as well as decrease sensory overload and distraction. Careful attention to aesthetic and environmental detail is an important nursing consideration related to improving appetite.

Problems with bowel control may be alleviated by implementation of a bowel-training program. A high-fiber diet (see Table 37-10) and adequate fluid (2000 to 3000 ml/day), as well as the selected dietary inclusions, should be given unless contraindicated. The client should be placed on a bedpan, assisted to a bedside commode, or walked to the bathroom at a regular time each day to assist with reestablishment of bowel regularity. A good time to establish this pattern is within 30 minutes after breakfast each day, which takes advantage of the gastrocolic reflex. If the client's usual bowel habits differ from this pattern, efforts should be made to adhere to the individual timing. Stool expanders and stool softeners are often used in addition to diet and habit retraining.

If these techniques are ineffective in reestablishing bowel regularity, a glycerin suppository may be inserted 15 to 30 minutes before the usual evacuation time. This stimulates the anorectal reflex and can often be discontinued when a regular pattern is reestablished. A suppository that produces chemical stimulation (e.g., Dulcolax) is used only if a glycerin suppository is ineffective. Dulcolax may cause uncomfortable abdominal cramping in older clients.

GENITOURINARY SYSTEM. If the client is unable to monitor urination, the nurse should assist with this activity. An indwelling catheter is not practical for long-term use because of the possibility of urinary tract infection and later problems with reestablishing bladder control. Incontinence often results from the client's inability to make elimination needs known. Nursing measures aimed at maintaining urinary continence include palpating the bladder regularly to assess for bladder distention and offering the commode, bedpan, or urinal every 2 hours around the clock. In addition, the nurse should ensure that the client maintains a high fluid intake during the day. Assumption of the usual position for urination (standing for a man and sitting for a woman) and application of pressure over the bladder area often aid in urination.

The use of fluid restriction or incontinent briefs or keeping of a urinal in place at all times are only temporary

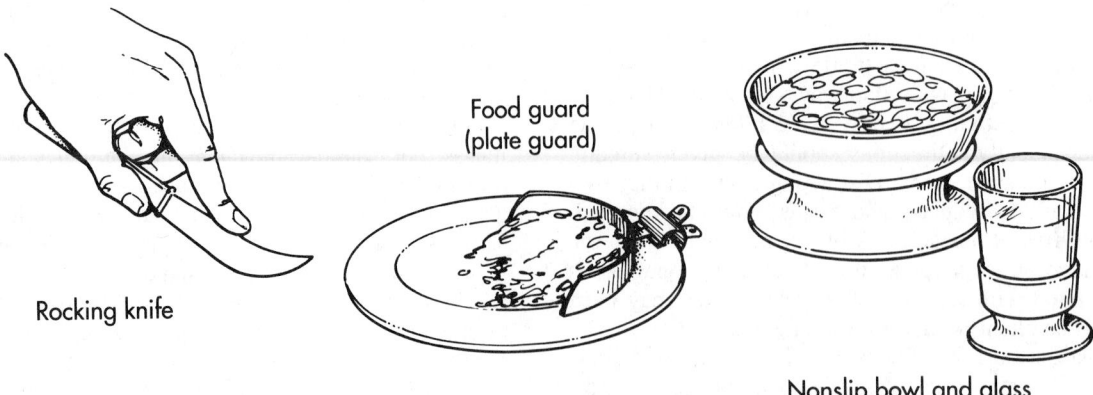

Rocking knife

Food guard (plate guard)

Nonslip bowl and glass

Fig. 53-8   Assistive devices for eating.

measures to reduce the occurrence or effects of incontinence. Long-term use of these measures discourages continence and can lead to dehydration and skin problems. Intermittent catheterization or external devices may be used for short periods until bladder retraining can be attempted.

If the client is unable to regain bladder control, a serious care problem develops. A coordinated retraining program by all members of the nursing staff is a major nursing responsibility. Until bladder and bowel control are attained, further rehabilitation efforts are hampered.

A client who has had a stroke may be concerned about loss of sexual function. Many are comfortable in expressing their fears if the nurse provides an atmosphere in which sexuality can be discussed.[15] The nurse sometimes has to initiate the conversation. Fear that sexual activity will bring on another stroke, alternative positions for intercourse, and the possibility of impotence are common concerns. Impotence, if it occurs, is more likely to result from psychological factors than neurological deficits.

COMMUNICATION PROBLEMS. Speech and language deficits constitute one of the most difficult problems for the social system to handle. Speech therapy is only a partial answer. The nurse needs to be a role model for the client's family when communicating with the aphasic client (see Table 53-8). The client needs frequent, meaningful, verbal stimulation. A common phenomenon is the client who does not read the cue cards with *dog* and *cat* written on them but can read a menu. The client perceives this well-meaning intervention as a childish game and refuses to play. A better approach for the nurse and the client's family is to talk about the activities of daily living that are familiar to the client. The client should always be allowed sufficient time to answer. A relaxed atmosphere should be maintained, and the client should not be pressured to respond. Reinforcing the use of simple responses such as "yes" or "no" may give the client enough confidence to tackle more difficult communication.

SENSORY/PERCEPTUAL PROBLEMS. Clients who have had strokes often exhibit emotional reactions that are not appropriate to the situation, as well as perceptual deficits. The type of response depends on the location of the stroke. Clients with a stroke on the right side of the brain are more likely to have difficulty judging position, distance, and rate of movement. Moreover, they tend to deny these difficulties and are assertive in tackling unfamiliar tasks. Clients may appear apathetic or unduly cheerful. They may fail to correlate spatial-perceptual problems with their inability to perform certain activities, such as getting the wheelchair through a wide doorway. They should be supervised in all activities before being allowed to pursue them independently. Directions should be given verbally and broken into small steps. Distracting clutter in the environment should be reduced, and rooms should be kept well lighted and free of obstacles. A mirror may help orient the client in relation to the environment. One-sided neglect is more common with left hemiplegia. The nurse may need to remind the client to care for the affected side.

A stroke in the left hemisphere often results in depression, inappropriate or exaggerated mood swings, or both. This emotional lability is upsetting and embarrassing to both the client and the family. The client may be unable to control emotions and may burst into tears or laughter. The behavior is out of context and often unrelated to the underlying emotional state of the client. Inappropriate behavior can be alleviated by distraction. The client is usually uncomfortable with this lack of control and will appreciate the intervention. The family needs to be counseled that inappropriate behavior is not a purposeful act by the client. Punitive acts such as shaming, scolding, or embarrassing the client are to be avoided.

COPING PROBLEMS. In addition to the psychological problems secondary to neurological deficit, the client with a stroke may need to be assisted to cope with permanent loss of function secondary to the stroke. Clients often go through all the stages associated with grief and mourning. Many clients are plagued by long-term depression, which may manifest itself with symptoms of anxiety; loss of energy, weight, and appetite; and sleep disturbances. Inability to resume prestroke role tasks is often a cause of depression. In addition, the time and energy required to perform previously simple tasks can result in anger and frustration.

The family and friends of a client who has had a stroke also need assistance from the nurse. The poststroke physical, mental, and emotional capabilities of the client may differ markedly from those of the prestroke person. Family members need to understand the true significance of residual stroke damage so that they can make realistic plans regarding both their own and the client's welfare.

It is a nursing responsibility to instruct the caregivers regarding the client's exercise, diet, activity, bowel and bladder activities, skin care, and oral hygiene. A public health referral promotes continuity of care and provides a support system for the family.

In their communication with the client and in the rest of their relationship, family members tend to develop patterns of interaction. These are sometimes detrimental to the long-term health of the client. For example, family members may respond by keeping the client in the dependent sick role. At the opposite extreme, family members may reject the client's illness because they expect prestroke behavior. The preferred solution is a compromise between these two ends of the continuum.

Family members have to cope with three aspects of the client's behavior. First, they must recognize those changes that are secondary to neurological deficits and that cannot be changed. Second, they must cope with the client's response to the losses at the same time that they are dealing with their own response. Third, they must deal with behavior that they have reinforced in the early stages of the illness. For example, the client may be reluctant to resume dressing, and the family may unconsciously reinforce the behavior by continuing to help with the dressing process. This response is due both to lack of knowledge and to guilt feelings. Internal dialogues demonstrate the latter: "He wouldn't have had the stroke if I had been a better wife," "I should have made her see the doctor." Consequently, family members may be hesitant to assert themselves because they are afraid of causing another stroke.

Family therapy is a helpful adjunct to a rehabilitation

program. The family needs support and reassurance. Open-ended statements such as "I imagine this is pretty confusing" may help the family express their feelings. In addition, family members need accurate and complete information about the disease and the treatment. They also need assistance in problem solving in this crisis period. In some settings, stroke support groups are used to help clients and their families deal with the realities of disability and share coping strategies.[16,17]

DISCHARGE PLANNING. Discharge planning should begin as early as possible during hospitalization. Once hospital care is no longer required the family may need assistance in arranging transfer to an intermediate-care facility. This transfer may be temporary or permanent, depending on the condition of the client and the situation of the primary care provider.

The care provider needs instruction and practice in necessary areas of care while the client is hospitalized. This allows for support and encouragement as well as opportunities for feedback. Adjustments in the home environment, such as removal of a door to accommodate a wheelchair, can be made before discharge.

Specific areas for instruction related to home care of the stroke client include exercise and ambulation techniques; dietary requirements; recognition of signs indicating the possibility of another stroke, such as headache, vertigo, numbness, and visual disturbances; understanding of emotional lability and the possibility of depression; medication routine; and time, place, and frequency of follow-up activities, such as occupational therapy and physical therapy.

Community resources can be an asset to clients and their families. The National Stroke Association provides information, resources, and referral services, as well as a quarterly newsletter on stroke.[18] The American Heart Association has information about stroke, hypertension, diet, exercise, and assistive devices. It also sponsors self-help groups in many locales. The Easter Seal Society may provide wheelchairs and other assistive devices. Other local groups are often available to aid with meals and transportation. Referral to a community health nurse promotes continuity of care.

C ase Study

ACUTE STROKE

Earl, a 61-year-old man, had a left hemisphere thrombotic stroke 4 days ago. Hypertension was diagnosed about 10 years ago, but he stopped taking the antihypertensive medication because he felt so well and disliked taking pills. He had not been to any physician until admitted to the hospital with the stroke. He describes himself as a healthy, active man. He owns his own accounting business and was on the job as an accountant when he had the stroke. He plays golf two to three times a week and is active in family and church activities. He is married and the father of three grown children.

Earl's neurological deficits after the stroke include weakness on the right side of the body, sensory impairment, mild aphasia consisting primarily of word-finding difficulty, and a right homonymous hemianopsia. His blood pressure since admission to the hospital has been consistently 130/90 to 150/95.

Discussion Questions

1. What is the relationship between stroke and hypertension?
2. How can a recurrence of Earl's stroke be prevented?
3. What behavioral style is anticipated with a stroke in the left hemisphere of the brain?
4. How can the nurse assist Earl and his wife to cope with their situation?
5. What nursing measures may be used to help Earl compensate for the visual field cut?
6. What factors should be considered in evaluation of Earl's potential to benefit from transfer to an intensive inpatient rehabilitation setting? When should he be transferred to the rehabilitation setting?
7. What community resources are available to help Earl and his wife to deal with their situation?

R eview Questions

The number of the question corresponds to the same-numbered objective at the beginning of the chapter.

1. Which of the following clients is most likely to have a stroke?
   a. a black 65-year-old man with hypertension
   b. a white 20-year-old woman on oral contraceptives
   c. an obese 15-year-old Native American adolescent
   d. an Asian 35-year-old woman who smokes
2. Which of the following is the *most* potent regulator of cerebral blood flow?
   a. oxygen
   b. carbon dioxide
   c. bicarbonate
   d. lactic acid
3. In which of the following sites is an atherosclerotic plaque most likely to develop?
   a. left ventricle of the heart
   b. bifurcation of the carotid artery
   c. aortic arch
   d. ophthalmic artery
4. A stroke due to thrombosis
   a. is associated with hypertension
   b. occurs following activity
   c. is usually fatal within 4 to 6 weeks
   d. is associated with cardiac dysfunction
5. A right-sided hemiplegia may be caused by a lesion in the
   a. lateral spinothalamic tract
   b. motor area of the left frontal lobe
   c. medial superior area of the paracentral lobule
   d. posterolateral nucleus of the thalamus
6. In the diagnosis of stroke, arteriography is used to determine the
   a. site and size of the infarction
   b. patency of the cerebrovascular system
   c. presence of increased ICP
   d. presence of blood in the CSF
7. For a client with a TIA the goal of therapy is the
   a. prevention of stroke

b. reduction of disability
c. reduction of cerebral edema
d. prevention of complications

8. For a stroke client with hemiplegia the nurse positions each joint
   a. higher than the proximal joint
   b. lower than the proximal joint
   c. at the same level as the proximal joint
   d. at the same level as the distal joint

9. Bowel training after a stroke includes all of the following interventions *except*
   a. adequate fluid intake
   b. assisting of client to toilet or commode at regular time daily
   c. enema every other day
   d. high-fiber diet

10. The most common response of the stroke client to the change in body image is
    a. denial
    b. depression
    c. disassociation
    d. intellectualization

REFERENCES

1. Boss BJ, Heath J, and Sunderland PM: Alterations of neurologic function. In McCance KL and Huether SE, eds: Pathophysiology, St Louis, 1990, Mosby–Year Book, Inc.
2. Whisnant JP: Classification of cerebrovascular diseases, III, Stroke 21:637-676, 1990.
3. Dawson T: Be stroke smart, Denver, 1987, National Stroke Association.
4. Kuller LH: Incidence rates of stroke in the eighties: the end of the decline of stroke? Stroke 20:841-843, 1989.
5. US Public Health Service, National Institutes of Health: Stroke: hope through research, Pub No 83-222, Washington, DC, 1983, US Government Printing Office.
6. Toole JF: Cerebrovascular disorders, ed 3, New York, 1984, Raven Press.
7. Wolfe PA: Transient ischemic attacks: locating the source, Hosp Pract 20:41, 1985.
8. Fode NC: Carotid endarterectomy: nursing care and controversies, J Neurosci Nurs 22:25-31, 1990.
9. Hahn K: Left vs right: what a difference the side makes in stroke, Nursing 87 9:44, 1987.
10. McDonald E: Aneurysmal subarachnoid hemorrhage, J Neurosci Nurs 21:313-321, 1989.
11. Emick-Herring B and Wood P: A team approach to neurologically based swallowing disorders, Rehabil Nurs 15:126-132, 1990.
12. Mumma C, ed: Rehabilitation nursing concepts and practice: a core curriculum, ed 2, Evanston, Ill, 1987, Rehabilitation Nursing Foundation.
13. Bobath B: Adult hemiplegia: evaluation and treatment, London, 1978, Heinemann.
14. Passarella PM and Lewis N: Nursing application of Bobath principles in stroke care, J Neurosci Nurs 19:106-109, 1987.
15. Burgener S and Logan G: Sexuality concerns of the post stroke patient, Rehabil Nurs 14:178-181, 195, 1989.
16. Pasquarello MA: Developing, implementing and evaluating a stroke recovery group, Rehabil Nurs 15:26-29, 1990.
17. Pierce LL and Salter JP: Stroke support group: a reality, Rehabil Nurs 13:189-190, 197, 1988.
18. The road ahead: a stroke recovery guide, Denver, 1986, National Stroke Association.

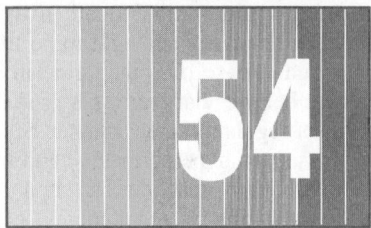
Nursing Role in Management
Chronic Neurological Problems

Judith M. Ozuna

1. Explain the potential impact of chronic neurological disease on physical and psychological well-being.
2. Compare and contrast muscle-contraction, migraine, and cluster headaches in terms of etiology, clinical manifestations, and treatment.
3. Describe the etiology, clinical manifestations, diagnostic studies, and management of epilepsy, multiple sclerosis, Parkinson's disease, and myasthenia gravis.
4. Explain the nursing role in the acute and chronic care of a client with a chronic neurological disease.
5. Describe the clinical manifestations and management of amyotrophic lateral sclerosis, Huntington's chorea, and muscular dystrophy.
6. Identify common physical complications in a person who is immobilized by chronic neurological disease.
7. Outline the major goals of treatment for the client with a chronic, progressive neurological disease.

Management of chronic neurological disease can be challenging for both clients and health care providers. Many neurological disorders involve progressive deterioration in physical and/or mental capabilities, which can be devastating to the client and the family. The client may experience psychological upheaval in the form of depression, fear, anxiety, anger, or withdrawal. This is compounded by changes in body image and self-esteem. In addition, the physical disabilities that result from degenerative disease necessitate varying and sometimes extreme alterations in lifestyle, which add to the emotional trauma of the client. Families are torn between their sense of obligation to care for the ill person and the need to lead their own lives. They are simultaneously pushed and pulled by feelings of guilt, love, despair, hope, resentment, and empathy.

The challenge of chronic neurological illness is equally great for health care providers. Many of these diseases have no cure, so health care professionals can only attempt to alleviate physical symptoms, prevent complications, assist clients in maximizing self-care abilities in the face of neurological deficits, and help them in the difficult task of adjusting to their illness. Nurses can and should greatly influence these aspects of management.

Reviewed by Janice S. Smith, R.N., M.S., Professor of Nursing, Front Range Community College, Westminister, Colorado.

HEADACHE

Headache is probably the most common type of pain experienced by human beings. Of all persons with headache, the majority have *functional* headaches of benign vascular or muscle-contraction origin; the remainder have *organic* headaches caused by significant intracranial or extracranial disease.

Not all tissues of the cranium are sensitive to pain. The pain-sensitive structures in the head that can cause headache are the intracranial and extracranial blood vessels, the venous sinuses, portions of the dura (near large blood vessels), muscles of the scalp and neck, cranial nerves V, VII, IX, and X, and cervical nerves II and III. Pain can result from (1) vascular stretching and dilatation, displacement of cerebral contents, inflammation, and direct pressure on cranial and cervical contents; (2) sustained contraction of skeletal scalp and neck muscles; and (3) noxious stimulation from diseases of the eyes, nose, ears, and sinuses.

Chronic headache of benign origin is the most common and perhaps least effectively treated physical disorder. The history and neurological examination are diagnostic keys.

Types

Muscle-contraction headache. Headache due to sustained contraction of the head and neck muscles has been

called *muscle-contraction, tension, psychogenic,* and *rheumatic* headache. It is considered the most difficult to treat.

Etiology. It is generally accepted that the pain of muscle-tension headache is a result of sustained contraction of skeletal muscles in the neck, scalp, and jaws. However, this may not fully explain the genesis of muscle-contraction headache in its chronic form. Some researchers believe that migraine and muscle-contraction headaches are similar in that the clinical features of each form of chronic headache cannot be fully explained by disturbance of vascular or muscular structures alone. In some clients, severe muscle-contraction headache can produce a pulsatory pain similar to that of migraine.[1]

Some clients may have actual structural alterations in muscle, joint, or connective tissues, which contribute to headache pain. One of the most common causes of headaches is contraction of the cervical muscles as a manifestation of emotional stress. Resolution of the underlying stress may be therapeutic for the headache.

Clinical manifestations. There is no prodrome (early manifestation of impending disease) in tension headache. The pain is usually bilateral, occurring most often in the back of the neck. It usually does not interfere with sleep. The pain is often described as a tight, squeezing, bandlike pressure. It is sustained, chronic, dull, and persistent. It may last weeks, months, or even years. Many clients can have a combination of migraine and muscle-contraction headaches, with features of both headaches occurring simultaneously. Persons with migraine may experience muscle-contraction headaches between migraine attacks.

Diagnostic studies. Careful history taking is probably the most important diagnostic tool for muscle-contraction headache. Electromyography (EMG) may reveal sustained contraction of neck, scalp, or facial muscles, but many clients may not show increased muscle tension with this test, even when the test is done during the actual headache. Conversely, clients with diagnosed migraine headaches may show increased muscle tension on EMG. If muscle-contraction headache is present during physical examination, increased resistance to passive movement of the head and tenderness of the head and neck may be found.

Migraine. Some migraine headaches start in adolescence. Females are affected more frequently than males. A family history of migraine can be found in 65% of persons with migraine. Although migraine has often been associated with persons who are high achievers and who suppress expressions of aggression and hostility, no single personality type describes all clients who experience migraine headache.

Etiology. Some researchers believe that migraine headache has a vascular origin and involves the intracranial and extracranial arteries of the head. Some studies support the classic theory of migraine, which is that the prodromal or aural phase is associated with decreased blood flow and vasoconstriction and that the headache phase is associated with increased blood flow and vasodilatation. Recent evidence suggests that a mechanism other than vasoconstriction may be involved in the prodrome of migraine. Other researchers support a neurogenic theory, which postulates that neuronal imbalance causes blood vessel spasm leading to headache.[2]

Increased platelet aggregation found in the circulation during the prodromal phase is thought to be triggered by a stress response and release of epinephrine in some cases. Some researchers believe that there is a profound instability of blood vessel regulation mechanisms. Studies suggest that the dilated artery is hyperpermeable and involved in a sterile local inflammatory reaction.[3] Several vasoconstrictive substances, including catecholamines, histamine, serotonin, peptide kinins, and prostaglandins, have been implicated in this process. Accumulation of these substances around the artery may sensitize it to pain.

Clinical manifestations. There are two major types of migraine, classic and common. *Common* migraine is the most common type of migraine. The prodrome is not sharply defined, and it can involve psychic disturbances, gastrointestinal (GI) upset, and changes in fluid balance. The prodrome may precede the headache by several hours or days. The headache itself may last several hours or days.

The other type of migraine is *classic migraine,* which occurs in only 10% of migraine headache episodes. The sharply defined prodrome may last 10 to 30 minutes before the headache begins and may include sensory dysfunction (e.g., visual field defects, tingling or burning sensations, or paresthesias), motor dysfunction (e.g., weakness, paralysis), dizziness, confusion, and even loss of consciousness. The classic preheadache symptom is perception of flashing lights in one quadrant of the visual field, often referred to as *scintillating scotomata.* This type of migraine usually peaks in 1 hour and may last several hours.

Clinical manifestations that occur in both classic and common migraine are generalized edema, irritability, pallor, nausea and vomiting, and sweating. During the headache phase, persons with migraine tend to "hibernate"; that is, they seek shelter from noise, light, odors, people, and problems. The headache is described as a steady, throbbing pain that is synchronous with the pulse. Although the headache is usually unilateral, it may switch to the opposite side in another episode. The diagnosis of migraine is usually made from the history. The neurological and other diagnostic examinations are often normal.

Cluster headache. Cluster headache is sometimes associated with migraine headache because of its similar vascular origin. Cluster headache occurs less frequently than migraine by a ratio of 1:10. Cluster headache is more frequent in men than in women by a ratio of 5:1. The onset is usually between the ages of 30 and 60 years. It occurs predominantly in young men.

Etiology. Although the vasodilatation in cluster headache is similar to that of migraine headache, the pathophysiology is not the same. There is no decrease in plasma serotonin level as there is in migraine, but there is an increase in plasma histamine concentration during the cluster headache. Neither the cause nor the pathophysiology of cluster headache is fully known. However, it is clear that paroxysmal recurring discharge of the parasympathetic nervous system is involved.

Clinical manifestations. The headache has an abrupt onset, usually without a prodrome. It peaks in 5 minutes and lasts 30 to 90 minutes. It may recur several times a day over several days and it usually affects the upper face,

periobital region, and forehead on one side of the face and head. The headache may not recur for months or years. Signs of parasympathetic discharge accompany the headache, and they include conjunctivitis, increased lacrimation (tearing), and nasal congestion on the side of the headache. A partial Horner's syndrome may be seen. This involves constriction of the pupil and ptosis (drooping) of the eyelid on the affected side. The headache is described as deep, steady, and boring but not throbbing, which may imply involvement of larger blood vessels. Attacks commonly occur on awakening from a nap or from a night's sleep. They can occur during sleep and often wake the person after a few hours of sleep.

Unlike the person with migraine, who seeks isolation and quiet, the person with a cluster headache paces the floor, cries out, does bizarre things, and resents being touched. The client with a cluster headache does not experience the systemic manifestations that accompany a migraine headache, such as nausea or vomiting. As with migraine, there are usually no complications.

Diagnostic studies. The diagnosis of cluster headache is primarily based on the history. However, a computerized tomography (CT) scan with contrast dye and cerebral angiography may be performed to rule out aneurysm, tumor, and infection.

Other headaches. Although migraine, cluster, and muscle-contraction headaches are by far the most common, other types of headache can occur. They may be the first symptom of a more serious illness. Headache can accompany subarachnoid hemorrhage; brain tumor; other intracranial masses; arteritis; vascular abnormalities; trigeminal neuralgia (tic douloureux); diseases of the eyes, nose, and teeth; and systemic illness (e.g., bacteremia, carbon monoxide poisoning, mountain sickness, polycythemia vera). The mechanism for pain is traction or inflammation of the pain-sensitive structures in the head. The symptoms vary greatly. Because of the variety of causes of headache, clinical evaluation must be thorough. It should include evaluation of personality, life adjustment, environment, and family situation as well as a comprehensive evaluation of physical status.

Therapeutic Management

If no disease is found, therapy is directed toward the functional type of headache. Table 54-1 outlines the general workup for a client with headache to rule out any intracranial or extracranial disease. Table 54-2 compares muscle-contraction headache, migraine, and cluster headache. Table 54-3 summarizes the current therapies for symptomatic and therapeutic relief of common headaches. Because drug therapy has not been totally successful, holistic therapies (affecting both mind and body) have been developed and have proved effective in both muscle-contraction and vascular headaches. These therapies include meditation, yoga, biofeedback, and muscle-relaxation training.

Biofeedback involves the use of physiological monitoring equipment to give the client information regarding muscle tension and peripheral blood flow (skin temperature of the hand). The client is trained to relax the muscles and raise hand temperature and is given reinforcement (op-

Table 54-1 Diagnostic Workup for Client with Headache

Complete history
Clinical examination (often negative)
  Inspection for local infections
  Palpation for tenderness, hardened arteries, bony swellings
  Auscultation for bruits over major arteries
Routine laboratory studies to rule out underlying causes of headache
  CBC
  Electrolytes
  Urinalysis
  Serological studies
X-ray film of sinuses
Special studies (e.g., CT scan, angiography, EMG, electroencephalography) for structural disease

CBC, Complete blood count.

erant conditioning) in accomplishing these physiological alterations.

Other treatments for muscle-contraction headache include physical therapy (e.g., massage, hot packs, cervical collar), injection of local anesthetic into spastic muscles, and correction of faulty posture. Acupuncture, acupressure, and hypnosis are successful innovative therapies, although acupuncture and acupressure provide only temporary relief. Most clients can benefit from psychotherapy aimed at helping them recognize conflicts and deal with them more effectively.

Pharmacological Management

Drug treatment for muscle-contraction headache usually involves a nonnarcotic analgesic (e.g., aspirin, acetaminophen) used alone or in combination with a sedative, a muscle relaxant, a tranquilizer, or codeine. However, many of these drugs have potentially dangerous side effects. Clients should be cautioned about long-term use of aspirin and aspirin combination drugs because they can cause gastric bleeding and coagulation abnormalities in susceptible persons. Long-term use of Fiorinal should be avoided because it contains a barbiturate, which may be habit forming, in addition to aspirin. Drugs containing acetaminophen (Tylenol, Phenaphen, Midrin) can cause liver damage with chronic use. Narcotics and tricyclic antidepressants (benzodiazepines) can cause addiction and habituation.

Drug treatment of the acute migraine attack is aimed at preventing the painful dilatation of the cranial blood vessels. Ergotamine tartrate (Cafergot) is considered the most effective drug for this. Ergotamine inhibits the reuptake of neuronally liberated norepinephrine into storage sites of the postganglionic nerve terminal of the sympathetic nervous system. This allows more norepinephrine to attach to α-adrenergic sites on smooth muscle in the artery wall, thereby causing prolonged vasoconstriction of cranial vessels. Relief of headache with ergotamine treatment usually confirms the diagnosis of vascular headache. Ergotamine can be administered orally, sublingually, parenterally, rec-

Table 54-2 Muscle-Contraction, Migraine, and Cluster Headaches

Site	Quality	Frequency	Duration	Time and Mode of Onset	Associated Symptoms
MUSCLE-CONTRACTION					
Bilateral, bandlike at base of skull, in face, or both	Constant, squeezing tightness	Dull, persistent, no specific pattern	Intermittent for months or years	Absence of relationship to time	Palpable neck and shoulder muscles, stiff neck, tenderness
MIGRAINE					
Unilateral (in 60% of cases), possible switching of sides, commonly anterior	Throbbing, synchronous with pulse	Periodic	Continuous for hours or days	Possible prodrome	Nausea and vomiting, edema, irritability, sweating, photophobia; prodrome of sensory, motor, or psychic phenomena
CLUSTER					
Unilateral, upward or downward radiation from one eye	Severe, bone crushing	Months or years between attacks, with attacks occurring in clusters of one to three times a day over 4 to 8 wk	30 to 90 minutes	Nocturnal onset, possible awakening of person after nap or few hours of sleep	Vasomotor symptoms such as facial flushing or pallor, unilateral lacrimation, ptosis, and coryza

Table 54-3

 Diagnostic and Therapeutic Management: Headache

DIAGNOSTIC

Muscle-contraction
  History of neck and head tenderness
  Resistance to movement
  EMG
Migraine
  History
Cluster
  History
  Thermography

THERAPEUTIC
Symptomatic

Muscle-contraction
  Nonnarcotic analgesics (aspirin, acetaminophen, ibuprofen)
  Analgesic combinations (Fiorinal)
  Muscle relaxants
Migraine
  Nonnarcotic analgesics (aspirin, acetaminophen)
  α-Adrenergic blockers (ergotamine tartrate)
  Analgesic combinations
Cluster
  α-Adrenergic blockers (ergotamine tartrate)
  Intranasal lidocaine

THERAPEUTIC—cont'd
Prophylactic

Muscle-contraction
  Tricyclic antidepressants (doxepin, amitriptyline)
  β-Adrenergic blockers (propranolol)
  Biofeedback
  Muscle-relaxation training
  Psychotherapy
Migraine
  β-Adrenergic blockers (propranolol)
  Serotonin antagonists (methylsergide)
  Calcium channel blockers
  Antidepressants (amitriptyline, imipramine)
  Biofeedback
  Yoga
  Meditation
Cluster
  α-Adrenergic blockers (ergotamine tartrate)
  Serotonin antagonists (methylsergide)
  Steroids (prednisone)
  Lithium

tally, or by inhalation. The usual dosage is 1 to 2 mg (oral, rectal) at the onset of the headache, followed by 2 mg within 1 hour. No more than 6 mg is given for any single attack. Other drugs that may relieve migraine headache include Fiorinal, Midrin, aspirin, acetaminophen (Tylenol, Datril), meperidine (Demerol), and codeine.

Because cluster headaches are so brief, there is not sufficient time for drugs to be absorbed. Inhalation of pure oxygen often aborts the headache. Ergotamine tartrate and methysergide, a serotonin inhibitor, may be used prophylactically when the cluster headache recurs at a known time.

A variety of drugs are used to prevent further migraine attacks. These drugs are taken during the interval between attacks rather than during the actual headache. Propranolol is the first choice for prophylaxis of migraine. Propranolol, a β-adrenergic blocking agent, prevents arterial vasoconstriction and inhibits platelet aggregation and adhesiveness. Tricyclic antidepressants, calcium channel blockers, clonidine, thiazides, and other antihypertensive drugs may also be used prophylactically for very severe or very frequent migraine headaches.

■ Nursing Management of Headache

Nursing assessment

Subjective and objective data that should be obtained from a person with headache are presented in Table 54-4. Because the history provides the key to assessment of headache, it should include specific details of the headache itself, such as location and type of pain, onset, frequency, duration, relation to events (emotional, psychological, physical), and time of day. Information about previous illnesses, surgery, trauma, allergies, family history, and response to medication should also be obtained. The nurse can suggest that the client keep a diary of headache episodes with specific details. This type of record can be of great help in determining the type of headache as well as the precipitating events.

Nursing diagnoses

Nursing diagnoses specific to the client with headache include, but are not limited to, the following:

1. Chronic pain related to headache
2. Anxiety related to lack of knowledge of headache etiology and treatment and uncertainty of occurrence of headache

Table 54-4

 Nursing Assessment of the Client With Headaches

SUBJECTIVE DATA

History
Positive family history, hypertension, seizures, cancer, recent fall, trauma, cranial infection, craniotomy; cerebrovascular accident; asthma or allergies; mental illness; relationship of headache to overwork, fatigue, menstruation, depression, anxiety, stress, exercise, travel, bright lights, other noxious environmental stimuli; ingestion of alcohol, caffeine, cheese, chocolate, monosodium glutamate, lunch meats, sausage, hot dogs, onions, avocados

Medications
Use of hydralazine, bromides, nitroglycerin, ergotamine (withdrawal), indomethacin (Indocin), oral contraceptives, over-the-counter or prescription remedies

General
Fever, malaise, insomnia, weakness, eye strain, anorexia

Pain
Migraine: Unilateral, severe, throbbing (possible switching of sides)
Cluster: Unilateral and severe, nocturnal
Muscle tension: Bilateral, bandlike, dull and persistent, base of skull
Sinus: Frontal and facial, gradual onset, worsening in morning, dull pain and pressure
Posttraumatic: Severe, chronic, localized or generalized; increase with coughing, position changes, emotional disturbances
Meningeal: Severe and generalized, radiation to neck
Temporal arteritis: Severe, throbbing, burning; temporal area
Brain tumor: Generalized, intense and steady, association with neurological deficits

SUBJECTIVE DATA—cont'd

Respiratory
Nasal congestion, discharge (sinusitis)
Gastrointestinal
Nausea and vomiting (migraine prodrome), projectile vomiting (brain tumor)
Neurological
Visual disturbances with migraine or brain tumor; photophobia with migraine or meningeal; ptosis, unilateral lacrimation with cluster; vertigo, irritability, poor concentration with posttraumatic
Musculoskeletal
Nuchal rigidity (meningeal, muscle tension)

OBJECTIVE DATA

General
Anxiety, apprehension
Integumentary
Cluster: diaphoresis, pallor, facial flushing with cheek edema; *migraine prodrome:* generalized edema
Cardiovascular
Carotid bruits
Neurological
Brain tumor: papilledema, gait disturbances; *meningeal:* paresthesias, confusion, loss of consciousness; *cluster:* Horner's syndrome
Possible findings
Possible evidence of disease, deformity, or infection on magnetic resonance imaging, cerebral arteriogram, lumbar puncture, electroencephelogram, EMG, skull x-ray studies; nonspecific CT scan

3. Ineffective individual coping related to chronic pain behavior
4. Hopelessness related to chronic pain, alteration of lifestyle, and ineffective treatment modalities

Nursing interventions

Clients with chronic headache present a great challenge to health care providers. Their headaches often result from inability to cope with daily stresses. The most effective therapy may be to help clients examine their lifestyle, recognize stressful situations, and learn to cope with them more appropriately. Precipitating factors can be identified, and ways of avoiding them can be developed. Daily exercise, relaxation periods, and socializing can be encouraged, since each can help reduce recurrence of headache. The nurse can suggest alternative ways of handling the pain of headache through practices such as relaxation, meditation, yoga, and self-hypnosis.

Besides analgesics and analgesic combination drugs for symptomatic relief of headache, clients should be encouraged to use relaxation techniques because they are effective in muscle-contraction and vascular headaches. Migraine sufferers often need a quiet, dimly lighted environment. Massage and moist hot packs to the neck and head can help clients with muscle-contraction headache.

The client should learn about the medications prescribed for prophylactic and symptomatic treatment of headache and should be able to describe the purpose, action, dosage, and side effects of the medication. To prevent accidental overdose, the client should make a written note of each dose of medication or headache remedy.

SEIZURE DISORDERS AND EPILEPSY

A seizure is a sudden alteration in normal brain activity that causes distinctive changes in behavior and body function. Seizures are frequently symptoms of an underlying illness. They may accompany a variety of disorders, or they may occur spontaneously without any apparent cause. Seizures resulting from systemic and metabolic disturbances are not considered epilepsy if the seizures cease when the underlying problem is corrected. In the adult, metabolic disturbances that cause seizures include acidosis, electrolyte imbalance, hypoglycemia, hypoxia, alcohol and barbiturate withdrawal, dehydration, and water intoxication. Extracranial disorders that can cause seizures are heart, lung, liver, and kidney disease, systemic lupus erythematosus, diabetes, hypertension, and septicemia.

Epilepsy connotes spontaneously recurring seizures. There are an estimated 1 to 2 million persons with epilepsy in the United States, and 80% experience their first seizure before the age of 20. After this age the incidence decreases.

Etiology

The most common causes of epilepsy during the first 6 months of life are severe birth injury, congenital defects involving the central nervous system (CNS), infections, and inborn errors of metabolism. Between the ages of 2 and 20 the primary factors are birth injury, infection, trauma, and genetic factors. From ages 20 to 30, epilepsy usually occurs as the result of structural lesions, such as trauma, brain tumors, or vascular disease. After the age of 50 the primary causes of epilepsy are cerebrovascular lesions and metastatic brain tumors. Although many causes of epilepsy have been identified, three fourths of all epilepsy cases cannot be attributed to a specific cause and are termed *idiopathic*.

The role of heredity in the etiology of epilepsy has been difficult to determine because of the problem of separating hereditary from environmental or acquired influences. However, it is known that certain normal and abnormal electroencephalogram (EEG) patterns are genetically transmitted. It has been determined that typical absence seizures (petit mal epilepsy) are inherited as an irregular autosomal dominant trait.[4] Some families carry a predisposition to epilepsy in the form of an inherently low threshold to seizure-producing stimuli, such as trauma, disease, and high fever. For example, an inherently low seizure threshold may explain the reason some persons develop seizures after a head injury or similar insult, whereas others do not.

Pathophysiology

Seizures are paroxysmal, uncontrolled electrical discharges of neurons in the brain that interrupt normal function. The specific clinical manifestations of a seizure are determined by the site of the electrical disturbance. Seizures can be the result of a variety of physical alterations. Because the brain transmits information by electrical and chemical processes, anything that disrupts these processes can cause a seizure. Researchers have found that in recurring seizures (epilepsy) a group of abnormal neurons (*seizure focus*) seem to undergo spontaneous firing. This firing spreads by physiological pathways to involve adjacent or distant areas of the brain. If this activity spreads to involve the whole brain, a generalized seizure occurs. The factor that causes this abnormal firing is not clear. Anything that depolarizes the nerve cell dendrites or the cell membrane induces a tendency to spontaneous firing. Often the area of the brain from which the epileptic activity arises is found to have scar tissue (gliosis). The scarring is thought to interfere with the normal chemical and structural environment of the brain neurons, making them more likely to fire abnormally.

It appears that repetitive electrical discharges from an epileptic focus in experimental animals can produce long-lasting and possibly permanent changes in neuron excitability, both locally and in distant areas of the brain. This effect is called *kindling*, and it presents an interesting and important implication for epilepsy in human beings: seizures can beget more seizures. Clinical experience indicates that the longer a person goes without good seizure control, the less likely the seizures are to be controlled. Therefore a vigorous attempt must be made to control recurring seizures.

Clinical Manifestations

The preferred method of classifying seizures is the International Classification System proposed by Gastaut in 1970 and revised in 1981 (Table 54-5).[5,6] It is based on the clinical and EEG manifestations of seizures. In this system, seizures are divided into two major classes, gener-

Table 54-5 International Classification of Epileptic Seizures

Partial seizures (local onset)
  Simple partial seizures (no impairment of consciousness)
    With motor symptoms
    With somatosensory or special sensory symptoms
    With autonomic symptoms
    With psychic symptoms
  Complex partial seizures (impairment of consciousness)
    Simple partial seizures with progression to impairment
      of consciousness
      With no other features
      With features of simple partial seizures
      With automatisms
    Impairment of consciousness at onset
      With no other features
      With features of simple partial seizures
      With automatisms
Generalized seizures (bilaterally symmetrical and without local onset)
  Absence seizures, atypical absence seizures
  Myoclonic seizures
  Clonic seizures
  Tonic seizures
  Tonic-clonic seizures
  Atonic seizures
Unclassified epileptic seizures (inadequate or incomplete data)

Modified from Commission on Classification and Terminology of the International League against Epilepsy: Proposal for revised clinical and electroencephalographic classification of epileptic seizures, Epilepsia 22:489-501, 1981.

alized and partial. Depending on the type, a seizure may progress through several phases, including *prodromal* signs or activity, which precedes a seizure; *aural*, or sensory warning; *ictal*, or full seizure; and *postictal*, or period of recovery after the seizure.

Generalized seizures. Generalized seizures are characterized by bilateral synchronous epileptic discharge in the brain from the onset of the seizure. Because the entire brain is affected at the onset of the seizures, there is no warning or aura. The person loses consciousness for a few seconds to several minutes.

Clonic-tonic seizures. The most common generalized seizure is the generalized tonic-clonic, or grand mal, seizure. This seizure is characterized by loss of consciousness and a fall to the ground if upright, followed by stiffening of the body (tonic phase) for 10 to 20 seconds and subsequent jerking of the extremities (clonic phase) for another 30 to 40 seconds. Cyanosis, excessive salivation, tongue or cheek biting, and incontinence may accompany the seizure.

In the postictal phase the person usually has muscle soreness, is very tired, and may sleep for several hours. Some persons may not feel normal for several hours or days after a seizure. The client has no memory of the seizure activity.

Typical absence seizures. The absence (petit mal) seizure usually occurs only in children and rarely continues beyond adolescence. It may cease altogether as the child matures, or it may evolve into another type of seizure. The typical clinical manifestation is a brief staring spell that lasts only a few seconds, so it often occurs unnoticed. There may be an extremely brief loss of consciousness. When untreated, the seizures may occur up to 100 times a day.

The EEG demonstrates a three-per-second (Hz) spike-and-wave pattern that is unique to this type of seizure. Absence seizures can often be precipitated by hyperventilation and flashing lights.

Atypical absence seizures. Another type of generalized seizure is the staring spell accompanied by other signs and symptoms, including brief warnings, peculiar behavior during the seizure, and/or confusion after the seizure. The EEG demonstrates atypical spike-and-wave patterns, usually greater or less than 3 Hz.

Other types. Other generalized seizures are myoclonic and akinetic seizures. A myoclonic seizure is characterized by a sudden, excessive jerk of the body or extremities. The jerk may be forceful enough to hurl the person to the ground. These seizures are very brief and may occur in clusters. The terms *akinetic* (arrest of movement), *atonic* (loss of tone), and *astatic* (loss of balance) have been used interchangeably to describe drop attacks or falling spells. This type of seizure involves a paroxysmal loss of muscle tone and begins quite suddenly with the person falling to the ground. Consciousness has usually returned by the time the person hits the ground, and normal activity can be resumed immediately. Persons with this type of seizure are at great risk of head injury and often have to wear protective helmets. A less severe akinetic seizure involves brief loss of muscle tone without falling.

Partial seizures. Partial (focal) seizures are another major class of the International Classification System. Partial seizures begin in a specific region of the cortex, as indicated by the EEG and usually by the clinical manifestations. For example, if the discharging focus is located in the medial aspect of the postcentral gyrus, the person may experience paresthesias and tingling or numbness in the leg on the side opposite the focus. If the discharging focus is located in the part of the brain that governs a particular function, sensory, motor, cognitive, and emotional phenomena may occur.

Partial seizures may be confined to one side of the brain and remain partial or focal in nature, or they may spread to involve the entire brain, culminating in generalized tonic-clonic seizure. Any tonic-clonic seizure preceded by an aura or warning is a partial seizure that secondarily generalizes. Many tonic-clonic seizures that appear to be generalized from the outset may actually be secondarily generalized seizures, but the preceding partial component may be so brief that it is undetected by the client, the observer, or even the EEG. Unlike the primary generalized tonic-clonic seizure, the secondarily generalized seizure may result in transient residual neurological deficit postictally. This is referred to as *Todd's paralysis* (focal paresis); it resolves after varying lengths of time.

Partial seizures are further divided into those with simple motor or sensory phenomena and those with complex symptoms (also called *temporal lobe*, or *psychomotor*, seizures). Simple partial seizures with elementary symptoms do not involve loss of consciousness and rarely last longer than 1 minute. They may involve motor, sensory, or autonomic phenomena or a combination of these. The terms *focal motor, focal sensory*, and *Jacksonian* have been used to describe seizures of the simple partial type.

Partial seizures with complex symptoms can involve a variety of behavioral, emotional, affective, and cognitive functions. The location of the discharging focus is usually in the temporal lobe; hence the term *temporal lobe seizure*. These seizures usually last longer than 1 minute and are frequently followed by a period of postictal confusion. Partial complex seizures are distinct from simple partial (focal motor, focal sensory) seizures in that they involve some alteration in consciousness. The sole manifestation may be clouding of consciousness or a confused state without any motor or sensory components. This type of attack is sometimes called *temporal lobe absence*. There is rarely the complete loss of consciousness that is typical of the generalized absence attack; nor does the person snap back to the preseizure state as does the person who has had a generalized absence attack.

The most common complex partial seizure involves lip smacking and *automatisms* (repetitive movements that may not be appropriate). These are often called *psychomotor seizures*. The person may continue an activity that was initiated before the seizure, such as counting out change or picking items from a grocery shelf but, after the seizure, does not remember the activity performed during the seizure. Other automatisms are less organized, such as picking at clothing, fumbling with objects (real or imaginary), or simply walking away.

A variety of psychosensory symptoms may occur during a partial complex seizure, including distortions of visual or auditory sensations and vertigo. There may be alterations in memory, such as a feeling of having experienced an event before *(déjà vu)*, or alterations in thought processes, such as forced thinking.

Alterations in sexual functioning can vary from hyposexuality to hypersexuality. Many clients with temporal lobe seizures have decreased sexual drive or are impotent. However, some may experience sexual sensations during their seizures. This is because the abnormal electrical activity arises from the brain centers responsible for these sensations. Some experience increased sexual drive just after a seizure. In addition, some antiepileptic medications can cause a decrease in sexual drive because of sedation. Others can cause impotence.

Complications

Physical. *Status epilepticus* is the most serious complication of epilepsy. This is a state in which seizures recur in rapid succession and the person does not regain consciousness or normal function between seizures. Status epilepticus can involve any type of seizure. During repeated seizures the brain uses more energy than can be supplied. Neurons become exhausted and cease to function. Perma-

nent brain damage may result. Grand mal status epilepticus is the most dangerous because it can cause ventilatory insufficiency, hypoxemia, cardiac dysrhythmias, hyperthermia, and systemic acidosis, all of which can be fatal.

Another complication of epilepsy is severe injury and even death due to trauma suffered during a seizure. Persons who lose consciousness during a seizure are at greatest risk of this. Death can result from head injury incurred in a fall, from drowning in the bathtub, or from severe burns.

Psychosocial. Perhaps the most common complication of epilepsy is the effect it has on a person's lifestyle. Although attitudes have improved in recent years, epilepsy still carries a social stigma.[7] It used to be associated with supernatural powers, possession by the devil, and insanity. Today the stigma probably exists because the characteristics of seizures are in direct conflict with modern societal values of self-control, conformity, and independence. The person with epilepsy may experience discrimination in employment and educational opportunities. Transportation may be difficult because of legal sanctions against driving in some states. The person may develop inadequate methods of coping.

Diagnostic Studies

The most useful diagnostic tool is an accurate and comprehensive description of the seizures and the person's health history. The EEG is a useful diagnostic adjuvant to the history but only if it shows abnormalities. Unfortunately, only a small percentage of persons with epilepsy have abnormal EEGs the first time the test is done. Several EEGs often need to be done before abnormalities are detected. Abnormal discharges may not occur during the 30 to 40 minutes of EEG sampling and may never indicate an abnormality. The EEG is not foolproof. Some persons who do not have epilepsy have abnormal EEGs; many with epilepsy have normal EEGs. Abnormal findings help to determine the seizure type and to pinpoint the seizure focus.

Plain skull x-ray studies, CT scan, MRI, radionuclide brain scans, cerebral angiography, and position emission tomography are also used in selected clinical situations.

Therapeutic Management

Most seizures do not require professional emergency medical care because they are self-limiting and rarely cause bodily injury. However, if several seizures occur in succession without the client regaining consciousness between seizures *(status epilepticus)*, if significant bodily harm occurs, or if the event is a first-time seizure, medical care should be sought immediately. Table 54-6 summarizes prehospital care of the client with a generalized tonic-clonic seizure, the seizure most likely to warrant professional emergency medical care.

The diagnostic and therapeutic management of seizure disorders is summarized in Table 54-7. Epilepsy is treated primarily with antiepileptic medication. Therapy is aimed at preventing seizures, since cure is not possible. Medications generally act by stabilizing nerve cell membranes and preventing spread of the epileptic discharge. Alternative

Table 54-6

Prehospital Emergency Care of the Client with Seizures*

Etiology: Idiopathic, head trauma, traumatic birth injury, drug overdose, hypertensive crisis, stroke, meningitis, cardiac arrest, fluid and electrolyte imbalance, hypoglycemia, septicemia, brain tumors, psychiatric disorders, high fevers, medical disorders (e.g., heart, liver, lung, and kidney disease, systemic lupus erythematosus)

CLINICAL MANIFESTATIONS

Aura hallucinations, peculiar sensations that precede seizure
Loss of consciousness
Tonic phase—continuous muscle contractions
Hypertonic phase—extreme muscular rigidity lasting 5 to 15 seconds
Clonic phase—ridigity and relaxation alternate in rapid succession
Loss of bowel and bladder control
Increased pulse rate
Postseizure stupor
Confusion and headache

MANAGEMENT

Stay with client until seizure has passed.
Protect client from injury during hypertonic, clonic, and tonic phases.
Establish and maintain an adequate airway.
Never try to force an airway between a client's clenched teeth.
Be prepared to assist with ventilations if client does not breathe spontaneously after seizure.
Suction as needed.
Monitor vital signs.
Establish an IV infusion with large-gauge needle.
Prepare for possible vomiting; insert a nasogastric tube to decompress the stomach.
Remove or loosen any tight clothing.
Do not restrain the client.
Protect the client's privacy.
Reassure and reorient the client after seizure.
Transport immediately to hospital.

*See Chapter 59 for a general discussion on measures related to prehospital emergency care.

Table 54-7

Diagnostic and Therapeutic Management: Seizures

DIAGNOSTIC
Complete history and physical examination
 Birth and development history
 Significant illnesses and injuries
 Family history
 Febrile seizures
 Comprehensive neurological assessment
Seizure history
 Precipitating factors
 Antecedent events
 Seizure description (including onset, duration, frequency, postictal state)
Diagnostic studies
 CBC, urinalysis, electrolytes, blood urea nitrogen, fasting blood glucose
 Lumbar puncture
 CT scan
 EEG

THERAPEUTIC
Antiepileptic medication*
Surgery†
Psychosocial counseling

CBC, Complete blood count.
*See Table 54-9.
†See Table 54-8.

therapies for epilepsy are surgical removal of the epileptic focus and biofeedback or operant conditioning in selected cases.

Although 70% of seizures are controlled by medication, a significant number of persons with epilepsy are candidates for surgical intervention. Surgery may be considered to control intractable seizures, to prevent cerebral degeneration due to repeated seizures, to prevent toxic syndromes from long-term use of antiepileptic drugs, and to improve quality of life.[8]

Not all types of epilepsy benefit from surgery (Table 54-8). The benefits of surgery include cessation of seizures or reduction in frequency. An extensive preoperative evaluation is important, including continuous EEG monitoring and other specific tests to ensure precise localization. Before surgery is performed, three absolute requirements must be met: (1) diagnosis of epilepsy must be confirmed; (2) there must have been an adequate trial of drug therapy without satisfactory results; and (3) the electroclinical syndrome must be defined.[8]

Biofeedback to control seizures is aimed at teaching the client to maintain a certain brain-wave frequency that is refractory to seizure activity. This method is still in the experimental stage.

Pharmacological Management

The primary goal of antiepileptic drug therapy is to obtain maximum seizure control with a minimum of toxic side effects. The principle of drug management is to begin with a single drug and increase the dosage until a therapeutic serum level is reached. Serum levels of the drug should be monitored regularly. The therapeutic range for each drug indicates the serum level above which most clients experience toxic side effects and below which most continue to have seizures. If seizure control is not achieved with a single drug, a second drug is added.

The primary drugs for treatment of generalized tonic-

Table 54-8 Surgical Procedures for Epilepsy

Type of Seizure	Surgical Procedure	Results
Complex partial seizure of temporal lobe origin	Resectioning of epileptogenic tissue	Absence of seizures 5 years postoperatively (55%-70%)
Partial seizures of frontal lobe origin	Resectioning of epileptogenic tissue (if in resectable area)	Absence of seizures 5 years postoperatively (30%-50%)
Generalized seizures (Lennox-Gastaut syndrome or drop attacks)	Sectioning of corpus callosum	Persistence of seizures, less violent, less frequent, less disabling events
Intractable unilateral multifocal epilepsy associated with infantile hemiplegia	Hemispherectomy or callosotomy	Reduction in seizure frequency and type, improvement in behavior

Table 54-9 Antiepileptic Drugs and Drug Interactions

Drug	Known Drug Interactions
GENERALIZED TOXIC-CLONIC AND PARTIAL SEIZURES	
Phenytoin (Dilantin)	Aspirin, benzodiazepines, bishydroxycoumarin, carbamazepine, cimetidine, clonazepam, coumarin, chloramphenicol, dexamethasone, disulfiram, ethosuximide, ethanol, isoniazid, methylphenidate, phenothiazines, phenylbutazone, valproic acid, propoxyphene, phenobarbital, tolbutamide, trazodone, birth control pills
Carbamazepine (Tegretol)	Phenytoin, ethosuximide, erythromycin, propoxyphene, primidone, divalproex sodium, birth control pills, calcium channel blockers
Phenobarbital	Bishydroxycoumarin, clonazepam, diazepam, dextropropoxyphene, carbamazepine, chlorpromazine, desipramine, phenothiazines, phenylbutazone, phenytoin, divalproex sodium, birth control pills
Primidone (Mysoline)	Isoniazid, same as phenobarbital interactions
ABSENCE, AKINETIC, AND MYOCLONIC SEIZURES	
Ethosuximide (Zarontin)	None
Divalproex sodium (Depakote)	Clonazepam, phenytoin, phenobarbital, ethosuximide, carbamazepine, aspirin, antacids
Clonazepam (Klonopin)	Divalproex sodium
Phenobarbital	Same as above

clonic and partial seizures are phenytoin (Dilantin), carbamazepine (Tegretol), phenobarbital, primidone (Mysoline), and divalproex sodium (Depakote). The primary drugs for treatment of absence, akinetic, and myoclonic seizures are ethosuximide (Zarontin), divalproex sodium (Depakote), and clonazepam (Klonopin). (Table 54-9 summarizes the known interactions of the major antiepileptic drugs.) Because many of these drugs (e.g., phenytoin, phenobarbital, ethosuximide) have a long half-life, they can be given in once- or twice-daily doses. This aids medication-taking compliance by simplifying the drug regimen and avoiding the need to take medication at work or school. These drugs should not be discontinued abruptly because this can precipitate seizures.

Toxic side effects of antiepileptic drugs involve the CNS and include diplopia, drowsiness, ataxia, and mental slowing. Neurological assessment for dose-related toxicity involves testing the eyes for nystagmus. Mild nystagmus confirms that the drug is being taken. If it is associated with diplopia, the dosage may have to be decreased. Hand and gait coordination should be assessed as well as cognitive functioning and general alertness.

Idiosyncratic side effects involve organs outside the CNS. These include the skin (rashes), gingivae (hypertrophy), bone marrow (blood dyscrasias), liver, and kidneys. Nurses should be knowledgeable about these side effects so that clients can be informed and proper treatment can be instituted. A common idiosyncratic side effect of phenytoin is hypertrophy of the gingivae, especially in children and young adults. This can be limited by good dental hygiene, including regular toothbrushing and flossing. If extensive, the hypertrophied gingival tissue may have to be surgically removed (gingivectomy), and phenytoin may have to be replaced by another antiepileptic drug.

Table 54-10

Nursing Assessment of the Client with Seizures

SUBJECTIVE DATA

History
Positive family history, previous seizures, birth defects or injuries, anoxic episodes; CNS trauma, tumors, or infections; hypertension and cerebrovascular disease; metabolic disorders, alcoholism; exposure to metals and carbon monoxide; hepatic, renal failure; fever; pregnancy, systemic lupus erythematosus

Medications
Compliance with antiseizure medications; barbiturate or alcohol withdrawal; use and overdose of cocaine, amphetamines, lidocaine, theophylline, penicillin, lithium, phenothiazines, tricyclic antidepressants

General
Weakness, fatigue, mood or behavioral changes hours or days before seizure

Pain
Headaches, muscle pain (postictal), abdominal pain

Gastrointestinal
Nausea and vomiting, diarrhea

Neurological
Frequency, duration, manifestations of seizures; aura; mentation changes

Muscular
Muscle soreness (postictal)

OBJECTIVE DATA

General
Precipitating factors, including severe metabolic acidosis or alkalosis, hyperkalemia, hypoglycemia, dehydration or water intoxication

OBJECTIVE DATA—cont'd

Integumentary
Bitter tongue, soft-tissue damage, cyanosis, diaphoresis (postictal)

Cardiovascular
Hypertension, tachycardia (ictal)

Gastrointestinal
Incontinence, gingival hyperplasia from phenytoin (Dilantin), excessive salivation

Urinary
Incontinence

Neurological
Generalized
Tonic-clonic: Loss of consciousness and postural tone, dilated pupils, hyperventilation, then apnea; possible airway occlusion; postictal phase
Absence: Altered consciousness (5 to 30 seconds), minor facial motor activity
Partial
Complex: Altered consciousness with inappropriate behaviors, automatisms, amnesia of event
Simple: Aura, consciousness, focal sensory, motor, cognitive, or emotional phenomena (focal motor); unilateral "marching" motor seizure (Jacksonian)

Musculoskeletal
Paresthesia or paralysis (postictal)

Possible findings
Positive toxic screen and high alcohol level; altered serum electrolytes; acidosis or alkalosis, very low blood glucose level, elevated blood urea nitrogen, serum creatinine, liver function tests, ammonia; abnormal CT or MRI of head, lumbar puncture; seizure activity on EEG

▪ Nursing Management of Seizures

Nursing assessment

Subjective and objective data that should be obtained from a person with a seizure disorder are presented in Table 54-10. Data related to a specific seizure episode can be obtained from a witness.

Nursing diagnoses

Nursing diagnoses are determined when the problem and the etiological factors are supported by clinical data. Nursing diagnoses related to seizures may include, but are not limited to, those presented in Table 54-11.

Nursing interventions

Health promotion and maintenance. Many cases of epilepsy can be prevented by promotion of general safety measures, such as wearing of helmets in situations involving risk of head injury. Improved prenatal, labor, and delivery care has reduced fetal trauma and hypoxia and thereby reduced brain damage leading to epilepsy. Children with fever should be treated quickly to avoid high temperatures, which may cause seizures.

Clients with epilepsy should practice good general health habits (proper diet, adequate rest, and exercise). They should be helped to identify events or situations that precipitate their seizures and should be given suggestions for avoiding them or handling them better. Clients should avoid excessive alcohol intake, fatigue, and loss of sleep. They should be helped to handle stress constructively.

Acute intervention. Nurses caring for hospitalized epileptic clients or clients who have had seizures as a result of metabolic factors have several responsibilities, including observation and treatment of the seizure, education, and psychosocial intervention. Table 54-11 summarizes the nursing care for the client with seizures.

When a seizure occurs, the nurse should carefully observe and record details of the event because the diagnosis and subsequent treatment often rest solely on the seizure description. All aspects of the seizure should be noted. What events preceded the seizure? When did the seizure occur? How long did each phase (aura, if any; ictus, or seizure; postictal period) last? What occurred during each

Table 54-11

NURSING CARE PLAN FOR THE CLIENT WITH SEIZURES

Defining Characteristics	Nursing Interventions	Evaluation Criteria

NURSING DIAGNOSIS: Ineffective breathing patterns related to neuromuscular impairment secondary to tonic phase of seizure or during postictal period

Abnormal respiratory rate, rhythm, or depth; nasal flaring; change in pulse (rate, rhythm, quality); dyspnea, shortness of breath; cyanosis, pallor, diaphoresis; absence of or abnormal breath sounds	Loosen constricting clothing. Assess breathing pattern, observing for labored respiration, tachypnea, bradypnea, dyspnea, apnea, cyanosis. Provide manual ventilation when necessary. Insert oral airway only after seizure activity has ceased. Administer oxygen when needed. Be prepared to assist with endotracheal intubation. Be prepared to obtain arterial blood gases.	Clear breath sounds, appropriate rate, rhythm, and depth

NURSING DIAGNOSIS: Ineffective airway clearance related to tracheobronchial obstruction

Ineffective cough, inability to remove secretions, absence of or abnormal breath sounds, abnormal respiratory rate, rhythm, or depth	Observe for signs of airway constriction. If vomiting occurs, turn client's head gently to side and remove as much vomitus as possible after the seizure. Suction airway if necessary. Administer oxygen when needed. Be prepared to assist with endotracheal intubation. Be prepared to obtain arterial blood gases. Establish and maintain patent airway.	Absence of airway obstruction, clear breath sounds

NURSING DIAGNOSIS: High risk for injury related to seizure activity and subsequent impaired physical mobility secondary to postictal weakness or paralysis

Trauma to mouth, cheek, tongue, lips; abrasions, bruises; broken bones; burns; drowning; weakness/ paralysis of one side of body (Todd paralysis), ataxia, fatigue, lethargy	Do not permit smoking in bed. If client has experienced frequent seizures recently, take axillary rather than oral temperature. If client anticipates a seizure may occur, assist to a safe location or position. Remain calm with client. Use seizure precautions as appropriate. Remove potentially harmful objects from surrounding area. Gently guide arm or leg movements to prevent injury during a seizure. Refrain from moving or restraining client during a seizure. Assist in determining whether operation of a motor vehicle or dangerous machinery is appropriate for client. Assist with activities of daily living as necessary after a seizure. Encourage mobility as tolerated. Provide information about the hazards of immobility.	Absence of injury, verbalization of knowledge of potential for injury during seizure

Modified from Santilli N and Sierzant TL: Advances in the treatment of epilepsy, J Neurosci Nurs 19:141-155, 1987.

Table 54-11

 NURSING CARE PLAN FOR THE CLIENT WITH SEIZURES—cont'd

Defining Characteristics	Nursing Interventions	Evaluation Criteria

NURSING DIAGNOSIS: **Impaired verbal communication related to transient aphasia secondary to postictal state**

Aphasia or dysphasia, dysarthria, confusion	Explain possible transient aphasia to client and family. Communicate in slow simple statements in postictal state. Provide written documentation of communication.	Evidence of adequate communication, achievement of needs

NURSING DIAGNOSIS: **Ineffective individual coping related to perceived loss of control, denial of diagnosis, or misconceptions regarding disease**

Verbalizations about not having epilepsy, lack of truth telling regarding seizure frequency, noncompliant behavior (driving or other high-risk behaviors in face of frequent seizures)	Explore reasons for denial. Implement and individualize teaching plan about causes and mechanisms of seizures, effectiveness of drugs in controlling seizures, inaccuracy of myths about epilepsy, avoidance of precipitating factors, state law regarding driving, pros and cons of medical ID tags, moderation in drinking and eating, exposure to stress, and avoidance of hazardous activities.	Acceptance of disorder as evidenced by using word *epilepsy* to describe illness and admitting seizures when they occur

NURSING DIAGNOSIS: **Self-concept disturbance related to diagnosis of epilepsy**

Anxiety, fear, social isolation, depression, role disturbance, altered family dynamics	Develop long-term plan to deal with developmental issues. Provide information about possible overprotection, community resources, and social stigmas that may be encountered. Assist client with explaining seizures and management to friends, school personnel, and employers. Advise client about employment counseling and job retraining. Discuss client's views about self in relation to seizures. Determine effect of seizures on daily activities and other activities important to client. Encourage client to focus on positive aspects of life. Provide information on referral to a neuropsychologist, psychologist, or social worker if indicated.	Sharing of feelings about diagnosis, identification of positive aspects about self, appropriate interactions with others, attainment and maintenance of high self-concept

NURSING DIAGNOSIS: **Altered health maintenance related to lack of knowledge about management of epilepsy**

Verbalization of deficiency in knowledge or skill, inaccurate perception of health status, failure to correctly perform desired or prescribed health behavior, noncompliance with prescribed health behavior, exhibition or expression of psychological alteration (e.g., anxiety, depression) resulting from misinformation or lack of information	Provide education about seizure activity and therapeutic management, including diagnosis and treatment, lifestyle adjustments, and community resources.	Demonstration by client and family of knowledge of health maintenance activities related to epilepsy, optimal seizure control, therapeutic drug levels, compliance with appointments and other recommendations

phase? Both subjective data (usually the only type of data in the aural phase) and objective data are important. Objective data should include the exact onset of the seizure (which body part was affected first and how), the course and nature of the seizure activity (loss of consciousness, tongue biting, automatisms, stiffening, jerking, total lack of muscle tone), what body parts were involved and in what sequence, and what autonomic signs were present (dilated pupils, excessive saliva, altered breathing, cyanosis, flushing, diaphoresis, incontinence). Assessment of the postictal period should include a detailed description of the level of consciousness, vital signs, memory loss, muscle soreness, speech disorders (aphasia, dysarthria), weakness or paralysis, sleep period, and the duration of each.

A seizure can be a frightening experience for the client and for others who may witness it. The nurse should assess the level of their understanding and provide information about how and why the event occurred. This is an excellent opportunity for the nurse to dispel many common misconceptions about seizures.

Chronic management. Prevention of recurring seizures is the major goal in the treatment of epilepsy. Because idiopathic epilepsy cannot be cured, medication must be taken regularly and continuously, often for a lifetime. The nurse should ensure that the client knows this, as well as the specifics of the medication regimen and what to do if a dose is missed. Usually the dose should be made up if the omission is remembered within 24 hours. The client should be cautioned not to adjust medications without professional guidance because this can increase seizure frequency and even cause status epilepticus. The client should be encouraged to report any medication side effects and to keep regular appointments with the health care provider.

Nurses should teach family members and significant others the first-aid treatment of tonic-clonic seizures. They should be reminded that it is not necessary to call an ambulance or send a person to the hospital after a single seizure unless the seizure is prolonged, another seizure immediately follows, or extensive injury has occurred.

Perhaps the greatest challenge that epilepsy presents to the client is adjusting to the personal limitations imposed by the illness. Discrimination in employment is the most serious problem facing the person with epilepsy. Clients can be informed that the Rehabilitation Act of 1973 was designed to protect handicapped persons (including those with epilepsy) from discrimination in employment. For issues relating to job discrimination, clients can be referred to the State Human Rights Commission or the State Department of Vocational Rehabilitation.

A variety of other resources can be offered to the client with epilepsy who has a specific problem. If the nurse believes that associating with others who have epilepsy can be beneficial, the client can be referred to the local chapter of the Epilepsy Foundation of America (EFA), a voluntary agency that offers a variety of services to clients with epilepsy. The client who is also a veteran can be referred to a Veterans Administration Hospital that provides comprehensive care.

The client should be informed that medical-alert brace-

lets, necklaces, and identification cards are available through the EFA, local pharmacies, or companies specializing in identification devices. However, the use of these medical identification tags is optional. Some clients have found them beneficial, but others have found them to be more a burden than a help because they prefer not to be identified as epileptic.

Social workers and welfare agencies can help with financial problems and living arrangements. The state services for those who have developmental disabilities can offer assistance with job placement and training for clients whose seizures are not well controlled. It can offer sheltered housing and provide funding for special needs, such as medical and psychological evaluation and transportation. State agencies specializing in vocational rehabilitation services can offer vocational assessment, counseling, funding for training, and assistance with job placement. They can also offer financial assistance for transportation and medical costs that are necessary for vocational rehabilitation or job maintenance. If intensive psychological counseling is needed, the nurse can refer the client to a community mental health center.

The client should be encouraged to learn more about epilepsy through self-education materials. The EFA provides several information pamphlets. Many agencies that offer services to epileptic persons, as well as local chapters of the organization, have these available as teaching aids.

MULTIPLE SCLEROSIS
Significance

Multiple sclerosis (MS) is a chronic, progressive, degenerative disorder of the CNS. This autoimmune disease affects 6 to 14 persons per 100,000 in the southern United States and 30 to 80 per 100,000 in the northern United States. It is considered a disease of young adults, with onset usually between 20 and 40 years of age. Women are affected more often than men.[1]

MS primarily affects white persons of northern European descent, which means that the disease is associated with certain environmental and familial factors. Incidence is highest in the temperate zones of the globe (between 45° and 65° latitude), especially northern Europe, Canada, and the northern United States. It is also associated with the place of birth. Someone born and raised in one of the regions listed who moves to a warmer climate (nearer the equator) after the age of 15 carries the same risk of MS as others in the country of origin. Blacks and Asians have a lower incidence of MS than whites.

As with many other immunologically mediated diseases, susceptibility to MS appears to be associated with certain major histocompatibility antigens (see Chapter 8). Human leukocyte antigen (HLA) studies in large groups of persons with MS show the existence of a genetic predisposition to the disease, primarily associated with DR2 and B7 antigens.[1]

The concept of precipitating factors is controversial. It is possible that their association with MS is pure chance. Possible precipitating factors include infection, physical injury, emotional stress, excessive fatigue, pregnancy, and lowered state of health.

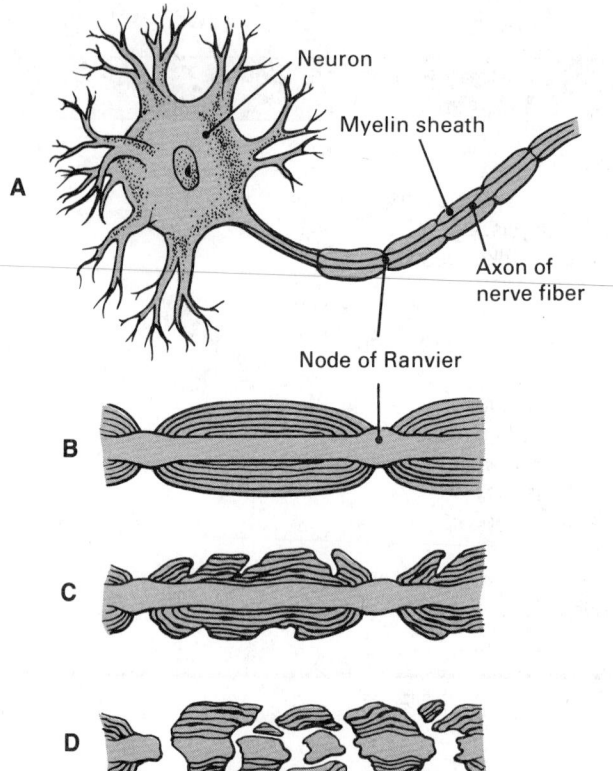

Fig. 54-1 **A,** Normal nerve cell with myelin sheath. **B,** Normal axon. **C,** Myelin breakdown. **D,** Myelin totally disrupted; axon not functioning.

Pathophysiology

MS is characterized by demyelination in the CNS. The primary neuropathological condition is an inflammatory demyelinating process that consists of loss of myelin, disappearance of oligodendrocytes (cells that make myelin), and the proliferation of astrocytes. These changes result in characteristic plaque formation, or sclerosis, scattered throughout multiple regions of the CNS. Initially the myelin sheaths of the neurons in the brain and spinal cord are attacked (Fig. 54-1, *A* and *B*). An inflammatory process accompanies the destruction of myelin. Early in the disease the myelin sheath is damaged, but the nerve fiber is not affected and nerve impulses are still transmitted (Fig. 54-1, *C*). At this point the client may complain of noticeable impairment of function (e.g., weakness). However, the myelin can regenerate and the symptoms can disappear, resulting in a remission.

As the disease progresses, the myelin becomes totally disrupted and the axon becomes involved (Fig. 54-1, *D*). Myelin is replaced by glial scar tissue, which forms hard, sclerotic plaques in multiple regions of the CNS. Without myelin, nerve impulses slow down, and with destruction of nerve axons, impulses are totally blocked, resulting in permanent loss of function. In many chronic lesions, demyelination continues with progressive loss of nerve function.

The disease process has a spotty distribution in the CNS. Therefore the signs and symptoms vary over time.

The disease is characterized by chronic progressive deterioration in some persons and by remissions and exacerbations in others. With repeated exacerbations, however, progressive scarring of myelin occurs, and the overall trend is progressive deterioration in neurological function.

Etiology

The basic cause is unknown, although research findings suggest MS is related to infectious (viral), immunological, and genetic factors. It is likely that the lesions in MS may be initiated by extrinsic factors (e.g., a viral agent) but perpetuated as a result of intrinsic factors (e.g., faulty immunoregulation). Autoantigens may be liberated from CNS tissue as a result of viral infection in persons who lack specific gene products to eliminate the virus and thus lead to the development of autoantibodies that react with normal white matter of the CNS.[9]

Whether the principal effector cells that mediate demyelination are T cells or macrophages is unknown. It is known that there is decreased T-suppressor cell activity in persons with active disease, especially before exacerbations. Demyelination in chronic, active plaques may be attributable to several immunological mechanisms.[9]

Clinical Manifestations

Because the onset is often insidious and gradual, with vague symptoms that occur intermittently over months or years, the disease may not be diagnosed until long after the onset of the first symptom. The clinical manifestations vary according to the areas of the CNS involved. Some clients have severe, long-lasting symptoms early in the course of the disease. Others may experience only occasional and mild symptoms for several years after onset.

Common signs and symptoms include motor, sensory, cerebellar, and emotional phenomena. Motor symptoms include weakness or paralysis of limbs, trunk, or head; diplopia; scanning speech; and spasticity of muscles that are chronically affected. Sensory symptoms include numbness and tingling and other paresthesias, patchy blindness (scotomas), blurred vision, vertigo, tinnitus, and decreased hearing. Cerebellar signs include nystagmus, ataxia, dysarthria, and dysphagia. Bowel and bladder function can be affected if the sclerotic plaque is located in areas of the CNS that control elimination. Problems with defecation usually involve constipation rather than fecal incontinence.

Urinary problems are variable. A common problem in MS clients is a spastic (uninhibited) bladder. This indicates a lesion above the second sacral nerve, which cuts off suprasegmental inhibiting influences on bladder contractility. As a result, the bladder has a small capacity for urine, and its contractions are unchecked. This is accompanied by urinary urgency and frequency and results in dribbling or incontinence. A flaccid (hypotonic) bladder indicates a lesion in the reflex arc governing bladder function. The bladder has a large capacity for urine because there is no sensation or desire to void, no pressure, and no pain. Consequently there is urinary retention, but urgency and frequency may also occur with this type of lesion. Urinary problems cannot be adequately diagnosed and treated unless urodynamic studies are done.

Sexual dysfunction occurs in many persons with MS.[10] Physiological impotence may result from spinal cord involvement in men. Women may experience decreased libido, difficulty with orgasmic response, painful intercourse, and decreased vaginal lubrication. Diminished sensation can prevent normal sexual response in both sexes. The emotional effects of chronic illness and loss of self-esteem also contribute to loss of sexual response.

Although intellectual functioning generally remains intact, emotional stability may be affected. Persons may be easily angered, depressed, or euphoric. Signs and symptoms of MS are aggravated or triggered by physical and emotional trauma, fatigue, and infection.

The average life expectancy after onset of symptoms is more than 25 years. The leading causes of death are related to respiratory and urinary infections and complications of decubitus ulcers. The life expectancy of persons with MS is about 80% that of the general population.

Diagnostic Studies

Because there is no definitive diagnostic test for MS, diagnosis is based primarily on history and clinical manifestations. Certain laboratory tests are currently used as adjuncts to the clinical examination. In some clients, CSF analysis may show an increase in lymphocytes during the active phase of the disease and an increase in oligoclonal immunoglobulin G (IgG). Sensory-evoked responses are often delayed in persons with MS because of decreased nerve conduction from the eye and the ear to the brain. CT scans and MRI may be helpful, since sclerotic plaques as small as 3 to 4 mm in diameter can be detected. Characteristic white-matter lesions scattered through the brain or spinal cord are evident on such scans.

Therapeutic Management

Because there is no cure for MS, therapeutic management is aimed at treating the disease process and providing symptomatic relief (Table 54-12). The disease process is treated with certain drugs and the symptoms are controlled with a variety of medications and other forms of therapy. Spasticity is primarily treated with antispasmodic drugs. However, surgery (e.g., neurectomy, rhizotomy, cordotomy) or dorsal-column electrical stimulation may be required. Intention tremor that becomes unmanageable with medication is sometimes treated by stereotactic surgery on the thalamus. This involves selective destruction of the ventrolateral nucleus in the thalamus. Neurological dysfunction sometimes improves with physical therapy, speech therapy, and hypothermia, which normalizes body temperature if it is above normal. Plasmapheresis for treating MS is currently under investigation at some medical centers (see Chapter 8).

Pharmacological Management

ACTH and prednisone are helpful in rapidly improving acute exacerbations, probably by reducing edema and acute inflammation at the site of demyelination. However, this does not necessarily affect the ultimate outcome or degree of residual neurological impairment from the attack. Immunosuppressive drugs, such as azathioprine (Imuran)

Table 54-12

Diagnostic and Therapeutic Management: Multiple Sclerosis

DIAGNOSTIC

History and physical examination
CSF analysis
Sensory-evoked response
CT scan, MRI scan

THERAPEUTIC

Drugs
  Antiinflammatory
  Immunosuppressive
  Anticholinergic
  Cholinergic
  Antispasmodic
Surgery
  Thalamotomy (unmanageable tremor)
  Neurectomy, rhizotomy, cordotomy (unmanageable spasticity)

CSF, Cerebrospinal fluid.

and cyclophosphamide (Cytoxan), have been tried, but they have not shown clear-cut beneficial effects in controlled studies. Table 54-13 summarizes the drugs that are commonly used for symptomatic treatment of MS.

Nutritional Considerations

Various nutritional measures that have been advocated in the management of MS include megavitamin therapy (vitamin B_{12}, vitamin C) and diets of high-fat, low-fat, and gluten-free food and raw food or vegetables. These particular dietary measures have not come into widespread use because of lack of proof of their effectiveness.

A nutritious, well-balanced diet is essential. Although there is no standard prescribed diet, a high-protein diet with supplementary vitamins is often advocated. A diet high in roughage may help relieve the problem of constipation. Vitamins are merely supplemental and not curative.

■ Nursing Management of Multiple Sclerosis

Nursing assessment

Subjective and objective data that should be obtained from a person with multiple sclerosis are presented in Table 54-14.

Nursing diagnoses

Nursing diagnoses are determined when the problem and the etiological factors are supported by clinical data. Nursing diagnoses related to MS may include, but are not limited to, those listed in Table 54-15.

Nursing interventions

Acute intervention. The most common reasons for hospitalization of the client with MS are diagnostic workup and treatment of an acute exacerbation of complications such as bladder dysfunction. During the diagnostic phase

Table 54-13 Drugs for Symptomatic Treatment of Multiple Sclerosis

Drug	Symptoms Relieved	Precautions	Side Effects	Educational Needs
CORTICOSTEROIDS				
ACTH, prednisone, dexamethasone, hydrocortisone	Exacerbations	Widespread effects on many enzymes and metabolic processes, few adverse effects with use for less than 1 month at a time	Edema, mental changes (euphoria), weight gain, redistribution of body fat*	Restrict salt intake. Do not abruptly stop therapy. Know drug interactions.
CHOLINERGICS				
Bethanicol chloride (Urecholine), neostigmine methylsulfate (Prostigmine)	Urinary retention (flaccid bladder)	History of hypotension, cardiac dysfunction, allergies, hyperthyroidism, stomach and intestinal problems; contraindication with adrenergic drugs (antiasthmatic drugs) because of possible induction of serious asthma attack (urecholine only)	Hypotension, diarrhea, diaphoresis, salivation, muscle weakness	Consult physician before using other drugs.
ANTICHOLINERGICS				
Propantheline bromide (Pro-Banthine), oxybutynin chloride (Ditropan)	Urinary frequency† and urgency (spastic bladder)	History of glaucoma, prostatic hypertrophy, cardiac dysfunction, intestinal obstruction	Dry mouth, blurred vision, constipation, hypertension, flushing, urinary retention (too high of dose)	Consult physician before using other drugs, especially sleeping aids, antihistamines (possibly leading to potentiated effect).
MUSCLE RELAXANTS				
Diazepam (Valium)	Spasticity	History of narrow-angle glaucoma	Drowsiness, ataxia, fatigue	Avoid driving and similar activities because of CNS-depressant effects. Be aware of addictive potential; avoid long-term use. Avoid concomitant use of phenothiazines, narcotics, barbiturates, MAO inhibitors, other antidepressants.
Baclofen (Lioresal)	Spasticity	History of hypersensitivity and renal damage, contraindication in pregnancy, possible exacerbation of seizures in clients with epilepsy	Drowsiness	Do not abruptly stop therapy (possibly leading to hallucinations). Avoid driving and similar activities because of sedative effect. Avoid use with other CNS depressants; take with food or milk.

*See Chapter 42 for effects of long-term steroid therapy.
†Urodynamic studies must be done before institution of therapy because clients with MS have multiple lesions and type of bladder dysfunction cannot be diagnosed from symptoms alone.

Continued.

Table 54-13 Drugs for Symptomatic Treatment of Multiple Sclerosis—cont'd

Drug	Symptoms Relieved	Precautions	Side Effects	Educational Needs
MUSCLE RELAXANTS—cont'd				
Dantrolene (Dantrium)	Spasticity	History of respiratory or cardiac dysfunction, possible induction of abnormal liver function or hepatitis, contraindication with estrogen therapy because of predisposition to hepatotoxicity	Drowsiness, dizziness, malaise, fatigue, diarrhea	Avoid driving. Avoid use with tranquilizers and alcohol (possibly causing photosensitivity).

Table 54-14

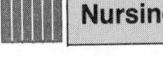 **Nursing Assessment of the Client with Multiple Sclerosis**

SUBJECTIVE DATA

History
Positive family history, ethnicity, recent or past viral infections or vaccinations, residence in cold or temperate climates, recent physical or emotional stress, pregnancy, infections, exposure to heat
Medications
Use of and compliance in taking steroids (e.g., ACTH, prednisone), immunosuppressants, anticholinergics, muscle relaxants
General
Weakness and fatigue aggravated by heat, weight loss, vertigo, mood swings
Pain
Eye, back, legs, joint pain; painful muscle spasms
Gastrointestinal
Dysphagia, constipation, difficulty in chewing
Urinary
Frequency, urgency, retention
Reproductive
Impotence, decreased libido

SUBJECTIVE DATA—cont'd

Neurological
Tingling and numbness, blurred or lost vision, diplopia
Musculoskeletal
Generalized muscular weakness

OBJECTIVE DATA

General
Apathy, inattentiveness
Integumentary
Pressure sores
Neurological
Scanning speech, nystagmus, ataxia, tremor, spasticity, hyperreflexia, tinnitus and decreased hearing, poor coordination
Musculoskeletal
Muscular weakness, paresis, paralysis, spasms, foot dragging, dysarthria
Possible findings
Reduction in T-suppressor cells, demyelinating lesions on CT and MRI scans, increased lymphocytes and IgG on examination of cerebrospinal fluid

the nurse has an important role in reassuring the client that even though there is a tentative diagnosis of MS, certain diagnostic studies must be made to rule out other neurological disorders. The nurse needs to assist the client in dealing with the anxiety caused by a diagnosis of disabling illness. Clients with recently diagnosed MS may need assistance with the grieving process.

During an acute exacerbation the client is often immobile and confined to bed for 2 to 3 weeks. The focus of nursing intervention at this phase is to prevent major hazards of immobility, such as respiratory and urinary tract infections and decubitus ulcers (for specific measures, see Table 54-15).

Chronic management. Chronic management is aimed at (1) helping the client adjust to the illness, (2) teaching how to avoid factors that precipitate exacerbations, (3) maximizing self-care in light of current neurological deficits, and (4) meeting the needs for activities of daily living. The main goal is to keep the client active and maximally functional.

Physical therapy is an important measure for keeping the client as functionally active as possible. The purpose of therapy is to relieve spasticity, increase coordination, and train the client to substitute nonaffected muscles for impaired ones. An especially beneficial type of physical therapy is water exercise (Fig. 54-2). Water gives buoy-

Table 54-15

 NURSING CARE PLAN FOR THE CLIENT WITH MULTIPLE SCLEROSIS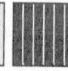

Defining Characteristics	Nursing Interventions	Evaluation Criteria

NURSING DIAGNOSIS: Ineffective airway clearance related to impaired ability to cough

Ineffective cough, inability to remove secretions, abnormal breath sounds, dyspnea, shortness of breath	Encourage and assist with coughing and deep breathing q 4 hr while client is awake. Turn client at least q 2 hr. Protect from infectious illnesses of clients, staff, family. Have client in upright position for eating.	Absence of infections, clear breath sounds, effective cough

NURSING DIAGNOSIS: Impaired physical mobility related to muscle weakness or paralysis and muscle spasticity

Weakness or paralysis, inability to ambulate, intermittent muscle spasms, pain associated with muscle spasms	Use assistive devices as indicated. Do range-of-motion exercises at least bid. Encourage and assist with ambulation and transfer as indicated. Change position of client, if bedridden, at least q 2 hr. Administer medication as ordered. Perform stretching exercises every shift.	Demonstration of use of adaptive devices to increase mobility and minimize potential for injury, maintenance or increase of strength of unaffected limbs, decreased duration of muscle spasms

NURSING DIAGNOSIS: Self-care deficit related to muscle spasticity and uncompensated neuromuscular deficits

Inability to perform some or all activities of daily living	Assess self-care problems. Promote use of appropriate assistive devices. Counsel regarding need for homemaker services. Perform or assist with activities of daily living only as indicated. Encourage independence when appropriate.	Optimal level of functioning

NURSING DIAGNOSIS: High risk for impaired skin integrity related to immobility, sensorimotor deficits, and inadequate nutrition

Red skin, open sores	Assess skin every shift. Turn client at least q 2 hr. Keep bed free of crumbs. Use circular massage of bony prominences with each turning. Provide high-protein diet. Cleanse back and buttocks if client is incontinent.	Skin intact and free of redness

NURSING DIAGNOSIS: Sensory/perceptual alteration related to visual disturbances

Blurred vision, decreased visual acuity, visual field defects, diplopia	Orient client to environment. Patch eyes q 4 hr. Assess visual acuity monthly. Maintain safe environment— side rails up, bed in low position. Indicate visual impairment on chart, Kardex, and over bed.	Satisfactory visual function for activities of daily living with minimal risk of injury

NURSING DIAGNOSIS: Altered patterns of urinary elimination (retention) related to sensorimotor deficits and/or inadequate fluid intake

Posturination residual > 50 ml, dribbling, bladder distention	Administer medications as ordered. Follow intermittent catheterization protocol. Use Credé's maneuver or reflex stimulation (manual stimulation). Monitor fluid intake of 3000 ml/day. Teach client signs and symptoms of urinary tract infection.	Urination each shift with residual < 50 ml

Continued.

Table 54-15

 NURSING CARE PLAN FOR THE CLIENT WITH MULTIPLE SCLEROSIS—cont'd

Defining Characteristics	Nursing Interventions	Evaluation Criteria
NURSING DIAGNOSIS: Altered patterns of urinary elimination (incontinence) related to sensorimotor deficits and/or possible urinary tract infection		
Incontinence, urgency, frequency	Administer medications as ordered. Initiate bladder-training program. Ensure that client is protected and will not be embarrassed by incontinence. Assess for urinary tract infection. Monitor fluid intake of 3000 ml/day.	Urinary continence
NURSING DIAGNOSIS: Constipation related to immobility, inadequate fluid intake, improper diet, and neuromuscular impairment		
Hard and formed stool, decreased bowel sounds, infrequent or absent bowel movements, feelings of rectal fullness, straining and pain on defecation, palpable impaction	Turn client regularly. Maintain activity to individual tolerance. Maintain fluid intake (3000 ml/day). Use prune juice at some time of day. Encourage high-residue diet. Administer stool softeners, suppositories as ordered. Initiate and maintain bowel program.	Return and maintenance of usual bowel habits
NURSING DIAGNOSIS: Sexual dysfunction related to uncompensated neuromuscular deficits		
Impotence, verbalization of problem, dissatisfaction with sex role, limitations on sexual performance, decreased libido	Initiate sexual counseling if indicated. Suggest alternative methods of sexual gratification.	Perception of satisfactory sexual functioning
NURSING DIAGNOSIS: Self-concept disturbance related to prolonged debilitating condition		
Feelings of inadequacy, depression, fatigue	Focus on remaining abilities and maintaining independence. Assist client in grieving process.	Maintenance of realistic self-concept in relation to disease
NURSING DIAGNOSIS: Altered family processes related to changing family roles, potential financial problems, and fluctuating physical condition		
Strained family relations, ineffective communication, verbalization of financial concerns	Facilitate open communication among family members. Promote problem-solving. Refer for family and financial counseling, if indicated. Educate family regarding fluctuating nature of disease.	Open communication among family members, seeking of outside assistance when indicated, maintenance of adequate care of ill member

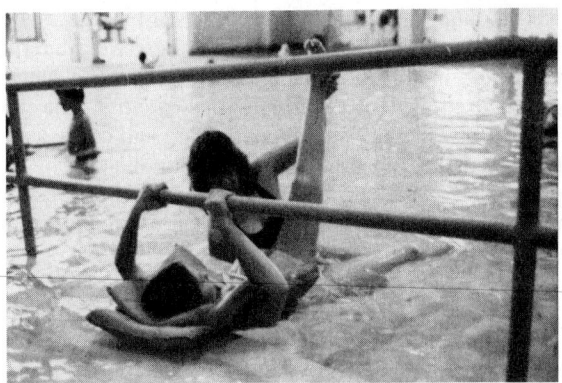

Fig. 54-2 Water therapy provides exercise and recreation for the client with a chronic neurological disease.

ancy to the body and allows the client to perform activities that would normally be impossible. In water the client experiences more control over the body.

Client education should focus on building general resistance to illness. This includes avoiding fatigue, extremes of heat and cold, and exposure to infection. The last factor involves avoiding exposure to ill persons and cold climates, as well as vigorous and early treatment of infection when it does occur. It is important to teach the client to (1) achieve a good balance of exercise and rest, (2) eat nutritious and well-balanced meals, and (3) avoid the hazards of immobility (contractures and pressure sores). Clients should know their treatment regimens, the side effects of medications and how to watch for them, and drug interactions with over-the-counter medications. The client should consult a health care provider before taking nonprescription medications.

The client with MS and the family must make many emotional adjustments because of the unpredictability of the disease, the need to change lifestyles, and the challenge of avoiding or decreasing precipitating factors. The National Multiple Sclerosis Society and its local chapters can offer a variety of services to meet the needs of clients with MS.

PARKINSON'S DISEASE

Parkinsonism is a syndrome that consists of slowness in the initiation and execution of movement (bradykinesia), increased muscle tonus (rigidity), tremor, and impaired postural reflexes. Parkinson's disease, a form of parkinsonism, is named after James Parkinson, who in 1817 wrote a classic essay on "shaking palsy," a disease whose cause is still unknown today. Many other disorders resemble this disease, but their causes are known. These include drug-induced parkinsonism, postencephalitic parkinsonism, and arteriosclerotic parkinsonism. The pathophysiology of these disorders, with the exception of drug-induced parkinsonism, is the same. There is injury or impairment of the dopamine-producing cells of the substantia nigra in the midbrain. The substantia nigra is part of the extrapyramidal system, which influences the initiation, modulation, and completion of movement and regulates unconscious automatic movements (see Chapter 50). In cases of drug-

induced parkinsonism the dopamine receptors in the brain are blocked.

Significance

About 500,000 persons in the United States have Parkinson's disease. About 1% of the population over the age of 50 years is affected.[1] The disease shows no gender, socioeconomic, or cultural preference, and symptoms most commonly occur after the age of 50. The average age of the client with Parkinson's disease is 65 years. There is no apparent genetic cause and no known cure. The disease rarely occurs in the black population.

Etiology and Pathophysiology

There are many causes of parkinsonism. Encephalitis lethargica, or type A encephalitis, has been clearly associated with the onset of parkinsonism. However, the incidence of postencephalitic parkinsonism has dwindled since the 1920s, when there was a large outbreak of this infectious illness. Parkinsonlike symptoms have followed intoxication with a variety of chemicals, including carbon monoxide and manganese (among copper miners) and an analogue of meperidine (MPTP). Drug-induced parkinsonism can follow reserpine, methyldopa, haloperidol, and phenothiazine therapy. Although clients with cerebrovascular disease may have parkinsonlike symptoms, there is little evidence that parkinsonism is caused by arteriosclerosis. Distinguishing arteriosclerosis from true Parkinson's disease is important for prognostic purposes. Clients with the former do not respond as well to treatment and are more likely to experience side effects of drug therapy. Most clients with parkinsonism have the degenerative or idiopathic form, for which the term *Parkinson's disease* is usually reserved.

The pathology of Parkinson's disease is associated with degeneration of the dopamine-producing neurons in the substantia nigra of the midbrain (Fig. 54-3). It is hypothesized that there is normally a balance between the effects of acetylcholine (ACh) and dopamine in the basal ganglia. Any shift in the balance of activity (increase in effects of ACh or decrease in effects of dopamine) seems to lead to parkinsonlike symptoms. Dopamine is a neurotransmitter that is essential for normal functioning of the extrapyramidal system, including control of posture, support, and voluntary motion. Levels of enzymes and dopamine metabolites are reduced. Postmortem cross sections of the midbrain show loss of the normal melanin pigment in the substantia nigra and loss of nerve cells there and elsewhere in the brain. In addition, deficient amounts of gamma-aminobutyric acid, serotonin, and norepinephrine have been found in the basal ganglia as well as in the substantia nigra.

Clinical Manifestations

The onset of Parkinson's disease is gradual and insidious, with a gradual progression and a prolonged course. In the beginning stages, only a mild tremor, a slight limp, or a decreased arm swing may be evident. Later in the disease the client may have a shuffling, propulsive gait with arms flexed and loss of postural reflexes. In some persons

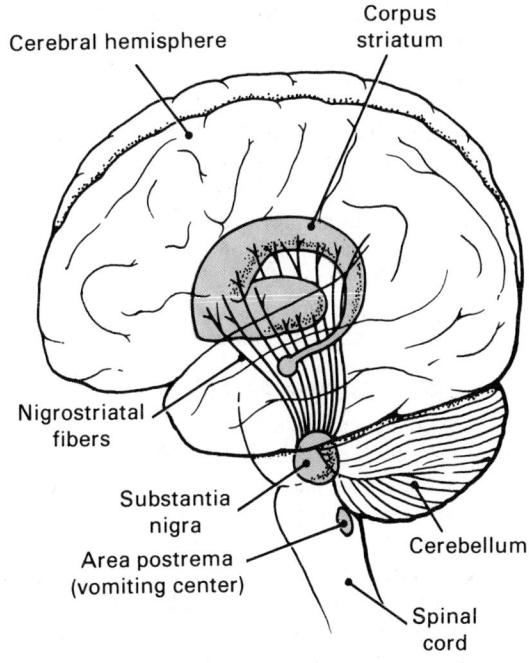

Fig. 54-3 Left-sided view of the human brain showing the substantia nigra and the corpus striatum *(shaded area)* lying deep within the cerebral hemisphere. Nerve fibers extend upward from the substantia nigra, divide into many branches, and carry dopamine to all regions of the corpus striatum.

there may be a slight change in speech patterns. None of these alone is sufficient evidence for a diagnosis of the disease.

Because there is no specific diagnostic test for Parkinson's disease, the diagnosis is based solely on the history and the clinical features. A firm diagnosis can be made only when there are at least two of the three characteristic signs of the classic triad: tremor, rigidity, and bradykinesia (slow or retarded movement). Although dementia occurs in up to 40% of persons with Parkinson's disease, intellectual impairment does not occur in the majority of clients.[11] The ultimate confirmation of Parkinson's disease is a positive response to antiparkinsonian medication.

Tremor. Tremor, often the first sign, may be minimal initially, so the client is the only one who notices it. This tremor can affect handwriting, causing it to become smaller, particularly toward the end of words *(micrographia)*. Parkinsonian tremor is more prominent at rest and is aggravated by emotional stress or increased concentration. The hand tremor is described as "pill rolling" because the thumb and forefinger appear to move in a rotary fashion as if rolling a pill, coin, or other small object. Tremor can involve the diaphragm, tongue, lips, and jaw but rarely causes shaking of the head. Unfortunately, in many persons a benign essential tremor has mistakenly been diagnosed as Parkinson's disease. Essential tremor occurs during voluntary movement, has a more rapid frequency than Parkinsonian tremor, and is familial.

Rigidity. Rigidity, the second sign of the triad, is increased resistance to passive motion when the limbs are moved through their range of motion. Parkinsonian rigidity is typified by a jerky quality, as if there were intermittent catches in the movement of a cogwheel, when the joint is moved. This is called *cogwheel rigidity*. The rigidity is due to sustained muscle contraction and consequently elicits a complaint of muscle soreness, tired and achy feelings, or pain in the head, upper body, spine, or legs. Another consequence of rigidity is slowness of movement, since it inhibits the smooth alternation of contraction and relaxation in opposing muscle groups (e.g., the biceps and triceps).

Bradykinesia. Bradykinesia is particularly evident in the loss of automatic movements, which is secondary to the physical and chemical alteration of the basal ganglia and related structures in the extrapyramidal portion of the CNS. In the unaffected client, automatic movements are involuntary and occur subconsciously. They include blinking of the eyelids, swinging of the arms while walking, swallowing of saliva, self-expression with facial and hand movements, and minor movements of postural adjustment. The client with Parkinson's disease does not execute these movements, and there is a lack of spontaneous activity. This accounts for the stooped posture, masked facies ("deadpan" expression), drooling of saliva, and shuffling gait *(festination)* that are characteristic of a person with this disease. In addition, there is difficulty initiating movement. Movements such as getting out of a chair cannot be executed unless they are consciously willed.

Complications

Many of the complications of Parkinson's disease are caused by the decomposition and loss of spontaneity of movement. Swallowing may become very difficult (dysphagia) in severe cases, leading to malnutrition or aspiration. General debilitation may lead to pneumonia, urinary tract infections, and skin breakdown. Mobility is greatly decreased. The gait slows, and turning is especially difficult. The gait is usually composed of rapid, short, shuffling ministeps. The posture is that of the "old man" image, with the head and trunk bent forward and the legs constantly flexed (Fig. 54-4). The lack of mobility may lead to constipation, ankle edema, and, more seriously, contractures. Orthostatic hypotension may occur in some persons, and along with loss of postural reflexes, may result in falls or other injury. Bothersome complications include seborrhea (increased oily secretion of the sebaceous glands of the skin), dandruff, excessive sweating, conjunctivitis, difficulty in reading, insomnia, incontinence, and depression.

Many of the apparent complications of Parkinson's disease are due to side effects of medication, particularly levodopa. Dyskinesias (e.g., athetosis of the neck) and weakness and akinesia (total immobility) may cause problems. These complications become apparent after prolonged levodopa therapy when the therapeutic index decreases.

Therapeutic Management

Because there is no cure for Parkinson's disease, therapeutic management (Table 54-16) is aimed at relieving the symptoms. Antiparkinsonian drugs either enhance dopa-

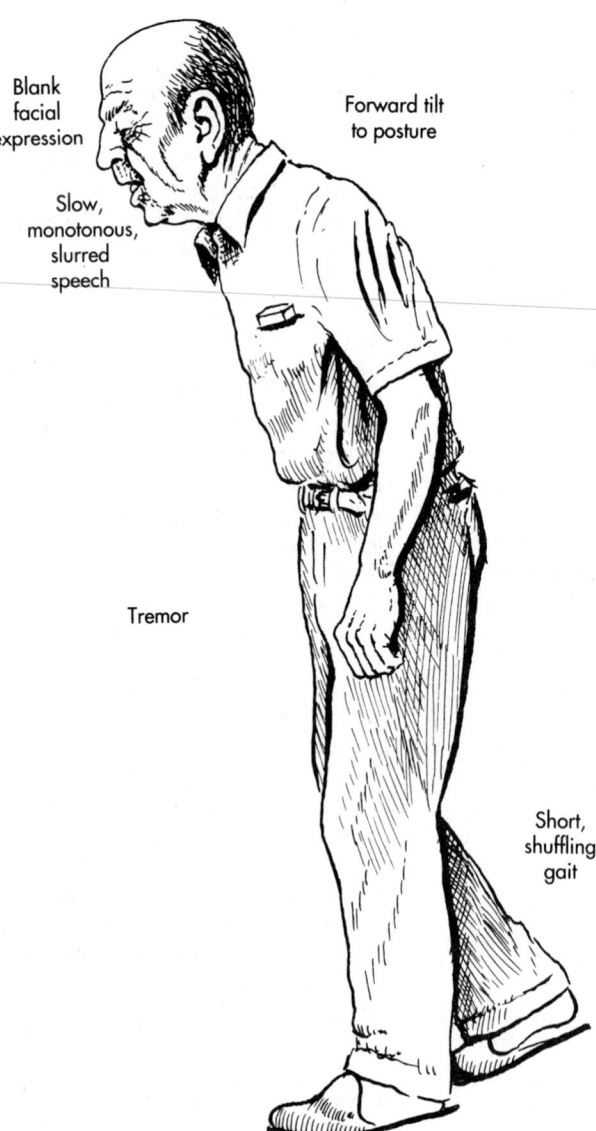

Blank facial expression

Forward tilt to posture

Slow, monotonous, slurred speech

Tremor

Short, shuffling gait

Fig. 54-4 Characteristic appearance of client with Parkinson's disease. (From Rudy E: Advanced neurological and neurosurgical nursing, St Louis, 1984, The CV Mosby Co, p 269.)

mine secretion or supply (dopaminergic) or antagonize or block the effects of the overactive cholinergic neurons in the striatum (anticholinergic).

The only other treatment for Parkinson's disease is cryothalamectomy or stereotaxic thalamotomy for correction of severe unilateral tremor. Surgical treatment is most effective in younger clients. The greater risk of complications and residual neurological deficits preclude the use of this treatment in older clients with more severe disease. Because the long-term benefits of surgery vary, the role of surgical intervention is limited.

Transplantation of adrenal tissue into the caudate nucleus in an attempt to provide viable dopamine-producing cells to the brain has had disappointing results.[12] The use of fetal tissue for this same purpose has promise. However, the use of federal funds for this type of research has been banned.

Table 54-16

Diagnostic and Therapeutic Management: Parkinson's Disease

DIAGNOSTIC

History
Physical examination
  Tremor
  Rigidity
  Bradykinesia
Positive response to antiparkinsonian medication*
Ruling out of side effects of phenothiazines, reserpine, benzodiazepines, haloperidol

THERAPEUTIC

Antiparkinsonian medication
Surgical destruction of ventrolateral nucleus of the thalamus

*See Table 54-17.

Pharmacological Management

Pharmacotherapy of Parkinson's disease is aimed at correcting an imbalance of neurotransmitters within the CNS characterized by relative dopamine deficiency and ACh excess in the corpus striatum. Levodopa with carbidopa (Sinemet) is often the first drug to be used. Levodopa is a precursor of dopamine and can cross the blood-brain barrier. It is converted to dopamine in the basal ganglia. Sinemet is the preferred drug in the biochemical sense because it contains carbidopa, an agent that inhibits the enzyme dopa-decarboxylase (which breaks down L-dopa before it reaches the brain). The net result is that more L-dopa reaches the brain, and therefore less drug is needed. Bromocriptine activates dopamine receptors and has antiparkinsonian properties. It may be used as an adjuvant drug. In addition to these major drug types, antihistamines are sometimes used to relieve tremor and rigidity. The antiviral agent amantadine (Symmetrel) is also an effective antiparkinsonian drug, although its mechanism of action is not known. A new drug, selegiline (Eldepryl), has been reported by some to delay the progression of early Parkinson's disease.[13] However, other clinicians have reported less encouraging results.[14] Table 54-17 summarizes the drugs commonly used in Parkinson's disease, the symptoms they relieve, and their common side effects. The use of only one drug is preferred, since there are fewer side effects and the medication is easier to adjust than when several drugs are used. Excessive amounts of dopaminergic drugs can lead to paradoxical intoxication (aggravation rather than relief of symptoms). Anticholinergic drugs may cause impaired erection and failure of ejaculation.

Nutritional Considerations

Diet is of major importance to the client with Parkinson's disease because malnutrition and constipation can be serious consequences of inadequate nutrition. Clients who have dysphagia and bradykinesia need appetizing foods

Table 54-17 Drugs for Symptomatic Treatment of Parkinsonism

Drug	Symptoms Relieved	Side Effects and Precautions
Dopaminergic		
Levodopa (L-dopa)	Bradykinesia, tremor, rigidity	Nausea, dyskinesia, hypotension, palpitations, dysrhythmias; agitation, hallucinations, confusion (in older clients); avoidance of vitamin pills and diet high in vitamin B_6 (reversal of effect of levodopa); contraindication with narrow-angle glaucoma
Levodopa/carbidopa (Sinemet)	Bradykinesia, tremor, rigidity	Less nausea but greater chance of dyskinesia, confusion, hallucinations; periodic check of BUN, SGOT, WBCs, Hct; contraindications of melanoma, narrow-angle glaucoma, combination with MAO inhibitors, reserpine, methyldopa, guanethidine, antipsychotics
Bromocriptine mesylate (Parlodel)	Bradykinesia, tremor, rigidity	Orthostatic hypotension, nausea, vomiting, toxic psychosis, limb edema, phlebitis, dizziness, headache, insomnia
Amantadine (Symmetrel)	Rigidity, akinesia	Nervousness, insomnia, confusion, hallucinations, dry mouth, nausea, edema, orthostatic hypotension
Anticholinergic		
Trihexyphenidyl (Artane), cycrimine (Pagitane), procyclidine (Kemadrin), benztropine mesylate (Cogentin), biperiden (Akineton)	Tremor	Dry mouth, blurred vision, constipation, delirium, anxiety, agitation, hallucinations; avoidance of drugs with similar actions, including over-the-counter drugs containing scopolamine or antihistamines (e.g., Sominex), antispasmodics (e.g., Donnatal, Bellergal), tricyclic antidepressants (Tofranil, Elavil, Norpramin, Vivactil)
Antihistaminic		
Diphenhydramine (Benadryl), orphenadrine (Disipal), chlorphenoxamine (Phenoxene), phenindamine (Thephorin)	Tremor, rigidity	Sedation, same precautions as for anticholinergic drugs
MAO-B inhibitor		
Selegiline (Eldepryl)	Bradykinesia, rigidity, tremor	Similar to dopaminergic drugs

BUN, Blood urea nitrogen; *SGOT,* serum glutamic-oxaloacetic transaminase; *WBCs,* white blood cells; *Hct,* hematocrit.

that are easily chewed and swallowed. The diet should contain adequate roughage and fruit to avoid constipation. Food should be cut into bite-sized pieces *before* it is served, and it should be served on a warmed plate to preserve its appeal. Eating six small meals a day may be less exhausting than eating three large meals a day. Ample time should be planned for eating to avoid frustration and encourage independence.

■ Nursing Management of Parkinson's Disease

Nursing assessment

Subjective and objective data that should be obtained from a person with Parkinson's disease are presented in Table 54-18.

Nursing diagnoses

When the problem and the etiological factors are supported by clinical data, nursing diagnoses can be determined. Nursing diagnoses related to Parkinson's disease may include, but are not limited to, those in Table 54-19.

Nursing interventions

Promotion of physical exercise and a well-balanced diet are major concerns for nursing care. Exercise can limit the consequences of decreased mobility such as muscle atrophy, contractures, and constipation. The American Parkinson's Disease Association publishes a booklet, *Home Exercises for Patients with Parkinson's Disease*, that illustrates a variety of exercises; it can be used by family members as well as health professionals.

Table 54-18

Nursing Assessment of the Client with Parkinson's Disease

SUBJECTIVE DATA	OBJECTIVE DATA
History	*General*
CNS trauma, cerebrovascular disorders, syphilis, exposure to metals and carbon monoxide, encephalitis	Blank (masked) facies, slow and monotonous speech, infrequent blinking
Medication	*Integumentary*
Use of major tranquilizers, especially haloperidol (Haldol) and phenothiazines, reserpine, methyldopa	Seborrhea
General	*Cardiovascular*
Depression, nervousness, mood swings, weight loss, fatigue	Postural hypotension
Pain	*Gastrointestinal*
Diffuse pain in legs, shoulders, neck, back, and hips; muscle soreness and cramping	Drooling
Integumentary	*Neurological*
Excessive sweating	Tremor at rest, first in hands (pill-rolling), later in legs, arms, face, and tongue; aggravation of tremor with anxiety, absence in sleep; shuffling gait; poor coordination; subtle dementia
Gastrointestinal	*Musculoskeletal*
Excessive salivation, dysphagia, constipation	"Cogwheel" rigidity, dysarthria, bradykinesia, contractures, stooped posture
Neurological	*Possible findings*
Handwriting deterioration (micrographia), loss of dexterity	Lack of specific tests, diagnosis on basis of history and physical findings
Musculoskeletal	
Difficulty in initiation of movements, frequent falls	

Table 54-19

NURSING CARE PLAN FOR THE CLIENT WITH PARKINSON'S DISEASE

Defining Characteristics	Nursing Interventions	Evaluation Criteria
NURSING DIAGNOSIS: Impaired physical mobility related to rigidity, tremor, bradykinesia, and akinesia		
Rigidity, tremor, bradykinesia, akinesia, cogwheeling, difficulty in initiation of volitional movements, shuffling gait	Assist with ambulation. Perform range-of-motion exercises to all extremities. Consult physical therapist or occupational therapist for aids to facilitate activities of daily living and safe ambulation. Evaluate tremor in relation to medication. Assist with fine and gross motor activities as needed. Teach aides to assist with mobility by instructing client to step over imaginary line, rock from side to side to initiate leg movement. Remove environmental barriers.	Maximal safe ambulation, maintenance of joint mobility
NURSING DIAGNOSIS: Self-care deficit related to parkinsonian symptoms		
Inability to perform activities of daily living, need for assistive devices	Encourage client's independence with activities of daily living within limits of mobility. Arrange client's room for optimal self-care. Establish time frame to allow client to complete care. Provide assistance as needed. Arrange occupational therapy consultation. Offer emotional support.	Optimal independence in activities of daily living

Modified from Lannon MC and others: Comprehensive care of the patient with Parkinson's disease, J Neurosci Nurs 18:122-131, 1986.

Continued.

Table 54-19

 NURSING CARE PLAN FOR THE CLIENT WITH PARKINSON'S DISEASE—cont'd

Defining Characteristics	Nursing Interventions	Evaluation Criteria
NURSING DIAGNOSIS: Impaired verbal and written communication related to dysarthria and tremor or bradykinesia, respectively		
Decreased volume, slow and slurred speech, inability to move facial muscles, decreased tongue mobility, micrographia, inability to write	Allow sufficient time for communication. Assist with diaphragmatic speech. Encourage deep breaths before speaking. Consult speech therapist. Provide alternative communication methods. Massage client's facial and neck muscles.	Development of method of communication to meet needs
NURSING DIAGNOSIS: Constipation related to immobility		
Hardened and formed stool, decreased bowel sounds, reported discomfort, nausea, decreased appetite	Increase fluid intake to 3 L/day. Increase fiber in diet with every meal. Increase mobility to tolerance. Give stool softeners, laxatives, suppositories as needed.	Return and maintenance of usual bowel habits
NURSING DIAGNOSIS: Sleep pattern disturbance related to medication side effects (hallucinations), anxiety, rigidity, and muscle discomfort		
Poor sleep history, inability to sleep uninterrupted, nightmares, vivid dreams or hallucinations, anxiety, rigidity or muscle discomfort	Provide quiet environment for sleep. Turn and position client for comfort. Provide passive range-of-motion exercises to extremities to alleviate rigidity. Provide daytime stimulus to maintain wakefulness. Offer support if hallucinations are present to decrease anxiety. Give sleep medications as ordered.	Verbalization of feeling rested on awakening
NURSING DIAGNOSIS: Altered nutrition: less than body requirements related to dysphagia		
Difficulty in swallowing and chewing, inadequate secretion clearance, drooling, decreased gag reflex	Carefully monitor swallowing ability during medication administration and mealtime. Report any difficulty to physician. Provide soft-solid and thick-liquid diet; avoid thin liquids. Massage client's facial and neck muscles before meals. Maintain client in upright position for all meals. Consult speech therapist and dietitian. Maintain caloric counts and weekly weights. Provide tonsil tip suction for increased secretions.	Maintenance of nutritional status and body weight
NURSING DIAGNOSIS: Activity intolerance related to rigidity, tremor, and immobility		
Boredom, lack of participation, restlessness, depression, hostility	Encourage ventilation of feelings. Determine preferred diversional activities. Adapt difficult activities when possible. Initiate new feasible activities such as reading. Be creative.	Engagement in diversional activities, verbalization of feelings

Modified from Lannon MC and others: Comprehensive care of the patient with Parkinson's disease, J Neurosci Nurs 18:122-131, 1986.

A physical therapist may be consulted to design an exercise program aimed at strengthening muscles. Overall muscle tone as well as specific exercises to strengthen muscles involved with speaking and swallowing should be included. Although exercise will not halt the progress of the disease, it will bring the client's motor function to an optimal level.

Because Parkinson's disease is a chronic degenerative disorder with no acute exacerbations, nurses should note that health teaching and nursing care are directed toward maintenance of good health, encouragement of independence, and avoidance of complications such as contractures.

Problems secondary to bradykinesia can be alleviated by relatively simple measures. The following are helpful hints for clients who tend to "freeze" while walking: consciously think about stepping over imaginary or real lines on the floor, drop rice kernels and step over them, rock from side to side, lift the toes when stepping, take one step backward and two steps forward. The client should be assessed for the possibility of L-dopa overdose because it is a common cause of akinesia ("freezing"). A brief period of dyskinesia, usually athetosis of the neck, should alert the nurse to this possibility.

Getting out of a chair can be facilitated by using an upright chair with arms and placing the back legs on small (2-inch) blocks. Other aspects of the environment can be altered. Rugs and excess furniture can be removed to avoid stumbling. An ottoman can be used to elevate the legs and avoid dependent-ankle edema. Clothing can be simplified by the use of slip-on shoes and Velcro hook and loop fasteners or zippers on clothing instead of buttons and hooks. An elevated toilet seat can facilitate getting on and off the toilet. The nurse should work closely with the client's family in exploring creative adaptations that allow the greatest amount of independence and self-care.

MYASTHENIA GRAVIS

Myasthenia gravis (MG) is a disease of the neuromuscular junction characterized by fluctuating weakness of certain skeletal muscle groups. Prevalence is estimated to be from 43 to 84 persons per million.[1] The peak age at onset in women is 20 to 30 years. Women are affected slightly more often than men, although a majority of persons with both thymoma and myasthenia (15% to 20% of all persons with myasthenia) are men over the age of 50.

Etiology and Pathophysiology

MG is an autoimmune process that results in a reduced number of ACh receptor sites at the neuromuscular junction. This prevents ACh molecules from attaching and causing muscle contraction. Anti-ACh receptor antibodies are detectable in the serum of 70% to 85% of clients with MG. Loss of muscle strength is the result of the abnormal antibodies, which speed the breakdown of ACh, block ACh binding sites, and possibly damage neuromuscular junctions.

Thymoma (neoplasm of the thymus gland) is found in about 10% of clients, and 80% of the remaining clients show a striking degree of thymus hyperplasia.[1] Antibodies to the ACh receptors are formed by the thymus gland and peripheral lymphoid organs and attack most of the receptor sites of the neuromuscular junction. Although a viral infection is suspected as precipitating an attack, a single specific cause for all myasthenia has not been found.

Clinical Manifestations

The primary feature of MG is easy fatigability of skeletal muscle during activity. Strength is usually restored after a period of rest. The muscles most often involved are those used for moving the eyes and eyelids, chewing, swallowing, speaking, and breathing. The cell bodies of the neurons for these muscles are located in the brainstem.

The muscles are generally strongest in the morning and become exhausted with continued activity. Consequently, by the end of the day, muscle fatigue is prominent.

The first manifestations of MG in 90% of cases are ptosis (drooping eyelid) and diplopia. Facial mobility and expression can be impaired. There may be difficulty in chewing and swallowing food. Speech is affected, and the voice often fades after a long conversation. The muscles of the trunk and limbs are less often affected. Of these, the proximal muscles of the neck, shoulder, and hip are more often affected than the distal muscles. No signs of neural disorder accompany MG; there is no sensory loss, reflexes are normal, and muscle atrophy is rare.

The course of this disease is highly variable. Some persons may have short-term remissions, others may stabilize, and others may have severe progressive involvement. Restricted ocular myasthenia, usually seen only in men, has a good prognosis. Exacerbations of myasthenia can be precipitated by emotional stress, pregnancy, menses, secondary illness, trauma, temperature extremes, hypokalemia, ingestion of drugs with neuromuscular blocking properties, and surgery. In some cases the onset of myasthenia occurs after one of these events.

Complications

The major complications of MG result from muscle weakness in areas that affect swallowing and breathing. An acute exacerbation of this type is sometimes called *myasthenic crisis*. Aspiration, respiratory insufficiency, and respiratory infection are the major complications.

Diagnostic Studies

The simplest diagnostic test for myasthenia is to have the client look at the ceiling for 2 to 3 minutes. There will be an increased droop of the eyelids, so that the person can barely keep the eyes open. After a brief rest the eyes can open again. Other tests may be used if the diagnosis is still in doubt. EMG may show a decrementing response to repeated stimulation of the hand muscles, indicative of muscle fatigability. Use of pharmacological agents may also aid in the diagnosis. The Tensilon test in a client with MG reveals improved muscle contractility after intravenous (IV) injection of edrophonium chloride (Tensilon chloride). This test also aids in the diagnosis of *cholinergic crisis* (secondary to overdose of neostigmine). In this condition, Tensilon (a cholinergic agent) does not improve muscle weakness but may actually increase it. Atropine should be readily available to counteract Tensilon effects when it is used diagnostically.

Therapeutic Management

The major therapies for MG are anticholinesterase drugs, alternate-day corticosteroids, nonsteroid immunosuppressants, and plasmapheresis. Removal of the thymus gland results in improvement in 85% of clients.[15] Surgery is indicated for clients with thymoma and practically all clients with uncomplicated MG who are less than 50 years of age and who, after a period of treatment with anticholinesterase drugs, are responding poorly and requiring increasing doses of medication.[1] The thymus gland in the

Table 54-20

 Diagnostic and Therapeutic Management: Myasthenia Gravis

DIAGNOSTIC

History
Physical examination
    Fatigability with prolonged upward gaze (2-3 min)
    Muscle weakness
EMG
Tensilon test

THERAPEUTIC

Drugs
    Anticholinesterase agents
    Corticosteroids
    Immunosuppressive agents
Surgery (thymectomy)
Plasmapheresis

client with MG appears to enhance the production of ACh receptor antibodies. Table 54-20 lists these therapies.

Plasmapheresis is a relatively new therapy for MG and was first reported in 1976. This procedure involves separation of plasma from blood by a machine called a *cell separator,* which is connected to the client by a vascular cannula similar to a dialysis cannula. This process supposedly "cleans" the plasma of myasthenia antibodies. Plasmapheresis can yield short-term improvement in symptoms, but it is expensive and inconvenient for many clients (see Chapter 8).

Pharmacological Management

One class of drug for treatment of MG is the anticholinesterase group. Neostigmine (Prostigmin) and pyridostigmine (Mestinon) are the most successful drugs of this group. The anticholinesterase drugs improve myasthenic weakness by inhibiting the destruction of ACh by acetylcholinesterase, thus facilitating transmission of impulses across the neuromuscular junction. Tailoring the dose to avoid a myasthenic or a cholinergic crisis often presents a clinical challenge. Corticosteroids (specifically prednisone) that shrink lymphatic tissue and suppress immunity may be helpful. Cytotoxic drugs such as azathioprine (Imuran) and cyclophosphamide (Cytoxan) may also be used for immunosuppression.

Many drugs are contraindicated or must be used with caution in clients with MG. Classes of drug that should be cautiously evaluated before use include corticosteroids, anesthetics, antidysrhythmics, antibiotics, quinine, antipsychotics, barbiturates and sedative-hypnotics, cathartics, diuretics, narcotics, muscle relaxants, thyroid preparations, and tranquilizers.

■ Nursing Management of Myasthenia Gravis

Nursing assessment

The nurse can assess the severity of MG by asking the client about fatigability, what body parts are affected, and how severely they are affected. The client's coping abilities and understanding of the disorder should also be assessed. Some persons become so fatigued that they are no longer able to work or even ambulate.

Objective data should include respiratory rate and depth, blood gas analyses, pulmonary function tests, and evidence of respiratory distress in clients with acute myasthenic crisis. Muscle strength of all face and limb muscles should be assessed, as should swallowing, speech (volume and clarity), and cough and gag reflexes.

Nursing diagnoses

Nursing diagnoses specific to the client with MG include, but are not limited to, the following:

1. Ineffective breathing patterns and airway clearance related to intercostal muscle weakness and impaired cough and gag reflexes
2. Impaired verbal communication related to weakness of the larynx, lips, mouth, pharynx, and jaw
3. Altered nutrition: less than body requirements related to impaired swallowing, weakness, and inability to prepare food or feed self
4. Sensory/perceptual visual alterations related to ptosis, decreased eye movements, and dysconjugate gaze
5. Self-care deficit related to muscle weakness and fatigability
6. Body-image disturbance related to inability to maintain usual lifestyle and role responsibilities.

Nursing interventions

Clients with MG who are admitted to the hospital usually have a respiratory tract infection or are in an acute myasthenic crisis. Nursing care is aimed at maintaining adequate ventilation, continuing drug therapy, and watching for side effects of therapy. The nurse must be able to distinguish cholinergic from myasthenic crisis (Table 54-21), since the causes and treatment of the two differ greatly.

As with other chronic illnesses, rehabilitative care focuses on the neurological deficits and their impact on daily living. A good diet that can be chewed and swallowed easily should be prescribed. Semisolid foods may be easier to eat than solids or liquids. Scheduling doses of medication so that peak action is reached at mealtime may make eating less difficult. Diversional activities that require little physical effort and match the interests of the client should be arranged. Education should focus on the importance of following the medical regimen, on potential adverse reactions to specific drugs, on planning activities of daily living to avoid fatigue, on the availability of community resources, and on complications of the disease and therapy (crisis conditions) and what to do about them. Contact with the MG Society or an MG support group may be very helpful and should be explored.

ALZHEIMER'S DISEASE

Alzheimer's disease is a type of dementia that is characterized by progressive deterioration in mental functioning and orientation. Until recently, chronological age was the main factor in distinguishing presenile and senile dementia of the Alzheimer type. Current practice now favors using the single category—dementia of the Alzheimer

Table 54-21 Myasthenic Crisis and Cholinergic Crisis

Causes	Differential Diagnosis
MYASTHENIC CRISIS	
Exacerbation after precipitating factors or failure to take medication as prescribed, too low a dose	Improved strength after IV administration of anticholinesterase drugs; increased weakness of skeletal muscle, manifesting as ptosis, bulbar signs (e.g., difficulty in swallowing, difficulty in articulating words), dyspnea
CHOLINERGIC CRISIS	
Overdose of anticholinesterase drugs that blocks ACh receptor sites, remission (spontaneous or after thymectomy)	Weakness within 1 hour after ingestion of anticholinesterase; increased weakness of skeletal muscle, manifesting as ptosis, bulbar signs, dyspnea; effects on smooth muscle, including pupillary miosis, salivation, diarrhea, nausea or vomiting, abdominal cramps, increase in bronchial secretions, salivation, sweating, or lacrimation

Table 54-22 Major Causes of Progressive Dementia

Senile dementia, Alzheimer type	50%
Multiinfarct (arteriosclerotic)	10%
Combination of senile dementia and multiinfarct	15%
Communicating hydrocephalus	
Alcoholic or posttraumatic	
Huntington's chorea	15%
Intracranial mass lesions	
Uncommon or combination with other causes	10%

Chronic drug use, Creutzfeldt-Jakob disease, metabolic (thyroid, liver, nutritional), degenerative (spinocerebellar, amyotrophic lateral sclerosis, parkinsonism, multiple sclerosis, Pick's disease, Wilson's disease, epilepsy), AIDS dementia, static postanoxic dementia

Modified from Andreoli TE and others: Cecil essentials of medicine, ed 2, Philadelphia, 1990, WB Saunders Co, p 687.
AIDS, Acquired immunodeficiency syndrome.

type (DAT)—to indicate that the disease process is the same, regardless of the age of the client.

DAT is increasingly recognized as one of the major health problems in the United States, particularly for persons over 65 years of age. It accounts for more than half of the cases of dementia (about 1 to 2 million cases). The major causes of progressive dementia are listed in Table 54-22.

Etiology and Pathophysiology

Although no single cause for DAT has been found, there are several models that have been proposed on the basis of scientific research. These etiological models suggest DAT may be caused by genetic factors, abnormal protein in the brain, inadequate cerebral blood flow, decreased ACh, infectious agents, and environmental toxins.[16] Major research efforts are currently under way to further explore the possible causes of DAT.

Structural changes associated with DAT include neurofibrillary tangles and senile plaques in the cerebral cortex and hippocampus. There is also an excessive loss of neurons, particularly in regions essential for memory and cognition.

Clinical Manifestations

An initial sign of DAT is subtle deterioration in memory. Inevitably this progresses to more profound memory loss that interferes with the client's ability to function. Recent events and new information cannot be recalled. Personal hygiene deteriorates, as does the ability to maintain attention. Later in the disease, long-term memories cannot be recalled, and clients lose the ability to recognize family members. Eventually the ability to communicate and to perform activities of daily living is lost. The progression of deterioration, which eventually leads to death, varies but can last as long as 20 years.

It is critical that DAT be distinguished from depression, a clinically similar condition, because depression is potentially reversible and often responds to appropriate treatment. A careful assessment can distinguish the two clinical conditions. Table 54-23 lists the clinical manifestations of depression and dementia to aid in proper diagnosis.

Diagnostic Studies

The diagnosis of DAT is a diagnosis of exclusion. When all other possible conditions that can cause mental impairment have been ruled out and the manifestations of dementia persist, the diagnosis of DAT can be made.

A CT or an MRI scan may show brain atrophy and enlarged ventricles in the later stages of the disease, although this finding occurs in other diseases and can also be seen in normal persons. Neuropsychological testing can help document the degree of cognitive dysfunction in the early stages. The definitive diagnosis of DAT can be made only at autopsy, when the presence of neurofibrillary tangles is

Table 54-23 Differentiation of Depression and Alzheimer's-Type Dementia

Onset	Psychiatric History	Mental Status	Sleep Disturbance	Somatic Complaints	Self-Image	Suicidal Ideation	Treatment	Weight Loss
DEPRESSION								
Abrupt (weeks)	Prior depression common	Pervasive dysphoria Normal or impaired cognition Variable performance Variable memory disturbance	Initial and early-morning insomnia	Often multiple	Poor	Present	High effectiveness of antidepressants	Yes, with appetite disturbance
DEMENTIA								
Insidious	Usually no history	Flattening of affect Impaired cognition Stable performance Effects on memory	Frequent awakenings	Often none	Normal	Absent	Very limited usefulness of antidepressants	No

Modified from Billig N and others: Diagnostic dilemma: is it dementia? Patient Care 1:198, 1989.

Table 54-24 Pharmacological Management of Alzheimer's Disease

Manifestation	Drugs	Adverse Side Effects
Depression	Tricyclic antidepressants (e.g., nortriptyline [Aventyl, Pamelor], amitryptiline [Elavil], imipramine [Tofranil], doxepin [Sinequan])	Orthostatic hypotension, sedation, dry mouth, constipation, urinary retention, blurry vision
	Nontricyclic antidepressant (e.g., trazodone [Desyrel])	Dry mouth, sedation, confusion
Psychoses and behavioral disturbances	Neuroleptics or antipsychotics (e.g., loxapine, haloperidol [Haldol])	Sedation, extrapyramidal effects, orthostatic hypotension, tardive dyskinesia
	Benzodiazepines (e.g., oxazepam [Serax], diazepam [Valium])	Sedation, confusion, disinhibition with paradoxical agitation, unsteady gait, dysarthria, incoordination
Anxiety	Benzodiazepines	Same as in psychoses and behavioral disturbances
Sleep disturbances	Benzodiazepines, neuroleptics	Same as in psychoses and behavioral disturbances

observed. There is no known treatment to stop the progression of the disease.

Therapeutic and Pharmacological Management

The therapeutic management of DAT is aimed at controlling the undesirable symptoms that the client may exhibit. Table 54-24 details the manifestation of symptoms, the usual pharmacological management, and the possible adverse side effects of the prescribed drugs. It is important to be aware that these drugs do not alter the course of the disease.

Many other forms of drug therapy, such as hyperbaric oxygen, routine and megadose vitamins, herbs, algae in the form of manna, and chelation, have been used. None have proved beneficial. Drugs such as physostigmine and other cholinesterase inhibitors have been used to treat the

Table 54-25

Nursing Assessment of the Client with Alzheimer's Disease

SUBJECTIVE DATA

History
Positive family history, repeated head trauma, exposure to metals (especially aluminum), previous CNS infection
Medications
Use of any drug to mitigate symptoms (e.g., tranquilizers, hypnotics, antidepressants)
General
Fatigue, depression, emotional lability
Neurological
Forgetfulness, inability to cope with complex situations, difficulty with problem solving (early signs)

OBJECTIVE DATA

General
Advanced: Poor hygiene, inability to perform activities of daily living, anorexia, malnutrition, weight loss, incontinence
Neurological
Early: Loss of recent memory; disorientation to date and time; flat affect; lack of spontaneity; impaired abstraction, cognition, and judgment; loss of remote memory; restlessness and agitation; inability to recognize family and friends; nocturnal wandering; repetitive behavior; loss of social graces; stubbornness, paranoia, belligerence
Advanced: Aphasia, agnosia, alexia (inability to understand written language), seizures
Possible findings
Diagnosis by exclusion, cerebral cortical atrophy on CT scan, poor scores on mental status tests

---

cholinergic system and to enhance ACh and prevent its breakdown in the nerve ending. The effectiveness of these drugs has been variable, and research is ongoing.[17]

▪ Nursing Management of Alzheimer's Disease

Nursing assessment

Subjective and objective data that should be obtained from a person with Alzheimer's disease are presented in Table 54-25.

Nursing diagnoses

Nursing diagnoses are determined when the problem and the etiological factors are supported by clinical data. Nursing diagnoses for Alzheimer's disease may include, but are not limited to, those listed in Table 54-26.

Nursing interventions

Although there is no current effective treatment for DAT, there is a need for ongoing monitoring of both the client with DAT and the client's caregiver. It is an important nursing responsibility to work collaboratively with the client's physician to manage symptoms effectively as they change over time. Nursing interventions are aimed at enhancing functional ability, providing for environmental

safety, and providing emotional support and respite care for the constant demands placed on caregivers.

Table 54-26 presents a nursing care plan for the client with Alzheimer's disease. The nurse is often responsible for teaching the caregiver to perform the many caregiving tasks that are required by this type of client. The nurse must consider both the person with DAT and the caregiver as clients with overlapping but unique problems. To aid in identifying the many problems of the caregiver, Table 54-27 presents a nursing care plan for the caregiver of a person with Alzheimer's disease.

Adult day care is one of the options available to the caregivers of a person with Alzheimer's disease. Although programs vary in size, structure, physical environment, and degree of experience of staff, the common goals of all day care programs are to provide respite for the family and protective services for the client.

The middle stage of the disease is probably the most beneficial time for adult day-care when the person with DAT can still benefit from stimulating activities that encourage independence and decision making in a protective environment. The client returns home tired, content, less frustrated, and ready to be with the family. The respite from the demands of care allows the family to be more responsive to the client's needs.

Although adult day-care may delay the transition, the demands on the caregiver generally exceed the resources, and the person with DAT is placed in an institutional setting. Special units to care for persons with DAT are becoming increasingly prevalent in long-term care settings. The nursing care needs of the person with DAT change as the disease progresses, emphasizing the need for regular assessment, monitoring, and support. Regardless of the setting, the severity of the symptoms and the amount of care required intensify over time.

Persons with DAT are subject to acute and other chronic illnesses. Their inability to communicate health symptoms and problems places the responsibility for assessment and diagnosis on caregivers and health professionals. Hospitalization of the person with DAT can be a traumatic event for both the client and the caregiver and can precipitate a crisis. Hospitalization often taxes the limited reserve resources of the person with DAT to the point where adaptation is no longer possible, and the disease seems to worsen quickly.

DAT is a devastating disease that disrupts all aspects of personal and family life. Support groups such as the Alzheimer's Disease and Related Disorders Association (ADRDA) have been formed throughout the United States to provide an atmosphere of understanding and to give current information about the disease itself and related topics such as safety, legal, ethical, and financial issues. Nurses often receive personal and professional satisfaction in participating in such support groups.

OTHER NEUROLOGICAL DISORDERS
Amyotrophic Lateral Sclerosis

Loss of motor neurons is the major morphological change in amyotrophic lateral sclerosis (ALS), a rare progressive neurological disease that usually leads to death in

Table 54-26

 NURSING CARE PLAN FOR THE CLIENT WITH ALZHEIMER'S DISEASE

Defining Characteristics	Nursing Interventions	Evaluation Criteria
NURSING DIAGNOSIS: Total self-care deficit related to memory deficit, neuromuscular impairment, inability to recognize function of grooming equipment, and inability to distinguish appropriate from inappropriate patterns of dressing, grooming, eating, and toileting		
Inability to independently and appropriately dress, bathe, groom, or toilet	Assess specific self-care deficit and determine probable cause. Verbally remind (cue) client of appropriate activity. Demonstrate use of equipment (e.g., toothbrush, hairbrush, washcloth). Lay out clothing daily. Continue to assess self-care capabilities and deficits, intervening when necessary. Toilet and change incontinence brief as scheduled. Ensure adequate food and fluid intake by directing client to feed self or by feeding client if necessary.	Cleanliness and exhibition of adequate hygiene, appropriate dressing and grooming, adequate amounts of nutritious foods, establishment of satisfactory toileting routine
NURSING DIAGNOSIS: Sleep pattern disturbance related to physical discomfort, environmental changes, excessive napping secondary to inability to initiate activities, and lack of physical activity		
Erratic sleep patterns, nighttime wandering, daytime sleepiness	Ensure that client's physical needs are met related to bedtime (e.g., client toileted, comfortable room temperature, quiet environment). Adapt usual nightly habits such as bedtime, night lights, warm milk. Reassure wakened client and reorient in soft, soothing tone. ("It is nighttime. It is time to go back to bed.") Prevent client from taking excessive naps. Identify and initiate appropriate daytime diversional activities. Plan and implement periods of physical activity during the day.	Reasonable periods of uninterrupted rest at appropriate times
NURSING DIAGNOSIS: Altered health maintenance related to impaired communication ability, short-term memory deficit, and cognitive impairment		
Inability to monitor health status	Complete physical assessment on admission. Monitor physical status. Assess any acute changes in behavior promptly and refer for adequate workup. Use simple questions requiring "yes" or "no" answers when questioning client. Point directly to body parts when attempting to ascertain site of discomfort or pain.	Prompt diagnosis and treatment of acute illness, maintenance of optimal physical health status
NURSING DIAGNOSIS: High risk for injury related to impaired judgment, possible gait instability, muscle weakness, and sensory/perceptual alteration		
Bruises, abrasions, broken bones, burns	Monitor activity. Maintain environment free from safety hazards, such as cluttered walkways, slippery floors, matches, high water temperatures, medications, possibility of wandering. Assess and record extent of physical limitation, if any. Provide assistance when necessary. Incorporate ambulation into care plan. Plan and implement periods of safe activity during the day.	Absence of accidental injuries

Modified from care plan developed by Marilyn Papier Williams, San Francisco.

Table 54-26

	NURSING CARE PLAN FOR THE CLIENT WITH ALZHEIMER'S DISEASE—cont'd	

Defining Characteristics	Nursing Interventions	Evaluation Criteria

NURSING DIAGNOSIS: **High risk for violence related to sensory overload, misinterpretation of environmental stimuli, lack of appropriate coping mechanisms, and unfamiliar environment**

| Acting out behavior, verbal threats, agitation | Prevent sensory overload. Avoid giving client tasks that prove frustrating. Ensure adequate sleep and rest periods. Provide opportunities for client to vent anxiety and frustration. Observe and document in detail any catastrophic reaction and precipitating events. Document interventions that eliminate this behavior. | Absence of self-directed or other-directed physical trauma |

NURSING DIAGNOSIS: **Ineffective individual coping related to depression in response to diagnosis of Alzheimer's disease**

| Depression, withdrawal, fatigue, social isolation | Assess for possibility and extent of depression. Provide opportunity for client to verbalize feelings. Facilitate communication between client and family. Provide appropriate diversional activities. Allow client to make decisions regarding self-care and environment when possible. Refer for further evaluation and counseling if indicated. | Feeling of value as individual |

2 to 6 years. This disease became known as *Lou Gehrig's disease* when the famous baseball player was stricken with it in the early 1940s. The onset is between the ages of 40 and 70 years, and twice as many men as women are affected.

For unknown reasons, motor neurons in the brainstem and spinal cord gradually degenerate. The dead motor neuron cannot produce or transport vital signals to muscle. Consequently, electrical and chemical messages originating in the brain never reach the muscles to activate them.

The primary symptoms are weakness of the upper extremities, dysarthria, and dysphagia. Muscle wasting and fasciculations result from the denervation of muscles and lack of stimulation and use. Death usually results from respiratory infection secondary to compromised respiratory function. Unfortunately, there is no cure and no treatment for ALS. This illness is devastating because the client remains cognitively intact while wasting away. The challenge of nursing care is to support the client's cognitive and emotional functions by providing diversional activities such as reading and human companionship.

Huntington's Disease

Huntington's disease is a genetically transmitted, autosomal dominant disorder that affects both men and women of all races. The offspring of a person with this disease have a 50% risk of inheriting it.

Like Parkinson's disease, the pathology of Huntington's disease involves the basal ganglia and the extrapyramidal system. However, instead of a deficiency of dopamine,

Huntington's disease involves a deficiency of the neurotransmitters ACh and γ-aminobutyric acid (GABA). The net effect is an excess of dopamine, which leads to symptoms opposite those of parkinsonism. The clinical manifestations, the onset of which is between the ages of 35 and 45 years, are characterized by abnormal and excessive involuntary movements *(chorea)*. These are writhing, twisting movements of the face, limbs, and body. The movements get worse as the disease progresses. Facial movements involving speech, chewing, and swallowing are affected and may cause aspiration and malnutrition. The gait deteriorates, and ambulation eventually becomes impossible. Perhaps the most devastating deterioration is in mental functions, which include intellectual decline, emotional lability, and psychotic behavior. Death usually occurs 10 to 20 years after the onset of symptoms.

Because there is no cure, therapeutic management is palliative. Antipsychotic, antidepressant, and antichorea medications are prescribed and have some effect. However, they do not alter the course of the disease. This disease presents a great challenge to health care professionals. The goal of nursing management is to provide the most comfortable environment possible for the client and the family by maintaining physical safety, treating the physical symptoms, and providing emotional and psychological support. Genetic counseling is very important.

Muscular Dystrophy

The many types of muscular dystrophy (MD) are all progressive, hereditary, degenerative diseases of skeletal

Table 54-27

NURSING CARE PLAN FOR THE CAREGIVER OF THE CLIENT WITH ALZHEIMER'S DISEASE

Defining Characteristics	Nursing Interventions	Evaluation Criteria

NURSING DIAGNOSIS: Ineffective individual coping related to unrelieved caregiving responsibilities, inadequate or underdeveloped support systems, perceived powerlessness, fatigue secondary to interrupted sleep pattern, and lack of knowledge regarding coping strategies and strategies for behavioral management and relaxation techniques

| Fatigue, verbalization of inability to cope, inability to meet needs, make decisions, ask for help; frequent illness, accidents; inappropriate defense mechanisms | Assess health status of caregiver. Refer for medical evaluation when appropriate. Instruct in relaxation and effective coping strategies. Assess knowledge of Alzheimer's disease process and management techniques. Assist caregiver in defining problem areas and assist with problem-solving techniques. Instruct in management of problem behaviors, referring for medical management when indicated. Evaluate client's readiness and motivation to use community resources. | Verbalization of confidence in ability to cope effectively with long-term caregiving responsibilities |

NURSING DIAGNOSIS: Social isolation related to diminishing social relationships secondary to unrelieved caregiving responsibilities, behavioral problems of client with Alzheimer's disease, and underdeveloped social support system

| Feelings of abandonment and uselessness, behavior changes (irritability, hypoactivity, depression, withdrawal), eating changes, inability to make decisions or concentrate | Assess past social network and diversional activities. Assess social support system of family and willingness and ability to participate in care. Assist in planning respite care through this system or formal community resources to enable caregiver to continue with important activities and social contacts. Refer to social services for realistic appraisal of financial resources for respite care and for linkage to community resources. Provide information regarding available support groups (e.g., Alzheimer's Disease and Related Disorders Association). | Satisfactory contact with significant others or members of a support group |

NURSING DIAGNOSIS: Anxiety related to uncertain outcome, perceived powerlessness, possible change in role functioning, erratic behavioral patterns of the person with Alzheimer's disease, high risk for injury secondary to possible violent reactions of client, and financial insecurity

| Autonomic changes (e.g., tachycardia, hypertension), apprehension, helplessness, fear, irritability, cognitive changes (e.g., forgetfulness, inability to concentrate) | Assess past roles of client with Alzheimer's disease and of caregiver. Document changes in functional expectations and refer to community resources or provide instruction as needed. Assess knowledge of behavioral management techniques and instruct as appropriate. Assist caregiver in problem-solving techniques; assist in looking at possible causes of catastrophic reactions as well as indications of agitation, which may indicate their onset. Refer to social services as indicated for complete list of community resources and possible sources of financial aid. | Decreased anxiety, sense of control of situation |

NURSING DIAGNOSIS: High risk for altered health maintenance related to unrelieved caretaking responsibilities, fatigue, and chronic stress

| Failure to care for self | Assess physical and emotional health status of caregiver. Collaborate with caregiver in planning interventions in major identified problem areas. Refer for additional evaluation if indicated. Assist with planning of continued care of client so that caregiver's personal health needs can be pursued. Stress need for maintaining own health. | Optimal health |

Table 54-27

NURSING CARE PLAN FOR THE CAREGIVER OF THE CLIENT WITH ALZHEIMER'S DISEASE—cont'd		
Defining Characteristics	**Nursing Interventions**	**Evaluation Criteria**

NURSING DIAGNOSIS: High risk for ineffective family coping related to chronic and deteriorating nature of Alzheimer's disease, feelings of helplessness and hopelessness, increasing financial hardship, and disappearing support systems

Verbalization of lack of help and hope in caring for family member, concern over finances, deteriorating emotional and physical health of caregiver	Encourage family to discuss caregiving situation with one another. Provide information on community resources to relieve stress and facilitate coping, such as day care, support groups, counseling, and respite care. Encourage and support family in their caregiving efforts. Refer for aid with financial concerns. Provide information on nature and course of Alzheimer's disease.	No evidence of destructive coping behaviors

muscle. There is no involvement of the nerves; rather, the problem is within the muscle fibers themselves. For unknown reasons, a genetic abnormality induces degeneration of muscle fibers. The common feature of MD is symmetrical muscle weakness and atrophy. There is no treatment for MD, and as in ALS, the client experiences progressive muscle weakness and wasting. Therapeutic management is purely symptomatic. Quinine, procainamide, and phenytoin can relieve myotonia, although side effects may outweigh the benefits of drug therapy. Surgical procedures, such as fasciotomy or tendon lengthening, and leg braces may preserve ambulation for several additional years. Complications include fractures, respiratory infections, and cardiac decompensation. Nursing care should be directed toward maintenance of normal daily activity as much as possible and avoidance of contractures, skeletal deformities, and obesity.

C ase Study

EPILEPSY

Mr. G. has been having partial simple and secondarily generalized tonic-clonic seizures. His medical records indicate that he has been free of seizures for several months. He is admitted to the hospital for treatment of lacerations after reportedly having a seizure at his job as a gas station attendant. He denies having had a seizure and says he just fell and hurt himself. His serum anticonvulsant level is well below the therapeutic range. His wife states that Mr. G. has had several seizures in his sleep over the past month. She says he denies having them, even though they wake him up and cause him to be incontinent and to injure his tongue. He still drives a car.

Discussion Questions

1. What is the pathogenesis of the type of epilepsy Mr. G. has?
2. What is the probable reason for Mr. G. having these recent seizures?

3. What kind of seizure is Mr. G. having in his sleep?
4. What psychological defense mechanism is Mr. G. exhibiting?
5. How would you counsel Mr. G. and his wife?

C ase Study

PARKINSON'S DISEASE

Mr. L. noticed that he required a progressively longer time to perform his usual daily activities. His family observed that he had problems getting in and out of chairs. They also found it difficult to interpret his facial expressions because they did not seem to reflect his mood. Customers on the phone frequently had to ask him to repeat words.

Mr. L. consulted his physician, who prescribed antiparkinsonian medication. However, he is now having problems with nausea and visual hallucinations at night and he is still having some difficulty dressing himself.

Discussion Questions

1. What is the pathogenesis of Parkinson's disease?
2. What are the typical symptoms of this disease?
3. How many symptoms have to be present before the diagnosis is made?
4. In relation to the communication problem, how should Mr. L. and his family be counseled?
5. How should the side effects of antiparkinsonian medication be handled?
6. What suggestions should be made to Mr. L. and his family about dressing himself?

R eview Questions

The number of the question corresponds to the same-numbered objective at the beginning of the chapter.

1. Chronic neurological disease often involves

   a. long-term use of medication
   b. progressive physical deterioration
   c. a and b
   d. a surgical cure

2. Which of the following statements is correct?
   a. Migraine headache involves contraction of the scalp and neck muscles.
   b. Muscle-contraction headache is described as a throbbing, usually unilateral pain.
   c. The prodrome of migraine is associated with vasoconstriction, and the actual headache is associated with vasodilatation.
   d. Cluster headache is associated with recurrent discharge of the sympathetic nervous system.

3. The triad of symptoms common in Parkinson's disease is
   a. diplopia, tremor, bradykinesia
   b. tremor, rigidity, bradykinesia
   c. spasticity, diplopia, tremor
   d. ataxia, drowsiness, dysarthria

4. Nursing intervention for the client with MS is aimed at management of
   a. incontinence, depression, spasticity
   b. incontinence, hallucinations, tremor
   c. bradykinesia, rigidity, tremor
   d. rigidity, incontinence, diplopia

5. The most common cause of death in ALS is
   a. cerebral infarction
   b. renal failure
   c. pulmonary embolus
   d. respiratory infection

6. Common physical complications of a person who is immobilized by chronic neurological disease are
   a. constipation, skin breakdown
   b. contractures, pneumonia
   c. urinary tract infections
   d. all the above

7. A major goal of treatment for the client with a chronic, progressive neurological disease is
   a. continuation of usual lifestyle
   b. cure
   c. adjustment by client and family to the disease
   d. total remission of the disease

REFERENCES

1. Adams RA and Victor M: Principles of neurology, New York, 1988, McGraw-Hill Book Co, Inc.
2. Kirn T: Discussion, ideas abound in migraine research, consensus remains elusive, JAMA 257:9-13, 1987.
3. Whitney CM and Daroff KB: An approach to migraine, J Neurosci Nurs 20:284-289, 1988.
4. Metrakos K and Metrakos JD: Genetics of convulsive disorders: II, genetic and centrenecephalic epilepsy, Neurology 11:474-483, 1961.
5. Gastaut H: Clinical and electroencephalographical classification of epileptic seizures, Epilepsia 11:102-113, 1970.
6. Commission on Classification and Terminology of the International League Against Epilepsy: Proposal for the revised clinical and electroencephalographic classification of epileptic seizures, Epilepsia 22:249-501, 1981.
7. Caveness WF, Meritt HH, and Gallup GH Jr: A survey of attitudes toward epilepsy in 1974 with an indication of trends over the past 25 years, Epilepsia 15:523-536, 1974.
8. National Institutes of Health Consensus Conference: Surgery for epilepsy, JAMA 264:729, 1990.
9. Rodrigues M: Multiple sclerosis: basic concepts and hypothesis, Mayo Clin Proc 64:570-576, 1989.
10. Erkickson RP, Lie MR, and Wineinger MA: Rehabilitation in multiple sclerosis, Mayo Clin Proc 64:818-828, 1989.
11. Cummings JL: The dementias of Parkinson's disease: prevalence, characteristics, neurology, and comparison with dementia of the Alzheimer type, Eur Neurol 28(suppl 1):5-23, 1988.
12. Gash DM and Sladek JR: Neural transplantation: problems and prospects—where do we go from here? Mayo Clin Proc 64:3363-3367, 1989.
13. The Parkinson's Study Group: Effect of deprenyl on the progression of disability in early Parkinson's disease, N Engl J Med 321:1264-1371, 1989.
14. Elizan TS and others: Selegine use to prevent progression of Parkinson's disease, Arch Neurol 46:1275, 1989.
15. Andreoli TE and others: Cecil essentials of medicine, ed 2, Philadelphia, 1990, WB Saunders Co, p 761.
16. Wurtman RJ: Alzheimer's disease, Sci Am 252:62-68, 1985.
17. Ashford JW, Sherman KA, and Kumar V: Advances in Alzheimer therapy: cholinesterase inhibitors, Neurobiol Aging 10:99-105, 1989.

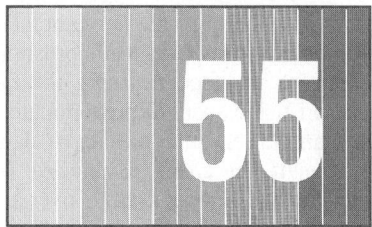

CHAPTER

55

Nursing Role in Management
Peripheral Nerve and Spinal Cord Problems

Connie A. Walleck

L earning Objectives

1. Explain the causes, clinical manifestations, and therapeutic and nursing management of the client with trigeminal neuralgia and Bell's palsy.
2. Explain the cause, clinical manifestations, and treatment of Guillain-Barré syndrome, botulism, tetanus, and neurosyphilis.
3. Describe the risk population and significance of spinal cord injury.
4. Define the classification of spinal cord injury and associated manifestations.
5. Describe the clinical manifestations and therapeutic and nursing management of spinal cord shock.

6. Compare the experimental and conventional therapeutic management of a client with a spinal cord injury.
7. Correlate the clinical manifestations of spinal cord injury with the level of disruption and rehabilitation potential.
8. Describe the nursing management for the major physical and psychological problems for the client with a spinal cord injury.
9. Explain the types, clinical manifestations, and therapeutic and nursing management of spinal cord tumors.

Cranial nerve disorders are most commonly classified as peripheral neuropathies. The cranial nerves become peripheral nerves as they exit the skull. The disorders usually involve the motor, sensory, or both branches of a single nerve (*mononeuropathies*). Causes of cranial nerve problems include tumors, trauma, infections, inflammatory processes, and idiopathic (unknown) causes. Two common cranial nerve disorders are trigeminal neuralgia (tic douloureux) and acute peripheral facial paralysis (Bell's palsy).

Another group of diseases called *polyneuropathies* affect multiple peripheral nerves. They have more generalized symptoms involving many nerves and are related to infectious processes and metabolic and chemical toxins. Examples of polyneuropathies include Guillain-Barré syndrome, botulism, tetanus, and neurosyphilis.

Spinal cord injuries are devastating to clients and can occur at any level of the spinal cord. They most commonly occur at the cervical and lumbar areas. The problems and complex therapeutic and nursing management of the client with spinal cord injuries are also discussed.

SPECIFIC CRANIAL NERVE DISORDERS
Trigeminal Neuralgia

Pathophysiology. Trigeminal neuralgia (tic douloureux) is a relatively common cranial nerve disorder affecting approximately 2% of the population. It is more commonly seen in women and usually begins in the fifth or sixth decade of life. The trigeminal nerve is the fifth cranial nerve (CN V) and has both motor and sensory *branches*. Only the sensory branches are involved in trigeminal neuralgia, primarily the maxillary branches (Fig. 55-1).[1]

Although no specific cause has been identified, nerve compression by tortuous arteries of the posterior fossa blood vessels, demyelinating plaques, the herpes virus infection, and a brain stem infarct have been suggested as initiating pathological events.[2] The effectiveness of antiepileptic drug therapy in shortening or suppressing the du-

Reviewed by Marylou Muwaswes, R.N., M.S., Assistant Clinical Professor, Department of Physiological Nursing, University of California, San Francisco, San Francisco, California.

1615

ration of an attack suggests a similar cell membrane defect as in epilepsy.

Clinical manifestations. The classic feature of trigeminal neuralgia is an abrupt onset of paroxysms of excruciating pain described as burning, knifelike, or a lightninglike shock in the lips, upper or lower gum, cheek, or side of the nose. Intense pain, twitching, grimacing, and frequent blinking and tearing of the eye occur during the acute attack (giving rise to the term *tic*). The attacks are usually brief, lasting seconds to 2 or 3 minutes, and are generally unilateral. Recurrences are unpredictable; they may occur several times a day or weeks or months apart. After the refractory (pain-free) period, a phenomenon known as *clustering* can occur that is characterized by a cycle of pain and refractoriness that continue for hours. As the client ages, remissions decrease.

The painful episodes are usually initiated by a triggering mechanism of light cutaneous stimulation at a specific point along the distribution of the nerve branches. Precipitating stimuli include chewing, teeth brushing, a hot or cold blast of air on the face, washing the face, or even talking; touch and tickle seem to predominate as causative factors rather than the sensation of pain or changes in temperature. As a result, the client may not eat properly, neglect hygienic practices, wear a cloth over the face, and withdraw from interaction with other individuals. Fortunately, the attacks are rarely nocturnal, and sleep is not interrupted. The client may sleep excessively as a means of coping with the pain.

Although this condition is considered benign, the severity of the pain and the disruption of lifestyle can result in almost total physical and psychological dysfunction or even suicide.

Therapeutic management. The physician must rule out other problems with similar manifestations such as other forms of facial and cephalic neuralgias as well as pain aris-

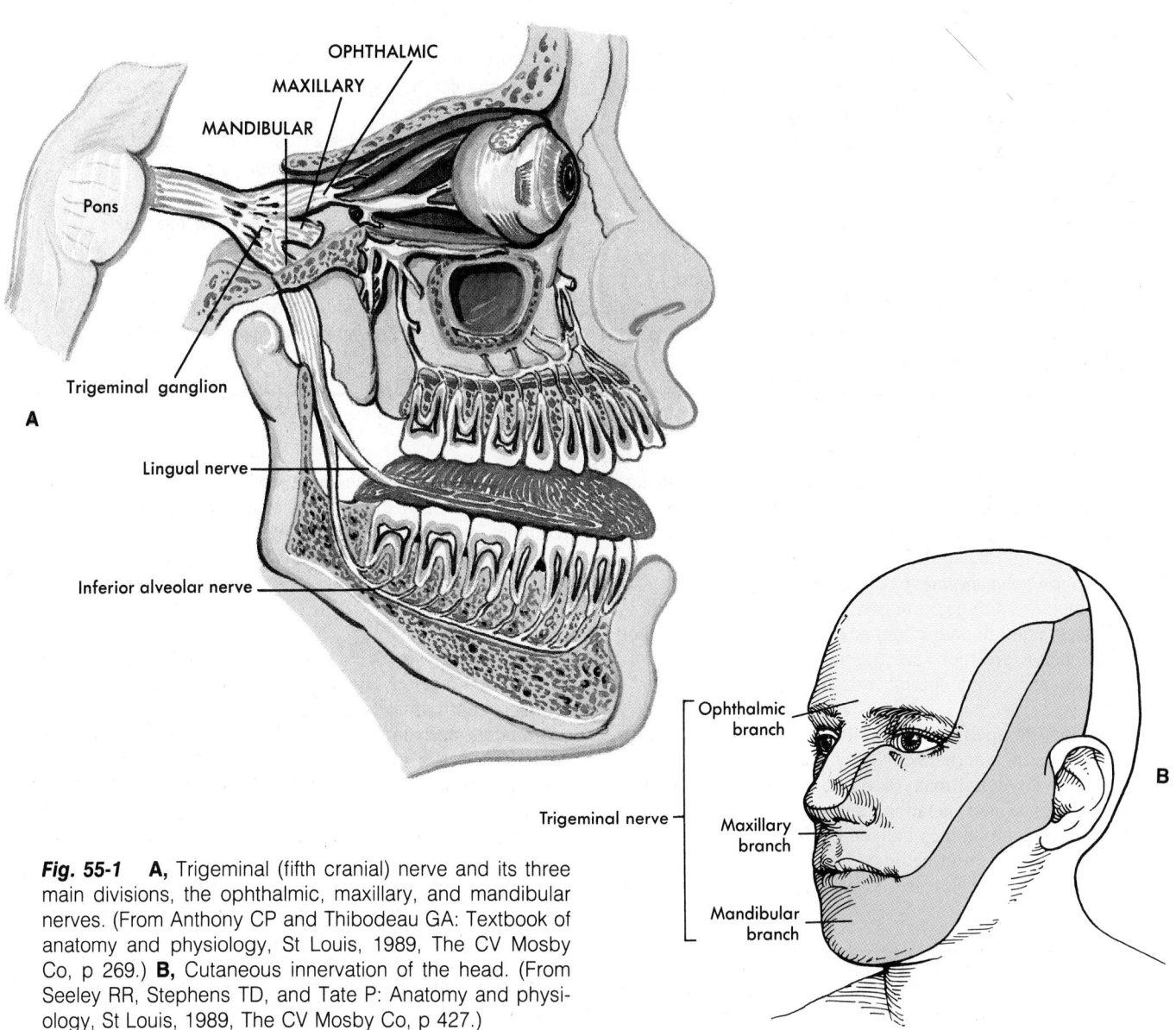

Fig. 55-1 **A,** Trigeminal (fifth cranial) nerve and its three main divisions, the ophthalmic, maxillary, and mandibular nerves. (From Anthony CP and Thibodeau GA: Textbook of anatomy and physiology, St Louis, 1989, The CV Mosby Co, p 269.) **B,** Cutaneous innervation of the head. (From Seeley RR, Stephens TD, and Tate P: Anatomy and physiology, St Louis, 1989, The CV Mosby Co, p 427.)

ing from the sinuses, teeth, and jaws. A complete neurological assessment is usually done, although results are usually normal. Once the diagnosis is made, the goal of treatment is relief of pain either medically or surgically (Table 55-1). The majority of clients obtain adequate relief through anticonvulsant drugs such as diphenylhydantoin (Dilantin) and carbamazepine (Tegretol). These drugs may prevent an acute attack or cause a remission of symptoms. These drugs may cause bone marrow suppression, leading to blood abnormalities, and routine complete blood cell (CBC) counts are required. Unfortunately, these drugs

may lose their effectiveness and are not a permanent solution. Some clients may seek help repeatedly by numerous visits to otolaryngologists or therapies such as acupuncture and megavitamins.

Local nerve blocking with local anesthetics is another treatment possibility. Local nerve blocking results in complete anesthesia of the area supplied by the injected branches. Relief of pain is only temporary, lasting from 6 to 18 months. This treatment is usually tolerated well by older adults.

Biofeedback is another form of pain control. For clients who are alert enough to understand the simple equipment and who can learn to use the feedback of one of their physiological parameters, biofeedback offers an innovative approach to the control of the pain. In addition to controlling the pain, the clients also experience a strong sense of personal control by mastering the process and altering certain body functions.

Surgical interventions. If a therapeutic regimen is not effective, surgical relief is available (Table 55-2). Percutaneous radiofrequency rhizotomy and microvascular decompression afford the greatest relief of pain. Percutaneous radiofrequency rhizotomy consists of placing a needle into the trigeminal rootlets that are adjacent to the pons and destroying the area by means of a radiofrequency current. This can result in anesthesia of the face, although some degree of sensation may be retained. Before surgery, injection of a lidocaine nerve block is recommended. This trial period allows the client to experience the effectiveness of the treatment and the local anesthesia of the face, which some may find intolerable. Irritation or inadvertent destruction of the ophthalmic branches of the nerve can result in loss of the corneal reflex. Microvascular decompression of the trigeminal nerve is accomplished by displacing and repositioning blood vessels that appear to be compressing the nerve at the root-entry zone where it exits

Table 55-1

Diagnostic and Therapeutic Management: Trigeminal Neuralgia

DIAGNOSTIC

History and physical examination
Brain scan or computerized tomography scan
Audiological evaluation
Electromyography
Spinal tap
Arteriography
Posterior myelography
Magnetic resonance imaging

THERAPEUTIC

Anticonvulsant therapy (e.g., diphenylhydantoin and carbamazepine)
Local nerve blocking
Biofeedback
Surgical intervention*

*See Table 55-2.

Table 55-2 Surgical Intervention for Trigeminal Neuralgia

Procedure	Technique	Benefit
PERIPHERAL		
Alcohol or phenol injection into one or more branches of trigeminal nerve	Dehydration of nerve	Complete anesthesia of affected area for 6 to 18 mo
Avulsion or resection of peripheral branches of facial nerve	Preganglionic sectioning of sensory portion	Permanent effect, appropriate procedure for poor surgical risk
INTRACRANIAL		
Retrogasserian rhizotomy	Temporal craniotomy (sectioning of sensory root in middle cranial fossa)	Permanent anesthesia (with adeptness, corneal reflex, touch)
Suboccipital craniotomy	Sectioning of sensory root of posterior fossa	Permanent anesthesia
Percutaneous radiofrequency rhizotomy	Destruction of sensory fibers by low-voltage current	Total pain relief, sparing of touch and corneal reflex, few residual problems
Microvascular decompression (Janetta procedure)	Lifting of artery pressing on nerve root in posterior fossa with wedge of sponge, leading to removal of pressure at nerve-root entry zone	Permanent pain relief without loss of sensation

the pons. This procedure relieves pain without residual sensory loss but is potentially dangerous, as is any surgery in the posterior fossa. It may be poorly tolerated in older adults because of the manipulation of the brainstem resulting in blood pressure fluctuations. Such fluctuations can be dangerous if the cardiovascular system is already compromised.

■ Nursing Management of Trigeminal Neuralgia

Nursing assessment

Assessment of the nature of the attacks, the triggering factors, and pain management techniques help the nurse plan for client care. The nursing assessment should include the client's nutritional status, hygiene (especially oral), and behavior (including withdrawal). Evaluation of the degree of pain and its effects on the client's lifestyle, drug history, emotional state, and suicidal tendencies are other important factors.

Nursing diagnoses

Nursing diagnoses specific to the client with trigeminal neuralgia include, but are not limited to, the following:

1. Acute pain related to the inflammation or compression of the trigeminal nerve
2. Altered nutrition: less than body requirements related to fear of eating causing pain
3. Anxiety related to uncertainty of timing and initiating event of pain and uncertainty regarding effectiveness of pain-relieving factors
4. Social isolation related to anxiety over pain attacks and desire to maintain nonstimulating environment

Nursing interventions

Acute intervention. Pain relief is primarily obtained by administration of recommended drug therapy. The nurse should monitor the client's response and note any side effects. The nurse should avoid strong narcotics such as morphine because of the potential for addiction over time. Moderate use of propoxyphene (Darvon) or pentazocine (Talwin) is acceptable. Alternative pain relief measures such as biofeedback or pain clinics should be explored for the client who is not a surgical candidate and whose pain is not controlled by other therapeutic measures. Careful assessment of pain history and drug dependency can assist with appropriate interventions.

Environmental management is essential to lessen triggering stimuli. The room should be kept at an even, moderate temperature and free of drafts. A private room is preferred during the acute period. The nurse must use care to avoid touching the client's face or jarring the bed. Many clients prefer to carry out their own care, fearing that they will be inadvertently injured by someone else.

The nurse should instruct the client about the importance of nutrition, hygiene, and oral care, conveying understanding if previous neglect is apparent. The nurse should provide lukewarm water and soft cloths or cotton saturated with solutions not requiring rinsing for cleansing the face. Small, very soft bristled toothbrush or warm mouthwash assists in promoting oral care. Hygiene activities are best carried out after medication or analgesics have been given.

The client will probably not engage in extensive conversation during the acute period. Alternative communication methods such as paper and pencil should be provided.

Food should be high in protein, calories, and easy to chew. It should be served lukewarm and offered frequently. The diet should be individualized according to personal, cultural, and religious preferences. Insertion of a nasogastric tube on the unaffected side may be necessary when the condition is severe.

If surgery is planned, the nurse is responsible for the preoperative teaching and instruction related to diagnostic studies to rule out other problems such as acoustic neuroma and neoplasms. The nurse may also need to reinforce the surgeon's instructions related to postoperative expectations; appropriate teaching of postoperative activities depends on whether a craniotomy or a local procedure is planned. Clients need to know that they will be awake during local procedures so that they can cooperate when corneal and ciliary reflexes and facial sensations are checked.

After the operation the client's pain is compared to the preoperative level. The corneal reflex, extraocular muscles, hearing, and facial nerve are evaluated frequently (see Chapter 50). General postoperative nursing care after a craniotomy is appropriate if intracranial surgery was performed (see Chapter 52). Diet and ambulation should be increased according to client progress or specific orders.

In the radiofrequency percutaneous electrocoagulation procedure an ice pack is applied to the jaw on the operative side for 3 to 5 hours. To avoid injuring the mouth, the client should not chew on the operative side until sensation has returned.

Chronic management. In pharmacological treatment the client needs instruction regarding the dosage and side effects of medications. Regular follow-up care should be planned. Although relief of pain may be complete, the client should be encouraged to keep environmental stimuli to a moderate level and to use stress reduction methods. Herpes simplex (cold sores) can occur from manipulation of the gasserian ganglion. Treatment consists of topical antiviral agents such as acyclovir (see Chapter 17).

Long-term management after surgical intervention depends on the residual effects of the type of procedure. If anesthesia is present or the corneal reflex is altered, the client should be taught to (1) chew on the unaffected side, (2) avoid hot foods or beverages that can burn the mucous membranes, (3) check the oral cavity after meals to remove food particles, (4) practice meticulous oral hygiene and continue with semiannual dental visits, (5) protect the face against extremes of temperature, (6) use an electric razor, and (7) wear protective eye shield.

The client may have developed protective practices to prevent pain and may need counseling or psychiatric assistance in personality readjustment, especially in reestablishing personal relationships. Some persons grieve the loss of the pain, especially if it had a special significance such as relieving guilt or anxiety. Occasionally clients may have used their pain to manipulate family members and friends and may not adjust after successful relief of pain. Careful management in the rehabilitative period can prevent "phantom pain" (see Chapter 50).

Bell's Palsy

Pathophysiology. Bell's palsy (peripheral facial paralysis, acute benign cranial polyneuritis) is a disorder characterized by a disruption of the motor branches of the facial nerve (CN VII) on one side of the face in the absence of any other disease such as a stroke. It can affect any age group, but it is more commonly seen in the 20- to 40-year age range. The cause is still unknown, but current theories suggest that the herpes simplex virus may cause inflammation and demyelination of the nerve. Mumps and emotional trauma with resultant vasoconstriction from the stress response have also been suggested as causes.[3]

The onset of Bell's palsy is often accompanied by an outbreak of herpes vesicles in or around the ear. Bell's palsy is considered benign, with full recovery after 3 to 4 months in about 85% of clients, especially if treatment is instituted immediately. A small number of clients may have some residual effects. Failure to show spontaneous recovery after 6 months indicates that the problem is probably not Bell's palsy.

Clinical manifestations and complications. The paralysis of the motor branches of the facial nerve typically results in a flaccidity of the affected side of the face, with drooping of the mouth accompanied by drooling. An inability to close the bottom eyelid, with an upward movement of the eyeball when closure is attempted, is also evident. A widened palpebral fissure, flattening of the nasolabial fold, and inability to smile, frown, or whistle are also common. Unilateral loss of taste is common. Decreased muscle movement may alter chewing ability, and although some clients may experience a loss of tearing, many clients complain of excessive tearing. The muscle weakness causes the lower lid to turn out, allowing overflow of normal tear production. Pain may be present behind the ear on the affected side, especially before the onset of paralysis.

Interventions are primarily supportive until the client has a return of function. Complications can include psychological withdrawal because of changes in body image, malnutrition and dehydration, mucous membrane trauma, muscle stretching, and facial spasms and contractures.

Therapeutic management. Diagnosis of Bell's palsy and the prognosis are indicated by (1) observation of the typical pattern of onset and signs, (2) testing of percutaneous nerve excitability, and (3) a Schirmer tear test for the presence of decreasing tearing on the affected side. The use of the Schirmer tear test is controversial because other factors can affect tearing. Corticosteroids, especially prednisone, are started immediately, and the best results are obtained if corticosteroids are initiated before paralysis is complete. When the client improves to the point that the corticosteroids are no longer necessary, they should be tapered off over a 2-week period. Usually the steroid treatment decreases the edema and pain, but mild analgesics can be used if necessary. Electromyographic (EMG) biofeedback is a successful modality for some clients with Bell's palsy.[4] Stimulation may maintain muscle tone and prevent atrophy. Vasodilators have been used to stimulate and promote circulation to the affected area. Care is primarily focused on relief of symptoms and prevention of complications.

■ Nursing Management of Bell's Palsy

Nursing assessment

Early recognition of the possibility of Bell's palsy is important. Because herpes simplex is a possible etiological factor, any person who is prone to herpes simplex should be alerted to seek health care if pain occurs in or around the ear. Assessment of facial muscles for any signs of weakness should also be done (see Chapter 50). Careful recording of assessment data provides information related to progress of the syndrome.

Nursing diagnoses

The nursing diagnoses specific to the client with Bell's palsy include, but are not limited to, the following:
1. Pain related to the inflammation of CN VII
2. Altered nutrition: less than body requirements related to inability to chew secondary to muscle weakness
3. High risk for trauma to the eye related to inability to blink
4. Body-image disturbance related to change in facial appearance secondary to facial muscle weakness

Nursing interventions

Mild analgesics can relieve pain. Hot wet packs can reduce the discomfort of herpetic lesions and aid circulation and relieve pain. The face should be protected from cold and drafts because trigeminal hyperesthesia may accompany the syndrome. Maintenance of good nutrition is important. The client should be taught to chew on the opposite (functional) side of the mouth to avoid trapping food and to improve taste. Thorough oral hygiene must be carried out after each meal to prevent the development of parotitis and dental cavities from accumulated residual food.

Dark glasses may be worn for protective and cosmetic reasons. Artificial tears (methylcellulose) should be instilled frequently during the day to prevent drying of the cornea. Ointment and an impermeable eye shield can be used at night to retain moisture, or the eye should be taped shut (see Chapter 15).

A facial sling may be helpful to support affected muscles, improve lip alignment, and facilitate eating. Vigorous massage can break down tissues, but gentle upward massage has psychological benefits even if physical effects other than the maintenance of circulation are questionable. When function begins to return, active facial exercises are performed several times a day.

The change in physical appearance as a result of Bell's palsy can be devastating. The client needs to be reassured that a stroke did not occur and that chances for a full recovery are good. The client's need for privacy should be respected, especially during meals, but the nurse's assistance in the client's adjustment to the physical changes should not be delayed. Enlisting support from family and friends is important. If the altered facial appearance is permanent, more intensive counseling may be indicated.[5]

POLYNEUROPATHIES
Guillain-Barré Syndrome

Pathophysiology. Guillain-Barré syndrome (Landry-Guillain-Barré-Strohl syndrome, infectious polyneuropathy, ascending polyneuropathic paralysis) is an acute, rap-

idly progressing, and potentially fatal form of polyneuritis. It affects the peripheral nervous system resulting in loss of myelin (a segmental demyelination) and in edema and inflammation of the affected nerves, causing a lack of neurotransmission to the periphery. The etiology of this disorder is unknown, but it is believed to be a cell-mediated autoimmune reaction directed at the peripheral nerves. The syndrome is frequently preceded by an immune-inciting event such as a viral illness, trauma, surgery, viral immunizations, or lymphoproliferative neoplasms. These stimuli are thought to cause a limited malfunctioning of the immune system, which sensitizes T lymphocytes to the client's myelin, causing myelin damage. Demyelination that stops or slows transmission of nerve impulses occurs. The muscle innervated by the damaged peripheral nerves undergoes denervation and atrophy. The lymphocytes are basically normal and return to complete functioning after the illness.

The syndrome affects both genders equally, and it is more commonly seen in adults aged 20 to 50 years, although it is observed in all age groups.[6] Some evidence has associated the occurrence of Guillain-Barré syndrome with the swine flu vaccine. During the mass screening against the swine flu in 1976 an eight to ten times greater incidence of the syndrome occurred in individuals who were immunized. It is not known whether to attribute this increase to the specific vaccine or whether the increase would also have occurred with other vaccines.[7] With adequate supportive care, the mortality rate for this syndrome can be as low as 5%.

Recently a chronic form of Guillain-Barré syndrome has been described in which the paralysis evolves more slowly. An apparent relapsing of symptoms occurs, with no involvement of respiratory function or cranial nerves. The client with this type of polyneuritis generally does not have a full recovery.[8]

Clinical manifestations and complications. Symptoms usually develop 1 to 3 weeks after an upper respiratory or gastrointestinal (GI) infection. Weakness of the lower extremities (evolving more or less symmetrically) occurs over hours to days to weeks, usually peaking about the fourteenth day. Distal muscles are more severely affected. Paresthesia (numbness and tingling) is frequent, and paralysis usually follows in the extremities. Hypotonia and areflexia are common, persistent symptoms. Objective sensory loss is variable, with deep sensibility more affected than superficial sensations.

Autonomic nervous function is rarely altered, but changes can occur. The syndrome of autonomic hyperreflexia with sinus tachycardia, severe hypertension, and anhydrosis (absence of sweating) can be seen occasionally with urinary or fecal retention.

Progression of the syndrome to include the lower brainstem involves the facial, abducens, optic, hypoglossal, trigeminal, and vagus nerves (CN VII, VI, III, XII, V, and X, respectively). This involvement manifests itself through facial weakness, extraocular eye movement difficulties, dysphagia, and paresthesia of the face.

The most serious complication of this syndrome is respiratory failure, which occurs as the paralysis progresses to the nerves that stimulate the thoracic area. Constant monitoring of the respiratory system by checking respiratory rate, depth, and forced vital capacity provides information about the need for immediate intervention. Respiratory or urinary tract infections may occur. Fever is generally the first sign of infection, and treatment is directed at the infecting organism. Immobility from the paralysis can cause problems such as ileus development, muscle atrophy, deep vein thrombosis, pulmonary emboli, skin breakdown, orthostatic hypotension, and nutritional deficiencies.

Therapeutic management. Diagnosis is based primarily on the client's history and clinical signs. Cerebrospinal fluid is normal initially, but after 7 to 10 days shows a markedly elevated protein level to 700 mg/100 dl (700 mg %, with normal protein being 15-45 mg %). EMG and nerve conduction studies are markedly abnormal in the affected extremities.

Therapeutic management is aimed at supportive care, particularly ventilatory support, during the acute phase. Corticosteroids and ACTH are used to suppress the immune response. Plasmapheresis is being used in an attempt to remove antibodies that may be present and shorten the course of the disease.

Monitoring blood pressure and cardiac rate and rhythm is also important during the acute phase because transient cardiac dysrhythmias have been reported. Autonomic dysfunction is common and usually takes the form of tachycardia. Hypotension secondary to the muscle atony may occur in severe cases. Vasopressor agents and volume expanders may be needed to treat the low blood pressure.

■ Nursing Management of Guillain-Barré Syndrome

Assessment of the client is the most important aspect of nursing care during the acute phase. The nurse needs to monitor the ascending paralysis, assess respiratory function, monitor arterial blood gases (ABGs), and assess the gag, corneal, and swallowing reflexes during the routine assessment.

The objective of therapy is to support body systems until recovery. Respiratory failure and infection are serious threats. Monitoring the vital capacity and ABGs is essential. If the vital capacity drops to less than 800 ml or the ABGs deteriorate, a tracheostomy may be done so that the client can be mechanically ventilated (see Chapter 23). Meticulous suctioning technique is needed to prevent infection whether the client has an endotracheal tube or tracheostomy. Thorough bronchial hygiene and chest physiotherapy help clear secretions and prevent respiratory deterioration. If fever develops, sputum cultures should be obtained to identify whether the respiratory tract is the source of the pathogen. Appropriate antibiotic therapy is then initiated.

A communications system must be established with the use of the client's available abilities. This is extremely difficult if the disease progresses to involvement of the cranial nerves. At the peak of a severe episode the client may be incapable of communication. The nurse must explain all procedures before doing them and reassure the client

that muscle function will return to some part of the body so that needs and desires can be communicated.

Urinary retention is common for a few days. Intermittent catheterization is preferred to an indwelling catheter to avoid urinary tract infections. Physiotherapy is indicated very early to help counter the hazards of immobility. Passive range-of-motion exercises and attention to body position help maintain function and prevent contractures. Nutritional needs must be met in spite of possible problems associated with gastric dilatation, ileus development, and aspiration potential if the gag reflex is lost. Initially, tube feedings or hyperalimentation may be used to ensure adequate caloric intake. Fluid and electrolytes that are used to ensure adequate caloric intake must be monitored carefully to prevent electrolyte imbalances and the possible occurrence of antidiuretic hormone (ADH) secretion dysfunction.

Throughout the course of the illness, the nurse should provide support and encouragement to the family and client. Because residual problems and relapses are uncommon except in the chronic form of the disease, complete recovery can be anticipated even though it is generally a slow process taking months or years if axonal degeneration occurs.

Botulism

Pathophysiology. Botulism is the most serious type of food poisoning. It is caused by GI absorption of the neurotoxin produced by *Clostridium botulinum*. This organism can grow in any food contaminated with the spores. Improper home canning of foods is often the cause. It is thought that the neurotoxin destroys or inhibits the neurotransmission of acetylcholine at the myoneural junction, resulting in disturbed muscle innervation. Symptoms are usually nausea, vomiting, and abdominal cramps, generally within 12 to 36 hours after consumption of the contaminated food. Neurological manifestations develop slowly (4 to 8 days). They include difficulty in convergence of the eyes, photophobia followed by ptosis, and paralysis of extraocular muscles and result in blurred vision, dry mouth, sore throat and difficulty in swallowing, ileus, mild muscle weakness, and respiratory symptoms that can rapidly deteriorate to respiratory arrest.

Because botulism is a reportable disease, local, state, and federal health agencies, particularly the Centers for Disease Control in Atlanta, should be notified.

Therapeutic management. The initial treatment of botulism is intravenous (IV) administration of botulinum antitoxin. Before administration of the antitoxin, possible sensitivity should be assessed by instillation of a drop of antitoxin in one eye. A rapidly occurring conjunctivitis indicates sensitivity, in which case the antitoxin is not given.

The GI tract is purged by laxatives, high colonic enemas, and gastric lavage to decrease absorption of the toxin. Prophylactic penicillin may be ordered to halt the release of toxin in the GI tract.

■ Nursing Management of Botulism

The nurse should educate the public to be alert to situations that may result in botulism. Particular attention should be given to foods with a low acid content, which supports germination and the production of botulin, a deadly poison. These foods include fish, vichyssoise, and peppers. All varieties of spores are destroyed by boiling for 10 minutes or maintaining at a temperature of 80° C for 30 minutes. Specific suggestions related to the preparation, storage, and use of food include the following[9]:

1. In home canning, the equipment manufacturer's directions should be followed. Only fresh fruits and vegetables with questionable spots removed should be used. All containers and utensils need to be cleansed, and the seal on the can or jar must be airtight. Canned foods should be stored properly in a cool, dry place.
2. A can with a swollen end should never be used; the swelling may be caused by gases from *C. botulinum*.
3. If the food is forcefully expelled when a container is opened, it should be discarded immediately and the contents should not be tasted.
4. If the contents of a can look or smell bad after opening, the can should be discarded without tasting of the contents.

Lye should be added to suspicious materials, and they should be stored for 24 hours before burying to destroy bacteria and toxins and to prevent further contamination. Materials may be flushed down the toilet or deposited in the garbage disposal if a large amounts of water is used.

Nursing care during the acute illness is similar to that for Guillain-Barré syndrome. Supportive nursing interventions include rest, activities to maintain respiratory function, adequate nutrition, and prevention of loss of muscle mass. Because the recovery process is slow, the client may develop problems related to a feeling of helplessness, boredom, and low morale.

Tetanus

Pathophysiology. Tetanus is an extremely severe polyradiculitis and polyneuritis affecting spinal and cranial nerves. It results from the effects of the neurotoxin released by the anaerobic bacillus *C. tetani*. Afferent stimuli produce an exaggerated response because of suppression of spinal and brainstem neurons by tetanus exotoxin that blocks postsynaptic inhibition. The host must be susceptible (i.e., not effectively immunized).[10] The spores of the bacillus are present in soil, garden mold, and manure and gain entry into the body through a traumatic or suppurative wound that provides an appropriate low-oxygen environment for them to mature and produce toxin. Other possible sources include dental infection, injections of heroin, human and animal bites, abortion, pregnancy, frostbite, compound fractures, and gunshot wounds. The incubation period is usually 7 days but can range from 1 to 54 days, with symptoms frequently appearing after the original wound is healed. In general, the longer the incubation period, the milder the illness and the better the prognosis.[11]

Worldwide, the number of cases per year is estimated to be 1 million. Only 147 cases of tetanus were reported in the United States from 1985 to 1986.[12] Mortality rates vary according to age, with infants and persons more than

60 years of age most seriously affected. Overall, mortality rates range from 45% to 55%.

Clinical manifestations. Manifestations of tetanus include a prickly sensation in the jaw muscles, which stimulates excessive yawning early in the disease. Within 24 hours the jaw muscles become tender and stiff (lockjaw). Generalized tonic spasms occur because of the lack of reciprocal innervation and dysphagia. As the disease progresses, the neck muscles, back, and extremities become progressively rigid. In severe forms, continuous tonic convulsions may occur with *opisthotonus* (extreme arching of the back and retraction of the head). Laryngeal and respiratory spasms cause apnea and anoxia. Additional effects are manifested by overstimulation of the sympathetic nervous system including profuse diaphoresis, labile hypertension, episodic tachycardia, hyperthermia, and cardiac dysrhythmias.[11] The slightest noise, jarring motion, or bright light can set off the convulsion. Mortality is almost 100% in the severe form. Residual injury such as vertebral fracture, muscular contraction, and brain damage because of hypoxia may remain.

Therapeutic management. The therapeutic management of tetanus includes administration of tetanus toxoid booster (Td) and tetanus immune globulin (TIG) before the onset of symptoms to neutralize circulating toxins. Once neurological signs have appeared, these injections are ineffective because the neurotoxin is permanently fixed as soon as it is attached to the neuromuscular end plate.[13]

Serum electrolytes, complete blood cell count (CBC), albumin, clotting factors, glucose, and ABGs are monitored. Cardiac function is monitored by electrocardiogram (ECG) and auscultation. As larger numbers of nerve cells are attacked, their inhibitory control over muscle activity decreases with development of symptoms. Control of spasms is essential and is managed by deep sedation, usually with diazepam, barbiturates, or chlorpromazine. A 10-day course of penicillin is recommended.

A tracheostomy is usually performed early and the client is maintained on mechanical ventilation. If sedation does not control seizures, skeletal-muscle-paralyzing drugs such as tubocurare are used. Pain is relieved by means of codeine or meperidine, often with the addition of promethazine. Antibiotics may be given to prevent secondary infections. Nutrition is maintained through IV or nasogastric feeding. Even with the best of care, the mortality rate is 50%. Those who recover have a long convalescence that includes extensive physiotherapy.

■ Nursing Management of Tetanus

Health teaching is aimed at ensuring tetanus prophylaxis, which is the most important factor influencing the incidence of this disease. Tetanus prevention and immunization protocols are summarized in Table 55-3. Clients should be taught that immediate thorough cleansing of all wounds with soap and water is important in the prevention of tetanus. If an open wound occurs and the client has not been immunized within 10 years, the primary care provider should be contacted so that a tetanus booster can be given.

If equine tetanus antitoxin is to be used, the client should be tested for sensitivity. Administration of equine

Table 55-3 Tetanus Prevention and Immunization Protocols

Prior Vaccinations with Td		Clean, Minor Wounds		All Other Wounds	
Total Number	Years Since Last Dose	Td	TIG	Td	TIG
≥3	<5	No	No	No	No
≥3	5-10	No	No	Yes	No
≥3	>10	Yes	No	Yes	No
≤2, unknown	—	Yes	No	Yes	Yes

Modified from Mandell GL, Douglas RG, and Bennett JE, eds: Principles and practice of infectious diseases, ed 3, New York, 1990, Churchill Livingstone, p 1846.

antitoxin is not recommended if sensitivity occurs; anaphylactic shock is potentially life threatening and desensitization is ineffective. The side effects of routine administration of the antitoxin are mild and include a sore arm, swelling at the site, and itching. Serious side effects rarely occur. Routine administration of a booster shot to an adequately immunized client can cause extreme arm swelling, lymphadenopathy, and severe hypersensitivity.

All clients should receive a written record of immunizations and be encouraged to complete their active immunization schedule. The client's immunization history should be accurately recorded to protect the client and care providers.

The acute nursing management of the client with tetanus is aimed at supportive care based on treatment of manifestations. The client should be placed in a quiet, darkened room insulated against noise. Nursing care should be administered with the utmost caution to avoid triggering spasms. Nursing care related to tracheostomy and mechanical ventilation is given as appropriate. Problems related to bowel and bladder function and immobility must be managed.

The client needs support during the acute phase because the fear of death is real. The family also needs support and explanations.

Neurosyphilis

Neurosyphilis (tertiary syphilis) is an infection of any part of the nervous system by the organism *Treponema pallidum*. It is the result of untreated or inadequately treated syphilis (see Chapter 47). The organism can invade the central nervous system (CNS) within a few months of the original infection. Except for causing some changes in the cerebrospinal fluid including increased white blood cells (WBCs) and protein and positive serological reaction, the organism lies dormant for years. Although not contagious, untreated neurosyphilis can be fatal. Penicillin therapy is effective for syphilitic meningitis, but the neurological deficits remain.

Late neurosyphilis results from degenerative changes in the spinal cord (tabes dorsalis) and brainstem (general paresis). *Tabes dorsalis* (progressive locomotor ataxia) is characterized by vague, sharp pains in the legs; ataxia; "slapping" gait; loss of proprioception and deep tendon re-

flexes; and zones of hyperesthesia. Charcot's joints, which are characterized by enlargement, bone destruction, and hypermobility, also occur as a result of effusion and edema.

Dementia paralytica is an ongoing spirochetal meningoencephalitis that causes a general dissolution of mental and physical capabilities. It may mimic a number of major or minor psychoses. Management includes treatment with penicillin, symptomatic care, and protection from physical injury.

SPINAL CORD TRAUMA
Significance

The manifestations of spinal cord injury are generally the direct result of trauma that causes cord compression, ischemia, edema, and possible cord transection. Before World War II, the life expectancy for the person with a spinal cord injury was only 10 years from the onset of injury. Presently, even the very young client with a spinal cord injury can anticipate a long life. The cause of premature death in the client with quadriplegia is usually related to respiratory involvement, but prognosis for life is generally only about 5 years less than for persons of the same age without spinal cord injury.

Health care providers often consider spinal cord disability to be one of the most devastating of physical disabilities. However, clients with spinal cord injury are remarkably resourceful, with impressive resilience and an ability to work out new patterns of living and coping.[14,15] Staff members often underestimate the client's potential for independence. Misplaced sympathy and overidentification can compromise the nurse's attempt to give the involved and complex care required by the injured person for optimal rehabilitation. Recovery is prolonged, and nurses must learn to gauge progress in inches rather than miles. Skilled, persistent care draws on every known nursing intervention until the client achieves a maximal level of independence.

The disruption of individual growth and development, altered family dynamics, economic loss in terms of absence from work, and the high cost of rehabilitation and/or maintenance make spinal cord trauma a devastating problem. Initial rehabilitation for a person with a spinal cord injury is approximately $30,000, depending on the geographical location. In 1987, the U.S. Armed Forces estimate that the care for military personnel with spinal cord injuries approached $1 billion.[16] New spinal cord injury affects 10,000 persons in the United States each year.[16]

Although many clients with spinal cord injuries can care for themselves with minimal assistance, a larger number are confined to nursing homes, care centers, and rehabilitation units. Clients with quadriplegia spend an average of 25 days per year in the hospital, whereas clients with paraplegia spend 15 days.[16] The loss to the work force in terms of human potential is inestimable.

Etiology

The high-risk population for spinal cord injury is primarily young adult males between the ages of 15 and 30 and those who are impulsive or risk takers in daily living. A history of numerous injuries before the cord injury is common. A high correlation exists between alcohol and drug abuse and spinal cord injury. Others listed at high risk for spinal cord injury include motorcyclists, sky divers, football players, police officers, divers, and military personnel. In decreasing order of prevalence, the causes of spinal cord injury include automobile accidents, diving, falls on stairs, industrial accidents, gunshot wounds, and many sports activities.[16] The resulting spinal cord injury can be due to cord compression by bone displacement, interruption of blood supply to the cord, or traction resulting from pulling on the cord.

Classification

Spinal cord injuries are classified by the mechanism of injury, level of injury, or degree of injury. The major mechanisms of injury are flexion, flexion-rotation, hyperextension, extension-rotation, or compression (Fig. 55-2). The flexion injury that includes dislocation is the most unstable of all injuries because the ligamentous structures that stabilize the spine are torn. This injury is most often implicated in severe neurological deficits.

The level of injury may be cervical, thoracic, or lumbar. Cervical and lumbar injuries are most common because these levels are associated with the greatest flexibility and movement.

The degree of spinal cord involvement may be either complete of incomplete (partial). Complete cord involvement results in flaccid paralysis and total loss of sensory and motor function below the level of lesion (injury). This loss can result in irreversible damage to the spinal cord. If the cervical cord is involved, paralysis of all four extremities resulting in quadriplegia occurs. If the thoracic or lumbar cord is damaged, the result is paraplegia. Figure 55-3 shows affected structures and functions at different levels of cord injury.

Incomplete cord lesion involvement (partial transection) results in a mixed loss of voluntary motor activity and sensation and leaves some tracts intact. The degree of sensory and motor loss varies depending on the level of the lesion and reflects the specific nerve tracts damaged and those spared. Four syndromes are associated with incomplete lesions.[17] Damage in the cervical central cord is termed *central cord syndrome,* which is characterized by microscopic hemorrhage and edema to the central cord (Fig. 55-4, *A*). Motor weakness is present in both the upper and lower extremities, but the weakness is much greater in the upper extremities than in the lower ones. It may change to a progressive lesion. Sensory dysfunction varies according to the site of injury or lesion. Bladder dysfunction is common. This syndrome is frequently a result of hyperextension of an osteoarthritic spine. The extent of recovery depends on the resolution of edema and the intactness of the spinal cord tracts.

Anterior cord syndrome is characterized by injury resulting in an acute compression of the anterior portion of the spinal cord, often a flexion injury (Fig. 55-4, *B*). The spinal cord lesion is in the anterior two thirds of the cord. Compression is usually caused by a disk or bony fragment; it may also be caused by actual destruction of the anterior cord by an anterior spinal artery occlusion caused by ischemia or thrombus. Manifestations include immediate ante-

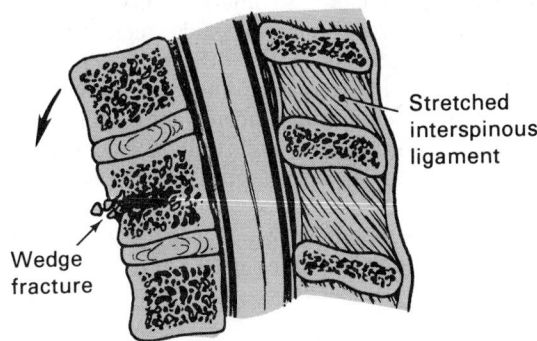

Stretched interspinous ligament

Wedge fracture

Flexion injury

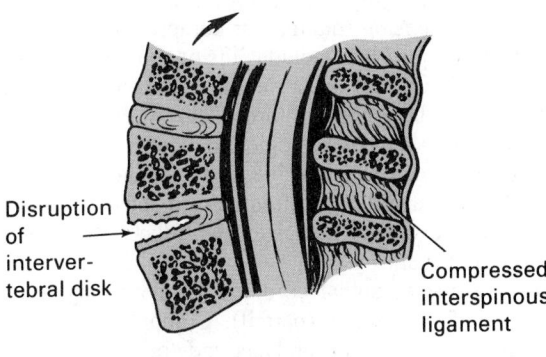

Disruption of intervertebral disk

Compressed interspinous ligament

Extension injury

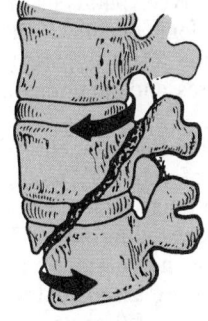

Displacement of vertebrae with fracture of 2 vertebral bodies and 1 disk

Flexion-rotation injury

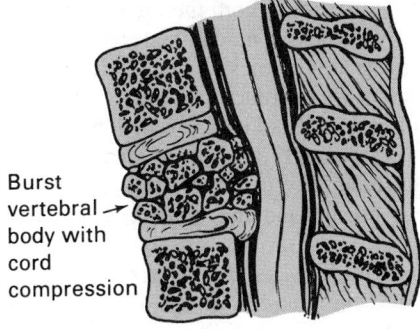

Burst vertebral body with cord compression

Compression injury

Fig. 55-2 Mechanisms of spinal injury.

rior paralysis that is complete from the injury or compression down. Hypoesthesia (decreased sensation) and decreased pain sensation occur below the level of injury.

Because the posterior cord tracts are not injured, sensations of touch, position, vibration, and motion remain intact. Dorsal column function is preserved. If the syndrome is caused by the compression of the anterior cord from bony fragments, surgical decompression is indicated.

Brown-Sequard syndrome is a result of transection or lesion of one half of the spinal cord (Fig. 55-4, *C*). This syndrome is characterized by a loss of motor function (paralysis) and position and vibratory sense, as well as vasomotor paralysis on the same side (ipsilateral) and below the hemisection. The opposite (contralateral) side of the hemisection has loss of pain and temperature sensation below the level of the lesion or hemisection.

Less commonly seen is the *posterior cord syndrome*. This syndrome results from compression or damage to the posterior part of the spinal cord that contains the sensory neurons and position-sense capabilities.

Pathophysiology

Initial injury. The spinal cord is extremely tough and is rarely torn or transected by direct trauma. The complete cord dissolution (previously thought to be transection) in severe trauma is related to autodestruction of the cord. Shortly after the injury, petechial hemorrhages are noted in the central gray matter of the cord. This is followed in 1 to 2 hours by extravasation of red blood cells (RBCs), fluid, and polymorphonuclear leukocytes that extend throughout the gray matter.[18] Vascular stasis occurs, and the endothelium of vessel walls is damaged. Hemorrhage, edema, and metabolites act together to produce ischemia, which progresses to necrotic destruction of the cord. The resulting hypoxia reduces the oxygen tension below the level that meets the metabolic needs of the cord. Lactate metabolites and a gross increase in norepinephrine are noted. In toxic doses, norepinephrine causes vasospasms, hypoxia, and subsequent necrosis. Unfortunately, the spinal cord has minimal ability to adapt to vasospasm by means of increased flow from anastomotic areas. By 4 hours after the injury this process has progressed to coagulation necrosis of up to 40% of the gray matter and adjacent white matter.[19]

By 24 hours after the injury the destructive process has progressed to where the spinal cord is composed mainly of necrotic tissue and aggregated RBCs, with only a small rim of identifiable white matter.[19] Edema secondary to the inflammatory response is particularly harmful because of lack of space for tissue expansion. The resultant compression of the cord and extension of edema above and below the injury therefore increases the ischemic damage. The end result is no different than mechanical severance of the cord.

The hemorrhagic necrosis causes the lesion to be complete after 48 hours, and any function of nerves that arise in and pass through this level is destroyed. Because additional edema extends the level of injury beyond the immediate level of destruction for 72 hours to 1 week, the exact extent of injury cannot be determined before that time.

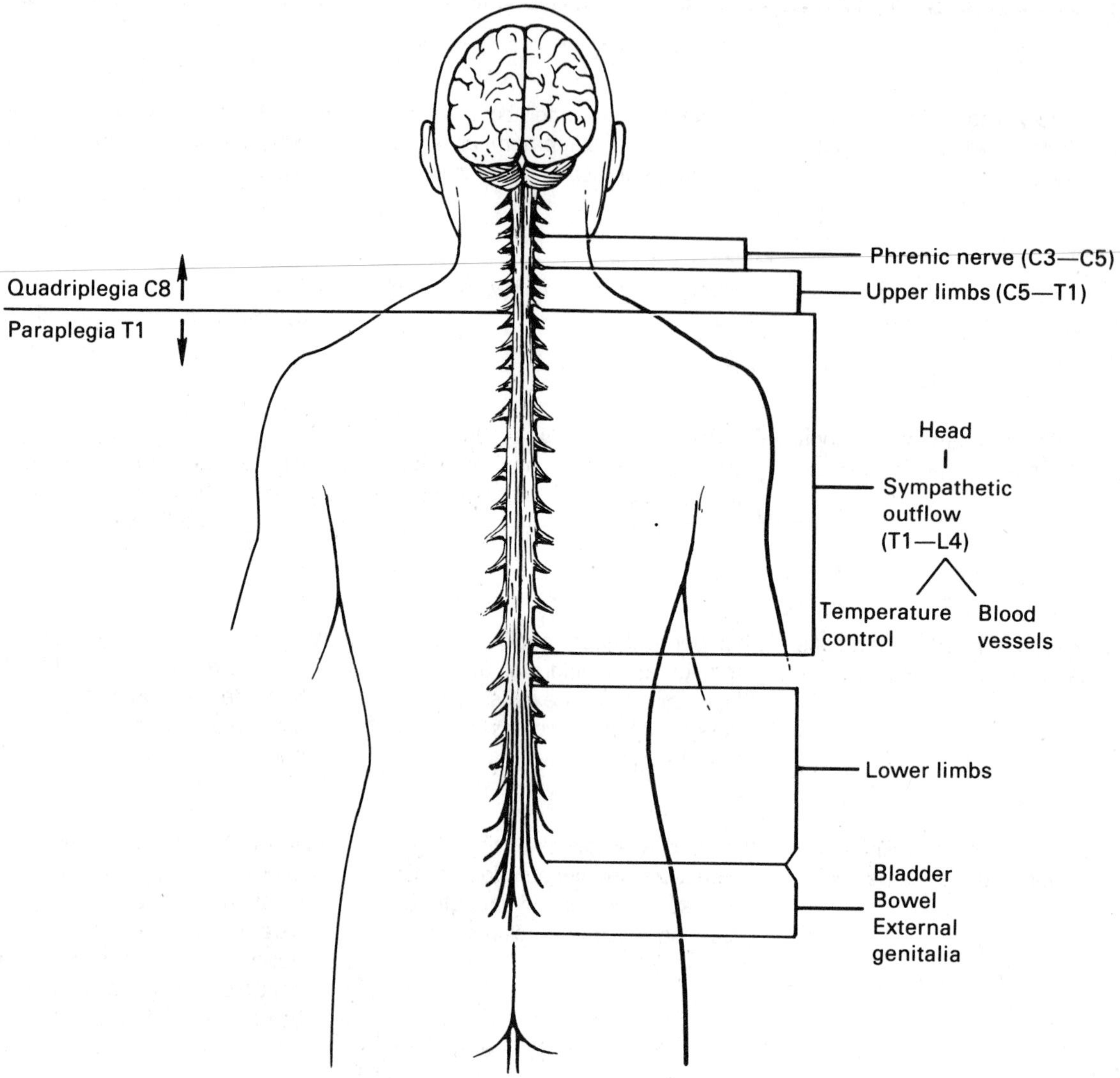

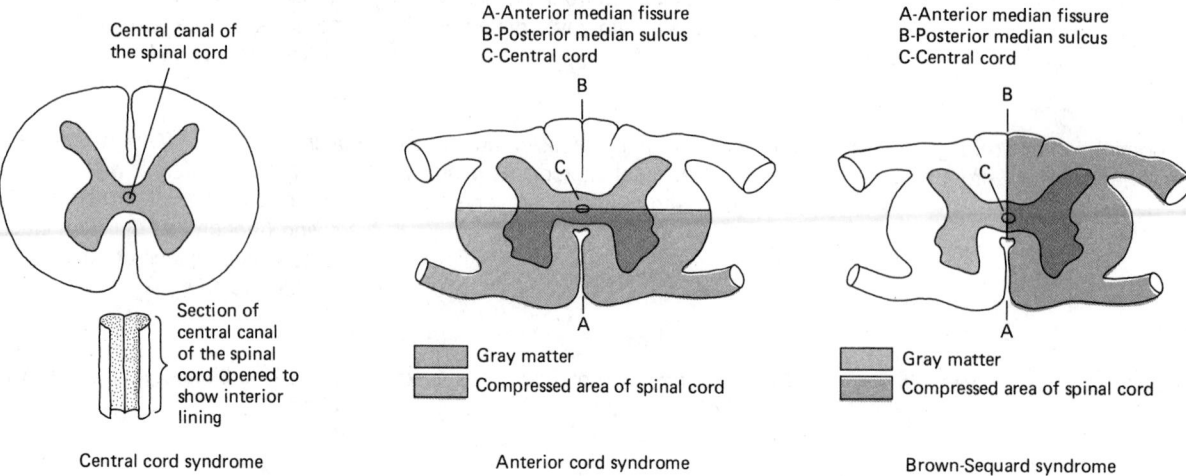

Quadriplegia C8

Paraplegia T1

Phrenic nerve (C3—C5)

Upper limbs (C5—T1)

Head

Sympathetic outflow (T1—L4)

Temperature control   Blood vessels

Lower limbs

Bladder
Bowel
External genitalia

Fig. 55-3   Symptoms, degree of paralysis, and potential for rehabilitation depend on the level of the lesion.

Central canal of the spinal cord

Section of central canal of the spinal cord opened to show interior lining

Central cord syndrome

A-Anterior median fissure
B-Posterior median sulcus
C-Central cord

B

C

A

Gray matter

Compressed area of spinal cord

Anterior cord syndrome

A-Anterior median fissure
B-Posterior median sulcus
C-Central cord

B

C

A

Gray matter

Compressed area of spinal cord

Brown-Sequard syndrome

Fig. 55-4   Three syndromes associated with incomplete cord lesions.

Table 55-4 Functional Level of Spinal Cord Disruption and Rehabilitation Potential

Autonomic	Movement Remaining	Rehabilitation Potential
QUADRIPLEGIA		
C1-C3		
Usually fatal injury, vagus domination of heart, respiration, blood vessels, all organs below injury	Movement in neck and above, loss of innervation to diaphragm, absence of independent respiratory function	Ability to drive electric wheelchair equipped with portable respirator by using chin control or mouth stick, lack of bowel and bladder control
C4		
Vagus domination of heart, respirations, and all vessels and organs below injury	Sensation and movement above neck	Ability to drive electric wheelchair by using chin control or mouth stick, lack of bowel and bladder control
C5		
Vagus domination of heart, respirations, and all vessels and organs below injury	Full neck, partial shoulder, back, biceps; gross elbow, inability to roll over or use hands; decreased respiratory reserve	Ability to drive electric wheelchair with mobile hand supports, ability to use powered hand splints (in some clients), lack of bowel and bladder control
C6		
Vagus domination of heart, respirations, and all vessels and organs below injury	Shoulder and upper back abduction and rotation at shoulder, full biceps to elbow flexion, wrist extension, weak grasp of thumb, decreased respiratory reserve	Ability to assist with transfer and perform some self-care, feed self with hand devices, push wheelchair on smooth, flat surface; lack of bowel and bladder control
C7-C8		
Vagus domination of heart, respirations, and all vessels and organs below injury	All triceps to elbow extension, finger extensors and flexors, good grasp with some decreased strength, decreased respiratory reserve	Ability to transfer self to wheelchair, roll over and sit up in bed, push self on most surfaces, perform most self-care; independent use of wheelchair; ability to drive car with powered hand controls (in some clients); lack of bowel and bladder control
PARAPLEGIA		
T1-T6		
Sympathetic innervation to heart, vagus domination of rest	Full innervation of upper extremities, back, essential intrinsic muscles of hand; full strength and dexterity of grasp; decreased trunk stability, decreased respiratory reserve	Full independence in self-care and in wheelchair, ability to drive car with hand controls (in most clients), ability to use full body brace for exercise but not for functional ambulation, lack of bowel and bladder control
T6-T12		
Vagus domination only of leg vessels, GI and genitourinary organs	Full, stable thoracic muscles and upper back; functional intercostals, resulting in increased respiratory reserve	Full independent use of wheelchair; ability to stand erect with full body brace, ambulate on crutches with swing (though gait difficult); inability to climb stairs; lack of bowel and bladder control
L1-L2		
Vagus domination of leg vessels	Varying control of legs and pelvis, instability of lower back	Good sitting balance, full use of wheelchair
L3-L4		
Partial domination of leg vessels, GI and genitourinary organs	Quadriceps and hip flexors, absence of hamstring function, flail ankles	Completely independent ambulation with short leg braces and canes, inability to stand for long periods, bladder and bowel continence

Spinal shock. In addition to the discrete damage at the trauma site, the entire cord below the level of the lesion fails to function, resulting in spinal shock characterized by hypotension, bradycardia, and warm, dry extremities. Spinal shock usually occurs at the time of injury and results in immediate depression of all cord functions in response to severe damage to the cord. The onset of spinal shock causes the client to have a complete loss of motor and sensory activity below the level of the lesion. Loss of sympathetic innervations causes peripheral vasodilatation, venous pooling, and a decreased cardiac output. These symptoms are generally associated with a cervical or high thoracic injury.

Spinal shock generally lasts for 7 to 10 days after onset. Indications that spinal shock has ended include spasticity, reflex emptying of the bladder, and hyperreflexia. After resolution of spinal shock, active rehabilitation can begin.

Clinical Manifestations

Manifestations are related to the level of injury and the degree of injury. The client with an incomplete lesion may demonstrate a mixture of symptoms. The higher the injury, the more serious are the sequelae because of the proximity of the cervical cord to the medulla and brainstem. Movement and rehabilitation potential related to specific locations of the spinal cord injury are described in Table 55-4. In general, sensory function closely parallels motor function at all levels.

The types of accidents causing spinal cord trauma can also result in head injury. The client should therefore be assessed for signs of concussion and increased intracranial pressure (see Chapter 52). In addition, a careful assessment for musculoskeletal injuries and trauma to internal organs should be performed. Because there are no muscle, bone, or visceral sensations, the only clue to internal trauma with hemorrhage may be a rapidly falling hematocrit level.

Therapeutic Management

The initial goals for the client with a spinal cord injury are to sustain life and prevent further cord damage. Table 55-5 outlines the prehospital care of the client with a spinal cord injury. Systemic and spinal cord shock must be treated. For injury at the cervical level, all body systems must be maintained until the full extent of the damage can be evaluated. Treatment of a spinal cord injury may be therapeutic or surgical. Therapeutic management for the client with a cervical injury is described in Table 55-6. The systemic support required by the client is less intense for thoracic and lumbar injuries. Respiratory care is not as

Table 55-5

 Prehospital Emergency Care of the Client with a Spinal Cord Injury*

Etiology: Squeezed, stretched, torn, or severed spinal cord from vertebral displacement due to crushing compression, flexion, hypertension, or flexion-rotation injuries

CLINICAL MANIFESTATIONS

Pain, tenderness, deformities, or muscle spasms adjacent to vertebral column
Numbness, paresthesias
Weakness or heaviness in limbs
Weakness, paralysis, or flaccidity of muscles
Cuts and bruises over head, face, neck, or back
Hypotension without other signs of shock
Diaphragmatic breathing
Priapism
Absence of signs and symptoms

MANAGEMENT

Maintain patent airway; assist with respirations if necessary; *do not* hyperextend neck to establish airway.
Note position and general appearance of client.
If back or neck injury is suspected, immobilize client and stabilize head and neck.
Start IV line with large-gauge needle.
Administer oxygen.
Monitor vital signs.
Treat any other injuries.
Transport on back board; treat persons suspected of having a spinal injury as if one were present.
Watch for nausea and vomiting; be prepared to suction.

*See Chapter 59 for a general discussion on measures related to prehospital emergency care.

Table 55-6

 Diagnostic and Therapeutic Management: Cervical Cord Injury

DIAGNOSTIC

Complete neurological examination
ABGs
Electrolytes, glucose, hemoglobin, and hematocrit levels
Urinalysis
Anteroposterior and lateral spine x-ray studies
CT scan
Myelography
MRI
EMG to measure evoked potentials

THERAPEUTIC

Immobilization of vertebral column by skeletal traction
Maintenance of heart rate (e.g., atropine) and blood pressure (e.g., dopamine)
Corticosteroid therapy to reduce edema
Insertion of nasogastric tube
Intubation (if indicated by ABGs)
Oxygen by high-humidity mask
Indwelling urinary catheter
Administration of IV fluids with moderate fluid restriction first 72 hr

CT, Computerized tomography; *MRI,* magnetic resonance imaging.

intense, and bradycardia is not a problem. Specific problems are treated symptomatically.

Surgical Interventions

The decision to perform surgery on a client with a spinal cord injury often depends on the preference of a particular clinician. Surgery is necessary when there is continued compression of the spinal cord by extrinsic forces. Surgery stabilizes the spinal column. In general, accepted criteria for early surgery include (1) evidence of cord compression, (2) progressive neurological deficit, (3) compound fracture of the vertebra (bony fragments may dislodge and penetrate the cord), (4) penetrating wounds of the spinal cord or surrounding structures, and (5) a bone fragment in the spinal cord.[20]

The more common surgical procedures include decompression laminectomy by anterior cervical and thoracic approaches with fusion, posterior laminectomy with the use of acrylic wire mesh and fusion, and insertion of Harrington rods with correction and stabilization of thoracic deformities. (Specific surgical and nursing interventions for these techniques are discussed in Chapter 57.)

Experimental Methods

The management of spinal cord injury has changed dramatically in recent years. Although many experimental methods are used, the prognosis for the client with indirect trauma has improved. Methods presently being tested are as follows[21]:

1. *Myelotomy:* The cord is opened, and blood, edema, and metabolites are drained.
2. *Norepinephrine counteractants:* These agents counteract the effects of norepinephrine when they are injected within 15 minutes of the injury and are effective only at toxic levels. They include α-methyltyrosine (AMT), which prevents hemorrhagic necrosis; reserpine, which depletes catecholamines in peripheral nerves and the CNS; levodopa, which competes with norepinephrine for nerve cell receptor sites; and steroids, which maintain vascular integrity, protect cellular membranes during decreased perfusion, and reduce edema.
3. *Hypothermia:* This method involves perfusion of the cord with 10° C normal saline solution, which slows the neural enzymatic processes and reduces cellular metabolic rates and oxygen requirements.
4. *Hyperbaric oxygen:* In a hyperbaric chamber the client breathes pure oxygen under increased atmospheric pressure. This results in increased oxygen to tissues and facilitates penetration of oxygen into hypoxic areas.
5. *Naloxone:* This drug counteracts the effects of catecholamine and endorphin release and is given during the first hour of injury.
6. *Thyrotropin-releasing hormone:* This agent is used to increase the metabolism and perfusion in the cord.

Pharmacological Management

Vasopressor agents employed in the acute phase are useful adjuvants to treatment. The goal is to maintain the mean arterial pressure at a level greater than 90 mm Hg so that perfusion to the spinal cord is improved. Dopamine is the drug of choice.

Pharmacological properties of drug metabolism are altered in spinal cord injury; therefore drug interactions may occur. For example, propoxyphene (Darvon) is believed to enhance vasodilatation and possibly aggravate orthostatic hypotension, as well as act as an analgesic. The result may enhance already existing problems in the neurologically disabled client. Drug-induced sedation can also mask a decreasing level of consciousness.

Pharmacological agents are used to treat specific autonomic dysfunctions such as GI hyperactivity, bleeding, bradycardia, orthostatic hypotension, inadequate emptying of the bladder, and autonomic dysreflexia. The nurse must observe the response to these drugs and provide specific interventions when adverse reactions are seen.

Complications

Immediate postinjury problems include (1) maintaining a patent airway, adequate ventilation, and adequate circulating blood volume and (2) preventing extension of cord damage.

Respiratory system. Cervical injury or fracture above the level of C4 presents special problems because of the total loss of respiratory function. Mechanical ventilation is required to keep the client alive; however, most of these clients will die. Injury or fracture below the level of C4 results in diaphragmatic breathing if the phrenic nerve is functioning. Hypoventilation almost always occurs with diaphragmatic respirations because of the decrease in vital capacity and tidal volume.

Cervical fractures or severe injuries cause a paralysis of abdominal musculature and frequently intercostal musculature; therefore, the client cannot cough effectively enough to remove secretions, leading to atelectasis and pneumonia. An artificial airway provides direct access for pathogens, and bronchial hygiene and chest physiotherapy are extremely important. In multiple trauma a neurogenic pulmonary edema may result from the sudden changes in thoracic pressures at the time of the injury. Pulmonary edema may also be due to fluid overload.

Cardiovascular system. Any cord transection above the level of T5 abolishes the influence of the sympathetic nervous system; consequently, bradycardia and hypotension occur. Close cardiac monitoring of slight bradycardia may show a stable cardiac condition. In marked bradycardia, appropriate medications to increase the heart rate and prevent hypoxemia are necessary.

The loss of the influence of the sympathetic nervous system results in vasodilatation, decreasing the venous return of blood to the heart, which results in a decrease in cardiac output and subsequent hypotension. IV fluids may resolve the problem, or vasopressor drugs may be required.

Renal system. Urinary retention is a common development in acute spinal injuries and spinal shock. The bladder is hyperirritable, with a loss of inhibition of reflex from the brain. Consequently, the client urinates small amounts frequently. The bladder becomes distended because of inadequate emptying. Urinary retention increases the chance

of infection. In addition, urinary calculi are likely to develop in a distended bladder retaining urine. Catheterization is indicated. Initially, an indwelling catheter is used, but intermittent catheterization should begin when spinal shock is over.

Gastrointestinal system. If the cord transection has occurred above the level of T5, the loss of sympathetic innervation may lead to the development of an ileus or gastric distention. A nasogastric tube for intermittent suctioning may relieve the gastric distention, and standard treatment is used for an ileus. The development of biochemical stress ulcers is a common occurrence due to excessive release of hydrochloric acid in the stomach. H_2 blockers are frequently used to prevent the occurrence of these ulcers during the initial extreme body stress. Antacids can also be used. Intraabdominal bleeding may occur and is difficult to diagnose because no subjective signs such as pain, tenderness, and guarding are observed. Continued hypotension in spite of vigorous treatment may be the only indication of bleeding. Expanding girth of the abdomen may also be noted. Another GI problem is the development of a fecal impaction due to lack of regularly emptying of the rectum.

Other systems. A major consequence of lack of movement is the deterioration of denervated skin, which can occur very quickly and lead to major infection or sepsis. A certain degree of muscle atrophy occurs during the flaccid paralysis state, whereas contractures tend to occur during the spastic state.

Poikilothermism is the adjustment of the body temperature to the room temperature. This occurs in spinal cord injuries because the interruption of the sympathetic nervous system prevents its temperature-controlling fibers from sending impulses that reach the hypothalamus and because there is minimal or no movement to generate heat.

Metabolic needs. Correcting an existing acid-base disturbance and maintaining acid-base balance promote the function of other body systems. Nasogastric suctioning may lead to alkalosis, and decreased perfusion may lead to acidosis. Electrolyte levels must be monitored until a normal diet is resumed and suctioning is discontinued. A positive nitrogen balance and a high-protein diet help prevent skin breakdown and infections and help decrease the rate of muscle atrophy.

▪ Nursing Management of Spinal Cord Injury

Nursing assessment

Subjective and objective data that should be obtained from the client with spinal cord injury are presented in Table 55-7. Other diagnostic studies add valuable information needed to design an appropriate plan of care (Table 55-7).

Nursing diagnoses

Nursing diagnosis for the client with spinal cord injury depends on the severity of the injury and the level of dysfunction. The nursing diagnoses in Table 55-8 are those associated with a client with a complete cervical cord injury.

Nursing interventions

Health promotion and maintenance. Nursing interventions include identification of the risk population, counsel-

Table 55-7

 Nursing Assessment of the Client with a Spinal Cord Injury

SUBJECTIVE DATA

History
Automobile, sports, industrial accidents; falls, gunshot wounds
General
Fear
Pain
Presence of pain at or above the level of injury
Respiratory
Dyspnea, inability to breathe adequately
Neurological
Loss of power, movement, sensation below level of injury; numbness, tingling, burning, twitching of extremities

OBJECTIVE DATA

General
Depression, anger, denial, anxiety, poikilothermism
Integumentary
Pallor or cyanosis, cool skin, lack of perspiration in affected area
Respiratory
Lesions at C1 to C3: apnea, inability to cough; lesions at C4: poor cough, diaphragmatic breathing, hypoventilation; lesions at C5 to T6: decreased respiratory reserve; cyanosis possible
Cardiovascular
Lesions above T5: bradycardia, hypotension, postural hypotension, absence of vasomotor tone, confusion
Gastrointestinal
Decreased or absent bowel sounds (for paralytic ileus in lesions above T5), abdominal distention, constipation, incontinence, fecal impaction
Urinary
Retention (for lesions between T1, L2)
Reproductive
Priapism, loss of sexual function
Neurological
Complete: Flaccid paralysis and anesthesia below level of injury resulting in quadriplegia (for lesions above C-8) or paraplegia (for lesions below C-8), hyperactive deep tendon reflexes, bilaterally positive Babinski's test
Incomplete: Mixed loss of voluntary motor activity and sensations
Musculoskeletal
Muscle atrophy (in flaccid state), contractures (in spastic state)
Possible findings
Location of level and type of bony involvement on spinal x-ray series; lesion, edema, compression on CT and MRI scans; positive finding on myelogram

CT, Computerized tomography; *MRI,* magnetic resonance imaging.

Table 55-8

 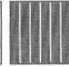

NURSING CARE PLAN FOR THE CLIENT WITH A SPINAL CORD INJURY*

Defining Characteristics	Nursing Interventions	Evaluation Criteria

NURSING DIAGNOSIS: Impaired gas exchange related to muscle fatigue and retained secretions

Decreased oxygen content, increased carbon dioxide concentration, cyanosis, fatigue	Maintain a patent airway. Assess respiratory parameters at least q 2 hr initially. Monitor ABGs at least q 4 hr. Provide aggressive pulmonary toilet, including chest physical therapy and quad-assist coughing q 4 hr. Assess strength of cough at least q 4 hr. Provide rest periods to prevent fatigue. Suction as necessary. Note skin color.	ABGs within normal limits, normal chest x-ray film, clear lungs on auscultation; absence of respiratory distress

NURSING DIAGNOSIS: Decreased cardiac output related to venous pooling of blood and immobility

Hypotension, tachycardia, restlessness, oliguria, decreased central venous and pulmonary artery pressures	Monitor blood pressure and pulse at least q 4 hr initially. Monitor cardiac rhythm. Administer dopamine or other vasopressor agent to maintain mean blood pressure > 80 mm Hg. Apply pneumatic compression devices to calves and/or antiembolism stockings. Perform range of motion to all extremities at least q 8 hr. Measure pulmonary capillary wedge pressure and cardiac output as ordered.	Adequate cardiac output as measured by thermodilution technique, stable blood pressure and pulse, absence of cyanosis and dysrhythmias; prevention of complications such as venous thrombosis or pulmonary emboli

NURSING DIAGNOSIS: Impaired skin integrity related to immobility and poor tissue perfusion

Reddened skin over bony prominences and pin and tong sites	Inspect all skin areas, especially over bony prominences, at least q 2 hr. Observe area around pins or tongs for signs of breakdown of infection at least every shift. Turn client at least q 2 hr. Use low air-loss bed, kinetic treatment table, or other specialty care devices as needed. Ensure adequate nutritional intake. Wash and dry client's skin thoroughly.	Intact skin

NURSING DIAGNOSIS: Constipation related to the injury, inadequate fluid intake, diet low in roughage, and immobility

Lack of bowel movement for more than 2 days, decreased bowel sounds, palpable impaction, hard stool or stool incontinence	Auscultate bowel sounds at least q 4 hr. Monitor abdominal distention. Note any nausea and vomiting; check gastric secretions for pH level. Administer antacids as ordered. Administer stool softeners. Begin bowel program as soon as bowel sounds return and include suppository every other day. Check for impaction every day. Teach client and family the bowel program. Ensure adequate food and fluid intake.	Restoration of GI function, establishment of bowel evacuation program, bowel movement at least every other day

NURSING DIAGNOSIS: Altered patterns of urinary elimination: retention related to injury and limited fluid intake

Lack of urine output, bladder distention, involuntary emptying of bladder (after spinal shock)	Palpate bladder for distention. Insert indwelling catheter during acute phase. Begin intermittent catheterization program when appropriate. Maintain accurate intake and output records. Encourage fluids (2-4 L/day). Send urine for culture at least once a week. Monitor BUN, creatinine levels, and WBC count. Measure urine specific gravity and pH. Teach client and family intermittent catherization using a clean technique. Teach Credé maneuver.	Prevention of urinary retention and infection, ability to perform catheterization or Credé's maneuver to empty bladder

BUN, Blood urea nitrogen.
*This care plan is suitable for a client with a high cervical injury due to flexion-rotation. It can be modified for clients with less severe problems.

Table 55-8

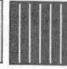

NURSING CARE PLAN FOR THE CLIENT WITH A SPINAL CORD INJURY*—cont'd

Defining Characteristics	Nursing Interventions	Evaluation Criteria

NURSING DIAGNOSIS: Impaired physical mobility related to spinal cord injury, vertebral column instability, or forced immobilization by traction

Defining Characteristics	Nursing Interventions	Evaluation Criteria
Inability to move purposefully, limited muscle strength, impaired coordination, impaired perception of position or presence of body parts	Check traction to ensure that frames are secure, and properly aligned and that weights are hanging free. Promote good pulmonary function. Turn client as ordered. Perform full range of motion to all extremities several times a day. Use splints as appropriate to prevent contractures and promote functional positioning. Assess motor and sensory function at least q 4 hr initially. Mobilize client as quickly as it is appropriate to do so.	Prevention or minimization of complications of immobility

NURSING DIAGNOSIS: Acute pain related to muscle spasm

Defining Characteristics	Nursing Interventions	Evaluation Criteria
Report of pain, mask of pain	Assess type, location, and degree of pain. Change client's position as appropriate. Medicate with antispasmodic agents as ordered and analgesics as needed. Use relaxation therapy to assist in decreasing spasms. Avoid sudden movements that can produce spasm.	Minimal complaints of discomfort, control of muscle spasms

NURSING DIAGNOSIS: Self-care deficit: total related to paralysis

Defining Characteristics	Nursing Interventions	Evaluation Criteria
Inability to feed, bathe, turn, toilet, or dress	Bathe and feed client. Encourage independence as appropriate. Give frequent rest periods after activity.	Achievement of all care needs, performance of rehabilitation to maximize self-care potential

NURSING DIAGNOSIS: Altered nutrition: less than body requirements related to paralytic ileus, need for increased intake of nutrients, and inability to eat independently

Defining Characteristics	Nursing Interventions	Evaluation Criteria
Weight loss >2.5 kg of admission weight, decreased serum albumin	Force fluids (2-4 L/day). Ensure enteral feedings given as ordered during acute phase. If client is eating, encourage high-protein, high-carbohydrate, high-calorie diet with high bulk. Allow client to select foods. Encourage family to bring in foods client likes. Take time when feeding client. Keep a caloric count and weigh client at least weekly.	Weight loss < 4.5 kg of admission weight

NURSING DIAGNOSIS: Sexual dysfunction related to inability to achieve erection or perceived pelvic sensations and lack of knowledge of alternate means of achieving sexual satisfaction

Defining Characteristics	Nursing Interventions	Evaluation Criteria
Inability to achieve erection or perceive pelvic sensation, verbalization of lack of knowledge of how to achieve sexual satisfaction	Establish an honest, caring relationship with client and sexual partner. Provide accurate information about effects of spinal cord injury on sexual functioning. Encourage questions. Suggest alternate methods and use of assistive devices to achieve sexual satisfaction. Discuss reflexogenic erection with men and vaginal lubrication techniques with women. Suggest that client discuss possibility of penile prosthesis with physician. Encourage client to be relaxed and unhurried during sexual activity. Refer for sexual counseling if indicated.	Expression of satisfaction with sexual activities, knowledge about variety of ways to achieve sexual expression

Continued.

Table 55-8

NURSING CARE PLAN FOR THE CLIENT WITH A SPINAL CORD INJURY*—cont'd

Defining Characteristics	Nursing Interventions	Evaluation Criteria
NURSING DIAGNOSIS: High risk for injury related to sensory deficit and lack of self-protective abilities		
Documentation loss of sensation below level of injury	Assess environment for potentially injurious situations. Use side rails. Pad side rails. Turn and transfer client carefully with adequate assistance. Assess skin every shift. Turn client q 2 hr. Answer call light promptly. Anticipate client's needs.	Absence of injuries
NURSING DIAGNOSIS: Altered family processes related to change in function of ill family member		
Poor communication patterns among family members, use of ineffective coping techniques (e.g., shouting, blaming, isolation), unwillingness of family members to assist with client care	Assess family dynamics related to roles and responsibilities. Encourage open communication among family members regarding long-term planning to meet client's needs, including financial aspects. Assist family members to understand client's feelings. Assist family members to develop an action plan to meet client's needs. Refer if appropriate.	Maximizing of family strengths, achievement of client's needs
NURSING DIAGNOSIS: High risk for ineffective individual coping related to loss of control over bodily functions and altered lifestyle secondary to quadriplegia		
Prolonged use of inappropriate defense mechanisms, inability to accept permanence of prognosis, refusal to use available support services	Listen to client, noting tone of voice and facial expression. Offer support and acceptance of feelings. Assist client with problem solving. Teach client relaxation techniques. Encourage use of support systems to discuss concerns. Provide information. Teach client healthy coping behaviors.	Verbalization of ability to cope with effects of spinal cord injury, use of appropriate problem-solving techniques, active participant in care planning
NURSING DIAGNOSIS: Body-image disturbance related to quadriplegia		
Expression of anger or other negative feelings, refusal to discuss changes in function, participate in social contacts, look at body	Establish a trusting relationship. Encourage discussion of feelings. Allow client to grieve. Provide accurate information about body functions. Maintain privacy as necessary. Encourage social interaction. Assist family members in supporting client. Make referral for counseling as needed.	Expression of feelings about self, working through feelings to adaptation, beginning of acceptance of altered physical abilities

*This care plan is suitable for a client with a high cervical injury due to flexion-rotation. It can be modified for clients with less severe problems.

ing, and education. Support of local legislation related to seat-belt use in cars, helmets for motorcyclists, child-safety seats, and tougher penalties for drunk-driving offenses are a professional responsibility. A coordinated community program for the training of emergency personnel is essential.

Acute intervention. High cervical injury due to flexion-rotation is the most complex spinal cord injury. Interventions for this type of injury can be modified for clients with less severe problems.

EMERGENCY ROOM CARE. After stabilization at the accident scene the person is transferred to a medical facility (see Chapter 59). A thorough assessment is done to specifically evaluate the degree of deficit and to establish the level and degree of injury. A history is obtained, with emphasis on how the accident occurred and the degree of disruption as perceived by the client immediately after the accident. Assessment involves testing muscle groups rather than individual muscles. Muscle groups should be tested with and against gravity, alone and against resistance, and on both

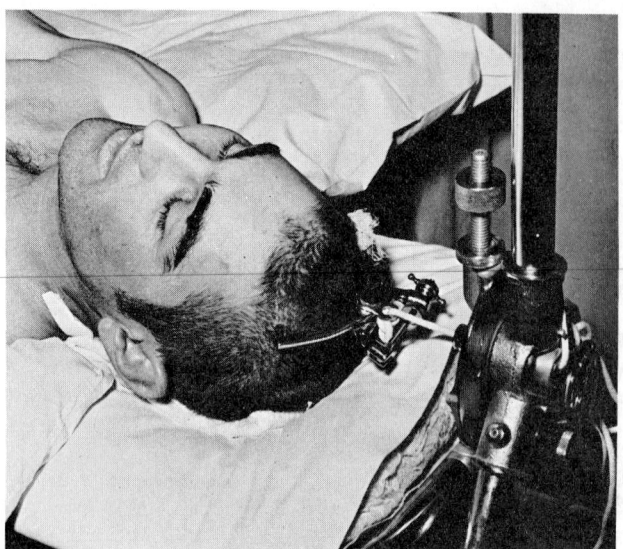

Fig. 55-5 Cervical traction is attached to tongs inserted in the skull. (Courtesy Orthopedic Frame Company, Kalamazoo, Mich.)

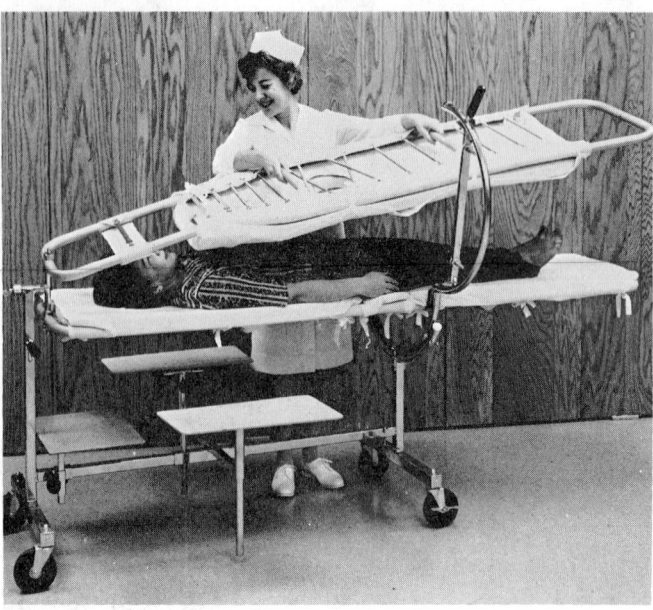

Fig. 55-6 Stryker frame. (Courtesy Orthopedic Frame Company, Kalamazoo, Mich.)

sides of the body. Spontaneous movement should be noted. The client should be asked to move legs and then hands, spread fingers, extend wrists, and shrug shoulders. After assessment of motor status, a sensory examination including touch and pain as tested by pin prick should be carried out, starting at the toes and working upward. If time and conditions permit, position sense and vibration can also be assessed.

An x-ray examination is done to document the injury. The client must be handled carefully before and during the x-ray procedure to prevent further injury. Respiratory, cardiac, and GI function should be monitored closely. The client may go directly to surgery following initial immobilization and stabilization or to the intensive care unit (ICU) for monitoring and management.

IMMOBILIZATION. Proper immobilization of the neck involves the maintenance of a neutral or extension position. Sandbags can be used to stabilize the neck to prevent flexion and extension of the cervical spine. The body should always be correctly aligned, and turning should be performed so that the client is moved as a unit to prevent movement of the spine. For cervical injuries, skeletal traction is usually provided by Crutchfield, Gardner-Wells, or another type of skull tongs (Fig. 55-5). Traction is provided by a rope that is extended from the center of the tongs over a pulley and that has weights attached at the end. Traction must be maintained at all times. One disadvantage of skull tongs is that the skull pins can be easily displaced. If this occurs, the head should be held in a neutral or extended position and help should be summoned. Sandbags can be positioned to stabilize the head and the physician reinserts the tongs (see Chapter 57).

Infection at the sites of tong insertion is another potential problem. Preventive care includes (1) dressing the sites daily after cleansing the area with an antiseptic solution

Table 55-9 Guidelines for the Use of Turning Frames*

1. Explain to client and family the purpose of the turning frame.
2. Properly secure all equipment, IV tubing, catheters, and respiratory tubing.
3. Periodically check equipment (e.g., for intactness of mattress, lacing, tautness).
4. Maintain alignment with full complement of equipment (e.g., rest wings).
5. Place client prone for meals, being careful to note respiratory problems and provide for expectoration if necessary.
6. Maintain sensory stimulation when client is prone (e.g., provide reading materials, fluid).
7. Place client supine for bowel program. Use accessory equipment for increased visual stimuli (e.g., prism glasses, mirrors).
8. Maintain constant traction, using special caution during turning of client.
9. Although this equipment was designed to be used by fewer personnel, always have an assistant.

*For specific guidelines, refer to operating manuals or the hospital procedure manual.

such as povidone-iodine (Betadine) and (2) applying an antibiotic ointment that acts as a mechanical barrier to the entrance of bacteria.

Special frames and beds are often used in the management of the client with a spinal cord injury (Table 55-9). Equipment includes the Stryker frame (Fig. 55-6), the Kinetic therapy Rotorest bed (Fig. 55-7), and less frequently,

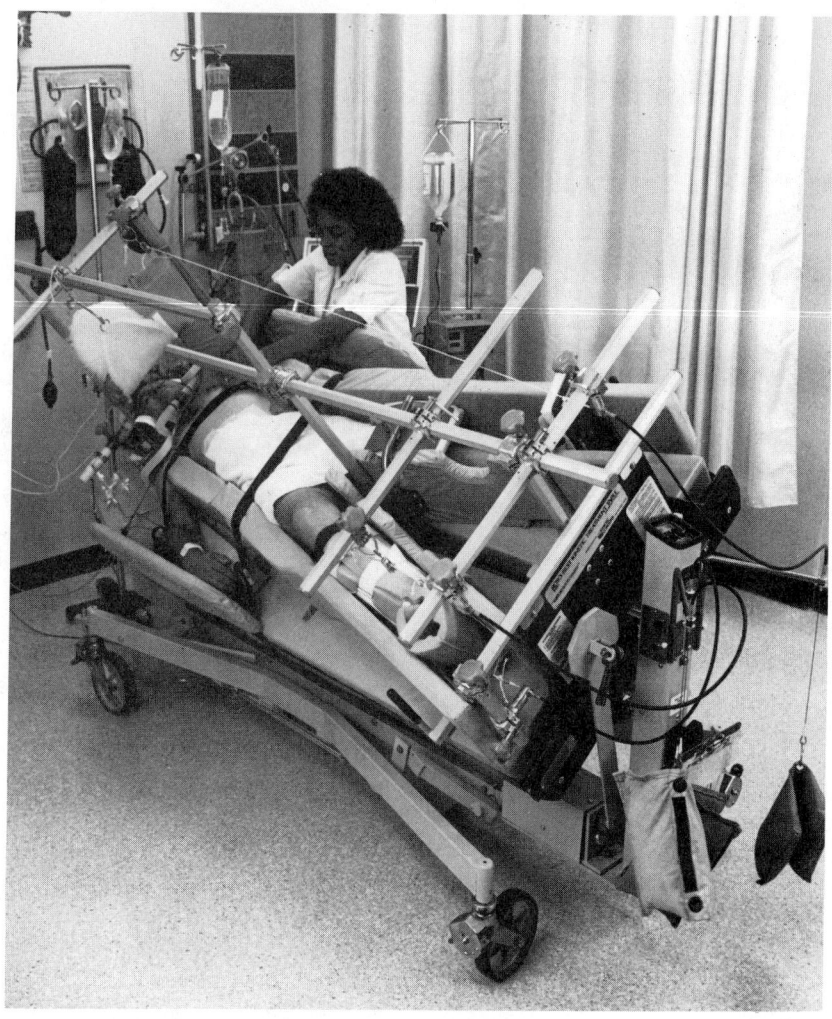

Fig. 55-7 Kinetic therapy treatment table (Rotorest bed).

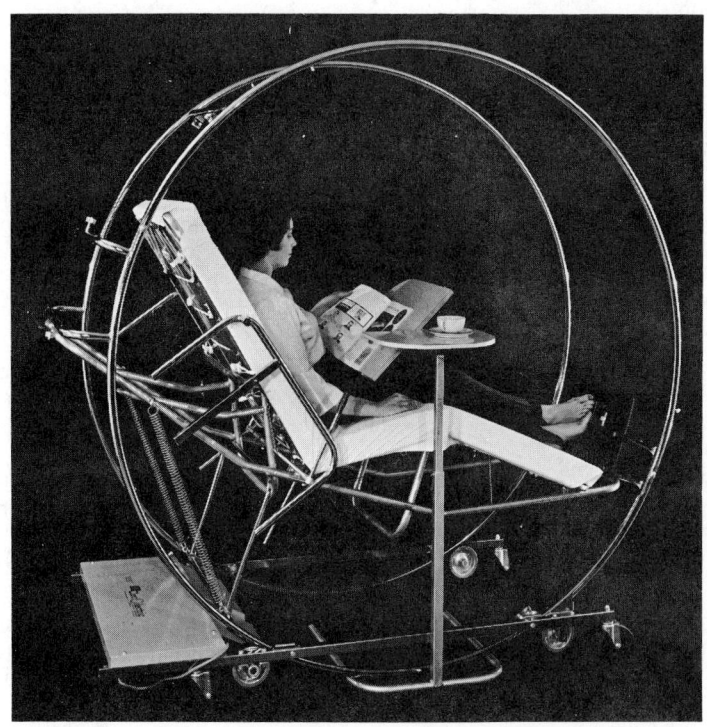

Fig. 55-8 Circo-electric bed. (Courtesy Orthopedic Frame Company, Kalamazoo, Mich.)

the Circo-electric bed (Fig. 55-8). The Stryker frame uses a side-to-side lateral turn. The Kinetic therapy Rotorest bed is new, and it uses a continual side-to-side slow rotation with the client in constant motion. The bed prevents pressure sores, cardiopulmonary complications, muscle wasting, bone demineralization, urinary stasis, and calculi. The therapeutic benefit of the Circo-electric bed has been questioned because of increased spinal bone movement and spinal compression, such as from axial loading in the vertical position.[22]

A physician should be available the first time the client is turned. The turn should be continued even if the client faints. Some clients never adjust to the use of a turning frame, so other techniques for position change need to be planned.

Depending on the type of injury and therapeutic interventions, the tongs and traction may be removed in 2 to 4 weeks after injury. In a stable injury, halo traction may be applied as soon as 5 days after the injury. The removal of traction and application of a collar or halo traction device allows the client to be more mobile and to be able to begin active rehabilitation. The halo apparatus applies cervical traction by means of a jacketlike arrangement that allows greater mobility and wheelchair activity than other traction systems.

Immobilization of the neck of the client with a spinal cord injury prevents further injury, but the effects of immobility are profound. The lack of any movement greatly increases catabolism and produces dysfunction in body organs because of decreased or absent innervation. The paralysis and accompanying psychological stress cause a lifelong problem related to nitrogen balance.

Meticulous skin care is critical because decreased sensation and circulation make the client particularly susceptible to skin breakdown. Tilt-table activities should be started as soon as possible to retard problems related to the supine position.[23]

RESPIRATORY DYSFUNCTION. During the first 48 hours after injury, edema may increase the level of dysfunction, and respiratory distress may occur. If the client is exhausted from labored breathing or if ABGs deteriorate (indicating inadequate oxygenation), endotracheal intubation or tracheostomy and mechanical ventilation should be initiated. Respiratory arrest is a possibility that requires careful monitoring of the respiratory system, and prompt action should it occur. All nurses who care for clients with spinal cord injuries should be competent at performing cardiopulmonary resuscitation. Pneumonia and atelectasis are potential problems because of the loss of vital capacity and the loss of intercostal and abdominal muscles, leaving only diaphragmatic breathing, pooled secretions, and ineffectual coughing. Nasal stuffiness and bronchospasms also present problems.

The nurse should regularly assess (1) breath sounds, (2) ABGs, (3) tidal volume, (4) vital capacity, (5) skin color, (6) breathing patterns (especially the use of accessory muscles), (7) subjective comments about the ability to breathe, and (8) the amount and color of sputum. A Pao_2 (partial pressure of oxygen in arterial blood) above 60 mm Hg and a $Paco_2$ (partial pressure of carbon dioxide in arterial

blood) below 45 mm Hg are acceptable values in a client with uncomplicated quadriplegia. The nurse should note the effect of the prone position because it can significantly reduce vital capacity and result in respiratory arrest. A client who is unable to count to 10 out loud without taking a breath needs immediate attention.

In addition to monitoring activities, the nurse can intervene in maintaining ventilation. Oxygen is administered until ABGs stabilize. Chest physiotherapy and quad-assist coughing facilitate the raising of secretions. Quad-assist coughing stimulates the action of the ineffective abdominal muscles during the expiratory phase of a cough. The nurse places a fist or the heel of a hand between the umbilicus and xiphoid process and exerts firm pressure to the area. Tracheal suctioning should be performed when indicated by auscultation of rales or rhonchi. Incentive spirometry, "blow bottles," and intermittent positive-pressure breathing are additional techniques to improve the client's respiratory status (see Chapters 21 and 22).

CARDIOVASCULAR INSTABILITY. Because of unopposed vagal response, the heart rate is slowed, often to below 60 beats per minute (bpm). Any increase in vagal stimulation such as turning or suctioning can result in cardiac arrest. Loss of sympathetic tone in peripheral vessels results in chronic low blood pressure with potential postural hypotension. Lack of muscle tone to aid venous return can result in sluggish blood flow and predispose the client to deep-vein thrombosis.

Vital signs need to be assessed frequently. If bradycardia is symptomatic, a medication such as atropine is administered. A temporary pacemaker may be inserted in some instances. Hypotension is managed with a vasopressor agent such as dopamine and fluid replacement.

If the client is on a circular electric bed, care must be exercised during the first few turnings. Turning should be done slowly, and the client should be observed closely. Vital signs should be monitored every 5 minutes. If the client faints, the nurse needs to complete the turn until the client is lying flat. The physician may order gradual elevation. The client is usually anxious until adjusted to the new sensations, but the nurse should heed complaints of vertigo, heart palpitations, and shortness of breath. Stryker frames are often preferred because there is less alteration of vascular dynamics. The legs should be wrapped to the thighs with elastic bandages or antiembolism stockings to prevent thromboemboli and to promote venous return. These leg wraps need to be removed every 8 hours for skin care. The use of alternate compression devices for the calves is advocated, and they need to be applied as soon as possible after admission and maintained throughout the hospitalization. An abdominal binder may also be beneficial. The nurse should also perform range-of-motion exercises and heel-cord stretching regularly. The calves of the legs should be assessed every shift for signs of deep vein thrombosis.

If blood loss has occurred from other injuries, the hemoglobin and hematocrit levels should be monitored and blood should be administered according to protocol. The nurse also needs to monitor the client for indications of hypovolemic shock secondary to hemorrhage.

FLUID AND NUTRITIONAL MAINTENANCE. During the first 48 to 72 hours after the injury the GI tract may stop functioning (paralytic ileus) and a nasogastric tube must then be inserted. Because the client cannot have oral intake, fluid and electrolyte needs must be carefully monitored. Specific solutions and additives are ordered based on individual requirements. Once bowel sounds are present or flatus is passed, oral food and fluids can gradually be introduced. If the client is unable to resume eating within 3 to 4 days, total parenteral nutrition may be started to provide nutritional support (see Chapter 35).

Because of severe catabolism, a high-protein, high-caloric diet is necessary. Calcium may be restricted if serum levels are high. Experts vary on the efficacy of milk to balance the nitrogen depletion. Many fear the potential for renal calculi, and most agree that some restriction of milk is necessary beyond the intermediate state of recovery.[24]

Increased roughage should be included to promote bowel function. Some clients experience anorexia, which can be due to psychological depression, boredom with institutional food, or discomfort at being fed (often by a hurried nurse). Some clients have a normally small appetite. Occasionally, refusal to eat is used as a means of maintaining control over the environment because of diminished or absent body control. If the client is not eating adequately, the cause should be thoroughly assessed. On the basis of this assessment, a contract may be made with the client regarding diet that uses mutual goal setting. This gives the client increased control of the situation and often results in improved nutritional intake. General measures such as providing a pleasant eating environment, allowing adequate time to eat (including any self-feeding the client can achieve), encouraging the family to bring in special foods, and planning social rewards for eating may be useful. A caloric count should be kept, and the client's weekly weight needs to be recorded as a means for evaluating progress. If feasible, the client should participate in recording caloric intake. The nurse should avoid allowing the client's nutritional intake to become the basis for a power struggle.

The client is usually maintained on a fluid restriction of 1800 to 2000 ml/day to facilitate a bladder training program. Urinary output is monitored closely.

BOWEL AND BLADDER MANAGEMENT. Urine is retained because of the loss of autonomic and reflex control of the bladder and sphincter. Because there is no sensation of fullness, overdistention of the bladder can result in reflux into the kidney with eventual kidney failure or even rupture of the bladder. Consequently an indwelling catheter is usually inserted as soon as possible after injury. Its patency must be ensured by irrigation and frequent inspection. In some institutions a physician's order is required for this procedure. Strict aseptic technique for catheter care is essential to avoid introducing infection. After the client is stabilized, the best means of managing long-term urinary functions is assessed. In general, the client is started on an intermittent catheterization program.

Urinary tract infections are a common problem. A large fluid intake and the liberal use of juices such as cranberry, grape, and apple are planned to prevent infections. These juices leave an acid ash in the urine, which discourages bacterial growth. Citrus juices are used sparingly. Ascorbic acid and a urinary antiseptic such as methenamine mandelate (Mandelamine) are sometimes given. The pH of the urine should be tested daily to evaluate acidity. If the appearance or odor of the urine is suspicious, a specimen is sent for culture.

Constipation is generally a problem during spinal shock because no voluntary or involuntary evacuation of the bowels exists. Suppositories are used in combination with a laxative to assist in bowel evacuation. Enemas are used only if absolutely necessary because they can overdistend the rectum and create problems for initiating an effective bowel program.

TEMPERATURE CONTROL. Because there is no vasoconstriction, piloerection, or heat loss through perspiration below the level of injury, temperature control is largely external to the client. Therefore the nurse monitors the environment closely to maintain an appropriate temperature. Body temperature is monitored regularly. The client is not overloaded with covers or unduly exposed (such as during bathing). If an infection develops, more extensive means of temperature control such as a cooling blanket may be necessary.

STRESS ULCERS. Ulcers are a problem to the client with a cord injury because of the physiological response to severe trauma and psychological stress. Peak incidence is 6 to 14 days after injury. Stool and gastric content are tested daily for blood, and the hematocrit is observed for a slow drop. If steroids are given, they should be accompanied by antacids and/or food. Drugs such as cimetidine (Tagamet) and propantheline bromide (Pro-Banthine) may be given prophylactically to decrease the secretion of hydrochloric acid.

SENSORY DEPRIVATION. The nurse must compensate for the client's absent sensation to prevent sensory deprivation. This is done by stimulating the client above the level of injury. Conversation, music, strong aromas, and interesting flavors should be a part of the nursing care plan. Prism glasses are provided so that the client can read and watch television. Every effort should be made to prevent the client from withdrawing from the environment.

Rehabilitative and chronic management. The physiological and psychological rehabilitation of the person with spinal cord injury is complex and involved. With physical and psychological care and intensive and specialized rehabilitation, the client with a spinal cord injury learns to function at the highest level of wellness. Special rehabilitation centers are available where clients must demonstrate adequate motivation for self-care to be admitted.

Many of the problems identified in the acute period become chronic and continue throughout life. Rehabilitation focuses on refined retraining of physiological processes. Braces, electronic wheelchairs, and mechanical apparatuses are used to maximize the client's remaining function. The client with high cervical spinal cord injury has greatly increased mobility with electronic diaphragmatic pacemakers and the Bantam respirator. Although rehabilitation and the special equipment required are costly, many programs are funded by the state and federal government.

If clients can be successfully brought through the acute period, their lives can be fuller and richer than previously believed possible. Like other persons who have been close to death, some clients find that their lives are richer and more meaningful than before the injury. Unfortunately, other clients may not have such a positive future outlook. The nurse has a pivotal role in the coordinated efforts of the health team to influence a positive outcome.

GRIEF. Clients with spinal cord injuries are aware of the extent of injury but also feel an overwhelming sense of loss. They are no longer in control but must depend on others for activities of daily living and for life-sustaining measures. Clients may believe that they are useless and burdens to their families. At a stage when independence is often of the greatest importance developmentally, they are totally dependent on others.

The client's response and recovery differ in some important aspects from those experiencing loss from amputation or terminal illness. First, regression can and does occur at different stages. The usual 2-year period for healthy adjustment to loss cannot be applied to the client with spinal cord injury. Working through grief is a difficult, lifelong process with which the client needs support and encouragement. With recent advances in rehabilitation, it is usual for the client to be independent physically and discharged from the rehabilitation center before completion of the grief process. Another phenomenon involves that of

triggering experiences — new experiences such as marriage may recall earlier unresolved difficulties. Depending on the success of previous grief work, the new demand for grief work may be shortened or prolonged.

The goal of recovery is related more to adjustment than to acceptance. Adjustment implies the ability to go on with living with certain limitations. Some severely disabled persons have a more meaningful life after the injury.

Although the client who is cooperative and accepting is easier to treat, the nurse should expect a wide fluctuation of emotions from a client with a spinal cord injury. It is often the nursing staff that has difficulty accepting the client's limitation.[24] Depression may not be a component of the recovery process. Societal norms allow depression after severe loss and almost impose it on those confronted with death or radical lifestyle changes. However, every client may not experience depression. Staff members must learn to not impose their needs to feel sorry for the client and expect the client to respond appropriately.[25]

The nurse's role in grief work is to allow mourning as a component of the rehabilitation process. Table 55-10 summarizes the mourning process and appropriate nursing interventions. During the shock and denial stage the nurse reassures the client and stresses the expertise of the entire health care team. During the anger stage, the nurse assists the client in achievement of control over the environment, particularly by allowing the client's input into the plan of

Table 55-10   Mourning Process and Nursing Interventions in Spinal Cord Injury

Client Behavior	Nursing Interventions
SHOCK AND DENIAL	
Struggle for survival, complete dependence, excessive sleep, withdrawal, fantasies, unrealistic expectations	Use meticulous nursing care. Be honest. Use simple diagrams to explain injury. Encourage client to begin long road to recovery.
ANGER	
Refusal to discuss paralysis, decreased self-esteem, manipulation, hostile and abusive language	Place client in room with another client with spinal cord injury further along in rehabilitation process; encourage self-care. Coordinate care with client. Support family members; prevent alleviation of guilt by supporting dependency. Use humor liberally. Allow client outbursts. Do not allow fixation.
DEPRESSION	
Sadness, pessimism, anorexia, nightmares, insomnia, agitation, psychomotor retardation, "blues," suicidal preoccupation, refusal to participate in any self-care activities	Encourage family involvement and resources. Plan graded steps in rehabilitation to give success with minimal opportunity for frustration. Give cheerful and willing assistance with activities of daily living. Avoid sympathy. Use firm kindness.
ADJUSTMENT	
Planning for the future, active participation in therapy, finding of personal meaning in experience and continuation of growth, return to premorbid personality	Remember that clients with spinal cord injuries have individual personalities. Balance support systems to encourage independence. Set goals with client input. Emphasize potentials as achieved by others. Avoid use of cliches.

care. The nurse should not respond to anger or manipulation or become involved with a power struggle with the client. As self-care abilities increase, the client's independence increases.

The client's family also requires counseling to avoid promoting dependency in the client through guilt or misplaced sympathy. The family is also experiencing an intense grieving process. A support group of family members and friends can help increase family members' knowledge and participation in the grieving process, physical difficulties, rehabilitation plan, and the meaning of the disability in society.

During the stage of depression, the nurse must keep a sense of humor and be patient and persistent. Sympathy is not helpful. The client should be treated in an adult manner and involved in decision making about care, but the nurse must insist that the care is performed. A primary nurse relationship is helpful, but the nurse needs some relief from the intense stress of continual interaction with the client. Staff planning and sessions in which staff members can express their feelings are helpful in providing consistency of care. To achieve the stage of adjustment, the client needs continual support throughout the rehabilitation in the forms of acceptance, affection, and caring. The nurse must be attentive when the client needs to talk and sensitive to needs at the various stages of the grief process.

REFLEXES. Once spinal cord shock is resolved, the return of reflexes may complicate rehabilitation. Lacking control from the higher brain centers, reflexes are inappropriate and often excessive. Erections can occur from a variety of stimuli, causing embarrassment and discomfort. Spasms ranging from mild twitches to convulsive movements below the level of the lesion may also occur. This reflex activity may be interpreted by the client or family as a return of function, and the nurse must tactfully explain the reason for the activity. The client may be informed of the positive use of these reflexes in sexual, bowel, and bladder retraining. Spasms may be relieved with the use of warm baths, whirlpool treatments, antispasmodics, and muscle relaxants. Peak spasticity occurs after 2 years, and if it is severe, destruction of the reflexes (chordotomy) may be necessary. This compromises retraining and should be done as a last resort.

AUTONOMIC DYSREFLEXIA. Autonomic dysreflexia (hyperreflexia) is a massive uncompensated cardiovascular reaction of the sympathetic division of the autonomic nervous system to visceral stimulation that occurs in clients with spinal cord lesions above T7. The condition is a life-threatening situation that requires immediate resolution.

The most common precipating cause is a distended bladder or rectum, although any sensory stimulation may cause autonomic dysreflexia. Contraction of the bladder or rectum, stimulation of the skin, or stimulation of the pain receptors may also cause autonomic hyperreflexia. Manifestations include hypertension (up to 300 mm Hg systolic), blurred vision, throbbing headache, marked diaphoresis above the level of the lesion, bradycardia (30 to 40 bpm), piloerection (erection of body hair) as a result of pilomotor spasm, nasal congestion, and nausea.

The pathology of autonomic dysreflexia involves the stimulation of sensory receptors below the level of the cord lesion. The intact autonomic system reacts with a reflex arteriolar spasm that increases blood pressure. Baroreceptors in cerebral vessels, the carotid sinus, and the aorta sense the hypertension and stimulate the parasympathetic system. The heart rate is decreased, but the visceral and peripheral vessels do not dilate because efferent impulses cannot pass through the cord lesion.

Nursing interventions in this serious emergency are elevation of the head of the bed 45 degrees, notification of the physician, and assessment to determine the cause. Abdominal palpation for a distended bladder is performed very gently to avoid increasing the stimulus. Immediate catheterization to relieve the distention may be necessary. Catheter irrigation performed very slowly and gently may open a plugged catheter, or a new catheter may be inserted. A digital rectal examination should be performed only after application of an anesthetic ointment to decrease rectal stimulation and to prevent an increase of symptoms. The nurse should remove all skin stimuli such as constrictive clothing and tight shoes. If symptoms persist after the source has been relieved, an α-adrenergic blocker such as phentolamine (Regitine) or an arteriolar vasodilator such as hydralazine (Apresoline) may be given. A low spinal anesthetic to block stimulation may be a lifesaving measure.[25] Careful monitoring must continue until the vital signs stabilize.

Clients and their families need to be taught the causes and symptoms of autonomic dysreflexia. They need to understand the life-threatening nature of this dysfunction and know how to relieve the cause.

SEXUALITY. Because the majority of clients with spinal cord injuries are men between the ages of 18 and 35 years, sexual rehabilitation is a major issue. To work with these clients, the nurse must have an awareness and an acceptance of personal sexuality as well as knowledge of human sexual responses. When discussing sexual potential, the nurse should use scientific terminology rather than slang whenever possible. Knowledge of the level of the lesion is needed to understand the client's potential for orgasm, erection, and fertility and the client's capacity for sexual satisfaction (Table 55-11). All clients with spinal cord injuries generally lack perineal sensation during intercourse regardless of the type of lesion.

Reflex sexual function capability is possible if the client has an upper motor neuron lesion. The presence of tone in the external rectal sphincter indicates an upper motor lesion. The absence of external rectal sphincter tone, bulbocavernosus reflex, or both indicates that the client has lower motor neuron involvement and is capable of areflexic sexual function.

The type of lesion determines the physical sexual response. Men with upper motor neuron lesions may have reflexogenic erections that are produced by reflex activity or external stimuli or that occur spontaneously. These spontaneous erections are often short lived and uncontrolled and cannot be maintained or summoned at a time of coitus. Orgasm and ejaculation are usually not possible for men with a complete upper motor neuron lesion.

Most clients with a complete lower motor neuron lesion

Table 55-11   Potential for Sexual Activity in Men with Spinal Cord Injuries

Erection	Ejaculation	Orgasm
UPPER MOTOR NEURON		
Complete		
Frequent (93%), reflexogenic only	Rare	Absent
Incomplete		
Most frequent (99%), reflexogenic (80%), reflexogenic and psychogenic (19%)	Less frequent (32%), after reflexogenic erection (74%), after psychogenic erection (26%)	Present (if ejaculation occurs)
LOWER MOTOR NEURON		
Complete		
Infrequent (26%)	Infrequent (18%)	Present (if ejaculation occurs)
Incomplete		
Psychogenic and reflexogenic	Frequent (70%), after psychogenic and reflexogenic erections	Present (if ejaculation occurs)

are unable to have either psychogenic or reflexogenic erections. They do not produce sperm. Clients with incomplete lower motor neuron lesions have the highest possibility of successful psychogenic erection with ejaculation. Studies suggest that up to 10% of these clients are fertile.

The woman of childbearing age with a spinal cord injury usually remains fertile, although orgasmic ability is lost. The injury does not affect the ability to become pregnant or to deliver through the normal birth canal.

Sexual rehabilitation for both men and women should begin informally after the acute phase of the injury has passed. Questions such as "Have you had an erection since your accident?" or "Have your menstrual periods continued since the accident?" are nonthreatening ways to introduce the topic of sexual functioning. The male client may pose a question such as, "Can I ever be a man again?"

Open discussion with the client is essential. This important aspect of rehabilitation should be handled by someone specially trained in sexual counseling. Unless this type of training has occurred the nurse should not attempt to direct the plan for sexual rehabilitation.

The properly trained nurse works with the client and partner to provide support during new relationships, with the emphasis on open communication. The nurse's educational role requires respect for every couple's personal standards of religious and cultural beliefs. Alternative

methods of obtaining sexual satisfaction such as oral-genital sex (cunnilingus and fellatio) may be suggested. Explicit films (e.g., *Touching*) may also be used. This film demonstrates the sexual activities of a client with paraplegia and a normal partner.[26] Graphics should be used cautiously because they may be too limiting or focus too much on the mechanics of sex rather than the relationship.

Sexual activities may require more planning and be less spontaneous than before the injury. For example, an attendant may need to undress the client and remove equipment.

Care should be taken not to dislodge the indwelling catheter during sexual activity. If a Texas catheter is used, it should be removed before sexual activity and the client should refrain from fluids. The bowel program should include evacuation the morning of sexual activity. The partner should be informed that an accident is always possible. Illustrations for teaching management of urinary equipment are available.[26] The woman may need a water-soluble lubricant to supplement inadequate vaginal secretions and facilitate vaginal penetration.

Menses may temporarily cease for as long as 6 months. If sexual activity is resumed, protection against an unplanned pregnancy is necessary. A normal pregnancy may be complicated by urinary tract infections, anemia, and autonomic dysreflexia. Because uterine contractions are not felt, a precipitate delivery is always a danger. In men, fertility is reduced because of decreased number and motility of sperm. For male clients desiring children, alternative methods include adoption and artificial insemination.

A relaxed atmosphere with wine, music, and perfume creates an attractive environment. Ample time for caressing, fondling, and kissing is essential. The partners should be encouraged to explore each other's erogenous areas such as the lips, neck, and ears, which can arouse psychogenic erection or orgasm. Few demands should be made initially.

NEUROGENIC BLADDER. Once spinal cord shock and the resulting bladder atony are resolved, the bladder is neurogenic. A neurogenic bladder is any type of bladder dysfunction related to abnormal or absent bladder innervation. It may lead to a residual urine problem, stone disease, or infection and is often associated with progressive renal deterioration. It is frequently associated with urinary incontinence. The network of fibers of the detrusor muscle forms the muscular wall of the bladder. The trigone is a small rectangular area near the bladder neck sometimes called the *internal sphincter*. The urogenital diaphragm or baseplate encircles the urethral opening completely and is sometimes called the *external sphincter*. Depending on the lesion, a neurogenic bladder may have no reflex detrusor contractions (areflexic, flaccid) or may have hyperactive reflex detrusor contractions (hyperreflexic, spastic). Common symptoms of a neurogenic bladder include urgency, frequency, incontinence, inability to void, and characteristics of obstruction.

Neurogenic bladder can be classified according to reflex detrusor activity, intravesical filling pressure, and continence function. Types of neurogenic bladder include the following:

1. *Uninhibited neurogenic bladder:* This lesion is due to a defect in the corticoregulatory tracts. The uninhibited neurogenic bladder behaves as though no inhibitions influenced the time and place of voiding. The newborn child has this type of bladder. It may occur after cerebrovascular accident and in clients with multiple sclerosis, syphilis, brain trauma, or brain tumor. The usual symptoms include increased frequency, urgency, and incontinence.

2. *Reflex neurogenic bladder:* The bladder behaves as part of the spinal reflex arc with no connection to the brain. The lesion affects sensory and motor tracts to and from the higher nerves above the conus medullaris and is occasionally seen in clients with multiple sclerosis and pernicious anemia. Symptoms are loss of voluntary control of the detrusor and sphincter muscles, urinary frequency, urgency, and lack of sensation of bladder filling.

3. *Autonomous neurogenic bladder:* The bladder behaves autonomously, as if it were completely cut off from the brain and spinal cord. It is seen in clients with spina bifida or myelomeningocele and in cases of trauma or neoplasm involving the conus medullaris, cauda equina, or pelvic nerves. It is occasionally seen after exenterating types of radical pelvic surgery and occasionally with a herniated intervertebral disk. These clients cannot initiate micturition in a normal way, and they may be incontinent.

4. *Motor paralytic bladder:* Motor paralytic bladder (lower motor neuron) acts as if there were paralysis of all motor function. It is seen in clients with poliomyelitis or herniated intervertebral disks. It is also seen with traumas or neoplasms involving the second, third, and fourth sacral roots (parasympathetic fibers). Symptoms may be similar to those seen in a client with outlet obstruction. If sensations are intact, the client feels the painful distention and hesitancy. There is no control of micturition, resulting in overdistention of the bladder and overflow incontinence.

5. *Sensory paralytic bladder:* This bladder is seen in clients with diabetes mellitus, tabes dorsalis, pernicious anemia, or multiple sclerosis. It is caused by damage to only the sensory limb of the bladder spinal reflex arc. The bladder acts as if there were paralysis of all sensory modalities. There are no particular symptoms except for poor bladder sensation, infrequent voiding, and large urine volume when the detrusor muscle ultimately decompensates.

The client with a spinal cord injury and a neurogenic bladder requires a comprehensive program to manage bladder function. The program should include the following:

1. *Diagnostic evaluation:* After the client's overall condition is stable with evidence of neurological reflexes, a cystometrogram, an IV pyelogram, and a urine culture are taken.

2. *Pharmacological:* Drugs to increase the strength of bladder contractions (detrusor), acidify the urine, and relax the urethral sphincter are administered.

3. *Nutrition:* A low-calcium diet (1 g/day) is advocated to reduce the possibility of kidney and bladder stones.

4. *Fluids:* A fluid intake of 1800 to 2000 ml/day must be maintained to prevent stone formation and to ensure adequate urine flow.

5. *Urine drainage:* The method used for urinary drainage depends on the condition of the client; the preference of the physician, nursing staff, and client; and the policy of the institution. Numerous drainage methods are possible, including reflex training, indwelling catheter, intermittent catheterization, urinary diversion surgery, and artificial sphincter.

With the return of the reflex arc, bladder function may be a reflex. However, because of the interruption in the pathways to the brain, the client has no control over urination, which results in a bladder with a small capacity, hyperirritable detrusor muscle and sphincter, and loss of inhibition of the reflex by the brain. The client or the nurse can use techniques such as the Credé and Valsalva maneuvers or a rectal stretch to facilitate complete emptying of the bladder. The Credé maneuver involves the exertion by the nurse or client of downward pressure over the bladder with a pumping motion. This maneuver may require a physician's order in some settings because it has the potential of stimulating autonomic dysreflexia in clients with upper motor neuron disease. In the Valsalva maneuver, the client inhales deeply, holds a breath, and bears down. The rectal stretch is the insertion of a gloved finger into the rectum, gently pulling to exert pressure on the sphincter to cause relaxation of the perineal floor. Combining the Valsalva maneuver with rectal stretch results in more complete emptying of the bladder. The client should be regularly assessed for residual urine after reflex bladder emptying. The goal of neurogenic bladder management is to attain a "balanced bladder" in which the residual urine is no more than 20% of the client's average bladder capacity, generally below 100 ml.[27] Many drugs affect urinary retention and indicate reassessment for residual. The ultimate goal for this technique is for the client to not need a catheter.

The long-term use of an indwelling catheter should be carefully evaluated because of the associated high incidence of urinary tract infection, fistula formation, and diverticula. Adequate fluid intake and patency of the catheter should be ensured. The frequency of catheter changing ranges from 1 week to 1 month, depending on the type of catheter used and agency policy.

Intermittent catheterization is the recommended method of bladder management (see Chapter 40). Nursing assessment is important in selecting the time interval between catheterizations. Initially, catheterization is done every 4 hours. If less than 200 ml of urine is drained, the time interval may be extended. If 500 ml or more of urine is obtained, the time interval is shortened. An overdistended bladder causes ischemia, which predisposes tissues to bacterial invasion and infection. Clients often experience diuresis at a regular time during a 24-hour period, which may necessitate an extra catheterization. The number of intermittent catheterizations per day is usually five or six.

Urinary diversion surgery may be necessary if the client has repeated urinary tract infections with renal involve-

ment or repeated stones or if therapeutic intervention has been unsuccessful (see Table 40-21). Surgeries such as perineal ureterostomy, cystotomy, vesicotomy, and anterior urethral transportation may be considered.

ARTIFICIAL SPHINCTER. The use of a surgically implanted artificial sphincter may be appropriate for some clients. The device is implanted with an inflatable cuff around the urethra or bladder neck. A pump mechanism that allows the client to activate the device for urination is implanted superficially. Other components regulate pressure and fluid flow within the system. One or two operations are necessary for instillation, and risks of complications include urethral erosion and scar tissue formation.[28] Clients may not remain totally dry even with the device in place.

BOWEL EVACUATION. Bowel evacuation needs careful management in the client with a spinal cord injury because voluntary control of this function may be lost. The usual measures for preventing constipation include a high-fiber diet and adequate fluid intake (see Table 37-10). In addition, suppositories or digital stimulation by the nurse or client may be necessary. Digital stimulation, with the Valsalva maneuver and a regular schedule, facilitates regularity.

In general, a bowel movement every other day is considered adequate. However, preinjury patterns should be considered. Incontinence can result from too much stool softener or a fecal impaction. Careful recording of bowel movements including amount, time, and consistency is important to the overall success of the program.

SPINAL CORD TUMORS
Pathophysiology

Tumors that affect the spinal cord account for 0.5% to 1% of all neoplasms. These tumors are classified as primary (arising from some component of cord, dura, nerves, or vessels), secondary (due to intraspinal extension from the vertebrae, neck, or thoracic abdominal tumors), and metastatic (from primary growths in the breast, thyroid, lung, kidney, and other sites). The thoracic and lumbar spine, including the sacrum, are the most commonly affected bones and are seen as extradural, intradural-extramedullary, and intradural-intramedullary tumors (Fig. 55-9, Table 55-12). Neurofibromas, meningiomas, gliomas, and hemangiomas are the most frequently occurring neoplasms.

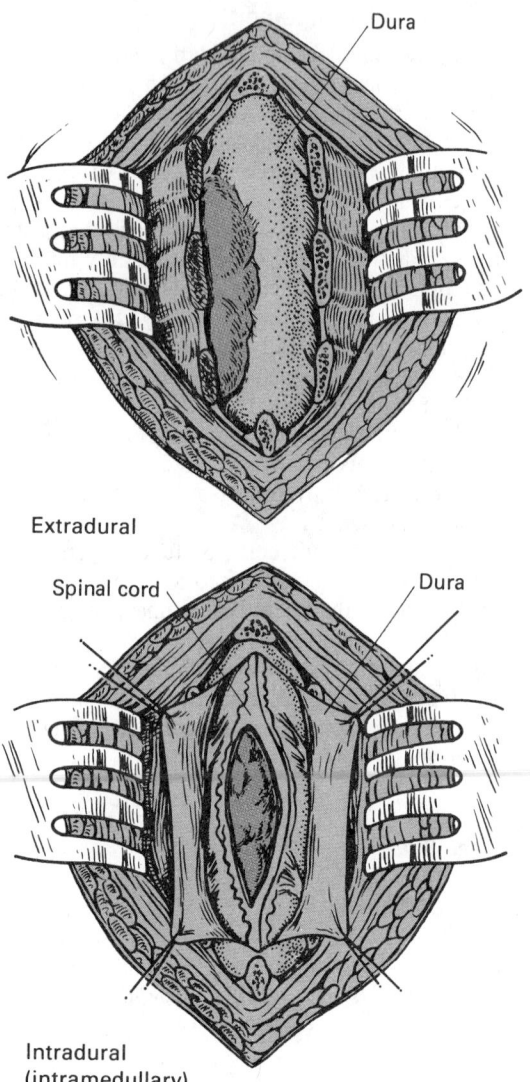

Extradural

Intradural
(intramedullary)

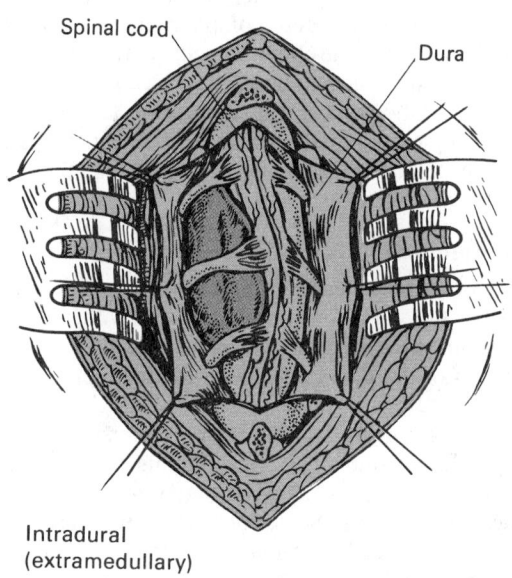

Intradural
(extramedullary)

Fig. 55-9 Types of spinal cord tumors.

Table 55-12 Classification of Spinal Cord Tumors

Type	Incidence	Treatment	Prognosis
Extradural (from bones of spine, in extradural space, or in paraspinal tissue)	20%-50% of all intraspinal tumors, mostly malignant metastatic lesions	Relief of cord pressure by surgical laminectomy, radiation, chemotherapy, or combination approach	Poor
Intradural extramedullary (within dura mater outside cord)	Most frequent of intradural tumors (40%), mostly benign meningiomas and neurofibromas	Complete surgical removal of tumor (if possible), partial removal followed by radiation	Usually very good if lack of damage to cord from compression
Intradural intramedullary	Least frequent of intradural tumors (5%-10%)	Partial surgical removal, radiation therapy (resulting in only temporary improvement)	Very poor

Because many of these tumors are slow growing, their symptoms stem from the mechanical effects of slow compression and irritation of nerve roots, displacement of the cord, and/or gradual obstruction of the vascular supply. The slowness of growth does not cause autodestruction as in traumatic lesions; therefore complete functional restoration is possible when the tumor is removed, except in the intradural-intramedullary tumors.

Most metastatic tumors are extradural lesions.[29] Tumors that commonly metastasize to the spinal epidural space are those that spread to bone, such as carcinomas of the breast, lung, prostate, and kidney.

Clinical Manifestations

The most common early symptom of a spinal cord tumor outside the cord is pain in the back with radiations simulating intercostal neuralgia, angina, or herpes zoster. The location of the pain depends on the level of compression, and the pain worsens with activity, coughing, straining, and lying down. Sensory disruption is later manifested by coldness, numbness, and tingling in an extremity or in several extremities, slowly progressing upward until it reaches the level of the lesion. Impaired sensation of pain, temperature, and light touch precedes a deficit in vibration and position sense that may progress to complete anesthesia. Motor weakness accompanies the sensory disturbances and consists of slowly increasing clumsiness, weakness, and spasticity. The sensory and motor disturbances are ipsilateral to the lesion. Sphincter disturbances are marked by urgency with difficulty in starting to urinate and progressing to retention with overflow incontinence.

Manifestations of intradural spinal tumor develop as progressive damage to the long spinal tracts, producing paralysis, sensory loss, and bladder dysfunction. Pain can be severe as a result of compression of spinal roots or vertebrae.

Extradural tumors are seen early on routine spinal x-ray films, whereas intradural and intramedullary tumors require myelography for detection. Spinal fluid analysis may reveal tumor cells.

The cord is decompressed after removal of the tumor by a laminectomy (see Chapter 57). More than 85% of primary neoplasms are benign and can be completely resected; 90% of clients recover without residual problems.

Therapeutic Management

Compression of the spinal cord is an emergency. Relief of the ischemia related to the compression is the goal of therapy. Corticosteroids are generally prescribed immediately to relieve tumor-related edema. Dexamethasone is usually used, often in large doses (up to 100 mg initially).

Treatment for nearly all spinal cord tumors is surgical removal. The exception is the metastatic tumor that is sensitive to radiation and that has caused only minimal neurological deficits in the client.[29] In general, tumors of the extradural or intradural-extramedullary group can be completely removed surgically. Intramedullary tumors offer a less favorable prognosis; however, exploration and removal is usually attempted.

Radiation therapy after the operation is fairly effective. Maximum permissible tissue dose is given over 6 to 8 weeks. Chemotherapy has also been used in conjunction with radiation therapy.

Relief of pain and return of function are the ultimate goals of treatment. Nurses need to be aware of the neurological status of the client before and after treatment. Ensuring that the client receives pain medication as needed is an important nursing responsibility. Depending on the amount of neurological dysfunction exhibited, the client may need to be cared for as though recovering from a spinal cord injury (see Table 55-8).

C ase Study

SPINAL CORD INJURY

John M., a 22-year-old man, sustained a fractured neck at the level of C5 when he ran his motorcycle into a guard rail on the highway. This was John's third accident in the past 2 years. He had sustained a fractured femur and was hospitalized for 22

days in a similar accident 6 months earlier. His wife of 4 years has just come home from the hospital with their third child. John is an unemployed sheet-metal worker.

John is admitted directly to the ICU, and the neurosurgeon puts in Crutchfield tongs with 20 lb of traction. As he arrives, John says to the nurse, "Tell the doctor to hurry, I'm going to be late for a motorcycle race." John has no movement or sensation below his neck.

Discussion Questions

1. What does the nurse say to John in response to his comment?
2. What are the first activities when John arrives in the ICU?
3. What physiological problems are anticipated from his injury?
4. What psychological problems are anticipated?
5. What questions need to be asked to plan long-range care?
6. How can the nurse best help his wife at this time?
7. What data need to be collected regarding the wife's needs?

R eview Questions

The number of the question corresponds to the same-numbered objective at the beginning of the chapter.

1. The client with trigeminal neuralgia presents with
   a. flaccid muscles of the neck
   b. vertigo, nausea, and vomiting
   c. paroxysms of excruciating facial pain
   d. dysphagia and respiratory distress
2. Which of the following is *not* true of Guillain-Barré syndrome?
   a. Cerebrospinal fluid may show increased protein.
   b. It is only mildly contagious.
   c. The onset of symptoms is gradual.
   d. Respiratory failure is a major cause of death.
3. The person most likely to sustain a spinal cord injury is a
   a. 30-year-old woman
   b. 50-year-old client with diabetes
   c. 42-year-old police officer
   d. 19-year-old man
4. The mechanism of spinal cord injury resulting in the most unstable injury is
   a. flexion-rotation
   b. flexion
   c. extension-rotation
   d. extension
5. Which of the following statements is true about the pathophysiology of indirect spinal cord trauma?
   a. The cord is very delicate and is readily transected by indirect trauma.
   b. Hemorrhage, edema, and excessive metabolites produce ischemia and progressive necrotic destruction.
   c. Oxygen tension in the cord is usually normal.
   d. The injury process starts in the white matter.
6. The reason norepinephrine counteractants for spinal cord injury are still not effective is that
   a. the dosage has not been determined
   b. clients are refusing the treatment
   c. they need to be injected within 15 minutes of injury
   d. the effect of all drugs is unknown
7. A client with an injury at the C6 level will be able to
   a. assist with transfer activities
   b. repair watches for a living
   c. walk with braces
   d. catheterize self
8. The initial nursing intervention for the client exhibiting symptoms of autonomic dysreflexia is to
   a. elevate the head of the bed 45 degrees
   b. increase the rate of IV infusion
   c. notify the attending physician
   d. retake the blood pressure in 5 minutes
9. Spinal cord tumors are usually
   a. fast growing
   b. slow growing
   c. untreatable
   d. rapidly fatal

REFERENCES

1. Fromm GH: Trigeminal neuralgia and related disorders, Crit Care Clin 7:305-319, 1989.
2. Andreoli TE and others: Cecil essentials of medicine, ed 2, Philadelphia, 1990, WB Saunders Co, p 712.
3. Cummings C: Nursing management of adults with peripheral and cranial nerve disorders. In Beare PG and Myers JL, eds: Principles and practice of adult health nursing, St Louis, 1990, Mosby–Year Book, Inc.
4. Watkinson PC: EMG biofeedback treatment for Bell's palsy, J Oral Rehabil 15:353-359, 1988.
5. Blaney GG: Alteration in peripheral senses. In Mitchell PH and others, eds: AACN's neuroscience nursing, Norwalk Conn, 1988, Appleton & Lange, pp 351-392.
6. Andreoli TE and others: Cecil essentials of medicine, ed 2, Philadelphia, 1990, WB Saunders Co, p 756.
7. Kurtzke JF: Neuroepidemiology, Ann Neurol 16:265, 1984.
8. Barohn RJ and others: Chronic inflammatory demyelinating polyradiculoneuropathy, Arch Neurol 46:878-884, 1989.
9. MacDonald KL: The changing epidemiology of adult botulism in the United States, Am J Epidemiol 124:794-799, 1986.
10. Sullivan M and Jackson BS: Tetanus: a case presentation, Focus Crit Care 11:39, 1984.
11. Chamberlain C: Admission diagnoses: rule out tetanus, Focus Crit Care 16:473, 1989.
12. Mandell GL, Douglas RG, and Bennett JE, eds: Principles and practice of infectious disease, ed 3, New York, 1990, Churchill Livingstone.
13. Mitchell PH and others, eds: Common neurologic health problems: the phenomena of neuroscience medicine, Norwich, Conn, 1988, Appleton & Lange, p 96.
14. Davis ME: Spinal cord injured adolescents and young adults: the meaning of body change, J Adv Nurs 14:389-396, 1989.
15. Dunnum L: Life satisfaction and spinal cord injury: the patient perspective, J Neurosci Nurs 22:43-47, 1990.
16. Albin MS and White RJ: Epidemiology, physiopathology, and experimental therapeutics in spinal cord injury. In Albin MS, ed: Acute spinal cord injury, Philadelphia, 1987, WB Saunders Co, pp 441-442.
17. Walleck CA: Spinal cord injury. In Cardona VD and others, eds: From resuscitation through rehabilitation, Philadelphia, 1988, WB Saunders Co, p 432.

18. Hickey JV: The clinical practice of neurological and neurosurgical nursing, ed 2, Philadelphia, 1986, JB Lippincott Co, p 389.

19. Carol MP and Ducker TB: Spinal cord injury and spinal shock syndrome. In Siegel JH, ed: Trauma, emergency surgery and critical care, New York, 1987, Churchill Livingstone, p 949.

20. Bergman TA and Seljeskog EL: Management of thoracolumbar and lumbar spine injuries. In Youmans JR, ed: Neurological surgery, ed 3, Philadelphia, 1990, WB Saunders Co, p 2419.

21. Gilbert J: Critical care management of the patient with acute spinal cord injury. In Albin M, ed: Acute spinal cord injury, Philadelphia, 1987, WB Saunders Co, pp 553-556.

22. Borkowski C: A comparison of pulmonary complications in spinal cord injured patients treated—two modes of spinal immobilization, J Neurosurg Nurs 21:79-85, 1989.

23. Fegone SF: Cardiovascular and hemodynamic response to tilting and standing in tetraplegic patients: a review, Paraplegia 22:99, 1984.

24. Mandjak-McCanon K: Rehabilitation of the patient with spinal cord injury, Trauma Quarterly 4:45, 1988.

25. Hartshern JC and Golsey M: Abrupt alterations in mobility. In Mitchell PH and others, eds: AACN's neuroscience nursing, Norwich, Conn, 1988, Appleton & Lange, pp 314-315.

26. Spica MM: Sexual counseling standards for the spinal cord-injured, J Neurosci Nurs 21:56-60, 1989.

27. O'Shaughnessy EJ, Traynor CD, and Berni R: Micturition monitor as an aid to management of neurogenic bladder, Arch Phys Med Rehabil 64:317, 1983.

28. Strawbridge LR and others: Augmentation cystoplasty and the artificial genitourinary sphincter, J Urol 142:297-301, 1989.

29. Simeone FA: Spinal cord tumors in adults. In Youmans JR, ed: Neurological surgery, ed 3, Philadelphia, 1990, WB Saunders Co, pp 3538-3541.

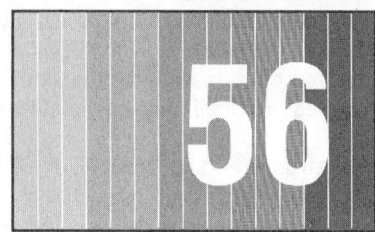

CHAPTER

56

Nursing Assessment

Musculoskeletal System

Susan C. Ruda

L earning Objectives

1. Describe the gross anatomical and microscopic structures of bone.
2. Explain the classification system of joints and movements at synovial joints.
3. Describe the functions of cartilage, muscles, ligaments, tendons, fascia, and bursae.
4. Describe age-related changes in the musculoskeletal system and differences in assessment findings.
5. Identify the significant subjective and objective data related to the musculoskeletal system that should be obtained from a client.

6. Describe the appropriate techniques used in the physical assessment of the musculoskeletal system.
7. Differentiate normal from common abnormal findings of a physical assessment of the musculoskeletal system.
8. Describe the purpose, significance of results, and nursing responsibilities related to diagnostic studies of the musculoskeletal system.

The ability to perform complex and precise movements permits human beings to interact and adapt to the environment. Proper functioning of the musculoskeletal system makes such movements possible. The musculoskeletal system is the largest organ system of the human body. It consists of bones, muscles, joints, cartilage, ligaments, tendons, fascia, and bursae.

The musculoskeletal system is particularly vulnerable to external environmental forces. These forces can cause alteration in the structure of bone or soft connective tissue, resulting in functional disruption. The consequences may be deformity, alteration of body image, alteration in mobility, pain, or permanent disability. These problems often produce long-term health problems that interfere with activities of daily living and the quality of life.

STRUCTURES AND FUNCTIONS OF THE MUSCULOSKELETAL SYSTEM
Bone

Function. The main functions of the musculoskeletal system are support, protection of vital organs, movement,

and mineral storage.[1] Bone forms the body's supporting framework. Without this support, the body would collapse. A second function of the musculoskeletal system is protection of vital organs and tissues. For example, the skull protects the brain, the vertebrae protect the spinal cord, and the rib cage protects the lungs and heart. Bones serve as a point of attachment for muscles; muscles are anchored to bones by tendons. Bone acts as a lever for muscles, and joints serve as fulcrums. Movement occurs as a result of muscle contractions applied to these levers. Bone also serves as a site for storage of inorganic minerals such as calcium and phosphorus. Cancellous bone contains hematopoietic tissue for production of blood cells.

Gross structure. Bone is a dynamic tissue that changes form and substance continually. It is composed of organic (collagen) and inorganic material (calcium, phosphate). Internal and external growth and remodeling are continuous processes.

Bone is classified according to structure as *compact* (dense) or *cancellous* (spongy). In compact bone, haversian systems fit closely together, giving a dense consistency to the bone structure. In cancellous bone there are many open spaces between thin processes and networks of bone tissue that are filled with either red or yellow marrow.

Reviewed by Peggy Mayfield, M.S.N., R.N.C., Adult Nurse Practitioner, Associate Professor Emeritus, Harris College of Nursing, Texas Christian University, Fort Worth, Texas.

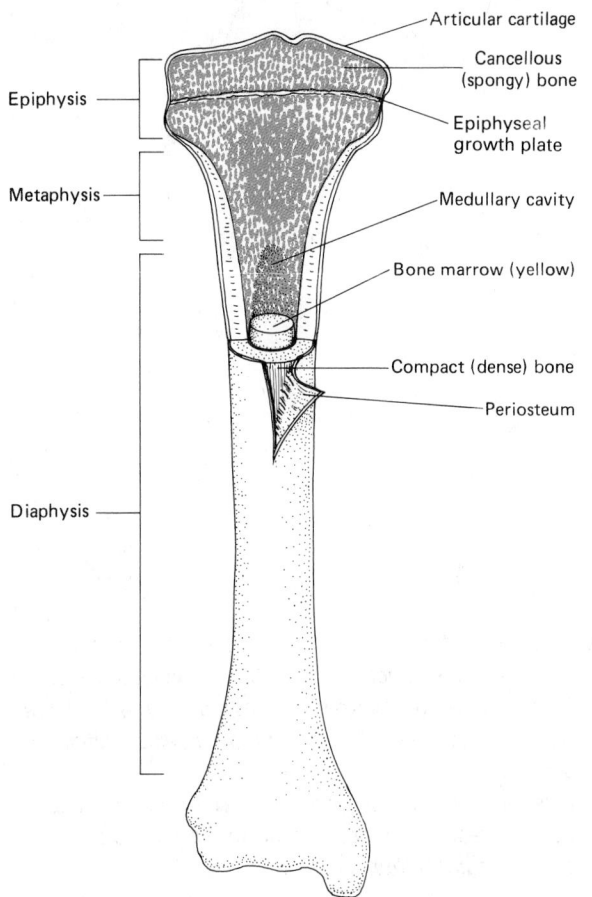

Fig. 56-1 Anatomical structure of a typical long bone.

The anatomical structure of bone can best be visualized by the typical long bone (e.g., femur) (Fig. 56-1). Each long bone consists of an epiphysis, articular cartilage, a diaphysis, periosteum, and a medullary (marrow) cavity.

The *epiphysis* is located at each end of a long bone and is composed of cancellous bone. It is the location for muscle attachment and provides stability for the joint. *Articular cartilage* covers the ends of the bone and provides smooth surfaces for joint movement.

The *diaphysis* is the main shaft of bone. It provides the bone with structural support and is composed of compact bone. The *metaphysis* is the flared area between the epiphysis and the diaphysis. During bone development it contains the growth zones. In the adult the metaphysis is joined to the epiphysis. The *epiphyseal plate* in children is the cartilaginous area that actively produces bone and results in longitudinal growth. In the adult, this plate hardens to mature bone, and longitudinal growth ceases.

The *periosteum* is fibrous connective tissue that covers the bone. Musculotendinous fibers attach to the outer layer of the periosteum. The inner layer of the periosteum contains osteoblasts (bone-forming cells), which are essential for transverse bone growth and fracture repair.

The *medullary* (marrow) *cavity* is in the center of the diaphysis. In the adult the medullary cavity of long bones contains yellow bone marrow. In the growing child, red bone marrow in the medullary cavity is actively involved in hematopoiesis. In the adult, hematopoiesis normally occurs only in the red bone marrow of the skull, ribs, sternum, vertebrae, and proximal ends of the humerus and femur.

Microscopic structure. The three types of bone cells are osteoblasts, osteocytes, and osteoclasts. *Osteoblasts* synthesize organic bone matrix and are the basic bone-forming cells. *Osteocytes* are the mature bone cells. *Osteoclasts* are involved in resorption of bone tissue and participate in bone remodeling. Bone is a special kind of connective tissue in which organic matter has become mineralized. The structural unit of compact bone is the haversian system (Fig. 56-2). It consists of lamellae, which are concentric layers of calcified collagen matrix that enclose a long canal (haversian system). The main function of the haversian system is to transport blood to bone tissue. Blood vessels from the periosteum go through Volkmann's canals to the blood vessels of the haversian system.

Osteocytes lie in small spaces called *lacunae* between lamellae. *Canaliculi* (tiny canals) extend from lacunae to connect the osteocytes to one another and to the haversian system.

Types. The skeleton consists of 206 bones that are classified according to shape as long, short, flat, or irregular.

Long bones are characterized by a central shaft and two epiphyseal ends (Fig. 56-1). Examples include the femur, humerus, and radius. *Short bones* are characterized by cancellous bone covered by a thin layer of compact bone. Examples include the carpals and tarsals.

Flat bones are characterized by two layers of compact bone separated by a layer of cancellous bone. Examples include the ribs, skull, scapula, and sternum. The spaces in the cancellous bone contain bone marrow. *Irregular bones* have a variety of shapes and sizes. Examples include the vertebrae, sacrum, and mandible.

Joints

Bones are connected to one another by means of structures called *joints* (articulations). Rigid bone can change position and permits movement by the action of joints. Joints are commonly classified according to their degree of movement (Fig. 56-3).

The diarthrodial (synovial) type, the most common joint, consists of a cavity between the articular surfaces of the bones that make up the joint (Fig. 56-4). The ends of the bone are covered with articular (hyaline) cartilage. A capsule of connective tissue called the *fibrous capsule* joins the two bones together, forming a cavity. The capsule is lined by a synovium, or synovial membrane, which secretes a thick synovial fluid to lubricate the joint and reduce friction. Types of diarthrodial joints are shown in Fig. 56-5.

Cartilage

Cartilage is a rigid connective tissue that supports soft tissue and provides the articular surfaces for joint movement. It protects underlying tissues. The cartilage that makes up the epiphyseal plate is also essential for the growth of long bones before physical maturity is reached.

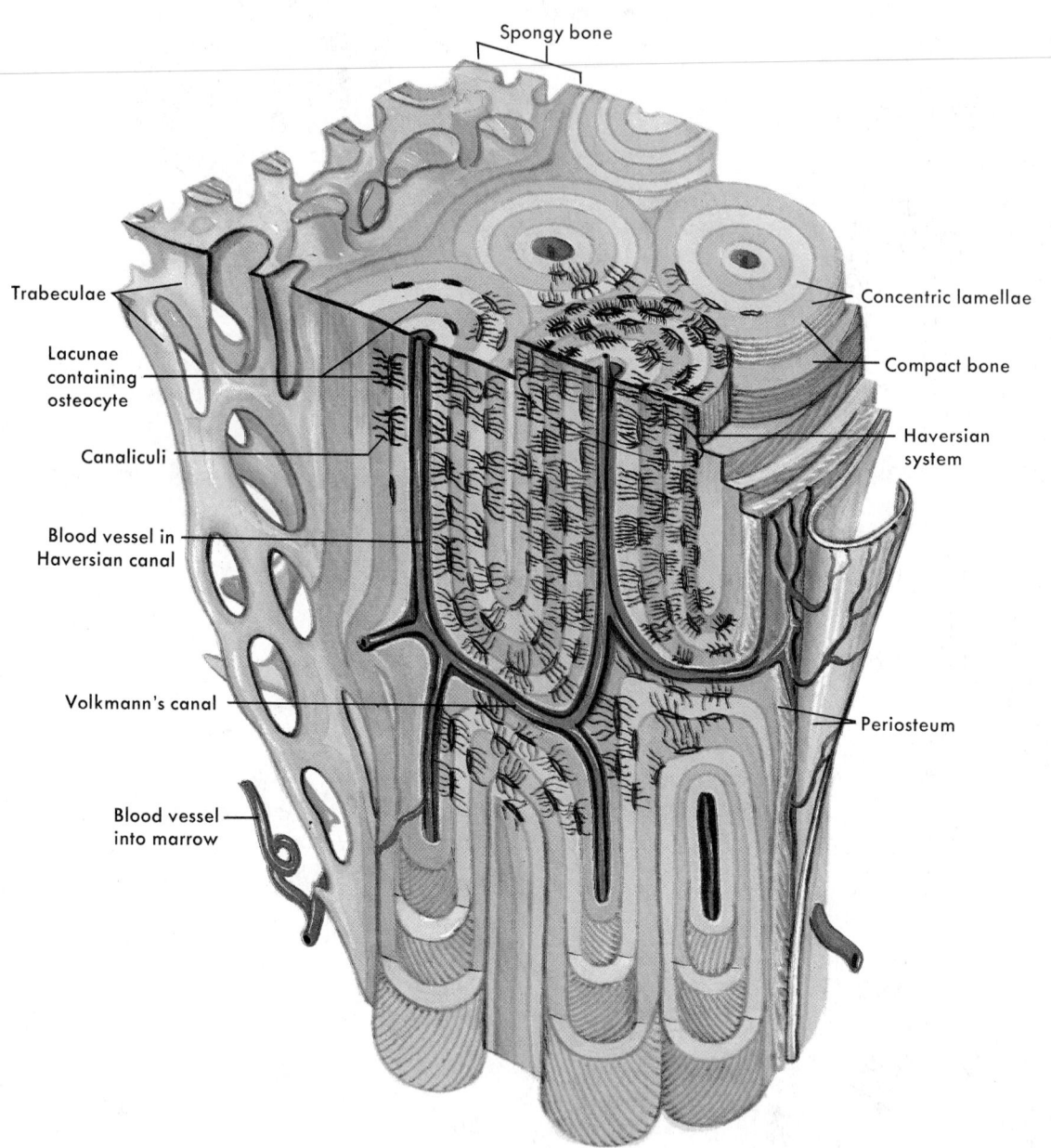

Fig. 56-2 Structure of bone showing haversian system. (From Thibodeau G: Anatomy and physiology, ed 12 St Louis, 1987, Times Mirror/Mosby College Publishing, p 93.)

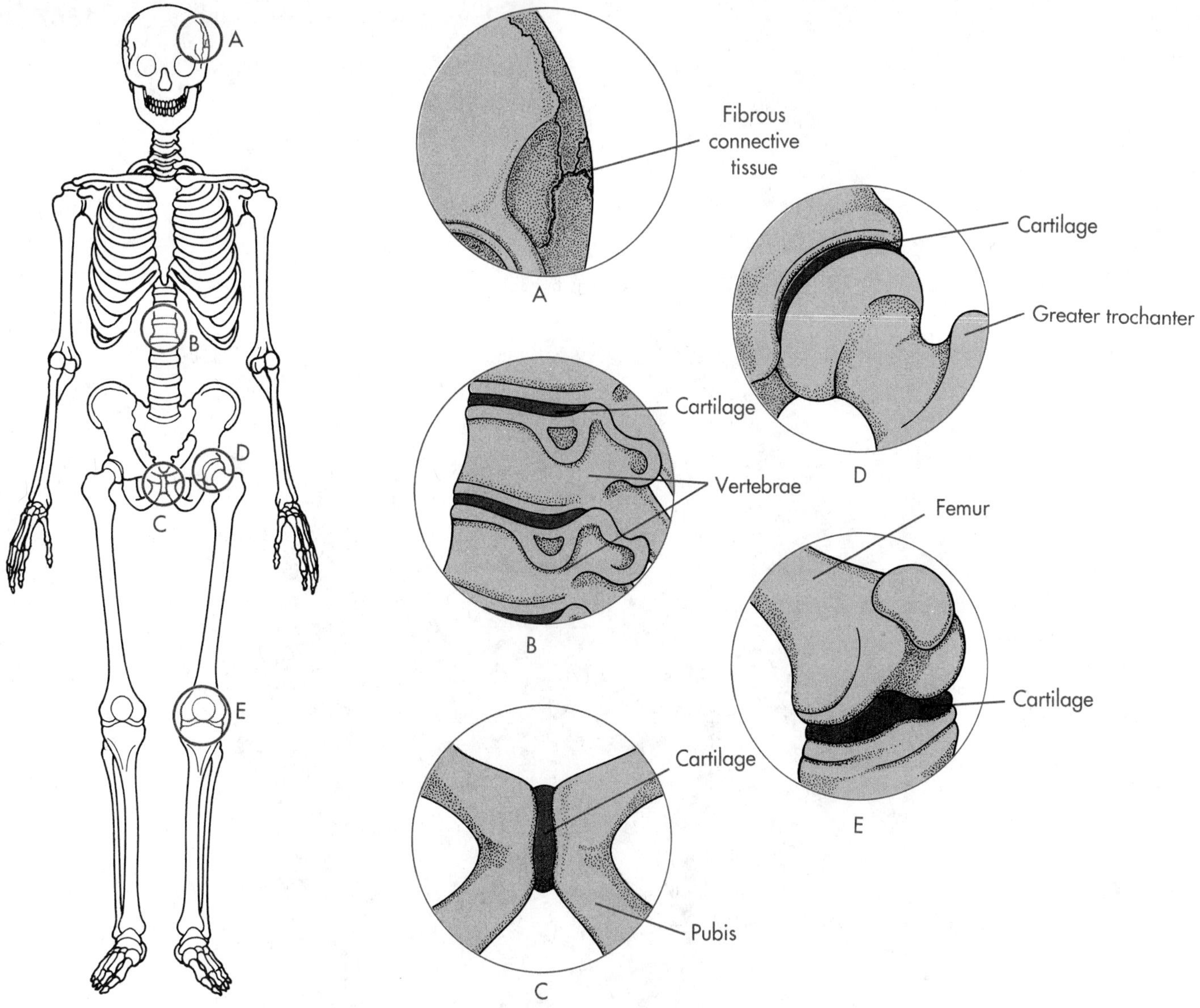

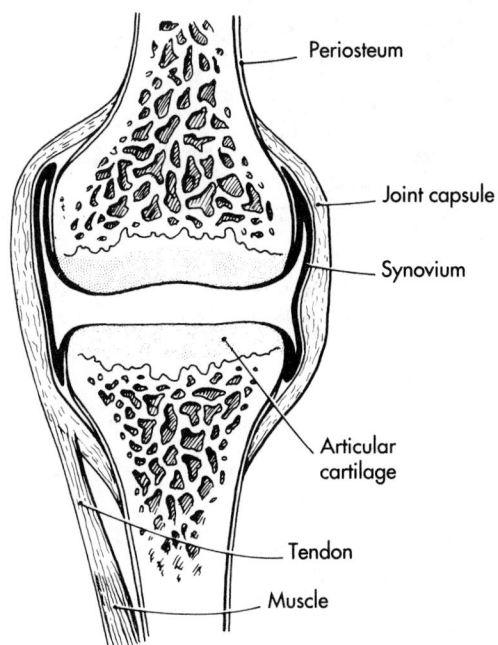

Fig. 56-3 Classification of joints. *A, B,* and *C* are synarthrotic (immovable) and amphiarthrotic (slightly movable) joints. *D* and *E* are diarthrotic (freely movable) joints.

Fibrous connective tissue

Cartilage

Greater trochanter

Cartilage

Vertebrae

Femur

Cartilage

Cartilage

Pubis

A

B

C

D

E

Periosteum

Joint capsule

Synovium

Articular cartilage

Tendon

Muscle

Fig. 56-4 Normal diarthrodial joint of the knee. (From Price S and Wilson L: Pathophysiology: clinical concepts of disease processes, ed 4, St Louis, 1991, Mosby–Year Book, Inc.)

Joint	Movement	Examples	Illustration
Hinge joint	Flexion, extension	Elbow joint (shown), interphalangeal joints, knee joint	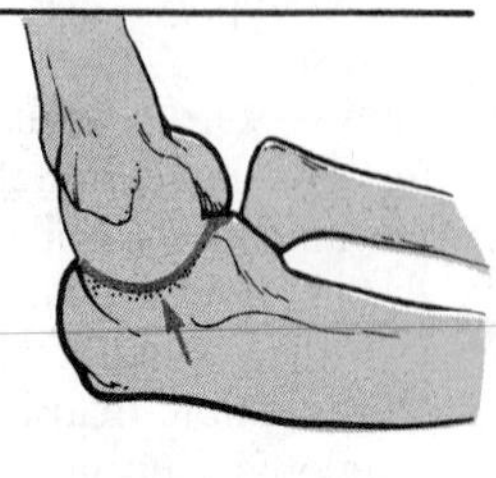
Ball and socket (syn.: spheroidal)	Flexion, extension; adduction, abduction; circumduction	Shoulder (shown), hip	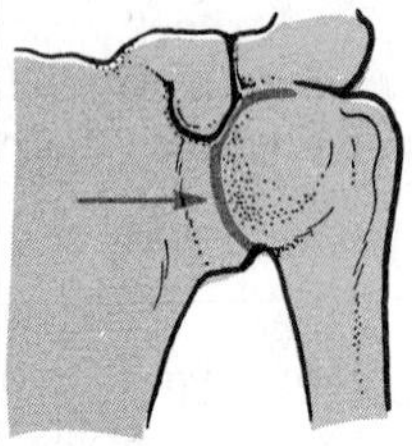
Pivot (syn.: rotary)	Rotation	Atlas-axis, proximal radioulnar joint (shown)	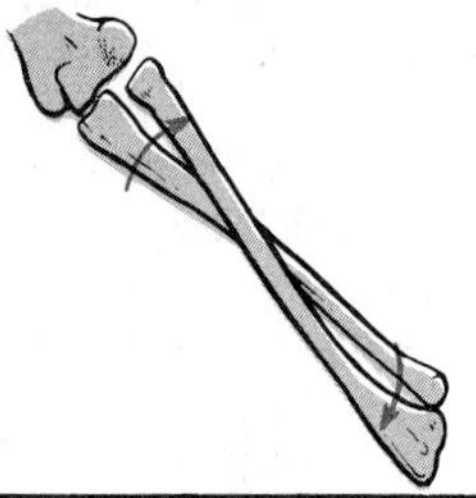
Condyloid	Flexion, extension; abduction, adduction; circumduction	Wrist joint (between radial and carpals) (shown)	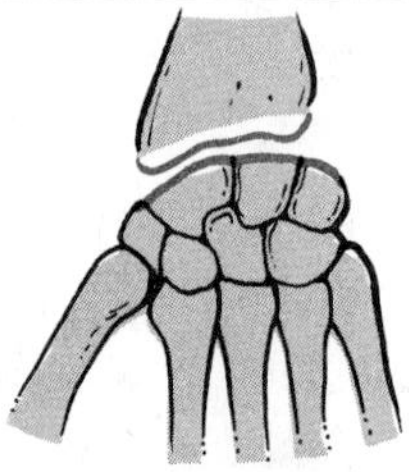
Saddle	Flexion, extension; abduction, adduction; circumduction, thumb-finger opposition	Carpometacarpal joint of thumb	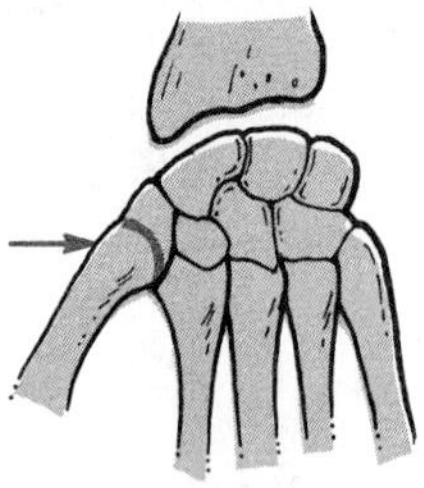
Gliding	One surface moves over another surface	Between tarsal bones, sacroiliac joint, between articular processes of vertebrae, between carpal bones (shown)	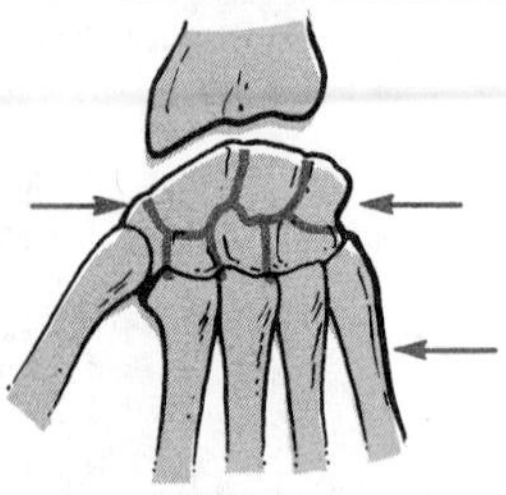

Fig. 56-5   Types of diarthrodial joints.

Cartilage is avascular and nourished by the diffusion of material from capillaries in adjacent connective tissue. Cartilage cells are slow to reproduce because of the lack of a direct blood supply. Therefore damaged cartilage heals slowly.

The three types of cartilage tissue are *hyaline, elastic,* and *fibrous.* Hyaline cartilage, the most common, contains a moderate amount of collagen fibers. It is found in the trachea, bronchi, nose, and articular surfaces of bones. Elastic cartilage, which contains collagen and elastic fibers, is more flexible than hyaline cartilage. It is found in the ear, epiglottis, and larynx. Fibrocartilage, which consists mostly of collagen fibers, is a very tough tissue that often functions as a shock absorber. It is found between vertebral disks and in the knee. Fibrocartilage also forms a protective cushion between the bones of the pelvic girdle.

Soft-Tissue Structures

Muscle

Types. The three types of muscle tissue are *cardiac* (branching), *smooth* (nonstriated), and *skeletal* (striated) muscle. Cardiac muscle is found in the heart. Smooth muscle is found in the walls of hollow structures such as the gastrointestinal (GI) tract, urinary bladder, uterus, and blood vessels. The function of both cardiac and smooth muscle is controlled by involuntary stimulation of the autonomic nervous system and cannot normally be controlled by conscious effort. Most skeletal muscles are attached to

bone. Contractions of skeletal muscle account for movement of the body and can be controlled voluntarily.

Structure. The structural unit of muscle is the muscle cell, which is also called a *muscle fiber.* Muscle is composed of numerous fibers bound together by connective tissue. Skeletal muscle fibers are multinucleated cylinders that range in length from several millimeters to several centimeters. Muscle fibers are composed of myofibrils, which in turn are made up of filaments.

Under a microscope, skeletal muscle shows alternating banding, which accounts for the striated appearance.[2] This appearance is due to a repeating pattern of filaments seen in the myofibrils. The sarcomere is the contractile unit of the myofibril. Each sarcomere contains myosin (thick) filaments and actin (thin) filaments. The arrangement of the thin and thick filaments accounts for the banding. As thick and thin filaments slide past each other, the sarcomeres shorten and muscle contraction occurs.

Contractions. Skeletal muscle contractions are of various types and are responsible for the two functions of posture and movement. *Isometric* contractions increase the tension within a muscle but do not produce movement. Repeated isometric contractions make muscles grow larger and stronger. *Isotonic* contractions produce movement. *Tonic* contractions do not produce movement but hold muscles in position and thus maintain posture.

Skeletal muscle produces three other types of contractions that have little to do with functional posture and

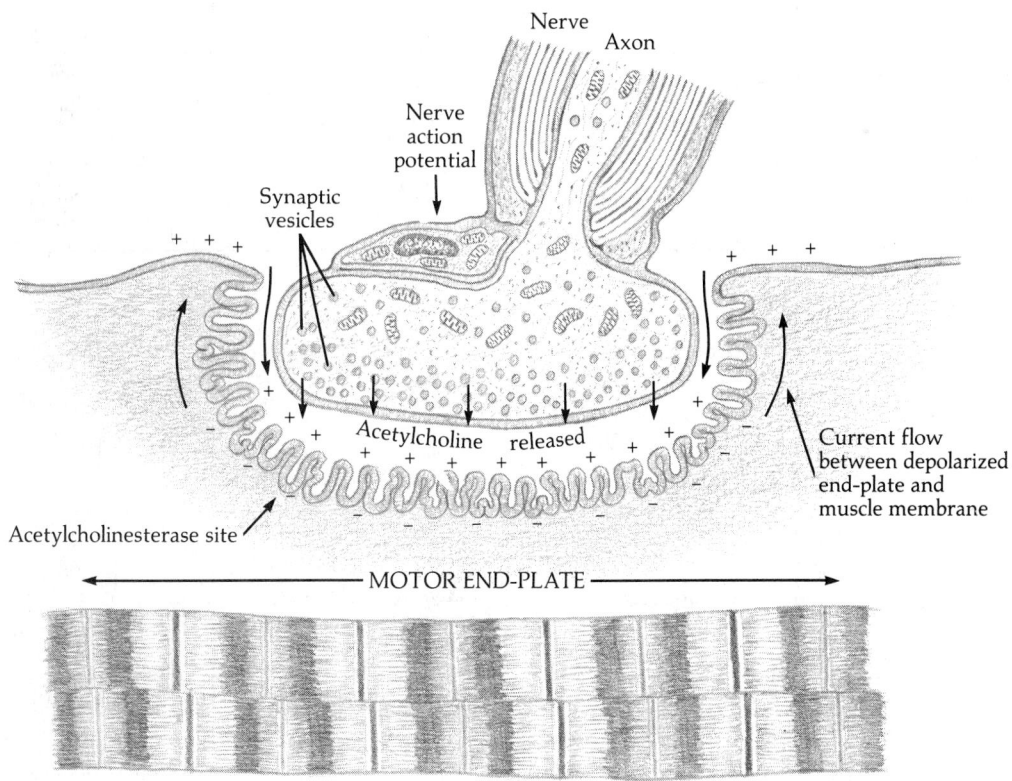

Fig. 56-6 Neuromuscular junction. (From Thompson J and others: Mosby's manual of clinical nursing, ed 2, St Louis, 1989, The CV Mosby Co.)

movement. They are a *twitch* contraction—a quick, jerky contraction in response to a single stimulus; a *tetanic* contraction—a more sustained twitch; and a *treppe* contraction—an increasingly stronger contraction in response to repeated stimulation.

The types of skeletal muscle contractions help explain the major benefits of exercise. These include looking and feeling better, improved posture, greater muscle control and strength, better muscle tone, less fatigue, and improved heart and lung function.

Neuromuscular junction. Skeletal muscles require a nerve supply to contract.[3] The nerve cell and the muscle fibers it supplies are called a *motor unit*. The junction between the axon of the nerve cell and the muscle cell it supplies is called the *myoneural* or *neuromuscular junction* (Fig. 56-6).

When acetylcholine is released from the motor end plate of the neuron, it diffuses across the neuromuscular junction and travels into the muscle fibers. In response to this stimulation, the sarcoplasmic reticulum releases calcium ions into the cytoplasm. The presence of these ions triggers the contraction in the myofibrils.

Energy source. The energy source used in muscle fiber contractions comes from adenosine triphosphate (ATP). ATP is synthesized by cellular oxidative metabolism in numerous mitochondria located close to the myofibrils. A second energy source is creatine phosphate, which can easily be converted to ATP. Creatine phosphate is synthesized and stored in muscle tissue.

Ligaments and tendons. Ligaments and tendons are both composed of dense, fibrous connective tissue. This type of connective tissue contains large numbers of collagen fibers that are closely packed. Tendons attach muscles to bones. They are an extension of the muscle sheath that attaches to the periosteum. Ligaments connect bones to bones at joints (e.g., the knee joint). They permit movement while providing stability.

Fibrous connective tissue has a relatively poor blood supply. Although the tissue can repair itself after injury, it is usually a slow process. For example, a sprain may require a long time to heal despite the minor nature of the injury.

Fascia. *Fascia* is the term used for layers of connective tissue. It is classified as either superficial or deep. Superficial fascia is the loose connective tissue located immediately under the skin. Deep fascia (dense, fibrous connective tissue) is found around muscle, between muscles, and around the bundles that bind nerves and blood vessels together.

Fascia separates one muscle from another to permit independent muscle action. It allows gliding of one muscle over another. In addition, fascia provides strength to muscle tissues.

Bursae. Bursae are small sacs of connective tissue lined with synovial membrane and synovial fluid. They are commonly located at joints and prevent friction. Bursae function as cushions to relieve pressure between the moving parts. They are found between the patella and the skin (prepatellar bursa), between the olecranon process and the skin (olecranon bursa), between the head of the humerus

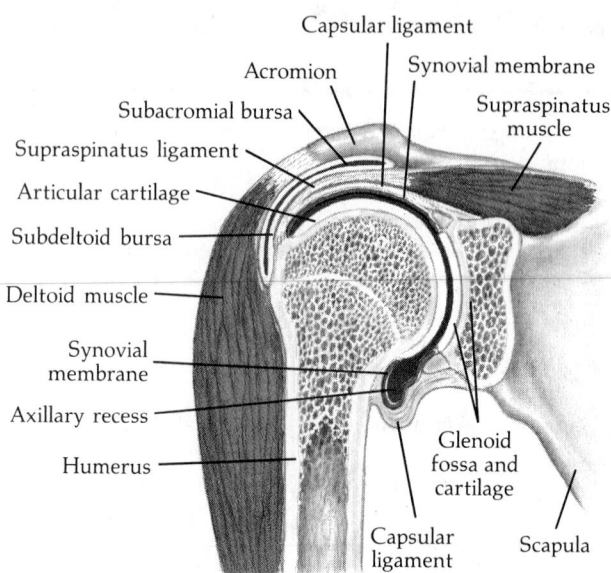

Fig. 56-7 Bursae of the shoulder joint. (From Thompson J and others: Mosby's manual of clinical nursing, ed 2, St Louis, 1989, The CV Mosby Co.)

and the acromion process (subacromial bursa), and between the lower portion of the gluteus maximus muscle and the bony ischial tuberosity (submuscular bursa) (Fig. 56-7). Bursitis (inflammation of the bursa) may be due to mechanical injury to the bursa or excessive use of a joint. "Tennis elbow" is a form of bursitis involving the olecranon process.

Effects of Aging

Many of the functional problems of older adults are due to problems of the musculoskeletal system. Impairment of various parts of the musculoskeletal system may be insidious in early adulthood. Obvious signs of musculoskeletal impairment may not appear until later. These changes can alter posture, function, and gait.[4]

In addition to the usual musculoskeletal assessment with a particular emphasis on exercise practices, the nurse should determine the impact of age-related changes of the musculoskeletal system on the functional status of the older client (Table 56-1). Functional limitations that are accepted by older adults as a normal part of aging can often be halted or reversed with appropriate interventions. Table 56-2 lists age-related changes of the musculoskeletal system and differences in assessment findings.

ASSESSMENT OF THE MUSCULOSKELETAL SYSTEM
Subjective Data

Health history. The health history serves as a basis for physical and laboratory assessments by offering insight to the nurse on specific areas that should be examined. Correct diagnosis depends on an accurate client history and a thorough examination. A musculoskeletal assessment can be made on a specific body part, as part of a general physical examination, or as an examination in itself. Judgment

Table 56-1 Prevention of Age-Related Musculoskeletal Problems

Action	Rationale
Use of ramps in buildings and at street corners instead of steps	Stair-walking motion may create enough stress on fragile bones to cause a hip fracture. Use of ramps may prevent falls.
Elimination of scatter rugs in the home	These are notorious for causing falls and fractures.
Response to pain and discomfort of osteoarthritis	
Resting in reclining position	Osteoarthritis is seen on x-ray film of most persons over the age of 50 and causes pain. Rest is the most useful way to decrease its discomfort.
Use of plain or enteric-coated aspirin or ibuprofen	Aspirin and other antiinflammatory drugs diminish inflammation of joints and hence reduce pain.
Use of a walker or cane to help with walking	Assistance decreases stress on inflamed joints and thus decreases discomfort.
Eating amount and kind of foods to prevent excess weight gain	Obesity adds stress to bones, which may predispose client to fractures.
Regular and frequent exercise	
Activities of daily living	Activities of daily living provide range-of-motion exercise, which should be done four times a day; 100% range of motion is not as critical as the ability to perform normal activities.
Hobbies (e.g., jigsaw puzzles, needlework, model building)	These exercise distal joints and prevent stiffness.
Walking short distances daily with shoes that give good support	Some weight-bearing exercise is essential and should be done two or three times daily. Good shoes provide for safety and promote comfort.
Gradual initiation of all activities	Starting gradually promotes optimal coordination. When a client slowly rises to a standing position, dizziness and hence falls and fractures can be prevented.

Table 56-2

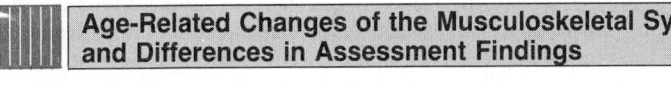 **Age-Related Changes of the Musculoskeletal System and Differences in Assessment Findings**

Changes	Differences in Assessment Findings
MUSCLE	
Decreased number and diameter of muscle cells, replacement of muscle cells by fibrous connective tissue	Decreased muscle strength and bulk, abdominal protrusion
Loss of elasticity in ligaments and cartilage	Decreased fine motor activity, decreased agility
Reduction in ability to store glycogen derived from carbohydrates, decreased ability to release glycogen as quick energy in time of stress	Slowed reaction times, slowing of most muscle reflexes, decreased endurance
JOINTS	
Erosion of articular cartilage, possible direct contact between bone ends	Manifestations of osteoarthritis, joint stiffness, possible crepitation on movement of joints, pain on range-of-motion movements
Overgrowth of bone around joint margins (osteophytes)	Heberden's nodes in fingers (especially in women), limited mobility in affected joints
Loss of water from disks between vertebrae, narrowing of joint vertebral spaces	Loss of height, kyphosis, back pain
BONE	
Decrease in bone mass	Dowager's hump (kyphosis)

must be used in selecting all or part of the components of the musculoskeletal history and physical examination on the basis of the client's presenting problem. Accidents often result in trauma to the musculoskeletal system and require a thorough assessment. If the injury is serious or life threatening, only pertinent information related to the accident is obtained, and a thorough assessment is deferred.

Complaints that should alert the nurse to obtain subjective and objective data related to the musculoskeletal system include pain, joint swelling, decreasing strength, change in size of an extremity or muscle, deformity, spasms, crepitation, changes in sensation, stiffness, and changes in gait.

Past health history

PEDIATRIC AND ADULT ILLNESSES. Certain illnesses are known to affect the musculoskeletal system either directly or indirectly. The client should be questioned specifically about a history of tuberculosis, poliomyelitis, diabetes mellitus, gout, inflammatory and degenerative arthritis, rickets, osteomalacia, scurvy, osteomyelitis or soft-tissue infection, fungal infection of the bones or joints, and neuromuscular disabilities. If the client has a history of any of these problems, a detailed account should be obtained (see Chapter 3). In addition, the client should be questioned about possible sources of secondary bacterial infection such as ears, tonsils, teeth, sinuses, or genitourinary tract.

IMMUNIZATIONS. The client should be specifically questioned about immunizations related to tetanus and polio. The date and reaction to a tuberculin skin test should also be obtained. Failure to be properly immunized or tested can result in serious musculoskeletal problems.

HOSPITALIZATION. Information should be obtained about hospitalizations that were necessitated by a musculoskeletal problem. The reason for the hospitalization, the date and duration, and the treatment should be carefully documented. Specifics of any surgical procedure and the postoperative course should also be obtained. The client should also be questioned about emergency treatment related to musculoskeletal disorders and injuries.

INJURIES. The list of minor and major injuries of the musculoskeletal system can be extensive in the client who is a good historian. It includes documentation of fractures, sprains, strains, and dislocations. The information should be recorded chronologically and should include the following:

1. Circumstances related to the injury
2. Diagnostic evaluations
3. Methods of treatment
4. Duration of treatment
5. Current status related to the injury
6. Need for assistive devices
7. Interference with activities of daily living

MEDICATION HISTORY. The client should be questioned carefully regarding prescription and over-the-counter drugs used to treat a musculoskeletal problem. Information on the reason for taking the medication, its name, the dose and frequency, length of time it was taken, its effect, and any side effects should be obtained. Specific inquiry should be made related to skeletal muscle relaxants, antirheumatoid agents, salicylates, nonsteroidal antiinflam-

matory agents, systemic steroids, and narcotics. The client should be questioned about GI distress or a bleeding ulcer if antiinflammatory agents have been taken.

In addition to drugs taken for treatment of a musculoskeletal problem, the client should be questioned about drugs that can have detrimental effects on this system. These drugs include anticonvulsants (osteomalacia), phenothiazines (gait disturbances), steroids (abnormal fat distribution and muscle weakness), and potassium-depleting diuretics (cramps and muscle weakness). Amphetamines and caffeine can cause a generalized increase in motor activity. Older women should be questioned about menopause and the use of postmenopausal hormone replacement therapy.

ALLERGIES. Food or contact allergies are of little consequence in relation to musculoskeletal problems. However, the general malaise often associated with allergic reactions may manifest in musculoskeletal stiffness and lethargy. Allergic reactions to drugs used to treat musculoskeletal problems can interfere with therapy, and an alternative treatment method may have to be used if the allergic reaction is severe.

Family history.
A three-generation family history should be obtained for rheumatoid arthritis, degenerative arthritis, gout, and scoliosis, since these problems have a familial predisposition.

Social and personal history.
Because each client is unique, all areas of the history must be considered. However, several areas of the client profile are particularly important to explore in depth.

OCCUPATION. Extremes of activity related to occupation can affect the musculoskeletal system. A sedentary occupation does not allow for maintaining muscle flexibility and strength. Jobs that require extreme effort and use of the body for heavy lifting and pushing can result in damage to the joints and supporting structures of the body. The nurse should inquire about occupationally related injuries to the musculoskeletal system, the amount of time lost from work, and the treatments used.

EXERCISE AND RECREATION. A detailed account of the type, duration, and frequency of activities related to exercise and recreation should be obtained and assessed regarding adequacy. This information is readily obtained when the client recounts a typical day. Daily, weekend, and seasonal patterns should be compared because occasional or sporadic exercise can be more problematic than regular exercise.

SAFETY PRACTICES. Specific questions should be asked about the safety practices of the client as they relate to the job environment, recreation, and exercise. For example, if the client is a jogger, the type of shoes worn and the jogging surface used should be investigated. The high incidence of trauma to the musculoskeletal system requires a careful investigation of the area of safety practices. Identification of problems in this area directs the need for client education.

DIET. The client's account of a typical day's diet can provide clues to two areas of concern in relation to the musculoskeletal system. Obesity predisposes people to ligamentous instability, particularly in the lower back region.

It also adds stress to weight-bearing joints. The maintenance of normal weight should be a goal for client education.

Abnormal nutritional states can predispose individuals to musculoskeletal problems such as osteoporosis, rickets, and osteomalacia. Adequate amounts of vitamins C and D, calcium, and protein are essential for a healthy, intact musculoskeletal system.

Review of systems. The review of systems is the final step in acquiring subjective data before beginning the physical examination. The client should be asked to describe any problems related to muscle pains or spasms, joint pain, redness or swelling, stiffness, backache, limitation of movement, weakness, clumsiness, crepitus, or any change in the bones or joints that causes trouble with daily activities. Any positive response must be carefully investigated and documented, including the psychological effect of the disability or deformity.

Objective Data

Physical examination. The primary methods used in the physical examination of the musculoskeletal system include inspection and palpation. The data gathered from a careful health history provide the nurse with clues about areas on which to concentrate the examination.

Inspection. Inspection begins during the nurse's initial contact with the client. The nurse should observe the client for any apparent asymmetry and for sitting and standing posture, gait, general body build, and configuration of the muscles. The nurse should be particularly aware of limitations in the client's ability to perform activities of daily living such as dressing, toileting, and eating.

The condition of the skin is observed for general color, scars, or overt signs of previous injury or operations. A systematic inspection is performed starting at the head and neck and proceeding to the upper extremities, the lower extremities, and finally the back. Although the order is not of great importance, the regular use of a systematic approach is important to avoid missing important aspects of the examination. The nurse should specifically inspect for joint motion and asymmetry of movement, swelling, deformity, masses, and evidence of limb-length or muscle-size discrepancies. The client's opposite body part is used for comparison when an abnormality is suspected.

Palpation. Any area that has aroused concern because of a subjective complaint or has been noted on inspection should be carefully palpated. The examiner's hands should be warm to prevent muscle spasm, which can interfere with identification of essential landmarks or soft-tissue structures. Palpation of the soft tissues, including muscles and joints, enables the examiner to evaluate skin temperature, local tenderness, swelling, and crepitation. It is important to establish the relationship of adjacent structures and to evaluate the general contour, abnormal prominences, and local landmarks. The usual sequence is to begin at the neck and proceed cephalocaudally (head to tail) to examine the neck, shoulders, elbows, wrists, hands, back, hips, knees, ankles, and feet. The different types of palpation are usually performed concurrently.

MOVEMENT. When examining joint movement, the nurse must carefully evaluate passive and active joint range of

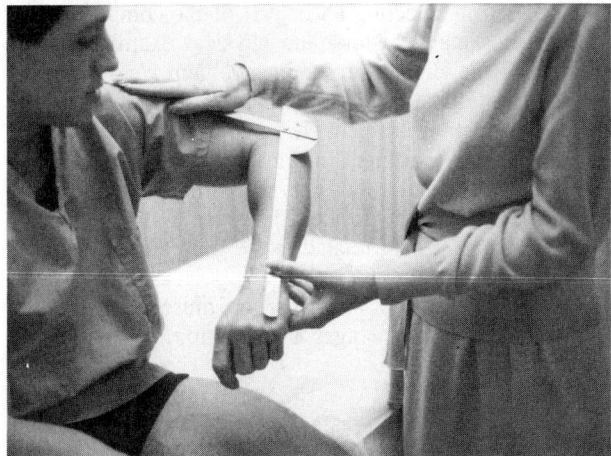

Fig. 56-8 Measurement of joint motion with a goniometer.

Table 56-3 Movement at Synovial Joints

Movement	Description
Flexion	Bending of joint that decreases angle between two bones, shortening of muscle length
Extension	Bending of joint that increases angle between two bones
Hyperextension	Extension in which angle exceeds 180 degrees
Abduction	Movement of part away from midline
Adduction	Movement of part toward midline
Pronation	Turning of palm downward or sole outward
Supination	Turning of palm upward or sole inward
Circumduction	Combination of flexion, extension, abduction, and adduction resulting in circular motion of body part
Rotation	Movement about longitudinal axis
Inversion	Turning of sole inward toward midline
Eversion	Turning of sole outward away from midline

motion. Active motion occurs as the result of the client's own movement of the musculature. It is usually examined first. Passive motion occurs as the result of movement of the extremity by the examiner. Normally the active and passive joint motions are similar. Caution is required when testing passive joint motion because of the possibility of injury to the underlying soft-tissue structures. Manipulations must cease immediately when pain or resistance is encountered. Specific degrees of range of motion of all joints are usually not measured unless a musculoskeletal problem has been identified. Joint motion is most accurately measured by a goniometer, which measures the amount of bending or angles of the joints (Fig. 56-8).

A less accurate but valuable assessment is to compare the range of motion of one extremity with the range of motion on the opposite side. The common movements at syn-

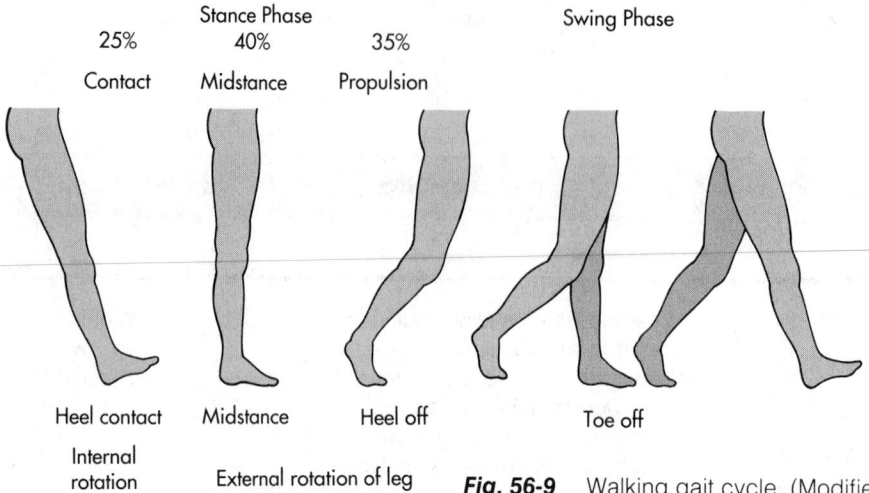

Stance Phase

| 25% | 40% | 35% | Swing Phase |
| Contact | Midstance | Propulsion | |

Heel contact   Midstance   Heel off   Toe off

Internal rotation of leg   External rotation of leg

Pronation   Supination

Fig. 56-9   Walking gait cycle. (Modified from Arnheim DD: Modern principles of athletic training, ed 7, St Louis, 1988, The CV Mosby Co.)

Table 56-4   Muscle Strength Scale

0—No detection of muscular contraction
1—A barely detectable flicker or trace of contraction
2—Active movement of body part with elimination of gravity
3—Active movement against gravity
4—Active movement against gravity and some resistance
5—Active movement against full resistance without evident fatigue (normal muscle strength)

Modified from Bates, B: A guide to physical examination and history taking, ed 4, Philadelphia, 1987, JB Lippincott Co.

Table 56-5   Normal Physical Assessment of Musculoskeletal System

Full range of motion of all joints
No joint swelling, deformity, or crepitation
Normal spinal curvatures
No tenderness on palpation of spine
No muscle atrophy or asymmetry
Muscle strength of 100%

---

ovial joints and the ones most commonly tested for joint motion are listed in Table 56-3.

MEASUREMENT. Limb length and circumferential measurement of muscle mass are often determined when subjective problems or length discrepancies are noted. For example, leg length measurements are obtained when gait disorders are observed. Limb length is measured between two bony prominences and compared with the similar measurement of the opposite extremity. Muscle mass is measured in any muscle that appears to have undergone hypertrophy or atrophy, and it is compared to the opposite extremity. Muscle mass is measured circumferentially at the largest area of the mass. When recording measurements, the nurse should record the exact location at which the measurements were obtained (e.g., the quadriceps muscle is measured 15 cm above the patella). This informs the next examiner of the exact area to be measured and ensures consistency in future examinations.

MUSCLE-STRENGTH TESTING. The strength of individual muscles or groups of muscles is graded in performance of movements during contraction against applied resistance (Table 56-4). The examiner should instruct the client to apply resistance to the force exerted by the examiner. For example, if the examiner tries to pull the bent arm down, the client should try to raise it. Muscle strength should also be compared to the strength of the opposite extremity.

Subtle variations in muscle strength may be noted when comparing the client's dominant side to the nondominant side.

GAIT. The nurse assesses gait by having the client walk across the room and back. The normal gait is divided into two separate phases, the stance phase and the swing phase (Fig. 56-9). The two occur simultaneously: while one limb is in stance phase, the other is in swing phase.

OTHER. Table 56-5 is an example of how to record a normal physical assessment of the musculoskeletal system. Common abnormal assessment findings of the musculoskeletal system are presented in Table 56-6.

DIAGNOSTIC STUDIES
Radiological Studies

The most common diagnostic study used to assess musculoskeletal problems is an x-ray examination. Radiological studies are important to establish the presence of a musculoskeletal problem and to follow its progress and the effectiveness of treatment.

A standard x-ray study is a film produced by the action of x rays emitted from a cathode tube diphotosensitive surface. X-ray films can be thought of as shadows of structures, particularly bony structures. Bones are more dense than other tissues and do not allow the x ray to penetrate. The standard x-ray film develops dense areas as white.

The anteroposterior and lateral views are the most commonly used standard x-ray perspectives. Because disk and

Table 56-6

 Common Assessment Abnormalities of the Musculoskeletal System

Finding	Description	Possible Etiology and Significance
Ankylosis	Scarring within a joint leading to stiffness or fixation	Chronic joint inflammation
Atrophy	Wasting of muscle, characterized by decrease in circumference and flabby appearance and resulting in decrease in function and muscle tone	Prolonged disuse, contraction, immobilization, muscle denervation
Contracture	Resistance to movement of muscle or joint as result of fibrosis of supporting soft tissues	Shortening of muscle or ligament structure, tightness of soft tissue, immobilization, incorrect positioning
Crepitation	Crackling sound or grating sensation as result of friction between bones	Fracture, chronic inflammation, dislocation
Effusion	Escape of fluid into body part, possibly with swelling and pain	Trauma, especially to knee
Felon	Purulent bacterial infection of pulp space (tissue mass) of distal phalanx of finger	Minor hand injury, puncture wound, laceration
Ganglion	Small, fluid-filled cyst usually on dorsal surface of wrist and foot	Degeneration of connective tissue close to tendons and joints leading to formation of small cysts
Hypertrophy	Increase in size of muscle as result of enlargement of existing cells	Exercise, increased androgens, increased stimulation or use
Kyphosis (round back)	Anteroposterior or forward bending of spine with convexity of curve in posterior direction, common in thoracic and sacral levels	Poor posture, tuberculosis, chronic arthritis, growth disturbance of vertebral epiphysis, osteoporosis
Lordosis	Deformity of spine resulting in anteroposterior curvature with concavity in posterior direction; common in lumbar spine	Secondary to other deformities of spine, muscular dystrophy, obesity, flexion contraction of hip, congenital dislocation of hip
Pes planus	Flatfoot	Congenital condition, muscle paralysis, mild cerebral palsy, early muscular dystrophy
Scoliosis	Deformity resulting in lateral curvature of spine	Idiopathic and/or congenital condition, fracture or dislocation, osteomalacia, functional condition
Subluxation	Partial dislocation of joint	Instability of joint capsule and supporting ligaments (e.g., from trauma, arthritis)
Valgus	Angulation of bone away from midline	Alteration in gait, pain, abnormal erosion of articular cartilage
Varus	Angulation of bone toward midline	Alteration in gait, pain, abnormal erosion of articular cartilage

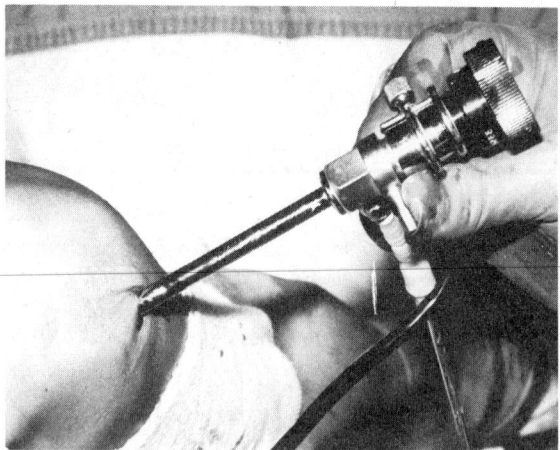

Fig. 56-10   Arthroscopy of a joint.

cartilage structures are not visible on standard x-ray films, special x rays (diskograms, arthrograms) involving the use of contrast media can be used to visualize them. MRI may also be used.

Arthroscopy

Endoscopy of the joints involves the use of an arthroscope for direct visualization of the interior of a joint cavity. It is performed in the operating room under sterile conditions. After local or general anesthesia has been administered, a large-bore needle is inserted into the joint pouch, and the joint is distended with saline solution (Fig. 56-10). The arthroscope is inserted, and the joint cavity is examined. Photographs or videotapes can be made through the scope, and a biopsy of the synovium or cartilage can be obtained. The procedure is particularly useful in the diagnosis of disorders of the knee and shoulder. It can also be used in joints such as the wrist and ankle. Minor tears in cartilage and other repairs can be made through the arthroscope, thus eliminating the need for a more extensive surgical procedure.

Arthrocentesis and Synovial Fluid Analysis

An arthrocentesis procedure is usually performed to obtain synovial fluid for examination. It may also be used to instill medications and remove fluid to relieve pain. After the skin has been cleaned, a local anesthetic is instilled. An 18-gauge or larger needle is inserted into the joint, and fluid is aspirated. The appropriate container must be readily available for laboratory analysis of the aspirated fluid.

The fluid is examined grossly for volume, color, clarity, viscosity, and mucin clot formation. Normal synovial fluid is clear, light yellow, and scanty (1 to 3 ml). Fluid from a septic joint may be purulent and thick or gray and thin. In gout the fluid may be whitish yellow. Blood may be aspirated if there is hemarthrosis. The mucin clot test indicates the character of the protein portion of the synovial fluid. Normally a white, ropelike mucin clot is formed. In an inflammatory process the clot breaks apart easily and fragments.

The fluid is examined microscopically for cell count and identification of the cells. The normal white blood cell (WBC) count is less than 200 cells/ml and no bacteria are found. The WBC count and protein are increased in an inflammatory process. The presence of uric acid crystals may indicate gout.

Muscle Enzymes

Muscle enzymes are released from injured or dead muscle cells. Determinations of muscle enzyme values are used to distinguish between muscle weakness that is due to nerve innervation problems and dystrophic disease of the muscle itself. The level of enzymes reflects the progress of the disorder and the effectiveness of treatment. Serum glutamic-oxaloacetic transaminase (also known as *aspartate aminotransferase*) levels are the least sensitive indicators of muscle disease, and creatine phosphokinase levels are the most sensitive.

Serological Studies

Approximately 85% of people with rheumatoid arthritis have an autoantibody known as *rheumatoid factor* in their serum. This factor is an anti-γ-globulin factor. The test used to determine the presence of this antibody is the latex fixation test. Latex particles are coated with denatured immunoglobulin G. If serum containing rheumatoid factor is mixed with these latex particles, it reacts with the latex particles and causes agglutination.

Other diagnostic studies of the musculoskeletal system are summarized in Table 56-7.

R | ***eview Questions***

The number of the question corresponds to the same-numbered objective at the beginning of the chapter.

1. Which of the following statements best describes the diaphysis?
   a. end of long bone
   b. main shaft of long bone
   c. flared area of long bone
   d. fibrous covering of bone
2. The type of synovial joint permitting the greatest degree of movement is the
   a. hinge joint
   b. pivot joint
   c. ball-and-socket joint
   d. gliding joint
3. The main function of ligaments is to
   a. attach muscles to muscles
   b. attach muscles to bones
   c. attach bones to bones
   d. support underlying muscle tissue
4. Narrowing of joint vertebral spaces in older adults can result in
   a. kyphosis
   b. decreased muscle bulk
   c. decreased endurance
   d. slowed reaction time
5. A musculoskeletal problem that often has a familial predisposition is

Text continued on p. 1662.

Table 56-7

Diagnostic Studies of the Musculoskeletal System

Study	Description and Purpose	Nursing Responsibility
RADIOLOGICAL		
Standard roentgenogram	An x-ray film is done to determine density and texture of bone. Study evaluates structural or functional changes of bones and joints. In anteroposterior view, x-ray beam passes from front to back, allowing one-dimensional view; lateral position provides two-dimensional view.	Avoid excessive exposure of client and self. Before procedure, remove any radiopaque objects that can interfere with results. Explain procedure to client.
Arthrogram	Study involves injection of contrast medium and/or air into joint cavity, which permits visualization of joint structures. Joint movement is followed with series of x-rays.	Assess client for possible allergy to contrast medium. Explain procedure. Prepare area to be injected aseptically. Inject contrast dye into joint structure using sterile technique.
Diskogram	An x-ray film of cervical or lumbar intervertebral disk is done after injection of contrast dye into nucleus pulposus. Study permits visualization of intervertebral disk abnormalities.	Same as for arthrogram.
Laminagram (tomogram)	Multiple x-ray views of body region are focused at successively deeper layers of tissue lying in predetermined planes. Study focuses on certain tissues, eliminating or blurring surrounding structures. Technique is useful in locating bone destruction, small body cavities, foreign bodies, and lesions overshadowed by opaque structures.	Explain procedure to client.
Sinogram	An x-ray film is made after injection of contrast dye into sinus tract (deep draining wound). Study visualizes course of sinus and tissues involved.	Same as for arthrogram.
Computerized tomography (CT) scan	An x-ray beam is used with a computer to provide a three-dimensional picture. It is used to identify soft-tissue abnormalities, bony abnormalities, and various musculoskeletal trauma.	Explain procedure to client. Inform client that procedure is painless. Inform client of importance of remaining still during procedure.
Magnetic resonance imaging (MRI)	Radiowaves and magnetic field are used to view soft tissue. Study is especially useful in the diagnosis of avascular necrosis, disk disease, tumors, osteomyelitis, ligament tears. Client is placed inside scanning chamber.	Explain procedure to client. Inform client that it is painless. Be aware that it is contraindicated in clients with aneurysm clips, metallic implants, pacemakers, electronic devices, hearing aids, shrapnel, and extreme obesity. Ensure that client has no metal on clothing (e.g., snaps, zippers, jewelry, credit cards). Convert IV to heparin lock. Inform client of importance of remaining still throughout examination. Inform clients who are claustrophobic that they may experience symptoms during examination. Administer antianxiety agent (if indicated and ordered).

Table 56-7

 Diagnostic Studies of the Musculoskeletal System—cont'd

Study	Description and Purpose	Nursing Responsibility
BONE MASS MEASUREMENTS		
Radiogrammetry, radiodensitometry	Study evaluates bone mass of metacarpals. A very low dose of radiation is used.	Explain procedure to client. Inform client that procedure is painless.
Single-photon absorptiometry	Low-dose radiation scanner measures mostly peripheral cortical bone at distal radius or midradius. Study is not useful for follow-up because of slow changes in cortical bone.	Same as above.
Dual-photon absorptiometry	Technique measures mixed trabecular and cortical bones at sites such as hip and lumbar spine. It can be used to calculate total body calcium concentration.	Same as above.
Computerized tomography scan	Scan measures almost pure trabecular bone. High radiation dose and higher errors of measurement are disadvantages. It is useful for following up effects of treatment.	Same as above.
RADIOISOTOPE STUDIES		
Bone scan	Technique involves injection of radioisotope (usually sodium pertechnate) that is taken up by bone. Camera scans entire body (front and back), and recording is made on paper. Degree of uptake is related to blood flow to bone. Increased uptake is seen in osteomyelitis, osteoporosis, and primary and metastatic malignant lesions and with certain fractures.	Explain procedure to client. Give calculated dose of radioisotope 2 hr before procedure. Ensure that bladder is emptied before scan. Inform client that procedure requires 1 hr while client lies supine and that no pain or harm will result from isotopes. Be aware that no follow-up scans are required.
ENDOSCOPY		
Arthroscopy	Study involves insertion of arthroscope into joint (usually knee) for visualization of structure and contents. It can be used for exploratory surgery (removal of loose bodies and biopsy) and for diagnosis of abnormalities of meniscus, articular cartilage, ligaments, or joint capsule.	Explain procedure to client. Inform client that procedure is performed in OR with strict asepsis and that either local or general anesthesia is used. After procedure, cover wound with sterile dressing. Wrap leg from midthigh to midcalf with compression dressing for 24 hr. Instruct client to limit activity for a few days.
MINERAL METABOLISM		
Alkaline phosphatase	This enzyme is produced by osteoblasts of bone and is needed for mineralization of organic bone matrix. Elevated levels are found in healing fractures, bone cancers, osteoporosis, osteomalacia, and Paget's disease. *Normal finding* is 5-13 King-Armstrong units, 2-5 Bodansky units, 3-10 Gutman units.	Explain procedure to client. Obtain blood samples by venipuncture. Observe venipuncture site for bleeding or hematoma formation. Inform client that procedure does not require fasting.

Continued.

Table 56-7

Diagnostic Studies of the Musculoskeletal System—cont'd

Study	Description and Purpose	Nursing Responsibility
MINERAL METABOLISM—cont'd		
Calcium	Bone is primary organ for calcium storage. Calcium provides bone with rigid consistency. Decreased level is found in osteomalacia, renal disease, and hypoparathyroidism; increased level is found in hyperparathyroidism, bone tumors, and acute osteoporosis. *Normal finding* is 9-11 mg/dl, 4.5-5.5 mEq/L.	Explain procedure to client. Observe venipuncture site for bleeding or hematoma formation. Inform client that procedure does not require fasting.
Phosphorus	Amount present is directly related to calcium metabolism. Decreased level is found in osteomalacia; increased level is found in chronic renal disease, healing fractures, osteolytic metastatic tumor. *Normal finding* is 2.8-4.5 mg/dl.	Explain procedure to client. Observe venipuncture site for bleeding or hematoma formation. Inform client that procedure does not require fasting.
SEROLOGICAL		
Rheumatoid factor (RF)	Study assesses presence of autoantibody (rheumatoid factor) in serum. Factor is not specific for rheumatoid arthritis and is seen in other connective tissue diseases as well as small percentage of normal population. *Normal finding* is negative or titer <1:20.	Explain procedure to client. Observe venipuncture site for bleeding or hematoma formation. Inform client that procedure does not require fasting.
Erythrocyte sedimentation rate (ESR)	Study is nonspecific index of inflammation. Study measures rapidity with which red blood cells settle out of unclotted blood in 1 hr. Results are influenced by physiological factors as well as diseases. Elevated levels are seen with any inflammatory process (especially rheumatoid arthritis, rheumatic fever, and respiratory infections). *Normal finding* is <20 mm/hr.	Explain procedure to client. Observe venipuncture site for bleeding or hematoma formation. Inform client that procedure does not require fasting.
Lupus erythematosus cells	Lupus erythematosus cells are seen in about 80% of cases of lupus erythematosus. Normally no lupus erythematosus cells are present.	Obtain blood from client and have blood smear made on slide.
Antinuclear antibody (ANA)	Study assesses presence of antibodies capable of destroying nucleus of body's tissue cells. Finding is positive in 95% of clients with lupus erythematosus and may also be positive in individuals with scleroderma or rheumatoid arthritis and in small percentage of normal population.	Explain procedure to client. Observe venipuncture site for bleeding or hematoma formation. Inform client that procedure does not require fasting.
Anti-DNA	Study detects serum antibodies that react with DNA. It is most specific test for systemic lupus erythematosus.	Explain procedure to client. Observe venipuncture site for bleeding or hematoma formation. Inform client that procedure does not require fasting.

*See Chapter 7.

Table 56-7

Diagnostic Studies of the Musculoskeletal System—cont'd

Study	Description and Purpose	Nursing Responsibility
SEROLOGICAL—cont'd		
Complement	Complement, a normal body protein, is essential to both immune and inflammatory reactions.* Complement components used up in these reactions are depleted. Subsequent test applied to serum yields little or no serum complement components. Complement depletions may be found in clients with rheumatoid arthritis or systemic lupus erythematosus.	Explain procedure to client. Observe venipuncture site for bleeding or hematoma formation. Inform client that procedure does not require fasting.
Uric acid	End product of purine metabolism is normally excreted in urine. Although not specific, levels are usually elevated in gout. *Normal findings* are 4.5-6.5 mg/dl (men) and 2.5-5.5 mg/dl (women).	Explain procedure to client. Observe venipuncture site for bleeding or hematoma formation. Inform client that procedure does not require fasting.
MUSCLE ENZYMES		
Creatine phosphokinase (CPK)	Highest concentration is found in skeletal muscle. Increased values are found in progressive muscular dystrophy, polymyositis, and traumatic injuries. *Normal findings* are 5-55 U/L (men) and 5-35 U/L (women).	Explain procedure to client. Observe venipuncture site for bleeding or hematoma formation. Inform client that procedure does not require fasting.
Aldolase	Study is useful in monitoring muscular dystrophy and dermatomyositis. *Normal finding* is 1.0-7.5 U/L.	Explain procedure to client. Observe venipuncture site for bleeding or hematoma formation. Inform client that procedure does not require fasting.
Serum glutamic oxaloacetic transaminase (SGOT) or aspartate aminotransferase (AST)	Enzyme is found in skeletal muscle but is primarily an enzyme of cardiac and hepatic cells. *Normal finding* is 15-45 U/L.	Explain procedure to client. Observe venipuncture site for bleeding or hematoma formation. Inform client that procedure does not require fasting.
INVASIVE PROCEDURES		
Arthrocentesis	Incision or puncture of joint capsule is done to obtain samples of synovial fluid from within joint cavity or to remove excess fluid. Local anesthesia and aseptic preparation is used before needle is inserted into joint and fluid aspirated. Study is useful in diagnosis of joint inflammation.	Explain procedure to client. Inform client that procedure is usually done at bedside or in examination room. Send samples of synovial fluid to laboratory for examination (if indicated). After procedure apply compression dressing and have client rest joint for 8-24 hr. Observe for leakage of blood or fluid on dressing.

Continued.

Table 56-7

Diagnostic Studies of the Musculoskeletal System—cont'd		
Study	**Description and Purpose**	**Nursing Responsibility**
INVASIVE PROCEDURES—cont'd		
Electromyogram	Study evaluates electrical potential associated with skeletal muscle contraction. Long, small-gauge needles are inserted into certain muscles. Needle probes are attached to leads that feed information to electromyogram machine. Recordings of electrical activity of muscle are traced on audiotransmitter as well as on oscilloscope and recording paper. Study is useful in providing information related to lower motor neuron dysfunction and primary muscle diseases.	Inform client that procedure is usually done in electromyogram laboratory while client lies supine on special table. Keep client awake to cooperate with voluntary movement. Inform client that procedure involves some discomfort from needle insertion. Avoid administration of stimulants and sedatives 24 hr before procedure.
MISCELLANEOUS		
Thermography	Technique uses infrared detector, which measures degree of heat radiating from skin surface. Study is useful in investigation of cause of inflamed joints and in following up client's response to antiinflammatory drug therapy.	Inform client that procedure is painless and noninvasive.
Plethysmography	Study records variations in volume and pressure of blood passing through tissues. Test is nonspecific and quantitative.	Inform client that procedure is painless and noninvasive.

    a. osteomalacia
    b. arthritis
    c. osteomyelitis
    d. poliomyelitis
6. Limb length is determined by
    a. measuring circumferentially at the largest muscle mass
    b. having the client bend from the waist
    c. measuring between two bony prominences on a limb
    d. having the shortest distance as the baseline
7. Wasting of a muscle is called
    a. contracture
    b. effusion
    c. atrophy
    d. osteoporosis
8. Serum alkaline phosphatase levels are usually elevated in
    a. severe muscle damage
    b. metabolic disorders of the bone
    c. increased osteoblast activity
    d. general body response to trauma

REFERENCES

1. Thibodeau GA: Anatomy and physiology, St Louis, 1987, Times Mirror/Mosby College Publishing, p 141.
2. Berne RM and Levy MN: Physiology, St Louis, 1988, The CV Mosby Co, p 315.
3. Spence AP: Basic human anatomy, Menlo Park, Calif., 1986, Benjamin/Cummings Publishing, p 184.
4. Esberger KK and Hughes ST, eds: Nursing care of the aged, Norwalk, Conn, 1989, Appleton & Lange, p 153.

CHAPTER

57

Nursing Role in Management
Musculoskeletal Problems

Susan C. Ruda

L *earning Objectives*

1. *Explain the pathophysiology, clinical manifestations, and management of soft-tissue injuries, including strains, sprains, dislocations, subluxations, bursitis, carpal tunnel syndrome, and muscle spasms.*
2. *Describe the sequential events involved in fracture healing.*
3. *Describe common complications associated with fracture injury and fracture healing.*
4. *Differentiate among open reduction, closed reduction, traction, and plaster immobilization regarding purpose, complications, and nursing management.*
5. *Explain the neurovascular assessment of an injured extremity.*
6. *Describe the therapeutic and nursing management of clients with specific fractures.*
7. *Describe the pathophysiological basis for and the management of osteomyelitis.*
8. *Describe the indications and therapeutic and nursing management for an amputation.*
9. *Describe the pathophysiology, clinical manifestations, and treatment of neoplasms of the bone.*
10. *Describe the causes and characteristics of acute and chronic low back pain.*
11. *Describe the conservative and surgical treatments of low back pain.*
12. *Describe the postoperative nursing management of a client who has undergone spinal surgery.*
13. *Explain the causes and management of common foot disorders.*
14. *Describe the pathophysiology, clinical manifestations, and management of metabolic bone diseases.*

The most common cause of musculoskeletal problems is injury from accidents resulting in fracture, dislocations, and associated soft-tissue injuries. Although most of these injuries are not fatal, the cost in terms of pain, disability, medical expense, and lost wages is enormous. For all ages, accidents are exceeded only by diseases of the heart, malignant neoplasms, and strokes as the cause of death. Accidents are the leading cause of death in children and young adults.

The nurse has an important role in educating the public in the basic principles of safety and accident prevention. The morbidity associated with accidents can be significantly reduced if people are aware of environmental hazards, use existing safety equipment, and apply safety and traffic rules. In the industrial setting the nurse should stress

the use of appropriate safety equipment and avoidance of hazardous working situations.

In the home environment, falls account for many musculoskeletal injuries. Preventive education should be directed toward the importance of wearing of shoes with functional soles and heels, avoidance of wet or slippery surfaces, careful placement of throw rugs, and removal of obstacles from the pathway of high-risk individuals such as persons with gait instability or visual or cognitive impairment.

SOFT-TISSUE INJURIES

Soft-tissue injuries include sprains, strains, dislocations, and subluxations. These common injuries are usually caused by trauma. The increase in the number of people who maintain a regular fitness program or participate in sports is believed to contribute to the increased incidence of soft-tissue injuries and inflammatory responses of the musculoskeletal system.[1]

Reviewed by Peggy M. Mayfield, M.S.N., R.N.C., Adult Nurse Practitioner, Associate Professor Emeritus, Harris College of Nursing, Texas Christian University, Fort Worth, Texas.

1663

Sprains and Strains

Sprains and strains are the two most common types of injury affecting the musculoskeletal system. These injuries are usually associated with abnormal stretching forces that may occur during vigorous activities.

A *sprain* is classified according to the number of ligament fibers torn. It is also classified according to the severity of the tear as first degree (minor tears), second degree, or third degree (almost complete). This injury affects the joint capsule and synovial membrane as well as the ligaments. Because these areas are rich in nerve endings, the injury can be quite painful. A *strain* is a stretching of a muscle and its fascial sheath.

Minor sprains and strains are usually self-limiting, and full function usually returns within 3 to 6 weeks. A severe sprain can result in an avulsion fracture, in which the ligament pulls loose a fragment of bone. Alternatively, the joint structure may become unstable and result in dislocation. At the time of injury, hemarthrosis (bleeding into a joint space or cavity) or disruption of the synovial lining may occur. An acute strain may involve rupture of a muscle.

X-ray films of the affected part are usually taken to rule out fracture or widening of the joint structure. Surgical repair may be necessary if the injury is significant enough to produce severe disruption of ligamentous or muscle structures, fracture, or dislocation.

■ Nursing Management of Sprains and Strains

Nursing assessment

The clinical manifestations of sprains and strains are similar and include pain, edema, decrease in function, and bruising. Pain aggravated by continued use is common. Edema develops in the injured area because of minute hemorrhages within the disrupted tissues and the ensuing inflammatory response. The client usually recounts a history of traumatic injury or recent exercise activity.

Nursing diagnoses

Nursing diagnoses specific to the client with a sprain or strain include, but are not limited to, the following:
1. Pain related to edema, muscle spasm, ineffective pain relief and/or comfort measures
2. Impaired physical mobility related to pain, activity restriction, or an immobilization device

Nursing interventions

The use of elastic support bandages or adhesive tape wrapping before beginning a vigorous activity is believed to reduce the occurrence of sprains. However, some physicians do not support preventive wrapping or taping. Stretching and warming-up exercises before vigorous activity also help prevent strains. Preconditioning exercise protects an inherently weak joint, since slow stretching is tolerated better by biological tissues than is quick stretching. Warm-up exercises "prelengthen" potentially strained tissues by avoiding the quick stretch often encountered in sports. Warm-up exercises also increase the temperature of muscle, which increases the speed of cell metabolism and the speed of nerve impulse transmission. The increased metabolism contributes to better oxygenation of muscle fiber during work. Stretching is also believed to improve ki-

Table 57-1

Prehospital Emergency Care of the Client with an Acute Soft-Tissue Injury*

Possible etiologies: Falls, direct blows, forced flexion or hyperextension, twisting forces

CLINICAL MANIFESTATIONS

Swelling
Ecchymosis
Tenderness
Pain
Loss of use or inability to bear weight (if lower extremity involved)
Muscle spasms
Abnormal extremity length (dislocation)

MANAGEMENT

Assess neurological and circulatory status of involved limb.
Elevate involved limb.
Apply compression bandage.
Apply cold pack or compress to affected area.
Immobilize affected extremity.
Do not allow weight-bearing of the involved limb (if lower extremity involved).

*See Chapter 59 for a general discussion on measures related to prehospital emergency care.

nesthetic awareness, thus lessening the chance of uncoordinated movement.

If an injury occurs, the immediate care focuses on (1) limitation of movement and use, (2) elevation of the affected extremity, and (3) protection of the extremity (Table 57-1). Cold in several forms can be used to produce hypothermia to the involved part. Physiological changes that occur in soft tissue as a result of the use of cold include vasoconstriction, reduction in transmission of nerve impulses, and reduction in conduction velocity.[2] These changes result in analgesia and anesthesia, reduction of muscle spasm without changes in muscular strength or endurance, reduction of local edema and inflammation, and reduction of local metabolic requirements. Few unwanted side effects accompany the use of cold to treat a soft-tissue injury. Cold is most useful when applied immediately after the injury has occurred. Mild analgesia may be necessary to manage client discomfort.

After the acute phase (which usually lasts 24 to 48 hours), warm, moist heat can be applied to the affected part to reduce swelling and provide comfort. The client is encouraged to use the limb provided that the joint is protected from assuming the position of injury by means such as casting, taping, and splinting. Movement of the joint surfaces maintains cartilage nutrition, and muscle contraction speeds circulation and phagocytosis of the hematoma.

Dislocation and Subluxation

A *dislocation* is a severe injury of the ligamentous structures that surround a joint. It results in the complete

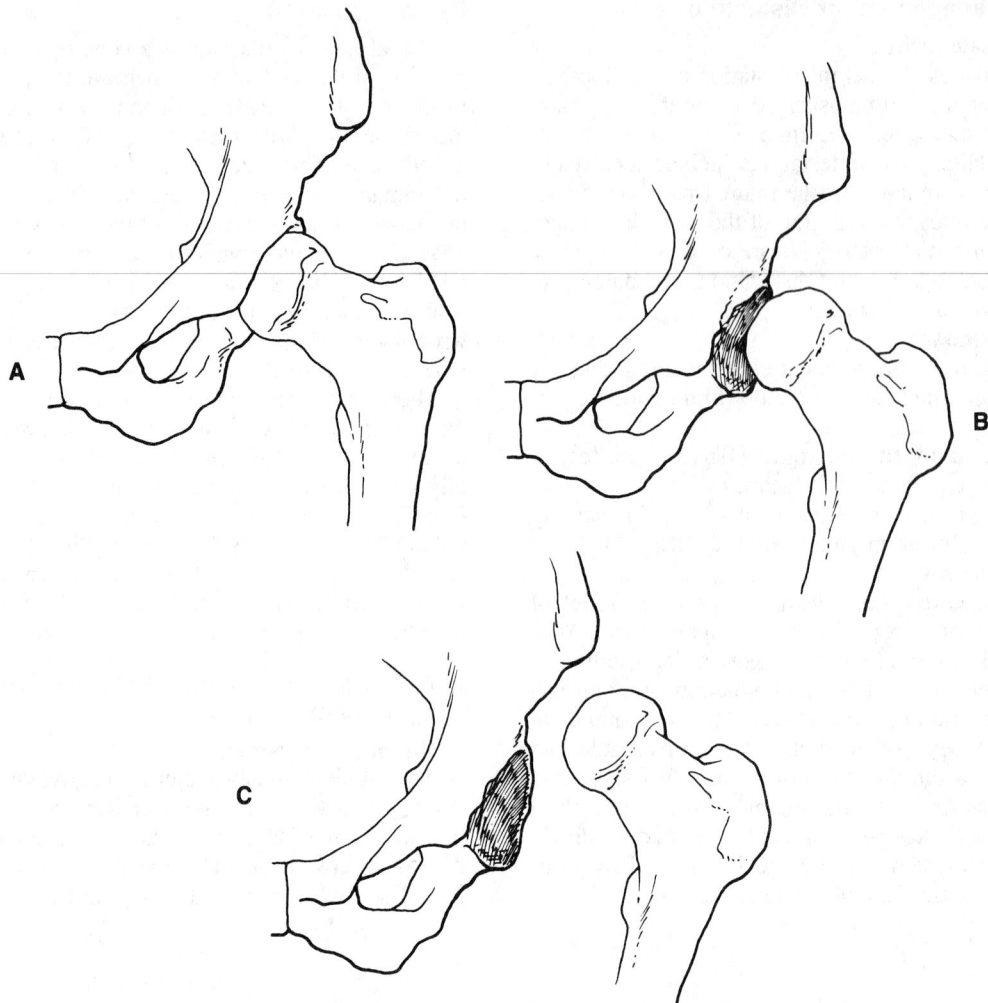

Fig. 57-1 Soft-tissue injury of the hip. **A,** Normal. **B,** Subluxation. **C,** Dislocation. (From Price S and Wilson L: Pathophysiology: clinical concepts of disease processes, ed 4, St Louis, 1992, Mosby–Year Book, Inc.)

displacement or separation of the articular surfaces of the joint. A *subluxation* is a partial or incomplete displacement of the joint surface. The clinical manifestations of a subluxation are similar to those of a dislocation but are less severe. Treatment of subluxation is similar to that of a dislocation but subluxation requires less healing time.

Dislocations characteristically result from overwhelming forces transmitted to the joint that cause a disruption of the soft tissues of the joint. The joints most frequently dislocated in the upper extremity include the thumb, elbow, and shoulder. In the lower extremity, the hip is vulnerable to dislocation occurring as a result of severe trauma, often associated with motor vehicle accidents (Fig. 57-1).

Radiological studies are performed to determine the extent of shifting of the involved structures. The joint may also be aspirated to determine the presence of fat cells. If fat cells from the exposed marrow are found in the synovial fluid, an intraarticular fracture is present.

A dislocation requires prompt intervention. The longer the joint remains unreduced, the greater is the possibility of avascular necrosis (bone cell death as a result of inadequate blood supply). The hip joint is particularly susceptible to avascular necrosis. The first goal of therapeutic management is to realign the dislocated portion of the joint in its original anatomical position. This can be accomplished by a closed reduction, which may be performed under either local or general anesthesia. Anesthesia is often necessary to produce muscle relaxation so that the bones can be manipulated. In some situations, open reduction may be necessary. After reduction the extremity is usually immobilized by taping or use of a sling to allow the torn ligaments and capsular tissue time to heal. Observation is indicated for the client with a posterior sternoclavicular dislocation because delayed intrathoracic complications, such as pneumothorax or subclavian vessel injury, may occur.[3]

■ Nursing Management of Dislocations

Nursing assessment

The most obvious clinical manifestation of a dislocation is asymmetry of the musculoskeletal contour. For example, if a hip is dislocated, the limb is shorter on the affected side. Additional manifestations include local pain, tenderness, loss of function of the injured part, and swelling of the soft tissues in the region of the joint. The major complications of a dislocated joint are open joint injuries, intraarticular fractures, fracture dislocation, and damage to adjacent neurovascular tissue.

Nursing diagnoses

Nursing diagnoses for the client experiencing a dislocation or subluxation include, but are not limited to, the following:

1. Pain related to edema, muscle spasm, ineffective pain relief and/or comfort measures
2. Impaired physical mobility related to pain, activity restrictions, or an immobilization device

Nursing interventions

Nursing care is directed toward symptomatic relief of pain and support and protection of the injured joint. After the joint has been immobilized, motion is usually restricted. A carefully regulated rehabilitation program can prevent the formation of contractures. The client must not stretch the joint beyond its limits. The torn capsule and ligament heal in a shortened position with fibrous scar tissue that is not as strong as the original tissue. Therefore a carefully regulated exercise program is required to slowly and methodically restore the joint to its original range of motion without causing another dislocation.

Carpal Tunnel Syndrome

Carpal tunnel syndrome is a condition caused by compression of the median nerve beneath the transverse carpal ligament within the narrow confines of the carpal tunnel located at the wrist (Fig. 57-2). This condition is frequently due to pressure from trauma or edema caused by inflammation of a tendon (tenosynovitis), neoplasm, rheumatoid synovial disease, or soft-tissue masses such as ganglia. Carpal tunnel syndrome occurs most frequently in middle-aged or postmenopausal women and in persons who are employed in occupations that require continuous wrist movement (e.g., butchers, computer operators, secretaries, carpenters).

Therapeutic management is directed toward relieving the underlying cause of the nerve compression. The early symptoms associated with carpal tunnel syndrome can usually be relieved by placing the hand and wrist at rest by immobilizing them in a hand splint. If the cause is inflammation, injection of hydrocortisone directly into the carpal tunnel may provide relief. If the problem continues, the median nerve may have to be surgically decompressed by longitudinal division of the transverse carpal ligament.

■ Nursing Management of Carpal Tunnel Syndrome

Nursing assessment

The clinical manifestations are weakness, pain and numbness of the hand, impaired sensation in the distribution of the median nerve, and clumsiness in performing fine hand movements. Holding the wrist in acute flexion for 60 seconds produces tingling and numbness over the

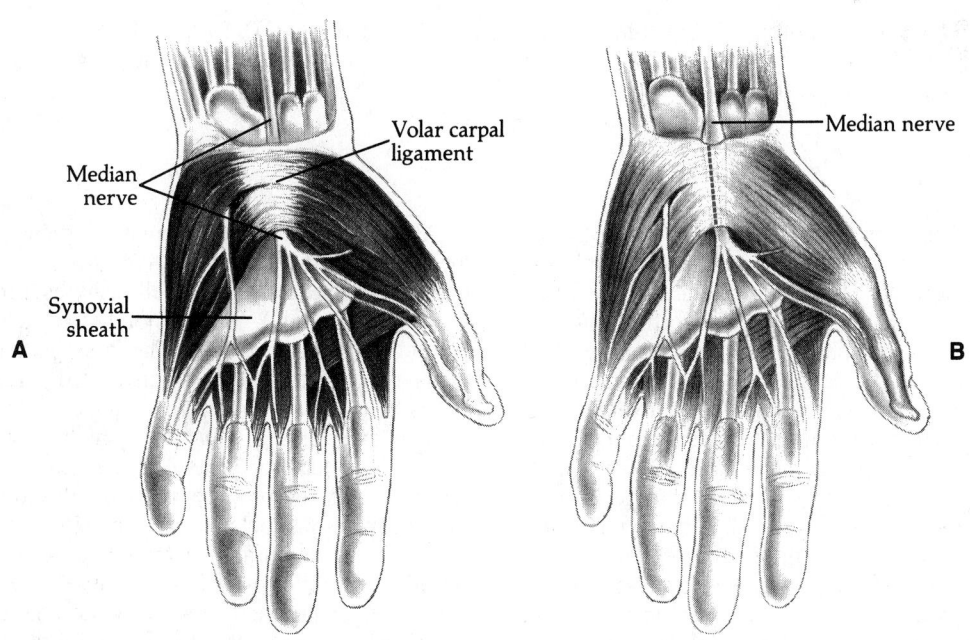

Fig. 57-2 **A,** Wrist structures involved in carpal syndrome. **B,** Decompression of median nerve. (From Thompson JC and others: Mosby's manual of clinical nursing, ed 2, St Louis, 1989, The CV Mosby Co, p 435.)

distribution of the median nerve, the palmar surface of the thumb, the index finger, the middle finger, and part of the ring finger. This is a positive Phalen's sign. In late stages, atrophy of the thenar muscles occurs. This syndrome can result in recurrent pain and eventual dysfunction of the hand.

Nursing diagnoses

Nursing diagnoses of the client with carpal tunnel syndrome include, but are not limited to, the following:

1. Pain related to ineffective pain relief and/or comfort measures or nerve compression
2. Impaired physical mobility related to pain, weakness
3. High risk for injury related to impaired sensation and clumsiness of the involved hand

Nursing interventions

Nursing care of the client with carpal tunnel syndrome usually occurs in the office or outpatient setting. Comfort should be maintained by use of medication to relieve pain and splints to protect the area. The client may be required to consider occupational changes because of discomfort and sensory and functional changes. If surgery is performed, the neurovascular status of the hand should be evaluated regularly. The client should be instructed in the appropriate assessments to perform at home, since the surgery is done on an outpatient basis.

Meniscus Injury

Meniscus injuries are closely associated with ligament sprains and commonly occur in young athletes engaged in sports such as basketball, rugby, football, soccer, and hockey. These activities produce a rotational stress when the knee is in a flexed position and the foot is fixed. A blow to the knee can cause the meniscus to be trapped between the femoral condyles and the plateau of the tibia, resulting in a torn meniscus (Fig. 57-3). There is a causal relationship between occupations that require working in a squatting or kneeling position and meniscus injuries.

An arthrogram, arthroscopy, or both can diagnose knee problems. Magnetic resonance imaging (MRI) is beneficial in confirming the diagnosis before arthroscopy is used. It has eliminated the use of an arthrogram as a diagnostic tool in many cases. In addition to precision diagnosis, arthroscopy can be performed to surgically remove damaged intraarticular structures or to repair structures such as the meniscus or cruciate ligament through miniature incisions.[4,5]

Initial treatment includes exercises aimed at strengthening the stability of the knee, such as straight-leg raising. The knee may also be unlocked by manipulation, followed by use of a removable splint. If conservative treatment is not effective in relieving symptoms, surgical excision of the meniscus (meniscectomy) may be necessary.

■ Nursing Management of Meniscus Injury

Nursing assessment

Meniscus injuries alone do not usually cause chronic edema because cartilage is avascular and aneural. However, a torn meniscus may be suspected when local tenderness or pain is reported. Pain is elicited by abduction or adduction of the leg at the knee. The usual clinical feature is a feeling by the client that the knee is unstable and may click and lock periodically. Quadriceps atrophy is evident if the injury has been present for some time. Degenerative joint disease can occur if a damaged, roughened meniscus is not surgically removed.

Nursing diagnoses

Nursing diagnoses of the client with a meniscus injury include, but are not limited to, the following:

1. Pain related to ineffective pain relief and/or comfort measures and failure to seek treatment
2. Impaired physical mobility related to pain and knee instability

Nursing interventions

Examination of the acutely injured knee should occur within 24 hours of injury. Initial care of this type of injury involves application of ice, immobilization, and protected weight-bearing.[6]

Bursitis

Bursae are closed sacs that are lined with synovial membrane and contain a small amount of synovial fluid. They are located beneath the skin at sites of friction, as between tendons, bones, and overlying joints. A bursa may

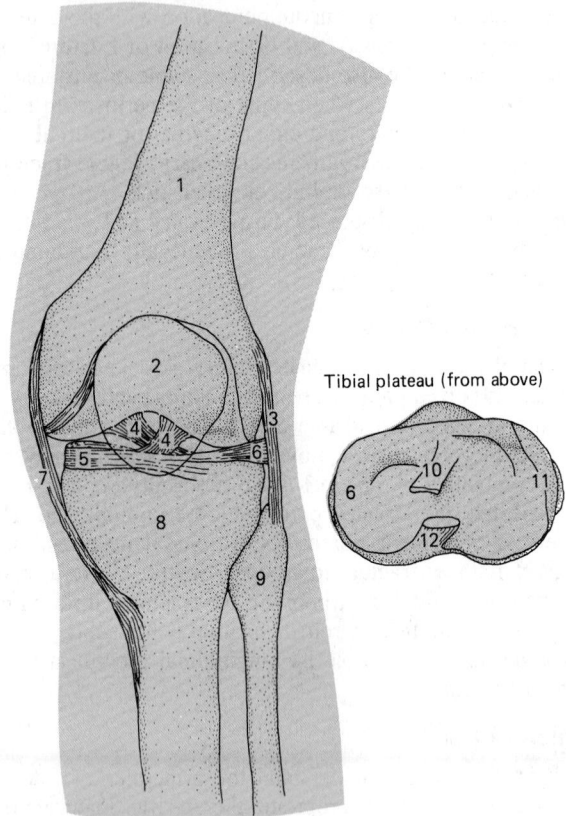

Fig. 57-3 Front view of injured knee with torn medial meniscus. *1*, Femur; *2*, patella; *3*, lateral collateral ligament; *4*, cruciate ligaments; *5*, medial meniscus; *6*, lateral meniscus; *7*, ruptured medial collateral ligament; *8*, tibia; *9*, fibula; *10*, anterior cruciate ligament; *11*, torn medial meniscus; *12*, posterior cruciate ligament. (Courtesy Eli Lilly, Indianapolis.)

Tibial plateau (from above)

become inflamed (bursitis) from repeated or excessive trauma or with friction, gout, rheumatoid arthritis, or infection. The primary clinical manifestations of bursitis are pain and swelling as a result of edema in the affected part. Sites at which bursitis commonly occurs include the hand, knee, trochanters, shoulder, and elbow.

Attempts are made to determine and correct the cause of the bursitis. Rest is often the only treatment needed. The affected part may be immobilized in a compression dressing or plaster splint. Aspiration of the bursal fluid and injection of hydrocortisone may be necessary. If the bursa wall has become thickened and continues to interfere with normal joint function, surgical excision (bursectomy) may be necessary. For example, subacromial bursal thickening causes pain and loss of range of motion on abduction of the shoulder. Septic bursae usually require surgical drainage.

Muscle Spasms

Local muscle spasms are a common condition often associated with overdoing everyday activities. Injury to a muscle stimulates free nerve endings, resulting in muscle excitation and spasms. The spasms produce additional pain, and a repetitive cycle is established. The clinical manifestations of muscle spasms of local origin include local pain, palpable muscle mass in spasm, tenderness, diminished range of motion of the affected site, and limitation of daily activities.

A careful history should be taken, and a physical examination should be performed to rule out central nervous system (CNS) problems. Muscle spasms can be managed with drug therapy, physical therapy, or both. A physical therapy program may include use of heat, supervised exercise, massage, hydrotherapy, local heat-producing applications, ultrasound (deep heat), manipulation, and bracing. Drugs used for treatment of local muscle spasms include analgesics, tranquilizers, and muscle relaxants.

■ Nursing Management of Acute Soft-Tissue Injuries

The major nursing responsibility for acute soft-tissue injury involves client education related to care of the injured part. This teaching often takes place in an outpatient setting, which is where most soft-tissue injuries are diagnosed and treated. The client should be instructed to reduce swelling by applying ice, which causes vasoconstriction. Initially, ice should be applied intermittently for the first 24 hours. Ice applications should not exceed 20 to 30 minutes per application, allowing a "warm-down" time of 10 to 15 minutes between applications. Leaving ice on the skin too long causes reflex vasodilation. Cold application to muscle in spasm for more than 1 hour also increases the spasm. The ice applications should be cold enough to produce reddening of the skin (hyperemia) followed by blanching and sensory anesthesia. Both ice and commercial cold packs can be made colder by wrapping them in a wet towel. Most clients can be taught to do this themselves.

After the swelling has stabilized, warm, moist heat can be applied several times daily to provide comfort and aid

in regaining joint mobility. Heat applications should also not exceed 20 to 30 minutes, allowing a "cool-down" time between applications. Heat can be applied in the form of a wrap or soak, depending on the area affected. The temperature of the water should not exceed 37.8° C (100° F). Prolonged heat application slows circulation rather than enhances it. Heat should be avoided during the first 24 to 48 hours, since the resulting vasodilatation increases edema and also increases any active hemorrhaging.

Use of an elastic bandage provides support and limits edema. The client should be carefully instructed on the application of an elastic bandage to prevent circulatory impairment. Pain relief can usually be obtained with the use of mild analgesic agents such as aspirin, ibuprofen, and acetaminophen. Rest for the injured part also aids in prompt recovery (see Table 57-1).

FRACTURES
Classification and Etiology

A fracture is a disruption or break in the continuity of the structure of bone. Traumatic injuries account for the majority of fractures, although some fractures are caused by a disease process (pathological fractures). Fractures are described and classified according to (1) type (Fig. 57-4), (2) communication or noncommunication with the external environment (Fig. 57-5), and (3) location of fracture (Fig. 57-6). Fractures are also described as stable or unstable. A *stable fracture* occurs when some of the periosteum is intact across the fracture and either external or internal fixation has rendered the fragments stationary. Stable fractures are usually transverse, spiral, or greenstick. An *unstable fracture* is grossly displaced during injury and is a site of poor fixation. Unstable fractures are usually comminuted or oblique.

Clinical Manifestations

The client's history indicates injury associated with immediate localized pain, decreased function, and inability to use the affected part (Table 57-2). The client guards and protects the part against movement. The fracture may not be accompanied by obvious bone deformity. If a fracture is suspected, the affected part should be immobilized. Unnecessary movement increases soft-tissue damage and may convert a closed fracture to an open fracture. Careful management is particularly important for fractures through the epiphyseal plate in children. If fixation is not solid, the entire long bone may cease its longitudinal growth at all or part of the plate.

Fracture Healing

It is important to understand the principles of fracture healing to provide appropriate therapeutic interventions (Fig. 57-7). The reparative process of bone healing (called *union*) occurs in the following stages:

1. *Fracture hematoma:* When a fracture occurs, bleeding and edema precede the development of a hematoma, which surrounds the ends of the fragments. The hematoma is extravasated blood that changes from a liquid to a semisolid clot.
2. *Granulation tissue:* During this stage, active phago-

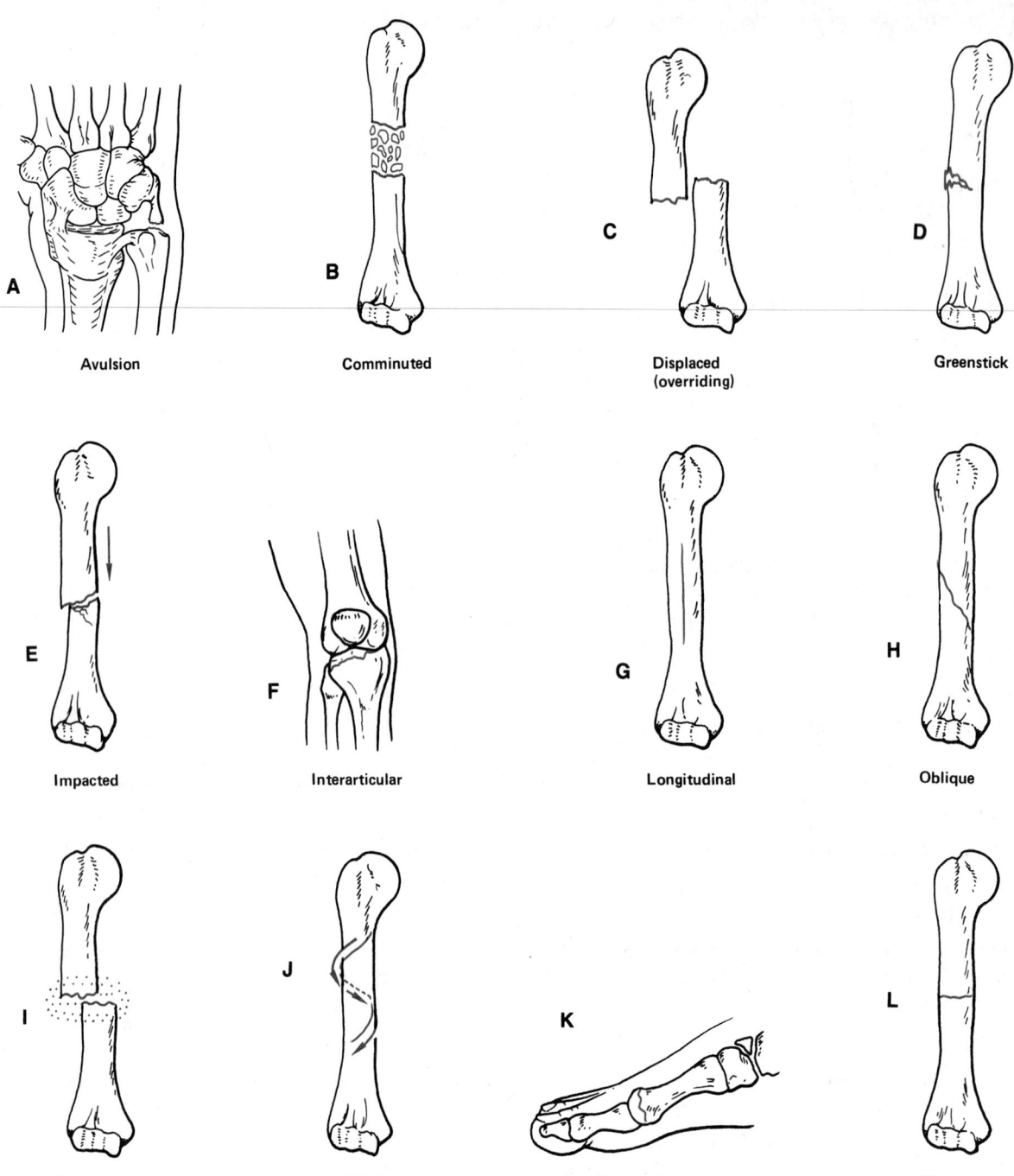

Fig. 57-4 Types of fractures. **A,** An avulsion is a fracture of bone resulting from the strong pulling effect of tendons or ligaments at the bone attachment. **B,** A comminuted fracture is a fracture with more than two fragments. The smaller fragments appear to be floating. **C,** A displaced (overriding) fracture involves a displaced fracture fragment that is overriding the other bone fragment. The periosteum is disrupted on both sides. **D,** A greenstick fracture is an incomplete fracture with one side splintered and the other side bent. The periosteum is not torn away from the bone. **E,** An impacted fracture is a comminuted fracture in which more than two fragments are driven into each other. **F,** An interarticular fracture is a fracture extending to the articular surface of the bone. **G,** A longitudinal fracture is an incomplete fracture in which the fracture line runs along the axis of the bone. The periosteum is not torn away from the bone. **H,** An oblique fracture is a fracture in which the line of the fracture extends in an oblique direction. **I,** A pathological fracture is a spontaneous fracture at the site of a bone disease. **J,** A spiral fracture is a fracture in which the line of the fracture extends in a spiral direction along the shaft of the bone. **K,** A stress fracture is a fracture occurring at the site of a muscle attachment. It is caused by a sudden, violent force or repeated, prolonged stress. **L,** A transverse fracture is a fracture in which the line of the fracture extends across the bone shaft at a right angle to the longitudinal axis.

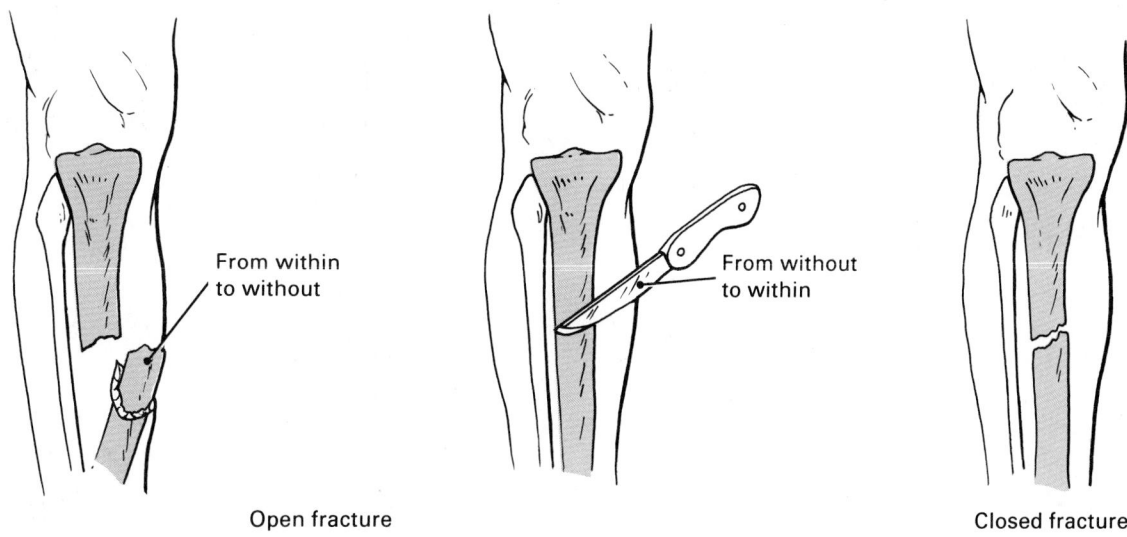

Fig. 57-5 Fracture classification according to communication.

Table 57-2 Clinical Manifestations of Fracture

Cause	Significance
EDEMA AND SWELLING	
Disruption of soft tissues or bleeding into surrounding tissues	Unchecked swelling in close space can occlude circulation and damage nerves.
PAIN AND TENDERNESS	
Muscle spasm as result of involuntary reflex action of muscle, direct tissue trauma, increased pressure on sensory nerve, movement of fracture parts	Pain and tenderness encourage splinting of fracture with reduction in motion of injured area.
MUSCLE SPASM	
Protective response to injury and fracture	Muscle spasms may displace nondisplaced fracture or prevent it from reducing spontaneously.
DEFORMITY	
Abnormal position of bone as result of original forces of injury and action of muscles pulling fragment into abnormal position	Deformity is cardinal sign of fracture; if uncorrected, it may result in problems with bony union and restoration of function of injured part.
ECCHYMOSIS	
Discoloration of skin as result of extravasation of blood in subcutaneous tissues	Ecchymosis usually appears several days after injury and may appear distal to injury. The nurse should reassure client that process is normal.
LOSS OF FUNCTION	
Disruption of bone, preventing functional use	Fracture must be managed properly to ensure restoration of function.
CREPITATION	
Grating or crunching together of bony fragments, producing palpable or audible crunching sensation	Examination for crepitation may increase chance for nonunion if bone ends are allowed to move excessively.

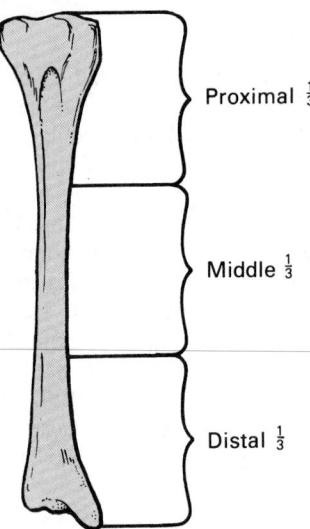

Fig. 57-6   Fracture classification according to location.

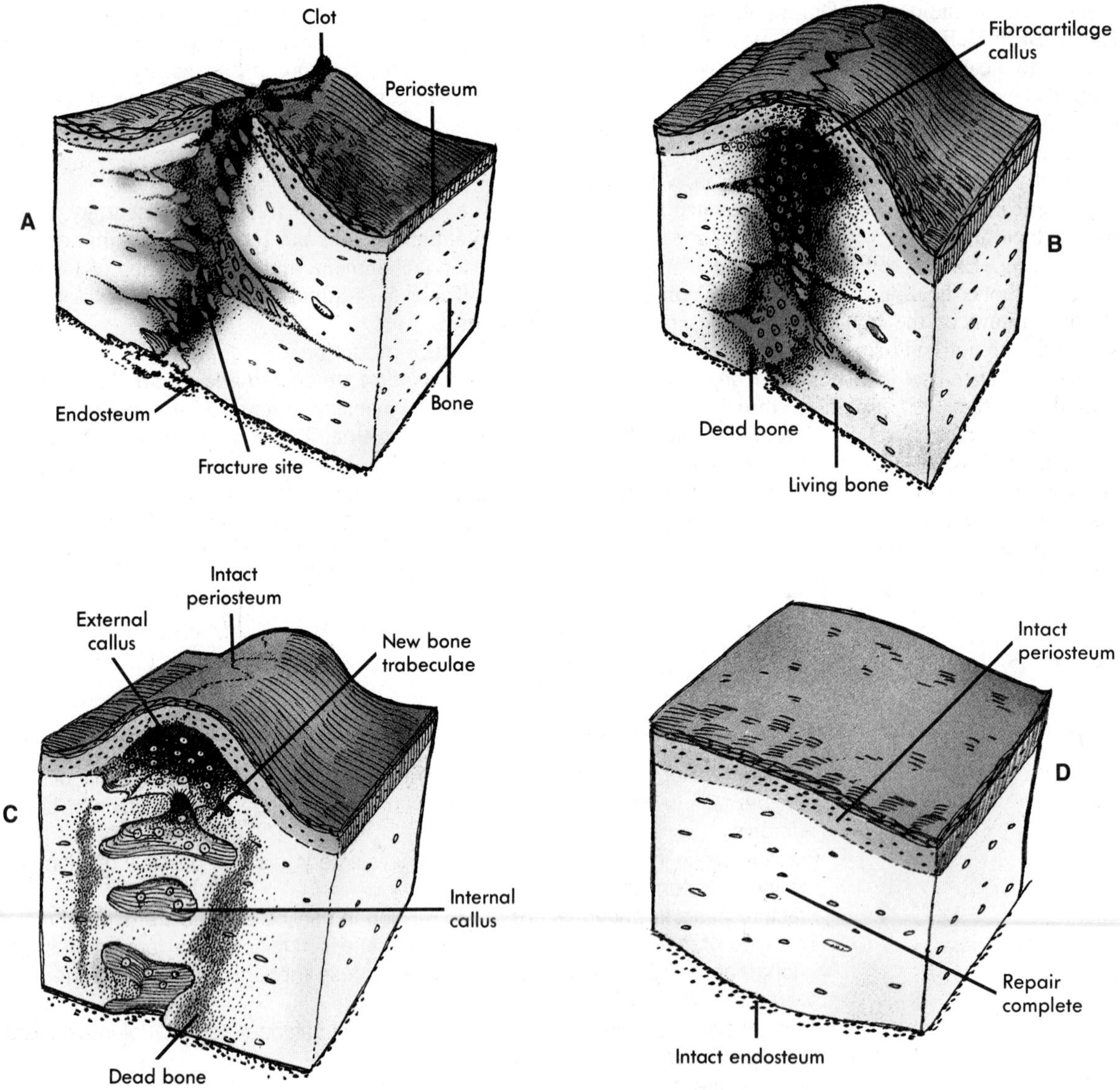

Proximal ⅓

Middle ⅓

Distal ⅓

Fig. 57-7   Healing process of a fracture. **A,** Bone fracture with blood clot formation. **B,** Fibrocartilage callus forms between bone fragments, closing the wound and attaching the fragments. **C,** Cancellous bone replaces the fibrocartilage callus. **D,** Bone is remodeled and the cancellous bone is replaced by compact bone. Healing is complete. (From Seeley RR, Stephens TD, and Tate P: Anatomy and Physiology, St Louis, 1989, Times Mirror/Mosby College Publishing, p 150.)

cytosis absorbs the products of local necrosis. The hematoma changes into new tissue known as *granulation tissue*. Granulation tissue (consisting of young blood vessels, fibroblasts, and osteoblasts) produces a new bone substance called *osteoid*.

3. *Callus formation:* As minerals are deposited in the osteoid, it forms an unorganized network of bone that is woven about the fracture parts. Callus is primarily composed of cartilage, osteoblasts, calcium, and phosphorus. It usually begins to appear by the end of the first week after injury. Evidence of callus formation can be verified by x-ray studies.

4. *Ossification:* Ossification of the callus begins within 2 to 3 weeks after the fracture and continues until the fracture has healed. This stage is marked by ossification of the callus that is sufficient enough to prevent movement at the fracture site when the bones are gently stressed. However, the fracture is still evident on radiograph. During this stage of clinical union the client can be converted from skeletal traction to a cast or the cast can be removed to allow mobility.

5. *Consolidation:* As callus continues to develop, the distance between bone fragments diminishes and eventually closes. This stage is called *consolidation*, and ossification continues. It can be equated with radiographical union.

6. *Remodeling:* Excess cells are absorbed in the final stage of bone healing, and union is completed. Gradual return of the injured bone to its preinjury structural strength and shape occurs. Remodeling of bone is enhanced as it responds to physical stress. Initially, stress is provided through exercise. Weight-bearing is gradually introduced. New bone is deposited in sites subjected to stress and resorbed at areas in which there is little stress. Radiographical union occurs when there is radiographical evidence of complete bony union.

Many factors such as age, initial displacement of the fracture, site of the fracture, and blood supply to the area influence the time required for healing to be complete. Healing may be disrupted or delayed if blood supply is not adequate, if immobilization is poor, if infection develops, or if traction is excessive. Healing time for fractures increases with age. For example, an uncomplicated midshaft fracture of the femur heals in 3 weeks in a newborn and requires 20 weeks to heal in an adult. Table 57-3 summarizes skeletal complications of fracture healing.

Fracture healing may not occur in the expected time *(delayed union)* or may not occur at all *(nonunion)*. The ossification process is arrested by causes such as inadequate immobilization and reduction, excess movement, infection, and poor nutrition.

Electrical stimulation is used successfully to stimulate bone healing. The electric current acts by modifying cell behavior so that fibrocartilage in the nonunion fracture gap is calcified, vascularized, and replaced by bone.[7] The electrodes are semiinvasive, noninvasive, or surgically implanted. Client motivation and ability must be high because the treatment takes up to 10 hours a day for 3 to 6 months.[8]

Therapeutic Management

The overall goals of fracture treatment are (1) anatomical realignment of bone fragments, (2) immobilization to maintain realignment, and (3) restoration of function of the part. Table 57-4 summarizes therapeutic management of fractures.

Fracture reduction

Manipulation or closed reduction. Manipulation is a nonsurgical, manual realignment of bones to their previous anatomical position. Traction and countertraction are manually applied to the bone fragments to restore position, length, and alignment. Closed reduction is usually performed under local or general anesthesia. After reduction or manipulation the injured part is immobilized by

Table 57-3 Complications of Fracture Healing

Problem	Description
Delayed union	Fracture healing progresses more slowly than expected; healing eventually occurs.
Nonunion	Fracture fails to heal properly despite treatment, resulting in fibrous union or pseudoarthrosis.
Malunion	Fracture heals in expected time but in unsatisfactory position, possibly resulting in deformity or dysfunction.
Angulation	Fracture heals in abnormal position in relation to midline of structure (type of malunion).
Pseudoarthrosis	This type of malunion occurs at fracture site in which false joint is formed on shaft of long bones. It is a fracture site that failed to fuse (neoarthrosis). Each bone end is covered with fibrous scar tissue.
Posttraumatic osteoporosis	This condition represents loss of mineral (bone substance) as result of immobilization and/or disuse.
Refracture	New fracture occurs through original fracture site.
Myositis ossificans	This condition is a response to muscle hemorrhage caused by trauma. The hematoma ossifies. Response may occur in arm, elbow, and thigh.

casting or traction to maintain alignment until healing occurs.

Open reduction. Open reduction is the correction of bone alignment through a surgical incision. It may include internal fixation of the fracture with the use of rods, wire, screws, pins, intramedullary rods, or nails. The type and location of the fracture, as well as the result of attempted closed reduction by means of traction, influence the decision to use open reduction. The chief disadvantages of this form of treatment are the possibility of infection and the complications associated with general anesthesia.

If open reduction and internal fixation is used, early initiation of range of motion of the joint is indicated. Machines that provide continuous passive motion to various joints are now available. Use of such machines can result in prevention of intraarticular adhesions, faster reconstruction of the subchondral bone plate, and possibly better healing of the articular cartilage. Ultimately, the development of posttraumatic degenerative arthritis may be reduced.

Traction. Traction devices apply a pulling force on the fractured extremity and result in realignment. The force can be applied through adhesive applied directly to the skin (*skin traction*) or through a metal pin or wire inserted directly into or through a bone (*skeletal traction*). Traction has several therapeutic purposes: (1) to reduce, align, and immobilize fractures until bony union occurs; (2) to lessen, prevent, or correct deformity associated with bone injury and muscle disease; and (3) to reduce muscle spasms in fracture of a long bone or back injury.

When traction is used to treat fractures, the forces are usually exerted on the distal fragment to obtain alignment with the proximal fragment. Several types of traction are used for this purpose (Table 57-5). Fracture alignment depends on the correct positioning and alignment of the client while the traction forces remain constant. For extremity traction to be effective, forces must be pulling in the opposite direction (*countertraction*) to prevent the client from sliding to the end of the bed. Countertraction may be achieved by elevating the end of the bed 8 to 12 inches and by using the weight of the client's own body.

Fracture immobilization

External fixation. External fixation of fractures is achieved by means of a cast or an external fixator. Casting is a common treatment after closed reduction has been performed. It allows the client to perform many normal activities of daily living while providing sufficient immobilization to ensure stability. Major cast materials include fiberglass, plaster of Paris, polyurethane, thermoplastic resins, and thermolabile plastic.

Plaster of Paris continues to be the material most widely used for casting. It consists of anhydrous calcium sulfate embedded in gauze. After immersion in water, it is wrapped and molded around the affected part (Fig. 57-8). The strength of the cast is determined by the number of layers of plaster bandage and the technique of application. As the cast dries, it recrystallizes and hardens. Heat is generated during the drying process. Increased edema as a result of the increased circulation may occur as a result of heat produced by the drying cast. After the cast is completely dry, it is strong and firm and can withstand stresses. The plaster is hard within 15 minutes, so the client can move around without problems. It is not strong enough for weight-bearing until it is dry (after about 24 to 48 hours).

Thermolabile plastic (Orthoplast) and *thermoplastic resins* (Hexcelite) are molded to fit the torso or extremity after being heated in warm water. Polyurethane, which is formed from polyester and cotton fabric impregnated with a chemical, is water activated by immersion in cool water to start the chemical process. Casts made of fiberglass tape are frequently used because they are lightweight and relatively waterproof and support earlier mobilization. They are appropriate in cases in which severe edema is not present or when multiple cast changes are not anticipated.

An *external fixator* is a metallic device used to compress fracture fragments and to immobilize reduced fractures when cast and traction are not appropriate. The external gear holds fragments in place much like surgically implanted internal devices do. The external fixator is attached directly to the bones by percutaneous pins (Fig. 57-9). Assessment for pin loosening and infection is critical. Infection signaled by exudate, redness, tenderness, and pain may require removal of the device. An external fixator used to treat fractures with associated soft-tissue trauma facilitates wound care.

Internal fixation. Internal fixation devices are surgically inserted at the time of realignment. They are biologically

---

Table 57-4

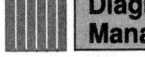

Diagnostic and Therapeutic Management: Fractures

DIAGNOSTIC

History and physical examination
X-ray examination

THERAPEUTIC

Fracture reduction

Manipulation
Open reduction
Closed reduction
Traction devices
    Skin traction
    Skeletal traction

Fracture immobilization

External casting and/or external fixation
Internal fixation devices
Maintenance traction

Open fractures

Surgical debridement
Tetanus immunization
Prophylactic antibiotic therapy
Immobilization

Table 57-5 Common Types of Traction

Type	Indications	Nursing Implications	
SKIN			
Buck's	Type is used for many conditions affecting hip, femur, knee, or back. It is generally used for temporary immobilization and stabilization of fractured hips or fractures of the femoral shaft. It can be unilateral or bilateral.	Assess for nerve and circulatory disturbances caused by circumferential bandages, especially over bony prominences, and for skin necrosis, an allergic reaction to the adhesive material, rotation of the extremity, and constant traction and counter-traction forces.	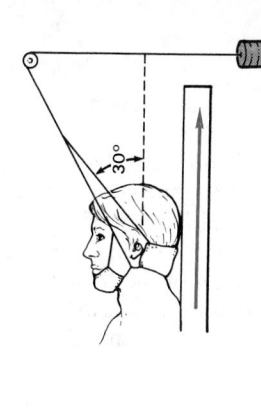
Russell's	Type is used for fractures of femur, hip, and certain knee problems.	Same as above. Assess knee sling for smoothness and an overly tight edge. Because the arrangement of this traction may vary, be aware of initial set-up and maintain it.	
Bryant's	Type is used for fractures of the femur, fractures in small children, and stabilization of hip joints in children under 2 yr or 30 lb in weight.	Be aware that with traction in place, buttocks should just clear the mattress. Check for undue pressure over the outer head and neck of fibula, dorsum of foot, Achilles tendon, scapulae, and shoulders. Check that bandages or boot has not slipped. Be aware that these are usually removed for skin care and assessment every 8 hr.	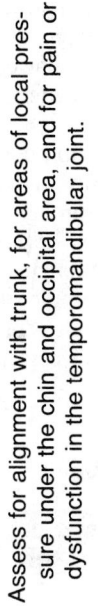 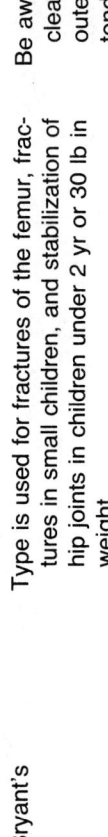
CIRCUMFERENTIAL			
Head halter	Type is used for soft-tissue disorders and degenerative disk disease of the cervical spine. It is not commonly used for unstable fractures of the cervical spine.	Assess for alignment with trunk, for areas of local pressure under the chin and occipital area, and for pain or dysfunction in the temporomandibular joint.	

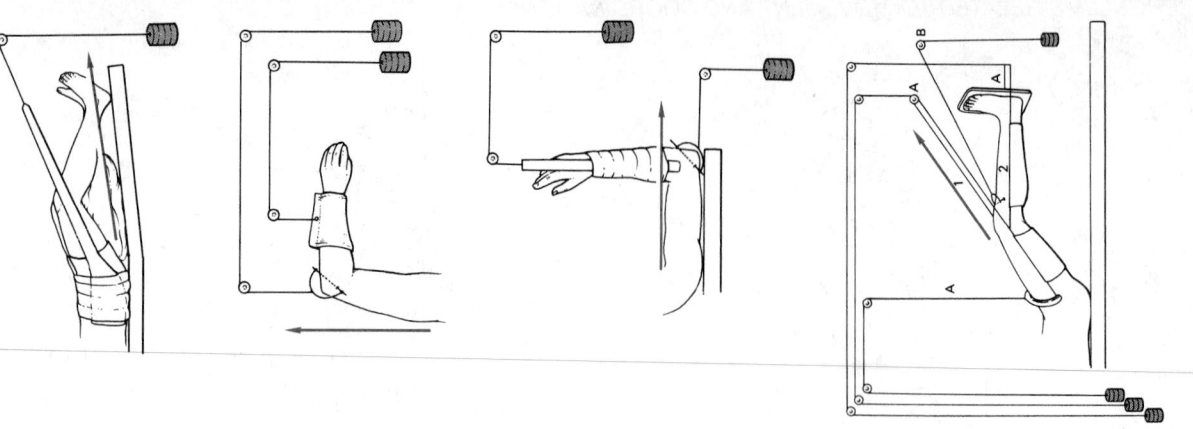

SKELETAL

Pelvic

Type is used for sciatica, muscle spasms (low back), and minor fractures of the lower spine.

Check for security of the pelvic belt. Check frequently for skin irritation over iliac crests. Use measure to prevent a skin breakdown. Check and adjust pelvic belt straps so that they are unrestricted and equal in length. Secure the straps with adhesive tape. Use a footboard to prevent footdrop. Maintain the correct angle of pull of the traction. Be aware that the physician orders the type of countertraction.

Overhead arm (90°-90°)

Type is commonly used for immobilization of fractures and dislocations of the upper arm and shoulder.

Be aware that the shoulder and elbow joint are maintained at 90° angles.

Lateral arm

Type is commonly used in immobilization of fractures and dislocations of the upper arm and shoulder.

Balanced suspension traction

Type is used for injury or fracture of the femoral shaft of the femur, acetabulum, hip, lower leg, or any combination of these.

Be aware that type uses half-ring Thomas splint (1) and Pearson attachment (2) and that suspension of the extremity (A) and direct skeletal traction (B) are applied. Be aware that type allows raising of the buttocks off the bed for bedpan use and skin care without altering the line of traction. Use nursing assessments so that countertraction is maintained (e.g., position client high in bed so that feet do not press on foot of bed, do not elevate the head of the bed more that 25° if it causes continual movement toward foot of the bed). Encourage self-help in client's performance of activities of daily living, movement in bed with help of trapeze, and flexion and extension of affected foot to prevent footdrop. Assess and care for skin of the groin (ischial) area, sacrum, and scapulae. Inspect the pin site and perform pin site care according to hospital policy.

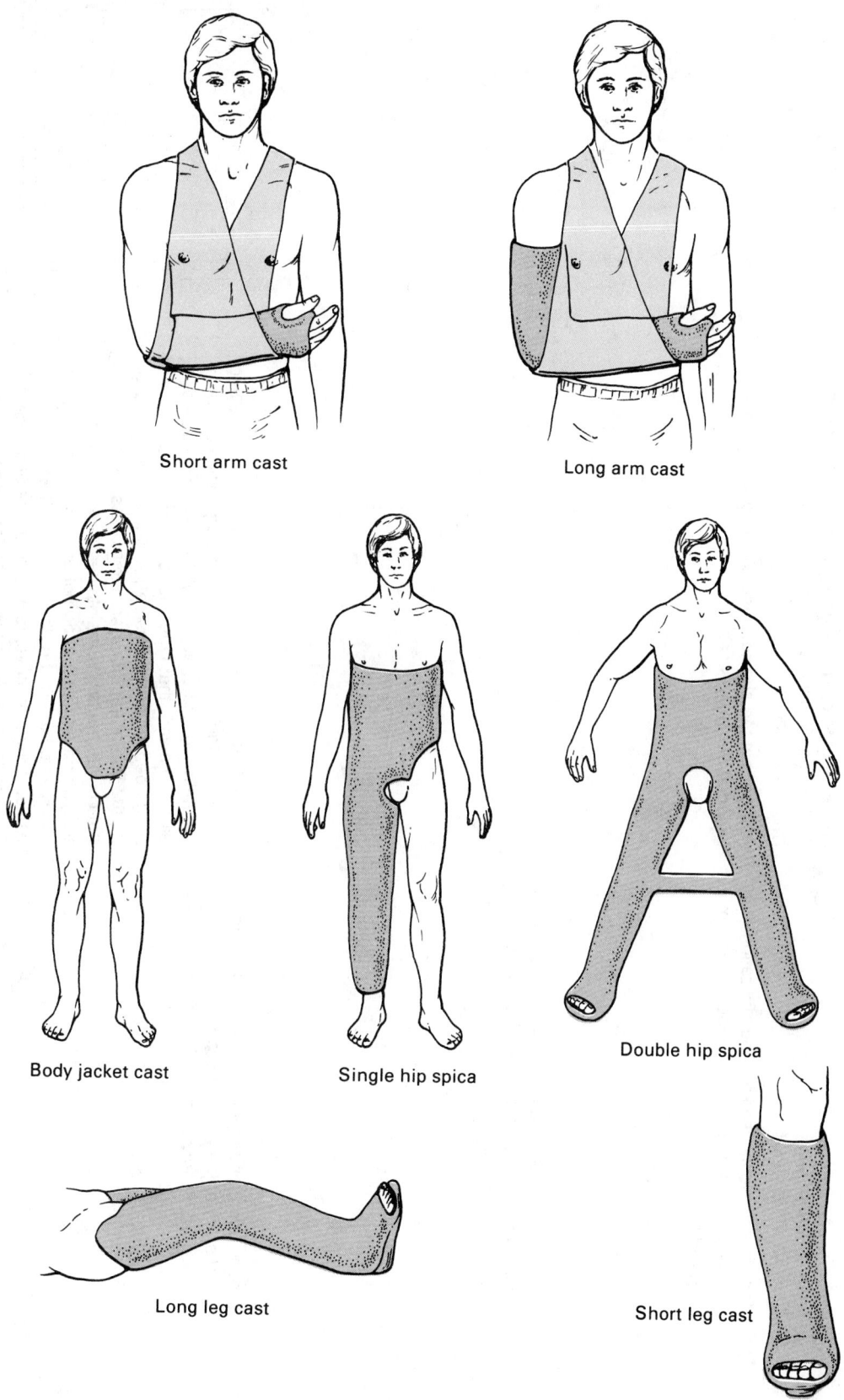

Short arm cast

Long arm cast

Body jacket cast

Single hip spica

Double hip spica

Long leg cast

Short leg cast

Fig. 57-8 Common casts used in treatment of disorders of the musculoskeletal system.

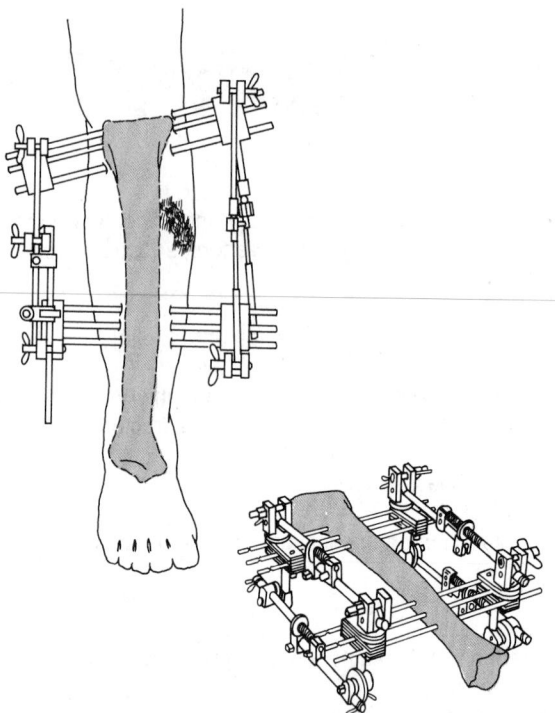

Fig. 57-9 External fixator attached to bones of lower extremity. Note open wound, external fixator in *lower right corner*. (External fixator courtesy Zimmer, Inc, Warsaw, In.)

inert devices that are used to realign and maintain bony fragments. Proper alignment is evaluated by x-ray studies at regular intervals.

Maintenance traction. Maintenance traction is initiation or continuation of traction and countertraction. A continuous pulling force can be applied directly to bone with wires and pins (skeletal traction) or can be applied indirectly by weights that are attached to the skin with adhesive straps or boots (skin traction). Skin traction is usually applied directly to the extremity with the use of adhesive material that is wrapped circumferentially with a bandage or a special garment with straps that is attached to a rope with a weight. Skin traction is applied for a short time and usually consists of not more than 7 to 10 lb of traction weight because of skin intolerance to pressure. Skeletal traction is usually indicated when the traction forces are expected to exceed 10 lb or when traction will be used for a long time. Use of too much weight to maintain traction can result in delayed union or nonunion. The major disadvantages of skeletal traction are infection in the area of bone in which the skeletal pin has been inserted and the consequences of prolonged immobility necessitated by skeletal traction.

Open fracture. Tetanus prevention should be ensured with use of tetanus toxoid or tetanus antitoxin for a client who has not been immunized. A broad-spectrum antibiotic is usually used prophylactically. A decision as to whether to close the wound or leave it open is based on the degree of contamination and the time elapsed before initiation of treatment.

The overall long-term goal of treatment is the correction of the fracture and return of the client to the preinjury level of functioning as soon as possible. Discharge planning should include referral to the appropriate human service agency for assistance in the transition to the home environment.

Pharmacological Management

Clients with fractures often experience varying degrees of pain associated with muscle spasms. These spasms are caused by involuntary reflexes that result from the muscle injury. Medications such as muscle relaxants are often prescribed for relief of the pain associated with muscle spasms.

Medications used primarily as muscle relaxants include carisoprodol (Rela, Soma), chlorphenesin carbamate (Maolate), chlorzoxazone (Paraflex), dantrolene sodium (Dantrium), cyclobenzaprine (Flexeril), metaxalone (Skelaxin), methocarbamol (Robaxin), mephenesin (Atensin), orphenadrine (Disipal), and styramate (Sinaxar). Medications that combine sedative action with muscle relaxant properties include chlormezanone (Trancopal), diazepam (Valium), meprobamate (Equanil, Miltown), and tybamate (Solacen, Tybatran).

Common side effects associated with muscle relaxants are drowsiness, lassitude, headache, weakness, fatigue, blurred vision, ataxia, and GI upset. Hypersensitivity reactions may include skin rash or pruritus. Ingestion of large doses of muscle relaxants may cause hypotension, tachycardia, or respiratory depression. The possible habituating effects associated with long-term use and the potential for abuse must be carefully considered.

Some physicians do not believe in prescribing muscle relaxants for relief of muscle spasms. Their rationale is that the reflex spasm will continue as long as the precipitating pain persists. If the pain is controlled by use of appropriate analgesia, the muscle spasms cease.

Nutritional Considerations

Proper nutrition is an essential component of the reparative process in injured tissue. An adequate energy source is needed to promote muscle strength and tone, build endurance, and enhance ambulation and gait-training skills. The client's dietary requirements must include ample protein (e.g., 1 g per kilogram of body weight), vitamins (especially B and C), and calcium to ensure optimal soft-tissue and bone healing. Low serum protein levels and vitamin C deficiencies interfere with tissue healing. Immobility and callus formation alter calcium needs. Three well-balanced meals a day usually provide the necessary nutrients. The well-balanced diet should be supplemented by a fluid intake of 2000 to 3000 ml/day to promote optimal bladder and bowel function. Adequate fluid and a high-fiber diet prevent constipation (see Table 37-10). If immobilized in a body jacket or hip spica bandage, the client should be instructed not to overeat to avoid pressure and cramping.

Table 57-6

Prehospital Emergency Care of the Client with a Fractured Extremity*

Possible etiologies: Falls, direct blows, forced flexion or hyperextension, twisting forces, pathological conditions, violent muscle contractions (seizures)

CLINICAL MANIFESTATIONS

Deformity or unnatural position of affected limb
Swelling and discoloration (ecchymosis)
Muscle spasm
Tenderness and pain
Loss of use
Numbness, tingling, loss of distal pulses
Grating and crepitus
Exposure of bone

MANAGEMENT

Assess airway, breathing, and circulation.
Assess client for any bleeding sites.
Immobilize joints above and below fracture site by splinting extremity.
Check pulses distal to injury before and after splinting.
Elevate injured limb (if possible).
Do not attempt to straighten fractured or dislocated joints.
Do not manipulate bone ends that may be protruding.
Apply cold pack or compresses to affected area.

*See Chapter 59 for a general discussion on measures related to prehospital emergency care.

Nursing Management of Fractures

Nursing assessment

A brief history of the accident, mechanism of injury, and the position in which the victim was found can be obtained from the client and witnesses. As soon as possible, the client should be transported to an emergency room where thorough assessment and treatment can be initiated (Table 57-6). Subjective and objective data that should be obtained from an individual with a fracture are presented in Table 57-7.

Special emphasis must be focused on the region distal to the site of injury. The involved extremity should be compared with the uninvolved extremity. Clinical findings must be documented before fracture treatment is initiated to avoid doubts about whether a problem discovered later was missed during the original examination or was caused by the treatment. Misdiagnosis may result from failure to consider clinical procedures as the cause of a client's complaints.[9]

Nursing diagnoses

Nursing diagnoses are determined when the problem and etiological factors are supported by clinical data. Nursing diagnoses related to fractures may include, but are not limited to, those presented in Table 57-8.

Nursing interventions

Acute intervention. Clients with fractures may be treated in an emergency room or physician's office and re-

Table 57-7

Nursing Assessment of the Client with a Fracture

SUBJECTIVE DATA

History
Circumstances surrounding injury, including sudden force or trauma, long-term repetitive forces (cause of stress fracture)
Medications
Use of analgesics (and achievement of relief)
Pain
Sudden and severe pain in location of injury, chronic pain that increases with activity (in stress fracture)
Neurological
Pain, numbness, tingling
Musculoskeletal
Loss of motion and sensation, muscle spasms

OBJECTIVE DATA

General
Apprehension, bleeding, guarding of injured site
Integumentary
Skin lacerations, color changes, bleeding into soft tissues (ecchymosis)
Cardiovascular
Reduced or absent pulse distal to injury, edema, delayed capillary refill, pallor, hematoma
Musculoskeletal
Restricted or lost function of affected part, local deformities, abnormal angulation, shortening, rotation, crepitation, muscle weakness
Neurological
Paresthesias, decreased sensation
Possible findings
Location and extent of fractures on radiograph, bone scans, tomograms, CT or MRI scans

---

leased to home care, or they may require hospitalization for varying amounts of time. Specific nursing measures depend on the type of treatment used and the setting in which clients are placed.

PREOPERATIVE MANAGEMENT. If surgical intervention is required to treat the fracture, clients need preoperative preparation. In addition to the usual preoperative nursing measures (see Chapter 11), the nurse should inform clients of the type of immobilization device that will be used and the expected activity limitations. Clients must be assured that their needs will be met by the nursing staff until they can again meet their needs. Assurance that pain medication will be available, if needed, is often beneficial.

Proper skin preparation is an important part of preoperative preparation. The protocol for skin preparation varies among agencies and may be the responsibility of the nurse. The aim of skin preparation is to clean the skin and remove debris and hair to reduce the possibility of infection. Careful attention to this preoperative treatment can influence the postoperative course.

Table 57-8

NURSING CARE PLAN FOR THE CLIENT WITH A FRACTURE

Defining Characteristics	Nursing Interventions	Evaluation Criteria
NURSING DIAGNOSIS: Potential complication: compartment syndrome related to nerve compression		
Pain in affected extremity that is unrelieved by medication, paresthesias, pallor, diminished pulse	Elevate extremity above heart level. Apply ice compresses as ordered. Assess nerve and vascular status of affected extremity q 2 hr. Notify physician immediately if client complains of increasing pain that is unrelieved by medication.	Normal neurovascular examination
NURSING DIAGNOSIS: Pain related to edema, movement of bone fragments, muscle spasms, and ineffective pain relief and/or comfort measures		
Pain descriptors, guarding; altered time perception; behaviors indicative of pain such as moaning, crying, restlessness, altered muscle tone, autonomic responses, decreased activity	Gently and correctly position fractured extremity. Assess site for constriction or pressure caused by immobilization apparatus. Give client analgesics and/or muscle relaxants as indicated.	Reduction or absence of pain
NURSING DIAGNOSIS: High risk for infection related to disruption of skin integrity and presence of environmental pathogens secondary to open fracture or external fixation pins		
Disruption of skin, increase in environmental exposure	Use sterile technique when providing pin or wound care or when performing dressing change. Observe for wound drainage. Obtain culture of wound. Administer antibiotics as ordered. Monitor temperature q 2 hr. Isolate client to prevent dissemination of pathogen or cross-contamination of wound, if indicated.	No evidence of wound infection
NURSING DIAGNOSIS: Activity intolerance related to prolonged immobility		
Verbal reports of fatigue or weakness, abnormal physiological responses to activity	Encourage active range-of-motion exercise of joints not immobilized. Perform resistance exercises of unaffected extremities. Plan rest periods between activities. Encourage client participation in activities of daily living and exercises. Monitor vital signs during activity.	Normal physiological responses to activity
NURSING DIAGNOSIS: High risk for impaired skin integrity related to immobility and presence of cast		
Immobilization device (cast, traction, splint), altered circulation (edema), lack of position changes	Examine potential pressure areas regularly. Petal cast edges. Turn client q 2 hr. Keep bed free of wrinkles and crumbs. Assess exposed skin areas of traction sites for signs of infection or irritation. Seek medical attention if cast becomes loose and permits rotation or flexion or causes skin abrasion. Instruct client not to insert items into cast.	No evidence of skin breakdown

Continued.

Table 57-8

NURSING CARE PLAN FOR THE CLIENT WITH A FRACTURE—cont'd		
Defining Characteristics	**Nursing Interventions**	**Evaluation Criteria**

NURSING DIAGNOSIS: **Impaired physical mobility related to lack of knowledge regarding changed mobility patterns and limited range of motion**

Inaccurate follow-through of previous instructions	Teach gait-training principles to client (nonweight-bearing gait status unless otherwise ordered by physician): sit with feet over edge of bed, stand with no weight on affected extremity, measure and adjust crutches. Start client's gait training on parallel bars. Ensure client's gait is compatible with weight-bearing status. Cooperate with physical therapist regarding exercise and gait training. Explain importance of activity of affected extremity as tolerated. Reinforce exercise program as prescribed by physician.	Demonstration of mobility with assistive device

NURSING DIAGNOSIS: **Altered health maintenance related to lack of knowledge regarding muscle atrophy, exercise program, and cast care**

Questioning of long-term effect of casting and cast care, activity restrictions	Instruct client on home care measures related to exercise, cast care, and prevention of complications. Plan for follow-up care with physician. Explain factors that contribute to atrophy. Emphasize relationship of activity to muscle atrophy.	Minimal loss of muscle bulk of affected extremity, verbalization of confidence in ability to follow prescribed discharge plan

POSTOPERATIVE MANAGEMENT. In general, postoperative nursing care and management is directed toward monitoring vital signs and applying the general principles of postoperative nursing care (see Chapter 13). Frequent neurovascular assessments of the affected extremity are necessary to detect subtle changes. Any limitations of movement or activity related to turning, positioning, and extremity support should be monitored closely. Pain and discomfort can be minimized through correct alignment and positioning. Dressings or casts should be carefully observed for any overt signs of bleeding or drainage. An acceptable method of detecting increases in bleeding is to draw a circle on the cast around an area of drainage, noting the date and time. An increase in size of the drainage area should be reported. If a wound-drainage system is in place, the patency of the system and the volume of drainage should be assessed at least once each shift. Whenever the contents of a drainage system are measured or emptied, the nurse should use sterile technique to avoid contamination. Additional nursing responsibilities depend on the type of immobilization used.

CAST CARE. Immediately after a cast is applied, there is a short period of exothermic reaction during which heat is released from the plaster. The client should be alerted to this occurrence, since it can increase edema. Evaporation of water and dissipation of heat from the cast can be hastened by exposing the cast to room air. A fresh cast should never be covered with a blanket because air cannot circulate and heat builds up in the cast. The client should be turned every 2 hours to reduce continuous pressure and to promote even drying of the cast. The drying process is usually complete within 24 to 72 hours. During the drying period the cast should not be subjected to any wetness, soiling, or abnormal stresses that can cause weakening or a break. It should be carefully handled with the palms of the hands rather than with the fingertips to avoid indentations that will dry and become potential pressure areas. Once the cast is thoroughly dry, the edge should be finished to avoid skin irritation (Fig. 57-10).

Regardless of the type of material of which it is made, a cast can interfere with circulation and nerve function because it is applied too tightly or because of excessive edema after application. Thus frequent neurovascular assessments of the immobilized extremity are critical. The client needs to be educated about signs of cast complication so that they can be reported promptly. Elevation of the extremity above the heart level to promote venous return and applications of ice to control or prevent edema are measures frequently used during the initial phase of immobilization. The nurse should instruct the client to exercise joints above and below the cast. Pulling out cast padding and scratching or placing foreign objects inside the cast should be forbidden because it predisposes the client to skin breakdown within the cast.

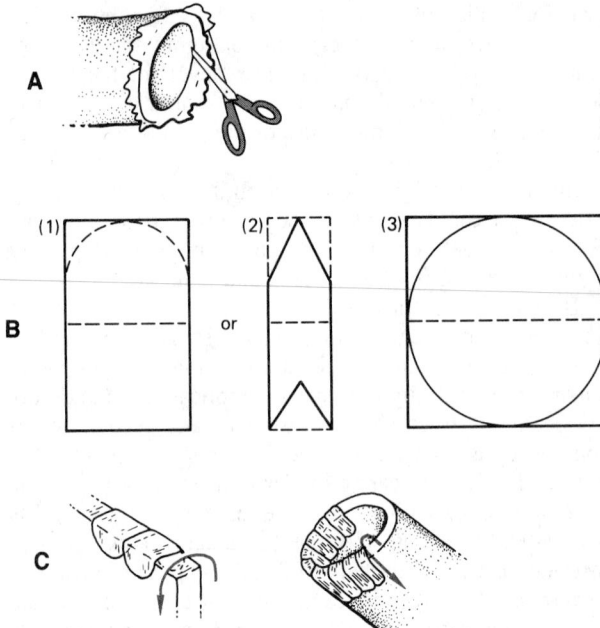

Fig. 57-10 Finishing edges of plaster cast with waterproof adhesive strips. **A,** The cast must be thoroughly dry. The nurse trims the excess sheet wadding and stretches the stockinette over the cast edge (when possible). **B,** Several strips (petals) of waterproof adhesive tape (2-inch-wide strips for wide areas and 1-inch-wide strips for small areas, each 1 inch long) are made in advance. **C,** The uncut end of the tape is placed beneath the cast edge. The petal is brought forward over the cast edge. Each succeeding petal overlaps the previous one by ½ inch, ensuring a smooth cast edge. A family member can help, and this can be done at home as needed.

If the client is immobilized as a result of the fracture, the nurse must plan care to prevent the occurrence of constipation and renal calculi. Constipation can be prevented by the maintenance of a high fluid intake and a diet high in bulk and roughage. If these measures are not effective in maintaining the client's normal bowel pattern, stool softeners, laxatives, or suppositories may be necessary. Maintaining a regular time for elimination in spite of bed rest is effective in promoting regularity.

Renal calculi can develop as a result of bone demineralization caused by immobilization. The resulting hypercalcemia causes a rise in urine pH and stone formation resulting from the precipitation of calcium. Unless contraindicated, a fluid intake of 2100 to 2800 ml/day is recommended. Cranberry juice is often recommended to acidify the urine and discourage the development of stones.

Rapid deconditioning of the circulatory system can occur as a result of bedrest. Unless contraindicated, these effects can be diminished by permitting clients to sit on the side of the bed, allowing their lower limbs to dangle over the bedside, and by performing standing transfers. When clients are allowed to increase activity, careful evaluation should be made to assess for orthostatic hypotension.

TYPES OF CASTS. Immobilization of an acute fracture or soft-tissue injury of the upper extremity is frequently accomplished by use of (1) the sugar-tong splint, (2) the short arm cast, and (3) the long arm cast. The *sugar-tong splint* is used for acute wrist injuries. Multiple layers of plaster splints are applied to the padded forearm, beginning at the phalangeal joints of the hand and extending up the dorsal aspect of the forearm around the distal humerus and then extending down the volar aspect of the forearm to the distal palmar crease. The splinting material is wrapped with either elastic bandage or bias stocking. The major advantage of the sugar-tong cast is prevention of the circumferential effects of a nonelastic cylinder.

The *short arm cast* is frequently used for the treatment of stable wrist or metacarpal injuries. An aluminum finger splint can be fabricated into the short arm cast for treatment of phalangeal injuries. The short arm cast is a circular plaster cast extending from the distal palmar area to the proximal forearm. This cast provides wrist immobilization and permits unrestricted elbow motion.

The *long arm cast* is commonly used for stable forearm or elbow fractures and stable wrist fractures. It is similar to the short arm cast but extends to the proximal humerus, restricting motion in the wrist and elbow. Nursing measures should be directed toward supporting the extremity and reducing the effects of edema by maintaining extremity elevation with a sling. When a sling is used, the nurse must ensure that the axillary region is well padded to prevent skin maceration associated with direct skin-to-skin contact. Placement of the sling should not place undue stress on the neck. Movement of the fingers should be encouraged to enhance the pumping action of veins to decrease edema. The nurse should also encourage the client to actively move nonimmobilized joints of the upper extremity to prevent stiffness and contractures.

The *body jacket cast* is used for immobilization and support for stable spine injuries of the thoracic or lumbar spine or after spinal surgery. This cast is applied around the chest and abdomen and extends from above the nipple line to the pubis. After application of the cast, the nurse must assess the client for the development of a cast syndrome. This condition occurs if the body cast is applied too tightly and the cast compresses the superior mesenteric artery against the duodenum. The client generally complains of abdominal pain, abdominal pressure, nausea, and vomiting. Treatment includes gastric decompression with a nasogastric tube and suction. The cast may need to be removed or split. Nursing assessment also includes observation of respiratory status, bowel and bladder function, and areas of pressure over the bony prominences, especially the iliac crest. During the time required for the cast to dry, the nurse should reposition the client every 2 to 3 hours to promote even cast drying and to relieve pressure and discomfort.

The *hip spica cast* is commonly used in the treatment of femoral fractures. The purpose of the hip spica cast is to immobilize the affected extremity and the trunk securely. It includes two separate casts joined together: (1) the body jacket and (2) the long leg cast. The location of the femoral fracture determines whether the unaffected extremity

has to be immobilized to restrict rotation of the pelvis and possible hip motion. The hip spica cast extends from above the nipple line to the base of the foot (single spica) and may include the opposite extremity up to an area above the knee (spica and a half) or both extremities (double spica). The nurse should assess the client for the same problems associated with the body jacket cast. During the initial drying stage the client should not be placed in the prone position because the cast may break. The client should be slightly turned from side to side and supported with pillows. When the client is repositioned, the support bar joining the thighs must never be used to assist in moving the client, since the bar can break and cause cast disruption. After the cast has dried, the nurse, with assistance, can turn the client to the prone position and provide pillow support under the chest and the immobilized extremity. Skin care around the cast edges and the areas not encompassed by plaster is very important to prevent any pressure sores. The nurse needs to instruct the client in the positioning activities required to get on and off the fracture bedpan. After the hip spica cast has dried sufficiently, the client is instructed in ambulation techniques by the physical therapist.

Injuries to the lower extremity are frequently immobilized by either a *long leg cast* or a *short leg cast*. The usual indications for applying a long leg cast are an unstable ankle fracture, soft-tissue injuries, a fractured tibia, and knee injuries. The cast usually extends from the base of the toes to the groin and gluteal crease. The short leg cast can be used for a variety of conditions but is usually used for stable ankle and foot injuries. After the application of a lower-extremity cast, the extremity should be elevated with pillows above the heart level for the first 24 hours. After the initial phase the cast should not be placed in a dependent position because of the possibility of excessive edema.

Initially, no weight can be put on the injured extremity. Later, a walking heel or cast shoe can be added to the cast. The nurse should observe for signs of pressure, especially in the regions of the fibular head and malleoli.

Because many fractures are casted in an outpatient setting, the client often requires only a short hospitalization or none at all. Therefore client education is an important nursing responsibility to prevent complications. In addition to specific instructions for cast care and recognition of complications, the nurse should encourage the client to contact the clinic or care provider if questions arise. (Table 57-9 summarizes client instructions for cast care.) The nurse should validate the client's understanding of these instructions before discharge from the clinic or hospital.

TRACTION. The nurse is responsible for client comfort and safety while traction is used and for ensuring proper functioning of the traction equipment. The equipment should be regularly examined for frayed ropes, loose knots, ropes out of the groove of the pulley, pulley clamps not fastened firmly to the bed frame, and weights not hanging freely.

When slings are used with traction, the nurse should inspect the skin area that is exposed in and near the sling regularly. Pressure over a bony prominence or a wrinkled area can impair blood flow, causing injury to the peripheral neurovascular structures. Skeletal traction pin sites must be observed for signs of infection. Pin-site care varies according to the preference of the physician but usually includes regular removal of exudate with peroxide, rinsing of pin sites with sterile saline solution, drying of the area with sterile gauze, and application of antibiotic ointment. External rotation of the hip can occur when skin traction is used on the lower extremity. The nurse can correct this position by placing a pillow, sandbag, or rolled-up drawsheet along the outer aspect of the femur. Whenever traction is used, the nurse should ensure that the client's body is always correctly aligned.

To offset some of the problems associated with prolonged immobility, the nurse should discuss specific activity with the physician. If exercise is permitted, the nurse should encourage participation by the client in a simple exercise regimen including the following[10,11]:

1. Participation in feeding and bathing activities
2. Use of the trapeze bar to get on and off the bedpan and for change of linens
3. Performance of simple range-of-motion exercises of all unaffected joints several times a day
4. Performance of isometric exercises and deep-breathing exercises several times a day
5. Change of position frequently to prevent pressure sores

Active exercises that move joints through the range of motion are the preferred activity, if allowed. Frequent exercise of the trunk and extremities is an excellent stimulus to deep breathing.

Table 57-9 Client Instructions for Cast Care

Do not
Get cast wet.*
Remove any padding.
Insert any foreign object inside cast.
Bear weight on new cast for 48 hr.
Cover cast with plastic for prolonged periods.
Do
Check with physician before getting cast wet.
Dry cast thoroughly after exposure to water†:
  Blot dry with towel.
  Use hair dryer on low setting until cast is thoroughly dry.
Elevate extremity above level of heart for first 48 hr.
Move joints above and below cast regularly.
Apply ice directly over fracture site for first 24 hr (avoid getting cast wet by keeping ice in plastic bag and protecting cast with cloth).
Report signs of possible problems to health care provider:
  Increasing pain
  Swelling associated with pain and discoloration of toes or fingers
  Pain during motion
  Burning or tingling under cast
Keep appointment to have fracture and cast checked.

---

*Plaster of Paris cast.
†Synthetic cast.

Complications

The majority of fractures heal without complications. If death occurs after a fracture, it is usually the result of damage to underlying organs and soft tissue or of certain complications of the fracture. Complications of fractures may be direct or indirect. Direct complications include problems with bone union, avascular necrosis, and bone infection. Indirect complications of fractures are associated with blood vessel and nerve damage resulting in conditions such as compartment syndrome, venous thrombosis, fat embolism, and traumatic or hypovolemic shock. Although most musculoskeletal injuries are not life threatening, open fractures accompanied by severe blood loss and fractures that damage vital organs are medical emergencies requiring immediate attention.

Infection. Open fractures and soft-tissue injuries have a high incidence of infection. An open fracture usually results from the impact of severe external forces. The soft-tissue injury often has more serious consequences than the fracture. Devitalized and contaminated tissue is an ideal medium for many common pathogens, including gas-forming bacilli. Treatment of infections is costly in terms of extended nursing and medical care, treatment, and loss of client income.

Therapeutic management. Open fractures require surgical intervention. The wound is cleaned by extensive irrigation, usually with sterile normal saline solution, and any gross contaminants are mechanically removed. Contused, contaminated, and devitalized tissue such as muscle, subcutaneous fat, skin, and fragments of bone are surgically excised *(debridement)*. The extent of the soft-tissue damage determines whether the wound will be closed at the time of surgery, whether closed suction drainage will be used, and whether skin grafting will be necessary. Depending on the location and extent of the fracture, reduction may be maintained by a plaster cast or by traction. During surgery the open wound may be irrigated with antibiotic solution. During the postoperative phase the client may have antibiotics administered intravenously, intramuscularly, or orally, usually for 7 to 10 days. Antibiotics used in conjunction with aggressive surgical management have greatly reduced the occurrence of infection.

Compartment syndrome. Compartment syndrome is the compression of structures within a defined area formed by fascial walls and is a result of secondary edema. Development of a compartment syndrome requires immediate attention. Normally there is some increase in edema as a result of soft-tissue injury in the general region of the injury. If edema continues, there may be an increase of pressure within the closed spaces of the tissue compartments formed by the nonelastic fascia. This can create sufficient pressure to obstruct venous circulation and cause arterial occlusion, resulting in inadequate circulation to the extremity or ischemia. As ischemia continues, muscle and nerve cells are destroyed and fibrotic tissue replaces the healthy tissue. Contracture and loss of function can occur.[12] Untreated compartment syndrome can result in permanent hyperesthesia and motor weakness.[13]

Compartment syndrome is associated with fractures or extensive soft-tissue damage in an extremity. The forearm

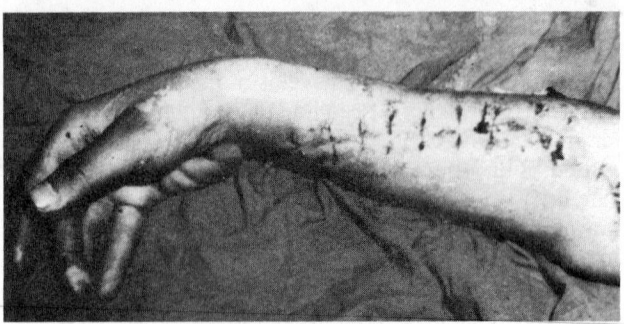

Fig. 57-11 Volkmann's ischemic contracture of the forearm secondary to a supracondylar fracture of the humerus. Note the incision line of an unsuccessful fasciotomy.

and lower leg are the most common sites of compartment syndrome. Fractures of the distal humerus and proximal tibia are the most common fractures associated with compartment syndrome. In the upper extremity, this condition is referred to as *Volkmann's contracture* (Fig. 57-11) and in the lower extremity as *anterior compartment syndrome,* although the underlying pathology is similar.

Clinical manifestations. The earliest sign of a developing compartment syndrome is progressive pain distal to the injury that is not relieved by the usual analgesics. The overlying skin may appear normal because surface vessels are not occluded. In addition to inability to actively extend the digits, pain results from passive extension of the digits. Other symptoms that develop as the condition progresses include numbness and tingling, loss of sensation, loss of function, pallor, coolness of the extremity, and diminished or absent peripheral pulses. Absence of a peripheral pulse is an ominous sign that indicates severe disturbance of circulation. Regular neurovascular assessments should be performed on all clients with injury of the distal humerus or proximal tibia or soft-tissue disruption in these areas. Infection as a result of tissue necrosis is the most common complication. It can be due to delayed decompression, inadequate release of the wound, or delayed closure of a fasciotomy.

Because of the possibility of muscle damage, urine output should be assessed. Myoglobin, which is released from damaged muscle cells, can be trapped in renal tubules because of its high molecular weight. Common signs of myoglobinuria are (1) dark urine associated with a positive benzidine test in the absence of hematuria and (2) the manifestations associated with acute renal failure (see Chapter 41).

Therapeutic management. Prompt, accurate diagnosis of compartment syndrome is critical. Prevention or early recognition is the key. The extremity should be elevated and ice should be applied to enhance venous return and decrease edema. It may be necessary to remove or loosen the bandage or cast or to reduce poundage on traction to prevent edema formation. It may also be necessary to relieve compression and restore blood supply by surgically incising the fascia *(fasciotomy)*. If compartment syndrome is untreated, amputation may be necessary to combat sepsis.

Death may result if compartment syndrome remains untreated.[13]

Venous thrombosis. The veins of the lower extremities and pelvis are highly susceptible to thrombus formation after fracture injury. Precipitating factors are venous stasis caused by incorrectly applied casts or traction, local pressure on a vein, or prolonged bed rest. Venous stasis is aggravated by inactivity of the muscles that normally assist in the pumping action of venous return of blood in the extremities. In addition to wearing antiembolism (compression) stockings and using mechanical compression devices, the client should be instructed to move the fingers or toes of the affected extremity against resistance and to perform range-of-motion exercises on all unaffected extremities. Because of the high risk of venous thrombosis in the immobile client, the physician may order prophylactic antiembolic medication such as aspirin, warfarin, or heparin (see Chapter 32).

Fat embolism. Fat emboli, which are often associated with fractures of long bones, are a contributory factor in many deaths associated with fractures. The fractures that most frequently cause fat embolism are those of the femur, tibia, and pelvis. There are two theories related to the origin of fat emboli. The *mechanical theory* suggests that fat is released from the marrow of injured bone. It is driven out by an increase in intramedullary pressures and transmitted through draining veins to pulmonary capillaries where it lodges. Some fat droplets traverse the capillary bed to enter systemic circulation and embolize to other sites. The *biochemical theory* postulates that catecholamines released at the time of trauma mobilize lipids from the adipose tissue and cause loss of chylomicron emulsion stability.[14] The chylomicrons form large fat globules that lodge in the lungs. This is possibly due to some biochemical change initiated by the injury. The tissues of the lungs, brain, heart, kidneys, and skin are most frequently affected.

Clinical manifestations. Initial manifestations of fat embolism usually occur 12 to 72 hours after injury.[15] The fat globules transported to the lungs cause a hemorrhagic interstitial pneumonitis that produces symptoms of adult respiratory distress syndrome, such as chest pain, tachypnea, cyanosis, dyspnea, apprehension, tachycardia, and decreased partial pressure of oxygen (Pao_2). All of these symptoms are caused by poor oxygen exchange. The changes in the mental state as a result of hypoxemia are very important. Memory loss, restlessness, confusion, elevated temperature, and headache prompt further investigation so that CNS involvement is not mistaken for alcohol withdrawal. The continued change in level of consciousness and petechiae located around the neck, anterior chest wall, axilla, buccal membrane of the mouth, and conjunctiva of the eye help distinguish between the two. Petechiae result from intravascular thromboses caused by decreased oxygenation.

The clinical course of a fat embolism may be brief and acute. Frequently the client expresses a feeling of impending disaster. In a short time, skin color changes from pallor to cyanosis, and the client may become comatose. No specific laboratory examinations are available to aid in the diagnosis. However, certain diagnostic abnormalities may be present. These include fat cells in the urine or sputum, a decrease of the Pao_2 to less than 60 mm Hg, and a decrease in the platelet count. A chest x-ray examination may reveal areas of pulmonary infiltrate or multiple areas of consolidation. This is sometimes referred to as the *snowstorm effect.*

Therapeutic management. Careful immobilization of a long bone fracture is believed to be helpful in reducing the occurrence of fat embolism. Use of steroids to prevent fat embolism is currently under investigation.[14]

Although there is no specific treatment for fat embolism, oxygen is administered to treat hypoxia. Steroids, anticoagulants, and low-molecular-weight dextran are beneficial in conjunction with the maintenance of alveolar gas exchange.[16] Intubation or intermittent positive-pressure breathing may be considered if a satisfactory Pao_2 cannot be obtained with supplemental oxygen alone. Management is essentially symptom-related and supportive. It includes restriction of fluid intake, correction of acidosis, and replacement of any blood loss. Coughing and deep breathing should be encouraged. The client should be repositioned as little as possible before fracture immobilization because of the danger of dislodging more fat droplets into the general circulation. Some clients may develop pulmonary edema, adult respiratory distress syndrome, or both, leading to an increased risk of mortality.

Rehabilitative Management

Psychosocial problems. Short-range rehabilitative goals are directed toward the transition from dependence to independence in performing simple activities of daily living and preservation or increase of strength and endurance. Long-range rehabilitative goals are aimed at preventing problems associated with musculoskeletal injury (Table 57-10). An important part of nursing care during the rehabilitative phase is assisting the client to adjust to any problems caused by the injury (e.g., separation from family, financial impact of medical care, loss of income from inability to work). The nurse must exhibit gentleness, support, and encouragement and should actively listen to the client's fears.

Progressive ambulation. The physical therapist often assumes primary responsibility for directing the client during the strengthening phase of care. The nurse must know the overall goals of the physical therapist in relation to the client's abilities, needs, and tolerance. Mobility training and instruction in the use of assistive aids constitute one of the major areas of responsibility of the physical therapist. The client with lower-extremity dysfunction is usually started in mobility training when able to sit in bed and dangle the feet over the side. This activity should be done two or three times per day for 10 to 15 minutes, with the nurse assisting as necessary. As endurance increases, the client is instructed in the techniques of transferring from bed to chair. Progressive ambulation is usually started with parallel bars and progresses to ambulatory assistive devices. When the client begins to ambulate, the nurse must know the weight-bearing allowed for the affected extremity and the correct technique if the client is using an assistance device. There are different degrees of weight-bearing ambulation: (1) nonweight-bearing ambulation, (2) partial-

Table 57-10 Problems Associated with Injury of the Musculoskeletal System

MUSCLE ATROPHY

Decreased muscle mass normally occurs as a result of disuse following prolonged immobilization. An isometric muscle-strengthening exercise regimen within the confines of the immobilization device assists in reducing the amount of atrophy. Muscle atrophy interferes with and prolongs the rehabilitation process.

CONTRACTURE

Abnormal muscle shortening is due to improper support and positioning of a joint. This results from an imbalance of muscle or ligament, which adaptively adjusts to a shortened position in the region of a joint. This condition can be prevented by frequent position change, correct body alignment, and active-passive range-of-motion exercises several times a day. Contracture of a joint immobilized for a long time with a cast is common. Intervention requires gradual and progressive stretching of the muscles or ligaments in the region of the joint.

FOOT DROP

Plantar-flexed position of the foot occurs when the Achilles tendon on the foot shortens because it has been allowed to assume an unsupported position. This may signify damage to the peroneal nerve. Nursing management of the client with long-term injuries must include measures of prevention by supporting the foot in dorsiflexion. Once foot drop has developed, ambulation and gait training may be significantly hindered.

PAIN

Frequently associated with fractures, edema, and muscle spasm, pain varies in intensity from mild to severe and is usually described as aching, dull, burning, throbbing, sharp, or deep. Important causal factors of pain include incorrect positioning and alignment of the extremity, incorrect support of the extremity, sudden movement of the extremity, an immobilization device that is applied too tightly or in an incorrect position, constrictive dressings, motion occurring at the fracture site, and psychosocial factors. Pain is a valuable assessment guide, and the underlying causes should be determined so that corrective nursing action can be taken before analgesics are administered.

MUSCLE SPASMS

These are caused by involuntary muscle contraction after fracture and may last as long as several weeks. Pain associated with muscle spasms is often intense. The duration varies from several seconds to several minutes. Nursing measures to reduce the intensity of the muscle spasms are similar to the corrective actions for pain control. The area involved in muscle spasms should not be massaged.

---

weight-bearing ambulation, and (3) full-weight-bearing ambulation.

Assistive devices. Devices for ambulation range from a cane, which can relieve up to 40% of the weight normally borne by a lower limb, to a walker or crutches, which allow complete nonweight-bearing ambulation. The decision about which device is appropriate for a client involves the need for maximum stability and safety versus maneuverability, which is required in small spaces such as bathrooms and buses. The decision is made more easily by discussing with clients the requirements of their lifestyles and by determining the device with which each client feels most secure and independent.

The technique for using assistive devices varies. The involved limb is usually advanced at the same time or immediately after the advance of the device. The uninvolved limb is advanced last. In almost all cases, canes are held in the hand opposite the involved extremity.

The common gait patterns with assistive devices are the following:
1. *Two-point gait:* Crutch on one side advances simultaneously with the opposite foot; gait is also used with cane ambulation.
2. *Four-point gait:* A slower version of the two-point gait, each "point" is advanced separately.
3. *Swing-to gait:* Both crutches are advanced together, followed by the lifting of both lower limbs to the same place; this gait is also used with walkers.
4. *Swing-through gait:* This gait is similar to the swing-to gait, but the client swings the body past the crutches.

A belt can be placed around the client's waist to provide stability during the learning stages. The nurse should discourage the client from reaching for furniture or relying on another person for support. When there is inadequate upper-limb strength or poorly fitted crutches, the client bears weight at the axilla rather than at the hands, endangering the neurovascular bundle that passes across the axilla. If verbal coaching does not correct the problem, the client should be kept from further ambulation until strength is adequate.

Clients who must ambulate without weight-bearing require sufficient upper-limb strength to lift their own weight at each step. Since the muscles of the shoulder girdle are not accustomed to this work, they require vigorous and diligent training in preparation for this task. Push-ups and pull-ups using the overhead trapeze bar and lifting of weights develop the triceps and biceps. Straight leg raises and quadriceps-setting exercises strengthen the quadriceps.

Counseling and referrals. During the rehabilitative process the client's family assumes an important role in the provision and follow-through of long-term care plans. The family must be instructed in the techniques of strength and endurance exercises, assistance with mobility training, and promoting activities that enhance the quality of daily living. Sexual counseling should be included in discharge planning. Unless nurses have specific preparation for sexual health counseling, they should remember that wrong answers are usually more harmful than no answers. For referral purposes, nurses must know whether sexual activity is compatible with the degree of injury and whether any restrictions are imposed by an immobilization or support device.

Colles' Fracture

A Colles' fracture is a fracture of the distal radius and is one of the most common fractures in adults. The styloid process of the ulna may be involved as well. The injury usually occurs when the client attempts to break a fall with the hand open. This type of fracture most frequently occurs in a woman over the age of 50 whose bones are osteoporotic. The clinical manifestations of Colles' fracture are pain in the immediate area of injury, pronounced swelling, and dorsal displacement of the distal fragment (dinner-fork deformity). The major complication associated with a Colles' fracture is vascular insufficiency as a result of edema.

A Colles' fracture is usually managed by closed manipulation of the fracture and immobilization by either a sugar-tong splint or a long arm cast. The elbow must be immobilized to prevent supination and pronation. Nursing management should include measures to prevent or reduce edema and accurate neurovascular assessment. Support and protection of the extremity should be provided, along with encouragement of active movement of the thumb and fingers. This type of movement helps reduce edema and increases venous return. The client should be instructed to perform active movements of the shoulder to prevent stiffness or contracture.

Fracture of the Humerus

Fractures involving the shaft of the humerus are a common injury among young and middle-aged adults. The prominent clinical manifestations are an obvious displacement of the humerus shaft, shortened extremity, abnormal mobility, and pain (Fig. 57-12). The major complications associated with fracture of the humerus are radial nerve injury and vascular injury to the brachial artery as a result of laceration, transection, or spasm.

The treatment for a fracture of the humerus depends on the location and displacement of the fracture. Treatment may include a hanging arm cast or the sling and swathe—a type of immobilization that prevents glenohumeral movement. The swathe encircles the trunk and humerus as an additional binder. It is also used for surgical repair of the shoulder and shoulder dislocation.

When these devices are used, the head of the bed must be elevated to assist gravity in reducing the fracture. The arm should be allowed to hang when the client is sitting

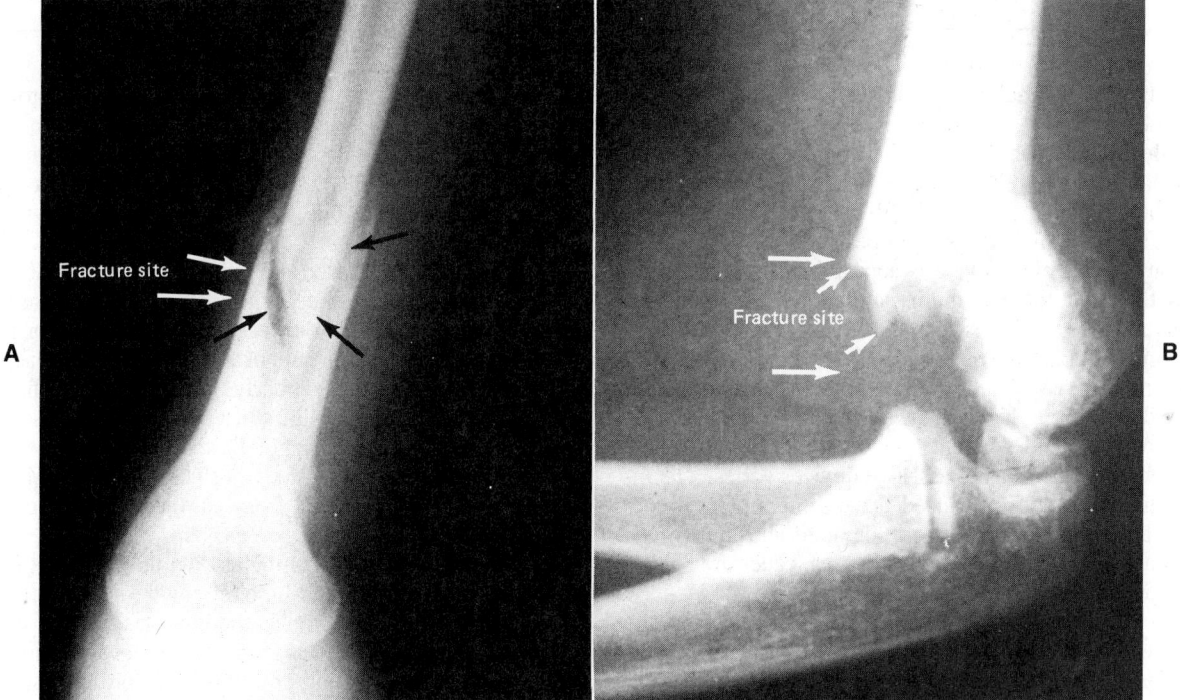

Fig. 57-12 **A,** Supracondylar fracture of the humerus. This type of injury results in the formation of a large hematoma. **B,** Fracture of distal shaft of humerus.

and standing. Nursing care should include measures to protect the axilla and prevent skin maceration. Skin or skeletal traction may also be used for purposes of reduction and immobilization.

During the rehabilitative phase an exercise program geared toward improving strength and motion of the injured extremity is extremely important. This should include assisted motion of the hand and fingers. The shoulder can also be exercised if the fracture is stable.

Fracture of the Pelvis

Pelvic fractures are usually caused by vehicular accidents. Older adult clients may sustain this injury from a fall. Although only 3% of all fractures are pelvic fractures, this type of injury accounts for 5% to 20% of the mortality from fractures. Preoccupation with associated injuries at the time of an accident may result in neglect of pelvic injuries. Pelvic fractures may cause serious intraabdominal injury such as colon laceration, paralytic ileus, intrapelvic hemorrhage, and rupture of the urethra or bladder.

Physical examination demonstrates local swelling, tenderness, deformity, and ecchymosis. The neurovascular status of the lower extremities and manifestations of associated injuries should be assessed. Pelvic fractures are diagnosed and classified by x-ray study. They may range from simple undisplaced fractures to more serious fracture dislocations with the potential for serious complications.

Treatment of a pelvic fracture depends on the severity of the injury. Bed rest for stable pelvic fractures is maintained from a few days to 6 weeks. More complex fractures may be treated with pelvic slings, skeletal traction, hip spica casts, open reduction, or a combination of these methods. Extreme care in handling or moving the client is important to prevent serious injury from a displaced fracture fragment. Because pelvic fracture can damage other organs, appropriate assessments are important in early nursing activities for this client.

The client should be turned only when specifically ordered by the physician. Back care is provided while the client is raised from the bed by independent use of the trapeze or with adequate assistance. Weight-bearing on the affected side should be avoided until healing is complete. If the pelvic fracture is undisplaced, the client is usually allowed to ambulate using a walker or crutches to distribute the weight-bearing between the upper and lower extremities. Elimination needs may require the use of an indwelling catheter in female clients if a pelvic sling is used.

Fracture of the Hip

Hip fractures are a common form of trauma in older adults. There are 147,000 to 227,000 hip fractures annually. A hip fracture may be expected to occur in one third of women and one sixth of men older than 65 years.[17] Fractures that occur within the capsule are called *intracapsular* fractures. Intracapsular fractures are further identified by a name taken from their specific location: (1) subcapital, (2) transcervical, and (3) basilar neck. These fractures are often associated with osteoporosis and minor trauma. *Extracapsular* fractures occur below the capsule and are termed *intertrochanteric* if they occur in a region

between the greater and lesser trochanter. They are termed *subtrochanteric* if they occur in the region below the trochanter (Fig. 57-13). Extracapsular fractures are usually caused by severe direct trauma or a fall.

Clinical manifestations. The clinical manifestations of hip fractures are external rotation, shortening of the affected extremity, and severe pain and tenderness in the region of the fracture site. Displaced femoral neck fractures cause serious disruption of the blood supply to the femoral head, which can result in avascular necrosis.

Therapeutic management. Surgical repair is the preferred method of managing intracapsular and extracapsular hip fractures. Surgical treatment permits the client to be out of bed sooner and prevents the major complications associated with immobility. In contrast, treatment with traction requires 12 to 16 weeks of immobilization for healing to occur, even if the blood supply to the region is intact. Initially the affected extremity may be temporarily immobilized by either Buck's or Russell traction until the client's physical condition is stabilized and surgery can be performed. Traction also helps relieve painful muscle spasms.

The intracapsular fracture is slow to heal because of interruptions in blood supply. When avascular necrosis appears imminent, the surgeon may elect to resect the femoral head and neck and insert a femoral head prosthesis. A variety of devices in the forms of compression screws and plates, nails, and pins are available to the surgeon for the purpose of repairing hip fracture by pinning. Intracapsular fractures are usually repaired with the use of a hip prosthesis (Fig. 57-14, *A*), and extracapsular fractures are usually pinned (Fig. 57-14, *B*). The principles of client care for these procedures are similar (Table 57-11).

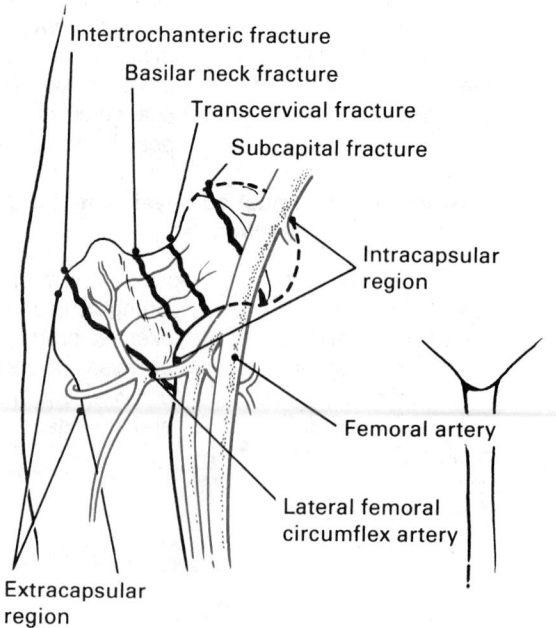

Fig. 57-13 Femur with location of various types of fracture.

Table 57-11

NURSING CARE PLAN FOR THE CLIENT WITH FRACTURE OF THE HIP

Defining Characteristics	Nursing Interventions	Evaluation Criteria

NURSING DIAGNOSIS: Pain related to edema, movement of bone fragments, muscle spasms, and ineffective pain relief and/or comfort measures

Pain descriptors, guarding, altered time perception; behaviors indicative of pain such as moaning, crying, restlessness; altered muscle tone, autonomic responses; lack of mobility	Align and position extremity and client correctly. Use gentleness when positioning or turning. Maintain constant traction forces. Administer analgesics as indicated.	Decrease in or absence of pain

NURSING DIAGNOSIS: High risk for disuse syndrome related to immobility secondary to fractured hip

Fractured bone, immobility, abnormal assessment findings related to all body systems	Foster activity to tolerance. Provide adequate hydration, nutrition, diversion. Plan passive and active range of motion and deep-breathing exercises. Turn client q 2 hr.	Absence of skin breakdown, absence of evidence of pulmonary infection or restriction of joint motion, adequate circulatory status, return of preinjury bowel status, adequate urinary output, maintenance of orientation and alertness

NURSING DIAGNOSIS: Potential complication: thromboembolic phenomenon related to immobility

Altered circulation, positive Homans' sign, edema, redness, calf pain, dyspnea, tachycardia, chest pain, petechiae	Monitor client for signs and symptoms of thromboembolic phenomenon. Apply antiembolism stockings to unaffected lower extremity. Teach resistive range of motion of unaffected extremities, especially ankle plantar flexion against footboard. With assistance, change client's position by using trapeze bar or opposite side rail every 1-2 hr.	Absence of evidence of thrombosis or embolism

NURSING DIAGNOSIS: Impaired physical mobility related to decreased muscle strength, casting, pinning, or traction

Inability to purposefully move within physical environment, limited joint range of motion, decreased muscle strength, mobility restrictions, inability to bear weight, presence of immobilizing device	Cooperate with physical therapist in muscle-strengthening program. Teach and assist client in exercise program; include resistive strengthening exercises of uninvolved lower and both upper limbs, elbow extension, shoulder depressors, and knee and hip extension.	Sufficient muscle strength to participate in gait-training program, restoration of optimal mobility

Table 57-11

 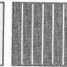

Defining Characteristics	Nursing Interventions	Evaluation Criteria
NURSING DIAGNOSIS: High risk for wound infection related to exposure to environmental pathogens and surgical procedure		
Inadequate primary and secondary defenses, trauma, increased environmental exposure	Assess wound site for erythema and drainage. Monitor temperature. Obtain wound culture, if indicated. Administer antibiotics as ordered. Use sterile technique when changing dressings or providing wound care.	Absence of evidence of wound infection, normal temperature
NURSING DIAGNOSIS: Self-care deficit: altered ambulation related to lack of knowledge regarding ambulation		
Inability to ambulate with proper, safe technique	Increase activities as tolerated. Assist client in standing at side of bed. Encourage quadriceps exercises, arm-strengthening exercises, and abdominal and gluteal contraction exercises. Instruct client about ambulatory training program. Be aware that nonweight-bearing status of involved extremity must be maintained unless changed by an order from physician. Get client out of bed and into chair, usually within 24 to 48 hours after surgery. Instruct and assist client with transfer from bed to chair. Instruct and assist client in use of ambulatory assistive devices. Explain ambulation program. Explain and demonstrate getting up and transfer and pivot activities. Teach use of ambulatory assistive device with nonweight-bearing gait.	Optimal level of function with ambulatory assistive device
NURSING DIAGNOSIS: Altered thought processes related to pain medication, change of environment, bed rest, social isolation, and decreased vision or hearing		
Impairment of ability to recall previous events, attention span, perception, judgment, and decision-making ability	Orient client to place and reason for hospitalization. Encourage visits by family and friends to provide familiar contacts. Keep side rails up if a family or staff member is not present. Keep light on at night. Minimize pain. Give careful explanation of procedures. Reinforce instructions as necessary.	Maintenance of orientation
NURSING DIAGNOSIS: Self-esteem disturbance related to uncertain future, perceived helplessness, and possible self-care deficits		
Expressions of hopelessness, despair; inability to concentrate on reading, writing, conversation; misdirected anger; extreme dependency on others	Ambulate client as prescribed and tolerated. Allow as much independence and decision making as possible. Talk about future activities with a positive attitude. Involve client and family in planning care. Plan for discharge needs.	Maintenance of optimistic attitude about recovery
NURSING DIAGNOSIS: Impaired home maintenance management related to injury, surgery, and lack of knowledge of postdischarge care		
Verbalization of concern by client or caregiver regarding ability to care for client after discharge, unavailable support system, observation of lack of knowledge regarding postdischarge care	Assess home environment. Teach client and family about proper ambulation, diet, medications, wound care, and physician follow-up. Inform about symptoms to report to physician such as fever, pain, cognitive changes. Refer for home care as needed.	Verbalization of confidence in ability to manage care postdischarge by client and family

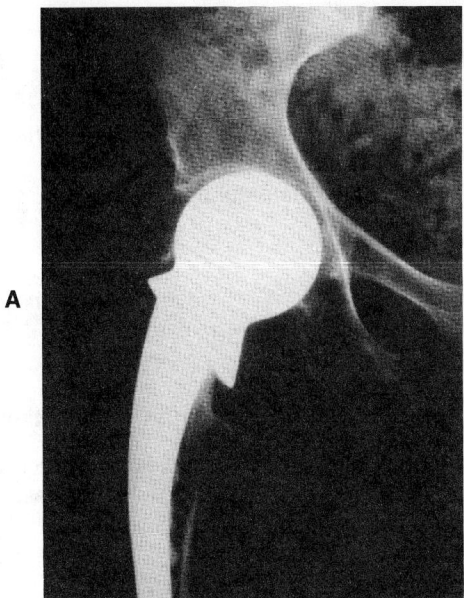

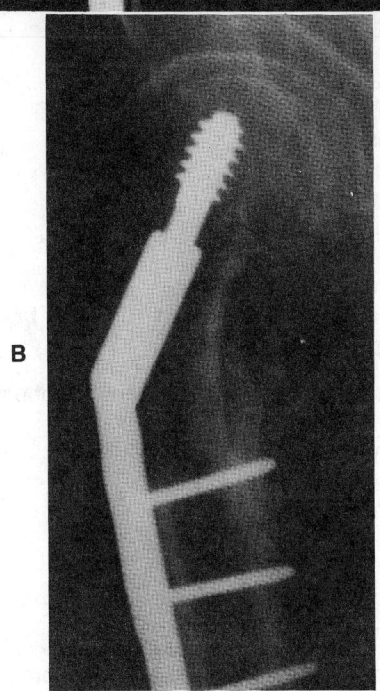

Fig. 57-14 Types of internal fixation. **A,** Femoral head prosthesis. **B,** Type of hip nail. (From Thompson JC and others: Mosby's manual of clinical nursing, St Louis, 1989, The CV Mosby Co, p 463.)

Preoperative management. Because older adults are most prone to hip fractures, chronic health problems must often be considered when planning treatment. Diabetes mellitus, hypertension, cardiac decompensation, and arthritis are chronic problems that may complicate clinical status. Surgery may be delayed until the client's general health improves.

Before surgery, severe muscle spasms can increase pain. These spasms are managed by appropriate medica-

tions, comfortable positioning unless contraindicated, and properly adjusted traction if it is being used.

Careful preoperative client education can affect future mobility. The client should know the method and frequency for exercising the unaffected leg and both arms. The client should also be shown how to use the trapeze bar and the opposite side rail to assist in changing positions. Ambulation usually begins by the second postoperative day. Practice in getting out of bed and transferring to a chair should be discussed and demonstrated before surgery. The family should be informed about the client's weight-bearing status after surgery. Plans for discharge should be discussed, and arrangements should be initiated well before the actual discharge date.

Postoperative management. The initial postoperative management of a client after surgical repair of hip fracture is similar to that for any geriatric surgical client: the nurse monitors vital signs and intake and output, supervises respiratory activities such as deep breathing and coughing, administers pain medication cautiously, and observes the dressing for signs of bleeding and infection.

In the early postoperative period there is a potential for impairment of circulation, movement, and sensation. The nurse should assess the client's toes for (1) ability to move, (2) warmth and pink color, (3) numbness or tingling, and (4) edema. Edema, which may develop after the client is out of bed, is alleviated by elevation of the leg whenever the client is in a chair. The pain resulting from poor alignment of the affected extremity can be prevented by keeping pillows (or an abductor splint) between the knees when the client is turning to either side. Sandbags and pillows are also used to prevent external rotation.

The physical therapist usually supervises active assistance exercises for the affected extremity and ambulation when the surgeon permits it. The nurse needs to monitor the client's ambulation status for proper crutch walking or use of the walker. The client must be able to use crutches or a walker before discharge.

If the hip fracture has been treated by insertion of a femoral-head prosthesis, measures to prevent dislocation must always be used (Table 57-12). The client and family must be fully aware of positions and activities that favor dislocation (flexion adduction or internal rotation). Many daily activities may reproduce these positions (e.g., putting on shoes and socks, crossing the legs or feet while seated, assuming the side-lying position incorrectly, standing up or sitting down while the body is flexed relative to the chair, sitting on low seats). Until the soft tissue surrounding the hip has healed sufficiently to stabilize the prosthesis these activities must be avoided, usually for at least 6 weeks. Sudden severe pain and extreme external rotation indicate prosthesis displacement.

In addition to teaching the client and family how to prevent prosthesis dislocation, the nurse should (1) place a large pillow between the client's legs when turning, (2) keep leg abductor splints on the client except when bathing, (3) avoid extreme hip flexion, and (4) avoid turning the client on the affected side unless approved by the surgeon.

If the hip fracture is treated by pinning, dislocation pre-

Table 57-12 Client Instructions for Femoral-Head Prosthesis

Do not

Force hip into more than 90 degrees of flexion.*

Force hip into adduction.

Force hip into internal rotation.

Cross legs.

Put on own shoes or stockings until 8 weeks after surgery.

Sit on chairs without arms to aid rising to a standing position.*

Do

Use toilet elevator on toilet seat.*

Place chair inside shower or tub and remain seated while washing.

Use pillow between legs for first 8 weeks after surgery when lying on "good" side or when supine.*

Keep hip in neutral, straight position when sitting, walking, or lying.*

Notify surgeon if severe pain, deformity, or loss of function occurs.*

Inform dentist of presence of prosthesis before dental work so that prophylactic antibiotics can be given.

*These precautions also apply after a hip pinning.

cautions are not necessary. The client is usually encouraged to be out of bed on the first postoperative day. Weight-bearing on the involved extremity is not allowed until radiographical examination indicates adequate healing, usually within 3 to 5 months.

Complications associated with femoral neck fracture include nonunion, avascular necrosis, and degenerative arthritis. As a result of an intertrochanteric fracture, the affected leg may be shortened.

The nurse must assist both the client and the family in adjusting to the restrictions and dependence imposed by the hip fracture. Depression can easily occur, but creative nursing care and awareness of the problem can do much to prevent it. The client and family may need to be informed about community referral services that can assist in the postdischarge rehabilitation phase. Hospitalization averages 7 to 10 days. Regular follow-up care for after discharge should be arranged.

Femoral Shaft Fracture

Femoral shaft fracture is a common injury occurring particularly in young adults. Severe direct force is required to produce this injury, since the femur can bend approximately 2 inches before an actual fracture occurs. The force exerted to cause the fracture frequently causes damage to the adjacent soft-tissue structures, which may be more serious than the bone injury. Displacement of the fracture fragments frequently results in open fracture and increased soft-tissue damage. This can result in considerable blood loss.

The clinical manifestations of a fracture of the femoral shaft are usually obvious. They include marked deformity and angulation, shortening of the extremity, inability to

move either the hip or knee, and pain. The common complications associated with fracture of the femoral shaft include fat embolism, nerve and vascular injury, and problems associated with union, open fracture, and soft-tissue damage.

Initial management is directed toward stabilization of the client and immobilization of the fracture. Treatment may consist of tibial pinning with balanced skeletal traction. Traction continues for 8 to 12 weeks. The nurse must encourage the client to perform exercises and range-of-motion activities for the uninvolved extremities and joints. The physician determines when active exercise can be instituted on the affected extremity. When there is sufficient clinical evidence of bone union, a hip spica cast may be applied.

Internal fixation is another way to manage a femoral fracture. It is carried out with the use of an intramedullary rod or compression plate. Internal fixation is frequently the preferred treatment because it reduces hospital stay and the complications associated with prolonged bed rest. Other indications for internal fixation are failure to obtain satisfactory reduction by nonsurgical methods and multiple associated injuries. During the postoperative phase the surgically repaired femur may be supported by suspension traction for 3 to 4 days to prevent excessive movement of the extremity and to control rotation; nonweight-bearing gait training is then begun.

Promotion and maintenance of strength in the affected extremity usually include gluteal and quadriceps exercises. It is important to ensure performance of range-of-motion and strengthening exercises for all uninvolved extremities in preparation for ambulation. The client may be immobilized in a hip spica cast and gradually progress to an articulating cast brace or may be allowed to begin nonweight-bearing activities with an ambulatory assistive device. Full weight-bearing is usually restricted until there is radiological evidence of bony union of the fracture fragments.

Fracture of the Tibia

The tibia is vulnerable to injury because it lacks anterior muscle covering, but strong force is required to produce a fractured tibia. As a result, soft-tissue damage, devascularization, and open fracture are frequent. Other complications associated with tibial fractures are compartment syndrome, fat embolism, problems associated with bony union, and possible infection associated with open fracture.

The recommended management for closed tibial fracture is closed reduction followed by immobilization in a long leg cast. Open reduction may be achieved with a compression plate. With either method of reduction, emphasis is placed on maintaining the strength of the quadriceps, since delayed union is frequent.

The neurovascular status of the affected extremity must be assessed at least every 2 hours during the first 48 hours. Clients are instructed to perform active range-of-motion exercises with all uninvolved extremities as well as exercises for the upper extremities to build the strength required for crutch walking. When the physician has determined that clients are ready for gait training, they are in-

structed in the principles of crutch walking. If the fracture is stable, partial weight-bearing is usually permissible. Compression across a stable fracture site stimulates healing. However, an unstable tibial fracture may permit only nonweight-bearing gait such as the swing-through gait. When fracture healing has progressed sufficiently (about 2 to 4 weeks), a walking heel is applied to the cast and full weight-bearing is allowed.

Stable Vertebral Fractures

A stable fracture of the vertebral column is usually caused by motor vehicle accidents, falls, diving, or athletic injuries. A stable fracture is one in which the fracture or the fragment is not likely to move or cause spinal cord damage. This type of injury is frequently confined to the anterior element (vertebral body) of the spinal column in the lumbar region. It involves the cervical and thoracic regions less frequently. The vertebral bodies are usually protected from displacement by the intact spinal ligaments.

Most clients with spinal fractures have stable fractures and experience only brief periods of disability. If the ligamentous structures are significantly disrupted, however, dislocation of the vertebral structures may occur, resulting in instability and injury to the spinal cord (unstable fracture). The most common injury to the vertebral body is the compression type of fracture caused by excessive vertical load, such as a severe fall on the buttocks or injury resulting from sudden flexion that forces the spine beyond its normal range of motion. The most serious complication of vertebral fractures is fracture displacement, which can cause damage to the spinal cord (see Chapter 55). Although stable vertebral fractures are not associated with abnormal spinal cord pathology, all spinal injuries should initially be considered unstable and potentially serious.

The client usually complains of pain and tenderness in the affected region of the spine. Compression fractures are associated with a gibbous deformity (flexion angulation localized to one vertebral level). This deformity may be noted during the physical examination. Bowel and bladder dysfunction may be an indication of a temporary interruption of the sympathetic nervous system or injury to the spinal cord.

The overall goal in management of stable fractures of a vertebral body is to keep the spine in good alignment until union has been accomplished. Many nursing interventions are aimed at assessing for the possibility of spinal cord trauma. Vital signs, color, and bowel and bladder function should be evaluated regularly, as should the motor and sensory status of the peripheral nerves distal to the injured region. Any deterioration in the client's neurovascular status should be reported promptly.

Treatment includes support, heat, and traction. The client is usually placed in a standard hospital bed with firm support from the mattress or a bedboard. The aim is to support the spinal cord, relax muscles, and release any compression on nerve roots. Heat and traction may be used to relieve muscle spasms resulting from the fracture, and traction may be used to reduce and immobilize fracture fragments. A trapeze bar is not usually allowed because its use disrupts alignment and immobilization. Both

an upright position and turning of the torso are prohibited. When turning, the client should be taught to keep the spine straight by turning shoulders and pelvis together. Nursing assistance is necessary for the client to turn in this "log-rolling" fashion.

Several days after the initial injury, the physician may apply a specially constructed orthotic device, a jacket cast, or a removable corset if there is no evidence of neurological deficit. This immobilizes the spine in the fracture area but allows client mobility. The client is discharged after (1) regaining ambulation skills, (2) learning care of the cast or orthotic device, and (3) learning how to cope with interferences in safety and security imposed by injury and treatment.

Facial Fractures

Any bone of the face can be fractured as a result of trauma. The primary concern after a facial injury is to establish and maintain a patent airway and to provide adequate ventilation by removal of foreign material and blood and by suctioning. An artificial airway (tracheostomy) may be needed if a patent airway cannot be maintained. Hemorrhage is controlled by pressure packing, and a physician fixates the fracture. Table 57-13 describes the clinical manifestations of more common facial fractures.

Concurrent soft-tissue injury often makes assessment of a facial injury difficult. Oral and maxillofacial examinations should be performed after the client has been stabilized and any life-threatening situations have been treated.

An x-ray film documents the extent of the injury. Computerized tomography (CT) imaging is most valuable for midface injuries. The CT scan can demonstrate air or hemorrhage in the cranium, orbits, and soft tissues.[18]

Injury to the eye must be suspected when a facial injury occurs, particularly if the injury is near the orbit. Unless a global rupture is suspected (because the globe is soft to palpation), the eyes should be measured for intraocular pressure.[19] If the intraocular pressure is elevated or uneven, the client should be seen by an ophthalmologist.

Specific treatment of a facial fracture depends on the site and extent of the fracture and the associated soft tissue injury. Immobilization and/or stabilization may be necessary. (Mandibular fractures are discussed in Chapter 34.)

Table 57-13 Clinical Manifestations of Facial Fractures

Fracture	Clinical Manifestation
Frontal bone	Rapid edema that may mask underlying fractures
Periorbital	Possible frontal sinus involvement
Nasal	Displacement of nasal bones, epistaxis
Zygomatic arch	Depression of zygomatic arch
Maxilla	Segmental motion of maxilla
Mandible	Dental fractures, bleeding, limited motion of mandible

The client who sustains a facial fracture requires sensitive nursing care, since alteration in appearance after the trauma may be drastic. Edema and discoloration subside with time, but concurrent soft-tissue injuries may result in permanent scarring. Attention to maintenance of a patent airway and adequate nutrition are ongoing concerns of the nurse throughout the recovery period.

OSTEOMYELITIS
Etiology and Pathophysiology

Osteomyelitis is an infection of bone by direct or indirect invasion by an organism. Direct entry results from contamination as a result of an open fracture or surgical intervention. Indirect inoculation results from a bloodborne infection from a distant site such as infected tonsils or furuncles. The most common infecting organism is *Staphylococcus aureus*. Gram-negative bacteria alone or mixed with gram-positive organisms account for one third to one half of the pathogenic strains.[20] The course and virulence of osteomyelitis are influenced by the blood supply to the affected bone. The widespread use of antibiotics in conjunction with surgical treatment has significantly reduced the mortality rate associated with osteomyelitis. The incidence and morbidity rates remain relatively unchanged, however, because new, drug-resistant strains of organisms have developed.

The *indirect-entry* variety of osteomyelitis (also called *hematogenous*) most frequently affects growing bone in boys and is associated with local trauma. The most common sites of indirect-entry osteomyelitis are the long bones of the leg, although any bone can be involved.

The *direct-entry* type of osteomyelitis can occur at any age when there is an open wound. After gaining entrance to the bone by way of arterial supply, the bacteria lodge in an area of bone in which circulation slows, usually the metaphysis. The locus of bacteria grows, resulting in an increase in pressure because of the nonexpanding container of tubular bone. This increasing pressure eventually leads to ischemia and vascular compromise. Once ischemia occurs, the bone dies. The area of devitalized bone eventually separates from the surrounding living bone, forming *sequestra*. These sequestra form havens for bacteria, and chronic osteomyelitis develops.

Once formed, a sequestrum continues to be an infected island of bone, surrounded by pus and unreachable by any bloodborne antibiotics or leukocytes. It enlarges and serves as a source of bacteria for metastasis to other sites, including the lungs and brain. Two situations are possible. The sequestrum may extrude through a defect in tubular bone; however, this is hindered by the formation of new bone laid down by the elevated periosteum called *involucrum*. Once outside the bone, the sequestrum may revascularize and undergo removal by normal defense processes. The other possibility is surgical removal. Unless resolved naturally or surgically, the necrotic sequestrum may develop a sinus tract, resulting in chronic wound drainage.

Wound culture determines the causative organism. A bone or tissue biopsy may also be necessary to determine the causative agent. The client's blood cultures are frequently positive. An elevated leukocyte count and sedimentation rate may also be found. Radiological signs suggestive of osteomyelitis usually do not appear until 10 to 21 days after the appearance of clinical symptoms, by which time the disease will have progressed. Radionuclide bone scans can establish the diagnosis within 24 to 72 hours.

Acute osteomyelitis refers to the initial infection or an infection of less than 1 month in duration. *Chronic osteomyelitis* refers to a bone infection that persists for longer than 4 weeks or an infection that has failed to respond to the initial course of antibiotic therapy.

Chronic osteomyelitis can represent either a continuous, persistent problem or a process of exacerbations and quiescence. It results from inadequately treated acute osteomyelitis. Pus accumulates, causing ischemia of the bone. Over time, granulation tissue turns to scar tissue. This avascular scar tissue provides an ideal site for bacterial growth and is impenetrable to antibiotics.

Therapeutic Management

Vigorous antibiotic therapy is the treatment of choice for acute osteomyelitis, as long as ischemia has not occurred. Wound cultures should be taken before antibiotic therapy is initiated so that specific antibiotic therapy can be determined by sensitivity studies. If antibiotic therapy is not started early in the course of the illness, surgical decompression is usually necessary to relieve pressure within the bone and prevent ischemia. Some type of immobilization for the affected part is usually indicated. Oral antibiotic therapy is usually continued for 4 to 8 weeks after discharge.

The most serious and potentially fatal complication of osteomyelitis is the development of overwhelming sepsis from metastasis of bacteria to other sites. Pathophysiological fractures may occur through weakened, devitalized bone. Soft tissue and bone healing occur slowly in the presence of infection, and subsequent deformity of the extremity may develop.

Treatment for chronic osteomyelitis includes surgical removal of poorly vascularized tissue and dead bone as well as extended use of antibiotics. After surgical debridement of devitalized and infected tissue, the wound may be closed, and a suction irrigation system for removal of any devitalized tissues remaining in the wound area is inserted. Regional perfusion involving constant irrigation of the affected bone with antibiotics is usually initiated. Hyperbaric oxygen therapy may be attempted when available.

Treatment for chronic osteomyelitis previously involved an extended hospital stay for intravenous (IV) antibiotic treatment or stabilization of the client and discharge with IV antibiotics. Oral antibiotics have not been successful due to poor penetration into organic bone. Currently, two new oral antibiotics, enoxacin and ciprofloxacin, are being used successfully to treat osteomyelitis, and they show good bone penetration.[21] Enoxacin is an investigational drug awaiting approval by the Food and Drug Administration.

Saucerization, a type of decompression surgery, removes a window (saucer) of bone to decrease pressure. Skin and bone grafting may be necessary if destruction is

extensive.[22] Antibiotic-impregnated beads may be surgically implanted at the time of debridement to combat the infection.[23] Infection and bone destruction may be so extensive that amputation of the extremity is necessary to preserve life.

■ Nursing Management of Osteomyelitis

The nursing management of the client with osteomyelitis is challenging and demanding. Often a prolonged hospital stay is required to ensure adequate treatment.

Nursing assessment

The clinical manifestations of osteomyelitis are systemic and local. Subjective and objective data that should be obtained from an individual with osteomyelitis are presented in Table 57-14.

Nursing diagnoses

Nursing diagnoses are determined when the problem and etiological factors are supported by clinical data. Nursing diagnoses related to osteomyelitis may include, but are not limited to, those presented in Table 57-15.

Nursing interventions

The involved extremity should be handled carefully to avoid excessive manipulation that increases pain and can possibly cause pathological fractures. Various types of

---

Table 57-14

Nursing Assessment of the Client with Osteomyelitis

SUBJECTIVE DATA

History
Bone trauma, open fracture, bone surgery, open and/or
  puncture wounds, other acute infections (e.g., strep
  throat, bacterial pneumonia, sinusitis, skin or tooth infec-
  tions, chronic urinary tract infections)
Medications
IV drug abuse, use of analgesics and antibiotics
General
Fever, chills, weakness, malaise
Pain
Increase in pain with movement of affected bone
Musculoskeletal
Muscle spasms around infected bone

OBJECTIVE DATA

General
Restlessness, irritability; high, spiking temperatures
Integumentary
Diaphoresis, erythema over infected bone
Musculoskeletal
Local tenderness, edema, warmth; restricted movement;
  wound drainage; spontaneous fractures
Possible findings
Leukocytosis, positive blood and wound cultures, elevated
  erythrocyte sedimentation rate; rarefaction with presence
  of sequestrum and involucrum on radiographs and radio-
  nuclide bone scans

---

sterile dressings are used to contain the exudate from draining wounds. Besides protecting the wound area, dressings are also used as adjuncts in the mechanical debridement of devitalized tissue from the wound site when they are removed. Types of dressings used include dry, sterile dressings, dressings saturated in saline or antibiotic solution, and wet-to-dry dressings. Soiled dressings should be handled carefully to prevent cross-contamination of the wound or spread of the infection to other clients. When the dressing is changed, sterile technique is essential; it should always include sterile dressing sets, gloves, and surgical cap, gown, and mask to reduce wound contamination from external sources.

Good body alignment and frequent position changes prevent complications and promote comfort. Flexion deformity, especially of the hip or knee, is a common sequela of osteomyelitis of the lower extremity because the client frequently positions the affected extremity in a flexed position to promote comfort. This can cause contracture, which may progress to a deformity. Foot drop can develop quickly in the lower extremity if the foot is not correctly supported. A splint is frequently applied to the involved extremity in an attempt to maintain immobilization, support, and comfort. The client should be instructed to avoid any activities such as exercise or heat application that increase circulation and serve as stimuli to the spread of infection.

Clients are frightened and discouraged because of the serious nature of the disease, systemic illness, pain, and the length and cost of treatment. Continued psychological support is an integral part of nursing management.

If the osteomyelitis becomes chronic, clients need physical and psychological support for a prolonged period. They may become suspicious and hostile toward the care providers when treatment plans do not effect a cure. Well-informed clients are better able to participate in decisions and cooperate in treatment plans.

AMPUTATION

During the past 20 years, major advances have been made in surgical amputation techniques, prosthetic design, and rehabilitation programs. These advances are enabling amputees to return to productive and satisfying social roles. There are an estimated 400,000 amputees in the United States, with an annual increase of 20,000. The middle and older age groups have the highest incidence of amputation because of the effects of peripheral vascular disease, especially atherosclerosis and diabetes mellitus. Traumatic injury is the usual cause for amputation in the younger adult. Amputation is required more often in persons engaged in hazardous occupations. The incidence in men is greater, since men are more often involved in such occupations.

Clinical Indications

The clinical features that indicate the need for an amputation depend on the underlying diseases or traumas. Common indications for amputation include circulatory impairment resulting from a peripheral vascular disorder, traumatic and thermal injuries, malignant tumors, uncontrolled

Table 57-15

 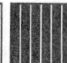

NURSING CARE PLAN FOR THE CLIENT WITH OSTEOMYELITIS

Defining Characteristics	Nursing Interventions	Evaluation Criteria
NURSING DIAGNOSIS: Pain related to ineffective pain control and/or comfort measures and inflammatory process secondary to infection		
Pain descriptors, guarding; altered time perception; behaviors indicative of pain such as moaning, crying, restlessness; altered muscle tone, autonomic responses; decreased activity	Avoid activities that increase circulation, such as exercise or application of heat. Use gentle handling and support when moving extremity. Maintain client's body in correct alignment and positioning. Keep client in bed. Avoid jarring bed. Use bed cradle if covers cause discomfort. Give analgesics as indicated.	Decrease in or absence of pain
NURSING DIAGNOSIS: High risk for hyperthermia related to infection		
Fever, restlessness, diaphoresis, chills, altered time perception, confusion	Take temperature q 4 hr. Provide comfort with cool environment, light clothing and bedding, antipyretic drugs as ordered, and sponge bath or tub bath. Prevent dehydration from insensible fluid loss by offering fluids every hr and by observing skin turgor and moistness of mucous membranes.	Normal temperature, minimal discomfort, absence of chilling or dehydration, evidence of effective antibiotic therapy
NURSING DIAGNOSIS: Fluid volume excess related to inflammatory process and immobility		
Edema, redness, warmth in affected area	Measure circumference of affected extremity daily. Elevate affected extremity unless contraindicated. Assess peripheral pulse of affected extremity every shift.	Decrease in or absence of edema in affected extremity
NURSING DIAGNOSIS: High risk for infection transmission related to contaminated wound drainage		
Open, draining wound; inadequate asepsis by health care providers	Follow hospital procedures for isolation techniques if indicated. Use proper technique for dressing changes and disposal of soiled dressings.	Absence of transmission of infection
NURSING DIAGNOSIS: Ineffective individual coping related to isolation, hospitalization, immobility, perceived powerlessness, and uncertain outcome		
Expressions of hopelessness; inability to concentrate on writing, reading, conversation; continual questioning of self-worth, withdrawal from others; misdirected anger; irritability; extreme dependency on others	Allow client and family to participate in care and decision making. Encourage client to verbalize concerns. Keep client informed of treatment plans and progress. Teach healthy coping behaviors. Visit client frequently and provide diversion.	Optimistic attitude toward recovery, demonstration of effective coping strategies
NURSING DIAGNOSIS: Impaired physical mobility related to limited use of affected extremity secondary to pain and edema		
Inability or unwillingness to move purposefully within environment	Assist client as needed. Increase mobility as ordered and tolerated. Provide support and encouragement.	Consistent increase in mobility and range of motion with minimal pain or discomfort

Continued.

Table 57-15

 NURSING CARE PLAN FOR THE CLIENT WITH OSTEOMYELITIS—cont'd

Defining Characteristics	Nursing Interventions	Evaluation Criteria
NURSING DIAGNOSIS: Impaired home management related to lack of knowledge regarding long-term management of osteomyelitis		
Verbalization of concern regarding home care by client or family members, need to learn new knowledge or skills for home management	Provide information and instruction regarding wound care, aseptic technique, and dressing disposal. Review medication regimen including schedule, name, dosage, purpose, and side effects. Stress importance of proper diet, rest, physician follow-up, and physical rehabilitation.	Verbalization of confidence in ability to carry out home management routine by client and/or family member, demonstration of ability to perform necessary procedures such as sterile dressing change

Table 57-16

 Diagnostic and Therapeutic Management: Amputation

DIAGNOSTIC

Physical examination
    Physical appearance of soft tissues
    Skin temperature
    Sensory function
    Presence of peripheral pulses
Arteriography
Thermography
Plethysmography
Transcutaneous ultrasonic Doppler recordings

THERAPEUTIC
Medical

Appropriate management of underlying disease process
Stabilization of trauma victim

Surgical

Appropriate type of amputation, leaving as long a stump as
    possible
Stump management
    Immediate prosthetic fitting
    Delayed prosthetic fitting

Rehabilitation

Coordination of prosthesis-fitting and gait-training activities
Coordination of muscle-strengthening and physical therapy
    regimens

or widespread infection of the extremity, and congenital disorders. These conditions may manifest as loss of sensation, inadequate circulation, pallor, sweating, and local or systemic infection. Although pain is often present, it is not usually the primary reason for an amputation. The underlying problem dictates whether the amputation is performed as elective or emergency surgery.

Therapeutic Management

The types of diagnostic studies to be done depend on the underlying problem that makes the amputation necessary. The white blood cell (WBC) count is often elevated, indicating infection. Vascular studies such as arteriography provide information about circulatory status of the extremity. The potential for revascularization surgery rather than amputation can be assessed on the basis of vascular studies. If the amputation is considered elective, the client's general health is carefully monitored. Chronic illnesses and infection are monitored closely. The client and family should be helped to understand the need for the amputation and be assured that rehabilitation can result in an active, useful life. If the amputation is done on an emergency basis as a result of trauma, the management is physically and emotionally more complicated (Table 57-16).

The goal of amputation surgery is to preserve extremity length and function. This improves the possibility of good prosthetic, cosmetic, and functional satisfaction. (Levels of amputation of upper and lower extremities are illustrated in Fig. 57-15.) The type of amputation depends on the reason for the surgery. A *closed amputation* is performed to create a weight-bearing stump; an anterior skin flap with dissected soft-tissue padding covers the bone stump. The skin flap is sutured posteriorly so that it will not be in a position to bear weight. Special care is necessary to prevent the accumulation of drainage, which can

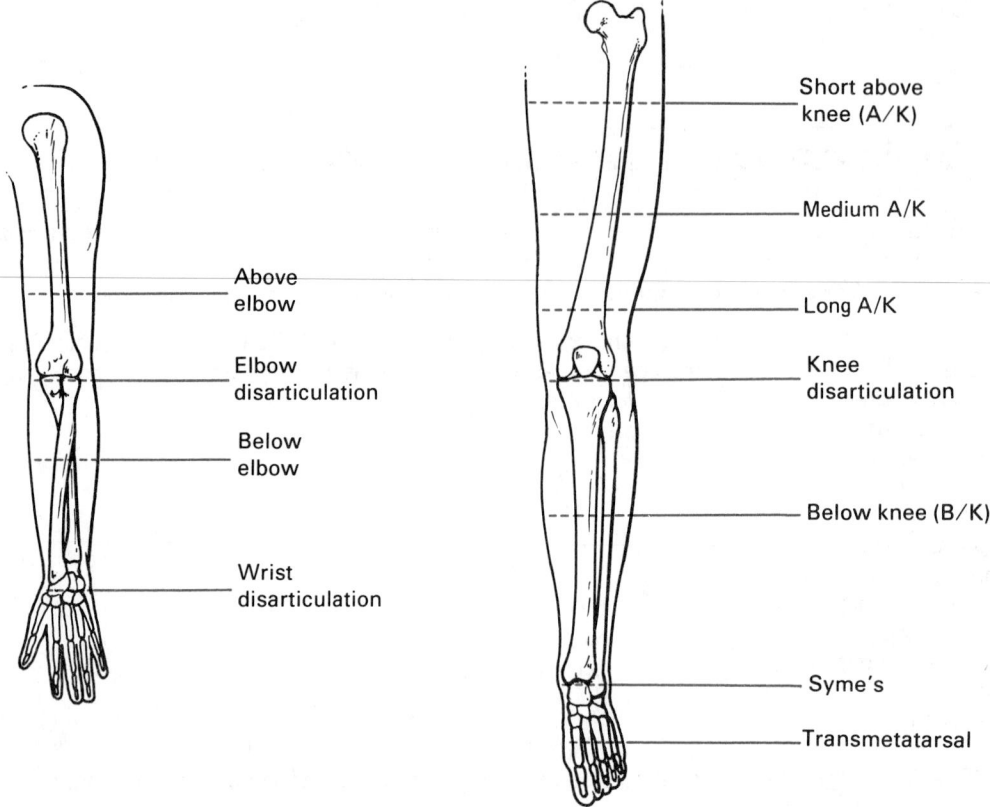

Fig. 57-15 Location and description of amputation sites of the upper and lower extremity.

produce pressure and harbor infection. *Disarticulation* is an amputation performed through a joint.

An *open amputation* leaves a stump surface that is not covered with skin. This type of surgery is generally indicated for control of actual or potential infection. The wound is usually closed later by a second surgical procedure or closed by skin traction surrounding the stump. This type of amputation is often referred to as a *guillotine amputation.*

■ Nursing Management of Amputation

Nursing assessment

Preexisting illnesses must be adequately assessed, since most amputations are performed because of neurological and/or vascular deficits. Assessment of the neurological and vascular status is an important part of this assessment process (see Chapters 26 and 50).

Nursing diagnoses

Nursing diagnoses are determined when the problem and etiological factors are supported by clinical data. Nursing diagnoses related to the client with an amputation may include, but are not limited to, those presented in Table 57-17.

Nursing interventions

Health promotion and maintenance. Most lower-limb amputations result from peripheral vascular disease, and most upper-limb amputations result from severe trauma.

This knowledge directs client education related to prevention of amputation. Control of causative illnesses such as peripheral vascular disease, diabetes mellitus, chronic osteomyelitis, and skin ulcers can eliminate or delay the need for amputation. Clients with these problems need to be taught to carefully examine their lower extremities daily for signs of impending problems. If clients cannot assume this responsibility, a family member should be instructed on the procedure. Clients and their families need to be instructed to report to the health care provider immediately if problems such as change in skin color or temperature, decrease or absence of sensation, tingling, pain, and the presence of a lesion occur.

Instruction in proper safety precautions in recreation and in the performance of hazardous work is a nursing responsibility of major importance. Preventing limb mutilation and subsequent amputation is one of the serious consequences of trauma avoided through such instruction.

Acute intervention. The nurse must recognize the tremendous psychological and social implications of a lower-limb amputation for the client. The disruption in body image caused by an amputation often causes a client to go through psychological stages similar to the grieving process. Allowing the client to go through a period of depression and recognizing it as a normal consequence of the amputation may do much to aid the client's acceptance of the amputation. The client's family must also be helped to

Table 57-17

 NURSING CARE PLAN FOR THE CLIENT WITH AN AMPUTATION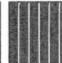

Defining Characteristics	Nursing Interventions	Evaluation Criteria
NURSING DIAGNOSIS: Body-image disturbance related to amputation and impaired mobility		
Verbalization of concerns about change in lifestyle, negative feelings about body, feelings of helplessness, hopelessness, powerlessness; change in social involvement or social relationships; preoccupation with loss of body part; refusal to verify actual change in body; refusal to touch or look at involved area	Provide psychological support, active listening, and encouragement. Assist client to be as independent as possible.	Acceptance of changed body image
NURSING DIAGNOSIS: High risk for impaired skin integrity related to immobility, improperly fitting prosthesis, and disease process		
Reddened skin area, verbalization of pain or discomfort in area, altered sensation, presence of prosthesis	Examine potential pressure areas regularly. Apply only clean, dry wrap to affected extremity; use proper technique. Change position regularly.	Absence of evidence of skin breakdown
NURSING DIAGNOSIS: Pain related to phantom limb sensation, surgical procedure, and ineffective comfort measures		
Pain descriptors, guarding; altered time perception, behaviors indicative of pain such as moaning, crying, restlessness; altered muscle tone, autonomic responses	Administer analgesics as ordered. Apply transcutaneous electrical nerve stimulation unit. Encourage position changes. Provide opportunities for distraction.	Reduction or absence of pain
NURSING DIAGNOSIS: Impaired physical mobility related to amputation of lower limb and decreased muscle strength secondary to immobility		
Inability to move purposefully within physical environment, limited joint range of motion, decreased muscle strength, mobility restrictions	Teach gait-training principles. Adjust prosthesis as needed.	Resumption of normal gait pattern, arm movements

Table 57-17

NURSING CARE PLAN FOR THE CLIENT WITH AN AMPUTATION—cont'd

Defining Characteristics	Nursing Interventions	Evaluation Criteria
NURSING DIAGNOSIS: Activity intolerance related to prolonged immobility, weakness, and fatigue		
Verbal reports of fatigue or weakness, abnormal physiological responses to activity	Encourage active range-of-motion exercise of joints. Perform resistive exercises for unaffected extremities. Plan progressive increase in activity with frequent rest periods. Encourage active participation in activities of daily living and exercises. Provide positive support. Monitor vital signs during activity.	Normal physiological response to activity
NURSING DIAGNOSIS: High risk for impaired physical mobility related to joint contractures secondary to improper positioning and immobility		
Malaligned stump, inability to move stump through range of motion	Plan regular range-of-motion exercises. Position stump in correct alignment. Perform passive or active exercises. Instruct client in exercise techniques.	No decrease in range of motion of extremities
NURSING DIAGNOSIS: High risk for trauma from falling related to change in center of balance, physical weakness, and impaired mobility secondary to amputation		
Impairment of judgement, previous trauma, lack of safety precautions, inability to adapt to loss of limb	Teach client gait-training principles. Offer assistance as needed. Provide safe environment. Teach muscle-strengthening exercises.	Absence of falls or other incidents of trauma
NURSING DIAGNOSIS: Ineffective individual coping related to effects of amputation on lifestyle		
Verbalization of inability to cope, anxiety, fear, anger, irritability, tension; inability to meet role expectations; altered societal participation; ineffective or inappropriate use of defense mechanisms; change in usual communication patterns; excess food intake, alcohol consumption, smoking; digestive, appetite disturbance; chronic fatigue or disturbance in sleep pattern	Explain factors that may contribute to development of maladaptive coping behavior. Describe and role play use of therapeutic coping skills and activities that enhance self-esteem and social interaction.	Absence of development of chronic sick-role behavior, use of positive coping strategies

work through the process to arrive at a realistic and positive attitude about the future. The reasons for an amputation and the rehabilitation potential depend on age, diagnosis, occupation, personality, resources, and support systems.

PREOPERATIVE CARE. Before surgery, the nurse should reinforce information the client and family have received about the reasons for the amputation, the proposed prosthesis, and the mobility training program. In addition to the usual preoperative instructions, the client undergoing an amputation has special education needs. To meet these needs, the nurse must know the level of amputation, the type of postsurgical dressing to be applied, and the type of prosthesis planned. The client should receive instruction in the performance of upper-extremity exercises such as push-ups in bed or in a wheelchair to promote arm strength. This is essential for later crutch walking and gait training. If possible, the nurse should instruct the client in the technique of crutch walking and the type of gait that will be used after surgery and during gait training with the prosthesis. General postoperative nursing care should be discussed, including positioning, support, and stump care. If a compression bandage is to be used after surgery, the client should be instructed about its purpose and how it will be applied. If an immediate prosthesis is planned, the general ambulation program should be discussed.

Clients need to be warned that they may feel as though their amputated limbs are still present after surgery. This *phantom sensation* (a sensation of aching, tingling, or itching in the amputated limb) usually disappears but may cause clients grave concern unless they are forewarned. The difference between phantom limb pain and phantom sensation should be distinguished for the client (see Chapter 51). As recovery and ambulation progress, phantom limb sensation usually subsides.

POSTOPERATIVE CARE. General postoperative care for the client who has had an amputation depends largely on the client's general state of health, the reason for the amputation, and the client's age. Nursing care must be individualized on the basis of these factors. For example, an older adult client needs particularly careful monitoring of respiratory status; a victim of a motorcycle accident may need careful neurological monitoring.

Basic goals of nursing care for a client who has undergone an amputation are to assist the client in the grieving process and regaining function and to prevent complications such as infection and contractures. Hemorrhage is another possible complication after amputation. Regular assessment of the surgical area is essential.

If an immediate postoperative prosthesis has been applied, the nurse must monitor vital signs carefully, since the surgical site is heavily covered and may not be visible.

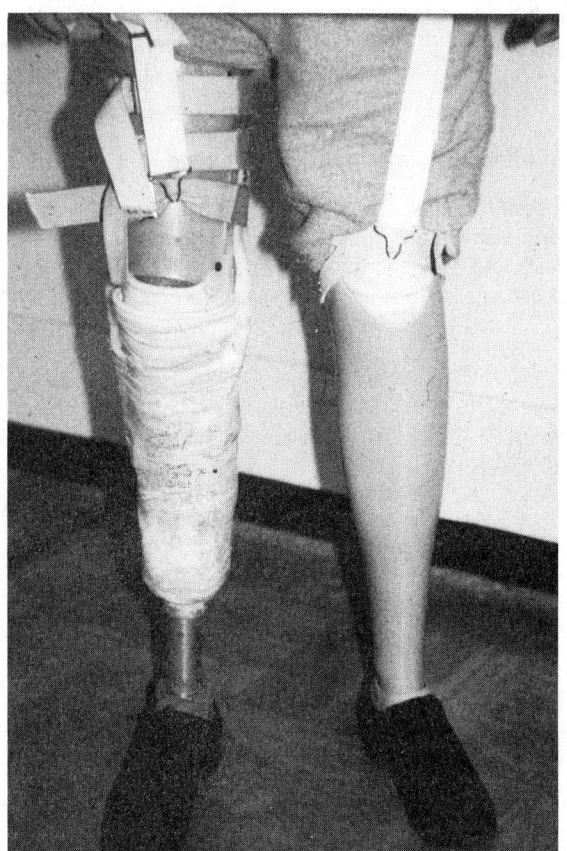

Fig. 57-16 Two types of prosthesis. Patellar tendon-bearing type, below-the-knee prosthesis with cuff suspension *(left)*. Early-fitting below-the-knee rigid plaster dressing with pylon *(right)*.

A surgical tourniquet must always be available for emergency use. If hemorrhage occurs, the surgeon should be notified immediately and efforts to control the hemorrhage should begin at once.

The surgeon must decide the type of prosthetic fitting that will be used after surgery. The *immediate prosthetic fitting,* often called the *immediate postsurgical fitting* or the *immediate postoperative fitting,* is done in the operating room after the amputation. A rigid plastic bandage is applied around the closed stump with a prosthetic pylon and foot-ankle assembly (Fig. 57-16). While the client is still anesthetized, the prosthetic pylon and ankle-foot assembly are aligned and adjusted to provide a smooth gait and to avoid excessive pressure on the stump area. A strap is placed on the proximal anterior surface of the rigid plaster bandage and attached to a waistband to prevent slippage. The main advantages of this device are reduction of edema and the psychological benefit of early ambulation. A disadvantage is the inability to directly visualize the surgical site.

The *delayed prosthetic fitting* may be the best choice for certain clients. Clients who have had amputations above the knee or below the elbow, older adults, debilitated individuals, and those with infection usually have delayed prosthetic fittings. The appropriate time for use of a prosthesis depends on satisfactory healing of the stump as well as on the general condition of the client. A temporary prosthesis may be used for partial weight-bearing once the sutures are removed. Barring any problems, clients can bear full weight on permanent prostheses by 3 months after amputation.

Not all clients are candidates for a prosthesis. It is important that the surgeon discuss ambulation possibilities frankly with the client and family. The seriously ill or debilitated client may not have the energy required to use a prosthesis. Mobility with a wheelchair may be the most realistic goal for this type of client.

Therapeutic management also includes the direction and coordination of the rehabilitation program for the amputee. Success depends on the physical and emotional health of the client. Chronic illness and debility complicate aggressive rehabilitation efforts.

Flexion contractures may delay the rehabilitation process. The most common and debilitating contracture is hip flexion. Hip adduction contracture is rare. Clients should avoid sitting in a chair with hips flexed for long intervals to prevent flexion contractures. Unless specifically contraindicated, clients should lie on their abdomens for 30 minutes three to four times each day and position the hips in extension while prone.

Proper stump bandaging fosters shaping and modeling for eventual prosthesis fitting (Fig. 57-17). The physician usually orders a compression bandage to be applied immediately after surgery to support the soft tissues, reduce edema, hasten healing, minimize pain, and promote stump shrinkage and maturation. This bandage may be an elastic roll applied to the stump or a stump shrinker—an elastic stocking that fits over the stump and lower trunk area.[24]

The compression bandage is initially worn at all times except during physical therapy and bathing. The bandage is taken off and reapplied several times daily, and care is taken so that it is applied snugly but not so tight as to interfere with circulation. Shrinker bandages should be washed and changed daily. After the stump has matured, it is bandaged only when the client is not wearing the prosthesis. The client should be instructed to avoid dangling the stump over the bedside to minimize edema formation.

As the client's overall condition improves, the nurse begins instruction in the principles and techniques of transferring from bed to chair and back. Active exercises and conditioning are essential in developing ambulation skills. The exercise regimen is normally started under the supervision of the physician and the physical therapist. The nurse must have a clear understanding of the exercise regimen to reinforce it and ensure that the exercises are performed correctly. Active range-of-motion exercises of all joints should be started as soon after surgery as the client's pain tolerance and medical status permit. In preparation for mobility, the client needs to increase triceps strength, shoulder depressors, and lower-limb support and to learn balance of the altered body. The loss of the weight of a limb requires adaptation of the client's proprioceptive mechanisms to prevent falls and frustration.

Crutch walking is started as soon as clients are physically able. If they have had immediate postsurgical fittings, orders related to weight-bearing must be carefully followed to avoid disruption of the skin flap and delay of the training process. Initial periods of ambulation should not exceed 5 minutes to prevent edema.

Before discharge the client and family need careful instruction related to stump care, ambulation, prevention of contractures, recognition of complications, exercise, and follow-up care. Table 57-18 outlines appropriate stump care.

Rehabilitative management. When the stump has healed satisfactorily and is well molded, the client is ready for fitting a prosthesis. Matching a client with a suitable prosthesis involves many factors, including age, general health, intelligence, motivation, occupation, and finances. After the physician makes the recommendation, the client is referred to a prosthetist, who initially makes a mold of the stump and measures landmarks for the fabrication of the prosthesis. The molded stump socket allows the stump to fit snugly into the prosthesis. The stump is covered with a stump sock to ensure good fit and prevent skin breakdown. The stump may continue to shrink, causing a loose fit, in which case a new socket has to be fabricated. The client may need to have the prosthesis adjusted to prevent rubbing and friction between the stump and the socket. Excessive movement of a loose prosthesis can cause severe skin irritation and breakdown.

The prosthesis is fitted by the prosthetist, who may also train the amputee to use it. It is important for the nurse to be familiar with the training program to encourage and assist the client. Learning to use a prosthesis is frustrating, and the client may easily become discouraged. The nurse must continually offer support until the client is able to manage alone.

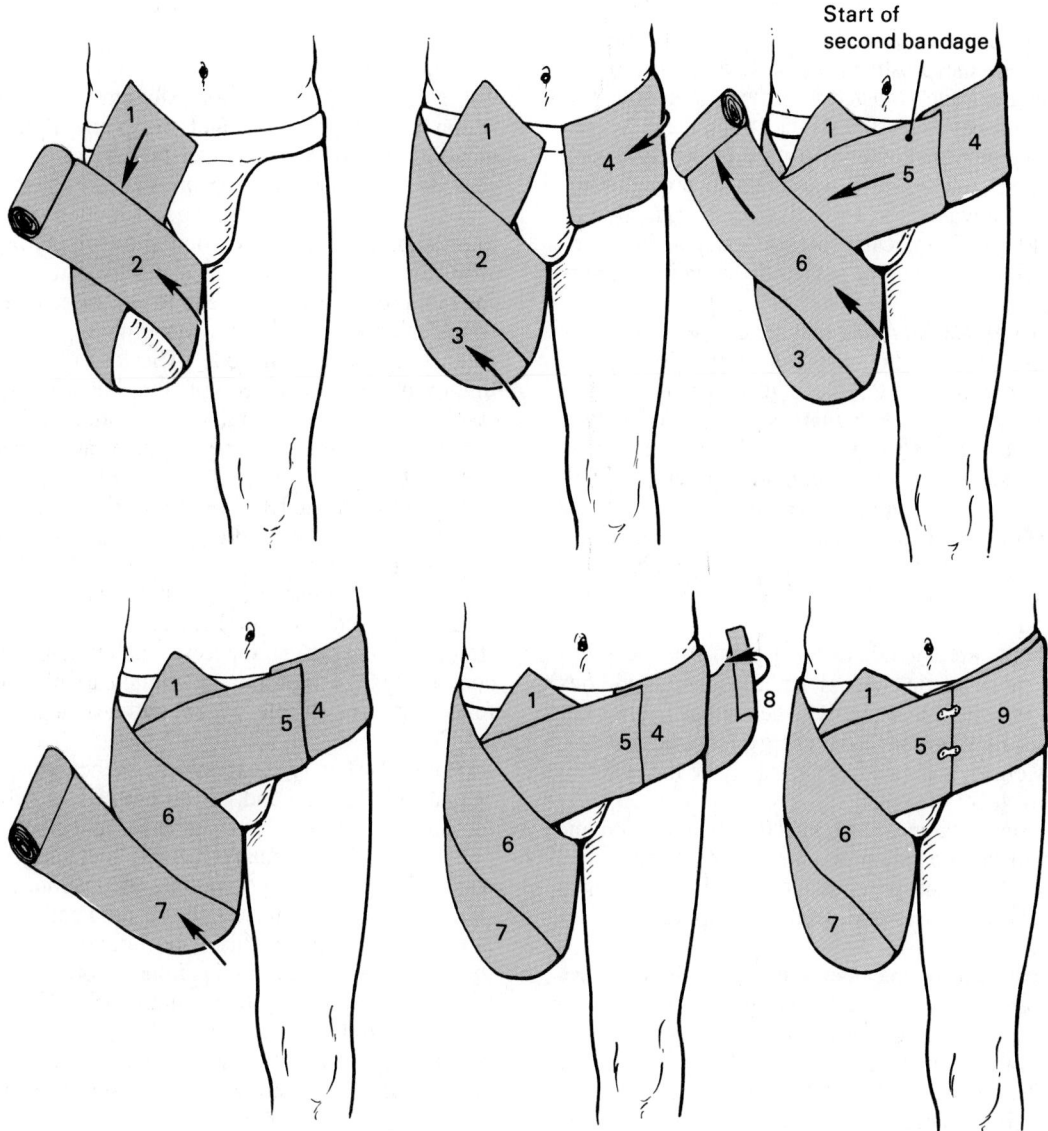

Fig. 57-17 Stump bandaging for the above-the-knee stump. Figure-eight style covers progressive areas of stump. Two bandages are required.

Table 57-18 Client Instruction for Stump Care

Inspect the stump daily for signs of skin irritation, especially redness.

Discontinue use of the prosthesis if an irritation develops. Have the area checked before resuming use of the prosthesis.

Wash thoroughly each night with warm water and a bacteriostatic soap. Rinse thoroughly and dry gently. Expose the stump to air for 20 minutes.

Do not use any substance such as lotions, alcohol, powders, or oil unless prescribed by the physician.

If a stump sock is worn, wear only the one supplied by the prosthetist. Change daily. Launder in a mild soap, squeeze, and lay flat to dry.

Artificial limbs become an integral part of the client's body image. Proper care ensures their long life and useful functioning. The client should be instructed to clean the socket daily with a mild soap and rinse thoroughly to remove irritants. The leather and metal parts of the prosthesis should not get wet. The client should be encouraged to have regular maintenance of the prosthesis performed. Consideration of the condition of the shoe is also necessary. A badly worn shoe alters the gait and may cause damage to the prosthesis.

The long-term goal of a return to normal activity may not be achieved in the hospital setting. Referral to a community health nurse can foster optimal physical and emotional adjustment.

SPECIAL CONSIDERATIONS IN UPPER-LIMB AMPUTATION. The emotional implications of an upper-limb amputation are often more devastating than those for lower-limb amputation. The enforced dependency brought about by one-handedness is both frustrating and humiliating to many clients. Because most upper-extremity amputations result from trauma, the client has also not had the opportunity to adjust psychologically to an amputation or to participate in the decision-making process.

Both immediate and delayed prosthetic fittings are possible for the below-the-elbow amputee. Prosthetic fitting is delayed for the above-the-elbow amputee. The usual functional prosthesis is the arm and hook. A cosmetic hand is available but has limited functional value. As with the lower-limb prosthesis, client motivation and endurance are major factors in a satisfactory outcome.

BONE CANCER

Primary malignant bone neoplasms are rare in adults and account for less than 1% of all deaths attributed to cancer. They are characterized by their rapid metastasis and bone destruction. Primary neoplasms occur most frequently in clients during childhood through young adulthood.

Multiple Myeloma

In adults, multiple myeloma (plasma cell myeloma) is the most frequently occurring primary tumor that arises in bone. It is a malignant neoplasm of plasma cells causing widespread infiltration and destruction of bone marrow and cortex, which produces osteolytic lesions throughout the skeletal system (see Chapter 26). The most commonly involved bones are those with active marrow, such as the axial skeleton, sternum, ribs, spine, clavicles, skull, pelvis, and long bones.[25]

Back pain is the most common symptom. As the bones become affected by proliferating plasma cells, painful destruction of bone cortex leads to generalized bone weakening. This may cause spontaneous fracture or collapse. Continued destruction of normal marrow components, increased red blood cell (RBC) destruction, renal failure, blood loss, and marrow suppression induced by chemotherapy cause the development of anemia and thrombocytopenia. During the course of the disease, there is a tendency to bleed because of platelet deficiency and dysfunction. Pronounced anemia, increased debility, and increasing pain are also common. In addition to the presence of proliferating neoplastic plasma cells, multiple myeloma is also characterized by the presence of abnormal immunoglobulins in the blood serum. The high concentration of protein increases the viscosity of the blood, impeding peripheral circulation and causing problems in the eyes, heart, kidneys, and digits. Repeated plasmapheresis may be indicated (see Chapter 8).

Multiple myeloma occurs most frequently in older adult men and blacks.[26] It has an insidious onset, and the lesions often remain localized for an extended time before disseminating. The client's history usually indicates progressive weakness, malaise, vague bone pains (particularly in the lower back), weight loss, and periods of immobility.

The diagnosis of multiple myeloma is confirmed by biopsy or bone marrow aspiration. The clinical features include multiple lytic bone lesions, hypercalcemia, azotemia, monoclonal serum spike, Bence Jones proteinuria, and a bone marrow largely replaced by plasma cells. Radiographical examination of the axial skeleton usually reveals destructive osteolytic defects that appear as punched-out areas. Bence Jones protein in the urine is indicative of multiple myeloma but is not found in the urine of all clients with the disease.

The overall prognosis is poor because by the time diagnosis has been confirmed, the disease has usually invaded the axial skeleton. The median life expectancy for the untreated client is approximately 17 months and for the treated client, from 26 months to not more than 5 years. The most common causes of death are compression of the spinal cord as a result of pathological fractures of the vertebrae, chronic renal failure, progressive anemia, and secondary infection.

Chemotherapeutic treatment of multiple myeloma has limited usefulness; it is primarily directed toward suppressing plasma cell growth by use of melphalen (Alkeran), cyclophosphamide (Cytoxan), doxorubicin (Adriamycin), and methotrexate (Amethopterin). Steroids are commonly

used in conjunction with melphalan and cyclophosphamide. Steroid therapy increases the client's susceptibility to infection.

Osteogenic Sarcoma

Osteogenic sarcoma (osteosarcoma) is a primary neoplasm of bone that is extremely malignant and is characterized by rapid growth and metastasis. It usually occurs in the metaphyseal region of the long bones of the extremities, particularly in the regions of the distal femur, proximal tibia, and proximal humerus. Osteogenic sarcoma has its highest incidence in persons between 10 and 25 years of age and occurs most commonly in males.

The clinical manifestations of osteogenic sarcoma are usually associated with a past history of minor injury and gradual onset of pain and swelling. The injury does not cause the neoplasm but serves to bring the preexisting condition to medical attention. The neoplasm grows rapidly and produces a noticeable increase in the size of the general region, which can restrict joint motion if the lesion is close to a joint structure. The diagnosis is confirmed by biopsied tissue specimens, elevation of serum alkaline phosphates and calcium levels, and radiographical findings.

Amputation combined with irradiation and chemotherapy is usually the treatment of choice. Limb-salvage surgical procedures in combination with irradiation and chemotherapy are being used more frequently with recurrence rates similar to those for amputation.[27] Early metastasis to the lungs is responsible for a poor prognosis and the survival rate of 15% to 20%.

Osteoclastoma

True osteoclastoma (giant cell tumor) is a malignant, destructive neoplasm that arises in the cancellous ends of long bones in young adults. Some variant giant cell tumors that have been put in this class of neoplasm are usually benign. Giant cell tumors most commonly occur between the ages of 20 and 35. The common sites are the distal end of the femur, proximal tibia, and distal radius. The giant cell tumor is a locally destructive lesion, the growth of which extends from a few months to several years. The clinical manifestations are usually swelling, local pain, and some disturbances in joint function. Radiographical evidence of giant cell tumor is variable but usually reveals local areas of bone destruction and eventual expansion of the bone ends. Treatment initially includes biopsy to establish the diagnosis, followed by surgical curettage of the lesion with bone grafting. After treatment there is a greater than 50% chance of recurrence. Recurrent giant cell tumors may subsequently make amputation necessary. Advances in chemotherapy have recently improved overall statistics.

Ewing's Sarcoma

Ewing's sarcoma is the third most common primary malignant neoplasm of bone, occurring most frequently in male clients under the age of 30. This neoplasm is characterized by rapid growth within the medullary cavity of long bone, especially the femur and tibia, and early metastasis. The most frequent site of metastasis is the lungs.

Ewing's sarcoma has a poor prognosis, with a survival rate estimated at only 5%. Common manifestations are progressive local pain, swelling, palpable soft-tissue mass, noticeable increase in size of the affected part, fever, and leukocytosis. Initially, radiographical evidence usually indicates periosteal elevation, which indicates extensive areas of bone destruction. Treatment usually involves radiation therapy and surgical resection or amputation. Chemotherapeutic agents commonly used are cyclophosphamide (Cytoxan), dactinomycin, vincristine (Oncovin), methotrexate, and doxorubicin (Adriamycin). New chemotherapeutic techniques hold the promise of improvement in survival rates.

Metastatic Lesions

The most common type of malignant bone tumor occurs as a result of metastasis from a primary tumor. Common sites for the primary tumor include the breast, intestinal tract, lungs, prostate, kidney, ovary, and thyroid. The metastatic lesion is commonly found in the spine, pelvis, or ribs. Pathological fractures at the site of metastasis are common, owing to weakening of the involved bone.

Once a primary lesion has been identified, bone scans are often done to detect metastatic lesions before they are visible on x-ray film. Treatment is palliative and consists of pain management and irradiation. Prognosis is poor.

■ Nursing Management of Bone Cancer

Nursing assessment

The client with bone cancer should be assessed for the location and severity of pain. Weakness that is due to anemia and increased debility may also be noted. Swelling at the involved site and decreased joint function, depending on the tumor site, should also be monitored.

Nursing diagnoses

Nursing diagnoses related to the client with bone cancer include, but are not limited to, the following:

1. Pain related to disease process, swelling, and inadequate pain relief and/or comfort measures
2. Impaired physical mobility related to disease process, pain, weakness, and debility
3. Body-image disturbance related to possible amputation, deformity, swelling, and effects of chemotherapy
4. Dysfunctional grieving related to poor prognosis of the disease
5. High risk for injury: pathological fractures related to disease process and inadequate handling or positioning of affected body part

Nursing interventions

Health promotion and maintenance. The nurse needs to teach the public to recognize the warning signs of bone cancer, including swelling, pain of unexplained origin, limitation of joint function, and changes in skin temperature. As with all forms of cancer, health promotion should stress the importance of periodic health examinations.

Acute intervention. Nursing care of the client with a malignant bone neoplasm does not differ significantly from the care given to the client with a malignant disease of any

body part. However, special attention is required to reduce the complications associated with prolonged bed rest and to prevent pathological fractures. The client is often reluctant to participate in therapeutic activities due to weakness and fear of pain. Regular rest periods should be provided between therapeutic activities. Careful handling of the affected extremity is important to prevent pathological fractures.

Chronic management. The nurse must be able to assist the client in accepting the guarded prognosis associated with neoplasms of the bone. Inability to accomplish age-specific developmental tasks can increase the frustrations with this condition. General principles related to cancer nursing are applicable (see Chapter 9). Special attention is necessary for the problems of pain and dysfunction, chemotherapy, and specific surgery such as cord decompression and amputation.

LOW BACK PAIN
Etiology and Pathophysiology

Low back pain is common and has probably affected every adult at least once during a lifetime. In industry, low back pain is responsible for more lost working hours than any other medical condition and represents one of the nation's costliest health problems. Each year about 18 million visits are made to physicians for treatment of this condition. Pain in the lumbar region is a common problem because this area (1) bears most of the weight of the body, (2) is the most flexible region of the spinal column, (3) contains nerve roots that are vulnerable to injury or disease, and (4) has an inherently poor biomechanical structure.

Low back pain is most often due to a musculoskeletal problem. However, other causes such as metabolic, circulatory, gynecological, urological, or psychological problems, which may refer pain to the lower back, must not be overlooked. The causes of low back pain of musculoskeletal origin include (1) acute lumbosacral strain, (2) instability of lumbosacral bony mechanism, (3) osteoarthritis of the lumbosacral vertebrae, (4) intervertebral disk degeneration, and (5) herniation of the intervertebral disk. Of these, the most common cause is mechanical strain of paravertebral muscles. Herniation of the nucleus pulposus is another common cause of low back pain.

Acute Low Back Pain

Acute low back pain is usually associated with some type of activity that causes undue stress on the tissues of the lower back. Often symptoms do not appear at the time of injury but develop later because of gradual buildup of paravertebral muscle spasms. Few definitive diagnostic abnormalities are present with paravertebral muscle strain. The straight-leg raise test may produce pain in the lumbar area without radiation along the sciatic nerve.

Therapeutic management. If the muscle spasms are not severe, the client may be treated on an outpatient basis with analgesics, muscle relaxants, and/or use of a corset.[28] A corset prevents rotation, flexion, and extension of the lower back.

If the spasms and pain are severe, a period of hospitalization may be necessary. Since paravertebral muscle spasms are worse when the client is upright, bed rest is the primary treatment for acute low back pain. Bathroom privileges are usually allowed. Bed rest is maintained until the client can move and turn from side to side with minimal discomfort. At this time, gradually increasing activity is initiated. Complete bed rest for the client usually lasts 5 to 10 days.

If conservative treatment is ineffective and the cause of the pain is nerve-root irritation, an epidural steroid injection may be performed. A needle is inserted into the epidural space under fluoroscopy, and steroid and a local anesthetic are injected. Epidural steroids decrease pain, speed return of function, and improve objective neurological signs. These injections appear to be most effective in clients with acute rather than chronic pain and clients with radicular pain who are not candidates for surgery. Typically, epidural injections can be repeated up to three times within 1 year.

■ Nursing Management of Acute Low Back Pain
Nursing assessment
Subjective and objective data that should be obtained from the client with low back pain are summarized in Table 57-19.
Nursing diagnoses
Nursing diagnoses are determined when the problem and etiological factors are supported by clinical data. Nursing diagnoses related to low back pain may include, but are not limited to, those presented in Table 57-20.
Nursing interventions
Health promotion and maintenance. The nurse is a significant role model and teacher for clients with low back problems. As a role model, the nurse should use proper body mechanics at all times. Proper body mechanics should be a primary consideration when teaching clients and care providers transfer and turning techniques. The nurse should assess the client's use of body mechanics and offer advice when activities that can produce back strain are used (Table 57-21).

Some physicians refer clients with back pain to a program called "Back School." It is a formal program usually taught by health professionals such as physicians, nurses, and physical therapists. It is designed to teach the client how to minimize the back pain and avoid repeat episodes of low back pain.

Clients are also advised to maintain appropriate weight. Excess body weight places extra stress on the lower back and weakens the abdominal muscles that support the lower back.

The position assumed while sleeping is also important in preventing low back pain. Sleeping in a prone position should be avoided because it produces excessive lumbar lordosis, placing excessive stress on the lower back. A firm mattress is recommended. The client should sleep in either a supine or side-lying position with the knees and hips flexed to prevent unnecessary stress on support muscles, ligamentous structures, and lumbosacral joints.

Table 57-19

Nursing Assessment of the Client with Low Back Pain

SUBJECTIVE DATA

History
Acute or chronic lumbosacral strain, osteoarthritis, degenerative disk disease, obesity, occupation, activity level, relationship of pain to activity
Medications
Use of analgesics, muscle relaxants, nonsteroidal antiinflammatory drugs, steroids, over-the-counter remedies
General
Poor posture
Pain
Pain in back, buttocks, or leg associated with walking, turning, straining, coughing, leg raising
Neurological
Numbness, tingling of legs, feet, toes
Musculoskeletal
Muscle spasms

OBJECTIVE DATA

General
Guarding
Neurological
Depressed or absent Achilles tendon reflex
Musculoskeletal
Tense, tight paravertebral muscles on palpation, decreased range of motion of spine
Possible findings
Localization of site of lesion on myelogram and CT scan, determination of muscular disorder on electromyography

---

Acute intervention. The primary nursing responsibilities in acute low back pain are to assist the client to maintain bed rest, promote comfort, and educate the client about the disease process. Whether the client is at home or hospitalized, measures to ensure bedrest should be enforced. Other nursing interventions related to acute low back pain are summarized in Table 57-20. Use of analgesics, nonsteroidal antiinflammatory agents, and muscle relaxants to promote comfort is incorporated into the plan of care.

Muscle-strengthening exercises may be part of the management plan. Although the actual exercises are often taught by the physical therapist, it is the nurse's responsibility to ensure that the client understands the type and frequency of exercise prescribed, as well as the rationale for the program.

Chronic management. The goal of management is to make an episode of acute low back pain an isolated incident. If the lumbosacral mechanism is unstable, repeated episodes can be anticipated. The lumbosacral spine may be unable to meet the demands placed on it without strain because of factors such as obesity, poor posture, poor muscular support, advancing age, or local trauma. Intervention is aimed at strengthening the supporting muscles by exercise and use of a corset to limit extremes of movement. In addition, weight reduction decreases the mechanical demands of the lower back.

Persistent use of poor body mechanics may result in repeated episodes of low back pain. If the strain is work related, occupational counseling may be necessary. The frustration, pain, and disability imposed on the client with low back pain problems require emotional support and understanding care by the nurse.

Chronic Low Back Pain

Pathophysiology. The causes of chronic low back pain include degenerative disk disease, lack of physical exercise, obesity, structural and postural abnormalities, and systemic disease. Structural degeneration of the intervertebral disk results in degenerative disk disease manifested by low back pain. This degeneration can also occur in the cervical spine area. The degeneration results in intervertebral narrowing and a lessening of the efficiency of the intervertebral disks in acting as shock absorbers. This inefficiency causes small tears in the annulus fibrosus, which predisposes the client to herniated nucleus pulposus. As the stresses on the degenerated disk continue and eventually exceed the strength of the disk, herniation of the intervertebral disk may result. Nuclear material from the intervertebral disk herniates, causing compression or tension on a lumbar or sacral spinal nerve root (Fig. 57-18).

Clinical manifestations. The most characteristic feature of a herniated intervertebral disk is back pain with associated buttock and leg pain along the distribution of the sciatic nerve. (Specific manifestations that are based on the level of lumbar disk herniation are summarized in Table 57-22.) The straight-leg-raise test may be positive, and back and/or leg pain may be reproduced by raising the leg and flexing the foot at 90 degrees. Low back pain from other causes may not be accompanied by leg pain.

Reflexes may be depressed or absent, depending on the spinal nerve root involved, and numbness or tingling in the toes and feet may be felt by the client. If the disk ruptures in the cervical area, the clinical manifestations are stiff neck, shoulder pain radiating to the hand, and paresthesias and sensory disturbances of the hand.

Diagnostic studies. A myelogram, MRI, or CT scan is helpful in localizing the site of herniation. A diskogram may be necessary if other methods of diagnosis are unsuccessful. An electromyograph (EMG) of the lower extremities can be performed to determine the severity of nerve irritation caused by herniation (see Table 56-7).

Therapeutic management. Degenerative disk disease is managed conservatively with pelvic traction, rest, limitation of extremes of spinal movement (corset), local heat, ultrasound, transcutaneous electrical nerve stimulation, and antiinflammatory medication.[21] If herniation of the disk occurs, more aggressive treatment is indicated (Table 57-23). Conservative treatment sometimes results in a

Table 57-20

 NURSING CARE PLAN FOR THE CLIENT WITH LOW BACK PAIN

Defining Characteristics	Nursing Interventions	Evaluation Criteria
NURSING DIAGNOSIS: Acute pain related to specific physical problem, muscle spasms, and ineffective comfort measures		
Pain descriptors, guarding; altered time perception; behaviors indicative of pain such as moaning, crying, restlessness; altered muscle tone, autonomic responses; palpable muscle spasm; decreased physical activity	Enforce bed rest. Keep head of bed elevated 20 degrees and knee of bed flexed (William's position). Maintain pelvic traction, correctly aligned, as ordered. Examine skin for pressure over iliac crest. Apply moist heat to lower back. Administer analgesics and/or muscle relaxants as ordered; document effect. Monitor motor strength, reflexes, and sensory status.	Reduction or absence of pain and muscle spasms
NURSING DIAGNOSIS: Constipation related to immobility, inadequate fluids, and pain medications		
Reduced frequency of bowel movement, hard and formed stools, decrease in quantity, palpable mass, report of feeling of pressure on rectum, report of feeling of fullness, abdominal cramps, impaired appetite, nausea	Provide high-bulk, high-fiber diet. Administer stool softeners as ordered. Monitor bowel movements. Maintain adequate hydration. Monitor fluid intake.	Regular bowel movement, absence of pain associated with straining
NURSING DIAGNOSIS: Impaired physical mobility related to pain		
Limited active joint range of motion, movement restrictions, pain, muscle spasms	Have client perform range-of-motion exercises daily. Start ambulation program slowly and progress with assistance. Avoid having client bend, sit, or lift. Report leg or back pain and change in sensation.	Unrestricted gait, ambulation within normal limits
NURSING DIAGNOSIS: Body-image disturbance related to impaired mobility and chronic pain		
Concern about change in lifestyle, negative feelings about body, change in social involvement or relationships; feelings of helplessness, hopelessness, powerlessness	Provide psychological support, active listening, and encouragement. Assist client in becoming as independent as possible.	Positive self-concept

Continued.

Table 57-20

NURSING CARE PLAN FOR THE CLIENT WITH LOW BACK PAIN—cont'd

Defining Characteristics	Nursing Interventions	Evaluation Criteria

Chronic management

NURSING DIAGNOSIS: Chronic pain related to lack of knowledge regarding pain management techniques

Verbal report or evidence of pain longer than 6 months in duration, fear of reinjury, physical and social withdrawal, altered ability to continue previous activities, weight changes, anorexia, changes in sleep pattern	Instruct client and family about home care and alternative methods of pain control, including use of heat, transcutaneous electrical nerve stimulation unit, and massage. Avoid strenuous activities, which increase pain. Assist in identifying activities that exacerbate pain and develop plans to prevent pain.	Development of effective methods of managing pain

NURSING DIAGNOSIS: Altered health maintenance related to lack of knowledge regarding posture, body mechanics, and weight reduction

Lack of necessary knowledge to participate in treatment plan, inadequate understanding or inaccurate follow-through of previous instructions	Assess body mechanics. Instruct client on proper body mechanics and use of firm mattress or bedboard. Assess for development of joint contracture or instability and decreasing muscle strength. Refer to physical therapist for low back exercises. Encourage activity and ambulation within limitations. Maintain client's position of correct anatomical alignment. Teach about weight reduction if indicated.	Use of proper body mechanics at all times, weight within normal limits, maintenance of activity and ambulation

NURSING DIAGNOSIS: Ineffective individual coping related to effects of chronic pain on lifestyle

Verbalization of inability to cope, anxiety, fear, anger, irritability, tension; inability to meet role expectations; altered societal participation; ineffective or inappropriate use of defense mechanisms; change in usual communication patterns; excess food intake, alcohol consumption, smoking; digestive, bowel, appetite disturbances; chronic fatigue or sleep-pattern disturbance	Explain factors that may contribute to development of maladaptive coping behavior. Explain how to develop therapeutic coping skills and activities that enhance self-esteem and social interaction.	No development of chronic sick-role behavior

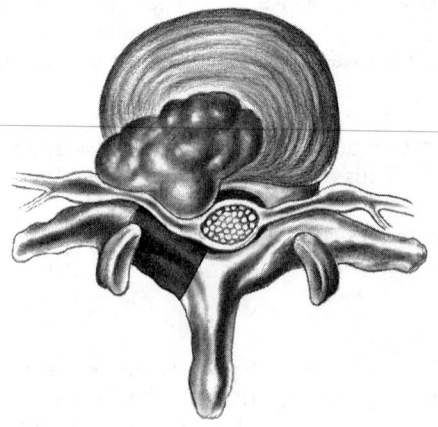

Fig. 57-18 Herniated nucleus pulposus. (From Thompson JC and others: Mosby's manual of clinical nursing, St Louis, 1989, The CV Mosby Co, p 469.)

Table 57-21 Client Instructions for Low Back Problems

Do not	*Do*
Lean forward without bending knees.	Prevent lower back from straining forward by placing a foot on a step or stool during prolonged standing.
Lift anything above level of elbows.	Sleep in a side-lying position with knees and hips bent.
Stand in one position for prolonged time.	Sleep on back with a lift under knees and legs or on back with 10-inch-high pillow under knees to flex hips and knees.
Sleep on abdomen or on back or side with legs out straight.	Sit in a chair with knees higher than hips and support arms on chair or knees.
Exercise without consulting health care provider if you have severe pain.	Exercise 15 minutes in the morning and 15 minutes in the evening regularly. Begin exercises with a 2- to 3-minute warming-up period by moving arms and legs, by alternately relaxing and tightening muscles. Exercise slowly with smooth movements as directed by a physical therapist.
Exceed prescribed amount and type of exercises without consulting health care provider.	Avoid chilling during and after exercising.
	Maintain appropriate body weight.
	Use a lumbar roll or pillow for sitting.

Table 57-22 Neurological Assessment of Lumbar Disk Herniation*

Intervertebral Level	Subjective Pain	Affected Reflex	Motor Function	Sensation
L3 - L4	Back to buttocks to posterior thigh to inner calf	Patellar	Quadriceps, anterior tibialis	Inner aspect of lower leg, anterior part of thigh
L4 - L5	Back to buttocks to dorsum of foot and big toe	None	Anterior tibialis, extensor hallucis longus, gluteus medius	Dorsum of foot and big toe
L5 - S1	Back to buttocks to sole of foot and heel	Achilles	Gastrocnemius, hamstring, gluteus maximus	Heel and lateral foot

*A disk herniation is occasionally so extensive that pressure on more than one nerve root results.

Table 57-23

Diagnostic and Therapeutic Management: Herniated Intervertebral Disk

DIAGNOSTIC

History
Physical examination with emphasis on neurological deficits and straight-leg raising
CT scan
MRI
Myelogram
Diskogram
EMG
Somatosensory-evoked potential

THERAPEUTIC
Conservative

Absolute bed rest
Medication
    Analgesics
    Antiinflammatory agents
    Muscle relaxants
Diathermy and local heat
Pelvic traction

Surgical

Laminectomy with or without spinal fusion
Chemonucleolysis
Diskectomy
Percutaneous lateral diskectomy
Spinal fusion with or without instrumentation

---

healing over of the herniated area with a decrease in the pain of the nerve-root irritation. Complete bedrest is often encouraged during this phase. Traction may be used to decrease muscle spasms. Once the symptoms subside, back-strengthening exercises are begun. The client should be educated in principles of good body mechanics. Extremes

of flexion and torsion are strongly discouraged. Most clients with herniated disks recover with a conservative treatment plan. However, if conservative treatment is unsuccessful, surgery may be indicated.

Chemonucleolysis, a procedure in which chymopapain is injected directly into the disk, may be considered by the physician. Chymopapain, an enzyme that decreases the water-binding properties of the disk, is injected and dissolves the herniated portion of the disk. Appropriate selection criteria for chemonucleolysis should be used to ensure success of the procedure. Selection criteria include radiation of pain to the leg, failure of a conservative treatment program, documented herniated disk by diagnostic tests, positive straight-leg-raise test, absence of allergy to papaya derivatives, and no previous chemonucleolysis injection.

The procedure is performed in the operating room. The client is usually discharged the next day. The client should be cautioned that severe muscle spasms may be experienced after the procedure. These may last several days to weeks. The client should also be informed that pain relief from the procedure is usually not immediate. The long-term effects of this procedure are being investigated.

Surgical interventions. A *percutaneous diskectomy* is a surgical procedure using a tube that is passed through the retroperitoneal soft tissues to the lateral border of the disk with the aid of fluoroscopy. The herniated portion of the disk is shaved and removed in small portions.[28] No incision is made and minimal blood loss occurs during a percutaneous diskectomy. The long-term effects of this procedure are being investigated.

A *diskectomy* is another type of surgical procedure that may be performed to decompress the nerve root. It involves the partial removal of the lamina. *Microsurgical diskectomy* is a version of the standard diskectomy in which the surgeon uses a microscope to allow better visualization of the disk and disk space during surgery to aid in the removal of the herniated portion.[28]

The traditional and most common procedure performed is a *laminectomy*. It involves the surgical excision of part of the posterior arch of the vertebra (referred to as the *lamina*) to gain access to part or all of the protruding disk. A

laminectomy may be performed in combination with a diskectomy.

A *spinal fusion* may be performed if an unstable bony mechanism is present. The spine is stabilized by creating an ankylosis (fusion) of contiguous vertebrae with a bone graft from the client's fibula or iliac crest or from donated bone. If vertebral instability exists, metal fixation with rods, plates, or screws may be performed at the time of spinal surgery to provide more stability and decrease vertebral motion.

■ Nursing Management of Spinal Surgery

Acute intervention

Clients who have undergone spinal surgery require vigilant routine postoperative care. Nursing intervention is also aimed at maintaining proper alignment of the spine at all times until healing has occurred. Flat bedrest may be maintained for 1 to 2 days depending on the surgeon's preference. Logrolling clients when turning is essential to maintain proper body alignment. Pillows can be used under the thighs of each leg when clients are supine and between the legs when they are in side-lying positions to provide comfort and ensure alignment.

Severe muscle spasms in the surgical area can be controlled with medication and with correct turning and positioning. The client often fears turning or any movement that increases pain by straining the surgical area. The nurse must offer reassurance that proper technique is being used to maintain body alignment. Sufficient staff should be available to move the client without undue pain or strain on staff members or the client.

Because the spinal canal may be unintentionally entered during surgery, there is potential for spinal fluid leakage. Severe headache or leakage of spinal fluid should be reported immediately. Cerebrospinal fluid appears clear on the dressing. It has a high glucose concentration and is positive for glucose when a dipstick test is done. The amount and characteristics of drainage should be noted by the nurse.

Frequent monitoring of neurological signs is a routine postoperative nursing responsibility after spinal surgery. Movement of arms and legs and responses to tests of sensation should be unchanged when compared to the preoperative status. Table 57-24 summarizes a lumbar laminectomy check appropriate for the client who has undergone back surgery. This check is repeated every 2 to 4 hours during the first 48 hours after surgery, and findings are compared with the preoperative assessment. Sensations such as numbness and tingling may not be relieved immediately after surgery. Any new muscle weakness or paresthesias should be documented and reported to the surgeon immediately.

Interference with bowel function may occur for several days and requires careful monitoring to prevent constipation and distention. Paralytic ileus can be evaluated by noting whether the client is passing flatus, is nauseated, has a flat, soft abdomen, and has bowel sounds.

Loss of sphincter tone or bladder tone may be indicative of nerve damage. Incontinence or difficulty in evacuation

Table 57-24 Lumbar Laminectomy Assessment

SENSATION*

Assess sensation of extremities.
Assess for feelings of numbness and tingling.

MOVEMENT*

Assess ability to move all extremities.

MUSCLE STRENGTH*

Assess for any motor weakness of the extremities.

CIRCULATION

Assess client's extremities for pulses, warmth, color.

WOUND

Assess dressing for drainage and note amount, color, characteristics.

PAIN

Document location of the pain.
Ask client to rate the pain on a scale of 1 to 10, with *1* being no pain and *10* being worst pain.
Evaluate pain after analgesia has been administered.

---

*Postoperative findings should be compared to preoperative assessments. It is not unusual for the client to continue to experience these symptoms after surgery. Symptoms gradually decrease over several months.

of the bowel or bladder must be monitored closely and reported to the surgeon.

Activity prescriptions vary with surgeons, but the client who has had a laminectomy usually ambulates early in the postoperative period. It is a nursing responsibility to know the specific orders related to activity for any given client.

In addition to the nursing care appropriate for a client who has had a laminectomy, there are other nursing responsibilities if the client has also had a spinal fusion. Because a bone graft is involved, the postoperative healing time is prolonged compared to that of a laminectomy. Immobilization over an extended time is necessary. A rigid orthosis ("thoracic-lumbar-sacral orthosis or chair-back brace") is often used during the period of immobilization. Some surgeons require that the client be taught to put it on and take it off by logrolling in bed, whereas others allow their clients to apply the brace in a sitting or standing position. The nurse should verify the preferred method before initiating this activity. The extended immobilization required by a spinal fusion carries with it all the potential problems related to this inactive state.

In addition to the primary surgical site, the donor site for the bone graft must be regularly assessed. The donor site may cause greater postoperative pain than the fused area. The donor site is bandaged with a pressure dressing to prevent excessive bleeding. If the donor site is the fib-

Table 57-25   Common Foot Problems

Disorder	Definition	Treatment
COMMON DISORDERS		
Forefoot		
Hallux valgus (bunion)	Painful deformity of large toe consisting of lateral angulation of large toe toward second toe, bony enlargement of medial side of first metatarsal head, and formation of bursa or callus over bony enlargement	Conservative treatment includes wearing shoes with wide forefoot or "bunion pocket" and use of bunion pads to relieve pressure on bursal sac. Surgical treatment is removal of bursal sac and bony enlargement and correction of lateral angulation of large toe.
Hallux rigidus	Painful stiffness of first metatarsophalangeal joint due to osteoarthritis or local trauma	Conservative treatment includes intraarticular corticosteroids and passive manual stretching of first metatarsophalangeal joint. A shoe with a stiff sole decreases pain in the joint during walking. Surgical treatment is joint fusion or arthroplasty with silicone rubber implant.
Hammertoe	Deformity of second toe, including dorsiflexion of metatarsophalangeal joint, plantar flexion of proximal interphalangeal joint and callus on dorsum of proximal interphalangeal joint and end of involved toe; complaints due to hammertoe including burning on bottom of foot and pain and difficulty in walking when wearing shoes	Conservative treatment consists of passive manual stretching of proximal interphalangeal joint and use of metatarsal arch support. Surgical correction consists of resection of base of middle phalanx and head of proximal phalanx and bringing raw bone ends together. Kirschner wire maintains straight position.
Morton's neuroma (Morton's toe or plantar neuroma)	Neuroma in web space between third and fourth metatarsal heads, causing sharp sudden attacks of pain and burning sensations	Surgical excision is the usual treatment.
Midfoot		
Pes planus (flatfoot)	Breakdown or lowering of metatarsal arch, causing pain in foot or leg or referred pain to other parts of body	Symptoms are relieved by use of resilient longitudinal arch supports. Surgical treatment consists of triple arthrodesis, fusion of subtalar joint.
Pes cavus	Elevation of longitudinal arch of foot resulting from contracture or plantar fascia or bony deformity of arch	Treatment is manipulation and casting (in clients younger than 6 years of age); surgical correction is necessary if it interferes with ambulation (in clients older than 6 years of age).
Hindfoot		
Painful heels	Complaint of heel pain with weight-bearing, common cause of plantar bursitis or calcaneal spur in adult	Corticosteroids are injected locally into inflamed bursa and sponge rubber heel cushion is used; surgical excision of bursa or spur is performed.

Table 57-25 Common Foot Problems—cont'd

Disorder	Definition	Treatment
LOCAL PROBLEMS		
Corn	Localized thickening of skin caused by continual pressure over bony prominences, especially metatarsal head, frequently causing localized pain	Corn is softened with warm water or preparations containing salicylic acid and trimmed with razor blade or scalpel. Pressure on bony prominences caused by shoes is relieved.
Soft corn	Painful lesion caused by bony prominence of one toe pressing against adjacent toe, usual location in web space between toes, softness due to secretions keeping web space relatively moist.	Pain is relieved by placing cotton between toes to separate them. Surgical treatment is excision of projecting bone spur.
Callus	Similar formation to corn but covering of wider area and usual location on weight-bearing part of foot	Same as for corn.
Plantar wart	Painful papillomatous growth caused by virus that may occur on any part of skin on sole of foot	Excision with electrocoagulation or surgical removal is done; ultrasound may also be used.

ula, neurovascular assessments of the extremity are a routine postoperative nursing responsibility.

Table 57-20 summarizes principles that should be reviewed with the client before discharge from the hospital. Any restrictions on activity such as exercise should be clarified with the physician. If the surgery involved the cervical spine, the nurse must be alert for symptoms of cord edema such as respiratory distress and a worsening neurological status in the upper extremities. After surgery, the client's neck is immobilized in a soft or hard cervical collar.

Chronic management

As the bone graft heals, the client needs to adjust to the permanent immobility imposed by surgery within that area. Instruction in proper body mechanics is essential and should be evaluated during the hospital stay. The client should be instructed to avoid sitting or standing for prolonged periods. Activities that should be encouraged include walking, lying down, and shifting weight from one foot to the other when standing. The client should learn to mentally think through an activity before starting any potentially injurious task such as bending, lifting, or stooping. The thighs and knees, rather than the back, should be used to absorb the shock of activity and movement. A firm mattress or bedboard is essential.

COMMON FOOT PROBLEMS

The foot is the platform that provides support for the weight of the body and absorbs considerable shock in ambulation. It is a complicated structure composed of bony structures, muscles, tendons, and ligaments. It can be affected by (1) congenital conditions, (2) structural weakness, (3) traumatic injuries, and (4) systemic conditions such as diabetes mellitus and rheumatoid arthritis. Abnormalities of the foot affect more than 80 million persons in the United States. Much of the pain, deformity, and disability associated with foot disorders can be directly attributed to or accentuated by improperly fitting shoes, which cause crowding and angulation of the toes and inhibition of the normal movement of foot muscles. The purpose of footwear is to (1) provide support, foot stability, shock absorption, and a foundation for orthoses; (2) increase friction with the walking surface; and (3) treat foot abnormalities.[29] (Table 57-25 summarizes common foot problems and their treatment.)

■ Nursing Management of Common Foot Problems

Health promotion and maintenance

Well-constructed and properly fitted shoes are essential for healthy, pain-free feet. Fashion styles, especially women's, often influence selection of footwear instead of considerations of comfort and support. Client education should stress the importance of having a shoe that conforms to the foot rather than to current fashion trends. The shoe must be long enough and wide enough to prevent crowding of the toes and forcing of the great toe into a position of hallux valgus. At the metatarsal head the width of the shoe should be sufficient to allow free movement of the foot muscles and permit bending of the toes. The shank of the shoe should be rigid enough to give optimal support. The height of the heel should be realistic in relation to the purpose for which the shoe is worn. Ideally, the heel of the shoe should not rise more than 1 inch higher than the forefoot support.

Foot care should include daily hygienic care and the wearing of clean stockings or socks. Stockings should be long enough to avoid wrinkling and the development of pressure areas. Trimming toenails straight across helps prevent ingrown toenails and reduces the possibility of infection. Persons with impaired circulation or diabetes mellitus require detailed instruction to prevent serious complications associated with blisters, pressure areas, and infections (see Table 43-18).

Acute intervention

Many foot problems require surgery. When surgery is performed, the foot is usually immobilized by a bulky dressing, short leg cast, slipper (plastic) cast, or a platform "shoe" that fits over the dressing and has a rigid sole. The foot should be elevated with the heel off the bed to help reduce discomfort and prevent edema. The neurovascular status should be assessed frequently during the immediate postoperative period. Depending on the type of surgery, pins or wires may extend through the toes, or a protective splint that extends over the end of the foot may be in place. Care must be taken not to jar these devices and cause pain. The devices may interfere with or preclude assessment for movement. The nurse should be aware that sensation may be difficult to evaluate, since postoperative pain can interfere with the client's ability to differentiate pain caused by the surgical procedure from pain resulting from nerve pressure or circulatory impairment.

The type and extent of surgery determine the type of ambulation allowed. Crutches may be necessary. The client may experience pain or a throbbing sensation when starting ambulation. The nurse should reinforce instructions given by the physical therapist and ensure that the client does not develop a faulty gait pattern such as walking on the heels in an attempt to avoid excessive pain or pressure. The nurse must reinforce the importance of walking with an erect posture and with proper weight distribution. Dysfunction of gait or continued pain should be reported to the physician. The nurse should instruct the client on the importance of frequent rest periods with the feet elevated.

METABOLIC DISEASE OF BONE

Normal bone metabolism depends on adequate intake, absorption, and use of calcium, phosphorus, protein, and vitamins. When there is dysfunction in one of these critical factors, generalized reduction of bone mass may result.

Osteomalacia

Osteomalacia is an uncommon disorder of adult bone associated with vitamin D deficiency, resulting in decalcification and softening of bone. This disease is the same as rickets in children except that the epiphyseal growth plates are closed in the adult. Vitamin D is required for the absorption of calcium from the intestines. Insufficient vitamin D intake can interfere with the normal mineralization of bone, causing failure or insufficient calcification of bone, which results in softening of bone and deformities. Etiological factors in the development of osteomalacia include lack of exposure to ultraviolet rays, GI malabsorption, chronic diarrhea, pregnancy, and kidney disease.

The most common clinical feature of osteomalacia is persistent skeletal pain. Other clinical manifestations include progressive muscular weakness, weight loss, and progressive deformities of the spine (kyphosis) or extremities. Fractures are common and demonstrate delayed healing when they occur.

Common laboratory findings associated with osteomalacia are decreased serum calcium and phosphorus levels and elevated serum alkaline phosphates. Radiographical examination may demonstrate the effects of generalized bone demineralization, especially loss of calcium in bones of the pelvis and the presence of associated bone deformity. Looser's transformation zones (ribbons of decalcification in bone found on x-ray film) are diagnostic of osteomalacia.

Therapeutic management of osteomalacia is directed toward correction of the underlying cause. Vitamin D is usually supplemented, and the client often shows dramatic response. Calcium and phosphorus intake may also be supplemented.

Osteoporosis

Osteoporosis is a condition in which there is a decrease in total bone mass. It is a crippling, painful bone disease that is the major cause of fractures in postmenopausal women and older adults in general.[30] Osteoporosis is increasing in incidence because more people are surviving to an older age.[31] The loss of bone substance causes the bone to become mechanically weakened and prone to either spontaneous fractures or fractures from minimal trauma. At least 15 million persons in the United States have some degree of osteoporosis. In the United States, the total cost of osteoporosis in terms of medical care, nursing home fees, and loss of income was estimated to exceed 8 billion dollars.[32] Demographic risk factors for osteoporosis are female gender, increasing age, white race, oophorectomy, prolonged immobility, and insufficient dietary calcium. Increased risk is associated with cigarette smoking and alcoholism, and decreased risk is associated with adequate physical activity and fluoride and vitamin D ingestion.

Adults normally begin losing bone between 30 and 40 years of age. When bone loss (resorption) exceeds bone formation and bones fracture under common, everyday stress, the condition becomes known as *osteoporosis*. Although resorption affects the entire skeletal system, osteoporosis occurs most commonly in the bones of the spine, hips, and wrists. Over time, wedging and fractures of the vertebrae produce gradual loss of height, and a humped back known as *dowager's hump* or *kyphosis* develops. The usual first signs are back pain or spontaneous fractures.

This disease often goes unnoticed because it cannot be detected by conventional radiography until more than 25% to 40% of calcium in the bone is lost; it is usually evident when the client is 60 to 65 years of age. Serum calcium, phosphorus, and alkaline phosphatase levels remain normal, although alkaline phosphatase may be elevated after a

fracture. (Table 56-7 lists bone mass studies that are useful in diagnosing osteoporosis.)

Osteoporosis is eight times more common in women than in men for several reasons: (1) Women have lower calcium intake than men throughout their lives (men between 15 and 50 years of age consume twice as much calcium as women). (2) Women have less bone mass because of their generally smaller frame size. (3) Resorption begins at an earlier age in women and is accelerated at menopause. (4) Pregnancy and breast-feeding deplete a woman's skeletal reserve unless calcium intake is adequate. (5) Longevity increases the likelihood of osteoporosis, and women live longer than men.

Many medications are known to decrease calcium retention. This list includes aluminum-containing antacids, caffeine, corticosteroids, nicotine, and tetracycline. At the time a medicine is prescribed, the client should be informed of this possible side effect.

Specific diseases associated with osteoporosis include intestinal malabsorption, kidney disease, rheumatoid arthritis, advanced alcoholism, cirrhosis of the liver, and diabetes mellitus.[17]

Prevention of osteoporosis focuses on adequate calcium intake (1000 mg/day in premenopausal women and postmenopausal women taking estrogen and 1500 mg/day in postmenopausal women who are not receiving supplemental estrogen) and regular exercise to strengthen bones. If dietary intake of calcium is inadequate, supplemental calcium should be taken (Table 57-26). Calcium supplementation inhibits age-related bone loss; however, no new bone is formed. Foods that are high in calcium include whole and skim milk, yogurt, turnip greens, cottage cheese, ice cream, sardines, and spinach.

Estrogen therapy after menopause is used to prevent osteoporosis. It has been shown to increase the risk of endometrial cancer; however, recent research indicates that this can be prevented by a combination therapy with the use of a cyclic estrogen-progesterone regimen (see Chapter 48).[34] Although the exact mechanism for the protective function of estrogen is not known, it is believed that estrogen sensitizes the skeleton to the effects of parathyroid hormone, leading to decreased bone resorption.[33] Estrogen replacement continues to have significant beneficial effects for 10 to 15 years after menopause.[31]

Table 57-26 Sources of Calcium

Food	Calcium (mg)	Food	Calcium (mg)
1 cup milk		1 med stalk cooked broccoli	158
Buttermilk	285	1 cup cooked spinach	200
Chocolate	284	1 cup cooked mustard greens	193
Whole	291	1 cup turnip greens	252
Low-fat	300	1 cup cooked collard greens with stems	289
Skim	302	1 cup bok choy	250
Half and half	254	1 cup kale	206
Evaporated, canned	657		
Egg nog	330	**BONUS SOURCES**	
		1 cup almonds	304
1 oz cheese		1 cup hazelnuts	240
American	174	1 tbs blackstrap molasses	137
Blue	150		
Brie	52	**POOR SOURCES**	
Camembert	110	Egg	28
Cheddar	130	1 cup cabbage	44
Cottage	130	1 oz cream cheese	23
Mozzarella	207	3 oz beef, pork, poultry	10
Parmesan	390	Apple, banana	10
Swiss	272	½ grapefruit	20
8 oz yogurt	415	1 med potato	14
1 cup ice cream	176	1 med carrot	14
Soft serve	272	¼ head lettuce	27
3 oz seafood			
Salmon	167		
Sardines with bones	372		
Shrimp	98		
Oysters	113		

Etidronate disodium (stedronate), a biphosphonate that inhibits osteoclast-mediated bone resorption, is currently under investigation as a treatment for osteoporosis. Intermittent cyclical therapy with etidronate significantly increases vertebral bone mass and decreases the rate of vertebral fracture in women with postmenopausal osteoporosis.[35,36]

The same measures used to prevent osteoporosis—weight-bearing exercise and adequate calcium intake—are also beneficial in treating osteoporosis. Although loss of bone mass cannot be significantly reversed, further loss can be prevented if the three-part program is followed.

Efforts are made to keep clients with osteoporosis ambulatory to prevent further loss of bone substance as a result of immobility. Treatment also involves protecting areas of potential pathological fractures; for example, a corset can be used by the client to prevent vertebral collapse.

Paget's Disease

Paget's disease (osteitis deformans) is a skeletal bone disorder in which there is excessive bone removal and replacement with associated skeletal deformity. It occurs most often after the fourth decade of life and most commonly in men. It is characterized by deformities of bone caused by unexplained abnormal regeneration and resorption of bone, fibrotic changes, and remodeling with structurally uneven bone. The regions of the skeleton commonly affected are the pelvis, long bones, spine, and cranium.

In milder forms of Paget's disease, clients may remain free of symptoms, and the disease may be discovered incidentally on radiographic examination. The initial clinical manifestations are usually insidious development of skeletal pain (which may progress to severe intractable pain), complaints of fatigue, and progressive development of bowlegs. Clients may complain that they are becoming shorter or that their heads are becoming larger. The serum alkaline phosphatase is markedly elevated in advanced forms of the disease. Radiographic examination reveals that the normal contour of the affected bone is curved and the bone cortex is thickened, especially the weight-bearing bones and cranium. Pathological fracture is the most common complication of Paget's disease and may be the first indication of the disease. Other complications include malignant osteosarcoma, chondrosarcoma, or fibrosarcoma. Therapeutic management of Paget's disease is usually limited to symptomatic and supportive care and correction of secondary deformities by either surgical intervention or braces. Bone resorption, relief of acute symptoms, and lowering of the serum alkaline phosphatase levels may be significantly influenced by the administration of calcitonin, which inhibits osteoclastic activity. Resistance to calcitonin therapy may occur.[36] Diphosphonates and their derivatives also inhibit the activity of Paget's disease.[37] Radiation therapy and local surgical procedures such as periosteal stripping may be used for the control of the client's pain.

■ Nursing Management of Metabolic Bone Diseases

Because metabolic bone disorders increase the possibility of pathological fractures, the nurse must use extreme caution when the client is turned or moved. It is important to keep the client as active as possible to retard demineralization of bone resulting from disuse or extended immobilization. A supervised exercise program is an essential part of the treatment program. If the client's condition permits, ambulation without causing fatigue must be encouraged.

A firm mattress should be used to provide back support and to relieve pain. The client may be required to wear a corset or light brace to relieve back pain and provide support when in the upright position. The client should be proficient in the correct application of such devices and know how to regularly examine areas of the skin for friction damage. Activities such as lifting and twisting should be discouraged. Good body mechanics are essential. Analgesics and muscle relaxants may be administered to relieve pain. A properly balanced nutritional program is very important in the management of metabolic disorders of bone, especially pertaining to vitamin D, calcium, and protein, which are necessary to ensure the availability of the components for bone formation. Prevention measures such as client education, use of an assistive device, and environmental changes should be actively pursued to prevent falls and subsequent fractures.

C *ase Study*

FRACTURE

Henry A., a 30-year-old man, was seen in the emergency room after an auto accident. His right lower extremity was splinted with a cardboard splint and large bulky dressing. Avulsion of soft tissue on the anterolateral aspect of the tibia was present with obvious deformity, marked swelling, and ecchymosis in the region of the injury. The client complained of severe pain.

Discussion Questions

1. What is the appropriate nursing neurovascular assessment of the injured extremity?
2. What is the difference between an open fracture and a closed fracture?
3. What are the probable therapeutic and nursing interventions to prevent infection?
4. What specific nursing activities should the nurse carry out to alleviate this client's pain?
5. What are the stages of healing that will occur as this fracture heals?

R *eview Questions*

The number of the question corresponds to the same-numbered objective at the beginning of the chapter.

1. Which statement most accurately describes a strain?
   a. musculotendinous injury caused by use of the structure beyond its capacity

b. overstretching of ligament fibers in the region of a joint

c. minor injury of muscle tissues caused by blunt trauma

d. torsional stress applied to the musculotendinous unit, which causes hemarthrosis

2. The remodeling phase of bone healing is characterized by

a. absence of movement at the fracture site

b. conforming of the callus mass to the contour of the bone

c. radiographical evidence of bony union

d. gradual return of the structural strength and shape of the injured bone

3. Pseudoarthrosis is a type of nonunion that is characterized by

a. fracture healing in an abnormal position

b. failure of the fracture to heal in spite of surgical intervention

c. formation of fibrous tissue at the fracture site that permits movement

d. slow healing

4. Instruction of the client in care of the cast should include

a. awareness of signs of developing peripheral nerve and vascular complications

b. hazards of walking on a new cast

c. joint exercise above and below the plaster immobilization device

d. all the above

5. Changes in pain that may indicate a neurovascular problem include

a. increase in pain

b. decrease in pain

c. absence of pain

d. all the above

6. The major complication associated with fracture of the humerus is

a. radial nerve injury

b. nonunion

c. bursitis

d. carpal tunnel syndrome

7. The most common infecting organism associated with osteomyelitis is

a. streptococci

b. *Escherichia coli*

c. *Staphylococcus aureus*

d. *Proteus* organisms

8. During the postoperative period the client with an amputation should be instructed that the amputated extremity should not be positioned in a flexed position because

a. this position promotes thrombosis formation

b. unnecessary movement of the extremity can cause wound separation

c. the flexed position can promote flexion contracture

d. this position increases pain and edema

9. Osteogenic sarcoma is characterized by

a. rapid growth and early metastasis

b. rapid destruction of plasma cells

c. destruction of red marrow within the medullary cavity

d. slow growth that can be controlled by chemotherapy

10. The most common cause of acute low back pain is

a. osteoarthritis of the lumbosacral spine

b. acute lumbosacral strain

c. herniated nucleus pulposus

d. degenerative disk disease

11. A major nursing responsibility related to prevention of low back pain is the teaching of

a. proper body mechanics

b. use of a foam rubber mattress

c. sleeping on the stomach

d. traction application

12. Important nursing interventions after a laminectomy include

a. maintenance of proper body alignment

b. prevention of constipation and distention

c. assessing for paralytic ileus

d. all the above

13. Lateral angulation of the great toe in relation to the first metatarsal head is a condition of the foot known as

a. hallux rigidus

b. hallux varus

c. hallux valgus

d. none of the above

14. A common cause of bone pain associated with osteoporosis is

a. increased bone formation

b. repeated microscopic fractures

c. decreased blood supply

d. compression of nerves

REFERENCES

1. Thompson JM and others, eds: Mosby's manual of clinical nursing, ed 2, St Louis, 1989, The CV Mosby Co, p 375.

2. Appenzeller O, ed: Sports medicine: fitness, training, injuries, ed 3, Baltimore, 1988, Urban & Schwarzenberg, pp 447-448.

3. Menke JS: Pitfalls in orthopedic trauma: part 1: the upper extremity, Emerg Med Clin North Am 21:66, 1989.

4. McCollister Evarts C, ed: Surgery of the musculoskeletal system, ed 2, New York, 1990, Churchill Livingstone, p 227.

5. Fullerton LR Jr: Arthroscopy: when and where to use it, Postgrad Med 81:127, 1987.

6. Appenzeller O, ed: Sports medicine: fitness, training, injuries, ed 3, Baltimore, 1988, Urban & Schwarzenberg, p 377.

7. Sneed NV and Van Breet: Treating ununited fractures with electricity: nursing implications, Gerontol Nurs 16:26-31, 1990.

8. Chapman MW, ed: Operative orthopaedics, Philadelphia, 1988, JB Lippincott Co, pp 510-511.

9. Moore MN: Orthopedic pitfalls in emergency medicine, South Med J 81:371, 1988.

10. Harper CM and Lyles YM: Physiology and complications of bed rest, J Am Geriatr Soc 36:1052, 1988.

11. Thompson JM and others, eds: Mosby's manual of clinical nursing, ed 2, St Louis, 1989, The CV Mosby Co, p 452.

12. Lavin RJ: The high-pressure demands of compartment syndrome, RN 52:23, 1989.

13. Proehl JA: Compartment syndrome, J Emerg Nurs 14:284, 1988.

14. Mims BC: Fat embolism syndrome: a variant of ARDS, Orthop Nurs 8:22-24, 1989.

15. Bolhoffner BR and Spiegel PG: Prevention of medical complications in orthopedic trauma, Clin Orthop 222:108, 1987.

16. McCollister Evarts C, ed: Surgery of the musculoskeletal system, ed 2, New York, 1990, Churchill Livingston, pp 46-47.

17. Rudy DR: Osteoporosis: overcoming a costly and debilitating disease, Postgrad Med 86:151-153, 1989.

18. Fonesca RJ and Walker RV: Oral and maxillofacial trauma, Philadelphia, 1991, WB Saunders Co.

19. Ocular injury in orbital fractures, J Emerg Med 21:83-85, 1989.

20. Gentry L: Approach to the patient with chronic osteomyelitis. In Remington JS and Schwartz JS, eds: Current clinical topics in infectious diseases, New York, 1987, McGraw-Hill Book Co, Inc.

21. Martin ME: Oral antibiotics for treatment of patients with osteomyelitis, Orthop Nurs 8:35-38, 1989.

22. McCollister Evarts C, ed: Surgery of the musculoskeletal system, ed 2, New York, 1990, Churchill Livingston, p 4352.

23. McCollister Evarts C, ed: Surgery of the musculoskeletal system, ed 2, New York, 1990, Churchill Livingston, p 4363.

24. McCollister Evarts C, ed: Surgery of the musculoskeletal system, ed 2, New York, 1990, Churchill Livingston, p 5205.

25. Mirra JM, ed: Bone tumors: clinical, radiologic, and pathologic correlations, Philadelphia, 1989, Lea & Febiger, p 1122.

26. Boffetta P, Stellman SK, and Garfinkel L: A case-control study of multiple myeloma nested in the American Cancer Society prospective study, Int J Cancer 43:554, 1989.

27. Simon MA: Current concepts review: limb salvage for osteosarcoma, J Bone Joint Surg 70A:307, 1988.

28. Salmond SW and others, eds: Core curriculum for orthopaedic nursing, ed 2, Pitman, NJ, 1991, Jannetti, pp 367-371.

29. McPoil TG Jr: Footwear, Phys Ther 68:1857, 1988.

30. Barth RW and Lane JM: Osteoporosis, Orthop Clin North Am 19:845, 1988.

31. Petitti DB and Sidney S: Hip fracture in women, Clin Orthop 246:150, 1989.

32. Bauer RL: Assessing osteoporosis, Hosp Pract 26:23, 1991.

33. Riggs L and Melton JL III, eds: Osteoporosis: etiology, diagnosis, and management, New York, 1988, Raven Press, pp 392-394.

34. McCollister Evarts C, ed: Surgery of the musculoskeletal system, ed 2, New York, 1990, Churchill Livingston, p 187.

35. Watts NB and others: Intermittent cyclical etidronate treatment of postmenopausal osteoporosis, N Engl J Med 323:73-79, 1990.

36. Storm T and others: Effect of intermittent cyclical etidronate therapy on bone mass and fracture rate in women with postmenopausal osteoporosis, N Engl J Med 322:1265-1271, 1990.

37. Hamdy RC: Paget's disease of bone, Hosp Pract 25:33-41, 1990.

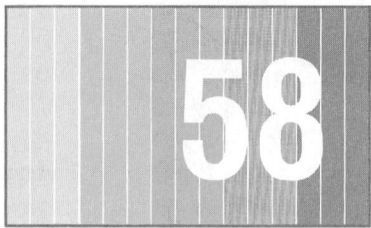

CHAPTER

58

Nursing Role in Management
Arthritis and Other Rheumatic Disorders

Gayle Ziegler Casterline

L earning Objectives

1. *Describe the pathophysiology, clinical manifestations, and therapeutic management of osteoarthritis, rheumatoid arthritis, gout, systemic lupus erythematosus, and systemic sclerosis.*
2. *Describe the clinical manifestations and management of juvenile rheumatoid arthritis, HLA-associated rheumatic diseases, septic arthritis, polymyositis, and dermatomyositis.*
3. *Describe the sequence of events leading to joint destruction in osteoarthritis and rheumatoid arthritis.*
4. *Compare osteoarthritis with inflammatory joint disease related to clinical manifestations, treatment, and prognosis.*
5. *Identify the nursing role in the conservative management of arthritis and related rheumatic problems.*
6. *Describe the types of reconstructive surgery associated with arthritis and related rheumatic problems.*
7. *Identify the preoperative and postoperative teaching and management of the client with reconstructive surgery associated with arthritis and related rheumatic problems.*
8. *Describe the pharmacological interventions and nursing considerations associated with arthritis and related rheumatic problems.*
9. *Identify psychological and social problems of the client with rheumatic disease and the appropriate nursing interventions necessary to meet the needs of the client with chronic rheumatic disease.*
10. *Identify the importance of the team approach to comprehensive management of rheumatic diseases.*

OSTEOARTHRITIS

Osteoarthritis (OA), also known as *degenerative joint disease,* is a slowly progressive, noninflammatory disorder of mobile joints, particularly weight-bearing articulations, and is characterized by degeneration of articular cartilage. The damage from OA is confined to the joints and surrounding tissues. OA may be primary or secondary; the cause of primary OA is unknown. Although both are influenced by multiple factors (metabolic, mechanical, genetic, and chemical), secondary OA has an identifiable precipitating event, such as previous fractures, infection, or congenital deformities, that is believed to predispose the person to later degenerative changes.[1]

Reviewed by Janice Smith Pigg, B.S.N., R.N., M.S., Nurse Consultant, Rheumatology, Director, Musculoskeletal Service, Columbia Hospital, Milwaukee, Wisconsin.

Significance

It is estimated that more than 40 million Americans have some evidence of OA. Nearly 90% of people more than 40 years of age exhibit typical changes on x-ray films. More than one third of these persons have clinical manifestations, including pain, stiffness, and limited range of motion (ROM). The spectrum of severity is wide, ranging from annoying and uncomfortable symptoms to significantly disabling disease. The incidence of OA increases with age. Men and women are affected equally.

Etiology and Pathophysiology

Degenerative changes over time cause the normally smooth, white, translucent joint cartilage to become yellow and opaque, with rough surfaces and areas of malacia (softening). As the layers of cartilage become thinner, bony surfaces are closer together. As the cartilage breaks down, fissures may appear and fragments of cartilage be-

come loose. Secondary inflammation of the synovial membrane may follow. As the articular surface becomes totally denuded of cartilage, subchondral bone increases in density and becomes sclerotic (eburnated). New bone (osteophyte) is formed at joint margins and at the attachment sites of ligaments and tendons.

There are several theories concerning the cause of cartilage deterioration. The enzyme hyaluronidase, which is normally found in the synovial fluid, may be responsible for digestion of proteoglycans through cracks in the surface layer of articular cartilage. Another theory suggests that inadequate nutrition of the cartilage may result in cartilage degeneration. Because cartilage is avascular, nutrients are provided by the synovial fluid. It has been demonstrated that deterioration of cartilage is an active process. DNA synthesis, which is normally absent in adult articular cartilage, is active in OA tissue and appears to be proportional to disease severity.[2]

Specific predisposing factors such as excessive use of or stress on a joint have been identified as accelerating osteoarthritic changes, such as in the knees of football players and the feet and ankles of ballet dancers. Genetic factors are demonstrated in generalized OA by Heberden's nodes. It appears to involve a single autosomal gene, dominant in women and recessive in men.

Other factors that influence the development of OA include congenital structural defects (e.g., Legg-Calvé-Perthes disease, genu varum), metabolic disturbances (e.g., diabetes mellitus, acromegaly), repeated intraarticular hemorrhage (e.g., hemophilia), neuropathic arthropathies, and inflammatory and septic arthritis.

Clinical Manifestations

Systemic. Constitutional symptoms such as fatigue or fever are not present in OA. Other organ involvement is absent as well, which is an important differentiation between OA and inflammatory joint disorders such as rheumatoid arthritis.

Joints. Articular manifestations are related to the particular joint involved. The client has pain on motion and weight-bearing that is generally relieved by rest. In advanced disease sleep may be disrupted by night pain. As cartilage (which does not contain nerve endings) is worn away, direct irritation and pressure occur on the nerves of subchondral bones. Pain is most often caused by soft tissue structure surrounding the joint becoming swollen or stretched, not by the arthritic joint itself.[3] Increasing pain is accompanied by progressive loss of function. Overall body coordination and posture may be affected as a result of the pain and loss of mobility.

Unlike pain, which is typically provoked by activity, joint stiffness occurs after periods of rest or static position. The client's symptoms are often aggravated by rising humidity and falling barometric pressure. Crepitation on joint motion and malalignment of the extremity may be noted on physical examination. Advanced disease is complicated by gross deformity and subluxation caused by deterioration of cartilage, collapse of subchondral bone, and extensive bony overgrowth.

Joints are usually affected asymmetrically. The joints

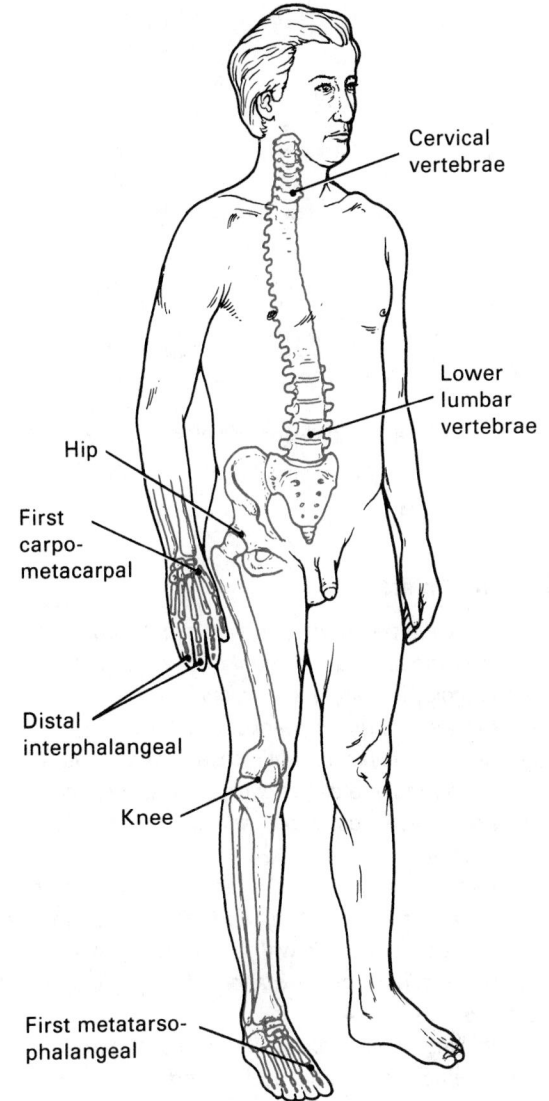

Fig. 58-1 Joints most frequently involved in OA.

most frequently involved are the distal interphalangeal joints of the fingers, first carpometacarpal joint, hips, knees, first metatarsophalangeal joint, and lower lumbar and cervical vertebrae (Fig. 58-1). Degenerative changes are rarely seen in metacarpophalangeal joints, wrists, elbows, or shoulders.

Nodules. Heberden's nodes are another common manifestation of OA, particularly in women with primary OA. These nodes are reactive bony overgrowths located at the distal interphalangeal joints (Fig. 58-2). Heberden's nodes are palpable protuberances that are often associated with flexion and lateral deviation of the distal phalanx, occur more frequently in women, and tend to appear in families. Bouchard's nodes, seen less commonly in OA, involve the proximal interphalangeal joints.

Heberden's nodes and Bouchard's nodes may present with redness, swelling, tenderness, and aching. They often begin in one finger and spread to others. Although there is usually no significant loss of function caused by the bony

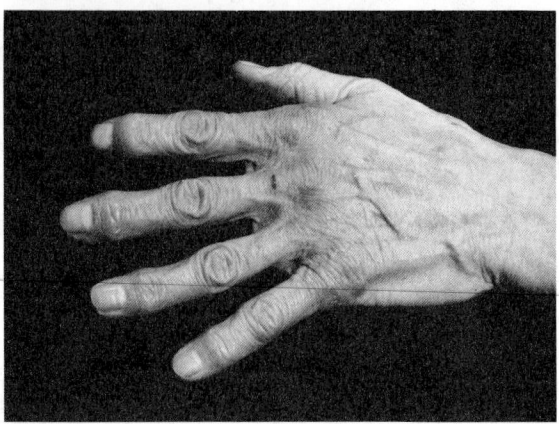

Fig. 58-2 Left hand of a 71-year-old woman with OA and Heberden's nodes.

Table 58-1

Diagnostic and Therapeutic Management: Osteoarthritis

DIAGNOSTIC

Complete history and physical examination
X-ray exam of involved joints
ESR
Synovial fluid analysis

THERAPEUTIC

Rest and joint protection
Heat, cold, exercise
Mild analgesia
Assistive devices
Stress management
Orthopedic surgery
   Debridement
   Arthrodesis
   Arthroplasty
   Osteotomy
   Total joint replacement

enlargements, clients are often distressed by the resulting disfigurement of their hands. Little can be done to prevent the occurrence of these nodes.

Hips. OA of the hips (malum coxae senilis) may be extremely disabling. Congenital or structural abnormalities are frequent causes. This problem occurs more frequently in men than in women and may be unilateral or bilateral. Hip pain may be perceived as pain in the groin, buttock, or medial side of the thigh or knee, so the client may find it difficult to localize the problem correctly. Pain on motion or on weight-bearing may become progressively severe, and pain on rest may ensue. Sitting down is difficult, as is rising from a chair when the hips are lower than the knees. The client learns to sit in a high seat with firm support and arm rests. Eventually, loss of ROM is significant, with marked limitation of extension and internal rotation.

Knees. Softening of the posterior surface of the patella (chondromalacia patellae) is seen most commonly in young people. Degeneration of the weight-bearing surfaces of the femoral and tibial condyles is usually seen in older women and is associated with limitation of motion, crepitus, and flexion deformity.

Vertebral column. OA in the spine may produce localized symptoms of stiffness and pain. Degenerative disease of the intervertebral disks results as the nucleus pulposus deteriorates, becoming brittle and inelastic. Herniation of the degenerating nucleus most often occurs posteriorly or laterally, compressing a nerve root and causing muscle spasm or radicular pain. Another type of OA of the vertebral column involves development of degenerative disease of the intervertebral (apophyseal) joints, which generally follows disk disease by a number of years. Marginal osteophytes (spurs) also appear at vertebral attachments of the anulus, periosteum, and longitudinal ligaments. These osteophytes may fuse and limit ROM, or they may press against intervertebral foramina, producing symptoms of nerve root compression. Osteophyte formation in the posterior aspect of the cervical spine may rarely produce vascular compression and insufficiency, resulting in intermittent dizziness, visual disturbances, headaches, and ataxia.

Diagnostic Studies

In late disease, x-ray films show joint space narrowing, bony sclerosis, spur formation, and in some cases subluxation. X-ray changes do not always correlate with the client's degree of pain. Degenerative disease is often evident on x-ray film, but the client is completely free of symptoms. Conversely, some clients have severe pain with only moderate x-ray changes. No specific laboratory abnormalities are useful in the diagnosis of OA. The erythrocyte sedimentation rate (ESR) is normal except in instances of erosive OA, in which moderate elevation may be noted. Synovial fluid aspirated from an involved joint may be increased in volume but is clear yellow and viscous. Analysis of the fluid reveals little or no sign of inflammation.

Therapeutic Management

There are no specific therapies for the management of OA. Therapy is aimed at pain control, prevention of progression and disability, and restoration of joint function (Table 58-1). Once the diagnosis is confirmed, the client should be assured that OA is likely to remain confined to a few joints and does not generally cause crippling. If joint destruction is extensive and pain is severe, surgery may be an option.

Pharmacological Management

Aspirin is the most commonly used drug for the treatment of OA. It is generally prescribed in larger than usual doses and is given on a regular basis. In addition to relieving pain, aspirin reduces inflammation and consequently reduces swelling, stiffness, and possibly joint damage. Aspirin may cause ringing in the ears and slight deafness. These symptoms disappear if the dosage is reduced. Gas-

trointestinal (GI) problems related to aspirin can be alleviated by giving the drug with meals or a full glass of water, by the use of antacids, or by taking of enteric-coated aspirin or aspirin with an antacid preparation. Because drug absorption is slowed when taken with food, the dose of aspirin may need to be increased to be effective.

Nonsteroidal antiinflammatory drugs (NSAIDs) are particularly beneficial for persons who are intolerant to aspirin or who do not respond adequately. Newer agents are available that offer the advantage of a once- or twice-daily regimen. The need to take fewer drugs during the day encourages increased compliance (see Table 58-6 for drug management). When given in equivalent antiinflammatory dosages, all NSAIDs are comparable.[4] Individual responses and side effects to any drug, however, are variable. Aspirin should not be used in combination with NSAIDs. Intraarticular injections of corticosteroids are used to treat a symptomatic flare. Systemic use of corticosteroids should be avoided because it may accelerate the disease process.

Nutritional Considerations

There is no specific diet for OA except that which maintains optimal health. However, if the client is obese, a weight reduction program becomes an important part of the total treatment plan. Body weight is magnified five times through the hips and three times through the knees. The additional strain of extra pounds can greatly increase pain and loss of function in OA. In addition, heavy thighs lead to malalignment at the knee, increasing wear on the medial aspect. (Chapter 35 discusses ways to assist the client in obtaining and maintaining ideal body weight.)

■ Nursing Management of Osteoarthritis

Nursing assessment

Nursing assessment of the client with OA should include careful documentation of the nature, location, severity, and frequency of joint pain and stiffness and the extent to which it affects the client's ability to perform activities of daily living. Successful and unsuccessful pain-relieving practices should be noted. The nurse should examine the affected joint or joints and note tenderness, swelling, limitation of movement, and crepitation. It is useful to compare the involved joint with the same joint on the opposite side of the body if that joint is not affected.

Nursing diagnoses

Nursing diagnoses specific to the client with OA include, but are not limited to, the following:

1. Pain related to physical activity and lack of knowledge of pain self-management techniques
2. High risk for sleep pattern disturbance related to pain
3. Impaired physical mobility related to weakness, stiffness, and/or pain on ambulation
4. Self-care deficit related to joint deformity and pain with activity
5. Altered nutrition: more than body requirements related to intake in excess of energy output
6. Self-esteem disturbance related to changing social and work roles
7. Stiffness related to inactivity

Nursing interventions

Health promotion and maintenance. Prevention of primary OA is not possible; however, preventive education may include elimination of excessive strain by reduction of occupational and recreational hazards and nutritional counseling for weight reduction. Community education may include proper body mechanics of lifting and good posture. Athletic instruction and physical fitness programs should include safety measures that protect and reduce trauma to the joint structures. Congenital conditions such as Legg-Calvé-Perthes disease that are known to predispose to development of OA should be treated promptly.

Acute intervention. The person with OA is most troubled by pain, stiffness, limitation of function, and the frustration of coping with these physical difficulties daily. The older adult may believe that OA is an inevitable part of the aging process and that nothing can be done to ease the discomfort and related disability.

The client may be hospitalized for treatment if persistent pain or a disabling deformity is present. More often, the client is treated by a personal physician or rheumatologist. The goals of therapy are to relieve pain, protect joints from further stress, and restore mechanical function and alignment.

Medications are administered for the relief of pain and inflammation, if present. Other interventions found to be successful by the client in relieving pain, such as massage, heat, cold, or a programmed exercise regimen, should also be used. A physical therapist can provide valuable assistance in planning an exercise program.

The nurse should assist the client with activities of daily living as necessary and provide planned rest periods during the day. Allowing sufficient time for the client to flex stiff joints and to perform other warm-up activities before initiating activities can reduce temporary stiffness. Proper body alignment should be maintained at all times. If used, cervical traction should be properly applied and maintained.

Client education related to OA is an important nursing responsibility that should be carried out regardless of the care setting. Areas to include in the educational program are nature and management of the disease, medication management, correct posture and body mechanics, correct use of assistive devices such as a cane or walker, principles of joint protection (Table 58-2) and energy conservation, and a therapeutic exercise program. Home management goals must be individualized to meet the client's

Table 58-2 Client Education for Joint Protection

Maintain good posture and proper body mechanics.
Maintain normal weight.
Use assistive devices, if indicated.
Avoid positions of deviation and stress.
Find less stressful ways to perform tasks.
Avoid tasks that cause pain.
Develop organizing and pacing techniques.
Avoid forceful repetitive movements.

needs, and family and social supports should be included in goal setting and education.

Chronic management. After diagnosis of OA and the initial educational efforts the nurse needs to assist the client in developing long-term strategies in managing the disease. The client needs to be assured that OA is a localized disease and that severe deforming arthritis is not the usual course.

Safety measures in the home and work environment are important. These measures include activities such as removal of scatter rugs, provision of rails at stairs and bathtub, use of night-lights, and the use of well-fitting supportive shoes. Assistive devices such as canes, walkers, elevated toilet seats, and grab bars to reduce joint load and ensure safety may also be helpful.

Splints may be prescribed to rest and stabilize painful or inflamed joints. Soft collars and/or cervical traction may be used for a home therapy program for cervical OA. Stiff, painful hands can be relieved by warm water soaking, contrast baths, or paraffin. If swelling is more diffuse, stretch gloves can be worn at night to provide relief. Sexual counseling helps the client and spouse to enjoy physical closeness by learning to adapt positions, alter timing, and increase awareness of partner's needs.

Management of the chronic pain and loss of function of affected joints continue to be a primary concern. Nonpharmacological techniques such as meditation, relaxation, and biofeedback are particularly suited to nursing intervention of pain and to assisting the client in developing alternative coping strategies. Many different approaches must often be used before a successful pain-relieving combination is found. Over time a successful combination may fail and new approaches to pain relief must be sought. Nursing interventions should assist the client and family to overcome the feelings of helplessness and frustration in managing this chronic illness. The correct combination of pacing technique, heat application, joint protection, exercise, and medication can restore self-esteem and encourage confidence. The benefits of an aerobic exercise program such as walking or aerobic aquatics have been documented.[5]

RHEUMATOID ARTHRITIS

Rheumatoid arthritis (RA) is a chronic, systemic disease characterized by recurrent inflammation of the diarthrodial joints and related structures. It is frequently accompanied by a variety of extraarticular manifestations, such as rheumatoid nodules, arteritis, neuropathy, scleritis, pericarditis, lymphadenopathy, and splenomegaly.[6] RA is characterized by periods of remission and exacerbation of disease activity. The course of illness varies, ranging from episodes of illness separated by periods of remission to a more continuous, progressive disease. Death from RA is rare.

Significance

Of the approximately 6 million Americans who have RA, 75% are women. There are no geographical or racial predispositions. Although RA can occur at any age, it most often occurs in women of childbearing age.[7] In terms of its potential for chronic disability, RA is the most serious form of arthritis and is considered a significant national health problem.

Etiology

The cause of RA remains unknown. Whether a single causative factor is responsible or multiple factors are involved is unclear. Several etiologies are possible:

1. *Infection:* Research continues to probe the possibility of specific infectious pathogens, particularly viruses, which may trigger the process.

2. *Autoimmunity:* RA is characterized by the presence of autoantibodies against immunoglobulin G (IgG). Although no virus particles have been identified, it is likely that an antigenic stimulus such as a virus leads to the formation of the abnormal IgG. The autoantibodies to this altered IgG are known as *rheumatoid factors,* and they combine with IgG to form immune complexes that deposit in the joints, blood vessels, and pleura. Complement is activated and an inflammatory response results (see Chapter 7). Neutrophils are attracted to the site of inflammation and release proteolytic enzymes that can damage articular cartilage and basement membranes of blood vessels and pleura.

   Joint changes are characterized by chronic inflammation with the presence of inflammatory cells and mediators that result in persistent immunological activity. The infiltrating T cells and macrophages are activated and release a variety of cytokines, including interleukin-1 and interleukin-2, tumor necrosis factor, colony-stimulating factor, and interleukin-6 (see Table 8-4).[8] The activity of these cytokines accounts for many of the features of rheumatoid synovitis, including the synovial tissue inflammation, synovial proliferation, cartilage and bone damage, and systemic manifestations of RA.

3. *Genetic factors:* Certain familial factors may influence the expression of the disease. An increased prevalence of a human leukocyte antigen (HLA) known as the *HLA-DR4* occurs in persons with RA. It is possible that these HLA antigens and perhaps other genetic susceptibility to an unidentified environmental factor, such as a virus, initiate the disease process (see Chapter 8).

4. *Other factors:* Metabolic and biochemical abnormalities, nutritional and environmental factors, and occupational and psychosocial influences may play a part in the cause and/or expression of the disease, but their contribution is entirely speculative.

Pathophysiology

The pathogenesis of RA is more clearly understood than its etiology. If unarrested, the disease progresses through four stages:

1. *First stage:* The unknown etiological factor initiates joint inflammation, or synovitis, with swelling of the synovial lining membrane and production of excess synovial fluid.

2. *Second stage:* Pannus (granulation inflammatory tissue) is formed at the juncture of synovium and car-

Table 58-3 Comparison of Rheumatoid Arthritis and Osteoarthritis

Parameter	Rheumatoid Arthritis	Osteoarthritis
Age	Young and middle-aged	Usually >40 yr of age
Gender	Female more often than male	Same incidence
Weight	Weight loss	Usually overweight
Illness	Systemic manifestations	Local joint manifestation
Affected joints	PIPs, MCPs, MTPs, wrists, elbows, shoulders, knees, hips, cervical spine	DIPs, first CMCs, thumbs, first MTPs, knees, spine, hips; asymmetrical, one or more joints
Effusions	Common	Uncommon
Nodules	Present	Heberden's nodes
Synovial fluid	Inflammatory	Noninflammatory
X-ray films	Osteoporosis, narrowing, erosions	Osteophytes, subchondral cysts, sclerosis
Anemia	Common	Uncommon
Rheumatoid factor	Positive	Negative
Sedimentation rate	Elevated	Normal

CMC, Carpometacarpal; *DIP,* distal interphalangeal; *MCP,* metacarpophalangeal; *MTP,* metatarsophalangeal; *PIP,* proximal interphalangeal.

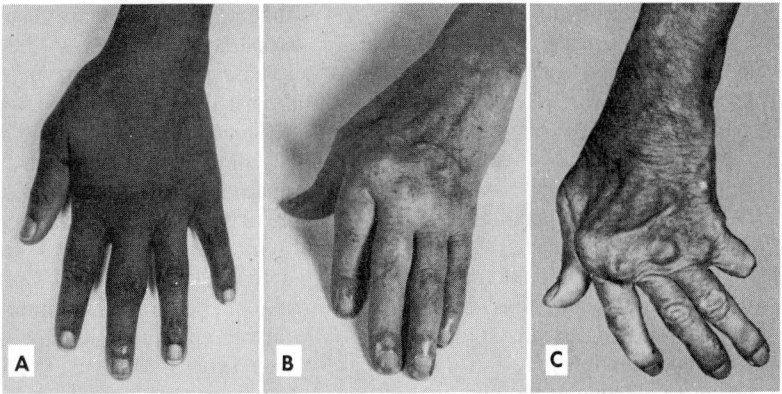

Fig. 58-3 RA of the hand. **A,** Early stage. **B,** Moderate involvement. **C,** Advanced stage.

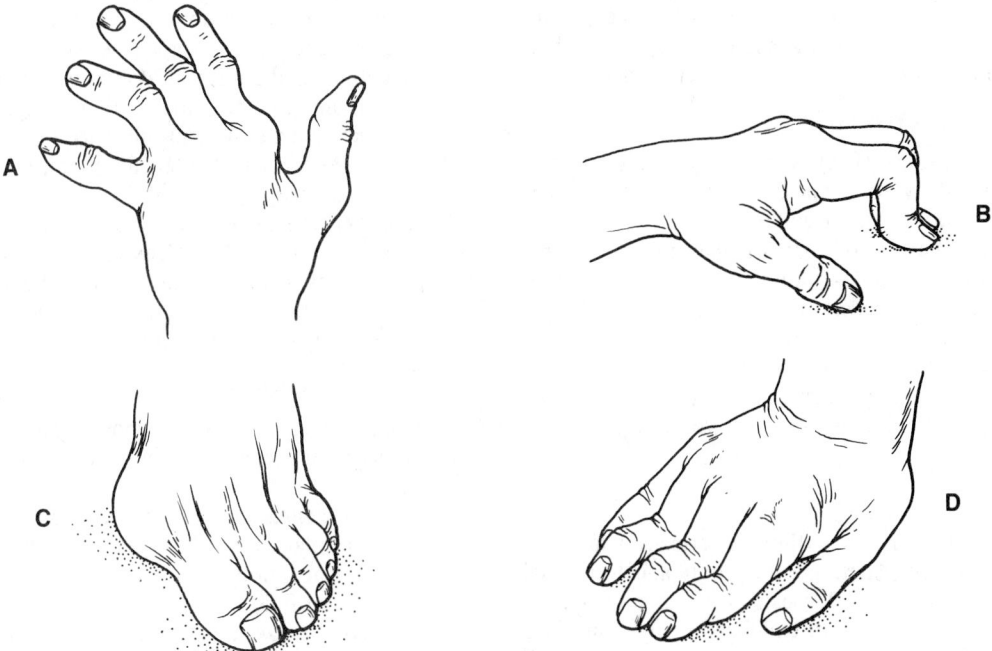

Fig. 58-4 Typical deformities of rheumatoid arthritis. **A,** Ulnar drift. **B,** Boutonniere. **C,** Hallux valgus. **D,** Swan-neck deformity.

tilage. This extends over the surface of the articular cartilage and eventually invades the joint capsule and subchondral bone.

3. *Third stage:* Tough fibrous connective tissue replaces pannus, occluding the joint space. Fibrous ankylosis results in decreased joint motion, malalignment, and deformity.

4. *Fourth stage:* As fibrous tissue calcifies, bony ankylosis may result in total joint immobilization.

Clinical Manifestations

Joints. RA typically develops insidiously. Nonspecific manifestations such as fatigue, anorexia, weight loss, and generalized stiffness may precede the onset of arthritic complaints. The stiffness becomes more localized after weeks to months. Some clients report a history of a precipitating stressful event such as infection, overwork, childbirth, surgery, or emotional upset. However, no data correlate these events and the onset of RA.

Specific articular involvement is manifested clinically by pain, stiffness, limitation of motion, and signs of inflammation (heat, swelling, and tenderness). Joint symptoms are generally bilaterally symmetrical and frequently affect small joints of the hands (proximal interphalangeal and metacarpophalangeal) and feet (metatarsophalangeal) as well as larger peripheral joints, including wrists, elbows, shoulders, knees, hips, ankles, and the jaw. The cervical spine may be affected, but the axial spine is generally spared. Early shoulder involvement is common in the older adult. Table 58-3 compares the manifestations of RA and OA.

The client characteristically has stiffness on arising in the morning and after periods of inactivity. This morning stiffness (gel phenomenon) usually lasts for 30 minutes to several hours or more, depending on disease activity. Metacarpal and proximal interphalangeal joints are typically swollen. The fingers may become spindle shaped from synovial hypertrophy and thickening of the joint capsule (Fig. 58-3). Joints become tender, painful, and warm to the touch. The pain is more pronounced on motion, varies in intensity, and may not be proportional to the degree of inflammation. Tenosynovitis frequently affects the extensor and flexor tendons around the wrists, producing symptoms of carpal tunnel syndrome (see Chapter 57) and making it difficult to grasp objects.

As disease activity progresses, inflammation and fibrosis of the joint capsule and supporting structures may lead to deformity and disability. Atrophy of muscles and destruction of tendons around the joint cause one articular surface to slip past the other (subluxation). Typical deformities of the hand include "ulnar drift," "swan neck," and boutonniere deformities (Fig. 58-4). Metatarsal-head subluxation and hallux valgus (bunion) may cause pain and walking disability.

Extraarticular manifestations. Rheumatoid nodules are present in 25% of all clients with RA and are probably the most common extraarticular finding. Small-vessel vasculitis is considered to be the initiating event in the formation of these nodules. They appear subcutaneously as firm, nontender masses and are usually found on olecranon bur-

sae, or along the extensor surface of the forearm. Nodules at the base of the spine and back of the head are common in older adults due to longer periods at rest. Nodules develop insidiously and can persist or regress spontaneously. They are usually not removed unless they are creating a problem because of the high probability of recurrence. Nodules may also appear on the eye or lungs; these indicate active disease and a poor prognosis.

Vasculitis (inflammation of blood vessels) may be responsible for a variety of systemic complications, including peripheral neuropathy, myopathy, cardiopulmonary involvement, and ischemic ulcerations of the skin. Fig. 58-5 shows the variety of extraarticular manifestations of RA.

Complications

Potential complications include infection, osteoporosis, amyloidosis, and Sjögren's syndrome. Spinal cord compression may occur from instability of articulations in the cervical spine.

Diagnostic Studies

Although no single laboratory test is conclusive, several findings are helpful in diagnosing RA in conjunction with the history and physical examination.[9] Moderate anemia is common. The ESR is elevated in 85% of clients and is useful in monitoring the response to therapy. Serum rheumatoid factor, a circulating antibody of the IgM class, is present in titers greater than 1:160 in nearly 80% of cases. Antinuclear antibody and lupus cell tests may be positive in a smaller percentage of clients.

Synovial fluid analysis may show increased volume and turbidity but decreased viscosity. The white blood cell (WBC) count is elevated (often as high as $30,000/\mu l$) and consists predominantly of polymorphonuclear leukocytes. Inflammatory changes in the synovium can be confirmed by tissue biopsy.

X-ray findings (which are not specifically diagnostic) may reveal only bone demineralization and soft-tissue swelling during the first 6 months of the disease. Later, narrowing of the joint space, destruction of articular cartilage, erosion, subluxation, and deformity are present. Malalignment and ankylosis occur in advanced disease. Table 58-4 describes the anatomical stages of RA.

Therapeutic Management

Therapeutic management of RA begins with a comprehensive program of pharmacotherapy and education. It is useful to view the drug therapy for RA with a "pyramid approach" that starts with mild antiinflammatory agents such as aspirin to disease-remitting agents such as penicellamine. Physical comfort is promoted by NSAIDs and rest. The client and family are educated about the disease process and home management needs. Responsible compliance with medications includes correct administration, reporting of side effects, and frequent medical and laboratory follow-up visits. Physical therapy maintains joint motion and muscle strength. Occupational therapy develops upper extremity function and encourages joint protection through the use of splinting, pacing techniques, and assistive devices.

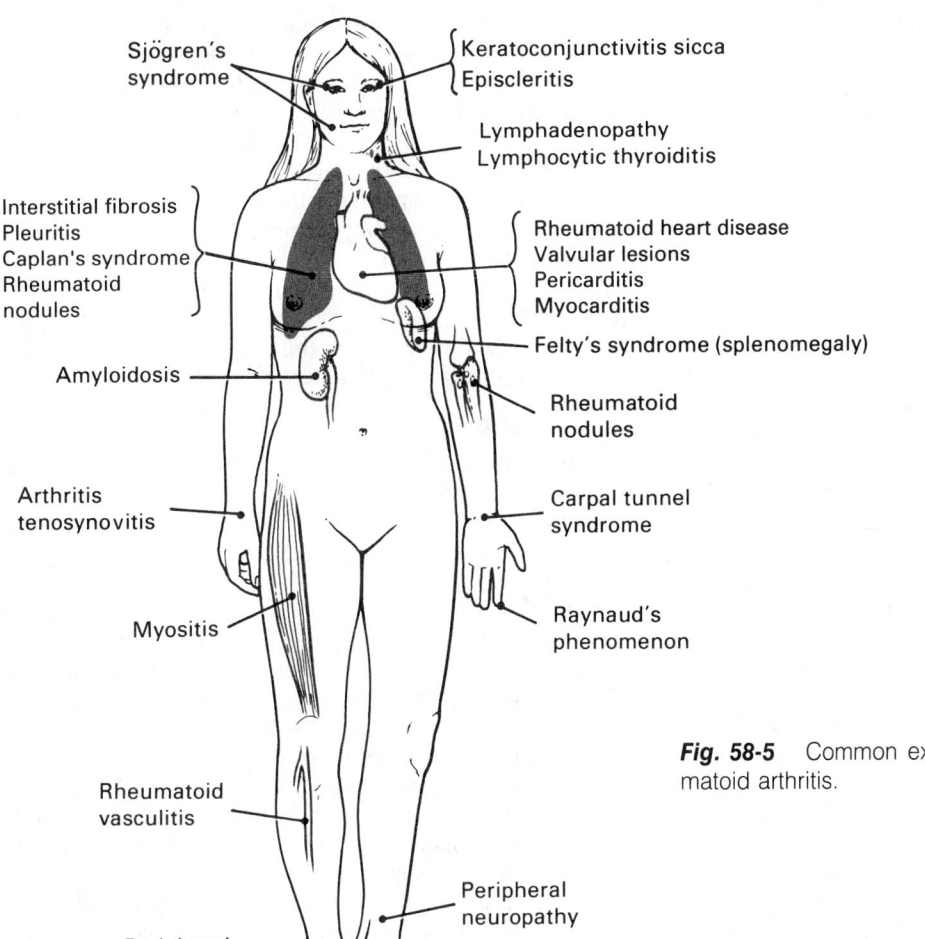

Sjögren's syndrome

Keratoconjunctivitis sicca
Episcleritis

Lymphadenopathy
Lymphocytic thyroiditis

Interstitial fibrosis
Pleuritis
Caplan's syndrome
Rheumatoid nodules

Rheumatoid heart disease
Valvular lesions
Pericarditis
Myocarditis

Felty's syndrome (splenomegaly)

Amyloidosis

Rheumatoid nodules

Arthritis tenosynovitis

Carpal tunnel syndrome

Myositis

Raynaud's phenomenon

Rheumatoid vasculitis

Peripheral neuropathy

Peripheral edema

Fig. 58-5 Common extraarticular manifestations of rheumatoid arthritis.

Table 58-4 American Rheumatism Association Anatomical Stages

Stage I—Early
No destructive changes on x-ray film, possible x-ray evidence of osteoporosis

Stage II—Moderate
X-ray evidence of osteoporosis, with or without slight bone or cartilage destruction, no joint deformities (although possibly limited joint mobility), adjacent muscle atrophy, possible presence of extraarticular soft tissue lesions (e.g., nodules, tenovaginitis)

Stage III—Severe
X-ray evidence of cartilage and bone destruction, in addition to osteoporosis; joint deformity, such as subluxation, ulnar deviation, or hyperextension, without fibrous or bony ankylosis; extensive muscle atrophy; possible presence of extraarticular soft tissue lesions (e.g., nodules, tenovaginitis)

Stage IV—Terminal
Fibrous or bony ankylosis, criteria of stage III

*Modified from Steinbrocker O, Traeger CH, and Batterman RC: Therapeutic criteria in rheumatoid arthritis, J Am Med Assoc 140:659-662, 1949.

An individualized treatment plan considers the nature of the disease activity, joint function, age, gender, family and social roles, and response to previous treatment (Table 58-5). Therapy emphasizes both the physical and the psychological problems resulting from arthritis. A caring, long-term relationship with arthritis health professionals promotes client self-esteem and hope and discourages the use of unproven remedies, which waste money and time.

Pharmacological Management

The foundation for the pharmacological treatment of RA is aspirin at dosages adequate to maintain an antiinflammatory effect (Table 58-6). To maintain this antiinflammatory action, aspirin is used in high dosages of 4 to 6 g/day (10 to 18 tablets) in divided doses to obtain a blood level of 15 to 30 mg/dl. Enteric-coated aspirin is often used to prevent gastric irritation. Enteric-coated tablets have a special covering to prevent their disintegration in the stomach. More recently, NSAIDs have been used when the client is intolerant to high doses of aspirin. Several NSAIDs such as piroxicam (Feldene) and sulindac (Clinoril), which are taken only once or twice a day in an effort to improve compliance, are now available.

Remission-inducing agents include antimalarials, peni-

Table 58-5

Diagnostic and Therapeutic Management: Rheumatoid Arthritis

DIAGNOSTIC

Complete history and physical examination
Laboratory studies
  Complete blood cell count
  ESR
  Protein electrophoresis
  Latex agglutination test for rheumatoid factor
  Antinuclear antibodies
Joint x-ray examination
Synovial fluid analysis

THERAPEUTIC

General
  Education, including disease process and management
  Nutrition
  General health measures

THERAPEUTIC—cont'd

Physical
  Rest, including local joint, systemic, and emotional
  Therapeutic exercise
  Joint protection and energy conservation
Pharmacotherapy
  NSAIDs
  Disease-modifying drugs such as hydroxychloroquine,
    gold, penicillamine
  Intraarticular or systemic corticosteroids
  Cytotoxic drugs (e.g., azathioprine, methotrexate, cyclo-
    phosphamide)
Orthopedic surgery, especially reconstructive joint replace-
  ment

Table 58-6 Pharmacological Management of Rheumatic Disorders

Drug	Mechanisms of Action	Common Side Effects	Nursing Considerations
SALICYLATES			
Aspirin, salsalate (Disalcid)	Antiinflammatory analgesic, antipyretic effect	GI irritation (ulcer and hemorrhage), hypersensitivity, salicylism (nausea, tinnitus, dizziness, hyperpnea), prolonged bleeding time	When drug is taken for antiinflammatory effect, discontinue if pain decreases. Administer drug with food, milk, antacids as prescribed, or full glass of water or use enteric-coated aspirin. Report signs of bleeding, (e.g., tarry stool, bruising, petechiae, melena).
NONSTEROIDAL ANTIINFLAMMATORY DRUGS			
Ibuprofen (Motrin)	Antiinflammatory analgesic	GI irritation, dizziness, rash	Report signs of bleeding, edema, skin rashes, persistent headaches, or visual disturbances.
Naproxen (Naprosyn, Anaprox)	Antiinflammatory analgesic	GI irritation, headache, tinnitus, pruritus	Check renal and hepatic function periodically in long-term therapy. Use cautiously in clients with GI, renal, or cardiac disease and in those with bleeding disorders.
Piroxicam (Feldene)	Antiinflammatory analgesic	GI irritation, allergic reactions	
Indomethacin (Indocin)	Antiinflammatory analgesic	GI irritation, headache, visual disturbances	
Sulindac (Clinoril)	Antiinflammatory analgesic	GI irritation, rash, dizziness, headache	
Tolmetin sodium (Tolectin)	Antiinflammatory analgesic	GI irritation, dizziness, rash, tinnitus	
Diclofenac (Voltaren)	Antiinflammatory analgesic	GI irritation, headache, dizziness	
Meclofenamate (Meclomen)		Diarrhea, pyrosis, flatulence, dizziness	

Continued.

Table 58-6 Pharmacological Management of Rheumatic Disorders—cont'd

Drug	Mechanism of Action	Common Side Effects	Nursing Considerations
CORTICOSTEROIDS			
Intraarticular injections			
Methylprednisolone acetate (Depo-Medrol)	Antiinflammatory analgesic	Suppression of local infection, local osteoporosis or neuropathic arthropathy from repeated injection	Use strict aseptic technique as joint fluid is removed and steroids are injected. Inform client that joint may feel worse immediately after injection.
Triamcinolone hexacetonide (Aristospan)	Antiinflammatory analgesic		Inform client that improvement lasts weeks to months after injection and that weight bearing should be minimized for 2-6 wk after injection.
Systemic			
Hydrocortisone sodium succinate (Solu-Cortef)	Antiinflammatory	Cushing's syndrome, including fluid retention, GI irritation, osteoporosis, hypertension, diabetes mellitus, acne, menstrual irregularities, hirsutism, risk of infection, bruising, iridocyclitis in children	Use only when symptoms persist with less potent antiinflammatory drugs or in life-threatening situations. Administer for limited time only, tapering dose slowly. Be aware that exacerbation of symptoms occurs with abrupt withdrawal. Monitor blood pressure, weight, CBC, and potassium. Limit salt intake. Report signs of infection. Instruct client to report corticosteroid use to surgeon or dentist to avoid postoperative adrenal insufficiency.
Methylprednisolone succinate sodium (Solu-Medrol)	Antiinflammatory		
Dexamethasone (Decadron)	Antiinflammatory		
Prednisone	Antiinflammatory		
Triamcinolone (Aristocort)	Antiinflammatory		
IMMUNOSUPPRESSIVE			
Azathioprine (Imuran)	Unknown, suppression of autoimmune mechanism	GI irritation and ulceration, alopecia, oral lesions, dermatitis, blood dyscrasia, bone marrow depression	Be aware that therapy is limited to clients not responsive to conventional therapy. Be aware of teratogenic potential that cautions against use for children or adults of childbearing age. Monitor CBC and urinalysis values.
Cyclophosphamide (Cytoxan)	Unknown, suppression of autoimmune mechanism	GI irritation and ulceration, alopecia, oral lesions, dermatitis, blood dyscrasia, bone marrow depression	Be aware that therapy is limited to clients not responsive to conventional therapy. Monitor CBC and urinalysis values. Be aware of teratogenic potential that cautions against use for children or adults of childbearing age. Inform client that contraception should be used during therapy.
Methotrexate	Unknown, disease-modifying effect	GI irritation, photosensitivity, oral lesions, hepatic toxicity, blood dyscrasia, infertility	Monitor CBC and liver function values. Instruct client to avoid alcoholic beverages and report signs of jaundice. Be aware of teratogenic potential that cautions against use for children or adults of childbearing age. Inform client that contraception should be used during and 3 mo after treatment.

Table 58-6 Pharmacological Management of Rheumatic Disorders—cont'd

Drug	Mechanism of Action	Common Side Effects	Nursing Considerations
REMISSION-INDUCING AGENTS			
Chrysotherapy			
Gold sodium thiomalate (Myochrysine), aurothioglucose (Solganal), auranofin (Ridaura)	Unknown, inflammatory-suppressive effect	Dermatitis, pruritus, stomatitis, blood dyscrasia, nephrotoxicity, diarrhea	Test blood and urine regularly. Check urine for blood and protein before each dose and delay injection until negative. Mix drug well and give deep intramuscular injection in buttocks. Inform client that symptomatic improvement is not expected for 3-6 mo and that therapy may be continued indefinitely. Institute new oral therapy with bulking agents. Do not taper oral dosage; be aware that laboratory testing is less frequent with oral drug. Instruct client to not become pregnant while receiving chrysotherapy.
Antimalarials			
Chloroquine phosphate (Aralen) Hydroxychloroquine sulfate (Plaquenil sulfate)	Unknown, disease-modifying effect	Asymptomatic retinopathy, corneal opacity, headache, dizziness, GI irritation, blood dyscrasia, pruritus	Inform client that ophthalmologic examination including slit lamp studies is required every 3-6 mo. Instruct client to take drug with meals, milk, or antacid as prescribed, to report all skin eruptions and visual disturbances, and to avoid excessive sun exposure. Be aware that drugs are contraindicated for clients with psoriasis. Monitor CBC and liver function values periodically. Instruct client to discuss condition with physician before pregnancy and breastfeeding.
Other			
Penicillamine (Cuprimine)	Unknown, disease-modifying effect	Blood dyscrasia, glomerulonephropathy	Give drug on empty stomach before meals (not with). Monitor CBC, urinalysis, and liver function values. Report fever, sore throat, chills, bruising, or bleeding. Be aware that drug is contraindicated with gold therapy. Instruct client to not become pregnant while taking drug.

cillamine, methotrexate, and gold therapy. Antimalarials may be prescribed for clients with persistent arthritis but take 4 to 6 months for effects to become evident. The possibility of rare irreversible retinal degeneration caused by deposition of these drugs in the pigment layer of the retina requires ophthalmological examination at 4- to 6-month intervals.[10] Gold (chrysotherapy) and penicillamine may be recommended for clients whose disease activity continues despite antiinflammatory therapy. These drugs should be considered only when the client understands the cumulative effect and is willing to commit to a lengthy treatment regimen, including frequent laboratory evaluations. The exact mechanism for the effectiveness of gold and penicillamine in the treatment of RA is not known.[11] Oral methotrexate appears to be a disease-modifying drug that has been reported as an effective treatment in RA.[12] The rapid antiinflammatory effect of methotrexate reduces clinical symptoms in days to weeks, whereas gold therapy must accumulate for 4 to 6 months for a full therapeutic effect. Methotrexate therapy requires frequent laboratory follow-up. The duration of safe treatment and the incidence of long-term hepatic and/or lung disease continue to be investigated.

Cytotoxic drugs such as cyclophosphamide, azathioprine, and methotrexate suppress aberrant inflammation and immune-mediated reactions that are responsible for the tissue damage in RA without markedly suppressing the normal host defense mechanisms. These drugs, also referred to as *immunosuppressives,* are generally used in flares when clear-cut danger of irreversible organ system dysfunction is present.

Corticosteroid therapy can be used several ways to achieve disease control. It may be used intraarticularly for a flare in one or two joints. Pain in the joint may increase for 1 to 2 days after injection because of the irritation by the medication. Pain and swelling are usually relieved for 1 to 6 weeks.

Bridge therapy (5 mg orally of the prescribed corticosteroid for 4 to 6 weeks) is used until one of the longer-acting drugs, such as hydroxychloroquine, gold, or D-penicillamine, has been taken long enough to suppress disease activity. *Burst corticosteroid therapy* describes high-dose (60 mg) corticosteroid used for a severe articular flare, which is then quickly tapered in 10 to 14 days. *Pulse therapy* (Solu-Medrol, at dosages of no more than 1 g/day intravenously for 3 days) is used to achieve fast control of inflammation and results in fewer side effects over the long term by the taking of a smaller daily dose. Regardless of the regimen, high-dose and/or long-term corticosteroid therapy results in drug dependency and serious side effects (see Chapter 44).

Nutritional Considerations

There is no special diet for RA; however, balanced nutrition is important. The fatigue, pain, depression, limited endurance, and limitation of mobility that may accompany RA may interfere with the client's appetite and ability to shop for and prepare food. Clients are vulnerable to fad claims for improvement through health foods and vitamins. Daily dietary supplementation with omega-3 fatty acids has been reported to decrease the number of tender joints and to prolong onset of fatigue. However, the effects are modest and the treatment requires further investigation for approval by the U.S. Food and Drug Administration.[13] A sensible weight-loss program should be undertaken by the obese client to relieve stress on affected joints.

Limited salt intake may help minimize weight gain caused by sodium retention if the client is taking corticosteroids. Steroids also increase the appetite, resulting in a higher caloric intake. Even the most compliant client becomes distressed as Cushing's syndrome symptoms—moon face and redistribution of fatty tissue to the trunk—change body appearances. The client must be encouraged to continue a balanced diet and not to alter corticosteroid dose or stop therapy abruptly. Weight slowly adjusts to normal several months after cessation of therapy.

■ Nursing Management of Rheumatoid Arthritis
Nursing assessment
Subjective and objective data that should be obtained from the client with RA are presented in Table 58-7.

Table 58-7

Nursing Assessment of the Client with Rheumatoid Arthritis

SUBJECTIVE DATA

History
Positive family history, viral infections, remissions and exacerbations, precipitating factors (e.g., emotional upset, infections, overwork, childbirth, surgery)
Medications
Use of aspirin, corticosteroids, NSAIDs, gold salts, penicillamine
General
Fever, weight loss, fatigue
Gastrointestinal
Dry mucous membranes of mouth and pharynx, melena
Neurological
Paresthesias of hands and feet, numbness, tingling, loss of sensation
Musculoskeletal
Morning stiffness and joint swelling, muscle weakness, symmetrical joint pain and aching that increases with motion or stress on joint

OBJECTIVE DATA

General
Lymphadenopathy
Integumentary
Keratoconjunctivitis, subcutaneous rheumatoid nodules (on forearm, elbows), skin ulcers, shiny, taut skin over involved joints
Cardiovascular
Symmetrical pallor and cyanosis of fingers (Raynaud's phenomenon)
Gastrointestinal
Splenomegaly (Felty's syndrome)
Musculoskeletal
Symmetrical joint involvement with swelling, erythema, heat, tenderness, and deformities; Bouchard's nodes (enlargement of proximal phalangeal and metacarpophalangeal joints); limitation of joint movement; muscle contractures; osteoporosis, muscle atrophy
Possible findings
Positive rheumatoid factor, elevated ESR; soft tissue swelling on MRI; osteoporosis, joint space narrowing, and bony erosion on radiographs

Nursing diagnoses
Nursing diagnoses related to RA may include, but are not limited to, those presented in Table 58-8.
Nursing interventions
Health promotion and maintenance. Prevention of RA is not possible at this time. However, community education programs should include information concerning the symptoms of RA to promote early diagnosis and treat-

Table 58-8

NURSING CARE PLAN FOR THE CLIENT WITH RHEUMATOID ARTHRITIS

Defining Characteristics	Nursing Interventions	Evaluation Criteria
NURSING DIAGNOSIS: Pain related to joint inflammation, overuse of joint, and ineffective pain and/or comfort measures		
Communication of pain descriptors, guarding behavior, and limited joint function; hot, swollen, painful joints; limited motion	Encourage decreased activity, increased rest, and supportive resting splints for affected joints. Teach self-administration of antiinflammatory medications as prescribed, including names, actions, side effects, dose, and administration of prescribed drugs; use of heat and cold therapy to reduce pain and swelling; use of daily rest periods; protective techniques that limit stress to joints; avoidance of undue physical and emotional stress; and nonpharmacological pain strategies (e.g., meditation, yoga).	Decreased pain, swelling, and erythema of joints
NURSING DIAGNOSIS: Altered mobility related to joint pain, stiffness, and swelling		
Limitation of joint motion, strength, and endurance; inability to perform routine activities of daily living	Apply moist heat (e.g., paraffin bath, hot packs, warm shower). Encourage ROM exercises; reduce frequency if pain and swelling are present. Schedule morning care and procedures later in the day after morning stiffness subsides. Assist with daily hygienic care. Teach client to use assistive devices to promote independence. Encourage joint protection and pacing techniques.	Increased ROM and function, decreased stiffness, independent care
NURSING DIAGNOSIS: Fatigue related to exacerbation of disease activity, anemia, drug side effects, muscle atrophy, sleep disturbance, or depression		
Weakness, decreased activity tolerance, increased joint pain, anemia, poor sleep habits, reduced appetite, irritability, sadness, hopelessness, poor posture	Balance activity with rest periods. Encourage regular general physical exercise such as walking, bicycling, or swimming. Review nutrition and sleep patterns. Refer for psychological counseling and coping strategies.	Improved stamina and endurance, better-quality sleep and eating habits, positive affect
NURSING DIAGNOSIS: Altered nutrition: less than body requirements related to fatigue, pain, treatment, and/or self-care deficit		
Weight loss, anemia, loss of appetite, stomatitis, gastritis or dyspepsia	Assess medications and treatments for GI side effects. Take diet history and teach basic four nutrition groups. Assess client's ability to shop for and prepare food. Use assistance devices that make preparation and eating easier and less painful.	Stable weight and good appetite
NURSING DIAGNOSIS: Joint deformity related to disease activity, noncompliance, and lack of knowledge of contracture prevention		
Ulnar deviation, muscle contracture, limited ROM	Instruct client on correct application of resting splints, selection of properly fitting footwear, maintenance of proper posture and body alignment, and selection and use of assistive devices. Assist client to develop less stressful ways to do tasks and protect joints. Encourage compliance with prescribed treatment and daily ROM exercises.	Minimal deformity, optimal function, proper body alignment

Continued.

Table 58-8

 NURSING CARE PLAN FOR THE CLIENT WITH RHEUMATOID ARTHRITIS—cont'd

Defining Characteristics	Nursing Interventions	Evaluation Criteria
NURSING DIAGNOSIS: Body-image disturbance related to chronic disease activity, long-term treatment program, deformities, stiffness, and inability to perform usual activities		
Social withdrawal, flat affect, altered self-concept, reduced sexual interest, lack of social support	Allow client to ventilate feelings about disease. Offer psychological support to client and family. Assist client to recognize need for regular therapeutic management and to resist false advertising and unproven remedies. Provide sexual counseling. Reassure client of self-worth. Assess client's knowledge of disease. Plan and initiate program of education on basis of client readiness. Include client's family in discussion of laboratory tests and procedures. Evaluate client's understanding through verbalization and demonstration.	Acceptance of body changes and maintenance of interest in life
NURSING DIAGNOSIS: Altered family processes related to client's inability to function secondary to chronic illness and treatment regimen		
Changes in family, social, and occupational roles; dysfunctional dynamics; loss of work status, economic resources	Help client and family to identify appropriate coping strategies for adjusting to changes in function and role responsibilities. Refer client to community vocational centers for job modifications and/or retraining. Encourage professional family counseling.	Successful adjustment of client and family to disease activity, vocational rehabilitation or modification
NURSING DIAGNOSIS: Self-care deficit (partial to total) related to disease progression, weakness, and contracture		
Inability to perform one or more activities of daily living.	Assess client's ability to perform activities of daily living and assist client with them as necessary. Provide assistive devices or refer to occupational therapist where appropriate. Allow client to pace activities.	Independent or assisted achievement of activities of daily living

ment. Many publications for the public are available through the Arthritis Foundation.*

Acute intervention. The primary objectives in the management of RA are reduction of inflammation, relief of pain, preservation of joint function, and prevention or correction of joint deformity. These may be approached by a comprehensive program of daily antiinflammatory medication, rest, joint protection, therapeutic heat, exercise, and thorough client and family education. The nurse is an integral member of the health team, working closely with the physician, physical and occupational therapists, and social worker to restore function and to help the client make lifestyle adjustments to chronic illness (Fig. 58-6).

The client with newly diagnosed RA may be hospitalized for control of acute inflammation, evaluation of systemic involvement, and comprehensive education by the health team. Hospitalization may also be necessary for cli-

ents with extraarticular complications or advanced disease requiring reconstructive surgery for disabling deformities.

Nursing intervention begins with a careful assessment of physical needs (joint pain, swelling, ROM, and general health status), psychosocial needs (family support, sexual satisfaction, emotional stress, financial constraints, vocation and career limitations), and environmental needs (transportation, home/work modifications). After the identification of problems and potential problems, a carefully planned program for rehabilitation and education can be coordinated by the nurse for the health care team.

Suppression of inflammation is most effectively achieved through the administration of antiinflammatory and/or remittive agents. Careful attention to timing sustains the salicylate level and reduces early-morning stiffness. Client and family education centers around the action and side effects of each drug prescribed and the importance of laboratory monitoring when necessary. Many clients with RA are taking many different drugs. The nurse must assist the client in making the drug regimen as clear

---

*Arthritis Foundation, 1314 Spring Street NW, Atlanta, GA 30309.

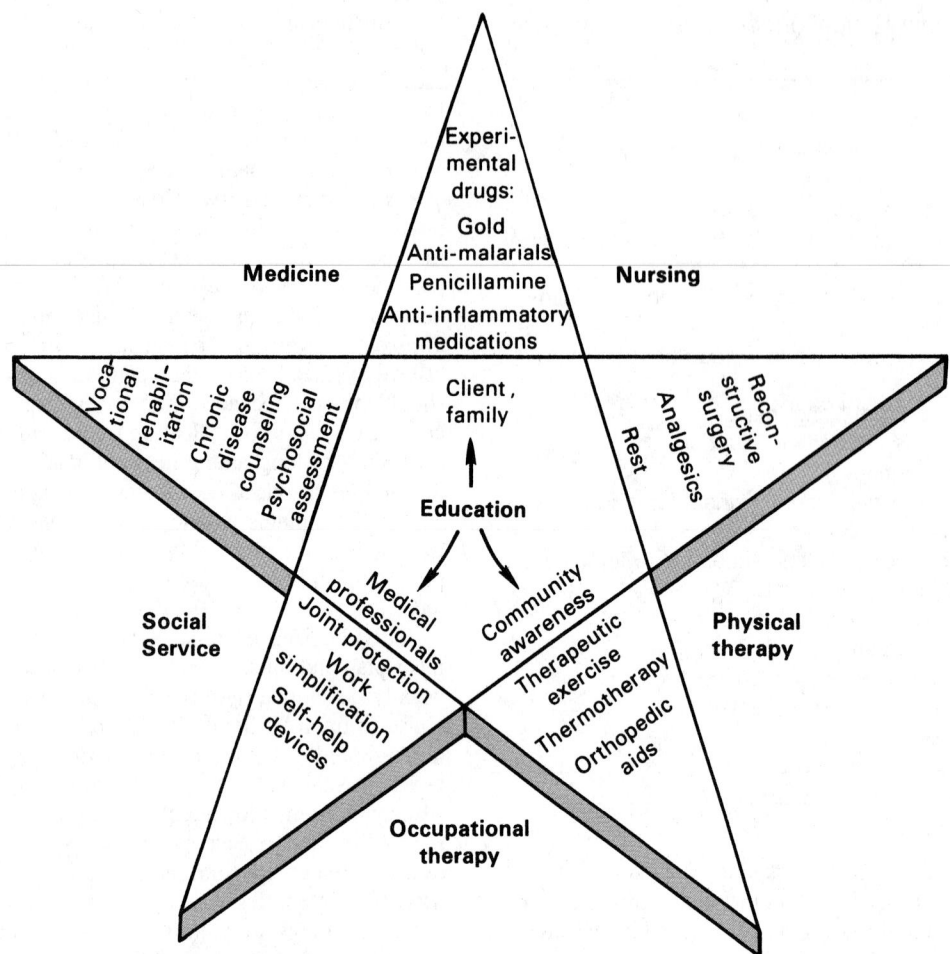

Fig. 58-6 Team approach to the management of rheumatoid arthritis.

and simple as possible. High-dose intravenous (IV) corticosteroids (pulse therapy) require careful observation for changes in blood pressure, peripheral edema, and signs of congestive heart failure.

Nonpharmacological relief of pain includes the use of therapeutic heat and cold, rest, relaxation techniques, joint protection (Tables 58-2 and 58-9), biofeedback, transcutaneous electrical nerve stimulation, and hypnosis. Assessment for individual differences and preference allows the nurse to help the client and family set goals that promote optimal comfort.

Lightweight splints are sometimes used to rest an inflamed joint and prevent deformity from muscle spasms and contractures. These splints should be removed, skin care given, ROM exercises performed, and splints reapplied as prescribed.[13] The occupational therapist may help to identify self-help devices that can assist in the activities of daily living.

Morning care and procedures should be planned around the client's morning stiffness and may need to be delayed. Sitting or standing in a warm shower, sitting in a tub with warm towels around the shoulders, or simply soaking the hands in a basin of warm water may help to relieve joint stiffness and allow the client to comfortably perform the activities of daily living. Careful skin care should be offered, particularly if the client is confined to bed.

The professional nurse acts as liaison among the client, family, and other members of the health team, coordinating services and evaluating the client's understanding of the total home management program (see Table 58-8).

Chronic management

REST. Regularly scheduled rest periods alternated throughout the day help relieve fatigue and pain and minimize excessive weight-bearing. The amount of rest necessary varies according to the severity of the disease and each client's limitations. Total bed rest is rarely necessary and should be avoided to prevent stiffness and immobility. Even a client with mild disease may require daytime rest in addition to 8 to 10 hours of sleep at night. The nurse should help the client identify ways to modify daily activities because overexertion can lead to fatigue and a flare-up in disease activity. Clients should rest *before* becoming exhausted. The nurse should assist the client in pacing and setting priorities on activities on the basis of realistic goals. Sitting rather than standing should be encouraged.

Good body alignment while resting is important. A firm mattress or bedboard should be used. Positions of exten-

Table 58-9 Client Education for Protection of Small Joints

Avoid positions of deformity.
  Press water from a sponge instead of wringing.
  Do not use pillows under knees.
Use strongest joint available for any task.
  When rising from chair, push with palms rather than fingers.
  Carry laundry basket in both arms rather than with fingers.
Distribute weight over many joints instead of stressing a few.
  Slide objects instead of lifting them.
  Hold packages close to body for support.
Change positions frequently.
  Do not hold book or grip steering wheel for long periods without resting.
  Avoid grasping pencil or cutting vegetables with knife for extended periods.
Avoid repetitious movements.
  Do not knit for long periods.
  Rest between rooms when vacuuming.
Modify chores to avoid stress on joints.
  Avoid heavy tasks.
  Sit on stool instead of standing.

sion should be encouraged, and positions of flexion should be avoided. Lying prone for ½ hour twice daily is recommended. Pillows should never be placed under the knees. A small, flat pillow may be used under the head. Splints and casts may be helpful in maintaining proper alignment, especially when joint inflammation is present.

JOINT PROTECTION. Protecting joints from stress is as important as taking medications regularly. Nursing intervention includes helping the client identify ways to modify tasks. Each client needs to learn less stressful ways to accomplish routine activities. The emphasis is on changing the way the task is done and on work-simplification techniques.

Energy conservation requires careful planning. Work should be done in short periods with scheduled rest breaks to avoid fatigue. Chores should be spread through the week rather than concentrated (e.g., all cleaning is not done on the weekend). Activities should be organized to avoid running up and down stairs. Carts should be used to carry things. Materials used often should be stored in a convenient, easily reached area. Time-saving devices (e.g., electric can opener) should be used if possible. Chores should be delegated to other family members.

The nurse should instruct the client with arthritis in activities that protect the small joints from stress. Observation of the client performing tasks at work, in the hospital, and in the home identifies activities that need to be revised. Joint-saving activities should be reinforced. Table 58-9 lists sample activities that protect small joints.

Client independence may be reinforced by occupational therapy with assistive devices that help simplify tasks; built-up utensils, buttonhooks, modified drawer handles, lightweight plastic dishes, and raised toilet seats are examples. Wearing clothing with buttons or a zipper down the front instead of the back makes dressing easier. The nurse can refer the client to the *Arthritis Foundation Self-Help Manual* for additional suggestions related to self-care.[14]

DAILY HEAT AND EXERCISE. Heat and cold therapy help to relieve stiffness, pain, and muscle spasm. Application of ice may be beneficial in an acute episode, and moist heat appears to offer better relief of chronic stiffness. Superficial heat sources such as heating pads, moist hot packs, paraffin baths, whirlpool baths, and warm baths or showers relieve stiffness before therapeutic exercises; the modality should be selected according to disease severity, ease of application, and cost. Heat and cold can be used as often as desired as long as the heat application does not exceed 20 minutes at one time and the cold application does not exceed 10 minutes at one time.[15] The nurse should alert the client to the possibility of a burn, especially if a heat-producing liniment is used with another external heat device.

Individualized exercise is an integral part of the treatment plan and must be carefully balanced. This program is usually developed by a physical therapist and includes exercise to improve flexibility, strength, and endurance. The nurse should be aware of the program to foster compliance and to ensure that the exercises are being done correctly. Inadequate joint movement can result in progressive joint immobility and muscle weakness; too much exercise can result in increased pain, inflammation, and joint destruction. If only one leg is painful, a cane can be used for relief. If both legs are painful, a walker can be used. A platform-wheeled walker is preferred to minimize strain on hands and wrists.

Gentle ROM exercises are usually done daily to keep the joints functional. The nurse needs to emphasize that usual daily activities *do not* provide adequate exercise to maintain joint motion. Careful adherence to the prescribed exercise program should be a prime goal of the teaching program. The client should have the opportunity to practice the exercises with supervision. Many clients enjoy aquatic exercises in a warm pool (25° C to 28° C [78° F to 83° F]), which allows easier ROM because of the buoyancy of the water.[16]

If the client is having an acute inflammatory episode, the joints are at risk for damage from overaggressive exercise. One or two repetitions of ROM exercises are sufficient until the acute episode subsides.

PSYCHOLOGICAL SUPPORT. Self-management and adherence to an individualized home program are contingent on a thorough understanding of RA, the nature and course of the disease, and the objectives of treatment. In addition, the client's perception of the disease and value system must be considered. The client should be able to recognize false advertising and unproved remedies despite claims of cure and relief of chronic pain. Information should be verified with health professionals and reliable community agencies.

A treatment program tailored to individual problems and lifestyle increases adherence. The nurse can help the

client recognize common fears and concerns faced by all clients living with a chronic illness. Evaluation of the family support system is important. The client is constantly threatened by problems of limited function and fatigue, loss of self-esteem, altered body image, and fear of disability and deformity. Alterations in sexuality should be discussed. Financial planning may be necessary. Community resources such as the Visiting Nurse Association, homemaker services, and vocational rehabilitation may be considered. Self-help groups are beneficial for some clients. Self-management classes are available in many communities.

JUVENILE-ONSET CHRONIC ARTHRITIS

Juvenile-onset chronic arthritis (JCA), the major rheumatic disease of youth since rheumatic fever has been controlled, is defined as RA beginning before 16 years of age and may be classified on the basis of the type of onset: systemic, pauciarticular, and polyarticular.[17] The last form most closely resembles adult RA; the others may represent other types of arthritis with onset during childhood. Children as young as 6 months of age may be affected, with the peak ages at onset between 1 and 5 years and again between 9 and 12 years. Prognosis is generally favorable, with nearly 70% of children having few or no inflammatory symptoms by adulthood. Residual deformity, however, may be a severe problem for some clients.

JCA may occur with arthritis confined to one joint *(pauciarticular)* or several *(polyarticular)*. Children most often do not complain of joint pain but may assume a position of flexion to minimize pain, carefully limit movement, or refuse to walk at all. A more constitutional variant known as *Still's disease* (systemic onset) occurs with high-spiking fever, vague arthralgias, generalized rash, hepatosplenomegaly, lymphadenopathy, and pleuritis or pericarditis. Complications of JCA include retarded growth and development and chronic, asymptomatic (and at times vision-threatening) eye inflammation.

Criteria for the diagnosis of JCA require persistent arthritis of one or more joints for at least 6 consecutive weeks, provided certain other similar disorders are ruled out. High-spiking fever, rheumatoid rash, generalized lymphadenopathy, and splenomegaly are more common in children than in adults with RA.[18] Leukocytosis is common, whereas rheumatoid factor is present in only 15% of those affected. Aspirin suppresses inflammation in the majority of cases. Chrysotherapy can be used for arthritis unresponsive to aspirin. Steroids are avoided when possible.

Nursing intervention requires an individualized written home program with emphasis on compliance. The family is best counseled about the course and prognosis of their child's arthritis according to the onset classification. Daily participation in a planned physical training program encourages full ROM and muscle strengthening and does not strain affected joints. Swimming, bicycling, and dance therapy are better than running, jumping, and kicking. Growth and development should be documented. Slit-lamp ophthalmological examinations must be done routinely for those clients at highest risk to develop ocular complications (pauciarticular group).

The school nurse should be involved in the child's care. Early-morning classes and stair climbing may be difficult for the child with arthritis. Parents are encouraged to treat the child as normally as possible, avoiding infantilizing or overprotection. An experienced multidisciplinary health care team can help the child and family meet the challenges of social and personality development. A family-oriented rather than a child-oriented approach is critical for the optimal management of JCA.[18]

HLA-ASSOCIATED RHEUMATIC DISEASE

Tissue typing is used in the field of human organ transplantation because specific tissue factors called *histocompatibility antigens* are responsible for the acceptance or rejection of a donor organ. These antigens reside on the cell surfaces of all nucleated cells and were first described on leukocytes; hence they were called *human leukocyte antigens*. It soon became apparent that there was an association between a number of autoimmune diseases and HLA antigens (see Table 8-17). An unusually high frequency of HLA-B27 is found in ankylosing spondylitis, psoriatic arthritis, and Reiter's syndrome, known as the *seronegative spondyloarthritides*.[19] Detection of this marker is an important aid to early diagnosis of these diseases.

Ankylosing Spondylitis

Ankylosing spondylitis (AS or Marie-Strümpell disease) is a chronic inflammatory disease that primarily affects the sacroiliac joints, apophyseal and costovertebral joints of the spine, and adjacent soft tissues. Approximately 90% of white clients with AS are positive for HLA-B27. The disease typically appears in adolescence or young adulthood.

AS may be equally prevalent in both sexes, but progressive disease is more common in men. Because women tend to have more peripheral joint involvement, the diagnosis is often delayed or missed.[20] There appears to be a definite familial tendency, and the disease is unusual in blacks.

Etiology and pathophysiology. The cause of AS is unknown. Genetic predisposition appears to play an important role in the disease pathogenesis, but the precise mechanisms are unknown. Environmental factors and infectious agents are also suspected. Inflammation in joints and adjacent tissue causes the formation of granulation tissue, eroding vertebral margins and resulting in spondylitis. Calcification tends to follow the inflammation process, leading to bony ankylosis.

Clinical manifestations and complications. The client typically has lower back pain, stiffness, and limitation of motion that is worse during the night and in the morning but improves with mild activity. General constitutional features such as fever, fatigue, anorexia, and weight loss are rarely present. Other symptoms depend on the stage of the disease and may include peripheral arthritis of the shoulders, hips, and knees and occasional ocular inflammation (iritis).

Involvement of costovertebral joints leads to a decrease in chest expansion. Advancing kyphosis leads to a bent-over posture, and compensating hip-flexion contractures may occur. Atlantoaxial subluxation of the cervical spine

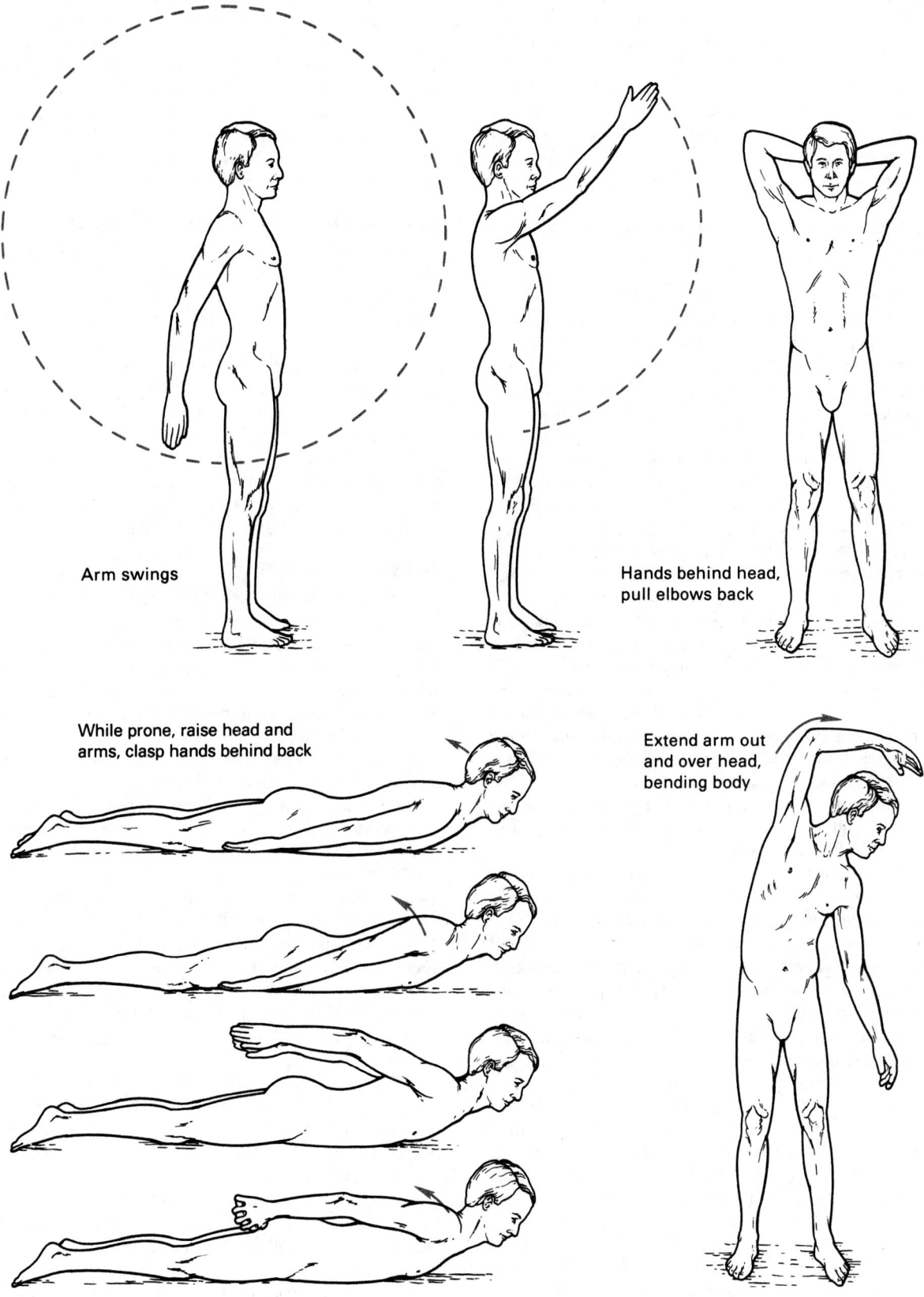

Arm swings

Hands behind head, pull elbows back

While prone, raise head and arms, clasp hands behind back

Extend arm out and over head, bending body

Fig. 58-7 Typical chest-cage stretching and deep chest breathing exercises for ankylosing spondylitis.

is a rare but serious complication resulting in spinal cord or brainstem compression. Extraskeletal involvement may include iritis, aortic valvular regurgitation, and apical pulmonary fibrosis.

Diagnostic studies. Changes on x-ray films may not become apparent for months to years after the onset of symptoms. When abnormalities are present, they include sacroiliac joints that show pseudowidening of the joint space and later obliteration with ankylosis. New bone formation (syndesmophytes) may be spotty or generalized (classic "bamboo spine"). The ESR and alkaline phosphatase and creatinine phosphokinase levels are usually elevated. Tissue typing is positive for HLA-B27 in the majority of clients.

Therapeutic management. Prevention of AS is not possible; however, families with diagnosed HLA-B27–positive rheumatic diseases should be alert to signs of lower back pain and arthritis symptoms.

Therapeutic management is aimed at maintaining maximal skeletal mobility. Proper posture is important in all activities. Although drugs do not halt the progression of the disease, drugs such as phenylbutazone and indomethacin can provide pain relief, which makes proper posture easier. Surgery to correct extreme flexion deformities may be performed in certain cases. A total hip replacement is done for clients with crippling hip ankylosis.

■ Nursing Management of Ankylosing Spondylitis

Nursing responsibilities for the client with AS include education about the nature of the disease and principles of therapy. The degree of limitation of motion should be assessed for baseline data. Pain should be managed by appropriate medication as well as by heat, massage, and gentle exercise. A continuing physical therapy program incorporating gentle, graded stretching and strengthening exercises must be followed by the client to prevent deformity and preserve ROM. Excessive physical exertion during periods of active inflammation should be discouraged. The client must understand the importance of a home management program and should demonstrate proper use of medications, local heat, and exercise. Proper positioning at rest is essential. The mattress should be firm, and pillows must be avoided. The client should sleep on the back and avoid positions that encourage flexion deformity. Postural training must include emphasis on avoiding forward flexion (e.g., leaning over a desk), heavy lifting, and prolonged walking, standing, or sitting. Application of moist heat should be followed by ROM exercises and daily chest expansion and deep-breathing exercises (Fig. 58-7). Sports that facilitate natural stretching, such as swimming and racquet games, should be encouraged. Family counseling and vocational rehabilitation are important.

Psoriatic Arthritis

Psoriatic arthritis can be defined as an association of clinically apparent psoriasis with inflammatory polyarthritis (see Chapter 17). Psoriatic skin changes may precede or follow articular symptoms. Approximately 10% to 15% of persons with psoriasis have such an arthritis, which is generally mild, with intermittent flare-ups affecting only a few peripheral joints. However, a severe erosive form indistinguishable from RA is also seen. Clients with psoriasis are subject to spondylitis, associated with an 80% frequency of HLA-B27 positivity. Hyperuricemia often accompanies the disease. Forms of treatment include splinting, joint protection, and physical therapy. Although gold has recently been used with success for the treatment of psoriatic arthritis, methotrexate continues to be one of the most effective agents for both cutaneous and articular manifestations.

Reiter's Syndrome

Reiter's syndrome is a self-limiting disease associated with arthritis, urethritis, conjunctivitis, and mucocutaneous lesions.[21] Although the exact etiology is unknown, Reiter's syndrome appears to be a reactive arthritis after certain enteric (e.g., *Shigella*) or venereal (*Chlamydia trachomatis*) infections. The disease usually affects males, and 85% of clients with Reiter's are positive for HLA-B27, which is evidence for a genetic component of the disease. Few other laboratory abnormalities occur. Arthritis tends to be asymmetrical, frequently involving the weight-bearing joints of the lower extremities and sometimes the lower part of the back.

These arthralgias usually begin 1 to 3 weeks after the appearance of the initial infection. The full attack may be accompanied by fever and other constitutional complaints, including anorexia with considerable weight loss, and may prove highly debilitating.

Soft-tissue manifestations commonly include Achilles tendinitis. Prognosis is favorable, with most clients recovering after 2 to 16 weeks. Lesions heal without a trace, and many clients have complete remission with full joint function. Half the clients, however, have recurring acute attacks; others follow a chronic course, having continued synovitis and progression of x-ray changes closely resembling those of AS. Progressive disease may result in major disability. Treatment is symptomatic. Joint inflammation is treated with NSAIDs.

SEPTIC ARTHRITIS

Septic arthritis (infectious or bacterial arthritis) is caused by invasion of the joint cavity with microorganisms. Various bacteria are commonly responsible, including *Staphylococcus aureus*, *Streptococcus hemolyticus*, *Diplococcus pneumoniae*, and *Neisseria gonorrhoeae*. Factors increasing the risk of such infections include previous joint trauma or arthritic disease, diseases of decreased host resistance such as leukemia and diabetes mellitus, treatment with corticosteroids or immunosuppressive drugs, and serious chronic illness. Infants, young children, and older adults appear to be more frequently affected by the infectious arthritides, with the exception of gonococcal arthritis, which affects sexually active young adults. A site of active infection is often responsible for bacteremia (microorganisms reaching the bloodstream), leading to hematogenous seeding of joints.

Inflammation of the joint cavity causes severe pain, erythema, and swelling of one or several joints. Fever

and/or shaking chills often accompany articular symptoms. Precise diagnosis is made by aspiration of the joint and culture of the synovial fluid. Nonspecific blood findings include peripheral blood leukocytosis and an elevated ESR. Intraarticular injection of antibiotics is avoided.

Septic arthritis is a medical emergency that requires prompt diagnosis and treatment to prevent joint destruction. Treatment is immediate administration of an appropriate antibiotic administered parenterally. Open surgical drainage may be required. Nursing intervention includes careful observation of the progression of joint inflammation. Immobilization of affected joints to control pain is often achieved by resting splints or traction. Gentle ROM exercises should be done. Pain and fever should be monitored and treated appropriately. Strict aseptic technique should be used during assistance with joint aspiration procedures. The necessity of antibiotics should be explained, and the importance of their continued use should be stressed. Support should be offered to the client requiring repeated arthrocentesis or operative drainage. The extent of joint damage is generally related to the invading microorganism and the time between infection onset and initiation of treatment.

LYME DISEASE

Lyme disease is a spirochetal infection transmitted by the bite of an infected tick, first identified in Lyme, Conn., after an unusual clustering of arthritis in children.[22] The disease is recognized worldwide. Lyme disease is spreading faster than any other infectious disease except human immunodeficiency viral infections.[23] The tick is no bigger than a poppy seed and typically feeds on mice, dogs, cats, cows, horses, raccoons, deer, and people. The peak season for human infection is during the summer months.

Early symptoms include flulike chills, fever, headache, fatigue, dizziness, and migratory joint pain. In most cases a characteristic "bull's eye" lesion appears, which begins as a red macule or papule and expands to form a large circular erythematous border with a pale center. If not treated, Lyme disease can progress in several weeks or months to debilitating arthritis, cardiac damage, and neurological symptoms such as encephalitis, facial palsy, and seizures.

Diagnosis can be made by detecting elevated antibody titers to *Borrelia burgdorferi*, but serological determinations must be interpreted with caution because of the frequency of false-positive and false-negative results. Effective antibiotic therapy includes amoxicillin for children and doxycycline or tetracycline for adults. Ceftriaxone is used intravenously to treat persistent neurological abnormalities. Treatment of Lyme disease during pregnancy is controversial. A vaccine is not available at this time. Public education for the prevention of Lyme disease is outlined in Table 58-10.

GOUT

Gout is characterized by recurrent attacks of acute arthritis in association with increased levels of serum uric acid. It may be classified as primary or secondary. In *primary gout* a hereditary error of purine metabolism leads to

Table 58-10   Client Education for Prevention of Lyme Disease

Avoid walking through tall grasses and low brush.
Mow grass and remove brush along paths, buildings, and campsites.
Move wood piles and bird feeders away from house.
Wear long pants or nylon tights of tightly woven, light-colored fabric so that ticks can be easily seen.
Tuck pants into boots or long socks, tuck long-sleeved shirts into pants, and wear closed shoes when hiking.
Check often for ticks crawling from legs to open skin.
Thoroughly inspect and wash clothes.
Spray insect repellant containing DEET on skin or permethrin on clothes, especially on lower extremities.
Have pets wear tick collars, inspect them often, and do not allow them on furniture or beds.
Remove attached ticks with tweezers (not fingers). Grasp tick's mouth parts as close to skin as possible and gently pull straight out. Do not twist or jerk.
Dispose of tick in alcohol or flush down toilet. Do not crush with fingers.
Wash bitten area with soap and water and apply antiseptic. Wash hands.
See a doctor immediately if flulike symptoms or "bull's eye" rash appears within a few weeks after removal of tick.

Table 58-11   Associated Conditions Leading to Hyperuricemia

Obesity	Malignant disease
Diabetes mellitus	Sickle cell anemia
Hyperlipidemia	Cytotoxic drugs
Hypertension	Intrinsic renal disease
Atherosclerosis	Drug-induced renal impairment
Myeloproliferative disorders	Acidosis or ketosis

the overproduction or retention of uric acid. *Secondary gout* may be related to another acquired disorder (Table 58-11) or may be the result of medications known to inhibit uric acid excretion. Secondary gout may also be caused by medications that increase the rate of cell death, such as the chemotherapeutic agents used in treating leukemia.

Significance

Primary gout occurs predominantly (90%) in middle-aged men, with almost no incidence in premenopausal women. Frequency of hyperuricemia is increased in the families of clients with primary gout. Although some races have been identified as having a low incidence of gout, people of the same race living in another country may exhibit higher mean serum uric acid levels, indicating that both genetic and environmental factors contribute to the pathophysiology.

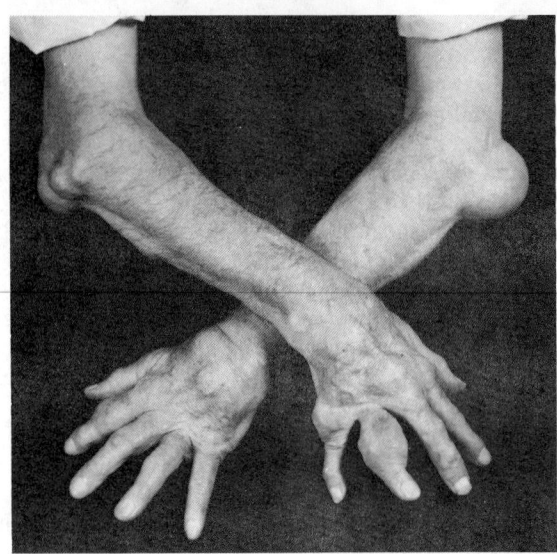

Fig. 58-8 Tophaceous gout.

Etiology and Pathophysiology

Uric acid represents the major end product of the catabolism of purines and is primarily excreted by the kidneys. Thus hyperuricemia may be the result of increased purine synthesis, decreased renal excretion, or both. About half the clients with primary gout can be shown to produce excessive amounts of uric acid. Folklore has long associated excesses of food and drink with acute attacks of gouty arthritis. Although high dietary intake of purine alone has relatively little effect on uric acid levels, it is clear that hyperuricemia may result from prolonged fasting or excessive drinking because of increased production of keto acids, which then inhibit normal renal excretion of uric acid.

Clinical Manifestations

In the acute phase, gouty arthritis may occur in one or more joints but usually less than four. Affected joints may appear dusky or cyanotic and are extremely tender. Inflammation of the great toe *(podagra)* is most commonly the initial involvement and occurs in 75% of all clients. Other joints affected are the midtarsal, ankle, knee, and wrist joints and the olecranon bursa. Acute gouty arthritis is usually precipitated by events such as trauma, surgery, alcohol ingestion, or systemic infection. Onset of symptoms is usually rapid, with swelling and pain peaking within several hours, often accompanied by low-grade fever. Individual attacks usually subside, treated or untreated, in 2 to 10 days. The affected joint returns entirely to normal, and clients are often free of symptoms between attacks.

Chronic gout is characterized by multiple joint involvement and deposits of sodium urate crystals *(tophi)*. These are typically seen in the synovium, subchondral bone, olecranon bursa, and vertebrae; along tendons; and in the skin and cartilage (Fig. 58-8). Tophi are rarely present at the time of the initial attack and are generally noted only many years after the onset of disease.

The severity of gouty arthritis is variable. The clinical course may consist of infrequent mild attacks or multiple severe episodes associated with a slowly progressive disability. In general, the higher the serum uric acid level, the earlier the appearance of tophi and the greater the tendency toward more frequent and severe episodes of acute gout. An elevated serum uric acid alone does not indicate gout, even when joint symptoms are present, because high serum uric acid is found in a variety of diseases. Gout can be diagnosed unequivocally only when urate crystals are found in joint fluid.

Complications

Chronic inflammation may result in joint deformity. Destruction of the cartilage may predispose the joint to secondary OA. Tophaceous deposits may be large and unsightly and may perforate overlying skin, producing draining sinuses that often become secondarily infected. Excessive uric acid excretion may lead to kidney stone formation. Pyelonephritis associated with intrarenal sodium urate deposits and obstruction may contribute to renal disease.

Diagnostic Studies

The diagnosis can be established by finding monosodium urate monohydrate crystals in the synovial fluid of an inflamed joint or tophus.[24] Serum uric acid levels are almost always elevated to 8 mg/dl or higher. Specimens for 24-hour urine uric acid levels are obtained to control for daily fluctuations in urate concentrations and are important in determining whether the client undersecretes or overproduces uric acid. Hyperuricemia is not specifically diagnostic of gout because increased levels may be related to a variety of drugs or may exist as a totally asymptomatic abnormality in the general population.

Therapeutic Management

Therapeutic management of gout (Table 58-12) has several goals. The first is to terminate an acute attack. This is accomplished by the use of an antiinflammatory agent such as colchicine. Future attacks are prevented by a maintenance dose of colchicine, weight reduction if necessary, avoidance of alcohol and high-purine foods, and the use of drugs to reduce the serum urate concentration.

Treatment is also aimed at preventing the formation of uric-acid kidney stones and other associated conditions such as hypertriglyceridemia and hypertension.

Pharmacological Management

Acute gouty arthritis is treated with one of three types of antiinflammatory agents: colchicine, NSAIDs, or corticosteroids. Corticosteroids should be reserved for cases in which colchicine or NSAIDs are contraindicated or ineffective.

Although medication does not prevent recurrent attacks of gout, it can control its symptoms in 75% of gout attacks, particularly with prompt treatment. Oral administration of colchicine generally produces dramatic pain relief within 24 to 48 hours. Colchicine has diagnostic merit in that a good response to treatment gives further evidence

Table 58-12

 Diagnostic and Therapeutic Management: Gout

DIAGNOSTIC

History and physical examination
Family history of gout
Presence of monosodium urate monohydrate crystals in synovial fluid
Elevated serum uric acid levels
24-hr urine for uric acid levels

THERAPEUTIC

Bed rest and joint immobilization
Local application of heat or cold
Joint aspiration and intraarticular corticosteroids
Analgesics
Drug therapy (e.g., colchicine, probenecid, allopurinol)

---

for the diagnosis of gout. Prophylactic doses of colchicine reduce the frequency of attacks but do not alter the serum uric acid level.

For many years the standard therapy for hyperuricemia has been a uricosuric drug (e.g., probenecid), which acts by increasing urinary uric acid excretion by inhibiting tubular reabsorption of urates. Aspirin inactivates the effect of uricosurics, resulting in urate retention, and should be avoided while clients are taking probenecid and other uricosuric drugs. Acetaminophen can be used safely if analgesia is required.

Adequate urine volume must be maintained to prevent precipitation of uric acid in the renal tubules. Allopurinol (Zyloprim), which blocks the production of uric acid, may control the serum level and is particularly useful in clients with uric acid stones or renal impairment in whom uricosuric drugs may be ineffective or dangerous. Regardless of which drug or combination of drugs is prescribed, it is essential that the concentration of serum urate be checked regularly to monitor the effectiveness of treatment.

Nutritional Considerations

Dietary restrictions may include limiting the use of alcohol and of foods high in purine (see Table 40-12). However, medication can generally control the situation without necessitating these limitations. Obese clients should be instructed in a carefully planned weight-reduction program.

■ Nursing Management of Gout

Acute gouty arthritis may be prevented by maintenance of the serum uric acid at normal levels. Nursing intervention is directed at supportive care of the inflamed joints. Bed rest may be appropriate, with affected joints properly immobilized. The limitation of motion and degree of pain should be assessed. Treatment effectiveness should be documented. Special care is taken to avoid causing pain to an inflamed joint by careless handling. Involvement of a lower extremity may require use of a cradle or footboard to protect the painful area from the weight of bed clothes.

The client and the family should understand that hyperuricemia and gouty arthritis are chronic problems that can be controlled but that adherence to a treatment program is necessary to achieve this goal. Thorough explanations should be given concerning the importance of drug therapy. The client should be able to demonstrate knowledge of precipitating factors that may cause an attack, including alcohol, overindulgence, starvation (fasting), medication (aspirin, diuretics), and major medical events (surgery, myocardial infarction). The need for periodic determination of blood uric acid levels should be stressed. All clients should understand the importance of moderation in their intake of calories, purines, and alcohol.

SYSTEMIC LUPUS ERYTHEMATOSUS

Systemic lupus erythematosus (SLE) is a chronic multisystem inflammatory disease of connective tissue that often involves the skin, joints, serous membranes (pleura, pericardium), kidney, hematological system, and central nervous system (CNS).[25] SLE is characterized by its variability within and among persons, with a chronic unpredictable course of exacerbations of disease activity alternating with periods of remission. The clinical presentation of SLE ranges from a mild to a serious illness with a tendency to acute, occasionally fatal exacerbations precipitated by several factors.

Significance

The true incidence of SLE is uncertain, but the rate appears to be increasing. It is unknown whether this increase is a reflection of heightened physician awareness or a true increase in frequency.[26] The general prevalence of SLE is approximately 1 in 2100.[27] Females have a higher incidence (about 5:1) than males. The disease is observed three times more often in black than in white women.[27]

Etiology and Pathophysiology

The etiology of SLE is unknown. However, three factors that play roles in the pathophysiology of SLE are (1) immunological processes, (2) genetic predisposition, and (3) environmental influences. SLE is a disorder of immunological regulation. Pathophysiology depends on autoimmune reactions directed against constituents of the cell nucleus, particularly DNA. In SLE, autoantibodies are produced against nuclear antigens (DNA, histones, ribonucleoproteins, and nucleolar), cytoplasmic antigens (ribosomal and cardiolipin), and blood cell surface antigens (WBCs, red blood cells [RBCs], platelets, and granulocytes). When autoantibodies bind to their specific antigens, complement activation occurs with the sequelae of destruction of cells or basement membranes and subsequent inflammation. The specific manifestations of SLE depend on which cell types or organs are involved.

The overaggressive antibody response is related to B-cell hyperactivity accompanied by multiple abnormalities in immunoregulation. Examples of this include decreased T-suppressor cells and diminished interleukin-2 production.[28]

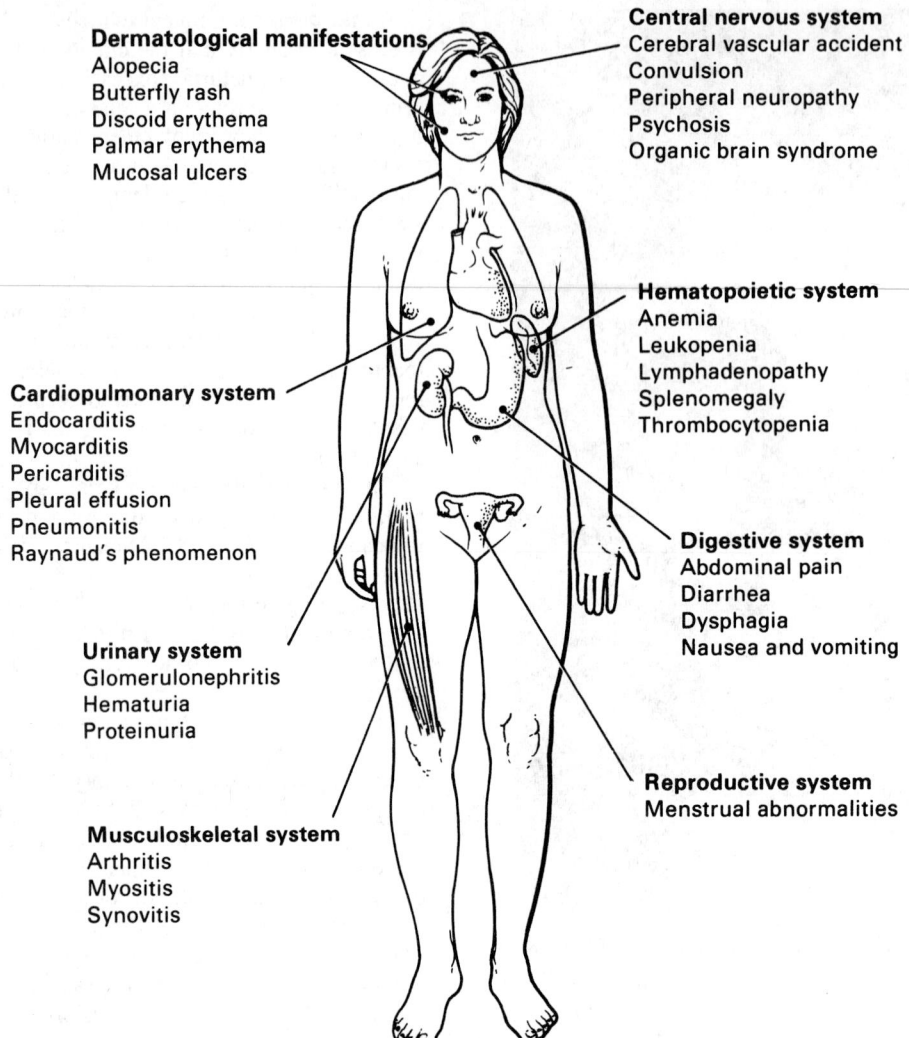

Dermatological manifestations
Alopecia
Butterfly rash
Discoid erythema
Palmar erythema
Mucosal ulcers

Central nervous system
Cerebral vascular accident
Convulsion
Peripheral neuropathy
Psychosis
Organic brain syndrome

Hematopoietic system
Anemia
Leukopenia
Lymphadenopathy
Splenomegaly
Thrombocytopenia

Cardiopulmonary system
Endocarditis
Myocarditis
Pericarditis
Pleural effusion
Pneumonitis
Raynaud's phenomenon

Digestive system
Abdominal pain
Diarrhea
Dysphagia
Nausea and vomiting

Urinary system
Glomerulonephritis
Hematuria
Proteinuria

Reproductive system
Menstrual abnormalities

Musculoskeletal system
Arthritis
Myositis
Synovitis

Fig. 58-9 Multisystem involvement in SLE.

The importance of heredity in the development and expression of SLE has been supported by recognition of familial clustering and the identification of genetic markers.[29] The major histocompatibility complexes HLA-DR2 and HLA-DR3 show significant associations with SLE.

Gonadal hormones are known to play a role in the etiology of SLE. Healthy women are more immunologically reactive than healthy men because estrogens augment immune regulation and androgens suppress it.[30] Onset or exacerbation of disease symptoms sometimes occurs after the onset of menarche, with the use of oral contraceptives, and during and after pregnancy.

Environmental influences on the expression of SLE include certain drugs, ultraviolet light, viral infection, and stress. Drug-induced SLE is generally mild and remits when the offending drug is discontinued.[31]

Clinical Manifestations and Complications

SLE is extremely variable in its severity, ranging from a relatively mild disorder to a rapidly progressive one af-

fecting many organ systems (Fig. 58-9). There is no characteristic pattern of progressive organ involvement, nor is it predictable which systems may become affected. SLE is characterized by alternating periods of remission and exacerbation. General constitutional complaints include fever, weight loss, and excessive fatigue and may precede an exacerbation of disease activity.

Dermatological manifestations. The most common cutaneous feature of SLE is an erythematous rash that can occur on the face, neck, and extremities. The classic butterfly rash, which is distributed across the bridge of the nose and cheeks, occurs in about 40% of clients (Fig. 58-10). The rash may appear as discoid (coinlike) lesions or as a diffuse maculopapular rash; it may occur anywhere on the body but is most frequently seen on the face and chest. A small group of clients have persistent lesions, photosensitivity, and mild systemic disease, and test positive for SS-A (Ro) antibodies. This syndrome is referred to as *subacute cutaneous lupus.*[32]

Exposure to sunlight and to other sources of ultraviolet

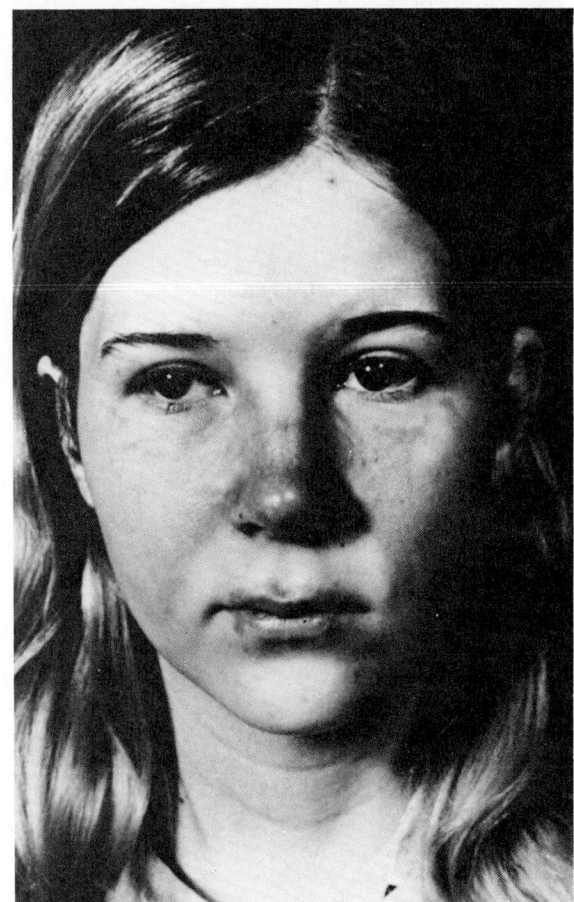

Fig. 58-10 Malar erythema across nose and cheeks in woman with SLE.

radiation can cause a severe skin reaction and may precipitate a flare-up of disease activity in persons who are photosensitive. Ulcers of the oral or nasopharyngeal membranes occur in up to one third of clients with SLE. Transient diffuse or patchy hair loss (alopecia) is common, with or without underlying scalp lesions. The hair eventually grows back.

Musculoskeletal problems. Polyarthralgia with morning stiffness is often the client's first complaint and may precede the onset of multisystem disease by many years. Arthritis occurs in 95% of all clients with SLE at some time in the disease course. Joint symptoms are typically migratory, producing pain without objective signs of inflammation. Lupus-related arthritis is generally nonerosive, but it may cause deformities such as swan neck, ulnar deviation, and subluxation with hyperlaxity of the joints.

Cardiopulmonary involvement. Pericarditis is present in nearly one fourth of clients with SLE and is usually associated with myocardial disease. Clients treated with corticosteroids have a higher incidence of atherosclerosis. Pleurisy with or without effusion is seen in nearly 50% of clients at some time during the illness, and pulmonary function studies are abnormal in 90%. Raynaud's phenomenon occurs in 20% of clients (see Chapter 32).

Renal disease. Clinical evidence of renal involvement is present in nearly half the clients with SLE and includes microscopic hematuria, excessive cellular casts in the urine sediment, proteinuria, and elevation of serum creatinine level. Kidney involvement varies in degree but may eventually end in renal failure. Regardless of whether renal manifestations are evident, nearly all clients with SLE show renal histological abnormalities in renal biopsy studies or autopsy results. Nephritis is the leading cause of death in clients with SLE.[33]

Clinical factors, including blood pressure, urinalysis, serum creatinine levels, serum complement levels, and autoantibodies to double-stranded DNA, should be monitored carefully and frequently over prolonged periods because renal involvement in the early stages is usually asymptomatic.

Central nervous system disease. CNS involvement ranks close behind kidney disease and infection as a leading cause of death in SLE. Seizures are the most common neurological manifestation and occur in as many as 15% of clients with SLE by the time of diagnosis. They may be of the grand mal, petit mal, or psychomotor type and are generally controlled by corticosteroids or anticonvulsant therapy.

Organic brain syndrome, another recognized CNS manifestation of SLE, is characterized by disordered thought processes, disorientation, memory deficits, and psychiatric symptoms such as severe depression and psychosis. Recovery from organic brain disease is expected, although some residual impairment may result. Occasionally a cerebrovascular accident (stroke) or aseptic meningitis may be attributable to SLE. It is difficult to diagnose neuropsychiatric SLE from non-SLE neurological problems.[34]

Infection. Clients with SLE appear to have increased susceptibility to infections, possibly related to defects in their ability to phagocytize invading bacteria, deficiencies in production of antibodies, and the immunosuppressive effect of many antiinflammatory drugs. Infection, a major cause of death, has an incidence of 30%. Pneumonia is most common. Any fever should be considered serious because it may indicate an underlying infectious process rather than lupus activity alone.

Diagnostic Studies

The diagnosis of SLE is based on the history, physical examination, and laboratory findings (Table 58-13). A variety of abnormalities may be present in the blood of clients with SLE, including elevated ESR, increase in γ-globulin levels, anemia, decreased WBC and platelet counts, electrocardiogram (ECG) or chest x-ray evidence of pericarditis or pleural effusion, and a biological false-positive serological test for syphilis. Abnormalities in urine sediment (cellular casts, proteinuria), reduced serum complement, and tissue specimens demonstrating changes compatible with SLE are other confirmatory findings.

Autoantibodies directed against nuclear antigens (ANA) have been detected in 99% of persons with SLE. Although extremely sensitive, ANA is not specific for SLE because it is present in 5% of normal persons and 38% of all persons more than 60 years of age. Anti-double-stranded DNA is found most commonly in SLE and rarely seen in

Table 58-13 Criteria for Systemic Lupus Erythematosus*

Malar rash
Discoid rash
Photosensitivity
Oral ulcers
Arthritis: Nonerosive, involvement of ≥ two joints
Serositis: Pleuritis or pericarditis
Renal disorder: Proteinuria or cellular
Neurological disorder: Seizures or psychosis
Hematological disorder: Hemolytic anemia, leukopenia, lymphopenia, or thrombocytopenia
Immunological disorder: Positive lupus cell preparation; antibodies to native DNA or antibody to Sm nuclear antigen false-positive serological test for syphilis
Antinuclear antigen

---

*A person is classified as having SLE if four or more of the criteria are present, serially or simultaneously, during any interval of observation. Revised criteria by a subcommittee of the American College of Rheumatology are used for the purpose of *classification* in population surveys, *not* for the diagnosis of individual clients.

Table 58-14

 Diagnostic and Therapeutic Management: Systemic Lupus Erythematosus

DIAGNOSTIC

History and physical examination
Lupus cell preparation
Antibodies
  Native DNA
  Sm nuclear antigen
  ANA titer
Complete blood cell count
Urinalysis
X-ray film of affected joints
Chest x-ray film
Complement levels (CH_{50}, C3)
ECG

THERAPEUTIC

NSAIDs
Antimalarials
Corticosteroids for exacerbations and severe disease
Immunosuppressive drugs (e.g., cyclophosphamide)

---

other rheumatic diseases. Anti-Sm antibody, an antibody to the Smith nuclear antigen, is a definitive serological marker for SLE and is not demonstrated in other rheumatic diseases.[35]

Therapeutic Management

The rate of spontaneous remission in SLE is high. Corticosteroids remain the mainstay for clients with more severe illness. Their use should be reserved for acute generalized exacerbation or serious organ involvement, although a reduced maintenance dosage is sometimes used. Immunosuppressive drugs may be used for clients who are resistant to corticosteroid therapy (see Table 58-14). Efficacy of treatment is most appropriately monitored by serial serum complement levels and anti-DNA titers.

The better prognosis of SLE may be the result of earlier diagnosis, prompt recognition of serious organ involvement, and better therapeutic regimens. Survival is influenced by several factors, including age, race, gender, socioeconomic status, accompanying morbid conditions, and severity of disease. For example, childhood-onset SLE accounts for nearly 20% of all cases and has a higher incidence of nephritis (up to 80%) than in other age groups, adversely influencing prognosis. The overall 15-year survival rate is estimated at about 90%.

Pharmacological Management

Therapeutic programs for SLE are prescribed to control inflammation and depend almost entirely on disease activity. Aspirin or other NSAIDs may reduce mild symptoms such as fever and arthritic complaints. GI upset and tinnitus, which are recognized adverse effects of these agents, should be reported. Antimalarial drugs such as hydroxychloroquine sulfate (Plaquenil) may be used to improve skin problems, but eye examinations must be scheduled periodically during this therapy because visual loss is a rare but serious side effect. Topical steroid preparations and intralesional steroid injections are effective treatments for skin lesions.

Corticosteroids are potent antiinflammatory medications used for acute generalized exacerbations of SLE and for the treatment of serious involvement of vital organs, including hematological abnormalities. As clinical and laboratory values improve, the dosages are gradually tapered.

Client education must include indications for use and proper administration of steroids and possible side effects (see Chapter 44). The client should understand that abrupt cessation may precipitate recurrence of disease activity. Immunosuppressive drug therapy such as azathioprine (Imuran) and cyclophosphamide (Cytoxan) is occasionally used in life-threatening situations for clients unresponsive to more conservative treatment.

■ Nursing Management of Systemic Lupus Erythematosus

Nursing assessment

As in the majority of rheumatic diseases, the chronic and unpredictable nature of SLE presents many challenges to clients and families. The physical, psychological, and sociocultural problems associated with the long-term management of SLE require the varied approaches and skills of the multidisciplinary health care team.

Subjective and objective data that should be obtained from a client with SLE are presented in Table 58-15. The extent to which pain and fatigue influence activities of daily living must be evaluated. A developmental approach focuses on age-appropriate educational and counseling concerns, such as personal relationships, family planning, occupational responsibilities, and recreational activities.

Table 58-15

Nursing Assessment of the Client with Systemic Lupus Erythematosus

SUBJECTIVE DATA	OBJECTIVE DATA
History	*General*
Positive family history, age, sex, race, remissions and exacerbation triggers, including overexposure to UV light, staphylococcal or viral infections, physical or psychological stress, x-ray exposure	Lymphadenopathy, periorbital edema, anxiety, mania
Medications	*Integumentary*
Use of hydralazine, isoniazid, anticonvulsants (possibly causing symptoms of SLE), corticosteroids, NSAIDs	Alopecia, keratoconjunctivitis, malar "butterfly" rash, palmar and/or discoid erythema, urticaria, purpura or petechiae, leg ulcers
General	*Respiratory*
Fatigue, fever, malaise, weight loss, depression, insomnia, frequent infections	Pleural friction rub
Pain	*Cardiovascular*
Headache, polyarthralgias, chest pain (pericardial, pleuritic), abdominal pain	Vasculitis, pericardial friction rub; hypertension, edema, dysrhythmias, murmurs, bilateral, symmetrical pallor and cyanosis of fingers (Raynaud's phenomenon)
Integumentary	*Gastrointestinal*
Photosensitivity with rash	Painless oral and pharyngeal ulcers, hepatosplenomegaly
Respiratory	*Neurological*
Nasal ulcers	Facial weakness, peripheral neuropathies, papilledema, dysarthria, confusion, hallucination, disorientation, psychosis, seizures, aphasia, hemiparesis
Gastrointestinal	*Musculoskeletal*
Oral ulcers, xerostomia (salivary gland dryness), dysphagia, nausea or vomiting, diarrhea or constipation	Myopathy, myositis, arthritis
Urinary	*Possible findings*
Hematuria, decreased urine output	Positive lupus cell preparation, elevated ANA titers, presence of anti-DNA and Sm-nuclear antibodies, decreased T-suppressor cell count
Reproductive	
Amenorrhea, irregular menstrual periods	
Neurological	
Visual disturbances, vertigo	
Musculoskeletal	
Morning stiffness, joint pain and swelling	

Nursing diagnoses

Nursing diagnoses are determined when the problem and etiological factors are supported by clinical data. Nursing diagnoses related to SLE may include, but are not limited to, those presented in Table 58-16.

Nursing interventions

Acute intervention. Prevention of SLE is not possible at this time. Education of health professionals and the community may promote a clearer understanding of the disease and earlier diagnosis and treatment.

During an exacerbation, clients may become abruptly and dramatically ill. Nursing intervention includes accurately recording the severity of symptoms and documenting response to therapy. Fever pattern, joint inflammation, limitation of motion, location and degree of discomfort, and fatigability should be specifically assessed.[36] The client's weight and fluid intake and output should be monitored because of the fluid-retention effect of steroids and the possibility of renal failure. Careful collection of 24-hour urine for protein may be required. The nurse should observe for signs of bleeding that result from drug therapy, such as pallor, skin bruising, petechiae, or tarry stools.

Careful assessment of neurological status includes observation for visual disturbances, headaches, personality changes, and forgetfulness. Psychosis may indicate CNS disease or may be the effect of corticosteroid therapy. Irritation of the nerves of the extremities (peripheral neuropathy) may produce numbness, tingling, and weakness of the hands and feet. Less frequently a stroke may result.

The nurse must explain the nature of the disease and modes of therapy and prepare the client for numerous diagnostic procedures. Emotional support for the client and family is essential.

Chronic management. Nursing interventions must emphasize health teaching and home management. The client must be taught to live *with* the disease, not *for* it.

The client must understand that even perfect adherence to the treatment plan is not a guarantee against exacerbation because the course of the disease is unpredictable. However, a variety of factors may encourage exacerbation, such as fatigue, sun exposure, emotional stress, infection, drugs, and surgery. Nursing interventions should be directed toward assisting the client and family to eliminate or minimize exposure to precipitating factors.[25] Client

Table 58-16

 NURSING CARE PLAN FOR THE CLIENT WITH SYSTEMIC LUPUS ERYTHEMATOSUS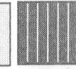

Defining Characteristics	Nursing Interventions	Evaluation Criteria
NURSING DIAGNOSIS: Fatigue related to disease process		
Lack of energy, inability to maintain routine	Assist client to prioritize activities to establish preferred daily routine. Analyze energy level patterns to use in planning daily activities. Teach energy conservation techniques such as sitting at kitchen sink, enlisting aid of others. Include family in planning. Teach stress-reducing techniques such as meditation, yoga.	Satisfaction with completion of priority activities, practicing of pacing of activities, verbalization of having more energy
NURSING DIAGNOSIS: Pain related to disease process and inadequate comfort measures		
Complaints of joint pain, lack of relief from pain-relieving measures; reduction of activity to avoid exacerbating pain	Provide for periods of rest. Administer analgesia as ordered. Monitor effect. Teach joint protection measures.* Apply heat or cold as needed. Use nonpharmacological pain interventions such as relaxation and visual imagery.	Satisfaction with pain relief measures, increased activity
NURSING DIAGNOSIS: Potential complication: increased inflammatory response related to exacerbation of disease process		
Problems associated with any affected body system (e.g., edema, hypertension, seizures, mental status, pain and joint swelling, dyspnea, cyanosis, oral and skin lesions)	Assess and monitor body systems regularly through vital signs, physical examination, laboratory studies, and client's subjective comments about health. Report alterations suggestive of a problem to physician. Teach client signs and symptoms to observe for and what to report to physician. Encourage ongoing medical follow-up.	Early report of problems and timely initiation of treatment, verbalization of areas in need of ongoing assessment
NURSING DIAGNOSIS: Body-image disturbance related to change in physical appearance		
Verbalization of dissatisfaction with physical appearance, lack of participation in hygiene and grooming practices, isolation, refusal to see friends and family	Discuss realistic expectations of physical changes with client. Encourage interest in hygiene and grooming. Teach ways to use cosmetics creatively. Encourage discussion about feelings.	Increased self-interest and participation in self-care, expression of positive comments about self
NURSING DIAGNOSIS: Impaired skin integrity related to photosensitivity, skin rash, and alopecia		
Rash anywhere on body, butterfly rash on face, alopecia, areas of ulceration on fingertips, complaints of urticaria and photosensitivity	Assess and monitor location and progression of rash. Administer medications and apply ointments as ordered. Keep skin clean and dry. Avoid unprescribed ointments. Discuss need to avoid sun exposure and use of SPF 15 when outdoors.	Continued avoidance of sun and use of sunscreens, absence of open skin lesions
NURSING DIAGNOSIS: Activity intolerance related to arthralgia, weakness, and fatigue		
Inability or unwillingness to ambulate or engage in physical activity, dyspnea, abnormal response to activity (e.g., increased pulse, respiratory rate)	Pace activities and allow periods of rest between activities. Encourage client to assist in setting activity schedule. Monitor vital signs when ambulating. Provide bed rest during exacerbation. Increase activities slowly. Provide ROM exercises q 4 hr to unaffected joints. Encourage use of assistive devices.	Expression of satisfaction with activity pattern, sufficient activities to avoid problems related to immobility, pacing of activities to level of tolerance

SPF, Sun protection factor.
*See Tables 58-2 and 58-9.

Continued.

Table 58-16

NURSING CARE PLAN FOR THE CLIENT WITH SYSTEMIC LUPUS ERYTHEMATOSUS—cont'd

Defining Characteristics	Nursing Interventions	Evaluation Criteria
NURSING DIAGNOSIS: Altered nutrition: less than body requirements related to anorexia, fatigue, oral ulcerations, and immunosuppressive therapy		
Weight loss, poor appetite, inability or unwillingness to eat adequate food to meet nutritional requirements, nausea, vomiting	Assess food preferences and include them in meal planning when possible. Offer small, frequent meals. Provide good oral hygiene before and after meals. Monitor pertinent laboratory values such as hemoglobin, electrolytes, and protein levels. Encourage family to bring in favorite foods.	Absence of weight loss, intake of sufficient quantity and quality of food to meet daily needs
NURSING DIAGNOSIS: Altered health maintenance related to lack of knowledge of long-term management of disease		
Questioning about SLE or incorrect answers to questions by client or family, use of unproven remedies	Teach client about disease process, including chronic management. Include family in teaching activities. Discuss need to wear Medical-Alert bracelet. Inform client of availability of assistance from Lupus Foundation and Arthritis Foundation.	Expression of confidence in ability to manage SLE over time and in home environment

understanding and cooperation are important to this goal. Client and family education should include the following:

1. Education on the disease process
2. Names of medications and actions, side effects, dosage, and administration
3. Energy-conservation and pacing techniques
4. Daily heat and exercise program (for arthralgia)
5. Avoidance of physical and emotional stress, overexposure to ultraviolet light, and unnecessary exposure to infection
6. Regular medical and laboratory follow-up
7. Marital counseling, if necessary
8. Referral resources to community and health care agencies

LUPUS AND PREGNANCY. SLE is diagnosed in the majority of women during the childbearing years. For the best outcome, pregnancy should be planned with the cooperation of the primary physician and obstetrician at a point when the disease activity is minimal. Only women with serious renal, cardiac, or CNS involvement should be counseled against pregnancy. Exacerbation is common during the postpartum period. Therapeutic abortion offers the same risk of postdelivery exacerbation as carrying the fetus to term.

Fetal risks include increased rates of miscarriage, prematurity, and stillbirth. Neonatal lupus is an uncommon occurrence, characterized by rash, transient lupus antibodies, and/or congenital complete heart block. SS-A antibodies in the mother appear to be associated with complete heart block in the fetus. Antiphospholipid antibodies may be predictive of placental insufficiency and thrombosis and have been correlated with repeated miscarriage and intrauterine fetal death.[37] Regular clinical and laboratory monitoring is essential for the pregnant woman with SLE.

PSYCHOSOCIAL ISSUES. Many psychosocial issues confront the client with SLE. Disease onset may be vague, and SLE is often undiagnosed for long periods of time. Most people have either never heard of SLE or have heard of the disease through an association with a friend or relative who had a poor outcome. The nurse should counsel the client and family that SLE has a good prognosis for the majority of persons. Men are often embarrassed that they have a "women's disease." Families are anxious about hereditary aspects and want to know whether their children will also have SLE. Many young couples require pregnancy and sexual counseling. Young people making decisions about marriage and careers worry about how SLE will interfere with their plans. The nurse may need to educate teachers and work personnel.

The obvious physical effects of skin rashes, discoid lesions, and alopecia may cause social isolation for the client with SLE, yet pain and fatigue are cited most frequently as interfering with quality living. Friends and relatives are confused by the client's complaints of transient joint pain and overwhelming fatigue. Pacing techniques and relaxation therapy can help keep the client actively involved. Daily planning should include recreational as well as occupational activities. Children and young adults find sun restrictions and physical limitations particularly difficult to follow. SLE also has a negative effect on the client's self-esteem and body image.[38] Nursing interventions assist the client in developing and accomplishing reasonable goals toward improving mobility, energy levels, and self-esteem.

SYSTEMIC SCLEROSIS

Systemic sclerosis (SS), or scleroderma, is a disorder of connective tissue characterized by fibrotic, degenerative,

and occasionally inflammatory changes in the skin, blood vessels, synovium, skeletal muscle, and internal organs. Skin thickening and tightening are the cardinal features. The disease may range from a diffuse cutaneous thickening with rapidly progressive and fatal visceral involvement to a more benign variant called *CREST* syndrome (*c*alcinosis, *R*aynaud's phenomenon, *e*sophageal hypomotility, *s*clerodactyly (skin change of the fingers) and *t*elangiectasia (maculelike angioma on the skin).[39]

Significance

SS affects women three times more frequently than men, with the female/male ratio increasing to 15:1 during the childbearing years. SS has been reported in all races. Although symptoms may begin at any time, the usual age at onset is between 30 and 50 years. SS affects approximately 700,000 people in the United States.[39]

Etiology and Pathophysiology

The exact cause of SS remains unclear. Microvascular and immunological abnormalities continue to be investigated. Widespread systemic disease may be the result of primary vessel injury or immune dysregulation. Disruption of the cell is followed by platelet aggregation, myointimal cell proliferation, and fibrosis. These changes produce decreased elasticity, stenosis, and occlusion of vessels.[40]

Clinical Manifestations

Raynaud's phenomenon. Raynaud's phenomenon (paroxysmal vasospasm of the digits) occurs in nearly 98% of clients with SS and is the most common initial complaint in CREST syndrome. Clients have diminished blood flow to fingers and toes on exposure to cold (blanching or white phase), followed by cyanosis as hemoglobin releases oxygen to the tissues (blue phase) and then erythema on rewarming (red phase). The color changes are often accompanied by numbness and tingling. Raynaud's phenomenon may precede the onset of systemic disease by months, years, or even decades.

Skin and joint changes. Symmetrical painless swelling or thickening of the skin of the fingers and hands may progress to diffuse scleroderma of the trunk. In CREST syndrome skin thickening is generally limited to the fingers and face. The skin loses elasticity and becomes taut and shiny, producing the typical expressionless facies with tightly pursed lips (Fig. 58-11). Flexion contractures and atrophy of soft tissue may give the hands a clawlike appearance. Polyarthralgias and morning stiffness may be early symptoms. Tendon friction rubs may be present.

Internal organ involvement. Esophageal hypomotility causes frequent reflux of gastric acid, causing heartburn, and substernal dysphagia for solid foods. If swallowing becomes difficult, the client often decreases food intake and loses weight. GI complaints may also include abdominal distention, diarrhea, malodorous floating stools (malabsorption syndrome) as a result of small-bowel disease, and constipation secondary to colonic involvement.

Lung involvement includes pleural thickening and pulmonary fibrosis on x-ray film as well as pulmonary function abnormalities. Pulmonary hypertension is seen almost exclusively in CREST syndrome.

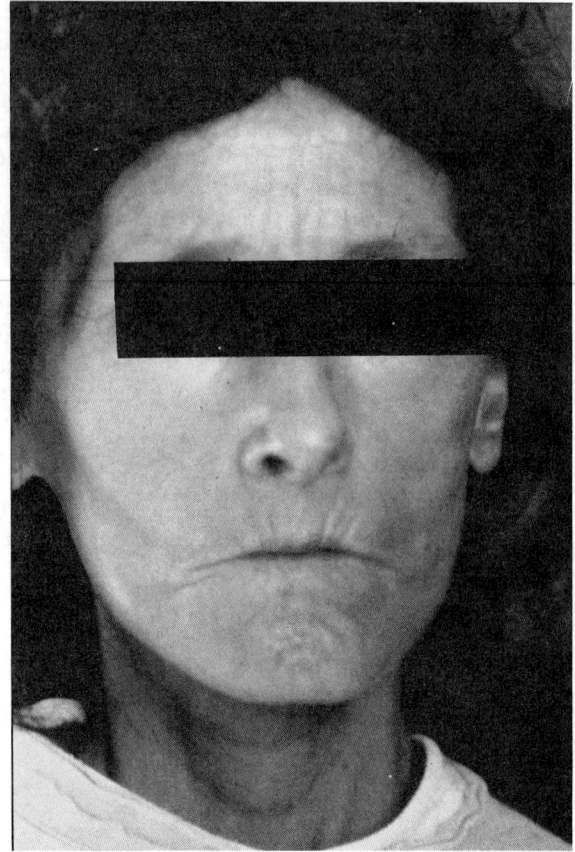

Fig. 58-11   Woman with systemic sclerosis.

Primary heart disease consists of pericarditis, pericardial effusion, and cardiac dysrhythmias. Myocardial fibrosis resulting in congestive failure occurs most frequently in those persons with diffuse SS.

Renal disease is a major cause of death in SS. Malignant arterial hypertension associated with rapidly progressive and irreversible renal insufficiency is often present. Recent improvements in dialysis, bilateral nephrectomy in clients with uncontrollable hypertension, and the advent of kidney transplantation have offered some hope to clients with renal failure.

Prognosis

The disease course of SS is variable. Persons with CREST syndrome have limited disability and the longest survival rates, although they are at higher risk for pulmonary arterial hypertension. Myocardial and renal involvement adversely affect the outcome in diffuse disease.

Diagnostic Studies

Blood studies may reveal a mildly elevated ESR and occasionally hypergammaglobinemia. The presence of ANA is observed in almost all persons with SS. Autoantibody Scl-70 has been reported in diffuse SS; anticentromere antibody has a marked specificity for the CREST syndrome. Nail-bed capillary microscopy characteristically shows capillary loop dilatation with limited disease and dilatation with avascular area in clients with diffuse dis-

ease.[41] If renal involvement is present, urinalysis may show proteinuria, microscopic hematuria, and casts. X-ray evidence of subcutaneous calcification, digital tuft resorption, distal esophageal hypomotility, and/or bilateral pulmonary fibrosis are diagnostic of SS. Pulmonary function studies reveal decreased vital capacity and diffusion capacity for carbon monoxide. Skin biopsy shows dermal collagen thickening, condensation, or homogenization.

Therapeutic Management

The therapeutic management of SS (Table 58-17) offers no specific treatment with long-range effect. It is directed toward attempts to prevent or treat secondary complications of involved organs. Various drugs such as antiinflammatory agents, D-penicillamine, and colchicine have been used with varying degrees of success.

Physical therapy helps maintain joint mobility and preserve muscle strength. Occupational therapy assists the client in maintaining functional abilities. Esophageal reflux may be treated by periodic dilatation of the esophagus. Raynaud's phenomenon may be temporarily relieved by thoracic sympathectomy.

Pharmacological Management

No specific drugs or combination of drugs have been proved effective as treatment for SS. Corticosteroids are generally reserved for clients with myositis or overlap syndromes (e.g., mixed connective tissue disease). Penicillamine (Cuprimine) increases the solubility of dermal collagen and causes thinning of the skin in some clients but has several potentially serious side effects. Colchicine has recently been used to inhibit the accumulation of collagen, but evidence is still insufficient to prove its therapeutic worth. The use of immunosuppressive agents is under investigation (Fig. 58-12).

Supportive measures include oral vasodilating drugs and intraarterial injections of reserpine. Calcium channel blockers (nifedipine, diltiazem) are the treatment of choice for Raynaud's phenomenon. Infected ulcers of the fingertips may be treated by soaking with hyaluronidase and using bacterial antibiotic ointment. Joint symptoms may be relieved by aspirin and other NSAIDs. Antacids may be useful for heartburn. Tetracycline and other broad-spectrum antibiotics may improve intestinal malabsorption. Combinations of antihypertensive medications, including hydralazine, minoxidil, captopril, propranolol, and methyldopa, have been used in the treatment of hypertension and renal failure.

■ Nursing Management of Systemic Sclerosis

Because prevention is not possible, nursing intervention often begins during a hospitalization for diagnostic purposes. Vital signs, weight, intake and output, respiratory function, and limitation of joint motion should be assessed daily as indicated by specific symptoms. Emotional stress and air conditioning may aggravate Raynaud's phenomenon. These clients should not have finger stick blood testing done because of compromised circulation and poor

---

Table 58-17

Diagnostic and Therapeutic Management: Systemic Sclerosis

DIAGNOSTIC

History and physical examination
Serological testing
Nail-bed capillary microscopy
X-ray films of chest, hands, GI tract
Skin and/or visceral biopsy

THERAPEUTIC

Vasodilator and antihypertensive drugs
Antiinflammatory agents, colchicine, D-penicillamine
Physical therapy
Antacids

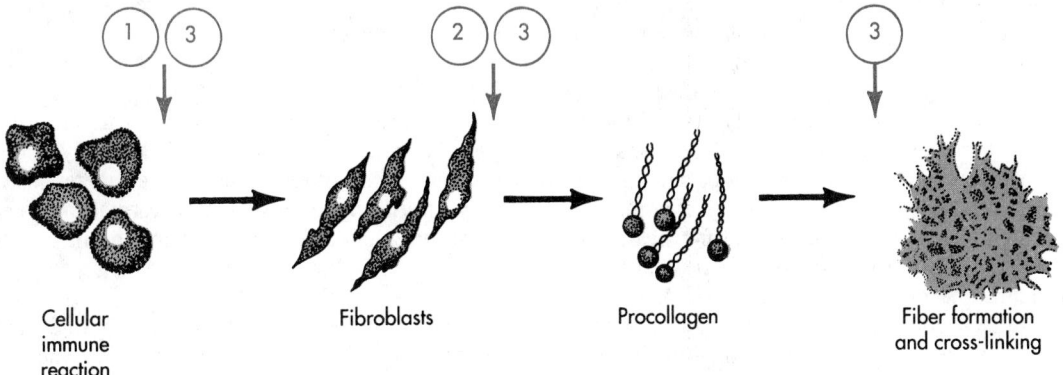

Fig. 58-12 Immune mechanisms in the pathogenesis of skin thickening in SS. The proposed locations of action of *1,* immunosuppressive agents; *2,* colchicine; and *3,* D-penicillamine are indicated. (From McCarty DJ: Arthritis and allied conditions: a textbook of rheumatology, ed 11, Philadelphia, 1989, Lea & Febiger, p 1140.)

digital healing. Diagnostic studies should be thoroughly explained. The nurse may help the client to resolve feelings of helplessness by educating the client about the illness and encouraging active participation in planning care.[42]

Health teaching is a major nursing concern as the client and family begin to live with this unusual disease. Obvious changes in the face and hands lead to poor self-image and loss of mobility and function. The client must actively carry out therapeutic exercises at home. The nurse should reinforce heat therapy, the use of assistive devices, and organization of activities to preserve strength and reduce disability.

Hands and feet should be protected from cold exposure and possible burns or cuts that might heal slowly. Smoking should be avoided because of its vasoconstricting effect. Signs of infection should be reported. Lotions may help to alleviate skin dryness and cracking but must be rubbed in for an unusually long time because of the thickness of the skin. Dysphagia may be reduced by eating small, frequent meals, chewing carefully and slowly, and drinking fluids. Heartburn may be minimized by using antacids 45 to 60 minutes after each meal and by sitting upright for 30 to 45 minutes after eating. Using additional pillows or raising the head of the bed on blocks may help to reduce nocturnal esophageal reflux.

Job modifications are often necessary: stair climbing, typing, writing, and cold exposure may pose particular problems. The client may become socially withdrawn as skin tightening alters the appearance of the face and hands. Some people need to wear gloves to protect fingertip ulcers and to provide extra warmth. Sensitive areas on fingertips resulting from ulcers or calcinosis may require padded utensils or special assistive devices to reduce discomfort. Dining out may become a socially embarrassing event because of the client's small mouth, difficult in swallowing, and reflux make eating less enjoyable. Daily oral hygiene must be emphasized, or neglect may lead to increased tooth and gingival problems. The client needs a dentist who can deal with a small oral aperture. Psychological support reduces stress and may positively influence peripheral motor response. Biofeedback training and relaxation techniques have been reported to reduce tension, improve sleeping habits, and actually raise digital temperature.

Sexual dysfunction resulting from body changes, pain, muscular weakness, limited mobility, decreased self-esteem, and decreased vaginal secretions may require sensitive counseling by the nurse. Specific suggestions based on individual client assessment should be offered.[43]

POLYMYOSITIS AND DERMATOMYOSITIS

Polymyositis and dermatomyositis are diffuse inflammatory myopathies of striated muscle, producing symmetrical weakness primarily in the proximal muscles of the pelvic and shoulder girdle. Dermatomyositis is distinguished by the presence of a characteristic skin rash. Both disorders have been classified according to treatment response and prognostic considerations.[44]

Polymyositis and dermatomyositis occur twice as frequently in women as in men, except for childhood dermat-

omyositis or myositis associated with neoplasia. Onset of the disease occurs most frequently in the fifth and sixth decades of life.[34] The incidence is slightly greater than that of muscular dystrophy in adults. In cases of dermatomyositis, especially among older persons, the frequency of malignancy appears to be increased.

Etiology and Pathophysiology

The exact cause of polymyositis and dermatomyositis is unknown. Theories include presence of an infectious agent, a hypersensitivity response, and cell-mediated immune system abnormalities. Close association with neoplastic disease suggests an autoimmune reaction. Histopathological study typically reveals the presence of inflammatory infiltrates, degeneration, regeneration, necrosis, and fibrosis of muscle fibers.

Clinical Manifestations and Complications

Muscular. The client usually has an insidious onset of proximal muscle weakness, primarily of the shoulders, neck, and pelvic girdle, and has difficulty rising from a chair or bathtub, climbing stairs, combing the hair, or reaching into a high cupboard. Neck muscles may become so weak that the client is unable to raise the head from the pillow. Muscle discomfort or tenderness is uncommon. Muscle examination reveals inability to move against resistance or even gravity. Weak pharyngeal muscles may produce proximal dysphagia (regurgitation of fluids through the nose) and dysphonia (nasal or hoarse voice).

Dermal. The typical skin rash appears as a dusky erythema of the face, neck, shoulders, anterior part of the chest, upper part of the back, and arms and occurs in nearly 40% of clients with muscular disease. A heliotrope (lavender hue) rash over the eyelids and periorbital edema are nearly pathognomic for dermatomyositis. The rash is prominent on the extensor surfaces of the forearms, elbows, knuckles, periungual areas, knees, and ankles. Scaling is a characteristic feature and may easily be confused with that of psoriasis or seborrheic dermatitis. Hyperemia and telangiectases are often present at the nail beds.

Other. Nearly half of the clients with polymyositis have mild or transient arthritis and/or Raynaud's phenomenon. Cotton wool patches can occur in the retina. Calcinosis, contractures, and muscle atrophy may occur with advanced disease. Aspiration pneumonia may result from weak pharyngeal muscles. Childhood dermatomyositis appears to have a more progressive, crippling course, and dermatomyositis diagnosed in men older than 40 years of age is more frequently associated with concurrent malignant disease. In severe cases, deglutition impairment and cardiorespiratory complications, such as pulmonary fibrosis and conduction defects, contribute to mortality.

Diagnostic Studies

Elevations in serum muscle enzymes (creatine kinase, aldolase, and aspartate aminotransferase) are most valuable in determining diagnosis and response to treatment. Circulating antibodies designated Pm-1 and Jo-1 have been identified in the sera of persons with polymyositis and myositis associated with SS.[35] Elevation of ESR is expected

with active disease. The electromyogram (EMG) shows polyphasic, short-duration potentials, fibrillation, and positive-spike waves. Muscle biopsy reveals necrosis, degeneration, regeneration, and interstitial chronic inflammatory cell infiltration (primary lymphocytes).

Therapeutic Management

Polymyositis and dermatomyositis can be treated with some success by the use of corticosteroids and, occasionally, immunosuppressive drugs. Improvement is generally achieved with prompt institution of corticosteroid therapy, and dosage is usually reduced as clinical improvement is noted. Relapses are common. Topical steroids may be applied to the skin rash. Clients who respond poorly to corticosteroids may improve with immunosuppressives (e.g., intermittent IV or daily oral cyclophosphamide). Corticosteroid therapy may cause potassium, which is necessary for normal muscle contraction, to be released from damaged muscle cells and to be lost in the urine. Supplemental dietary potassium (e.g., from orange juice, bananas) is encouraged. Steroid-induced myopathy may complicate long-term therapy. Immunosuppressive agents such as methotrexate, azathioprine, and cyclophosphamide are used for their corticosteroid-sparing effect, allowing functional improvement with reduction in corticosteroid dosage.

Physical therapy can be helpful and should be tailored to the activity of the disease. Massage and passive movement are appropriate during active disease, with more aggressive exercises reserved for periods when disease activity is minimal, as evidenced by low serum enzyme levels.

A careful search for possible malignant lesions should be undertaken for the client more than 40 years of age. If malignant disease is found, it should be treated appropriately (see Chapter 9). Complete remission of dermatomyositis may occur if the malignant lesion is removed.

◼ Nursing Management of Polymyositis and Dermatomyositis

Although prevention is not possible, greater recognition of polymyositis and its insidious onset resembling muscular dystrophy may favorably influence prognosis by more rapid diagnosis and institution of therapy.

Nursing interventions should include assessment of muscular weakness and limitation of motion. The nurse promotes bed rest and assists the client with activities of daily living when extreme weakness is present. Special attention is provided at mealtime to prevent aspiration. The nature of the disease and modes of therapy should be thoroughly reviewed, and the diagnostic tests should be explained. Understanding that the benefits of therapy are often delayed is important; for example, weakness may increase during the first few weeks of corticosteroid therapy.

The client should have a thorough understanding of the chronic nature of this disorder, the usefulness and the side effects of all prescribed medications, and the importance of regular medical care and serial laboratory testing. The nurse should provide guidelines for conserving energy by means of organizing activities and pacing techniques. Daily ROM exercises are encouraged to prevent contrac-

tures, and when active inflammation is not evident, muscle-strengthening (repetitive) exercises may be started.

Overlapping Forms of Connective Tissue Disease

Clients having a combination of clinical features of several rheumatic diseases are described as having *overlapping* or *mixed* connective tissue disease.[45] Although this combination was believed to be a distinct clinical disorder, follow-up revealed evolution primarily to SLE or SS. This early undifferentiated or transitional form of connective tissue disease has a typical serological pattern, including high titer of speckled ANA, high levels of antibody to ribonuclease-sensitive extractable nuclear antibody, and autoantibodies to ribonucleoprotein.

SJÖGREN'S SYNDROME

Sjögren's syndrome is characterized by autoantibodies to two protein-RNA complexes termed *SS-A/Ro* and *SS-B/La*. The manifestations are caused by inflammation and dysfunction of the exocrine glands, particularly the salivary and lacrimal glands.[46]

More than 90% of the clients are women, and half have RA or another connective tissue disease. Dry mouth can complicate the differential diagnosis in older women. Decreased tearing leads to a "gritty" sensation in the eye, burning, and photosensitivity. Dry mouth produces buccal membrane fissures, dysphagia, and frequent dental caries. Dry nasal and respiratory passages are common and can result in a cough. Often the parotid glands are enlarged. Other exocrine glands may also be affected; for example, vaginal dryness may lead to dyspareunia.

Histological study reveals lymphocyte infiltration of salivary and lacrimal glands, but the disease may become more generalized and involve lymph nodes, bone marrow, and visceral organs (pseudolymphoma). Extraglandular proliferation may become frankly malignant (e.g., lymphoma). Rheumatoid and antinuclear factors are present in the majority of clients. Anemia, leukopenia, hypergammaglobulinemia, and elevated ESR are usually found.

Ophthalmological examination (Schirmer test), salivary flow rates, and lower lip biopsy of minor salivary glands confirm the diagnosis. The treatment is symptomatic, including (1) artificial tears instillation as often as necessary to maintain adequate hydration and lubrication, (2) surgical punctal occlusion, and (3) increased fluids with meals. Dental hygiene is important. Increased humidity at home may reduce respiratory infections. Vaginal lubrication with a water-soluble product such as K-Y jelly lubricant may increase comfort during intercourse. Corticosteroids and immunosuppressive drugs are indicated for treatment of pseudolymphoma.

RHEUMATIC DISEASE IN OLDER CLIENTS

The prevalence of rheumatic disease in older adults is high, and the disease is accompanied by problems unique to this age group. The most problematic areas related to rheumatic disease in older adults include the following:

1. The high incidence of OA expected in older adults often keeps the clinician from considering the presence of other rheumatic diseases.

2. Age alone causes changes in serological profiles, making interpretation of laboratory values such as rheumatoid factors more difficult.
3. Multidrug regimens common to the older adult can result in iatrogenic arthritis.
4. Nonorganic musculoskeletal pain syndromes and weakness may relate to depressive reactions and physical inactivity.
5. Rheumatic diseases that commonly manifest in younger adults can present in older clients, often in milder form.
6. Residual effects of rheumatic disease present for long periods must be managed.[47]

A major concern of treatment in the older client relates to the use of corticosteroid therapy. Steroid-induced osteopenia adds to the problem of age- and inactivity-related osteoporosis and can increase the occurrence of pathological fractures, especially compression fractures of vertebrae. Steroid-induced myopathy can be minimized or prevented by an age-appropriate exercise program. Although important for all age groups, an adequate support system for the older client is a critical factor in compliance with the management program, which should include nutritional planning, exercise, general health maintenance, and appropriate pharmacotherapy.

COMMON JOINT SURGICAL PROCEDURES

Joint surgery dates back to 1891, when hip, finger, and thumb joints were implanted. In the following years the technology of joint replacement was actively pursued. Rejection of the prosthesis material and loosening of the parts were two persistent problems. The discovery of Vitallium, an alloy, and methylmethacrylate cement to fix the prosthesis in place were significant advances in the field of joint surgery. Since that time, improvements have been made in prosthetic design, materials, and surgical techniques.

Indications

Joint surgery may be indicated for conditions related to trauma, arthritic processes, or other painful conditions resulting in functional disability. Surgery is aimed at relieving pain, improving joint motion, correcting deformity and malalignment, reducing vertical loads and shear stresses, and removing intraarticular causes of erosion.[48]

Pain is one of the primary reasons for joint surgery. In addition to the effects of chronic pain on the physical and emotional well-being of the client, any movement of the painful joint is often avoided. If this lack of movement is not corrected, contraction with limitation of motion often occurs. Limitation of motion at any joint can be demonstrated on physical examination and by joint space narrowing on radiological examination.

There may also be a slow loss of cartilage in affected joints, which may be related to loss of motion. Synovitis can cause tendon damage, resulting in rupture or subluxation of the joint and subsequent loss of function. Continuing disease activity may cause loss of cartilage and bony surface and result in mechanical barriers to movement requiring surgical intervention.

Types

Synovectomy. Synovectomy (removal of synovial membrane) is used as a prophylactic measure and as a palliative treatment of RA. Removal of synovial membrane, thought to be the location of the basic pathological changes in joint destruction, helps prevent further damage. A synovectomy is best performed early in the disease process to prevent serious destruction of joint surfaces. Removal of the thickened synovium prevents extension of the inflammatory process into the adjacent cartilage, ligaments, and tendons.

It is impossible to surgically remove all the synovium in a joint. The underlying disease process is still present and will again affect the regenerating synovium. However, the disease appears to be milder after synovectomy, and definite improvement in pain, weight-bearing, and ROM can be expected. Common sites for this surgery include the knees, elbow, wrist, and fingers.

Osteotomy. An osteotomy is performed by cutting a bone to change its alignment and thereby correct deformity, relieve pain, and shift the load to a less damaged area of the joint. The knee and hip joints are the most common sites. Currently, osteotomy is considered an important alternative to total joint arthroplasty in persons less than 50 years of age. Long-term results are generally good, with excellent pain relief, improved function, and maintenance of physiological joint motion and stability. A functional ROM must be present preoperatively because some motion may be lost after surgery. It is used in OA and chronic RA mainly after a joint becomes ankylosed in a nonfunctional position. The postoperative care is similar to the treatment of an internal fixation of a fracture at a comparable site (see Chapter 57). The osteotomy is usually fixed by internal measures such as wire, screws and plates, bone grafts, or fixation material.

Debridement. Debridement is the removal of degenerative debris such as loose bodies, osteophytes, joint debris, and degenerated menisci from a joint. This procedure is usually performed on the knee. A functional ROM is necessary preoperatively because some joint motion may be lost. Open debridement often results in prolonged convalescence and knee stiffness, which are particularly problematic for the older adult. Advances in arthroscopic techniques, which eliminate the need for a surgical incision, are changing associated morbidity and recovery time.

Arthroplasty. Arthroplasty is the reconstruction or replacement of a joint. This surgical procedure is performed to relieve pain, improve or maintain ROM, and correct deformity—conditions that can result from OA, RA, avascular necrosis, congenital deformities or dislocations, and other systemic problems. There are several types of arthroplasty, including replacement of part of a joint, surgical reshaping of the bones of the joints, and total joint replacement. Innovative procedures and prosthetic devices offer exciting possibilities for future reconstructive joint surgery (Fig. 58-13). Replacement arthroplasty is available for the elbow, shoulder, phalangeal joints of the fingers, hip, knee, and ankle.

The major problem related to arthroplasty is loosening of the implants, usually caused by a problem of the ce-

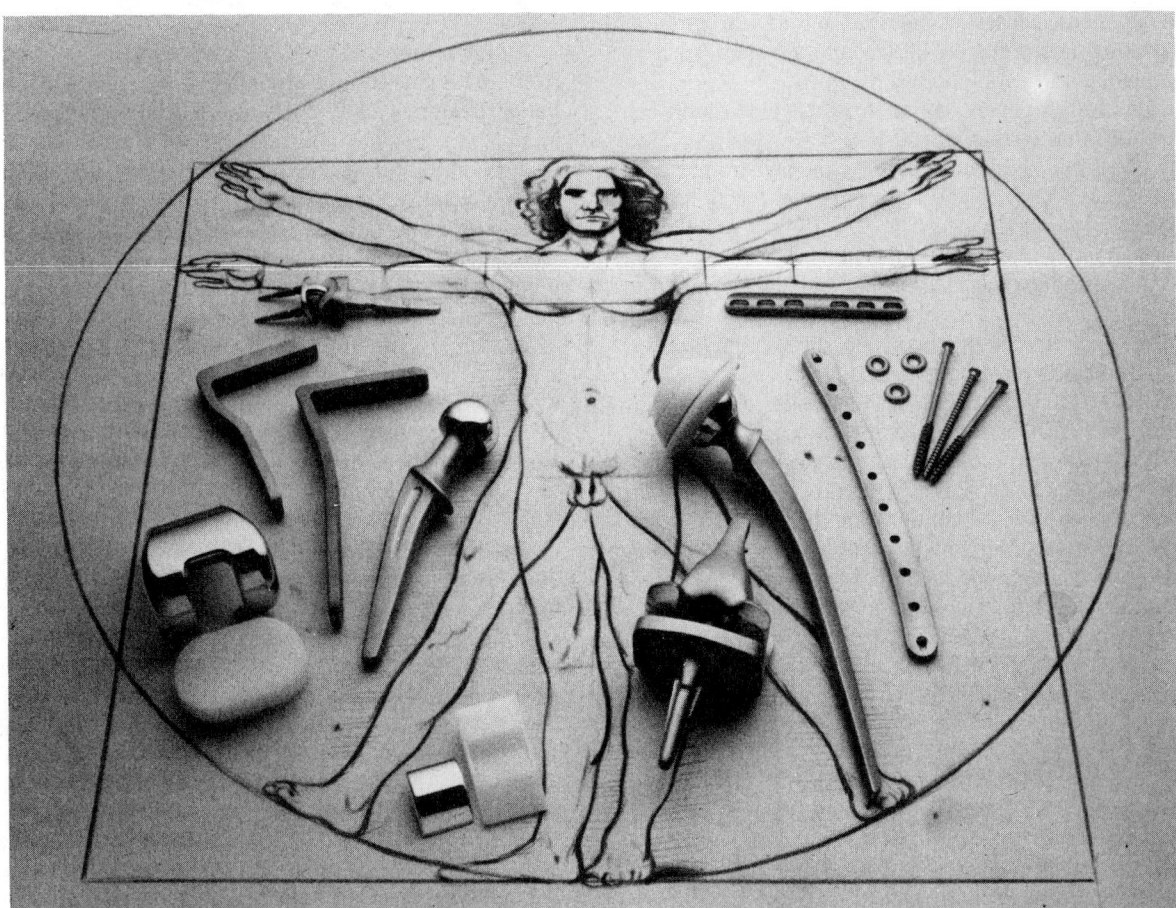

Fig. 58-13 Vitallium alloy joint replacements.

ment, polymethylmethacrylate, and its bond with the bone. The use of cemented versus noncemented implants is controversial.[47] Traditionally, methylmethacrylate, a grout that interlocks components by filling in interstices, has been used. High rates of loosening prompted interest in wedging implants into bone and eliminating cement completely. Porous-surface implants allow bone ingrowth for biological fixation. A third possibility involves implantation of a cementless cup and a cemented femoral component. Choice of a method depends on client age and activity and surgeon preference.

Hip. Hip reconstruction is frequently used in the treatment of clients with RA and OA as well as for fractures of the hip. This surgery is usually performed on clients more than 60 years of age. It is occasionally done in younger clients, but the long-term effects and durability of the joint have not been established. It is also done on clients who have had previously unsuccessful surgery for fracture repair. (For a detailed discussion of the client undergoing a total hip replacement, see Chapter 57.)

Knee. Unremitting pain as a result of severe destructive deterioration of the knee joint is the main indication for knee arthroplasty. The presence of osteoporosis may necessitate bone grafting to augment defects and to correct bone deficiencies. Either part or all of the knee joint may be replaced with a metal and plastic prosthetic device. Great emphasis is placed on postoperative exercising,

which requires a high degree of motivation on the part of the client because of the pain involved. Within 2 to 5 days after surgery the client is instructed to perform quadricep-setting exercises and straight-leg raising. Active flexion exercises through the use of a passive-motion machine postoperatively promotes earlier joint mobility and shortens hospitalization. Weight-bearing is begun when the client can use a walker or crutches.

Finger joints. A silicone rubber arthroplastic device is used to help restore function in the fingers of the client with RA. The goal of hand surgery is primarily to restore function related to grasp, pinch, stability, and strength rather than to correct cosmetic deformity. The metacarpophalangeal and proximal interphalangeal joints are most commonly involved. Ulnar deviation is often present, which results in severe functional limitations of the hand. Before surgery the client is instructed in hand exercises including flexion, extension, abduction, and adduction of the fingers. Postoperatively, the hand is kept elevated with a bulky dressing in place. The operative area and the hand should be checked for sensation, temperature, pulse, and signs of infection. Once the dressing is removed, a guided splinting program is initiated. The success of the surgery depends largely on the postoperative treatment plan, which is often carried out under the direction of an occupational therapist. The client is discharged with splints to use while sleeping and hand exercises to perform for 10 to 12 weeks

at least three to four times a day. The client is also instructed to avoid lifting heavy objects.

Elbows and shoulders. Although available, total replacement of elbow and shoulder joints is not as common as other forms of arthroplasty. Shoulder replacements are used in clients with severe pain because of RA, OA, necrosis, or an old trauma. The shoulder replacement is usually considered if the client has adequate surrounding muscle strength and bone stock. If joint replacement is necessary for both elbow and shoulder, the elbow is usually done first because a severely painful elbow interferes with the shoulder rehabilitation program.

Significant pain relief has been achieved in all diagnostic groups, with 90% of clients having no pain at rest or minimal pain with activity. Functional improvements have resulted in better hygiene and increased ability to perform activities of daily living in most clients. Rehabilitation is longer and more difficult than with other joint surgeries.

Arthrodesis. Arthrodesis is the surgical fusion of a joint. This procedure relieves pain and provides a stable joint by eliminating the ROM of a particular joint. The fusion is usually accomplished by removal of the articular hyaline cartilage and the addition of bone grafts across the joint surface. The affected joint must be immobilized until bone healing has occurred.

Common areas of fusion are the wrist, ankle, cervical spine, and lumbar spine. It must be stressed to the client that the fused joint will have no motion. Arthrodesis is usually considered after other forms of surgical intervention such as synovectomy, osteotomy, and arthroplasty have been unsuccessful.

Complications

Deep infection is a serious complication of joint surgery, particularly joint replacement surgery. The most common causative organisms are gram-positive aerobic streptococci and staphylococci. The conservative estimate of the current incidence of deep infection after joint replacement surgery is 1%.[47] In these instances the infection almost always leads to pain and septic loosening, generally requiring extensive surgery. Removal of the prosthesis from the infected joint causes large skeletal defects, extremity shortening, and marked disability. Although reoperation is possible, it takes longer, is more complicated, and more often results in loosening.

Efforts to reduce the incidence of deep infection include the use of specially designed hypersterile operating rooms with laminar air flow and prophylactic antibiotic administration. Administration of the drug begins immediately before surgery and continues for 24 to 48 hours postoperatively.

Deep vein thrombosis is another potentially serious complication after selected joint surgeries, particularly those involving the lower extremities. Prophylaxis such as aspirin, warfarin, or pneumatic compression of the legs is usually instituted in these clients. Clients may be followed postoperatively with venous plethysmography to detect proximal deep vein thrombosis, the source of most pulmonary emboli. The peak incidence of pulmonary embolus is on the fourth postoperative day.[48]

Therapeutic Management

Preoperative evaluation. As surgical techniques and care improve, more clients with chronic diseases such as RA are being considered as surgical candidates. Because joint surgery is usually elective, the preoperative status of the client must be carefully evaluated. The primary goal of preoperative evaluation is to identify risk factors associated with preoperative complications related to the client, the type of surgery, the skill of the surgeon and other care providers, and the type and duration of anesthesia. Once potential risk factors are identified, specific actions can be instituted to reduce such risks. Specific risk factors, including a history of urinary tract infection, thrombophlebitis, pulmonary embolus, hypocoagulability, peptic ulcer disease, or pneumonia, should be explored. Any infection should be treated preoperatively. Anticipated dental work should be completed before surgery.

If lower-extremity surgery is planned, the arms and shoulders need to be evaluated to determine whether they can manipulate crutches or a walker. If hip surgery is anticipated, the knees must be evaluated to determine whether they are stable enough to effectively support the body's weight postoperatively. Balance and equilibrium should be adequate to allow unimpeded postoperative recovery.

Artificial joint recipients need to commit themselves to a lifestyle that is compatible with the intrinsic capabilities of the prosthetic components so that prosthesis longevity can be maximized.

Careful timing and preparation of the client are important for surgery on the client with RA. Specific management decisions need to be made concerning the following courses of action:

1. Adjusting antirheumatic drug therapy
2. Ordering supplemental corticosteroid coverage for clients who are taking or have recently discontinued corticosteroids
3. Assessing the need for prophylactic therapy for venous thromboembolism
4. Assessing the need for prophylactic antimicrobial therapy

The client with RA should be strong constitutionally, preferably with a low ESR, and should be watched for postoperative anemia. Iron preparations may be given preoperatively. Clients who have been receiving prolonged steroid therapy must be monitored carefully because they may be susceptible to shock after surgery due to adrenal insufficiency.

Postoperative management. Postoperatively, the surgeon is concerned with nerve function and circulatory status. In general, the affected joint is exercised as early as possible, and ambulation is encouraged. Specific details regarding exercise and ambulation vary among surgeons, so detailed directions should be requested.

■ Nursing Management of Joint Surgery

The nursing management of the client undergoing joint surgery includes preoperative and postoperative activities. Preoperatively, the nurse should reinforce the surgeon's explanation of the intended procedure and help the client set realistic expectations. It is important that the client un-

Table 58-18

NURSING CARE PLAN FOR THE CLIENT UNDERGOING JOINT SURGERY

Defining Characteristics	Nursing Interventions	Evaluation Criteria

Acute intervention

NURSING DIAGNOSIS: Impaired physical mobility related to pain, stiffness, and surgical procedure

Difficulty in ambulating; reluctance, unwillingness, or inability to participate in physical rehabilitation; guarded movement; expression of fear about ambulating	Begin exercise program as directed. Cooperate with physical therapist to increase client compliance. Give pain medication before exercise.	Functional ROM of operated joint

NURSING DIAGNOSIS: Pain related to surgical procedure, edema, and ineffective pain or comfort measures

Expression of verbal and nonverbal cues related to pain such as moaning, crying, guarding; withdrawal, apprehension; expression of dissatisfaction with pain control	Assess factors that precipitate and relieve pain. Give pain medication as ordered. Monitor effect. Use nursing measures to relieve pain, such as massage, positioning, distraction.	Minimal pain on movement of operated joint, expression of satisfaction with pain relief measures

NURSING DIAGNOSIS: High risk for infection related to exposure of joint during surgery, presence of environmental pathogen, and ineffective prophylaxis

Fever, purulent drainage and redness at wound site, increased pain, elevated WBC count	Monitor vital signs q 4 hr. Assess dressing for amount and character of drainage q 4 hr. Assess level of pain. Use strict aseptic technique for dressing changes.	No evidence of infection (e.g., fever, increased pain, drainage)

NURSING DIAGNOSIS: High risk for injury: falls related to weakness, fatigue, orthostatic hypotension, pain, gait instability, and use of assistive device

Unsteady gait, weakness, and lightheadedness; improper use of assistive device when upright	Assess for predisposing factors. Assess client's readiness to ambulate. Assist as necessary with ambulation. Assess environment for fall potential and alter as indicated. Schedule pain medication administration to maximize effectiveness during ambulation. Provide supervised practice with assistive devices.	Absence of falls

NURSING DIAGNOSIS: Potential complication: dislocation of prosthesis related to improper movement or activity and infection

Pain in affected joint, loss of function, shortening or malalignment of extremity	Instruct client on safe positions and activities. Use assistive devices (e.g., raised toilet seat) as indicated. Reinforce instructions of physical therapists. Teach signs of dislocation to report (e.g., pain, loss of function, deformity).	Absence of joint dislocation

NURSING DIAGNOSIS: Potential complication: nerve or circulatory impairment related to edema

Anesthesia, paresthesia, coldness, pallor, excessive pain, swelling of affected extremity or body area	Assess nerve and circulatory status q 1 hr first 24 hr, then every 2-4 hr. Notify surgeon immediately if abnormalities are noted. Initiate measures to minimize edema such as cold packs and elevation of affected part.	No evidence of nerve or circulatory impairment

Table 58-18

NURSING CARE PLAN FOR THE CLIENT UNDERGOING JOINT SURGERY—cont'd

Defining Characteristics	Nursing Interventions	Evaluation Criteria
NURSING DIAGNOSIS: Self-care deficit related to restrictions imposed by joint surgery, pain, weakness		
Inability or unwillingness to perform part or all of activities of daily living	Assess client's ability to perform activities of daily living. Assist as necessary. Ensure all basic needs are met. Assure client of your willingness to assist with activities of daily living postoperatively. Assure client that self-care abilities will be resumed with time.	Independent or assisted achievement of needs of activities of daily living
NURSING DIAGNOSIS: Altered health maintenance related to lack of knowledge of follow-up care		
Expression of concern with ability to care for self after discharge, frequent questioning about follow-up care, lack of plan for follow-up care	Instruct client on usual follow-up protocol, including activity limitations, medications, follow-up visit, signs to observe related to infection, dislocation. Make clear to client that joint surgery does not alter underlying disease process. Assist client to identify activities that require modification. Refer for vocational counseling if indicated.	Expression of confidence in ability to manage self-care after discharge and to make necessary lifestyle changes
NURSING DIAGNOSIS: High risk for ineffective individual coping related to unrealistic expectations, limited physical activity, and inadequate support system		
Expression of inability to cope; use of inappropriate coping mechanisms such as anger, crying, withdrawal, isolation; high anxiety level; inadequate support system	Discuss realistic postoperative expectations with client. Identify possible areas requiring adjustments. Initiate visiting nurse referral. Assess support system and enhance if necessary. Teach client replacement coping techniques if indicated. Encourage realistic appraisal of present situation and attempt to problem solve.	Acceptance and adjustment to limitations of function and strength, use of positive coping mechanisms

derstand and accept the limitations of the proposed surgery and realize that it will not remove the underlying disease process. Client activities such as exercises, turning, coughing, and deep breathing should be explained and opportunities for practice provided. The client should be reassured that pain relief will be available if necessary. A preoperative visit from a physical therapist can explain in detail the postoperative exercise program, measure for crutches or other assistive devices, let the client see the tilt table if one is indicated, and introduce the client to the various elements of rehabilitation. The nurse's role in the therapy program can be explained for the client. The spirit of respect and cooperation displayed between the physical therapist and the nurse can do much to reassure an anxious client.

The nurse should begin discussion of discharge planning with the client and family. The family should be instructed to examine the home for any obstacles that may cause a fall, such as scatter rugs and electric cords. The duration of the hospital stay and the expected postoperative events should be discussed so that the client and family can plan ahead. Walking, golf (without carrying clubs), and social dancing are not discouraged, but unnecessary

stair climbing, hiking, tennis, skiing, and running are generally forbidden. Specific nursing interventions related to joint surgery are summarized in Table 58-18.

The general postoperative care for a surgical client is appropriate (see Chapter 13). The nerve and circulatory status of the operated areas should be assessed every hour for the first 24 hours. Anesthesia, paresthesia, coldness, pallor, excessive pain, and swelling should be reported immediately to the surgeon. Specific directions related to activity and positioning should be followed carefully. Nursing measures for pain control such as massage, positioning, and distraction should be used in addition to pain medication. Careful timing of exercise activity to follow pain medication improves client cooperation in the necessary procedures. The family is encouraged to accompany the client to the physical therapy department to observe the exercise program and to offer support and encouragement. The nurse should consult regularly with the physical therapist on ways to implement the exercise program on the nursing unit.

The nurse should be alert for the possible need for referral before discharge. A social worker may be able to assist the client with transportation and financial concerns. A

visiting nurse can ease the transition from hospital to home and provide both physical and emotional support to the client and family. Because many surgical procedures require long-term exercise programs, the visiting nurse can monitor this program and assess and refer any problems that arise.

The client should be instructed on specific complications to report, including infection (e.g., fever, increased pain, and drainage) and dislocation of the prosthesis (pain, loss of function, shortening or malalignment of an extremity). The client should clearly understand the need to continue medical supervision for the underlying disease process and the need for postoperative follow-up by the surgeon.

C ase Study

RHEUMATOID ARTHRITIS

Mrs. M. is a 36-year-old, obese, white woman who has RA. She has three children 4, 7, and 10 years of age. Her husband Jack is a truck driver who works nights. About a year ago she noticed that her hands and feet were painful and some of the small joints were swollen. Some mornings she found it rather difficult to get out of bed because she felt generally tired and stiff. She also thought at times that she was running a slight fever. Only when her symptoms began to interfere with her activities to such an extent that her friends began to notice did she seek help. By this time she was having increased pain and stiffness, and her hands at times were so swollen that she could not open jars or work in the yard without great difficulty. Mrs. M. was admitted to the hospital for examination and a comprehensive treatment program. She stated on admission that she had arthritis but did not know what type. Her medication program consisted of naproxen (Naprosyn), 500 mg twice daily. Oral gold therapy was being considered. She was wearing a copper bracelet that her neighbor gave her on hearing of her recent diagnosis of arthritis. She also stated that for the past year she had been taking "arthritis strength" Anacin that she saw advertised on television for "aches and pains of arthritis" because her symptoms sounded similar.

Discussion Questions

1. How might the nurse explain the pathology of RA to Mrs. M?
2. What manifestations did Mrs. M. have that suggested the diagnosis of RA?
3. What results may be expected of gold therapy? What are the nursing responsibilities related to gold therapy?
4. What are some suggestions that may be offered concerning home management and joint protection?
5. How can the nurse help Mrs. M. to recognize ineffective, unproved methods of treatment?
6. What other sources of information regarding arthritis might the nurse suggest to Mrs. M.?

R eview Questions

The number of the question corresponds to the same-numbered objective at the beginning of the chapter.

1. A common manifestation of OA is
   a. fever
   b. fatigue
   c. pain
   d. elevated ESR
2. The most common site of muscle weakness in polymyositis is the
   a. chest and thorax
   b. shoulder and pelvic girdle
   c. upper legs and hips
   d. knees and ankles
3. The final stage in the pathology of RA is
   a. fibrous ankylosis
   b. pannus formation
   c. bony ankylosis
   d. synovitis
4. OA is characterized by
   a. systemic joint manifestations
   b. morning stiffness and evening pain
   c. presence of sepsis
   d. anemia
5. When caring for the client with SLE, the nurse should
   a. observe for CNS involvement
   b. monitor and record fever pattern
   c. assess limitation of movement
   d. all the above
6. The purpose of a synovectomy is to
   a. prevent further joint damage
   b. ankylose a joint
   c. correct a deformity
   d. replace a joint
7. Before surgery the client with RA should have
   a. a cardiovascular and respiratory assessment
   b. a low ESR
   c. an assessment of steroid use
   d. all the above
8. Drugs commonly used in the treatment of RA include all the following *except*
   a. penicillamine
   b. antibiotics
   c. aspirin
   d. corticosteroids
9. The primary goal of nursing intervention for a client with a rheumatic disease is
   a. weight loss
   b. absence of pain
   c. maximal self-care
   d. gainful employment
10. Effective interdisciplinary arthritis health-care team functioning includes
    a. collaboration and feedback
    b. formal and informal communication
    c. evaluation of client outcomes
    d. all the above

REFERENCES

1. Funk JR, MacBriar BR, and Peterson AF: Tibial osteotomy, Orthop Nurs 9:29-34, 1990.
2. Cook TDV, Bennett EL, and Ohno O: Identification of immunoglobulins and complement components in articular collagenous tissues of patients with idiopathic osteoarthroses. In Nuki G, ed: The aetiopathogenesis of osteoarthroses, Kent, UK, 1980, Pitman Medical.

3. Kale SA and Raymond MK: Osteoarthritis: the patient centered approach, Consultant 30:24-29, 1990.
4. Hochberg M: NSAIDs: patterns of usage and side effects, Hosp Pract 24:167-174, 1989.
5. Minor MA and others: Efficacy of physical conditioning exercise in patients with rheumatoid arthritis and osteoarthritis, Arthritis Rheum 32:1396-1405, 1989.
6. Zvaifler NJ: Etiology and pathogenesis of rheumatoid arthritis. In McCarty DJ, ed: Arthritis and allied conditions, ed 11, Philadelphia, 1989, Lea & Febiger, p 659.
7. Medsger TA and Masi AT: Epidemiology of the rheumatic diseases. In McCarty DJ, ed: Arthritis and allied conditions, ed 11, Philadelphia, 1989, Lea & Febiger, p 16.
8. Tirestein G and Zvaifler N: The pathogenesis of rheumatoid arthritis. In Pesetsy DS and others, eds: Immunology of rheumatic disease, Rheum Dis Clin North Am 13:447-453, 1987.
9. Arnett FC and others: The American Rheumatism Association 1987 revised criteria for the classification of RA, Arthritis Rheum 31:315-324, 1988.
10. Maksymowychio C and Russell AS: Antimalarials in rheumatology: efficacy and safety, Semin Arthritis Rheum 16:196, 1987.
11. McEvoy GK and others, eds: American hospital formulary service, Bethesda, Md, 1990, American Society of Hospital Pharmacists.
12. Kremer JM and Lee JK: A long-term prospective study of the use of methotrexate in rheumatoid arthritis: update after a mean of 53 months, Arthritis Rheum 31:577-584, 1988.
13. Kremer JM and others: Fish-oil fatty acid supplementation in active RA, Ann Intern Med 106:497-503, 1987.
14. Guide to independent living for people with arthritis, Atlanta, 1988, Arthritis Foundation.
15. Mirabelli L: Caring for patients with rheumatoid arthritis, Nursing 9:67-72, 1990.
16. McDuffie FC and Boutaugh M: Pool exercise for people with arthritis, Clin Rheum Pract 3:168-169, 1985.
17. Cassidy JT and others: A study of classification criteria for a diagnosis of juvenile rheumatoid arthritis, Arthritis Rheum 29:274-281, 1986.
18. Calabrog J: Juvenile rheumatoid arthritis. In Katz WA, ed: Diagnosis and management of rheumatic diseases, ed 2, Philadelphia, 1988, JB Lippincott Co, pp 396-408.
19. Arnett FC: Seronegative spondyarthropathies, Bull Rheum Dis 37:1-12, 1987.
20. Bluestone R: Atypical ankylosing spondylitis, Hosp Pract 24:88, 1989.
21. Calin A: Reactive arthritis and Reiter's syndrome. In Katz WA, ed: Diagnosis and management of rheumatic diseases, ed 2, Philadelphia, 1988, JB Lippincott Co, pp 440-447.
22. Steere AC: Lyme disease, N Engl J Med 321:586-596, 1989.
23. Zwolski K: Lyme disease, Orthop Nurs 9:10-17, 1990.
24. McCarty DJ: Intractable gouty arthritis, Hosp Pract June 15, 1987, p 195.
25. Wallace DJ and Dubois EJ, eds: Dubois' lupus erythematosus, ed 3, Philadelphia, 1987, Lea & Febiger.
26. Masi AT and Medsger TA Jr: Epidemiology of the rheumatic diseases. In McCarty DJ, ed: Arthritis and allied conditions, ed 11, Philadelphia, 1989, Lea & Febiger, p 16.
27. Andreoli TE and others, eds: Cecil essentials of medicine, ed 2, Philadelphia, 1990, WB Saunders Co, p 643.
28. Talal N: Etiology of SLE. In Wallace DJ and Dubois EJ, eds: Dubois' lupus erythematosus, ed 3, Philadelphia, 1987, Lea & Febiger.
29. Arnett FC: Familial SLE, the HLA system and the genetics of lupus erythematosus. In Wallace DJ and Dubois EJ, eds: Dubois' lupus erythematosus, ed 3, Philadelphia, 1987, Lea & Febiger.
30. Lahita RG and others: Abnormal estrogen and androgen metabolism in the human with SLE, Am J Kidney Dis 2(suppl 1):206, 1982.
31. Hess E: Drug-related lupus, N Engl J Med 318:1460-1462, 1988.

32. Callen JP and Klein J: Subacute cutaneous lupus erythematosus, Arthritis Rheum 31:1007-1013, 1988.
33. Hahn BH: Lupus nephritis: therapeutic decisions, Hosp Pract Mar 30, 1990, p 89.
34. Gladman DD and Urowitz MB: Morbidity in SLE, J Rheumatol 14(suppl 13):223-226, 1987.
35. Wilson MR: Antinuclear antibodies and anticytoplasmic antibodies in SLE. In Wallace DJ and Dubois EJ, eds: Dubois' lupus erythematosus, ed 3, Philadelphia, 1987, Lea & Febiger.
36. Krupp LB and others: The fatigue severity scale: application to patients with multiple sclerosis and systemic lupus erythematosus, Arch Neurol 46:1121-1123, 1989.
37. Alarcon-Segoveci D: Pathogenetic potential of antiphospholipid antibodies, J Rheumatol 15:890-892, 1988.
38. Cornwell CJ and Schmitt MH: Perceived health status, self-esteem and body image in women with rheumatoid arthritis or systemic lupus erythematosus, Res Nurs Health 13:99-107, 1990.
39. Larabee JH: Progressive systemic sclerosis: part I—the disease and medical management, ANNA 16:489-493, 1990.
40. Leroy EC and Lomeo R: The spectrum of scleroderma I, Hosp Pract Oct 30, 1989, pp 33-40.
41. Leroy EC and Lomeo R: The spectrum of scleroderma II, Hosp Pract Nov 15, 1989, pp 65-72.
42. Ziegler G: Systemic lupus erythematosus and systemic sclerosis, Nurs Clin North Am 19:673-695, 1984.
43. Larrabee JH and others: Progressive systemic sclerosis: part 2—nursing management, ANNA 16:495-498, 1989.
44. Hochberg MC, Feldman D, and Stevens MB: Adult onset polymyositis/dermatomyositis: an analysis of clinical and laboratory features and survival in 76 patients with a review of the literature, Semin Arthritis Rheum 15:168-178, 1986.
45. Leroy EC and Medsger TA Jr: The spectrum of scleroderma-related syndromes: primer on the rheumatic diseases, ed 9, Atlanta, 1988, Arthritis Foundation.
46. Andreoli TE and others: Cecil essentials of medicine, ed 2, Philadelphia, 1990, WB Saunders Co, pp 647-648.
47. Grelsamer R: Medical complications in patients with joint replacements, Hosp Pract July 15, 1988, pp 164-172.
48. Sledge CB and Poss R: Surgical management of arthritis: primer on the rheumatic diseases, ed 9, Atlanta, 1988, Arthritis Foundation.

SECTION IX REFERENCES
BOOKS

Byrne TN and Waxman SG: Spinal cord compression: diagnosis and principles of management, Philadelphia, 1990, FA Davis Co.

Cohen GD: The brain in human aging, New York, 1990, Springer Publishing Co.

Dittmar SS: Rehabilitation nursing: process and application, St Louis, 1989, The CV Mosby Co.

Errico TJ, Bauer RD, and Waugh T, eds: Spinal trauma, Philadelphia, 1991, JB Lippincott Co.

Ferrer-Brechner T, ed: Common problems in pain management, Chicago, 1990, Year Book Medical Publishers.

Hamdy RC and others: Alzheimer's disease: a handbook for caregivers, St Louis, 1990, Mosby–Year Book, Inc.

Hertling D and Kessler RM: Management of common musculoskeletal disorders: physical therapy principles and methods, ed 2, Philadelphia, 1990, JB Lippincott Co.

Hopkins A, ed: Headache: problems in diagnosis and management, Philadelphia, 1988, WB Saunders Co.

Kaplan PE and Tanner ED: Musculoskeletal pain and disability, Norwalk, Conn, 1989, Appleton & Lange.

Kelly WN: Textbook of rheumatology, ed 3, Philadelphia, 1989, WB Saunders Co.

Layfer LF, Petasnick J, and Katz RS: Rheumatologic disorders, Philadelphia, 1988, WB Saunders Co.

Lechtenberg R: Seizure recognition and treatment, New York, 1990, Churchill Livingstone, Inc.

McCaffery M and Beebe A: Pain: clinical manual for nursing practice, St Louis, 1989, The CV Mosby Co.

McCarty DJ, ed: Arthritis and allied conditions: a textbook of rheumatology, ed 11, Philadelphia, 1989, Lea & Febiger.

Merritt HH and Rowland LP: Merritt's textbook of neurology, ed 8, Philadelphia, 1989, Lea & Febiger.

Prentice WE: Rehabilitation techniques in sports medicine, St Louis, 1990, Mosby–Year Book, Inc.

Reckling FW, Reckling JB, and Mohn MP, eds: Orthopaedic anatomy and surgical approaches, St Louis, 1990, Mosby–Year Book, Inc.

Salcman M, ed: Neurologic emergencies: recognition and management, ed 2, New York, 1990, Raven Press.

Sherman OH and Minkoff J, eds: Arthroscopic surgery, Baltimore, 1990, Williams & Wilkins.

Sinaki M, Dale DA, and Hurley DL: Living with osteoporosis: guidelines for women before and after diagnosis, St Louis, 1988, The CV Mosby Co.

Symon L, Thomas DGT, and Clark K, eds: Neurosurgery, ed 4, Boston, 1989, Butterworth Publishers.

Umphred DA, ed: Neurological rehabilitation, ed 2, St Louis, 1990, Mosby–Year Book, Inc.

Zuckerman JC, ed: Comprehensive care of orthopaedic injuries in the elderly, Baltimore, 1990, Urban & Schwarzenberg, Inc.

JOURNALS

Acorn S and Andersen S: Depression in multiple sclerosis: critique of the research literature, J Neurosci Nurs 22:209, 1990.

Ammons AM: Cerebral injuries and intracranial hemorrhages as a result of trauma, Nurs Clin North Am 25:23, 1990.

Borkowski C: A comparison of pulmonary complications in spinal cord-injured patients treated with two modes of spinal immobilization, J Neurosci Nurs 21:79, 1989.

Boss BJ and Brewer L: Syncope: neuroscience nursing assessment based on an understanding of underlying pathophysiological mechanisms, J Neurosci Nurs 20:245, 1988.

Brassell MP: Pharmacologic management of rheumatic diseases, Orthop Nurs 85:43, 1988.

Buckwalter KC, Abraham IL, and Neundorfer MM: Alzheimer's disease: involving nursing in the development and implementation of health care for patients and families, Nurs Clin North Am 23:1, 1988.

Buelow JM and Jamieson D: Potential for altered nutritional status in the stroke patient, Rehabil Nurs 15:260, 1990.

Burgener S and Logan G: Sexuality concerns of the post-stroke patient, Rehabil Nurs 14:178, 1989.

Chamberlain A: Arthritis: social problems and practical solutions, Nurs Times 85:36, 1989.

Chicano LA: Humanistic aspects of sexuality as related to spinal cord injury, J Neurosci Nurs 21:366, 1989.

Dicks B: Treatment of pain in the cancer patient: the role of the nurse, Recent Results Cancer Res 108:33, 1988.

Dillehay RC and Sandys MR: Caregivers for Alzheimer's patients: what we are learning from research, Int J Aging Hum Dev 30:263, 1990.

Dunnum L: Life satisfaction and spinal cord injury: the patient perspective, J Neurosci Nurs 22:43, 1990.

Fabiszewski KJ: Alzheimer's disease: overview and progression, J Adv Med Surg Nurs 1:1, 1989.

Finocchiaro DN and Herzfeld ST: Understanding autonomic dysreflexia, Am J Nurs 90:56, 1990.

Grabbe LL and Brown LB: Identifying neurologic complications of A.I.D.S., Nursing 19:66, 1989.

Guin P: Standardized nursing care plans for acute care SCI: improved documentation, SCI Nurs 7:4, 1990.

Harper J: Use of steroids in cerebral edema: therapeutic implications, Heart Lung 17:70, 1988.

Holm K and Hedricks C: Immobility and bone loss in the aging adult, Crit Care Nurs Q 12:46, 1989.

Hughes MC: Critical care nursing for the patient with a spinal cord injury, Crit Care Nurs Clin North Am 2:33, 1990.

Johnson L: Operative management of unstable pelvic fractures, Orthop Nurs 8:21, 1989.

Keller C and others: Psychological responses in aphasia: theoretical considerations and nursing implications, J Neurosci Nurs 21:290, 1989.

Killen JM: Role stabilization in families after spinal cord injury, Rehabil Nurs 15:19, 1990.

Kirby NA: The individual with high quadriplegia, Nurs Clin North Am 24:179, 1989.

Kirkevold M: Caring for stroke patients: heavy or exciting? Image J Nurs Sch 22:79, 1990.

Leisifer D: Monitoring pain control and charting, Crit Care Clin 6:283, 1990.

MacDonald E: Aneurysmal subarachnoid hemorrhage, J Neurosci Nurs 21:313, 1989.

Mahon-Darby J and others: Powerlessness in cervical spinal cord injury patients, Dimens Crit Care Nurs 7:346, 1988.

Mendius RA: Female sexuality and spinal cord injury, SCI Nurs 6:68, 1989.

Mims BC: Fat embolism syndrome: a variant of ARDS (continuing education credit), Orthop Nurs 8:22, 1989.

Morgante LA, Madonna MG, and Pokoluk R: Research and treatment in multiple sclerosis: implications for nursing practice, J Neurosci Nurs 21:285, 1989.

Neatherlin JS: Creutzfeldt-Jakob disease, J Neurosci Nurs 20:309, 1988.

Nelson AL: Patients' perspectives of a spinal cord injury unit, SCI Nurs 7:44, 1990.

Olson B and Ustanko L: Self-care needs of patients in the halo brace, Orthop Nurs 9:27, 1990.

Pallett PJ: A conceptual framework for studying family caregiver burden in Alzheimer's-type dementia, Image J Nurs Sch 22:52, 1990.

Palmer M and Wyness MA: Positioning and handling: important considerations in the care of the severely head-injured patient, J Neurosci Nurs 20:42, 1988.

Patterson C and LeClair JK: Acute decompensation in dementia: recognition and management, Geriatrics 44:20, 1989.

Paxquarello MA: Developing, implementing, and evaluating a stroke recovery group, Rehabil Nurs 15:26, 1990.

Printz-Feddersen V: Group process effect on caregiver burden, J Neurosci Nurs 22:164, 1990.

Redheffer GM and Bailey M: Assessing and splinting fractures: emergency photo guide, Nursing 19:51, 1989.

Richmond TS: Spinal cord injury, Nurs Clin North Am 25:57, 1990.

Romito D: A critical path for CVA patients, Rehabil Nurs 15:153, 1990.

Scherer P: How AIDS attacks the brain, Am J Nurs 90:44, 1990.

Scherer P: How HIV attacks the peripheral nervous system, Am J Nurs 90:66, 1990.

Simon JM: A multidisciplinary approach to chronic pain, Rehabil Nurs 14:23, 1989.

Snelling J: The role of the family in relation to chronic pain: review of the literature, J Adv Nurs 15:771, 1990.

Spaulding JM and others: Total ankle arthroplasty: a procedural review, AORN J 48:201, 1988.

Spica MM: Sexual counseling standards for the spinal cord-injured, J Neurosci Nurs 21:56, 1989.

Sullivan J: Brain resuscitation: nursing interventions, Crit Care Nurs Clin North Am 1:155, 1989.

Tanner DC, Gerstenberger DL, and Keller CS: Guidelines for treatment of chronic depression in the aphasic patient, Rehabil Nurs 14:77, 1989.

Ulmer DB: Special needs of the young spinal cord injured patient in a nursing home, SCI Nurs 7:27, 1990.

Vernon GM: Parkinson's disease, J Neurosci Nurs 21:273, 1989.

Whitney CM and Daroff RB: An approach to migraine, J Neurosci Nurs 20:284, 1988.

Wilkie DJ: Cancer pain management: state-of-the-art nursing care, Nurs Clin North Am 25:331, 1990.

Witte M: Pain control, J Gerontol Nurs 15:32, 1989.

ORGANIZATIONS

American Association of Neuroscience Nurses
218 North Jefferson Street, #204
Chicago, IL 60606
Arthritis Foundation
1314 Spring Street, NW
Atlanta, GA 30309
Association of Rehabilitation Nurses
5700 Old Orchard Road, First floor
Skokie, IL 60077
National Association of Orthopaedic Nurses, Inc.
North Woodbury Road, Box 56
Pitman, NJ 08071
National Institute of Neurological and Communicative Disorders and Stroke
9000 Rockville Pike
Bethesda, MD 20892
National Parkinson Foundation
Bob Hope Road
Miami, FL 33136
Parkinson's Disease Foundation
William Black Medical Research Building
Columbia Presbyterian Medical Center
650 West 168th Street
New York, NY 10032

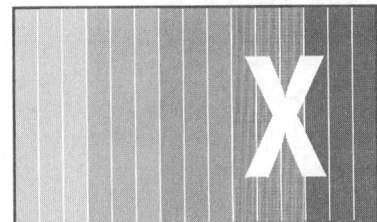

SECTION

X

PROBLEMS IN SPECIAL SITUATIONS

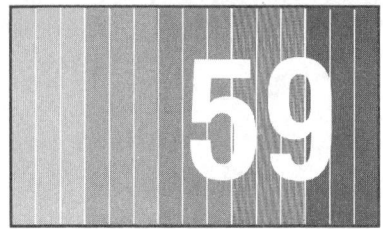

CHAPTER 59

Nursing Role in Management
Selected Emergency Situations*

Jacqueline Rhoads

Rapid developments in the treatment of medical and traumatic emergencies were seen in the 1970s. Technological advances, organized prehospital care, and specific training programs in emergency medicine and nursing combined to decrease the morbidity and mortality rates of emergency victims significantly. The advent of urgent care centers has given the client more choices in deciding how health care needs are to be met. Full-service emergency departments in acute-care hospitals now treat predominantly emergency victims who have a high probability of serious morbidity or death.

For clarity, emergencies are often divided into two groups: medical emergencies and traumatic emergencies. *Medical emergencies* are defined as all acute physiological crises that are not directly caused by a traumatic impact to the body and generally do not require surgical intervention. *Traumatic emergencies* are physiological crises that are directly caused by impact to the body and generally require surgical intervention.

EMERGENCY CARE OVERVIEW

Advances in medical technology, the development of medical equipment (e.g., cardiac monitoring, Heimlich valves, orthopedic traction) tailored to be used in prehospital situations (e.g., in field care, on ambulances) and specific training for physicians and nurses have done much to improve the care of emergency victims. Paraprofessionals such as emergency medical technicians (EMT-Bs) and paramedics (EMT-Ps) are also specially trained to deliver appropriate prehospital emergency care. This addition to the health care team has greatly increased the likelihood of survival for emergency victims until they reach a hospital emergency department. Sophisticated transportation systems, some of which use small planes and helicopters, have been developed to ensure rapid transport of the emergency victim to definitive treatment. Many of these programs employ nurses to deliver prehospital care.

Emergency Medical Service System

Emergency care is the responsibility of the community as well as the medical facilities providing the care. Congress passed the Emergency Medical Services Acts in 1973 and amended them in 1976 and 1979. These acts gave communities incentives and federal money to develop regional emergency medical services (EMS) systems nationwide. The purpose of an EMS system is to integrate the use of personnel, facilities, and equipment for the coordinated delivery of emergency care over specific geographical areas. These systems were mandated to provide for individual emergency care as well as for care required during natural and other large-scale disasters. The 15 mandatory requirements of an EMS system are the following:

1. Provision of personnel
2. Training of personnel
3. Communications
4. Transportation

Reviewed by Sharon Gavin Fought, R.N., Ph.D., Assistant Professor, Department of Physiological Nursing, University of Washington, Seattle, Washington and Amanda Conley, R.N., B.S.N., C.E.N., Clinical Coordinator, Emergency Department and Air Ambulance, Presbyterian Hospital, Albuquerque, New Mexico.

*The recognition of a life-threatening illness or injury is a critical aspect of emergency care. This chapter focuses on specific medical and traumatic emergency conditions not discussed elsewhere in this book. A complete list of emergency care tables can be found on the back inside cover.

5. Categorization of facilities
6. Critical care units
7. Use of public safety agencies
8. Consumer participation
9. Accessibility of care for all without reference to ability to pay
10. Transfer of clients
11. Standard medical record keeping
12. Consumer information and education
13. Independent review and evaluation
14. Disaster linkage
15. Mutual aid agreements

Good Samaritan Act

Most states have a Good Samaritan act to protect physicians, nurses, and EMTs from legal action that can result from their attempts to render aid to persons who need medical assistance. This legislation is meant to encourage the offer of emergency care by health care providers without fear of reprisal. The first Good Samaritan Act was passed in California, and it states that practitioners are not held liable for their actions as long as they do not do anything that can be defined as grossly negligent or that constitutes willful misconduct.[1]

The Good Samaritan Act does not protect an individual from negligence. Negligence occurs when practitioners render first aid outside their scope of practice or the standards expected of their practice. Negligence can also occur if practitioners willfully choose not to respond to calls for medical aid and this results in serious injuries.

Emergency Nursing

The integrated nature of the EMS system has affected the roles that health care workers assume while delivering emergency care. There is a great deal of overlap among medical, nursing, and paramedical roles. The division of labor depends on levels of training, state and county laws, and the community standard of care.

Emergency nursing is one of the most challenging specialties in the field of health care. This specialty requires that the nurse, whether in the hospital emergency department or at the emergency site, use a scientific knowledge base, effective communication and clinical skills, and the nursing process to care for clients' and families' physiological and emotional needs. The principles of crisis intervention as well as the actual use of emergency skills are important to the victim and family in the emotion-laden, stressful environment of an emergency situation. Rapid assessment, history taking, appropriate intervention, and emotional support for the family and victim occur in a very short time.

The emergency nurse must also take part in health promotion by teaching clients about accident prevention and basic emergency care in the home. Public awareness can greatly reduce the number of accidents and morbidity and mortality rates in emergencies that go untreated before the victim's arrival at an emergency care facility. The emergency nurse needs to be aware of clients who regularly or consistently return to the hospital with injuries. They may be accident prone or the victims of battering.

ASSESSMENT OF THE EMERGENCY VICTIM

Recognition of a life-threatening illness or injury is one of the most important aspects of emergency care. Before the medical differential diagnosis, the recognition of dangerous clinical signs and symptoms and the initiation of actions to reverse or avert a crisis are mandatory. Therefore initial contact with the client requires the taking of a brief, accurate history and the performance of a rapid, thorough assessment.

History Taking

The history of the accident or illness is important because it can provide clues to the cause of the crisis and suggest specific assessment needs. The client may be unable to give a history, but family, friends, and witnesses can frequently give accurate information. The history should include the following questions:

1. What is the chief complaint? What caused the person to seek attention?
2. How long ago did the incident occur? How long ago did the client become ill?
3. Where did the accident occur? Where did the client become ill?
4. Describe the accident or illness. How did it happen?
5. What has happened since the onset of the illness/injury?
   a. Has the client been moved?
   b. What emergency care was started at the scene of the incident?
   c. What are the client's subjective complaints?
   d. What are witnesses' (if any) descriptions of the client's behavior since the onset?
   e. What are the details of the EMS report?
6. What is the client's health care history?
   a. Allergies
   b. Medications
   c. Past health history (especially cardiac and respiratory conditions and diabetes)
   d. Last meal
   e. Events preceding illness/injury
   f. Pregnancy status
   g. Last tetanus toxoid vaccine

Interview Technique

Obtaining an accurate history in an emergency situation depends on the nurse's interviewing skills. The nurse should avoid using medical jargon and leading the client. For example, "Does the pain in your chest radiate down your left arm?" is a poor question because it suggests a location to the client. A better question is, "Where is your pain?"

The nurse must remain nonjudgmental toward historians or risk losing important information. "Listening" to nonverbal communication is as important to a complete history as verbal responses to questions. Clients and families who are emotionally distraught by a crisis may not give accurate information. There are also situations in which historians wish to protect themselves or someone else. For example, a woman who has stabbed her husband may be unwilling to discuss the events that led to the situation.

The nurse needs to verify confusing and conflicting information with other family members and/or witnesses and to remember that questions should be asked in a manner that will enable clients and families to respond readily.

Assessment Process

Because emergencies require rapid intervention, the physical assessment process must begin as the history is being taken. The initial assessment takes in the client as a whole and the environment as well, including personal interactions. People who seek help in an emergency room are usually in states of crisis. Entry into the EMS system is often an intimidating, frightening experience. People do not have the opportunity to prepare for coping with an emergency in the same way that they prepare for an anticipated hospitalization. Included with the fear of what is happening to them are the fear and anxiety associated with placing themselves under the care of total strangers. There is little time for the client, the family, and the nurse to develop relationships. The entire range of crisis behaviors (e.g., crying, expressions of anger, dazed attitude) are seen by EMS personnel. Nurses must realize that suspicious behaviors that may be exhibited by clients and families is not directed at them but rather are normal reactions under the circumstances. People need to know what the nurse is doing for them. It is the responsibility of the emergency personnel to maintain open communication throughout the history and assessment period.

Certain behaviors should alert the emergency department nurse to potential problems. Inconsistent histories given by several family members may signal a problem such as physical abuse. The client who curses, verbally abuses the nurse, or shows anger or acting out behavior may be severely hypoxic, intoxicated, or have a serious head injury. As the assessment proceeds, the nurse must continue to observe behaviors and interactions along with physical signs.

Assessment is a continual process that is often repeated at regular intervals to detect any changes in the client's status. Some general principles of assessment are to do the following:

1. *Make* the assessment quickly.
2. *Conduct* the assessment systematically.
3. *Compare* the assessment findings with the history.
4. *Listen* for client complaints, abnormal breathing, breath sounds, heart sounds, and bowel sounds.
5. *Look* at skin color and body movements, and observe for the presence of blood.
6. *Feel* for deformities and areas that elicit pain.
7. *Smell* for breath odors such as alcohol, acetone, and gasoline and for chemical odors on clothes.

Primary survey. Assessment of an individual client begins with the primary survey—airway, breathing, and circulation (Table 59-1). This whole process should only take approximately 2 minutes. If problems are identified as life threatening at any time during the survey, appropriate therapeutic interventions should be started immediately.[2]

Airway. Nearly all immediate deaths of trauma victims occur because of airway problems caused by obstruction by the tongue, saliva, blood, or vomitus. In any emer-

---

Table 59-1   Primary Survey of an Emergency Client

AIRWAY

Clear airway.
Open airway (observe cervical spine precautions).
Use appropriate airway adjuncts if necessary.

BREATHING

Assess ventilation.
   Look for chest movements associated with breathing.
   Listen for air being expired through nose and mouth.
   Feel for air being expired.
Observe and count rate of respiration.
Note color of nail beds, mucous membranes, skin.
Give supplemental oxygen via appropriate delivery system.
If there is head trauma, hyperventilate with 100% oxygen.
Have suction readily available.
Anticipate emesis and avoid possibility of aspiration.
Auscultate lungs.
If client is not breathing, ventilate.*

CIRCULATION

Check carotid and/or femoral pulse.
Use chest compression, if necessary.
Assess color, temperature, and moisture of skin.
Check capillary refill.
Start at least two large-bore intravenous lines.
Assess for external bleeding.
Control external bleeding.
   Apply direct pressure.
   If bleeding continues, apply pressure to arteries proximal to injury.

---

*See Table 30-14.

---

gency situation the airway should always be the most important part of the primary survey. If the airway is not maintained, obstruction of air flow occurs and hypoxia and death can result.

Any client with significant upper-body injuries or face, head, or neck trauma should always be suspected of having possible cervical spine trauma. If the client has an obstructed airway, use of the jaw thrust maneuver (Fig. 59-1) while cervical spine stabilization is maintained is the only acceptable method for opening the client's airway.

When this has been accomplished, the mouth and nose need to be checked for fractured teeth, avulsions of skin or mucous membranes, blood, and vomitus. If any of these are present, they should be carefully removed to ensure a patent airway. The nurse should pay special attention to note any facial bone fractures or displacement that can also obstruct the client's airway.

Airway maintenance should progress rapidly from the least to the most invasive method.[3] The airway may be maintained by simple insertion of an oral airway to prevent posterior displacement of the tongue. A nasotracheal or oral tracheal tube may also be indicated (see Chapter 20).

Breathing. Securing adequate air flow through the upper airway does not ensure adequate ventilation. The in-

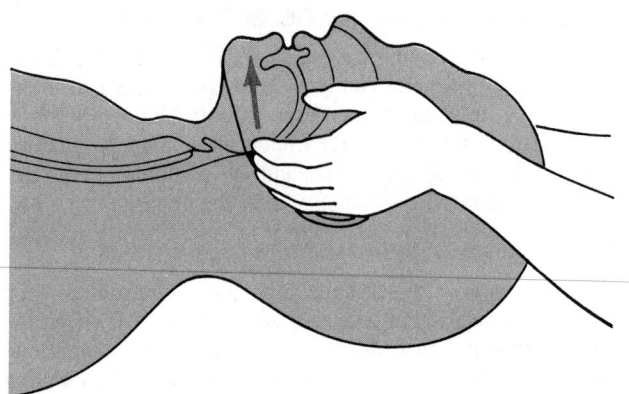

Fig. 59-1 Jaw-thrust maneuver is the only widely recommended procedure for use on unconscious clients with possible neck or spinal injuries. The client should be lying supine with the rescuer kneeling at the top of the head. The rescuer should carefully reach forward and gently place one hand on each side of the client's chin at the lateral angles of the lower jaw. The client's head should be stabilized with the rescuer's forearms, then the jaw pushed forward while pressure is applied with the index fingers.

tegrity of the chest wall, symmetry, discoloration, and bilateral equal expansion should be noted (see Chapter 21). Alterations may be due to fractured ribs, pneumothorax, or penetrating injury and can be easily assessed at the same time that the client's breathing is evaluated. Every injured client has an unpredictable increased oxygen demand. *Every trauma victim needs supplemental oxygen.*

Circulation. The components of the circulatory system are an effective pump (heart), intact blood vessels, and adequate blood volume. Taking these components into consideration, the nurse should begin by checking the carotid and/or femoral pulse. Peripheral pulses may be absent as a result of direct injury or vasoconstriction (from stimulation of the sympathetic nervous system). Delayed capillary refill (longer than 2 seconds) at the nail beds or at the thenar eminence is one of the most significant signs indicating the possible presence of shock. External bleeding is assessed and controlled, and pressure is applied to arteries proximal to the injury if bleeding continues (Fig. 59-2).

Secondary survey. During the primary survey, care is taken to correct any life-threatening airway, breathing, or circulation problems as quickly as possible. Once this has been accomplished, a secondary survey is initiated. For maximum effectiveness, the client's clothes must be removed while the nurse takes care to keep the client's head and neck stable, especially if a facial, head, or neck injury is suspected. This secondary survey should only take 1 to 2 minutes and should start from the client's head and move downward to the toes; the condition of the client's back should be especially noted. The secondary survey should cover a thorough health history of the client as well as a comprehensive physical assessment (Table 59-2).

The secondary survey begins with the head and neck. The client's level of consciousness is assessed. If consciousness is decreased, the cause must be sought. For example, the client may have epilepsy or be under the influ-

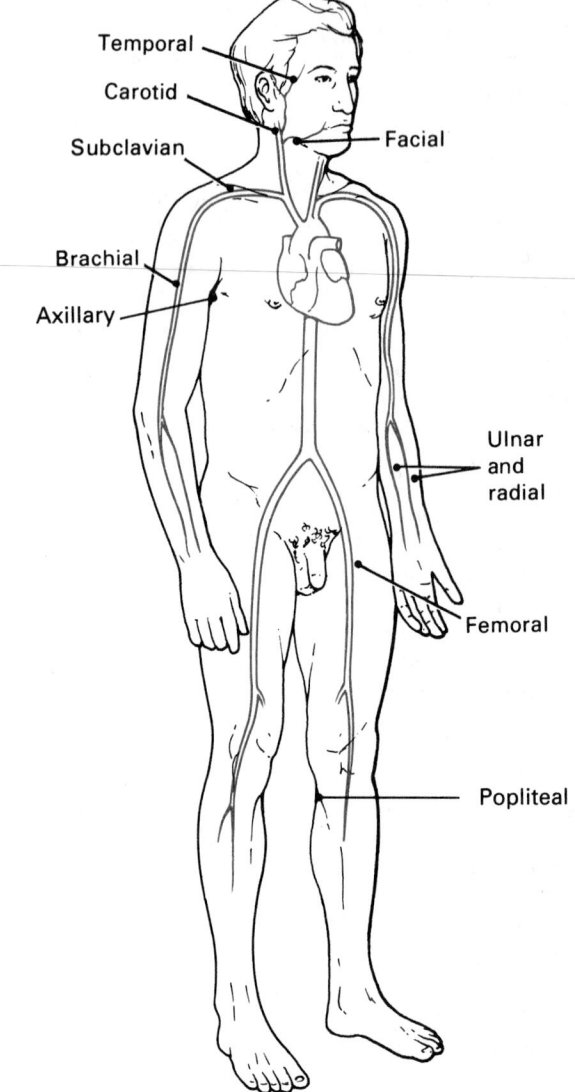

Fig. 59-2 Pressure points for control of hemorrhage.

ence of alcohol or drugs. The pupil size and reaction to light are recorded. The head is palpated for deformities, swelling, hematomas, and areas of softness, as well as for pain. Neck examination includes palpation and visualization of the trachea to determine that it is in the midline and not deviated to the left or right; a deviated trachea may signal a life-threatening tension pneumothorax. Pain in the cervical spine area may signify fracture of a cervical vertebra. The cervical spine *must* be protected.

The physical assessment continues with the chest, spine, abdomen, pelvis, and extremities. Each region is checked for symmetry, motion, external signs of illness or injury (e.g., open wounds), hematomas, and altered skin color and rashes; each region is also palpated for deformities and pain. The front of the client's body is assessed first, and then the client is turned over so that the back can be assessed. Regardless of the victim's chief complaint, a thorough assessment and an accurate history are critical in an emergency situation.[4]

Table 59-2 Secondary Survey of an
Emergency Victim

HEAD AND NECK

Level of consciousness*
Pupil size and reaction to light
Examination of eyes, ears, nose, and mouth
  Bleeding
  Foreign bodies
  Drainage
  Pain
  Cyanosis
Examination of head
  Lacerations
  Depressions of cranial or facial bones
  Contusions
  Pain
Examination of neck
  Stiffness
  Pain in cervical vertebrae
  Tracheal deviations
  Distended neck veins
  Bleeding or edema
  Difficulty in swallowing
  Bruising

CHEST AND SPINE

Anterior and posterior symmetry of chest wall
Motion (equal movement with respiration)
External signs of injury of illness
  Petechiae
  Signs of external injury
  Bleeding
  Cyanosis
  Pain
  Respiratory distress
  Breath sounds
  Pain or deformity of vertebrae

ABDOMEN AND PELVIS

Symmetry of external abdominal wall and bony structures
External signs of injury of illness (e.g., bruising, lacerations, punctures)
Type (localized or rebound) and location of pain
Bowel sounds
Rigidity or distention of abdomen
Genitalia (obvious injury)
Rectal bleeding

EXTREMITIES

Signs of external injury
Bleeding and lacerations
Deformities
Pain
Movement and strength in arms and legs
Sensation in each limb
Color of skin
Presence and quality of peripheral pulses

*See Table 52-2.

MEDICAL AND TRAUMATIC EMERGENCIES

Care of clients who have a medical or traumatic emergency brings with it a challenge and commitment to intervene under time constraints, especially if the client's life is in jeopardy. It is extremely important to *rapidly* identify the primary problem, understand its pathology, and develop a plan of care to quickly treat the client.

Environmental Medical Emergencies

Emergency care personnel are often confronted with specific medical emergencies that occur because of exposure to extremes of heat or cold. These environmental encounters are often serious and carry considerable risk for clients. Greater interest in recreational activities with older participants, competitive athletics, and underwater exploration have increased the number of environmental emergencies seen in emergency centers today.

Heat injury. Heat illness often occurs because of strenuous activities in hot or humid environments, the wearing of clothing that interferes with perspiration, high fevers, endocrine problems, obesity, and alcohol or drug problems. The basic mechanisms of heat illness are increased heat production, perspiration, and peripheral blood flow and salt and water evaporation. These mechanisms increase the metabolic rate and muscle activity.

Heat stress increases cardiac output to compensate for the increased peripheral blood flow. Dehydration occurs because of the increased sweating and evaporation of sweat that results in loss of salt and water. The end result may be heat cramps, heat exhaustion, or heat stroke.

Heat cramps are brief, intermittent, severe muscle cramps occurring in large muscle groups that are fatigued by heavy work. The cramps tend to occur after exercise. They are usually seen in individuals who are not acclimated to heat, who sweat profusely, and who replace fluid lost with salt-poor solutions. Heat cramps seem to be related to salt deficiency and are rapidly relieved by administration of salt solutions. Manifestations and treatment of heat cramps are presented in Table 59-3.

Heat exhaustion or *heat prostration* is due to prolonged exposure to heat, resulting in severe dehydration. It is usually seen in people who have engaged in sports or strenuous exercise in hot, humid weather but can also occur in sedentary people. Two types of heat exhaustion can occur: water depletion and salt depletion. *Water-depletion* heat exhaustion results from inadequate fluid replacement by persons exposed to hot environments. Poor water intake results in dehydration, hypernatremia, increased core temperature, increased pulse rate, decreased sweating, and altered level of consciousness as a result of progressive central nervous system (CNS) deterioration.

Salt-depletion heat exhaustion takes longer to develop than water-depletion heat exhaustion. It occurs when a person perspires excessively and drinks adequate water but has no salt intake. Clinical findings include hyponatremia, low urinary sodium, low chloride concentration, and normal body temperature.[5]

Most cases of heat exhaustion involve loss of water and salt, and clients quickly recover with a cool environment and fluid replacement. Decisions regarding the type of

Table 59-3 Clinical Manifestations and Management of Heat Cramps, Heat Exhaustion, and Heat Stroke

Clinical Manifestations	Management
HEAT CRAMPS	
Severe pain and cramps in lower-extremity muscles and abdomen, faintness, dizziness, weakness, profuse sweating	Increase sodium chloride intake by giving salty liquids, IV infusion. Encourage rest. Move client to cool environment.
HEAT EXHAUSTION	
Pale skin, profuse sweating, nausea and vomiting, rapid weak pulse, lowered blood pressure, dilatation of pupils, transient loss of consciousness, malaise, total body weakness	Place client in cooler environment. Loosen clothing. Apply cold compresses. Elevate legs above heart level. Replace fluids.
HEAT STROKE	
Elevated temperature (39.4° C to 41.1° C; 103° F to 106° F), reddish flush to skin, hot and dry skin, initial elevation of blood pressure, bounding pulse, rapid and irregular respirations, agitation, weakness, dizziness, nausea and vomiting, decreased level of consciousness, coma	Reduce body temperature rapidly (e.g., with ice bath, air conditioner). Monitor rectal temperature. Administer chlorpromazine or diazepam to reduce shivering. Elevate head of bed. Hospitalize client. Provide oxygen, IV fluid replacement, and supportive care.

fluid and electrolyte replacement depend on the electrolyte laboratory results, blood urea nitrogen (BUN), and hematocrit. Clients with severe electrolyte and water deficiencies require intravenous (IV) solutions to reestablish normal balance.

Although uncommon, *heat stroke* is the most serious of the three emergencies and results in death if left untreated. Older adults and individuals with diabetes mellitus or chronic renal, cardiovascular, or pulmonary disease are particularly vulnerable. Heat stroke is common during periods of prolonged heat and high humidity. The onset may be rapid or gradual.

In heat emergencies, increased environmental temperature accompanied by profuse diaphoresis raises the body temperature rapidly. When this occurs, the body's oxygen requirement is increased. The respiratory rate increases to meet this demand. The heart rate also increases to meet tissue demands for a higher oxygen level. These physiological responses to heat continue to raise the body temperature. Clients with diseased cardiac or pulmonary systems cannot tolerate the increased demand. Regardless of the body's effort to compensate, it cannot generate adequate oxygen levels. The nurse needs to note whether a client has any condition that decreases the ability to compensate for increased oxygen needs.

Clients who are on certain drug regimens are at greater risk of experiencing heat emergencies and the nurse should ask about the client's use of these regimens. Diuretic therapy, anticholinergics, and phototoxic drugs such as phenothiazines, thiazides, antihistamines, tolbutamide (Orinase), chlorpropamide (Diabinese), and certain antibiotics increase the risk of heat emergencies. Alcohol increases metabolic heat production and causes impairment in judgment, placing the user at greater risk during periods of high temperature.

Whenever a person demonstrates an altered level of consciousness, the body temperature should be taken. In

Table 59-4 Methods of Lowering Body Temperature

Removal of clothing	Gastric lavage
Oral administration of cool fluids (if client is alert)	Alcohol sponge baths (used with caution)
Ice packs over major blood vessels	Evaporative cooling (e.g., fans, skin wetting)
Peritoneal lavage with cold liquid	Cardiopulmonary bypass*
Rectal enemas	

*In extreme emergencies.

the field the oral or axillary route is practical; the nurse should take care to assess the client's level of consciousness before inserting an oral thermometer. In the emergency room (ER) a tympanic rectal thermometer or probe is preferred to continuously monitor core temperature.

If the temperature indicates that the client has hyperthermia (40.6° C [105° F]), cooling procedures should be started immediately (Table 59-4). In the field, all clothing should be removed, and the client should be placed in a cool area. Cold liquid should be splashed on the client, and if a fan is available, it should be used to keep the air circulating over the client's body. Commercial cold packs or ice (properly covered) can be applied to large superficial vessel areas such as the neck and the inguinal and axillary areas. In the ER, cooling blankets and evaporative cooling can be used. Severe shivering may occur. Care should be taken to control the shivering because it can increase the metabolic rate, oxygen consumption, and body temperature.

Hypotension is very common in heat injuries as a result of the shunting of blood through dilated skin vessels. The heart increases its output, but the body's needs are not

met. Fluid replacement should be carefully monitored. This can be done through a central venous pressure line and monitoring of vital signs. The client should be carefully monitored for metabolic acidosis, via serial arterial blood gases (ABGs), as well as for other laboratory data abnormalities.

After appropriate treatment, client teaching must be aimed at preventing recurrence of the emergency. Clients who are taking phototoxic drugs should be warned that these drugs make them very susceptible to heat emergencies.

Cold-related emergencies. *Hypothermia* is defined as a core temperature of less than 35° C (95° F) as a result of exposure to cold. It occurs when the heat produced by the body is less than the amount of body heat lost to the environment. Heat is lost as radiant energy from the body in large amounts through the head and thorax and through respiration. As heat is lost, the peripheral vascular system constricts in an attempt to conserve heat. If clothing is wet, evaporation speeds heat loss. Wind also speeds heat loss by lowering the environmental temperature, which increases the heat requirement. The body produces heat largely through caloric intake. As cold temperatures persist, shivering and movement are the body's only mechanisms for producing heat. However, these mechanisms also speed heat loss.

Any core temperature below 32° C (90° F) is considered severe and potentially life threatening. Hypothermia can occur in cases of near drowning. People who engage in winter sports or become lost in wilderness areas where night temperatures are low are also susceptible to hypothermia. Other groups at risk are alcoholics, homeless people, and older adults. Alcohol causes peripheral vasodilatation, making individuals more susceptible to the cold. People who live on the street may not have sufficient protection to cope with sudden drops in temperature. Older adults may lower their furnace thermostats to reduce the cost of heating their homes or apartments. In addition, decreased subcutaneous fat makes older adults more susceptible to the effects of a cold environment; thus, they have an impaired ability to increase heat production and decrease heat loss.

Clinical manifestations of progressively worsening hypothermia include shivering, slow and/or slurred speech, amnesia, loss of muscle coordination, drowsiness, acidosis, dysrhythmias, and coma. Clients may not shiver if the heat loss occurred slowly. Unconsciousness generally occurs when the core body temperature decreases to 29° C (84° F). Hypothermia must be assessed with the use of core temperature measurements—ABGs, electrocardiogram (ECG), and vital signs. Special thermometers are required to register low body temperatures. Blood pressure, pulse rate, and respiratory rate are frequently decreased.

Treatment of hypothermia is aimed at rewarming the client, correcting the dehydration and acidosis, maintaining clear upper and lower airways, and treating cardiac dysrhythmias (Table 59-5). The client should be moved to a warm, dry environment and should be handled and stimulated as little as possible. Damp clothing should be removed, and warm blankets should be placed around the

Table 59-5

 Prehospital Emergency Care of the Client with Hypothermia

Etiology: Prolonged exposure to cold, prolonged immersion, excessive perspiration, inadequate clothing relative to environmental temperature, any situation in which the body loses more heat than it produces

CLINICAL MANIFESTATIONS

Shivering
Sleepiness
Apathy
Listlessness
Unconsciousness
Decreased respiratory rate
Decreased pulse rate
Decreased temperature

MANAGEMENT

Get the client out of cold environment or wet clothing.
Apply warming materials such as blankets, heating pads, or hot water bottles. If far from hospital, immerse client in tub of warm water at 40.5° C (105° F).
Monitor vital signs.
Maintain airway and administer heated oxygen. Assist with ventilations if client is not breathing at an adequate respiratory rate.
Start IV line with warm 5% dextrose in Ringer's lactate solution and be prepared to give emergency drugs.
Do not rub body parts vigorously if frostbite is suspected.
Monitor cardiac rhythm.

client. Rectal or tympanic temperatures, heart rate, respiratory rate, ECG findings, blood pressure, and urinary output via urinary catheter must be monitored frequently. Serum glucose must be monitored hourly until the client is stable. Drug therapy may consist of administration of sodium bicarbonate and dextrose according to laboratory results until rewarming is complete. (An IV should be started with a large-bore needle.) Rapid core rewarming is accomplished by means of one or all of the following: (1) hot drinks, (2) IV warm fluids, (3) circulating water bath at 40° C, (4) 100% warm, humidified oxygen by bag or mask, (5) peritoneal lavage with heated normal saline solution (42° C [107.6° F]), (6) mediastinal lavage with heated saline solution, and (7) gastric lavage with heated saline solution. Internal (core) rewarming is a quicker method that is used to treat severely hypothermic clients.[6] Rewarming should not be too rapid. The client needs to be continuously monitored, and advanced life support should be available if the need arises.

After the emergency, the nurse should teach the client how to avoid future problems. People should not travel to high elevations or venture out into cold temperatures unless they are prepared with extra clothing that is warm and dry, high-sugar foods for extra calories, and a plan for survival if an accident occurs.

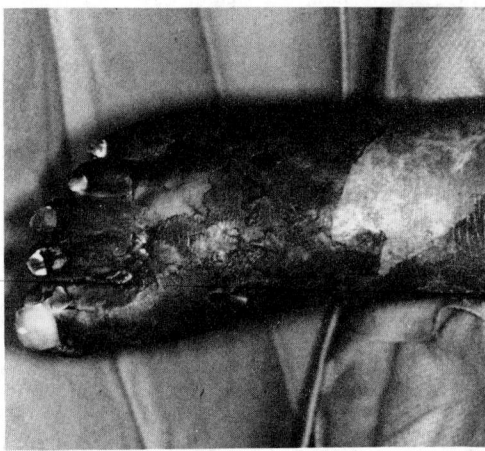

Fig. 59-3 Third-degree frostbite of the foot. Because nutrient vessels to the toes are protected by little subcutaneous tissue, these digits became ischemic and eventually required amputation. (From Moore EE and others: Early care of the injured patient, ed 4, Philadelphia, 1990, BC Decker, p 309).

Table 59-6 Signs and Symptoms of Frostbite

MILD INJURY	DEEP INJURY
Bright red and warm	Deep purple and cool
Pain	Minimal pain
Paresthesias	Small hemorrhagic vesicles
Rapid onset of edema	Slow onset of edema
Large vesicles (early)	Demarcation and mummification of deep structures
Superficial eschar (later)	

Modified from Moore EE and others: Early care of the injured patient, ed 4, Philadelphia, 1990, BC Decker, p 309.

Frostbite. Frostbite occurs in the same situations that produce hypothermia. When a portion of the body is exposed to freezing temperatures for a prolonged period, frostbite may occur (Fig. 59-3). Ears, nose, fingers, and toes are the most susceptible. The manifestations of frostbite range from numbness and tingling to evidence of necrosis (Table 59-6). Necrosis is related to the mechanical effects of ice crystals, loss of cellular water, and microvascular thrombosis.

Emergency management requires moderately rapid rewarming of the affected part, such as by submersion of the extremity in a water bath at approximately 43° C (110° F). Massage should never be used because it may increase tissue damage. All clothes and jewelry that constrict the frozen extremity should be removed. Any blisters should be left intact. The client should not be allowed to smoke cigarettes because of their vasoconstricting effect. Gentle exercise to increase blood flow should be encouraged. Efforts need to be made to promote normal blood circulation until definitive care can begin. Once the frostbitten limb has been rewarmed, treatment is conservative and usually

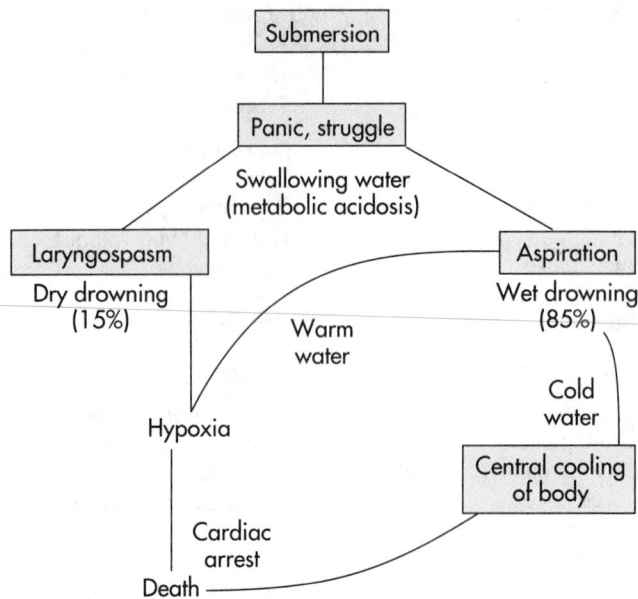

Fig. 59-4 Progression of a drowning incident. (From Auerback P and Geehr E: Management of wilderness and environmental emergencies, ed 2, St Louis, 1989, The CV Mosby Co, p 915.)

consists of bed rest, elevation of the injured part, tetanus toxoid administration, and use of antibiotics if infection is suspected. If a person with frostbite is left untreated or if treatment is not successful, frostbite may result in amputation of the affected part.

Drowning and near drowning. Drowning accounts for approximately 8000 deaths each year in the United States, and this number is rising because of the increased population, increasing use of swimming pools, and substance abuse. It is the fourth most common cause of accidental death among males 1 to 34 years of age and females 9 to 15 years of age. Children under 4 years of age account for 40% of all drownings.[7]

Drowning is defined as death from suffocation after submersion in water or other fluid media. *Near drowning* implies that the victim did not die but survived for at least 24 hours after suffocation by submersion in water. *Immersion syndrome* is sudden death that occurs as a result of sudden immersion in cold water. Sudden death is triggered by vagally induced dysrhythmias. Drowning typically begins with an attempt to hold the breath. As carbon monoxide builds up, hypoxia progresses and is followed by profound air hunger and panic (Fig. 59-4). Gasping inspirations cause either aspiration of fluid (wet drowning) or laryngospasm (dry drowning).

Acute asphyxia is present in most near-drowning victims, regardless of whether they have aspirated water. Laryngeal spasm may prevent aspiration. Victims who do not aspirate water have a better prognosis because fluid and acid-base imbalances are less severe. (Clinical manifestations of near drowning are presented in Table 59-7.)

Near-drowning victims have recovered with no long-term effects after having been submerged in cold water for

Table 59-7 Clinical Manifestations
of Near Drowning

PULMONARY	CARDIOVASCULAR
Hypoxia	Dysrhythmias
Lung injury, resulting in decreased surfactant	Cardiogenic shock
	Hypovolemia (salt water)
Fluid in alveoli	Transient hypervolemia (fresh water)
Atelectasis	
Pneumonia	Decreased hematocrit (fresh water)
Pulmonary edema	
NEUROLOGICAL	**METABOLIC**
Lethargy	Acidosis (respiratory and/or metabolic)
Drowsiness	
Decreased level of consciousness	Hyperkalemia
	Hypernatremia (salt water)
Seizures	
Coma	

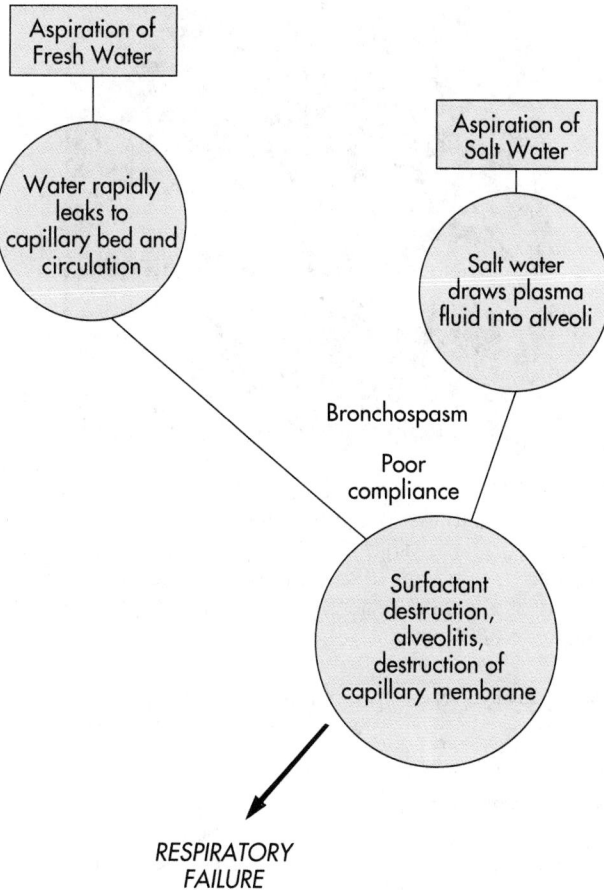

Fig. 59-5 Pulmonary effects of water aspiration. (From Auerback P and Geehr E: Management of wilderness and environmental emergencies, ed 2, St Louis, 1989, The CV Mosby Co, p 915.)

up to 40 minutes.[8] Aggressive resuscitation efforts and the mammalian diving reflex apparently combine to improve survival possibilities for these victims. Cold water lowers the body's demand for oxygen. The mammalian diving reflex induces apnea, bradycardia, and significant peripheral vasoconstriction. Blood flow is redistributed to the heart, lungs, and brain—the organs with the highest tissue oxygen requirements. The diving reflex is primarily seen in children.

Although the amount of water aspirated may be small, the osmotic gradient of the fluid causes fluid imbalances in the body. Because fresh water is hypotonic, it is rapidly absorbed into the circulatory system. Salt water is hypertonic and draws fluid from the circulation into interstitial tissue and the alveoli. Additional fluid is frequently swallowed by the near-drowning victim. Large amounts of fresh water are rapidly absorbed via the gastrointestinal (GI) system, causing hypervolemia. However, the most important life-threatening consequence of near drowning is hypoxia. Respiratory failure commonly follows submersion incidents and is a result of fluid-filled and poorly ventilated alveoli (Fig. 59-5).

The body attempts to compensate for the hypoxic state by shunting more of its blood to the lungs. This can result in pulmonary edema because of the increased pulmonary pressures and shunted volume. Hypoxemia worsens as blood continues to be shunted through alveoli that are not oxygenated. Metabolic acidosis results from anaerobic metabolism. Compensatory mechanisms attempt to preserve organ and tissue integrity. In immersion hypothermia, the CNS slows the metabolic rate and thereby decreases the hypoxic effects. If prolonged, this response can lead to cardiac irregularities and potentially life-threatening dysrhythmias.

Prehospital care of the drowning victim is presented in Table 59-8. Initial evaluation of the victim at the scene involves assessment of airway, cervical spine, breathing,

and circulation. At the scene of the near drowning, no attempt should be made to drain fluid from the victim's lungs because it is fruitless, can result in time delay, and is potentially life threatening to the victim.

Because near-drowning victims have a good chance of surviving, therapy is vigorous and is directed at correcting hypoxia, acid-base imbalances, and fluid imbalances; supporting basic physiological functions; and moderate rewarming (if severe hypothermia is present). An IV (lactated Ringer's or normal saline solution) should be started for the delivery of emergency medications, and all clients should be carefully monitored by ECG to detect any life-threatening dysrhythmias. If the client was submerged in cold water, special note of the core body temperature is imperative, and attempts to rewarm the client should be made.

Emesis is a constant threat because the client may have swallowed large amounts of water. Special care should be taken to prevent aspiration by suctioning the oral pharynx if the client starts to vomit. If the client is unresponsive, a nasogastric tube should be inserted to decompress the stomach to remove swallowed air and prevent the aspiration of vomitus and debris. Special care should be applied to the client's cervical spine. All near-drowning victims

Table 59-8

Prehospital Emergency Care of the Near-Drowning Client

Etiology: Exhaustion while swimming, loss of control or support, entrapment or entanglement by objects in water

CLINICAL MANIFESTATIONS

Panic
Inefficient breathing
Decreased buoyancy
Exhaustion
Loss of consciousness
Cardiac arrest

MANAGEMENT

Do not remove victim from water. Keep victim floating supine until a backboard or other rigid support is available.
Clear airway of water, debris, and vomitus.
Keep head and neck supported (e.g., with backboard).
Begin rescue breathing as soon as possible. Do not wait until client is out of the water to resuscitate.
Assess for possible cervical neck injury.
Treat for hypothermia.
Administer oxygen by mask (8-10 L/min).
Intubate if client is tachypneic or dyspneic with cyanosis.
Be prepared to suction oral pharynx.

---

carry a high risk of cervical spine injury. High-flow oxygen (100%), warmed and humidified, is initiated for all clients through either mask, ambu bag, or endotracheal tube. ABGs are used to determine the degree of hypoxia, and chest x-ray studies are used to determine the pulmonary status.

If pulmonary edema is present or if alveoli are collapsing, mechanical ventilation with positive end-expiratory pressure or continuous positive airway pressure may be used to improve gas exchange across the alveolar-capillary membrane (see Chapter 23). Ventilation and oxygenation are the primary means of treating acidosis. Mannitol or furosemide (Lasix) may be given to decrease the amount of free water and to treat cerebral edema.

The level of consciousness is carefully monitored by the use of a neurological check sheet and the Glasgow Coma Scale (see Table 52-2). Deterioration in neurological status may indicate cerebral edema, increased hypoxia, or profound acidosis. Near-drowning victims may also have head injuries that may cause prolonged alterations in the level of consciousness when other monitored parameters are returning to normal.

All victims of near drowning (no matter how mild the episode appears) should be brought to the hospital for at least 4 to 6 hours of observation. Delayed pulmonary edema, pneumonia, and cerebral edema are not uncommon complications.[9] Clients may be allowed to go home after this time if they are completely free of symptoms and if adequate medical follow-up can be guaranteed.

Poisonings

A poison is any chemical that harms the body. In the United States there are more than 1 million cases of poisoning annually. Poisonings may be accidental or purposeful, as in the case of suicide attempts. The nurse must be nonjudgmental during the initial interview with the client; the accuracy of the history may depend on the nurse's ability to remain neutral. This is especially true when interviewing persons who have attempted suicide or parents who have carelessly left poisonous agents easily available to children. Many poison histories are not accurate. The history should include the type of poisoning present, the amount of toxin exposure, the length of time since the exposure occurred, symptoms that have appeared since the poisoning, and health history (including allergies and present medications being taken by the client). If contact is made with clients before their arrival in the ER, they should be instructed to bring the poison container to the hospital.

Poisonings may be of the surface or topical type or may involve inhalation, ingestion, or injection. Once in the body, poisons can result in damage in several ways. The actual effect and extent of damage caused by a poison depend on the nature of the poison, its concentration, and sometimes the way in which it enters the body. Common poison substances are presented in Table 59-9.

Surface toxins. Surface or topical poisons may damage the skin. Most are corrosives or irritants that are slowly absorbed into body tissues and the bloodstream. Included in this group are many of the insecticides and agricultural chemicals in common use. Initially, the corrosive chemicals may damage only the skin. Then they continue to damage tissues and are absorbed by the body, causing widespread damage. Surface toxins must be washed from the client with copious amounts of water as soon as possible. Special attention must be given to those body areas that serve as pockets collecting the toxin, such as the ears and the navel. All contaminated clothes should be removed, and the affected areas should be washed again.

Inhaled toxins. Inhaled poisons take the form of gases, vapors, and sprays. Many of these substances are in common use in homes, industry, and agriculture. These poisons include carbon monoxide (from car exhaust, wood burning stoves, and furnaces), ammonia, chlorine, gases produced from volatile liquid chemicals (including many industrial solvents), and insect sprays. Inhaled toxins are difficult to treat and may result in hoarseness, chemical pneumonitis, and pulmonary edema. Appropriate treatment includes removing victims from the toxin source, keeping them quiet, administering oxygen, and observing for respiratory distress.

Ingested toxins. Ingested toxins are common and may range from an overdose of medication to food poisoning. Some toxins require immediate induction of vomiting; others contraindicate this action. The local poison control center should be called if one is available. In general, induction of vomiting is contraindicated in the following circumstances: (1) ingestion of strong bases or acids (e.g., drain cleaners, ammonia, toilet bowl cleaners) or low-viscosity petroleum products (e.g., kerosene, gasoline) be-

Table 59-9 Common Poison Substances

Poison	Manifestations	Treatment
Acetaminophen (Tylenol)	Nausea and vomiting, anorexia, malaise, diaphoresis, liver abnormalities	Activated charcoal, *N*-acetylcysteine
Acids and alkalis *Acids:* toilet bowl cleaners, antirust compounds; *alkalis:* drain cleaners, dishwashing detergents, ammonia	Excess salivation, dysphagia, epigastric pain, pneumonitis, burns of mouth, esophagus, and stomach	Immediate dilution (water, milk), glucocorticords (for alkali burns), contraindication for gastric emptying
Alcohol*		
Aspirin and aspirin-containing medications	Increased respiratory rate, respiratory alkalosis, headache, vertigo, tinnitus, sweating, nausea, electrolyte imbalances	Gastric emptying, activated charcoal, alkaline diuresis, supportive care
Bleaches	Irritation of lips, mouth, and eyes, superficial injury to esophagus; chemical pneumonia and pulmonary edema	Washing of exposed skin and eyes, dilution with water and milk, gastric lavage, prevention of vomiting and aspiration
Carbon monoxide	Dyspnea, headache, tachypnea, confusion, impaired judgment, cyanosis, respiratory depression	Removal from source, administration of 100% oxygen
Cyanide	Headache, faintness, vertigo, tachycardia, hypertension, nausea and vomiting, almond odor to breath	Amyl nitrate, sodium nitrate, sodium thiosulfate, oxygen
Ethylene glycol	Sweet aromatic odor to breath, nausea and vomiting, slurred speech, ataxia, lethargy, respiratory depression	Gastric lavage, activated charcoal, supportive care
Iron	Vomiting (often bloody), diarrhea (often bloody), fever, hyperglycemia, lethargy, hypotension, seizures, coma	Ipecac-induced vomiting, gastric lavage, chelation therapy (deferoxamine)
Nonsteroidal antiinflammatory drugs	Gastroenteritis, abdominal pain, drowsiness, nystagmus, hepatic damage	Induced emesis, activated charcoal, cathartics
Tricyclic antidepressants (e.g., amitriptyline, imipramine)	In low doses: anticholinergic effects, agitation, hypertension, tachycardia; in high doses: CNS depression, respiratory depression, seizures, hypotension	Activated charcoal, gastric lavage, supportive care, contraindication for induced emesis
Alcohol, barbiturates, benzodiazepines, cocaine, hallucinogens, stimulants*		

*See Chapter 60.

cause vomiting can cause aspiration and severe damage to the esophagus, (2) absence of gag reflex, (3) unconsciousness, and (4) seizures. If none of these conditions exists, vomiting should be induced even if the ingestion occurred several hours earlier. Vomiting can be induced by giving the adult victim 30 ml syrup of ipecac by mouth, followed by 600 to 900 ml of oral fluid. The dose may be repeated once if necessary. All gastric contents should be saved for laboratory analysis. Another method of removing the toxin is insertion of a large nasogastric or orogastric tube into the client's stomach and lavage with at least 3 L saline solution.

Treatment of the poison victim is directed toward removing the toxin from the body, supporting the body systems until the crisis is past, and administering an antidote if the poison is known and if a specific antidote to it exists. Frequently the specific poison that caused the crisis is not known. Supportive care must be given regardless of whether an antidote is available. The so-called universal antidote (a mixture of burnt toast, magnesium oxide, and tannic acid) has no place in emergency poison management; it is a waste of precious time to give this worthless mixture. If the client has ingested strong bases or acids or petroleum products, one or two glasses of milk or water can be drunk unless directed otherwise. Dilution is contraindicated when the client has ingested medicinal substances because water can actually speed absorption. Table 59-10 describes selected common poisons with their specific antidotes.

Because many ingested poisons can be absorbed in the lower GI tract, an alert client may become comatose and critically ill at a later time. Cathartics and activated charcoal are used to decrease the possibility of GI absorption. Activated charcoal is given orally or through a large naso-

Table 59-10 Antidotes for Common Poisons

Poison	Antidote
Carbon monoxide	Oxygen
Cyanide	Cyanide kit, including amyl nitrite, sodium nitrite, sodium thiosulfate
Organophosphate insecticides (e.g., parathion, malathion)	Atropine, 2-PAM (pralidoxime), physostigmine
Diphenhydramine (Benadryl), atropine, potato leaves, tricyclic antidepressants	Diazepam (Valium) and phenytoin (Dilantin) as adjunct treatment
Phenothiazines, haloperidol	Diphenhydramine (Benadryl)
Narcotic ingestion	Naloxone (Narcan)
Methanol, ethylene glycol (antifreeze)	Ethanol
Acetaminophen	*N*-Acetylcysteine
Heavy metals	Penicillamine, disodium edetate

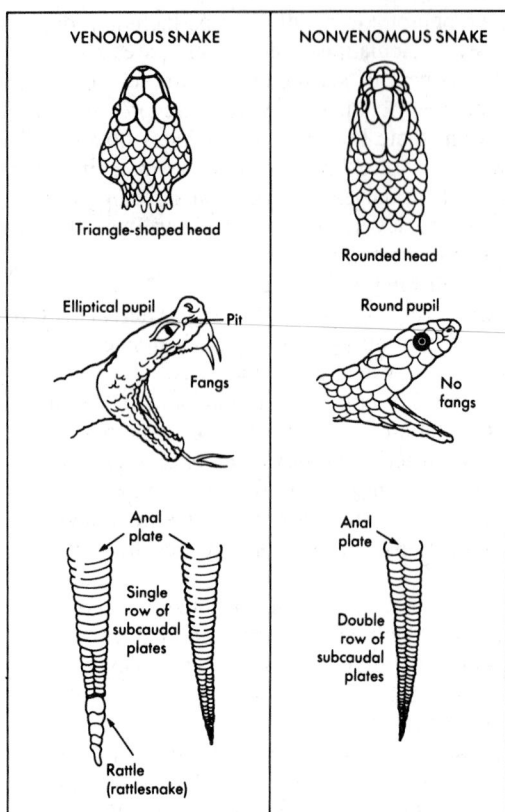

Fig. 59-6 Venomous and nonvenomous snakes. (From Rosen P and others: Emergency medicine, vol 1, ed 2, St Louis, 1988, The CV Mosby Co.)

gastric or orogastric tube and then removed from the gastric tract by vomiting or aspiration of stomach contents via the tube. It has no known contraindications and can absorb a number of poisons from the GI tract.

Activated charcoal does not absorb ethanol, alkali, iron, boric acid, methanol, or cyanide. Cathartics are used to decrease toxicity by moving poisons through the GI system rapidly, thereby reducing absorption. Magnesium-containing cathartics are contraindicated in pesticide poisonings.

Food poisoning is also a type of poison ingestion (see Chapter 34). Frequently a large number of people become ill after the ingestion of the same contaminated food. This can help speed identification of the toxic agent. Food poisoning may be caused by chemicals in the food or by bacterial toxins. Chemical food poisons include antimony (from gray-enameled utensils), cadmium (caused by acid liquids in cadmium-plated containers), sodium cyanide (cockroach poison), and zinc (caused by cooking or storing acid foods in galvanized iron containers). These poisons cause GI symptoms that develop within a few minutes to 2 hours. Bacterial sources of food poisoning include *Clostridium botulinum* (found in improperly canned vegetables and preserved meat and fish), salmonellae (found in food contaminated by rat feces, the housefly, and human carriers), and staphylococci (found in contaminated milk, mayonnaise, and cream).

Treatment of food poisoning is supportive and directed toward relief of symptoms. Botulism is the most severe form and causes respiratory paralysis and death if untreated (see Chapter 55). Salmonellae and staphylococci poisoning cause severe GI distress (nausea, vomiting, and diarrhea).

Injected toxins

Insect bites. Insect bites, especially from bees, yellow jackets, hornets, and wasps, can cause an anaphylactic re-

action in a hypersensitive person (see Chapter 8). The stinger of the insect is often left in the skin after the bite and continues to release venom. The stinger should be removed by a scraping motion with a fingernail, knife, or needle; tweezers may cause more venom to be released by squeezing the stinger.

Local treatment of bites consists of applications of cool compresses or solutions and antipruritic lotions or oral antihistamines. Persons known to be allergic to insects should carry emergency insect-bite kits that contain epinephrine.

Snakebite. Poisonous snakes in the United States include rattlesnakes, copperheads, moccasins (pit vipers), and coral snakes (Fig. 59-6). It is important for the nurse to become familiar with the types and identifying characteristics of poisonous snakes in the region of the country in which the emergency facility is located.

Various toxic properties of venom determine the degree of pathology. Local reactions to snakebite are intense, burning pain and rapidly developing edema, sometimes accompanied by bleeding. Sloughing of the tissue may also occur around the area of the bite. Generalized toxic reactions from snake venom include nausea and vomiting, dizziness, tachycardia, muscle fasciculations, GI bleeding, and respiratory problems. Envenomation by a coral snake

may have neurotoxic manifestations including drowsiness, weakness, fasciculations, and muscle paresis.

The treatment of snakebite is controversial. Some general principles of emergency care are presented in Table 59-11. Immediate hospital care includes obtaining laboratory studies for blood typing and cross-matching, complete blood count, urinalysis, coagulation screening tests, BUN, blood glucose level, and serum electrolytes. Other measures include the following:

1. Establishing an IV line
2. Measuring and recording circumference of the injured extremity every 30 to 60 minutes
3. Testing for antivenin sensitivity
4. Administering tetanus prophylaxis if the client's immunization is not current (see Table 55-3)
5. Administering prophylactic antibiotics
6. Administering IV antivenin because it is the only specific treatment for snake venom poisoning
7. Maintaining respiration by mechanical or other means

Follow-up care of snakebite may require debridement or fasciotomy. Contracture formation and amputation are common events after snakebite. Very young and very old persons are most vulnerable.

Spider bites

BLACK WIDOW SPIDER. Venomous spider bites occur most commonly by the black widow spider or the brown recluse spider. The black widow spider bite may be accompanied by a momentary sharp pain. The pain is often not felt until 15 minutes to 1 hour after the bite when the client complains of a dull, crampy pain in the bite area. This pain eventually spreads throughout the body. The abdomen becomes boardlike, and the waves of pain become excruciating, causing the client to turn, toss, and cry. The black widow spider injects a neurotoxin that produces diffuse central and peripheral nervous excitement, hyperactive reflexes, muscle spasms, hypertension, and vasoconstriction. Respirations are often labored. Nausea, vomiting, headache, diaphoresis, and paresthesias of the hands and feet may also be present. Because the bite itself is not prominent, victims are often thought to have an abdominal catastrophe such as perforated ulcer, appendicitis, or pancreatitis.

First aid involves cleansing the wound and administering tetanus toxoid; antivenin is used if the symptoms are severe. Calcium gluconate and muscle relaxants are used to treat muscle spasms. The symptoms run their course in several hours, although mild recurrences for 2 to 3 days are common. The client usually recovers in a week with no complications.

BROWN RECLUSE SPIDER. These spiders inject a venom that is known to cause skin necrosis and severe hemolysis. Local manifestations include burning, itching, pain, and bleb (blister) and erythema formation that can eventually develop into necrotic lesions. Systemic manifestations may include fever, myalgias, rash, hemolysis, shock, hemorrhage, and pulmonary edema. Hemolysis may lead to hemoglobinuria, renal failure, and death. This bite is especially dangerous to the young and to older adults.

Treatment depends on the severity of the bite. If the client is relatively free of symptoms, no treatment is necessary. If bleb or bullae formation, intense pain, and signs of rapidly progressive ischemia and necrosis are present, treatment is necessary. Treatment measures include cool or ice compresses, tetanus prophylaxis, elevation of the affected extremity, surgical debridement, and antibiotics for prevention of a secondary infection. Clients with systemic manifestations should be hospitalized and monitored for signs of hemolysis, disseminated intravascular coagulation, and acute renal failure. Systemic glucocorticoids are sometimes used during the acute phase of the resulting illness.

Human bites.

Human bites are associated with a high incidence of serious disabling complications. The main complication is infection that is due to the injection of oral bacterial flora, most commonly *Staphylococcus aureus* and streptococci. Infections occur in approximately 50% of all reported cases in which victims have not sought medical intervention within 24 hours of the injury.[10] If the human bite is deep, there can be significant damage to the tissue with hematoma formation and deep invasion of oral flora. When a human bite occurs, there is usually a retraction of skin with edema that causes a trapping of organisms of the oral flora and results in a serious infection. Treatment usually involves aggressive cleansing of the bite, debridement, prophylactic antibiotics, and tetanus prophylaxis. The wound should be left open to heal. Depending on the location of the human bite, x-ray examination may be indicated.

Table 59-11

Prehospital Emergency Care of a Client with a Snakebite

Etiology: Injection of toxin into blood stream

CLINICAL MANIFESTATIONS

Fang marks
Progressive swelling
Nausea and vomiting
Paresthesias
Burning pain
Ecchymoses

MANAGEMENT

Avoid panic and reassure the client.
Kill snake or remove client from area.
Immobilize affected part.
Reduce any physical activity.
Remove any rings, bracelets, or other constricting items on the bitten extremity.
Place a wide constricting band above or proximal to the bite, being sure not to restrict arterial blood flow.
Do not put the injured part in ice or use ice packs, since further tissue damage may occur.
Do not incise and suction the wound, since greater tissue damage may occur.
Attempt to identify the snake and bring it to ER.

Animal bites. Approximately 500,000 to 2 million animal bites are reported each year in the United States. Most of these bites are dog bites (80%) and cat bites (8% to 15%). Rodents, monkeys, and squirrels account for less than 10%.[10]

The most significant problems associated with animal bites are infection and the mechanical destruction of skin, muscle, tendons, blood vessels, and bone. The bite injury may be a simple laceration, a crush injury, a puncture wound, or a tearing or avulsion of the tissue. The potential complications from animal bites include serious infections; fractures; tendon, ligament, or nerve damage; and gross body-image changes.

The initial management of an animal bite is the same as that for any type of emergency—the maintenance of an adequate airway, especially if the bite is near or on the neck or face. Control of bleeding with maintenance of adequate circulation is the next step in the management of care. Careful inspection of the wound follows; special attention is given to tissue integrity and location of nerves, tendons, blood vessels, ligaments, joints, and organs that may be affected by the bite. The wound should be cleaned with saline-solution irrigations, antibiotics should be administered, and tetanus prophylaxis should be given. Wound exploration, removal of foreign matter, and debridement may be indicated.

One of the most important considerations in the treatment of animal bites is whether rabies prophylaxis is indicated. Although rabies rarely affects human beings in the United States, every year approximately 25,000 persons receive rabies prophylaxis.[3] Rabies is transmitted when the virus is introduced into open cuts or wounds. If rabies is known to be present or is suspected of being present, the animal should be captured. Any animal exhibiting abnormal behavior or suspected of being rabid should be killed, and the brain should be examined by fluorescent antibodies for rabies. Rabies prophylaxis may involve passive immunization with rabies immune globulin or active immunization with antirabies vaccine. Indications for rabies prophylaxis include (1) a bite from a wild animal, (2) an unprovoked attack by a dog that cannot be examined for rabies for 10 days, and (3) a bite from an animal observed to develop signs of rabies.

Nurse's role in education. The nurse must be aware of the responsibility of educating the public to the dangers of poisonous substances and insect or animal bites in the hope of preventing these types of emergencies. Initial treatment measures should be taught to the public, since early treatment can save lives. Parents should know the types of poisons they routinely keep in their homes and how to store them properly out of the reach of small children. All homes should have syrup of ipecac available to induce emesis without delay after acute poisoning has occurred. People who work around dangerous substances should be taught how to decontaminate one another if an accident occurs. People should be made aware of means to treat insect and animal bites until medical care can be obtained. Poison control centers are available in communities 24 hours a day to give poison information and treatment referral assistance to consumers and health care profes-

sionals. Everyone should have the telephone number of the local poison control center. These centers give poison treatment information over the telephone that is specifically focused on prehospital care.

Abdominal Injuries

Injuries to the abdominal area most often occur as a result of *blunt trauma* (e.g., motor vehicle accident) or *penetrating injuries,* which are primarily from gunshot wounds or stab wounds to the abdomen.[12] (Blunt trauma is most common.) Regardless of whether it is a blunt or penetrating injury, the result is often the same—damage to or alteration of the internal organs.

Common injuries of the abdomen include lacerated liver, ruptured spleen, pancreatic trauma, mesenteric artery tears, diaphragmatic rupture, urinary bladder rupture, great vessel tears, renal injury, and stomach or intestinal rupture. These injuries may result in massive blood loss and hypovolemic shock. Surgery must be performed as early as possible to repair the damaged organs and to stop the bleeding. Common sequelae to intraabdominal trauma are peritonitis and massive infection, particularly when the bowel is perforated.

Clinical manifestations of abdominal trauma are (1) guarding and splinting of the abdominal wall; (2) a hard, distended abdomen (indicating intraabdominal bleeding); (3) decreased or absent bowel sounds; (4) contusions, abrasions, or bruising over the abdomen; (5) abdominal pain; (6) pain over the scapula caused by irritation of the phrenic nerve by free blood in the abdomen; (7) hematemesis or hematuria; and (8) signs of hypovolemic shock. An ecchymotic discoloration around the umbilicus (Cullen's sign) can indicate intraabdominal or retroperitoneal hemorrhage.

Intraabdominal injuries are often associated with low rib fractures, fractured femur, fractured pelvis, and thoracic injury. If any of these injuries are present, the client should be observed for abdominal trauma.

Specific diagnostic procedures include a complete blood count, urinalysis, x-ray examination of the abdomen, computerized tomography (CT) scan, and peritoneal lavage. In the peritoneal lavage procedure the abdomen below the umbilicus is locally anesthetized, and a large angiocatheter or peritoneal dialysis catheter is inserted into the abdomen. A syringe is attached to the catheter, and an attempt is made to gently aspirate any blood. A liter of saline solution is then infused into the abdomen and drained. The fluid is observed for gross abnormalities, especially blood, and is sent to the laboratory for microscopic evaluation. Positive findings include any of the following: (1) red blood cell count greater than $100,000/\mu l$, (2) white blood cell count greater than $500/\mu l$; (3) high amylase level; and (4) presence of bacteria, bile, or fecal material. If the results are positive, immediate surgery is indicated. If the results are negative, continued observation of the client is warranted. An impaled object should never be removed until skilled care is available. Removal may cause further injury and bleeding.

Emergency care of the victim of intraabdominal trauma focuses on fluid replacement and prevention of hypovole-

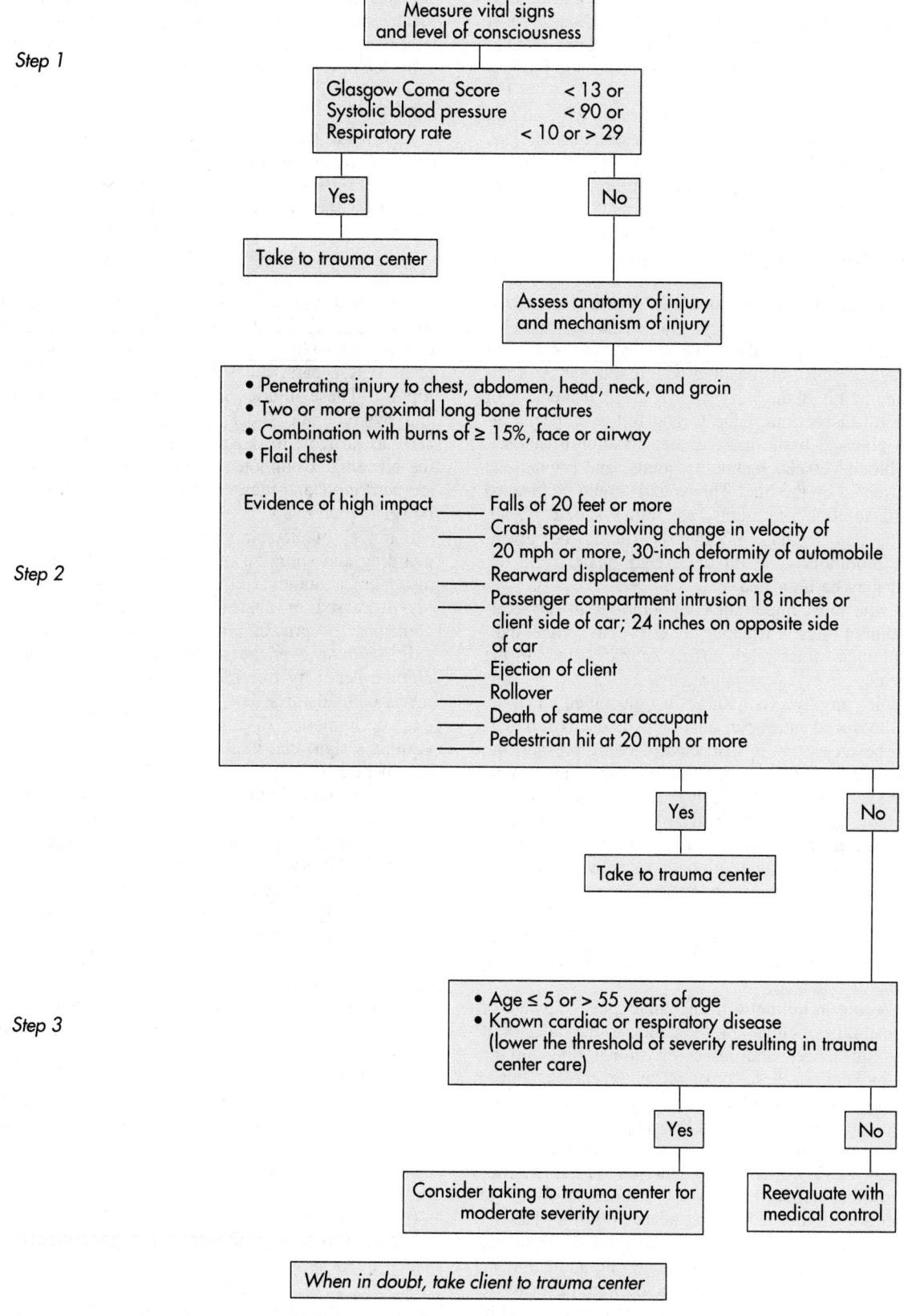

Fig. 59-7 Triage decision algorithm. The ACS Committee on Trauma criteria for direct transport of clients to a trauma center. (From American College of Surgeons, Hospital and prehospital resources for optimal care of the injured patient, Chicago, 1986, American College of Surgeons.)

mic shock (see Table 37-15). IV lines are started, and volume expanders or blood is given if the client is hypotensive. A nasogastric tube is inserted to decompress the stomach and prevent the aspiration of vomitus. No pain medication is given because analgesics can mask the progression of clinical manifestations.

Regardless of the mechanism of injury, physical evidence of abdominal trauma in a client who is hemodynamically unstable mandates immediate laparotomy. In other cases the indications for laparotomy must be correlated with the mechanism of injury. For example, if an individual has a gunshot wound or impaled object, surgery is usually indicated.

TRIAGE

Triage (sorting) is a method of managing emergency or disaster situations by sorting clients according to their need for treatment or transport so that the greatest number of lives are saved. Triage needs to be used whenever the needs for care exceed the resources available.[13] A triage system identifies and categorizes the victims so that the most critically injured (those with the most life-threatening injuries) are treated first. The process involves constant reassessment of the casualties as the situation changes (Fig. 59-7).

With triage principles, high priority is given to hemorrhage, respiratory insufficiency, and altered level of consciousness. Intermediate priority is given to closed fractures and minor burns. A low priority is given to ambulatory victims with minor tissue injuries or with dazed affect and no apparent physical injuries. (The case study offers a basis for applying the principles of triage and emergency management.)

DEATH IN THE EMERGENCY ROOM

Unfortunately, there are a number of emergency victims who do not benefit from all the skill, expertise, and technology available in the ER. People do die. It is important for emergency nurses to be able to deal with their own feelings about sudden death so that they can help families and loved ones begin the grieving process.

The emergency nurse should recognize the importance of certain hospital rituals in preparing the bereaved to grieve, such as collecting the belongings, arranging for an autopsy, viewing the body, and making mortuary arrangements. The death must seem real so that the loved ones can begin to grieve. This will assist the loved ones to accept the death. The emergency nurse cannot afford to forget the surviving loved ones after a death in the ER.

C *ase Study*

MULTIPLE-TRAUMA SITUATION

Vehicle 1 is traveling south at a speed of 40 mph. The driver does not yield for the red light and is hit by vehicle 2, which is traveling west at 45 mph. By the time the police arrive at the scene, a crowd has gathered with many angry motorists honking their horns because traffic is blocked in four directions.

There are four victims of the accident. Victim A is walking around aimlessly and appears dazed. He has a small hematoma above his right eye with no other apparent injuries. He denies loss of consciousness and is oriented.

Victim B is still in the car. She is conscious but pinned by the dashboard and door. She complains of pain in her left arm and leg with limited movement. She has an open wound on her left leg, and there is a noticeable amount of blood on the floor of the car.

Victim C is unconscious and sprawled over the hood of the car, having been thrown through the windshield. She has multiple lacerations over her face, a depression over the left frontal bone, and profuse bleeding from the mouth and nose. Her eyes are swollen shut. She is still breathing and has a palpable, weak pulse of 60.

Victim D is unconscious and has no apparent injuries. He is still sitting in the car with his seat belt strapped. However, he is not breathing, is cyanotic, and has a weak, thready pulse. The rescuers removed his lower denture plate but could not find his upper plate. They are unable to breathe into his lungs.

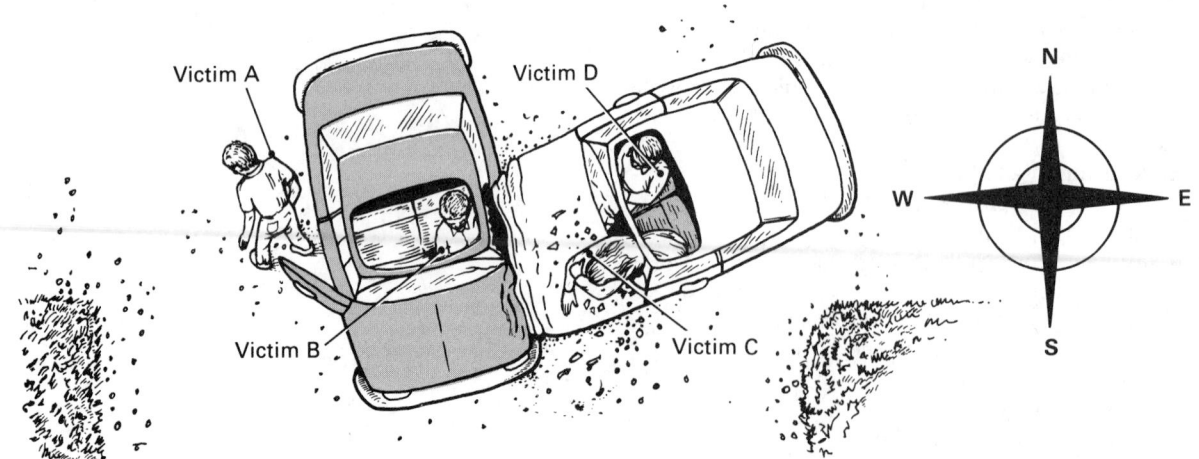

Multiple-trauma situation resulting from traffic accident.

Discussion Questions

1. What injuries may victims A and B have?
2. What precautions should be taken in removing victim B from the car?
3. What is the significance of victim C not wearing a seat belt?
4. What are possible causes of unconsciousness in victim C? What injuries may she have?
5. What probably caused the obstructed airway in victim D? What are the steps to clear an obstructed airway?
6. How are the principles of triage applied in this situation?

R eview Questions

The number of the question corresponds to the same-numbered objective at the beginning of the chapter.

1. A differentiating feature between medical and traumatic emergencies is that
   a. medical emergencies are not as life threatening as traumatic emergencies
   b. medical emergencies are situational and not physiological crises
   c. traumatic emergencies are caused by a direct impact to the body
   d. traumatic emergencies always require surgical intervention
2. Which of the following is *not* part of an EMS system?
   a. public information campaign
   b. transportation system
   c. disaster preparedness
   d. rehabilitative care facility
3. An important principle of history taking in emergency situations is to
   a. obtain history after giving emergency care
   b. record history before giving care
   c. verify history with family members or friends
   d. ask leading questions to facilitate the process
4. Which of the following should be done before making an assessment of an emergency victim?
   a. make sure client is breathing
   b. obtain verbal permission to give care
   c. obtain written permission to give care
   d. leave emergency scene to summon help
5. A person who has overdosed on aspirin is brought unconscious to the emergency room. Initial treatment is to
   a. wait for an antidote
   b. give the universal antidote
   c. give syrup of ipecac
   d. aspirate stomach with large nasogastric or orogastric tube
6. The primary purpose of peritoneal lavage is to
   a. dialyze toxic substances out of the body
   b. remove ascitic fluid
   c. remove foreign particles
   d. assess for internal bleeding

REFERENCES

1. Hafen B and Karren K: Prehospital emergency care and crisis intervention, ed 3, Austin, TX, 1989, Morton Publishers.
2. Sheehy SB and others: Manual of clinical trauma care, St Louis, 1989, The CV Mosby Co.
3. Moore EE and others: Early care of the injured patient, ed 4, Philadelphia, 1990, BC Decker.
4. Beaver BM: Care of the multiple trauma victim: the first hour, Nurs Clin North Am 25:11-21, 1990.
5. Yarbrough B and Hubbard R: Heat related illness. In Auerbach P and Geehr E: Management of wilderness and environmental emergencies, ed 2, St Louis, 1989, The CV Mosby Co, pp 119-138.
6. Danzl D and others: Accidental hypothermia. In Auerbach P and Geehr E: Management of wilderness and environmental emergencies, ed 2, St Louis, 1989, The CV Mosby Co, pp 35-65.
7. Stewart R: Submersion incidents. In Auerbach P and Geehr E: Management of wilderness and environmental emergencies, ed 2, St Louis, 1989, The CV Mosby Co, pp 907-932.
8. Siebake H and others: Survival after 40 minutes submersion without cerebral sequelae, Lancet 1:1275-1277, 1975.
9. Lee G: Flight nursing: principles and practice, St Louis, 1991, Mosby–Year Book, Inc, pp 469-488.
10. Callaham M: Wild and domestic animal attack. In Auerbach P and Geehr E: Management of wilderness and environmental emergencies, ed 2, St Louis, 1989, The CV Mosby Co, pp 684-721.
11. Sullivan J and Wingert W: Reptile bites. In Auerbach P and Geehr E: Management of wilderness and environmental emergencies, ed 2, St Louis, 1989, The CV Mosby Co, pp 480-510.
12. Grant HD and others: Brady emergency care, Englewood Cliffs, NJ, 1990, Brady.
13. Sullivan R: Triage: a subspecialty of emergency nursing, Emphasis Nurs 3:26-33, 1989.

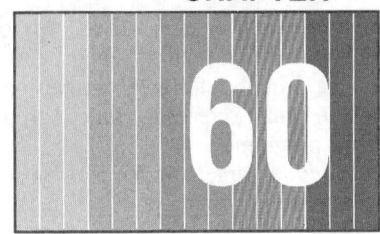

CHAPTER 60

Nursing Role in Management
Drug Abuse and Dependence

Patsy L. Orth Duphorne

Alcohol and drug abuse have become a major threat to the health and welfare of populations throughout the world. Patterns of drug abuse are so pervasive in society today that they have led to a declaration of "war on drugs."

The consequences of alcohol and drug abuse place a heavy burden on the resources in society. Individuals who

Reviewed by Patricia Long, R.N., Ed.D., C.S., C.A.R.N., Associate Professor, Chairperson, Department of Family and Community Health Nursing, School of Nursing, State University of New York at Stony Brook, New York; Psychotherapist in Private Practice.

abuse drugs, including alcohol, place a heavy demand on the health care system because they typically use many more health care resources than other clients.[1] Approximately 25% of hospitalized clients have alcohol-related problems.[2] Emergency department visits for cocaine overdose have increased 200% within the past decade.[3] Nurses are in critical positions to recognize signs and symptoms of drug abuse and dependence and to initiate appropriate case management.

This chapter addresses a number of patterns of alcohol and drug abuse and the nurse's role in health promotion and management of client care. It focuses on the nature of

addiction, the recognition of the signs and symptoms of drug abuse and dependence, and the treatment of health-related problems. Current issues of drug abuse among high-risk populations and problems of codependency and chemical dependence in nurses are also presented.

PREVENTION AND HEALTH PROMOTION

The beginning of the 1990s has revealed a major shift related to drug abuse from an emphasis on treatment to a broader health care perspective that incorporates prevention activities. Prevention efforts include a public health approach that focuses on the interactions of the host, agent (drug), and environment. Strategies are aimed at change of the environment as well as individual behavior.

The focus of *primary prevention* is health promotion. It targets nondrug users or individuals with minimal drug exposure. Prevention at this level involves collective or group participation and action to influence social policy and develop social responsibility. The nurse's role is to serve as educator, resource, role model, and agent of change. Examples of primary prevention include measures to change the environment such as legislation on the minimum drinking age, laws concerning drinking and driving, and measures to change individual behaviors such as the training of peer educators in schools, mass media campaigns, and community-based programs.

Secondary prevention targets individuals who are "at risk" for the development of a problem because of family drug history, occupation, ethnic or racial background, or lifestyle. The focus of secondary prevention is health supervision and protection that involves early identification and treatment of individuals who use drugs occasionally or frequently and who show signs of abuse. Special high-risk populations have been targeted and include Native Americans, Hispanic males, Alaskan natives, and blacks. Children of alcoholics are also considered high risk, as are many health professionals such as nurses, physicians, pharmacists, and dentists. The nurse's role is to facilitate

the development of drug-free alternatives, to provide early detection through screening, and to support early intervention and treatment through referral. Examples of secondary prevention include health screening clinics and peer or employee assistance programs.

Tertiary prevention targets individuals who have already been identified as having a problem and usually have the diagnosis of *substance abuse dependent* or *substance dependent*. They may be involved with the health care system in an acute stage, a chronic stage, or a recovery stage of the illness. The focus of tertiary prevention is to control and monitor the illness. The nurse's role is to provide direct client care, to promote interdisciplinary collaboration, and to work with community health systems. Examples of tertiary prevention include symptom management, health education, support groups (e.g., Alcoholics Anonymous, Alanon, Narcotics Anonymous), and relapse prevention plans.

Relapse prevention is a behavioral approach that identifies environmental cues that trigger relapse. It assists the recovering individual in the development of coping strategies and increased self-efficacy or personal confidence for managing high-risk situations. Although it has been used primarily in work with alcoholics, it may be useful in the prevention of other relapse situations.

Patterns of drug use may be viewed within a prevention framework (Fig. 60-1). As patterns of dependence become firmly established, individuals have less chance for reversing these patterns without treatment and rehabilitation. Nurses need to use this information to assess clients' patterns of drug use to incorporate appropriate prevention strategies into case management. Health promotion strategies are listed in Table 60-1.

MODELS OF ADDICTION

Models are useful in directing treatment and planning prevention, education, and research activities. Theories and research related to alcohol use are responsible for the

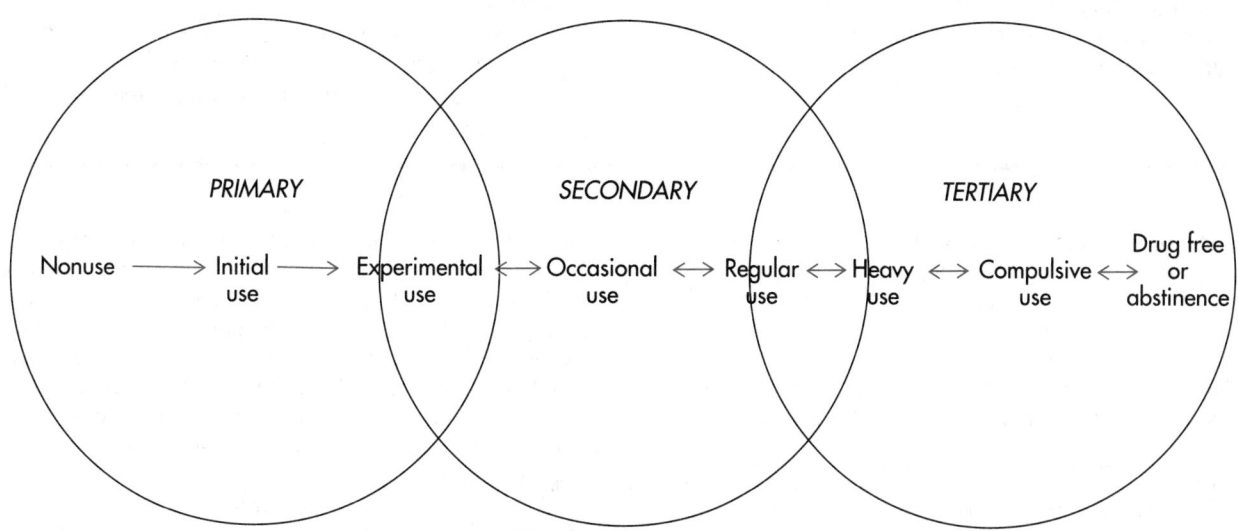

Fig. 60-1 Drug use patterns and prevention framework.

development of most of the models that have been applied to drug addiction in general. The *disease model* or *medical model* legitimized alcohol addiction as an illness and removed the element of blame from the addict. The *biopsychosocial model* integrates current research findings and promotes a holistic approach. The *public health model* expands the focus of concern to the community and implies a multifaceted approach to the problem. Specific information on these and other models of addiction is presented in Table 60-2.

Terminology

Terminology used to describe components of addiction is confusing due to conflicting philosophies, different application of terms, and terms that are emotionally charged. Commonly accepted definitions are listed in Table 60-3. *Abuse* refers to a deviation from a norm and varies according to each society. *Psychological dependence* occurs with all abused drugs and serves as a primary reinforcer for

Table 60-1   Health Promotion Strategies Related to Drug Addiction

Recognition of nurse's attitudes, beliefs, and values related to addiction
Assessment of nurse's patterns of drug use
Education of public and nurses about addiction
Identification of individuals at risk
Identification of early signs and symptoms of addiction
Activities to effect social change
Use of knowledge about drug use and abuse in health education of clients
Use of knowledge of compulsive and dependent behavior in teaching health maintenance

Modified from American Nurses' Association, Drug and Alcohol Nursing Association, and National Nurses Society on Addiction: The care of clients with addictions, Kansas City, Mo, 1987, American Nurses' Association.

Table 60-2   Models of Addiction

Premise	Causal Factors	Treatment Focus	Nursing Implications
MORAL			
Abuse is sin and/or crime.	Weak will	None	Assess stigma of "addict" label.
	Lack of control	Legal (jail)	Educate about addiction process.
	Immorality	Morals	Reinforce responsibility without attaching blame.
	Individual blame	Social sanctions (e.g., "Just Say No")	Support peer resistance skills and abstinence.
MEDICAL AND DISEASE			
Alcoholism is a chronic, progressive disease.	Biochemical differences (opiate receptor sites, metabolic abnormalities, endorphins), genetic transmission (e.g., alcoholism)	Physical symptoms Related illnesses Control of progression Intervention for drug treatment, rehabilitation—abstinence, relapse	Identify signs and symptoms. Recognize related illnesses. Educate about stages, including relapse. Refer for treatment and support groups.
PSYCHODYNAMIC			
Addiction is related to unmet intrapersonal or interpersonal needs or emotional and mental problems.	Personality traits, "addictive personality," defense mechanisms, personality disorder, neurosis, depression, anxiety Family dysfunction	Psychotherapy Group therapy Family therapy	Assist in increasing self-esteem, communication skills, and coping and social skills. Assess emotional problems. Refer for treatment.
BIOPSYCHOSOCIAL			
Addiction is a multidimensional problem, not the result of a single factor.	Biological Psychological Social	Comprehensive—basis on role of family, culture, society in problem and solution	Assess all dimensions. Include family. Help to build social support network. Assist to increase functioning in all areas. Promote healthy lifestyle.

Continued.

Table 60-2 Models of Addiction—cont'd

Premise	Causal Factors	Treatment Focus	Nursing Implications
SOCIAL LEARNING			
Addiction is a maladaptive habit or learned behavior.	Skill deficits Expectancies (relief of tension) Poor modeling	Cognitive therapy, behavioral therapy, skill training, self-control training	Teach coping and assertiveness skills. Identify antecedents ("triggers"). Link triggers with consequences. Encourage self-responsibility. Provide positive reinforcement of healthy coping. Guide relapse prevention.
SOCIOCULTURAL			
Addiction reflects conflicts and issues in society.	Role strain Family problems Socioeconomic conditions Rituals, practices, taboos Unclear cultural norms Changing cultures Mixed social messages	Traditions, values, beliefs; peer pressure; role/job satisfaction; separation from family	Support traditions. Clarify norms. Increase awareness of mixed messages. Assist in increasing problem-solving skills. Address codependency issues. Empower to make healthy choices.
PUBLIC HEALTH			
Addiction is based on interactions of host, agent, and environment.	Host: high risk, poor self-control and coping skills Agent: type of drug, frequency of use, route of administration, availability Environment: family, friends, community resources, media	Multifaceted (medical, emotional, and social problems), risk appraisal, genetic counseling, self-control training, social action	Assess risk factors. Provide information and assist with skills. Empower for social responsibility.

Table 60-3 Definitions Related to Addictive Behavior

Addiction: Pattern of loss of control of use or compulsive use followed by continued use in spite of adverse consequences

Loss of control: Inability to stop drug or alcohol use after initial dose

Abuse: Pattern of abnormal or pathological use resulting in physical, emotional, or social impairment

Tolerance: Need to continually increase the amount of drug to obtain the desired effect or to maintain a certain drug dose to function

Withdrawal: Predictable progression of symptoms or "rebound" action in response to decreased drug dose

Dependence: Process of psychological and physiological addiction characterized by tolerance and the development of withdrawal symptoms when dose is decreased or stopped

Craving: Subjective need for drug, usually experienced after decreased use or abstinence

Abstinence: Refraining from drug or alcohol use

Detoxification: Process of ridding the body of drug and its effects

Relapse: Process of readdiction involving thoughts, feelings, and behaviors that lead to reuse of drug during recovery period

continued drug use. Most drugs that are abused produce some form of *physiological dependence,* which varies from a mild to a severe degree. *Tolerance* develops after repeated use and is seen more rapidly with some drugs, such as cocaine. Tolerance may occur in the absence of addiction and may develop for one aspect of a drug's action and not another. *Reverse tolerance* refers to a decrease in the amount of a drug needed to obtain the desired effect. This is due to the slowing of metabolism as a result of liver damage and usually occurs in advanced stages of addiction.

Characteristics

Addictions have certain common features (Table 60-4). These characteristics may be present in the initiation and/or maintenance of patterns of alcohol and drug abuse and dependence. The nurse needs to recognize the importance of these features in contributing to the complex problems of addiction.

Addictive Process

The length of time required to move from casual use to dependence involves many factors related to the host, agent, and environment. The type of drug, frequency of use, amount of drug used, route of administration, health of the user, and support for drug use from friends or family members *(enabling)* affect the development of an addiction. Repeated intravenous (IV) use of heroin or cocaine can produce addiction in a few days or weeks, although it generally takes years and heavy periods of drinking to develop an addiction to alcohol.

The process of addiction may be thought of as a cycle that is self-reinforcing (Fig. 60-2). Interruptions in the cycle may be due to inaccessibility of the drug, decrease in the amount, attempts to control drug use, or entrance into treatment. This may precipitate withdrawal symptoms in physically dependent individuals. Rapid reinstatement of the cycle occurs during relapse.

Classification and Diagnoses

Diagnoses of addictions are based on the criteria developed by the American Psychiatric Association in the *Diagnostic and Statistical Manual of Mental Disorders.* The classification includes two categories: *psychoactive substance use disorders* and *psychoactive substance–induced*

Table 60-4   Common Characteristics of Addiction

Excessive and compulsive use
Impulsive behaviors
Powerful immediate reinforcement
Feelings of depression, helplessness, dependence
Defenses, including denial, projection, manipulation
Low frustration tolerance
Poor body image, low self-esteem
Tendency to relapse
Family dysfunction
Lack of social support (unrelated to drug use)
Chronic or terminal illness related to abuse patterns (e.g., cirrhosis)

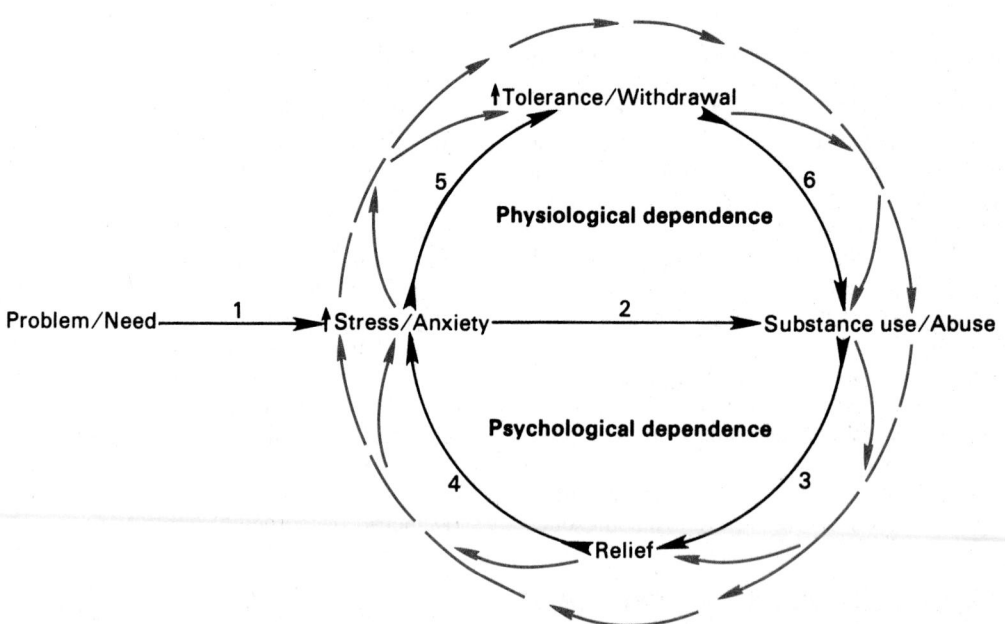

Fig. 60-2   The addictive cycle. Step 1: The problem or need arouses stress or anxiety and is dealt with through substance use. Steps 2 to 4: The cycle of substance use, relief, and recurring stress or anxiety is repeated until psychological dependence is established. Interrupting the cycle brings about anxiety but not physical symptoms. Steps 5 to 6: Physiological dependence usually follows psychological dependence. Withdrawal symptoms follow abstinence. Interruptions in the cycle are indicated by a *broken line.*

Table 60-5 Diagnostic Criteria for Psychoactive Substance Dependence and Abuse

SUBSTANCE DEPENDENCE*

1. Substance often taken in larger amounts or over a longer period than the person intended
2. Persistent desire or one or more unsuccessful efforts to cut down or control substance use
3. A great deal of time spent in activities necessary to get the substance (e.g., theft), taking the substance (e.g., chain smoking), or recovering from its effects
4. Frequent intoxication or withdrawal symptoms when expected to fulfill major role obligations at work, school, or home (e.g., does not go to work because hung over, goes to school or work "high," intoxicated while taking care of children), or uses substance when physically hazardous (e.g., drives when intoxicated)
5. Important social, occupational, or recreational activities given up or reduced because of substance use
6. Continued substance use despite knowledge of persistent or recurrent social, psychological, or physical problem that is caused or exacerbated by use of the substance (e.g., continued use of heroin despite family arguments about it, cocaine-induced depression, or exacerbation of an ulcer with drinking)
7. Marked tolerance: Need for markedly increased amounts of the substance (i.e., at least a 50% increase) to achieve intoxication or desired effect or markedly diminished effect with continued use of the same amount
8. Characteristic withdrawal symptoms†
9. Substance often taken to relieve or avoid withdrawal symptoms†

SUBSTANCE ABUSE‡

1. Continued use despite knowledge of a persistent or recurrent social, occupational, psychological, or physical problem that is caused or exacerbated by use of the psychoactive substance
2. Recurrent use in situations in which use is physically hazardous (e.g., driving while intoxicated)

Modified from American Psychiatric Association: Diagnostic & statistical manual of mental disorders, ed 3, rev, Washington, DC, 1987, American Psychiatric Association

*At least three of the criteria are met, and some symptoms have persisted for at least 1 month or have occurred repeatedly over a longer period to fit this classification.

†These items may not apply to marijuana, hallucinogens, or phencyclidine (PCP).

‡At least one of the criteria is met, some symptoms of the disturbance have persisted for at least 1 month or have occurred repeatedly over a longer period, and the criteria for substance dependence have never been met.

organic mental disorders. The former refers to patterns of abuse and dependence associated with maladaptive behavioral changes (Table 60-5). The latter refers to the primary central nervous system (CNS) effects of intoxication, withdrawal, delirium, dementia, delusional disorder, amnesic disorder, hallucinosis, and mood disorder. Criteria for the diagnosis of alcoholism have also been compiled by the National Council on Alcoholism.[4] Major and minor clinical, physiological, behavioral, and laboratory indicators of alcoholism are identified and differentiated among early, middle, and late stages.

Nursing diagnoses assist nurses in the organization and management of client problems. Specific nursing diagnoses are useful in caring for individuals who have problems related to alcohol and drug abuse. The National Nurses Society on Addictions and the American Nurses' Association have identified several relevant nursing diagnoses (Table 60-6).

PATTERNS OF DRUG ABUSE AND DEPENDENCE

Patterns of abuse and dependence lead to physical and emotional symptoms and maladaptive behavioral changes that indicate pathological drug use. These patterns are complicated by the frequent use of multiple drugs. Age appears to be a factor in multiple drug abuse. It is reported that 80% of alcoholics under the age of 30 are addicted to at least one other drug.[5] Over 80% of cocaine addicts are

reported to be also addicted to alcohol, and 50% of cocaine addicts are also addicted to cannabis.[6]

Patterns of dependence may result from three types of multiple drug use—mixed addiction, dual addiction, or cross tolerance. *Mixed addiction* occurs when an individual alternates use of one class of drugs with another to alleviate or counteract the effects of the original drug (e.g., alternate use of "uppers" like cocaine with "downers" like alcohol or heroin). *Dual addiction* refers to the use of drugs that have similar effects (e.g., alcohol and barbiturates). This term has also been used to indicate an addiction to more than one drug. *Cross tolerance* is a type of dependence that occurs after tolerance has developed for one drug (e.g., diazepam [Valium] or chlordiazepoxide [Librium]), and the use of other drugs in the same class precipitates similar effects of tolerance (e.g., meperidine [Demerol] or morphine).[7]

A separate diagnosis for each drug is usually made in cases of multiple drug use, if specific criteria are met for each individual drug. If not, a diagnosis of multiple substance abuse or dependence may be made. Any stimulant, depressant, or hallucinogen may be abused, and most have a high potential for dependence. The most important drug-related determinants of potential for abuse and dependence are the dose, the manner of use, and the duration of action. The drug is only one component in addiction, and factors related to the individual and the environment also

Table 60-6   List of Nursing Diagnoses for
Addicted Clients

BIOLOGICAL RESPONSES

Sensory/perceptual alterations
High risk for injury
Self-care deficit
Sexual dysfunction
High risk for infection
Sleep pattern disturbance
Altered nutrition: less than body requirements
Pain
Altered growth and development

COGNITIVE RESPONSES

Altered thought processes
Noncompliance

PSYCHOSOCIAL RESPONSES

Impaired verbal communication
Ineffective individual coping
Self-esteem disturbance
Anxiety
Social isolation
Altered family processes
Altered parenting
Altered growth and development
High risk for violence
Fear

SPIRITUAL RESPONSES

Spiritual distress
Powerlessness
Hopelessness
Dysfunctional grieving

Modified from American Nurses' Association and National Nurses'
Society on Addictions: Standards of addictions nursing practice with
selected diagnoses and criteria, Kansas City, Mo, 1988, American
Nurses' Association.

play important roles in initiating and maintaining patterns
of abuse and dependence.

STIMULANTS

The two most prevalent stimulants are nicotine and caffeine. However, amphetamines and cocaine are the stimulants that lead to the most serious types of abuse. The most
potent stimulant of natural origin is cocaine. The amphetamine group includes amphetamine (Benzedrine), dextro-
amphetamine (Dexedrine), and methamphetamine (Des-
oxyn), also known as *speed*. Phenmetrazine (Preludin) and
methylphenidate (Ritalin) are also stimulants that may be
abused. Other drugs in this category are benzphetamine
(Didrex), diethylpropion (Tenuate), fenfluramine (Pondi-
min), mazindol (Sanorex), phendimetrazine (Anorex, Ad-
phen), and phentermine (Fastin, Ionamin), which are anorectic drugs.[8]

Amphetamines

Etiology. Amphetamines were developed in the 1930s
as a substitute for ephedrine. Amphetamine was found to
be a potent bronchodilator and useful in inhalers. It was
also found to be effective in the treatment of narcolepsy, a
disorder characterized by falling asleep without warning
and by hyperactivity in children. Currently, methylphenidate (Ritalin) is primarily used in the treatment of hyperactivity in children, and phenmetrazine (Preludin) is used as
an appetite suppressant.

As amphetamine use became more tightly controlled
through prescriptions, "look-alike" pills that are identical
in appearance to amphetamines and illicit methamphetamine (e.g., "crank," "crystal") became popular. These
pseudostimulants, which contain large amounts of caffeine
along with ephedrine and phenylpropanolamine, have been
cited as causes for some deaths.[15] Recently, "act-alikes,"
less potent forms with no resemblance to amphetamines,
have appeared in states prohibiting look-alikes. Use of
crank and "ice," a smokable form of methamphetamine,
has increased in some parts of the country.

Clinical manifestations of abuse. Amphetamines affect the CNS and have adrenergic (sympathomimetic) effects on the sympathetic branch of the autonomic nervous
system. They follow the pattern of CNS stimulation that
begins with feelings of euphoria and excitement and continues with effects on the cardiovascular, respiratory, and
heat-regulating systems. These drugs affect the catecholamine system, producing an excess of neurotransmitters
that lead to a "fight or flight" reaction.[16]

The primary effects of stimulants are listed in Table
60-7 and may also include dilated pupils, diaphoresis,
smooth-muscle relaxation, and an increase in metabolic
rates. Users may initially use these drugs to increase alertness or concentration, improve performance, relieve fatigue, or control weight. They come to rely on the euphoric effects of feeling more powerful, more decisive,
and self-possessed. These drugs may also lead to unpleasant feelings of irritability, fear, and anxiety. An increased
dose tends to precipitate rapid mood swings, hallucinations, racing thoughts, feeling of being out of control or
aggressive, and compulsive or meaningless behaviors.

Amphetamines are primarily taken orally, and peak effects occur within 2 to 3 hours; complete elimination occurs within 2 days.[9] Effects are generally intensified by IV
injection of the drug, which produces a "rush" or "flash,"
an almost immediate intense burst of energy and related
feelings. Frequent or heavy IV use may lead to a psychosis
that mimics schizophrenia or mania. Individuals on a
speed binge may have injected as much as 1000 mg every
2 to 3 hours.[8] Smoking of these drugs produces a similar
instantaneous effect and is believed to be the most rapid,
intense response route. Intranasal ingestion (*snorting*) has
the longest effect because of local constriction of blood
vessels.[10]

Two patterns of use may be observed—daily and episodic. Episodic use includes *binging*, which entails continuous use of high doses in a short time (48 hours) and ends
only when the user collapses or runs out of the drug.[11]
Binge patterns are very common and often represent a shift

Table 60-7 Effects of Frequently Abused Drugs

Drug	Psychological Effects	Physiological Effects	Effects of Overdose	Withdrawal Syndrome
STIMULANTS				
Cocaine, amphetamines, methylphenidate, phenmetrazine, other stimulants	Elation, psychomotor agitation, grandiosity, talkativeness, ↑ alertness, mood swings	Dilated pupils, ↑ blood pressure, ↑ TPR, diaphoresis, nausea, vomiting, insomnia, loss of appetite	Agitation, increased body temperature, hallucinations, convulsions, possible death	Severely depressed mood, prolonged sleep, apathy, irritability, disorientation
DEPRESSANTS				
Chloral hydrate, barbiturates, methaqualone, benzodiazepines, alcohol	Disorientation, euphoria, emotional lability, ↑ sexual and aggressive drives with intoxication (↓ with increased doses), talkativeness	Slurred speech, staggering, constricted pupils, ↓ respirations, sedation, nausea	Shallow respiration, cold and clammy skin, weak and rapid pulse, coma, possible death	Anxiety, insomnia, tremors, delirium, convulsions, possible death
NARCOTICS				
Opium, morphine, codeine, heroin, methadone, other narcotics	Euphoria, ↓ sexual and aggressive drives	↓ Respiratory rate, nausea, "nodding out," insensitivity to pain, constricted pupils	Slow and shallow breathing, clammy skin, constricted pupils, coma, possible death	Watery eyes, runny nose, yawning, loss of appetite, tremors, panic, chills and sweating, cramps, nausea
HALLUCINOGENS				
LSD, psilocybin, mescaline, peyote, amphetamine variants, phencyclidine	Hallucinations, illusions, altered body and time perception, mood swings, suspiciousness, confusion, anxiety, panic, intense emotions, depersonalization	Lack of coordination, dilated pupils, ↑ blood pressure, tremors, blurred vision, nausea, dizziness, ↓ weakness response to pain	More prolonged episodes, possibly resembling psychotic states	N/A
CANNABIS				
Marijuana, tetrahydrocannabinol, hashish	Euphoria, impaired memory and attention, relaxation, poor judgment, apathy, abrupt mood changes, slowed time sensation	↑ Appetite, tachycardia, reddened eyes	Fatigue, paranoia; hallucinogenlike psychotic state (at very high doses)	Insomnia, hyperactivity (rare syndrome)
INHALANTS				
Glues, aerosols, cleaning solutions, nail polish removers, lighter fluids, paints and paint thinners, other petroleum products, halothane, nitrous oxide, amyl nitrite, butyl nitrite	Giddiness, lightheadedness, decreased inhibitions, floating sensation, illusions, clouding of thoughts, drowsiness, amnesia	Eye irritation, sensitivity to light, double vision, ringing in ears, irritation in lining of nose and mouth, cough, nausea, vomiting, diarrhea, faint heart beat, cardiac irregularities or dysrhythmias	Anxiety, mental impairment, depressed respiration, cardiac dysrhythmias, sudden death	No clinically relevant syndrome, development of tolerance likely at high doses

↑, Increased; *TPR*, temperature, pulse, respirations; ↓, decreased; *LSD*, lysergic acid diethylamide; *N/A*, no data available.

from daily use. A binge period is followed by a "crash" or an intense "down" type of depression and the physical symptoms associated with coming off of a "run" (i.e., withdrawal).

Tolerance develops rapidly with these drugs and leads to an intense craving, even in the absence of euphoria. Physical dependence has been recognized but is characterized more by psychological manifestations than physical ones. Certain mental abnormalities may develop as a result of high doses. Early signs may include bruxism (grinding of teeth), touching and picking the face and extremities, repetitious movements, suspiciousness, and a sense of being watched.[8]

Toxic reactions to stimulants are usually dose related and refer to increasing levels of stimulation, sometimes described as "overamping," which may culminate in massive overdose and death. Reactions from high doses are characterized by paranoia with auditory and visual hallucinations. A sublethal overdose may be recognized by symptoms of headache, dizziness, agitation, hostility, tremor, panic, flushed skin, chest pain with palpitations, diaphoresis, vomiting, and abdominal cramps. Without medical intervention, death may occur as the result of seizures, cardiovascular collapse, and hyperthermia. Physical exertion increases the risk of toxicity and may contribute to sudden death even when moderate amounts of the drug are used.[8]

Stimulant withdrawal follows a pattern of rebound depression and is characterized by depression, irritability, anxiety, fatigue, insomnia or hypersomnia, or psychomotor agitation. Symptoms peak in about 2 to 4 days and last for more than 24 hours after the drug has been stopped.[11] Suicidal thoughts, anxiety, and extreme tenseness may persist for weeks or months.

Therapeutic management. Clients generally seek treatment for medical complications such as panic reactions or temporary psychosis related to intoxication, overdose, or withdrawal. Overdose has also been termed *acute poisoning*. Primary features of amphetamine intoxication are maladaptive behavioral changes such as fighting, manifestations of grandiosity, hypervigilance, psychomotor agitation, impaired judgment, and social or occupational dysfunction. Physical symptoms may include dilated pupils, elevated blood pressure, tachycardia, perspiration or chills, and nausea and vomiting. Agitation is usually the first symptom, and it can develop rapidly into a potentially fatal condition. Other symptoms may be decreased appetite, sleep disorders, chest pain, tremors, delirium, dizziness, respiratory paralysis, and cardiac dysrhythmias.

Amphetamine intoxication may be self-limiting within 24 hours. Treatment is directed toward symptoms and support. The use of benzodiazepines has been effective. Acute intoxication requires careful observation to prevent symptoms from developing into a medical emergency. It is also important to assess the individual's mental status to assist in differentiating drug-induced depression and psychoses from psychiatric disorders.[12]

The nurse must recognize signs and symptoms of drug intoxication and ask questions about types of drugs used, frequency of use, dose or amount, route of administration, and time of last use. Accurate assessment is the key to intervention. A drug screen should be ordered to confirm the type of drug and level of toxicity. The nurse should take a comprehensive health history focusing on preexisting problems with cardiovascular, respiratory, neurological, renal, or hepatic systems such as pseudocholinesterase deficiency, which may indicate clients who are particularly sensitive to the toxic effects of the drug.

Prehospital management of drug overdose involves checking the individual's level of consciousness, respiration, and circulation; calling for help or medical assistance, if needed; establishing the *ABCs* (airway, breathing, circulation); eliciting information about the substance or substances (name, route, when taken, period of time taken, amount taken); eliciting information about the individual's health history including state before overdose; calling poison control; and administering an agent such as ipecac to induce vomiting. After the individual is transported to the hospital, gastric lavage may be initiated and activated charcoal may be given. Emergency room nursing care for drug overdose is basically supportive and involves securing an airway, administering oxygen, placing the client in Trendelenburg's position, administering muscle relaxants or barbiturates or diazepam as needed, and monitoring vital signs.[13]

Management of withdrawal involves assessment and monitoring of symptoms with particular attention to suicidal thoughts and complications from multiple drug use. The primary aims of management of withdrawal are to control symptoms, decrease craving, and establish a basis for recovery. Before inpatient treatment begins, withdrawal should be managed. Specific approaches to management include providing active support, encouraging adequate nutrition including vitamin supplements, maintaining adequate fluid balance, recommending aerobic exercise if there are no medical contraindications, and teaching relaxation techniques and the use of nutritional aids such as milk, cheese, and tryptophan to promote sleep. Drugs that may be helpful during this period include amantadine, bromocriptine, and levodopa to decrease craving; neuroleptics or some benzodiazepines to relieve "crash" symptoms; and desipramine (Norpramin), imipramine (Tofranil), or trazodone (Desyrel) to prevent relapse.[14]

Cocaine

Etiology. Cocaine is a white powder (40%-60% pure) that is mixed (cut) with sugars, local anesthetics, and stimulants. Because of its anesthetic and vasocontrictive qualities, it had been used for eye, nose, and throat surgery but has generally been replaced by safer drugs. The prevalence of the use of cocaine has recently been surpassed by the widespread use of "crack," a cocaine alkaloid that gets its name from the popping sound the crystals make when heated. Crack has grown in popularity with adolescents because it is cheap, readily available, and easy to use and has an increased purity over cocaine (90% to 95%).[15]

Clinical manifestations of abuse. Cocaine mimics the effects of amphetamines except that it has a more rapid onset and a shorter duration of action. With cocaine the main euphoria effect lasts only 15 to 40 minutes or about one fourth of the duration of amphetamines.[13] It is easily ab-

sorbed from all sites and rapidly absorbed across all mucous membranes and into the bloodstream within 3 minutes. It is metabolized in the liver and eliminated by the kidneys; metabolites remain in the urine for 24 to 36 hours.[12]

The most common route of administration is intranasally, although it may be used parenterally, orally, vaginally, sublingually, and rectally; it may also be smoked. The most rapid routes of administration are IV and inhalational (smoking). When taken IV or inhaled, cocaine's effects are felt within 1 minute and last about 20 minutes.[16]

Addiction can develop from any route of administration. Collapse and scarring of the veins at the injection site may occur as a result of "shooting up." With intranasal use, the nasal septum and mucosa may be damaged, leading to nasal sores, decreased olfaction, chronic sinusitis, perforation, and collapse of the nose or septal necrosis (Fig. 60-3). Cocaine "runny nose" or chronic rhinitis is common with long-term intranasal use. Frequent sniffing and increased susceptibility to upper respiratory infections are common symptoms of cocaine abuse.

Users who experience personality changes are described as being "coked out." Anxiety, restlessness, and extreme irritability may signal the onset of a toxic psychosis. Cocaine psychosis is characterized by tactile hallucinations of bugs crawling under the skin (formication) and scratches on arms, legs, or chest, which may indicate attempts to dig out the bugs. This psychosis is shorter than the psychosis observed with amphetamine abuse.

Medical complications are directly related to the route of administration, type of cocaine and adulterants, dose, and individual vulnerabilities. They may include cellulitis, wound abscess, hepatitis, acquired immunodeficiency syndrome (AIDS), seizures, myocardial infarction, cardiac dysrhythmias, sudden cardiac death, rhabdomyolysis (skeletal muscle injury), acute renal failure, acute respiratory distress, pulmonary edema, asthma, abruptio placentae, premature onset of labor, and bilateral loss of eyebrow and eyelash hair (from inhalation of hot vapors).

Infants whose mothers used cocaine during pregnancy are at higher risk for intrauterine growth retardation, lower birth weight, smaller head circumference, decreased length, lower Apgar scores, neurobehavioral impairment, some congenital abnormalities, and sudden infant death syndrome (SIDS).[24]

Frequent causes of death associated with cocaine abuse include cerebral hemorrhage, respiratory failure, and cardiovascular collapse. There is no margin of safety with use of cocaine, and there is no antidote for toxicity. Repeated use appears to lower the level of toxicity ("kindling"), especially for seizures.[12]

Overdose occurs more frequently with IV use, smoking "freebase," or "body packing." Freebasing is the process of extracting the alkaloid form from cocaine hydrochloride, producing crack and rock. Freebase can be smoked in

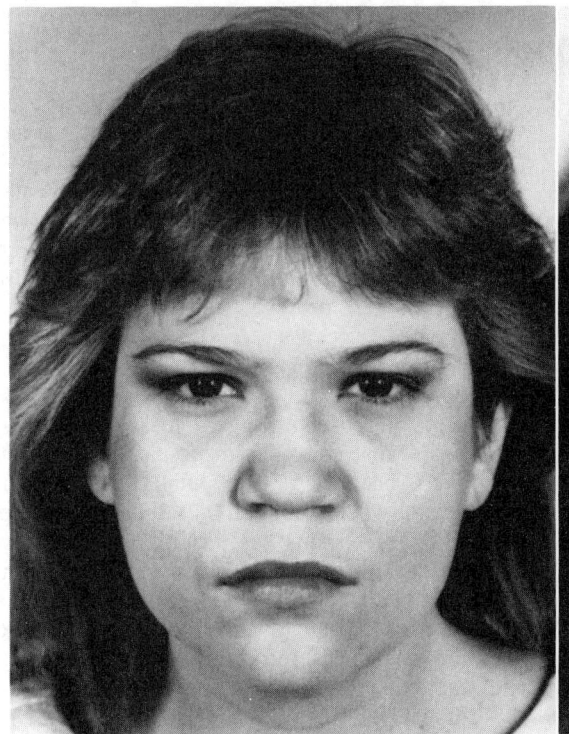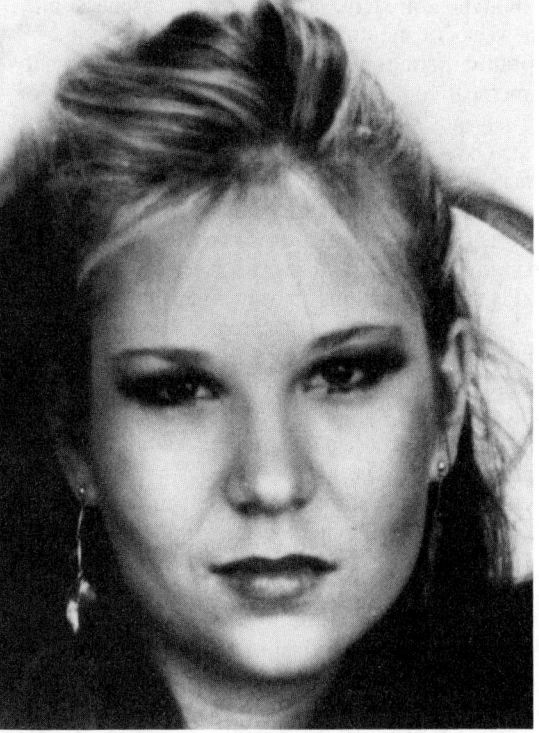

Fig. 60-3 Cocaine nose: nasal collapse—before and after cocaine use. (From Deutsch HL and Millard DR: A new cocaine abuse complex, Arch Otolaryngol Head Neck Surg 115:236, 1989.)

a cigarette with tobacco or heated and inhaled through a water pipe. The effects are very short, lasting about 15 to 20 minutes compared with the effects of snorting, which may last 1½ hours.[12] "Body packing" is a form of smuggling packets of cocaine across borders in the intestines. If the packets burst, a toxic reaction and death occur unless immediate medical intervention is available.

Crack in the form of chips, chunks, or rocks is the most potent form of the drug and produces the most dramatic high and the most rapid addiction. Because crack is inhaled, it is absorbed more rapidly (2 to 3 seconds) as a result of the larger surface area in the lungs compared with that of the nasal mucosa. Consequently, crack produces a more intense effect and withdrawal. Pulmonary damage from smoking crack may be evident with black or dark brown sputum.[13]

Therapeutic management. Cocaine abuse and dependence have become growing concerns in emergency rooms and drug treatment programs. The picture of the addict may be complicated by cocaine abusers' frequent use of alcohol, marijuana, or heroin. The addict may use drugs such as chlordiazepoxide, diazepam, lorazepam (Ativan), or alprazolam (Xanax) to minimize unpleasant effects of withdrawal. Cocaine combined with heroin is called *speedball* and cocaine combined with PCP is called *space base*. One of the most dangerous combinations is cocaine and alcohol because it increases the risk of induced liver injury.[17]

Individuals who are addicted to cocaine do not seek treatment initially for drug abuse but rather for problems with sleep, appetite, depression, sinusitis, respiratory infections, chest pain, or migrainelike headaches. Specific

clues that should alert the nurse to cocaine abuse or dependence are included in Table 60-8. Clients are usually hesitant to admit to illegal drug use. They need to know the importance of providing an accurate drug history, which will be confidential. Questions about drug use patterns need to be stated in a direct, nonjudgmental manner.

Management of cocaine intoxication, overdose, and withdrawal is handled in the same manner as that for amphetamines. Fatal cocaine poisoning has occurred because of adrenergic crisis that resulted in seizures, hyperthermia, coma, and cardiac failure. The cocaine ("Casey Jones") reaction may be seen as an accelerated onset and progression of symptoms through phases of stimulation and depression (Table 60-9). The pattern of the cocaine reaction usually involves an early stimulation phase that resolves in 20 minutes, but symptoms can progress rapidly to depression,

Table 60-8 Signs Indicative of Cocaine Abuse or Dependence

Chronic nasal congestion	History of abruptio placentae,
Cold symptoms	premature labor, spontane-
Epistaxis	ous abortion, impotence,
Unexplained weight loss	decreased libido
Chest pain	Depression or suicide threats
Dyspnea	Behavior changes or mood
Severe headache	shifts
Dizziness	Needle tracks with pale center
Palpitations	

Table 60-9 Fatal Cocaine Poisoning

Central Nervous System	Cardiovascular System	Respiratory System
EARLY STIMULATION		
Euphoria, elation, talkativeness, irritability, emotional lability, stereotyped movements, tremor, sudden headache, small-muscle twitching, "cocaine bugs," "snowlights," paranoid-type psychosis, feelings of impending doom, ↑ temperature	Variable pulse, ↑ BP, skin pallor, premature ventricular contractions	↑ Respiratory rate and depth, dyspnea
ADVANCED STIMULATION		
↓ Stimuli response, convulsions, ↑ deep-tendon reflexes, incontinence	↑ Pulse; ↑ BP; cerebral hemorrhage; ↓ cardiac output; ventricular dysrhythmias; hypotension; rapid, weak, irregular pulse; cyanosis	Gasping, rapid respiration; Cheyne-Stokes respiration; progressive hypoxia
DEPRESSION		
Flaccid muscle paralysis, fixed dilated pupils, coma, depressed reflexes, loss of vital functions, death	Ventricular fibrillation, circulatory collapse, generalized cyanosis, cardiac arrest, death	Agonal breaths, respiratory failure, pulmonary edema, death

↑, Increased; *BP*, blood pressure; ↓, decreased.
Modified from Gay GR: Clinical management of acute and chronic cocaine poisoning, Ann Emerg Med 11:562-572, 1982.

Table 60-10

 NURSING CARE PLAN FOR THE CLIENT WITH COCAINE POISONING

Defining Characteristics	Nursing Interventions	Evaluation Criteria
NURSING DIAGNOSIS: Anxiety related to increased CNS stimulation		
Increased pulse rate, palpitations, hyperventilation, talkativeness, fearfulness, irritability, emotional lability, tremor, chest pains, confusion, disorientation, paranoid-type psychosis, feelings of losing control or going crazy	Continuously monitor vital signs. Explain procedures. Provide safe, secure environment. Reduce level of anxiety with comfort measures and medications, if indicated. Decrease delusions and agitation by decreasing stimuli (if possible). Reinforce reality orientation. Use calm approach.	Decreased physiological and psychological manifestations of anxiety; discussion of feelings of anxiety, dread, and helplessness; acknowledgement of toxic effects of cocaine
NURSING DIAGNOSIS: Total self-care deficit related to advanced CNS stimulation progressing to CNS depression		
Self-feeding, self-bathing, self-dressing, or self-toileting deficits or inability to perform any self-care activities	Assess self-care deficits. Provide assistance as needed and explain procedures. Monitor vital signs. As client recovers, reassess ability to participate in self-care. Refer to occupational therapist to relearn skills, if indicated. Provide opportunities for self-care and hope of recovery to previous level of functioning.	Absence of seizures, alertness, proper orientation, increased level of functioning of vital systems, ability to perform self-care activities
NURSING DIAGNOSIS: Fluid volume deficit related to diaphoresis and hypermetabolic state		
Dry throat, thirst, decreased urinary output, fluid output greater than intake, dry skin and mucous membranes, decreased skin turgor, nausea, vomiting, confusion, dizziness, diaphoresis, hemorrhage, hyperthermia, increased pulse rate	Monitor fluid intake and output. Assess for dehydration. Start IV lines with large-bore needles for one or more fluid resuscitations with normal saline and lactated Ringer's solution. Monitor vital signs. Provide cooling blanket, ice packs, or ice water sponge for elevated temperature, if indicated. Monitor serum electrolytes, BUN, urine and serum osmolalities, creatinine clearance, hematocrit, and hemoglobin. Consider additional fluid losses associated with vomiting, diarrhea, fever. Give sips of 5% glucose solution. Administer IV ammonium chloride to acidify urine.	Absence of manifestations of dehydration, maintenance of intake of at least 1500 ml/day (oral fluids) and output of at least 1000-1500 ml/day, vital signs and lab work within normal limits; clear sensorium, absence of vomiting, hemorrhage, diarrhea
NURSING DIAGNOSIS: Situational low self-esteem related to addictive behavior or cocaine abuse		
Self-destructive behavior associated with cocaine abuse, isolation, negative self-talk, anger, despair, powerlessness, hopelessness, sadness, depression, self-neglect, apathy, denial, noncompliance with treatment	Assess emotional status. Assist in identifying and expressing feelings. Provide support and reassurance for short term and recovery. Support use of effective coping mechanisms to deal with crisis. Assist client in identifying responsibility and control in situation. Mobilize current support system. Assist client in management of specific problems (e.g., hospitalization, depression). Refer to treatment program, counseling, support group, or other resource.	Expression of feelings of self-worth, identification of positive aspects of self, expression of positive outlook for future, ability to analyze own behavior associated with cocaine abuse and its consequences

BUN, Blood urea nitrogen; *ACLS,* advanced cardiac life support.

Table 60-10

NURSING CARE PLAN FOR THE CLIENT WITH COCAINE POISONING—cont'd

Defining Characteristics	Nursing Interventions	Evaluation Criteria

NURSING DIAGNOSIS: **Potential complications: neurological, cardiovascular, and respiratory problems related to the direct toxic action of cocaine on tissues and its potentiation of the effects of norephinephrine and epinephrine**

Compromised vital signs, seizures, altered level of consciousness and motor activity, dysrhythmias, vascular collapse, cerebral vascular accident, congestive heart failure, hypoxia, adult respiratory distress syndrome, cardiopulmonary arrest	Monitor neurological status, including level of consciousness. Take seizure precautions. Provide airway management and ventilation support. Continuously monitor vital signs. Keep open IV lines. Administer medications aggressively, as indicated. Put client in 30-degree Trendelenburg's position when indicated. Employ ACLS measures, if indicated.	Resolution of crisis with no further complications, return to normal status of vital functioning

NURSING DIAGNOSIS: **High risk for self-directed violence related to cocaine abuse**

Compulsive focus of attention on cocaine, low self-esteem, hopelessness, acute agitation, depression, suicidal thoughts, poor impulse control, helplessness, lack of support systems, hallucinations, proneness to violence	Assess risk for self-destruction (motivation for stopping drug use). Assist client in building self-esteem with caring, empathic approach. Assess support systems. Assist client in contacting members of support systems. Help client develop positive coping mechanisms. Initiate health teaching and referral for treatment or counseling when crisis is resolved.	Abstinence from further drug use, seeking of treatment for cocaine abuse, development of effective coping mechanisms in handling stress, no apparent risk of self-harm

and total collapse of body systems may occur within 2 to 3 minutes.

Effective treatment of seizures and hyperthermia is vital to prevent the progression of symptoms. Aggressive treatment and advanced physical assessment skills are required to manage multisystem failure and promote positive outcomes. Ammonium chloride may be used to acidify the urine and to increase the rate of excretion. Drugs may be useful but are usually avoided unless absolutely necessary to control seizures or other life-threatening conditions.

Critical care management by the nurse means close monitoring of neurological status, level of consciousness, seizure precautions, pulmonary assessment, and airway management in addition to continuous physical assessment. Even after client status improves, intensive nursing care is necessary to monitor for neurological, pulmonary, and cardiovascular changes and signs or symptoms of infection, blood dyscrasias, or other complications (Table 60-10).

Special problems. There is growing concern and recognition of the role of cocaine in both accidental and violent crime–related trauma. One study found that 75% of clients who were admitted to a large trauma center had positive results of screens for illicit drugs or prescription

drugs with abuse potential. Of the clients with positive results of drug screens, 73% were positive for cocaine, indicating recent use. A strong positive relationship was found between cocaine use and violent crime–related injury.[18] This implies that a large number of trauma victims may be under the influence of cocaine and need to be carefully assessed for signs and symptoms of overdose, withdrawal, and medical complications that could lead to adverse interactions with drugs used in the management of pain, injuries, or surgical intervention. Drugs like cocaine can have adverse interactions with certain drugs such as halothane, cyclopropane, and trichloroethylene, which are used during general anesthesia. During the surgical recovery period, nurses should be alert for clients who may exhibit signs and symptoms of drug interactions with pain medications or anesthesia or exhibit symptoms of withdrawal.

Engaging an individual who is addicted to cocaine in treatment is very difficult because of the intense craving for the drug and a strong denial that "cocaine is not addicting" or that the individual can control it. Often various forms of leverage such as family threats, loss of job or professional license, legal action, or major health consequences provide sufficient motivation for an individual to enter a treatment program. Although many drug abusers

Table 60-11 Warning Signs of Relapse

Apprehension about well-being
Defensiveness and denial
Loneliness and isolation
Periods of confusion and restlessness
Easiness to anger
Irregular eating and sleeping habits
Feelings of powerlessness, helplessness, depression
Development of "don't care" attitude
Wishful thinking and fantasizing
Loss of daily structure

Table 60-12 Depressants

SEDATIVE-HYPNOTICS	ALCOHOL
Chloral hydrate	Ethanol
Barbiturates	Methanol
Amobarbital (Amytal)*	Ethylene glycol
Butabarbital (Butisol)*	Isopropyl alcohol
Talbutal (Lotusate)*	
Pentobarbital (Nembutal)†	**OPIATE NARCOTICS**
Secobarbital (Seconal)†	Opium
Phenobarbital (Luminal)‡	Morphine
Benzodiazepines	Codeine
Lorazepam (Ativan)*	Heroin
Flurazepam (Dalmane)‡	Hydrocodone (Hycodan)
Diazepam (Valium)‡	Hydromorphone (Dilaudid)
Chlordiazepoxide (Librium)‡	Meperidine (Demerol)
Alprazolam (Xanax)*	Methadone (Dolophine)
Oxazepam (Serax)*	Oxymorphone (Numorphan)
Chlorazepate (Tranxene)‡	Fentanyl (Sublimaze)
Midazolam (Versed)†	Pentazocine (Talwin)
Triazolam (Halcion)†	Oxycodone (Percodan)
Halazepam (Paxipam)‡	Propoxyphene (Darvon)
Temazepam (Restoril)*	Acetaminophen with oxycodone (Tylox)
Methaqualone (Quaalude, Parest, Sopor)	
Glutethimide (Doriden)	
Meprobamate (Equanil, Miltown)	
Methyprylon (Noludar)	
Ethchlorvynol (Placidyl)	

*Intermediate acting.
†Short acting.
‡Long acting.

can be effectively treated in outpatient programs, inpatient programs should be recommended for some. This includes those who use IV or freebase cocaine compulsively, are physically dependent on other addictive drugs, have a serious medical or emotional problem, have a severe impairment of psychosocial functioning, have a destructive pattern of drug use, are resistant to treatment, or have failed previous outpatient programs.[19]

A structured inpatient program may be desirable during early recovery to provide a support system until the addict is able to develop coping skills and resources to resist drug use and begin working toward a drug-free lifestyle. Complete abstinence from drugs is important, since the use of another drug can trigger craving for cocaine and result in relapse because of paired associations with previous cocaine use. Relapse prevention is an essential component of any recovery program and includes behavioral, cognitive, educational, and self-control techniques. The individual needs to identify specific high-risk situations that are likely to lead to drug use and to practice ways to avoid or deal with these situations. Conditioned urges and drug cravings are consistently extinguished by substituting other activities for drug use. Clients are taught to recognize early warning signs that serve as "setups" for drug use (Table 60-11). Negative consequences of the drugs are recalled to counteract distorted memories of the drug euphoria. Temporary relapses are presented as opportunities for learning to minimize feelings of failure and to assist the individual to continue with abstinence. The individual also learns ways to reduce stress and live a balanced lifestyle.

DEPRESSANTS

Drugs categorized as depressants have common psychological effects and the ability to produce sedation and other major depressant effects (Table 60-12). Drugs in this category have also been called *hypnotics, anxiolytics, antianxiety agents,* and *narcotics.* Antipsychotics are not considered CNS depressants and are not physically addictive. They are seldom used to produce a state of euphoria.

With the exception of alcohol and some federally regulated drugs, most CNS depressants are medically useful. Alcohol is also a major depressant and the most widely used substance in the category. It is frequently used in combination with barbiturates or benzodiazepines as well as stimulants and hallucinogens. Depressants have been used frequently with stimulants to produce an upper-downer effect or to "mellow out" the effect of stimulants.

Drugs other than alcohol in this category may be prescribed for relief of anxiety, insomnia, pain, symptoms of withdrawal from alcohol, or as anticonvulsants or anesthetic agents. These drugs have been widely recognized for their abuse potential, which leads to rapid tolerance, dependency, and medical emergencies involving overdoses and withdrawal.

Sedative-Hypnotics

Etiology. The discovery of sedative-hypnotics resulted from a search for a "safer" nonaddicting drug. Each new discovery was heralded as safer than the previous one, but over time, each drug has been found to be capable of abuse and addiction. Chloral hydrate and paraldehyde were two of the earliest drugs used for their sedating effects. They were generally replaced when barbituates were introduced. The barbiturates are frequently responsible for accidental overdoses and are often used to commit suicide, especially in combination with alcohol.

Glutethemide (Doriden) was believed to be a safe barbiturate substitute but was found to be quite deadly because

of the long duration of its effects, which made it difficult to reverse overdoses. Placidyl is also believed to be dangerous because of its delayed metabolism. Meprobamate (Miltown, Equanil) or "happy pills" rapidly became popular as minor tranquilizers and as muscle relaxants. Methaqualone (Quaalude, Parest, Sopor) was also introduced as a sleeping pill but soon became widely abused as a "love drug" (aphrodisiac) and is no longer available by prescription.

Benzodiazepines were considered more selective as antianxiety agents with less drowsiness and a larger margin of safety than the barbiturates. Chlordiazepoxide (Librium), diazepam (Valium), and alprazolam (Xanax) have been the most popular benzodiazepines. As concern increased about overuse and abuse of these drugs, other antianxiety agents have been developed such as buspirone (BuSpar), which is not sedating, does not cause functional impairment, and is not believed to cause physical dependence.

Two patterns of abuse and dependence have been recognized with sedative-hypnotics. The first pattern begins with prescription use of the drug for treatment of anxiety or insomnia. Subsequently, the client increases the dose and frequency of use without medical advice or indication. The second, more common pattern involves illegal sources, which often begins with intermittent use by teenagers or young adults at parties to get "high" and leads to daily use and rapid tolerance.

Clinical manifestations of abuse. Sedative-hypnotics act primarily on the CNS. They depress cardiac and respiratory function and are largely metabolized in the liver and excreted in the urine. Benzodiazepines are thought to act by increasing the inhibitory neural effects of the neurotransmitter γ-aminobutyric acid.

The effects of this group of drugs are dose related (Table 60-7). With low doses, sedation and calming effects occur, whereas with high doses, they act as hypnotics and sleep is induced. They decrease the time needed to fall asleep, increase total sleep time, but decrease the amount of REM (rapid eye movement) sleep or dream sleep. Excessive amounts produce an initial euphoria and a state of intoxication similar to alcohol intoxication, including impaired judgment, slurred speech, and loss of motor coordination.

Tolerance develops rapidly with a narrowing margin of safety between the intoxicating effects and the lethal dose. Accidental overdoses may occur because of differences in tolerance. Tolerance develops to the sedative effects, requiring higher doses to achieve euphoria. The tolerance may not have developed to the brain-stem-depressant effects, so an increased dose may trigger hypotension and respiratory depression resulting in death.

Barbiturates and benzodiazepines may be classified on the basis of their length of action as short, intermediate, or long acting. Generally, the short-acting barbiturates are more likely to lead to dependence and abuse than are the long-acting benzodiazepines. The benzodiazepines have a slower onset and a longer duration of effect.

The benzodiazepines affect the limbic system to decrease anxiety without producing sedation at low doses. Although they are believed to have a wide margin of safety, they are not without adverse reactions, including rebound anxiety and insomnia with short-acting drugs and confusion and memory loss with long-acting drugs. They should be used cautiously in individuals who are older, who have organic brain disorders, or who are taking other drugs such as narcotics, antidepressants, antipsychotics, antihypertensives, antihistamines, other sedative-hypnotics, or alcohol. They may also cause depression, paradoxical excitement in children or older adults, sexual dysfunction, hypotension, and respiratory depression.[28]

The symptoms of mild to moderate overdose are similar to those of alcohol intoxication. The presenting signs of severe overdose include coma; cold, clammy skin; weak, rapid pulse; and slow, rapid, shallow respirations. Death may result from cardiac or respiratory arrest.

Manifestations of withdrawal from benzodiazepines include nausea and/or vomiting, muscle cramps, diaphoresis, increased sensitivity to light and sound, anxiety, dysphoria, tachycardia, hypertension, convulsions, and coarse tremors of hands, tongue, and eyelids.[20] The withdrawal syndrome may be a medical emergency, since it may progress from minor symptoms within the first 24 hours and lead to convulsions, delirium, psychoses, and respiratory and cardiac arrest. Symptoms of major withdrawal peak on the second or third day for short-acting barbiturates, benzodiazepines, and meprobamate and on the seventh or eighth day for long-acting barbiturates and benzodiazepines. Withdrawal symptoms tend to be more intense with short-acting drugs.

Therapeutic management. There are no known antagonists to counteract the effects of these drugs. Emergency life support measures must be taken in cases of overdose. In addition to the symptoms associated with overdose and withdrawal, there can be complications associated with the route of administration. These may include cellulitis, vascular complications, serum hepatitis, endocarditis, pneumonia, tetanus, other bacterial infections, and AIDS.

Treatment of dependent individuals must include a gradual withdrawal of the drug. Most individuals who have been abusing large amounts of these drugs need to be hospitalized to manage symptoms of withdrawal safely. Withdrawal from sedatives, especially barbiturates, can be fatal. Withdrawal from benzodiazepines may be less severe. The most common treatment approach is the use of pentobarbital (Nembutal) to determine the degree of dependence and the use of phenobarbital in graduated doses for detoxification.[21]

Nursing management includes ensuring safety, preventing injury, and halting the progression of symptoms. Specific nursing approaches include careful monitoring of vital signs and levels of orientation and providing reassurance and orientation as needed. Clients who have overdosed must be treated aggressively and may require dialysis to decrease the drug level and to prevent irreversible CNS depressant effects and death. It is important to avoid the use of any CNS stimulants in the treatment of overdose.

Alcohol

Etiology. Three main patterns of alcohol abuse or dependence exist. One pattern consists of consuming large amounts on a daily basis. A second pattern consists of

Table 60-13 Risk Factors Related to Alcoholism

History of alcoholism in family
History of total abstinence
Broken or disrupted home
Last or near last child in large family
Female relatives with history of recurrent depression
Heavy smoking
Member of specific cultural groups
    Irish
    Scandinavian
    Native American
    Eskimo

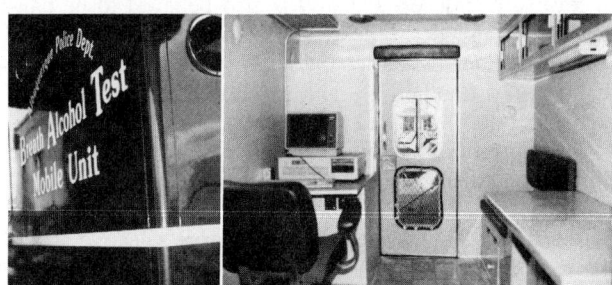

Fig. 60-4 **A,** Breath alcohol test mobile unit and **B,** intox-ilyzer (breathalyzer) used by police departments to measure blood alcohol levels. (Courtesy Albuquerque Police Department, Albuquerque, NM.)

drinking large amounts on weekends. A third pattern consists of binge drinking of large amounts for weeks or months with long intervening periods of sobriety. The average alcoholic has alternating periods of abstinence and heavy drinking. The course of dependence generally occurs over a period of 5 to 30 years and may be preceded by stages of heavy social drinking and alcohol abuse in which multiple medical, legal, social, and occupational complications are experienced.[22]

Types of drinking behavior in alcoholics have also been identified. A gamma type or "loss of control" style of drinking that involves tolerance, craving, and withdrawal symptoms is the most common type and is frequently seen in members of Alcoholics Anonymous. Recently, two types of alcoholism have been identified that result from genetic predisposition. Type I (milieu limited) may be found in both genders, has a late onset (after the age of 25), and is environmentally provoked but involves genetic factors. Type II (male-limited) is highly heritable, has an early onset (before the age of 25), has limited environmental influences, and is associated with serious law-breaking.[2]

Alcohol dependence and abuse are frequently associated with use and abuse of cannabis, cocaine, heroin, amphetamines, and sedative-hypnotics, particularly in adolescents and adults under the age of 30. The combination of alcohol and benzodiazepines is more common in middle age. The onset of drinking for males usually occurs in the late teens or twenties, with the first hospitalization in the late thirties or forties and symptoms of dependence after 45 years of age. The onset of drinking for females occurs later and is usually associated with a history of a mood disorder.[19] Hospitalization and symptoms of dependence may occur at an earlier age for women because of a more rapid progression of effects. Women tend to be solitary drinkers and combine alcohol with other drugs.

Risk factors include a family history of alcoholism or recurrent depressions, which may have been observed in grandparents, aunts, uncles, parents, or siblings. Daughters, as well as sons, of alcoholic fathers are at risk for the development of problems with alcohol. Increasing attention has been given to the children of alcoholics and the problems that they may experience as adults. Risk factors related to alcoholism are summarized in Table 60-13.

Clinical manifestations of abuse. Alcohol depresses the CNS; it crosses the blood-brain barrier and interacts with brain cell membranes, affecting specific proteins in the function of certain neurotransmitters such as γ-aminobutyric acid. Alcohol requires no digestion, since it is absorbed from the stomach and the small intestine. Alcohol is almost completely metabolized in the body and has a slow oxidation rate. The absorption rate can be decreased by food in the stomach, especially protein and fats or plain water mixed with alcohol. The rate is increased by mixing alcohol with soda water or by strong emotions. When large amounts are ingested, 10% to 15% may be eliminated unchanged from the kidneys, lungs, and skin.

The liver is the site of oxidation. The alcohol dehydrogenase system breaks alcohol down with the help of enzymes. If the enzymes are not able to work, acetaldehyde builds up in the system, and a disulfiram ethanol reaction or "Antabuse" reaction occurs. The rate of oxidation is approximately one drink per hour (7 g equals 7 ml of 100% alcohol). Alcohol (5% to 15%) is also excreted directly through the lungs, perspiration, and urine.[10] The catalase system and the microsomol enzyme oxidase system also assist in the metabolism of alcohol.

Alcohol's effects are directly proportional to the blood alcohol concentration (BAC). Because alcohol is evenly distributed in the body through the bloodstream, the BAC can be correlated with psychophysiological effects on the body. Alcohol may be measured within 15 to 20 minutes of ingestion, peaks in 60 to 90 minutes, and is excreted in 12 to 24 hours (Fig. 60-4). BAC is affected by the amount consumed, drinking rate, body composition (percent fat content), drink concentration, and hormones. For the nonalcoholic drinker, the BAC is fairly predictable. At higher levels of BAC, there is a narrow margin of safety between anesthesia and lethality[23] (Table 60-14).

Alcohol has a biphasic effect: at low doses it acts as a behavioral stimulant, and at high doses it acts as a depressant. Alcohol has a direct or indirect effect on every organ and system within the body. The organ most affected is the liver; toxic effects cause episodic problems with hepatitis and cirrhosis. Other primary target organs are the pancreas, the heart, and bone marrow. The endocrine, gas-

Table 60-14 Blood Alcohol Concentration

BAC (mg%)*	Psychophysiological Effect
20	Light and moderate drinkers begin to feel some effects. Approximate BAC is reached after one drink.
40	Most people begin to feel relaxed.
60	Judgment is mildly impaired. People are less able to make rational decisions about their capabilities (e.g., to drive).
80	Definite impairment of muscle coordination and driving skills occurs. Person is legally drunk in some states.
100	Clear deterioration of reaction time and control is observed. Person is legally drunk in most states.
120	Vomiting occurs unless this level is reached slowly.
150	Balance and movement are impaired. Equivalent of a half pint of whiskey is circulating in the bloodstream.
300	Many people lose consciousness.
400	Most people lose consciousness and some die.
450	Breathing stops; person eventually dies.

Modified from Miller WR and Munoz RF: How to control your drinking, Englewood Cliffs, NJ, 1976, Prentice-Hall, p 11.

*Blood alcohol concentration is generally recorded in milligrams of alcohol per deciliter (mg/dl) of blood, or milligrams percent (mg%). BAC is determined by how much alcohol is consumed, how fast it is consumed, and the person's weight.

trointestinal (GI), and immune systems are also important targets. Indirect effects are associated with metabolic changes that include hypoglycemia, fluid and electrolyte imbalances, hyperuricemia, low magnesium and phosphate levels, lactic acidosis, respiratory acidosis, and ketoacidosis.

Alcohol is an immunosuppressant that increases the risks for tuberculosis, viral infection, and cancer (oral, head, neck, liver, pancreas, stomach, colorectum.) It is associated with hypertension and an increased risk for coronary artery disease, stroke, myocardial infarction, and sudden cardiac death. Alcohol also has a teratogenic effect on the fetus as early as the third week of pregnancy. Fetal alcohol effects have been identified in a number of children of alcoholics. Long-term follow-up of children with fetal alcohol syndrome as adolescents showed that the effects are permanent.

Alcohol may cause mental confusion and memory problems and a number of alcohol-associated organic mental disorders, including Wernicke-Korsakoff syndrome. Wernicke's encephalopathy develops within days to weeks. It has early symptoms of vomiting, nystagmus, difficulty concentrating, polyneuropathy, and a sense of unreality. It is reversible with the administration of thiamine, but it may progress to Korsakoff's psychosis (alcohol amnestic disorder), coma, and death. Korsakoff's psychosis is irreversible and involves an inability to recall or assimilate new information but is not accompanied by dementia or delirium.[24]

Intoxication is evident with increasing BAC and represents the four stages of anesthesia. It may be mild, moderate, or severe, and it may result in coma. Intoxication is also evident in behavioral and physical changes. Behavioral changes include aggressiveness, impaired judgment, impaired attention, irritability, euphoria, depression, and emotional lability. Physical signs include slurred speech, incoordination, unsteady gait, nystagmus, and flushed face. Long-term alcoholics are able to mask the signs because of developed tolerance.

Major indicators of alcoholism are a physical disease related to alcohol use (e.g., cirrhosis), alcohol withdrawal, physical tolerance, a belief of an inability to control drinking, and continued abusive drinking in spite of known hazards. Blackouts (periods for which an individual has no memory but was conscious) are an early sign of abuse and a probable sign of alcoholism. Psychological signs of alcoholism include depression, frequent references to drinking, relief drinking for negative feelings or physical or social discomforts, and the use of defense mechanisms, such as denial, projection, rationalization, all-or-none thinking, and avoidance to minimize the consequences and to maintain the drinking behavior. Behavioral signs associated with alcoholism reflect impaired functioning as a result of drinking in the areas of family relationships, employment, and legal or social situations. As the disease progresses, the individual becomes more focused on drinking activities to the exclusion of all else.

Alcohol withdrawal is a state of CNS hyperactivity and irritability, or rebound reaction, to a marked decrease (20% BAC) in consumption or cessation of alcohol after periods of frequent or prolonged heavy drinking. Hangovers, which appear early in alcohol use, are replaced by symptoms of withdrawal. Four characteristic signs of withdrawal are gross tremor, grand mal seizures, hallucinosis, and delirium tremens (DTs).[25] (Hallucinosis is a sensory perceptual problem in which the individual is aware that the experience is not real.)

Most alcoholics experience a mild or minor withdrawal syndrome in the first 8 to 12 hours after the last drink. Some individuals progress to a major syndrome or DTs, which include more disorientation, visual or auditory hallucinations, and increased autonomic hyperactivity without seizures. Death may be caused by hyperthermia, peripheral circulatory collapse, or cardiac failure.

Diagnostic studies. Early recognition and identification of clients with alcohol-related problems is critical to successful treatment outcomes. The nurse must be aware of the wide range of signs and symptoms of alcohol abuse and dependence. The nurse in the medical-surgical setting needs to operate from a high level of suspicion to accurately assist in screening clients and to assess responses to questions and treatments (Fig. 60-5).

A quick assessment for alcohol and drug emergency conditions is essential for all incoming clients, regardless of age or condition, and particularly for accident or trauma victims (Table 60-15). A thorough psychosocial assess-

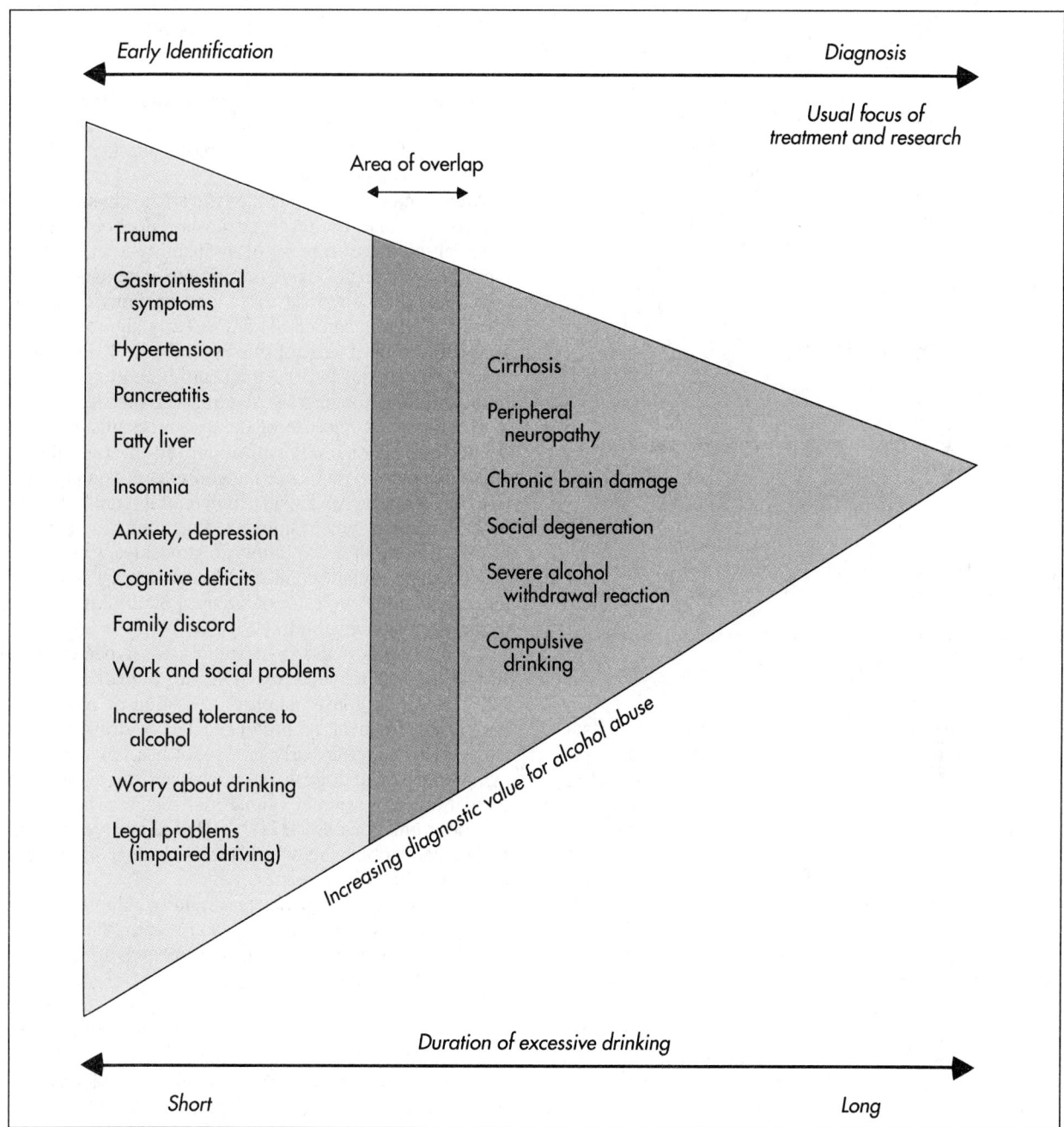

Fig. 60-5 Early recognition of alcohol-related illnesses and other problems. (From Skinner HA: Early intervention for alcohol and drug problems: core issues for medical education, Aust Drug Alcohol Rev 5:69-74, 1986.)

Table 60-15 Assessment Guide for Alcohol and Drug Emergency Conditions

Aspects affecting impending withdrawal

When did you have your last drink?

When did you start your last drinking bout?

What have you been drinking during this last drinking episode?

How much alcohol did you consume each day during your last drinking episode?

In the past, what reactions have you experienced when you stopped drinking?

☐ Tremors   ☐ Seizures

☐ Hearing or seeing things   ☐ Other_____

☐ DTs

Have you ever taken Dilantin or any other drug for seizures?

What other medications, if any, are you currently taking?

☐ Prescription   ☐ Over the counter   ☐ Street drugs

Are you allergic to any drugs?

Potential emergency conditions

Do you have any chronic health problems?

☐ Diabetes   ☐ Stomach

☐ Lung   ☐ Liver

☐ Heart   ☐ Other_____

Have you recently experienced any of the following?

☐ Pain   ☐ Difficulty keeping your balance

☐ Bleeding

☐ Breathing problems   ☐ Double vision

☐ Vomiting   ☐ Periods of confusion

☐ Diarrhea   ☐ Other

Have you recently been injured?

☐ Fight   ☐ Fall

☐ Auto crash   ☐ Other_____

Modified from Estes NJ, Smith-DiJulio K, and Heinemann ME: Nursing diagnosis of the alcoholic person, St Louis, 1980, The CV Mosby Co, p 106.

ment must be done, when indicated, and it should cover drinking history and current health and social problems. It is essential to obtain information about current and past alcohol and drug use patterns.

The way in which the nurse poses questions and the nonverbal messages conveyed about clients affect their willingness to respond.[25] The nurse must use an open and nonjudgmental approach and stress the importance of having an accurate alcohol and drug history for the health care team to provide effective care and prevent any unexpected complications.[26]

Clients' use of denial should not be viewed as a major roadblock but as an opportunity to provide them with new information about their condition and the effects and consequences of alcohol use. Denial may be circumvented by asking indirect questions such as, "How often has drinking caused you pain?" The nursing diagnosis of "ineffective denial" addresses some useful outcome criteria and interventions (Table 60-16).

Some useful screening tools include the Alcohol Use Disorders Identification Test (AUDIT) (a 10-item questionnaire to identify early-stage problem drinkers), the Short Michigan Alcoholism Screening Test (MAST) (a 13-item tool), and the CAGE questionnaire (a four-item mnemonic tool) (Tables 60-17 and 60-18).[27-29]

Laboratory tests that may provide evidence of alcoholism are liver function tests, complete blood count, fasting blood sugar, blood urea nitrogen, serum electrolytes, urinalysis, serology, stool sample for occult blood, electrocardiogram, and chest x-ray film. Biochemical markers include blood levels of γ-glutamyltransferase (GGT), aspartate serum aminotransaminase (AST), alkaline phosphatase, and mean corpuscular volume.

Therapeutic management. Initial treatment is aimed at detoxification and stabilization of the client's condition. The most frequent emergency room problems related to alcohol are accidents and toxic reactions. Toxic reactions occur as the result of combining alcohol with another drug and may lead to respiratory and circulatory failure without adequate intervention. Naloxone (Narcan), an opiate antagonist, may be given if opiates have been used with alcohol. Toxicology screens identify types of drugs (including alcohol) and levels present. Methanol (wood alcohol), ethylene glycol (antifreeze), and isopropyl alcohol (rubbing alcohol) may be found in accidental overdoses or suicide attempts involving the homeless, older adults, children, or poor individuals.

Acute alcohol intoxication may present as an emergency; it is important to obtain an accurate history and to check vital signs and proceed with the ABCs if necessary. Body temperature needs to be assessed in addition to pulse rate. Generally, the pulse rate is normal in uncomplicated intoxication but elevated in withdrawal. Hypotension may be a sign of occult bleeding. Clients who are hypoglycemic should be given thiamine before they receive dextrose to prevent Wernicke's encephalopathy.

A rapid physical examination including a neurological status should focus on signs of dehydration, hypertension, head or spinal trauma, infection, liver disease, and myopathy or rhabdomyolysis. Seizures may occur and are managed with an anticonvulsant such as diazepam or phenobarbital. It is critical to continue assessments until the BAC has decreased to at least 100 mg% and until any associated disorders or injuries have been ruled out. A satisfactory BAC is usually reached within 6 to 8 hours.

Alcohol withdrawal or detoxification is the first step in the management of the disease. The goals of treatment for withdrawal are to prevent the progression of symptoms, to provide for the safety and comfort of clients, and to engage them in long-term treatment. Clients need to be carefully assessed, since alcohol withdrawal may be life threatening. Most of the life-threatening conditions occur during the first few days of withdrawal. Generally, acute withdrawal lasts for 3 to 5 days. The Clinical Institute Withdrawal Assessment of Alcohol (CIWA-A) scale is a reliable and practical tool for evaluating the severity of alcohol withdrawal.[30]

Individuals experiencing withdrawal may also be suffering from other illnesses, underlying conditions, or trauma. The most common severe manifestations are hallucinations

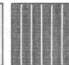

Table 60-16

NURSING CARE PLAN FOR THE CLIENT WITH DENIAL OF ALCOHOL OR DRUG ABUSE

Defining Characteristics	Nursing Interventions	Evaluation Criteria

NURSING DIAGNOSIS: Ineffective denial related to refusal to acknowledge substance abuse or dependency

Defining Characteristics	Nursing Interventions	Evaluation Criteria
Delay in seeking or refusal of health care to detriment of health, lack of perception of personal relevance of symptoms or danger, self-treatment, minimization of symptoms, lack of admittance of impact of disease on life, inappropriate affect, blaming of others for problems, use of rationalization or intellectualization	Present facts regarding the nature of alcoholism and drug addiction. Help client focus on present, *not* on the reasons for the problem. Assist client in identifying and altering patterns of substance abuse (e.g., explain medical consequences). Do *not* argue about whether client is an "alcoholic" or "abuser" or allow client to use blame of others, rationalization, or intellectualization. Assist client in identifying effect of substance abuse on life and significant others (i.e., motivation to stop abuse). Support insight on behaviors and consequences. Help client to express affect in acceptable manner. Assist client to improve self-esteem. Instill a sense of hope. Discuss alternative coping strategies, that is, anticipation of stressful events, development of problem-solving and assertiveness skills. Assist client in resocialization and building support system, including groups (e.g., Alcoholics Anonymous, Narcotics Anonymous). Assist client in achieving abstinence (e.g., set short-term goals, evaluate negative consequences). Initiate referral as indicated.	Ability to explain psychological and physiological effects of alcohol and drug use, admission of alcohol and drug abuse problem, expression of sense of hope, use of alternative coping mechanisms to relieve stress, recognition of need for continued treatment

---

Table 60-17   Short Michigan Alcoholism Screening Test

		Yes	No
1.	Do you feel you are a normal drinker? (A normal drinker is a person who drinks less than or as much as most other people) (No)*	Yes_____	No_____
2.	Does your wife, husband, a parent, or other near relative ever worry or complain about your drinking? (Yes)	Yes_____	No_____
3.	Do you ever feel guilty about your drinking? (Yes)	Yes_____	No_____
4.	Do friends and relatives think you are a normal drinker? (One who drinks less than or no more than most other people) (No)	Yes_____	No_____
5.	Are you able to stop drinking when you want to? (No)	Yes_____	No_____
6.	Have you ever attended a meeting of Alcoholics Anonymous (for your personal concerns about your own drinking) (Yes)	Yes_____	No_____
7.	Has drinking ever created problems between you and your wife, husband, a parent, or other near relative? (Yes)	Yes_____	No_____
8.	Have you ever gotten into trouble at work because of drinking? (Yes)	Yes_____	No_____
9.	Have you ever neglected your obligations, your family, or your work for two or more days in a row because you were drinking? (Yes)	Yes_____	No_____
10.	Have you ever gone to anyone for help about your drinking? (Yes)	Yes_____	No_____
11.	Have you ever been in a hospital because of your drinking? (Yes)	Yes_____	No_____
12.	Have you ever been arrested for drunken driving, driving while intoxicated, or driving under the influence of alcohol? (Yes)	Yes_____	No_____
13.	Have you ever been arrested, even for a few hours, because of other drunken behavior? (Yes)	Yes_____	No_____

From Selzer M, Vinokur A, and van Roojen L: A self-administered short alcoholism screening test (SMAST), J Stud Alcohol 36:86, 1975.
*Alcoholism-indicating responses appear in parentheses.
Scoring: 0-1, nonalcoholic; 2, possibly alcoholic; 3 or more, alcoholic.

Table 60-18   The CAGE Questionnaire*

C Have you ever felt you should *cut* down on your drinking?

A Have people *annoyed* you by criticizing your drinking?

G Have you ever felt bad or *guilty* about your drinking?

E Have you ever had a drink first thing in the morning to steady your nerves or get rid of a hangover (*eye-opener*)?

From Mayfield D, and others: The CAGE questionnaire: validation of a new alcoholism screening instrument, Am J Psychiatry 131:1121, 1974.
*A score of two or three "yes" responses strongly suggests alcoholism.

and grand mal seizures. The progression of withdrawal to DTs can be prevented by prompt early treatment (Table 60-19). A quiet, calm environment is important to prevent exacerbation of symptoms. The use of restraints, IVs, and side rails should be avoided whenever possible. Supportive care is needed to ensure adequate rest and nutrition. It is important not to overhydrate clients, particularly individuals with renal or cardiac disease, since overhydration could lead to sudden dysrhythmias. The majority of clients improve without medical treatment.

Medications may be useful in decreasing symptoms, increasing levels of comfort, and decreasing the risk of convulsions and DTs. Benzodiazepines are the most effective agent in preventing and treating alcohol withdrawal seizures and DTs; in addition, three newer agents have also been promising, β-adrenergic blockers (atenolol), clonidine, and calcium channel blockers. Clients who are intoxicated with rising BACs should not be given other depressants because of their additive effects. Inadequate treatment of alcohol withdrawal may precipitate more severe stages of the current withdrawal and produce more severe symptoms in future withdrawals.

Special problems. A *protracted withdrawal syndrome,* "dry drunk," or protracted abstinence withdrawal may occur as a delayed reaction after abstinence and the normal period of withdrawal. The individual exhibits signs of anxiety, irritability, hostility, depression, insomnia, or fatigue, which last 3 weeks to 3 months. This should not be confused with an acute withdrawal syndrome that follows a drinking episode with falling BAC. Although these symptoms may precipitate a relapse, they do not occur as the result of a "slip." Treatment may include the use of anxiolytics, antidepressants, antipsychotics, or β-adrenergic blockers.

Although cessation of drinking is the short-term goal that is accomplished through detoxification and the withdrawal process, social rehabilitation and prolonged abstinence are the primary long-term goals. The aim of intervention is to assist the client to see the adverse consequences of drinking and to make appropriate lifestyle changes. The earlier an individual engages in treatment, the greater are the chances of recovery. A formal intervention process may be planned and implemented if an individual's situation is critical and if that person is unwilling or unable to recognize a problem with alcohol. This consists of a planned meeting by concerned friends, family, and co-workers who confront the individual with their observations and how the drinking behavior has affected them personally; they insist that the individual enter treatment.

A variety of inpatient and outpatient treatment programs are available. There is no evidence that inpatient programs are more effective than outpatient programs. The needs of each client should be matched to the particular goals and approaches of a treatment program.

Aftercare services are very important to sustain the individual in recovery. These may include family counseling, group meetings, and/or individual counseling. The family and the work environment are critical in assisting individuals in recovery to return to healthy patterns of functioning. A number of drugs have been used as adjuncts in aftercare programs, including agents that repress the desire to drink such as bromocriptine and naltrexone and agents that prevent drinking by causing aversive consequences when alcohol is consumed such as disulfiram (Antabuse).

Spontaneous remission can occur for approximately one fourth of alcoholics.[10] Vailliant[22] describes the natural healing processes of alcoholics in which others, including health care professionals, provide the care and understanding to decrease suffering and the risk of mortality until self-healing occurs.

Drug interactions with alcohol. The interaction of other substances with alcohol may produce four different effects—antagonistic, additive, synergistic, and cross-tolerant. *Antagonistic* effects occur when the effect of either substance is blocked or decreased. These effects are seen with the antialcohols, some hypoglycemics, and some antibiotics. The disulfiram-ethanol reaction occurs within 5 to 10 minutes of drinking alcohol in individuals taking Antabuse. It may produce flushing, headache, bounding pulse, diaphoresis, nausea, vomiting, and vasomotor collapse with orthostatic hypotension.[31]

Additive effects are enhanced effects of two substances that equal the combined effects of both substances. Drugs that interact with alcohol in this manner include antihypertensives, antihistamines, marijuana, antianginals (nitrates), and analgesics (salicylates). Alcohol taken with aspirin may exacerbate GI bleeding. Cardiovascular drugs and alcohol may cause digitalis toxicity. Alcohol and nitrates may lead to postural hypotension, faintness, and loss of consciousness.

Synergistic effects are the most dangerous, since the combined effects of the two drugs are multiplied. Substances that interact in this manner with alcohol include the barbiturates, benzodiazepines, meprobamate, chloral hydrate, paraldehyde, narcotics, and anesthetics. Most of these substances potentiate depressant effects and often lead to respiratory failure and death. Alcohol may produce either a synergistic or an antagonistic effect when used with antidepressants.

Cross-tolerance is increased sensitivity to the effects of other substances in similar drug categories. Once sensitized to certain drugs, a greater amount of those drugs is

Table 60-19

 NURSING CARE PLAN FOR THE CLIENT IN ALCOHOL WITHDRAWAL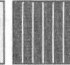

Defining Characteristics	Nursing Interventions	Evaluation Criteria
NURSING DIAGNOSIS: High risk for injury related to sensorimotor deficits, seizure activity, and confusion		
Impaired mobility— unsteady gait, sensory deficits, tremors; impaired judgment, disorientation; seizure activity	Monitor vital signs every 3 min to 1 hr, especially increased pulse rate. Use side rails. Assist with walking and personal hygiene. Provide support and reassurance. Use seizure precautions. Administer benzodiazepines, vitamins, anticonvulsants as ordered.	Absence of falls or injuries, decrease in tremors and psychomotor activity, absence of seizures
NURSING DIAGNOSIS: Sensory/perceptual alterations related to sensory overload		
Inaccurate interpretation of environmental stimuli, disorientation in time or place or about people, anxious, fearful, auditory or visual hallucinations	Stay with client. Provide quiet, nonstimulating, well-lit environment. Orient to nurse and environment with each contact. Use calm, matter-of-fact approach. Explain procedures and what is expected. Do not reinforce fears or hallucinations by agreeing or disagreeing. Present reality clearly with "I" statements.	Absence of hallucinations, maintenance of contact with reality, proper orientation to person, place, time
NURSING DIAGNOSIS: Pain related to symptoms of withdrawal from alcohol		
Communications of discomfort, increased pulse, tachypnea, diaphoresis, tremors, seizures, nausea and vomiting, difficulty in sleeping, restlessness	Provide medications to relieve symptoms (e.g., benzodiazepines) as ordered. Provide comfort measures, decrease stimuli. Teach relaxation techniques.	Sense of well-being, comfort; normal vital signs; absence of tremors, nausea, vomiting; increase in appetite, ability to sleep
NURSING DIAGNOSIS: Ineffective individual coping related to lack of knowledge of problem-solving and assertiveness skills		
Inappropriate use of alcohol and other drugs, inability to problem solve, depression, suicidal thoughts, association of anger or guilt with managing stressors	Assist client to express negative thoughts and feelings (sadness, hopelessness, anger, guilt). Assess degree of depression and suicidal or homicidal thoughts or poor impulse control. Make referral if indicated. Teach steps of problem solving. Assist client in practicing assertive responses to stressful situations.	Decrease in depression, increase in expression of thoughts and feelings, problem-solving ability, assertiveness

Table 60-19

 NURSING CARE PLAN FOR THE CLIENT IN ALCOHOL WITHDRAWAL—cont'd

Defining Characteristics	Nursing Interventions	Evaluation Criteria
NURSING DIAGNOSIS: Sleep pattern disturbance related to increased CNS stimulation		
Feelings of fear, restlessness, agitation, hallucinations, mood alterations, fatigue, dozing, difficulty falling or remaining asleep	Monitor sleep pattern. Identify contributing factors. Reduce or eliminate environmental distractions (lights, noise) and interruptions. Provide comfort measures—bedtime routine, bathing, snacks, massage, music, reading. Assist with relaxation activities (e.g., walking, simple exercises), if client is able. Decrease potential for injury during sleep (e.g., use night lights, low bed).	Ability to describe factors that prevent or inhibit sleep, use of techniques to induce or maintain sleep, normal sleep patterns and rested feeling after sleep
NURSING DIAGNOSIS: High risk for violence related to alcohol or drug abuse and/or depression		
Feelings of fear, suicidal or homicidal thoughts, hallucinations, environmental misperceptions, poor impulse control, panic	Assess level of risk. Provide safe environment on the basis of risk level, including informing staff of risk. Use medications or restraints if necessary. Communicate expectation of need to maintain control of behavior (no harm to self or others). Use clear, simple language. Express concern and hope that client will feel better. Provide reassurance that feelings are temporary.	No exhibition of self-destructive or violent behavior, maintenance of control over behavior, acceptance of help, use of effective coping mechanisms to handle stress
NURSING DIAGNOSIS: Altered health maintenance related to lack of knowledge of progression of alcoholism and its effects and relapse prevention		
Inappropriate use of alcohol and other drugs; inaccurate or lack of knowledge of signs and symptoms of alcoholism, nature of disease, effect on body; repeated relapses; inability to maintain sobriety	Provide educational information to client and family about alcoholism—development, effects, and consequences. Teach early warning signs of relapse. Assist client in rehearsing responses to stressful situations or triggers to drinking. Provide names of resources to call for help. Support abstinence and participation in support groups (e.g., Alcoholics Anonymous). Refer to treatment program or counseling, if indicated.	Recognition of signs and symptoms of disease, knowledge of warning signs of relapse, plan for seeking help at first sign of relapse, abstinence from alcohol, regular participation in support groups

required to obtain the same effect. Alcohol is cross-tolerant to other depressants, including opiates, anticonvulsants, and anesthetics. Acute intoxication increases the effects of anticonvulsants and anticoagulants, and long-term alcohol use decreases the effects of anticonvulsants and anticoagulants.

Surgical interventions. Special precautions must be taken for clients who are intoxicated or alcohol dependent and require surgery. Alcoholic shock as a cause of a decreased pulse and a high BAC may be overlooked in an accident victim. The client may be taken to surgery to stop internal bleeding because of the decreased pulse.[32] Many persons are undiagnosed as alcoholics at the time of admission for surgery. Health problems such as malnutrition, dehydration, and infection may need to be treated before surgery can be performed. Clients who are alcohol dependent but have no alcohol in their systems usually require an *increased* level of anesthesia because of cross-tolerance. The intoxicated individual needs a *decreased* level of anesthesia because of the synergistic effect of the alcohol present in the system.

Whenever possible, surgery is postponed until the BAC is less than 200 mg%. In individuals with a BAC over 150 mg% a synergistic effect occurs with anesthesia. Clients with a BAC over 250 mg% present a significantly increased surgical risk and mortality rate.[32] Acute withdrawal and DTs may be triggered by surgery and the cessation of alcohol consumption. Surgery should be delayed for at least 48 to 72 hours, if possible, or IV alcohol may be given if immediate surgery is required to avoid this reaction. Alcohol interferes with pulmonary function and may be associated with increased incidence of hepatic dysfunction, poor wound healing, and metabolic abnormalities that can affect the outcome of surgery. Vital signs, including body temperature, must be closely monitored to identify signs of withdrawal, possible infections, and system failure.

Opiates

Opium is an extract harvested from the poppy, *Papaver somniferum.* The primary nonsynthetic narcotics that are alkaloids of opium primarily include morphine and codeine. Thebaine is a major alkaloid of another variety of poppy and is converted to codeine, hydrocodone, oxycodone, oxymorphone, nalbuphine, naloxone, and the Bentley compounds. Semisynthetic narcotics include heroin, hydromorphone (Dilaudid), oxycodone, etorphine, and diprenorphine. Synthetic narcotics include meperidine (Demerol), methadone, levo-α-acetylmethadol, and propoxyphene (Darvon). Narcotic antagonists include naloxone (Narcan) and nalorphine (Nalline).

Etiology. Patterns of opium abuse may be seen in medical abusers or individuals who misuse analgesics in a medical setting, street abusers, or abusers who get methadone legally. Initial use in teens or young adults begins with peer-group encouragement to get high and may include use of a combination of drugs, which may continue after opioid use is established.

Clinical manifestations of abuse. Opiates are CNS depressants and have been found to act on neurotransmitters.

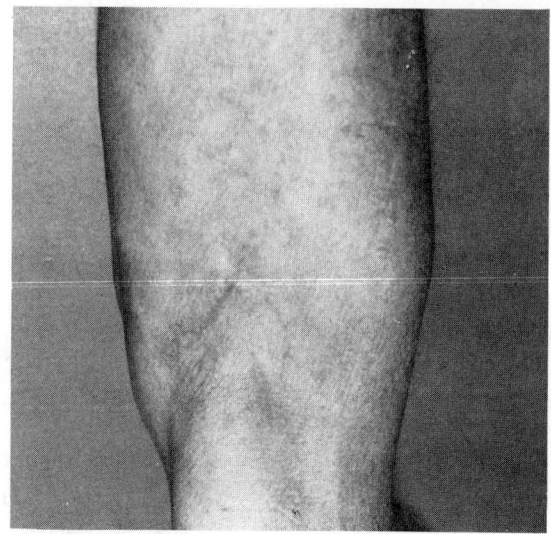

Fig. 60-6 IV drug use. The V-shaped track mark in the antecubital fossa is darkened due to increased use and scarring.

Endogenous opiates, endorphins and enkephalins, have been discovered in the brain, pituitary gland, and adrenal gland, and they appear to regulate pain perception. Opiates are detoxified in the liver and excreted in urine and bile. Most of the metabolites, with the exception of methadone, are excreted within 24 hours but may be found in the urine for up to 48 hours.[33]

Narcotics are the most effective medicines to relieve intense pain and are also useful as cough suppressants (antitussives) and to treat intestinal disorders such as colic and diarrhea. Narcotics are usually prescribed for oral use or intramuscular injection. As drugs of abuse, they are sniffed, smoked, or self-administered by subcutaneous ("skin-popping") or IV ("mainlining") injection (Fig. 60-6).

Heroin is rapidly converted to morphine in the body. The standard guideline for producing analgesia is 10 mg morphine. By comparison, 3 to 4 mg morphine is roughly equivalent to 1 to 2 mg heroin, 0.5 mg hydromorphone (Dilaudid), 20 mg meperidine, and 30 mg codeine.[34] Hydromorphone is shorter acting, more sedating than morphine, and two to eight times as potent. Percodan is aspirin plus oxycodone. Etorphine (a Bentley compound) is more than 1000 times as potent as morphine.[15]

Abuse of methadone commonly causes overdose. It is as potent as morphine, but addiction occurs at a lower level than with morphine and has longer-lasting effects. Methadone does not produce sedation; it is a powerful antitussive and spasmolytic. Propoxyphene (Darvon), which is related to methadone, is less dependence producing and less effective as an analgesic. Levo-α-acetylmethadol is related to methadone and is currently under investigation.

The primary effects of narcotics are analgesia, drowsiness, changes in mood, and at high doses, clouding of mental functioning (see Table 60-7). Relief of suffering may provide a short-term euphoria. However, initial ef-

fects are frequently unpleasant. Effects include pinpoint pupils, reduced vision, apathy, decreased physical activity, constipation, nausea, vomiting, and even respiratory depression. There is usually no loss of motor coordination or slurred speech as observed in use of other depressants. IV use usually causes a "kick" or "rush" of feelings in the lower abdomen, along with warm skin flushing, an intoxicated feeling, euphoria, and decreased respiratory rate, peristalsis, and pupil size. The narcotics lead to a rapid tolerance and physical dependence after short-term use.

The signs of opioid intoxication may be seen within 2 to 5 minutes of IV use, beginning with euphoria and progressing to lethargy, somnolence, apathy, and dysphoria. Pupil constriction is present unless anoxia occurs with severe overdose, which leads to pupil dilatation. Unintentional overdose frequently occurs with illicit use of narcotics because of the unpredictability in potency and purity. Some narcotic overdoses may be actual suicide attempts. Signs of overdose include decreased respiration, blue lips, pale or blue skin, pinpoint pupils, hyperemia, recent needle marks, pulmonary edema, cardiac dysrhythmias, and/or convulsions. Death is usually due to respiratory depression and pulmonary and/or cerebral edema.

Withdrawal from opioids occurs with cessation of prolonged moderate to heavy use or decreased amount or the administration of an antagonist along with at least three of the following symptoms: craving, nausea or vomiting, muscle aches, lacrimation or rhinorrhea, pupillary dilatation, piloerection ("gooseflesh") or perspiration, diarrhea, yawning, fever, or insomnia. Generally, within 12 hours of the last dose there is physical discomfort followed by a restless sleep ("yen"), flulike symptoms, and craving. The onset of withdrawal begins at the time of the next usual dose and ranges from 4 to 6 hours for heroin to a day or longer for methadone. The kicking movements sometimes observed in clients in withdrawal are responsible for the phrase "kicking the habit." Individuals may be suicidal during withdrawal.

The severity of withdrawal is related to the degree of dependence, but it usually runs its course in 96 hours. Protracted abstinence may occur after withdrawal. Symptoms may recur for 6 to 8 months. Physical dependence may not always indicate drug abuse. Clients who receive therapeutic doses of narcotics may develop tolerance and dependence. However, when the medical conditions are resolved, the opiate is no longer needed.[35]

Medical complications may be due to the route of administration. Street heroin, which is often cut with quinine, has vasodilator effects when given IV and may lead to tetanus and tissue abscesses if administered subcutaneously (Fig. 60-7).

Therapeutic management. The short-term prognosis for narcotic addicts is very poor due to high relapse rates. The long-term prognosis is better because addicts in their 30's and 40's tend to burn-out or stop drug use. Studies indicate that treatment programs must last at least 6 months to have a significant impact on drug use.[36]

Overdose of opiates may be a medical emergency and the ABCs of cardiopulmonary resuscitation must be followed. An adequate airway must be established, vital

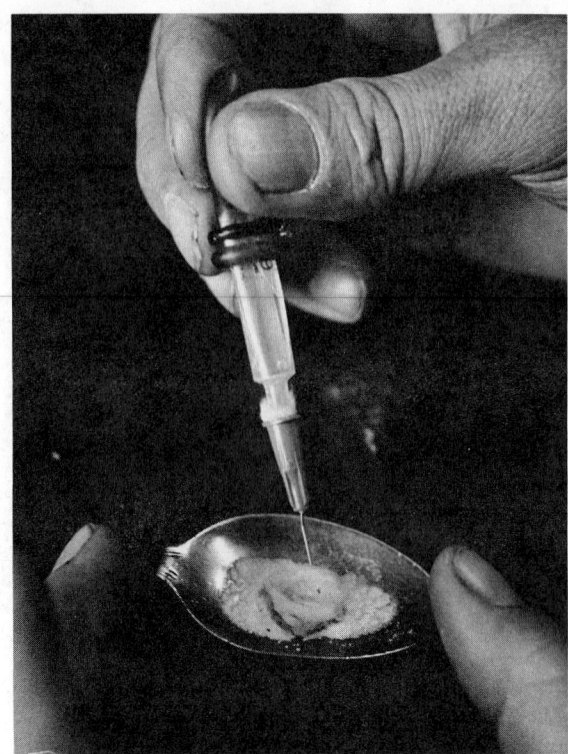

Fig. 60-7 Heroin use. (From Ray O and Ksir C: Drugs, society and human behavior, St Louis, 1990, Mosby–Year Book, Inc.)

signs must be monitored, aspiration must be prevented, and IV fluids must be started. Problems such as hypotension, dysrhythmias, and pulmonary edema are treated appropriately. Laboratory work must be done to investigate possible mixed drug ingestion. A narcotic antagonist such as naloxone, nalorphine, or levallorphan should be given before any irreversible brain anoxia develops. Vital signs provide important clues of withdrawal or infections. Precautionary tetanus immunizations are often given.

Treatment of withdrawal is related to symptoms and may not require any medication. One of the goals of treatment for opiate addicts is to assist them in maintaining a relative comfort level to engage them in a rehabilitation program. A flowsheet of symptom severity and treatment is often used for inpatient treatment programs. It is important to perform a medical examination and to take an adequate history to identify concurrent health problems and the degree of dependence.

Symptoms may be reduced by the administration of opiates in decreasing amounts over 2 weeks. Methadone is often recommended for oral use, but any opiate may be administered. Withdrawal from methadone results in fewer physical symptoms and is less severe than withdrawal from opiates. Nonopiates may also be administered for detoxification and include clonidine (Catapres) and the benzodiazepines for heroin withdrawal. A cocktail of medications such as carisoprodol (Soma), prochlorperazine (Compazine), and pentazocine (Talwin) may be effective.

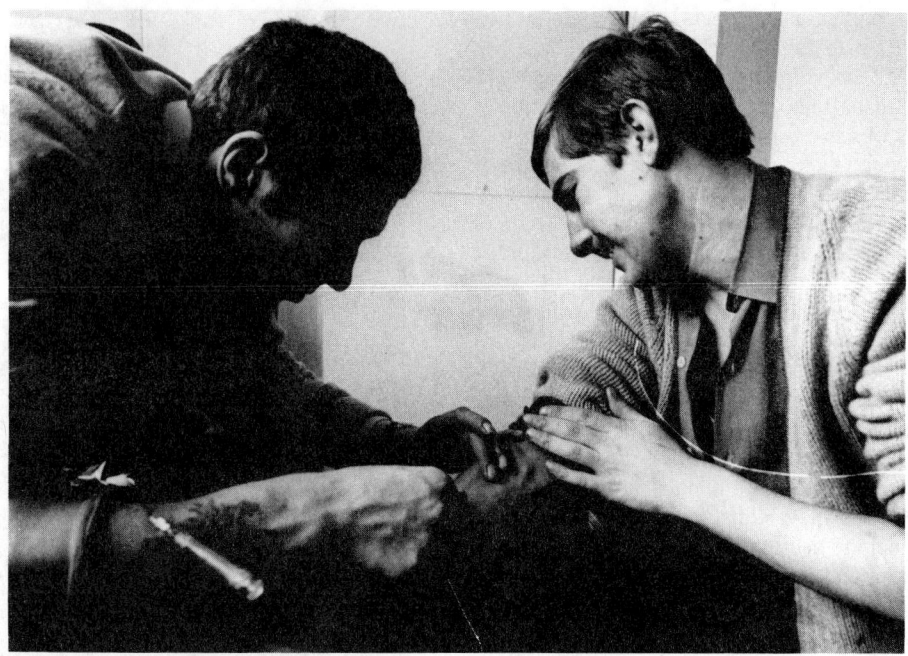

Fig. 60-8   Shooting up. Sharing needles and syringes and other contaminated "works" has increased the spread of HIV. (From Ray O and Ksir C: Drugs, society and human behavior, St Louis, 1990, Mosby–Year Book, Inc.)

In addition, acupuncture and hypnosis have also been used for relief of withdrawal symptoms.

Complications that are associated with opiate addiction include AIDS, abscesses, tetanus, malaria, hepatitis, gastric ulcers, dysrhythmias, endocarditis, anemias, electrolyte abnormalities, bone and joint infections, eye ground abnormalities, kidney failure, muscle destruction, pneumonia, lung abscesses, tuberculosis, bronchospasm and wheezing, stroke, lymphadenopathy, abnormal sexual function, and depression.

Methadone is a federally regulated synthetic narcotic that may be used in detoxification and maintenance programs for heroin addicts. Methadone maintenance is supportive therapy that is most effective when provided in addition to education and counseling programs. Methadone has been beneficial for some individuals and is the most effective method of decreasing the risk of heroin use and the most promising available treatment for IV narcotic users seeking treatment.

Opioid antagonists reverse the effect of opioid narcotics and may precipitate symptoms of withdrawal in dependent individuals. They prevent euphoria and protect against dependence. They produce analgesia and have been used to diagnose narcotic dependence. They have been used very effectively in reversing the respiratory depression associated with narcotic overdose. The most commonly administered opioid antagonists are nalorphine (Nalline) and naloxone (Narcan). Opioid agonist-antagonist agents have both analgesic and opiate-antagonist effects. Examples of these drugs include pentazocine (Talwin), buprenorphine (Temgesic), butorphanol (Stadol), nalbuphine (Nubain), and fentanyl (Sublimaze).[37]

Special problems. Opiate abusers have been found to begin initial use of tobacco and alcohol and move on to marijuana and a combination of other drugs. They return to alcohol abuse when their primary drug of choice is not available. Abusers in medical settings are usually individuals who are middle class, females, and/or individuals with pain syndromes who are frequently on more than one prescription drug. Health care professionals have the highest rate of abuse of analgesics of any middle-class population. Job stresses, interference of work with family life, long hours, and availability of drugs are considered contributing factors.

Pure heroin addiction is rare; heroin addicts usually also abuse alcohol and other nonopiate drugs. Over the past 20 years a shift in patterns of IV drug abuse from heroin to cocaine has occurred. Approximately 25% of all individuals with AIDS are IV drug abusers who compose the second largest "at risk" group for human immunodeficiency virus (HIV) infections. The number of IV drug users with AIDS is doubling almost every year.[8] This population is at risk, not only because of needle sharing but also because of the immunocompromising effects of opiate drugs. Heroin users have been found to have a higher incidence of infections, especially those associated with needle use (Figure 60-8). Drug use tends to reduce safe sex practices, which also increases the risk of contracting AIDS. Drug abuse treatment has been found to limit the spread of HIV infection by decreasing the prevalence of IV drug use and by decreasing regular drug use that impairs the immune system.

Patterns of abuse of more than one substance develop more rapidly in adolescents who tend to use several drugs

concurrently. The issue of codependence in the family needs to be addressed, along with alcohol and drug use by other family members. Families may enable teenagers' drug use either directly by giving them money or indirectly by denying the problem or being afraid to confront them. The typical pattern is a progression of stages of drug use beginning with cigarettes and alcohol and moving to marijuana and then cocaine, hallucinogens, and opiates. Most drug use is initiated with the involvement of at least one legal drug. A very rapid progression of cocaine abuse (usually within months) occurs in adolescents.[38]

HALLUCINOGENS

A number of psychoactive substances that are either natural or synthetic act to produce a change in level of consciousness, alter mood, and induce hallucinations. These drugs are classified as hallucinogens and include cannabis, peyote and mescaline, DOM or STP (2,5-dimethyl-4-methylamphetamine), DOB (4-bromo homolog of DOM), MDA (methylene dioxyamphetamine), MDMA (methylene dioxymethylamphetamine—also called "ecstasy"), psilocybin and psilocin, lysergic acid diethylamide (LSD), phencyclidine, and inhalants. Cannabis, phencyclidine, and inhalants are sometimes categorized separately, because pure hallucinations are seldom observed with use of these drugs.

Cannabis

Etiology. The cannabis group includes substances with psychoactive ingredients derived from the cannabis, or hemp, plant or chemically similar synthetic substances. The three drugs of this group that are most commonly found in the United States are marijuana, hashish, and hashish oil. Many chemicals or cannabinoids are synthesized from the cannabis plant. δ-9-Tetrahydrocannabinol (THC) is believed to be responsible for most of the psychoactive effects. Marijuana, which is derived from the dried leaves and flowering tops of the plant, is a less potent source of THC than hashish, which is a rich resinous secretion of the plant. Hashish oil, a dark viscous extraction of the plant, has a much higher percent of THC. A drop or two of hashish oil on a cigarette has the same effect as a marijuana "joint."

THC has been used to treat tetanus, migraine, postpartum psychoses, insomnia, gonorrhea, and opium addiction. Although a number of potential benefits have been reported, the only established uses are for resistant glaucoma, for the control of nausea from cancer chemotherapy, and for temporary treatment of acute asthma attacks.

Patterns of use vary from occasional to long-term, habitual use. Generally, it is the first illegal drug that is used by young people, with the exception of alcohol. Peer influence is considered the strongest predictor of use. Occasional users are more common, and they tend to smoke in groups. Daily use may lead to compulsive or all-day, everyday use.

Clinical manifestations of abuse. The mechanism of action of cannabis is uncertain, but it is believed to involve interaction with lipid components of the cell membranes. It is metabolized in the liver, is fat-soluble and stored in body fats, and has a half-life of 7 to 8 days. It is excreted as metabolites in feces and urine. Metabolites may be detectable days to weeks after brief exposures to marijuana. Tolerance occurs to many effects. Physiological dependence may develop with long-term heavy use. A mild cross-tolerance to alcohol develops. Marijuana has low toxicity, and there are no known lethal doses with its use.[10]

The effects of use depend on the dose, route of administration, personality of user, previous drug experience, user's expectations, and setting of use. Marijuana is used to cope with negative feelings; to avoid distress, boredom, and emptiness; and to self-medicate certain conditions such as affective disorders, personality disorders, and schizophrenia. Marijuana may be ingested by smoking or eating or, rarely, IV injection. It is usually smoked, and the peak plasma level occurs within 10 minutes. The most prominent effects occur in 20 to 30 minutes, and intoxication lasts from 2 to 3 hours.[10]

The most prominently affected organs appear to be the brain, the cardiovascular system, and the lungs (see Table 60-7). Most changes are reversible. Signs of intoxication include euphoria, anxiety, suspiciousness or paranoid ideation, sensation of slowed time, impaired judgment, social withdrawal, redness of conjunctiva, increased appetite (for sweets), dry mouth, and tachycardia. Problems of habitual users include impaired short-term memory, visual hallucinations (from high doses), decreased motor coordination, tremors, increased heart and respiratory rates, increased sexual arousal, and sleepiness. Marijuana use may precipitate seizures in persons with epilepsy, psychotic episodes in persons with schizophrenia, and ketoacidosis in persons with diabetes.

Acute problems range from anxiety reactions to panic attacks or psychotic episodes. Panic attacks usually occur in first-time users who are not familiar with the drug or its effects. Symptoms of panic reactions include anxiety, fear of losing control or going crazy, and fear of physical illness. Flashbacks, or reexperiencing of intense drug experiences, are time limited and involve a change in time sense or a feeling of slowed thinking. A toxic reaction that involves an organic brain syndrome or paranoia may occur. Psychotic symptoms may manifest temporarily as paranoia or hallucinations. An organic brain syndrome with a temporary clouding of mental processes may also be observed. If withdrawal symptoms are present, they are very limited and usually mild. High-dose compulsive use is believed to be associated with an amotivational syndrome in some individuals, but it is difficult to attribute a cause and effect relationship.

Medical problems associated with marijuana use are generally mild and transient. Some more serious potential problems have been reported with heavy use. These include bronchitis, increased rates of precancerous lesions in the lungs, sinusitis, pharyngitis, acute memory impairment, increased risk of cardiac problems for individuals with heart disease, depression of the immune system, and alterations in the reproductive and endocrine systems and in cell metabolism. Marijuana is widely used by individuals who are at high risk for AIDS. Some authorities sus-

pect that it alters the immune status and increases susceptibility to retrovirus infections and eventually the development of AIDS.[39]

Therapeutic management. Acute reactions, including intoxication and withdrawal, are usually mild and time limited. Individuals may be treated for toxic reactions to a combination of drugs that includes marijuana or may seek treatment for panic reactions. Most approaches depend on the characteristics and severity of symptoms. Treatment is directed toward relief of symptoms, and the administration of drugs is avoided if possible. It is important to do a physical examination and a toxicology screen and to take a thorough history. The approach is basically the same for treating panic, flashbacks, and toxic reactions. The main interventions are to provide support and reassurance to the client by explaining what is happening. A psychosis may be uncovered after the use of marijuana. The client should understand that the level of intoxication may fluctuate over several days as metabolites are released.

Individuals with cannabis intoxication or other acute problems related to cannabis use are seldom hospitalized and may be assisted in recovery by provision of a quiet environment and adequate support and reassurance. Long-term users may seek treatment for annoying symptoms rather than drug use. They may need assistance in achieving abstinence and may experience changes in their mental functioning, alertness, memory, and motivation. As with other drug use, maintaining abstinence usually entails changes in values, lifestyles, and friends.

LSD, DMT, Mescaline, and Related Substances

Etiology. Hallucinogens may be natural (such as peyote) or synthetically produced (such as LSD). Peyote or mescaline are plant products of cacti and psilocybin from fungi. Most of these substances are taken orally and introduced to adolescents by experimentation among peer groups. Some individuals find the experience unpleasant and stop use; others continue to use the drug episodically. Few individuals use these drugs daily. These drugs interfere with the ability to function effectively. Therefore with these drugs, abuse is observed more commonly than actual dependence patterns.

Clinical manifestations of abuse. The mechanism of action of these substances is unknown but is believed to be associated with the neurotransmitter serotonin. Tolerance develops rapidly with recurrent use, which necessitates use of larger doses, but tolerance disappears after use is stopped. Cross-tolerance may be found for most of the hallucinogens, including LSD, mescaline, and psilocybin, but does not extend to marijuana. Psychological dependence occurs with hallucinogens, but no significant withdrawal syndrome indicating physiological dependence is evident.

These drugs produce a change in the level of consciousness and distort the perception of reality. Senses of time, distance, and direction may be disrupted. Vivid psychedelic effects that sharpen senses and distort stimuli, including altered body images, occur. The individual may "hear" colors and "see" sounds (synesthesia). Illusions, visual hallucinations, and delusions are frequently observed with higher doses but may occur at low doses.

Hallucinogenic drugs produce a state of excitement of the CNS that alters mood and causes either euphoria or depression (see Table 60-7). Euphoria is usually present. If depression occurs and is severe, a mood disorder may develop and a suicide attempt may be made. Impaired thinking, problem solving, and judgment are common and can lead to impulsive acts and accidents. Acute anxiety, restlessness, and sleeplessness are also common. Most symptoms of use are related to sensory perception changes and psychological effects. Physical symptoms reflect adrenalinelike or adrenergic effects. They include dilated pupils, flushed face, fine tremor, increased blood pressure, elevated blood sugar levels, increased body temperature, blurred vision, tachycardia, palpitations, diaphoresis, and incoordination.

Hallucinogen intoxication or hallucinosis includes these perceptual changes. As with other types of hallucinogens, the response of the user is heavily influenced by the dose, the expectation of the user, the individual's personality, and the setting of use. The individual attributes all effects to the drug. Users may fear losing their minds or may have paranoid thoughts, which may lead (in some cases) to a delusional disorder or an acute psychotic disorder. The onset of symptoms of hallucinosis usually occurs within an hour of use and may last from 8 to 12 hours for LSD or from 1 hour to 3 days with other hallucinogens.

Mild and transitory flashbacks are common after hallucinogen use, but only severe forms are given the diagnosis of posthallucinogen perception disorder. In addition to hallucinations, other kinds of flashbacks may include feelings of depersonalization or recurrent distress. These experiences include intensified colors, flashes of color, false perceptions of movement, or halos around objects. They may be triggered by entering of a darkened area, falling asleep, use of cannabis or phenothiazine, or an acute physical or personal crisis.

LSD is a very potent drug that is produced from lysergic acid and that causes hallucinations at low doses. It may be purchased as a powder, solution, capsule or tablet, thin squares of gelatin ("window panes"), or it may be dissolved on sugar cubes or pieces of blotting paper ("blotter acid"). It is usually taken orally but may be taken subcutaneously or IV, or smoked with tobacco.

Mescaline or peyote is the second most widely used hallucinogen, and it is produced from the buttons of the peyote cactus. It is ground into a powder and taken orally. It may also be produced synthetically. Mescaline has a slower onset of action than LSD and may produce nausea and vomiting in the user.

Psilocybin is an active ingredient of "sacred" or "magic" mushrooms. It produces hallucinations similar to those of mescaline and LSD. It is taken orally and has a rapid onset. It can also be made synthetically.

DOM or STP ("serenity, tranquility, peace") is a synthetic drug similar to amphetamine and mescaline in structure and to LSD in its effects; however, it is less potent than LSD. Related drugs include DOB, MDA, and MDMA ("ecstasy," "C"). These are taken orally but may be "snorted" or injected IV. Many of the amphetamine derivatives are not federally controlled substances and there-

fore have been produced as "designer drugs" and sold as hallucinogens.

Other less potent hallucinogens include nutmeg, morning glory seeds, catnip and locoweed, nitrous oxide, and amyl or butyl nitrite. Nitrous oxide or "laughing gas" is used medically by dentists and obstetricians and as a propellant in canned whipped cream. Frequent use of nitrous oxide may result in a paranoid psychosis. Amyl and butyl nitrite are potent vasodilators that have been used in the treatment of angina. They have been used by persons who are homosexual to postpone and enhance orgasm.

Therapeutic management. Emergency problems most commonly related to abuse of LSD type of drugs are panic reactions, flashbacks, and toxic reactions. Panic reactions are a type of "bad trip" generally experienced by individuals with limited previous exposure to these drugs. The emotional dysphoria lasts for the duration of the drug's action. Treatment approaches are directed toward providing reassurance to the user, educating and orienting the user, and providing consistent verbal contact in a supportive and nonthreatening environment. Hospitalization and medications are generally not necessary. An antianxiety drug such as diazepam or chlordiazepoxide may be given if needed. A careful drug and psychosocial history are important in identifying concurrent alcohol or drug use or psychiatric problems. Because many hallucinogens are not what they are claimed to be, users may not know what substances they have taken.

Flashbacks are generally approached in the same manner. It is important that the use of marijuana, antihistamines, and stimulants be avoided in the treatment of flashbacks. Toxic reactions usually have a rapid onset and clear within 24 hours except for reactions to STP or PCP. Approaches follow the same outline that is used for panic reactions, with close monitoring of vital signs and ABCs to deal with life-threatening emergencies such as convulsions and hyperthermia. A physical assessment that includes a neurological examination should be done. Any psychosis or organic brain syndrome is treated symptomatically until it resolves or until an underlying problem is identified. An amotivational syndrome has been described for long-term hallucinogen abusers.

PCP

Etiology. PCP was developed as a general anesthetic but serious side effects including agitation, hallucinations, confusion, and delirium caused its use to be discontinued. It is a white crystalline powder that also comes in tablets, capsules, and liquid. It is commonly sprinkled on leafy material such as parsley or oregano and smoked. It may also be taken orally or IV or inhaled. It is usually first encountered as a contaminant of other illegal substances and is frequently misrepresented as mescaline, LSD, or THC.

PCP is believed to pose a greater risk than any other drug of abuse except crack. It is usually taken episodically in binges or "runs" rather than daily. Abuse or dependence develops after a minimal exposure to PCP. Patterns of use tend to increase with age, and the average user is 20 to 30 years of age. There have been some signs that use of PCP may be decreasing in prevalence.[10]

Clinical manifestations of abuse. Sympathomimetic or cholinergic effects, such as perspiring, flushing, drooling, and pupil constriction, occur with the use of PCP. It is not clear whether tolerance or withdrawal symptoms develop. Some believe that tolerance may occur with some actions. PCP is metabolized in the liver, but only a small amount is excreted in the urine. In addition, PCP has a long half-life.

PCP induces feelings of strength, power, invulnerability, and psychic numbing. The high that occurs with intoxication resembles drunkenness in which balance is affected and the user has a sensation of bouncing or floating. In addition to these effects, the user may experience psychomotor agitation, belligerence, physical aggressiveness, impulsiveness, and unpredictability. More bizarre and violent behavior occurs with PCP than with amphetamines or LSD. Behavior with the use of PCP may mimic paranoid schizophrenia or manic states. Behavioral toxicity is dose related and ranges from mild intoxication to lethal overdoses. Physical symptoms may include nystagmus, hypertension, numbness, ataxia, dysarthria, muscle rigidity, seizures, and hyperacusis (see Table 60-7).

Therapeutic management. Emergency problems associated with the use of PCP include confusion, paranoia, violent outbursts, and hallucinations. Toxicology tests of blood and urine are necessary to correctly identify use of this drug. Approaches are the same as those for the treatment of other hallucinogens and include reassurance, education, avoidance of medications, support of vital functions, and treatment of symptoms. Symptoms of toxic reactions may appear at low oral doses and may take 2 to 6 weeks to clear. Acidification of the urine assists in the excretion of PCP. Severe reactions that are not rapidly cleared may require hospitalization. A narrow margin exists between mild intoxication and a life-threatening reaction. A high rate of relapse is found in long-term users.

Inhalants

Etiology. Inhalants are volatile compounds or hydrocarbons found in commercial or industrial substances and cleaning solvents. The most frequently abused agents are glues, aerosols, cleaning solutions, nail polish removers, lighter fluids, paints and paint thinners, typewriter correction fluid, and gasoline. Carbon tetrachloride, toluene, and acetone are some of the common ingredients. Most compounds contain a mixture of psychoactive substances.

Patterns of use may begin with children 9 to 13 years old who are usually part of a peer group that may also use alcohol and cannabis. Young children may use inhalants several times a week, whereas young adults may become intoxicated every day. Inhalant use increases over time until inhalants become the drug of choice. Inhalants are generally used with peers. Factors frequently associated with inhalant use include family dysfunction, school or work adjustment problems, and legal problems. Minority youth living in economically depressed areas are especially prone to abuse of inhalants. Most adolescents who use inhalants stop using them after several years and may select another drug. Another high-risk group is industrial workers who work with volatile substances on a long-term basis and who may develop a dependence.

Intoxicating vapors are commonly taken in by soaking a rag in the substance and applying it to the nose and mouth. Other methods include placing the substance in a paper or plastic bag and inhaling the gases, inhaling directly from containers, or spraying aerosols into the nose or mouth. Use of plastic bags has frequently been associated with suffocation.

Clinical manifestations of abuse. Inhalant use causes signs of confusion and generalized CNS depression, leading to a mild state of anesthesia. Metabolism of most substances occurs in the liver and kidneys. Tolerance of higher doses develops rapidly but may reflect increased use and preference for higher levels of intoxication rather than true tolerance. Withdrawal symptoms have not been substantiated.

The high often starts within 5 minutes of use and has a short duration with symptoms lasting for only an hour and a half. The effects of such a high are similar to those observed with the use of alcohol and barbituates, beginning with decreased inhibitory effects that later become more inhibitory. Inhalant intoxication is often associated with symptoms of aggressiveness, impulsiveness, and impaired judgment. Physical signs may include dizziness, nystagmus, incoordination, slurred speech, unsteady gait, lethargy, depressed reflexes, psychomotor retardation, tremor, generalized muscle weakness, blurred vision or diplopia, stupor or coma, and euphoria. Inhalant users may be identified by a rash around the nose and mouth, breath odors, or residue on hands, face, or clothing. Light sensitivity, eye irritation, ringing in the ears, and irritation to the nose, throat, and lungs may also be present. Complaints may include nausea, vomiting, diarrhea, and headache.

Therapeutic management. The most common emergency problems are toxic reactions, organic brain syndromes, and medical complications. Toxic reactions occur very rapidly and may be life threatening enough to cause sudden death as a result of respiratory depression or cardiac dysrhythmias. The individual who has a toxic reaction may also exhibit some degree of mental impairment and anxiety. Treatment is symptom related, and acute life support is provided to control dysrhythmias and aid respirations. Treatment also includes offering supportive care as for other depressant and hallucinogen toxic reactions.

Organic brain syndrome usually has a rapid onset of disorientation and confusion but usually clears within hours. Treatment consists of providing a supportive environment, decreasing stimuli, offering reassurance and reality orientation, and providing for the safety of the individual during angry outbursts. Medical complications are not common but may occur with increased risk for long-term abusers. These include cardiac irregularities or dysrhythmias, hepatitis, liver failure, impairment of lung function, aplastic anemia, skeletal muscle weakness, GI upset, peripheral neuropathies, possible permanent CNS damage, and possible abnormalities in infants born to users.

SPECIAL POPULATIONS WITH ADDICTIVE PROBLEMS
Homeless

It is now believed that between 20% to 45% of the homeless population have alcohol-related problems.[40]

Conditions of homelessness compound the usual problems of alcohol abuse and include problems such as exposure to the elements, infectious diseases, nutritional deficiencies, trauma, frostbite, peripheral vascular disorders, physical debilitation, infestations, and tuberculosis. Alcoholism may have played a significant role in leading to a homeless situation. Some of this population may have been married or had strong social networks before a progressive deterioration as a result of alcohol abuse. Mental illness and drug abuse have been found to coexist in a significant number of homeless people.[41]

Women Alcoholics

Women drink significantly less than men and have fewer alcohol-related problems. However, there has been a recent increase in the number of drinking-related problems among women in their 20's and early 30's. Heavy drinking begins for most women after health problems have occurred. Gastric metabolism of alcohol in nonalcoholic women is lower than in men; that is, one drink is more potent for women and produces a greater effect.[42] One study identified the following profile for women alcoholics: a history of hospitalizations for alcohol-related illnesses, addictions to other drugs such as antidepressants and tranquilizers, problems with sex-role identity, problems with control, limited coping skills, a masculine sex-role identity, and affective disorders.[43] Women alcoholics develop liver disease and have a higher mortality rate at an earlier age than men. There also appears to be a link between bulimia and alcoholism in women. Alcoholism has a telescoping effect in women with a later onset and more rapid progression. Treatment programs that address the specific needs of women are needed for outcomes to be successful.

Older Adult Alcoholics

People over 65 years of age consume less alcohol than younger adults and generally have a lower prevalence of alcohol abuse. Older adults are at high risk for adverse health effects of alcohol. They may drink more frequently in smaller amounts. Alcohol may have a greater effect on older adults as a result of decreased metabolism, greater cellular sensitivity, and interactions with medications and illnesses. The most common presenting problems are usually medical or psychiatric illnesses, including alcohol-associated organic mental disorder. Other common alcohol-related problems in older adults include falls, trauma, malnutrition, insomnia, GI bleeding, cardiovascular disorders, stroke, depression, and dementia. The nurse needs to be alert to the possibility of abuse in this population group.

Alcohol dependence in older adults may have an early or a late onset. It may develop in response to a sudden loss or illness. Screening of older adults for alcohol dependence is important in making an association with a medical illness; it is important to determine if a problem exists and if drinking is a health risk. One screening method is called "giving patients the *heat*" and asks four open-ended questions: *H*ow do you use alcohol? Have you *e*ver thought you used alcohol to *e*xcess? Has *a*nyone else ever thought you used too much? Have you ever had any *t*rouble resulting from your use? A positive response or a response that raises suspicion should be followed up by a complete his-

tory of substance use. Cognitive impairment is frequently present with alcohol abuse among older adults. Older adults tend to experience a more severe withdrawal than younger individuals and require higher doses of sedation.[44]

Adult Children of Alcoholics

An estimated 28 million adult children of alcoholics (ACOAs) live in the United States.[45] Some studies indicate that ACOAs are found in large numbers in nursing and other helping professions. The child of an alcoholic may develop a codependent pattern of relating to the alcoholic to survive. Traits of ACOAs include guessing at what is normal behavior, judging themselves without mercy, having difficulty with intimate relationships, and being extremely responsible or irresponsible. They have problems with the need for control, approval seeking, lack of authenticity, low self-esteem, and difficulty in establishing trust and healthy relationships. They neglect fun and pleasure, repress feelings, and avoid necessary conflict. ACOAs experience extensive free-floating anxiety, excessive feelings of guilt and shame, and compulsions or addictive behaviors. They are at high risk for chemical dependence. A number of community support groups have been developed to address specific problems of ACOAs.[46]

CURRENT ISSUES
Codependency

The term *codependency* had its roots in describing relationships of family members, particularly spouses of alcoholic husbands or wives. It allowed family members to acknowledge their own feelings in the situation and to begin to look at their own dysfunctional behaviors in the relationship. Codependency relates to a number of other addictions and has been generalized to refer to dysfunctional relationships that are not associated with chemical dependency. It is a process that keeps individuals "out of touch" with themselves by being preoccupied with others to the exclusion of their own needs. It develops from rigid family systems with unspoken rules and roles that lead to dysfunctional patterns of living and problem solving. Learned rules such as not talking about problems serve to shut down thoughts and feelings. Roles that children learn within the family are enabler, hero, scapegoat, lost child, and mascot. These roles and the rules that accompany them become patterns of relating that children take with them into adulthood.

Low self-esteem is the core of codependency. Individuals who are codependent borrow their feelings of self-worth from others by taking on others' feelings as their own. Progressive stages of codependency and recovery have been identified. The recovery process is based on self-care and involves the process of grieving, learning to set boundaries, recognizing shame and guilt, acquiring the skill of reparenting oneself, and initiating daily affirmations such as, "I am a worthwhile person."[47]

Nurses and other caretakers may readily become involved in helping relationships that trigger classic characteristics of codependency. These may include feeling responsible for all aspects of another's life, neglecting their own needs, being overcommited and overworked, acting on another's behalf or solving others' problems, seeking

perfectionism, denying anything painful, and being unable or unwilling to share information about themselves. Recovery for the nurse means first recognizing this behavior pattern and then being willing to make some changes. Change is usually best facilitated by involvement with outside resources such as a self-help group (e.g., Codependents Anonymous, Al-Anon, Adult Children of Alcoholics), therapist, or therapy group.

Chemical Dependence in Nurses

Because of widespread denial and the "conspiracy of silence," chemical dependency has not been addressed as a professional issue until the past decade. Historically, nurses who were suspected of addiction were fired; this has been called the "throw-away nurse syndrome."[48] The American Nurses' Association responded to the need to help the helper by passing a resolution in 1982 advocating rehabilitation for nurses who are chemically dependent and the establishment of assistance programs by the state nurses' association.

The National Nurses Society on Addictions (NNSA) produced a position paper on impaired nurses, established a national network of resources, and created a model diversion program to assist states in developing programs. The goals of programs are to protect the safety of the public, to maintain the integrity of the profession, and to ensure that the nurse is offered the possibility of treatment and rehabilitation before being fired or before the license to practice is revoked. Essential components of these programs include education, intervention, referral to appropriate treatment, monitoring of recovery, and support for reentry into practice. Types of programs include diversion programs through the state board of nursing, which allow nurses to maintain their licenses and ability to practice while being monitored through recovery, state nurses' association peer assistance programs, and employee assistance programs.

The prevalence of chemical dependence among nurses is unknown. Approximately 6% to 8% (120,000 to 160,000) of the registered nurse population has an alcohol- or drug-related problem.[49] A number of contributing factors have been identified, including the caretaker mentality, which is a characteristic of codependency. Nurses frequently operate with a number of false perceptions and beliefs such as that taking of drugs solves problems or that knowledge of drugs provides automatic immunity to drug problems.

Nurses frequently lack the knowledge and understanding of addiction and of how to recognize early behavioral clues. Nursing education has not adequately provided knowledge of prevention strategies, interventions, advances in research and treatments, or skills needed to work with clients (or co-workers) in every area of nursing. Many nurses' working knowledge is based on public stereotypes and clinical experiences with difficult alcohol and drug abusers.

Signs and symptoms of chemical dependence related to work performance may be apparent in personality and behavior changes, job performance changes, and time and attendance changes (Table 60-20).[50] Nurses often enable chemical dependence to continue among co-workers by

Table 60-20 Clues to Recognize the Chemically Dependent Nurse*

Alcoholic Nurse	Drug-Addicted Nurse
PERSONALITY AND BEHAVIOR CHANGES	
More irritable with clients and co-workers	Extreme and rapid mood swings
Withdrawal	Constant wearing of long sleeves
Mood swings	Suspicious behavior concerning controlled substances
Lunch alone	Signing out of more controlled drugs than anyone else
Isolation, desire to work nights	Frequent spills or breakage
Inappropriate responses	Waiting until alone to open narcotics cabinet
Elaborate excuses for behavior	Constant volunteering as medicine nurse
Unkempt appearance	
Evidence of blackouts	
JOB PERFORMANCE CHANGES	
Less production of work	Too many medication errors
Difficulty in meeting deadlines	Spillage of too many controlled drugs or breakage of too
Illogical or sloppy charting procedures	many vials
Frequent errors	Illogical or sloppy charting procedures
TIME AND ATTENDANCE CHANGES	
Increased absenteeism	Frequent absence from unit
Long lunch hours	Early arrival at work and delay of departure from work
Absence from floor without explanation	Loitering at work even when not on duty
Contact by telephone to request compensatory time at beginning of shift	Abundant use of sick leave

Modified from The regulatory management of the chemically dependent nurse, Chicago, 1987, National Council of State Boards of Nursing, Inc, Nursing Practice and Standards Committee, pp 10-11.
*These symptoms need documentation; some documentation will be anecdotal.

covering up mistakes or tardiness, making excuses for another nurse's behavior, repeatedly helping someone complete an assignment, or simply ignoring obvious signs and symptoms. Helping chemically dependent nurses requires sharing observations and concerns with the nurse and supervisor to provide the means for rehabilitation. Caring about nurses who are in trouble because of drug and alcohol abuse may be a painful process for the co-worker. It involves self-awareness, confrontation, patience, and support and belief in the nurse's recovery. Nurses who have travelled the road to recovery and regained control over their lives can offer insight to other nurses and hope for those whose lives and health have been affected by unhealthy patterns of drug and alcohol use.

C *ase Study*

COCAINE TOXICITY

Mr. C. is a 34-year-old man who was admitted to the unit from the emergency room where he presented with chest pain, tachycardia, dizziness, nausea, and severe migrainelike headache. He was extremely nervous and irritable and insisted that he was having a heart attack and needed to see a cardiologist. Mr. C. denied any previous history of angina or myocardial infarction. The only significant findings include a history of chronic sinusitis, nasal sores, frequent upper respiratory infections, and a recent weight loss of 20 lb. His girlfriend brought Mr. C. to the hospital. She related that

they had been at a party earlier in the evening, that they had been drinking and smoking some pot, and that Mr. C. had snorted some cocaine with his friends. She was concerned about his increasing need for cocaine over the past few months and had noticed a change in his personality; he was more irritable, seclusive, and restless. She hoped he would get help for his drug problem before it became worse.

Mr. C. is the oldest of three siblings. His parents are living and well. His father is a recovering alcoholic. No other significant family history was noted.

On admission, Mr. C. appeared pale and diaphoretic, exhibited tremors, and was apprehensive. Blood pressure was 210/110, pulse was 100, respiration was 30, and temperature was 38.9° C (102° F).

Discussion Questions

1. What other information is needed to assess Mr. C.'s condition?
2. How should questions regarding these areas be addressed?
3. What other clues should the nurse be alert for in assessing this client's drug use?
4. What emergency conditions need to be carefully monitored?
5. What medical conditions should be considered?
6. What nursing diagnoses are useful in planning care?
7. What nursing interventions support these diagnoses?
8. How would effectiveness of the interventions be evaluated?
9. What is the best way to approach Mr. C. to engage him in a treatment program?

R eview Questions

The number of the question corresponds to the same-numbered objective at the beginning of the chapter.

1. Primary prevention activities are aimed at
   a. early identification and treatment of frequent drug users
   b. collective action to influence social policy and develop social responsibility
   c. control and monitoring of addicted persons
   d. prevention of relapses for recovering persons
2. The nurse's assessment of personal patterns of drug use is a health promotion strategy that supports the nurse's position as
   a. educator
   b. resource
   c. role model
   d. change agent
3. The public health model of addiction directs nurses to
   a. recognize related illnesses
   b. assess emotional problems
   c. support traditions, values, and beliefs
   d. assess risk factors
4. A pattern of abnormal or pathophysiological use resulting in physical, emotional, or social impairment is known as
   a. abuse
   b. dependence
   c. tolerance
   d. loss of control
5. One of the most compelling reasons leading to continued drug use is
   a. poor body image
   b. powerful immediate gratification
   c. family dysfunction
   d. poor social skills
6. Interruptions in the addictive cycle after the development of tolerance generally precipitate
   a. loss of control
   b. decreased tolerance
   c. withdrawal symptoms
   d. no change in condition
7. Diagnostic criteria for psychoactive substance dependence may include all of the following *except*
   a. great deal of time spent in activities necessary to get the substance
   b. recurrent use in situations in which use is physically hazardous
   c. frequent intoxication or withdrawal symptoms
   d. marked tolerance
8. A nursing diagnosis that represents a biological response and that is frequently used with addicted clients is
   a. knowledge deficit
   b. ineffective denial
   c. sensory/perceptual alteration
   d. grief
9. A withdrawal syndrome that is characterized by a severely depressed mood, prolonged sleep, apathy, irritability, and disorientation is associated with dependence on
   a. stimulants
   b. depressants
   c. narcotics
   d. cannabis
10. Clients with drug-related problems (intoxication, toxicity, withdrawal) usually seek treatment for
    a. medical complications
    b. detoxification
    c. addiction
    d. finding another drug source
11. The key to an initial effective nursing intervention in case management of clients with problems associated with drug use is
    a. offering education on addiction
    b. providing a quiet, nonstimulating atmosphere
    c. carrying out an accurate assessment
    d. assisting with reality orientation
12. Trauma clients, particularly those with violent crime–related injuries, should be assessed for use of which of these?
    a. cannabis
    b. cocaine
    c. LSD
    d. codeine
13. Which statement is true about older adults?
    a. They generally consume more alcohol than younger adults.
    b. They tend to experience a less severe alcohol withdrawal than younger adults.
    c. Those who abuse alcohol are at higher risk for physical abuse.
    d. Cognitive impairment is seldom present with alcohol abuse among older adults.
14. Nurses may be enablers by
    a. fostering assertiveness in clients
    b. seeking solutions to clients' problems
    c. assisting clients to identify their feelings
    d. confronting clients' denial
15. Factors contributing to chemical dependence among nurses include all of the following *except*
    a. caretaker mentality
    b. belief that drugs solve problems
    c. lack of knowledge of addiction
    d. recognition of early behavioral clues
16. Helping chemically dependent nurses means
    a. covering for nurses until they are better
    b. confronting nurses and assisting them to get treatment
    c. ignoring signs and symptoms until they are obvious
    d. removing the nurses from position of direct client care

REFERENCES

1. Williams GD and others: Demographic trends, alcohol abuse and alcoholism, Alcohol Health Res World, Spring 1987, p 80.
2. Nuckols CC and Greeson J: Cocaine addiction—assessment and intervention, Nurs Clin North Am 24:33-43, 1989.

3. Gold MS, Smith DE, and Olden K: Cocaine: helping patients avoid the end of the line, Pract J Prim Care Phys Emer Med Rep pp 1-8 1985.

4. Criteria Committee, National Council on Alcoholism: Criteria for the diagnosis of alcoholism, Ann Intern Med 77:249, 1972.

5. Galizio M and Maish SA: Determinants of substance abuse, New York, 1985, Plenum Publishing Corp, pp 383-424.

6. Miller NS and Gold MS: Suggestions for changes in DSM-III-R criteria for substance use disorders, Am J Drug Alcohol Abuse 15:228, 1989.

7. Naegle MA: Substance abuse. In Birckhead LM, ed: Psychiatric/mental health nursing: the therapeutic use of self, New York, 1989, JB Lippincott Co, p 436.

8. United States Department of Justice: Drugs of abuse, Washington, DC, 1989, US Government Printing Office.

9. Ray O and Ksir C: Drugs, society, and human behavior, ed 5, St Louis, 1990, Times Mirror/Mosby College Publishing, p 118.

10. Schuckit MD: Drug and alcohol abuse: a clinical guide to diagnosis and treatment, ed 3, New York, 1989, Plenum Publishing Corp, p 98.

11. American Psychiatric Association: Diagnostic and statistical manual of mental disorders, ed 3, rev, Washington, DC, 1987, American Psychiatric Association, p 175.

12. Cregler LL: Adverse health consequences of cocaine abuse, J Natl Med Assoc 81:34, 1989.

13. Gawin FH: Cocaine abuse and addiction, J Fam Pract 29:195, 1989.

14. Kosten TR: Pharmacotherapeutic interventions for cocaine abuse—matching patients to treatments, J Nerv Ment Dis 177:384-385, 1989.

15. Bowser BB: Crack and AIDS: an ethnographic impression, J Natl Med Assoc 81:538-540, 1989.

16. VanDette JM and Cornish LA: Drug review: medical complications of illicit cocaine use, Clin Pharm 8:402, 1989.

17. Robert SM and others: Alcohol and cocaine-induced liver injury, Alcohol Health Res World 20:22-25, 1987.

18. Lindenbaum GA and others: Patterns of alcohol and drug abuse in an urban trauma center: the increasing role of cocaine abuse, J Trauma 29:1654-1658, 1989.

19. Washton AM: Nonpharmacologic treatment of cocaine abuse, Psychiatr Clin North Am 9:564, 1986.

20. Todd B: Disabling anxiety, Geriatr Nurs (New York) 9:152, 154, 156, 1989.

21. Schatzberg AF and Cole JO: Manual of clinical psychopharmacology, Washington, DC, 1986, American Psychiatric Press, pp 234-236.

22. Vaillant GE: The natural history of alcoholism, Cambridge, Mass, 1983, Harvard University Press, p 310.

23. Ray OS: Drugs, society and human behavior, St Louis, 1983, The CV Mosby Co, p 167.

24. Lerner WD, Marx JA, and Mathews JJ: Alcoholic emergencies, Patient Care, May 30, 1988, p 114 (insert).

25. Tweed SH: Identifying the alcoholic client, Nurs Clin North Am 24:17, 1989.

26. Bartek JK and others: Nurse-identified problems in the management of alcoholic patients, J Stud Alcohol 49:62-70, 1988.

27. Babor TF and others: AUDIT: the alcohol use disorders identification test: guidelines for use in primary health care, Geneva, 1989, World Health Organization.

28. Selzer M, Vinokur A, and Van Roojen L: A self-administered short alcoholism screening test (SMAST), J Stud Alcohol 36:86, 1975.

29. Mayfield DG, McLeod G, and Hall P: The CAGE questionnaire: validation of a new alcoholism screening instrument, Am J Psychiatry 131:1121-1123, 1974.

Department of Health and Human Services, Public Health Service, ADAMHA, NIAAA: Research on promising pharmacotherapies for alcoholism, Washington, DC, 1990, US Government Printing Office.

31. Gitlow SE and Peyser HS, eds: Alcoholism—a practical treatment guide, ed 2, New York, 1988, Grune & Stratton, pp 231-232.

32. Estes NJ and Heinemann ME: Alcoholism: development, consequences, and interventions, ed 3, St Louis, 1986, The CV Mosby Co, p 341.

33. Jaffe JH: Drug addiction and drug abuse. In Gilman AG and others, eds: The pharmacological basis of therapeutics, ed 7, New York, 1985, Macmillan Publishing Co, pp 532-581.

34. Woods JH and Winger G: Opioids, receptors, and abuse liability. In: Miltzer HY, ed: Psychopharmacology: the third generation of progress, New York, 1987, Raven Press, pp 1555-1564.

35. Platt JJ: Heroin addiction: theory, research and treatment, ed 2, Malabar, Fla, 1986, RE Krieger Publishing Co, Inc, p 64.

36. Hubbard RL and others: Role of drug-abuse treatment in limiting the spread of AIDS, Rev Infect Dis 10:383, 1988.

37. Casey AF and Parfett RT: Opioid analgesics: chemistry and receptors, New York, 1986, Plenum Publishing Corp, pp 1, 31.

38. Semlitz L and Gold MS: Adolescent drug abuse: diagnosis, treatment, and prevention, Psychiatr Clin North Am 9:455, 459-462, 466, 1986.

39. Friedman H and others: Drugs of abuse and virus susceptibility. In Bridge TP and others, eds: Psychological, neuropsychiatric, and substance abuse aspects of AIDS, New York, 1988, Raven Press, p 126.

40. Lubran BG: Alcohol-related problems among the homeless: NIAAA's response, Alcohol Health Res World 11:4, 1987.

41. Wright JD and others: Ailments and alcohol: health status among the drinking homeless, Alcohol Health Res World 11:22-27, 1987.

42. Seligmann J: The alcohol gender gap—women feel it faster, Newsweek, Jan 22, 1990, p 53.

43. Joyce C: The woman alcoholic, AJN 89:1314-1316, 1989.

44. Willenbring ML: Organic mental disorders associated with heavy drinking and alcohol dependence, Clin Geriatr Med 4:882-884, 1988.

45. Leerhsen C and Namuth T: Alcohol and the family, Newsweek, Jan 18, 1988, p 62.

46. Fischer KE: Adult children of alcoholics: implications for the nursing profession, Nurs Forum 4:159-163, 1987-1988.

47. Zerwekh J and Michaels B: Co-dependency: assessment and recovery, Nurs Clin North Am 24:109-120, 1989.

48. Sullivan E, Bissell L, and Williams E: Chemical dependency in nursing: the deadly diversion, Menlo Park, Calif, 1988, Addison-Wesley Pub Co.

49. American Nurses' Association: Impaired nursing practice (media backgrounder), ANA News, Kansas City, Mo, Mar 1987, American Nurses' Association.

50. The regulatory management of the chemically dependent nurse, National Council of State Boards of Nursing, Inc, Nursing Practice and Standards Committee, Chicago, 1987, monograph.

SECTION X REFERENCES

BOOKS

Bosker G and others: Geriatric emergency medicine, St Louis, 1990, Mosby–Year Book, Inc.

Committee on Trauma, American College of Surgeons: Early care of the injured patient, ed 4, St Louis, 1990, Mosby–Year Book, Inc.

Dernocolur KB: Street sense: communication, safety, and control, ed 2, Englewood Cliffs, NJ, 1990, Prentice-Hall, Inc.

Estes NJ and Heinemann ME: Alcoholism: development, consequences and interventions, ed 3, St Louis, 1986, The CV Mosby Co.

Grant HD, Murray RH Jr, and Bergeron JD: Brady emergency care, ed 5, Englewood Cliffs, NJ, 1990, Prentice-Hall, Inc.

Haack MR and Hughes TL, eds: Addiction in the nursing profession: approaches to intervention and recovery, New York, 1989, Springer Publishing Co.

Lee G, ed: Flight nursing: principles and practice, St Louis, 1991, Mosby–Year Book, Inc.

Mancini ME: Pocket manual of emergency nursing procedures, St Louis, 1988, The CV Mosby Co.

Mancini ME and Klein J: Decision making in trauma nursing, St Louis, 1990, Mosby–Year Book, Inc.

Nuckols CC: Cocaine—from dependency to recovery, ed 2, Blue Ridge Summit, Penn, 1989, TAB Books, Inc.

Parcel GS and Rinear CE: Basic emergency care of the sick and injured, ed 4, St Louis, 1989, The CV Mosby Co.

Rosen P, Barkin RM, and Sternbach GL: Principles of emergency medicine, St Louis, 1990, Mosby–Year Book, Inc.

Schwartz GR: Emergency medicine: the essential update, Philadelphia, 1989, WB Saunders Co.

Sheehy SAB, Marvin JA, and Jimmerson CL: Manual of clinical trauma care: the first hour, St Louis, 1989, The CV Mosby Co.

Sheehy SB: Mosby's manual of emergency care, ed 3, St Louis, 1990, Mosby–Year Book, Inc.

Slacman M, ed: Neurological emergencies: recognition and management, ed 2, New York, 1990, Raven Press.

Trunkey DD and Lewis FR: Current therapy of trauma, vol 3, ed 3, St Louis, 1990, Mosby–Year Book, Inc.

JOURNALS

Boyd-Monk H: Eye trauma: a close-up on emergency care, RN 52:22, 1989.

Cermak TL, Hunt T, and Keene BWT: Codependency: more than a catchword, Patient Care 23:131, 1989.

Compton P: Drug abuse—a self-care deficit, J Psychosocial Nurs 27:22, 1989.

Cooper JR: Methadone treatment and acquired immunodeficiency syndrome, JAMA 262:1664, 1989.

Cooper K: Drug overdose, AJN 89:1146, 1989.

Davidson DM: Cardiovascular effects of alcohol, West J Med 151:430, 1989.

Dubiel D: Action stat! Cocaine overdose, Nursing 20:33, 1990.

Ettinger NA and Albin RJ: A review of the respiratory effects of smoking cocaine, Am J Med 87:664, 1989.

Fraser S and Atkins J: Survivors' recollections of helpful and unhelpful emergency nurse activities surrounding sudden death of a loved one, JEN 16:13, 1990.

Gaspares L and Noone J: Managing emergencies, Nursing 19:96, 1989.

Green P: The chemically dependent nurse, Nurs Clin North Am 24:81, 1989.

Hahn RA and others: Prevalance of HIV infection among intravenous drug users in the U.S., JAMA 261:2677, 1989.

Hall SF and Wray LM: Codependency: nurses who give too much, AJN 89:1456, 1989.

Heinemann ME and Hoffman AL: Nurse educators look at alcohol education for the profession, Alcohol Health Res World 13:48, 1989.

Herron DG and Nance J: Emergency department nursing management of patients with orthopedic fractures resulting from motor vehicle accidents, Nurs Clin North Am 25:71, 1990.

Higgins R: Cocaine abuse: what every emergency nurse should know, J Emerg Nurs 15:318, 1989.

Horsburgh CR, Anderson Jr, and Boyko EJ: Increased incidence of infections in intravenous drug users, Infect Control Hosp Epidemiol 10:211, 1989.

Huggins B: Trauma physiology, Nurs Clin North Am 25:1, 1990.

Leiker TL: The role of the addictions nurse specialist in the general hospital setting, Nurs Clin North Am 24:137, 1989.

McKinley MG: Near drowning: a nursing challenge, Crit Care Nurse 9:52, 1989.

Naegle MA: Patterns and implications of drug use by students of nursing, NSNA Imprint 36:84, 1989.

Nelson NP and Beckel J: Patient care guidelines: near-drowning, JEN 16:119, 1990.

Quinn-Larson J and Pickard MR: The impaired nursing student, Nurse Educator 14:36, 1989.

Rich J: Action Stat! Acute alcohol intoxication, Nursing 19:33, 1989.

Roberts SS: A marker gene for alcoholism? J NIH Res 2:25, 1990.

Sedlak S and Mace D: Hidden problems with bleeding in trauma patients, J Emerg Nurs 15:422, 1989.

Vandegaer F: Cocaine—the deadliest addiction, Nursing 19:72, 1989.

Voorhees LA: Dealing with chemical dependency, AAOHN J 37:1, 1989.

Wallen J and Noble JA: Alcoholism treatment in general hospitals, J Stud Alcohol 50:301, 1989.

Weinman SA: Methanol poisoning in the emergency department, J Emerg Nurs 16:137, 1990.

Willis D and Harbit MD: A fatal attraction: cocaine related subarachnoid hemorrhage, J Neurosci Nurs 21:171, 1989.

ORGANIZATIONS

Alcohol, Drug Abuse, and Mental Health Administration
Public Health Service
5600 Fishers Lane
Rockville, MD 20857

Alcoholics Anonymous
General Service Office
Grand Central Station
Box 459
New York, NY 10164-0459

American Red Cross
National Headquarters
17 and D Streets, NW
Washington, DC 20006

Cocaine Anonymous World Services
3740 Overland Avenue, Suite G
Los Angeles, CA 90034

Cocaine/Crack Action Helpline
1-800-888-9383

Crack Abuse 24-Hour Hotline
1-800-444-9999

Drugs Anonymous
P.O. Box 473
Ansonia Station
New York, NY 10023

Emergency Nurses Association
230 East Ohio
Chicago, IL 60611

National Council on Alcoholism
12 West 21st Street
New York, NY 10010

National Nurses Society on Addictions
5700 Old Orchard Road, First floor
Skokie, IL 60077

Nurses Alliance for the Prevention of Nuclear War
339 Lafayette Street, Room 202
New York, NY 10012

Overeaters Anonymous
P.O. Box 92870
Los Angeles, CA 90009

APPENDIX

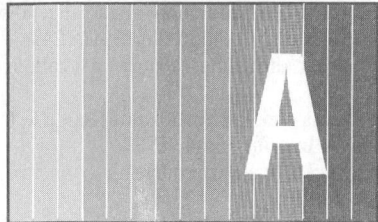

Nursing Diagnoses

HEALTH-PERCEPTION–HEALTH-MANAGEMENT PATTERN

Altered health maintenance
Health seeking behaviors (specify)
Noncompliance (specify)
High risk for infection
High risk for injury (trauma)
High risk for poisoning
High risk for suffocation
Altered protection

NUTRITIONAL-METABOLIC PATTERN

Altered nutrition: high risk for more than body requirements
Altered nutrition: more than body requirements
Altered nutrition: less than body requirements
Ineffective breastfeeding
Effective breastfeeding
Impaired swallowing
High risk for aspiration
Altered oral mucous membrane
Potential fluid volume deficit
Fluid volume deficit (actual) (1)
Fluid volume deficit (actual) (2)
Fluid volume excess
High risk for impaired skin integrity
Impaired skin integrity
Impaired tissue integrity
High risk for altered body temperature
Ineffective thermoregulation
Hyperthermia
Hypothermia

ELIMINATION PATTERN

Constipation
Colonic constipation
Perceived constipation
Diarrhea
Bowel incontinence
Altered urinary elimination pattern
Functional incontinence
Reflex incontinence
Stress incontinence
Urge incontinence
Total incontinence
Urinary retention

ACTIVITY-EXERCISE PATTERN

Potential activity intolerance
Activity intolerance (specify level)

Fatigue
Impaired physical mobility (specify level)
High risk for disuse syndrome
Total self-care deficit (specify level)
Self-bathing—hygiene deficit (specify level)
Self-dressing—grooming deficit (specify level)
Self-feeding deficit (specify level)
Self-toileting deficit (specify level)
Diversional activity deficit
Impaired home maintenance management (mild, moderate, severe, potential, chronic)
Ineffective airway clearance
Ineffective breathing pattern
Impaired gas exchange
Decreased cardiac output
Altered tissue perfusion (specify)
Dysreflexia
Altered growth and development

SLEEP-REST PATTERN

Sleep-pattern disturbance

COGNITIVE-PERCEPTUAL PATTERN

Pain
Chronic pain
Sensory/perceptual alteration: input deficit
Sensory/perceptual alteration: input excess
Unilateral neglect
Knowledge deficit (specify)
Impaired thought processes
Decisional conflict (specify)

SELF-PERCEPTION–SELF-CONCEPT PATTERN

Fear (specify focus)
Anxiety
Hopelessness
Powerlessness (severe, moderate, low)
Self-esteem disturbance
Chronic low self-esteem
Situational low self-esteem
Body-image disturbance
Personal identity disturbance

ROLE-RELATIONSHIP PATTERN

Anticipatory grieving
Dysfunctional grieving
Disturbance in role performance
Social isolation
Impaired social interaction

Altered family processes
High risk for altered parenting
Altered parenting
Parental role conflict
Impaired verbal communication
High risk for violence

SEXUALITY-REPRODUCTIVE PATTERN

Sexual dysfunction
Altered sexuality patterns
Rape trauma syndrome
Rape trauma syndrome: compound reaction
Rape trauma syndrome: silent reaction

COPING–STRESS-TOLERANCE PATTERN

Ineffective coping (individual)
Defensive coping
Ineffective denial
Impaired adjustment
Post-trauma response
Family coping: potential for growth
Ineffective family coping: compromised
Ineffective family coping: disabling

VALUE-BELIEF PATTERN

Spiritual distress (distress of human spirit)

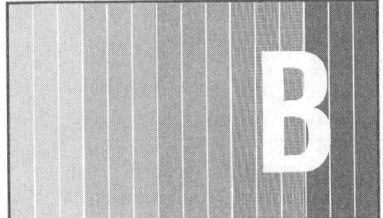

Laboratory Values

Cecilia C. Dail
Beth Runnels
Sally D. Sperry

The tables in this appendix list some of the most common tests, their normal values, and possible etiologies of abnormal values. Laboratory values may vary with different techniques and/or different laboratories. Possible etiologies are presented in alphabetic order. Abbreviations appearing in the tables are defined as follows:

$<$ = less than
$>$ = greater than
g = gram
L = liter
mEq = milliequivalent
ml = milliliter
dl = deciliter
mm Hg = millimeter of mercury
fl = femtoliter
mm = millimeter

mg = milligram (10^{-3})
μg = microgram (one millionth of a gram) (10^{-6})
ng = nanogram (one billionth of a gram)(10^{-9})
pg = picogram (one trillionth of a gram) (10^{-12})
μU = microunit
μl = microliter
IU = international unit
mOsm = milliosmole
U = unit
μmol = micromole
nmol = nanomole
mmol = millimole
pmol = picomole
kPa = kilopascal
μkat = microkatal

Table B-1 Serum, Plasma, and Whole Blood Chemistries

| Test | Normal Values | | Possible Etiology | |
	Conventional Units	SI Units	Higher	Lower
Acetone			Diabetic acidosis, high-fat diet, low-carbohydrate diet, starvation	
Quantitative	0.3-2.0 mg/dl	52-344 μmol/L		
Qualitative	Negative	Same as conventional units		
Albumin	3.5-5.0 g/dl	507-725 μmol/L	Dehydration	Chronic liver disease, malabsorption, malnutrition, nephrotic syndrome
Aldolase	1.0-7.5 U/L	Same as conventional units	Skeletal muscle disease	Renal disease
α-Amino acid nitrogen	3.5-5.5 mg/dl	2.5-3.9 mmol/L	Infectious hepatitis, poisoning from carbon tetrachloride, arsenic, chloroform	Bacterial pneumonia, insulin administration
α-1-Antitrypsin	200-400 mg/dl	2.0-4.0 g/L	Acute and chronic inflammation, arthritis, stress syndrome	Chronic lung disease (early onset), malnutrition, nephrotic syndrome
α-1-Fetoprotein	<25 ng/ml	<25 μg/L	Cancer of testes and ovaries, carcinoma of liver	
α-Hydroxybutyric dehydrogenase (α-HBD)	72-184 U/L (method dependent)	Same as conventional units	Hemolytic anemia, leukemia, malignant melanoma, muscular dystrophy, myocardial infarction, nephrotic syndrome	
Ammonia	30-70 μg/dl	17.6-41.1 μmol/L	Severe liver disease	
Amylase	25-125 U/L (method dependent)	Same as conventional units	Acute and chronic pancreatitis, mumps (salivary gland disease), perforated ulcers	Acute alcoholism, cirrhosis of liver, extensive destruction of pancreas
Ascorbic acid	0.4-2.0 mg/dl	23-114 μmol/L	Excessive ingestion of vitamin C	Connective tissue disorders, hepatic disease, renal disease, rheumatic fever, vitamin C deficiency
Bicarbonate	20-30 mEq/L	20-30 mmol/L	Compensated respiratory acidosis, metabolic alkalosis	Compensated respiratory alkalosis, metabolic acidosis
Bilirubin			Biliary obstruction, impaired liver function, hemolytic anemia, pernicious anemia, prolonged fasting	
Total	0.2-1.3 mg/dl	3.4-22.0 μmol/L		
Indirect	0.1-1.0 mg/dl	1.7-17 μmol/L		
Direct	0.1-0.3 mg/dl	1.7-5.1 μmol/L		
Blood gases*				
Arterial pH	7.35-7.45	Same as conventional units	Alkalosis	Acidosis
Venous pH	7.35-7.45	Same as conventional units		
Arterial P_{CO_2}	35-45 mm Hg	4.67-6.00 kPa	Compensated metabolic alkalosis	Compensated metabolic acidosis
Venous P_{CO_2}	42-52 mm Hg	5.60-6.93 kPa	Respiratory acidosis	Respiratory alkalosis
Arterial P_{O_2}	75-100 mm Hg	10.0-13.33 kPa	Administration of high concentration of oxygen	Chronic lung disease, decreased cardiac output
Venous P_{O_2}	30-50 mm Hg	4.0-6.67 kPa		

*Because arterial blood gases are influenced by altitude, the value for P_{O_2} decreases as altitude increases. The lower value is normal for an altitude of 1 mile.

Continued.

Table B-1 Serum, Plasma, and Whole Blood Chemistries—cont'd

Test	Normal Values		Possible Etiology	
	Conventional Units	**SI Units**	**Higher**	**Lower**
Calcium	9-11 mg/dl (4.5-5.5 mEq/L)	2.25-2.74 mmol/L	Acute osteoporosis, hyperparathyroidism, vitamin D intoxication, multiple myeloma	Acute pancreatitis, hypoparathyroidism, liver disease, malabsorption syndrome, renal failure, vitamin D deficiency
Carbon dioxide (CO$_2$ content)	20-30 mEq/L	20-30 mmol/L	Same as bicarbonate	
Carotene	50-200 μg/dl	0.93-3.70 μmol/L	Cystic fibrosis, hypothyroidism, pancreatic insufficiency	Dietary deficiency, malabsorption disorders
Chloride	95-105 mEq/L	95-105 mmol/L	Cardiac decompensation, metabolic acidosis, respiratory alkalosis, steroid therapy, uremia	Addison's disease, diarrhea, metabolic alkalosis, respiratory acidosis, vomiting
Cholesterol	140-220 mg/dl (age dependent)	3.6-5.7 mmol/L	Biliary obstruction, hypothyroidism, idiopathic hypercholesterolemia, renal disease, uncontrolled diabetes	Extensive liver disease, hyperthyroidism, malnutrition, steroid therapy
HDL (high-density lipoproteins)				
Male	>45 mg/dl	> 1.2 mmol/L		
Female	>55 mg/dl	> 1.4 mmol/L		
LDL (low-density lipoproteins)	<130 mg/dl	< 3.4 mmol/L		
Cholinesterase (RBC)	0.65-1.00 pH 4-10 U/L	Same as conventional units	Exercise	Acute infections, insecticide intoxication, liver disease, muscular dystrophy
Pseudocholinesterase (plasma)		Same as conventional units		
Copper	80-150 μg/dl	12.6-23.6 μmol/L	Cirrhosis, female on contraceptives	Wilson's disease
Cortisol	8 AM: 5-25 μg/dl 8 PM: <10 μg/dl	0.14-0.69 μmol/L <0.28 μmol/L	Cushing's syndrome, pancreatitis, stress	Adrenal insufficiency, panhypopituitary states
Creatine	0.2-1.0 mg/dl	15.3-76.3 μmol/L	Active rheumatoid arthritis, biliary obstruction, hyperthyroidism, renal disorders, severe muscle disease	Diabetes mellitus
Creatine phosphokinase (CPK) or creatine kinase (CK)			Musculoskeletal injury or disease, myocardial infarction, severe myocarditis, exercise, numerous intramuscular injections, brain damage	
Male	<160 U/L	Same as conventional units		
Female	<130 U/L (method dependent)	Same as conventional units		
Creatinine	0.5-1.5 mg/dl	44-133 μmol/L	Severe renal disease	
Ferritin (serum)	20-300 ng/ml	20-300 μg/L	Sideroblastic anemia, infection, inflammation, liver disease	Iron deficiency anemia
Folic acid (folate)	3-25 ng/ml	7-57 nmol/L		Alcoholism, hemolytic anemia, inadequate diet, malabsorption syndrome, megaloblastic anemia

RBC, Red blood cell.

Table B-1   Serum, Plasma, and Whole Blood Chemistries—cont'd

Test	Normal Values		Possible Etiology	
	Conventional Units	**SI Units**	**Higher**	**Lower**
Glucose, fasting	70-120 mg/dl	3.89-6.66 mmol/L	Acute stress, cerebral lesions, Cushing's disease, diabetes mellitus, hyperthyroidism, pancreatic insufficiency	Addison's disease, hepatic disease, hypothyroidism, insulin overdosage, pancreatic tumor, pituitary hypofunction, postgastrectomy dumping syndrome
Glucose tolerance (GTT)			Diabetes mellitus	Hyperinsulinism
Fasting	70-120 mg/dl	3.89-6.66 mmol/L		
30 min	30-60 mg/dl above fasting	1.67-3.33 mmol/L		
60 min	20-50 mg/dl above fasting	1.11-2.78 mmol/L		
120 min	5-15 mg/dl above fasting	0.28-0.83 mmol/L		
180 min	Fasting level or lower	Fasting level or lower		
Haptoglobin	70-200 mg/dl	0.7-2.0 g/L	Infectious and inflammatory processes, malignant neoplasms	Hemolytic anemia, mononucleosis, toxoplasmosis, chronic liver disease
Insulin	4-24 µU/ml	29-172 pmol/L	Acromegaly, adenoma of islet cells, untreated mild case of type II diabetes	Diabetes mellitus, obesity
Iron, total	50-150 µg/dl	9.0-26.9 µmol/L	Excessive RBC destruction	Iron-deficiency anemia
Iron-binding capacity	250-410 µg/dl	45-73 µmol/L	Iron-deficient state, oral contraceptives, polycythemia	Cancer, chronic infections, pernicious anemia, uremia
Lactic acid	5-20 mg/dl	0.56-2.2 mmol/L	Acidosis, congestive heart failure, shock	
Lactic dehydrogenase (LDH)	95-200 U/L 80-120 U (Wacker)	Same as conventional units	Congestive heart failure, hemolytic disorders, hepatitis, metastatic cancer of liver, myocardial infarction, pernicious anemia, pulmonary embolus, skeletal muscle damage	
Lactic dehydrogenase isoenzymes				
LDH_1	20%-35%	0.20-0.35	Myocardial infarction, pernicious anemia	
LDH_2	30%-40%	0.30-0.40	Pulmonary embolus, sickle cell crisis	
LDH_3	15%-25%	0.15-0.25	Malignant lymphoma, pulmonary embolus	
LDH_4	0%-10%	0-0.10	Lupus erythematosus, pulmonary infarction	
LDH_5	4%-12%	0.04-0.12	Congestive heart failure, hepatitis, pulmonary embolus and infarction, skeletal muscle damage	

Continued.

Table B-1 Serum, Plasma, and Whole Blood Chemistries—cont'd

Test	Normal Values		Possible Etiology	
	Conventional Units	**SI Units**	**Higher**	**Lower**
Lipase	0.2-1.5 U/ml	Same as conventional units	Acute pancreatitis, hepatic disorders, perforated peptic ulcer	
Magnesium	1.5-2.5 mEq/L	0.75-1.25 mmol/L	Addison's disease, hypothyroidism, renal failure	Chronic alcoholism, hyperparathyroidism, hyperthyroidism, hypoparathyroidism, severe malabsorption
Osmolality	285-295 mOsm/kg	Same as conventional units	Chronic renal disease, diabetes mellitus	Addison's disease, diuretic therapy
Oxygen saturation (arterial)	95%-98%	0.95-0.98 saturated	Polycythemia	Anemia, cardiac decompensation, respiratory disorders
pH	See blood gases			
Phenylalanine	0-2 mg/dl	0-121 μmol/L	Phenylketonuria	
Phosphatase, acid	0.11-0.60 U/L (method dependent)	Same as conventional units	Advanced Paget's disease, cancer of prostate, hyperparathyroidism	
Phosphatase, alkaline	25-90 U/L (method and age dependent)	Same as conventional units	Bone diseases, marked hyperparathyroidism, obstruction of biliary system, rickets	Excessive vitamin D ingestion, hypothyroidism, milk-alkali syndrome
Phosphorus, inorganic	2.8-4.5 mg/dl	0.90-1.45 mmol/L	Healing fractures, hypoparathyroidism, renal disease, vitamin D intoxication	Diabetes mellitus, hyperparathyroidism, vitamin D deficiency
Potassium	3.5-5.5 mEq/L	3.5-5.5 mmol/L	Addison's disease, diabetic ketosis, massive tissue destruction, renal failure	Cushing's syndrome, diarrhea (severe), diuretic therapy, gastrointestinal fistula, pyloric obstruction, starvation, vomiting
Proteins			Burns, cirrhosis (globulin fraction), dehydration	Congenital agammaglobulinemia, liver disease, malabsorption
Total	6.0-8.0 g/dl	60-80 g/L		
Albumin	3.5-5.0 g/dl	35-50 g/L		
Globulin	2-3.5 g/dl	20-35 g/L		
Albumin/globulin ratio	1.5:1-2.5:1	Same as conventional units	Multiple myeloma (globulin fraction), shock, vomiting	Malnutrition, nephrotic syndrome, proteinuria, renal disease, severe burns
Renin			Renal hypertension, volume decrease (e.g., hemorrhage)	Increased salt intake, primary aldosteronism
Supine position	1.4-2.9 ng/ml/hr	0.39-0.81 ng/L·sec		
Upright position	0.4-4.5 ng/ml/hr	0.11-1.25 ng/L·sec		
Sodium	135-145 mEq/L	135-145 mmol/L	Dehydration, impaired renal function, primary aldosteronism, steroid therapy	Addison's disease, diabetic ketoacidosis, diuretic therapy, excessive loss from gastrointestinal tract, excessive perspiration, water intoxication

Table B-1   Serum, Plasma, and Whole Blood Chemistries—cont'd

| Test | Normal Values | | Possible Etiology | |
	Conventional Units	SI Units	Higher	Lower
Testosterone				
Male	400-1200 ng/dl	13.9-41.6 nmol/L		Hypofunction of testes
Female	25-90 ng/dl	0.87-3.1 nmol/L	Polycystic ovary, virilizing tumors	
T_4 (thyroxine)	5-12 μg/dl	64-154 nmol/L	Hyperthyroidism, thyroiditis	Cretinism, hypothyroidism, myxedema
T_3 uptake	25%-35%	0.25-0.35	Hyperthyroidism, metastatic neoplasms	Hypothyroidism, pregnancy
T_3 (triiodothyronine)	110-230 ng/dl	1.7-3.5 nmol/L	Hyperthyroidism	
Thyroid-stimulating hormone (TSH)	0.3-5.4 μU/ml	0.3-5.4 mU/L	Myxedema, primary hypothyroidism	Secondary hypothyroidism
Transaminases				
Serum glutamic-oxaloacetic (SGOT) or aspartate aminotransferase (AST)	7-40 U/L	0.12-0.67 μkat/L	Liver disease, myocardial infarction, pulmonary infarction, acute hepatitis	
Serum glutamic-pyruvic (SGPT) or alanine aminotransferase (ALT)	5-36 U/L	0.08-0.6 μkat/L	Liver disease, shock	
Triglycerides	40-150 mg/dl	0.45-1.69 mmol/L	Diabetes mellitus, hyperlipidemia, hypothyroidism, liver disease	Malnutrition
Urea nitrogen (BUN)	10-30 mg/dl	1.8-7.1 mmol/L	Increase in protein catabolism (fever, stress), renal disease, urinary tract infection	Malnutrition, severe liver damage
Uric acid			Gout, gross tissue destruction, high-protein weight reduction diet, leukemia, renal failure, eclampsia	Administration of uricosuric drugs
Male	4.5-6.5 mg/dl	149-327 μmol/L		
Female	2.5-5.5 mg/dl	268-387 μmol/L		
Vitamin A	15-60 μg/dl	0.52-2.09 μmol/L	Excess ingestion of vitamin A	Vitamin A deficiency
Vitamin B_{12}	200-1000 pg/ml	148-738 pmol/L	Myeloid leukemia	Extreme vegetarianism, malabsorption syndrome, pernicious anemia, total or partial gastrectomy
Zinc	50-150 μg/dl	7.6-22.9 μmol/L		Alcoholic cirrhosis

Table B-2 Hematology

Test	Normal Values		Possible Etiology	
	Conventional Units	SI Units	Higher	Lower
Bleeding time (Ivy) (Simplate)	1-6 min 3.0-9.5 min	60-360 sec 180-570 sec	Defective platelet function, thrombocytopenia, von Willebrand disease, aspirin ingestion	
Activated partial thromboplastin time (APTT)	30-45 sec*	Same as conventional units	Deficiency of factors I, II, V, VIII, IX and X, XI, XII; hemophilia, liver disease, heparin therapy	
Prothrombin time (Protime, PT)	12-15 sec*	Same as conventional units	Anticoagulant therapy, deficiency of factors I, II, V, VII, and X, inadequate vitamin K in diet, liver disease	
Fibrinogen	200-400 mg/dl	2.0-4.0 g/L	Burns (after first 36 hr), inflammatory disease	Burns (during first 36 hr), DIC, severe liver disease
Fibrin degradation products	<10 mg/L		Acute DIC, massive hemorrhage, primary fibrinolysis	
Erythrocyte count (altitude dependent)			Dehydration, high altitudes, polycythemia vera, severe diarrhea	Anemia, leukemia, posthemorrhage
Male	$4.5\text{-}6.0 \times 10^6/\mu l$	$4.5\text{-}6.0 \times 10^{12}/L$		
Female	$4.0\text{-}5.0 \times 10^6/\mu l$	$4.0\text{-}5.0 \times 10^{12}/L$		
Mean corpuscular volume (MCV)	82-98 fl	Same as conventional units	Macrocytic anemia	Microcytic anemia
Mean corpuscular hemoglobin (MCH)	27-33 pg	Same as conventional units	Macrocytic anemia	Microcytic anemia
Mean corpuscular hemoglobin concentration (MCHC)	32%-36%	0.32-0.36	Spherocytosis	Hypochromic anemia
Erythrocyte sedimentation rate (ESR)			Moderate increase: acute hepatitis, myocardial infarction, rheumatoid arthritis; marked increase: acute and severe bacterial infections, malignancies, pelvic inflammatory disease	Malaria Severe liver disease Sickle cell anemia
Male	<15 mm/hr	Same as conventional units		
Female	<20 mm/hr	Same as conventional units		

DIC, Disseminated intravascular coagulation; *RBC,* red blood cell; *COPD,* chronic obstructive pulmonary disease.
*Values depend on reagent used.
†Components of complete blood count (CBC).

Table B-2 Hematology—cont'd

Test	Normal Values		Possible Etiology	
	Conventional Units	SI Units	Higher	Lower
Hematocrit (altitude dependent)†			Dehydration, high altitudes, polycythemia	Anemia, hemorrhage, overhydration
Male	40%-54%	0.40-0.54		
Female	38%-47%	0.38-0.47		
Hemoglobin (altitude dependent)†			COPD, high altitudes, polycythemia	Anemia, hemorrhage
Male	13.5-18.0 g/dl	135-180 g/L		
Female	12.0-16.0 g/dl	120-160 g/L		
Platelet count (thrombocytes)†	150,000-400,000/μl	150-400 × 10⁹/L	Acute infections, chronic granulocytic leukemia, chronic pancreatitis, cirrhosis, collagen disorders, polycythemia, postsplenectomy	Acute leukemia, DIC, thrombocytopenic purpura
Reticulocyte count	0.5%-1.5% of RBC	0.005-0.015 of RBC	Hemolytic anemia, polycythemia vera	Hypoproliferative anemia, macrocytic anemia, microcytic anemia
White blood cell count†	4-11,000/μl	4.0-11.0 × 10⁹/L	Inflammatory and infectious processes, leukemia	Aplastic anemia, side effects of chemotherapy and irradiation
WBC Differential				
Segmented neutrophils	50%-70%	0.50-0.70	Bacterial infections, collagen diseases, Hodgkin's disease	Aplastic anemia, viral infections
Band neutrophils	0%-8%	0-0.08	Acute infections	
Lymphocytes	20%-40%	0.20-0.40	Chronic infections, lymphocytic leukemia, mononucleosis, viral infections	Adrenocortical steroid therapy, Hodgkin's disease, whole body irradiation
Monocytes	4%-8%	0.04-0.08	Chronic inflammatory disorders, malaria, monocytic leukemia	
Eosinophils	0%-4%	0-0.04	Allergic reactions, eosinophilic and chronic granulocytic leukemia, parasitic disorders	Steroid therapy
Basophils	0%-2%	0-0.02	Acute severe infections, myeloproliferative diseases	Anaphylactic reaction
Sickle cell preparation	Negative	Same as conventional units	Sickle cell anemia	
Lupus erythematosus (LE preparation)	Absence of LE cells	Same as conventional units	Lupus erythematosus, rheumatoid arthritis	

Table B-3 Serology-Immunology

Test	Normal Values		Possible Etiology	
	Conventional Units	**SI Units**	**Higher**	**Lower**
Antinuclear antibody (ANA)	Negative or titer <1:10	Same as conventional units	Chronic hepatitis, rheumatoid arthritis, scleroderma, systemic lupus erythematosus	
Anti-DNA antibody	Negative or titer <1:10 or <20% binding	Same as conventional units	Systemic lupus erythematosus	
Anti-RNP	Negative	Same as conventional units	Mixed connective tissue disease, rheumatoid arthritis, systemic lupus erythematosus, Sjögren's syndrome, scleroderma	
Anti-Sm	Negative	Same as conventional units	Systemic lupus erythematosus	
Antistreptolysin-O (ASO)	≤166 Todd units	Same as conventional units	Acute glomerulonephritis, rheumatic fever, streptococcal infection	
C-reactive protein (CRP)	Negative or ≤1.2 mg/dl	Same as conventional units	Acute infections, any inflammatory condition, widespread malignancy	
Carcinoembryonic antigen (CEA)	≤2.5 ng/ml	≤2.5 μg/L	Carcinoma of colon, liver, pancreas; chronic cigarette smoking; inflammatory bowel disease; other cancers	
Complement components				
C1q	11-21 mg/dl	0.11-0.21 g/L		Acute glomerulonephritis, systemic lupus erythematosus, rheumatoid arthritis, subacute bacterial endocarditis, serum sickness
C3	80-180 mg/dl	0.8-1.8 g/L		
C4	15-50 mg/dl	0.15-0.5 g/L		
Coombs' or Anti-human globulin (AHG)			Acquired hemolytic anemia, anti-Rh antibodies in pregnant women, blood incompatibilities, presence of irregular antibody serum, transfusion reaction	
Direct	Negative	Same as conventional units		
Indirect	Negative			

RNP, Ribonuclear protein; *RPR*, rapid plasma reagin test; *VDRL*, venereal disease research laboratory test; *CSF*, colony-stimulating factor.

Table B-3 Serology-Immunology—cont'd

Test	Normal Values		Possible Etiology	
	Conventional Units	SI Units	Higher	Lower
Fluorescent treponemal antibody (FTA-ABS)	Nonreactive	Same as conventional units	Syphilis	
Hepatitis A antibody (IgM)	Negative	Same as conventional units	Hepatitis A	
Hepatitis B surface antigen (HB$_s$Ag)	Negative	Same as conventional units	Hepatitis B	
Immunoglobulin				
IgA	90-400 mg/dl	0.9-4.0 g/L	IgA myeloma, chronic liver disease, chronic infection, rheumatoid arthritis, autoimmune disorders	Burns, hereditary telangiectasia, malabsorption syndromes
IgD	0.5-12 mg/dl	5-120 mg/L	Chronic infection, connective tissue disease	
IgE	<1 mg/dl	<10 mg/L	Anaphylactic shock, atopic disease (allergies), parasite infections	
IgG	650-1800 mg/dl	6.5-18.0 g/L	Infections—acute and chronic, hepatitis, IgG monoclonal gammopathy, systemic lupus erythematosus	Congenital deficiencies, acquired deficiencies, nephrotic syndromes, burns, immunosuppression
IgM	55-300 mg/dl	0.5-3.0 g/L	Acute infections, rheumatoid arthritis, liver disease	Congenital and acquired antibody deficiencies, lymphocytic leukemia, protein-losing enteropathies
Monospot or monotest	Negative	Same as conventional units	Infectious mononucleosis	
Rheumatoid factor (RA factor)	Negative or titer <1:20	Same as conventional units	Rheumatoid arthritis, Sjögren's syndrome, systemic lupus erythematosus	
RPR	Nonreactive	Same as conventional units	Syphilis	
VDRL-CSF	Nonreactive	Same as conventional units	Syphilis	
Thyroid antibodies	≤1:10 titer	Same as conventional units	Hashimoto's thyroiditis, thyroid carcinoma, early hypothyroidism, pernicious anemia, systemic lupus erythematosus, Graves' disease	

Table B-4 Urine Chemistry

Test	Specimen	Conventional Units	SI Units	Possible Etiology Higher	Possible Etiology Lower
Acetone	Random	Negative	Same as conventional units	Diabetes mellitus, high-fat and low-carbohydrate diets, starvation states	
Aldosterone	24 hr	2-26 µg/day	5.5-72.1 nmol/day	Primary aldosteronism: adrenocortical tumors; secondary aldosteronism: cardiac failure, cirrhosis, large dose of ACTH, salt depletion	ACTH deficiency, Addison's disease, corticosteroid therapy
Amylase	24 hr	1-17 U/day	Same as conventional units	Acute pancreatitis	
Bence Jones protein	Random	Negative	Same as conventional units	Multiple myeloma, biliary duct obstruction	
Bilirubin	Random	Negative	Same as conventional units	Hepatitis	
Calcium	24 hr	100-250 mg/day	2.5-6.3 mmol/day	Bone tumor, hyperparathyroidism, milk-alkali syndrome	Hypoparathyroidism, malabsorption of calcium and vitamin D
Catecholamines	24 hr			Pheochromocytoma, progressive muscular dystrophy	
Epinephrine		<20 µg/day	<118 nmol/day		
Norepinephrine		<100 µg/day	<591 nmol/day		
Chloride	24 hr	110-250 mEq/day	110-250 mmol/day	Addison's disease	Burns, excess perspiration, vomiting, diarrhea, menstruation
Copper	24 hr	<30 µg/day	<0.5 µmol/day	Cirrhosis, Wilson's disease	
Coproporphyrin	24 hr	50-200 µg/day	76-305 nmol/day	Lead poisoning, oral contraceptive use, poliomyelitis	
Creatine	24 hr	<100 mg/day	<763 µmol/day	Carcinoma of liver, hyperthyroidism, diabetes, Addison's disease, infections, burns, muscular dystrophy, skeletal muscle atrophy	Hypothyroidism
Creatinine	24 hr	0.8-2.0 g/day	7.1-17.7 mmol/day	Anemia, leukemia, muscular atrophy, salmonellae	Renal disease
Creatinine clearance	24 hr	85-135 ml/min	1.42-2.25 ml/sec		Renal disease
Estrogens	24 hr				
Female				Gonadal or adrenal tumor	Agenesis of ovaries, endocrine disturbance, ovarian dysfunction
Ovulation peak		28-100 µg/day	104-370 nmol/day		
Luteal peak		22-80 µg/day	81-296 nmol/day		
Pregnancy		Up to 45,000 µg/day	Up to 166,455 nmol/day		
Menopause		1.4-19.6 µg/day	5.2-72.5 nmol/day		
Male		5-18 µg/day	18-67 nmol/day		
Glucose	Random	Negative	Same as conventional units	Diabetes mellitus, low renal threshold for glucose resorption, physiological stress, pituitary disorders	

ACTH, Corticotropin.

Table B-4 Urine Chemistry—cont'd

Test	Specimen	Normal Values Conventional Units	Normal Values SI Units	Possible Etiology Higher	Possible Etiology Lower
Hemoglobin	Random	Negative	Same as conventional units	Extensive burns, glomerulonephritis, hemolytic anemias, hemolytic transfusion reaction	
17-Hydroxy-corticosteroids	24 hr			Adrenal cancer, Cushing's syndrome	Addison's disease, hypofunction of anterior pituitary
Male		3.5-12 mg/day	9.7-33 μmol/day		
Female		3-10 mg/day	8.3-28 μmol/day		
5-Hydroxyindoleacetic 24 hr acid (5-HIAA)		2-9 mg/day	10.5-47.1 μmol/day	Malignant carcinoid syndrome	
17-Ketosteroids	24 hr			Autonomous tumor of adrenals, Cushing's syndrome, adrenal hyperplasia, interstitial cell tumor of testes, hyperpituitarism, severe stress	Adrenal cortical insufficiency, diabetes mellitus, hypogonadism, hypopituitarism
Male		10-22 mg/day	35-76 μmol/day		
Female		6-16 mg/day	20.8-55 μmol/day		
Ketone bodies	24 hr	20-50 mg/day	0.34-0.86 mmol/day	Marked ketonuria	
Lead	24 hr	<100 μg/day	<0.48 μmol/day	Lead poisoning	
Metanephrine	24 hr	<1.3 mg/day	<7.1 μmol/day	Pheochromocytoma	
Myoglobin	Random	Negative	Same as conventional units	Crushing injuries, electric shock, extreme physical exertion	
pH	Random	4.0-8.0	Same as conventional units	Chronic renal failure, compensatory phase of alkalosis, salicylate intoxication, vegetable diet	Compensatory phase of acidosis, dehydration, emphysema
Phenylpyruvic acid	Random	Negative	Same as conventional units	Phenylketonuria	
Phosphorus, inorganic	24 hr	0.9-1.3 g/day	29-42 mmol/day	Fever, hypoparathyroidism, nervous exhaustion, rickets, tuberculosis	Acute infections, nephritis
Porphobilinogen	Random	Negative	Same as conventional units	Acute intermittent porphyria, liver disorders	
Protein (dipstick)	Random	Negative	Same as conventional units	Congestive heart failure, nephritis, nephrosis, physiological stress	
Protein (quantitative)	24 hr	<150 mg/day	<0.15 g/day	Cardiac failure, inflammatory processes of urinary tract, nephritis, nephrosis, toxemia of pregnancy	
Sodium	24 hr	40-250 mEq/day	40-250 mmol/day	Acute tubular necrosis	Hyponatremia
Specific gravity	Random	1.003-1.030	Same as conventional units	Albuminuria, dehydration, glycosuria	Diabetes insipidus
Titratable acidity	24 hr	20-50 mEq/day	Same as conventional units	Metabolic acidosis	Metabolic alkalosis
Uric acid	24 hr	250-750 mg/day	1.5-4.5 mmol/day	Gout, leukemia	Nephritis

Continued.

Table B-4 Urine Chemistry—cont'd

Test	Specimen	Normal Values Conventional Units	SI Units	Possible Etiology Higher	Lower
Urobilinogen	24 hr Random	0.5-4.0 mg/day <1.0 Erhlich unit	0.8-6.8 μmol/day Same as conventional units	Hemolytic disease, hepatic parenchymal cell damage, liver disease	Complete obstruction of bile duct
Uroporphyrins	Random	Negative	Same as conventional units	Porphyria	
Vanillylmandelic acid	24 hr	1-8 mg/day 1.5-7 μg/mg creatine	5-40 μmol/day	Pheochromocytoma	

Table B-5 Gastric Analysis

Test	Normal Values Conventional Units	SI Units	Possible Etiology Higher	Lower
Basal				
Free hydrochloric acid	0-30 mEq/L	Same conventional units	Hypermotility of stomach	Pernicious anemia
Total acidity	15-45 mEq/L	Same conventional units	Gastric and duodenal ulcers	Gastric carcinoma
Combined acidity	10-15 mEq/L	Same conventional units	Zollinger-Ellison syndrome	Severe gastritis
Poststimulation				
Free hydrochloric acid	10-130 mEq/L	Same conventional units		
Total acidity	20-150 mEq/L	Same conventional units		

Table B-6 Fecal Analysis

Test	Normal Values Conventional Units	SI Units	Possible Etiology Higher	Lower
Fecal fat	<6 g/24 hr	<21 mmol/day	Chronic pancreatic disease, obstruction of common bile duct, malabsorption syndrome	
Urobilinogen	30-220 mg/100 g of stool	51-372 μmol/100 g of stool	Hemolytic anemias	Complete biliary obstruction
Mucus	Negative	Same as conventional units	Mucous colitis, spastic constipation	
Pus	Negative	Same as conventional units	Chronic bacillary dysentery, chronic ulcerative colitis, localized abscesses	
Blood*	Negative	Same as conventional units	Anal fissures, hemorrhoids, malignant tumor, peptic ulcer, ulcerative colitis	
Color				
Brown			Various color depending on diet	
Clay			Biliary obstruction or presence of barium sulfate	
Tarry			More than 100 ml of blood in GI tract	
Red			Blood in large intestine	
Black			Blood in upper gastrointestinal tract or iron medication	

*Ingestion of meat may produce false-positive results. Client may be placed on a meat-free diet for 3 days before the test.

Table B-7 Cerebrospinal Fluid Analysis

Test	Normal Values Conventional Units	SI Units	Possible Etiology Higher	Lower
Pressure	60-150 mm	Same as conventional units	Hemorrhage, intracranial tumor, meningitis	Head injury, spinal tumor, subdural hematoma
Blood	Negative	Same as conventional units	Intracranial hemorrhage	
Cell count (age dependent)				
WBC	0-8 cells/μl	$0\text{-}8 \times 10^6$/L	Inflammation or infections of CNS	
RBC	0	0×10^6/L		
Chloride	100-130 mEq/L	100-130 mmol/L	Uremia	Bacterial infections of CNS (meningitis, encephalitis)
Glucose	45-75 mg/dl	2.5-4.2 mmol/L	Diabetes mellitus, viral infections of CNS	Bacterial infections and tuberculosis of CNS
Protein				
Lumbar	15-45 mg/dl	0.15-0.45 g/L	Guillain-Barré syndrome, poliomyelitis, traumatic tap	
Cisternal	15-25 mg/dl	0.15-0.25 g/L	Syphilis of CNS	
Ventricular	5-15 mg/dl	0.05-0.15 g/L	Acute meningitis, brain tumor, chronic infections, multiple sclerosis	

WBC, White blood cell; *RBC*, red blood cell; *CNS*, central nervous system.

Table B-8 Toxicology of Common Drugs

Drug	Therapeutic Level		Toxic Level	
	Conventional Units	**SI Units**	**Conventional Units**	**SI Units**
Acetaminophen (Tylenol)	1-2 mg/dl	66-132 µmol/L	>5 mg/dl	>330 µmol/L
Barbiturates				
Short acting	1-2 mg/dl	Dependent on composition of mixture	>5 mg/dl	
Intermediate acting	1-5 mg/dl		>10 mg/dl	
Long acting	15-35 mg/dl		>40 mg/dl	
Carbon monoxide (carboxyhemoglobin)				
Normal values	<5% saturation of hemoglobin	<0.05	Symptoms with >20% saturation	>0.20
Urban nonsmokers	<5% saturation of hemoglobin	<0.05		
Rural nonsmokers	0.5%-2% saturation of hemoglobin	0.005-0.02		
Smokers	5%-9% saturation of hemoglobin	0.05-0.09		
Heavy smokers	>9% saturation of hemoglobin	>0.09		
Chlordiazepoxide (Librium)	0.05-5.0 mg/L	2-17 µmol/L	>10 µg/ml	>33 µmol/L
Chlorpromazine (Thorazine)	0.5 µg/ml	1.6 µmol/L	>2.0 µg/ml	>6.3 µmol/L
Diazepam (Valium)	0.10-0.25 mg/L	0.35-0.88 µmol/L	>1.0 mg/L ≥2.0 mg/L (lethal)	>3.5 µmol/L
Digitalis preparations				
Digoxin	0.8-2.4 ng/ml	1.0-3.1 nmol/L	>2.5 ng/ml	>2.6 nmol/L
Digitoxin	14-30 ng/ml	18-39 nmol/L	>30 ng/ml	>39 nmol/L
Dilantin	10-20 mg/L	40-80 µmol/L	>30 mg/L	>120 µmol/L
Gentamicin (Garamycin)				
Peak	4-10 mg/L	9-22 µmol/L	>10 mg/L	>22 µmol/L
Trough	<2 mg/L	<4 mmol/L	>2 mg/L	>4 µmol/L
Meperidine (Dermerol)	20-200 µg/dl	2.83-8.09 µmol/L	>200 g/dl	>8.09 µmol/L
Propranolol (Inderal)	50-100 ng/ml	192-386 nmol/L	>200 ng/ml	>771 nmol/L
Salicylates	15-20 mg/dl	1.09-1.45 mmol/L	>20 mg/dl >60 mg/dl (lethal)	>1.45 mmol/L >4.34 mmol/L
Alcohol (ethanol)*				

*See Table 60-14.

Answer Key to Review Questions

CHAPTER 1

1. a
2. d
3. b
4. d
5. a
6. a
7. c

CHAPTER 2

1. a
2. c
3. d
4. b
5. d
6. b
7. a
8. b

CHAPTER 3

1. b
2. b
3. b
4. d
5. a
6. d

CHAPTER 4

1. b
2. d
3. c
4. d
5. c
6. d
7. d

CHAPTER 5

1. b
2. c
3. c
4. a
5. a
6. d

7. b
8. c

CHAPTER 6

1. c
2. b
3. c
4. b
5. b
6. b
7. b
8. a
9. c
10. c
11. c
12. b

CHAPTER 7

1. a
2. c
3. b
4. c
5. d
6. b
7. d
8. a
9. c
10. b

CHAPTER 8

1. d
2. d
3. b
4. a
5. d
6. c
7. d
8. c
9. b
10. b
11. a
12. c
13. a
14. d

CHAPTER 9

1. d
2. a
3. c
4. a
5. c
6. b
7. d
8. d
9. d
10. b
11. d
12. a
13. d
14. a
15. c

CHAPTER 10

1. c
2. b
3. b
4. b
5. a
6. c
7. d
8. d
9. a

CHAPTER 11

1. b
2. b
3. c
4. a
5. a
6. c
7. a
8. d
9. b

CHAPTER 12

1. b
2. a
3. c
4. a

5. a
6. b
7. d
8. b

CHAPTER 13

1. b
2. b
3. b
4. a
5. c
6. a

CHAPTER 14

1. b
2. d
3. a
4. a
5. b
6. d
7. c

CHAPTER 15

1. c
2. a
3. c
4. b
5. b
6. b
7. d
8. a
9. b
10. d
11. c

CHAPTER 16

1. d
2. b
3. a
4. b
5. c
6. a
7. a

8. b
9. a

CHAPTER 17

1. b
2. a
3. d
4. a
5. d
6. c
7. b
8. b
9. c
10. c
11. a

CHAPTER 18

1. c
2. b
3. a
4. c
5. b
6. c
7. c
8. a
9. b
10. b
11. d
12. c

CHAPTER 19

1. c
2. b
3. b
4. a
5. c
6. d
7. a
8. c
9. d
10. d

CHAPTER 20

1. d
2. c
3. a
4. d
5. b
6. c
7. a
8. c

CHAPTER 21

1. c
2. a
3. c

4. d
5. c
6. a
7. b
8. a
9. a
10. a
11. d
12. d
13. c
14. a
15. b

CHAPTER 22

1. b
2. b
3. d
4. a
5. c
6. b

CHAPTER 23

1. d
2. a
3. b
4. b
5. a
6. c
7. d

CHAPTER 24

1. c
2. a
3. b
4. c
5. c
6. a
7. d

CHAPTER 25

1. c
2. d
3. b
4. d
5. c
6. c
7. d
8. a
9. b
10. d
11. c
12. d
13. c
14. b
15. c
16. c
17. a

CHAPTER 26

1. c
2. b
3. a
4. d
5. c
6. a
7. b
8. a
9. c
10. d

CHAPTER 27

1. a
2. c
3. b
4. a
5. d
6. a
7. d
8. a
9. b
10. b
11. d
12. c
13. d

CHAPTER 28

1. b
2. d
3. c
4. b
5. a
6. c
7. d
8. c
9. d
10. c
11. d
12. a
13. b

CHAPTER 29

1. b
2. a
3. a
4. b
5. c
6. b

CHAPTER 30

1. d
2. d
3. b
4. d

5. b
6. a

CHAPTER 31

1. a
2. d
3. c
4. a
5. d
6. a
7. b
8. b
9. a
10. d

CHAPTER 32

1. a
2. d
3. d
4. c
5. a
6. b
7. a
8. b
9. c
10. c
11. c
12. d

CHAPTER 33

1. b
2. c
3. d
4. a
5. b
6. d
7. a
8. a

CHAPTER 34

1. a
2. a
3. d
4. b
5. b
6. c
7. d
8. b
9. b
10. c
11. a

CHAPTER 35

1. c
2. d
3. c

4. c
5. b
6. a

CHAPTER 36

1. c
2. a
3. a
4. a
5. b
6. c

CHAPTER 37

1. b
2. c
3. a
4. c
5. a
6. d
7. a
8. d
9. b
10. a
11. a
12. a
13. a
14. a
15. d

CHAPTER 38

1. b
2. d
3. b
4. c
5. b
6. a
7. c
8. d
9. c
10. b
11. a

CHAPTER 39

1. b
2. c
3. b
4. d
5. c
6. c
7. b

CHAPTER 40

1. b
2. b
3. c
4. c

5. b
6. b
7. a
8. a
9. d
10. d
11. c
12. c

CHAPTER 41

1. b
2. b
3. d
4. c
5. b
6. b
7. c
8. c
9. b
10. c
11. c

CHAPTER 42

1. c
2. b
3. d
4. a
5. c
6. d
7. c
8. b
9. d

CHAPTER 43

1. b
2. a
3. b
4. b
5. d
6. c
7. c

CHAPTER 44

1. a
2. d
3. b
4. d
5. b
6. d
7. a
8. d
9. c

CHAPTER 45

1. c
2. d

3. b
4. c
5. a
6. b
7. c
8. c

CHAPTER 46

1. d
2. a
3. a
4. d
5. c
6. b
7. c

CHAPTER 47

1. a
2. d
3. b
4. b
5. a
6. a
7. b
8. b

CHAPTER 48

1. c
2. c
3. d
4. b
5. b
6. c
7. a
8. d
9. b
10. c
11. d
12. d
13. b
14. a
15. d

CHAPTER 49

1. d
2. b
3. d
4. d

CHAPTER 50

1. c
2. a
3. d
4. b
5. d
6. d

7. c
8. a
9. c
10. b
11. c

CHAPTER 51

1. d
2. c
3. b
4. a
5. d
6. c
7. a
8. a
9. c

CHAPTER 52

1. c
2. b
3. d
4. d
5. b
6. c
7. d
8. a
9. c
10. a
11. c
12. d
13. d
14. d
15. b

CHAPTER 53

1. a
2. b
3. b
4. c
5. b
6. b
7. a
8. a
9. c
10. b

CHAPTER 54

1. c
2. c
3. b
4. a
5. d
6. d
7. c

CHAPTER 55

1. c
2. c
3. d
4. b
5. d
6. c
7. a
8. a
9. b

CHAPTER 56

1. b
2. c
3. c
4. a
5. b
6. c
7. c
8. c

CHAPTER 57

1. a
2. d
3. c
4. d
5. d
6. a
7. c
8. c
9. a
10. b
11. a
12. d
13. c
14. b

CHAPTER 58

1. c
2. b

3. c
4. b
5. d
6. a
7. d
8. b
9. c
10. d

CHAPTER 59

1. c
2. d
3. c
4. a
5. d
6. d

CHAPTER 60

1. b
2. c
3. d
4. a
5. b
6. c
7. b
8. c
9. a
10. a
11. c
12. b
13. c
14. b
15. d
16. b

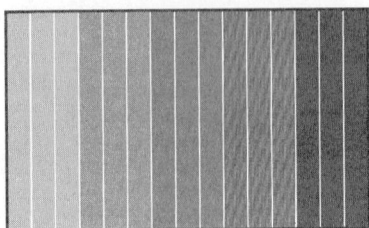

Index

Page numbers in italics indicate illustrations; *t* indicates tables.

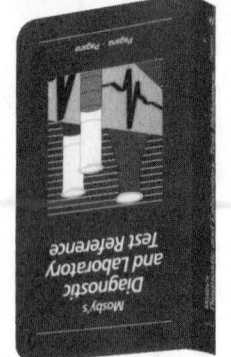
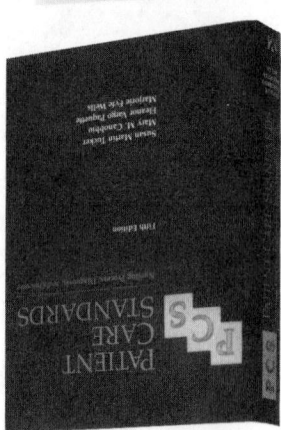
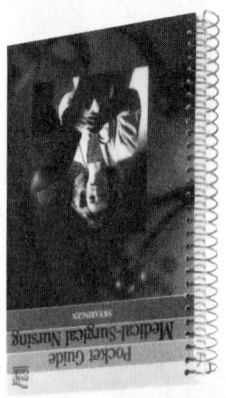
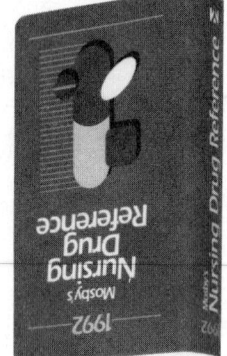